REFERENCE BOOK
Use in Reference
Department ONLY

P9-CNE-992

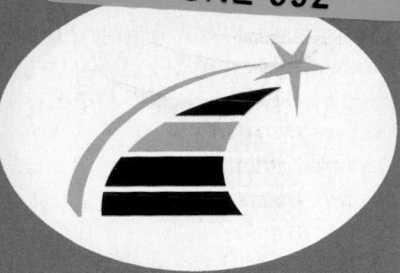

Trust Carol J. Buck
for your certification review needs!

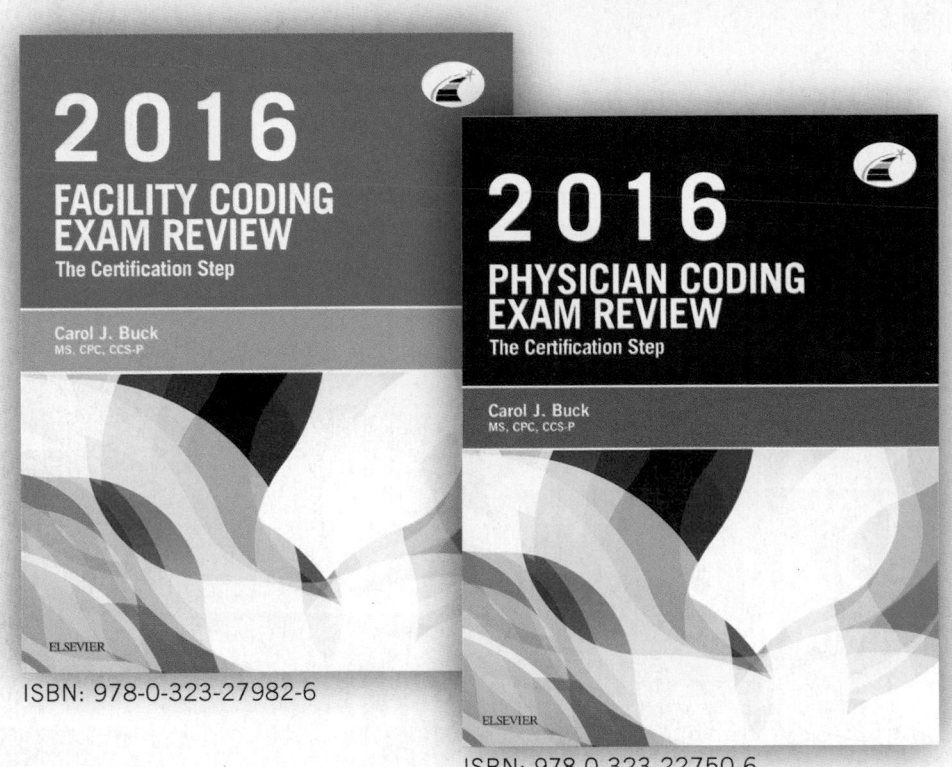

ISBN: 978-0-323-27982-6

ISBN: 978-0-323-22750-6

Everything you need to prepare for certification exams

Study key topics with concentrated reviews

Practice tests that mimic the real certification exams

Order today!

- Order securely at **www.elsevier.com.**
- Call toll-free **1-800-545-2522.**
- Visit your **local bookstore.**

ELSEVIER

CERT-01

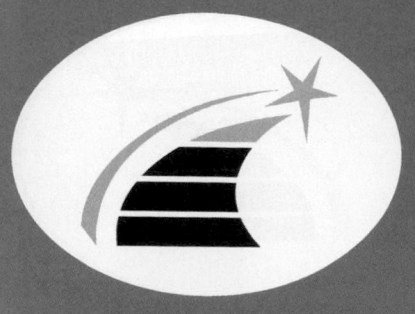

Trust Carol J. Buck and Elsevier for all your professional coding needs!

Available packaged with AMA's CPT

Standard Edition
ISBN: 978-0-323-38989-1

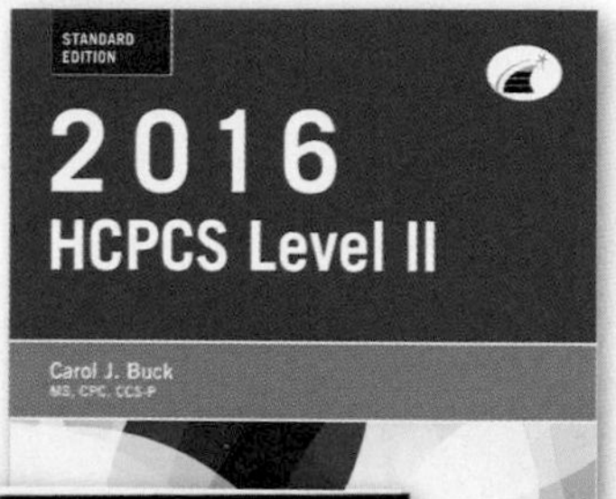

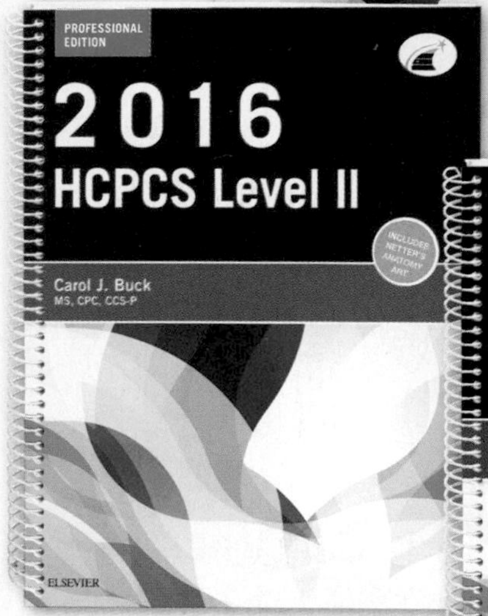

2016 HCPCS Level II
Carol J. Buck
MS, CPC, CCS-P

Standard Edition
ISBN: 978-1-4557-7496-8

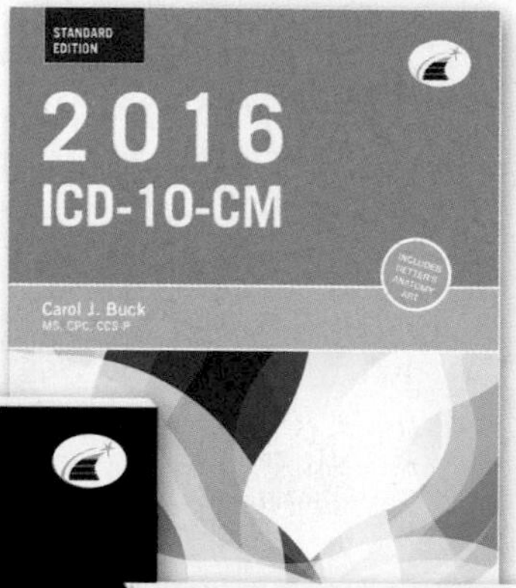

2016 ICD-10-CM
Carol J. Buck
MS, CPC, CCS-P

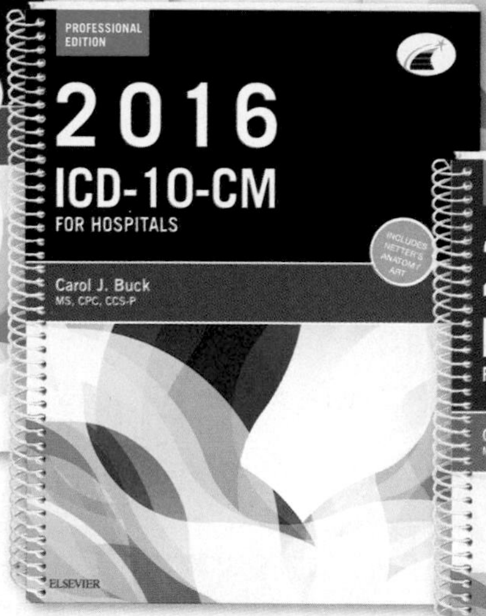

2016 HCPCS Level II
Carol J. Buck
MS, CPC, CCS-P

Standard Edition
ISBN: 978-1-4557-7495-1

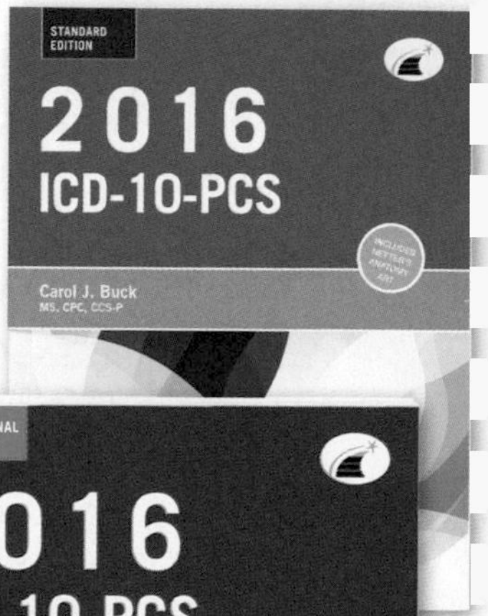

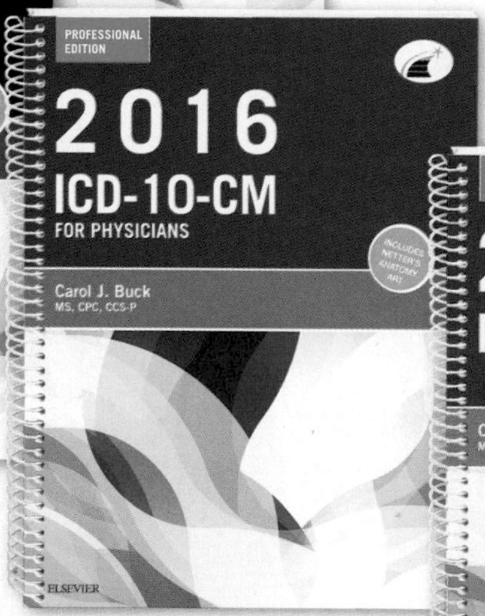

2016 ICD-10-PCS
Carol J. Buck
MS, CPC, CCS-P

2016 ICD-10-CM FOR HOSPITALS
Carol J. Buck
MS, CPC, CCS-P

2016 ICD-10-CM FOR PHYSICIANS
Carol J. Buck
MS, CPC, CCS-P

2016 ICD-10-PCS
Carol J. Buck
MS, CPC, CCS-P

ISBN: 978-0-323-38983-9
HCPCS Level II
Professional Edition

ISBN: 978-0-323-27975-8
ICD-10-CM Hospital
Professional Edition

ISBN: 978-0-323-27976-5
ICD-10-CM Physician
Professional Edition

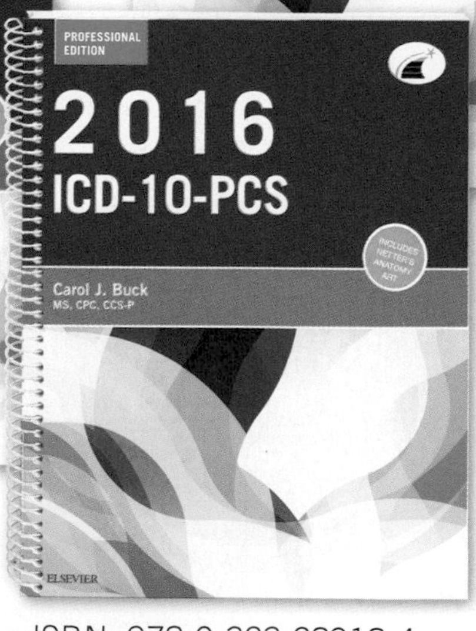

ISBN: 978-0-323-28918-4
ICD-10-PCS
Professional Edition

Order today! Call 1-800-545-2522; order at www.elsevier.com; or visit your bookstore.

NHP-012

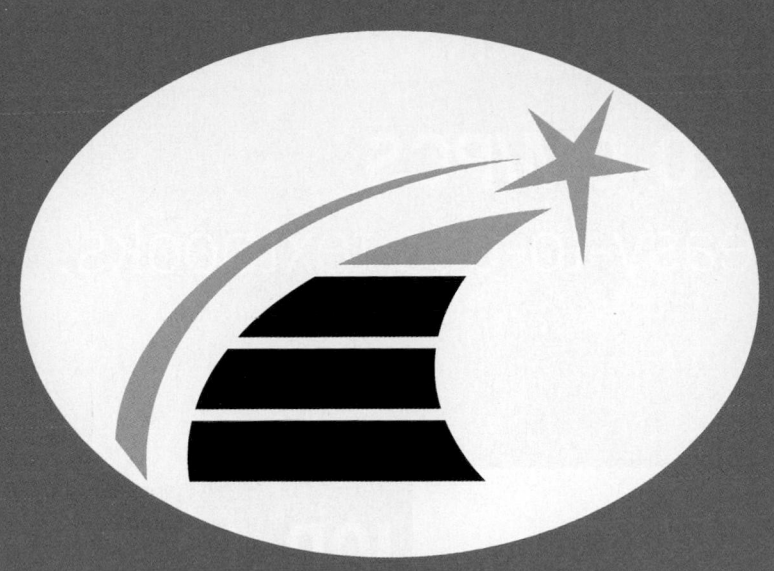

Step 4:
Professional Resources

"Nothing is particularly hard if you divide it into small jobs."

— Henry Ford

As you reach higher and more specialized levels of coding, we want to applaud you for taking this step in your career. You won't be disappointed. Specialized coders are like rare gems—**they are harder to find and greatly valued** in the profession.

— Carol J. Buck,
MS, CPC, CCS-P

— Jackie L. Grass,
CPC

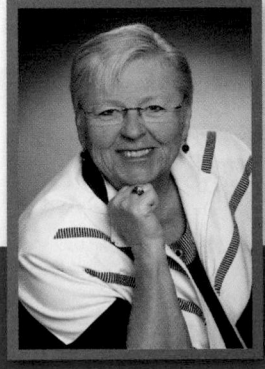
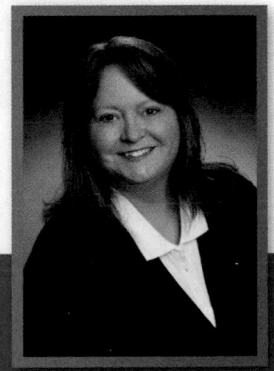

Track your progress!

See the checklist in the back of this book to learn more about your steps toward coding success!

BB-04

Learn ICD-10-CM/PCS
with these easy-to-use textbooks.

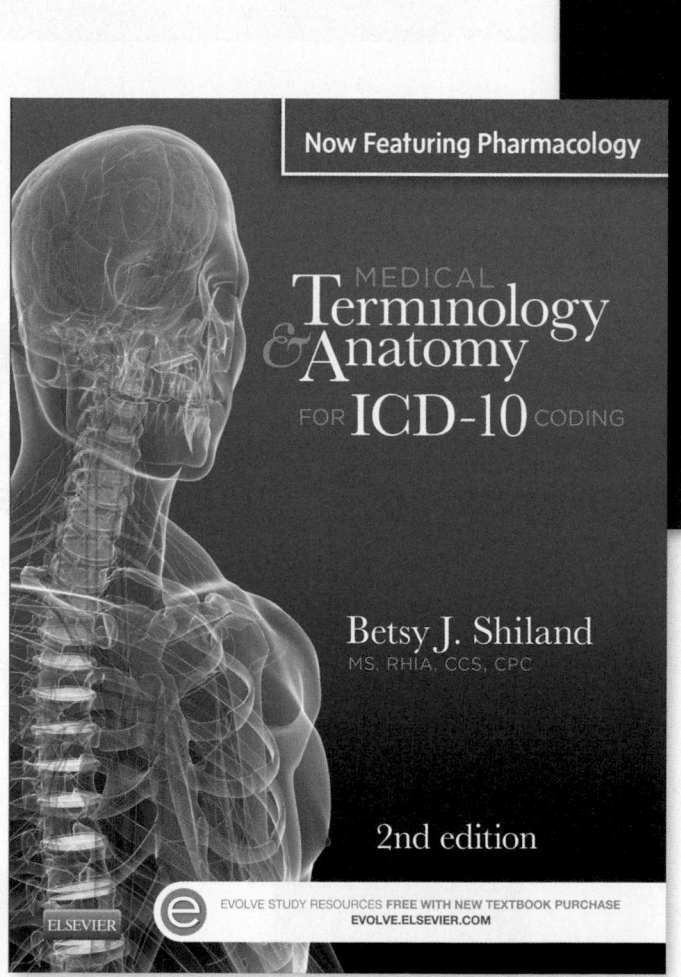

Lovaasen: ICD-10-CM/PCS Coding:
Theory and Practice, 2016 Edition
ISBN: 978-0-323-38993-8

Shiland: Medical Terminology & Anatomy
for ICD-10 Coding, Second Edition
ISBN: 978-0-323-26017-6

Order today!
- Order securely at **www.elsevier.com.**
- Call toll-free **1-800-545-2522.**
- Visit your **local bookstore.**

ELSEVIER

LB-01

PROFESSIONAL
EDITION

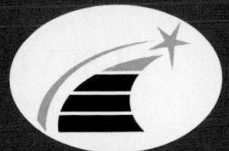

2016
ICD-10-CM
FOR PHYSICIANS

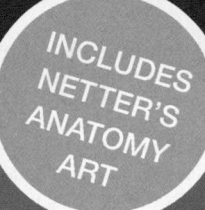

INCLUDES
NETTER'S
ANATOMY
ART

Carol J. Buck
MS, CPC, CCS-P

Former Program Director
Medical Secretary Programs
Northwest Technical College
East Grand Forks, Minnesota

ELSEVIER

ELSEVIER

3251 Riverport Lane
St. Louis, Missouri 63043

2016 ICD-10-CM PHYSICIAN EDITION

ISBN: 978-0-323-27976-5
eISBN: 978-0-323-29184-2

Copyright © 2016 Elsevier Inc. All Rights Reserved.

Some material was previously published.

No part of this publication may be reproduced or transmitted in any form or by any means, electronic or mechanical, including photocopying, recording, or any information storage and retrieval system, without permission in writing from the publisher. Details on how to seek permission, further information about the Publisher's permissions policies and our arrangements with organizations such as the Copyright Clearance Center and the Copyright Licensing Agency can be found at our website: www.elsevier.com/permissions.

This book and the individual contributions contained in it are protected under copyright by the Publisher (other than as may be noted herein).

Notice

Knowledge and best practice in this field are constantly changing. As new research and experience broaden our understanding, changes in research methods, professional practices, or medical treatment may become necessary.

Practitioners and researchers must always rely on their own experience and knowledge in evaluating and using any information, methods, compounds, or experiments described herein. In using such information or methods they should be mindful of their own safety and the safety of others, including parties for whom they have a professional responsibility.

With respect to any drug or pharmaceutical products identified, readers are advised to check the most current information provided (i) on procedures featured or (ii) by the manufacturer of each product to be administered, to verify the recommended dose or formula, the method and duration of administration, and contraindications. It is the responsibility of practitioners, relying on their own experience and knowledge of their patients, to make diagnoses, to determine dosages and the best treatment for each individual patient, and to take all appropriate safety precautions.

To the fullest extent of the law, neither the Publisher nor the authors, contributors, or editors, assume any liability for any injury and/or damage to persons or property as a matter of products liability, negligence or otherwise, or from any use or operation of any methods, products, instructions, or ideas contained in the material herein.

Library of Congress Cataloging-in-Publication Data

Buck, Carol J., author.
  2016 ICD-10-CM for physicians professional edition / Carol J. Buck.
    p. ; cm.
  ICD-10-CM for physicians professional edition
  ISBN 978-0-323-27976-5 (spiral bound : alk. paper) -- ISBN 978-0-323-29184-2 (eISBN)
  I. Title. II. Title: ICD-10-CM for physicians professional edition.
  [DNLM: 1. International statistical classification of diseases and related health problems. 10th revision.
Clinical modification. 2. Disease--classification. 3. Clinical Coding--standards. 4. International
Classification of Diseases. 5. Medical Records--classification. 6. Physicians. WB 15]
  RB115
  616.001'2--dc23

                                                                                    2015023074

Director, Private Sector Education & Professional/References: Jeanne R. Olson
Content Development Manager: Luke Held
Publishing Services Manager: Jeffrey Patterson
Project Manager: Lisa A. P. Bushy
Senior Designer: Julia Dummitt

Printed in Canada

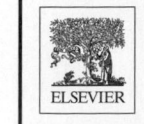 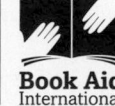 Working together to grow libraries in developing countries

www.elsevier.com • www.bookaid.org

Last digit is the print number: 9 8 7 6 5 4 3 2 1

DEVELOPMENT OF THIS EDITION

Editorial Consultant

Jenna Price
President
Price Editorial Services, LLC
St. Louis, Missouri

Query Team

Patricia Cordy Henricksen, MS, CHCA, CPC-I, CPC, CCP-P, ASC-PM
Auditing and Coding Educator
Soterion Medical Services
Lexington, Kentucky

Jackie L. Grass, CPC
Coding and Reimbursement Specialist
Grand Forks, North Dakota

Kathleen Buchda, CPC, CPMA
Revenue Recognition
New Richmond, Wisconsin

Elsevier/MC Strategies Revenue Cycle, Coding and Compliance Staff

"Experts in providing e-learning on revenue cycle, coding and compliance."

Deborah Neville, RHIA, CCS-P
Director

Lynn-Marie D. Wozniak, MS, RHIT
Content Manager

Sandra L. Macica, MS, RHIA, CCS, ROCC
Product Specialist

Therese M. Jorwic, MPH, RHIA, CCS, CCS-P, FAHIMA
Product Specialist

Received
DEC 2015
Acquisitions
C.U. Library

Campbell University Library
Buies Creek, NC 27506

Received

CONTENTS

GUIDE TO USING THE 2016 ICD-10-CM FOR PHYSICIANS

Medical coding has long been a part of the health care profession. Through the years medical coding systems have become more complex and extensive. Today, medical coding is an intricate and immense process that is present in every health care setting. The increased use of electronic submissions for health care services only increases the need for coders who understand the coding process.

2016 ICD-10-CM for Physicians, Professional Edition was developed to help meet the needs of coding professionals at all levels by offering a comprehensive coding text at a reasonable price.

All material strictly adheres to the latest government versions available at the time of printing. Updates from the *Definitions of Medicare Code Edits* (MCE) will be posted to the companion website (www. codingupdates.com) when available.

Illustrations and Items

The ICD-10-CM Tabular List contains illustrations, pictures, and items to assist you in understanding difficult terminology, diseases/conditions, or coding in a specific category. Items are always printed in ▆▆▆▆ ink so that the added material is not mistaken for official notations or instructions. ▆▆▆▆ ink is used for other annotations in the text. Your ideas on what other descriptions or illustrations should be in future editions of this text are always appreciated.

Instructional Notations

Includes Notes

Includes

The word 'Includes' appears immediately under certain categories to further define, or give examples of, the content of the category.

Excludes Notes

The ICD-10-CM has two types of excludes notes. Each note has a different definition for use, but they are both similar in that they indicate that codes excluded from each other are independent of each other.

Excludes1

A type 1 Excludes note is a pure excludes. It means "NOT CODED HERE!" An Excludes1 note indicates that the code excluded should never be used at the same time as the code above the Excludes1 note. An Excludes1 is for use when two conditions cannot occur together, such as a congenital form versus an acquired form of the same condition.

Excludes2

A type 2 Excludes note represents "NOT INCLUDED HERE." An Excludes2 note indicates that the condition excluded is not part of the condition it is excluded from but a patient may have both conditions at the same time. When an Excludes2 note appears under a code, it is acceptable to use both the code and the excluded code together.

Code First/Use Additional Code notes (etiology/manifestation paired codes)

Certain conditions have both an underlying etiology and multiple body system manifestations due to the underlying etiology. For such conditions the ICD-10-CM has a coding convention that requires the underlying condition be sequenced first, followed by the manifestation. Wherever such a combination exists, there is a "use additional code" note at the etiology note, and a "code first" note at the manifestation code. These instructional notes indicate the proper sequencing order of the codes, etiology followed by manifestation.

In most cases the manifestation codes will have in the code title, "in diseases classified elsewhere." Codes with this title are a component of the etiology/manifestation convention. The code title indicates that it is a manifestation code. "In diseases classified elsewhere" codes are never permitted to be used as first-listed or principal diagnosis codes. They must be used in conjunction with an underlying condition code, and they must be listed following the underlying condition.

Use additional

The words indicate an instructional note that another code may be needed.

Code first

The words indicate an instructional note that directs the coder to sequence the underlying condition before the manifestation.

Code also

A "code also" note instructs that two codes may be required to fully describe a condition, but the sequencing of the two codes is discretionary, depending on the severity of the conditions and the reason for the encounter.

Unspecified

The highlight indicates that although the code is valid as a principal (first-listed) diagnosis, it is not as specific as other codes without the highlight.

7th characters and placeholder X

For codes less than 6 characters that require a 7th character a placeholder X should be assigned for all characters less than 6. The 7th character must always be the 7th character of a code.

Annotated

Throughout the manual, revisions, additions, and deleted codes or words are indicated by the following symbols:

⟵▥ **Revised:** Revisions within the line or code from the previous edition are indicated by the arrow.

◀ **New:** Additions to the previous edition are indicated by the triangle.

~~deleted~~ **Deleted:** Deletions from the previous edition are struck through.

ICD-10-CM Tabular List Symbols

● **Use Additional Character(s):** The red stop sign cautions that the code requires additional character(s) to ensure the greatest specificity.

X For codes less than 6 characters that require a 7th character, a placeholder X should be assigned for all characters less than 6. The 7th character must always be the 7th character of a code.

OGCR The *Official Guidelines for Coding and Reporting* symbol includes the placement of a portion of a guideline as that guideline pertains to the code by which it is located. The complete OGCR are located in Part I.

▶ **Manifestation Code:** Describes the manifestation of an underlying disease, not the disease itself, and therefore should not be assigned as a principal diagnosis, according to the *Definitions of Medicare Code Edits, Version 32* (MCE).

Age conflict: The *Definitions of Medicare Code Edits* (MCE) detects inconsistencies between a patient's age and diagnosis. For example, a 5-year-old patient with benign prostatic hypertrophy or a 78-year-old pregnant female.

The diagnosis is clinically and virtually impossible in a patient of the stated age. Therefore, either the diagnosis or the age is presumed to be incorrect. There are four age categories for diagnoses in the *Definitions of Medicare Code Edits, Version 32* (MCE):

N • Newborn. Age of 0 years; a subset of diagnoses intended only for newborns and neonates (e.g., fetal distress, perinatal jaundice).

P • Pediatric. Age range is 0-17 years inclusive (e.g., Reye's syndrome, routine child health exam).

M • Maternity. Age range is 12-55 years inclusive (e.g., diabetes in pregnancy, antepartum pulmonary complication).

A • Adult. Age range is 15-124 years inclusive (e.g., senile delirium, mature cataract).

♀♂ **Sex conflict:** *Definitions of Medicare Code Edits, Version 32* (MCE) detects inconsistencies between a patient's sex and any diagnosis or procedure on the patient's record. For example, a male patient with cervical cancer (diagnosis) or a female patient with a prostatectomy (procedure). In both instances, the indicated diagnosis or the procedure conflicts with the stated sex of the patient. Therefore, either the patient's diagnosis, procedure, or sex is presumed to be incorrect.

SYMBOLS AND CONVENTIONS

ICD-10-CM Tabular

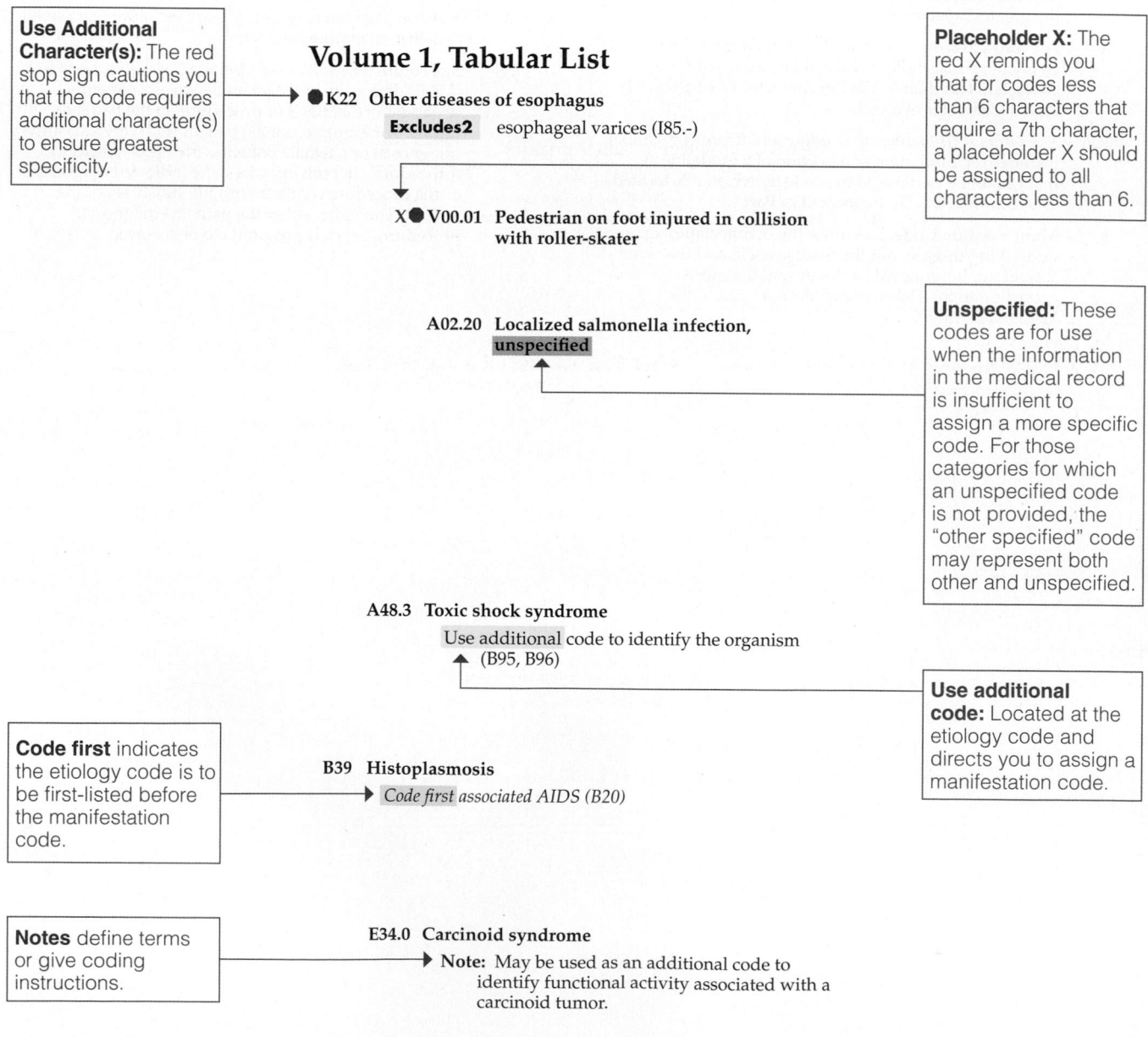

Use Additional Character(s): The red stop sign cautions you that the code requires additional character(s) to ensure greatest specificity.

Volume 1, Tabular List

● **K22** **Other diseases of esophagus**

 Excludes2 esophageal varices (I85.-)

X ● **V00.01** **Pedestrian on foot injured in collision with roller-skater**

A02.20 **Localized salmonella infection, unspecified**

A48.3 **Toxic shock syndrome**

 Use additional code to identify the organism (B95, B96)

B39 **Histoplasmosis**

 Code first associated AIDS (B20)

E34.0 **Carcinoid syndrome**

 Note: May be used as an additional code to identify functional activity associated with a carcinoid tumor.

Placeholder X: The red X reminds you that for codes less than 6 characters that require a 7th character, a placeholder X should be assigned to all characters less than 6.

Unspecified: These codes are for use when the information in the medical record is insufficient to assign a more specific code. For those categories for which an unspecified code is not provided, the "other specified" code may represent both other and unspecified.

Use additional code: Located at the etiology code and directs you to assign a manifestation code.

Code first indicates the etiology code is to be first-listed before the manifestation code.

Notes define terms or give coding instructions.

Codes or index entries are for purposes of illustration only and may not be current.

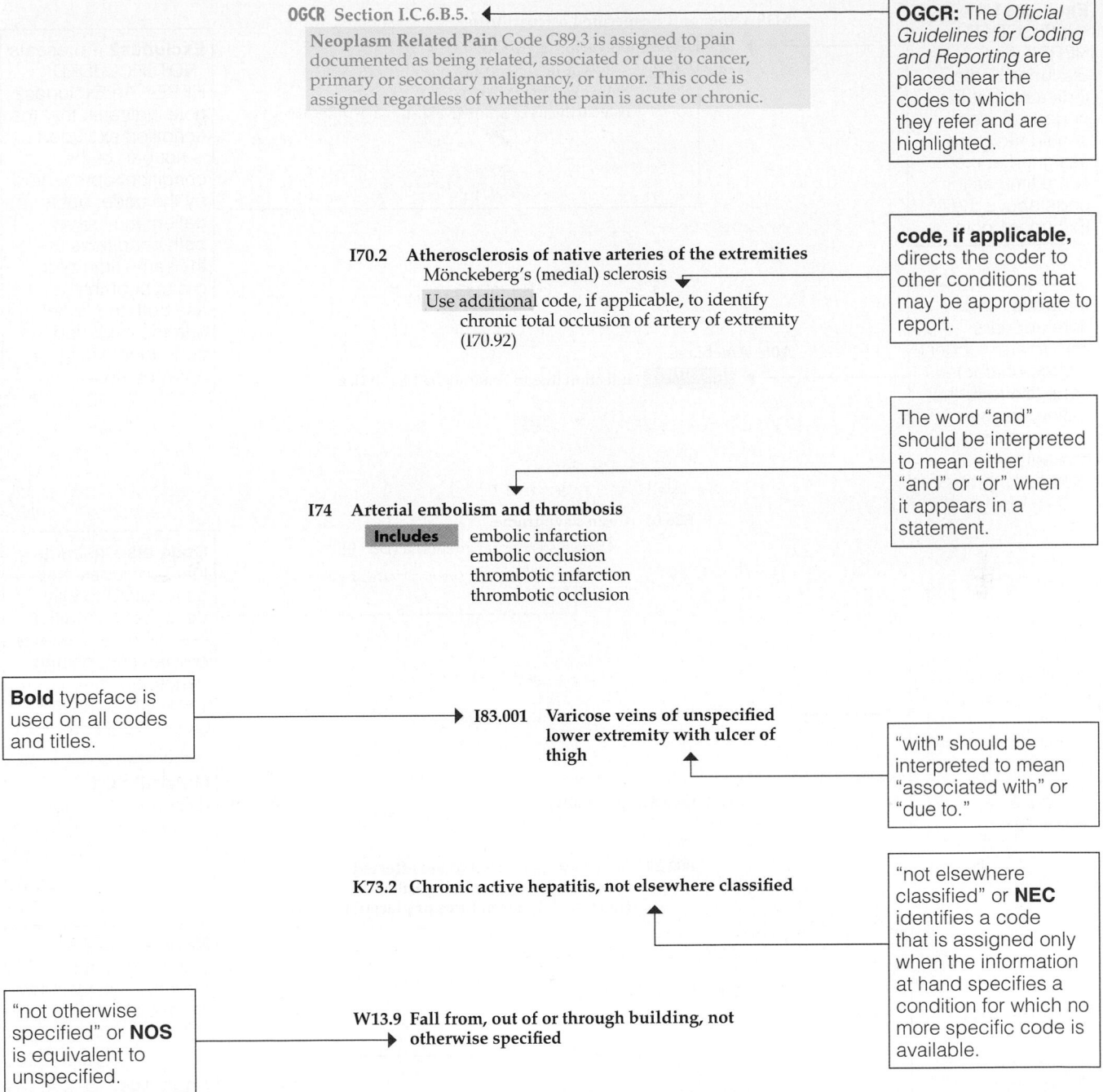

OGCR Section I.C.6.B.5.

Neoplasm Related Pain Code G89.3 is assigned to pain documented as being related, associated or due to cancer, primary or secondary malignancy, or tumor. This code is assigned regardless of whether the pain is acute or chronic.

OGCR: The *Official Guidelines for Coding and Reporting* are placed near the codes to which they refer and are highlighted.

I70.2 **Atherosclerosis of native arteries of the extremities**
Mönckeberg's (medial) sclerosis

Use additional code, if applicable, to identify chronic total occlusion of artery of extremity (I70.92)

code, if applicable, directs the coder to other conditions that may be appropriate to report.

The word "and" should be interpreted to mean either "and" or "or" when it appears in a statement.

I74 **Arterial embolism and thrombosis**
Includes embolic infarction
embolic occlusion
thrombotic infarction
thrombotic occlusion

Bold typeface is used on all codes and titles.

I83.001 **Varicose veins of unspecified lower extremity with ulcer of thigh**

"with" should be interpreted to mean "associated with" or "due to."

"not elsewhere classified" or **NEC** identifies a code that is assigned only when the information at hand specifies a condition for which no more specific code is available.

K73.2 **Chronic active hepatitis, not elsewhere classified**

"not otherwise specified" or **NOS** is equivalent to unspecified.

W13.9 **Fall from, out of or through building, not otherwise specified**

Codes or index entries are for purposes of illustration only and may not be current.

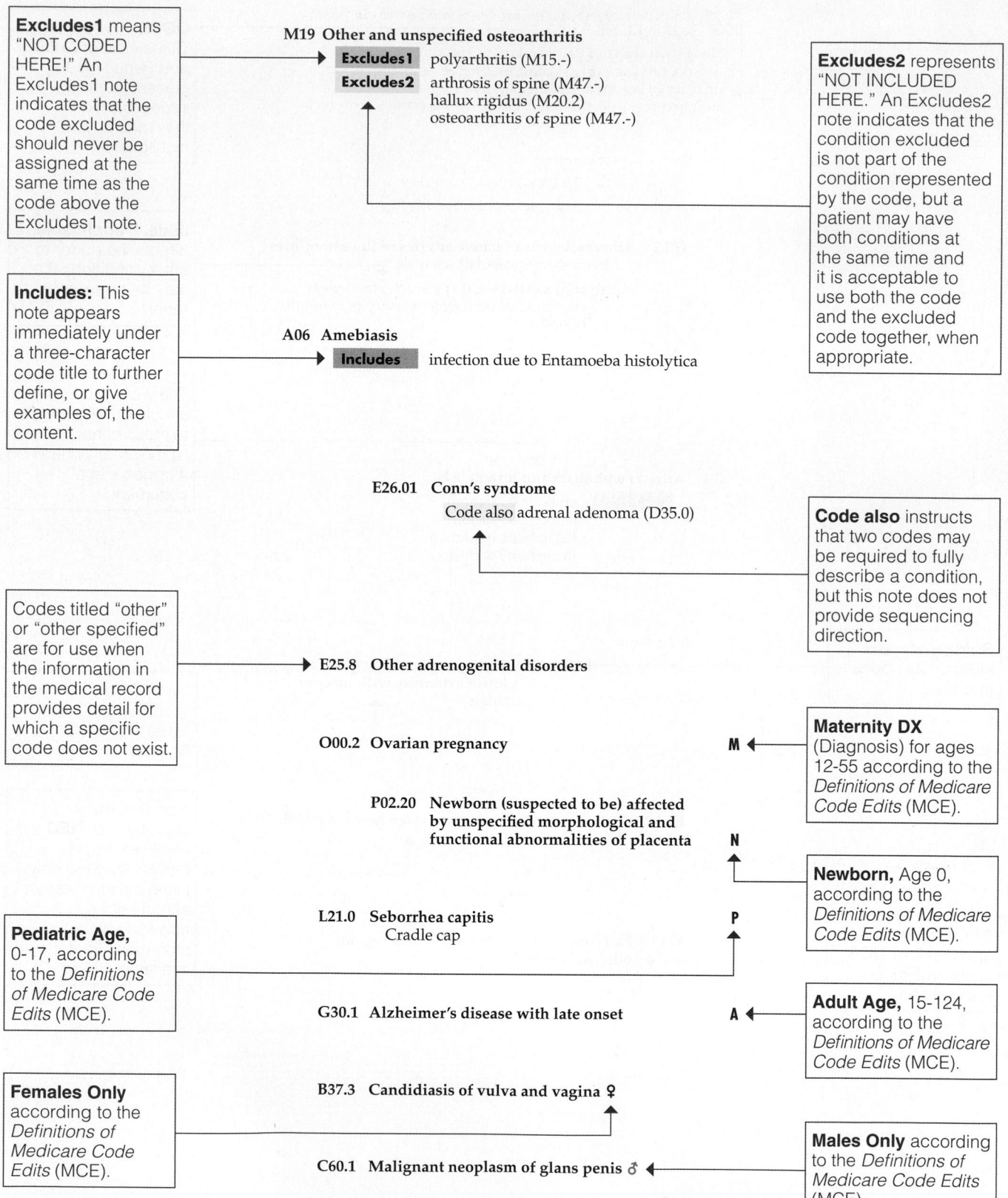

Excludes1 means "NOT CODED HERE!" An Excludes1 note indicates that the code excluded should never be assigned at the same time as the code above the Excludes1 note.

M19 Other and unspecified osteoarthritis
   Excludes1   polyarthritis (M15.-)
   Excludes2   arthrosis of spine (M47.-)
                    hallux rigidus (M20.2)
                    osteoarthritis of spine (M47.-)

Excludes2 represents "NOT INCLUDED HERE." An Excludes2 note indicates that the condition excluded is not part of the condition represented by the code, but a patient may have both conditions at the same time and it is acceptable to use both the code and the excluded code together, when appropriate.

Includes: This note appears immediately under a three-character code title to further define, or give examples of, the content.

A06 Amebiasis
   Includes   infection due to Entamoeba histolytica

E26.01   Conn's syndrome
         Code also adrenal adenoma (D35.0)

Code also instructs that two codes may be required to fully describe a condition, but this note does not provide sequencing direction.

Codes titled "other" or "other specified" are for use when the information in the medical record provides detail for which a specific code does not exist.

E25.8   Other adrenogenital disorders

O00.2   Ovarian pregnancy   M

Maternity DX (Diagnosis) for ages 12-55 according to the *Definitions of Medicare Code Edits* (MCE).

P02.20   Newborn (suspected to be) affected by unspecified morphological and functional abnormalities of placenta   N

Newborn, Age 0, according to the *Definitions of Medicare Code Edits* (MCE).

L21.0   Seborrhea capitis
        Cradle cap   P

Pediatric Age, 0-17, according to the *Definitions of Medicare Code Edits* (MCE).

G30.1   Alzheimer's disease with late onset   A

Adult Age, 15-124, according to the *Definitions of Medicare Code Edits* (MCE).

Females Only according to the *Definitions of Medicare Code Edits* (MCE).

B37.3   Candidiasis of vulva and vagina ♀

C60.1   Malignant neoplasm of glans penis ♂

Males Only according to the *Definitions of Medicare Code Edits* (MCE).

Codes or index entries are for purposes of illustration only and may not be current.

▶ H22   *Disorders of iris and ciliary body in diseases classified elsewhere*

   Code first *underlying disease, such as:*
      gout (M1A-, M10.-)

Manifestation
according to the
*Definitions of
Medicare Code
Edits* (MCE).

G14   **Postpolio syndrome**
   Includes   Postpolio myelitic syndrome
   Excludes1 sequelae of poliomyelitis (B91)

Codes or index entries are for purposes of illustration only and may not be current.

Alphabetic Index

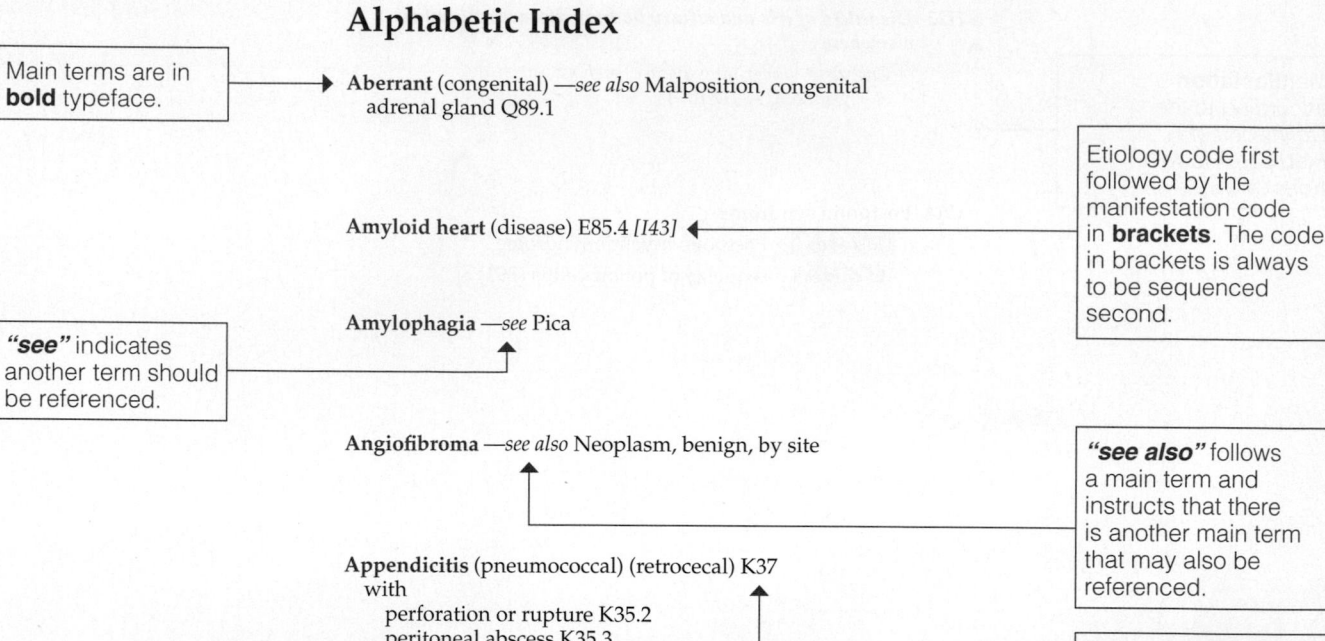

Main terms are in **bold** typeface.

Aberrant (congenital) —*see also* Malposition, congenital
   adrenal gland Q89.1

Etiology code first followed by the manifestation code in **brackets**. The code in brackets is always to be sequenced second.

Amyloid heart (disease) E85.4 *[I43]*

Amylophagia —*see* Pica

"see" indicates another term should be referenced.

Angiofibroma —*see also* Neoplasm, benign, by site

"see also" follows a main term and instructs that there is another main term that may also be referenced.

Appendicitis (pneumococcal) (retrocecal) K37
   with
      perforation or rupture K35.2
      peritoneal abscess K35.3

A default code is listed next to the main term and represents that condition most commonly associated with the main term. If a condition is documented in a medical record without any additional information, such as acute or chronic, the default code should be assigned.

Codes or index entries are for purposes of illustration only and may not be current.

PART I

Introduction

ICD-10-CM Official Guidelines for Coding and Reporting 2016

Narrative changes appear in **bold** text
Items <u>underlined</u> have been moved within the guidelines since the 2014 version
Italics are used to indicate revisions to heading changes

The Centers for Medicare and Medicaid Services (CMS) and the National Center for Health Statistics (NCHS), two departments within the U.S. Federal Government's Department of Health and Human Services (DHHS) provide the following guidelines for coding and reporting using the International Classification of Diseases, 10th Revision, Clinical Modification (ICD-10-CM). These guidelines should be used as a companion document to the official version of the ICD-10-CM as published on the NCHS website. The ICD-10-CM is a morbidity classification published by the United States for classifying diagnoses and reason for visits in all health care settings. The ICD-10-CM is based on the ICD-10, the statistical classification of disease published by the World Health Organization (WHO).

These guidelines have been approved by the four organizations that make up the Cooperating Parties for the ICD-10-CM: the American Hospital Association (AHA), the American Health Information Management Association (AHIMA), CMS, and NCHS.

These guidelines are a set of rules that have been developed to accompany and complement the official conventions and instructions provided within the ICD-10-CM itself. The instructions and conventions of the classification take precedence over guidelines. These guidelines are based on the coding and sequencing instructions in the Tabular List and Alphabetic Index of ICD-10-CM, but provide additional instruction. Adherence to these guidelines when assigning ICD-10-CM diagnosis codes is required under the Health Insurance Portability and Accountability Act (HIPAA). The diagnosis codes (Tabular List and Alphabetic Index) have been adopted under HIPAA for all healthcare settings. A joint effort between the healthcare provider and the coder is essential to achieve complete and accurate documentation, code assignment, and reporting of diagnoses and procedures. These guidelines have been developed to assist both the healthcare provider and the coder in identifying those diagnoses that are to be reported. The importance of consistent, complete documentation in the medical record cannot be overemphasized. Without such documentation accurate coding cannot be achieved. The entire record should be reviewed to determine the specific reason for the encounter and the conditions treated.

The term encounter is used for all settings, including hospital admissions. In the context of these guidelines, the term provider is used throughout the guidelines to mean physician or any qualified health care practitioner who is legally accountable for establishing the patient's diagnosis. Only this set of guidelines, approved by the Cooperating Parties, is official.

The guidelines are organized into sections. Section I includes the structure and conventions of the classification and general guidelines that apply to the entire classification, and chapter-specific guidelines that correspond to the chapters as they are arranged in the classification. Section II includes guidelines for selection of principal diagnosis for non-outpatient settings. Section III includes guidelines for reporting additional diagnoses in non-outpatient settings. Section IV is for outpatient coding and reporting. It is necessary to review all sections of the guidelines to fully understand all of the rules and instructions needed to code properly.

ICD-10-CM Official Guidelines for Coding and Reporting

Section I. Conventions, general coding guidelines and chapter specific guidelines

A. Conventions for the ICD-10-CM
1. The Alphabetic Index and Tabular List
2. Format and Structure:
3. Use of codes for reporting purposes
4. Placeholder character
5. 7th Characters
6. Abbreviations
   a. Alphabetic Index abbreviations
   b. Tabular List abbreviations
7. Punctuation
8. Use of "and"
9. Other and Unspecified codes
   a. "Other" codes
   b. "Unspecified" codes
10. Includes Notes
11. Inclusion terms
12. Excludes Notes
    a. Excludes1
    b. Excludes2
13. Etiology/manifestation convention ("code first", "use additional code" and "in diseases classified elsewhere" notes)
14. "And"
15. "With"
16. "See" and "See Also"
17. "Code also note"
18. Default codes

B. General Coding Guidelines
1. Locating a code in the ICD-10-CM
2. Level of Detail in Coding
3. Code or codes from A00.0 through T88.9, Z00-Z99.8
4. Signs and symptoms
5. Conditions that are an integral part of a disease process
6. Conditions that are not an integral part of a disease process
7. Multiple coding for a single condition
8. Acute and Chronic Conditions
9. Combination Code
10. Sequela (Late Effects)
11. Impending or Threatened Condition
12. Reporting Same Diagnosis Code More than Once
13. Laterality
14. Documentation for BMI, Non-pressure ulcers and Pressure Ulcer Stages
15. Syndromes
16. Documentation of Complications of Care
17. Borderline Diagnosis
18. Use of Sign/Symptom/Unspecified Codes

C. Chapter-Specific Coding Guidelines
1. Chapter 1: Certain Infectious and Parasitic Diseases (A00-B99)
   a. Human Immunodeficiency Virus (HIV) Infections
   b. Infectious agents as the cause of diseases classified to other chapters
   c. Infections resistant to antibiotics
   d. Sepsis, Severe Sepsis, and Septic Shock
   e. Methicillin Resistant *Staphylococcus aureus* (MRSA) Conditions
2. Chapter 2: Neoplasms (C00-D49)
   a. Treatment directed at the malignancy
   b. Treatment of secondary site
   c. Coding and sequencing of complications
   d. Primary malignancy previously excised
   e. Admissions/Encounters involving chemotherapy, immunotherapy and radiation therapy
   f. Admission/encounter to determine extent of malignancy
   g. Symptoms, signs, and abnormal findings listed in Chapter 18 associated with neoplasms
   h. Admission/encounter for pain control/management
   i. Malignancy in two or more noncontiguous sites
   j. Disseminated malignant neoplasm, unspecified
   k. Malignant neoplasm without specification of site
   l. Sequencing of neoplasm codes
   m. Current malignancy versus personal history of malignancy
   n. Leukemia, Multiple Myeloma, and Malignant Plasma Cell Neoplasms in remission versus personal history
   o. Aftercare following surgery for neoplasm
   p. Follow-up care for completed treatment of a malignancy
   q. Prophylactic organ removal for prevention of malignancy
   r. Malignant neoplasm associated with transplanted organ
3. Chapter 3: Disease of the blood and blood-forming organs and certain disorders involving the immune mechanism (D50-D89)
4. Chapter 4: Endocrine, Nutritional, and Metabolic Diseases (E00-E89)
   a. Diabetes mellitus
5. Chapter 5: Mental, Behavioral and Neurodevelopmental disorders (F01 – F99)
   a. Pain disorders related to psychological factors
   b. Mental and behavioral disorders due to psychoactive substance use
6. Chapter 6: Diseases of the Nervous System (G00-G99)
   a. Dominant/nondominant side
   b. Pain - Category G89
7. Chapter 7: Diseases of the Eye and Adnexa (H00-H59)
   a. Glaucoma
8. Chapter 8: Diseases of the Ear and Mastoid Process (H60-H95)
9. Chapter 9: Diseases of the Circulatory System (I00-I99)
   a. Hypertension
   b. Atherosclerotic Coronary Artery Disease and Angina
   c. Intraoperative and Postprocedural Cerebrovascular Accident
   d. Sequelae of Cerebrovascular Disease
   e. Acute myocardial infarction (AMI)

10. Chapter 10: Diseases of the Respiratory System (J00-J99)
    a. Chronic Obstructive Pulmonary Disease [COPD] and Asthma
    b. Acute Respiratory Failure
    c. Influenza due to certain identified influenza viruses
    d. Ventilator associated Pneumonia
11. Chapter 11: Diseases of the Digestive System (K00-K95)
12. Chapter 12: Diseases of the Skin and Subcutaneous Tissue (L00-L99)
    a. Pressure ulcer stage codes
13. Chapter 13: Diseases of the Musculoskeletal System and Connective Tissue (M00-M99)
    a. Site and laterality
    b. Acute traumatic versus chronic or recurrent musculoskeletal conditions
    c. Coding of Pathologic Fractures
    d. Osteoporosis
14. Chapter 14: Diseases of Genitourinary System (N00-N99)
    a. Chronic kidney disease
15. Chapter 15: Pregnancy, Childbirth, and the Puerperium (O00-O9A)
    a. General Rules for Obstetric Cases
    b. Selection of OB Principal or First-listed Diagnosis
    c. Pre-existing conditions versus conditions due to the pregnancy
    d. Pre-existing hypertension in pregnancy
    e. Fetal Conditions Affecting the Management of the Mother
    f. HIV Infection in Pregnancy, Childbirth and the Puerperium
    g. Diabetes mellitus in pregnancy
    h. Long term use of insulin
    i. Gestational (pregnancy induced) diabetes
    j. Sepsis and septic shock complicating abortion, pregnancy, childbirth and the puerperium
    k. Puerperal sepsis
    l. Alcohol and tobacco use during pregnancy, childbirth and the puerperium
    m. Poisoning, toxic effects, adverse effects and underdosing in a pregnant patient
    n. Normal Delivery, Code O80
    o. The Peripartum and Postpartum Periods
    p. Code O94, Sequelae of complication of pregnancy, childbirth, and the puerperium
    q. Termination of Pregnancy and Spontaneous abortions
    r. Abuse in a pregnant patient
16. Chapter 16: Certain Conditions Originating in the Perinatal Period (P00-P96)
    a. General Perinatal Rules
    b. Observation and Evaluation of Newborns for Suspected Conditions not Found
    c. Coding Additional Perinatal Diagnoses
    d. Prematurity and Fetal Growth Retardation
    e. Low birth weight and immaturity status
    f. Bacterial Sepsis of Newborn
    g. Stillbirth
17. Chapter 17: Congenital malformations, deformations, and chromosomal abnormalities (Q00-Q99)
18. Chapter 18: Symptoms, signs, and abnormal clinical and laboratory findings, not elsewhere classified (R00-R99)
    a. Use of symptom codes
    b. Use of a symptom code with a definitive diagnosis code
    c. Combination codes that include symptoms
    d. Repeated falls
    e. Coma scale
    f. Functional quadriplegia
    g. SIRS due to Non-Infectious Process
    h. Death NOS
19. Chapter 19: Injury, poisoning, and certain other consequences of external causes (S00-T88)
    a. Application of 7th Characters in Chapter 19
    b. Coding of Injuries
    c. Coding of Traumatic Fractures
    d. Coding of Burns and Corrosions
    e. Adverse Effects, Poisoning, Underdosing and Toxic Effects
    f. Adult and child abuse, neglect and other maltreatment
    g. Complications of care
20. Chapter 20: External Causes of Morbidity (V00-Y99)
    a. General External Cause Coding Guidelines
    b. Place of Occurrence Guideline
    c. Activity Code
    d. Place of Occurrence, Activity, and Status Codes Used with other External Cause Code
    e. If the Reporting Format Limits the Number of External Cause Codes
    f. Multiple External Cause Coding Guidelines
    g. Child and Adult Abuse Guideline
    h. Unknown or Undetermined Intent Guideline
    i. Sequelae (Late Effects) of External Cause Guidelines
    j. Terrorism Guidelines
    k. External cause status
21. Chapter 21: Factors influencing health status and contact with health services (Z00-Z99)
    a. Use of Z codes in any healthcare setting
    b. Z Codes indicate a reason for an encounter
    c. Categories of Z Codes

Section II. Selection of Principal Diagnosis

A. Codes for symptoms, signs, and ill-defined conditions
B. Two or more interrelated conditions, each potentially meeting the definition for principal diagnosis
C. Two or more diagnoses that equally meet the definition for principal diagnosis
D. Two or more comparative or contrasting conditions
E. A symptom(s) followed by contrasting/comparative diagnoses
F. Original treatment plan not carried out
G. Complications of surgery and other medical care
H. Uncertain Diagnosis

I. Admission from Observation Unit
1. Admission Following Medical Observation
2. Admission Following Post-Operative Observation
J. Admission from Outpatient Surgery
K. Admissions/Encounters for Rehabilitation

Section III. Reporting Additional Diagnoses

A. Previous conditions
B. Abnormal findings
C. Uncertain Diagnosis

Section IV. Diagnostic Coding and Reporting Guidelines for Outpatient Services

A. Selection of first-listed condition
1. Outpatient Surgery
2. Observation Stay
B. Codes from A00.0 through T88.9, Z00-Z99
C. Accurate reporting of ICD-10-CM diagnosis codes
D. Codes that describe symptoms and signs
E. Encounters for circumstances other than a disease or injury
F. Level of Detail in Coding
1. ICD-10-CM codes with 3, 4, 5, 6, or 7 characters
2. Use of full number of characters required for a code
G. ICD-10-CM code for the diagnosis, condition, problem, or other reason for encounter/visit
H. Uncertain diagnosis
I. Chronic diseases
J. Code all documented conditions that coexist
K. Patients receiving diagnostic services only
L. Patients receiving therapeutic services only
M. Patients receiving preoperative evaluations only
N. Ambulatory surgery
O. Routine outpatient prenatal visits
P. Encounters for general medical examinations with abnormal findings
Q. Encounters for routine health screenings

Appendix I: Present on Admission Reporting Guidelines

Section I. Conventions, general coding guidelines and chapter specific guidelines

The conventions, general guidelines and chapter-specific guidelines are applicable to all health care settings unless otherwise indicated. The conventions and instructions of the classification take precedence over guidelines.

A. **Conventions for the ICD-10-CM**
The conventions for the ICD-10-CM are the general rules for use of the classification independent of the guidelines. These conventions are incorporated within the Alphabetic Index and Tabular List of the ICD-10-CM as instructional notes.

1. **The Alphabetic Index and Tabular List**
The ICD-10-CM is divided into the Alphabetic Index, an alphabetical list of terms and their corresponding code, and the Tabular List, a structured list of codes divided into chapters based on body system or condition. The Alphabetic Index consists of the following parts: the Index of Diseases and Injury, the Index of External Causes of Injury, the Table of Neoplasms and the Table of Drugs and Chemicals.
See Section I.C2. General guidelines
See Section I.C.19. Adverse effects, poisoning, underdosing and toxic effects

2. **Format and Structure:**
The ICD-10-CM Tabular List contains categories, subcategories and codes. Characters for categories, subcategories and codes may be either a letter or a number. All categories are 3 characters. A three-character category that has no further subdivision is equivalent to a code. Subcategories are either 4 or 5 characters. Codes may be 3, 4, 5, 6 or 7 characters. That is, each level of subdivision after a category is a subcategory. The final level of subdivision is a code. Codes that have applicable 7th characters are still referred to as codes, not subcategories. A code that has an applicable 7th character is considered invalid without the 7th character.
The ICD-10-CM uses an indented format for ease in reference

3. **Use of codes for reporting purposes**
For reporting purposes only codes are permissible, not categories or subcategories, and any applicable 7th character is required.

4. **Placeholder character**
The ICD-10-CM utilizes a placeholder character "X". The "X" is used as a placeholder at certain codes to allow for future expansion. An example of this is at the poisoning, adverse effect and underdosing codes, categories T36-T50. Where a placeholder exists, the X must be used in order for the code to be considered a valid code.

5. **7th Characters**
Certain ICD-10-CM categories have applicable 7th characters. The applicable 7th character is required for all codes within the category, or as the notes in the Tabular List instruct. The 7th character must always be the 7th character in the data field. If a code that requires a 7th character is not 6 characters, a placeholder X must be used to fill in the empty characters.

6. **Abbreviations**
a. **Alphabetic Index abbreviations**
NEC "Not elsewhere classifiable"
This abbreviation in the Alphabetic Index represents "other specified". When a specific code is not available for a condition the Alphabetic Index directs the coder to the "other specified" code in the Tabular List.
NOS "Not otherwise specified"
This abbreviation is the equivalent of unspecified.

GUIDELINES (ICD-10-CM)

b. **Tabular List abbreviations**

NEC "Not elsewhere classifiable"
This abbreviation in the Tabular List represents "other specified". When a specific code is not available for a condition the Tabular List includes an NEC entry under a code to identify the code as the "other specified" code.

NOS "Not otherwise specified"
This abbreviation is the equivalent of unspecified.

7. **Punctuation**

[ ] Brackets are used in the Tabular List to enclose synonyms, alternative wording or explanatory phrases. Brackets are used in the Alphabetic Index to identify manifestation codes.

( ) Parentheses are used in both the Alphabetic Index and Tabular List to enclose supplementary words that may be present or absent in the statement of a disease or procedure without affecting the code number to which it is assigned. The terms within the parentheses are referred to as nonessential modifiers. The nonessential modifiers in the Alphabetic Index to Diseases apply to subterms following a main term except when a nonessential modifier and a subentry are mutually exclusive, the subentry takes precedence. For example, in the ICD-10-CM Alphabetic Index under the main term Enteritis, "acute" is a nonessential modifier and "chronic" is a subentry. In this case, the nonessential modifier "acute" does not apply to the subentry "chronic".

: Colons are used in the Tabular List after an incomplete term which needs one or more of the modifiers following the colon to make it assignable to a given category.

8. **Use of "and".**

See Section I.A.14. Use of the term "And"

9. **Other and Unspecified codes**

a. **"Other" codes**

Codes titled "other" or "other specified" are for use when the information in the medical record provides detail for which a specific code does not exist. Alphabetic Index entries with NEC in the line designate "other" codes in the Tabular List. These Alphabetic Index entries represent specific disease entities for which no specific code exists so the term is included within an "other" code.

b. **"Unspecified" codes**

Codes titled "unspecified" are for use when the information in the medical record is insufficient to assign a more specific code. For those categories for which an unspecified code is not provided, the "other specified" code may represent both other and unspecified.

See Section I.B.18 Use of Signs/Symptom/Unspecified Codes

10. **Includes Notes**

This note appears immediately under a three-character code title to further define, or give examples of, the content of the category.

11. **Inclusion terms**

List of terms is included under some codes. These terms are the conditions for which that code is to be used. The terms may be synonyms of the code title, or, in the case of "other specified" codes, the terms are a list of the various conditions assigned to that code. The inclusion terms are not necessarily exhaustive. Additional terms found only in the Alphabetic Index may also be assigned to a code.

12. **Excludes Notes**

The ICD-10-CM has two types of excludes notes. Each type of note has a different definition for use but they are all similar in that they indicate that codes excluded from each other are independent of each other.

a. **Excludes1**

A type 1 Excludes note is a pure excludes note. It means "NOT CODED HERE!" An Excludes1 note indicates that the code excluded should never be used at the same time as the code above the Excludes1 note. An Excludes1 is used when two conditions cannot occur together, such as a congenital form versus an acquired form of the same condition.

b. **Excludes2**

A Type 2 Excludes note represents "Not included here". An excludes2 note indicates that the condition excluded is not part of the condition represented by the code, but a patient may have both conditions at the same time. When an Excludes2 note appears under a code, it is acceptable to use both the code and the excluded code together, when appropriate.

13. **Etiology/manifestation convention ("code first", "use additional code" and "in diseases classified elsewhere" notes)**

Certain conditions have both an underlying etiology and multiple body system manifestations due to the underlying etiology. For such conditions, the ICD-10-CM has a coding convention that requires the underlying condition be sequenced first followed by the manifestation. Wherever such a combination exists, there is a "use additional code" note at the etiology code, and a "code first" note at the manifestation code. These instructional notes indicate the proper sequencing order of the codes, etiology followed by manifestation.

In most cases the manifestation codes will have in the code title, "in diseases classified elsewhere." Codes with this title are a component of the etiology/ manifestation convention. The code title indicates that it is a manifestation code. "In diseases classified elsewhere" codes are never permitted to be used as first-listed or principal diagnosis codes. They must be used in conjunction with an underlying condition code and they must be listed following the underlying condition. See category F02, Dementia in other diseases classified elsewhere, for an example of this convention.

There are manifestation codes that do not have "in diseases classified elsewhere" in the title. For such codes, there is a "use additional code" note at the etiology code and a "code first" note at the manifestation code and the rules for sequencing apply.

In addition to the notes in the Tabular List, these conditions also have a specific Alphabetic Index entry structure. In the Alphabetic Index both conditions are listed together with the etiology code first followed by the manifestation codes in brackets. The code in brackets is always to be sequenced second.

An example of the etiology/manifestation convention is dementia in Parkinson's disease. In the Alphabetic Index, code G20 is listed first, followed by code F02.80 or F02.81 in brackets. Code G20 represents the underlying etiology, Parkinson's disease, and must be sequenced first, whereas codes F02.80 and F02.81 represent the manifestation of dementia in diseases classified elsewhere, with or without behavioral disturbance.

"Code first" and "Use additional code" notes are also used as sequencing rules in the classification for certain codes that are not part of an etiology/manifestation combination.

See Section I.B.7. Multiple coding for a single condition.

14. "And"

The word "and" should be interpreted to mean either "and" or "or" when it appears in a title.

For example, cases of "tuberculosis of bones", "tuberculosis of joints" and "tuberculosis of bones and joints" are classified to subcategory A18.0, Tuberculosis of bones and joints.

15. "With"

The word "with" should be interpreted to mean "associated with" or "due to" when it appears in a code title, the Alphabetic Index, or an instructional note in the Tabular List.

The word "with" in the Alphabetic Index is sequenced immediately following the main term, not in alphabetical order.

16. "See" and "See Also"

The "see" instruction following a main term in the Alphabetic Index indicates that another term should be referenced. It is necessary to go to the main term referenced with the "see" note to locate the correct code.

A "see also" instruction following a main term in the Alphabetic Index instructs that there is another main term that may also be referenced that may provide additional Alphabetic Index entries that may be useful. It is not necessary to follow the "see also" note when the original main term provides the necessary code.

17. "Code also note"

A "code also" note instructs that two codes may be required to fully describe a condition, but this note does not provide sequencing direction.

18. Default codes

A code listed next to a main term in the ICD-10-CM Alphabetic Index is referred to as a default code. The default code represents that condition that is most commonly associated with the main term, or is the unspecified code for the condition. If a condition is documented in a medical record (for example, appendicitis) without any additional information, such as acute or chronic, the default code should be assigned.

B. General Coding Guidelines

1. Locating a code in the ICD-10-CM

To select a code in the classification that corresponds to a diagnosis or reason for visit documented in a medical record, first locate the term in the Alphabetic Index, and then verify the code in the Tabular List. Read and be guided by instructional notations that appear in both the Alphabetic Index and the Tabular List.

It is essential to use both the Alphabetic Index and Tabular List when locating and assigning a code. The Alphabetic Index does not always provide the full code. Selection of the full code, including laterality and any applicable 7th character can only be done in the Tabular List. A dash (-) at the end of an Alphabetic Index entry indicates that additional characters are required. Even if a dash is not included at the Alphabetic Index entry, it is necessary to refer to the Tabular List to verify that no 7th character is required.

2. Level of Detail in Coding

Diagnosis codes are to be used and reported at their highest number of characters available.

ICD-10-CM diagnosis codes are composed of codes with 3, 4, 5, 6 or 7 characters. Codes with three characters are included in ICD-10-CM as the heading of a category of codes that may be further subdivided by the use of fourth and/or fifth characters and/or sixth characters, which provide greater detail.

A three-character code is to be used only if it is not further subdivided. A code is invalid if it has not been coded to the full number of characters required for that code, including the 7th character, if applicable.

3. Code or codes from A00.0 through T88.9, Z00-Z99.8

The appropriate code or codes from A00.0 through T88.9, Z00-Z99.8 must be used to identify diagnoses, symptoms, conditions, problems, complaints or other reason(s) for the encounter/visit.

4. Signs and symptoms

Codes that describe symptoms and signs, as opposed to diagnoses, are acceptable for reporting purposes when a related definitive diagnosis has not been established (confirmed) by the provider.

Chapter 18 of ICD-10-CM, Symptoms, Signs, and Abnormal Clinical and Laboratory Findings, Not Elsewhere Classified (codes R00.0 - R99) contains many, but not all codes for symptoms.
See Section I.B.18 Use of Signs/Symptom/ Unspecified Codes

5. Conditions that are an integral part of a disease process
Signs and symptoms that are associated routinely with a disease process should not be assigned as additional codes, unless otherwise instructed by the classification.

6. Conditions that are not an integral part of a disease process
Additional signs and symptoms that may not be associated routinely with a disease process should be coded when present.

7. Multiple coding for a single condition
In addition to the etiology/manifestation convention that requires two codes to fully describe a single condition that affects multiple body systems, there are other single conditions that also require more than one code. "Use additional code" notes are found in the Tabular List at codes that are not part of an etiology/manifestation pair where a secondary code is useful to fully describe a condition. The sequencing rule is the same as the etiology/manifestation pair, "use additional code" indicates that a secondary code should be added.

For example, for bacterial infections that are not included in chapter 1, a secondary code from category B95, Streptococcus, Staphylococcus, and Enterococcus, as the cause of diseases classified elsewhere, or B96, Other bacterial agents as the cause of diseases classified elsewhere, may be required to identify the bacterial organism causing the infection. A "use additional code" note will normally be found at the infectious disease code, indicating a need for the organism code to be added as a secondary code.

"Code first" notes are also under certain codes that are not specifically manifestation codes but may be due to an underlying cause. When there is a "code first" note and an underlying condition is present, the underlying condition should be sequenced first.

"Code, if applicable, any causal condition first", notes indicate that this code may be assigned as a principal diagnosis when the causal condition is unknown or not applicable. If a causal condition is known, then the code for that condition should be sequenced as the principal or first-listed diagnosis.

Multiple codes may be needed for sequela, complication codes and obstetric codes to more fully describe a condition. See the specific guidelines for these conditions for further instruction.

8. Acute and Chronic Conditions
If the same condition is described as both acute (subacute) and chronic, and separate subentries exist in the Alphabetic Index at the same indentation level, code both and sequence the acute (subacute) code first.

9. Combination Code
A combination code is a single code used to classify:
   Two diagnoses, or
   A diagnosis with an associated secondary process (manifestation)
      A diagnosis with an associated complication
   Combination codes are identified by referring to subterm entries in the Alphabetic Index and by reading the inclusion and exclusion notes in the Tabular List.

Assign only the combination code when that code fully identifies the diagnostic conditions involved or when the Alphabetic Index so directs. Multiple coding should not be used when the classification provides a combination code that clearly identifies all of the elements documented in the diagnosis. When the combination code lacks necessary specificity in describing the manifestation or complication, an additional code should be used as a secondary code.

10. Sequela (Late Effects)
A sequela is the residual effect (condition produced) after the acute phase of an illness or injury has terminated. There is no time limit on when a sequela code can be used. The residual may be apparent early, such as in cerebral infarction, or it may occur months or years later, such as that due to a previous injury. **Examples of sequela include: scar formation resulting from a burn, deviated septum due to a nasal fracture, and infertility due to tubal occlusion from old tuberculosis.** Coding of sequela generally requires two codes sequenced in the following order: the condition or nature of the sequela is sequenced first. The sequela code is sequenced second.

An exception to the above guidelines are those instances where the code for the sequela is followed by a manifestation code identified in the Tabular List and title, or the sequela code has been expanded (at the fourth, fifth or sixth character levels) to include the manifestation(s). The code for the acute phase of an illness or injury that led to the sequela is never used with a code for the late effect.
See Section I.C.9. Sequelae of cerebrovascular disease
See Section I.C.15. Sequelae of complication of pregnancy, childbirth and the puerperium
See Section I.C.19. Application of 7th characters for Chapter 19

11. Impending or Threatened Condition
Code any condition described at the time of discharge as "impending" or "threatened" as follows:
   If it did occur, code as confirmed diagnosis.
   If it did not occur, reference the Alphabetic Index to determine if the condition has a subentry term for "impending" or "threatened" and also reference main term entries for "Impending" and for "Threatened."
   If the subterms are listed, assign the given code.
   If the subterms are not listed, code the existing underlying condition(s) and not the condition described as impending or threatened.

GUIDELINES (ICD-10-CM)

12. **Reporting Same Diagnosis Code More than Once**
Each unique ICD-10-CM diagnosis code may be reported only once for an encounter. This applies to bilateral conditions when there are no distinct codes identifying laterality or two different conditions classified to the same ICD-10-CM diagnosis code.

13. **Laterality**
Some ICD-10-CM codes indicate laterality, specifying whether the condition occurs on the left, right or is bilateral. If no bilateral code is provided and the condition is bilateral, assign separate codes for both the left and right side. If the side is not identified in the medical record, assign the code for the unspecified side.

14. **Documentation for BMI, Non-pressure ulcers and Pressure Ulcer Stages**
For the Body Mass Index (BMI), depth of non-pressure chronic ulcers and pressure ulcer stage codes, code assignment may be based on medical record documentation from clinicians who are not the patient's provider (i.e., physician or other qualified healthcare practitioner legally accountable for establishing the patient's diagnosis), since this information is typically documented by other clinicians involved in the care of the patient (e.g., a dietitian often documents the BMI and nurses often documents the pressure ulcer stages). However, the associated diagnosis (such as overweight, obesity, or pressure ulcer) must be documented by the patient's provider. If there is conflicting medical record documentation, either from the same clinician or different clinicians, the patient's attending provider should be queried for clarification.

The BMI codes should only be reported as secondary diagnoses. As with all other secondary diagnosis codes, the BMI codes should only be assigned when they meet the definition of a reportable additional diagnosis (see Section III, Reporting Additional Diagnoses).

15. **Syndromes**
Follow the Alphabetic Index guidance when coding syndromes. In the absence of Alphabetic Index guidance, assign codes for the documented manifestations of the syndrome. Additional codes for manifestations that are not an integral part of the disease process may also be assigned when the condition does not have a unique code.

16. **Documentation of Complications of Care**
Code assignment is based on the provider's documentation of the relationship between the condition and the care or procedure. The guideline extends to any complications of care, regardless of the chapter the code is located in. It is important to note that not all conditions that occur during or following medical care or surgery are classified as complications. There must be a cause-and-effect relationship between the care provided and the condition, and an indication in the documentation that it is a complication. Query the provider for clarification, if the complication is not clearly documented.

17. **Borderline Diagnosis**
If the provider documents a "borderline" diagnosis at the time of discharge, the diagnosis is coded as confirmed, unless the classification provides a specific entry (e.g., borderline diabetes). If a borderline condition has a specific index entry in ICD-10-CM, it should be coded as such. Since borderline conditions are not uncertain diagnoses, no distinction is made between the care setting (inpatient versus outpatient). Whenever the documentation is unclear regarding a borderline condition, coders are encouraged to query for clarification.

18. **Use of Sign/Symptom/Unspecified Codes**
Sign/symptom and "unspecified" codes have acceptable, even necessary, uses. While specific diagnosis codes should be reported when they are supported by the available medical record documentation and clinical knowledge of the patient's health condition, there are instances when signs/symptoms or unspecified codes are the best choices for accurately reflecting the healthcare encounter. Each healthcare encounter should be coded to the level of certainty known for that encounter.

If a definitive diagnosis has not been established by the end of the encounter, it is appropriate to report codes for sign(s) and/or symptom(s) in lieu of a definitive diagnosis. When sufficient clinical information isn't known or available about a particular health condition to assign a more specific code, it is acceptable to report the appropriate "unspecified" code (e.g., a diagnosis of pneumonia has been determined, but not the specific type). Unspecified codes should be reported when they are the codes that most accurately reflect what is known about the patient's condition at the time of that particular encounter. It would be inappropriate to select a specific code that is not supported by the medical record documentation or conduct medically unnecessary diagnostic testing in order to determine a more specific code.

C. **Chapter-Specific Coding Guidelines**
In addition to general coding guidelines, there are guidelines for specific diagnoses and/or conditions in the classification. Unless otherwise indicated, these guidelines apply to all health care settings. Please refer to Section II for guidelines on the selection of principal diagnosis.

1. **Chapter 1: Certain Infectious and Parasitic Diseases (A00-B99)**

a. **Human Immunodeficiency Virus (HIV) Infections**

1) **Code only confirmed cases**
Code only confirmed cases of HIV infection/illness. This is an exception to the hospital inpatient guideline Section II, H.

In this context, "confirmation" does not require documentation of positive serology or culture for HIV; the provider's diagnostic statement that the patient is HIV positive, or has an HIV-related illness is sufficient.

2) Selection and sequencing of HIV codes

(a) Patient admitted for HIV-related condition

If a patient is admitted for an HIV-related condition, the principal diagnosis should be B20, Human immunodeficiency virus [HIV] disease followed by additional diagnosis codes for all reported HIV-related conditions.

(b) Patient with HIV disease admitted for unrelated condition

If a patient with HIV disease is admitted for an unrelated condition (such as a traumatic injury), the code for the unrelated condition (e.g., the nature of injury code) should be the principal diagnosis. Other diagnoses would be B20 followed by additional diagnosis codes for all reported HIV-related conditions.

(c) Whether the patient is newly diagnosed

Whether the patient is newly diagnosed or has had previous admissions/encounters for HIV conditions is irrelevant to the sequencing decision.

(d) Asymptomatic human immunodeficiency virus

Z21, Asymptomatic human immunodeficiency virus [HIV] infection status, is to be applied when the patient without any documentation of symptoms is listed as being "HIV positive," "known HIV," "HIV test positive," or similar terminology. Do not use this code if the term "AIDS" is used or if the patient is treated for any HIV-related illness or is described as having any condition(s) resulting from his/her HIV positive status; use B20 in these cases.

(e) Patients with inconclusive HIV serology

Patients with inconclusive HIV serology, but no definitive diagnosis or manifestations of the illness, may be assigned code R75, Inconclusive laboratory evidence of human immunodeficiency virus [HIV].

(f) Previously diagnosed HIV-related illness

Patients with any known prior diagnosis of an HIV-related illness should be coded to B20. Once a patient has developed an HIV-related illness, the patient should always be assigned code B20 on every subsequent admission/encounter. Patients previously diagnosed with any HIV illness (B20) should never be assigned to R75 or Z21, Asymptomatic human immunodeficiency virus [HIV] infection status.

(g) HIV Infection in Pregnancy, Childbirth and the Puerperium

During pregnancy, childbirth or the puerperium, a patient admitted (or presenting for a health care encounter) because of an HIV-related illness should receive a principal diagnosis code of O98.7-, Human immunodeficiency [HIV] disease complicating pregnancy, childbirth and the puerperium, followed by B20 and the code(s) for the HIV-related illness(es). Codes from Chapter 15 always take sequencing priority.

Patients with asymptomatic HIV infection status admitted (or presenting for a health care encounter) during pregnancy, childbirth, or the puerperium should receive codes of O98.7- and Z21.

(h) Encounters for testing for HIV

If a patient is being seen to determine his/her HIV status, use code Z11.4, Encounter for screening for human immunodeficiency virus [HIV]. Use additional codes for any associated high risk behavior.

If a patient with signs or symptoms is being seen for HIV testing, code the signs and symptoms. An additional counseling code Z71.7, Human immunodeficiency virus [HIV] counseling, may be used if counseling is provided during the encounter for the test.

When a patient returns to be informed of his/her HIV test results and the test result is negative, use code Z71.7, Human immunodeficiency virus [HIV] counseling.

If the results are positive, see previous guidelines and assign codes as appropriate.

b. Infectious agents as the cause of diseases classified to other chapters

Certain infections are classified in chapters other than Chapter 1 and no organism is identified as part of the infection code. In these instances, it is necessary to use an additional code from Chapter 1 to identify the organism. A code from category B95, Streptococcus, Staphylococcus, and Enterococcus as the cause of diseases classified to other chapters, B96, Other bacterial agents as the cause of diseases classified to other chapters, or B97, Viral agents as the cause of diseases classified to other chapters, is to be used as an additional code to identify the organism. An instructional note will be found at the infection code advising that an additional organism code is required.

c. Infections resistant to antibiotics

Many bacterial infections are resistant to current antibiotics. It is necessary to identify all infections documented as antibiotic resistant. Assign a code from category Z16, Resistance to antimicrobial drugs, following the infection code only if the infection code does not identify drug resistance.

d. Sepsis, Severe Sepsis, and Septic Shock

1) Coding of Sepsis and Severe Sepsis

(a) Sepsis

For a diagnosis of sepsis, assign the appropriate code for the underlying systemic infection. If the type of infection or causal organism is not further specified, assign code A41.9, Sepsis, unspecified organism.

A code from subcategory R65.2, Severe sepsis, should not be assigned unless severe sepsis or an associated acute organ dysfunction is documented.

(i) Negative or inconclusive blood cultures and sepsis
Negative or inconclusive blood cultures do not preclude a diagnosis of sepsis in patients with clinical evidence of the condition, however, the provider should be queried.

(ii) Urosepsis
The term urosepsis is a nonspecific term. It is not to be considered synonymous with sepsis. It has no default code in the Alphabetic Index. Should a provider use this term, he/she must be queried for clarification.

(iii) Sepsis with organ dysfunction
If a patient has sepsis and associated acute organ dysfunction or multiple organ dysfunction (MOD), follow the instructions for coding severe sepsis.

(iv) Acute organ dysfunction that is not clearly associated with the sepsis
If a patient has sepsis and an acute organ dysfunction, but the medical record documentation indicates that the acute organ dysfunction is related to a medical condition other than the sepsis, do not assign a code from subcategory R65.2, Severe sepsis. An acute organ dysfunction must be associated with the sepsis in order to assign the severe sepsis code. If the documentation is not clear as to whether an acute organ dysfunction is related to the sepsis or another medical condition, query the provider.

(b) Severe sepsis
The coding of severe sepsis requires a minimum of 2 codes: first a code for the underlying systemic infection, followed by a code from subcategory R65.2, Severe sepsis. If the causal organism is not documented, assign code A41.9, Sepsis, unspecified organism, for the infection. Additional code(s) for the associated acute organ dysfunction are also required.

Due to the complex nature of severe sepsis, some cases may require querying the provider prior to assignment of the codes.

2) Septic shock

(a) Septic shock generally refers to circulatory failure associated with severe sepsis, and therefore, it represents a type of acute organ dysfunction.

For all cases of septic shock, the code for the systemic infection should be sequenced first, followed by code R65.21, Severe sepsis with septic shock or code T81.12, Postprocedural septic shock. Any additional codes for the other acute organ dysfunctions should also be assigned. As noted in the sequencing instructions in the Tabular List, the code for septic shock cannot be assigned as a principal diagnosis.

3) Sequencing of severe sepsis
If severe sepsis is present on admission, and meets the definition of principal diagnosis, the underlying systemic infection should be assigned as principal diagnosis followed by the appropriate code from subcategory R65.2 as required by the sequencing rules in the Tabular List. A code from subcategory R65.2 can never be assigned as a principal diagnosis.

When severe sepsis develops during an encounter (it was not present on admission) the underlying systemic infection and the appropriate code from subcategory R65.2 should be assigned as secondary diagnoses.

Severe sepsis may be present on admission but the diagnosis may not be confirmed until sometime after admission. If the documentation is not clear whether severe sepsis was present on admission, the provider should be queried.

4) Sepsis and severe sepsis with a localized infection
If the reason for admission is both sepsis or severe sepsis and a localized infection, such as pneumonia or cellulitis, a code(s) for the underlying systemic infection should be assigned first and the code for the localized infection should be assigned as a secondary diagnosis. If the patient has severe sepsis, a code from subcategory R65.2 should also be assigned as a secondary diagnosis. If the patient is admitted with a localized infection, such as pneumonia, and sepsis/severe sepsis doesn't develop until after admission, the localized infection should be assigned first, followed by the appropriate sepsis/severe sepsis codes.

5) Sepsis due to a postprocedural infection

(a) Documentation of causal relationship
As with all postprocedural complications, code assignment is based on the provider's documentation of the relationship between the infection and the procedure.

(b) Sepsis due to a postprocedural infection
For such cases, the postprocedural infection code, such as, T80.2, Infections following infusion, transfusion, and therapeutic injection, T81.4, Infection following a procedure, T88.0, Infection following immunization, or O86.0, Infection of obstetric surgical wound, should be coded first, followed by the code for the specific infection. If the patient has severe sepsis the appropriate code from subcategory R65.2 should also be assigned with the additional code(s) for any acute organ dysfunction.

(c) Postprocedural infection and postprocedural septic shock

In cases where a postprocedural infection has occurred and has resulted in severe sepsis the code for the precipitating complication such as code T81.4, Infection following a procedure, or O86.0, Infection of obstetrical surgical wound should be coded first followed by code R65.**20**, Severe sepsis without septic shock. **A Code for the systemic infection should also be assigned.**

If a postprocedural infection has resulted in postprocedural septic shock, the code for the precipitating complication such as code T81.4, Infection following a procedure, or O86.0, Infection of obstetrical surgical wound should be coded first followed by code T81.12-, Postprocedural septic shock. A code for the systemic infection should also be assigned.

6) Sepsis and severe sepsis associated with a noninfectious process (condition)

In some cases a noninfectious process (condition), such as trauma, may lead to an infection which can result in sepsis or severe sepsis. If sepsis or severe sepsis is documented as associated with a noninfectious condition, such as a burn or serious injury, and this condition meets the definition for principal diagnosis, the code for the noninfectious condition should be sequenced first, followed by the code for the resulting infection. If severe sepsis is present, a code from subcategory R65.2 should also be assigned with any associated organ dysfunction(s) codes. It is not necessary to assign a code from subcategory R65.1, Systemic inflammatory response syndrome (SIRS) of non-infectious origin, for these cases.

If the infection meets the definition of principal diagnosis it should be sequenced before the non-infectious condition. When both the associated non-infectious condition and the infection meet the definition of principal diagnosis either may be assigned as principal diagnosis.

Only one code from category R65, Symptoms and signs specifically associated with systemic inflammation and infection, should be assigned. Therefore, when a non-infectious condition leads to an infection resulting in severe sepsis, assign the appropriate code from subcategory R65.2, Severe sepsis. Do not additionally assign a code from subcategory R65.1, Systemic inflammatory response syndrome (SIRS) of non-infectious origin.

See Section I.C.18. SIRS due to non-infectious process

7) Sepsis and septic shock complicating abortion, pregnancy, childbirth, and the puerperium

See Section I.C.15. Sepsis and septic shock complicating abortion, pregnancy, childbirth and the puerperium

8) Newborn sepsis

See Section I.C.16. f. Bacterial sepsis of Newborn

e. Methicillin Resistant Staphylococcus aureus (MRSA) Conditions

1) Selection and sequencing of MRSA codes

(a) Combination codes for MRSA infection

When a patient is diagnosed with an infection that is due to methicillin resistant *Staphylococcus aureus* (MRSA), and that infection has a combination code that includes the causal organism (e.g., sepsis, pneumonia) assign the appropriate combination code for the condition (e.g., code A41.02, Sepsis due to Methicillin resistant Staphylococcus aureus or code J15.212, Pneumonia due to Methicillin resistant Staphylococcus aureus). Do not assign code B95.62, Methicillin resistant Staphylococcus aureus infection as the cause of diseases classified elsewhere, as an additional code because the combination code includes the type of infection and the MRSA organism. Do not assign a code from subcategory Z16.11, Resistance to penicillins, as an additional diagnosis.

See Section C.1. for instructions on coding and sequencing of sepsis and severe sepsis.

(b) Other codes for MRSA infection

When there is documentation of a current infection (e.g., wound infection, stitch abscess, urinary tract infection) due to MRSA, and that infection does not have a combination code that includes the causal organism, assign the appropriate code to identify the condition along with code B95.62, Methicillin resistant Staphylococcus aureus infection as the cause of diseases classified elsewhere for the MRSA infection. Do not assign a code from subcategory Z16.11, Resistance to penicillins.

(c) Methicillin susceptible Staphylococcus aureus (MSSA) and MRSA colonization

The condition or state of being colonized or carrying MSSA or MRSA is called colonization or carriage, while an individual person is described as being colonized or being a carrier. Colonization means that MSSA or MSRA is present on or in the body without necessarily causing illness. A positive MRSA colonization test might be documented by the provider as "MRSA screen positive" or "MRSA nasal swab positive".

Assign code Z22.322, Carrier or suspected carrier of Methicillin resistant Staphylococcus aureus, for patients documented as having MRSA colonization. Assign code Z22.321, Carrier or suspected carrier of Methicillin susceptible Staphylococcus aureus, for patient documented as having MSSA colonization. Colonization is not necessarily indicative of a disease process or as the cause of a specific condition the patient may have unless documented as such by the provider.

(d) MRSA colonization and infection

If a patient is documented as having both MRSA colonization and infection during a hospital admission, code Z22.322, Carrier or suspected carrier of Methicillin resistant Staphylococcus aureus, and a code for the MRSA infection may both be assigned.

GUIDELINES (ICD-10-CM)

2. Chapter 2: Neoplasms (C00-D49)
General guidelines

Chapter 2 of the ICD-10-CM contains the codes for most benign and all malignant neoplasms. Certain benign neoplasms, such as prostatic adenomas, may be found in the specific body system chapters. To properly code a neoplasm it is necessary to determine from the record if the neoplasm is benign, in-situ, malignant, or of uncertain histologic behavior. If malignant, any secondary (metastatic) sites should also be determined.

Primary malignant neoplasms overlapping site boundaries

A primary malignant neoplasm that overlaps two or more contiguous (next to each other) sites should be classified to the subcategory/ code .8 ('overlapping lesion'), unless the combination is specifically indexed elsewhere. For multiple neoplasms of the same site that are not contiguous such as tumors in different quadrants of the same breast, codes for each site should be assigned.

Malignant neoplasm of ectopic tissue

Malignant neoplasms of ectopic tissue are to be coded to the site of origin mentioned, e.g., ectopic pancreatic malignant neoplasms involving the stomach are coded to pancreas, unspecified (C25.9).

The neoplasm table in the Alphabetic Index should be referenced first. However, if the histological term is documented, that term should be referenced first, rather than going immediately to the Neoplasm Table, in order to determine which column in the Neoplasm Table is appropriate. For example, if the documentation indicates "adenoma," refer to the term in the Alphabetic Index to review the entries under this term and the instructional note to "see also neoplasm, by site, benign." The table provides the proper code based on the type of neoplasm and the site. It is important to select the proper column in the table that corresponds to the type of neoplasm. The Tabular List should then be referenced to verify that the correct code has been selected from the table and that a more specific site code does not exist.

See Section I.C.21. Factors influencing health status and contact with health services, Status, for information regarding Z15.0, codes for genetic susceptibility to cancer.

a. Treatment directed at the malignancy

If the treatment is directed at the malignancy, designate the malignancy as the principal diagnosis.

The only exception to this guideline is if a patient admission/encounter is solely for the administration of chemotherapy, immunotherapy or radiation therapy, assign the appropriate Z51.— code as the first-listed or principal diagnosis, and the diagnosis or problem for which the service is being performed as a secondary diagnosis.

b. Treatment of secondary site

When a patient is admitted because of a primary neoplasm with metastasis and treatment is directed toward the secondary site only, the secondary neoplasm is designated as the principal diagnosis even though the primary malignancy is still present.

c. Coding and sequencing of complications

Coding and sequencing of complications associated with the malignancies or with the therapy thereof are subject to the following guidelines:

1) Anemia associated with malignancy

When admission/encounter is for management of an anemia associated with the malignancy, and the treatment is only for anemia, the appropriate code for the malignancy is sequenced as the principal or first-listed diagnosis followed by the appropriate code for the anemia (such as code D63.0, Anemia in neoplastic disease).

2) Anemia associated with chemotherapy, immunotherapy and radiation therapy

When the admission/encounter is for management of an anemia associated with an adverse effect of the administration of chemotherapy or immunotherapy and the only treatment is for the anemia, the anemia code is sequenced first followed by the appropriate codes for the neoplasm and the adverse effect (T45.1X5, Adverse effect of antineoplastic and immunosuppressive drugs).

When the admission/encounter is for management of an anemia associated with an adverse effect of radiotherapy, the anemia code should be sequenced first, followed by the appropriate neoplasm code and code Y84.2, Radiological procedure and radiotherapy as the cause of abnormal reaction of the patient, or of later complication, without mention of misadventure at the time of the procedure.

3) Management of dehydration due to the malignancy

When the admission/encounter is for management of dehydration due to the malignancy and only the dehydration is being treated (intravenous rehydration), the dehydration is sequenced first, followed by the code(s) for the malignancy.

4) Treatment of a complication resulting from a surgical procedure

When the admission/encounter is for treatment of a complication resulting from a surgical procedure, designate the complication as the principal or first-listed diagnosis if treatment is directed at resolving the complication.

d. Primary malignancy previously excised

When a primary malignancy has been previously excised or eradicated from its site and there is no further treatment directed to that site and there is no evidence of any existing primary malignancy, a code from category Z85, Personal history of malignant neoplasm, should be used to indicate the former site of the malignancy. Any mention of extension, invasion, or metastasis to another site is coded as a secondary malignant neoplasm to that site. The secondary site may be the principal or first-listed with the Z85 code used as a secondary code.

e. **Admissions/Encounters involving chemotherapy, immunotherapy and radiation therapy**

   1) **Episode of care involves surgical removal of neoplasm**

When an episode of care involves the surgical removal of a neoplasm, primary or secondary site, followed by adjunct chemotherapy or radiation treatment during the same episode of care, the code for the neoplasm should be assigned as principal or first-listed diagnosis.

   2) **Patient admission/encounter solely for administration of chemotherapy, immunotherapy and radiation therapy**

If a patient admission/encounter is solely for the administration of chemotherapy, immunotherapy or radiation therapy assign code Z51.0, Encounter for antineoplastic radiation therapy, or Z51.11, Encounter for antineoplastic chemotherapy, or Z51.12, Encounter for antineoplastic immunotherapy as the first-listed or principal diagnosis. If a patient receives more than one of these therapies during the same admission more than one of these codes may be assigned, in any sequence.

The malignancy for which the therapy is being administered should be assigned as a secondary diagnosis.

   3) **Patient admitted for radiation therapy, chemotherapy or immunotherapy and develops complications**

When a patient is admitted for the purpose of radiotherapy, immunotherapy or chemotherapy and develops complications such as uncontrolled nausea and vomiting or dehydration, the principal or first-listed diagnosis is Z51.0, Encounter for antineoplastic radiation therapy, or Z51.11, Encounter for antineoplastic chemotherapy, or Z51.12, Encounter for antineoplastic immunotherapy followed by any codes for the complications.

f. **Admission/encounter to determine extent of malignancy**

When the reason for admission/encounter is to determine the extent of the malignancy, or for a procedure such as paracentesis or thoracentesis, the primary malignancy or appropriate metastatic site is designated as the principal or first-listed diagnosis, even though chemotherapy or radiotherapy is administered.

g. **Symptoms, signs, and abnormal findings listed in Chapter 18 associated with neoplasms**

Symptoms, signs, and ill-defined conditions listed in Chapter 18 characteristic of, or associated with, an existing primary or secondary site malignancy cannot be used to replace the malignancy as principal or first-listed diagnosis, regardless of the number of admissions or encounters for treatment and care of the neoplasm.

See section I.C.21. Factors influencing health status and contact with health services, Encounter for prophylactic organ removal.

h. **Admission/encounter for pain control/ management**

See Section I.C.6. for information on coding admission/ encounter for pain control/management.

i. **Malignancy in two or more noncontiguous sites**

A patient may have more than one malignant tumor in the same organ. These tumors may represent different primaries or metastatic disease, depending on the site. Should the documentation be unclear, the provider should be queried as to the status of each tumor so that the correct codes can be assigned.

j. **Disseminated malignant neoplasm, unspecified**

Code C80.0, Disseminated malignant neoplasm, unspecified, is for use only in those cases where the patient has advanced metastatic disease and no known primary or secondary sites are specified. It should not be used in place of assigning codes for the primary site and all known secondary sites.

k. **Malignant neoplasm without specification of site**

Code C80.1, Malignant (primary) neoplasm, unspecified, equates to Cancer, unspecified. This code should only be used when no determination can be made as to the primary site of a malignancy. This code should rarely be used in the inpatient setting.

l. **Sequencing of neoplasm codes**

   1) **Encounter for treatment of primary malignancy**

If the reason for the encounter is for treatment of a primary malignancy, assign the malignancy as the principal/first-listed diagnosis. The primary site is to be sequenced first, followed by any metastatic sites.

   2) **Encounter for treatment of secondary malignancy**

When an encounter is for a primary malignancy with metastasis and treatment is directed toward the metastatic (secondary) site(s) only, the metastatic site(s) is designated as the principal/ first-listed diagnosis. The primary malignancy is coded as an additional code.

   3) **Malignant neoplasm in a pregnant patient**

When a pregnant woman has a malignant neoplasm, a code from subcategory O9A.1-, Malignant neoplasm complicating pregnancy, childbirth, and the puerperium, should be sequenced first, followed by the appropriate code from Chapter 2 to indicate the type of neoplasm.

   4) **Encounter for complication associated with a neoplasm**

When an encounter is for management of a complication associated with a neoplasm, such as dehydration, and the treatment is only for the complication, the complication is coded first, followed by the appropriate code(s) for the neoplasm.

GUIDELINES (ICD-10-CM)

The exception to this guideline is anemia. When the admission/encounter is for management of an anemia associated with the malignancy, and the treatment is only for anemia, the appropriate code for the malignancy is sequenced as the principal or first-listed diagnosis followed by code D63.0, Anemia in neoplastic disease.

5) Complication from surgical procedure for treatment of a neoplasm

When an encounter is for treatment of a complication resulting from a surgical procedure performed for the treatment of the neoplasm, designate the complication as the principal/first-listed diagnosis. See guideline regarding the coding of a current malignancy versus personal history to determine if the code for the neoplasm should also be assigned.

6) Pathologic fracture due to a neoplasm

When an encounter is for a pathological fracture due to a neoplasm, and the focus of treatment is the fracture, a code from subcategory M84.5, Pathological fracture in neoplastic disease, should be sequenced first, followed by the code for the neoplasm.

If the focus of treatment is the neoplasm with an associated pathological fracture, the neoplasm code should be sequenced first, followed by a code from M84.5 for the pathological fracture.

m. Current malignancy versus personal history of malignancy

When a primary malignancy has been excised but further treatment, such as an additional surgery for the malignancy, radiation therapy or chemotherapy is directed to that site, the primary malignancy code should be used until treatment is completed.

When a primary malignancy has been previously excised or eradicated from its site, there is no further treatment (of the malignancy) directed to that site, and there is no evidence of any existing primary malignancy, a code from category Z85, Personal history of malignant neoplasm, should be used to indicate the former site of the malignancy.

See Section I.C.21. Factors influencing health status and contact with health services, History (of)

n. Leukemia, Multiple Myeloma, and Malignant Plasma Cell Neoplasms in remission versus personal history

The categories for leukemia, and category C90, Multiple myeloma and malignant plasma cell neoplasms, have codes indicating whether or not the leukemia has achieved remission. There are also codes Z85.6, Personal history of leukemia, and Z85.79, Personal history of other malignant neoplasms of lymphoid, hematopoietic and related tissues. If the documentation is unclear, as to whether the leukemia has achieved remission, the provider should be queried.

See Section I.C.21. Factors influencing health status and contact with health services, History (of)

o. Aftercare following surgery for neoplasm

See Section I.C.21. Factors influencing health status and contact with health services, Aftercare

p. Follow-up care for completed treatment of a malignancy

See Section I.C.21. Factors influencing health status and contact with health services, Follow-up

q. Prophylactic organ removal for prevention of malignancy

See Section I.C. 21, Factors influencing health status and contact with health services, Prophylactic organ removal

r. Malignant neoplasm associated with transplanted organ

A malignant neoplasm of a transplanted organ should be coded as a transplant complication. Assign first the appropriate code from category T86.-, Complications of transplanted organs and tissue, followed by code C80.2, Malignant neoplasm associated with transplanted organ. Use an additional code for the specific malignancy.

3. Chapter 3: Disease of the blood and blood-forming organs and certain disorders involving the immune mechanism (D50-D89)

Reserved for future guideline expansion

4. Chapter 4: Endocrine, Nutritional, and Metabolic Diseases (E00-E89)

a. Diabetes mellitus

The diabetes mellitus codes are combination codes that include the type of diabetes mellitus, the body system affected, and the complications affecting that body system. As many codes within a particular category as are necessary to describe all of the complications of the disease may be used. They should be sequenced based on the reason for a particular encounter. Assign as many codes from categories E08 – E13 as needed to identify all of the associated conditions that the patient has.

1) Type of diabetes

The age of a patient is not the sole determining factor, though most type 1 diabetics develop the condition before reaching puberty. For this reason type 1 diabetes mellitus is also referred to as juvenile diabetes.

2) Type of diabetes mellitus not documented

If the type of diabetes mellitus is not documented in the medical record the default is E11.-, Type 2 diabetes mellitus.

3) Diabetes mellitus and the use of insulin

If the documentation in a medical record does not indicate the type of diabetes but does indicate that the patient uses insulin, code E11, Type 2 diabetes mellitus, should be assigned. Code Z79.4, Long-term (current) use of insulin, should also be assigned to indicate that the patient uses insulin. Code Z79.4 should not be assigned if insulin is given temporarily to bring a type 2 patient's blood sugar under control during an encounter.

4) Diabetes mellitus in pregnancy and gestational diabetes

See Section I.C.15. Diabetes mellitus in pregnancy.
See Section I.C.15. Gestational (pregnancy induced) diabetes

5) Complications due to insulin pump malfunction

(a) Underdose of insulin due to insulin pump failure

An underdose of insulin due to an insulin pump failure should be assigned to a code from subcategory T85.6, Mechanical complication of other specified internal and external prosthetic devices, implants and grafts, that specifies the type of pump malfunction, as the principal or first-listed code, followed by code T38.3X6-, Underdosing of insulin and oral hypoglycemic [antidiabetic] drugs. Additional codes for the type of diabetes mellitus and any associated complications due to the underdosing should also be assigned.

(b) Overdose of insulin due to insulin pump failure

The principal or first-listed code for an encounter due to an insulin pump malfunction resulting in an overdose of insulin, should also be T85.6-, Mechanical complication of other specified internal and external prosthetic devices, implants and grafts, followed by code T38.3X1-, Poisoning by insulin and oral hypoglycemic [antidiabetic] drugs, accidental (unintentional).

6) Secondary diabetes mellitus

Codes under categories E08, Diabetes mellitus due to underlying condition, E09, Drug or chemical induced diabetes mellitus and E13, Other specified diabetes mellitus, identify complications/manifestations associated with secondary diabetes mellitus. Secondary diabetes is always caused by another condition or event (e.g., cystic fibrosis, malignant neoplasm of pancreas, pancreatectomy, adverse effect of drug, or poisoning).

(a) Secondary diabetes mellitus and the use of insulin

For patients who routinely use insulin, code Z79.4, Long-term (current) use of insulin, should also be assigned. Code Z79.4 should not be assigned if insulin is given temporarily to bring a patient's blood sugar under control during an encounter.

(b) Assigning and sequencing secondary diabetes codes and its causes

The sequencing of the secondary diabetes codes in relationship to codes for the cause of the diabetes is based on the Tabular List instructions for categories E08, E09 and E13.

(i) Secondary diabetes mellitus due to pancreatectomy For postpancreatectomy diabetes mellitus (lack of insulin due to the surgical removal of all or part of the pancreas), assign code E89.1, Postprocedural hypoinsulinemia. Assign a code from category E13 and a code from subcategory Z90.41-, Acquired absence of pancreas, as additional codes.

(ii) Secondary diabetes due to drugs Secondary diabetes may be caused by an adverse effect of correctly administered medications, poisoning or sequela of poisoning.

See section I.C.19.e for coding of adverse effects and poisoning, and section I.C.20 for external cause code reporting.

5. Chapter 5: Mental, Behavioral and Neurodevelopmental disorders (F01 – F99)

a. Pain disorders related to psychological factors

Assign code F45.41, for pain that is exclusively related to psychological disorders. As indicated by the Excludes 1 note under category G89, a code from category G89 should not be assigned with code F45.41

Code F45.42, Pain disorders with related psychological factors, should be used with a code from category G89, Pain, not elsewhere classified, if there is documentation of a psychological component for a patient with acute or chronic pain.

See Section I.C.6. Pain

c. Mental and behavioral disorders due to psychoactive substance use

1) In Remission

Selection of codes for "in remission" for categories F10-F19, Mental and behavioral disorders due to psychoactive substance use (categories F10-F19 with -.21) requires the provider's clinical judgment. The appropriate codes for "in remission" are assigned only on the basis of provider documentation (as defined in the Official Guidelines for Coding and Reporting).

2) Psychoactive Substance Use, Abuse And Dependence

When the provider documentation refers to use, abuse and dependence of the same substance (e.g. alcohol, opioid, cannabis, etc.), only one code should be assigned to identify the pattern of use based on the following hierarchy:

- If both use and abuse are documented, assign only the code for abuse
- If both abuse and dependence are documented, assign only the code for dependence
- If use, abuse and dependence are all documented, assign only the code for dependence
- If both use and dependence are documented, assign only the code for dependence.

3) Psychoactive Substance Use

As with all other diagnoses, the codes for psychoactive substance use (F10.9-, F11.9-, F12.9-, F13.9-, F14.9-, F15.9-, F16.9-) should only be assigned based on provider documentation and when they meet the definition of a reportable diagnosis (see Section III, Reporting Additional Diagnoses). The codes are to be used only when the psychoactive substance use is associated

GUIDELINES (ICD-10-CM)

with a mental or behavioral disorder, and such a relationship is documented by the provider.

6. **Chapter 6: Diseases of the Nervous System (G00-G99)**

a. **Dominant/nondominant side**

Codes from category G81, Hemiplegia and hemiparesis, and subcategories, G83.1, Monoplegia of lower limb, G83.2, Monoplegia of upper limb, and G83.3, Monoplegia, unspecified, identify whether the dominant or nondominant side is affected. Should the affected side be documented, but not specified as dominant or nondominant, and the classification system does not indicate a default, code selection is as follows:

- For ambidextrous patients, the default should be dominant.
- If the left side is affected, the default is non-dominant.
- If the right side is affected, the default is dominant.

b. **Pain - Category G89**

1) **General coding information**

Codes in category G89, Pain, not elsewhere classified, may be used in conjunction with codes from other categories and chapters to provide more detail about acute or chronic pain and neoplasm-related pain, unless otherwise indicated below.

If the pain is not specified as acute or chronic, post-thoracotomy, postprocedural, or neoplasm-related, do not assign codes from category G89.

A code from category G89 should not be assigned if the underlying (definitive) diagnosis is known, unless the reason for the encounter is pain control/management and not management of the underlying condition.

When an admission or encounter is for a procedure aimed at treating the underlying condition (e.g., spinal fusion, kyphoplasty), a code for the underlying condition (e.g., vertebral fracture, spinal stenosis) should be assigned as the principal diagnosis. No code from category G89 should be assigned.

(a) **Category G89 Codes as Principal or First-Listed Diagnosis**

Category G89 codes are acceptable as principal diagnosis or the first-listed code:

- When pain control or pain management is the reason for the admission/encounter (e.g., a patient with displaced intervertebral disc, nerve impingement and severe back pain presents for injection of steroid into the spinal canal). The underlying cause of the pain should be reported as an additional diagnosis, if known.
- When a patient is admitted for the insertion of a neurostimulator for pain control, assign the appropriate pain code as the principal or first-listed diagnosis. When an admission or encounter is for a procedure aimed at treating the underlying condition and a

neurostimulator is inserted for pain control during the same admission/encounter, a code for the underlying condition should be assigned as the principal diagnosis and the appropriate pain code should be assigned as a secondary diagnosis.

(b) **Use of Category G89 Codes in Conjunction with Site Specific Pain Codes**

(i) **Assigning Category G89 and Site-Specific Pain Codes**

Codes from category G89 may be used in conjunction with codes that identify the site of pain (including codes from chapter 18) if the category G89 code provides additional information. For example, if the code describes the site of the pain, but does not fully describe whether the pain is acute or chronic, then both codes should be assigned.

(ii) **Sequencing of Category G89 Codes with Site-Specific Pain Codes**

The sequencing of category G89 codes with site-specific pain codes (including chapter 18 codes), is dependent on the circumstances of the encounter/admission as follows:

- If the encounter is for pain control or pain management, assign the code from category G89 followed by the code identifying the specific site of pain (e.g., encounter for pain management for acute neck pain from trauma is assigned code G89.11, Acute pain due to trauma, followed by code M54.2, Cervicalgia, to identify the site of pain).
- If the encounter is for any other reason except pain control or pain management, and a related definitive diagnosis has not been established (confirmed) by the provider, assign the code for the specific site of pain first, followed by the appropriate code from category G89.

2) **Pain due to devices, implants and grafts**
See Section I.C.19. Pain due to medical devices

3) **Postoperative Pain**

The provider's documentation should be used to guide the coding of postoperative pain, as well as *Section III. Reporting Additional Diagnoses* and *Section IV. Diagnostic Coding and Reporting in the Outpatient Setting.*

The default for post-thoracotomy and other postoperative pain not specified as acute or chronic is the code for the acute form.

Routine or expected postoperative pain immediately after surgery should not be coded.

(a) **Postoperative pain not associated with specific postoperative complication**

Postoperative pain not associated with a specific postoperative complication is assigned to the appropriate postoperative pain code in category G89.

(b) Postoperative pain associated with specific postoperative complication

Postoperative pain associated with a specific postoperative complication (such as painful wire sutures) is assigned to the appropriate code(s) found in Chapter 19, Injury, poisoning, and certain other consequences of external causes. If appropriate, use additional code(s) from category G89 to identify acute or chronic pain (G89.18 or G89.28).

4) Chronic pain

Chronic pain is classified to subcategory G89.2. There is no time frame defining when pain becomes chronic pain. The provider's documentation should be used to guide use of these codes.

5) Neoplasm Related Pain

Code G89.3 is assigned to pain documented as being related, associated or due to cancer, primary or secondary malignancy, or tumor. This code is assigned regardless of whether the pain is acute or chronic.

This code may be assigned as the principal or first-listed code when the stated reason for the admission/encounter is documented as pain control/pain management. The underlying neoplasm should be reported as an additional diagnosis.

When the reason for the admission/encounter is management of the neoplasm and the pain associated with the neoplasm is also documented, code G89.3 may be assigned as an additional diagnosis. It is not necessary to assign an additional code for the site of the pain.

See Section I.C.2 for instructions on the sequencing of neoplasms for all other stated reasons for the admission/ encounter (except for pain control/pain management).

6) Chronic pain syndrome

Central pain syndrome (G89.0) and chronic pain syndrome (G89.4) are different than the term "chronic pain," and therefore codes should only be used when the provider has specifically documented this condition.

See Section I.C.5. Pain disorders related to psychological factors

7. **Chapter 7: Diseases of the Eye and Adnexa (H00-H59)**

   a. **Glaucoma**

   1) **Assigning Glaucoma Codes**

   Assign as many codes from category H40, Glaucoma, as needed to identify the type of glaucoma, the affected eye, and the glaucoma stage.

   2) **Bilateral glaucoma with same type and stage**

   When a patient has bilateral glaucoma and both eyes are documented as being the same type and stage, and there is a code for bilateral glaucoma, report only the code for the type of glaucoma, bilateral, with the seventh character for the stage.

   When a patient has bilateral glaucoma and both eyes are documented as being the same type and stage, and the classification does not provide a code for bilateral glaucoma (i.e. subcategories H40.10, H40.11 and H40.20) report only one code for the type of glaucoma with the appropriate seventh character for the stage.

   3) **Bilateral glaucoma stage with different types or stages**

   When a patient has bilateral glaucoma and each eye is documented as having a different type or stage, and the classification distinguishes laterality, assign the appropriate code for each eye rather than the code for bilateral glaucoma.

   When a patient has bilateral glaucoma and each eye is documented as having a different type, and the classification does not distinguish laterality (i.e. subcategories H40.10, H40.11 and H40.20), assign one code for each type of glaucoma with the appropriate seventh character for the stage.

   When a patient has bilateral glaucoma and each eye is documented as having the same type, but different stage, and the classification does not distinguish laterality (i.e. subcategories H40.10, H40.11 and H40.20), assign a code for the type of glaucoma for each eye with the seventh character for the specific glaucoma stage documented for each eye.

   4) **Patient admitted with glaucoma and stage evolves during the admission**

   If a patient is admitted with glaucoma and the stage progresses during the admission, assign the code for highest stage documented.

   5) **Indeterminate stage glaucoma**

   Assignment of the seventh character "4" for "indeterminate stage" should be based on the clinical documentation. The seventh character "4" is used for glaucomas whose stage cannot be clinically determined. This seventh character should not be confused with the seventh character "0", unspecified, which should be assigned when there is no documentation regarding the stage of the glaucoma.

8. **Chapter 8: Diseases of the Ear and Mastoid Process (H60-H95)**

   Reserved for future guideline expansion

9. **Chapter 9: Diseases of the Circulatory System (I00-I99)**

   a. **Hypertension**

   1) **Hypertension with Heart Disease**

   Heart conditions classified to I50.- or I51.4-I51.9, are assigned to, a code from category I11, Hypertensive heart disease, when a causal relationship is stated (due to hypertension) or implied (hypertensive). Use an additional code from category I50, Heart failure, to identify the type of heart failure in those patients with heart failure.

   The same heart conditions (I50.-, I51.4-I51.9) with hypertension, but without a stated causal relationship, are coded separately. Sequence according to the circumstances of the admission/ encounter.

GUIDELINES (ICD-10-CM)

2) Hypertensive Chronic Kidney Disease

Assign codes from category I12, Hypertensive chronic kidney disease, when both hypertension and a condition classifiable to category N18, Chronic kidney disease (CKD), are present. Unlike hypertension with heart disease, ICD-10-CM presumes a cause-and-effect relationship and classifies chronic kidney disease with hypertension as hypertensive chronic kidney disease.

The appropriate code from category N18 should be used as a secondary code with a code from category I12 to identify the stage of chronic kidney disease.

See Section I.C.14. Chronic kidney disease.

If a patient has hypertensive chronic kidney disease and acute renal failure, an additional code for the acute renal failure is required.

3) Hypertensive Heart and Chronic Kidney Disease

Assign codes from combination category I13, Hypertensive heart and chronic kidney disease, when both hypertensive kidney disease and hypertensive heart disease are stated in the diagnosis. Assume a relationship between the hypertension and the chronic kidney disease, whether or not the condition is so designated. If heart failure is present, assign an additional code from category I50 to identify the type of heart failure.

The appropriate code from category N18, Chronic kidney disease, should be used as a secondary code with a code from category I13 to identify the stage of chronic kidney disease.

See Section I.C.14. Chronic kidney disease.

The codes in category I13, Hypertensive heart and chronic kidney disease, are combination codes that include hypertension, heart disease and chronic kidney disease. The Includes note at I13 specifies that the conditions included at I11 and I12 are included together in I13. If a patient has hypertension, heart disease and chronic kidney disease then a code from I13 should be used, not individual codes for hypertension, heart disease and chronic kidney disease, or codes from I11 or I12.

For patients with both acute renal failure and chronic kidney disease an additional code for acute renal failure is required.

4) Hypertensive Cerebrovascular Disease

For hypertensive cerebrovascular disease, first assign the appropriate code from categories I60-I69, followed by the appropriate hypertension code.

5) Hypertensive Retinopathy

Subcategory H35.0, Background retinopathy and retinal vascular changes, should be used with a code from category I10 – I15, Hypertensive disease to include the systemic hypertension. The sequencing is based on the reason for the encounter.

6) Hypertension, Secondary

Secondary hypertension is due to an underlying condition. Two codes are required: one to identify the underlying etiology and one from category I15 to identify the hypertension. Sequencing of codes is determined by the reason for admission/encounter.

7) Hypertension, Transient

Assign code R03.0, Elevated blood pressure reading without diagnosis of hypertension, unless patient has an established diagnosis of hypertension. Assign code O13.-, Gestational [pregnancy-induced] hypertension without significant proteinuria, or O14.-, Pre-eclampsia, for transient hypertension of pregnancy.

8) Hypertension, Controlled

This diagnostic statement usually refers to an existing state of hypertension under control by therapy. Assign the appropriate code from categories I10-I15, Hypertensive diseases.

9) Hypertension, Uncontrolled

Uncontrolled hypertension may refer to untreated hypertension or hypertension not responding to current therapeutic regimen. In either case, assign the appropriate code from categories I10-I15, Hypertensive diseases.

b. Atherosclerotic Coronary Artery Disease and Angina

ICD-10-CM has combination codes for atherosclerotic heart disease with angina pectoris. The subcategories for these codes are I25.11, Atherosclerotic heart disease of native coronary artery with angina pectoris and I25.7, Atherosclerosis of coronary artery bypass graft(s) and coronary artery of transplanted heart with angina pectoris.

When using one of these combination codes it is not necessary to use an additional code for angina pectoris. A causal relationship can be assumed in a patient with both atherosclerosis and angina pectoris, unless the documentation indicates the angina is due to something other than the atherosclerosis.

If a patient with coronary artery disease is admitted due to an acute myocardial infarction (AMI), the AMI should be sequenced before the coronary artery disease.

See Section I.C.9. Acute myocardial infarction (AMI)

c. Intraoperative and Postprocedural Cerebrovascular Accident

Medical record documentation should clearly specify the cause-and-effect relationship between the medical intervention and the cerebrovascular accident in order to assign a code for intraoperative or postprocedural cerebrovascular accident.

Proper code assignment depends on whether it was an infarction or hemorrhage and whether it occurred intraoperatively or postoperatively. If it was a cerebral hemorrhage, code assignment depends on the type of procedure performed.

d. Sequelae of Cerebrovascular Disease

1) Category I69, Sequelae of Cerebrovascular disease

Category I69 is used to indicate conditions classifiable to categories I60-I67 as the causes of sequela (neurologic deficits), themselves classified elsewhere. These "late effects" include neurologic deficits that persist after initial onset of conditions classifiable to categories I60-I67. The neurologic deficits caused by cerebrovascular disease may be present from the onset or may arise at any time after the onset of the condition classifiable to categories I60-I67.

Codes from category I69, Sequelae of cerebrovascular disease, that specify hemiplegia, hemiparesis and monoplegia identify whether the dominant or nondominant side is affected. Should the affected side be documented, but not specified as dominant or nondominant, and the classification system does not indicate a default, code selection is as follows:

- For ambidextrous patients, the default should be dominant.
- If the left side is affected, the default is non-dominant.
- If the right side is affected, the default is dominant.

2) Codes from category I69 with codes from I60-I67

Codes from category I69 may be assigned on a health care record with codes from I60-I67, if the patient has a current cerebrovascular disease and deficits from an old cerebrovascular disease.

3) Codes from category I69 and Personal history of transient ischemic attack (TIA) and cerebral infarction (Z86.73)

Codes from category I69 should not be assigned if the patient does not have neurologic deficits.

See Section I.C.21. 4. History (of) for use of personal history codes

e. Acute myocardial infarction (AMI)

1) ST elevation myocardial infarction (STEMI) and non ST elevation myocardial infarction (NSTEMI)

The ICD-10-CM codes for acute myocardial infarction (AMI) identify the site, such as anterolateral wall or true posterior wall. Subcategories I21.0-I21.2 and code I21.3 are used for ST elevation myocardial infarction (STEMI). Code I21.4, Non-ST elevation (NSTEMI) myocardial infarction, is used for non ST elevation myocardial infarction (NSTEMI) and nontransmural MIs.

If NSTEMI evolves to STEMI, assign the STEMI code. If STEMI converts to NSTEMI due to thrombolytic therapy, it is still coded as STEMI.

For encounters occurring while the myocardial infarction is equal to, or less than, four weeks old, including transfers to another acute setting or a postacute setting, and the patient requires continued care for the myocardial infarction, codes from category I21 may continue to be reported. For encounters after the 4 week time frame and the patient is still receiving care related to the myocardial infarction, the appropriate aftercare code should be assigned, rather than a code from category I21. For old or healed myocardial infarctions not requiring further care, code I25.2, Old myocardial infarction, may be assigned.

2) Acute myocardial infarction, unspecified

Code I21.3, ST elevation (STEMI) myocardial infarction of unspecified site, is the default for unspecified acute myocardial infarction. If only STEMI or transmural MI without the site is documented, assign code I21.3.

3) AMI documented as nontransmural or subendocardial but site provided

If an AMI is documented as nontransmural or subendocardial, but the site is provided, it is still coded as a subendocardial AMI.

See Section I.C.21.3 for information on coding status post administration of tPA in a different facility within the last 24 hours.

4) Subsequent acute myocardial infarction

A code from category I22, Subsequent ST elevation (STEMI) and non ST elevation (NSTEMI) myocardial infarction, is to be used when a patient who has suffered an AMI has a new AMI within the 4 week time frame of the initial AMI. A code from category I22 must be used in conjunction with a code from category I21. The sequencing of the I22 and I21 codes depends on the circumstances of the encounter.

10. Chapter 10: Diseases of the Respiratory System (J00-J99)

a. Chronic Obstructive Pulmonary Disease [COPD] and Asthma

1) Acute exacerbation of chronic obstructive bronchitis and asthma

The codes in categories J44 and J45 distinguish between uncomplicated cases and those in acute exacerbation. An acute exacerbation is a worsening or a decompensation of a chronic condition. An acute exacerbation is not equivalent to an infection superimposed on a chronic condition, though an exacerbation may be triggered by an infection.

b. Acute Respiratory Failure

1) Acute respiratory failure as principal diagnosis

A code from subcategory J96.0, Acute respiratory failure, or subcategory J96.2, Acute and chronic respiratory failure, may be assigned as a principal diagnosis when it is the condition established after study to be chiefly responsible for occasioning the admission to the hospital, and the selection is supported by the Alphabetic Index and Tabular List. However, chapter-specific coding guidelines (such as obstetrics, poisoning, HIV, newborn) that provide sequencing direction take precedence.

2) Acute respiratory failure as secondary diagnosis

Respiratory failure may be listed as a secondary diagnosis if it occurs after admission, or if it is

GUIDELINES (ICD-10-CM)

present on admission, but does not meet the definition of principal diagnosis.

3) Sequencing of acute respiratory failure and another acute condition

When a patient is admitted with respiratory failure and another acute condition, (e.g., myocardial infarction, cerebrovascular accident, aspiration pneumonia), the principal diagnosis will not be the same in every situation. This applies whether the other acute condition is a respiratory or nonrespiratory condition. Selection of the principal diagnosis will be dependent on the circumstances of admission. If both the respiratory failure and the other acute condition are equally responsible for occasioning the admission to the hospital, and there are no chapter-specific sequencing rules, the guideline regarding two or more diagnoses that equally meet the definition for principal diagnosis *(Section II, C.)* may be applied in these situations.

If the documentation is not clear as to whether acute respiratory failure and another condition are equally responsible for occasioning the admission, query the provider for clarification.

c. Influenza due to certain identified influenza viruses

Code only confirmed cases of influenza due to certain identified influenza viruses (category J09), and due to other identified influenza virus (category J10). This is an exception to the hospital inpatient guideline Section II, H. (Uncertain Diagnosis).

In this context, "confirmation" does not require documentation of positive laboratory testing specific for avian or other novel influenza A or other identified influenza virus. However, coding should be based on the provider's diagnostic statement that the patient has avian influenza, or other novel influenza A, for category J09, or has another particular identified strain of influenza, such as H1N1 or H3N2, but not identified as novel or variant, for category J10.

If the provider records "suspected" or "possible" or "probable" avian influenza, or novel influenza, or other identified influenza, then the appropriate influenza code from category J11, Influenza due to unidentified influenza virus, should be assigned. A code from category J09, Influenza due to certain identified influenza viruses, should not be assigned nor should a code from category J10, Influenza due to other identified influenza virus.

d. Ventilator associated Pneumonia

1) Documentation of Ventilator associated Pneumonia

As with all procedural or postprocedural complications, code assignment is based on the provider's documentation of the relationship between the condition and the procedure.

Code J95.851, Ventilator associated pneumonia, should be assigned only when the provider has documented ventilator associated pneumonia (VAP). An additional code to identify the organism

(e.g., Pseudomonas aeruginosa, code B96.5) should also be assigned. Do not assign an additional code from categories J12-J18 to identify the type of pneumonia.

Code J95.851 should not be assigned for cases where the patient has pneumonia and is on a mechanical ventilator and the provider has not specifically stated that the pneumonia is ventilator-associated pneumonia. If the documentation is unclear as to whether the patient has a pneumonia that is a complication attributable to the mechanical ventilator, query the provider.

2) Ventilator associated Pneumonia Develops after Admission

A patient may be admitted with one type of pneumonia (e.g., code J13, Pneumonia due to Streptococcus pneumonia) and subsequently develop VAP. In this instance, the principal diagnosis would be the appropriate code from categories J12-J18 for the pneumonia diagnosed at the time of admission. Code J95.851, Ventilator associated pneumonia, would be assigned as an additional diagnosis when the provider has also documented the presence of ventilator associated pneumonia.

11. Chapter 11: Diseases of the Digestive System (K00-K95)

Reserved for future guideline expansion

12. Chapter 12: Diseases of the Skin and Subcutaneous Tissue (L00-L99)

a. Pressure ulcer stage codes

1) Pressure ulcer stages

Codes from category L89, Pressure ulcer, are combination codes that identify the site of the pressure ulcer as well as the stage of the ulcer.

The ICD-10-CM classifies pressure ulcer stages based on severity, which is designated by stages 1-4, unspecified stage and unstageable.

Assign as many codes from category L89 as needed to identify all the pressure ulcers the patient has, if applicable.

2) Unstageable pressure ulcers

Assignment of the code for unstageable pressure ulcer (L89.--0) should be based on the clinical documentation. These codes are used for pressure ulcers whose stage cannot be clinically determined (e.g., the ulcer is covered by eschar or has been treated with a skin or muscle graft) and pressure ulcers that are documented as deep tissue injury but not documented as due to trauma. This code should not be confused with the codes for unspecified stage (L89.--9). When there is no documentation regarding the stage of the pressure ulcer, assign the appropriate code for unspecified stage (L89.--9).

3) Documented pressure ulcer stage

Assignment of the pressure ulcer stage code should be guided by clinical documentation of the stage or documentation of the terms found in the Alphabetic Index. For clinical terms describing the stage that are not found in the Alphabetic Index, and there is no documentation of the stage, the provider should be queried.

4) Patients admitted with pressure ulcers documented as healed
No code is assigned if the documentation states that the pressure ulcer is completely healed.

5) Patients admitted with pressure ulcers documented as healing
Pressure ulcers described as healing should be assigned the appropriate pressure ulcer stage code based on the documentation in the medical record. If the documentation does not provide information about the stage of the healing pressure ulcer, assign the appropriate code for unspecified stage.

If the documentation is unclear as to whether the patient has a current (new) pressure ulcer or if the patient is being treated for a healing pressure ulcer, query the provider.

6) Patient admitted with pressure ulcer evolving into another stage during the admission
If a patient is admitted with a pressure ulcer at one stage and it progresses to a higher stage, assign the code for the highest stage reported for that site.

13. Chapter 13: Diseases of the Musculoskeletal System and Connective Tissue (M00-M99)

a. Site and laterality
Most of the codes within Chapter 13 have site and laterality designations. The site represents the bone, joint or the muscle involved. For some conditions where more than one bone, joint or muscle is usually involved, such as osteoarthritis, there is a "multiple sites" code available. For categories where no multiple site code is provided and more than one bone, joint or muscle is involved, multiple codes should be used to indicate the different sites involved.

1) Bone versus joint
For certain conditions, the bone may be affected at the upper or lower end, (e.g., avascular necrosis of bone, M87, Osteoporosis, M80, M81). Though the portion of the bone affected may be at the joint, the site designation will be the bone, not the joint.

b. Acute traumatic versus chronic or recurrent musculoskeletal conditions
Many musculoskeletal conditions are a result of previous injury or trauma to a site, or are recurrent conditions. Bone, joint or muscle conditions that are the result of a healed injury are usually found in chapter 13. Recurrent bone, joint or muscle conditions are also usually found in chapter 13. Any current, acute injury should be coded to the appropriate injury code from chapter 19. Chronic or recurrent conditions should generally be coded with a code from chapter 13. If it is difficult to determine from the documentation in the record which code is best to describe a condition, query the provider.

c. Coding of Pathologic Fractures
7th character A is for use as long as the patient is receiving active treatment for the fracture. Examples of active treatment are: surgical treatment,

emergency department encounter, evaluation and **continuing** treatment by **the same or a different** physician. **While the patient may be seen by a new or different provider over the course of treatment for a pathological fracture, assignment of the 7th character is based on whether the patient is undergoing active treatment and not whether the provider is seeing the patient for the first time.**

7th character, D is to be used for encounters after the patient has completed active treatment. The other 7th characters, listed under each subcategory in the Tabular List, are to be used for subsequent encounters for treatment of problems associated with the healing, such as malunions, nonunions, and sequelae.

Care for complications of surgical treatment for fracture repairs during the healing or recovery phase should be coded with the appropriate complication codes.

See Section I.C.19. Coding of traumatic fractures.

d. Osteoporosis
Osteoporosis is a systemic condition, meaning that all bones of the musculoskeletal system are affected. Therefore, site is not a component of the codes under category M81, Osteoporosis without current pathological fracture. The site codes under category M80, Osteoporosis with current pathological fracture, identify the site of the fracture, not the osteoporosis.

1) Osteoporosis without pathological fracture
Category M81, Osteoporosis without current pathological fracture, is for use for patients with osteoporosis who do not currently have a pathologic fracture due to the osteoporosis, even if they have had a fracture in the past. For patients with a history of osteoporosis fractures, status code Z87.310, Personal history of (healed) osteoporosis fracture, should follow the code from M81.

2) Osteoporosis with current pathological fracture
Category M80, Osteoporosis with current pathological fracture, is for patients who have a current pathologic fracture at the time of an encounter. The codes under M80 identify the site of the fracture. A code from category M80, not a traumatic fracture code, should be used for any patient with known osteoporosis who suffers a fracture, even if the patient had a minor fall or trauma, if that fall or trauma would not usually break a normal, healthy bone.

14. Chapter 14: Diseases of Genitourinary System (N00-N99)

a. Chronic kidney disease

1) Stages of chronic kidney disease (CKD)
The ICD-10-CM classifies CKD based on severity. The severity of CKD is designated by stages 1-5. Stage 2, code N18.2, equates to mild CKD; stage 3, code N18.3, equates to moderate CKD; and stage 4, code N18.4, equates to severe CKD. Code N18.6, End stage renal disease (ESRD), is assigned when the provider has documented end-stage-renal disease (ESRD).

GUIDELINES (ICD-10-CM)

If both a stage of CKD and ESRD are documented, assign code N18.6 only.

2) Chronic kidney disease and kidney transplant status

Patients who have undergone kidney transplant may still have some form of chronic kidney disease CKD because the kidney transplant may not fully restore kidney function. Therefore, the presence of CKD alone does not constitute a transplant complication. Assign the appropriate N18 code for the patient's stage of CKD and code Z94.0, Kidney transplant status. If a transplant complication such as failure or rejection or other transplant complication is documented, see section I.C.19.g for information on coding complications of a kidney transplant. If the documentation is unclear as to whether the patient has a complication of the transplant, query the provider.

3) Chronic kidney disease with other conditions

Patients with CKD may also suffer from other serious conditions, most commonly diabetes mellitus and hypertension. The sequencing of the CKD code in relationship to codes for other contributing conditions is based on the conventions in the Tabular List.

See I.C.9. Hypertensive chronic kidney disease.
See I.C.19. Chronic kidney disease and kidney transplant complications.

15. Chapter 15: Pregnancy, Childbirth, and the Puerperium (O00-O9A)

a. General Rules for Obstetric Cases

1) Codes from chapter 15 and sequencing priority

Obstetric cases require codes from chapter 15, codes in the range O00-O9A, Pregnancy, Childbirth, and the Puerperium. Chapter 15 codes have sequencing priority over codes from other chapters. Additional codes from other chapters may be used in conjunction with chapter 15 codes to further specify conditions. Should the provider document that the pregnancy is incidental to the encounter, then code Z33.1, Pregnant state, incidental, should be used in place of any chapter 15 codes. It is the provider's responsibility to state that the condition being treated is not affecting the pregnancy.

2) Chapter 15 codes used only on the maternal record

Chapter 15 codes are to be used only on the maternal record, never on the record of the newborn.

3) Final character for trimester

The majority of codes in Chapter 15 have a final character indicating the trimester of pregnancy. The timeframes for the trimesters are indicated at the beginning of the chapter. If trimester is not a component of a code it is because the condition always occurs in a specific trimester, or the concept of trimester of pregnancy is not applicable. Certain codes have characters for only certain trimesters because the condition does not occur in all trimesters, but it may occur in more than just one.

Assignment of the final character for trimester should be based on the provider's documentation of the trimester (or number of weeks) for the current admission/encounter. This applies to the assignment of trimester for pre-existing conditions as well as those that develop during or are due to the pregnancy. The provider's documentation of the number of weeks may be used to assign the appropriate code identifying the trimester.

Whenever delivery occurs during the current admission, and there is an "in childbirth" option for the obstetric complication being coded, the "in childbirth" code should be assigned.

4) Selection of trimester for inpatient admissions that encompass more than one trimester

In instances when a patient is admitted to a hospital for complications of pregnancy during one trimester and remains in the hospital into a subsequent trimester, the trimester character for the antepartum complication code should be assigned on the basis of the trimester when the complication developed, not the trimester of the discharge. If the condition developed prior to the current admission/encounter or represents a pre-existing condition, the trimester character for the trimester at the time of the admission/encounter should be assigned.

5) Unspecified trimester

Each category that includes codes for trimester has a code for "unspecified trimester." The "unspecified trimester" code should rarely be used, such as when the documentation in the record is insufficient to determine the trimester and it is not possible to obtain clarification.

6) 7th character for Fetus Identification

Where applicable, a 7th character is to be assigned for certain categories (O31, O32, O33.3 - O33.6, O35, O36, O40, O41, O60.1, O60.2, O64, and O69) to identify the fetus for which the complication code applies.

Assign 7th character "0":
- For single gestations
- When the documentation in the record is insufficient to determine the fetus affected and it is not possible to obtain clarification.
- When it is not possible to clinically determine which fetus is affected.

b. Selection of OB Principal or First-listed Diagnosis

1) Routine outpatient prenatal visits

For routine outpatient prenatal visits when no complications are present, a code from category Z34, Encounter for supervision of normal pregnancy, should be used as the first-listed diagnosis. These codes should not be used in conjunction with chapter 15 codes.

2) Prenatal outpatient visits for high-risk patients

For routine prenatal outpatient visits for patients with high-risk pregnancies, a code from category O09, Supervision of high-risk pregnancy, should be used as the first-listed diagnosis. Secondary chapter 15 codes may be used in conjunction with these codes if appropriate.

3) Episodes when no delivery occurs
In episodes when no delivery occurs, the principal diagnosis should correspond to the principal complication of the pregnancy which necessitated the encounter. Should more than one complication exist, all of which are treated or monitored, any of the complications codes may be sequenced first.

4) When a delivery occurs
When a delivery occurs, the principal diagnosis should correspond to the main circumstances or complication of the delivery. In cases of cesarean delivery, the selection of the principal diagnosis should be the condition established after study that was responsible for the patient's admission. If the patient was admitted with a condition that resulted in the performance of a cesarean procedure, that condition should be selected as the principal diagnosis. If the reason for the admission/encounter was unrelated to the condition resulting in the cesarean delivery, the condition related to the reason for the admission/encounter should be selected as the principal diagnosis.

5) Outcome of delivery
A code from category Z37, Outcome of delivery, should be included on every maternal record when a delivery has occurred. These codes are not to be used on subsequent records or on the newborn record.

c. Pre-existing conditions versus conditions due to the pregnancy
Certain categories in Chapter 15 distinguish between conditions of the mother that existed prior to pregnancy (pre-existing) and those that are a direct result of pregnancy. When assigning codes from Chapter 15, it is important to assess if a condition was pre-existing prior to pregnancy or developed during or due to the pregnancy in order to assign the correct code.

Categories that do not distinguish between pre-existing and pregnancy-related conditions may be used for either. It is acceptable to use codes specifically for the puerperium with codes complicating pregnancy and childbirth if a condition arises postpartum during the delivery encounter.

d. Pre-existing hypertension in pregnancy
Category O10, Pre-existing hypertension complicating pregnancy, childbirth and the puerperium, includes codes for hypertensive heart and hypertensive chronic kidney disease. When assigning one of the O10 codes that includes hypertensive heart disease or hypertensive chronic kidney disease, it is necessary to add a secondary code from the appropriate hypertension category to specify the type of heart failure or chronic kidney disease.

See Section I.C.9. Hypertension.

e. Fetal Conditions Affecting the Management of the Mother
1) Codes from categories O35 and O36
Codes from categories O35, Maternal care for known or suspected fetal abnormality and damage, and O36, Maternal care for other fetal problems, are assigned only when the fetal condition is actually responsible for modifying the management of the mother, i.e., by requiring diagnostic studies, additional observation, special care, or termination of pregnancy. The fact that the fetal condition exists does not justify assigning a code from this series to the mother's record.

2) In utero surgery
In cases when surgery is performed on the fetus, a diagnosis code from category O35, Maternal care for known or suspected fetal abnormality and damage, should be assigned identifying the fetal condition. Assign the appropriate procedure code for the procedure performed.

No code from Chapter 16, the perinatal codes, should be used on the mother's record to identify fetal conditions. Surgery performed in utero on a fetus is still to be coded as an obstetric encounter.

f. HIV Infection in Pregnancy, Childbirth and the Puerperium
During pregnancy, childbirth or the puerperium, a patient admitted because of an HIV-related illness should receive a principal diagnosis from subcategory O98.7-, Human immunodeficiency [HIV] disease complicating pregnancy, childbirth and the puerperium, followed by the code(s) for the HIV-related illness(es).

Patients with asymptomatic HIV infection status admitted during pregnancy, childbirth, or the puerperium should receive codes of O98.7- and Z21, Asymptomatic human immunodeficiency virus [HIV] infection status.

g. Diabetes mellitus in pregnancy
Diabetes mellitus is a significant complicating factor in pregnancy. Pregnant women who are diabetic should be assigned a code from category O24, Diabetes mellitus in pregnancy, childbirth, and the puerperium, first, followed by the appropriate diabetes code(s) (E08-E13) from Chapter 4.

h. Long term use of insulin
Code Z79.4, Long-term (current) use of insulin, should also be assigned if the diabetes mellitus is being treated with insulin.

i. Gestational (pregnancy induced) diabetes
Gestational (pregnancy induced) diabetes can occur during the second and third trimester of pregnancy in women who were not diabetic prior to pregnancy. Gestational diabetes can cause complications in the pregnancy similar to those of pre-existing diabetes mellitus. It also puts the woman at greater risk of developing diabetes after the pregnancy. Codes for gestational diabetes are in subcategory O24.4, Gestational

diabetes mellitus. No other code from category O24, Diabetes mellitus in pregnancy, childbirth, and the puerperium, should be used with a code from O24.4.

The codes under subcategory O24.4 include diet controlled and insulin controlled. If a patient with gestational diabetes is treated with both diet and insulin, only the code for insulin-controlled is required.

Code Z79.4, Long-term (current) use of insulin, should not be assigned with codes from subcategory O24.4.

An abnormal glucose tolerance in pregnancy is assigned a code from subcategory O99.81, Abnormal glucose complicating pregnancy, childbirth, and the puerperium.

j. Sepsis and septic shock complicating abortion, pregnancy, childbirth and the puerperium

When assigning a chapter 15 code for sepsis complicating abortion, pregnancy, childbirth, and the puerperium, a code for the specific type of infection should be assigned as an additional diagnosis. If severe sepsis is present, a code from subcategory R65.2, Severe sepsis, and code(s) for associated organ dysfunction(s) should also be assigned as additional diagnoses.

k. Puerperal sepsis

Code O85, Puerperal sepsis, should be assigned with a secondary code to identify the causal organism (e.g., for a bacterial infection, assign a code from category B95-B96, Bacterial infections in conditions classified elsewhere). A code from category A40, Streptococcal sepsis, or A41, Other sepsis, should not be used for puerperal sepsis. If applicable, use additional codes to identify severe sepsis (R65.2-) and any associated acute organ dysfunction.

l. Alcohol and tobacco use during pregnancy, childbirth and the puerperium

1) Alcohol use during pregnancy, childbirth and the puerperium

Codes under subcategory O99.31, Alcohol use complicating pregnancy, childbirth, and the puerperium, should be assigned for any pregnancy case when a mother uses alcohol during the pregnancy or postpartum. A secondary code from category F10, Alcohol related disorders, should also be assigned to identify manifestations of the alcohol use.

2) Tobacco use during pregnancy, childbirth and the puerperium

Codes under subcategory O99.33, Smoking (tobacco) complicating pregnancy, childbirth, and the puerperium, should be assigned for any pregnancy case when a mother uses any type of tobacco product during the pregnancy or postpartum. A secondary code from category F17, Nicotine dependence, should also be assigned to identify the type of nicotine dependence.

m. Poisoning, toxic effects, adverse effects and underdosing in a pregnant patient

A code from subcategory O9A.2, Injury, poisoning and certain other consequences of external causes complicating pregnancy, childbirth, and the puerperium, should be sequenced first, followed by the appropriate injury, poisoning, toxic effect, adverse effect or underdosing code, and then the additional code(s) that specifies the condition caused by the poisoning, toxic effect, adverse effect or underdosing.

See Section I.C.19. Adverse effects, poisoning, underdosing and toxic effects.

n. Normal Delivery, Code O80

1) Encounter for full term uncomplicated delivery

Code O80 should be assigned when a woman is admitted for a full-term normal delivery and delivers a single, healthy infant without any complications antepartum, during the delivery, or postpartum during the delivery episode. Code O80 is always a principal diagnosis. It is not to be used if any other code from chapter 15 is needed to describe a current complication of the antenatal, delivery, or perinatal period. Additional codes from other chapters may be used with code O80 if they are not related to or are in any way complicating the pregnancy.

2) Uncomplicated delivery with resolved antepartum complication

Code O80 may be used if the patient had a complication at some point during the pregnancy, but the complication is not present at the time of the admission for delivery.

3) Outcome of delivery for O80

Z37.0, Single live birth, is the only outcome of delivery code appropriate for use with O80.

o. The Peripartum and Postpartum Periods

1) Peripartum and Postpartum periods

The postpartum period begins immediately after delivery and continues for six weeks following delivery. The peripartum period is defined as the last month of pregnancy to five months postpartum.

2) Peripartum and postpartum complication

A postpartum complication is any complication occurring within the six-week period.

3) Pregnancy-related complications after 6 week period

Chapter 15 codes may also be used to describe pregnancy-related complications after the peripartum or postpartum period if the provider documents that a condition is pregnancy related.

4) Admission for routine postpartum care following delivery outside hospital

When the mother delivers outside the hospital prior to admission and is admitted for routine postpartum care and no complications are noted, code Z39.0, Encounter for care and examination of mother immediately after delivery, should be assigned as the principal diagnosis.

5) Pregnancy associated cardiomyopathy
Pregnancy associated cardiomyopathy, code O90.3, is unique in that it may be diagnosed in the third trimester of pregnancy but may continue to progress months after delivery. For this reason, it is referred to as peripartum cardiomyopathy. Code O90.3 is only for use when the cardiomyopathy develops as a result of pregnancy in a woman who did not have pre-existing heart disease.

p. Code O94, Sequelae of complication of pregnancy, childbirth, and the puerperium

1) Code O94
Code O94, Sequelae of complication of pregnancy, childbirth, and the puerperium, is for use in those cases when an initial complication of a pregnancy develops a sequelae requiring care or treatment at a future date.

2) After the initial postpartum period
This code may be used at any time after the initial postpartum period.

3) Sequencing of Code O94
This code, like all sequela codes, is to be sequenced following the code describing the sequelae of the complication.

q. Termination of Pregnancy and Spontaneous abortions

1) Abortion with Liveborn Fetus
When an attempted termination of pregnancy results in a liveborn fetus assign code Z33.2, Encounter for elective termination of pregnancy and a code from category Z37, Outcome of Delivery.

2) Retained Products of Conception following an abortion
Subsequent encounters for retained products of conception following a spontaneous abortion or elective termination of pregnancy are assigned the appropriate code from category O03, Spontaneous abortion, or codes O07.4, Failed attempted termination of pregnancy without complication and Z33.2, Encounter for elective termination of pregnancy. This advice is appropriate even when the patient was discharged previously with a discharge diagnosis of complete abortion.

3) Complications leading to abortion
Codes from Chapter 15 may be used as additional codes to identify any documented complications of the pregnancy in conjunction with codes in categories in O07 and O08.

r. Abuse in a pregnant patient
For suspected or confirmed cases of abuse of a pregnant patient, a code(s) from subcategories O9A.3, Physical abuse complicating pregnancy, childbirth, and the puerperium, O9A.4, Sexual abuse complicating pregnancy, childbirth, and the puerperium, and O9A.5, Psychological abuse complicating pregnancy, childbirth, and the puerperium, should be sequenced first, followed by the appropriate codes (if applicable) to identify any associated current injury due to physical abuse, sexual abuse, and the perpetrator of abuse.
See Section I.C.19. Adult and child abuse, neglect and other maltreatment.

16. Chapter 16: Certain Conditions Originating in the Perinatal Period (P00-P96)
For coding and reporting purposes the perinatal period is defined as before birth through the 28th day following birth. The following guidelines are provided for reporting purposes

a. General Perinatal Rules

1) Use of Chapter 16 Codes
Codes in this chapter are never for use on the maternal record. Codes from Chapter 15, the obstetric chapter, are never permitted on the newborn record. Chapter 16 codes may be used throughout the life of the patient if the condition is still present.

2) Principal Diagnosis for Birth Record
When coding the birth episode in a newborn record, assign a code from category Z38, Liveborn infants according to place of birth and type of delivery, as the principal diagnosis. A code from category Z38 is assigned only once, to a newborn at the time of birth. If a newborn is transferred to another institution, a code from category Z38 should not be used at the receiving hospital.

A code from category Z38 is used only on the newborn record, not on the mother's record.

3) Use of Codes from other Chapters with Codes from Chapter 16
Codes from other chapters may be used with codes from chapter 16 if the codes from the other chapters provide more specific detail. Codes for signs and symptoms may be assigned when a definitive diagnosis has not been established. If the reason for the encounter is a perinatal condition, the code from chapter 16 should be sequenced first.

4) Use of Chapter 16 Codes after the Perinatal Period
Should a condition originate in the perinatal period, and continue throughout the life of the patient, the perinatal code should continue to be used regardless of the patient's age.

5) Birth process or community acquired conditions
If a newborn has a condition that may be either due to the birth process or community acquired and the documentation does not indicate which it is, the default is due to the birth process and the code from Chapter 16 should be used. If the condition is community-acquired, a code from Chapter 16 should not be assigned.

6) Code all clinically significant conditions
All clinically significant conditions noted on routine newborn examination should be coded. A condition is clinically significant if it requires:
- clinical evaluation; or
- therapeutic treatment; or
- diagnostic procedures; or

- extended length of hospital stay; or
- increased nursing care and/or monitoring; or
- has implications for future health care needs

Note: The perinatal guidelines listed above are the same as the general coding guidelines for "additional diagnoses", except for the final point regarding implications for future health care needs. Codes should be assigned for conditions that have been specified by the provider as having implications for future health care needs.

b. Observation and Evaluation of Newborns for Suspected Conditions not Found

Reserved for future expansion

c. Coding Additional Perinatal Diagnoses

1) Assigning codes for conditions that require treatment

Assign codes for conditions that require treatment or further investigation, prolong the length of stay, or require resource utilization.

2) Codes for conditions specified as having implications for future health care needs

Assign codes for conditions that have been specified by the provider as having implications for future health care needs.

Note: This guideline should not be used for adult patients.

d. Prematurity and Fetal Growth Retardation

Providers utilize different criteria in determining prematurity. A code for prematurity should not be assigned unless it is documented. Assignment of codes in categories P05, Disorders of newborn related to slow fetal growth and fetal malnutrition, and P07, Disorders of newborn related to short gestation and low birth weight, not elsewhere classified, should be based on the recorded birth weight and estimated gestational age. Codes from category P05 should not be assigned with codes from category P07.

When both birth weight and gestational age are available, two codes from category P07 should be assigned, with the code for birth weight sequenced before the code for gestational age.

e. Low birth weight and immaturity status

Codes from category P07, Disorders of newborn related to short gestation and low birth weight, not elsewhere classified, are for use for a child or adult who was premature or had a low birth weight as a newborn and this is affecting the patient's current health status.

See Section I.C.21. Factors influencing health status and contact with health services, Status.

f. Bacterial Sepsis of Newborn

Category P36, Bacterial sepsis of newborn, includes congenital sepsis. If a perinate is documented as having sepsis without documentation of congenital or community acquired, the default is congenital and a code from category P36 should be assigned. If the P36 code includes the causal organism, an additional code from category B95, Streptococcus, Staphylococcus, and Enterococcus as the cause of diseases classified elsewhere, or B96, Other bacterial agents as the cause of diseases classified elsewhere, should not be assigned. If the P36 code does not include the causal organism, assign an additional code from category B96. If applicable, use additional codes to identify severe sepsis (R65.2-) and any associated acute organ dysfunction.

g. Stillbirth

Code P95, Stillbirth, is only for use in institutions that maintain separate records for stillbirths. No other code should be used with P95. Code P95 should not be used on the mother's record.

17. Chapter 17: Congenital malformations, deformations, and chromosomal abnormalities (Q00-Q99)

Assign an appropriate code(s) from categories Q00-Q99, Congenital malformations, deformations, and chromosomal abnormalities when a malformation/deformation or chromosomal abnormality is documented. A malformation/deformation/or chromosomal abnormality may be the principal/first-listed diagnosis on a record or a secondary diagnosis.

When a malformation/deformation/or chromosomal abnormality does not have a unique code assignment, assign additional code(s) for any manifestations that may be present.

When the code assignment specifically identifies the malformation/deformation/or chromosomal abnormality, manifestations that are an inherent component of the anomaly should not be coded separately. Additional codes should be assigned for manifestations that are not an inherent component.

Codes from Chapter 17 may be used throughout the life of the patient. If a congenital malformation or deformity has been corrected, a personal history code should be used to identify the history of the malformation or deformity. Although present at birth, malformation/deformation/or chromosomal abnormality may not be identified until later in life. Whenever the condition is diagnosed by the physician, it is appropriate to assign a code from codes Q00-Q99.

For the birth admission, the appropriate code from category Z38, Liveborn infants, according to place of birth and type of delivery, should be sequenced as the principal diagnosis, followed by any congenital anomaly codes, Q00-Q99.

18. Chapter 18: Symptoms, signs, and abnormal clinical and laboratory findings, not elsewhere classified (R00-R99)

Chapter 18 includes symptoms, signs, abnormal results of clinical or other investigative procedures, and ill-defined conditions regarding which no diagnosis classifiable elsewhere is recorded. Signs and symptoms that point to a specific diagnosis have been assigned to a category in other chapters of the classification.

a. Use of symptom codes

Codes that describe symptoms and signs are acceptable for reporting purposes when a related definitive diagnosis has not been established (confirmed) by the provider.

GUIDELINES (ICD-10-CM)

b. Use of a symptom code with a definitive diagnosis code

Codes for signs and symptoms may be reported in addition to a related definitive diagnosis when the sign or symptom is not routinely associated with that diagnosis, such as the various signs and symptoms associated with complex syndromes. The definitive diagnosis code should be sequenced before the symptom code.

Signs or symptoms that are associated routinely with a disease process should not be assigned as additional codes, unless otherwise instructed by the classification.

c. Combination codes that include symptoms

ICD-10-CM contains a number of combination codes that identify both the definitive diagnosis and common symptoms of that diagnosis. When using one of these combination codes, an additional code should not be assigned for the symptom.

d. Repeated falls

Code R29.6, Repeated falls, is for use for encounters when a patient has recently fallen and the reason for the fall is being investigated.

Code Z91.81, History of falling, is for use when a patient has fallen in the past and is at risk for future falls. When appropriate, both codes R29.6 and Z91.81 may be assigned together.

e. Coma scale

The coma scale codes (R40.2-) can be used in conjunction with traumatic brain injury codes, acute cerebrovascular disease or sequelae of cerebrovascular disease codes. These codes are primarily for use by trauma registries, but they may be used in any setting where this information is collected. The coma scale codes should be sequenced after the diagnosis code(s).

These codes, one from each subcategory, are needed to complete the scale. The 7th character indicates when the scale was recorded. The 7th character should match for all three codes.

At a minimum, report the initial score documented on presentation at your facility. This may be a score from the emergency medicine technician (EMT) or in the emergency department. If desired, a facility may choose to capture multiple coma scale scores.

Assign code R40.24, Glasgow coma scale, total score, when only the total score is documented in the medical record and not the individual score(s).

f. Functional quadriplegia

Functional quadriplegia (code R53.2) is the lack of ability to use one's limbs or to ambulate due to extreme debility. It is not associated with neurologic deficit or injury, and code R53.2 should not be used for cases of neurologic quadriplegia. It should only be assigned if functional quadriplegia is specifically documented in the medical record.

g. SIRS due to Non-Infectious Process

The systemic inflammatory response syndrome (SIRS) can develop as a result of certain non-infectious disease processes, such as trauma, malignant neoplasm, or pancreatitis. When SIRS is documented with a noninfectious condition, and no subsequent infection is documented, the code for the underlying condition, such as an injury, should be assigned, followed by code R65.10, Systemic inflammatory response syndrome (SIRS) of non-infectious origin without acute organ dysfunction, or code R65.11, Systemic inflammatory response syndrome (SIRS) of non-infectious origin with acute organ dysfunction. If an associated acute organ dysfunction is documented, the appropriate code(s) for the specific type of organ dysfunction(s) should be assigned in addition to code R65.11. If acute organ dysfunction is documented, but it cannot be determined if the acute organ dysfunction is associated with SIRS or due to another condition (e.g., directly due to the trauma), the provider should be queried.

h. Death NOS

Code R99, Ill-defined and unknown cause of mortality, is only for use in the very limited circumstance when a patient who has already died is brought into an emergency department or other healthcare facility and is pronounced dead upon arrival. It does not represent the discharge disposition of death.

19. **Chapter 19: Injury, poisoning, and certain other consequences of external causes (S00-T88)**

   a. Application of 7th Characters in Chapter 19

   Most categories in chapter 19 have a 7th character requirement for each applicable code. Most categories in this chapter have three 7th character values (with the exception of fractures): A, initial encounter, D, subsequent encounter and S, sequela. Categories for traumatic fractures have additional 7th character values. **While the patient may be seen by a new or different provider over the course of treatment for an injury, assignment of the 7th character is based on whether the patient is undergoing active treatment and not whether the provider is seeing the patient for the first time.**

   For complication codes, active treatment refers to treatment for the condition described by the code, even though it may be related to an earlier precipitating problem. For example, code T84.50XA, Infection and inflammatory reaction due to unspecified internal joint prosthesis, initial encounter, is used when active treatment is provided for the infection, even though the condition relates to the prosthetic device, implant or graft that was placed at a previous encounter.

   7th character "A", initial encounter is used while the patient is receiving active treatment for the condition. Examples of active treatment are: surgical treatment, emergency department encounter, and evaluation and **continuing** treatment by **the same or a different** physician.

   7th character "D" subsequent encounter is used for encounters after the patient has received active treatment of the condition and is receiving routine care for the condition during the healing or recovery phase. Examples of subsequent care are:

cast change or removal, **an x-ray to check healing status of fracture,** removal of external or internal fixation device, medication adjustment, other aftercare and follow up visits following treatment of the injury or condition.

The aftercare Z codes should not be used for aftercare for conditions such as injuries or poisonings, where 7th characters are provided to identify subsequent care. For example, for aftercare of an injury, assign the acute injury code with the 7th character "D" (subsequent encounter).

7th character "S", sequela, is for use for complications or conditions that arise as a direct result of a condition, such as scar formation after a burn. The scars are sequelae of the burn. When using 7th character "S", it is necessary to use both the injury code that precipitated the sequela and the code for the sequela itself. The "S" is added only to the injury code, not the sequela code. The 7th character "S" identifies the injury responsible for the sequela. The specific type of sequela (e.g. scar) is sequenced first, followed by the injury code.

See Section I.B.10. Sequelae, (Late Effects)

b. Coding of Injuries

When coding injuries, assign separate codes for each injury unless a combination code is provided, in which case the combination code is assigned. Code T07, Unspecified multiple injuries should not be assigned in the inpatient setting unless information for a more specific code is not available. Traumatic injury codes (S00-T14.9) are not to be used for normal, healing surgical wounds or to identify complications of surgical wounds.

The code for the most serious injury, as determined by the provider and the focus of treatment, is sequenced first.

1) Superficial injuries

Superficial injuries such as abrasions or contusions are not coded when associated with more severe injuries of the same site.

2) Primary injury with damage to nerves/ blood vessels

When a primary injury results in minor damage to peripheral nerves or blood vessels, the primary injury is sequenced first with additional code(s) for injuries to nerves and spinal cord (such as category S04), and/or injury to blood vessels (such as category S15). When the primary injury is to the blood vessels or nerves, that injury should be sequenced first.

c. Coding of Traumatic Fractures

The principles of multiple coding of injuries should be followed in coding fractures. Fractures of specified sites are coded individually by site in accordance with both the provisions within categories S02, S12, S22, S32, S42, S49, S52, S59, S62, S72, S79, S82, S89, S92 and the level of detail furnished by medical record content.

A fracture not indicated as open or closed should be coded to closed. A fracture not indicated whether displaced or not displaced should be coded to displaced.

More specific guidelines are as follows:

1) Initial vs. Subsequent Encounter for Fractures

Traumatic fractures are coded using the appropriate 7th character for initial encounter (A, B, C) while the patient is receiving active treatment for the fracture. Examples of active treatment are: surgical treatment, emergency department encounter, and evaluation and **continuing (ongoing)** treatment by **the same or a different** physician. The appropriate 7th character for initial encounter should also be assigned for a patient who delayed seeking treatment for the fracture or nonunion.

Fractures are coded using the appropriate 7th character for subsequent care for encounters after the patient has completed active treatment of the fracture and is receiving routine care for the fracture during the healing or recovery phase. Examples of fracture aftercare are: cast change or removal, **an x-ray to check healing status of fracture,** removal of external or internal fixation device, medication adjustment, and follow-up visits following fracture treatment.

Care for complications of surgical treatment for fracture repairs during the healing or recovery phase should be coded with the appropriate complication codes.

Care of complications of fractures, such as malunion and nonunion, should be reported with the appropriate 7th character for subsequent care with nonunion (K, M, N,) or subsequent care with malunion (P, Q, R).

Malunion/nonunion: The appropriate 7th character for initial encounter should also be assigned for a patient who delayed seeking treatment for the fracture or nonunion.

A code from category M80, not a traumatic fracture code, should be used for any patient with known osteoporosis who suffers a fracture, even if the patient had a minor fall or trauma, if that fall or trauma would not usually break a normal, healthy bone.

See Section I.C.13. Osteoporosis.

The aftercare Z codes should not be used for aftercare for traumatic fractures. For aftercare of a traumatic fracture, assign the acute fracture code with the appropriate 7th character.

2) Multiple fractures sequencing

Multiple fractures are sequenced in accordance with the severity of the fracture.

d. Coding of Burns and Corrosions

The ICD-10-CM makes a distinction between burns and corrosions. The burn codes are for thermal burns, except sunburns, that come from a heat source, such as a fire or hot appliance. The burn codes are also for burns resulting from electricity and radiation. Corrosions are burns due to chemicals. The guidelines are the same for burns and corrosions.

Current burns (T20-T25) are classified by depth, extent and by agent (X code). Burns are classified by depth as first degree (erythema), second degree (blistering), and third degree (full-thickness involvement). Burns of the eye and internal organs (T26-T28) are classified by site, but not by degree.

1) Sequencing of burn and related condition codes

Sequence first the code that reflects the highest degree of burn when more than one burn is present.

   a. When the reason for the admission or encounter is for treatment of external multiple burns, sequence first the code that reflects the burn of the highest degree.

   b. When a patient has both internal and external burns, the circumstances of admission govern the selection of the principal diagnosis or first-listed diagnosis.

   c. When a patient is admitted for burn injuries and other related conditions such as smoke inhalation and/or respiratory failure, the circumstances of admission govern the selection of the principal or first-listed diagnosis.

2) Burns of the same local site

Classify burns of the same local site (three-character category level, T20-T28) but of different degrees to the subcategory identifying the highest degree recorded in the diagnosis.

3) Non-healing burns

Non-healing burns are coded as acute burns.
Necrosis of burned skin should be coded as a non-healed burn.

4) Infected Burn

For any documented infected burn site, use an additional code for the infection.

5) Assign separate codes for each burn site

When coding burns, assign separate codes for each burn site. Category T30, Burn and corrosion, body region unspecified is extremely vague and should rarely be used.

6) Burns and Corrosions Classified According to Extent of Body Surface Involved

Assign codes from category T31, Burns classified according to extent of body surface involved, or T32, Corrosions classified according to extent of body surface involved, when the site of the burn is not specified or when there is a need for additional data. It is advisable to use category T31 as additional coding when needed to provide data for evaluating burn mortality, such as that needed by burn units. It is also advisable to use category T31 as an additional code for reporting purposes when there is mention of a third-degree burn involving 20 percent or more of the body surface.

Categories T31 and T32 are based on the classic "rule of nines" in estimating body surface involved: head and neck are assigned nine percent, each arm nine percent, each leg 18 percent, the anterior trunk 18 percent, posterior trunk 18 percent, and genitalia one percent. Providers may change these percentage assignments where necessary to accommodate infants and children who have proportionately larger heads than adults, and patients who have large buttocks, thighs, or abdomen that involve burns.

7) Encounters for treatment of sequela of burns

Encounters for the treatment of the late effects of burns or corrosions (i.e., scars or joint contractures) should be coded with a burn or corrosion code with the 7th character "S" for sequela.

8) Sequelae with a late effect code and current burn

When appropriate, both a code for a current burn or corrosion with 7th character "A" or "D" and a burn or corrosion code with 7th character "S" may be assigned on the same record (when both a current burn and sequelae of an old burn exist). Burns and corrosions do not heal at the same rate and a current healing wound may still exist with sequela of a healed burn or corrosion.

See Section I.B.10. Sequela, (Late Effects)

9) Use of an external cause code with burns and corrosions

An external cause code should be used with burns and corrosions to identify the source and intent of the burn, as well as the place where it occurred.

e. Adverse Effects, Poisoning , Underdosing and Toxic Effects

Codes in categories T36-T65 are combination codes that include the substance that was taken as well as the intent. No additional external cause code is required for poisonings, toxic effects, adverse effects and underdosing codes.

1) Do not code directly from the Table of Drugs

Do not code directly from the Table of Drugs and Chemicals. Always refer back to the Tabular List.

2) Use as many codes as necessary to describe

Use as many codes as necessary to describe completely all drugs, medicinal or biological substances.

3) If the same code would describe the causative agent

If the same code would describe the causative agent for more than one adverse reaction, poisoning, toxic effect or underdosing, assign the code only once.

4) If two or more drugs, medicinal or biological substances

If two or more drugs, medicinal or biological substances are reported, code each individually unless a combination code is listed in the Table of Drugs and Chemicals.

5) The occurrence of drug toxicity is classified in ICD-10-CM as follows:

(a) Adverse Effect

When coding an adverse effect of a drug that has been correctly prescribed and properly administered, assign the appropriate code for the nature of the adverse effect followed by the appropriate code for the adverse effect of the drug (T36-T50). The code for the drug should have a 5th or 6th character "5" (for example

T36.0X5-) Examples of the nature of an adverse effect are tachycardia, delirium, gastrointestinal hemorrhaging, vomiting, hypokalemia, hepatitis, renal failure, or respiratory failure.

(b) Poisoning

When coding a poisoning or reaction to the improper use of a medication (e.g., overdose, wrong substance given or taken in error, wrong route of administration), first assign the appropriate code from categories T36-T50. The poisoning codes have an associated intent as their 5th or 6th character (accidental, intentional self-harm, assault and undetermined). Use additional code(s) for all manifestations of poisonings.

If there is also a diagnosis of abuse or dependence of the substance, the abuse or dependence is assigned as an additional code.

Examples of poisoning include:

    (i) Error was made in drug prescription Errors made in drug prescription or in the administration of the drug by provider, nurse, patient, or other person.

    (ii) Overdose of a drug intentionally taken If an overdose of a drug was intentionally taken or administered and resulted in drug toxicity, it would be coded as a poisoning.

    (iii) Nonprescribed drug taken with correctly prescribed and properly administered drug.
If a nonprescribed drug or medicinal agent was taken in combination with a correctly prescribed and properly administered drug, any drug toxicity or other reaction resulting from the interaction of the two drugs would be classified as a poisoning.

    (iv) Interaction of drug(s) and alcohol. When a reaction results from the interaction of a drug(s) and alcohol, this would be classified as poisoning.

See Section I.C.4. if poisoning is the result of insulin pump malfunctions.

(c) Underdosing

Underdosing refers to taking less of a medication than is prescribed by a provider or a manufacturer's instruction. For underdosing, assign the code from categories T36-T50 (fifth or sixth character "6").

Codes for underdosing should never be assigned as principal or first-listed codes. If a patient has a relapse or exacerbation of the medical condition for which the drug is prescribed because of the reduction in dose, then the medical condition itself should be coded.

Noncompliance (Z91.12-, Z91.13-) or complication of care (Y63.6-Y63.9) codes are to be used with an underdosing code to indicate intent, if known.

(d) Toxic Effects

When a harmful substance is ingested or comes in contact with a person, this is classified as a toxic effect. The toxic effect codes are in categories T51-T65.

Toxic effect codes have an associated intent: accidental, intentional self-harm, assault and undetermined.

f. Adult and child abuse, neglect and other maltreatment

Sequence first the appropriate code from categories T74.- (Adult and child abuse, neglect and other maltreatment, confirmed) or T76.- (Adult and child abuse, neglect and other maltreatment, suspected) for abuse, neglect and other maltreatment, followed by any accompanying mental health or injury code(s).

If the documentation in the medical record states abuse or neglect it is coded as confirmed (T74.-). It is coded as suspected if it is documented as suspected (T76.-).

For cases of confirmed abuse or neglect an external cause code from the assault section (X92-Y08) should be added to identify the cause of any physical injuries. A perpetrator code (Y07) should be added when the perpetrator of the abuse is known. For suspected cases of abuse or neglect, do not report external cause or perpetrator code.

If a suspected case of abuse, neglect or mistreatment is ruled out during an encounter code Z04.71, Encounter for examination and observation following alleged physical adult abuse, ruled out, or code Z04.72, Encounter for examination and observation following alleged child physical abuse, ruled out, should be used, not a code from T76.

If a suspected case of alleged rape or sexual abuse is ruled out during an encounter code Z04.41, Encounter for examination and observation following alleged physical adult abuse, ruled out, or code Z04.42, Encounter for examination and observation following alleged rape or sexual abuse, ruled out, should be used, not a code from T76.

See Section I.C.15. Abuse in a pregnant patient.

g. Complications of care

1) General guidelines for complications of care

(a) Documentation of complications of care

See Section I.B.16. for information on documentation of complications of care.

2) Pain due to medical devices

Pain associated with devices, implants or grafts left in a surgical site (for example painful hip prosthesis) is assigned to the appropriate code(s) found in Chapter 19, Injury, poisoning, and certain other consequences of external causes. Specific codes for pain due to medical devices are found in the T code section of the ICD-10-CM. Use additional code(s) from category G89 to identify

GUIDELINES (ICD-10-CM)

acute or chronic pain due to presence of the device, implant or graft (G89.18 or G89.28).

3) Transplant complications

(a) Transplant complications other than kidney

Codes under category T86, Complications of transplanted organs and tissues, are for use for both complications and rejection of transplanted organs. A transplant complication code is only assigned if the complication affects the function of the transplanted organ. Two codes are required to fully describe a transplant complication: the appropriate code from category T86 and a secondary code that identifies the complication.

Pre-existing conditions or conditions that develop after the transplant are not coded as complications unless they affect the function of the transplanted organs.

See I.C.21. for transplant organ removal status
See I.C.2. for malignant neoplasm associated with transplanted organ.

(b) Kidney transplant complications

Patients who have undergone kidney transplant may still have some form of chronic kidney disease (CKD) because the kidney transplant may not fully restore kidney function. Code T86.1- should be assigned for documented complications of a kidney transplant, such as transplant failure or rejection or other transplant complication. Code T86.1- should not be assigned for post kidney transplant patients who have chronic kidney (CKD) unless a transplant complication such as transplant failure or rejection is documented. If the documentation is unclear as to whether the patient has a complication of the transplant, query the provider.

Conditions that affect the function of the transplanted kidney, other than CKD, should be assigned a code from subcategory T86.1, Complications of transplanted organ, Kidney, and a secondary code that identifies the complication.

For patients with CKD following a kidney transplant, but who do not have a complication such as failure or rejection, *see section I.C.14. Chronic kidney disease and kidney transplant status.*

4) Complication codes that include the external cause

As with certain other T codes, some of the complications of care codes have the external cause included in the code. The code includes the nature of the complication as well as the type of procedure that caused the complication. No external cause code indicating the type of procedure is necessary for these codes.

5) Complications of care codes within the body system chapters

Intraoperative and postprocedural complication codes are found within the body system chapters with codes specific to the organs and structures of that body system. These codes should be sequenced first, followed by a code(s) for the specific complication, if applicable.

20. Chapter 20: External Causes of Morbidity (V00-Y99)

The external causes of morbidity codes should never be sequenced as the first-listed or principal diagnosis.

External cause codes are intended to provide data for injury research and evaluation of injury prevention strategies. These codes capture how the injury or health condition happened (cause), the intent (unintentional or accidental; or intentional, such as suicide or assault), the place where the event occurred the activity of the patient at the time of the event, and the person's status (e.g., civilian, military).

There is no national requirement for mandatory ICD-10-CM external cause code reporting. Unless a provider is subject to a state-based external cause code reporting mandate or these codes are required by a particular payer, reporting of ICD-10-CM codes in Chapter 20, External Causes of Morbidity, is not required. In the absence of a mandatory reporting requirement, providers are encouraged to voluntarily report external cause codes, as they provide valuable data for injury research and evaluation of injury prevention strategies.

a. General External Cause Coding Guidelines

1) Used with any code in the range of A00.0-T88.9, Z00-Z99

An external cause code may be used with any code in the range of A00.0-T88.9, Z00-Z99, classification that is a health condition due to an external cause. Though they are most applicable to injuries, they are also valid for use with such things as infections or diseases due to an external source, and other health conditions, such as a heart attack that occurs during strenuous physical activity.

2) External cause code used for length of treatment

Assign the external cause code, with the appropriate 7th character (initial encounter, subsequent encounter or sequela) for each encounter for which the injury or condition is being treated.

Most categories in chapter 20 have a 7th character requirement for each applicable code. Most categories in this chapter have three 7th character values: A, initial encounter, D, subsequent encounter and S, sequela. While the patient may be seen by a new or different provider over the course of treatment for an injury or condition, assignment of the 7th character for external cause should match the 7th character of the code assigned for the associated injury or condition for the encounter.

3) Use the full range of external cause codes

Use the full range of external cause codes to completely describe the cause, the intent, the place of occurrence and if applicable, the activity of the patient at the time of the event, and the patient's status, for all injuries, and other health conditions due to an external cause.

4) Assign as many external cause codes as necessary

Assign as many external cause codes as necessary to fully explain each cause. If only one external code can be recorded, assign the code most related to the principal diagnosis.

5) The selection of the appropriate external cause code

The selection of the appropriate external cause code is guided by the Alphabetic Index of External Causes and by Inclusion and Exclusion notes in the Tabular List.

6) External cause code can never be a principal diagnosis

An external cause code can never be a principal (first-listed) diagnosis.

7) Combination external cause codes

Certain of the external cause codes are combination codes that identify sequential events that result in an injury, such as a fall which results in striking against an object. The injury may be due to either event or both. The combination external cause code used should correspond to the sequence of events regardless of which caused the most serious injury.

8) No external cause code needed in certain circumstances

No external cause code from Chapter 20 is needed if the external cause and intent are included in a code from another chapter (e.g. T36.0X1- Poisoning by penicillins, accidental (unintentional)).

b. Place of Occurrence Guideline

Codes from category Y92, Place of occurrence of the external cause, are secondary codes for use after other external cause codes to identify the location of the patient at the time of injury or other condition.

Generally, a place of occurrence code is **assigned** only once, at the initial encounter for treatment. **However, in the rare instance that a new injury occurs during hospitalization, an additional place of occurrence code may be assigned.** No 7th characters are used for Y92. Only one code from Y92 should be recorded on a medical record.

Do not use place of occurrence code Y92.9 if the place is not stated or is not applicable.

c. Activity Code

Assign a code from category Y93, Activity code, to describe the activity of the patient at the time the injury or other health condition occurred.

An activity code is used only once, at the initial encounter for treatment. Only one code from Y93 should be recorded on a medical record.

The activity codes are not applicable to poisonings, adverse effects, misadventures or sequela.

Do not assign Y93.9, Unspecified activity, if the activity is not stated.

A code from category Y93 is appropriate for use with external cause and intent codes if identifying the activity provides additional information about the event.

d. Place of Occurrence, Activity, and Status Codes Used with other External Cause Code

When applicable, place of occurrence, activity, and external cause status codes are sequenced after the main external cause code(s). Regardless of the number of external cause codes assigned, there should be only one place of occurrence code, one activity code, and one external cause status code assigned to an encounter.

e. If the Reporting Format Limits the Number of External Cause Codes

If the reporting format limits the number of external cause codes that can be used in reporting clinical data, report the code for the cause/intent most related to the principal diagnosis. If the format permits capture of additional external cause codes, the cause/intent, including medical misadventures, of the additional events should be reported rather than the codes for place, activity, or external status.

f. Multiple External Cause Coding Guidelines

More than one external cause code is required to fully describe the external cause of an illness or injury. The assignment of external cause codes should be sequenced in the following priority:

If two or more events cause separate injuries, an external cause code should be assigned for each cause. The first-listed external cause code will be selected in the following order:

External codes for child and adult abuse take priority over all other external cause codes.
See Section I.C.19., Child and Adult abuse guidelines.

External codes for terrorism events take priority over all other external cause codes except child and adult abuse.

External cause codes for cataclysmic events take priority over all other external cause codes except child and adult abuse and terrorism.

External cause codes for transport accidents take priority over all other external cause codes except cataclysmic events, child and adult abuse and terrorism.

Activity and external cause status codes are assigned following all causal (intent) external cause codes.

The first-listed external cause code should correspond to the cause of the most serious diagnosis due to an assault, accident, or self-harm, following the order of hierarchy listed above.

g. Child and Adult Abuse Guideline

Adult and child abuse, neglect and maltreatment are classified as assault. Any of the assault codes may be used to indicate the external cause of any injury resulting from the confirmed abuse.

For confirmed cases of abuse, neglect and maltreatment, when the perpetrator is known, a code from Y07, Perpetrator of maltreatment and neglect, should accompany any other assault codes.

See Section I.C.19. Adult and child abuse, neglect and other maltreatment

h. Unknown or Undetermined Intent Guideline

If the intent (accident, self-harm, assault) of the cause of an injury or other condition is unknown or unspecified, code the intent as accidental intent. All transport accident categories assume accidental intent.

1) Use of undetermined intent

External cause codes for events of undetermined intent are only for use if the documentation in the record specifies that the intent cannot be determined.

i. Sequelae (Late Effects) of External Cause Guidelines

1) Sequelae external cause codes

Sequela are reported using the external cause code with the 7th character "S" for sequela. These codes should be used with any report of a late effect or sequela resulting from a previous injury.

See Section I.B.10. Sequela, (Late Effects)

2) Sequela external cause code with a related current injury

A sequela external cause code should never be used with a related current nature of injury code.

3) Use of sequela external cause codes for subsequent visits

Use a late effect external cause code for subsequent visits when a late effect of the initial injury is being treated. Do not use a late effect external cause code for subsequent visits for follow-up care (e.g., to assess healing, to receive rehabilitative therapy) of the injury when no late effect of the injury has been documented.

j. Terrorism Guidelines

1) Cause of injury identified by the Federal Government (FBI) as terrorism

When the cause of an injury is identified by the Federal Government (FBI) as terrorism, the first-listed external cause code should be a code from category Y38, Terrorism. The definition of terrorism employed by the FBI is found at the inclusion note at the beginning of category Y38. Use additional code for place of occurrence (Y92.-). More than one Y38 code may be assigned if the injury is the result of more than one mechanism of terrorism.

2) Cause of an injury is suspected to be the result of terrorism

When the cause of an injury is suspected to be the result of terrorism a code from category Y38 should not be assigned. Suspected cases should be classified as assault.

3) Code Y38.9, Terrorism, secondary effects

Assign code Y38.9, Terrorism, secondary effects, for conditions occurring subsequent to the terrorist event. This code should not be assigned for conditions that are due to the initial terrorist act.

It is acceptable to assign code Y38.9 with another code from Y38 if there is an injury due to the initial terrorist event and an injury that is a subsequent result of the terrorist event.

k. External cause status

A code from category Y99, External cause status, should be assigned whenever any other external cause code is assigned for an encounter, including an Activity code, except for the events noted below. Assign a code from category Y99, External cause status, to indicate the work status of the person at the time the event occurred. The status code indicates whether the event occurred during military activity, whether a non-military person was at work, whether an individual including a student or volunteer was involved in a non-work activity at the time of the causal event.

A code from Y99, External cause status, should be assigned, when applicable, with other external cause codes, such as transport accidents and falls. The external cause status codes are not applicable to poisonings, adverse effects, misadventures or late effects.

Do not assign a code from category Y99 if no other external cause codes (cause, activity) are applicable for the encounter.

An external cause status code is used only once, at the initial encounter for treatment. Only one code from Y99 should be recorded on a medical record.

Do not assign code Y99.9, Unspecified external cause status, if the status is not stated.

21. Chapter 21: Factors influencing health status and contact with health services (Z00-Z99)

Note: The chapter specific guidelines provide additional information about the use of Z codes for specified encounters.

a. Use of Z codes in any healthcare setting

Z codes are for use in any healthcare setting. Z codes may be used as either a first-listed (principal diagnosis code in the inpatient setting) or secondary code, depending on the circumstances of the encounter. Certain Z codes may only be used as first-listed or principal diagnosis.

b. Z Codes indicate a reason for an encounter

Z codes are not procedure codes. A corresponding procedure code must accompany a Z code to describe any procedure performed.

c. Categories of Z Codes

1) Contact/Exposure

Category Z20 indicates contact with, and suspected exposure to, communicable diseases. These codes are for patients who do not show any sign or symptom of a disease but are suspected to have been exposed to it by close personal contact with an infected individual or are in an area where a disease is epidemic.

Category Z77, **Other contact with and (suspected) exposures hazardous to health,** indicates contact with and suspected exposures hazardous to health.

Contact/exposure codes may be used as a first-listed code to explain an encounter for testing, or, more commonly, as a secondary code to identify a potential risk.

2) Inoculations and vaccinations

Code Z23 is for encounters for inoculations and vaccinations. It indicates that a patient is being seen to receive a prophylactic inoculation against a disease. Procedure codes are required to identify the actual administration of the injection and the type(s) of immunizations given. Code Z23 may be used as a secondary code if the inoculation is given as a routine part of preventive health care, such as a well-baby visit.

3) Status

Status codes indicate that a patient is either a carrier of a disease or has the sequelae or residual of a past disease or condition. This includes such things as the presence of prosthetic or mechanical devices resulting from past treatment. A status code is informative, because the status may affect the course of treatment and its outcome. A status code is distinct from a history code. The history code indicates that the patient no longer has the condition.

A status code should not be used with a diagnosis code from one of the body system chapters, if the diagnosis code includes the information provided by the status code. For example, code Z94.1, Heart transplant status, should not be used with a code from subcategory T86.2, Complications of heart transplant. The status code does not provide additional information. The complication code indicates that the patient is a heart transplant patient.

For encounters for weaning from a mechanical ventilator, assign a code from subcategory J96.1, Chronic respiratory failure, followed by code Z99.11, Dependence on respirator [ventilator] status.

The status Z codes/categories are:

Z14   Genetic carrier
Genetic carrier status indicates that a person carries a gene, associated with a particular disease, which may be passed to offspring who may develop that disease. The person does not have the disease and is not at risk of developing the disease.

Z15   Genetic susceptibility to disease Genetic susceptibility indicates that a person has a gene that increases the risk of that person developing the disease.

Codes from category Z15 should not be used as principal or first-listed codes. If the patient has the condition to which he/she is susceptible, and that condition is the reason for the encounter, the code for the current condition should be sequenced first. If the patient is being seen for follow-up after completed treatment for this condition, and the condition no longer exists, a follow-up code should be sequenced first, followed by the appropriate personal history and genetic susceptibility codes. If the purpose of the encounter is genetic counseling associated with procreative management, code Z31.5, Encounter for genetic counseling, should be assigned as the first-listed code, followed by a code from category Z15. Additional codes should be assigned for any applicable family or personal history.

Z16   Resistance to antimicrobial drugs
This code indicates that a patient has a condition that is resistant to antimicrobial drug treatment. Sequence the infection code first.

Z17   Estrogen receptor status

Z18   Retained foreign body fragments

Z21   Asymptomatic HIV infection status This code indicates that a patient has tested positive for HIV but has manifested no signs or symptoms of the disease.

Z22   Carrier of infectious disease Carrier status indicates that a person harbors the specific organisms of a disease without manifest symptoms and is capable of transmitting the infection.

Z28.3   Underimmunization status

Z33.1   Pregnant state, incidental This code is a secondary code only for use when the pregnancy is in no way complicating the reason for visit. Otherwise, a code from the obstetric chapter is required.

Z66   Do not resuscitate
This code may be used when it is documented by the provider that a patient is on do not resuscitate status at any time during the stay.

Z67   Blood type

Z68   Body mass index (BMI)

Z74.01   Bed confinement status

Z76.82   Awaiting organ transplant status

Z78   Other specified health status
Code Z78.1, Physical restraint status, may be used when it is documented by the provider that a patient has been put in restraints during the current encounter. Please note that this code should not be reported when it is documented by the provider that a patient is temporarily restrained during a procedure.

Z79   Long-term (current) drug therapy
Codes from this category indicate a patient's continuous use of a prescribed drug (including such things as aspirin therapy) for the long-term treatment of a condition or for prophylactic use. It is not for use for patients who have addictions to drugs. This subcategory is not for use of medications for detoxification or maintenance programs to prevent withdrawal symptoms in patients with drug dependence (e.g., methadone maintenance for opiate dependence). Assign the appropriate code for the drug dependence instead.

Assign a code from Z79 if the patient is receiving a medication for an extended period as a prophylactic measure (such as for the prevention of deep vein thrombosis) or as treatment of a chronic condition (such as arthritis) or a disease requiring a lengthy course of treatment (such as cancer). Do not assign a code from category Z79 for medication being administered for a brief period of time to treat an acute illness or injury (such as a course of antibiotics to treat acute bronchitis).

Z88   Allergy status to drugs, medicaments and biological substances Except: Z88.9, Allergy status to unspecified drugs, medicaments and biological substances status

Z89   Acquired absence of limb

Z90   Acquired absence of organs, not elsewhere classified

Z91.0- Allergy status, other than to drugs and biological substances

Z92.82 Status post administration of tPA (rtPA) in a different facility within the last 24 hours prior to admission to a current facility Assign code Z92.82, Status post administration of tPA (rtPA) in a different facility within the last 24 hours prior to admission to current facility, as a secondary diagnosis when a patient is received by transfer into a facility and documentation indicates they were administered tissue plasminogen activator (tPA) within the last 24 hours prior to admission to the current facility. This guideline applies even if the patient is still receiving the tPA at the time they are received into the current facility. The appropriate code for the condition for which the tPA was administered (such as cerebrovascular disease or myocardial infarction) should be assigned first. Code Z92.82 is only applicable to the receiving facility record and not to the transferring facility record.

Z93   Artificial opening status

Z94   Transplanted organ and tissue status

Z95   Presence of cardiac and vascular implants and grafts

Z96   Presence of other functional implants

Z97   Presence of other devices

Z98   Other postprocedural states

Assign code Z98.85, Transplanted organ removal status, to indicate that a transplanted organ has been previously removed. This code should not be assigned for the encounter in which the transplanted organ is removed. The complication necessitating removal of the transplant organ should be assigned for that encounter.

See section I.C.19. for information on the coding of organ transplant complications.

Z99   Dependence on enabling machines and devices, not elsewhere classified

Note: Categories Z89-Z90 and Z93-Z99 are for use only if there are no complications or malfunctions of the organ or tissue replaced, the amputation site or the equipment on which the patient is dependent.

4) History (of)

There are two types of history Z codes, personal and family. Personal history codes explain a patient's past medical condition that no longer exists and is not receiving any treatment, but that has the potential for recurrence, and therefore may require continued monitoring.

Family history codes are for use when a patient has a family member(s) who has had a particular disease that causes the patient to be at higher risk of also contracting the disease.

Personal history codes may be used in conjunction with follow-up codes and family history codes may be used in conjunction with screening codes to explain the need for a test or procedure. History codes are also acceptable on any medical record regardless of the reason for visit. A history of an illness, even if no longer present, is important information that may alter the type of treatment ordered.

The history Z code categories are:

Z80   Family history of primary malignant neoplasm

Z81   Family history of mental and behavioral disorders

Z82   Family history of certain disabilities and chronic diseases (leading to disablement)

Z83   Family history of other specific disorders

Z84   Family history of other conditions

Z85   Personal history of malignant neoplasm

Z86   Personal history of certain other diseases

Z87   Personal history of other diseases and conditions

Z91.4- Personal history of psychological trauma, not elsewhere classified

Z91.5   Personal history of self-harm

Z91.8- Other specified personal risk factors, not elsewhere classified
        Exception:
        Z91.83, Wandering in diseases classified elsewhere

Z92   Personal history of medical treatment Except: Z92.0, Personal history of contraception Except: Z92.82, Status post administration of tPA (rtPA) in a different facility within the last 24 hours prior to admission to a current facility

5) Screening

Screening is the testing for disease or disease precursors in seemingly well individuals so that early detection and treatment can be provided for those who test positive for the disease (e.g., screening mammogram).

The testing of a person to rule out or confirm a suspected diagnosis because the patient has some sign or symptom is a diagnostic examination, not a screening. In these cases, the sign or symptom is used to explain the reason for the test.

A screening code may be a first-listed code if the reason for the visit is specifically the screening exam. It may also be used as an additional code if the screening is done during an office visit for other health problems. A screening code is not necessary if the screening is inherent to a routine examination, such as a pap smear done during a routine pelvic examination.

Should a condition be discovered during the screening then the code for the condition may be assigned as an additional diagnosis.

The Z code indicates that a screening exam is planned. A procedure code is required to confirm that the screening was performed.

The screening Z codes/categories:

Z11 Encounter for screening for infectious and parasitic diseases

Z12 Encounter for screening for malignant neoplasms

Z13 Encounter for screening for other diseases and disorders Except: Z13.9, Encounter for screening, unspecified

Z36 Encounter for antenatal screening for mother

6) Observation

There are two observation Z code categories. They are for use in very limited circumstances when a person is being observed for a suspected condition that is ruled out. The observation codes are not for use if an injury or illness or any signs or symptoms related to the suspected condition are present. In such cases the diagnosis/symptom code is used with the corresponding external cause code.

The observation codes are to be used as principal diagnosis only. Additional codes may be used in addition to the observation code but only if they are unrelated to the suspected condition being observed.

Codes from subcategory Z03.7 Encounter for suspected maternal and fetal conditions ruled out, may either be used as a first-listed or as an additional code assignment depending on the case. They are for use in very limited circumstances on a maternal record when an encounter is for a suspected maternal or fetal condition that is ruled out during that encounter (for example, a maternal or fetal condition may be suspected due to an abnormal test result). These codes should not be used when the condition is confirmed. In those cases, the confirmed condition should be coded. In addition, these codes are not for use if an illness or any signs or symptoms related to the suspected condition or problem are present. In such cases the diagnosis/symptom code is used.

Additional codes may be used in addition to the code from subcategory Z03.7, but only if they are unrelated to the suspected condition being evaluated.

Codes from subcategory Z03.7 may not be used for encounters for antenatal screening of mother. *See Section I.C.21. Screening.*

For encounters for suspected fetal condition that are inconclusive following testing and evaluation, assign the appropriate code from category O35, O36, O40 or O41.

The observation Z code categories:

Z03 Encounter for medical observation for suspected diseases and conditions ruled out

Z04 Encounter for examination and observation for other reasons Except: Z04.9, Encounter for examination and observation for unspecified reason

7) Aftercare

Aftercare visit codes cover situations when the initial treatment of a disease has been performed and the patient requires continued care during the healing or recovery phase, or for the long-term consequences of the disease. The aftercare Z code should not be used if treatment is directed at a current, acute disease. The diagnosis code is to be used in these cases.

Exceptions to this rule are codes Z51.0, Encounter for antineoplastic radiation therapy, and codes from subcategory Z51.1, Encounter for antineoplastic chemotherapy and immunotherapy. These codes are to be first-listed, followed by the diagnosis code when a patient's encounter is solely to receive radiation therapy, chemotherapy, or immunotherapy for the treatment of a neoplasm. If the reason for the encounter is more than one type of antineoplastic therapy, code Z51.0 and a code from subcategory Z51.1 may be assigned together, in which case one of these codes would be reported as a secondary diagnosis.

The aftercare Z codes should also not be used for aftercare for injuries. For aftercare of an injury, assign the acute injury code with the appropriate 7th character (for subsequent encounter).

The aftercare codes are generally first-listed to explain the specific reason for the encounter. An aftercare code may be used as an additional code when some type of aftercare is provided in addition to the reason for admission and no diagnosis code is applicable. An example of this would be the closure of a colostomy during an encounter for treatment of another condition.

Aftercare codes should be used in conjunction with other aftercare codes or diagnosis codes to provide better detail on the specifics of an aftercare encounter visit, unless otherwise directed by the classification. Should a patient receive multiple types of antineoplastic therapy during the same encounter, code Z51.0, Encounter for antineoplastic radiation therapy, and codes from subcategory Z51.1, Encounter for antineoplastic chemotherapy and immunotherapy, may be used together on a record. The sequencing of multiple aftercare codes depends on the circumstances of the encounter.

Certain aftercare Z code categories need a secondary diagnosis code to describe the resolving condition or sequelae. For others, the condition is included in the code title.

Additional Z code aftercare category terms include fitting and adjustment, and attention to artificial openings.

Status Z codes may be used with aftercare Z codes to indicate the nature of the aftercare. For

GUIDELINES (ICD-10-CM)

example code Z95.1, Presence of aortocoronary bypass graft, may be used with code Z48.812, Encounter for surgical aftercare following surgery on the circulatory system, to indicate the surgery for which the aftercare is being performed. A status code should not be used when the aftercare code indicates the type of status, such as using Z43.0, Encounter for attention to tracheostomy, with Z93.0, Tracheostomy status.

The aftercare Z category/codes:

Z42　Encounter for plastic and reconstructive surgery following medical procedure or healed injury

Z43　Encounter for attention to artificial openings

Z44　Encounter for fitting and adjustment of external prosthetic device

Z45　Encounter for adjustment and management of implanted device

Z46　Encounter for fitting and adjustment of other devices

Z47　Orthopedic aftercare

Z48　Encounter for other postprocedural aftercare

Z49　Encounter for care involving renal dialysis

Z51　Encounter for other aftercare

8) Follow-up

The follow-up codes are used to explain continuing surveillance following completed treatment of a disease, condition, or injury. They imply that the condition has been fully treated and no longer exists. They should not be confused with aftercare codes, or injury codes with a 7th character for subsequent encounter, that explain ongoing care of a healing condition or its sequelae. Follow-up codes may be used in conjunction with history codes to provide the full picture of the healed condition and its treatment. The follow-up code is sequenced first, followed by the history code.

A follow-up code may be used to explain multiple visits. Should a condition be found to have recurred on the follow-up visit, then the diagnosis code for the condition should be assigned in place of the follow-up code.

The follow-up Z code categories:

Z08　Encounter for follow-up examination after completed treatment for malignant neoplasm

Z09　Encounter for follow-up examination after completed treatment for conditions other than malignant neoplasm

Z39　Encounter for maternal postpartum care and examination

9) Donor

Codes in category Z52, Donors of organs and tissues, are used for living individuals who are donating blood or other body tissue. These codes are only for individuals donating for others, not for self-donations. They are not used to identify cadaveric donations.

10) Counseling

Counseling Z codes are used when a patient or family member receives assistance in the aftermath of an illness or injury, or when support is required in coping with family or social problems. They are not used in conjunction with a diagnosis code when the counseling component of care is considered integral to standard treatment.

The counseling Z codes/categories:

Z30.0-　Encounter for general counseling and advice on contraception

Z31.5　Encounter for genetic counseling

Z31.6-　Encounter for general counseling and advice on procreation

Z32.2　Encounter for childbirth instruction

Z32.3　Encounter for childcare instruction

Z69　Encounter for mental health services for victim and perpetrator of abuse

Z70　Counseling related to sexual attitude, behavior and orientation

Z71　Persons encountering health services for other counseling and medical advice, not elsewhere classified

Z76.81　Expectant mother prebirth pediatrician visit

11) Encounters for Obstetrical and Reproductive Services

See Section I.C.15. Pregnancy, Childbirth, and the Puerperium, for further instruction on the use of these codes.

Z codes for pregnancy are for use in those circumstances when none of the problems or complications included in the codes from the Obstetrics chapter exist (a routine prenatal visit or postpartum care). Codes in category Z34, Encounter for supervision of normal pregnancy, are always first listed and are not to be used with any other code from the OB chapter.

Codes in category Z3A, Weeks of gestation, may be assigned to provide additional information about the pregnancy.

The date of the admission should be used to determine weeks of gestation for inpatient admissions that encompass more than one gestational week.

The outcome of delivery, category Z37, should be included on all maternal delivery records. It is always a secondary code. Codes in category Z37 should not be used on the newborn record.

Z codes for family planning (contraceptive) or procreative management and counseling should be included on an obstetric record either during the pregnancy or the postpartum stage, if applicable.

Z codes/categories for obstetrical and reproductive services:

Z30　Encounter for contraceptive management

Z31　Encounter for procreative management

Z32.2　Encounter for childbirth instruction

Z32.3　Encounter for childcare instruction

Z33　Pregnant state

Z34　Encounter for supervision of normal pregnancy

Z36   Encounter for antenatal screening of
        mother
Z3A   Weeks of gestation
Z37   Outcome of delivery
Z39   Encounter for maternal postpartum care
        and examination
Z76.81 Expectant mother prebirth pediatrician
        visit

12) Newborns and Infants

*See Section I.C.16. Newborn (Perinatal) Guidelines, for
further instruction on the use of these codes.*

Newborn Z codes/categories:

Z76.1   Encounter for health supervision and
        care of foundling
Z00.1- Encounter for routine child health
        examination
Z38   Liveborn infants according to place of
        birth and type of delivery

13) Routine and administrative examinations

The Z codes allow for the description of encounters
for routine examinations, such as, a general
check-up, or, examinations for administrative
purposes, such as, a pre-employment physical. The
codes are not to be used if the examination is for
diagnosis of a suspected condition or for treatment
purposes. In such cases the diagnosis code is
used. During a routine exam, should a diagnosis
or condition be discovered, it should be coded
as an additional code. Pre-existing and chronic
conditions and history codes may also be included
as additional codes as long as the examination is
for administrative purposes and not focused on
any particular condition.

Some of the codes for routine health
examinations distinguish between "with" and
"without" abnormal findings. Code assignment
depends on the information that is known at the
time the encounter is being coded. For example, if
no abnormal findings were found during the
examination, but the encounter is being coded
before test results are back, it is acceptable to assign
the code for "without abnormal findings." When
assigning a code for "with abnormal findings,"
additional code(s) should be assigned to identify
the specific abnormal finding(s).

Pre-operative examination and pre-procedural
laboratory examination Z codes are for use only in
those situations when a patient is being cleared for
a procedure or surgery and no treatment is given.

The Z codes/categories for routine and
administrative examinations:

Z00   Encounter for general examination
        without complaint, suspected or
        reported diagnosis
Z01   Encounter for other special examination
        without complaint, suspected or
        reported diagnosis
Z02   Encounter for administrative
        examination
        Except: Z02.9, Encounter for
        administrative examinations, unspecified
Z32.0- Encounter for pregnancy test

14) Miscellaneous Z codes

The miscellaneous Z codes capture a number of
other health care encounters that do not fall into
one of the other categories. Certain of these codes
identify the reason for the encounter; others are
for use as additional codes that provide useful
information on circumstances that may affect a
patient's care and treatment.

Prophylactic Organ Removal

For encounters specifically for prophylactic removal
of an organ (such as prophylactic removal of breasts
due to a genetic susceptibility to cancer or a family
history of cancer), the principal or first-listed code
should be a code from category Z40, Encounter for
prophylactic surgery, followed by the appropriate
codes to identify the associated risk factor (such as
genetic susceptibility or family history).

If the patient has a malignancy of one site and is
having prophylactic removal at another site to
prevent either a new primary malignancy or
metastatic disease, a code for the malignancy
should also be assigned in addition to a code from
subcategory Z40.0, Encounter for prophylactic
surgery for risk factors related to malignant
neoplasms. A Z40.0 code should not be assigned if
the patient is having organ removal for treatment
of a malignancy, such as the removal of the testes
for the treatment of prostate cancer.

Miscellaneous Z codes/categories:

Z28   Immunization not carried out
        Except: Z28.3, Underimmunization
        status
Z40   Encounter for prophylactic surgery
Z41   Encounter for procedures for purposes
        other than remedying health state
        Except: Z41.9, Encounter for procedure
        for purposes other than remedying
        health state, unspecified
Z53   Persons encountering health services for
        specific procedures and treatment, not
        carried out
Z55   Problems related to education and
        literacy
Z56   Problems related to employment and
        unemployment
Z57   Occupational exposure to risk factors
Z58   Problems related to physical
        environment
Z59   Problems related to housing and
        economic circumstances
Z60   Problems related to social environment
Z62   Problems related to upbringing
Z63   Other problems related to primary
        support group, including family
        circumstances
Z64   Problems related to certain psychosocial
        circumstances
Z65   Problems related to other psychosocial
        circumstances
Z72   Problems related to lifestyle
Z73   Problems related to life management
        difficulty

Z74 Problems related to care provider dependency Except: Z74.01, Bed confinement status

Z75 Problems related to medical facilities and other health care

Z76.0 Encounter for issue of repeat prescription

Z76.3 Healthy person accompanying sick person

Z76.4 Other boarder to healthcare facility

Z76.5 Malingerer [conscious simulation]

Z91.1- Patient's noncompliance with medical treatment and regimen

Z91.83 Wandering in diseases classified elsewhere

Z91.89 Other specified personal risk factors, not elsewhere classified

15) Nonspecific Z codes

Certain Z codes are so non-specific, or potentially redundant with other codes in the classification, that there can be little justification for their use in the inpatient setting. Their use in the outpatient setting should be limited to those instances when there is no further documentation to permit more precise coding. Otherwise, any sign or symptom or any other reason for visit that is captured in another code should be used.

Nonspecific Z codes/categories:

Z02.9 Encounter for administrative examinations, unspecified

Z04.9 Encounter for examination and observation for unspecified reason

Z13.9 Encounter for screening, unspecified

Z41.9 Encounter for procedure for purposes other than remedying health state, unspecified

Z52.9 Donor of unspecified organ or tissue

Z86.59 Personal history of other mental and behavioral disorders

Z88.9 Allergy status to unspecified drugs, medicaments and biological substances status

Z92.0 Personal history of contraception

16) Z Codes That May Only be Principal/First-Listed Diagnosis

The following Z codes/categories may only be reported as the principal/first-listed diagnosis, except when there are multiple encounters on the same day and the medical records for the encounters are combined:

Z00 Encounter for general examination without complaint, suspected or reported diagnosis

Z01 Encounter for other special examination without complaint, suspected or reported diagnosis

Z02 Encounter for administrative examination

Z03 Encounter for medical observation for suspected diseases and conditions ruled out

Z04 Encounter for examination and observation for other reasons

Z33.2 Encounter for elective termination of pregnancy

Z31.81 Encounter for male factor infertility in female patient

Z31.82 Encounter for Rh incompatibility status

Z31.83 Encounter for assisted reproductive fertility procedure cycle

Z31.84 Encounter for fertility preservation procedure

Z34 Encounter for supervision of normal pregnancy

Z39 Encounter for maternal postpartum care and examination

Z38 Liveborn infants according to place of birth and type of delivery

Z42 Encounter for plastic and reconstructive surgery following medical procedure or healed injury

Z51.0 Encounter for antineoplastic radiation therapy

Z51.1- Encounter for antineoplastic chemotherapy and immunotherapy

Z52 Donors of organs and tissues Except: Z52.9, Donor of unspecified organ or tissue

Z76.1 Encounter for health supervision and care of foundling

Z76.2 Encounter for health supervision and care of other healthy infant and child

Z99.12 Encounter for respirator [ventilator] dependence during power failure

Section II. Selection of Principal Diagnosis

The circumstances of inpatient admission always govern the selection of principal diagnosis. The principal diagnosis is defined in the Uniform Hospital Discharge Data Set (UHDDS) as "that condition established after study to be chiefly responsible for occasioning the admission of the patient to the hospital for care."

The UHDDS definitions are used by hospitals to report inpatient data elements in a standardized manner. These data elements and their definitions can be found in the July 31, 1985, Federal Register (Vol. 50, No, 147), pp. 31038-40.

Since that time the application of the UHDDS definitions has been expanded to include all nonoutpatient settings (acute care, short term, long term care and psychiatric hospitals; home health agencies; rehab facilities; nursing homes, etc).

In determining principal diagnosis, coding conventions in the ICD-10-CM, the Tabular List and Alphabetic Index take precedence over these official coding guidelines.

(See Section I.A., Conventions for the ICD-10-CM)

The importance of consistent, complete documentation in the medical record cannot be overemphasized. Without such documentation the application of all coding guidelines is a difficult, if not impossible, task.

A. Codes for symptoms, signs, and ill-defined conditions

Codes for symptoms, signs, and ill-defined conditions from Chapter 18 are not to be used

GUIDELINES (ICD-10-CM)

GUIDELINES (ICD-10-CM)

as principal diagnosis when a related definitive diagnosis has been established.

B. Two or more interrelated conditions, each potentially meeting the definition for principal diagnosis.

When there are two or more interrelated conditions (such as diseases in the same ICD-10-CM chapter or manifestations characteristically associated with a certain disease) potentially meeting the definition of principal diagnosis, either condition may be sequenced first, unless the circumstances of the admission, the therapy provided, the Tabular List, or the Alphabetic Index indicate otherwise.

C. Two or more diagnoses that equally meet the definition for principal diagnosis

In the unusual instance when two or more diagnoses equally meet the criteria for principal diagnosis as determined by the circumstances of admission, diagnostic workup and/or therapy provided, and the Alphabetic Index, Tabular List, or another coding guidelines does not provide sequencing direction, any one of the diagnoses may be sequenced first.

D. Two or more comparative or contrasting conditions.

In those rare instances when two or more contrasting or comparative diagnoses are documented as "either/or" (or similar terminology), they are coded as if the diagnoses were confirmed and the diagnoses are sequenced according to the circumstances of the admission. If no further determination can be made as to which diagnosis should be principal, either diagnosis may be sequenced first.

E. A symptom(s) followed by contrasting/ comparative diagnoses
GUIDELINE HAS BEEN DELETED EFFECTIVE OCTOBER 1, 2014

F. Original treatment plan not carried out

Sequence as the principal diagnosis the condition, which after study occasioned the admission to the hospital, even though treatment may not have been carried out due to unforeseen circumstances.

G. Complications of surgery and other medical care

When the admission is for treatment of a complication resulting from surgery or other medical care, the complication code is sequenced as the principal diagnosis. If the complication is classified to the T80-T88 series and the code lacks the necessary specificity in describing the complication, an additional code for the specific complication should be assigned.

H. Uncertain Diagnosis

If the diagnosis documented at the time of discharge is qualified as "probable", "suspected", "likely", "questionable", "possible", or "still to be ruled out", or other similar terms indicating uncertainty, code the condition as if it existed or was established. The bases for these guidelines are

the diagnostic workup, arrangements for further workup or observation, and initial therapeutic approach that correspond most closely with the established diagnosis.

Note: This guideline is applicable only to inpatient admissions to short-term, acute, long-term care and psychiatric hospitals.

I. Admission from Observation Unit

1. Admission Following Medical Observation

When a patient is admitted to an observation unit for a medical condition, which either worsens or does not improve, and is subsequently admitted as an inpatient of the same hospital for this same medical condition, the principal diagnosis would be the medical condition which led to the hospital admission.

2. Admission Following Post-Operative Observation

When a patient is admitted to an observation unit to monitor a condition (or complication) that develops following outpatient surgery, and then is subsequently admitted as an inpatient of the same hospital, hospitals should apply the Uniform Hospital Discharge Data Set (UHDDS) definition of principal diagnosis as "that condition established after study to be chiefly responsible for occasioning the admission of the patient to the hospital for care."

J. Admission from Outpatient Surgery

When a patient receives surgery in the hospital's outpatient surgery department and is subsequently admitted for continuing inpatient care at the same hospital, the following guidelines should be followed in selecting the principal diagnosis for the inpatient admission:

- If the reason for the inpatient admission is a complication, assign the complication as the principal diagnosis.
- If no complication, or other condition, is documented as the reason for the inpatient admission, assign the reason for the outpatient surgery as the principal diagnosis.
- If the reason for the inpatient admission is another condition unrelated to the surgery, assign the unrelated condition as the principal diagnosis.

K. Admissions/Encounters for Rehabilitation

When the purpose for the admission/encounter is rehabilitation, sequence first the code for the condition for which the service is being performed. For example, for an admission/encounter for rehabilitation for right-sided dominant hemiplegia following a cerebrovascular infarction, report code I69.351, Hemiplegia and hemiparesis following cerebral infarction affecting right dominant side, as the first-listed or principal diagnosis.

If the condition for which the rehabilitation service is no longer present, report the appropriate aftercare code as the first-listed or principal diagnosis. For example, if a patient with severe degenerative osteoarthritis of the hip, underwent hip replacement and the current encounter/ admission is for rehabilitation, report code Z47.1, Aftercare following joint replacement surgery, as the first-listed or principal diagnosis.

See Section I.C.21.c.7, Factors influencing health states and contact with health services, Aftercare.

Section III. Reporting Additional Diagnoses

GENERAL RULES FOR OTHER (ADDITIONAL) DIAGNOSES

For reporting purposes the definition for "other diagnoses" is interpreted as additional conditions that affect patient care in terms of requiring:

clinical evaluation; or
therapeutic treatment; or
diagnostic procedures; or
extended length of hospital stay; or
increased nursing care and/or monitoring.

The UHDDS item #11-b defines Other Diagnoses as "all conditions that coexist at the time of admission, that develop subsequently, or that affect the treatment received and/or the length of stay. Diagnoses that relate to an earlier episode which have no bearing on the current hospital stay are to be excluded." UHDDS definitions apply to inpatients in acute care, short-term, long term care and psychiatric hospital setting. The UHDDS definitions are used by acute care short-term hospitals to report inpatient data elements in a standardized manner. These data elements and their definitions can be found in the July 31, 1985, Federal Register (Vol. 50, No, 147), pp. 31038-40.

Since that time the application of the UHDDS definitions has been expanded to include all nonoutpatient settings (acute care, short term, long term care and psychiatric hospitals; home health agencies; rehab facilities; nursing homes, etc). The following guidelines are to be applied in designating "other diagnoses" when neither the Alphabetic Index nor the Tabular List in ICD-10-CM provide direction. The listing of the diagnoses in the patient record is the responsibility of the attending provider.

A. Previous conditions

If the provider has included a diagnosis in the final diagnostic statement, such as the discharge summary or the face sheet, it should ordinarily be coded. Some providers include in the diagnostic statement resolved conditions or diagnoses and status-post procedures from previous admission that have no bearing on the current stay. Such conditions are not to be reported and are coded only if required by hospital policy.

However, history codes (categories Z80-Z87) may be used as secondary codes if the historical condition or family history has an impact on current care or influences treatment.

B. Abnormal findings

Abnormal findings (laboratory, x-ray, pathologic, and other diagnostic results) are not coded and reported unless the provider indicates their clinical significance. If the findings are outside the normal range and the attending provider has ordered other tests to evaluate the condition or prescribed treatment, it is appropriate to ask the provider whether the abnormal finding should be added.

Please note: This differs from the coding practices in the outpatient setting for coding encounters for diagnostic tests that have been interpreted by a provider.

C. Uncertain Diagnosis

If the diagnosis documented at the time of discharge is qualified as "probable", "suspected", "likely", "questionable", "possible", or "still to be ruled out" or other similar terms indicating uncertainty, code the condition as if it existed or was established. The bases for these guidelines are the diagnostic workup, arrangements for further workup or observation, and initial therapeutic approach that correspond most closely with the established diagnosis.

Note: This guideline is applicable only to inpatient admissions to short-term, acute, long-term care and psychiatric hospitals.

Section IV. Diagnostic Coding and Reporting Guidelines for Outpatient Services

These coding guidelines for outpatient diagnoses have been approved for use by hospitals/ providers in coding and reporting hospital-based outpatient services and provider-based office visits.

Information about the use of certain abbreviations, punctuation, symbols, and other conventions used in the ICD-10-CM Tabular List (code numbers and titles), can be found in Section IA of these guidelines, under "Conventions Used in the Tabular List." Section I.B. contains general guidelines that apply to the entire classification. Section I.C. contains chapter-specific guidelines that correspond to the chapters as they are arranged in the classification. Information about the correct sequence to use in finding a code is also described in Section I.

The terms encounter and visit are often used interchangeably in describing outpatient service contacts and, therefore, appear together in these guidelines without distinguishing one from the other.

Though the conventions and general guidelines apply to all settings, coding guidelines for outpatient and provider reporting of diagnoses will vary in a number of instances from those for inpatient diagnoses, recognizing that:

The Uniform Hospital Discharge Data Set (UHDDS) definition of principal diagnosis applies only to inpatients in acute, short-term, long-term care and psychiatric hospitals.

Coding guidelines for inconclusive diagnoses (probable, suspected, rule out, etc.) were developed for inpatient reporting and do not apply to outpatients.

A. Selection of first-listed condition

In the outpatient setting, the term first-listed diagnosis is used in lieu of principal diagnosis.

In determining the first-listed diagnosis the coding conventions of ICD-10-CM, as well as the general and disease specific guidelines take precedence over the outpatient guidelines.

Diagnoses often are not established at the time of the initial encounter/visit. It may take two or more visits before the diagnosis is confirmed.

The most critical rule involves beginning the search for the correct code assignment through the Alphabetic Index. Never begin searching initially in the Tabular List as this will lead to coding errors.

1. Outpatient Surgery

When a patient presents for outpatient surgery (same day surgery), code the reason for the surgery as the first-listed diagnosis (reason for the encounter), even if the surgery is not performed due to a contraindication.

2. Observation Stay

When a patient is admitted for observation for a medical condition, assign a code for the medical condition as the first-listed diagnosis.

When a patient presents for outpatient surgery and develops complications requiring admission to observation, code the reason for the surgery as the first reported diagnosis (reason for the encounter), followed by codes for the complications as secondary diagnoses.

B. Codes from A00.0 through T88.9, Z00-Z99

The appropriate code(s) from A00.0 through T88.9, Z00-Z99 must be used to identify diagnoses, symptoms, conditions, problems, complaints, or other reason(s) for the encounter/visit.

C. Accurate reporting of ICD-10-CM diagnosis codes

For accurate reporting of ICD-10-CM diagnosis codes, the documentation should describe the patient's condition, using terminology which includes specific diagnoses as well as symptoms, problems, or reasons for the encounter. There are ICD-10-CM codes to describe all of these.

D. Codes that describe symptoms and signs

Codes that describe symptoms and signs, as opposed to diagnoses, are acceptable for reporting purposes when a diagnosis has not been established (confirmed) by the provider. Chapter 18 of ICD-10-CM, Symptoms, Signs, and Abnormal Clinical and Laboratory Findings Not Elsewhere Classified (codes R00-R99) contain many, but not all codes for symptoms.

E. Encounters for circumstances other than a disease or injury

ICD-10-CM provides codes to deal with encounters for circumstances other than a disease or injury. The Factors Influencing Health Status and Contact with Health Services codes (Z00-Z99) are provided to deal with occasions when circumstances other than a disease or injury are recorded as diagnosis or problems.

See Section I.C.21. Factors influencing health status and contact with health services.

F. Level of Detail in Coding

1. ICD-10-CM codes with 3, 4, 5, 6 or 7 characters

ICD-10-CM is composed of codes with 3, 4, 5, 6 or 7 characters. Codes with three characters are included in ICD-10-CM as the heading of a category of codes that may be further subdivided by the use of fourth, fifth, sixth or seventh characters to provide greater specificity.

2. Use of full number of characters required for a code

A three-character code is to be used only if it is not further subdivided. A code is invalid if it has not been coded to the full number of characters required for that code, including the 7th character, if applicable.

G. ICD-10-CM code for the diagnosis, condition, problem, or other reason for encounter/visit

List first the ICD-10-CM code for the diagnosis, condition, problem, or other reason for encounter/visit shown in the medical record to be chiefly responsible for the services provided. List additional codes that describe any coexisting conditions. In some cases the first-listed diagnosis may be a symptom when a diagnosis has not been established (confirmed) by the physician.

H. Uncertain diagnosis

Do not code diagnoses documented as "probable", "suspected," "questionable," "rule out," or "working diagnosis" or other similar terms indicating uncertainty. Rather, code the condition(s) to the highest degree of certainty for that encounter/visit, such as symptoms, signs, abnormal test results, or other reason for the visit.

Please note: This differs from the coding practices used by short-term, acute care, long-term care and psychiatric hospitals.

I. Chronic diseases

Chronic diseases treated on an ongoing basis may be coded and reported as many times as the patient receives treatment and care for the condition(s)

J. Code all documented conditions that coexist

Code all documented conditions that coexist at the time of the encounter/visit, and require or affect patient care treatment or management. Do not code conditions that were previously treated and no longer exist. However, history codes (categories Z80-Z87) may be used as secondary codes if the historical condition or family history has an impact on current care or influences treatment.

K. Patients receiving diagnostic services only

For patients receiving diagnostic services only during an encounter/visit, sequence first the diagnosis, condition, problem, or other reason for encounter/visit shown in the medical record to be chiefly responsible for the outpatient services provided during the encounter/visit. Codes for other diagnoses (e.g., chronic conditions) may be sequenced as additional diagnoses.

For encounters for routine laboratory/radiology testing in the absence of any signs, symptoms, or associated diagnosis, assign Z01.89, Encounter for other specified special examinations. If routine testing is performed during the same encounter as a test to evaluate a sign, symptom, or diagnosis, it is appropriate to assign both the Z code and the code describing the reason for the non-routine test.

For outpatient encounters for diagnostic tests that have been interpreted by a physician, and the final report is available at the time of coding, code any confirmed or definitive diagnosis(es) documented in the interpretation. Do not code related signs and symptoms as additional diagnoses.

Please note: This differs from the coding practice in the hospital inpatient setting regarding abnormal findings on test results.

L. **Patients receiving therapeutic services only**
For patients receiving therapeutic services only during an encounter/visit, sequence first the diagnosis, condition, problem, or other reason for encounter/visit shown in the medical record to be chiefly responsible for the outpatient services provided during the encounter/visit. Codes for other diagnoses (e.g., chronic conditions) may be sequenced as additional diagnoses.

The only exception to this rule is that when the primary reason for the admission/encounter is chemotherapy or radiation therapy, the appropriate Z code for the service is listed first, and the diagnosis or problem for which the service is being performed listed second.

M. **Patients receiving preoperative evaluations only**
For patients receiving preoperative evaluations only, sequence first a code from subcategory Z01.81, Encounter for pre-procedural examinations, to describe the pre-op consultations. Assign a code for the condition to describe the reason for the surgery as an additional diagnosis. Code also any findings related to the pre-op evaluation.

N. **Ambulatory surgery**
For ambulatory surgery, code the diagnosis for which the surgery was performed. If the postoperative diagnosis is known to be different from the preoperative diagnosis at the time the diagnosis is confirmed, select the postoperative diagnosis for coding, since it is the most definitive.

O. **Routine outpatient prenatal visits**
See Section I.C.15. Routine outpatient prenatal visits.

P. **Encounters for general medical examinations with abnormal findings**
The subcategories for encounters for general medical examinations, Z00.0-, provide codes for with and without abnormal findings. Should a general medical examination result in an abnormal finding, the code for general medical examination with abnormal finding should be assigned as the first-listed diagnosis. A secondary code for the abnormal finding should also be coded.

Q. **Encounters for routine health screenings**
See Section I.C.21. Factors influencing health status and contact with health services, Screening

Appendix I
Present on Admission Reporting Guidelines

Introduction

These guidelines are to be used as a supplement to the *ICD-10-CM Official Guidelines for Coding and Reporting* to facilitate the assignment of the Present on Admission (POA) indicator for each diagnosis and external cause of injury code reported on claim forms (UB-04 and 837 Institutional).

These guidelines are not intended to replace any guidelines in the main body of the *ICD-10-CM Official Guidelines for Coding and Reporting*. The POA guidelines are not intended to provide guidance on when a condition should be coded, but rather, how to apply the POA indicator to the final set of diagnosis codes that have been assigned in accordance with Sections I, II, and III of the official coding guidelines. Subsequent to the assignment of the ICD-10-CM codes, the POA indicator should then be assigned to those conditions that have been coded.

As stated in the Introduction to the ICD-10-CM Official Guidelines for Coding and Reporting, a joint effort between the healthcare provider and the coder is essential to achieve complete and accurate documentation, code assignment, and reporting of diagnoses and procedures. The importance of consistent, complete documentation in the medical record cannot be overemphasized. Medical record documentation from any provider involved in the care and treatment of the patient may be used to support the determination of whether a condition was present on admission or not. In the context of the official coding guidelines, the term "provider" means a physician or any qualified healthcare practitioner who is legally accountable for establishing the patient's diagnosis.

These guidelines are not a substitute for the provider's clinical judgment as to the determination of whether a condition was/was not present on admission. The provider should be queried regarding issues related to the linking of signs/symptoms, timing of test results, and the timing of findings.

General Reporting Requirements

All claims involving inpatient admissions to general acute care hospitals or other facilities that are subject to a law or regulation mandating collection of present on admission information.

Present on admission is defined as present at the time the order for inpatient admission occurs—conditions that develop during an outpatient encounter, including emergency department, observation, or outpatient surgery, are considered as present on admission.

POA indicator is assigned to principal and secondary diagnoses (as defined in Section II of the Official Guidelines for Coding and Reporting) and the external cause of injury codes.

Issues related to inconsistent, missing, conflicting or unclear documentation must still be resolved by the provider.

If a condition would not be coded and reported based on UHDDS definitions and current official coding guidelines, then the POA indicator would not be reported.

Reporting Options

Y - Yes

N - No

U - Unknown

W - Clinically undetermined

Unreported/Not used - (Exempt from POA reporting)

Reporting Definitions

Y = present at the time of inpatient admission

N = not present at the time of inpatient admission

U = documentation is insufficient to determine if condition is present on admission

W = provider is unable to clinically determine whether condition was present on admission or not

Timeframe for POA Identification and Documentation

There is no required timeframe as to when a provider (per the definition of "provider" used in these guidelines) must identify or document a condition to be present on admission. In some clinical situations, it may not be possible for a provider to make a definitive diagnosis (or a condition may not be recognized or reported by the patient) for a period of time after admission. In some cases it may be several days before the provider arrives at a definitive diagnosis. This does not mean that the condition was not present on admission. Determination of whether the condition was present on admission or not will be based on the applicable POA guideline as identified in this document, or on the provider's best clinical judgment.

If at the time of code assignment the documentation is unclear as to whether a condition was present on admission or not, it is appropriate to query the provider for clarification.

Assigning the POA Indicator

Condition is on the "Exempt from Reporting" list

Leave the "present on admission" field blank if the condition is on the list of ICD-10-CM codes for which this field is not applicable. This is the only circumstance in which the field may be left blank.

POA Explicitly Documented

Assign Y for any condition the provider explicitly documents as being present on admission.

Assign N for any condition the provider explicitly documents as not present at the time of admission.

Conditions diagnosed prior to inpatient admission

Assign "Y" for conditions that were diagnosed prior to admission (example: hypertension, diabetes mellitus, asthma)

Conditions diagnosed during the admission but clearly present before admission

Assign "Y" for conditions diagnosed during the admission that were clearly present but not diagnosed until after admission occurred.

Diagnoses subsequently confirmed after admission are considered present on admission if at the time of admission they are documented as suspected, possible, rule out, differential diagnosis, or constitute an underlying cause of a symptom that is present at the time of admission.

Condition develops during outpatient encounter prior to inpatient admission

Assign Y for any condition that develops during an outpatient encounter prior to a written order for inpatient admission.

Documentation does not indicate whether condition was present on admission

Assign "U" when the medical record documentation is unclear as to whether the condition was present on admission. "U" should not be routinely assigned and used only in very limited circumstances. Coders are encouraged to query the providers when the documentation is unclear.

Documentation states that it cannot be determined whether the condition was or was not present on admission

Assign "W" when the medical record documentation indicates that it cannot be clinically determined whether or not the condition was present on admission.

Chronic condition with acute exacerbation during the admission

If a single code identifies both the chronic condition and the acute exacerbation, see POA guidelines pertaining to combination codes.

If a single code only identifies the chronic condition and not the acute exacerbation (e.g., acute exacerbation of chronic leukemia), assign "Y."

Conditions documented as possible, probable, suspected, or rule out at the time of discharge

If the final diagnosis contains a possible, probable, suspected, or rule out diagnosis, and this diagnosis was based on signs, symptoms or clinical findings suspected at the time of inpatient admission, assign "Y."

If the final diagnosis contains a possible, probable, suspected, or rule out diagnosis, and this diagnosis was based on signs, symptoms or clinical findings that were not present on admission, assign "N".

Conditions documented as impending or threatened at the time of discharge

If the final diagnosis contains an impending or threatened diagnosis, and this diagnosis is based on symptoms or clinical findings that were present on admission, assign "Y".

If the final diagnosis contains an impending or threatened diagnosis, and this diagnosis is based on symptoms or clinical findings that were not present on admission, assign "N".

Acute and Chronic Conditions

Assign "Y" for acute conditions that are present at time of admission and N for acute conditions that are not present at time of admission.

Assign "Y" for chronic conditions, even though the condition may not be diagnosed until after admission.

If a single code identifies both an acute and chronic condition, see the POA guidelines for combination codes.

Combination Codes

Assign "N" if any part of the combination code was not present on admission (e.g., COPD with acute exacerbation and the exacerbation was not present on admission; gastric ulcer that does not start bleeding until after admission; asthma patient develops status asthmaticus after admission).

Assign "Y" if all parts of the combination code were present on admission (e.g., patient with acute prostatitis admitted with hematuria).

If the final diagnosis includes comparative or contrasting diagnoses, and both were present, or suspected, at the time of admission, assign "Y".

For infection codes that include the causal organism, assign "Y" if the infection (or signs of the infection) was present on admission, even though the culture results may not be known until after admission (e.g., patient is admitted with pneumonia and the provider documents pseudomonas as the causal organism a few days later).

Same Diagnosis Code for Two or More Conditions

When the same ICD-10-CM diagnosis code applies to two or more conditions during the same encounter (e.g. two separate conditions classified to the same ICD-10-CM diagnosis code):

Assign "Y" if all conditions represented by the single ICD-10-CM code were present on admission (e.g. bilateral unspecified age-related cataracts).

Assign "N" if any of the conditions represented by the single ICD-10-CM code was not present on admission (e.g. traumatic secondary and recurrent hemorrhage and seroma is assigned to a single code T79.2, but only one of the conditions was present on admission).

Obstetrical conditions

Whether or not the patient delivers during the current hospitalization does not affect assignment of the POA indicator. The determining factor for POA assignment is whether the pregnancy complication or obstetrical condition described by the code was present at the time of admission or not.

If the pregnancy complication or obstetrical condition was present on admission (e.g., patient admitted in preterm labor), assign "Y".

If the pregnancy complication or obstetrical condition was not present on admission (e.g., 2nd degree laceration during delivery, postpartum hemorrhage that occurred during current hospitalization, fetal distress develops after admission), assign "N".

If the obstetrical code includes more than one diagnosis and any of the diagnoses identified by the code were not present on admission assign "N".

(e.g., Category O11, Pre-existing hypertension with pre-eclampsia)

Perinatal conditions

Newborns are not considered to be admitted until after birth. Therefore, any condition present at birth or that developed in utero is considered present at admission and should be assigned "Y". This includes conditions that occur during delivery (e.g., injury during delivery, meconium aspiration, exposure to streptococcus B in the vaginal canal).

Congenital conditions and anomalies

Assign "Y" for congenital conditions and anomalies except for categories Q00-Q99, Congenital anomalies, which are on the exempt list. Congenital conditions are always considered present on admission.

External cause of injury codes

Assign "Y" for any external cause code representing an external cause of morbidity that occurred prior to inpatient admission (e.g., patient fell out of bed at home, patient fell out of bed in emergency room prior to admission).

Assign "N" for any external cause code representing an external cause of morbidity that occurred during inpatient hospitalization (e.g., patient fell out of hospital bed during hospital stay, patient experienced an adverse reaction to a medication administered after inpatient admission).

GUIDELINES (ICD-10-CM)

Categories and Codes
Exempt from Diagnosis Present on Admission Requirement

Note: "Diagnosis present on admission" for these code categories are exempt because they represent circumstances regarding the healthcare encounter or factors influencing health status that do not represent a current disease or injury or are always present on admission

B90-B94, Sequelae of infectious and parasitic diseases

E64, Sequelae of malnutrition and other nutritional deficiencies

I25.2, Old myocardial infarction

I69, Sequelae of cerebrovascular disease

O09, Supervision of high risk pregnancy

O66.5, Attempted application of vacuum extractor and forceps

O80, Encounter for full-term uncomplicated delivery

O94, Sequelae of complication of pregnancy, childbirth, and the puerperium

P00, Newborn (suspected to be) affected by maternal conditions that may be unrelated to present pregnancy

Q00 - Q99, Congenital malformations, deformations and chromosomal abnormalities

S00-T88.9, Injury, poisoning and certain other consequences of external causes with 7th character representing subsequent encounter or sequela

V00-V09, Pedestrian injured in transport accident

Except V00.81-, Accident with wheelchair (powered)

V00.83-, Accident with motorized mobility scooter

V10-V19, Pedal cycle rider injured in transport accident

V20-V29, Motorcycle rider injured in transport accident

V30-V39, Occupant of three-wheeled motor vehicle injured in transport accident

V40-V49, Car occupant injured in transport accident

V50-V59, Occupant of pick-up truck or van injured in transport accident

V60-V69, Occupant of heavy transport vehicle injured in transport accident

V70-V79, Bus occupant injured in transport accident

V80-V89, Other land transport accidents

V90-V94, Water transport accidents

V95-V97, Air and space transport accidents

V98-V99, Other and unspecified transport accidents

W09, Fall on and from playground equipment

W14, Fall from tree

W15, Fall from cliff

W17.0, Fall into well

W17.1, Fall into storm drain or manhole

W18.01, Striking against sports equipment with subsequent fall

W21, Striking against or struck by sports equipment

W30, Contact with agricultural machinery

W31, Contact with other and unspecified machinery

W32-W34, Accidental handgun discharge and malfunction

W35- W40, Exposure to inanimate mechanical forces

W52, Crushed, pushed or stepped on by crowd or human stampede

W56, Contact with nonvenomous marine animal

W58, Contact with crocodile or alligator

W61, Contact with birds (domestic) (wild)

W62, Contact with nonvenomous amphibians

W89, Exposure to man-made visible and ultraviolet light

X02, Exposure to controlled fire in building or structure

X03, Exposure to controlled fire, not in building or structure

X04, Exposure to ignition of highly flammable material

X52, Prolonged stay in weightless environment

X71, Intentional self-harm by drowning and submersion

Except X71.0-, Intentional self-harm by drowning and submersion while in bath tub

X72, Intentional self-harm by handgun discharge

X73, Intentional self-harm by rifle, shotgun and larger firearm discharge

X74, Intentional self-harm by other and unspecified firearm and gun discharge

X75, Intentional self-harm by explosive material

X76, Intentional self-harm by smoke, fire and flames

X77, Intentional self-harm by steam, hot vapors and hot objects

X81, Intentional self-harm by jumping or lying in front of moving object

X82, Intentional self-harm by crashing of motor vehicle

X83, Intentional self-harm by other specified means

Y03, Assault by crashing of motor vehicle

Y07, Perpetrator of assault, maltreatment and neglect

Y08.8, Assault by strike by sports equipment

Y21, Drowning and submersion, undetermined intent

Y22, Handgun discharge, undetermined intent

Y23, Rifle, shotgun and larger firearm discharge, undetermined intent

Y24, Other and unspecified firearm discharge, undetermined intent

Y30, Falling, jumping or pushed from a high place, undetermined intent

Y32, Assault by crashing of motor vehicle, undetermined intent

Y37, Military operations

Y36, Operations of war

Y92, Place of occurrence of the external cause

Y93, Activity code

Y99, External cause status

GUIDELINES (ICD-10-CM)

Z00, Encounter for general examination without complaint, suspected or reported diagnosis

Z01, Encounter for other special examination without complaint, suspected or reported diagnosis

Z02, Encounter for administrative examination

Z03, Encounter for medical observation for suspected diseases and conditions ruled out

Z08, Encounter for follow-up examination following completed treatment for malignant neoplasm

Z09, Encounter for follow-up examination after completed treatment for conditions other than malignant neoplasm

Z11, Encounter for screening for infectious and parasitic diseases

Z11.8, Encounter for screening for other infectious and parasitic diseases

Z12, Encounter for screening for malignant neoplasms

Z13, Encounter for screening for other diseases and disorders

Z13.4, Encounter for screening for certain developmental disorders in childhood

Z13.5, Encounter for screening for eye and ear disorders

Z13.6, Encounter for screening for cardiovascular disorders

Z13.83, Encounter for screening for respiratory disorder NEC

Z13.89, Encounter for screening for other disorder

Z13.89, Encounter for screening for other disorder

Z14, Genetic carrier

Z15, Genetic susceptibility to disease

Z17, Estrogen receptor status

Z18, Retained foreign body fragments

Z22, Carrier of infectious disease

Z23, Encounter for immunization

Z28, Immunization not carried out and underimmunization status

Z28.3, Underimmunization status

Z30, Encounter for contraceptive management

Z31, Encounter for procreative management

Z34, Encounter for supervision of normal pregnancy

Z36, Encounter for antenatal screening of mother

Z37, Outcome of delivery

Z38, Liveborn infants according to place of birth and type of delivery

Z39, Encounter for maternal postpartum care and examination

Z41, Encounter for procedures for purposes other than remedying health state

Z42, Encounter for plastic and reconstructive surgery following medical procedure or healed injury

Z43, Encounter for attention to artificial openings

Z44, Encounter for fitting and adjustment of external prosthetic device

Z45, Encounter for adjustment and management of implanted device

Z46, Encounter for fitting and adjustment of other devices

Z47.8, Encounter for other orthopedic aftercare

Z49, Encounter for care involving renal dialysis

Z51, Encounter for other aftercare

Z51.5, Encounter for palliative care

Z51.8, Encounter for other specified aftercare

Z52, Donors of organs and tissues

Z59, Problems related to housing and economic circumstances

Z63, Other problems related to primary support group, including family circumstances

Z65, Problems related to other psychosocial circumstances

Z65.8, Other specified problems related to psychosocial circumstances

Z67.1 - Z67.9, Blood type

Z68, Body mass index (BMI)

Z72, Problems related to lifestyle

Z74.01, Bed confinement status

Z76, Persons encountering health services in other circumstances

Z77.110- Z77.128, Environmental pollution and hazards in the physical environment

Z78, Other specified health status

Z79, Long term (current) drug therapy

Z80, Family history of primary malignant neoplasm

Z81, Family history of mental and behavioral disorders

Z82, Family history of certain disabilities and chronic diseases (leading to disablement)

Z83, Family history of other specific disorders

Z84, Family history of other conditions

Z85, Personal history of primary malignant neoplasm

Z86, Personal history of certain other diseases

Z87, Personal history of other diseases and conditions

Z87.828, Personal history of other (healed) physical injury and trauma

Z87.891, Personal history of nicotine dependence

Z88, Allergy status to drugs, medicaments and biological substances

Z89, Acquired absence of limb

Z90.710, Acquired absence of both cervix and uterus

Z91.0, Allergy status, other than to drugs and biological substances

Z91.4, Personal history of psychological trauma, not elsewhere classified

Z91.5, Personal history of self-harm

Z91.8, Other specified risk factors, not elsewhere classified

Z92, Personal history of medical treatment

Z93, Artificial opening status

Z94, Transplanted organ and tissue status

Z95, Presence of cardiac and vascular implants and grafts

Z97, Presence of other devices

Z98, Other postprocedural states

Z99, Dependence on enabling machines and devices, not elsewhere classified

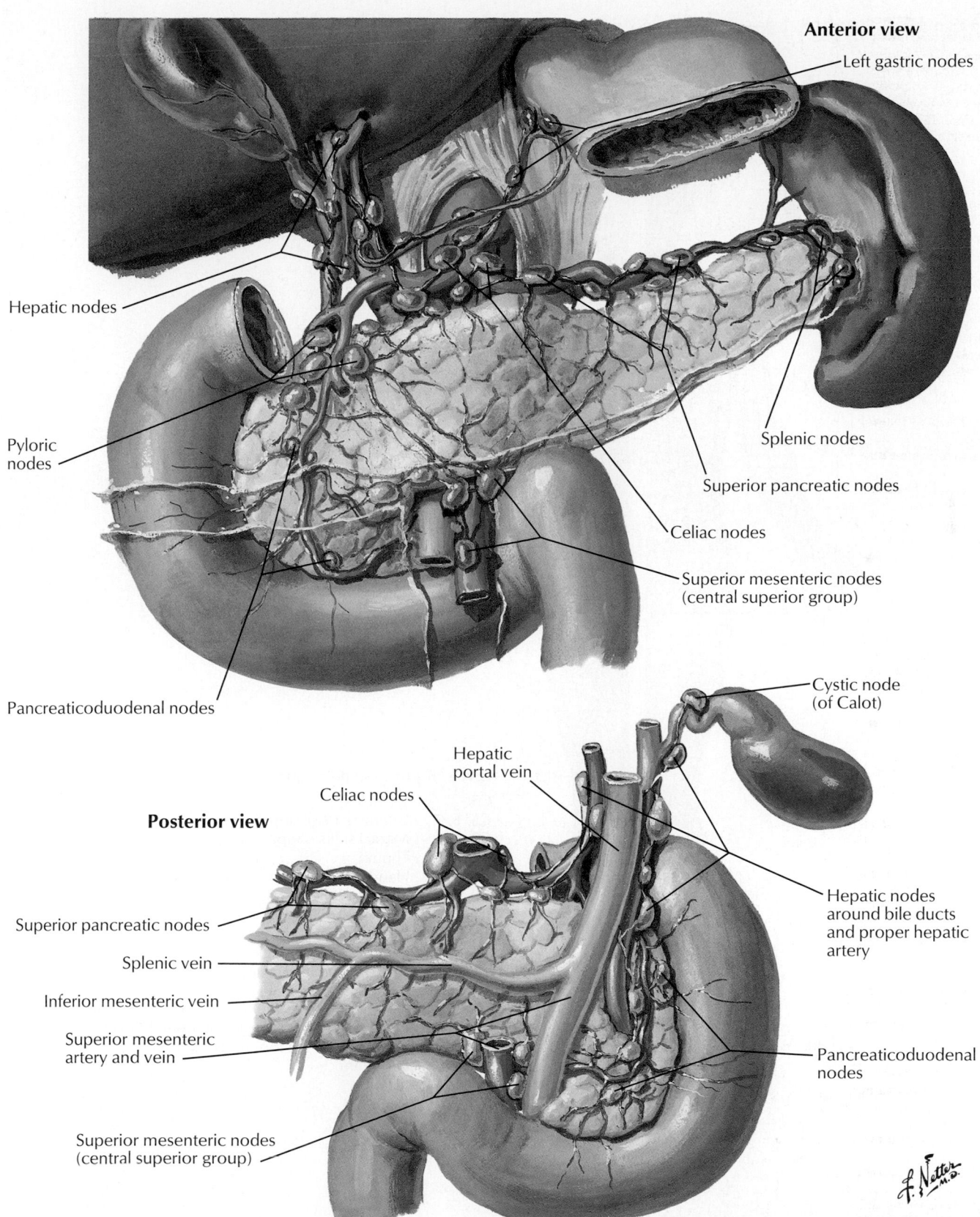

Anterior view

Left gastric nodes

Hepatic nodes

Pyloric nodes

Splenic nodes

Superior pancreatic nodes

Celiac nodes

Superior mesenteric nodes (central superior group)

Pancreaticoduodenal nodes

Cystic node (of Calot)

Hepatic portal vein

Celiac nodes

Posterior view

Superior pancreatic nodes

Splenic vein

Inferior mesenteric vein

Superior mesenteric artery and vein

Superior mesenteric nodes (central superior group)

Hepatic nodes around bile ducts and proper hepatic artery

Pancreaticoduodenal nodes

Plate 315 Lymph Vessels and Nodes of Pancreas. (Netter: Atlas of Human Anatomy, 4 ed, 2006, Saunders.)

NETTER'S ANATOMY ILLUSTRATIONS

NETTER'S ANATOMY ILLUSTRATIONS

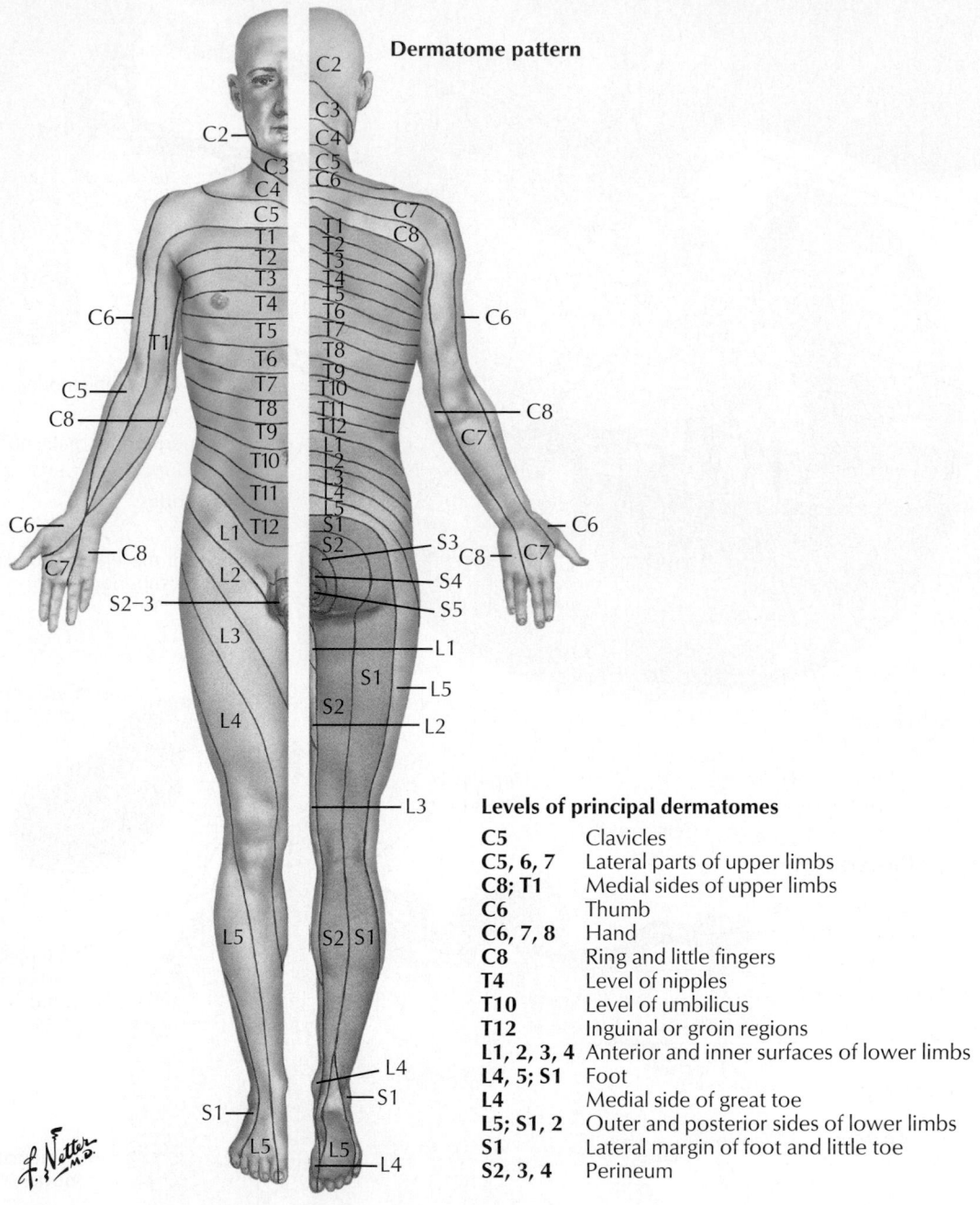

Dermatome pattern

Levels of principal dermatomes

C5	Clavicles
C5, 6, 7	Lateral parts of upper limbs
C8; T1	Medial sides of upper limbs
C6	Thumb
C6, 7, 8	Hand
C8	Ring and little fingers
T4	Level of nipples
T10	Level of umbilicus
T12	Inguinal or groin regions
L1, 2, 3, 4	Anterior and inner surfaces of lower limbs
L4, 5; S1	Foot
L4	Medial side of great toe
L5; S1, 2	Outer and posterior sides of lower limbs
S1	Lateral margin of foot and little toe
S2, 3, 4	Perineum

Plate 164 Dermatomes. (Netter: Atlas of Human Anatomy, 4 ed, 2006, Saunders.)

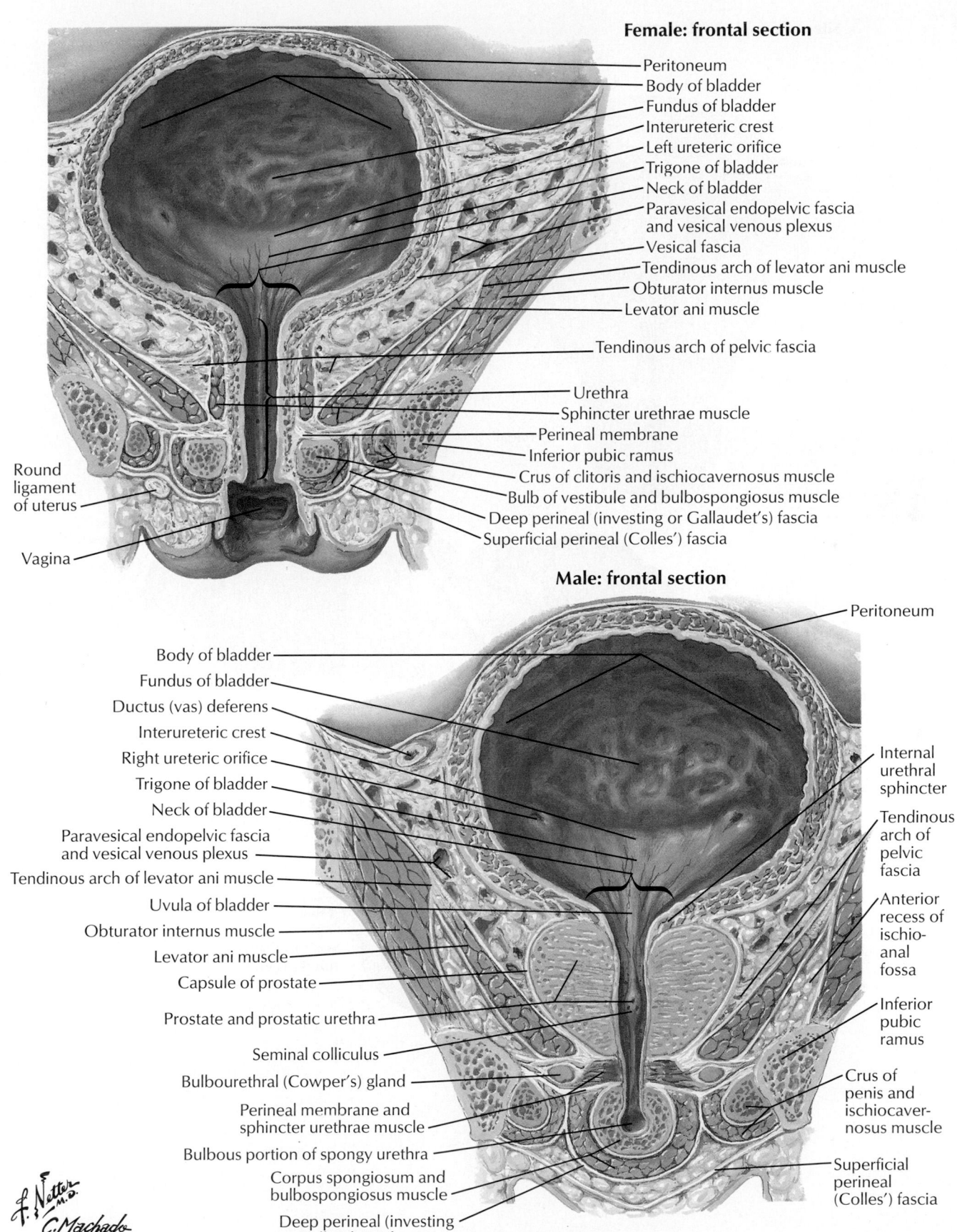

Female: frontal section

- Peritoneum
- Body of bladder
- Fundus of bladder
- Interureteric crest
- Left ureteric orifice
- Trigone of bladder
- Neck of bladder
- Paravesical endopelvic fascia and vesical venous plexus
- Vesical fascia
- Tendinous arch of levator ani muscle
- Obturator internus muscle
- Levator ani muscle
- Tendinous arch of pelvic fascia
- Urethra
- Sphincter urethrae muscle
- Perineal membrane
- Inferior pubic ramus
- Crus of clitoris and ischiocavernosus muscle
- Bulb of vestibule and bulbospongiosus muscle
- Deep perineal (investing or Gallaudet's) fascia
- Superficial perineal (Colles') fascia

Round ligament of uterus

Vagina

Male: frontal section

- Body of bladder
- Fundus of bladder
- Ductus (vas) deferens
- Interureteric crest
- Right ureteric orifice
- Trigone of bladder
- Neck of bladder
- Paravesical endopelvic fascia and vesical venous plexus
- Tendinous arch of levator ani muscle
- Uvula of bladder
- Obturator internus muscle
- Levator ani muscle
- Capsule of prostate
- Prostate and prostatic urethra
- Seminal colliculus
- Bulbourethral (Cowper's) gland
- Perineal membrane and sphincter urethrae muscle
- Bulbous portion of spongy urethra
- Corpus spongiosum and bulbospongiosus muscle
- Deep perineal (investing or Gallaudet's) fascia

- Peritoneum
- Internal urethral sphincter
- Tendinous arch of pelvic fascia
- Anterior recess of ischio-anal fossa
- Inferior pubic ramus
- Crus of penis and ischiocavernosus muscle
- Superficial perineal (Colles') fascia

Plate 366   Urinary Bladder: Female and Male. (Netter: Atlas of Human Anatomy, 4 ed, 2006, Saunders.)

NETTER'S ANATOMY ILLUSTRATIONS

Sites of ectopic implantation

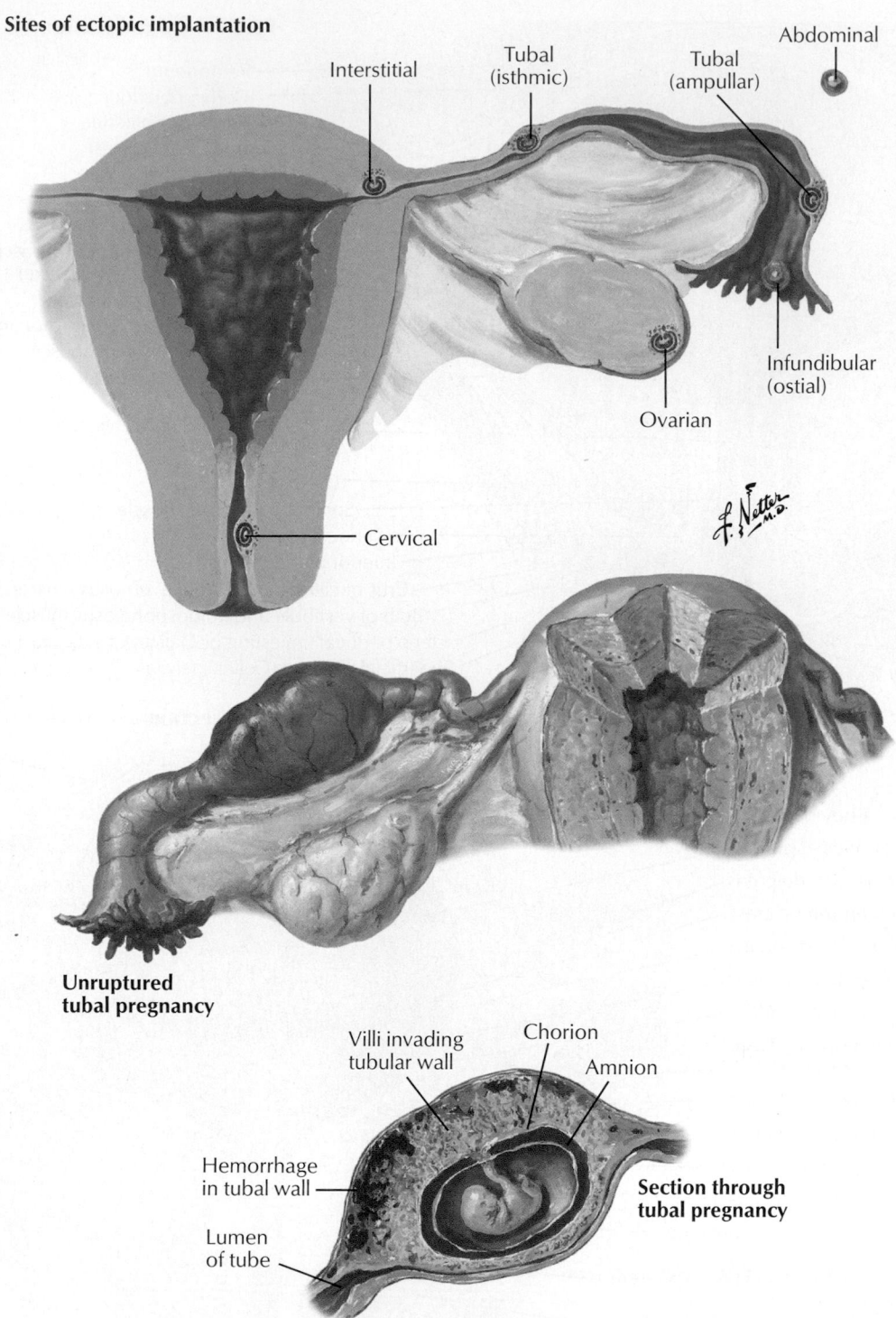

Interstitial

Tubal (isthmic)

Tubal (ampullar)

Abdominal

Infundibular (ostial)

Ovarian

Cervical

Unruptured tubal pregnancy

Villi invading tubular wall

Chorion

Amnion

Hemorrhage in tubal wall

Section through tubal pregnancy

Lumen of tube

Plate 375 Ectopic Pregnancy. (Netter: Atlas of Human Anatomy, 4 ed, 2006, Saunders.)

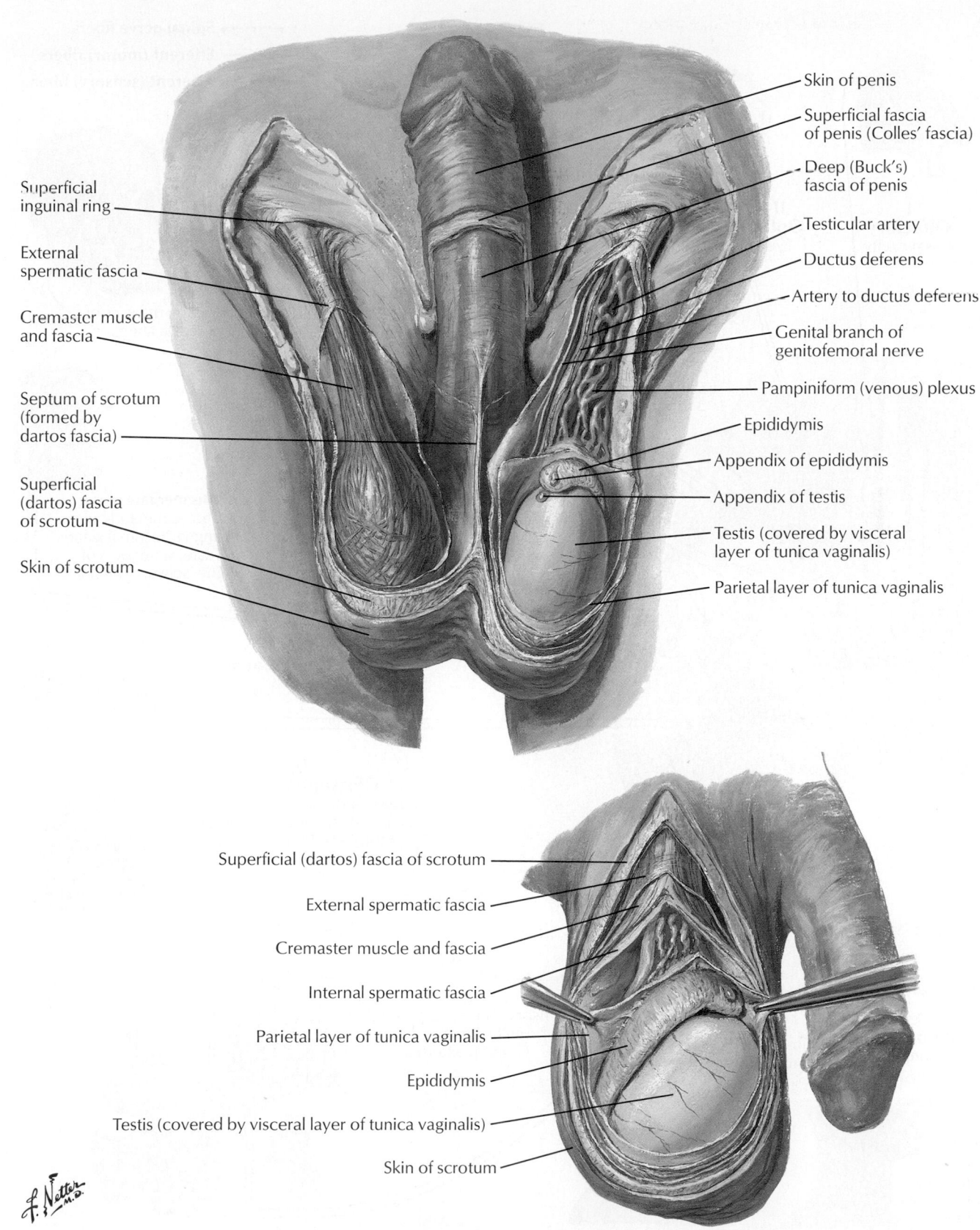

Skin of penis

Superficial fascia of penis (Colles' fascia)

Deep (Buck's) fascia of penis

Testicular artery

Ductus deferens

Artery to ductus deferens

Genital branch of genitofemoral nerve

Pampiniform (venous) plexus

Epididymis

Appendix of epididymis

Appendix of testis

Testis (covered by visceral layer of tunica vaginalis)

Parietal layer of tunica vaginalis

Superficial inguinal ring

External spermatic fascia

Cremaster muscle and fascia

Septum of scrotum (formed by dartos fascia)

Superficial (dartos) fascia of scrotum

Skin of scrotum

Superficial (dartos) fascia of scrotum

External spermatic fascia

Cremaster muscle and fascia

Internal spermatic fascia

Parietal layer of tunica vaginalis

Epididymis

Testis (covered by visceral layer of tunica vaginalis)

Skin of scrotum

Plate 387 Scrotum and Contents. (Netter: Atlas of Human Anatomy, 4 ed, 2006, Saunders.)

NETTER'S ANATOMY ILLUSTRATIONS

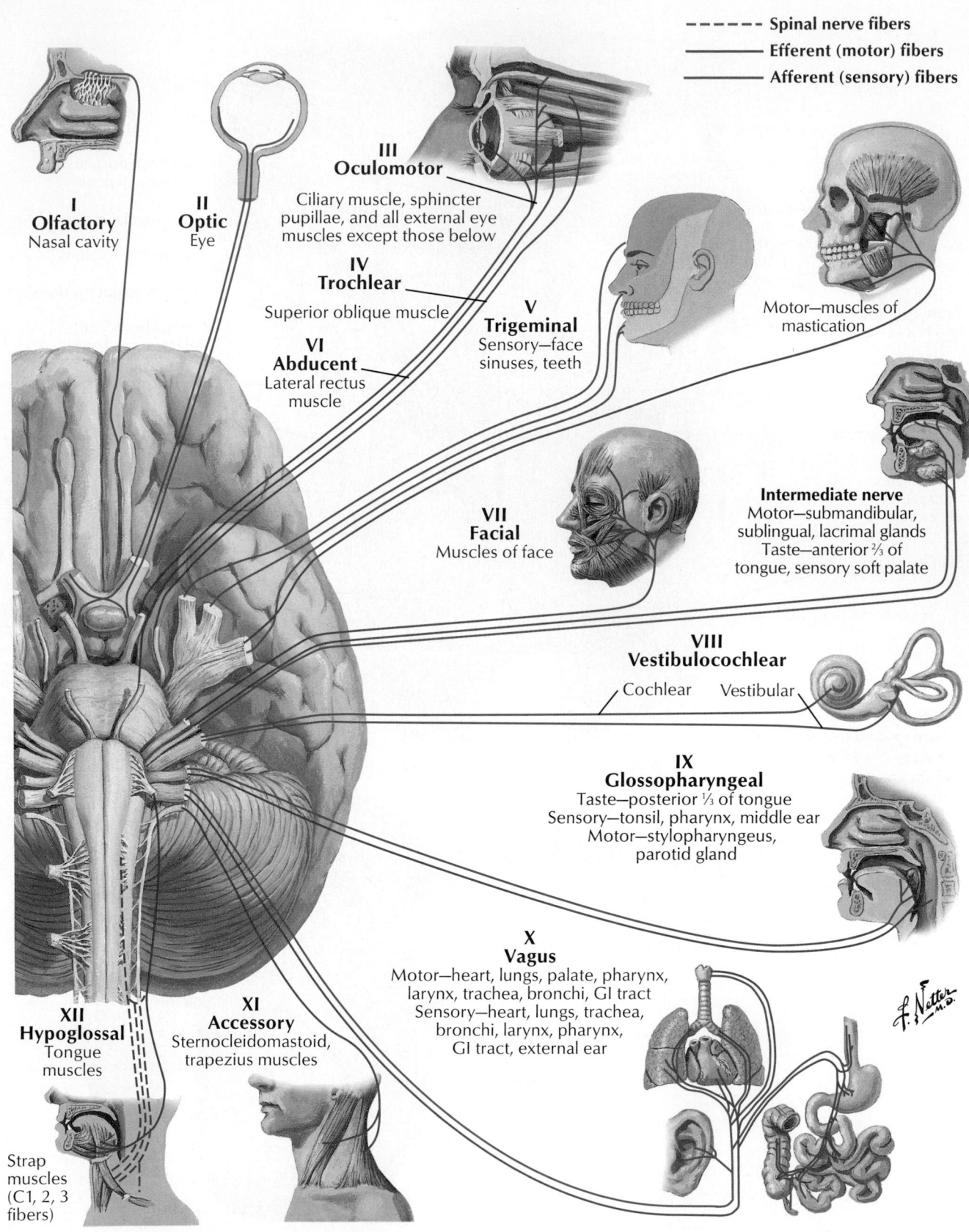

- - - - - Spinal nerve fibers
———— Efferent (motor) fibers
———— Afferent (sensory) fibers

I
Olfactory
Nasal cavity

II
Optic
Eye

III
Oculomotor
Ciliary muscle, sphincter pupillae, and all external eye muscles except those below

IV
Trochlear
Superior oblique muscle

VI
Abducent
Lateral rectus muscle

V
Trigeminal
Sensory—face sinuses, teeth

Motor—muscles of mastication

VII
Facial
Muscles of face

Intermediate nerve
Motor—submandibular, sublingual, lacrimal glands
Taste—anterior ⅔ of tongue, sensory soft palate

VIII
Vestibulocochlear

Cochlear   Vestibular

IX
Glossopharyngeal
Taste—posterior ⅓ of tongue
Sensory—tonsil, pharynx, middle ear
Motor—stylopharyngeus, parotid gland

X
Vagus
Motor—heart, lungs, palate, pharynx, larynx, trachea, bronchi, GI tract
Sensory—heart, lungs, trachea, bronchi, larynx, pharynx, GI tract, external ear

XII
Hypoglossal
Tongue muscles

XI
Accessory
Sternocleidomastoid, trapezius muscles

Strap muscles (C1, 2, 3 fibers)

Plate 118   Cranial Nerves (Motor and Sensory Distribution): Schema. (Netter: Atlas of Human Anatomy, 4 ed, 2006, Saunders.)

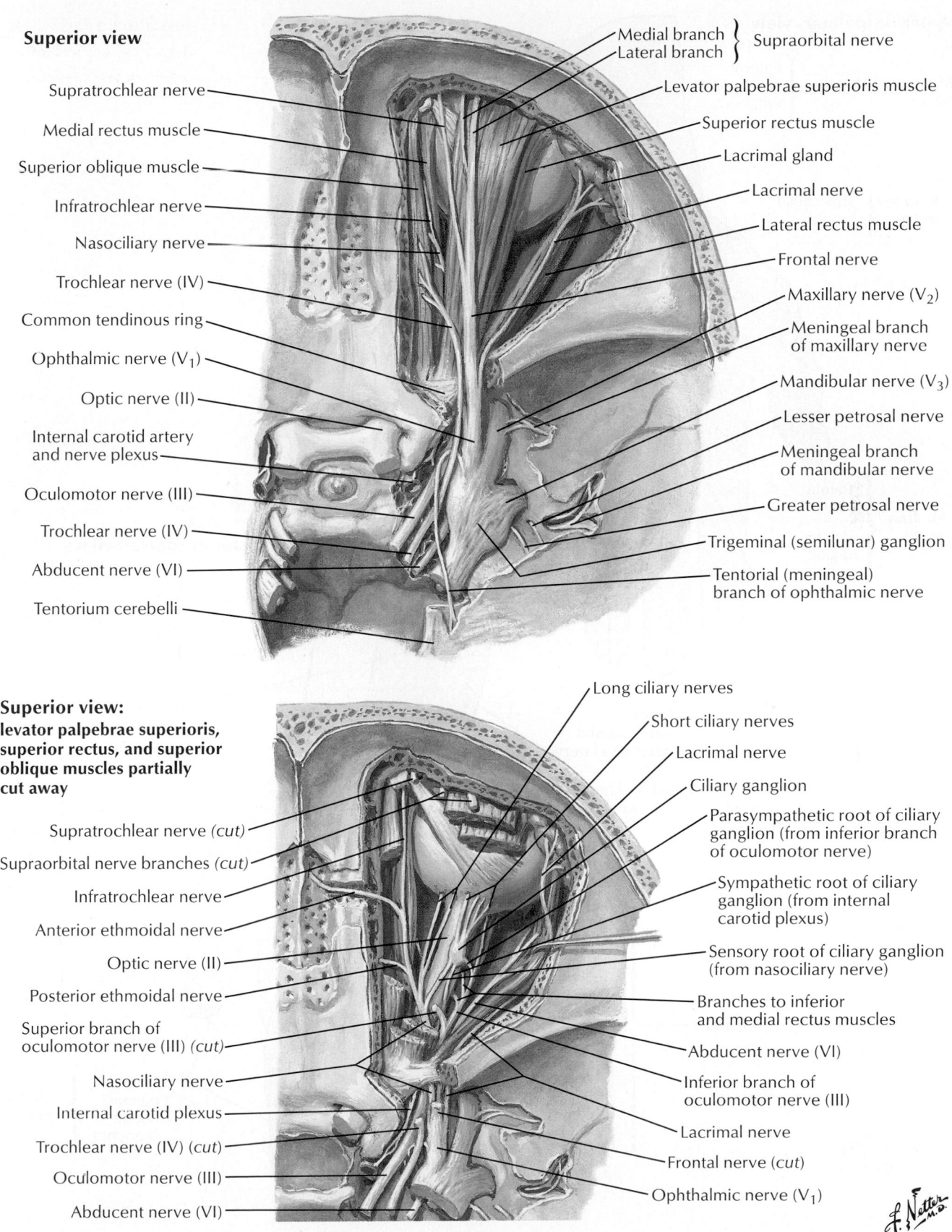

Superior view

- Supratrochlear nerve
- Medial rectus muscle
- Superior oblique muscle
- Infratrochlear nerve
- Nasociliary nerve
- Trochlear nerve (IV)
- Common tendinous ring
- Ophthalmic nerve (V₁)
- Optic nerve (II)
- Internal carotid artery and nerve plexus
- Oculomotor nerve (III)
- Trochlear nerve (IV)
- Abducent nerve (VI)
- Tentorium cerebelli

- Medial branch } Supraorbital nerve
- Lateral branch
- Levator palpebrae superioris muscle
- Superior rectus muscle
- Lacrimal gland
- Lacrimal nerve
- Lateral rectus muscle
- Frontal nerve
- Maxillary nerve (V₂)
- Meningeal branch of maxillary nerve
- Mandibular nerve (V₃)
- Lesser petrosal nerve
- Meningeal branch of mandibular nerve
- Greater petrosal nerve
- Trigeminal (semilunar) ganglion
- Tentorial (meningeal) branch of ophthalmic nerve

Superior view:
levator palpebrae superioris, superior rectus, and superior oblique muscles partially cut away

- Supratrochlear nerve (cut)
- Supraorbital nerve branches (cut)
- Infratrochlear nerve
- Anterior ethmoidal nerve
- Optic nerve (II)
- Posterior ethmoidal nerve
- Superior branch of oculomotor nerve (III) (cut)
- Nasociliary nerve
- Internal carotid plexus
- Trochlear nerve (IV) (cut)
- Oculomotor nerve (III)
- Abducent nerve (VI)

- Long ciliary nerves
- Short ciliary nerves
- Lacrimal nerve
- Ciliary ganglion
- Parasympathetic root of ciliary ganglion (from inferior branch of oculomotor nerve)
- Sympathetic root of ciliary ganglion (from internal carotid plexus)
- Sensory root of ciliary ganglion (from nasociliary nerve)
- Branches to inferior and medial rectus muscles
- Abducent nerve (VI)
- Inferior branch of oculomotor nerve (III)
- Lacrimal nerve
- Frontal nerve (cut)
- Ophthalmic nerve (V₁)

f. Netter
M.D.

Plate 86 Nerves of Orbit. (Netter: Atlas of Human Anatomy, 4 ed, 2006, Saunders.)

NETTER'S ANATOMY ILLUSTRATIONS

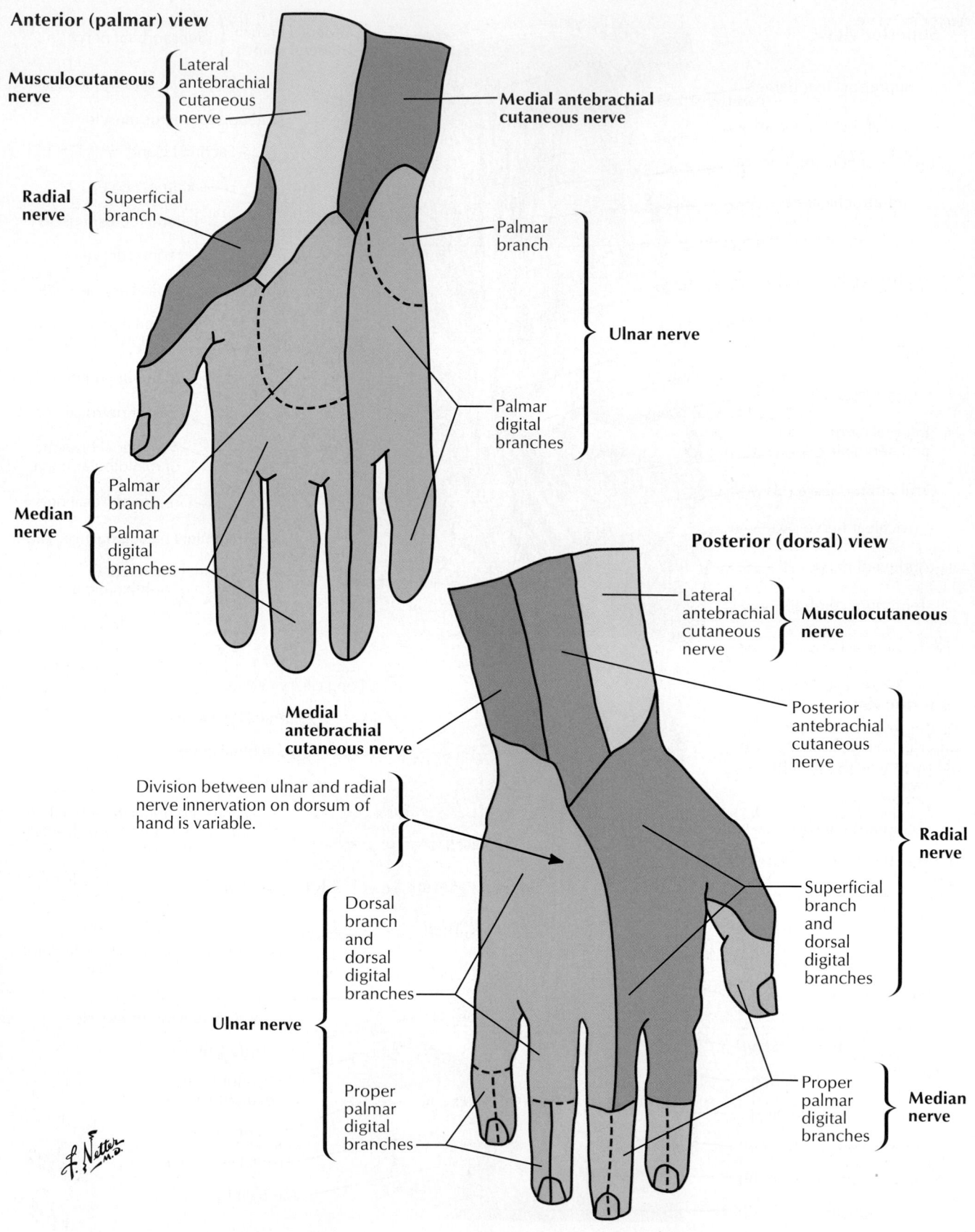

Anterior (palmar) view

Musculocutaneous nerve — Lateral antebrachial cutaneous nerve

Medial antebrachial cutaneous nerve

Radial nerve — Superficial branch

Palmar branch

Ulnar nerve

Palmar digital branches

Median nerve — Palmar branch / Palmar digital branches

Posterior (dorsal) view

Lateral antebrachial cutaneous nerve — **Musculocutaneous nerve**

Medial antebrachial cutaneous nerve

Posterior antebrachial cutaneous nerve

Division between ulnar and radial nerve innervation on dorsum of hand is variable.

Radial nerve

Superficial branch and dorsal digital branches

Ulnar nerve — Dorsal branch and dorsal digital branches

Proper palmar digital branches

Proper palmar digital branches — **Median nerve**

NETTER'S ANATOMY ILLUSTRATIONS

Plate 472 Cutaneous Innervation of Wrist and Hand. (Netter: Atlas of Human Anatomy, 4 ed, 2006, Saunders.)

Anterior view

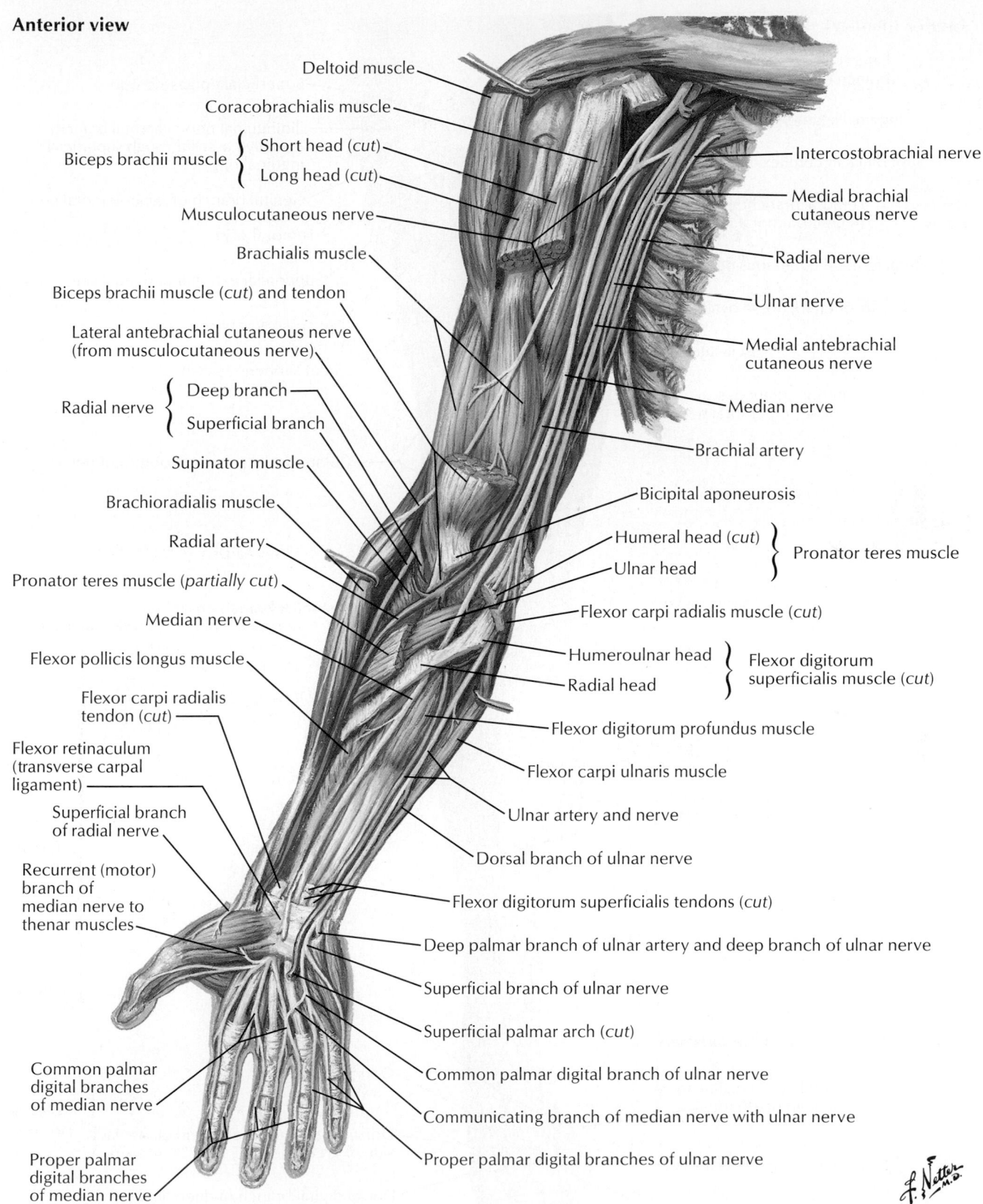

Deltoid muscle

Coracobrachialis muscle

Biceps brachii muscle {
Short head (*cut*)
Long head (*cut*)

Musculocutaneous nerve

Brachialis muscle

Biceps brachii muscle (*cut*) and tendon

Lateral antebrachial cutaneous nerve
(from musculocutaneous nerve)

Radial nerve {
Deep branch
Superficial branch

Supinator muscle

Brachioradialis muscle

Radial artery

Pronator teres muscle (*partially cut*)

Median nerve

Flexor pollicis longus muscle

Flexor carpi radialis
tendon (*cut*)

Flexor retinaculum
(transverse carpal
ligament)

Superficial branch
of radial nerve

Recurrent (motor)
branch of
median nerve to
thenar muscles

Common palmar
digital branches
of median nerve

Proper palmar
digital branches
of median nerve

Intercostobrachial nerve

Medial brachial
cutaneous nerve

Radial nerve

Ulnar nerve

Medial antebrachial
cutaneous nerve

Median nerve

Brachial artery

Bicipital aponeurosis

Humeral head (*cut*) }
Ulnar head
Pronator teres muscle

Flexor carpi radialis muscle (*cut*)

Humeroulnar head }
Radial head
Flexor digitorum
superficialis muscle (*cut*)

Flexor digitorum profundus muscle

Flexor carpi ulnaris muscle

Ulnar artery and nerve

Dorsal branch of ulnar nerve

Flexor digitorum superficialis tendons (*cut*)

Deep palmar branch of ulnar artery and deep branch of ulnar nerve

Superficial branch of ulnar nerve

Superficial palmar arch (*cut*)

Common palmar digital branch of ulnar nerve

Communicating branch of median nerve with ulnar nerve

Proper palmar digital branches of ulnar nerve

Plate 473 Arteries and Nerves of Upper Limb. (Netter: Atlas of Human Anatomy, 4 ed, 2006, Saunders.)

NETTER'S ANATOMY ILLUSTRATIONS

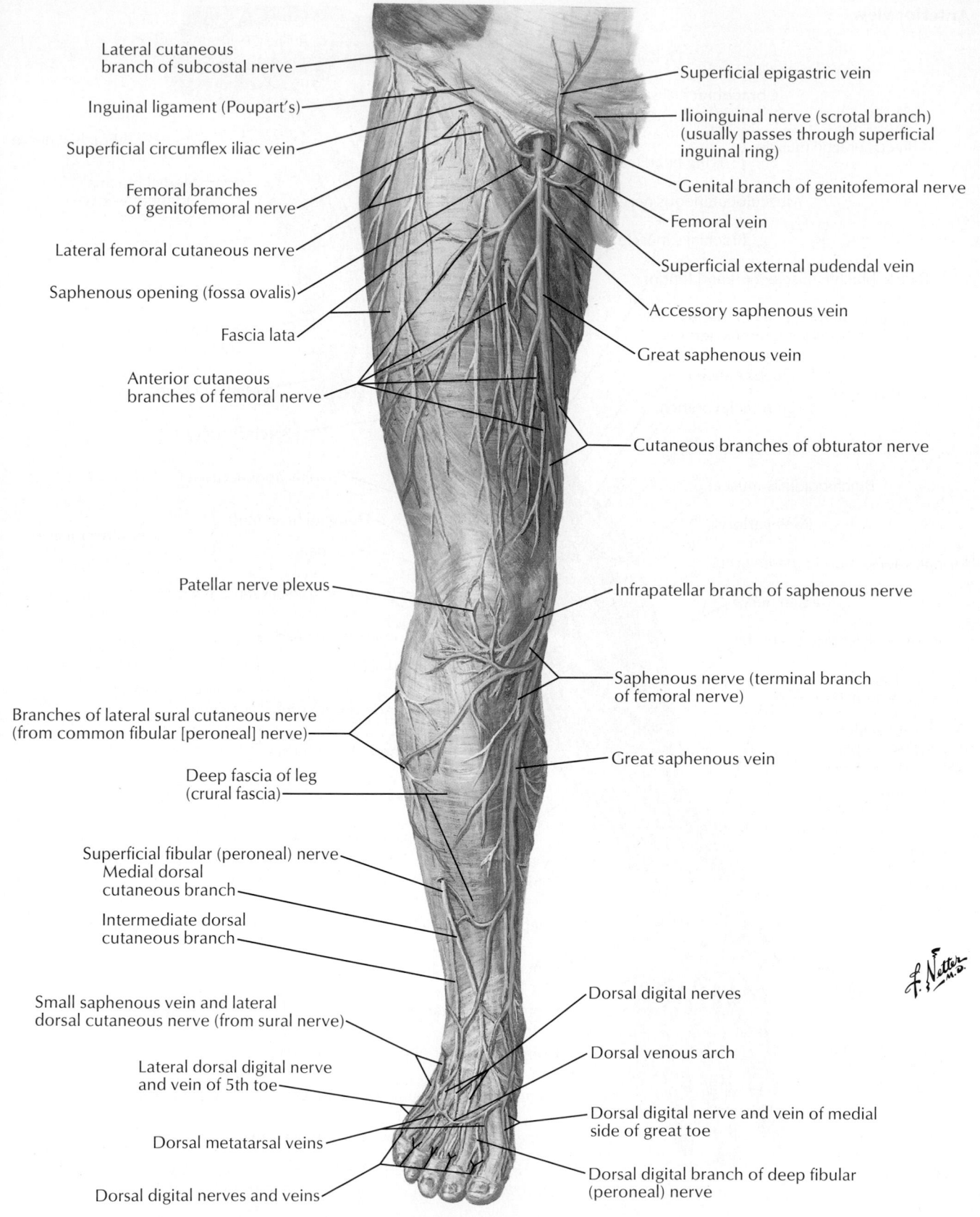

Lateral cutaneous branch of subcostal nerve

Inguinal ligament (Poupart's)

Superficial circumflex iliac vein

Femoral branches of genitofemoral nerve

Lateral femoral cutaneous nerve

Saphenous opening (fossa ovalis)

Fascia lata

Anterior cutaneous branches of femoral nerve

Patellar nerve plexus

Branches of lateral sural cutaneous nerve (from common fibular [peroneal] nerve)

Deep fascia of leg (crural fascia)

Superficial fibular (peroneal) nerve Medial dorsal cutaneous branch

Intermediate dorsal cutaneous branch

Small saphenous vein and lateral dorsal cutaneous nerve (from sural nerve)

Lateral dorsal digital nerve and vein of 5th toe

Dorsal metatarsal veins

Dorsal digital nerves and veins

Superficial epigastric vein

Ilioinguinal nerve (scrotal branch) (usually passes through superficial inguinal ring)

Genital branch of genitofemoral nerve

Femoral vein

Superficial external pudendal vein

Accessory saphenous vein

Great saphenous vein

Cutaneous branches of obturator nerve

Infrapatellar branch of saphenous nerve

Saphenous nerve (terminal branch of femoral nerve)

Great saphenous vein

Dorsal digital nerves

Dorsal venous arch

Dorsal digital nerve and vein of medial side of great toe

Dorsal digital branch of deep fibular (peroneal) nerve

Plate 544   Superficial Nerves and Veins of Lower Limb: Anterior View. (Netter: Atlas of Human Anatomy, 4 ed, 2006, Saunders.)

NETTER'S ANATOMY ILLUSTRATIONS

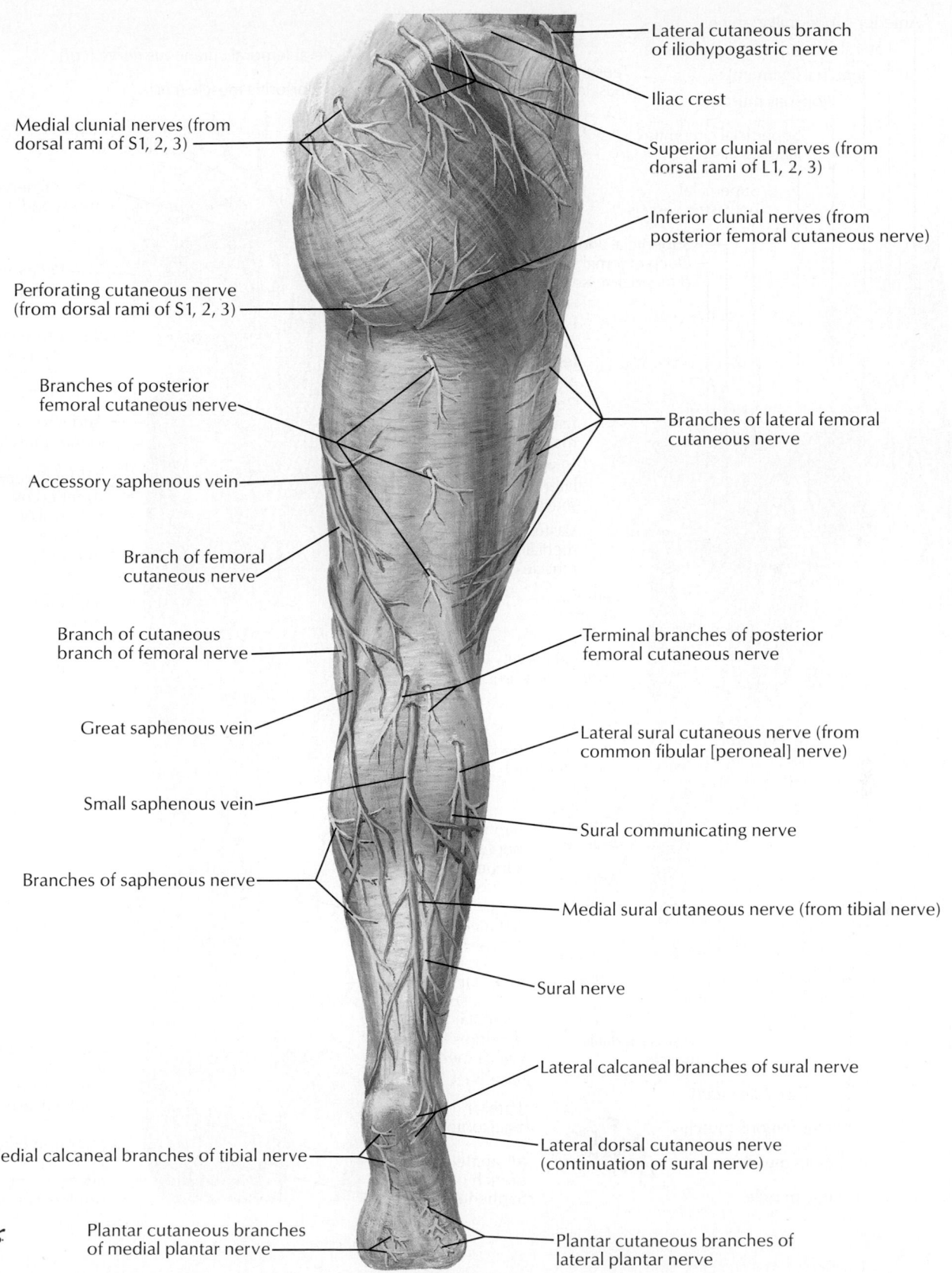

Lateral cutaneous branch of iliohypogastric nerve

Iliac crest

Superior clunial nerves (from dorsal rami of L1, 2, 3)

Inferior clunial nerves (from posterior femoral cutaneous nerve)

Medial clunial nerves (from dorsal rami of S1, 2, 3)

Perforating cutaneous nerve (from dorsal rami of S1, 2, 3)

Branches of posterior femoral cutaneous nerve

Accessory saphenous vein

Branch of femoral cutaneous nerve

Branches of lateral femoral cutaneous nerve

Branch of cutaneous branch of femoral nerve

Great saphenous vein

Terminal branches of posterior femoral cutaneous nerve

Lateral sural cutaneous nerve (from common fibular [peroneal] nerve)

Small saphenous vein

Sural communicating nerve

Branches of saphenous nerve

Medial sural cutaneous nerve (from tibial nerve)

Sural nerve

Lateral calcaneal branches of sural nerve

Medial calcaneal branches of tibial nerve

Lateral dorsal cutaneous nerve (continuation of sural nerve)

Plantar cutaneous branches of medial plantar nerve

Plantar cutaneous branches of lateral plantar nerve

Plate 545   Superficial Nerves and Veins of Lower Limb: Posterior View. (Netter: Atlas of Human Anatomy, 4 ed, 2006, Saunders.)

NETTER'S ANATOMY ILLUSTRATIONS

NETTER'S ANATOMY ILLUSTRATIONS

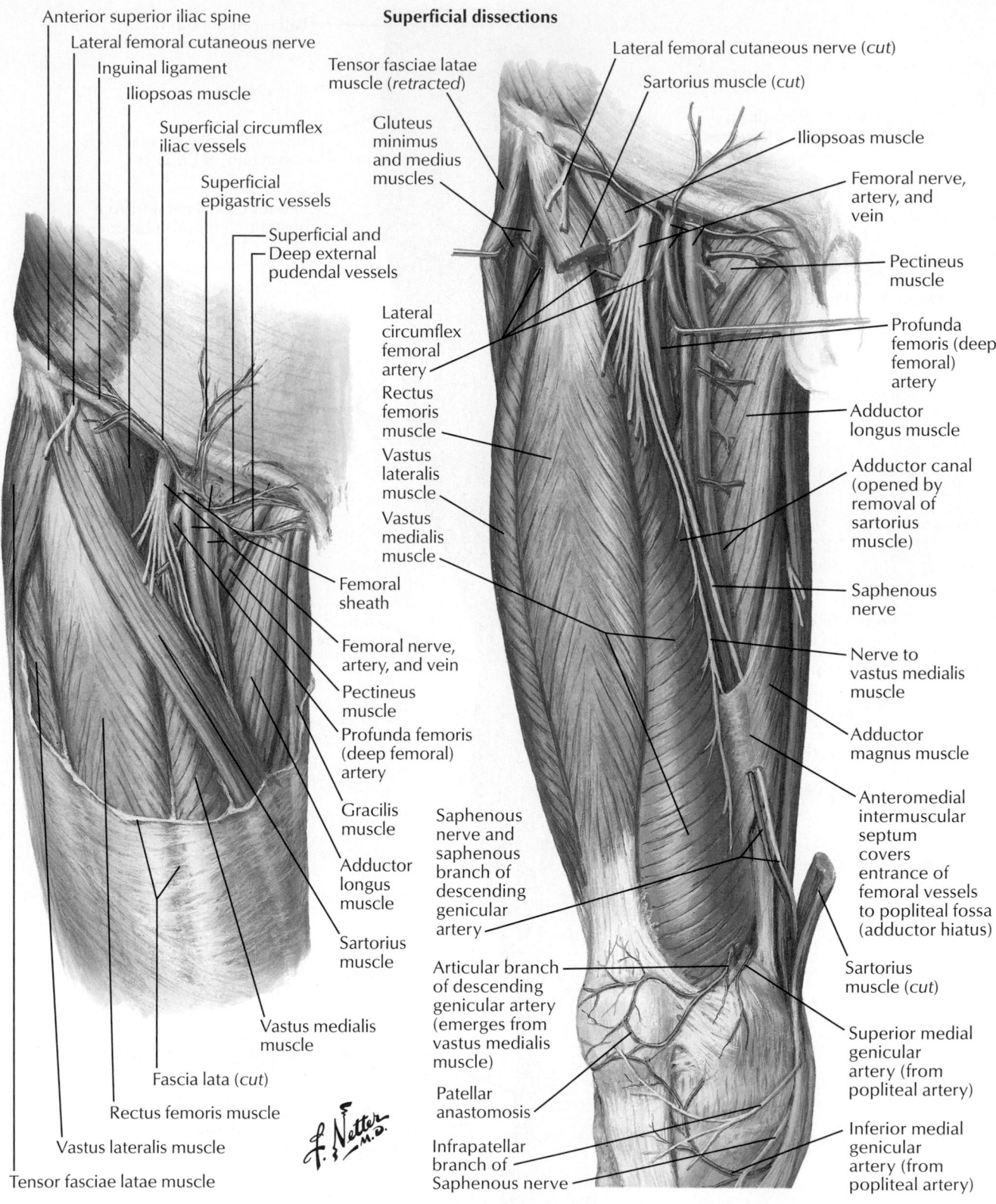

Superficial dissections

Anterior superior iliac spine
Lateral femoral cutaneous nerve
Inguinal ligament
Iliopsoas muscle
Superficial circumflex iliac vessels
Superficial epigastric vessels
Superficial and Deep external pudendal vessels

Tensor fasciae latae muscle (*retracted*)
Gluteus minimus and medius muscles
Lateral circumflex femoral artery
Rectus femoris muscle
Vastus lateralis muscle
Vastus medialis muscle
Femoral sheath
Femoral nerve, artery, and vein
Pectineus muscle
Profunda femoris (deep femoral) artery
Gracilis muscle
Adductor longus muscle
Sartorius muscle
Vastus medialis muscle
Fascia lata (*cut*)
Rectus femoris muscle
Vastus lateralis muscle
Tensor fasciae latae muscle

Lateral femoral cutaneous nerve (*cut*)
Sartorius muscle (*cut*)
Iliopsoas muscle
Femoral nerve, artery, and vein
Pectineus muscle
Profunda femoris (deep femoral) artery
Adductor longus muscle
Adductor canal (opened by removal of sartorius muscle)
Saphenous nerve
Nerve to vastus medialis muscle
Adductor magnus muscle
Anteromedial intermuscular septum covers entrance of femoral vessels to popliteal fossa (adductor hiatus)
Sartorius muscle (*cut*)
Superior medial genicular artery (from popliteal artery)
Inferior medial genicular artery (from popliteal artery)

Saphenous nerve and saphenous branch of descending genicular artery
Articular branch of descending genicular artery (emerges from vastus medialis muscle)
Patellar anastomosis
Infrapatellar branch of Saphenous nerve

F. Netter M.D.

Plate 500 Arteries and Nerves of Thigh: Anterior Views. (Netter: Atlas of Human Anatomy, 4 ed, 2006, Saunders.)

60

Deep dissection

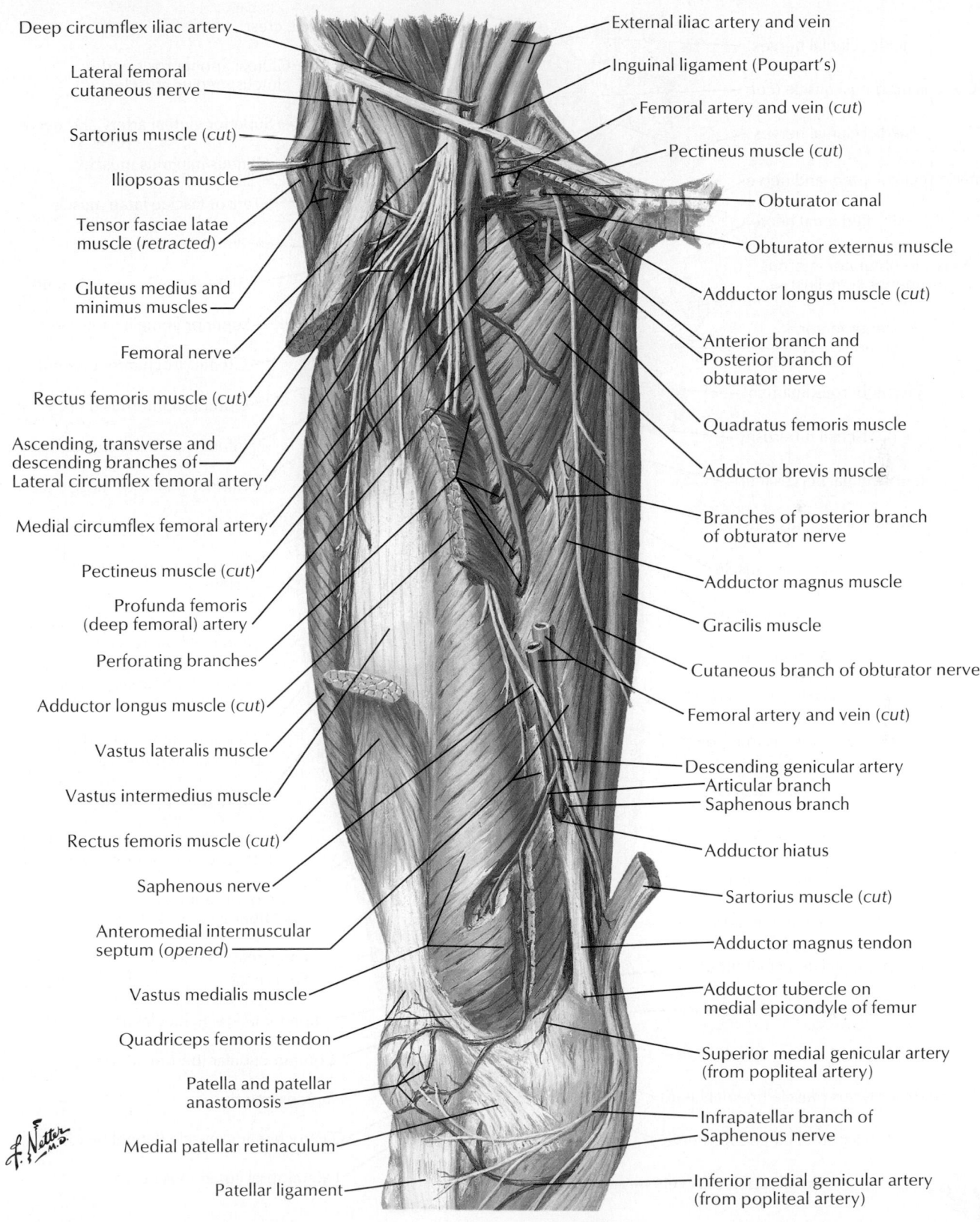

Deep circumflex iliac artery

Lateral femoral cutaneous nerve

Sartorius muscle (*cut*)

Iliopsoas muscle

Tensor fasciae latae muscle (*retracted*)

Gluteus medius and minimus muscles

Femoral nerve

Rectus femoris muscle (*cut*)

Ascending, transverse and descending branches of Lateral circumflex femoral artery

Medial circumflex femoral artery

Pectineus muscle (*cut*)

Profunda femoris (deep femoral) artery

Perforating branches

Adductor longus muscle (*cut*)

Vastus lateralis muscle

Vastus intermedius muscle

Rectus femoris muscle (*cut*)

Saphenous nerve

Anteromedial intermuscular septum (*opened*)

Vastus medialis muscle

Quadriceps femoris tendon

Patella and patellar anastomosis

Medial patellar retinaculum

Patellar ligament

External iliac artery and vein

Inguinal ligament (Poupart's)

Femoral artery and vein (*cut*)

Pectineus muscle (*cut*)

Obturator canal

Obturator externus muscle

Adductor longus muscle (*cut*)

Anterior branch and Posterior branch of obturator nerve

Quadratus femoris muscle

Adductor brevis muscle

Branches of posterior branch of obturator nerve

Adductor magnus muscle

Gracilis muscle

Cutaneous branch of obturator nerve

Femoral artery and vein (*cut*)

Descending genicular artery
Articular branch
Saphenous branch

Adductor hiatus

Sartorius muscle (*cut*)

Adductor magnus tendon

Adductor tubercle on medial epicondyle of femur

Superior medial genicular artery (from popliteal artery)

Infrapatellar branch of Saphenous nerve

Inferior medial genicular artery (from popliteal artery)

Plate 501 Arteries and Nerves of Thigh: Posterior View. (Netter: Atlas of Human Anatomy, 4 ed, 2006, Saunders.)

61

Deep dissection

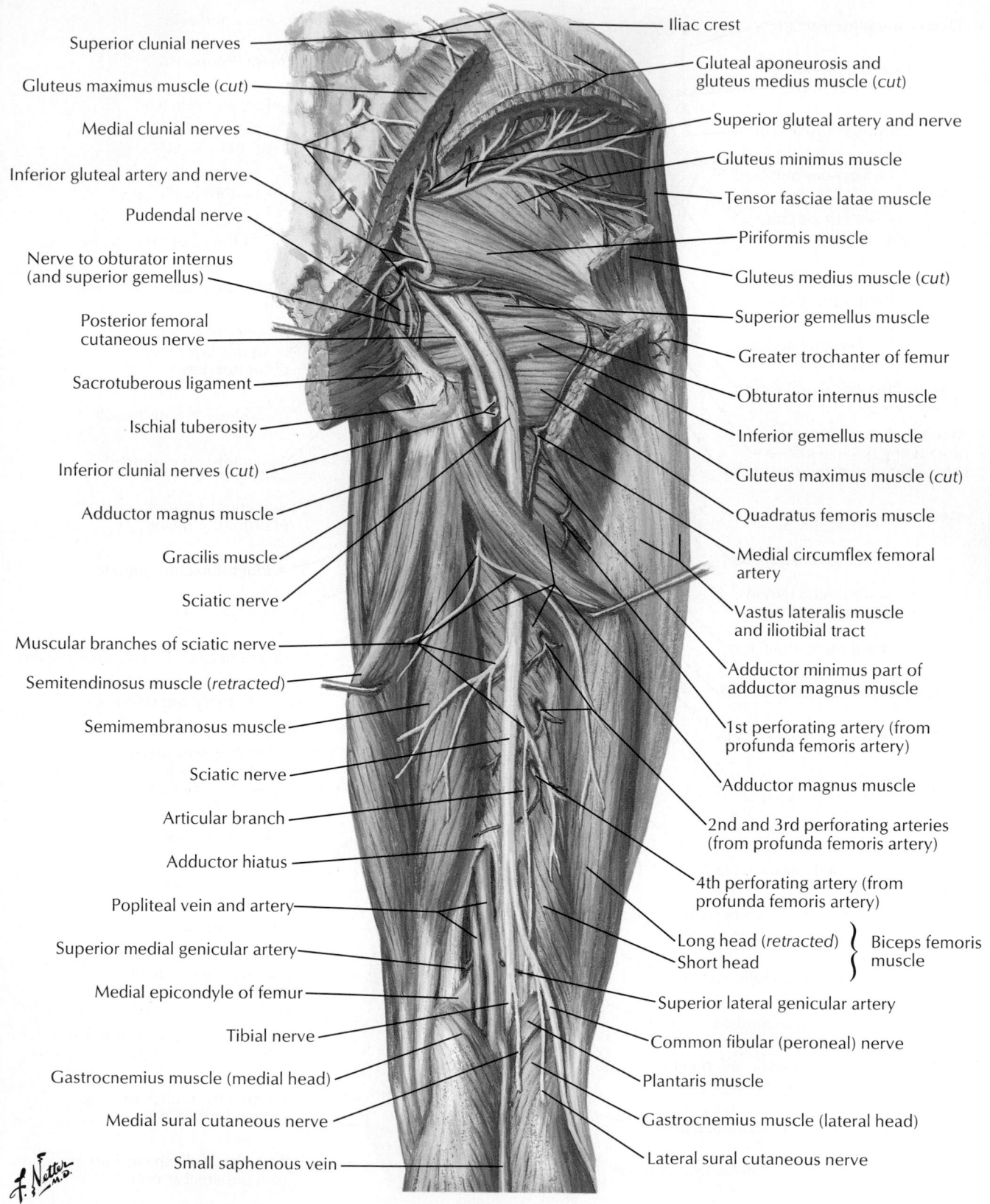

Superior clunial nerves

Gluteus maximus muscle (*cut*)

Medial clunial nerves

Inferior gluteal artery and nerve

Pudendal nerve

Nerve to obturator internus (and superior gemellus)

Posterior femoral cutaneous nerve

Sacrotuberous ligament

Ischial tuberosity

Inferior clunial nerves (*cut*)

Adductor magnus muscle

Gracilis muscle

Sciatic nerve

Muscular branches of sciatic nerve

Semitendinosus muscle (*retracted*)

Semimembranosus muscle

Sciatic nerve

Articular branch

Adductor hiatus

Popliteal vein and artery

Superior medial genicular artery

Medial epicondyle of femur

Tibial nerve

Gastrocnemius muscle (medial head)

Medial sural cutaneous nerve

Small saphenous vein

Iliac crest

Gluteal aponeurosis and gluteus medius muscle (*cut*)

Superior gluteal artery and nerve

Gluteus minimus muscle

Tensor fasciae latae muscle

Piriformis muscle

Gluteus medius muscle (*cut*)

Superior gemellus muscle

Greater trochanter of femur

Obturator internus muscle

Inferior gemellus muscle

Gluteus maximus muscle (*cut*)

Quadratus femoris muscle

Medial circumflex femoral artery

Vastus lateralis muscle and iliotibial tract

Adductor minimus part of adductor magnus muscle

1st perforating artery (from profunda femoris artery)

Adductor magnus muscle

2nd and 3rd perforating arteries (from profunda femoris artery)

4th perforating artery (from profunda femoris artery)

Long head (*retracted*) ⎫
Short head ⎭ Biceps femoris muscle

Superior lateral genicular artery

Common fibular (peroneal) nerve

Plantaris muscle

Gastrocnemius muscle (lateral head)

Lateral sural cutaneous nerve

NETTER'S ANATOMY ILLUSTRATIONS

Plate 502 Arteries and Nerves of Thigh: Posterior View. (Netter: Atlas of Human Anatomy, 4 ed, 2006, Saunders.)

Horizontal section

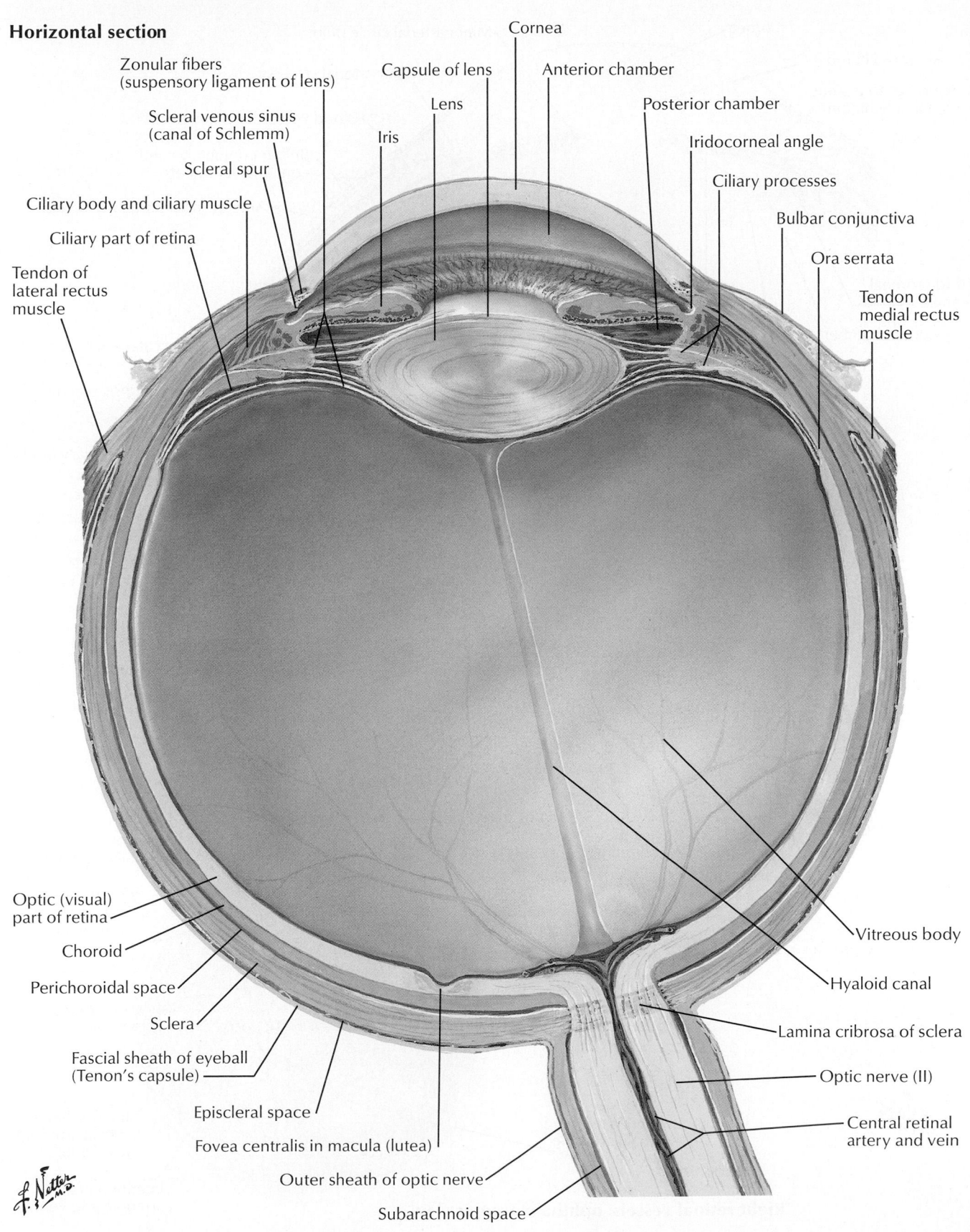

Zonular fibers
(suspensory ligament of lens)

Scleral venous sinus
(canal of Schlemm)

Scleral spur

Ciliary body and ciliary muscle

Ciliary part of retina

Tendon of
lateral rectus
muscle

Iris

Capsule of lens

Lens

Cornea

Anterior chamber

Posterior chamber

Iridocorneal angle

Ciliary processes

Bulbar conjunctiva

Ora serrata

Tendon of
medial rectus
muscle

Optic (visual)
part of retina

Choroid

Perichoroidal space

Sclera

Fascial sheath of eyeball
(Tenon's capsule)

Episcleral space

Fovea centralis in macula (lutea)

Outer sheath of optic nerve

Subarachnoid space

Vitreous body

Hyaloid canal

Lamina cribrosa of sclera

Optic nerve (II)

Central retinal
artery and vein

NETTER'S ANATOMY ILLUSTRATIONS

Plate 87   Eyeball. (Netter: Atlas of Human Anatomy, 4 ed, 2006, Saunders.)

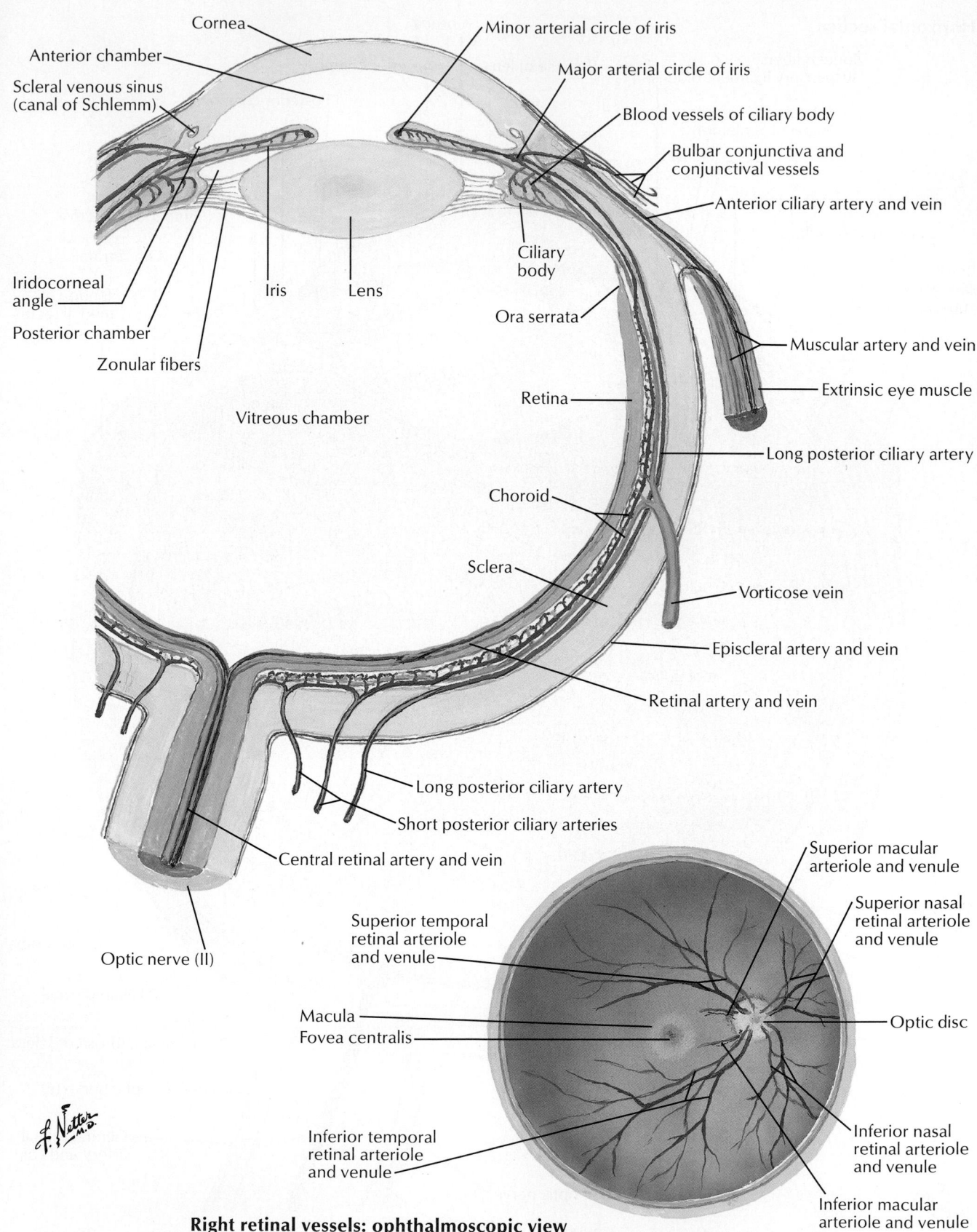

Cornea

Anterior chamber

Scleral venous sinus
(canal of Schlemm)

Iridocorneal
angle

Posterior chamber

Zonular fibers

Iris

Lens

Vitreous chamber

Minor arterial circle of iris

Major arterial circle of iris

Blood vessels of ciliary body

Bulbar conjunctiva and
conjunctival vessels

Anterior ciliary artery and vein

Ciliary
body

Ora serrata

Retina

Choroid

Sclera

Muscular artery and vein

Extrinsic eye muscle

Long posterior ciliary artery

Vorticose vein

Episcleral artery and vein

Retinal artery and vein

Long posterior ciliary artery

Short posterior ciliary arteries

Central retinal artery and vein

Optic nerve (II)

Superior macular
arteriole and venule

Superior temporal
retinal arteriole
and venule

Superior nasal
retinal arteriole
and venule

Macula

Fovea centralis

Optic disc

Inferior temporal
retinal arteriole
and venule

Inferior nasal
retinal arteriole
and venule

Inferior macular
arteriole and venule

Right retinal vessels: ophthalmoscopic view

Plate 90 Intrinsic Arteries and Veins of Eye. (Netter: Atlas of Human Anatomy, 4 ed, 2006, Saunders.)

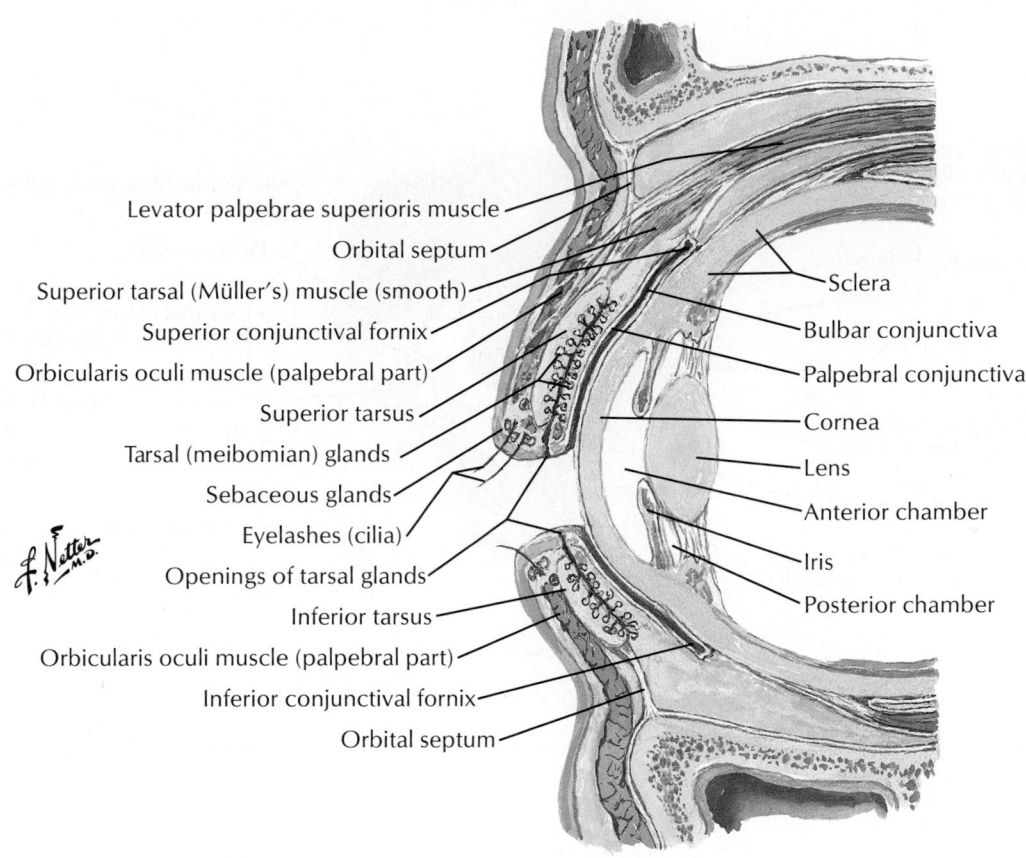

Levator palpebrae superioris muscle

Orbital septum

Superior tarsal (Müller's) muscle (smooth)

Superior conjunctival fornix

Orbicularis oculi muscle (palpebral part)

Superior tarsus

Tarsal (meibomian) glands

Sebaceous glands

Eyelashes (cilia)

Openings of tarsal glands

Inferior tarsus

Orbicularis oculi muscle (palpebral part)

Inferior conjunctival fornix

Orbital septum

Sclera

Bulbar conjunctiva

Palpebral conjunctiva

Cornea

Lens

Anterior chamber

Iris

Posterior chamber

Plate 81, Middle Eyelids. (Netter: Atlas of Human Anatomy, 4 ed, 2006, Saunders.)

Superior palpebral conjunctiva: tarsal (meibomian) glands shining through

Seen through cornea { Pupil / Iris }

Corneoscleral junction (corneal limbus)

Bulbar conjunctiva over sclera

Inferior conjunctival fornix

Inferior palpebral conjunctiva: tarsal glands shining through

Superior lacrimal papilla and punctum

Plica semilunaris

Lacrimal caruncle in lacrimal lake (lacus lacrimalis)

Inferior lacrimal papilla and punctum

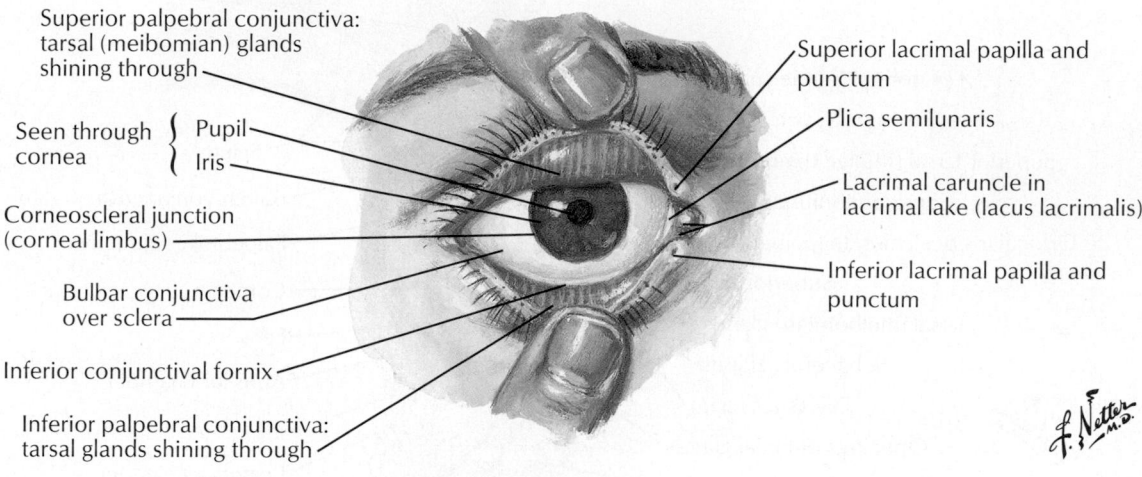

F. Netter, M.D.

Plate 81, Upper Eyelid. (Netter: Atlas of Human Anatomy, 4 ed, 2006, Saunders.)

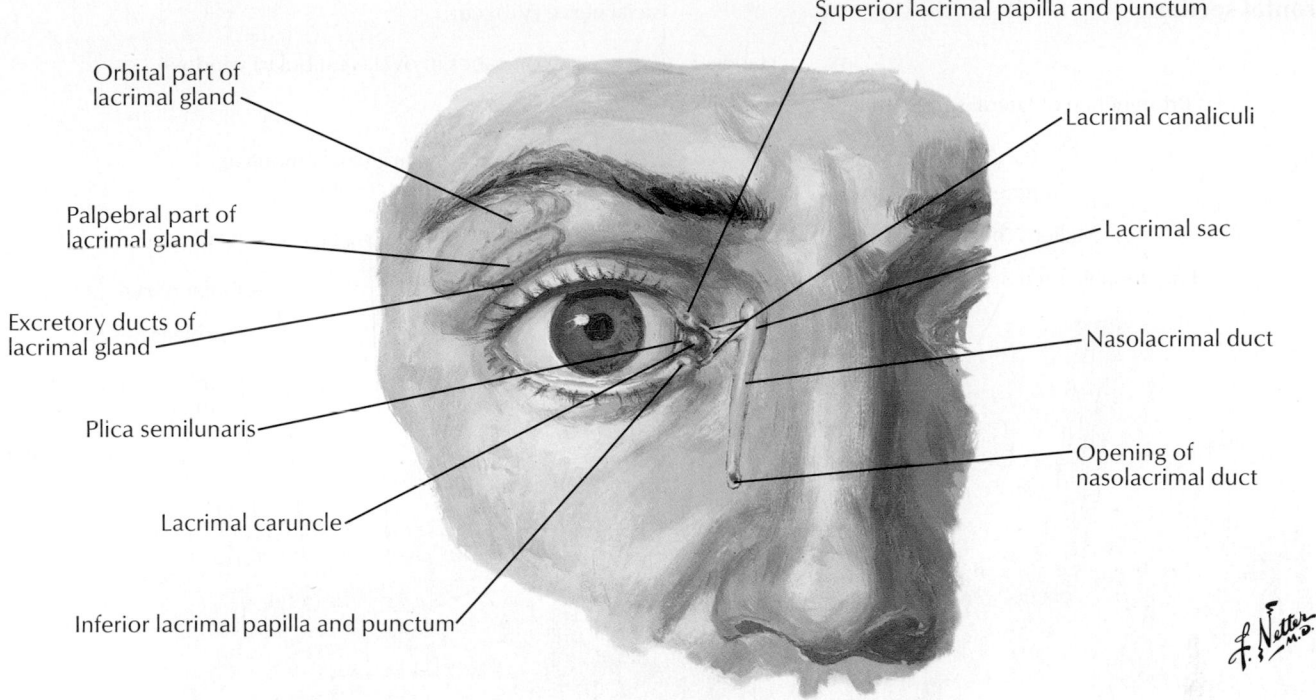

Orbital part of lacrimal gland

Palpebral part of lacrimal gland

Excretory ducts of lacrimal gland

Plica semilunaris

Lacrimal caruncle

Inferior lacrimal papilla and punctum

Superior lacrimal papilla and punctum

Lacrimal canaliculi

Lacrimal sac

Nasolacrimal duct

Opening of nasolacrimal duct

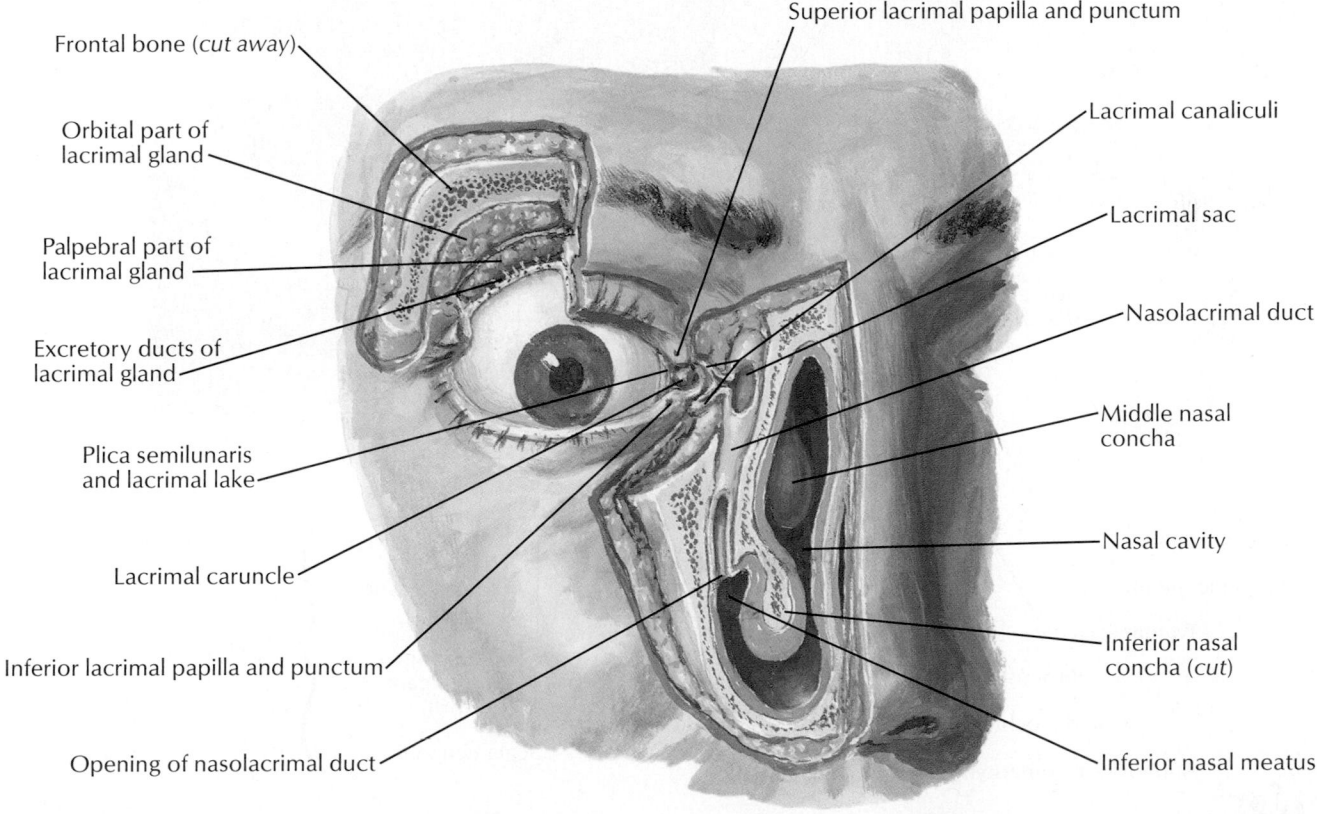

Frontal bone (*cut away*)

Orbital part of lacrimal gland

Palpebral part of lacrimal gland

Excretory ducts of lacrimal gland

Plica semilunaris and lacrimal lake

Lacrimal caruncle

Inferior lacrimal papilla and punctum

Opening of nasolacrimal duct

Superior lacrimal papilla and punctum

Lacrimal canaliculi

Lacrimal sac

Nasolacrimal duct

Middle nasal concha

Nasal cavity

Inferior nasal concha (*cut*)

Inferior nasal meatus

Plate 82   Lacrimal Apparatus. (Netter: Atlas of Human Anatomy, 4 ed, 2006, Saunders.)

Frontal section

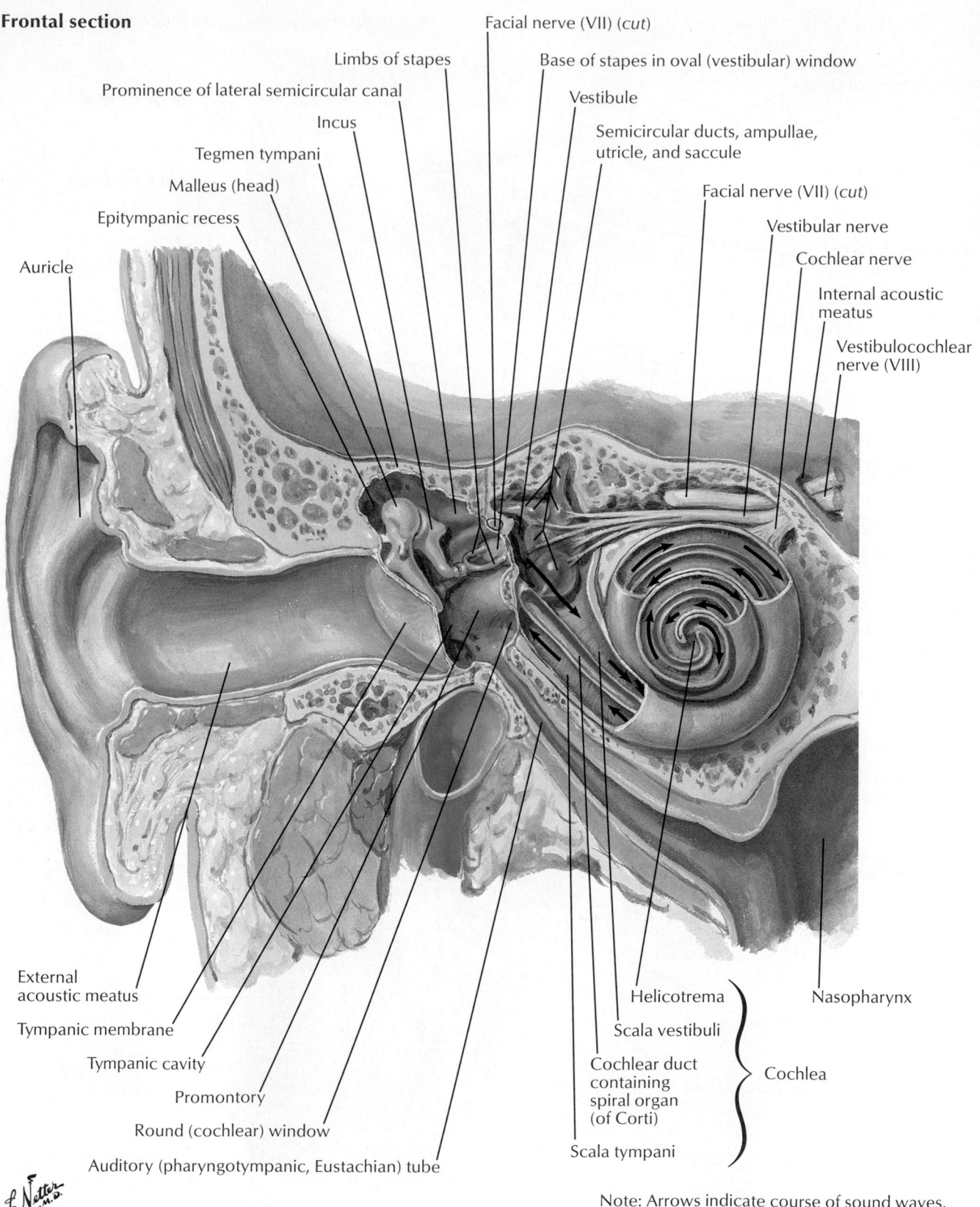

Facial nerve (VII) (*cut*)

Limbs of stapes

Base of stapes in oval (vestibular) window

Prominence of lateral semicircular canal

Vestibule

Incus

Semicircular ducts, ampullae, utricle, and saccule

Tegmen tympani

Malleus (head)

Facial nerve (VII) (*cut*)

Epitympanic recess

Vestibular nerve

Cochlear nerve

Auricle

Internal acoustic meatus

Vestibulocochlear nerve (VIII)

External acoustic meatus

Helicotrema

Nasopharynx

Tympanic membrane

Scala vestibuli

Tympanic cavity

Cochlear duct containing spiral organ (of Corti)

Cochlea

Promontory

Round (cochlear) window

Scala tympani

Auditory (pharyngotympanic, Eustachian) tube

Note: Arrows indicate course of sound waves.

NETTER'S ANATOMY ILLUSTRATIONS

Plate 92 Pathway of Sound Reception. (Netter: Atlas of Human Anatomy, 4 ed, 2006, Saunders.)

Medial wall of tympanic cavity: lateral view

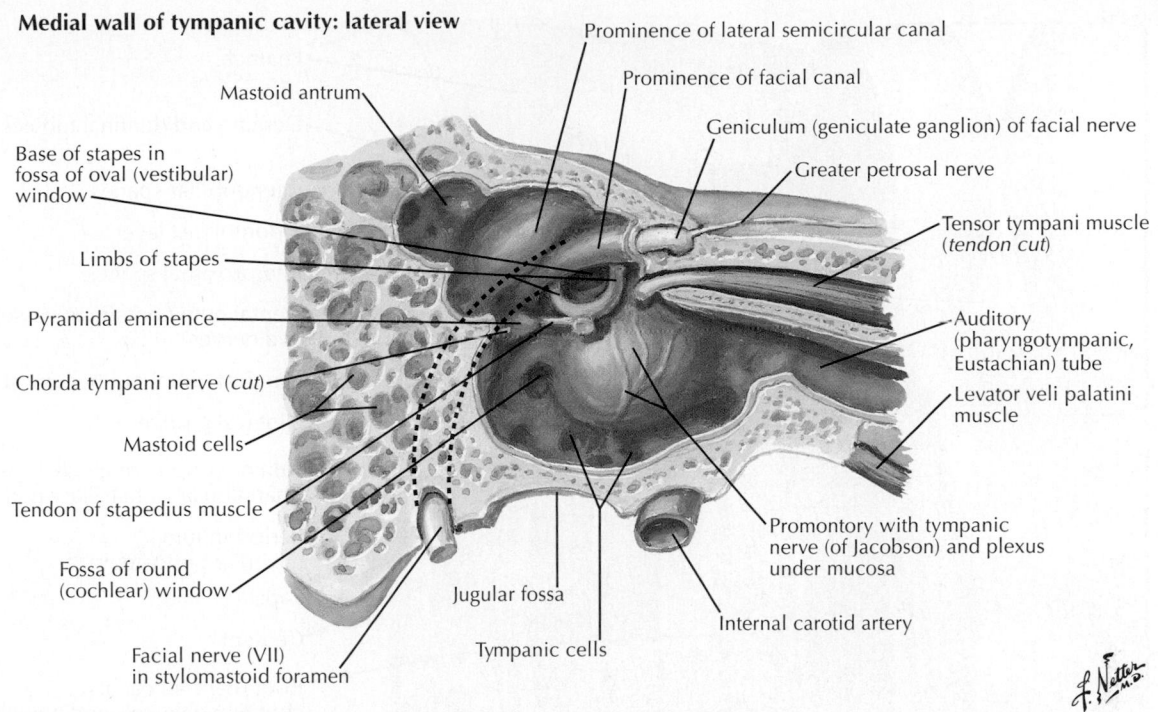

Mastoid antrum

Prominence of lateral semicircular canal

Prominence of facial canal

Geniculum (geniculate ganglion) of facial nerve

Greater petrosal nerve

Base of stapes in fossa of oval (vestibular) window

Limbs of stapes

Pyramidal eminence

Chorda tympani nerve (*cut*)

Mastoid cells

Tendon of stapedius muscle

Fossa of round (cochlear) window

Facial nerve (VII) in stylomastoid foramen

Jugular fossa

Tympanic cells

Tensor tympani muscle (*tendon cut*)

Auditory (pharyngotympanic, Eustachian) tube

Levator veli palatini muscle

Promontory with tympanic nerve (of Jacobson) and plexus under mucosa

Internal carotid artery

Plate 94 Tympanic Cavity. (Netter: Atlas of Human Anatomy, 4 ed, 2006, Saunders.)

Otoscopic view of right tympanic membrane

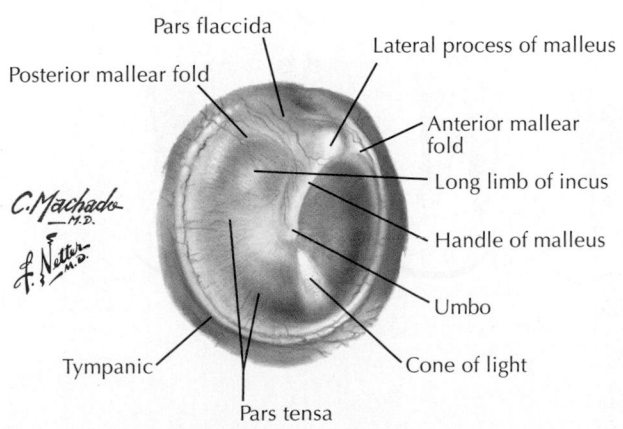

Pars flaccida

Posterior mallear fold

Lateral process of malleus

Anterior mallear fold

Long limb of incus

Handle of malleus

Umbo

Cone of light

Tympanic

Pars tensa

Plate 93 Tympanic Cavity. (Netter: Atlas of Human Anatomy, 4 ed, 2006, Saunders.)

Dissected right bony labyrinth (otic capsule): membranous labyrinth removed

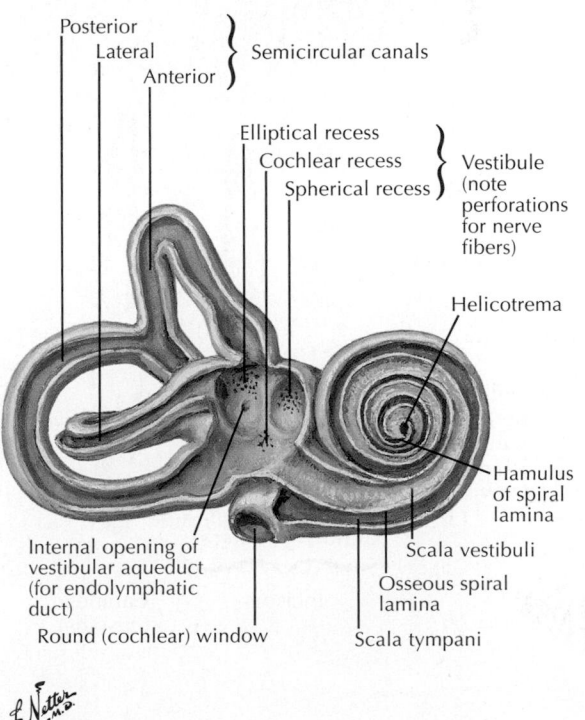

Posterior

Lateral

Anterior

Semicircular canals

Elliptical recess

Cochlear recess

Spherical recess

Vestibule (note perforations for nerve fibers)

Helicotrema

Hamulus of spiral lamina

Scala vestibuli

Osseous spiral lamina

Scala tympani

Internal opening of vestibular aqueduct (for endolymphatic duct)

Round (cochlear) window

Plate 95 Bony Membranous Labyrinth. (Netter: Atlas of Human Anatomy, 4 ed, 2006, Saunders.)

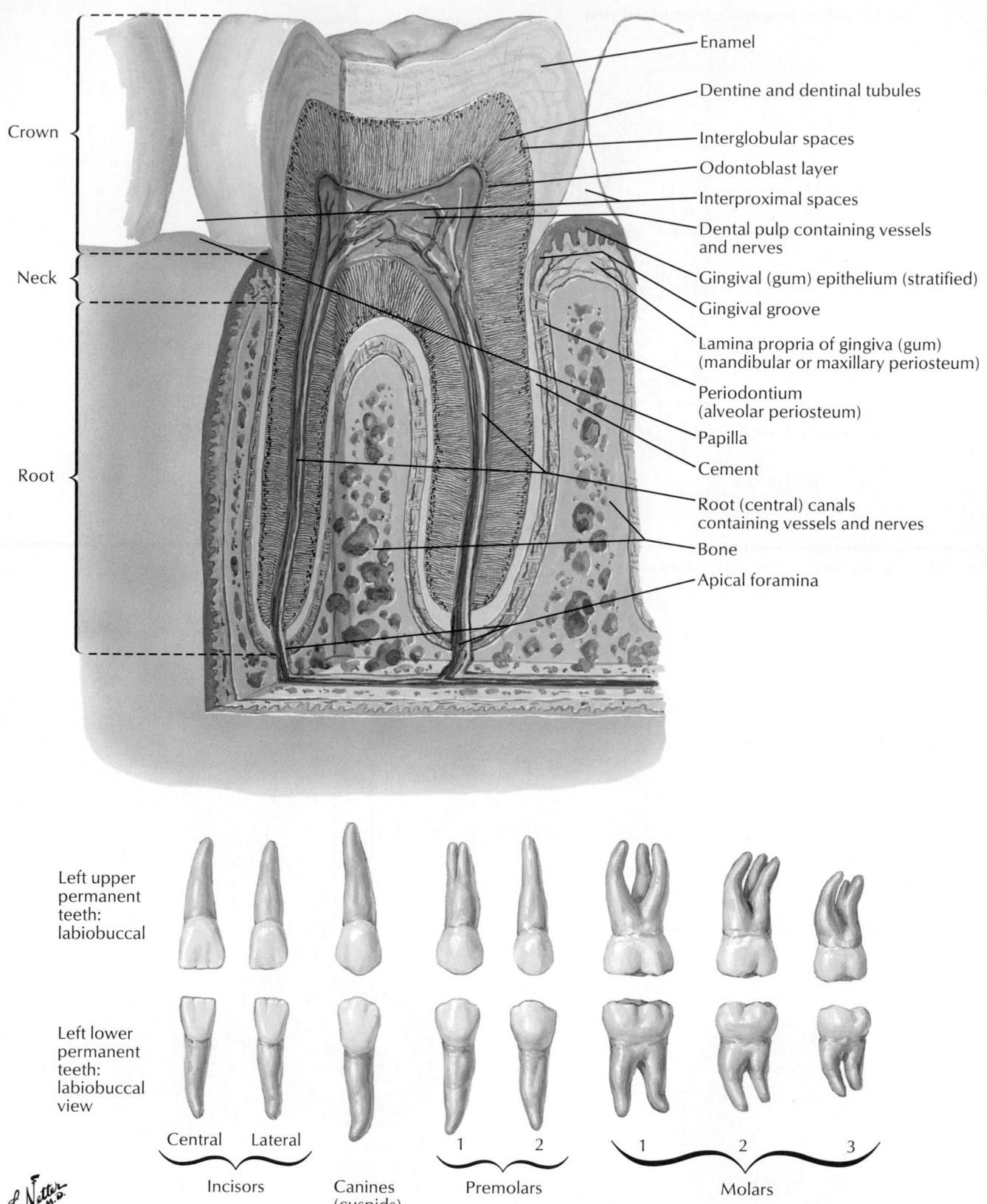

Crown

Neck

Root

Enamel

Dentine and dentinal tubules

Interglobular spaces

Odontoblast layer

Interproximal spaces

Dental pulp containing vessels and nerves

Gingival (gum) epithelium (stratified)

Gingival groove

Lamina propria of gingiva (gum) (mandibular or maxillary periosteum)

Periodontium (alveolar periosteum)

Papilla

Cement

Root (central) canals containing vessels and nerves

Bone

Apical foramina

Left upper permanent teeth: labiobuccal

Left lower permanent teeth: labiobuccal view

Central   Lateral

Incisors

Canines (cuspids)

1   2

Premolars

1   2   3

Molars

Plate 57 Teeth. (Netter: Atlas of Human Anatomy, 4 ed, 2006, Saunders.)

Tongue

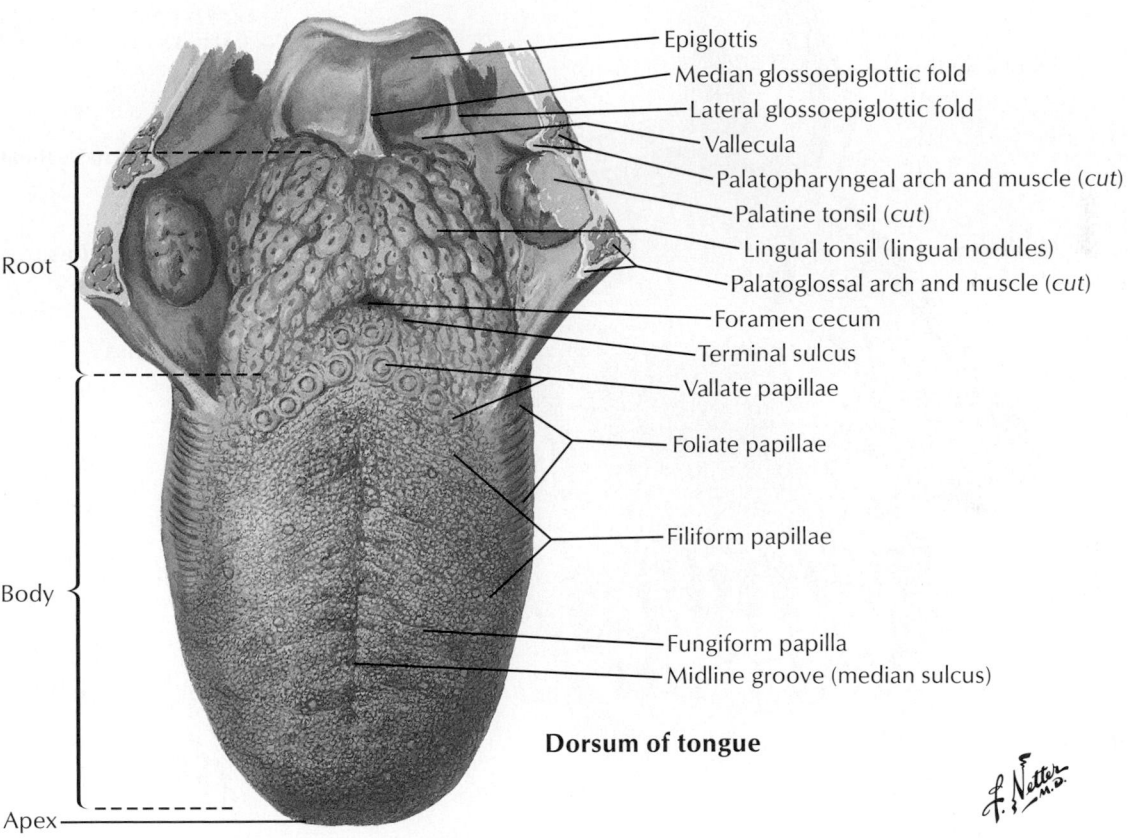

Epiglottis

Median glossoepiglottic fold

Lateral glossoepiglottic fold

Vallecula

Palatopharyngeal arch and muscle (*cut*)

Palatine tonsil (*cut*)

Lingual tonsil (lingual nodules)

Palatoglossal arch and muscle (*cut*)

Foramen cecum

Terminal sulcus

Vallate papillae

Foliate papillae

Filiform papillae

Fungiform papilla

Midline groove (median sulcus)

Root

Body

Apex

Dorsum of tongue

Plate 58   Tongue. (Netter: Atlas of Human Anatomy, 4 ed, 2006, Saunders.)

NETTER'S ANATOMY ILLUSTRATIONS

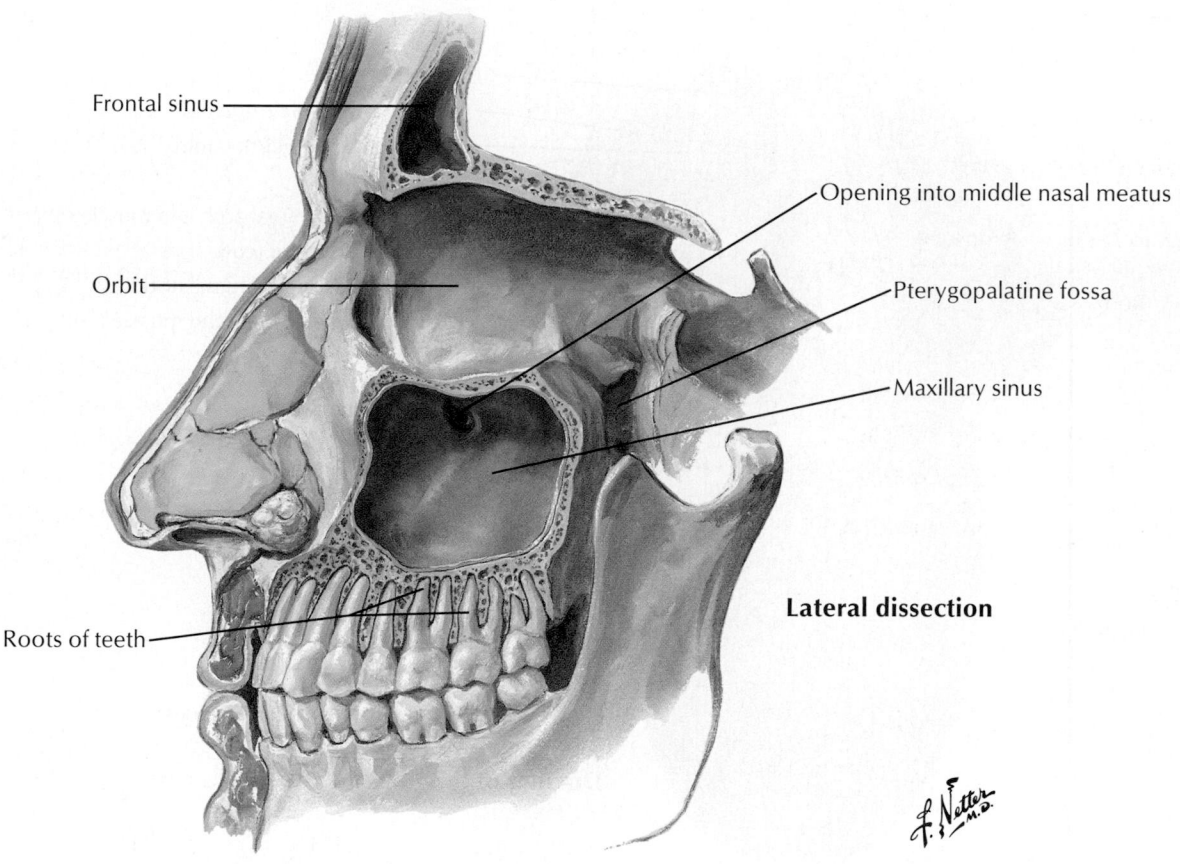

Frontal sinus

Orbit

Roots of teeth

Opening into middle nasal meatus

Pterygopalatine fossa

Maxillary sinus

Lateral dissection

Plate 49 Paranasal Sinuses. (Netter: Atlas of Human Anatomy, 4 ed, 2006, Saunders.)

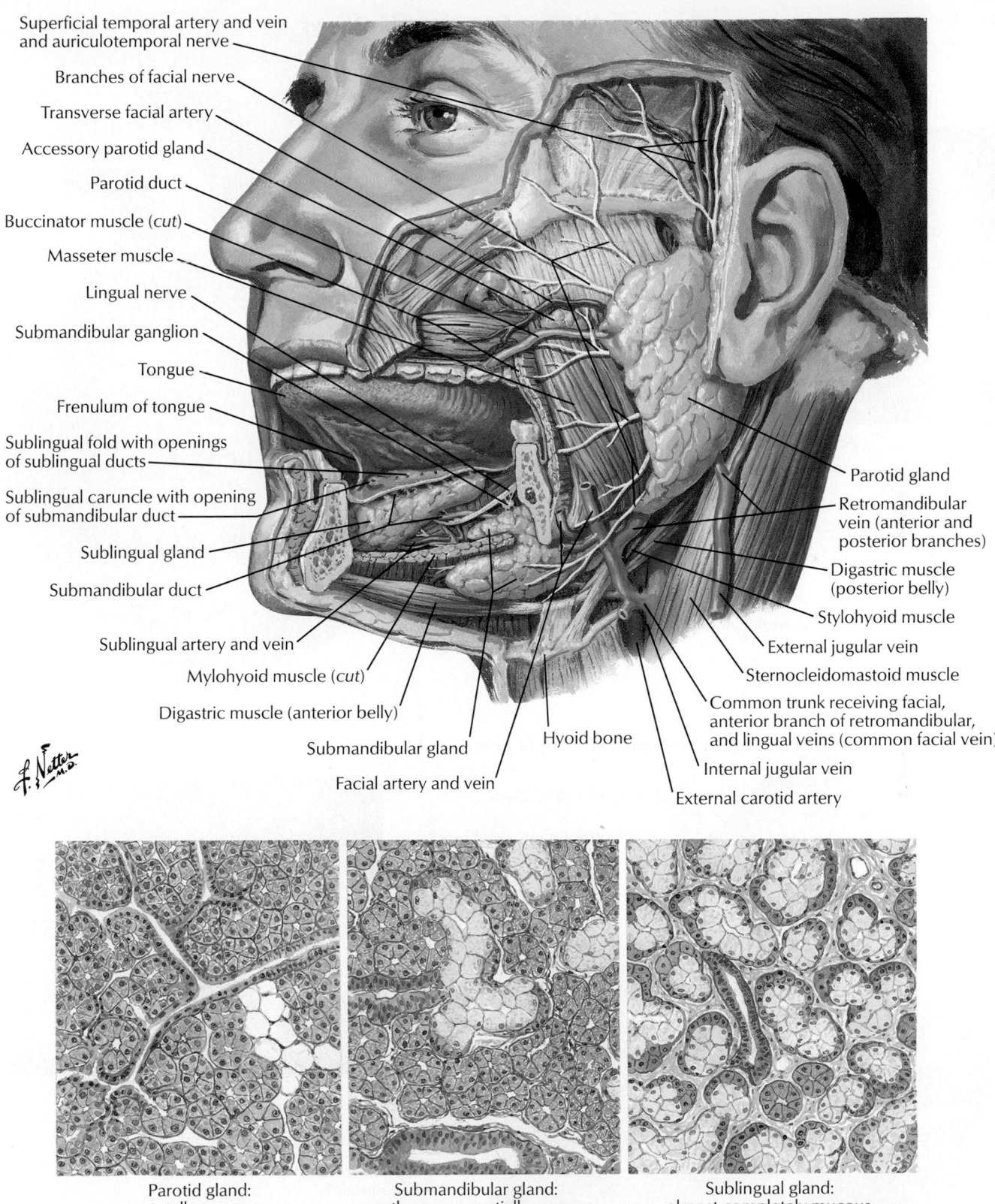

Superficial temporal artery and vein and auriculotemporal nerve

Branches of facial nerve

Transverse facial artery

Accessory parotid gland

Parotid duct

Buccinator muscle (cut)

Masseter muscle

Lingual nerve

Submandibular ganglion

Tongue

Frenulum of tongue

Sublingual fold with openings of sublingual ducts

Sublingual caruncle with opening of submandibular duct

Sublingual gland

Submandibular duct

Sublingual artery and vein

Mylohyoid muscle (cut)

Digastric muscle (anterior belly)

Submandibular gland

Facial artery and vein

Hyoid bone

Parotid gland

Retromandibular vein (anterior and posterior branches)

Digastric muscle (posterior belly)

Stylohyoid muscle

External jugular vein

Sternocleidomastoid muscle

Common trunk receiving facial, anterior branch of retromandibular, and lingual veins (common facial vein)

Internal jugular vein

External carotid artery

Parotid gland: totally serous

Submandibular gland: mostly serous, partially mucous

Sublingual gland: almost completely mucous

Plate 61 Salivary Glands. (Netter: Atlas of Human Anatomy, 4 ed, 2006, Saunders.)

Coronary Arteries: Arteriographic Views

Right coronary artery: left anterior oblique view

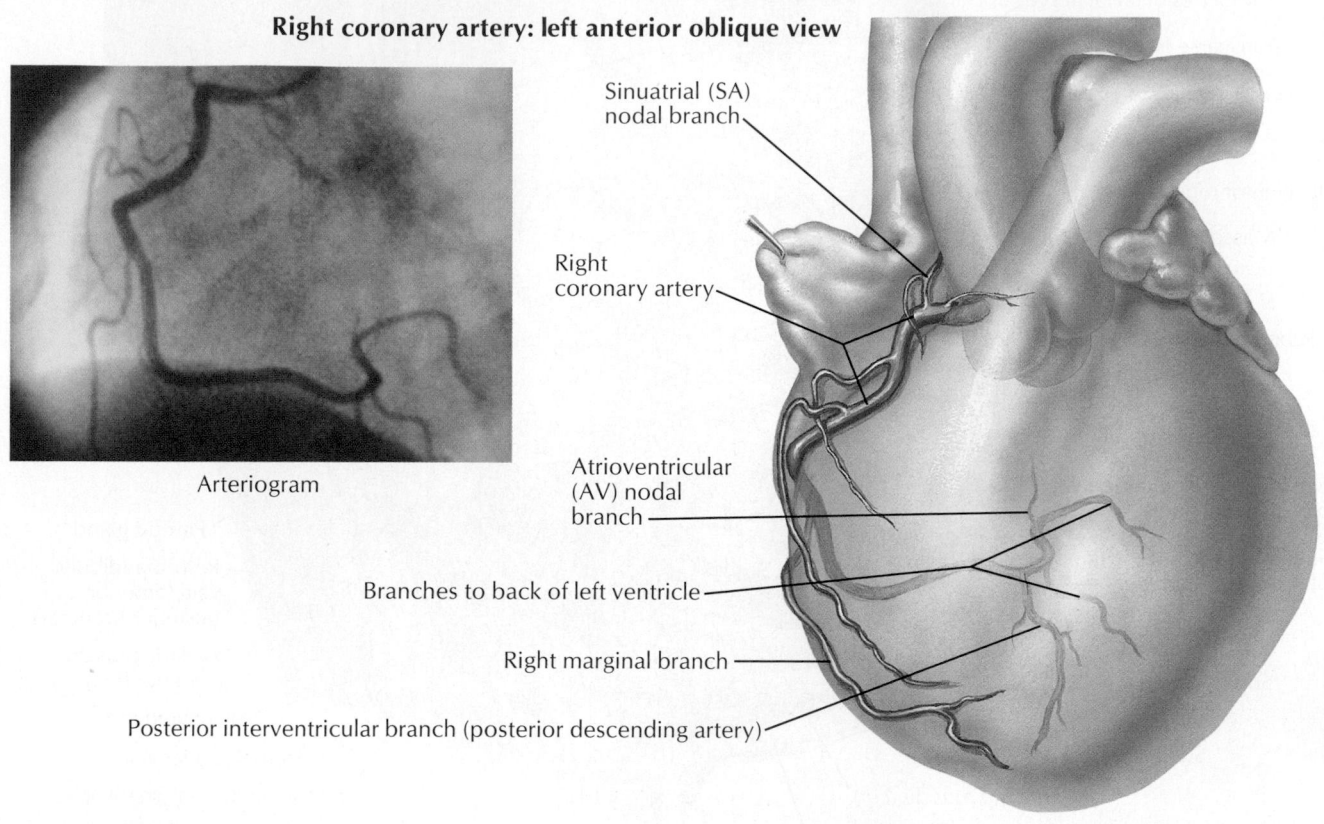

Arteriogram

Sinuatrial (SA) nodal branch

Right coronary artery

Atrioventricular (AV) nodal branch

Branches to back of left ventricle

Right marginal branch

Posterior interventricular branch (posterior descending artery)

Right coronary artery: right anterior oblique view

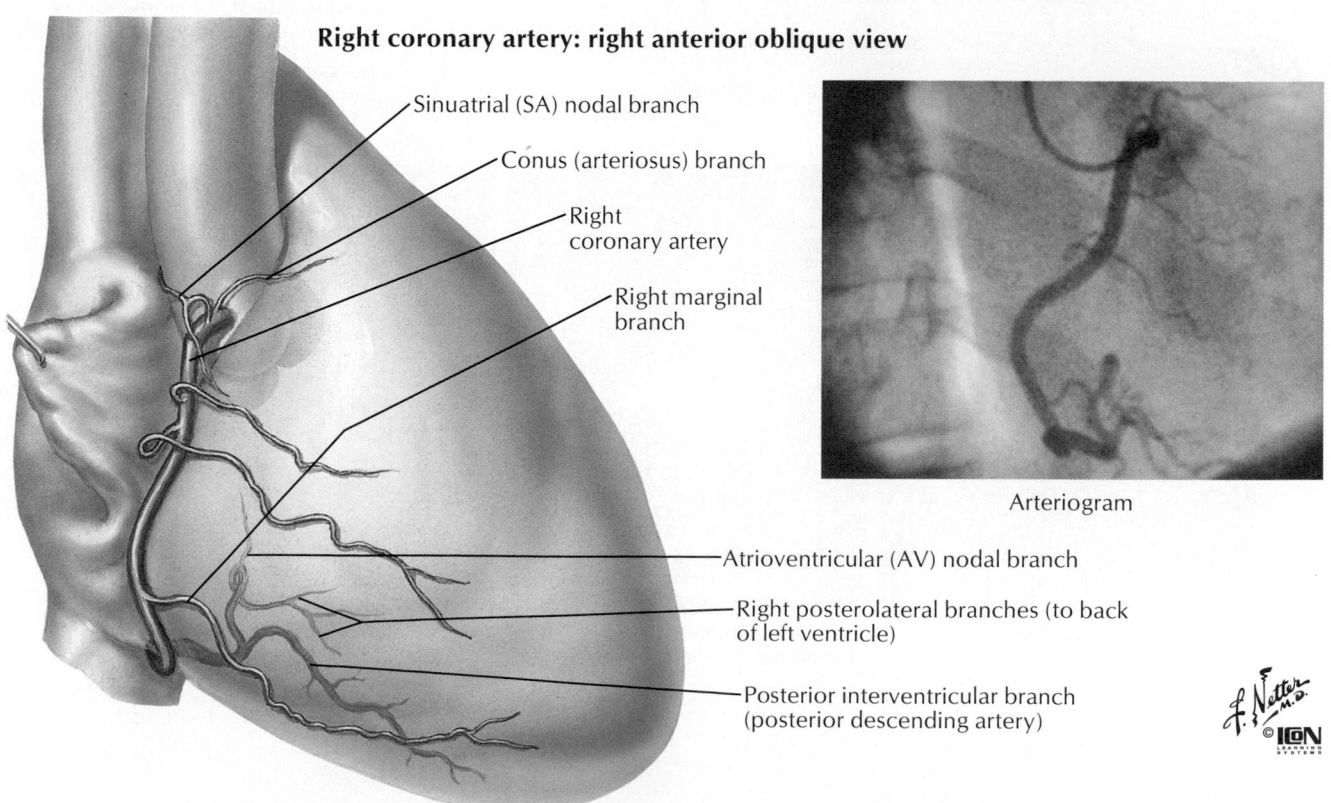

Sinuatrial (SA) nodal branch

Conus (arteriosus) branch

Right coronary artery

Right marginal branch

Arteriogram

Atrioventricular (AV) nodal branch

Right posterolateral branches (to back of left ventricle)

Posterior interventricular branch (posterior descending artery)

Plate 218 Coronary Arteries: Arteriographic Views. (Netter: Atlas of Human Anatomy, 4 ed, 2006, Saunders.)

Left coronary artery: left anterior oblique view

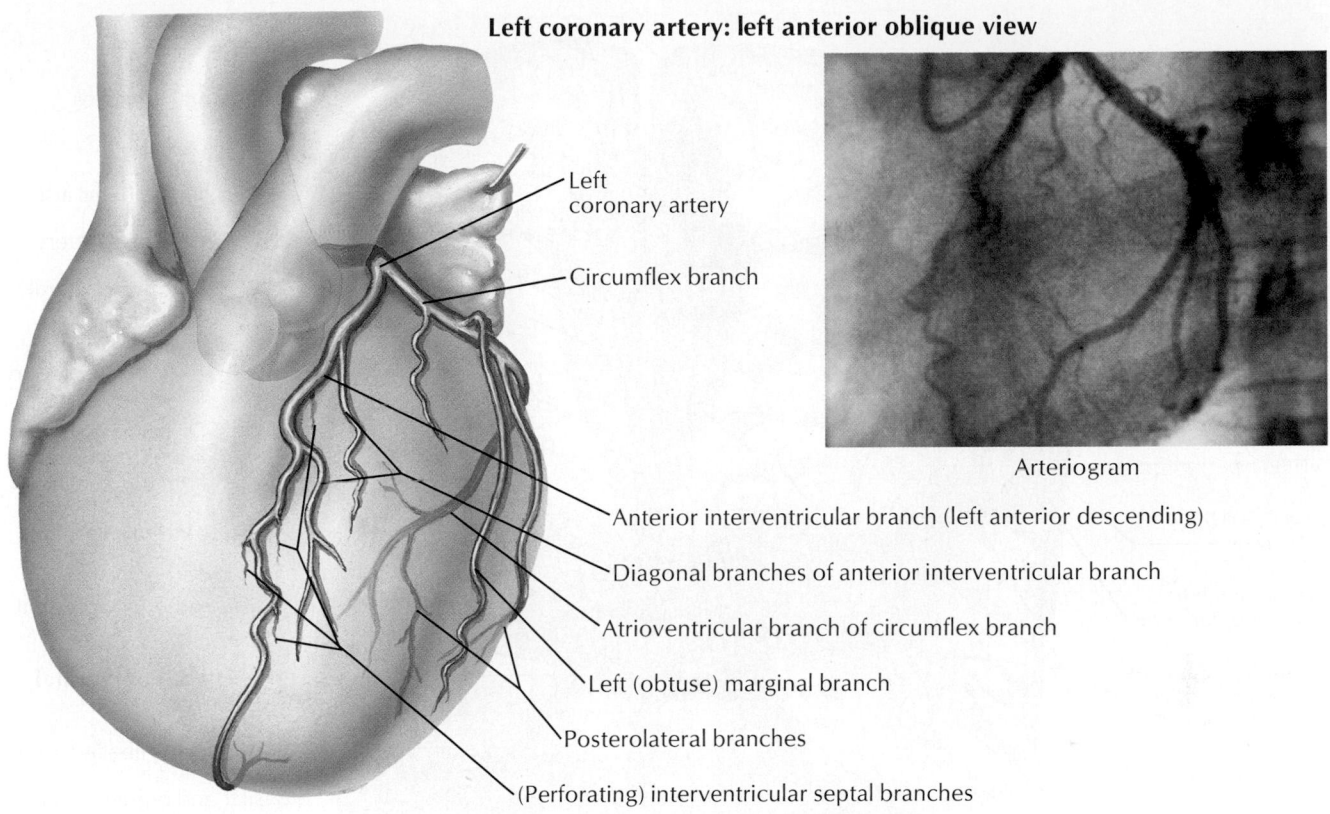

Left coronary artery

Circumflex branch

Arteriogram

Anterior interventricular branch (left anterior descending)

Diagonal branches of anterior interventricular branch

Atrioventricular branch of circumflex branch

Left (obtuse) marginal branch

Posterolateral branches

(Perforating) interventricular septal branches

Left coronary artery: right anterior oblique view

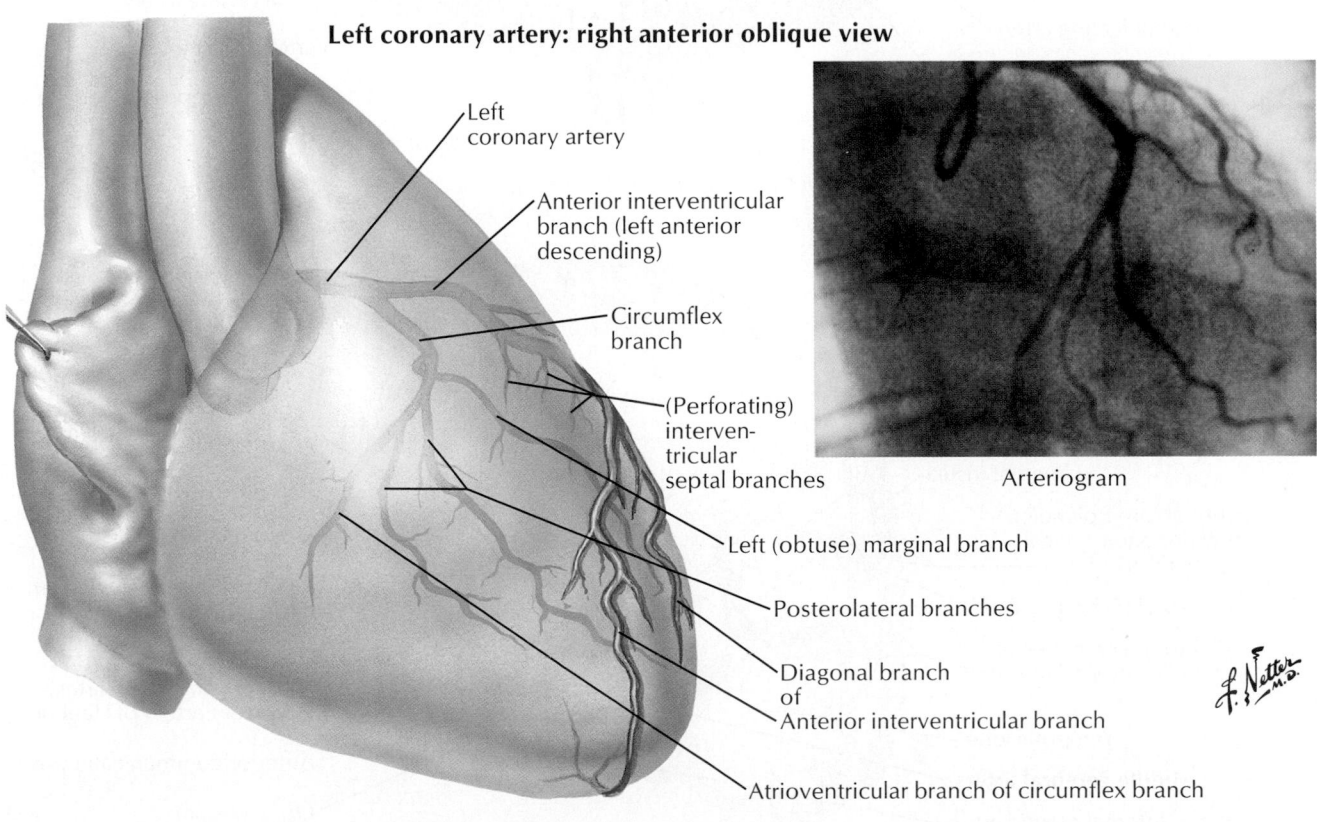

Left coronary artery

Anterior interventricular branch (left anterior descending)

Circumflex branch

(Perforating) interventricular septal branches

Arteriogram

Left (obtuse) marginal branch

Posterolateral branches

Diagonal branch of Anterior interventricular branch

Atrioventricular branch of circumflex branch

NETTER'S ANATOMY ILLUSTRATIONS

Plate 219 Coronary Arteries: Arteriographic Views. (Netter: Atlas of Human Anatomy, 4 ed, 2006, Saunders.)

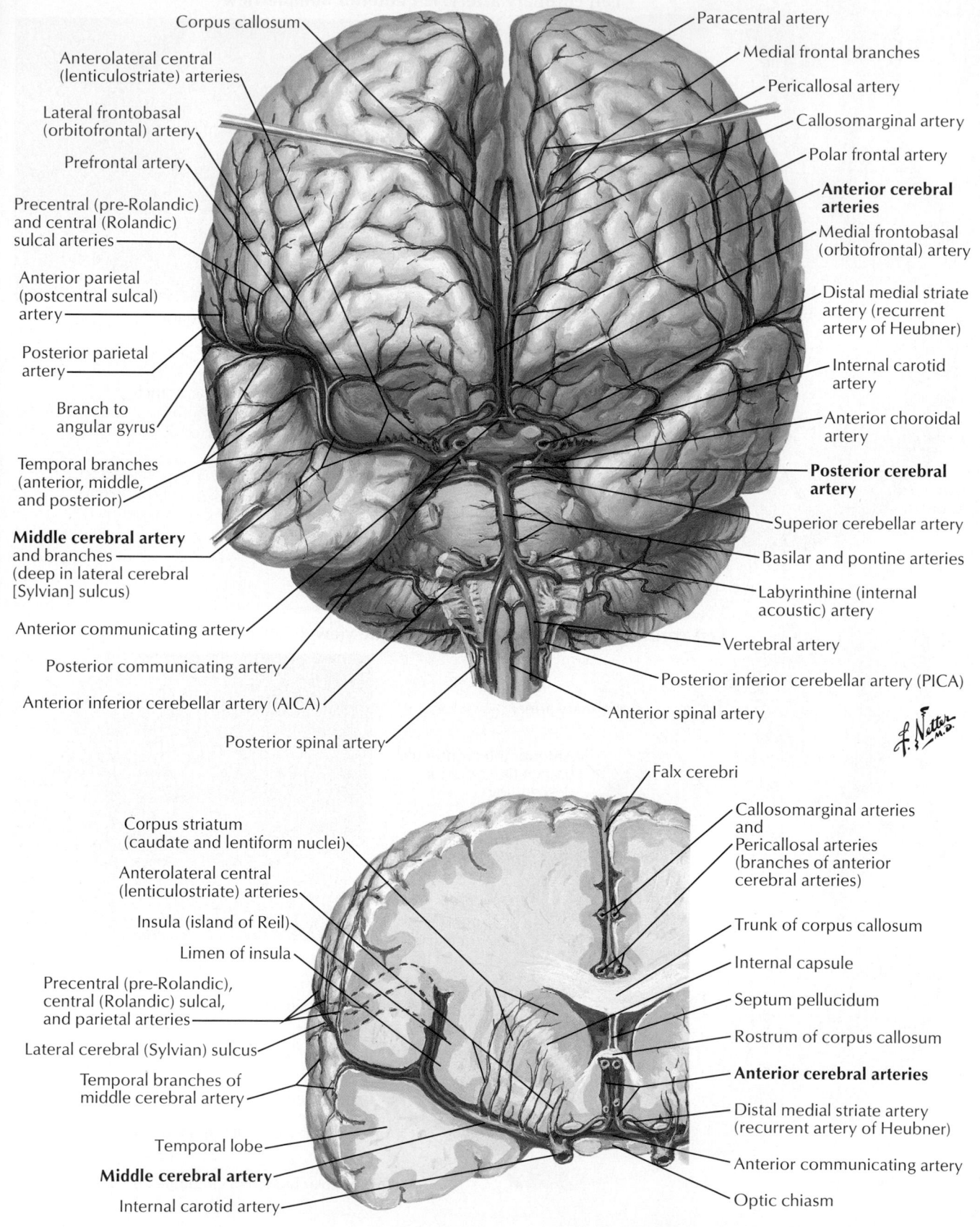

Corpus callosum

Anterolateral central (lenticulostriate) arteries

Lateral frontobasal (orbitofrontal) artery

Prefrontal artery

Precentral (pre-Rolandic) and central (Rolandic) sulcal arteries

Anterior parietal (postcentral sulcal) artery

Posterior parietal artery

Branch to angular gyrus

Temporal branches (anterior, middle, and posterior)

Middle cerebral artery and branches (deep in lateral cerebral [Sylvian] sulcus)

Anterior communicating artery

Posterior communicating artery

Anterior inferior cerebellar artery (AICA)

Posterior spinal artery

Paracentral artery

Medial frontal branches

Pericallosal artery

Callosomarginal artery

Polar frontal artery

Anterior cerebral arteries

Medial frontobasal (orbitofrontal) artery

Distal medial striate artery (recurrent artery of Heubner)

Internal carotid artery

Anterior choroidal artery

Posterior cerebral artery

Superior cerebellar artery

Basilar and pontine arteries

Labyrinthine (internal acoustic) artery

Vertebral artery

Posterior inferior cerebellar artery (PICA)

Anterior spinal artery

Falx cerebri

Corpus striatum (caudate and lentiform nuclei)

Anterolateral central (lenticulostriate) arteries

Insula (island of Reil)

Limen of insula

Precentral (pre-Rolandic), central (Rolandic) sulcal, and parietal arteries

Lateral cerebral (Sylvian) sulcus

Temporal branches of middle cerebral artery

Temporal lobe

Middle cerebral artery

Internal carotid artery

Callosomarginal arteries and Pericallosal arteries (branches of anterior cerebral arteries)

Trunk of corpus callosum

Internal capsule

Septum pellucidum

Rostrum of corpus callosum

Anterior cerebral arteries

Distal medial striate artery (recurrent artery of Heubner)

Anterior communicating artery

Optic chiasm

Plate 141 Arteries of Brain: Frontal View and Section. (Netter: Atlas of Human Anatomy, 4 ed, 2006, Saunders.)

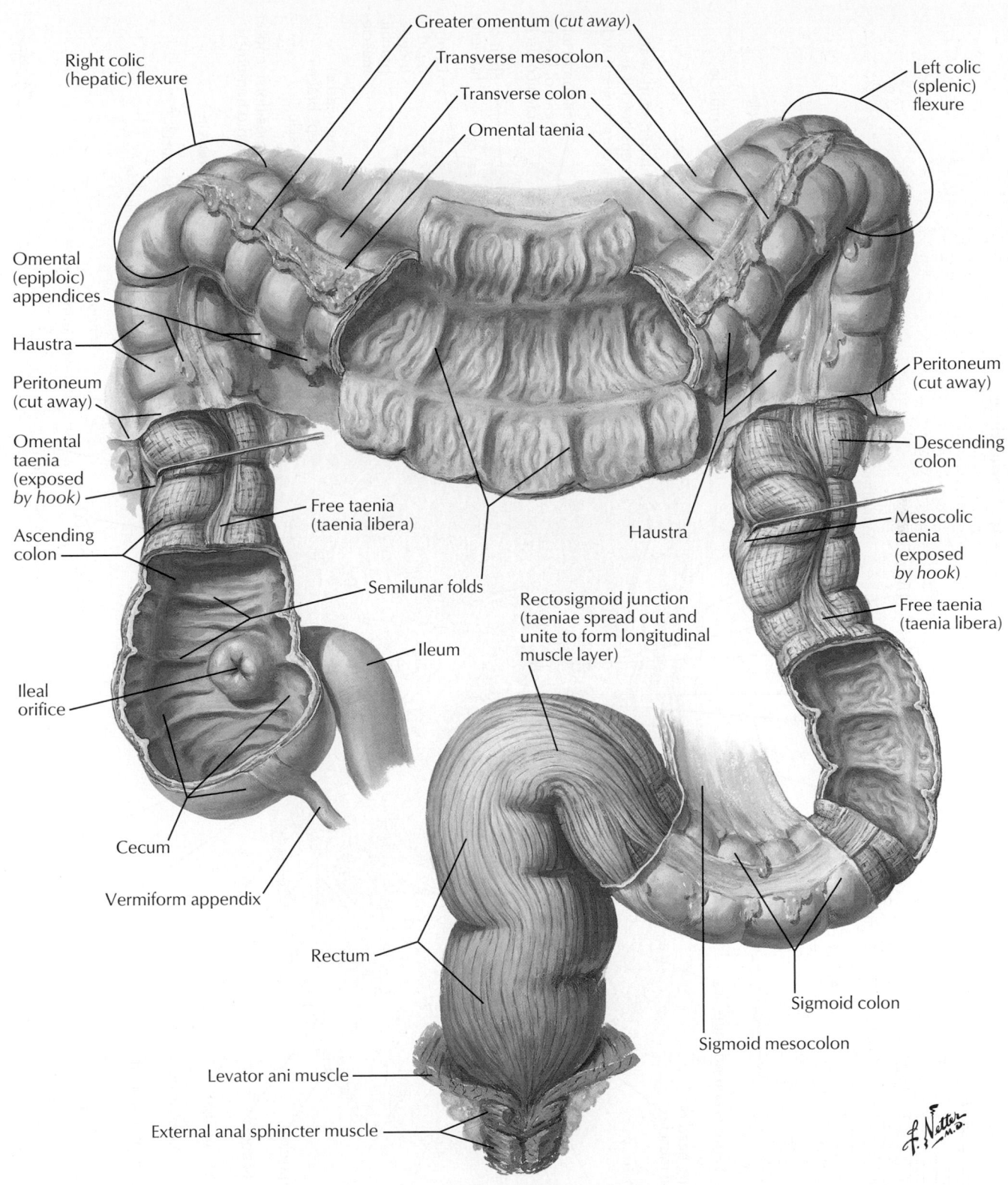

Right colic
(hepatic) flexure

Greater omentum (*cut away*)

Transverse mesocolon

Transverse colon

Omental taenia

Left colic
(splenic)
flexure

Omental
(epiploic)
appendices

Haustra

Peritoneum
(cut away)

Omental
taenia
(exposed
by hook)

Ascending
colon

Ileal
orifice

Cecum

Vermiform appendix

Free taenia
(taenia libera)

Semilunar folds

Ileum

Haustra

Peritoneum
(cut away)

Descending
colon

Mesocolic
taenia
(exposed
by hook)

Free taenia
(taenia libera)

Rectosigmoid junction
(taeniae spread out and
unite to form longitudinal
muscle layer)

Rectum

Levator ani muscle

External anal sphincter muscle

Sigmoid colon

Sigmoid mesocolon

NETTER'S ANATOMY ILLUSTRATIONS

Plate 284 Mucosa and Musculature of Large Intestine. (Netter: Atlas of Human Anatomy, 4 ed, 2006, Saunders.)

Transverse Section: T3–4 Intervertebral Disc, Manubrium

Plate 244

T3–4

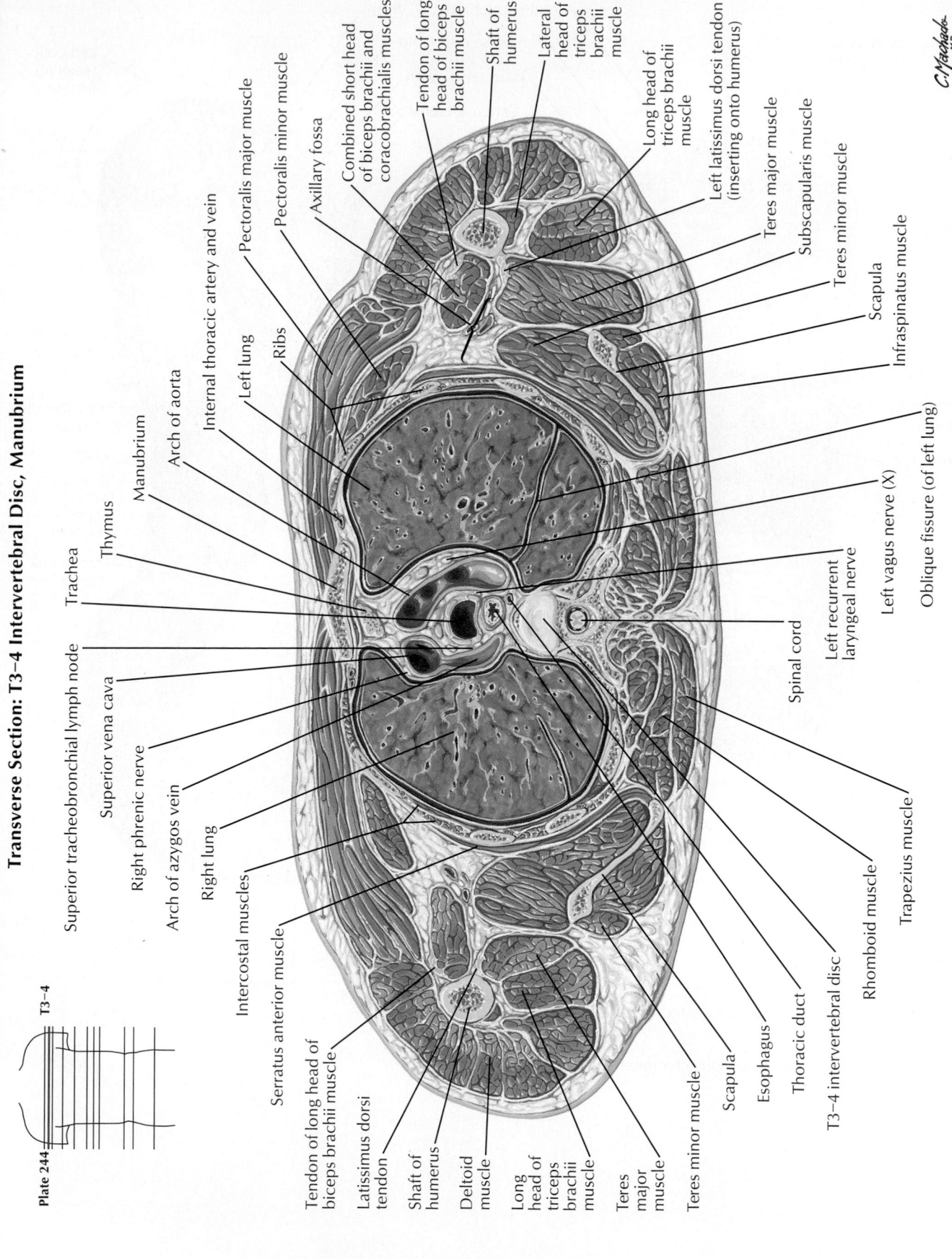

Trachea

Thymus

Manubrium

Arch of aorta

Internal thoracic artery and vein

Left lung

Ribs

Pectoralis minor muscle

Pectoralis major muscle

Axillary fossa

Combined short head of biceps brachii and coracobrachialis muscles

Tendon of long head of biceps brachii muscle

Shaft of humerus

Lateral head of triceps brachii muscle

Long head of triceps brachii muscle

Left latissimus dorsi tendon (inserting onto humerus)

Teres major muscle

Subscapularis muscle

Teres minor muscle

Scapula

Infraspinatus muscle

Superior tracheobronchial lymph node

Superior vena cava

Right phrenic nerve

Arch of azygos vein

Right lung

Intercostal muscles

Serratus anterior muscle

Tendon of long head of biceps brachii muscle

Latissimus dorsi tendon

Shaft of humerus

Deltoid muscle

Long head of triceps brachii muscle

Teres major muscle

Teres minor muscle

Scapula

Esophagus

Thoracic duct

T3–4 intervertebral disc

Rhomboid muscle

Trapezius muscle

Left recurrent laryngeal nerve

Left vagus nerve (X)

Oblique fissure (of left lung)

Spinal cord

Plate 244 Cross Section of Thorax at T3-4 Disc Level. (Netter: Atlas of Human Anatomy, 4 ed, 2006, Saunders.)

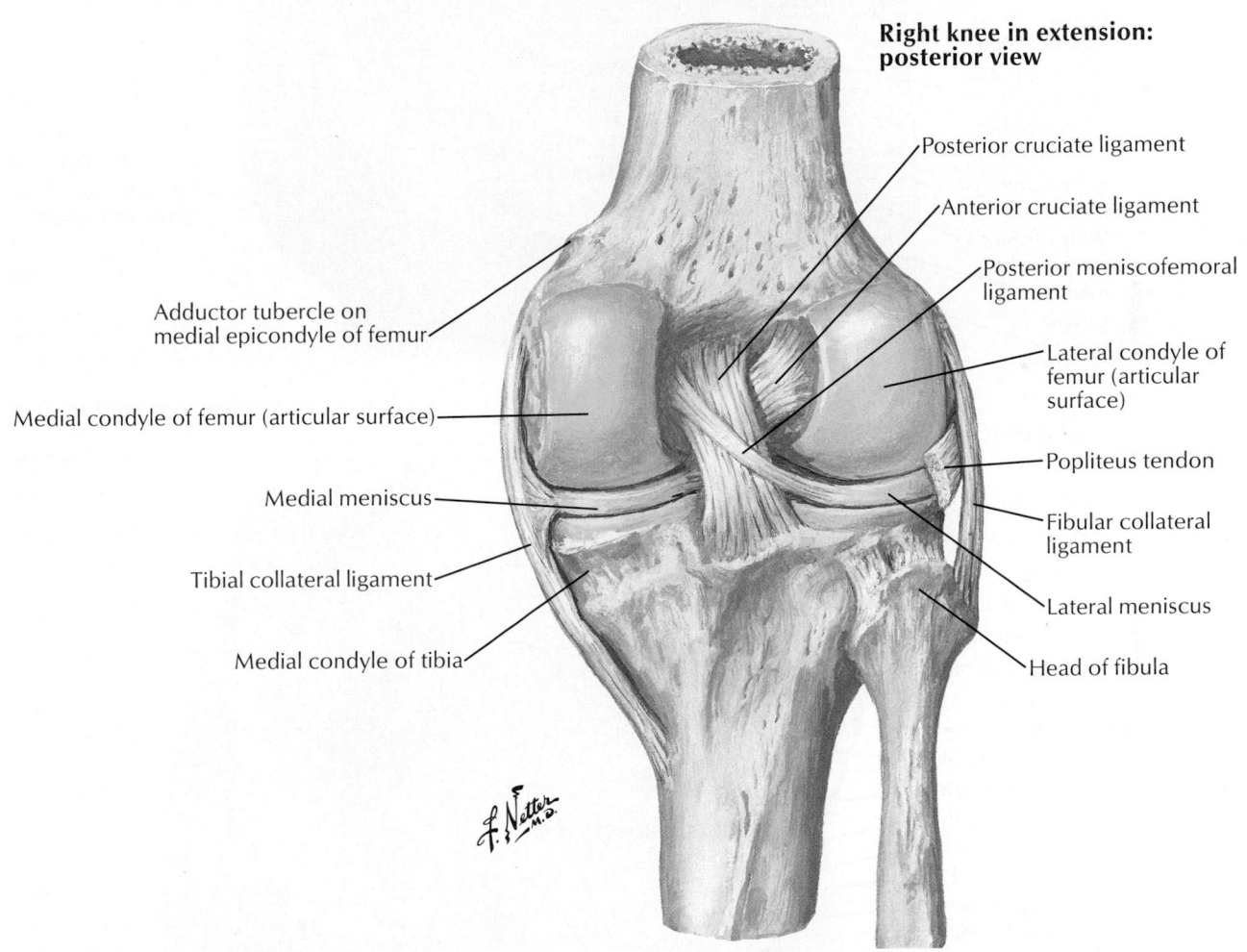

Right knee in extension: posterior view

Posterior cruciate ligament

Anterior cruciate ligament

Posterior meniscofemoral ligament

Adductor tubercle on medial epicondyle of femur

Lateral condyle of femur (articular surface)

Medial condyle of femur (articular surface)

Popliteus tendon

Medial meniscus

Fibular collateral ligament

Tibial collateral ligament

Lateral meniscus

Medial condyle of tibia

Head of fibula

Plate 509 Knee: Cruciate and Collateral Ligaments. (Netter: Atlas of Human Anatomy, 4 ed, 2006, Saunders.)

79

NETTER'S ANATOMY ILLUSTRATIONS

NETTER'S ANATOMY ILLUSTRATIONS

Paramedian (sagittal) dissection

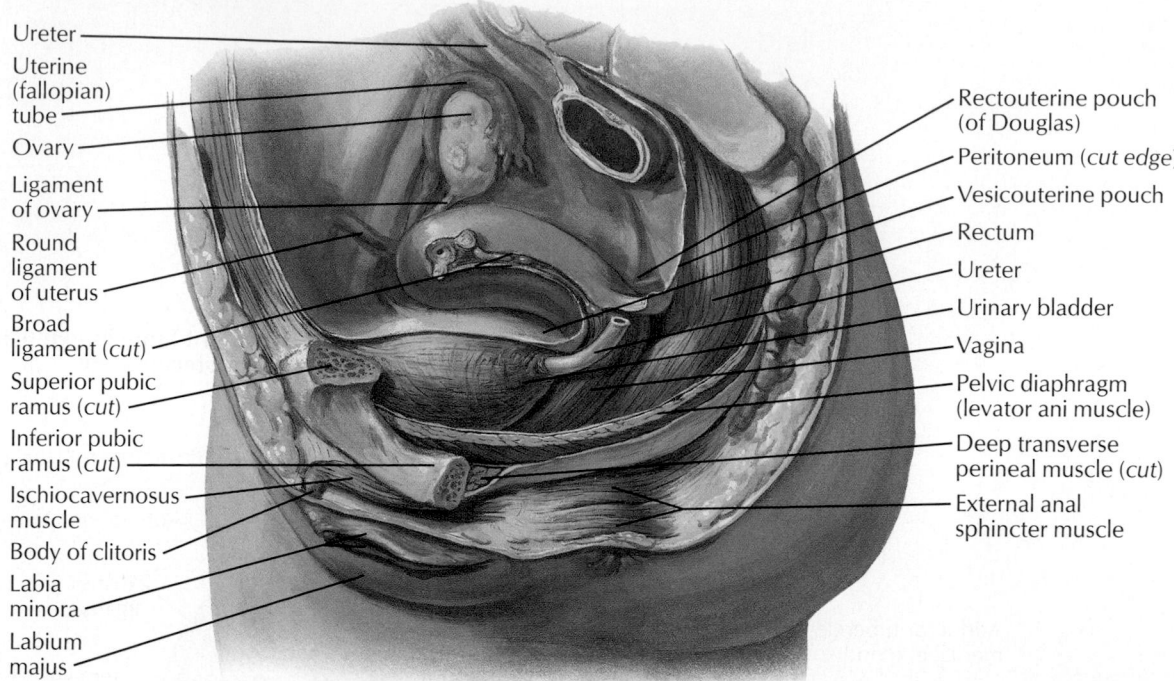

Ureter

Uterine (fallopian) tube

Ovary

Ligament of ovary

Round ligament of uterus

Broad ligament (*cut*)

Superior pubic ramus (*cut*)

Inferior pubic ramus (*cut*)

Ischiocavernosus muscle

Body of clitoris

Labia minora

Labium majus

Rectouterine pouch (of Douglas)

Peritoneum (*cut edge*)

Vesicouterine pouch

Rectum

Ureter

Urinary bladder

Vagina

Pelvic diaphragm (levator ani muscle)

Deep transverse perineal muscle (*cut*)

External anal sphincter muscle

Median (sagittal) section

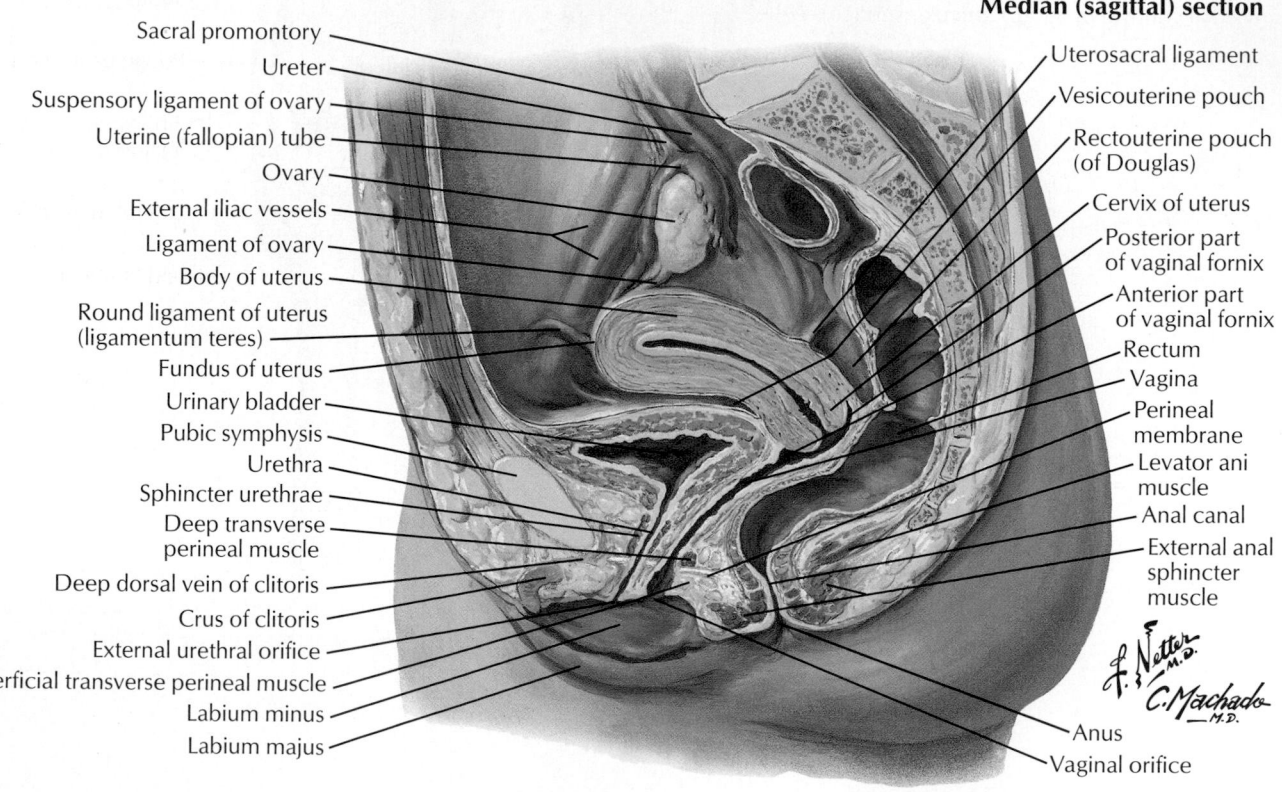

Sacral promontory

Ureter

Suspensory ligament of ovary

Uterine (fallopian) tube

Ovary

External iliac vessels

Ligament of ovary

Body of uterus

Round ligament of uterus (ligamentum teres)

Fundus of uterus

Urinary bladder

Pubic symphysis

Urethra

Sphincter urethrae

Deep transverse perineal muscle

Deep dorsal vein of clitoris

Crus of clitoris

External urethral orifice

Superficial transverse perineal muscle

Labium minus

Labium majus

Uterosacral ligament

Vesicouterine pouch

Rectouterine pouch (of Douglas)

Cervix of uterus

Posterior part of vaginal fornix

Anterior part of vaginal fornix

Rectum

Vagina

Perineal membrane

Levator ani muscle

Anal canal

External anal sphincter muscle

Anus

Vaginal orifice

Plate 360   Pelvic Viscera and Perineum: Female. (Netter: Atlas of Human Anatomy, 4 ed, 2006, Saunders.)

Alphabetic Index

A

Aarskog's syndrome Q87.1
Abandonment —see Maltreatment
Abasia (-astasia) (hysterical) F44.4
Abderhalden-Kaufmann-Lignac syndrome
  (cystinosis) E72.04
Abdomen, abdominal —see also condition
  acute R10.0
  angina K55.1
  muscle deficiency syndrome Q79.4
Abdominalgia —see Pain, abdominal
Abduction contracture, hip or other joint —see
  Contraction, joint
Aberrant (congenital) —see also Malposition,
  congenital
  adrenal gland Q89.1
  artery (peripheral) Q27.8
    basilar NEC Q28.1
    cerebral Q28.3
    coronary Q24.5
    digestive system Q27.8
    eye Q15.8
    lower limb Q27.8
    precerebral Q28.1
    pulmonary Q25.79
    renal Q27.2
    retina Q14.1
    specified site NEC Q27.8
    subclavian Q27.8
    upper limb Q27.8
    vertebral Q28.1
  breast Q83.8
  endocrine gland NEC Q89.2
  hepatic duct Q44.5
  pancreas Q45.3
  parathyroid gland Q89.2
  pituitary gland Q89.2
  sebaceous glands, mucous membrane,
    mouth, congenital Q38.6
  spleen Q89.09
  subclavian artery Q27.8
  thymus (gland) Q89.2
  thyroid gland Q89.2
  vein (peripheral) NEC Q27.8
    cerebral Q28.3
    digestive system Q27.8
    lower limb Q27.8
    precerebral Q28.1
    specified site NEC Q27.8
    upper limb Q27.8
Aberration
  distantal —see Disturbance, visual
  mental F99
Abetalipoproteinemia E78.6
Abiotrophy R68.89
Ablatio, ablation
  retinae —see Detachment, retina
Ablepharia, ablepharon Q10.3
Abnormal, abnormality, abnormalities —see
  also Anomaly
  acid-base balance (mixed) E87.4
  albumin R77.0
  alphafetoprotein R77.2
  alveolar ridge K08.9
  anatomical relationship Q89.9
  apertures, congenital, diaphragm
    Q79.1
  auditory perception H93.29-
    diplacusis —see Diplacusis
    hyperacusis —see Hyperacusis
    recruitment —see Recruitment, auditory
    threshold shift —see Shift, auditory
      threshold
  autosomes Q99.9
    fragile site Q95.5
  basal metabolic rate R94.8
  biosynthesis, testicular androgen
    E29.1
  bleeding time R79.1

Abnormal, abnormality, abnormalities —
  (Continued)
  blood level (of)
    cobalt R79.0
    copper R79.0
    iron R79.0
    lithium R78.89
    magnesium R79.0
    mineral NEC R79.0
    zinc R79.0
  blood pressure
    elevated R03.0
    low reading (nonspecific) R03.1
  blood sugar R73.09
  blood-gas level R79.81
  bowel sounds R19.15
    absent R19.11
    hyperactive R19.12
  brain scan R94.02
  breathing R06.9
  caloric test R94.138
  cerebrospinal fluid R83.9
    cytology R83.6
    drug level R83.2
    enzyme level R83.0
    hormones R83.1
    immunology R83.4
    microbiology R83.5
    nonmedicinal level R83.3
    specified type NEC R83.8
  chemistry, blood R79.9
    C-reactive protein R79.82
    drugs —see Findings, abnormal, in
      blood
    gas level R79.81
    minerals R79.0
    pancytopenia D61.818
    PTT R79.1
    specified NEC R79.89
    toxins —see Findings, abnormal, in
      blood
  chest sounds (friction) (rales) R09.89
  chromosome, chromosomal Q99.9
    with more than three X chromosomes,
      female Q97.1
    analysis result R89.8
      bronchial washings R84.8
      cerebrospinal fluid R83.8
      cervix uteri NEC R87.89
      nasal secretions R84.8
      nipple discharge R89.8
      peritoneal fluid R85.89
      pleural fluid R84.8
      prostatic secretions R86.8
      saliva R85.89
      seminal fluid R86.8
      sputum R84.8
      synovial fluid R89.8
      throat scrapings R84.8
      vagina R87.89
      vulva R87.89
      wound secretions R89.8
    dicentric replacement Q93.2
    ring replacement Q93.2
    sex Q99.8
      female phenotype Q97.9
        specified NEC Q97.8
      male phenotype Q98.9
        specified NEC Q98.8
      structural male Q98.6
    specified NEC Q99.8
  clinical findings NEC R68.89
  coagulation D68.9
    newborn, transient P61.6
    profile R79.1
    time R79.1
  communication —see Fistula
  conjunctiva, vascular H11.41-
  coronary artery Q24.5
  cortisol-binding globulin E27.8

Abnormal, abnormality, abnormalities —
  (Continued)
  course, eustachian tube Q17.8
  creatinine clearance R94.4
  cytology
    anus R85.619
      atypical squamous cells cannot
        exclude high grade squamous
        intraepithelial lesion (ASC-H)
        R85.611
      atypical squamous cells of
        undetermined significance
        (ASC-US) R85.610
      cytologic evidence of malignancy
        R85.614
      high grade squamous intraepithelial
        lesion (HGSIL) R85.613
      human papillomavirus (HPV) DNA
        test
        high risk positive R85.81
        low risk postive R85.82
      inadequate smear R85.615
      low grade squamous intraepithelial
        lesion (LGSIL) R85.612
      satisfactory anal smear but lacking
        transformation zone R85.616
      specified NEC R85.618
      unsatisfactory smear R85.615
    female genital organs —see Abnormal,
      Papanicolaou (smear)
  dark adaptation curve H53.61
  dentofacial NEC —see Anomaly, dentofacial
  development, developmental Q89.9
    central nervous system Q07.9
  diagnostic imaging
    abdomen, abdominal region NEC
      R93.5
    biliary tract R93.2
    breast R92.8
    central nervous system NEC R90.89
    cerebrovascular NEC R90.89
    coronary circulation R93.1
    digestive tract NEC R93.3
    gastrointestinal (tract) R93.3
    genitourinary organs R93.8
    head R93.0
    heart R93.1
    intrathoracic organ NEC R93.8
    limbs R93.6
    liver R93.2
    lung (field) R91.8
    musculoskeletal system NEC R93.7
    retroperitoneum R93.5
    site specified NEC R93.8
    skin and subcutaneous tissue R93.8
    skull R93.0
    urinary organs R93.4
  direction, teeth, fully erupted M26.30
  ear ossicles, acquired NEC H74.39-
    ankylosis —see Ankylosis, ear ossicles
    discontinuity —see Discontinuity, ossicles,
      ear
    partial loss —see Loss, ossicles, ear
      (partial)
  Ebstein Q22.5
  echocardiogram R93.1
  echoencephalogram R90.81
  echogram —see Abnormal, diagnostic
    imaging
  electrocardiogram [ECG] [EKG] R94.31
  electroencephalogram [EEG] R94.01
  electrolyte —see Imbalance, electrolyte
  electromyogram [EMG] R94.131
  electro-oculogram [EOG] R94.110
  electrophysiological intracardiac studies
    R94.39
  electroretinogram [ERG] R94.111
  erythrocytes
    congenital, with perinatal jaundice D58.9
  feces (color) (contents) (mucus) R19.5

◀ New   ◀▥ Revised   ~~deleted~~ Deleted

Abnormal, abnormality, abnormalities —
(Continued)
  finding —see Findings, abnormal, without
      diagnosis
  fluid
    amniotic —see Abnormal, specimen,
        specified
    cerebrospinal —see Abnormal,
        cerebrospinal fluid
    peritoneal —see Abnormal, specimen,
        digestive organs
    pleural —see Abnormal, specimen,
        respiratory organs
    synovial —see Abnormal, specimen,
        specified
    thorax (bronchial washings) (pleural
        fluid) —see Abnormal, specimen,
        respiratory organs
    vaginal —see Abnormal, specimen, female
        genital organs
  form
    teeth K00.2
    uterus —see Anomaly, uterus
  function studies
    auditory R94.120
    bladder R94.8
    brain R94.09
    cardiovascular R94.30
    ear R94.128
    endocrine NEC R94.7
    eye NEC R94.118
    kidney R94.4
    liver R94.5
    nervous system
      central NEC R94.09
      peripheral NEC R94.138
    pancreas R94.8
    placenta R94.8
    pulmonary R94.2
    special senses NEC R94.128
    spleen R94.8
    thyroid R94.6
    vestibular R94.121
  gait —see Gait
    hysterical F44.4
  gastrin secretion E16.4
  globulin R77.1
    cortisol-binding E27.8
    thyroid-binding E07.89
  glomerular, minor (see also N00-N07 with
      fourth character .0) N05.0
  glucagon secretion E16.3
  glucose tolerance (test) (non-fasting)
      R73.09
  gravitational (G) forces or states (effect of)
      T75.81
  hair (color) (shaft) L67.9
    specified NEC L67.8
  hard tissue formation in pulp (dental)
      K04.3
  head movement R25.0
  heart
    rate R00.9
      specified NEC R00.8
    shadow R93.1
    sounds NEC R01.2
  hemoglobin (disease) (see also Disease,
      hemoglobin) D58.2
    trait —see Trait, hemoglobin, abnormal
  histology NEC R89.7
  immunological findings R89.4
    in serum R76.9
      specified NEC R76.8
  increase in appetite R63.2
  involuntary movement —see Abnormal,
      movement, involuntary
  jaw closure M26.51
  karyotype R89.8
  kidney function test R94.4
  knee jerk R29.2
  leukocyte (cell) (differential) NEC D72.9

Abnormal, abnormality, abnormalities —
(Continued)
  liver
  loss of
    height R29.890
    weight R63.4
  mammogram NEC R92.8
    calcification (calculus) R92.1
    microcalcification R92.0
  Mantoux test R76.11
  movement (disorder) —see also Disorder,
      movement
    head R25.0
    involuntary R25.9
      fasciculation R25.3
      of head R25.0
      spasm R25.2
      specified type NEC R25.8
      tremor R25.1
  myoglobin (Aberdeen) (Annapolis) R89.7
  neonatal screening P09
  oculomotor study R94.113
  palmar creases Q82.8
  Papanicolaou (smear)
    anus R85.619
      atypical squamous cells cannot
          exclude high grade squamous
          intraepithelial lesion (ASC-H)
          R85.611
      atypical squamous cells of undetermined
          significance (ASC-US) R85.610
      cytologic evidence of malignancy
          R85.614
      high grade squamous intraepithelial
          lesion (HGSIL) R85.613
      human papillomavirus (HPV)
          DNA test
          high risk positive R85.81
          low risk postive R85.82
      inadequate smear R85.615
      low grade squamous intraepithelial
          lesion (LGSIL) R85.612
      satisfactory anal smear but lacking
          transformation zone R85.616
      specified NEC R85.618
      unsatisfactory smear R85.615
    bronchial washings R84.6
    cerebrospinal fluid R83.6
    cervix R87.619
      atypical squamous cells cannot
          exclude high grade squamous
          intraepithelial lesion (ASC-H)
          R87.611
      atypical squamous cells of undetermined
          significance (ASC-US) R87.610
      cytologic evidence of malignancy
          R87.614
      high grade squamous intraepithelial
          lesion (HGSIL) R87.613
      inadequate smear R87.615
      low grade squamous intraepithelial
          lesion (LGSIL) R87.612
      non-atypical endometrial cells
          R87.618
      satisfactory cervical smear but
          lacking transformation zone
          R87.616
      specified NEC R87.618
      thin preparaton R87.619
      unsatisfactory smear R87.615
    nasal secretions R84.6
    nipple discharge R89.6
    peritoneal fluid R85.69
    pleural fluid R84.6
    prostatic secretions R86.6
    saliva R85.69
    seminal fluid R86.6
    sites NEC R89.6
    sputum R84.6
    synovial fluid R89.6
    throat scrapings R84.6

Abnormal, abnormality, abnormalities —
(Continued)
  Papanicolaou (smear) (Continued)
    vagina R87.629
      atypical squamous cells cannot
          exclude high grade squamous
          intraepithelial lesion (ASC-H)
          R87.621
      atypical squamous cells of
          undetermined significance
          (ASC-US) R87.620
      cytologic evidence of malignancy
          R87.624
      high grade squamous intraepithelial
          lesion (HGSIL) R87.623
      inadequate smear R87.625
      low grade squamous intraepithelial
          lesion (LGSIL) R87.622
      specified NEC R87.628
      thin preparation R87.629
      unsatisfactory smear R87.625
    vulva R87.69
    wound secretions R89.6
  partial thromboplastin time (PTT) R79.1
  pelvis (bony) —see Deformity, pelvis
  percussion, chest (tympany) R09.89
  periods (grossly) —see Menstruation
  phonocardiogram R94.39
  plantar reflex R29.2
  plasma
    protein R77.9
      specified NEC R77.8
    viscosity R70.1
  pleural (folds) Q34.0
  posture R29.3
  product of conception O02.9
    specified type NEC O02.89
  prothrombin time (PT) R79.1
  pulmonary
    artery, congenital Q25.79
    function, newborn P28.89
    test results R94.2
  pulsations in neck R00.2
  pupillary H21.56-
    function (reaction) (reflex) —see Anomaly,
        pupil, function
  radiological examination —see Abnormal,
      diagnostic imaging
  red blood cell (s) (morphology) (volume)
      R71.8
  reflex —see Reflex
  renal function test R94.4
  response to nerve stimulation R94.130
  retinal correspondence H53.31
  retinal function study R94.111
  rhythm, heart —see also Arrhythmia
  saliva —see Abnormal, specimen, digestive
      organs
  scan
    kidney R94.4
    liver R93.2
    thyroid R94.6
  secretion
    gastrin E16.4
    glucagon E16.3
  semen, seminal fluid —see Abnormal,
      specimen, male genital organs
  serum level (of)
    acid phosphatase R74.8
    alkaline phosphatase R74.8
    amylase R74.8
    enzymes R74.9
      specified NEC R74.8
    lipase R74.8
    triacylglycerol lipase R74.8
  shape
    gravid uterus —see Anomaly, uterus
  sinus venosus Q21.1
  size, tooth, teeth K00.2
  spacing, tooth, teeth, fully erupted
      M26.30

Abnormal, abnormality, abnormalities — *(Continued)*
specimen
digestive organs (peritoneal fluid) (saliva) R85.9
cytology R85.69
drug level R85.2
enzyme level R85.0
histology R85.7
hormones R85.1
immunology R85.4
microbiology R85.5
nonmedicinal level R85.3
specified type NEC R85.89
female genital organs (secretions) (smears) R87.9
cytology R87.69
cervix R87.619
human papillomavirus (HPV) DNA test
high risk positive R87.810
low risk positive R87.820
inadequate (unsatisfactory) smear R87.615
non-atypical endometrial cells R87.618
specified NEC R87.618
vagina R87.629
human papillomavirus (HPV) DNA test
high risk positive R87.811
low risk positive R87.821
inadequate (unsatisfactory) smear R87.625
vulva R87.69
drug level R87.2
enzyme level R87.0
histological R87.7
hormones R87.1
immunology R87.4
microbiology R87.5
nonmedicinal level R87.3
specified type NEC R87.89
male genital organs (prostatic secretions) (semen) R86.9
cytology R86.6
drug level R86.2
enzyme level R86.0
histological R86.7
hormones R86.1
immunology R86.4
microbiology R86.5
nonmedicinal level R86.3
specified type NEC R86.8
nipple discharge —*see* Abnormal, specimen, specified
respiratory organs (bronchial washings) (nasal secretions) (pleural fluid) (sputum) R84.9
cytology R84.6
drug level R84.2
enzyme level R84.0
histology R84.7
hormones R84.1
immunology R84.4
microbiology R84.5
nonmedicinal level R84.3
specified type NEC R84.8
specified organ, system and tissue NOS R89.9
cytology R89.6
drug level R89.2
enzyme level R89.0
histology R89.7
hormones R89.1
immunology R89.4
microbiology R89.5
nonmedicinal level R89.3
specified type NEC R89.8
synovial fluid —*see* Abnormal, specimen, specified

Abnormal, abnormality, abnormalities — *(Continued)*
specimen *(Continued)*
thorax (bronchial washings) (pleural fluids) —*see* Abnormal, specimen, respiratory organs
vagina (secretion) (smear) R87.629
vulva (secretion) (smear) R87.69
wound secretion —*see* Abnormal, specimen, specified
spermatozoa —*see* Abnormal, specimen, male genital organs
sputum (amount) (color) (odor) R09.3
stool (color) (contents) (mucus) R19.5
bloody K92.1
guaiac positive R19.5
synchondrosis Q78.8
thermography (*see also* Abnormal, diagnostic imaging) R93.8
thyroid-binding globulin E07.89
tooth, teeth (form) (size) K00.2
toxicology (findings) R78.9
transport protein E88.09
tumor marker NEC R97.8
ultrasound results —*see* Abnormal, diagnostic imaging
umbilical cord complicating delivery O69.9
urination NEC R39.19
urine (constituents) R82.90
bile R82.2
cytological examination R82.8
drugs R82.5
fat R82.0
glucose R81
heavy metals R82.6
hemoglobin R82.3
histological examination R82.8
ketones R82.4
microbiological examination (culture) R82.7
myoglobin R82.1
positive culture R82.7
protein —*see* Proteinuria
specified substance NEC R82.99
chromoabnormality NEC R82.91
substances nonmedical R82.6
uterine hemorrhage —*see* Hemorrhage, uterus
vectorcardiogram R94.39
visually evoked potential (VEP) R94.112
white blood cells D72.9
specified NEC D72.89
X-ray examination —*see* Abnormal, diagnostic imaging
Abnormity (any organ or part) —*see* Anomaly
Abocclusion M26.29
hemolytic disease (newborn) P55.1
incompatibility reaction ABO —*see* Complication (s), transfusion, incompatibility reaction, ABO
Abolition, language R48.8
Aborter, habitual or recurrent —*see* Loss (of), pregnancy, recurrent
Abortion (complete) (spontaneous) O03.9
with
retained products of conception - see Abortion, incomplete
attempted (elective) (failed) O07.4
complicated by O07.30
afibrinogenemia O07.1
cardiac arrest O07.36
chemical damage of pelvic organ (s) O07.34
circulatory collapse O07.31
cystitis O07.38
defibrination syndrome O07.1
electrolyte imbalance O07.33
embolism (air) (amniotic fluid) (blood clot) (fat) (pulmonary) (septic) (soap) O07.2
endometritis O07.0

Abortion *(Continued)*
attempted *(Continued)*
complicated by *(Continued)*
genital tract and pelvic infection O07.0
hemolysis O07.1
hemorrhage (delayed) (excessive) O07.1
infection
genital tract or pelvic O07.0
urinary tract tract O07.38
intravascular coagulation O07.1
laceration of pelvic organ (s) O07.34
metabolic disorder O07.33
oliguria O07.32
oophoritis O07.0
parametritis O07.0
pelvic peritonitis O07.0
perforation of pelvic organ (s) O07.34
renal failure or shutdown O07.32
salpingitis or salpingo-oophoritis O07.0
sepsis O07.37
shock O07.31
specified condition NEC O07.39
tubular necrosis (renal) O07.32
uremia O07.32
urinary tract infection O07.38
venous complication NEC O07.35
embolism (air) (amniotic fluid) (blood clot) (fat) (pulmonary) (septic) (soap) O07.2
complicated (by) (following) O03.80
afibrinogenemia O03.6
cardiac arrest O03.86
chemical damage of pelvic organ (s) O03.84
circulatory collapse O03.81
cystitis O03.88
defibrination syndrome O03.6
electrolyte imbalance O03.83
embolism (air) (amniotic fluid) (blood clot) (fat) (pulmonary) (septic) (soap) O03.7
endometritis O03.5
genital tract and pelvic infection O03.5
hemolysis O03.6
hemorrhage (delayed) (excessive) O03.6
infection
genital tract or pelvic O03.5
urinary tract O03.88
intravascular coagulation O03.6
laceration of pelvic organ (s) O03.84
metabolic disorder O03.83
oliguria O03.82
oophoritis O03.5
parametritis O03.5
pelvic peritonitis O03.5
perforation of pelvic organ (s) O03.84
renal failure or shutdown O03.82
salpingitis or salpingo-oophoritis O03.5
sepsis O03.87
shock O03.81
specified condition NEC O03.89
tubular necrosis (renal) O03.82
uremia O03.82
urinary tract infection O03.88
venous complication NEC O03.85
embolism (air) (amniotic fluid) (blood clot) (fat) (pulmonary) (septic) (soap) O03.7
failed —*see* Abortion, attempted
habitual or recurrent N96
with current abortion —*see* categories O03-O06
without current pregnancy N96
care in current pregnancy O26.2-
incomplete (spontaneous) O03.4
complicated (by) (following) O03.30
afibrinogenemia O03.1
cardiac arrest O03.36
chemical damage of pelvic organ (s) O03.34
circulatory collapse O03.31
cystitis O03.38

◀ New ◀▥ Revised ~~deleted~~ Deleted

Abortion (*Continued*)
  incomplete (*Continued*)
    complicated (*Continued*)
      defibrination syndrome O03.1
      electrolyte imbalance O03.33
      embolism (air) (amniotic fluid) (blood
        clot) (fat) (pulmonary) (septic)
        (soap) O03.2
      endometritis O03.0
      genital tract and pelvic infection O03.0
      hemolysis O03.1
      hemorrhage (delayed) (excessive)
        O03.1
      infection
        genital tract or pelvic O03.0
        urinary tract O03.38
      intravascular coagulation O03.1
      laceration of pelvic organ (s) O03.34
      metabolic disorder O03.33
      oliguria O03.32
      oophoritis O03.0
      parametritis O03.0
      pelvic peritonitis O03.0
      perforation of pelvic organ (s) O03.34
      renal failure or shutdown O03.32
      salpingitis or salpingo-oophoritis O03.0
      sepsis O03.37
      shock O03.31
      specified condition NEC O03.39
      tubular necrosis (renal) O03.32
      uremia O03.32
      urinary infection O03.38
      venous complication NEC O03.35
        embolism (air) (amniotic fluid) (blood
          clot) (fat) (pulmonary) (septic)
          (soap) O03.2
  induced (encounter for) Z33.2
    complicated by O04.80
      afibrinogenemia O04.6
      cardiac arrest O04.86
      chemical damage of pelvic organ (s)
        O04.84
      circulatory collapse O04.81
      cystitis O04.88
      defibrination syndrome O04.6
      electrolyte imbalance O04.83
      embolism (air) (amniotic fluid) (blood
        clot) (fat) (pulmonary) (septic)
        (soap) O04.7
      endometritis O04.5
      genital tract and pelvic infection O04.5
      hemolysis O04.6
      hemorrhage (delayed) (excessive)
        O04.6
      infection
        genital tract or pelvic O04.5
        urinary tract O04.88
      intravascular coagulation O04.6
      laceration of pelvic organ (s) O04.84
      metabolic disorder O04.83
      oliguria O04.82
      oophoritis O04.5
      parametritis O04.5
      pelvic peritonitis O04.5
      perforation of pelvic organ (s) O04.84
      renal failure or shutdown O04.82
      salpingitis or salpingo-oophoritis O04.5
      sepsis O04.87
      shock O04.81
      specified condition NEC O04.89
      tubular necrosis (renal) O04.82
      uremia O04.82
      urinary tract infection O04.88
      venous complication NEC O04.85
        embolism (air) (amniotic fluid) (blood
          clot) (fat) (pulmonary) (septic)
          (soap) O04.7
  missed O02.1
  spontaneous —*see* Abortion (complete)
    (spontaneous)
    threatened O20.0

Abortion (*Continued*)
  threatened (spontaneous) O20.0
  tubal O00.1
Abortus fever A23.1
Aboulomania F60.7
Abrami's disease D59.8
Abramov-Fiedler myocarditis (acute isolated
  myocarditis) I40.1
Abrasion T14.8
  abdomen, abdominal (wall) S30.811
  alveolar process S00.512
  ankle S90.51-
  antecubital space —*see* Abrasion, elbow
  anus S30.817
  arm (upper) S40.81-
  auditory canal —*see* Abrasion, ear
  auricle —*see* Abrasion, ear
  axilla —*see* Abrasion, arm
  back, lower S30.810
  breast S20.11-
  brow S00.81
  buttock S30.810
  calf —*see* Abrasion, leg
  canthus —*see* Abrasion, eyelid
  cheek S00.81
    internal S00.512
  chest wall —*see* Abrasion, thorax
  chin S00.81
  clitoris S30.814
  cornea S05.0-
  costal region —*see* Abrasion, thorax
  dental K03.1
  digit (s)
    foot —*see* Abrasion, toe
    hand —*see* Abrasion, finger
  ear S00.41-
  elbow S50.31-
  epididymis S30.813
  epigastric region S30.811
  epiglottis S10.11
  esophagus (thoracic) S27.818
    cervical S10.11
  eyebrow —*see* Abrasion, eyelid
  eyelid S00.21-
  face S00.81
  finger (s) S60.41-
    index S60.41-
    little S60.41-
    middle S60.41-
    ring S60.41-
  flank S30.811
  foot (except toe (s) alone) S90.81-
    toe —*see* Abrasion, toe
  forearm S50.81-
    elbow only —*see* Abrasion, elbow
  forehead S00.81
  genital organs, external
    female S30.816
    male S30.815
  groin S30.811
  gum S00.512
  hand S60.51-
  head S00.91
    ear —*see* Abrasion, ear
    eyelid —*see* Abrasion, eyelid
    lip S00.511
    nose S00.31
    oral cavity S00.512
    scalp S00.01
    specified site NEC S00.81
  heel —*see* Abrasion, foot
  hip S70.21-
  inguinal region S30.811
  interscapular region S20.419
  jaw S00.81
  knee S80.21-
  labium (majus) (minus) S30.814
  larynx S10.11
  leg (lower) S80.81-
    knee —*see* Abrasion, knee
    upper —*see* Abrasion, thigh

Abrasion (*Continued*)
  lip S00.511
  lower back S30.810
  lumbar region S30.810
  malar region S00.81
  mammary —*see* Abrasion, breast
  mastoid region S00.81
  mouth S00.512
  nail
    finger —*see* Abrasion, finger
    toe —*see* Abrasion, toe
  nape S10.81
  nasal S00.31
  neck S10.91
    specified site NEC S10.81
    throat S10.11
  nose S00.31
  occipital region S00.01
  oral cavity S00.512
  orbital region —*see* Abrasion, eyelid
  palate S00.512
  palm —*see* Abrasion, hand
  parietal region S00.01
  pelvis S30.810
  penis S30.812
  perineum
    female S30.814
    male S30.810
  periocular area —*see* Abrasion, eyelid
  phalanges
    finger —*see* Abrasion, finger
    toe —*see* Abrasion, toe
  pharynx S10.11
  pinna —*see* Abrasion, ear
  popliteal space —*see* Abrasion, knee
  prepuce S30.812
  pubic region S30.810
  pudendum
    female S30.816
    male S30.815
  sacral region S30.810
  scalp S00.01
  scapular region —*see* Abrasion, shoulder
  scrotum S30.813
  shin —*see* Abrasion, leg
  shoulder S40.21-
  skin NEC T14.8
  sternal region S20.319
  submaxillary region S00.81
  submental region S00.81
  subungual
    finger (s) —*see* Abrasion, finger
    toe (s) —*see* Abrasion, toe
  supraclavicular fossa S10.81
  supraorbital S00.81
  temple S00.81
  temporal region S00.81
  testis S30.813
  thigh S70.31-
  thorax, thoracic (wall) S20.91
    back S20.41-
    front S20.31-
  throat S10.11
  thumb S60.31-
  toe (s) (lesser) S90.416
    great S90.41-
  tongue S00.512
  tooth, teeth (dentifrice) (habitual) (hard
    tissues) (occupational) (ritual)
    (traditional) K03.1
  trachea S10.11
  tunica vaginalis S30.813
  tympanum, tympanic membrane —*see*
    Abrasion, ear
  uvula S00.512
  vagina S30.814
  vocal cords S10.11
  vulva S30.814
  wrist S60.81-
Abrism —*see* Poisoning, food, noxious,
  plant

◀ New   ◀||| Revised   ~~deleted~~ Deleted

Abruptio placentae O45.9-
  with
    afibrinogenemia O45.01-
    coagulation defect O45.00-
      specified NEC O45.09-
    disseminated intravascular coagulation
      O45.02-
    hypofibrinogenemia O45.01-
    specified NEC O45.8-
Abruption, placenta —*see* Abruptio placentae
Abscess (connective tissue) (embolic) (fistulous)
  (infective) (metastatic) (multiple)
  (pernicious) (pyogenic) (septic) L02.91
  with
    diverticular disease (intestine) K57.80
      with bleeding K57.81
      large intestine K57.20
        with
          bleeding K57.21
          small intestine K57.40
            with bleeding K57.41
      small intestine K57.00
        with
          bleeding K57.01
          large intestine K57.40
            with bleeding K57.41
    lymphangitis - code by site under
      Abscess
  abdomen, abdominal
    cavity K65.1
    wall L02.211
  abdominopelvic K65.1
  accessory sinus —*see* Sinusitis
  adrenal (capsule) (gland) E27.8
  alveolar K04.7
    with sinus K04.6
  amebic A06.4
    brain (and liver or lung abscess) A06.6
    genitourinary tract A06.82
    liver (without mention of brain or lung
      abscess) A06.4
    lung (and liver) (without mention of brain
      abscess) A06.5
    specified site NEC A06.89
    spleen A06.89
  anerobic A48.0
  ankle —*see* Abscess, lower limb
  anorectal K61.2
  antecubital space —*see* Abscess, upper limb
  antrum (chronic) (Highmore) —*see* Sinusitis,
    maxillary
  anus K61.0
  apical (tooth) K04.7
    with sinus (alveolar) K04.6
  appendix K35.3
  areola (acute) (chronic) (nonpuerperal) N61
    puerperal, postpartum or gestational —*see*
      Infection, nipple
  arm (any part) —*see* Abscess, upper limb
  artery (wall) I77.89
  atheromatous I77.2
  auricle, ear —*see* Abscess, ear, external
  axilla (region) L02.41-
    lymph gland or node L04.2
  back (any part, except buttock) L02.212
  Bartholin's gland N75.1
    with
      abortion —*see* Abortion, by type
        complicated by, sepsis
      ectopic or molar pregnancy O08.0
      following ectopic or molar pregnancy
        O08.0
  Bezold's —*see* Mastoiditis, acute
  bilharziasis B65.1
  bladder (wall) —*see* Cystitis, specified type
    NEC
  bone (subperiosteal) —*see also* Osteomyelitis,
    specified type NEC
    accessory sinus (chronic) —*see* Sinusitis
    chronic or old —*see* Osteomyelitis, chronic
    jaw (lower) (upper) M27.2

Abscess (Continued)
  bone (Continued)
    mastoid —*see* Mastoiditis, acute,
      subperiosteal
    petrous —*see* Petrositis
    spinal (tuberculous) A18.01
      nontuberculous —*see* Osteomyelitis,
        vertebra
  bowel K63.0
  brain (any part) (cystic) (otogenic) G06.0
    amebic (with abscess of any other site)
      A06.6
    gonococcal A54.82
    pheomycotic (chromomycotic) B43.1
    tuberculous A17.81
  breast (acute) (chronic) (nonpuerperal) N61
    newborn P39.0
    puerperal, postpartum, gestational —*see*
      Mastitis, obstetric, purulent
  broad ligament N73.2
    acute N73.0
    chronic N73.1
  Brodie's (localized) (chronic) M86.8X-
  bronchi J98.09
  buccal cavity K12.2
  bulbourethral gland N34.0
  bursa M71.00
    ankle M71.07-
    elbow M71.02-
    foot M71.07-
    hand M71.04-
    hip M71.05-
    knee M71.06-
    multiple sites M71.09
    pharyngeal J39.1
    shoulder M71.01-
    specified site NEC M71.08
    wrist M71.03-
  buttock L02.31
  canthus —*see* Blepharoconjunctivitis
  cartilage —*see* Disorder, cartilage, specified
    type NEC
  cecum K35.3
  cerebellum, cerebellar G06.0
    sequelae G09
  cerebral (embolic) G06.0
    sequelae G09
  cervical (meaning neck) L02.11
    lymph gland or node L04.0
  cervix (stump) (uteri) —*see* Cervicitis
  cheek (external) L02.01
    inner K12.2
  chest J86.9
    with fistula J86.0
    wall L02.213
  chin L02.01
  choroid —*see* Inflammation, chorioretinal
  circumtonsillar J36
  cold (lung) (tuberculous) —*see also*
    Tuberculosis, abscess, lung
    articular —*see* Tuberculosis, joint
  colon (wall) K63.0
  colostomy K94.02
  conjunctiva —*see* Conjunctivitis, acute
  cornea H16.31-
  corpus
    cavernosum N48.21
    luteum —*see* Oophoritis
  Cowper's gland N34.0
  cranium G06.0
  cul-de-sac (Douglas') (posterior) —*see*
    Peritonitis, pelvic, female
  cutaneous —*see* Abscess, by site
  dental K04.7
    with sinus (alveolar) K04.6
  dentoalveolar K04.7
    with sinus K04.6
  diaphragm, diaphragmatic K65.1
  Douglas' cul-de-sac or pouch —*see*
    Peritonitis, pelvic, female
  Dubois A50.59

Abscess (Continued)
  ear (middle) —*see also* Otitis, media,
    suppurative
    acute —*see* Otitis, media, suppurative,
      acute
    external H60.0-
  entamebic —*see* Abscess, amebic
  enterostomy K94.12
  epididymis N45.4
  epidural G06.2
    brain G06.0
    spinal cord G06.1
  epiglottis J38.7
  epiploon, epiploic K65.1
  erysipelatous —*see* Erysipelas
  esophagus K20.8
  ethmoid (bone) (chronic) (sinus) J32.2
  external auditory canal —*see* Abscess, ear,
    external
  extradural G06.2
    brain G06.0
      sequelae G09
    spinal cord G06.1
  extraperitoneal K68.19
  eye —*see* Endophthalmitis, purulent
  eyelid H00.03-
  face (any part, except ear, eye and nose)
    L02.01
  fallopian tube —*see* Salpingitis
  fascia M72.8
  fauces J39.1
  fecal K63.0
  femoral (region) —*see* Abscess, lower
    limb
  filaria, filarial —*see* Infestation, filarial
  finger (any) —*see also* Abscess, hand
    nail —*see* Cellulitis, finger
  foot L02.61-
  forehead L02.01
  frontal sinus (chronic) J32.1
  gallbladder K81.0
  genital organ or tract
    female (external) N76.4
    male N49.9
      multiple sites N49.8
      specified NEC N49.8
  gestational mammary O91.11-
  gestational subareolar O91.11-
  gingival K05.21
  gland, glandular (lymph) (acute) —*see*
    Lymphadenitis, acute
  gluteal (region) L02.31
  gonorrheal —*see* Gonococcus
  groin L02.214
  gum K05.21
  hand L02.51-
  head NEC L02.811
    face (any part, except ear, eye and nose)
      L02.01
  heart —*see* Carditis
  heel —*see* Abscess, foot
  helminthic —*see* Infestation, helminth
  hepatic (cholangitic) (hematogenic)
    (lymphogenic) (pylephlebitic) K75.0
    amebic A06.4
  hip (region) —*see* Abscess, lower limb
  ileocecal K35.3
  ileostomy (bud) K94.12
  iliac (region) L02.214
    fossa K35.3
  infraclavicular (fossa) —*see* Abscess, upper
    limb
  inguinal (region) L02.214
    lymph gland or node L04.1
  intestine, intestinal NEC K63.0
    rectal K61.1
  intra-abdominal (*see also* Abscess,
    peritoneum) K65.1
    postoperative T81.4
    retroperitoneal K68.11
  intracranial G06.0

Abscess (Continued)

intramammary —see Abscess, breast
intraorbital —see Abscess, orbit
intraperitoneal K65.1
intrasphincteric (anus) K61.4
intraspinal G06.1
intratonsillar J36
ischiorectal (fossa) K61.3
jaw (bone) (lower) (upper) M27.2
joint —see Arthritis, pyogenic or pyemic
  spine (tuberculous) A18.01
    nontuberculous —see Spondylopathy, infective
kidney N15.1
  with calculus N20.0
    with hydronephrosis N13.6
  puerperal (postpartum) O86.21
knee —see also Abscess, lower limb
  joint M00.9
labium (majus) (minus) N76.4
lacrimal
  caruncle —see Inflammation, lacrimal, passages, acute
  gland —see Dacryoadenitis
  passages (duct) (sac) —see Inflammation, lacrimal, passages, acute
lacunar N34.0
larynx J38.7
lateral (alveolar) K04.7
  with sinus K04.6
leg (any part) —see Abscess, lower limb
lens H27.8
lingual K14.0
  tonsil J36
lip K13.0
Littre's gland N34.0
liver (cholangitic) (hematogenic) (lymphogenic) (pylephlebitic) (pyogenic) K75.0
  amebic (due to Entamoeba histolytica) (dysenteric) (tropical) A06.4
    with
      brain abscess (and liver or lung abscess) A06.6
      lung abscess A06.5
loin (region) L02.211
lower limb L02.41-
lumbar (tuberculous) A18.01
  nontuberculous L02.212
lung (miliary) (putrid) J85.2
  with pneumonia J85.1
    due to specified organism (see Pneumonia, in (due to))
  amebic (with liver abscess) A06.5
    with
      brain abscess A06.6
      pneumonia A06.5
lymph, lymphatic, gland or node (acute) —see also Lymphadenitis, acute
  mesentery I88.0
malar M27.2
mammary gland —see Abscess, breast
marginal, anus K61.0
mastoid —see Mastoiditis, acute
maxilla, maxillary M27.2
  molar (tooth) K04.7
    with sinus K04.6
  premolar K04.7
  sinus (chronic) J32.0
mediastinum J85.3
meibomian gland —see Hordeolum
meninges G06.2
mesentery, mesenteric K65.1
mesosalpinx —see Salpingitis
mons pubis L02.215
mouth (floor) K12.2
muscle —see Myositis, infective
myocardium I40.0
nabothian (follicle) —see Cervicitis
nasal J32.9
nasopharyngeal J39.1

Abscess (Continued)

navel L02.216
  newborn P38.9
    with mild hemorrhage P38.1
    without hemorrhage P38.9
neck (region) L02.11
  lymph gland or node L04.0
nephritic —see Abscess, kidney
nipple N61
  associated with
    lactation —see Pregnancy, complicated by,
    pregnancy —see Pregnancy, complicated by
nose (external) (fossa) (septum) J34.0
  sinus (chronic) —see Sinusitis
omentum K65.1
operative wound T81.4
orbit, orbital —see Cellulitis, orbit
otogenic G06.0
ovary, ovarian (corpus luteum) —see Oophoritis
oviduct —see Oophoritis
palate (soft) K12.2
  hard M27.2
palmar (space) —see Abscess, hand
pancreas (duct) —see Pancreatitis, acute
parafrenal N48.21
parametric, parametrium N73.2
  acute N73.0
  chronic N73.1
paranephric N15.1
parapancreatic —see Pancreatitis, acute
parapharyngeal J39.0
pararectal K61.1
parasinus —see Sinusitis
parauterine (see also Disease, pelvis, inflammatory) N73.2
paravaginal —see Vaginitis
parietal region (scalp) L02.811
parodontal K05.21
parotid (duct) (gland) K11.3
  region K12.2
pectoral (region) L02.213
pelvis, pelvic
  female —see Disease, pelvis, inflammatory
  male, peritoneal K65.1
penis N48.21
  gonococcal (accessory gland) (periurethral) A54.1
perianal K61.0
periapical K04.7
  with sinus (alveolar) K04.6
periappendicular K35.3
pericardial I30.1
pericecal K35.3
pericemental K05.21
pericholecystic —see Cholecystitis, acute
pericoronal K05.21
peridental K05.21
perimetric (see also Disease, pelvis, inflammatory) N73.2
perinephric, perinephritic —see Abscess, kidney
perineum, perineal (superficial) L02.215
  urethra N34.0
periodontal (parietal) K05.21
  apical K04.7
periosteum, periosteal —see also Osteomyelitis, specified type NEC
  with osteomyelitis —see also Osteomyelitis, specified type NEC
    acute —see Osteomyelitis, acute
    chronic —see Osteomyelitis, chronic
peripharyngeal J39.0
peripleuritic J86.9
  with fistula J86.0
periprostatic N41.2
perirectal K61.1
perirenal (tissue) —see Abscess, kidney
perisinuous (nose) —see Sinusitis

Abscess (Continued)

peritoneum, peritoneal (perforated) (ruptured) K65.1
  with appendicitis K35.3
  pelvic
    female —see Peritonitis, pelvic, female
    male K65.1
  postoperative T81.4
  puerperal, postpartum, childbirth O85
  tuberculous A18.31
peritonsillar J36
perityphlic K35.3
periureteral N28.89
periurethral N34.0
  gonococcal (accessory gland) (periurethral) A54.1
periuterine (see also Disease, pelvis, inflammatory) N73.2
perivesical —see Cystitis, specified type NEC
petrous bone —see Petrositis
phagedenic NOS L02.91
  chancroid A57
pharynx, pharyngeal (lateral) J39.1
pilonidal L05.01
pituitary (gland) E23.6
pleura J86.9
  with fistula J86.0
popliteal —see Abscess, lower limb
postcecal K35.3
postlaryngeal J38.7
postnasal J34.0
postoperative (any site) T81.4
  retroperitoneal K68.11
postpharyngeal J39.0
posttonsillar J36
post-typhoid A01.09
pouch of Douglas —see Peritonitis, pelvic, female
premammary —see Abscess, breast
prepatellar —see Abscess, lower limb
prostate N41.2
  gonococcal (acute) (chronic) A54.22
psoas muscle K68.12
puerperal - code by site under Puerperal, abscess
pulmonary —see Abscess, lung
pulp, pulpal (dental) K04.0
rectovaginal septum K63.0
rectovesical —see Cystitis, specified type NEC
rectum K61.1
renal —see Abscess, kidney
retina —see Inflammation, chorioretinal
retrobulbar —see Abscess, orbit
retrocecal K65.1
retrolaryngeal J38.7
retromammary —see Abscess, breast
retroperitoneal NEC K68.19
  postprocedural K68.11
retropharyngeal J39.0
retrouterine —see Peritonitis, pelvic, female
retrovesical —see Cystitis, specified type NEC
root, tooth K04.7
  with sinus (alveolar) K04.6
round ligament (see also Disease, pelvis, inflammatory) N73.2
rupture (spontaneous) NOS L02.91
sacrum (tuberculous) A18.01
  nontuberculous M46.28
salivary (duct) (gland) K11.3
scalp (any part) L02.811
scapular —see Osteomyelitis, specified type NEC
sclera —see Scleritis
scrofulous (tuberculous) A18.2
scrotum N49.2
seminal vesicle N49.0
septal, dental K04.7
  with sinus (alveolar) K04.6
serous —see Periostitis
shoulder (region) —see Abscess, upper limb
sigmoid K63.0

Abscess *(Continued)*
  sinus (accessory) (chronic) (nasal) —*see also*
      Sinusitis
    intracranial venous (any) G06.0
  Skene's duct or gland N34.0
  skin —*see* Abscess, by site
  specified site NEC L02.818
  spermatic cord N49.1
  sphenoidal (sinus) (chronic) J32.3
  spinal cord (any part) (staphylococcal) G06.1
    tuberculous A17.81
  spine (column) (tuberculous) A18.01
    epidural G06.1
    nontuberculous —*see* Osteomyelitis,
        vertebra
  spleen D73.3
    amebic A06.89
  stitch T81.4
  subarachnoid G06.2
    brain G06.0
    spinal cord G06.1
  subareolar —*see* Abscess, breast
  subcecal K35.3
  subcutaneous —*see also* Abscess, by site
    pheomycotic (chromomycotic) B43.2
  subdiaphragmatic K65.1
  subdural G06.2
    brain G06.0
      sequelae G09
    spinal cord G06.1
  subgaleal L02.811
  subhepatic K65.1
  sublingual K12.2
    gland K11.3
  submammary —*see* Abscess, breast
  submandibular (region) (space) (triangle)
      K12.2
    gland K11.3
  submaxillary (region) L02.01
    gland K11.3
  submental L02.01
    gland K11.3
  subperiosteal —*see* Osteomyelitis, specified
      type NEC
  subphrenic K65.1
    postoperative T81.4
  suburethral N34.0
  sudoriparous L75.8
  supraclavicular (fossa) —*see* Abscess, upper
      limb
  suprapelvic, acute N73.0
  suprarenal (capsule) (gland) E27.8
  sweat gland L74.8
  tear duct —*see* Inflammation, lacrimal,
      passages, acute
  temple L02.01
  temporal region L02.01
  temporosphenoidal G06.0
  tendon (sheath) M65.00
    ankle M65.07-
    foot M65.07-
    forearm M65.03-
    hand M65.04-
    lower leg M65.06-
    pelvic region M65.05-
    shoulder region M65.01-
    specified site NEC M65.08
    thigh M65.05-
    upper arm M65.02-
  testis N45.4
  thigh —*see* Abscess, lower limb
  thorax J86.9
    with fistula J86.0
  throat J39.1
  thumb —*see also* Abscess, hand
    nail —*see* Cellulitis, finger
  thymus (gland) E32.1
  thyroid (gland) E06.0
  toe (any) —*see also* Abscess, foot
    nail —*see* Cellulitis, toe
  tongue (staphylococcal) K14.0

Abscess *(Continued)*
  tonsil (s) (lingual) J36
  tonsillopharyngeal J36
  tooth, teeth (root) K04.7
    with sinus (alveolar) K04.6
    supporting structures NEC K05.21
  trachea J39.8
  trunk L02.219
    abdominal wall L02.211
    back L02.212
    chest wall L02.213
    groin L02.214
    perineum L02.215
    umbilicus L02.216
  tubal —*see* Salpingitis
  tuberculous —*see* Tuberculosis, abscess
  tubo-ovarian —*see* Salpingo-oophoritis
  tunica vaginalis N49.1
  umbilicus L02.216
  upper
    limb L02.41-
    respiratory J39.8
  urethral (gland) N34.0
  urinary N34.0
  uterus, uterine (wall) —*see also* Endometritis
    ligament (*see also* Disease, pelvis,
        inflammatory) N73.2
    neck —*see* Cervicitis
  uvula K12.2
  vagina (wall) —*see* Vaginitis
  vaginorectal —*see* Vaginitis
  vas deferens N49.1
  vermiform appendix K35.3
  vertebra (column) (tuberculous) A18.01
    nontuberculous —*see* Osteomyelitis,
        vertebra
  vesical —*see* Cystitis, specified type NEC
  vesico-uterine pouch —*see* Peritonitis, pelvic,
      female
  vitreous (humor) —*see* Endophthalmitis,
      purulent
  vocal cord J38.3
  von Bezold's —*see* Mastoiditis, acute
  vulva N76.4
  vulvovaginal gland N75.1
  web space —*see* Abscess, hand
  wound T81.4
  wrist —*see* Abscess, upper limb
Absence (of) (organ or part) (complete or
    partial)
  adrenal (gland) (congenital) Q89.1
    acquired E89.6
  albumin in blood E88.09
  alimentary tract (congenital) Q45.8
    upper Q40.8
  alveolar process (acquired) —*see* Anomaly,
      alveolar
  ankle (acquired) Z89.44-
  anus (congenital) Q42.3
    with fistula Q42.2
  aorta (congenital) Q25.4
  appendix, congenital Q42.8
  arm (acquired) Z89.20-
    above elbow Z89.22-
      congenital (with hand present) —*see*
          Agenesis, arm, with hand present
          and hand —*see* Agenesis, forearm,
              and hand
    below elbow Z89.21-
      congenital (with hand present) —*see*
          Agenesis, arm, with hand present
          and hand —*see* Agenesis, forearm,
              and hand
    congenital —*see* Defect, reduction, upper
        limb
    shoulder (following explantation of
        shoulder joint prosthesis) (joint) (with
        or without presence of antibiotic-
        impregnated cement spacer) Z89.23-
    congenital (with hand present) —*see*
        Agenesis, arm, with hand present

Absence *(Continued)*
  artery (congenital) (peripheral) Q27.8
    brain Q28.3
    coronary Q24.5
    pulmonary Q25.79
    specified NEC Q27.8
    umbilical Q27.0
  atrial septum (congenital) Q21.1
  auditory canal (congenital) (external) Q16.1
  auricle (ear), congenital Q16.0
  bile, biliary duct, congenital Q44.5
  bladder (acquired) Z90.6
    congenital Q64.5
  bowel sounds R19.11
  brain Q00.0
    part of Q04.3
  breast (s) (and nipple (s)) (acquired) Z90.1-
    congenital Q83.8
  broad ligament Q50.6
  bronchus (congenital) Q32.4
  canaliculus lacrimalis, congenital Q10.4
  cerebellum (vermis) Q04.3
  cervix (acquired) (with uterus) Z90.710
    with remaining uterus Z90.712
    congenital Q51.5
  chin, congenital Q18.8
  cilia (congenital) Q10.3
    acquired —*see* Madarosis
  clitoris (congenital) Q52.6
  coccyx, congenital Q76.49
  cold sense R20.8
  congenital
    lumen —*see* Atresia
    organ or site NEC —*see* Agenesis
    septum —*see* Imperfect, closure
  corpus callosum Q04.0
  cricoid cartilage, congenital Q31.8
  diaphragm (with hernia), congenital Q79.1
  digestive organ (s) or tract, congenital
      Q45.8
    acquired NEC Z90.49
    upper Q40.8
  ductus arteriosus Q28.8
  duodenum (acquired) Z90.49
    congenital Q41.0
  ear, congenital Q16.9
    acquired H93.8-
    auricle Q16.0
    external Q16.0
    inner Q16.5
    lobe, lobule Q17.8
    middle, except ossicles Q16.4
      ossicles Q16.3
    ossicles Q16.3
  ejaculatory duct (congenital) Q55.4
  endocrine gland (congenital) NEC Q89.2
    acquired E89.89
  epididymis (congenital) Q55.4
    acquired Z90.79
  epiglottis, congenital Q31.8
  esophagus (congenital) Q39.8
    acquired (partial) Z90.49
  eustachian tube (congenital) Q16.2
  extremity (acquired) Z89.9
    congenital Q73.0
    knee (following explantation of knee joint
        prosthesis) (joint) (with or without
        presence of antibiotic-impregnated
        cement spacer) Z89.52-
    lower (above knee) Z89.619
      below knee Z89.51-
    upper —*see* Absence, arm
  eye (acquired) Z90.01
    congenital Q11.1
    muscle (congenital) Q10.3
  eyeball (acquired) Z90.01
  eyelid (fold) (congenital) Q10.3
    acquired Z90.01
  face, specified part NEC Q18.8
  fallopian tube (s) (acquired) Z90.79
    congenital Q50.6

◀ New　　◀▥ Revised　　deleted Deleted

Absence *(Continued)*
  family member (causing problem in home)
    NEC *(see also* Disruption, family)
    Z63.32
  femur, congenital —*see* Defect, reduction,
    lower limb, longitudinal, femur
  fibrinogen (congenital) D68.2
    acquired D65
  finger (s) (acquired) Z89.02-
    congenital —*see* Agenesis, hand
  foot (acquired) Z89.43-
    congenital —*see* Agenesis, foot
  forearm (acquired) —*see* Absence, arm, below
    elbow
  gallbladder (acquired) Z90.49
    congenital Q44.0
  gamma globulin in blood D80.1
    hereditary D80.0
  genital organs
    acquired (female) (male) Z90.79
    female, congenital Q52.8
      external Q52.71
      internal NEC Q52.8
    male, congenital Q55.8
  genitourinary organs, congenital NEC
    female Q52.8
    male Q55.8
  globe (acquired) Z90.01
    congenital Q11.1
  glottis, congenital Q31.8
  hand and wrist (acquired) Z89.11-
    congenital —*see* Agenesis, hand
  head, part (acquired) NEC Z90.09
  heat sense R20.8
  hip (following explantation of hip joint
    prosthesis) (joint) (with or without
    presence of antibiotic-impregnated
    cement spacer) Z89.62-
  hymen (congenital) Q52.4
  ileum (acquired) Z90.49
    congenital Q41.2
  immunoglobulin, isolated NEC D80.3
    IgA D80.2
    IgG D80.3
    IgM D80.4
  incus (acquired) —*see* Loss, ossicles, ear
    congenital Q16.3
  inner ear, congenital Q16.5
  intestine (acquired) (small) Z90.49
    congenital Q41.9
      specified NEC Q41.8
    large Z90.49
      congenital Q42.9
        specified NEC Q42.8
  iris, congenital Q13.1
  jejunum (acquired) Z90.49
    congenital Q41.1
  joint
    acquired
      hip (following explantation of hip
        joint prosthesis) (with or without
        presence of antibiotic-impregnated
        cement spacer) Z89.62-
      knee (following explantation of knee
        joint prosthesis) (with or without
        presence of antibiotic-impregnated
        cement spacer) Z89.52-
      shoulder (following explantation of
        shoulder joint prosthesis) (with
        or without presence of antibiotic-
        impregnated cement spacer)
        Z89.23-
    congenital NEC Q74.8
  kidney (s) (acquired) Z90.5
    congenital Q60.2
      bilateral Q60.1
      unilateral Q60.0
  knee (following explantation of knee joint
    prosthesis) (joint) (with or without
    presence of antibiotic-impregnated
    cement spacer) Z89.52-

Absence *(Continued)*
  labyrinth, membranous Q16.5
  larynx (congenital) Q31.8
    acquired Z90.02
  leg (acquired) (above knee) Z89.61-
    below knee (acquired) Z89.51-
    congenital —*see* Defect, reduction, lower
      limb
  lens (acquired) —*see also* Aphakia
    congenital Q12.3
    post cataract extraction Z98.4-
  limb (acquired) —*see* Absence, extremity
  lip Q38.6
  liver (congenital) Q44.7
  lung (fissure) (lobe) (bilateral) (unilateral)
    (congenital) Q33.3
    acquired (any part) Z90.2
  menstruation —*see* Amenorrhea
  muscle (congenital) (pectoral) Q79.8
    ocular Q10.3
  neck, part Q18.8
  neutrophil —*see* Agranulocytosis
  nipple (s) (with breast (s)) (acquired)
    Z90.1-
    congenital Q83.2
  nose (congenital) Q30.1
    acquired Z90.09
  organ
    of Corti, congenital Q16.5
    or site, congenital NEC Q89.8
      acquired NEC Z90.89
  osseous meatus (ear) Q16.4
  ovary (acquired)
    bilateral Z90.722
    congenital
      bilateral Q50.02
      unilateral Q50.01
    unilateral Z90.721
  oviduct (acquired)
    bilateral Z90.722
    congenital Q50.6
    unilateral Z90.721
  pancreas (congenital) Q45.0
    acquired Z90.410
      complete Z90.410
      partial Z90.411
      total Z90.410
  parathyroid gland (acquired)
    E89.2
    congenital Q89.2
  patella, congenital Q74.1
  penis (congenital) Q55.5
    acquired Z90.79
  pericardium (congenital) Q24.8
  pituitary gland (congenital) Q89.2
    acquired E89.3
  prostate (acquired) Z90.79
    congenital Q55.4
  pulmonary valve Q22.0
  punctum lacrimale (congenital) Q10.4
  radius, congenital —*see* Defect, reduction,
    upper limb, longitudinal, radius
  rectum (congenital) Q42.1
    with fistula Q42.0
    acquired Z90.49
  respiratory organ NOS Q34.9
  rib (acquired) Z90.89
    congenital Q76.6
  sacrum, congenital Q76.49
  salivary gland (s), congenital Q38.4
  scrotum, congenital Q55.29
  seminal vesicles (congenital) Q55.4
    acquired Z90.79
  septum
    atrial (congenital) Q21.1
    between aorta and pulmonary artery
      Q21.4
    ventricular (congenital) Q20.4
  sex chromosome
    female phenotype Q97.8
    male phenotype Q98.8

Absence *(Continued)*
  skull bone (congenital) Q75.8
    with
      anencephaly Q00.0
      encephalocele —*see* Encephalocele
      hydrocephalus Q03.9
        with spina bifida —*see* Spina
          bifida, by site, with
          hydrocephalus
      microcephaly Q02
  spermatic cord, congenital Q55.4
  spine, congenital Q76.49
  spleen (congenital) Q89.01
    acquired Z90.81
  sternum, congenital Q76.7
  stomach (acquired) (partial) Z90.3
    congenital Q40.2
  superior vena cava, congenital
    Q26.8
  teeth, tooth (congenital) K00.0
    acquired (complete) K08.109
      class I K08.101
      class II K08.102
      class III K08.103
      class IV K08.104
      due to
        caries K08.139
          class I K08.131
          class II K08.132
          class III K08.133
          class IV K08.134
        periodontal disease K08.129
          class I K08.121
          class II K08.122
          class III K08.123
          class IV K08.124
        specified NEC K08.199
          class I K08.191
          class II K08.192
          class III K08.193
          class IV K08.194
        trauma K08.119
          class I K08.111
          class II K08.112
          class III K08.113
          class IV K08.114
      partial K08.409
        class I K08.401
        class II K08.402
        class III K08.403
        class IV K08.404
        due to
          caries K08.439
            class I K08.431
            class II K08.432
            class III K08.433
            class IV K08.434
          periodontal disease K08.429
            class I K08.421
            class II K08.422
            class III K08.423
            class IV K08.424
          specified NEC K08.499
            class I K08.491
            class II K08.492
            class III K08.493
            class IV K08.494
          trauma K08.419
            class I K08.411
            class II K08.412
            class III K08.413
            class IV K08.414
  tendon (congenital) Q79.8
  testis (congenital) Q55.0
    acquired Z90.79
  thumb (acquired) Z89.01-
    congenital —*see* Agenesis, hand
  thymus gland Q89.2
  thyroid (gland) (acquired) E89.0
    cartilage, congenital Q31.8
    congenital E03.1

◀ New   ◀⁞⁞ Revised   ~~deleted~~ Deleted

Absence *(Continued)*
  toe (s) (acquired) Z89.42-
    with foot —*see* Absence, foot and
      ankle
    congenital —*see* Agenesis, foot
    great Z89.41-
  tongue, congenital Q38.3
  trachea (cartilage), congenital Q32.1
  transverse aortic arch, congenital
    Q25.4
  tricuspid valve Q22.4
  umbilical artery, congenital Q27.0
  upper arm and forearm with hand present,
    congenital —*see* Agenesis, arm, with
    hand present
  ureter (congenital) Q62.4
    acquired Z90.6
  urethra, congenital Q64.5
  uterus (acquired) Z90.710
    with cervix Z90.710
    with remaining cervical stump
      Z90.711
    congenital Q51.0
  uvula, congenital Q38.5
  vagina, congenital Q52.0
  vas deferens (congenital) Q55.4
    acquired Z90.79
  vein (peripheral) congenital NEC
    Q27.8
    cerebral Q28.3
    digestive system Q27.8
    great Q26.8
    lower limb Q27.8
    portal Q26.5
    precerebral Q28.1
    specified site NEC Q27.8
    upper limb Q27.8
  vena cava (inferior) (superior), congenital
    Q26.8
  ventricular septum Q20.4
  vertebra, congenital Q76.49
  vulva, congenital Q52.71
  wrist (acquired) Z89.12-
Absorbent system disease I87.8
Absorption
  carbohydrate, disturbance K90.4
  chemical —*see* Table of Drugs and
    Chemicals
    through placenta (newborn) P04.9
      environmental substance P04.6
      nutritional substance P04.5
      obstetric anesthetic or analgesic drug
        P04.0
  drug NEC —*see* Table of Drugs and
    Chemicals
    addictive
      through placenta (newborn) P04.49
        cocaine P04.41
    medicinal
      through placenta (newborn) P04.1
    through placenta (newborn) P04.1
      obstetric anesthetic or analgesic drug
        P04.0
  fat, disturbance K90.4
    pancreatic K90.3
  noxious substance —*see* Table of Drugs and
    Chemicals
  protein, disturbance K90.4
  starch, disturbance K90.4
  toxic substance —*see* Table of Drugs and
    Chemicals
  uremic —*see* Uremia
Abstinence symptoms, syndrome
  alcohol F10.239
    with delirium F10.231
  cocaine F14.23
  neonatal P96.1
  nicotine —*see* Dependence, drug, nicotine,
    with, withdrawal
  opioid F11.93
    with dependence F11.23

Abstinence symptoms, syndrome *(Continued)*
  psychoactive NEC F19.939
    with
      delirium F19.931
      dependence F19.239
        with
          delirium F19.231
          perceptual disturbance F19.232
        uncomplicated F19.230
      perceptual disturbance F19.932
    uncomplicated F19.930
  sedative F13.939
    with
      delirium F13.931
      dependence F13.239
        with
          delirium F13.231
          perceptual disturbance F13.232
        uncomplicated F13.230
      perceptual disturbance F13.932
    uncomplicated F13.930
  stimulant NEC F15.93
    with dependence F15.23
Abulia R68.89
Abulomania F60.7
Abuse
  adult —*see* Maltreatment, adult
    as reason for
      couple seeking advice (including
        offender) Z63.0
  alcohol (non-dependent) F10.10
    with
      anxiety disorder F10.180
      intoxication F10.129
        with delirium F10.121
        uncomplicated F10.120
      mood disorder F10.14
      other specified disorder F10.188
      psychosis F10.159
        delusions F10.150
        hallucinations F10.151
      sexual dysfunction F10.181
      sleep disorder F10.182
      unspecified disorder F10.19
    counseling and surveillance Z71.41
  amphetamine (or related substance) —*see*
    Abuse, drug, stimulant NEC
  analgesics (non-prescribed) (over the counter)
    F55.8
  antacids F55.0
  antidepressants —*see* Abuse, drug,
    psychoactive NEC
  anxiolytic —*see* Abuse, drug, sedative
  barbiturates —*see* Abuse, drug, sedative
  caffeine —*see* Abuse, drug, stimulant NEC
  cannabis, cannabinoids —*see* Abuse, drug,
    cannabis
  child —*see* Maltreatment, child
  cocaine —*see* Abuse, drug, cocaine
  drug NEC (non-dependent) F19.10
    with sleep disorder F19.182
    amphetamine type —*see* Abuse, drug,
      stimulant NEC
    analgesics (non-prescribed) (over the
      counter) F55.8
    antacids F55.0
    antidepressants —*see* Abuse, drug,
      psychoactive NEC
    anxiolytics —*see* Abuse, drug, sedative
    barbiturates —*see* Abuse, drug, sedative
    caffeine —*see* Abuse, drug, stimulant NEC
    cannabis F12.10
      with
        anxiety disorder F12.180
        intoxication F12.129
          with
            delirium F12.121
            perceptual disturbance
              F12.122
          uncomplicated F12.120
        other specified disorder F12.188

Abuse *(Continued)*
  drug NEC *(Continued)*
    cannabis *(Continued)*
      with *(Continued)*
        psychosis F12.159
          delusions F12.150
          hallucinations F12.151
        unspecified disorder F12.19
    cocaine F14.10
      with
        anxiety disorder F14.180
        intoxication F14.129
          with
            delirium F14.121
            perceptual disturbance F14.122
          uncomplicated F14.120
        mood disorder F14.14
        other specified disorder F14.188
        psychosis F14.159
          delusions F14.150
          hallucinations F14.151
        sexual dysfunction F14.181
        sleep disorder F14.182
        unspecified disorder F14.19
    counseling and surveillance Z71.51
    hallucinogen F16.10
      with
        anxiety disorder F16.180
        flashbacks F16.183
        intoxication F16.129
          with
            delirium F16.121
            perceptual disturbance F16.122
          uncomplicated F16.120
        mood disorder F16.14
        other specified disorder F16.188
        perception disorder, persisting F16.183
        psychosis F16.159
          delusions F16.150
          hallucinations F16.151
        unspecified disorder F16.19
    hashish —*see* Abuse, drug, cannabis
    herbal or folk remedies F55.1
    hormones F55.3
    hypnotics —*see* Abuse, drug, sedative
    inhalant F18.10
      with
        anxiety disorder F18.180
        dementia, persisting F18.17
        intoxication F18.129
          with delirium F18.121
          uncomplicated F18.120
        mood disorder F18.14
        other specified disorder F18.188
        psychosis F18.159
          delusions F18.150
          hallucinations F18.151
        unspecified disorder F18.19
    laxatives F55.2
    LSD —*see* Abuse, drug, hallucinogen
    marihuana —*see* Abuse, drug, cannabis
    morphine type (opioids) —*see* Abuse, drug,
      opioid
    opioid F11.10
      with
        intoxication F11.129
          with
            delirium F11.121
            perceptual disturbance F11.122
          uncomplicated F11.120
        mood disorder F11.14
        other specified disorder F11.188
        psychosis F11.159
          delusions F11.150
          hallucinations F11.151
        sexual dysfunction F11.181
        sleep disorder F11.182
        unspecified disorder F11.19
    PCP (phencyclidine) (or related
      substance) —*see* Abuse, drug,
      hallucinogen

◀ New   ◀▥ Revised   ~~deleted~~ Deleted

Abuse (*Continued*)
drug NEC (*Continued*)
psychoactive NEC F19.10
with
amnestic disorder F19.16
anxiety disorder F19.180
dementia F19.17
intoxication F19.129
with
delirium F19.121
perceptual disturbance
F19.122
uncomplicated F19.120
mood disorder F19.14
other specified disorder F19.188
psychosis F19.159
delusions F19.150
hallucinations F19.151
sexual dysfunction F19.181
sleep disorder F19.182
unspecified disorder F19.19
sedative, hypnotic or anxiolytic F13.10
with
anxiety disorder F13.180
intoxication F13.129
with delirium F13.121
uncomplicated F13.120
mood disorder F13.14
other specified disorder F13.188
psychosis F13.159
delusions F13.150
hallucinations F13.151
sexual dysfunction F13.181
sleep disorder F13.182
unspecified disorder F13.19
solvent —*see* Abuse, drug, inhalant
steroids F55.3
stimulant NEC F15.10
with
anxiety disorder F15.180
intoxication F15.129
with
delirium F15.121
perceptual disturbance F15.122
uncomplicated F15.120
mood disorder F15.14
other specified disorder F15.188
psychosis F15.159
delusions F15.150
hallucinations F15.151
sexual dysfunction F15.181
sleep disorder F15.182
unspecified disorder F15.19
tranquilizers —*see* Abuse, drug, sedative
vitamins F55.4
hallucinogens —*see* Abuse, drug, hallucinogen
hashish —*see* Abuse, drug, cannabis
herbal or folk remedies F55.1
hormones F55.3
hypnotic —*see* Abuse, drug, sedative
inhalant —*see* Abuse, drug, inhalant
laxatives F55.2
LSD —*see* Abuse, drug, hallucinogen
marihuana —*see* Abuse, drug, cannabis
morphine type (opioids) —*see* Abuse, drug, opioid
non-psychoactive substance NEC F55.8
antacids F55.0
folk remedies F55.1
herbal remedies F55.1
hormones F55.3
laxatives F55.2
steroids F55.3
vitamins F55.4
opioids —*see* Abuse, drug, opioid
PCP (phencyclidine) (or related substance) — *see* Abuse, drug, hallucinogen
physical (adult) (child) —*see* Maltreatment
psychoactive substance —*see* Abuse, drug, psychoactive NEC

Abuse (*Continued*)
psychological (adult) (child) —*see* Maltreatment
sedative —*see* Abuse, drug, sedative
sexual —*see* Maltreatment
solvent —*see* Abuse, drug, inhalant
steroids F55.3
vitamins F55.4
Acalculia R48.8
developmental F81.2
Acanthamebiasis (with) B60.10
conjunctiva B60.12
keratoconjunctivitis B60.13
meningoencephalitis B60.11
other specified B60.19
Acanthocephaliasis B83.8
Acanthocheilonemiasis B74.4
Acanthocytosis E78.6
Acantholysis L11.9
Acanthosis (acquired) (nigricans) L83
benign Q82.8
congenital Q82.8
seborrheic L82.1
inflamed L82.0
tongue K14.3
Acapnia E87.3
Acarbia E87.2
Acardia, acardius Q89.8
Acardiacus amorphus Q89.8
Acardiotrophia I51.4
Acariasis B88.0
scabies B86
Acarodermatitis (urticarioides) B88.0
Acarophobia F40.218
Acatalasemia, acatalasia E80.3
Acathisia (drug induced) G25.71
Accelerated atrioventricular conduction I45.6
Accentuation of personality traits (type A) Z73.1
Accessory (congenital)
adrenal gland Q89.1
anus Q43.4
appendix Q43.4
atrioventricular conduction I45.6
auditory ossicles Q16.3
auricle (ear) Q17.0
biliary duct or passage Q44.5
bladder Q64.79
blood vessels NEC Q27.9
coronary Q24.5
bone NEC Q79.8
breast tissue, axilla Q83.1
carpal bones Q74.0
cecum Q43.4
chromosome (s) NEC (nonsex) Q92.9
with complex rearrangements NEC Q92.5
seen only at prometaphase Q92.8
13 —*see* Trisomy, 13
18 —*see* Trisomy, 18
21 —*see* Trisomy, 21
partial Q92.9
sex
female phenotype Q97.8
coronary artery Q24.5
cusp (s), heart valve NEC Q24.8
pulmonary Q22.3
cystic duct Q44.5
digit (s) Q69.9
ear (auricle) (lobe) Q17.0
endocrine gland NEC Q89.2
eye muscle Q10.3
eyelid Q10.3
face bone (s) Q75.8
fallopian tube (fimbria) (ostium) Q50.6
finger (s) Q69.0
foreskin N47.8
frontonasal process Q75.8

Accessory (*Continued*)
gallbladder Q44.1
genital organ (s)
female Q52.8
external Q52.79
internal NEC Q52.8
male Q55.8
genitourinary organs NEC Q89.8
female Q52.8
male Q55.8
hallux Q69.2
heart Q24.8
valve NEC Q24.8
pulmonary Q22.3
hepatic ducts Q44.5
hymen Q52.4
intestine (large) (small) Q43.4
kidney Q63.0
lacrimal canal Q10.6
leaflet, heart valve NEC Q24.8
ligament, broad Q50.6
liver Q44.7
duct Q44.5
lobule (ear) Q17.0
lung (lobe) Q33.1
muscle Q79.8
navicular of carpus Q74.0
nervous system, part NEC Q07.8
nipple Q83.3
nose Q30.8
organ or site not listed —*see* Anomaly, by site
ovary Q50.31
oviduct Q50.6
pancreas Q45.3
parathyroid gland Q89.2
parotid gland (and duct) Q38.4
pituitary gland Q89.2
preauricular appendage Q17.0
prepuce N47.8
renal arteries (multiple) Q27.2
rib Q76.6
cervical Q76.5
roots (teeth) K00.2
salivary gland Q38.4
sesamoid bones Q74.8
foot Q74.2
hand Q74.0
skin tags Q82.8
spleen Q89.09
sternum Q76.7
submaxillary gland Q38.4
tarsal bones Q74.2
teeth, tooth K00.1
tendon Q79.8
thumb Q69.1
thymus gland Q89.2
thyroid gland Q89.2
toes Q69.2
tongue Q38.3
tooth, teeth K00.1
tragus Q17.0
ureter Q62.5
urethra Q64.79
urinary organ or tract NEC Q64.8
uterus Q51.2
vagina Q52.10
valve, heart NEC Q24.8
pulmonary Q22.3
vertebra Q76.49
vocal cords Q31.8
vulva Q52.79
Accident
birth —*see* Birth, injury
cardiac —*see* Infarct, myocardium
cerebral I63.9
cerebrovascular (embolic) (ischemic) (thrombotic) I63.9
aborted I63.9
hemorrhagic —*see* Hemorrhage, intracranial, intracerebral

Accident (Continued)
  cerebrovascular (Continued)
    old (without sequelae) Z86.73
      with sequelae (of) —see Sequelae,
        infarction, cerebral
    coronary —see Infarct, myocardium
    craniovascular I63.9
    vascular, brain I63.9
Accidental —see condition
Accommodation (disorder) —see also condition
  hysterical paralysis of F44.89
  insufficiency of H52.4
  paresis —see Paresis, of accommodation
  spasm —see Spasm, of accommodation
Accouchement —see Delivery
Accreta placenta O43.21-
Accretio cordis (nonrheumatic) I31.0
Accretions, tooth, teeth K03.6
Acculturation difficulty Z60.3
Accumulation secretion, prostate N42.89
Acephalia, acephalism, acephalus, acephaly Q00.0
Acephalobrachia monster Q89.8
Acephalochirus monster Q89.8
Acephalogaster Q89.8
Acephalostomus monster Q89.8
Acephalothorax Q89.8
Acerophobia F40.298
Acetonemia R79.89
  in Type 1 diabetes E10.10
    with coma E10.11
Acetonuria R82.4
Achalasia (cardia) (esophagus) K22.0
  congenital Q39.5
  pylorus Q40.0
  sphincteral NEC K59.8
Ache (s) —see Pain
Acheilia Q38.6
Achillobursitis —see Tendinitis, Achilles
Achillodynia —see Tendinitis, Achilles
Achlorhydria, achlorhydric (neurogenic) K31.83
  anemia D50.8
  diarrhea K31.83
  psychogenic F45.8
  secondary to vagotomy K91.1
Achluophobia F40.228
Acholia K82.8
Acholuric jaundice (familial)
  (splenomegalic) —see also Spherocytosis
  acquired D59.8
Achondrogenesis Q77.0
Achondroplasia (osteosclerosis congenita) Q77.4
Achroma, cutis L80
Achromat (ism), achromatopsia (acquired) (congenital) H53.51
Achromia, congenital —see Albinism
Achromia parasitica B36.0
Achylia gastrica K31.89
  psychogenic F45.8
Acid
  burn —see Corrosion
  deficiency
    amide nicotinic E52
    ascorbic E54
    folic E53.8
    nicotinic E52
    pantothenic E53.8
  intoxication E87.2
  peptic disease K30
  phosphatase deficiency E83.39
  stomach K30
    psychogenic F45.8
Acidemia E87.2
  argininosuccinic E72.22
  isovaleric E71.110
  metabolic (newborn) P19.9
    first noted before onset of labor P19.0
    first noted during labor P19.1
    noted at birth P19.2

Acidemia (Continued)
  methylmalonic E71.120
  pipecolic E72.3
  propionic E71.121
Acidity, gastric (high) K30
  psychogenic F45.8
Acidocytopenia —see Agranulocytosis
Acidocytosis D72.1
Acidopenia —see Agranulocytosis
Acidosis (lactic) (respiratory) E87.2
  in Type 1 diabetes E10.10
    with coma E10.11
  kidney, tubular N25.89
  lactic E87.2
  metabolic NEC E87.2
    with respiratory acidosis E87.4
    late, of newborn P74.0
  mixed metabolic and respiratory,
    newborn P84
  newborn P84
  renal (hyperchloremic) (tubular)
    N25.89
  respiratory E87.2
    complicated by
      metabolic
        acidosis E87.4
        alkalosis E87.4
Aciduria
  argininosuccinic E72.22
  glutaric (type I) E72.3
    type II E71.313
    type III E71.5-
  orotic (congenital) (hereditary) (pyrimidine
    deficiency) E79.8
    anemia D53.0
Acladiosis (skin) B36.0
Aclasis, diaphyseal Q78.6
Acleistocardia Q21.1
Aclusion —see Anomaly, dentofacial,
  malocclusion
Acne L70.9
  artificialis L70.8
  atrophica L70.2
  cachecticorum (Hebra) L70.8
  conglobata L70.1
  cystic L70.0
  decalvans L66.2
  excoriée des jeunes filles L70.5
  frontalis L70.2
  indurata L70.0
  infantile L70.4
  keloid L73.0
  lupoid L70.2
  necrotic, necrotica (miliaris) L70.2
  neonatal L70.4
  nodular L70.0
  occupational L70.8
  picker's L70.5
  pustular L70.0
  rodens L70.2
  rosacea L71.9
  specified NEC L70.8
  tropica L70.3
  varioliformis L70.2
  vulgaris L70.0
Acnitis (primary) A18.4
Acosta's disease T70.29
Acoustic —see condition
Acousticophobia F40.298
Acquired —see also condition
  immunodeficiency syndrome
    (AIDS) B20
Acrania Q00.0
Acroangiodermatitis I78.9
Acroasphyxia, chronic I73.89
Acrobystitis N47.7
Acrocephalopolysyndactyly Q87.0
Acrocephalosyndactyly Q87.0
Acrocephaly Q75.0
Acrochondrohyperplasia —see Syndrome,
  Marfan's

Acrocyanosis I73.8
  newborn P28.2
    meaning transient blue hands and feet -
      omit code
Acrodermatitis L30.8
  atrophicans (chronica) L90.4
  continua (Hallopeau) L40.2
  enteropathica (hereditary) E83.2
  Hallopeau's L40.2
  infantile papular L44.4
  perstans L40.2
  pustulosa continua L40.2
  recalcitrant pustular L40.2
Acrodynia —see Poisoning, mercury
Acromegaly, acromegalia E22.0
Acromelalgia I73.81
Acromicria, acromikria Q79.8
Acronyx L60.0
Acropachy, thyroid —see Thyrotoxicosis
Acroparesthesia (simple) (vasomotor) I73.89
Acropathy, thyroid —see Thyrotoxicosis
Acrophobia F40.241
Acroposthitis N47.7
Acroscleriasis, acroscleroderma,
  acrosclerosis —see Sclerosis, systemic
Acrosphacelus I96
Acrospiroma, eccrine —see Neoplasm, skin,
  benign
Acrostealgia —see Osteochondropathy
Acrotrophodynia —see Immersion
ACTH ectopic syndrome E24.3
Actinic —see condition
Actinobacillosis, actinobacillus A28.8
  mallei A24.0
  muris A25.1
Actinomyces israelii (infection) —see
  Actinomycosis
Actinomycetoma (foot) B47.1
Actinomycosis, actinomycotic A42.9
  with pneumonia A42.0
  abdominal A42.1
  cervicofacial A42.2
  cutaneous A42.89
  gastrointestinal A42.1
  pulmonary A42.0
  sepsis A42.7
  specified site NEC A42.89
Actinoneuritis G62.82
Action, heart
  disorder I49.9
  irregular I49.9
    psychogenic F45.8
Activated protein C resistance D68.51
Active —see condition
Acute —see also condition
  abdomen R10.0
  gallbladder —see Cholecystitis, acute
Acyanotic heart disease (congenital) Q24.9
Acystia Q64.5
Adair-Dighton syndrome (brittle bones and
  blue sclera, deafness) Q78.0
Adamantinoblastoma —see Ameloblastoma
Adamantinoma —see also Cyst, calcifying
  odontogenic
  long bones C40.90
    lower limb C40.2-
    upper limb C40.0-
  malignant C41.1
    jaw (bone) (lower) C41.1
      upper C41.0
  tibial C40.2-
Adamantoblastoma —see Ameloblastoma
Adams-Stokes (-Morgagni) **disease or**
  syndrome I45.9
Adaption reaction —see Disorder, adjustment
Addiction (see also Dependence) F19.20
  alcohol, alcoholic (ethyl) (methyl) (wood)
    (without remission) F10.20
    with remission F10.21
  drug —see Dependence, drug

Addiction *(Continued)*
  ethyl alcohol (without remission) F10.20
    with remission F10.21
  heroin —*see* Dependence, drug, opioid
  methyl alcohol (without remission) F10.20
    with remission F10.21
  methylated spirit (without remission) F10.20
    with remission F10.21
  morphine(-like substances) —*see*
    Dependence, drug, opioid
  nicotine —*see* Dependence, drug, nicotine
  opium and opioids —*see* Dependence, drug,
    opioid
  tobacco —*see* Dependence, drug, nicotine
Addisonian crisis E27.2
Addison's
  anemia (pernicious) D51.0
  disease (bronze) or syndrome E27.1
    tuberculous A18.7
  keloid L94.0
Addison-Biermer anemia (pernicious) D51.0
Addison-Schilder complex E71.528
Additional —*see also* Accessory
  chromosome (s) Q99.8
    21 —*see* Trisomy, 21
  sex —*see* Abnormal, chromosome, sex
Adduction contracture, hip or other joint —*see*
  Contraction, joint
Adenitis —*see also* Lymphadenitis
  acute, unspecified site L04.9
  axillary I88.9
    acute L04.2
    chronic or subacute I88.1
  Bartholin's gland N75.8
  bulbourethral gland —*see* Urethritis
  cervical I88.9
    acute L04.0
    chronic or subacute I88.1
  chancroid (Hemophilus ducreyi) A57
  chronic, unspecified site I88.1
  Cowper's gland —*see* Urethritis
  due to Pasteurella multocida (p. septica)
    A28.0
  epidemic, acute B27.09
  gangrenous L04.9
  gonorrheal NEC A54.89
  groin I88.9
    acute L04.1
    chronic or subacute I88.1
  infectious (acute) (epidemic) B27.09
  inguinal I88.9
    acute L04.1
    chronic or subacute I88.1
  lymph gland or node, except mesenteric
    I88.9
    acute —*see* Lymphadenitis, acute
    chronic or subacute I88.1
  mesenteric (acute) (chronic) (nonspecific)
    (subacute) I88.0
  parotid gland (suppurative) —*see*
    Sialoadenitis
  salivary gland (any) (suppurative) —*see*
    Sialoadenitis
  scrofulous (tuberculous) A18.2
  Skene's duct or gland —*see* Urethritis
  strumous, tuberculous A18.2
  subacute, unspecified site I88.1
  sublingual gland (suppurative) —*see*
    Sialoadenitis
  submandibular gland (suppurative) —*see*
    Sialoadenitis
  submaxillary gland (suppurative) —*see*
    Sialoadenitis
  tuberculous —*see* Tuberculosis, lymph gland
  urethral gland —*see* Urethritis
  Wharton's duct (suppurative) —*see*
    Sialoadenitis
Adenoacanthoma —*see* Neoplasm, malignant,
  by site
Adenoameloblastoma —*see* Cyst, calcifying
  odontogenic

Adenocarcinoid (tumor) —*see* Neoplasm,
  malignant, by site
Adenocarcinoma —*see also* Neoplasm,
  malignant, by site
  acidophil
    specified site —*see* Neoplasm, malignant,
      by site
    unspecified site C75.1
  adrenal cortical C74.0-
  alveolar —*see* Neoplasm, lung, malignant
  apocrine
    breast —*see* Neoplasm, breast, malignant
    in situ
      breast D05.8-
      specified site NEC —*see* Neoplasm, skin,
        in situ
      unspecified site D04.9
    specified site NEC —*see* Neoplasm, skin,
      malignant
    unspecified site C44.99
  basal cell
    specified site —*see* Neoplasm, skin,
      malignant
    unspecified site C08.9
  basophil
    specified site —*see* Neoplasm, malignant,
      by site
    unspecified site C75.1
  bile duct type C22.1
    liver C22.1
    specified site NEC —*see* Neoplasm,
      malignant, by site
    unspecified site C22.1
  bronchiolar —*see* Neoplasm, lung, malignant
  bronchioloalveolar —*see* Neoplasm, lung,
    malignant
  ceruminous C44.29-
  cervix, in situ (*see also* Carcinoma, cervix
    uteri, in situ) D06.9
  chromophobe
    specified site —*see* Neoplasm, malignant,
      by site
    unspecified site C75.1
  diffuse type
    specified site —*see* Neoplasm, malignant,
      by site
    unspecified site C16.9
  duct
    infiltrating
      with Paget's disease —*see* Neoplasm,
        breast, malignant
      specified site —*see* Neoplasm,
        malignant, by site
      unspecified site (female) C50.91-
        male C50.92-
    specified site —*see* Neoplasm, malignant,
      by site
    unspecified site
      female C56.9
      male C61
  eosinophil
    specified site —*see* Neoplasm, malignant,
      by site
    unspecified site C75.1
  follicular
    with papillary C73
    moderately differentiated C73
    specified site —*see* Neoplasm, malignant,
      by site
    trabecular C73
    unspecified site C73
    well differentiated C73
  Hurthle cell C73
  in
    adenomatous
      polyposis coli C18.9
  infiltrating duct
    with Paget's disease —*see* Neoplasm,
      breast, malignant
    specified site —*see* Neoplasm, malignant,
      by site

Adenocarcinoma *(Continued)*
  infiltrating duct *(Continued)*
    unspecified site (female) C50.91-
      male C50.92-
  inflammatory
    specified site —*see* Neoplasm, malignant,
      by site
    unspecified site (female) C50.91-
      male C50.92-
  intestinal type
    specified site —*see* Neoplasm, malignant,
      by site
    unspecified site C16.9
  intracystic papillary
  intraductal
    breast D05.1-
    noninfiltrating
      breast D05.1-
      papillary
        with invasion
          specified site —*see* Neoplasm,
            malignant, by site
          unspecified site (female)
            C50.91-
            male C50.92-
        breast D05.1-
        specified site NEC —*see* Neoplasm, in
          situ, by site
        unspecified site D05.1-
      specified site NEC —*see* Neoplasm, in
        situ, by site
      unspecified site D05.1-
    papillary
      with invasion
        specified site —*see* Neoplasm,
          malignant, by site
        unspecified site (female) C50.91-
          male C50.92-
      breast D05.1-
      specified site —*see* Neoplasm, in situ,
        by site
      unspecified site D05.1-
    specified site NEC —*see* Neoplasm, in situ,
      by site
    unspecified site D05.1-
  islet cell
    with exocrine, mixed
      specified site —*see* Neoplasm,
        malignant, by site
      unspecified site C25.9
    pancreas C25.4
    specified site NEC —*see* Neoplasm,
      malignant, by site
    unspecified site C25.4
  lobular
    in situ
      breast D05.0-
      specified site NEC —*see* Neoplasm, in
        situ, by site
      unspecified site D05.0-
    specified site —*see* Neoplasm, malignant,
      by site
    unspecified site (female) C50.91-
      male C50.92-
  mucoid —*see also* Neoplasm, malignant, by
    site
    cell
      specified site —*see* Neoplasm,
        malignant, by site
      unspecified site C75.1
  nonencapsulated sclerosing C73
  papillary
    with follicular C73
    follicular variant C73
    intraductal (noninfiltrating)
      with invasion
        specified site —*see* Neoplasm,
          malignant, by site
        unspecified site (female) C50.91-
          male C50.92-
      breast D05.1-

Adenocarcinoma *(Continued)*
　papillary *(Continued)*
　　intraductal *(Continued)*
　　　specified site NEC —*see* Neoplasm, in situ, by site
　　　unspecified site D05.1-
　　serous
　　　specified site —*see* Neoplasm, malignant, by site
　　　unspecified site C56.9
　papillocystic
　　specified site —*see* Neoplasm, malignant, by site
　　unspecified site C56.9
　pseudomucinous
　　specified site —*see* Neoplasm, malignant, by site
　　unspecified site C56.9
　renal cell C64-
　sebaceous —*see* Neoplasm, skin, malignant, by site
　serous —*see also* Neoplasm, malignant, by site
　　papillary
　　　specified site —*see* Neoplasm, malignant, by site
　　　unspecified site C56.9
　sweat gland —*see* Neoplasm, skin, malignant
　water-clear cell C75.0
Adenocarcinoma-in-situ —*see also* Neoplasm, in situ, by site
　breast D05.9-
Adenofibroma
　clear cell —*see* Neoplasm, benign, by site
　endometrioid D27.9
　　borderline malignancy D39.10
　　malignant C56-
　mucinous
　　specified site —*see* Neoplasm, benign, site
　　unspecified site D27.9
　papillary
　　specified site —*see* Neoplasm, benign, by site
　　unspecified site D27.9
　prostate —*see* Enlargement, enlarged, prostate
　serous
　　specified site —*see* Neoplasm, benign, by site
　　unspecified site D27.9
　specified site —*see* Neoplasm, benign, by site
　unspecified site D27.9
Adenofibrosis
　breast —*see* Fibroadenosis, breast
　endometrioid N80.0
Adenoiditis (chronic) J35.02
　with tonsillitis J35.03
　acute J03.90
　　recurrent J03.91
　　specified organism NEC J03.80
　　　recurrent J03.81
　　staphylococcal J03.80
　　　recurrent J03.81
　　streptococcal J03.00
　　　recurrent J03.01
Adenoids —*see* condition
Adenolipoma —*see* Neoplasm, benign, by site
Adenolipomatosis, Launois-Bensaude E88.89
Adenolymphoma
　specified site —*see* Neoplasm, benign, by site
　unspecified site D11.9
Adenoma —*see also* Neoplasm, benign, by site
　acidophil
　　specified site —*see* Neoplasm, benign, site
　　unspecified site D35.2
　acidophil-basophil, mixed
　　specified site —*see* Neoplasm, benign, by site
　　unspecified site D35.2

Adenoma *(Continued)*
　adrenal (cortical) D35.00
　　clear cell D35.00
　　compact cell D35.00
　　glomerulosa cell D35.00
　　heavily pigmented variant D35.00
　　mixed cell D35.00
　alpha-cell
　　pancreas D13.7
　　specified site NEC —*see* Neoplasm, benign, by site
　　unspecified site D13.7
　alveolar D14.30
　apocrine
　　breast D24-
　　specified site NEC —*see* Neoplasm, skin, benign, by site
　　unspecified site D23.9
　basal cell D11.9
　basophil
　　specified site —*see* Neoplasm, benign, by site
　　unspecified site D35.2
　basophil-acidophil, mixed
　　specified site —*see* Neoplasm, benign, site
　　unspecified site D35.2
　beta-cell
　　pancreas D13.7
　　specified site NEC —*see* Neoplasm, benign, by site
　　unspecified site D13.7
　bile duct D13.4
　　common D13.5
　　extrahepatic D13.5
　　intrahepatic D13.4
　　specified site NEC —*see* Neoplasm, benign, by site
　　unspecified site D13.4
　black D35.00
　bronchial D38.1
　　cylindroid type —*see* Neoplasm, lung, malignant
　ceruminous D23.2-
　chief cell D35.1
　chromophobe
　　specified site —*see* Neoplasm, benign, by site
　　unspecified site D35.2
　colloid
　　specified site —*see* Neoplasm, benign, by site
　　unspecified site D34
　duct
　eccrine, papillary —*see* Neoplasm, skin, benign
　endocrine, multiple
　　single specified site —*see* Neoplasm, uncertain behavior, by site
　　two or more specified sites D44-
　　unspecified site D44.9
　endometrioid —*see also* Neoplasm, benign
　　borderline malignancy —*see* Neoplasm, uncertain behavior, by site
　eosinophil
　　unspecified site D35.2
　fetal
　　specified site —*see* Neoplasm, benign, by site
　　unspecified site D34
　follicular
　　specified site —*see* Neoplasm, benign, by site
　　unspecified site D34
　hepatocellular D13.4
　Hurthle cell D34
　islet cell
　　pancreas D13.7
　　specified site NEC —*see* Neoplasm, benign, by site
　　unspecified site D13.7

Adenoma *(Continued)*
　liver cell D13.4
　macrofollicular
　　specified site —*see* Neoplasm, benign, by site
　　unspecified site D34
　malignant, malignum —*see* Neoplasm, malignant, by site
　microcystic
　　pancreas D13.7
　　specified site NEC —*see* Neoplasm, benign, by site
　　unspecified site D13.7
　microfollicular
　　specified site —*see* Neoplasm, benign, by site
　　unspecified site D34
　mucoid cell
　　specified site —*see* Neoplasm, benign, by site
　　unspecified site D35.2
　multiple endocrine
　　single specified site —*see* Neoplasm, uncertain behavior, by site
　　two or more specified sites D44-
　　unspecified site D44.9
　nipple D24-
　papillary —*see also* Neoplasm, benign, by site
　　eccrine —*see* Neoplasm, skin, benign, by site
　Pick's tubular
　　specified site —*see* Neoplasm, benign, by site
　　unspecified site
　　　female D27.9
　　　male D29.20
　pleomorphic
　　carcinoma in —*see* Neoplasm, salivary gland, malignant
　　　specified site —*see* Neoplasm, malignant, by site
　　　unspecified site C08.9
　polypoid —*see also* Neoplasm, benign
　　adenocarcinoma in —*see* Neoplasm, malignant, by site
　　adenocarcinoma in situ —*see* Neoplasm, in situ, by site
　prostate —*see* Neoplasm, benign, prostate
　rete cell D29.20
　sebaceous —*see* Neoplasm, skin, benign
　Sertoli cell
　　specified site —*see* Neoplasm, benign, by site
　　unspecified site
　　　female D27.9
　　　male D29.20
　skin appendage —*see* Neoplasm, skin, benign
　sudoriferous gland —*see* Neoplasm, skin, benign
　sweat gland —*see* Neoplasm, skin, benign
　testicular
　　unspecified site
　　　female D27.9
　　　male D29.20
　tubular —*see also* Neoplasm, benign, by site
　　adenocarcinoma in —*see* Neoplasm, malignant, by site
　　adenocarcinoma in situ —*see* Neoplasm, in situ, by site
　　Pick's
　　　specified site —*see* Neoplasm, benign
　　　unspecified site
　　　　female D27.9
　　　　male D29.20
　tubulovillous —*see also* Neoplasm, benign, by site
　　adenocarcinoma in —*see* Neoplasm, malignant, by site
　　adenocarcinoma in situ —*see* Neoplasm, in situ, by site

◀ New　　◀▥ Revised　　~~deleted~~ Deleted

Adenoma (Continued)
villous —see Neoplasm, uncertain behavior, by site
adenocarcinoma in —see Neoplasm, malignant, by site
adenocarcinoma in situ —see Neoplasm, in situ, by site
water-clear cell D35.1
Adenomatosis
endocrine (multiple) E31.20
single specified site —see Neoplasm, uncertain behavior, by site
erosive of nipple D24-
pluriendocrine —see Adenomatosis, endocrine
pulmonary D38.1
malignant —see Neoplasm, lung, malignant
specified site —see Neoplasm, benign, by site
unspecified site D12.6
Adenomatous
goiter (nontoxic) E04.9
with hyperthyroidism —see Hyperthyroidism, with, goiter, nodular
toxic —see Hyperthyroidism, with, goiter, nodular
Adenomyoma —see also Neoplasm, benign, by site
prostate —see Enlarged, prostate
Adenomyometritis N80.0
Adenomyosis N80.0
Adenopathy (lymph gland) R59.9
generalized R59.1
inguinal R59.0
localized R59.0
mediastinal R59.0
mesentery R59.0
syphilitic (secondary) A51.49
tracheobronchial R59.0
tuberculous A15.4
primary (progressive) A15.7
tuberculous —see also Tuberculosis, lymph gland
tracheobronchial A15.4
primary (progressive) A15.7
Adenosalpingitis —see Salpingitis
Adenosarcoma —see Neoplasm, malignant, by site
Adenosclerosis I88.8
Adenosis (sclerosing) **breast** —see Fibroadenosis, breast
Adenovirus, as cause of disease classified elsewhere B97.0
Adentia (complete) (partial) —see Absence, teeth
Adherent —see also Adhesions
labia (minora) N90.89
pericardium (nonrheumatic) I31.0
rheumatic I09.2
placenta (with hemorrhage) O72.0
without hemorrhage O73.0
prepuce, newborn N47.0
scar (skin) L90.5
tendon in scar L90.5
Adhesions, adhesive (postinfective) K66.0
with intestinal obstruction K56.5
abdominal (wall) —see Adhesions, peritoneum
appendix K38.8
bile duct (common) (hepatic) K83.8
bladder (sphincter) N32.89
bowel —see Adhesions, peritoneum
cardiac I31.0
rheumatic I09.2
cecum —see Adhesions, peritoneum
cervicovaginal N88.1
congenital Q52.8
postpartal O90.89
old N88.1
cervix N88.1
ciliary body NEC —see Adhesions, iris

Adhesions, adhesive (Continued)
clitoris N90.89
colon —see Adhesions, peritoneum
common duct K83.8
congenital —see also Anomaly, by site
fingers —see Syndactylism, complex, fingers
omental, anomalous Q43.3
peritoneal Q43.3
tongue (to gum or roof of mouth) Q38.3
conjunctiva (acquired) H11.21-
congenital Q15.8
cystic duct K82.8
diaphragm —see Adhesions, peritoneum
due to foreign body —see Foreign body
duodenum —see Adhesions, peritoneum
ear
middle H74.1-
epididymis N50.8
epidural —see Adhesions, meninges
epiglottis J38.7
eyelid H02.59
female pelvis N73.6
gallbladder K82.8
globe H44.89
heart I31.0
rheumatic I09.2
ileocecal (coil) —see Adhesions, peritoneum
ileum —see Adhesions, peritoneum
intestine —see also Adhesions, peritoneum
with obstruction K56.5
intra-abdominal —see Adhesions, peritoneum
iris H21.50-
anterior H21.51-
goniosynechiae H21.52-
posterior H21.54-
to corneal graft T85.89
joint —see Ankylosis
knee M23.8X
temporomandibular M26.61
labium (majus) (minus), congenital Q52.5
liver —see Adhesions, peritoneum
lung J98.4
mediastinum J98.5
meninges (cerebral) (spinal) G96.12
congenital Q07.8
tuberculous (cerebral) (spinal) A17.0
mesenteric —see Adhesions, peritoneum
nasal (septum) (to turbinates) J34.89
ocular muscle —see Strabismus, mechanical
omentum —see Adhesions, peritoneum
ovary N73.6
congenital (to cecum, kidney or omentum) Q50.39
paraovarian N73.6
pelvic (peritoneal)
female N73.6
postprocedural N99.4
male —see Adhesions, peritoneum
postpartal (old) N73.6
tuberculous A18.17
penis to scrotum (congenital) Q55.8
periappendiceal —see also Adhesions, peritoneum
pericardium (nonrheumatic) I31.0
focal I31.8
rheumatic I09.2
tuberculous A18.84
pericholecystic K82.8
perigastric —see Adhesions, peritoneum
periovarian N73.6
periprostatic N42.89
perirectal —see Adhesions, peritoneum
perirenal N28.89
peritoneum, peritoneal (postinfective) (postprocedural) K66.0
with obstruction (intestinal) K56.5
congenital Q43.3
pelvic, female N73.6
postprocedural N99.4

Adhesions, adhesive (Continued)
peritoneum, peritoneal (Continued)
postpartal, pelvic N73.6
to uterus N73.6
peritubal N73.6
periureteral N28.89
periuterine N73.6
perivesical N32.89
perivesicular (seminal vesicle) N50.8
pleura, pleuritic J94.8
tuberculous NEC A15.6
pleuropericardial J94.8
postoperative (gastrointestinal tract) K66.0
with obstruction K91.3
due to foreign body accidentally left in wound —see Foreign body, accidentally left during a procedure
pelvic peritoneal N99.4
urethra —see Stricture, urethra, postprocedural
vagina N99.2
postpartal, old (vulva or perineum) N90.89
preputial, prepuce N47.5
pulmonary J98.4
pylorus —see Adhesions, peritoneum
sciatic nerve —see Lesion, nerve, sciatic
seminal vesicle N50.8
shoulder (joint) —see Capsulitis, adhesive
sigmoid flexure —see Adhesions, peritoneum
spermatic cord (acquired) N50.8
congenital Q55.4
spinal canal G96.12
stomach —see Adhesions, peritoneum
subscapular —see Capsulitis, adhesive
temporomandibular M26.61
tendinitis —see also Tenosynovitis, specified type NEC
shoulder —see Capsulitis, adhesive
testis N44.8
tongue, congenital (to gum or roof of mouth) Q38.3
acquired K14.8
trachea J39.8
tubo-ovarian N73.6
tunica vaginalis N44.8
uterus N73.6
internal N85.6
to abdominal wall N73.6
vagina (chronic) N89.5
postoperative N99.2
vitreomacular H43.82-
vitreous H43.89
vulva N90.89
Adiaspiromycosis B48.8
Adie (-Holmes) **pupil or syndrome** —see Anomaly, pupil, function, tonic pupil
Adiponecrosis neonatorum P83.8
Adiposis —see also Obesity
cerebralis E23.6
dolorosa E88.2
Adiposity —see also Obesity
heart —see Degeneration, myocardial
localized E65
Adiposogenital dystrophy E23.6
Adjustment
disorder —see Disorder, adjustment
implanted device —see Encounter (for), adjustment (of)
prosthesis, external —see Fitting
reaction —see Disorder, adjustment
Administration of tPA (rtPA) in a different facility within the last 24 hours prior to admission to current facility Z92.82
Admission (for) —see also Encounter (for)
adjustment (of)
artificial
arm Z44.00-
complete Z44.01-
partial Z44.02-
eye Z44.2

Admission (*Continued*)
  adjustment (*Continued*)
    artificial (*Continued*)
      leg Z44.10-
        complete Z44.11-
        partial Z44.12-
    brain neuropacemaker Z46.2
      implanted Z45.42
    breast
      implant Z45.81
      prosthesis (external) Z44.3
    colostomy belt Z46.89
    contact lenses Z46.0
    cystostomy device Z46.6
    dental prosthesis Z46.3
    device NEC
      abdominal Z46.89
      implanted Z45.89
        cardiac Z45.09
          defibrillator (with synchronous
            cardiace pacemaker) Z45.02
          pacemaker Z45.018
            pulse generator Z45.010
        hearing device Z45.328
          bone conduction Z45.320
          cochlear Z45.321
        infusion pump Z45.1
        nervous system Z45.49
          CSF drainage Z45.41
          hearing device —*see* Admission,
            adjustment, device, implanted,
            hearing device
          neuropacemaker Z45.42
          visual substitution Z45.31
        specified NEC Z45.89
        vascular access Z45.2
        visual substitution Z45.31
      nervous system Z46.2
        implanted —*see* Admission,
          adjustment, device, implanted,
          nervous system
      orthodontic Z46.4
      prosthetic Z44.9
        arm —*see* Admission, adjustment,
          artificial, arm
        breast Z44.3
        dental Z46.3
        eye Z44.2
        leg —*see* Admission, adjustment,
          artificial, leg
        specified type NEC Z44.8
    substitution
      auditory Z46.2
        implanted —*see* Admission,
          adjustment, device, implanted,
          hearing device
      nervous system Z46.2
        implanted —*see* Admission,
          adjustment, device, implanted,
          nervous system
      visual Z46.2
        implanted Z45.31
      urinary Z46.6
    hearing aid Z46.1
      implanted —*see* Admission, adjustment,
        device, implanted, hearing device
    ileostomy device Z46.89
    intestinal appliance or device NEC
      Z46.89
    neuropacemaker (brain) (peripheral nerve)
      (spinal cord) Z46.2
      implanted Z45.42
    orthodontic device Z46.4
    orthopedic (brace) (cast) (device) (shoes)
      Z46.89
    pacemaker
      cardiac Z45.018
        pulse generator Z45.010
      nervous system Z46.2
        implanted Z45.42
    portacath (port-a-cath) Z45.2

Admission (*Continued*)
  adjustment (*Continued*)
    prosthesis Z44.9
      arm —*see* Admission, adjustment,
        artificial, arm
      breast Z44.3
      dental Z46.3
      eye Z44.2
      leg —*see* Admission, adjustment,
        artificial, leg
      specified NEC Z44.8
      spectacles Z46.0
    aftercare (*see also* Aftercare) Z51.89
      postpartum
        immediately after delivery Z39.0
        routine follow-up Z39.2
      radiation therapy (antineoplastic) Z51.0
    attention to artificial opening (of) Z43.9
      artificial vagina Z43.7
      colostomy Z43.3
      cystostomy Z43.5
      enterostomy Z43.4
      gastrostomy Z43.1
      ileostomy Z43.2
      jejunostomy Z43.4
      nephrostomy Z43.6
      specified site NEC Z43.8
        intestinal tract Z43.4
        urinary tract Z43.6
      tracheostomy Z43.0
      ureterostomy Z43.6
      urethrostomy Z43.6
    breast augmentation or reduction Z41.1
    breast reconstruction following mastectomy
      Z42.1
    change of
      dressing (nonsurgical) Z48.00
      neuropacemaker device (brain) (peripheral
        nerve) (spinal cord) Z46.2
        implanted Z45.42
      surgical dressing Z48.01
    circumcision, ritual or routine (in absence of
      diagnosis) Z41.2
    clinical research investigation (control)
      (normal comparison) (participant)
      Z00.6
    contraceptive management Z30.9
    cosmetic surgery NEC Z41.1
    counseling (*see also* Counseling)
      dietary Z71.3
      HIV Z71.7
      human immunodeficiency virus Z71.7
      nonattending third party Z71.0
      procreative management NEC Z31.69
    delivery, full-term, uncomplicated O80
      cesarean, without indication O82
    dietary surveillance and counseling Z71.3
    ear piercing Z41.3
    examination at health care facility (adult) (*see*
      also Examination) Z00.00
      with abnormal findings Z00.01
      clinical research investigation (control)
        (normal comparison) (participant)
        Z00.6
      dental Z01.20
        with abnormal findings Z01.21
      donor (potential) Z00.5
      ear Z01.10
        with abnormal findings NEC
          Z01.118
      eye Z01.00
        with abnormal findings Z01.01
      general, specified reason NEC Z00.8
      hearing Z01.10
        with abnormal findings NEC
          Z01.118
      postpartum checkup Z39.2
      psychiatric (general) Z00.8
        requested by authority Z04.6
      vision Z01.00
        with abnormal findings Z01.01

Admission (*Continued*)
  fitting (of)
    artificial
      arm —*see* Admission, adjustment,
        artificial, arm
      eye Z44.2
      leg —*see* Admission, adjustment,
        artificial, leg
    brain neuropacemaker Z46.2
      implanted Z45.42
    breast prosthesis (external) Z44.3
    colostomy belt Z46.89
    contact lenses Z46.0
    cystostomy device Z46.6
    dental prosthesis Z46.3
    dentures Z46.3
    device NEC
      abdominal Z46.89
      nervous system Z46.2
        implanted —*see* Admission,
          adjustment, device, implanted,
          nervous system
      orthodontic Z46.4
      prosthetic Z44.9
        breast Z44.3
        dental Z46.3
        eye Z44.2
      substitution
        auditory Z46.2
          implanted —*see* Admission,
            adjustment, device, implanted,
            hearing device
        nervous system Z46.2
          implanted —*see* Admission,
            adjustment, device, implanted,
            nervous system
        visual Z46.2
          implanted Z45.31
    hearing aid Z46.1
    ileostomy device Z46.89
    intestinal appliance or device NEC
      Z46.89
    neuropacemaker (brain) (peripheral nerve)
      (spinal cord) Z46.2
      implanted Z45.42
    orthodontic device Z46.4
    orthopedic device (brace) (cast) (shoes)
      Z46.89
    prosthesis Z44.9
      arm —*see* Admission, adjustment,
        artificial, arm
      breast Z44.3
      dental Z46.3
      eye Z44.2
      leg —*see* Admission, adjustment,
        artificial, leg
      specified type NEC Z44.8
      spectacles Z46.0
  follow-up examination Z09
  intrauterine device management Z30.431
    initial prescription Z30.014
  mental health evaluation Z00.8
    requested by authority Z04.6
  observation —*see* Observation
  Papanicolaou smear, cervix Z12.4
    for suspected malignant neoplasm
      Z12.4
  plastic and reconstructive surgery following
    medical procedure or healed injury
    NEC Z42.8
  plastic surgery, cosmetic NEC Z41.1
  postpartum observation
    immediately after delivery Z39.0
    routine follow-up Z39.2
  poststerilization (for restoration) Z31.0
    aftercare Z31.42
  procreative management Z31.9
  prophylactic (measure)
    organ removal Z40.00
      breast Z40.01
      ovary Z40.02

◀ New   ◀▯ Revised   ~~deleted~~ Deleted

Admission (*Continued*)
  prophylactic (*Continued*)
    organ removal (*Continued*)
      specified organ NEC Z40.09
      testes Z40.09
    vaccination Z23
  psychiatric examination (general) Z00.8
    requested by authority Z04.6
  radiation therapy (antineoplastic) Z51.0
  reconstructive surgery following medical
    procedure or healed injury NEC
    Z42.8
  removal of
    cystostomy catheter Z43.5
    drains Z48.03
    dressing (nonsurgical) Z48.00
    intrauterine contraceptive device Z30.432
    neuropacemaker (brain) (peripheral nerve)
      (spinal cord) Z46.2
      implanted Z45.42
    staples Z48.02
    surgical dressing Z48.01
    sutures Z48.02
    ureteral stent Z46.6
  respirator [ventilator] use during power
    failure Z99.12
  restoration of organ continuity
    (poststerilization) Z31.0
    aftercare Z31.42
  sensitivity test —*see also* Test, skin
    allergy NEC Z01.82
    Mantoux Z11.1
  tuboplasty following previous sterilization
    Z31.0
    aftercare Z31.42
  vasoplasty following previous sterilization
    Z31.0
    aftercare Z31.42
  vision examination Z01.00
    with abnormal findings Z01.01
  waiting period for admission to other facility
    Z75.1
Adnexitis (suppurative) —*see*
  Salpingo-oophoritis
Adolescent X-linked adrenoleukodystrophy
  E71.521
Adrenal (gland) —*see* condition
Adrenalism, tuberculous A18.7
Adrenalitis, adrenitis E27.8
  autoimmune E27.1
  meningococcal, hemorrhagic A39.1
Adrenarche, premature E27.0
Adrenocortical syndrome —*see* Cushing's,
  syndrome
Adrenogenital syndrome E25.9
  acquired E25.8
  congenital E25.0
  salt loss E25.0
Adrenogenitalism, congenital E25.0
Adrenoleukodystrophy E71.529
  neonatal E71.511
  X-linked E71.529
    Addison only phenotype E71.528
    Addison-Schilder E71.528
    adolescent E71.521
    adrenomyeloneuropathy E71.522
    childhood cerebral E71.520
    other specified E71.528
Adrenomyeloneuropathy E71.522
Adventitious bursa —*see* Bursopathy, specified
  type NEC
Adverse effect —*see* Table of Drugs and
  Chemicals, categories T36-T50, with 6th
  character 5
Advice —*see* Counseling
Adynamia (episodica) (hereditary) (periodic)
  G72.3
Aeration lung imperfect, newborn —*see*
  Atelectasis
Aerobullosis T70.3
Aerocele —*see* Embolism, air

Aerodermectasia
  subcutaneous (traumatic) T79.7
Aerodontalgia T70.29
Aeroembolism T70.3
Aerogenes capsulatus infection A48.0
Aero-otitis media T70.0
Aerophagy, aerophagia (psychogenic) F45.8
Aerophobia F40.228
Aerosinusitis T70.1
Aerotitis T70.0
Affection —*see* Disease
Afibrinogenemia (*see also* Defect, coagulation)
  D68.8
  acquired D65
  congenital D68.2
  following ectopic or molar pregnancy O08.1
  in abortion —*see* Abortion, by type,
    complicated by, afibrinogenemia
  puerperal O72.3
African
  sleeping sickness B56.9
  tick fever A68.1
  trypanosomiasis B56.9
    gambian B56.0
    rhodesian B56.1
Aftercare (*see also* Care) Z51.89
  following surgery (for) (on)
    amputation Z47.81
    attention to
      drains Z48.03
      dressings (nonsurgical) Z48.00
        surgical Z48.01
      sutures Z48.02
    circulatory system Z48.812
    delayed (planned) wound closure Z48.1
    digestive system Z48.815
    explantation of joint prosthesis (staged
      procedure)
      hip Z47.32
      knee Z47.33
      shoulder Z47.31
    genitourinary system Z48.816
    joint replacement Z47.1
    neoplasm Z48.3
    nervous system Z48.811
    oral cavity Z48.814
    organ transplant
      bone marrow Z48.290
      heart Z48.21
      heart-lung Z48.280
      kidney Z48.22
      liver Z48.23
      lung Z48.24
      multiple organs NEC Z48.288
      specified NEC Z48.298
    orthopedic NEC Z47.89
    planned wound closure Z48.1
    removal of internal fixation device Z47.2
    respiratory system Z48.813
    scoliosis Z47.82
    sense organs Z48.810
    skin and subcutaneous tissue Z48.817
    specified body system
      circulatory Z48.812
      digestive Z48.815
      genitourinary Z48.816
      nervous Z48.811
      oral cavity Z48.814
      respiratory Z48.813
      sense organs Z48.810
      skin and subcutaneous tissue Z48.817
      teeth Z48.814
    specified NEC Z48.89
    spinal Z48.89
    teeth Z48.814
  fracture — code to fracture with seventh
    character D
  involving
    removal of
      drains Z48.03
      dressings (nonsurgical) Z48.00

Aftercare (*Continued*)
  involving (*Continued*)
    removal of (*Continued*)
      staples Z48.02
      surgical dressings Z48.01
      sutures Z48.02
    neuropacemaker (brain) (peripheral nerve)
      (spinal cord) Z46.2
      implanted Z45.42
    orthopedic NEC Z47.89
    postprocedural —*see* Aftercare, following
      surgery
After-cataract —*see* Cataract, secondary
Agalactia (primary) O92.3
  elective, secondary or therapeutic O92.5
Agammaglobulinemia (acquired (secondary))
  (nonfamilial) D80.1
  with
    immunoglobulin-bearing B-lymphocytes
      D80.1
    lymphopenia D81.9
  autosomal recessive (Swiss type) D80.0
  Bruton's X-linked D80.0
  common variable (CVAgamma) D80.1
  congenital sex-linked D80.0
  hereditary D80.0
  lymphopenic D81.9
  Swiss type (autosomal recessive) D80.0
  X-linked (with growth hormone deficiency)
    (Bruton) D80.0
Aganglionosis (bowel) (colon) Q43.1
Age (old) —*see* Senility
Agenesis
  adrenal (gland) Q89.1
  alimentary tract (complete) (partial) NEC
    Q45.8
    upper Q40.8
  anus, anal (canal) Q42.3
    with fistula Q42.2
  aorta Q25.4
  appendix Q42.8
  arm (complete) Q71.0-
    with hand present Q71.1-
  artery (peripheral) Q27.9
    brain Q28.3
    coronary Q24.5
    pulmonary Q25.79
    specified NEC Q27.8
    umbilical Q27.0
  auditory (canal) (external) Q16.1
  auricle (ear) Q16.0
  bile duct or passage Q44.5
  bladder Q64.5
  bone Q79.9
  brain Q00.0
    part of Q04.3
  breast (with nipple present) Q83.8
    with absent nipple Q83.0
  bronchus Q32.4
  canaliculus lacrimalis Q10.4
  carpus —*see* Agenesis, hand
  cartilage Q79.9
  cecum Q42.8
  cerebellum Q04.3
  cervix Q51.5
  chin Q18.8
  cilia Q10.3
  circulatory system, part NOS Q28.9
  clavicle Q74.0
  clitoris Q52.6
  coccyx Q76.49
  colon Q42.9
    specified NEC Q42.8
  corpus callosum Q04.0
  cricoid cartilage Q31.8
  diaphragm (with hernia) Q79.1
  digestive organ (s) or tract (complete)
    (partial) NEC Q45.8
    upper Q40.8
  ductus arteriosus Q28.8
  duodenum Q41.0

Agenesis (*Continued*)
ear Q16.9
auricle Q16.0
lobe Q17.8
ejaculatory duct Q55.4
endocrine (gland) NEC Q89.2
epiglottis Q31.8
esophagus Q39.8
eustachian tube Q16.2
eye Q11.1
adnexa Q15.8
eyelid (fold) Q10.3
face
bones NEC Q75.8
specified part NEC Q18.8
fallopian tube Q50.6
femur —*see* Defect, reduction, lower limb, longitudinal, femur
fibula —*see* Defect, reduction, lower limb, longitudinal, fibula
finger (complete) (partial) —*see* Agenesis, hand
foot (and toes) (complete) (partial) Q72.3-
forearm (with hand present) —*see* Agenesis, arm, with hand present
and hand Q71.2-
gallbladder Q44.0
gastric Q40.2
genitalia, genital (organ (s))
female Q52.8
external Q52.71
internal NEC Q52.8
male Q55.8
glottis Q31.8
hair Q84.0
hand (and fingers) (complete) (partial) Q71.3-
heart Q24.8
valve NEC Q24.8
pulmonary Q22.0
hepatic Q44.7
humerus —*see* Defect, reduction, upper limb
hymen Q52.4
ileum Q41.2
incus Q16.3
intestine (small) Q41.9
large Q42.9
specified NEC Q42.8
iris (dilator fibers) Q13.1
jaw M26.09
jejunum Q41.1
kidney (s) (partial) Q60.2
bilateral Q60.1
unilateral Q60.0
labium (majus) (minus) Q52.71
labyrinth, membranous Q16.5
lacrimal apparatus Q10.4
larynx Q31.8
leg (complete) Q72.0-
with foot present Q72.1-
lower leg (with foot present) —*see* Agenesis, leg, with foot present
and foot Q72.2-
lens Q12.3
limb (complete) Q73.0
lower —*see* Agenesis, leg
upper —*see* Agenesis, arm
lip Q38.0
liver Q44.7
lung (fissure) (lobe) (bilateral) (unilateral) Q33.3
mandible, maxilla M26.09
metacarpus —*see* Agenesis, hand
metatarsus —*see* Agenesis, foot
muscle Q79.8
eyelid Q10.3
ocular Q15.8
musculoskeletal system NEC Q79.8
nail (s) Q84.3
neck, part Q18.8
nerve Q07.8
nervous system, part NEC Q07.8

Agenesis (*Continued*)
nipple Q83.2
nose Q30.1
nuclear Q07.8
organ
of Corti Q16.5
or site not listed —*see* Anomaly, by site
osseous meatus (ear) Q16.1
ovary
bilateral Q50.02
unilateral Q50.01
oviduct Q50.6
pancreas Q45.0
parathyroid (gland) Q89.2
parotid gland (s) Q38.4
patella Q74.1
pelvic girdle (complete) (partial) Q74.2
penis Q55.5
pericardium Q24.8
pituitary (gland) Q89.2
prostate Q55.4
punctum lacrimale Q10.4
radioulnar —*see* Defect, reduction, upper limb
radius —*see* Defect, reduction, upper limb, longitudinal, radius
rectum Q42.1
with fistula Q42.0
renal Q60.2
bilateral Q60.1
unilateral Q60.0
respiratory organ NEC Q34.8
rib Q76.6
roof of orbit Q75.8
round ligament Q52.8
sacrum Q76.49
salivary gland Q38.4
scapula Q74.0
scrotum Q55.29
seminal vesicles Q55.4
septum
atrial Q21.1
between aorta and pulmonary artery Q21.4
ventricular Q20.4
shoulder girdle (complete) (partial) Q74.0
skull (bone) Q75.8
with
anencephaly Q00.0
encephalocele —*see* Encephalocele
hydrocephalus Q03.9
with spina bifida —*see* Spina bifida, by site, with hydrocephalus
microcephaly Q02
spermatic cord Q55.4
spinal cord Q06.0
spine Q76.49
spleen Q89.01
sternum Q76.7
stomach Q40.2
submaxillary gland (s) (congenital) Q38.4
tarsus —*see* Agenesis, foot
tendon Q79.8
testicle Q55.0
thymus (gland) Q89.2
thyroid (gland) E03.1
cartilage Q31.8
tibia —*see* Defect, reduction, lower limb, longitudinal, tibia
tibiofibular —*see* Defect, reduction, lower limb, specified type NEC
toe (and foot) (complete) (partial) —*see* Agenesis, foot
tongue Q38.3
trachea (cartilage) Q32.1
ulna —*see* Defect, reduction, upper limb, longitudinal, ulna
upper limb —*see* Agenesis, arm
ureter Q62.4
urethra Q64.5
urinary tract NEC Q64.8

Agenesis (*Continued*)
uterus Q51.0
uvula Q38.5
vagina Q52.0
vas deferens Q55.4
vein (s) (peripheral) Q27.9
brain Q28.3
great NEC Q26.8
portal Q26.5
vena cava (inferior) (superior) Q26.8
vermis of cerebellum Q04.3
vertebra Q76.49
vulva Q52.71
Ageusia R43.2
Agitated —*see* condition
Agitation R45.1
Aglossia (congenital) Q38.3
Aglossia-adactylia syndrome Q87.0
Aglycogenosis E74.00
Agnosia (body image) (other senses) (tactile) R48.1
developmental F88
verbal R48.1
auditory R48.1
developmental F80.2
developmental F80.2
visual (object) R48.3
Agoraphobia F40.00
with panic disorder F40.01
without panic disorder F40.02
Agrammatism R48.8
Agranulocytopenia —*see* Agranulocytosis
Agranulocytosis (chronic) (cyclical) (genetic) (infantile) (periodic) (pernicious) (*see also* Neutropenia) D70.9
congenital D70.0
cytoreductive cancer chemotherapy sequela D70.1
drug-induced D70.2
due to cytoreductive cancer chemotherapy D70.1
due to infection D70.3
secondary D70.4
drug-induced D70.2
due to cytoreductive cancer chemotherapy D70.1
Agraphia (absolute) R48.8
with alexia R48.0
developmental F81.81
Ague (dumb) —*see* Malaria
Agyria Q04.3
Ahumada-del Castillo syndrome E23.0
Aichomophobia F40.298
AIDS (related complex) B20
Ailment heart —*see* Disease, heart
Ailurophobia F40.218
Ainhum (disease) L94.6
AIPHI (acute idiopathic pulmonary hemorrhage in infants (over 28 days old)) R04.81
Air
anterior mediastinum J98.2
compressed, disease T70.3
conditioner lung or pneumonitis J67.7
embolism (artery) (cerebral) (any site) T79.0
with ectopic or molar pregnancy O08.2
due to implanted device NEC —*see* Complications, by site and type, specified NEC
following
abortion —*see* Abortion by type, complicated by, embolism
ectopic or molar pregnancy O08.2
infusion, therapeutic injection or transfusion T80.0
in pregnancy, childbirth or puerperium —*see* Embolism, obstetric
traumatic T79.0
hunger, psychogenic F45.8
rarefied, effects of —*see* Effect, adverse, high altitude
sickness T75.3

Airplane sickness T75.3
Akathisia (drug-induced) (treatment- induced) G25.71
  neuroleptic induced (acute) G25.71
Akinesia R29.898
Akinetic mutism R41.89
Akureyri's disease G93.3
Alactasia, congenital E73.0
Alagille's syndrome Q44.7
Alastrim B03
Albers-Schönberg syndrome Q78.2
Albert's syndrome —see Tendinitis, Achilles
Albinism, albino E70.30
  with hematologic abnormality E70.339
    Chédiak-Higashi syndrome E70.330
    Hermansky-Pudlak syndrome E70.331
    other specified E70.338
  I E70.320
  II E70.321
  ocular E70.319
    autosomal recessive E70.311
    other specified E70.318
    X-linked E70.310
  oculocutaneous E70.329
    other specified E70.328
    tyrosinase (ty) negative E70.320
    tyrosinase (ty) positive E70.321
  other specified E70.39
Albinismus E70.30
Albright (-McCune)(-Sternberg) syndrome Q78.1
Albuminous —see condition
Albuminuria, albuminuric (acute) (chronic) (subacute) (see also Proteinuria) R80.9
  complicating pregnancy —see Proteinuria, gestational
    with
      gestational hypertension —see Pre-eclampsia
      pre-existing hypertension —see Hypertension, complicating pregnancy, pre-existing, with, pre-eclampsia
  gestational —see Proteinuria, gestational
    with
      gestational hypertension —see Pre-eclampsia
      pre-existing hypertension —see Hypertension, complicating pregnancy, pre-existing, with, pre-eclampsia
  orthostatic R80.2
  postural R80.2
  pre-eclamptic —see Pre-eclampsia
  scarlatinal A38.8
Albuminurophobia F40.298
Alcaptonuria E70.29
Alcohol, alcoholic, alcohol-induced
  addiction (without remission) F10.20
    with remission F10.21
  amnestic disorder, persisting F10.96
    with dependence F10.26
  brain syndrome, chronic F10.97
    with dependence F10.27
  cardiopathy I42.6
  counseling and surveillance Z71.41
    family member Z71.42
  delirium (acute) (tremens) (withdrawal) F10.231
    with intoxication F10.921
      in
        abuse F10.121
        dependence F10.221
  dementia F10.97
    with dependence F10.27
  deterioration F10.97
    with dependence F10.27
  hallucinosis (acute) F10.951
    in
      abuse F10.151
      dependence F10.251

Alcohol, alcoholic, alcohol-induced (Continued)
  insanity F10.959
  intoxication (acute) (without dependence) F10.129
    with
      delirium F10.121
      dependence F10.229
        with delirium F10.221
        uncomplicated F10.220
      uncomplicated F10.120
  jealousy F10.988
  Korsakoff's, Korsakov's, Korsakow's F10.26
  liver K70.9
    acute —see Disease, liver, alcoholic, hepatitis
  mania (acute) (chronic) F10.959
  paranoia, paranoid (type) psychosis F10.950
  pellagra E52
  poisoning, accidental (acute) NEC —see Table of Drugs and Chemicals, alcohol, poisoning
  psychosis —see Psychosis, alcoholic
  withdrawal (without convulsions) F10.239
    with delirium F10.231
Alcoholism (chronic) (without remission) F10.20
  with
    psychosis —see Psychosis, alcoholic
    remission F10.21
  Korsakov's F10.96
    with dependence F10.26
Alder (-Reilly) anomaly or syndrome (leukocyte granulation) D72.0
Aldosteronism E26.9
  familial (type I) E26.02
  glucocorticoid-remediable E26.02
  primary (due to (bilateral) adrenal hyperplasia) E26.09
  primary NEC E26.09
  secondary E26.1
  specified NEC E26.89
Aldosteronoma D44.10
Aldrich(-Wiskott) syndrome (eczema-thrombocytopenia) D82.0
Alektorophobia F40.218
Aleppo boil B55.1
Aleukemic —see condition Aleukia
  congenital D70.0
  hemorrhagica D61.9
    congenital D61.09
  splenica D73.1
Alexia R48.0
  developmental F81.0
  secondary to organic lesion R48.0
Algoneurodystrophy M89.00
  ankle M89.07-
  foot M89.07-
  forearm M89.03-
  hand M89.04-
  lower leg M89.06-
  multiple sites M89.0-
  shoulder M89.01-
  specified site NEC M89.08
  thigh M89.05-
  upper arm M89.02-
Algophobia F40.298
Alienation, mental —see Psychosis
Alkalemia E87.3
Alkalosis E87.3
  metabolic E87.3
    with respiratory acidosis E87.4
  respiratory E87.3
Alkaptonuria E70.29
Allen-Masters syndrome N83.8
Allergy, allergic (reaction) (to) T78.40
  air-borne substance NEC (rhinitis) J30.89
  alveolitis (extrinsic) J67.9
    due to
      Aspergillus clavatus J67.4
      Cryptostroma corticale J67.6

Allergy, allergic (Continued)
  alveolitis (Continued)
    due to (Continued)
      organisms (fungal, thermophilic actinomycete) growing in ventilation (air conditioning) systems J67.7
    specified type NEC J67.8
  anaphylactic reaction or shock T78.2
  angioneurotic edema T78.3
  animal (dander) (epidermal) (hair) (rhinitis) J30.81
  bee sting (anaphylactic shock) —see Toxicity, venom, arthropod, bee
  biological —see Allergy, drug
  colitis K52.2
  dander (animal) (rhinitis) J30.81
  dandruff (rhinitis) J30.81
  dental restorative material (existing) K08.55
  dermatitis —see Dermatitis, contact, allergic
  diathesis —see History, allergy
  drug, medicament & biological (any) (external) (internal) T78.40
    correct substance properly administered —see Table of Drugs and Chemicals, by drug, adverse effect
    wrong substance given or taken NEC (by accident) —see Table of Drugs and Chemicals, by drug, poisoning
  due to pollen J30.1
  dust (house) (stock) (rhinitis) J30.89
    with asthma —see Asthma, allergic extrinsic
  eczema —see Dermatitis, contact, allergic
  epidermal (animal) (rhinitis) J30.81
  feathers (rhinitis) J30.89
  food (any) (ingested) NEC T78.1
    anaphylactic shock —see Shock, anaphylactic, due to food
    dermatitis —see Dermatitis, due to, food
    dietary counseling and surveillance Z71.3
    in contact with skin L23.6
    rhinitis J30.5
    status (without reaction) Z91.018
      eggs Z91.012
      milk products Z91.011
      peanuts Z91.010
      seafood Z91.013
      specified NEC Z91.018
  gastrointestinal K52.2
  grain J30.1
  grass (hay fever) (pollen) J30.1
    asthma —see Asthma, allergic extrinsic
  hair (animal) (rhinitis) J30.81
  history (of) —see History, allergy
  horse serum —see Allergy, serum
  inhalant (rhinitis) J30.89
    pollen J30.1
  kapok (rhinitis) J30.89
  medicine —see Allergy, drug
  milk protein K52.2
  nasal, seasonal due to pollen J30.1
  pneumonia J82
  pollen (any) (hay fever) J30.1
    asthma —see Asthma, allergic extrinsic
  primrose J30.1
  primula J30.1
  purpura D69.0
  ragweed (hay fever) (pollen) J30.1
    asthma —see Asthma, allergic extrinsic
  rose (pollen) J30.1
  seasonal NEC J30.2
  Senecio jacobae (pollen) J30.1
  serum (see also Reaction, serum) T80.69
    anaphylactic shock T80.59
  shock (anaphylactic) T78.2
    due to
      administration of blood and blood products T80.51

Allergy, allergic *(Continued)*
  shock *(Continued)*
    due to *(Continued)*
      adverse effect of correct medicinal
        substance properly administered
        T88.6
      immunization T80.52
      serum NEC T80.59
      vaccination T80.52
    specific NEC T78.49
  tree (any) (hay fever) (pollen) J30.1
    asthma —*see* Asthma, allergic extrinsic
  upper respiratory J30.9
  urticaria L50.0
  vaccine —*see* Allergy, serum
  wheat —*see* Allergy, food
Allescheriasis B48.2
Alligator skin disease Q80.9
Allocheiria, allochiria R20.8
Almeida's disease —*see*
  Paracoccidioidomycosis
Alopecia (hereditaria) (seborrheica) L65.9
  androgenic L64.9
    drug-induced L64.0
    specified NEC L64.8
  areata L63.9
    ophiasis L63.2
    specified NEC L63.8
    totalis L63.0
    universalis L63.1
  cicatricial L66.9
    specified NEC L66.8
  circumscripta L63.9
  congenital, congenitalis Q84.0
  due to cytotoxic drugs NEC L65.8
  mucinosa L65.2
  postinfective NEC L65.8
  postpartum L65.0
  premature L64.8
  specific (syphilitic) A51.32
  specified NEC L65.8
  syphilitic (secondary) A51.32
  totalis (capitis) L63.0
  universalis (entire body) L63.1
  X-ray L58.1
Alpers' disease G31.81
Alpine sickness T70.29
Alport syndrome Q87.81
ALTE (apparent life threatening event) in
  newborn and infant R68.13
Alteration (of), **Altered**
  awareness, transient R40.4
  mental status R41.82
  pattern of family relationships affecting child
    Z62.898
  sensation
    following
      cerebrovascular disease I69.998
        cerebral infarction I69.398
        intracerebral hemorrhage I69.198
        nontraumatic intracranial hemorrhage
          NEC I69.298
        specified disease NEC I69.898
        subarachnoid hemorrhage I69.098
Alternating —*see* condition
Altitude, high (effects) —*see* Effect, adverse,
  high altitude
Aluminosis (of lung) J63.0
Alveolitis
  allergic (extrinsic) —*see* Pneumonitis,
    hypersensitivity
  due to
    Aspergillus clavatus J67.4
    Cryptostroma corticale J67.6
  fibrosing (cryptogenic) (idiopathic) J84.112
  jaw M27.3
  sicca dolorosa M27.3
Alveolus, alveolar —*see* condition
Alymphocytosis D72.810
  thymic (with immunodeficiency) D82.1
Alymphoplasia, thymic D82.1

Alzheimer's disease or sclerosis —*see* Disease,
  Alzheimer's
Amastia (with nipple present) Q83.8
  with absent nipple Q83.0
Amathophobia F40.228
Amaurosis (acquired) (congenital) —*see also*
  Blindness
  fugax G45.3
  hysterical F44.6
  Leber's congenital H35.50
  uremic —*see* Uremia
Amaurotic idiocy (infantile) (juvenile) (late) E75.4
Amaxophobia F40.248
Ambiguous genitalia Q56.4
Amblyopia (congenital) (ex anopsia) (partial)
  (suppression) H53.00-
  anisometropic —*see* Amblyopia, refractive
  deprivation H53.01-
  hysterical F44.6
  nocturnal —*see also* Blindness, night
    vitamin A deficiency E50.5
  refractive H53.02-
  strabismic H53.03-
  tobacco H53.8
  toxic NEC H53.8
  uremic —*see* Uremia
Ameba, amebic (histolytica) —*see also*
  Amebiasis
  abscess (liver) A06.4
Amebiasis A06.9
  with abscess —*see* Abscess, amebic
  acute A06.0
  chronic (intestine) A06.1
    with abscess —*see* Abscess, amebic
  cutaneous A06.7
  cutis A06.7
  cystitis A06.81
  genitourinary tract NEC A06.82
  hepatic —*see* Abscess, liver, amebic
  intestine A06.0
  nondysenteric colitis A06.2
  skin A06.7
  specified site NEC A06.89
Ameboma (of intestine) A06.3
Amelia Q73.0
  lower limb —*see* Agenesis, leg
  upper limb —*see* Agenesis, arm
Ameloblastoma —*see also* Cyst, calcifying
  odontogenic
  long bones C40.9-
    lower limb C40.2-
    upper limb C40.0-
  malignant C41.1
    jaw (bone) (lower) C41.1
      upper C41.0
  tibial C40.2-
Amelogenesis imperfecta K00.5
  nonhereditaria (segmentalis) K00.4
Amenorrhea N91.2
  hyperhormonal E28.8
  primary N91.0
  secondary N91.1
Amentia —*see* Disability, intellectual
  Meynert's (nonalcoholic) F04
American
  leishmaniasis B55.2
  mountain tick fever A93.2
Ametropia —*see* Disorder, refraction
Amianthosis J61
Amimia R48.8
Amino-acid disorder E72.9
  anemia D53.0
Aminoacidopathy E72.9
Aminoaciduria E72.9
Amnes (t)ic syndrome (post-traumatic) F04
  induced by
    alcohol F10.96
      with dependence F10.26
    psychoactive NEC F19.96
      with
        abuse F19.16
        dependence F19.26

Amnes (t)ic syndrome *(Continued)*
  induced by *(Continued)*
    sedative F13.96
      with dependence F13.26
Amnesia R41.3
  anterograde R41.1
  auditory R48.8
  dissociative F44.0
  hysterical F44.0
  postictal in epilepsy —*see* Epilepsy
  psychogenic F44.0
  retrograde R41.2
  transient global G45.4
Amnion, amniotic —*see* condition
Amnionitis —*see* Pregnancy, complicated by
Amok F68.8
Amoral traits F60.89
Ampulla
  lower esophagus K22.8
  phrenic K22.8
Amputation —*see also* Absence, by site,
  acquired
  neuroma (postoperative) (traumatic) —*see*
    Complications, amputation stump,
    neuroma
  stump (surgical)
    abnormal, painful, or with complication
      (late) —*see* Complications,
      amputation stump
    healed or old NOS Z89.9
  traumatic (complete) (partial)
    arm (upper) (complete) S48.91-
      at
        elbow S58.01-
          partial S58.02-
        shoulder joint (complete) S48.01-
          partial S48.02-
      between
        elbow and wrist (complete) S58.11-
          partial S58.12-
        shoulder and elbow (complete) S48.11-
          partial S48.12-
      partial S48.92-
    breast (complete) S28.21-
      partial S28.22-
    clitoris (complete) S38.211
      partial S38.212
    ear (complete) S08.11-
      partial S08.12-
    finger (complete) (metacarpophalangeal)
      S68.11-
      index S68.11-
      little S68.11-
      middle S68.11-
      partial S68.12-
        index S68.12-
        little S68.12-
        middle S68.12-
        ring S68.12-
      ring S68.11-
      thumb —*see* Amputation, traumatic,
        thumb
      transphalangeal (complete) S68.61-
        index S68.61-
        little S68.61-
        middle S68.61-
        partial S68.62-
          index S68.62-
          little S68.62-
          middle S68.62-
          ring S68.62-
        ring S68.61-
    foot (complete) S98.91-
      at ankle level S98.01-
        partial S98.02-
      midfoot S98.31-
        partial S98.32-
      partial S98.92-
    forearm (complete) S58.91-
      at elbow level (complete) S58.01-
        partial S58.02-

◀ New   ◀▥ Revised   ~~deleted~~ Deleted

Amputation *(Continued)*
traumatic *(Continued)*
forearm *(Continued)*
between elbow and wrist (complete) S58.11-
partial S58.12-
partial S58.92-
genital organ (s) (external)
female (complete) S38.211
partial S38.212
male
penis (complete) S38.221
partial S38.222
scrotum (complete) S38.231
partial S38.232
testes (complete) S38.231
partial S38.232
hand (complete) (wrist level) S68.41-
finger (s) alone —*see* Amputation, traumatic, finger
partial S68.42-
thumb alone —*see* Amputation, traumatic, thumb
transmetacarpal (complete) S68.71-
partial S68.72-
head
ear —*see* Amputation, traumatic, ear
nose (partial) S08.812
complete S08.811
part S08.89
scalp S08.0
hip (and thigh) (complete) S78.91-
at hip joint (complete) S78.01-
partial S78.02-
between hip and knee (complete) S78.11-
partial S78.12-
partial S78.92-
labium (majus) (minus) (complete) S38.21-
partial S38.21-
leg (lower) S88.91-
at knee level S88.01-
partial S88.02-
between knee and ankle S88.11-
partial S88.12-
partial S88.92-
nose (partial) S08.812
complete S08.811
penis (complete) S38.221
partial S38.222
scrotum (complete) S38.231
partial S38.232
shoulder —*see* Amputation, traumatic, arm
at shoulder joint —*see* Amputation, traumatic, arm, at shoulder joint
testes (complete) S38.231
partial S38.232
thigh —*see* Amputation, traumatic, hip
thorax, part of S28.1
breast —*see* Amputation, traumatic, breast
thumb (complete) (metacarpophalangeal) S68.01-
partial S68.02-
transphalangeal (complete) S68.51-
partial S68.52-
toe (lesser) S98.13-
great S98.11-
partial S98.12-
more than one S98.21-
partial S98.22-
partial S98.14-
vulva (complete) S38.211
partial S38.212
Amputee (bilateral) (old) Z89.9
Amsterdam dwarfism Q87.1
Amusia R48.8
developmental F80.89
Amyelencephalus, amyelencephaly Q00.0
Amyelia Q06.0
Amygdalitis —*see* Tonsillitis
Amygdalolith J35.8

Amyloid heart (disease) E85.4 *[I43]*
Amyloidosis (generalized) (primary) E85.9
with lung involvement E85.4 *[J99]*
familial E85.2
genetic E85.2
heart E85.4 *[I43]*
hemodialysis-associated E85.3
liver E85.4 *[K77]*
localized E85.4
neuropathic heredofamilial E85.1
non-neuropathic heredofamilial E85.0
organ limited E85.4
Portuguese E85.1
pulmonary E85.4 *[J99]*
secondary systemic E85.3
skin (lichen) (macular) E85.4 *[L99]*
specified NEC E85.8
subglottic E85.4 *[J99]*
Amylopectinosis (brancher enzyme deficiency) E74.03
Amylophagia —*see* Pica
Amyoplasia congenita Q79.8
Amyotonia M62.89
congenita G70.2
Amyotrophia, amyotrophy, amyotrophic G71.8
congenita Q79.8
diabetic —*see* Diabetes, amyotrophy
lateral sclerosis G12.21
neuralgic G54.5
spinal progressive G12.21
Anacidity, gastric K31.83
psychogenic F45.8
Anaerosis of newborn P28.89
Analbuminemia E88.09
Analgesia —*see* Anesthesia
Analphalipoproteinemia E78.6
Anaphylactic
purpura D69.0
shock or reaction —*see* Shock, anaphylactic
Anaphylactoid shock or reaction —*see* Shock, anaphylactic
Anaphylactoid syndrome of pregnancy O88.01-
Anaphylaxis —*see* Shock, anaphylactic
Anaplasia cervix (*see also* Dysplasia, cervix) N87.9
Anaplasmosis, human A77.49
Anarthria R47.1
Anasarca R60.1
cardiac —*see* Failure, heart, congestive
lung J18.2
newborn P83.2
nutritional E43
pulmonary J18.2
renal N04.9
Anastomosis
aneurysmal —*see* Aneurysm
arteriovenous ruptured brain I60.8
intestinal K63.89
complicated NEC K91.89
involving urinary tract N99.89
retinal and choroidal vessels (congenital) Q14.8
Anatomical narrow angle H40.03-
Ancylostoma, ancylostomiasis (braziliense) (caninum) (ceylanicum) (duodenale) B76.0
Necator americanus B76.1
Andersen's disease (glycogen storage) E74.09
Anderson-Fabry disease E75.21
Andes disease T70.29
Andrews' disease (bacterid) L08.89
Androblastoma
benign
specified site —*see* Neoplasm, benign, by site
unspecified site
female D27.9
male D29.20

Androblastoma *(Continued)*
malignant
specified site —*see* Neoplasm, malignant, by site
unspecified site
female C56.9
male C62.90
specified site —*see* Neoplasm, uncertain behavior, by site
tubular
with lipid storage
specified site —*see* Neoplasm, benign, by site
unspecified site
female D27.9
male D29.20
specified site —*see* Neoplasm, benign, by site
unspecified site
female D27.9
male D29.20
unspecified site
female D39.10
male D40.10
Androgen insensitivity syndrome (*see also* Syndrome, androgen insensitivity) E34.50
Androgen resistance syndrome (*see also* Syndrome, androgen insensitivity) E34.50
Android pelvis Q74.2
with disproportion (fetopelvic) O33.3
causing obstructed labor O65.3
Androphobia F40.290
Anectasis, pulmonary (newborn) —*see* Atelectasis
Anemia (essential) (general) (hemoglobin deficiency) (infantile) (primary) (profound) D64.9
with (due to) (in)
disorder of
anaerobic glycolysis D55.2
pentose phosphate pathway D55.1
koilonychia D50.9
achlorhydric D50.8
achrestic D53.1
Addison (-Biermer) (pernicious) D51.0
agranulocytic —*see* Agranulocytosis
amino-acid-deficiency D53.0
aplastic D61.9
congenital D61.09
drug-induced D61.1
due to
drugs D61.1
external agents NEC D61.2
infection D61.2
radiation D61.2
idiopathic D61.3
red cell (pure) D60.9
chronic D60.0
congenital D61.01
specified type NEC D60.8
transient D60.1
specified type NEC D61.89
toxic D61.2
aregenerative
congenital D61.09
asiderotic D50.9
atypical (primary) D64.9
Baghdad spring D55.0
Balantidium coli A07.0
Biermer's (pernicious) D51.0
blood loss (chronic) D50.0
acute D62
bothriocephalus B70.0 *[D63.8]*
brickmaker's B76.9 *[D63.8]*
cerebral I67.89
childhood D58.9
chlorotic D50.8
chronic
blood loss D50.0
hemolytic D58.9
idiopathic D59.9
simple D53.9

Anemia *(Continued)*
  chronica congenita aregenerativa D61.09
  combined system disease NEC D51.0 *[G32.0]*
    due to dietary vitamin B12 deficiency
      D51.3 *[G32.0]*
  complicating pregnancy, childbirth
      or puerperium —*see* Pregnancy,
      complicated by (management affected
      by), anemia
  congenital P61.4
    aplastic D61.09
    due to isoimmunization NOS P55.9
    dyserythropoietic, dyshematopoietic
      D64.4
    following fetal blood loss P61.3
    Heinz body D58.2
    hereditary hemolytic NOS D58.9
    pernicious D51.0
    spherocytic D58.0
  Cooley's (erythroblastic) D56.1
  cytogenic D51.0
  deficiency D53.9
    2, 3 diphosphoglycurate mutase D55.2
    2, 3 PG D55.2
    6 phosphogluconate dehydrogenase
      D55.1
    6-PGD D55.1
    amino-acid D53.0
    combined B12 and folate D53.1
    enzyme D55.9
      drug-induced (hemolytic) D59.2
      glucose-6-phosphate dehydrogenase
        (G6PD) D55.0
      glycolytic D55.2
      nucleotide metabolism D55.3
      related to hexose monophosphate
        (HMP) shunt pathway NEC D55.1
      specified type NEC D55.8
    erythrocytic glutathione D55.1
    folate D52.9
      dietary D52.0
      drug-induced D52.1
    folic acid D52.9
      dietary D52.0
      drug-induced D52.1
    G SH D55.1
    G6PD D55.0
    GGS-R D55.1
    glucose-6-phosphate dehydrogenase D55.0
    glutathione reductase D55.1
    glyceraldehyde phosphate dehydrogenase
      D55.2
    hexokinase D55.2
    iron D50.9
      secondary to blood loss (chronic) D50.0
    nutritional D53.9
      with
        poor iron absorption D50.8
        specified deficiency NEC D53.8
    phosphofructo-aldolase D55.2
    phosphoglycerate kinase D55.2
    PK D55.2
    protein D53.0
    pyruvate kinase D55.2
    transcobalamin II D51.2
    triose-phosphate isomerase D55.2
    vitamin B12 NOS D51.9
      dietary D51.3
      due to
        intrinsic factor deficiency D51.0
        selective vitamin B12 malabsorption
          with proteinuria D51.1
      pernicious D51.0
      specified type NEC D51.8
  Diamond-Blackfan (congenital hypoplastic)
    D61.01
  dibothriocephalus B70.0 *[D63.8]*
  dimorphic D53.1
  diphasic D53.1
  Diphyllobothrium (Dibothriocephalus) B70.0
    [D63.8]

Anemia *(Continued)*
  due to (in) (with)
    antineoplastic chemotherapy D64.81
    blood loss (chronic) D50.0
      acute D62
    chemotherapy, antineoplastic D64.81
    chronic disease classified elsewhere NEC
      D63.8
    chronic kidney disease D63.1
    deficiency
      amino-acid D53.0
      copper D53.8
      folate (folic acid) D52.9
        dietary D52.0
        drug-induced D52.1
      molybdenum D53.8
      protein D53.0
      zinc D53.8
    dietary vitamin B12 deficiency D51.3
    disorder of
      glutathione metabolism D55.1
      nucleotide metabolism D55.3
    drug —*see* Anemia, by type —*see also* Table
      of Drugs and Chemicals
    end stage renal disease D63.1
    enzyme disorder D55.9
    fetal blood loss P61.3
    fish tapeworm (D latum) infestation B70.0
      [D63.8]
    hemorrhage (chronic) D50.0
      acute D62
    impaired absorption D50.9
    loss of blood (chronic) D50.0
      acute D62
    myxedema E03.9 *[D63.8]*
    Necator americanus B76.1 *[D63.8]*
    prematurity P61.2
    selective vitamin B12 malabsorption with
      proteinuria D51.1
    transcobalamin II deficiency D51.2
  Dyke-Young type (secondary) (symptomatic)
    D59.1
  dyserythropoietic (congenital) D64.4
  dyshematopoietic (congenital) D64.4
  Egyptian B76.9 *[D63.8]*
  elliptocytosis —*see* Elliptocytosis
  enzyme-deficiency, drug-induced D59.2
  epidemic (*see also* Ancylostomiasis) B76.9
    [D63.8]
  erythroblastic
    familial D56.1
    newborn (*see also* Disease, hemolytic) P55.9
    of childhood D56.1
  erythrocytic glutathione deficiency D55.1
  erythropoietin-resistant anemia (EPO
      resistant anemia) D63.1
  Faber's (achlorhydric anemia) D50.9
  factitious (self-induced blood letting) D50.0
  familial erythroblastic D56.1
  Fanconi's (congenital pancytopenia) D61.09
  favism D55.0
  fish tapeworm (D. latum) infestation B70.0
    [D63.8]
  folate (folic acid) deficiency D52.9
  glucose-6-phosphate dehydrogenase (G6PD)
    deficiency D55.0
  glutathione-reductase deficiency D55.1
  goat's milk D52.0
  granulocytic —*see* Agranulocytosis
  Heinz body, congenital D58.2
  hemolytic D58.9
    acquired D59.9
      with hemoglobinuria NEC D59.6
      autoimmune NEC D59.1
      infectious D59.4
      specified type NEC D59.8
      toxic D59.4
    acute D59.9
      due to enzyme deficiency specified type
        NEC D55.8
    Lederer's D59.1

Anemia *(Continued)*
  hemolytic *(Continued)*
    autoimmune D59.1
      drug-induced D59.0
    chronic D58.9
      idiopathic D59.9
    cold type (secondary) (symptomatic) D59.1
    congenital (spherocytic) —*see*
        Spherocytosis
    due to
      cardiac conditions D59.4
      drugs (nonautoimmune) D59.2
        autoimmune D59.0
      enzyme disorder D55.9
        drug-induced D59.2
      presence of shunt or other internal
        prosthetic device D59.4
    familial D58.9
    hereditary D58.9
      due to enzyme disorder D55.9
        specified type NEC D55.8
      specified type NEC D58.8
    idiopathic (chronic) D59.9
    mechanical D59.4
    microangiopathic D59.4
    nonautoimmune D59.4
      drug-induced D59.2
    nonspherocytic
      congenital or hereditary NEC D55.8
        glucose-6-phosphate dehydrogenase
          deficiency D55.0
        pyruvate kinase deficiency D55.2
        type
          I D55.1
          II D55.2
      type
        I D55.1
        II D55.2
    secondary D59.4
      autoimmune D59.1
    specified (hereditary) type NEC D58.8
    Stransky-Regala type (*see also*
        Hemoglobinopathy) D58.8
    symptomatic D59.4
      autoimmune D59.1
    toxic D59.4
    warm type (secondary) (symptomatic)
      D59.1
  hemorrhagic (chronic) D50.0
    acute D62
  Herrick's D57.1
  hexokinase deficiency D55.2
  hookworm B76.9 *[D63.8]*
  hypochromic (idiopathic) (microcytic)
    (normoblastic) D50.9
    due to blood loss (chronic) D50.0
      acute D62
    familial sex-linked D64.0
    pyridoxine-responsive D64.3
    sideroblastic, sex-linked D64.0
  hypoplasia, red blood cells D61.9
    congenital or familial D61.01
  hypoplastic (idiopathic) D61.9
    congenital or familial (of childhood)
      D61.01
  hypoproliferative (refractive) D61.9
  idiopathic D64.9
    aplastic D61.3
    hemolytic, chronic D59.9
  in (due to) (with)
    chronic kidney disease D63.1
    end stage renal disease D63.1
    failure, kidney (renal) D63.1
    neoplastic disease (*see also* Neoplasm)
      D63.0
  intertropical (*see also* Ancylostomiasis)
    D63.8
  iron deficiency D50.9
    secondary to blood loss (chronic) D50.0
      acute D62
    specified type NEC D50.8

◀ New   ◀═ Revised   ~~deleted~~ Deleted

Anemia (*Continued*)
Joseph-Diamond-Blackfan (congenital hypoplastic) D61.01
Lederer's (hemolytic) D59.1
leukoerythroblastic D61.82
macrocytic D53.9
  nutritional D52.0
  tropical D52.8
malarial (*see also* Malaria) B54 [*D63.8*]
malignant (progressive) D51.0
malnutrition D53.9
marsh (*see also* Malaria) B54 [*D63.8*]
Mediterranean (with other hemoglobinopathy) D56.9
megaloblastic D53.1
  combined B12 and folate deficiency D53.1
  hereditary D51.1
  nutritional D52.0
  orotic aciduria D53.0
  refractory D53.1
  specified type NEC D53.1
megalocytic D53.1
microcytic (hypochromic) D50.9
  due to blood loss (chronic) D50.0
    acute D62
  familial D56.8
microdrepanocytosis D57.40
microelliptopoikilocytic (Rietti-Greppi-Micheli) D56.9
miner's B76.9 [*D63.8*]
myelodysplastic D46.9
myelofibrosis D75.81
myelogenous D64.89
myelopathic D64.89
myelophthisic D61.82
myeloproliferative D47.Z9
newborn P61.4
  due to
    ABO (antibodies, isoimmunization, maternal/fetal incompatibility) P55.1
    Rh (antibodies, isoimmunization, maternal/fetal incompatibility) P55.0
  following fetal blood loss P61.3
  posthemorrhagic (fetal) P61.3
nonspherocytic hemolytic —*see* Anemia, hemolytic, nonspherocytic
normocytic (infectional) D64.9
  due to blood loss (chronic) D50.0
    acute D62
  myelophthisic D61.82
nutritional (deficiency) D53.9
  with
    poor iron absorption D50.8
    specified deficiency NEC D53.8
  megaloblastic D52.0
of prematurity P61.2
orotaciduric (congenital) (hereditary) D53.0
osteosclerotic D64.89
ovalocytosis (hereditary) —*see* Elliptocytosis
paludal (*see also* Malaria) B54 [*D63.8*]
pernicious (congenital) (malignant) (progressive) D51.0
pleochromic D64.89
  of sprue D52.8
posthemorrhagic (chronic) D50.0
  acute D62
  newborn P61.3
postoperative (postprocedural)
  due to (acute) blood loss D62
    chronic blood loss D50.0
  specified NEC D64.9
postpartum O90.81
pressure D64.89
progressive D64.9
  malignant D51.0
  pernicious D51.0
protein-deficiency D53.0
pseudoleukemica infantum D64.89

Anemia (*Continued*)
pure red cell D60.9
  congenital D61.01
pyridoxine-responsive D64.3
pyruvate kinase deficiency D55.2
refractory D46.4
  with
    excess of blasts D46.20
      1 (RAEB 1) D46.21
      2 (RAEB 2) D46.22
      in transformation (RAEB T) —*see* Leukemia, acute myeloblastic
    hemochromatosis D46.1
    sideroblasts (ring) (RARS) D46.1
  without ring sideroblasts, so stated D46.0
  without sideroblasts without excess of blasts D46.0
  megaloblastic D53.1
  sideroblastic D46.1
  sideropenic D50.9
Rietti-Greppi-Micheli D56.9
scorbutic D53.2
secondary to
  blood loss (chronic) D50.0
    acute D62
  hemorrhage (chronic) D50.0
    acute D62
semiplastic D61.89
sickle-cell —*see* Disease, sickle-cell
sideroblastic D64.3
  hereditary D64.0
  hypochromic, sex-linked D64.0
  pyridoxine-responsive NEC D64.3
  refractory D46.1
  secondary (due to)
    disease D64.1
    drugs and toxins D64.2
  specified type NEC D64.3
sideropenic (refractory) D50.9
  due to blood loss (chronic) D50.0
    acute D62
simple chronic D53.9
specified type NEC D64.89
spherocytic (hereditary) —*see* Spherocytosis
splenic D64.89
splenomegalic D64.89
stomatocytosis D58.8
syphilitic (acquired) (late) A52.79 [*D63.8*]
target cell D64.89
thalassemia D56.9
thrombocytopenic —*see* Thrombocytopenia
toxic D61.2
tropical B76.9 [*D63.8*]
  macrocytic D52.8
tuberculous A18.89 [*D63.8*]
vegan D51.3
vitamin
  B6-responsive D64.3
  B12 deficiency (dietary) pernicious D51.0
von Jaksch's D64.89
Witts' (achlorhydric anemia) D50.8
Anemophobia F40.228
Anencephalus, anencephaly Q00.0
Anergasia —*see* Psychosis, organic
Anesthesia, anesthetic R20.0
complication or reaction NEC (*see also* Complications, anesthesia) T88.59
  due to
    correct substance properly administered —*see* Table of Drugs and Chemicals, by drug, adverse effect
    overdose or wrong substance given —*see* Table of Drugs and Chemicals, by drug, poisoning
cornea H18.81-
dissociative F44.6
functional (hysterical) F44.6
hyperesthetic, thalamic G89.0
hysterical F44.6
local skin lesion R20.0

Anesthesia, anesthetic (*Continued*)
sexual (psychogenic) F52.1
shock (due to) T88.2
skin R20.0
testicular N50.9
Anetoderma (maculosum) (of) L90.8
Jadassohn-Pellizzari L90.2
Schweniger-Buzzi L90.1
Aneurin deficiency E51.9
Aneurysm (anastomotic) (artery) (cirsoid) (diffuse) (false) (fusiform) (multiple) (saccular) I72.9
abdominal (aorta) I71.4
  ruptured I71.3
  syphilitic A52.01
aorta, aortic (nonsyphilitic) I71.9
  abdominal I71.4
    ruptured I71.3
  arch I71.2
    ruptured I71.1
  arteriosclerotic I71.9
    ruptured I71.8
  ascending I71.2
    ruptured I71.1
  congenital Q25.4
  descending I71.9
    abdominal I71.4
      ruptured I71.3
    ruptured I71.8
    thoracic I71.2
      ruptured I71.1
  ruptured I71.8
  sinus, congenital Q25.4
  syphilitic A52.01
  thoracic I71.2
    ruptured I71.1
  thoracoabdominal I71.6
    ruptured I71.5
  thorax, thoracic (arch) I71.2
    ruptured I71.1
  transverse I71.2
    ruptured I71.1
  valve (heart) (*see also* Endocarditis, aortic) I35.8
arteriosclerotic I72.9
  cerebral I67.1
    ruptured —*see* Hemorrhage, intracranial, subarachnoid
arteriovenous (congenital) —*see also* Malformation, arteriovenous
  acquired I77.0
  brain I67.1
  coronary I25.41
  pulmonary I28.0
  brain Q28.2
    ruptured I60.8
  peripheral —*see* Malformation, arteriovenous, peripheral
  precerebral vessels Q28.0
  specified site NEC —*see also* Malformation, arteriovenous
    acquired I77.0
basal —*see* Aneurysm, brain
berry (congenital) (nonruptured) I67.1
  ruptured I60.7
brain I67.1
  arteriosclerotic I67.1
    ruptured —*see* Hemorrhage, intracranial, subarachnoid
  arteriovenous (congenital) (nonruptured) Q28.2
    acquired I67.1
      ruptured I60.8
    ruptured I60.8
  berry (congenital) (nonruptured) I67.1
    ruptured (*see also* Hemorrhage, intracranial, subarachnoid) I60.7
  congenital Q28.3
    ruptured I60.7
  meninges I67.1
    ruptured I60.8

Aneurysm (Continued)
  brain (Continued)
    miliary (congenital) (nonruptured) I67.1
      ruptured (see also Hemorrhage,
        intracranial, subarachnoid) I60.7
    mycotic I33.0
    ruptured —see Hemorrhage, intracranial,
      subarachnoid
    syphilitic (hemorrhage) A52.05
  cardiac (false) (see also Aneurysm, heart)
    I25.3
  carotid artery (common) (external) I72.0
    internal (intracranial) I67.1
      extracranial portion I72.0
    ruptured into brain I60.0-
    syphilitic A52.09
      intracranial A52.05
  cavernous sinus I67.1
    arteriovenous (congenital) (nonruptured)
      Q28.3
      ruptured I60.8
  celiac I72.8
  central nervous system, syphilitic A52.05
  cerebral —see Aneurysm, brain
  chest —see Aneurysm, thorax
  circle of Willis I67.1
    congenital Q28.3
      ruptured I60.6
    ruptured I60.6
  common iliac artery I72.3
  congenital (peripheral) Q27.8
    brain Q28.3
      ruptured I60.7
    coronary Q24.5
    digestive system Q27.8
    lower limb Q27.8
    pulmonary Q25.79
    retina Q14.1
    specified site NEC Q27.8
    upper limb Q27.8
  conjunctiva —see Abnormality, conjunctiva,
    vascular
  conus arteriosus —see Aneurysm, heart
  coronary (arteriosclerotic) (artery) I25.41
    arteriovenous, congenital Q24.5
    congenital Q24.5
    ruptured —see Infarct, myocardium
    syphilitic A52.06
    vein I25.89
  cylindroid (aorta) I71.9
    ruptured I71.8
    syphilitic A52.01
  ductus arteriosus Q25.0
  endocardial, infective (any valve) I33.0
  femoral (artery) (ruptured) I72.4
  gastroduodenal I72.8
  gastroepiploic I72.8
  heart (wall) (chronic or with a stated duration
    of over 4 weeks) I25.3
    valve —see Endocarditis
  hepatic I72.8
  iliac (common) (artery) (ruptured) I72.3
  infective I72.9
    endocardial (any valve) I33.0
  innominate (nonsyphilitic) I72.8
    syphilitic A52.09
  interauricular septum —see Aneurysm, heart
  interventricular septum —see Aneurysm,
    heart
  intrathoracic (nonsyphilitic) I71.2
    ruptured I71.1
    syphilitic A52.01
  lower limb I72.4
  lung (pulmonary artery) I28.1
  mediastinal (nonsyphilitic) I72.8
    syphilitic A52.09
  miliary (congenital) I67.1
    ruptured —see Hemorrhage, intracerebral,
      subarachnoid, intracranial
  mitral (heart) (valve) I34.8
  mural —see Aneurysm, heart

Aneurysm (Continued)
  mycotic I72.9
    endocardial (any valve) I33.0
    ruptured, brain —see Hemorrhage,
      intracerebral, subarachnoid
  myocardium —see Aneurysm, heart
  neck I72.0
  pancreaticoduodenal I72.8
  patent ductus arteriosus Q25.0
  peripheral NEC I72.8
    congenital Q27.8
      digestive system Q27.8
      lower limb Q27.8
      specified site NEC Q27.8
      upper limb Q27.8
  popliteal (artery) (ruptured) I72.4
  precerebral, congenital (nonruptured)
    Q28.1
  pulmonary I28.1
    arteriovenous Q25.72
      acquired I28.0
    syphilitic A52.09
    valve (heart) —see Endocarditis,
      pulmonary
  racemose (peripheral) I72.9
    congenital —see Aneurysm,
      congenital
  radial I72.1
  Rasmussen NEC A15.0
  renal (artery) I72.2
  retina —see also Disorder, retina,
    microaneurysms
    congenital Q14.1
    diabetic —see Diabetes, microaneurysms,
      retinal
  sinus of Valsalva Q25.4
  specified NEC I72.8
  spinal (cord) I72.8
    syphilitic (hemorrhage) A52.09
  splenic I72.8
  subclavian (artery) (ruptured)
    I72.8
    syphilitic A52.09
  superior mesenteric I72.8
  syphilitic (aorta) A52.01
    central nervous system A52.05
    congenital (late) A50.54 [I79.0]
    spine, spinal A52.09
  thoracoabdominal (aorta) I71.6
    ruptured I71.5
    syphilitic A52.01
  thorax, thoracic (aorta) (arch) (nonsyphilitic)
    I71.2
    ruptured I71.1
    syphilitic A52.01
  traumatic (complication) (early),
    specified site —see Injury,
    blood vessel
  tricuspid (heart) (valve) I07.8
  ulnar I72.1
  upper limb (ruptured) I72.1
  valve, valvular —see Endocarditis
  visceral NEC I72.8
  venous (see also Varix) I86.8
    congenital Q27.8
      digestive system Q27.8
      lower limb Q27.8
      specified site NEC Q27.8
      upper limb Q27.8
  ventricle —see Aneurysm, heart
  visceral NEC I72.8
Angelman syndrome Q93.5
Anger R45.4
Angiectasis, angiectopia I99.8
Angiitis I77.6
  allergic granulomatous M30.1
  hypersensitivity M31.0
  necrotizing M31.9
    specified NEC M31.8
  nervous system, granulomatous
    I67.7

Angina (attack) (cardiac) (chest) (heart)
  (pectoris) (syndrome) (vasomotor)
  I20.9
  with
    atherosclerotic heart disease —see
      Arteriosclerosis, coronary
      (artery)
    documented spasm I20.1
  abdominal K55.1
  accelerated —see Angina, unstable
  agranulocytic —see Agranulocytosis
  angiospastic —see Angina, with documented
    spasm
  aphthous B08.5
  crescendo —see Angina, unstable
  croupous J05.0
  cruris I73.9
  de novo effort —see Angina, unstable
  diphtheritic, membranous A36.0
  equivalent I20.8
  exudative, chronic J37.0
  following acute myocardial infarction
    I23.7
  gangrenous diphtheritic A36.0
  intestinal K55.1
  Ludovici K12.2
  Ludwig's K12.2
  malignant diphtheritic A36.0
  membranous J05.0
    diphtheritic A36.0
    Vincent's A69.1
  mesenteric K55.1
  monocytic —see Mononucleosis, infectious
  of effort —see Angina, specified NEC
  phlegmonous J36
    diphtheritic A36.0
  post-infarctional I23.7
  pre-infarctional —see Angina, unstable
  Prinzmetal —see Angina, with documented
    spasm
  progressive —see Angina, unstable
  pseudomembranous A69.1
  pultaceous, diphtheritic A36.0
  spasm-induced —see Angina, with
    documented spasm
  specified NEC I20.8
  stable I20.9
  stenocardia —see Angina, specified NEC
  stridulous, diphtheritic A36.2
  tonsil J36
  trachealis J05.0
  unstable I20.0
  variant —see Angina, with documented
    spasm
  Vincent's A69.1
  worsening effort —see Angina, unstable
Angioblastoma —see Neoplasm, connective
  tissue, uncertain behavior
Angiocholecystitis —see Cholecystitis, acute
Angiocholitis (see also Cholecystitis, acute)
  K83.0
Angiodysgenesis spinalis G95.19
Angiodysplasia (cecum) (colon) K55.20
  with bleeding K55.21
  duodenum (and stomach) K31.819
    with bleeding K31.811
  stomach (and duodenum) K31.819
    with bleeding K31.811
Angioedema (allergic) (any site) (with urticaria)
  T78.3
  hereditary D84.1
Angioendothelioma —see Neoplasm, uncertain
  behavior, by site
  benign D18.00
    intra-abdominal D18.03
    intracranial D18.02
    skin D18.01
    specified site NEC D18.09
  bone —see Neoplasm, bone, malignant
  Ewing's —see Neoplasm, bone, malignant
Angioendotheliomatosis C85.8-

◄ New   ◄▥ Revised   ~~deleted~~ Deleted

Angiofibroma —*see also* Neoplasm, benign, by site
  juvenile
    specified site —*see* Neoplasm, benign, by site
    unspecified site D10.6
Angiohemophilia (A) (B) D68.0
Angioid streaks (choroid) (macula) (retina) H35.33
Angiokeratoma —*see* Neoplasm, skin, benign
  corporis diffusum E75.21
Angioleiomyoma —*see* Neoplasm, connective tissue, benign
Angiolipoma —*see also* Lipoma
  infiltrating —*see* Lipoma
Angioma —*see also* Hemangioma, by site
  capillary I78.1
  hemorrhagicum hereditaria I78.0
  intra-abdominal D18.03
  intracranial D18.02
  malignant —*see* Neoplasm, connective tissue, malignant
  plexiform D18.00
    intra-abdominal D18.03
    intracranial D18.02
    skin D18.01
    specified site NEC D18.09
  senile I78.1
  serpiginosum L81.7
  skin D18.01
  specified site NEC D18.09
  spider I78.1
  stellate I78.1
  venous Q28.3
Angiomatosis Q82.8
  bacillary A79.89
  encephalotrigeminal Q85.8
  hemorrhagic familial I78.0
  hereditary familial I78.0
  liver K76.4
Angiomyolipoma —*see* Lipoma
Angiomyoliposarcoma —*see* Neoplasm, connective tissue, malignant
Angiomyoma —*see* Neoplasm, connective tissue, benign
Angiomyosarcoma —*see* Neoplasm, connective tissue, malignant
Angiomyxoma —*see* Neoplasm, connective tissue, uncertain behavior
Angioneurosis F45.8
Angioneurotic edema (allergic) (any site) (with urticaria) T78.3
  hereditary D84.1
Angiopathia, angiopathy I99.9
  cerebral I67.9
    amyloid E85.4 [I68.0]
  diabetic (peripheral) —*see* Diabetes, angiopathy
  peripheral I73.9
    diabetic —*see* Diabetes, angiopathy
    specified type NEC I73.89
  retinae syphilitica A52.05
  retinalis (juvenilis)
    diabetic —*see* Diabetes, retinopathy
    proliferative —*see* Retinopathy, proliferative
Angiosarcoma —*see also* Neoplasm, connective tissue, malignant
  liver C22.3
Angiosclerosis —*see* Arteriosclerosis
Angiospasm (peripheral) (traumatic) (vessel) I73.9
  brachial plexus G54.0
  cerebral G45.9
  cervical plexus G54.2
  nerve
    arm —*see* Mononeuropathy, upper limb
      axillary G54.0
      median —*see* Lesion, nerve, median
      ulnar —*see* Lesion, nerve, ulnar
    axillary G54.0

Angiospasm (Continued)
  nerve (Continued)
    leg —*see* Mononeuropathy, lower limb
    median —*see* Lesion, nerve, median
    plantar —*see* Lesion, nerve, plantar
    ulnar —*see* Lesion, nerve, ulnar
Angiospastic disease or edema I73.9
Angiostrongyliasis
  due to
    Parastrongylus
      cantonensis B83.2
      costaricensis B81.3
  intestinal B81.3
Anguillulosis —*see* Strongyloidiasis
Angulation
  cecum —*see* Obstruction, intestine
  coccyx (acquired) (*see also* subcategory) M43.8
    congenital NEC Q76.49
  femur (acquired) —*see also* Deformity, limb, specified type NEC, thigh
    congenital Q74.2
  intestine (large) (small) —*see* Obstruction, intestine
  sacrum (acquired) (*see also* subcategory) M43.8
    congenital NEC Q76.49
  sigmoid (flexure) —*see* Obstruction, intestine
  spine —*see* Dorsopathy, deforming, specified NEC
  tibia (acquired) —*see also* Deformity, limb, specified type NEC, lower leg
    congenital Q74.2
  ureter N13.5
    with infection N13.6
  wrist (acquired) —*see also* Deformity, limb, specified type NEC, forearm
    congenital Q74.0
Angulus infectiosus (lips) K13.0
Anhedonia R45.84
Anhidrosis L74.4
Anhydration, anhydremia E86.0
  with
    hypernatremia E87.0
    hyponatremia E87.1
Anhydremia E86.0
  with
    hypernatremia E87.0
    hyponatremia E87.1
Anidrosis L74.4
Aniridia (congenital) Q13.1
Anisakiasis (infection) (infestation) B81.0
Anisakis larvae infestation B81.0
Aniseikonia H52.32
Anisocoria (pupil) H57.02
  congenital Q13.2
Anisocytosis R71.8
Anisometropia (congenital) H52.31
Ankle —*see* condition
Ankyloblepharon (eyelid) (acquired) —*see also* Blepharophimosis
  filiforme (adnatum) (congenital) Q10.3
  total Q10.3
Ankyloglossia Q38.1
Ankylosis (fibrous) (osseous) (joint) M24.60
  ankle M24.67-
  arthrodesis status Z98.1
  cricoarytenoid (cartilage) (joint) (larynx) J38.7
  dental K03.5
  ear ossicles H74.31-
  elbow M24.62-
  foot M24.67-
  hand M24.64-
  hip M24.65-
  incostapedial joint (infectional) —*see* Ankylosis, ear ossicles
  jaw (temporomandibular) M26.61
  knee M24.66-
  lumbosacral (joint) M43.27
  postoperative (status) Z98.1
  produced by surgical fusion, status Z98.1
  sacro-iliac (joint) M43.28

Ankylosis (Continued)
  shoulder M24.61-
  spine (joint) —*see also* Fusion, spine
    spondylitic —*see* Spondylitis, ankylosing
  surgical Z98.1
  temporomandibular M26.61
  tooth, teeth (hard tissues) K03.5
  wrist M24.63-
Ankylostoma —*see* Ancylostoma
Ankylostomiasis —*see* Ancylostomiasis
Ankylurethria —*see* Stricture, urethra
Annular —*see also* condition
  detachment, cervix N88.8
  organ or site, congenital NEC —*see* Distortion
  pancreas (congenital) Q45.1
Anodontia (complete) (partial) (vera) K00.0
  acquired K08.10
Anomaly, anomalous (congenital) (unspecified type) Q89.9
  abdominal wall NEC Q79.59
  acoustic nerve Q07.8
  adrenal (gland) Q89.1
  Alder (-Reilly) (leukocyte granulation) D72.0
  alimentary tract Q45.9
    upper Q40.9
  alveolar M26.70
    hyperplasia M26.79
      mandibular M26.72
      maxillary M26.71
    hypoplasia M26.79
      mandibular M26.74
      maxillary M26.73
    ridge (process) M26.79
    specified NEC M26.79
  ankle (joint) Q74.2
  anus Q43.9
  aorta (arch) NEC Q25.4
    coarctation (preductal) (postductal) Q25.1
  aortic cusp or valve Q23.9
  appendix Q43.8
  apple peel syndrome Q41.1
  aqueduct of Sylvius Q03.0
    with spina bifida —*see* Spina bifida, with hydrocephalus
  arm Q74.0
  arteriovenous NEC
    coronary Q24.5
    gastrointestinal Q27.33
      acquired —*see* Angiodysplasia
  artery (peripheral) Q27.9
    basilar NEC Q28.1
    cerebral Q28.3
    coronary Q24.5
    digestive system Q27.8
    eye Q15.8
    great Q25.9
      specified NEC Q25.8
    lower limb Q27.8
    peripheral Q27.9
      specified NEC Q27.8
    pulmonary NEC Q25.79
    renal Q27.2
    retina Q14.1
    specified site NEC Q27.8
    subclavian Q27.8
    umbilical Q27.0
    upper limb Q27.8
    vertebral NEC Q28.1
  aryteno-epiglottic folds Q31.8
  atrial
    bands or folds Q20.8
    septa Q21.1
  atrioventricular
    excitation I45.6
    septum Q21.0
  auditory canal Q17.8
  auricle
    ear Q17.8
      causing impairment of hearing Q16.9
    heart Q20.8
  Axenfeld's Q15.0

Anomaly, anomalous *(Continued)*
back Q89.9
band
  atrial Q20.8
  heart Q24.8
  ventricular Q24.8
Bartholin's duct Q38.4
biliary duct or passage Q44.5
bladder Q64.70
  absence Q64.5
  diverticulum Q64.6
  exstrophy Q64.10
    cloacal Q64.12
    extroversion Q64.19
    specified type NEC Q64.19
    supravesical fissure Q64.11
  neck obstruction Q64.31
  specified type NEC Q64.79
bone Q79.9
  arm Q74.0
  face Q75.9
  leg Q74.2
  pelvic girdle Q74.2
  shoulder girdle Q74.0
  skull Q75.9
    with
      anencephaly Q00.0
      encephalocele —*see* Encephalocele
      hydrocephalus Q03.9
        with spina bifida —*see* Spina bifida,
          by site, with hydrocephalus
      microcephaly Q02
brain (multiple) Q04.9
  vessel Q28.3
breast Q83.9
broad ligament Q50.6
bronchus Q32.4
bulbus cordis Q21.9
bursa Q79.9
canal of Nuck Q52.4
canthus Q10.3
capillary Q27.9
cardiac Q24.9
  chambers Q20.9
    specified NEC Q20.8
  septal closure Q21.9
    specified NEC Q21.8
  valve NEC Q24.8
    pulmonary Q22.3
cardiovascular system Q28.8
carpus Q74.0
caruncle, lacrimal Q10.6
cascade stomach Q40.2
cauda equina Q06.3
cecum Q43.9
cerebral Q04.9
  vessels Q28.3
cervix Q51.9
Chédiak-Higashi(-Steinbrinck) (congenital
  gigantism of peroxidase granules)
  E70.330
cheek Q18.9
chest wall Q67.8
  bones Q76.9
chin Q18.9
chordae tendineae Q24.8
choroid Q14.3
  plexus Q07.8
chromosomes, chromosomal Q99.9
  D (1) —*see* condition, chromosome 13
  E (3) —*see* condition, chromosome 18
  G —*see* condition, chromosome 21
  sex
    female phenotype Q97.8
    gonadal dysgenesis (pure) Q99.1
    Klinefelter's Q98.4
    male phenotype Q98.9
    Turner's Q96.9
  specified NEC Q99.8
cilia Q10.3
circulatory system Q28.9

Anomaly, anomalous *(Continued)*
clavicle Q74.0
clitoris Q52.6
coccyx Q76.49
colon Q43.9
common duct Q44.5
communication
  coronary artery Q24.5
  left ventricle with right atrium Q21.0
concha (ear) Q17.3
connection
  portal vein Q26.5
  pulmonary venous Q26.4
    partial Q26.3
    total Q26.2
  renal artery with kidney Q27.2
cornea (shape) Q13.4
coronary artery or vein Q24.5
cranium —*see* Anomaly, skull
cricoid cartilage Q31.8
cystic duct Q44.5
dental
  alveolar —*see* Anomaly, alveolar
  arch relationship M26.20
    specified NEC M26.29
dentofacial M26.9
  alveolar —*see* Anomaly, alveolar
  dental arch relationship M26.20
    specified NEC M26.29
  functional M26.50
    specified NEC M26.59
  jaw-cranial base relationship M26.10
    asymmetry M26.12
      maxillary M26.11
    specified type NEC M26.19
  jaw size M26.00
    macrogenia M26.05
    mandibular
      hyperplasia M26.03
      hypoplasia M26.04
    maxillary
      hyperplasia M26.01
      hypoplasia M26.02
    microgenia M26.06
    specified type NEC M26.09
  malocclusion M26.4
    dental arch relationship NEC M26.29
    jaw-cranial base relationship —*see*
      Anomaly, dentofacial, jaw-cranial
      base relationship
    jaw size —*see* Anomaly, dentofacial, jaw
      size
  specified type NEC M26.89
  temporomandibular joint M26.60
    adhesions M26.61
    ankylosis M26.61
    arthralgia M26.62
    articular disc M26.63
    specified type NEC M26.69
  tooth position, fully erupted M26.30
    specified NEC M26.39
dermatoglyphic Q82.8
diaphragm (apertures) NEC Q79.1
digestive organ (s) or tract Q45.9
  lower Q43.9
  upper Q40.9
distance, interarch (excessive) (inadequate)
  M26.25
distribution, coronary artery Q24.5
ductus
  arteriosus Q25.0
  botalli Q25.0
duodenum Q43.9
dura (brain) Q04.9
  spinal cord Q06.9
ear (external) Q17.9
  causing impairment of hearing Q16.9
  inner Q16.5
  middle (causing impairment of hearing)
    Q16.4
    ossicles Q16.3

Anomaly, anomalous *(Continued)*
Ebstein's (heart) (tricuspid valve) Q22.5
ectodermal Q82.9
Eisenmenger's (ventricular septal defect)
  Q21.8
ejaculatory duct Q55.4
elbow Q74.0
endocrine gland NEC Q89.2
epididymis Q55.4
epiglottis Q31.8
esophagus Q39.9
eustachian tube Q17.8
eye Q15.9
  anterior segment Q13.9
    specified NEC Q13.89
  posterior segment Q14.9
    specified NEC Q14.8
  ptosis (eyelid) Q10.0
  specified NEC Q15.8
eyebrow Q18.8
eyelid Q10.3
  ptosis Q10.0
face Q18.9
  bone (s) Q75.9
fallopian tube Q50.6
fascia Q79.9
femur NEC Q74.2
fibula NEC Q74.2
finger Q74.0
fixation, intestine Q43.3
flexion (joint) NOS Q74.9
  hip or thigh Q65.89
foot NEC Q74.2
  varus (congenital) Q66.3
foramen
  Botalli Q21.1
  ovale Q21.1
forearm Q74.0
forehead Q75.8
form, teeth K00.2
fovea centralis Q14.1
frontal bone —*see* Anomaly, skull
gallbladder (position) (shape) (size)
  Q44.1
Gartner's duct Q52.4
gastrointestinal tract Q45.9
genitalia, genital organ (s) or system
  female Q52.9
    external Q52.70
    internal NOS Q52.9
  male Q55.9
    hydrocele P83.5
    specified NEC Q55.8
genitourinary NEC
  female Q52.9
  male Q55.9
Gerbode Q21.0
glottis Q31.8
granulation or granulocyte, genetic
  (constitutional) (leukocyte) D72.0
gum Q38.6
gyri Q07.9
hair Q84.2
hand Q74.0
hard tissue formation in pulp K04.3
head —*see* Anomaly, skull
heart Q24.9
  auricle Q20.8
  bands or folds Q24.8
  fibroelastosis cordis I42.4
  obstructive NEC Q22.6
  patent ductus arteriosus (Botalli) Q25.0
  septum Q21.9
    auricular Q21.1
    interatrial Q21.1
    interventricular Q21.0
      with pulmonary stenosis or atresia,
        dextraposition of aorta and
        hypertrophy of right ventricle
        Q21.3
    specified NEC Q21.8

Anomaly, anomalous *(Continued)*
  heart *(Continued)*
    septum *(Continued)*
      ventricular Q21.0
        with pulmonary stenosis or atresia, dextraposition of aorta and hypertrophy of right ventricle Q21.3
      tetralogy of Fallot Q21.3
      valve NEC Q24.8
        aortic
          bicuspid valve Q23.1
          insufficiency Q23.1
          stenosis Q23.0
            subaortic Q24.4
        mitral
          insufficiency Q23.3
          stenosis Q23.2
        pulmonary Q22.3
          atresia Q22.0
          insufficiency Q22.2
          stenosis Q22.1
            infundibular Q24.3
            subvalvular Q24.3
        tricuspid
          atresia Q22.4
          stenosis Q22.4
      ventricle Q20.8
  heel NEC Q74.2
  Hegglin's D72.0
  hemianencephaly Q00.0
  hemicephaly Q00.0
  hemicrania Q00.0
  hepatic duct Q44.5
  hip NEC Q74.2
  hourglass stomach Q40.2
  humerus Q74.0
  hydatid of Morgagni
    female Q50.5
    male (epididymal) Q55.4
      testicular Q55.29
  hymen Q52.4
  hypersegmentation of neutrophils, hereditary D72.0
  hypophyseal Q89.2
  ileocecal (coil) (valve) Q43.9
  ileum Q43.9
  ilium NEC Q74.2
  integument Q84.9
    specified NEC Q84.8
  interarch distance (excessive) (inadequate) M26.25
  intervertebral cartilage or disc Q76.49
  intestine (large) (small) Q43.9
    with anomalous adhesions, fixation or malrotation Q43.3
  iris Q13.2
  ischium NEC Q74.2
  jaw —*see* Anomaly, dentofacial
    alveolar —*see* Anomaly, alveolar
  jaw-cranial base relationship —*see* Anomaly, dentofacial, jaw-cranial base relationship
  jejunum Q43.8
  joint Q74.9
    specified NEC Q74.8
  Jordan's D72.0
  kidney (s) (calyx) (pelvis) Q63.9
    artery Q27.2
    specified NEC Q63.8
  Klippel-Feil (brevicollis) Q76.1
  knee Q74.1
  labium (majus) (minus) Q52.70
  labyrinth, membranous Q16.5
  lacrimal apparatus or duct Q10.6
  larynx, laryngeal (muscle) Q31.9
    web (bed) Q31.0
  lens Q12.9
  leukocytes, genetic D72.0
    granulation (constitutional) D72.0
  lid (fold) Q10.3

Anomaly, anomalous *(Continued)*
  ligament Q79.9
    broad Q50.6
    round Q52.8
  limb Q74.9
    lower NEC Q74.2
      reduction deformity —*see* Defect, reduction, lower limb
    upper Q74.0
  lip Q38.0
  liver Q44.7
    duct Q44.5
  lower limb NEC Q74.2
  lumbosacral (joint) (region) Q76.49
    kyphosis —*see* Kyphosis, congenital
    lordosis —*see* Lordosis, congenital
  lung (fissure) (lobe) Q33.9
  mandible —*see* Anomaly, dentofacial
  maxilla —*see* Anomaly, dentofacial
  May (-Hegglin) D72.0
  meatus urinarius NEC Q64.79
  meningeal bands or folds Q07.9
    constriction of Q07.8
    spinal Q06.9
  meninges Q07.9
    cerebral Q04.8
    spinal Q06.9
  meningocele Q05.9
  mesentery Q45.9
  metacarpus Q74.0
  metatarsus NEC Q74.2
  middle ear Q16.4
    ossicles Q16.3
  mitral (leaflets) (valve) Q23.9
    insufficiency Q23.3
    specified NEC Q23.8
    stenosis Q23.2
  mouth Q38.6
  Müllerian —*see also* Anomaly, by site
    uterus NEC Q51.818
  multiple NEC Q89.7
  muscle Q79.9
    eyelid Q10.3
  musculoskeletal system, except limbs Q79.9
  myocardium Q24.8
  nail Q84.6
  narrowness, eyelid Q10.3
  nasal sinus (wall) Q30.8
  neck (any part) Q18.9
  nerve Q07.9
    acoustic Q07.8
    optic Q07.8
  nervous system (central) Q07.9
  nipple Q83.9
  nose, nasal (bones) (cartilage) (septum) (sinus) Q30.9
    specified NEC Q30.8
  ocular muscle Q15.8
  omphalomesenteric duct Q43.0
  opening, pulmonary veins Q26.4
  optic
    disc Q14.2
    nerve Q07.8
  opticociliary vessels Q13.2
  orbit (eye) Q10.7
  organ Q89.9
    of Corti Q16.5
  origin
    artery
      innominate Q25.8
      pulmonary Q25.79
      renal Q27.2
      subclavian Q25.8
  osseous meatus (ear) Q16.1
  ovary Q50.39
  oviduct Q50.6
  palate (hard) (soft) NEC Q38.5
  pancreas or pancreatic duct Q45.3
  papillary muscles Q24.8
  parathyroid gland Q89.2
  paraurethral ducts Q64.79

Anomaly, anomalous *(Continued)*
  parotid (gland) Q38.4
  patella Q74.1
  Pelger-Huët (hereditary hyposegmentation) D72.0
  pelvic girdle NEC Q74.2
  pelvis (bony) NEC Q74.2
    rachitic E64.3
  penis (glans) Q55.69
  pericardium Q24.8
  peripheral vascular system Q27.9
  Peter's Q13.4
  pharynx Q38.8
  pigmentation L81.9
    congenital Q82.8
  pituitary (gland) Q89.2
  pleural (folds) Q34.0
  portal vein Q26.5
    connection Q26.5
  position, tooth, teeth, fully erupted M26.30
    specified NEC M26.39
  precerebral vessel Q28.1
  prepuce Q55.69
  prostate Q55.4
  pulmonary Q33.9
    artery NEC Q25.79
    valve Q22.3
      atresia Q22.0
      insufficiency Q22.2
      specified type NEC Q22.3
      stenosis Q22.1
        infundibular Q24.3
        subvalvular Q24.3
    venous connection Q26.4
      partial Q26.3
      total Q26.2
  pupil Q13.2
    function H57.00
      anisocoria H57.02
      Argyll Robertson pupil H57.01
      miosis H57.03
      mydriasis H57.04
      specified type NEC H57.09
      tonic pupil H57.05-
  pylorus Q40.3
  radius Q74.0
  rectum Q43.9
  reduction (extremity) (limb)
    femur (longitudinal) —*see* Defect, reduction, lower limb, longitudinal, femur
    fibula (longitudinal) —*see* Defect, reduction, lower limb, longitudinal, fibula
    lower limb —*see* Defect, reduction, lower limb
    radius (longitudinal) —*see* Defect, reduction, upper limb, longitudinal, radius
    tibia (longitudinal) —*see* Defect, reduction, lower limb, longitudinal, tibia
    ulna (longitudinal) —*see* Defect, reduction, upper limb, longitudinal, ulna
    upper limb —*see* Defect, reduction, upper limb
  refraction —*see* Disorder, refraction
  renal Q63.9
    artery Q27.2
    pelvis Q63.9
      specified NEC Q63.8
  respiratory system Q34.9
    specified NEC Q34.8
  retina Q14.1
  rib Q76.6
    cervical Q76.5
  Rieger's Q13.81
  rotation —*see* Malrotation
    hip or thigh Q65.89
  round ligament Q52.8
  sacroiliac (joint) NEC Q74.2

Anomaly, anomalous (*Continued*)
sacrum NEC Q76.49
  kyphosis —*see* Kyphosis, congenital
  lordosis —*see* Lordosis, congenital
saddle nose, syphilitic A50.57
salivary duct or gland Q38.4
scapula Q74.0
scrotum —*see* Malformation, testis and
  scrotum
sebaceous gland Q82.9
seminal vesicles Q55.4
sense organs NEC Q07.8
sex chromosomes NEC —*see also* Anomaly,
  chromosomes
  female phenotype Q97.8
  male phenotype Q98.9
shoulder (girdle) (joint) Q74.0
sigmoid (flexure) Q43.9
simian crease Q82.8
sinus of Valsalva Q25.4
skeleton generalized Q78.9
skin (appendage) Q82.9
skull Q75.9
  with
    anencephaly Q00.0
    encephalocele —*see* Encephalocele
    hydrocephalus Q03.9
      with spina bifida —*see* Spina bifida, by
        site, with hydrocephalus
    microcephaly Q02
specified organ or site NEC Q89.8
spermatic cord Q55.4
spine, spinal NEC Q76.49
  column NEC Q76.49
    kyphosis —*see* Kyphosis, congenital
    lordosis —*see* Lordosis, congenital
  cord Q06.9
  nerve root Q07.8
spleen Q89.09
  agenesis Q89.01
stenonian duct Q38.4
sternum NEC Q76.7
stomach Q40.3
submaxillary gland Q38.4
tarsus NEC Q74.2
tendon Q79.9
testis —*see* Malformation, testis and
  scrotum
thigh NEC Q74.2
thorax (wall) Q67.8
  bony Q76.9
throat Q38.8
thumb Q74.0
thymus gland Q89.2
thyroid (gland) Q89.2
  cartilage Q31.8
tibia NEC Q74.2
  saber A50.56
toe Q74.2
tongue Q38.3
tooth, teeth K00.9
  eruption K00.6
  position, fully erupted M26.30
  spacing, fully erupted M26.30
trachea (cartilage) Q32.1
tragus Q17.9
tricuspid (leaflet) (valve) Q22.9
  atresia or stenosis Q22.4
  Ebstein's Q22.5
Uhl's (hypoplasia of myocardium, right
  ventricle) Q24.8
ulna Q74.0
umbilical artery Q27.0
union
  cricoid cartilage and thyroid cartilage
    Q31.8
  thyroid cartilage and hyoid bone
    Q31.8
  trachea with larynx Q31.8
upper limb Q74.0
urachus Q64.4

Anomaly, anomalous (*Continued*)
ureter Q62.8
  obstructive NEC Q62.39
    cecoureterocele Q62.32
    orthotopic ureterocele Q62.31
urethra Q64.70
  absence Q64.5
  double Q64.74
  fistula to rectum Q64.73
  obstructive Q64.39
    stricture Q64.32
  prolapse Q64.71
  specified type NEC Q64.79
urinary tract Q64.9
uterus Q51.9
  with only one functioning horn
    Q51.4
uvula Q38.5
vagina Q52.4
valleculae Q31.8
valve (heart) NEC Q24.8
  coronary sinus Q24.5
  inferior vena cava Q24.8
  pulmonary Q22.3
  sinus coronario Q24.5
  venae cavae inferioris Q24.8
vas deferens Q55.4
vascular Q27.9
  brain Q28.3
  ring Q25.4
vein (s) (peripheral) Q27.9
  brain Q28.3
  cerebral Q28.3
  coronary Q24.5
  developmental Q28.3
  great Q26.9
    specified NEC Q26.8
vena cava (inferior) (superior) Q26.9
venous —*see* Anomaly, vein (s)
  venous return Q26.8
ventricular
  bands or folds Q24.8
  septa Q21.0
vertebra Q76.49
  kyphosis —*see* Kyphosis, congenital
  lordosis —*see* Lordosis, congenital
vesicourethral orifice Q64.79
vessel (s) Q27.9
  optic papilla Q14.2
  precerebral Q28.1
vitelline duct Q43.0
vitreous body or humor Q14.0
vulva Q52.70
wrist (joint) Q74.0
Anomia R48.8
Anonychia (congenital) Q84.3
  acquired L60.8
Anophthalmos, anophthalmus (congenital)
  (globe) Q11.1
  acquired Z90.01
Anopia, anopsia H53.46-
  quadrant H53.46-
Anorchia, anorchism, anorchidism Q55.0
Anorexia R63.0
  hysterical F44.89
  nervosa F50.00
    atypical F50.9
    binge-eating type F50.2
      with purging F50.02
    restricting type F50.01
Anorgasmy, psychogenic (female)
  F52.31
  male F52.32
Anosmia R43.0
  hysterical F44.6
  postinfectional J39.8
Anosognosia R41.89
Anosteoplasia Q78.9
Anovulatory cycle N97.0
Anoxemia R09.02
  newborn P84

Anoxia (pathological) R09.02
altitude T70.29
cerebral G93.1
  complicating
    anesthesia (general) (local) or other
      sedation T88.59
      in labor and delivery O74.3
      in pregnancy O29.21-
      postpartum, puerperal O89.2
    delivery (cesarean) (instrumental)
      O75.4
  during a procedure G97.81
  newborn P84
  resulting from a procedure G97.82
due to
  drowning T75.1
  high altitude T70.29
heart —*see* Insufficiency, coronary
intrauterine P84
myocardial —*see* Insufficiency, coronary
newborn P84
spinal cord G95.11
systemic (by suffocation) (low content in
  atmosphere) —*see* Asphyxia,
  traumatic
Anteflexion —*see* Anteversion
Antenatal
care (normal pregnancy) Z34.90
screening (encounter for) of mother
  Z36
Antepartum —*see* condition
Anterior —*see* condition
Antero-occlusion M26.220
Anteversion
cervix —*see* Anteversion, uterus
femur (neck), congenital Q65.89
uterus, uterine (cervix) (postinfectional)
  (postpartal, old) N85.4
  congenital Q51.818
  in pregnancy or childbirth —*see* Pregnancy,
    complicated by
Anthophobia F40.228
Anthracosilicosis J60
Anthracosis (lung) (occupational) J60
lingua K14.3
Anthrax A22.9
with pneumonia A22.1
cerebral A22.8
colitis A22.2
cutaneous A22.0
gastrointestinal A22.2
inhalation A22.1
intestinal A22.2
meningitis A22.8
pulmonary A22.1
respiratory A22.1
sepsis A22.7
specified manifestation NEC A22.8
Anthropoid pelvis Q74.2
with disproportion (fetopelvic) O33.0
Anthropophobia F40.10
generalized F40.11
Antibodies, maternal (blood group) —*see*
  Isoimmunization, affecting management
  of pregnancy
anti-D —*see* Isoimmunization, affecting
  management of pregnancy, Rh
newborn P55.0
Antibody
anticardiolipin R76.0
  with
    hemorrhagic disorder D68.312
    hypercoagulable state D68.61
antiphosphatidylglycerol R76.0
  with
    hemorrhagic disorder D68.312
    hypercoagulable state D68.61
antiphosphatidylinositol R76.0
  with
    hemorrhagic disorder D68.312
    hypercoagulable state D68.61

◀ New   ⬅ Revised   ~~deleted~~ Deleted

Antibody (*Continued*)
   antiphosphatidylserine R76.0
      with
         hemorrhagic disorder D68.312
         hypercoagulable state D68.61
      antiphospholipid R76.0
      with
         hemorrhagic disorder D68.312
         hypercoagulable state D68.61
Anticardiolipin syndrome D68.61
Anticoagulant, circulating (intrinsic) (*see also* -
      Disorder, hemorrhagic) D68.318
   drug-induced (extrinsic) (*see also* - Disorder,
      hemorrhagic) D68.32
Antidiuretic hormone syndrome E22.2
Antimonial cholera —*see* Poisoning,
      antimony
Antiphospholipid
   antibody
      with hemorrhagic disorder D68.312
      syndrome D68.61
Antisocial personality F60.2
Antithrombinemia —*see* Circulating
      anticoagulants
Antithromboplastinemia D68.318
Antithromboplastinogenemia D68.318
Antitoxin complication or reaction —*see*
      Complications, vaccination
Antlophobia F40.228
Antritis J32.0
   maxilla J32.0
      acute J01.00
         recurrent J01.01
   stomach K29.60
      with bleeding K29.61
Antrum, antral —*see* condition
Anuria R34
   calculous (impacted) (recurrent) (*see also*
         Calculus, urinary) N20.9
   following
      abortion —*see* Abortion by type
            complicated by, renal failure
      ectopic or molar pregnancy O08.4
   newborn P96.0
   postprocedural N99.0
   postrenal N13.8
   traumatic (following crushing) T79.5
Anus, anal —*see* condition
Anusitis K62.89
Anxiety F41.9
   depression F41.8
   episodic paroxysmal F41.0
   generalized F41.1
   hysteria F41.8
   neurosis F41.1
   panic type F41.0
   reaction F41.1
   separation, abnormal (of childhood) F93.0
   specified NEC F41.8
   state F41.1
Aorta, aortic —*see* condition
Aortectasia —*see* Ectasia, aorta
   with aneurysm —*see* Aneurysm, aorta
Aortitis (nonsyphilitic) (calcific) I77.6
   arteriosclerotic I70.0
   Doehle-Heller A52.02
   luetic A52.02
   rheumatic —*see* Endocarditis, acute,
         rheumatic
   specific (syphilitic) A52.02
   syphilitic A52.02
      congenital A50.54 [I79.1]
Apathetic thyroid storm —*see* Thyrotoxicosis
Apathy R45.3
Apeirophobia F40.228
Apepsia K30
   psychogenic F45.8
Aperistalsis, esophagus K22.0
Apertognathia M26.29
Apert's syndrome Q87.0
Aphagia R13.0
   psychogenic F50.9

Aphakia (acquired) (postoperative) H27.0-
      congenital Q12.3
Aphasia (amnestic) (global) (nominal)
      (semantic) (syntactic) R47.01
   acquired, with epilepsy (Landau-Kleffner
         syndrome) —*see* Epilepsy, specified
         NEC
   auditory (developmental) F80.2
   developmental (receptive type) F80.2
      expressive type F80.1
      Wernicke's F80.2
   following
      cerebrovascular disease I69.920
         cerebral infarction I69.320
         intracerebral hemorrhage I69.120
         nontraumatic intracranial hemorrhage
            NEC I69.220
         specified disease NEC I69.820
         subarachnoid hemorrhage I69.020
   primary progressive G31.01 [F02.80]
      with behavioral disturbance G31.01
         [F02.81]
   progressive isolated G31.01 [F02.80]
      with behavioral disturbance G31.01
         [F02.81]
   sensory F80.2
   syphilis, tertiary A52.19
   Wernicke's (developmental) F80.2
Aphonia (organic) R49.1
   hysterical F44.4
   psychogenic F44.4
Aphthae, aphthous —*see also* condition
   Bednar's K12.0
   cachectic K14.0
   epizootic B08.8
   fever B08.8
   oral (recurrent) K12.0
   stomatitis (major) (minor) K12.0
   thrush B37.0
   ulcer (oral) (recurrent) K12.0
      genital organ (s) NEC
         female N76.6
         male N50.8
      larynx J38.7
Apical —*see* condition
Apiphobia F40.218
Aplasia —*see also* Agenesis
   abdominal muscle syndrome Q79.4
   alveolar process (acquired) —*see* Anomaly,
         alveolar
      congenital Q38.6
   aorta (congenital) Q25.4
   axialis extracorticalis (congenita) E75.29
   bone marrow (myeloid) D61.9
      congenital D61.01
   brain Q00.0
      part of Q04.3
   bronchus Q32.4
   cementum K00.4
   cerebellum Q04.3
   cervix (congenital) Q51.5
   congenital pure red cell D61.01
   corpus callosum Q04.0
   cutis congenita Q84.8
   erythrocyte congenital D61.01
   extracortical axial E75.29
   eye Q11.1
   fovea centralis (congenital) Q14.1
   gallbladder, congenital Q44.0
   iris Q13.1
   labyrinth, membranous Q16.5
   limb (congenital) Q73.8
      lower —*see* Defect, reduction, lower
         limb
      upper —*see* Agenesis, arm
   lung, congenital (bilateral) (unilateral)
         Q33.3
   pancreas Q45.0
   parathyroid-thymic D82.1
   Pelizaeus-Merzbacher E75.29
   penis Q55.5
   prostate Q55.4

Aplasia (*Continued*)
   red cell (with thymoma) D60.9
      acquired D60.9
         due to drugs D60.9
      adult D60.9
      chronic D60.0
      congenital D61.01
      constitutional D61.01
      due to drugs D60.9
      hereditary D61.01
      of infants D61.01
      primary D61.01
      pure D61.01
         due to drugs D60.9
      specified type NEC D60.8
      transient D60.1
   round ligament Q52.8
   skin Q84.8
   spermatic cord Q55.4
   spleen Q89.01
   testicle Q55.0
   thymic, with immunodeficiency D82.1
   thyroid (congenital) (with myxedema)
         E03.1
   uterus Q51.0
   ventral horn cell Q06.1
Apnea, apneic (of) (spells) R06.81
   newborn NEC P28.4
      obstructive P28.4
      sleep (central) (obstructive) (primary)
         P28.3
   prematurity P28.4
   sleep G47.30
      central (primary) G47.31
         in conditions classified elsewhere
            G47.37
      obstructive (adult) (pediatric) G47.33
      primary central G47.31
      specified NEC G47.39
Apneumatosis, newborn P28.0
Apocrine metaplasia (breast) —*see* Dysplasia,
      mammary, specified type NEC
Apophysitis (bone) —*see also*
      Osteochondropathy
   calcaneus M92.8
   juvenile M92.9
Apoplectiform convulsions (cerebral ischemia)
      I67.82
Apoplexia, apoplexy, apoplectic
   adrenal A39.1
   heart (auricle) (ventricle) —*see* Infarct,
         myocardium
   heat T67.0
   hemorrhagic (stroke) —*see* Hemorrhage,
         intracranial
   meninges, hemorrhagic —*see* Hemorrhage,
         intracranial, subarachnoid
   uremic N18.9 [I68.8]
Appearance
   bizarre R46.1
   specified NEC R46.89
   very low level of personal hygiene R46.0
Appendage
   epididymal (organ of Morgagni) Q55.4
   intestine (epiploic) Q43.8
   preauricular Q17.0
   testicular (organ of Morgagni) Q55.29
Appendicitis (pneumococcal) (retrocecal) K37
   with
      perforation or rupture K35.2
      peritoneal abscess K35.3
      peritonitis NEC K35.3
         generalized (with perforation or
               rupture) K35.2
         localized (with perforation or rupture)
               K35.3
   acute (catarrhal) (fulminating) (gangrenous)
         (obstructive) (retrocecal) (suppurative)
         K35.80
      with
         peritoneal abscess K35.3

A

Appendicitis (*Continued*)
  acute (*Continued*)
    with (*Continued*)
      peritonitis NEC K35.3
        generalized (with perforation or rupture) K35.2
        localized (with perforation or rupture) K35.3
      specified NEC K35.89
    amebic A06.89
    chronic (recurrent) K36
    exacerbation —*see* Appendicitis, acute
    gangrenous —*see* Appendicitis, acute
    healed (obliterative) K36
    interval K36
    neurogenic K36
    obstructive K36
    recurrent K36
    relapsing K36
    subacute (adhesive) K36
    subsiding K36
    suppurative —*see* Appendicitis, acute
    tuberculous A18.32
Appendicopathia oxyurica B80
Appendix, appendicular —*see also* condition
  epididymis Q55.4
  Morgagni
    female Q50.5
    male (epididymal) Q55.4
      testicular Q55.29
  testis Q55.29
Appetite
  depraved —*see* Pica
  excessive R63.2
  lack or loss (*see also* Anorexia) R63.0
    nonorganic origin F50.8
    psychogenic F50.8
  perverted (hysterical) —*see* Pica
Apple peel syndrome Q41.1
Apprehension state F41.1
Apprehensiveness, abnormal F41.9
Approximal wear K03.0
Apraxia (classic) (ideational) (ideokinetic) (ideomotor) (motor) (verbal) R48.2
  following
    cerebrovascular disease I69.990
      cerebral infarction I69.390
      intracerebral hemorrhage I69.190
      nontraumatic intracranial hemorrhage NEC I69.290
      specified disease NEC I69.890
      subarachnoid hemorrhage I69.090
  oculomotor, congenital H51.8
Aptyalism K11.7
Apudoma —*see* Neoplasm, uncertain behavior, by site
Aqueous misdirection H40.83-
Arabicum elephantiasis —*see* Infestation, filarial
Arachnitis —*see* Meningitis
Arachnodactyly —*see* Syndrome, Marfan's
Arachnoiditis (acute) (adhesive) (basal) (brain) (cerebrospinal) —*see* Meningitis
Arachnophobia F40.210
Arboencephalitis, Australian A83.4
Arborization block (heart) I45.5
ARC (AIDS-related complex) B20
Arches —*see* condition
Arcuate uterus Q51.810
Arcuatus uterus Q51.810
Arcus (cornea) **senilis** —*see* Degeneration, cornea, senile
Arc-welder's lung J63.4
Areflexia R29.2
Areola —*see* condition
Argentaffinoma —*see also* Neoplasm, uncertain behavior, by site
  malignant —*see* Neoplasm, malignant, by site
  syndrome E34.0
Argininemia E72.21

Arginosuccinic aciduria E72.22
Argyll Robertson phenomenon, pupil or syndrome (syphilitic) A52.19
  atypical H57.09
  nonsyphilitic H57.09
Argyria, argyriasis
  conjunctival H11.13-
  from drug or medicament —*see* Table of Drugs and Chemicals, by substance
Argyrosis, conjunctival H11.13-
Arhinencephaly Q04.1
Ariboflavinosis E53.0
Arm —*see* condition
Arnold-Chiari disease, obstruction or syndrome (type II) Q07.00
  with
    hydrocephalus Q07.02
      with spina bifida Q07.03
    spina bifida Q07.01
      with hydrocephalus Q07.03
  type III —*see* Encephalocele
  type IV Q04.8
Aromatic amino-acid metabolism disorder E70.9
  specified NEC E70.8
Arousals, confusional G47.51
Arrest, arrested
  cardiac I46.9
    complicating
      abortion —*see* Abortion, by type, complicated by, cardiac arrest
      anesthesia (general) (local) or other sedation —*see* Table of Drugs and Chemicals, by drug
      in labor and delivery O74.2
      in pregnancy O29.11-
        postpartum, puerperal O89.1
      delivery (cesarean) (instrumental) O75.4
    due to
      cardiac condition I46.2
      specified condition NEC I46.8
    intraoperative I97.71-
    newborn P29.81
    postprocedural I97.12-
      obstetric procedure O75.4
  cardiorespiratory —*see* Arrest, cardiac
  circulatory —*see* Arrest, cardiac
  deep transverse O64.0
  development or growth
    bone —*see* Disorder, bone, development or growth
    child R62.50
    tracheal rings Q32.1
  epiphyseal
    complete
      femur M89.15-
      humerus M89.12-
      tibia M89.16-
      ulna M89.13-
    forearm M89.13-
      specified NEC M89.13-
      ulna —*see* Arrest, epiphyseal, by type, ulna
    lower leg M89.16-
      specified NEC M89.168
      tibia —*see* Arrest, epiphyseal, by type, tibia
    partial
      femur M89.15-
      humerus M89.12-
      tibia M89.16-
      ulna M89.13-
      specified NEC M89.18
  granulopoiesis —*see* Agranulocytosis
  growth plate —*see* Arrest, epiphyseal
  heart —*see* Arrest, cardiac
  legal, anxiety concerning Z65.3
  physeal —*see* Arrest, epiphyseal
  respiratory R09.2
    newborn P28.81
  sinus I45.5

Arrest, arrested (*Continued*)
  spermatogenesis (complete) —*see* Azoospermia
    incomplete —*see* Oligospermia
  transverse (deep) O64.0
Arrhenoblastoma
  benign
    specified site —*see* Neoplasm, benign, by site
    unspecified site
      female D27.9
      male D29.20
  malignant
    specified site —*see* Neoplasm, malignant, by site
    unspecified site
      female C56.9
      male C62.90
  specified site —*see* Neoplasm, uncertain behavior, by site
  unspecified site
    female D39.10
    male D40.10
Arrhythmia (auricle)(cardiac) (juvenile) (nodal) (reflex)(sinus)(supraventricular) (transitory)(ventricle) I49.9
  block I45.9
  extrasystolic I49.49
  newborn
    bradycardia P29.12
      occurring before birth P03.819
        before onset of labor P03.810
        during labor P03.811
    tachycardia P29.11
  psychogenic F45.8
  specified NEC I49.8
  vagal R55
  ventricular re-entry I47.0
Arrillaga-Ayerza syndrome (pulmonary sclerosis with pulmonary hypertension) I27.0
Arsenical pigmentation L81.8
  from drug or medicament —*see* Table of Drugs and Chemicals
Arsenism —*see* Poisoning, arsenic
Arterial —*see* condition
Arteriofibrosis —*see* Arteriosclerosis
Arteriolar sclerosis —*see* Arteriosclerosis
Arteriolith —*see* Arteriosclerosis
Arteriolitis I77.6
  necrotizing, kidney I77.5
  renal —*see* Hypertension, kidney
Arteriolosclerosis —*see* Arteriosclerosis
Arterionephrosclerosis —*see* Hypertension, kidney
Arteriopathy I77.9
Arteriosclerosis, arteriosclerotic (diffuse) (obliterans) (of) (senile) (with calcification) I70.90
  aorta I70.0
  arteries of extremities —*see* Arteriosclerosis, extremities
  brain I67.2
  bypass graft
    coronary —*see* Arteriosclerosis, coronary, bypass graft
    extremities —*see* Arteriosclerosis, extremities, bypass graft
  cardiac —*see* Disease, heart, ischemic, atherosclerotic
  cardiopathy —*see* Disease, heart, ischemic, atherosclerotic
  cardiorenal —*see* Hypertension, cardiorenal
  cardiovascular —*see* Disease, heart, ischemic, atherosclerotic
  carotid (*see also* Occlusion, artery, carotid) I65.2-
  central nervous system I67.2
  cerebral I67.2
  cerebrovascular I67.2

◀ New   ◀|||| Revised   ~~deleted~~ Deleted

Arteriosclerosis, arteriosclerotic *(Continued)*
 coronary (artery) I25.10
  bypass graft I25.810
   with
    angina pectoris I25.709
     with documented spasm I25.701
     specified type NEC I25.708
     unstable I25.700
    ischemic chest pain I25.709
   autologous artery I25.810
    with
     angina pectoris I25.729
      with documented spasm I25.721
      specified type I25.728
      unstable I25.720
     ischemic chest pain I25.729
   autologous vein I25.810
    with
     angina pectoris I25.719
      with documented spasm I25.711
      specified type I25.718
      unstable I25.710
     ischemic chest pain I25.719
   nonautologous biological I25.810
    with
     angina pectoris I25.739
      with documented spasm I25.731
      specified type I25.738
      unstable I25.730
     ischemic chest pain I25.739
   specified type NEC I25.810
    with
     angina pectoris I25.799
      with documented spasm I25.791
      specified type I25.798
      unstable I25.790
     ischemic chest pain I25.799
  due to
   calcified coronary lesion (severely) I25.84
   lipid rich plaque I25.83
  native vessel
   with
    angina pectoris I25.119
     with documented spasm I25.111
     specified type NEC I25.118
     unstable I25.110
    ischemic chest pain I25.119
  transplanted heart I25.811
   bypass graft I25.812
    with
     angina pectoris I25.769
      with documented spasm I25.761
      specified type I25.768
      unstable I25.760
     ischemic chest pain I25.769
   native coronary artery I25.811
    with
     angina pectoris I25.759
      with documented spasm I25.751
      specified type I25.758
      unstable I25.750
     ischemic chest pain I25.759
 extremities (native arteries) I70.209
  bypass graft I70.309
   autologous vein graft I70.409
    leg I70.409
     with
      gangrene (and intermittent claudication, rest pain and ulcer) I70.469
      intermittent claudication I70.419
      rest pain (and intermittent claudication) I70.429

Arteriosclerosis, arteriosclerotic *(Continued)*
 extremities *(Continued)*
  bypass graft *(Continued)*
   autologous vein graft *(Continued)*
    leg *(Continued)*
     bilateral I70.403
      with
       gangrene (and intermittent claudication, rest pain and ulcer) I70.463
       intermittent claudication I70.413
       rest pain (and intermittent claudication) I70.423
      specified type NEC I70.493
     left I70.402
      with
       gangrene (and intermittent claudication, rest pain and ulcer) I70.462
       intermittent claudication I70.412
       rest pain (and intermittent claudication) I70.422
       ulceration (and intermittent claudication and rest pain) I70.449
        ankle I70.443
        calf I70.442
        foot site NEC I70.445
        heel I70.444
        lower leg NEC I70.448
        midfoot I70.444
        thigh I70.441
      specified type NEC I70.492
     right I70.401
      with
       gangrene (and intermittent claudication, rest pain and ulcer) I70.461
       intermittent claudication I70.411
       rest pain (and intermittent claudication) I70.421
       ulceration (and intermittent claudication and rest pain) I70.439
        ankle I70.433
        calf I70.432
        foot site NEC I70.435
        heel I70.434
        lower leg NEC I70.438
        midfoot I70.434
        thigh I70.431
      specified type NEC I70.491
     specified type NEC I70.499
    specified NEC I70.408
     with
      gangrene (and intermittent claudication, rest pain and ulcer) I70.468
      intermittent claudication I70.418
      rest pain (and intermittent claudication) I70.428
      ulceration (and intermittent claudication and rest pain) I70.45
     specified type NEC I70.498
   leg I70.309
    with
     gangrene (and intermittent claudication, rest pain and ulcer) I70.369
     intermittent claudication I70.319
     rest pain (and intermittent claudication) I70.329
    bilateral I70.303
     with
      gangrene (and intermittent claudication, rest pain and ulcer) I70.363

Arteriosclerosis, arteriosclerotic *(Continued)*
 extremities *(Continued)*
  bypass graft *(Continued)*
   leg *(Continued)*
    bilateral *(Continued)*
     with *(Continued)*
      intermittent claudication I70.313
      rest pain (and intermittent claudication) I70.323
     specified type NEC I70.393
    left I70.302
     with
      gangrene (and intermittent claudication, rest pain and ulcer) I70.362
      intermittent claudication I70.312
      rest pain (and intermittent claudication) I70.322
      ulceration (and intermittent claudication and rest pain) I70.349
       ankle I70.343
       calf I70.342
       foot site NEC I70.345
       heel I70.344
       lower leg NEC I70.348
       midfoot I70.344
       thigh I70.341
     specified type NEC I70.392
    right I70.301
     with
      gangrene (and intermittent claudication, rest pain and ulcer) I70.361
      intermittent claudication I70.311
      rest pain (and intermittent claudication) I70.321
      ulceration (and intermittent claudication and rest pain) I70.339
       ankle I70.333
       calf I70.332
       foot site NEC I70.335
       heel I70.334
       lower leg NEC I70.338
       midfoot I70.334
       thigh I70.331
     specified type NEC I70.391
    specified type NEC I70.399
   nonautologous biological graft I70.509
    leg I70.509
     with
      gangrene (and intermittent claudication, rest pain and ulcer) I70.569
      intermittent claudication I70.519
      rest pain (and intermittent claudication) I70.529
     bilateral I70.503
      with
       gangrene (and intermittent claudication, rest pain and ulcer) I70.563
       intermittent claudication I70.513
       rest pain (and intermittent claudication) I70.523
      specified type NEC I70.593
     left I70.502
      with
       gangrene (and intermittent claudication, rest pain and ulcer) I70.562
       intermittent claudication I70.512
       rest pain (and intermittent claudication) I70.522

Arteriosclerosis, arteriosclerotic *(Continued)*
  extremities *(Continued)*
    bypass graft *(Continued)*
      nonautologous biological graft
          (Continued)
        leg *(Continued)*
          left *(Continued)*
            with *(Continued)*
              ulceration (and intermittent
                  claudication and rest
                  pain) I70.549
                ankle I70.543
                calf I70.542
                foot site NEC I70.545
                heel I70.544
                lower leg NEC I70.548
                midfoot I70.544
                thigh I70.541
              specified type NEC I70.592
          right I70.501
            with
              gangrene (and intermittent
                  claudication, rest pain
                  and ulcer) I70.561
              intermittent claudication
                  I70.511
              rest pain (and intermittent
                  claudication) I70.521
              ulceration (and intermittent
                  claudication and rest
                  pain) I70.539
                ankle I70.533
                calf I70.532
                foot site NEC I70.535
                heel I70.534
                lower leg NEC I70.538
                midfoot I70.534
                thigh I70.531
              specified type NEC I70.591
          specified type NEC I70.599
        specified NEC I70.508
          with
            gangrene (and intermittent
                claudication, rest pain and
                ulcer) I70.568
            intermittent claudication I70.518
            rest pain (and intermittent
                claudication) I70.528
            ulceration (and intermittent
                claudication and rest pain)
                I70.55
          specified type NEC I70.598
      nonbiological graft I70.609
        leg I70.609
          with
            gangrene (and intermittent
                claudication, rest pain and
                ulcer) I70.669
            intermittent claudication
                I70.619
            rest pain (and intermittent
                claudication) I70.629
          bilateral I70.603
            with
              gangrene (and intermittent
                  claudication, rest pain
                  and ulcer) I70.663
              intermittent claudication
                  I70.613
              rest pain (and intermittent
                  claudication) I70.623
            specified type NEC I70.693
          left I70.602
            with
              gangrene (and intermittent
                  claudication, rest pain
                  and ulcer) I70.662
              intermittent claudication
                  I70.612
              rest pain (and intermittent
                  claudication) I70.622

Arteriosclerosis, arteriosclerotic *(Continued)*
  extremities *(Continued)*
    bypass graft *(Continued)*
      nonbiological graft *(Continued)*
        leg *(Continued)*
          left *(Continued)*
            with *(Continued)*
              ulceration (and intermittent
                  claudication and rest
                  pain) I70.649
                ankle I70.643
                calf I70.642
                foot site NEC I70.645
                heel I70.644
                lower leg NEC I70.648
                midfoot I70.644
                thigh I70.641
              specified type NEC I70.692
          right I70.601
            with
              gangrene (and intermittent
                  claudication, rest pain
                  and ulcer) I70.661
              intermittent claudication
                  I70.611
              rest pain (and intermittent
                  claudication) I70.621
              ulceration (and intermittent
                  claudication and rest
                  pain) I70.639
                ankle I70.633
                calf I70.632
                foot site NEC I70.635
                heel I70.634
                lower leg NEC I70.638
                midfoot I70.634
                thigh I70.631
              specified type NEC I70.691
          specified type NEC I70.699
        specified NEC I70.608
          with
            gangrene (and intermittent
                claudication, rest pain and
                ulcer) I70.668
            intermittent claudication
                I70.618
            rest pain (and intermittent
                claudication) I70.628
            ulceration (and intermittent
                claudication and rest pain)
                I70.65
          specified type NEC I70.698
      specified graft NEC I70.709
        leg I70.709
          with
            gangrene (and intermittent
                claudication, rest pain and
                ulcer) I70.769
            intermittent claudication
                I70.719
            rest pain (and intermittent
                claudication) I70.729
          bilateral I70.703
            with
              gangrene (and intermittent
                  claudication, rest pain
                  and ulcer) I70.763
              intermittent claudication
                  I70.713
              rest pain (and intermittent
                  claudication) I70.723
            specified type NEC I70.793
          left I70.702
            with
              gangrene (and intermittent
                  claudication, rest pain
                  and ulcer) I70.762
              intermittent claudication
                  I70.712
              rest pain (and intermittent
                  claudication) I70.722

Arteriosclerosis, arteriosclerotic *(Continued)*
  extremities *(Continued)*
    bypass graft *(Continued)*
      specified graft NEC *(Continued)*
        leg *(Continued)*
          left *(Continued)*
            with *(Continued)*
              ulceration (and intermittent
                  claudication and rest
                  pain) I70.749
                ankle I70.743
                calf I70.742
                foot site NEC I70.745
                heel I70.744
                lower leg NEC I70.748
                midfoot I70.744
                thigh I70.741
              specified type NEC I70.792
          right I70.701
            with
              gangrene (and intermittent
                  claudication, rest pain
                  and ulcer) I70.761
              intermittent claudication
                  I70.711
              rest pain (and intermittent
                  claudication) I70.721
              ulceration (and intermittent
                  claudication and rest
                  pain) I70.739
                ankle I70.733
                calf I70.732
                foot site NEC I70.735
                heel I70.734
                lower leg NEC I70.738
                midfoot I70.734
                thigh I70.731
              specified type NEC I70.791
          specified type NEC I70.799
        specified NEC I70.708
          with
            gangrene (and intermittent
                claudication, rest pain and
                ulcer) I70.768
            intermittent claudication
                I70.718
            rest pain (and intermittent
                claudication) I70.728
            ulceration (and intermittent
                claudication and rest pain)
                I70.75
          specified type NEC I70.798
      specified NEC I70.308
        with
          gangrene (and intermittent
              claudication, rest pain and
              ulcer) I70.368
          intermittent claudication I70.318
          rest pain (and intermittent
              claudication) I70.328
          ulceration (and intermittent
              claudication and rest pain)
              I70.35
        specified type NEC I70.398
    leg I70.209
      with
        gangrene (and intermittent
            claudication, rest pain and ulcer)
            I70.269
        intermittent claudication I70.219
        rest pain (and intermittent
            claudication) I70.229
      bilateral I70.203
        with
          gangrene (and intermittent
              claudication, rest pain and
              ulcer) I70.263
          intermittent claudication I70.213
          rest pain (and intermittent
              claudication) I70.223
        specified type NEC I70.293

◄ New   ◄▦ Revised   ~~deleted~~ Deleted

Arteriosclerosis, arteriosclerotic (*Continued*)
extremities (*Continued*)
leg (*Continued*)
left I70.202
with
gangrene (and intermittent
claudication, rest pain and
ulcer) I70.262
intermittent claudication I70.212
rest pain (and intermittent
claudication) I70.222
ulceration (and intermittent
claudication and rest pain)
I70.249
ankle I70.243
calf I70.242
foot site NEC I70.245
heel I70.244
lower leg NEC I70.248
midfoot I70.244
thigh I70.241
specified type NEC I70.292
right I70.201
with
gangrene (and intermittent
claudication, rest pain and
ulcer) I70.261
intermittent claudication I70.211
rest pain (and intermittent
claudication) I70.221
ulceration (and intermittent
claudication and rest pain)
I70.239
ankle I70.233
calf I70.232
foot site NEC I70.235
heel I70.234
lower leg NEC I70.238
midfoot I70.234
thigh I70.231
specified type NEC I70.291
specified type NEC I70.299
specified site NEC I70.208
with
gangrene (and intermittent
claudication, rest pain and ulcer)
I70.268
intermittent claudication I70.218
rest pain (and intermittent
claudication) I70.228
ulceration (and intermittent
claudication and rest pain)
I70.25
specified type NEC I70.298
generalized I70.91
heart (disease) —*see* Arteriosclerosis,
coronary (artery)
kidney —*see* Hypertension, kidney
medial —*see* Arteriosclerosis, extremities
mesenteric (artery) K55.1
Mönckeberg's —*see* Arteriosclerosis,
extremities
myocarditis I51.4
peripheral (of extremities) —*see*
Arteriosclerosis, extremities
pulmonary (idiopathic) I27.0
renal (arterioles) —*see also* Hypertension,
kidney
artery I70.1
retina (vascular) I70.8 [H35.0-]
specified artery NEC I70.8
spinal (cord) G95.19
vertebral (artery) I67.2
Arteriospasm I73.9
Arteriovenous —*see* condition
Arteritis I77.6
allergic M31.0
aorta (nonsyphilitic) I77.6
syphilitic A52.02
aortic arch M31.4
brachiocephalic M31.4

Arteritis (*Continued*)
brain I67.7
syphilitic A52.04
cerebral I67.7
in
diseases classified elsewhere I68.2
systemic lupus erythematosus M32.19
listerial A32.89
syphilitic A52.04
tuberculous A18.89
coronary (artery) I25.89
rheumatic I01.8
chronic I09.89
syphilitic A52.06
cranial (left) (right), giant cell M31.6
deformans —*see* Arteriosclerosis
giant cell NEC M31.6
with polymyalgia rheumatica M31.5
necrosing or necrotizing M31.9
specified NEC M31.8
nodosa M30.0
obliterans —*see* Arteriosclerosis
pulmonary I28.8
rheumatic —*see* Fever, rheumatic
senile —*see* Arteriosclerosis
suppurative I77.2
syphilitic (general) A52.09
brain A52.04
coronary A52.06
spinal A52.09
temporal, giant cell M31.6
young female aortic arch syndrome M31.4
Artery, arterial —*see also* condition
abscess I77.89
single umbilical Q27.0
Arthralgia (allergic) —*see also* Pain, joint
in caisson disease T70.3
temporomandibular M26.62
Arthritis, arthritic (acute) (chronic)
(nonpyogenic) (subacute) M19.90
allergic —*see* Arthritis, specified form NEC
ankylosing (crippling) (spine) —*see also*
Spondylitis, ankylosing
sites other than spine —*see* Arthritis,
specified form NEC
atrophic —*see* Osteoarthritis
spine —*see* Spondylitis, ankylosing
back —*see* Spondylopathy, inflammatory
blennorrhagic (gonococcal) A54.42
Charcot's —*see* Arthropathy, neuropathic
diabetic —*see* Diabetes, arthropathy,
neuropathic
syringomyelic G95.0
chylous (filarial) (*see also* category M01) B74.9
climacteric (any site) NEC —*see* Arthritis,
specified form NEC
crystal (-induced) —*see* Arthritis, in, crystals
deformans —*see* Osteoarthritis
degenerative —*see* Osteoarthritis
due to or associated with
acromegaly E22.0
brucellosis —*see* Brucellosis
caisson disease T70.3
diabetes —*see* Diabetes, arthropathy
dracontiasis (*see also* category M01) B72
enteritis NEC
regional —*see* Enteritis, regional
erysipelas (*see also* category M01) A46
erythema
epidemic A25.1
nodosum L52
filariasis NOS B74.9
glanders A24.0
helminthiasis (*see also* category M01) B83.9
hemophilia D66 [M36.2]
Henoch-(Schönlein) purpura D69.0 [M36.4]
human parvovirus (*see also* category M01)
B97.6
infectious disease NEC —*see* category M01
leprosy (*see also* category M01) (*see also*
Leprosy) A30.9

Arthritis, arthritic (*Continued*)
due to or associated with (*Continued*)
Lyme disease A69.23
mycobacteria (*see also* category M01)
A31.8
parasitic disease NEC (*see also* category
M01) B89
paratyphoid fever (*see also* category M01)
(*see also* Fever, paratyphoid) A01.4
rat bite fever (*see also* category M01)
A25.1
regional enteritis —*see* Enteritis, regional
respiratory disorder NOS J98.9
serum sickness (*see also* Reaction, serum)
T80.69
syringomyelia G95.0
typhoid fever A01.04
epidemic erythema A25.1
febrile —*see* Fever, rheumatic
gonococcal A54.42
gouty (acute) —*see* Gout, idiopathic
in (due to)
acromegaly (*see also* subcategory M14.8-)
E22.0
amyloidosis (*see also* subcategory M14.8-)
E85.4
bacterial disease (*see also* subcategory M01)
A49.9
Behçet's syndrome M35.2
caisson disease (*see also* subcategory
M14.8-) T70.3
coliform bacilli (Escherichia coli) —*see*
Arthritis, in, pyogenic organism NEC
crystals M11.9
dicalcium phosphate —*see* Arthritis, in,
crystals, specified type NEC
hydroxyapatite M11.0-
pyrophosphate —*see* Arthritis, in,
crystals, specified type NEC
specified type NEC M11.80
ankle M11.87-
elbow M11.82-
foot joint M11.87-
hand joint M11.84-
hip M11.85-
knee M11.86-
multiple sites M11.8-
shoulder M11.81-
vertebrae M11.88
wrist M11.83-
dermatoarthritis, lipoid E78.81
dracontiasis (dracunculiasis) (*see also*
category M01) B72
endocrine disorder NEC (*see also*
subcategory M14.8-) E34.9
enteritis, infectious NEC (*see also* category
M01) A09
specified organism NEC (*see also*
category M01) A08.8
erythema
multiforme (*see also* subcategory M14.8-)
L51.9
nodosum (*see also* subcategory M14.8-)
L52
gout —*see* Gout, idiopathic
helminthiasis NEC (*see also* category M01)
B83.9
hemochromatosis (*see also* subcategory
M14.8-) E83.118
hemoglobinopathy NEC D58.2 [M36.3]
hemophilia NEC D66 [M36.2]
Hemophilus influenzae M00.8- [B96.3]
Henoch(-Schönlein) purpura D69.0 [M36.4]
hyperparathyroidism NEC (*see also*
subcategory M14.8-) E21.3
hypersensitivity reaction NEC T78.49
[M36.4]
hypogammaglobulinemia (*see also*
subcategory M14.8-) D80.1
hypothyroidism NEC (*see also* subcategory
M14.8-) E03.9

Arthritis, arthritic (*Continued*)
  in (*Continued*)
    infection —*see* Arthritis, pyogenic or pyemic
      spine —*see* Spondylopathy, infective
    infectious disease NEC —*see* category M01
    leprosy (*see also* category M01) A30.9
    leukemia NEC C95.9- [*M36.1*]
    lipoid dermatoarthritis E78.81
    Lyme disease A69.23
    Mediterranean fever, familial (*see also* subcategory M14.8-) E85.0
    Meningococcus A39.83
    metabolic disorder NEC (*see also* subcategory M14.8-) E88.9
    multiple myelomatosis C90.0- [*M36.1*]
    mumps B26.85
    mycosis NEC (*see also* category M01) B49
    myelomatosis (multiple) C90.0- [*M36.1*]
    neurological disorder NEC G98.0
    ochronosis (*see also* subcategory M14.8-) E70.29
    O'nyong-nyong (*see also* category M01) A92.1
    parasitic disease NEC (*see also* category M01) B89
    paratyphoid fever (*see also* category M01) A01.4
    Pseudomonas —*see* Arthritis, pyogenic, bacterial NEC
    psoriasis L40.50
    pyogenic organism NEC —*see* Arthritis, pyogenic, bacterial NEC
    Reiter's disease —*see* Reiter's disease
    respiratory disorder NEC (*see also* subcategory M14.8-) J98.9
    reticulosis, malignant (*see also* subcategory M14.8-) C86.0
    rubella B06.82
    Salmonella (arizonae) (cholerae-suis) (enteritidis) (typhimurium) A02.23
    sarcoidosis D86.86
    specified bacteria NEC —*see* Arthritis, pyogenic, bacterial NEC
    sporotrichosis B42.82
    syringomyelia G95.0
    thalassemia NEC D56.9 [*M36.3*]
    tuberculosis —*see* Tuberculosis, arthritis
    typhoid fever A01.04
    urethritis, Reiter's —*see* Reiter's disease
    viral disease NEC (*see also* category M01) B34.9
  infectious or infective —*see also* Arthritis, pyogenic or pyemic
    spine —*see* Spondylopathy, infective
  juvenile M08.90
    with systemic onset —*see* Still's disease
    ankle M08.97-
    elbow M08.92-
    foot joint M08.97-
    hand joint M08.94-
    hip M08.95-
    knee M08.96-
    multiple site M08.99
    pauciarticular M08.40
      ankle M08.47-
      elbow M08.42-
      foot joint M08.47-
      hand joint M08.44-
      hip M08.45-
      knee M08.46-
      shoulder M08.41-
      vertebrae M08.48
      wrist M08.43-
    psoriatic L40.54
    rheumatoid —*see* Arthritis, rheumatoid, juvenile
    shoulder M08.91-

Arthritis, arthritic (*Continued*)
  juvenile (*Continued*)
    specified type NEC M08.80
      ankle M08.87-
      elbow M08.82-
      foot joint M08.87-
      hand joint M08.84-
      hip M08.85-
      knee M08.86-
      multiple site M08.89
      shoulder M08.81-
      specified joint NEC M08.88
      vertebrae M08.88
      wrist M08.83-
    vertebra M08.98
    wrist M08.93-
  meaning osteoarthritis —*see* Osteoarthritis
  meningococcal A39.83
  menopausal (any site) NEC —*see* Arthritis, specified form NEC
  mutilans (psoriatic) L40.52
  mycotic NEC (*see also* category M01) B49
  neuropathic (Charcot) —*see* Arthropathy, neuropathic
    diabetic —*see* Diabetes, arthropathy, neuropathic
    nonsyphilitic NEC G98.0
    syringomyelic G95.0
  ochronotic (*see also* subcategory M14.8-) E70.29
  palindromic (any site) —*see* Rheumatism, palindromic
  pneumococcal M00.10
    ankle M00.17-
    elbow M00.12-
    foot joint —*see* Arthritis, pneumococcal, ankle
    hand joint M00.14-
    hip M00.15-
    knee M00.16-
    multiple site M00.19
    shoulder M00.11-
    vertebra M00.18
    wrist M00.13-
  postdysenteric —*see* Arthropathy, postdysenteric
  postmeningococcal A39.84
  postrheumatic, chronic —*see* Arthropathy, postrheumatic, chronic
  primary progressive —*see also* Arthritis, specified form NEC
    spine —*see* Spondylitis, ankylosing
  psoriatic L40.50
  purulent (any site except spine) —*see* Arthritis, pyogenic or pyemic
    spine —*see* Spondylopathy, infective
  pyogenic or pyemic (any site except spine) M00.9
    bacterial NEC M00.80
      ankle M00.87-
      elbow M00.82-
      foot joint —*see* Arthritis, pyogenic, bacterial NEC, ankle
      hand joint M00.84-
      hip M00.85-
      knee M00.86-
      multiple site M00.89
      shoulder M00.81-
      vertebra M00.88
      wrist M00.83-
    pneumococcal —*see* Arthritis, pneumococcal
    spine —*see* Spondylopathy, infective
    staphylococcal —*see* Arthritis, staphylococcal
    streptococcal —*see* Arthritis, streptococcal NEC
    pneumococcal —*see* Arthritis, pneumococcal
  reactive —*see* Reiter's disease
  rheumatic —*see also* Arthritis, rheumatoid
    acute or subacute —*see* Fever, rheumatic

Arthritis, arthritic (*Continued*)
  rheumatoid M06.9
    with
      carditis —*see* Rheumatoid, carditis
      endocarditis —*see* Rheumatoid, carditis
      heart involvement NEC —*see* Rheumatoid, carditis
      lung involvement —*see* Rheumatoid, lung
      myocarditis —*see* Rheumatoid, carditis
      myopathy —*see* Rheumatoid, myopathy
      pericarditis —*see* Rheumatoid, carditis
      polyneuropathy —*see* Rheumatoid, polyneuropathy
      rheumatoid factor —*see* Arthritis, rheumatoid, seropositive
      splenoadenomegaly and leukopenia — *see* Felty's syndrome
      vasculitis —*see* Rheumatoid, vasculitis
      visceral involvement NEC —*see* Rheumatoid, arthritis, with involvement of organs NEC
    juvenile (with or without rheumatoid factor) M08.00
      ankle M08.07-
      elbow M08.02-
      foot joint M08.07-
      hand joint M08.04-
      hip M08.05-
      knee M08.06-
      multiple site M08.09
      shoulder M08.01-
      vertebra M08.08
      wrist M08.03-
    seronegative M06.00
      ankle M06.07-
      elbow M06.02-
      foot joint M06.07-
      hand joint M06.04-
      hip M06.05-
      knee M06.06-
      multiple sites M06.09
      shoulder M06.01-
      vertebra M06.08
      wrist M06.03-
    seropositive M05.9
      without organ involvement M05.70
        ankle M05.77-
        elbow M05.72-
        foot joint M05.77-
        hand joint M05.74-
        hip M05.75-
        knee M05.76-
        multiple sites M05.79
        shoulder M05.71-
        vertebra —*see* Spondylitis, ankylosing
        wrist M05.73-
    specified NEC M05.80
      ankle M05.87-
      elbow M05.82-
      foot joint M05.87-
      hand joint M05.84-
      hip M05.85-
      knee M05.86-
      multiple sites M05.89
      shoulder M05.81-
      vertebra —*see* Spondylitis, ankylosing
      wrist M05.83-
    specified type NEC M06.80
      ankle M06.87-
      elbow M06.82-
      foot joint M06.87-
      hand joint M06.84-
      hip M06.85-
      knee M06.86-
      multiple site M06.89
      shoulder M06.81-
      vertebra M06.88
      wrist M06.83-
    spine —*see* Spondylitis, ankylosing
  rubella B06.82

◀ New   ◀||| Revised   ~~deleted~~ Deleted

Arthritis, arthritic (Continued)
scorbutic (see also subcategory M14.8-) E54
senile or senescent —see Osteoarthritis
septic (any site except spine) —see Arthritis, pyogenic or pyemic
spine —see Spondylopathy, infective
serum (nontherapeutic) (therapeutic) —see Arthropathy, postimmunization
specified form NEC M13.80
  ankle M13.87-
  elbow M13.82-
  foot joint M13.87-
  hand joint M13.84-
  hip M13.85-
  knee M13.86-
  multiple site M13.89
  shoulder M13.81-
  specified joint NEC M13.88
  wrist M13.83-
spine —see also Spondylopathy, inflammatory
  infectious or infective NEC —see Spondylopathy, infective
  Marie-Strümpell —see Spondylitis, ankylosing
  pyogenic —see Spondylopathy, infective
  rheumatoid —see Spondylitis, ankylosing
  traumatic (old) —see Spondylopathy, traumatic
  tuberculous A18.01
staphylococcal M00.00
  ankle M00.07-
  elbow M00.02-
  foot joint —see Arthritis, staphylococcal, ankle
  hand joint M00.04-
  hip M00.05-
  knee M00.06-
  multiple site M00.09
  shoulder M00.01-
  vertebra M00.08
  wrist M00.03-
streptococcal NEC M00.20
  ankle M00.27-
  elbow M00.22-
  foot joint —see Arthritis, streptococcal, ankle
  hand joint M00.24-
  hip M00.25-
  knee M00.26-
  multiple site M00.29
  shoulder M00.21-
  vertebra M00.28
  wrist M00.23-
suppurative —see Arthritis, pyogenic or pyemic
syphilitic (late) A52.16
  congenital A50.55 [M12.80]
syphilitica deformans (Charcot) A52.16
temporomandibular M26.69
toxic of menopause (any site) —see Arthritis, specified form NEC
transient —see Arthropathy, specified form NEC
traumatic (chronic) —see Arthropathy, traumatic
tuberculous A18.02
  spine A18.01
uratic —see Gout, idiopathic
urethritica (Reiter's) —see Reiter's disease
vertebral —see Spondylopathy, inflammatory
villous (any site) —see Arthropathy, specified form NEC
Arthrocele —see Effusion, joint
Arthrodesis status Z98.1
Arthrodynia —see also Pain, joint
Arthrodysplasia Q74.9
Arthrofibrosis, joint —see Ankylosis
Arthrogryposis (congenital) Q68.8
  multiplex congenita Q74.3
Arthrokatadysis M24.7

Arthropathy (see also Arthritis) M12.9
Charcot's —see Arthropathy, neuropathic
  diabetic —see Diabetes, arthropathy, neuropathic
  syringomyelic G95.0
cricoarytenoid J38.7
crystal (-induced) —see Arthritis, in, crystals
diabetic NEC —see Diabetes, arthropathy
distal interphalangeal, psoriatic L40.51
enteropathic M07.60
  ankle M07.67-
  elbow M07.62-
  foot joint M07.67-
  hand joint M07.64-
  hip M07.65-
  knee M07.66-
  multiple site M07.69
  shoulder M07.61-
  vertebra M07.68
  wrist M07.63-
following intestinal bypass M02.00
  ankle M02.07-
  elbow M02.02-
  foot joint M02.07-
  hand joint M02.04-
  hip M02.05-
  knee M02.06-
  multiple site M02.09
  shoulder M02.01-
  vertebra M02.08
  wrist M02.03-
gouty —see also Gout, idiopathic
  in (due to)
    Lesch-Nyhan syndrome E79.1 [M14.8-]
    sickle-cell disorders D57- [M14.8-]
hemophilic NEC D66 [M36.2]
  in (due to)
    hyperparathyroidism NEC E21.3 [M14.8-]
    metabolic disease NOS E88.9 [M14.8-]
in (due to)
  acromegaly E22.0 [M14.8-]
  amyloidosis E85.4 [M14.8-]
  blood disorder NOS D75.9 [M36.3]
  diabetes —see Diabetes, arthropathy
  endocrine disease NOS E34.9 [M14.8-]
  erythema
    multiforme L51.9 [M14.8-]
    nodosum L52 [M14.8-]
  hemochromatosis E83.118 [M14.8-]
  hemoglobinopathy NEC D58.2 [M36.3]
  hemophilia NEC D66 [M36.2]
  Henoch-Schönlein purpura D69.0 [M36.4]
  hyperthyroidism E05.90 [M14.8-]
  hypothyroidism E03.9 [M14.8-]
  infective endocarditis I33.0 [M12.80]
  leukemia NEC C95.9- [M36.1]
  malignant histiocytosis C96.A [M36.1]
  metabolic disease NOS E88.9 [M14.8-]
  multiple myeloma C90.0- [M36.1]
  neoplastic disease NOS (see also Neoplasm) D49.9 [M36.1]
  nutritional deficiency (see also subcategory M14.8-) E63.9
  psoriasis NOS L40.50
  sarcoidosis D86.86
  syphilis (late) A52.77
    congenital A50.55 [M12.80]
  thyrotoxicosis (see also subcategory M14.8-) E05.90
  ulcerative colitis K51.90 [M07.60]
  viral hepatitis (postinfectious) NEC B19.9 [M12.80]
  Whipple's disease (see also subcategory M14.8-) K90.81
Jaccoud —see Arthropathy, postrheumatic, chronic
juvenile —see Arthritis, juvenile
  psoriatic L40.54
mutilans (psoriatic) L40.52

Arthropathy (Continued)
neuropathic (Charcot) M14.60
  ankle M14.67-
  diabetic —see Diabetes, arthropathy, neuropathic
  elbow M14.62-
  foot joint M14.67-
  hand joint M14.64-
  hip M14.65-
  knee M14.66-
  multiple site M14.69
  nonsyphilitic NEC G98.0
  shoulder M14.61-
  syringomyelic G95.0
  vertebra M14.68
  wrist M14.63-
ostopulmonary —see Osteoarthropathy, hypertrophic, specified NEC
postdysenteric M02.10
  ankle M02.17-
  elbow M02.12-
  foot joint M02.17-
  hand joint M02.14-
  hip M02.15-
  knee M02.16-
  multiple site M02.19
  shoulder M02.11-
  vertebra M02.18
  wrist M02.13-
postimmunization M02.20
  ankle M02.27-
  elbow M02.22-
  foot joint M02.27-
  hand joint M02.24-
  hip M02.25-
  knee M02.26-
  multiple site M02.29
  shoulder M02.21-
  vertebra M02.28
  wrist M02.23-
postinfectious NEC B99 [M12.80]
  in (due to)
    enteritis due to Yersinia enterocolitica A04.6 [M12.80]
    syphilis A52.77
    viral hepatitis NEC B19.9 [M12.80]
postrheumatic, chronic (Jaccoud) M12.00
  ankle M12.07-
  elbow M12.02-
  foot joint M12.07-
  hand joint M12.04-
  hip M12.05-
  knee M12.06-
  multiple site M12.09
  shoulder M12.01-
  specified joint NEC M12.08
  vertebrae M12.08
  wrist M12.03-
psoriatic NEC L40.59
  interphalangeal, distal L40.51
reactive M02.9
  in (due to)
    infective endocarditis I33.0 [M02.9]
  specified type NEC M02.80
    ankle M02.87-
    elbow M02.82-
    foot joint M02.87-
    hand joint M02.84-
    hip M02.85-
    knee M02.86-
    multiple site M02.89
    shoulder M02.81-
    vertebra M02.88
    wrist M02.83-
specified form NEC M12.80
  ankle M12.87-
  elbow M12.82-
  foot joint M12.87-
  hand joint M12.84-
  hip M12.85-
  knee M12.86-
  multiple site M12.89

Arthropathy (Continued)
  specified form NEC (Continued)
    shoulder M12.81-
    specified joint NEC M12.88
    vertebrae M12.88
    wrist M12.83-
  syringomyelic G95.0
  tabes dorsalis A52.16
  tabetic A52.16
  transient —see Arthropathy, specified form
    NEC
  traumatic M12.50
    ankle M12.57-
    elbow M12.52-
    foot joint M12.57-
    hand joint M12.54-
    hip M12.55-
    knee M12.56-
    multiple site M12.59
    shoulder M12.51-
    specified joint NEC M12.58
    vertebrae M12.58
    wrist M12.53-
Arthropyosis —see Arthritis, pyogenic or pyemic
Arthrosis (deformans) (degenerative) (localized)
  (see also Osteoarthritis) M19.90
  spine —see Spondylosis
Arthus' phenomenon or reaction T78.41
  due to
    drug —see Table of Drugs and Chemicals,
      by drug
Articular —see condition
Articulation, reverse (teeth) M26.24
Artificial
  insemination complication —see
    Complications, artificial, fertilization
  opening status (functioning) (without
    complication) Z93.9
    anus (colostomy) Z93.3
    colostomy Z93.3
    cystostomy Z93.50
      appendico-vesicostomy Z93.52
      cutaneous Z93.51
      specified NEC Z93.59
    enterostomy Z93.4
    gastrostomy Z93.1
    ileostomy Z93.2
    intestinal tract NEC Z93.4
    jejunostomy Z93.4
    nephrostomy Z93.6
    specified site NEC Z93.8
    tracheostomy Z93.0
    ureterostomy Z93.6
    urethrostomy Z93.6
    urinary tract NEC Z93.6
    vagina Z93.8
    vagina status Z93.8
Arytenoid —see condition
Asbestosis (occupational) J61
ASC-H (atypical squamous cells cannot exclude
  high grade squamous intraepithelial lesion
  on cytologic smear)
  anus R85.611
  cervix R87.611
  vagina R87.621
ASC-US (atypical squamous cells of
  undetermined significance on cytologic
  smear)
  anus R85.610
  cervix R87.610
  vagina R87.620
Ascariasis B77.9
  with
    complications NEC B77.89
    intestinal complications B77.0
    pneumonia, pneumonitis B77.81
Ascaridosis, ascaridiasis —see Ascariasis
Ascaris (infection) (infestation)
  (lumbricoides) —see Ascariasis
Ascending —see condition
Aschoff's bodies —see Myocarditis, rheumatic

Ascites (abdominal) R18.8
  cardiac I50.9
  chylous (nonfilarial) I89.8
    filarial —see Infestation, filarial
  due to
    cirrhosis, alcoholic K70.31
    hepatitis
      alcoholic K70.11
      chronic active K71.51
    S. japonicum B65.2
  heart I50.9
  malignant R18.0
  pseudochylous R18.8
  syphilitic A52.74
  tuberculous A18.31
Aseptic —see condition
Asherman's syndrome N85.6
Asialia K11.7
Asiatic cholera —see Cholera
Asimultagnosia (simultanagnosia) R48.3
Askin's tumor —see Neoplasm, connective
  tissue, malignant
Asocial personality F60.2
Asomatognosia R41.4
Aspartylglucosaminuria E77.1
Asperger's disease or syndrome F84.5
Aspergilloma —see Aspergillosis
Aspergillosis (with pneumonia) B44.9
  bronchopulmonary, allergic B44.81
  disseminated B44.7
  generalized B44.7
  pulmonary NEC B44.1
    allergic B44.81
    invasive B44.0
  specified NEC B44.89
  tonsillar B44.2
Aspergillus (flavus) (fumigatus) (infection)
  (terreus) —see Aspergillosis
Aspermatogenesis —see Azoospermia
Aspermia (testis) —see Azoospermia
Asphyxia, asphyxiation (by) R09.01
  antenatal P84
  birth P84
  bunny bag —see Asphyxia, due to,
    mechanical threat to breathing, trapped
    in bed clothes
  crushing S28.0
  drowning T75.1
  gas, fumes, or vapor —see Table of Drugs and
    Chemicals
  inhalation —see Inhalation
  intrauterine P84
  local I73.00
    with gangrene I73.01
  mucus —see also Foreign body, respiratory
    tract, causing asphyxia
  newborn P84
  pathological R09.01
  postnatal P84
    mechanical —see Asphyxia, due to,
      mechanical threat to breathing
  prenatal P84
  reticularis R23.1
  strangulation —see Asphyxia, due to,
    mechanical threat to breathing
  submersion T75.1
  traumatic T71.9
    due to
      crushed chest S28.0
      foreign body (in) —see Foreign body,
        respiratory tract, causing asphyxia
      low oxygen content of ambient air T71.20
      due to
        being trapped in
          low oxygen environment T71.29
            in car trunk T71.221
              circumstances undetermined
                T71.224
              done with intent to harm by
                another person T71.223
                self T71.222

Asphyxia, asphyxiation (Continued)
  traumatic (Continued)
    due to (Continued)
      low oxygen content of ambient air
        (Continued)
        due to (Continued)
          being trapped in (Continued)
            low oxygen environment
              (Continued)
              in refrigerator T71.231
                circumstances undetermined
                  T71.234
                done with intent to harm by
                  another person T71.233
                  self T71.232
        cave-in T71.21
      mechanical threat to breathing
        (accidental) T71.191
      circumstances undetermined T71.194
      done with intent to harm by
        another person T71.193
      self T71.192
      hanging T71.161
        circumstances undetermined
          T71.164
        done with intent to harm by
          another person T71.163
        self T71.162
      plastic bag T71.121
        circumstances undetermined
          T71.124
        done with intent to harm by
          another person T71.123
        self T71.122
      smothering
        in furniture T71.151
          circumstances undetermined
            T71.154
          done with intent to harm by
            another person T71.153
          self T71.152
        under
          another person's body T71.141
            circumstances undetermined
              T71.144
            done with intent to harm
              T71.143
          pillow T71.111
            circumstances undetermined
              T71.114
            done with intent to harm by
              another person T71.113
              self T71.112
      trapped in bed clothes T71.131
        circumstances undetermined
          T71.134
        done with intent to harm by
          another person T71.133
        self T71.132
  vomiting, vomitus —see Foreign body,
    respiratory tract, causing asphyxia
Aspiration
  amniotic (clear) fluid (newborn) P24.10
    with
      pneumonia (pneumonitis) P24.11
      respiratory symptoms P24.11
  blood
    newborn (without respiratory symptoms)
      P24.20
      with
        pneumonia (pneumonitis) P24.21
        respiratory symptoms P24.21
      specified age NEC —see Foreign body,
        respiratory tract
  bronchitis J69.0
  food or foreign body (with asphyxiation) —
    see Asphyxia, food
  liquor (amnii) (newborn) P24.10
    with
      pneumonia (pneumonitis) P24.11
      respiratory symptoms P24.11

◀ New   ◀⫿⫿ Revised   ~~deleted~~ Deleted

Aspiration *(Continued)*
meconium (newborn) (without respiratory symptoms) P24.00
with
pneumonitis (pneumonitis) P24.01
respiratory symptoms P24.01
milk (newborn) (without respiratory symptoms) P24.30
with
pneumonia (pneumonitis) P24.31
respiratory symptoms P24.31
specified age NEC —*see* Foreign body, respiratory tract
mucus —*see also* Foreign body, by site, causing asphyxia
newborn P24.10
with
pneumonia (pneumonitis) P24.11
respiratory symptoms P24.11
neonatal P24.9
specific NEC (without respiratory symptoms) P24.80
with
pneumonia (pneumonitis) P24.81
respiratory symptoms P24.81
newborn P24.9
specific NEC (without respiratory symptoms) P24.80
with
pneumonia (pneumonitis) P24.81
respiratory symptoms P24.81
pneumonia J69.0
pneumonitis J69.0
syndrome of newborn —*see* Aspiration, by substance, with pneumonia
vernix caseosa (newborn) P24.80
with
pneumonia (pneumonitis) P24.81
respiratory symptoms P24.81
vomitus —*see also* Foreign body, respiratory tract
newborn (without respiratory symptoms) P24.30
with
pneumonia (pneumonitis) P24.31
respiratory symptoms P24.31
Asplenia (congenital) Q89.01
postsurgical Z90.81
Assam fever B55.0
Assault, sexual —*see* Maltreatment
Assmann's focus NEC A15.0
Astasia (-abasia) (hysterical) F44.4
Asteatosis cutis L85.3
Astereognosia, astereognosis R48.1
Asterixis R27.8
in liver disease K71.3
Asteroid hyalitis —*see* Deposit, crystalline
Asthenia, asthenic R53.1
cardiac (*see also* Failure, heart) I50.9
psychogenic F45.8
cardiovascular (*see also* Failure, heart) I50.9
psychogenic F45.8
heart (*see also* Failure, heart) I50.9
psychogenic F45.8
nervous F48.8
neurocirculatory F45.8
neurotic F48.8
psychogenic F48.8
psychoneurotic F48.8
psychophysiologic F48.8
reaction (psychophysiologic) F48.8
senile R54
Asthenopia —*see also* Discomfort, visual
hysterical F44.6
psychogenic F44.6

Asthenospermia —*see* Abnormal, specimen, male genital organs
Asthma, asthmatic (bronchial) (catarrh) (spasmodic) J45.909
with
chronic obstructive bronchitis J44.9
with
acute lower respiratory infection J44.0
exacerbation (acute) J44.1
chronic obstructive pulmonary disease J44.9
with
acute lower respiratory infection J44.0
exacerbation (acute) J44.1
exacerbation (acute) J45.901
hay fever —*see* Asthma, allergic extrinsic
rhinitis, allergic —*see* Asthma, allergic extrinsic
status asthmaticus J45.902
allergic extrinsic J45.909
with
exacerbation (acute) J45.901
status asthmaticus J45.902
atopic —*see* Asthma, allergic extrinsic
cardiac —*see* Failure, ventricular, left
cardiobronchial I50.1
childhood J45.909
with
exacerbation (acute) J45.901
status asthmaticus J45.902
chronic obstructive J44.9
with
acute lower respiratory infection J44.0
exacerbation (acute) J44.1
collier's J60
cough variant J45.991
detergent J69.8
due to
detergent J69.8
inhalation of fumes J68.3
eosinophilic J82
extrinsic, allergic —*see* Asthma, allergic extrinsic
grinder's J62.8
hay —*see* Asthma, allergic extrinsic
heart I50.1
idiosyncratic —*see* Asthma, nonallergic
intermittent (mild) J45.20
with
exacerbation (acute) J45.21
status asthmaticus J45.22
intrinsic, nonallergic —*see* Asthma, nonallergic
Kopp's E32.8
late-onset J45.909
with
exacerbation (acute) J45.901
status asthmaticus J45.902
mild intermittent J45.20
with
exacerbation (acute) J45.21
status asthmaticus J45.22
mild persistent J45.30
with
exacerbation (acute) J45.31
status asthmaticus J45.32
Millar's (laryngismus stridulus) J38.5
miner's J60
mixed J45.909
with
exacerbation (acute) J45.901
status asthmaticus J45.902
moderate persistent J45.40
with
exacerbation (acute) J45.41
status asthmaticus J45.42

Asthma, asthmatic *(Continued)*
nervous —*see* Asthma, nonallergic
nonallergic (intrinsic) J45.909
with
exacerbation (acute) J45.901
status asthmaticus J45.902
persistent
mild J45.30
with
exacerbation (acute) J45.31
status asthmaticus J45.32
moderate J45.40
with
exacerbation (acute) J45.41
status asthmaticus J45.42
severe J45.50
with
exacerbation (acute) J45.51
status asthmaticus J45.52
platinum J45.998
pneumoconiotic NEC J64
potter's J62.8
predominantly allergic J45.909
psychogenic F54
pulmonary eosinophilic J82
red cedar J67.8
Rostan's I50.1
sandblaster's J62.8
sequoiosis J67.8
severe persistent J45.50
with
exacerbation (acute) J45.51
status asthmaticus J45.52
specified NEC J45.998
stonemason's J62.8
thymic E32.8
tuberculous —*see* Tuberculosis, pulmonary
Wichmann's (laryngismus stridulus) J38.5
wood J67.8
Astigmatism (compound) (congenital) H52.20-
irregular H52.21-
regular H52.22-
Astraphobia F40.220
Astroblastoma
specified site —*see* Neoplasm, malignant, by site
unspecified site C71.9
Astrocytoma (cystic)
anaplastic
specified site —*see* Neoplasm, malignant, by site
unspecified site C71.9
fibrillary
specified site —*see* Neoplasm, malignant, by site
unspecified site C71.9
fibrous
specified site —*see* Neoplasm, malignant, by site
unspecified site C71.9
gemistocytic
specified site —*see* Neoplasm, malignant, by site
unspecified site C71.9
juvenile
specified site —*see* Neoplasm, malignant, by site
unspecified site C71.9
pilocytic
specified site —*see* Neoplasm, malignant, by site
unspecified site C71.9
piloid
specified site —*see* Neoplasm, malignant, by site
unspecified site C71.9
protoplasmic
specified site —*see* Neoplasm, malignant, by site
unspecified site C71.9

Astrocytoma *(Continued)*
  specified site NEC —*see* Neoplasm,
      malignant, by site
  subependymal D43.2
    giant cell
      specified site —*see* Neoplasm, uncertain
          behavior, by site
      unspecified site D43.2
    specified site —*see* Neoplasm, uncertain
        behavior, by site
    unspecified site D43.2
  unspecified site C71.9
Astroglioma
  specified site —*see* Neoplasm, malignant, by
      site
  unspecified site C71.9
Asymbolia R48.8
Asymmetry —*see also* Distortion
  between native and reconstructed breast N65.1
  face Q67.0
  jaw (lower) —*see* Anomaly, dentofacial, jaw-
      cranial base relationship, asymmetry
Asynergia, asynergy R27.8
  ventricular I51.89
Asystole (heart) —*see* Arrest, cardiac
At risk
  for falling Z91.81
Ataxia, ataxy, ataxic R27.0
  acute R27.8
  brain (hereditary) G11.9
  cerebellar (hereditary) G11.9
    with defective DNA repair G11.3
    alcoholic G31.2
    early-onset G11.1
    in
      alcoholism G31.2
      myxedema E03.9 *[G13.2]*
      neoplastic disease (*see also* Neoplasm)
          D49.9 *[G13.1]*
      specified disease NEC G32.81
    late-onset (Marie's) G11.2
  cerebral (hereditary) G11.9
  congenital nonprogressive G11.0
  family, familial —*see* Ataxia, hereditary
  following
    cerebrovascular disease I69.993
      cerebral infarction I69.393
      intracerebral hemorrhage I69.193
      nontraumatic intracranial hemorrhage
          NEC I69.293
      specified disease NEC I69.893
      subarachnoid hemorrhage I69.093
  Friedreich's (heredofamilial) (cerebellar)
      (spinal) G11.1
  gait R26.0
    hysterical F44.4
  general R27.8
  gluten M35.9 *[G32.81]*
    with celiac disease K90.0 *[G32.81]*
  hereditary G11.9
    with neuropathy G60.2
    cerebellar —*see* Ataxia, cerebellar
    spastic G11.4
    specified NEC G11.8
    spinal (Friedreich's) G11.1
  heredofamilial —*see* Ataxia, hereditary
  Hunt's G11.1
  hysterical F44.4
  locomotor (progressive) (syphilitic) (partial)
      (spastic) A52.11
    diabetic —*see* Diabetes, ataxia
  Marie's (cerebellar) (heredofamilial) (late-
      onset) G11.2
  nonorganic origin F44.4
  nonprogressive, congenital G11.0
  psychogenic F44.4
  Roussy-Lévy G60.0
  Sanger-Brown's (hereditary) G11.2
  spastic hereditary G11.4
  spinal
    hereditary (Friedreich's) G11.1
    progressive (syphilitic) A52.11

Ataxia, ataxy, ataxic *(Continued)*
  spinocerebellar, X-linked recessive G11.1
  telangiectasia (Louis-Bar) G11.3
Ataxia-telangiectasia (Louis-Bar) G11.3
Atelectasis (massive) (partial) (pressure)
    (pulmonary) J98.11
  newborn P28.10
    due to resorption P28.11
    partial P28.19
    primary P28.0
    secondary P28.19
  primary (newborn) P28.0
  tuberculous —*see* Tuberculosis, pulmonary
Atelocardia Q24.9
Atelomyelia Q06.1
Atheroembolism
  of
    extremities
      lower I75.02-
      upper I75.01-
    kidney I75.81
    specified NEC I75.89
Atheroma, atheromatous (*see also*
    Arteriosclerosis) I70.90
  aorta, aortic I70.0
    valve (*see also* Endocarditis, aortic) I35.8
  aorto-iliac I70.0
  artery —*see* Arteriosclerosis
  basilar (artery) I67.2
  carotid (artery) (common) (internal) I67.2
  cerebral (arteries) I67.2
  coronary (artery) I25.10
    with angina pectoris —*see* Arteriosclerosis,
        coronary (artery)
  degeneration —*see* Arteriosclerosis
  heart, cardiac —*see* Disease, heart, ischemic,
      atherosclerotic
  mitral (valve) I34.8
  myocardium, myocardial —*see* Disease, heart,
      ischemic, atherosclerotic
  pulmonary valve (heart) (*see also*
      Endocarditis, pulmonary) I37.8
  tricuspid (heart) (valve) I36.8
  valve, valvular —*see* Endocarditis
  vertebral (artery) I67.2
Atheromatosis —*see* Arteriosclerosis
Atherosclerosis —*see also* Arteriosclerosis
  coronary
    artery I25.10
      with angina pectoris —*see*
          Arteriosclerosis, coronary (artery),
      due to
        calcified coronary lesion (severely)
            I25.84
        lipid rich plaque I25.83
    transplanted heart I25.811
      bypass graft I25.812
        with angina pectoris —*see*
            Arteriosclerosis, coronary (artery)
      native coronary artery I25.811
        with angina pectoris —*see*
            Arteriosclerosis, coronary (artery)
Athetosis (acquired) R25.8
  bilateral (congenital) G80.3
  congenital (bilateral) (double) G80.3
  double (congenital) G80.3
  unilateral R25.8
Athlete's
  foot B35.3
  heart I51.7
Athrepsia E41
Athyrea (acquired) —*see also* Hypothyroidism
  congenital E03.1
Atonia, atony, atonic
  bladder (sphincter) (neurogenic) N31.2
  capillary I78.8
  cecum K59.8
    psychogenic F45.8
  colon —*see* Atony, intestine
  congenital P94.2
  esophagus K22.8

Atonia, atony, atonic *(Continued)*
  intestine K59.8
    psychogenic F45.8
  stomach K31.89
    neurotic or psychogenic F45.8
  uterus (during labor) O62.2
    with hemorrhage (postpartum) O72.1
    postpartum (with hemorrhage) O72.1
      without hemorrhage O75.89
Atopy —*see* History, allergy
Atransferrinemia, congenital E88.09
Atresia, atretic
  alimentary organ or tract NEC Q45.8
    upper Q40.8
  ani, anus, anal (canal) Q42.3
    with fistula Q42.2
  aorta (arch) (ring) Q25.2
  aortic (orifice) (valve) Q23.0
    arch Q25.2
    congenital with hypoplasia of ascending
        aorta and defective development of
        left ventricle (with mitral stenosis)
        Q23.4
    in hypoplastic left heart syndrome Q23.4
  aqueduct of Sylvius Q03.0
    with spina bifida —*see* Spina bifida, with
        hydrocephalus
  artery NEC Q27.8
    cerebral Q28.3
    coronary Q24.5
    digestive system Q27.8
    eye Q15.8
    lower limb Q27.8
    pulmonary Q25.5
    specified site NEC Q27.8
    umbilical Q27.0
    upper limb Q27.8
  auditory canal (external) Q16.1
  bile duct (common) (congenital) (hepatic)
      Q44.2
    acquired —*see* Obstruction, bile duct
  bladder (neck) Q64.39
    obstruction Q64.31
  bronchus Q32.4
  cecum Q42.8
  cervix (acquired) N88.2
    congenital Q51.828
    in pregnancy or childbirth —*see* Anomaly,
        cervix, in pregnancy or childbirth
        causing obstructed labor O65.5
  choana Q30.0
  colon Q42.9
    specified NEC Q42.8
  common duct Q44.2
  cricoid cartilage Q31.8
  cystic duct Q44.2
    acquired K82.8
      with obstruction K82.0
  digestive organs NEC Q45.8
  duodenum Q41.0
  ear canal Q16.1
  ejaculatory duct Q55.4
  epiglottis Q31.8
  esophagus Q39.0
    with tracheoesophageal fistula Q39.1
  eustachian tube Q17.8
  fallopian tube (congenital) Q50.6
    acquired N97.1
  follicular cyst N83.0
  foramen of
    Luschka Q03.1
      with spina bifida —*see* Spina bifida, with
          hydrocephalus
    Magendie Q03.1
      with spina bifida —*see* Spina bifida, with
          hydrocephalus
  gallbladder Q44.1
  genital organ
    external
      female Q52.79
      male Q55.8

◀ New   ◀▥ Revised   ~~deleted~~ Deleted

Atresia, atretic *(Continued)*
  genital organ *(Continued)*
    internal
      female Q52.8
      male Q55.8
  glottis Q31.8
  gullet Q39.0
    with tracheoesophageal fistula Q39.1
  heart valve NEC Q24.8
    pulmonary Q22.0
    tricuspid Q22.4
  hymen Q52.3
    acquired (postinfective) N89.6
  ileum Q41.2
  intestine (small) Q41.9
    large Q42.9
      specified NEC Q42.8
  iris, filtration angle Q15.0
  jejunum Q41.1
  lacrimal apparatus Q10.4
  larynx Q31.8
  meatus urinarius Q64.33
  mitral valve Q23.2
    in hypoplastic left heart syndrome
      Q23.4
  nares (anterior) (posterior) Q30.0
  nasopharynx Q34.8
  nose, nostril Q30.0
    acquired J34.89
  organ or site NEC Q89.8
  osseous meatus (ear) Q16.1
  oviduct (congenital) Q50.6
    acquired N97.1
  parotid duct Q38.4
    acquired K11.8
  pulmonary (artery) Q25.5
    valve Q22.0
  pulmonic Q22.0
  pupil Q13.2
  rectum Q42.1
    with fistula Q42.0
  salivary duct Q38.4
    acquired K11.8
  sublingual duct Q38.4
    acquired K11.8
  submandibular duct Q38.4
    acquired K11.8
  submaxillary duct Q38.4
    acquired K11.8
  thyroid cartilage Q31.8
  trachea Q32.1
  tricuspid valve Q22.4
  ureter Q62.10
    pelvic junction Q62.11
    vesical orifice Q62.12
  ureteropelvic junction Q62.11
  ureterovesical orifice Q62.12
  urethra (valvular) Q64.39
    stricture Q64.32
  urinary tract NEC Q64.8
  uterus Q51.818
    acquired N85.8
  vagina (congenital) Q52.4
    acquired (postinfectional) (senile)
      N89.5
  vas deferens Q55.3
  vascular NEC Q27.8
    cerebral Q28.3
    digestive system Q27.8
    lower limb Q27.8
    specified site NEC Q27.8
    upper limb Q27.8
  vein NEC Q27.8
    digestive system Q27.8
    great Q26.8
    lower limb Q27.8
    portal Q26.5
    pulmonary Q26.3
    specified site NEC Q27.8
    upper limb Q27.8
  vena cava (inferior) (superior) Q26.8

Atresia, atretic *(Continued)*
  vesicourethral orifice Q64.31
  vulva Q52.79
    acquired N90.5
Atrichia, atrichosis —*see* Alopecia
Atrophia —*see also* Atrophy
  cutis senilis L90.8
    due to radiation L57.8
  gyrata of choroid and retina H31.23
  senilis R54
    dermatological L90.8
      due to radiation (nonionizing) (solar)
        L57.8
  unguium L60.3
    congenita Q84.6
Atrophie blanche (en plaque) (de Milian) L95.0
Atrophoderma, atrophodermia (of) L90.9
  diffusum (idiopathic) L90.4
  maculatum L90.8
    et striatum L90.8
      due to syphilis A52.79
    syphilitic A51.39
  neuriticum L90.8
  Pasini and Pierini L90.3
  pigmentosum Q82.1
  reticulatum symmetricum faciei L66.4
  senile L90.8
    due to radiation (nonionizing) (solar) L57.8
  vermiculata (cheeks) L66.4
Atrophy, atrophic (of)
  adrenal (capsule) (gland) E27.49
    primary (autoimmune) E27.1
  alveolar process or ridge (edentulous) K08.20
  anal sphincter (disuse) N81.84
  appendix K38.8
  arteriosclerotic —*see* Arteriosclerosis
  bile duct (common) (hepatic) K83.8
  bladder N32.89
    neurogenic N31.8
  blanche (en plaque) (of Milian) L95.0
  bone (senile) NEC —*see also* Disorder, bone,
      specified type NEC
    due to
      tabes dorsalis (neurogenic) A52.11
  brain (cortex) (progressive) G31.9
    frontotemporal circumscribed G31.01
      [F02.80]
      with behavioral disturbance G31.01
        [F02.81]
    senile NEC G31.1
  breast N64.2
    obstetric —*see* Disorder, breast, specified
        type NEC
  buccal cavity K13.79
  cardiac —*see* Degeneration, myocardial
  cartilage (infectional) (joint) —*see* Disorder,
      cartilage, specified NEC
  cerebellar —*see* Atrophy, brain
  cerebral —*see* Atrophy, brain
  cervix (mucosa) (senile) (uteri) N88.8
    menopausal N95.8
  Charcot-Marie-Tooth G60.0
  choroid (central) (macular) (myopic) (retina)
      H31.10-
    diffuse secondary H31.12-
    gyrate H31.23
    senile H31.11-
  ciliary body —*see* Atrophy, iris
  conjunctiva (senile) H11.89
  corpus cavernosum N48.89
  cortical —*see* Atrophy, brain
  cystic duct K82.8
  Déjérine-Thomas G23.8
  disuse NEC —*see* Atrophy, muscle
  Duchenne-Aran G12.21
  ear H93.8-
  edentulous alveolar ridge K08.20
  endometrium (senile) N85.8
    cervix N88.8
  enteric K63.89
  epididymis N50.8

Atrophy, atrophic *(Continued)*
  eyeball —*see* Disorder, globe, degenerated
      condition, atrophy
  eyelid (senile) —*see* Disorder, eyelid,
      degenerative
  facial (skin) L90.9
  fallopian tube (senile) N83.32
    with ovary N83.33
  fascioscapulohumeral (Landouzy- Déjérine)
      G71.0
  fatty, thymus (gland) E32.8
  gallbladder K82.8
  gastric K29.40
    with bleeding K29.41
  gastrointestinal K63.89
  glandular I89.8
  globe H44.52-
  gum K06.0
  hair L67.8
  heart (brown) —*see* Degeneration, myocardial
  hemifacial Q67.4
    Romberg G51.8
  infantile E41
    paralysis, acute —*see* Poliomyelitis,
        paralytic
  intestine K63.89
  iris (essential) (progressive) H21.26-
    specified NEC H21.29
  kidney (senile) (terminal) (*see also* Sclerosis,
      renal) N26.1
    congenital or infantile Q60.5
      bilateral Q60.4
      unilateral Q60.3
    hydronephrotic —*see* Hydronephrosis
  lacrimal gland (primary) H04.14-
    secondary H04.15-
  Landouzy-Déjérine G71.0
  laryngitis, infective J37.0
  larynx J38.7
  Leber's optic (hereditary) H47.22
  lip K13.0
  liver (yellow) K72.90
    with coma K72.91
    acute, subacute K72.00
      with coma K72.01
    chronic K72.10
      with coma K72.11
  lung (senile) J98.4
  macular (dermatological) L90.8
    syphilitic, skin A51.39
      striated A52.79
  mandible (edentulous) K08.20
    minimal K08.21
    moderate K08.22
    severe K08.23
  maxilla K08.20
    minimal K08.24
    moderate K08.25
    severe K08.26
  muscle, muscular (diffuse) (general)
      (idiopathic) (primary) M62.50
    ankle M62.57-
    Duchenne-Aran G12.21
    foot M62.57-
    forearm M62.53-
    hand M62.54-
    infantile spinal G12.0
    lower leg M62.56-
    multiple sites M62.59
    myelopathic —*see* Atrophy, muscle, spinal
    myotonic G71.11
    neuritic G58.9
    neuropathic (peroneal) (progressive) G60.0
    pelvic (disuse) N81.84
    peroneal G60.0
    progressive (bulbar) G12.21
      adult G12.1
      infantile (spinal) G12.0
      spinal G12.9
        adult G12.1
        infantile G12.0

Atrophy, atrophic (Continued)
  muscle, muscular (Continued)
    pseudohypertrophic G71.0
    shoulder region M62.51-
    specified site NEC M62.58
    spinal G12.9
      adult form G12.1
      Aran-Duchenne G12.21
      childhood form, type II G12.1
      distal G12.1
      hereditary NEC G12.1
      infantile, type I (Werdnig- Hoffmann) G12.0
      juvenile form, type III (Kugelberg-Welander) G12.1
      progressive G12.21
      scapuloperoneal form G12.1
      specified NEC G12.8
    syphilitic A52.78
    thigh M62.55-
    upper arm M62.52-
  myocardium —see Degeneration, myocardial
  myometrium (senile) N85.8
    cervix N88.8
  myopathic NEC —see Atrophy, muscle
  myotonia G71.11
  nail L60.3
  nasopharynx J31.1
  nerve —see also Disorder, nerve
    abducens —see Strabismus, paralytic, sixth nerve
    accessory G52.8
    acoustic or auditory —see subcategory H93.3
    cranial G52.9
      eighth (auditory) —see subcategory H93.3
      eleventh (accessory) G52.8
      fifth (trigeminal) G50.8
      first (olfactory) G52.0
      fourth (trochlear) —see Strabismus, paralytic, fourth nerve
      second (optic) H47.20
      sixth (abducens) —see Strabismus, paralytic, sixth nerve
      tenth (pneumogastric) (vagus) G52.2
      third (oculomotor) —see Strabismus, paralytic, third nerve
      twelfth (hypoglossal) G52.3
    hypoglossal G52.3
    oculomotor —see Strabismus, paralytic, third nerve
    olfactory G52.0
    optic (papillomacular bundle)
      syphilitic (late) A52.15
        congenital A50.44
    pneumogastric G52.2
    trigeminal G50.8
    trochlear —see Strabismus, paralytic, fourth nerve
    vagus (pneumogastric) G52.2
  neurogenic, bone, tabetic A52.11
  nutritional E41
  old age R54
  olivopontocerebellar G23.8
  optic (nerve) H47.20
    glaucomatous H47.23-
    hereditary H47.22
    primary H47.21-
    specified type NEC H47.29-
    syphilitic (late) A52.15
      congenital A50.44
  orbit H05.31-
  ovary (senile) N83.31
    with fallopian tube N83.33
  oviduct (senile) —see Atrophy, fallopian tube
  palsy, diffuse (progressive) G12.22
  pancreas (duct) (senile) K86.8
  parotid gland K11.0
  pelvic muscle N81.84
  penis N48.89

Atrophy, atrophic (Continued)
  pharynx J39.2
  pluriglandular E31.8
    autoimmune E31.0
  polyarthritis M15.9
  prostate N42.89
  pseudohypertrophic (muscle) G71.0
  renal (see also Sclerosis, renal) N26.1
  retina, retinal (postinfectional) H35.89
  rhinitis J31.0
  salivary gland K11.0
  scar L90.5
  sclerosis, lobar (of brain) G31.09 [F02.80]
    with behavioral disturbance G31.09 [F02.81]
  scrotum N50.8
  seminal vesicle N50.8
  senile R54
    due to radiation (nonionizing) (solar) L57.8
  skin (patches) (spots) L90.9
    degenerative (senile) L90.8
    due to radiation (nonionizing) (solar) L57.8
    senile L90.8
  spermatic cord N50.8
  spinal (acute) (cord) G95.89
    muscular —see Atrophy, muscle, spinal
    paralysis G12.20
      acute —see Poliomyelitis, paralytic
      meaning progressive muscular atrophy G12.21
  spine (column) —see Spondylopathy, specified NEC
  spleen (senile) D73.0
  stomach K29.40
    with bleeding K29.41
  striate (skin) L90.6
    syphilitic A52.79
  subcutaneous L90.9
  sublingual gland K11.0
  submandibular gland K11.0
  submaxillary gland K11.0
  Sudeck's —see Algoneurodystrophy
  suprarenal (capsule) (gland) E27.49
    primary E27.1
  systemic affecting central nervous system in
      myxedema E03.9 [G13.2]
      neoplastic disease (see also Neoplasm) D49.9 [G13.1]
      specified disease NEC G13.8
  tarso-orbital fascia, congenital Q10.3
  testis N50.0
  thenar, partial —see Syndrome, carpal tunnel
  thymus (fatty) E32.8
  thyroid (gland) (acquired) E03.4
    with cretinism E03.1
    congenital (with myxedema) E03.1
  tongue (senile) K14.8
    papillae K14.4
  trachea J39.8
  tunica vaginalis N50.8
  turbinate J34.89
  tympanic membrane (nonflaccid) H73.82-
    flaccid H73.81-
  upper respiratory tract J39.8
  uterus, uterine (senile) N85.8
    cervix N88.8
    due to radiation (intended effect) N85.8
      adverse effect or misadventure N99.89
  vagina (senile) N95.2
  vas deferens N50.8
  vascular I99.8
  vertebra (senile) —see Spondylopathy, specified NEC
  vulva (senile) N90.5
  Werdnig-Hoffmann G12.0
  yellow —see Failure, hepatic

Attack, attacks
  with alteration of consciousness (with automatisms) —see Epilepsy, localization-related, symptomatic, with complex partial seizures
  without alteration of consciousness — see Epilepsy, localization-related, symptomatic, with simple partial seizures
  Adams-Stokes I45.9
  akinetic —see Epilepsy, generalized, specified NEC
  angina —see Angina
  atonic —see Epilepsy, generalized, specified NEC
  benign shuddering G25.83
  cataleptic —see Catalepsy
  coronary —see Infarct, myocardium
  cyanotic, newborn P28.2
  drop NEC R55
  epileptic —see Epilepsy
  heart —see infarct, myocardium
  hysterical F44.9
  jacksonian —see Epilepsy, localization-related, symptomatic, with simple partial seizures
  myocardium, myocardial —see Infarct, myocardium
  myoclonic —see Epilepsy, generalized, specified NEC
  panic F41.0
  psychomotor —see Epilepsy, localization-related, symptomatic, with complex partial seizures
  salaam —see Epilepsy, spasms
  schizophreniform, brief F23
  shuddering, benign G25.83
  Stokes-Adams I45.9
  syncope R55
  transient ischemic (TIA) G45.9
    specified NEC G45.8
  unconsciousness R55
    hysterical F44.89
  vasomotor R55
  vasovagal (paroxysmal) (idiopathic) R55
Attention (to)
  artificial
    opening (of) Z43.9
      digestive tract NEC Z43.4
        colon Z43.3
        ilium Z43.2
        stomach Z43.1
      specified NEC Z43.8
      trachea Z43.0
      urinary tract NEC Z43.6
        cystostomy Z43.5
        nephrostomy Z43.6
        ureterostomy Z43.6
        urethrostomy Z43.6
      vagina Z43.7
  colostomy Z43.3
  cystostomy Z43.5
  deficit disorder or syndrome F98.8
    with hyperactivity —see Disorder, attention-deficit hyperactivity
  gastrostomy Z43.1
  ileostomy Z43.2
  jejunostomy Z43.4
  nephrostomy Z43.6
  surgical dressings Z48.01
  sutures Z48.02
  tracheostomy Z43.0
  ureterostomy Z43.6
  urethrostomy Z43.6
Attrition
  gum K06.0
  tooth, teeth (excessive) (hard tissues) K03.0
Atypical, atypism —see also condition
  cells (on cytolgocial smear) (endocervical) (endometrial) (glandular)
    cervix R87.619
    vagina R87.629

◀ New   ◀‖‖ Revised   ~~deleted~~ Deleted

Atypical, atypism (*Continued*)
 cervical N87.9
 endometrium N85.9
  hyperplasia N85.00
 parenting situation Z62.9
Auditory —*see* condition
Aujeszky's disease B33.8
Aurantiasis, cutis E67.1
Auricle, auricular —*see also* condition
 cervical Q18.2
Auriculotemporal syndrome G50.8
Austin Flint murmur (aortic insufficiency) I35.1
Australian
 Q fever A78
 X disease A83.4
Autism, autistic (childhood) (infantile) F84.0
 atypical F84.9
Autodigestion R68.89
Autoerythrocyte sensitization (syndrome)
 D69.2
Autographism L50.3
Autoimmune
 disease (systemic) M35.9
 inhibitors to clotting factors D68.311
 lymphoproliferative syndrome [ALPS]
  D89.82
 thyroiditis E06.3
Autointoxication R68.89
Automatism G93.89
 with temporal sclerosis G93.81
 epileptic —*see* Epilepsy, localization- related,
  symptomatic, with complex partial
  seizures
 paroxysmal, idiopathic —*see* Epilepsy,
  localization-related, symptomatic, with
  complex partial seizures
Autonomic, autonomous
 bladder (neurogenic) N31.2
 hysteria seizure F44.5
Autosensitivity, erythrocyte D69.2
Autosensitization, cutaneous L30.2
Autosome —*see* condition by chromosome
 involved

Autotopagnosia R48.1
Autotoxemia R68.89
Autumn —*see* condition
Avellis' syndrome G46.8
Aversion
 oral R63.3
  newborn P92.-
  nonorganic origin F98.2
 sexual F52.1
Aviator's
 disease or sickness —*see* Effect, adverse, high
  altitude
 ear T70.0
Avitaminosis (multiple) (*see also* Deficiency,
  vitamin) E56.9
 B E53.9
  with
   beriberi E51.11
   pellagra E52
 B2 E53.0
 B6 E53.1
 B12 E53.8
 D E55.9
  with rickets E55.0
 G E53.0
 K E56.1
 nicotinic acid E52
AVNRT (atrioventricular nodal re-entrant
  tachycardia) I47.1
AVRT (atrioventricular nodal re-entrant
  tachycardia) I47.1
Avulsion (traumatic)
 blood vessel —*see* Injury, blood vessel
 bone —*see* Fracture, by site
 cartilage —*see also* Dislocation, by site
  symphyseal (inner), complicating delivery
   O71.6
 external site other than limb —*see* Wound,
  open, by site
 eye S05.7-
 head (intracranial)
  external site NEC S08.89
  scalp S08.0

Avulsion (*Continued*)
 internal organ or site —*see* Injury, by site
 joint —*see also* Dislocation, by site
  capsule —*see* Sprain, by site
 kidney S37.06-
 ligament —*see* Sprain, by site
 limb —*see also* Amputation, traumatic, by site
  skin and subcutaneous tissue —*see* Wound,
   open, by site
 muscle —*see* Injury, muscle
 nerve (root) —*see* Injury, nerve
 scalp S08.0
 skin and subcutaneous tissue —*see* Wound,
  open, by site
 spleen S36.032
 symphyseal cartilage (inner), complicating
  delivery O71.6
 tendon —*see* Injury, muscle
 tooth S03.2
Awareness of heart beat R00.2
Axenfeld's
 anomaly or syndrome Q15.0
 degeneration (calcareous) Q13.4
Axilla, axillary —*see also* condition
 breast Q83.1
Axonotmesis —*see* Injury, nerve
Ayerza's disease or syndrome (pulmonary
  artery sclerosis with pulmonary
  hypertension) I27.0
Azoospermia (organic) N46.01
 due to
  drug therapy N46.021
  efferent duct obstruction N46.023
  infection N46.022
  radiation N46.024
  specified cause NEC N46.029
  systemic disease N46.025
Azotemia R79.89
 meaning uremia N19
Aztec ear Q17.3
Azygos
 continuation inferior vena cava Q26.8
 lobe (lung) Q33.1

A

B

Baastrup's disease —*see* Kissing spine
Babesiosis B60.0
Babington's disease (familial hemorrhagic telangiectasia) I78.0
Babinski's syndrome A52.79
Baby
  crying constantly R68.11
  floppy (syndrome) P94.2
Bacillary —*see* condition
Bacilluria N39.0
Bacillus —*see also* Infection, bacillus
  abortus infection A23.1
  anthracis infection A22.9
  coli infection (*see also* Escherichia coli) B96.20
  Flexner's A03.1
  mallei infection A24.0
  Shiga's A03.0
  suipestifer infection —*see* Infection, salmonella
Back —*see* condition
Backache (postural) M54.9
  sacroiliac M53.3
  specified NEC M54.89
Backflow —*see* Reflux
Backward reading (dyslexia) F81.0
Bacteremia R78.81
  with sepsis —*see* Sepsis
Bactericholia —*see* Cholecystitis, acute
Bacterid, bacteride (pustular) L40.3
Bacterium, bacteria, bacterial
  agent NEC, as cause of disease classified elsewhere B96.89
  in blood —*see* Bacteremia
  in urine —*see* Bacteriuria
Bacteriuria, bacteruria N39.0
  asymptomatic N39.0
Bacteroides
  fragilis, as cause of disease classified elsewhere B96.6
Bad
  heart —*see* Disease, heart
  trip
    due to drug abuse —*see* Abuse, drug, hallucinogen
    due to drug dependence —*see* Dependence, drug, hallucinogen
Baelz's disease (cheilitis glandularis apostematosa) K13.0
Baerensprung's disease (eczema marginatum) B35.6
Bagasse disease or pneumonitis J67.1
Bagassosis J67.1
Baker's cyst —*see* Cyst, Baker's
Bakwin-Krida syndrome (craniometaphyseal dysplasia) Q78.5
Balancing side interference M26.56
Balanitis (circinata) (erosiva) (gangrenosa) (phagedenic) (vulgaris) N48.1
  amebic A06.82
  candidal B37.42
  due to Haemophilus ducreyi A57
  gonococcal (acute) (chronic) A54.09
  xerotica obliterans N48.0
Balanoposthitis N47.6
  gonococcal (acute) (chronic) A54.09
  ulcerative (specific) A63.8
Balanorrhagia —*see* Balanitis
Balantidiasis, balantidiosis A07.0
Bald tongue K14.4
Baldness —*see also* Alopecia
  male-pattern —*see* Alopecia, androgenic
Balkan grippe A78
Balloon disease —*see* Effect, adverse, high altitude
Balo's disease (concentric sclerosis) G37.5
Bamberger-Marie disease —*see* Osteoarthropathy, hypertrophic, specified type NEC
Bancroft's filariasis B74.0

Band (s)
  adhesive —*see* Adhesions, peritoneum
  anomalous or congenital —*see also* Anomaly, by site
    heart (atrial) (ventricular) Q24.8
    intestine Q43.3
    omentum Q43.3
  cervix N88.1
  constricting, congenital Q79.8
  gallbladder (congenital) Q44.1
  intestinal (adhesive) —*see* Adhesions, peritoneum
  obstructive
    intestine K56.5
    peritoneum K56.5
  periappendiceal, congenital Q43.3
  peritoneal (adhesive) —*see* Adhesions, peritoneum
  uterus N73.6
    internal N85.6
  vagina N89.5
Bandemia D72.825
Bandl's ring (contraction), complicating delivery O62.4
Bangkok hemorrhagic fever A91
Bang's disease (brucella abortus) A23.1
Bankruptcy, anxiety concerning Z59.8
Bannister's disease T78.3
  hereditary D84.1
Banti's disease or syndrome (with cirrhosis) (with portal hypertension) K76.6
Bar, median, prostate —*see* Enlargement, enlarged, prostate
Barcoo disease or rot —*see* Ulcer, skin
Barlow's disease E54
Barodontalgia T70.29
Baron Münchausen syndrome —*see* Disorder, factitious
Barosinusitis T70.1
Barotitis T70.0
Barotrauma T70.29
  odontalgia T70.29
  otitic T70.0
  sinus T70.1
Barraquer (-Simons) disease or syndrome (progressive lipodystrophy) E88.1
Barré-Guillain disease or syndrome G61.0
Barré-Liéou syndrome (posterior cervical sympathetic) M53.0
Barrel chest M95.4
Barrett's
  disease —*see* Barrett's, esophagus
  esophagus K22.70
    with dysplasia K22.719
      high grade K22.711
      low grade K22.710
    without dysplasia K22.70
  syndrome —*see* Barrett's, esophagus
  ulcer K22.10
    with bleeding K22.11
    without bleeding K22.10
Barth syndrome E78.71
Bársony (-Polgár) (-Teschendorf) syndrome (corkscrew esophagus) K22.4
Bartholinitis (suppurating) N75.8
  gonococcal (acute) (chronic) (with abscess) A54.1
Bartonellosis A44.9
  cutaneous A44.1
  mucocutaneous A44.1
  specified NEC A44.8
  systemic A44.0
Barton's fracture S52.56-
Bartter's syndrome E26.81
Basal —*see* condition
Basan's (hidrotic) ectodermal dysplasia Q82.4
Baseball finger —*see* Dislocation, finger
Basedow's disease (exophthalmic goiter) —*see* Hyperthyroidism, with, goiter
Basic —*see* condition
Basilar —*see* condition

Bason's (hidrotic) ectodermal dysplasia Q82.4
Basopenia —*see* Agranulocytosis
Basophilia D72.824
Basophilism (cortico-adrenal) (Cushing's) (pituitary) E24.0
Bassen-Kornzweig disease or syndrome E78.6
Bat ear Q17.5
Bateman's
  disease B08.1
  purpura (senile) D69.2
Bathing cramp T75.1
Bathophobia F40.248
Batten (-Mayou) disease E75.4
  retina E75.4 [H36]
Batten-Steinert syndrome G71.11
Battered —*see* Maltreatment
Battey Mycobacterium infection A31.0
Battle exhaustion F43.0
Battledore placenta O43.19-
Baumgarten-Cruveilhier cirrhosis, disease or syndrome K74.69
Bauxite fibrosis (of lung) J63.1
Bayle's disease (general paresis) A52.17
Bazin's disease (primary) (tuberculous) A18.4
Beach ear —*see* Swimmer's, ear
Beaded hair (congenital) Q84.1
Béal conjunctivitis or syndrome B30.2
Beard's disease (neurasthenia) F48.8
Beat (s)
  atrial, premature I49.1
  ectopic I49.49
  elbow —*see* Bursitis, elbow
  escaped, heart I49.49
  hand —*see* Bursitis, hand
  knee —*see* Bursitis, knee
  premature I49.40
    atrial I49.1
    auricular I49.1
    supraventricular I49.1
Beau's
  disease or syndrome —*see* Degeneration, myocardial
  lines (transverse furrows on fingernails) L60.4
Bechterev's syndrome —*see* Spondylitis, ankylosing
Beck's syndrome (anterior spinal artery occlusion) I65.8
Becker's
  cardiomyopathy I42.8
  disease
    idiopathic mural endomyocardial disease I42.3
    myotonia congenita, recessive form G71.12
  dystrophy G71.0
  pigmented hairy nevus D22.5
Beckwith-Wiedemann syndrome Q87.3
Bed confinement status Z74.01
Bed sore —*see* Ulcer, pressure, by site
Bedbug bite (s) —*see* Bite (s), by site, superficial, insect
Bedclothes, asphyxiation or suffocation by —*see* Asphyxia, traumatic, due to, mechanical, trapped
Bednar's
  aphthae K12.0
  tumor —*see* Neoplasm, malignant, by site
Bedridden Z74.01
Bedsore —*see* Ulcer, pressure, by site
Bedwetting —*see* Enuresis
Bee sting (with allergic or anaphylactic shock) —*see* Toxicity, venom, arthropod, bee
Beer drinker's heart (disease) I42.6
Begbie's disease (exophthalmic goiter) —*see* Hyperthyroidism, with, goiter
Behavior
  antisocial
    adult Z72.811
    child or adolescent Z72.810
  disorder, disturbance —*see* Disorder, conduct
  disruptive —*see* Disorder, conduct

◀ New   ⬅ Revised   ~~deleted~~ Deleted

Behavior *(Continued)*
drug seeking Z72.89
inexplicable R46.2
marked evasiveness R46.5
obsessive-compulsive R46.81
overactivity R46.3
poor responsiveness R46.4
self-damaging (life-style) Z72.89
sleep-incompatible Z72.821
slowness R46.4
specified NEC R46.89
strange (and inexplicable) R46.2
suspiciousness R46.5
type A pattern Z73.1
undue concern or preoccupation with
stressful events R46.6
verbosity and circumstantial detail obscuring
reason for contact R46.7
Behcet's disease or syndrome M35.2
Behr's disease —*see* Degeneration, macula
Beigel's disease or morbus (white piedra)
B36.2
Bejel A65
Bekhterev's syndrome —*see* Spondylitis,
ankylosing
Belching —*see* Eructation
Bell's
mania F30.8
palsy, paralysis G51.0
infant or newborn P11.3
spasm G51.3
Bence Jones albuminuria or proteinuria NEC
R80.3
Bends T70.3
Benedikt's paralysis or syndrome G46.3
Benign (*see also* condition)
prostatic hyperplasia —*see* Hyperplasia,
prostate
Bennett's fracture (displaced) S62.21-
Benson's disease —*see* Deposit, crystalline
Bent
back (hysterical) F44.4
nose M95.0
congenital Q67.4
Bereavement (uncomplicated) Z63.4
Bergeron's disease (hysterical chorea) F44.4
Berger's disease —*see* Nephropathy, IgA
Beriberi (dry) E51.11
heart (disease) E51.12
polyneuropathy E51.11
wet E51.12
involving circulatory system E51.11
Berlin's disease or edema (traumatic) S05.8X-
Berlock (berloque) dermatitis L56.2
Bernard-Horner syndrome G90.2
Bernard-Soulier disease or thrombopathia
D69.1
Bernhardt (-Roth) disease —*see*
Mononeuropathy, lower limb, meralgia
paresthetica
Bernheim's syndrome —*see* Failure, heart,
congestive
Bertielliasis B71.8
Berylliosis (lung) J63.2
Besnier-Boeck (-Schaumann) disease —*see*
Sarcoidosis
Besnier's
lupus pernio D86.3
prurigo L20.0
Bestiality F65.89
Best's disease H35.50
Beta-mercaptolactate-cysteine disulfiduria
E72.09
Betalipoproteinemia, broad or floating E78.2
Betting and gambling Z72.6
pathological (compulsive) F63.0
Bezoar T18.9
intestine T18.3
stomach T18.2
Bezold's abscess —*see* Mastoiditis, acute
Bianchi's syndrome R48.8

Bicornate or bicornis uterus Q51.3
in pregnancy or childbirth O34.59-
causing obstructed labor O65.5
Bicuspid aortic valve Q23.1
Biedl-Bardet syndrome Q87.89
Bielschowsky (-Jansky) disease E75.4
Biermer's (pernicious) anemia or disease D51.0
Biett's disease L93.0
Bifid (congenital)
apex, heart Q24.8
clitoris Q52.6
kidney Q63.8
nose Q30.2
patella Q74.1
scrotum Q55.29
toe NEC Q74.2
tongue Q38.3
ureter Q62.8
uterus Q51.3
uvula Q35.7
Biforis uterus (suprasimplex) Q51.3
Bifurcation (congenital)
gallbladder Q44.1
kidney pelvis Q63.8
renal pelvis Q63.8
rib Q76.6
tongue, congenital Q38.3
trachea Q32.1
ureter Q62.8
urethra Q64.74
vertebra Q76.49
Big spleen syndrome D73.1
Bigeminal pulse R00.8
Bilateral —*see* condition
Bile
duct —*see* condition
pigments in urine R82.2
Bilharziasis —*see also* Schistosomiasis
chyluria B65.0
cutaneous B65.3
galacturia B65.0
hematochyluria B65.0
intestinal B65.1
lipemia B65.9
lipuria B65.0
oriental B65.2
piarhemia B65.9
pulmonary NOS B65.9 *[J99]*
pneumonia B65.9 *[J17]*
tropical hematuria B65.0
vesical B65.0
Biliary —*see* condition
Bilirubin metabolism disorder E80.7
specified NEC E80.6
Bilirubinemia, familial nonhemolytic E80.4
Bilirubinuria R82.2
Biliuria R82.2
Bilocular stomach K31.2
Binswanger's disease I67.3
Biparta, bipartite
carpal scaphoid Q74.0
patella Q74.1
vagina Q52.10
Bird
face Q75.8
fancier's disease or lung J67.2
Birt-Hogg-Dube syndrome Q87.89
Birth
complications in mother —*see* Delivery,
complicated
compression during NOS P15.9
defect —*see* Anomaly
immature (less than 37 completed weeks) —
see Preterm, newborn
extremely (less than 28 completed
weeks) —*see* Immaturity, extreme
inattention, at or after —*see* Maltreatment,
child, neglect
injury NOS P15.9
basal ganglia P11.1
brachial plexus NEC P14.3

Birth *(Continued)*
injury NOS *(Continued)*
brain (compression) (pressure)
P11.2
central nervous system NOS P11.9
cerebellum P11.1
cerebral hemorrhage P10.1
external genitalia P15.5
eye P15.3
face P15.4
fracture
bone P13.9
specified NEC P13.8
clavicle P13.4
femur P13.2
humerus P13.3
long bone, except femur P13.3
radius and ulna P13.3
skull P13.0
spine P11.5
tibia and fibula P13.3
intracranial P11.2
laceration or hemorrhage P10.9
specified NEC P10.8
intraventricular hemorrhage P10.2
laceration
brain P10.1
by scalpel P15.8
peripheral nerve P14.9
liver P15.0
meninges
brain P11.1
spinal cord P11.5
nerve
brachial plexus P14.3
cranial NEC (except facial) P11.4
facial P11.3
peripheral P14.9
phrenic (paralysis) P14.2
paralysis
facial nerve P11.3
spinal P11.5
penis P15.5
rupture
spinal cord P11.5
scalp P12.9
scalpel wound P15.8
scrotum P15.5
skull NEC P13.1
fracture P13.0
specified type NEC P15.8
spinal cord P11.5
spine P11.5
spleen P15.1
sternomastoid (hematoma) P15.2
subarachnoid hemorrhage P10.3
subcutaneous fat necrosis P15.6
subdural hemorrhage P10.0
tentorial tear P10.4
testes P15.5
vulva P15.5
lack of care, at or after —*see* Maltreatment,
child, neglect
neglect, at or after —*see* Maltreatment, child,
neglect
palsy or paralysis, newborn, NOS (birth
injury) P14.9
premature (infant) —*see* Preterm,
newborn
shock, newborn P96.89
trauma —*see* Birth, injury
weight
4000 grams to 4499 grams P08.1
4500 grams or more P08.0
low (2499 grams or less) —*see* Low,
birthweight
extremely (999 grams or less) —*see* Low,
birthweight, extreme
Birthmark Q82.5
Bisalbuminemia E88.09
Biskra's button B55.1

◀ New   ◀ Revised   ~~deleted~~ Deleted

Bite (Continued)
  neck (Continued)
    superficial NEC S10.97
      insect S10.96
    throat S11.85
      superficial NEC S10.17
        insect S10.16
  nose (septum) (sinus) S01.25
    superficial NEC S00.37
      insect S00.36
  occipital region —see Bite, scalp
  oral cavity S01.552
    superficial NEC S00.572
      insect S00.562
  orbital region —see Bite, eyelid
  palate —see Bite, oral cavity
  palm —see Bite, hand
  parietal region —see Bite, scalp
  pelvis S31.050
    with penetration into retroperitoneal space
      S31.051
    superficial NEC S30.870
      insect S30.860
  penis S31.25
    superficial NEC S30.872
      insect S30.862
  perineum
    female —see Bite, vulva
    male —see Bite, pelvis
  periocular area (with or without lacrimal
    passages) —see Bite, eyelid
  phalanges
    finger —see Bite, finger
    toe —see Bite, toe
  pharynx S11.25
    superficial NEC S10.17
      insect S10.16
  pinna —see Bite, ear
  poisonous —see Venom
  popliteal space —see Bite, knee
  prepuce —see Bite, penis
  pubic region —see Bite, abdomen, wall
  rectovaginal septum —see Bite, vulva
  red bug B88.0
  reptile NEC —see also Venom, bite,
    reptile
    nonvenomous —see Bite, by site
    snake —see Venom, bite, snake
  sacral region —see Bite, back, lower
  sacroiliac region —see Bite, back, lower
  salivary gland —see Bite, oral cavity
  scalp S01.05
    superficial NEC S00.07
      insect S00.06
  scapular region —see Bite, shoulder
  scrotum S31.35
    superficial NEC S30.873
      insect S30.863
  sea-snake (venomous) —see Toxicity, venom,
    snake, sea snake
  shin —see Bite, leg
  shoulder S41.05-
    superficial NEC S40.27-
      insect S40.26-
  snake —see also Venom, bite, snake
    nonvenomous —see Bite, by site
  spermatic cord —see Bite, testis
  spider (venomous) —see Toxicity, venom,
    spider
    nonvenomous —see Bite, by site,
      superficial, insect
  sternal region —see Bite, thorax, front
  submaxillary region —see Bite, head,
    specified site NEC
  submental region —see Bite, head, specified
    site NEC
  subungual
    finger (s) —see Bite, finger
    toe —see Bite, toe
  superficial —see Bite, by site, superficial
  supraclavicular fossa S11.85

Bite (Continued)
  supraorbital —see Bite, head, specified site
    NEC
  temple, temporal region —see Bite, head,
    specified site NEC
  temporomandibular area —see Bite, cheek
  testis S31.35
    superficial NEC S30.873
      insect S30.863
  thigh S71.15-
    superficial NEC S70.37-
      insect S70.36-
  thorax, thoracic (wall) S21.95
    back S21.25-
      with penetration into thoracic cavity
        S21.45-
    breast —see Bite, breast
    front S21.15-
      with penetration into thoracic cavity
        S21.35-
    superficial NEC S20.97
      back S20.47-
      front S20.37-
      insect S20.96
        back S20.46-
        front S20.36-
  throat —see Bite, neck, throat
  thumb S61.05-
    with
      damage to nail S61.15-
    superficial NEC S60.37-
      insect S60.36-
  thyroid S11.15
    superficial NEC S10.87
      insect S10.86
  toe (s) S91.15-
    with
      damage to nail S91.25-
    great S91.15-
      with
        damage to nail S91.25-
    lesser S91.15-
      with
        damage to nail S91.25-
    superficial NEC S90.47-
      great S90.47-
      insect S90.46-
        great S90.46-
  tongue S01.552
  trachea S11.025
    superficial NEC S10.17
      insect S10.16
  tunica vaginalis —see Bite, testis
  tympanum, tympanic membrane —see Bite,
    ear
  umbilical region S31.155
  uvula —see Bite, oral cavity
  vagina —see Bite, vulva
  venomous —see Venom
  vocal cords S11.035
    superficial NEC S10.17
      insect S10.16
  vulva S31.45
    superficial NEC S30.874
      insect S30.864
  wrist S61.55-
    superficial NEC S60.87-
      insect S60.86-
Biting, cheek or lip K13.1
Biventricular failure (heart) I50.9
Björck (-Thorson) syndrome (malignant
  carcinoid) E34.0
Black
  death A20.9
  eye S00.1-
  hairy tongue K14.3
  heel (foot) S90.3-
  lung (disease) J60
  palm (hand) S60.22-
Blackfan-Diamond anemia or syndrome
  (congenital hypoplastic anemia) D61.01

Blackhead L70.0
Blackout R55
Bladder —see condition
Blast (air) (hydraulic) (immersion) (underwater)
  blindness S05.8X-
  injury
    abdomen or thorax —see Injury, by site
    ear (acoustic nerve trauma) —see Injury,
      nerve, acoustic, specified type NEC
  syndrome NEC T70.8
Blastoma —see Neoplasm, malignant, by site
  pulmonary —see Neoplasm, lung, malignant
Blastomycosis, blastomycotic B40.9
  Brazilian —see Paracoccidioidomycosis
  cutaneous B40.3
  disseminated B40.7
  European —see Cryptococcosis
  generalized B40.7
  keloidal B48.0
  North American B40.9
  primary pulmonary B40.0
  pulmonary B40.2
    acute B40.0
    chronic B40.1
  skin B40.3
  South American —see
    Paracoccidioidomycosis
  specified NEC B40.89
Bleb (s) R23.8
  emphysematous (lung) (solitary) J43.9
  endophthalmitis H59.43
  filtering (vitreous), after glaucoma surgery
    Z98.83
  inflamed (infected), postprocedural H59.40
    stage 1 H59.41
    stage 2 H59.42
    stage 3 H59.43
  lung (ruptured) J43.9
    congenital —see Atelectasis
    newborn P25.8
  subpleural (emphysematous) J43.9
Blebitis, postprocedural H59.40
  stage 1 H59.41
  stage 2 H59.42
  stage 3 H59.43
Bleeder (familial) (hereditary) —see Hemophilia
Bleeding —see also Hemorrhage
  anal K62.5
  anovulatory N97.0
  atonic, following delivery O72.1
  capillary I78.8
    puerperal O72.2
  contact (postcoital) N93.0
  due to uterine subinvolution N85.3
  ear —see Otorrhagia
  excessive, associated with menopausal onset
    N92.4
  familial —see Defect, coagulation
  following intercourse N93.0
  gastrointestinal K92.2
  hemorrhoids —see Hemorrhoids
  intermenstrual (regular) N92.3
    irregular N92.1
  intraoperative —see Complication,
    intraoperative, hemorrhage
  irregular N92.6
  menopausal N92.4
  newborn, intraventricular —see
    Newborn, affected by, hemorrhage,
    intraventricular
  nipple N64.59
  nose R04.0
  ovulation N92.3
  postclimacteric N95.0
  postcoital N93.0
  postmenopausal N95.0
  postoperative —see Complication,
    postprocedural, hemorrhage
  preclimacteric N92.4
  puberty (excessive, with onset of menstrual
    periods) N92.2

Bleeding *(Continued)*
rectum, rectal K62.5
newborn P54.2
tendencies —*see* Defect, coagulation
throat R04.1
tooth socket (post-extraction) K91.840
umbilical stump P51.9
uterus, uterine NEC N93.9
climacteric N92.4
dysfunctional of functional N93.8
menopausal N92.4
preclimacteric or premenopausal
N92.4
unrelated to menstrual cycle N93.9
vagina, vaginal (abnormal) N93.9
dysfunctional or functional N93.8
newborn P54.6
vicarious N94.89
Blennorrhagia, blennorrhagic —*see* Gonorrhea
Blennorrhea (acute) (chronic) —*see also*
Gonorrhea
inclusion (neonatal) (newborn) P39.1
lower genitourinary tract (gonococcal)
A54.00
neonatorum (gonococcal ophthalmia)
A54.31
Blepharelosis —*see* Entropion
Blepharitis (angularis) (ciliaris) (eyelid)
(marginal) (nonulcerative) H01.009
herpes zoster B02.39
left H01.006
lower H01.005
upper H01.004
right H01.003
lower H01.002
upper H01.001
squamous H01.029
left H01.026
lower H01.025
upper H01.024
right H01.023
lower H01.022
upper H01.021
ulcerative H01.019
left H01.016
lower H01.015
upper H01.014
right H01.013
lower H01.012
upper H01.011
Blepharochalasis H02.30
congenital Q10.0
left H02.36
lower H02.35
upper H02.34
right H02.33
lower H02.32
upper H02.31
Blepharoclonus H02.59
Blepharoconjunctivitis H10.50-
angular H10.52-
contact H10.53-
ligneous H10.51-
Blepharophimosis (eyelid) H02.529
congenital Q10.3
left H02.526
lower H02.525
upper H02.524
right H02.523
lower H02.522
upper H02.521
Blepharoptosis H02.40-
congenital Q10.0
mechanical H02.41-
myogenic H02.42-
neurogenic H02.43-
paralytic H02.43-
Blepharopyorrhea, gonococcal A54.39
Blepharospasm G24.5
drug induced G24.01
Blighted ovum O02.0

Blind —*see also* Blindness
bronchus (congenital) Q32.4
loop syndrome K90.2
congenital Q43.8
sac, fallopian tube (congenital) Q50.6
spot, enlarged —*see* Defect, visual field,
localized, scotoma, blind spot area
tract or tube, congenital NEC —*see* Atresia,
by site
Blindness (acquired) (congenital) (both eyes)
H54.0
blast S05.8X-
color —*see* Deficiency, color vision
concussion S05.8X-
cortical H47.619
left brain H47.612
right brain H47.611
day H53.11
due to injury (current episode) S05.9-
sequelae — code to injury with seventh
character S
eclipse (total) —*see* Retinopathy, solar
emotional (hysterical) F44.6
face H53.16
hysterical F44.6
legal (both eyes) (USA definition) H54.8
mind R48.8
night H53.60
abnormal dark adaptation curve H53.61
acquired H53.62
congenital H53.63
specified type NEC H53.69
vitamin A deficiency E50.5
one eye (other eye normal) H54.40
left (normal vision on right) H54.42
low vision on right H54.12
low vision, other eye H54.10
right (normal vision on left) H54.41
low vision on left H54.11
psychic R48.8
river B73.01
snow —*see* Photokeratitis
sun, solar —*see* Retinopathy, solar
transient —*see* Disturbance, vision, subjective,
loss, transient
traumatic (current episode) S05.9-
word (developmental) F81.0
acquired R48.0
secondary to organic lesion R48.0
Blister (nonthermal)
abdominal wall S30.821
alveolar process S00.522
ankle S90.52-
antecubital space —*see* Blister, elbow
anus S30.827
arm (upper) S40.82-
auditory canal —*see* Blister, ear
auricle —*see* Blister, ear
axilla —*see* Blister, arm
back, lower S30.820
beetle dermatitis L24.89
breast S20.12-
brow S00.82
calf —*see* Blister, leg
canthus —*see* Blister, eyelid
cheek S00.82
internal S00.522
chest wall —*see* Blister, thorax
chin S00.82
costal region —*see* Blister, thorax
digit (s)
foot —*see* Blister, toe
hand —*see* Blister, finger
due to burn —*see* Burn, by site, second degree
ear S00.42-
elbow S50.32-
epiglottis S10.12
esophagus, cervical S10.12
eyebrow —*see* Blister, eyelid
eyelid S00.22-
face S00.82

Blister *(Continued)*
fever B00.1
finger (s) S60.429
index S60.42-
little S60.42-
middle S60.42-
ring S60.42-
foot (except toe (s) alone) S90.82-
toe —*see* Blister, toe
forearm S50.82-
elbow only —*see* Blister, elbow
forehead S00.82
fracture - omit code
genital organ
female S30.826
male S30.825
gum S00.522
hand S60.52-
head S00.92
ear —*see* Blister, ear
eyelid —*see* Blister, eyelid
lip S00.521
nose S00.32
oral cavity S00.522
scalp S00.02
specified site NEC S00.82
heel —*see* Blister, foot
hip S70.22-
interscapular region S20.429
jaw S00.82
knee S80.22-
larynx S10.12
leg (lower) S80.82-
knee —*see* Blister, knee
upper —*see* Blister, thigh
lip S00.521
malar region S00.82
mammary —*see* Blister, breast
mastoid region S00.82
mouth S00.522
multiple, skin, nontraumatic R23.8
nail
finger —*see* Blister, finger
toe —*see* Blister, toe
nasal S00.32
neck S10.92
specified site NEC S10.82
throat S10.12
nose S00.32
occipital region S00.02
oral cavity S00.522
orbital region —*see* Blister, eyelid
palate S00.522
palm —*see* Blister, hand
parietal region S00.02
pelvis S30.820
penis S30.822
periocular area —*see* Blister, eyelid
phalanges
finger —*see* Blister, finger
toe —*see* Blister, toe
pharynx S10.12
pinna —*see* Blister, ear
popliteal space —*see* Blister, knee
scalp S00.02
scapular region —*see* Blister, shoulder
scrotum S30.823
shin —*see* Blister, leg
shoulder S40.22-
sternal region S20.329
submaxillary region S00.82
submental region S00.82
subungual
finger (s) —*see* Blister, finger
toe (s) —*see* Blister, toe
supraclavicular fossa S10.82
supraorbital S00.82
temple S00.82
temporal region S00.82
testis S30.823
thermal —*see* Burn, second degree, by site

◄ New ⬅ Revised ~~deleted~~ Deleted

B

Blister *(Continued)*
  thigh S70.32-
  thorax, thoracic (wall) S20.92
    back S20.42-
    front S20.32-
  throat S10.12
  thumb S60.32-
  toe (s) S90.42-
    great S90.42-
  tongue S00.522
  trachea S10.12
  tympanum, tympanic membrane —*see* Blister,
    ear
  upper arm —*see* Blister, arm (upper)
  uvula S00.522
  vagina S30.824
  vocal cords S10.12
  vulva S30.824
  wrist S60.82-
Bloating R14.0
Bloch-Sulzberger disease or syndrome Q82.3
Block, blocked
  alveolocapillary J84.10
  arborization (heart) I45.5
  arrhythmic I45.9
  atrioventricular (incomplete) (partial) I44.30
    with atrioventricular dissociation I44.2
    complete I44.2
      congenital Q24.6
    congenital Q24.6
    first degree I44.0
    second degree (types I and II) I44.1
    specified NEC I44.39
    third degree I44.2
    types I and II I44.1
  auriculoventricular —*see* Block,
    atrioventricular
  bifascicular (cardiac) I45.2
  bundle-branch (complete) (false) (incomplete)
    I45.4
    bilateral I45.2
    left I44.7
      with right bundle branch block I45.2
      hemiblock I44.60
        anterior I44.4
        posterior I44.5
      incomplete I44.7
        with right bundle branch block I45.2
    right I45.10
      with
        left bundle branch block I45.2
        left fascicular block I45.2
      specified NEC I45.19
    Wilson's type I45.19
  cardiac I45.9
  conduction I45.9
    complete I44.2
  fascicular (left) I44.60
    anterior I44.4
    posterior I44.5
    right I45.0
    specified NEC I44.69
  foramen Magendie (acquired) G91.1
    congenital Q03.1
      with spina bifida —*see* Spina bifida, by
        site, with hydrocephalus
  heart I45.9
    bundle branch I45.4
      bilateral I45.2
    complete (atrioventricular) I44.2
    congenital Q24.6
    first degree (atrioventricular) I44.0
    second degree (atrioventricular) I44.1
    specified type NEC I45.5
    third degree (atrioventricular) I44.2
  hepatic vein I82.0
  intraventricular (nonspecific) I45.4
    bundle branch
      bilateral I45.2
  kidney N28.9
    postcystoscopic or postprocedural N99.0

Block, blocked *(Continued)*
  Mobitz (types I and II) I44.1
  myocardial —*see* Block, heart
  nodal I45.5
  organ or site, congenital NEC —*see* Atresia,
    by site
  portal (vein) I81
  second degree (types I and II) I44.1
  sinoatrial I45.5
  sinoauricular I45.5
  third degree I44.2
  trifascicular I45.3
  tubal N97.1
  vein NOS I82.90
  Wenckebach (types I and II) I44.1
Blockage —*see* Obstruction
Blocq's disease F44.4
Blood
  constituents, abnormal R78.9
  disease D75.9
  donor —*see* Donor, blood
  dyscrasia D75.9
    with
      abortion —*see* Abortion, by type,
        complicated by, hemorrhage
      ectopic pregnancy O08.1
      molar pregnancy O08.1
    following ectopic or molar pregnancy
      O08.1
    newborn P61.9
    puerperal, postpartum O72.3
  flukes NEC —*see* Schistosomiasis
  in
    feces K92.1
      occult R19.5
    urine —*see* Hematuria
  mole O02.0
  occult in feces R19.5
  pressure
    decreased, due to shock following injury
      T79.4
    examination only Z01.30
    fluctuating I99.8
    high —*see* Hypertension
      borderline R03.0
      incidental reading, without diagnosis of
        hypertension R03.0
    low —*see also* Hypotension
      incidental reading, without diagnosis of
        hypotension R03.1
  spitting —*see* Hemoptysis
  staining cornea —*see* Pigmentation, cornea,
    stromal
  transfusion
    reaction or complication —*see*
      Complications, transfusion
  type
    A (Rh positive) Z67.10
      Rh negative Z67.11
    AB (Rh positive) Z67.30
      Rh negative Z67.31
    B (Rh positive) Z67.20
      Rh negative Z67.21
    O (Rh positive) Z67.40
      Rh negative Z67.41
    Rh (positive) Z67.90
      negative Z67.91
  vessel rupture —*see* Hemorrhage
  vomiting —*see* Hematemesis
Blood-forming organs, disease D75.9
Bloodgood's disease —*see* Mastopathy,
  cystic
Bloom (-Machacek)(-Torre) **syndrome**
  Q82.8
Blount's disease or osteochondrosis —*see*
  Osteochondrosis, juvenile, tibia
Blue
  baby Q24.9
  diaper syndrome E72.09
  dome cyst (breast) —*see* Cyst, breast
  dot cataract Q12.0

Blue *(Continued)*
  nevus D22.9
  sclera Q13.5
    with fragility of bone and deafness Q78.0
  toe syndrome I75.02-
Blueness —*see* Cyanosis
Blues, postpartal O90.6
  baby O90.6
Blurring, visual H53.8
Blushing (abnormal) (excessive) R23.2
BMI —*see* Body, mass index
Boarder, hospital NEC Z76.4
  accompanying sick person Z76.3
  healthy infant or child Z76.2
    foundling Z76.1
Bockhart's impetigo L01.02
Bodechtel-Guttman disease (subacute
  sclerosing panencephalitis) A81.1
Boder-Sedgwick syndrome (ataxia-
  telangiectasia) G11.3
Body, bodies
  Aschoff's —*see* Myocarditis, rheumatic
  asteroid, vitreous —*see* Deposit, crystalline
  cytoid (retina) —*see* Occlusion, artery, retina
  drusen (degenerative) (macula) (retinal) —*see*
    also Degeneration, macula, drusen
    optic disc —*see* Drusen, optic disc
  foreign —*see* Foreign body
  loose
    joint, except knee —*see* Loose, body, joint
      knee M23.4-
    sheath, tendon —*see* Disorder, tendon,
      specified type NEC
  mass index (BMI)
    adult
      19 or less Z68.1
      20.0-20.9 Z68.20
      21.0-21.9 Z68.21
      22.0-22.9 Z68.22
      23.0-23.9 Z68.23
      24.0-24.9 Z68.24
      25.0-25.9 Z68.25
      26.0-26.9 Z68.26
      27.0-27.9 Z68.27
      28.0-28.9 Z68.28
      29.0-29.9 Z68.29
      30.0-30.9 Z68.30
      31.0-31.9 Z68.31
      32.0-32.9 Z68.32
      33.0-33.9 Z68.33
      34.0-34.9 Z68.34
      35.0-35.9 Z68.35
      36.0-36.9 Z68.36
      37.0-37.9 Z68.37
      38.0-38.9 Z68.38
      39.0-39.9 Z68.39
      40.0-44.9 Z68.41
      45.0-49.9 Z68.42
      50.0-59.9 Z68.43
      60.0-69.9 Z68.44
      70 and over Z68.45
    pediatric
      5th percentile to less than 85th percentile
        for age Z68.52
      85th percentile to less than 95th
        percentile for age Z68.53
      greater than or equal to ninety-fifth
        percentile for age Z68.54
      less than fifth percentile for age Z68.51
  Mooser's A75.2
  rice —*see also* Loose, body, joint
    knee M23.4-
  rocking F98.4
Boeck's
  disease or sarcoid —*see* Sarcoidosis
  lupoid (miliary) D86.3
Boerhaave's syndrome (spontaneous
  esophageal rupture) K22.3
Boggy
  cervix N88.8
  uterus N85.8

Boil —see also Furuncle, by site
   Aleppo B55.1
   Baghdad B55.1
   Delhi B55.1
   lacrimal
      gland —see Dacryoadenitis
      passages (duct) (sac) —see Inflammation,
         lacrimal, passages, acute
   Natal B55.1
   orbit, orbital —see Abscess, orbit
   tropical B55.1
Bold hives —see Urticaria
Bombé, iris —see Membrane, pupillary
Bone —see condition
Bonnevie-Ullrich syndrome Q87.1
Bonnier's syndrome —see subcategory
   H81.8
Bonvale dam fever T73.3
Bony block of joint —see Ankylosis
BOOP (bronchiolitis obliterans organized
   pneumonia) J84.89
Borderline
   diabetes mellitus R73.09
   hypertension R03.0
   osteopenia M85.8-
   pelvis, with obstruction during labor
      O65.1
   personality F60.3
Borna disease A83.9
Bornholm disease B33.0
Boston exanthem A88.0
Botalli, ductus (patent) (persistent) Q25.0
Bothriocephalus latus infestation B70.0
Botulism (foodborne intoxication) A05.1
   infant A48.51
   non-foodborne A48.52
   wound A48.52
Bouba —see Yaws
Bouchard's nodes (with arthropathy) M15.2
Bouffée délirante F23
Bouillaud's disease or syndrome (rheumatic
   heart disease) I01.9
Bourneville's disease Q85.1
Boutonniere deformity (finger) —see
   Deformity, finger, boutonniere
Bouveret (-Hoffmann) syndrome (paroxysmal
   tachycardia) I47.9
Bovine heart —see Hypertrophy, cardiac
Bowel —see condition
Bowen's
   dermatosis (precancerous) —see Neoplasm,
      skin, in situ
   disease —see Neoplasm, skin, in situ
   epithelioma —see Neoplasm, skin, in situ
   type
      epidermoid carcinoma-in-situ —see
         Neoplasm, skin, in situ
      intraepidermal squamous cell carcinoma —
         see Neoplasm, skin, in situ
Bowing
   femur —see also Deformity, limb, specified
      type NEC, thigh
      congenital Q68.3
   fibula —see also Deformity, limb, specified
      type NEC, lower leg
      congenital Q68.4
   forearm —see Deformity, limb, specified type
      NEC, forearm
   leg (s), long bones, congenital Q68.5
   radius —see Deformity, limb, specified type
      NEC, forearm
   tibia —see also Deformity, limb, specified type
      NEC, lower leg
      congenital Q68.4
Bowleg (s) (acquired) M21.16-
   congenital Q68.5
   rachitic E64.3
Boyd's dysentery A03.2
Brachial —see condition
Brachycardia R00.1
Brachycephaly Q75.0

Bradley's disease A08.19
Bradyarrhythmia, cardiac I49.8
Bradycardia (sinoatrial) (sinus) (vagal) R00.1
   neonatal P29.12
   reflex G90.09
   tachycardia syndrome I49.5
Bradykinesia R25.8
Bradypnea R06.89
Bradytachycardia I49.5
Brailsford's disease or osteochondrosis —see
   Osteochondrosis, juvenile, radius
Brain —see also condition
   death G93.82
   syndrome —see Syndrome, brain
Branched-chain amino-acid disorder E71.2
Branchial —see condition
   cartilage, congenital Q18.2
Branchiogenic remnant (in neck) Q18.0
Brandt's syndrome (acrodermatitis
   enteropathica) E83.2
Brash (water) R12
Bravais-jacksonian epilepsy —see Epilepsy,
   localization-related, symptomatic, with
   simple partial seizures
Braxton Hicks contractions —see False, labor
Brazilian leishmaniasis B55.2
BRBPR K62.5
Break, retina (without detachment) H33.30-
   with retinal detachment —see Detachment,
      retina
   horseshoe tear H33.31-
   multiple H33.33-
   round hole H33.32-
Breakdown
   device, graft or implant (see also
      Complications, by site and type,
      mechanical) T85.618
      arterial graft NEC —see Complication,
         cardiovascular device, mechanical,
         vascular
      breast (implant) T85.41
      catheter NEC T85.618
         cystostomy T83.010
         dialysis (renal) T82.41
            intraperitoneal T85.611
         infusion NEC T82.514
            spinal (epidural) (subdural) T85.610
         urinary (indwelling) T83.018
      electronic (electrode) (pulse generator)
         (stimulator)
         bone T84.310
         cardiac T82.119
            electrode T82.110
            pulse generator T82.111
            specified type NEC T82.118
         nervous system —see Complication,
            prosthetic device, mechanical,
            electronic nervous system
            stimulator
         urinary —see Complication,
            genitourinary, device, urinary,
            mechanical
      fixation, internal (orthopedic) NEC —see
         Complication, fixation device,
         mechanical
      gastrointestinal —see Complications,
         prosthetic device, mechanical,
         gastrointestinal device
      genital NEC T83.418
         intrauterine contraceptive device T83.31
         penile prosthesis T83.410
      heart NEC —see Complication,
         cardiovascular device, mechanical
      joint prosthesis —see Complications...,
         joint prosthesis,internal, mechanical,
         by site
      ocular NEC —see Complications, prosthetic
         device, mechanical, ocular device
      orthopedic NEC —see Complication,
         orthopedic, device, mechanical
      specified NEC T85.618

Breakdown (Continued)
   device, graft or implant (Continued)
      sutures, permanent T85.612
         used in bone repair —see Complications,
            fixation device, internal
            (orthopedic), mechanical
      urinary NEC —see also Complication,
         genitourinary, device, urinary,
         mechanical
         graft T83.21
      vascular NEC —see Complication,
         cardiovascular device, mechanical
      ventricular intracranial shunt T85.01
   nervous F48.8
   perineum O90.1
   respirator J95.850
      specified NEC J95.859
   ventilator J95.850
      specified NEC J95.859
Breast —see also condition
   buds E30.1
      in newborn P96.89
   dense R92.2
   nodule N63
Breath
   foul R19.6
   holder, child R06.89
   holding spell R06.89
   shortness R06.02
Breathing
   labored —see Hyperventilation
   mouth R06.5
      causing malocclusion M26.5
   periodic R06.3
      high altitude G47.32
Breathlessness R06.81
Breda's disease —see Yaws
Breech presentation (mother) O32.1
   causing obstructed labor O64.1
   footling O32.8
      causing obstructed labor O64.8
   incomplete O32.8
      causing obstructed labor O64.8
Breisky's disease N90.4
Brennemann's syndrome I88.0
Brenner
   tumor (benign) D27.9
      borderline malignancy D39.1-
      malignant C56
      proliferating D39.1
Bretonneau's disease or angina A36.0
Breus' mole O02.0
Brevicollis Q76.49
Brickmakers' anemia B76.9 [D63.8]
Bridge, myocardial Q24.5
Bright red blood per rectum (BRBPR) K62.5
Bright's disease —see also Nephritis
   arteriosclerotic —see Hypertension, kidney
Brill (-Zinsser) disease (recrudescent typhus)
   A75.1
   flea-borne A75.2
   louse-borne A75.1
Brill-Symmers' disease C82.90
Brion-Kayser disease —see Fever, parathyroid
Briquet's disorder or syndrome F45.0
Brissaud's
   infantilism or dwarfism E23.0
   motor-verbal tic F95.2
Brittle
   bones disease Q78.0
   nails L60.3
      congenital Q84.6
Broad —see also condition
   beta disease E78.2
   ligament laceration syndrome N83.8
Broad- or floating-betalipoproteinemia
   E78.2
Brock's syndrome (atelectasis due to enlarged
   lymph nodes) J98.19
Brocq-Duhring disease (dermatitis
   herpetiformis) L13.0

◀ New   ⬅ Revised   d̶e̶l̶e̶t̶e̶d̶ Deleted

Brodie's abscess or disease M86.8X-
Broken
  arches —see also Deformity, limb, flat foot
  arm (meaning upper limb) —see Fracture, arm
  back —see Fracture, vertebra
  bone —see Fracture
  implant or internal device —see Complications, by site and type, mechanical
  leg (meaning lower limb) —see Fracture, leg
  nose S02.2
  tooth, teeth —see Fracture, tooth
Bromhidrosis, bromidrosis L75.0
Bromidism, bromism G92
  chronic (dependence) F13.20
  due to
    correct substance properly administered — see Table of Drugs and Chemicals, by drug, adverse effect
    overdose or wrong substance given or taken —see Table of Drugs and Chemicals, by drug, poisoning
Bromidrosiphobia F40.298
Bronchi, bronchial —see condition
Bronchiectasis (cylindrical) (diffuse) (fusiform) (localized) (saccular) J47.9
  with
    acute
      bronchitis J47.0
      lower respiratory infection J47.0
    exacerbation (acute) J47.1
  congenital Q33.4
  tuberculous NEC —see Tuberculosis, pulmonary
Bronchiolectasis —see Bronchiectasis
Bronchiolitis (acute) (infective) (subacute) J21.9
  with
    bronchospasm or obstruction J21.9
    influenza, flu or grippe —see Influenza, with, respiratory manifestations NEC
  chemical (chronic) J68.4
    acute J68.0
  chronic (fibrosing) (obliterative) J44.9
  due to
    external agent —see Bronchitis, acute, due to
    human metapneumovirus J21.1
    respiratory syncytial virus J21.0
    specified organism NEC J21.8
  fibrosa obliterans J44.9
  influenzal —see Influenza, with, respiratory manifestations NEC
  obliterans J42
    with organizing pneumonia (BOOP) J84.89
  obliterative (chronic) (subacute) J44.9
    due to chemicals, gases, fumes or vapors (inhalation) J68.4
    due to fumes or vapors J68.4
  respiratory, interstitial lung disease J84.115
Bronchitis (diffuse) (fibrinous) (hypostatic) (infective) (membranous) J40
  with
    influenza, flu or grippe —see Influenza, with, respiratory manifestations NEC
    obstruction (airway) (lung) J44.9
    tracheitis (15 years of age and above) J40
      acute or subacute J20.9
      chronic J42
      under 15 years of age J20.9
  acute or subacute (with bronchospasm or obstruction) J20.9
    with
      bronchiectasis J47.0
      chronic obstructive pulmonary disease J44.0
      chemical (due to gases, fumes or vapors) J68.0

Bronchitis (Continued)
  acute or subacute (Continued)
    due to
      fumes or vapors J68.0
      Haemophilus influenzae J20.1
      Mycoplasma pneumoniae J20.0
      radiation J70.0
      specified organism NEC J20.8
      Streptococcus J20.2
      virus
        coxsackie J20.3
        echovirus J20.7
        parainfluenzae J20.4
        respiratory syncytial J20.5
        rhinovirus J20.6
      viral NEC J20.8
  allergic (acute) J45.909
    with
      exacerbation (acute) J45.901
      status asthmaticus J45.902
  arachidic T17.528
  aspiration (due to fumes or vapors) J68.0
  asthmatic J45.9
    chronic J44.9
      with
        acute lower respiratory infection J44.0
        exacerbation (acute) J44.1
  capillary —see Pneumonia, broncho
  caseous (tuberculous) A15.5
  Castellani's A69.8
  catarrhal (15 years of age and above) J40
    acute —see Bronchitis, acute
    chronic J41.0
    under 15 years of age J20.9
  chemical (acute) (subacute) J68.0
    chronic J68.4
    due to fumes or vapors J68.0
      chronic J68.4
  chronic J42
    with
      airways obstruction J44.9
      tracheitis (chronic) J42
    asthmatic (obstructive) J44.9
    catarrhal J41.0
    chemical (due to fumes or vapors) J68.4
    due to
      chemicals, gases, fumes or vapors (inhalation) J68.4
      radiation J70.1
      tobacco smoking J41.0
    emphysematous J44.9
    mucopurulent J41.1
    non-obstructive J41.0
    obliterans J44.9
    obstructive J44.9
    purulent J41.1
    simple J41.0
  croupous —see Bronchitis, acute
  due to gases, fumes or vapors (chemical) J68.0
  emphysematous (obstructive) J44.9
  exudative —see Bronchitis, acute
  fetid J41.1
  grippal —see Influenza, with, respiratory manifestations NEC
  in those under 15 years age —see Bronchitis, acute
    chronic —see Bronchitis, chronic
  influenzal —see Influenza, with, respiratory manifestations NEC
  mixed simple and mucopurulent J41.8
  moulder's J62.8
  mucopurulent (chronic) (recurrent) J41.1
    acute or subacute J20.9
    simple (mixed) J41.8
  obliterans (chronic) J44.9
  obstructive (chronic) (diffuse) J44.9
  pituitous J41.1
  pneumococcal, acute or subacute J20.2
  pseudomembranous, acute or subacute —see Bronchitis, acute

Bronchitis (Continued)
  purulent (chronic) (recurrent) J41.1
    acute or subacute —see Bronchitis, acute
  putrid J41.1
  senile (chronic) J42
  simple and mucopurulent (mixed) J41.8
  smokers' J41.0
  spirochetal NEC A69.8
  subacute —see Bronchitis, acute
  suppurative (chronic) J41.1
    acute or subacute —see Bronchitis, acute
  tuberculous A15.5
  under 15 years of age —see Bronchitis, acute
    chronic —see Bronchitis, chronic
  viral NEC, acute or subacute (see also Bronchitis, acute) J20.8
Bronchoalveolitis J18.0
Bronchoaspergillosis B44.1
Bronchocele meaning goiter E04.0
Broncholithiasis J98.09
  tuberculous NEC A15.5
Bronchomalacia J98.09
  congenital Q32.2
Bronchomycosis NOS B49 [J99]
  candidal B37.1
Bronchopleuropneumonia —see Pneumonia, broncho
Bronchopneumonia —see Pneumonia, broncho
Bronchopneumonitis —see Pneumonia, broncho
Bronchopulmonary —see condition
Bronchopulmonitis —see Pneumonia, broncho
Bronchorrhagia (see Hemoptysis)
Bronchorrhea J98.09
  acute J20.9
  chronic (infective) (purulent) J42
Bronchospasm (acute) J98.01
  with
    bronchiolitis, acute J21.9
    bronchitis, acute (conditions in J20) —see Bronchitis, acute
  due to external agent —see condition, respiratory, acute, due to
  exercise induced J45.990
Bronchospirochetosis A69.8
  Castellani A69.8
Bronchostenosis J98.09
Bronchus —see condition
Brontophobia F40.220
Bronze baby syndrome P83.8
Brooke's tumor —see Neoplasm, skin, benign
Brown enamel of teeth (hereditary) K00.5
Brown's sheath syndrome H50.61-
Brown-Séquard disease, paralysis or syndrome G83.81
Bruce sepsis A23.0
Brucellosis (infection) A23.9
  abortus A23.1
  canis A23.3
  dermatitis A23.9
  melitensis A23.0
  mixed A23.8
  sepsis A23.9
    melitensis A23.0
    specified NEC A23.8
  suis A23.2
Bruck-de Lange disease Q87.1
Bruck's disease —see Deformity, limb
Brugsch's syndrome Q82.8
Bruise (skin surface intact) —see also Contusion
  with
    open wound —see Wound, open
  internal organ —see Injury, by site
  newborn P54.5
  scalp, due to birth injury, newborn P12.3
  umbilical cord O69.5
Bruit (arterial) R09.89
  cardiac R01.1
Brush burn —see Abrasion, by site
Bruton's X-linked agammaglobulinemia D80.0

Bruxism
  psychogenic F45.8
  sleep related G47.63
Bubbly lung syndrome P27.0
Bubo I88.8
  blennorrhagic (gonococcal) A54.89
  chancroidal A57
  climatic A55
  due to Haemophilus ducreyi A57
  gonococcal A54.89
  indolent (nonspecific) I88.8
  inguinal (nonspecific) I88.8
    chancroidal A57
    climatic A55
    due to H. ducreyi A57
    infective I88.8
  scrofulous (tuberculous) A18.2
  soft chancre A57
  suppurating —see Lymphadenitis, acute
  syphilitic (primary) A51.0
    congenital A50.07
  tropical A55
  virulent (chancroidal) A57
Bubonic plague A20.0
Bubonocele —see Hernia, inguinal
Buccal —see condition
Buchanan's disease or osteochondrosis
    M91.0
Buchem's syndrome (hyperostosis corticalis)
    M85.2
Bucket-handle fracture or tear (semilunar
    cartilage) —see Tear, meniscus
Budd-Chiari syndrome (hepatic vein
    thrombosis) I82.0
Budgerigar fancier's disease or lung
    J67.2
Buds
  breast E30.1
    in newborn P96.89
Buerger's disease (thromboangiitis obliterans)
    I73.1
Bulbar —see condition
Bulbus cordis (left ventricle) (persistent)
    Q21.8
Bulimia (nervosa) F50.2
  atypical F50.9
  normal weight F50.9
Bulky
  stools R19.5
  uterus N85.2
Bulla (e) R23.8
  lung (emphysematous) (solitary) J43.9
    newborn P25.8
Bullet wound —see also Wound, open
  fracture - code as Fracture, by site
  internal organ —see Injury, by site
Bundle
  branch block (complete) (false)
      (incomplete) —see Block, bundle-branch
  of His —see condition
Bunion —see Deformity, toe, hallux valgus
Buphthalmia, buphthalmos (congenital)
    Q15.0
Burdwan fever B55.0
Bürger-Grütz disease or syndrome
    E78.3
Buried
  penis (congenital) Q55.64
    acquired N48.83
  roots K08.3
Burke's syndrome K86.8
Burkitt
  cell leukemia C91.0-
  lymphoma (malignant) C83.7-
    small noncleaved, diffuse C83.7-
    spleen C83.77
    undifferentiated C83.7-
  tumor C83.7-
  type
    acute lymphoblastic leukemia C91.0-
    undifferentiated C83.7-

Burn (electricity) (flame) (hot gas, liquid or hot
    object) (radiation) (steam) (thermal) T30.0
  abdomen, abdominal (muscle) (wall) T21.02
    first degree T21.12
    second degree T21.22
    third degree T21.32
  above elbow T22.039
    first degree T22.139
    left T22.032
      first degree T22.132
      second degree T22.232
      third degree T22.332
    right T22.031
      first degree T22.131
      second degree T22.231
      third degree T22.331
    second degree T22.239
    third degree T22.339
  acid (caustic) (external) (internal) —see
      Corrosion, by site
  alimentary tract NEC T28.2
    esophagus T28.1
    mouth T28.0
    pharynx T28.0
  alkaline (caustic) (external) (internal) —see
      Corrosion, by site
  ankle T25.019
    first degree T25.119
    left T25.012
      first degree T25.112
      second degree T25.212
      third degree T25.312
    multiple with foot —see Burn, lower, limb,
        multiple, ankle and foot
    right T25.011
      first degree T25.111
      second degree T25.211
      third degree T25.311
    second degree T25.219
    third degree T25.319
  anus —see Burn, buttock
  arm (lower) (upper) —see Burn, upper, limb
  axilla T22.049
    first degree T22.149
    left T22.042
      first degree T22.142
      second degree T22.242
      third degree T22.342
    right T22.041
      first degree T22.141
      second degree T22.241
      third degree T22.341
    second degree T22.249
    third degree T22.349
  back (lower) T21.04
    first degree T21.14
    second degree T21.24
    third degree T21.34
    upper T21.03
      first degree T21.13
      second degree T21.23
      third degree T21.33
  blisters - code as Burn, second degree, by site
  breast (s) —see Burn, chest wall
  buttock (s) T21.05
    first degree T21.15
    second degree T21.25
    third degree T21.35
  calf T24.039
    first degree T24.139
    left T24.032
      first degree T24.132
      second degree T24.232
      third degree T24.332
    right T24.031
      first degree T24.131
      second degree T24.231
      third degree T24.331
    second degree T24.239
    third degree T24.339
  canthus (eye) —see Burn, eyelid

Burn (Continued)
  caustic acid or alkaline —see Corrosion, by
      site
  cervix T28.3
  cheek T20.06
    first degree T20.16
    second degree T20.26
    third degree T20.36
  chemical (acids) (alkalines) (caustics)
      (external) (internal) —see Corrosion,
      by site
  chest wall T21.01
    first degree T21.11
    second degree T21.21
    third degree T21.31
  chin T20.03
    first degree T20.13
    second degree T20.23
    third degree T20.33
  colon T28.2
  conjunctiva (and cornea) —see Burn, cornea
  cornea (and conjunctiva) T26.1-
    chemical —see Corrosion, cornea
  corrosion (external) (internal) —see
      Corrosion, by site
  deep necrosis of underlying tissue - code as
      Burn, third degree, by site
  dorsum of hand T23.069
    first degree T23.169
    left T23.062
      first degree T23.162
      second degree T23.262
      third degree T23.362
    right T23.061
      first degree T23.161
      second degree T23.261
      third degree T23.361
    second degree T23.269
    third degree T23.369
  due to ingested chemical agent —see
      Corrosion, by site
  ear (auricle) (external) (canal) T20.01
    first degree T20.11
    second degree T20.21
    third degree T20.31
  elbow T22.029
    first degree T22.129
    left T22.022
      first degree T22.122
      second degree T22.222
      third degree T22.322
    right T22.021
      first degree T22.121
      second degree T22.221
      third degree T22.321
    second degree T22.229
    third degree T22.329
  epidermal loss - code as Burn, second degree,
      by site
  erythema, erythematous - code as Burn, first
      degree, by site
  esophagus T28.1
  extent (percentage of body surface)
    less than 10 percent T31.0
    10-19 percent T31.10
      with 0-9 percent third degree burns
          T31.10
      with 10-19 percent third degree burns
          T31.11
    20-29 percent T31.20
      with 0-9 percent third degree burns
          T31.20
      with 10-19 percent third degree burns
          T31.21
      with 20-29 percent third degree burns
          T31.22
    30-39 percent T31.30
      with 0-9 percent third degree burns
          T31.30
      with 10-19 percent third degree burns
          T31.31

Burn (*Continued*)
  extent (*Continued*)
    30-39 percent (*Continued*)
      with 20-29 percent third degree burns
        T31.32
      with 30-39 percent third degree burns
        T31.33
    40-49 percent T31.40
      with 0-9 percent third degree burns T31.40
      with 10-19 percent third degree burns
        T31.41
      with 20-29 percent third degree burns
        T31.42
      with 30-39 percent third degree burns
        T31.43
      with 40-49 percent third degree burns
        T31.44
    50-59 percent T31.50
      with 0-9 percent third degree burns T31.50
      with 10-19 percent third degree burns
        T31.51
      with 20-29 percent third degree burns
        T31.52
      with 30-39 percent third degree burns
        T31.53
      with 40-49 percent third degree burns
        T31.54
      with 50-59 percent third degree burns
        T31.55
    60-69 percent T31.60
      with 0-9 percent third degree burns T31.60
      with 10-19 percent third degree burns
        T31.61
      with 20-29 percent third degree burns
        T31.62
      with 30-39 percent third degree burns
        T31.63
      with 40-49 percent third degree burns
        T31.64
      with 50-59 percent third degree burns
        T31.65
      with 60-69 percent third degree burns
        T31.66
    70-79 percent T31.70
      with 0-9 percent third degree burns T31.70
      with 10-19 percent third degree burns
        T31.71
      with 20-29 percent third degree burns
        T31.72
      with 30-39 percent third degree burns
        T31.73
      with 40-49 percent third degree burns
        T31.74
      with 50-59 percent third degree burns
        T31.75
      with 60-69 percent third degree burns
        T31.76
      with 70-79 percent third degree burns
        T31.77
    80-89 percent T31.80
      with 0-9 percent third degree burns T31.80
      with 10-19 percent third degree burns
        T31.81
      with 20-29 percent third degree burns
        T31.82
      with 30-39 percent third degree burns
        T31.83
      with 40-49 percent third degree burns
        T31.84
      with 50-59 percent third degree burns
        T31.85
      with 60-69 percent third degree burns
        T31.86
      with 70-79 percent third degree burns
        T31.87
      with 80-89 percent third degree burns
        T31.88
    90 percent or more T31.90
      with 0-9 percent third degree burns T31.90
      with 10-19 percent third degree burns
        T31.91

Burn (*Continued*)
  extent (*Continued*)
    90 percent or more (*Continued*)
      with 20-29 percent third degree burns
        T31.92
      with 30-39 percent third degree burns
        T31.93
      with 40-49 percent third degree burns
        T31.94
      with 50-59 percent third degree burns
        T31.95
      with 60-69 percent third degree burns
        T31.96
      with 70-79 percent third degree burns
        T31.97
      with 80-89 percent third degree burns
        T31.98
      with 90 percent or more third degree
        burns T31.99
  extremity —*see* Burn, limb
  eye (s) and adnexa T26.4-
    with resulting rupture and destruction of
      eyeball T26.2-
    conjunctival sac —*see* Burn, cornea
    cornea —*see* Burn, cornea
    lid —*see* Burn, eyelid
    periocular area —*see* Burn, eyelid
    specified site NEC T26.3-
  eyeball —*see* Burn, eye
  eyelid (s) T26.0-
    chemical —*see* Corrosion, eyelid
  face —*see* Burn, head
  finger T23.029
    first degree T23.129
    left T23.022
      first degree T23.122
      second degree T23.222
      third degree T23.322
    multiple sites (without thumb) T23.039
      with thumb T23.049
        first degree T23.149
        left T23.042
          first degree T23.142
          second degree T23.242
          third degree T23.342
        right T23.041
          first degree T23.141
          second degree T23.241
          third degree T23.341
        second degree T23.249
        third degree T23.349
      first degree T23.139
      left T23.032
        first degree T23.132
        second degree T23.232
        third degree T23.332
      right T23.031
        first degree T23.131
        second degree T23.231
        third degree T23.331
      second degree T23.239
      third degree T23.339
    right T23.021
      first degree T23.121
      second degree T23.221
      third degree T23.321
    second degree T23.229
    third degree T23.329
  flank —*see* Burn, abdominal wall
  foot T25.029
    first degree T25.129
    left T25.022
      first degree T25.122
      second degree T25.222
      third degree T25.322
    multiple with ankle —*see* Burn, lower,
      limb, multiple, ankle and foot
    right T25.021
      first degree T25.121
      second degree T25.221
      third degree T25.321

Burn (*Continued*)
  foot (*Continued*)
    second degree T25.229
    third degree T25.329
  forearm T22.019
    first degree T22.119
    left T22.012
      first degree T22.112
      second degree T22.212
      third degree T22.312
    right T22.011
      first degree T22.111
      second degree T22.211
      third degree T22.311
    second degree T22.219
    third degree T22.319
  forehead T20.06
    first degree T20.16
    second degree T20.26
    third degree T20.36
  fourth degree - code as Burn, third degree,
    by site
  friction —*see* Burn, by site
  from swallowing caustic or corrosive
    substance NEC —*see* Corrosion,
    by site
  full thickness skin loss - code as Burn, third
    degree, by site
  gastrointestinal tract NEC T28.2
    from swallowing caustic or corrosive
      substance T28.7
  genital organs
    external
      female T21.07
        first degree T21.17
        second degree T21.27
        third degree T21.37
      male T21.06
        first degree T21.16
        second degree T21.26
        third degree T21.36
    internal T28.3
      from caustic or corrosive substance
        T28.8
  groin —*see* Burn, abdominal wall
  hand (s) T23.009
    back —*see* Burn, dorsum of hand
    finger —*see* Burn, finger
    first degree T23.109
    left T23.002
      first degree T23.102
      second degree T23.202
      third degree T23.302
    multiple sites with wrist T23.099
      first degree T23.199
      left T23.092
        first degree T23.192
        second degree T23.292
        third degree T23.392
      right T23.091
        first degree T23.191
        second degree T23.291
        third degree T23.391
      second degree T23.299
      third degree T23.399
    palm —*see* Burn, palm
    right T23.001
      first degree T23.101
      second degree T23.201
      third degree T23.301
    second degree T23.209
    third degree T23.309
    thumb —*see* Burn, thumb
  head (and face) (and neck) T20.00
    cheek —*see* Burn, cheek
    chin —*see* Burn, chin
    ear —*see* Burn, ear
    eye (s) only —*see* Burn, eye
    first degree T20.10
    forehead —*see* Burn, forehead
    lip —*see* Burn, lip

Burn (*Continued*)
head (*Continued*)
multiple sites T20.09
first degree T20.19
second degree T20.29
third degree T20.39
neck —*see* Burn, neck
nose —*see* Burn, nose
scalp —*see* Burn, scalp
second degree T20.20
third degree T20.30
hip (s) —*see* Burn, lower, limb
inhalation —*see* Burn, respiratory tract
caustic or corrosive substance (fumes) —*see*
Corrosion, respiratory tract
internal organ (s) T28.40
alimentary tract T28.2
esophagus T28.1
eardrum T28.41
esophagus T28.1
from caustic or corrosive substance
(swallowing) NEC —*see* Corrosion,
by site
genitourinary T28.3
mouth T28.0
pharynx T28.0
respiratory tract —*see* Burn, respiratory
tract
specified organ NEC T28.49
interscapular region —*see* Burn, back, upper
intestine (large) (small) T28.2
knee T24.029
first degree T24.129
left T24.022
first degree T24.122
second degree T24.222
third degree T24.322
right T24.021
first degree T24.121
second degree T24.221
third degree T24.321
second degree T24.229
third degree T24.329
labium (majus) (minus) —*see* Burn, genital
organs, external, female
lacrimal apparatus, duct, gland or sac —*see*
Burn, eye, specified site NEC
larynx T27.0
with lung T27.1
leg (s) (lower) (upper) —*see* Burn, lower,
limb
lightning —*see* Burn, by site
limb (s)
lower (except ankle or foot alone) —*see*
Burn, lower, limb
upper —*see* Burn, upper limb
lip (s) T20.02
first degree T20.12
second degree T20.22
third degree T20.32
lower
back —*see* Burn, back
limb T24.009
ankle —*see* Burn, ankle
calf —*see* Burn, calf
first degree T24.109
foot —*see* Burn, foot
hip —*see* Burn, thigh
knee —*see* Burn, knee
left T24.002
first degree T24.102
second degree T24.202
third degree T24.302
multiple sites, except ankle and foot
T24.099
ankle and foot T25.099
first degree T25.199
left T25.092
first degree T25.192
second degree T25.292
third degree T25.392

Burn (*Continued*)
lower (*Continued*)
limb (*Continued*)
multiple sites, except ankle and foot
(*Continued*)
ankle and foot (*Continued*)
right T25.091
first degree T25.191
second degree
T25.291
third degree T25.391
second degree T25.299
third degree T25.399
first degree T24.199
left T24.092
first degree T24.192
second degree T24.292
third degree T24.392
right T24.091
first degree T24.191
second degree
T24.291
third degree T24.391
second degree T24.299
third degree T24.399
right T24.001
first degree T24.101
second degree T24.201
third degree T24.301
second degree T24.209
thigh —*see* Burn, thigh
third degree T24.309
toe —*see* Burn, toe
lung (with larynx and trachea)
T27.1
mouth T28.0
neck T20.07
first degree T20.17
second degree T20.27
third degree T20.37
nose (septum) T20.04
first degree T20.14
second degree T20.24
third degree T20.34
ocular adnexa —*see* Burn, eye
orbit region —*see* Burn, eyelid
palm T23.059
first degree T23.159
left T23.052
first degree T23.152
second degree T23.252
third degree T23.352
right T23.051
first degree T23.151
second degree T23.251
third degree T23.351
second degree T23.259
third degree T23.359
partial thickness - code as Burn,
unspecified degree, by site
pelvis —*see* Burn, trunk
penis —*see* Burn, genital organs,
external, male
perineum
female —*see* Burn, genital organs,
external, female
male —*see* Burn, genital organs,
external, male
periocular area —*see* Burn, eyelid
pharynx T28.0
rectum T28.2
respiratory tract T27.3
larynx —*see* Burn, larynx
specified part NEC T27.2
trachea —*see* Burn, trachea
sac, lacrimal —*see* Burn, eye, specified site
NEC
scalp T20.05
first degree T20.15
second degree T20.25
third degree T20.35

Burn (*Continued*)
scapular region T22.069
first degree T22.169
left T22.062
first degree T22.162
second degree T22.262
third degree T22.362
right T22.061
first degree T22.161
second degree T22.261
third degree T22.361
second degree T22.269
third degree T22.369
sclera —*see* Burn, eye, specified site NEC
scrotum —*see* Burn, genital organs, external,
male
shoulder T22.059
first degree T22.159
left T22.052
first degree T22.152
second degree T22.252
third degree T22.352
right T22.051
first degree T22.151
second degree T22.251
third degree T22.351
second degree T22.259
third degree T22.359
stomach T28.2
temple —*see* Burn, head
testis —*see* Burn, genital organs, external, male
thigh T24.019
first degree T24.119
left T24.012
first degree T24.112
second degree T24.212
third degree T24.312
right T24.011
first degree T24.111
second degree T24.211
third degree T24.311
second degree T24.219
third degree T24.319
thorax (external) —*see* Burn, trunk
throat (meaning pharynx) T28.0
thumb (s) T23.019
first degree T23.119
left T23.012
first degree T23.112
second degree T23.212
third degree T23.312
multiple sites with fingers T23.049
first degree T23.149
left T23.042
first degree T23.142
second degree T23.242
third degree T23.342
right T23.041
first degree T23.141
second degree T23.241
third degree T23.341
second degree T23.249
third degree T23.349
right T23.011
first degree T23.111
second degree T23.211
third degree T23.311
second degree T23.219
third degree T23.319
toe T25.039
first degree T25.139
left T25.032
first degree T25.132
second degree T25.232
third degree T25.332
right T25.031
first degree T25.131
second degree T25.231
third degree T25.331
second degree T25.239
third degree T25.339

◀ New ◀▥ Revised ~~deleted~~ Deleted

Burn (Continued)
  tongue T28.0
  tonsil (s) T28.0
  trachea T27.0
    with lung T27.1
  trunk T21.00
    abdominal wall —see Burn, abdominal
      wall
    anus —see Burn, buttock
    axilla —see Burn, upper limb
    back —see Burn, back
    breast —see Burn, chest wall
    buttock —see Burn, buttock
    chest wall —see Burn, chest wall
    first degree T21.10
    flank —see Burn, abdominal wall
    genital
      female —see Burn, genital organs,
        external, female
      male —see Burn, genital organs, external,
        male
    groin —see Burn, abdominal wall
    interscapular region —see Burn, back,
      upper
    labia —see Burn, genital organs, external,
      female
    lower back —see Burn, back
    penis —see Burn, genital organs, external,
      male
    perineum
      female —see Burn, genital organs,
        external, female
      male —see Burn, genital organs, external,
        male
    scapula region —see Burn, scapular
      region
    scrotum —see Burn, genital organs,
      external, male
    second degree T21.20
    specified site NEC T21.09
      first degree T21.19
      second degree T21.29
      third degree T21.39
    testes —see Burn, genital organs, external,
      male
    third degree T21.30
    upper back —see Burn, back, upper
    vulva —see Burn, genital organs, external,
      female
  unspecified site with extent of body surface
    involved specified
    less than 10 percent T31.0
    10-19 percent (0-9 percent third degree)
      T31.10
      with 10-19 percent third degree T31.11
    20-29 percent (0-9 percent third degree)
      T31.20
      with
        10-19 percent third degree T31.21
        20-29 percent third degree T31.22
    30-39 percent (0-9 percent third degree)
      T31.30
      with
        10-19 percent third degree T31.31
        20-29 percent third degree T31.32
        30-39 percent third degree T31.33
    40-49 percent (0-9 percent third degree)
      T31.40
      with
        10-19 percent third degree T31.41
        20-29 percent third degree T31.42
        30-39 percent third degree T31.43
        40-49 percent third degree T31.44
    50-59 percent (0-9 percent third degree)
      T31.50
      with
        10-19 percent third degree T31.51
        20-29 percent third degree T31.52
        30-39 percent third degree T31.53
        40-49 percent third degree T31.54
        50-59 percent third degree T31.55

Burn (Continued)
  unspecified site with extent of body surface
    involved specified (Continued)
    60-69 percent (0-9 percent third degree)
      T31.60
      with
        10-19 percent third degree T31.61
        20-29 percent third degree T31.62
        30-39 percent third degree T31.63
        40-49 percent third degree T31.64
        50-59 percent third degree T31.65
        60-69 percent third degree T31.66
    70-79 percent (0-9 percent third degree)
      T31.70
      with
        10-19 percent third degree T31.71
        20-29 percent third degree T31.72
        30-39 percent third degree T31.73
        40-49 percent third degree T31.74
        50-59 percent third degree T31.75
        60-69 percent third degree T31.76
        70-79 percent third degree T31.77
    80-89 percent (0-9 percent third degree)
      T31.80
      with
        10-19 percent third degree T31.81
        20-29 percent third degree T31.82
        30-39 percent third degree T31.83
        40-49 percent third degree T31.84
        50-59 percent third degree T31.85
        60-69 percent third degree T31.86
        70-79 percent third degree T31.87
        80-89 percent third degree T31.88
    90 percent or more (0-9 percent third
      degree) T31.90
      with
        10-19 percent third degree T31.91
        20-29 percent third degree T31.92
        30-39 percent third degree T31.93
        40-49 percent third degree T31.94
        50-59 percent third degree T31.95
        60-69 percent third degree T31.96
        70-79 percent third degree T31.97
        80-89 percent third degree T31.98
        90-99 percent third degree T31.99
  upper limb T22.00
    above elbow —see Burn, above elbow
    axilla —see Burn, axilla
    elbow —see Burn, elbow
    first degree T22.10
    forearm —see Burn, forearm
    hand —see Burn, hand
    interscapular region —see Burn, back,
      upper
    multiple sites T22.099
      first degree T22.199
      left T22.092
        first degree T22.192
        second degree T22.292
        third degree T22.392
      right T22.091
        first degree T22.191
        second degree T22.291
        third degree T22.391
      second degree T22.299
      third degree T22.399
    scapular region —see Burn, scapular region
    second degree T22.20
    shoulder —see Burn, shoulder
    third degree T22.30
    wrist —see Burn, wrist
  uterus T28.3
  vagina T28.3
  vulva —see Burn, genital organs, external,
    female
  wrist T23.079
    first degree T23.179
    left T23.072
      first degree T23.172
      second degree T23.272
      third degree T23.372

Burn (Continued)
  wrist (Continued)
    multiple sites with hand T23.099
      first degree T23.199
      left T23.092
        first degree T23.192
        second degree T23.292
        third degree T23.392
      right T23.091
        first degree T23.191
        second degree T23.291
        third degree T23.391
      second degree T23.299
      third degree T23.399
    right T23.071
      first degree T23.171
      second degree T23.271
      third degree T23.371
    second degree T23.279
    third degree T23.379
Burnett's syndrome E83.52
Burning
  feet syndrome E53.9
  sensation R20.8
  tongue K14.6
Burn-out (state) Z73.0
Burns' disease or osteochondrosis —see
  Osteochondrosis, juvenile, ulna
Bursa —see condition
Bursitis M71.9
  Achilles —see Tendinitis, Achilles
  adhesive —see Bursitis, specified NEC
  ankle —see Enthesopathy, lower limb, ankle,
    specified type NEC
  calcaneal —see Enthesopathy, foot, specified
    type NEC
  collateral ligament, tibial —see Bursitis, tibial
    collateral
  due to use, overuse, pressure —see also
    Disorder, soft tissue, due to use,
    specified type NEC
  specified NEC —see Disorder, soft tissue,
    due to use, specified NEC
  Duplay's M75.0
  elbow NEC M70.3-
    olecranon M70.2-
  finger —see Disorder, soft tissue, due to use,
    specified type NEC, hand
  foot —see Enthesopathy, foot, specified type
    NEC
  gonococcal A54.49
  gouty —see Gout, idiopathic
  hand M70.1-
  hip NEC M70.7-
    trochanteric M70.6-
  infective NEC M71.10
    abscess —see Abscess, bursa
    ankle M71.17-
    elbow M71.12-
    foot M71.17-
    hand M71.14-
    hip M71.15-
    knee M71.16-
    multiple sites M71.19
    shoulder M71.11-
    specified site NEC M71.18
    wrist M71.13-
  ischial —see Bursitis, hip
  knee NEC M70.5-
    prepatellar M70.4-
  occupational NEC —see also Disorder, soft
    tissue, due to, use
  olecranon —see Bursitis, elbow, olecranon
  pharyngeal J39.1
  popliteal —see Bursitis, knee
  prepatellar M70.4-
  radiohumeral M77.8
  rheumatoid M06.20
    ankle M06.27-
    elbow M06.22-
    foot joint M06.27-

Bursitis *(Continued)*
  rheumatoid *(Continued)*
    hand joint M06.24-
    hip M06.25-
    knee M06.26-
    multiple site M06.29
    shoulder M06.21-
    vertebra M06.28
    wrist M06.23-
  scapulohumeral —*see* Bursitis, shoulder
  semimembranous muscle (knee) —*see*
    Bursitis, knee
  shoulder M75.5-
    adhesive —*see* Capsulitis, adhesive
  specified NEC M71.50
    ankle M71.57-
    due to use, overuse or pressure —*see*
      Disorder, soft tissue, due to, use
    elbow M71.52-
    foot M71.57-
    hand M71.54-
    hip M71.55-
    knee M71.56-
    shoulder —*see* Bursitis, shoulder
    specified site NEC M71.58

Bursitis *(Continued)*
  specified NEC *(Continued)*
    tibial collateral M76.4-
    wrist M71.53-
  subacromial —*see* Bursitis, shoulder
  subcoracoid —*see* Bursitis, shoulder
  subdeltoid —*see* Bursitis, shoulder
  syphilitic A52.78
  Thornwaldt, Tornwaldt J39.2
  tibial collateral —*see* Bursitis, tibial collateral
  toe —*see* Enthesopathy, foot, specified type
    NEC
  trochanteric (area) —*see* Bursitis, hip,
    trochanteric
  wrist —*see* Bursitis, hand
Bursopathy M71.9
  specified type NEC M71.80
    ankle M71.87-
    elbow M71.82-
    foot M71.87-
    hand M71.84-
    hip M71.85-
    knee M71.86-
    multiple sites M71.89
    shoulder M71.81-

Bursopathy *(Continued)*
  specified type NEC *(Continued)*
    specified site NEC M71.88
    wrist M71.83-
Burst stitches or sutures (complication of
  surgery) T81.31
  external operation wound T81.31
  internal operation wound T81.32
Buruli ulcer A31.1
Bury's disease L95.1
Buschke's
  disease B45.3
  scleredema —*see* Sclerosis, systemic
Busse-Buschke disease B45.3
Buttock —*see* condition
Button
  Biskra B55.1
  Delhi B55.1
  oriental B55.1
Buttonhole deformity (finger) —*see* Deformity,
  finger, boutonniere
Bwamba fever A92.8
Byssinosis J66.0
Bywaters' syndrome T79.5

C

Cachexia R64
  cancerous R64
  cardiac —see Disease, heart
  dehydration E86.0
    with
      hypernatremia E87.0
      hyponatremia E87.1
  due to malnutrition R64
  exophthalmic —see Hyperthyroidism
  heart —see Disease, heart
  hypophyseal E23.0
  hypopituitary E23.0
  lead —see Poisoning, lead
  malignant R64
  marsh —see Malaria
  nervous F48.8
  old age R54
  paludal —see Malaria
  pituitary E23.0
  renal N28.9
  saturnine —see Poisoning, lead
  senile R54
  Simmonds' E23.0
  splenica D73.0
  strumipriva E03.4
  tuberculous NEC —see Tuberculosis
Café au lait spots L81.3
Caffey's syndrome Q78.8
Caisson disease T70.3
Cake kidney Q63.1
Caked breast (puerperal, postpartum)
    O92.79
Calabar swelling B74.3
Calcaneal spur —see Spur, bone, calcaneal
Calcaneo-apophysitis M92.8
Calcareous —see condition
Calcicosis J62.8
Calciferol (vitamin D) deficiency E55.9
  with rickets E55.0
Calcification
  adrenal (capsule) (gland) E27.49
    tuberculous E35 [B90.8]
  aorta I70.0
  artery (annular) —see Arteriosclerosis
  auricle (ear) —see Disorder, pinna, specified
    type NEC
  basal ganglia G23.8
  bladder N32.89
    due to Schistosoma hematobium B65.0
  brain (cortex) —see Calcification, cerebral
  bronchus J98.09
  bursa M71.40
    ankle M71.47-
    elbow M71.42-
    foot M71.47-
    hand M71.44-
    hip M71.45-
    knee M71.46-
    multiple sites M71.49
    shoulder M75.3-
    specified site NEC M71.48
    wrist M71.43-
  cardiac —see Degeneration, myocardial
  cerebral (cortex) G93.89
    artery I67.2
  cervix (uteri) N88.8
  choroid plexus G93.89
  conjunctiva —see Concretion, conjunctiva
  corpora cavernosa (penis) N48.89
  cortex (brain) —see Calcification, cerebral
  dental pulp (nodular) K04.2
  dentinal papilla K00.4
  falx cerebri G96.19
  gallbladder K82.8
  general E83.59
  heart —see also Degeneration, myocardial
    valve —see Endocarditis
  idiopathic infantile arterial (IIAC) Q28.8

Calcification (Continued)
  intervertebral cartilage or disc
    (postinfective) —see Disorder, disc,
    specified NEC
  intracranial —see Calcification, cerebral
  joint —see Disorder, joint, specified type
    NEC
  kidney N28.89
    tuberculous N29 [B90.1]
  larynx (senile) J38.7
  lens —see Cataract, specified NEC
  lung (active) (postinfectional) J98.4
    tuberculous B90.9
  lymph gland or node (postinfectional) I89.8
    tuberculous (see also Tuberculosis, lymph
      gland) B90.8
  mammographic R92.1
  massive (paraplegic) —see Myositis,
    ossificans, in, quadriplegia
  medial —see Arteriosclerosis, extremities
  meninges (cerebral) (spinal) G96.19
  metastatic E83.59
  Mönckeberg's —see Arteriosclerosis,
    extremities
  muscle M61.9
    due to burns —see Myositis, ossificans, in,
      burns
    paralytic —see Myositis, ossificans, in,
      quadriplegia
    specified type NEC M61.40
      ankle M61.47-
      foot M61.47-
      forearm M61.43-
      hand M61.44-
      lower leg M61.46-
      multiple sites M61.49
      pelvic region M61.45-
      shoulder region M61.41-
      specified site NEC M61.48
      thigh M61.45-
      upper arm M61.42-
  myocardium, myocardial —see Degeneration,
    myocardial
  ovary N83.8
  pancreas K86.8
  penis N48.89
  periarticular —see Disorder, joint, specified
    type NEC
  pericardium (see also Pericarditis) I31.1
  pineal gland E34.8
  pleura J94.8
    postinfectional J94.8
    tuberculous NEC B90.9
  pulpal (dental) (nodular) K04.2
  sclera H15.89
  spleen D73.89
  subcutaneous L94.2
  suprarenal (capsule) (gland) E27.49
  tendon (sheath) —see also Tenosynovitis,
    specified type NEC
    with bursitis, synovitis or tenosynovitis —
      see Tendinitis, calcific
  trachea J39.8
  ureter N28.89
  vitreous —see Deposit, crystalline
Calcified —see Calcification
Calcinosis (interstitial) (tumoral) (universalis)
    E83.59
  with Raynaud's phenomenon, esophageal
    dysfunction, sclerodactyly,
    telangiectasia (CREST syndrome)
    M34.1
  circumscripta (skin) L94.2
  cutis L94.2
Calciphylaxis (see also Calcification, by site)
    E83.59
Calcium
  deposits —see Calcification, by site
  metabolism disorder E83.50
  salts or soaps in vitreous —see Deposit,
    crystalline

Calciuria R82.99
Calculi —see Calculus
Calculosis, intrahepatic —see Calculus, bile
    duct
Calculus, calculi, calculous
  ampulla of Vater —see Calculus, bile duct
  anuria (impacted) (recurrent) (see also
    Calculus, urinary) N20.9
  appendix K38.1
  bile duct (common) (hepatic) K80.50
    with
      calculus of gallbladder —see Calculus,
        gallbladder and bile duct
      cholangitis K80.30
        with
          cholecystitis —see Calculus, bile
            duct, with cholecystitis
          obstruction K80.31
        acute K80.32
          with
            chronic cholangitis K80.36
              with obstruction K80.37
            obstruction K80.33
        chronic K80.34
          with
            acute cholangitis K80.36
              with obstruction K80.37
            obstruction K80.35
      cholecystitis (with cholangitis) K80.40
        with obstruction K80.41
        acute K80.42
          with
            chronic cholecystitis K80.46
              with obstruction K80.47
            obstruction K80.43
        chronic K80.44
          with
            acute cholecystitis K80.46
              with obstruction K80.47
            obstruction K80.45
      obstruction K80.51
  biliary —see also Calculus, gallbladder
    specified NEC K80.80
      with obstruction K80.81
  bilirubin, multiple —see Calculus,
    gallbladder
  bladder (encysted) (impacted) (urinary)
    (diverticulum) N21.0
  bronchus J98.09
  calyx (kidney) (renal) —see Calculus, kidney
  cholesterol (pure) (solitary) —see Calculus,
    gallbladder
  common duct (bile) —see Calculus, bile duct
  conjunctiva —see Concretion, conjunctiva
  cystic N21.0
    duct —see Calculus, gallbladder
  dental (subgingival) (supragingival)
    K03.6
  diverticulum
    bladder N21.0
    kidney N20.0
  epididymis N50.8
  gallbladder K80.20
    with
      bile duct calculus —see Calculus,
        gallbladder and bile duct
      cholecystitis K80.10
        with obstruction K80.11
        acute K80.00
          with
            chronic cholecystitis K80.12
              with obstruction K80.13
            obstruction K80.01
        chronic K80.10
          with
            acute cholecystitis K80.12
              with obstruction K80.13
            obstruction K80.11
      specified NEC K80.18
        with obstruction K80.19
      obstruction K80.21

Calculus, calculi, calculous (Continued)
  gallbladder and bile duct K80.70
    with
      cholecystitis K80.60
        with obstruction K80.61
        acute K80.62
          with
            chronic cholecystitis K80.66
              with obstruction K80.67
              obstruction K80.63
        chronic K80.64
          with
            acute cholecystitis K80.66
              with obstruction K80.67
              obstruction K80.65
      obstruction K80.71
  hepatic (duct) —see Calculus, bile duct
  hepatobiliary K80.80
    with obstruction K80.81
  ileal conduit N21.8
  intestinal (impaction) (obstruction) K56.49
  kidney (impacted) (multiple) (pelvis)
    (recurrent) (staghorn) N20.0
    with calculus, ureter N20.2
    congenital Q63.8
  lacrimal passages —see Dacryolith
  liver (impacted) —see Calculus, bile duct
  lung J98.4
  mammographic R92.1
  nephritic (impacted) (recurrent) —see
    Calculus, kidney
  nose J34.89
  pancreas (duct) K86.8
  parotid duct or gland K11.5
  pelvis, encysted —see Calculus, kidney
  prostate N42.0
  pulmonary J98.4
  pyelitis (impacted) (recurrent) N20.0
    with hydronephrosis N13.2
  pyelonephritis (impacted) (recurrent) —see
    category N20
    with hydronephrosis N13.2
  renal (impacted) (recurrent) —see Calculus,
    kidney
  salivary (duct) (gland) K11.5
  seminal vesicle N50.8
  staghorn —see Calculus, kidney
  Stensen's duct K11.5
  stomach K31.89
  sublingual duct or gland K11.5
    congenital Q38.4
  submandibular duct, gland or region K11.5
  submaxillary duct, gland or region K11.5
  suburethral N21.8
  tonsil J35.8
  tooth, teeth (subgingival) (supragingival)
    K03.6
  tunica vaginalis N50.8
  ureter (impacted) (recurrent) N20.1
    with calculus, kidney N20.2
      with hydronephrosis N13.2
        with infection N13.6
  urethra (impacted) N21.1
  urinary (duct) (impacted) (passage) (tract)
    N20.9
    with hydronephrosis N13.2
      with infection N13.6
    in (due to)
    lower N21.9
      specified NEC N21.8
  vagina N89.8
  vesical (impacted) N21.0
  Wharton's duct K11.5
  xanthine E79.8 [N22]
Calicectasis N28.89
Caliectasis N28.89
California
  disease B38.9
  encephalitis A83.5
Caligo cornea —see Opacity, cornea, central
Callositas, callosity (infected) L84

Callus (infected) L84
  bone —see Osteophyte
    excessive, following fracture - code as
      Sequelae of fracture
Calorie deficiency or malnutrition (see also
  Malnutrition) E46
Calvé-Perthes disease —see Legg-Calve-Perthes
  disease
Calvé's disease —see Osteochondrosis, juvenile,
  spine
Calvities —see Alopecia, androgenic
Cameroon fever —see Malaria
Camptocormia (hysterical) F44.4
Camurati-Engelmann syndrome Q78.3
Canal —see also condition
  atrioventricular common Q21.2
Canaliculitis (lacrimal) (acute) (subacute)
  H04.33-
  Actinomyces A42.89
  chronic H04.42-
Canavan's disease E75.29
Canceled procedure (surgical) Z53.9
  because of
    contraindication Z53.09
      smoking Z53.01
    left against medical advice (AMA) Z53.21
    patient's decision Z53.20
      for reasons of belief or group pressure
        Z53.1
      specified reason NEC Z53.29
    specified reason NEC Z53.8
Cancer —see also Neoplasm, by site, malignant
  bile duct type, liver C22.1
  blood —see Leukemia
  breast (see also Neoplasm, breast, malignant)
    C50.91-
  hepatocellular C22.0
  lung (see also Neoplasm, lung, malignant)
    C34.90-
  ovarian (see also Neoplasm, ovary, malignant)
    C56.9-
  unspecified site (primary) C80.1
Cancer (o)**phobia** F45.29
Cancerous —see Neoplasm, malignant, by site
Cancrum oris A69.0
Candidiasis, candidal B37.9
  balanitis B37.42
  bronchitis B37.1
  cheilitis B37.83
  congenital P37.5
  cystitis B37.41
  disseminated B37.7
  endocarditis B37.6
  enteritis B37.82
  esophagitis B37.81
  intertrigo B37.2
  lung B37.1
  meningitis B37.5
  mouth B37.0
  nails B37.2
  neonatal P37.5
  onychia B37.2
  oral B37.0
  osteomyelitis B37.89
  otitis externa B37.84
  paronychia B37.2
  perionyxis B37.2
  pneumonia B37.1
  proctitis B37.82
  pulmonary B37.1
  pyelonephritis B37.49
  sepsis B37.7
  skin B37.2
  specified site NEC B37.89
  stomatitis B37.0
  systemic B37.7
  urethritis B37.41
  urogenital site NEC B37.49
  vagina B37.3
  vulva B37.3
  vulvovaginitis B37.3

Candidid L30.2
Candidosis —see Candidiasis
Candiru infection or infestation B88.8
Canities (premature) L67.1
  congenital Q84.2
Canker (mouth) (sore) K12.0
  rash A38.9
Cannabinosis J66.2
Canton fever A75.9
Cantrell's syndrome Q87.89
Capillariasis (intestinal) B81.1
  hepatic B83.8
Capillary —see condition
Caplan's syndrome —see Rheumatoid, lung
Capsule —see condition
Capsulitis (joint) —see also Enthesopathy
  adhesive (shoulder) M75.0-
  hepatic K65.8
  labyrinthine —see Otosclerosis, specified NEC
  thyroid E06.9
Caput
  crepitus Q75.8
  medusae I86.8
  succedaneum P12.81
Car sickness T75.3
Carapata (disease) A68.0
Carate —see Pinta
Carbon lung J60
Carbuncle L02.93
  abdominal wall L02.231
  anus K61.0
  auditory canal, external —see Abscess, ear,
    external
  auricle ear —see Abscess, ear, external
  axilla L02.43-
  back (any part) L02.232
  breast N61
  buttock L02.33
  cheek (external) L02.03
  chest wall L02.233
  chin L02.03
  corpus cavernosum N48.21
  ear (any part) (external) (middle) —see
    Abscess, ear, external
  external auditory canal —see Abscess, ear,
    external
  eyelid —see Abscess, eyelid
  face NEC L02.03
  femoral (region) —see Carbuncle, lower limb
  finger —see Carbuncle, hand
  flank L02.231
  foot L02.63-
  forehead L02.03
  genital —see Abscess, genital
  gluteal (region) L02.33
  groin L02.234
  hand L02.53-
  head NEC L02.831
  heel —see Carbuncle, foot
  hip —see Carbuncle, lower limb
  kidney —see Abscess, kidney
  knee —see Carbuncle, lower limb
  labium (majus) (minus) N76.4
  lacrimal
    gland —see Dacryoadenitis
    passages (duct) (sac) —see Inflammation,
      lacrimal, passages, acute
  leg —see Carbuncle, lower limb
  lower limb L02.43-
  malignant A22.0
  navel L02.236
  neck L02.13
  nose (external) (septum) J34.0
  orbit, orbital —see Abscess, orbit
  palmar (space) —see Carbuncle, hand
  partes posteriores L02.33
  pectoral region L02.233
  penis N48.21
  perineum L02.235
  pinna —see Abscess, ear, external
  popliteal —see Carbuncle, lower limb

Carbuncle (Continued)
  scalp L02.831
  seminal vesicle N49.0
  shoulder —see Carbuncle, upper limb
  specified site NEC L02.838
  temple (region) L02.03
  thumb —see Carbuncle, hand
  toe —see Carbuncle, foot
  trunk L02.239
    abdominal wall L02.231
    back L02.232
    chest wall L02.233
    groin L02.234
    perineum L02.235
    umbilicus L02.236
  umbilicus L02.236
  upper limb L02.43-
  urethra N34.0
  vulva N76.4
Carbunculus —see Carbuncle
Carcinoid (tumor) —see Tumor, carcinoid
Carcinoidosis E34.0
Carcinoma (malignant) —see also Neoplasm, by
    site, malignant
  acidophil
    specified site —see Neoplasm, malignant,
      by site
    unspecified site C75.1
  acidophil-basophil, mixed
    specified site —see Neoplasm, malignant,
      by site
    unspecified site C75.1
  adnexal (skin) —see Neoplasm, skin,
    malignant
  adrenal cortical C74.0-
  alveolar —see Neoplasm, lung, malignant
    cell —see Neoplasm, lung, malignant
  ameloblastic C41.1
    upper jaw (bone) C41.0
  apocrine
    breast —see Neoplasm, breast, malignant
    specified site NEC —see Neoplasm, skin,
      malignant
    unspecified site C44.99
  basal cell (pigmented) (see also Neoplasm,
    skin, malignant) C44.91
    fibro-epithelial —see Neoplasm, skin,
      malignant
    morphea —see Neoplasm, skin, malignant
    multicentric —see Neoplasm, skin,
      malignant
  basaloid
  basal-squamous cell, mixed —see Neoplasm,
    skin, malignant
  basophil
    specified site —see Neoplasm, malignant,
      by site
    unspecified site C75.1
  basophil-acidophil, mixed
    specified site —see Neoplasm, malignant,
      by site
    unspecified site C75.1
  basosquamous —see Neoplasm, skin,
    malignant
  bile duct
    with hepatocellular, mixed C22.0
    liver C22.1
    specified site NEC —see Neoplasm,
      malignant, by site
    unspecified site C22.1
  branchial or branchiogenic C10.4
  bronchial or bronchogenic —see Neoplasm,
    lung, malignant
  bronchiolar —see Neoplasm, lung, malignant
  bronchioloalveolar —see Neoplasm, lung,
    malignant
  C cell
    specified site —see Neoplasm, malignant,
      by site
    unspecified site C73
  ceruminous C44.29-

Carcinoma (Continued)
  cervix uteri
    in situ D06.9
      endocervix D06.0
      exocervix D06.1
      specified site NEC D06.7
  chorionic
    specified site —see Neoplasm, malignant,
      by site
    unspecified site
      female C58
      male C62.90
  chromophobe
    specified site —see Neoplasm, malignant,
      by site
    unspecified site C75.1
  cloacogenic
    specified site —see Neoplasm, malignant,
      by site
    unspecified site C21.2
  diffuse type
    specified site —see Neoplasm, malignant,
      by site
    unspecified site C16.9
  duct (cell)
    with Paget's disease —see Neoplasm,
      breast, malignant
    infiltrating
      with lobular carcinoma (in situ)
        specified site —see Neoplasm,
          malignant, by site
        unspecified site (female) C50.91-
          male C50.92-
      specified site —see Neoplasm,
        malignant, by site
      unspecified site (female) C50.91-
        male C50.92-
  ductal
    with lobular
      specified site —see Neoplasm,
        malignant, by site
      unspecified site (female) C50.91-
        male C50.92-
  ductular, infiltrating
    specified site —see Neoplasm, malignant,
      by site
    unspecified site (female) C50.91-
      male C50.92-
  embryonal
    liver C22.7
  endometrioid
    specified site —see Neoplasm, malignant,
      by site
    unspecified site
      female C56.9
      male C61
  eosinophil
    specified site —see Neoplasm, malignant,
      by site
    unspecified site C75.1
  epidermoid —see also Neoplasm, skin
      malignant
    in situ, Bowen's type —see Neoplasm, skin,
      in situ
  fibroepithelial, basal cell —see Neoplasm,
    skin, malignant
  follicular
    with papillary (mixed) C73
    moderately differentiated C73
    pure follicle C73
    specified site —see Neoplasm, malignant,
      by site
    trabecular C73
    unspecified site C73
    well differentiated C73
  generalized, with unspecified primary site
    C80.0
  glycogen-rich —see Neoplasm, breast,
    malignant
  granulosa cell C56-
  hepatic cell C22.0

Carcinoma (Continued)
  hepatocellular C22.0
    with bile duct, mixed C22.0
    fibrolamellar C22.0
  hepatocholangiolitic C22.0
  Hurthle cell C73
  in
    adenomatous
      polyposis coli C18.9
    pleomorphic adenoma —see Neoplasm,
      salivary glands, malignant
    situ —see Carcinoma-in-situ
  infiltrating
    duct
      with lobular
        specified site —see Neoplasm,
          malignant, by site
        unspecified site (female) C50.91-
          male C50.92-
      with Paget's disease —see Neoplasm,
        breast, malignant
      specified site —see Neoplasm,
        malignant
      unspecified site (female) C50.91-
        male C50.92-
    ductular
      specified site —see Neoplasm,
        malignant
      unspecified site (female) C50.91-
        male C50.92-
    lobular
      specified site —see Neoplasm,
        malignant
      unspecified site (female) C50.91-
        male C50.92-
  inflammatory
    specified site —see Neoplasm, malignant
    unspecified site (female) C50.91-
      male C50.92-
  intestinal type
    specified site —see Neoplasm, malignant,
      by site
    unspecified site C16.9
  intracystic
    noninfiltrating —see Neoplasm, in situ,
      by site
  intraductal (noninfiltrating)
    with Paget's disease —see Neoplasm,
      breast, malignant
    breast D05.1-
    papillary
      with invasion
        specified site —see Neoplasm,
          malignant, by site
        unspecified site (female) C50.91-
          male C50.92-
      breast D05.1-
      specified site NEC —see Neoplasm,
        in situ, by site
      unspecified site (female) D05.1-
    specified site NEC —see Neoplasm,
      in situ, by site
    unspecified site (female) D05.1-
  intraepidermal —see Neoplasm, in situ
    squamous cell, Bowen's type —see
      Neoplasm, skin, in situ
  intraepithelial —see Neoplasm, in situ,
      by site
    squamous cell —see Neoplasm, in situ,
      by site
  intraosseous C41.1
    upper jaw (bone) C41.0
  islet cell
    with exocrine, mixed
      specified site —see Neoplasm,
        malignant, by site
      unspecified site C25.9
    pancreas C25.4
    specified site NEC —see Neoplasm,
      malignant, by site
    unspecified site C25.4

Carcinoma (Continued)
  juvenile, breast —see Neoplasm, breast,
    malignant
  large cell
    small cell
      specified site —see Neoplasm,
        malignant, by site
      unspecified site C34.90
  Leydig cell (testis)
    specified site —see Neoplasm, malignant,
      by site
    unspecified site
      female C56.9
      male C62.90
  lipid-rich (female) C50.91-
    male C50.92-
  liver cell C22.0
  liver NEC C22.7
  lobular (infiltrating)
    with intraductal
      specified site —see Neoplasm,
        malignant, by site
      unspecified site (female) C50.91-
        male C50.92-
    noninfiltrating
      breast D05.0-
      specified site NEC —see Neoplasm, in
        situ, by site
      unspecified site D05.0-
    specified site —see Neoplasm, malignant,
      by site
    unspecified site (female) C50.91-
      male C50.92-
  medullary
    with
      amyloid stroma
        specified site —see Neoplasm,
          malignant, by site
        unspecified site C73
      lymphoid stroma
        specified site —see Neoplasm,
          malignant, by site
        unspecified site (female) C50.91-
          male C50.92-
  Merkel cell C4A.9
    anal margin C4A.51
    anal skin C4A.51
    canthus C4A.1-
    ear and external auricular canal C4A.2-
    external auricular canal C4A.2-
    eyelid, including canthus C4A.1-
    face C4A.30
      specified NEC C4A.39
    hip C4A.7-
    lip C4A.0
    lower limb, including hip C4A.7-
    neck C4A.4
    nodal presentation C7B.1
    nose C4A.31
    overlapping sites C4A.8
    perianal skin C4A.51
    scalp C4A.4
    secondary C7B.1
    shoulder C4A.6-
    skin of breast C4A.52
    trunk NEC C4A.59
    upper limb, including shoulder C4A.6-
    visceral metastatic C7B.1
  metastatic —see Neoplasm, secondary
  metatypical —see Neoplasm, skin, malignant
  morphea, basal cell —see Neoplasm, skin,
    malignant
  mucoid
    cell
      specified site —see Neoplasm,
        malignant, by site
      unspecified site C75.1
  neuroendocrine —see also Tumor,
    neuroendocrine
    high grade, any site C7A.1
    poorly differentiated, any site C7A.1

Carcinoma (Continued)
  nonencapsulated sclerosing C73
  noninfiltrating
    intracystic —see Neoplasm, in situ, by site
    intraductal
      breast D05.1-
      papillary
        breast D05.1-
        specified site NEC —see Neoplasm, in
          situ, by site
        unspecified site D05.1-
      specified site —see Neoplasm, in situ,
        by site
      unspecified site D05.1-
    lobular
      breast D05.0-
      specified site NEC —see Neoplasm, in
        situ, by site
      unspecified site (female) D05.0-
  oat cell
    specified site —see Neoplasm, malignant,
      by site
    unspecified site C34.90
  odontogenic C41.1
    upper jaw (bone) C41.0
  papillary
    with follicular (mixed) C73
    follicular variant C73
    intraductal (noninfiltrating)
      with invasion
        specified site —see Neoplasm,
          malignant, by site
        unspecified site (female) C50.91-
          male C50.92-
      breast D05.1-
      specified site NEC —see Neoplasm, in
        situ, by site
      unspecified site D05.1-
    serous
      specified site —see Neoplasm,
        malignant, by site
      surface
        specified site —see Neoplasm,
          malignant, by site
        unspecified site C56.9
      unspecified site C56.9
  papillocystic
    specified site —see Neoplasm, malignant,
      by site
    unspecified site C56.9
  parafollicular cell
    specified site —see Neoplasm, malignant,
      by site
    unspecified site C73
  pilomatrix —see Neoplasm, skin, malignant
  pseudomucinous
    specified site —see Neoplasm, malignant,
      by site
    unspecified site C56.9
  renal cell C64-
  Schmincke —see Neoplasm, nasopharynx,
    malignant
  Schneiderian
    specified site —see Neoplasm, malignant,
      by site
    unspecified site C30.0
  sebaceous —see Neoplasm, skin, malignant
  secondary —see also Neoplasm, secondary,
    by site
    Merkel cell C7B.1
  secretory, breast —see Neoplasm, breast,
    malignant
  serous
    papillary
      specified site —see Neoplasm,
        malignant, by site
      unspecified site C56.9
    surface, papillary
      specified site —see Neoplasm,
        malignant, by site
      unspecified site C56.9

Carcinoma (Continued)
  Sertoli cell
    specified site —see Neoplasm, malignant,
      by site
    unspecified site C62.90
      female C56.9
      male C62.90
  skin appendage —see Neoplasm, skin,
    malignant
  small cell
    fusiform cell
      specified site —see Neoplasm,
        malignant, by site
      unspecified site C34.90
    intermediate cell
      specified site —see Neoplasm,
        malignant, by site
      unspecified site C34.90
    large cell
      specified site —see Neoplasm,
        malignant, by site
      unspecified site C34.90
  solid
    with amyloid stroma
      specified site —see Neoplasm,
        malignant, by site
      unspecified site C73
    microinvasive
      specified site —see Neoplasm,
        malignant, by site
      unspecified site C53.9
  sweat gland —see Neoplasm, skin,
    malignant
  theca cell C56.-
  thymic C37
  unspecified site (primary) C80.1
  water-clear cell C75.0
Carcinoma-in-situ —see also Neoplasm, in situ,
  by site
  breast NOS D05.9-
    specified type NEC D05.8-
  epidermoid —see also Neoplasm, in situ, by
    site
    with questionable stromal invasion
      cervix D06.9
      specified site NEC —see Neoplasm, in
        situ, by site
      unspecified site D06.9
    Bowen's type —see Neoplasm, skin,
      in situ
  intraductal
    breast D05.1-
    specified site NEC —see Neoplasm, in situ,
      by site
    unspecified site D05.1-
  lobular
    with
      infiltrating duct
        breast (female) C50.91-
          male C50.92-
        specified site NEC —see Neoplasm,
          malignant
        unspecified site (female) C50.91-
          male C50.92-
      intraductal
        breast D05.8-
        specified site NEC —see Neoplasm, in
          situ, by site
        unspecified site (female) D05.8-
    breast D05.0-
    specified site NEC —see Neoplasm, in situ,
      by site
    unspecified site D05.0-
  squamous cell —see also Neoplasm, in situ,
    by site
    with questionable stromal invasion
      cervix D06.9
      specified site NEC —see Neoplasm, in
        situ, by site
      unspecified site D06.9
Carcinomaphobia F45.29

◀ New   ◀▥ Revised   ~~deleted~~ Deleted

Carcinomatosis C80.0
  peritonei C78.6
  unspecified site (primary) (secondary) C80.0
Carcinosarcoma —see Neoplasm, malignant,
    by site
  embryonal —see Neoplasm, malignant, by
    site
Cardia, cardial —see condition
Cardiac —see also condition
  death, sudden —see Arrest, cardiac
  pacemaker
    in situ Z95.0
    management or adjustment Z45.018
  tamponade I31.4
Cardialgia —see Pain, precordial
Cardiectasis —see Hypertrophy, cardiac
Cardiochalasia K21.9
Cardiomalacia I51.5
Cardiomegalia glycogenica diffusa E74.02 [I43]
Cardiomegaly —see also Hypertrophy, cardiac
  congenital Q24.8
  glycogen E74.02 [I43]
  idiopathic I51.7
Cardiomyoliposis I51.5
Cardiomyopathy (familial) (idiopathic) I42.9
  alcoholic I42.6
  amyloid E85.4 [I43]
  arteriosclerotic —see Disease, heart, ischemic,
    atherosclerotic
  beriberi E51.12
  cobalt-beer I42.6
  congenital I42.4
  congestive I42.0
  constrictive NOS I42.5
  dilated I42.0
  due to
    alcohol I42.6
    beriberi E51.12
    cardiac glycogenosis E74.02 [I43]
    drugs I42.7
    external agents NEC I42.7
    Friedreich's ataxia G11.1
    myotonia atrophica G71.11 [I43]
    progressive muscular dystrophy G71.0
  glycogen storage E74.02 [I43]
  hypertensive —see Hypertension, heart
  hypertrophic (nonobstructive) I42.2
    obstructive I42.1
      congenital Q24.8
  in
    Chagas' disease (chronic) B57.2
      acute B57.0
    sarcoidosis D86.85
  ischemic I25.5
  metabolic E88.9 [I43]
    thyrotoxic E05.90 [I43]
      with thyroid storm E05.91 [I43]
  newborn I42.8
    congenital I42.4
  nutritional E63.9 [I43]
    beriberi E51.12
  obscure of Africa I42.8
  peripartum O90.3
  postpartum O90.3
  restrictive NEC I42.5
  rheumatic I09.0
  secondary I42.9
  stress induced I51.81
  takotsubo I51.81
  thyrotoxic E05.90 [I43]
    with thyroid storm E05.91 [I43]
  toxic NEC I42.7
  tuberculous A18.84
  viral B33.24
Cardionephritis —see Hypertension,
    cardiorenal
Cardionephropathy —see Hypertension,
    cardiorenal
Cardionephrosis —see Hypertension,
    cardiorenal
Cardiopathia nigra I27.0

Cardiopathy (see also Disease, heart) I51.9
  idiopathic I42.9
  mucopolysaccharidosis E76.3 [I52]
Cardiopericarditis —see Pericarditis
Cardiophobia F45.29
Cardiorenal —see condition
Cardiorrhexis —see Infarct, myocardium
Cardiosclerosis —see Disease, heart, ischemic,
    atherosclerotic
Cardiosis —see Disease, heart
Cardiospasm (esophagus) (reflex) (stomach)
    K22.0
  congenital Q39.5
    with megaesophagus Q39.5
Cardiostenosis —see Disease, heart
Cardiosymphysis I31.0
Cardiovascular —see condition
Carditis (acute) (bacterial) (chronic) (subacute)
    I51.89
  meningococcal A39.50
  rheumatic —see Disease, heart, rheumatic
  rheumatoid —see Rheumatoid, carditis
  viral B33.20
Care (of) (for) (following)
  child (routine) Z76.2
  family member (handicapped) (sick)
    creating problem for family Z63.6
    provided away from home for holiday
      relief Z75.5
    unavailable, due to
      absence (person rendering care)
        (sufferer) Z74.2
      inability (any reason) of person
        rendering care Z74.2
  foundling Z76.1
  holiday relief Z75.5
  improper —see Maltreatment
  lack of (at or after birth) (infant) —see
    Maltreatment, child, neglect
  lactating mother Z39.1
  palliative Z51.5
  postpartum
    immediately after delivery Z39.0
    routine follow-up Z39.2
  respite Z75.5
  unavailable, due to
    absence of person rendering care
      Z74.2
    inability (any reason) of person
      rendering care Z74.2
  well-baby Z76.2
Caries
  bone NEC A18.03
  dental K02.9
    arrested (coronal) (root) K02.3
    chewing surface
      limited to enamel K02.51
      penetrating into dentin K02.52
      penetrating into pulp K02.53
    coronal surface
      chewing surface
        limited to enamel K02.51
        penetrating into dentin K02.52
        penetrating into pulp K02.53
      pit and fissure surface
        limited to enamel K02.51
        penetrating into dentin K02.52
        penetrating into pulp K02.53
      smooth surface
        limited to enamel K02.61
        penetrating into dentin K02.62
        penetrating into pulp K02.63
    pit and fissure surface
      limited to enamel K02.51
      penetrating into dentin K02.52
      penetrating into pulp K02.53
    root K02.7
    smooth surface
      limited to enamel K02.61
      penetrating into dentin K02.62
      penetrating into pulp K02.63

Caries (Continued)
  external meatus —see Disorder, ear, external,
    specified type NEC
  hip (tuberculous) A18.02
  initial (tooth)
    chewing surface K02.51
    pit and fissure surface K02.51
    smooth surface K02.61
  knee (tuberculous) A18.02
  labyrinth —see subcategory H83.8
  limb NEC (tuberculous) A18.03
  mastoid process (chronic) —see Mastoiditis,
    chronic
    tuberculous A18.03
  middle ear —see subcategory H74.8
  nose (tuberculous) A18.03
  orbit (tuberculous) A18.03
  ossicles, ear —see Abnormal, ear ossicles
  petrous bone —see Petrositis
  root (dental) (tooth) K02.7
  sacrum (tuberculous) A18.01
  spine, spinal (column) (tuberculous) A18.01
  syphilitic A52.77
    congenital (early) A50.02 [M90.80]
  tooth, teeth —see Caries, dental
  tuberculous A18.03
  vertebra (column) (tuberculous) A18.01
Carious teeth —see Caries, dental
Carneous mole O02.0
Carnitine insufficiency E71.40
Carotid body or sinus syndrome G90.01
Carotidynia G90.01
Carotinemia (dietary) E67.1
Carotinosis (cutis) (skin) E67.1
Carpal tunnel syndrome —see Syndrome,
    carpal tunnel
Carpenter's syndrome Q87.0
Carpopedal spasm —see Tetany
Carr-Barr-Plunkett syndrome Q97.1
Carrier (suspected) of
  amebiasis Z22.1
  bacterial disease NEC Z22.39
    diphtheria Z22.2
    intestinal infectious NEC Z22.1
      typhoid Z22.0
    meningococcal Z22.31
    sexually transmitted Z22.4
    specified NEC Z22.39
    staphylococcal (Methicillin susceptible)
      Z22.321
      Methicillin resistant Z22.322
    streptococcal Z22.338
      group B Z22.330
    typhoid Z22.0
  cholera Z22.1
  diphtheria Z22.2
  gastrointestinal pathogens NEC Z22.1
  genetic Z14.8
    cystic fibrosis Z14.1
    hemophilia A (asymptomatic) Z14.01
      symptomatic Z14.02
  gonorrhea Z22.4
  HAA (hepatitis Australian-antigen) Z22.59
  HB (c)(s)-AG Z22.51
  hepatitis (viral) Z22.50
    Australia-antigen (HAA) Z22.59
    B surface antigen (HBsAg) Z22.51
      with acute delta- (super)infection
        B17.0
    C Z22.52
    specified NEC Z22.59
  human T-cell lymphotropic virus type-1
    (HTLV-1) infection Z22.6
  infectious organism Z22.9
    specified NEC Z22.8
  meningococci Z22.31
  Salmonella typhosa Z22.0
  serum hepatitis —see Carrier, hepatitis
  staphylococci (Methicillin susceptible)
    Z22.321
    Methicillin resistant Z22.322

Carrier of *(Continued)*
  streptococci Z22.338
    group B Z22.330
  syphilis Z22.4
  typhoid Z22.0
  venereal disease NEC Z22.4
Carrion's disease A44.0
Carter's relapsing fever (Asiatic) A68.1
Cartilage —*see* condition
Caruncle (inflamed)
  conjunctiva (acute) —*see* Conjunctivitis, acute
  labium (majus) (minus) N90.89
  lacrimal —*see* Inflammation, lacrimal,
    passages
  myrtiform N89.8
  urethral (benign) N36.2
Cascade stomach K31.2
Caseation lymphatic gland (tuberculous) A18.2
Cassidy (-Scholte) **syndrome** (malignant
  carcinoid) E34.0
Castellani's disease A69.8
Castration, traumatic, male S38.231
Casts in urine R82.99
Cat
  cry syndrome Q93.4
  ear Q17.3
  eye syndrome Q92.8
Catabolism, senile R54
Catalepsy (hysterical) F44.2
  schizophrenic F20.2
Cataplexy (idiopathic) —*see* - Narcolepsy
Cataract (cortical) (immature) (incipient) H26.9
  with
    neovascularization —*see* Cataract,
     complicated
  age-related —*see* Cataract, senile
  anterior
    and posterior axial embryonal Q12.0
    pyramidal Q12.0
  associated with
    galactosemia E74.21 *[H28]*
    myotonic disorders G71.19 *[H28]*
  blue Q12.0
  central Q12.0
  cerulean Q12.0
  complicated H26.20
    with
      neovascularization H26.21-
      ocular disorder H26.22-
      glaucomatous flecks H26.23-
  congenital Q12.0
  coraliform Q12.0
  coronary Q12.0
  crystalline Q12.0
  diabetic —*see* Diabetes, cataract
  drug-induced H26.3-
  due to
    ocular disorder —*see* Cataract, complicated
    radiation H26.8
  electric H26.8
  extraction status Z98.4-
  glass-blower's H26.8
  heat ray H26.8
  heterochromic —*see* Cataract, complicated
  hypermature —*see* Cataract, senile,
    morgagnian type
  in (due to)
    chronic iridocyclitis —*see* Cataract,
     complicated
    diabetes —*see* Diabetes, cataract
    endocrine disease E34.9 *[H28]*
    eye disease —*see* Cataract, complicated
    hypoparathyroidism E20.9 *[H28]*
    malnutrition-dehydration E46 *[H28]*
    metabolic disease E88.9 *[H28]*
    myotonic disorders G71.19 *[H28]*
    nutritional disease E63.9 *[H28]*
  infantile —*see* Cataract, presenile
  irradiational —*see* Cataract, specified NEC
  juvenile —*see* Cataract, presenile
  malnutrition-dehydration E46 *[H28]*

Cataract *(Continued)*
  morgagnian —*see* Cataract, senile,
    morgagnian type
  myotonic G71.19 *[H28]*
  myxedema E03.9 *[H28]*
  nuclear
    embryonal Q12.0
    sclerosis —*see* Cataract, senile, nuclear
  presenile H26.00-
    combined forms H26.06-
    cortical H26.01-
    lamellar —*see* Cataract, presenile, cortical
    nuclear H26.03-
    specified NEC H26.09
    subcapsular polar (anterior) H26.04-
      posterior H26.05-
    zonular —*see* Cataract, presenile, cortical
  secondary H26.40
    Soemmering's ring H26.41-
    specified NEC H26.49-
    to eye disease —*see* Cataract, complicated
  senile H25.9
    brunescens —*see* Cataract, senile, nuclear
    combined forms H25.81-
    coronary —*see* Cataract, senile, incipient
    cortical H25.01-
    hypermature —*see* Cataract, senile,
     morgagnian type
    incipient (mature) (total) H25.09-
     cortical —*see* Cataract, senile, cortical
     subcapsular —*see* Cataract, senile,
      subcapsular
    morgagnian type (hypermature) H25.2-
    nuclear (sclerosis) H25.1-
    polar subcapsular (anterior) (posterior) —
     see Cataract, senile, incipient
    punctate —*see* Cataract, senile, incipient
    specified NEC H25.89
    subcapsular polar (anterior) H25.03-
     posterior H25.04-
  snowflake —*see* Diabetes, cataract
  specified NEC H26.8
  toxic —*see* Cataract, drug-induced
  traumatic H26.10-
    localized H26.11-
    partially resolved H26.12-
    total H26.13-
  zonular (perinuclear) Q12.0
Cataracta —*see also* Cataract
  brunescens —*see* Cataract, senile, nuclear
  centralis pulverulenta Q12.0
  cerulea Q12.0
  complicata —*see* Cataract, complicated
  congenita Q12.0
  coralliformis Q12.0
  coronaria Q12.0
  diabetic —*see* Diabetes, cataract
  membranacea
    accreta —*see* Cataract, secondary
    congenita Q12.0
  nigra —*see* Cataract, senile, nuclear
  sunflower —*see* Cataract, complicated
Catarrh, catarrhal (acute) (febrile) (infectious)
  (inflammation) (*see also* condition) J00
  bronchial —*see* Bronchitis
  chest —*see* Bronchitis
  chronic J31.0
  due to congenital syphilis A50.03
  enteric —*see* Enteritis
  eustachian H68.009
  fauces —*see* Pharyngitis
  gastrointestinal —*see* Enteritis
  gingivitis K05.00
    nonplaque induced K05.01
    plaque induced K05.00
  hay —*see* Fever, hay
  intestinal —*see* Enteritis
  larynx, chronic J37.0
  liver B15.9
    with hepatic coma B15.0
  lung —*see* Bronchitis

Catarrh, catarrhal *(Continued)*
  middle ear, chronic —*see* Otitis, media,
    nonsuppurative, chronic, serous
  mouth K12.1
  nasal (chronic) —*see* Rhinitis
  nasobronchial J31.1
  nasopharyngeal (chronic) J31.1
    acute J00
  pulmonary —*see* Bronchitis
  spring (eye) (vernal) —*see* Conjunctivitis,
    acute, atopic
  summer (hay) —*see* Fever, hay
  throat J31.2
  tubotympanal —*see also* Otitis, media,
    nonsuppurative
    chronic —*see* Otitis, media,
     nonsuppurative, chronic, serous
Catatonia (schizophrenic) F20.2
Catatonic
  disorder due to known physiologic condition
    F06.1
  schizophrenia F20.2
  stupor R40.1
Cat-scratch —*see also* Abrasion
  disease or fever A28.1
Cauda equina —*see* condition
Cauliflower ear M95.1-
Causalgia (upper limb) G56.4-
  lower limb G57.7-
Cause
  external, general effects T75.89
Caustic burn —*see* Corrosion, by site
Cavare's disease (familial periodic paralysis)
  G72.3
Cave-in, injury
  crushing (severe) —*see* Crush
  suffocation —*see* Asphyxia, traumatic, due to
    low oxygen, due to cave-in
Cavernitis (penis) N48.29
Cavernositis N48.29
Cavernous —*see* condition
Cavitation of lung —*see also* Tuberculosis,
  pulmonary
  nontuberculous J98.4
Cavities, dental —*see* Caries, dental
Cavity
  lung —*see* Cavitation of lung
  optic papilla Q14.2
  pulmonary —*see* Cavitation of lung
Cavovarus foot, congenital Q66.1
Cavus foot (congenital) Q66.7
  acquired —*see* Deformity, limb, foot, specified
    NEC
Cazenave's disease L10.2
Cecitis K52.9
  with perforation, peritonitis, or rupture K65.8
Cecum —*see* condition
Celiac
  artery compression syndrome I77.4
  disease K90.0
  infantilism K90.0
Cell (s), **cellular** —*see also* condition
  in urine R82.99
Cellulitis (diffuse) (phlegmonous) (septic)
  (suppurative) L03.90
  abdominal wall L03.311
  anaerobic A48.0
  ankle —*see* Cellulitis, lower limb
  anus K61.0
  arm —*see* Cellulitis, upper limb
  auricle (ear) —*see* Cellulitis, ear
  axilla L03.11-
  back (any part) L03.312
  broad ligament
    acute N73.0
  buttock L03.317
  cervical (meaning neck) L03.221
  cervix (uteri) —*see* Cervicitis
  cheek (external) L03.211
    internal K12.2
  chest wall L03.313

◀ New   ◀◀◀ Revised   ~~deleted~~ Deleted

Cellulitis *(Continued)*
chronic L03.90
clostridial A48.0
corpus cavernosum N48.22
digit
  finger —*see* Cellulitis, finger
  toe —*see* Cellulitis, toe
Douglas' cul-de-sac or pouch
  acute N73.0
drainage site (following operation) T81.4
ear (external) H60.1-
eosinophilic (granulomatous) L98.3
erysipelatous —*see* Erysipelas
external auditory canal —*see* Cellulitis, ear
eyelid —*see* Abscess, eyelid
face NEC L03.211
finger (intrathecal) (periosteal)
  (subcutaneous) (subcuticular) L03.01-
foot —*see* Cellulitis, lower limb
gangrenous —*see* Gangrene
genital organ NEC
  female (external) N76.4
  male N49.9
    multiple sites N49.8
    specified NEC N49.8
gluteal (region) L03.317
gonococcal A54.89
groin L03.314
hand —*see* Cellulitis, upper limb
head NEC L03.811
  face (any part, except ear, eye and nose)
    L03.211
heel —*see* Cellulitis, lower limb
hip —*see* Cellulitis, lower limb
jaw (region) L03.211
knee —*see* Cellulitis, lower limb
labium (majus) (minus) —*see* Vulvitis
lacrimal passages —*see* Inflammation,
  lacrimal, passages
larynx J38.7
leg —*see* Cellulitis, lower limb
lip K13.0
lower limb L03.11-
  toe —*see* Cellulitis, toe
mouth (floor) K12.2
multiple sites, so stated L03.90
nasopharynx J39.1
navel L03.316
  newborn P38.9
    with mild hemorrhage P38.1
    without hemorrhage P38.9
neck (region) L03.221
nose (septum) (external) J34.0
orbit, orbital H05.01-
palate (soft) K12.2
pectoral (region) L03.313
pelvis, pelvic (chronic)
  female (*see also* Disease, pelvis,
    inflammatory) N73.2
    acute N73.0
  following ectopic or molar pregnancy
    O08.0
  male K65.0
penis N48.22
perineal, perineum L03.315
perirectal K61.1
peritonsillar J36
periurethral N34.0
periuterine (*see also* Disease, pelvis,
  inflammatory) N73.2
  acute N73.0
pharynx J39.1
rectum K61.1
retroperitoneal K68.9
round ligament
  acute N73.0
scalp (any part) L03.811
scrotum N49.2
seminal vesicle N49.0
shoulder —*see* Cellulitis, upper limb
specified site NEC L03.818

Cellulitis *(Continued)*
submandibular (region) (space) (triangle)
  K12.2
  gland K11.3
submaxillary (region) K12.2
  gland K11.3
thigh —*see* Cellulitis, lower limb
thumb (intrathecal) (periosteal)
  (subcutaneous) (subcuticular) —*see*
  Cellulitis, finger
toe (intrathecal) (periosteal) (subcutaneous)
  (subcuticular) L03.03-
tonsil J36
trunk L03.319
  abdominal wall L03.311
  back (any part) L03.312
  buttock L03.317
  chest wall L03.313
  groin L03.314
  perineal, perineum L03.315
  umbilicus L03.316
tuberculous (primary) A18.4
umbilicus L03.316
upper limb L03.11-
  axilla —*see* Cellulitis, axilla
  finger —*see* Cellulitis, finger
  thumb —*see* Cellulitis, finger
vaccinal T88.0
vocal cord J38.3
vulva —*see* Vulvitis
wrist —*see* Cellulitis, upper limb
Cementoblastoma, benign —*see* Cyst,
  calcifying odontogenic
Cementoma —*see* Cyst, calcifying odontogenic
Cementoperiostitis —*see* Periodontitis
Cementosis K03.4
Central auditory processing disorder H93.25
Central pain syndrome G89.0
Cephalematocele, cephal (o)hematocele
  newborn P52.8
    birth injury P10.8
  traumatic —*see* Hematoma, brain
Cephalematoma, cephalhematoma (calcified)
  newborn (birth injury) P12.0
  traumatic —*see* Hematoma, brain
Cephalgia, cephalalgia —*see also* Headache
  histamine G44.009
    intractable G44.001
    not intractable G44.009
  trigeminal autonomic (TAC) NEC G44.099
    intractable G44.091
    not intractable G44.099
Cephalic —*see* condition
Cephalitis —*see* Encephalitis
Cephalocele —*see* Encephalocele
Cephalomenia N94.89
Cephalopelvic —*see* condition
Cerclage (with cervical incompetence) **in**
  pregnancy —*see* Incompetence, cervix, in
  pregnancy
Cerebellitis —*see* Encephalitis
Cerebellum, cerebellar —*see* condition
Cerebral —*see* condition
Cerebritis —*see* Encephalitis
Cerebro-hepato-renal syndrome Q87.89
Cerebromalacia —*see* Softening, brain
  sequelae of cerebrovascular disease I69.398
Cerebroside lipidosis E75.22
Cerebrospasticity (congenital) G80.1
Cerebrospinal —*see* condition
Cerebrum —*see* condition
Ceroid-lipofuscinosis, neuronal E75.4
Cerumen (accumulation) (impacted) H61.2-
Cervical —*see also* condition
  auricle Q18.2
  dysplasia in pregnancy —*see* Abnormal,
    cervix, in pregnancy or childbirth
  erosion in pregnancy —*see* Abnormal, cervix,
    in pregnancy or childbirth
  fibrosis in pregnancy —*see* Abnormal, cervix,
    in pregnancy or childbirth

Cervical *(Continued)*
  fusion syndrome Q76.1
  rib Q76.5
  shortening (complicating pregnancy)
    O26.87-
Cervicalgia M54.2
Cervicitis (acute) (chronic) (nonvenereal)
  (senile (atrophic)) (subacute) (with
  ulceration) N72
  with
    abortion —*see* Abortion, by type
      complicated by genital tract and
      pelvic infection
    ectopic pregnancy O08.0
    molar pregnancy O08.0
  chlamydial A56.09
  gonococcal A54.03
  herpesviral A60.03
  puerperal (postpartum) O86.11
  syphilitic A52.76
  trichomonal A59.09
  tuberculous A18.16
Cervicocolpitis (emphysematosa) (*see also*
  Cervicitis) N72
Cervix —*see* condition
Cesarean delivery, previous, affecting
  management of pregnancy O34.21
Céstan (-Chenais) paralysis or syndrome
  G46.3
Céstan-Raymond syndrome I65.8
Cestode infestation B71.9
  specified type NEC B71.8
Cestodiasis B71.9
Chabert's disease A22.9
Chacaleh E53.8
Chafing L30.4
Chagas' (-Mazza) disease (chronic) B57.2
  with
    cardiovascular involvement NEC B57.2
    digestive system involvement B57.30
      megacolon B57.32
      megaesophagus B57.31
      other specified B57.39
    megacolon B57.32
    megaesophagus B57.31
    myocarditis B57.2
    nervous system involvement B57.40
      meningitis B57.41
      meningoencephalitis B57.42
      other specified B57.49
    specified organ involvement NEC B57.5
  acute (with) B57.1
    cardiovascular NEC B57.0
    myocarditis B57.0
Chagres fever B50.9
Chairridden Z74.09
Chalasia (cardiac sphincter) K21.9
Chalazion H00.19
  left H00.16
    lower H00.15
    upper H00.14
  right H00.13
    lower H00.12
    upper H00.11
Chalcosis —*see also* Disorder, globe,
  degenerative, chalcosis
  cornea —*see* Deposit, cornea
  crystalline lens —*see* Cataract, complicated
  retina H35.89
Chalicosis (pulmonum) J62.8
Chancre (any genital site) (hard) (hunterian)
  (mixed) (primary) (seronegative)
  (seropositive) (syphilitic) A51.0
  congenital A50.07
  conjunctiva NEC A51.2
  Ducrey's A57
  extragenital A51.2
  eyelid A51.2
  lip A51.2
  nipple A51.2
  Nisbet's A57

Chancre (Continued)
of
carate A67.0
pinta A67.0
yaws A66.0
palate, soft A51.2
phagedenic A57
simple A57
soft A57
bubo A57
palate A51.2
urethra A51.0
yaws A66.0
Chancroid (anus) (genital) (penis) (perineum) (rectum) (urethra) (vulva) A57
Chandler's disease (osteochondritis dissecans, hip) —see Osteochondritis, dissecans, hip
Change (s) (in) (of) —see also Removal
arteriosclerotic —see Arteriosclerosis
bone —see also Disorder, bone
diabetic —see Diabetes, bone change
bowel habit R19.4
cardiorenal (vascular) —see Hypertension, cardiorenal
cardiovascular —see Disease, cardiovascular
circulatory I99.9
cognitive (mild) (organic) R41.89
color, tooth, teeth
during formation K00.8
posteruptive K03.7
contraceptive device Z30.433
corneal membrane H18.30
Bowman's membrane fold or rupture H18.31-
Descemet's membrane
fold H18.32-
rupture H18.33-
coronary —see Disease, heart, ischemic
degenerative, spine or vertebra —see Spondylosis
dental pulp, regressive K04.2
dressing (nonsurgical) Z48.00
surgical Z48.01
heart —see Disease, heart
hip joint —see Derangement, joint, hip
hyperplastic larynx J38.7
hypertrophic
nasal sinus J34.89
turbinate, nasal J34.3
upper respiratory tract J39.8
indwelling catheter Z46.6
inflammatory —see also Inflammation
sacroiliac M46.1
job, anxiety concerning Z56.1
joint —see Derangement, joint
life —see Menopause
mental status R41.82
minimal (glomerular) (see also N00-N07 with fourth character .0) N05.0
myocardium, myocardial —see Degeneration, myocardial - of life —see Menopause
pacemaker Z45.018
pulse generator Z45.010
personality (enduring) F68.8
due to (secondary to)
general medical condition F07.0
secondary (nonspecific) F60.89
regressive, dental pulp K04.2
renal —see Disease, renal
retina H35.9
myopic H44.2-
sacroiliac joint M53.3
senile (see also condition) R54
sensory R20.8
skin R23.9
acute, due to ultraviolet radiation L56.9
specified NEC L56.8
chronic, due to nonionizing radiation L57.9
specified NEC L57.8
cyanosis R23.0
flushing R23.2

Change (Continued)
skin (Continued)
pallor R23.1
petechiae R23.3
specified change NEC R23.8
swelling —see Mass, localized
texture R23.4
trophic
arm —see Mononeuropathy, upper limb
leg —see Mononeuropathy, lower limb
vascular I99.9
vasomotor I73.9
voice R49.9
psychogenic F44.4
specified NEC R49.8
Changing sleep-work schedule, affecting sleep G47.26
Changuinola fever A93.1
Chapping skin T69.8
Charcot-Marie-Tooth disease, paralysis or syndrome G60.0
Charcot's
arthropathy —see Arthropathy, neuropathic
cirrhosis K74.3
disease (tabetic arthropathy) A52.16
joint (disease) (tabetic) A52.16
diabetic —see Diabetes, with, arthropathy
syringomyelic G95.0
syndrome (intermittent claudication) I73.9
CHARGE association Q89.8
Charley-horse (quadriceps) M62.831
traumatic (quadriceps) S76.11-
Charlouis' disease —see Yaws
Cheadle's disease E54
Checking (of)
cardiac pacemaker (battery) (electrode (s)) Z45.018
pulse generator Z45.010
intrauterine contraceptive device Z30.431
Check-up —see Examination
Chédiak-Higashi (-Steinbrinck) **syndrome** (congenital gigantism of peroxidase granules) E70.330
Cheek —see condition
Cheese itch B88.0
Cheese-washer's lung J67.8
Cheese-worker's lung J67.8
Cheilitis (acute) (angular) (catarrhal) (chronic) (exfoliative) (gangrenous) (glandular) (infectional) (suppurative) (ulcerative) (vesicular) K13.0
actinic (due to sun) L56.8
other than from sun L59.8
candidal B37.83
Cheilodynia K13.0
Cheiloschisis —see Cleft, lip
Cheilosis (angular) K13.0
with pellagra E52
due to
vitamin B2 (riboflavin) deficiency E53.0
Cheiromegaly M79.89
Cheiropompholyx L30.1
Cheloid —see Keloid
Chemical burn —see Corrosion, by site
Chemodectoma —see Paraganglioma, nonchromaffin
Chemosis, conjunctiva —see Edema, conjunctiva
Chemotherapy (session) (for)
cancer Z51.11
neoplasm Z51.11
Cherubism M27.8
Chest —see condition
Cheyne-Stokes breathing (respiration) R06.3
Chiari's
disease or syndrome (hepatic vein thrombosis) I82.0
malformation
type I G93.5
type II —see Spina bifida
net Q24.8

Chicago disease B40.9
Chickenpox —see Varicella
Chiclero ulcer or sore B55.1
Chigger (infestation) B88.0
Chignon (disease) B36.8
newborn (from vacuum extraction) (birth injury) P12.1
Chilaiditi's syndrome (subphrenic displacement, colon) Q43.3
Chilblain (s) (lupus) T69.1
Child
custody dispute Z65.3
Childbirth —see Delivery
Childhood
cerebral X-linked adrenoleukodystrophy E71.520
period of rapid growth Z00.2
Chill (s) R68.83
with fever R50.9
without fever R68.83
congestive in malarial regions B54
Chilomastigiasis A07.8
Chimera 46,XX/46,XY Q99.0
Chin —see condition
Chinese dysentery A03.9
Chionophobia F40.228
Chitral fever A93.1
Chlamydia, chlamydial A74.9
cervicitis A56.09
conjunctivitis A74.0
cystitis A56.01
endometritis A56.11
epididymitis A56.19
female
pelvic inflammatory disease A56.11
pelviperitonitis A56.11
orchitis A56.19
peritonitis A74.81
pharyngitis A56.4
proctitis A56.3
psittaci (infection) A70
salpingitis A56.11
sexually-transmitted infection NEC A56.8
specified NEC A74.89
urethritis A56.01
vulvovaginitis A56.02
Chlamydiosis —see Chlamydia
Chloasma (skin) (idiopathic) (symptomatic) L81.1
eyelid H02.719
hyperthyroid E05.90 [H02.719]
with thyroid storm E05.91 [H02.719]
left H02.716
lower H02.715
upper H02.714
right H02.713
lower H02.712
upper H02.711
Chloroma C92.3-
Chlorosis D50.9
Egyptian B76.9 [D63.8]
miner's B76.9 [D63.8]
Chlorotic anemia D50.8
Chocolate cyst (ovary) N80.1
Choked
disc or disk —see Papilledema
on food, phlegm, or vomitus NOS —see Foreign body, by site
while vomiting NOS —see Foreign body, by site
Chokes (resulting from bends) T70.3
Choking sensation R09.89
Cholangiectasis K83.8
Cholangiocarcinoma
with hepatocellular carcinoma, combined C22.0
liver C22.1
specified site NEC —see Neoplasm, malignant, by site
unspecified site C22.1

◀ New ◀▥▥ Revised ~~deleted~~ Deleted

Cholangiohepatitis K83.8
  due to fluke infestation B66.1
Cholangiohepatoma C22.0
Cholangiolitis (acute) (chronic) (extrahepatic)
    (gangrenous) (intrahepatic) K83.0
  paratyphoidal —see Fever, paratyphoid
  typhoidal A01.09
Cholangioma D13.4
  malignant —see Cholangiocarcinoma
Cholangitis (ascending) (primary) (recurrent)
    (sclerosing) (secondary) (stenosing)
    (suppurative) K83.0
  with calculus, bile duct —see Calculus, bile
    duct, with cholangitis
  chronic nonsuppurative destructive K74.3
Cholecystectasia K82.8
Cholecystitis K81.9
  with
    calculus, stones in
      bile duct (common) (hepatic) —
        see Calculus, bile duct, with
        cholecystitis
      cystic duct —see Calculus, gallbladder,
        with cholecystitis
      gallbladder —see Calculus, gallbladder,
        with cholecystitis
      choledocholithiasis —see Calculus, bile
        duct, with cholecystitis
      cholelithiasis —see Calculus, gallbladder,
        with cholecystitis
  acute (emphysematous) (gangrenous)
    (suppurative) K81.0
    with
      calculus, stones in
        cystic duct —see Calculus,
          gallbladder, with cholecystitis,
          acute
        gallbladder —see Calculus,
          gallbladder, with cholecystitis,
          acute
        choledocholithiasis —see Calculus, bile
          duct, with cholecystitis, acute
        cholelithiasis —see Calculus,
          gallbladder, with cholecystitis,
          acute
      chronic cholecystitis K81.2
        with gallbladder calculus K80.12
          with obstruction K80.13
  chronic K81.1
    with acute cholecystitis K81.2
      with gallbladder calculus K80.12
        with obstruction K80.13
  emphysematous (acute) —see Cholecystitis,
    acute
  gangrenous —see Cholecystitis, acute
  paratyphoidal, current A01.4
  suppurative —see Cholecystitis, acute
  typhoidal A01.09
Cholecystolithiasis —see Calculus, gallbladder
Choledochitis (suppurative) K83.0
Choledocholith —see Calculus, bile duct
Choledocholithiasis (common duct) (hepatic
    duct) —see Calculus, bile duct
  cystic —see Calculus, gallbladder
  typhoidal A01.09
Cholelithiasis (cystic duct) (gallbladder)
    (impacted) (multiple) —see Calculus,
    gallbladder
  bile duct (common) (hepatic) —see Calculus,
    bile duct
  hepatic duct —see Calculus, bile duct
  specified NEC K80.80
    with obstruction K80.81
Cholemia —see also Jaundice
  familial (simple) (congenital) E80.4
  Gilbert's E80.4
Choleperitoneum, choleperitonitis K65.3
Cholera (Asiatic) (epidemic) (malignant)
    A00.9
  antimonial —see Poisoning, antimony
  classical A00.0

Cholera (Continued)
  due to Vibrio cholerae 01 A00.9
    biovar cholerae A00.0
    biovar eltor A00.1
    el tor A00.1
  el tor A00.1
Cholerine —see Cholera
Cholestasis NEC K83.1
  with hepatocyte injury K71.0
  due to total parenteral nutrition (TPN) K76.89
  pure K71.0
Cholesteatoma (ear) (middle) (with reaction)
    H71.9-
  attic H71.0-
  external ear (canal) H60.4-
  mastoid H71.2-
  postmastoidectomy cavity (recurrent) —see
    Complications, postmastoidectomy,
    recurrent cholesteatoma
  recurrent (postmastoidectomy) —see
    Complications, postmastoidectomy,
    recurrent cholesteatoma
  tympanum H71.1-
Cholesteatosis, diffuse H71.3-
Cholesteremia E78.0
Cholesterin in vitreous —see Deposit,
    crystalline
Cholesterol
  deposit
    retina H35.89
    vitreous —see Deposit, crystalline
  elevated (high) E78.0
    with elevated (high) triglycerides E78.2
    screening for Z13.220
  imbibition of gallbladder K82.4
Cholesterolemia (essential) (familial)
    (hereditary) (pure) E78.0
Cholesterolosis, cholesterosis (gallbladder)
    K82.4
  cerebrotendinous E75.5
Cholocolic fistula K82.3
Choluria R82.2
Chondritis M94.8X9
  aurical H61.03-
  costal (Tietze's) M94.0
  external ear H61.03-
  patella, posttraumatic —see Chondromalacia,
    patella
  pinna H61.03-
  purulent M94.8X-
  tuberculous NEC A18.02
    intervertebral A18.01
Chondroblastoma —see also Neoplasm, bone,
    benign
  malignant —see Neoplasm, bone, malignant
Chondrocalcinosis M11.20
  ankle M11.27-
  elbow M11.22-
  familial M11.10
    ankle M11.17-
    elbow M11.12-
    foot joint M11.17-
    hand joint M11.14-
    hip M11.15-
    knee M11.16-
    multiple site M11.19
    shoulder M11.11-
    vertebrae M11.18
    wrist M11.13-
  foot joint M11.27-
  hand joint M11.24-
  hip M11.25-
  knee M11.26-
  multiple site M11.29
  shoulder M11.21-
  specified type NEC M11.20
    ankle M11.27-
    elbow M11.22-
    foot joint M11.27-
    hand joint M11.24-
    hip M11.25-

Chondrocalcinosis (Continued)
  specified type NEC (Continued)
    knee M11.26-
    multiple site M11.29
    shoulder M11.21-
    vertebrae M11.28
    wrist M11.23-
  vertebrae M11.28
  wrist M11.23-
Chondrodermatitis nodularis helicis or
    anthelicis —see Perichondritis, ear
Chondrodysplasia Q78.9
  with hemangioma Q78.4
  calcificans congenita Q77.3
  fetalis Q77.4
  metaphyseal (Jansen's) (McKusick's)
    (Schmid's) Q78.5
  punctata Q77.3
Chondrodystrophy, chondrodystrophia
    (familial) (fetalis) (hypoplastic) Q78.9
  calcificans congenita Q77.3
  myotonic (congenital) G71.13
  punctata Q77.3
Chondroectodermal dysplasia Q77.6
Chondrogenesis imperfecta Q77.4
Chondrolysis M94.35-
Chondroma —see also Neoplasm, cartilage,
    benign
  juxtacortical —see Neoplasm, bone, benign
  periosteal —see Neoplasm, bone, benign
Chondromalacia (systemic) M94.20
  acromioclavicular joint M94.21-
  ankle M94.27-
  elbow M94.22-
  foot joint M94.27-
  glenohumeral joint M94.21-
  hand joint M94.24-
  hip M94.25-
  knee M94.26-
    patella M22.4-
  multiple sites M94.29
  patella M22.4-
  rib M94.28
  sacroiliac joint M94.259
  shoulder M94.21-
  sternoclavicular joint M94.21-
  vertebral joint M94.28
  wrist M94.23-
Chondromatosis —see also Neoplasm, cartilage,
    uncertain behavior
  internal Q78.4
Chondromyxosarcoma —see Neoplasm,
    cartilage, malignant
Chondro-osteodysplasia (Morquio-Brailsford
    type) E76.219
Chondro-osteodystrophy E76.29
Chondro-osteoma —see Neoplasm, bone,
    benign
Chondropathia tuberosa M94.0
Chondrosarcoma —see Neoplasm, cartilage,
    malignant
  juxtacortical —see Neoplasm, bone, malignant
  mesenchymal —see Neoplasm, connective
    tissue, malignant
  myxoid —see Neoplasm, cartilage, malignant
Chordee (nonvenereal) N48.89
  congenital Q54.4
  gonococcal A54.09
Chorditis (fibrinous) (nodosa) (tuberosa) J38.2
Chordoma —see Neoplasm, vertebral (column),
    malignant
Chorea (chronic) (gravis) (posthemiplegic)
    (senile) (spasmodic) G25.5
  with
    heart involvement I02.0
      active or acute (conditions in I01-) I02.0
        rheumatic I02.9
          with valvular disorder I02.0
    rheumatic heart disease (chronic) (inactive)
      (quiescent) — code to rheumatic heart
      condition involved

Chorea (Continued)
  drug-induced G25.4
  habit F95.8
  hereditary G10
  Huntington's G10
  hysterical F44.4
  minor I02.9
    with heart involvement I02.0
  progressive G25.5
    hereditary G10
  rheumatic (chronic) I02.9
    with heart involvement I02.0
  Sydenham's I02.9
    with heart involvement —see Chorea, with
      rheumatic heart disease
    nonrheumatic G25.5
Choreoathetosis (paroxysmal) G25.5
Chorioadenoma (destruens) D39.2
Chorioamnionitis O41.12-
Chorioangioma D26.7
Choriocarcinoma —see Neoplasm, malignant,
  by site
  combined with
    embryonal carcinoma —see Neoplasm,
      malignant, by site
    other germ cell elements —see Neoplasm,
      malignant, by site
    teratoma —see Neoplasm, malignant, by
      site
  specified site —see Neoplasm, malignant, by
    site
  unspecified site
    female C58
    male C62.90
Chorioencephalitis (acute) (lymphocytic)
  (serous) A87.2
Chorioepithelioma —see Choriocarcinoma
Choriomeningitis (acute) (lymphocytic)
  (serous) A87.2
Chorionepithelioma —see Choriocarcinoma
Chorioretinitis —see also Inflammation,
  chorioretinal
  disseminated —see also Inflammation,
    chorioretinal, disseminated
    in neurosyphilis A52.19
  Egyptian B76.9 [D63.8]
  focal —see also Inflammation, chorioretinal,
    focal
  histoplasmic B39.9 [H32]
  in (due to)
    histoplasmosis B39.9 [H32]
    syphilis (secondary) A51.43
      late A52.71
    toxoplasmosis (acquired) B58.01
      congenital (active) P37.1 [H32]
    tuberculosis A18.53
  juxtapapillary, juxtapapillaris —see
    Inflammation, chorioretinal, focal,
    juxtapapillary
  leprous A30.9 [H32]
  miner's B76.9 [D63.8]
  progressive myopia (degeneration) H44.2-
  syphilitic (secondary) A51.43
    congenital (early) A50.01 [H32]
      late A50.32
    late A52.71
  tuberculous A18.53
Chorioretinopathy, central serous H35.71-
Choroid —see condition
Choroideremia H31.21
Choroiditis —see Chorioretinitis
Choroidopathy —see Disorder, choroid
Choroidoretinitis —see Chorioretinitis
Choroidoretinopathy, central serous —see
  Chorioretinopathy, central serous
Christian-Weber disease M35.6
Christmas disease D67
Chromaffinoma —see also Neoplasm, benign,
  by site
  malignant —see Neoplasm, malignant, by site
Chromatopsia —see Deficiency, color vision

Chromhidrosis, chromidrosis L75.1
Chromoblastomycosis —see Chromomycosis
Chromoconversion R82.91
Chromomycosis B43.9
  brain abscess B43.1
  cerebral B43.1
  cutaneous B43.0
  skin B43.0
  specified NEC B43.8
  subcutaneous abscess or cyst B43.2
Chromophytosis B36.0
Chromosome —see condition by chromosome
    involved
  D (1) —see condition, chromosome 13
  E (3) —see condition, chromosome 18
  G —see condition, chromosome 21
Chromotrichomycosis B36.8
Chronic —see condition
  fracture —see Fracture, pathological
Churg-Strauss syndrome M30.1
Chyle cyst, mesentery I89.8
Chylocele (nonfilarial) I89.8
  filarial (see also Infestation, filarial) B74.9
    [N51]
  tunica vaginalis N50.8
    filarial (see also Infestation, filarial) B74.9
      [N51]
Chylomicronemia (fasting) (with
    hyperprebetalipoproteinemia) E78.3
Chylopericardium I31.3
  acute I30.9
Chylothorax (nonfilarial) I89.8
  filarial (see also Infestation, filarial) B74.9
    [J91.8]
Chylous —see condition
Chyluria (nonfilarial) R82.0
  due to
    bilharziasis B65.0
    Brugia (malayi) B74.1
      timori B74.2
    schistosomiasis (bilharziasis) B65.0
    Wuchereria (bancrofti) B74.0
  filarial —see Infestation, filarial
Cicatricial (deformity) —see Cicatrix
Cicatrix (adherent) (contracted) (painful)
    (vicious) (see also Scar) L90.5
  adenoid (and tonsil) J35.8
  alveolar process M26.79
  anus K62.89
  auricle —see Disorder, pinna, specified type
    NEC
  bile duct (common) (hepatic) K83.8
  bladder N32.89
  bone —see Disorder, bone, specified type
    NEC
  brain G93.89
  cervix (postoperative) (postpartal) N88.1
  common duct K83.8
  cornea H17.9
    tuberculous A18.59
  duodenum (bulb), obstructive K31.5
  esophagus K22.2
  eyelid —see Disorder, eyelid function
  hypopharynx J39.2
  lacrimal passages —see Obstruction, lacrimal
  larynx J38.7
  lung J98.4
  middle ear —see subcategory H74.8
  mouth K13.79
  muscle M62.89
    with contracture —see Contraction, muscle
      NEC
  nasopharynx J39.2
  palate (soft) K13.79
  penis N48.89
  pharynx J39.2
  prostate N42.89
  rectum K62.89
  retina —see Scar, chorioretinal
  semilunar cartilage —see Derangement,
    meniscus

Cicatrix (Continued)
  seminal vesicle N50.8
  skin L90.5
    infected L08.89
    postinfective L90.5
    tuberculous B90.8
  specified site NEC L90.5
  throat J39.2
  tongue K14.8
  tonsil (and adenoid) J35.8
  trachea J39.8
  tuberculous NEC B90.9
  urethra N36.8
  uterus N85.8
  vagina N89.8
    postoperative N99.2
  vocal cord J38.3
  wrist, constricting (annular) L90.5
CIDP (chronic inflammatory demyelinating
    polyneuropathy) G61.81
CIN —see Neoplasia, intraepithelial, cervix
Cinchonism —see Deafness, ototoxic
  correct substance properly administered —see
    Table of Drugs and Chemicals, by drug,
    adverse effect
  overdose or wrong substance given or
    taken —see Table of Drugs and
    Chemicals, by drug, poisoning
Circle of Willis —see condition
Circular —see condition
Circulating anticoagulants (see also - Disorder,
    hemorrhagic) D68.318
  due to drugs (see also - Disorder,
    hemorrhagic) D68.32
  following childbirth O72.3
Circulation
  collateral, any site I99.8
  defective (lower extremity) I99.8
    congenital Q28.9
  embryonic Q28.9
  failure (peripheral) R57.9
    newborn P29.89
  fetal, persistent P29.3
  heart, incomplete Q28.9
Circulatory system —see condition
Circulus senilis (cornea) —see Degeneration,
    cornea, senile
Circumcision (in absence of medical indication)
    (ritual) (routine) Z41.2
Circumscribed —see condition
Circumvallate placenta O43.11-
Cirrhosis, cirrhotic (hepatic) (liver) K74.60
  alcoholic K70.30
    with ascites K70.31
  atrophic —see Cirrhosis, liver
  Baumgarten-Cruveilhier K74.69
  biliary (cholangiolitic) (cholangitic)
    (hypertrophic) (obstructive)
    (pericholangiolitic) K74.5
    due to
      Clonorchiasis B66.1
      flukes B66.3
    primary K74.3
    secondary K74.4
  cardiac (of liver) K76.1
  Charcot's K74.3
  cholangiolitic, cholangitic, cholestatic
    (primary) K74.3
  congestive K76.1
  Cruveilhier-Baumgarten K74.69
  cryptogenic (liver) K74.69
  due to
    hepatolenticular degeneration E83.01
    Wilson's disease E83.01
    xanthomatosis E78.2
  fatty K76.0
    alcoholic K70.0
  Hanot's (hypertrophic) K74.3
  hepatic —see Cirrhosis, liver
  hypertrophic K74.3
  Indian childhood K74.69

◀ New   ◀══ Revised   ~~deleted~~ Deleted

Cirrhosis, cirrhotic *(Continued)*
kidney —*see* Sclerosis, renal
Laennec's K70.30
  with ascites K70.31
  alcoholic K70.30
    with ascites K70.31
  nonalcoholic K74.69
liver K74.60
  alcoholic K70.30
    with ascites K70.31
    fatty K70.0
  congenital P78.81
  syphilitic A52.74
lung (chronic) J84.10
macronodular K74.69
  alcoholic K70.30
    with ascites K70.31
micronodular K74.69
  alcoholic K70.30
    with ascites K70.31
mixed type K74.69
monolobular K74.3
nephritis —*see* Sclerosis, renal
nutritional K74.69
  alcoholic K70.30
    with ascites K70.31
obstructive —*see* Cirrhosis, biliary
ovarian N83.8
pancreas (duct) K86.8
pigmentary E83.110
portal K74.69
  alcoholic K70.30
    with ascites K70.31
postnecrotic K74.69
  alcoholic K70.30
    with ascites K70.31
pulmonary J84.10
renal —*see* Sclerosis, renal
spleen D73.2
stasis K76.1
Todd's K74.3
unilobar K74.3
xanthomatous (biliary) K74.5
  due to xanthomatosis (familial) (metabolic)
    (primary) E78.2
Cistern, subarachnoid R93.0
Citrullinemia E72.23
Citrullinuria E72.23
Civatte's disease or poikiloderma
  L57.3
Clam digger's itch B65.3
Clammy skin R23.1
Clap —*see* Gonorrhea
Clarke-Hadfield syndrome (pancreatic
  infantilism) K86.8
Clark's paralysis G80.9
Clastothrix L67.8
Claude Bernard-Horner syndrome
  G90.2
  traumatic —*see* Injury, nerve, cervical
    sympathetic
Claude's disease or syndrome G46.3
Claudicatio venosa intermittens I87.8
Claudication, intermittent I73.9
  cerebral (artery) G45.9
  spinal cord (arteriosclerotic) G95.19
    syphilitic A52.09
  venous (axillary) I87.8
Claustrophobia F40.240
Clavus (infected) L84
Clawfoot (congenital) Q66.89
  acquired —*see* Deformity, limb, clawfoot
Clawhand (acquired) —*see also* Deformity, limb,
  clawhand
  congenital Q68.1
Clawtoe (congenital) Q66.89
  acquired —*see* Deformity, toe, specified
    NEC
Clay eating —*see* Pica
Cleansing of artificial opening —*see* Attention
  to, artificial, opening

Cleft (congenital) —*see also* Imperfect,
    closure
alveolar process M26.79
branchial (cyst) (persistent) Q18.2
cricoid cartilage, posterior Q31.8
lip (unilateral) Q36.9
  with cleft palate Q37.9
    hard Q37.1
      with soft Q37.5
    soft Q37.3
      with hard Q37.5
  bilateral Q36.0
    with cleft palate Q37.8
      hard Q37.0
        with soft Q37.4
      soft Q37.2
        with hard Q37.4
  median Q36.1
nose Q30.2
palate Q35.9
  with cleft lip (unilateral) Q37.9
    bilateral Q37.8
  hard Q35.1
    with
      cleft lip (unilateral) Q37.1
        bilateral Q37.0
      soft Q35.5
        with cleft lip (unilateral) Q37.5
          bilateral Q37.4
  medial Q35.5
  soft Q35.3
    with
      cleft lip (unilateral) Q37.3
        bilateral Q37.2
      hard Q35.5
        with cleft lip (unilateral) Q37.5
          bilateral Q37.4
penis Q55.69
scrotum Q55.29
thyroid cartilage Q31.8
uvula Q35.7
Cleidocranial dysostosis Q74.0
Cleptomania F63.2
Clicking hip (newborn) R29.4
Climacteric (female) —*see also* Menopause
  arthritis (any site) NEC —*see* Arthritis,
    specified form NEC
  depression (single episode) F32.8
  male (symptoms) (syndrome) NEC N50.8
  paranoid state F22
  polyarthritis NEC —*see* Arthritis, specified
    form NEC
  symptoms (female) N95.1
Clinical research investigation (clinical trial)
    (control subject) (normal comparison)
    (participant) Z00.6
Clitoris —*see* condition **Cloaca** (persistent)
  Q43.7
Clonorchiasis, clonorchis infection (liver)
  B66.1
Clonus R25.8
Closed bite M26.29
Clostridium (C.) **perfringens, as cause of**
    disease classified elsewhere B96.7
Closure
  congenital, nose Q30.0
  cranial sutures, premature Q75.0
  defective or imperfect NEC —*see* Imperfect,
    closure
  fistula, delayed —*see* Fistula
  foramen ovale, imperfect Q21.1
  hymen N89.6
  interauricular septum, defective Q21.1
  interventricular septum, defective Q21.0
  lacrimal duct —*see also* Stenosis, lacrimal,
    duct
    congenital Q10.5
  nose (congenital) Q30.0
    acquired M95.0
  of artificial opening —*see* Attention to,
    artificial, opening

Closure *(Continued)*
primary angle, without glaucoma damage
  H40.06-
vagina N89.5
valve —*see* Endocarditis
vulva N90.5
Clot (blood) —*see also* Embolism
artery (obstruction) (occlusion) —*see*
  Embolism
bladder N32.89
brain (intradural or extradural) —*see*
  Occlusion, artery, cerebral
circulation I74.9
heart —*see also* Infarct, myocardium
  not resulting in infarction I24.0
vein —*see* Thrombosis
Clouded state R40.1
epileptic —*see* Epilepsy, specified NEC
paroxysmal —*see* Epilepsy, specified NEC
Cloudy antrum, antra J32.0
Clouston's (hidrotic) **ectodermal dysplasia**
  Q82.4
Clubbed nail pachydermoperiostosis M89.40
  [L62]
Clubbing of finger (s) (nails) R68.3
Clubfinger R68.3
  congenital Q68.1
Clubfoot (congenital) Q66.89
  acquired —*see* Deformity, limb, clubfoot
  equinovarus Q66.0
  paralytic —*see* Deformity, limb, clubfoot
Clubhand (congenital) (radial) Q71.4-
  acquired —*see* Deformity, limb, clubhand
Clubnail R68.3
  congenital Q84.6
Clump, kidney Q63.1
Clumsiness, clumsy child syndrome F82
Cluttering F98.81
Clutton's joints A50.51 [M12.80]
Coagulation, intravascular (diffuse)
    (disseminated) —*see also* Defibrination
    syndrome
  complicating abortion —*see* Abortion, by
    type, complicated by, intravascular
    coagulation
  following ectopic or molar pregnancy O08.1
Coagulopathy —*see also* Defect, coagulation
  consumption D65
  intravascular D65
    newborn P60
Coalition
  calcaneo-scaphoid Q66.89
  tarsal Q66.89
Coalminer's
  elbow —*see* Bursitis, elbow, olecranon
  lung or pneumoconiosis J60
Coalworker's lung or pneumoconiosis J60
Coarctation
  aorta (preductal) (postductal) Q25.1
  pulmonary artery Q25.71
Coated tongue K14.3
Coats' disease (exudative retinopathy) —*see*
  Retinopathy, exudative
Cocainism —*see* Dependence, drug, cocaine
Coccidioidomycosis B38.9
  cutaneous B38.3
  disseminated B38.7
  generalized B38.7
  meninges B38.4
  prostate B38.81
  pulmonary B38.2
    acute B38.0
    chronic B38.1
  skin B38.3
  specified NEC B38.89
Coccidioidosis —*see* Coccidioidomycosis
Coccidiosis (intestinal) A07.3
Coccydynia, coccygodynia M53.3
Coccyx —*see* condition
Cochin-China diarrhea K90.1
Cockayne's syndrome Q87.1

Cocked up toe —see Deformity, toe, specified NEC
Cock's peculiar tumor L72.3
Codman's tumor —see Neoplasm, bone, benign
Coenurosis B71.8
Coffee-worker's lung J67.8
Cogan's syndrome H16.32-
  oculomotor apraxia H51.8
Coitus, painful (female) N94.1
  male N53.12
  psychogenic F52.6
Cold J00
  with influenza, flu, or grippe —see Influenza, with, respiratory manifestations NEC
  agglutinin disease or hemoglobinuria (chronic) D59.1
  bronchial —see Bronchitis
  chest —see Bronchitis
  common (head) J00
  effects of T69.9
    specified effect NEC T69.8
  excessive, effects of T69.9
    specified effect NEC T69.8
  exhaustion from T69.8
  exposure to T69.9
    specified effect NEC T69.8
  head J00
  injury syndrome (newborn) P80.0
  on lung —see Bronchitis
  rose J30.1
  sensitivity, auto-immune D59.1
  virus J00
Coldsore B00.1
Colibacillosis A49.8
  as the cause of other disease (see also Escherichia coli) B96.20
  generalized A41.50
Colic (bilious) (infantile) (intestinal) (recurrent) (spasmodic) R10.83
  abdomen R10.83
    psychogenic F45.8
  appendix, appendicular K38.8
  bile duct —see Calculus, bile duct
  biliary —see Calculus, bile duct
  common duct —see Calculus, bile duct
  cystic duct —see Calculus, gallbladder
  Devonshire NEC —see Poisoning, lead
  gallbladder —see Calculus, gallbladder
  gallstone —see Calculus, gallbladder
    gallbladder or cystic duct —see Calculus, gallbladder
  hepatic (duct) —see Calculus, bile duct
  hysterical F45.8
  kidney N23
  lead NEC —see Poisoning, lead
  mucous K58.9
    with diarrhea K58.0
    psychogenic F54
  nephritic N23
  painter's NEC —see Poisoning, lead
  pancreas K86.8
  psychogenic F45.8
  renal N23
  saturnine NEC —see Poisoning, lead
  ureter N23
  urethral N36.8
    due to calculus N21.1
  uterus NEC N94.89
    menstrual —see Dysmenorrhea
  worm NOS B83.9
Colicystitis —see Cystitis
Colitis (acute) (catarrhal) (chronic) (noninfective) (hemorrhagic) (see also Enteritis) K52.9
  allergic K52.2
  amebic (acute) (see also Amebiasis) A06.0
    nondysenteric A06.2
  anthrax A22.2
  bacillary —see Infection, Shigella
  balantidial A07.0
  Clostridium difficile A04.7

Colitis (Continued)
  coccidial A07.3
  collagenous K52.89
  cystica superficialis K52.89
  dietary counseling and surveillance (for) Z71.3
  dietetic K52.2
  drug-induced K52.1
  due to radiation K52.0
  eosinophilic K52.82
  food hypersensitivity K52.2
  giardial A07.1
  granulomatous —see Enteritis, regional, large intestine
  infectious —see Enteritis, infectious
  ischemic K55.9
    acute (fulminant) (subacute) K55.0
    chronic K55.1
    due to mesenteric artery insufficiency K55.1
    fulminant (acute) K55.0
  left sided K51.50
    with
      abscess K51.514
      complication K51.519
        specified NEC K51.518
      fistula K51.513
      obstruction K51.512
      rectal bleeding K51.511
  lymphocytic K52.89
  membranous
    psychogenic F54
  microscopic (collagenous) (lymphocytic) K52.89
  mucous —see Syndrome, irritable, bowel
    psychogenic F54
  noninfective K52.9
    specified NEC K52.89
  polyposa —see Polyp, colon, inflammatory
  protozoal A07.9
  pseudomembranous A04.7
  pseudomucinous —see Syndrome, irritable, bowel
  regional —see Enteritis, regional, large intestine
  segmental —see Enteritis, regional, large intestine
  septic —see Enteritis, infectious
  spastic K58.9
    with diarrhea K58.0
    psychogenic F54
  staphylococcal A04.8
    foodborne A05.0
  subacute ischemic K55.0
  thromboulcerative K55.0
  toxic NEC K52.1
    due to Clostridium difficile A04.7
  transmural —see Enteritis, regional, large intestine
  trichomonal A07.8
  tuberculous (ulcerative) A18.32
  ulcerative (chronic) K51.90
    with
      complication K51.919
        abscess K51.914
        fistula K51.913
        obstruction K51.912
        rectal bleeding K51.911
        specified complication NEC K51.918
    enterocolitis —see Enterocolitis, ulcerative
    ileocolitis —see Ileocolitis, ulcerative
    mucosal proctocolitis —see Proctocolitis, mucosal
    proctitis —see Proctitis, ulcerative
    pseudopolyposis —see Polyp, colon, inflammatory
    psychogenic F54
    rectosigmoiditis —see Rectosigmoiditis, ulcerative

Colitis (Continued)
  ulcerative (Continued)
    specified type NEC K51.80
      with
        complication K51.819
          abscess K51.814
          fistula K51.813
          obstruction K51.812
          rectal bleeding K51.811
          specified complication NEC K51.818
Collagenosis, collagen disease (nonvascular) (vascular) M35.9
  cardiovascular I42.8
  reactive perforating L87.1
  specified NEC M35.8
Collapse R55
  adrenal E27.2
  cardiorespiratory R57.0
  cardiovascular R57.0
    newborn P29.89
  circulatory (peripheral) R57.9
    during or after labor and delivery O75.1
    following ectopic or molar pregnancy O08.3
    newborn P29.89
  during or
    after labor and delivery O75.1
    resulting from a procedure, not elsewhere classified T81.10
  external ear canal —see Stenosis, external ear canal
  general R55
  heart —see Disease, heart
  heat T67.1
  hysterical F44.89
  labyrinth, membranous (congenital) Q16.5
  lung (massive) (see also Atelectasis) J98.19
    pressure due to anesthesia (general) (local) or other sedation T88.2
      during labor and delivery O74.1
      in pregnancy O29.02-
      postpartum, puerperal O89.09
  myocardial —see Disease, heart
  nervous F48.8
  neurocirculatory F45.8
  nose M95.0
  postoperative T81.10
  pulmonary (see also Atelectasis) J98.19
    newborn —see Atelectasis
  trachea J39.8
  tracheobronchial J98.09
  valvular —see Endocarditis
  vascular (peripheral) R57.9
    during or after labor and delivery O75.1
    following ectopic or molar pregnancy O08.3
    newborn P29.89
  vertebra M48.50-
    cervical region M48.52-
    cervicothoracic region M48.53-
    in (due to)
      metastasis —see Collapse, vertebra, in, specified disease NEC
      osteoporosis (see also Osteoporosis) M80.88
        cervical region M80.88
        cervicothoracic region M80.88
        lumbar region M80.88
        lumbosacral region M80.88
        multiple sites M80.88
        occipito-atlanto-axial region M80.88
        sacrococcygeal region M80.88
        thoracic region M80.88
        thoracolumbar region M80.88
      specified disease NEC M48.50-
        cervical region M48.52-
        cervicothoracic region M48.53-
        lumbar region M48.56-
        lumbosacral region M48.57-
        occipito-atlanto-axial region M48.51-

Collapse (*Continued*)
  vertebra (*Continued*)
    in (*Continued*)
      specified disease NEC (*Continued*)
        sacrococcygeal region M48.58-
          thoracic region M48.54-
          thoracolumbar region M48.55-
      lumbar region M48.56-
      lumbosacral region M48.57-
      occipito-atlanto-axial region M48.51-
      sacrococcygeal region M48.58-
      thoracic region M48.54-
      thoracolumbar region M48.55-
Collateral —*see also* condition
  circulation (venous) I87.8
  dilation, veins I87.8
Colles' fracture S52.53-
Collet (-Sicard) **syndrome** G52.7
Collier's asthma or lung J60
Collodion baby Q80.2
Colloid nodule (of thyroid) (cystic) E04.1
Coloboma (iris) Q13.0
  eyelid Q10.3
  fundus Q14.8
  lens Q12.2
  optic disc (congenital) Q14.2
    acquired H47.31-
Coloenteritis —*see* Enteritis
Colon —*see* condition
Colonization
  MRSA (Methicillin resistant Staphylococcus aureus) Z22.322
  MSSA (Methicillin susceptible Staphylococcus aureus) Z22.321
  status —*see* Carrier (suspected) of
Coloptosis K63.4
Color blindness —*see* Deficiency, color vision
Colostomy
  attention to Z43.3
  fitting or adjustment Z46.89
  malfunctioning K94.03
  status Z93.3
Colpitis (acute) —*see* Vaginitis
Colpocele N81.5
Colpocystitis —*see* Vaginitis
Colpospasm N94.2
Column, spinal, vertebral —*see* condition
Coma R40.20
  with
    motor response (none) R40.231
      abnormal R40.233
      extension R40.232
      flexion withdrawal R40.234
      localizes pain R40.235
      obeys commands R40.236
    opening of eyes (never) R40.211
      in response to
        pain R40.212
        sound R40.213
      spontaneous R40.214
    verbal response (none) R40.221
      confused conversation R40.224
      inappropriate words R40.223
      incomprehensible words R40.222
      oriented R40.225
  eclamptic —*see* Eclampsia
  epileptic —*see* Epilepsy
  Glasgow, scale score —*see* Glasgow coma scale
  hepatic —*see* Failure, hepatic, by type, with coma
  hyperglycemic (diabetic) —*see* Diabetes, coma
  hyperosmolar (diabetic) —*see* Diabetes, coma
  hypoglycemic (diabetic) —*see* Diabetes, coma, hypoglycemic
    nondiabetic E15
  in diabetes —*see* Diabetes, coma
  insulin-induced —*see* Coma, hypoglycemic
  myxedematous E03.5
  newborn P91.5
  persistent vegetative state R40.3

Coma (*Continued*)
  specified NEC, without documented Glasgow coma scale score, or with partial Glasgow coma scale score reported R40.244
Comatose —*see* Coma
Combat fatigue F43.0
Combined —*see* condition
Comedo, comedones (giant) L70.0
Comedocarcinoma —*see also* Neoplasm, breast, malignant
  noninfiltrating
    breast D05.8-
    specified site —*see* Neoplasm, in situ, by site
    unspecified site D05.8-
Comedomastitis —*see* Ectasia, mammary duct
Comminuted fracture - code as Fracture, closed
Common
  arterial trunk Q20.0
  atrioventricular canal Q21.2
  atrium Q21.1
  cold (head) J00
  truncus (arteriosus) Q20.0
  variable immunodeficiency —*see* Immunodeficiency, common variable
  ventricle Q20.4
Commotio, commotion (current)
  brain —*see* Injury, intracranial, concussion
  cerebri —*see* Injury, intracranial, concussion
  retinae S05.8X-
  spinal cord —*see* Injury, spinal cord, by region
  spinalis —*see* Injury, spinal cord, by region
Communication
  between
    base of aorta and pulmonary artery Q21.4
    left ventricle and right atrium Q20.5
    pericardial sac and pleural sac Q34.8
    pulmonary artery and pulmonary vein, congenital Q25.72
  congenital between uterus and digestive or urinary tract Q51.7
Compartment syndrome (deep) (posterior) (traumatic) T79.A0
  abdomen T79.A3
  lower extremity (hip, buttock, thigh, leg, foot, toes) T79.A2
  nontraumatic
    abdomen M79.A3
    lower extremity (hip, buttock, thigh, leg, foot, toes) M79.A2-
    specified site NEC M79.A9
    upper extremity (shoulder, arm, forearm, wrist, hand, fingers) M79.A1-
  specified site NEC T79.A9
  upper extremity (shoulder, arm, forearm, wrist, hand, fingers) T79.A1
Compensation
  failure —*see* Disease, heart
  neurosis, psychoneurosis —*see* Disorder, factitious
Complaint —*see also* Disease
  bowel, functional K59.9
    psychogenic F45.8
  intestine, functional K59.9
    psychogenic F45.8
  kidney —*see* Disease, renal
  miners' J60
Complete —*see* condition
Complex
  Addison-Schilder E71.528
  cardiorenal —*see* Hypertension, cardiorenal
  Costen's M26.69
  disseminated mycobacterium avium-intracellulare (DMAC) A31.2
  Eisenmenger's (ventricular septal defect) I27.89
  hypersexual F52.8
  jumped process, spine —*see* Dislocation, vertebra

Complex (*Continued*)
  primary, tuberculous A15.7
  Schilder-Addison E71.528
  subluxation (vertebral) M99.19
    abdomen M99.19
    acromioclavicular M99.17
    cervical region M99.11
    cervicothoracic M99.11
    costochondral M99.18
    costovertebral M99.18
    head region M99.10
    hip M99.15
    lower extremity M99.16
    lumbar region M99.13
    lumbosacral M99.13
    occipitocervical M99.10
    pelvic region M99.15
    pubic M99.15
    rib cage M99.18
    sacral region M99.14
    sacrococcygeal M99.14
    sacroiliac M99.14
    specified NEC M99.19
    sternochondral M99.18
    sternoclavicular M99.17
    thoracic region M99.12
    thoracolumbar M99.12
    upper extremity M99.17
  Taussig-Bing (transposition, aorta and overriding pulmonary artery) Q20.1
Complication (s) (from) (of)
  accidental puncture or laceration during a procedure (of) —*see* Complications, intraoperative (intraprocedural), puncture or laceration
  amputation stump (surgical) (late) NEC T87.9
    dehiscence T87.81
    infection or inflammation T87.40
      lower limb T87.4-
      upper limb T87.4-
    necrosis T87.50
      lower limb T87.5-
      upper limb T87.5-
    neuroma T87.30
      lower limb T87.3-
      upper limb T87.3-
    specified type NEC T87.89
  anastomosis (and bypass) —*see also* Complications, prosthetic device or implant
    intestinal (internal) NEC K91.89
      involving urinary tract N99.89
    urinary tract (involving intestinal tract) N99.89
    vascular —*see* Complications, cardiovascular device or implant
  anesthesia, anesthetic (*see also* Anesthesia, complication) T88.59
    brain, postpartum, puerperal O89.2
    cardiac
      in
        labor and delivery O74.2
        pregnancy O29.19-
      postpartum, puerperal O89.1
    central nervous system
      in
        labor and delivery O74.3
        pregnancy O29.29-
      postpartum, puerperal O89.2
    difficult or failed intubation T88.4
      in pregnancy O29.6-
    failed sedation (conscious) (moderate) during procedure T88.52
    hyperthermia, malignant T88.3
    hypothermia T88.51
    intubation failure T88.4
    malignant hyperthermia T88.3

Complication (*Continued*)
  anesthesia, anesthetic (*Continued*)
    pulmonary
      in
        labor and delivery O74.1
        pregnancy NEC O29.09-
        postpartum, puerperal O89.09
    shock T88.2
    spinal and epidural
      in
        labor and delivery NEC O74.6
          headache O74.5
        pregnancy NEC O29.5X-
        postpartum, puerperal NEC O89.5
          headache O89.4
  anti-reflux device —*see* Complications,
    esophageal anti-reflux device
  aortic (bifurcation) graft —*see* Complications,
    graft, vascular
  aortocoronary (bypass) graft —*see*
    Complications, coronary artery (bypass)
    graft
  aortofemoral (bypass) graft —*see*
    Complications, extremity artery
    (bypass) graft
  arteriovenous
    fistula, surgically created T82.9
      embolism T82.818
      fibrosis T82.828
      hemorrhage T82.838
      infection or inflammation T82.7
      mechanical
        breakdown T82.510
        displacement T82.520
        leakage T82.530
        malposition T82.520
        obstruction T82.590
        perforation T82.590
        protrusion T82.590
      pain T82.848
      specified type NEC T82.898
      stenosis T82.858
      thrombosis T82.868
    shunt, surgically created T82.9
      embolism T82.818
      fibrosis T82.828
      hemorrhage T82.838
      infection or inflammation T82.7
      mechanical
        breakdown T82.511
        displacement T82.521
        leakage T82.531
        malposition T82.521
        obstruction T82.591
        perforation T82.591
        protrusion T82.591
      pain T82.848
      specified type NEC T82.898
      stenosis T82.858
      thrombosis T82.868
  arthroplasty —*see* Complications, joint
    prosthesis
  artificial
    fertilization or insemination N98.9
      attempted introduction (of)
        embryo in embryo transfer N98.3
        ovum following in vitro fertilization
          N98.2
      hyperstimulation of ovaries N98.1
      infection N98.0
      specified NEC N98.8
    heart T82.9
      embolism T82.817
      fibrosis T82.827
      hemorrhage T82.837
      infection or inflammation T82.7
      mechanical
        breakdown T82.512
        displacement T82.522
        leakage T82.532
        malposition T82.522

Complication (*Continued*)
  artificial (*Continued*)
    heart (*Continued*)
      mechanical (*Continued*)
        obstruction T82.592
        perforation T82.592
        protrusion T82.592
      pain T82.847
      specified type NEC T82.897
      stenosis T82.857
      thrombosis T82.867
    opening
      cecostomy —*see* Complications,
        colostomy
      colostomy —*see* Complications,
        colostomy
      cystostomy —*see* Complications,
        cystostomy
      enterostomy —*see* Complications,
        enterostomy
      gastrostomy —*see* Complications,
        gastrostomy
      ileostomy —*see* Complications,
        enterostomy
      jejunostomy —*see* Complications,
        enterostomy
      nephrostomy —*see* Complications,
        stoma, urinary tract
      tracheostomy —*see* Complications,
        tracheostomy
      ureterostomy —*see* Complications,
        stoma, urinary tract
      urethrostomy —*see* Complications,
        stoma, urinary tract
  balloon implant or device
    gastrointestinal T85.9
      embolism T85.81
      fibrosis T85.82
      hemorrhage T85.83
      infection and inflammation
        T85.79
      pain T85.84
      specified type NEC T85.89
      stenosis T85.85
      thrombosis T85.86
    vascular (counterpulsation) T82.9
      embolism T82.818
      fibrosis T82.828
      hemorrhage T82.838
      infection or inflammation T82.7
      mechanical
        breakdown T82.513
        displacement T82.523
        leakage T82.533
        malposition T82.523
        obstruction T82.593
        perforation T82.593
        protrusion T82.593
      pain T82.848
      specified type NEC T82.898
      stenosis T82.858
      thrombosis T82.868
  bariatric procedure
    gastric band procedure K95.09
      infection K95.01
    specified procedure NEC K95.89
      infection K95.81
  bile duct implant (prosthetic) T85.9
    embolism T85.81
    fibrosis T85.82
    hemorrhage T85.83
    infection and inflammation T85.79
    mechanical
      breakdown T85.510
      displacement T85.520
      malfunction T85.510
      malposition T85.520
      obstruction T85.590
      perforation T85.590
      protrusion T85.590
      specified NEC T85.590

Complication (*Continued*)
  bile duct implant (*Continued*)
    pain T85.84
    specified type NEC T85.89
    stenosis T85.85
    thrombosis T85.86
  bladder device (auxiliary) —*see*
    Complications, genitourinary, device or
    implant, urinary system
  bleeding (postoperative) —*see* Complication,
    postoperative, hemorrhage
    intraoperative —*see* Complication,
      intraoperative, hemorrhage
  blood vessel graft —*see* Complications, graft,
    vascular
  bone
    device NEC T84.9
      embolism T84.81
      fibrosis T84.82
      hemorrhage T84.83
      infection or inflammation T84.7
      mechanical
        breakdown T84.318
        displacement T84.328
        malposition T84.328
        obstruction T84.398
        perforation T84.398
        protrusion T84.398
      pain T84.84
      specified type NEC T84.89
      stenosis T84.85
      thrombosis T84.86
    graft —*see* Complications, graft, bone
    growth stimulator (electrode) —*see*
      Complications, electronic stimulator
      device, bone
    marrow transplant —*see* Complications,
      transplant, bone, marrow
  brain neurostimulator (electrode) —*see*
    Complications, electronic stimulator
    device, brain
  breast implant (prosthetic) T85.9
    capsular contracture T85.44
    embolism T85.81
    fibrosis T85.82
    hemorrhage T85.83
    infection and inflammation
      T85.79
    mechanical
      breakdown T85.41
      displacement T85.42
      leakage T85.43
      malposition T85.42
      obstruction T85.49
      perforation T85.49
      protrusion T85.49
      specified NEC T85.49
    pain T85.84
    specified type NEC T85.89
    stenosis T85.85
    thrombosis T85.86
  bypass —*see also* Complications, prosthetic
    device or implant
    aortocoronary —*see* Complications,
      coronary artery (bypass) graft
    arterial —*see also* Complications, graft,
      vascular
    extremity —*see* Complications, extremity
      artery (bypass) graft
  cardiac —*see also* Disease, heart
    device, implant or graft T82.9
      embolism T82.817
      fibrosis T82.827
      hemorrhage T82.837
      infection or inflammation T82.7
      valve prosthesis T82.6
      mechanical
        breakdown T82.519
          specified device NEC T82.518
        displacement T82.529
          specified device NEC T82.528

Complication (*Continued*)
  cardiac (*Continued*)
    device, implant or graft (*Continued*)
      mechanical (*Continued*)
        leakage T82.539
          specified device NEC T82.538
        malposition T82.529
          specified device NEC T82.528
        obstruction T82.599
          specified device NEC T82.598
        perforation T82.599
          specified device NEC T82.598
        protrusion T82.599
          specified device NEC T82.598
      pain T82.847
      specified type NEC T82.897
      stenosis T82.857
      thrombosis T82.867
  cardiovascular device, graft or implant T82.9
    aortic graft —*see* Complications, graft, vascular
    arteriovenous
      fistula, artificial —*see* Complication, arteriovenous, fistula, surgically created
      shunt —*see* Complication, arteriovenous, shunt, surgically created
    artificial heart —*see* Complication, artificial, heart
    balloon (counterpulsation) device —*see* Complication, balloon implant, vascular
    carotid artery graft —*see* Complications, graft, vascular
    coronary bypass graft —*see* Complication, coronary artery (bypass) graft
    dialysis catheter (vascular) —*see* Complication, catheter, dialysis
    electronic T82.9
      electrode T82.9
        embolism T82.817
        fibrosis T82.827
        hemorrhage T82.837
        infection T82.7
        mechanical
          breakdown T82.110
          displacement T82.120
          leakage T82.190
          obstruction T82.190
          perforation T82.190
          protrusion T82.190
          specified type NEC T82.190
        pain T82.847
        specified NEC T82.897
        stenosis T82.857
        thrombosis T82.867
      embolism T82.817
      fibrosis T82.827
      hemorrhage T82.837
      infection T82.7
      mechanical
        breakdown T82.119
        displacement T82.129
        leakage T82.199
        obstruction T82.199
        perforation T82.199
        protrusion T82.199
        specified type NEC T82.199
      pain T82.847
      pulse generator T82.9
        embolism T82.817
        fibrosis T82.827
        hemorrhage T82.837
        infection T82.7
        mechanical
          breakdown T82.111
          displacement T82.121
          leakage T82.191
          obstruction T82.191
          perforation T82.191

Complication (*Continued*)
  cardiovascular device, graft or implant (*Continued*)
    electronic (*Continued*)
      pulse generator (*Continued*)
        mechanical (*Continued*)
          protrusion T82.191
          specified type NEC T82.191
        pain T82.847
        specified NEC T82.897
        stenosis T82.857
        thrombosis T82.867
      specified condition NEC T82.897
      specified device NEC T82.9
        embolism T82.817
        fibrosis T82.827
        hemorrhage T82.837
        infection T82.7
        mechanical
          breakdown T82.118
          displacement T82.128
          leakage T82.198
          obstruction T82.198
          perforation T82.198
          protrusion T82.198
          specified type NEC T82.198
        pain T82.847
        specified NEC T82.897
        stenosis T82.857
        thrombosis T82.867
      stenosis T82.857
      thrombosis T82.867
    extremity artery graft —*see* Complication, extremity artery (bypass) graft
    femoral artery graft —*see* Complication, extremity artery (bypass) graft
    heart
      transplant —*see* Complication, transplant, heart
      valve —*see* Complication, prosthetic device, heart valve
        graft —*see* Complication, heart, valve, graft
    heart-lung transplant —*see* Complication, transplant, heart, with lung
    infection or inflammation T82.7
    umbrella device —*see* Complication, umbrella device, vascular
    vascular graft (or anastomosis) —*see* Complication, graft, vascular
  carotid artery (bypass) graft —*see* Complications, graft, vascular
  catheter (device) NEC —*see also* Complications, prosthetic device or implant
    cystostomy T83.9
      embolism T83.81
      fibrosis T83.82
      hemorrhage T83.83
      infection and inflammation T83.59
      mechanical
        breakdown T83.010
        displacement T83.020
        leakage T83.030
        malposition T83.020
        obstruction T83.090
        perforation T83.090
        protrusion T83.090
        specified NEC T83.090
      pain T83.84
      specified type NEC T83.89
      stenosis T83.85
      thrombosis T83.86
    dialysis (vascular) T82.9
      embolism T82.818
      fibrosis T82.828
      hemorrhage T82.838
      infection and inflammation T82.7
      intraperitoneal —*see* Complications, catheter, intraperitoneal

Complication (*Continued*)
  catheter NEC (*Continued*)
    dialysis (*Continued*)
      mechanical
        breakdown T82.41
        displacement T82.42
        leakage T82.43
        malposition T82.42
        obstruction T82.49
        perforation T82.49
        protrusion T82.49
      pain T82.848
      specified type NEC T82.898
      stenosis T82.858
      thrombosis T82.868
    epidural infusion T85.9
      embolism T85.81
      fibrosis T85.82
      hemorrhage T85.83
      infection and inflammation T85.79
      mechanical
        breakdown T85.610
        displacement T85.620
        leakage T85.630
        malfunction T85.610
        malposition T85.620
        obstruction T85.690
        perforation T85.690
        protrusion T85.690
        specified NEC T85.690
      pain T85.84
      specified type NEC T85.89
      stenosis T85.85
      thrombosis T85.86
    intraperitoneal dialysis T85.9
      embolism T85.81
      fibrosis T85.82
      hemorrhage T85.83
      infection and inflammation T85.71
      mechanical
        breakdown T85.611
        displacement T85.621
        leakage T85.631
        malfunction T85.611
        malposition T85.621
        obstruction T85.691
        perforation T85.691
        protrusion T85.691
        specified NEC T85.691
      pain T85.84
      specified type NEC T85.89
      stenosis T85.85
      thrombosis T85.86
    intravenous infusion T82.9
      embolism T82.818
      fibrosis T82.828
      hemorrhage T82.838
      infection or inflammation T82.7
      mechanical
        breakdown T82.514
        displacement T82.524
        leakage T82.534
        malposition T82.524
        obstruction T82.594
        perforation T82.594
        protrusion T82.594
      pain T82.848
      specified type NEC T82.898
      stenosis T82.858
      thrombosis T82.868
    subdural infusion T85.9
      embolism T85.81
      fibrosis T85.82
      hemorrhage T85.83
      infection and inflammation T85.79
      mechanical
        breakdown T85.610
        displacement T85.620
        leakage T85.630
        malfunction T85.610
        malposition T85.620

Complication (Continued)
  catheter NEC (Continued)
    subdural infusion (Continued)
      mechanical (Continued)
        obstruction T85.690
        perforation T85.690
        protrusion T85.690
        specified NEC T85.690
      pain T85.84
      specified type NEC T85.89
      stenosis T85.85
      thrombosis T85.86
    urethral, indwelling T83.9
      displacement T83.028
      embolism T83.81
      fibrosis T83.82
      hemorrhage T83.83
      infection and inflammation T83.51
      leakage T83.038
      malposition T83.028
      mechanical
        breakdown T83.018
      obstruction (mechanical) T83.098
      pain T83.84
      perforation T83.098
      protrusion T83.098
      specified type NEC T83.098
      stenosis T83.85
      thrombosis T83.86
    urinary (indwelling) —see Complications, catheter, urethral, indwelling
  cecostomy (stoma) —see Complications, colostomy
  cesarean delivery wound NEC O90.89
    disruption O90.0
    hematoma O90.2
    infection (following delivery) O86.0
  chemotherapy (antineoplastic) NEC T88.7
  chin implant (prosthetic) —see Complication, prosthetic device or implant, specified NEC
  circulatory system I99.8
    intraoperative I97.88
    postprocedural I97.89
      following cardiac surgery I97.19-
        postcardiotomy syndrome I97.0
      hypertension I97.3
      lymphedema after mastectomy I97.2
      postcardiotomy syndrome I97.0
      specified NEC I97.89
  colostomy (stoma) K94.00
    hemorrhage K94.01
    infection K94.02
    malfunction K94.03
    mechanical K94.03
    specified complication NEC K94.09
  contraceptive device, intrauterine —see Complications, intrauterine, contraceptive device
  cord (umbilical) —see Complications, umbilical cord
  corneal graft —see Complications, graft, cornea
  coronary artery (bypass) graft T82.9
    atherosclerosis —see Arteriosclerosis, coronary (artery)
    embolism T82.818
    fibrosis T82.828
    hemorrhage T82.838
    infection and inflammation T82.7
    mechanical
      breakdown T82.211
      displacement T82.212
      leakage T82.213
      malposition T82.212
      obstruction T82.218
      perforation T82.218
      protrusion T82.218
      specified NEC T82.218
    pain T82.848
    specified type NEC T82.897

Complication (Continued)
  coronary artery graft (Continued)
    stenosis T82.858
    thrombosis T82.868
  counterpulsation device (balloon), intra-aortic —see Complications, balloon implant, vascular
  cystostomy (stoma) N99.518
    catheter —see Complications, catheter, cystostomy
    hemorrhage N99.510
    infection N99.511
    malfunction N99.512
    specified type NEC N99.518
  delivery (see also Complications, obstetric) O75.9
    procedure (instrumental) (manual) (surgical) O75.4
    specified NEC O75.89
  dialysis (peritoneal) (renal) —see also Complications, infusion
    catheter (vascular) —see Complication, catheter, dialysis
      peritoneal, intraperitoneal —see Complications, catheter, intraperitoneal
  dorsal column (spinal) neurostimulator —see Complications, electronic stimulator device, spinal cord
  drug NEC T88.7
  ear procedure —see also Disorder, ear
    intraoperative H95.88-
      hematoma —see Complications, intraoperative, hemorrhage (hematoma) (of), ear
      hemorrhage —see Complications, intraoperative, hemorrhage (hematoma) (of), ear
      laceration —see Complications, intraoperative, puncture or laceration..., ear
      specified NEC H95.88-
    postoperative H95.89-
      external ear canal stenosis H95.81-
      hematoma —see Complications, postprocedural, hemorrhage (hematoma) (of), ear
      hemorrhage —see Complications, postprocedural, hemorrhage (hematoma) (of), ear
      postmastoidectomy —see Complications, postmastoidectomy
      specified NEC H95.89-
  ectopic pregnancy O08.9
    damage to pelvic organs O08.6
    embolism O08.2
    genital infection O08.0
    hemorrhage (delayed) (excessive) O08.1
    metabolic disorder O08.5
    renal failure O08.4
    shock O08.3
    specified type NEC O08.0
    venous complication NEC O08.7
  electronic stimulator device
    bladder (urinary) —see Complications, electronic stimulator device, urinary
    bone T84.9
      breakdown T84.310
      displacement T84.320
      embolism T84.81
      fibrosis T84.82
      hemorrhage T84.83
      infection or inflammation T84.7
      malfunction T84.310
      malposition T84.320
      mechanical NEC T84.390
      obstruction T84.390
      pain T84.84
      perforation T84.390
      protrusion T84.390
      specified type NEC T84.89

Complication (Continued)
  electronic stimulator device (Continued)
    bone (Continued)
      stenosis T84.85
      thrombosis T84.86
    brain T85.9
      embolism T85.81
      fibrosis T85.82
      hemorrhage T85.83
      infection and inflammation T85.79
      mechanical
        breakdown T85.110
        displacement T85.120
        leakage T85.190
        malposition T85.120
        obstruction T85.190
        perforation T85.190
        protrusion T85.190
        specified NEC T85.190
      pain T85.84
      specified type NEC T85.89
      stenosis T85.85
      thrombosis T85.86
    cardiac (defibrillator) (pacemaker) —see Complications, cardiovascular device or implant, electronic
    muscle T84.9
      breakdown T84.418
      displacement T84.428
      embolism T84.81
      fibrosis T84.82
      hemorrhage T84.83
      infection or inflammation T84.7
      mechanical NEC T84.498
      pain T84.84
      specified type NEC T84.89
      stenosis T84.85
      thrombosis T84.86
    nervous system T85.9
      brain —see Complications, electronic stimulator device, brain
      embolism T85.81
      fibrosis T85.82
      hemorrhage T85.83
      infection and inflammation T85.79
      mechanical
        breakdown T85.118
        displacement T85.128
        leakage T85.199
        malposition T85.128
        obstruction T85.199
        perforation T85.199
        protrusion T85.199
        specified NEC T85.199
      pain T85.84
      peripheral nerve —see Complications, electronic stimulator device, peripheral nerve
      specified type NEC T85.89
      spinal cord —see Complications, electronic stimulator device, spinal cord
      stenosis T85.85
      thrombosis T85.86
    peripheral nerve T85.9
      embolism T85.81
      fibrosis T85.82
      hemorrhage T85.83
      infection and inflammation T85.79
      mechanical
        breakdown T85.111
        displacement T85.121
        leakage T85.191
        malposition T85.121
        obstruction T85.191
        perforation T85.191
        protrusion T85.191
        specified NEC T85.191
      pain T85.84
      specified type NEC T85.89
      stenosis T85.85
      thrombosis T85.86

Complication (*Continued*)
  electronic stimulator device (*Continued*)
    spinal cord T85.9
      embolism T85.81
      fibrosis T85.82
      hemorrhage T85.83
      infection and inflammation
        T85.79
      mechanical
        breakdown T85.112
        displacement T85.122
        leakage T85.192
        malposition T85.122
        obstruction T85.192
        perforation T85.192
        protrusion T85.192
        specified NEC T85.192
      pain T85.84
      specified type NEC T85.89
      stenosis T85.85
      thrombosis T85.86
    urinary T83.9
      embolism T83.81
      fibrosis T83.82
      hemorrhage T83.83
      infection and inflammation T83.59
      mechanical
        breakdown T83.110
        displacement T83.120
        malposition T83.120
        perforation T83.190
        protrusion T83.190
        specified NEC T83.190
      pain T83.84
      specified type NEC T83.89
      stenosis T83.85
      thrombosis T83.86
  electroshock therapy T88.9
    specified NEC T88.8
  endocrine E34.9
    postprocedural
      adrenal hypofunction E89.6
      hypoinsulinemia E89.1
      hypoparathyroidism E89.2
      hypopituitarism E89.3
      hypothyroidism E89.0
      ovarian failure E89.40
        asymptomatic E89.40
        symptomatic E89.41
      specified NEC E89.89
      testicular hypofunction E89.5
  endodontic treatment NEC M27.59
  enterostomy (stoma) K94.10
    hemorrhage K94.11
    infection K94.12
    malfunction K94.13
    mechanical K94.13
    specified complication NEC K94.19
  episiotomy, disruption O90.1
  esophageal anti-reflux device T85.9
    embolism T85.81
    fibrosis T85.82
    hemorrhage T85.83
    infection and inflammation T85.79
    mechanical
      breakdown T85.511
      displacement T85.521
      malfunction T85.511
      malposition T85.521
      obstruction T85.591
      perforation T85.591
      protrusion T85.591
      specified NEC T85.591
    pain T85.84
    specified type NEC T85.89
    stenosis T85.85
    thrombosis T85.86
  esophagostomy K94.30
    hemorrhage K94.31
    infection K94.32
    malfunction K94.33

Complication (*Continued*)
  esophagostomy (*Continued*)
    mechanical K94.33
    specified complication NEC K94.39
  extracorporeal circulation T80.90
  extremity artery (bypass) graft T82.9
    arteriosclerosis —*see* Arteriosclerosis,
      extremities, bypass graft
    embolism T82.818
    fibrosis T82.828
    hemorrhage T82.838
    infection and inflammation T82.7
    mechanical
      breakdown T82.318
        femoral artery T82.312
      displacement T82.328
        femoral artery T82.322
      leakage T82.338
        femoral artery T82.332
      malposition T82.328
        femoral artery T82.322
      obstruction T82.398
        femoral artery T82.392
      perforation T82.398
        femoral artery T82.392
      protrusion T82.398
        femoral artery T82.392
    pain T82.848
    specified type NEC T82.898
    stenosis T82.858
    thrombosis T82.868
  eye H57.9
    corneal graft —*see* Complications, graft,
      cornea
    implant (prosthetic) T85.9
      embolism T85.81
      fibrosis T85.82
      hemorrhage T85.83
      infection and inflammation T85.79
      mechanical
        breakdown T85.318
        displacement T85.328
        leakage T85.398
        malposition T85.328
        obstruction T85.398
        perforation T85.398
        protrusion T85.398
        specified NEC T85.398
      pain T85.84
      specified type NEC T85.89
      stenosis T85.85
      thrombosis T85.86
    intraocular lens —*see* Complications,
      intraocular lens
    orbital prosthesis —*see* Complications,
      orbital prosthesis
  female genital N94.9
    device, implant or graft NEC —*see*
      Complications, genitourinary, device
      or implant, genital tract
  femoral artery (bypass) graft —*see*
      Complication, extremity artery (bypass)
      graft
  fixation device, internal (orthopedic) T84.9
    infection and inflammation T84.60
      arm T84.61-
        humerus T84.61-
        radius T84.61-
        ulna T84.61-
      leg T84.629
        femur T84.62-
        fibula T84.62-
        tibia T84.62-
      specified site NEC T84.69
      spine T84.63
    mechanical
      breakdown
        limb T84.119
          carpal T84.210
          femur T84.11-
          fibula T84.11-

Complication (*Continued*)
  fixation device, internal (*Continued*)
    mechanical (*Continued*)
      breakdown (*Continued*)
        limb (*Continued*)
          humerus T84.11-
          metacarpal T84.210
          metatarsal T84.213
          phalanx
            foot T84.213
            hand T84.210
          radius T84.11-
          tarsal T84.213
          tibia T84.11-
          ulna T84.11-
          specified bone NEC T84.218
          spine T84.216
      displacement
        limb T84.129
          carpal T84.220
          femur T84.12-
          fibula T84.12-
          humerus T84.12-
          metacarpal T84.220
          metatarsal T84.223
          phalanx
            foot T84.223
            hand T84.220
          radius T84.12-
          tarsal T84.223
          tibia T84.12-
          ulna T84.12-
          specified bone NEC T84.228
          spine T84.226
      malposition —*see* Complications,
        fixation device, internal,
        mechanical, displacement
      obstruction —*see* Complications, fixation
        device, internal, mechanical,
        specified type NEC
      perforation —*see* Complications, fixation
        device, internal, mechanical,
        specified type NEC
      protrusion —*see* Complications, fixation
        device, internal, mechanical,
        specified type NEC
      specified type NEC
        limb T84.199
          carpal T84.290
          femur T84.19-
          fibula T84.19-
          humerus T84.19-
          metacarpal T84.290
          metatarsal T84.293
          phalanx
            foot T84.293
            hand T84.290
          radius T84.19-
          tarsal T84.293
          tibia T84.19-
          ulna T84.19-
          specified bone NEC T84.298
          vertebra T84.296
    specified type NEC T84.89
    embolism T84.81
    fibrosis T84.82
    hemorrhage T84.83
    pain T84.84
    specified complication NEC T84.89
    stenosis T84.85
    thrombosis T84.86
  following
    acute myocardial infarction NEC I23.8
      aneurysm (false) (of cardiac wall) (of
        heart wall) (ruptured) I23.3
      angina I23.7
      atrial
        septal defect I23.1
        thrombosis I23.6
      cardiac wall rupture I23.3
      chordae tendinae rupture I23.4

Complication (*Continued*)
  following (*Continued*)
    acute myocardial infarction NEC
        (*Continued*)
      defect
        septal
          atrial (heart) I23.1
          ventricular (heart) I23.2
        hemopericardium I23.0
        papillary muscle rupture I23.5
        rupture
          cardiac wall I23.3
            with hemopericardium
                I23.0
          chordae tendineae I23.4
          papillary muscle I23.5
        specified NEC I23.8
        thrombosis
          atrium I23.6
          auricular appendage I23.6
          ventricle (heart) I23.6
        ventricular
          septal defect I23.2
          thrombosis I23.6
    ectopic or molar pregnancy O08.9
      cardiac arrest O08.81
      sepsis O08.82
      specified type NEC O08.89
      urinary tract infection O08.83
    termination of pregnancy —*see* Abortion
  gastrointestinal K92.9
    bile duct prosthesis —*see* Complications,
        bile duct implant
    esophageal anti-reflux device —*see*
        Complications, esophageal
        anti-reflux device
    postoperative
      colostomy —*see* Complications,
          colostomy
      dumping syndrome K91.1
      enterostomy —*see* Complications,
          enterostomy
      gastrostomy —*see* Complications,
          gastrostomy
      malabsorption NEC K91.2
      obstruction K91.3
      postcholecystectomy syndrome
          K91.5
      specified NEC K91.89
      vomiting after GI surgery K91.0
    prosthetic device or implant
      bile duct prosthesis —*see* Complications,
          bile duct implant
      esophageal anti-reflux device —*see*
          Complications, esophageal anti-
          reflux device
      specified type NEC
        embolism T85.81
        fibrosis T85.82
        hemorrhage T85.83
        mechanical
          breakdown T85.518
          displacement T85.528
          malfunction T85.518
          malposition T85.528
          obstruction T85.598
          perforation T85.598
          protrusion T85.598
          specified NEC T85.598
        pain T85.84
        specified complication NEC
            T85.89
        stenosis T85.85
        thrombosis T85.86
  gastrostomy (stoma) K94.20
    hemorrhage K94.21
    infection K94.22
    malfunction K94.23
    mechanical K94.23
    specified complication NEC
        K94.29

Complication (*Continued*)
  genitourinary
    device or implant T83.9
      genital tract T83.9
        infection or inflammation T83.6
        intrauterine contraceptive device —*see*
            Complications, intrauterine,
            contraceptive device
        mechanical —*see* Complications, by
            device, mechanical
        mesh —*see* Complications, mesh
        penile prosthesis —*see* Complications,
            prosthetic device, penile
        specified type NEC T83.89
          embolism T83.81
          fibrosis T83.82
          hemorrhage T83.83
          pain T83.84
          specified complication NEC T83.89
          stenosis T83.85
          thrombosis T83.86
        vaginal mesh —*see* Complications,
            mesh
      urinary system T83.9
        cystostomy catheter —*see*
            Complication, catheter,
            cystostomy
        electronic stimulator —*see*
            Complications, electronic
            stimulator device, urinary
        indwelling urethral catheter —*see*
            Complications, catheter, urethral,
            indwelling
        infection or inflammation T83.59
          indwelling urinary catheter T83.51
        kidney transplant —*see* Complication,
            transplant, kidney
        organ graft —*see* Complication, graft,
            urinary organ
        specified type NEC T83.89
          embolism T83.81
          fibrosis T83.82
          hemorrhage T83.83
          mechanical T83.198
            breakdown T83.118
            displacement T83.128
            malfunction T83.118
            malposition T83.128
            obstruction T83.198
            perforation T83.198
            protrusion T83.198
            specified NEC T83.198
          pain T83.84
          specified complication NEC
              T83.89
          stenosis T83.85
          thrombosis T83.86
        sphincter implant —*see*
            Complications, implant, urinary
            sphincter
    postprocedural
      pelvic peritoneal adhesions N99.4
      renal failure N99.0
      specified NEC N99.89
      stoma —*see* Complications, stoma,
          urinary tract
      urethral stricture —*see* Stricture, urethra,
          postprocedural
    vaginal
      adhesions N99.2
      vault prolapse N99.3
  graft (bypass) (patch) —*see also*
      Complications, prosthetic device or
      implant
    aorta —*see* Complications, graft,
        vascular
    arterial —*see* Complication, graft,
        vascular
    bone T86.839
      failure T86.831
      infection T86.832

Complication (*Continued*)
  graft (*Continued*)
    bone (*Continued*)
      mechanical T84.318
        breakdown T84.318
        displacement T84.328
        protrusion T84.398
        specified type NEC T84.398
      rejection T86.830
      specified type NEC T86.838
    carotid artery —*see* Complications, graft,
        vascular
    cornea T86.849
      failure T86.841
      infection T86.842
      mechanical T85.398
        breakdown T85.318
        displacement T85.328
        protrusion T85.398
        specified type NEC T85.398
      rejection T86.840
      retroprosthetic membrane T85.398
      specified type NEC T86.848
    femoral artery (bypass) —*see* Complication,
        extremity artery (bypass) graft
    genital organ or tract —*see* Complications,
        genitourinary, device or implant,
        genital tract
    muscle T84.9
      breakdown T84.410
      displacement T84.420
      embolism T84.81
      fibrosis T84.82
      hemorrhage T84.83
      infection and inflammation T84.7
      mechanical NEC T84.490
      pain T84.84
      specified type NEC T84.89
      stenosis T84.85
      thrombosis T84.86
    nerve —*see* Complication, prosthetic device
        or implant, specified NEC
    skin —*see* Complications, prosthetic device
        or implant, skin graft
    tendon T84.9
      breakdown T84.410
      displacement T84.420
      embolism T84.81
      fibrosis T84.82
      hemorrhage T84.83
      infection and inflammation T84.7
      mechanical NEC T84.490
      pain T84.84
      specified type NEC T84.89
      stenosis T84.85
      thrombosis T84.86
    urinary organ T83.9
      embolism T83.81
      fibrosis T83.82
      hemorrhage T83.83
      infection and inflammation T83.59
        indwelling urinary catheter T83.51
      mechanical
        breakdown T83.21
        displacement T83.22
        leakage T83.23
        malposition T83.22
        obstruction T83.29
        perforation T83.29
        protrusion T83.29
        specified NEC T83.29
      pain T83.84
      specified type NEC T83.89
      stenosis T83.85
      thrombosis T83.86
    vascular T82.9
      embolism T82.818
      femoral artery —*see* Complication,
          extremity artery (bypass) graft
      fibrosis T82.828
      hemorrhage T82.838

◀ New   ◀ Revised   ~~deleted~~ Deleted

Complication (*Continued*)
  graft (*Continued*)
    vascular (*Continued*)
      mechanical
        breakdown T82.319
          aorta (bifurcation) T82.310
          carotid artery T82.311
          specified vessel NEC T82.318
        displacement T82.329
          aorta (bifurcation) T82.320
          carotid artery T82.321
          specified vessel NEC T82.328
        leakage T82.339
          aorta (bifurcation) T82.330
          carotid artery T82.331
          specified vessel NEC T82.338
        malposition T82.329
          aorta (bifurcation) T82.320
          carotid artery T82.321
          specified vessel NEC T82.328
        obstruction T82.399
          aorta (bifurcation) T82.390
          carotid artery T82.391
          specified vessel NEC T82.398
        perforation T82.399
          aorta (bifurcation) T82.390
          carotid artery T82.391
          specified vessel NEC T82.398
        protrusion T82.399
          aorta (bifurcation) T82.390
          carotid artery T82.391
          specified vessel NEC T82.398
      pain T82.848
      specified complication NEC T82.898
      stenosis T82.858
      thrombosis T82.868
  heart I51.9
    assist device
      infection and inflammation T82.7
    following acute myocardial infarction —
      see Complications, following, acute
      myocardial infarction
    postoperative —*see* Complications,
      circulatory system
    transplant —*see* Complication, transplant,
      heart
      and lung (s) —*see* Complications,
        transplant, heart, with lung
    valve
      graft (biological) T82.9
        embolism T82.817
        fibrosis T82.827
        hemorrhage T82.837
        infection and inflammation T82.7
        mechanical T82.228
          breakdown T82.221
          displacement T82.222
          leakage T82.223
          malposition T82.222
          obstruction T82.228
          perforation T82.228
          protrusion T82.228
        pain T82.847
        specified type NEC T82.897
        stenosis T82.857
        thrombosis T82.867
      prosthesis T82.9
        embolism T82.817
        fibrosis T82.827
        hemorrhage T82.837
        infection or inflammation T82.6
        mechanical T82.09
          breakdown T82.01
          displacement T82.02
          leakage T82.03
          malposition T82.02
          obstruction T82.09
          perforation T82.09
          protrusion T82.09

Complication (*Continued*)
  heart (*Continued*)
    valve (*Continued*)
      prosthesis (*Continued*)
        pain T82.847
        specified type NEC T82.897
          mechanical T82.09
        stenosis T82.857
        thrombosis T82.867
  hematoma
    intraoperative —*see* Complication,
      intraoperative, hemorrhage
    postprocedural —*see* Complication,
      postprocedural, hemorrhage
  hemodialysis —*see* Complications,
    dialysis
  hemorrhage
    intraoperative —*see* Complication,
      intraoperative, hemorrhage
    postprocedural —*see* Complication,
      postprocedural, hemorrhage
  ileostomy (stoma) —*see* Complications,
    enterostomy
  immunization (procedure) —*see*
    Complications, vaccination
  implant —*see also* Complications, by site and
    type
    urinary sphincter T83.9
      embolism T83.81
      fibrosis T83.82
      hemorrhage T83.83
      infection and inflammation T83.59
      mechanical
        breakdown T83.111
        displacement T83.121
        leakage T83.191
        malposition T83.121
        obstruction T83.191
        perforation T83.191
        protrusion T83.191
        specified NEC T83.191
      pain T83.84
      specified type NEC T83.89
      stenosis T83.85
      thrombosis T83.86
  infusion (procedure) T80.90
    air embolism T80.0
    blood —*see* Complications, transfusion
    catheter —*see* Complications, catheter
    infection T80.29
    pump —*see* Complications, cardiovascular,
      device or implant
    sepsis T80.29
    serum reaction (*see also* Reaction, serum)
      T80.69
      anaphylactic shock (*see also* Shock,
        anaphylactic) T80.59
    specified type NEC T80.89
  inhalation therapy NEC T81.81
  injection (procedure) T80.90
    drug reaction —*see* Reaction, drug
    infection T80.29
    sepsis T80.29
    serum (prophylactic) (therapeutic) —*see*
      Complications, vaccination
    specified type NEC T80.89
    vaccine (any) —*see* Complications,
      vaccination
  inoculation (any) —*see* Complications,
    vaccination
  insulin pump
    infection and inflammation T85.72
    mechanical
      breakdown T85.614
      displacement T85.624
      leakage T85.633
      malposition T85.624
      obstruction T85.694
      perforation T85.694
      protrusion T85.694
      specified NEC T85.694

Complication (*Continued*)
  intestinal pouch NEC K91.858
  intraocular lens (prosthetic) T85.9
    embolism T85.81
    fibrosis T85.82
    hemorrhage T85.83
    infection and inflammation T85.79
    mechanical
      breakdown T85.21
      displacement T85.22
      malposition T85.22
      obstruction T85.29
      perforation T85.29
      protrusion T85.29
      specified NEC T85.29
    pain T85.84
    specified type NEC T85.89
    stenosis T85.85
    thrombosis T85.86
  intraoperative (intraprocedural)
    cardiac arrest
      during cardiac surgery I97.710
      during other surgery I97.711
    cardiac functional disturbance NEC
      during cardiac surgery I97.790
      during other surgery I97.791
    hemorrhage (hematoma) (of)
      circulatory system organ or structure
        during cardiac bypass I97.411
        during cardiac catheterization I97.410
        during other circulatory system
          procedure I97.418
        during other procedure I97.42
      digestive system organ
        during procedure on digestive system
          K91.61
        during procedure on other organ
          K91.62
      ear
        during procedure on ear and mastoid
          process H95.21
        during procedure on other organ
          H95.22
      endocrine system organ or structure
        during procedure on endocrine
          system organ or structure E36.01
        during procedure on other organ
          E36.02
      eye and adnexa
        during ophthalmic procedure H59.11-
        during other procedure H59.12-
      genitourinary organ or structure
        during procedure on genitourinary
          organ or structure N99.61
        during procedure on other organ
          N99.62
      mastoid process
        during procedure on ear and mastoid
          process H95.21
        during procedure on other organ
          H95.22
      musculoskeletal structure
        during musculoskeletal surgery
          M96.810
        during non-orthopedic surgery
          M96.811
        during orthopedic surgery M96.810
      nervous system
        during a nervous system procedure
          G97.31
        during other procedure G97.32
      respiratory system
        during other procedure J95.62
        during procedure on respiratory
          system organ or structure
          J95.61
      skin and subcutaneous tissue
        during a dermatologic procedure
          L76.01
        during a procedure on other organ
          L76.02

Complication (Continued)
  intraoperative (Continued)
    hemorrhage (Continued)
      spleen
        during a procedure on other organ
          D78.02
        during a procedure on the spleen
          D78.01
    puncture or laceration (accidental)
      (unintentional) (of)
      brain
        during a nervous system procedure
          G97.48
        during other procedure G97.49
      circulatory system organ or structure
        during circulatory system procedure
          I97.51
        during other procedure I97.52
      digestive system
        during procedure on digestive system
          K91.71
        during procedure on other organ
          K91.72
      ear
        during procedure on ear and mastoid
          process H95.31
        during procedure on other organ
          H95.32
      endocrine system organ or structure
        during procedure on endocrine
          system organ or structure E36.11
        during procedure on other organ
          E36.12
      eye and adnexa
        during ophthalmic procedure H59.21-
        during other procedure H59.22-
      genitourinary organ or structure
        during procedure on genitourinary
          organ or structure N99.71
        during procedure on other organ
          N99.72
      mastoid process
        during procedure on ear and mastoid
          process H95.31
        during procedure on other organ
          H95.32
      musculoskeletal structure
        during musculoskeletal surgery
          M96.820
        during non-orthopedic surgery
          M96.821
        during orthopedic surgery M96.820
      nervous system
        during a nervous system procedure
          G97.48
        during other procedure G97.49
      respiratory system
        during other procedure J95.72
        during procedure on respiratory
          system organ or structure J95.71
      skin and subcutaneous tissue
        during a dermatologic procedure
          L76.11
        during a procedure on other organ
          L76.12
      spleen
        during a procedure on other organ
          D78.12
        during a procedure on the spleen
          D78.11
    specified NEC
      circulatory system I97.88
      digestive system K91.81
      ear H95.88
      endocrine system E36.8
      eye and adnexa H59.88
      genitourinary system N99.81
      mastoid process H95.88
      musculoskeletal structure M96.89
      nervous system G97.81
      respiratory system J95.88

Complication (Continued)
  intraoperative (Continued)
    specified NEC (Continued)
      skin and subcutaneous tissue L76.81
      spleen D78.81
  intraperitoneal catheter (dialysis)
    (infusion) —see Complications, catheter,
    intraperitoneal
  intrauterine
    contraceptive device
      embolism T83.81
      fibrosis T83.82
      hemorrhage T83.83
      infection and inflammation T83.6
      mechanical
        breakdown T83.31
        displacement T83.32
        malposition T83.32
        obstruction T83.39
        perforation T83.39
        protrusion T83.39
        specified NEC T83.39
      pain T83.84
      specified type NEC T83.89
      stenosis T83.85
      thrombosis T83.86
    procedure (fetal), to newborn P96.5
  jejunostomy (stoma) —see Complications,
    enterostomy
  joint prosthesis, internal T84.9
    breakage (fracture) T84.01-
    dislocation T84.02-
    fracture T84.01-
    infection or inflammation T84.50
      hip T84.5-
      knee T84.5-
      specified joint NEC T84.59
    instability T84.02-
    malposition —see Complications, joint
      prosthesis, mechanical,
      displacement
    mechanical
      breakage, broken T84.01-
      dislocation T84.02-
      fracture T84.01-
      instability T84.02-
      leakage —see Complications, joint
        prosthesis, mechanical, specified
        NEC
      loosening T84.039
        hip T84.03-
        knee T84.03-
        specified joint NEC T84.038
      obstruction —see Complications, joint
        prosthesis, mechanical, specified
        NEC
      perforation —see Complications, joint
        prosthesis, mechanical, specified
        NEC
      periprosthetic
        fracture T84.049
          hip T84.04-
          knee T84.04-
          other specified joint T84.048
        osteolysis T84.059
          hip T84.05-
          knee T84.05-
          other specified joint T84.058
      protrusion —see Complications, joint
        prosthesis, mechanical, specified
        NEC
      specified complication NEC T84.099
        hip T84.09-
        knee T84.09-
        other specified joint T84.098
      subluxation T84.02-
      wear of articular bearing surface
        T84.069
        hip T84.06-
        knee T84.06-
        other specified joint T84.068

Complication (Continued)
  joint prosthesis, internal (Continued)
    specified joint NEC T84.89
      embolism T84.81
      fibrosis T84.82
      hemorrhage T84.83
      pain T84.84
      specified complication NEC T84.89
      stenosis T84.85
      thrombosis T84.86
      subluxation T84.02-
  kidney transplant —see Complications,
    transplant, kidney
  labor O75.9
    specified NEC O75.89
  liver transplant (immune or nonimmune) —
    see Complications, transplant, liver
  lumbar puncture G97.1
    cerebrospinal fluid leak G97.0
    headache or reaction G97.1
  lung transplant —see Complications,
    transplant, lung
    and heart —see Complications, transplant,
      lung, with heart
  male genital N50.9
    device, implant or graft —see
      Complications, genitourinary, device
      or implant, genital tract
    postprocedural or postoperative —see
      Complications, genitourinary,
      postprocedural
    specified NEC N99.89
  mastoid (process) procedure
    intraoperative H95.88-
      hematoma —see Complications,
        intraoperative, hemorrhage
        (hematoma) (of), mastoid
        process
      hemorrhage —see Complications,
        intraoperative, hemorrhage
        (hematoma) (of), mastoid
        process
      laceration —see Complications,
        intraoperative, puncture or
        laceration..., mastoid process
      specified NEC H95.88-
    postmastoidectomy —see Complications,
      postmastoidectomy
    postoperative H95.89-
      external ear canal stenosis H95.81-
      hematoma —see Complications...,
        postprocedural, hemorrhage
        (hematoma) (of), mastoid
        process
      hemorrhage —see Complications...,
        postprocedural, hemorrhage
        (hematoma) (of), mastoid
        process
      postmastoidectomy —see Complications,
        postmastoidectomy
      specified NEC H95.89-
  mastoidectomy cavity —see Complications,
    postmastoidectomy
  mechanical —see Complications, by site and
    type, mechanical
  medical procedures (see also Complication(s),
    intraoperative) T88.9
  metabolic E88.9
    postoperative E89.89
    specified NEC E89.89
  molar pregnancy NOS O08.9
    damage to pelvic organs O08.6
    embolism O08.2
    genital infection O08.0
    hemorrhage (delayed) (excessive)
      O08.1
    metabolic disorder O08.5
    renal failure O08.4
    shock O08.3
    specified type NEC O08.0
    venous complication NEC O08.7

◀ New   ◀ Revised   deleted Deleted

Complication (*Continued*)
  musculoskeletal system —*see also*
    Complication, intraoperative
    (intraprocedural), by site
    device, implant or graft NEC —*see*
      Complications, orthopedic, device or
      implant
    internal fixation (nail) (plate) (rod) —*see*
      Complications, fixation device,
      internal
    joint prosthesis —*see* Complications, joint
      prosthesis
    postoperative (postprocedural) M96.89
      with osteoporosis —*see* Osteoporosis
      fracture following insertion of device —
        see Fracture, following insertion of
        orthopedic implant, joint prosthesis
        or bone plate
      joint instability after prosthesis removal
        M96.89
      lordosis M96.4
      postlaminectomy syndrome NEC
        M96.1
        kyphosis M96.3
      pseudarthrosis M96.0
      specified complication NEC M96.89
    post radiation M96.89
      kyphosis M96.3
      scoliosis M96.5
      specified complication NEC M96.89
  nephrostomy (stoma) —*see* Complications,
    stoma, urinary tract, external NEC
  nervous system G98.8
    central G96.9
    device, implant or graft —*see also*
      Complication, prosthetic device or
      implant, specified NEC
      electronic stimulator (electrode (s)) —
        see Complications, electronic
        stimulator device
      ventricular shunt —*see* Complications,
        ventricular shunt
    electronic stimulator (electrode (s)) —*see*
      Complications, electronic stimulator
      device
    postprocedural G97.82
      intracranial hypotension G97.2
      specified NEC G97.82
      spinal fluid leak G97.0
    newborn, due to intrauterine (fetal)
      procedure P96.5
  nonabsorbable (permanent) sutures —*see*
    Complication, sutures, permanent
  obstetric O75.9
    procedure (instrumental) (manual)
      (surgical) specified NEC O75.4
    specified NEC O75.89
    surgical wound NEC O90.89
      hematoma O90.2
      infection O86.0
  ocular lens implant —*see* Complications,
    intraocular lens
  ophthalmologic
    postprocedural bleb —*see* Blebitis
  orbital prosthesis T85.9
    embolism T85.81
    fibrosis T85.82
    hemorrhage T85.83
    infection and inflammation T85.79
    mechanical
      breakdown T85.31-
      displacement T85.32-
      malposition T85.32-
      obstruction T85.39-
      perforation T85.39-
      protrusion T85.39-
      specified NEC T85.39-
    pain T85.84
    specified type NEC T85.89
    stenosis T85.85
    thrombosis T85.86

Complication (*Continued*)
  organ or tissue transplant (partial) (total) —
    see Complications, transplant
  orthopedic —*see also* Disorder, soft tissue
    device or implant T84.9
      bone
        device or implant —*see* Complication,
          bone, device NEC
        graft —*see* Complication, graft, bone
      breakdown T84.418
      displacement T84.428
      electronic bone stimulator —*see*
        Complications, electronic
        stimulator device, bone
      embolism T84.81
      fibrosis T84.82
      fixation device —*see* Complication,
        fixation device, internal
      hemorrhage T84.83
      infection or inflammation T84.7
      joint prosthesis —*see* Complication, joint
        prosthesis, internal
      malfunction T84.418
      malposition T84.428
      mechanical NEC T84.498
      muscle graft —*see* Complications, graft,
        muscle
      obstruction T84.498
      pain T84.84
      perforation T84.498
      protrusion T84.498
      specified complication NEC T84.89
      stenosis T84.85
      tendon graft —*see* Complications, graft,
        tendon
      thrombosis T84.86
    fracture (following insertion of device) —
      see Fracture, following insertion of
      orthopedic implant, joint prosthesis
      or bone plate
    postprocedural M96.89
      fracture —*see* Fracture, following
        insertion of orthopedic implant,
        joint prosthesis or bone plate
      postlaminectomy syndrome NEC
        M96.1
        kyphosis M96.3
        lordosis M96.4
      postradiation
        kyphosis M96.2
        scoliosis M96.5
      pseudarthrosis post-fusion M96.0
      specified type NEC M96.89
  pacemaker (cardiac) —*see* Complications,
    cardiovascular device or implant,
    electronic
  pancreas transplant —*see* Complications,
    transplant, pancreas
  penile prosthesis (implant) —*see*
    Complications, prosthetic device,
    penile
  perfusion NEC T80.90
  perineal repair (obstetrical) NEC O90.89
    disruption O90.1
    hematoma O90.2
    infection (following delivery) O86.0
  phototherapy T88.9
    specified NEC T88.8
  postmastoidectomy NEC H95.19-
    cyst, mucosal H95.13-
    granulation H95.12-
    inflammation, chronic H95.11-
    recurrent cholesteatoma H95.0-
  postoperative —*see* Complications,
    postprocedural
    circulatory —*see* Complications, circulatory
      system
    ear —*see* Complications, ear
    endocrine —*see* Complications,
      endocrine
    eye —*see* Complications, eye

Complication (*Continued*)
  postoperative (*Continued*)
    lumbar puncture G97.1
      cerebrospinal fluid leak G97.0
    nervous system (central) (peripheral) —*see*
      Complications, nervous system
    respiratory system —*see* Complications,
      respiratory system
  postprocedural —*see also* Complications,
    surgical procedure
    cardiac arrest
      following cardiac surgery I97.120
      following other surgery I97.121
    cardiac functional disturbance NEC
      following cardiac surgery I97.190
      following other surgery I97.191
    cardiac insufficiency
      following cardiac surgery I97.110
      following other surgery I97.111
    chorioretinal scars following retinal
      surgery H59.81-
    following cataract surgery
      cataract (lens) fragments H59.02-
      cystoid macular edema H59.03-
      specified NEC H59.09-
      vitreous (touch) syndrome H59.01-
    heart failure
      following cardiac surgery I97.130
      following other surgery I97.131
    hemorrhage (hematoma) (of)
      circulatory system organ or structure
        following a cardiac bypass I97.611
        following a cardiac catheterization
          I97.610
        following other circulatory system
          procedure I97.618
        following other procedure I97.62
      digestive system
        following procedure on digestive
          system K91.840
        following procedure on other organ
          K91.841
      ear
        following other procedure H95.42
        following procedure on ear and
          mastoid process H95.41
      endocrine system
        following endocrine system
          procedure E89.810
        following other procedure
          E89.811
      eye and adnexa
        following ophthalmic procedure
          H59.31-
        following other procedure H59.32-
      genitourinary organ or structure
        following procedure on
          genitourinary organ or
          structure N99.820
        following procedure on other organ
          N99.821
      mastoid process
        following other procedure H95.42
        following procedure on ear and
          mastoid process H95.41
      musculoskeletal structure
        following musculoskeletal surgery
          M96.830
        following non-orthopedic surgery
          M96.831
        following orthopedic surgery
          M96.830
      nervous system
        following a nervous system procedure
          G97.51
        following other procedure G97.52
      respiratory system
        following other procedure J95.831
        following procedure on respiratory
          system organ or structure
          J95.830

Complication *(Continued)*
  postprocedural *(Continued)*
    hemorrhage *(Continued)*
      skin and subcutaneous tissue
        following a dermatologic procedure
          L76.21
        following a procedure on other organ
          L76.22
      spleen
        following procedure on other organ
          D78.22
        following procedure on the spleen
          D78.21
    specified NEC
      circulatory system I97.89
      digestive K91.89
      ear H95.89
      endocrine E89.89
      eye and adnexa H59.89
      genitourinary N99.89
      mastoid process H95.89
      metabolic E89.89
      musculoskeletal structure M96.89
      nervous system G97.82
      respiratory system J95.89
      skin and subcutaneous tissue L76.82
      spleen D78.89
  pregnancy NEC —*see* Pregnancy,
    complicated by
  prosthetic device or implant T85.9
    bile duct —*see* Complications, bile duct
      implant
    breast —*see* Complications, breast implant
    cardiac and vascular NEC —*see*
      Complications, cardiovascular
      device or implant
    corneal transplant —*see* Complications,
      graft, cornea
    electronic nervous system stimulator —*see*
      Complications, electronic stimulator
      device
    epidural infusion catheter —*see*
      Complications, catheter, epidural
    esophageal anti-reflux device —*see*
      Complications, esophageal anti-reflux
      device
    genital organ or tract —*see* Complications,
      genitourinary, device or implant,
      genital tract
    heart valve —*see* Complications, heart,
      valve, prosthesis
    infection or inflammation T85.79
      intestine transplant T86.892
      liver transplant T86.43
      lung transplant T86.812
      pancreas transplant T86.892
      skin graft T86.822
    intraocular lens —*see* Complications,
      intraocular lens
    intraperitoneal (dialysis) catheter —
      see Complications, catheter,
      intraperitoneal
    joint —*see* Complications, joint prosthesis,
      internal
    mechanical NEC T85.698
      dialysis catheter (vascular) —*see also*
        Complication, catheter, dialysis,
        mechanical
        peritoneal —*see* Complication,
          catheter, intraperitoneal,
          mechanical
      gastrointestinal device T85.598
      ocular device T85.398
      subdural (infusion) catheter T85.690
      suture, permanent T85.692
        that for bone repair —*see*
          Complications, fixation device,
          internal (orthopedic), mechanical
    ventricular shunt
      breakdown T85.01
      displacement T85.02
      leakage T85.03

Complication *(Continued)*
  prosthetic device or implant *(Continued)*
    mechanical NEC *(Continued)*
      ventricular shunt *(Continued)*
        malposition T85.02
        obstruction T85.09
        perforation T85.09
        protrusion T85.09
        specified NEC T85.09
    mesh
      erosion (to surrounding organ or tissue)
        T83.718
        vaginal (into pelvic floor muscles)
          T83.711
      exposure (into surrounding organ or
        tissue) T83.728
        vaginal (into vagina) (through vaginal
          wall) T83.721
    orbital —*see* Complications, orbital
      prosthesis
    penile T83.9
      embolism T83.81
      fibrosis T83.82
      hemorrhage T83.83
      infection and inflammation T83.6
      mechanical
        breakdown T83.410
        displacement T83.420
        leakage T83.490
        malposition T83.420
        obstruction T83.490
        perforation T83.490
        protrusion T83.490
        specified NEC T83.490
      pain T83.84
      specified type NEC T83.89
      stenosis T83.85
      thrombosis T83.86
    prosthetic materials NEC
      erosion (to surrounding organ or tissue)
        T83.718
        vaginal (into pelvic floor muscles)
          T83.711
      exposure (into surrounding organ or
        tissue) T83.728
        vaginal (into vagina) (through vaginal
          wall) T83.721
    skin graft T86.829
      artificial skin or decellularized
        allodermis
        embolism T85.81
        fibrosis T85.82
        hemorrhage T85.83
        infection and inflammation T85.79
        mechanical
          breakdown T85.613
          displacement T85.623
          malfunction T85.613
          malposition T85.623
          obstruction T85.693
          perforation T85.693
          protrusion T85.693
          specified NEC T85.693
        pain T85.84
        specified type NEC T85.89
        stenosis T85.85
        thrombosis T85.86
      failure T86.821
      infection T86.822
      rejection T86.820
      specified NEC T86.828
    specified NEC T85.9
      embolism T85.81
      fibrosis T85.82
      hemorrhage T85.83
      infection and inflammation T85.79
      mechanical
        breakdown T85.618
        displacement T85.628
        leakage T85.638
        malfunction T85.618
        malposition T85.628

Complication *(Continued)*
  prosthetic device or implant *(Continued)*
    specified NEC *(Continued)*
      mechanical *(Continued)*
        obstruction T85.698
        perforation T85.698
        protrusion T85.698
        specified NEC T85.698
      pain T85.84
      specified type NEC T85.89
      stenosis T85.85
      thrombosis T85.86
    subdural infusion catheter —*see*
      Complications, catheter, subdural
    sutures —*see* Complications, sutures
    urinary organ or tract NEC —*see*
      Complications, genitourinary, device
      or implant, urinary system
    vascular —*see* Complications,
      cardiovascular device or implant
    ventricular shunt —*see* Complications,
      ventricular shunt (device)
  puerperium —*see* Puerperal
  puncture, spinal G97.1
    cerebrospinal fluid leak G97.0
    headache or reaction G97.1
  pyelogram N99.89
  radiation
    kyphosis M96.2
    scoliosis M96.5
  reattached
    extremity (infection) (rejection)
      lower T87.1X-
      upper T87.0X-
    specified body part NEC T87.2
  reconstructed breast
    asymmetry between native and
      reconstructed breast N65.1
    deformity N65.0
    disproportion between native and
      reconstructed breast N65.1
    excess tissue N65.0
    misshappen N65.0
  reimplant NEC —*see also* Complications,
    prosthetic device or implant
    limb (infection) (rejection) —*see*
      Complications, reattached,
      extremity
    organ (partial) (total) —*see* Complications,
      transplant
    prosthetic device NEC —*see* Complications,
      prosthetic device
  renal N28.9
    allograft —*see* Complications, transplant,
      kidney
    dialysis —*see* Complications, dialysis
  respirator
    mechanical J95.850
      specified NEC J95.859
  respiratory system J98.9
    device, implant or graft —*see*
      Complication, prosthetic device or
      implant, specified NEC
    lung transplant —*see* Complications,
      prosthetic device or implant, lung
      transplant
    postoperative J95.89
      air leak J95.812
      Mendelson's syndrome (chemical
        pneumonitis) J95.4
      pneumothorax J95.811
      pulmonary insufficiency (acute) (after
        nonthoracic surgery) J95.2
        chronic J95.3
        following thoracic surgery J95.1
      respiratory failure (acute) J95.821
        acute and chronic J95.822
      specified NEC J95.89
      subglottic stenosis J95.5
      tracheostomy complication —*see*
        Complications, tracheostomy
  therapy T81.89

◀ New   ◀▥ Revised   ~~deleted~~ Deleted

Complication (*Continued*)
sedation during labor and delivery
O74.9
  cardiac O74.2
  central nervous system O74.3
  pulmonary NEC O74.1
shunt —*see also* Complications, prosthetic
  device or implant
  arteriovenous —*see* Complications,
    arteriovenous, shunt
  ventricular (communicating) —*see*
    Complications, ventricular shunt
skin
  graft T86.829
    failure T86.821
    infection T86.822
    rejection T86.820
    specified type NEC T86.828
spinal
  anesthesia —*see* Complications, anesthesia,
    spinal
  catheter (epidural) (subdural) —*see*
    Complications, catheter
  puncture or tap G97.1
    cerebrospinal fluid leak G97.0
    headache or reaction G97.1
stent
  bile duct —*see* Complications, bile duct
    prosthesis
  urinary T83.9
    embolism T83.81
    fibrosis T83.82
    hemorrhage T83.83
    infection and inflammation T83.59
    mechanical
      breakdown T83.112
      displacement T83.122
      leakage T83.192
      malposition T83.122
      obstruction T83.192
      perforation T83.192
      protrusion T83.192
      specified NEC T83.192
    pain T83.84
    specified type NEC T83.89
    stenosis T83.85
    thrombosis T83.86
stoma
  digestive tract
    colostomy —*see* Complications,
      colostomy
    enterostomy —*see* Complications,
      enterostomy
    esophagostomy —*see* Complications,
      esophagostomy
    gastrostomy —*see* Complications,
      gastrostomy
  urinary tract N99.538
    cystostomy —*see* Complications,
      cystostomy
    external NOS N99.528
      hemorrhage N99.520
      infection N99.521
      malfunction N99.522
      specified type NEC N99.528
    hemorrhage N99.530
    infection N99.531
    malfunction N99.532
    specified type NEC N99.538
stomach banding —*see* Complication (s),
  bariatric procedure
stomach stapling —*see* Complication (s),
  bariatric procedure
surgical material, nonabsorbable —*see*
  Complication, suture, permanent
surgical procedure (on) T81.9
  amputation stump (late) —*see*
    Complications, amputation
    stump
  cardiac —*see* Complications, circulatory
    system

Complication (*Continued*)
surgical procedure (*Continued*)
  cholesteatoma, recurrent —*see*
    Complications, postmastoidectomy,
    recurrent cholesteatoma
  circulatory (early) —*see* Complications,
    circulatory system
  digestive system —*see* Complications,
    gastrointestinal
  dumping syndrome (postgastrectomy)
    K91.1
  ear —*see* Complications, ear
  elephantiasis or lymphedema I97.89
    postmastectomy I97.2
  emphysema (surgical) T81.82
  endocrine —*see* Complications, endocrine
  eye —*see* Complications, eye
  fistula (persistent postoperative) T81.83
  foreign body inadvertently left in wound
    (sponge) (suture) (swab) —*see*
    Foreign body, accidentally left during
    a procedure
  gastrointestinal —*see* Complications,
    gastrointestinal
  genitourinary NEC N99.89
  hematoma
    intraoperative —*see* Complication,
      intraoperative, hemorrhage
    postprocedural —*see* Complication,
      postprocedural, hemorrhage
  hemorrhage
    intraoperative —*see* Complication,
      intraoperative, hemorrhage
    postprocedural —*see* Complication,
      postprocedural, hemorrhage
  hepatic failure K91.82
  hyperglycemia (postpancreatectomy) E89.1
  hypoinsulinemia (postpancreatectomy)
    E89.1
  hypoparathyroidism
    (postparathyroidectomy) E89.2
  hypopituitarism (posthypophysectomy)
    E89.3
  hypothyroidism (post-thyroidectomy)
    E89.0
  intestinal obstruction K91.3
  intracranial hypotension following
    ventricular shunting
    (ventriculostomy) G97.2
  lymphedema I97.89
    postmastectomy I97.2
  malabsorption (postsurgical) NEC K91.2
    osteoporosis —*see* Osteoporosis,
      postsurgical malabsorption
  mastoidectomy cavity NEC —*see*
    Complications, postmastoidectomy
  metabolic E89.89
    specified NEC E89.89
  musculoskeletal —*see* Complications,
    musculoskeletal system
  nervous system (central) (peripheral) —*see*
    Complications, nervous system
  ovarian failure E89.40
    asymptomatic E89.40
    symptomatic E89.41
  peripheral vascular —*see* Complications,
    surgical procedure, vascular
  postcardiotomy syndrome I97.0
  postcholecystectomy syndrome K91.5
  postcommissurotomy syndrome I97.0
  postgastrectomy dumping syndrome
    K91.1
  postlaminectomy syndrome NEC M96.1
    kyphosis M96.3
  postmastectomy lymphedema syndrome
    I97.2
  postmastoidectomy cholesteatoma —*see*
    Complications, postmastoidectomy,
    recurrent cholesteatoma
  postvagotomy syndrome K91.1
  postvalvulotomy syndrome I97.0

Complication (*Continued*)
surgical procedure (*Continued*)
  pulmonary insufficiency (acute) J95.2
    chronic J95.3
    following thoracic surgery J95.1
  reattached body part —*see* Complications,
    reattached
  respiratory —*see* Complications,
    respiratory system
  shock (hypovolemic) T81.19
  spleen (postoperative) D78.89
    intraoperative D78.81
  stitch abscess T81.4
  subglottic stenosis (postsurgical) J95.5
  testicular hypofunction E89.5
  transplant —*see* Complications, organ or
    tissue transplant
  urinary NEC N99.89
  vaginal vault prolapse (posthysterectomy)
    N99.3
  vascular (peripheral)
    artery T81.719
      mesenteric T81.710
      renal T81.711
      specified NEC T81.718
    vein T81.72
  wound infection T81.4
suture, permanent (wire) NEC T85.9
  with repair of bone —*see* Complications,
    fixation device, internal
  embolism T85.81
  fibrosis T85.82
  hemorrhage T85.83
  infection and inflammation T85.79
  mechanical
    breakdown T85.612
    displacement T85.622
    malfunction T85.612
    malposition T85.622
    obstruction T85.692
    perforation T85.692
    protrusion T85.692
    specified NEC T85.692
  pain T85.84
  specified type NEC T85.89
  stenosis T85.85
  thrombosis T85.86
tracheostomy J95.00
  granuloma J95.09
  hemorrhage J95.01
  infection J95.02
  malfunction J95.03
  mechanical J95.03
  obstruction J95.03
  specified type NEC J95.09
  tracheo-esophageal fistula J95.04
transfusion (blood) (lymphocytes) (plasma)
  T80.92
  air embolism T80.0
  circulatory overload E87.71
  febrile nonhemolytic transfusion reaction
    R50.84
  hemochromatosis E83.111
  hemolysis T80.89
  hemolytic reaction (antigen unspecified)
    T80.919
  incompatibility reaction (antigen
    unspecified) T80.919
    ABO T80.30
      delayed serologic (DSTR) T80.39
      hemolytic transfusion reaction
        (HTR) (unspecified time after
        transfusion) T80.319
        acute (AHTR) (less than 24 hours
          after transfusion) T80.310
        delayed (DHTR) (24 hours or more
          after transfusion) T80.311
      specified NEC T80.39
    acute (antigen unspecified) T80.910
    delayed (antigen unspecified) T80.911
    delayed serologic (DSTR) T80.89

Complication *(Continued)*
  transfusion *(Continued)*
    incompatibility reaction *(Continued)*
      Non-ABO (minor antigens (Duffy) (Kell)
        (Kidd) (Lewis) (M) (N) (P) (S)) T80.
        A0
      delayed serologic (DSTR) T80.A9
      hemolytic transfusion reaction
        (HTR) (unspecified time after
        transfusion) T80.A19
      acute (AHTR) (less than 24 hours
        after transfusion) T80.A10
      delayed (DHTR) (24 hours or more
        after transfusion) T80.A11
      specified NEC T80.A9
      Rh (antigens (C) (c) (D) (E) (e)) (factor)
        T80.40
      delayed serologic (DSTR) T80.49
      hemolytic transfusion reaction
        (HTR) (unspecified time after
        transfusion) T80.419
      acute (AHTR) (less than 24 hours
        after transfusion) T80.410
      delayed (DHTR) (24 hours or more
        after transfusion) T80.411
      specified NEC T80.49
    infection T80.29
      acute T80.22
    reaction NEC T80.89
    sepsis T80.29
    shock T80.89
  transplant T86.90
    bone T86.839
      failure T86.831
      infection T86.832
      rejection T86.830
      specified type NEC T86.838
    bone marrow T86.00
      failure T86.02
      infection T86.03
      rejection T86.01
      specified type NEC T86.09
    cornea T86.849
      failure T86.841
      infection T86.842
      rejection T86.840
      specified type NEC T86.848
    failure T86.92
    heart T86.20
      with lung T86.30
        cardiac allograft vasculopathy T86.290
        failure T86.32
        infection T86.33
        rejection T86.31
        specified type NEC T86.39
      failure T86.22
      infection T86.23
      rejection T86.21
      specified type NEC T86.298
    infection T86.93
    intestine T86.859
      failure T86.851
      infection T86.852
      rejection T86.850
      specified type NEC T86.858
    kidney T86.10
      failure T86.12
      infection T86.13
      rejection T86.11
      specified type NEC T86.19
    liver T86.40
      failure T86.42
      infection T86.43
      rejection T86.41
      specified type NEC T86.49
    lung T86.819
      with heart T86.30
        failure T86.32
        infection T86.33
        rejection T86.31
        specified type NEC T86.39

Complication *(Continued)*
  transplant *(Continued)*
    lung *(Continued)*
      failure T86.811
      infection T86.812
      rejection T86.810
      specified type NEC T86.818
    malignant neoplasm C80.2
    pancreas T86.899
      failure T86.891
      infection T86.892
      rejection T86.890
      specified type NEC T86.898
    peripheral blood stem cells T86.5
    post-transplant lymphoproliferative
      disorder (PTLD) D47.Z1
    rejection T86.91
    skin T86.829
      failure T86.821
      infection T86.822
      rejection T86.820
      specified type NEC T86.828
    specified
      tissue T86.899
        failure T86.891
        infection T86.892
        rejection T86.890
        specified type NEC T86.898
      type NEC T86.99
    stem cell (from peripheral blood) (from
      umbilical cord) T86.5
    umbilical cord stem cells T86.5
  trauma (early) T79.9
    specified NEC T79.8
  ultrasound therapy NEC T88.9
  umbilical cord NEC
    complicating delivery O69.9
      specified NEC O69.89
  umbrella device, vascular T82.9
    embolism T82.818
    fibrosis T82.828
    hemorrhage T82.838
    infection or inflammation T82.7
    mechanical
      breakdown T82.515
      displacement T82.525
      leakage T82.535
      malposition T82.525
      obstruction T82.595
      perforation T82.595
      protrusion T82.595
    pain T82.848
    specified type NEC T82.898
    stenosis T82.858
    thrombosis T82.868
  urethral catheter —*see* Complications,
    catheter, urethral, indwelling
  vaccination T88.1
    anaphylaxis NEC T80.52
    arthropathy —*see* Arthropathy,
      postimmunization
    cellulitis T88.0
    encephalitis or encephalomyelitis
      G04.02
    infection (general) (local) NEC T88.0
    meningitis G03.8
    myelitis G04.89
    protein sickness T80.62
    rash T88.1
    reaction (allergic) T88.1
      serum T80.62
    sepsis T88.0
    serum intoxication, sickness, rash,
      or other serum reaction NEC
      T80.62
      anaphylactic shock T80.52
    shock (allergic) (anaphylactic) T80.52
    vaccinia (generalized) (localized) T88.1
  vas deferens device or implant —*see*
    Complications, genitourinary, device or
    implant, genital tract

Complication *(Continued)*
  vascular I99.9
    device or implant T82.9
      embolism T82.818
      fibrosis T82.828
      hemorrhage T82.838
      infection or inflammation T82.7
      mechanical
        breakdown T82.519
          specified device NEC T82.518
        displacement T82.529
          specified device NEC T82.528
        leakage T82.539
          specified device NEC T82.538
        malposition T82.529
          specified device NEC T82.528
        obstruction T82.599
          specified device NEC T82.598
        perforation T82.599
          specified device NEC T82.598
        protrusion T82.599
          specified device NEC T82.598
      pain T82.848
      specified type NEC T82.898
      stenosis T82.858
      thrombosis T82.868
    dialysis catheter —*see* Complication,
      catheter, dialysis
    following infusion, therapeutic injection or
      transfusion T80.1
    graft T82.9
      embolism T82.818
      fibrosis T82.828
      hemorrhage T82.838
      mechanical
        breakdown T82.319
          aorta (bifurcation) T82.310
          carotid artery T82.311
          specified vessel NEC T82.318
        displacement T82.329
          aorta (bifurcation) T82.320
          carotid artery T82.321
          specified vessel NEC T82.328
        leakage T82.339
          aorta (bifurcation) T82.330
          carotid artery T82.331
          specified vessel NEC T82.338
        malposition T82.329
          aorta (bifurcation) T82.320
          carotid artery T82.321
          specified vessel NEC T82.328
        obstruction T82.399
          aorta (bifurcation) T82.390
          carotid artery T82.391
          specified vessel NEC T82.398
        perforation T82.399
          aorta (bifurcation) T82.390
          carotid artery T82.391
          specified vessel NEC T82.398
        protrusion T82.399
          aorta (bifurcation) T82.390
          carotid artery T82.391
          specified vessel NEC T82.398
      pain T82.848
      specified complication NEC T82.898
      stenosis T82.858
      thrombosis T82.868
    postoperative —*see* Complications,
      postoperative, circulatory
  vena cava device (filter) (sieve) (umbrella) —
    see Complications, umbrella device,
    vascular
  ventilation therapy NEC T81.81
  ventilator
    mechanical J95.850
      specified NEC J95.859
  ventricular (communicating) shunt (device)
    T85.9
    embolism T85.81
    fibrosis T85.82
    hemorrhage T85.83

◀ New   ◀▥ Revised   ~~deleted~~ Deleted

Complication (Continued)
  ventricular shunt (Continued)
    infection and inflammation T85.79
    mechanical
      breakdown T85.01
      displacement T85.02
      leakage T85.03
      malposition T85.02
      obstruction T85.09
      perforation T85.09
      protrusion T85.09
      specified NEC T85.09
    pain T85.84
    specified type NEC T85.89
    stenosis T85.85
    thrombosis T85.86
  wire suture, permanent (implanted) —see
    Complications, suture, permanent
Compressed air disease T70.3
Compression
  with injury - code by Nature of injury
  artery I77.1
    celiac, syndrome I77.4
  brachial plexus G54.0
  brain (stem) G93.5
    due to
      contusion (diffuse) —see Injury,
        intracranial, diffuse
        focal —see Injury, intracranial, focal
      injury NEC —see Injury, intracranial,
        diffuse
      traumatic —see Injury, intracranial,
        diffuse
  bronchus J98.09
  cauda equina G83.4
  celiac (artery) (axis) I77.4
  cerebral —see Compression, brain
  cervical plexus G54.2
  cord
    spinal —see Compression, spinal
    umbilical —see Compression, umbilical
      cord
  cranial nerve G52.9
    eighth —see subcategory H93.3
    eleventh G52.8
    fifth G50.8
    first G52.0
    fourth —see Strabismus, paralytic, fourth
      nerve
    ninth G52.1
    second —see Disorder, nerve, optic
    seventh G52.8
    sixth —see Strabismus, paralytic, sixth
      nerve
    tenth G52.2
    third —see Strabismus, paralytic, third
      nerve
    twelfth G52.3
  diver's squeeze T70.3
  during birth (newborn) P15.9
  esophagus K22.2
  eustachian tube —see Obstruction, eustachian
    tube, cartilaginous
  facies Q67.1
  fracture —see Fracture
  heart —see Disease, heart
  intestine —see Obstruction, intestine
  laryngeal nerve, recurrent G52.2
    with paralysis of vocal cords and larynx
      J38.00
      bilateral J38.02
      unilateral J38.01
  lumbosacral plexus G54.1
  lung J98.4
  lymphatic vessel I89.0
  medulla —see Compression, brain
  nerve (see also Disorder, nerve) G58.9
    arm NEC —see Mononeuropathy, upper
      limb
    axillary G54.0
    cranial —see Compression, cranial nerve

Compression (Continued)
  nerve (Continued)
    leg NEC —see Mononeuropathy, lower
      limb
    median (in carpal tunnel) —see Syndrome,
      carpal tunnel
    optic —see Disorder, nerve, optic
    plantar —see Lesion, nerve, plantar
    posterior tibial (in tarsal tunnel) —see
      Syndrome, tarsal tunnel
    root or plexus NOS (in) G54.9
      intervertebral disc disorder NEC —
        see Disorder, disc, with,
        radiculopathy
      with myelopathy —see Disorder, disc,
        with, myelopathy
      neoplastic disease (see also Neoplasm)
        D49.9 [G55]
      spondylosis —see Spondylosis, with
        radiculopathy
    sciatic (acute) —see Lesion, nerve, sciatic
    sympathetic G90.8
    traumatic —see Injury, nerve
    ulnar —see Lesion, nerve, ulnar
    upper extremity NEC —see
      Mononeuropathy, upper limb
  spinal (cord) G95.20
    by displacement of intervertebral disc
      NEC —see also Disorder, disc, with,
      myelopathy
    nerve root NOS G54.9
      due to displacement of intervertebral
        disc NEC —see Disorder, disc, with,
        radiculopathy
      with myelopathy —see Disorder, disc,
        with, myelopathy
    specified NEC G95.29
    spondylogenic (cervical) (lumbar,
      lumbosacral) (thoracic) —see
      Spondylosis, with myelopathy
      NEC
      anterior —see Syndrome, anterior, spinal
        artery, compression
      traumatic —see Injury, spinal cord, by
        region
  subcostal nerve (syndrome) —see
    Mononeuropathy, upper limb, specified
    NEC
  sympathetic nerve NEC G90.8
  syndrome T79.5
  trachea J39.8
  ulnar nerve (by scar tissue) —see Lesion,
    nerve, ulnar
  umbilical cord
    complicating delivery O69.2
      cord around neck O69.1
      prolapse O69.0
      specified NEC O69.2
  ureter N13.5
  vein I87.1
  vena cava (inferior) (superior) I87.1
Compulsion, compulsive
  gambling F63.0
  neurosis F42
  personality F60.5
  states F42
  swearing F42
    in Gilles de la Tourette's syndrome
      F95.2
  tics and spasms F95.9
Concato's disease (pericardial polyserositis)
  A19.9
  nontubercular I31.1
  pleural —see Pleurisy, with effusion
Concavity chest wall M95.4
Concealed penis Q55.69
Concern (normal) about sick person in family
  Z63.6
Concrescence (teeth) K00.2
Concretio cordis I31.1
  rheumatic I09.2

Concretion —see also Calculus
  appendicular K38.1
  canaliculus —see Dacryolith
  clitoris N90.89
  conjunctiva H11.12-
  eyelid —see Disorder, eyelid, specified type
    NEC
  lacrimal passages —see Dacryolith
  prepuce (male) N47.8
  salivary gland (any) K11.5
  seminal vesicle N50.8
  tonsil J35.8
Concussion (brain) (cerebral) (current) S06.0X-
  blast (air) (hydraulic) (immersion)
    (underwater)
      abdomen or thorax —see Injury, blast, by
        site
      ear with acoustic nerve injury —see Injury,
        nerve, acoustic, specified type NEC
  cauda equina S34.3
  conus medullaris S34.02
  ocular S05.8X-
  spinal (cord)
    cervical S14.0
    lumbar S34.01
    sacral S34.02
    thoracic S24.0
  syndrome F07.81
Condition —see Disease
Conditions arising in the perinatal period —
  see Newborn, affected by
Conduct disorder —see Disorder, conduct
Condyloma A63.0
  acuminatum A63.0
  gonorrheal A54.09
  latum A51.31
  syphilitic A51.31
    congenital A50.07
  venereal, syphilitic A51.31
Conflagration —see also Burn
  asphyxia (by inhalation of gases, fumes or
    vapors) —see also Table of Drugs and
    Chemicals T59.9-
Conflict (with) —see also Discord
  family Z73.9
  marital Z63.0
    involving divorce or estrangement Z63.5
  parent-child Z62.820
    parent-adopted child Z62.821
    parent-biological child Z62.820
    parent-foster child Z62.822
  social role NEC Z73.5
Confluent —see condition
Confusion, confused R41.0
  epileptic F05
  mental state (psychogenic) F44.89
  psychogenic F44.89
  reactive (from emotional stress, psychological
    trauma) F44.89
Confusional arousals G47.51
Congelation T69.9
Congenital —see also condition
  aortic septum Q25.4
  intrinsic factor deficiency D51.0
  malformation —see Anomaly
Congestion, congestive
  bladder N32.89
  bowel K63.89
  brain G93.89
  breast N64.59
  bronchial J98.09
  catarrhal J31.0
  chest R09.89
  chill, malarial —see Malaria
  circulatory NEC I99.8
  duodenum K31.89
  eye —see Hyperemia, conjunctiva
  facial, due to birth injury P15.4
  general R68.89
  glottis J37.0
  heart —see Failure, heart, congestive

Congestion, congestive (*Continued*)
  hepatic K76.1
  hypostatic (lung) —*see* Edema, lung
  intestine K63.89
  kidney N28.89
  labyrinth —*see* subcategory H83.8
  larynx J37.0
  liver K76.1
  lung R09.89
    active or acute —*see* Pneumonia
  malaria, malarial —*see* Malaria
  nasal R09.81
  nose R09.81
  orbit, orbital —*see also* Exophthalmos
    inflammatory (chronic) —*see* Inflammation,
      orbit
  ovary N83.8
  pancreas K86.8
  pelvic, female N94.89
  pleural J94.8
  prostate (active) N42.1
  pulmonary —*see* Congestion, lung
  renal N28.89
  retina H35.81
  seminal vesicle N50.1
  spinal cord G95.19
  spleen (chronic) D73.2
  stomach K31.89
  trachea —*see* Tracheitis
  urethra N36.8
  uterus N85.8
    with subinvolution N85.3
  venous (passive) I87.8
  viscera R68.89
Congestive —*see* Congestion
Conical
  cervix (hypertrophic elongation) N88.4
  cornea —*see* Keratoconus
  teeth K00.2
Conjoined twins Q89.4
Conjugal maladjustment Z63.0
  involving divorce or estrangement Z63.5
Conjunctiva —*see* condition
Conjunctivitis (staphylococcal) (streptococcal)
    NOS H10.9
  Acanthamoeba B60.12
  acute H10.3-
    atopic H10.1-
    chemical (*see also* Corrosion, cornea) H10.21-
    mucopurulent H10.02-
      follicular H10.01-
    pseudomembranous H10.22-
    serous except viral H10.23-
      viral —*see* Conjunctivitis, viral
    toxic H10.21-
  adenoviral (acute) (follicular) B30.1
  allergic (acute) —*see* Conjunctivitis, acute,
    atopic
    chronic H10.45
      vernal H10.44
  anaphylactic —*see* Conjunctivitis, acute,
    atopic
  Apollo B30.3
  atopic (acute) —*see* Conjunctivitis, acute,
    atopic
  Béal's B30.2
  blennorrhagic (gonococcal) (neonatorum)
    A54.31
  chemical (acute) (*see also* Corrosion, cornea)
    H10.21-
  chlamydial A74.0
    due to trachoma A71.1
    neonatal P39.1
  chronic (nodosa) (petrificans) (phlyctenular)
    H10.40-
    allergic H10.45
      vernal H10.44
    follicular H10.43-
    giant papillary H10.41-
    simple H10.42-
    vernal H10.44

Conjunctivitis (*Continued*)
  coxsackievirus 24 B30.3
  diphtheritic A36.86
  due to
    dust —*see* Conjunctivitis, acute, atopic
    filariasis B74.9
    mucocutaneous leishmaniasis B55.2
  enterovirus type 70 (hemorrhagic) B30.3
  epidemic (viral) B30.9
    hemorrhagic B30.3
  gonococcal (neonatorum) A54.31
  granular (trachomatous) A71.1
    sequelae (late effect) B94.0
  hemorrhagic (acute) (epidemic) B30.3
  herpes zoster B02.31
  in (due to)
    Acanthamoeba B60.12
    adenovirus (acute) (follicular) B30.1
    Chlamydia A74.0
    coxsackievirus 24 B30.3
    diphtheria A36.86
    enterovirus type 70 (hemorrhagic) B30.3
    filariasis B74.9
    gonococci A54.31
    herpes (simplex) virus B00.53
      zoster B02.31
    infectious disease NEC B99
    meningococci A39.89
    mucocutaneous leishmaniasis B55.2
    rosacea L71.9
    syphilis (late) A52.71
    zoster B02.31
  inclusion A74.0
  infantile P39.1
    gonococcal A54.31
  Koch-Weeks' —*see* Conjunctivitis, acute,
    mucopurulent
  light —*see* Conjunctivitis, acute, atopic
  ligneous —*see* Blepharoconjunctivitis,
    ligneous
  meningococcal A39.89
  mucopurulent —*see* Conjunctivitis, acute,
    mucopurulent
  neonatal P39.1
    gonococcal A54.31
  Newcastle B30.8
  of Béal B30.2
  parasitic
    filariasis B74.9
    mucocutaneous leishmaniasis B55.2
  Parinaud's H10.89
  petrificans H10.89
  rosacea L71.9
  specified NEC H10.89
  swimming-pool B30.1
  trachomatous A71.1
    acute A71.0
    sequelae (late effect) B94.0
  traumatic NEC H10.89
  tuberculous A18.59
  tularemic A21.1
  tularensis A21.1
  viral B30.9
    due to
      adenovirus B30.1
      enterovirus B30.3
    specified NEC B30.8
Conjunctivochalasis H11.82-
Connective tissue —*see* condition
Conn's syndrome E26.01
Conradi (-Hunermann) **disease** Q77.3
Consanguinity Z84.3
  counseling Z71.89
Conscious simulation (of illness) Z76.5
Consecutive —*see* condition
Consolidation lung (base) —*see* Pneumonia,
    lobar
Constipation (atonic) (neurogenic) (simple)
    (spastic) K59.00
  drug-induced —*see* Table of Drugs and
    Chemicals

Constipation (*Continued*)
  outlet dysfunction K59.02
  psychogenic F45.8
  slow transit K59.01
  specified NEC K59.09
Constitutional —*see also* condition
  substandard F60.7
Constitutionally substandard F60.7
Constriction —*see also* Stricture
  auditory canal —*see* Stenosis, external ear
    canal
  bronchial J98.09
  duodenum K31.5
  esophagus K22.2
  external
    abdomen, abdominal (wall) S30.841
    alveolar process S00.542
    ankle S90.54-
    antecubital space —*see* Constriction,
      external, forearm
    arm (upper) S40.84-
    auricle —*see* Constriction, external, ear
    axilla —*see* Constriction, external, arm
    back, lower S30.840
    breast S20.14-
    brow S00.84
    buttock S30.840
    calf —*see* Constriction, external, leg
    canthus —*see* Constriction, external, eyelid
    cheek S00.84
      internal S00.542
    chest wall —*see* Constriction, external,
      thorax
    chin S00.84
    clitoris S30.844
    costal region —*see* Constriction, external,
      thorax
    digit (s)
      foot —*see* Constriction, external, toe
      hand —*see* Constriction, external, finger
    ear S00.44-
    elbow S50.34-
    epididymis S30.843
    epigastric region S30.841
    esophagus, cervical S10.14
    eyebrow —*see* Constriction, external, eyelid
    eyelid S00.24-
    face S00.84
    finger (s) S60.44-
      index S60.44-
      little S60.44-
      middle S60.44-
      ring S60.44-
    flank S30.841
    foot (except toe (s) alone) S90.84-
      toe —*see* Constriction, external, toe
    forearm S50.84-
      elbow only —*see* Constriction, external,
        elbow
    forehead S00.84
    genital organs, external
      female S30.846
      male S30.845
    groin S30.841
    gum S00.542
    hand S60.54-
    head S00.94
      ear —*see* Constriction, external, ear
      eyelid —*see* Constriction, external, eyelid
      lip S00.541
      nose S00.34
      oral cavity S00.542
      scalp S00.04
      specified site NEC S00.84
    heel —*see* Constriction, external, foot
    hip S70.24-
    inguinal region S30.841
    interscapular region S20.449
    jaw S00.84
    knee S80.24-
    labium (majus) (minus) S30.844

◀ New   ◀⊞ Revised   ~~deleted~~ Deleted

Constriction (*Continued*)
external (*Continued*)
larynx S10.14
leg (lower) S80.84-
knee —*see* Constriction, external, knee
upper —*see* Constriction, external, thigh
lip S00.541
lower back S30.840
lumbar region S30.840
malar region S00.84
mammary —*see* Constriction, external, breast
mastoid region S00.84
mouth S00.542
nail
finger —*see* Constriction, external, finger
toe —*see* Constriction, external, toe
nasal S00.34
neck S10.94
specified site NEC S10.84
throat S10.14
nose S00.34
occipital region S00.04
oral cavity S00.542
orbital region —*see* Constriction, external, eyelid
palate S00.542
palm —*see* Constriction, external, hand
parietal region S00.04
pelvis S30.840
penis S30.842
perineum
female S30.844
male S30.840
periocular area —*see* Constriction, external, eyelid
phalanges
finger —*see* Constriction, external, finger
toe —*see* Constriction, external, toe
pharynx S10.14
pinna —*see* Constriction, external, ear
popliteal space —*see* Constriction, external, knee
prepuce S30.842
pubic region S30.840
pudendum
female S30.846
male S30.845
sacral region S30.840
scalp S00.04
scapular region —*see* Constriction, external, shoulder
scrotum S30.843
shin —*see* Constriction, external, leg
shoulder S40.24-
sternal region S20.349
submaxillary region S00.84
submental region S00.84
subungual
finger (s) —*see* Constriction, external, finger
toe (s) —*see* Constriction, external, toe
supraclavicular fossa S10.84
supraorbital S00.84
temple S00.84
temporal region S00.84
testis S30.843
thigh S70.34-
thorax, thoracic (wall) S20.94
back S20.44-
front S20.34-
throat S10.14
thumb S60.34-
toe (s) (lesser) S90.44-
great S90.44-
tongue S00.542
trachea S10.14
tunica vaginalis S30.843
uvula S00.542

Constriction (*Continued*)
external (*Continued*)
vagina S30.844
vulva S30.844
wrist S60.84-
gallbladder —*see* Obstruction, gallbladder
intestine —*see* Obstruction, intestine
larynx J38.6
congenital Q31.8
specified NEC Q31.8
subglottic Q31.1
organ or site, congenital NEC —*see* Atresia, by site
prepuce (acquired) (congenital) N47.1
pylorus (adult hypertrophic) K31.1
congenital or infantile Q40.0
newborn Q40.0
ring dystocia (uterus) O62.4
spastic —*see also* Spasm
ureter N13.5
ureter N13.5
with infection N13.6
urethra —*see* Stricture, urethra
visual field (peripheral) (functional) —*see* Defect, visual field
Constrictive —*see* condition
Consultation
without complaint or sickness Z71.9
feared complaint unfounded Z71.1
specified reason NEC Z71.89
medical —*see* Counseling, medical
religious Z71.81
specified reason NEC Z71.89
spiritual Z71.81
Consumption —*see* Tuberculosis
Contact (with) —*see also* Exposure (to)
acariasis Z20.7
AIDS virus Z20.6
air pollution Z77.110
algae and algae toxins Z77.121
algae bloom Z77.121
anthrax Z20.810
aromatic (hazardous) compounds NEC Z77.028
aromatic amines Z77.020
aromatic dyes NOS Z77.028
arsenic Z77.010
asbestos Z77.090
bacterial disease NEC Z20.818
benzene Z77.021
blue-green algae bloom Z77.121
body fluids (potentially hazardous) Z77.21
brown tide Z77.121
chemicals (chiefly nonmedicinal) (hazardous) NEC Z77.098
cholera Z20.09
chromium compounds Z77.018
communicable disease Z20.9
bacterial NEC Z20.818
specified NEC Z20.89
viral NEC Z20.828
cyanobacteria bloom Z77.121
dyes Z77.098
Escherichia coli (E. coli) Z20.01
fiberglass —*see* Table of Drugs and Chemicals, fiberglass
German measles Z20.4
gonorrhea Z20.2
hazardous metals NEC Z77.018
hazardous substances NEC Z77.29
hazards in the physical environment NEC Z77.128
hazards to health NEC Z77.9
HIV Z20.6
HTLV-III/LAV Z20.6
human immunodeficiency virus (HIV) Z20.6
infection Z20.9
specified NEC Z20.89
infestation (parasitic) NEC Z20.7
intestinal infectious disease NEC Z20.09
Escherichia coli (E. coli) Z20.01

Contact (*Continued*)
lead Z77.011
meningococcus Z20.811
mold (toxic) Z77.120
nickel dust Z77.018
noise Z77.122
parasitic disease Z20.7
pediculosis Z20.7
pfiesteria piscicida Z77.121
poliomyelitis Z20.89
pollution
air Z77.110
environmental NEC Z77.118
soil Z77.112
water Z77.111
polycyclic aromatic hydrocarbons Z77.028
rabies Z20.3
radiation, naturally occurring NEC Z77.123
radon Z77.123
red tide (Florida) Z77.121
rubella Z20.4
sexually-transmitted disease Z20.2
smallpox (laboratory) Z20.89
syphilis Z20.2
tuberculosis Z20.1
uranium Z77.012
varicella Z20.820
venereal disease Z20.2
viral disease NEC Z20.828
viral hepatitis Z20.5
water pollution Z77.111
Contamination, food —*see* Intoxication, foodborne
Contraception, contraceptive
advice Z30.09
counseling Z30.09
device (intrauterine) (in situ) Z97.5
causing menorrhagia T83.83
checking Z30.431
complications —*see* Complications, intrauterine, contraceptive device
in place Z97.5
initial prescription Z30.014
reinsertion Z30.433
removal Z30.432
replacement Z30.433
emergency (postcoital) Z30.012
initial prescription Z30.019
injectable Z30.013
intrauterine device Z30.014
pills Z30.011
postcoital (emergency) Z30.012
specified type NEC Z30.018
subdermal implantable Z30.019
maintenance Z30.40
examination Z30.8
injectable Z30.42
intrauterine device Z30.431
pills Z30.41
specified type NEC Z30.49
subdermal implantable Z30.49
management Z30.9
specified NEC Z30.8
postcoital (emergency) Z30.012
prescription Z30.019
repeat Z30.40
sterilization Z30.2
surveillance (drug) —*see* Contraception, maintenance
Contraction (s), **contracture, contracted**
Achilles tendon —*see also* Short, tendon, Achilles
congenital Q66.89
amputation stump (surgical) (flexion) (late) next proximal joint T87.89
anus K59.8
bile duct (common) (hepatic) K83.8
bladder N32.89
neck or sphincter N32.0
bowel, cecum, colon or intestine, any part — *see* Obstruction, intestine

Contraction, contracture, contracted
(Continued)
　Braxton Hicks —*see* False, labor
　breast implant, capsular T85.44
　bronchial J98.09
　burn (old) —*see* Cicatrix
　cervix —*see* Stricture, cervix
　cicatricial —*see* Cicatrix
　conjunctiva, trachomatous, active A71.1
　　sequelae (late effect) B94.0
　Dupuytren's M72.0
　eyelid —*see* Disorder, eyelid function
　fascia (lata) (postural) M72.8
　　Dupuytren's M72.0
　　palmar M72.0
　　plantar M72.2
　finger NEC —*see also* Deformity, finger
　　congenital Q68.1
　　joint —*see* Contraction, joint, hand
　flaccid —*see* Contraction, paralytic
　gallbladder K82.0
　heart valve —*see* Endocarditis
　hip —*see* Contraction, joint, hip
　hourglass
　　bladder N32.89
　　　congenital Q64.79
　　gallbladder K82.0
　　　congenital Q44.1
　　stomach K31.89
　　　congenital Q40.2
　　　psychogenic F45.8
　　uterus (complicating delivery) O62.4
　hysterical F44.4
　internal os —*see* Stricture, cervix
　joint (abduction) (acquired) (adduction)
　　　(flexion) (rotation) M24.50
　　ankle M24.57-
　　congenital NEC Q68.8
　　　hip Q65.89
　　elbow M24.52-
　　foot joint M24.57-
　　hand joint M24.54-
　　hip M24.55-
　　　congenital Q65.89
　　hysterical F44.4
　　knee M24.56-
　　shoulder M24.51-
　　wrist M24.53-
　kidney (granular) (secondary) N26.9
　　congenital Q63.8
　　hydronephritic —*see* Hydronephrosis
　　　Page N26.2
　　pyelonephritic —*see* Pyelitis, chronic
　　tuberculous A18.11
　ligament —*see also* Disorder, ligament
　　congenital Q79.8
　muscle (postinfective) (postural) NEC M62.40
　　with contracture of joint —*see* Contraction,
　　　joint
　　ankle M62.47-
　　congenital Q79.8
　　　sternocleidomastoid Q68.0
　　extraocular —*see* Strabismus
　　eye (extrinsic) —*see* Strabismus
　　foot M62.47-
　　forearm M62.43-
　　hand M62.44-
　　hysterical F44.4
　　ischemic (Volkmann's) T79.6
　　lower leg M62.46-
　　multiple sites M62.49
　　pelvic region M62.45-
　　posttraumatic —*see* Strabismus, paralytic
　　psychogenic F45.8
　　　conversion reaction F44.4
　　shoulder region M62.41-
　　specified site NEC M62.48
　　thigh M62.45-
　　upper arm M62.42-
　neck —*see* Torticollis
　ocular muscle —*see* Strabismus

Contraction, contracture, contracted
(Continued)
　organ or site, congenital NEC —*see* Atresia,
　　by site
　outlet (pelvis) —*see* Contraction, pelvis
　palmar fascia M72.0
　paralytic
　　joint —*see* Contraction, joint
　　muscle —*see also* Contraction, muscle NEC
　　　ocular —*see* Strabismus, paralytic
　pelvis (acquired) (general) M95.5
　　with disproportion (fetopelvic) O33.1
　　　causing obstructed labor O65.1
　　　inlet O33.2
　　　mid-cavity O33.3
　　　outlet O33.3
　plantar fascia M72.2
　premature
　　atrium I49.1
　　auriculoventricular I49.49
　　heart I49.49
　　junctional I49.2
　　supraventricular I49.1
　　ventricular I49.3
　prostate N42.89
　pylorus NEC —*see also* Pylorospasm
　　psychogenic F45.8
　rectum, rectal (sphincter) K59.8
　ring (Bandl's) (complicating delivery) O62.4
　scar —*see* Cicatrix
　spine —*see* Dorsopathy, deforming
　sternocleidomastoid (muscle), congenital
　　Q68.0
　stomach K31.89
　　hourglass K31.89
　　　congenital Q40.2
　　　psychogenic F45.8
　　psychogenic F45.8
　tendon (sheath) M62.40
　　with contracture of joint —*see* Contraction,
　　　joint
　　Achilles —*see* Short, tendon, Achilles
　　ankle M62.47-
　　　Achilles —*see* Short, tendon, Achilles
　　foot M62.47-
　　forearm M62.43-
　　hand M62.44-
　　lower leg M62.46-
　　multiple sites M62.49
　　neck M62.48
　　pelvic region M62.45-
　　shoulder region M62.41-
　　specified site NEC M62.48
　　thigh M62.45-
　　thorax M62.48
　　trunk M62.48
　　upper arm M62.42-
　toe —*see* Deformity, toe, specified NEC
　ureterovesical orifice (postinfectional) N13.5
　　with infection N13.6
　urethra —*see also* Stricture, urethra
　　orifice N32.0
　uterus N85.8
　　abnormal NEC O62.9
　　clonic (complicating delivery) O62.4
　　dyscoordinate (complicating delivery) O62.4
　　hourglass (complicating delivery) O62.4
　　hypertonic O62.4
　　hypotonic NEC O62.2
　　inadequate
　　　primary O62.0
　　　secondary O62.1
　　incoordinate (complicating delivery) O62.4
　　poor O62.2
　　tetanic (complicating delivery) O62.4
　vagina (outlet) N89.5
　vesical N32.89
　　neck or urethral orifice N32.0
　visual field —*see* Defect, visual field,
　　generalized
　Volkmann's (ischemic) T79.6

Contusion (skin surface intact) T14.8
　abdomen, abdominal (muscle) (wall) S30.1
　adnexa, eye NEC S05.8X-
　adrenal gland S37.812
　alveolar process S00.532
　ankle S90.0-
　antecubital space —*see* Contusion, forearm
　anus S30.3
　arm (upper) S40.02-
　　lower (with elbow) —*see* Contusion,
　　　forearm
　auditory canal —*see* Contusion, ear
　auricle —*see* Contusion, ear
　axilla —*see* Contusion, arm, upper
　back —*see also* Contusion, thorax, back
　　lower S30.0
　bile duct S36.13
　bladder S37.22
　bone NEC T14.8
　brain (diffuse) —*see* Injury, intracranial, diffuse
　　focal —*see* Injury, intracranial, focal
　brainstem S06.38-
　breast S20.0-
　broad ligament S37.892
　brow S00.83
　buttock S30.0
　canthus, eye S00.1-
　cauda equina S34.3
　cerebellar, traumatic S06.37-
　cerebral S06.33-
　　left side S06.32-
　　right side S06.31-
　cheek S00.83
　　internal S00.532
　chest (wall) —*see* Contusion, thorax
　chin S00.83
　clitoris S30.23
　colon —*see* Injury, intestine, large, contusion
　common bile duct S36.13
　conjunctiva S05.1-
　　with foreign body (in conjunctival sac) —
　　　see Foreign body, conjunctival sac
　conus medullaris (spine) S34.139
　cornea —*see* Contusion, eyeball
　　with foreign body —*see* Foreign body,
　　　cornea
　corpus cavernosum S30.21
　cortex (brain) (cerebral) —*see* Injury,
　　intracranial, diffuse
　　focal —*see* Injury, intracranial, focal
　costal region —*see* Contusion, thorax
　cystic duct S36.13
　diaphragm S27.802
　duodenum S36.420
　ear S00.43-
　elbow S50.0-
　　with forearm —*see* Contusion, forearm
　epididymis S30.22
　epigastric region S30.1
　epiglottis S10.0
　esophagus (thoracic) S27.812
　　cervical S10.0
　eyeball S05.1-
　eyebrow S00.1-
　eyelid (and periocular area) S00.1-
　face NEC S00.83
　fallopian tube S37.529
　　bilateral S37.522
　　unilateral S37.521
　femoral triangle S30.1
　finger (s) S60.00
　　with damage to nail (matrix) S60.10
　　index S60.02-
　　　with damage to nail S60.12-
　　little S60.05-
　　　with damage to nail S60.15-
　　middle S60.03-
　　　with damage to nail S60.13-
　　ring S60.04-
　　　with damage to nail S60.14-
　　thumb —*see* Contusion, thumb

◀ New　◀⁗ Revised　~~deleted~~ Deleted

Contusion (Continued)
- flank S30.1
- foot (except toe (s) alone) S90.3-
  - toe —see Contusion, toe
- forearm S50.1-
  - elbow only —see Contusion, elbow
- forehead S00.83
- gallbladder S36.122
- genital organs, external
  - female S30.202
  - male S30.201
- globe (eye) —see Contusion, eyeball
- groin S30.1
- gum S00.532
- hand S60.22-
  - finger (s) —see Contusion, finger
  - wrist —see Contusion, wrist
- head S00.93
  - ear —see Contusion, ear
  - eyelid —see Contusion, eyelid
  - lip S00.531
  - nose S00.33
  - oral cavity S00.532
  - scalp S00.03
  - specified part NEC S00.83
- heel —see Contusion, foot
- hepatic duct S36.13
- hip S70.0-
- ileum S36.428
- iliac region S30.1
- inguinal region S30.1
- interscapular region S20.229
- intra-abdominal organ S36.92
  - colon —see Injury, intestine, large, contusion
  - liver S36.112
  - pancreas —see Contusion, pancreas
  - rectum S36.62
  - small intestine —see Injury, intestine, small, contusion
  - specified organ NEC S36.892
  - spleen —see Contusion, spleen
  - stomach S36.32
- iris (eye) —see Contusion, eyeball
- jaw S00.83
- jejunum S36.428
- kidney S37.01-
  - major (greater than 2 cm) S37.02-
  - minor (less than 2 cm) S37.01-
- knee S80.0-
- labium (majus) (minus) S30.23
- lacrimal apparatus, gland or sac S05.8X-
- larynx S10.0
- leg (lower) S80.1-
  - knee —see Contusion, knee
- lens —see Contusion, eyeball
- lip S00.531
- liver S36.112
- lower back S30.0
- lumbar region S30.0
- lung S27.329
  - bilateral S27.322
  - unilateral S27.321
- malar region S00.83
- mastoid region S00.83
- membrane, brain —see Injury, intracranial, diffuse
  - focal —see Injury, intracranial, focal
- mesentery S36.892
- mesosalpinx S37.892
- mouth S00.532
- muscle —see Contusion, by site
- nail
  - finger —see Contusion, finger, with damage to nail
  - toe —see Contusion, toe, with damage to nail
- nasal S00.33
- neck S10.93
  - specified site NEC S10.83
  - throat S10.0

Contusion (Continued)
- nerve —see Injury, nerve
- newborn P54.5
- nose S00.33
- occipital
  - lobe (brain) —see Injury, intracranial, diffuse
    - focal —see Injury, intracranial, focal
  - region (scalp) S00.03
- orbit (region) (tissues) S05.1-
- ovary S37.429
  - bilateral S37.422
  - unilateral S37.421
- palate S00.532
- pancreas S36.229
  - body S36.221
  - head S36.220
  - tail S36.222
- parietal
  - lobe (brain) —see Injury, intracranial, diffuse
    - focal —see Injury, intracranial, focal
  - region (scalp) S00.03
- pelvic organ S37.92
  - adrenal gland S37.812
  - bladder S37.22
  - fallopian tube —see Contusion, fallopian tube
  - kidney —see Contusion, kidney
  - ovary —see Contusion, ovary
  - prostate S37.822
  - specified organ NEC S37.892
  - ureter S37.12
  - urethra S37.32
  - uterus S37.62
- pelvis S30.0
- penis S30.21
- perineum
  - female S30.23
  - male S30.0
- periocular area S00.1-
- peritoneum S36.81
- periurethral tissue —see Contusion, urethra
- pharynx S10.0
- pinna —see Contusion, ear
- popliteal space —see Contusion, knee
- prepuce S30.21
- prostate S37.822
- pubic region S30.1
- pudendum
  - female S30.202
  - male S30.201
- quadriceps femoris —see Contusion, thigh
- rectum S36.62
- retroperitoneum S36.892
- round ligament S37.892
- sacral region S30.0
- scalp S00.03
  - due to birth injury P12.3
- scapular region —see Contusion, shoulder
- sclera —see Contusion, eyeball
- scrotum S30.22
- seminal vesicle S37.892
- shoulder S40.01-
- skin NEC T14.8
- small intestine —see Injury, intestine, small, contusion
- spermatic cord S30.22
- spinal cord —see Injury, spinal cord, by region
  - cauda equina S34.3
  - conus medullaris S34.139
- spleen S36.029
  - major S36.021
  - minor S36.020
- sternal region S20.219
- stomach S36.32
- subconjunctival S05.1-
- subcutaneous NEC T14.8

Contusion (Continued)
- submaxillary region S00.83
- submental region S00.83
- subperiosteal NEC T14.8
- subungual
  - finger —see Contusion, finger, with damage to nail
  - toe —see Contusion, toe, with damage to nail
- supraclavicular fossa S10.83
- supraorbital S00.83
- suprarenal gland S37.812
- temple (region) S00.83
- temporal
  - lobe (brain) —see Injury, intracranial, diffuse
    - focal —see Injury, intracranial, focal
  - region S00.83
- testis S30.22
- thigh S70.1-
- thorax (wall) S20.20
  - back S20.22-
  - front S20.21-
- throat S10.0
- thumb S60.01-
  - with damage to nail S60.11-
- toe (s) (lesser) S90.12-
  - with damage to nail S90.22-
  - great S90.11-
    - with damage to nail S90.21-
    - specified type NEC S90.221
- tongue S00.532
- trachea (cervical) S10.0
  - thoracic S27.52
- tunica vaginalis S30.22
- tympanum, tympanic membrane —see Contusion, ear
- ureter S37.12
- urethra S37.32
- urinary organ NEC S37.892
- uterus S37.62
- uvula S00.532
- vagina S30.23
- vas deferens S37.892
- vesical S37.22
- vocal cord (s) S10.0
- vulva S30.23
- wrist S60.21-
Conus (congenital) (any type) Q14.8
- cornea —see Keratoconus
- medullaris syndrome G95.81
Conversion hysteria, neurosis or reaction F44.9
Converter, tuberculosis (test reaction) R76.11
Conviction (legal), **anxiety concerning** Z65.0
- with imprisonment Z65.1
Convulsions (idiopathic) (see also Seizure (s)) R56.9
- apoplectiform (cerebral ischemia) I67.82
- benign neonatal (familial) —see Epilepsy, generalized, idiopathic
- dissociative F44.5
- epileptic —see Epilepsy
- epileptiform, epileptoid —see Seizure, epileptiform
- ether (anesthetic) —see Table of Drugs and Chemicals, by drug
- febrile R56.00
  - with status epilepticus G40.901
  - complex R56.01
    - with status epilepticus G40.901
  - simple R56.00
- hysterical F44.5
- infantile P90
  - epilepsy —see Epilepsy
- jacksonian —see Epilepsy, localization-related, symptomatic, with simple partial seizures
- myoclonic G25.3
- neonatal, benign (familial) —see Epilepsy, generalized, idiopathic
- newborn P90

Convulsions *(Continued)*
  obstetrical (nephritic) (uremic) —*see*
    Eclampsia
  paretic A52.17
  post traumatic R56.1
  psychomotor —*see* Epilepsy, localization-
    related, symptomatic, with complex
    partial seizures
  recurrent R56.9
  reflex R25.8
  scarlatinal A38.8
  tetanus, tetanic —*see* Tetanus
  thymic E32.8
Convulsive —*see also* Convulsions
Cooley's anemia D56.1
Coolie itch B76.9
Cooper's
  disease —*see* Mastopathy, cystic
  hernia —*see* Hernia, abdomen, specified site
    NEC
Copra itch B88.0
Coprophagy F50.8
Coprophobia F40.298
Coproporphyria, hereditary E80.29
Cor
  biloculare Q20.8
  bovis, bovinum —*see* Hypertrophy, cardiac
  pulmonale (chronic) I27.81
    acute I26.09
  triatriatum, triatrium Q24.2
  triloculare Q20.8
    biatrium Q20.4
    biventriculare Q21.1
Corbus' disease (gangrenous balanitis) N48.1
Cord —*see also* condition
  around neck (tightly) (with compression)
    complicating delivery O69.1
  bladder G95.89
    tabetic A52.19
Cordis ectopia Q24.8
Corditis (spermatic) N49.1
Corectopia Q13.2
Cori's disease (glycogen storage) E74.03
Corkhandler's disease or lung J67.3
Corkscrew esophagus K22.4
Corkworker's disease or lung J67.3
Corn (infected) L84
Cornea —*see also* condition
  donor Z52.5
  plana Q13.4
Cornelia de Lange syndrome Q87.1
Cornu cutaneum L85.8
Cornual gestation or pregnancy O00.8
Coronary (artery) —*see* condition
Coronavirus, as cause of disease classified
  elsewhere B97.29
  SARS-associated B97.21
Corpora —*see also* condition
  amylacea, prostate N42.89
  cavernosa —*see* condition
Corpulence —*see* Obesity
Corpus —*see* condition
Corrected transposition Q20.5
Corrosion (injury) (acid) (caustic) (chemical)
  (lime) (external) (internal) T30.4
  abdomen, abdominal (muscle) (wall) T21.42
    first degree T21.52
    second degree T21.62
    third degree T21.72
  above elbow T22.439
    first degree T22.539
    left T22.432
      first degree T22.532
      second degree T22.632
      third degree T22.732
    right T22.431
      first degree T22.531
      second degree T22.631
      third degree T22.731
    second degree T22.639
    third degree T22.739

Corrosion *(Continued)*
  alimentary tract NEC T28.7
  ankle T25.419
    first degree T25.519
    left T25.412
      first degree T25.512
      second degree T25.612
      third degree T25.712
    multiple with foot —*see* Corrosion,
      lower, limb, multiple, ankle
      and foot
    right T25.411
      first degree T25.511
      second degree T25.611
      third degree T25.711
    second degree T25.619
    third degree T25.719
  anus —*see* Corrosion, buttock
  arm (s) (meaning upper limb (s)) —*see*
    Corrosion, upper limb
  axilla T22.449
    first degree T22.549
    left T22.442
      first degree T22.542
      second degree T22.642
      third degree T22.742
    right T22.441
      first degree T22.541
      second degree T22.641
      third degree T22.741
    second degree T22.649
    third degree T22.749
  back (lower) T21.44
    first degree T21.54
    second degree T21.64
    third degree T21.74
    upper T21.43
      first degree T21.53
      second degree T21.63
      third degree T21.73
  blisters - code as Corrosion, second degree,
    by site
  breast (s) —*see* Corrosion, chest wall
  buttock (s) T21.45
    first degree T21.55
    second degree T21.65
    third degree T21.75
  calf T24.439
    first degree T24.539
    left T24.432
      first degree T24.532
      second degree T24.632
      third degree T24.732
    right T24.431
      first degree T24.531
      second degree T24.631
      third degree T24.731
    second degree T24.639
    third degree T24.739
  canthus (eye) —*see* Corrosion,
    eyelid
  cervix T28.8
  cheek T20.46
    first degree T20.56
    second degree T20.66
    third degree T20.76
  chest wall T21.41
    first degree T21.51
    second degree T21.61
    third degree T21.71
  chin T20.43
    first degree T20.53
    second degree T20.63
    third degree T20.73
  colon T28.7
  conjunctiva (and cornea) —*see* Corrosion,
    cornea
  cornea (and conjunctiva) T26.6-
  deep necrosis of underlying tissue -
    code as Corrosion, third degree,
    by site

Corrosion *(Continued)*
  dorsum of hand T23.469
    first degree T23.569
    left T23.462
      first degree T23.562
      second degree T23.662
      third degree T23.762
    right T23.461
      first degree T23.561
      second degree T23.661
      third degree T23.761
    second degree T23.669
    third degree T23.769
  ear (auricle) (external) (canal)
    T20.41
    drum T28.91
    first degree T20.51
    second degree T20.61
    third degree T20.71
  elbow T22.429
    first degree T22.529
    left T22.422
      first degree T22.522
      second degree T22.622
      third degree T22.722
    right T22.421
      first degree T22.521
      second degree T22.621
      third degree T22.721
    second degree T22.629
    third degree T22.729
  entire body —*see* Corrosion, multiple
    body regions
  epidermal loss - code as Corrosion,
    second degree, by site
  epiglottis T27.4
  erythema, erythematous - code
    as Corrosion, first degree,
    by site
  esophagus T28.6
  extent (percentage of body surface)
    less than 10 percent T32.0
    10-19 percent (0-9 percent third degree)
      T32.10
      with 10-19 percent third degree
        T32.11
    20-29 percent (0-9 percent third degree)
      T32.20
      with
        10-19 percent third degree T32.21
        20-29 percent third degree T32.22
    30-39 percent (0-9 percent third degree)
      T32.30
      with
        10-19 percent third degree T32.31
        20-29 percent third degree T32.32
        30-39 percent third degree T32.33
    40-49 percent (0-9 percent third degree)
      T32.40
      with
        10-19 percent third degree T32.41
        20-29 percent third degree T32.42
        30-39 percent third degree T32.43
        40-49 percent third degree T32.44
    50-59 percent (0-9 percent third degree)
      T32.50
      with
        10-19 percent third degree T32.51
        20-29 percent third degree T32.52
        30-39 percent third degree T32.53
        40-49 percent third degree T32.54
        50-59 percent third degree T32.55
    60-69 percent (0-9 percent third degree)
      T32.60
      with
        10-19 percent third degree T32.61
        20-29 percent third degree T32.62
        30-39 percent third degree T32.63
        40-49 percent third degree T32.64
        50-59 percent third degree T32.65
        60-69 percent third degree T32.66

◀ New   ⬅ Revised   ~~deleted~~ Deleted

Corrosion *(Continued)*
  lower *(Continued)*
    limb *(Continued)*
      multiple sites, except ankle and foot *(Continued)*
        ankle and foot *(Continued)*
          right T25.491
            first degree T25.591
            second degree T25.691
            third degree T25.791
          second degree T25.699
          third degree T25.799
        first degree T24.599
        left T24.492
          first degree T24.592
          second degree T24.692
          third degree T24.792
        right T24.491
          first degree T24.591
          second degree T24.691
          third degree T24.791
        second degree T24.699
        third degree T24.799
      right T24.401
        first degree T24.501
        second degree T24.601
        third degree T24.701
      second degree T24.609
      thigh —*see* Corrosion, thigh
      third degree T24.709
  lung (with larynx and trachea) T27.5
  mouth T28.5
  neck T20.47
    first degree T20.57
    second degree T20.67
    third degree T20.77
  nose (septum) T20.44
    first degree T20.54
    second degree T20.64
    third degree T20.74
  ocular adnexa —*see* Corrosion, eye
  orbit region —*see* Corrosion, eyelid
  palm T23.459
    first degree T23.559
    left T23.452
      first degree T23.552
      second degree T23.652
      third degree T23.752
    right T23.451
      first degree T23.551
      second degree T23.651
      third degree T23.751
    second degree T23.659
    third degree T23.759
  partial thickness - code as Corrosion, unspecified degree, by site
  pelvis —*see* Corrosion, trunk
  penis —*see* Corrosion, genital organs, external, male
  perineum
    female —*see* Corrosion, genital organs, external, female
    male —*see* Corrosion, genital organs, external, male
  periocular area —*see* Corrosion, eyelid
  pharynx T28.5
  rectum T28.7
  respiratory tract T27.7
    larynx —*see* Corrosion, larynx
    specified part NEC T27.6
    trachea —*see* Corrosion, larynx
  sac, lacrimal —*see* Corrosion, eye, specified site NEC
  scalp T20.45
    first degree T20.55
    second degree T20.65
    third degree T20.75

Corrosion *(Continued)*
  scapular region T22.469
    first degree T22.569
    left T22.462
      first degree T22.562
      second degree T22.662
      third degree T22.762
    right T22.461
      first degree T22.561
      second degree T22.661
      third degree T22.761
    second degree T22.669
    third degree T22.769
  sclera —*see* Corrosion, eye, specified site NEC
  scrotum —*see* Corrosion, genital organs, external, male
  shoulder T22.459
    first degree T22.559
    left T22.452
      first degree T22.552
      second degree T22.652
      third degree T22.752
    right T22.451
      first degree T22.551
      second degree T22.651
      third degree T22.751
    second degree T22.659
    third degree T22.759
  stomach T28.7
  temple —*see* Corrosion, head
  testis —*see* Corrosion, genital organs, external, male
  thigh T24.419
    first degree T24.519
    left T24.412
      first degree T24.512
      second degree T24.612
      third degree T24.712
    right T24.411
      first degree T24.511
      second degree T24.611
      third degree T24.711
    second degree T24.619
    third degree T24.719
  thorax (external) —*see* Corrosion, trunk
  throat (meaning pharynx) T28.5
  thumb (s) T23.419
    first degree T23.519
    left T23.412
      first degree T23.512
      second degree T23.612
      third degree T23.712
    multiple sites with fingers T23.449
      first degree T23.549
      left T23.442
        first degree T23.542
        second degree T23.642
        third degree T23.742
      right T23.441
        first degree T23.541
        second degree T23.641
        third degree T23.741
      second degree T23.649
      third degree T23.749
    right T23.411
      first degree T23.511
      second degree T23.611
      third degree T23.711
    second degree T23.619
    third degree T23.719
  toe T25.439
    first degree T25.539
    left T25.432
      first degree T25.532
      second degree T25.632
      third degree T25.732
    right T25.431
      first degree T25.531
      second degree T25.631
      third degree T25.731

Corrosion *(Continued)*
  toe *(Continued)*
    second degree T25.639
    third degree T25.739
  tongue T28.5
  tonsil (s) T28.5
  total body —*see* Corrosion, multiple body regions
  trachea T27.4
    with lung T27.5
  trunk T21.40
    abdominal wall —*see* Corrosion, abdominal wall
    anus —*see* Corrosion, buttock
    axilla —*see* Corrosion, upper limb
    back —*see* Corrosion, back
    breast —*see* Corrosion, chest wall
    buttock —*see* Corrosion, buttock
    chest wall —*see* Corrosion, chest wall
    first degree T21.50
    flank —*see* Corrosion, abdominal wall
    genital
      female —*see* Corrosion, genital organs, external, female
      male —*see* Corrosion, genital organs, external, male
    groin —*see* Corrosion, abdominal wall
    interscapular region —*see* Corrosion, back, upper
    labia —*see* Corrosion, genital organs, external, female
    lower back —*see* Corrosion, back
    penis —*see* Corrosion, genital organs, external, male
    perineum
      female —*see* Corrosion, genital organs, external, female
      male —*see* Corrosion, genital organs, external, male
    scapular region —*see* Corrosion, upper limb
    scrotum —*see* Corrosion, genital organs, external, male
    second degree T21.60
    shoulder —*see* Corrosion, upper limb
    specified site NEC T21.49
      first degree T21.59
      second degree T21.69
      third degree T21.79
    testes —*see* Corrosion, genital organs, external, male
    third degree T21.70
    upper back —*see* Corrosion, back, upper
    vagina T28.8
    vulva —*see* Corrosion, genital organs, external, female
  unspecified site with extent of body surface involved specified
    less than 10 percent T32.0
    10-19 percent (0-9 percent third degree) T32.10
      with 10-19 percent third degree T32.11
    20-29 percent (0-9 percent third degree) T32.20
      with
        10-19 percent third degree T32.21
        20-29 percent third degree T32.22
    30-39 percent (0-9 percent third degree) T32.30
      with
        10-19 percent third degree T32.31
        20-29 percent third degree T32.32
        30-39 percent third degree T32.33
    40-49 percent (0-9 percent third degree) T32.40
      with
        10-19 percent third degree T32.41
        20-29 percent third degree T32.42
        30-39 percent third degree T32.43
        40-49 percent third degree T32.44

Corrosion *(Continued)*
unspecified site with extent of body surface
involved specified *(Continued)*
50-59 percent (0-9 percent third degree)
T32.50
with
10-19 percent third degree T32.51
20-29 percent third degree T32.52
30-39 percent third degree T32.53
40-49 percent third degree T32.54
50-59 percent third degree T32.55
60-69 percent (0-9 percent third degree)
T32.60
with
10-19 percent third degree T32.61
20-29 percent third degree T32.62
30-39 percent third degree T32.63
40-49 percent third degree T32.64
50-59 percent third degree T32.65
60-69 percent third degree T32.66
70-79 percent (0-9 percent third degree)
T32.70
with
10-19 percent third degree T32.71
20-29 percent third degree T32.72
30-39 percent third degree T32.73
40-49 percent third degree T32.74
50-59 percent third degree T32.75
60-69 percent third degree T32.76
70-79 percent third degree T32.77
80-89 percent (0-9 percent third degree)
T32.80
with
10-19 percent third degree T32.81
20-29 percent third degree T32.82
30-39 percent third degree T32.83
40-49 percent third degree T32.84
50-59 percent third degree T32.85
60-69 percent third degree T32.86
70-79 percent third degree T32.87
80-89 percent third degree T32.88
90 percent or more (0-9 percent third
degree) T32.90
with
10-19 percent third degree T32.91
20-29 percent third degree T32.92
30-39 percent third degree T32.93
40-49 percent third degree T32.94
50-59 percent third degree T32.95
60-69 percent third degree T32.96
70-79 percent third degree T32.97
80-89 percent third degree T32.98
90-99 percent third degree T32.99
upper limb (axilla) (scapular region) T22.40
above elbow —*see* Corrosion, above
elbow
axilla —*see* Corrosion, axilla
elbow —*see* Corrosion, elbow
first degree T22.50
forearm —*see* Corrosion, forearm
hand —*see* Corrosion, hand
interscapular region —*see* Corrosion, back,
upper
multiple sites T22.499
first degree T22.599
left T22.492
first degree T22.592
second degree T22.692
third degree T22.792
right T22.491
first degree T22.591
second degree T22.691
third degree T22.791
second degree T22.699
third degree T22.799
scapular region —*see* Corrosion, scapular
region
second degree T22.60
shoulder —*see* Corrosion, shoulder
third degree T22.70
wrist —*see* Corrosion, hand

Corrosion *(Continued)*
uterus T28.8
vagina T28.8
vulva —*see* Corrosion, genital organs,
external, female
wrist T23.479
first degree T23.579
left T23.472
first degree T23.572
second degree T23.672
third degree T23.772
multiple sites with hand T23.499
first degree T23.599
left T23.492
first degree T23.592
second degree T23.692
third degree T23.792
right T23.491
first degree T23.591
second degree T23.691
third degree T23.791
second degree T23.699
third degree T23.799
right T23.471
first degree T23.571
second degree T23.671
third degree T23.771
second degree T23.679
third degree T23.779
Corrosive burn —*see* Corrosion
Corsican fever —*see* Malaria
Cortical —*see* condition
Cortico-adrenal —*see* condition
Coryza (acute) J00
with grippe or influenza —*see* Influenza,
with, respiratory manifestations
NEC
syphilitic
congenital (chronic) A50.05
Costen's syndrome or complex M26.69
Costiveness —*see* Constipation
Costochondritis M94.0
Cot death R99
Cotard's syndrome F22
Cotia virus B08.8
Cotton wool spots (retinal) H35.81
Cotungo's disease —*see* Sciatica
Cough (affected) (chronic) (epidemic) (nervous)
R05
with hemorrhage —*see* Hemoptysis
bronchial R05
with grippe or influenza —*see* Influenza,
with, respiratory manifestations
NEC
functional F45.8
hysterical F45.8
laryngeal, spasmodic R05
psychogenic F45.8
smokers' J41.0
tea taster's B49
Counseling (for) Z71.9
abuse NEC
perpetrator Z69.82
victim Z69.81
alcohol abuser Z71.41
family Z71.42
child abuse
nonparental
perpetrator Z69.021
victim Z69.020
parental
perpetrator Z69.011
victim Z69.010
consanguinity Z71.89
contraceptive Z30.09
dietary Z71.3
drug abuser Z71.51
family member Z71.52
family Z71.89
fertility preservation (prior to cancer therapy)
(prior to removal of gonads) Z31.62

Counseling *(Continued)*
for non-attending third party Z71.0
related to sexual behavior or orientation
Z70.2
genetic NEC Z31.5
health (advice) (education) (instruction) —*see*
Counseling, medical
human immunodeficiency virus (HIV)
Z71.7
impotence Z70.1
insulin pump use Z46.81
medical (for) Z71.9
boarding school resident Z59.3
consanguinity Z71.89
feared complaint and no disease found
Z71.1
human immunodeficiency virus (HIV)
Z71.7
institutional resident Z59.3
on behalf of another Z71.0
related to sexual behavior or orientation
Z70.2
person living alone Z60.2
specified reason NEC Z71.89
natural family planning
procreative Z31.61
to avoid pregnancy Z30.02
perpetrator (of)
abuse NEC Z69.82
child abuse
non-parental Z69.021
parental Z69.011
rape NEC Z69.82
spousal abuse Z69.12
procreative NEC Z31.69
fertility preservation (prior to cancer
therapy) (prior to removal of
gonads) Z31.62
using natural family planning
Z31.61
promiscuity Z70.1
rape victim Z69.81
religious Z71.81
sex, sexual (related to) Z70.9
attitude (s) Z70.0
behavior or orientation Z70.1
combined concerns Z70.3
non-responsiveness Z70.1
on behalf of third party Z70.2
specified reason NEC Z70.8
specified reason NEC Z71.89
spiritual Z71.81
spousal abuse (perpetrator) Z69.12
victim Z69.11
substance abuse Z71.89
alcohol Z71.41
drug Z71.51
tobacco Z71.6
tobacco use Z71.6
use (of)
insulin pump Z46.81
victim (of)
abuse Z69.81
child abuse
by parent Z69.010
non-parental Z69.020
rape NEC Z69.81
Coupled rhythm R00.8
Couvelaire syndrome or uterus (complicating
delivery) O45.8X-
Cowperitis —*see* Urethritis
Cowper's gland —*see* condition
Cowpox B08.010
due to vaccination T88.1
Coxa
magna M91.4-
plana M91.2-
valga (acquired) —*see also* Deformity, limb,
specified type NEC, thigh
congenital Q65.81
sequelae (late effect) of rickets E64.3

Coxa *(Continued)*
  vara (acquired) —*see also* Deformity, limb,
    specified type NEC, thigh
      congenital Q65.82
      sequelae (late effect) of rickets E64.3
Coxalgia, coxalgic (nontuberculous) —*see also*
  Pain, joint, hip
    tuberculous A18.02
Coxitis —*see* Monoarthritis, hip
Coxsackie (virus) (infection) B34.1
  as cause of disease classified elsewhere B97.11
  carditis B33.20
  central nervous system NEC A88.8
  endocarditis B33.21
  enteritis A08.39
  meningitis (aseptic) A87.0
  myocarditis B33.22
  pericarditis B33.23
  pharyngitis B08.5
  pleurodynia B33.0
  specific disease NEC B33.8
Crabs, meaning pubic lice B85.3
Crack baby P04.41
Cracked nipple N64.0
  associated with
    lactation O92.13
      pregnancy O92.11-
      puerperium O92.12
Cracked tooth K03.81
Cradle cap L21.0
Craft neurosis F48.8
Cramp (s) R25.2
  abdominal —*see* Pain, abdominal
  bathing T75.1
  colic R10.83
    psychogenic F45.8
  due to immersion T75.1
  fireman T67.2
  heat T67.2
  immersion T75.1
  intestinal —*see* Pain, abdominal
    psychogenic F45.8
  leg, sleep related G47.62
  limb (lower) (upper) NEC R25.2
    sleep related G47.62
  linotypist's F48.8
    organic G25.89
  muscle (limb) (general) R25.2
    due to immersion T75.1
    psychogenic F45.8
  occupational (hand) F48.8
    organic G25.89
  salt-depletion E87.1
  sleep related, leg G47.62
  stoker's T67.2
  swimmer's T75.1
  telegrapher's F48.8
    organic G25.89
  typist's F48.8
    organic G25.89
  uterus N94.89
    menstrual —*see* Dysmenorrhea
  writer's F48.8
    organic G25.89
Cranial —*see* condition
Craniocleidodysostosis Q74.0
Craniofenestria (skull) Q75.8
Craniolacunia (skull) Q75.8
Craniopagus Q89.4
Craniopathy, metabolic M85.2
Craniopharyngeal —*see* condition
Craniopharyngioma D44.4
Craniorachischisis (totalis) Q00.1
Cranioschisis Q75.8
Craniostenosis Q75.0
Craniosynostosis Q75.0
Craniotabes (cause unknown) M83.8
  neonatal P96.3
  rachitic E64.3
  syphilitic A50.56
Cranium —*see* condition

Craw-craw —*see* Onchocerciasis
Creaking joint —*see* Derangement, joint,
  specified type NEC
Creeping
  eruption B76.9
  palsy or paralysis G12.22
Crenated tongue K14.8
Creotoxism A05.9
Crepitus
  caput Q75.8
  joint —*see* Derangement, joint, specified type
    NEC
Crescent or conus choroid, congenital Q14.3
CREST syndrome M34.1
Cretin, cretinism (congenital) (endemic)
  (nongoitrous) (sporadic) E00.9
  pelvis
    with disproportion (fetopelvic) O33.0
      causing obstructed labor O65.0
  type
    hypothyroid E00.1
    mixed E00.2
    myxedematous E00.1
    neurological E00.0
Creutzfeldt-Jakob disease or syndrome (with
  dementia) A81.00
  familial A81.09
  iatrogenic A81.09
  specified NEC A81.09
  sporadic A81.09
  variant (vCJD) A81.01
Crib death R99
Cribriform hymen Q52.3
Cri-du-chat syndrome Q93.4
Crigler-Najjar disease or syndrome E80.5
Crime, victim of Z65.4
Crimean hemorrhagic fever A98.0
Criminalism F60.2
Crisis
  abdomen R10.0
  acute reaction F43.0
  addisonian E27.2
  adrenal (cortical) E27.2
  celiac K90.0
  Dietl's N13.8
  emotional —*see also* Disorder, adjustment
    acute reaction to stress F43.0
    specific to childhood and adolescence
      F93.8
  glaucomatocyclitic —*see* Glaucoma,
    secondary, inflammation
  heart —*see* Failure, heart
  nitritoid I95.2
    correct substance properly administered —
      see Table of Drugs and Chemicals, by
      drug, adverse effect
    overdose or wrong substance given or
      taken —*see* Table of Drugs and
      Chemicals, by drug, poisoning
  oculogyric H51.8
    psychogenic F45.8
  Pel's (tabetic) A52.11
  psychosexual identity F64.2
  renal N28.0
  sickle-cell D57.00
    with
      acute chest syndrome D57.01
      splenic sequestration D57.02
  state (acute reaction) F43.0
  tabetic A52.11
  thyroid —*see* Thyrotoxicosis with thyroid
    storm
  thyrotoxic —*see* Thyrotoxicosis with thyroid
    storm
Crocq's disease (acrocyanosis) I73.89
Crohn's disease —*see* Enteritis, regional
Crooked septum, nasal J34.2
Cross syndrome E70.328
Crossbite (anterior) (posterior) M26.24
Cross-eye —*see* Strabismus, convergent
  concomitant

Croup, croupous (catarrhal) (infectious)
  (inflammatory) (nondiphtheritic) J05.0
  bronchial J20.9
  diphtheritic A36.2
  false J38.5
  spasmodic J38.5
    diphtheritic A36.2
  stridulous J38.5
    diphtheritic A36.2
Crouzon's disease Q75.1
Crowding, tooth, teeth, fully erupted M26.31
CRST syndrome M34.1
Cruchet's disease A85.8
Cruelty in children —*see also* Disorder,
  conduct
Crural ulcer —*see* Ulcer, lower limb
Crush, crushed, crushing T14.8
  abdomen S38.1
  ankle S97.0-
  arm (upper) (and shoulder) S47.-
  axilla —*see* Crush, arm
  back, lower S38.1
  buttock S38.1
  cheek S07.0
  chest S28.0
  cranium S07.1
  ear S07.0
  elbow S57.0-
  extremity
    lower
      ankle —*see* Crush, ankle
      below knee —*see* Crush, leg
      foot —*see* Crush, foot
      hip —*see* Crush, hip
      knee —*see* Crush, knee
      thigh —*see* Crush, thigh
      toe —*see* Crush, toe
    upper
      below elbow S67.9-
      elbow —*see* Crush, elbow
      finger —*see* Crush, finger
      forearm —*see* Crush, forearm
      hand —*see* Crush, hand
      thumb —*see* Crush, thumb
      upper arm —*see* Crush, arm
      wrist —*see* Crush, wrist
  face S07.0
  finger (s) S67.1-
    with hand (and wrist) —*see* Crush, hand,
      specified site NEC
    index S67.19-
    little S67.19-
    middle S67.19-
    ring S67.19-
    thumb —*see* Crush, thumb
  foot S97.8-
    toe —*see* Crush, toe
  forearm S57.8-
  genitalia, external
    female S38.002
      vagina S38.03
      vulva S38.03
    male S38.001
      penis S38.01
      scrotum S38.02
      testis S38.02
  hand (except fingers alone) S67.2-
    with wrist S67.4-
  head S07.9
    specified NEC S07.8
  heel —*see* Crush, foot
  hip S77.0-
    with thigh S77.2-
  internal organ (abdomen, chest, or pelvis)
    NEC T14.8
  knee S87.0-
  labium (majus) (minus) S38.03
  larynx S17.0
  leg (lower) S87.8-
    knee —*see* Crush, knee
  lip S07.0

◀ New   ⬅ Revised   ~~deleted~~ Deleted

Crush, crushed, crushing (Continued)
  lower
    back S38.1
    leg —see Crush, leg
  neck S17.9
  nerve —see Injury, nerve
  nose S07.0
  pelvis S38.1
  penis S38.01
  scalp S07.8
  scapular region —see Crush, arm
  scrotum S38.02
  severe, unspecified site T14.8
  shoulder (and upper arm) —see Crush, arm
  skull S07.1
  syndrome (complication of trauma) T79.5
  testis S38.02
  thigh S77.1-
    with hip S77.2-
  throat S17.8
  thumb S67.0-
    with hand (and wrist) —see Crush, hand, specified site NEC
  toe (s) S97.10-
    great S97.11-
    lesser S97.12-
  trachea S17.0
  vagina S38.03
  vulva S38.03
  wrist S67.3-
    with hand S67.4-
Crusta lactea L21.0
Crusts R23.4
Crutch paralysis —see Injury, brachial plexus
Cruveilhier-Baumgarten cirrhosis, disease or syndrome K74.69
Cruveilhier's atrophy or disease G12.8
Crying (constant) (continuous) (excessive)
  child, adolescent, or adult R45.83
  infant (baby) (newborn) R68.11
Cryofibrinogenemia D89.2
Cryoglobulinemia (essential) (idiopathic) (mixed) (primary) (purpura) (secondary) (vasculitis) D89.1
  with lung involvement D89.1 [J99]
Cryptitis (anal) (rectal) K62.89
Cryptococcosis, cryptococcus (infection) (neoformans) B45.9
  bone B45.3
  cerebral B45.1
  cutaneous B45.2
  disseminated B45.7
  generalized B45.7
  meningitis B45.1
  meningocerebralis B45.1
  osseous B45.3
  pulmonary B45.0
  skin B45.2
  specified NEC B45.8
Cryptopapillitis (anus) K62.89
Cryptophthalmos Q11.2
  syndrome Q87.0
Cryptorchid, cryptorchism, cryptorchidism Q53.9
  bilateral Q53.20
    abdominal Q53.21
    perineal Q53.22
  unilateral Q53.10
    abdominal Q53.11
    perineal Q53.12
Cryptosporidiosis A07.2
  hepatobiliary B88.8
  respiratory B88.8
Cryptostromosis J67.6
Crystalluria R82.99
Cubitus
  congenital Q68.8
  valgus (acquired) M21.0-
    congenital Q68.8
    sequelae (late effect) of rickets E64.3

Cubitus (Continued)
  varus (acquired) M21.1-
    congenital Q68.8
    sequelae (late effect) of rickets E64.3
Cultural deprivation or shock Z60.3
Curling esophagus K22.4
Curling's ulcer —see Ulcer, peptic, acute
Curschmann (-Batten) (-Steinert) **disease or syndrome** G71.11
Curse, Ondine's —see Apnea, sleep
Curvature
  organ or site, congenital NEC —see Distortion
  penis (lateral) Q55.61
  Pott's (spinal) A18.01
  radius, idiopathic, progressive (congenital) Q74.0
  spine (acquired) (angular) (idiopathic) (incorrect) (postural) —see Dorsopathy, deforming
    congenital Q67.5
    due to or associated with
      Charcot-Marie-Tooth disease (see also subcategory M49.8) G60.0
      osteitis
        deformans M88.88
        fibrosa cystica (see also subcategory M49.8) E21.0
      tuberculosis (Pott's curvature) A18.01
    sequelae (late effect) of rickets E64.3
    tuberculous A18.01
Cushingoid due to steroid therapy E24.2
  correct substance properly administered —see Table of Drugs and Chemicals, by drug, adverse effect
  overdose or wrong substance given or taken —see Table of Drugs and Chemicals, by drug, poisoning
Cushing's
  syndrome or disease E24.9
    drug-induced E24.2
    iatrogenic E24.2
    pituitary-dependent E24.0
    specified NEC E24.8
  ulcer —see Ulcer, peptic, acute
Cusp, Carabelli - omit code
Cut (external) —see also Laceration
  muscle —see Injury, muscle
Cutaneous —see also condition
  hemorrhage R23.3
  larva migrans B76.9
Cutis —see also condition
  hyperelastica Q82.8
    acquired L57.4
  laxa (hyperelastica) —see Dermatolysis
  marmorata R23.8
  osteosis L94.2
  pendula —see Dermatolysis
  rhomboidalis nuchae L57.2
  verticis gyrata Q82.8
    acquired L91.8
Cyanosis R23.0
  due to
    patent foramen botalli Q21.1
    persistent foramen ovale Q21.1
  enterogenous D74.8
  paroxysmal digital —see Raynaud's disease
    with gangrene I73.01
  retina, retinal H35.89
Cyanotic heart disease I24.9
  congenital Q24.9
Cycle
  anovulatory N97.0
  menstrual, irregular N92.6
Cyclencephaly Q04.9
Cyclical vomiting (see also Vomiting, cyclical) G43.A0
  psychogenic F50.8
Cyclitis (see also Iridocyclitis) H20.9
  chronic —see Iridocyclitis, chronic
  Fuchs' heterochromic H20.81-
  granulomatous —see Iridocyclitis, chronic

Cyclitis (Continued)
  lens-induced —see Iridocyclitis, lens-induced
  posterior H30.2-
Cycloid personality F34.0
Cyclophoria H50.54
Cyclopia, cyclops Q87.0
Cyclopism Q87.0
Cyclosporiasis A07.4
Cyclothymia F34.0
Cyclothymic personality F34.0
Cyclotropia H50.41-
Cylindroma —see also Neoplasm, malignant, by site
  eccrine dermal —see Neoplasm, skin, benign
  skin —see Neoplasm, skin, benign
Cylindruria R82.99
Cynanche
  diphtheritic A36.2
  tonsillaris J36
Cynophobia F40.218
Cynorexia R63.2
Cyphosis —see Kyphosis
Cyprus fever —see Brucellosis
Cyst (colloid) (mucous) (simple) (retention)
  adenoid (infected) J35.8
  adrenal gland E27.8
    congenital Q89.1
  air, lung J98.4
  allantoic Q64.4
  alveolar process (jaw bone) M27.40
  amnion, amniotic O41.8X-
  anterior
    chamber (eye) —see Cyst, iris
    nasopalatine K09.1
  antrum J34.1
  anus K62.89
  apical (tooth) (periodontal) K04.8
  appendix K38.8
  arachnoid, brain (acquired) G93.0
    congenital Q04.6
  arytenoid J38.7
  Baker's M71.2-
    ruptured M66.0
    tuberculous A18.02
  Bartholin's gland N75.0
  bile duct (common) (hepatic) K83.5
  bladder (multiple) (trigone) N32.89
  blue dome (breast) —see Cyst, breast
  bone (local) NEC M85.60
    aneurysmal M85.50
      ankle M85.57-
      foot M85.57-
      forearm M85.53-
      hand M85.54-
      jaw M27.49
      lower leg M85.56-
      multiple site M85.59
      neck M85.58
      rib M85.58
      shoulder M85.51-
      skull M85.58
      specified site NEC M85.58
      thigh M85.55-
      toe M85.57-
      upper arm M85.52-
      vertebra M85.58
    solitary M85.40
      ankle M85.47-
      fibula M85.46-
      foot M85.47-
      hand M85.44-
      humerus M85.42-
      jaw M27.49
      neck M85.48
      pelvis M85.45-
      radius M85.43-
      rib M85.48
      shoulder M85.41-
      skull M85.48
      specified site NEC M85.48

Cyst *(Continued)*
  bone NEC *(Continued)*
    solitary *(Continued)*
      tibia M85.46-
      toe M85.47-
      ulna M85.43-
      vertebra M85.48
    specified type NEC M85.60
      ankle M85.67-
      foot M85.67-
      forearm M85.63-
      hand M85.64-
      jaw M27.40
        developmental (nonodontogenic)
          K09.1
          odontogenic K09.0
        latent M27.0
      lower leg M85.66-
      multiple site M85.69
      neck M85.68
      rib M85.68
      shoulder M85.61-
      skull M85.68
      specified site NEC M85.68
      thigh M85.65-
      toe M85.67-
      upper arm M85.62-
      vertebra M85.68
  brain (acquired) G93.0
    congenital Q04.6
    hydatid B67.99 *[G94]*
    third ventricle (colloid), congenital Q04.6
  branchial (cleft) Q18.0
  branchiogenic Q18.0
  breast (benign) (blue dome) (pedunculated)
    (solitary) N60.0-
    involution —*see* Dysplasia, mammary,
      specified type NEC
    sebaceous —*see* Dysplasia, mammary,
      specified type NEC
  broad ligament (benign) N83.8
  bronchogenic (mediastinal) (sequestration)
    J98.4
    congenital Q33.0
  buccal K09.8
  bulbourethral gland N36.8
  bursa, bursal NEC M71.30
    with rupture —*see* Rupture, synovium
    ankle M71.37-
    elbow M71.32-
    foot M71.37-
    hand M71.34-
    hip M71.35-
    multiple sites M71.39
    pharyngeal J39.2
    popliteal space —*see* Cyst, Baker's
    shoulder M71.31-
    specified site NEC M71.38
    wrist M71.33-
  calcifying odontogenic D16.5
    upper jaw (bone) (maxilla) D16.4
  canal of Nuck (female) N94.89
    congenital Q52.4
  canthus —*see* Cyst, conjunctiva
  carcinomatous —*see* Neoplasm, malignant,
    by site
  cauda equina G95.89
  cavum septi pellucidi —*see* Cyst, brain
  celomic (pericardium) Q24.8
  cerebellopontine (angle) —*see* Cyst, brain
  cerebellum —*see* Cyst, brain
  cerebral —*see* Cyst, brain
  cervical lateral Q18.1
  cervix NEC N88.8
    embryonic Q51.6
    nabothian N88.8
  chiasmal optic NEC —*see* Disorder, optic,
    chiasm
  chocolate (ovary) N80.1
  choledochus, congenital Q44.4
  chorion O41.8X-

Cyst *(Continued)*
  choroid plexus G93.0
  ciliary body —*see* Cyst, iris
  clitoris N90.7
  colon K63.89
  common (bile) duct K83.5
  congenital NEC Q89.8
    adrenal gland Q89.1
    epiglottis Q31.8
    esophagus Q39.8
    fallopian tube Q50.4
    kidney Q61.00
      more than one (multiple) Q61.02
        specified as polycystic Q61.3
          adult type Q61.2
          infantile type NEC Q61.19
            collecting duct dilation Q61.11
      solitary Q61.01
    larynx Q31.8
    liver Q44.6
    lung Q33.0
    mediastinum Q34.1
    ovary Q50.1
    oviduct Q50.4
    periurethral (tissue) Q64.79
    prepuce Q55.69
    salivary gland (any) Q38.4
    sublingual Q38.6
    submaxillary gland Q38.6
    thymus (gland) Q89.2
    tongue Q38.3
    ureterovesical orifice Q62.8
    vulva Q52.79
  conjunctiva H11.44-
  cornea H18.89-
  corpora quadrigemina G93.0
  corpus
    albicans N83.29
    luteum (hemorrhagic) (ruptured) N83.1
  Cowper's gland (benign) (infected) N36.8
  cranial meninges G93.0
  craniobuccal pouch E23.6
  craniopharyngeal pouch E23.6
  cystic duct K82.8
  Cysticercus —*see* Cysticercosis
  Dandy-Walker Q03.1
    with spina bifida —*see* Spina bifida
  dental (root) K04.8
    developmental K09.0
    eruption K09.0
    primordial K09.0
  dentigerous (mandible) (maxilla) K09.0
  dermoid —*see* Neoplasm, benign, by site
    with malignant transformation C56.-
    implantation
      external area or site (skin) NEC L72.0
      iris —*see* Cyst, iris, implantation
      vagina N89.8
      vulva N90.7
    mouth K09.8
    oral soft tissue K09.8
    sacrococcygeal —*see* Cyst, pilonidal
  developmental K09.1
    odontogenic K09.0
    oral region (nonodontogenic) K09.1
    ovary, ovarian Q50.1
  dura (cerebral) G93.0
    spinal G96.19
  ear (external) Q18.1
  echinococcal —*see* Echinococcus
  embryonic
    cervix uteri Q51.6
    fallopian tube Q50.4
    vagina Q51.6
  endometrium, endometrial (uterus) N85.8
    ectopic —*see* Endometriosis
  enterogenous Q43.8
  epidermal, epidermoid (inclusion) (*see also*
    Cyst, skin) L72.0
    mouth K09.8
    oral soft tissue K09.8

Cyst *(Continued)*
  epididymis N50.3
  epiglottis J38.7
  epiphysis cerebri E34.8
  epithelial (inclusion) L72.0
  epoophoron Q50.5
  eruption K09.0
  esophagus K22.8
  ethmoid sinus J34.1
  external female genital organs NEC
    N90.7
  eye NEC H57.8
    congenital Q15.8
  eyelid (sebaceous) H02.829
    infected —*see* Hordeolum
    left H02.826
      lower H02.825
      upper H02.824
    right H02.823
      lower H02.822
      upper H02.821
  fallopian tube N83.8
    congenital Q50.4
  fimbrial (twisted) Q50.4
  fissural (oral region) K09.1
  follicle (graafian) (hemorrhagic) N83.0
    nabothian N88.8
  follicular (atretic) (hemorrhagic) (ovarian)
    N83.0
    dentigerous K09.0
    odontogenic K09.0
    skin L72.9
      specified NEC L72.8
  frontal sinus J34.1
  gallbladder K82.8
  ganglion —*see* Ganglion
  Gartner's duct Q52.4
  gingiva K09.0
  gland of Moll —*see* Cyst, eyelid
  globulomaxillary K09.1
  graafian follicle (hemorrhagic) N83.0
  granulosal lutein (hemorrhagic) N83.1
  hemangiomatous D18.00
    intra-abdominal D18.03
    intracranial D18.02
    skin D18.01
    specified site NEC D18.09
  hydatid (*see also* Echinococcus) B67.90
    brain B67.99 *[G94]*
    liver (*see also* Cyst, liver, hydatid) B67.8
    lung NEC B67.99 *[J99]*
    Morgagni
      female Q50.5
      male (epididymal) Q55.4
        testicular Q55.29
    specified site NEC B67.99
  hymen N89.8
    embryonic Q52.4
  hypopharynx J39.2
  hypophysis, hypophyseal (duct) (recurrent)
    E23.6
    cerebri E23.6
  implantation (dermoid)
    external area or site (skin) NEC L72.0
    iris —*see* Cyst, iris, implantation
    vagina N89.8
    vulva N90.7
  incisive canal K09.1
  inclusion (epidermal) (epithelial)
    (epidermoid) (squamous) L72.0
    not of skin - code under Cyst, by site
  intestine (large) (small) K63.89
  intracranial —*see* Cyst, brain
  intraligamentous —*see also* Disorder,
    ligament
    knee —*see* Derangement, knee
  intrasellar E23.6
  iris H21.309
    exudative H21.31-
    idiopathic H21.30-
    implantation H21.32-

◀ New   ◀▥ Revised   ~~deleted~~ Deleted

Cyst *(Continued)*
  iris *(Continued)*
    parasitic H21.33-
    pars plana (primary) H21.34-
      exudative H21.35-
  jaw (bone) M27.40
    aneurysmal M27.49
    developmental (odontogenic) K09.0
    fissural K09.1
    hemorrhagic M27.49
    traumatic M27.49
  joint NEC —*see* Disorder, joint, specified type
    NEC
  kidney (acquired) N28.1
    calyceal —*see* Hydronephrosis
    congenital Q61.00
      more than one (multiple) Q61.02
        specified as polycystic Q61.3
          adult type (autosomal dominant)
            Q61.2
          infantile type (autosomal recessive)
            NEC Q61.19
            collecting duct dilation Q61.11
    pyelogenic —*see* Hydronephrosis
    simple N28.1
    solitary (single) Q61.01
      acquired N28.1
  labium (majus) (minus) N90.7
    sebaceous N90.7
  lacrimal —*see also* Disorder, lacrimal system,
    specified NEC
    gland H04.13-
    passages or sac —*see* Disorder, lacrimal
      system, specified NEC
  larynx J38.7
  lateral periodontal K09.0
  lens H27.8
    congenital Q12.8
  lip (gland) K13.0
  liver (idiopathic) (simple) K76.89
    congenital Q44.6
    hydatid B67.8
      granulosus B67.0
      multilocularis B67.5
  lung J98.4
    congenital Q33.0
    giant bullous J43.9
  lutein N83.1
  lymphangiomatous D18.1
  lymphoepithelial, oral soft tissue K09.8
  macula —*see* Degeneration, macula, hole
  malignant —*see* Neoplasm, malignant, by site
  mammary gland —*see* Cyst, breast
  mandible M27.40
    dentigerous K09.0
    radicular K04.8
  maxilla M27.40
    dentigerous K09.0
    radicular K04.8
  medial, face and neck Q18.8
  median
    anterior maxillary K09.1
    palatal K09.1
  mediastinum, congenital Q34.1
  meibomian (gland) —*see* Chalazion
    infected —*see* Hordeolum
  membrane, brain G93.0
  meninges (cerebral) G93.0
    spinal G96.19
  meniscus, knee —*see* Derangement, knee,
    meniscus, cystic
  mesentery, mesenteric K66.8
    chyle I89.8
  mesonephric duct
    female Q50.5
    male Q55.4
  milk N64.89
  Morgagni (hydatid)
    female Q50.5
    male (epididymal) Q55.4
      testicular Q55.29
  mouth K09.8

Cyst *(Continued)*
  Müllerian duct Q50.4
    appendix testis Q55.29
    cervix Q51.6
    fallopian tube Q50.4
    female Q50.4
    male Q55.29
    prostatic utricle Q55.4
    vagina (embryonal) Q52.4
  multilocular (ovary) D39.10
    benign —*see* Neoplasm, benign, by site
  myometrium N85.8
  nabothian (follicle) (ruptured) N88.8
  nasoalveolar K09.1
  nasolabial K09.1
  nasopalatine (anterior) (duct) K09.1
  nasopharynx J39.2
  neoplastic —*see* Neoplasm, uncertain
    behavior, by site
    benign —*see* Neoplasm, benign, by site
  nervous system NEC G96.8
  neuroenteric (congenital) Q06.8
  nipple —*see* Cyst, breast
  nose (turbinates) J34.1
    sinus J34.1
  odontogenic, developmental K09.0
  omentum (lesser) K66.8
    congenital Q45.8
  ora serrata —*see* Cyst, retina, ora serrata
  oral
    region K09.9
      developmental (nonodontogenic) K09.1
        specified NEC K09.8
    soft tissue K09.9
      specified NEC K09.8
  orbit H05.81-
  ovary, ovarian (twisted) N83.20
    adherent N83.20
    chocolate N80.1
    corpus
      albicans N83.29
      luteum (hemorrhagic) N83.1
    dermoid D27.9
    developmental Q50.1
    due to failure of involution NEC N83.20
    endometrial N80.1
    follicular (graafian) (hemorrhagic) N83.0
    hemorrhagic N83.20
    in pregnancy or childbirth O34.8-
      with obstructed labor O65.5
    multilocular D39.10
    pseudomucinous D27.9
    retention N83.29
    serous N83.20
    specified NEC N83.29
    theca lutein (hemorrhagic) N83.1
    tuberculous A18.18
  oviduct N83.8
  palate (median) (fissural) K09.1
  palatine papilla (jaw) K09.1
  pancreas, pancreatic (hemorrhagic) (true) K86.2
    congenital Q45.2
    false K86.3
  paralabral
    hip M24.85-
    shoulder S43.43-
  paramesonephric duct Q50.4
    female Q50.4
    male Q55.29
  paranephric N28.1
  paraphysis, cerebri, congenital Q04.6
  parasitic B89
  parathyroid (gland) E21.4
  paratubal N83.8
  paraurethral duct N36.8
  paroophoron Q50.5
  parotid gland K11.6
  parovarian Q50.5
  pelvis, female N94.89
    in pregnancy or childbirth O34.8-
      causing obstructed labor O65.5

Cyst *(Continued)*
  penis (sebaceous) N48.89
  periapical K04.8
  pericardial (congenital) Q24.8
    acquired (secondary) I31.8
  pericoronal K09.0
  periodontal K04.8
    lateral K09.0
  peripelvic (lymphatic) N28.1
  peritoneum K66.8
    chylous I89.8
  periventricular, acquired, newborn P91.1
  pharynx (wall) J39.2
  pilar L72.11
  pilonidal (infected) (rectum) L05.91
    with abscess L05.01
    malignant C44.59-
  pituitary (duct) (gland) E23.6
  placenta O43.19-
  pleura J94.8
  popliteal —*see* Cyst, Baker's
  porencephalic Q04.6
    acquired G93.0
  postanal (infected) —*see* Cyst, pilonidal
  postmastoidectomy cavity (mucosal) —*see*
    Complications, postmastoidectomy, cyst
  preauricular Q18.1
  prepuce N47.4
    congenital Q55.69
  primordial (jaw) K09.0
  prostate N42.83
  pseudomucinous (ovary) D27.9
  pupillary, miotic H21.27-
  radicular (residual) K04.8
  radiculodental K04.8
  ranular K11.8
  Rathke's pouch E23.6
  rectum (epithelium) (mucous) K62.89
  renal —*see* Cyst, kidney
  residual (radicular) K04.8
  retention (ovary) N83.29
    salivary gland K11.6
  retina H33.19-
    ora serrata H33.11-
    parasitic H33.12-
  retroperitoneal K68.9
  sacrococcygeal (dermoid) —*see* Cyst,
    pilonidal
  salivary gland or duct (mucous extravasation
    or retention) K11.6
  Sampson's N80.1
  sclera H15.89
  scrotum L72.9
    sebaceous L72.3
  sebaceous (duct) (gland) L72.3
    breast —*see* Dysplasia, mammary, specified
      type NEC
    eyelid —*see* Cyst, eyelid
    genital organ NEC
      female N94.89
      male N50.8
    scrotum L72.3
  semilunar cartilage (knee) (multiple) —*see*
    Derangement, knee, meniscus, cystic
  seminal vesicle N50.8
  serous (ovary) N83.20
  sinus (accessory) (nasal) J34.1
  Skene's gland N36.8
  skin L72.9
    breast —*see* Dysplasia, mammary, specified
      type NEC
    epidermal, epidermoid L72.0
    epithelial L72.0
    eyelid —*see* Cyst, eyelid
    genital organ NEC
      female N90.7
      male N50.8
    inclusion L72.0
    scrotum L72.9
    sebaceous L72.3
    sweat gland or duct L74.8

◀ New   ◀▥ Revised   ~~deleted~~ Deleted

Cystathionine synthase deficiency E72.11
Cystathioninemia E72.19
Cystathioninuria E72.19
Cystic —*see also* condition
  breast (chronic) —*see* Mastopathy, cystic
  corpora lutea (hemorrhagic) N83.1
  duct —*see* condition
  eyeball (congenital) Q11.0
  fibrosis —*see* Fibrosis, cystic
  kidney (congenital) Q61.9
    adult type Q61.2
    infantile type NEC Q61.19
      collecting duct dilatation Q61.11
    medullary Q61.5
  liver, congenital Q44.6
  lung disease J98.4
    congenital Q33.0
  mastitis, chronic —*see* Mastopathy, cystic
  medullary, kidney Q61.5
  meniscus —*see* Derangement, knee,
      meniscus, cystic
  ovary N83.20
Cysticercosis, cysticerciasis B69.9
  with
    epileptiform fits B69.0
    myositis B69.81
  brain B69.0
  central nervous system B69.0
  cerebral B69.0
  ocular B69.1
  specified NEC B69.89
Cysticercus cellulose infestation —*see*
    Cysticercosis
Cystinosis (malignant) E72.04
Cystinuria E72.01
Cystitis (exudative) (hemorrhagic) (septic)
    (suppurative) N30.90
  with
    fibrosis —*see* Cystitis, chronic, interstitial
    hematuria N30.91
    leukoplakia —*see* Cystitis, chronic,
        interstitial
    malakoplakia —*see* Cystitis, chronic,
        interstitial
    metaplasia —*see* Cystitis, chronic,
        interstitial
    prostatitis N41.3
  acute N30.00
    with hematuria N30.01
    of trigone N30.30
      with hematuria N30.31
  allergic —*see* Cystitis, specified type NEC
  amebic A06.81
  bilharzial B65.9 [N33]

Cystitis (Continued)
  blennorrhagic (gonococcal) A54.01
  bullous —*see* Cystitis, specified type NEC
  calculous N21.0
  chlamydial A56.01
  chronic N30.20
    with hematuria N30.21
    interstitial N30.10
      with hematuria N30.11
    of trigone N30.30
      with hematuria N30.31
    specified NEC N30.20
      with hematuria N30.21
  cystic (a) —*see* Cystitis, specified type NEC
  diphtheritic A36.85
  echinococcal
    granulosus B67.39
    multilocularis B67.69
  emphysematous —*see* Cystitis, specified type
      NEC
  encysted —*see* Cystitis, specified type NEC
  eosinophilic —*see* Cystitis, specified type
      NEC
  follicular —*see* Cystitis, of trigone
  gangrenous —*see* Cystitis, specified type NEC
  glandularis —*see* Cystitis, specified type NEC
  gonococcal A54.01
  incrusted —*see* Cystitis, specified type NEC
  interstitial (chronic) —*see* Cystitis, chronic,
      interstitial
  irradiation N30.40
    with hematuria N30.41
  irritation —*see* Cystitis, specified type NEC
  malignant —*see* Cystitis, specified type NEC
  of trigone N30.30
    with hematuria N30.31
  panmural —*see* Cystitis, chronic, interstitial
  polyposa —*see* Cystitis, specified type NEC
  prostatic N41.3
  puerperal (postpartum) O86.22
  radiation —*see* Cystitis, irradiation
  specified type NEC N30.80
    with hematuria N30.81
  subacute —*see* Cystitis, chronic
  submucous —*see* Cystitis, chronic, interstitial
  syphilitic (late) A52.76
  trichomonal A59.03
  tuberculous A18.12
  ulcerative —*see* Cystitis, chronic, interstitial
Cystocele (-urethrocele)
  female N81.10
    with prolapse of uterus —*see* Prolapse,
        uterus
    lateral N81.12

Cystocele (Continued)
  female (Continued)
    midline N81.11
    paravaginal N81.12
  in pregnancy or childbirth O34.8-
    causing obstructed labor O65.5
  male N32.89
Cystolithiasis N21.0
Cystoma —*see also* Neoplasm, benign, by site
  endometrial, ovary N80.1
  mucinous
    specified site —*see* Neoplasm, benign, by
        site
    unspecified site D27.9
  serous
    specified site —*see* Neoplasm, benign, by
        site
    unspecified site D27.9
  simple (ovary) N83.29
Cystoplegia N31.2
Cystoptosis N32.89
Cystopyelitis —*see* Pyelonephritis
Cystorrhagia N32.89
Cystosarcoma phyllodes D48.6-
  benign D24-
  malignant —*see* Neoplasm, breast, malignant
Cystostomy
  attention to Z43.5
  complication —*see* Complications,
      cystostomy
  status Z93.50
    appendico-vesicostomy Z93.52
    cutaneous Z93.51
    specified NEC Z93.59
Cystourethritis —*see* Urethritis
Cystourethrocele —*see also* Cystocele
  female N81.10
    with uterine prolapse —*see* Prolapse,
        uterus
    lateral N81.12
    midline N81.11
    paravaginal N81.12
  male N32.89
Cytomegalic inclusion disease
  congenital P35.1
Cytomegalovirus infection B25.9
Cytomycosis (reticuloendothelial) B39.4
Cytopenia D75.9
  refractory
    with multilineage dysplasia D46.A
      and ring sideroblasts (RCMD RS) D46.B
Czerny's disease (periodic hydrarthrosis of the
    knee) —*see* Effusion, joint, knee

D

Daae (-Finsen) disease (epidemic pleurodynia) B33.0
Dabney's grip B33.0
Da Costa's syndrome F45.8
Dacryoadenitis, dacryadenitis H04.00-
 acute H04.01-
 chronic H04.02-
Dacryocystitis H04.30-
 acute H04.32-
 chronic H04.41-
 neonatal P39.1
 phlegmonous H04.31-
 syphilitic A52.71
  congenital (early) A50.01
 trachomatous, active A71.1
  sequelae (late effect) B94.0
Dacryocystoblenorrhea —*see* Inflammation, lacrimal, passages, chronic
Dacryocystocele —*see* Disorder, lacrimal system, changes
Dacryolith, dacryolithiasis H04.51-
Dacryoma —*see* Disorder, lacrimal system, changes
Dacryopericystitis —*see* Dacryocystitis
Dacryops H04.11-
Dacryostenosis —*see also* Stenosis, lacrimal
 congenital Q10.5
Dactylitis
 bone —*see* Osteomyelitis
 sickle-cell D57.00
  Hb C D57.219
  Hb SS D57.00
  specified NEC D57.819
 skin L08.9
 syphilitic A52.77
 tuberculous A18.03
Dactylolysis spontanea (ainhum) L94.6
Dactylosymphysis Q70.9
 fingers —*see* Syndactylism, complex, fingers
 toes —*see* Syndactylism, complex, toes
Damage
 arteriosclerotic —*see* Arteriosclerosis
 brain (nontraumatic) G93.9
  anoxic, hypoxic G93.1
   resulting from a procedure G97.82
  child NEC G80.9
  due to birth injury P11.2
 cardiorenal (vascular) —*see* Hypertension, cardiorenal
 cerebral NEC —*see* Damage, brain
 coccyx, complicating delivery O71.6
 coronary —*see* Disease, heart, ischemic
 eye, birth injury P15.3
 liver (nontraumatic) K76.9
  alcoholic K70.9
  due to drugs —*see* Disease, liver, toxic
  toxic —*see* Disease, liver, toxic
 medication T88.7
 pelvic
  joint or ligament, during delivery O71.6
  organ NEC
   during delivery O71.5
   following ectopic or molar pregnancy O08.6
 renal —*see* Disease, renal
 subendocardium, subendocardial —*see* Degeneration, myocardial
 vascular I99.9
Dana-Putnam syndrome (subacute combined sclerosis with pernicious anemia) —*see* Degeneration, combined
Danbolt (-Cross) syndrome (acrodermatitis enteropathica) E83.2
Dandruff L21.0
Dandy-Walker syndrome Q03.1
 with spina bifida —*see* Spina bifida
Danlos' syndrome Q79.6

Darier (-White) disease (congenital) Q82.8
 meaning erythema annulare centrifugum L53.1
Darier-Roussy sarcoid D86.3
Darling's disease or histoplasmosis B39.4
Darwin's tubercle Q17.8
Dawson's (inclusion body) encephalitis A81.1
De Beurmann (-Gougerot) disease B42.1
De la Tourette's syndrome F95.2
De Lange's syndrome Q87.1
De Morgan's spots (senile angiomas) I78.1
De Quervain's
 disease (tendon sheath) M65.4
 syndrome E34.51
 thyroiditis (subacute granulomatous thyroiditis) E06.1
De Toni-Fanconi (-Debré) syndrome E72.09
 with cystinosis E72.04
Dead
 fetus, retained (mother) O36.4
  early pregnancy O02.1
 labyrinth —*see* subcategory H83.2
 ovum, retained O02.0
Deaf nonspeaking NEC H91.3
Deafmutism (acquired) (congenital) NEC H91.3
 hysterical F44.6
 syphilitic, congenital (*see also* subcategory H94.8) A50.09
Deafness (acquired) (complete) (hereditary) (partial) H91.9-
 with blue sclera and fragility of bone Q78.0
 auditory fatigue —*see* Deafness, specified type NEC
 aviation T70.0
  nerve injury —*see* Injury, nerve, acoustic, specified type NEC
 boilermaker's —*see* subcategory H83.3
 central —*see* Deafness, sensorineural
 conductive H90.2
  and sensorineural, mixed H90.8
   bilateral H90.6
  bilateral H90.0
  unilateral H90.1-
 congenital H90.5
  with blue sclera and fragility of bone Q78.0
 due to toxic agents —*see* Deafness, ototoxic
 emotional (hysterical) F44.6
 functional (hysterical) F44.6
 high frequency H91.9-
 hysterical F44.6
 low frequency H91.9-
 mental R48.8
 mixed conductive and sensorineural H90.8
  bilateral H90.6
  unilateral H90.7-
 nerve —*see* Deafness, sensorineural
 neural —*see* Deafness, sensorineural
 noise-induced —*see also* subcategory H83.3
  nerve injury —*see* Injury, nerve, acoustic, specified type NEC
 nonspeaking H91.3
 ototoxic —*see* subcategory H91.0
 perceptive —*see* Deafness, sensorineural
 psychogenic (hysterical) F44.6
 sensorineural H90.5
  and conductive, mixed H90.8
   bilateral H90.6
  bilateral H90.3
  unilateral H90.4-
 sensory —*see* Deafness, sensorineural
 specified type NEC —*see* subcategory H91.8
 sudden (idiopathic) H91.2-
 syphilitic A52.15
 transient ischemic H93.01-
 traumatic —*see* Injury, nerve, acoustic, specified type NEC
 word (developmental) H93.25

Death (cause unknown) (of) (unexplained) (unspecified cause) R99
 brain G93.82
 cardiac (sudden) (with successful resuscitation) — code to underlying disease
  family history of Z82.41
  personal history of Z86.74
 family member (assumed) Z63.4
Debility (chronic) (general) (nervous) R53.81
 congenital or neonatal NOS P96.9
 nervous R53.81
 old age R54
 senile R54
Débove's disease (splenomegaly) R16.1
Decalcification
 bone —*see* Osteoporosis
 teeth K03.89
Decapsulation, kidney N28.89
Decay
 dental —*see* Caries, dental
 senile R54
 tooth, teeth —*see* Caries, dental
Deciduitis (acute)
 following ectopic or molar pregnancy O08.0
Decline (general) —*see* Debility
 cognitive, age-associated R41.81
Decompensation
 cardiac (acute) (chronic) —*see* Disease, heart
 cardiovascular —*see* Disease, cardiovascular
 heart —*see* Disease, heart
 hepatic —*see* Failure, hepatic
 myocardial (acute) (chronic) —*see* Disease, heart
 respiratory J98.8
Decompression sickness T70.3
Decrease (d)
 absolute neutrophile count —*see* Neutropenia
 blood
  platelets —*see* Thrombocytopenia
  pressure R03.1
   due to shock following injury T79.4
    operation T81.19
 estrogen E28.39
  postablative E89.40
   asymptomatic E89.40
   symptomatic E89.41
 fragility of erythrocytes D58.8
 function
  lipase (pancreatic) K90.3
  ovary in hypopituitarism E23.0
  parenchyma of pancreas K86.8
  pituitary (gland) (anterior) (lobe) E23.0
   posterior (lobe) E23.0
 functional activity R68.89
 glucose R73.09
 hematocrit R71.0
 hemoglobin R71.0
 leukocytes D72.819
  specified NEC D72.818
 libido R68.82
 lymphocytes D72.810
 platelets D69.6
 respiration, due to shock following injury T79.4
 sexual desire R68.82
 tear secretion NEC —*see* Syndrome, dry eye
 tolerance
  fat K90.4
  glucose R73.09
  pancreatic K90.3
  salt and water E87.8
 vision NEC H54.7
 white blood cell count D72.819
  specified NEC D72.818
Decubitus (ulcer) —*see* Ulcer, pressure, by site
 cervix N86
Deepening acetabulum —*see* Derangement, joint, specified type NEC, hip

◀ New ◀||| Revised ~~deleted~~ Deleted

Defect, defective Q89.9
  3-beta-hydroxysteroid dehydrogenase E25.0
  11-hydroxylase E25.0
  21-hydroxylase E25.0
  abdominal wall, congenital Q79.59
  antibody immunodeficiency D80.9
  aorticopulmonary septum Q21.4
  atrial septal (ostium secundum type) Q21.1
    following acute myocardial infarction (current complication) I23.1
    ostium primum type Q21.2
  atrioventricular
    canal Q21.2
    septum Q21.2
  auricular septal Q21.1
  bilirubin excretion NEC E80.6
  biosynthesis, androgen (testicular) E29.1
  bulbar septum Q21.0
  catalase E80.3
  cell membrane receptor complex (CR3) D71
  circulation I99.9
    congenital Q28.9
    newborn Q28.9
  coagulation (factor) (*see also* Deficiency, factor) D68.9
    with
      ectopic pregnancy O08.1
      molar pregnancy O08.1
    acquired D68.4
    antepartum with hemorrhage —*see* Hemorrhage, antepartum, with coagulation defect
    due to
      liver disease D68.4
      vitamin K deficiency D68.4
    hereditary NEC D68.2
    intrapartum O67.0
    newborn, transient P61.6
    postpartum O72.3
    specified type NEC D68.8
  complement system D84.1
  conduction (heart) I45.9
    bone —*see* Deafness, conductive
  congenital, organ or site not listed —*see* Anomaly, by site
  coronary sinus Q21.1
  cushion, endocardial Q21.2
  degradation, glycoprotein E77.1
  dental bridge, crown, fillings —*see* Defect, dental restoration
  dental restoration K08.50
    specified NEC K08.59
  dentin (hereditary) K00.5
  Descemet's membrane, congenital Q13.89
  developmental —*see also* Anomaly
    cauda equina Q06.3
  diaphragm
    with elevation, eventration or hernia —*see* Hernia, diaphragm
    congenital Q79.1
      with hernia Q79.0
      gross (with hernia) Q79.0
  ectodermal, congenital Q82.9
  Eisenmenger's Q21.8
  enzyme
    catalase E80.3
    peroxidase E80.3
  esophagus, congenital Q39.9
  extensor retinaculum M62.89
  fibrin polymerization D68.2
  filling
    bladder R93.4
    kidney R93.4
    stomach R93.3
    ureter R93.4
  Gerbode Q21.0
  glycoprotein degradation E77.1
  Hageman (factor) D68.2
  hearing —*see* Deafness
  high grade F70
  interatrial septal Q21.1

Defect, defective (*Continued*)
  interauricular septal Q21.1
  interventricular septal Q21.0
    with dextroposition of aorta, pulmonary stenosis and hypertrophy of right ventricle Q21.3
    in tetralogy of Fallot Q21.3
  learning (specific) —*see* Disorder, learning
  lymphocyte function antigen-1 (LFA-1) D84.0
  lysosomal enzyme, post-translational modification E77.0
  major osseous M89.70
    ankle M89.77-
    carpus M89.74-
    clavicle M89.71-
    femur M89.75-
    fibula M89.76-
    fingers M89.74-
    foot M89.77-
    forearm M89.73-
    hand M89.74-
    humerus M89.72-
    lower leg M89.76-
    metacarpus M89.74-
    metatarsus M89.77-
    multiple sites M89.79
    pelvic region M89.75-
    pelvis M89.75-
    radius M89.73-
    scapula M89.71-
    shoulder region M89.71-
    specified NEC M89.78
    tarsus M89.77-
    thigh M89.75-
    tibia M89.76-
    toes M89.77-
    ulna M89.73-
  mental —*see* Disability, intellectual
  modification, lysosomal enzymes, post-translational E77.0
  obstructive, congenital
    renal pelvis Q62.39
    ureter Q62.39
      atresia —*see* Atresia, ureter
      cecoureterocele Q62.32
      megaureter Q62.2
      orthotopic ureterocele Q62.31
  osseous, major M89.70
    ankle M89.77-
    carpus M89.74-
    clavicle M89.71-
    femur M89.75-
    fibula M89.76-
    fingers M89.74-
    foot M89.77-
    forearm M89.73-
    hand M89.74-
    humerus M89.72-
    lower leg M89.76-
    metacarpus M89.74-
    metatarsus M89.77-
    multiple sites M89.9
    pelvic region M89.75-
    pelvis M89.75-
    radius M89.73-
    scapula M89.71-
    shoulder region M89.71-
    specified NEC M89.78
    tarsus M89.77-
    thigh M89.75-
    tibia M89.76-
    toes M89.77-
    ulna M89.73-
  osteochondral NEC (*see also* Deformity) M95.8-
  ostium
    primum Q21.2
    secundum Q21.1
  peroxidase E80.3
  placental blood supply —*see* Insufficiency, placental

Defect, defective (*Continued*)
  platelets, qualitative D69.1
    constitutional D68.0
  postural NEC, spine —*see* Dorsopathy, deforming
  reduction
    limb Q73.8
      lower Q72.9-
        absence —*see* Agenesis, leg
        foot —*see* Agenesis, foot
        longitudinal
          femur Q72.4-
          fibula Q72.6-
          tibia Q72.5-
        specified type NEC Q72.89-
        split foot Q72.7-
      specified type NEC Q73.8
      upper Q71.9-
        absence —*see* Agenesis, arm
        forearm —*see* Agenesis, forearm
        hand —*see* Agenesis, hand
        lobster-claw hand Q71.6-
        longitudinal
          radius Q71.4-
          ulna Q71.5-
        specified type NEC Q71.89-
    renal pelvis Q63.8
      obstructive Q62.39
  respiratory system, congenital Q34.9
  restoration, dental K08.50
    specified NEC K08.59
  retinal nerve bundle fibers H35.89
  septal (heart) NOS Q21.9
    acquired (atrial) (auricular) (ventricular) (old) I51.0
    atrial Q21.1
      concurrent with acute myocardial infarction —*see* Infarct, myocardium
      following acute myocardial infarction (current complication) I23.1
    ventricular (*see also* Defect, ventricular septal) Q21.0
  sinus venosus Q21.1
  speech R47.9
    developmental F80.9
    specified NEC R47.89
  Taussig-Bing (aortic transposition and overriding pulmonary artery) Q20.1
  teeth, wedge K03.1
  vascular (local) I99.9
    congenital Q27.9
  ventricular septal Q21.0
    concurrent with acute myocardial infarction —*see* Infarct, myocardium
    following acute myocardial infarction (current complication) I23.2
    in tetralogy of Fallot Q21.3
  vision NEC H54.7
  visual field H53.40
    bilateral
      heteronymous H53.47
      homonymous H53.46-
    generalized contraction H53.48-
    localized
      arcuate H53.43-
      scotoma (central area) H53.41-
        blind spot area H53.42-
      sector H53.43-
      specified type NEC H53.45-
  voice R49.9
    specified NEC R49.8
  wedge, tooth, teeth (abrasion) K03.1
Deferentitis N49.1
  gonorrheal (acute) (chronic) A54.23
Defibrination (syndrome) D65
  antepartum —*see* Hemorrhage, antepartum, with coagulation defect, disseminated intravascular coagulation
  following ectopic or molar pregnancy O08.1
  intrapartum O67.0

Defibrination (*Continued*)
  newborn P60
  postpartum O72.3
Deficiency, deficient
  3-beta hydroxysteroid dehydrogenase E25.0
  11-hydroxylase E25.0
  21-hydroxylase E25.0
  5-alpha reductase (with male
      pseudohermaphroditism) E29.1
  abdominal muscle syndrome Q79.4
  AC globulin (congenital) (hereditary) D68.2
    acquired D68.4
  accelerator globulin (Ac G) (blood) D68.2
  acid phosphatase E83.39
  activating factor (blood) D68.2
  adenosine deaminase (ADA) D81.3
  aldolase (hereditary) E74.19
  alpha-1-antitrypsin E88.01
  amino-acids E72.9
  anemia —*see* Anemia
  aneurin E51.9
  antibody with
    hyperimmunoglobulinemia D80.6
    near-normal immunoglobins D80.6
  antidiuretic hormone E23.2
  anti-hemophilic
    factor (A) D66
      B D67
      C D68.1
    globulin (AHG) NEC D66
  antithrombin (antithrombin III) D68.59
  ascorbic acid E54
  attention (disorder) (syndrome) F98.8
    with hyperactivity —*see* Disorder,
      attention-deficit hyperactivity
  autoprothrombin
    I D68.2
    II D67
    C D68.2
  beta-glucuronidase E76.29
  biotin E53.8
  biotin-dependent carboxylase D81.819
  biotinidase D81.810
  brancher enzyme (amylopectinosis) E74.03
  C1 esterase inhibitor (C1-INH) D84.1
  calciferol E55.9
    with
      adult osteomalacia M83.8
      rickets —*see* Rickets
  calcium (dietary) E58
  calorie, severe E43
    with marasmus E41
      and kwashiorkor E42
  cardiac —*see* Insufficiency, myocardial
  carnitine E71.40
    due to
      hemodialysis E71.43
      inborn errors of metabolism E71.42
      Valproic acid therapy E71.43
    iatrogenic E71.43
    muscle palmityltransferase E71.314
    primary E71.41
    secondary E71.448
  carotene E50.9
  central nervous system G96.8
  ceruloplasmin (Wilson) E83.01
  choline E53.8
  Christmas factor D67
  chromium E61.4
  clotting (blood) (*see also* Deficiency,
    coagulation factor) D68.9
  clotting factor NEC (hereditary) (*see also*
    Deficiency, factor) D68.2
  coagulation NOS D68.9
    with
      ectopic pregnancy O08.1
      molar pregnancy O08.1
    acquired (any) D68.4
    antepartum hemorrhage —*see*
      Hemorrhage, antepartum, with
      coagulation defect

Deficiency, deficient (*Continued*)
  coagulation NOS (*Continued*)
    clotting factor NEC (*see also* Deficiency,
      factor) D68.2
    due to
      hyperprothrombinemia D68.4
      liver disease D68.4
      vitamin K deficiency D68.4
    newborn, transient P61.6
    postpartum O72.3
    specified NEC D68.8
  cognitive F09
  color vision H53.50
    achromatopsia H53.51
    acquired H53.52
    deuteranomaly H53.53
    protanomaly H53.54
    specified type NEC H53.59
    tritanomaly H53.55
  combined glucocorticoid and
    mineralocorticoid E27.49
  contact factor D68.2
  copper (nutritional) E61.0
  corticoadrenal E27.40
    primary E27.1
  craniofacial axis Q75.0
  cyanocobalamin E53.8
  debrancher enzyme (limit dextrinosis) E74.03
  dehydrogenase
    long chain/very long chain acyl CoA
      E71.310
    medium chain acyl CoA E71.311
    short chain acyl CoA E71.312
  diet E63.9
  dihydropyrimidine dehydrogenase (DPD)
    E88.89
  disaccharidase E73.9
  edema —*see* Malnutrition, severe
  endocrine E34.9
  energy-supply —*see* Malnutrition
  enzymes, circulating NEC E88.09
  ergosterol E55.9
    with
      adult osteomalacia M83.8
      rickets —*see* Rickets
  essential fatty acid (EFA) E63.0
  factor —*see also* Deficiency, coagulation
    Hageman D68.2
    I (congenital) (hereditary) D68.2
    II (congenital) (hereditary) D68.2
    IX (congenital) (functional) (hereditary)
      (with functional defect) D67
    multiple (congenital) D68.8
      acquired D68.4
    V (congenital) (hereditary) D68.2
    VII (congenital) (hereditary) D68.2
    VIII (congenital) (functional) (hereditary)
      (with functional defect) D66
      with vascular defect D68.0
    X (congenital) (hereditary) D68.2
    XI (congenital) (hereditary) D68.1
    XII (congenital) (hereditary) D68.2
    XIII (congenital) (hereditary) D68.2
  femoral, proximal focal (congenital) —
    see Defect, reduction, lower limb,
    longitudinal, femur
  fibrin-stabilizing factor (congenital)
    (hereditary) D68.2
    acquired D68.4
  fibrinase D68.2
  fibrinogen (congenital) (hereditary) D68.2
    acquired D65
  folate E53.8
  folic acid E53.8
  foreskin N47.3
  fructokinase E74.11
  fructose 1,6-diphosphatase E74.19
  fructose-1-phosphate aldolase E74.19
  galactokinase E74.29
  galactose-1-phosphate uridyl transferase
    E74.29

Deficiency, deficient (*Continued*)
  gammaglobulin in blood D80.1
    hereditary D80.0
  glass factor D68.2
  glucocorticoid E27.49
    mineralocorticoid E27.49
  glucose-6-phosphatase E74.01
  glucose-6-phosphate dehydrogenase anemia
    D55.0
  glucuronyl transferase E80.5
  glycogen synthetase E74.09
  gonadotropin (isolated) E23.0
  growth hormone (idiopathic) (isolated) E23.0
  Hageman factor D68.2
  hemoglobin D64.9
  hepatophosphorylase E74.09
  homogentisate 1,2-dioxygenase E70.29
  hormone
    anterior pituitary (partial) NEC E23.0
      growth E23.0
    growth (isolated) E23.0
    pituitary E23.0
    testicular E29.1
  hypoxanthine-(guanine)-
    phosphoribosyltransferase (HG-PRT)
    (total HG-PRT) E79.1
  immunity D84.9
    cell-mediated D84.8
      with thrombocytopenia and eczema
        D82.0
    combined D81.9
    humoral D80.9
    IgA (secretory) D80.2
    IgG D80.3
    IgM D80.4
  immuno —*see* Immunodeficiency
  immunoglobulin, selective
    A (IgA) D80.2
    G (IgG) (subclasses) D80.3
    M (IgM) D80.4
  inositol (B complex) E53.8
  intrinsic
    factor (congenital) D51.0
    sphincter N36.42
      with urethral hypermobility N36.43
  iodine E61.8
    congenital syndrome —*see* Syndrome,
      iodine-deficiency, congenital
  iron E61.1
    anemia D50.9
  kalium E87.6
  kappa-light chain D80.8
  labile factor (congenital) (hereditary) D68.2
    acquired D68.4
  lacrimal fluid (acquired) —*see also* Syndrome,
    dry eye
    congenital Q10.6
  lactase
    congenital E73.0
    secondary E73.1
  Laki-Lorand factor D68.2
  lecithin cholesterol acyltransferase E78.6
  lipocaic K86.8
  lipoprotein (familial) (high density) E78.6
  liver phosphorylase E74.09
  lysosomal alpha-1, 4 glucosidase E74.02
  magnesium E61.2
  major histocompatibility complex
    class I D81.6
    class II D81.7
  manganese E61.3
  menadione (vitamin K) E56.1
    newborn P53
  mental (familial) (hereditary) —*see* Disability,
    intellectual
  methylenetetrahydrofolate reductase
    (MTHFR) E72.12
  mineral NEC E61.8
  mineralocorticoid E27.49
    with glucocorticoid E27.49
  molybdenum (nutritional) E61.5

◀ New   ⬅ Revised   ~~deleted~~ Deleted

Deficiency, deficient (*Continued*)
moral F60.2
multiple nutrient elements E61.7
muscle
  carnitine (palmityltransferase) E71.314
  phosphofructokinase E74.09
myoadenylate deaminase E79.2
myocardial —*see* Insufficiency, myocardial
myophosphorylase E74.04
NADH diaphorase or reductase (congenital) D74.0
NADH-methemoglobin reductase (congenital) D74.0
natrium E87.1
niacin (amide) (-tryptophan) E52
nicotinamide E52
nicotinic acid E52
number of teeth —*see* Anodontia
nutrient element E61.9
  multiple E61.7
  specified NEC E61.8
nutrition, nutritional E63.9
  sequelae —*see* Sequelae, nutritional deficiency
  specified NEC E63.8
ornithine transcarbamylase E72.4
ovarian E28.39
oxygen —*see* Anoxia
pantothenic acid E53.8
parathyroid (gland) E20.9
perineum (female) N81.89
phenylalanine hydroxylase E70.1
phosphoenolpyruvate carboxykinase E74.4
phosphofructokinase E74.19
phosphomannomutase E74.8
phosphomannose isomerase E74.8
phosphomannosyl mutase E74.8
phosphorylase kinase, liver E74.09
pituitary hormone (isolated) E23.0
plasma thromboplastin
  antecedent (PTA) D68.1
  component (PTC) D67
platelet NEC D69.1
  constitutional D68.0
polyglandular E31.8
  autoimmune E31.0
potassium (K) E87.6
prepuce N47.3
proaccelerin (congenital) (hereditary) D68.2
  acquired D68.4
proconvertin factor (congenital) (hereditary) D68.2
  acquired D68.4
protein (*see also* Malnutrition) E46
  anemia D53.0
  C D68.59
  S D68.59
prothrombin (congenital) (heredItary) D68.2
  acquired D68.4
Prower factor D68.2
pseudocholinesterase E88.09
PTA (plasma thromboplastin antecedent) D68.1
PTC (plasma thromboplastin component) D67
purine nucleoside phosphorylase (PNP) D81.5
pyracin (alpha) (beta) E53.1
pyridoxal E53.1
pyridoxamine E53.1
pyridoxine (derivatives) E53.1
pyruvate
  carboxylase E74.4
  dehydrogenase E74.4
riboflavin (vitamin B2) E53.0
salt E87.1
secretion
  ovary E28.39
  salivary gland (any) K11.7
  urine R34
selenium (dietary) E59
serum antitrypsin, familial E88.01

Deficiency, deficient (*Continued*)
short stature homeobox gene (SHOX)
  with
    dyschondrosteosis Q78.8
    short stature (idiopathic) E34.3
    Turner's syndrome Q96.9
sodium (Na) E87.1
SPCA (factor VII) D68.2
sphincter, intrinsic N36.42
  with urethral hypermobility N36.43
stable factor (congenital) (hereditary) D68.2
  acquired D68.4
Stuart-Prower (factor X) D68.2
sucrase E74.39
sulfatase E75.29
sulfite oxidase E72.19
thiamin, thiaminic (chloride) E51.9
  beriberi (dry) E51.11
    wet E51.12
thrombokinase D68.2
  newborn P53
thyroid (gland) —*see* Hypothyroidism
tocopherol E56.0
tooth bud K00.0
transcobalamine II (anemia) D51.2
vanadium E61.6
vascular I99.9
vasopressin E23.2
viosterol —*see* Deficiency, calciferol
vitamin (multiple) NOS E56.9
  A E50.9
    with
      Bitot's spot (corneal) E50.1
      follicular keratosis E50.8
      keratomalacia E50.4
      manifestations NEC E50.8
      night blindness E50.5
      scar of cornea, xerophthalmic E50.6
      xeroderma E50.8
      xerophthalmia E50.7
      xerosis
        conjunctival E50.0
          and Bitot's spot E50.1
        cornea E50.2
          and ulceration E50.3
    sequelae E64.1
  B (complex) NOS E53.9
    with
      beriberi (dry) E51.11
        wet E51.12
      pellagra E52
  B1 NOS E51.9
    beriberi (dry) E51.11
      with circulatory system manifestations E51.11
        wet E51.12
  B12 E53.8
  B2 (riboflavin) E53.0
  B6 E53.1
  C E54
    sequelae E64.2
  D E55.9
    with
      adult osteomalacia M83.8
      rickets —*see* Rickets
    25-hydroxylase E83.32
  E E56.0
  folic acid E53.8
  G E53.0
  group B E53.9
    specified NEC E53.8
  H (biotin) E53.8
  K E56.1
    of newborn P53
  nicotinic E52
  P E56.8
  PP (pellagra-preventing) E52
  specified NEC E56.8
  thiamin E51.9
    beriberi —*see* Beriberi
zinc, dietary E60

Deficit —*see also* Deficiency
attention and concentration R41.840
  disorder —*see* Attention, deficit
cognitive communication R41.841
cognitive NEC R41.89
  following
    cerebral infarction I69.31
    cerebrovascular disease I69.91
      specified disease NEC I69.81
    intracerebral hemorrhage I69.11
    nontraumatic intracranial hemorrhage NEC I69.21
    subarachnoid hemorrhage I69.01
concentration R41.840
executive function R41.844
frontal lobe R41.844
neurologic NEC R29.818
ischemic
  reversible (RIND) I63.9
    prolonged (PRIND) I63.9
oxygen R09.02
prolonged reversible ischemic neurologic (PRIND) I63.9
psychomotor R41.843
visuospatial R41.842
Deflection
radius —*see* Deformity, limb, specified type NEC, forearm
septum (acquired) (nasal) (nose) J34.2
spine —*see* Curvature, spine
turbinate (nose) J34.2
Defluvium
capillorum —*see* Alopecia
ciliorum —*see* Madarosis
unguium L60.8
Deformity Q89.9
abdomen, congenital Q89.9
abdominal wall
  acquired M95.8
  congenital Q79.59
acquired (unspecified site) M95.9
adrenal gland Q89.1
alimentary tract, congenital Q45.9
  upper Q40.9
ankle (joint) (acquired) —*see also* Deformity, limb, lower leg
  abduction —*see* Contraction, joint, ankle
  congenital Q68.8
  contraction —*see* Contraction, joint, ankle
  specified type NEC —*see* Deformity, limb, foot, specified NEC
anus (acquired) K62.89
  congenital Q43.9
aorta (arch) (congenital) Q25.4
  acquired I77.89
aortic
  arch, acquired I77.89
  cusp or valve (congenital) Q23.8
    acquired (*see also* Endocarditis, aortic) I35.8
arm (acquired) (upper) —*see also* Deformity, limb, upper arm
  congenital Q68.8
  forearm —*see* Deformity, limb, forearm
artery (congenital) (peripheral) NOS Q27.9
  acquired I77.89
  coronary (acquired) I25.9
    congenital Q24.5
  umbilical Q27.0
atrial septal Q21.1
auditory canal (external) (congenital) —*see also* Malformation, ear, external
  acquired —*see* Disorder, ear, external, specified type NEC
auricle
  ear (congenital) —*see also* Malformation, ear, external
    acquired —*see* Disorder, pinna, deformity
back —*see* Dorsopathy, deforming

Deformity *(Continued)*

bile duct (common) (congenital) (hepatic) Q44.5
  acquired K83.8
biliary duct or passage (congenital) Q44.5
  acquired K83.8
bladder (neck) (trigone) (sphincter) (acquired) N32.89
  congenital Q64.79
bone (acquired) NOS M95.9
  congenital Q79.9
  turbinate M95.0
brain (congenital) Q04.9
  acquired G93.89
  reduction Q04.3
breast (acquired) N64.89
  congenital Q83.9
  reconstructed N65.0
bronchus (congenital) Q32.4
  acquired NEC J98.09
bursa, congenital Q79.9
canaliculi (lacrimalis) (acquired) *—see also* Disorder, lacrimal system, changes
  congenital Q10.6
canthus, acquired *—see* Disorder, eyelid, specified type NEC
capillary (acquired) I78.8
cardiovascular system, congenital Q28.9
caruncle, lacrimal (acquired) *—see also* Disorder, lacrimal system, changes
  congenital Q10.6
cascade, stomach K31.2
cecum (congenital) Q43.9
  acquired K63.89
cerebral, acquired G93.89
  congenital Q04.9
cervix (uterus) (acquired) NEC N88.8
  congenital Q51.9
cheek (acquired) M95.2
  congenital Q18.9
chest (acquired) (wall) M95.4
  congenital Q67.8
  sequelae (late effect) of rickets E64.3
chin (acquired) M95.2
  congenital Q18.9
choroid (congenital) Q14.3
  acquired H31.8
  plexus Q07.8
    acquired G96.19
cicatricial *—see* Cicatrix
cilia, acquired *—see* Disorder, eyelid, specified type NEC
clavicle (acquired) M95.8
  congenital Q68.8
clitoris (congenital) Q52.6
  acquired N90.89
clubfoot *—see* Clubfoot
coccyx (acquired) *—see* subcategory M43.8
colon (congenital) Q43.9
  acquired K63.89
concha (ear), congenital *—see also* Malformation, ear, external
  acquired *—see* Disorder, pinna, deformity
cornea (acquired) H18.70
  congenital Q13.4
  descemetocele *—see* Descemetocele
  ectasia *—see* Ectasia, cornea
  specified NEC H18.79-
  staphyloma *—see* Staphyloma, cornea
coronary artery (acquired) I25.9
  congenital Q24.5
cranium (acquired) *—see* Deformity, skull
cricoid cartilage (congenital) Q31.8
  acquired J38.7
cystic duct (congenital) Q44.5
  acquired K82.8
Dandy-Walker Q03.1
  with spina bifida *—see* Spina bifida
diaphragm (congenital) Q79.1
  acquired J98.6
digestive organ NOS Q45.9

Deformity *(Continued)*

ductus arteriosus Q25.0
duodenal bulb K31.89
duodenum (congenital) Q43.9
  acquired K31.89
dura *—see* Deformity, meninges
ear (acquired) *—see also* Disorder, pinna, deformity
  congenital (external) Q17.9
    internal Q16.5
    middle Q16.4
      ossicles Q16.3
    ossicles Q16.3
ectodermal (congenital) NEC Q84.9
ejaculatory duct (congenital) Q55.4
  acquired N50.8
elbow (joint) (acquired) *—see also* Deformity, limb, upper arm
  congenital Q68.8
  contraction *—see* Contraction, joint, elbow
endocrine gland NEC Q89.2
epididymis (congenital) Q55.4
  acquired N50.8
epiglottis (congenital) Q31.8
  acquired J38.7
esophagus (congenital) Q39.9
  acquired K22.8
eustachian tube (congenital) NEC Q17.8
eye, congenital Q15.9
eyebrow (congenital) Q18.8
eyelid (acquired) *—see also* Disorder, eyelid, specified type NEC
  congenital Q10.3
face (acquired) M95.2
  congenital Q18.9
fallopian tube, acquired N83.8
femur (acquired) *—see* Deformity, limb, specified type NEC, thigh
fetal
  with fetopelvic disproportion O33.7
  causing obstructed labor O66.3
finger (acquired) M20.00-
  boutonniere M20.02-
  congenital Q68.1
  flexion contracture *—see* Contraction, joint, hand
  mallet finger M20.01-
  specified NEC M20.09-
  swan-neck M20.03-
flexion (joint) (acquired) *(see also* Deformity, limb, flexion) M21.20
  congenital NOS Q74.9
  hip Q65.89
foot (acquired) *—see also* Deformity, limb, lower leg
  cavovarus (congenital) Q66.1
  congenital NOS Q66.9
    specified type NEC Q66.89
  specified type NEC *—see* Deformity, limb, foot, specified NEC
  valgus (congenital) Q66.6
    acquired *—see* Deformity, valgus, ankle
  varus (congenital) NEC Q66.3
    acquired *—see* Deformity, varus, ankle
forearm (acquired) *—see also* Deformity, limb, forearm
  congenital Q68.8
forehead (acquired) M95.2
  congenital Q75.8
frontal bone (acquired) M95.2
  congenital Q75.8
gallbladder (congenital) Q44.1
  acquired K82.8
gastrointestinal tract (congenital) NOS Q45.9
  acquired K63.89
genitalia, genital organ (s) or system NEC
  female (congenital) Q52.9
    acquired N94.89
    external Q52.70
  male (congenital) Q55.9
    acquired N50.8

Deformity *(Continued)*

globe (eye) (congenital) Q15.8
  acquired H44.89
gum, acquired NEC K06.8
hand (acquired) *—see* Deformity, limb, hand
  congenital Q68.1
head (acquired) M95.2
  congenital Q75.8
heart (congenital) Q24.9
  septum Q21.9
    auricular Q21.1
    ventricular Q21.0
  valve (congenital) NEC Q24.8
    acquired *—see* Endocarditis
heel (acquired) *—see* Deformity, foot
hepatic duct (congenital) Q44.5
  acquired K83.8
hip (joint) (acquired) *—see also* Deformity, limb, thigh
  congenital Q65.9
  due to (previous) juvenile osteochondrosis *—see* Coxa, plana
  flexion *—see* Contraction, joint, hip
hourglass *—see* Contraction, hourglass
humerus (acquired) M21.82-
  congenital Q74.0
hypophyseal (congenital) Q89.2
ileocecal (coil) (valve) (acquired) K63.89
  congenital Q43.9
ileum (congenital) Q43.9
  acquired K63.89
ilium (acquired) M95.5
  congenital Q74.2
integument (congenital) Q84.9
intervertebral cartilage or disc (acquired) *—see* Disorder, disc, specified NEC
intestine (large) (small) (congenital) NOS Q43.9
  acquired K63.89
intrinsic minus or plus (hand) *—see* Deformity, limb, specified type NEC, forearm
iris (acquired) H21.89
  congenital Q13.2
ischium (acquired) M95.5
  congenital Q74.2
jaw (acquired) (congenital) M26.9
joint (acquired) NEC M21.90
  congenital Q68.8
  elbow M21.92-
  hand M21.94-
  hip M21.95-
  knee M21.96-
  shoulder M21.92-
  wrist M21.93-
kidney (s) (calyx) (pelvis) (congenital) Q63.9
  acquired N28.89
  artery (congenital) Q27.2
    acquired I77.89
Klippel-Feil (brevicollis) Q76.1
knee (acquired) NEC *—see also* Deformity, limb, lower leg
  congenital Q68.2
labium (majus) (minus) (congenital) Q52.79
  acquired N90.89
lacrimal passages or duct (congenital) NEC Q10.6
  acquired *—see* Disorder, lacrimal system, changes
larynx (muscle) (congenital) Q31.8
  acquired J38.7
  web (glottic) Q31.0
leg (upper) (acquired) NEC *—see also* Deformity, limb, thigh
  congenital Q68.8
  lower leg *—see* Deformity, limb, lower leg
lens (acquired) H27.8
  congenital Q12.9
lid (fold) (acquired) *—see also* Disorder, eyelid, specified type NEC
  congenital Q10.3

◀ New   ◀▥ Revised   ~~deleted~~ Deleted

Deformity (Continued)
- ligament (acquired) —see Disorder, ligament
  - congenital Q79.9
- limb (acquired) M21.90
  - clawfoot M21.53-
  - clawhand M21.51-
  - clubfoot M21.54-
  - clubhand M21.52-
  - congenital, except reduction deformity Q74.9
  - flat foot M21.4-
  - flexion M21.20
    - ankle M21.27-
    - elbow M21.22-
    - finger M21.24-
    - hip M21.25-
    - knee M21.26
    - shoulder M21.21-
    - toe M21.27-
    - wrist M21.23-
  - foot
    - claw —see Deformity, limb, clawfoot
    - club —see Deformity, limb, clubfoot
    - drop M21.37-
    - flat —see Deformity, limb, flat foot
    - specified NEC M21.6X-
  - forearm M21.93-
  - hand M21.94-
  - lower leg M21.96-
  - specified type NEC M21.80
    - forearm M21.83-
    - lower leg M21.86-
    - thigh M21.85-
    - upper arm M21.82-
  - thigh M21.95-
  - unequal length M21.70
    - short site is
      - femur M21.75-
      - fibula M21.76-
      - humerus M21.72-
      - radius M21.73-
      - tibia M21.76-
      - ulna M21.73-
  - upper arm M21.92-
  - valgus —see Deformity, valgus
  - varus —see Deformity, varus
  - wrist drop M21.33-
- lip (acquired) NEC K13.0
  - congenital Q38.0
- liver (congenital) Q44.7
  - acquired K76.89
- lumbosacral (congenital) (joint) (region) Q76.49
  - acquired —see subcategory M43.8
  - kyphosis —see Kyphosis, congenital
  - lordosis —see Lordosis, congenital
- lung (congenital) Q33.9
  - acquired J98.4
- lymphatic system, congenital Q89.9
- Madelung's (radius) Q74.0
- mandible (acquired) (congenital) M26.9
- maxilla (acquired) (congenital) M26.9
- meninges or membrane (congenital) Q07.9
  - cerebral Q04.8
    - acquired G96.19
  - spinal cord (congenital) G96.19
    - acquired G96.19
- metacarpus (acquired) —see Deformity, limb, forearm
  - congenital Q74.0
- metatarsus (acquired) —see Deformity, foot
  - congenital Q66.9
- middle ear (congenital) Q16.4
  - ossicles Q16.3
- mitral (leaflets) (valve) I05.8
  - parachute Q23.2
  - stenosis, congenital Q23.2
- mouth (acquired) K13.79
  - congenital Q38.6
- multiple, congenital NEC Q89.7

Deformity (Continued)
- muscle (acquired) M62.89
  - congenital Q79.9
    - sternocleidomastoid Q68.0
- musculoskeletal system (acquired) M95.9
  - congenital Q79.9
  - specified NEC M95.8
- nail (acquired) L60.8
  - congenital Q84.6
- nasal —see Deformity, nose
- neck (acquired) M95.3
  - congenital Q18.9
    - sternocleidomastoid Q68.0
- nervous system (congenital) Q07.9
- nipple (congenital) Q83.9
  - acquired N64.89
- nose (acquired) (cartilage) M95.0
  - bone (turbinate) M95.0
  - congenital Q30.9
    - bent or squashed Q67.4
  - saddle M95.0
    - syphilitic A50.57
  - septum (acquired) J34.2
    - congenital Q30.8
  - sinus (wall) (congenital) Q30.8
    - acquired M95.0
  - syphilitic (congenital) A50.57
    - late A52.73
- ocular muscle (congenital) Q10.3
  - acquired —see Strabismus, mechanical
- opticociliary vessels (congenital) Q13.2
- orbit (eye) (acquired) H05.30
  - atrophy —see Atrophy, orbit
  - congenital Q10.7
  - due to
    - bone disease NEC H05.32-
    - trauma or surgery H05.33-
  - enlargement —see Enlargement, orbit
  - exostosis —see Exostosis, orbit
- organ of Corti (congenital) Q16.5
- ovary (congenital) Q50.39
  - acquired N83.8
- oviduct, acquired N83.8
- palate (congenital) Q38.5
  - acquired M27.8
  - cleft (congenital) —see Cleft, palate
- pancreas (congenital) Q45.3
  - acquired K86.8
- parathyroid (gland) Q89.2
- parotid (gland) (congenital) Q38.4
  - acquired K11.8
- patella (acquired) —see Disorder, patella, specified NEC
- pelvis, pelvic (acquired) (bony) M95.5
  - with disproportion (fetopelvic) O33.0
    - causing obstructed labor O65.0
  - congenital Q74.2
  - rachitic sequelae (late effect) E64.3
- penis (glans) (congenital) Q55.69
  - acquired N48.89
- pericardium (congenital) Q24.8
  - acquired —see Pericarditis
- pharynx (congenital) Q38.8
  - acquired J39.2
- pinna, acquired —see also Disorder, pinna, deformity
  - congenital Q17.9
- pituitary (congenital) Q89.2
- posture —see Dorsopathy, deforming
- prepuce (congenital) Q55.69
  - acquired N47.8
- prostate (congenital) Q55.4
  - acquired N42.89
- pupil (congenital) Q13.2
  - acquired —see Abnormality, pupillary
- pylorus (congenital) Q40.3
  - acquired K31.89
- rachitic (acquired), old or healed E64.3
- radius (acquired) —see also Deformity, limb, forearm
  - congenital Q68.8

Deformity (Continued)
- rectum (congenital) Q43.9
  - acquired K62.89
- reduction (extremity) (limb), congenital (see also condition and site) Q73.8
  - brain Q04.3
  - lower —see Defect, reduction, lower limb
  - upper —see Defect, reduction, upper limb
- renal —see Deformity, kidney
- respiratory system (congenital) Q34.9
- rib (acquired) M95.4
  - congenital Q76.6
  - cervical Q76.5
- rotation (joint) (acquired) —see Deformity, limb, specified site NEC
  - congenital Q74.9
  - hip —see Deformity, limb, specified type NEC, thigh
    - congenital Q65.89
- sacroiliac joint (congenital) Q74.2
  - acquired —see subcategory M43.8
- sacrum (acquired) —see subcategory M43.8
- saddle
  - back —see Lordosis
  - nose M95.0
    - syphilitic A50.57
- salivary gland or duct (congenital) Q38.4
  - acquired K11.8
- scapula (acquired) M95.8
  - congenital Q68.8
- scrotum (congenital) —see also Malformation, testis and scrotum
  - acquired N50.8
- seminal vesicles (congenital) Q55.4
  - acquired N50.8
- septum, nasal (acquired) J34.2
- shoulder (joint) (acquired) —see Deformity, limb, upper arm
  - congenital Q74.0
  - contraction —see Contraction, joint, shoulder
- sigmoid (flexure) (congenital) Q43.9
  - acquired K63.89
- skin (congenital) Q82.9
- skull (acquired) M95.2
  - congenital Q75.8
    - with
      - anencephaly Q00.0
      - encephalocele —see Encephalocele
      - hydrocephalus Q03.9
        - with spina bifida —see Spina bifida, by site, with hydrocephalus
      - microcephaly Q02
- soft parts, organs or tissues (of pelvis)
  - in pregnancy or childbirth NEC O34.8-
    - causing obstructed labor O65.5
- spermatic cord (congenital) Q55.4
  - acquired N50.8
  - torsion —see Torsion, spermatic cord
- spinal —see Dorsopathy, deforming
  - column (acquired) —see Dorsopathy, deforming
  - congenital Q67.5
  - cord (congenital) Q06.9
    - acquired G95.89
  - nerve root (congenital) Q07.9
- spine (acquired) —see also Dorsopathy, deforming
  - congenital Q67.5
  - rachitic E64.3
  - specified NEC —see Dorsopathy, deforming, specified NEC
- spleen
  - acquired D73.89
  - congenital Q89.09
- Sprengel's (congenital) Q74.0
- sternocleidomastoid (muscle), congenital Q68.0
- sternum (acquired) M95.4
  - congenital NEC Q76.7

Deformity *(Continued)*
stomach (congenital) Q40.3
  acquired K31.89
submandibular gland (congenital) Q38.4
submaxillary gland (congenital) Q38.4
  acquired K11.8
talipes —*see* Talipes
testis (congenital) —*see also* Malformation,
  testis and scrotum
  acquired N44.8
    torsion —*see* Torsion, testis
thigh (acquired) —*see also* Deformity, limb,
  thigh
  congenital NEC Q68.8
thorax (acquired) (wall) M95.4
  congenital Q67.8
  sequelae of rickets E64.3
thumb (acquired) —*see also* Deformity, finger
  congenital NEC Q68.1
thymus (tissue) (congenital) Q89.2
thyroid (gland) (congenital) Q89.2
  cartilage Q31.8
    acquired J38.7
tibia (acquired) —*see also* Deformity, limb,
  specified type NEC, lower leg
  congenital NEC Q68.8
  saber (syphilitic) A50.56
toe (acquired) M20.6-
  congenital Q66.9
  hallux rigidus M20.2-
  hallux valgus M20.1-
  hallux varus M20.3-
  hammer toe M20.4-
  specified NEC M20.5X-
tongue (congenital) Q38.3
  acquired K14.8
tooth, teeth K00.2
trachea (rings) (congenital) Q32.1
  acquired J39.8
transverse aortic arch (congenital) Q25.4
tricuspid (leaflets) (valve) I07.8
  atresia or stenosis Q22.4
  Ebstein's Q22.5
trunk (acquired) M95.8
  congenital Q89.9
ulna (acquired) —*see also* Deformity, limb,
  forearm
  congenital NEC Q68.8
urachus, congenital Q64.4
ureter (opening) (congenital) Q62.8
  acquired N28.89
urethra (congenital) Q64.79
  acquired N36.8
urinary tract (congenital) Q64.9
  urachus Q64.4
uterus (congenital) Q51.9
  acquired N85.8
uvula (congenital) Q38.5
vagina (acquired) N89.8
  congenital Q52.4
valgus NEC M21.00
  ankle M21.07-
  elbow M21.02-
  hip M21.05-
  knee M21.06-
valve, valvular (congenital) (heart) Q24.8
  acquired —*see* Endocarditis
varus NEC M21.10
  ankle M21.17-
  elbow M21.12-
  hip M21.15
  knee M21.16-
  tibia —*see* Osteochondrosis, juvenile, tibia
vas deferens (congenital) Q55.4
  acquired N50.8
vein (congenital) Q27.9
  great Q26.9
vertebra —*see* Dorsopathy, deforming
vertical talus (congenital) Q66.80
  left foot Q66.82
  right foot Q66.81

Deformity *(Continued)*
vesicourethral orifice (acquired) N32.89
  congenital NEC Q64.79
vessels of optic papilla (congenital) Q14.2
visual field (contraction) —*see* Defect, visual
  field
vitreous body, acquired H43.89
vulva (congenital) Q52.79
  acquired N90.89
wrist (joint) (acquired) —*see also* Deformity,
  limb, forearm
  congenital Q68.8
  contraction —*see* Contraction, joint, wrist
Degeneration, degenerative
adrenal (capsule) (fatty) (gland) (hyaline)
  (infectional) E27.8
amyloid (*see also* Amyloidosis) E85.9
anterior cornua, spinal cord G12.29
anterior labral S43.49-
aorta, aortic I70.0
  fatty I77.89
aortic valve (heart) —*see* Endocarditis, aortic
arteriovascular —*see* Arteriosclerosis
artery, arterial (atheromatous) (calcareous) —
  see also Arteriosclerosis
  cerebral, amyloid E85.4 *[I68.0]*
  medial —*see* Arteriosclerosis, extremities
articular cartilage NEC —*see* Derangement,
  joint, articular cartilage, by site
atheromatous —*see* Arteriosclerosis
basal nuclei or ganglia G23.9
  specified NEC G23.8
bone NEC —*see* Disorder, bone, specified
  type NEC
brachial plexus G54.0
brain (cortical) (progressive) G31.9
  alcoholic G31.2
  arteriosclerotic I67.2
  childhood G31.9
    specified NEC G31.89
  cystic G31.89
    congenital Q04.6
  in
    alcoholism G31.2
    beriberi E51.2
    cerebrovascular disease I67.9
    congenital hydrocephalus Q03.9
      with spina bifida —*see also* Spina
        bifida
    Fabry-Anderson disease E75.21
    Gaucher's disease E75.22
    Hunter's syndrome E76.1
    lipidosis
      cerebral E75.4
      generalized E75.6
    mucopolysaccharidosis —*see*
      Mucopolysaccharidosis
    myxedema E03.9 *[G32.89]*
    neoplastic disease (*see also* Neoplasm)
      D49.6 *[G32.89]*
    Niemann-Pick disease E75.249 *[G32.89]*
    sphingolipidosis E75.3 *[G32.89]*
    vitamin B12 deficiency E53.8 *[G32.89]*
  senile NEC G31.1
breast N64.89
Bruch's membrane —*see* Degeneration,
  choroid
capillaries (fatty) I78.8
  amyloid E85.8 *[I79.8]*
cardiac —*see also* Degeneration, myocardial
  valve, valvular —*see* Endocarditis
cardiorenal —*see* Hypertension, cardiorenal
cardiovascular —*see also* Disease,
  cardiovascular
  renal —*see* Hypertension, cardiorenal
cerebellar NOS G31.9
  alcoholic G31.2
  primary (hereditary) (sporadic) G11.9
cerebral —*see* Degeneration, brain
cerebrovascular I67.9
  due to hypertension I67.4

Degeneration, degenerative *(Continued)*
cervical plexus G54.2
cervix N88.8
  due to radiation (intended effect) N88.8
    adverse effect or misadventure N99.89
chamber angle H21.21-
changes, spine or vertebra —*see* Spondylosis
chorioretinal —*see also* Degeneration, choroid
  hereditary H31.20
choroid (colloid) (drusen) H31.10-
  atrophy —*see* Atrophy, choroidal
  hereditary —*see* Dystrophy, choroidal,
    hereditary
ciliary body H21.22-
cochlear —*see* subcategory H83.8
combined (spinal cord) (subacute) E53.8
  [G32.0]
  with anemia (pernicious) D51.0 *[G32.0]*
    due to dietary vitamin B12 deficiency
      D51.3 *[G32.0]*
  in (due to)
    vitamin B12 deficiency E53.8 *[G32.0]*
      anemia D51.9 *[G32.0]*
conjunctiva H11.10
  concretions —*see* Concretion, conjunctiva
  deposits —*see* Deposit, conjunctiva
  pigmentations —*see* Pigmentation,
    conjunctiva
  pinguecula —*see* Pinguecula
  xerosis —*see* Xerosis, conjunctiva
cornea H18.40
  calcerous H18.43
    band keratopathy H18.42-
  familial, hereditary —*see* Dystrophy, cornea
  hyaline (of old scars) H18.49
  keratomalacia —*see* Keratomalacia
  nodular H18.45-
  peripheral H18.46-
  senile H18.41-
  specified type NEC H18.49
cortical (cerebellar) (parenchymatous) G31.89
  alcoholic G31.2
  diffuse, due to arteriopathy I67.2
corticobasal G31.85
cutis L98.8
  amyloid E85.4 *[L99]*
dental pulp K04.2
disc disease —*see* Degeneration,
  intervertebral disc NEC
dorsolateral (spinal cord) —*see* Degeneration,
  combined
extrapyramidal G25.9
eye, macular —*see also* Degeneration, macula
  congenital or hereditary —*see* Dystrophy,
    retina
facet joints —*see* Spondylosis
fatty
  liver NEC K76.0
    alcoholic K70.0
grey matter (brain) (Alpers') G31.81
heart —*see also* Degeneration, myocardial
  amyloid E85.4 *[I43]*
  atheromatous —*see* Disease, heart,
    ischemic, atherosclerotic
  ischemic —*see* Disease, heart, ischemic
hepatolenticular (Wilson's) E83.01
hepatorenal K76.7
hyaline (diffuse) (generalized)
  localized —*see* Degeneration, by site
infrapatellar fat pad M79.4
intervertebral disc NOS
  with
    myelopathy —*see* Disorder, disc, with,
      myelopathy
    radiculitis or radiculopathy —*see*
      Disorder, disc, with, radiculopathy
  cervical, cervicothoracic —*see* Disorder,
    disc, cervical, degeneration
    with
      myelopathy —*see* Disorder, disc,
        cervical, with myelopathy

◀ New   ◀ Revised   ~~deleted~~ Deleted

Degeneration, degenerative *(Continued)*
  intervertebral disc NOS *(Continued)*
    cervical, cervicothoracic *(Continued)*
      with *(Continued)*
        neuritis, radiculitis or
          radiculopathy —*see* Disorder,
          disc, cervical, with neuritis
    lumbar region M51.36
      with
        myelopathy M51.06
        neuritis, radiculitis, radiculopathy or
          sciatica M51.16
    lumbosacral region M51.37
      with
        neuritis, radiculitis, radiculopathy or
          sciatica M51.17
    sacrococcygeal region M53.3
    thoracic region M51.34
      with
        myelopathy M51.04
        neuritis, radiculitis, radiculopathy
          M51.14
    thoracolumbar region M51.35
      with
        myelopathy M51.05
        neuritis, radiculitis, radiculopathy
          M51.15
  intestine, amyloid E85.4
  iris (pigmentary) H21.23-
  ischemic —*see* Ischemia
  joint disease —*see* Osteoarthritis
  kidney N28.89
    amyloid E85.4 *[N29]*
    cystic, congenital Q61.9
    fatty N28.89
    polycystic Q61.3
      adult type (autosomal dominant) Q61.2
      infantile type (autosomal recessive) NEC
        Q61.19
      collecting duct dilatation Q61.11
  Kuhnt-Junius (*see also* Degeneration, macula)
    H35.32
  lens —*see* Cataract
  lenticular (familial) (progressive) (Wilson's)
    (with cirrhosis of liver) E83.01
  liver (diffuse) NEC K76.89
    amyloid E85.4 *[K77]*
    cystic K76.89
      congenital Q44.6
    fatty NEC K76.0
      alcoholic K70.0
    hypertrophic K76.89
    parenchymatous, acute or subacute
      K72.00
      with coma K72.01
    pigmentary K76.89
    toxic (acute) K71.9
  lung J98.4
  lymph gland I89.8
    hyaline I89.8
  macula, macular (acquired) (age-related)
    (senile) H35.30
    angioid streaks H35.33
    atrophic age-related H35.31
    congenital or hereditary —*see* Dystrophy,
      retina
    cystoid H35.35-
    drusen H35.36-
    exudative H35.32
    hole H35.34-
    nonexudative H35.31
    puckering H35.37-
    toxic H35.38-
  membranous labyrinth, congenital (causing
    impairment of hearing) Q16.5
  meniscus —*see* Derangement, meniscus
  mitral —*see* Insufficiency, mitral
  Mönckeberg's —*see* Arteriosclerosis,
    extremities
  motor centers, senile G31.1
  multi-system G90.3

Degeneration, degenerative *(Continued)*
  mural —*see* Degeneration, myocardial
  muscle (fatty) (fibrous) (hyaline)
    (progressive) M62.89
    heart —*see* Degeneration, myocardial
  myelin, central nervous system G37.9
  myocardial, myocardium (fatty) (hyaline)
    (senile) I51.5
    with rheumatic fever (conditions in I00)
      I09.0
      active, acute or subacute I01.2
        with chorea I02.0
      inactive or quiescent (with chorea)
        I09.0
    hypertensive —*see* Hypertension, heart
    rheumatic —*see* Degeneration, myocardial,
      with rheumatic fever
    syphilitic A52.06
  nasal sinus (mucosa) J32.9
    frontal J32.1
    maxillary J32.0
  nerve —*see* Disorder, nerve
  nervous system G31.9
    alcoholic G31.2
    amyloid E85.4 *[G99.8]*
    autonomic G90.9
    fatty G31.89
    specified NEC G31.89
  nipple N64.89
  olivopontocerebellar (hereditary) (familial)
    G23.8
  osseous labyrinth —*see* subcategory H83.8
  ovary N83.8
    cystic N83.20
    microcystic N83.20
  pallidal pigmentary (progressive) G23.0
  pancreas K86.8
    tuberculous A18.83
  penis N48.89
  pigmentary (diffuse) (general)
    localized —*see* Degeneration, by site
    pallidal (progressive) G23.0
  pineal gland E34.8
  pituitary (gland) E23.6
  popliteal fat pad M79.4
  posterolateral (spinal cord) —*see*
    Degeneration, combined
  pulmonary valve (heart) I37.8
  pulp (tooth) K04.2
  pupillary margin H21.24-
  renal —*see* Degeneration, kidney
  retina H35.9
    hereditary (cerebroretinal) (congenital)
      (juvenile) (macula) (peripheral)
      (pigmentary) —*see* Dystrophy, retina
    Kuhnt-Junius (*see also* Degeneration,
      macula) H35.32
    macula (cystic) (exudative) (hole)
      (nonexudative) (pseudohole) (senile)
      (toxic) —*see* Degeneration, macula
    peripheral H35.40
      lattice H35.41-
      microcystoid H35.42-
      paving stone H35.43-
      secondary
        pigmentary H35.45-
        vitreoretinal H35.46-
      senile reticular H35.44-
    pigmentary (primary) —*see also* Dystrophy,
      retina
      secondary —*see* Degeneration, retina,
        peripheral, secondary
    posterior pole —*see* Degeneration, macula
  saccule, congenital (causing impairment of
    hearing) Q16.5
  senile R54
    brain G31.1
    cardiac, heart or myocardium —*see*
      Degeneration, myocardial
    motor centers G31.1
    vascular —*see* Arteriosclerosis

Degeneration, degenerative *(Continued)*
  sinus (cystic) —*see also* Sinusitis
    polypoid J33.1
  skin L98.8
    amyloid E85.4 *[L99]*
    colloid L98.8
  spinal (cord) G31.89
    amyloid E85.4 *[G32.89]*
    combined (subacute) —*see* Degeneration,
      combined
    dorsolateral —*see* Degeneration, combined
    familial NEC G31.89
    fatty G31.89
    funicular —*see* Degeneration, combined
    posterolateral —*see* Degeneration,
      combined
    subacute combined —*see* Degeneration,
      combined
    tuberculous A17.81
  spleen D73.0
    amyloid E85.4 *[D77]*
  stomach K31.89
  striatonigral G23.2
  suprarenal (capsule) (gland) E27.8
  synovial membrane (pulpy) —*see* Disorder,
    synovium, specified type NEC
  tapetoretinal —*see* Dystrophy, retina
  thymus (gland) E32.8
    fatty E32.8
  thyroid (gland) E07.89
  tricuspid (heart) (valve) I07.9
  tuberculous NEC —*see* Tuberculosis
  turbinate J34.89
  uterus (cystic) N85.8
  vascular (senile) —*see* Arteriosclerosis
    hypertensive —*see* Hypertension
  vitreoretinal, secondary —*see* Degeneration,
    retina, peripheral, secondary,
    vitreoretinal
  vitreous (body) H43.81-
  Wallerian —*see* Disorder, nerve
  Wilson's hepatolenticular E83.01
Deglutition
  paralysis R13.0
    hysterical F44.4
  pneumonia J69.0
Degos' disease I77.89
Dehiscence (of)
  amputation stump T87.81
  cesarean wound O90.0
  closure of
    cornea T81.31
    craniotomy T81.32
    fascia (muscular) (superficial) T81.32
    internal organ or tissue T81.32
    laceration (external) (internal) T81.33
    ligament T81.32
    mucosa T81.31
    muscle or muscle flap T81.32
    ribs or rib cage T81.32
    skin and subcutaneous tissue (full-
      thickness) (superficial) T81.31
    skull T81.32
    sternum (sternotomy) T81.32
    tendon T81.32
    traumatic laceration (external) (internal)
      T81.33
  episiotomy O90.1
  operation wound NEC T81.31
    external operation wound (superficial)
      T81.31
    internal operation wound (deep)
      T81.32
  perineal wound (postpartum) O90.1
  traumatic injury wound repair T81.33
  wound T81.30
    traumatic repair T81.33
Dehydration E86.0
  hypertonic E87.0
  hypotonic E87.1
  newborn P74.1

Déjérine-Roussy syndrome G93.89
Déjérine-Sottas disease or neuropathy
    (hypertrophic) G60.0
Déjérine-Thomas atrophy G23.8
Delay, delayed
  any plane in pelvis
    complicating delivery O66.9
  birth or delivery NOS O63.9
  closure, ductus arteriosus (Botalli) P29.3
  coagulation —see Defect, coagulation
  conduction (cardiac) (ventricular) I45.9
  delivery, second twin, triplet, etc O63.2
  development R62.50
    global F88
    intellectual (specific) F81.9
    language F80.9
      due to hearing loss F80.4
    learning F81.9
    pervasive F84.9
    physiological R62.50
      specified stage NEC R62.0
    reading F81.0
    sexual E30.0
    speech F80.9
      due to hearing loss F80.4
    spelling F81.81
  gastric emptying K30
  menarche E30.0
  menstruation (cause unknown) N91.0
  milestone R62.0
  passage of meconium (newborn) P76.0
  primary respiration P28.9
  puberty (constitutional) E30.0
  separation of umbilical cord P96.82
  sexual maturation, female E30.0
  sleep phase syndrome G47.21
  union, fracture —see Fracture, by site
  vaccination Z28.9
Deletion (s)
  autosome Q93.9
    identified by fluorescence in situ
      hybridization (FISH) Q93.89
    identified by in situ hybridization (ISH)
      Q93.89
  chromosome
    with complex rearrangements NEC Q93.7
    part of NEC Q93.5
    seen only at prometaphase Q93.89
    short arm
      4 Q93.3
      5p Q93.4
      22q11.2 Q93.81
    specified NEC Q93.89
  long arm chromosome 18 or 21 Q93.89
    with complex rearrangements NEC
      Q93.7
  microdeletions NEC Q93.88
Delhi boil or button B55.1
Delinquency (juvenile) (neurotic) F91.8
  group Z72.810
Delinquent immunization status Z28.3
Delirium, delirious (acute or subacute) (not
    alcohol or drug-induced) (with dementia)
    R41.0
  alcoholic (acute) (tremens) (withdrawal)
    F10.921
    with intoxication F10.921
    in
      abuse F10.121
      dependence F10.221
  due to (secondary to)
    alcohol
      intoxication F10.921
      in
        abuse F10.121
        dependence F10.221
      withdrawal F10.231
    amphetamine intoxication F15.921
    in
      abuse F15.121
      dependence F15.221

Delirium, delirious (Continued)
  due to (Continued)
    anxiolytic
      intoxication F13.921
      in
        abuse F13.121
        dependence F13.221
      withdrawal F13.231
    cannabis intoxication (acute) F12.921
    in
      abuse F12.121
      dependence F12.221
    cocaine intoxication (acute) F14.921
    in
      abuse F14.121
      dependence F14.221
    general medical condition F05
    hallucinogen intoxication F16.921
    in
      abuse F16.121
      dependence F16.221
    hypnotic
      intoxication F13.921
      in
        abuse F13.121
        dependence F13.221
      withdrawal F13.231
    inhalant intoxication (acute) F18.921
    in
      abuse F18.121
      dependence F18.221
    multiple etiologies F05
    opioid intoxication (acute) F11.921
    in
      abuse F11.121
      dependence F11.221
    phencyclidine intoxication (acute) F16.921
    in
      abuse F16.121
      dependence F16.221
    psychoactive substance NEC intoxication
      (acute) F19.921
    in
      abuse F19.121
      dependence F19.221
    sedative
      intoxication F13.921
      in
        abuse F13.121
        dependence F13.221
      withdrawal F13.231
    unknown etiology F05
  exhaustion F43.0
  hysterical F44.89
  postprocedural (postoperative) F05
  puerperal F05
  thyroid —see Thyrotoxicosis with thyroid
    storm
  traumatic —see Injury, intracranial
  tremens (alcohol-induced) F10.231
    sedative-induced F13.231
Delivery (childbirth) (labor)
  arrested active phase O62.1
  cesarean (for)
    without indication O82
    abnormal
      pelvis (bony) (deformity) (major) NEC
        with disproportion (fetopelvic)
        O33.0
        with obstructed labor O65.0
      presentation or position O32.9
    abruptio placentae (see also Abruptio
      placentae) 045.9-
    acromion presentation O32.2
    atony, uterus O62.2
    breech presentation O32.1
      incomplete O32.8
    brow presentation O32.3
    cephalopelvic disproportion O33.9
    cerclage O34.3-
    chin presentation O32.3

Delivery (Continued)
  cesarean (Continued)
    cicatrix of cervix O34.4-
    contracted pelvis (general)
      inlet O33.2
      outlet O33.3
    cord presentation or prolapse O69.0
    cystocele O34.8-
    deformity (acquired) (congenital)
      pelvic organs or tissues NEC O34.8-
      pelvis (bony) NEC O33.0
    disproportion NOS O33.9
    eclampsia —see Eclampsia
    face presentation O32.3
    failed
      forceps O66.5
      induction of labor O61.9
        instrumental O61.1
        mechanical O61.1
        medical O61.0
        specified NEC O61.8
        surgical O61.1
      trial of labor NOS O66.40
        following previous cesarean delivery
          O66.41
      vacuum extraction O66.5
      ventouse O66.5
    fetal-maternal hemorrhage O43.01-
    hemorrhage (intrapartum) O67.9
      with coagulation defect O67.0
      specified cause NEC O67.8
    high head at term O32.4
    hydrocephalic fetus O33.6
    incarceration of uterus O34.51-
    incoordinate uterine action O62.4
    increased size, fetus O33.5
    inertia, uterus O62.2
      primary O62.0
      secondary O62.1
    lateroversion, uterus O34.59-
    mal lie O32.9
    malposition
      fetus O32.9
      pelvic organs or tissues NEC O34.8-
      uterus NEC O34.59-
    malpresentation NOS O32.9
    oblique presentation O32.2
    occurring after 37 completed weeks of
      gestation but before 39 completed
      weeks gestation due to (spontaneous)
      onset of labor O75.82
    oversize fetus O33.5
    pelvic tumor NEC O34.8-
    placenta previa O44.1-
      without hemorrhage O44.0-
    placental insufficiency O36.51-
    planned, occurring after 37 completed
      weeks of gestation but before 39
      completed weeks gestation due to
      (spontaneous) onset of labor O75.82
    polyp, cervix O34.4-
      causing obstructed labor O65.5
    poor dilatation, cervix O62.0
    pre-eclampsia O14.9-
      mild O14.0-
      moderate O14.0-
      severe
        with hemolysis, elevated liver
          enzymes and low platelet count
          (HELLP) O14.2-
    previous
      cesarean delivery O34.21
      surgery (to)
        cervix O34.4-
        gynecological NEC O34.8-
        rectum O34.7-
        uterus O34.29
        vagina O34.6-
    prolapse
      arm or hand O32.2
      uterus O34.52-

◄ New   ◄ Revised   deleted Deleted

Delivery *(Continued)*
  cesarean *(Continued)*
    prolonged labor NOS O63.9
    rectocele O34.8-
    retroversion
      uterus O34.53-
    rigid
      cervix O34.4-
      pelvic floor O34.8-
      perineum O34.7-
      vagina O34.6-
      vulva O34.7-
    sacculation, pregnant uterus O34.59-
    scar (s)
      cervix O34.4-
      cesarean delivery O34.21
      uterus O34.29
    Shirodkar suture in situ O34.3-
    shoulder presentation O32.2
    stenosis or stricture, cervix O34.4-
    streptococcus B carrier state O99.824
    transverse presentation or lie O32.2
    tumor, pelvic organs or tissues NEC
      O34.8-
      cervix O34.4-
    umbilical cord presentation or prolapse
      O69.0
  completely normal case O80
  complicated O75.9
    by
      abnormal, abnormality (of)
        forces of labor O62.9
          specified type NEC O62.8
        glucose O99.814
        uterine contractions NOS O62.9
      abruptio placentae *(see also* Abruptio
        placentae) O45.9-
      abuse
        physical O9A.32
        psychological O9A.52
        sexual O9A.42
      adherent placenta O72.0
        without hemorrhage O73.0
      alcohol use O99.314
      anemia (pre-existing) O99.02
      anesthetic death O74.8
      annular detachment of cervix O71.3
      atony, uterus O62.2
      attempted vacuum extraction and
        forceps O66.5
      Bandl's ring O62.4
      bariatric surgery status O99.844
      biliary tract disorder O26.62
      bleeding *—see* Delivery, complicated by,
        hemorrhage
      blood disorder NEC O99.12
      cervical dystocia (hypotonic) O62.2
        primary O62.0
        secondary O62.1
      circulatory system disorder O99.42
      compression of cord (umbilical) NEC
        O69.2
      condition NEC O99.89
      contraction, contracted ring O62.4
      cord (umbilical)
        around neck
          with compression O69.1
          without compression O69.81
        bruising O69.5
        complication O69.9
          specified NEC O69.89
        compression NEC O69.2
        entanglement O69.2
          without compression O69.82
        hematoma O69.5
        presentation O69.0
        prolapse O69.0
        short O69.3
        thrombosis (vessels) O69.5
        vascular lesion O69.5
      Couvelaire uterus O45.8X-

Delivery *(Continued)*
  complicated *(Continued)*
    by *(Continued)*
      damage to (injury to) NEC
        perineum O71.82
        periurethral tissue O71.82
        vulva O71.82
      delay following rupture of membranes
        (spontaneous) *—see* Pregnancy,
        complicated by, premature rupture
        of membranes
      depressed fetal heart tones O76
      diabetes O24.92
        gestational O24.429
          diet controlled O24.420
          insulin controlled O24.424
        pre-existing O24.32
          specified NEC O24.82
          type 1 O24.02
          type 2 O24.12
      diastasis recti (abdominis) O71.89
      dilatation
        bladder O66.8
        cervix incomplete, poor or slow O62.0
      disease NEC O99.89
      disruptio uteri *—see* Delivery,
        complicated by, rupture, uterus
      drug use O99.324
      dysfunction, uterus NOS O62.9
        hypertonic O62.4
        hypotonic O62.2
          primary O62.0
          secondary O62.1
        incoordinate O62.4
      eclampsia O15.1
      embolism (pulmonary) *—see* Embolism,
        obstetric
      endocrine, nutritional or metabolic
        disease NEC O99.284
      failed
        attempted vaginal birth after previous
          cesarean delivery O66.41
        induction of labor O61.9
          instrumental O61.1
          mechanical O61.1
          medical O61.0
          specified NEC O61.8
          surgical O61.1
        trial of labor O66.40
      female genital mutilation O65.5
      fetal
        abnormal acid-base balance O68
        acidemia O68
        acidosis O68
        alkalosis O68
        death, early O02.1
        deformity O66.3
        heart rate or rhythm (abnormal) (non-
          reassuring) O76
        hypoxia O77.8
        stress O77.9
          due to drug administration O77.1
          electrocardiographic evidence of
            O77.8
          specified NEC O77.8
          ultrasound evidence of O77.8
      fever during labor O75.2
      gastric banding status O99.844
      gastric bypass status O99.844
      gastrointestinal disease NEC
        O99.62
      gestational diabetes O24.429
        diet controlled O24.420
        insulin (and diet) controlled
          O24.424
      gonorrhea O98.22
      hematoma O71.7
        ischial spine O71.7
        pelvic O71.7
        vagina O71.7
        vulva or perineum O71.7

Delivery *(Continued)*
  complicated *(Continued)*
    by *(Continued)*
      hemorrhage (uterine) O67.9
        associated with
          afibrinogenemia O67.0
          coagulation defect O67.0
          hyperfibrinolysis O67.0
          hypofibrinogenemia O67.0
        due to
          low-lying placenta O44.1-
          placenta previa O44.1-
          premature separation of placenta
            (normally implanted) *(see also*
            Abruptio placentae) O45.9-
          retained placenta O72.0
          uterine leiomyoma O67.8
        placenta NEC O67.8
        postpartum NEC (atonic) (immediate)
          O72.1
          with retained or trapped placenta
            O72.0
          delayed O72.2
          secondary O72.2
          third stage O72.0
      hourglass contraction, uterus O62.4
      hypertension, hypertensive (pre-
        existing) *—see* Hypertension,
        complicated by, childbirth (labor)
      hypotension O26.5-
      incomplete dilatation (cervix) O62.0
      incoordinate uterus contractions
        O62.4
      inertia, uterus O62.2
        during latent phase of labor O62.0
        primary O62.0
        secondary O62.1
      infection (maternal) O98.92
        carrier state NEC O99.834
        gonorrhea O98.22
        human immunodeficiency virus (HIV)
          O98.72
        sexually transmitted NEC O98.32
        specified NEC O98.82
        syphilis O98.12
        tuberculosis O98.02
        viral hepatitis O98.42
        viral NEC O98.52
      injury (to mother) *(see also* Delivery,
        complicated, by, damage to)
        O71.9
        nonobstetric O9A.22
          caused by abuse *—see* Delivery,
            complicated by, abuse
      intrauterine fetal death, early O02.1
      inversion, uterus O71.2
      laceration (perineal) O70.9
        anus (sphincter) O70.4
          with third degree laceration
            O70.2
            with mucosa O70.3
          without third degree laceration
            O70.4
        bladder (urinary) O71.5
        bowel O71.5
        cervix (uteri) O71.3
        fourchette O70.0
        hymen O70.0
        labia O70.0
        pelvic
          floor O70.1
          organ NEC O71.5
        perineum, perineal O70.9
          first degree O70.0
          fourth degree O70.3
          muscles O70.1
          second degree O70.1
          skin O70.0
          slight O70.0
          third degree O70.2
        peritoneum (pelvic) O71.5

Delivery (Continued)
  complicated (Continued)
    by (Continued)
      laceration (Continued)
        rectovaginal (septum) (without
            perineal laceration) O71.4
          with perineum O70.2
            with anal or rectal mucosa
                O70.3
        specified NEC O71.89
        sphincter ani —see Delivery,
            complicated, by, laceration, anus
            (sphincter)
        urethra O71.5
        uterus O71.81
          before labor O71.81
        vagina, vaginal (deep) (high) (without
            perineal laceration) O71.4
          with perineum O70.0
          muscles, with perineum O70.1
        vulva O70.0
      liver disorder O26.62
      malignancy O9A.12
      malnutrition O25.2
      malposition, malpresentation
        without obstruction O32.9 —see
            also Delivery, complicated by,
            obstruction
        breech O32.1
        compound O32.6
        face (brow) (chin) O32.3
        footling O38.8
        high head O32.4
        oblique O32.2
        specified NEC O32.8
        transverse O32.2
        unstable lie O32.0
      placenta (with hemorrhage) O44.1-
        without hemorrhage O44.0-
      uterus or cervix O65.5
      meconium in amniotic fluid O77.0
      mental disorder NEC O99.344
      metrorrhexis —see Delivery, complicated
          by, rupture, uterus
      nervous system disorder O99.354
      obesity (pre-existing) O99.214
      obesity surgery status O99.844
      obstetric trauma O71.9
        specified NEC O71.89
      obstructed labor
        due to
          breech (complete) (frank)
              presentation O64.1
            incomplete O64.8
          brow presenation O64.3
          buttock presentation O64.1
          chin presentation O64.2
          compound presentation O64.5
          contracted pelvis O65.1
          deep transverse arrest O64.0
          deformed pelvis O65.0
          dystocia (fetal) O66.9
            due to
              conjoined twins O66.3
              fetal
                abnormality NEC O66.3
                ascites O66.3
                hydrops O66.3
                meningomyelocele O66.3
                sacral teratoma O66.3
                tumor O66.3
              hydrocephalic fetus O66.3
            shoulder O66.0
          face presentation O64.2
          fetopelvic disproportion O65.4
          footling presentation O64.8
          impacted shoulders O66.0
          incomplete rotation of fetal head
              O64.0
          large fetus O66.2
          locked twins O66.1

Delivery (Continued)
  complicated (Continued)
    by (Continued)
      obstructed labor (Continued)
        due to (Continued)
          malposition O64.9
            specified NEC O64.8
          malpresentation O64.9
            specified NEC O64.8
          multiple fetuses NEC O66.6
          pelvic
            abnormality (maternal) O65.9
              organ O65.5
                specified NEC O65.8
            contraction
              inlet O65.2
              mid-cavity O65.3
              outlet O65.3
          persistent (position)
            occipitoiliac O64.0
            occipitoposterior O64.0
            occipitosacral O64.0
            occipitotransverse O64.0
          prolapsed arm O64.4
          shoulder presentation O64.4
        specified NEC O66.8
      pathological retraction ring, uterus
          O62.4
      penetration, pregnant uterus by
          instrument O71.1
      perforation —see Delivery, complicated
          by, laceration
      placenta, placental
        ablatio (see also Abruptio placentae)
            O45.9-
        abnormality O43.9-
          specified NEC O43.89-
        abruptio (see also Abruptio placentae)
            O45.9-
        accreta O43.21-
        adherent (with hemorrhage) O72.0
          without hemorrhage O73.0
        detachment (premature) (see also
            Abruptio placentae) O45.9-
        disorder O43.9-
          specified NEC O43.89-
        hemorrhage NEC O67.8
        increta O43.22-
        low (implantation) O44.1-
          without hemorrhage O44.0-
        malformation O43.10-
        malposition O44.1-
          without hemorrhage O44.0-
        percreta O43.23-
        previa (central) (lateral) (low)
            (marginal) (partial) (total) O44.1-
          without hemorrhage O44.0-
        retained (with hemorrhage) O72.0
          without hemorrhage O73.0
        separation (premature) O45.9-
          specified NEC O45.8X-
        vicious insertion O44.1-
      precipitate labor O62.3
      premature rupture, membranes (see
          also Pregnancy, complicated by,
          premature rupture of membranes)
          O42.90
      prolapse
        arm or hand O32.2
        cord (umbilical) O69.0
        foot or leg O32.8
        uterus O34.52-
      prolonged labor O63.9
        first stage O63.0
        second stage O63.1
      protozoal disease (maternal) O98.62
      respiratory disease NEC O99.52
      retained membranes or portions of
          placenta O72.2
        without hemorrhage O73.1
      retarded birth O63.9

Delivery (Continued)
  complicated (Continued)
    by (Continued)
      retention of secundines (with
          hemorrhage) O72.0
        without hemorrhage O73.0
        partial O72.2
          without hemorrhage O73.1
      rupture
        bladder (urinary) O71.5
        cervix O71.3
        pelvic organ NEC O71.5
        urethra O71.5
        uterus (during or after labor) O71.1
          before labor O71.0-
      separation, pubic bone (symphysis
          pubis) O71.6
      shock O75.1
      shoulder presentation O64.4
      skin disorder NEC O99.72
      spasm, cervix O62.4
      stenosis or stricture, cervix O65.5
      streptococcus B carrier state O99.824
      subluxation of symphysis (pubis) O26.72
      syphilis (maternal) O98.12
      tear —see Delivery, complicated by,
          laceration
      tetanic uterus O62.4
      trauma (obstetrical) (see also Delivery,
          complicated, by, damage to) O71.9
        non-obstetric O9A.22
        periurethral O71.82
        specified NEC O71.89
      tuberculosis (maternal) O98.02
      tumor, pelvic organs or tissues NEC
          O65.5
      umbilical cord around neck
        with compression O69.1
        without compression O69.81
      uterine inertia O62.2
        during latent phase of labor O62.0
        primary O62.0
        secondary O62.1
      vasa previa O69.4
      velamentous insertion of cord O43.12-
    specified complication NEC O75.89
  delayed NOS O63.9
    following rupture of membranes
        artificial O75.5
    second twin, triplet, etc. O63.2
  forceps, low following failed vacuum
      extraction O66.5
  missed (at or near term) O36.4
  normal O80
  obstructed —see Delivery, complicated by,
      obstruction
  precipitate O62.3
  preterm (see also Pregnancy, complicated by,
      preterm labor) O60.10
  spontaneous O80
  term pregnancy NOS O80
  uncomplicated O80
  vaginal, following previous cesarean delivery
      O34.21
Delusions (paranoid) —see Disorder, delusional
Dementia (degenerative (primary)) (old age)
    (persisting) F03.90
  with
    aggressive behavior F03.91
    behavioral disturbance F03.91
    combative behavior F03.91
    Lewy bodies G31.83 [F02.80]
      with behavioral disturbance G31.83
          [F02.81]
    Parkinson's disease G20 [F02.80]
      with behavioral disturbance G20
          [F02.81]
    Parkinsonism G31.83 [F02.80]
      with behavioral disturbance G31.83
          [F02.81]
    violent behavior F03.91

184

Dementia *(Continued)*
alcoholic F10.97
with dependence F10.27
Alzheimer's type —*see* Disease, Alzheimer's
arteriosclerotic —*see* Dementia, vascular
atypical, Alzheimer's type —*see* Disease,
Alzheimer's, specified NEC
congenital —*see* Disability, intellectual
frontal (lobe) G31.09 *[F02.80]*
with behavioral disturbance G31.09
[F02.81]
frontotemporal G31.09 *[F02.80]*
with behavioral disturbance G31.09
[F02.81]
specified NEC G31.09 *[F02.80]*
with behavioral disturbance G31.09
[F02.81]
in (due to)
alcohol F10.97
with dependence F10.27
Alzheimer's disease —*see* Disease,
Alzheimer's
arteriosclerotic brain disease —*see*
Dementia, vascular
cerebral lipidoses E75.- *[F02.80]*
with behavioral disturbance
E75.- *[F02.81]*
Creutzfeldt-Jakob disease *(see also*
Creutzfeldt-Jakob disease or
syndrome (with dementia)) A81.00
epilepsy G40.- *[F02.80]*
with behavioral disturbance
G40.- *[F02.81]*
hepatolenticular degeneration E83.01
[F02.80]
with behavioral disturbance E83.01
[F02.81]
human immunodeficiency virus (HIV)
disease B20 *[F02.80]*
with behavioral disturbance B20
[F02.81]
Huntington's disease or chorea G10
hypercalcemia E83.52 *[F02.80]*
with behavioral disturbance E83.52
[F02.81]
hypothyroidism, acquired E03.9 *[F02.80]*
with behavioral disturbance E03.9
[F02.81]
due to iodine deficiency E01.8
[F02.80]
with behavioral disturbance E01.8
[F02.81]
inhalants F18.97
with dependence F18.27
multiple
etiologies F03
sclerosis G35 *[F02.80]*
with behavioral disturbance G35
[F02.81]
neurosyphilis A52.17 *[F02.80]*
with behavioral disturbance A52.17
[F02.81]
juvenile A50.49 *[F02.80]*
with behavioral disturbance A50.49
[F02.81]
niacin deficiency E52 *[F02.80]*
with behavioral disturbance E52
[F02.81]
paralysis agitans G20 *[F02.80]*
with behavioral disturbance G20
[F02.81]
Parkinson's disease G20 *[F02.80]*
pellagra E52 *[F02.80]*
with behavioral disturbance E52
[F02.81]
Pick's G31.01 *[F02.80]*
with behavioral disturbance G31.01
[F02.81]
polyarteritis nodosa M30.0 *[F02.80]*
with behavioral disturbance M30.0
[F02.81]

Dementia *(Continued)*
in *(Continued)*
psychoactive drug F19.97
with dependence F19.27
inhalants F18.97
with dependence F18.27
sedatives, hypnotics or anxiolytics
F13.97
with dependence F13.27
sedatives, hypnotics or anxiolytics F13.97
with dependence F13.27
systemic lupus erythematosus
M32.- *[F02.80]*
with behavioral disturbance
M32.- *[F02.81]*
trypanosomiasis
African B56.9 *[F02.80]*
with behavioral disturbance B56.9
[F02.81]
unknown etiology F03
vitamin B12 deficiency E53.8 *[F02.80]*
with behavioral disturbance E53.8
[F02.81]
volatile solvents F18.97
with dependence F18.27
infantile, infantilis F84.3
Lewy body G31.83 *[F02.80]*
with behavioral disturbance G31.83
[F02.81]
multi-infarct —*see* Dementia, vascular
paralytica, paralytic (syphilitic) A52.17
[F02.80]
with behavioral disturbance A52.17
[F02.81]
juvenilis A50.45
paretic A52.17
praecox —*see* Schizophrenia
presenile F03
Alzheimer's type —*see* Disease,
Alzheimer's, early onset
primary degenerative F03
progressive, syphilitic A52.17
senile F03
with acute confusional state F05
Alzheimer's type —*see* Disease,
Alzheimer's, late onset
depressed or paranoid type F03
vascular (acute onset) (mixed) (multi-infarct)
(subcortical) F01.50
with behavioral disturbance F01.51
Demineralization, bone —*see* Osteoporosis
Demodex folliculorum (infestation) B88.0
Demophobia F40.248
Demoralization R45.3
Demyelination, demyelinization
central nervous system G37.9
specified NEC G37.8
corpus callosum (central) G37.1
disseminated, acute G36.9
specified NEC G36.8
global G35
in optic neuritis G36.0
Dengue (classical) (fever) A90
hemorrhagic A91
sandfly A93.1
Dennie-Marfan syphilitic syndrome
A50.45
Dens evaginatus, in dente or invaginatus
K00.2
Dense breasts R92.2
Density
increased, bone (disseminated) (generalized)
(spotted) —*see* Disorder, bone, density
and structure, specified type NEC
lung (nodular) J98.4
Dental —*see also* condition
examination Z01.20
with abnormal findings Z01.21
restoration
aesthetically inadequate or displeasing
K08.56

Dental *(Continued)*
restoration *(Continued)*
defective K08.50
specified NEC K08.59
failure of marginal integrity K08.51
failure of periodontal anatomical integrity
K08.54
Dentia praecox K00.6
Denticles (pulp) K04.2
Dentigerous cyst K09.0
Dentin
irregular (in pulp) K04.3
opalescent K00.5
secondary (in pulp) K04.3
sensitive K03.89
Dentinogenesis imperfecta K00.5
Dentinoma —*see* Cyst, calcifying odontogenic
Dentition (syndrome) K00.7
delayed K00.6
difficult K00.7
precocious K00.6
premature K00.6
retarded K00.6
Dependence (on) (syndrome) F19.20
with remission F19.21
alcohol (ethyl) (methyl) (without remission)
F10.20
with
amnestic disorder, persisting F10.26
anxiety disorder F10.280
dementia, persisting F10.27
intoxication F10.229
with delirium F10.221
uncomplicated F10.220
mood disorder F10.24
psychotic disorder F10.259
with
delusions F10.250
hallucinations F10.251
remission F10.21
sexual dysfunction F10.281
sleep disorder F10.282
specified disorder NEC F10.288
withdrawal F10.239
with
delirium F10.231
perceptual disturbance F10.232
uncomplicated F10.230
counseling and surveillance Z71.41
amobarbital —*see* Dependence, drug,
sedative
amphetamine (s) (type) —*see* Dependence,
drug, stimulant NEC
amytal (sodium) —*see* Dependence, drug,
sedative
analgesic NEC F55.8
anesthetic (agent) (gas) (general) (local)
NEC —*see* Dependence, drug,
psychoactive NEC
anxiolytic NEC —*see* Dependence, drug,
sedative
barbital (s) —*see* Dependence, drug, sedative
barbiturate (s) (compounds) (drugs
classifiable to T42) —*see* Dependence,
drug, sedative
benzedrine —*see* Dependence, drug,
stimulant NEC
bhang —*see* Dependence, drug, cannabis
bromide (s) NEC —*see* Dependence, drug,
sedative
caffeine —*see* Dependence, drug, stimulant
NEC
cannabis (sativa) (indica) (resin) (derivatives)
(type) —*see* Dependence, drug, cannabis
chloral (betaine) (hydrate) —*see* Dependence,
drug, sedative
chlordiazepoxide —*see* Dependence, drug,
sedative
coca (leaf) (derivatives) —*see* Dependence,
drug, cocaine
cocaine —*see* Dependence, drug, cocaine

Dependence (Continued)

codeine —see Dependence, drug, opioid
combinations of drugs F19.20
dagga —see Dependence, drug, cannabis
demerol —see Dependence, drug, opioid
dexamphetamine —see Dependence, drug,
    stimulant NEC
dexedrine —see Dependence, drug, stimulant
    NEC
dextromethorphan —see Dependence, drug,
    opioid
dextromoramide —see Dependence, drug,
    opioid
dextro-nor-pseudo-ephedrine —see
    Dependence, drug, stimulant NEC
dextrorphan —see Dependence, drug, opioid
diazepam —see Dependence, drug, sedative
dilaudid —see Dependence, drug, opioid
D-lysergic acid diethylamide —see
    Dependence, drug, hallucinogen
drug NEC F19.20
    with sleep disorder F19.282
    cannabis F12.20
        with
            anxiety disorder F12.280
            intoxication F12.229
                with
                    delirium F12.221
                    perceptual disturbance F12.222
                uncomplicated F12.220
            other specified disorder F12.288
            psychosis F12.259
                delusions F12.250
                hallucinations F12.251
            unspecified disorder F12.29
        in remission F12.21
    cocaine F14.20
        with
            anxiety disorder F14.280
            intoxication F14.229
                with
                    delirium F14.221
                    perceptual disturbance F14.222
                uncomplicated F14.220
            mood disorder F14.24
            other specified disorder F14.288
            psychosis F14.259
                delusions F14.250
                hallucinations F14.251
            sexual dysfunction F14.281
            sleep disorder F14.282
            unspecified disorder F14.29
            withdrawal F14.23
        in remission F14.21
        withdrawal symptoms in newborn P96.1
    counseling and surveillance Z71.51
    hallucinogen F16.20
        with
            anxiety disorder F16.280
            flashbacks F16.283
            intoxication F16.229
                with delirium F16.221
                uncomplicated F16.220
            mood disorder F16.24
            other specified disorder F16.288
            perception disorder, persisting F16.283
            psychosis F16.259
                delusions F16.250
                hallucinations F16.251
            unspecified disorder F16.29
        in remission F16.21
    in remission F19.21
    inhalant F18.20
        with
            anxiety disorder F18.280
            dementia, persisting F18.27
            intoxication F18.229
                with delirium F18.221
                uncomplicated F18.220
            mood disorder F18.24
            other specified disorder F18.288

Dependence (Continued)
drug NEC (Continued)
    inhalant (Continued)
        with (Continued)
            psychosis F18.259
                delusions F18.250
                hallucinations F18.251
            unspecified disorder F18.29
        in remission F18.21
    nicotine F17.200
        with disorder F17.209
            remission F17.201
            specified disorder NEC F17.208
            withdrawal F17.203
        chewing tobacco F17.220
            with disorder F17.229
                remission F17.221
                specified disorder NEC F17.228
                withdrawal F17.223
        cigarettes F17.210
            with disorder F17.219
                remission F17.211
                specified disorder NEC F17.218
                withdrawal F17.213
        specified product NEC F17.290
            with disorder F17.299
                remission F17.291
                specified disorder NEC F17.298
                withdrawal F17.293
    opioid F11.20
        with
            intoxication F11.229
                with
                    delirium F11.221
                    perceptual disturbance F11.222
                uncomplicated F11.220
            mood disorder F11.24
            other specified disorder F11.288
            psychosis F11.259
                delusions F11.250
                hallucinations F11.251
            sexual dysfunction F11.281
            sleep disorder F11.282
            unspecified disorder F11.29
            withdrawal F11.23
        in remission F11.21
    psychoactive NEC F19.20
        with
            amnestic disorder F19.26
            anxiety disorder F19.280
            dementia F19.27
            intoxication F19.229
                with
                    delirium F19.221
                    perceptual disturbance
                        F19.222
                uncomplicated F19.220
            mood disorder F19.24
            other specified disorder F19.288
            psychosis F19.259
                delusions F19.250
                hallucinations F19.251
            sexual dysfunction F19.281
            sleep disorder F19.282
            unspecified disorder F19.29
            withdrawal F19.239
                with
                    delirium F19.231
                    perceptual disturbance
                        F19.232
                uncomplicated F19.230
    sedative, hypnotic or anxiolytic F13.20
        with
            amnestic disorder F13.26
            anxiety disorder F13.280
            dementia, persisting F13.27
            intoxication F13.229
                with delirium F13.221
                uncomplicated F13.220
            mood disorder F13.24
            other specified disorder F13.288

Dependence (Continued)
drug NEC (Continued)
    sedative, hypnotic or anxiolytic (Continued)
        with (Continued)
            psychosis F13.259
                delusions F13.250
                hallucinations F13.251
            sexual dysfunction F13.281
            sleep disorder F13.282
            unspecified disorder F13.29
            withdrawal F13.239
                with
                    delirium F13.231
                    perceptual disturbance F13.232
                uncomplicated F13.230
        in remission F13.21
    stimulant NEC F15.20
        with
            anxiety disorder F15.280
            intoxication F15.229
                with
                    delirium F15.221
                    perceptual disturbance F15.222
                uncomplicated F15.220
            mood disorder F15.24
            other specified disorder F15.288
            psychosis F15.259
                delusions F15.250
                hallucinations F15.251
            sexual dysfunction F15.281
            sleep disorder F15.282
            unspecified disorder F15.29
            withdrawal F15.23
        in remission F15.21
    ethyl
        alcohol (without remission) F10.20
            with remission F10.21
        bromide —see Dependence, drug,
            sedative
        carbamate F19.20
        chloride F19.20
        morphine —see Dependence, drug, opioid
    ganja —see Dependence, drug, cannabis
    glue (airplane) (sniffing) —see Dependence,
        drug, inhalant
    glutethimide —see Dependence, drug,
        sedative
    hallucinogenics —see Dependence, drug,
        hallucinogen
    hashish —see Dependence, drug, cannabis
    hemp —see Dependence, drug, cannabis
    heroin (salt) (any) —see Dependence, drug,
        opioid
    hypnotic NEC —see Dependence, drug,
        sedative
    Indian hemp —see Dependence, drug,
        cannabis
    inhalants —see Dependence, drug, inhalant
    khat —see Dependence, drug, stimulant NEC
    laudanum —see Dependence, drug, opioid
    LSD (-25) (derivatives) —see Dependence,
        drug, hallucinogen
    luminal —see Dependence, drug, sedative
    lysergic acid —see Dependence, drug,
        hallucinogen
    maconha —see Dependence, drug, cannabis
    marihuana —see Dependence, drug, cannabis
    meprobamate —see Dependence, drug,
        sedative
    mescaline —see Dependence, drug,
        hallucinogen
    methadone —see Dependence, drug, opioid
    methamphetamine (s) —see Dependence,
        drug, stimulant NEC
    methaqualone —see Dependence, drug,
        sedative
    methyl
        alcohol (without remission) F10.20
            with remission F10.21
        bromide —see Dependence, drug, sedative
        morphine —see Dependence, drug, opioid

◀ New ◀▦ Revised ~~deleted~~ Deleted

Dependence *(Continued)*
  methyl *(Continued)*
    phenidate —*see* Dependence, drug, stimulant NEC
    sulfonal —*see* Dependence, drug, sedative
  morphine (sulfate) (sulfite) (type) —*see* Dependence, drug, opioid
  narcotic (drug) NEC —*see* Dependence, drug, opioid
  nembutal —*see* Dependence, drug, sedative
  neraval —*see* Dependence, drug, sedative
  neravan —*see* Dependence, drug, sedative
  neurobarb —*see* Dependence, drug, sedative
  nicotine —*see* Dependence, drug, nicotine
  nitrous oxide F19.20
  nonbarbiturate sedatives and tranquilizers
      with similar effect —*see* Dependence, drug, sedative
  on
    artificial heart (fully implantable) (mechanical) Z95.812
    aspirator Z99.0
    care provider (because of) Z74.9
      impaired mobility Z74.09
      need for
        assistance with personal care Z74.1
        continuous supervision Z74.3
      no other household member able to render care Z74.2
      specified reason NEC Z74.8
    machine Z99.89
      enabling NEC Z99.89
      specified type NEC Z99.89
    renal dialysis (hemodialysis) (peritoneal) Z99.2
    respirator Z99.11
    ventilator Z99.11
    wheelchair Z99.3
  opiate —*see* Dependence, drug, opioid
  opioids —*see* Dependence, drug, opioid
  opium (alkaloids) (derivatives) (tincture) —*see* Dependence, drug, opioid
  oxygen (long-term) (supplemental) Z99.81
  paraldehyde —*see* Dependence, drug, sedative
  paregoric —*see* Dependence, drug, opioid
  PCP (phencyclidine) (*see also* Abuse, drug, hallucinogen) F16.20
  pentobarbital —*see* Dependence, drug, sedative
  pentobarbitone (sodium) —*see* Dependence, drug, sedative
  pentothal —*see* Dependence, drug, sedative
  peyote —*see* Dependence, drug, hallucinogen
  phencyclidine (PCP) (and related substances) (*see also* Abuse, drug, hallucinogen) F16.20
  phenmetrazine —*see* Dependence, drug, stimulant NEC
  phenobarbital —*see* Dependence, drug, sedative
  polysubstance F19.20
  psilocibin, psilocin, psilocyn, psilocyline —*see* Dependence, drug, hallucinogen
  psychostimulant NEC —*see* Dependence, drug, stimulant NEC
  secobarbital —*see* Dependence, drug, sedative
  seconal —*see* Dependence, drug, sedative
  sedative NEC —*see* Dependence, drug, sedative
  specified drug NEC —*see* Dependence, drug
  stimulant NEC —*see* Dependence, drug, stimulant NEC
  substance NEC —*see* Dependence, drug
  supplemental oxygen Z99.81
  tobacco —*see* Dependence, drug, nicotine
    counseling and surveillance Z71.6
  tranquilizer NEC —*see* Dependence, drug, sedative
  vitamin B6 E53.1
  volatile solvents —*see* Dependence, drug, inhalant

Dependency
  care-provider Z74.9
  passive F60.7
  reactions (persistent) F60.7
Depersonalization (in neurotic state) (neurotic) (syndrome) F48.1
Depletion
  extracellular fluid E86.9
  plasma E86.1
  potassium E87.6
    nephropathy N25.89
  salt or sodium E87.1
    causing heat exhaustion or prostration T67.4
    nephropathy N28.9
  volume NOS E86.9
Deployment (current) (military) status Z56.82
  in theater or in support of military war, peacekeeping and humanitarian operations Z56.82
  personal history of Z91.82
    military war, peacekeeping and humanitarian deployment (current or past conflict) Z91.82
  returned from Z91.82
Depolarization, premature I49.40
  atrial I49.1
  junctional I49.2
  specified NEC I49.49
  ventricular I49.3
Deposit
  bone in Boeck's sarcoid D86.89
  calcareous, calcium —*see* Calcification
  cholesterol
    retina H35.89
    vitreous (body) (humor) —*see* Deposit, crystalline
  conjunctiva H11.11-
  cornea H18.00-
    argentous H18.02-
    due to metabolic disorder H18.03-
    Kayser-Fleischer ring H18.04-
    pigmentation —*see* Pigmentation, cornea
  crystalline, vitreous (body) (humor) H43.2-
  hemosiderin in old scars of cornea —*see* Pigmentation, cornea, stromal
  metallic in lens —*see* Cataract, specified NEC
  skin R23.8
  tooth, teeth (betel) (black) (green) (materia alba) (orange) (tobacco) K03.6
  urate, kidney —*see* Calculus, kidney
Depraved appetite —*see* Pica
Depressed
  HDL cholesterol E78.6
Depression (acute) (mental) F32.9
  agitated (single episode) F32.2
  anaclitic —*see* Disorder, adjustment
  anxiety F41.8
    persistent F34.1
  arches —*see also* Deformity, limb, flat foot
  atypical (single episode) F32.8
  basal metabolic rate R94.8
  bone marrow D75.89
  central nervous system R09.2
  cerebral R29.818
    newborn P91.4
  cerebrovascular I67.9
  chest wall M95.4
  climacteric (single episode) F32.8
  endogenous (without psychotic symptoms) F33.2
    with psychotic symptoms F33.3
  functional activity R68.89
  hysterical F44.89
  involutional (single episode) F32.8
  major F32.9
    with psychotic symptoms F32.3
    recurrent —*see* Disorder, depressive, recurrent
  manic-depressive —*see* Disorder, depressive, recurrent

Depression *(Continued)*
  masked (single episode) F32.8
  medullary G93.89
  menopausal (single episode) F32.8
  metatarsus —*see* Depression, arches
  monopolar F33.9
  nervous F34.1
  neurotic F34.1
  nose M95.0
  postnatal F53
  postpartum F53
  post-psychotic of schizophrenia F32.8
  post-schizophrenic F32.8
  psychogenic (reactive) (single episode) F32.9
  psychoneurotic F34.1
  psychotic (single episode) F32.3
    recurrent F33.3
  reactive (psychogenic) (single episode) F32.9
    psychotic (single episode) F32.3
  recurrent —*see* Disorder, depressive, recurrent
  respiratory center G93.89
  seasonal —*see* Disorder, depressive, recurrent
  senile F03

  severe, single episode F32.2
  situational F43.21
  skull Q67.4
  specified NEC (single episode) F32.8
  sternum M95.4
  visual field —*see* Defect, visual field
  vital (recurrent) (without psychotic symptoms) F33.2
    with psychotic symptoms F33.3
    single episode F32.2
Deprivation
  cultural Z60.3
  effects NOS T73.9
    specified NEC T73.8
  emotional NEC Z65.8
    affecting infant or child —*see* Maltreatment, child, psychological
  food T73.0
  protein —*see* Malnutrition
  sleep Z72.820
  social Z60.4
    affecting infant or child —*see* Maltreatment, child, psychological
  specified NEC T73.8
  vitamins —*see* Deficiency, vitamin
  water T73.1
Derangement
  ankle (internal) —*see* Derangement, joint, ankle
  cartilage (articular) NEC —*see* Derangement, joint, articular cartilage, by site
    recurrent —*see* Dislocation, recurrent
  cruciate ligament, anterior, current injury —*see* Sprain, knee, cruciate, anterior
  elbow (internal) —*see* Derangement, joint, elbow
  hip (joint) (internal) (old) —*see* Derangement, joint, hip
  joint (internal) M24.9
    ankylosis —*see* Ankylosis
    articular cartilage M24.10
      ankle M24.17-
      elbow M24.12-
      foot M24.17-
      hand M24.14-
      hip M24.15-
      knee NEC M23.9-
      loose body —*see* Loose, body
      shoulder M24.11-
      wrist M24.13-
    contracture —*see* Contraction, joint
    current injury —*see also* Dislocation
      knee, meniscus or cartilage —*see* Tear, meniscus

Derangement (Continued)
  joint (Continued)
    dislocation
      pathological —see Dislocation,
        pathological
      recurrent —see Dislocation, recurrent
    knee —see Derangement, knee
    ligament —see Disorder, ligament
    loose body —see Loose, body
    recurrent —see Dislocation, recurrent
    specified type NEC M24.80
      ankle M24.87-
      elbow M24.82-
      foot joint M24.87-
      hand joint M24.84-
      hip M24.85-
      shoulder M24.81-
      wrist M24.83-
    temporomandibular M26.69
  knee (recurrent) M23.9-
    ligament disruption, spontaneous
        M23.60-
      anterior cruciate M23.61-
      capsular M23.67-
      instability, chronic M23.5-
      lateral collateral M23.64-
      medial collateral M23.63-
      posterior cruciate M23.62-
    loose body M23.4-
    meniscus M23.30-
      cystic M23.00-
        lateral M23.002
          anterior horn M23.04-
          posterior horn M23.05-
          specified NEC M23.06-
        medial M23.005
          anterior horn M23.01-
          posterior horn M23.02-
          specified NEC M23.03-
      degenerate —see Derangement, knee,
          meniscus, specified NEC
      detached —see Derangement, knee,
          meniscus, specified NEC
      due to old tear or injury M23.20-
        lateral M23.20-
          anterior horn M23.24-
          posterior horn M23.25-
          specified NEC M23.26-
        medial M23.20-
          anterior horn M23.21-
          posterior horn M23.22-
          specified NEC M23.23-
      retained —see Derangement, knee,
          meniscus, specified NEC
      specified NEC M23.30-
        lateral M23.30-
          anterior horn M23.34-
          posterior horn M23.35-
          specified NEC M23.36-
        medial M23.30-
          anterior horn M23.31-
          posterior horn M23.32-
          specified NEC M23.33-
      old M23.8X-
      specified NEC —see subcategory M23.8
  low back NEC —see Dorsopathy, specified
      NEC
  meniscus —see Derangement, knee,
      meniscus
  mental —see Psychosis
  patella, specified NEC —see Disorder,
      patella, derangement NEC
  semilunar cartilage (knee) —see
      Derangement, knee, meniscus,
      specified NEC
  shoulder (internal) —see Derangement,
      joint, shoulder
Dercum's disease E88.2
Derealization (neurotic) F48.1
Dermal —see condition
Dermaphytid —see Dermatophytosis

Dermatitis (eczematous) L30.9
  ab igne L59.0
  acarine B88.0
  actinic (due to sun) L57.8
    other than from sun L59.8
  allergic —see Dermatitis, contact, allergic
  ambustionis, due to burn or scald —see Burn
  amebic A06.7
  ammonia L22
  arsenical (ingested) L27.8
  artefacta L98.1
    psychogenic F54
  atopic L20.9
    psychogenic F54
    specified NEC L20.89
  autoimmune progesterone L30.8
  berlock, berloque L56.2
  blastomycotic B40.3
  blister beetle L24.89
  bullous, bullosa L13.9
    mucosynechial, atrophic L12.1
    seasonal L30.8
    specified NEC L13.8
  calorica L59.0
    due to burn or scald —see Burn
  caterpillar L24.89
  cercarial B65.3
  combustionis L59.0
    due to burn or scald —see Burn
  congelationis T69.1
  contact (occupational) L25.9
    allergic L23.9
      due to
        adhesives L23.1
        cement L23.5
        chemical products NEC L23.5
        chromium L23.0
        cosmetics L23.2
        dander (cat) (dog) L23.81
        drugs in contact with skin L23.3
        dyes L23.4
        food in contact with skin L23.6
        hair (cat) (dog) L23.81
        insecticide L23.5
        metals L23.0
        nickel L23.0
        plants, non-food L23.7
        plastic L23.5
        rubber L23.5
        specified agent NEC L23.89
      due to
        cement L25.3
        chemical products NEC L25.3
        cosmetics L25.0
        dander (cat) (dog) L23.81
        drugs in contact with skin L25.1
        dyes L25.2
        food in contact with skin L25.4
        hair (cat) (dog) L23.81
        plants, non-food L25.5
        specified agent NEC L25.8
      irritant L24.9
        due to
          cement L25.3
          chemical products NEC L24.5
          cosmetics L24.3
          detergents L24.0
          drugs in contact with skin L24.4
          food in contact with skin L24.6
          oils and greases L24.1
          plants, non-food L24.7
          solvents L24.2
          specified agent NEC L24.89
  contusiformis L52
  diabetic —see E08-E13 with .620
  diaper L22
  diphtheritica A36.3
  dry skin L85.3
  due to
    acetone (contact) (irritant) L24.2
    acids (contact) (irritant) L24.5

Dermatitis (Continued)
  due to (Continued)
    adhesive (s) (allergic) (contact) (plaster)
        L23.1
      irritant L24.5
    alcohol (irritant) (skin contact) (substances in
        category T51) L24.2
      taken internally L27.8
    alkalis (contact) (irritant) L24.5
    arsenic (ingested) L27.8
    carbon disulfide (contact) (irritant) L24.2
    caustics (contact) (irritant) L24.5
    cement (contact) L25.3
    cereal (ingested) L27.2
    chemical (s) NEC L25.3
      taken internally L27.8
    chlorocompounds L24.2
    chromium (contact) (irritant) L24.81
    coffee (ingested) L27.2
    cold weather L30.8
    cosmetics (contact) L25.0
      allergic L23.2
      irritant L24.3
    cyclohexanes L24.2
    dander (cat) (dog) L23.81
    Demodex species B88.0
    Dermanyssus gallinae B88.0
    detergents (contact) (irritant) L24.0
    dichromate L24.81
    drugs and medicaments (generalized)
        (internal use) L27.0
      external —see Dermatitis, due to, drugs,
        in contact with skin
      in contact with skin L25.1
        allergic L23.3
        irritant L24.4
      localized skin eruption L27.1
      specified substance —see Table of Drugs
        and Chemicals
    dyes (contact) L25.2
      allergic L23.4
      irritant L24.89
    epidermophytosis —see Dermatophytosis
    esters L24.2
    external irritant NEC L24.9
    fish (ingested) L27.2
    flour (ingested) L27.2
    food (ingested) L27.2
      in contact with skin L25.4
    fruit (ingested) L27.2
    furs (allergic) (contact) L23.81
    glues —see Dermatitis, due to, adhesives
    glycols L24.2
    greases NEC (contact) (irritant) L24.1
    hair (cat) (dog) L23.81
    hot
      objects and materials —see Burn
      weather or places L59.0
    hydrocarbons L24.2
    infrared rays L59.8
    ingestion, ingested substance L27.9
      chemical NEC L27.8
      drugs and medicaments —see
        Dermatitis, due to, drugs
      food L27.2
      specified NEC L27.8
    insecticide in contact with skin L24.5
    internal agent L27.9
      drugs and medicaments (generalized) —
        see Dermatitis, due to, drugs
      food L27.2
    irradiation —see Dermatitis, due to,
        radioactive substance
    ketones L24.2
    lacquer tree (allergic) (contact) L23.7
    light (sun) NEC L57.8
      acute L56.8
      other L59.8
    Liponyssoides sanguineus B88.0
    low temperature L30.8
    meat (ingested) L27.2

◄ New   ◄|||| Revised   ~~deleted~~ Deleted

Dermatitis *(Continued)*
  due to *(Continued)*
    metals, metal salts (contact) (irritant) L24.81
    milk (ingested) L27.2
    nickel (contact) (irritant) L24.81
    nylon (contact) (irritant) L24.5
    oils NEC (contact) (irritant) L24.1
    paint solvent (contact) (irritant) L24.2
    petroleum products (contact) (irritant) (substances in T52) L24.2
    plants NEC (contact) L25.5
      allergic L23.7
      irritant L24.7
    plasters (adhesive) (any) (allergic) (contact) L23.1
      irritant L24.5
    plastic (contact) L25.3
    preservatives (contact) —*see* Dermatitis, due to, chemical, in contact with skin
    primrose (allergic) (contact) L23.7
    primula (allergic) (contact) L23.7
    radiation L59.8
      nonionizing (chronic exposure) L57.8
      sun NEC L57.8
        acute L56.8
    radioactive substance L58.9
      acute L58.0
      chronic L58.1
    radium L58.9
      acute L58.0
      chronic L58.1
    ragweed (allergic) (contact) L23.7
    Rhus (allergic) (contact) (diversiloba) (radicans) (toxicodendron) (venenata) (verniciflua) L23.7
    rubber (contact) L24.5
    Senecio jacobaea (allergic) (contact) L23.7
    solvents (contact) (irritant) (substances in categories T52) L24.2
    specified agent NEC (contact) L25.8
      allergic L23.89
      irritant L24.89
    sunshine NEC L57.8
      acute L56.8
    tetrachlorethylene (contact) (irritant) L24.2
    toluene (contact) (irritant) L24.2
    turpentine (contact) L24.2
    ultraviolet rays (sun NEC) (chronic exposure) L57.8
      acute L56.8
    vaccine or vaccination L27.0
      specified substance —*see* Table of Drugs and Chemicals
    varicose veins —*see* Varix, leg, with, inflammation
    X-rays L58.9
      acute L58.0
      chronic L58.1
  dyshydrotic L30.1
  dysmenorrheica N94.6
  escharotica —*see* Burn
  exfoliative, exfoliativa (generalized) L26
    neonatorum L00
  eyelid —*see also* Dermatosis, eyelid
    allergic H01.119
      left H01.116
        lower H01.115
        upper H01.114
      right H01.113
        lower H01.112
        upper H01.111
    contact —*see* Dermatitis, eyelid, allergic
    due to
      Demodex species B88.0
      herpes (zoster) B02.39
        simplex B00.59

Dermatitis *(Continued)*
  eyelid *(Continued)*
    eczematous H01.139
      left H01.136
        lower H01.135
        upper H01.134
      right H01.133
        lower H01.132
        upper H01.131
  facta, factitia, factitial L98.1
    psychogenic F54
  flexural NEC L20.82
  friction L30.4
  fungus B36.9
    specified type NEC B36.8
  gangrenosa, gangrenous infantum L08.0
  harvest mite B88.0
  heat L59.0
  herpesviral, vesicular (ear) (lip) B00.1
  herpetiformis (bullous) (erythematous) (pustular) (vesicular) L13.0
    juvenile L12.2
    senile L12.0
  hiemalis L30.8
  hypostatic, hypostatica —*see* Varix, leg, with, inflammation
  infectious eczematoid L30.3
  infective L30.3
  irritant —*see* Dermatitis, contact, irritant
  Jacquet's (diaper dermatitis) L22
  Leptus B88.0
  lichenified NEC L28.0
  medicamentosa (generalized) (internal use) —*see* Dermatitis, due to drugs
  mite B88.0
  multiformis L13.0
    juvenile L12.2
  napkin L22
  neurotica L13.0
  nummular L30.0
  papillaris capillitii L73.0
  pellagrous E52
  perioral L71.0
  photocontact L56.2
  polymorpha dolorosa L13.0
  pruriginosa L13.0
  pruritic NEC L30.8
  psychogenic F54
  purulent L08.0
  pustular
    contagious B08.02
    subcorneal L13.1
  pyococcal L08.0
  pyogenica L08.0
  repens L40.2
  Ritter's (exfoliativa) L00
  Schamberg's L81.7
  schistosome B65.3
  seasonal bullous L30.8
  seborrheic L21.9
    infantile L21.1
    specified NEC L21.8
  sensitization NOS L23.9
  septic L08.0
  solare L57.8
  specified NEC L30.8
  stasis I87.2
    with varicose ulcer —*see* Varix, leg, with ulcer, with inflammation
    due to postthrombotic syndrome —*see* Syndrome, postthrombotic
  suppurative L08.0
  traumatic NEC L30.4
  trophoneurotica L13.0
  ultraviolet (sun) (chronic exposure) L57.8
    acute L56.8
  varicose —*see* Varix, leg, with, inflammation
  vegetans L10.1
  verrucosa B43.0
  vesicular, herpesviral B00.1

Dermatoarthritis, lipoid E78.81
Dermatochalasis, eyelid H02.839
  left H02.836
    lower H02.835
    upper H02.834
  right H02.833
    lower H02.832
    upper H02.831
Dermatofibroma (lenticulare) —*see* Neoplasm, skin, benign
  protuberans —*see* Neoplasm, skin, uncertain behavior
Dermatofibrosarcoma (pigmented) (protuberans) —*see* Neoplasm, skin, malignant
Dermatographia L50.3
Dermatolysis (exfoliativa) (congenital) Q82.8
  acquired L57.4
  eyelids —*see* Blepharochalasis
  palpebrarum —*see* Blepharochalasis
  senile L57.4
Dermatomegaly NEC Q82.8
Dermatomucosomyositis M33.10
  with
    myopathy M33.12
    respiratory involvement M33.11
    specified organ involvement NEC M33.19
Dermatomycosis B36.9
  furfuracea B36.0
  specified type NEC B36.8
Dermatomyositis (acute) (chronic) —*see also* Dermatopolymyositis
  in (due to) neoplastic disease (*see also* Neoplasm) D49.9 *[M36.0]*
Dermatoneuritis of children —*see* Poisoning, mercury
Dermatophilosis A48.8
Dermatophytid L30.2
Dermatophytide —*see* Dermatophytosis
Dermatophytosis (epidermophyton) (infection) (Microsporum) (tinea) (Trichophyton) B35.9
  beard B35.0
  body B35.4
  capitis B35.0
  corporis B35.4
  deep-seated B35.8
  disseminated B35.8
  foot B35.3
  granulomatous B35.8
  groin B35.6
  hand B35.2
  nail B35.1
  perianal (area) B35.6
  scalp B35.0
  specified NEC B35.8
Dermatopolymyositis M33.90
  with
    myopathy M33.92
    respiratory involvement M33.91
    specified organ involvement NEC M33.99
  in neoplastic disease (*see also* Neoplasm) D49.9 *[M36.0]*
  juvenile M33.00
    with
      myopathy M33.02
      respiratory involvement M33.01
      specified organ involvement NEC M33.09
  specified NEC M33.10
    myopathy M33.12
    respiratory involvement M33.11
    specified organ involvement NEC M33.19
Dermatopolyneuritis —*see* Poisoning, mercury
Dermatorrhexis Q79.6
  acquired L57.4
Dermatosclerosis —*see also* Scleroderma
  localized L94.0

Dermatosis L98.9
　Andrews' L08.89
　Bowen's —see Neoplasm, skin, in situ
　bullous L13.9
　　specified NEC L13.8
　exfoliativa L26
　eyelid (noninfectious)
　　dermatitis —see Dermatitis, eyelid
　　discoid lupus erythematosus —see Lupus,
　　　erythematosus, eyelid
　　xeroderma —see Xeroderma, acquired,
　　　eyelid
　factitial L98.1
　febrile neutrophilic L98.2
　gonococcal A54.89
　herpetiformis L13.0
　　juvenile L12.2
　linear IgA L13.8
　menstrual NEC L98.8
　neutrophilic, febrile L98.2
　occupational —see Dermatitis, contact
　papulosa nigra L82.1
　pigmentary L81.9
　　progressive L81.7
　　Schamberg's L81.7
　psychogenic F54
　purpuric, pigmented L81.7
　pustular, subcorneal L13.1
　transient acantholytic L11.1
Dermographia, dermographism L50.3
Dermoid (cyst) —see also Neoplasm, benign,
　　by site
　with malignant transformation C56-
　due to radiation (nonionizing) L57.8
Dermopathy
　infiltrative with thyrotoxicosis —see
　　Thyrotoxicosis
　nephrogenic fibrosing L90.8
Dermophytosis —see Dermatophytosis
Descemetocele H18.73-
Descemet's membrane —see condition
Descending —see condition
Descensus uteri —see Prolapse, uterus
Desert
　rheumatism B38.0
　sore —see Ulcer, skin
Desertion (newborn) —see Maltreatment
Desmoid (extra-abdominal) (tumor) —see
　　Neoplasm, connective tissue, uncertain
　　behavior
　abdominal D48.1
Despondency F32.9
Desquamation, skin R23.4
Destruction, destructive —see also Damage
　articular facet —see also Derangement, joint,
　　specified type NEC
　　knee M23.8X-
　　vertebra —see Spondylosis
　bone —see also Disorder, bone, specified type
　　NEC
　　syphilitic A52.77
　joint —see also Derangement, joint, specified
　　type NEC
　　sacroiliac M53.3
　rectal sphincter K62.89
　septum (nasal) J34.89
　tuberculous NEC —see Tuberculosis
　tympanum, tympanic membrane
　　(nontraumatic) —see Disorder,
　　tympanic membrane, specified
　　NEC
　vertebral disc —see Degeneration,
　　intervertebral disc
Destructiveness —see also Disorder, conduct
　adjustment reaction —see Disorder,
　　adjustment
Desultory labor O62.2
Detachment
　cartilage —see Sprain
　cervix, annular N88.8
　　complicating delivery O71.3

Detachment (Continued)
　choroid (old) (postinfectional) (simple)
　　(spontaneous) H31.40-
　　hemorrhagic H31.41-
　　serous H31.42-
　ligament —see Sprain
　meniscus (knee) —see also Derangement,
　　knee, meniscus, specified NEC
　　current injury —see Tear, meniscus
　　due to old tear or injury —see
　　　Derangement, knee, meniscus, due
　　　to old tear
　retina (without retinal break) (serous) H33.2-
　　with retinal:
　　　break H33.00-
　　　　giant H33.03-
　　　　multiple H33.02-
　　　　single H33.01-
　　　dialysis H33.04-
　　pigment epithelium —see Degeneration,
　　　retina, separation of layers, pigment
　　　epithelium detachment
　　rhegmatogenous —see Detachment, retina,
　　　with retinal, break
　　specified NEC H33.8
　　total H33.05-
　　traction H33.4-
　vitreous (body) H43.81
Detergent asthma J69.8
Deterioration
　epileptic F06.8
　general physical R53.81
　heart, cardiac —see Degeneration, myocardial
　mental —see Psychosis
　myocardial, myocardium —see Degeneration,
　　myocardial
　senile (simple) R54
Deuteranomaly (anomalous trichromat) H53.53
Deuteranopia (complete) (incomplete) H53.53
Development
　abnormal, bone Q79.9
　arrested R62.50
　　bone —see Arrest, development or growth,
　　　bone
　　child R62.50
　　due to malnutrition E45
　defective, congenital —see also Anomaly, by
　　site
　　cauda equina Q06.3
　　left ventricle Q24.8
　　　in hypoplastic left heart syndrome
　　　　Q23.4
　　valve Q24.8
　　　pulmonary Q22.3
　delayed (see also Delay, development) R62.50
　　arithmetical skills F81.2
　　language (skills) (expressive) F80.1
　　learning skill F81.9
　　mixed skills F88
　　motor coordination F82
　　reading F81.0
　　specified learning skill NEC F81.89
　　speech F80.9
　　spelling F81.81
　　written expression F81.81
　imperfect, congenital —see also Anomaly, by
　　site
　　heart Q24.9
　　lungs Q33.6
　incomplete
　　bronchial tree Q32.4
　　organ or site not listed —see Hypoplasia,
　　　by site
　　respiratory system Q34.9
　sexual, precocious NEC E30.1
　tardy, mental (see also Disability, intellectual)
　　F79
Developmental —see condition
　testing, child —see Examination, child
Devergie's disease (pityriasis rubra pilaris)
　L44.0

Deviation (in)
　conjugate palsy (eye) (spastic) H51.0
　esophagus (acquired) K22.8
　eye, skew H51.8
　midline (jaw) (teeth) (dental arch) M26.29
　　specified site NEC —see Malposition
　nasal septum J34.2
　　congenital Q67.4
　opening and closing of the mandible M26.53
　organ or site, congenital NEC —see
　　Malposition, congenital
　septum (nasal) (acquired) J34.2
　　congenital Q67.4
　sexual F65.9
　　bestiality F65.89
　　erotomania F52.8
　　exhibitionism F65.2
　　fetishism, fetishistic F65.0
　　　transvestism F65.1
　　frotteurism F65.81
　　masochism F65.51
　　multiple F65.89
　　necrophilia F65.89
　　nymphomania F52.8
　　pederosis F65.4
　　pedophilia F65.4
　　sadism, sadomasochism F65.52
　　satyriasis F52.8
　　specified type NEC F65.89
　　transvestism F64.1
　　voyeurism F65.3
　teeth, midline M26.29
　trachea J39.8
　ureter, congenital Q62.61
Device
　cerebral ventricle (communicating) in situ
　　Z98.2
　contraceptive —see Contraceptive, device
　drainage, cerebrospinal fluid, in situ Z98.2
Devic's disease G36.0
Devil's
　grip B33.0
　pinches (purpura simplex) D69.2
Devitalized tooth K04.99
Devonshire colic —see Poisoning, lead
Dextraposition, aorta Q20.3
　in tetralogy of Fallot Q21.3
Dextrinosis, limit (debrancher enzyme
　　deficiency) E74.03
Dextrocardia (true) Q24.0
　with
　　complete transposition of viscera Q89.3
　　situs inversus Q89.3
Dextrotransposition, aorta Q20.3
d-glycericacidemia E72.59
Dhat syndrome F48.8
Dhobi itch B35.6
Di George's syndrome D82.1
Di Guglielmo's disease C94.0-
Diabetes, diabetic (mellitus) (sugar) E11.9
　with
　　amyotrophy E11.44
　　arthropathy NEC E11.618
　　autonomic (poly)neuropathy E11.43
　　cataract E11.36
　　Charcot's joints E11.610
　　chronic kidney disease E11.22
　　circulatory complication NEC E11.59
　　complication E11.8
　　　specified NEC E11.69
　　dermatitis E11.620
　　foot ulcer E11.621
　　gangrene E11.52
　　gastroparesis E11.43
　　glomerulonephrosis, intracapillary E11.21
　　glomerulosclerosis, intercapillary E11.21
　　hyperglycemia E11.65
　　hyperosmolarity E11.00
　　　with coma E11.01
　　hypoglycemia E11.649
　　　with coma E11.641

Diabetes, diabetic *(Continued)*
  with *(Continued)*
    kidney complications NEC E11.29
    Kimmelstiel-Wilson disease E11.21
    loss of protective sensation (LOPS) —*see*
      Diabetes, by type, with neuropathy
    mononeuropathy E11.41
    myasthenia E11.44
    necrobiosis lipoidica E11.620
    nephropathy E11.21
    neuralgia E11.42
    neurologic complication NEC E11.49
    neuropathic arthropathy E11.610
    neuropathy E11.40
    ophthalmic complication NEC E11.39
    oral complication NEC E11.638
    periodontal disease E11.630
    peripheral angiopathy E11.51
      with gangrene E11.52
    polyneuropathy E11.42
    renal complication NEC E11.29
    renal tubular degeneration E11.29
    retinopathy E11.319
      with macular edema E11.311
      nonproliferative E11.329
        with macular edema E11.321
        mild E11.329
          with macular edema E11.321
        moderate E11.339
          with macular edema E11.331
        severe E11.349
          with macular edema E11.341
      proliferative E11.359
        with macular edema E11.351
    skin complication NEC E11.628
    skin ulcer NEC E11.622
  bronzed E83.110
  complicating pregnancy —*see* Pregnancy,
    complicated by, diabetes
  dietary counseling and surveillance Z71.3
  due to drug or chemical E09.9
    with
      amyotrophy E09.44
      arthropathy NEC E09.618
      autonomic (poly)neuropathy E09.43
      cataract E09.36
      Charcot's joints E09.610
      chronic kidney disease E09.22
      circulatory complication NEC E09.59
      complication E09.8
        specified NEC E09.69
      dermatitis E09.620
      foot ulcer E09.621
      gangrene E09.52
      gastroparesis E09.43
      glomerulonephrosis, intracapillary
        E09.21
      glomerulosclerosis, intercapillary E09.21
      hyperglycemia E09.65
      hyperosmolarity E09.00
        with coma E09.01
      hypoglycemia E09.649
        with coma E09.641
      ketoacidosis E09.10
        with coma E09.11
      kidney complications NEC E09.29
      Kimmelstiel-Wilson disease E09.21
      mononeuropathy E09.41
      myasthenia E09.44
      necrobiosis lipoidica E09.620
      nephropathy E09.21
      neuralgia E09.42
      neurologic complication NEC E09.49
      neuropathic arthropathy E09.610
      neuropathy E09.40
      ophthalmic complication NEC E09.39
      oral complication NEC E09.638
      periodontal disease E09.630
      peripheral angiopathy E09.51
        with gangrene E09.52
      polyneuropathy E09.42

Diabetes, diabetic *(Continued)*
  due to drug or chemical *(Continued)*
    with *(Continued)*
      renal complication NEC E09.29
      renal tubular degeneration E09.29
      retinopathy E09.319
        with macular edema E09.311
        nonproliferative E09.329
          with macular edema E09.321
          mild E09.329
            with macular edema E09.321
          moderate E09.339
            with macular edema E09.331
          severe E09.349
            with macular edema E09.341
        proliferative E09.359
          with macular edema E09.351
      skin complication NEC E09.628
      skin ulcer NEC E09.622
  due to underlying condition E08.9
    with
      amyotrophy E08.44
      arthropathy NEC E08.618
      autonomic (poly)neuropathy E08.43
      cataract E08.36
      Charcot's joints E08.610
      chronic kidney disease E08.22
      circulatory complication NEC E08.59
      complication E08.8
        specified NEC E08.69
      dermatitis E08.620
      foot ulcer E08.621
      gangrene E08.52
      gastroparesis E08.43
      glomerulonephrosis, intracapillary
        E08.21
      glomerulosclerosis, intercapillary
        E08.21
      hyperglycemia E08.69
      hyperosmolarity E08.00
        with coma E08.01
      hypoglycemia E08.649
        with coma E08.641
      ketoacidosis E08.10
        with coma E08.11
      kidney complications NEC E08.29
      Kimmelstiel-WIlson disease E08.21
      mononeuropathy E08.41
      myasthenia E08.44
      necrobiosis lipoidica E08.620
      nephropathy E08.21
      neuralgia E08.42
      neurologic complication NEC E08.49
      neuropathic arthropathy E08.610
      neuropathy E08.40
      ophthalmic complication NEC
        E08.39
      oral complication NEC E08.638
      periodontal disease E08.630
      peripheral angiopathy E08.51
        with gangrene E08.52
      polyneuropathy E08.42
      renal complication NEC E08.29
      renal tubular degeneration E08.29
      retinopathy E08.319
        with macular edema E08.311
        nonproliferative E08.329
          with macular edema E08.321
          mild E08.329
            with macular edema E08.321
          moderate E08.339
            with macular edema E08.331
          severe E08.349
            with macular edema E08.341
        proliferative E08.359
          with macular edema E08.351
      skin complication NEC E08.628
      skin ulcer NEC E08.622
  gestational (in pregnancy) O24.419
    affecting newborn P70.0
    diet-controlled O24.410

Diabetes, diabetic *(Continued)*
  gestational *(Continued)*
    in childbirth O24.429
      diet-controlled O24.420
      insulin (and diet) controlled
        O24.424
    insulin (and diet) controlled
      O24.414
    puerperal O24.439
      diet-controlled O24.430
      insulin (and diet) controlled O24.434
  hepatogenous E13.9
  inadequately controlled — code to Diabetes,
    by type, with hyperglycemia
  insipidus E23.2
    nephrogenic N25.1
    pituitary E23.2
    vasopressin resistant N25.1
  insulin dependent — code to type of
    diabetes
  juvenile-onset —*see* Diabetes, type 1
  ketosis-prone —*see* Diabetes, type 1
  latent R73.09
  neonatal (transient) P70.2
  non-insulin dependent — code to type of
    diabetes
  out of control — code to Diabetes, by type,
    with hyperglycemia
  phosphate E83.39
  poorly controlled — code to Diabetes, by
    type, with hyperglycemia
  postpancreatectomy —*see* Diabetes, specified
    type NEC
  postprocedural —*see* Diabetes, specified type
    NEC
  secondary diabetes mellitus NEC —*see*
    Diabetes, specified type NEC
  specified type NEC E13.9
    with
      amyotrophy E13.44
      arthropathy NEC E13.618
      autonomic (poly)neuropathy E13.43
      cataract E13.36
      Charcot's joints E13.610
      chronic kidney disease E13.22
      circulatory complication NEC E13.59
      complication E13.8
        specified NEC E13.69
      dermatitis E13.620
      foot ulcer E13.621
      gangrene E13.52
      gastroparesis E13.43
      glomerulonephrosis, intracapillary
        E13.21
      glomerulosclerosis, intercapillary
        E13.21
      hyperglycemia E13.65
      hyperosmolarity E13.00
        with coma E13.01
      hypoglycemia E13.649
        with coma E13.641
      ketoacidosis E13.10
        with coma E13.11
      kidney complications NEC E13.29
      Kimmelstiel-Wilson disease E13.21
      mononeuropathy E13.41
      myasthenia E13.44
      necrobiosis lipoidica E13.620
      nephropathy E13.21
      neuralgia E13.42
      neurologic complication NEC E13.49
      neuropathic arthropathy E13.610
      neuropathy E13.40
      ophthalmic complication NEC E13.39
      oral complication NEC E13.638
      periodontal disease E13.630
      peripheral angiopathy E13.51
        with gangrene E13.52
      polyneuropathy E13.42
      renal complication NEC E13.29
      renal tubular degeneration E13.29

Diastasis *(Continued)*
 muscle *(Continued)*
  pelvic region M62.05-
  shoulder region M62.01-
  specified site NEC M62.08
  thigh M62.05-
  upper arm M62.02-
 recti (abdomen)
  complicating delivery O71.89
  congenital Q79.59
Diastema, tooth, teeth, fully erupted M26.32
Diastematomyelia Q06.2
Diataxia, cerebral G80.4
Diathesis
 allergic —*see* History, allergy
 bleeding (familial) D69.9
 cystine (familial) E72.00
 gouty —*see* Gout
 hemorrhagic (familial) D69.9
  newborn NEC P53
 spasmophilic R29.0
Diaz's disease or osteochondrosis (juvenile)
  (talus) —*see* Osteochondrosis, juvenile,
  tarsus
Dibothriocephalus, dibothriocephaliasis
  (latus) (infection) (infestation) B70.0
 larval B70.1
Dicephalus, dicephaly Q89.4
Dichotomy, teeth K00.2
Dichromat, dichromatopsia (congenital) —*see*
  Deficiency, color vision
Dichuchwa A65
Dicroceliasis B66.2
Didelphia, didelphys —*see* Double uterus
Didymytis N45.1
 with orchitis N45.3
Dietary
 inadequacy or deficiency E63.9
 surveillance and counseling Z71.3
Dietl's crisis N13.8
Dieulafoy lesion (hemorrhagic)
 duodenum K31.82
 esophagus K22.8
 intestine (colon) K63.81
 stomach K31.82
Difficult, difficulty (in)
 acculturation Z60.3
 feeding R63.3
  newborn P92.9
   breast P92.5
   specified NEC P92.8
  nonorganic (infant or child) F98.29
 intubation, in anesthesia T88.4
 mechanical, gastroduodenal stoma K91.89
  causing obstruction K91.3
 reading (developmental) F81.0
  secondary to emotional disorders F93.9
 spelling (specific) F81.81
  with reading disorder F81.89
  due to inadequate teaching Z55.8
 swallowing —*see* Dysphagia
 walking R26.2
 work
  conditions NEC Z56.5
  schedule Z56.3
Diffuse —*see* condition
DiGeorge's syndrome (thymic hypoplasia)
  D82.1
Digestive —*see* condition
Dihydropyrimidine dehydrogenase disease
  (DPD) E88.89
Diktyoma —*see* Neoplasm, malignant, by site
Dilaceration, tooth K00.4
Dilatation
 anus K59.8
  venule —*see* Hemorrhoids
 aorta (focal) (general) —*see* Ectasia, aorta
  with aneurysm —*see* Aneurysm, aorta
 artery —*see* Aneurysm
 bladder (sphincter) N32.89
  congenital Q64.79

Dilatation *(Continued)*
 blood vessel I99.8
 bronchial J47.9
  with
   exacerbation (acute) J47.1
   lower respiratory infection J47.0
 calyx (due to obstruction) —*see*
   Hydronephrosis
 capillaries I78.8
 cardiac (acute) (chronic) —*see also*
   Hypertrophy, cardiac
  congenital Q24.8
   valve NEC Q24.8
    pulmonary Q22.3
  valve —*see* Endocarditis
 cavum septi pellucidi Q06.8
 cervix (uteri) —*see also* Incompetency,
   cervix
  incomplete, poor, slow complicating
   delivery O62.0
 colon K59.3
  congenital Q43.1
  psychogenic F45.8
 common duct (acquired) K83.8
  congenital Q44.5
 cystic duct (acquired) K82.8
  congenital Q44.5
 duct, mammary —*see* Ectasia, mammary
   duct
 duodenum K59.8
 esophagus K22.8
  congenital Q39.5
  due to achalasia K22.0
 eustachian tube, congenital Q17.8
 gallbladder K82.8
 gastric —*see* Dilatation, stomach
 heart (acute) (chronic) —*see also* Hypertrophy,
   cardiac
  congenital Q24.8
  valve —*see* Endocarditis
 ileum K59.8
  psychogenic F45.8
 jejunum K59.8
  psychogenic F45.8
 kidney (calyx) (collecting structures) (cystic)
   (parenchyma) (pelvis) (idiopathic)
   N28.89
 lacrimal passages or duct —*see* Disorder,
   lacrimal system, changes
 lymphatic vessel I89.0
 mammary duct —*see* Ectasia, mammary
   duct
 Meckel's diverticulum (congenital) Q43.0
  malignant —*see* Table of Neoplasms, small
   intestine, malignant
 myocardium (acute) (chronic) —*see*
   Hypertrophy, cardiac organ or site,
   congenital NEC —*see* Distortion
 pancreatic duct K86.8
 pericardium —*see* Pericarditis
 pharynx J39.2
 prostate N42.89
 pulmonary
  artery (idiopathic) I28.8
  valve, congenital Q22.3
 pupil H57.04
 rectum K59.3
 saccule, congenital Q16.5
 salivary gland (duct) K11.8
 sphincter ani K62.89
 stomach K31.89
  acute K31.0
  psychogenic F45.8
 submaxillary duct K11.8
 trachea, congenital Q32.1
 ureter (idiopathic) N28.82
  congenital Q62.2
  due to obstruction N13.4
 urethra (acquired) N36.8
 vasomotor I73.9
 vein I86.8

Dilatation *(Continued)*
 ventricular, ventricle (acute) (chronic) —*see*
   also Hypertrophy, cardiac
  cerebral, congenital Q04.8
 venule NEC I86.8
 vesical orifice N32.89
Dilated, dilation —*see* Dilatation
Diminished, diminution
 hearing (acuity) —*see* Deafness
 sense or sensation (cold) (heat) (tactile)
   (vibratory) R20.8
 vision NEC H54.7
 vital capacity R94.2
Diminuta taenia B71.0
Dimitri-Sturge-Weber disease Q85.8
Dimple
 parasacral, pilonidal or postanal —*see* Cyst,
   pilonidal
Dioctophyme renalis (infection) (infestation)
   B83.8
Dipetalonemiasis B74.4
Diphallus Q55.69
Diphtheria, diphtheritic (gangrenous)
   (hemorrhagic) A36.9
 carrier (suspected) Z22.2
 cutaneous A36.3
 faucial A36.0
 infection of wound A36.3
 laryngeal A36.2
 myocarditis A36.81
 nasal, anterior A36.89
 nasopharyngeal A36.1
 neurological complication A36.89
 pharyngeal A36.0
 specified site NEC A36.89
 tonsillar A36.0
Diphyllobothriasis (intestine) B70.0
 larval B70.1
Diplacusis H93.22-
Diplegia (upper limbs) G83.0
 congenital (cerebral) G80.8
 facial G51.0
 lower limbs G82.20
 spastic G80.1
Diplococcus, diplococcal —*see* condition
Diplopia H53.2
Dipsomania F10.20
 with
  psychosis —*see* Psychosis, alcoholic
  remission F10.21
Dipylidiasis B71.1
Direction, teeth, abnormal, fully erupted
   M26.30
Dirofilariasis B74.8
Dirt-eating child F98.3
Disability, disabilities
 heart —*see* Disease, heart
 intellectual F79
  with
   autistic features F84.9
   mild (I.Q. 50-69) F70
   moderate (I.Q. 35-49) F71
   profound (I.Q. under 20) F73
   severe (I.Q. 20-34) F72
   specified level NEC F78
  knowledge acquisition F81.9
  learning F81.9
  limiting activities Z73.6
  spelling, specific F81.81
Disappearance of family member Z63.4
Disarticulation —*see* Amputation
 meaning traumatic amputation —*see*
   Amputation, traumatic
Discharge (from)
 abnormal finding in —*see* Abnormal,
   specimen
 breast (female) (male) N64.52
 diencephalic autonomic idiopathic —*see*
   Epilepsy, specified NEC
 ear —*see also* Otorrhea
  blood —*see* Otorrhagia

Discharge *(Continued)*
excessive urine R35.8
nipple N64.52
penile R36.9
postnasal R09.82
prison, anxiety concerning Z65.2
urethral R36.9
without blood R36.0
hematospermia R36.1
vaginal N89.8
Discitis, diskitis M46.40
cervical region M46.42
cervicothoracic region M46.43
lumbar region M46.46
lumbosacral region M46.47
multiple sites M46.49
occipito-atlanto-axial region M46.41
pyogenic —*see* Infection, intervertebral
disc, pyogenic
sacrococcygeal region M46.48
thoracic region M46.44
thoracolumbar region M46.45
Discoid
meniscus (congenital) Q68.6
semilunar cartilage (congenital) —*see*
Derangement, knee, meniscus,
specified NEC
Discoloration
nails L60.8
teeth (posteruptive) K03.7
during formation K00.8
Discomfort
chest R07.89
visual H53.14-
Discontinuity, ossicles, ear
H74.2-
Discord (with)
boss Z56.4
classmates Z55.4
counselor Z64.4
employer Z56.4
family Z63.8
fellow employees Z56.4
in-laws Z63.1
landlord Z59.2
lodgers Z59.2
neighbors Z59.2
probation officer Z64.4
social worker Z64.4
teachers Z55.4
workmates Z56.4
Discordant connection
atrioventricular (congenital) Q20.5
ventriculoarterial Q20.3
Discrepancy
centric occlusion maximum intercuspation
M26.55
leg length (acquired) —*see* Deformity, limb,
unequal length
congenital —*see* Defect, reduction, lower
limb
uterine size date O26.84-
Discrimination
ethnic Z60.5
political Z60.5
racial Z60.5
religious Z60.5
sex Z60.5
Disease, diseased —*see also* Syndrome
absorbent system I87.8
acid-peptic K30
Acosta's T70.29
Adams-Stokes (-Morgagni) (syncope with
heart block) I45.9
Addison's anemia (pernicious) D51.0
adenoids (and tonsils) J35.9
adrenal (capsule) (cortex) (gland) (medullary)
E27.9
hyperfunction E27.0
specified NEC E27.8
ainhum L94.6

Disease, diseased *(Continued)*
airway
obstructive, chronic J44.9
due to
cotton dust J66.0
specific organic dusts NEC J66.8
reactive —*see* Asthma
akamushi (scrub typhus) A75.3
Albers-Schönberg (marble bones) Q78.2
Albert's —*see* Tendinitis, Achilles
alimentary canal K63.9
alligator-skin Q80.9
acquired L85.0
alpha heavy chain C88.3
alpine T70.29
altitude T70.20
alveolar ridge
edentulous K06.9
specified NEC K06.8
alveoli, teeth K08.9
Alzheimer's G30.9 *[F02.80]*
with behavioral disturbance G30.9
[F02.81]
early onset G30.0 *[F02.80]*
with behavioral disturbance G30.0
[F02.81]
late onset G30.1 *[F02.80]*
with behavioral disturbance G30.1
[F02.81]
specified NEC G30.8 *[F02.80]*
with behavioral disturbance G30.8
[F02.81]
amyloid —*see* Amyloidosis
Andersen's (glycogenosis IV) E74.09
Andes T70.29
Andrews' (bacterid) L08.89
angiospastic I73.9
cerebral G45.9
vein I87.8
anterior
chamber H21.9
horn cell G12.29
antiglomerular basement membrane
(anti-GBM) antibody M31.0
tubulo-interstitial nephritis N12
antral —*see* Sinusitis, maxillary
anus K62.9
specified NEC K62.89
aorta (nonsyphilitic) I77.9
syphilitic NEC A52.02
aortic (heart) (valve) I35.9
rheumatic I06.9
Apollo B30.3
aponeuroses —*see* Enthesopathy
appendix K38.9
specified NEC K38.8
aqueous (chamber) H21.9
Arnold-Chiari —*see* Arnold-Chiari disease
arterial I77.9
occlusive —*see* Occlusion, by site
due to stricture or stenosis I77.1
arteriocardiorenal —*see* Hypertension,
cardiorenal
arteriolar (generalized) (obliterative)
I77.9
arteriorenal —*see* Hypertension, kidney
arteriosclerotic —*see also* Arteriosclerosis
cardiovascular —*see* Disease, heart,
ischemic, atherosclerotic
coronary (artery) —*see* Disease, heart,
ischemic, atherosclerotic
heart —*see* Disease, heart, ischemic,
atherosclerotic
artery I77.9
cerebral I67.9
coronary I25.10
with angina pectoris —*see*
Arteriosclerosis, coronary
(artery),
arthropod-borne NOS (viral) A94
specified type NEC A93.8

Disease, diseased *(Continued)*
atticoantral, chronic H66.20
left H66.22
with right H66.23
right H66.21
with left H66.23
auditory canal —*see* Disorder, ear, external
auricle, ear NEC —*see* Disorder, pinna
Australian X A83.4
autoimmune (systemic) NOS M35.9
hemolytic (cold type) (warm type) D59.1
drug-induced D59.0
thyroid E06.3
aviator's —*see* Effect, adverse, high altitude
Ayala's Q78.5
Ayerza's (pulmonary artery sclerosis with
pulmonary hypertension) I27.0
Babington's (familial hemorrhagic
telangiectasia) I78.0
bacterial A49.9
specified NEC A48.8
zoonotic A28.9
specified type NEC A28.8
Baelz's (cheilitis glandularis apostematosa)
K13.0
bagasse J67.1
balloon —*see* Effect, adverse, high altitude
Bang's (brucella abortus) A23.1
Bannister's T78.3
barometer makers' —*see* Poisoning, mercury
Barraquer (-Simons') (progressive
lipodystrophy) E88.1
Barrett's —*see* Barrett's, esophagus
Bartholin's gland N75.9
basal ganglia G25.9
degenerative G23.9
specified NEC G23.8
specified NEC G25.89
Basedow's (exophthalmic goiter) —*see*
Hyperthyroidism, with, goiter (diffuse)
Bateman's B08.1
Batten-Steinert G71.11
Battey A31.0
Beard's (neurasthenia) F48.8
Becker
idiopathic mural endomyocardial I42.3
myotonia congenita G71.12
Begbie's (exophthalmic goiter) —*see*
Hyperthyroidism, with, goiter (diffuse)
behavioral, organic F07.9
Beigel's (white piedra) B36.2
Benson's —*see* Deposit, crystalline
Bernard-Soulier (thrombopathy) D69.1
Bernhardt (-Roth) —*see* Mononeuropathy,
lower limb, meralgia paresthetica
Biermer's (pernicious anemia) D51.0
bile duct (common) (hepatic) K83.9
with calculus, stones —*see* Calculus, bile
duct
specified NEC K83.8
biliary (tract) K83.9
specified NEC K83.8
Billroth's —*see* Spina bifida
bird fancier's J67.2
black lung J60
bladder N32.9
in (due to)
schistosomiasis (bilharziasis) B65.0 *[N33]*
specified NEC N32.89
bleeder's D66
blood D75.9
forming organs D75.9
vessel I99.9
Bloodgood's —*see* Mastopathy, cystic
Bodechtel-Guttmann (subacute sclerosing
panencephalitis) A81.1
bone —*see also* Disorder, bone
aluminum M83.4
fibrocystic NEC
jaw M27.49
bone-marrow D75.9

◀ New ◀▦ Revised ~~deleted~~ Deleted

Disease, diseased *(Continued)*
Borna A83.9
Bornholm (epidemic pleurodynia) B33.0
Bouchard's (myopathic dilatation of the stomach) K31.0
Bouillaud's (rheumatic heart disease) I01.9
Bourneville (-Brissaud) (tuberous sclerosis) Q85.1
Bouveret (-Hoffmann) (paroxysmal tachycardia) I47.9
bowel K63.9
  functional K59.9
    psychogenic F45.8
brain G93.9
  arterial, artery I67.9
  arteriosclerotic I67.2
  congenital Q04.9
  degenerative —*see* Degeneration, brain
  inflammatory —*see* Encephalitis
  organic G93.9
    arteriosclerotic I67.2
  parasitic NEC B71.9 *[G94]*
  senile NEC G31.1
  specified NEC G93.89
breast (*see also* Disorder, breast) N64.9
  cystic (chronic) —*see* Mastopathy, cystic
  fibrocystic —*see* Mastopathy, cystic
  Paget's
    female, unspecified side C50.91-
    male, unspecified side C50.92-
  specified NEC N64.89
Breda's —*see* Yaws
Bretonneau's (diphtheritic malignant angina) A36.0
Bright's —*see* Nephritis
  arteriosclerotic —*see* Hypertension, kidney
Brill's (recrudescent typhus) A75.1
Brill-Zinsser (recrudescent typhus) A75.1
Brion-Kayser —*see* Fever, paratyphoid
broad
  beta E78.2
  ligament (noninflammatory) N83.9
    inflammatory —*see* Disease, pelvis, inflammatory
    specified NEC N83.8
Brocq-Duhring (dermatitis herpetiformis) L13.0
Brocq's
  meaning
    dermatitis herpetiformis L13.0
    prurigo L28.2
bronchopulmonary J98.4
bronchus NEC J98.09
bronze Addison's E27.1
  tuberculous A18.7
budgerigar fancier's J67.2
Buerger's (thromboangiitis obliterans) I73.1
bullous L13.9
  chronic of childhood L12.2
  specified NEC L13.8
Bürger-Grütz (essential familial hyperlipemia) E78.3
bursa —*see* Bursopathy
caisson T70.3
California —*see* Coccidioidomycosis
capillaries I78.9
  specified NEC I78.8
Carapata A68.0
cardiac —*see* Disease, heart
cardiopulmonary, chronic I27.9
cardiorenal (hepatic) (hypertensive) (vascular) —*see* Hypertension, cardiorenal
cardiovascular (atherosclerotic) I25.10
  with angina pectoris —*see* Arteriosclerosis, coronary (artery),
  congenital Q28.9
  hypertensive —*see* Hypertension, heart
  newborn P29.9
    specified NEC P29.89

Disease, diseased *(Continued)*
cardiovascular *(Continued)*
  renal (hypertensive) —*see* Hypertension, cardiorenal
  syphilitic (asymptomatic) A52.00
cartilage —*see* Disorder, cartilage
Castellani's A69.8
cat-scratch A28.1
Cavare's (familial periodic paralysis) G72.3
cecum K63.9
celiac (adult) (infantile) K90.0
cellular tissue L98.9
central core G71.2
cerebellar, cerebellum —*see* Disease, brain
cerebral —*see also* Disease, brain
  degenerative —*see* Degeneration, brain
cerebrospinal G96.9
cerebrovascular I67.9
  acute I67.89
    embolic I63.4-
    thrombotic I63.3-
  arteriosclerotic I67.2
  specified NEC I67.89
cervix (uteri) (noninflammatory) N88.9
  inflammatory —*see* Cervicitis
  specified NEC N88.8
Chabert's A22.9
Chandler's (osteochondritis dissecans, hip) —*see* Osteochondritis, dissecans, hip
Charlouis —*see* Yaws
Chédiak-Steinbrinck (-Higashi) (congenital gigantism of peroxidase granules) E70.330
chest J98.9
Chiari's (hepatic vein thrombosis) I82.0
Chicago B40.9
Chignon B36.8
chigo, chigoe B88.1
childhood granulomatous D71
Chinese liver fluke B66.1
chlamydial A74.9
  specified NEC A74.89
cholecystic K82.9
choroid H31.9
  specified NEC H31.8
Christmas D67
chronic bullous of childhood L12.2
chylomicron retention E78.3
ciliary body H21.9
  specified NEC H21.89
circulatory (system) NEC I99.8
  newborn P29.9
  syphilitic A52.00
    congenital A50.54
coagulation factor deficiency (congenital) —*see* Defect, coagulation
coccidioidal —*see* Coccidioidomycosis
cold
  agglutinin or hemoglobinuria D59.1
    paroxysmal D59.6
  hemagglutinin (chronic) D59.1
collagen NOS (nonvascular) (vascular) M35.9
  specified NEC M35.8
colon K63.9
  functional K59.9
    congenital Q43.2
  ischemic K55.0
combined system —*see* Degeneration, combined
compressed air T70.3
Concato's (pericardial polyserositis) A19.9
  nontubercular I31.1
  pleural —*see* Pleurisy, with effusion
conjunctiva H11.9
  chlamydial A74.0
  specified NEC H11.89
  viral B30.9
    specified NEC B30.8

Disease, diseased *(Continued)*
connective tissue, systemic (diffuse) M35.9
  in (due to)
    hypogammaglobulinemia D80.1 *[M36.8]*
    ochronosis E70.29 *[M36.8]*
  specified NEC M35.8
Conor and Bruch's (boutonneuse fever) A77.1
Cooper's —*see* Mastopathy, cystic
Cori's (glycogenosis III) E74.03
corkhandler's or corkworker's J67.3
cornea H18.9
  specified NEC H18.89-
coronary (artery) —*see* Disease, heart, ischemic, atherosclerotic
  congenital Q24.5
  ostial, syphilitic (aortic) (mitral) (pulmonary) A52.03
corpus cavernosum N48.9
  specified NEC N48.89
Cotugno's —*see* Sciatica
coxsackie (virus) NEC B34.1
cranial nerve NOS G52.9
Creutzfeldt-Jakob —*see* Creutzfeldt-Jakob disease or syndrome
Crocq's (acrocyanosis) I73.89
Crohn's —*see* Enteritis, regional
Curschmann G71.11
cystic
  breast (chronic) —*see* Mastopathy, cystic
  kidney, congenital Q61.9
  liver, congenital Q44.6
  lung J98.4
    congenital Q33.0
cytomegalic inclusion (generalized) B25.9
  with pneumonia B25.0
  congenital P35.1
cytomegaloviral B25.9
  specified NEC B25.8
Czerny's (periodic hydrarthrosis of the knee) —*see* Effusion, joint, knee
Daae (-Finsen) (epidemic pleurodynia) B33.0
Darling's —*see* Histoplasmosis capsulati
Débove's (splenomegaly) R16.1
deer fly —*see* Tularemia
Degos' I77.8
demyelinating, demyelinizating (nervous system) G37.9
  multiple sclerosis G35
  specified NEC G37.8
dense deposit (*see also* N00-N07 with fourth character .6) N05.6
deposition, hydroxyapatite —*see* Disease, hydroxyapatite deposition
de Quervain's (tendon sheath) M65.4
  thyroid (subacute granulomatous thyroiditis) E06.1
Devergie's (pityriasis rubra pilaris) L44.0
Devic's G36.0
diaphorase deficiency D74.0
diaphragm J98.6
diarrheal, infectious NEC A09
digestive system K92.9
  specified NEC K92.89
disc, degenerative —*see* Degeneration, intervertebral disc
discogenic —*see also* Displacement, intervertebral disc NEC
  with myelopathy —*see* Disorder, disc, with, myelopathy
diverticular —*see* Diverticula
Dubois (thymus) A50.59 *[E35]*
Duchenne-Griesinger G71.0
Duchenne's
  muscular dystrophy G71.0
  pseudohypertrophy, muscles G71.0
ductless glands E34.9
Duhring's (dermatitis herpetiformis) L13.0
duodenum K31.9
  specified NEC K31.89
Dupré's (meningism) R29.1
Dupuytren's (muscle contracture) M72.0

Disease, diseased *(Continued)*
  Durand-Nicholas-Favre (climatic bubo) A55
  Duroziez's (congenital mitral stenosis) Q23.2
  ear —*see* Disorder, ear
  Eberth's —*see* Fever, typhoid
  Ebola (virus) A98.4
  Ebstein's heart Q22.5
  Echinococcus —*see* Echinococcus
  echovirus NEC B34.1
  Eddowes' (brittle bones and blue sclera)
      Q78.0
  edentulous (alveolar) ridge K06.9
      specified NEC K06.8
  Edsall's T67.2
  Eichstedt's (pityriasis versicolor) B36.0
  Ellis-van Creveld (chondroectodermal
      dysplasia) Q77.6
  end stage renal (ESRD) N18.6
      due to hypertension I12.0
  endocrine glands or system NEC E34.9
  endomyocardial (eosinophilic) I42.3
  English (rickets) E55.0
  enteroviral, enterovirus NEC B34.1
      central nervous system NEC A88.8
  epidemic B99.9
      specified NEC B99.8
  epididymis N50.9
  Erb (-Landouzy) G71.0
  Erdheim-Chester (ECD) E88.89
  esophagus K22.9
      functional K22.4
      psychogenic F45.8
      specified NEC K22.8
  Eulenburg's (congenital paramyotonia)
      G71.19
  eustachian tube —*see* Disorder, eustachian
      tube
  external
      auditory canal —*see* Disorder, ear, external
      ear —*see* Disorder, ear, external
  extrapyramidal G25.9
      specified NEC G25.89
  eye H57.9
      anterior chamber H21.9
      inflammatory NEC H57.8
      muscle (external) —*see* Strabismus
      specified NEC H57.8
      syphilitic —*see* Oculopathy, syphilitic
  eyeball H44.9
      specified NEC H44.89
  eyelid —*see* Disorder, eyelid
      specified NEC —*see* Disorder, eyelid,
          specified type NEC
  eyeworm of Africa B74.3
  facial nerve (seventh) G51.9
      newborn (birth injury) P11.3
  Fahr (of brain) G23.8
  Fahr Volhard (of kidney) I12.-
  fallopian tube (noninflammatory) N83.9
      inflammatory —*see* Salpingo-oophoritis
      specified NEC N83.8
  familial periodic paralysis G72.3
  Fanconi's (congenital pancytopenia) D61.09
  fascia NEC —*see also* Disorder, muscle
      inflammatory —*see* Myositis
      specified NEC M62.89
  Fauchard's (periodontitis) —*see* Periodontitis
  Favre-Durand-Nicolas (climatic bubo) A55
  Fede's K14.0
  Feer's —*see* Poisoning, mercury
  female pelvic inflammatory (*see also* Disease,
      pelvis, inflammatory) N73.9
      syphilitic (secondary) A51.42
      tuberculous A18.17
  Fernels' (aortic aneurysm) I71.9
  fibrocaseous of lung —*see* Tuberculosis,
      pulmonary
  fibrocystic —*see* Fibrocystic disease
  Fiedler's (leptospiral jaundice) A27.0
  fifth B08.3
  file-cutter's —*see* Poisoning, lead

Disease, diseased *(Continued)*
  fish-skin Q80.9
      acquired L85.0
  Flajani (-Basedow) (exophthalmic goiter) —
      see Hyperthyroidism, with, goiter
      (diffuse)
  flax-dresser's J66.1
  fluke —*see* Infestation, fluke
  foot and mouth B08.8
  foot process N04.9
  Forbes' (glycogenosis III) E74.03
  Fordyce-Fox (apocrine miliaria) L75.2
  Fordyce's (ectopic sebaceous glands) (mouth)
      Q38.6
  Forestier's (rhizomelic pseudopolyarthritis)
      M35.3
      meaning ankylosing hyperostosis —*see*
          Hyperostosis, ankylosing
  Fothergill's
      neuralgia —*see* Neuralgia, trigeminal
      scarlatina anginosa A38.9
  Fournier (gangrene) N49.3
      female N76.89
  fourth B08.8
  Fox (-Fordyce) (apocrine miliaria) L75.2
  Francis' —*see* Tularemia
  Franklin C88.2
  Frei's (climatic bubo) A55
  Friedreich's
      combined systemic or ataxia G11.1
      myoclonia G25.3
  frontal sinus —*see* Sinusitis, frontal
  fungus NEC B49
  Gaisböck's (polycythemia hypertonica) D75.1
  gallbladder K82.9
      calculus —*see* Calculus, gallbladder
      cholecystitis —*see* Cholecystitis
      cholesterolosis K82.4
      fistula —*see* Fistula, gallbladder
      hydrops K82.1
      obstruction —*see* Obstruction, gallbladder
      perforation K82.2
      specified NEC K82.8
  gamma heavy chain C88.2
  Gamna's (siderotic splenomegaly) D73.2
  Gamstorp's (adynamia episodica hereditaria)
      G72.3
  Gandy-Nanta (siderotic splenomegaly) D73.2
  ganister J62.8
  gastric —*see* Disease, stomach
  gastroesophageal reflux (GERD) K21.9
      with esophagitis K21.0
  gastrointestinal (tract) K92.9
      amyloid E85.4
      functional K59.9
          psychogenic F45.8
      specified NEC K92.89
  Gee (-Herter) (-Heubner) (-Thaysen)
      (nontropical sprue) K90.0
  genital organs
      female N94.9
      male N50.9
  Gerhardt's (erythromelalgia) I73.81
  Gibert's (pityriasis rosea) L42
  Gierke's (glycogenosis I) E74.01
  Gilles de la Tourette's (motor-verbal tic) F95.2
  gingiva K06.9
      specified NEC K06.8
  gland (lymph) I89.9
  Glanzmann's (hereditary hemorrhagic
      thrombasthenia) D69.1
  glass-blower's (cataract) —*see* Cataract,
      specified NEC
      salivary gland hypertrophy K11.1
  Glisson's —*see* Rickets
  globe H44.9
      specified NEC H44.89
  glomerular —*see also* Glomerulonephritis
      with edema —*see* Nephrosis
      acute —*see* Nephritis, acute
      chronic —*see* Nephritis, chronic

Disease, diseased *(Continued)*
  glomerular *(Continued)*
      minimal change N05.0
      rapidly progressive N01.9
  glycogen storage E74.00
      Andersen's E74.09
      Cori's E74.03
      Forbes' E74.03
      generalized E74.00
      glucose-6-phosphatase deficiency E74.01
      heart E74.02 *[I43]*
      hepatorenal E74.09
      Hers' E74.09
      liver and kidney E74.09
      McArdle's E74.04
      muscle phosphofructokinase E74.09
      myocardium E74.02 *[I43]*
      Pompe's E74.02
      Tauri's E74.09
      type 0 E74.09
      type I E74.01
      type II E74.02
      type III E74.03
      type IV E74.09
      type V E74.04
      type VI-XI E74.09
      Von Gierke's E74.01
  Goldstein's (familial hemorrhagic
      telangiectasia) I78.0
  gonococcal NOS A54.9
  graft-versus-host (GVH) D89.813
      acute D89.810
      acute on chronic D89.812
      chronic D89.811
  grainhandler's J67.8
  granulomatous (childhood) (chronic) D71
  Graves' (exophthalmic goiter) —*see*
      Hyperthyroidism, with, goiter
      (diffuse)
  Griesinger's —*see* Ancylostomiasis
  Grisel's M43.6
  Gruby's (tinea tonsurans) B35.0
  Guillain-Barré G61.0
  Guinon's (motor-verbal tic) F95.2
  gum K06.9
  gynecological N94.9
  H (Hartnup's) E72.02
  Haff —*see* Poisoning, mercury
  Hageman (congenital factor XII deficiency)
      D68.2
  hair (color) (shaft) L67.9
      follicles L73.9
          specified NEC L73.8
  Hamman's (spontaneous mediastinal
      emphysema) J98.2
  hand, foot and mouth B08.4
  Hansen's —*see* Leprosy
  Hantavirus, with pulmonary manifestations
      B33.4
      with renal manifestations A98.5
  Harada's H30.81-
  Hartnup (pellagra-cerebellar ataxia-renal
      aminoaciduria) E72.02
  Hart's (pellagra-cerebellar ataxia-renal
      aminoaciduria) E72.02
  Hashimoto's (struma lymphomatosa)
      E06.3
  Hb —*see* Disease, hemoglobin
  heart (organic) I51.9
      with
          pulmonary edema (acute) (*see also*
              Failure, ventricular, left) I50.1
          rheumatic fever (conditions in I00)
              active I01.9
                  with chorea I02.0
                  specified NEC I01.8
              inactive or quiescent (with chorea)
                  I09.9
                  specified NEC I09.89
      amyloid E85.4 *[I43]*
      aortic (valve) I35.9

◀ New   ◀━ Revised   ~~deleted~~ Deleted

Disease, diseased *(Continued)*
heart *(Continued)*
arteriosclerotic or sclerotic (senile) —
see Disease, heart, ischemic,
atherosclerotic
artery, arterial —*see* Disease, heart,
ischemic, atherosclerotic
beer drinkers' I42.6
beriberi (wet) E51.12
black I27.0
congenital Q24.9
cyanotic Q24.9
specified NEC Q24.8
coronary —*see* Disease, heart, ischemic
cryptogenic I51.9
fibroid —*see* Myocarditis
functional I51.89
psychogenic F45.8
glycogen storage E74.02 *[143]*
gonococcal A54.83
hypertensive —*see* Hypertension, heart
hyperthyroid *(see also* Hyperthyroidism)
E05.90 *[143]*
with thyroid storm E05.91 *[143]*
ischemic (chronic or with a stated duration
of over 4 weeks) I25.9
atherosclerotic (of) I25.10
with angina pectoris —*see*
Arteriosclerosis, coronary
(artery)
coronary artery bypass graft —*see*
Arteriosclerosis, coronary
(artery),
cardiomyopathy I25.5
diagnosed on ECG or other special
investigation, but currently
presenting no symptoms I25.6
silent I25.6
specified form NEC I25.89
kyphoscoliotic I27.1
meningococcal A39.50
endocarditis A39.51
myocarditis A39.52
pericarditis A39.53
mitral I05.9
specified NEC I05.8
muscular —*see* Degeneration,
myocardial
psychogenic (functional) F45.8
pulmonary (chronic) I27.9
in schistosomiasis B65.9 *[152]*
specified NEC I27.89
rheumatic (chronic) (inactive) (old)
(quiescent) (with chorea) I09.9
active or acute I01.9
with chorea (acute) (rheumatic)
(Sydenham's) I02.0
specified NEC I09.89
senile —*see* Myocarditis
syphilitic A52.06
aortic A52.03
aneurysm A52.01
congenital A50.54 *[152]*
thyrotoxic *(see also* Thyrotoxicosis) E05.90
[143]
with thyroid storm E05.91 *[143]*
valve, valvular (obstructive)
(regurgitant) —*see also* Endocarditis
congenital NEC Q24.8
pulmonary Q22.3
vascular —*see* Disease, cardiovascular
heavy chain NEC C88.2
alpha C88.3
gamma C88.2
mu C88.2
Hebra's
pityriasis
maculata et circinata L42
rubra pilaris L44.0
prurigo L28.2
hematopoietic organs D75.9

Disease, diseased *(Continued)*
hemoglobin or Hb
abnormal (mixed) NEC D58.2
with thalassemia D56.9
AS genotype D57.3
Bart's D56.0
C (Hb-C) D58.2
with other abnormal hemoglobin NEC
D58.2
elliptocytosis D58.1
Hb-S D57.2-
sickle-cell D57.2-
thalassemia D56.8
Constant Spring D58.2
D (Hb-D) D58.2
E (Hb-E) D58.2
E-beta thalassemia D56.5
elliptocytosis D58.1
H (Hb-H) (thalassemia) D56.0
with other abnormal hemoglobin NEC
D56.9
Constant Spring D56.0
I thalassemia D56.9
M D74.0
S or SS D57.1
SC D57.2-
SD D57.8-
SE D57.8-
spherocytosis D58.0
unstable, hemolytic D58.2
hemolytic (newborn) P55.9
autoimmune (cold type) (warm type) D59.1
drug-induced D59.0
due to or with
incompatibility
ABO (blood group) P55.1
blood (group) (Duffy) (K(ell)) (Kidd)
(Lewis) (M) (S) NEC P55.8
Rh (blood group) (factor) P55.0
Rh negative mother P55.0
specified type NEC P55.8
unstable hemoglobin D58.2
hemorrhagic D69.9
newborn P53
Henoch (-Schönlein) (purpura nervosa)
D69.0
hepatic —*see* Disease, liver
hepatobiliary K83.9
toxic K71.9
hepatolenticular E83.01
heredodegenerative NEC
spinal cord G95.89
herpesviral, disseminated B00.7
Hers' (glycogenosis VI) E74.09
Herter (-Gee) (-Heubner) (nontropical sprue)
K90.0
Heubner-Herter (nontropical sprue) K90.0
high fetal gene or hemoglobin thalassemia
D56.9
Hildenbrand's —*see* Typhus
hip (joint) M25.9
congenital Q65.89
suppurative M00.9
tuberculous A18.02
His (-Werner) (trench fever) A79.0
Hodgson's I71.2
ruptured I71.1
Holla —*see* Spherocytosis
hookworm B76.9
specified NEC B76.8
host-versus-graft D89.813
acute D89.810
acute on chronic D89.812
chronic D89.811
human immunodeficiency virus (HIV) B20
Huntington's G10
Hutchinson's (cheiropompholyx) —*see*
Hutchinson's disease
hyaline (diffuse) (generalized)
membrane (lung) (newborn) P22.0
adult J80

Disease, diseased *(Continued)*
hydatid —*see* Echinococcus
hydroxyapatite deposition M11.00
ankle M11.07-
elbow M11.02-
foot joint M11.07-
hand joint M11.04-
hip M11.05-
knee M11.06-
multiple site M11.09
shoulder M11.01-
vertebra M11.08
wrist M11.03-
hyperkinetic —*see* Hyperkinesia
hypertensive —*see* Hypertension
hypophysis E23.7
Iceland G93.3
I-cell E77.0
immune D89.9
immunoproliferative (malignant) C88.9
small intestinal C88.3
specified NEC C88.8
inclusion B25.9
salivary gland B25.9
infectious, infective B99.9
congenital P37.9
specified NEC P37.8
viral P35.9
specified type NEC P35.8
specified NEC B99.8
inflammatory
penis N48.29
abscess N48.21
cellulitis N48.22
prepuce N47.7
balanoposthitis N47.6
tubo-ovarian —*see* Salpingo-oophoritis
intervertebral disc —*see also* Disorder, disc
with myelopathy —*see* Disorder, disc, with,
myelopathy
cervical, cervicothoracic —*see* Disorder,
disc, cervical
with
myelopathy —*see* Disorder, disc,
cervical, with myelopathy
neuritis, radiculitis or
radiculopathy —*see* Disorder,
disc, cervical, with neuritis
specified NEC —*see* Disorder, disc,
cervical, specified type NEC
lumbar (with)
myelopathy M51.06
neuritis, radiculitis, radiculopathy or
sciatica M51.16
specified NEC M51.86
lumbosacral (with)
neuritis, radiculitis, radiculopathy or
sciatica M51.17
specified NEC M51.87
specified NEC —*see* Disorder, disc,
specified NEC
thoracic (with)
myelopathy M51.04
neuritis, radiculitis or radiculopathy
M51.14
specified NEC M51.84
thoracolumbar (with)
myelopathy M51.05
neuritis, radiculitis or radiculopathy
M51.15
specified NEC M51.85
intestine K63.9
functional K59.9
psychogenic F45.8
specified NEC K59.8
organic K63.9
protozoal A07.9
specified NEC K63.89
iris H21.9
specified NEC H21.89
iron metabolism or storage E83.10

Disease, diseased (*Continued*)
island (scrub typhus) A75.3
itai-itai —*see* Poisoning, cadmium
Jakob-Creutzfeldt —*see* Creutzfeldt- Jakob disease or syndrome
jaw M27.9
  fibrocystic M27.49
  specified NEC M27.8
jigger B88.1
joint —*see also* Disorder, joint
  Charcot's —*see* Arthropathy, neuropathic (Charcot)
  degenerative —*see* Osteoarthritis
    multiple M15.9
    spine —*see* Spondylosis
  hypertrophic —*see* Osteoarthritis
  sacroiliac M53.3
  specified NEC —*see* Disorder, joint, specified type NEC
  spine NEC —*see* Dorsopathy
  suppurative —*see* Arthritis, pyogenic or pyemic
Jourdain's (acute gingivitis) K05.00
  nonplaque induced K05.01
  plaque induced K05.00
Kaschin-Beck (endemic polyarthritis) M12.10
  ankle M12.17-
  elbow M12.12-
  foot joint M12.17-
  hand joint M12.14-
  hip M12.15-
  knee M12.16-
  multiple site M12.19
  shoulder M12.11-
  vertebra M12.18
  wrist M12.13-
Katayama B65.2
Kedani (scrub typhus) A75.3
Keshan E59
kidney (functional) (pelvis) N28.9
  chronic N18.9
    hypertensive —*see* Hypertension, kidney
    stage 1 N18.1
    stage 2 (mild) N18.2
    stage 3 (moderate) N18.3
    stage 4 (severe) N18.4
    stage 5 N18.5
  complicating pregnancy —*see* Pregnancy, complicated by, renal disease
  cystic (congenital) Q61.9
  diabetic - see E08-E13 with .22
  fibrocystic (congenital) Q61.8
  hypertensive —*see* Hypertension, kidney
  in (due to)
    schistosomiasis (bilharziasis) B65.9 [*N29*]
  multicystic Q61.4
  polycystic Q61.3
    adult type Q61.2
    childhood type NEC Q61.19
      collecting duct dilatation Q61.11
Kimmelstiel (-Wilson) (intercapillary polycystic (congenital) glomerulosclerosis) —*see* E08-E13 with .21
Kimura D21.9
  specified site (see Neoplasm, connective tissue benign)
Kinnier Wilson's (hepatolenticular degeneration) E83.01
kissing —*see* Mononucleosis, infectious
Klebs' (*see also* Glomerulonephritis) N05.-
Klippel-Feil (brevicollis) Q76.1
Köhler-Pellegrini-Stieda (calcification, knee joint) —*see* Bursitis, tibial collateral
Kok Q89.8
König's (osteochondritis dissecans) —*see* Osteochondritis, dissecans
Korsakoff's (nonalcoholic) F04
  alcoholic F10.96
    with dependence F10.26
Kostmann's (infantile genetic agranulocytosis) D70.0

Disease, diseased (*Continued*)
kuru A81.81
Kyasanur Forest A98.2
labyrinth, ear —*see* Disorder, ear, inner
lacrimal system —*see* Disorder, lacrimal system
Lafora's —*see* Epilepsy, generalized, idiopathic
Lancereaux-Mathieu (leptospiral jaundice) A27.0
Landry's G61.0
Larrey-Weil (leptospiral jaundice) A27.0
larynx J38.7
legionnaires' A48.1
  nonpneumonic A48.2
Lenegre's I44.2
lens H27.9
  specified NEC H27.8
Lev's (acquired complete heart block) I44.2
Lewy body (dementia) G31.83 [*F02.80*]
  with behavioral disturbance G31.83 [*F02.81*]
Lichtheim's (subacute combined sclerosis with pernicious anemia) D51.0
Lightwood's (renal tubular acidosis) N25.89
Lignac's (cystinosis) E72.04
lip K13.0
lipid-storage E75.6
  specified NEC E75.5
Lipschütz's N76.6
liver (chronic) (organic) K76.9
  alcoholic (chronic) K70.9
    acute —*see* Disease, liver, alcoholic, hepatitis
    cirrhosis K70.30
      with ascites K70.31
    failure K70.40
      with coma K70.41
    fatty liver K70.0
    fibrosis K70.2
    hepatitis K70.10
      with ascites K70.11
    sclerosis K70.2
  cystic, congenital Q44.6
  drug-induced (idiosyncratic) (toxic) (predictable) (unpredictable) —*see* Disease, liver, toxic
  end stage K72.90
    due to hepatitis —*see* Hepatitis
  fatty, nonalcoholic (NAFLD) K76.0
    alcoholic K70.0
  fibrocystic (congenital) Q44.6
  fluke
    Chinese B66.1
    oriental B66.1
    sheep B66.3
  glycogen storage E74.09 [*K77*]
  in (due to)
    schistosomiasis (bilharziasis) B65.9 [*K77*]
  inflammatory K75.9
    alcoholic K70.1
    specified NEC K75.89
  polycystic (congenital) Q44.6
  toxic K71.9
    with
      cholestasis K71.0
      cirrhosis (liver) K71.7
      fibrosis (liver) K71.7
      focal nodular hyperplasia K71.8
      hepatic granuloma K71.8
      hepatic necrosis K71.10
        with coma K71.11
      hepatitis NEC K71.6
        acute K71.2
        chronic
          active K71.50
            with ascites K71.51
          lobular K71.4
          persistent K71.3
        lupoid K71.50
          with ascites K71.51

Disease, diseased (*Continued*)
liver (*Continued*)
  toxic (*Continued*)
    with (*Continued*)
      peliosis hepatis K71.8
      veno-occlusive disease (VOD) of liver K71.8
  veno-occlusive K76.5
Lobo's (keloid blastomycosis) B48.0
Lobstein's (brittle bones and blue sclera) Q78.0
Ludwig's (submaxillary cellulitis) K12.2
lumbosacral region M53.87
lung J98.4
  black J60
  congenital Q33.9
  cystic J98.4
    congenital Q33.0
  fibroid (chronic) —*see* Fibrosis, lung
  fluke B66.4
    oriental B66.4
  in
    amyloidosis E85.4 [*J99*]
    sarcoidosis D86.0
    Sjögren's syndrome M35.02
    systemic
      lupus erythematosus M32.13
      sclerosis M34.81
  interstitial J84.9
    of childhood, specified NEC J84.848
    respiratory bronchiolitis J84.115
    specified NEC J84.89
  obstructive (chronic) J44.9
    with
      acute
        bronchitis J44.0
        exacerbation NEC J44.1
        lower respiratory infection J44.0
      alveolitis, allergic J67.9
      asthma J44.9
      bronchiectasis J47.9
        with
          exacerbation (acute) J47.1
          lower respiratory infection J47.0
      bronchitis J44.9
        with
          exacerbation (acute) J44.1
          lower respiratory infection J44.0
      emphysema J44.9
      hypersensitivity pneumonitis J67.9
    decompensated J44.1
      with
        exacerbation (acute) J44.1
  polycystic J98.4
    congenital Q33.0
  rheumatoid (diffuse) (interstitial) —*see* Rheumatoid, lung
Lutembacher's (atrial septal defect with mitral stenosis) Q21.1
Lyme A69.20
lymphatic (gland) (system) (channel) (vessel) I89.9
lymphoproliferative D47.9
  specified NEC D47.Z9
  T-gamma D47.Z9
  X-linked D82.3
Magitot's M27.2
malarial —*see* Malaria
malignant —*see also* Neoplasm, malignant, by site
Manson's B65.1
maple bark J67.6
maple-syrup-urine E71.0
Marburg (virus) A98.3
Marion's (bladder neck obstruction) N32.0
Marsh's (exophthalmic goiter) —*see* Hyperthyroidism, with, goiter (diffuse)
mastoid (process) —*see* Disorder, ear, middle
Mathieu's (leptospiral jaundice) A27.0
Maxcy's A75.2

◀ New   ⬅ Revised   ~~deleted~~ Deleted

Disease, diseased *(Continued)*
  McArdle (-Schmid-Pearson) (glycogenosis V) E74.04
  mediastinum J98.5
  medullary center (idiopathic) (respiratory) G93.89
  Meige's (chronic hereditary edema) Q82.0
  meningococcal —*see* Infection, meningococcal
  mental F99
    organic F09
  mesenchymal M35.9
  mesenteric embolic K55.0
  metabolic, metabolism E88.9
    bilirubin E80.7
  metal-polisher's J62.8
  metastatic (*see also* Neoplasm, secondary, by site) C79.9
  microvascular — code to condition
  microvillus
    atrophy Q43.8
    inclusion (MVD) Q43.8
  middle ear —*see* Disorder, ear, middle
  Mikulicz' (dryness of mouth, absent or decreased lacrimation) K11.8
  Milroy's (chronic hereditary edema) Q82.0
  Minamata —*see* Poisoning, mercury
  minicore G71.2
  Minor's G95.19
  Minot's (hemorrhagic disease, newborn) P53
  Minot-von Willebrand-Jürgens (angiohemophilia) D68.0
  Mitchell's (erythromelalgia) I73.81
  mitral (valve) I05.9
    nonrheumatic I34.9
  mixed connective tissue M35.1
  moldy hay J67.0
  Monge's T70.29
  Morgagni-Adams-Stokes (syncope with heart block) I45.9
  Morgagni's (syndrome) (hyperostosis frontalis interna) M85.2
  Morton's (with metatarsalgia) —*see* Lesion, nerve, plantar
  Morvan's G60.8
  motor neuron (bulbar) (familial) (mixed type) (spinal) G12.20
    amyotrophic lateral sclerosis G12.21
    progressive bulbar palsy G12.22
    specified NEC G12.29
  moyamoya I67.5
  mu heavy chain disease C88.2
  multicore G71.2
  muscle —*see also* Disorder, muscle
    inflammatory —*see* Myositis
    ocular (external) —*see* Strabismus
  musculoskeletal system, soft tissue —*see also* Disorder, soft tissue
    specified NEC —*see* Disorder, soft tissue, specified type NEC
  mushroom workers' J67.5
  mycotic B49
  myelodysplastic, not classified C94.6
  myeloproliferative, not classified C94.6
    chronic D47.1
  myocardium, myocardial (*see also* Degeneration, myocardial) I51.5
    primary (idiopathic) I42.9
  myoneural G70.9
  Naegeli's D69.1
  nails L60.9
    specified NEC L60.8
  Nairobi (sheep virus) A93.8
  nasal J34.9
  nemaline body G71.2
  nerve —*see* Disorder, nerve
  nervous system G98.8
    autonomic G90.9
    central G96.9
      specified NEC G96.8
    congenital Q07.9
    parasympathetic G90.9

Disease, diseased *(Continued)*
  nervous system *(Continued)*
    specified NEC G98.8
    sympathetic G90.9
    vegetative G90.9
  neuromuscular system G70.9
  Newcastle B30.8
  Nicolas (-Durand)-Favre (climatic bubo) A55
  nipple N64.9
    Paget's C50.01-
      female C50.01-
      male C50.02-
  Nishimoto (-Takeuchi) I67.5
  nonarthropod-borne NOS (viral) B34.9
    enterovirus NEC B34.1
  nonautoimmune hemolytic D59.4
    drug-induced D59.2
  Nonne-Milroy-Meige (chronic hereditary edema) Q82.0
  nose J34.9
  nucleus pulposus —*see* Disorder, disc
  nutritional E63.9
  oast-house-urine E72.19
  ocular
    herpesviral B00.50
    zoster B02.30
  obliterative vascular I77.1
  Ohara's —*see* Tularemia
  Opitz's (congestive splenomegaly) D73.2
  Oppenheim-Urbach (necrobiosis lipoidica diabeticorum) —*see* E08-E13 with .620
  optic nerve NEC —*see* Disorder, nerve, optic
    orbit —*see* Disorder, orbit
  Oriental liver fluke B66.1
  Oriental lung fluke B66.4
  Ormond's N13.5
  Oropouche virus A93.0
  Osler-Rendu (familial hemorrhagic telangiectasia) I78.0
  osteofibrocystic E21.0
  Otto's M24.7
  outer ear —*see* Disorder, ear, external
  ovary (noninflammatory) N83.9
    cystic N83.20
    inflammatory —*see* Salpingo-oophoritis
    polycystic E28.2
    specified NEC N83.8
  Owren's (congenital) —*see* Defect, coagulation
  pancreas K86.9
    cystic K86.2
    fibrocystic E84.9
    specified NEC K86.8
  panvalvular I08.9
    specified NEC I08.8
  parametrium (noninflammatory) N83.9
  parasitic B89
    cerebral NEC B71.9 *[G94]*
    intestinal NOS B82.9
    mouth B37.0
    skin NOS B88.9
    specified type —*see* Infestation
    tongue B37.0
  parathyroid (gland) E21.5
    specified NEC E21.4
  Parkinson's G20
  parodontal K05.6
  Parrot's (syphilitic osteochondritis) A50.02
  Parry's (exophthalmic goiter) —*see* Hyperthyroidism, with, goiter (diffuse)
  Parson's (exophthalmic goiter) —*see* Hyperthyroidism, with, goiter (diffuse)
  Paxton's (white piedra) B36.2
  pearl-worker's —*see* Osteomyelitis, specified type NEC
  Pellegrini-Stieda (calcification, knee joint) — *see* Bursitis, tibial collateral
  pelvis, pelvic
    female NOS N94.9
      specified NEC N94.89
    gonococcal (acute) (chronic) A54.24

Disease, diseased *(Continued)*
  pelvis, pelvic *(Continued)*
    inflammatory (female) N73.9
      acute N73.0
      chronic N73.1
      specified NEC N73.8
      syphilitic (secondary) A51.42
        late A52.76
      tuberculous A18.17
    organ, female N94.9
    peritoneum, female NEC N94.89
  penis N48.9
    inflammatory N48.29
      abscess N48.21
      cellulitis N48.22
    specified NEC N48.89
  periapical tissues NOS K04.90
  periodontal K05.6
    specified NEC K05.5
  periosteum —*see* Disorder, bone, specified type NEC
  peripheral
    arterial I73.9
    autonomic nervous system G90.9
    nerves —*see* Polyneuropathy
    vascular NOS I73.9
  peritoneum K66.9
    pelvic, female NEC N94.89
    specified NEC K66.8
  persistent mucosal (middle ear) H66.20
    left H66.22
      with right H66.23
    right H66.21
      with left H66.23
  Petit's —*see* Hernia, abdomen, specified site NEC
  pharynx J39.2
    specified NEC J39.2
  Phocas' —*see* Mastopathy, cystic
  photochromogenic (acid-fast bacilli) (pulmonary) A31.0
    nonpulmonary A31.9
  Pick's G31.01 *[F02.80]*
    with behavioral disturbance G31.01 *[F02.81]*
  pigeon fancier's J67.2
  pineal gland E34.8
  pink —*see* Poisoning, mercury
  Pinkus' (lichen nitidus) L44.1
  pinworm B80
  Piry virus A93.8
  pituitary (gland) E23.7
  pituitary-snuff-taker's J67.8
  pleura (cavity) J94.9
    specified NEC J94.8
  pneumatic drill (hammer) T75.21
  Pollitzer's (hidradenitis suppurativa) L73.2
  polycystic
    kidney or renal Q61.3
      adult type Q61.2
      childhood type NEC Q61.19
        collecting duct dilatation Q61.11
    liver or hepatic Q44.6
    lung or pulmonary J98.4
      congenital Q33.0
    ovary, ovaries E28.2
    spleen Q89.09
  polyethylene T84.05-
  Pompe's (glycogenosis II) E74.02
  Posadas-Wernicke B38.9
  Potain's (pulmonary edema) —*see* Edema, lung
  prepuce N47.8
    inflammatory N47.7
      balanoposthitis N47.6
  Pringle's (tuberous sclerosis) Q85.1
  prion, central nervous system A81.9
    specified NEC A81.89
  prostate N42.9
    specified NEC N42.89

Disease, diseased *(Continued)*
  protozoal B64
    acanthamebiasis —*see* Acanthamebiasis
    African trypanosomiasis —*see* African
      trypanosomiasis
    babesiosis B60.0
    Chagas disease —*see* Chagas disease
    intestine, intestinal A07.9
    leishmaniasis —*see* Leishmaniasis
    malaria —*see* Malaria
    naegleriasis B60.2
    pneumocystosis B59
    specified organism NEC B60.8
    toxoplasmosis —*see* Toxoplasmosis
  pseudo-Hurler's E77.0
  psychiatric F99
  psychotic —*see* Psychosis
  Puente's (simple glandular cheilitis)
    K13.0
  puerperal *(see also* Puerperal) O90.89
  pulmonary —*see also* Disease, lung
    artery I28.9
    chronic obstructive J44.9
      with
        acute bronchitis J44.0
        exacerbation (acute) J44.1
        lower respiratory infection (acute)
          J44.0
      decompensated J44.1
        with
          exacerbation (acute) J44.1
    heart I27.9
      specified NEC I27.89
    hypertensive (vascular) I27.0
    valve I37.9
      rheumatic I09.89
  pulp (dental) NOS K04.90
  pulseless M31.4
  Putnam's (subacute combined sclerosis with
    pernicious anemia) D51.0
  Pyle (-Cohn) (craniometaphyseal dysplasia)
    Q78.5
  ragpicker's or ragsorter's A22.1
  Raynaud's —*see* Raynaud's disease
  reactive airway —*see* Asthma
  Reclus' (cystic) —*see* Mastopathy,
    cystic
  rectum K62.9
    specified NEC K62.89
  Refsum's (heredopathia atactica
    polyneuritiformis) G60.1
  renal (functional) (pelvis) *(see also* Disease,
    kidney) N28.9
    with
      edema —*see* Nephrosis
      glomerular lesion —*see*
        Glomerulonephritis
        with edema —*see* Nephrosis
      interstitial nephritis N12
    acute N28.9
    chronic *(see also* Disease, kidney, chronic)
      N18.9
    cystic, congenital Q61.9
    diabetic —*see* E08-E13 with .22
    end-stage (failure) N18.6
      due to hypertension I12.0
    fibrocystic (congenital) Q61.8
    hypertensive —*see* Hypertension,
      kidney
    lupus M32.14
    phosphate-losing (tubular) N25.0
    polycystic (congenital) Q61.3
      adult type Q61.2
      childhood type NEC Q61.19
        collecting duct dilatation Q61.11
    rapidly progressive N01.9
    subacute N01.9
  Rendu-Osler-Weber (familial hemorrhagic
    telangiectasia) I78.0
  renovascular (arteriosclerotic) —*see*
    Hypertension, kidney

Disease, diseased *(Continued)*
  respiratory (tract) J98.9
    acute or subacute NOS J06.9
      due to
        chemicals, gases, fumes or vapors
          (inhalation) J68.3
        external agent J70.9
          specified NEC J70.8
        radiation J70.0
        smoke inhalation J70.5
      noninfectious J39.8
    chronic NOS J98.9
      due to
        chemicals, gases, fumes or vapors
          J68.4
        external agent J70.9
          specified NEC J70.8
        radiation J70.1
      newborn P27.9
        specified NEC P27.8
    due to
      chemicals, gases, fumes or vapors J68.9
        acute or subacute NEC J68.3
        chronic J68.4
      external agent J70.9
        specified NEC J70.8
    newborn P28.9
      specified type NEC P28.89
    upper J39.9
      acute or subacute J06.9
      noninfectious NEC J39.8
      specified NEC J39.8
      streptococcal J06.9
  retina, retinal H35.9
    Batten's or Batten-Mayou E75.4 *[H36]*
    specified NEC H35.89
  rheumatoid —*see* Arthritis, rheumatoid
  rickettsial NOS A79.9
    specified type NEC A79.89
  Riga (-Fede) (cachectic aphthae) K14.0
  Riggs' (compound periodontitis) —*see*
    Periodontitis
  Ritter's L00
  Rivalta's (cervicofacial actinomycosis)
    A42.2
  Robles' (onchocerciasis) B73.01
  Roger's (congenital interventricular septal
    defect) Q21.0
  Rosenthal's (factor XI deficiency) D68.1
  Ross River B33.1
  Rossbach's (hyperchlorhydria) K30
  Rotes Quérol —*see* Hyperostosis, ankylosing
  Roth (-Bernhardt) —*see* Mononeuropathy,
    lower limb, meralgia paresthetica
  Runeberg's (progressive pernicious anemia)
    D51.0
  sacroiliac NEC M53.3
  salivary gland or duct K11.9
    inclusion B25.9
    specified NEC K11.8
    virus B25.9
  sandworm B76.9
  Schimmelbusch's —*see* Mastopathy, cystic
  Schmorl's —*see* Schmorl's disease or nodes
  Schönlein (-Henoch) (purpura rheumatica)
    D69.0
  Schottmüller's —*see* Fever, paratyphoid
  Schultz's (agranulocytosis) —*see*
    Agranulocytosis
  Schwalbe-Ziehen-Oppenheim G24.1
  Schwartz-Jampel G71.13
  sclera H15.9
    specified NEC H15.89
  scrofulous (tuberculous) A18.2
  scrotum N50.9
  sebaceous glands L73.9
  semilunar cartilage, cystic —*see also*
    Derangement, knee, meniscus, cystic
  seminal vesicle N50.9
  serum NEC *(see also* Reaction, serum)
    T80.69

Disease, diseased *(Continued)*
  sexually transmitted A64
    anogenital
      herpesviral infection —*see* Herpes,
        anogenital
      warts A63.0
    chancroid A57
    chlamydial infection —*see* Chlamydia
    gonorrhea —*see* Gonorrhea
    granuloma inguinale A58
    specified organism NEC A63.8
    syphilis —*see* Syphilis
    trichomoniasis —*see* Trichomoniasis
  Sézary C84.1-
  shimamushi (scrub typhus) A75.3
  shipyard B30.0
  sickle-cell D57.1
    with crisis (vasoocclusive pain) D57.00
      with
        acute chest syndrome D57.01
        splenic sequestration D57.02
    elliptocytosis D57.8-
    Hb-C D57.20
      with crisis (vasoocclusive pain) D57.219
        with
          acute chest syndrome D57.211
          splenic sequestration D57.212
      without crisis D57.20
    Hb-SD D57.80
      with crisis D57.819
        with
          acute chest syndrome D57.811
          splenic sequestration D57.812
    Hb-SE D57.80
      with crisis D57.819
        with
          acute chest syndrome D57.811
          splenic sequestration D57.812
    specified NEC D57.80
      with crisis D57.819
        with
          acute chest syndrome D57.811
          splenic sequestration D57.812
    spherocytosis D57.80
      with crisis D57.819
        with
          acute chest syndrome D57.811
          splenic sequestration D57.812
    thalassemia D57.40
      with crisis (vasoocclusive pain) D57.419
        with
          acute chest syndrome D57.411
          splenic sequestration D57.412
      without crisis D57.40
  silo-filler's J68.8
    bronchitis J68.0
    pneumonitis J68.0
    pulmonary edema J68.1
  simian B B00.4
  Simons' (progressive lipodystrophy) E88.1
  sin nombre virus B33.4
  sinus —*see* Sinusitis
  Sirkari's B55.0
  sixth B08.20
    due to human herpesvirus 6 B08.21
    due to human herpesvirus 7 B08.22
  skin L98.9
    due to metabolic disorder NEC E88.9
      [L99]
    specified NEC L98.8
  slim (HIV) B20
  small vessel I73.9
  Sneddon-Wilkinson (subcorneal pustular
    dermatosis) L13.1
  South African creeping B88.0
  spinal (cord) G95.9
    congenital Q06.9
    specified NEC G95.89
  spine —*see also* Spondylopathy
    joint —*see* Dorsopathy
    tuberculous A18.01

◀ New ◀▥▥ Revised ~~deleted~~ Deleted

Disease, diseased (Continued)
spinocerebellar (hereditary) G11.9
    specified NEC G11.8
spleen D73.9
    amyloid E85.4 [D77]
    organic D73.9
    polycystic Q89.09
    postinfectional D73.89
sponge-diver's —see Toxicity, venom, marine animal, sea anemone
Startle Q89.8
Steinert's G71.11
Sticker's (erythema infectiosum) B08.3
Stieda's (calcification, knee joint) —see Bursitis, tibial collateral
Stokes' (exophthalmic goiter) —see Hyperthyroidism, with, goiter (diffuse)
Stokes-Adams (syncope with heart block) I45.9
stomach K31.9
    functional, psychogenic F45.8
    specified NEC K31.89
stonemason's J62.8
storage
    glycogen —see Disease, glycogen storage
    mucopolysaccharide —see Mucopolysaccharidosis
striatopallidal system NEC G25.89
Stuart-Prower (congenital factor X deficiency) D68.2
Stuart's (congenital factor X deficiency) D68.2
subcutaneous tissue —see Disease, skin
supporting structures of teeth K08.9
    specified NEC K08.8
suprarenal (capsule) (gland) E27.9
    hyperfunction E27.0
    specified NEC E27.8
sweat glands L74.9
    specified NEC L74.8
Sweeley-Klionsky E75.21
Swift (-Feer) —see Poisoning, mercury
swimming-pool granuloma A31.1
Sylvest's (epidemic pleurodynia) B33.0
sympathetic nervous system G90.9
synovium —see Disorder, synovium
syphilitic —see Syphilis
systemic tissue mast cell C96.2
tanapox (virus) B08.71
Tangier E78.6
Tarral-Besnier (pityriasis rubra pilaris) L44.0
Tauri's E74.09
tear duct —see Disorder, lacrimal system
tendon, tendinous —see also Disorder, tendon
    nodular —see Trigger finger
terminal vessel I73.9
testis N50.9
thalassemia Hb-S —see Disease, sickle-cell, thalassemia
Thaysen-Gee (nontropical sprue) K90.0
Thomsen G71.12
throat J39.2
    septic J02.0
thromboembolic —see Embolism
thymus (gland) E32.9
    specified NEC E32.8
thyroid (gland) E07.9
    heart (see also Hyperthyroidism) E05.90 [I43]
        with thyroid storm E05.91 [I43]
    specified NEC E07.89
Tietze's M94.0
tongue K14.9
    specified NEC K14.8
tonsils, tonsillar (and adenoids) J35.9
tooth, teeth K08.9
    hard tissues K03.9
        specified NEC K03.89
    pulp NEC K04.99
    specified NEC K08.8
Tourette's F95.2
trachea NEC J39.8

Disease, diseased (Continued)
tricuspid I07.9
    nonrheumatic I36.9
triglyceride-storage E75.5
trophoblastic —see Mole, hydatidiform
tsutsugamushi A75.3
tube (fallopian) (noninflammatory) N83.9
    inflammatory —see Salpingitis
    specified NEC N83.8
tuberculous NEC —see Tuberculosis
tubo-ovarian (noninflammatory) N83.9
    inflammatory —see Salpingo-oophoritis
    specified NEC N83.8
tubotympanic, chronic —see Otitis, media, suppurative, chronic, tubotympanic
tubulo-interstitial N15.9
    specified NEC N15.8
tympanum —see Disorder, tympanic membrane
Uhl's Q24.8
Underwood's (sclerema neonatorum) P83.0
Unverricht (-Lundborg) —see Epilepsy, generalized, idiopathic
Urbach-Oppenheim (necrobiosis lipoidica diabeticorum) —see E08-E13 with .620
ureter N28.9
    in (due to)
        schistosomiasis (bilharziasis) B65.0 [N29]
urethra N36.9
    specified NEC N36.8
urinary (tract) N39.9
    bladder N32.9
        specified NEC N32.89
    specified NEC N39.8
uterus (noninflammatory) N85.9
    infective —see Endometritis
    inflammatory —see Endometritis
    specified NEC N85.8
uveal tract (anterior) H21.9
    posterior H31.9
vagabond's B85.1
vagina, vaginal (noninflammatory) N89.9
    inflammatory NEC N76.89
    specified NEC N89.8
valve, valvular I38
    multiple I08.9
        specified NEC I08.8
van Creveld-von Gierke (glycogenosis I) E74.01
vas deferens N50.9
vascular I99.9
    arteriosclerotic —see Arteriosclerosis
    ciliary body NEC —see Disorder, iris, vascular
    hypertensive —see Hypertension
    iris NEC —see Disorder, iris, vascular
    obliterative I77.1
        peripheral I73.9
    occlusive I99.8
    peripheral (occlusive) I73.9
        in diabetes mellitus —see E08-E13 with .51
vasomotor I73.9
vasospastic I73.9
vein I87.9
venereal (see also Disease, sexually transmitted) A64
    chlamydial NEC A56.8
        anus A56.3
        genitourinary NOS A56.2
        pharynx A56.4
        rectum A56.3
    fifth A55
    sixth A55
    specified nature or type NEC A63.8
vertebra, vertebral —see also Spondylopathy
    disc —see Disorder, disc
vibration —see Vibration, adverse effects

Disease, diseased (Continued)
viral, virus (see also Disease, by type of virus) B34.9
    arbovirus NOS A94
    arthropod-borne NOS A94
    congenital P35.9
        specified NEC P35.8
    Hanta (with renal manifestations) (Dobrava) (Puumala) (Seoul) A98.5
        with pulmonary manifestations (Andes) (Bayou) (Bermejo) (Black Creek Canal) (Choclo) (Juquitiba) (Laguna negra) (Lechiguanas) (New York) (Oran) (Sin nombre) B33.4
    Hantaan (Korean hemorrhagic fever) A98.5
    human immunodeficiency (HIV) B20
    Kunjin A83.4
    nonarthropod-borne NOS B34.9
    Powassan A84.8
    Rocio (encephalitis) A83.6
    Sin nombre (Hantavirus) (cardio)-pulmonary syndrome B33.4
    Tahyna B33.8
    vesicular stomatitis A93.8
vitreous H43.9
    specified NEC H43.89
vocal cord J38.3
Volkmann's, acquired T79.6
von Eulenburg's (congenital paramyotonia) G71.19
von Gierke's (glycogenosis I) E74.01
von Graefe's —see Strabismus, paralytic, ophthalmoplegia, progressive
von Willebrand (-Jürgens) (angiohemophilia) D68.0
Vrolik's (osteogenesis imperfecta) Q78.0
vulva (noninflammatory) N90.9
    inflammatory NEC N76.89
    specified NEC N90.89
Wallgren's (obstruction of splenic vein with collateral circulation) I87.8
Wassilieff's (leptospiral jaundice) A27.0
wasting NEC R64
    due to malnutrition E41
Waterhouse-Friderichsen A39.1
Wegner's (syphilitic osteochondritis) A50.02
Weil's (leptospiral jaundice of lung) A27.0
Weir Mitchell's (erythromelalgia) I73.81
Werdnig-Hoffmann G12.0
Wermer's E31.21
Werner-His (trench fever) A79.0
Werner-Schultz (neutropenic splenomegaly) D73.81
Wernicke-Posadas B38.9
whipworm B79
white blood cells D72.9
    specified NEC D72.89
white matter R90.82
white-spot, meaning lichen sclerosus et atrophicus L90.0
    penis N48.0
    vulva N90.4
Wilkie's K55.1
Wilkinson-Sneddon (subcorneal pustular dermatosis) L13.1
Willis' —see Diabetes
Wilson's (hepatolenticular degeneration) E83.01
woolsorter's A22.1
yaba monkey tumor B08.72
yaba pox (virus) B08.72
zoonotic, bacterial A28.9
    specified type NEC A28.8
Disfigurement (due to scar) L90.5
Disgerminoma —see Dysgerminoma
DISH (diffuse idiopathic skeletal hyperostosis) —see Hyperostosis, ankylosing
Disinsertion, retina —see Detachment, retina
Dislocatable hip, congenital Q65.6

Dislocation (articular)
  with fracture —*see* Fracture
  acromioclavicular (joint) S43.10-
    with displacement
      100%-200% S43.12-
      more than 200% S43.13-
    inferior S43.14-
    posterior S43.15-
  ankle S93.0-
  astragalus —*see* Dislocation, ankle
  atlantoaxial S13.121
  atlantooccipital S13.111
  atloidooccipital S13.111
  breast bone S23.29
  capsule, joint code by site under Dislocation
  carpal (bone) —*see* Dislocation, wrist
  carpometacarpal (joint) NEC S63.05-
    thumb S63.04-
  cartilage (joint) - code by site under
    Dislocation
  cervical spine (vertebra) —*see* Dislocation,
    vertebra, cervical
  chronic —*see* Dislocation, recurrent
  clavicle —*see* Dislocation, acromioclavicular
    joint
  coccyx S33.2
  congenital NEC Q68.8
  coracoid —*see* Dislocation, shoulder
  costal cartilage S23.29
  costochondral S23.29
  cricoarytenoid articulation S13.29
  cricothyroid articulation S13.29
  dorsal vertebra —*see* Dislocation, vertebra,
    thoracic
  ear ossicle —*see* Discontinuity, ossicles, ear
  elbow S53.10-
    congenital Q68.8
    pathological —*see* Dislocation, pathological
      NEC, elbow
    radial head alone —*see* Dislocation, radial
      head
    recurrent —*see* Dislocation, recurrent,
      elbow
    traumatic S53.10-
      anterior S53.11-
      lateral S53.14-
      medial S53.13-
      posterior S53.12-
      specified type NEC S53.19-
  eye, nontraumatic —*see* Luxation, globe
  eyeball, nontraumatic —*see* Luxation, globe
  femur
    distal end —*see* Dislocation, knee
    proximal end —*see* Dislocation, hip
  fibula
    distal end —*see* Dislocation, ankle
    proximal end —*see* Dislocation, knee
  finger S63.25-
    index S63.25-
    interphalangeal S63.27-
      distal S63.29-
        index S63.29-
        little S63.29-
        middle S63.29-
        ring S63.29-
      index S63.27-
      little S63.27-
      middle S63.27-
      proximal S63.28-
        index S63.28-
        little S63.28-
        middle S63.28-
        ring S63.28-
      ring S63.27-
    little S63.25-
    metacarpophalangeal S63.26-
      index S63.26-
      little S63.26-
      middle S63.26-
      ring S63.26-
    middle S63.25-

Dislocation (*Continued*)
  finger (*Continued*)
    recurrent —*see* Dislocation, recurrent,
      finger
    ring S63.25-
    thumb —*see* Dislocation, thumb
  foot S93.30-
    recurrent —*see* Dislocation, recurrent,
      foot
    specified site NEC S93.33-
    tarsal joint S93.31-
    tarsometatarsal joint S93.32-
    toe —*see* Dislocation, toe
  fracture —*see* Fracture
  glenohumeral (joint) —*see* Dislocation,
    shoulder
  glenoid —*see* Dislocation, shoulder
  habitual —*see* Dislocation, recurrent
  hip S73.00-
    anterior S73.03-
      obturator S73.02-
    central S73.04-
    congenital (total) Q65.2
      bilateral Q65.1
      partial Q65.5
        bilateral Q65.4
        unilateral Q65.3-
      unilateral Q65.0-
    developmental M24.85-
    pathological —*see* Dislocation, pathological
      NEC, hip
    posterior S73.01-
    recurrent —*see* Dislocation, recurrent, hip
  humerus, proximal end —*see* Dislocation,
    shoulder
  incomplete —*see* Subluxation, by site
  incus —*see* Discontinuity, ossicles, ear
  infracoracoid —*see* Dislocation, shoulder
  innominate (pubic junction) (sacral junction)
    S33.39
    acetabulum —*see* Dislocation, hip
  interphalangeal (joint (s))
    finger S63.279
      distal S63.29-
        index S63.29-
        little S63.29-
        middle S63.29-
        ring S63.29-
      index S63.27-
      little S63.27-
      middle S63.27-
      proximal S63.28-
        index S63.28-
        little S63.28-
        middle S63.28-
        ring S63.28-
      ring S63.27-
    foot or toe —*see* Dislocation, toe
    thumb S63.12-
      distal joint S63.14-
      proximal joint S63.13-
  jaw (cartilage) (meniscus) S03.0
  joint prosthesis —*see* Complications, joint
    prosthesis, mechanical, displacement,
    by site
  knee S83.106
    cap —*see* Dislocation, patella
    congenital Q68.2
    old M23.8X-
    patella —*see* Dislocation, patella
    pathological —*see* Dislocation, pathological
      NEC, knee
    proximal tibia
      anteriorly S83.11-
      laterally S83.14-
      medially S83.13-
      posteriorly S83.12-
    recurrent —*see also* Derangement, knee,
      specified NEC
    specified type NEC S83.19-
  lacrimal gland H04.16-

Dislocation (*Continued*)
  lens (complete) H27.10-
    anterior H27.12-
    congenital Q12.1
    ocular implant —*see* Complications,
      intraocular lens
    partial H27.11-
    posterior H27.13-
    traumatic S05.8X-
  ligament code by site under Dislocation
  lumbar (vertebra) —*see* Dislocation, vertebra,
    lumbar
  lumbosacral (vertebra) —*see also* Dislocation,
    vertebra, lumbar
    congenital Q76.49
  mandible S03.0
  meniscus (knee) —*see* Tear, meniscus
    other sites code by site under Dislocation
  metacarpal (bone)
    distal end —*see* Dislocation, finger
    proximal end S63.06-
  metacarpophalangeal (joint)
    finger S63.26-
      index S63.26-
      little S63.26-
      middle S63.26-
      ring S63.26-
    thumb S63.11-
  metatarsal (bone) —*see* Dislocation, foot
  metatarsophalangeal (joint (s)) —*see*
    Dislocation, toe
  midcarpal (joint) S63.03-
  midtarsal (joint) —*see* Dislocation, foot
  neck S13.20
    specified site NEC S13.29
    vertebra —*see* Dislocation, vertebra,
      cervical
  nose (septal cartilage) S03.1
  occipitoatloid S13.111
  old —*see* Derangement, joint, specified type
    NEC
  ossicles, ear —*see* Discontinuity, ossicles,
    ear
  partial —*see* Subluxation, by site
  patella S83.006
    congenital Q74.1
    lateral S83.01-
    recurrent (nontraumatic) M22.0-
      incomplete M22.1-
    specified type NEC S83.09-
  pathological NEC M24.30
    ankle M24.37-
    elbow M24.32-
    foot joint M24.37-
    hand joint M24.34-
    hip M24.35-
    knee M24.36-
    lumbosacral joint —*see* subcategory
      M53.2
    pelvic region —*see* Dislocation,
      pathological, hip
    sacroiliac —*see* subcategory M53.2
    shoulder M24.31-
    wrist M24.33-
  pelvis NEC S33.30
    specified NEC S33.39
  phalanx
    finger or hand —*see* Dislocation, finger
    foot or toe —*see* Dislocation, toe
  prosthesis, internal —*see* Complications,
    prosthetic device, by site, mechanical
  radial head S53.006
    anterior S53.01-
    posterior S53.02-
    specified type NEC S53.09-
  radiocarpal (joint) S63.02-
  radiohumeral (joint) —*see* Dislocation, radial
    head
  radioulnar (joint)
    distal S63.01-
    proximal —*see* Dislocation, elbow

◀ New   ⬅ Revised   ~~deleted~~ Deleted

Dislocation *(Continued)*
radius
  distal end —*see* Dislocation, wrist
  proximal end —*see* Dislocation, radial
    head
recurrent M24.40
  ankle M24.47-
  elbow M24.42-
  finger M24.44-
  foot joint M24.47-
  hand joint M24.44-
  hip M24.45-
  knee M24.46-
    patella —*see* Dislocation, patella,
      recurrent
  patella —*see* Dislocation, patella, recurrent
  sacroiliac —*see* subcategory M53.2
  shoulder M24.41-
  toe M24.47-
  vertebra *(see also* subcategory) M43.5
    atlantoaxial M43.4
      with myelopathy M43.3
  wrist M24.43-
rib (cartilage) S23.29
sacrococcygeal S33.2
sacroiliac (joint) (ligament) S33.2
  congenital Q74.2
  recurrent —*see* subcategory M53.2
sacrum S33.2
scaphoid (bone) (hand) (wrist) —*see*
    Dislocation, wrist
  foot —*see* Dislocation, foot
scapula —*see* Dislocation, shoulder, girdle,
    scapula
semilunar cartilage, knee —*see* Tear, meniscus
septal cartilage (nose) S03.1
septum (nasal) (old) J34.2
sesamoid bone code by site under Dislocation
shoulder (blade) (ligament) (joint) (traumatic)
    S43.006
  acromioclavicular —*see* Dislocation,
    acromioclavicular
  chronic —*see* Dislocation, recurrent,
    shoulder
  congenital Q68.8
  girdle S43.30-
    scapula S43.31-
    specified site NEC S43.39-
  humerus S43.00-
    anterior S43.01-
    inferior S43.03-
    posterior S43.02-
  pathological —*see* Dislocation, pathological
    NEC, shoulder
  recurrent —*see* Dislocation, recurrent,
    shoulder
  specified type NEC S43.08-
spine
  cervical —*see* Dislocation, vertebra, cervical
  congenital Q76.49
  due to birth trauma P11.5
  lumbar —*see* Dislocation, vertebra, lumbar
  thoracic —*see* Dislocation, vertebra,
    thoracic
spontaneous —*see* Dislocation, pathological
sternoclavicular (joint) S43.206
  anterior S43.21-
  posterior S43.22-
sternum S23.29
subglenoid —*see* Dislocation, shoulder
symphysis pubis S33.4
talus —*see* Dislocation, ankle
tarsal (bone (s)) (joint (s)) —*see* Dislocation,
    foot
tarsometatarsal (joint (s)) —*see* Dislocation,
    foot
temporomandibular (joint) S03.0
thigh, proximal end —*see* Dislocation, hip
thorax S23.20
  specified site NEC S23.29
  vertebra —*see* Dislocation, vertebra

Dislocation *(Continued)*
thumb S63.10-
  interphalangeal joint —*see* Dislocation,
    interphalangeal (joint), thumb
  metacarpophalangeal joint —*see*
    Dislocation, metacarpophalangeal
    (joint), thumb
thyroid cartilage S13.29
tibia
  distal end —*see* Dislocation, ankle
  proximal end —*see* Dislocation, knee
tibiofibular (joint)
  distal —*see* Dislocation, ankle
  superior —*see* Dislocation, knee
toe (s) S93.106
  great S93.10-
    interphalangeal joint S93.11-
    metatarsophalangeal joint S93.12-
  interphalangeal joint S93.119
  lesser S93.106
    interphalangeal joint S93.11-
    metatarsophalangeal joint S93.12-
  metatarsophalangeal joint S93.12-
tooth S03.2
trachea S23.29
ulna
  distal end S63.07-
  proximal end —*see* Dislocation, elbow
ulnohumeral (joint) —*see* Dislocation, elbow
vertebra (articular process) (body)
    (traumatic)
  cervical S13.101
    atlantoaxial joint S13.121
    atlantooccipital joint S13.111
    atloidooccipital joint S13.111
    joint between
      C0 and C1 S13.111
      C1 and C2 S13.121
      C2 and C3 S13.131
      C3 and C4 S13.141
      C4 and C5 S13.151
      C5 and C6 S13.161
      C6 and C7 S13.171
      C7 and T1 S13.181
    occipitoatloid joint S13.111
  congenital Q76.49
  lumbar S33.101
    joint between
      L1 and L2 S33.111
      L2 and L3 S33.121
      L3 and L4 S33.131
      L4 and L5 S33.141
  nontraumatic —*see* Displacement,
    intervertebral disc
  partial —*see* Subluxation, by site
  recurrent NEC —*see* subcategory
    M43.5
  thoracic S23.101
    joint between
      T1 and T2 S23.111
      T2 and T3 S23.121
      T3 and T4 S23.123
      T4 and T5 S23.131
      T5 and T6 S23.133
      T6 and T7 S23.141
      T7 and T8 S23.143
      T8 and T9 S23.151
      T9 and T10 S23.153
      T10 and T11 S23.161
      T11 and T12 S23.163
      T12 and L1 S23.171
wrist (carpal bone) S63.006
  carpometacarpal joint —*see* Dislocation,
    carpometacarpal (joint)
  distal radioulnar joint —*see* Dislocation,
    radioulnar (joint), distal
  metacarpal bone, proximal —*see*
    Dislocation, metacarpal (bone),
    proximal end
  midcarpal —*see* Dislocation, midcarpal
    (joint)

Dislocation *(Continued)*
wrist *(Continued)*
  radiocarpal joint —*see* Dislocation,
    radiocarpal (joint)
  recurrent —*see* Dislocation, recurrent,
    wrist
  specified site NEC S63.09-
  ulna —*see* Dislocation, ulna, distal end
xiphoid cartilage S23.29
Disorder (of) —*see also* Disease
acantholytic L11.9
  specified NEC L11.8
acute
  psychotic —*see* Psychosis, acute
  stress F43.0
adjustment (grief) F43.20
  with
    anxiety F43.22
      with depressed mood F43.23
    conduct disturbance F43.24
      with emotional disturbance
        F43.25
    depressed mood F43.21
      with anxiety F43.23
    other specified symptom F43.29
adrenal (capsule) (gland) (medullary)
    E27.9
  specified NEC E27.8
adrenogenital E25.9
  drug-induced E25.8
  iatrogenic E25.8
  idiopathic E25.8
adult personality (and behavior) F69
  specified NEC F68.8
affective (mood) —*see* Disorder, mood
aggressive, unsocialized F91.1
alcohol-related F10.99
  with
    amnestic disorder, persisting
      F10.96
    anxiety disorder F10.980
    dementia, persisting F10.97
    intoxication F10.929
      with delirium F10.921
      uncomplicated F10.920
    mood disorder F10.94
    other specified F10.988
    psychotic disorder F10.959
      with
        delusions F10.950
        hallucinations F10.951
    sexual dysfunction F10.981
    sleep disorder F10.982
allergic —*see* Allergy
alveolar NEC J84.09
amino-acid
  cystathioninuria E72.19
  cystinosis E72.04
  cystinuria E72.01
  glycinuria E72.09
  homocystinuria E72.11
  metabolism —*see* Disturbance,
    metabolism, amino-acid
    specified NEC E72.8
  neonatal, transitory P74.8
  renal transport NEC E72.09
  transport NEC E72.09
amnesic, amnestic
  alcohol-induced F10.96
    with dependence F10.26
  due to (secondary to) general medical
    condition F04
  psychoactive NEC-induced F19.96
    with
      abuse F19.16
      dependence F19.26
  sedative, hypnotic or anxiolytic-
    induced F13.96
    with dependence F13.26
anaerobic glycolysis with anemia
    D55.2

Disorder *(Continued)*
  anxiety F41.9
    due to (secondary to)
      alcohol F10.980
      amphetamine F15.980
        in
          abuse F15.180
          dependence F15.280
      anxiolytic F13.980
        in
          abuse F13.180
          dependence F13.280
      caffeine F15.980
        in
          abuse F15.180
          dependence F15.280
      cannabis F12.980
        in
          abuse F12.180
          dependence F12.280
      cocaine F14.980
        in
          abuse F14.180
          dependence F14.180
      general medical condition F06.4
      hallucinogen F16.980
        in
          abuse F16.180
          dependence F16.280
      hypnotic F13.980
        in
          abuse F13.180
          dependence F13.280
      inhalant F18.980
        in
          abuse F18.180
          dependence F18.280
      phencyclidine F16.980
        in
          abuse F16.180
          dependence F16.280
      psychoactive substance NEC
          F19.980
        in
          abuse F19.180
          dependence F19.280
      sedative F13.980
        in
          abuse F13.180
          dependence F13.280
      volatile solvents F18.980
        in
          abuse F18.180
          dependence F18.280
    generalized F41.1
    mixed
      with depression (mild) F41.8
      specified NEC F41.3
    organic F06.4
    phobic F40.9
      of childhood F40.8
    specified NEC F41.8
  aortic valve —*see* Endocarditis, aortic
  aromatic amino-acid metabolism E70.9
    specified NEC E70.8
  arteriole NEC I77.89
  artery NEC I77.89
  articulation —*see* Disorder, joint
  attachment (childhood)
    disinhibited F94.2
    reactive F94.1
  attention-deficit hyperactivity (adolescent)
      (adult) (child) F90.9
    combined type F90.2
    hyperactive type F90.1
    inattentive type F90.0
    specified type NEC F90.8
  attention-deficit without hyperactivity
      (adolescent) (adult) (child) F90.0
  auditory processing (central) H93.25
  autistic F84.0

Disorder *(Continued)*
  autonomic nervous system G90.9
    specified NEC G90.8
  avoidant, child or adolescent F40.10
  balance
    acid-base E87.8
      mixed E87.4
    electrolyte E87.8
    fluid NEC E87.8
  behavioral (disruptive) —*see* Disorder,
      conduct
  beta-amino-acid metabolism E72.8
  bile acid and cholesterol metabolism
      E78.70
    Barth syndrome E78.71
    other specified E78.79
    Smith-Lemli-Opitz syndrome E78.72
  bilirubin excretion E80.6
  binocular
    movement H51.9
      convergence
        excess H51.12
        insufficiency H51.11
      internuclear ophthalmoplegia —*see*
          Ophthalmoplegia, internuclear
      palsy of conjugate gaze H51.0
      specified type NEC H51.8
    vision NEC —*see* Disorder, vision,
        binocular
  bipolar (I) F31.9
    current episode
      depressed F31.9
        with psychotic features F31.5
        without psychotic features
            F31.30
          mild F31.31
          moderate F31.32
          severe (without psychotic features)
              F31.4
          with psychotic features
              F31.5
      hypomanic F31.0
      manic F31.9
        with psychotic features F31.2
        without psychotic features F31.10
          mild F31.11
          moderate F31.12
          severe (without psychotic features)
              F31.13
          with psychotic features F31.2
      mixed F31.60
        mild F31.61
        moderate F31.62
        severe (without psychotic features)
            F31.63
        with psychotic features F31.64
      severe depression (without psychotic
          features) F31.4
        with psychotic features F31.5
    II F31.81
    in remission (currently) F31.70
      in full remission
        most recent episode
          depressed F31.76
          hypomanic F31.72
          manic F31.74
          mixed F31.78
      in partial remission
        most recent episode
          depressed F31.75
          hypomanic F31.71
          manic F31.73
          mixed F31.77
    organic F06.30
    single manic episode F30.9
      mild F30.11
      moderate F30.12
      severe (without psychotic symptoms)
          F30.13
        with psychotic symptoms F30.2
    specified NEC F31.89

Disorder *(Continued)*
  bladder N32.9
    functional NEC N31.9
    in schistosomiasis B65.0 *[N33]*
    specified NEC N32.89
  bleeding D68.9
  blood D75.9
    in congenital early syphilis A50.09 *[D77]*
  body dysmorphic F45.22
  bone M89.9
    continuity M84.9
      specified type NEC M84.80
        ankle M84.87-
        fibula M84.86-
        foot M84.87-
        hand M84.84-
        humerus M84.82-
        neck M84.88
        pelvis M84.859
        radius M84.83-
        rib M84.88
        shoulder M84.81-
        skull M84.88
        thigh M84.85-
        tibia M84.86-
        ulna M84.83-
        vertebra M84.88
    density and structure M85.9
      cyst —*see also* Cyst, bone, specified type
          NEC
        aneurysmal —*see* Cyst, bone,
            aneurysmal
        solitary —*see* Cyst, bone, solitary
      diffuse idiopathic skeletal
          hyperostosis —*see* Hyperostosis,
          ankylosing
      fibrous dysplasia (monostotic) —*see*
          Dysplasia, fibrous, bone
      fluorosis —*see* Fluorosis, skeletal
      hyperostosis of skull M85.2
      osteitis condensans —*see* Osteitis,
          condensans
      specified type NEC M85.8-
        ankle M85.87-
        foot M85.87-
        forearm M85.83-
        hand M85.84-
        lower leg M85.86-
        multiple sites M85.89
        neck M85.88
        rib M85.88
        shoulder M85.81-
        skull M85.88
        thigh M85.85-
        upper arm M85.82-
        vertebra M85.88
    development and growth NEC
        M89.20
      carpus M89.24-
      clavicle M89.21-
      femur M89.25-
      fibula M89.26-
      finger M89.24-
      humerus M89.22-
      ilium M89.259
      ischium M89.259
      metacarpus M89.24-
      metatarsus M89.27-
      multiple sites M89.29
      neck M89.28
      radius M89.23-
      rib M89.28
      scapula M89.21-
      skull M89.28
      tarsus M89.27-
      tibia M89.26-
      toe M89.27-
      ulna M89.23-
      vertebra M89.28
    specified type NEC M89.8X-
  brachial plexus G54.0

◄ New ◄◄ Revised ~~deleted~~ Deleted

Disorder *(Continued)*
disc *(Continued)*
cervical *(Continued)*
with *(Continued)*
neuritis, radiculitis or radiculopathy
M50.10
C2-C3 M50.11
C3-C4 M50.11
C4-C5 M50.12
C5-C6 M50.12
C6-C7 M50.12
C7-T1 M50.13
cervicothoracic region M50.13
high cervical region M50.11
mid-cervical region M50.12
C2-C3 M50.91
C3-C4 M50.91
C4-C5 M50.92
C5-C6 M50.92
C6-C7 M50.92
C7-T1 M50.93
cervicothoracic region M50.93
degeneration M50.30
C2-C3 M50.31
C3-C4 M50.31
C4-C5 M50.32
C5-C6 M50.32
C6-C7 M50.32
C7-T1 M50.33
cervicothoracic region M50.33
high cervical region M50.31
mid-cervical region M50.32
displacement M50.20
C2-C3 M50.21
C3-C4 M50.21
C4-C5 M50.22
C5-C6 M50.22
C6-C7 M50.22
C7-T1 M50.23
cervicothoracic region M50.23
high cervical region M50.21
mid-cervical region M50.22
high cervical region M50.91
mid-cervical region M50.92
specified type NEC M50.80
C2-C3 M50.81
C3-C4 M50.81
C4-C5 M50.82
C5-C6 M50.82
C6-C7 M50.82
C7-T1 M50.83
cervicothoracic region M50.83
high cervical region M50.81
mid-cervical region M50.82
specified NEC
lumbar region M51.86
lumbosacral region M51.87
sacrococcygeal region M53.3
thoracic region M51.84
thoracolumbar region M51.85
disinhibited attachment (childhood)
F94.2
disintegrative, childhood NEC F84.3
disruptive behavior F98.9
dissocial personality F60.2
dissociative F44.9
affecting
motor function F44.4
and sensation F44.7
sensation F44.6
and motor function F44.7
brief reactive F43.0
due to (secondary to) general medical
condition F06.8
mixed F44.7
organic F06.8
other specified NEC F44.89
double heterozygous sickling —*see* Disease,
sickle-cell
dream anxiety F51.5
drug induced hemorrhagic D68.32

Disorder *(Continued)*
drug related F19.99
abuse —*see* Abuse, drug
dependence —*see* Dependence,
drug
dysmorphic body F45.1
dysthymic F34.1
ear H93.9-
bleeding —*see* Otorrhagia
deafness —*see* Deafness
degenerative H93.09-
discharge —*see* Otorrhea
external H61.9-
auditory canal stenosis —*see* Stenosis,
external ear canal
exostosis —*see* Exostosis, external ear
canal
impacted cerumen —*see* Impaction,
cerumen
otitis —*see* Otitis, externa
perichondritis —*see* Perichondritis,
ear
pinna —*see* Disorder, pinna
specified type NEC H61.89-
in diseases classified elsewhere
H62.8X-
inner H83.9-
vestibular dysfunction —*see* Disorder,
vestibular function
middle H74.9-
adhesive H74.1-
ossicle —*see* Abnormal, ear ossicles
polyp —*see* Polyp, ear (middle)
specified NEC, in diseases classified
elsewhere H75.8-
postprocedural —*see* Complications, ear,
procedure
specified NEC, in diseases classified
elsewhere H94.8-
eating (adult) (psychogenic) F50.9
anorexia —*see* Anorexia
bulimia F50.2
child F98.29
pica F98.3
rumination disorder F98.21
pica F50.8
childhood F98.3
electrolyte (balance) NEC E87.8
with
abortion —*see* Abortion by type
complicated by specified condition
NEC
ectopic pregnancy O08.5
molar pregnancy O08.5
acidosis (metabolic) (respiratory)
E87.2
alkalosis (metabolic) (respiratory)
E87.3
elimination, transepidermal L87.9
specified NEC L87.8
emotional (persistent) F34.9
of childhood F93.9
specified NEC F93.8
endocrine E34.9
postprocedural E89.89
specified NEC E89.89
erectile (male) (organic) (*see also*
Dysfunction, sexual, male, erectile)
N52.9
nonorganic F52.21
erythematous —*see* Erythema
esophagus K22.9
functional K22.4
psychogenic F45.8
eustachian tube H69.9-
infection —*see* Salpingitis, eustachian
obstruction —*see* Obstruction, eustachian
tube
patulous —*see* Patulous, eustachian
tube
specified NEC H69.8-

Disorder *(Continued)*
extrapyramidal G25.9
in diseases classified elsewhere —*see*
category G26
specified type NEC G25.89
eye H57.9
postprocedural —*see* Complication,
postprocedural, eye
eyelid H02.9
cyst —*see* Cyst, eyelid
degenerative H02.70
chloasma —*see* Chloasma, eyelid
madarosis —*see* Madarosis
specified type NEC H02.79
vitiligo —*see* Vitiligo, eyelid
xanthelasma —*see* Xanthelasma
dermatochalasis —*see* Dermato-chalasis
edema —*see* Edema, eyelid
elephantiasis —*see* Elephantiasis, eyelid
foreign body, retained —*see* Foreign body,
retained, eyelid
function H02.59
abnormal innervation syndrome —*see*
Syndrome, abnormal innervation
blepharochalasis —*see* Blepharochalasis
blepharoclonus —*see* Blepharoclonus
blepharophimosis —*see*
Blepharophimosis
blepharoptosis —*see* Blepharoptosis
lagophthalmos —*see* Lagophthalmos
lid retraction —*see* Retraction, lid
hypertrichosis —*see* Hypertrichosis, eyelid
specified type NEC H02.89
vascular H02.879
left H02.876
lower H02.875
upper H02.874
right H02.873
lower H02.872
upper H02.871
factitious F68.10
with predominantly
physical symptoms F68.12
with psychological symptoms F68.13
psychological symptoms F68.11
with physical symptoms F68.13
factor, coagulation —*see* Defect, coagulation
fatty acid
metabolism E71.30
specified NEC E71.39
oxidation
LCAD E71.310
MCAD E71.311
SCAD E71.312
specified deficiency NEC E71.318
feeding (infant or child) (*see also* Disorder,
eating) R63.3-
feigned (with obvious motivation) Z76.5
without obvious motivation —*see* Disorder,
factitious
female
hypoactive sexual desire F52.0
orgasmic F52.31
sexual arousal F52.22
fibroblastic M72.9
specified NEC M72.8
fluency
adult onset F98.5
childhood onset F80.81
following
cerebral infarction I69.323
cerebrovascular disease I69.923
specified disease NEC I69.823
intracerebral hemorrhage I69.123
nontraumatic intracranial hemorrhage
NEC I69.223
subarachnoid hemorrhage I69.023
in conditions classified elsewhere R47.82
fluid balance E87.8
follicular (skin) L73.9
specified NEC L73.8

◀ New   ◀▥▥ Revised   ~~deleted~~ Deleted

Disorder (Continued)
  fructose metabolism E74.10
    essential fructosuria E74.11
    fructokinase deficiency E74.11
    fructose-1, 6-diphosphatase deficiency E74.19
    hereditary fructose intolerance E74.12
    other specified E74.19
  functional polymorphonuclear neutrophils D71
  gallbladder, biliary tract and pancreas in diseases classified elsewhere K87
  gamma-glutamyl cycle E72.8
  gastric (functional) K31.9
    motility K30
    psychogenic F45.8
    secretion K30
  gastrointestinal (functional) NOS K92.9
    newborn P78.9
    psychogenic F45.8
  gender-identity or -role F64.9
    childhood F64.2
    effect on relationship F66
    of adolescence or adulthood (nontranssexual) F64.1
    specified NEC F64.8
    uncertainty F66
  genitourinary system
    female N94.9
    male N50.9
    psychogenic F45.8
  globe H44.9
    degenerated condition H44.50
      absolute glaucoma H44.51-
      atrophy H44.52-
      leucocoria H44.53-
    degenerative H44.30
      chalcosis H44.31-
      myopia H44.2-
      siderosis H44.32-
      specified type NEC H44.39-
    endophthalmitis —see Endophthalmitis
    foreign body, retained —see Foreign body, intraocular, old, retained
    hemophthalmos —see Hemophthalmos
    hypotony H44.40
      due to
        ocular fistula H44.42-
          specified disorder NEC H44.43-
      flat anterior chamber H44.41-
      primary H44.44-
    luxation —see Luxation, globe
    specified type NEC H44.89
  glomerular (in) N05.9
    amyloidosis E85.4 [N08]
    cryoglobulinemia D89.1 [N08]
    disseminated intravascular coagulation D65 [N08]
    Fabry's disease E75.21 [N08]
    familial lecithin cholesterol acyltransferase deficiency E78.6 [N08]
    Goodpasture's syndrome M31.0
    hemolytic-uremic syndrome D59.3
    Henoch (-Schönlein) purpura D69.0 [N08]
    malariae malaria B52.0
    microscopic polyangiitis M31.7 [N08]
    multiple myeloma C90.0- [N08]
    mumps B26.83
    schistosomiasis B65.9 [N08]
    sepsis NEC A41.- [N08]
      streptococcal A40.- [N08]
    sickle-cell disorders D57.- [N08]
    strongyloidiasis B78.9 [N08]
    subacute bacterial endocarditis I33.0 [N08]
    syphilis A52.75
    systemic lupus erythematosus M32.14
    thrombotic thrombocytopenic purpura M31.1 [N08]
    Waldenström macroglobulinemia C88.0 [N08]
    Wegener's granulomatosis M31.31

Disorder (Continued)
  gluconeogenesis E74.4
  glucosaminoglycan metabolism — see Disorder, metabolism, glucosaminoglycan
  glycine metabolism E72.50
    d-glycericacidemia E72.59
    hyperhydroxyprolinemia E72.59
    hyperoxaluria E72.53
    hyperprolinemia E72.59
    non-ketotic hyperglycinemia E72.51
    oxalosis E72.53
    oxaluria E72.53
    sarcosinemia E72.59
    trimethylaminuria E72.52
  glycoprotein metabolism E77.9
    specified NEC E77.8
  habit (and impulse) F63.9
    involving sexual behavior NEC F65.9
    specified NEC F63.89
  heart action I49.9
  hematological D75.9
    newborn (transient) P61.9
      specified NEC P61.8
  hematopoietic organs D75.9
  hemorrhagic NEC D69.9
    drug-induced D68.32
    due to
      extrinsic circulating anticoagulants D68.32
      increase in
        anti-IIa D68.32
        anti-Xa D68.32
      intrinsic
        circulating anticoagulants D68.318
        increase in
          antithrombin D68.318
          anti-VIIIa D68.318
          anti-IXa D68.318
          anti-XIa D68.318
    following childbirth O72.3
  hemostasis —see Defect, coagulation
  histidine metabolism E70.40
    histidinemia E70.41
    other specified E70.49
  hyperkinetic —see Disorder, attention-deficit hyperactivity
  hyperleucine-isoleucinemia E71.19
  hypervalinemia E71.19
  hypoactive sexual desire F52.0
  hypochondriacal F45.20
    body dysmorphic F45.22
    neurosis F45.21
    other specified F45.29
  identity
    dissociative F44.81
    of childhood F93.8
  immune mechanism (immunity) D89.9
    specified type NEC D89.89
  impaired renal tubular function N25.9
    specified NEC N25.89
  impulse (control) F63.9
  inflammatory
    pelvic, in diseases classified elsewhere — see category N74
    penis N48.29
      abscess N48.21
      cellulitis N48.22
  integument, newborn P83.9
    specified NEC P83.8
  intermittent explosive F63.81
  internal secretion pancreas —see Increased, secretion, pancreas, endocrine
  intestine, intestinal
    carbohydrate absorption NEC E74.39
      postoperative K91.2
    functional NEC K59.9
      postoperative K91.89
    psychogenic F45.8
    vascular K55.9
      chronic K55.1
      specified NEC K55.8

Disorder (Continued)
  intraoperative (intraprocedural) —see Complications, intraoperative
  involuntary emotional expression (IEED) F48.2
  iris H21.9
    adhesions —see Adhesions, iris
    atrophy —see Atrophy, iris
    chamber angle recession —see Recession, chamber angle
    cyst —see Cyst, iris
    degeneration —see Degeneration, iris
    in diseases classified elsewhere H22
    iridodialysis —see Iridodialysis
    iridoschisis —see Iridoschisis
    miotic pupillary cyst —see Cyst, pupillary
    pupillary
      abnormality —see Abnormality, pupillary
      membrane —see Membrane, pupillary
    specified type NEC H21.89
    vascular NEC H21.1X-
  iron metabolism E83.10
    specified NEC E83.19
  isovaleric acidemia E71.110
  jaw, developmental M27.0
    temporomandibular —see Anomaly, dentofacial, temporomandibular joint
  joint M25.9
    derangement —see Derangement, joint
    effusion —see Effusion, joint
    fistula —see Fistula, joint
    hemarthrosis —see Hemarthrosis
    instability —see Instability, joint
    osteophyte —see Osteophyte
    pain —see Pain, joint
    psychogenic F45.8
    specified type NEC M25.80
      ankle M25.87-
      elbow M25.82-
      foot joint M25.87-
      hand joint M25.84-
      hip M25.85-
      knee M25.86-
      shoulder M25.81-
      wrist M25.83-
    stiffness —see Stiffness, joint
  ketone metabolism E71.32
  kidney N28.9
    functional (tubular) N25.9
    in
      schistosomiasis B65.9 [N29]
    tubular function N25.9
      specified NEC N25.89
  lacrimal system H04.9
    changes H04.69
      fistula —see Fistula, lacrimal
    gland H04.19
      atrophy —see Atrophy, lacrimal gland
      cyst —see Cyst, lacrimal, gland
      dacryops —see Dacryops
      dislocation —see Dislocation, lacrimal gland
      dry eye syndrome —see Syndrome, dry eye
      infection —see Dacryoadenitis
      granuloma —see Granuloma, lacrimal
      inflammation —see Inflammation, lacrimal
      obstruction —see Obstruction, lacrimal
    specified NEC H04.89
  lactation NEC O92.79
  language (developmental) F80.9
    expressive F80.1
    mixed receptive and expressive F80.2
    receptive F80.2
  late luteal phase dysphoric N94.89
  learning (specific) F81.9
    acalculia R48.8
    alexia R48.0
    mathematics F81.2
    reading F81.0

Disorder *(Continued)*
  learning *(Continued)*
    specified NEC F81.89
    spelling F81.81
    written expression F81.81
  lens H27.9
    aphakia —*see* Aphakia
    cataract —*see* Cataract
    dislocation —*see* Dislocation, lens
    specified type NEC H27.8
  ligament M24.20
    ankle M24.27-
    attachment, spine —*see* Enthesopathy, spinal
    elbow M24.22-
    foot joint M24.27-
    hand joint M24.24-
    hip M24.25-
    knee —*see* Derangement, knee, specified
      NEC
    shoulder M24.21-
    vertebra M24.28
    wrist M24.23-
  ligamentous attachments —*see also*
    Enthesopathy
    spine —*see* Enthesopathy, spinal
  lipid
    metabolism, congenital E78.9
    storage E75.6
    specified NEC E75.5
  lipoprotein
    deficiency (familial) E78.6
    metabolism E78.9
    specified NEC E78.89
  liver K76.9
    malarial B54 [K77]
  low back —*see also* Dorsopathy, specified
    NEC
  lumbosacral
    plexus G54.1
    root (nerve) NEC G54.4
  lung, interstitial, drug-induced J70.4
    acute J70.2
    chronic J70.3
  lymphoproliferative, post-transplant (PTLD)
    D47.Z1
  lysine and hydroxylysine metabolism E72.3
  male
    erectile (organic) (*see also* Dysfunction,
      sexual, male, erectile) N52.9
      nonorganic F52.21
    hypoactive sexual desire F52.0
    orgasmic F52.32
  manic F30.9
    organic F06.33
  mastoid —*see also* Disorder, ear, middle
    postprocedural —*see* Complications, ear,
      procedure
  meniscus —*see* Derangement, knee, meniscus
  menopausal N95.9
    specified NEC N95.8
  menstrual N92.6
    psychogenic F45.8
    specified NEC N92.5
  mental (or behavioral) (nonpsychotic) F99
    due to (secondary to)
      amphetamine
        due to drug abuse —*see* Abuse, drug,
          stimulant
        due to drug dependence —*see*
          Dependence, drug, stimulant
      brain disease, damage and dysfunction
        F09
      caffeine use
        due to drug abuse —*see* Abuse, drug,
          stimulant
        due to drug dependence —*see*
          Dependence, drug, stimulant
      cannabis use
        due to drug abuse —*see* Abuse, drug,
          cannabis
        due to drug dependence —*see*
          Dependence, drug, cannabis

Disorder *(Continued)*
  mental *(Continued)*
    due to *(Continued)*
      general medical condition F09
      sedative or hypnotic use
        due to drug abuse —*see* Abuse, drug,
          sedative
        due to drug dependence —*see*
          Dependence, drug, sedative
      tobacco (nicotine) use —*see* Dependence,
        drug, nicotine
    following organic brain damage F07.9
      frontal lobe syndrome F07.0
      personality change F07.0
      postconcussional syndrome F07.81
      specified NEC F07.89
    infancy, childhood or adolescence F98.9
    neurotic —*see* Neurosis
    organic or symptomatic F09
    presenile, psychotic F03
    problem NEC
    psychoneurotic —*see* Neurosis
    psychotic —*see* Psychosis
    puerperal F53
    senile, psychotic NEC F03
  metabolic, amino acid, transitory, newborn
    P74.8
  metabolism NOS E88.9
    amino-acid E72.9
      aromatic E70.9
        albinism —*see* Albinism
        histidine E70.40
          histidinemia E70.41
          other specified E70.49
        hyperphenylalaninemia E70.1
          classical phenylketonuria E70.0
        other specified E70.8
        tryptophan E70.5
        tyrosine E70.20
          hypertyrosinemia E70.21
          other specified E70.29
      branched chain E71.2
        3-methylglutaconic aciduria E71.111
        hyperleucine-isoleucinemia E71.19
        hypervalinemia E71.19
        isovaleric acidemia E71.110
        maple syrup urine disease E71.0
        methylmalonic acidemia E71.120
        organic aciduria NEC E71.118
        other specified E71.19
        proprionate NEC E71.128
        proprionic acidemia E71.121
      glycine E72.50
        d-glycericacidemia E72.59
        hyperhydroxyprolinemia E72.59
        hyperoxaluria E72.53
        hyperprolinemia E72.59
        non-ketotic hyperglycinemia E72.51
        other specified E72.59
        sarcosinemia E72.59
        trimethylaminuria E72.52
      hydroxylysine E72.3
      lysine E72.3
      ornithine E72.4
      other specified E72.8
        beta-amino acid E72.8
        gamma-glutamyl cycle E72.8
      straight-chain E72.8
      sulfur-bearing E72.10
        homocystinuria E72.11
        methylenetetrahydrofolate reductase
          deficiency E72.12
        other specified E72.19
    bile acid and cholesterol metabolism
      E78.70
    bilirubin E80.7
      specified NEC E80.6
    calcium E83.50
      hypercalcemia E83.52
      hypocalcemia E83.51
      other specified E83.59

Disorder *(Continued)*
  metabolism NOS *(Continued)*
    carbohydrate E74.9
      specified NEC E74.8
    cholesterol and bile acid metabolism
      E78.70
    congenital E88.9
    copper E83.00
      specified type NEC E83.09
      Wilson's disease E83.01
    cystinuria E72.01
    fructose E74.10
    galactose E74.20
    glucosaminoglycan E76.9
      mucopolysaccharidosis —*see*
        Mucopolysaccharidosis
      specified NEC E76.8
    glutamine E72.8
    glycine E72.50
    glycogen storage (hepatorenal) E74.09
    glycoprotein E77.9
      specified NEC E77.8
    glycosaminoglycan E76.9
      specified NEC E76.8
    in labor and delivery O75.89
    iron E83.10
    isoleucine E71.19
    leucine E71.19
    lipoid E78.9
    lipoprotein E78.9
      specified NEC E78.89
    magnesium E83.40
      hypermagnesemia E83.41
      hypomagnesemia E83.42
      other specified E83.49
    mineral E83.9
      specified NEC E83.89
    mitochondrial E88.40
      MELAS syndrome E88.41
      MERRF syndrome (myoclonic epilepsy
        associated with ragged-red fibers)
        E88.42
      other specified E88.49
    ornithine E72.4
    phosphatases E83.30
    phosphorus E83.30
      acid phosphatase deficiency
        E83.39
      hypophosphatasia E83.39
      hypophosphatemia E83.39
        familial E83.31
      other specified E83.39
      pseudovitamin D deficiency
        E83.32
    plasma protein NEC E88.09
    porphyrin —*see* Porphyria
    postprocedural E89.89
      specified NEC E89.89
    purine E79.9
      specified NEC E79.8
    pyrimidine E79.9
      specified NEC E79.8
    pyruvate E74.4
    serine E72.8
    sodium E87.8
    specified NEC E88.89
    threonine E72.8
    valine E71.19
    zinc E83.2
  methylmalonic acidemia E71.120
  micturition NEC R39.19
    feeling of incomplete emptying
      R39.14
    hesitancy R39.11
    poor stream R39.12
    psychogenic F45.8
    split stream R39.13
    straining R39.16
    urgency R39.15
  mitochondrial metabolism E88.40
  mitral (valve) —*see* Endocarditis, mitral

◀ New ◀▥ Revised ~~deleted~~ Deleted

Disorder (*Continued*)
mixed
 anxiety and depressive F41.8
 of scholastic skills (developmental)
   F81.89
 receptive expressive language F80.2
mood F39
 bipolar —*see* Disorder, bipolar
 depressive —*see* Disorder, depressive
 due to (secondary to)
  alcohol F10.94
  amphetamine F15.94
   in
    abuse F15.14
    dependence F15.24
  anxiolytic F13.94
   in
    abuse F13.14
    dependence F13.24
  cocaine F14.94
   in
    abuse F14.14
    dependence F14.24
  general medical condition F06.30
  hallucinogen F16.94
   in
    abuse F16.14
    dependence F16.24
  hypnotic F13.94
   in
    abuse F13.14
    dependence F13.24
  inhalant F18.94
   in
    abuse F18.14
    dependence F18.24
  opioid F11.94
   in
    abuse F11.14
    dependence F11.24
  phencyclidine (PCP) F16.94
   in
    abuse F16.14
    dependence F16.24
  physiological condition F06.30
   with
    depressive features F06.31
    major depressive-like episode
      F06.32
    manic features F06.33
    mixed features F06.34
  psychoactive substance NEC F19.94
   in
    abuse F19.14
    dependence F19.24
  sedative F13.94
   in
    abuse F13.14
    dependence F13.24
  volatile solvents F18.94
   in
    abuse F18.14
    dependence F18.24
 manic episode F30.9
  with psychotic symptoms F30.2
  without psychotic symptoms
    F30.10
   mild F30.11
   moderate F30.12
   severe F30.13
  in remission (full) F30.4
   partial F30.3
  specified type NEC F30.8
 organic F06.30
  right hemisphere F07.89
 persistent F34.9
  cyclothymia F34.0
  dysthymia F34.1
  specified type NEC F34.8
 recurrent F39
 right hemisphere organic F07.89

Disorder (*Continued*)
movement G25.9
 drug-induced G25.70
  akathisia G25.71
  specified NEC G25.79
 hysterical F44.4
 in diseases classified elsewhere —*see*
   category G26
 periodic limb G47.61
  sleep related G47.61
 sleep related NEC G47.69
 specified NEC G25.89
 stereotyped F98.4
 treatment-induced G25.9
multiple personality F44.81
muscle M62.9
 attachment, spine —*see* Enthesopathy,
   spinal
 in trichinellosis —*see* Trichinellosis, with
   muscle disorder
 psychogenic F45.8
 specified type NEC M62.89
 tone, newborn P94.9
  specified NEC P94.8
muscular
 attachments —*see also* Enthesopathy
  spine —*see* Enthesopathy, spinal
 urethra N36.44
musculoskeletal system, soft tissue —*see*
   Disorder, soft tissue
 postprocedural M96.89
 psychogenic F45.8
myoneural G70.9
 due to lead G70.1
 specified NEC G70.89
 toxic G70.1
myotonic NEC G71.19
nail, in diseases classified elsewhere L62
neck region NEC —*see* Dorsopathy, specified
   NEC
nerve G58.9
 abducent NEC —*see* Strabismus, paralytic,
   sixth nerve
 accessory G52.8
 acoustic —*see* subcategory H93.3
 auditory —*see* subcategory H93.3
 auriculotemporal G50.8
 axillary G54.0
 cerebral —*see* Disorder, nerve, cranial
 cranial G52.9
  eighth —*see* subcategory H93.3
  eleventh G52.8
  fifth G50.9
  first G52.0
  fourth NEC —*see* Strabismus, paralytic,
    fourth nerve
  multiple G52.7
  ninth G52.1
  second NEC —*see* Disorder, nerve, optic
  seventh NEC G51.8
  sixth NEC —*see* Strabismus, paralytic,
    sixth nerve
  specified NEC G52.8
  tenth G52.2
  third NEC —*see* Strabismus, paralytic,
    third nerve
  twelfth G52.3
 entrapment —*see* Neuropathy, entrapment
 facial G51.9
  specified NEC G51.8
 femoral —*see* Lesion, nerve, femoral
 glossopharyngeal NEC G52.1
 hypoglossal G52.3
 intercostal G58.0
 lateral
  cutaneous of thigh —*see*
    Mononeuropathy, lower limb,
    meralgia paresthetica
  popliteal —*see* Lesion, nerve, popliteal
 lower limb —*see* Mononeuropathy, lower
   limb

Disorder (*Continued*)
nerve (*Continued*)
 medial popliteal —*see* Lesion, nerve,
   popliteal, medial
 median NEC —*see* Lesion, nerve,
   median
 multiple G58.7
 oculomotor NEC —*see* Strabismus,
   paralytic, third nerve
 olfactory G52.0
 optic NEC H47.09-
  hemorrhage into sheath —*see*
    Hemorrhage, optic nerve
  ischemic H47.01-
 peroneal —*see* Lesion, nerve, popliteal
 phrenic G58.8
 plantar —*see* Lesion, nerve, plantar
 pneumogastric G52.2
 posterior tibial —*see* Syndrome, tarsal
   tunnel
 radial —*see* Lesion, nerve, radial
 recurrent laryngeal G52.2
 root G54.9
  cervical G54.2
  lumbosacral G54.1
  specified NEC G54.8
  thoracic G54.3
 sciatic NEC —*see* Lesion, nerve, sciatic
 specified NEC G58.8
  lower limb —*see* Mononeuropathy,
    lower limb, specified NEC
  upper limb —*see* Mononeuropathy,
    upper limb, specified NEC
 sympathetic G90.9
 tibial —*see* Lesion, nerve, popliteal,
   medial
 trigeminal G50.9
  specified NEC G50.8
 trochlear NEC —*see* Strabismus, paralytic,
   fourth nerve
 ulnar —*see* Lesion, nerve, ulnar
 upper limb —*see* Mononeuropathy, upper
   limb
 vagus G52.2
nervous system G98.8
 autonomic (peripheral) G90.9
  specified NEC G90.8
 central G96.9
  specified NEC G96.8
 parasympathetic G90.9
 specified NEC G98.8
 sympathetic G90.9
 vegetative G90.9
neurohypophysis NEC E23.3
neurological NEC R29.818
neuromuscular G70.9
 hereditary NEC G71.9
 specified NEC G70.89
 toxic G70.1
neurotic F48.9
 specified NEC F48.8
neutrophil, polymorphonuclear D71
nicotine use —*see* Dependence, drug,
   nicotine
nightmare F51.5
nose J34.9
 specified NEC J34.89
obsessive-compulsive F42
odontogenesis NOS K00.9
opioid use
 with
  opioid-induced psychotic disorder
    F11.959
   with
    delusions F11.950
    hallucinations F11.951
 due to drug abuse —*see* Abuse, drug,
   opioid
 due to drug dependence —*see* Dependence,
   drug, opioid
oppositional defiant F91.3

Disorder *(Continued)*
  optic
    chiasm H47.49
      due to
        inflammatory disorder H47.41
        neoplasm H47.42
        vascular disorder H47.43
    disc H47.39-
      coloboma —*see* Coloboma, optic disc
      drusen —*see* Drusen, optic disc
      pseudopapilledema —*see*
          Pseudopapilledema
      radiations —*see* Disorder, visual, pathway
      tracts —*see* Disorder, visual, pathway
    orbit H05.9
      cyst —*see* Cyst, orbit
      deformity —*see* Deformity, orbit
      edema —*see* Edema, orbit
      enophthalmos —*see* Enophthalmos
      exophthalmos —*see* Exophthalmos
      hemorrhage —*see* Hemorrhage, orbit
      inflammation —*see* Inflammation, orbit
      myopathy —*see* Myopathy, extraocular
          muscles
      retained foreign body —*see* Foreign body,
          orbit, old
      specified type NEC H05.89
    organic
      anxiety F06.4
      catatonic F06.1
      delusional F06.2
      dissociative F06.8
      emotionally labile (asthenic) F06.8
      mood (affective) F06.30
      schizophrenia-like F06.2
    orgasmic (female) F52.31
      male F52.32
    ornithine metabolism E72.4
    overanxious F41.1
      of childhood F93.8
    pain
      with related psychological factors F45.42
      exclusively related to psychological factors
          F45.41
    pancreatic internal secretion E16.9
      specified NEC E16.8
    panic F41.0
      with agoraphobia F40.01
    papulosquamous L44.9
      in diseases classified elsewhere L45
      specified NEC L44.8
    paranoid F22
      induced F24
      shared F24
    parathyroid (gland) E21.5
      specified NEC E21.4
    parietoalveolar NEC J84.09
    paroxysmal, mixed R56.9
    patella M22.9-
      chondromalacia —*see* Chondromalacia,
          patella
      derangement NEC M22.3X-
      recurrent
        dislocation —*see* Dislocation, patella,
            recurrent
        subluxation —*see* Dislocation, patella,
            recurrent, incomplete
      specified NEC M22.8X-
    patellofemoral M22.2X-
    pentose phosphate pathway with anemia
        D55.1
    perception, due to hallucinogens F16.983
      in
        abuse F16.183
        dependence F16.283
    peripheral nervous system NEC G64
    peroxisomal E71.50
      biogenesis
        neonatal adrenoleukodystrophy E71.511
        specified disorder NEC E71.518
        Zellweger syndrome E71.510

Disorder *(Continued)*
  peroxisomal *(Continued)*
    rhizomelic chondrodysplasia punctata
        E71.540
    specified form NEC E71.548
      group 1 E71.518
      group 2 E71.53
      group 3 E71.542
    X-linked adrenoleukodystrophy
        E71.529
      adolescent E71.521
      adrenomyeloneuropathy E71.522
      childhood E71.520
      specified form NEC E71.528
    Zellweger-like syndrome E71.541
  persistent
    (somatoform) pain F45.41
    affective (mood) F34.9
  personality (*see also* Personality) F60.9
    affective F34.0
    aggressive F60.3
    amoral F60.2
    anankastic F60.5
    antisocial F60.2
    anxious F60.6
    asocial F60.2
    asthenic F60.7
    avoidant F60.6
    borderline F60.3
    change (secondary) due to general medical
        condition F07.0
    compulsive F60.5
    cyclothymic F34.0
    dependent (passive) F60.7
    depressive F34.1
    dissocial F60.2
    emotional instability F60.3
    expansive paranoid F60.0
    explosive F60.3
    following organic brain damage
        F07.9
    histrionic F60.4
    hyperthymic F34.0
    hypothymic F34.1
    hysterical F60.4
    immature F60.89
    inadequate F60.7
    labile F60.3
    mixed (nonspecific) F60.89
    moral deficiency F60.2
    narcissistic F60.81
    negativistic F60.89
    obsessional F60.5
    obsessive (-compulsive) F60.5
    organic F07.9
    overconscientious F60.5
    paranoid F60.0
    passive (-dependent) F60.7
    passive-aggressive F60.89
    pathological NEC F60.9
    pseudosocial F60.2
    psychopathic F60.2
    schizoid F60.1
    schizotypal F21
    self-defeating F60.7
    specified NEC F60.89
    type A F60.5
    unstable (emotional) F60.3
  pervasive, developmental F84.9
  phobic anxiety, childhood F40.8
  phosphate-losing tubular N25.0
  pigmentation L81.9
    choroid, congenital Q14.3
    diminished melanin formation L81.6
    iron L81.8
    specified NEC L81.8
  pinna (noninfective) H61.10-
    deformity, acquired H61.11-
    hematoma H61.12-
    perichondritis —*see* Perichondritis, ear
    specified type NEC H61.19-

Disorder *(Continued)*
  pituitary gland E23.7
    iatrogenic (postprocedural) E89.3
    specified NEC E23.6
  platelets D69.1
  plexus G54.9
    specified NEC G54.8
  polymorphonuclear neutrophils D71
  porphyrin metabolism —*see* Porphyria
  postconcussional F07.81
  posthallucinogen perception F16.983
    in
      abuse F16.183
      dependence F16.283
  postmenopausal N95.9
    specified NEC N95.8
  postprocedural (postoperative) —*see*
      Complications, postprocedural
  post-transplant lymphoproliferative D47.z1
  post-traumatic stress (PTSD) F43.10
    acute F43.11
    chronic F43.12
  premenstrual dysphoric (PMDD) N94.3
  prepuce N47.8
  propionic acidemia E71.121
  prostate N42.9
    specified NEC N42.89
  psychogenic NOS (*see also* condition) F45.9
    anxiety F41.8
    appetite F50.9
    asthenic F48.8
    cardiovascular (system) F45.8
    compulsive F42
    cutaneous F54
    depressive F32.9
    digestive (system) F45.8
    dysmenorrheic F45.8
    dyspneic F45.8
    endocrine (system) F54
    eye NEC F45.8
    feeding —*see* Disorder, eating
    functional NEC F45.8
    gastric F45.8
    gastrointestinal (system) F45.8
    genitourinary (system) F45.8
    heart (function) (rhythm) F45.8
    hyperventilatory F45.8
    hypochondriacal —*see* Disorder,
        hypochondriacal
    intestinal F45.8
    joint F45.8
    learning F81.9
    limb F45.8
    lymphatic (system) F45.8
    menstrual F45.8
    micturition F45.8
    monoplegic NEC F44.4
    motor F44.4
    muscle F45.8
    musculoskeletal F45.8
    neurocirculatory F45.8
    obsessive F42
    occupational F48.8
    organ or part of body NEC F45.8
    paralytic NEC F44.4
    phobic F40.9
    physical NEC F45.8
    rectal F45.8
    respiratory (system) F45.8
    rheumatic F45.8
    sexual (function) F52.9
    skin (allergic) (eczematous) F54
    sleep F51.9
    specified part of body NEC F45.8
    stomach F45.8
  psychological F99
    associated with
      disease classified elsewhere F54
      sexual
        development F66
        relationship F66
        uncertainty about gender identity F66

◀ New   ◀▥ Revised   ~~deleted~~ Deleted

Disorder (Continued)
psychomotor NEC F44.4
  hysterical F44.4
psychoneurotic —see also Neurosis
  mixed NEC F48.8
psychophysiologic —see Disorder,
  somatoform
psychosexual F65.9
  development F66
  identity of childhood F64.2
psychosomatic NOS —see Disorder,
  somatoform
  multiple F45.0
  undifferentiated F45.1
psychotic —see Psychosis
  transient (acute) F23
puberty E30.9
  specified NEC E30.8
pulmonary (valve) —see Endocarditis,
  pulmonary
purine metabolism E79.9
pyrimidine metabolism E79.9
pyruvate metabolism E74.4
reactive attachment (childhood) F94.1
reading R48.0
  developmental (specific) F81.0
receptive language F80.2
receptor, hormonal, peripheral (see also
  Syndrome, androgen insensitivity)
  E34.50
recurrent brief depressive F33.8
reflex R29.2
refraction H52.7
  aniseikonia H52.32
  anisometropia H52.31
  astigmatism —see Astigmatism
  hypermetropia —see Hypermetropia
  myopia —see Myopia
  presbyopia H52.4
  specified NEC H52.6
relationship F68.8
  due to sexual orientation F66
REM sleep behavior G47.52
renal function, impaired (tubular) N25.9
resonance R49.9
  specified NEC R49.8
respiratory function, impaired —see also
  Failure, respiration
  postprocedural —see Complication,
   postoperative, respiratory system
  psychogenic F45.8
retina H35.9
  angioid streaks H35.33
  changes in vascular appearance H35.01-
  degeneration —see Degeneration, retina
  dystrophy (hereditary) —see Dystrophy,
   retina
  edema H35.81
  hemorrhage —see Hemorrhage, retina
  ischemia H35.82
  macular degeneration —see Degeneration,
   macula
  microaneurysms H35.04-
  microvascular abnormality NEC
   H35.09
  neovascularization —see
   Neovascularization, retina
  retinopathy —see Retinopathy
  separation of layers H35.70
   central serous chorioretinopathy
    H35.71-
   pigment epithelium detachment (serous)
    H35.72-
    hemorrhagic H35.73-
  specified type NEC H35.89
  telangiectasis —see Telangiectasis, retina
  vasculitis —see Vasculitis, retina
retroperitoneal K68.9
right hemisphere organic affective F07.89
rumination (infant or child) F98.21
sacrum, sacrococcygeal NEC M53.3

Disorder (Continued)
schizoaffective F25.9
  bipolar type F25.0
  depressive type F25.1
  manic type F25.0
  mixed type F25.0
  specified NEC F25.8
schizoid of childhood F84.5
schizophreniform F20.81
  brief F23
schizotypal (personality) F21
secretion, thyrocalcitonin E07.0
seizure (see also Epilepsy) G40.909
  intractable G40.919
   with status epilepticus G40.911
semantic pragmatic F80.89
  with autism F84.0
sense of smell R43.1
  psychogenic F45.8
separation anxiety, of childhood F93.0
sexual
  arousal, female F52.22
  aversion F52.1
  function, psychogenic F52.9
  maturation F66
  nonorganic F52.9
  preference (see also Deviation, sexual) F65.9
   fetishistic transvestism F65.1
  relationship F66
shyness, of childhood and adolescence
  F40.10
sibling rivalry F93.8
sickle-cell (sickling) (homozygous) —see
  Disease, sickle-cell
  heterozygous D57.3
  specified type NEC D57.8-
  trait D57.3
sinus (nasal) J34.9
  specified NEC J34.89
skin L98.9
  atrophic L90.9
   specified NEC L90.8
  granulomatous L92.9
   specified NEC L92.8
  hypertrophic L91.9
   specified NEC L91.8
  infiltrative NEC L98.6
  newborn P83.9
   specified NEC P83.8
  psychogenic (allergic) (eczematous)
   F54
sleep G47.9
  breathing-related —see Apnea, sleep
  circadian rhythm G47.20
   advance sleep phase type G47.22
   delayed sleep phase type G47.21
   due to
    alcohol
     abuse F10.182
     dependence F10.282
     use F10.982
    amphetamines
     abuse F15.182
     dependence F15.282
     use F15.982
    caffeine
     abuse F15.182
     dependence F15.282
     use F15.982
    cocaine
     abuse F14.182
     dependence F14.282
     use F14.982
    drug NEC
     abuse F19.182
     dependence F19.282
     use F19.982
    opioid
     abuse F11.182
     dependence F11.282
     use F11.982

Disorder (Continued)
sleep (Continued)
  circadian rhythm (Continued)
   due to (Continued)
    psychoactive substance NEC
     abuse F19.182
     dependence F19.282
     use F19.982
    sedative, hypnotic, or anxiolytic
     abuse F13.182
     dependence F13.282
     use F13.982
    stimulant NEC
     abuse F15.182
     dependence F15.282
     use F15.982
   free running type G47.24
   in conditions classified elsewhere
    G47.27
   irregular sleep wake type G47.23
   jet lag type G47.25
   shift work type G47.26
   specified NEC G47.29
  due to
   alcohol
    abuse F10.182
    dependence F10.282
    use F10.982
   amphetamine
    abuse F15.182
    dependence F15.282
    use F15.982
   anxiolytic
    abuse F13.182
    dependence F13.282
    use F13.982
   caffeine
    abuse F15.182
    dependence F15.282
    use F15.982
   cocaine
    abuse F14.182
    dependence F14.282
    use F14.982
   drug NEC
    abuse F19.182
    dependence F19.282
    use F19.982
   hypnotic
    abuse F13.182
    dependence F13.282
    use F13.982
   opioid
    abuse F11.182
    dependence F11.282
    use F11.982
   psychoactive substance NEC
    abuse F19.182
    dependence F19.282
    use F19.982
   sedative
    abuse F13.182
    dependence F13.282
    use F13.982
   stimulant NEC
    abuse F15.182
    dependence F15.282
    use F15.982
  emotional F51.9
  excessive somnolence —see Hypersomnia
  hypersomnia type —see Hypersomnia
  initiating or maintaining —see Insomnia
  nightmares F51.5
  nonorganic F51.9
   specified NEC F51.8
  parasomnia type G47.50
  specified NEC G47.8
  terrors F51.4
  walking F51.3
sleep-wake pattern or schedule —see
  Disorder, sleep, circadian rhythm

Disorder *(Continued)*
  social
    anxiety of childhood F40.10
    functioning in childhood F94.9
      specified NEC F94.8
  soft tissue M79.9
    ankle M79.9
    due to use, overuse and pressure
        M70.90
      ankle M70.97-
      bursitis —*see* Bursitis
      foot M70.97-
      forearm M70.93-
      hand M70.94-
      lower leg M70.96-
      multiple sites M70.99
      pelvic region M70.95-
      shoulder region M70.91-
      specified site NEC M70.98
      specified type NEC M70.80
        ankle M70.87-
        foot M70.87-
        forearm M70.83-
        hand M70.84-
        lower leg M70.86-
        multiple sites M70.89
        pelvic region M70.85-
        shoulder region M70.81-
        specified site NEC M70.88
        thigh M70.85-
        upper arm M70.82-
      thigh M70.95-
      upper arm M70.92-
    foot M79.9
    forearm M79.9
    hand M79.9
    lower leg M79.9
    multiple sites M79.9
    occupational —*see* Disorder, soft tissue,
        due to use, overuse and pressure
    pelvic region M79.9
    shoulder region M79.9
    specified type NEC M79.89
    thigh M79.9
    upper arm M79.9
  somatization F45.0
  somatoform F45.9
    pain (persistent) F45.41
    somatization (multiple) (long-lasting) F45.0
    specified NEC F45.8
    undifferentiated F45.1
  somnolence, excessive —*see* Hypersomnia
  specific
    arithmetical F81.2
    developmental, of motor F82
    reading F81.0
    speech and language F80.9
    spelling F81.81
    written expression F81.81
  speech R47.9
    articulation (functional) (specific) F80.0
    developmental F80.9
    specified NEC R47.89
  spelling (specific) F81.81
  spine —*see also* Dorsopathy
    ligamentous or muscular attachments,
        peripheral —*see* Enthesopathy, spinal
    specified NEC —*see* Dorsopathy, specified
        NEC
  stereotyped, habit or movement F98.4
  stomach (functional) —*see* Disorder, gastric
  stress F43.9
    post-traumatic F43.10
      acute F43.11
      chronic F43.12
  sulfur-bearing amino-acid metabolism
      E72.10
  sweat gland (eccrine) L74.9
    apocrine L75.9
      specified NEC L75.8
    specified NEC L74.8

Disorder *(Continued)*
  synovium M67.90
    acromioclavicular M67.91-
    ankle M67.97-
    elbow M67.92-
    foot M67.97-
    forearm M67.93-
    hand M67.94-
    hip M67.95-
    knee M67.96-
    multiple sites M67.99
    rupture —*see* Rupture, synovium
    shoulder M67.91-
    specified type NEC M67.80
      acromioclavicular M67.81-
      ankle M67.87-
      elbow M67.82-
      foot M67.87-
      hand M67.84-
      hip M67.85-
      knee M67.86-
      multiple sites M67.89
      wrist M67.83-
    synovitis —*see* Synovitis
    upper arm M67.92-
    wrist M67.93-
  temperature regulation, newborn P81.9
    specified NEC P81.8
  temporomandibular joint —*see* Anomaly,
      dentofacial, temporomandibular joint
  tendon M67.90
    acromioclavicular M67.91-
    ankle M67.97-
    contracture —*see* Contracture, tendon
    elbow M67.92-
    foot M67.97-
    forearm M67.93-
    hand M67.94-
    hip M67.95-
    knee M67.96-
    multiple sites M67.99
    rupture —*see* Rupture, tendon
    shoulder M67.91-
    specified type NEC M67.80
      acromioclavicular M67.81-
      ankle M67.87-
      elbow M67.82-
      foot M67.87-
      hand M67.84-
      hip M67.85-
      knee M67.86-
      multiple sites M67.89
      trunk M67.88
      wrist M67.83-
    synovitis —*see* Synovitis
    tendinitis —*see* Tendinitis
    tenosynovitis —*see* Tenosynovitis
    trunk M67.98
    upper arm M67.92-
    wrist M67.93-
  thoracic root (nerve) NEC G54.3
  thyrocalcitonin hypersecretion E07.0
  thyroid (gland) E07.9
    function NEC, neonatal, transitory P72.2
    iodine-deficiency related E01.8
    specified NEC E07.89
  tic —*see* Tic
  tooth K08.9
    development K00.9
      specified NEC K00.8
    eruption K00.6
  Tourette's F95.2
  trance and possession F44.89
  tricuspid (valve) —*see* Endocarditis,
      tricuspid
  tryptophan metabolism E70.5
  tubular, phosphate-losing N25.0
  tubulo-interstitial (in)
    brucellosis A23.9 *[N16]*
    cystinosis E72.04
    diphtheria A36.84

Disorder *(Continued)*
  tubulo-interstitial *(Continued)*
    glycogen storage disease E74.00 *[N16]*
    leukemia NEC C95.9- *[N16]*
    lymphoma NEC C85.9- *[N16]*
    mixed cryoglobulinemia D89.1 *[N16]*
    multiple myeloma C90.0- *[N16]*
    Salmonella infection A02.25
    sarcoidosis D86.84
    sepsis A41.9 *[N16]*
      streptococcal A40.9 *[N16]*
    systemic lupus erythematosus M32.15
    toxoplasmosis B58.83
    transplant rejection T86.91 *[N16]*
    Wilson's disease E83.01 *[N16]*
  tubulo-renal function, impaired N25.9
    specified NEC N25.89
  tympanic membrane H73.9-
    atrophy —*see* Atrophy, tympanic
        membrane
    infection —*see* Myringitis
    perforation —*see* Perforation, tympanum
    specified NEC H73.89-
  unsocialized aggressive F91.1
  urea cycle metabolism E72.20
    argininemia E72.21
    arginosuccinic aciduria E72.22
    citrullinemia E72.23
    ornithine transcarbamylase deficiency
        E72.4
    other specified E72.29
  ureter (in) N28.9
    schistosomiasis B65.0 *[N29]*
    tuberculosis A18.11
  urethra N36.9
    specified NEC N36.8
  urinary system N39.9
    specified NEC N39.8
  valve, heart
    aortic —*see* Endocarditis, aortic
    mitral —*see* Endocarditis, mitral
    pulmonary —*see* Endocarditis, pulmonary
    rheumatic
      aortic —*see* Endocarditis, aortic,
          rheumatic
      mitral —*see* Endocarditis, mitral
      pulmonary —*see* Endocarditis,
          pulmonary, rheumatic
      tricuspid —*see* Endocarditis, tricuspid
    tricuspid —*see* Endocarditis, tricuspid
  vestibular function H81.9-
    specified NEC —*see* subcategory H81.8
    in diseases classified elsewhere H82.-
    vertigo —*see* Vertigo
  vision, binocular H53.30
    abnormal retinal correspondence H53.31
    diplopia H53.2
    fusion with defective stereopsis H53.32
    simultaneous perception H53.33
    suppression H53.34
  visual
    cortex
      blindness H47.619
        left brain H47.612
        right brain H47.611
      due to
        inflammatory disorder H47.629
          left brain H47.622
          right brain H47.621
        neoplasm H47.639
          left brain H47.632
          right brain H47.631
        vascular disorder H47.649
          left brain H47.642
          right brain H47.641
    pathway H47.9
      due to
        inflammatory disorder H47.51-
        neoplasm H47.52-
        vascular disorder H47.53-
      optic chiasm —*see* Disorder, optic, chiasm

◀ New   ◀▦ Revised   ~~deleted~~ Deleted

Disorder (Continued)
  vitreous body H43.9
    crystalline deposits —see Deposit, crystalline
    degeneration —see Degeneration, vitreous
    hemorrhage —see Hemorrhage, vitreous
    opacities —see Opacity, vitreous
    prolapse —see Prolapse, vitreous
    specified type NEC H43.89
  voice R49.9
    specified type NEC R49.8
  volatile solvent use
    due to drug abuse —see Abuse, drug, inhalant
    due to drug dependence —see Dependence, drug, inhalant
  white blood cells D72.9
    specified NEC D72.89
  withdrawing, child or adolescent F40.10
Disorientation R41.0
Displacement, displaced
  acquired traumatic of bone, cartilage, joint, tendon NEC —see Dislocation
  adrenal gland (congenital) Q89.1
  appendix, retrocecal (congenital) Q43.8
  auricle (congenital) Q17.4
  bladder (acquired) N32.89
    congenital Q64.19
  brachial plexus (congenital) Q07.8
  brain stem, caudal (congenital) Q04.8
  canaliculus (lacrimalis), congenital Q10.6
  cardia through esophageal hiatus (congenital) Q40.1
  cerebellum, caudal (congenital) Q04.8
  cervix —see Malposition, uterus
  colon (congenital) Q43.3
  device, implant or graft (see also Complications, by site and type, mechanical) T85.628
    arterial graft NEC —see Complication, cardiovascular device, mechanical, vascular
    breast (implant) T85.42
    catheter NEC T85.628
      dialysis (renal) T82.42
        intraperitoneal T85.621
      infusion NEC T82.524
        spinal (epidural) (subdural) T85.620
      urinary (indwelling) T83.028
        cystostomy T83.020
    electronic (electrode) (pulse generator) (stimulator) —see Complication, electronic stimulator
    fixation, internal (orthopedic) NEC —see Complication, fixation device, mechanical
    gastrointestinal —see Complications, prosthetic device, mechanical, gastrointestinal device
    genital NEC T83.428
      intrauterine contraceptive device T83.32
      penile prosthesis T83.420
    heart NEC —see Complication, cardiovascular device, mechanical
    joint prosthesis —see Complications, joint prosthesis, mechanical
    ocular —see Complications, prosthetic device, mechanical, ocular device
    orthopedic NEC —see Complication, orthopedic, device or graft, mechanical
    specified NEC T85.628
    urinary NEC —see also Complication, genitourinary, device, urinary, mechanical
      graft T83.22
    vascular NEC —see Complication, cardiovascular device, mechanical
  ventricular intracranial shunt T85.02

Displacement, displaced (Continued)
  electronic stimulator
    bone T84.320
    cardiac —see Complications, cardiac device, electronic
    nervous system —see Complication, prosthetic device, mechanical, electronic nervous system stimulator
    urinary —see Complications, electronic stimulator, urinary
  esophageal mucosa into cardia of stomach, congenital Q39.8
  esophagus (acquired) K22.8
    congenital Q39.8
  eyeball (acquired) (lateral) (old) —see Displacement, globe
    congenital Q15.8
    current —see Avulsion, eye
  fallopian tube (acquired) N83.4
    congenital Q50.6
    opening (congenital) Q50.6
  gallbladder (congenital) Q44.1
  gastric mucosa (congenital) Q40.2
  globe (acquired) (old) (lateral) H05.21-
    current —see Avulsion, eye
  heart (congenital) Q24.8
    acquired I51.89
  hymen (upward) (congenital) Q52.4
  intervertebral disc NEC
    with myelopathy —see Disorder, disc, with, myelopathy
    cervical, cervicothoracic (with) M50.20
      myelopathy —see Disorder, disc, cervical, with myelopathy
      neuritis, radiculitis or radiculopathy —see Disorder, disc, cervical, with neuritis
    due to trauma —see Dislocation, vertebra
    lumbar region M51.26
      with
        neuritis, radiculitis, radiculopathy or sciatica M51.16
    lumbosacral region M51.27
      with
        myelopathy M51.07
        neuritis, radiculitis, radiculopathy or sciatica M51.17
    sacrococcygeal region M53.3
    thoracic region M51.24
      with
        myelopathy M51.04
        neuritis, radiculitis, radiculopathy M51.14
    thoracolumbar region M51.25
      with
        myelopathy M51.05
        neuritis, radiculitis, radiculopathy M51.15
  intrauterine device T83.32
  kidney (acquired) N28.83
    congenital Q63.2
  lachrymal, lacrimal apparatus or duct (congenital) Q10.6
  lens, congenital Q12.1
  macula (congenital) Q14.1
  Meckel's diverticulum Q43.0
    malignant —see Table of Neoplasms, small intestine, malignant
  nail (congenital) Q84.6
    acquired L60.8
  opening of Wharton's duct in mouth Q38.4
  organ or site, congenital NEC —see Malposition, congenital
  ovary (acquired) N83.4
    congenital Q50.39
    free in peritoneal cavity (congenital) Q50.39
    into hernial sac N83.4

Displacement, displaced (Continued)
  oviduct (acquired) N83.4
    congenital Q50.6
  parathyroid (gland) E21.4
  parotid gland (congenital) Q38.4
  punctum lacrimale (congenital) Q10.6
  sacro-iliac (joint) (congenital) Q74.2
    current injury S33.2
    old —see subcategory M53.2
  salivary gland (any) (congenital) Q38.4
  spleen (congenital) Q89.09
  stomach, congenital Q40.2
  sublingual duct Q38.4
  tongue (downward) (congenital) Q38.3
  tooth, teeth, fully erupted M26.30
    horizontal M26.33
    vertical M26.34
  trachea (congenital) Q32.1
  ureter or ureteric opening or orifice (congenital) Q62.62
  uterine opening of oviducts or fallopian tubes Q50.6
  uterus, uterine —see Malposition, uterus
  ventricular septum Q21.0
    with rudimentary ventricle Q20.4
Disproportion
  between native and reconstructed breast N65.1
  fiber-type G71.2
Disruptio uteri —see Rupture, uterus
Disruption (of)
  ciliary body NEC H21.89
  closure of
    cornea T81.31
    craniotomy T81.32
    fascia (muscular) (superficial) T81.32
    internal organ or tissue T81.32
    laceration (external) (internal) T81.33
    ligament T81.32
    mucosa T81.31
    muscle or muscle flap T81.32
    ribs or rib cage T81.32
    skin and subcutaneous tissue (full-thickness) (superficial) T81.31
    skull T81.32
    sternum (sternotomy) T81.32
    tendon T81.32
    traumatic laceration (external) (internal) T81.33
  family Z63.8
    due to
      absence of family member due to military deployment Z63.31
      absence of family member NEC Z63.32
      alcoholism and drug addiction in family Z63.72
      bereavement Z63.4
      death (assumed) or disappearance of family member Z63.4
      divorce or separation Z63.5
      drug addiction in family Z63.72
      return of family member from military deployment (current or past conflict) Z63.71
      stressful life events NEC Z63.79
  iris NEC H21.89
  ligament (s) —see also Sprain
    knee
      current injury —see Dislocation, knee
      old (chronic) —see Derangement, knee, ligament, instability, chronic
      spontaneous NEC —see Derangement, knee, disruption ligament
  ossicular chain —see Discontinuity, ossicles, ear
  pelvic ring (stable) S32.810
    unstable S32.811
  traumatic injury wound repair T81.33

Disruption *(Continued)*
 wound T81.30
  episiotomy O90.1
  operation T81.31
   cesarean O90.0
   external operation wound (superficial)
    T81.31
   internal operation wound (deep)
    T81.32
  perineal (obstetric) O90.1
  traumatic injury repair T81.33
Dissatisfaction with
 employment Z56.9
 school environment Z55.4
Dissecting —*see* condition
Dissection
 aorta I71.00
  abdominal I71.02
  thoracic I71.01
  thoracoabdominal I71.03
 artery
  carotid I77.71
  cerebral (nonruptured) I67.0
   ruptured —*see* Hemorrhage, intracranial,
    subarachnoid
  coronary I25.42
  iliac I77.72
  renal I77.73
  specified NEC I77.79
  vertebral I77.74
 traumatic —*see* Wound, open, by site
 vascular I99.8
 wound —*see* Wound, open
Disseminated —*see* condition
Dissociation
 auriculoventricular or atrioventricular (AV)
   (any degree) (isorhythmic) I45.89
  with heart block I44.2
 interference I45.89
Dissociative reaction, state F44.9
Dissolution, vertebra —*see* Osteoporosis
Distension, distention
 abdomen R14.0
 bladder N32.89
 cecum K63.89
 colon K63.89
 gallbladder K82.8
 intestine K63.89
 kidney N28.89
 liver K76.89
 seminal vesicle N50.8
 stomach K31.89
  acute K31.0
  psychogenic F45.8
 ureter —*see* Dilatation, ureter
 uterus N85.8
Distoma hepaticum infestation B66.3
Distomiasis B66.9
 bile passages B66.3
 hemic B65.9
 hepatic B66.3
  due to Clonorchis sinensis B66.1
 intestinal B66.5
 liver B66.3
  due to Clonorchis sinensis B66.1
 lung B66.4
 pulmonary B66.4
Distomolar (fourth molar) K00.1
Disto-occlusion (Division I) (Division II)
  M26.212
Distortion (s) (congenital)
 adrenal (gland) Q89.1
 arm NEC Q68.8
 bile duct or passage Q44.5
 bladder Q64.79
 brain Q04.9
 cervix (uteri) Q51.9
 chest (wall) Q67.8
  bones Q76.8
 clavicle Q74.0
 clitoris Q52.6

Distortion *(Continued)*
 coccyx Q76.49
 common duct Q44.5
 coronary Q24.5
 cystic duct Q44.5
 ear (auricle) (external) Q17.3
  inner Q16.5
  middle Q16.4
   ossicles Q16.3
 endocrine NEC Q89.2
 eustachian tube Q17.8
 eye (adnexa) Q15.8
 face bone (s) NEC Q75.8
 fallopian tube Q50.6
 femur NEC Q68.8
 fibula NEC Q68.8
 finger (s) Q68.1
 foot Q66.9
 genitalia, genital organ (s)
  female Q52.8
   external Q52.79
   internal NEC Q52.8
 gyri Q04.8
 hand bone (s) Q68.1
 heart (auricle) (ventricle) Q24.8
  valve (cusp) Q24.8
 hepatic duct Q44.5
 humerus NEC Q68.8
 hymen Q52.4
 intrafamilial communications
   Z63.8
 jaw NEC M26.89
 labium (majus) (minus) Q52.79
 leg NEC Q68.8
 lens Q12.8
 liver Q44.7
 lumbar spine Q76.49
  with disproportion O33.8
   causing obstructed labor O65.0
 lumbosacral (joint) (region) Q76.49
  kyphosis —*see* Kyphosis, congenital
  lordosis —*see* Lordosis, congenital
 nerve Q07.8
 nose Q30.8
 organ
  of Corti Q16.5
  or site not listed —*see* Anomaly, by site
   ossicles, ear Q16.3
 oviduct Q50.6
 pancreas Q45.3
 parathyroid (gland) Q89.2
 pituitary (gland) Q89.2
 radius NEC Q68.8
 sacroiliac joint Q74.2
 sacrum Q76.49
 scapula Q74.0
 shoulder girdle Q74.0
 skull bone (s) NEC Q75.8
  with
   anencephalus Q00.0
   encephalocele —*see* Encephalocele
   hydrocephalus Q03.9
    with spina bifida —*see* Spina bifida,
     with hydrocephalus
   microcephaly Q02
 spinal cord Q06.8
 spine Q76.49
  kyphosis —*see* Kyphosis, congenital
  lordosis —*see* Lordosis, congenital
 spleen Q89.09
 sternum NEC Q76.7
 thorax (wall) Q67.8
  bony Q76.8
 thymus (gland) Q89.2
 thyroid (gland) Q89.2
 tibia NEC Q68.8
 toe (s) Q66.9
 tongue Q38.3
 trachea (cartilage) Q32.1
 ulna NEC Q68.8
 ureter Q62.8

Distortion *(Continued)*
 urethra Q64.79
  causing obstruction Q64.39
 uterus Q51.9
 vagina Q52.4
 vertebra Q76.49
  kyphosis —*see* Kyphosis, congenital
  lordosis —*see* Lordosis, congenital
 visual —*see also* Disturbance, vision
  shape and size H53.15
 vulva Q52.79
 wrist (bones) (joint) Q68.8
Distress
 abdomen —*see* Pain, abdominal
 acute respiratory (adult) (child) J80
 epigastric R10.13
 fetal P84
  complicating pregnancy —*see* Stress, fetal
 gastrointestinal (functional) K30
  psychogenic F45.8
 intestinal (functional) NOS K59.9
  psychogenic F45.8
 maternal, during labor and delivery
   O75.0
 respiratory R06.00
  adult J80
  child J80
  newborn P22.9
   specified NEC P22.8
  orthopnea R06.01
  psychogenic F45.8
  shortness of breath R06.02
  specified type NEC R06.09
Distribution vessel, atypical Q27.9
 coronary artery Q24.5
 precerebral Q28.1
Distichiasis L68.8
Districhiasis L68.8
Disturbance (s) —*see also* Disease
 absorption K90.9
  calcium E58
  carbohydrate K90.4
  fat K90.4
   pancreatic K90.3
  protein K90.4
  starch K90.4
  vitamin —*see* Deficiency, vitamin
 acid-base equilibrium E87.8
  mixed E87.4
 activity and attention (with hyperkinesis) —
   see Disorder, attention-deficit
   hyperactivity
 amino acid transport E72.00
 assimilation, food K90.9
 auditory nerve, except deafness —*see*
   subcategory H93.3
 behavior —*see* Disorder, conduct
 blood clotting (mechanism) (*see also* Defect,
   coagulation) D68.9
 cerebral
  nerve —*see* Disorder, nerve, cranial
  status, newborn P91.9
   specified NEC P91.8
 circulatory I99.9
 conduct (*see also* Disorder, conduct)
   F91.9
  adjustment reaction —*see* Disorder,
    adjustment
  compulsive F63.9
  disruptive F91.9
  hyperkinetic —*see* Disorder, attention-
    deficit hyperactivity
  socialized F91.2
  specified NEC F91.8
  unsocialized F91.1
 coordination R27.8
 cranial nerve —*see* Disorder, nerve,
   cranial
 deep sensibility —*see* Disturbance,
   sensation
 digestive K30
  psychogenic F45.8

Disturbance *(Continued)*
electrolyte —*see also* Imbalance, electrolyte
  newborn, transitory P74.4
    hyperammonemia P74.6
    potassium balance P74.3
    sodium balance P74.2
    specified type NEC P74.4
emotions specific to childhood and
    adolescence F93.9
  with
    anxiety and fearfulness NEC F93.8
    elective mutism F94.0
    oppositional disorder F91.3
    sensitivity (withdrawal) F40.10
    shyness F40.10
    social withdrawal F40.10
  involving relationship problems F93.8
  mixed F93.8
  specified NEC F93.8
endocrine (gland) E34.9
  neonatal, transitory P72.9
    specified NEC P72.8
equilibrium R42
fructose metabolism E74.10
gait —*see* Gait
  hysterical F44.4
  psychogenic F44.4
gastrointestinal (functional) K30
  psychogenic F45.8
habit, child F98.9
hearing, except deafness and tinnitus —*see*
    Abnormal, auditory perception
heart, functional (conditions in I44-I50)
  due to presence of (cardiac) prosthesis
    I97.19-
  postoperative I97.89
    cardiac surgery I97.19-
hormones E34.9
innervation uterus (parasympathetic)
    (sympathetic) N85.8
keratinization NEC
  gingiva K05.10
    nonplaque induced K05.11
    plaque induced K05.10
  lip K13.0
  oral (mucosa) (soft tissue) K13.29
  tongue K13.29
learning (specific) —*see* Disorder,
    learning
memory —*see* Amnesia
  mild, following organic brain damage
    F06.8
mental F99
  associated with diseases classified
    elsewhere F54
metabolism E88.9
  with
    abortion —*see* Abortion, by type with
        other specified complication
    ectopic pregnancy O08.5
    molar pregnancy O08.5
  amino-acid E72.9
    aromatic E70.9
    branched-chain E71.2
    straight-chain E72.8
    sulfur-bearing E72.10
  ammonia E72.20
  arginine E72.21
  arginosuccinic acid E72.22
  carbohydrate E74.9
  cholesterol E78.9
  citrulline E72.23
  cystathionine E72.19
  general E88.9
  glutamine E72.8
  histidine E70.40
  homocystine E72.19
  hydroxylysine E72.3
  in labor or delivery O75.89
  iron E83.10
  lipoid E78.9

Disturbance *(Continued)*
metabolism *(Continued)*
  lysine E72.3
  methionine E72.19
  neonatal, transitory P74.9
    calcium and magnesium P71.9
      specified type NEC P71.8
    carbohydrate metabolism P70.9
      specified type NEC P70.8
    specified NEC P74.8
  ornithine E72.4
  phosphate E83.39
  sodium NEC E87.8
  threonine E72.8
  tryptophan E70.5
  tyrosine E70.20
  urea cycle E72.20
motor R29.2
nervous, functional R45.0
neuromuscular mechanism (eye), due to
    syphilis A52.15
nutritional E63.9
  nail L60.3
ocular motion H51.9
  psychogenic F45.8
oculogyric H51.8
  psychogenic F45.8
oculomotor H51.9
  psychogenic F45.8
olfactory nerve R43.1
optic nerve NEC —*see* Disorder, nerve,
    optic
oral epithelium, including tongue NEC
    K13.29
perceptual due to
  alcohol withdrawal F10.232
  amphetamine intoxication F15.922
    in
      abuse F15.122
      dependence F15.222
  anxiolytic withdrawal F13.232
  cannabis intoxication (acute) F12.922
    in
      abuse F12.122
      dependence F12.222
  cocaine intoxication (acute) F14.922
    in
      abuse F14.122
      dependence F14.222
  hypnotic withdrawal F13.232
  opioid intoxication (acute) F11.922
    in
      abuse F11.122
      dependence F11.222
  phencyclidine intoxication (acute)
      F19.922
    in
      abuse F19.122
      dependence F19.222
  sedative withdrawal F13.232
personality (pattern) (trait) (*see also* Disorder,
    personality) F60.9
  following organic brain damage
      F07.9
polyglandular E31.9
  specified NEC E31.8
potassium balance, newborn P74.3
psychogenic F45.9
psychomotor F44.4
psychophysical visual H53.16
pupillary —*see* Anomaly, pupil, function
reflex R29.2
rhythm, heart I49.9
salivary secretion K11.7
sensation (cold) (heat) (localization) (tactile
    discrimination) (texture) (vibratory)
    NEC R20.9
  hysterical F44.6
  skin R20.9
    anesthesia R20.0
    hyperesthesia R20.3

Disturbance *(Continued)*
sensation *(Continued)*
  skin *(Continued)*
    hypoesthesia R20.1
    paresthesia R20.2
    specified type NEC R20.8
  smell R43.9
    and taste (mixed) R43.8
    anosmia R43.0
    parosmia R43.1
    specified NEC R43.8
  taste R43.9
    and smell (mixed) R43.8
    parageusia R43.2
    specified NEC R43.8
sensory —*see* Disturbance, sensation
situational (transient) —*see also* Disorder,
    adjustment
  acute F43.0
sleep G47.9
  nonorganic origin F51.9
smell —*see* Disturbance, sensation,
    smell
sociopathic F60.2
sodium balance, newborn P74.2
speech R47.9
  developmental F80.9
  specified NEC R47.89
stomach (functional) K31.9
sympathetic (nerve) G90.9
taste —*see* Disturbance, sensation,
    taste
temperature
  regulation, newborn P81.9
    specified NEC P81.8
  sense R20.8
    hysterical F44.6
tooth
  eruption K00.6
  formation K00.4
  structure, hereditary NEC K00.5
touch —*see* Disturbance, sensation
vascular I99.9
  arteriosclerotic —*see* Arteriosclerosis
vasomotor I73.9
vasospastic I73.9
vision, visual H53.9
  following
    cerebral infarction I69.398
    cerebrovascular disease I69.998
      specified NEC I69.898
    intracerebral hemorrhage I69.198
    nontraumatic intracranial hemorrhage
        NEC I69.298
    specified disease NEC I69.898
    subarachnoid hemorrhage I69.098
  psychophysical H53.16
  specified NEC H53.8
  subjective H53.10
    day blindness H53.11
    discomfort H53.14-
    distortions of shape and size H53.15
    loss
      sudden H53.13-
      transient H53.12-
    specified type NEC H53.19
voice R49.9
  psychogenic F44.4
  specified NEC R49.8
Diuresis R35.8
Diver's palsy, paralysis or squeeze T70.3
Diverticulitis (acute) K57.92
  bladder —*see* Cystitis
  ileum —*see* Diverticulitis, intestine, small
  intestine K57.92
    with
      abscess, perforation or peritonitis
          K57.80
        with bleeding K57.81
      bleeding K57.93
    congenital Q43.8

Diverticulitis (Continued)
- intestine (Continued)
  - large K57.32
    - with
      - abscess, perforation or peritonitis K57.20
        - with bleeding K57.21
      - bleeding K57.33
    - small intestine K57.52
      - with
        - abscess, perforation or peritonitis K57.40
          - with bleeding K57.41
        - bleeding K57.53
  - small K57.12
    - with
      - abscess, perforation or peritonitis K57.00
        - with bleeding K57.01
      - bleeding K57.13
    - large intestine K57.52
      - with
        - abscess, perforation or peritonitis K57.40
          - with bleeding K57.41
        - bleeding K57.53

Diverticulosis K57.90
- with bleeding K57.91
- large intestine K57.30
  - with
    - bleeding K57.31
    - small intestine K57.50
      - with bleeding K57.51
- small intestine K57.10
  - with
    - bleeding K57.11
    - large intestine K57.50
      - with bleeding K57.51

Diverticulum, diverticula (multiple) K57.90
- appendix (noninflammatory) K38.2
- bladder (sphincter) N32.3
  - congenital Q64.6
- bronchus (congenital) Q32.4
  - acquired J98.09
- calyx, calyceal (kidney) N28.89
- cardia (stomach) K31.4
- cecum —see Diverticulosis, intestine, large
  - congenital Q43.8
- colon —see Diverticulosis, intestine, large
  - congenital Q43.8
- duodenum —see Diverticulosis, intestine, small
  - congenital Q43.8
- epiphrenic (esophagus) K22.5
- esophagus (congenital) Q39.6
  - acquired (epiphrenic) (pulsion) (traction) K22.5
- eustachian tube —see Disorder, eustachian tube, specified NEC
- fallopian tube N83.8
- gastric K31.4
- heart (congenital) Q24.8
- ileum —see Diverticulosis, intestine, small
- jejunum —see Diverticulosis, intestine, small
- kidney (pelvis) (calyces) N28.89
  - with calculus —see Calculus, kidney
- Meckel's (displaced) (hypertrophic) Q43.0
  - malignant —see Table of Neoplasms, small intestine, malignant
- midthoracic K22.5
- organ or site, congenital NEC —see Distortion
- pericardium (congenital) (cyst) Q24.8
  - acquired I31.8
- pharyngoesophageal (congenital) Q39.6
  - acquired K22.5
- pharynx (congenital) Q38.7
- rectosigmoid —see Diverticulosis, intestine, large
  - congenital Q43.8
- rectum —see Diverticulosis, intestine, large
- Rokitansky's K22.5

Diverticulum, diverticula (Continued)
- seminal vesicle N50.8
- sigmoid —see Diverticulosis, intestine, large
  - congenital Q43.8
- stomach (acquired) K31.4
  - congenital Q40.2
- trachea (acquired) J39.8
- ureter (acquired) N28.89
  - congenital Q62.8
- ureterovesical orifice N28.89
- urethra (acquired) N36.1
  - congenital Q64.79
- ventricle, left (congenital) Q24.8
- vesical N32.3
  - congenital Q64.6
- Zenker's (esophagus) K22.5

Division
- cervix uteri (acquired) N88.8
- glans penis Q55.69
- labia minora (congenital) Q52.79
- ligament (partial or complete) (current) —see also Sprain
  - with open wound —see Wound, open
- muscle (partial or complete) (current) —see also Injury, muscle
  - with open wound —see Wound, open
- nerve (traumatic) —see Injury, nerve
- spinal cord —see Injury, spinal cord, by region
- vein I87.8

Divorce, causing family disruption Z63.5
Dix-Hallpike neurolabyrinthitis —see Neuronitis, vestibular
Dizziness R42
- hysterical F44.89
- psychogenic F45.8

DMAC (disseminated mycobacterium avium-intracellulare complex) A31.2
DNR (do not resuscitate) Z66
Doan-Wiseman syndrome (primary splenic neutropenia) —see Agranulocytosis
Doehle-Heller aortitis A52.02
Dog bite —see Bite
Dohle body panmyelopathic syndrome D72.0
Dolichocephaly Q67.2
Dolichocolon Q43.8
Dolichostenomelia —see Syndrome, Marfan's
Donohue's syndrome E34.8
Donor (organ or tissue) Z52.9
- blood (whole) Z52.000
  - autologous Z52.010
  - specified component (lymphocytes) (platelets) NEC Z52.008
    - autologous Z52.018
    - specified donor NEC Z52.098
  - specified donor NEC Z52.090
  - stem cells Z52.001
    - autologous Z52.011
    - specified donor NEC Z52.091
- bone Z52.20
  - autologous Z52.21
  - marrow Z52.3
  - specified type NEC Z52.29
- cornea Z52.5
- egg (Oocyte) Z52.819
  - age 35 and over Z52.812
    - anonymous recipient Z52.812
    - designated recipient Z52.813
  - under age 35 Z52.810
    - anonymous recipient Z52.810
    - designated recipient Z52.811
- kidney Z52.4
- liver Z52.6
- lung Z52.89
- lymphocyte —see Donor, blood, specified components NEC
- Oocyte —see Donor, egg
- platelets Z52.008
- potential, examination of Z00.5
- semen Z52.89

Donor (Continued)
- skin Z52.10
  - autologous Z52.11
  - specified type NEC Z52.19
- specified organ or tissue NEC Z52.89
- sperm Z52.89

Donovanosis A58
Dorsalgia M54.9
- psychogenic F45.41
- specified NEC M54.89
Dorsopathy M53.9
- deforming M43.9
  - specified NEC —see subcategory M43.8
- specified NEC M53.80
  - cervical region M53.82
  - cervicothoracic region M53.83
  - lumbar region M53.86
  - lumbosacral region M53.87
  - occipito-atlanto-axial region M53.81
  - sacrococcygeal region M53.88
  - thoracic region M53.84
  - thoracolumbar region M53.85
Double
- albumin E88.09
- aortic arch Q25.4
- auditory canal Q17.8
- auricle (heart) Q20.8
- bladder Q64.79
- cervix Q51.820
  - with doubling of uterus (and vagina) Q51.10
    - with obstruction Q51.11
- inlet ventricle Q20.4
- kidney with double pelvis (renal) Q63.0
- meatus urinarius Q64.75
- monster Q89.4
- outlet
  - left ventricle Q20.2
  - right ventricle Q20.1
- pelvis (renal) with double ureter Q62.5
- tongue Q38.3
- ureter (one or both sides) Q62.5
  - with double pelvis (renal) Q62.5
- urethra Q64.74
- urinary meatus Q64.75
- uterus Q51.2
  - with
    - doubling of cervix (and vagina) Q51.10
      - with obstruction Q51.11
  - in pregnancy or childbirth O34.59-
    - causing obstructed labor O65.5
- vagina Q52.10
  - with doubling of uterus (and cervix) Q51.10
    - with obstruction Q51.11
- vision H53.2
- vulva Q52.79
Douglas' pouch, cul-de-sac —see condition
Down syndrome Q90.9
- meiotic nondisjunction Q90.0
- mitotic nondisjunction Q90.1
- mosaicism Q90.1
- translocation Q90.2
DPD (dihydropyrimidine dehydrogenase deficiency) E88.89
Dracontiasis B72
Dracunculiasis, dracunculosis B72
Dream state, hysterical F44.89
Drepanocytic anemia —see Disease, sickle-cell
Dresbach's syndrome (elliptocytosis) D58.1
Dreschlera (hawaiiensis) (infection) B43.8
Dressler's syndrome I24.1
Drift, ulnar —see Deformity, limb, specified type NEC, forearm
Drinking (alcohol)
- excessive, to excess NEC (without dependence) F10.10
  - habitual (continual) (without remission) F10.20
    - with remission F10.21

Drip, postnasal (chronic) R09.82
  due to
    allergic rhinitis —*see* Rhinitis, allergic
    common cold J00
    gastroesophageal reflux —*see* Reflux,
      gastroesophageal
    nasopharyngitis —*see* Nasopharyngitis
    other known condition — code to
      condition
    sinusitis —*see* Sinusitis
Droop
  facial R29.810
    cerebrovascular disease I69.992
      cerebral infarction I69.392
      intracerebral hemorrhage I69.192
      nontraumatic intracranial hemorrhage
        NEC I69.292
      specified disease NEC I69.892
      subarachnoid hemorrhage I69.092
Drop (in)
  attack NEC R55
  finger —*see* Deformity, finger
  foot —*see* Deformity, limb, foot, drop
  hematocrit (precipitous) R71.0
  hemoglobin R71.0
  toe —*see* Deformity, toe, specified NEC
  wrist —*see* Deformity, limb, wrist drop
Dropped heart beats I45.9
Dropsy, dropsical —*see also* Hydrops
  abdomen R18.8
  brain —*see* Hydrocephalus
  cardiac, heart —*see* Failure, heart, congestive
  gangrenous —*see* Gangrene
  heart —*see* Failure, heart, congestive
  kidney —*see* Nephrosis
  lung —*see* Edema, lung
  newborn due to isoimmunization P56.0
  pericardium —*see* Pericarditis
Drowned, drowning (near) T75.1
Drowsiness R40.0
Drug
  abuse counseling and surveillance Z71.51
  addiction —*see* Dependence
  dependence —*see* Dependence
  habit —*see* Dependence
  harmful use —*see* Abuse, drug
  induced fever R50.2
  overdose —*see* Table of Drugs and Chemicals,
    by drug, poisoning
  poisoning —*see* Table of Drugs and
    Chemicals, by drug, poisoning
  resistant organism infection (*see also*
    Resistant, organism, to, drug) Z16.30
  therapy
    long term (current) (prophylactic) —*see*
      Therapy, drug long-term (current)
      (prophylactic)
    short term - omit code
  wrong substance given or taken in error —*see*
    Table of Drugs and Chemicals, by drug,
    poisoning
Drunkenness (without dependence) F10.129
  acute in alcoholism F10.229
  chronic (without remission) F10.20
    with remission F10.21
  pathological (without dependence) F10.129
    with dependence F10.229
  sleep F51.9
Drusen
  macula (degenerative) (retina) —*see*
    Degeneration, macula, drusen
  optic disc H47.32-
Dry, dryness —*see also* condition
  larynx J38.7
  mouth R68.2
    due to dehydration E86.0
  nose J34.89
  socket (teeth) M27.3
  throat J39.2
DSAP L56.5
Duane's syndrome H50.81-

Dubin-Johnson disease or syndrome E80.6
Dubois' disease (thymus gland) A50.59 *[E35]*
Dubowitz' syndrome Q87.1
Duchenne-Aran muscular atrophy G12.21
Duchenne-Griesinger disease G71.0
Duchenne's
  disease or syndrome
    motor neuron disease G12.22
    muscular dystrophy G71.0
  locomotor ataxia (syphilitic) A52.11
  paralysis
    birth injury P14.0
    due to or associated with
      motor neuron disease G12.22
      muscular dystrophy G71.0
Ducrey's chancre A57
Duct, ductus —*see* condition
Duhring's disease (dermatitis herpetiformis)
  L13.0
Dullness, cardiac (decreased) (increased) R01.2
Dumb ague —*see* Malaria
Dumbness —*see* Aphasia
Dumdum fever B55.0
Dumping syndrome (postgastrectomy) K91.1
Duodenitis (nonspecific) (peptic) K29.80
  with bleeding K29.81
Duodenocholangitis —*see* Cholangitis
Duodenum, duodenal —*see* condition
Duplay's bursitis or periarthritis —*see*
  Tendinitis, calcific, shoulder
Duplication, duplex —*see also* Accessory
  alimentary tract Q45.8
  anus Q43.4
  appendix (and cecum) Q43.4
  biliary duct (any) Q44.5
  bladder Q64.79
  cecum (and appendix) Q43.4
  cervix Q51.820
  chromosome NEC
    with complex rearrangements NEC
      Q92.5
    seen only at prometaphase Q92.8
  cystic duct Q44.5
  digestive organs Q45.8
  esophagus Q39.8
  frontonasal process Q75.8
  intestine (large) (small) Q43.4
  kidney Q63.0
  liver Q44.7
  pancreas Q45.3
  penis Q55.69
  respiratory organs NEC Q34.8
  salivary duct Q38.4
  spinal cord (incomplete) Q06.2
  stomach Q40.2
Dupré's disease (meningism) R29.1
Dupuytren's contraction or disease M72.0
Durand-Nicolas-Favre disease A55
Durotomy (inadvertent) (incidental) G97.41
Duroziez's disease (congenital mitral stenosis)
  Q23.2
Dutton's relapsing fever (West African) A68.1
Dwarfism E34.3
  achondroplastic Q77.4
  congenital E34.3
  constitutional E34.3
  hypochondroplastic Q77.4
  hypophyseal E23.0
  infantile E34.3
  Laron-type E34.3
  Lorain (-Levi) type E23.0
  metatropic Q77.8
  nephrotic-glycosuric (with
    hypophosphatemic rickets) E72.09
  nutritional E45
  pancreatic K86.8
  pituitary E23.0
  renal N25.0
  thanatophoric Q77.1
Dyke-Young anemia (secondary)
  (symptomatic) D59.1

Dysacusis —*see* Abnormal, auditory
  perception
Dysadrenocortism E27.9
  hyperfunction E27.0
Dysarthria R47.1
  following
    cerebral infarction I69.322
    cerebrovascular disease I69.922
      specified disease NEC I69.822
    intracerebral hemorrhage I69.122
    nontraumatic intracranial hemorrhage
      NEC I69.222
    subarachnoid hemorrhage I69.022
Dysautonomia (familial) G90.1
Dysbarism T70.3
Dysbasia R26.2
  angiosclerotica intermittens I73.9
  hysterical F44.4
  lordotica (progressiva) G24.1
  nonorganic origin F44.4
  psychogenic F44.4
Dysbetalipoproteinemia (familial) E78.2
Dyscalculia R48.8
  developmental F81.2
Dyschezia K59.00
Dyschondroplasia (with hemangiomata)
  Q78.4
Dyschromia (skin) L81.9
Dyscollagenosis M35.9
Dyscranio-pygo-phalangy Q87.0
Dyscrasia
  blood (with) D75.9
    antepartum hemorrhage —*see*
      Hemorrhage, antepartum, with
      coagulation defect
    intrapartum hemorrhage O67.0
    newborn P61.9
      specified type NEC P61.8
    puerperal, postpartum O72.3
  polyglandular, pluriglandular E31.9
Dysendocrinism E34.9
Dysentery, dysenteric (catarrhal) (diarrhea)
  (epidemic) (hemorrhagic) (infectious)
  (sporadic) (tropical) A09
  abscess, liver A06.4
  amebic (*see also* Amebiasis) A06.0
    with abscess —*see* Abscess, amebic
    acute A06.0
    chronic A06.1
  arthritis (*see also* category M01) A09
    bacillary (*see also* category M01) A03.9
  bacillary A03.9
    arthritis (*see also* category M01)
      A03.9
    Boyd A03.2
    Flexner A03.1
    Schmitz (-Stutzer) A03.0
    Shiga (-Kruse) A03.0
    Shigella A03.9
      boydii A03.2
      dysenteriae A03.0
      flexneri A03.1
      group A A03.0
      group B A03.1
      group C A03.2
      group D A03.3
      sonnei A03.3
      specified type NEC A03.8
    Sonne A03.3
    specified type NEC A03.8
  balantidial A07.0
  Balantidium coli A07.0
  Boyd's A03.2
  candidal B37.82
  Chilomastix A07.8
  Chinese A03.9
  coccidial A07.3
  Dientamoeba (fragilis) A07.8
  Embadomonas A07.8
  Entamoeba, entamebic —*see* Dysentery,
    amebic

Dysentery, dysenteric *(Continued)*
  Flexner-Boyd A03.2
  Flexner's A03.1
  Giardia lamblia A07.1
  Hiss-Russell A03.1
  Lamblia A07.1
  leishmanial B55.0
  malarial —*see* Malaria
  metazoal B82.0
  monilial B37.82
  protozoal A07.9
  Salmonella A02.0
  schistosomal B65.1
  Schmitz (-Stutzer) A03.0
  Shiga (-Kruse) A03.0
  Shigella NOS —*see* Dysentery, bacillary
  Sonne A03.3
  strongyloidiasis B78.0
  trichomonal A07.8
  viral *(see also* Enteritis, viral) A08.4
Dysequilibrium R42
Dysesthesia R20.8
  hysterical F44.6
Dysfibrinogenemia (congenital) D68.2
Dysfunction
  adrenal E27.9
    hyperfunction E27.0
  autonomic
    due to alcohol G31.2
    somatoform F45.8
  bladder N31.9
    neurogenic NOS —*see* Dysfunction,
      bladder, neuromuscular
    neuromuscular NOS N31.9
      atonic (motor) (sensory) N31.2
      autonomous N31.2
      flaccid N31.2
      nonreflex N31.2
      reflex N31.1
      specified NEC N31.8
      uninhibited N31.0
  bleeding, uterus N93.8
  cerebral G93.89
  colon K59.9
    psychogenic F45.8
  colostomy K94.03
  cystic duct K82.8
  cystostomy (stoma) —*see* Complications,
      cystostomy
  ejaculatory N53.19
    anejaculatory orgasm N53.13
    painful N53.12
    premature F52.4
    retarded N53.11
  endocrine NOS E34.9
  endometrium N85.8
  enterostomy K94.13
  gallbladder K82.8
  gastrostomy (stoma) K94.23
  gland, glandular NOS E34.9
  heart I51.89
  hemoglobin D75.89
  hepatic K76.89
  hypophysis E23.7
  hypothalamic NEC E23.3
  ileostomy (stoma) K94.13
  jejunostomy (stoma) K94.13
  kidney —*see* Disease, renal
  labyrinthine —*see* subcategory H83.2
  left ventricular, following sudden emotional
      stress I51.81
  liver K76.89
  male —*see* Dysfunction, sexual, male
  orgasmic (female) F52.31
    male F52.32
  ovary E28.9
    specified NEC E28.8
  papillary muscle I51.89
  parathyroid E21.4
  physiological NEC R68.89
    psychogenic F59

Dysfunction *(Continued)*
  pineal gland E34.8
  pituitary (gland) E23.3
  platelets D69.1
  polyglandular E31.9
    specified NEC E31.8
  psychophysiologic F59
  psychosexual F52.9
    with
      dyspareunia F52.6
      premature ejaculation F52.4
      vaginismus F52.5
  pylorus K31.9
  rectum K59.9
    psychogenic F45.8
  reflex (sympathetic) —*see* Syndrome, pain,
      complex regional I
  segmental —*see* Dysfunction, somatic
  senile R54
  sexual (due to) R37
    alcohol F10.981
    amphetamine F15.981
      in
        abuse F15.181
        dependence F15.281
    anxiolytic F13.981
      in
        abuse F13.181
        dependence F13.281
    cocaine F14.981
      in
        abuse F14.181
        dependence F14.281
    excessive sexual drive F52.8
    failure of genital response (male)
      F52.21
    female F52.22
    female N94.9
      aversion F52.1
      dyspareunia N94.1
        psychogenic F52.6
      frigidity F52.22
      nymphomania F52.8
      orgasmic F52.31
      psychogenic F52.9
        aversion F52.1
        dyspareunia F52.6
        frigidity F52.22
        nymphomania F52.8
        orgasmic F52.31
        vaginismus F52.5
      vaginismus N94.2
        psychogenic F52.5
    hypnotic F13.981
      in
        abuse F13.181
        dependence F13.281
    inhibited orgasm (female) F52.31
      male F52.32
    lack
      of sexual enjoyment F52.1
      or loss of sexual desire F52.0
    male N53.9
      anejaculatory orgasm N53.13
      ejaculatory N53.19
        painful N53.12
        premature F52.4
        retarded N53.11
      erectile N52.9
        drug induced N52.2
        due to
          disease classified elsewhere N52.1
          drug N52.2
        postoperative (postprocedural) N52.39
          following
            prostatectomy N52.34
              radical N52.31
            radical cystectomy N52.32
            urethral surgery N52.33
        psychogenic F52.21
        specified cause NEC N52.8

Dysfunction *(Continued)*
  sexual *(Continued)*
    male *(Continued)*
      erectile *(Continued)*
        vasculogenic
          arterial insufficiency N52.01
            with corporo-venous occlusive
              N52.03
          corporo-venous occlusive N52.02
            with arterial insufficiency
              N52.03
      impotence —*see* Dysfunction, sexual,
        male, erectile
      psychogenic F52.9
        aversion F52.1
        erectile F52.21
        orgasmic F52.32
        premature ejaculation F52.4
        satyriasis F52.8
        specified type NEC F52.8
      specified type NEC N53.8
    nonorganic F52.9
      specified NEC F52.8
    opioid F11.981
      in
        abuse F11.181
        dependence F11.281
    orgasmic dysfunction (female) F52.31
      male F52.32
    premature ejaculation F52.4
    psychoactive substances NEC F19.981
      in
        abuse F19.181
        dependence F19.281
    psychogenic F52.9
    sedative F13.981
      in
        abuse F13.181
        dependence F13.281
    sexual aversion F52.1
    vaginismus (nonorganic) (psychogenic)
      F52.5
  sinoatrial node I49.5
  somatic M99.09
    abdomen M99.09
    acromioclavicular M99.07
    cervical region M99.01
    cervicothoracic M99.01
    costochondral M99.08
    costovertebral M99.08
    head region M99.00
    hip M99.05
    lower extremity M99.06
    lumbar region M99.03
    lumbosacral M99.03
    occipitocervical M99.00
    pelvic region M99.05
    pubic M99.05
    rib cage M99.08
    sacral region M99.04
    sacrococcygeal M99.04
    sacroiliac M99.04
    specified NEC M99.09
    sternochondral M99.08
    sternoclavicular M99.07
    thoracic region M99.02
    thoracolumbar M99.02
    upper extremity M99.07
  somatoform autonomic F45.8
  stomach K31.89
    psychogenic F45.8
  suprarenal E27.9
    hyperfunction E27.0
  symbolic R48.9
    specified type NEC R48.8
  temporomandibular (joint) M26.69
    joint-pain syndrome M26.62
  testicular (endocrine) E29.9
    specified NEC E29.8
  thymus E32.9
  thyroid E07.9

◀ New   ◀▥ Revised   ~~deleted~~ Deleted

Dysfunction *(Continued)*
ureterostomy (stoma) —*see* Complications, stoma, urinary tract
urethrostomy (stoma) —*see* Complications, stoma, urinary tract
uterus, complicating delivery O62.9
hypertonic O62.4
hypotonic O62.2
primary O62.0
secondary O62.1
ventricular I51.9
with congestive heart failure I50.9-
left, reversible, following sudden emotional stress I51.81

Dysgenesis
gonadal (due to chromosomal anomaly) Q96.9
pure Q99.1
renal Q60.5
bilateral Q60.4
unilateral Q60.3
reticular D72.0
tidal platelet D69.3

Dysgerminoma
specified site —*see* Neoplasm, malignant, by site
unspecified site
female C56.9
male C62.90

Dysgeusia R43.2
Dysgraphia R27.8
Dyshidrosis, dysidrosis L30.1
Dyskaryotic cervical smear R87.619
Dyskeratosis L85.8
cervix —*see* Dysplasia, cervix
congenital Q82.8
uterus NEC N85.8
Dyskinesia G24.9
biliary (cystic duct or gallbladder) K82.8
drug induced
orofacial G24.01
esophagus K22.4
hysterical F44.4
intestinal K59.8
nonorganic origin F44.4
orofacial (idiopathic) G24.4
drug induced G24.01
psychogenic F44.4
subacute, drug induced G24.01
tardive G24.01
neuroleptic induced G24.01
trachea J39.8
tracheobronchial J98.09
Dyslalia (developmental) F80.0
Dyslexia R48.0
developmental F81.0
Dyslipidemia E78.5
depressed HDL cholesterol E78.6
elevated fasting triglycerides E78.1
Dysmaturity —*see also* Light for dates
pulmonary (newborn) (Wilson-Mikity) P27.0
Dysmenorrhea (essential) (exfoliative) N94.6
congestive (syndrome) N94.6
primary N94.4
psychogenic F45.8
secondary N94.5
Dysmetabolic syndrome X E88.81
Dysmetria R27.8
Dysmorphism (due to)
alcohol Q86.0
exogenous cause NEC Q86.8
hydantoin Q86.1
warfarin Q86.2
Dysmorphophobia (nondelusional) F45.22
delusional F22
Dysnomia R47.01
Dysorexia R63.0
psychogenic F50.8

Dysostosis
cleidocranial, cleidocranialis Q74.0
craniofacial Q75.1
Fairbank's (idiopathic familial generalized osteophytosis) Q78.9
mandibulofacial (incomplete) Q75.4
multiplex E76.01
oculomandibular Q75.5
Dyspareunia (female) N94.1
male N53.12
nonorganic F52.6
psychogenic F52.6
secondary N94.1
Dyspepsia R10.13
atonic K30
functional (allergic) (congenital) (gastrointestinal) (occupational) (reflex) K30
intestinal K59.8
nervous F45.8
neurotic F45.8
psychogenic F45.8
Dysphagia R13.10
cervical R13.19
following
cerebral infarction I69.391
cerebrovascular disease I69.991
specified NEC I69.891
intracerebral hemorrhage I69.191
nontraumatic intracranial hemorrhage NEC I69.291
specified disease NEC I69.891
subarachnoid hemorrhage I69.091
functional (hysterical) F45.8
hysterical F45.8
nervous (hysterical) F45.8
neurogenic R13.19
oral phase R13.11
oropharyngeal phase R13.12
pharyneal phase R13.13
pharyngoesophageal phase R13.14
psychogenic F45.8
sideropenic D50.1
spastica K22.4
specified NEC R13.19
Dysphagocytosis, congenital D71
Dysphasia R47.02
developmental
expressive type F80.1
receptive type F80.2
following
cerebrovascular disease I69.921
cerebral infarction I69.321
intracerebral hemorrhage I69.121
nontraumatic intracranial hemorrhage NEC I69.221
specified disease NEC I69.821
subarachnoid hemorrhage I69.021
Dysphonia R49.0
functional F44.4
hysterical F44.4
psychogenic F44.4
spastica J38.3
Dysphoria, postpartal O90.6
Dyspituitarism E23.3
Dysplasia —*see also* Anomaly
acetabular, congenital Q65.89
alveolar capillary, with vein misalignment J84.843
anus (histologically confirmed) (mild) (moderate) K62.82
severe D01.3
arrhythmogenic right ventricular I42.8
arterial, fibromuscular I77.3
asphyxiating thoracic (congenital) Q77.2
brain Q07.9
bronchopulmonary, perinatal P27.1
cervix (uteri) N87.9
mild N87.0
moderate N87.1
severe D06.9

Dysplasia *(Continued)*
chondroectodermal Q77.6
colon D12.6
craniometaphyseal Q78.5
dentinal K00.5
diaphyseal, progressive Q78.3
dystrophic Q77.5
ectodermal (anhidrotic) (congenital) (hereditary) Q82.4
hydrotic Q82.8
epithelial, uterine cervix —*see* Dysplasia, cervix
eye (congenital) Q11.2
fibrous
bone NEC (monostotic) M85.00
ankle M85.07-
foot M85.07-
forearm M85.03-
hand M85.04-
lower leg M85.06-
multiple site M85.09
neck M85.08
rib M85.08
shoulder M85.01-
skull M85.08
specified site NEC M85.08
thigh M85.05-
toe M85.07-
upper arm M85.02-
vertebra M85.08
diaphyseal, progressive Q78.3
jaw M27.8
polyostotic Q78.1
florid osseous —*see also* Cyst, calcifying odontogenic
high grade, focal D12.6
hip, congenital Q65.89
joint, congenital Q74.8
kidney Q61.4
multicystic Q61.4
leg Q74.2
lung, congenital (not associated with short gestation) Q33.6
mammary (gland) (benign) N60.9-
cyst (solitary) —*see* Cyst, breast
cystic —*see* Mastopathy, cystic
duct ectasia —*see* Ectasia, mammary duct
fibroadenosis —*see* Fibroadenosis, breast
fibrosclerosis —*see* Fibrosclerosis, breast
specified type NEC N60.8-
metaphyseal (Jansen's) (McKusick's) (Schmid's) Q78.5
muscle Q79.8
oculodentodigital Q87.0
periapical (cemental) (cemento-osseous) —*see* Cyst, calcifying odontogenic
periosteum —*see* Disorder, bone, specified type NEC
polyostotic fibrous Q78.1
prostate (*see also* Neoplasia, intraepithelial, prostate) N42.3
severe D07.5
renal Q61.4
multicystic Q61.4
retinal, congenital Q14.1
right ventricular, arrhythmogenic I42.8
septo-optic Q04.4
skin L98.8
spinal cord Q06.1
spondyloepiphyseal Q77.7
thymic, with immunodeficiency D82.1
vagina N89.3
mild N89.0
moderate N89.1
severe NEC D07.2
vulva N90.3
mild N90.0
moderate N90.1
severe NEC D07.1

Dyspnea (nocturnal) (paroxysmal) R06.00
  asthmatic (bronchial) J45.909
    with
      bronchitis J45.909
        with
          exacerbation (acute) J45.901
          status asthmaticus J45.902
        chronic J44.9
      exacerbation (acute) J45.901
      status asthmaticus J45.902
    cardiac —*see* Failure, ventricular, left
  cardiac —*see* Failure, ventricular, left
  functional F45.8
  hyperventilation R06.4
  hysterical F45.8
  newborn P28.89
  psychogenic F45.8
  shortness of breath R06.02
  specified type NEC R06.09
Dyspraxia R27.8
  developmental (syndrome) F82
Dysproteinemia E88.09
Dysreflexia, autonomic G90.4
Dysrhythmia
  cardiac I49.9
    newborn
      bradycardia P29.12
        occurring before birth P03.819
          before onset of labor P03.810
          during labor P03.811
      tachycardia P29.11
    postoperative I97.89
  cerebral or cortical —*see* Epilepsy
Dyssomnia —*see* Disorder, sleep
Dyssynergia
  biliary K83.8
  bladder sphincter N36.44
  cerebellaris myoclonica (Hunt's ataxia) G11.1
Dysthymia F34.1
Dysthyroidism E07.9
Dystocia O66.9
  affecting newborn P03.1
  cervical (hypotonic) O62.2
    affecting newborn P03.6
    primary O62.0
    secondary O62.1
  contraction ring O62.4
  fetal O66.9
    abnormality NEC O66.3
    conjoined twins O66.3
    oversize O66.2
  maternal O66.9
  positional O64.9
  shoulder (girdle) O66.0
    causing obstructed labor O66.0
  uterine NEC O62.4

Dystonia G24.9
  deformans progressiva G24.1
  drug induced NEC G24.09
    acute G24.02
    specified NEC G24.09
  familial G24.1
  idiopathic G24.1
    familial G24.1
    nonfamilial G24.2
    orofacial G24.4
  lenticularis G24.8
  musculorum deformans G24.1
  neuroleptic induced (acute) G24.02
  orofacial (idiopathic) G24.4
  oromandibular G24.4
    due to drug G24.01
  specified NEC G24.8
  torsion (familial) (idiopathic) G24.1
    acquired G24.8
    genetic G24.1
    symptomatic (nonfamilial) G24.2
Dystonic movements R25.8
Dystrophy, dystrophia
  adiposogenital E23.6
  Becker's type G71.0
  cervical sympathetic G90.2
  choroid (hereditary) H31.20
    central areolar H31.22
    choroideremia H31.21
    gyrate atrophy H31.23
    specified type NEC H31.29
  cornea (hereditary) H18.50
    endothelial H18.51
    epithelial H18.52
    granular H18.53
    lattice H18.54
    macular H18.55
    specified type NEC H18.59
  Duchenne's type G71.0
  due to malnutrition E45
  Erb's G71.0
  Fuchs' H18.51
  Gower's muscular G71.0
  hair L67.8
  infantile neuraxonal G31.89
  Landouzy-Déjérine G71.0
  Leyden-Möbius G71.0
  muscular G71.0
    benign (Becker type) G71.0
    congenital (hereditary) (progressive)
      (with specific morphological
      abnormalities of the muscle fiber)
      G71.0
      myotonic G71.11
    distal G71.0
    Duchenne type G71.0
    Emery-Dreifuss G71.0

Dystrophy, dystrophia *(Continued)*
  muscular *(Continued)*
    Erb type G71.0
    facioscapulohumeral G71.0
    Gower's G71.0
    hereditary (progressive) G71.0
    Landouzy-Déjérine type G71.0
    limb-girdle G71.0
    myotonic G71.11
    progressive (hereditary) G71.0
      Charcot-Marie (-Tooth) type
      G60.0
    pseudohypertrophic (infantile)
      G71.0
    severe (Duchenne type) G71.0
  myocardium, myocardial —*see*
    Degeneration, myocardial
  nail L60.3
    congenital Q84.6
  nutritional E45
  ocular G71.0
  oculocerebrorenal E72.03
  oculopharyngeal G71.0
  ovarian N83.8
  polyglandular E31.8
  reflex (neuromuscular) (sympathetic) —
    see Syndrome, pain, complex
    regional I
  retinal (hereditary) H35.50
    in
      lipid storage disorders E75.6
        [H36]
      systemic lipidoses E75.6 *[H36]*
    involving
      pigment epithelium H35.54
      sensory area H35.53
    pigmentary H35.52
    vitreoretinal H35.51
  Salzmann's nodular —*see* Degeneration,
    cornea, nodular
  scapuloperoneal G71.0
  skin NEC L98.8
  sympathetic (reflex) —*see* Syndrome, pain,
    complex regional I
    cervical G90.2
  tapetoretinal H35.54
  thoracic, asphyxiating Q77.2
  unguium L60.3
    congenital Q84.6
  vitreoretinal H35.51
  vulva N90.4
  yellow (liver) —*see* Failure, hepatic
Dysuria R30.0
  psychogenic F45.8

E

Eales' disease H35.06-
Ear —see also condition
  piercing Z41.3
  tropical B36.8
  wax (impacted) H61.20
    left H61.22
      with right H61.23
    right H61.21
      with left H61.23
Earache —see subcategory H92.0
Early satiety R68.81
Eaton-Lambert syndrome—see Syndrome,
  Lambert-Eaton
Eberth's disease (typhoid fever) A01.00
Ebola virus disease A98.4
Ebstein's anomaly or syndrome (heart) Q22.5
Eccentro-osteochondrodysplasia E76.29
Ecchondroma —see Neoplasm, bone, benign
Ecchondrosis D48.0
Ecchymosis R58
  conjunctiva —see Hemorrhage, conjunctiva
  eye (traumatic) —see Contusion, eyeball
  eyelid (traumatic) —see Contusion, eyelid
  newborn P54.5
  spontaneous R23.3
  traumatic —see Contusion
Echinocciasis —see Echinococcus
Echinococcosis —see Echinococcus
Echinococcus (infection) B67.90
  granulosus B67.4
    bone B67.2
    liver B67.0
    lung B67.1
    multiple sites B67.32
    specified site NEC B67.39
    thyroid B67.31 [E35]
  liver NOS B67.8
    granulosus B67.0
    multilocularis B67.5
  lung NEC B67.99
    granulosus B67.1
    multilocularis B67.69
  multilocularis B67.7
    liver B67.5
    multiple sites B67.61
    specified site NEC B67.69
  specified site NEC B67.99
    granulosus B67.39
    multilocularis B67.69
  thyroid NEC B67.99
    granulosus B67.31 [E35]
    multilocularis B67.69 [E35]
Echinorhynchiasis B83.8
Echinostomiasis B66.8
Echolalia R48.8
Echovirus, as cause of disease classified
  elsewhere B97.12
Eclampsia, eclamptic (coma) (convulsions)
  (delirium) (with hypertension) NEC O15.9
  during labor and delivery O15.1
  postpartum O15.2
  pregnancy O15.0-
  puerperal O15.2
Economic circumstances affecting care Z59.9
Economo's disease A85.8
Ectasia, ectasis
  annuloaortic I35.8
  aorta I77.819
    with aneurysm —see Aneurysm, aorta
    abdominal I77.811
    thoracic I77.810
    thoracoabdominal I77.812
  breast —see Ectasia, mammary duct
  capillary I78.8
  cornea H18.71-
  gastric antral vascular (GAVE) K31.819
    with hemorrhage K31.811
    without hemorrhage K31.819
  mammary duct N60.4-

Ectasia, ectasis (Continued)
  salivary gland (duct) K11.8
  sclera —see Sclerectasia
Ecthyma L08.0
  contagiosum B08.02
  gangrenosum L08.0
  infectiosum B08.02
Ectocardia Q24.8
Ectodermal dysplasia (anhidrotic) Q82.4
Ectodermosis crosiva pluriorificialis
    L51.1
Ectopic, ectopia (congenital)
  abdominal viscera Q45.8
    due to defect in anterior abdominal wall
      Q79.59
  ACTH syndrome E24.3
  adrenal gland Q89.1
  anus Q43.5
  atrial beats I49.1
  beats I49.49
    atrial I49.1
    ventricular I49.3
  bladder Q64.10
  bone and cartilage in lung Q33.5
  brain Q04.8
  breast tissue Q83.8
  cardiac Q24.8
  cerebral Q04.8
  cordis Q24.8
  endometrium —see Endometriosis
  gastric mucosa Q40.2
  gestation —see Pregnancy, by site
  heart Q24.8
  hormone secretion NEC E34.2
  kidney (crossed) (pelvis) Q63.2
  lens, lentis Q12.1
  mole —see Pregnancy, by site
  organ or site NEC —see Malposition,
    congenital
  pancreas Q45.3
  pregnancy —see Pregnancy, ectopic
  pupil —see Abnormality, pupillary
  renal Q63.2
  sebaceous glands of mouth Q38.6
  spleen Q89.09
  testis Q53.00
    bilateral Q53.02
    unilateral Q53.01
  thyroid Q89.2
  tissue in lung Q33.5
  ureter Q62.63
  ventricular beats I49.3
  vesicae Q64.10
Ectromelia Q73.8
  lower limb —see Defect, reduction, limb,
    lower, specified type NEC
  upper limb —see Defect, reduction, limb,
    upper, specified type NEC
Ectropion H02.109
  cervix N86
    with cervicitis N72
  congenital Q10.1
  eyelid (paralytic) H02.109
    cicatricial H02.119
      left H02.116
        lower H02.115
        upper H02.114
      right H02.113
        lower H02.112
        upper H02.111
    congenital Q10.1
    left H02.106
      lower H02.105
      upper H02.104
    mechanical H02.129
      left H02.126
        lower H02.125
        upper H02.124
      right H02.123
        lower H02.122
        upper H02.121

Ectropion (Continued)
  eyelid (Continued)
    right H02.103
      lower H02.102
      upper H02.101
    senile H02.139
      left H02.136
        lower H02.135
        upper H02.134
      right H02.133
        lower H02.132
        upper H02.131
    spastic H02.149
      left H02.146
        lower H02.145
        upper H02.144
      right H02.143
        lower H02.142
        upper H02.141
  iris H21.89
  lip (acquired) K13.0
    congenital Q38.0
  urethra N36.8
  uvea H21.89
Eczema (acute) (chronic) (erythematous)
    (fissum) (rubrum) (squamous) (see also
    Dermatitis) L30.9
  contact —see Dermatitis, contact
  dyshydrotic L30.1
  external ear —see Otitis, externa, acute,
    eczematoid
  flexural L20.82
  herpeticum B00.0
  hypertrophicum L28.0
  hypostatic —see Varix, leg, with,
    inflammation
  impetiginous L01.1
  infantile (due to any substance)
    L20.83
    intertriginous L21.1
    seborrheic L21.1
  intertriginous NEC L30.4
    infantile L21.1
  intrinsic (allergic) L20.84
  lichenified NEC L28.0
  marginatum (hebrae) B35.6
  pustular L30.3
  stasis —see Varix, leg, with, inflammation
  vaccination, vaccinatum T88.1
  varicose —see Varix, leg, with,
    inflammation
Eczematid L30.2
Eddowes (-Spurway) syndrome Q78.0
Edema, edematous (infectious) (pitting)
    (toxic) R60.9
  with nephritis —see Nephrosis
  allergic T78.3
  amputation stump (surgical) (sequelae
    (late effect)) T87.89
  angioneurotic (allergic) (any site) (with
    urticaria) T78.3
    hereditary D84.1
  angiospastic I73.9
  Berlin's (traumatic) S05.8X-
  brain (cytotoxic) (vasogenic) G93.6
    due to birth injury P11.0
      newborn (anoxia or hypoxia) P52.4
        birth injury P11.0
    traumatic —see Injury, intracranial,
      cerebral edema
  cardiac —see Failure, heart, congestive
  cardiovascular —see Failure, heart,
    congestive
  cerebral —see Edema, brain
  cerebrospinal —see Edema, brain
  cervix (uteri) (acute) N88.8
    puerperal, postpartum O90.89
  chronic hereditary Q82.0
  circumscribed, acute T78.3
    hereditary D84.1
  conjunctiva H11.42-

Edema, edematous *(Continued)*
  cornea H18.2-
    idiopathic H18.22-
    secondary H18.23-
      due to contact lens H18.21-
  due to
    lymphatic obstruction I89.0
    salt retention E87.0
  epiglottis —*see* Edema, glottis
  essential, acute T78.3
    hereditary D84.1
  extremities, lower —*see* Edema, legs
  eyelid NEC H02.849
    left H02.846
      lower H02.845
      upper H02.844
    right H02.843
      lower H02.842
      upper H02.841
  familial, hereditary Q82.0
  famine —*see* Malnutrition, severe
  generalized R60.1
  glottis, glottic, glottidis (obstructive) (passive)
        J38.4
    allergic T78.3
      hereditary D84.1
  heart —*see* Failure, heart, congestive
  heat T67.7
  hereditary Q82.0
  inanition —*see* Malnutrition, severe
  intracranial G93.6
  iris H21.89
  joint —*see* Effusion, joint
  larynx —*see* Edema, glottis
  legs R60.0
    due to venous obstruction I87.1
    hereditary Q82.0
  localized R60.0
    due to venous obstruction I87.1
  lower limbs —*see* Edema, legs
  lung J81.1
    with heart condition or failure —*see*
        Failure, ventricular, left
    acute J81.0
    chemical (acute) J68.1
      chronic J68.1
    chronic J81.1
      due to
        chemicals, gases, fumes or vapors
            (inhalation) J68.1
        external agent J70.9
          specified NEC J70.8
        radiation J70.1
    due to
      chemicals, fumes or vapors (inhalation)
          J68.1
      external agent J70.9
        specified NEC J70.8
      high altitude T70.29
      near drowning T75.1
      radiation J70.0
    meaning failure, left ventricle I50.1
  lymphatic I89.0
    due to mastectomy I97.2
  macula H35.81
    cystoid, following cataract surgery —*see*
        Complications, postprocedural,
        following cataract surgery
    diabetic —*see* Diabetes, by type, with,
        retinopathy, with macular edema
  malignant —*see* Gangrene, gas
  Milroy's Q82.0
  nasopharynx J39.2
  newborn P83.30
    hydrops fetalis —*see* Hydrops, fetalis
    specified NEC P83.39
  nutritional —*see also* Malnutrition, severe
    with dyspigmentation, skin and hair E40
  optic disc or nerve —*see* Papilledema
  orbit H05.22-
  pancreas K86.8

Edema, edematous *(Continued)*
  papilla, optic —*see* Papilledema
  penis N48.89
  periodic T78.3
    hereditary D84.1
  pharynx J39.2
  pulmonary —*see* Edema, lung
  Quincke's T78.3
    hereditary D84.1
  renal —*see* Nephrosis
  retina H35.81
    diabetic —*see* Diabetes, by type, with,
        retinopathy, with macular edema
  salt E87.0
  scrotum N50.8
  seminal vesicle N50.8
  spermatic cord N50.8
  spinal (cord) (vascular) (nontraumatic) G95.19
  starvation —*see* Malnutrition, severe
  stasis —*see* Hypertension, venous, (chronic)
  subglottic —*see* Edema, glottis
  supraglottic —*see* Edema, glottis
  testis N44.8
  tunica vaginalis N50.8
  vas deferens N50.8
  vulva (acute) N90.89
Edentulism —*see* Absence, teeth, acquired
Edsall's disease T67.2
Educational handicap Z55.9
  specified NEC Z55.8
Edward's syndrome —*see* Trisomy, 18
Effect, adverse
  abnormal gravitational (G) forces or states
      T75.81
  abuse —*see* Maltreatment
  air pressure T70.9
    specified NEC T70.8
  altitude (high) —*see* Effect, adverse, high
      altitude
  anesthesia (*see also* Anesthesia) T88.59
    in labor and delivery O74.9
    in pregnancy NEC O29.3-
    local, toxic
      in labor and delivery O74.4-
      postpartum, puerperal O89.3
    postpartum, puerperal O89.9
    specified NEC T88.59
      in labor and delivery O74.8
      postpartum, puerperal O89.8
    spinal and epidural T88.59
      headache T88.59
        in labor and delivery O74.5
        postpartum, puerperal O89.4
      specified NEC
        in labor and delivery O74.6
        postpartum, puerperal O89.5
  antitoxin —*see* Complications, vaccination
  atmospheric pressure T70.9
    due to explosion T70.8
    high T70.3
    low —*see* Effect, adverse, high altitude
    specified effect NEC T70.8
  biological, correct substance properly
      administered —*see* Effect, adverse, drug
  blood (derivatives) (serum) (transfusion) —
      see Complications, transfusion
  chemical substance —*see* Table of Drugs and
      Chemicals
  cold (temperature) (weather) T69.9
    chilblains T69.1
    frostbite —*see* Frostbite
    specified effect NEC T69.8
  drugs and medicaments T88.7
    specified drug —*see* Table of Drugs and
        Chemicals, by drug, adverse effect
    specified effect — code to condition
  electric current, electricity (shock) T75.4
    burn —*see* Burn
  exertion (excessive) T73.3
  exposure —*see* Exposure
  external cause NEC T75.89

Effect, adverse *(Continued)*
  foodstuffs T78.1
    allergic reaction —*see* Allergy, food
      causing anaphylaxis —*see* Shock,
        anaphylactic, due to food
    noxious —*see* Poisoning, food, noxious
  gases, fumes, or vapors T59.9-
    specified agent —*see* Table of Drugs and
        Chemicals
  glue (airplane) sniffing
    due to drug abuse —*see* Abuse, drug,
        inhalant
    due to drug dependence —*see* Dependence,
        drug, inhalant
  heat —*see* Heat
  high altitude NEC T70.29
    anoxia T70.29
    on
      ears T70.0
      sinuses T70.1
    polycythemia D75.1
  high pressure fluids T70.4
  hot weather —*see* Heat
  hunger T73.0
  immersion, foot —*see* Immersion
  immunization —*see* Complications,
      vaccination
  immunological agents —*see* Complications,
      vaccination
  infrared (radiation) (rays) NOS T66
    dermatitis or eczema L59.8
  infusion —*see* Complications, infusion
  lack of care of infants —*see* Maltreatment,
      child
  lightning —*see* Lightning
  medical care T88.9
    specified NEC T88.8
  medicinal substance, correct, properly
      administered —*see* Effect, adverse, drug
  motion T75.3
  noise, on inner ear —*see* subcategory H83.3
  overheated places —*see* Heat
  psychosocial, of work environment Z56.5
  radiation (diagnostic) (infrared) (natural
      source) (therapeutic) (ultraviolet)
      (X-ray) NOS T66
    dermatitis or eczema —*see* Dermatitis, due
        to, radiation
    fibrosis of lung J70.1
    pneumonitis J70.0
    pulmonary manifestations
      acute J70.0
      chronic J70.1
    skin L59.9
  radioactive substance NOS
    dermatitis or eczema —*see* Radiodermatitis
  reduced temperature T69.9
    immersion foot or hand —*see* Immersion
    specified effect NEC T69.8
  serum NEC (*see also* Reaction, serum)
      T80.69
  specified NEC T78.8
    external cause NEC T75.89
  strangulation —*see* Asphyxia, traumatic
  submersion T75.1
  thirst T73.1
  toxic —*see* Toxicity
  transfusion —*see* Complications, transfusion
  ultraviolet (radiation) (rays) NOS T66
    burn —*see* Burn
    dermatitis or eczema —*see* Dermatitis, due
        to, ultraviolet rays
      acute L56.8
  vaccine (any) —*see* Complications,
      vaccination
  vibration —*see* Vibration, adverse effects
  water pressure NEC T70.9
    specified NEC T70.8
  weightlessness T75.82
  whole blood —*see* Complications, transfusion
  work environment Z56.5

◄ New   ◄▦ Revised   ~~deleted~~ Deleted

Effect (s) (of) (from) —*see* Effect, adverse NEC
Effects, late —*see* Sequelae
Effluvium
  anagen L65.1
  telogen L65.0
Effort syndrome (psychogenic) F45.8
Effusion
  amniotic fluid —*see* Pregnancy, complicated
    by, prematue rupture of membranes
  brain (serous) G93.6
  bronchial —*see* Bronchitis
  cerebral G93.6
  cerebrospinal —*see also* Meningitis
    vessel G93.6
  chest —*see* Effusion, pleura
  chylous, chyliform (pleura) J94.0
  intracranial G93.6
  joint M25.40
    ankle M25.47-
    elbow M25.42-
    foot joint M25.47-
    hand joint M25.44-
    hip M25.45-
    knee M25.46-
    shoulder M25.41-
    specified joint NEC M25.48
    wrist M25.43-
  malignant pleural J91.0
  meninges —*see* Meningitis
  pericardium, pericardial (noninflammatory)
    I31.3
    acute —*see* Pericarditis, acute
  peritoneal (chronic) R18.8
  pleura, pleurisy, pleuritic, pleuropericardial
    J90
    chylous, chyliform J94.0
    due to systemic lupus erythematosis
      M32.13
    influenzal —*see* Influenza, with, respiratory
      manifestations NEC
    malignant J91.0
    newborn P28.89
    tuberculous NEC A15.6
      primary (progressive) A15.7
  spinal —*see* Meningitis
  thorax, thoracic —*see* Effusion, pleura
Egg shell nails L60.3
  congenital Q84.6
Egyptian splenomegaly B65.1
Ehlers-Danlos syndrome Q79.6
Ehrlichiosis A77.40
  due to
    E. chafeensis A77.41
    E. sennetsu A79.81
    specified organism NEC A77.49
Eichstedt's disease B36.0
Eisenmenger's
  complex or syndrome I27.89
  defect Q21.8
Ejaculation
  painful N53.12
  premature F52.4
  retarded N53.11
  retrograde N53.14
  semen, painful N53.12
    psychogenic F52.6
Ekbom's syndrome (restless legs) G25.81
Ekman's syndrome (brittle bones and blue
  sclera) Q78.0
Elastic skin Q82.8
  acquired L57.4
Elastofibroma —*see* Neoplasm, connective
  tissue, benign
Elastoma (juvenile) Q82.8
  Miescher's L87.2
Elastomyofibrosis I42.4
Elastosis
  actinic, solar L57.8
  atrophicans (senile) L57.4
  perforans serpiginosa L87.2
  senilis L57.4

Elbow —*see* condition
Electric current, electricity, effects (concussion)
  (fatal) (nonfatal) (shock) T75.4
  burn —*see* Burn
Electric feet syndrome E53.8
Electrocution T75.4
  from electroshock gun (taser) T75.4
Electrolyte imbalance E87.8
  with
    abortion —*see* Abortion by type,
      complicated by, electrolyte imbalance
    ectopic pregnancy O08.5
    molar pregnancy O08.5
Elephantiasis (nonfilarial) I89.0
  arabicum —*see* Infestation, filarial
  bancroftian B74.0
  congenital (any site) (hereditary) Q82.0
  due to
    Brugia (malayi) B74.1
      timori B74.2
    mastectomy I97.2
    Wuchereria (bancrofti) B74.0
  eyelid H02.859
    left H02.856
      lower H02.855
      upper H02.854
    right H02.853
      lower H02.852
      upper H02.851
  filarial, filariensis —*see* Infestation, filarial
  glandular I89.0
  graecorum A30.9
  lymphangiectatic I89.0
  lymphatic vessel I89.0
    due to mastectomy I97.2
  scrotum (nonfilarial) I89.0
  streptococcal I89.0
  surgical I97.89
    postmastectomy I97.2
  telangiectodes I89.0
  vulva (nonfilarial) N90.89
Elevated, elevation
  antibody titer R76.0
  basal metabolic rate R94.8
  blood pressure —*see also* Hypertension
    reading (incidental) (isolated) (nonspecific),
      no diagnosis of hypertension R03.0
  blood sugar R73.9
  body temperature (of unknown origin) R50.9
  C-reactive protein (CRP) R79.82
  cancer antigen 125 [CA 125] R97.1
  carcinoembryonic antigen [CEA] R97.0
  cholesterol E78.0
    with high triglycerides E78.2
  conjugate, eye H51.0
  diaphragm, congenital Q79.1
  erythrocyte sedimentation rate R70.0
  fasting glucose R73.01
  fasting triglycerides E78.1
  finding on laboratory examination —*see*
    Findings, abnormal, inconclusive,
    without diagnosis, by type of exam
  GFR (glomerular filtration rate) —*see*
    Findings, abnormal, inconclusive,
    without diagnosis, by type of exam
  glucose tolerance (oral) R73.02
  immunoglobulin level R76.8
  indoleacetic acid R82.5
  lactic acid dehydrogenase (LDH) level R74.0
  leukocytes D72.829
  lipoprotein a level E78.8
  liver function
    study R94.5
    test R79.89
      alkaline phosphatase R74.8
      aminotransferase R74.0
      bilirubin R17
      hepatic enzyme R74.8
      lactate dehydrogenase R74.0
  lymphocytes D72.820
  prostate specific antigen [PSA] R97.2

Elevated, elevation (*Continued*)
  Rh titer —*see* Complication (s), transfusion,
    incompatibility reaction, Rh (factor)
  scapula, congenital Q74.0
  sedimentation rate R70.0
  SGOT R74.0
  SGPT R74.0
  transaminase level R74.0
  triglycerides E78.1
    with high cholesterol E78.2
  tumor associated antigens [TAA] NEC
    R97.8
  tumor specific antigens [TSA] NEC R97.8
  urine level of
    17-ketosteroids R82.5
    catecholamine R82.5
    indoleacetic acid R82.5
    steroids R82.5
    vanillylmandelic acid (VMA) R82.5
  venous pressure I87.8
  white blood cell count D72.829
    specified NEC D72.828
Elliptocytosis (congenital) (hereditary) D58.1
  Hb C (disease) D58.1
  hemoglobin disease D58.1
  sickle-cell (disease) D57.8-
    trait D57.3
Ellison-Zollinger syndrome E16.4
Ellis-van Creveld syndrome
  (chondroectodermal dysplasia) Q77.6
Elongated, elongation (congenital) —*see also*
  Distortion
  bone Q79.9
  cervix (uteri) Q51.828
    acquired N88.4
    hypertrophic N88.4
  colon Q43.8
  common bile duct Q44.5
  cystic duct Q44.5
  frenulum, penis Q55.69
  labia minora (acquired) N90.6
  ligamentum patellae Q74.1
  petiolus (epiglottidis) Q31.8
  tooth, teeth K00.2
  uvula Q38.6
Eltor cholera A00.1
Emaciation (due to malnutrition) E41
Embadomoniasis A07.8
Embedded tooth, teeth K01.0
  root only K08.3
Embolic —*see* condition
Embolism (multiple) (paradoxical) I74.9
  air (any site) (traumatic) T79.0
    following
      abortion —*see* Abortion by type
        complicated by embolism
      ectopic pregnancy O08.2
      infusion, therapeutic injection or
        transfusion T80.0
      molar pregnancy O08.2
      procedure NEC
        artery T81.719
          mesenteric T81.710
          renal T81.711
          specified NEC T81.718
        vein T81.72
    in pregnancy, childbirth or puerperium —
      see Embolism, obstetric
  amniotic fluid (pulmonary) —*see also*
    Embolism, obstetric
    following
      abortion —*see* Abortion by type
        complicated by embolism
      ectopic pregnancy O08.2
      molar pregnancy O08.2
  aorta, aortic I74.10
    abdominal I74.09
      saddle I74.01
    bifurcation I74.09
    saddle I74.01
    thoracic I74.11

Embolism (*Continued*)
artery I74.9
  auditory, internal I65.8
  basilar —*see* Occlusion, artery, basilar
  carotid (common) (internal) —*see*
    Occlusion, artery, carotid
  cerebellar (anterior inferior) (posterior
    inferior) (superior) I66.3
  cerebral —*see* Occlusion, artery, cerebral
  choroidal (anterior) I66.8
  communicating posterior I66.8
  coronary —*see also* Infarct, myocardium
    not resulting in infarction I24.0
  extremity I74.4
    lower I74.3
    upper I74.2
  hypophyseal I66.8
  iliac I74.5
  limb I74.4
    lower I74.3
    upper I74.2
  mesenteric (with gangrene) K55.0
  ophthalmic —*see* Occlusion, artery, retina
  peripheral I74.4
  pontine I66.8
  precerebral —*see* Occlusion, artery,
    precerebral
  pulmonary —*see* Embolism, pulmonary
  renal N28.0
  retinal —*see* Occlusion, artery, retina
  septic I76
  specified NEC I74.8
  vertebral —*see* Occlusion, artery, vertebral
basilar (artery) I65.1
blood clot
  following
    abortion —*see* Abortion by type
      complicated by embolism
    ectopic or molar pregnancy O08.2
  in pregnancy, childbirth or puerperium —
    see Embolism, obstetric
brain —*see also* Occlusion, artery, cerebral
  following
    abortion —*see* Abortion by type
      complicated by embolism
    ectopic or molar pregnancy O08.2
  puerperal, postpartum, childbirth —*see*
    Embolism, obstetric
capillary I78.8
cardiac —*see also* Infarct, myocardium
  not resulting in infarction I24.0
carotid (artery) (common) (internal) —*see*
  Occlusion, artery, carotid
cavernous sinus (venous) —*see* Embolism,
  intracranial venous sinus
cerebral —*see* Occlusion, artery, cerebral
cholesterol —*see* Atheroembolism
coronary (artery or vein) (systemic) —*see*
  Occlusion, coronary
due to device, implant or graft —*see also*
  Complications, by site and type,
    specified NEC
  arterial graft NEC T82.818
  breast (implant) T85.81
  catheter NEC T85.81
    dialysis (renal) T82.818
      intraperitoneal T85.81
    infusion NEC T82.818
      spinal (epidural) (subdural) T85.81
    urinary (indwelling) T83.81
  electronic (electrode) (pulse generator)
    (stimulator)
    bone T84.81
    cardiac T82.817
    nervous system (brain) (peripheral
      nerve) (spinal) T85.81
    urinary T83.81
  fixation, internal (orthopedic) NEC T84.81
  gastrointestinal (bile duct) (esophagus)
    T85.81
  genital NEC T83.81

Embolism (*Continued*)
due to device, implant or graft (*Continued*)
  heart (graft) (valve) T82.817
  joint prosthesis T84.81
  ocular (corneal graft) (orbital implant)
    T85.81
  orthopedic (bone graft) NEC T86.838
  specified NEC T85.81
  urinary (graft) NEC T83.81
  vascular NEC T82.818
  ventricular intracranial shunt T85.81
extremities
  lower —*see* Embolism, vein, lower
    extremity
    arterial I74.3
  upper I74.2
eye H34.9
fat (cerebral) (pulmonary) (systemic) T79.1
  complicating delivery —*see* Embolism,
    obstetric
  following
    abortion —*see* Abortion by type
      complicated by embolism
    ectopic or molar pregnancy O08.2
following
  abortion —*see* Abortion by type
    complicated by embolism
  ectopic or molar pregnancy O08.2
  infusion, therapeutic injection or
    transfusion
    air T80.0
heart (fatty) —*see also* Infarct, myocardium
  not resulting in infarction I24.0
hepatic (vein) I82.0
in pregnancy, childbirth or puerperium —*see*
  Embolism, obstetric
intestine (artery) (vein) (with gangrene) K55.0
intracranial —*see also* Occlusion, artery,
  cerebral
  venous sinus (any) G08
    nonpyogenic I67.6
intraspinal venous sinuses or veins G08
  nonpyogenic G95.19
kidney (artery) N28.0
lateral sinus (venous) —*see* Embolism,
  intracranial, venous sinus
leg —*see* Embolism, vein, lower extremity
  arterial I74.3
longitudinal sinus (venous) —*see* Embolism,
  intracranial, venous sinus
lung (massive) —*see* Embolism, pulmonary
meninges I66.8
mesenteric (artery) (vein) (with gangrene)
  K55.0
obstetric (in) (pulmonary)
  childbirth O88.82
    air O88.02
    amniotic fluid O88.12
    blood clot O88.22
    fat O88.82
    pyemic O88.32
    septic O88.32
    specified type NEC O88.82
  pregnancy O88.81-
    air O88.01-
    amniotic fluid O88.11-
    blood clot O88.21-
    fat O88.81-
    pyemic O88.31-
    septic O88.31-
    specified type NEC O88.81-
  puerperal O88.83
    air O88.03
    amniotic fluid O88.13
    blood clot O88.23
    fat O88.83
    pyemic O88.33
    septic O88.33
    specified type NEC O88.83
ophthalmic —*see* Occlusion, artery, retina
penis N48.81

Embolism (*Continued*)
peripheral artery NOS I74.4
pituitary E23.6
popliteal (artery) I74.3
portal (vein) I81
postoperative, postprocedural
  artery T81.719
    mesenteric T81.710
    renal T81.711
    specified NEC T81.718
  vein T81.72
precerebral artery —*see* Occlusion, artery,
  precerebral
puerperal —*see* Embolism, obstetric
pulmonary (acute) (artery) (vein) I26.99
  with acute cor pulmonale I26.09
  chronic I27.82
  following
    abortion —*see* Abortion by type
      complicated by embolism
    ectopic or molar pregnancy O08.2
  healed or old Z86.711
  in pregnancy, childbirth or puerperium —
    see Embolism, obstetric
  personal history of Z86.711
  saddle I26.92
    with acute cor pulmonale I26.02
  septic I26.90
    with acute cor pulmonale I26.01
pyemic (multiple) I76
  following
    abortion —*see* Abortion by type
      complicated by embolism
    ectopic or molar pregnancy O08.2
  Hemophilus influenzae A41.3
  pneumococcal A40.3
    with pneumonia J13
  puerperal, postpartum, childbirth (any
    organism) —*see* Embolism, obstetric
  specified organism NEC A41.89
  staphylococcal A41.2
  streptococcal A40.9
renal (artery) N28.0
  vein I82.3
retina, retinal —*see* Occlusion, artery, retina
saddle
  abdominal aorta I74.01
  pulmonary artery I26.92
    with acute cor pulmonale I26.02
septic (arterial) I76
  complicating abortion —*see* Abortion, by
    type, complicated by, embolism
sinus —*see* Embolism, intracranial, venous
  sinus
soap complicating abortion —*see* Abortion,
  by type, complicated by, embolism
spinal cord G95.19
  pyogenic origin G06.1
spleen, splenic (artery) I74.8
upper extremity I74.2
vein (acute) I82.90
  antecubital I82.61-
    chronic I82.71-
  axillary I82.A1-
    chronic I82.A2-
  basilic I82.61-
    chronic I82.71-
  brachial I82.62-
    chronic I82.72-
  brachiocephalic (innominate) I82.290
    chronic I82.291
  cephalic I82.61-
    chronic I82.71-
  chronic I82.91
  deep (DVT) I82.40-
    calf I82.4Z-
      chronic I82.5Z-
    lower leg I82.4Z-
      chronic I82.5Z-
    thigh I82.4Y-
      chronic I82.5Y-

◀ New   ◀▥ Revised   ~~deleted~~ Deleted

Embolism *(Continued)*
  vein *(Continued)*
    deep *(Continued)*
      upper leg I82.4Y
        chronic I82.5y--
      femoral I82.41-
        chronic I82.51-
      iliac (iliofemoral) I82.42-
        chronic I82.52-
      innominate I82.290
        chronic I82.291
      internal jugular I82.C1-
        chronic I82.C2-
      lower extremity
        deep I82.40-
          chronic I82.50-
            specified NEC I82.49-
              chronic NEC I82.59-
        distal
          deep I82.4Z-
        proximal
          deep I82.4Y-
            chronic I82.5Y-
        superficial I82.81-
      popliteal I82.43-
        chronic I82.53-
      radial I82.62-
        chronic I82.72-
      renal I82.3
      saphenous (greater) (lesser) I82.81-
      specified NEC I82.890
        chronic NEC I82.891
      subclavian I82.B1-
        chronic I82.B2-
      thoracic NEC I82.290
        chronic I82.291
      tibial I82.44-
        chronic I82.54-
      ulnar I82.62-
        chronic I82.72-
      upper extremity I82.60-
        chronic I82.70-
        deep I82.62-
          chronic I82.72-
        superficial I82.61-
          chronic I82.71-
  vena cava
    inferior (acute) I82.220
      chronic I82.221
    superior (acute) I82.210
      chronic I82.211
  venous sinus G08
  vessels of brain —*see* Occlusion, artery,
    cerebral
Embolus —*see* Embolism
Embryoma —*see also* Neoplasm, uncertain
  behavior, by site
  benign —*see* Neoplasm, benign, by site
  kidney C64.-
  liver C22.0
  malignant —*see also* Neoplasm, malignant,
    by site
    kidney C64.-
    liver C22.0
    testis C62.9-
      descended (scrotal) C62.1-
      undescended C62.0-
  testis C62.9-
    descended (scrotal) C62.1-
    undescended C62.0-
Embryonic
  circulation Q28.9
  heart Q28.9
  vas deferens Q55.4
Embryopathia NOS Q89.9
Embryotoxon Q13.4
Emesis —*see* Vomiting
Emotional lability R45.86
Emotionality, pathological F60.3
Emotogenic disease —*see* Disorder,
  psychogenic

Emphysema (atrophic) (bullous) (chronic)
  (interlobular) (lung) (obstructive)
  (pulmonary) (senile) (vesicular)
  J43.9
  cellular tissue (traumatic) T79.7
    surgical T81.82
  centrilobular J43.2
  compensatory J98.3
  congenital (interstitial) P25.0
  conjunctiva H11.89
  connective tissue (traumatic) T79.7
    surgical T81.82
  due to chemicals, gases, fumes or vapors
    J68.4
  eyelid (s) —*see* Disorder, eyelid, specified
    type NEC
    surgical T81.82
    traumatic T79.7
  interstitial J98.2
    congenital P25.0
    perinatal period P25.0
  laminated tissue T79.7
    surgical T81.82
  mediastinal J98.2
    newborn P25.2
  orbit, orbital —*see* Disorder, orbit, specified
    type NEC
  panacinar J43.1
  panlobular J43.1
  specified NEC J43.8
  subcutaneous (traumatic) T79.7
    nontraumatic J98.2
    postprocedural T81.82
    surgical T81.82
  surgical T81.82
  thymus (gland) (congenital) E32.8
  traumatic (subcutaneous) T79.7
  unilateral J43.0
Empty nest syndrome Z60.0
Empyema (acute) (chest) (double) (pleura)
  (supradiaphragmatic) (thorax) J86.9
  with fistula J86.0
  accessory sinus (chronic) —*see* Sinusitis
  antrum (chronic) —*see* Sinusitis, maxillary
  brain (any part) —*see* Abscess, brain
  ethmoidal (chronic) (sinus) —*see* Sinusitis,
    ethmoidal
  extradural —*see* Abscess, extradural
  frontal (chronic) (sinus) —*see* Sinusitis,
    frontal
  gallbladder K81.0
  mastoid (process) (acute) —*see* Mastoiditis,
    acute
  maxilla, maxillary M27.2
    sinus (chronic) —*see* Sinusitis,
      maxillary
  nasal sinus (chronic) —*see* Sinusitis
  sinus (accessory) (chronic) (nasal) —*see*
    Sinusitis
  sphenoidal (sinus) (chronic) —*see* Sinusitis,
    sphenoidal
  subarachnoid —*see* Abscess, extradural
  subdural —*see* Abscess, subdural
  tuberculous A15.6
  ureter —*see* Ureteritis
  ventricular —*see* Abscess, brain
En coup de sabre lesion L94.1
Enamel pearls K00.2
Enameloma K00.2
Enanthema, viral B09
Encephalitis (chronic) (hemorrhagic)
  (idiopathic) (nonepidemic) (spurious)
  (subacute) G04.90
  acute (*see also* Encephalitis, viral) A86
    disseminated G04.00
      infectious G04.01
      noninfectious G04.81
      postimmunization (postvaccination)
        G04.02
      postinfectious G04.01
    inclusion body A85.8

Encephalitis *(Continued)*
  acute *(Continued)*
    necrotizing hemorrhagic G04.30
      postimmunization G04.32
      postinfectious G04.31
      specified NEC G04.39
  arboviral, arbovirus NEC A85.2
  arthropod-borne NEC (viral) A85.2
  Australian A83.4
  California (virus) A83.5
  Central European (tick-borne) A84.1
  Czechoslovakian A84.1
  Dawson's (inclusion body) A81.1
  diffuse sclerosing A81.1
  disseminated, acute G04.00
  due to
    cat scratch disease A28.1
    human immunodeficiency virus (HIV)
      disease B20 [G05.3]
    malaria —*see* Malaria
    rickettsiosis —*see* Rickettsiosis
    smallpox inoculation G04.02
    typhus —*see* Typhus
  Eastern equine A83.2
  endemic (viral) A86
  epidemic NEC (viral) A86
  equine (acute) (infectious) (viral) A83.9
    Eastern A83.2
    Venezuelan A92.2
    Western A83.1
  Far Eastern (tick-borne) A84.0
  following vaccination or other immunization
    procedure G04.02
  herpes zoster B02.0
  herpesviral B00.4
    due to herpesvirus 6 B10.01
    due to herpesvirus 7 B10.09
    specified NEC B10.09
  Ilheus (virus) A83.8
  in (due to)
    actinomycosis A42.82
    adenovirus A85.1
    African trypanosomiasis B56.9 [G05.3]
    Chagas' disease (chronic) B57.42
    cytomegalovirus B25.8
    enterovirus A85.0
    herpes (simplex) virus B00.4
      due to herpesvirus 6 B10.01
      due to herpesvirus 7 B10.09
      specified NEC B10.09
    infectious disease NEC B99 [G05.3]
    influenza —*see* Influenza, with,
      encephalopathy
    listeriosis A32.12
    measles B05.0
    mumps B26.2
    naegleriasis B60.2
    parasitic disease NEC B89 [G05.3]
    poliovirus A80.9 [G05.3]
    rubella B06.01
    syphilis
      congenital A50.42
      late A52.14
    systemic lupus erythematosus M32.19
    toxoplasmosis (acquired) B58.2
      congenital P37.1
    tuberculosis A17.82
    zoster B02.0
  inclusion body A81.1
  infectious (acute) (virus) NEC A86
  Japanese (B type) A83.0
  La Crosse A83.5
  lead —*see* Poisoning, lead
  lethargica (acute) (infectious) A85.8
  louping ill A84.8
  lupus erythematosus, systemic M32.19
  lymphatica A87.2
  Mengo A85.8
  meningococcal A39.81
  Murray Valley A83.4
  otitic NEC H66.40 [G05.3]

Encephalitis (Continued)
  parasitic NOS B71.9
  periaxial G37.0
  periaxialis (concentrica) (diffuse) G37.5
  postchickenpox B01.11
  postexanthematous NEC B09
  postimmunization G04.02
  postinfectious NEC G04.01
  postmeasles B05.0
  postvaccinal G04.02
  postvaricella B01.11
  postviral NEC A86
  Powassan A84.8
  Rasmussen G04.81
  Rio Bravo A85.8
  Russian
    autumnal A83.0
    spring-summer (taiga) A84.0
  saturnine —see Poisoning, lead
  specified NEC G04.81
  St. Louis A83.3
  subacute sclerosing A81.1
  summer A83.0
  suppurative G04.81
  tick-borne A84.9
  Torula, torular (cryptococcal) B45.1
  toxic NEC G92
  trichinosis B75 [G05.3]
  type
    B A83.0
    C A83.3
  van Bogaert's A81.1
  Venezuelan equine A92.2
  Vienna A85.8
  viral, virus A86
    arthropod-borne NEC A85.2
      mosquito-borne A83.9
        Australian X disease A83.4
        California virus A83.5
        Eastern equine A83.2
        Japanese (B type) A83.0
        Murray Valley A83.4
        specified NEC A83.8
        St. Louis A83.3
        type B A83.0
        type C A83.3
        Western equine A83.1
      tick-borne A84.9
        biundulant A84.1
        central European A84.1
        Czechoslovakian A84.1
        diphasic meningoencephalitis
          A84.1
        Far Eastern A84.0
        Russian spring-summer (taiga)
          A84.0
        specified NEC A84.8
      specified type NEC A85.8
    Western equine A83.1
Encephalocele Q01.9
  frontal Q01.0
  nasofrontal Q01.1
  occipital Q01.2
  specified NEC Q01.8
Encephalocystocele —see Encephalocele
Encephaloduroarteriomyosynangiosis
  (EDAMS) I67.5
Encephalomalacia (brain) (cerebellar)
  (cerebral) —see Softening, brain
Encephalomeningitis —see
  Meningoencephalitis
Encephalomeningocele —see Encephalocele
Encephalomeningomyelitis —see
  Meningoencephalitis
Encephalomyelitis (see also Encephalitis)
  G04.90
  acute disseminated G04.00
    infectious G04.01
    noninfectious G04.81
    postimmunization G04.02
    postinfectious G04.01

Encephalomyelitis (Continued)
  acute necrotizing hemorrhagic G04.30
    postimmunization G04.32
    postinfectious G04.31
    specified NEC G04.39
  benign myalgic G93.3
  equine A83.9
    Eastern A83.2
    Venezuelan A92.2
    Western A83.1
  in diseases classified elsewhere G05.3
  myalgic, benign G93.3
  postchickenpox B01.11
  postinfectious NEC G04.01
  postmeasles B05.0
  postvaccinal G04.02
  postvaricella B01.11
  rubella B06.01
  specified NEC G04.81
  Venezuelan equine A92.2
Encephalomyelocele —see Encephalocele
Encephalomyelomeningitis —see
  Meningoencephalitis
Encephalomyelopathy G96.9
Encephalomyeloradiculitis (acute) G61.0
Encephalomyeloradiculoneuritis (acute)
  (Guillain-Barré) G61.0
Encephalomyeloradiculopathy G96.9
Encephalopathia hyperbilirubinemica,
  newborn P57.9
  due to isoimmunization (conditions in P55)
    P57.0
Encephalopathy (acute) G93.40
  acute necrotizing hemorrhagic G04.30
    postimmunization G04.32
    postinfectious G04.31
    specified NEC G04.39
  alcoholic G31.2
  anoxic —see Damage, brain, anoxic
  arteriosclerotic I67.2
  centrolobar progressive (Schilder) G37.0
  congenital Q07.9
  degenerative, in specified disease NEC
    G32.89
  due to
    drugs (see also Table of Drugs and
      Chemicals) G92
  demyelinating callosal G37.1
  hepatic —see Failure, hepatic
  hyperbilirubinemic, newborn P57.9
    due to isoimmunization (conditions in P55)
      P57.0
  hypertensive I67.4
  hypoglycemic E16.2
  hypoxic —see Damage, brain, anoxic
  hypoxic ischemic P91.60
    mild P91.61
    moderate P91.62
    severe P91.63
  in (due to) (with)
    birth injury P11.1
    hyperinsulinism E16.1 [G94]
    influenza —see Influenza, with,
      encephalopathy
    lack of vitamin (see also Deficiency, vitamin)
      E56.9 [G32.89]
    neoplastic disease (see also Neoplasm)
      D49.9 [G13.1]
    serum (see also Reaction, serum) T80.69
    syphilis A52.17
    trauma (postconcussional) F07.81
      current injury —see Injury, intracranial
    vaccination G04.02
  lead —see Poisoning, lead
  metabolic G93.41
    drug induced G92
    toxic G92
  myoclonic, early, symptomatic —see Epilepsy,
    generalized, specified NEC
  necrotizing, subacute (Leigh) G31.82
  pellagrous E52 [G32.89]

Encephalopathy (Continued)
  portosystemic —see Failure, hepatic
  postcontusional F07.81
    current injury —see Injury, intracranial,
      diffuse
  posthypoglycemic (coma) E16.1 [G94]
  postradiation G93.89
  saturnine —see Poisoning, lead
  septic G93.41
  specified NEC G93.49
  spongioform, subacute (viral) A81.09
  toxic G92
    metabolic G92
  traumatic (postconcussional) F07.81
    current injury —see Injury, intracranial
  vitamin B deficiency NEC E53.9 [G32.89]
    vitamin B1 E51.2
  Wernicke's E51.2
Encephalorrhagia —see Hemorrhage,
  intracranial, intracerebral
Encephalosis, posttraumatic F07.81
Enchondroma —see also Neoplasm, bone,
  benign
Enchondromatosis (cartilaginous) (multiple)
  Q78.4
Encopresis R15.9
  functional F98.1
  nonorganic origin F98.1
  psychogenic F98.1
Encounter (with health service) (for) Z76.89
  adjustment and management (of)
    breast implant Z45.81
    implanted device NEC Z45.89
    myringotomy device (stent) (tube)
      Z45.82
  administrative purpose only Z02.9
    examination for
      adoption Z02.82
      armed forces Z02.3
      disability determination Z02.71
      driving license Z02.4
      employment Z02.1
      insurance Z02.6
      medical certificate NEC Z02.79
      paternity testing Z02.81
      residential institution admission
        Z02.2
      school admission Z02.0
      sports Z02.5
    specified reason NEC Z02.89
  aftercare —see Aftercare
  antenatal screening Z36
  assisted reproductive fertility procedure cycle
    Z31.83
  blood typing Z01.83
    Rh typing Z01.83
  breast augmentation or reduction Z41.1
  breast implant exchange (different material)
    (different size) Z45.81
  breast reconstruction following mastectomy
    Z42.1
  check-up —see Examination
  chemotherapy for neoplasm Z51.11
  colonoscopy, screening Z12.11
  counseling —see Counseling
  delivery, full-term, uncomplicated O80
    cesarean, without indication O82
  ear piercing Z41.3
  examination —see Examination
  expectant parent (s) (adoptive) pre-birth
    pediatrician visit Z76.81
  fertility preservation procedure (prior to
    cancer therapy) (prior to removal of
    gonads) Z31.84
  fitting (of) —see Fitting (and adjustment) (of)
  genetic
    counseling Z31.5
    testing —see Test, genetic
  hearing conservation and treatment Z01.12
  immunotherapy for neoplasm Z51.12
  in vitro fertilization cycle Z31.83

◀ New   ◀▥ Revised   ~~deleted~~ Deleted

Encounter (Continued)
  instruction (in)
    child care (postpartal) (prenatal) Z32.3
    childbirth Z32.2
    natural family planning
      procreative Z31.61
      to avoid pregnancy Z30.02
    insulin pump titration Z46.81
    joint prosthesis insertion following prior
        explantation of joint prosthesis (staged
        procedure)
      hip Z47.32
      knee Z47.33
      shoulder Z47.31
  laboratory (as part of a general medical
      examination) Z00.00
    with abnormal findings Z00.01
  mental health services (for)
    abuse NEC
      perpetrator Z69.82
      victim Z69.81
    child abuse
      nonparental
        perpetrator Z69.021
        victim Z69.020
      parental
        perpetrator Z69.011
        victim Z69.010
    spousal or partner abuse
      perpetrator Z69.12
      victim Z69.11
  observation (for) (ruled out)
    exposure to (suspected)
      anthrax Z03.810
      biological agent NEC Z03.818
  pediatrician visit, by expectant parent (s)
      (adoptive) Z76.81
  plastic and reconstructive surgery following
      medical procedure or healed injury
      NEC Z42.8
  pregnancy
    supervision of —see Pregnancy,
        supervision of
    test Z32.00
      result negative Z32.02
      result positive Z32.01
  radiation therapy (antineoplastic) Z51.0
  radiological (as part of a general medical
      examination) Z00.00
    with abnormal findings Z00.01
  reconstructive surgery following medical
      procedure or healed injury NEC Z42.8
  removal (of) —see also Removal
    artificial
      arm Z44.00-
        complete Z44.01-
        partial Z44.02-
      eye Z44.2-
      leg Z44.10-
        complete Z44.11-
        partial Z44.12-
    breast implant Z45.81
      tissue expander (without synchronous
          insertion of permanent implant)
          Z45.81
    device Z46.9
      specified NEC Z46.89
    external
      fixation device — code to fracture with
          seventh character D
      prosthesis, prosthetic device Z44.9
        breast Z44.3-
        specified NEC Z44.8
    implanted device NEC Z45.89
    insulin pump Z46.81
    internal fixation device Z47.2
    myringotomy device (stent) (tube) Z45.82
    nervous system device NEC Z46.2
      brain neuropacemaker Z46.2
      visual substitution device Z46.2
        implanted Z45.31

Encounter (Continued)
  removal (Continued)
    non-vascular catheter Z46.82
    orthodontic device Z46.4
    stent
      ureteral Z46.6
    urinary device Z46.6
  repeat cervical smear to confirm findings of
      recent normal smear following initial
      abnormal smear Z01.42
  respirator [ventilator] use during power
      failure (Z99.12)
  Rh typing Z01.83
  screening —see Screening
  specified NEC Z76.89
  sterilization Z30.2
  suspected condition, ruled out
    amniotic cavity and membrane Z03.71
    cervical shortening Z03.75
    fetal anomaly Z03.73
    fetal growth Z03.74
    maternal and fetal conditions NEC Z03.79
    oligohydramnios Z03.71
    placental problem Z03.72
    polyhydramnios Z03.71
  suspected exposure (to), ruled out
    anthrax Z03.810
    biological agents NEC Z03.818
  termination of pregnancy, elective Z33.2
  testing —see Test
  therapeutic drug level monitoring Z51.81
  titration, insulin pump Z46.81
  to determine fetal viability of pregnancy
      O36.80
  training
    insulin pump Z46.81
  X-ray of chest (as part of a general medical
      examination Z00.00)
    with abnormal findings Z00.01
Encystment —see Cyst
Endarteritis (bacterial, subacute) (infective)
      I77.6
  brain I67.7
  cerebral or cerebrospinal I67.7
  deformans —see Arteriosclerosis
  embolic —see Embolism
  obliterans —see also Arteriosclerosis
    pulmonary I28.8
  pulmonary I28.8
  retina —see Vasculitis, retina
  senile —see Arteriosclerosis
  syphilitic A52.09
    brain or cerebral A52.04
    congenital A50.54 [I79.8]
  tuberculous A18.89
Endemic —see condition
Endocarditis (chronic) (marantic) (nonbacterial)
      (thrombotic) (valvular) I38
  with rheumatic fever (conditions in I00)
    active —see Endocarditis, acute, rheumatic
    inactive or quiescent (with chorea) I09.1
  acute or subacute I33.9
    infective I33.0
    rheumatic (aortic) (mitral) (pulmonary)
        (tricuspid) I01.1
      with chorea (acute) (rheumatic)
          (Sydenham's) I02.0
  aortic (heart) (nonrheumatic) (valve) I35.8
    with
      mitral disease I08.0
        with tricuspid (valve) disease I08.3
        active or acute I01.1
          with chorea (acute) (rheumatic)
              (Sydenham's) I02.0
      rheumatic fever (conditions in I00)
        active —see Endocarditis, acute,
            rheumatic
        inactive or quiescent (with chorea)
            I06.9
      tricuspid (valve) disease I08.2
        with mitral (valve) disease I08.3

Endocarditis (Continued)
  aortic (Continued)
    acute or subacute I33.9
    arteriosclerotic I35.8
    rheumatic I06.9
      with mitral disease I08.0
        with tricuspid (valve) disease I08.3
        active or acute I01.1
          with chorea (acute) (rheumatic)
              (Sydenham's) I02.0
      active or acute I01.1
        with chorea (acute) (rheumatic)
            (Sydenham's) I02.0
      specified NEC I06.8
    specified cause NEC I35.8
    syphilitic A52.03
  arteriosclerotic I38
  atypical verrucous (Libman-Sacks) M32.11
  bacterial (acute) (any valve) (subacute) I33.0
  candidal B37.6
  congenital Q24.8
  constrictive I33.0
  Coxiella burnetii A78 [I39]
  Coxsackie B33.21
  due to
    prosthetic cardiac valve T82.6
    Q fever A78 [I39]
    Serratia marcescens I33.0
    typhoid (fever) A01.02
  gonococcal A54.83
  infectious or infective (acute) (any valve)
      (subacute) I33.0
  lenta (acute) (any valve) (subacute) I33.0
  Libman-Sacks M32.11
  listerial A32.82
  Löffler's I42.3
  malignant (acute) (any valve) (subacute) I33.0
  meningococcal A39.51
  mitral (chronic) (double) (fibroid) (heart)
      (inactive) (valve) (with chorea) I05.9
    with
      aortic (valve) disease I08.0
        with tricuspid (valve) disease I08.3
        active or acute I01.1
          with chorea (acute) (rheumatic)
              (Sydenham's) I02.0
      rheumatic fever (conditions in I00)
        active —see Endocarditis, acute,
            rheumatic
        inactive or quiescent (with chorea)
            I05.9
      tricuspid (valve) disease I08.1
        with aortic (valve) disease I08.3
    active or acute I01.1
      with chorea (acute) (rheumatic)
          (Sydenham's) I02.0
    bacterial I33.0
    arteriosclerotic I34.8
    nonrheumatic I34.8
      acute or subacute I33.9
    specified NEC I05.8
  monilial B37.6
  multiple valves I08.9
    specified disorders I08.8
  mycotic (acute) (any valve) (subacute) I33.0
  pneumococcal (acute) (any valve) (subacute)
      I33.0
  pulmonary (chronic) (heart) (valve) I37.8
    with rheumatic fever (conditions in I00)
      active —see Endocarditis, acute,
          rheumatic
      inactive or quiescent (with chorea)
          I09.89
        with aortic, mitral or tricuspid disease
            I08.8
    acute or subacute I33.9
      rheumatic I01.1
        with chorea (acute) (rheumatic)
            (Sydenham's) I02.0
    arteriosclerotic I37.8
    congenital Q22.2

Endocarditis *(Continued)*
  pulmonary *(Continued)*
    rheumatic (chronic) (inactive) (with chorea)
        I09.89
      active or acute I01.1
        with chorea (acute) (rheumatic)
            (Sydenham's) I02.0
      syphilitic A52.03
    purulent (acute) (any valve) (subacute) I33.0
    Q fever A78 *[I39]*
    rheumatic (chronic) (inactive) (with chorea)
        I09.1
      active or acute (aortic) (mitral)
          (pulmonary) (tricuspid) I01.1
        with chorea (acute) (rheumatic)
            (Sydenham's) I02.0
    rheumatoid —*see* Rheumatoid, carditis
    septic (acute) (any valve) (subacute) I33.0
    streptococcal (acute) (any valve) (subacute)
        I33.0
    subacute —*see* Endocarditis, acute
    suppurative (acute) (any valve) (subacute)
        I33.0
    syphilitic A52.03
    toxic I33.9
    tricuspid (chronic) (heart) (inactive)
        (rheumatic) (valve) (with chorea) I07.9
      with
        aortic (valve) disease I08.2
          mitral (valve) disease I08.3
        mitral (valve) disease I08.1
          aortic (valve) disease I08.3
        rheumatic fever (conditions in I00)
          active —*see* Endocarditis, acute,
              rheumatic
          inactive or quiescent (with chorea)
              I07.8
      active or acute I01.1
        with chorea (acute) (rheumatic)
            (Sydenham's) I02.0
    arteriosclerotic I36.8
    nonrheumatic I36.8
      acute or subacute I33.9
    specified cause, except rheumatic I36.8
    tuberculous —*see* Tuberculosis, endocarditis
    typhoid A01.02
    ulcerative (acute) (any valve) (subacute) I33.0
    vegetative (acute) (any valve) (subacute) I33.0
    verrucous (atypical) (nonbacterial)
        (nonrheumatic) M32.11
Endocardium, endocardial —*see also* condition
  cushion defect Q21.2
Endocervicitis —*see also* Cervicitis
  due to intrauterine (contraceptive) device
      T83.6
  hyperplastic N72
Endocrine —*see* condition
Endocrinopathy, pluriglandular E31.9
Endodontic
  overfill M27.52
  underfill M27.53
Endodontitis K04.0
Endomastoiditis —*see* Mastoiditis
Endometrioma N80.9
Endometriosis N80.9
  appendix N80.5
  bladder N80.8
  bowel N80.5
  broad ligament N80.3
  cervix N80.0
  colon N80.5
  cul-de-sac (Douglas') N80.3
  exocervix N80.0
  fallopian tube N80.2
  female genital organ NEC N80.8
  gallbladder N80.8
  in scar of skin N80.6
  internal N80.0
  intestine N80.5
  lung N80.8
  myometrium N80.0

Endometriosis *(Continued)*
  ovary N80.1
  parametrium N80.3
  pelvic peritoneum N80.3
  peritoneal (pelvic) N80.3
  rectovaginal septum N80.4
  rectum N80.5
  round ligament N80.3
  skin (scar) N80.6
  specified site NEC N80.8
  stromal D39.0
  umbilicus N80.8
  uterus (internal) N80.0
  vagina N80.4
  vulva N80.8
Endometritis (decidual) (nonspecific)
    (purulent) (senile) (atrophic) (suppurative)
    N71.9
  with ectopic pregnancy O08.0
  acute N71.0
  blenorrhagic (gonococcal) (acute) (chronic)
      A54.24
  cervix, cervical (with erosion or ectropion) —
      see also Cervicitis
    hyperplastic N72
  chlamydial A56.11
  chronic N71.1
  following
    abortion —*see* Abortion by type
        complicated by genital infection
    ectopic or molar pregnancy O08.0
  gonococcal, gonorrheal (acute) (chronic)
      A54.24
  hyperplastic (*see also* Hyperplasia,
      endometrial) N85.00-
    cervix N72
  puerperal, postpartum, childbirth O86.12
  subacute N71.0
  tuberculous A18.17
Endometrium —*see* condition
Endomyocardiopathy, South African I42.3
Endomyocarditis —*see* Endocarditis
Endomyofibrosis I42.3
Endomyometritis —*see* Endometritis
Endopericarditis —*see* Endocarditis
Endoperineuritis —*see* Disorder, nerve
Endophlebitis —*see* Phlebitis
Endophthalmia —*see* Endophthalmitis,
    purulent
Endophthalmitis (acute) (infective) (metastatic)
    (subacute) H44.009
  bleb associated H59.4 —*see also* Bleb,
      inflamed (infected), postprocedural
  gonorrheal A54.39
  in (due to)
    cysticercosis B69.1
    onchocerciasis B73.01
    toxocariasis B83.0
  panuveitis —*see* Panuveitis
  parasitic H44.12-
  purulent H44.00-
    panophthalmitis —*see* Panophthalmitis
    vitreous abscess H44.02-
  specified NEC H44.19
  sympathetic —*see* Uveitis, sympathetic
Endosalpingioma D28.2
Endosalpingiosis N94.89
Endosteitis —*see* Osteomyelitis
Endothelioma, bone —*see* Neoplasm, bone,
    malignant
Endotheliosis (hemorrhagic infectional) D69.8
Endotoxemia — code to condition
Endotrachelitis —*see* Cervicitis
Engelmann (-Camurati) **syndrome** Q78.3
English disease —*see* Rickets
Engman's disease L30.3
Engorgement
  breast N64.59
    newborn P83.4
    puerperal, postpartum O92.79
  lung (passive) —*see* Edema, lung

Engorgement *(Continued)*
  pulmonary (passive) —*see* Edema, lung
  stomach K31.89
  venous, retina —*see* Occlusion, retina, vein,
      engorgement
Enlargement, enlarged —*see also* Hypertrophy
  adenoids J35.2
    with tonsils J35.3
  alveolar ridge K08.8
    congenital —*see* Anomaly, alveolar
  apertures of diaphragm (congenital) Q79.1
  gingival K06.1
  heart, cardiac —*see* Hypertrophy, cardiac
  lacrimal gland, chronic H04.03-
  liver —*see* Hypertrophy, liver
  lymph gland or node R59.9
    generalized R59.1
    localized R59.0
  orbit H05.34-
  organ or site, congenital NEC —*see* Anomaly,
      by site
  parathyroid (gland) E21.0
  pituitary fossa R93.0
  prostate N40.0
    with lower urinary tract symptoms (LUTS)
        N40.1
    without lower urinary tract symptoms
        (LUTS) N40.0
  sella turcica R93.0
  spleen —*see* Splenomegaly
  thymus (gland) (congenital) E32.0
  thyroid (gland) —*see* Goiter
  tongue K14.8
  tonsils J35.1
    with adenoids J35.3
  uterus N85.2
Enophthalmos H05.40-
  due to
    orbital tissue atrophy H05.41-
    trauma or surgery H05.42-
Enostosis M27.8
Entamebic, entamebiasis —*see* Amebiasis
Entanglement
  umbilical cord (s) O69.2
    with compression O69.2
      without compression O69.82
    around neck (with compression) O69.1
      without compression O69.81
    of twins in monoamniotic sac O69.2
Enteralgia —*see* Pain, abdominal
Enteric —*see* condition
Enteritis (acute) (diarrheal) (hemorrhagic)
    (noninfective) (septic) K52.9
  adenovirus A08.2
  aertrycke infection A02.0
  allergic K52.2
  amebic (acute) A06.0
    with abscess —*see* Abscess, amebic
    chronic A06.1
      with abscess —*see* Abscess, amebic
      nondysenteric A06.2
    nondysenteric A06.2
  astrovirus A08.32
  bacillary NOS A03.9
  bacterial A04.9
    specified NEC A04.8
  calicivirus A08.31
  candidal B37.82
  Chilomastix A07.8
  choleriformis A00.1
  chronic (noninfectious) K52.9
    ulcerative —*see* Colitis, ulcerative
  cicatrizing (chronic) —*see* Enteritis, regional,
      small intestine
  Clostridium
    botulinum (food poisoning) A05.1
    difficile A04.7
  coccidial A07.3
  coxsackie virus A08.39
  dietetic K52.2
  drug-induced K52.1

◄ New ◄▦ Revised ~~deleted~~ Deleted

Enteritis (Continued)
  due to
    astrovirus A08.32
    calicivirus A08.31
    coxsackie virus A08.39
    drugs K52.1
    echovirus A08.39
    enterovirus NEC A08.39
    food hypersensitivity K52.2
    infectious organism (bacterial) (viral) —see
      Enteritis, infectious
    torovirus A08.39
    Yersinia enterocolitica A04.6
  echovirus A08.39
  eltor A00.1
  enterovirus NEC A08.39
  eosinophilic K52.81
  epidemic (infectious) A09
  fulminant K55.0
  gangrenous —see Enteritis, infectious
  giardial A07.1
  infectious NOS A09
    due to
      adenovirus A08.2
      Aerobacter aerogenes A04.8
      Arizona (bacillus) A02.0
      bacteria NOS A04.9
        specified NEC A04.8
      Campylobacter A04.5
      Clostridium difficile A04.7
      Clostridium perfringens A04.8
      Enterobacter aerogenes A04.8
      enterovirus A08.39
      Escherichia coli A04.4
        enteroaggregative A04.4
        enterohemorrhagic A04.3
        enteroinvasive A04.2
        enteropathogenic A04.0
        enterotoxigenic A04.1
        specified NEC A04.4
      specified
        bacteria NEC A04.8
        virus NEC A08.39
      Staphylococcus A04.8
      virus NEC A08.4
        specified type NEC A08.39
      Yersinia enterocolitica A04.6
    specified organism NEC A08.8
  influenzal —see Influenza, with, digestive
    manifestations
  ischemic K55.9
    acute K55.0
    chronic K55.1
  microsporidial A07.8
  mucomembranous, myxomembranous —see
    Syndrome, irritable bowel
  mucous —see Syndrome, irritable bowel
  necroticans A05.2
  necrotizing of newborn —see Enterocolitis,
    necrotizing, in newborn
  neurogenic —see Syndrome, irritable
    bowel
  newborn necrotizing —see Enterocolitis,
    necrotizing, in newborn
  noninfectious K52.9
  norovirus A08.11
  parasitic NEC B82.9
  paratyphoid (fever) —see Fever, paratyphoid
  protozoal A07.9
    specified NEC A07.8
  radiation K52.0
  regional (of) K50.90
    with
      complication K50.919
        abscess K50.914
        fistula K50.913
        intestinal obstruction K50.912
        rectal bleeding K50.911
        specified complication NEC K50.918
    colon —see Enteritis, regional, large
      intestine

Enteritis (Continued)
  regional (Continued)
    duodenum —see Enteritis, regional, small
      intestine
    ileum —see Enteritis, regional, small
      intestine
    jejunum —see Enteritis, regional, small
      intestine
    large bowel —see Enteritis, regional, large
      intestine
    large intestine (colon) (rectum) K50.10
      with
        complication K50.119
          abscess K50.114
          fistula K50.113
          intestinal obstruction K50.112
          rectal bleeding K50.111
          small intestine (duodenum) (ileum)
            (jejunum) involvement K50.80
            with
              complication K50.819
                abscess K50.814
                fistula K50.813
                intestinal obstruction
                  K50.812
                rectal bleeding K50.811
                specified complication NEC
                  K50.818
          specified complication NEC K50.118
    rectum —see Enteritis, regional, large
      intestine
    small intestine (duodenum) (ileum)
      (jejunum) K50.00
      with
        complication K50.019
          abscess K50.014
          fistula K50.013
          intestinal obstruction K50.012
          large intestine (colon) (rectum)
            involvement K50.80
            with
              complication K50.819
                abscess K50.814
                fistula K50.813
                intestinal obstruction
                  K50.812
                rectal bleeding K50.811
                specified complication NEC
                  K50.818
          rectal bleeding K50.011
          specified complication NEC
            K50.018
  rotaviral A08.0
  Salmonella, salmonellosis (arizonae)
    (cholerae-suis) (enteritidis)
    (typhimurium) A02.0
  segmental —see Enteritis, regional
  septic A09
  Shigella —see Infection, Shigella
  small round structured NEC A08.19
  spasmodic, spastic —see Syndrome, irritable
    bowel
  staphylococcal A04.8
    due to food A05.0
  torovirus A08.39
  toxic NEC K52.1
    due to Clostridium difficile A04.7
  trichomonal A07.8
  tuberculous A18.32
  typhosa A01.00
  ulcerative (chronic) —see Colitis, ulcerative
  viral A08.4
    adenovirus A08.2
    enterovirus A08.39
    Rotavirus A08.0
    small round structured NEC A08.19
    specified NEC A08.39
    virus specified NEC A08.39
Enterobiasis B80
Enterobius vermicularis (infection) (infestation)
  B80

Enterocele —see also Hernia, abdomen
  pelvic, pelvis (acquired) (congenital)
    N81.5
  vagina, vaginal (acquired) (congenital)
    NEC N81.5
Enterocolitis (see also Enteritis) K52.9
  due to Clostridium difficile A04.7
  fulminant ischemic K55.0
  granulomatous —see Enteritis, regional
  hemorrhagic (acute) K55.0
    chronic K55.1
  infectious NEC A09
  ischemic K55.9
  necrotizing
    due to Clostridium difficile A04.7
    in newborn P77.9
      stage 1 (without pneumatosis, without
        perforation) P77.1
      stage 2 (with pneumatosis, without
        perforation) P77.2
      stage 3 (with pneumatosis, with
        perforation) P77.3
    noninfectious K52.9
    newborn —see Enterocolitis, necrotizing, in
      newborn
  pseudomembranous (newborn) A04.7
  radiation K52.0
    newborn —see Enterocolitis, necrotizing, in
      newborn
  ulcerative (chronic) —see Pancolitis,
    ulcerative (chronic)
Enterogastritis —see Enteritis
Enteropathy K63.9
  gluten-sensitive K90.0
  hemorrhagic, terminal K55.0
  protein-losing K90.4
Enteroperitonitis —see Peritonitis
Enteroptosis K63.4
Enterorrhagia K92.2
Enterospasm —see also Syndrome, irritable,
  bowel
  psychogenic F45.8
Enterostenosis —see also Obstruction, intestine
  K56.69
Enterostomy
  complication —see Complication,
    enterostomy
  status Z93.4
Enterovirus, as cause of disease classified
  elsewhere B97.10
  coxsackievirus B97.11
  echovirus B97.12
  other specified B97.19
Enthesopathy (peripheral) M77.9
  Achilles tendinitis —see Tendinitis,
    Achilles
  ankle and tarsus M77.9
    specified type NEC —see Enthesopathy,
      foot, specified type NEC
  anterior tibial syndrome M76.81-
  calcaneal spur —see Spur, bone, calcaneal
  elbow region M77.8
    lateral epicondylitis —see Epicondylitis,
      lateral
    medial epicondylitis —see Epicondylitis,
      medial
  foot NEC M77.9
    metatarsalgia —see Metatarsalgia
    specified type NEC M77.5-
  forearm M77.9
  gluteal tendinitis —see Tendinitis, gluteal
  hand M77.9
  hip —see Enthesopathy, lower limb, specified
    type NEC
  iliac crest spur —see Spur, bone, iliac crest
  iliotibial band syndrome —see Syndrome,
    iliotibial band
  knee —see Enthesopathy, lower limb, lower
    leg, specified type NEC
  lateral epicondylitis —see Epicondylitis,
    lateral

Enthesopathy (Continued)
　lower limb (excluding foot) M76.9
　　Achilles tendinitis —see Tendinitis, Achilles
　　anterior tibial syndrome M76.81-
　　gluteal tendinitis —see Tendinitis, gluteal
　　iliac crest spur —see Spur, bone, iliac crest
　　iliotibial band syndrome —see Syndrome,
　　　　iliotibial band
　　patellar tendinitis —see Tendinitis, patellar
　　pelvic region —see Enthesopathy, lower
　　　limb, specified type NEC
　　peroneal tendinitis —see Tendinitis,
　　　peroneal
　　posterior tibial syndrome M76.82-
　　psoas tendinitis —see Tendinitis, psoas
　　shoulder M77.9
　　specified type NEC M76.89-
　　tibial collateral bursitis —see Bursitis, tibial
　　　collateral
　medial epicondylitis —see Epicondylitis,
　　medial
　multiple sites M77.9
　patellar tendinitis —see Tendinitis, patellar
　pelvis M77.9
　periarthritis of wrist —see Periarthritis,
　　wrist
　peroneal tendinitis —see Tendinitis,
　　peroneal
　posterior tibial syndrome M76.82-
　psoas tendinitis —see Tendinitis, psoas
　shoulder region —see Lesion, shoulder
　specified site NEC M77.9
　specified type NEC M77.8
　spinal M46.00
　　cervical region M46.02
　　cervicothoracic region M46.03
　　lumbar region M46.06
　　lumbosacral region M46.07
　　multiple sites M46.09
　　occipito-atlanto-axial region M46.01
　　sacrococcygeal region M46.08
　　thoracic region M46.04
　　thoracolumbar region M46.05
　tibial collateral bursitis —see Bursitis, tibial
　　collateral
　upper arm M77.9
　wrist and carpus NEC M77.8
　　calcaneal spur —see Spur, bone, calcaneal
　　periarthritis of wrist —see Periarthritis,
　　　wrist
Entomophobia F40.218
Entomophthoromycosis B46.8
Entrance, air into vein —see Embolism, air
Entrapment, nerve —see Neuropathy,
　entrapment
Entropion (eyelid) (paralytic) H02.009
　cicatricial H02.019
　　left H02.016
　　　lower H02.015
　　　upper H02.014
　　right H02.013
　　　lower H02.012
　　　upper H02.011
　congenital Q10.2
　left H02.006
　　lower H02.005
　　upper H02.004
　mechanical H02.029
　　left H02.026
　　　lower H02.025
　　　upper H02.024
　　right H02.023
　　　lower H02.022
　　　upper H02.021
　right H02.003
　　lower H02.002
　　upper H02.001
　senile H02.039
　　left H02.036
　　　lower H02.035
　　　upper H02.034

Entropion (Continued)
　senile (Continued)
　　right H02.033
　　　lower H02.032
　　　upper H02.031
　　spastic H02.049
　　　left H02.046
　　　　lower H02.045
　　　　upper H02.044
　　　right H02.043
　　　　lower H02.042
　　　　upper H02.041
Enucleated eye (traumatic, current) S05.7-
Enuresis R32
　functional F98.0
　habit disturbance F98.0
　nocturnal N39.44
　　psychogenic F98.0
　nonorganic origin F98.0
　psychogenic F98.0
Eosinopenia —see Agranulocytosis
Eosinophilia (allergic) (hereditary) (idiopathic)
　(secondary) D72.1
　with
　　angiolymphoid hyperplasia (ALHE)
　　　D18.01
　infiltrative J82
　Löffler's J82
　peritoneal —see Peritonitis, eosinophilic
　pulmonary NEC J82
　tropical (pulmonary) J82
Eosinophilia-myalgia syndrome M35.8
Ependymitis (acute) (cerebral) (chronic)
　(granular) —see Encephalomyelitis
Ependymoblastoma
　specified site —see Neoplasm, malignant, by
　　site
　unspecified site C71.9
Ependymoma (epithelial) (malignant)
　anaplastic
　　specified site —see Neoplasm, malignant,
　　　by site
　　unspecified site C71.9
　benign
　　specified site —see Neoplasm, benign, by
　　　site
　　unspecified site D33.2
　myxopapillary D43.2
　　specified site —see Neoplasm, uncertain
　　　behavior, by site
　　unspecified site D43.2
　papillary D43.2
　　specified site —see Neoplasm, uncertain
　　　behavior, by site
　　unspecified site D43.2
　specified site —see Neoplasm, malignant, by
　　site
　unspecified site C71.9
Ependymopathy G93.89
Ephelis, ephelides L81.2
Epiblepharon (congenital) Q10.3
Epicanthus, epicanthic fold (eyelid)
　(congenital) Q10.3
Epicondylitis (elbow)
　lateral M77.1-
　medial M77.0-
Epicystitis —see Cystitis
Epidemic —see condition
Epidermidalization, cervix —see Dysplasia,
　cervix
Epidermis, epidermal —see condition
Epidermodysplasia verruciformis B07.8
Epidermolysis
　bullosa (congenital) Q81.9
　　acquired L12.30
　　　drug-induced L12.31
　　　specified cause NEC L12.35
　　dystrophica Q81.2
　　letalis Q81.1
　　simplex Q81.0
　　specified NEC Q81.8

Epidermolysis (Continued)
　necroticans combustiformis L51.2
　　due to drug —see Table of Drugs and
　　　Chemicals, by drug
Epidermophytid —see Dermatophytosis
Epidermophytosis (infected) —see
　Dermatophytosis
Epididymis —see condition
Epididymitis (acute) (nonvenereal) (recurrent)
　(residual) N45.1
　with orchitis N45.3
　blennorrhagic (gonococcal) A54.23
　caseous (tuberculous) A18.15
　chlamydial A56.19
　filarial (see also Infestation, filarial) B74.9
　　[N51]
　gonococcal A54.23
　syphilitic A52.76
　tuberculous A18.15
Epididymo-orchitis (see also Epididymitis)
　N45.3
Epidural —see condition
Epigastrium, epigastric —see condition
Epigastrocele —see Hernia, ventral
Epiglottis —see condition
Epiglottitis, epiglottiditis (acute) J05.10
　with obstruction J05.11
　chronic J37.0
Epignathus Q89.4
Epilepsia partialis continua (see also
　Kozhevnikof's epilepsy) G40.1-
Epilepsy, epileptic, epilepsia (attack)
　(cerebral) (convulsion) (fit) (seizure)
　G40.909

> Note: the following terms are to be
> considered equivalent to intractable:
> pharmacoresistant (pharmacologically
> resistant), treatment resistant, refractory
> (medically) and poorly controlled

　with
　　complex partial seizures —see Epilepsy,
　　　localization-related, symptomatic,
　　　with complex partial seizures
　　grand mal seizures on awakening —
　　　see Epilepsy, generalized, specified
　　　NEC
　　myoclonic absences —see Epilepsy,
　　　generalized, specified NEC
　　myoclonic-astatic seizures —see Epilepsy,
　　　generalized, specified NEC
　　simple partial seizures —see Epilepsy,
　　　localization-related, symptomatic,
　　　with simple partial seizures
　akinetic —see Epilepsy, generalized, specified
　　NEC
　benign childhood with centrotemporal EEG
　　spikes —see Epilepsy, localization-
　　related, idiopathic
　benign myoclonic in infancy G40.80-
　Bravais-jacksonian —see Epilepsy,
　　localization-related, symptomatic,
　　with simple partial seizures
　childhood
　　with occipital EEG paroxysms —see
　　　Epilepsy, localization-related,
　　　idiopathic
　　absence G40.A09
　　　intractable G40.A19
　　　　with status epilepticus G40.A11
　　　　without status epilepticus
　　　　　G40.A19
　　　not intractable G40.A09
　　　　with status epilepticus G40.A01
　　　　without status epilepticus
　　　　　G40.A09
　climacteric —see Epilepsy, specified NEC
　cysticercosis B69.0
　deterioration (mental) F06.8
　due to syphilis A52.19

◀ New　⬅ Revised　~~deleted~~ Deleted

Epilepsy, epileptic, epilepsia *(Continued)*
focal —*see* Epilepsy, localization-related, symptomatic, with simple partial seizures
generalized
  idiopathic G40.309
    intractable G40.319
      with status epilepticus G40.311
      without status epilepticus G40.319
    not intractable G40.309
      with status epilepticus G40.301
      without status epilepticus G40.309
  specified NEC G40.409
    intractable G40.419
      with status epilepticus G40.411
      without status epilepticus G40.419
    not intractable G40.409
      with status epilepticus G40.401
      without status epilepticus G40.409
impulsive petit mal —*see* Epilepsy, juvenile myoclonic
intractable G40.919
  with status epilepticus G40.911
  without status epilepticus G40.919
juvenile absence G40.A09
  intractable G40.A19
    with status epilepticus G40.A11
    without status epilepticus G40.A19
  not intractable G40.A09
    with status epilepticus G40.A01
    without status epilepticus G40.A09
juvenile myoclonic G40.B11
  intractable G40.B19
    with status epilepticus G40.B11
    without status epilepticus G40.B19
  not intractable G40.B09
    with status epilepticus G40.B01
    without status epilepticus G40.B09
localization-related (focal) (partial)
  idiopathic G40.009
    with seizures of localized onset G40.009
      intractable G40.019
        with status epilepticus G40.011
        without status epilepticus G40.019
      not intractable G40.009
        with status epilepticus G40.001
        without status epilepticus G40.009
  symptomatic
    with complex partial seizures G40.209
      intractable G40.219
        with status epilepticus G40.211
        without status epilepticus G40.219
      not intractable G40.209
        with status epilepticus G40.201
        without status epilepticus G40.209
    with simple partial seizures G40.109
      intractable G40.119
        with status epilepticus G40.111
        without status epilepticus G40.119
      not intractable G40.109
        with status epilepticus G40.101
        without status epilepticus G40.109
myoclonus, myoclonic (progressive) —*see* Epilepsy, generalized, specified NEC
not intractable G40.909
  with status epilepticus G40.901
  without status epilepticus G40.909
on awakening —*see* Epilepsy, generalized, specified NEC
parasitic NOS B71.9 *[G94]*
partialis continua (*see also* Kozhevnikof's epilepsy) G40.1-
peripheral —*see* Epilepsy, specified NEC
procursiva —*see* Epilepsy, localization-related, symptomatic, with simple partial seizures
progressive (familial) myoclonic —*see* Epilepsy, generalized, idiopathic

Epilepsy, epileptic, epilepsia *(Continued)*
reflex —*see* Epilepsy, specified NEC
related to
  alcohol G40.509
    not intractable G40.509
      with status epilepticus G40.501
      without status epilepticus G40.509
  drugs G40.509
    not intractable G40.509
      with status epilepticus G40.501
      without status epilepticus G40.509
  external causes G40.509
    not intractable G40.509
      with status epilepticus G40.501
      without status epilepticus G40.509
  hormonal changes G40.509
    not intractable G40.509
      with status epilepticus G40.501
      without status epilepticus G40.509
  sleep deprivation G40.509
    not intractable G40.509
      with status epilepticus G40.501
      without status epilepticus G40.509
  stress G40.509
    not intractable G40.509
      with status epilepticus G40.501
      without status epilepticus G40.509
somatomotor —*see* Epilepsy, localization-related, symptomatic, with simple partial seizures
somatosensory —*see* Epilepsy, localization-related, symptomatic, with simple partial seizures
spasms G40.822
  intractable G40.824
    with status epilepticus G40.823
    without status epilepticus G40.824
  not intractable G40.822
    with status epilepticus G40.821
    without status epilepticus G40.822
specified NEC G40.802
  intractable G40.804
    with status epilepticus G40.803
    without status epilepticus G40.804
  not intractable G40.802
    with status epilepticus G40.801
    without status epilepticus G40.802
syndromes
  generalized
    idiopathic G40.309
      intractable G40.319
        with status epilepticus G40.311
        without status epilepticus G40.319
      not intractable G40.309
        with status epilepticus G40.301
        without status epilepticus G40.309
    specified NEC G40.409
      intractable G40.419
        with status epilepticus G40.411
        without status epilepticus G40.419
      not intractable G40.409
        with status epilepticus G40.401
        without status epilepticus G40.409
    localization-related (focal) (partial)
      idiopathic G40.009
        with seizures of localized onset G40.009
          intractable G40.019
            with status epilepticus G40.011
            without status epilepticus G40.019
          not intractable G40.009
            with status epilepticus G40.001
            without status epilepticus G40.009
      symptomatic
        with complex partial seizures G40.209
          intractable G40.219
            with status epilepticus G40.211
            without status epilepticus G40.219

Epilepsy, epileptic, epilepsia *(Continued)*
syndromes *(Continued)*
  localization-related *(Continued)*
    symptomatic *(Continued)*
      with complex partial seizures *(Continued)*
        not intractable G40.209
          with status epilepticus G40.201
          without status epilepticus G40.209
      with simple partial seizures G40.109
        intractable G40.119
          with status epilepticus G40.111
          without status epilepticus G40.119
        not intractable G40.109
          with status epilepticus G40.101
          without status epilepticus G40.109
  specified NEC G40.802
    intractable G40.804
      with status epilepticus G40.803
      without status epilepticus G40.804
    not intractable G40.802
      with status epilepticus G40.801
      without status epilepticus G40.802
tonic (-clonic) —*see* Epilepsy, generalized, specified NEC
twilight F05
uncinate (gyrus) —*see* Epilepsy, localization-related, symptomatic, with complex partial seizures
Unverricht (-Lundborg) (familial myoclonic) —*see* Epilepsy, generalized, idiopathic
visceral —*see* Epilepsy, specified NEC
visual —*see* Epilepsy, specified NEC
Epiloia Q85.1
Epimenorrhea N92.0
Epipharyngitis —*see* Nasopharyngitis
Epiphora H04.20-
due to
  excess lacrimation H04.21-
  insufficient drainage H04.22-
Epiphyseal arrest —*see* Arrest, epiphyseal
Epiphyseolysis, epiphysiolysis —*see* Osteochondropathy
Epiphysitis —*see also* Osteochondropathy
juvenile M92.9
syphilitic (congenital) A50.02
Epiplocele —*see* Hernia, abdomen
Epiploitis —*see* Peritonitis
Epiplosarcomphalocele —*see* Hernia, umbilicus
Episcleritis (suppurative) H15.10-
in (due to)
  syphilis A52.71
  tuberculosis A18.51
nodular H15.12-
periodica fugax H15.11-
  angioneurotic —*see* Edema, angioneurotic
syphilitic (late) A52.71
tuberculous A18.51
Episode
affective, mixed F39
depersonalization (in neurotic state) F48.1
depressive F32.9
  major F32.9
    mild F32.0
    moderate F32.1
    severe (without psychotic symptoms) F32.2
      with psychotic symptoms F32.3
  recurrent F33.9
    brief F33.8
  specified NEC F32.8
hypomanic F30.8
manic F30.9
  with
    psychotic symptoms F30.2
    remission (full) F30.4
      partial F30.3
  without psychotic symptoms F30.10
    mild F30.11
    moderate F30.12

Episode *(Continued)*
  manic *(Continued)*
    without psychotic symptoms *(Continued)*
      severe (without psychotic symptoms) F30.13
        with psychotic symptoms F30.2
      other specified F30.8
      recurrent F31.89
    psychotic F23
      organic F06.8
    schizophrenic (acute) NEC, brief F23
Epispadias (female) (male) Q64.0
Episplenitis D73.89
Epistaxis (multiple) R04.0
  hereditary I78.0
  vicarious menstruation N94.89
Epithelioma (malignant) —*see also* Neoplasm, malignant, by site
  adenoides cysticum —*see* Neoplasm, skin, benign
  basal cell —*see* Neoplasm, skin, malignant
  benign —*see* Neoplasm, benign, by site
  Bowen's —*see* Neoplasm, skin, in situ
  calcifying, of Malherbe —*see* Neoplasm, skin, benign
  external site —*see* Neoplasm, skin, malignant
  intraepidermal, Jadassohn —*see* Neoplasm, skin, benign
  squamous cell —*see* Neoplasm, malignant, by site
Epitheliomatosis pigmented Q82.1
Epitheliopathy, multifocal placoid pigment H30.14-
Epithelium, epithelial —*see* condition
Epituberculosis (with atelectasis) (allergic) A15.7
Eponychia Q84.6
Epstein's
  nephrosis or syndrome —*see* Nephrosis
  pearl K09.8
Epulis (gingiva) (fibrous) (giant cell) K06.8
Equinia A24.0
Equinovarus (congenital) (talipes) Q66.0
  acquired —*see* Deformity, limb, clubfoot
Equivalent
  convulsive (abdominal) —*see* Epilepsy, specified NEC
  epileptic (psychic) —*see* Epilepsy, localization-related, symptomatic, with complex partial seizures
Erb (-Duchenne) **paralysis** (birth injury) (newborn) P14.0
Erb's
  disease G71.0
  palsy, paralysis (brachial) (birth) (newborn) P14.0
    spinal (spastic) syphilitic A52.17
  pseudohypertrophic muscular dystrophy G71.0
Erb-Goldflam disease or syndrome G70.00
  with exacerbation (acute) G70.01
  in crisis G70.01
Erdheim's syndrome (acromegalic macrospondylitis) E22.0
Erection, painful (persistent) —*see* Priapism
Ergosterol deficiency (vitamin D) E55.9
  with
    adult osteomalacia M83.8
    rickets —*see* Rickets
Ergotism —*see also* Poisoning, food, noxious, plant
  from ergot used as drug (migraine therapy) —*see* Table of Drugs and Chemicals
Erosio interdigitalis blastomycetica B37.2
Erosion
  artery I77.2
    without rupture I77.89
  bone —*see* Disorder, bone, density and structure, specified NEC
  bronchus J98.09

Erosion *(Continued)*
  cartilage (joint) —*see* Disorder, cartilage, specified type NEC
  cervix (uteri) (acquired) (chronic) (congenital) N86
    with cervicitis N72
  cornea (nontraumatic) —*see* Ulcer, cornea
    recurrent H18.83-
    traumatic —*see* Abrasion, cornea
  dental (idiopathic) (occupational) (due to diet, drugs or vomiting) K03.2
  duodenum, postpyloric —*see* Ulcer, duodenum
  esophagus K22.10
    with bleeding K22.11
  gastric —*see* Ulcer, stomach
  gastrojejunal —*see* Ulcer, gastrojejunal
  implanted mesh —*see* Complications, mesh
  intestine K63.3
  lymphatic vessel I89.8
  pylorus, pyloric (ulcer) —*see* Ulcer, stomach
  spine, aneurysmal A52.09
  stomach —*see* Ulcer, stomach
  teeth (idiopathic) (occupational) (due to diet, drugs or vomiting) K03.2
  urethra N36.8
  uterus N85.8
Erotomania F52.8
Error
  metabolism, inborn —*see* Disorder, metabolism
  refractive —*see* Disorder, refraction
Eructation R14.2
  nervous or psychogenic F45.8
Eruption
  creeping B76.9
  drug (generalized) (taken internally) L27.0
    fixed L27.1
    in contact with skin —*see* Dermatitis, due to drugs
    localized L27.1
  Hutchinson, summer L56.4
  Kaposi's varicelliform B00.0
  napkin L22
  polymorphous light (sun) L56.4
  recalcitrant pustular L13.8
  ringed R23.8
  skin (nonspecific) R21
    creeping (meaning hookworm) B76.9
    due to inoculation/vaccination (generalized) (*see also* Dermatitis, due to, vaccine) L27.0
      localized L27.1
    erysipeloid A26.0
    feigned L98.1
    Kaposi's varicelliform B00.0
    lichenoid L28.0
    meaning dermatitis —*see* Dermatitis
    toxic NEC L53.0
  tooth, teeth, abnormal (incomplete) (late) (premature) (sequence) K00.6
  vesicular R23.8
Erysipelas (gangrenous) (infantile) (newborn) (phlegmonous) (suppurative) A46
  external ear A46 *[H62.40]*
  puerperal, postpartum O86.89
Erysipeloid A26.9
  cutaneous (Rosenbach's) A26.0
  disseminated A26.8
  sepsis A26.7
  specified NEC A26.8
Erythema, erythematous (infectional) (inflammation) L53.9
  ab igne L59.0
  annulare (centrifugum) (rheumaticum) L53.1
  arthriticum epidemicum A25.1
  brucellum —*see* Brucellosis
  chronic figurate NEC L53.3
  chronicum migrans (Borrelia burgdorferi) A69.20
  diaper L22

Erythema, erythematous *(Continued)*
  due to
    chemical NEC L53.0
      in contact with skin L24.5
    drug (internal use) —*see* Dermatitis, due to, drugs
  elevatum diutinum L95.1
  endemic E52
  epidemic, arthritic A25.1
  figuratum perstans L53.3
  gluteal L22
  heat - code by site under Burn, first degree
  ichthyosiforme congenitum bullous Q80.3
  in diseases classified elsewhere L54
  induratum (nontuberculous) L52
    tuberculous A18.4
  infectiosum B08.3
  intertrigo L30.4
  iris L51.9
  marginatum L53.2
    in (due to) acute rheumatic fever I00
  medicamentosum —*see* Dermatitis, due to, drugs
  migrans A26.0
    chronicum A69.20
    tongue K14.1
  multiforme (major) (minor) L51.9
    bullous, bullosum L51.1
    conjunctiva L51.1
    nonbullous L51.0
    pemphigoides L12.0
    specified NEC L51.8
  napkin L22
  neonatorum P83.8
    toxic P83.1
  nodosum L52
    tuberculous A18.4
  palmar L53.8
  pernio T69.1
  rash, newborn P83.8
  scarlatiniform (recurrent) (exfoliative) L53.8
  solare L55.0
  specified NEC L53.8
  toxic, toxicum NEC L53.0
    newborn P83.1
  tuberculous (primary) A18.4
Erythematous, erythematosus —*see* condition
Erythermalgia (primary) I73.81
Erythralgia I73.81
Erythrasma L08.1
Erythredema (polyneuropathy) —*see* Poisoning, mercury
Erythremia (acute) C94.0-
  chronic D45
  secondary D75.1
Erythroblastopenia (*see also* Aplasia, red cell) D60.9
  congenital D61.01
Erythroblastophthisis D61.09
Erythroblastosis (fetalis) (newborn) P55.9
  due to
    ABO (antibodies) (incompatibility) (isoimmunization) P55.1
    Rh (antibodies) (incompatibility) (isoimmunization) P55.0
Erythrocyanosis (crurum) I73.89
Erythrocythemia —*see* Erythremia
Erythrocytosis (megalosplenic) (secondary) D75.1
  familial D75.0
  oval, hereditary —*see* Elliptocytosis
  secondary D75.1
  stress D75.1
Erythroderma (secondary) (*see also* Erythema) L53.9
  bullous ichthyosiform, congenital Q80.3
  desquamativum L21.1
  ichthyosiform, congenital (bullous) Q80.3
  neonatorum P83.8
  psoriaticum L40.8

◀ New ◀ Revised ~~deleted~~ Deleted

Erythrodysesthesia, palmar plantar (PPE) L27.1
Erythrogenesis imperfecta D61.09
Erythroleukemia C94.0-
Erythromelalgia I73.81
Erythrophagocytosis D75.89
Erythrophobia F40.298
Erythroplakia, oral epithelium, and tongue K13.29
Erythroplasia (Queyrat) D07.4
  specified site — see Neoplasm, skin, in situ
  unspecified site D07.4
Escherichia coli (E. coli), as cause of disease classified elsewhere B96.20
  non-O157 Shiga toxin-producing (with known O group) B96.22
  non-Shiga toxin-producing B96.29
  O157 with confirmation of Shiga toxin when H antigen is unknown, or is not H7 B96.21
  O157:H- (nonmotile) with confirmation of Shiga toxin B96.21
  O157:H7 with or without confirmation of Shiga toxin-production B96.21
  Shiga toxin-producing (with unspecified O group) (STEC) B96.23
  O157 B96.21
  O157:H7 with or without confirmation of Shiga toxin-production B96.21
  specified NEC B96.22
  specified NEC B96.29
Esophagismus K22.4
Esophagitis (acute) (alkaline) (chemical) (chronic) (infectional) (necrotic) (peptic) (postoperative) K20.9
  candidal B37.81
  due to gastrointestinal reflux disease K21.0
  eosinophilic K20.0
  reflux K21.0
  specified NEC K20.8
  tuberculous A18.83
  ulcerative K22.10
    with bleeding K22.11
Esophagocele K22.5
Esophagomalacia K22.8
Esophagospasm K22.4
Esophagostenosis K22.2
Esophagostomiasis B81.8
Esophagotracheal —see condition
Esophagus —see condition
Esophoria H50.51
  convergence, excess H51.12
  divergence, insufficiency H51.8
Esotropia —see Strabismus, convergent concomitant
Espundia B55.2
Essential —see condition
Esthesioneuroblastoma C30.0
Esthesioneurocytoma C30.0
Esthesioneuroepithelioma C30.0
Esthiomene A55
Estivo-autumnal malaria (fever) B50.9
Estrangement (marital) Z63.5
  parent-child NEC Z62.890
Estriasis —see Myiasis
Ethanolism —see Alcoholism
Etherism —see Dependence, drug, inhalant
Ethmoid, ethmoidal —see condition
Ethmoiditis (chronic) (nonpurulent) (purulent) —see also Sinusitis, ethmoidal
  influenzal —see Influenza, with, respiratory manifestations NEC
  Woakes' J33.1
Ethylism —see Alcoholism
Eulenburg's disease (congenital paramyotonia) G71.19
Eumycetoma B47.0
Eunuchoidism E29.1
  hypogonadotropic E23.0
European blastomycosis —see Cryptococcosis
Eustachian —see condition

Evaluation (for) (of)
  development state
    adolescent Z00.3
    period of
      delayed growth in childhood Z00.70
        with abnormal findings Z00.71
      rapid growth in childhood Z00.2
    puberty Z00.3
  growth and developmental state (period of rapid growth) Z00.2
    delayed growth Z00.70
      with abnormal findings Z00.71
  mental health (status) Z00.8
    requested by authority Z04.6
  period of
    delayed growth in childhood Z00.70
      with abnormal findings Z00.71
    rapid growth in childhood Z00.2
  suspected condition —see Observation
Evans syndrome D69.41
Event, apparent life threatening in newborn and infant (ALTE) R68.13
Eventration —see also Hernia, ventral
  colon into chest —see Hernia, diaphragm
  diaphragm (congenital) Q79.1
Eversion
  bladder N32.89
  cervix (uteri) N86
    with cervicitis N72
  foot NEC —see also Deformity, valgus, ankle
    congenital Q66.6
  punctum lacrimale (postinfectional) (senile) H04.52-
  ureter (meatus) N28.89
  urethra (meatus) N36.8
  uterus N81.4
Evidence
  cytologic
    of malignancy on anal smear R85.614
    of malignancy on cervical smear R87.614
    of malignancy on vaginal smear R87.624
Evisceration
  birth injury P15.8
  traumatic NEC
    eye —see Enucleated eye
Evulsion —see Avulsion
Ewing's sarcoma or tumor —see Neoplasm, bone, malignant
Examination (for) (following) (general) (of) (routine) Z00.00
  with abnormal findings Z00.01
  abuse, physical (alleged), ruled out
    adult Z04.71
    child Z04.72
  adolescent (development state) Z00.3
  alleged rape or sexual assault (victim), ruled out
    adult Z04.41
    child Z04.42
  allergy Z01.82
  annual (adult) (periodic) (physical) Z00.00
    with abnormal findings Z00.01
    gynecological Z01.419
      with abnormal findings Z01.411
  antibody response Z01.84
  blood —see Examination, laboratory
  blood pressure Z01.30
    with abnormal findings Z01.31
  cancer staging —see Neoplasm, malignant, by site
  cervical Papanicolaou smear Z12.4
    as part of routine gynecological examination Z01.419
      with abnormal findings Z01.411
  child (over 28 days old) Z00.129
    with abnormal findings Z00.121
    under 28 days old —see Newborn, examination
  clinical research control or normal comparison (control) (participant) Z00.6

Examination (Continued)
  contraceptive (drug) maintenance (routine) Z30.8
    device (intrauterine) Z30.431
  dental Z01.20
    with abnormal findings Z01.21
  developmental —see Examination, child
  donor (potential) Z00.5
  ear Z01.10
    with abnormal findings NEC Z01.118
  eye Z01.00
    with abnormal findings Z01.01
  following
    accident NEC Z04.3
      transport Z04.1
      work Z04.2
    assault, alleged, ruled out
      adult Z04.71
      child Z04.72
    motor vehicle accident Z04.1
    treatment (for) Z09
      combined NEC Z09
        fracture Z09
        malignant neoplasm Z08
      malignant neoplasm Z08
      mental disorder Z09
      specified condition NEC Z09
  follow-up (routine) (following) Z09
    chemotherapy NEC Z09
      malignant neoplasm Z08
    fracture Z09
    malignant neoplasm Z08
    postpartum Z39.2
    psychotherapy Z09
    radiotherapy NEC Z09
      malignant neoplasm Z08
    surgery NEC Z09
      malignant neoplasm Z08
  gynecological Z01.419
    with abnormal findings Z01.411
    for contraceptive maintenance Z30.8
  health —see Examination, medical
  hearing Z01.10
    with abnormal findings NEC Z01.118
    following failed hearing screening Z01.110
  immunity status testing Z01.84
  laboratory (as part of a general medical examination) Z00.00
    with abnormal findings Z00.01
    preprocedural Z01.812
  lactating mother Z39.1
  medical (adult) (for) (of) Z00.00
    with abnormal findings Z00.01
    administrative purpose only Z02.9
      specified NEC Z02.89
    admission to
      armed forces Z02.3
      old age home Z02.2
      prison Z02.89
      residential institution Z02.2
      school Z02.0
        following illness or medical treatment Z02.0
      summer camp Z02.89
    adoption Z02.82
    blood alcohol or drug level Z02.83
    camp (summer) Z02.89
    clinical research, normal subject (control) (participant) Z00.6
    control subject in clinical research (normal comparison) (participant) Z00.6
    donor (potential) Z00.5
    driving license Z02.4
    general (adult) Z00.00
      with abnormal findings Z00.01
    immigration Z02.89
    insurance purposes Z02.6
    marriage Z02.89
    medicolegal reasons NEC Z04.8
    naturalization Z02.89
    participation in sport Z02.5

Examination *(Continued)*
  medical *(Continued)*
    paternity testing Z02.81
    population survey Z00.8
    pre-employment Z02.1
    pre-operative —*see* Examination,
      pre-procedural
    pre-procedural
      cardiovascular Z01.810
      respiratory Z01.811
      specified NEC Z01.818
    preschool children
      for admission to school Z02.0
    prisoners
      for entrance into prison Z02.89
    recruitment for armed forces Z02.3
    specified NEC Z00.8
    sport competition Z02.5
  medicolegal reason NEC Z04.8
  newborn —*see* Newborn, examination
  pelvic (annual) (periodic) Z01.419
    with abnormal findings Z01.411
  period of rapid growth in childhood Z00.2
  periodic (adult) (annual) (routine) Z00.00
    with abnormal findings Z00.01
  physical (adult) —*see also* Examination,
    medical Z00.00
    sports Z02.5
  postpartum
    immediately after delivery Z39.0
    routine follow-up Z39.2
  pre-chemotherapy (antineoplastic) Z01.818
  prenatal (normal pregnancy) (*see also*
    Pregnancy, normal) Z34.9-
  pre-procedural (pre-operative)
    cardiovascular Z01.810
    laboratory Z01.812
    respiratory Z01.811
    specified NEC Z01.818
  prior to chemotherapy (antineoplastic)
    Z01.818
  psychiatric NEC Z00.8
    follow-up not needing further care Z09
    requested by authority Z04.6
  radiological (as part of a general medical
    examination) Z00.00
    with abnormal findings Z00.01
  repeat cervical smear to confirm findings of
    recent normal smear following initial
    abnormal smear Z01.42
  skin (hypersensitivity) Z01.82
  special (*see also* Examination, by type) Z01.89
    specified type NEC Z01.89
  specified type or reason NEC Z04.8
  teeth Z01.20
    with abnormal findings Z01.21
  urine —*see* Examination, laboratory
  vision Z01.00
    with abnormal findings Z01.01
Exanthem, exanthema —*see also* Rash
  with enteroviral vesicular stomatitis B08.4
  Boston A88.0
  epidemic with meningitis A88.0 *[G02]*
  subitum B08.20
    due to human herpesvirus 6 B08.21
    due to human herpesvirus 7 B08.22
  viral, virus B09
    specified type NEC B08.8
Excess, excessive, excessively
  alcohol level in blood R78.0
  androgen (ovarian) E28.1
  attrition, tooth, teeth K03.0
  carotene, carotin (dietary) E67.1
  cold, effects of T69.9
    specified effect NEC T69.8
  convergence H51.12
  crying
    in child, adolescent, or adult R45.83
    in infant R68.11
  development, breast N62
  divergence H51.8

Excess, excessive, excessively *(Continued)*
  drinking (alcohol) NEC (without
    dependence) F10.10
    habitual (continual) (without remission)
      F10.20
  eating R63.2
  estrogen E28.0
  fat —*see also* Obesity
    in heart —*see* Degeneration, myocardial
    localized E65
  foreskin N47.8
  gas R14.0
  glucagon E16.3
  heat —*see* Heat
  intermaxillary vertical dimension of fully
    erupted teeth M26.37
  interocclusal distance of fully erupted teeth
    M26.37
  kalium E87.5
  large
    colon K59.3
      congenital Q43.8
    infant P08.0
    organ or site, congenital NEC —*see*
      Anomaly, by site
  long
    organ or site, congenital NEC —*see*
      Anomaly, by site
  menstruation (with regular cycle) N92.0
    with irregular cycle N92.1
  napping Z72.821
  natrium E87.0
  number of teeth K00.1
  nutrient (dietary) NEC R63.2
  potassium (K) E87.5
  salivation K11.7
  secretion —*see also* Hypersecretion
    milk O92.6
    sputum R09.3
    sweat R61
  sexual drive F52.8
  short
    organ or site, congenital NEC —*see*
      Anomaly, by site
    umbilical cord in labor or delivery O69.3
  skin, eyelid (acquired) —*see* Blepharochalasis
    congenital Q10.3
  sodium (Na) E87.0
  spacing of fully erupted teeth M26.32
  sputum R09.3
  sweating R61
  thirst R63.1
    due to deprivation of water T73.1
  tuberosity of jaw M26.07
  vitamin
    A (dietary) E67.0
      administered as drug (prolonged
        intake) —*see* Table of Drugs and
        Chemicals, vitamins, adverse
        effect
      overdose or wrong substance given or
        taken —*see* Table of Drugs and
        Chemicals, vitamins, poisoning
    D (dietary) E67.3
      administered as drug (prolonged
        intake) —*see* Table of Drugs and
        Chemicals, vitamins, adverse
        effect
      overdose or wrong substance given or
        taken —*see* Table of Drugs and
        Chemicals, vitamins, poisoning
  weight
    gain R63.5
    loss R63.4
Excitability, abnormal, under minor stress
  (personality disorder) F60.3
Excitation
  anomalous atrioventricular I45.6
  psychogenic F30.8
  reactive (from emotional stress, psychological
    trauma) F30.8

Excitement
  hypomanic F30.8
  manic F30.9
  mental, reactive (from emotional stress,
    psychological trauma) F30.8
  state, reactive (from emotional stress,
    psychological trauma) F30.8
Excoriation (traumatic) —*see also* Abrasion
  neurotic L98.1
Exfoliation
  due to erythematous conditions according to
    extent of body surface involved L49.0
    10-19 percent of body surface L49.1
    20-29 percent of body surface L49.2
    30-39 percent of body surface L49.3
    40-49 percent of body surface L49.4
    50-59 percent of body surface L49.5
    60-69 percent of body surface L49.6
    70-79 percent of body surface L49.7
    80-89 percent of body surface L49.8
    90-99 percent of body surface L49.9
    less than 10 percent of body surface L49.0
  teeth, due to systemic causes K08.0
Exfoliative —*see* condition
Exhaustion, exhaustive (physical NEC) R53.83
  battle F43.0
  cardiac —*see* Failure, heart
  delirium F43.0
  due to
    cold T69.8
    excessive exertion T73.3
    exposure T73.2
    neurasthenia F48.8
  heart —*see* Failure, heart
  heat (*see also* Heat, exhaustion) T67.5
    due to
      salt depletion T67.4
      water depletion T67.3
  maternal, complicating delivery O75.81
  mental F48.8
  myocardium, myocardial —*see* Failure, heart
  nervous F48.8
  old age R54
  psychogenic F48.8
  psychosis F43.0
  senile R54
  vital NEC Z73.0
Exhibitionism F65.2
Exocervicitis —*see* Cervicitis
Exomphalos Q79.2
  meaning hernia —*see* Hernia, umbilicus
Exophoria H50.52
  convergence, insufficiency H51.11
  divergence, excess H51.8
Exophthalmos H05.2-
  congenital Q15.8
  constant NEC H05.24-
  displacement, globe —*see* Displacement,
    globe
  due to thyrotoxicosis (hyperthyroidism) —*see*
    Hyperthyroidism, with, goiter (diffuse)
  dysthyroid —*see* Hyperthyroidism, with,
    goiter (diffuse)
  goiter —*see* Hyperthyroidism, with, goiter
    (diffuse)
  intermittent NEC H05.25-
  malignant —*see* Hyperthyroidism, with,
    goiter (diffuse)
  orbital
    edema —*see* Edema, orbit
    hemorrhage —*see* Hemorrhage, orbit
  pulsating NEC H05.26-
  thyrotoxic, thyrotropic —*see*
    Hyperthyroidism, with, goiter (diffuse)
Exostosis —*see also* Disorder, bone
  cartilaginous —*see* Neoplasm, bone, benign
  congenital (multiple) Q78.6
  external ear canal H61.81-
  gonococcal A54.49
  jaw (bone) M27.8
  multiple, congenital Q78.6

◀ New   ◀||| Revised   ~~deleted~~ Deleted

Exostosis *(Continued)*
  orbit H05.35-
    osteocartilaginous —*see* Neoplasm, bone,
      benign
  syphilitic A52.77
Exotropia —*see* Strabismus, divergent
    concomitant
Explanation of
  investigation finding Z71.2
  medication Z71.89
Exposure (to) *(see also* Contact, with) T75.89
  acariasis Z20.7
  AIDS virus Z20.6
  air pollution Z77.110
  algae and algae toxins Z77.121
  algae bloom Z77.121
  anthrax Z20.810
  aromatic amines Z77.020
  aromatic (hazardous) compounds NEC
    Z77.028
  aromatic dyes NOS Z77.028
  arsenic Z77.010
  asbestos Z77.090
  bacterial disease NEC Z20.818
  benzene Z77.021
  blue-green algae bloom Z77.121
  body fluids (potentially hazardous) Z77.21
  brown tide Z77.121
  chemicals (chiefly nonmedicinal) (hazardous)
    NEC Z77.098
  cholera Z20.09
  chromium compounds Z77.018
  cold, effects of T69.9
    specified effect NEC T69.8
  communicable disease Z20.9
    bacterial NEC Z20.818
    specified NEC Z20.89
    viral NEC Z20.828
  cyanobacteria bloom Z77.121
  disaster Z65.5
  discrimination Z60.5
  dyes Z77.098
  effects of T73.9
  environmental tobacco smoke (acute)
    (chronic) Z77.22
  Escherichia coli (E. coli) Z20.01
  exhaustion due to T73.2
  fiberglass —*see* Table of Drugs and
    Chemicals, fiberglass
  German measles Z20.4
  gonorrhea Z20.2
  hazardous metals NEC Z77.018
  hazardous substances NEC Z77.29
  hazards in the physical environment NEC
    Z77.128
  hazards to health NEC Z77.9
  human immunodeficiency virus (HIV) Z20.6
  human T-lymphotropic virus type-1 (HTLV-1)
    Z20.89

Exposure *(Continued)*
  implanted
    mesh —*see* Complications, mesh
    prosthetic materials NEC —*see*
      Complications, prosthetic materials
      NEC
  infestation (parasitic) NEC Z20.7
  intestinal infectious disease NEC Z20.09
    Escherichia coli (E. coli) Z20.01
  lead Z77.011
  meningococcus Z20.811
  mold (toxic) Z77.120
  nickel dust Z77.018
  noise Z77.122
  occupational
    air contaminants NEC Z57.39
    dust Z57.2
    environmental tobacco smoke Z57.31
    extreme temperature Z57.6
    noise Z57.0
    radiation Z57.1
    risk factors Z57.9
      specified NEC Z57.8
    toxic agents (gases) (liquids) (solids)
      (vapors) in agriculture Z57.4
    toxic agents (gases) (liquids) (solids)
      (vapors) in industry NEC Z57.5
    vibration Z57.7
  parasitic disease NEC Z20.7
  pediculosis Z20.7
  persecution Z60.5
  pfiesteria piscicida Z77.121
  poliomyelitis Z20.89
  pollution
    air Z77.110
    environmental NEC Z77.118
    soil Z77.112
    water Z77.111
  polycyclic aromatic hydrocarbons Z77.028
  prenatal (drugs) (toxic chemicals) —*see*
    Newborn, affected by (suspected to
    be), noxious substances transmitted via
    placenta or breast milk
  rabies Z20.3
  radiation, naturally occurring NEC Z77.123
  radon Z77.123
  red tide (Florida) Z77.121
  rubella Z20.4
  second hand tobacco smoke (acute) (chronic)
    Z77.22
    in the perinatal period P96.81
  sexually-transmitted disease Z20.2
  smallpox (laboratory) Z20.89
  syphilis Z20.2
  terrorism Z65.4
  torture Z65.4
  tuberculosis Z20.1
  uranium Z77.012
  varicella Z20.820

Exposure *(Continued)*
  venereal disease Z20.2
  viral disease NEC Z20.828
  war Z65.5
  water pollution Z77.111
Exsanguination —*see* Hemorrhage
Exstrophy
  abdominal contents Q45.8
  bladder Q64.10
    cloacal Q64.12
    specified type NEC Q64.19
    supravesical fissure Q64.11
Extensive —*see* condition
Extra —*see also* Accessory
  marker chromosomes (normal individual)
    Q92.61
    in abnormal individual Q92.62
  rib Q76.6
    cervical Q76.5
Extrasystoles (supraventricular) I49.49
  atrial I49.1
  auricular I49.1
  junctional I49.2
  ventricular I49.3
Extrauterine gestation or pregnancy —*see*
    Pregnancy, by site
Extravasation
  blood R58
  chyle into mesentery I89.8
  pelvicalyceal N13.8
  pyelosinus N13.8
  urine (from ureter) R39.0
  vesicant agent
    antineoplastic chemotherapy T80.810
    other agent NEC T80.818
Extremity —*see* condition, limb
Extrophy —*see* Exstrophy
Extroversion
  bladder Q64.19
  uterus N81.4
    complicating delivery O71.2
    postpartal (old) N81.4
Extruded tooth (teeth) M26.34
Extrusion
  breast implant (prosthetic) T85.42
  eye implant (globe) (ball) T85.328
  intervertebral disc —*see* Displacement,
    intervertebral disc
  ocular lens implant (prosthetic) —*see*
    Complications, intraocular lens
  vitreous —*see* Prolapse, vitreous
Exudate
  pleural —*see* Effusion, pleura
  retina H35.89
Exudative —*see* condition
Eye, eyeball, eyelid —*see* condition
Eyestrain —*see* Disturbance, vision, subjective
Eyeworm disease of Africa B74.3

F

Faber's syndrome (achlorhydric anemia) D50.9
Fabry (-Anderson) **disease** E75.21
Faciocephalalgia, autonomic (*see also*
    Neuropathy, peripheral, autonomic)
    G90.09
Factor (s)
    psychic, associated with diseases classified
        elsewhere F54
    psychological
        affecting physical conditions F54
        or behavioral
            affecting general medical condition F54
            associated with disorders or diseases
                classified elsewhere F54
Fahr disease (of brain) G23.8
Fahr Volhard disease (of kidney) I12.-
Failure, failed
    abortion —*see* Abortion, attempted
    aortic (valve) I35.8
        rheumatic I06.8
    attempted abortion —*see* Abortion, attempted
    biventricular I50.9
    bone marrow —*see* Anemia, aplastic
    cardiac —*see* Failure, heart
    cardiorenal (chronic) I50.9
        hypertensive I13.2
    cardiorespiratory (*see also* Failure, heart)
        R09.2
    cardiovascular (chronic) —*see* Failure, heart
    cerebrovascular I67.9
    cervical dilatation in labor O62.0
    circulation, circulatory (peripheral) R57.9
        newborn P29.89
    compensation —*see* Disease, heart
    compliance with medical treatment or
        regimen —*see* Noncompliance
    congestive —*see* Failure, heart, congestive
    dental implant (endosseous) M27.69
        due to
            failure of dental prosthesis M27.63
            lack of attached gingiva M27.62
            occlusal trauma (poor prosthetic design)
                M27.62
            parafunctional habits M27.62
            periodontal infection (peri-implantitis)
                M27.62
            poor oral hygiene M27.62
        osseointegration M27.61
            due to
                complications of systemic disease
                    M27.61
                poor bone quality M27.61
            iatrogenic M27.61
        post-osseointegration
            biological M27.62
            due to complications of systemic disease
                M27.62
            iatrogenic M27.62
            mechanical M27.63
        pre-integration M27.61
        pre-osseointegration M27.61
        specified NEC M27.69
    descent of head (at term) of pregnancy
        (mother) O32.4
    endosseous dental implant —*see* Failure,
        dental implant
    engagement of head (term of pregnancy)
        (mother) O32.4
    erection (penile) (*see also* Dysfunction, sexual,
        male, erectile) N52.9
        nonorgqanic F52.21
    examination (s), anxiety concerning Z55.2
    expansion terminal respiratory units
        (newborn) (primary) P28.0
    forceps NOS (with subsequent cesarean
        delivery) O66.5
    gain weight (child over 28 days old) R62.51
        adult R62.7
        newborn P92.6

Failure, failed (*Continued*)
    genital response (male) F52.21
        female F52.22
    heart (acute) (senile) (sudden) I50.9
        with
            acute pulmonary edema —*see* Failure,
                ventricular, left
            decompensation —*see* Failure, heart,
                congestive
            dilatation —*see* Disease, heart
        arteriosclerotic I70.90
        biventricular I50.9
        combined left-right sided I50.9
        compensated I50.9
        complicating
            anesthesia (general) (local) or other
                sedation
                in labor and delivery O74.2
                in pregnancy O29.12-
                postpartum, puerperal O89.1
            delivery (cesarean) (instrumental) O75.4
        congestive (compensated)
            (decompensated) I50.9
            with rheumatic fever (conditions in I00)
                active I01.8
                inactive or quiescent (with chorea)
                    I09.81
            newborn P29.0
            rheumatic (chronic) (inactive) (with
                chorea) I09.81
                active or acute I01.8
                    with chorea I02.0
        decompensated I50.9
        degenerative —*see* Degeneration,
            myocardial
        diastolic (congestive) I50.30
            acute (congestive) I50.31
                and (on) chronic (congestive) I50.33
            chronic (congestive) I50.32
                and (on) acute (congestive) I50.33
            combined with systolic (congestive)
                I50.40
                acute (congestive) I50.41
                    and (on) chronic (congestive)
                        I50.43
                chronic (congestive) I50.42
                    and (on) acute (congestive) I50.43
        due to presence of cardiac prosthesis
            I97.13-
        following cardiac surgery I97.13-
        high output NOS I50.9
        hypertensive —*see* Hypertension, heart
        left (ventricular) —*see* Failure, ventricular,
            left
        low output (syndrome) NOS I50.9
        newborn P29.0
        organic —*see* Disease, heart
        peripartum O90.3
        postprocedural I97.13-
        rheumatic (chronic) (inactive) I09.9
        right (ventricular) (secondary to left
            heart failure) —*see* Failure, heart,
            congestive
        systolic (congestive) I50.20
            acute (congestive) I50.21
                and (on) chronic (congestive)
                    I50.23
            chronic (congestive) I50.22
                and (on) acute (congestive) I50.23
            combined with diastolic (congestive)
                I50.40
                acute (congestive) I50.41
                    and (on) chronic (congestive)
                        I50.43
                chronic (congestive) I50.42
                    and (on) acute (congestive)
                        I50.43
        thyrotoxic (*see also* Thyrotoxicosis)
            E05.90 [*I43*]
            with thyroid storm E05.91 [*I43*]
        valvular —*see* Endocarditis

Failure, failed (*Continued*)
    hepatic K72.90
        with coma K72.91
        acute or subacute K72.00
            with coma K72.01
            due to drugs K71.10
                with coma K71.11
        alcoholic (acute) (chronic) (subacute)
            K70.40
            with coma K70.41
        chronic K72.10
            with coma K72.11
            due to drugs (acute) (subacute) (chronic)
                K71.10
                with coma K71.11
        due to drugs (acute) (subacute) (chronic)
            K71.10
            with coma K71.11
        postprocedural K91.82
    hepatorenal K76.7
    induction (of labor) O61.9
        abortion —*see* Abortion, attempted
        by
            oxytocic drugs O61.0
            prostaglandins O61.0
        instrumental O61.1
        mechanical O61.1
        medical O61.0
        specified NEC O61.8
        surgical O61.1
    intubation during anesthesia T88.4
        in pregnancy O29.6-
        labor and delivery O74.7
        postpartum, puerperal O89.6
    involution, thymus (gland) E32.0
    kidney (*see also* Disease, kidney, chronic) N19
        acute (*see also* Failure, renal, acute) N17.9-
        diabetic - see E08-E13 with .22
    lactation (complete) O92.3
        partial O92.4
    Leydig's cell, adult E29.1
    liver —*see* Failure, hepatic
    menstruation at puberty N91.0
    mitral I05.8
    myocardial, myocardium (*see also* Failure,
        heart) I50.9
        chronic (*see also* Failure, heart, congestive)
            I50.9
        congestive (*see also* Failure, heart,
            congestive) I50.9
    orgasm (female) (psychogenic) F52.31
        male F52.32
    ovarian (primary) E28.39
        iatrogenic E89.40
            asymptomatic E89.40
            symptomatic E89.41
        postprocedural (postablative)
            (postirradiation) (postsurgical)
            E89.40
            asymptomatic E89.40
            symptomatic E89.41
    ovulation causing infertility N97.0
    polyglandular, autoimmune E31.0
    prosthetic joint implant —*see* Complications,
        joint prosthesis, mechanical,
        breakdown, by site
    renal N19
        with
            tubular necrosis (acute) N17.0
        acute N17.9
            with
                cortical necrosis N17.1
                medullary necrosis N17.2
                tubular necrosis N17.0
            specified NEC N17.8
        chronic N18.9
            hypertensive —*see* Hypertension,
                kidney
        congenital P96.0
        end stage (chronic) N18.6
            due to hypertension I12.0

◀ New   ◀|||| Revised   ~~deleted~~ Deleted

Failure, failed (Continued)
renal (Continued)
following
abortion —see Abortion by type
complicated by specified
condition NEC
crushing T79.5
ectopic or molar pregnancy O08.4
labor and delivery (acute) O90.4
hypertensive —see Hypertension,
kidney
postprocedural N99.0
respiration, respiratory J96.9
with
hypercapnia J96.92
hypoxia J96.91
acute J96.00
with
hypercapnia J96.02
hypoxia J96.01
acute and (on) chronic J96.20
with
hypercapnia J96.22
hypoxia J96.21
center G93.89
chronic J96.10
with
hypercapnia J96.12
hypoxia J96.11
newborn P28.5
postprocedural (acute) J95.821
acute and chronic J95.822
rotation
cecum Q43.3
colon Q43.3
intestine Q43.3
kidney Q63.2
sedation (conscious) (moderate) during
procedure T88.52
history of Z92.83
segmentation —see also Fusion
fingers —see Syndactylism, complex,
fingers
vertebra Q76.49
with scoliosis Q76.3
seminiferous tubule, adult E29.1
senile (general) R54
sexual arousal (male) F52.21
female F52.22
testicular endocrine function E29.1
to thrive (child over 28 days old)
R62.51
adult R62.7
newborn P92.6
transplant T86.92
bone T86.831
marrow T86.02
cornea T86.841
heart T86.22
with lung (s) T86.32
intestine T86.851
kidney T86.12
liver T86.42
lung (s) T86.811
with heart T86.32
pancreas T86.891
skin (allograft) (autograft) T86.821
specified organ or tissue NEC T86.891
stem cell (peripheral blood) (umbilical
cord) T86.5
trial of labor (with subsequent cesarean
delivery) O66.40
following previous cesarean delivery
O66.41
tubal ligation N99.89
urinary —see Disease, kidney, chronic
vacuum extraction NOS (with subsequent
cesarean delivery) O66.5
vasectomy N99.89
ventouse NOS (with subsequent cesarean
delivery) O66.5

Failure, failed (Continued)
ventricular (see also Failure, heart) I50.9
left I50.1
with rheumatic fever (conditions in I00)
active I01.8
with chorea I02.0
inactive or quiescent (with chorea)
I09.81
rheumatic (chronic) (inactive) (with
chorea) I09.81
active or acute I01.8
with chorea I02.0
right (see also Failure, heart, congestive)
I50.9
vital centers, newborn P91.8
Fainting (fit) R55
Fallen arches —see Deformity, limb, flat foot
Falling, falls (repeated) R29.6
any organ or part —see Prolapse
Fallopian
insufflation Z31.41
tube —see condition
Fallot's
pentalogy Q21.8
tetrad or tetralogy Q21.3
triad or trilogy Q22.3
False —see also condition
croup J38.5
joint —see Nonunion, fracture
labor (pains) O47.9
at or after 37 completed weeks of gestation
O47.1
before 37 completed weeks of gestation
O47.0-
passage, urethra (prostatic) N36.5
pregnancy F45.8
Family, familial —see also condition
disruption Z63.8
involving divorce or separation Z63.5
Li-Fraumeni (syndrome) Z15.01
planning advice Z30.09
problem Z63.9
specified NEC Z63.8
retinoblastoma C69.2-
Famine (effects of) T73.0
edema —see Malnutrition, severe
Fanconi (-de Toni)(-Debré) **syndrome** E72.09
with cystinosis E72.04
Fanconi's anemia (congenital pancytopenia)
D61.09
Farber's disease or syndrome E75.29
Farcy A24.0
Farmer's
lung J67.0
skin L57.8
Farsightedness —see Hypermetropia
Fascia —see condition
Fasciculation R25.3
Fasciitis M72.9
diffuse (eosinophilic) M35.4
infective M72.8
necrotizing M72.6
necrotizing M72.6
nodular M72.4
perirenal (with ureteral obstruction)
N13.5
with infection N13.6
plantar M72.2
specified NEC M72.8
traumatic (old) M72.8
current - code by site under Sprain
Fascioliasis B66.3
Fasciolopsis, fasciolopsiasis (intestinal)
B66.5
Fascioscapulohumeral myopathy G71.0
Fast pulse R00.0
Fat
embolism —see Embolism, fat
excessive —see also Obesity
in heart —see Degeneration, myocardial
in stool R19.5

Fat (Continued)
localized (pad) E65
heart —see Degeneration, myocardial
knee M79.4
retropatellar M79.4
necrosis
breast N64.1
mesentery K65.4
omentum K65.4
pad E65
knee M79.4
Fatigue R53.83
auditory deafness —see Deafness
chronic R53.82
combat F43.0
general R53.83
psychogenic F48.8
heat (transient) T67.6
muscle M62.89
myocardium —see Failure, heart
neoplasm-related R53.0
nervous, neurosis F48.8
operational F48.8
psychogenic (general) F48.8
senile R54
voice R49.8
Fatness —see Obesity
Fatty —see also condition
apron E65
degeneration —see Degeneration, fatty
heart (enlarged) —see Degeneration,
myocardial
liver NEC K76.0
alcoholic K70.0
nonalcoholic K76.0
necrosis —see Degeneration, fatty
Fauces —see condition
Fauchard's disease (periodontitis) —see
Periodontitis
Faucitis J02.9
Favism (anemia) D55.0
Favus —see Dermatophytosis
Fazio-Londe disease or syndrome
G12.1
Fear complex or reaction F40.9
Fear of —see Phobia
Feared complaint unfounded Z71.1
Febris, febrile —see also Fever
flava (see also Fever, yellow) A95.9
melitensis A23.0
pestis —see Plague
recurrens —see Fever, relapsing
rubra A38.9
Fecal
incontinence R15.9
smearing R15.1
soiling R15.1
urgency R15.2
Fecalith (impaction) K56.41
appendix K38.1
congenital P76.8
Fede's disease K14.0
**Feeble rapid pulse due to shock following
injury** T79.4
Feeble-minded F70
Feeding
difficulties R63.3
problem R63.3
newborn P92.9
specified NEC P92.8
nonorganic (adult) —see Disorder,
eating
Feeling (of)
foreign body in throat R09.89
Feer's disease —see Poisoning, mercury
Feet —see condition
Feigned illness Z76.5
Feil-Klippel syndrome (brevicollis) Q76.1
Feinmesser's (hidrotic) **ectodermal dysplasia**
Q82.4
Felinophobia F40.218

Felon —*see also* Cellulitis, digit
  with lymphangitis —*see* Lymphangitis, acute,
    digit
Felty's syndrome M05.00
  ankle M05.07-
  elbow M05.02-
  foot joint M05.07-
  hand joint M05.04-
  hip M05.05-
  knee M05.06-
  multiple site M05.09
  shoulder M05.01-
  vertebra —*see* Spondylitis, ankylosing
  wrist M05.03-
Female genital cutting status —*see* Female
  genital mutilation status (FGM)
Female genital mutilation status (FGM) N90.810
  specified NEC N90.818
  type I (clitorectomy status) N90.811
  type II (clitorectomy with excision of labia
    minora status) N90.812
  type III (infibulation status) N90.813
  type IV N90.818
Femur, femoral —*see* condition
Fenestration, fenestrated —*see also* Imperfect,
  closure
  aortico-pulmonary Q21.4
  cusps, heart valve NEC Q24.8
    pulmonary Q22.3
  pulmonic cusps Q22.3
Fernell's disease (aortic aneurysm) I71.9
Fertile eunuch syndrome E23.0
Fetid
  breath R19.6
  sweat L75.0
Fetishism F65.0
  transvestic F65.1
Fetus, fetal —*see also* condition
  alcohol syndrome (dysmorphic) Q86.0
  compressus O31.0-
  hydantoin syndrome Q86.1
  lung tissue P28.0
  papyraceous O31.0-
Fever (inanition) (of unknown origin)
  (persistent) (with chills) (with rigor) R50.9
  abortus A23.1
  Aden (dengue) A90
  African tick-borne A68.1
  American
    mountain (tick) A93.2
    spotted A77.0
  aphthous B08.8
  arbovirus, arboviral A94
    hemorrhagic A94
    specified NEC A93.8
  Argentinian hemorrhagic A96.0
  Assam B55.0
  Australian Q A78
  Bangkok hemorrhagic A91
  Barmah forest A92.8
  Bartonella A44.0
  bilious, hemoglobinuric B50.8
  blackwater B50.8
  blister B00.1
  Bolivian hemorrhagic A96.1
  Bonvale dam T73.3
  boutonneuse A77.1
  brain —*see* Encephalitis
  Brazilian purpuric A48.4
  breakbone A90
  Bullis A77.0
  Bunyamwera A92.8
  Burdwan B55.0
  Bwamba A92.8
  Cameroon —*see* Malaria
  Canton A75.9
  catarrhal (acute) J00
    chronic J31.0
  cat-scratch A28.1
  Central Asian hemorrhagic A98.0
  cerebral —*see* Encephalitis

Fever (Continued)
  cerebrospinal meningococcal A39.0
  Chagres B50.9
  Chandipura A92.8
  Changuinola A93.1
  Charcot's (biliary) (hepatic) (intermittent) —
    see Calculus, bile duct
  Chikungunya (viral) (hemorrhagic)
    A92.0
  Chitral A93.1
  Colombo —*see* Fever, paratyphoid
  Colorado tick (virus) A93.2
  congestive (remittent) —*see* Malaria
  Congo virus A98.0
  continued malarial B50.9
  Corsican —*see* Malaria
  Crimean-Congo hemorrhagic A98.0
  Cyprus —*see* Brucellosis
  dandy A90
  deer fly —*see* Tularemia
  dengue (virus) A90
    hemorrhagic A91
    sandfly A93.1
  desert B38.0
  drug induced R50.2
  due to
    conditions classified elsewhere
      R50.81
    heat T67.0
  enteric A01.00
  enteroviral exanthematous (Boston
    exanthem) A88.0
  ephemeral (of unknown origin) R50.9
  epidemic hemorrhagic A98.5
  erysipelatous —*see* Erysipelas
  estivo-autumnal (malarial) B50.9
  famine A75.0
  five day A79.0
  following delivery O86.4
  Fort Bragg A27.89
  gastroenteric A01.00
  gastromalarial —*see* Malaria
  Gibraltar —*see* Brucellosis
  glandular —*see* Mononucleosis, infectious
  Guama (viral) A92.8
  Haverhill A25.1
  hay (allergic) J30.1
    with asthma (bronchial) J45.909
      with
        exacerbation (acute) J45.901
        status asthmaticus J45.902
    due to
      allergen other than pollen J30.89
      pollen, any plant or tree J30.1
  heat (effects) T67.0
  hematuric, bilious B50.8
  hemoglobinuric (malarial) (bilious) B50.8
  hemorrhagic (arthropod-borne) NOS A94
    with renal syndrome A98.5
    arenaviral A96.9
      specified NEC A96.8
    Argentinian A96.0
    Bangkok A91
    Bolivian A96.1
    Central Asian A98.0
    Chikungunya A92.0
    Crimean-Congo A98.0
    dengue (virus) A91
    epidemic A98.5
    Junin (virus) A96.0
    Korean A98.5
    Kyasanur forest A98.2
    Machupo (virus) A96.1
    mite-borne A93.8
    mosquito-borne A92.8
    Omsk A98.1
    Philippine A91
    Russian A98.5
    Singapore A91
    Southeast Asia A91
    Thailand A91

Fever (Continued)
  hemorrhagic NOS (Continued)
    tick-borne NEC A93.8
    viral A99
      specified NEC A98.8
  hepatic —*see* Cholecystitis
  herpetic —*see* Herpes
  icterohemorrhagic A27.0
  Indiana A93.8
  infective B99.9
    specified NEC B99.8
  intermittent (bilious) —*see also* Malaria
    of unknown origin R50.9
    pernicious B50.9
  iodide R50.2
  Japanese river A75.3
  jungle —*see also* Malaria
    yellow A95.0
  Junin (virus) hemorrhagic A96.0
  Katayama B65.2
  kedani A75.3
  Kenya (tick) A77.1
  Kew Garden A79.1
  Korean hemorrhagic A98.5
  Lassa A96.2
  Lone Star A77.0
  Machupo (virus) hemorrhagic A96.1
  malaria, malarial —*see* Malaria
  Malta A23.9
  Marseilles A77.1
  marsh —*see* Malaria
  Mayaro (viral) A92.8
  Mediterranean (*see also* Brucellosis) A23.9
    familial E85.0
    tick A77.1
  meningeal —*see* Meningitis
  Meuse A79.0
  Mexican A75.2
  mianeh A68.1
  miasmatic —*see* Malaria
  mosquito-borne (viral) A92.9
    hemorrhagic A92.8
  mountain —*see also* Brucellosis
    meaning Rocky Mountain spotted fever
      A77.0
    tick (American) (Colorado) (viral) A93.2
  Mucambo (viral) A92.8
  mud A27.9
  Neapolitan —*see* Brucellosis
  neutropenic D70.9
  newborn P81.9
    environmental P81.0
  Nine-Mile A78
  non-exanthematous tick A93.2
  North Asian tick-borne A77.2
  Omsk hemorrhagic A98.1
  O'nyong-nyong (viral) A92.1
  Oropouche (viral) A93.0
  Oroya A44.0
  paludal —*see* Malaria
  Panama (malarial) B50.9
  Pappataci A93.1
  paratyphoid A01.4
    A A01.1
    B A01.2
    C A01.3
  parrot A70
  periodic (Mediterranean) E85.0
  persistent (of unknown origin) R50.9
  petechial A39.0
  pharyngoconjunctival B30.2
  Philippine hemorrhagic A91
  phlebotomus A93.1
  Piry (virus) A93.8
  Pixuna (viral) A92.8
  Plasmodium ovale B53.0
  polioviral (nonparalytic) A80.4
  Pontiac A48.2
  postimmunization R50.83
  postoperative R50.82
    due to infection T81.4

◀ New   ◀◀ Revised   ~~deleted~~ Deleted

Fever *(Continued)*
  posttransfusion R50.84
  postvaccination R50.83
  presenting with conditions classified
      elsewhere R50.81
  pretibial A27.89
  puerperal O86.4
  Q A78
  quadrilateral A78
  quartan (malaria) B52.9
  Queensland (coastal) (tick) A77.3
  quintan A79.0
  rabbit —*see* Tularemia
  rat-bite A25.9
    due to
        Spirillum A25.0
        Streptobacillus moniliformis A25.1
  recurrent —*see* Fever, relapsing
  relapsing (Borrelia) A68.9
    Carter's (Asiatic) A68.1
    Dutton's (West African) A68.1
    Koch's A68.9
    louse-borne A68.0
    Novy's
      louse-borne A68.0
      tick-borne A68.1
    Obermeyer's (European) A68.0
    tick-borne A68.1
  remittent (bilious) (congestive) (gastric) —*see*
      Malaria
  rheumatic (active) (acute) (chronic) (subacute)
      I00
    with central nervous system involvement
        I02.9
    active with heart involvement (*see*
        category) I01
    inactive or quiescent with
      cardiac hypertrophy I09.89
      carditis I09.9
      endocarditis I09.1
        aortic (valve) I06.9
          with mitral (valve) disease I08.0
        mitral (valve) I05.9
          with aortic (valve) disease I08.0
        pulmonary (valve) I09.89
        tricuspid (valve) I07.8
      heart disease NEC I09.89
      heart failure (congestive) (conditions in
          I50.9) I09.81
      left ventricular failure (conditions in
          I50.1) I09.81
      myocarditis, myocardial degeneration
          (conditions in I51.4) I09.0
      pancarditis I09.9
      pericarditis I09.2
  Rift Valley (viral) A92.4
  Rocky Mountain spotted A77.0
  rose J30.1
  Ross River B33.1
  Russian hemorrhagic A98.5
  San Joaquin (Valley) B38.0
  sandfly A93.1
  Sao Paulo A77.0
  scarlet A38.9
  seven day (leptospirosis) (autumnal)
      (Japanese) A27.89
    dengue A90
  shin-bone A79.0
  Singapore hemorrhagic A91
  solar A90
  Songo A98.5
  sore B00.1
  South African tick-bite A68.1
  Southeast Asia hemorrhagic A91
  spinal —*see* Meningitis
  spirillary A25.0
  splenic —*see* Anthrax
  spotted A77.9
    American A77.0
    Brazilian A77.0
    cerebrospinal meningitis A39.0

Fever *(Continued)*
  spotted *(Continued)*
    Colombian A77.0
    due to Rickettsia
      australis A77.3
      conorii A77.1
      rickettsii A77.0
      sibirica A77.2
      specified type NEC A77.8
    Ehrlichiosis A77.40
      due to
          E. chafeensis A77.41
          specified organism NEC A77.49
    Rocky Mountain A77.0
  steroid R50.2
  streptobacillary A25.1
  subtertian B50.9
  Sumatran mite A75.3
  sun A90
  swamp A27.9
  swine A02.8
  sylvatic, yellow A95.0
  Tahyna B33.8
  tertian —*see* Malaria, tertian
  Thailand hemorrhagic A91
  thermic T67.0
  three-day A93.1
  tick
    American mountain A93.2
    Colorado A93.2
    Kemerovo A93.8
    Mediterranean A77.1
    mountain A93.2
    nonxanthematous A93.2
    Quaranfil A93.8
  tick-bite NEC A93.8
  tick-borne (hemorrhagic) NEC A93.8
  trench A79.0
  tsutsugamushi A75.3
  typhogastric A01.00
  typhoid (abortive) (hemorrhagic)
      (intermittent) (malignant) A01.00
    complicated by
      arthritis A01.04
      heart involvement A01.02
      meningitis A01.01
      osteomyelitis A01.05
      pneumonia A01.03
      specified NEC A01.09
  typhomalarial —*see* Malaria
  typhus —*see* Typhus (fever)
  undulant —*see* Brucellosis
  unknown origin R50.9
  uveoparotid D86.89
  valley B38.0
  Venezuelan equine A92.2
  vesicular stomatitis A93.8
  viral hemorrhagic —*see* Fever, hemorrhagic,
      by type of virus
  Volhynian A79.0
  Wesselsbron (viral) A92.8
  West
    African B50.8
    Nile (viral) A92.30
      with
        complications NEC A92.39
        cranial nerve disorders A92.32
        encephalitis A92.31
        encephalomyelitis A92.31
        neurologic manifestation NEC
            A92.32
        optic neuritis A92.32
        polyradiculitis A92.32
  Whitmore's —*see* Melioidosis
  Wolhynian A79.0
  worm B83.9
  yellow A95.9
    jungle A95.0
    sylvatic A95.0
    urban A95.1
  Zika (viral) A92.8

Fibrillation
  atrial or auricular (established) I48.91
    chronic I48.2
    paroxysmal I48.0
    permanent I48.2
    persistent I48.1
  cardiac I49.8
  heart I49.8
  muscular M62.89
  ventricular I49.01
Fibrin
  ball or bodies, pleural (sac) J94.1
  chamber, anterior (eye) (gelatinous
      exudate) —*see* Iridocyclitis, acute
Fibrinogenolysis —*see* Fibrinolysis
Fibrinogenopenia D68.8
  acquired D65
  congenital D68.2
Fibrinolysis (hemorrhagic) (acquired) D65
  antepartum hemorrhage —*see* Hemorrhage,
      antepartum, with coagulation defect
  following
      abortion —*see* Abortion by type
          complicated by hemorrhage
      ectopic or molar pregnancy O08.1
  intrapartum O67.0
  newborn, transient P60
  postpartum O72.3
Fibrinopenia (hereditary) D68.2
  acquired D68.4
Fibrinopurulent —*see* condition
Fibrinous —*see* condition
Fibroadenoma
  cellular intracanalicular D24-
  giant D24-
  intracanalicular
    cellular D24-
    giant D24-
    specified site —*see* Neoplasm, benign, by
        site
    unspecified site D24-
  juvenile D24-
  pericanalicular
    specified site —*see* Neoplasm, benign, by
        site
    unspecified site D24-
  phyllodes D24-
  prostate D29.1
  specified site NEC —*see* Neoplasm, benign,
      by site
  unspecified site D24-
Fibroadenosis, breast (chronic) (cystic) (diffuse)
    (periodic) (segmental) N60.2-
Fibroangioma —*see also* Neoplasm, benign, by
    site
  juvenile
    specified site —*see* Neoplasm, benign, by
        site
    unspecified site D10.6
Fibrochondrosarcoma —*see* Neoplasm,
    cartilage, malignant
Fibrocystic
  disease —*see also* Fibrosis, cystic
    breast —*see* Mastopathy, cystic
    jaw M27.49
    kidney (congenital) Q61.8
    liver Q44.6
    pancreas E84.9
  kidney (congenital) Q61.8
Fibrodysplasia ossificans progressiva —*see*
    Myositis, ossificans, progressiva
Fibroelastosis (cordis) (endocardial)
    (endomyocardial) I42.4
Fibroid (tumor) —*see also* Neoplasm, connective
    tissue, benign
  disease, lung (chronic) —*see* Fibrosis, lung
  heart (disease) —*see* Myocarditis
  in pregnancy or childbirth O34.1-
    causing obstructed labor O65.5
  induration, lung (chronic) —*see* Fibrosis, lung
  lung —*see* Fibrosis, lung

Fibroid *(Continued)*
  pneumonia (chronic) —*see* Fibrosis, lung
  uterus D25.9
Fibrolipoma —*see* Lipoma
Fibroliposarcoma —*see* Neoplasm, connective
  tissue, malignant
Fibroma —*see also* Neoplasm, connective tissue,
  benign
  ameloblastic —*see* Cyst, calcifying
    odontogenic
  bone (nonossifying) —*see* Disorder, bone,
    specified type NEC
    ossifying —*see* Neoplasm, bone,
      benign
  cementifying —*see* Neoplasm, bone,
    benign
  chondromyxoid —*see* Neoplasm, bone,
    benign
  desmoplastic —*see* Neoplasm, connective
    tissue, uncertain behavior
  durum —*see* Neoplasm, connective tissue,
    benign
  fascial —*see* Neoplasm, connective tissue,
    benign
  invasive —*see* Neoplasm, connective tissue,
    uncertain behavior
  molle —*see* Lipoma
  myxoid —*see* Neoplasm, connective tissue,
    benign
  nasopharynx, nasopharyngeal (juvenile)
    D10.6
  nonosteogenic (nonossifying) —*see* Dysplasia,
    fibrous
  odontogenic (central) —*see* Cyst, calcifying
    odontogenic
  ossifying —*see* Neoplasm, bone, benign
  periosteal —*see* Neoplasm, bone, benign
  soft —*see* Lipoma
Fibromatosis M72.9
  abdominal —*see* Neoplasm, connective tissue,
    uncertain behavior
  aggressive —*see* Neoplasm, connective tissue,
    uncertain behavior
  congenital generalized —*see* Neoplasm,
    connective tissue, uncertain behavior
  Dupuytren's M72.0
  gingival K06.1
  palmar (fascial) M72.0
  plantar (fascial) M72.2
  pseudosarcomatous (proliferative)
    (subcutaneous) M72.4
  retroperitoneal D48.3
  specified NEC M72.8
Fibromyalgia M79.7
Fibromyoma —*see also* Neoplasm, connective
  tissue, benign
  uterus (corpus) —*see also* Leiomyoma, uterus
    in pregnancy or childbirth —*see* Fibroid, in
      pregnancy or childbirth
      causing obstructed labor O65.5
Fibromyositis M79.7
Fibromyxolipoma D17.9
Fibromyxoma —*see* Neoplasm, connective
  tissue, benign
Fibromyxosarcoma —*see* Neoplasm, connective
  tissue, malignant
Fibro-odontoma, ameloblastic —*see* Cyst,
  calcifying odontogenic
Fibro-osteoma —*see* Neoplasm, bone, benign
Fibroplasia, retrolental H35.17
Fibropurulent —*see* condition
Fibrosarcoma —*see also* Neoplasm, connective
  tissue, malignant
  ameloblastic C41.1
    upper jaw (bone) C41.0
  congenital —*see* Neoplasm, connective tissue,
    malignant
  fascial —*see* Neoplasm, connective tissue,
    malignant
  infantile —*see* Neoplasm, connective tissue,
    malignant

Fibrosarcoma *(Continued)*
  odontogenic C41.1
    upper jaw (bone) C41.0
  periosteal —*see* Neoplasm, bone, malignant
Fibrosclerosis
  breast N60.3-
  multifocal M35.5
  penis (corpora cavernosa) N48.6
Fibrosis, fibrotic
  adrenal (gland) E27.8
  amnion O41.8X-
  anal papillae K62.89
  arteriocapillary —*see* Arteriosclerosis
  bladder N32.89
    interstitial —*see* Cystitis, chronic,
      interstitial
    localized submucosal —*see* Cystitis,
      chronic, interstitial
    panmural —*see* Cystitis, chronic,
      interstitial
  breast —*see* Fibrosclerosis, breast
  capillary (*see also* Arteriosclerosis) I70.90
    lung (chronic) —*see* Fibrosis, lung
  cardiac —*see* Myocarditis
  cervix N88.8
  chorion O41.8X-
  corpus cavernosum (sclerosing) N48.6
  cystic (of pancreas) E84.9
    with
      distal intestinal obstruction syndrome
        E84.19
      fecal impaction E84.19
      intestinal manifestations NEC E84.19
      pulmonary manifestations E84.0
      specified manifestations NEC E84.8
  due to device, implant or graft (*see also*
    Complications, by site and type,
    specified NEC) T85.82
    arterial graft NEC T82.828
    breast (implant) T85.82
    catheter NEC T85.82
      dialysis (renal) T82.828
        intraperitoneal T85.82
      infusion NEC T82.828
        spinal (epidural) (subdural) T85.82
      urinary (indwelling) T83.82
    electronic (electrode) (pulse generator)
      (stimulator)
      bone T84.82
      cardiac T82.827
      nervous system (brain) (peripheral
        nerve) (spinal) T85.82
      urinary T83.82
    fixation, internal (orthopedic) NEC T84.82
    gastrointestinal (bile duct) (esophagus)
      T85.82
    genital NEC T83.82
    heart NEC T82.827
    joint prosthesis T84.82
    ocular (corneal graft) (orbital implant)
      NEC T85.82
    orthopedic NEC T84.82
    specified NEC T85.82
    urinary NEC T83.82
    vascular NEC T82.828
    ventricular intracranial shunt T85.82
  ejaculatory duct N50.8
  endocardium —*see* Endocarditis
  endomyocardial (tropical) I42.3
  epididymis N50.8
  eye muscle —*see* Strabismus, mechanical
  heart —*see* Myocarditis
  hepatic —*see* Fibrosis, liver
  hepatolienal (portal hypertension) K76.6
  hepatosplenic (portal hypertension) K76.6
  infrapatellar fat pad M79.4
  intrascrotal N50.8
  kidney N26.9
  liver K74.0
    with sclerosis K74.2
    alcoholic K70.2

Fibrosis, fibrotic *(Continued)*
  lung (atrophic) (chronic) (confluent)
    (massive) (perialveolar) (peribronchial)
    J84.10
    with
      anthracosilicosis J60
      anthracosis J60
      asbestosis J61
      bagassosis J67.1
      bauxite J63.1
      berylliosis J63.2
      byssinosis J66.0
      calcicosis J62.8
      chalicosis J62.8
      dust reticulation J64
      farmer's lung J67.0
      ganister disease J62.8
      graphite J63.3
      pneumoconiosis NOS J64
      siderosis J63.4
      silicosis J62.8
    capillary J84.10
    congenital P27.8
    diffuse (idiopathic) J84.10
      chemicals, gases, fumes or vapors
        (inhalation) J68.4
      interstitial J84.10
        acute J84.114
      talc J62.0
    following radiation J70.1
    idiopathic J84.112
    postinflammatory J84.10
    silicotic J62.8
    tuberculous —*see* Tuberculosis, pulmonary
  lymphatic gland I89.8
  median bar —*see* Hyperplasia, prostate
  mediastinum (idiopathic) J98.5
  meninges G96.19
  myocardium, myocardial —*see* Myocarditis
  ovary N83.8
  oviduct N83.8
  pancreas K86.8
  penis NEC N48.6
  pericardium I31.0
  perineum, in pregnancy or childbirth O34.7-
    causing obstructed labor O65.5
  pleura J94.1
  popliteal fat pad M79.4
  prostate (chronic) —*see* Hyperplasia, prostate
  pulmonary (*see also* Fibrosis, lung) J84.10
    congenital P27.8
    idiopathic J84.112
  rectal sphincter K62.89
  retroperitoneal, idiopathic (with ureteral
    obstruction) N13.5
    with infection N13.6
  sclerosing mesenteric (idiopathic) K65.4
  scrotum N50.8
  seminal vesicle N50.8
  senile R54
  skin L90.5
  spermatic cord N50.8
  spleen D73.89
    in schistosomiasis (bilharziasis) B65.9
      [D77]
  subepidermal nodular —*see* Neoplasm, skin,
    benign
  submucous (oral) (tongue) K13.5
  testis N44.8
    chronic, due to syphilis A52.76
  thymus (gland) E32.8
  tongue, submucous K13.5
  tunica vaginalis N50.8
  uterus (non-neoplastic) N85.8
  vagina N89.8
  valve, heart —*see* Endocarditis
  vas deferens N50.8
  vein I87.8
Fibrositis (periarticular) M79.7
  nodular, chronic (Jaccoud's) (rheumatoid) —
    see Arthropathy, postrheumatic, chronic

Fibrothorax J94.1
Fibrotic —*see* Fibrosis
Fibrous —*see* condition
Fibroxanthoma —*see also* Neoplasm, connective
    tissue, benign
  atypical —*see* Neoplasm, connective tissue,
    uncertain behavior
  malignant —*see* Neoplasm, connective tissue,
    malignant
Fibroxanthosarcoma —*see* Neoplasm,
    connective tissue, malignant
Fiedler's
  disease (icterohemorrhagic leptospirosis)
    A27.0
  myocarditis (acute) I40.1
Fifth disease B08.3
  venereal A55
Filaria, filarial, filariasis —*see* Infestation,
    filarial
Filatov's disease —*see* Mononucleosis,
    infectious
File-cutter's disease —*see* Poisoning, lead
Filling defect
  biliary tract R93.2
  bladder R93.4
  duodenum R93.3
  gallbladder R93.2
  gastrointestinal tract R93.3
  intestine R93.3
  kidney R93.4
  stomach R93.3
  ureter R93.4
Fimbrial cyst Q50.4
Financial problem affecting care NOS Z59.9
  bankruptcy Z59.8
  foreclosure on loan Z59.8
Findings, abnormal, inconclusive, without
    diagnosis —*see also* Abnormal
  17-ketosteroids, elevated R82.5
  acetonuria R82.4
  alcohol in blood R78.0
  anisocytosis R71.8
  antenatal screening of mother O28.9
    biochemical O28.1
    chromosomal O28.5
    cytological O28.2
    genetic O28.5
    hematological O28.0
    radiological O28.4
    specified NEC O28.8
    ultrasonic O28.3
  antibody titer, elevated R76.0
  anticardiolipin antibody R76.0
  antiphosphatidylglycerol antibody R76.0
  antiphosphatidylinositol antibody R76.0
  antiphosphatidylserine antibody R76.0
  antiphospholipid antibody R76.0
  bacteriuria N39.0
  bicarbonate E87.8
  bile in urine R82.2
  blood sugar R73.09
    high R73.9
    low (transient) E16.2
  body fluid or substance, specified NEC R88.8
  casts, urine R82.99
  catecholamines R82.5
  cells, urine R82.99
  chloride E87.8
  cholesterol E78.9
    high E78.0
      with high triglycerides E78.2
  chyluria R82.0
  cloudy
    dialysis effluent R88.0
    urine R82.90
  creatinine clearance R94.4
  crystals, urine R82.99
  culture
    blood R78.81
    positive —*see* Positive, culture
  echocardiogram R93.1

Findings, abnormal, inconclusive, without
    diagnosis (*Continued*)
  electrolyte level, urinary R82.99
  function study NEC R94.8
    bladder R94.8
    endocrine NEC R94.7
      thyroid R94.6
    kidney R94.4
    liver R94.5
    pancreas R94.8
    placenta R94.8
    pulmonary R94.2
    spleen R94.8
  gallbladder, nonvisualization R93.2
  glucose (tolerance test) (non-fasting)
    R73.09
  glycosuria R81
  heart
    shadow R93.1
    sounds R01.2
  hematinuria R82.3
  hematocrit drop (precipitous) R71.0
  hemoglobinuria R82.3
  human papillomavirus (HPV) DNA test
    positive
    cervix
      high risk R87.810
      low risk R87.820
    vagina
      high risk R87.811
      low risk R87.821
  in blood (of substance not normally found in
    blood) R78.9
    addictive drug NEC R78.4
    alcohol (excessive level) R78.0
    cocaine R78.2
    hallucinogen R78.3
    heavy metals (abnormal level) R78.79
    lead R78.71
    lithium (abnormal level) R78.89
    opiate drug R78.1
    psychotropic drug R78.5
    specified substance NEC R78.89
    steroid agent R78.6
  indoleacetic acid, elevated R82.5
  ketonuria R82.4
  lactic acid dehydrogenase (LDH) R74.0
  liver function test R79.89
  mammogram NEC R92.8
    calcification (calculus) R92.1
    inconclusive result (due to dense breasts)
      R92.2
    microcalcification R92.0
  mediastinal shift R93.8
  melanin, urine R82.99
  myoglobinuria R82.1
  neonatal screening P09
  nonvisualization of gallbladder R93.2
  odor of urine NOS R82.90
  Papanicolaou cervix R87.619
    non-atypical endometrial cells R87.618
  pneumoencephalogram R93.0
  poikilocytosis R71.8
  potassium (deficiency) E87.6
    excess E87.5
  PPD R76.11
  radiologic (X-ray) R93.8
    abdomen R93.5
    biliary tract R93.2
    breast R92.8
    gastrointestinal tract R93.3
    genitourinary organs R93.8
    head R93.0
    inconclusive due to excess body fat of
      patient R93.9
    intrathoracic organs NEC R93.1
    placenta R93.8
    retroperitoneum R93.5
    skin R93.8
    skull R93.0
    subcutaneous tissue R93.8

Findings, abnormal, inconclusive, without
    diagnosis (*Continued*)
  red blood cell (count) (morphology) (sickling)
    (volume) R71.8
  scan NEC R94.8
    bladder R94.8
    bone R94.8
    kidney R94.4
    liver R93.2
    lung R94.2
    pancreas R94.8
    placental R94.8
    spleen R94.8
    thyroid R94.6
  sedimentation rate, elevated R70.0
  SGOT R74.0
  SGPT R74.0
  sodium (deficiency) E87.1
    excess E87.0
  specified body fluid NEC R88.8
  stress test R94.39
  thyroid (function) (metabolic rate) (scan)
    (uptake) R94.6
  transaminase (level) R74.0
  triglycerides E78.9
    high E78.1
      with high cholesterol E78.2
  tuberculin skin test (without active
    tuberculosis) R76.11
  urine R82.90
    acetone R82.4
    bacteria N39.0
    bile R82.2
    casts or cells R82.99
    chyle R82.0
    culture positive R82.7
    glucose R81
    hemoglobin R82.3
    ketone R82.4
    sugar R81
  vanillylmandelic acid (VMA), elevated
    R82.5
  vectorcardiogram (VCG) R94.39
  ventriculogram R93.0
  white blood cell (count) (differential)
    (morphology) D72.9
  xerography R92.8
Finger —*see* condition
Fire, Saint Anthony's —*see* Erysipelas
Fire-setting
  pathological (compulsive) F63.1
Fish hook stomach K31.89
Fishmeal-worker's lung J67.8
Fissure, fissured
  anus, anal K60.2
    acute K60.0
    chronic K60.1
    congenital Q43.8
  ear, lobule, congenital Q17.8
  epiglottis (congenital) Q31.8
  larynx J38.7
    congenital Q31.8
  lip K13.0
    congenital —*see* Cleft, lip
  nipple N64.0
    associated with
      lactation O92.13
      pregnancy O92.11-
      puerperium O92.12
  nose Q30.2
  palate (congenital) —*see* Cleft, palate
  skin R23.4
  spine (congenital) —*see also* Spina bifida
    with hydrocephalus —*see* Spina bifida, by
      site, with hydrocephalus
  tongue (acquired) K14.5
    congenital Q38.3
Fistula (cutaneous) L98.8
  abdomen (wall) K63.2
    bladder N32.2
    intestine NEC K63.2

Fistula (*Continued*)
  abdomen (*Continued*)
    ureter N28.89
    uterus N82.5
  abdominorectal K63.2
  abdominosigmoidal K63.2
  abdominothoracic J86.0
  abdominouterine N82.5
    congenital Q51.7
  abdominovesical N32.2
  accessory sinuses —*see* Sinusitis
  actinomycotic —*see* Actinomycosis
  alveolar antrum —*see* Sinusitis, maxillary
  alveolar process K04.6
  anorectal K60.5
  antrobuccal —*see* Sinusitis, maxillary
  antrum —*see* Sinusitis, maxillary
  anus, anal (recurrent) (infectional) K60.3
    congenital Q43.6
      with absence, atresia and stenosis Q42.2
    tuberculous A18.32
  aorta-duodenal I77.2
  appendix, appendicular K38.3
  arteriovenous (acquired) (nonruptured) I77.0
    brain I67.1
      congenital Q28.2
        ruptured I60.8
      ruptured I60.8
    cerebral —*see* Fistula, arteriovenous, brain
    congenital (peripheral) —*see also*
      Malformation, arteriovenous
      brain Q28.2
        ruptured I60.8
      coronary Q24.5
      pulmonary Q25.72
    coronary I25.41
      congenital Q24.5
    pulmonary I28.0
      congenital Q25.72
    surgically created (for dialysis) Z99.2
      complication —*see* Complication,
        arteriovenous, fistula, surgically
        created
    traumatic —*see* Injury, blood vessel
  artery I77.2
  aural (mastoid) —*see* Mastoiditis, chronic
  auricle —*see also* Disorder, pinna, specified
    type NEC
    congenital Q18.1
  Bartholin's gland N82.8
  bile duct (common) (hepatic) K83.3
    with calculus, stones —*see* Calculus, bile
      duct
  biliary (tract) —*see* Fistula, bile duct
  bladder (sphincter) NEC (*see also* Fistula,
    vesico-) N32.2
    into seminal vesicle N32.2
  bone —*see also* Disorder, bone, specified type
    NEC
    with osteomyelitis, chronic —*see*
      Osteomyelitis, chronic, with draining
      sinus
  brain G93.89
    arteriovenous (acquired) I67.1
      congenital Q28.2
  branchial (cleft) Q18.0
  branchiogenous Q18.0
  breast N61
    puerperal, postpartum or gestational, due
      to mastitis (purulent) —*see* Mastitis,
      obstetric, purulent
  bronchial J86.0
  bronchocutaneous, bronchomediastinal,
    bronchopleural,
    bronchopleuromediastinal (infective)
    J86.0
    tuberculous NEC A15.5
  bronchoesophageal J86.0
    congenital Q39.2
      with atresia of esophagus Q39.1
  bronchovisceral J86.0

buccal cavity (infective) K12.2
cecosigmoidal K63.2
cecum K63.2
cerebrospinal (fluid) G96.0
cervical, lateral Q18.1
cervicoaural Q18.1
cervicosigmoidal N82.4
cervicovesical N82.1
cervix N82.8
chest (wall) J86.0
cholecystenteric —*see* Fistula, gallbladder
cholecystocolic —*see* Fistula, gallbladder
cholecystocolonic —*see* Fistula, gallbladder
cholecystoduodenal —*see* Fistula,
  gallbladder
cholecystogastric —*see* Fistula, gallbladder
cholecystointestinal —*see* Fistula,
  gallbladder
choledochoduodenal —*see* Fistula,
  bile duct
cholocolic K82.3
coccyx —*see* Sinus, pilonidal
colon K63.2
colostomy K94.09
common duct —*see* Fistula, bile duct
congenital, site not listed —*see* Anomaly, by
  site
coronary, arteriovenous I25.41
  congenital Q24.5
costal region J86.0
cul-de-sac, Douglas' N82.8
cystic duct —*see also* Fistula, gallbladder
  congenital Q44.5
dental K04.6
diaphragm J86.0
duodenum K31.6
ear (external) (canal) —*see* Disorder, ear,
  external, specified type NEC
enterocolic K63.2
enterocutaneous K63.2
enterouterine N82.4
  congenital Q51.7
enterovaginal N82.4
  congenital Q52.2
  large intestine N82.3
  small intestine N82.2
enterovesical N32.1
epididymis N50.8
  tuberculous A18.15
esophagobronchial J86.0
  congenital Q39.2
    with atresia of esophagus Q39.1
esophagocutaneous K22.8
esophagopleural-cutaneous J86.0
esophagotracheal J86.0
  congenital Q39.2
    with atresia of esophagus Q39.1
esophagus K22.8
  congenital Q39.2
    with atresia of esophagus Q39.1
ethmoid —*see* Sinusitis, ethmoidal
eyeball (cornea) (sclera) —*see* Disorder, globe,
  hypotony
eyelid H01.8
fallopian tube, external N82.5
fecal K63.2
  congenital Q43.6
from periapical abscess K04.6
frontal sinus —*see* Sinusitis, frontal
gallbladder K82.3
  with calculus, cholelithiasis, stones —*see*
    Calculus, gallbladder
gastric K31.6
gastrocolic K31.6
  congenital Q40.2
  tuberculous A18.32
gastroenterocolic K31.6
gastroesophageal K31.6
gastrojejunal K31.6
gastrojejunocolic K31.6

genital tract (female) N82.9
  specified NEC N82.8
  to intestine NEC N82.4
  to skin N82.5
hepatic artery-portal vein, congenital Q26.6
hepatopleural J86.0
hepatopulmonary J86.0
ileorectal or ileosigmoidal K63.2
ileovaginal N82.2
ileovesical N32.1
ileum K63.2
in ano K60.3
  tuberculous A18.32
inner ear (labyrinth) —*see* subcategory H83.1
intestine NEC K63.2
intestinocolonic (abdominal) K63.2
intestinoureteral N28.89
intestinouterine N82.4
intestinovaginal N82.4
  large intestine N82.3
  small intestine N82.2
intestinovesical N32.1
ischiorectal (fossa) K61.3
jejunum K63.2
joint M25.10
  ankle M25.17-
  elbow M25.12-
  foot joint M25.17-
  hand joint M25.14-
  hip M25.15-
  knee M25.16-
  shoulder M25.11-
  specified joint NEC M25.18
  tuberculous —*see* Tuberculosis, joint
  vertebrae M25.18
  wrist M25.13-
kidney N28.89
labium (majus) (minus) N82.8
labyrinth —*see* subcategory H83.1
lacrimal (gland) (sac) H04.61-
lacrimonasal duct —*see* Fistula, lacrimal
laryngotracheal, congenital Q34.8
larynx J38.7
lip K13.0
  congenital Q38.0
lumbar, tuberculous A18.01
lung J86.0
lymphatic I89.8
mammary (gland) N61
mastoid (process) (region) —*see* Mastoiditis,
  chronic
maxillary J32.0
medial, face and neck Q18.8
mediastinal J86.0
mediastinobronchial J86.0
mediastinocutaneous J86.0
middle ear —*see* subcategory H74.8
mouth K12.2
nasal J34.89
  sinus —*see* Sinusitis
nasopharynx J39.2
nipple N64.0
nose J34.89
oral (cutaneous) K12.2
  maxillary J32.0
  nasal (with cleft palate) —*see* Cleft, palate
orbit, orbital —*see* Disorder, orbit, specified
  type NEC
oroantral J32.0
oviduct, external N82.5
palate (hard) M27.8
pancreatic K86.8
pancreaticoduodenal K86.8
parotid (gland) K11.4
  region K12.2
penis N48.89
perianal K60.3
pericardium (pleura) (sac) —*see* Pericarditis
pericecal K63.2
perineorectal K60.4
perineosigmoidal K63.2

◀ New   ◀▥ Revised   ~~deleted~~ Deleted

Fistula *(Continued)*
  perineum, perineal (with urethral
    involvement) NEC N36.0
    tuberculous A18.13
    ureter N28.89
  perirectal K60.4
    tuberculous A18.32
  peritoneum K65.9
  pharyngoesophageal J39.2
  pharynx J39.2
    branchial cleft (congenital) Q18.0
  pilonidal (infected) (rectum) —*see* Sinus,
    pilonidal
  pleura, pleural, pleurocutaneous,
    pleuroperitoneal J86.0
    tuberculous NEC A15.6
  pleuropericardial I31.8
  portal vein-hepatic artery, congenital Q26.6
  postauricular H70.81-
  postoperative, persistent T81.83
    specified site —*see* Fistula, by site
  preauricular (congenital) Q18.1
  prostate N42.89
  pulmonary J86.0
    arteriovenous I28.0
      congenital Q25.72
    tuberculous —*see* Tuberculosis, pulmonary
  pulmonoperitoneal J86.0
  rectolabial N82.4
  rectosigmoid (intercommunicating) K63.2
  rectoureteral N28.89
  rectourethral N36.0
    congenital Q64.73
  rectouterine N82.4
    congenital Q51.7
  rectovaginal N82.3
    congenital Q52.2
    tuberculous A18.18
  rectovesical N32.1
    congenital Q64.79
  rectovesicovaginal N82.3
  rectovulval N82.4
    congenital Q52.79
  rectum (to skin) K60.4
    congenital Q43.6
      with absence, atresia and stenosis Q42.0
    tuberculous A18.32
  renal N28.89
  retroauricular —*see* Fistula, postauricular
  salivary duct or gland (any) K11.4
    congenital Q38.4
  scrotum (urinary) N50.8
    tuberculous A18.15
  semicircular canals —*see* subcategory H83.1
  sigmoid K63.2
    to bladder N32.1
  sinus —*see* Sinusitis
  skin L98.8
    to genital tract (female) N82.5
  splenocolic D73.89
  stercoral K63.2
  stomach K31.6
  sublingual gland K11.4
  submandibular gland K11.4
  submaxillary (gland) K11.4
    region K12.2
  thoracic J86.0
    duct I89.8
  thoracoabdominal J86.0
  thoracogastric J86.0
  thoracointestinal J86.0
  thorax J86.0
  thyroglossal duct Q89.2
  thyroid E07.89
  trachea, congenital (external) (internal) Q32.1
  tracheoesophageal J86.0
    congenital Q39.2
      with atresia of esophagus Q39.1
    following tracheostomy J95.04
  traumatic arteriovenous —*see* Injury, blood
    vessel, by site

Fistula *(Continued)*
  tuberculous - code by site under
    Tuberculosis
  typhoid A01.09
  umbilicourinary Q64.8
  urachus, congenital Q64.4
  ureter (persistent) N28.89
  ureteroabdominal N28.89
  ureterorectal N28.89
  ureterosigmoido-abdominal N28.89
  ureterovaginal N82.1
  ureterovesical N32.2
  urethra N36.0
    congenital Q64.79
    tuberculous A18.13
  urethroperineal N36.0
  urethroperineovesical N32.2
  urethrorectal N36.0
    congenital Q64.73
  urethroscrotal N50.8
  urethrovaginal N82.1
  urethrovesical N32.2
  urinary (tract) (persistent) (recurrent)
    N36.0
  uteroabdominal N82.5
    congenital Q51.7
  uteroenteric, uterointestinal N82.4
    congenital Q51.7
  uterorectal N82.4
    congenital Q51.7
  uteroureteric N82.1
  uterourethral Q51.7
  uterovaginal N82.8
  uterovesical N82.1
    congenital Q51.7
  uterus N82.8
  vagina (postpartal) (wall) N82.8
  vaginocutaneous (postpartal) N82.5
  vaginointestinal NEC N82.4
    large intestine N82.3
    small intestine N82.2
  vaginoperineal N82.5
  vasocutaneous, congenital Q55.7
  vesical NEC N32.2
  vesicoabdominal N32.2
  vesicocervicovaginal N82.1
  vesicocolic N32.1
  vesicocutaneous N32.2
  vesicoenteric N32.1
  vesicointestinal N32.1
  vesicometrorectal N82.4
  vesicoperineal N32.2
  vesicorectal N32.1
    congenital Q64.79
  vesicosigmoidal N32.1
  vesicosigmoidovaginal N82.3
  vesicoureteral N32.2
  vesicoureterovaginal N82.1
  vesicourethral N32.2
  vesicourethrorectal N32.1
  vesicouterine N82.1
    congenital Q51.7
  vesicovaginal N82.0
  vulvorectal N82.4
    congenital Q52.79
Fit R56.9
  epileptic —*see* Epilepsy
  fainting R55
  hysterical F44.5
  newborn P90
Fitting (and adjustment) (of)
  artificial
    arm —*see* Admission, adjustment, artificial,
      arm
    breast Z44.3
    eye Z44.2
    leg —*see* Admission, adjustment, artificial,
      leg
  automatic implantable cardiac defibrillator
    (with synchronous cardiac pacemaker)
    Z45.02

Fitting *(Continued)*
  brain neuropacemaker Z46.2
    implanted Z45.42
  cardiac defibrillator —*see* Fitting (and
    adjustment) (of), automatic implantable
    cardiac defibrillator
  catheter, non-vascular Z46.82
  colostomy belt Z46.89
  contact lenses Z46.0
  cystostomy device Z46.6
  defibrillator, cardiac —*see* Fitting (and
    adjustment) (of), automatic implantable
    cardiac defibrillator
  dentures Z46.3
  device NOS Z46.9
    abdominal Z46.89
    gastrointestinal NEC Z46.59
    implanted NEC Z45.89
    nervous system Z46.2
      implanted —*see* Admission, adjustment,
        device, implanted, nervous
        system
    orthodontic Z46.4
    orthoptic Z46.0
    orthotic Z46.89
    prosthetic (external) Z44.9
      breast Z44.3
      dental Z46.3
      eye Z44.2
      specified NEC Z44.8
    specified NEC Z46.89
    substitution
      auditory Z46.2
        implanted —*see* Admission,
          adjustment, device, implanted,
          hearing device
      nervous system Z46.2
        implanted —*see* Admission,
          adjustment, device, implanted,
          nervous system
      visual Z46.2
        implanted Z45.31
    urinary Z46.6
  gastric lap band Z46.51
  gastrointestinal appliance NEC Z46.59
  glasses (reading) Z46.0
  hearing aid Z46.1
  ileostomy device Z46.89
  insulin pump Z46.81
  intestinal appliance NEC Z46.89
  myringotomy device (stent) (tube) Z45.82
  neuropacemaker Z46.2
    implanted Z45.42
  non-vascular catheter Z46.82
  orthodontic device Z46.4
  orthopedic device (brace) (cast) (corset)
    (shoes) Z46.89
  pacemaker (cardiac) Z45.018
    nervous system (brain) (peripheral nerve)
      (spinal cord) Z46.2
      implanted Z45.42
    pulse generator Z45.010
  portacath (port-a-cath) Z45.2
  prosthesis (external) Z44.9
    arm —*see* Admission, adjustment, artificial,
      arm
    breast Z44.3
    dental Z46.3
    eye Z44.2
    leg —*see* Admission, adjustment, artificial,
      leg
    specified NEC Z44.8
  spectacles Z46.0
  wheelchair Z46.89
Fitzhugh-Curtis syndrome
  due to
    Chlamydia trachomatis A74.81
    Neisseria gonorrhorea (gonococcal
      peritonitis) A54.85
Fitz's syndrome (acute hemorrhagic
  pancreatitis) K85.8

Fixation
joint —*see* Ankylosis
larynx J38.7
stapes —*see* Ankylosis, ear ossicles
deafness —*see* Deafness, conductive
uterus (acquired) —*see* Malposition, uterus
vocal cord J38.3
Flabby ridge K06.8
Flaccid —*see also* condition
palate, congenital Q38.5
Flail
chest S22.5-
newborn (birth injury) P13.8
joint (paralytic) M25.20
ankle M25.27-
elbow M25.22-
foot joint M25.27-
hand joint M25.24-
hip M25.25-
knee M25.26-
shoulder M25.21-
specified joint NEC M25.28
wrist M25.23-
Flajani's disease —*see* Hyperthyroidism, with, goiter (diffuse)
Flap, liver K71.3
Flashbacks (residual to hallucinogen use) F16.283
Flat
chamber (eye) —*see* Disorder, globe, hypotony, flat anterior chamber
chest, congenital Q67.8
foot (acquired) (fixed type) (painful) (postural) —*see also* Deformity, limb, flat foot
congenital (rigid) (spastic (everted)) Q66.5-
rachitic sequelae (late effect) E64.3
organ or site, congenital NEC —*see* Anomaly, by site
pelvis M95.5
with disproportion (fetopelvic) O33.0
causing obstructed labor O65.0
congenital Q74.2
Flatau-Schilder disease G37.0
Flatback syndrome M40.30
lumbar region M40.36
lumbosacral region M40.37
thoracolumbar region M40.35
Flattening
head, femur M89.8X5
hip —*see* Coxa, plana
lip (congenital) Q18.8
nose (congenital) Q67.4
acquired M95.0
Flatulence R14.3
psychogenic F45.8
Flatus R14.3
vaginalis N89.8
Flax-dresser's disease J66.1
Flea bite —*see* Injury, bite, by site, superficial, insect
Flecks, glaucomatous (subcapsular) —*see* Cataract, complicated
Fleischer (-Kayser) **ring** (cornea) H18.04-
Fleshy mole O02.0
Flexibilitas cerea —*see* Catalepsy
Flexion
amputation stump (surgical) T87.89
cervix —*see* Malposition, uterus
contracture, joint —*see* Contraction, joint
deformity, joint (*see also* Deformity, limb, flexion) M21.20
hip, congenital Q65.89
uterus —*see also* Malposition, uterus
lateral —*see* Lateroversion, uterus
Flexner-Boyd dysentery A03.2
Flexner's dysentery A03.1
Flexure —*see* Flexion
Flint murmur (aortic insufficiency) I35.1
Floater, vitreous —*see* Opacity, vitreous

Floating
cartilage (joint) —*see also* Loose, body, joint
knee —*see* Derangement, knee, loose body
gallbladder, congenital Q44.1
kidney N28.89
congenital Q63.8
spleen D73.89
Flooding N92.0
Floor —*see* condition
Floppy
baby syndrome (nonspecific) P94.2
iris syndrome (intraoperative) (IFIS) H21.81
nonrheumatic mitral valve syndrome I34.1
Flu —*see also* Influenza
avian (*see also* Influenza, due to, identified novel influenza A virus) J09.X2
bird (*see also* Influenza, due to, identified novel influenza A virus) J09.X2
intestinal NEC A08.4
swine (viruses that normally cause infections in pigs) (*see also* Influenza, due to, identified novel influenza A virus) J09.X2
Fluctuating blood pressure I99.8
Fluid
abdomen R18.8
chest J94.8
heart —*see* Failure, heart, congestive
joint —*see* Effusion, joint
loss (acute) E86.9
with
hypernatremia E87.0
hyponatremia E87.1
lung —*see* Edema, lung
overload E87.70
specified NEC E87.79
peritoneal cavity R18.8
pleural cavity J94.8
retention R60.9
Flukes NEC —*see also* Infestation, fluke
blood NEC —*see* Schistosomiasis
liver B66.3
Fluor (vaginalis) N89.8
trichomonal or due to Trichomonas (vaginalis) A59.00
Fluorosis
dental K00.3
skeletal M85.10
ankle M85.17-
foot M85.17-
forearm M85.13-
hand M85.14-
lower leg M85.16-
multiple site M85.19
neck M85.18
rib M85.18
shoulder M85.11-
skull M85.18
specified site NEC M85.18
thigh M85.15-
toe M85.17-
upper arm M85.12-
vertebra M85.18
Flush syndrome E34.0
Flushing R23.2
menopausal N95.1
Flutter
atrial or auricular I48.92
atypical I48.4
type I I48.3
type II I48.4
typical I48.3
heart I49.8
atrial or auricular I48.92
atypical I48.4
type I I48.3
type II I48.4
typical I48.3
ventricular I49.02
ventricular I49.02

FNHTR (febrile nonhemolytic transfusion reaction) R50.84
Fochier's abscess - code by site under Abscess
Focus, Assmann's —*see* Tuberculosis, pulmonary
Fogo selvagem L10.3
Foix-Alajouanine syndrome G95.19
Fold, folds (anomalous) —*see also* Anomaly, by site
Descemet's membrane —*see* Change, corneal membrane, Descemet's, fold
epicanthic Q10.3
heart Q24.8
Folie à deux F24
Follicle
cervix (nabothian) (ruptured) N88.8
graafian, ruptured, with hemorrhage N83.0
nabothian N88.8
Follicular —*see* condition
Folliculitis (superficial) L73.9
abscedens et suffodiens L66.3
cyst N83.0
decalvans L66.2
deep —*see* Furuncle, by site
gonococcal (acute) (chronic) A54.01
keloid, keloidalis L73.0
pustular L01.02
ulerythematosa reticulata L66.4
Folliculome lipidique
specified site —*see* Neoplasm, benign, by site
unspecified site
female D27.9
male D29.20
Følling's disease E70.0
Follow-up —*see* Examination, follow-up
Fong's syndrome (hereditary osteo-onychodysplasia) Q78.5
Food
allergy L27.2
asphyxia (from aspiration or inhalation) —*see* Foreign body, by site
choked on —*see* Foreign body, by site
deprivation T73.0
specified kind of food NEC E63.8
intoxication —*see* Poisoning, food
lack of T73.0
poisoning —*see* Poisoning, food
rejection NEC —*see* Disorder, eating
strangulation or suffocation —*see* Foreign body, by site
toxemia —*see* Poisoning, food
Foot —*see* condition
Foramen ovale (nonclosure) (patent) (persistent) Q21.1
Forbes' glycogen storage disease E74.03
Fordyce-Fox disease L75.2
Fordyce's disease (mouth) Q38.6
Forearm —*see* condition
Foreign body
with
laceration —*see* Laceration, by site, with foreign body
puncture wound —*see* Puncture, by site, with foreign body
accidentally left following a procedure T81.509
aspiration T81.506
resulting in
adhesions T81.516
obstruction T81.526
perforation T81.536
specified complication NEC T81.596
cardiac catheterization T81.505
resulting in
acute reaction T81.60
aseptic peritonitis T81.61
specified NEC T81.69
adhesions T81.515
obstruction T81.525
perforation T81.535
specified complication NEC T81.595

◀ New ◀▬▬ Revised d̶e̶l̶e̶t̶e̶d̶ Deleted

Foreign body *(Continued)*
  accidentally left following a procedure
    (Continued)
    causing
      acute reaction T81.60
        aseptic peritonitis T81.61
        specified complication NEC T81.69
      adhesions T81.519
      aseptic peritonitis T81.61
      obstruction T81.529
      perforation T81.539
      specified complication NEC T81.599
    endoscopy T81.504
      resulting in
        adhesions T81.514
        obstruction T81.524
        perforation T81.534
        specified complication NEC T81.594
    immunization T81.503
      resulting in
        adhesions T81.513
        obstruction T81.523
        perforation T81.533
        specified complication NEC T81.593
    infusion T81.501
      resulting in
        adhesions T81.511
        obstruction T81.521
        perforation T81.531
        specified complication NEC T81.591
    injection T81.503
      resulting in
        adhesions T81.513
        obstruction T81.523
        perforation T81.533
        specified complication NEC T81.593
    kidney dialysis T81.502
      resulting in
        adhesions T81.512
        obstruction T81.522
        perforation T81.532
        specified complication NEC T81.592
    packing removal T81.507
      resulting in
        acute reaction T81.60
          aseptic peritonitis T81.61
          specified NEC T81.69
        adhesions T81.517
        obstruction T81.527
        perforation T81.537
        specified complication NEC T81.597
    puncture T81.506
      resulting in
        adhesions T81.516
        obstruction T81.526
        perforation T81.536
        specified complication NEC T81.596
    specified procedure NEC T81.508
      resulting in
        acute reaction T81.60
          aseptic peritonitis T81.61
          specified NEC T81.69
        adhesions T81.518
        obstruction T81.528
        perforation T81.538
        specified complication NEC T81.598
    surgical operation T81.500
      resulting in
        acute reaction T81.60
          aseptic peritonitis T81.61
          specified NEC T81.69
        adhesions T81.510
        obstruction T81.520
        perforation T81.530
        specified complication NEC T81.590
    transfusion T81.501
      resulting in
        adhesions T81.511
        obstruction T81.521
        perforation T81.531
        specified complication NEC T81.591

Foreign body *(Continued)*
  alimentary tract T18.9
    anus T18.5
    colon T18.4
    esophagus —*see* Foreign body, esophagus
    mouth T18.0
    multiple sites T18.8
    rectosigmoid (junction) T18.5
    rectum T18.5
    small intestine T18.3
    specified site NEC T18.8
    stomach T18.2
  anterior chamber (eye) S05.5-
  auditory canal —*see* Foreign body, entering
    through orifice, ear
  bronchus T17.508
    causing
      asphyxiation T17.500
        food (bone) (seed) T17.520
        gastric contents (vomitus) T17.510
        specified type NEC T17.590
      injury NEC T17.508
        food (bone) (seed) T17.528
        gastric contents (vomitus) T17.518
        specified type NEC T17.598
  canthus —*see* Foreign body, conjunctival sac
  ciliary body (eye) S05.5-
  conjunctival sac T15.1-
  cornea T15.0-
  entering through orifice
    accessory sinus T17.0
    alimentary canal T18.9
      multiple parts T18.8
      specified part NEC T18.8
    alveolar process T18.0
    antrum (Highmore's) T17.0
    anus T18.5
    appendix T18.4
    auditory canal —*see* Foreign body, entering
      through orifice, ear
    auricle —*see* Foreign body, entering
      through orifice, ear
    bladder T19.1
    bronchioles —*see* Foreign body, respiratory
      tract, specified site NEC
    bronchus (main) —*see* Foreign body,
      bronchus
    buccal cavity T18.0
    canthus (inner) —*see* Foreign body,
      conjunctival sac
    cecum T18.4
    cervix (canal) (uteri) T19.3
    colon T18.4
    conjunctival sac —*see* Foreign body,
      conjunctival sac
    cornea —*see* Foreign body, cornea
    digestive organ or tract NOS T18.9
      multiple parts T18.8
      specified part NEC T18.8
    duodenum T18.3
    ear (external) T16.-
    esophagus —*see* Foreign body, esophagus
    eye (external) NOS T15.9-
      conjunctival sac —*see* Foreign body,
        conjunctival sac
      cornea —*see* Foreign body, cornea
      specified part NEC T15.8-
    eyeball —*see also* Foreign body, entering
      through orifice, eye, specified part
      NEC
      with penetrating wound —*see* Puncture,
        eyeball
    eyelid —*see also* Foreign body, conjunctival
      sac
      with
        laceration —*see* Laceration, eyelid,
          with foreign body
        puncture —*see* Puncture, eyelid, with
          foreign body
        superficial injury —*see* Foreign body,
          superficial, eyelid

Foreign body *(Continued)*
  entering through orifice *(Continued)*
    gastrointestinal tract T18.9
      multiple parts T18.8
      specified part NEC T18.8
    genitourinary tract T19.9
      multiple parts T19.8
      specified part NEC T19.8
    globe —*see* Foreign body, entering through
      orifice, eyeball
    gum T18.0
    Highmore's antrum T17.0
    hypopharynx —*see* Foreign body, pharynx
    ileum T18.3
    intestine (small) T18.3
      large T18.4
    lacrimal apparatus (punctum) —*see*
      Foreign body, entering through
      orifice, eye, specified part NEC
    large intestine T18.4
    larynx —*see* Foreign body, larynx
    lung —*see* Foreign body, respiratory tract,
      specified site NEC
    maxillary sinus T17.0
    mouth T18.0
    nasal sinus T17.0
    nasopharynx —*see* Foreign body, pharynx
    nose (passage) T17.1
    nostril T17.1
    oral cavity T18.0
    palate T18.0
    penis T19.4
    pharynx —*see* Foreign body, pharynx
    piriform sinus —*see* Foreign body, pharynx
    rectosigmoid (junction) T18.5
    rectum T18.5
    respiratory tract —*see* Foreign body,
      respiratory tract
    sinus (accessory) (frontal) (maxillary)
      (nasal) T17.0
      piriform —*see* Foreign body, pharynx
    small intestine T18.3
    stomach T18.2
    suffocation by —*see* Foreign body, by site
    tear ducts or glands —*see* Foreign body,
      entering through orifice, eye,
      specified part NEC
    throat —*see* Foreign body, pharynx
    tongue T18.0
    tonsil, tonsillar (fossa) —*see* Foreign body,
      pharynx
    trachea —*see* Foreign body, trachea
    ureter T19.8
    urethra T19.0
    uterus (any part) T19.3
    vagina T19.2
    vulva T19.2
  esophagus T18.108
    causing
      injury NEC T18.108
        food (bone) (seed) T18.128
        gastric contents (vomitus) T18.118
        specified type NEC T18.198
      tracheal compression T18.100
        food (bone) (seed) T18.120
        gastric contents (vomitus) T18.110
        specified type NEC T18.190
  felling of, in throat R09.89
  fragment —*see* Retained, foreign body
    fragments (type of)
  genitourinary tract T19.9
    bladder T19.1
    multiple parts T19.8
    penis T19.4
    specified site NEC T19.8
    urethra T19.0
    uterus T19.3
      IUD Z97.5
    vagina T19.2
      contraceptive device Z97.5
    vulva T19.2

◀ New   ◀▥▥ Revised   ~~deleted~~ Deleted

Foreign body (*Continued*)
  superficial, without open wound (*Continued*)
    knee S80.25-
    labium (majus) (minus) S30.854
    larynx S10.15
    leg (lower) S80.85-
      knee —*see* Foreign body, superficial, knee
      upper —*see* Foreign body, superficial, thigh
    lip S00.551
    lower back S30.850
    lumbar region S30.850
    malar region S00.85
    mammary —*see* Foreign body, superficial, breast
    mastoid region S00.85
    mouth S00.552
    nail
      finger —*see* Foreign body, superficial, finger
      toe —*see* Foreign body, superficial, toe
    nape S10.85
    nasal S00.35
    neck S10.95
      specified site NEC S10.85
      throat S10.15
    nose S00.35
    occipital region S00.05
    oral cavity S00.552
    orbital region —*see* Foreign body, superficial, eyelid
    palate S00.552
    palm —*see* Foreign body, superficial, hand
    parietal region S00.05
    pelvis S30.850
    penis S30.852
    perineum
      female S30.854
      male S30.850
    periocular area —*see* Foreign body, superficial, eyelid
    phalanges
      finger —*see* Foreign body, superficial, finger
      toe —*see* Foreign body, superficial, toe
    pharynx S10.15
    pinna —*see* Foreign body, superficial, ear
    popliteal space —*see* Foreign body, superficial, knee
    prepuce S30.852
    pubic region S30.850
    pudendum
      female S30.856
      male S30.855
    sacral region S30.850
    scalp S00.05
    scapular region —*see* Foreign body, superficial, shoulder
    scrotum S30.853
    shin —*see* Foreign body, superficial, leg
    shoulder S40.25-
    sternal region S20.359
    submaxillary region S00.85
    submental region S00.85
    subungual
      finger (s) —*see* Foreign body, superficial, finger
      toe (s) —*see* Foreign body, superficial, toe
    supraclavicular fossa S10.85
    supraorbital S00.85
    temple S00.85
    temporal region S00.85
    testis S30.853
    thigh S70.35-
    thorax, thoracic (wall) S20.95
      back S20.45-
      front S20.35-
    throat S10.15
    thumb S60.35-

Foreign body (*Continued*)
  superficial, without open wound (*Continued*)
    toe (s) (lesser) S90.456
      great S90.45-
    tongue S00.552
    trachea S10.15
    tunica vaginalis S30.853
    tympanum, tympanic membrane —*see* Foreign body, superficial, ear
    uvula S00.552
    vagina S30.854
    vocal cords S10.15
    vulva S30.854
    wrist S60.85-
  swallowed T18.9
  trachea T17.408
    causing
      asphyxiation T17.400
        food (bone) (seed) T17.420
        gastric contents (vomitus) T17.410
        specified type NEC T17.490
      injury NEC T17.408
        food (bone) (seed) T17.428
        gastric contents (vomitus) T17.418
        specified type NEC T17.498
  type of fragment —*see* Retained, foreign body fragments (type of)
  vitreous (humor) S05.5-
Forestier's disease (rhizomelic pseudopolyarthritis) M35.3-
  meaning ankylosing hyperostosis —*see* Hyperostosis, ankylosing
Formation
  hyalin in cornea —*see* Degeneration, cornea
  sequestrum in bone (due to infection) —*see* Osteomyelitis, chronic
  valve
    colon, congenital Q43.8
    ureter (congenital) Q62.39
Formication R20.2
Fort Bragg fever A27.89
Fossa —*see also* condition
  pyriform —*see* condition
Foster-Kennedy syndrome H47.14-
Fothergill's
  disease (trigeminal neuralgia) —*see also* Neuralgia, trigeminal
  scarlatina anginosa A38.9
Foul breath R19.6
Foundling Z76.1
Fournier disease or gangrene N49.3
  female N76.89
Fourth
  cranial nerve —*see* condition
  molar K00.1
Foville's (peduncular) **disease or syndrome** G46.3
Fox (-Fordyce) **disease** (apocrine miliaria) L75.2
Fracture, burst —*see* Fracture, traumatic, by site
Fracture, chronic —*see* Fracture, pathological
Fracture, insufficiency —*see* Fracture, pathologic, by site
Fracture, pathological (pathologic) —*see also* Fracture, traumatic M84.40
  ankle M84.47-
  carpus M84.44-
  clavicle M84.41-
  dental implant M27.63
  dental restorative material K08.539
    with loss of material K08.531
    without loss of material K08.530
  due to
    neoplastic disease NEC (*see also* Neoplasm) M84.50
      ankle M84.57-
      carpus M84.54-
      clavicle M84.51-
      femur M84.55-
      fibula M84.56-
      finger M84.54-
      hip M84.559

Fracture, pathological (*Continued*)
  due to (*Continued*)
    neoplastic disease NEC (*Continued*)
      humerus M84.52-
      ilium M84.550
      ischium M84.550
      metacarpus M84.54-
      metatarsus M84.57-
      neck M84.58
      pelvis M84.550
      radius M84.53-
      rib M84.58
      scapula M84.51-
      skull M84.58
      specified site NEC M84.58
      tarsus M84.57-
      tibia M84.56-
      toe M84.57-
      ulna M84.53-
      vertebra M84.58
    osteoporosis M80.80
      disuse —*see* Osteoporosis, specified type NEC, with pathological fracture
      drug-induced —*see* Osteoporosis, drug induced, with pathological fracture
      idiopathic —*see* Osteoporosis, specified type NEC, with pathological fracture
      postmenopausal —*see* Osteoporosis, postmenopausal, with pathological fracture
      postoophorectomy —*see* Osteoporosis, postoophorectomy, with pathological fracture
      postsurgical malabsorption —*see* Osteoporosis, specified type NEC, with pathological fracture
      specified cause NEC —*see* Osteoporosis, specified type NEC, with pathological fracture
  specified disease NEC M84.60
    ankle M84.67-
    carpus M84.64-
    clavicle M84.61-
    femur M84.65-
    fibula M84.66-
    finger M84.64-
    hip M84.65-
    humerus M84.62-
    ilium M84.650
    ischium M84.650
    metacarpus M84.64-
    metatarsus M84.67-
    neck M84.68
    radius M84.63-
    rib M84.68
    scapula M84.61-
    skull M84.68
    tarsus M84.67-
    tibia M84.66-
    toe M84.67-
    ulna M84.63-
    vertebra M84.68
  femur M84.45-
  fibula M84.46-
  finger M84.44-
  hip M84.459
  humerus M84.42-
  ilium M84.454
  ischium M84.454
  joint prosthesis —*see* Complications, joint prosthesis, mechanical, breakdown, by site
  periprosthetic —*see* Complications, joint prosthesis, mechanical, periprosthesis, fracture, by site
  metacarpus M84.44-
  metatarsus M84.47-
  neck M84.48
  pelvis M84.454
  radius M84.43-

Fracture, pathological (*Continued*)
  restorative material (dental) K08.539
    with loss of material K08.531
    without loss of material K08.530
  rib M84.48
  scapula M84.41-
  skull M84.48
  tarsus M84.47-
  tibia M84.46-
  toe M84.47-
  ulna M84.43-
  vertebra M84.48
Fracture, traumatic (abduction) (adduction)
    (separation) (*see also* Fracture,
    pathological) T14.8
  acetabulum S32.40-
    column
      anterior (displaced) (iliopubic) S32.43-
        nondisplaced S32.436
      posterior (displaced) (ilioischial) S32.443
        nondisplaced S32.44-
    dome (displaced) S32.48-
      nondisplaced S32.48
    specified NEC S32.49-
    transverse (displaced) S32.45-
      with associated posterior wall fracture
        (displaced) S32.46-
        nondisplaced S32.46-
      nondisplaced S32.45-
    wall
      anterior (displaced) S32.41-
        nondisplaced S32.41-
      medial (displaced) S32.47-
        nondisplaced S32.47-
      posterior (displaced) S32.42-
        with associated transverse fracture
          (displaced) S32.46-
          nondisplaced S32.46-
        nondisplaced S32.42-
  acromion —*see* Fracture, scapula, acromial
    process
  ankle S82.899
    bimalleolar (displaced) S82.84-
      nondisplaced S82.84-
    lateral malleolus only (displaced) S82.6-
      nondisplaced S82.6-
    medial malleolus (displaced) S82.5-
      associated with Maisonneuve's
        fracture —*see* Fracture,
        Maisonneuve's
      nondisplaced S82.5-
    talus —*see* Fracture, tarsal, talus
    trimalleolar (displaced) S82.85-
      nondisplaced S82.85-
  arm (upper) —*see also* Fracture, humerus,
    shaft
    humerus —*see* Fracture, humerus
    radius —*see* Fracture, radius
    ulna —*see* Fracture, ulna
  astragalus —*see* Fracture, tarsal, talus
  atlas —*see* Fracture, neck, cervical vertebra,
    first
  axis —*see* Fracture, neck, cervical vertebra,
    second
  back —*see* Fracture, vertebra
  Barton's —*see* Barton's fracture
  base of skull —*see* Fracture, skull, base
  basicervical (basal) (femoral) S72.0
  Bennett's —*see* Bennett's fracture
  bimalleolar —*see* Fracture, ankle, bimalleolar
  blow-out S02.3
  bone NEC T14.8
    birth injury P13.9
    following insertion of orthopedic implant,
      joint prosthesis or bone plate —*see*
      Fracture, following insertion of
      orthopedic implant, joint prosthesis
      or bone plate
    in (due to) neoplastic disease NEC —*see*
      Fracture, pathological, due to,
      neoplastic disease

Fracture, traumatic (*Continued*)
  bone NEC (*Continued*)
    pathological (cause unknown) —*see*
      Fracture, pathological
  breast bone —*see* Fracture, sternum
  bucket handle (semilunar cartilage) —*see*
    Tear, meniscus
  burst —*see* Fracture, traumatic, by site
  calcaneus —*see* Fracture, tarsal, calcaneus
  carpal bone (s) S62.10-
    capitate (displaced) S62.13-
      nondisplaced S62.13-
    cuneiform —*see* Fracture, carpal bone,
      triquetrum
    hamate (body) (displaced) S62.143
      hook process (displaced) S62.15-
        nondisplaced S62.15-
      nondisplaced S62.14-
    larger multangular —*see* Fracture, carpal
      bones, trapezium
    lunate (displaced) S62.12-
      nondisplaced S62.12-
    navicular S62.00-
      distal pole (displaced) S62.01-
        nondisplaced S62.01-
      middle third (displaced) S62.02-
        nondisplaced S62.02-
      proximal third (displaced) S62.03-
        nondisplaced S62.03-
      volar tuberosity —*see* Fracture, carpal
        bones, navicular, distal pole
    os magnum —*see* Fracture, carpal bones,
      capitate
    pisiform (displaced) S62.16-
      nondisplaced S62.16-
    semilunar —*see* Fracture, carpal bones,
      lunate
    smaller multangular —*see* Fracture, carpal
      bones, trapezoid
    trapezium (displaced) S62.17-
      nondisplaced S62.17-
    trapezoid (displaced) S62.18-
      nondisplaced S62.18-
    triquetrum (displaced) S62.11-
      nondisplaced S62.11-
    unciform —*see* Fracture, carpal bones,
      hamate
  cervical —*see* Fracture, vertebra, cervical
  clavicle S42.00-
    acromial end (displaced) S42.03-
      nondisplaced S42.03-
    birth injury P13.4
    lateral end —*see* Fracture, clavicle, acromial
      end
    shaft (displaced) S42.02-
      nondisplaced S42.02-
    sternal end (anterior) (displaced) S42.01-
      nondisplaced S42.01-
      posterior S42.01-
  coccyx S32.2
  collapsed —*see* Collapse, vertebra
  collar bone —*see* Fracture, clavicle
  Colles' —*see* Colles' fracture
  compression, not due to trauma —*see*
    Collapse, vertebra
  coronoid process —*see* Fracture, ulna, upper
    end, coronoid process
  corpus cavernosum penis S39.840
  costochondral cartilage S23.41
  costochondral, costosternal junction —*see*
    Fracture, rib
  cranium —*see* Fracture, skull
  cricoid cartilage S12.8
  cuboid (ankle) —*see* Fracture, tarsal, cuboid
  cuneiform
    foot —*see* Fracture, tarsal, cuneiform
    wrist —*see* Fracture, carpal, triquetrum
  delayed union —*see* Delay, union, fracture
  dental restorative material K08.539
    with loss of material K08.531
    without loss of material K08.530

Fracture, traumatic (*Continued*)
  due to
    birth injury —*see* Birth, injury,
      fracture
    osteoporosis —*see* Osteoporosis,
      with fracture
  Dupuytren's —*see* Fracture, ankle, lateral
    malleolus
  elbow S42.40-
  ethmoid (bone) (sinus) —*see* Fracture, skull,
    base
  face bone S02.92
  fatigue —*see also* Fracture, stress
    vertebra M48.40
      cervical region M48.42
      cervicothoracic region M48.43
      lumbar region M48.46
      lumbosacral region M48.47
      occipito-atlanto-axial region M48.41
      sacrococcygeal region M48.48
      thoracic region M48.44
      thoracolumbar region M48.45
  femur, femoral S72.9-
    basicervical (basal) S72.0
    birth injury P13.2
    capital epiphyseal S79.01-
    condyles, epicondyles —*see* Fracture,
      femur, lower end
    distal end —*see* Fracture, femur,
      lower end
    epiphysis
      head —*see* Fracture, femur, upper end,
        epiphysis
      lower —*see* Fracture, femur, lower end,
        epiphysis
      upper —*see* Fracture, femur, upper end,
        epiphysis
    following insertion of implant, prosthesis
      or plate M96.66-
    head —*see* Fracture, femur, upper end,
      head
    intertrochanteric —*see* Fracture, femur,
      trochanteric
    intratrochanteric —*see* Fracture, femur,
      trochanteric
    lower end S72.40-
      condyle (displaced) S72.41-
        lateral (displaced) S72.42-
          nondisplaced S72.42-
        medial (displaced) S72.43-
          nondisplaced S72.43-
        nondisplaced S72.41-
      epiphysis (displaced) S72.44-
        nondisplaced S72.44-
      physeal S79.10-
        Salter-Harris
          Type I S79.11-
          Type II S79.12-
          Type III S79.13-
          Type IV S79.14-
        specified NEC S79.19-
      specified NEC S72.49-
      supracondylar (displaced) S72.45-
        with intracondylar extension
          (displaced) S72.46-
          nondisplaced S72.46-
        nondisplaced S72.45-
      torus S72.47-
    neck —*see* Fracture, femur, upper end,
      neck
    pertrochanteric —*see* Fracture, femur,
      trochanteric
    shaft (lower third) (middle third) (upper
      third) S72.30-
      comminuted (displaced) S72.35-
        nondisplaced S72.35-
      oblique (displaced) S72.33-
        nondisplaced S72.33-
      segmental (displaced) S72.36-
        nondisplaced S72.36-
      specified NEC S72.39-

◄ New   ◄▥ Revised   ~~deleted~~ Deleted

Fracture, traumatic *(Continued)*
femur, femoral *(Continued)*
shaft *(Continued)*
spiral (displaced) S72.34-
nondisplaced S72.34-
transverse (displaced) S72.32-
nondisplaced S72.32-
specified site NEC —*see* subcategory S72.8
subcapital (displaced) S72.01-
subtrochanteric (region) (section)
(displaced) S72.2-
nondisplaced S72.2-
transcervical —*see* Fracture, femur, upper
end, neck
transtrochanteric —*see* Fracture, femur,
trochanteric
trochanteric S72.10-
apophyseal (displaced) S72.13-
nondisplaced S72.13-
greater trochanter (displaced) S72.11-
nondisplaced S72.11-
intertrochanteric (displaced) S72.14-
nondisplaced S72.14-
lesser trochanter (displaced) S72.12-
nondisplaced S72.12-
upper end S72.00-
apophyseal (displaced) S72.13-
nondisplaced S72.13-
cervicotrochanteric —*see* Fracture,
femur, upper end, neck, base
epiphysis (displaced) S72.02-
nondisplaced S72.02-
head S72.05-
articular (displaced) S72.06-
nondisplaced S72.06-
specified NEC S72.09-
intertrochanteric (displaced) S72.14-
nondisplaced S72.14-
intracapsular S72.01-
midcervical (displaced) S72.03-
nondisplaced S72.03-
neck S72.00-
base (displaced) S72.04-
nondisplaced S72.04-
specified NEC S72.09-
pertrochanteric —*see* Fracture, femur,
upper end, trochanteric
physeal S79.00-
Salter-Harris type I S79.01-
specified NEC S79.09-
subcapital (displaced) S72.01-
subtrochanteric (displaced) S72.2-
nondisplaced S72.2-
transcervical —*see* Fracture, femur,
upper end, midcervical
trochanteric S72.10-
greater (displaced) S72.11-
nondisplaced S72.11-
lesser (displaced) S72.12-
nondisplaced S72.12-
fibula (shaft) (styloid) S82.40-
comminuted (displaced) S82.45-
nondisplaced S82.45-
following insertion of implant, prosthesis
or plate M96.67-
involving ankle or malleolus —*see*
Fracture, fibula, lateral malleolus
lateral malleolus (displaced) S82.6-
nondisplaced S82.6-
lower end
physeal S89.30-
Salter-Harris
Type I S89.31-
Type II S89.32-
specified NEC S89.39-
specified NEC S82.83-
torus S82.82-
oblique (displaced) S82.43-
nondisplaced S82.43-
segmental (displaced) S82.46-
nondisplaced S82.46-

Fracture, traumatic *(Continued)*
fibula *(Continued)*
specified NEC S82.49-
spiral (displaced) S82.44-
nondisplaced S82.44-
transverse (displaced) S82.42-
nondisplaced S82.42-
upper end
physeal S89.20-
Salter-Harris
Type I S89.21-
Type II S89.22-
specified NEC S89.29-
specified NEC S82.83-
torus S82.81-
finger (except thumb) S62.60-
distal phalanx (displaced) S62.63-
nondisplaced S62.66-
index S62.60-
distal phalanx (displaced) S62.63-
nondisplaced S62.66-
medial phalanx (displaced) S62.62-
nondisplaced S62.65-
proximal phalanx (displaced) S62.61-
nondisplaced S62.64-
little S62.60-
distal phalanx (displaced) S62.63-
nondisplaced S62.66-
medial phalanx (displaced) S62.62-
nondisplaced S62.65-
proximal phalanx (displaced) S62.61-
nondisplaced S62.64-
medial phalanx (displaced) S62.62-
nondisplaced S62.65-
middle S62.60-
distal phalanx (displaced) S62.63-
nondisplaced S62.66-
medial phalanx (displaced) S62.62-
nondisplaced S62.65-
proximal phalanx (displaced) S62.61-
nondisplaced S62.64-
proximal phalanx (displaced) S62.61-
nondisplaced S62.64-
ring S62.60-
distal phalanx (displaced) S62.63-
nondisplaced S62.66-
medial phalanx (displaced) S62.62-
nondisplaced S62.65-
proximal phalanx (displaced) S62.61-
nondisplaced S62.64-
thumb —*see* Fracture, thumb
following insertion (intraoperative)
(postoperative) of orthopedic implant,
joint prosthesis or bone plate M96.69
femur M96.66-
fibula M96.67-
humerus M96.62-
pelvis M96.65
radius M96.63-
specified bone NEC M96.69
tibia M96.67-
ulna M96.63-
foot S92.90-
astragalus —*see* Fracture, tarsal, talus
calcaneus —*see* Fracture, tarsal, calcaneus
cuboid —*see* Fracture, tarsal, cuboid
cuneiform —*see* Fracture, tarsal, cuneiform
metatarsal —*see* Fracture, metatarsal
navicular —*see* Fracture, tarsal, navicular
talus —*see* Fracture, tarsal, talus
tarsal —*see* Fracture, tarsal
toe —*see* Fracture, toe
forearm S52.9-
radius —*see* Fracture, radius
ulna —*see* Fracture, ulna
fossa (anterior) (middle) (posterior) S02.19
frontal (bone) (skull) S02.0
sinus S02.19
glenoid (cavity) (scapula) —*see* Fracture,
scapula, glenoid cavity
greenstick —*see* Fracture, by site

Fracture, traumatic *(Continued)*
hallux —*see* Fracture, toe, great
hand S62.9-
carpal —*see* Fracture, carpal bone
finger (except thumb) —*see* Fracture, finger
metacarpal —*see* Fracture, metacarpal
navicular (scaphoid) (hand) —*see* Fracture,
carpal bone, navicular
thumb —*see* Fracture, thumb
healed or old
with complications - code by Nature of the
complication
heel bone —*see* Fracture, tarsal, calcaneus
Hill-Sachs S42.29-
hip —*see* Fracture, femur, neck
humerus S42.30-
anatomical neck —*see* Fracture, humerus,
upper end
articular process —*see* Fracture, humerus,
lower end
capitellum —*see* Fracture, humerus, lower
end, condyle, lateral
distal end —*see* Fracture, humerus, lower
end
epiphysis
lower —*see* Fracture, humerus, lower
end, physeal
upper —*see* Fracture, humerus, upper
end, physeal
external condyle —*see* Fracture, humerus,
lower end, condyle, lateral
following insertion of implant, prosthesis
or plate M96.62-
great tuberosity —*see* Fracture, humerus,
upper end, greater tuberosity
intercondylar —*see* Fracture, humerus,
lower end
internal epicondyle —*see* Fracture,
humerus, lower end, epicondyle,
medial
lesser tuberosity —*see* Fracture, humerus,
upper end, lesser tuberosity
lower end S42.40-
condyle
lateral (displaced) S42.45-
nondisplaced S42.45-
medial (displaced) S42.46-
nondisplaced S42.46-
epicondyle
lateral (displaced) S42.43-
nondisplaced S42.43-
medial (displaced) S42.44-
incarcerated S42.44-
nondisplaced S42.44-
physeal S49.10-
Salter-Harris
Type I S49.11-
Type II S49.12-
Type III S49.13-
Type IV S49.14-
specified NEC S49.19-
specified NEC (displaced) S42.49-
nondisplaced S42.49-
supracondylar (simple) (displaced)
S42.41-
comminuted (displaced) S42.42-
nondisplaced S42.42-
nondisplaced S42.41-
torus S42.48-
transcondylar (displaced) S42.47-
nondisplaced S42.47-
proximal end —*see* Fracture, humerus,
upper end
shaft S42.30-
comminuted (displaced) S42.35-
nondisplaced S42.35-
greenstick S42.31-
oblique (displaced) S42.33-
nondisplaced S42.33-
segmental (displaced) S42.36-
nondisplaced S42.36-

Fracture, traumatic *(Continued)*
  humerus *(Continued)*
    shaft *(Continued)*
      specified NEC S42.39-
      spiral (displaced) S42.34-
        nondisplaced S42.34-
      transverse (displaced) S42.32-
        nondisplaced S42.32-
      supracondylar —*see* Fracture, humerus, lower end
      surgical neck —*see* Fracture, humerus, upper end, surgical neck
      trochlea —*see* Fracture, humerus, lower end, condyle, medial
      tuberosity —*see* Fracture, humerus, upper end
    upper end S42.20-
      anatomical neck —*see* Fracture, humerus, upper end, specified NEC
      articular head —*see* Fracture, humerus, upper end, specified NEC
      epiphysis —*see* Fracture, humerus, upper end, physeal
      greater tuberosity (displaced) S42.25-
        nondisplaced S42.25-
      lesser tuberosity (displaced) S42.26-
        nondisplaced S42.26-
      physeal S49.00-
        Salter-Harris
          Type I S49.01-
          Type II S49.02-
          Type III S49.03-
          Type IV S49.04-
        specified NEC S49.09-
      specified NEC (displaced) S42.29-
        nondisplaced S42.29-
      surgical neck (displaced) S42.21-
        four-part S42.24-
        nondisplaced S42.21-
        three-part S42.23-
        two-part (displaced) S42.22-
          nondisplaced S42.22-
      torus S42.27-
      transepiphyseal —*see* Fracture, humerus, upper end, physeal
  hyoid bone S12.8
  ilium S32.30-
    with disruption of pelvic ring —*see* Disruption, pelvic ring
    avulsion (displaced) S32.31-
      nondisplaced S32.31-
    specified NEC S32.39-
  impaction, impacted - code as Fracture, by site
  innominate bone —*see* Fracture, ilium
  instep —*see* Fracture, foot
  ischium S32.60-
    with disruption of pelvic ring —*see* Disruption, pelvic ring
    avulsion (displaced) S32.61-
      nondisplaced S32.61-
    specified NEC S32.69-
  jaw (bone) (lower) —*see* Fracture, mandible
    upper —*see* Fracture, maxilla
  joint prosthesis —*see* Complications, joint prosthesis, mechanical, breakdown, by site
    periprosthetic —*see* Complications, joint prosthesis, mechanical, periprosthesis, fracture, by site
  knee cap —*see* Fracture, patella
  larynx S12.8
  late effects —*see* Sequelae, fracture
  leg (lower) S82.9-
    ankle —*see* Fracture, ankle
    femur —*see* Fracture, femur
    fibula —*see* Fracture, fibula
    malleolus —*see* Fracture, ankle
    patella —*see* Fracture, patella
    specified site NEC S82.89-
    tibia —*see* Fracture, tibia

Fracture, traumatic *(Continued)*
  lumbar spine —*see* Fracture, vertebra, lumbar
  lumbosacral spine S32.9
  Maisonneuve's (displaced) S82.86-
    nondisplaced S82.86-
  malar bone *(see also* Fracture, maxilla) S02.400
  malleolus —*see* Fracture, ankle
  malunion —*see* Fracture, by site
  mandible (lower jawbone) S02.609
    alveolus S02.67
    angle (of jaw) S02.65
    body, unspecified S02.600
    condylar process S02.61
    coronoid process S02.63
    ramus, unspecified S02.64
    specified site NEC S02.69
    subcondylar process S02.62
    symphysis S02.66
  manubrium (sterni) S22.21
    dissociation from sternum S22.23
  march —*see* Fracture, traumatic, stress, by site
  maxilla, maxillary (bone) (sinus) (superior) (upper jaw) S02.401
    alveolus S02.42
    inferior —*see* Fracture, mandible
    LeFort I S02.411
    LeFort II S02.412
    LeFort III S02.413
  metacarpal S62.309
    base (displaced) S62.319
      nondisplaced S62.349
    fifth S62.30-
      base (displaced) S62.31-
        nondisplaced S62.34-
      neck (displaced) S62.33-
        nondisplaced S62.36-
      shaft (displaced) S62.32-
        nondisplaced S62.35-
      specified NEC S62.398
    first S62.20-
      base NEC (displaced) S62.23-
        nondisplaced S62.23-
      Bennett's —*see* Bennett's fracture
      neck (displaced) S62.25-
        nondisplaced S62.25-
      shaft (displaced) S62.24-
        nondisplaced S62.24-
      specified NEC S62.29-
    fourth S62.30-
      base (displaced) S62.31-
        nondisplaced S62.34-
      neck (displaced) S62.33-
        nondisplaced S62.36-
      shaft (displaced) S62.32-
        nondisplaced S62.35-
      specified NEC S62.39-
    neck (displaced) S62.33-
      nondisplaced S62.36-
    Rolando's —*see* Rolando's fracture
    second S62.30-
      base (displaced) S62.31-
        nondisplaced S62.34-
      neck (displaced) S62.33-
        nondisplaced S62.36-
      shaft (displaced) S62.32-
        nondisplaced S62.35-
      specified NEC S62.39-
    shaft (displaced) S62.32-
      nondisplaced S62.35-
    specified NEC S62.399
    third S62.30-
      base (displaced) S62.31-
        nondisplaced S62.34-
      neck (displaced) S62.33-
        nondisplaced S62.36-
      shaft (displaced) S62.32-
        nondisplaced S62.35-
      specified NEC S62.39-
  metastatic —*see* Fracture, pathological, due to, neoplastic disease —*see also* Neoplasm

Fracture, traumatic *(Continued)*
  metatarsal bone S92.30-
    fifth (displaced) S92.35-
      nondisplaced S92.35-
    first (displaced) S92.31-
      nondisplaced S92.31-
    fourth (displaced) S92.34-
      nondisplaced S92.34-
    second (displaced) S92.32-
      nondisplaced S92.32-
    third (displaced) S92.33-
      nondisplaced S92.33-
  Monteggia's —*see* Monteggia's fracture
  multiple
    hand (and wrist) NEC —*see* Fracture, by site
    ribs —*see* Fracture, rib, multiple
  nasal (bone (s)) S02.2
  navicular (scaphoid) (foot) —*see also* Fracture, tarsal, navicular
    hand —*see* Fracture, carpal, navicular
  neck S12.9
    cervical vertebra S12.9
      fifth (displaced) S12.400
        nondisplaced S12.401
        specified type NEC (displaced) S12.490
          nondisplaced S12.491
      first (displaced) S12.000
        burst (stable) S12.01
          unstable S12.02
        lateral mass (displaced) S12.040
          nondisplaced S12.041
        nondisplaced S12.001
        posterior arch (displaced) S12.030
          nondisplaced S12.031
        specified type NEC (displaced) S12.090
          nondisplaced S12.091
      fourth (displaced) S12.300
        nondisplaced S12.301
        specified type NEC (displaced) S12.390
          nondisplaced S12.391
      second (displaced) S12.100
        dens (anterior) (displaced) (type II) S12.110
          nondisplaced S12.112
          posterior S12.111
          specified type NEC (displaced) S12.120
            nondisplaced S12.121
        nondisplaced S12.101
        specified type NEC (displaced) S12.190
          nondisplaced S12.191
      seventh (displaced) S12.600
        nondisplaced S12.601
        specified type NEC (displaced) S12.690
          displaced S12.691
      sixth (displaced) S12.500
        nondisplaced S12.501
        specified type NEC (displaced) S12.590
          displaced S12.591
      third (displaced) S12.200
        nondisplaced S12.201
        specified type NEC (displaced) S12.290
          displaced S12.291
    hyoid bone S12.8
    larynx S12.8
    specified site NEC S12.8
    thyroid cartilage S12.8
    trachea S12.8
  neoplastic NEC —*see* Fracture, pathological, due to, neoplastic disease
  neural arch —*see* Fracture, vertebra
  newborn —*see* Birth, injury, fracture
  nontraumatic —*see* Fracture, pathological

◀ New ◀▥ Revised ~~deleted~~ Deleted

Fracture, traumatic (Continued)
nonunion —see Nonunion, fracture
nose, nasal (bone) (septum) S02.2
occiput —see Fracture, skull, base, occiput
odontoid process —see Fracture, neck,
    cervical vertebra, second
olecranon (process) (ulna) —see Fracture,
    ulna, upper end, olecranon process
orbit, orbital (bone) (region) S02.8
    floor (blow-out) S02.3
    roof S02.19
os
    calcis —see Fracture, tarsal, calcaneus
    magnum —see Fracture, carpal, capitate
    pubis —see Fracture, pubis
palate S02.8
parietal bone (skull) S02.0
patella S82.00-
    comminuted (displaced) S82.04-
      nondisplaced S82.04-
    longitudinal (displaced) S82.02-
      nondisplaced S82.02-
    osteochondral (displaced) S82.01-
      nondisplaced S82.01-
    specified NEC S82.09-
    transverse (displaced) S82.03-
      nondisplaced S82.03-
pedicle (of vertebral arch) —see Fracture,
    vertebra
pelvis, pelvic (bone) S32.9
    acetabulum —see Fracture, acetabulum
    circle —see Disruption, pelvic ring
    following insertion of implant, prosthesis
      or plate M96.65
    ilium —see Fracture, ilium
    ischium —see Fracture, ischium
    multiple
      with disruption of pelvic ring (circle) —
        see Disruption, pelvic ring
      without disruption of pelvic ring (circle)
        S32.82
    pubis —see Fracture, pubis
    sacrum —see Fracture, sacrum
    specified site NEC S32.89
phalanx
    foot —see Fracture, toe
    hand —see Fracture, finger
pisiform —see Fracture, carpal, pisiform
pond —see Fracture, skull
prosthetic device, internal —see
    Complications, prosthetic device, by
    site, mechanical
pubis S32.50-
    with disruption of pelvic ring —see
      Disruption, pelvic ring
    specified site NEC S32.59-
    superior rim S32.59-
radius S52.9-
    distal end —see Fracture, radius,
      lower end
    following insertion of implant, prosthesis
      or plate M96.63-
    head —see Fracture, radius, upper end,
      head
    lower end S52.50-
      Barton's —see Barton's fracture
      Colles' —see Colles' fracture
      extraarticular NEC S52.55-
      intraarticular NEC S52.57-
      physeal S59.20-
        Salter-Harris
          Type I S59.21-
          Type II S59.22-
          Type III S59.23-
          Type IV S59.24-
        specified NEC S59.29-
      Smith's —see Smith's fracture
      specified NEC S52.59-
      styloid process (displaced) S52.51-
        nondisplaced S52.51-
      torus S52.52-

Fracture, traumatic (Continued)
radius (Continued)
    neck —see Fracture, radius, upper end
    proximal end —see Fracture, radius, upper
      end
    shaft S52.30-
      bent bone S52.38-
      comminuted (displaced) S52.35-
        nondisplaced S52.35-
      Galeazzi's —see Galeazzi's fracture
      greenstick S52.31-
      oblique (displaced) S52.33-
        nondisplaced S52.33-
      segmental (displaced) S52.36-
        nondisplaced S52.36-
      specified NEC S52.39-
      spiral (displaced) S52.34-
        nondisplaced S52.34-
      transverse (displaced) S52.32-
        nondisplaced S52.32-
    upper end S52.10-
      head (displaced) S52.12-
        nondisplaced S52.12-
      neck (displaced) S52.13-
        nondisplaced S52.13-
      physeal S59.10-
        Salter-Harris
          Type I S59.11-
          Type II S59.12-
          Type III S59.13-
          Type IV S59.14-
        specified NEC S59.19-
      specified NEC S52.18-
      torus S52.11-
ramus
    inferior or superior, pubis —see Fracture,
      pubis
    mandible —see Fracture, mandible
restorative material (dental) K08.539
    with loss of material K08.531
    without loss of material K08.530
rib S22.3-
    with flail chest —see Flail, chest
    multiple S22.4-
      with flail chest —see Flail, chest
root, tooth —see Fracture, tooth
sacrum S32.10
    specified NEC S32.19
    Type
      1 S32.14
      2 S32.15
      3 S32.16
      4 S32.17
    Zone
      I S32.119
        displaced (minimally) S32.111
          severely S32.112
        nondisplaced S32.110
      II S32.129
        displaced (minimally) S32.121
          severely S32.122
        nondisplaced S32.120
      III S32.139
        displaced (minimally) S32.131
          severely S32.132
        nondisplaced S32.130
scaphoid (hand) —see also Fracture, carpal,
    navicular
    foot —see Fracture, tarsal, navicular
scapula S42.10-
    acromial process (displaced) S42.12-
      nondisplaced S42.12-
    body (displaced) S42.11-
      nondisplaced S42.11-
    coracoid process (displaced) S42.13-
      nondisplaced S42.13-
    glenoid cavity (displaced) S42.14-
      nondisplaced S42.14-
    neck (displaced) S42.15-
      nondisplaced S42.15-
    specified NEC S42.19-

Fracture, traumatic (Continued)
semilunar bone, wrist —see Fracture, carpal,
    lunate
sequelae —see Sequelae, fracture
sesamoid bone
    hand —see Fracture, carpal
    other - code by site under Fracture
shepherd's —see Fracture, tarsal, talus
shoulder (girdle) S42.9-
    blade —see Fracture, scapula
sinus (ethmoid) (frontal) S02.19
skull S02.91
    base S02.10
      occiput S02.119
        condyle S02.113
          type I S02.110
          type II S02.111
          type III S02.112
        specified NEC S02.118
      specified NEC S02.19
    birth injury P13.0
    frontal bone S02.0
    parietal bone S02.0
    specified site NEC S02.8
    temporal bone S02.19
    vault S02.0
Smith's —see Smith's fracture
sphenoid (bone) (sinus) S02.19
spine —see Fracture, vertebra
spinous process —see Fracture, vertebra
spontaneous (cause unknown) —see Fracture,
    pathological
stave (of thumb) —see Fracture, metacarpal,
    first
sternum S22.20
    with flail chest —see Flail, chest
    body S22.22
    manubrium S22.21
    xiphoid (process) S22.24
stress M84.30
    ankle M84.37-
    carpus M84.34-
    clavicle M84.31-
    femoral neck M84.359
    femur M84.35-
    fibula M84.36-
    finger M84.34-
    hip M84.359
    humerus M84.32-
    ilium M84.350
    ischium M84.350
    metacarpus M84.34-
    metatarsus M84.37-
    neck —see Fracture, fatigue, vertebra
    pelvis M84.350
    radius M84.33-
    rib M84.38
    scapula M84.31-
    skull M84.38
    tarsus M84.37-
    tibia M84.36-
    toe M84.37-
    ulna M84.33-
    vertebra —see Fracture, fatigue, vertebra
supracondylar, elbow —see Fracture,
    humerus, lower end, supracondylar
symphysis pubis —see Fracture, pubis
talus (ankle bone) —see Fracture, tarsal,
    talus
tarsal bone (s) S92.20-
    astragalus —see Fracture, tarsal, talus
    calcaneus S92.00-
      anterior process (displaced) S92.02-
        nondisplaced S92.02-
      body (displaced) S92.01-
        nondisplaced S92.01-
      extraarticular NEC (displaced)
        S92.05-
        nondisplaced S92.05-
      intraarticular (displaced) S92.06-
        nondisplaced S92.06-

Fracture, traumatic *(Continued)*
  tarsal bone *(Continued)*
    calcaneus *(Continued)*
      tuberosity (displaced) S92.04-
        avulsion (displaced) S92.03-
          nondisplaced S92.03-
        nondisplaced S92.04-
    cuboid (displaced) S92.21-
      nondisplaced S92.21-
    cuneiform
      intermediate (displaced) S92.23-
        nondisplaced S92.23-
      lateral (displaced) S92.22-
        nondisplaced S92.22-
      medial (displaced) S92.24-
        nondisplaced S92.24-
    navicular (displaced) S92.25-
      nondisplaced S92.25-
    scaphoid —*see* Fracture, tarsal,
        navicular
    talus S92.10-
      avulsion (displaced) S92.15-
        nondisplaced S92.15-
      body (displaced) S92.12-
        nondisplaced S92.12-
      dome (displaced) S92.14-
        nondisplaced S92.14-
      head (displaced) S92.12-
        nondisplaced S92.12-
      lateral process (displaced) S92.14-
        nondisplaced S92.14-
      neck (displaced) S92.11-
        nondisplaced S92.11-
      posterior process (displaced)
          S92.13-
        nondisplaced S92.13-
      specified NEC S92.19-
  temporal bone (styloid) S02.19
  thorax (bony) S22.9
    with flail chest —*see* Flail, chest
    rib S22.3-
      multiple S22.4-
        with flail chest —*see* Flail, chest
    sternum S22.20
      body S22.22
      manubrium S22.21
      xiphoid process S22.24
    vertebra (displaced) S22.009
      burst (stable) S22.001
        unstable S22.002
      eighth S22.069
        burst (stable) S22.061
          unstable S22.062
        specified type NEC S22.068
        wedge compression S22.060
      eleventh S22.089
        burst (stable) S22.081
          unstable S22.082
        specified type NEC S22.088
        wedge compression S22.080
      fifth S22.059
        burst (stable) S22.051
          unstable S22.052
        specified type NEC S22.058
        wedge compression S22.050
      first S22.019
        burst (stable) S22.011
          unstable S22.012
        specified type NEC S22.018
        wedge compression S22.010
      fourth S22.049
        burst (stable) S22.041
          unstable S22.042
        specified type NEC S22.048
        wedge compression S22.040
      ninth S22.079
        burst (stable) S22.071
          unstable S22.072
        specified type NEC S22.078
        wedge compression S22.070
      nondisplaced S22.001

Fracture, traumatic *(Continued)*
  thorax *(Continued)*
    vertebra *(Continued)*
      second S22.029
        burst (stable) S22.021
          unstable S22.022
        specified type NEC S22.028
        wedge compression S22.020
      seventh S22.069
        burst (stable) S22.061
          unstable S22.062
        specified type NEC S22.068
        wedge compression S22.060
      sixth S22.059
        burst (stable) S22.051
          unstable S22.052
        specified type NEC S22.058
        wedge compression S22.050
      specified type NEC S22.008
      tenth S22.079
        burst (stable) S22.071
          unstable S22.072
        specified type NEC S22.078
        wedge compression S22.070
      third S22.039
        burst (stable) S22.031
          unstable S22.032
        specified type NEC S22.038
        wedge compression S22.030
      twelfth S22.089
        burst (stable) S22.081
          unstable S22.082
        specified type NEC S22.088
        wedge compression S22.080
      wedge compression S22.000
  thumb S62.50-
    distal phalanx (displaced) S62.52-
      nondisplaced S62.52-
    proximal phalanx (displaced) S62.51-
      nondisplaced S62.51-
  thyroid cartilage S12.8
  tibia (shaft) S82.20-
    comminuted (displaced) S82.25-
      nondisplaced S82.25-
    condyles —*see* Fracture, tibia, upper end
    distal end —*see* Fracture, tibia, lower end
    epiphysis
      lower —*see* Fracture, tibia, lower end
      upper —*see* Fracture, tibia, upper end
    following insertion of implant, prosthesis
        or plate M96.67-
    head (involving knee joint) —*see* Fracture,
        tibia, upper end
    intercondyloid eminence —*see* Fracture,
        tibia, upper end
    involving ankle or malleolus —*see*
        Fracture, ankle, medial malleolus
    lower end S82.30-
      physeal S89.10-
        Salter-Harris
          Type I S89.11-
          Type II S89.12-
          Type III S89.13-
          Type IV S89.14-
          specified NEC S89.19-
      pilon (displaced) S82.87-
        nondisplaced S82.87-
      specified NEC S82.39-
      torus S82.31-
    malleolus —*see* Fracture, ankle, medial
        malleolus
    oblique (displaced) S82.23-
      nondisplaced S82.23-
    pilon —*see* Fracture, tibia, lower end,
        pilon
    proximal end —*see* Fracture, tibia, upper
        end
    segmental (displaced) S82.26-
      nondisplaced S82.26-
    specified NEC S82.29-
    spine —*see* Fracture, upper end, spine

Fracture, traumatic *(Continued)*
  tibia *(Continued)*
    spiral (displaced) S82.24-
      nondisplaced S82.24-
    transverse (displaced) S82.22-
      nondisplaced S82.22-
    tuberosity —*see* Fracture, tibia, upper end,
        tuberosity
    upper end S82.10-
      bicondylar (displaced) S82.14-
        nondisplaced S82.14-
      lateral condyle (displaced) S82.12-
        nondisplaced S82.12-
      medial condyle (displaced) S82.13-
        nondisplaced S82.13-
      physeal S89.00-
        Salter-Harris
          Type I S89.01-
          Type II S89.02-
          Type III S89.03-
          Type IV S89.04-
          specified NEC S89.09-
      plateau —*see* Fracture, tibia, upper end,
          bicondylar
      specified NEC S82.19-
      spine (displaced) S82.11-
        nondisplaced S82.11-
      torus S82.16-
      tuberosity (displaced) S82.15-
        nondisplaced S82.15-
  toe S92.91-
    great (displaced) S92.40-
      distal phalanx (displaced) S92.42-
        nondisplaced S92.42-
      nondisplaced S92.40-
      proximal phalanx (displaced) S92.41-
        nondisplaced S92.41-
      specified NEC S92.49-
    lesser (displaced) S92.50-
      distal phalanx (displaced) S92.53-
        nondisplaced S92.53-
      medial phalanx (displaced) S92.52-
        nondisplaced S92.52-
      nondisplaced S92.50-
      proximal phalanx (displaced) S92.51-
        nondisplaced S92.51-
      specified NEC S92.59-
  tooth (root) S02.5
  trachea (cartilage) S12.8
  transverse process —*see* Fracture, vertebra
  trapezium or trapezoid bone —*see* Fracture,
      carpal
  trimalleolar —*see* Fracture, ankle, trimalleolar
  triquetrum (cuneiform of carpus) —*see*
      Fracture, carpal, triquetrum
  trochanter —*see* Fracture, femur,
      trochanteric
  tuberosity (external) - code by site under
      Fracture
  ulna (shaft) S52.20-
    bent bone S52.28-
    coronoid process —*see* Fracture, ulna,
        upper end, coronoid process
    distal end —*see* Fracture, ulna, lower end
    following insertion of implant, prosthesis
        or plate M96.63-
    head S52.00-
    lower end S52.60-
      physeal S59.00-
        Salter-Harris
          Type I S59.01-
          Type II S59.02-
          Type III S59.03-
          Type IV S59.04-
          specified NEC S59.09-
      specified NEC S52.69-
      styloid process (displaced) S52.61-
        nondisplaced S52.61-
      torus S52.62-
    proximal end —*see* Fracture, ulna, upper
        end

◀ New   ◀▥ Revised   ~~deleted~~ Deleted

Fracture, traumatic (*Continued*)
  ulna (*Continued*)
    shaft S52.20-
      comminuted (displaced) S52.25-
        nondisplaced S52.25-
      greenstick S52.21-
      Monteggia's —*see* Monteggia's fracture
      oblique (displaced) S52.23-
        nondisplaced S52.23-
      segmental (displaced) S52.26-
        nondisplaced S52.26-
      specified NEC S52.29-
      spiral (displaced) S52.24-
        nondisplaced S52.24-
      transverse (displaced) S52.22-
        nondisplaced S52.22-
    upper end S52.00-
      coronoid process (displaced) S52.04-
        nondisplaced S52.04-
      olecranon process (displaced)
        S52.02-
        with intraarticular extension
          S52.03-
        nondisplaced S52.02-
          with intraarticular extension
            S52.03-
      specified NEC S52.09-
      torus S52.01-
  unciform —*see* Fracture, carpal, hamate
  vault of skull S02.0
  vertebra, vertebral (arch) (body) (column)
    (neural arch) (pedicle) (spinous process)
    (transverse process)
    atlas —*see* Fracture, neck, cervical vertebra,
      first
    axis —*see* Fracture, neck, cervical vertebra,
      second
    cervical (teardrop) S12.9
      axis —*see* Fracture, neck, cervical
        vertebra, second
      first (atlas) —*see* Fracture, neck, cervical
        vertebra, first
      second (axis) —*see* Fracture, neck,
        cervical vertebra, second
    chronic M84.48
    coccyx S32.2
    dorsal —*see* Fracture, thorax, vertebra
    lumbar S32.009
      burst (stable) S32.001
        unstable S32.002
      fifth S32.059
        burst (stable) S32.051
          unstable S32.052
        specified type NEC S32.058
        wedge compression S32.050
      first S32.019
        burst (stable) S32.011
          unstable S32.012
        specified type NEC S32.018
        wedge compression S32.010
      fourth S32.049
        burst (stable) S32.041
          unstable S32.042
        specified type NEC S32.048
        wedge compression S32.040
      second S32.029
        burst (stable) S32.021
          unstable S32.022
        specified type NEC S32.028
        wedge compression S32.020
      specified type NEC S32.008
      third S32.039
        burst (stable) S32.031
          unstable S32.032
        specified type NEC S32.038
        wedge compression S32.030
      wedge compression S32.000
    metastatic —*see* Collapse, vertebra, in,
      specified disease NEC —*see also*
      Neoplasm
    newborn (birth injury) P11.5

Fracture, traumatic (*Continued*)
  vertebra, vertebral (*Continued*)
    sacrum S32.10
      specified NEC S32.19
      Type
        1 S32.14
        2 S32.15
        3 S32.16
        4 S32.17
      Zone
        I S32.119
          displaced (minimally) S32.111
            severely S32.112
          nondisplaced S32.110
        II S32.129
          displaced (minimally) S32.121
            severely S32.122
          nondisplaced S32.120
        III S32.139
          displaced (minimally) S32.131
            severely S32.132
          nondisplaced S32.130
      thoracic —*see* Fracture, thorax, vertebra
    vertex S02.0
    vomer (bone) S02.2
    wrist S62.10-
      carpal —*see* Fracture, carpal bone
      navicular (scaphoid) (hand) —*see* Fracture,
        carpal, navicular
    xiphisternum, xiphoid (process) S22.24
    zygoma S02.442
Fragile, fragility
  autosomal site Q95.5
  bone, congenital (with blue sclera) Q78.0
  capillary (hereditary) D69.8
  hair L67.8
  nails L60.3
  non-sex chromosome site Q95.5
  X chromosome Q99.2
Fragilitas
  crinium L67.8
  ossium (with blue sclerae) (hereditary)
    Q78.0
  unguium L60.3
    congenital Q84.6
Fragments, cataract (lens), **following cataract**
  surgery H59.02-
  retained foreign body —*see* Retained, foreign
    body fragments (type of)
Frailty (frail) R54
  mental R41.81
Frambesia, frambesial (tropica) —*see also* Yaws
  initial lesion or ulcer A66.0
  primary A66.0
Frambeside
  gummatous A66.4
  of early yaws A66.2
Frambesioma A66.1
Franceschetti-Klein (-Wildervanck) **disease or**
  syndrome Q75.4
Francis' disease —*see* Tularemia
Franklin disease C88.2
Frank's essential thrombocytopenia D69.3
Fraser's syndrome Q87.0
Freckle (s) L81.2
  malignant melanoma in —*see* Melanoma
  melanotic (Hutchinson's) —*see* Melanoma,
    in situ
  retinal D49.81
Frederickson's hyperlipoproteinemia, type
  I and V E78.3
  IIA E78.0
  IIB and III E78.2
  IV E78.1
Freeman Sheldon syndrome Q87.0
Freezing —*see also* Effect, adverse, cold T69.9
Freiberg's disease (infraction of metatarsal
  head or osteochondrosis) —*see*
  Osteochondrosis, juvenile, metatarsus
Frei's disease A55
Fremitus, friction, cardiac R01.2

Frenum, frenulum
  external os Q51.828
  tongue (shortening) (congenital) Q38.1
Frequency micturition (nocturnal) R35.0
  psychogenic F45.8
Frey's syndrome
  auriculotemporal G50.8
  hyperhidrosis L74.52
Friction
  burn —*see* Burn, by site
  fremitus, cardiac R01.2
  precordial R01.2
  sounds, chest R09.89
Friderichsen-Waterhouse syndrome or disease
  A39.1
Friedländer's B (bacillus) **NEC** (*see also*
  condition) A49.8
Friedreich's
  ataxia G11.1
  combined systemic disease G11.1
  facial hemihypertrophy Q67.4
  sclerosis (cerebellum) (spinal cord)
    G11.1
Frigidity F52.22
Fröhlich's syndrome E23.6
Frontal —*see also* condition
  lobe syndrome F07.0
Frostbite (superficial) T33.90
  with
    partial thickness skin loss —*see* Frostbite
      (superficial), by site
    tissue necrosis T34.90
  abdominal wall T33.3
    with tissue necrosis T34.3
  ankle T33.81-
    with tissue necrosis T34.81-
  arm T33.4-
  with tissue necrosis T34.4-
    finger (s) —*see* Frostbite, finger
    hand —*see* Frostbite, hand
    wrist —*see* Frostbite, wrist
  ear T33.01-
    with tissue necrosis T34.01-
  face T33.09
    with tissue necrosis T34.09
  finger T33.53-
    with tissue necrosis T34.53-
  foot T33.82-
    with tissue necrosis T34.82-
  hand T33.52-
    with tissue necrosis T34.52-
  head T33.09
    with tissue necrosis T34.09
    ear —*see* Frostbite, ear
    nose —*see* Frostbite, nose
  hip (and thigh) T33.6-
    with tissue necrosis T34.6-
  knee T33.7-
    with tissue necrosis T34.7-
  leg T33.9-
    with tissue necrosis T34.9-
    ankle —*see* Frostbite, ankle
    foot —*see* Frostbite, foot
    knee —*see* Frostbite, knee
    lower T33.7-
      with tissue necrosis T34.7-
    thigh —*see* Frostbite, hip
    toe —*see* Frostbite, toe
  limb
    lower T33.99
      with tissue necrosis T34.99
    upper —*see* Frostbite, arm
  neck T33.1
    with tissue necrosis T34.1
  nose T33.02
    with tissue necrosis T34.02
  pelvis T33.3
    with tissue necrosis T34.3
  specified site NEC T33.99
    with tissue necrosis T34.99
  thigh —*see* Frostbite, hip

◀ New   ◀ Revised   ~~deleted~~ Deleted

Frostbite (Continued)
  thorax T33.2
    with tissue necrosis T34.2
  toes T33.83-
    with tissue necrosis T34.83-
  trunk T33.99
    with tissue necrosis T34.99
  wrist T33.51-
    with tissue necrosis T34.51-
Frotteurism F65.81
Frozen (see also Effect, adverse, cold) T69.9
  pelvis (female) N94.89
    male K66.8
  shoulder —see Capsulitis, adhesive
Fructokinase deficiency E74.11
Fructose 1,6 diphosphatase deficiency E74.19
Fructosemia (benign) (essential) E74.12
Fructosuria (benign) (essential) E74.11
Fuchs'
  black spot (myopic) H44.2-
  dystrophy (corneal endothelium) H18.51
  heterochromic cyclitis —see Cyclitis, Fuchs'
    heterochromic
Fucosidosis E77.1
Fugue R68.89
  dissociative F44.1
  hysterical (dissociative) F44.1
  postictal in epilepsy —see Epilepsy
  reaction to exceptional stress (transient)
    F43.0
Fulminant, fulminating —see condition
Functional —see also condition
  bleeding (uterus) N93.8
Functioning, intellectual, borderline R41.83
Fundus —see condition
Fungemia NOS B49
Fungus, fungous
  cerebral G93.89
  disease NOS B49
  infection —see Infection, fungus
Funiculitis (acute) (chronic) (endemic) N49.1
  gonococcal (acute) (chronic) A54.23
  tuberculous A18.15
Funnel
  breast (acquired) M95.4
    congenital Q67.6
    sequelae (late effect) of rickets E64.3
  chest (acquired) M95.4
    congenital Q67.6
    sequelae (late effect) of rickets E64.3
  pelvis (acquired) M95.5
    with disproportion (fetopelvic) O33.3
      causing obstructed labor O65.3
    congenital Q74.2
FUO (fever of unknown origin) R50.9
Furfur L21.0
  microsporon B36.0
Furrier's lung J67.8
Furrowed K14.5
  nail (s) (transverse) L60.4
    congenital Q84.6
  tongue K14.5
    congenital Q38.3
Furuncle L02.92
  abdominal wall L02.221
  ankle —see Furuncle, lower limb
  antecubital space —see Furuncle, upper limb
  anus K61.0
  arm —see Furuncle, upper limb

Furuncle (Continued)
  auditory canal, external —see Abscess, ear,
    external
  auricle (ear) —see Abscess, ear, external
  axilla (region) L02.42-
  back (any part) L02.222
  breast N61
  buttock L02.32
  cheek (external) L02.02
  chest wall L02.223
  chin L02.02
  corpus cavernosum N48.21
  ear, external —see Abscess, ear, external
  external auditory canal —see Abscess, ear,
    external
  eyelid —see Abscess, eyelid
  face L02.02
  femoral (region) —see Furuncle, lower limb
  finger —see Furuncle, hand
  flank L02.221
  foot L02.62-
  forehead L02.02
  gluteal (region) L02.32
  groin L02.224
  hand L02.52-
  head L02.821
    face L02.02
  hip —see Furuncle, lower limb
  kidney —see Abscess, kidney
  knee —see Furuncle, lower limb
  labium (majus) (minus) N76.4
  lacrimal
    gland —see Dacryoadenitis
    passages (duct) (sac) —see Inflammation,
      lacrimal, passages, acute
  leg (any part) —see Furuncle, lower limb
  lower limb L02.42-
  malignant A22.0
  mouth K12.2
  navel L02.226
  neck L02.12
  nose J34.0
  orbit, orbital —see Abscess, orbit
  palmar (space) —see Furuncle, hand
  partes posteriores L02.32
  pectoral region L02.223
  penis N48.21
  perineum L02.225
  pinna —see Abscess, ear, external
  popliteal —see Furuncle, lower limb
  prepatellar —see Furuncle, lower limb
  scalp L02.821
  seminal vesicle N49.0
  shoulder —see Furuncle, upper limb
  specified site NEC L02.828
  submandibular K12.2
  temple (region) L02.02
  thumb —see Furuncle, hand
  toe —see Furuncle, foot
  trunk L02.229
    abdominal wall L02.221
    back L02.222
    chest wall L02.223
    groin L02.224
    perineum L02.225
    umbilicus L02.226
  umbilicus L02.226
  upper limb L02.42-
  vulva N76.4

Furunculosis —see Furuncle
Fused —see Fusion, fused
Fusion, fused (congenital)
  astragaloscaphoid Q74.2
  atria Q21.1
  auditory canal Q16.1
  auricles, heart Q21.1
  binocular with defective stereopsis H53.32
  bone Q79.8
  cervical spine M43.22
  choanal Q30.0
  commissure, mitral valve Q23.2
  cusps, heart valve NEC Q24.8
    mitral Q23.2
    pulmonary Q22.1
    tricuspid Q22.4
  ear ossicles Q16.3
  fingers Q70.0-
  hymen Q52.3
  joint (acquired) —see also Ankylosis
    congenital Q74.8
  kidneys (incomplete) Q63.1
  labium (majus) (minus) Q52.5
  larynx and trachea Q34.8
  limb, congenital Q74.8
    lower Q74.2
    upper Q74.0
  lobes, lung Q33.8
  lumbosacral (acquired) M43.27
    arthrodesis status Z98.1
    congenital Q76.49
    postprocedural status Z98.1
  nares, nose, nasal, nostril (s) Q30.0
  organ or site not listed —see Anomaly,
    by site
  ossicles Q79.9
    auditory Q16.3
  pulmonic cusps Q22.1
  ribs Q76.6
  sacroiliac (joint) (acquired) M43.28
    arthrodesis status Z98.1
    congenital Q74.2
    postprocedural status Z98.1
  spine (acquired) NEC M43.20
    arthrodesis status Z98.1
    cervical region M43.22
    cervicothoracic region M43.23
    congenital Q76.49
    lumbar M43.26
    lumbosacral region M43.27
    occipito-atlanto-axial region M43.21
    postoperative status Z98.1
    sacrococcygeal region M43.28
    thoracic region M43.24
    thoracolumbar region M43.25
  sublingual duct with submaxillary duct at
    opening in mouth Q38.4
  testes Q55.1
  toes Q70.2
  tooth, teeth K00.2
  trachea and esophagus Q39.8
  twins Q89.4
  vagina Q52.4
  ventricles, heart Q21.0
  vertebra (arch) —see Fusion, spine
  vulva Q52.5
Fusospirillosis (mouth) (tongue) (tonsil)
  A69.1
Fussy baby R68.12

◀ New   ◀ Revised   ~~deleted~~ Deleted

G

Gain in weight (abnormal) (excessive) —*see also* Weight, gain
Gaisböck's disease (polycythemia hypertonica) D75.1
Gait abnormality R26.9
  ataxic R26.0
  falling R29.6
  hysterical (ataxic) (staggering) F44.4
  paralytic R26.1
  spastic R26.1
  specified type NEC R26.89
  staggering R26.0
  unsteadiness R26.81
  walking difficulty NEC R26.2
Galactocele (breast) N64.89
  puerperal, postpartum O92.79
Galactokinase deficiency E74.29
Galactophoritis N61
  gestational, puerperal, postpartum O91.2-
Galactorrhea O92.6
  not associated with childbirth N64.3
Galactosemia (classic) (congenital) E74.21
Galactosuria E74.29
Galacturia R82.0
  schistosomiasis (bilharziasis) B65.0
Galeazzi's fracture S52.37-
Galen's vein —*see* condition
Galeophobia F40.218
Gall duct —*see* condition
Gallbladder —*see also* condition
  acute K81.0
Gallop rhythm R00.8
Gallstone (colic) (cystic duct) (gallbladder) (impacted) (multiple) —*see also* Calculus, gallbladder
  with
    cholecystitis —*see* Calculus, gallbladder, with cholecystitis
  bile duct (common) (hepatic) —*see* Calculus, bile duct
  causing intestinal obstruction K56.3
  specified NEC K80.80
    with obstruction K80.81
Gambling Z72.6
  pathological (compulsive) F63.0
Gammopathy (of undetermined significance [MGUS]) D47.2
  associated with lymphoplasmacytic dyscrasia D47.2
  monoclonal D47.2
  polyclonal D89.0
Gamna's disease (siderotic splenomegaly) D73.1
Gamophobia F40.298
Gampsodactylia (congenital) Q66.7
Gamstorp's disease (adynamia episodica hereditaria) G72.3
Gandy-Nanta disease (siderotic splenomegaly) D73.1
Gang
  membership offenses Z72.810
Gangliocytoma D36.10
Ganglioglioma —*see* Neoplasm, uncertain behavior, by site
Ganglion (compound) (diffuse) (joint) (tendon (sheath)) M67.40
  ankle M67.47-
  foot M67.47-
  forearm M67.43-
  hand M67.44-
  lower leg M67.46-
  multiple sites M67.49
  of yaws (early) (late) A66.6
  pelvic region M67.45-
  periosteal —*see* Periostitis
  shoulder region M67.41-
  specified site NEC M67.48
  thigh region M67.45-
  tuberculous A18.09
  upper arm M67.42-
  wrist M67.43-

Ganglioneuroblastoma —*see* Neoplasm, nerve, malignant
Ganglioneuroma D36.10
  malignant —*see* Neoplasm, nerve, malignant
Ganglioneuromatosis D36.10
Ganglionitis
  fifth nerve —*see* Neuralgia, trigeminal
  gasserian (postherpetic) (postzoster) B02.21
  geniculate G51.1
    newborn (birth injury) P11.3
    postherpetic, postzoster B02.21
  herpes zoster B02.21
  postherpetic geniculate B02.21
Gangliosidosis E75.10
  GM1 E75.19
  GM2 E75.00
    other specified E75.09
    Sandhoff disease E75.01
    Tay-Sachs disease E75.02
  GM3 E75.19
  mucolipidosis IV E75.11
Gangosa A66.5
Gangrene, gangrenous (connective tissue) (dropsical) (dry) (moist) (skin) (ulcer) (*see also* Necrosis) I96
  with diabetes (mellitus) —*see* Diabetes, gangrene
  abdomen (wall) I96
  alveolar M27.3
  appendix K35.80
    with
      perforation or rupture K35.2
      peritoneal abscess K35.3
      peritonitis NEC K35.3
        generalized (with perforation or rupture) K35.2
        localized (with perforation or rupture) K35.3
  arteriosclerotic (general) (senile) —*see* Arteriosclerosis, extremities, with, gangrene
  auricle I96
  Bacillus welchii A48.0
  bladder (infectious) —*see* Cystitis, specified type NEC
  bowel, cecum, or colon —*see* Gangrene, intestine
  Clostridium perfringens or welchii A48.0
  cornea H18.89-
  corpora cavernosa N48.29
    noninfective N48.89
  cutaneous, spreading I96
  decubital —*see* Ulcer, pressure, by site
  diabetic (any site) —*see* Diabetes, gangrene
  emphysematous —*see* Gangrene, gas
  epidemic —*see* Poisoning, food, noxious, plant
  epididymis (infectional) N45.1
  erysipelas —*see* Erysipelas
  extremity (lower) (upper) I96
  Fournier N49.3
    female N76.89
  fusospirochetal A69.0
  gallbladder —*see* Cholecystitis, acute
  gas (bacillus) A48.0
    following
      abortion —*see* Abortion by type complicated by infection
      ectopic or molar pregnancy O08.0
  glossitis K14.0
  hernia —*see* Hernia, by site, with gangrene
  intestine, intestinal (hemorrhagic) (massive) K55.0
    with
      mesenteric embolism K55.0
      obstruction —*see* Obstruction, intestine
  laryngitis J04.0

Gangrene, gangrenous (Continued)
  limb (lower) (upper) I96
  lung J85.0
    spirochetal A69.8
  lymphangitis I89.1
  Meleney's (synergistic) —*see* Ulcer, skin
  mesentery K55.0
    with
      embolism K55.0
      intestinal obstruction —*see* Obstruction, intestine
  mouth A69.0
  ovary —*see* Oophoritis
  pancreas K85.9
  penis N48.29
    noninfective N48.89
  perineum I96
  pharynx —*see also* Pharyngitis
    Vincent's A69.1
  presenile I73.1
  progressive synergistic —*see* Ulcer, skin
  pulmonary J85.0
  pulpal (dental) K04.1
  quinsy J36
  Raynaud's (symmetric gangrene) I73.01
  retropharyngeal J39.2
  scrotum N49.3
    noninfective N50.8
  senile (atherosclerotic) —*see* Arteriosclerosis, extremities, with, gangrene
  spermatic cord N49.1
    noninfective N50.8
  spine I96
  spirochetal NEC A69.8
  spreading cutaneous I96
  stomatitis A69.0
  symmetrical I73.01
  testis (infectional) N45.2
    noninfective N44.8
  throat —*see also* Pharyngitis
    diphtheritic A36.0
    Vincent's A69.1
  thyroid (gland) E07.89
  tooth (pulp) K04.1
  tuberculous NEC —*see* Tuberculosis
  tunica vaginalis N49.1
    noninfective N50.8
  umbilicus I96
  uterus —*see* Endometritis
  uvulitis K12.2
  vas deferens N49.1
    noninfective N50.8
  vulva N76.89
Ganister disease J62.8
Ganser's syndrome (hysterical) F44.89
Gardner-Diamond syndrome (autoerythrocyte sensitization) D69.2
Gargoylism E76.01
Garré's disease, osteitis (sclerosing), **osteomyelitis** —*see* Osteomyelitis, specified type NEC
Garrod's pad, knuckle M72.1
Gartner's duct
  cyst Q52.4
  persistent Q50.6
Gas R14.3
  asphyxiation, inhalation, poisoning, suffocation NEC —*see* Table of Drugs and Chemicals
  excessive R14.0
  gangrene A48.0
    following
      abortion —*see* Abortion by type complicated by infection
      ectopic or molar pregnancy O08.0
  on stomach R14.0
  pains R14.1
Gastralgia —*see also* Pain, abdominal
Gastrectasis K31.0
  psychogenic F45.8
Gastric —*see* condition

Gastrinoma
  malignant
    pancreas C25.4
    specified site NEC —*see* Neoplasm,
      malignant, by site
    unspecified site C25.4
  specified site —*see* Neoplasm, uncertain
    behavior
  unspecified site D37.9
Gastritis (simple) K29.70
  with bleeding K29.71
  acute (erosive) K29.00
    with bleeding K29.01
  alcoholic K29.20
    with bleeding K29.21
  allergic K29.60
    with bleeding K29.61
  atrophic (chronic) K29.40
    with bleeding K29.41
  chronic (antral) (fundal) K29.50
    with bleeding K29.51
    atrophic K29.40
      with bleeding K29.41
    superficial K29.30
      with bleeding K29.31
  dietary counseling and surveillance Z71.3
  due to diet deficiency E63.9
  eosinophilic K52.81
  giant hypertrophic K29.60
    with bleeding K29.61
  granulomatous K29.60
    with bleeding K29.61
  hypertrophic (mucosa) K29.60
    with bleeding K29.61
  nervous F54
  spastic K29.60
    with bleeding K29.61
  specified NEC K29.60
    with bleeding K29.61
  superficial chronic K29.30
    with bleeding K29.31
  tuberculous A18.83
  viral NEC A08.4
Gastrocarcinoma —*see* Neoplasm, malignant,
  stomach
Gastrocolic —*see* condition
Gastrodisciasis, gastrodiscoidiasis B66.8
Gastroduodenitis K29.90
  with bleeding K29.91
  virus, viral A08.4
    specified type NEC A08.39
Gastrodynia —*see* Pain, abdominal
Gastroenteritis (acute) (chronic) (noninfectious)
    (*see also* Enteritis) K52.9
  allergic K52.2
  dietetic K52.2
  drug-induced K52.1
  due to
    Cryptosporidium A07.2
    drugs K52.1
    food poisoning —*see* Intoxication, foodborne
    radiation K52.0
  eosinophilic K52.81
  epidemic (infectious) A09
  food hypersensitivity K52.2
  infectious —*see* Enteritis, infectious
  influenzal —*see* Influenza, with
    gastroenteritis
  noninfectious K52.9
    specified NEC K52.89
  rotaviral A08.0
  Salmonella A02.0
  toxic K52.1
  viral NEC A08.4
    acute infectious A08.39
      type Norwalk A08.11
    infantile (acute) A08.39
    Norwalk agent A08.11
    rotaviral A08.0
    severe of infants A08.39
    specified type NEC A08.39

Gastroenteropathy (*see also* Gastroenteritis)
  K52.9
  acute, due to Norovirus A08.11
  acute, due to Norwalk agent A08.11
  infectious A09
Gastroenteroptosis K63.4
Gastroesophageal laceration-hemorrhage
  syndrome K22.6
Gastrointestinal —*see* condition
Gastrojejunal —*see* condition
Gastrojejunitis (*see also* Enteritis) K52.9
Gastrojejunocolic —*see* condition
Gastroliths K31.89
Gastromalacia K31.89
Gastroparalysis K31.84
  diabetic —*see* Diabetes, gastroparalysis
Gastroparesis K31.84
  diabetic —*see* Diabetes, by type, with
    gastroparesis
Gastropathy K31.9
  congestive portal K31.89
  erythematous K29.70
  exudative K90.89
  portal hypertensive K31.89
Gastroptosis K31.89
Gastrorrhagia K92.2
  psychogenic F45.8
Gastroschisis (congenital) Q79.3
Gastrospasm (neurogenic) (reflex) K31.89
  neurotic F45.8
  psychogenic F45.8
Gastrostaxis —*see* Gastritis, with bleeding
Gastrostenosis K31.89
Gastrostomy
  attention to Z43.1
  status Z93.1
Gastrosuccorrhea (continuous) (intermittent)
  K31.89
  neurotic F45.8
  psychogenic F45.8
Gatophobia F40.218
Gaucher's disease or splenomegaly (adult)
  (infantile) E75.22
Gee (-Herter)(-Thaysen) **disease** (nontropical
  sprue) K90.0
Gélineau's syndrome G47.419
  with cataplexy G47.411
Gemination, tooth, teeth K00.2
Gemistocytoma
  specified site —*see* Neoplasm, malignant, by
    site
  unspecified site C71.9
General, generalized —*see* condition
Genetic
  carrier (status)
    cystic fibrosis Z14.1
    hemophilia A (asymptomatic) Z14.01
      symptomatic Z14.02
    specified NEC Z14.8
  susceptibility to disease NEC Z15.89
    malignant neoplasm Z15.09
      breast Z15.01
      endometrium Z15.04
      ovary Z15.02
      prostate Z15.03
      specified NEC Z15.09
    multiple endocrine neoplasia Z15.81
Genital —*see* condition
Genito-anorectal syndrome A55
Genitourinary system —*see* condition
Genu
  congenital Q74.1
  extrorsum (acquired) —*see also* Deformity,
    varus, knee
    congenital Q74.1
    sequelae (late effect) of rickets E64.3
  introrsum (acquired) —*see also* Deformity,
    valgus, knee
    congenital Q74.1
    sequelae (late effect) of rickets E64.3
  rachitic (old) E64.3

Genu (*Continued*)
  recurvatum (acquired) —*see also* Deformity,
    limb, specified type NEC, lower leg
    congenital Q68.2
    sequelae (late effect) of rickets E64.3
  valgum (acquired) (knock-knee) M21.06-
    congenital Q74.1
    sequelae (late effect) of rickets E64.3
  varum (acquired) (bowleg) M21.16-
    congenital Q74.1
    sequelae (late effect) of rickets E64.3
Geographic tongue K14.1
Geophagia —*see* Pica
Geotrichosis B48.3
  stomatitis B48.3
Gephyrophobia F40.242
Gerbode defect Q21.0
GERD (gastroesophageal reflux disease)
  K21.9
Gerhardt's
  disease (erythromelalgia) I73.81
  syndrome (vocal cord paralysis)
    J38.00
    bilateral J38.02
    unilateral J38.01
German measles —*see also* Rubella
  exposure to Z20.4
Germinoblastoma (diffuse) C85.9-
  follicular C82.9-
Germinoma —*see* Neoplasm, malignant,
  by site
Gerontoxon —*see* Degeneration, cornea,
  senile
Gerstmann-Sträussler-Scheinker syndrome
  (GSS) A81.82
Gerstmann's syndrome R48.8
  developmental F81.2
Gestation (period) —*see also* Pregnancy
  ectopic —*see* Pregnancy, by site
  multiple O30.9-
    greater than quadruplets —*see* Pregnancy,
      multiple (gestation), specified NEC
    specified NEC —*see* Pregnancy, multiple
      (gestation), specified NEC
Gestational
  mammary abscess O91.11-
  purulent mastitis O91.11-
  subareolar abscess O91.11-
Ghon tubercle, primary infection A15.7
Ghost
  teeth K00.4
  vessels (cornea) H16.41-
Ghoul hand A66.3
Gianotti-Crosti disease L44.4
Giant
  cell
    epulis K06.8
    peripheral granuloma K06.8
  esophagus, congenital Q39.5
  kidney, congenital Q63.3
  urticaria T78.3
    hereditary D84.1
Giardiasis A07.1
Gibert's disease or pityriasis L42
Giddiness R42
  hysterical F44.89
  psychogenic F45.8
Gierke's disease (glycogenosis I) E74.01
Gigantism (cerebral) (hypophyseal) (pituitary)
  E22.0
  constitutional E34.4
Gilbert's disease or syndrome E80.4
Gilchrist's disease B40.9
Gilford-Hutchinson disease E34.8
Gilles de la Tourette's disease or syndrome
  (motor-verbal tic) F95.2
Gingivitis K05.10
  acute (catarrhal) K05.00
    necrotizing A69.1
    nonplaque induced K05.01
    plaque induced K05.00

◀ New   ◀▥ Revised   ~~deleted~~ Deleted

Gingivitis *(Continued)*
  chronic (desquamative) (hyperplastic)
      (simple marginal) (ulcerative) K05.10
    nonplaque induced K05.11
    plaque induced K05.10
  expulsiva —*see* Periodontitis
  necrotizing ulcerative (acute) A69.1
  pellagrous E52
    acute necrotizing A69.1
  Vincent's A69.1
Gingivoglossitis K14.0
Gingivopericementitis —*see* Periodontitis
Gingivosis —*see* Gingivitis, chronic
Gingivostomatitis K05.10
  herpesviral B00.2
  necrotizing ulcerative (acute) A69.1
Gland, glandular —*see* condition
Glanders A24.0
Glanzmann (-Naegeli) disease or
    thrombasthenia D69.1
Glasgow coma scale
  total score
    3-8 R40.243
    9-12 R40.242
    13-15 R40.241
Glass-blower's disease (cataract) —*see*
    Cataract, specified NEC
Glaucoma H40.9
  with
    increased episcleral venous pressure
        H40.81-
    pseudoexfoliation of lens —*see* Glaucoma,
        open angle, primary, capsular
  absolute H44.51-
  angle-closure (primary) H40.20-
    acute (attack) (crisis) H40.21-
    chronic H40.22-
    intermittent H40.23-
    residual stage H40.24-
  borderline H40.00-
  capsular (with pseudoexfoliation of lens) —
      see Glaucoma, open angle, primary,
      capsular
  childhood Q15.0
  closed angle —*see* Glaucoma, angle-closure
  congenital Q15.0
  corticosteroid-induced —*see* Glaucoma,
      secondary, drugs
  hypersecretion H40.82-
  in (due to)
    amyloidosis E85.4 *[H42]*
    aniridia Q13.1 *[H42]*
    concussion of globe —*see* Glaucoma,
        secondary, trauma
    dislocation of lens —*see* Glaucoma,
        secondary
    disorder of lens NEC —*see* Glaucoma,
        secondary
    drugs —*see* Glaucoma, secondary, drugs
    endocrine disease NOS E34.9 *[H42]*
    eye
      inflammation —*see* Glaucoma,
          secondary, inflammation
      trauma —*see* Glaucoma, secondary,
          trauma
    hypermature cataract —*see* Glaucoma,
        secondary
    iridocyclitis —*see* Glaucoma, secondary,
        inflammation
    lens disorder —*see* Glaucoma, secondary,
        Lowe's syndrome E72.03 *[H42]*
    metabolic disease NOS E88.9 *[H42]*
    ocular disorders NEC —*see* Glaucoma,
        secondary
    onchocerciasis B73.02
    pupillary block —*see* Glaucoma, secondary
    retinal vein occlusion —*see* Glaucoma,
        secondary
    Rieger's anomaly Q13.81 *[H42]*
    rubeosis of iris —*see* Glaucoma, secondary
    tumor of globe —*see* Glaucoma, secondary

Glaucoma *(Continued)*
  infantile Q15.0
  low tension —*see* Glaucoma, open angle,
      primary, low-tension
  malignant H40.83-
  narrow angle —*see* Glaucoma, angle-closure
  newborn Q15.0
  noncongestive (chronic) —*see* Glaucoma,
      open angle
  nonobstructive —*see* Glaucoma, open
      angle
  obstructive —*see also* Glaucoma,
      angle-closure
    due to lens changes —*see* Glaucoma,
        secondary
  open angle H40.10-
    primary H40.11-
      capsular (with pseudoexfoliation of lens)
          H40.14-
      low-tension H40.12-
      pigmentary H40.13-
      residual stage H40.15-
  phacolytic —*see* Glaucoma, secondary
  pigmentary —*see* Glaucoma, open angle,
      primary, pigmentary
  postinfectious —*see* Glaucoma, secondary,
      inflammation
  secondary (to) H40.5-
    drugs H40.6-
    inflammation H40.4-
    trauma H40.3-
  simple (chronic) H40.11
  simplex H40.11
  specified type NEC H40.89
  suspect H40.00-
  syphilitic A52.71
  traumatic —*see also* Glaucoma, secondary,
      trauma
    newborn (birth injury) P15.3
  tuberculous A18.59
Glaucomatous flecks (subcapsular) —*see*
    Cataract, complicated
Glazed tongue K14.4
Gleet (gonococcal) A54.01
Glénard's disease K63.4
Glioblastoma (multiforme)
  with sarcomatous component
    specified site —*see* Neoplasm, malignant,
        by site
    unspecified site C71.9
  giant cell
    specified site —*see* Neoplasm, malignant,
        by site
    unspecified site C71.9
  specified site —*see* Neoplasm, malignant, by
      site
  unspecified site C71.9
Glioma (malignant)
  astrocytic
    specified site —*see* Neoplasm, malignant,
        by site
    unspecified site C71.9
  mixed
    specified
      specified site —*see* Neoplasm, malignant,
          by site
      unspecified site C71.9
  nose Q30.8
  specified site NEC —*see* Neoplasm,
      malignant, by site
  subependymal D43.2
    specified site —*see* Neoplasm, uncertain
        behavior, by site
    unspecified site D43.2
  unspecified site C71.9
Gliomatosis cerebri C71.0
Glioneuroma —*see* Neoplasm, uncertain
    behavior, by site
Gliosarcoma
  specified site —*see* Neoplasm, malignant, by
      site
  unspecified site C71.9

Gliosis (cerebral) G93.89
  spinal G95.89
Glisson's disease —*see* Rickets
Globinuria R82.3
Globus (hystericus) F45.8
Glomangioma D18.00
  intra-abdominal D18.03
  intracranial D18.02
  skin D18.01
  specified site NEC D18.09
Glomangiomyoma D18.00
  intra-abdominal D18.03
  intracranial D18.02
  skin D18.01
  specified site NEC D18.09
Glomangiosarcoma —*see* Neoplasm, connective
    tissue, malignant
Glomerular
  disease in syphilis A52.75
  nephritis —*see* Glomerulonephritis
Glomerulitis —*see* Glomerulonephritis
Glomerulonephritis (*see also* Nephritis)
    N05.9
  with
    edema —*see* Nephrosis
    minimal change N05.0
    minor glomerular abnormality N05.0
  acute N00.9
  chronic N03.9
  crescentic (diffuse) NEC (*see also* N00-N07
      with fourth character .7) N05.7
  dense deposit (*see also* N00-N07 with fourth
      character .6) N05.6
  diffuse
    crescentic (*see also* N00-N07 with fourth
        character .7) N05.7
    endocapillary proliferative (*see also*
        N00N07 with fourth character .4)
        N05.4
    membranous (*see also* N00-N07 with fourth
        character .2) N05.2
    mesangial proliferative (*see also* N00N07
        with fourth character .3) N05.3
    mesangiocapillary (*see also* N00-N07 with
        fourth character .5) N05.5
    sclerosing N05.8
  endocapillary proliferative (diffuse) NEC (*see
      also* N00-N07 with fourth character .4)
      N05.4
  extracapillary NEC (*see also* N00-N07 with
      fourth character .7) N05.7
  focal (and segmental) (*see also* N00-N07 with
      fourth character .1) N05.1
  hypocomplementemic —*see*
      Glomerulonephritis,
      membranoproliferative
  IgA —*see* Nephropathy, IgA
  immune complex (circulating) NEC
      N05.8
  in (due to)
    amyloidosis E85.4 *[N08]*
    bilharziasis B65.9 *[N08]*
    cryoglobulinemia D89.1 *[N08]*
    defibrination syndrome D65 *[N08]*
    diabetes mellitus —*see* Diabetes,
        glomerulosclerosis
    disseminated intravascular coagulation
        D65 *[N08]*
    Fabry (-Anderson) disease E75.21 *[N08]*
    Goodpasture's syndrome M31.0
    hemolytic-uremic syndrome D59.3
    Henoch (-Schönlein) purpura D69.0
        [N08]
    lecithin cholesterol acyltransferase
        deficiency E78.6 *[N08]*
    microscopic polyangiitis M31.7 *[N08]*
    multiple myeloma C90.0- *[N08]*
    Plasmodium malariae B52.0
    schistosomiasis B65.9 *[N08]*
    sepsis A41.9- *[N08]*
      streptococcal A40- *[N08]*

Glomerulonephritis (Continued)
  in (Continued)
    sickle-cell disorders D57.- [N08]
    strongyloidiasis B78.9 [N08]
    subacute bacterial endocarditis I33.0
        [N08]
    syphilis (late) congenital A50.59 [N08]
    systemic lupus erythematosus M32.14
    thrombotic thrombocytopenic purpura
        M31.1 [N08]
    typhoid fever A01.09
    Waldenström macroglobulinemia C88.0
        [N08]
    Wegener's granulomatosis M31.31
  latent or quiescent N03.9
  lobular, lobulonodular —see
      Glomerulonephritis,
      membranoproliferative
  membranoproliferative (diffuse) (type 1
      or 3) (see also N00-N07 with fourth
      character .5) N05.5
    dense deposit (type 2) NEC (see also
        N00-N07 with fourth character .6)
        N05.6
  membranous (diffuse) NEC (see also N00-N07
      with fourth character .2) N05.2
  mesangial
    IgA/IgG —see Nephropathy, IgA
    proliferative (diffuse) NEC (see also
        N00-N07 with fourth character .3)
        N05.3
  mesangiocapillary (diffuse) NEC (see also
      N00-N07 with fourth character .5)
      N05.5
  necrotic, necrotizing NEC (see also N00-N07
      with fourth character .8) N05.8
  nodular —see Glomerulonephritis,
      membranoproliferative
  poststreptococcal NEC N05.9
    acute N00.9
    chronic N03.9
    rapidly progressive N01.9
  proliferative NEC (see also N00-N07 with
      fourth character .8) N05.8
    diffuse (lupus) M32.14
  rapidly progressive N01.9
  sclerosing, diffuse N05.8
  specified pathology NEC (see also N00-N07
      with fourth character .8) N05.8
  subacute N01.9
Glomerulopathy —see Glomerulonephritis
Glomerulosclerosis —see also Sclerosis,
    renal
  intercapillary (nodular) (with diabetes) —see
      Diabetes, glomerulosclerosis
  intracapillary —see Diabetes,
      glomerulosclerosis
Glossagra K14.6
Glossalgia K14.6
Glossitis (chronic superficial) (gangrenous)
    (Moeller's) K14.0
  areata exfoliativa K14.1
  atrophic K14.4
  benign migratory K14.1
  cortical superficial, sclerotic K14.0
  Hunter's D51.0
  interstitial, sclerous K14.0
  median rhomboid K14.2
  pellagrous E52
  superficial, chronic K14.0
Glossocele K14.8
Glossodynia K14.6
  exfoliativa K14.4
Glossoncus K14.8
Glossopathy K14.9
Glossophytia K14.3
Glossoplegia K14.8
Glossoptosis K14.8
Glossopyrosis K14.6
Glossotrichia K14.3
Glossy skin L90.8

Glottis —see condition
Glottitis (see also Laryngitis) J04.0
Glucagonoma
  pancreas
    benign D13.7
    malignant C25.4
    uncertain behavior D37.8
  specified site NEC
    benign —see Neoplasm, benign, by site
    malignant —see Neoplasm, malignant, by
        site
    uncertain behavior —see Neoplasm,
        uncertain behavior, by site
  unspecified site
    benign D13.7
    malignant C25.4
    uncertain behavior D37.8
Glucoglycinuria E72.51
Glucose-galactose malabsorption E74.39
Glue
  ear —see Otitis, media, nonsuppurative,
      chronic, mucoid
  sniffing (airplane) —see Abuse, drug,
      inhalant
    dependence —see Dependence, drug,
        inhalant
Glutaric aciduria E72.3
Glycinemia E72.51
Glycinuria (renal) (with ketosis) E72.09
Glycogen
  infiltration —see Disease, glycogen storage
  storage disease —see Disease, glycogen
      storage
Glycogenosis (diffuse) (generalized) —see also
    Disease, glycogen storage
  cardiac E74.02 [I43]
  diabetic, secondary —see Diabetes,
      glycogenosis, secondary
  pulmonary interstitial J84.842
Glycopenia E16.2
Glycosuria R81
  renal E74.8
Gnathostoma spinigerum (infection)
    (infestation), **gnathostomiasis** (wandering
    swelling) B83.1
Goiter (plunging) (substernal) E04.9
  with
    hyperthyroidism (recurrent) —see
        Hyperthyroidism, with, goiter
    thyrotoxicosis —see Hyperthyroidism,
        with, goiter
  adenomatous —see Goiter, nodular
  cancerous C73
  congenital (nontoxic) E03.0
    diffuse E03.0
    parenchymatous E03.0
    transitory, with normal functioning
        P72.0
  cystic E04.2
    due to iodine-deficiency E01.1
  due to
    enzyme defect in synthesis of thyroid
        hormone E07.1
    iodine-deficiency (endemic) E01.2
  dyshormonogenetic (familial) E07.1
  endemic (iodine-deficiency) E01.2
    diffuse E01.0
    multinodular E01.1
  exophthalmic —see Hyperthyroidism, with,
      goiter
  iodine-deficiency (endemic) E01.2
    diffuse E01.0
    multinodular E01.1
    nodular E01.1
  lingual Q89.2
  lymphadenoid E06.3
  malignant C73
  multinodular (cystic) (nontoxic) E04.2
    toxic or with hyperthyroidism E05.20
        with thyroid storm E05.21
  neonatal NEC P72.0

Goiter (Continued)
  nodular (nontoxic) (due to) E04.9
    with
        hyperthyroidism E05.20
            with thyroid storm E05.21
        thyrotoxicosis E05.20
            with thyroid storm E05.21
    endemic E01.1
    iodine-deficiency E01.1
    sporadic E04.9
    toxic E05.20
        with thyroid storm E05.21
  nontoxic E04.9
    diffuse (colloid) E04.0
    multinodular E04.2
    simple E04.0
    specified NEC E04.8
    uninodular E04.1
  simple E04.0
  toxic —see Hyperthyroidism, with, goiter
  uninodular (nontoxic) E04.1
    toxic or with hyperthyroidism E05.10
        with thyroid storm E05.11
Goiter-deafness syndrome E07.1
Goldberg syndrome Q89.8
Goldberg-Maxwell syndrome E34.51
Goldblatt's hypertension or kidney I70.1
Goldenhar (-Gorlin) **syndrome** Q87.0
Goldflam-Erb disease or syndrome G70.00
  with exacerbation (acute) G70.01
  in crisis G70.01
Goldscheider's disease Q81.8
Goldstein's disease (familial hemorrhagic
    telangiectasia) I78.0
Golfer's elbow —see Epicondylitis, medial
Gonadoblastoma
  specified site —see Neoplasm, uncertain
      behavior, by site
  unspecified site
    female D39.10
    male D40.10
Gonecystitis —see Vesiculitis
Gongylonemiasis B83.8
Goniosynechiae —see Adhesions, iris,
    goniosynechiae
Gonococcemia A54.86
Gonococcus, gonococcal (disease) (infection)
    (see also condition) A54.9
  anus A54.6
  bursa, bursitis A54.49
  conjunctiva, conjunctivitis (neonatorum)
      A54.31
  endocardium A54.83
  eye A54.30
    conjunctivitis A54.31
    iridocyclitis A54.32
    keratitis A54.33
    newborn A54.31
    other specified A54.39
  fallopian tubes (acute) (chronic) A54.24
  genitourinary (organ) (system) (tract) (acute)
      A54.00
    lower A54.00
        with abscess (accessory gland)
            (periurethral) A54.1
    upper (see also condition) A54.29
  heart A54.83
  iridocyclitis A54.32
  joint A54.42
  lymphatic (gland) (node) A54.89
  meninges, meningitis A54.81
  musculoskeletal A54.40
    arthritis A54.42
    osteomyelitis A54.43
    other specified A54.49
    spondylopathy A54.41
  pelviperitonitis A54.24
  pelvis (acute) (chronic) A54.24
  pharynx A54.5
  proctitis A54.6
  pyosalpinx (acute) (chronic) A54.24
  rectum A54.6

◀ New ◀═ Revised ~~deleted~~ Deleted

Gonococcus, gonococcal *(Continued)*
  skin A54.89
  specified site NEC A54.89
  tendon sheath A54.49
  throat A54.5
  urethra (acute) (chronic) A54.01
    with abscess (accessory gland)
      (periurethral) A54.1
  vulva (acute) (chronic) A54.02
Gonocytoma
  specified site —*see* Neoplasm, uncertain
    behavior, by site
  unspecified site
    female D39.10
    male D40.10
Gonorrhea (acute) (chronic) A54.9
  Bartholin's gland (acute) (chronic) (purulent)
    A54.02
    with abscess (accessory gland)
      (periurethral) A54.1
  bladder A54.01
  cervix A54.03
  conjunctiva, conjunctivitis (neonatorum)
    A54.31
  contact Z20.2
  Cowper's gland (with abscess) A54.1
  exposure to Z20.2
  fallopian tube (acute) (chronic) A54.24
  kidney (acute) (chronic) A54.21
  lower genitourinary tract A54.00
    with abscess (accessory gland)
      (periurethral) A54.1
  ovary (acute) (chronic) A54.24
  pelvis (acute) (chronic) A54.24
    female pelvic inflammatory disease A54.24
  penis A54.09
  prostate (acute) (chronic) A54.22
  seminal vesicle (acute) (chronic) A54.23
  specified site not listed (*see also* Gonococcus)
    A54.89
  spermatic cord (acute) (chronic) A54.23
  urethra A54.01
    with abscess (accessory gland)
      (periurethral) A54.1
  vagina A54.02
  vas deferens (acute) (chronic) A54.23
  vulva A54.02
Goodall's disease A08.19
Goodpasture's syndrome M31.0
Gopalan's syndrome (burning feet) E53.0
Gorlin-Chaudry-Moss syndrome Q87.0
Gottron's papules L94.4
Gougerot's syndrome (trisymptomatic) L81.7
Gougerot-Blum syndrome (pigmented
  purpuric lichenoid dermatitis) L81.7
Gougerot-Carteaud disease or syndrome
  (confluent reticulate papillomatosis) L83
Gouley's syndrome (constrictive pericarditis)
  I31.1
Goundou A66.6
Gout, chronic (*see also* Gout, gouty) M1A.9-
  drug-induced M1A.20
    ankle M1A.27-
    elbow M1A.22-
    foot joint M1A.27-
    hand joint M1A.24-
    hip M1A.25-
    knee M1A.26-
    multiple site M1A.29-
    shoulder M1A.21-
    vertebrae M1A.28
    wrist M1A.23-
  idiopathic M1A.00
    ankle M1A.07-
    elbow M1A.02-
    foot joint M1A.07-
    hand joint M1A.04-
    hip M1A.05-
    knee M1A.06-
    multiple site M1A.09
    shoulder M1A.01-

Gout, chronic *(Continued)*
  idiopathic *(Continued)*
    vertebrae M1A.08
    wrist M1A.03-
  in (due to) renal impairment M1A.30
    ankle M1A.37-
    elbow M1A.32-
    foot joint M1A.37-
    hand joint M1A.34-
    hip M1A.35-
    knee M1A.36-
    multiple site M1A.39
    shoulder M1A.31-
    vertebrae M1A.38
    wrist M1A.33-
  lead-induced M1A.10
    ankle M1A.17-
    elbow M1A.12-
    foot joint M1A.17-
    hand joint M1A.14-
    hip M1A.15-
    knee M1A.16-
    multiple site M1A.19
    shoulder M1A.11-
    vertebrae M1A.18
    wrist M1A.13-
  primary —*see* Gout, chronic, idiopathic
  saturnine —*see* Gout, chronic, lead-induced
  secondary NEC M1A.40
    ankle M1A.47-
    elbow M1A.42-
    foot joint M1A.47-
    hand joint M1A.44-
    hip M1A.45-
    knee M1A.46-
    multiple site M1A.49
    shoulder M1A.41-
    vertebrae M1A.48
    wrist M1A.43-
  syphilitic (*see also* subcategory M14.8-) A52.77
  tophi M1A.9
Gout, gouty (acute) (attack) (flare) (*see also*
  Gout, chronic) M10.9-
  drug-induced M10.20
    ankle M10.27-
    elbow M10.22-
    foot joint M10.27-
    hand joint M10.24-
    hip M10.25-
    knee M10.26-
    multiple site M10.29
    shoulder M10.21-
    vertebrae M10.28
    wrist M10.23-
  idiopathic M10.00
    ankle M10.07-
    elbow M10.02-
    foot joint M10.07-
    hand joint M10.04-
    hip M10.05-
    knee M10.06-
    multiple site M10.09
    shoulder M10.01-
    vertebrae M10.08
    wrist M10.03-
  in (due to) renal impairment M10.30
    ankle M10.37-
    elbow M10.32-
    foot joint M10.37-
    hand joint M10.34-
    hip M10.35-
    knee M10.36-
    multiple site M10.39
    shoulder M10.31-
    vertebrae M10.38
    wrist M10.33-
  lead-induced M10.10
    ankle M10.17-
    elbow M10.12-
    foot joint M10.17-
    hand joint M10.14-

Gout, gouty *(Continued)*
  lead-induced *(Continued)*
    hip M10.15-
    knee M10.16-
    multiple site M10.19
    shoulder M10.11-
    vertebrae M10.18
    wrist M10.13-
  primary —*see* Gout, idiopathic
  saturnine —*see* Gout, lead-induced
  secondary NEC M10.40
    ankle M10.47-
    elbow M10.42-
    foot joint M10.47-
    hand joint M10.44-
    hip M10.45-
    knee M10.46-
    multiple site M10.49
    shoulder M10.41-
    vertebrae M10.48
    wrist M10.43-
  syphilitic (*see also* subcategory M14.8-) A52.77
  tophi NEC —*see* Gout, chronic
Gower's
  muscular dystrophy G71.0
  syndrome (vasovagal attack) R55
Gradenigo's syndrome —*see* Otitis, media,
  suppurative, acute
Graefe's disease —*see* Strabismus, paralytic,
  ophthalmoplegia, progressive
Graft-versus-host disease D89.813
  acute D89.810
  acute on chronic D89.812
  chronic D89.811
Grain mite (itch) B88.0
Grainhandler's disease or lung J67.8
Grand mal —*see* Epilepsy, generalized,
  specified NEC
Grand multipara status only (not pregnant)
  Z64.1
  pregnant —*see* Pregnancy, complicated by,
    grand multiparity
Granite worker's lung J62.8
Granular —*see also* condition
  inflammation, pharynx J31.2
  kidney (contracting) —*see* Sclerosis, renal
  liver K74.69
Granulation tissue (abnormal) (excessive)
  L92.9
  postmastoidectomy cavity —*see*
    Complications, postmastoidectomy,
    granulation
Granulocytopenia (primary) (malignant) —*see*
  Agranulocytosis
Granuloma L92.9
  abdomen K66.8
    from residual foreign body L92.3
    pyogenicum L98.0
  actinic L57.5
  annulare (perforating) L92.0
  apical K04.5
  aural —*see* Otitis, externa, specified NEC
  beryllium (skin) L92.3
  bone
    eosinophilic C96.6
    from residual foreign body —*see*
      Osteomyelitis, specified type NEC
    lung C96.6
  brain (any site) G06.0
    schistosomiasis B65.9 [G07]
  canaliculus lacrimalis —*see* Granuloma,
    lacrimal
  candidal (cutaneous) B37.2
  cerebral (any site) G06.0
  coccidioidal (primary) (progressive) B38.7
    lung B38.1
    meninges B38.4
  colon K63.89
  conjunctiva H11.22-
  dental K04.5
  ear, middle —*see* Cholesteatoma

Granuloma (*Continued*)
  eosinophilic C96.6
    bone C96.6
    lung C96.6
    oral mucosa K13.4
    skin L92.2
  eyelid H01.8
  facial (e) L92.2
  foreign body (in soft tissue) NEC M60.20
    ankle M60.27-
    foot M60.27-
    forearm M60.23-
    hand M60.24-
    in operation wound —*see* Foreign body,
      accidentally left during a procedure
    lower leg M60.26-
    pelvic region M60.25-
    shoulder region M60.21-
    skin L92.3
    specified site NEC M60.28
    subcutaneous tissue L92.3
    thigh M60.25-
    upper arm M60.22-
  gangraenescens M31.2
  genito-inguinale A58
  giant cell (central) (reparative) (jaw) M27.1
    gingiva (peripheral) K06.8
  gland (lymph) I88.8
  hepatic NEC K75.3
    in (due to)
      berylliosis J63.2 [K77]
      sarcoidosis D86.89
  Hodgkin C81.9
  ileum K63.89
  infectious B99.9
    specified NEC B99.8
  inguinale (Donovan) (venereal) A58
  intestine NEC K63.89
  intracranial (any site) G06.0
  intraspinal (any part) G06.1
  iridocyclitis —*see* Iridocyclitis, chronic
  jaw (bone) (central) M27.1
    reparative giant cell M27.1
  kidney (*see also* Infection, kidney) N15.8
  lacrimal H04.81-
  larynx J38.7
  lethal midline (faciale (e)) M31.2
  liver NEC —*see* Granuloma, hepatic
  lung (infectious) —*see also* Fibrosis, lung
    coccidioidal B38.1
    eosinophilic C96.6
  Majocchi's B35.8
  malignant (facial (e)) M31.2
  mandible (central) M27.1
  midline (lethal) M31.2
  monilial (cutaneous) B37.2
  nasal sinus —*see* Sinusitis
  operation wound T81.89
    foreign body —*see* Foreign body,
      accidentally left during a procedure
    stitch T81.89
    talc —*see* Foreign body, accidentally left
      during a procedure
  oral mucosa K13.4
  orbit, orbital H05.11-
  paracoccidioidal B41.8
  penis, venereal A58
  periapical K04.5
  peritoneum K66.8
    due to ova of helminths NOS (*see also*
      Helminthiasis) B83.9 [K67]
  postmastoidectomy cavity —*see*
    Complications, postmastoidectomy,
    recurrent cholesteatoma
  prostate N42.89
  pudendi (ulcerating) A58
  pulp, internal (tooth) K03.3
  pyogenic, pyogenicum (of) (skin) L98.0
    gingiva K06.8
    maxillary alveolar ridge K04.5
    oral mucosa K13.4

Granuloma (*Continued*)
  rectum K62.89
  reticulohistiocytic D76.3
  rubrum nasi L74.8
  Schistosoma —*see* Schistosomiasis
  septic (skin) L98.0
  silica (skin) L92.3
  sinus (accessory) (infective) (nasal) —*see*
    Sinusitis
  skin L92.9
    from residual foreign body L92.3
    pyogenicum L98.0
  spine
    syphilitic (epidural) A52.19
    tuberculous A18.01
  stitch (postoperative) T81.89
  suppurative (skin) L98.0
  swimming pool A31.1
  talc —*see also* Granuloma, foreign body
    in operation wound —*see* Foreign body,
      accidentally left during a procedure
  telangiectaticum (skin) L98.0
  tracheostomy J95.09
  trichophyticum B35.8
  tropicum A66.4
  umbilicus L92.9
  urethra N36.8
  uveitis —*see* Iridocyclitis, chronic
  vagina A58
  venereum A58
  vocal cord J38.3
Granulomatosis L92.9
  lymphoid C83.8-
  miliary (listerial) A32.89
  necrotizing, respiratory M31.30
  progressive septic D71
  specified NEC L92.8
  Wegener's M31.30
    with renal involvement M31.31
Granulomatous tissue (abnormal) (excessive)
  L92.9
Granulosis rubra nasi L74.8
Graphite fibrosis (of lung) J63.3
Graphospasm F48.8
  organic G25.89
Grating scapula M89.8X1
Gravel (urinary) —*see* Calculus, urinary
Graves' disease —*see* Hyperthyroidism, with,
  goiter
Gravis —*see* condition
Grawitz tumor C64.-
Gray syndrome (newborn) P93.0
Grayness, hair (premature) L67.1
  congenital Q84.2
Green sickness D50.8
Greenfield's disease
  meaning
    concentric sclerosis (encephalitis periaxialis
      concentrica) G37.5
    metachromatic leukodystrophy E75.25
Greenstick fracture - code as Fracture,
  by site
Grey syndrome (newborn) P93.0
Grief F43.21
  prolonged F43.29
  reaction (*see also* Disorder, adjustment)
    F43.20
Griesinger's disease B76.9
Grinder's lung or pneumoconiosis J62.8
Grinding, teeth
  psychogenic F45.8
  sleep related G47.63
Grip
  Dabney's B33.0
  devil's B33.0
Grippe, grippal —*see also* Influenza
  Balkan A78
  summer, of Italy A93.1
Grisel's disease M43.6
Groin —*see* condition
Grooved tongue K14.5

Ground itch B76.9
Grover's disease or syndrome L11.1
Growing pains, children R29.898
Growth (fungoid) (neoplastic) (new) —*see also*
  Neoplasm
  adenoid (vegetative) J35.8
  benign —*see* Neoplasm, benign, by site
  malignant —*see* Neoplasm, malignant, by site
  rapid, childhood Z00.2
  secondary —*see* Neoplasm, secondary, by site
Gruby's disease B35.0
Gubler-Millard paralysis or syndrome G46.3
Guerin-Stern syndrome Q74.3
Guidance, insufficient anterior (occlusal)
  M26.54
Guillain-Barré disease or syndrome G61.0
  sequelae G65.0
Guinea worms (infection) (infestation) B72
Guinon's disease (motor-verbal tic) F95.2
Gull's disease E03.4
Gum —*see* condition
Gumboil K04.7
  with sinus K04.6
Gumma (syphilitic) A52.79
  artery A52.09
    cerebral A52.04
  bone A52.77
    of yaws (late) A66.6
  brain A52.19
  cauda equina A52.19
  central nervous system A52.3
  ciliary body A52.71
  congenital A50.59
  eyelid A52.71
  heart A52.06
  intracranial A52.19
  iris A52.71
  kidney A52.75
  larynx A52.73
  leptomeninges A52.19
  liver A52.74
  meninges A52.19
  myocardium A52.06
  nasopharynx A52.73
  neurosyphilitic A52.3
  nose A52.73
  orbit A52.71
  palate (soft) A52.79
  penis A52.76
  pericardium A52.06
  pharynx A52.73
  pituitary A52.79
  scrofulous (tuberculous) A18.4
  skin A52.79
  specified site NEC A52.79
  spinal cord A52.19
  tongue A52.79
  tonsil A52.73
  trachea A52.73
  tuberculous A18.4
  ulcerative due to yaws A66.4
  ureter A52.75
  yaws A66.4
    bone A66.6
Gunn's syndrome Q07.8
Gunshot wound —*see also* Wound, open
  fracture - code as Fracture, by site
  internal organs —*see* Injury, by site
Gynandrism Q56.0
Gynandroblastoma
  specified site —*see* Neoplasm, uncertain
    behavior, by site
  unspecified site
    female D39.10
    male D40.10
Gynecological examination (periodic) (routine)
  Z01.419
  with abnormal findings Z01.411
Gynecomastia N62
Gynephobia F40.291
Gyrate scalp Q82.8

◀ New   ⬛◀ Revised   ~~deleted~~ Deleted

H

H (Hartnup's) disease E72.02
Haas' disease or osteochondrosis (juvenile) (head of humerus) —*see* Osteochondrosis, juvenile, humerus
Habit, habituation
  bad sleep Z72.821
  chorea F95.8
  disturbance, child F98.9
  drug —*see* Dependence, drug
  irregular sleep Z72.821
  laxative F55.2
  spasm —*see* Tic
  tic —*see* Tic
Haemophilus (H.) influenzae, as cause of disease classified elsewhere B96.3
Haff disease —*see* Poisoning, mercury
Hageman's factor defect, deficiency or disease D68.2
Haglund's disease or osteochondrosis (juvenile) (os tibiale externum) —*see* Osteochondrosis, juvenile, tarsus
Hailey-Hailey disease Q82.8
Hair —*see also* condition
  plucking F63.3
    in stereotyped movement disorder F98.4
  tourniquet syndrome —*see also* Constriction, external, by site
    finger S60.44-
    penis S30.842
    thumb S60.34-
    toe S90.44-
Hairball in stomach T18.2
Hair-pulling, pathological (compulsive) F63.3
Hairy black tongue K14.3
Half vertebra Q76.49
Halitosis R19.6
Hallerman-Streiff syndrome Q87.0
Hallervorden-Spatz disease G23.0
Hallopeau's acrodermatitis or disease L40.2
Hallucination R44.3
  auditory R44.0
  gustatory R44.2
  olfactory R44.2
  specified NEC R44.2
  tactile R44.2
  visual R44.1
Hallucinosis (chronic) F28
  alcoholic (acute) F10.951
    in
      abuse F10.151
      dependence F10.251
  drug-induced F19.951
    cannabis F12.951
    cocaine F14.951
    hallucinogen F16.151
    in
      abuse F19.151
        cannabis F12.151
        cocaine F14.151
        hallucinogen F16.151
        inhalant F18.151
        opioid F11.151
        sedative, anxiolytic or hypnotic F13.151
        stimulant NEC F15.151
      dependence F19.251
        cannabis F12.251
        cocaine F14.251
        hallucinogen F16.251
        inhalant F18.251
        opioid F11.251
        sedative, anxiolytic or hypnotic F13.251
        stimulant NEC F15.251
    inhalant F18.951
    opioid F11.951
    sedative, anxiolytic or hypnotic F13.951
    stimulant NEC F15.951
  organic F06.0

Hallux
  deformity (acquired) NEC M20.5X-
  limitus M20.5X-
  malleus (acquired) NEC M20.3-
  rigidus (acquired) M20.2-
    congenital Q74.2
    sequelae (late effect) of rickets E64.3
  valgus (acquired) M20.1-
    congenital Q66.6
  varus (acquired) M20.3-
    congenital Q66.3
Halo, visual H53.19
Hamartoma, hamartoblastoma Q85.9
  epithelial (gingival), odontogenic, central or peripheral —*see* Cyst, calcifying odontogenic
Hamartosis Q85.9
Hamman-Rich syndrome J84.114
Hammer toe (acquired) NEC —*see also* Deformity, toe, hammer toe
  congenital Q66.89
  sequelae (late effect) of rickets E64.3
Hand —*see* condition
Hand-foot syndrome L27.1
Handicap, handicapped
  educational Z55.9
    specified NEC Z55.8
Hand-Schüller-Christian disease or syndrome C96.5
Hanging (asphyxia) (strangulation) (suffocation) —*see* Asphyxia, traumatic, due to mechanical threat
Hangnail —*see also* Cellulitis, digit
  with lymphangitis —*see* Lymphangitis, acute, digit
Hangover (alcohol) F10.129
Hanhart's syndrome Q87.0
Hanot-Chauffard (-Troisier) syndrome E83.19
Hanot's cirrhosis or disease K74.3
Hansen's disease —*see* Leprosy
Hantaan virus disease (Korean hemorrhagic fever) A98.5
Hantavirus disease (with renal manifestations) (Dobrava) (Puumala) (Seoul) A98.5
  with pulmonary manifestations (Andes) (Bayou) (Bermejo) (Black Creek Canal) (Choclo) (Juquitiba) (Laguna negra) (Lechiguanas) (New York) (Oran) (Sin nombre) B33.4
Happy puppet syndrome Q93.5
Harada's disease or syndrome H30.81-
Hardening
  artery —*see* Arteriosclerosis
  brain G93.89
Harelip (complete) (incomplete) —*see* Cleft, lip
Harlequin (newborn) Q80.4
Harley's disease D59.6
Harmful use (of)
  alcohol F10.10
  anxiolytics —*see* Abuse, drug, sedative
  cannabinoids —*see* Abuse, drug, cannabis
  cocaine —*see* Abuse, drug, cocaine
  drug —*see* Abuse, drug
  hallucinogens —*see* Abuse, drug, hallucinogen
  hypnotics —*see* Abuse, drug, sedative - opioids —*see* Abuse, drug, opioid
  PCP (phencyclidine) —*see* Abuse, drug, hallucinogen
  sedatives —*see* Abuse, drug, sedative
  stimulants NEC —*see* Abuse, drug, stimulant
Harris' lines —*see* Arrest, epiphyseal
Hartnup's disease E72.02
Harvester's lung J67.0
Harvesting ovum for in vitro fertilization Z31.83
Hashimoto's disease or thyroiditis E06.3
Hashitoxicosis (transient) E06.3
Hassal-Henle bodies or warts (cornea) H18.49
Haut mal —*see* Epilepsy, generalized, specified NEC

Haverhill fever A25.1
Hay fever (*see also* Fever, hay) J30.1
Hayem-Widal syndrome D59.8
Haygarth's nodes M15.8
Haymaker's lung J67.0
Hb (abnormal)
  Bart's disease D56.0
  disease —*see* Disease, hemoglobin
  trait —*see* Trait
Head —*see* condition
Headache R51
  allergic NEC G44.89
  associated with sexual activity G44.82
  chronic daily R51
  cluster G44.009
    chronic G44.029
      intractable G44.021
      not intractable G44.029
    episodic G44.019
      intractable G44.011
      not intractable G44.019
    intractable G44.001
    not intractable G44.009
  cough (primary) G44.83
  daily chronic R51
  drug-induced NEC G44.40
    intractable G44.41
    not intractable G44.40
  exertional (primary) G44.84
  histamine G44.009
    intractable G44.001
    not intractable G44.009
  hypnic G44.81
  lumbar puncture G97.1
  medication overuse G44.40
    intractable G44.41
    not intractable G44.40
  menstrual —*see* Migraine, menstrual
  migraine (type) (*see also* Migraine) G43.909
  nasal septum R51
  neuralgiform, short lasting unilateral, with conjunctival injection and tearing (SUNCT) G44.059
    intractable G44.051
    not intractable G44.059
  new daily persistent (NDPH) G44.52
  orgasmic G44.82
  periodic syndromes in adults and children G43.C0
    with refractory migraine G43.C1
      intractable G43.C1
      not intractable G43.C0
    without refractory migraine G43.C0
  postspinal puncture G97.1
  post-traumatic G44.309
    acute G44.319
      intractable G44.311
      not intractable G44.319
    chronic G44.329
      intractable G44.321
      not intractable G44.329
    intractable G44.301
    not intractable G44.309
  pre-menstrual —*see* Migraine, menstrual
  preorgasmic G44.82
  primary
    cough G44.83
    exertional G44.84
    stabbing G44.85
    thunderclap G44.53
  rebound G44.40
    intractable G44.41
    not intractable G44.40
  short lasting unilateral neuralgiform, with conjunctival injection and tearing (SUNCT) G44.059
    intractable G44.051
    not intractable G44.059
  specified syndrome NEC G44.89

◀ New ◀▥ Revised ~~deleted~~ Deleted

Headache (*Continued*)
spinal and epidural anesthesia - induced T88.59
in labor and delivery O74.5
in pregnancy O29.4-
postpartum, puerperal O89.4
spinal fluid loss (from puncture) G97.1
stabbing (primary) G44.85
tension (-type) G44.209
chronic G44.229
intractable G44.221
not intractable G44.229
episodic G44.219
intractable G44.211
not intractable G44.219
intractable G44.201
not intractable G44.209
thunderclap (primary) G44.53
vascular NEC G44.1
Healthy
infant
accompanying sick mother Z76.3
receiving care Z76.2
person accompanying sick person Z76.3
Hearing examination Z01.10
with abnormal findings NEC Z01.118
following failed hearing screening Z01.110
for hearing conservation and treatment Z01.12
Heart —*see* condition
Heart beat
abnormality R00.9
specified NEC R00.8
awareness R00.2
rapid R00.0
slow R00.1
Heartburn R12
psychogenic F45.8
Heat (effects) T67.9
apoplexy T67.0
burn (*see also* Burn) L55.9
collapse T67.1
cramps T67.2
dermatitis or eczema L59.0
edema T67.7
erythema - code by site under Burn, first degree
excessive T67.9
specified effect NEC T67.8
exhaustion T67.5
anhydrotic T67.3
due to
salt (and water) depletion T67.4
water depletion T67.3
with salt depletion T67.4
fatigue (transient) T67.6
fever T67.0
hyperpyrexia T67.0
prickly L74.0
prostration —*see* Heat, exhaustion
pyrexia T67.0
rash L74.0
specified effect NEC T67.8
stroke T67.0
sunburn —*see* Sunburn
syncope T67.1
Heavy-for-dates NEC (infant) (4000g to 4499g) P08.1
exceptionally (4500g or more) P08.0
Hebephrenia, hebephrenic (schizophrenia) F20.1
Heberden's disease or nodes (with arthropathy) M15.1
Hebra's
pityriasis L26
prurigo L28.2
Heel —*see* condition
Heerfordt's disease D86.89
Hegglin's anomaly or syndrome D72.0
Heilmeyer-Schoner disease D45
Heine-Medin disease A80.9

Heinz body anemia, congenital D58.2
Heliophobia F40.228
Heller's disease or syndrome F84.3
HELLP syndrome (hemolysis, elevated liver enzymes and low platelet count) O14.2-
Helminthiasis —*see also* Infestation, helminth
Ancylostoma B76.0
intestinal B82.0
mixed types (types classifiable to more than one of the titles B65.0-B81.3 and B81.8) B81.4
specified type NEC B81.8
mixed types (intestinal) (types classifiable to more than one of the titles B65.0-B81.3 and B81.8) B81.4
Necator (americanus) B76.1
specified type NEC B83.8
Heloma L84
Hemangioblastoma —*see* Neoplasm, connective tissue, uncertain behavior
malignant —*see* Neoplasm, connective tissue, malignant
Hemangioendothelioma —*see also* Neoplasm, uncertain behavior, by site
benign D18.00
intra-abdominal D18.03
intracranial D18.02
skin D18.01
specified site NEC D18.09
bone (diffuse) —*see* Neoplasm, bone, malignant
epithelioid —*see also* Neoplasm, uncertain behavior, by site
malignant —*see* Neoplasm, malignant, by site
malignant —*see* Neoplasm, connective tissue, malignant
Hemangiofibroma —*see* Neoplasm, benign, by site
Hemangiolipoma —*see* Lipoma
Hemangioma D18.00
arteriovenous D18.00
intra-abdominal D18.03
intracranial D18.02
skin D18.01
specified site NEC D18.09
capillary D18.00
intra-abdominal D18.03
intracranial D18.02
skin D18.01
specified site NEC D18.09
cavernous D18.00
intra-abdominal D18.03
intracranial D18.02
skin D18.01
specified site NEC D18.09
epithelioid D18.00
intra-abdominal D18.03
intracranial D18.02
skin D18.01
specified site NEC D18.09
histiocytoid D18.00
intra-abdominal D18.03
intracranial D18.02
skin D18.01
specified site NEC D18.09
infantile D18.00
intra-abdominal D18.03
intracranial D18.02
skin D18.01
specified site NEC D18.09
intra-abdominal D18.03
intracranial D18.02
intramuscular D18.00
intra-abdominal D18.03
intracranial D18.02
skin D18.01
specified site NEC D18.09
juvenile D18.00
malignant —*see* Neoplasm, connective tissue, malignant

Hemangioma (*Continued*)
plexiform D18.00
intra-abdominal D18.03
intracranial D18.02
skin D18.01
specified site NEC D18.09
racemose D18.00
intra-abdominal D18.03
intracranial D18.02
skin D18.01
specified site NEC D18.09
sclerosing —*see* Neoplasm, skin, benign
simplex D18.00
intra-abdominal D18.03
intracranial D18.02
skin D18.01
specified site NEC D18.09
skin D18.01
specified site NEC D18.09
venous D18.00
intra-abdominal D18.03
intracranial D18.02
skin D18.01
specified site NEC D18.09
verrucous keratotic D18.00
intra-abdominal D18.03
intracranial D18.02
skin D18.01
specified site NEC D18.09
Hemangiomatosis (systemic) I78.8
involving single site —*see* Hemangioma
Hemangiopericytoma —*see also* Neoplasm, connective tissue, uncertain behavior
benign —*see* Neoplasm, connective tissue, benign
malignant —*see* Neoplasm, connective tissue, malignant
Hemangiosarcoma —*see* Neoplasm, connective tissue, malignant
Hemarthrosis (nontraumatic) M25.00
ankle M25.07-
elbow M25.02-
foot joint M25.07-
hand joint M25.04-
hip M25.05-
in hemophilic arthropathy —*see* Arthropathy, hemophilic
knee M25.06-
shoulder M25.01-
specified joint NEC M25.08
traumatic —*see* Sprain, by site
vertebrae M25.08
wrist M25.03-
Hematemesis K92.0
with ulcer - code by site under Ulcer, with hemorrhage K27.4
newborn, neonatal P54.0
due to swallowed maternal blood P78.2
Hematidrosis L74.8
Hematinuria —*see also* Hemoglobinuria
malarial B50.8
Hematobilia K83.8
Hematocele
female NEC N94.89
with ectopic pregnancy O00.9
ovary N83.8
male N50.1
Hematochezia (*see also* Melena) K92.1
Hematochyluria —*see also* Infestation, filarial
schistosomiasis (bilharziasis) B65.0
Hematocolpos (with hematometra or hematosalpinx) N89.7
Hematocornea —*see* Pigmentation, cornea, stromal
Hematogenous —*see* condition
Hematoma (traumatic) (skin surface intact) —*see also* Contusion
with
injury of internal organs —*see* Injury, by site
open wound —*see* Wound, open
amputation stump (surgical) (late) T87.89

◀ New   ◀▥ Revised   ~~deleted~~ Deleted

Hematoma (*Continued*)
aorta, dissecting I71.00
  abdominal I71.02
  thoracic I71.01
  thoracoabdominal I71.03
aortic intramural —*see* Dissection, aorta
arterial (complicating trauma) —*see* Injury,
    blood vessel, by site
auricle —*see* Contusion, ear
  nontraumatic —*see* Disorder, pinna,
    hematoma
birth injury NEC P15.8
brain (traumatic)
  with
    cerebral laceration or contusion
        (diffuse) —*see* Injury, intracranial,
        diffuse
      focal —*see* Injury, intracranial,
        focal
    cerebellar, traumatic S06.37-
    intracerebral, traumatic —*see* Injury,
        intracranial, intracerebral
        hemorrhage
    newborn NEC P52.4
      birth injury P10.1
    nontraumatic —*see* Hemorrhage,
        intracranial
    subarachnoid, arachnoid, traumatic —*see*
        Injury, intracranial, subarachnoid
        hemorrhage
    subdural, traumatic —*see* Injury,
        intracranial, subdural hemorrhage
breast (nontraumatic) N64.89
broad ligament (nontraumatic) N83.7
  traumatic S37.892
cerebellar, traumatic S06.37-
cerebral —*see* Hematoma, brain
cerebrum S06.36-
  left S06.35-
  right S06.34-
cesarean delivery wound O90.2
complicating delivery (perineal) (pelvic)
    (vagina) (vulva) O71.7
corpus cavernosum (nontraumatic) N48.89
epididymis (nontraumatic) N50.1
epidural (traumatic) —*see* Injury, intracranial,
    epidural hemorrhage
  spinal —*see* Injury, spinal cord, by region
episiotomy O90.2
face, birth injury P15.4
genital organ NEC (nontraumatic)
  female (nonobstetric) N94.89
    traumatic S30.202
  male N50.1
    traumatic S30.201
internal organs —*see* Injury, by site
intracerebral, traumatic —*see* Injury,
    intracranial, intracerebral hemorrhage
intraoperative —*see* Complications,
    intraoperative, hemorrhage
labia (nontraumatic) (nonobstetric) N90.8
liver (subcapsular) (nontraumatic) K76.89
  birth injury P15.0
mediastinum —*see* Injury, intrathoracic
mesosalpinx (nontraumatic) N83.7
  traumatic S37.898
muscle - code by site under Contusion
nontraumatic
  muscle M79.81
  soft tissue M79.81
obstetrical surgical wound O90.2
orbit, orbital (nontraumatic) —*see also*
    Hemorrhage, orbit
  traumatic —*see* Contusion, orbit
pelvis (female) (nontraumatic) (nonobstetric)
    N94.89
  obstetric O71.7
  traumatic —*see* Injury, by site
penis (nontraumatic) N48.89
  birth injury P15.5
perianal (nontraumatic) K64.5

Hematoma (*Continued*)
perineal S30.23
  complicating delivery O71.7
perirenal —*see* Injury, kidney
pinna —*see* Contusion, ear
  nontraumatic —*see* Disorder, pinna,
    hematoma
placenta O43.89-
postoperative (postprocedural) —*see*
    Complication, postprocedural,
    hemorrhage
retroperitoneal (nontraumatic) K66.1
  traumatic S36.892
scrotum, superficial S30.22
  birth injury P15.5
seminal vesicle (nontraumatic) N50.1
  traumatic S37.892
spermatic cord (traumatic) S37.892
  nontraumatic N50.1
spinal (cord) (meninges) —*see also* Injury,
    spinal cord, by region
  newborn (birth injury) P11.5
spleen D73.5
  intraoperative —*see* Complications,
    intraoperative, hemorrhage, spleen
  postprocedural (postoperative) —*see*
    Complications, postprocedural,
    hemorrhage, spleen
sternocleidomastoid, birth injury P15.2
sternomastoid, birth injury P15.2
subarachnoid (traumatic) —*see* Injury,
    intracranial, subarachnoid hemorrhage
  newborn (nontraumatic) P52.5
    due to birth injury P10.3
  nontraumatic —*see* Hemorrhage,
    intracranial, subarachnoid
subdural (traumatic) —*see* Injury, intracranial,
    subdural hemorrhage
  newborn (localized) P52.8
    birth injury P10.0
  nontraumatic —*see* Hemorrhage,
    intracranial, subdural
superficial, newborn P54.5
testis (nontraumatic) N50.1
  birth injury P15.5
tunica vaginalis (nontraumatic) N50.1
umbilical cord, complicating delivery
    O69.5
uterine ligament (broad) (nontraumatic)
    N83.7
  traumatic S37.892
vagina (ruptured) (nontraumatic) N89.8
  complicating delivery O71.7
vas deferens (nontraumatic) N50.1
  traumatic S37.892
vitreous —*see* Hemorrhage, vitreous
vulva (nontraumatic) (nonobstetric)
    N90.89
  complicating delivery O71.7
  newborn (birth injury) P15.5
Hematometra N85.7
  with hematocolpos N89.7
Hematomyelia (central) G95.19
  newborn (birth injury) P11.5
  traumatic T14.8
Hematomyelitis G04.90
Hematoperitoneum —*see* Hemoperitoneum
Hematophobia F40.230
Hematopneumothorax (*see* Hemothorax)
Hematopoiesis, cyclic D70.4
Hematoporphyria —*see* Porphyria
Hematorachis, hematorrhachis G95.19
  newborn (birth injury) P11.5
Hematosalpinx N83.6
  with
    hematocolpos N89.7
    hematometra N85.7
      with hematocolpos N89.7
  infectional —*see* Salpingitis
Hematospermia R36.1
Hematothorax (*see* Hemothorax)

Hematuria R31.9
benign (familial) (of childhood) —*see also*
    Hematuria, idiopathic
  essential microscopic R31.1
due to sulphonamide, sulfonamide —*see* Table
    of Drugs and Chemicals, by drug
endemic (*see also* Schistosomiasis) B65.0
gross R31.0
idiopathic N02.9
  with glomerular lesion
    crescentic (diffuse) glomerulonephritis
        N02.7
    dense deposit disease N02.6
    endocapillary proliferative
        glomerulonephritis N02.4
    focal and segmental hyalinosis or
        sclerosis N02.1
    membranoproliferative (diffuse) N02.5
    membranous (diffuse) N02.2
    mesangial proliferative (diffuse) N02.3
    mesangiocapillary (diffuse) N02.5
    minor abnormality N02.0
    proliferative NEC N02.8
    specified pathology NEC N02.8
intermittent —*see* Hematuria, idiopathic
malarial B50.8
microscopic NEC R31.2
  benign essential R31.1
paroxysmal —*see also* Hematuria, idiopathic
  nocturnal D59.5
persistent —*see* Hematuria, idiopathic
recurrent —*see* Hematuria, idiopathic
tropical (*see also* Schistosomiasis) B65.0
tuberculous A18.13
Hemeralopia (day blindness) H53.11
  vitamin A deficiency E50.5
Hemi-akinesia R41.4
Hemianalgesia R20.0
Hemianencephaly Q00.0
Hemianesthesia R20.0
Hemianopia, hemianopsia (heteronymous)
    H53.47
  homonymous H53.46-
  syphilitic A52.71
Hemiathetosis R25.8
Hemiatrophy R68.89
  cerebellar G31.9
  face, facial, progressive (Romberg) G51.8
  tongue K14.8
Hemiballism (us) G25.5
Hemicardia Q24.8
Hemicephalus, hemicephaly Q00.0
Hemichorea G25.5
Hemicolitis, left —*see* Colitis, left sided
Hemicrania
  congenital malformation Q00.0
  continua G44.51
  meaning migraine (*see also* Migraine) G43.909
  paroxysmal G44.039
    chronic G44.049
      intractable G44.041
      not intractable G44.049
    episodic G44.039
      intractable G44.031
      not intractable G44.039
    intractable G44.031
    not intractable G44.039
Hemidystrophy —*see* Hemiatrophy
Hemiectromelia Q73.8
Hemihypalgesia R20.8
Hemihypesthesia R20.1
Hemi-inattention R41.4
Hemimelia Q73.8
  lower limb —*see* Defect, reduction, lower
    limb, specified type NEC
  upper limb —*see* Defect, reduction, upper
    limb, specified type NEC
Hemiparalysis —*see* Hemiplegia
Hemiparesis —*see* Hemiplegia
Hemiparesthesia R20.2
Hemiparkinsonism G20

Hemiplegia G81.9-
  alternans facialis G83.89
  ascending NEC G81.90
    spinal G95.89
  congenital (cerebral) G80.8
    spastic G80.2
  embolic (current episode) I63.4-
  flaccid G81.0-
  following
    cerebrovascular disease I69.959
      cerebral infarction I69.35-
        intracerebral hemorrhage I69.15-
        nontraumatic intracranial hemorrhage
          NEC I69.25-
        specified disease NEC I69.85-
        stroke NOS I69.35-
        subarachnoid hemorrhage I69.05-
  hysterical F44.4
  newborn NEC P91.8
    birth injury P11.9
  spastic G81.1-
    congenital G80.2
  thrombotic (current episode) I63.3
Hemisection, spinal cord —see Injury, spinal
    cord, by region
Hemispasm (facial) R25.2
Hemisporosis B48.8
Hemitremor R25.1
Hemivertebra Q76.49
  failure of segmentation with scoliosis Q76.3
  fusion with scoliosis Q76.3
Hemochromatosis E83.119
  with refractory anemia D46.1
  due to repeated red blood cell transfusion
    E83.111
  hereditary (primary) E83.110
  primary E83.110
  specified NEC E83.118
Hemoglobin —see also condition
  abnormal (disease) —see Disease,
    hemoglobin
  AS genotype D57.3
  Constant Spring D58.2
  E-beta thalassemia D56.5
  fetal, hereditary persistence (HPFH) D56.4
  H Constant Spring D56.0
  low NOS D64.9
  S (Hb S), heterozygous D57.3
Hemoglobinemia D59.9
  due to blood transfusion T80.89
  paroxysmal D59.6
    nocturnal D59.5
Hemoglobinopathy (mixed) D58.2
  with thalassemia D56.8
  sickle-cell D57.1
    with thalassemia D57.40
      with crisis (vasoocclusive pain)
        D57.419
        with
          acute chest syndrome D57.411
          splenic sequestration D57.412
      without crisis D57.40
Hemoglobinuria R82.3
  with anemia, hemolytic, acquired (chronic)
    NEC D59.6
  cold (agglutinin) (paroxysmal) (with
    Raynaud's syndrome) D59.6
  due to exertion or hemolysis NEC D59.6
  intermittent D59.6
  malarial B50.8
  march D59.6
  nocturnal (paroxysmal) D59.5
  paroxysmal (cold) D59.6
    nocturnal D59.5
Hemolymphangioma D18.1
Hemolysis
  intravascular
    with
      abortion —see Abortion, by type,
        complicated by, hemorrhage
      ectopic or molar pregnancy O08.1

Hemolysis (Continued)
  intravascular (Continued)
    with (Continued)
      hemorrhage
        antepartum —see Hemorrhage,
          antepartum, with coagulation
          defect
        intrapartum (see also Hemorrhage,
          complicating, delivery) O67.0
      postpartum O72.3
  neonatal (excessive) P58.9
    specified NEC P58.8
Hemolytic —see condition
Hemopericardium I31.2
  following acute myocardial infarction
    (current complication) I23.0
  newborn P54.8
  traumatic —see Injury, heart, with
    hemopericardium
Hemoperitoneum K66.1
  infectional K65.9
  traumatic S36.899
    with open wound —see Wound, open, with
      penetration into peritoneal cavity
Hemophilia (classical) (familial) (hereditary)
    D66
  A D66
  B D67
  C D68.1
  acquired D68.311
  autoimmune D68.311
  calcipriva (see also Defect, coagulation) D68.4
  nonfamilial (see also Defect, coagulation)
    D68.4
  secondary D68.311
  vascular D68.0
Hemophthalmos H44.81-
Hemopneumothorax —see also Hemothorax
  traumatic S27.2
Hemoptysis R04.2
  newborn P26.9
  tuberculous —see Tuberculosis, pulmonary
Hemorrhage, hemorrhagic (concealed) R58
  abdomen R58
  accidental antepartum —see Hemorrhage,
    antepartum
  acute idiopathic pulmonary, in infants
    R04.81
  adenoid J35.8
  adrenal (capsule) (gland) E27.49
    medulla E27.8
    newborn P54.4
  after delivery —see Hemorrhage, postpartum
  alveolar
    lung, newborn P26.8
    process K08.8
  alveolus K08.8
  amputation stump (surgical) T87.89
  anemia (chronic) D50.0
    acute D62
  antepartum (with) O46.90
    with coagulation defect O46.00-
      afibrinogenemia O46.01-
      disseminated intravascular coagulation
        O46.02-
      hypofibrinogenemia O46.01-
      specified defect NEC O46.09-
    before 20 weeks gestation O20.9
      specified type NEC O20.8
      threatened abortion O20.0
    due to
      abruptio placenta (see also Abruptio
        placentae) O45.9-
      leiomyoma, uterus —see Hemorrhage,
        antepartum, specified cause NEC
      placenta previa O44.1-
      specified cause NEC —see subcategory
        O46.8X-
  anus (sphincter) K62.5
  apoplexy (stroke) —see Hemorrhage,
    intracranial, intracerebral

Hemorrhage, hemorrhagic (Continued)
  arachnoid —see Hemorrhage, intracranial,
    subarachnoid
  artery R58
    brain —see Hemorrhage, intracranial,
      intracerebral
  basilar (ganglion) I61.0
  bladder N32.89
  bowel K92.2
    newborn P54.3
  brain (miliary) (nontraumatic) —see
    Hemorrhage, intracranial, intracerebral
    due to
      birth injury P10.1
      syphilis A52.05
    epidural or extradural (traumatic) —
      see Injury, intracranial, epidural
      hemorrhage
    newborn P52.4
      birth injury P10.1
    subarachnoid —see Hemorrhage,
      intracranial, subarachnoid
    subdural —see Hemorrhage, intracranial,
      subdural
  brainstem (nontraumatic) I61.3
    traumatic S06.38-
  breast N64.59
  bronchial tube —see Hemorrhage, lung
  bronchopulmonary —see Hemorrhage, lung
  bronchus —see Hemorrhage, lung
  bulbar I61.5
  capillary I78.8
    primary D69.8
  cecum K92.2
  cerebellar, cerebellum (nontraumatic) I61.4
    newborn P52.6
    traumatic S06.37-
  cerebral, cerebrum —see also Hemorrhage,
    intracranial, intracerebral
    lobe I61.1
    newborn (anoxic) P52.4
      birth injury P10.1
  cerebromeningeal I61.8
  cerebrospinal —see Hemorrhage, intracranial,
    intracerebral
  cervix (uteri) (stump) NEC N88.8
  chamber, anterior (eye) —see Hyphema
  childbirth —see Hemorrhage, complicating,
    delivery
  choroid H31.30-
    expulsive H31.31-
  ciliary body —see Hyphema
  cochlea —see subcategory H83.8
  colon K92.2
  complicating
    abortion —see Abortion, by type,
      complicated by, hemorrhage
    delivery O67.9
      associated with coagulation defect
        (afibrinogenemia) (DIC)
        (hyperfibrinolysis) O67.0
      specified cause NEC O67.8
    surgical procedure —see Hemorrhage,
      intraoperative
  conjunctiva H11.3-
    newborn P54.8
  cord, newborn (stump) P51.9
  corpus luteum (ruptured) cyst N83.1
  cortical (brain) I61.1
  cranial —see Hemorrhage, intracranial
  cutaneous R23.3
    due to autosensitivity, erythrocyte D69.2
    newborn P54.5
  delayed
    following ectopic or molar pregnancy
      O08.1
    postpartum O72.2
  diathesis (familial) D69.9
  disease D69.9
    newborn P53
    specified type NEC D69.8

◀ New   ⬅ Revised   ~~deleted~~ Deleted

Hemorrhage, hemorrhagic *(Continued)*
  due to or associated with
    afibrinogenemia or other coagulation
        defect (conditions in categories
        D65-D69)
      antepartum —*see* Hemorrhage,
          antepartum, with coagulation
          defect
      intrapartum O67.0
    dental implant M27.61
    device, implant or graft *(see also*
        Complications, by site and type,
        specified NEC) T85.83
      arterial graft NEC T82.838
      breast T85.83
      catheter NEC T85.83
        dialysis (renal) T82.838
          intraperitoneal T85.83
        infusion NEC T82.838
          spinal (epidural) (subdural) T85.83
        urinary (indwelling) T83.83
      electronic (electrode) (pulse generator)
          (stimulator)
        bone T84.83
        cardiac T82.837
        nervous system (brain) (peripheral
            nerve) (spinal) T85.83
        urinary T83.83
      fixation, internal (orthopedic) NEC T84.83
      gastrointestinal (bile duct) (esophagus)
          T85.83
      genital NEC T83.83
      heart NEC T82.837
      joint prosthesis T84.83
      ocular (corneal graft) (orbital implant)
          NEC T85.83
      orthopedic NEC T84.83
        bone graft T86.838
      specified NEC T85.83
      urinary NEC T83.83
      vascular NEC T82.838
      ventricular intracranial shunt T85.83
  duodenum, duodenal K92.2
    ulcer —*see* Ulcer, duodenum, with
        hemorrhage
  dura mater —*see* Hemorrhage, intracranial,
      subdural
  endotracheal —*see* Hemorrhage, lung
  epicranial subaponeurotic (massive), birth
      injury P12.2
  epidural (traumatic) —*see also* Injury,
      intracranial, epidural hemorrhage
    nontraumatic I62.1
  esophagus K22.8
    varix I85.01
      secondary I85.11
  excessive, following ectopic gestation
      (subsequent episode) O08.1
  extradural (traumatic) —*see* Injury,
      intracranial, epidural hemorrhage
    birth injury P10.8
    newborn (anoxic) (nontraumatic) P52.8
    nontraumatic I62.1
  eye NEC H57.8
    fundus —*see* Hemorrhage, retina
    lid —*see* Disorder, eyelid, specified type
        NEC
  fallopian tube N83.6
  fibrinogenolysis —*see* Fibrinolysis
  fibrinolytic (acquired) —*see* Fibrinolysis
  from
    ear (nontraumatic) —*see* Otorrhagia
    tracheostomy stoma J95.01
  fundus, eye —*see* Hemorrhage, retina
  funis —*see* Hemorrhage, umbilicus, cord
  gastric —*see* Hemorrhage, stomach
  gastroenteric K92.2
    newborn P54.3
  gastrointestinal (tract) K92.2
    newborn P54.3
  genital organ, male N50.1

Hemorrhage, hemorrhagic *(Continued)*
  genitourinary (tract) NOS R31.9
  gingiva K06.8
  globe (eye) —*see* Hemophthalmos
  graafian follicle cyst (ruptured) N83.0
  gum K06.8
  heart I51.89
  hypopharyngeal (throat) R04.1
  intermenstrual (regular) N92.3
    irregular N92.1
  internal (organs) NEC R58
    capsule I61.0
    ear —*see* subcategory H83.8
    newborn P54.8
  intestine K92.2
    newborn P54.3
  intra-abdominal R58
  intra-alveolar (lung), newborn P26.8
  intracerebral (nontraumatic) —*see*
      Hemorrhage, intracranial,
      intracerebral
  intracranial (nontraumatic) I62.9
    birth injury P10.9
    epidural, nontraumatic I62.1
    extradural, nontraumatic I62.1
    intracerebral (nontraumatic) (in) I61.9
      brain stem I61.3
      cerebellum I61.4
      hemisphere I61.2
        cortical (superficial) I61.1
        subcortical (deep) I61.0
      intraoperative
        during a nervous system procedure
            G97.31
        during other procedure G97.32
      intraventricular I61.5
      multiple localized I61.6
      newborn P52.4
        birth injury P10.1
      postprocedural
        following a nervous system procedure
            G97.51
        following other procedure
            G97.52
      specified NEC I61.8
      superficial I61.1
      traumatic (diffuse) —*see* Injury,
          intracranial, diffuse
      focal —*see* Injury, intracranial, focal
    newborn P52.9
      specified NEC P52.8
    subarachnoid (nontraumatic) (from)
        I60.9
      intracranial (cerebral) artery I60.7
        anterior communicating I60.2-
        basilar I60.4
        carotid siphon and bifurcation
            I60.0-
        communicating I60.7
          anterior I60.2-
          posterior I60.3-
        middle cerebral I60.1-
        posterior communicating I60.3-
        specified artery NEC I60.6
        vertebral I60.5-
      newborn P52.5
        birth injury P10.3
      specified NEC I60.8
      traumatic S06.6X-
    subdural (nontraumatic) I62.00
      acute I62.01
      birth injury P10.0
      chronic I62.03
      newborn (anoxic) (hypoxic) P52.8
        birth injury P10.0
      spinal G95.19
      subacute I62.02
      traumatic —*see* Injury, intracranial,
          subdural hemorrhage
    traumatic —*see* Injury, intracranial, focal
        brain injury

Hemorrhage, hemorrhagic *(Continued)*
  intramedullary NEC G95.19
  intraocular —*see* Hemophthalmos
  intraoperative, intraprocedural —*see*
      Complication, hemorrhage (hematoma),
      intraoperative (intraprocedural), by site
  intrapartum —*see* Hemorrhage, complicating,
      delivery
  intrapelvic
    female N94.89
    male K66.1
  intraperitoneal K66.1
  intrapontine I61.3
  intraprocedural —*see* Complication,
      hemorrhage (hematoma), intraoperative
      (intraprocedural), by site
  intrauterine N85.7
    complicating delivery (see also Hemorrhage,
        complicating, delivery) O67.9
    postpartum —*see* Hemorrhage, postpartum
  intraventricular I61.5
    newborn (nontraumatic) (see also Newborn,
        affected by, hemorrhage) P52.3
      due to birth injury P10.2
      grade
        1 P52.0
        2 P52.1
        3 P52.21
        4 P52.22
  intravesical N32.89
  iris (postinfectional) (postinflammatory)
      (toxic) —*see* Hyphema
  joint (nontraumatic) —*see* Hemarthrosis
  kidney N28.89
  knee (joint) (nontraumatic) —*see*
      Hemarthrosis, knee
  labyrinth —*see* subcategory H83.8
  lenticular striate artery I61.0
  ligature, vessel —*see* Hemorrhage,
      postoperative
  liver K76.89
  lung R04.89
    newborn P26.9
      massive P26.1
      specified NEC P26.8
    tuberculous —*see* Tuberculosis, pulmonary
  massive umbilical, newborn P51.0
  mediastinum —*see* Hemorrhage, lung
  medulla I61.3
  membrane (brain) I60.8
    spinal cord —*see* Hemorrhage, spinal cord
  meninges, meningeal (brain) (middle) I60.8
    spinal cord —*see* Hemorrhage, spinal cord
  mesentery K66.1
  metritis —*see* Endometritis
  mouth K13.79
  mucous membrane NEC R58
    newborn P54.8
  muscle M62.89
  nail (subungual) L60.8
  nasal turbinate R04.0
    newborn P54.8
  navel, newborn P51.9
  newborn P54.9
    specified NEC P54.8
  nipple N64.59
  nose R04.0
    newborn P54.8
  omentum K66.1
  optic nerve (sheath) H47.02-
  orbit, orbital H05.23-
  ovary NEC N83.8
  oviduct N83.6
  pancreas K86.8
  parathyroid (gland) (spontaneous) E21.4
  parturition —*see* Hemorrhage, complicating,
      delivery
  penis N48.89
  pericardium, pericarditis I31.2
  peritoneum, peritoneal K66.1
  peritonsillar tissue J35.8
    due to infection J36

Hemorrhage, hemorrhagic (*Continued*)
petechial R23.3
  due to autosensitivity, erythrocyte D69.2
pituitary (gland) E23.6
pleura —*see* Hemorrhage, lung
polioencephalitis, superior E51.2
polymyositis —*see* Polymyositis
pons, pontine I61.3
posterior fossa (nontraumatic) I61.8
  newborn P52.6
postmenopausal N95.0
postnasal R04.0
postoperative —*see* Complications,
  postprocedural, hemorrhage, by site
postpartum NEC (following delivery of
  placenta) O72.1
  delayed or secondary O72.2
  retained placenta O72.0
  third stage O72.0
pregnancy —*see* Hemorrhage, antepartum
preretinal —*see* Hemorrhage, retina
prostate N42.1
puerperal —*see* Hemorrhage, postpartum
  delayed or secondary O72.2
pulmonary R04.89
  newborn P26.9
    massive P26.1
    specified NEC P26.8
  tuberculous —*see* Tuberculosis, pulmonary
purpura (primary) D69.3
rectum (sphincter) K62.5
  newborn P54.2
recurring, following initial hemorrhage at
  time of injury T79.2
renal N28.89
respiratory passage or tract R04.9
  specified NEC R04.89
retina, retinal (vessels) H35.6-
  diabetic —*see* Diabetes, retinal, hemorrhage
retroperitoneal R58
scalp R58
scrotum N50.1
secondary (nontraumatic) R58
  following initial hemorrhage at time of
  injury T79.2
seminal vesicle N50.1
skin R23.3
  newborn P54.5
slipped umbilical ligature P51.8
spermatic cord N50.1
spinal (cord) G95.19
  newborn (birth injury) P11.5
spleen D73.5
  intraoperative —*see* Complications,
    intraoperative, hemorrhage, spleen
  postprocedural —*see* Complications,
    postprocedural, hemorrhage, spleen
stomach K92.2
  newborn P54.3
  ulcer —*see* Ulcer, stomach, with
    hemorrhage
subarachnoid (nontraumatic) —*see*
  Hemorrhage, intracranial, subarachnoid
subconjunctival —*see also* Hemorrhage,
  conjunctiva
  birth injury P15.3
subcortical (brain) I61.0
subcutaneous R23.3
subdiaphragmatic R58
subdural (acute) (nontraumatic) —*see*
  Hemorrhage, intracranial, subdural
subependymal
  newborn P52.0
    with intraventricular extension P52.1
      and intracerebral extension P52.22
subgaleal P12.1
subhyaloid —*see* Hemorrhage, retina
subperiosteal —*see* Disorder, bone, specified
  type NEC
subretinal —*see* Hemorrhage, retina
subtentorial —*see* Hemorrhage, intracranial,
  subdural

Hemorrhage, hemorrhagic (*Continued*)
subungual L60.8
suprarenal (capsule) (gland) E27.49
  newborn P54.4
tentorium (traumatic) NEC —*see*
  Hemorrhage, brain
  newborn (birth injury) P10.4
testis N50.1
third stage (postpartum) O72.0
thorax —*see* Hemorrhage, lung
throat R04.1
thymus (gland) E32.8
thyroid (cyst) (gland) E07.89
tongue K14.8
tonsil J35.8
trachea —*see* Hemorrhage, lung
tracheobronchial R04.89
  newborn P26.0
traumatic — code to specific injury
  cerebellar —*see* Hemorrhage, brain
  intracranial —*see* Hemorrhage, brain
  recurring or secondary (following initial
    hemorrhage at time of injury)
    T79.2
tuberculous NEC (*see also* Tuberculosis,
  pulmonary) A15.0
tunica vaginalis N50.1
ulcer - code by site under Ulcer, with
  hemorrhage K27.4
umbilicus, umbilical
  cord
    after birth, newborn P51.9
    complicating delivery O69.5
    newborn P51.9
      massive P51.0
      slipped ligature P51.8
    stump P51.9
urethra (idiopathic) N36.8
uterus, uterine (abnormal) N93.9
  climacteric N92.4
  complicating delivery —*see* Hemorrhage,
    complicating, delivery
  dysfunctional or functional N93.8
  intermenstrual (regular) N92.3
    irregular N92.1
  postmenopausal N95.0
  postpartum —*see* Hemorrhage,
    postpartum
  preclimacteric or premenopausal N92.4
  prepubertal N93.8
  pubertal N92.2
vagina (abnormal) N93.9
  newborn P54.6
vas deferens N50.1
vasa previa O69.4
ventricular I61.5
vesical N32.89
viscera NEC R58
  newborn P54.8
vitreous (humor) (intraocular) H43.1-
vulva N90.89

Hemorrhoids (bleeding) (without mention of
  degree) K64.9
1st degree (grade/stage I) (without prolapse
  outside of anal canal) K64.0
2nd degree (grade/stage II) (that
    prolapse with straining but retract
    spontaneously) K64.1
3rd degree (grade/stage III) (that prolapse
    with straining and require manual
    replacement back inside anal canal)
    K64.2
4th degree (grade/stage IV) (with prolapsed
    tissue that cannot be manually replaced)
    K64.3
complicating
  pregnancy O22.4
  puerperium O87.2
external K64.4
  with
    thrombosis K64.5

Hemorrhage, hemorrhagic (*Continued*)
internal (without mention of degree) K64.8
  prolapsed K64.8
  skin tags
    anus K64.4
    residual K64.4
  specified NEC K64.8
  strangulated (*see also* Hemorrhoids, by
    degree) K64.8
  thrombosed (*see also* Hemorrhoids, by degree)
    K64.5
  ulcerated (*see also* Hemorrhoids, by degree)
    K64.8
Hemosalpinx N83.6
with
  hematocolpos N89.7
  hematometra N85.7
    with hematocolpos N89.7
Hemosiderosis (dietary) E83.19
pulmonary, idiopathic E83.1 [*J84.03*]
transfusion T80.89
Hemothorax (bacterial) (nontuberculous)
  J94.2
newborn P54.8
traumatic S27.1
  with pneumothorax S27.2
tuberculous NEC A15.6
Henoch (-Schönlein) **disease or syndrome**
  (purpura) D69.0
Henpue, henpuye A66.6
Hepar lobatum (syphilitic) A52.74
Hepatalgia K76.89
Hepatitis K75.9
acute B17.9
  with coma K72.01
  with hepatic failure —*see* Failure, hepatic
  alcoholic —*see* Hepatitis, alcoholic
  infectious B15.9
    with hepatic coma B15.0
  viral B17.9
alcoholic (acute) (chronic) K70.10
  with ascites K70.11
amebic —*see* Abscess, liver, amebic
anicteric (viral) —*see* Hepatitis, viral
antigen-associated (HAA) —*see* Hepatitis, B
Australia-antigen (positive) —*see* Hepatitis, B
autoimmune K75.4
B B19.10
  with hepatic coma B19.11
  acute B16.9
    with
      delta-agent (coinfection) (without
        hepatic coma) B16.1
        with hepatic coma B16.0
      hepatic coma (without delta-agent
        coinfection) B16.2
  chronic B18.1
    with delta-agent B18.0
bacterial NEC K75.89
C (viral) B19.20
  with hepatic coma B19.21
  acute B17.10
    with hepatic coma B17.11
  chronic B18.2
catarrhal (acute) B15.9
  with hepatic coma B15.0
cholangiolitic K75.89
cholestatic K75.89
chronic K73.9
  active NEC K73.2
  lobular NEC K73.1
  persistent NEC K73.0
  specified NEC K73.8
cytomegaloviral B25.1
due to ethanol (acute) (chronic) —*see*
  Hepatitis, alcoholic
epidemic B15.9
  with hepatic coma B15.0
fulminant NEC (viral) —*see* Hepatitis, viral
granulomatous NEC K75.3
herpesviral B00.81

◀ New   ◀▬ Revised   ~~deleted~~ Deleted

Hepatitis (*Continued*)
history of
B Z86.19
C Z86.19
homologous serum —*see* Hepatitis, viral,
type B
in (due to)
mumps B26.81
toxoplasmosis (acquired) B58.1
congenital (active) P37.1 [*K77*]
infectious, infective (acute) (chronic)
(subacute) B15.9
with hepatic coma B15.0
inoculation —*see* Hepatitis, viral, type B
interstitial (chronic) K74.69
lupoid NEC K75.2
malignant NEC (with hepatic failure)
K72.90
with coma K72.91
neonatal giant cell P59.29
neonatal (idiopathic) (toxic) P59.29
newborn P59.29
postimmunization —*see* Hepatitis, viral,
type B
post-transfusion —*see* Hepatitis, viral, type B
reactive, nonspecific K75.2
serum —*see* Hepatitis, viral, type B
specified type NEC
with hepatic failure —*see* Failure, hepatic
syphilitic (late) A52.74
congenital (early) A50.08 [*K77*]
late A50.59 [*K77*]
secondary A51.45
toxic (*see also* Disease, liver, toxic) K71.6
tuberculous A18.83
viral, virus B19.9
with hepatic coma B19.0
acute B17.9
chronic B18.9
specified NEC B18.8
type
B B18.1
with delta-agent B18.0
C B18.2
congenital P35.3
coxsackie B33.8 [*K77*]
cytomegalic inclusion B25.1
in remission, any type — code to Hepatitis,
chronic, by type
non-A, non-B B17.8
specified type NEC (with or without coma)
B17.8
type
A B15.9
with hepatic coma B15.0
B B19.10
with hepatic coma B19.11
acute B16.9
with
delta-agent (coinfection) (without
hepatic coma) B16.1
with hepatic coma B16.0
hepatic coma (without delta-
agent coinfection) B16.2
chronic B18.1
with delta-agent B18.0
C B19.20
with hepatic coma B19.21
acute B17.10
with hepatic coma B17.11
chronic B18.2
E B17.2
non-A, non-B B17.8
Hepatization lung (acute) —*see* Pneumonia,
lobar
Hepatoblastoma C22.2
Hepatocarcinoma C22.0
Hepatocholangiocarcinoma C22.0
Hepatocholangioma, benign D13.4
Hepatocholangitis K75.89
Hepatolenticular degeneration E83.01

Hepatoma (malignant) C22.0
benign D13.4
embryonal C22.0
Hepatomegaly —*see also* Hypertrophy, liver
with splenomegaly R16.2
congenital Q44.7
in mononucleosis
gammaherpesviral B27.09
infectious specified NEC B27.89
Hepatoptosis K76.89
**Hepatorenal syndrome following labor and
delivery** O90.4
Hepatosis K76.89
Hepatosplenomegaly R16.2
hyperlipemic (Bürger-Grütz type) E78.3 [*K77*]
Hereditary —*see* condition
Heredodegeneration, macular —*see* Dystrophy,
retina
Heredopathia atactica polyneuritiformis G60.1
Heredosyphilis —*see* Syphilis, congenital
Herlitz' syndrome Q81.1
Hermansky-Pudlak syndrome E70.331
Hermaphrodite, hermaphroditism (true) Q56.0
46,XX with streak gonads Q99.1
46,XX/46,XY Q99.0
46,XY with streak gonads Q99.1
chimera 46,XX/46,XY Q99.0
Hernia, hernial (acquired) (recurrent) K46.9
with
gangrene —*see* Hernia, by site, with,
gangrene
incarceration —*see* Hernia, by site, with,
obstruction
irreducible —*see* Hernia, by site, with,
obstruction
obstruction —*see* Hernia, by site, with,
obstruction
strangulation —*see* Hernia, by site, with,
obstruction
abdomen, abdominal K46.9
with
gangrene (and obstruction) K46.1
obstruction K46.0
femoral —*see* Hernia, femoral
incisional —*see* Hernia, incisional
inguinal —*see* Hernia, inguinal
specified site NEC K45.8
with
gangrene (and obstruction) K45.1
obstruction K45.0
umbilical —*see* Hernia, umbilical
wall —*see* Hernia, ventral
appendix —*see* Hernia, abdomen
bladder (mucosa) (sphincter)
congenital (female) (male) Q79.51
female —*see* Cystocele
male N32.89
brain, congenital —*see* Encephalocele
cartilage, vertebra —*see* Displacement,
intervertebral disc
cerebral, congenital —*see also* Encephalocele
endaural Q01.8
ciliary body (traumatic) S05.2-
colon —*see* Hernia, abdomen
Cooper's —*see* Hernia, abdomen, specified
site NEC
crural —*see* Hernia, femoral
diaphragm, diaphragmatic K44.9
with
gangrene (and obstruction) K44.1
obstruction K44.0
congenital Q79.0
direct (inguinal) —*see* Hernia, inguinal
diverticulum, intestine —*see* Hernia,
abdomen
double (inguinal) —*see* Hernia, inguinal,
bilateral
due to adhesions (with obstruction) K56.5
epigastric (*see also* Hernia, ventral) K43.9
esophageal hiatus —*see* Hernia, hiatal
external (inguinal) —*see* Hernia, inguinal

Hernia, hernial (*Continued*)
fallopian tube N83.4
fascia M62.89
femoral K41.90
with
gangrene (and obstruction) K41.40
not specified as recurrent K41.40
recurrent K41.41
obstruction K41.30
not specified as recurrent K41.30
recurrent K41.31
bilateral K41.20
with
gangrene (and obstruction) K41.10
not specified as recurrent K41.10
recurrent K41.11
obstruction K41.00
not specified as recurrent K41.00
recurrent K41.01
not specified as recurrent K41.20
recurrent K41.21
not specified as recurrent K41.90
recurrent K41.91
unilateral K41.90
with
gangrene (and obstruction) K41.40
not specified as recurrent K41.40
recurrent K41.41
obstruction K41.30
not specified as recurrent K41.30
recurrent K41.31
not specified as recurrent K41.90
recurrent K41.91
foramen magnum G93.5
congenital Q01.8
funicular (umbilical) —*see also* Hernia,
umbilicus
spermatic (cord) —*see* Hernia, inguinal
gastrointestinal tract —*see* Hernia, abdomen
Hesselbach's —*see* Hernia, femoral, specified
site NEC
hiatal (esophageal) (sliding) K44.9
with
gangrene (and obstruction) K44.1
obstruction K44.0
congenital Q40.1
hypogastric —*see* Hernia, ventral
incarcerated —*see also* Hernia, by site, with
obstruction
with gangrene —*see* Hernia, by site, with
gangrene
incisional K43.92
with
gangrene (and obstruction) K43.1
obstruction K43.0
indirect (inguinal) —*see* Hernia, inguinal
inguinal (direct) (external) (funicular)
(indirect) (internal) (oblique) (scrotal)
(sliding) K40.90
with
gangrene (and obstruction) K40.40
not specified as recurrent K40.40
recurrent K40.41
obstruction K40.30
not specified as recurrent K40.30
recurrent K40.31
bilateral K40.20
with
gangrene (and obstruction)
K40.10
not specified as recurrent
K40.10
recurrent K40.11
obstruction K40.00
not specified as recurrent
K40.00
recurrent K40.01
not specified as recurrent K40.20
recurrent K40.21
not specified as recurrent K40.90
recurrent K40.91

Hernia, hernial *(Continued)*
  inguinal *(Continued)*
    unilateral K40.90
      with
        gangrene (and obstruction) K40.40
          not specified as recurrent K40.40
          recurrent K40.41
        obstruction K40.30
          not specified as recurrent K40.30
          recurrent K40.31
      not specified as recurrent K40.90
      recurrent K40.91
  internal —*see also* Hernia, abdomen
    inguinal —*see* Hernia, inguinal
  interstitial —*see* Hernia, abdomen
  intervertebral cartilage or disc —*see*
    Displacement, intervertebral disc
  intestine, intestinal —*see* Hernia, by site
  intra-abdominal —*see* Hernia, abdomen
  iris (traumatic) S05.2-
  irreducible —*see also* Hernia, by site, with
    obstruction
    with gangrene —*see* Hernia, by site, with
      gangrene
  ischiatic —*see* Hernia, abdomen, specified
    site NEC
  ischiorectal —*see* Hernia, abdomen, specified
    site NEC
  lens (traumatic) S05.2-
  linea (alba) (semilunaris) —*see* Hernia,
    ventral
  Littre's —*see* Hernia, abdomen
  lumbar —*see* Hernia, abdomen, specified site
    NEC
  lung (subcutaneous) J98.4
  mediastinum J98.5
  mesenteric (internal) —*see* Hernia, abdomen
  midline —*see* Hernia, ventral
  muscle (sheath) M62.89
  nucleus pulposus —*see* Displacement,
    intervertebral disc
  oblique (inguinal) —*see* Hernia, inguinal
  obstructive —*see also* Hernia, by site, with
    obstruction
    with gangrene —*see* Hernia, by site, with
      gangrene
  obturator —*see* Hernia, abdomen, specified
    site NEC
  omental —*see* Hernia, abdomen
  ovary N83.4
  oviduct N83.4
  paraesophageal —*see also* Hernia, diaphragm
    congenital Q40.1
  parastomal K43.5
    with
      gangrene (and obstruction) K43.4
      obstruction K43.3
  paraumbilical —*see* Hernia, umbilicus
  perineal —*see* Hernia, abdomen, specified
    site NEC
  Petit's —*see* Hernia, abdomen, specified site
    NEC
  postoperative —*see* Hernia, incisional
  pregnant uterus —*see* Abnormal, uterus in
    pregnancy or childbirth
  prevesical N32.89
  properitoneal —*see* Hernia, abdomen,
    specified site NEC
  pudendal —*see* Hernia, abdomen, specified
    site NEC
  rectovaginal N81.6
  retroperitoneal —*see* Hernia, abdomen,
    specified site NEC
  Richter's —*see* Hernia, abdomen, with
    obstruction
  Rieux's, Riex's —*see* Hernia, abdomen,
    specified site NEC
  sac condition (adhesion) (dropsy)
    (inflammation) (laceration)
    (suppuration) - code by site under
    Hernia

Hernia, hernial *(Continued)*
  sciatic —*see* Hernia, abdomen, specified site
    NEC
  scrotum, scrotal —*see* Hernia, inguinal
  sliding (inguinal) —*see also* Hernia,
    inguinal
    hiatus —*see* Hernia, hiatal
  spigelian —*see* Hernia, ventral
  spinal —*see* Spina bifida
  strangulated —*see also* Hernia, by site, with
    obstruction
    with gangrene —*see* Hernia, by site, with
      gangrene
  subxiphoid —*see* Hernia, ventral
  supra-umbilicus —*see* Hernia, ventral
  tendon —*see* Disorder, tendon, specified type
    NEC
  Treitz's (fossa) —*see* Hernia, abdomen,
    specified site NEC
  tunica vaginalis Q55.29
  umbilicus, umbilical K42.9
    with
      gangrene (and obstruction) K42.1
      obstruction K42.0
  ureter N28.89
  urethra, congenital Q64.79
  urinary meatus, congenital Q64.79
  uterus N81.4
    pregnant —*see* Abnormal, uterus in
      pregnancy or childbirth
  vaginal (anterior) (wall) —*see* Cystocele
  Velpeau's —*see* Hernia, femoral
  ventral K43.90
    with
      gangrene (and obstruction) K43.7
      obstruction K43.6
    incisional K43.2
      with
        gangrene (and obstruction) K43.1
        obstruction K43.0
    recurrent —*see* Hernia, incisional
    specified NEC K43.9
      with
        gangrene (and obstruction) K43.7
        obstruction K43.6
  vesical
    congenital (female) (male) Q79.51
    female —*see* Cystocele
    male N32.89
  vitreous (into wound) S05.2-
    into anterior chamber —*see* Prolapse,
      vitreous
Herniation —*see also* Hernia
  brain (stem) G93.5
  cerebral G93.5
  mediastinum J98.5
  nucleus pulposus —*see* Displacement,
    intervertebral disc
Herpangina B08.5
Herpes, herpesvirus, herpetic B00.9
  anogenital A60.9
    perianal skin A60.1
    rectum A60.1
    urogenital tract A60.00
      cervix A60.03
      male genital organ NEC A60.02
      penis A60.01
      specified site NEC A60.09
      vagina A60.04
      vulva A60.04
  blepharitis (zoster) B02.39
    simplex B00.59
  circinatus B35.4
    bullosus L12.0
  conjunctivitis (simplex) B00.53
    zoster B02.31
  cornea B02.33
  encephalitis B00.4
    due to herpesvirus 6 B10.01
    due to herpesvirus 7 B10.09
    specified NEC B10.09

Herpes, herpesvirus, herpetic *(Continued)*
  eye (zoster) B02.30
    simplex B00.50
  eyelid (zoster) B02.39
    simplex B00.59
  facialis B00.1
  febrilis B00.1
  geniculate ganglionitis B02.21
  genital, genitalis A60.00
    female A60.09
    male A60.02
  gestational, gestationis O26.4-
  gingivostomatitis B00.2
  human B00.9
    1 —*see* Herpes, simplex
    2 —*see* Herpes, simplex
    3 —*see* Varicella
    4 —*see* Mononucleosis, Epstein-Barr (virus)
    5 —*see* Disease, cytomegalic inclusion
      (generalized)
    6
      encephalitis B10.01
      specified NEC B10.81
    7
      encephalitis B10.09
      specified NEC B10.82
    8 B10.89
  infection NEC B10.89
    Kaposi's sarcoma associated B10.89
  iridocyclitis (simplex) B00.51
    zoster B02.32
  iris (vesicular erythema multiforme) L51.9
  iritis (simplex) B00.51
  Kaposi's sarcoma associated B10.89
  keratitis (simplex) (dendritic) (disciform)
    (interstitial) B00.52
    zoster (interstitial) B02.33
  keratoconjunctivitis (simplex) B00.52
    zoster B02.33
  labialis B00.1
  lip B00.1
  meningitis (simplex) B00.3
    zoster B02.1
  ophthalmicus (zoster) NEC B02.30
    simplex B00.50
  penis A60.01
  perianal skin A60.1
  pharyngitis, pharyngotonsillitis B00.2
  rectum A60.1
  scrotum A60.02
  sepsis B00.7
  simplex B00.9
    complicated NEC B00.89
    congenital P35.2
    conjunctivitis B00.53
    external ear B00.1
    eyelid B00.59
    hepatitis B00.81
    keratitis (interstitial) B00.52
    myleitis B00.82
    specified complication NEC B00.89
    visceral B00.89
  stomatitis B00.2
  tonsurans B35.0
  visceral B00.89
  vulva A60.04
  whitlow B00.89
  zoster (*see also* condition) B02.9
    auricularis B02.21
    complicated NEC B02.8
    conjunctivitis B02.31
    disseminated B02.7
    encephalitis B02.0
    eye(lid) B02.39
    geniculate ganglionitis B02.21
    keratitis (interstitial) B02.33
    meningitis B02.1
    myelitis B02.24
    neuritis, neuralgia B02.29
    ophthalmicus NEC B02.30
    oticus B02.21

◀ New   ◀ Revised   ~~deleted~~ Deleted

Herpes, herpesvirus, herpetic *(Continued)*
  zoster *(Continued)*
    polyneuropathy B02.23
    specified complication NEC B02.8
    trigeminal neuralgia B02.22
Herpesvirus (human) —*see* Herpes
Herpetophobia F40.218
Herrick's anemia —*see* Disease, sickle-cell
Hers' disease E74.09
Herter-Gee syndrome K90.0
Herxheimer's reaction R68.89
Hesitancy
  of micturition R39.11
  urinary R39.11
Hesselbach's hernia —*see* Hernia, femoral,
  specified site NEC
Heterochromia (congenital) Q13.2
  cataract —*see* Cataract, complicated
  cyclitis (Fuchs) —*see* Cyclitis, Fuchs'
    heterochromic
  hair L67.1
  iritis —*see* Cyclitis, Fuchs' heterochromic
  retained metallic foreign body
    (nonmagnetic) —*see* Foreign body,
    intraocular, old, retained
    magnetic —*see* Foreign body, intraocular,
    old, retained, magnetic
  uveitis —*see* Cyclitis, Fuchs' heterochromic
Heterophoria —*see* Strabismus, heterophoria
Heterophyes, heterophyiasis (small intestine)
  B66.8
Heterotopia, heterotopic —*see also* Malposition,
  congenital
  cerebralis Q04.8
Heterotropia —*see* Strabismus
Heubner-Herter disease K90.0
Hexadactylism Q69.9
HGSIL (cytology finding) (high grade
  squamous intraepithelial lesion on
  cytologic smear) (Pap smear finding)
  anus R85.613
  cervix R87.613
    biopsy (histology) finding — code to CIN
    II or CIN III
  vagina R87.623
    biopsy (histology) finding — code to VAIN
    II or VAIN III
Hibernoma —*see* Lipoma
Hiccup, hiccough R06.6
  epidemic B33.0
  psychogenic F45.8
Hidden penis (congenital) Q55.64
  acquired N48.83
Hidradenitis (axillaris) (suppurative) L73.2
Hidradenoma (nodular) —*see also* Neoplasm,
  skin, benign
  clear cell —*see* Neoplasm, skin, benign
  papillary —*see* Neoplasm, skin, benign
Hidrocystoma —*see* Neoplasm, skin, benign
High
  altitude effects T70.20
    anoxia T70.29
    on
      ears T70.0
      sinuses T70.1
    polycythemia D75.1
  arch
    foot Q66.7
    palate, congenital Q38.5
  arterial tension —*see* Hypertension
  basal metabolic rate R94.8
  blood pressure —*see also* Hypertension
    borderline R03.0
    reading (incidental) (isolated)
      (nonspecific), without diagnosis of
      hypertension R03.0
  cholesterol E78.0
    with high triglycerides E78.2
  diaphragm (congenital) Q79.1
  expressed emotional level within family Z63.8
  head at term O32.4

High *(Continued)*
  palate, congenital Q38.5
  risk
    infant NEC Z76.2
    sexual behavior (heterosexual) Z72.51
      bisexual Z72.53
      homosexual Z72.52
  temperature (of unknown origin) R50.9
  thoracic rib Q76.6
  triglycerides E78.1
    with high cholesterol E78.2
Hildenbrand's disease A75.0
Hilum —*see* condition
Hip —*see* condition
Hippel's disease Q85.8
Hippophobia F40.218
Hippus H57.09
Hirschsprung's disease or megacolon Q43.1
Hirsutism, hirsuties L68.0
Hirudiniasis
  external B88.3
  internal B83.4
Hiss-Russell dysentery A03.1
Histidinemia, histidinuria E70.41
Histiocytoma —*see also* Neoplasm, skin, benign
  fibrous —*see also* Neoplasm, skin, benign
    atypical —*see* Neoplasm, connective tissue,
      uncertain behavior
    malignant —*see* Neoplasm, connective
      tissue, malignant
Histiocytosis D76.3
  acute differentiated progressive C96.0
  Langerhans' cell NEC C96.6
    multifocal X
      multisystemic (disseminated) C96.0
      unisystemic C96.5
    pulmonary, adult (adult PLCH) J84.82
    unifocal (X) C96.6
  lipid, lipoid D76.3
    essential E75.29
  malignant C96.A
  mononuclear phagocytes NEC D76.1
    Langerhans' cells C96.6
  non-Langerhans cell D76.3
  polyostotic sclerosing D76.3
  sinus, with massive lymphadenopathy D76.3
  syndrome NEC D76.3
  X NEC C96.6
    acute (progressive) C96.0
    chronic C96.6
    multifocal C96.5
    multisystemic C96.0
    unifocal C96.6
Histoplasmosis B39.9
  with pneumonia NEC B39.2
  African B39.5
  American —*see* Histoplasmosis, capsulati
  capsulati B39.4
    disseminated B39.3
    generalized B39.3
    pulmonary B39.2
      acute B39.0
      chronic B39.1
  Darling's B39.4
  duboisii B39.5
  lung NEC B39.2
History
  family (of) —*see also* History, personal (of)
    alcohol abuse Z81.1
    allergy NEC Z84.89
    anemia Z83.2
    arthritis Z82.61
    asthma Z82.5
    blindness Z82.1
    cardiac death (sudden) Z82.41
    carrier of genetic disease Z84.81
    chromosomal anomaly Z82.79
    chronic
      disabling disease NEC Z82.8
      lower respiratory disease Z82.5
    colonic polyps Z83.71

History *(Continued)*
  family *(Continued)*
    congenital malformations and
      deformations Z82.79
      polycystic kidney Z82.71
    consanguinity Z84.3
    deafness Z82.2
    diabetes mellitus Z83.3
    disability NEC Z82.8
    disease or disorder (of)
      allergic NEC Z84.89
      behavioral NEC Z81.8
      blood and blood-forming organs Z83.2
      cardiovascular NEC Z82.49
      chronic disabling NEC Z82.8
      digestive Z83.79
      ear NEC Z83.52
      endocrine NEC Z83.49
      eye NEC Z83.518
        glaucoma Z83.511
      genitourinary NEC Z84.2
      glaucoma Z83.511
      hematological Z83.2
      immune mechanism Z83.2
      infectious NEC Z83.1
      ischemic heart Z82.49
      kidney Z84.1
      mental NEC Z81.8
      metabolic Z83.49
      musculoskeletal NEC Z82.69
      neurological NEC Z82.0
      nutritional Z83.49
      parasitic NEC Z83.1
      psychiatric NEC Z81.8
      respiratory NEC Z83.6
      skin and subcutaneous tissue NEC Z84.0
      specified NEC Z84.89
    drug abuse NEC Z81.3
    epilepsy Z82.0
    genetic disease carrier Z84.81
    glaucoma Z83.511
    hearing loss Z82.2
    human immunodeficiency virus (HIV)
      infection Z83.0
    Huntington's chorea Z82.0
    intellectual disability Z81.0
    leukemia Z80.6
    malignant neoplasm (of) NOS Z80.9
      bladder Z80.52
      breast Z80.3
      bronchus Z80.1
      digestive organ Z80.0
      gastrointestinal tract Z80.0
      genital organ Z80.49
        ovary Z80.41
        prostate Z80.42
        specified organ NEC Z80.49
        testis Z80.43
      hematopoietic NEC Z80.7
      intrathoracic organ NEC Z80.2
      kidney Z80.51
      lung Z80.1
      lymphatic NEC Z80.7
      ovary Z80.41
      prostate Z80.42
      respiratory organ NEC Z80.2
      specified site NEC Z80.8
      testis Z80.43
      trachea Z80.1
      urinary organ or tract Z80.59
        bladder Z80.52
        kidney Z80.51
    mental
      disorder NEC Z81.8
    multiple endocrine neoplasia (MEN)
      syndrome Z83.41
    osteoporosis Z82.62
    polycystic kidney Z82.71
    polyps (colon) Z83.71
    psychiatric disorder Z81.8
    psychoactive substance abuse NEC Z81.3

History *(Continued)*
  family *(Continued)*
    respiratory condition NEC Z83.6
      asthma and other lower respiratory
        conditions Z82.5
    self-harmful behavior Z81.8
    skin condition Z84.0
    specified condition NEC Z84.89
    stroke (cerebrovascular) Z82.3
    substance abuse NEC Z81.4
      alcohol Z81.1
      drug NEC Z81.3
      psychoactive NEC Z81.3
      tobacco Z81.2
    sudden cardiac death Z82.41
    tobacco abuse Z81.2
    violence, violent behavior Z81.8
    visual loss Z82.1
  personal (of) —*see also* History,
    family (of)
    abuse
      adult Z91.419
        physical and sexual Z91.410
        psychological Z91.411
      childhood Z62.819
        physical Z62.810
        psychological Z62.811
        sexual Z62.810
    alcohol dependence F10.21
    allergy (to) Z88.9
      analgesic agent NEC Z88.6
      anesthetic Z88.4
      antibiotic agent NEC Z88.1
      anti-infective agent NEC Z88.3
      contrast media Z91.041
      drugs, medicaments and biological
        substances Z88.9
        specified NEC Z88.8
      food Z91.018
        additives Z91.02
        eggs Z91.012
        milk products Z91.011
        peanuts Z91.010
        seafood Z91.013
        specified food NEC Z91.018
      insect Z91.038
        bee Z91.030
      latex Z91.040
      medicinal agents Z88.9
        specified NEC Z88.8
      narcotic agent NEC Z88.5
      nonmedicinal agents Z91.048
      penicillin Z88.0
      serum Z88.7
      specified NEC Z91.09
      sulfonamides Z88.2
      vaccine Z88.7
    anaphylactic shock Z87.892
    anaphylaxis Z87.892
    behavioral disorders Z86.59
    benign carcinoid tumor Z86.012
    benign neoplasm Z86.018
      brain Z86.011
      carcinoid Z86.012
      colonic polyps Z86.010
    brain injury (traumatic) Z87.820
    breast implant removal Z98.86
    calculi, renal Z87.442
    cancer —*see* History, personal (of),
      malignant neoplasm (of)
    cardiac arrest (death), successfully
      resuscitated Z86.74
    cerebral infarction without residual deficit
      Z86.73
    cervical dysplasia Z87.410
    chemotherapy for neoplastic condition
      Z92.21
    childhood abuse —*see* History, personal
      (of), abuse
    cleft lip (corrected) Z87.730
    cleft palate (corrected) Z87.730

History *(Continued)*
  personal *(Continued)*
    collapsed vertebra (healed) Z87.311
      due to osteoporosis Z87.310
    combat and operational stress reaction
      Z86.51
    congenital malformation (corrected)
      Z87.798
      circulatory system (corrected) Z87.74
      digestive system (corrected) NEC
        Z87.738
      ear (corrected) Z87.720
      eye (corrected) Z87.721
      face and neck (corrected) Z87.790
      genitourinary system (corrected) NEC
        Z87.718
      heart (corrected) Z87.74
      integument (corrected) Z87.76
      limb (s) (corrected) Z87.76
      musculoskeletal system (corrected)
        Z87.76
      neck (corrected) Z87.790
      nervous system (corrected) NEC
        Z87.728
      respiratory system (corrected) Z87.75
      sense organs (corrected) NEC Z87.728
      specified NEC Z87.798
    contraception Z92.0
    deployment (military) Z91.82
    diabetic foot ulcer Z86.31
    disease or disorder (of) Z87.898
      blood and blood-forming organs Z86.2
      circulatory system Z86.79
        specified condition NEC Z86.79
      connective tissue NEC Z87.39
      digestive system Z87.19
        colonic polyp Z86.010
        peptic ulcer disease Z87.11
        specified condition NEC Z87.19
      ear Z86.69
      endocrine Z86.39
        diabetic foot ulcer Z86.31
        gestational diabetes Z86.32
        specified type NEC Z86.39
      eye Z86.69
      genital (track) system NEC
        female Z87.42
        male Z87.438
      hematological Z86.2
      Hodgkin Z85.71
      immune mechanism Z86.2
      infectious Z86.19
        malaria Z86.13
        Methicillin resistant Staphylococcus
          aureus (MRSA) Z86.14
        poliomyelitis Z86.12
        specified NEC Z86.19
        tuberculosis Z86.11
      mental NEC Z86.59
      metabolic Z86.39
        diabetic foot ulcer Z86.31
        gestational diabetes Z86.32
        specified type NEC Z86.39
      musculoskeletal NEC Z87.39
      nervous system Z86.69
      nutritional Z86.39
      parasitic Z86.19
      respiratory system NEC Z87.09
      sense organs Z86.69
      skin Z87.2
      specified site or type NEC Z87.898
      subcutaneous tissue Z87.2
      trophoblastic Z87.59
      urinary system NEC Z87.448
    drug dependence —*see* Dependence, drug,
      by type, in remission
    drug therapy
      antineoplastic chemotherapy Z92.21
      estrogen Z92.23
      immunosupression Z92.25
      inhaled steroids Z92.240

History *(Continued)*
  personal *(Continued)*
    drug therapy *(Continued)*
      monoclonal drug Z92.22
      specified NEC Z92.29
      steroid Z92.241
      systemic steroids Z92.241
    dysplasia
      cervical Z87.410
      prostatic Z87.430
      vaginal Z87.411
      vulvar Z87.412
    embolism (venous) Z86.718
      pulmonary Z86.711
    encephalitis Z86.61
    estrogen therapy Z92.23
    extracorporeal membrane oxygenation
      (ECMO) Z92.81
    failed conscious sedation Z92.83
    failed moderate sedation Z92.83
    fall, falling Z91.81
    fracture (healed)
      fatigue Z87.312
      fragility Z87.310
      osteoporosis Z87.310
      pathological NEC Z87.311
      stress Z87.312
      traumatic Z87.81
    gestational diabetes Z86.32
    hepatitis
      B Z86.19
      C Z86.19
    Hodgkin disease Z85.71
    hyperthermia, malignant Z88.4
    hypospadias (corrected) Z87.710
    hysterectomy Z90.710
    immunosupression therapy Z92.25
    in situ neoplasm
      breast Z86.000
      cervix uteri Z86.001
      specified NEC Z86.008
    infection NEC Z86.19
      central nervous system Z86.61
      Methicillin resistant Staphylococcus
        aureus (MRSA) Z86.14
      urinary (tract) Z87.41
    injury NEC Z87.828
    in utero procedure during pregnancy
      Z98.870
    in utero procedure while a fetus
      Z98.871
    irradiation Z92.3
    kidney stones Z87.442
    leukemia Z85.6
    lymphoma (non-Hodgkin) Z85.72
    malignant melanoma (skin) Z85.820
    malignant neoplasm (of) Z85.9
      accessory sinuses Z85.22
      anus NEC Z85.048
        carcinoid Z85.040
      bladder Z85.51
      bone Z85.830
      brain Z85.841
      breast Z85.3
      bronchus NEC Z85.118
        carcinoid Z85.110
      carcinoid —*see* History, personal (of),
        malignant neoplasm, by site,
        carcinioid
      cervix Z85.41
      colon NEC Z85.038
        carcinoid Z85.030
      digestive organ Z85.00
        specified NEC Z85.09
      endocrine gland NEC Z85.858
      epididymis Z85.48
      esophagus Z85.01
      eye Z85.840
      gastrointestinal tract —*see* History,
        malignant neoplasm, digestive
        organ

◀ New   ◀▥ Revised   ~~deleted~~ Deleted

History (Continued)
  personal (Continued)
    malignant neoplasm (Continued)
      genital organ
        female Z85.40
          specified NEC Z85.44
        male Z85.45
          specified NEC Z85.49
      hematopoietic NEC Z85.79
      intrathoracic organ Z85.20-
      kidney NEC Z85.528
        carcinoid Z85.520
      large intestine NEC Z85.038
        carcinoid Z85.030
      larynx Z85.21
      liver Z85.05
      lung NEC Z85.118
        carcinoid Z85.110
      mediastinum Z85.29
      Merkel cell Z85.821
      middle ear Z85.22
      nasal cavities Z85.22
      nervous system NEC Z85.848
      oral cavity Z85.819
        specified site NEC Z85.818
      ovary Z85.43
      pancreas Z85.07
      pelvis Z85.53
      pharynx Z85.819
        specified site NEC Z85.818
      pleura Z85.29
      prostate Z85.46
      rectosigmoid junction NEC Z85.048
        carcinoid Z85.040
      rectum NEC Z85.048
        carcinoid Z85.040
      respiratory organ Z85.20
      sinuses, accessory Z85.22
      skin NEC Z85.828
        melanoma Z85.820
        Merkel cell Z85.821
      small intestine NEC Z85.068
        carcinoid Z85.060
      soft tissue Z85.831
      specified site NEC Z85.89
      stomach NEC Z85.028
        carcinoid Z85.020
      testis Z85.47
      thymus NEC Z85.238
        carcinoid Z85.230
      thyroid Z85.850
      tongue Z85.810
      trachea Z85.12
      ureter Z85.54
      urinary organ or tract Z85.50
        specified NEC Z85.59
      uterus Z85.42
    maltreatment Z91.89
    medical treatment NEC Z92.89
    melanoma (malignant) (skin) Z85.820
    meningitis Z86.61
    mental disorder Z86.59
    Merkel cell carcinoma (skin) Z85.821
    Methicillin resistant Staphylococcus aureus (MRSA) Z86.14
    military deployment Z91.82
    military war, peacekeeping and humanitarian deployment (current or past conflict) Z91.82
    myocardial infarction (old) I25.2
    neglect (in)
      adult Z91.412
      childhood Z62.812
    neoplasm
      benign Z86.018
        brain Z86.011
        colon polyp Z86.010
      in situ
        breast Z86.000
        cervix uteri Z86.001
        specified NEC Z86.008

History (Continued)
  personal (Continued)
    neoplasm (Continued)
      malignant —see History of, malignant neoplasm
      uncertain behavior Z86.03
    nephrotic syndrome Z87.441
    nicotine dependence Z87.891
    noncompliance with medical treatment or regimen —see Noncompliance
    nutritional deficiency Z86.39
    obstetric complications Z87.59
      childbirth Z87.59
      pregnancy Z87.59
      pre-term labor Z87.51
      puerperium Z87.59
    osteoporosis fractures Z87.31
    parasuicide (attempt) Z91.5
    physical trauma NEC Z87.828
      self-harm or suicide attempt Z91.5
    pneumonia (recurrent) Z87.01
    poisoning NEC Z91.89
      self-harm or suicide attempt Z91.5
    poor personal hygiene Z91.89
    preterm labor Z87.51
    procedure during pregnancy Z98.870
    procedure while a fetus Z98.871
    prolonged reversible ischemic neurologic deficit (PRIND) Z86.73
    prostatic dysplasia Z87.430
    psychiatric disorder NEC Z87.89
    psychological
      abuse
        adult Z91.411
        child Z62.811
      trauma, specified NEC Z91.49
    radiation therapy Z92.3
    removal
      implant
        breast Z98.86
    renal calculi Z87.442
    respiratory condition NEC Z87.09
    retained foreign body fully removed Z87.821
    risk factors NEC Z91.89
    self-harm Z91.5
    self-poisoning attempt Z91.5
    sex reassignment Z87.890
    sleep-wake cycle problem Z72.821
      specified NEC Z87.898
    steroid therapy (systemic) Z92.241
      inhaled Z92.240
    stroke without residual deficits Z86.73
    substance abuse NEC F10-F19 with fifth character 1
    sudden cardiac arrest Z86.74
    sudden cardiac death successfully resuscitated Z86.74
    suicide attempt Z91.5
    surgery NEC Z98.89
      sex reassignment Z87.890
      transplant —see Transplant
    thrombophlebitis Z86.72
    thrombosis (venous) Z86.718
      pulmonary Z86.711
    tobacco dependence Z87.891
    transient ischemic attack (TIA) without residual deficits Z86.73
    trauma (physical) NEC Z87.828
      psychological NEC Z91.49
      self-harm Z91.5
    traumatic brain injury Z87.820
    unhealthy sleep-wake cycle Z72.821
    urinary (recurrent) (tract) infection (s) Z87.440
    urinary calculi Z87.42
    vaginal dysplasia Z87.411
    venous thrombosis or embolism Z86.718
      pulmonary Z86.711
    vulvar dysplasia Z87.412

His-Werner disease A79.0
HIV (see also Human, immunodeficiency virus) B20
  laboratory evidence (nonconclusive) R75
  nonconclusive test (in infants) R75
  positive, seropositive Z21
Hives (bold) —see Urticaria
Hoarseness R49.0
Hobo Z59.0
Hodgkin disease —see Lymphoma, Hodgkin
Hodgson's disease I71.2
  ruptured I71.1
Hoffa-Kastert disease E88.89
Hoffa's disease E88.89
Hoffmann-Bouveret syndrome I47.9
Hoffmann's syndrome E03.9 [G73.7]
Hole (round)
  macula H35.34-
  retina (without detachment) —see Break, retina, round hole
    with detachment —see Detachment, retina, with retinal, break
Holiday relief care Z75.5
Hollenhorst's plaque —see Occlusion, artery, retina
Hollow foot (congenital) Q66.7
  acquired —see Deformity, limb, foot, specified NEC
Holoprosencephaly Q04.2
Holt-Oram syndrome Q87.2
Homelessness Z59.0
Homesickness —see Disorder, adjustment
Homocystinemia, homocystinuria E72.11
Homogentisate 1,2-dioxygenase deficiency E70.29
Homologous serum hepatitis (prophylactic) (therapeutic) —see Hepatitis, viral, type B
Honeycomb lung J98.4
  congenital Q33.0
Hooded
  clitoris Q52.6
  penis Q55.69
Hookworm (anemia) (disease) (infection) (infestation) B76.9
  specified NEC B76.8
Hordeolum (eyelid) (externum) (recurrent) H00.019
  internum H00.029
    left H00.026
      lower H00.025
      upper H00.024
    right H00.023
      lower H00.022
      upper H00.021
  left H00.016
    lower H00.015
    upper H00.014
  right H00.013
    lower H00.012
    upper H00.011
Horn
  cutaneous L85.8
  nail L60.2
    congenital Q84.6
Horner (-Claude Bernard) syndrome G90.2
  traumatic —see Injury, nerve, cervical sympathetic
Horseshoe kidney (congenital) Q63.1
Horton's headache or neuralgia G44.099
  intractable G44.091
  not intractable G44.099
Hospital hopper syndrome —see Disorder, factitious
Hospitalism in children —see Disorder, adjustment
Hostility R45.5
  towards child Z62.3
Hot flashes
  menopausal N95.1

Hourglass (contracture) —see also Contraction, hourglass
  stomach K31.89
    congenital Q40.2
    stricture K31.2
Household, housing circumstance affecting care Z59.9
  specified NEC Z59.8
Housemaid's knee —see Bursitis, prepatellar
Hudson (-Stähli) line (cornea) —see Pigmentation, cornea, anterior
Human
  bite (open wound) —see also Bite
    intact skin surface —see Bite, superficial
  herpesvirus —see Herpes
  immunodeficiency virus (HIV) disease (infection) B20
    asymptomatic status Z21
    contact Z20.6
    counseling Z71.7
    dementia B20 [F02.80]
      with behavioral disturbance B20 [F02.81]
    exposure to Z20.6
    laboratory evidence R75
    type-2 (HIV 2) as cause of disease classified elsewhere B97.35
  papillomavirus (HPV)
    DNA test positive
      high risk
        cervix R87.810
        vagina R87.811
      low risk
        cervix R87.820
        vagina R87.821
    screening for Z11.51
  T-cell lymphotropic virus
    type-1 (HTLV-I) infection B33.3
      as cause of disease classified elsewhere B97.33
      carrier Z22.6
    type-2 (HTLV-II) as cause of disease classified elsewhere B97.34
Humidifier lung or pneumonitis J67.7
Humiliation (experience) in childhood Z62.898
Humpback (acquired) —see Kyphosis
Hunchback (acquired) —see Kyphosis
Hunger T73.0
  air, psychogenic F45.8
Hungry bone syndrome E83.81
Hunner's ulcer —see Cystitis, chronic, interstitial
Hunter's
  glossitis D51.0
  syndrome E76.1
Huntington's disease or chorea G10
  with dementia G10 [F02.80]
    with behavioral disturbance G10 [F02.81]
Hunt's
  disease or syndrome (herpetic geniculate ganglionitis) B02.21
    dyssynergia cerebellaris myoclonica G11.1
    neuralgia B02.21
Hurler (-Scheie) disease or syndrome E76.02
Hurst's disease G36.1
Hurthle cell
  adenocarcinoma C73
  adenoma D34
  carcinoma C73
  tumor D34
Hutchinson-Boeck disease or syndrome —see Sarcoidosis
Hutchinson-Gilford disease or syndrome E34.8
Hutchinson's
  disease, meaning
    angioma serpiginosum L81.7
    pompholyx (cheiropompholyx) L30.1
    prurigo estivalis L56.4
    summer eruption or summer prurigo L56.4
    melanotic freckle —see Melanoma, in situ
    malignant melanoma in —see Melanoma

Hutchinson's (Continued)
  teeth or incisors (congenital syphilis) A50.52
  triad (congenital syphilis) A50.53
Hyalin plaque, sclera, senile H15.89
Hyaline membrane (disease) (lung) (pulmonary) (newborn) P22.0
Hyalinosis
  cutis (et mucosae) E78.89
  focal and segmental (glomerular) (see also N00-N07 with fourth character .1) N05.1
Hyalitis, hyalosis, asteroid —see also Deposit, crystalline
  syphilitic (late) A52.71
Hydatid
  cyst or tumor —see Echinococcus
  mole —see Hydatidiform mole
  Morgagni
    female Q50.5
    male (epididymal) Q55.4
    testicular Q55.29
Hydatidiform mole (benign) (complicating pregnancy) (delivered) (undelivered) O01.9
  classical O01.0
  complete O01.0
  incomplete O01.1
  invasive D39.2
  malignant D39.2
  partial O01.1
Hydatidosis —see Echinococcus
Hydradenitis (axillaris) (suppurative) L73.2
Hydradenoma —see Hidradenoma
Hydramnios O40.-
Hydrancephaly, hydranencephaly Q04.3
  with spina bifida —see Spina bifida, with hydrocephalus
Hydrargyrism NEC —see Poisoning, mercury
Hydrarthrosis —see also Effusion, joint
  gonococcal A54.42
  intermittent M12.40
    ankle M12.47-
    elbow M12.42-
    foot joint M12.47-
    hand joint M12.44-
    hip M12.45-
    knee M12.46-
    multiple site M12.49
    shoulder M12.41-
    specified joint NEC M12.48
    wrist M12.43-
  of yaws (early) (late) (see also subcategory M14.8-) A66.6
  syphilitic (late) A52.77
    congenital A50.55 [M12.80]
Hydremia D64.89
Hydrencephalocele (congenital) —see Encephalocele
Hydrencephalomeningocele (congenital) —see Encephalocele
Hydroa R23.8
  aestivale L56.4
  vacciniforme L56.4
Hydroadenitis (axillaris) (suppurative) L73.2
Hydrocalycosis —see Hydronephrosis
Hydrocele (spermatic cord) (testis) (tunica vaginalis) N43.3
  canal of Nuck N94.89
  communicating N43.2
    congenital P83.5
  congenital P83.5
  encysted N43.0
  female NEC N94.89
  infected N43.1
  newborn P83.5
  round ligament N94.89
  specified NEC N43.2
  spinalis —see Spina bifida
  vulva N90.89

Hydrocephalus (acquired) (external) (internal) (malignant) (recurrent) G91.9
  aqueduct Sylvius stricture Q03.0
  causing disproportion O33.6
    with obstructed labor O66.3
  communicating G91.0
  congenital (external) (internal) Q03.9
    with spina bifida Q05.4
      cervical Q05.0
      dorsal Q05.1
      lumbar Q05.2
      lumbosacral Q05.2
      sacral Q05.3
      thoracic Q05.1
      thoracolumbar Q05.1
    specified NEC Q03.8
  due to toxoplasmosis (congenital) P37.1
  foramen Magendie block (acquired) G91.1
    congenital (see also Hydrocephalus, congenital) Q03.1
  in (due to)
    infectious disease NEC B89 [G91.4]
    neoplastic disease NEC (see also Neoplasm) G91.4
    parasitic disease B89 [G91.4]
  newborn Q03.9
    with spina bifida —see Spina bifida, with hydrocephalus
  noncommunicating G91.1
  normal pressure G91.2
    secondary G91.0
  obstructive G91.1
  otitic G93.2
  post-traumatic NEC G91.3
  secondary G91.4
    post-traumatic G91.3
  specified NEC G91.8
  syphilitic, congenital A50.49
Hydrocolpos (congenital) N89.8
Hydrocystoma —see Neoplasm, skin, benign
Hydroencephalocele (congenital) —see Encephalocele
Hydroencephalomeningocele (congenital) —see Encephalocele
Hydrohematopneumothorax —see Hemothorax
Hydromeningitis —see Meningitis
Hydromeningocele (spinal) —see also Spina bifida
  cranial —see Encephalocele
Hydrometra N85.8
Hydrometrocolpos N89.8
Hydromicrocephaly Q02
Hydromphalos (since birth) Q45.8
Hydromyelia Q06.4
Hydromyelocele —see Spina bifida
Hydronephrosis (atrophic) (early) (functionless) (intermittent) (primary) (secondary) NEC N13.30
  with
    infection N13.6
    obstruction (by) (of)
      renal calculus N13.2
        with infection N13.6
      ureteral NEC N13.1
        with infection N13.6
        calculus N13.2
          with infection N13.6
      ureteropelvic junction (congenital) Q62.0
        with infection N13.6
      ureteral stricture NEC N13.1
        with infection N13.6
  congenital Q62.0
  specified type NEC N13.39
  tuberculous A18.11
Hydropericarditis —see Pericarditis
Hydropericardium —see Pericarditis
Hydroperitoneum R18.8
Hydrophobia —see Rabies
Hydrophthalmos Q15.0
Hydropneumohemothorax —see Hemothorax
Hydropneumopericarditis —see Pericarditis

Hydropneumopericardium —*see* Pericarditis
Hydropneumothorax J94.8
  traumatic —*see* Injury, intrathoracic, lung
  tuberculous NEC A15.6
Hydrops R60.9
  abdominis R18.8
  articulorum intermittens —*see* Hydrarthrosis,
    intermittent
  cardiac —*see* Failure, heart, congestive
  causing obstructed labor (mother) O66.3
  endolymphatic H81.0-
  fetal —*see* Pregnancy, complicated by,
    hydrops, fetalis
  fetalis P83.2
    due to
      ABO isoimmunization P56.0
      alpha thalassemia D56.0
      hemolytic disease P56.90
        specified NEC P56.99
      isoimmunization (ABO) (Rh) P56.0
      other specified nonhemolytic disease
        NEC P83.2
      Rh incompatibility P56.0
    during pregnancy —*see* Pregnancy,
      complicated by, hydrops, fetalis
  gallbladder K82.1
  joint —*see* Effusion, joint
  labyrinth H81.0
  newborn (idiopathic) P83.2
    due to
      ABO isoimmunization P56.0
      alpha thalassemia D56.0
      hemolytic disease P56.90
        specified NEC P56.99
      isoimmunization (ABO) (Rh) P56.0
      Rh incompatibility P56.0
  nutritional —*see* Malnutrition, severe
  pericardium —*see* Pericarditis
  pleura —*see* Hydrothorax
  spermatic cord —*see* Hydrocele
Hydropyonephrosis N13.6
Hydrorachis Q06.4
Hydrorrhea (nasal) J34.89
  pregnancy —*see* Rupture, membranes,
    premature
Hydrosadenitis (axillaris) (suppurative) L73.2
Hydrosalpinx (fallopian tube) (follicularis)
  N70.11
Hydrothorax (double) (pleura) J94.8
  chylous (nonfilarial) I89.8
    filarial (*see also* Infestation, filarial) B74.9
      [J91.8]
  traumatic —*see* Injury, intrathoracic
  tuberculous NEC (non primary) A15.6
Hydroureter (*see also* Hydronephrosis) N13.4
  with infection N13.6
  congenital Q62.39
Hydroureteronephrosis —*see* Hydronephrosis
Hydrourethra N36.8
Hydroxykynureninuria E70.8
Hydroxylysinemia E72.3
Hydroxyprolinemia E72.59
Hygiene, sleep
  abuse Z72.821
  inadequate Z72.821
  poor Z72.821
Hygroma (congenital) (cystic) D18.1
  praepatellare, prepatellar —*see* Bursitis,
    prepatellar
Hymen —*see* condition
Hymenolepis, hymenolepiasis (diminuta)
  (infection) (infestation) (nana) B71.0
Hypalgesia R20.8
Hyperacidity (gastric) K31.89
  psychogenic F45.8
Hyperactive, hyperactivity F90.9
  basal cell, uterine cervix —*see* Dysplasia,
    cervix
  bowel sounds R19.12
  cervix epithelial (basal) —*see* Dysplasia,
    cervix

Hyperactive, hyperactivity (*Continued*)
  child F90.9
    attention deficit —*see* Disorder, attention-
      deficit hyperactivity
  detrusor muscle N32.81
  gastrointestinal K31.89
    psychogenic F45.8
  nasal mucous membrane J34.3
  stomach K31.89
  thyroid (gland) —*see* Hyperthyroidism
Hyperacusis H93.23-
Hyperadrenalism E27.5
Hyperadrenocorticism E24.9
  congenital E25.0
  iatrogenic E24.2
    correct substance properly administered —
      see Table of Drugs and Chemicals, by
      drug, adverse effect
    overdose or wrong substance given or
      taken —*see* Table of Drugs and
      Chemicals, by drug, poisoning
  not associated with Cushing's syndrome
    E27.0
  pituitary-dependent E24.0
Hyperaldosteronism E26.9
  familial (type I) E26.02
  glucocorticoid-remediable E26.02
  primary (due to (bilateral) adrenal
    hyperplasia) E26.09
  primary NEC E26.09
  secondary E26.1
  specified NEC E26.89
Hyperalgesia R20.8
Hyperalimentation R63.2
  carotene, carotin E67.1
  specified NEC E67.8
  vitamin
    A E67.0
    D E67.3
Hyperaminoaciduria
  arginine E72.21
  cystine E72.01
  lysine E72.3
  ornithine E72.4
Hyperammonemia (congenital) E72.20
Hyperazotemia —*see* Uremia
Hyperbetalipoproteinemia (familial) E78.0
  with prebetalipoproteinemia E78.2
Hyperbilirubinemia
  constitutional E80.6
  familial conjugated E80.6
  neonatal (transient) —*see* Jaundice, newborn
Hypercalcemia, hypocalciuric, familial E83.52
Hypercalciuria, idiopathic E83.52
Hypercapnia R06.89
  newborn P84
Hypercarotenemia, hypercarotinemia (dietary)
  E67.1
Hypercementosis K03.4
Hyperchloremia E87.8
Hyperchlorhydria K31.89
  neurotic F45.8
  psychogenic F45.8
Hypercholesterinemia —*see*
  Hypercholesterolemia
Hypercholesterolemia (essential) (familial)
  (hereditary) (primary) (pure) E78.0
  with hyperglyceridemia, endogenous E78.2
  dietary counseling and surveillance Z71.3
Hyperchylia gastrica, psychogenic F45.8
Hyperchylomicronemia (familial) (primary)
  E78.3
  with hyperbetalipoproteinemia E78.3
Hypercoagulable (state) D68.59
  activated protein C resistance D68.51
  antithrombin (III) deficiency D68.59
  factor V Leiden mutation D68.51
  primary NEC D68.59
  protein C deficiency D68.59
  protein S deficiency D68.59
  prothrombin gene mutation D68.52

Hypercoagulable (*Continued*)
  secondary D68.69
  specified NEC D68.69
Hypercoagulation (state) D68.59
Hypercorticalism, pituitary-dependent E24.0
Hypercorticosolism —*see* Cushing's syndrome
Hypercorticosteronism E24.2
  correct substance properly administered —*see*
    Table of Drugs and Chemicals, by drug,
    adverse effect
  overdose or wrong substance given or
    taken —*see* Table of Drugs and
    Chemicals, by drug, poisoning
Hypercortisonism E24.2
  correct substance properly administered —*see*
    Table of Drugs and Chemicals, by drug,
    adverse effect
  overdose or wrong substance given or
    taken —*see* Table of Drugs and
    Chemicals, by drug, poisoning
Hyperekplexia Q89.8
Hyperelectrolytemia E87.8
Hyperemesis R11.10
  with nausea R11.2
  gravidarum (mild) O21.0
    with
      carbohydrate depletion O21.1
      dehydration O21.1
      electrolyte imbalance O21.1
      metabolic disturbance O21.1
    severe (with metabolic disturbance) O21.1
  projectile R11.12
  psychogenic F45.8
Hyperemia (acute) (passive) R68.89
  anal mucosa K62.89
  bladder N32.89
  cerebral I67.89
  conjunctiva H11.43-
  ear internal, acute —*see* subcategory
    H83.0
  enteric K59.8
  eye —*see* Hyperemia, conjunctiva
  eyelid (active) (passive) —*see* Disorder,
    eyelid, specified type NEC
  intestine K59.8
  iris —*see* Disorder, iris, vascular
  kidney N28.89
  labyrinth —*see* subcategory H83.0
  liver (active) K76.89
  lung (passive) —*see* Edema, lung
  pulmonary (passive) —*see* Edema, lung
  renal N28.89
  retina H35.89
  stomach K31.89
Hyperesthesia (body surface) R20.3
  larynx (reflex) J38.7
    hysterical F44.89
  pharynx (reflex) J39.2
    hysterical F44.89
Hyperestrogenism (drug-induced) (iatrogenic)
  E28.0
Hyperexplexia Q89.8
Hyperfibrinolysis —*see* Fibrinolysis
Hyperfructosemia E74.19
Hyperfunction
  adrenal cortex, not associated with Cushing's
    syndrome E27.0
    medulla E27.5
      adrenomedullary E27.5
    virilism E25.9
      congenital E25.0
  ovarian E28.8
  pancreas K86.8
  parathyroid (gland) E21.3
  pituitary (gland) (anterior) E22.9
    specified NEC E22.8
  polyglandular E31.1
  testicular E29.0
Hypergammaglobulinemia D89.2
  polyclonal D89.0
  Waldenström D89.0

Hypergastrinemia E16.4
Hyperglobulinemia R77.1
Hyperglycemia, hyperglycemic (transient)
R73.9
coma —see Diabetes, by type, with coma
postpancreatectomy E89.1
Hyperglyceridemia (endogenous) (essential)
(familial) (hereditary) (pure) E78.1
mixed E78.3
Hyperglycinemia (non-ketotic) E72.51
Hypergonadism
ovarian E28.8
testicular (primary) (infantile) E29.0
Hyperheparinemia D68.32
Hyperhidrosis, hyperidrosis R61
focal
primary L74.519
axilla L74.510
face L74.511
palms L74.512
soles L74.513
secondary L74.52
generalized R61
localized
primary L74.519
axilla L74.510
face L74.511
palms L74.512
soles L74.513
secondary L74.52
psychogenic F45.8
secondary R61
focal L74.52
Hyperhistidinemia E70.41
Hyperhomocysteinemia E72.11
Hyperhydroxyprolinemia E72.59
Hyperinsulinism (functional) E16.1
with
coma (hypoglycemic) E15
encephalopathy E16.1 [G94]
ectopic E16.1
therapeutic misadventure (from
administration of insulin) —see
subcategory T38.3
Hyperkalemia E87.5
Hyperkeratosis (see also Keratosis) L85.9
cervix N88.0
due to yaws (early) (late) (palmar or plantar)
A66.3
follicularis Q82.8
penetrans (in cutem) L87.0
palmoplantaris climacterica L85.1
pinta A67.1
senile (with pruritus) L57.0
universalis congenita Q80.8
vocal cord J38.3
vulva N90.4
Hyperkinesia, hyperkinetic (disease) (reaction)
(syndrome) (childhood) (adolescence) —
see also Disorder, attention-deficit
hyperactivity
heart I51.89
Hyperleucine-isoleucinemia E71.19
Hyperlipemia, hyperlipidemia E78.5
combined E78.2
familial E78.4
group
A E78.0
B E78.1
C E78.2
D E78.3
mixed E78.2
specified NEC E78.4
Hyperlipidosis E75.6
hereditary NEC E75.5
Hyperlipoproteinemia E78.5
Fredrickson's type
I E78.3
IIa E78.0
IIb E78.2
III E78.2

Hyperlipoproteinemia (Continued)
Fredrickson's type (Continued)
IV E78.1
V E78.3
low-density-lipoprotein-type (LDL) E78.0
very-low-density-lipoprotein-type (VLDL)
E78.1
Hyperlucent lung, unilateral J43.0
Hyperlysinemia E72.3
Hypermagnesemia E83.41
neonatal P71.8
Hypermenorrhea N92.0
Hypermethioninemia E72.19
Hypermetropia (congenital) H52.0-
Hypermobility, hypermotility
cecum —see Syndrome, irritable bowel
coccyx —see subcategory M53.2
colon —see Syndrome, irritable bowel
psychogenic F45.8
ileum K58.9
intestine (see also Syndrome, irritable bowel)
K58.9
psychogenic F45.8
meniscus (knee) —see Derangement, knee,
meniscus
scapula —see Instability, joint, shoulder
stomach K31.89
psychogenic F45.8
syndrome M35.7
urethra N36.41
with intrinsic sphincter deficiency N36.43
Hypernasality R49.21
Hypernatremia E87.0
Hypernephroma C64.-
Hyperopia —see Hypermetropia
Hyperorexia nervosa F50.2
Hyperornithinemia E72.4
Hyperosmia R43.1
Hyperosmolality E87.0
Hyperostosis (monomelic) —see also Disorder,
bone, density and structure, specified NEC
ankylosing (spine) M48.10
cervical region M48.12
cervicothoracic region M48.13
lumbar region M48.16
lumbosacral region M48.17
multiple sites M48.19
occipito-atlanto-axial region M48.11
sacrococcygeal region M48.18
thoracic region M48.14
thoracolumbar region M48.15
cortical (skull) M85.2
infantile M89.8X-
frontal, internal of skull M85.2
interna frontalis M85.2
skeletal, diffuse idiopathic —see
Hyperostosis, ankylosing
skull M85.2
congenital Q75.8
vertebral, ankylosing —see Hyperostosis,
ankylosing
Hyperovarism E28.8
Hyperoxaluria (primary) E72.53
Hyperparathyroidism E21.3
primary E21.0
secondary (renal) N25.81
non-renal E21.1
specified NEC E21.2
tertiary E21.2
Hyperpathia R20.8
Hyperperistalsis R19.2
psychogenic F45.8
Hyperpermeability, capillary I78.8
Hyperphagia R63.2
Hyperphenylalaninemia NEC E70.1
Hyperphoria (alternating) H50.53
Hyperphosphatemia E83.39
Hyperpiesis, hyperpiesia —see Hypertension
Hyperpigmentation —see also Pigmentation
melanin NEC L81.4
postinflammatory L81.0

Hyperpinealism E34.8
Hyperpituitarism E22.9
Hyperplasia, hyperplastic
adenoids J35.2
adrenal (capsule) (cortex) (gland) E27.8
with
sexual precocity (male) E25.9
congenital E25.0
virilism, adrenal E25.9
congenital E25.0
virilization (female) E25.9
congenital E25.0
congenital E25.0
salt-losing E25.0
adrenomedullary E27.5
angiolymphoid, eosinophilia (ALHE) D18.01
appendix (lymphoid) K38.0
artery, fibromuscular I77.3
bone —see also Hypertrophy, bone
marrow D75.89
breast —see also Hypertrophy, breast
ductal (atypical) N60.9-
C-cell, thyroid E07.0
cementation (tooth) (teeth) K03.4
cervical gland R59.0
cervix (uteri) (basal cell) (endometrium)
(polypoid) —see also Dysplasia, cervix
congenital Q51.828
clitoris, congenital Q52.6
denture K06.2
endocervicitis N72
endometrium, endometrial (adenomatous)
(benign) (cystic) (glandular) (glandular-
cystic) (polypoid) N85.00
with atypia N85.02
cervix —see Dysplasia, cervix
complex (without atypia) N85.01
simple (without atypia) N85.01
epithelial L85.9
focal, oral, including tongue K13.29
nipple N62
skin L85.9
tongue K13.29
vaginal wall N89.3
erythroid D75.89
fibromuscular of artery (carotid) (renal) I77.3
genital
female NEC N94.89
male N50.8
gingiva K06.1
glandularis cystica uteri (interstitialis) (see also
Hyperplasia, endometrial) N85.00-
gum K06.1
hymen, congenital Q52.4
irritative, edentulous (alveolar) K06.2
jaw M26.09
alveolar M26.79
lower M26.03
alveolar M26.72
upper M26.01
alveolar M26.71
kidney (congenital) Q63.3
labia N90.6
epithelial N90.3
liver (congenital) Q44.7
nodular, focal K76.89
lymph gland or node R59.9
mandible, mandibular M26.03
alveolar M26.72
unilateral condylar M27.8
maxilla, maxillary M26.01
alveolar M26.71
myometrium, myometrial N85.2
neuroendocrine cell, of infancy J84.841
nose
lymphoid J34.89
polypoid J33.9
oral mucosa (irritative) K13.6
organ or site, congenital NEC —see Anomaly,
by site
ovary N83.8

◀ New ◀≣ Revised ~~deleted~~ Deleted

Hyperplasia, hyperplastic (*Continued*)
palate, papillary (irritative) K13.6
pancreatic islet cells E16.9
alpha E16.8
with excess
gastrin E16.4
glucagon E16.3
beta E16.1
parathyroid (gland) E21.0
pharynx (lymphoid) J39.2
prostate (adenofibromatous) (nodular)
N40.0
with lower urinary tract symptoms (LUTS)
N40.1
without lower urinary tract symptoms
(LUTS) N40.0
renal artery I77.89
reticulo-endothelial (cell) D75.89
salivary gland (any) K11.1
Schimmelbusch's —*see* Mastopathy,
cystic
suprarenal capsule (gland) E27.8
thymus (gland) (persistent) E32.0
thyroid (gland) —*see* Goiter
tonsils (faucial) (infective) (lingual)
(lymphoid) J35.1
with adenoids J35.3
unilateral condylar M27.8
uterus, uterine N85.2
endometrium (glandular) (*see also*
Hyperplasia, endometrial)
N85.00-
vulva N90.6
epithelial N90.3
Hyperpnea —*see* Hyperventilation
Hyperpotassemia E87.5
Hyperprebetalipoproteinemia (familial)
E78.1
Hyperprolactinemia E22.1
Hyperprolinemia (type I) (type II) E72.59
Hyperproteinemia E88.09
**Hyperprothrombinemia, causing coagulation
factor deficiency** D68.4
Hyperpyrexia R50.9
heat (effects) T67.0
malignant, due to anesthetic T88.3
rheumatic —*see* Fever, rheumatic
unknown origin R50.9
Hyper-reflexia R29.2
Hypersalivation K11.7
Hypersecretion
ACTH (not associated with Cushing's
syndrome) E27.0
pituitary E24.0
adrenaline E27.5
adrenomedullary E27.5
androgen (testicular) E29.0
ovarian (drug-induced) (iatrogenic)
E28.1
calcitonin E07.0
catecholamine E27.5
corticoadrenal E24.9
cortisol E24.9
epinephrine E27.5
estrogen E28.0
gastric K31.89
psychogenic F45.8
gastrin E16.4
glucagon E16.3
hormone (s)
ACTH (not associated with Cushing's
syndrome) E27.0
pituitary E24.0
antidiuretic E22.2
growth E22.0
intestinal NEC E34.1
ovarian androgen E28.1
pituitary E22.9
testicular E29.0
thyroid stimulating E05.80
with thyroid storm E05.81

Hypersecretion (*Continued*)
insulin —*see* Hyperinsulinism
lacrimal glands —*see* Epiphora
medulloadrenal E27.5
milk O92.6
ovarian androgens E28.1
salivary gland (any) K11.7
thyrocalcitonin E07.0
upper respiratory J39.8
Hypersegmentation, leukocytic, hereditary
D72.0
**Hypersensitive, hypersensitiveness,
hypersensitivity** —*see also* Allergy
carotid sinus G90.01
colon —*see* Irritable, colon
drug T88.7
gastrointestinal K52.2
psychogenic F45.8
labyrinth —*see* subcategory H83.2
pain R20.8
pneumonitis —*see* Pneumonitis,
allergic
reaction T78.40
upper respiratory tract NEC J39.3
Hypersomnia (organic) G47.10
due to
alcohol
abuse F10.182
dependence F10.282
use F10.982
amphetamines
abuse F15.182
dependence F15.282
use F15.982
caffeine
abuse F15.182
dependence F15.282
use F15.982
cocaine
abuse F14.182
dependence F14.282
use F14.982
drug NEC
abuse F19.182
dependence F19.282
use F19.982
medical condition G47.14
mental disorder F51.13
opioid
abuse F11.182
dependence F11.282
use F11.982
psychoactive substance NEC
abuse F19.182
dependence F19.282
use F19.982
sedative, hypnotic, or anxiolytic
abuse F13.182
dependence F13.282
use F13.982
stimulant NEC
abuse F15.182
dependence F15.282
use F15.982
idiopathic G47.11
with long sleep time G47.11
without long sleep time G47.12
menstrual related G47.13
nonorganic origin F51.11
specified NEC F51.19
not due to a substance or known
physiological condition F51.11
specified NEC F51.19
primary F51.11
recurrent G47.13
specified NEC G47.19
Hypersplenia, hypersplenism D73.1
Hyperstimulation, ovaries (associated with
induced ovulation) N98.1
Hypersusceptibility —*see* Allergy
Hypertelorism (ocular) (orbital) Q75.2

Hypertension, hypertensive (accelerated)
(benign) (essential) (idiopathic)
(malignant) (systemic) I10
with
heart involvement (conditions in
I51.4-I51.9 due to hypertension) —*see*
Hypertension, heart
kidney involvement —*see* Hypertension,
kidney
benign, intracranial G93.2
borderline R03.0
cardiorenal (disease) I13.10
with heart failure I13.0
with stage 1 through stage 4 chronic
kidney disease I13.0
with stage 5 or end stage renal disease
I13.2
without heart failure I13.10
with stage 1 through stage 4 chronic
kidney disease I13.10
with stage 5 or end stage renal disease
I13.11
cardiovascular
disease (arteriosclerotic) (sclerotic) —*see*
Hypertension, heart
renal (disease) —*see* Hypertension,
cardiorenal
chronic venous —*see* Hypertension, venous
(chronic)
complicating
childbirth (labor) O10.92
with
heart disease O10.12
with renal disease O10.32
renal disease O10.22
with heart disease O10.32
essential O10.02
secondary O10.42
pregnancy O16.-
with edema (*see also* Pre-eclampsia) O14.9-
gestational (pregnancy induced)
(transient) (without proteinuria)
O13.-
with proteinuria O14.9-
mild pre-eclampsia O14.0-
moderate pre-eclampsia O14.0-
severe pre-eclampsia O14.1-
with hemolysis, elevated liver
enzymes and low platelet
count (HELLP) O14.2-
pre-existing O10.91-
with
heart disease O10.11-
with renal disease O10.31-
pre-eclampsia O11.-
renal disease O10.21-
with heart disease O10.31-
essential O10.01-
secondary O10.41-
puerperium pre-existing O10.93
with
heart disease O10.13
with renal disease O10.33
renal disease O10.23
with heart disease O10.33
essential O10.03
pregnancy-induced O13.9
secondary O10.43
due to
endocrine disorders I15.2
pheochromocytoma I15.2
renal disorders NEC I15.1
arterial I15.0
renovascular disorders I15.0
specified disease NEC I15.8
encephalopathy I67.4
gestational (without significant proteinuria)
(pregnancy-induced) (transient) O13.-
with significant proteinuria —*see*
Pre-eclampsia
Goldblatt's I70.1

◀ New   ⬅ Revised   ~~deleted~~ Deleted

Hypertrophy, hypertrophic (*Continued*)
metatarsus —*see* Hypertrophy, bone,
    metatarsus
mucous membrane
    alveolar ridge K06.2
      gum K06.1
    nose (turbinate) J34.3
muscle M62.89
muscular coat, artery I77.89
myocardium —*see also* Hypertrophy, cardiac
    idiopathic I42.2
myometrium N85.2
nail L60.2
    congenital Q84.5
nasal J34.89
    alae J34.89
    bone J34.89
    cartilage J34.89
    mucous membrane (septum) J34.3
    sinus J34.89
    turbinate J34.3
nasopharynx, lymphoid (infectional) (tissue)
    (wall) J35.2
nipple N62
organ or site, congenital NEC —*see* Anomaly,
    by site - ovary N83.8
palate (hard) M27.8
    soft K13.79
pancreas, congenital Q45.3
parathyroid (gland) E21.0
parotid gland K11.1
penis N48.89
pharyngeal tonsil J35.2
pharynx J39.2
    lymphoid (infectional) (tissue) (wall)
      J35.2
pituitary (anterior) (fossa) (gland) E23.6
prepuce (congenital) N47.8
    female N90.89
prostate —*see* Enlargement, enlarged,
    prostate
    congenital Q55.4
pseudomuscular G71.0
pylorus (adult) (muscle) (sphincter) K31.1
    congenital or infantile Q40.0
rectal, rectum (sphincter) K62.89
rhinitis (turbinate) J31.0
salivary gland (any) K11.1
    congenital Q38.4
scaphoid (tarsal) —*see* Hypertrophy, bone,
    tarsus
scar L91.0
scrotum N50.8
seminal vesicle N50.8
sigmoid —*see* Megacolon
skin L91.9
    specified NEC L91.8
spermatic cord N50.8
spleen —*see* Splenomegaly
spondylitis —*see* Spondylosis
stomach K31.89
sublingual gland K11.1
submandibular gland K11.1
suprarenal cortex (gland) E27.8
synovial NEC M67.20
    acromioclavicular M67.21-
    ankle M67.27-
    elbow M67.22-
    foot M67.27-
    hand M67.24-
    hip M67.25-
    knee M67.26-
    multiple sites M67.29
    specified site NEC M67.28
    wrist M67.23-
tendon —*see* Disorder, tendon, specified type
    NEC
testis N44.8
    congenital Q55.29
thymic, thymus (gland) (congenital)
    E32.0

Hypertrophy, hypertrophic (*Continued*)
thyroid (gland) —*see* Goiter
toe (congenital) Q74.2
    acquired —*see also* Deformity, toe, specified
      NEC
tongue K14.8
    congenital Q38.2
    papillae (foliate) K14.3
tonsils (faucial) (infective) (lingual)
    (lymphoid) J35.1
    with adenoids J35.3
tunica vaginalis N50.8
ureter N28.89
urethra N36.8
uterus N85.2
    neck (with elongation) N88.4
    puerperal O90.89
uvula K13.79
vagina N89.8
vas deferens N50.8
vein I87.8
ventricle, ventricular (heart) —*see also*
    Hypertrophy, cardiac
    congenital Q24.8
    in tetralogy of Fallot Q21.3
verumontanum N36.8
vocal cord J38.3
vulva N90.6
    stasis (nonfilarial) N90.6
Hypertropia H50.2-
Hypertyrosinemia E70.21
Hyperuricemia (asymptomatic) E79.0
Hypervalinemia E71.19
Hyperventilation (tetany) R06.4
hysterical F45.8
psychogenic F45.8
syndrome F45.8
Hypervitaminosis (dietary) NEC E67.8
A E67.0
    administered as drug (prolonged intake) —
      see Table of Drugs and Chemicals,
      vitamins, adverse effect
    overdose or wrong substance given or
      taken —*see* Table of Drugs and
      Chemicals, vitamins, poisoning
B6 E67.2
D E67.3
    administered as drug (prolonged intake) —
      see Table of Drugs and Chemicals,
      vitamins, adverse effect
    overdose or wrong substance given or
      taken —*see* Table of Drugs and
      Chemicals, vitamins, poisoning
K E67.8
    administered as drug (prolonged intake) —
      see Table of Drugs and Chemicals,
      vitamins, adverse effect
    overdose or wrong substance given or
      taken —*see* Table of Drugs and
      Chemicals, vitamins, poisoning
Hypervolemia E87.70
specified NEC E87.79
Hypesthesia R20.1
cornea —*see* Anesthesia, cornea
Hyphema H21.0-
traumatic S05.1-
Hypoacidity, gastric K31.89
psychogenic F45.8
Hypoadrenalism, hypoadrenia E27.40
primary E27.1
tuberculous A18.7
Hypoadrenocorticism E27.40
pituitary E23.0
primary E27.1
Hypoalbuminemia E88.09
Hypoaldosteronism E27.40
Hypoalphalipoproteinemia E78.6
Hypobarism T70.29
Hypobaropathy T70.29
Hypobetalipoproteinemia (familial)
    E78.6

Hypocalcemia E83.51
dietary E58
neonatal P71.1
    due to cow's milk P71.0
    phosphate-loading (newborn) P71.1
Hypochloremia E87.8
Hypochlorhydria K31.89
neurotic F45.8
psychogenic F45.8
Hypochondria, hypochondriac,
    hypochondriasis (reaction) F45.21
sleep F51.03
Hypochondrogenesis Q77.0
Hypochondroplasia Q77.4
Hypochromasia, blood cells D50.8
Hypodontia —*see* Anodontia
Hypoeosinophilia D72.89
Hypoesthesia R20.1
Hypofibrinogenemia D68.8
acquired D65
congenital (hereditary) D68.2
Hypofunction
adrenocortical E27.40
    drug-induced E27.3
    postprocedural E89.6
    primary E27.1
adrenomedullary, postprocedural E89.6
cerebral R29.818
corticoadrenal NEC E27.40
intestinal K59.8
labyrinth —*see* subcategory H83.2
ovary E28.39
pituitary (gland) (anterior) E23.0
testicular E29.1
    postprocedural (postsurgical)
      (postirradiation) (iatrogenic) E89.5
Hypogalactia O92.4
Hypogammaglobulinemia (*see also*
    Agammaglobulinemia) D80.1
hereditary D80.0
nonfamilial D80.1
transient, of infancy D80.7
Hypogenitalism (congenital) —*see*
    Hypogonadism
Hypoglossia Q38.3
Hypoglycemia (spontaneous) E16.2
coma E15
    diabetic —*see* Diabetes, coma
diabetic —*see* Diabetes, hypoglycemia
dietary counseling and surveillance Z71.3
drug-induced E16.0
    with coma (nondiabetic) E15
due to insulin E16.0
    with coma (nondiabetic) E15
    therapeutic misadventure —*see*
      subcategory T38.3
functional, nonhyperinsulinemic E16.1
iatrogenic E16.0
    with coma (nondiabetic) E15
in infant of diabetic mother P70.1
    gestational diabetes P70.0
infantile E16.1
leucine-induced E71.19
neonatal (transitory) P70.4
    iatrogenic P70.3
reactive (not drug-induced) E16.1
transitory neonatal P70.4
Hypogonadism
female E28.39
hypogonadotropic E23.0
male E29.1
ovarian (primary) E28.39
pituitary E23.0
testicular (primary) E29.1
Hypohidrosis, hypoidrosis L74.4
Hypoinsulinemia, postprocedural E89.1
Hypokalemia E87.6
Hypoleukocytosis —*see* Agranulocytosis
Hypolipoproteinemia (alpha) (beta) E78.6
Hypomagnesemia E83.42
neonatal P71.2

Hypomania, hypomanic reaction F30.8
Hypomenorrhea —*see* Oligomenorrhea
Hypometabolism R63.8
Hypomotility
  gastrointestinal (tract) K31.89
    psychogenic F45.8
  intestine K59.8
    psychogenic F45.8
  stomach K31.89
    psychogenic F45.8
Hyponasality R49.22
Hyponatremia E87.1
Hypo-osmolality E87.1
Hypo-ovarianism, hypo-ovarism E28.39
Hypoparathyroidism E20.9
  familial E20.8
  idiopathic E20.0
  neonatal, transitory P71.4
  postprocedural E89.2
  specified NEC E20.8
Hypoperfusion (in)
  newborn P96.89
Hypopharyngitis —*see* Laryngopharyngitis
Hypophoria H50.53
Hypophosphatemia, hypophosphatasia
    (acquired) (congenital) (renal) E83.39
  familial E83.31
Hypophyseal, hypophysis —*see also* condition
  dwarfism E23.0
  gigantism E22.0
Hypopiesis —*see* Hypotension
Hypopinealism E34.8
Hypopituitarism (juvenile) E23.0
  drug-induced E23.1
  due to
    hypophysectomy E89.3
    radiotherapy E89.3
  iatrogenic NEC E23.1
  postirradiation E89.3
  postpartum E23.0
  postprocedural E89.3
Hypoplasia, hypoplastic
  adrenal (gland), congenital Q89.1
  alimentary tract, congenital Q45.8
    upper Q40.8
  anus, anal (canal) Q42.3
    with fistula Q42.2
  aorta, aortic Q25.4
    ascending, in hypoplastic left heart
      syndrome Q23.4
    valve Q23.1
      in hypoplastic left heart syndrome
        Q23.4
  areola, congenital Q83.8
  arm (congenital) —*see* Defect, reduction,
    upper limb
  artery (peripheral) Q27.8
    brain (congenital) Q28.3
    coronary Q24.5
    digestive system Q27.8
    lower limb Q27.8
    pulmonary Q25.79
      functional, unilateral J43.0
    retinal (congenital) Q14.1
    specified site NEC Q27.8
    umbilical Q27.0
    upper limb Q27.8
  auditory canal Q17.8
    causing impairment of hearing Q16.9
  biliary duct or passage Q44.5
  bone NOS Q79.9
    face Q75.8
    marrow D61.9
      megakaryocytic D69.49
    skull —*see* Hypoplasia, skull
  brain Q02
    gyri Q04.3
    part of Q04.3
  breast (areola) N64.82
  bronchus Q32.4
  cardiac Q24.8

Hypoplasia, hypoplastic (*Continued*)
  carpus —*see* Defect, reduction, upper limb,
    specified type NEC
  cartilage hair Q78.5
  cecum Q42.8
  cementum K00.4
  cephalic Q02
  cerebellum Q04.3
  cervix (uteri), congenital Q51.821
  clavicle (congenital) Q74.0
  coccyx Q76.49
  colon Q42.9
    specified NEC Q42.8
  corpus callosum Q04.0
  cricoid cartilage Q31.2
  digestive organ (s) or tract NEC Q45.8
    upper (congenital) Q40.8
  ear (auricle) (lobe) Q17.2
    middle Q16.4
  enamel of teeth (neonatal) (postnatal)
    (prenatal) K00.4
  endocrine (gland) NEC Q89.2
  endometrium N85.8
  epididymis (congenital) Q55.4
  epiglottis Q31.2
  erythroid, congenital D61.01
  esophagus (congenital) Q39.8
  eustachian tube Q17.8
  eye Q11.2
  eyelid (congenital) Q10.3
  face Q18.8
    bone (s) Q75.8
  femur (congenital) —*see* Defect,
    reduction, lower limb, specified
    type NEC
  fibula (congenital) —*see* Defect,
    reduction, lower limb, specified
    type NEC
  finger (congenital) —*see* Defect,
    reduction, upper limb, specified
    type NEC
  focal dermal Q82.8
  foot —*see* Defect, reduction, lower limb,
    specified type NEC
  gallbladder Q44.0
  genitalia, genital organ (s)
    female, congenital Q52.8
      external Q52.79
      internal NEC Q52.8
    in adiposogenital dystrophy E23.6
  glottis Q31.2
  hair Q84.2
  hand (congenital) —*see* Defect, reduction,
    upper limb, specified type NEC
  heart Q24.8
  humerus (congenital) —*see* Defect,
    reduction, upper limb, specified
    type NEC
  intestine (small) Q41.9
    large Q42.9
      specified NEC Q42.8
  jaw M26.09
    alveolar M26.79
    lower M26.04
      alveolar M26.74
    upper M26.02
      alveolar M26.73
  kidney (s) Q60.5
    bilateral Q60.4
    unilateral Q60.3
  labium (majus) (minus), congenital Q52.79
  larynx Q31.2
  left heart syndrome Q23.4
  leg (congenital) —*see* Defect, reduction, lower
    limb
  limb Q73.8
    lower (congenital) —*see* Defect, reduction,
      lower limb
    upper (congenital) —*see* Defect, reduction,
      upper limb
  liver Q44.7

Hypoplasia, hypoplastic (*Continued*)
  lung (lobe) (not associated with short
    gestation) Q33.6
    associated with immaturity, low birth
      weight, prematurity, or short
      gestation P28.0
  mammary (areola), congenital Q83.8
  mandible, mandibular M26.04
    alveolar M26.74
    unilateral condylar M27.8
    maxillary M26.02
      alveolar M26.73
  medullary D61.9
  megakaryocytic D69.49
  metacarpus —*see* Defect, reduction, upper
    limb, specified type NEC
  metatarsus —*see* Defect, reduction, lower
    limb, specified type NEC
  muscle Q79.8
  nail (s) Q84.6
  nose, nasal Q30.1
  optic nerve H47.03-
  osseous meatus (ear) Q17.8
  ovary, congenital Q50.39
  pancreas Q45.0
  parathyroid (gland) Q89.2
  parotid gland Q38.4
  patella Q74.1
  pelvis, pelvic girdle Q74.2
  penis (congenital) Q55.62
  peripheral vascular system Q27.8
    digestive system Q27.8
    lower limb Q27.8
    specified site NEC Q27.8
    upper limb Q27.8
  pituitary (gland) (congenital) Q89.2
  pulmonary (not associated with short
    gestation) Q33.6
    artery, functional J43.0
    associated with short gestation P28.0
  radioulnar —*see* Defect, reduction, upper
    limb, specified type NEC
  radius —*see* Defect, reduction, upper limb
  rectum Q42.1
    with fistula Q42.0
  respiratory system NEC Q34.8
  rib Q76.6
  right heart syndrome Q22.6
  sacrum Q76.49
  scapula Q74.0
  scrotum Q55.1
  shoulder girdle Q74.0
  skin Q82.8
  skull (bone) Q75.8
    with
      anencephaly Q00.0
      encephalocele —*see* Encephalocele
      hydrocephalus Q03.9
        with spina bifida —*see* Spina bifida, by
          site, with hydrocephalus
      microcephaly Q02
  spinal (cord) (ventral horn cell) Q06.1
  spine Q76.49
  sternum Q76.7
  tarsus —*see* Defect, reduction, lower limb,
    specified type NEC
  testis Q55.1
  thymic, with immunodeficiency D82.1
  thymus (gland) Q89.2
    with immunodeficiency D82.1
  thyroid (gland) E03.1
    cartilage Q31.2
  tibiofibular (congenital) —*see* Defect,
    reduction, lower limb, specified type
    NEC
  toe —*see* Defect, reduction, lower limb,
    specified type NEC
  tongue Q38.3
  Turner's K00.4
  ulna (congenital) —*see* Defect, reduction,
    upper limb

◀ New   ◀ Revised   ~~deleted~~ Deleted

Hypoplasia, hypoplastic (*Continued*)
umbilical artery Q27.0
unilateral condylar M27.8
ureter Q62.8
uterus, congenital Q51.811
vagina Q52.4
vascular NEC peripheral Q27.8
brain Q28.3
digestive system Q27.8
lower limb Q27.8
specified site NEC Q27.8
upper limb Q27.8
vein (s) (peripheral) Q27.8
brain Q28.3
digestive system Q27.8
great Q26.8
lower limb Q27.8
specified site NEC Q27.8
upper limb Q27.8
vena cava (inferior) (superior) Q26.8
vertebra Q76.49
vulva, congenital Q52.79
zonule (ciliary) Q12.8
Hypopotassemia E87.6
Hypoproconvertinemia, congenital
(hereditary) D68.2
Hypoproteinemia E77.8
Hypoprothrombinemia (congenital)
(hereditary) (idiopathic) D68.2
acquired D68.4
newborn, transient P61.6
Hypoptyalism K11.7
Hypopyon (eye) (anterior chamber) —*see*
Iridocyclitis, acute, hypopyon
Hypopyrexia R68.0
Hyporeflexia R29.2
Hyposecretion
ACTH E23.0
antidiuretic hormone E23.2
ovary E28.39
salivary gland (any) K11.7
vasopressin E23.2
Hyposegmentation, leukocytic, hereditary
D72.0
Hyposiderinemia D50.9
Hypospadias Q54.9
balanic Q54.0
coronal Q54.0
glandular Q54.0
penile Q54.1
penoscrotal Q54.2

Hypospadias (*Continued*)
perineal Q54.3
specified NEC Q54.8
Hypospermatogenesis —*see* Oligospermia
Hyposplenism D73.0
Hypostasis pulmonary, passive —*see* Edema,
lung
Hypostatic —*see* condition
Hyposthenuria N28.89
Hypotension (arterial) (constitutional) I95.9
chronic I95.89
drug-induced I95.2
due to (of) hemodialysis I95.3
iatrogenic I95.89
idiopathic (permanent) I95.0
intracranial, following ventricular shunting
(ventriculostomy) G97.2
intra-dialytic I95.3
maternal, syndrome (following labor and
delivery) O26.5-
neurogenic, orthostatic G90.3
orthostatic (chronic) I95.1
due to drugs I95.2
neurogenic G90.3
postoperative I95.81
postural I95.1
specified NEC I95.89
Hypothermia (accidental) T68
due to anesthesia, anesthetic T88.51
low environmental temperature T68
neonatal P80.9
environmental (mild) NEC P80.8
mild P80.8
severe (chronic) (cold injury syndrome)
P80.0
specified NEC P80.8
not associated with low environmental
temperature R68.0
Hypothyroidism (acquired) E03.9
congenital (without goiter) E03.1
with goiter (diffuse) E03.0
due to
exogenous substance NEC E03.2
iodine-deficiency, acquired E01.8
subclinical E02
irradiation therapy E89.0
medicament NEC E03.2
P-aminosalicylic acid (PAS) E03.2
phenylbutazone E03.2
resorcinol E03.2
sulfonamide E03.2

Hypothyroidism (*Continued*)
due to (*Continued*)
surgery E89.0
thiourea group drugs E03.2
iatrogenic NEC E03.2
iodine-deficiency (acquired) E01.8
congenital —*see* Syndrome, iodine-
deficiency, congenital
subclinical E02
neonatal, transitory P72.2
postinfectious E03.3
postirradiation E89.0
postprocedural E89.0
postsurgical E89.0
specified NEC E03.8
subclinical, iodine-deficiency related E02
Hypotonia, hypotonicity, hypotony
bladder N31.2
congenital (benign) P94.2
eye —*see* Disorder, globe, hypotony
Hypotrichosis —*see* Alopecia
Hypotropia H50.2-
Hypoventilation R06.89
congenital central alveolar G47.35
sleep related
idiopathic nonobstructive alveolar G47.34
in conditions classified elsewhere G47.36
Hypovitaminosis —*see* Deficiency, vitamin
Hypovolemia E86.1
surgical shock T81.19
traumatic (shock) T79.4
Hypoxemia R09.02
newborn P84
sleep related, in conditions classified
elsewhere G47.36
Hypoxia (*see also* Anoxia) R09.02
cerebral, during a procedure NEC G97.81
postprocedural NEC G97.82
intrauterine P84
myocardial —*see* Insufficiency, coronary
newborn P84
sleep-related G47.34
Hypsarhythmia —*see* Epilepsy, generalized,
specified NEC
Hysteralgia, pregnant uterus O26.89-
Hysteria, hysterical (conversion) (dissociative
state) F44.9
anxiety F41.8
convulsions F44.5
psychosis, acute F44.9
Hysteroepilepsy F44.5

I

Ichthyoparasitism due to Vandellia cirrhosa B88.8
Ichthyosis (congenital) Q80.9
  acquired L85.0
  fetalis Q80.4
  hystrix Q80.8
  lamellar Q80.2
  lingual K13.29
  palmaris and plantaris Q82.8
  simplex Q80.0
  vera Q80.8
  vulgaris Q80.0
  X-linked Q80.1
Ichthyotoxism —*see* Poisoning, fish
  bacterial —*see* Intoxication, foodborne
Icteroanemia, hemolytic (acquired) D59.9
  congenital —*see* Spherocytosis
Icterus —*see also* Jaundice
  conjunctiva R17
  gravis, newborn P55.0
  hematogenous (acquired) D59.9
  hemolytic (acquired) D59.9
    congenital —*see* Spherocytosis
  hemorrhagic (acute) (leptospiral)
      (spirochetal) A27.0
    newborn P53
  infectious B15.9
    with hepatic coma B15.0
    leptospiral A27.0
    spirochetal A27.0
  neonatorum —*see* Jaundice, newborn
  newborn P59.9
  spirochetal A27.0
Ictus solaris, solis T67.0
Ideation
  homicidal R45.850
  suicidal R45.851
Identity disorder (child) F64.9
  gender role F64.2
  psychosexual F64.2
Idioglossia F80.0
Idiopathic —*see* condition
Idiot, idiocy (congenital) F73
  amaurotic (Bielschowsky(-Jansky)) (family)
      (infantile (late)) (juvenile (late)) (Vogt-
      Spielmeyer) E75.4
  microcephalic Q02
Id reaction (due to bacteria) L30.2
IgE asthma J45.909
IIAC (idiopathic infantile arterial calcification)
    Q28.8
Ileitis (chronic) (noninfectious) (*see also*
    Enteritis) K52.9
  backwash —*see* Pancolitis, ulcerative
      (chronic)
  infectious A09
  regional (ulcerative) —*see* Enteritis, regional,
      small intestine
  segmental —*see* Enteritis, regional
  terminal (ulcerative) —*see* Enteritis, regional,
      small intestine
Ileocolitis (*see also* Enteritis) K52.9
  infectious A09
  regional —*see* Enteritis, regional
Ileostomy
  attention to Z43.2
  malfunctioning K94.13
  status Z93.2
    with complication —*see* Complications,
        enterostomy
Ileotyphus —*see* Typhoid
Ileum —*see* condition
Ileus (bowel) (colon) (inhibitory) (intestine)
    K56.7
  adynamic K56.0
  due to gallstone (in intestine) K56.3
  duodenal (chronic) K31.5
  gallstone K56.3
  mechanical NEC K56.69

Ileus (*Continued*)
  meconium P76.0
    in cystic fibrosis E84.11
    meaning meconium plug (without cystic
        fibrosis) P76.0
  myxedema K59.8
  neurogenic K56.0
    Hirschsprung's disease or megacolon
        Q43.1
  newborn
    due to meconium P76.0
      in cystic fibrosis E84.11
      meaning meconium plug (without cystic
          fibrosis) P76.0
    transitory P76.1
  obstructive K56.69
  paralytic K56.0
Iliac —*see* condition
Iliotibial band syndrome M76.3-
Illiteracy Z55.0
Illness (*see also* Disease) R69
  manic-depressive —*see* Disorder, bipolar
Imbalance R26.89
  autonomic G90.8
  constituents of food intake E63.1
  electrolyte E87.8
    with
      abortion —*see* Abortion by type,
          complicated by, electrolyte
          imbalance
      molar pregnancy O08.5
    due to hyperemesis gravidarum O21.1
    following ectopic or molar pregnancy
        O08.5
    neonatal, transitory NEC P74.4
      potassium P74.3
      sodium P74.2
  endocrine E34.9
  eye muscle NOS H50.9
  hormone E34.9
  hysterical F44.4
  labyrinth —*see* subcategory H83.2
  posture R29.3
  protein-energy —*see* Malnutrition
  sympathetic G90.8
Imbecile, imbecility (I.Q. 35-49) F71
Imbedding, intrauterine device T83.39
Imbibition, cholesterol (gallbladder) K82.4
Imbrication, teeth, fully erupted M26.30
Imerslund (-Gräsbeck) **syndrome** D51.1
Immature —*see also* Immaturity
  birth (less than 37 completed weeks) —*see*
      Preterm, newborn
    extremely (less than 28 completed
        weeks) —*see* Immaturity, extreme
  personality F60.89
Immaturity (less than 37 completed weeks) —
    see also Preterm, newborn
  extreme of newborn (less than 28 completed
      weeks of gestation) (less than
      196 completed days of gestation)
      (unspecified weeks of gestation) P07.20
    gestational age
      23 completed weeks (23 weeks, 0 days
          through 23 weeks, 6 days) P07.22
      24 completed weeks (24 weeks, 0 days
          through 24 weeks, 6 days) P07.23
      25 completed weeks (25 weeks, 0 days
          through 25 weeks, 6 days) P07.24
      26 completed weeks (26 weeks, 0 days
          through 26 weeks, 6 days) P07.25
      27 completed weeks (27 weeks, 0 days
          through 27 weeks, 6 days) P07.26
      less than 23 completed weeks P07.21
  fetus or infant light-for-dates —*see*
      Light-for-dates
  lung, newborn P28.0
  organ or site NEC —*see* Hypoplasia
  pulmonary, newborn P28.0
  reaction F60.89
  sexual (female) (male), after puberty E30.0

Immersion T75.1
  foot T69.02-
  hand T69.01-
Immobile, immobility
  complete, due to severe physical disability or
      frailty R53.2
  intestine K59.8
  syndrome (paraplegic) M62.3
Immune reconstitution (inflammatory)
    syndrome [IRIS] D89.3
Immunization —*see also* Vaccination
  ABO —*see* Incompatibility, ABO
    in newborn P55.1
  complication —*see* Complications,
      vaccination
  encounter for Z23
  not done (not carried out) Z28.9
    because (of)
      acute illness of patient Z28.01
      allergy to vaccine (or component) Z28.04
      caregiver refusal Z28.82
      chronic illness of patient Z28.02
      contraindication NEC Z28.09
      group pressure Z28.1
      guardian refusal Z28.82
      immune compromised state of patient
          Z28.03
      parent refusal Z28.82
      patient's belief Z28.1
      patient had disease being vaccinated
          against Z28.81
      patient refusal Z28.21
      religious beliefs of patient Z28.1
      specified reason NEC Z28.89
        of patient Z28.29
      unspecified patient reason Z28.20
  Rh factor
    affecting management of pregnancy NEC
        O36.09-
      anti-D antibody O36.01-
    from transfusion —*see* Complication (s),
        transfusion, incompatibility reaction,
        Rh (factor)
Immunocytoma C83.0-
Immunodeficiency D84.9
  with
    adenosine-deaminase deficiency D81.3
    antibody defects D80.9
      specified type NEC D80.8
    hyperimmunoglobulinemia D80.6
    increased immunoglobulin M (IgM) D80.5
    major defect D82.9
      specified type NEC D82.8
    partial albinism D82.8
    short-limbed stature D82.2
    thrombocytopenia and eczema D82.0
  antibody with
    hyperimmunoglobulinemia D80.6
    near-normal immunoglobulins D80.6
  autosomal recessive, Swiss type D80.0
  combined D81.9
    biotin-dependent carboxylase D81.819
      biotinidase D81.810
      holocarboxylase synthetase D81.818
      specified type NEC D81.818
    severe (SCID) D81.9
      with
        low or normal B-cell numbers D81.2
        low T- and B-cell numbers D81.1
        reticular dysgenesis D81.0
    specified type NEC D81.89
  common variable D83.9
    with
      abnormalities of B-cell numbers and
          function D83.0
      autoantibodies to B- or T-cells D83.2
      immunoregulatory T-cell disorders
          D83.1
    specified type NEC D83.8
  following hereditary defective response to
      Epstein-Barr virus (EBV) D82.3

◀ New   ◀┅ Revised   ~~deleted~~ Deleted

Immunodeficiency (Continued)
  selective, immunoglobulin
    A (IgA) D80.2
    G (IgG) (subclasses) D80.3
    M (IgM) D80.4
  severe combined (SCID) D81.9
  specified type NEC D84.8
  X-linked, with increased IgM D80.5
Immunotherapy (encounter for)
  antineoplastic Z51.12
Impaction, impacted
  bowel, colon, rectum (see also Impaction, fecal) K56.49
    by gallstone K56.3
  calculus —see Calculus
  cerumen (ear) (external) H61.2-
  cuspid — see Impaction, tooth
  dental (same or adjacent tooth) K01.1
  fecal, feces K56.41
  fracture —see Fracture, by site
  gallbladder —see Calculus, gallbladder
  gallstone (s) —see Calculus, gallbladder
    bile duct (common) (hepatic) —see Calculus, bile duct
    cystic duct —see Calculus, gallbladder
    in intestine, with obstruction (any part) K56.3
  intestine (calculous) NEC (see also Impaction, fecal) K56.49
    gallstone, with ileus K56.3
  intrauterine device (IUD) T83.39
  molar —see Impaction, tooth
  shoulder, causing obstructed labor O66.0
  tooth, teeth K01.1
  turbinate J34.89
Impaired, impairment (function)
  auditory discrimination —see Abnormal, auditory perception
  cognitive, mild, so stated G31.84
  dual sensory Z73.82
  fasting glucose R73.01
  glucose tolerance (oral) R73.02
  hearing —see Deafness
  heart —see Disease, heart
  kidney N28.9
    disorder resulting from N25.9
      specified NEC N25.89
  liver K72.90
    with coma K72.91
  mastication K08.8
  mild cognitive, so stated G31.84
  mobility
    ear ossicles —see Ankylosis, ear ossicles
    requiring care provider Z74.09
  myocardium, myocardial —see Insufficiency, myocardial
  rectal sphincter R19.8
  renal (acute) (chronic) N28.9
    disorder resulting from N25.9
      specified NEC N25.89
  vision NEC H54.7
    both eyes H54.3
Impediment, speech R47.9
  psychogenic (childhood) F98.8
  slurring R47.81
  specified NEC R47.89
Impending
  coronary syndrome I20.0
  delirium tremens F10.239
  myocardial infarction I20.0
Imperception auditory (acquired) —see also Deafness
  congenital H93.25
Imperfect
  aeration, lung (newborn) NEC —see Atelectasis
  closure (congenital)
    alimentary tract NEC Q45.8
      lower Q43.8
      upper Q40.8
    atrioventricular ostium Q21.2

Imperfect (Continued)
  closure (Continued)
    atrium (secundum) Q21.1
    branchial cleft or sinus Q18.0
    choroid Q14.3
    cricoid cartilage Q31.8
    cusps, heart valve NEC Q24.8
      pulmonary Q22.3
    ductus
      arteriosus Q25.0
      Botalli Q25.0
    ear drum (causing impairment of hearing) Q16.4
    esophagus with communication to bronchus or trachea Q39.1
    eyelid Q10.3
    foramen
      botalli Q21.1
      ovale Q21.1
    genitalia, genital organ (s) or system
      female Q52.8
        external Q52.79
        internal NEC Q52.8
      male Q55.8
    glottis Q31.8
    interatrial ostium or septum Q21.1
    interauricular ostium or septum Q21.1
    interventricular ostium or septum Q21.0
    larynx Q31.8
    lip —see Cleft, lip
    nasal septum Q30.3
    nose Q30.2
    omphalomesenteric duct Q43.0
    optic nerve entry Q14.2
    organ or site not listed —see Anomaly, by site
    ostium
      interatrial Q21.1
      interauricular Q21.1
      interventricular Q21.0
    palate —see Cleft, palate
    preauricular sinus Q18.1
    retina Q14.1
    roof of orbit Q75.8
    sclera Q13.5
    septum
      aorticopulmonary Q21.4
      atrial (secundum) Q21.1
      between aorta and pulmonary artery Q21.4
      heart Q21.9
      interatrial (secundum) Q21.1
      interauricular (secundum) Q21.1
      interventricular Q21.0
        in tetralogy of Fallot Q21.3
      nasal Q30.3
      ventricular Q21.0
        with pulmonary stenosis or atresia, dextraposition of aorta, and hypertrophy of right ventricle Q21.3
        in tetralogy of Fallot Q21.3
    skull Q75.0
      with
        anencephaly Q00.0
        encephalocele —see Encephalocele
        hydrocephalus Q03.9
          with spina bifida —see Spina bifida, by site, with hydrocephalus
        microcephaly Q02
    spine (with meningocele) —see Spina bifida
    trachea Q32.1
    tympanic membrane (causing impairment of hearing) Q16.4
    uterus Q51.818
    vitelline duct Q43.0
  erection —see Dysfunction, sexual, male, erectile
  fusion —see Imperfect, closure
  inflation, lung (newborn) —see Atelectasis

Imperfect (Continued)
  posture R29.3
  rotation, intestine Q43.3
  septum, ventricular Q21.0
Imperfectly descended testis —see Cryptorchid
Imperforate (congenital) —see also Atresia
  anus Q42.3
    with fistula Q42.2
  cervix (uteri) Q51.828
  esophagus Q39.0
    with tracheoesophageal fistula Q39.1
  hymen Q52.3
  jejunum Q41.1
  pharynx Q38.8
  rectum Q42.1
    with fistula Q42.0
  urethra Q64.39
  vagina Q52.4
Impervious (congenital) —see also Atresia
  anus Q42.3
    with fistula Q42.2
  bile duct Q44.2
  esophagus Q39.0
    with tracheoesophageal fistula Q39.1
  intestine (small) Q41.9
    large Q42.9
      specified NEC Q42.8
  rectum Q42.1
    with fistula Q42.0
  ureter —see Atresia, ureter
  urethra Q64.39
Impetiginization of dermatoses L01.1
Impetigo (any organism) (any site) (circinate) (contagiosa) (simplex) (vulgaris) L01.00
  Bockhart's L01.02
  bullous, bullosa L01.03
  external ear L01.00 [H62.40]
  follicularis L01.02
  furfuracea L30.5
  herpetiformis L40.1
    nonobstetrical L40.1
  neonatorum L01.03
  nonbullous L01.01
  specified type NEC L01.09
  ulcerative L01.09
Impingement (on teeth)
  soft tissue
    anterior M26.81
    posterior M26.82
Implant, endometrial N80.9
Implantation
  anomalous —see Anomaly, by site
    ureter Q62.63
  cyst
    external area or site (skin) NEC L72.0
    iris —see Cyst, iris, implantation
    vagina N89.8
    vulva N90.7
  dermoid (cyst) —see Implantation, cyst
Impotence (sexual) N52.9
  counseling Z70.1
  organic origin (see also Dysfunction, sexual, male, erectile) N52.9
  psychogenic F52.21
Impression, basilar Q75.8
Imprisonment, anxiety concerning Z65.1
Improper care (child) (newborn) —see Maltreatment
Improperly tied umbilical cord (causing hemorrhage) P51.8
Impulsiveness (impulsive) R45.87
Inability to swallow —see Aphagia
Inaccessible, inaccessibility
  health care NEC Z75.3
    due to
      waiting period Z75.2
        for admission to facility elsewhere Z75.1
    other helping agencies Z75.4
Inactive —see condition

Inadequate, inadequacy
aesthetics of dental restoration K08.56
biologic, constitutional, functional, or social F60.7
development
child R62.50
genitalia
after puberty NEC E30.0
congenital
female Q52.8
external Q52.79
internal Q52.8
male Q55.8
lungs Q33.6
associated with short gestation P28.0
organ or site not listed —see Anomaly, by site
diet (causing nutritional deficiency) E63.9
eating habits Z72.4
environment, household Z59.1
family support Z63.8
food (supply) NEC Z59.4
hunger effects T73.0
functional F60.7
household care, due to
family member
handicapped or ill Z74.2
on vacation Z75.5
temporarily away from home Z74.2
technical defects in home Z59.1
temporary absence from home of person rendering care Z74.2
housing (heating) (space) Z59.1
income (financial) Z59.6
intrafamilial communication Z63.8
material resources Z59.9
mental —see Disability, intellectual
parental supervision or control of child Z62.0
personality F60.7
pulmonary
function R06.89
newborn P28.5
ventilation, newborn P28.5
sample of cytologic smear
anus R85.615
cervix R87.615
vagina R87.625
social F60.7
insurance Z59.7
skills NEC Z73.4
supervision of child by parent Z62.0
teaching affecting education Z55.8
welfare support Z59.7
Inanition R64
with edema —see Malnutrition, severe
due to
deprivation of food T73.0
malnutrition —see Malnutrition
fever R50.9
Inappropriate
change in quantitative human chorionic gonadotropin (hCG) in early pregnancy O02.81
diet or eating habits Z72.4
level of quantitative human chorionic gonadotropin (hCG) for gestational age in early pregnancy O02.81
secretion
antidiuretic hormone (ADH) (excessive) E22.2
deficiency E23.2
pituitary (posterior) E22.2
Inattention at or after birth —see Neglect
Incarceration, incarcerated
enterocele K46.0
gangrenous K46.1
epiplocele K46.0
gangrenous K46.1
exophthalmos K42.0
gangrenous K42.1

Incarceration, incarcerated (Continued)
hernia —see also Hernia, by site, with obstruction
with gangrene —see Hernia, by site, with gangrene
iris, in wound —see Injury, eye, laceration, with prolapse
lens, in wound —see Injury, eye, laceration, with prolapse
omphalocele K42.0
prison, anxiety concerning Z65.1
rupture —see Hernia, by site
sarcoepiplocele K46.0
gangrenous K46.1
sarcoepiplomphalocele K42.0
with gangrene K42.1
uterus N85.8
gravid O34.51-
causing obstructed labor O65.5
Incised wound
external —see Laceration
internal organs —see Injury, by site
Incision, incisional
hernia K43.2
with
gangrene (and obstruction) K43.1
obstruction K43.0
surgical, complication —see Complications, surgical procedure
traumatic
external —see Laceration
internal organs —see Injury, by site
Inclusion
azurophilic leukocytic D72.0
blennorrhea (neonatal) (newborn) P39.1
gallbladder in liver (congenital) Q44.1
Incompatibility
ABO
affecting management of pregnancy O36.11-
anti-A sensitization O36.11-
anti-B sensitization O36.19-
specified NEC O36.19-
infusion or transfusion reaction —see Complication (s), transfusion, incompatibility reaction, ABO
newborn P55.1
blood (group) (Duffy) (K(ell)) (Kidd) (Lewis) (M) (S) NEC
affecting management of pregnancy O36.11-
anti-A sensitization O36.11-
anti-B sensitization O36.19-
infusion or transfusion reaction T80.89
newborn P55.8
divorce or estrangement Z63.5
Rh (blood group) (factor) Z31.82
affecting management of pregnancy NEC O36.09-
anti-D antibody O36.01-
infusion or transfusion reaction —see Complication (s), transfusion, incompatibility reaction, Rh (factor)
newborn P55.0
rhesus —see Incompatibility, Rh
Incompetency, incompetent, incompetence
annular
aortic (valve) —see Insufficiency, aortic
mitral (valve) I34.0
pulmonary valve (heart) I37.1
aortic (valve) —see Insufficiency, aortic
cardiac valve —see Endocarditis
cervix, cervical (os) N88.3
in pregnancy O34.3-
chronotropic I45.89
with
autonomic dysfunction G90.8
ischemic heart disease I25.89
left ventricular dysfunction I51.89
sinus node dysfunction I49.8
esophagogastric (junction) (sphincter) K22.0

Incompetency, incompetent, incompetence (Continued)
mitral (valve) —see Insufficiency, mitral
pelvic fundus N81.89
pubocervical tissue N81.82
pulmonary valve (heart) I37.1
congenital Q22.3
rectovaginal tissue N81.83
tricuspid (annular) (valve) —see Insufficiency, tricuspid
valvular —see Endocarditis
congenital Q24.8
vein, venous (saphenous) (varicose) —see Varix, leg
Incomplete —see also condition
bladder, emptying R33.9
defecation R15.0
expansion lungs (newborn) NEC —see Atelectasis
rotation, intestine Q43.3
Inconclusive
diagnostic imaging due to excess body fat of patient R93.9
findings on diagnostic imaging of breast NEC R92.8
mammogram (due to dense breasts) R92.2
Incontinence R32
anal sphincter R15.9
feces R15.9
nonorganic origin F98.1
overflow N39.490
psychogenic F45.8
rectal R15.9
reflex N39.498
stress (female) (male) N39.3
and urge N39.46
urethral sphincter R32
urge N39.41
and stress (female) (male) N39.46
urine (urinary) R32
continuous N39.45
due to cognitive impairment, or severe physical disability or immobility R39.81
functional R39.81
mixed (stress and urge) N39.46
nocturnal N39.44
nonorganic origin F98.0
overflow N39.490
post dribbling N39.43
reflex N39.498
specified NEC N39.498
stress (female) (male) N39.3
and urge N39.46
total N39.498
unaware N39.42
urge N39.41
and stress (female) (male) N39.46
Incontinentia pigmenti Q82.3
Incoordinate, incoordination
esophageal-pharyngeal (newborn) —see Dysphagia
muscular R27.8
uterus (action) (contractions) (complicating delivery) O62.4
Increase, increased
abnormal, in development R63.8
androgens (ovarian) E28.1
anticoagulants (antithrombin) (anti-VIIIa) (anti-IXa) (anti-Xa) (anti-XIa) —see Circulating anticoagulants)
cold sense R20.8
estrogen E28.0
function
adrenal
cortex —see Cushing's, syndrome
medulla E27.5
pituitary (gland) (anterior) (lobe) E22.9
posterior E22.2
heat sense R20.8
intracranial pressure (benign) G93.2

◀ New   ◀▥ Revised   ~~deleted~~ Deleted

Increase, increased (Continued)
  permeability, capillaries I78.8
  pressure, intracranial G93.2
  secretion
    gastrin E16.4
    glucagon E16.3
    pancreas, endocrine E16.9
      growth hormone-releasing hormone
        E16.8
      pancreatic polypeptide E16.8
      somatostatin E16.8
      vasoactive-intestinal polypeptide
        E16.8
  sphericity, lens Q12.4
  splenic activity D73.1
  venous pressure I87.8
    portal K76.6
Increta placenta O43.22-
Incrustation, cornea, foreign body (lead)
  (zinc) —see Foreign body, cornea
Incyclophoria H50.54
Incyclotropia —see Cyclotropia
Indeterminate sex Q56.4
India rubber skin Q82.8
Indigestion (acid) (bilious) (functional) K30
  catarrhal K31.89
  due to decomposed food NOS A05.9
  nervous F45.8
  psychogenic F45.8
Indirect —see condition
Induratio penis plastica N48.6
Induration, indurated
  brain G93.89
  breast (fibrous) N64.51
    puerperal, postpartum O92.29
  broad ligament N83.8
  chancre
    anus A51.1
    congenital A50.07
    extragenital NEC A51.2
  corpora cavernosa (penis) (plastic) N48.6
  liver (chronic) K76.89
  lung (black) (chronic) (fibroid) (see also
    Fibrosis, lung) J84.10
    essential brown J84.03
  penile (plastic) N48.6
  phlebitic —see Phlebitis
  skin R23.4
Inebriety (without dependence) —see Alcohol,
  intoxication
Inefficiency, kidney N28.9
Inelasticity, skin R23.4
Inequality, leg (length) (acquired) —see also
  Deformity, limb, unequal length
  congenital —see Defect, reduction, lower
    limb
  lower leg —see Deformity, limb, unequal
    length
Inertia
  bladder (neurogenic) N31.2
  stomach K31.89
    psychogenic F45.8
  uterus, uterine during labor O62.2
    during latent phase of labor O62.0
    primary O62.0
    secondary O62.1
  vesical (neurogenic) N31.2
Infancy, infantile, infantilism —see also
  condition
  celiac K90.0
  genitalia, genitals (after puberty) E30.0
  Herter's (nontropical sprue) K90.0
  intestinal K90.0
  Lorain E23.0
  pancreatic K86.8
  pelvis M95.5
    with disproportion (fetopelvic) O33.1
      causing obstructed labor O65.1
  pituitary E23.0
  renal N25.0
  uterus —see Infantile, genitalia

Infant (s) —see also Infancy
  excessive crying R68.11
  irritable child R68.12
  lack of care —see Neglect
  liveborn (singleton) Z38.2
    born in hospital Z38.00
      by cesarean Z38.01
    born outside hospital Z38.1
    multiple NEC Z38.8
      born in hospital Z38.68
        by cesarean Z38.69
      born outside hospital Z38.7
    quadruplet Z38.8
      born in hospital Z38.63
        by cesarean Z38.64
      born outside hospital Z38.7
    quintuplet Z38.8
      born in hospital Z38.65
        by cesarean Z38.66
      born outside hospital Z38.7
    triplet Z38.8
      born in hospital Z38.61
        by cesarean Z38.62
      born outside hospital Z38.7
    twin Z38.5
      born in hospital Z38.30
        by cesarean Z38.31
      born outside hospital Z38.4
  of diabetic mother (syndrome of) P70.1
    gestational diabetes P70.0
Infantile —see also condition
  genitalia, genitals E30.0
  os, uterine E30.0
  penis E30.0
  testis E29.1
  uterus E30.0
Infantilism —see Infancy
Infarct, infarction
  adrenal (capsule) (gland) E27.49
  appendices epiploicae K55.0
  bowel K55.0
  brain (stem) —see Infarct, cerebral
  breast N64.89
  brewer's (kidney) N28.0
  cardiac —see Infarct, myocardium
  cerebellar —see Infarct, cerebral
  cerebral (see also Occlusion, artery cerebral or
    precerebral, with infarction) I63.9-
    aborted I63.9
    cortical I63.9
    due to
      cerebral venous thrombosis,
        nonpyogenic I63.6
      embolism
        cerebral arteries I63.4-
        precerebral arteries I63.1-
      occlusion NEC
        cerebral arteries I63.5-
        precerebral arteries I63.2-
      stenosis NEC
        cerebral arteries I63.5-
        precerebral arteries I63.2-
      thrombosis
        cerebral artery I63.3-
        precerebral artery I63.0-
    intraoperative
      during cardiac surgery I97.810
      during other surgery I97.811
    postprocedural
      following cardiac surgery I97.820
      following other surgery I97.821
    specified NEC I63.8
  colon (acute) (agnogenic) (embolic)
    (hemorrhagic) (nonocclusive)
    (nonthrombotic) (occlusive) (segmental)
    (thrombotic) (with gangrene) K55.0
  coronary artery —see Infarct, myocardium
  embolic —see Embolism
  fallopian tube N83.8
  gallbladder K82.8
  heart —see Infarct, myocardium

Infarct, infarction (Continued)
  hepatic K76.3
  hypophysis (anterior lobe) E23.6
  impending (myocardium) I20.0
  intestine (acute) (agnogenic) (embolic)
    (hemorrhagic) (nonocclusive)
    (nonthrombotic) (occlusive)
    (thrombotic) (with gangrene) K55.0
  kidney N28.0
  liver K76.3
  lung (embolic) (thrombotic) —see Embolism,
    pulmonary
  lymph node I89.8
  mesentery, mesenteric (embolic) (thrombotic)
    (with gangrene) K55.0
  muscle (ischemic) M62.20
    ankle M62.27-
    foot M62.27-
    forearm M62.23-
    hand M62.24-
    lower leg M62.26-
    pelvic region M62.25-
    shoulder region M62.21-
    specified site NEC M62.28
    thigh M62.25-
    upper arm M62.22-
  myocardium, myocardial (acute) (with stated
    duration of 4 weeks or less) I21.3
    diagnosed on ECG, but presenting no
      symptoms I25.2
    healed or old I25.2
    intraoperative
      during cardiac surgery I97.790
      during other surgery I97.791
    non-Q wave I21.4
    non-ST elevation (NSTEMI) I21.4
      subsequent I22.2
    nontransmural I21.4
    past (diagnosed on ECG or other
      investigation, but currently
      presenting no symptoms) I25.2
    postprocedural
      following cardiac surgery I97.190
      following other surgery I97.191
    Q wave (see also, Infarct, myocardium, by
      site) I21.3
    ST elevation (STEMI) I21.3
      anterior (anteroapical) (anterolateral)
        (anteroseptal) (Q wave) (wall)
        I21.09
        subsequent I22.0
      inferior (diaphragmatic) (inferolateral)
        (inferoposterior) (wall) NEC
        I21.19
        subsequent I22.1
      inferoposterior transmural (Q wave)
        I21.11
      involving
        coronary artery of anterior wall NEC
          I21.09
        coronary artery of inferior wall NEC
          I21.19
        diagonal coronary artery I21.02
        left anterior descending coronary
          artery I21.02
        left circumflex coronary artery I21.21
        left main coronary artery I21.01
        oblique marginal coronary artery
          I21.21
        right coronary artery I21.11
      lateral (apical-lateral) (basal-lateral)
        (high) I21.29
        subsequent I22.8
      posterior (posterobasal) (posterolateral)
        (posteroseptal) (true) I21.29
        subsequent I22.8
      septal I21.29
        subsequent I22.8
      specified NEC I21.29
        subsequent I22.8
      subsequent I22.9

Infarct, infarction *(Continued)*
- myocardium, myocardial *(Continued)*
  - subsequent (recurrent) (reinfarction) I22.9
    - anterior (anteroapical) (anterolateral) (anteroseptal) (wall) I22.0
    - diaphragmatic (wall) I22.1
    - inferior (diaphragmatic) (inferolateral) (inferoposterior) (wall) I22.1
    - lateral (apical-lateral) (basal-lateral) (high) I22.8
    - non-ST elevation (NSTEMI) I22.2
    - posterior (posterobasal) (posterolateral) (posteroseptal) (true) I22.8
    - septal I22.8
    - specified NEC I22.8
    - ST elevation I22.9
      - anterior (anteroapical) (anterolateral) (anteroseptal) (wall) I22.0
      - inferior (diaphragmatic) (inferolateral) (inferoposterior) (wall) I22.1
      - specified NEC I22.8
  - subendocardial I22.2
  - transmural I22.9
    - anterior (anteroapical) (anterolateral) (anteroseptal) (wall) I22.0
    - diaphragmatic (wall) I22.1
    - inferior (diaphragmatic) (inferolateral) (inferoposterior) (wall) I22.1
    - lateral (apical-lateral) (basal-lateral) (high) I22.8
    - posterior (posterobasal) (posterolateral) (posteroseptal) (true) I22.8
    - specified NEC I22.8
  - syphilitic A52.06
  - transmural I21.3
    - anterior (anteroapical) (anterolateral) (anteroseptal) (Q wave) (wall) NEC I21.09
    - inferior (diaphragmatic) (inferolateral) (inferoposterior) (Q wave) (wall) NEC I21.19
    - inferoposterior (Q wave) I21.11
    - lateral (apical-lateral) (basal-lateral) (high) NEC I21.29
    - posterior (posterobasal) (posterolateral) (posteroseptal) (true) NEC I21.29
    - septal NEC I21.29
    - specified NEC I21.29
- nontransmural I21.4
- omentum K55.0
- ovary N83.8
- pancreas K86.8
- papillary muscle —*see* Infarct, myocardium
- parathyroid gland E21.4
- pituitary (gland) E23.6
- placenta O43.81-
- prostate N42.89
- pulmonary (artery) (vein) (hemorrhagic) —*see* Embolism, pulmonary
- renal (embolic) (thrombotic) N28.0
- retina, retinal (artery) —*see* Occlusion, artery, retina
- spinal (cord) (acute) (embolic) (nonembolic) G95.11
- spleen D73.5
  - embolic or thrombotic I74.8
- subendocardial (acute) (nontransmural) I21.4
- suprarenal (capsule) (gland) E27.49
- testis N50.1
- thrombotic —*see also* Thrombosis
  - artery, arterial —*see* Embolism
- thyroid (gland) E07.89
- ventricle (heart) —*see* Infarct, myocardium

Infecting —*see* condition

Infection, infected, infective (opportunistic) B99.9
- with
  - drug resistant organism —*see* Resistance (to), drug —*see also* specific organism
  - lymphangitis —*see* Lymphangitis

Infection, infected, infective *(Continued)*
- with *(Continued)*
  - organ dysfunction (acute) R65.20
    - with septic shock R65.21
  - abscess (skin) - code by site under Abscess
- Absidia —*see* Mucormycosis
- Acanthamoeba —*see* Acanthamebiasis
- Acanthocheilonema (perstans) (streptocerca) B74.4
- accessory sinus (chronic) —*see* Sinusitis
- achorion —*see* Dermatophytosis
- Acremonium falciforme B47.0
- acromioclavicular M00.9
- Actinobacillus (actinomycetem-comitans) A28.8
  - mallei A24.0
  - muris A25.1
- Actinomadura B47.1
- Actinomyces (israelii) (*see also* Actinomycosis) A42.9
- Actinomycetales —*see* Actinomycosis
- actinomycotic NOS —*see* Actinomycosis
- adenoid (and tonsil) J03.90
  - chronic J35.02
- adenovirus NEC
  - as cause of disease classified elsewhere B97.0
  - unspecified nature or site B34.0
- aerogenes capsulatus A48.0
- aertrycke —*see* Infection, salmonella
- alimentary canal NOS —*see* Enteritis, infectious
- Allescheria boydii B48.2
- Alternaria B48.8
- alveolus, alveolar (process) K04.7
- Ameba, amebic (histolytica) —*see* Amebiasis
- amniotic fluid, sac or cavity O41.10-
  - chorioamnionitis O41.12-
  - placentitis O41.14-
- amputation stump (surgical) —*see* Complication, amputation stump, infection
- Ancylostoma (duodenalis) B76.0
- Anisakiasis, Anisakis larvae B81.0
- anthrax —*see* Anthrax
- antrum (chronic) —*see* Sinusitis, maxillary
- anus, anal (papillae) (sphincter) K62.89
- arbovirus (arbor virus) A94
  - specified type NEC A93.8
- artificial insemination N98.0
- Ascaris lumbricoides —*see* Ascariasis
- Ascomycetes B47.0
- Aspergillus (flavus) (fumigatus) (terreus) —*see* Aspergillosis
- atypical
  - acid-fast (bacilli) —*see* Mycobacterium, atypical
  - mycobacteria —*see* Mycobacterium, atypical
  - virus A81.9
    - specified type NEC A81.89
- auditory meatus (external) —*see* Otitis, externa, infective
- auricle (ear) —*see* Otitis, externa, infective
- axillary gland (lymph) L04.2
- Bacillus A49.9
  - abortus A23.1
  - anthracis —*see* Anthrax
  - Ducrey's (any location) A57
  - Flexner's A03.1
  - Friedländer's NEC A49.8
  - gas (gangrene) A48.0
  - mallei A24.0
  - melitensis A23.0
  - paratyphoid, paratyphosus A01.4
    - A A01.1
    - B A01.2
    - C A01.3
  - Shiga (-Kruse) A03.0
  - suipestifer —*see* Infection, salmonella
  - swimming pool A31.1

Infection, infected, infective *(Continued)*
- Bacillus *(Continued)*
  - typhosa A01.00
  - welchii —*see* Gangrene, gas
- bacterial NOS A49.9
  - as cause of disease classified elsewhere B96.89
    - Bacteroides fragilis [B. fragilis] B96.6
    - Clostridium perfringens [C. perfringens] B96.7
    - Enterobacter sakazakii B96.89
    - Enterococcus B95.2
    - Escherichia coli [E. coli] (*see also* Escherichia coli) B96.20
    - Helicobacter pylori [H.pylori] B96.81
    - Hemophilus influenzae [H. influenzae] B96.3
    - Klebsiella pneumoniae [K. pneumoniae] B96.1
    - Mycoplasma pneumoniae [M. pneumoniae] B96.0
    - Proteus (mirabilis) (morganii) B96.4
    - Pseudomonas (aeruginosa) (mallei) (pseudomallei) B96.5
    - Staphylococcus B95.8
      - aureus (methicillin susceptible) (MSSA) B95.61
        - methicillin resistant (MRSA) B95.62
      - specified NEC B95.7
    - Streptococcus B95.5
      - group A B95.0
      - group B B95.1
      - pneumoniae B95.3
      - specified NEC B95.4
    - Vibrio vulnificus B96.82
  - specified NEC A48.8
- Bacterium
  - paratyphosum A01.4
    - A A01.1
    - B A01.2
    - C A01.3
  - typhosum A01.00
- Bacteroides NEC A49.8
  - fragilis, as cause of disease classified elsewhere B96.6
- Balantidium coli A07.0
- Bartholin's gland N75.8
- Basidiobolus B46.8
- bile duct (common) (hepatic) —*see* Cholangitis
- bladder —*see* Cystitis
- Blastomyces, blastomycotic —*see also* Blastomycosis
  - brasiliensis —*see* Paracoccidioidomycosis
  - dermatitidis —*see* Blastomycosis
  - European —*see* Cryptococcosis
  - Loboi B48.0
  - North American B40.9
  - South American —*see* Paracoccidioidomycosis
- bleb, postprocedure —*see* Blebitis
- bone —*see* Osteomyelitis
- Bordetella —*see* Whooping cough
- Borrelia bergdorfi A69.20
- brain (*see also* Encephalitis) G04.90
  - membranes —*see* Meningitis
  - septic G06.0
  - meninges —*see* Meningitis, bacterial
- branchial cyst Q18.0
- breast —*see* Mastitis
- bronchus —*see* Bronchitis
- Brucella A23.9
  - abortus A23.1
  - canis A23.3
  - melitensis A23.0
  - mixed A23.8
  - specified NEC A23.8
  - suis A23.2
- Brugia (malayi) B74.1
  - timori B74.2
- bursa —*see* Bursitis, infective

◀ New ◀▦ Revised ~~deleted~~ Deleted

Infection, infected, infective *(Continued)*
buttocks (skin) L08.9
Campylobacter, intestinal A04.5
  as cause of disease classified elsewhere
    B96.81
Candida (albicans) (tropicalis) —*see*
  Candidiasis
candiru B88.8
Capillaria (intestinal) B81.1
  hepatica B83.8
  philippinensis B81.1
cartilage —*see* Disorder, cartilage, specified
  type NEC
catheter-related bloodstream (CRBSI) T80.211
cat liver fluke B66.0
cellulitis - code by site under Cellulitis
central line-associated T80.219
  bloodstream (CLABSI) T80.211
  specified NEC T80.218
Cephalosporium falciforme B47.0
cerebrospinal —*see* Meningitis
cervical gland (lymph) L04.0
cervix —*see* Cervicitis
cesarean delivery wound (puerperal) O86.0
cestodes —*see* Infestation, cestodes
chest J22
Chilomastix (intestinal) A07.8
Chlamydia, chlamydial A74.9
  anus A56.3
  genitourinary tract A56.2
    lower A56.00
    specified NEC A56.19
  lymphogranuloma A55
  pharynx A56.4
  psittaci A70
  rectum A56.3
  sexually transmitted NEC A56.8
cholera —*see* Cholera
Cladosporium
  bantianum (brain abscess) B43.1
  carrionii B43.0
  castellanii B36.1
  trichoides (brain abscess) B43.1
  werneckii B36.1
Clonorchis (sinensis) (liver) B66.1
Clostridium NEC
  bifermentans A48.0
  botulinum (food poisoning) A05.1
    infant A48.51
    wound A48.52
  difficile
    as cause of disease classified elsewhere
      B96.89
    foodborne (disease) A04.7
    gas gangrene A48.0
    necrotizing enterocolitis A04.7
    sepsis A41.4
  gas-forming NEC A48.0
  histolyticum A48.0
  novyi, causing gas gangrene A48.0
  oedematiens A48.0
  perfringens
    as cause of disease classified elsewhere
      B96.7
    due to food A05.2
    foodborne (disease) A05.2
    gas gangrene A48.0
    sepsis A41.4
  septicum, causing gas gangrene A48.0
  sordellii, causing gas gangrene A48.0
  welchii
    as cause of disease classified elsewhere
      B96.7
    foodborne (disease) A05.2
    gas gangrene A48.0
    necrotizing enteritis A05.2
    sepsis A41.4
Coccidioides (immitis) —*see*
  Coccidioidomycosis
colon —*see* Enteritis, infectious
colostomy K94.02

Infection, infected, infective *(Continued)*
common duct —*see* Cholangitis
congenital P39.9
  Candida (albicans) P37.5
  cytomegalovirus P35.1
  hepatitis, viral P35.3
  herpes simplex P35.2
  infectious or parasitic disease P37.9
    specified NEC P37.8
  listeriosis (disseminated) P37.2
  malaria NEC P37.4
    falciparum P37.3
  Plasmodium falciparum P37.3
  poliomyelitis P35.8
  rubella P35.0
  skin P39.4
  toxoplasmosis (acute) (subacute) (chronic)
    P37.1
  tuberculosis P37.0
  urinary (tract) P39.3
  vaccinia P35.8
  virus P35.9
    specified type NEC P35.8
Conidiobolus B46.8
coronavirus NEC B34.2
  as cause of disease classified elsewhere
    B97.29
  severe acute respiratory syndrome (SARS
    associated) B97.21
corpus luteum —*see* Salpingo-oophoritis
Corynebacterium diphtheriae —*see*
  Diphtheria
cotia virus B08.8
Coxiella burnetii A78
coxsackie —*see* Coxsackie
Cryptococcus neoformans —*see*
  Cryptococcosis
Cryptosporidium A07.2
Cunninghamella —*see* Mucormycosis
cyst —*see* Cyst
cystic duct (*see also* Cholecystitis) K81.9
Cysticercus cellulosae —*see* Cysticercosis
cytomegalovirus, cytomegaloviral B25.9
  congenital P35.1
  maternal, maternal care for (suspected)
    damage to fetus O35.3
  mononucleosis B27.10
    with
      complication NEC B27.19
      meningitis B27.12
      polyneuropathy B27.11
delta-agent (acute), in hepatitis B carrier
  B17.0
dental (pulpal origin) K04.7
Deuteromycetes B47.0
Dicrocoelium dendriticum B66.2
Dipetalonema (perstans) (streptocerca) B74.4
diphtherial —*see* Diphtheria
Diphyllobothrium (adult) (latum) (pacificum)
  B70.0
  larval B70.1
Diplogonoporus (grandis) B71.8
Dipylidium caninum B67.4
Dirofilaria B74.8
Dracunculus medinensis B72
Drechslera (hawaiiensis) B43.8
Ducrey Haemophilus (any location) A57
due to or resulting from
  artificial insemination N98.0
  central venous catheter T80.219
    bloodstream T80.211
    exit or insertion site T80.212
    localized T80.212
    port or reservoir T80.212
    specified NEC T80.218
    tunnel T80.212
  device, implant or graft (*see also*
    Complications, by site and type,
    infection or inflammation) T85.79
    arterial graft NEC T82.7
    breast (implant) T85.79

Infection, infected, infective *(Continued)*
due to or resulting from *(Continued)*
  device, implant or graft *(Continued)*
    catheter NEC T85.79
      dialysis (renal) T82.7
        intraperitoneal T85.71
      infusion NEC T82.7
        spinal (epidural) (subdural)
          T85.79
      urinary (indwelling) T83.51
    electronic (electrode) (pulse generator)
      (stimulator)
      bone T84.7
      cardiac T82.7
      nervous system (brain) (peripheral
        nerve) (spinal) T85.79
      urinary T83.59
    fixation, internal (orthopedic) NEC —*see*
      Complication, fixation device,
      infection
    gastrointestinal (bile duct) (esophagus)
      T85.79
    genital NEC T83.6
    heart NEC T82.7
      valve (prosthesis) T82.6
        graft T82.7
    joint prosthesis —*see* Complication, joint
      prosthesis, infection
    ocular (corneal graft) (orbital implant)
      NEC T85.79
    orthopedic NEC T84.7
    specified NEC T85.79
    urinary NEC T83.59
    vascular NEC T82.7
    ventricular intracranial shunt
      T85.79
  Hickman catheter T80.219
    bloodstream T80.211
    localized T80.212
    specified NEC T80.218
  immunization or vaccination T88.0
  infusion, injection or transfusion NEC
    T80.29
    acute T80.22
  injury NEC - code by site under Wound,
    open
  peripherally inserted central catheter
    (PICC) T80.219
    bloodstream T80.211
    localized T80.212
    specified NEC T80.218
  portacath (port-a-cath) T80.219
    bloodstream T80.211
    localized T80.212
    specified NEC T80.218
  surgery T81.4
  triple lumen catheter T80.219
    bloodstream T80.211
    localized T80.212
    specified NEC T80.218
  umbilical venous catheter T80.219
    bloodstream T80.211
    localized T80.212
    specified NEC T80.218
during labor NEC O75.3
ear (middle) —*see also* Otitis media
  external —*see* Otitis, externa, infective
  inner —*see* subcategory H83.0
Eberthella typhosa A01.00
Echinococcus —*see* Echinococcus
echovirus
  as cause of disease classified elsewhere
    B97.12
  unspecified nature or site B34.1
endocardium I33.0
endocervix —*see* Cervicitis
Entamoeba —*see* Amebiasis
enteric —*see* Enteritis, infectious
Enterobacter sakazakii B96.89
Enterobius vermicularis B80
enterostomy K94.12

Infection, infected, infective (*Continued*)
- enterovirus B34.1
  - as cause of disease classified elsewhere B97.10
    - coxsackievirus B97.11
    - echovirus B97.12
    - specified NEC B97.19
- Entomophthora B46.8
- Epidermophyton —*see* Dermatophytosis
- epididymis —*see* Epididymitis
- episiotomy (puerperal) O86.0
- Erysipelothrix (insidiosa) (rhusiopathiae) — *see* Erysipeloid
- erythema infectiosum B08.3
- Escherichia (E.) coli NEC A49.8
  - as cause of disease classified elsewhere (*see also* Escherichia coli) B96.20
  - congenital P39.8
    - sepsis P36.4
  - generalized A41.51
  - intestinal —*see* Enteritis, infectious, due to, Escherichia coli
- ethmoidal (chronic) (sinus) —*see* Sinusitis, ethmoidal
- eustachian tube (ear) —*see* Salpingitis, eustachian
- external auditory canal (meatus) NEC —*see* Otitis, externa, infective
- eye (purulent) —*see* Endophthalmitis, purulent
- eyelid —*see* Inflammation, eyelid
- fallopian tube —*see* Salpingo-oophoritis
- Fasciola (gigantica) (hepatica) (indica) B66.3
- Fasciolopsis (buski) B66.5
- filarial —*see* Infestation, filarial
- finger (skin) L08.9
  - nail L03.01-
    - fungus B35.1
- fish tapeworm B70.0
  - larval B70.1
- flagellate, intestinal A07.9
- fluke —*see* Infestation, fluke
- focal
  - teeth (pulpal origin) K04.7
  - tonsils J35.01
- Fonsecaea (compactum) (pedrosoi) B43.0
- food —*see* Intoxication, foodborne
- foot (skin) L08.9
  - dermatophytic fungus B35.3
- Francisella tularensis —*see* Tularemia
- frontal (sinus) (chronic) —*see* Sinusitis, frontal
- fungus NOS B49
  - beard B35.0
  - dermatophytic —*see* Dermatophytosis
  - foot B35.3
  - groin B35.6
  - hand B35.2
  - nail B35.1
  - pathogenic to compromised host only B48.8
  - perianal (area) B35.6
  - scalp B35.0
  - skin B36.9
    - foot B35.3
    - hand B35.2
    - toenails B35.1
- Fusarium B48.8
- gallbladder —*see* Cholecystitis
- gas bacillus —*see* Gangrene, gas
- gastrointestinal —*see* Enteritis, infectious
- generalized NEC —*see* Sepsis
- genital organ or tract
  - female —*see* Disease, pelvis, inflammatory
  - male N49.9
    - multiple sites N49.8
    - specified NEC N49.8
- Ghon tubercle, primary A15.7
- Giardia lamblia A07.1

Infection, infected, infective (*Continued*)
- gingiva (chronic) K05.10
  - acute K05.00
    - nonplaque induced K05.01
    - plaque induced K05.00
  - nonplaque induced K05.11
  - plaque induced K05.10
- glanders A24.0
- glenosporopsis B48.0
- Gnathostoma (spinigerum) B83.1
- Gongylonema B83.8
- gonococcal —*see* Gonococcus
- gram-negative bacilli NOS A49.9
- guinea worm B72
- gum (chronic) K05.10
  - acute K05.00
    - nonplaque induced K05.01
    - plaque induced K05.00
  - nonplaque induced K05.11
  - plaque induced K05.10
- Haemophilus —*see* Infection, Hemophilus
- heart —*see* Carditis
- Helicobacter pylori A04.8
  - as cause of disease classified elsewhere B96.81
- helminths B83.9
  - intestinal B82.0
    - mixed (types classifiable to more than one of the titles B65.0-B81.3 and B81.8) B81.4
    - specified type NEC B81.8
  - specified type NEC B83.8
- Hemophilus
  - aegyptius, systemic A48.4
  - ducrey (any location) A57
  - generalized A41.3
  - influenzae NEC A49.2
    - as cause of disease classified elsewhere B96.3
- herpes (simplex) —*see also* Herpes
  - congenital P35.2
  - disseminated B00.7
  - zoster B02.9
- herpesvirus, herpesviral —*see* Herpes
- Heterophyes (heterophyes) B66.8
- hip (joint) NEC M00.9
  - due to internal joint prosthesis
    - left T84.52
    - right T84.51
  - skin NEC L08.9
- Histoplasma —*see* Histoplasmosis
  - American B39.4
  - capsulatum B39.4
- hookworm B76.9
- human
  - papilloma virus A63.0
  - T-cell lymphotropic virus type-1 (HTLV-1) B33.3
- hydrocele N43.0
- Hymenolepis B71.0
- hypopharynx —*see* Pharyngitis
- inguinal (lymph) glands L04.1
  - due to soft chancre A57
- intervertebral disc, pyogenic M46.30
  - cervical region M46.32
  - cervicothoracic region M46.33
  - lumbar region M46.36
  - lumbosacral region M46.37
  - multiple sites M46.39
  - occipito-atlanto-axial region M46.31
  - sacrococcygeal region M46.38
  - thoracic region M46.34
  - thoracolumbar region M46.35
- intestine, intestinal —*see* Enteritis, infectious
  - specified NEC A08.8
- intra-amniotic affecting newborn NEC P39.2
- Isospora belli or hominis A07.3
- Japanese B encephalitis A83.0
- jaw (bone) (lower) (upper) M27.2
- joint NEC M00.9
  - due to internal joint prosthesis T84.50

Infection, infected, infective (*Continued*)
- kidney (cortex) (hematogenous) N15.9
  - with calculus N20.0
    - with hydronephrosis N13.6
  - following ectopic gestation O08.83
  - pelvis and ureter (cystic) N28.85
  - puerperal (postpartum) O86.21
  - specified NEC N15.8
- Klebsiella (K.) pneumoniae NEC A49.8
  - as cause of disease classified elsewhere B96.1
- knee (joint) NEC M00.9
  - due to internal joint prosthesis
    - left T84.54
    - right T84.53
  - joint M00.9
  - skin L08.9
- Koch's —*see* Tuberculosis
- labia (majora) (minora) (acute) —*see* Vulvitis
- lacrimal
  - gland —*see* Dacryoadenitis
  - passages (duct) (sac) —*see* Inflammation, lacrimal, passages
- lancet fluke B66.2
- larynx NEC J38.7
- leg (skin) NOS L08.9
- Legionella pneumophila A48.1
  - nonpneumonic A48.2
- Leishmania —*see also* Leishmaniasis
  - aethiopica B55.1
  - braziliensis B55.2
  - chagasi B55.0
  - donovani B55.0
  - infantum B55.0
  - major B55.1
  - mexicana B55.1
  - tropica B55.1
- lentivirus, as cause of disease classified elsewhere B97.31
- Leptosphaeria senegalensis B47.0
- Leptospira interrogans A27.9
  - autumnalis A27.89
  - canicola A27.89
  - hebdomadis A27.89
  - icterohaemorrhagiae A27.0
  - pomona A27.89
  - specified type NEC A27.89
- leptospirochetal NEC —*see* Leptospirosis
- Listeria monocytogenes —*see also* Listeriosis
  - congenital P37.2
- Loa loa B74.3
  - with conjunctival infestation B74.3
  - eyelid B74.3
- Loboa loboi B48.0
- local, skin (staphylococcal) (streptococcal) L08.9
  - abscess - code by site under Abscess
  - cellulitis - code by site under Cellulitis
  - specified NEC L08.89
  - ulcer —*see* Ulcer, skin
- Loefflerella mallei A24.0
- lung (*see also* Pneumonia) J18.9
  - atypical Mycobacterium A31.0
  - spirochetal A69.8
  - tuberculous —*see* Tuberculosis, pulmonary
  - virus —*see* Pneumonia, viral
- lymph gland —*see also* Lymphadenitis, acute
  - mesenteric I88.0
- lymphoid tissue, base of tongue or posterior pharynx, NEC (chronic) J35.03
- Madurella (grisea) (mycetomii) B47.0
- major
  - following ectopic or molar pregnancy O08.0
  - puerperal, postpartum, childbirth O85
- Malassezia furfur B36.0
- Malleomyces
  - mallei A24.0
  - pseudomallei (whitmori) —*see* Melioidosis

Infection, infected, infective (Continued)

mammary gland N61
Mansonella (ozzardi) (perstans) (streptocerca) B74.4
mastoid —see Mastoiditis
maxilla, maxillary M27.2
  sinus (chronic) —see Sinusitis, maxillary
mediastinum J98.5
Medina (worm) B72
meibomian cyst or gland —see Hordeolum
meninges —see Meningitis, bacterial
meningococcal (see also condition) A39.9
  adrenals A39.1
  brain A39.81
  cerebrospinal A39.0
  conjunctiva A39.89
  endocardium A39.51
  heart A39.50
    endocardium A39.51
    myocardium A39.52
    pericardium A39.53
  joint A39.83
  meninges A39.0
  meningococcemia A39.4
    acute A39.2
    chronic A39.3
  myocardium A39.52
  pericardium A39.53
  retrobulbar neuritis A39.82
  specified site NEC A39.89
mesenteric lymph nodes or glands NEC I88.0
Metagonimus B66.8
metatarsophalangeal M00.9
methicillin
  resistant Staphylococcus aureus (MRSA) A49.02
  susceptible Staphylococcus aureus (MSSA) A49.01
Microsporum, microsporic —see Dermatophytosis
mixed flora (bacterial) NEC A49.8
Monilia —see Candidiasis
Monosporium apiospermum B48.2
mouth, parasitic B37.0
Mucor —see Mucormycosis
muscle NEC —see Myositis, infective
mycelium NOS B49
mycetoma B47.9
  actinomycotic NEC B47.1
  mycotic NEC B47.0
Mycobacterium, mycobacterial —see Mycobacterium
Mycoplasma NEC A49.3
  pneumoniae, as cause of disease classified elsewhere B96.0
mycotic NOS B49
  pathogenic to compromised host only B48.8
  skin NOS B36.9
myocardium NEC I40.0
nail (chronic)
  with lymphangitis —see Lymphangitis, acute, digit
  finger L03.01-
    fungus B35.1
    ingrowing L60.0
  toe L03.03-
    fungus B35.1
nasal sinus (chronic) —see Sinusitis
nasopharynx —see Nasopharyngitis
navel L08.82
Necator americanus B76.1
Neisseria —see Gonococcus
Neotestudina rosatii B47.0
newborn P39.9
  intra-amniotic NEC P39.2
  skin P39.4
  specified type NEC P39.8

Infection, infected, infective (Continued)

nipple N61
  associated with
    lactation O91.03
    pregnancy O91.01-
    puerperium O91.02
Nocardia —see Nocardiosis
obstetrical surgical wound (puerperal) O86.0
Oesophagostomum (apiostomum) B81.8
Oestrus ovis —see Myiasis
Oidium albicans B37.9
Onchocerca (volvulus) —see Onchocerciasis -
  oncovirus, as cause of disease classified elsewhere B97.32
operation wound T81.4
Opisthorchis (felineus) (viverrini) B66.0
orbit, orbital —see Inflammation, orbit
orthopoxvirus NEC B08.09
ovary —see Salpingo-oophoritis
Oxyuris vermicularis B80
pancreas (acute) K85.9
  abscess —see Pancreatitis, acute
  specified NEC K85.8
papillomavirus, as cause of disease classified elsewhere B97.7
papovavirus NEC B34.4
Paracoccidioides brasiliensis —see Paracoccidioidomycosis
Paragonimus (westermani) B66.4
parainfluenza virus B34.8
parameningococcus NOS A39.9
parapoxvirus B08.60
  specified NEC B08.69
parasitic B89
Parastrongylus
  cantonensis B83.2
  costaricensis B81.3
  paratyphoid A01.4
    Type A A01.1
    Type B A01.2
    Type C A01.3
paraurethral ducts N34.2
parotid gland —see Sialoadenitis
parvovirus NEC B34.3
  as cause of disease classified elsewhere B97.6
Pasteurella NEC A28.0
  multocida A28.0
  pestis —see Plague
  pseudotuberculosis A28.0
  septica (cat bite) (dog bite) A28.0
  tularensis —see Tularemia
pelvic, female —see Disease, pelvis, inflammatory
Penicillium (marneffei) B48.4
penis (glans) (retention) NEC N48.29
periapical K04.5
peridental, periodontal K05.20
  generalized K05.22
  localized K05.21
perinatal period P39.9
  specified type NEC P39.8
perineal repair (puerperal) O86.0
periorbital —see Inflammation, orbit
perirectal K62.89
perirenal —see Infection, kidney
peritoneal —see Peritonitis
periureteral N28.89
Petriellidium boydii B48.2
pharynx —see also Pharyngitis
  coxsackievirus B08.5
  posterior, lymphoid (chronic) J35.03
Phialophora
  gougerotii (subcutaneous abscess or cyst) B43.2
  jeanselmei (subcutaneous abscess or cyst) B43.2
  verrucosa (skin) B43.0
Piedraia hortae B36.3

Infection, infected, infective (Continued)

pinta A67.9
  intermediate A67.1
  late A67.2
  mixed A67.3
  primary A67.0
pinworm B80
pityrosporum furfur B36.0
pleuro-pneumonia-like organism (PPLO) NEC A49.3
  as cause of disease classified elsewhere B96.0
pneumococcus, pneumococcal NEC A49.1
  as cause of disease classified elsewhere B95.3
  generalized (purulent) A40.3
    with pneumonia J13
Pneumocystis carinii (pneumonia) B59
Pneumocystis jiroveci (pneumonia) B59
port or reservoir T80.212
postoperative T81.4
postoperative wound T81.4
postprocedural T81.4
postvaccinal T88.0
prepuce NEC N47.7
  with penile inflammation N47.6
prion —see Disease, prion, central nervous system
prostate (capsule) —see Prostatitis
Proteus (mirabilis) (morganii) (vulgaris) NEC A49.8
  as cause of disease classified elsewhere B96.4
protozoal NEC B64
  intestinal A07.9
    specified NEC A07.8
  specified NEC B60.8
Pseudoallescheria boydii B48.2
Pseudomonas NEC A49.8
  as cause of disease classified elsewhere B96.5
  mallei A24.0
  pneumonia J15.1
  pseudomallei —see Melioidosis
puerperal O86.4
  genitourinary tract NEC O86.89
  major or generalized O85
  minor O86.4
  specified NEC O86.89
pulmonary —see Infection, lung
purulent —see Abscess
Pyrenochaeta romeroi B47.0
Q fever A78
rectum (sphincter) K62.89
renal —see also Infection, kidney
  pelvis and ureter (cystic) N28.85
reovirus, as cause of disease classified elsewhere B97.5
respiratory (tract) NEC J98.8
  acute J22
  chronic J98.8
  influenzal (upper) (acute) —see Influenza, with, respiratory manifestations NEC
  lower (acute) J22
    chronic —see Bronchitis, chronic
  rhinovirus J00
  syncytial virus, as cause of disease classified elsewhere B97.4
  upper (acute) NOS J06.9
    chronic J39.8
    streptococcal J06.9
    viral NOS J06.9
resulting from
  presence of internal prosthesis, implant, graft —see Complications, by site and type, infection
retortamoniasis A07.8
retroperitoneal NEC K68.9

Infection, infected, infective (*Continued*)
retrovirus B33.3
  as cause of disease classified elsewhere B97.30
    human
      immunodeficiency, type 2 (HIV 2) B97.35
      T-cell lymphotropic
        type I (HTLV-I) B97.33
        type II (HTLV-II) B97.34
    lentivirus B97.31
    oncovirus B97.32
    specified NEC B97.39
Rhinosporidium (seeberi) B48.1
rhinovirus
  as cause of disease classified elsewhere B97.89
  unspecified nature or site B34.8
Rhizopus —*see* Mucormycosis
rickettsial NOS A79.9
roundworm (large) NEC B82.0
  Ascariasis (*see also* Ascariasis) B77.9
rubella —*see* Rubella
Saccharomyces —*see* Candidiasis
salivary duct or gland (any) —*see* Sialoadenitis
Salmonella (aertrycke) (arizonae) (callinarum) (cholerae-suis) (enteritidis) (suipestifer) (typhimurium) A02.9
  with
    (gastro) enteritis A02.0
    sepsis A02.1
    specified manifestation NEC A02.8
  due to food (poisoning) A02.9
  hirschfeldii A01.3
  localized A02.20
    arthritis A02.23
    meningitis A02.21
    osteomyelitis A02.24
    pneumonia A02.22
    pyelonephritis A02.25
    specified NEC A02.29
  paratyphi A01.4
    A A01.1
    B A01.2
    C A01.3
  schottmuelleri A01.2
  typhi, typhosa —*see* Typhoid
Sarcocystis A07.8
scabies B86
Schistosoma —*see* Infestation, Schistosoma
scrotum (acute) NEC N49.2
seminal vesicle —*see* Vesiculitis
septic
  localized, skin —*see* Abscess
sheep liver fluke B66.3
Shigella A03.9
  boydii A03.2
  dysenteriae A03.0
  flexneri A03.1
  group
    A A03.0
    B A03.1
    C A03.2
    D A03.3
  Schmitz (-Stutzer) A03.0
  schmitzii A03.0
  shigae A03.0
  sonnei A03.3
  specified NEC A03.8
shoulder (joint) NEC M00.9
  due to internal joint prosthesis T84.59
  skin NEC L08.9
sinus (accessory) (chronic) (nasal) —*see also* Sinusitis
  pilonidal —*see* Sinus, pilonidal
  skin NEC L08.89
Skene's duct or gland —*see* Urethritis
skin (local) (staphylococcal) (streptococcal) L08.9
  abscess - code by site under Abscess

Infection, infected, infective (*Continued*)
skin (*Continued*)
  cellulitis - code by site under Cellulitis
  due to fungus B36.9
    specified type NEC B36.8
  mycotic B36.9
    specified type NEC B36.8
  newborn P39.4
  ulcer —*see* Ulcer, skin
slow virus A81.9
  specified NEC A81.89
Sparganum (mansoni) (proliferum) (baxteri) B70.1
specific —*see also* Syphilis
  to perinatal period —*see* Infection, congenital
specified NEC B99.8
spermatic cord NEC N49.1
sphenoidal (sinus) —*see* Sinusitis, sphenoidal
spinal cord NOS (*see also* Myelitis) G04.91
  abscess G06.1
  meninges —*see* Meningitis
  streptococcal G04.89
Spirillum A25.0
spirochetal NOS A69.9
  lung A69.8
  specified NEC A69.8
Spirometra larvae B70.1
spleen D73.89
Sporotrichum, Sporothrix (schenckii) —*see* Sporotrichosis
staphylococcal, unspecified site
  aureus (methicillin susceptible) (MSSA) A49.01
    methicillin resistant (MRSA) A49.02
  as cause of disease classified elsewhere B95.8
    aureus (methicillin susceptible) (MSSA) B95.61
      methicillin resistant (MRSA) B95.62
    specified NEC B95.7
  food poisoning A05.0
  generalized (purulent) A41.2
  pneumonia —*see* Pneumonia, staphylococcal
Stellantchasmus falcatus B66.8
streptobacillus moniliformis A25.1
streptococcal NEC A49.1
  as cause of disease classified elsewhere B95.5
  B genitourinary complicating
    childbirth O98.82
    pregnancy O98.81-
    puerperium O98.83
  congenital
    sepsis P36.10
      group B P36.0
      specified NEC P36.19
  generalized (purulent) A40.9
Streptomyces B47.1
Strongyloides (stercoralis) —*see* Strongyloidiasis
stump (amputation) (surgical) —*see* Complication, amputation stump, infection
subcutaneous tissue, local L08.9
suipestifer —*see* Infection, salmonella
swimming pool bacillus A31.1
Taenia —*see* Infestation, Taenia
Taeniarhynchus saginatus B68.1
tapeworm —*see* Infestation, tapeworm
tendon (sheath) —*see* Tenosynovitis, infective NEC
Ternidens diminutus B81.8
testis —*see* Orchitis
threadworm B80
throat —*see* Pharyngitis
thyroglossal duct K14.8

Infection, infected, infective (*Continued*)
toe (skin) L08.9
  cellulitis L03.03-
    fungus B35.1
  nail L03.03-
    fungus B35.1
tongue NEC K14.0
  parasitic B37.0
tonsil (and adenoid) (faucial) (lingual) (pharyngeal) —*see* Tonsillitis
tooth, teeth K04.7
  periapical K04.7
  peridental, periodontal K05.20
    generalized K05.22
    localized K05.21
  pulp K04.0
  socket M27.3
TORCH —*see* Infection, congenital without active infection P00.2
Torula histolytica —*see* Cryptococcosis
Toxocara (canis) (cati) (felis) B83.0
Toxoplasma gondii —*see* Toxoplasma
trachea, chronic J42
trematode NEC —*see* Infestation, fluke
trench fever A79.0
Treponema pallidum —*see* Syphilis
Trichinella (spiralis) B75
Trichomonas A59.9
  cervix A59.09
  intestine A07.8
  prostate A59.02
  specified site NEC A59.8
  urethra A59.03
  urogenitalis A59.00
  vagina A59.01
  vulva A59.01
Trichophyton, trichophytic —*see* Dermatophytosis
Trichosporon (beigelii) cutaneum B36.2
Trichostrongylus B81.2
Trichuris (trichiura) B79
Trombicula (irritans) B88.0
Trypanosoma
  brucei
    gambiense B56.0
    rhodesiense B56.1
  cruzi —*see* Chagas' disease
tubal —*see* Salpingo-oophoritis
tuberculous NEC —*see* Tuberculosis
tubo-ovarian —*see* Salpingo-oophoritis
tunica vaginalis N49.1
tunnel T80.212
tympanic membrane NEC —*see* Myringitis
typhoid (abortive) (ambulant) (bacillus) —*see* Typhoid
typhus A75.9
  flea-borne A75.2
  mite-borne A75.3
  recrudescent A75.1
  tick-borne A77.9
    African A77.1
    North Asian A77.2
umbilicus L08.82
ureter N28.86
urethra —*see* Urethritis
urinary (tract) N39.0
  bladder —*see* Cystitis
  complicating
    pregnancy O23.4-
      specified type NEC O23.3-
  kidney —*see* Infection, kidney
  newborn P39.3
  puerperal (postpartum) O86.20
  tuberculous A18.13
  urethra —*see* Urethritis
uterus, uterine —*see* Endometritis
vaccination T88.0
vaccinia not from vaccination B08.011
vagina (acute) —*see* Vaginitis
varicella B01.9
varicose veins —*see* Varix

◀ New   ◀ Revised   ~~deleted~~ Deleted

Infection, infected, infective (Continued)
vas deferens NEC N49.1
vesical —see Cystitis
Vibrio
  cholerae A00.0
    El Tor A00.1
  parahaemolyticus (food poisoning) A05.3
  vulnificus
    as cause of disease classified elsewhere
      B96.82
    foodborne intoxication A05.5
Vincent's (gum) (mouth) (tonsil) A69.1
virus, viral NOS B34.9
  adenovirus
    as cause of disease classified elsewhere
      B97.0
    unspecified nature or site B34.0
  arborvirus, arborvirus arthropod-borne A94
  as cause of disease classified elsewhere
    B97.89
    adenovirus B97.0
    coronavirus B97.29
      SARS-associated B97.21
    coxsackievirus B97.11
    echovirus B97.12
    enterovirus B97.10
      coxsackievirus B97.11
      echovirus B97.12
      specified NEC B97.19
    human
      immunodeficiency, type 2 (HIV 2)
        B97.35
      metapneumovirus B97.81
      T-cell lymphotropic,
        type I (HTLV-I) B97.33
        type II (HTLV-II) B97.34
    papillomavirus B97.7
    parvovirus B97.6
    reovirus B97.5
    respiratory syncytial B97.4
    retrovirus B97.30
      human
        immunodeficiency, type 2 (HIV 2)
          B97.35
        T-cell lymphotropic,
          type I (HTLV-I) B97.33
          type II (HTLV-II) B97.34
      lentivirus B97.31
      oncovirus B97.32
      specified NEC B97.39
    specified NEC B97.89
  central nervous system A89
    atypical A81.9
      specified NEC A81.89
    enterovirus NEC A88.8
      meningitis A87.0
    slow virus A81.9
      specified NEC A81.89
    specified NEC A88.8
  chest J98.8
  cotia B08.8
  coxsackie (see also Infection, coxsackie)
    B34.1
    as cause of disease classified elsewhere
      B97.11
  ECHO
    as cause of disease classified elsewhere
      B97.12
    unspecified nature or site B34.1
  encephalitis, tick-borne A84.9
  enterovirus, as cause of disease classified
    elsewhere B97.10
    coxsackievirus B97.11
    echovirus B97.12
    specified NEC B97.19
  exanthem NOS B09
  human metapneumovirus as cause of
    disease classified elsewhere B97.81
  human papilloma as cause of disease
    classified elsewhere B97.7
  intestine —see Enteritis, viral

Infection, infected, infective (Continued)
virus, viral NOS (Continued)
  respiratory syncytial
    as cause of disease classified elsewhere
      B97.4
    bronchopneumonia J12.1
    common cold syndrome J00
    nasopharyngitis (acute) J00
  rhinovirus
    as cause of disease classified elsewhere
      B97.89
    unspecified nature or site B34.8
  slow A81.9
    specified NEC A81.89
  specified type NEC B33.8
    as cause of disease classified elsewhere
      B97.89
    unspecified nature or site B34.8
  unspecified nature or site B34.9
  West Nile —see Virus, West Nile
vulva (acute) —see Vulvitis
West Nile —see Virus, West Nile
whipworm B79
worms B83.9
  specified type NEC B83.8
Wuchereria (bancrofti) B74.0
  malayi B74.1
  yatapoxvirus B08.70
    specified NEC B08.79
yeast (see also Candidiasis) B37.9
yellow fever —see Fever, yellow
Yersinia
  enterocolitica (intestinal) A04.6
  pestis —see Plague
  pseudotuberculosis A28.2
Zeis' gland —see Hordeolum
zoonotic bacterial NOS A28.9
Zopfia senegalensis B47.0
Infective, infectious —see condition
Infertility
female N97.9
  age-related N97.8
  associated with
    anovulation N97.0
    cervical (mucus) disease or anomaly
      N88.3
    congenital anomaly
      cervix N88.3
      fallopian tube N97.1
      uterus N97.2
      vagina N97.8
    dysmucorrhea N88.3
    fallopian tube disease or anomaly N97.1
    pituitary-hypothalamic origin E23.0
    specified origin NEC N97.8
    Stein-Leventhal syndrome E28.2
    uterine disease or anomaly N97.2
    vaginal disease or anomaly N97.8
  due to
    cervical anomaly N88.3
    fallopian tube anomaly N97.1
    ovarian failure E28.39
    Stein-Leventhal syndrome E28.2
    uterine anomaly N97.2
    vaginal anomaly N97.8
  nonimplantation N97.2
  origin
    cervical N88.3
    tubal (block) (occlusion) (stenosis)
      N97.1
    uterine N97.2
    vaginal N97.8
male N46.9
  azoospermia N46.01
    extratesticular cause N46.029
      drug therapy N46.021
      efferent duct obstruction N46.023
      infection N46.022
      radiation N46.024
      specified cause NEC N46.029
      systemic disease N46.025

Infertility (Continued)
male (Continued)
  oligospermia N46.11
    extratesticular cause N46.129
      drug therapy N46.121
      efferent duct obstruction N46.123
      infection N46.122
      radiation N46.124
      specified cause NEC N46.129
      systemic disease N46.125
  specified type NEC N46.8
Infestation B88.9
Acanthocheilonema (perstans) (streptocerca)
  B74.4
Acariasis B88.0
  demodex folliculorum B88.0
  sarcoptes scabiei B86
  trombiculae B88.0
Agamofilaria streptocerca B74.4
Ancylostoma, ankylostoma (braziliense)
  (caninum) (ceylanicum) (duodenale)
  B76.0
  americanum B76.1
  new world B76.1
Anisakis larvae, anisakiasis B81.0
arthropod NEC B88.2
Ascaris lumbricoides —see Ascariasis
Balantidium coli A07.0
beef tapeworm B68.1
Bothriocephalus (latus) B70.0
  larval B70.1
broad tapeworm B70.0
  larval B70.1
Brugia (malayi) B74.1
  timori B74.2
candiru B88.8
Capillaria
  hepatica B83.8
  philippinensis B81.1
cat liver fluke B66.0
cestodes B71.9
  diphyllobothrium —see Infestation,
    diphyllobothrium
  dipylidiasis B71.1
  hymenolepiasis B71.0
  specified type NEC B71.8
chigger B88.0
chigo, chigoe B88.1
Clonorchis (sinensis) (liver) B66.1
coccidial A07.3
crab-lice B85.3
Cysticercus cellulosae —see Cysticercosis
Demodex (folliculorum) B88.0
Dermanyssus gallinae B88.0
Dermatobia (hominis) —see Myiasis
Dibothriocephalus (latus) B70.0
  larval B70.1
Dicrocoelium dendriticum B66.2
Diphyllobothrium (adult) (latum) (intestinal)
  (pacificum) B70.0
  larval B70.1
Diplogonoporus (grandis) B71.8
Dipylidium caninum B67.4
Distoma hepaticum B66.3
dog tapeworm B67.4
Dracunculus medinensis B72
dragon worm B72
dwarf tapeworm B71.0
Echinococcus —see Echinococcus
Echinostomum ilocanum B66.8
Entamoeba (histolytica) —see Infection,
  Ameba
Enterobius vermicularis B80
eyelid
  in (due to)
    leishmaniasis B55.1
    loiasis B74.3
    onchocerciasis B73.09
    phthiriasis B85.3
  parasitic NOS B89
eyeworm B74.3

Infestation *(Continued)*
  Fasciola (gigantica) (hepatica) (indica) B66.3
  Fasciolopsis (buski) (intestine) B66.5
  filarial B74.9
    bancroftian B74.0
    conjunctiva B74.9
    due to
      Acanthocheilonema (perstans)
        (streptocerca) B74.4
      Brugia (malayi) B74.1
        timori B74.2
      Dracunculus medinensis B72
      guinea worm B72
      loa loa B74.3
      Mansonella (ozzardi) (perstans)
        (streptocerca) B74.4
      Onchocerca volvulus B73.00
        eye B73.00
        eyelid B73.09
      Wuchereria (bancrofti) B74.0
    Malayan B74.1
    ozzardi B74.4
    specified type NEC B74.8
  fish tapeworm B70.0
    larval B70.1
  fluke B66.9
    blood NOS —*see* Schistosomiasis
    cat liver B66.0
    intestinal B66.5
    lancet B66.2
    liver (sheep) B66.3
      cat B66.0
      Chinese B66.1
      due to clonorchiasis B66.1
      oriental B66.1
    lung (oriental) B66.4
    sheep liver B66.3
    specified type NEC B66.8
  fly larvae —*see* Myiasis
  Gasterophilus (intestinalis) —*see* Myiasis
  Gastrodiscoides hominis B66.8
  Giardia lamblia A07.1
  Gnathostoma (spinigerum) B83.1
  Gongylonema B83.8
  guinea worm B72
  helminth B83.9
    angiostrongyliasis B83.2
      intestinal B81.3
    gnathostomiasis B83.1
    hirudiniasis, internal B83.4
    intestinal B82.0
      angiostrongyliasis B81.3
      anisakiasis B81.0
      ascariasis —*see* Ascariasis
      capillariasis B81.1
      cysticercosis —*see* Cysticercosis
      diphyllobothriasis —*see* Infestation,
        diphyllobothriasis
      dracunculiasis B72
      echinococcus —*see* Echinococcosis
      enterobiasis B80
      filariasis —*see* Infestation, filarial
      fluke —*see* Infestation, fluke
      hookworm —*see* Infestation, hookworm
      mixed (types classifiable to more than
        one of the titles B65.0-B81.3 and
        B81.8) B81.4
      onchocerciasis —*see* Onchocerciasis
      schistosomiasis —*see* Infestation,
        schistosoma
      specified
        cestode NEC —*see* Infestation, cestode
          type NEC B81.8
      strongyloidiasis —*see* Strongyloidiasis
      taenia —*see* Infestation, taenia
      trichinellosis B75
      trichostrongyliasis B81.2
      trichuriasis B79
    specified type NEC B83.8
    syngamiasis B83.3
    visceral larva migrans B83.0

Infestation *(Continued)*
  Heterophyes (heterophyes) B66.8
  hookworm B76.9
    ancylostomiasis B76.0
    necatoriasis B76.1
    specified type NEC B76.8
  Hymenolepis (diminuta) (nana) B71.0
  intestinal NEC B82.9
  leeches (aquatic) (land) —*see* Hirudiniasis
  Leishmania —*see* Leishmaniasis
  lice, louse —*see* Infestation, Pediculus
  Linguatula B88.8
  Liponyssoides sanguineus B88.0
  Loa loa B74.3
    conjunctival B74.3
    eyelid B74.3
  louse —*see* Infestation, Pediculus
  maggots —*see* Myiasis
  Mansonella (ozzardi) (perstans) (streptocerca)
    B74.4
  Medina (worm) B72
  Metagonimus (yokogawai) B66.8
  microfilaria streptocerca —*see* Onchocerciasis
    eye B73.00
    eyelid B73.09
  mites B88.9
    scabic B86
  Monilia (albicans) —*see* Candidiasis
  mouth B37.0
  Necator americanus B76.1
  nematode NEC (intestinal) B82.0
    Ancylostoma B76.0
    conjunctiva NEC B83.9
    Enterobius vermicularis B80
    Gnathostoma spinigerum B83.1
    physaloptera B80
    specified NEC B81.8
    trichostrongylus B81.2
    trichuris (trichuria) B79
  Oesophagostomum (apiostomum) B81.8
  Oestrus ovis (*see also* Myiasis) B87.9
  Onchocerca (volvulus) —*see* Onchocerciasis
  Opisthorchis (felineus) (viverrini) B66.0
  orbit, parasitic NOS B89
  Oxyuris vermicularis B80
  Paragonimus (westermani) B66.4
  parasite, parasitic B89
    eyelid B89
    intestinal NOS B82.9
    mouth B37.0
    skin B88.9
    tongue B37.0
  Parastrongylus
    cantonensis B83.2
    costaricensis B81.3
  Pediculus B85.2
    body B85.1
    capitis (humanus) (any site) B85.0
    corporis (humanus) (any site) B85.1
    head B85.0
    mixed (classifiable to more than one of the
      titles B85.0-B85.3) B85.4
    pubis (any site) B85.3
  Pentastoma B88.8
  Phthirus (pubis) (any site) B85.3
    with any infestation classifiable to
      B85.0-B85.2 B85.4
  pinworm B80
  pork tapeworm (adult) B68.0
  protozoal NEC B64
    intestinal A07.9
      specified NEC A07.8
    specified NEC B60.8
  pubic, louse B85.3
  rat tapeworm B71.0
  red bug B88.0
  roundworm (large) NEC B82.0
    Ascariasis (*see also* Ascariasis) B77.9
  sandflea B88.1
  Sarcoptes scabiei B86
  scabies B86

Infestation *(Continued)*
  Schistosoma B65.9
    bovis B65.8
    cercariae B65.3
    haematobium B65.0
    intercalatum B65.8
    japonicum B65.2
    mansoni B65.1
    mattheei B65.8
    mekongi B65.8
    specified type NEC B65.8
    spindale B65.8
  screw worms —*see* Myiasis
  skin NOS B88.9
  Sparganum (mansoni) (proliferum) (baxteri)
    B70.1
    larval B70.1
  specified type NEC B88.8
  Spirometra larvae B70.1
  Stellantchasmus falcatus B66.8
  Strongyloides stercoralis —*see*
    Strongyloidiasis
  Taenia B68.9
    diminuta B71.0
    echinococcus —*see* Echinococcus
    mediocanellata B68.1
    nana B71.0
    saginata B68.1
    solium (intestinal form) B68.0
      larval form —*see* Cysticercosis
  Taeniarhynchus saginatus B68.1
  tapeworm B71.9
    beef B68.1
    broad B70.0
      larval B70.1
    dog B67.4
    dwarf B71.0
    fish B70.0
      larval B70.1
    pork B68.0
    rat B71.0
  Ternidens diminutus B81.8
  Tetranychus molestissimus B88.0
  threadworm B80
  tongue B37.0
  Toxocara (canis) (cati) (felis) B83.0
  trematode (s) NEC —*see* Infestation,
    fluke
  Trichinella (spiralis) B75
  Trichocephalus B79
  Trichomonas —*see* Trichomoniasis
  Trichostrongylus B81.2
  Trichuris (trichiura) B79
  Trombicula (irritans) B88.0
  Tunga penetrans B88.1
  Uncinaria americana B76.1
  Vandellia cirrhosa B88.8
  whipworm B79
  worms B83.9
    intestinal B82.0
  Wuchereria (bancrofti) B74.0
Infiltrate, infiltration
  amyloid (generalized) (localized) —*see*
    Amyloidosis
  calcareous NEC R89.7
    localized —*see* Degeneration, by site
  calcium salt R89.7
  cardiac
    fatty —*see* Degeneration, myocardial
    glycogenic E74.02 *[143]*
  corneal —*see* Edema, cornea
  eyelid —*see* Inflammation, eyelid
  glycogen, glycogenic —*see* Disease,
    glycogen storage
  heart, cardiac
    fatty —*see* Degeneration,
      myocardial
    glycogenic E74.02 *[143]*
  inflammatory in vitreous H43.89
  kidney N28.89
  leukemic —*see* Leukemia

◀ New   ◀▦ Revised   ~~deleted~~ Deleted

Infiltrate, infiltration *(Continued)*
  liver K76.89
    fatty —*see* Fatty, liver NEC
    glycogen *(see also* Disease, glycogen
        storage) E74.03 *[K77]*
  lung R91.8
    eosinophilic J82
  lymphatic *(see also* Leukemia, lymphatic)
      C91.9-
    gland I88.9
  muscle, fatty M62.89
  myocardium, myocardial
    fatty —*see* Degeneration, myocardial
    glycogenic E74.02 *[I43]*
  on chest x-ray R91.8
  pulmonary R91.8
    with eosinophilia J82
  skin (lymphocytic) L98.6
  thymus (gland) (fatty) E32.8
  urine R39.0
  vesicant agent
    antineoplastic chemotherapy T80.810
    other agent NEC T80.818
  vitreous body H43.89
Infirmity R68.89
  senile R54
Inflammation, inflamed, inflammatory (with
    exudation)
  abducent (nerve) —*see* Strabismus, paralytic,
      sixth nerve
  accessory sinus (chronic) —*see* Sinusitis
  adrenal (gland) E27.8
  alveoli, teeth M27.3
    scorbutic E54
  anal canal, anus K62.89
  antrum (chronic) —*see* Sinusitis, maxillary
  appendix —*see* Appendicitis
  arachnoid —*see* Meningitis
  areola N61
    puerperal, postpartum or gestational —*see*
        Infection, nipple
  areolar tissue NOS L08.9
  artery —*see* Arteritis
  auditory meatus (external) —*see* Otitis,
      externa
  Bartholin's gland N75.8
  bile duct (common) (hepatic) or passage —*see*
      Cholangitis
  bladder —*see* Cystitis
  bone —*see* Osteomyelitis
  brain —*see also* Encephalitis
    membrane —*see* Meningitis
  breast N61
    puerperal, postpartum, gestational —*see*
        Mastitis, obstetric
  broad ligament —*see* Disease, pelvis,
      inflammatory
  bronchi —*see* Bronchitis
  catarrhal J00
  cecum —*see* Appendicitis
  cerebral —*see also* Encephalitis
    membrane —*see* Meningitis
  cerebrospinal
    meningococcal A39.0
  cervix (uteri) —*see* Cervicitis
  chest J98.8
  chorioretinal H30.9-
    cyclitis —*see* Cyclitis
    disseminated H30.10-
      generalized H30.13-
      peripheral H30.12-
      posterior pole H30.11-
    epitheliopathy —*see* Epitheliopathy
    focal H30.00-
      juxtapapillary H30.01-
      macular H30.04-
      paramacular —*see* Inflammation,
          chorioretinal, focal, macular
      peripheral H30.03-
      posterior pole H30.02-
    specified type NEC H30.89-

Inflammation, inflamed, inflammatory
    (Continued)
  choroid —*see* Inflammation, chorioretinal
  chronic, postmastoidectomy cavity —*see*
      Complications, postmastoidectomy,
      inflammation
  colon —*see* Enteritis
  connective tissue (diffuse) NEC —*see*
      Disorder, soft tissue, specified type NEC
  cornea —*see* Keratitis
  corpora cavernosa N48.29
  cranial nerve —*see* Disorder, nerve, cranial
  Douglas' cul-de-sac or pouch (chronic) N73.0
  due to device, implant or graft —*see also*
      Complications, by site and type,
      infection or inflammation
    arterial graft T82.7
    breast (implant) T85.79
    catheter T85.79
      dialysis (renal) T82.7
        intraperitoneal T85.71
      infusion T82.7
        spinal (epidural) (subdural) T85.79
      urinary (indwelling) T83.51
    electronic (electrode) (pulse generator)
        (stimulator)
      bone T84.7
      cardiac T82.7
      nervous system (brain) (peripheral
          nerve) (spinal) T85.79
      urinary T83.59
    fixation, internal (orthopedic) NEC —*see*
        Complication, fixation device,
        infection
    gastrointestinal (bile duct) (esophagus)
        T85.79
    genital NEC T83.6
    heart NEC T82.7
      valve (prosthesis) T82.6
        graft T82.7
    joint prosthesis —*see* Complication, joint
        prosthesis, infection
    ocular (corneal graft) (orbital implant)
        NEC T85.79
    orthopedic NEC T84.7
    specified NEC T85.79
    urinary NEC T83.59
    vascular NEC T82.7
    ventricular intracranial shunt T85.79
  duodenum K29.80
    with bleeding K29.81
  dura mater —*see* Meningitis
  ear (middle) —*see also* Otitis, media
    external —*see* Otitis, externa
    inner —*see* subcategory H83.0
  epididymis —*see* Epididymitis
  esophagus K20.9
  ethmoidal (sinus) (chronic) —*see* Sinusitis,
      ethmoidal
  eustachian tube (catarrhal) —*see* Salpingitis,
      eustachian
  eyelid H01.9
    abscess —*see* Abscess, eyelid
    blepharitis —*see* Blepharitis
    chalazion —*see* Chalazion
    dermatosis (noninfectious) —*see*
        Dermatosis, eyelid
    hordeolum —*see* Hordeolum
    specified NEC H01.8
  fallopian tube —*see* Salpingo-oophoritis
  fascia —*see* Myositis
  follicular, pharynx J31.2
  frontal (sinus) (chronic) —*see* Sinusitis, frontal
  gallbladder —*see* Cholecystitis
  gastric —*see* Gastritis
  gastrointestinal —*see* Enteritis
  genital organ (internal) (diffuse)
    female —*see* Disease, pelvis, inflammatory
    male N49.9
      multiple sites N49.8
      specified NEC N49.8

Inflammation, inflamed, inflammatory
    (Continued)
  gland (lymph) —*see* Lymphadenitis
  glottis —*see* Laryngitis
  granular, pharynx J31.2
  gum K05.10
    nonplaque induced K05.11
    plaque induced K05.10
  heart —*see* Carditis
  hepatic duct —*see* Cholangitis
  ileoanal (internal) pouch K91.850
  ileum —*see also* Enteritis
    regional or terminal —*see* Enteritis,
        regional
  intestinal pouch K91.850
  intestine (any part) —*see* Enteritis
  jaw (acute) (bone) (chronic) (lower)
      (suppurative) (upper) M27.2
  joint NEC —*see* Arthritis
    sacroiliac M46.1
  kidney —*see* Nephritis
  knee (joint) M13.169
    tuberculous A18.02
  labium (majus) (minus) —*see* Vulvitis
  lacrimal
    gland —*see* Dacryoadenitis
    passages (duct) (sac) —*see also*
        Dacryocystitis
      canaliculitis —*see* Canaliculitis, lacrimal
  larynx —*see* Laryngitis
  leg NOS L08.9
  lip K13.0
  liver (capsule) —*see also* Hepatitis
    chronic K73.9
    suppurative K75.0
  lung (acute) —*see also* Pneumonia
    chronic J98.4
  lymphatic vessel —*see* Lymphangitis
  lymph gland or node —*see* Lymphadenitis
  maxilla, maxillary M27.2
    sinus (chronic) —*see* Sinusitis, maxillary
  membranes of brain or spinal cord —*see*
      Meningitis
  meninges —*see* Meningitis
  mouth K12.1
  muscle —*see* Myositis
  myocardium —*see* Myocarditis
  nasal sinus (chronic) —*see* Sinusitis
  nasopharynx —*see* Nasopharyngitis
  navel L08.82
  nerve NEC —*see* Neuralgia
  nipple N61
    puerperal, postpartum or gestational —*see*
        Infection, nipple
  nose —*see* Rhinitis
  oculomotor (nerve) —*see* Strabismus,
      paralytic, third nerve
  optic nerve —*see* Neuritis, optic
  orbit (chronic) H05.10
    acute H05.00
      abscess —*see* Abscess, orbit
      cellulitis —*see* Cellulitis, orbit
      osteomyelitis —*see* Osteomyelitis,
          orbit
      periostitis —*see* Periostitis, orbital
      tenonitis —*see* Tenonitis, eye
      granuloma —*see* Granuloma, orbit
      myositis —*see* Myositis, orbital
  ovary —*see* Salpingo-oophoritis
  oviduct —*see* Salpingo-oophoritis
  pancreas (acute) —*see* Pancreatitis
  parametrium N73.0
  parotid region L08.9
  pelvis, female —*see* Disease, pelvis,
      inflammatory
  penis (corpora cavernosa) N48.29
  perianal K62.89
  pericardium —*see* Pericarditis
  perineum (female) (male) L08.9
  perirectal K62.89
  peritoneum —*see* Peritonitis

Inflammation, inflamed, inflammatory
(Continued)
periuterine —*see* Disease, pelvis,
    inflammatory
perivesical —*see* Cystitis
petrous bone (acute) (chronic) —*see* Petrositis
pharynx (acute) —*see* Pharyngitis
pia mater —*see* Meningitis
pleura —*see* Pleurisy
polyp, colon (*see also* Polyp, colon,
    inflammatory) K51.40
prostate —*see also* Prostatitis
    specified type NEC N41.8
rectosigmoid —*see* Rectosigmoiditis
rectum (*see also* Proctitis) K62.89
respiratory, upper (*see also* Infection,
    respiratory, upper) J06.9
    acute, due to radiation J70.0
    chronic, due to external agent —*see*
        condition, respiratory, chronic, due to
    due to
        chemicals, gases, fumes or vapors
            (inhalation) J68.2
        radiation J70.1
retina —*see* Chorioretinitis
retrocecal —*see* Appendicitis
retroperitoneal —*see* Peritonitis
salivary duct or gland (any) (suppurative) —
    see Sialoadenitis
scorbutic, alveoli, teeth E54
scrotum N49.2
seminal vesicle —*see* Vesiculitis
sigmoid —*see* Enteritis
sinus —*see* Sinusitis
Skene's duct or gland —*see* Urethritis
skin L08.9
spermatic cord N49.1
sphenoidal (sinus) —*see* Sinusitis, sphenoidal
spinal
    cord —*see* Encephalitis
    membrane —*see* Meningitis
    nerve —*see* Disorder, nerve
spine —*see* Spondylopathy, inflammatory
spleen (capsule) D73.89
stomach —*see* Gastritis
subcutaneous tissue L08.9
suprarenal (gland) E27.8
synovial —*see* Tenosynovitis
tendon (sheath) NEC —*see* Tenosynovitis
testis —*see* Orchitis
throat (acute) —*see* Pharyngitis
thymus (gland) E32.8
thyroid (gland) —*see* Thyroiditis
tongue K14.0
tonsil —*see* Tonsillitis
trachea —*see* Tracheitis
trochlear (nerve) —*see* Strabismus, paralytic,
    fourth nerve
tubal —*see* Salpingo-oophoritis
tuberculous NEC —*see* Tuberculosis
tubo-ovarian —*see* Salpingo-oophoritis
tunica vaginalis N49.1
tympanic membrane —*see* Tympanitis
umbilicus, umbilical L08.82
uterine ligament —*see* Disease, pelvis,
    inflammatory
uterus (catarrhal) —*see* Endometritis
uveal tract (anterior) NOS —*see also*
    Iridocyclitis
    posterior —*see* Chorioretinitis
vagina —*see* Vaginitis
vas deferens N49.1
vein —*see also* Phlebitis
    intracranial or intraspinal (septic) G08
    thrombotic I80.9
        leg —*see* Phlebitis, leg
        lower extremity —*see* Phlebitis, leg
vocal cord J38.3
vulva —*see* Vulvitis
Wharton's duct (suppurative) —*see*
    Sialoadenitis

Inflation, lung, imperfect (newborn) —*see*
    Atelectasis
Influenza (bronchial) (epidemic) (respiratory
    (upper)) (unidentified influenza virus)
    J11.1
    with
        digestive manifestations J11.2
        encephalopathy J11.81
        enteritis J11.2
        gastroenteritis J11.2
        gastrointestinal manifestations J11.2
        laryngitis J11.1
        myocarditis J11.82
        otitis media J11.83
        pharyngitis J11.1
        pneumonia J11.00
            specified type J11.08
        respiratory manifestations NEC J11.1
        specified manifestation NEC J11.89
    A/H5N1 —*see also* Influenza, due to,
        identified novel influenza A virus J09.X2
    avian —*see also* Influenza, due to, identified
        novel influenza A virus J09.X2
    bird (*see also* Influenza, due to, identified
        novel influenza A virus) J09.X2
    novel (2009) H1N1 influenza (*see also*
        Influenza, due to, identified influenza
        virus NEC) J10.1
    novel influenza A/H1N1 (*see also* Influenza,
        due to, identified influenza virus NEC)
        J10.1
    due to
        avian (*see also* Influenza, due to, identified
            novel influenza A virus) J09.X2
        identified influenza virus NEC J10.1
            with
                digestive manifestations J10.2
                encephalopathy J10.81
                enteritis J10.2
                gastroenteritis J10.2
                gastrointestinal manifestations J10.2
                laryngitis J10.1
                myocarditis J10.82
                otitis media J10.83
                pharyngitis J10.1
                pneumonia (unspecified type) J10.00
                    with same identified influenza virus
                        J10.01
                    specified type NEC J10.08
                respiratory manifestations NEC J10.1
                specified manifestation NEC J10.89
        identified novel influenza A virus J09.X2
            with
                digestive manifestations J09.X3
                encephalopathy J09.X9
                enteritis J09.X3
                gastroenteritis J09.X3
                gastrointestinal manifestations
                    J09.X3
                laryngitis J09.X2
                myocarditis J09.X9
                otitis media J09.X9
                pharyngitis J09.X2
                pneumonia J09.X1
                respiratory manifestations NEC J09.X2
                specified manifestation NEC J09.X9
                upper respiratory symptoms J09.X2
        of other animal origin, not bird or swine (*see
            also* Influenza, due to, identified novel
            influenza A virus) J09.X2
        swine (viruses that normally cause infections
            in pigs) (*see also* Influenza, due to,
            identified novel influenza A virus) J09.
            X2
Influenza-like disease —*see* Influenza
Influenzal —*see* Influenza
Infraction, Freiberg's (metatarsal head) —*see*
    Osteochondrosis, juvenile, metatarsus
Infraeruption of tooth (teeth) M26.34
**Infusion complication, misadventure, or
    reaction** —*see* Complications, infusion

Ingestion
    chemical —*see* Table of Drugs and Chemicals,
        by substance, poisoning
    drug or medicament
        correct substance properly administered —
            see Table of Drugs and Chemicals, by
            drug, adverse effect
        overdose or wrong substance given or
            taken —*see* Table of Drugs and
            Chemicals, by drug, poisoning
    foreign body —*see* Foreign body, alimentary
        tract
    tularemia A21.3
Ingrowing
    hair (beard) L73.1
    nail (finger) (toe) L60.0
Inguinal —*see also* condition
    testicle Q53.9
        bilateral Q53.21
        unilateral Q53.11
Inhalation
    anthrax A22.1
    flame T27.3
    food or foreign body —*see* Foreign body, by
        site
    gases, fumes, or vapors NEC T59.9-
        specified agent —*see* Table of Drugs and
            Chemicals, by substance
    liquid or vomitus —*see* Asphyxia
    meconium (newborn) P24.00
        with
            with respiratory symptoms P24.01
            pneumonia (pneumonitis) P24.01
    mucus —*see* Asphyxia, mucus
    oil or gasoline (causing suffocation) —*see*
        Foreign body, by site
    smoke J70.5
        due to chemicals, gases, fumes and vapors
            J68.9
    steam —*see* Toxicity, vapors
    stomach contents or secretions —*see* Foreign
        body, by site
    due to anesthesia (general) (local) or other
        sedation T88.59
            in labor and delivery O74.0
            in pregnancy O29.01-
            postpartum, puerperal O89.01
Inhibition, orgasm
    female F52.31
    male F52.32
Inhibitor, systemic lupus erythematosus
    (presence of) D68.62
Iniencephalus, iniencephaly Q00.2
Injection, traumatic jet (air) (industrial) (water)
    (paint or dye) T70.4
Injury (*see also* specified injury type)
    T14.90
    abdomen, abdominal S39.91
        blood vessel —*see* Injury, blood vessel,
            abdomen
        cavity —*see* Injury, intra-abdominal
        contusion S30.1
        internal —*see* Injury, intra-abdominal
        intra-abdominal organ —*see* Injury,
            intra-abdominal
        nerve —*see* Injury, nerve, abdomen
        open —*see* Wound, open, abdomen
        specified NEC S39.81
        superficial —*see* Injury, superficial,
            abdomen
    Achilles tendon S86.00-
        laceration S86.02-
        specified type NEC S86.09-
        strain S86.01-
    acoustic, resulting in deafness —*see* Injury,
        nerve, acoustic
    adrenal (gland) S37.819
        contusion S37.812
        laceration S37.813
        specified type NEC S37.818
    alveolar (process) S09.93

◀ New ◀◀ Revised ~~deleted~~ Deleted

Injury *(Continued)*
  ankle S99.91-
    contusion —*see* Contusion, ankle
    dislocation —*see* Dislocation, ankle
    fracture —*see* Fracture, ankle
    nerve —*see* Injury, nerve, ankle
    open —*see* Wound, open, ankle
    specified type NEC S99.81-
    sprain —*see* Sprain, ankle
    superficial —*see* Injury, superficial, ankle
  anterior chamber, eye —*see* Injury, eye, specified site NEC
  anus —*see* Injury, abdomen
  aorta (thoracic) S25.00
    abdominal S35.00
      laceration (minor) (superficial) S35.01
        major S35.02
      specified type NEC S35.09
    laceration (minor) (superficial) S25.01
      major S25.02
    specified type NEC S25.09
  arm (upper) S49.9-
    blood vessel —*see* Injury, blood vessel, arm
    contusion —*see* Contusion, arm, upper
    fracture —*see* Fracture, humerus
    lower —*see* Injury, forearm
    muscle —*see* Injury, muscle, shoulder
    nerve —*see* Injury, nerve, arm
    open —*see* Wound, open, arm
    specified type NEC S49.8-
    superficial —*see* Injury, superficial, arm
  artery (complicating trauma) —*see also* Injury, blood vessel, by site
    cerebral or meningeal —*see* Injury, intracranial
  auditory canal (external) (meatus) S09.91
  auricle, auris, ear S09.91
  axilla —*see* Injury, shoulder
  back —*see* Injury, back, lower
  bile duct S36.13
  birth —*see also* Birth, injury P15.9
  bladder (sphincter) S37.20
    at delivery O71.5
    contusion S37.22
    laceration S37.23
    obstetrical trauma O71.5
    specified type NEC S37.29
  blast (air) (hydraulic) (immersion) (underwater) NEC T14.8
    acoustic nerve trauma —*see* Injury, nerve, acoustic
    bladder —*see* Injury, bladder
    brain —*see* Concussion
    colon —*see* Injury, intestine, large, blast injury
    ear (primary) S09.31-
      secondary S09.39-
    generalized T70.8
    lung —*see* Injury, intrathoracic, lung, blast injury
    multiple body organs T70.8
    peritoneum S36.81
    rectum S36.61
    retroperitoneum S36.898
    small intestine S36.419
      duodenum S36.410
      specified site NEC S36.418
    specified
      intra-abdominal organ NEC S36.898
      pelvic organ NEC S37.899
  blood vessel NEC T14.8
    abdomen S35.9-
      aorta —*see* Injury, aorta, abdominal
      celiac artery —*see* Injury, blood vessel, celiac artery
      iliac vessel —*see* Injury, blood vessel, iliac

Injury *(Continued)*
  blood vessel NEC *(Continued)*
    abdomen *(Continued)*
      laceration S35.91
      mesenteric vessel —*see* Injury, mesenteric
      portal vein —*see* Injury, blood vessel, portal vein
      renal vessel —*see* Injury, blood vessel, renal
      specified vessel NEC S35.8X-
      splenic vessel —*see* Injury, blood vessel, splenic
      vena cava —*see* Injury, vena cava, inferior
    ankle —*see* Injury, blood vessel, foot
    aorta (abdominal) (thoracic) —*see* Injury, aorta
    arm (upper) NEC S45.90-
      forearm —*see* Injury, blood vessel, forearm
      laceration S45.91-
      specified
        site NEC S45.80-
          laceration S45.81-
          specified type NEC S45.89-
        type NEC S45.99-
      superficial vein S45.30-
        laceration S45.31-
        specified type NEC S45.39-
    axillary
      artery S45.00-
        laceration S45.01-
        specified type NEC S45.09-
      vein S45.20-
        laceration S45.21-
        specified type NEC S45.29-
    azygos vein —*see* Injury, blood vessel, thoracic, specified site NEC
    brachial
      artery S45.10-
        laceration S45.11-
        specified type NEC S45.19-
      vein S45.20-
        laceration S45.219
        specified type NEC S45.29-
    carotid artery (common) (external) (internal, extracranial) S15.00-
      internal, intracranial S06.8-
      laceration (minor) (superficial) S15.01-
        major S15.02-
      specified type NEC S15.09-
    celiac artery S35.219
      branch S35.299
        laceration (minor) (superficial) S35.291
          major S35.292
        specified NEC S35.298
      laceration (minor) (superficial) S35.211
        major S35.212
      specified type NEC S35.218
    cerebral —*see* Injury, intracranial
    deep plantar —*see* Injury, blood vessel, plantar artery
    digital (hand) —*see* Injury, blood vessel, finger
    dorsal
      artery (foot) S95.00-
        laceration S95.01-
        specified type NEC S95.09-
      vein (foot) S95.20-
        laceration S95.21-
        specified type NEC S95.29-
    due to accidental laceration during procedure —*see* Laceration, accidental complicating surgery
    extremity —*see* Injury, blood vessel, limb
    femoral
      artery (common) (superficial) S75.00-
        laceration (minor) (superficial) S75.01-
          major S75.02-
        specified type NEC S75.09-

Injury *(Continued)*
  blood vessel NEC *(Continued)*
    femoral *(Continued)*
      vein (hip level) (thigh level) S75.10-
        laceration (minor) (superficial) S75.11-
          major S75.12-
        specified type NEC S75.19-
    finger S65.50-
      index S65.50-
        laceration S65.51-
        specified type NEC S65.59-
      laceration S65.51-
      little S65.50-
        laceration S65.51-
        specified type NEC S65.59-
      middle S65.50-
        laceration S65.51-
        specified type NEC S65.59-
      specified type NEC S65.59-
      thumb —*see* Injury, blood vessel, thumb
    foot S95.90-
      dorsal
        artery —*see* Injury, blood vessel, dorsal, artery
        vein —*see* Injury, blood vessel, dorsal, vein
      laceration S95.91-
      plantar artery —*see* Injury, blood vessel, plantar artery
      specified
        site NEC S95.80-
          laceration S95.81-
          specified type NEC S95.89-
        specified type NEC S95.99-
    forearm S55.90-
      laceration S55.91-
      radial artery —*see* Injury, blood vessel, radial artery
      specified
        site NEC S55.80-
          laceration S55.81-
          specified type NEC S55.89-
        type NEC S55.99-
      ulnar artery —*see* Injury, blood vessel, ulnar artery
      vein S55.20-
        laceration S55.21-
        specified type NEC S55.29-
    gastric
      artery —*see* Injury, mesenteric, artery, branch
      vein —*see* Injury, blood vessel, abdomen
    gastroduodenal artery —*see* Injury, mesenteric, artery, branch
    greater saphenous vein (lower leg level) S85.30-
      hip (and thigh) level S75.20-
        laceration (minor) (superficial) S75.21-
          major S75.22-
        specified type NEC S75.29-
      laceration S85.31-
      specified type NEC S85.39-
    hand (level) S65.90-
      finger —*see* Injury, blood vessel, finger
      laceration S65.91-
      palmar arch —*see* Injury, blood vessel, palmar arch
      radial artery —*see* Injury, blood vessel, radial artery, hand
      specified
        site NEC S65.80-
          laceration S65.81-
          specified type NEC S65.89-
        type NEC S65.99-
      thumb —*see* Injury, blood vessel, thumb
      ulnar artery —*see* Injury, blood vessel, ulnar artery, hand
    head S09.0
      intracranial —*see* Injury, intracranial
      multiple S09.0

Injury *(Continued)*
    blood vessel NEC *(Continued)*
        hepatic
            artery —*see* Injury, mesenteric, artery
            vein —*see* Injury, vena cava, inferior
        hip S75.90-
            femoral artery —*see* Injury, blood vessel,
                femoral, artery
            femoral vein —*see* Injury, blood vessel,
                femoral, vein
            greater saphenous vein —*see* Injury,
                blood vessel, greater saphenous,
                hip level
            laceration S75.91-
            specified
                site NEC S75.80-
                    laceration S75.81-
                    specified type NEC S75.89-
                type NEC S75.99-
        hypogastric (artery) (vein) —*see* Injury,
            blood vessel, iliac
        iliac S35.5-
            artery S35.51-
            specified vessel NEC S35.5-
            uterine vessel —*see* Injury, blood vessel,
                uterine
            vein S35.51-
        innominate —*see* Injury, blood vessel,
            thoracic, innominate
        intercostal (artery) (vein) —*see* Injury,
            blood vessel, thoracic, intercostal
        jugular vein (external) S15.20-
            internal S15.30-
                laceration (minor) (superficial)
                    S15.31-
                    major S15.32-
                specified type NEC S15.39-
            laceration (minor) (superficial) S15.21-
                major S15.22-
            specified type NEC S15.29-
        leg (level) (lower) S85.90-
            greater saphenous —*see* Injury, blood
                vessel, greater saphenous
            laceration S85.91-
            lesser saphenous —*see* Injury, blood
                vessel, lesser saphenous
            peroneal artery —*see* Injury, blood
                vessel, peroneal artery
            popliteal
                artery —*see* Injury, blood vessel,
                    popliteal, artery
                vein —*see* Injury, blood vessel,
                    popliteal, vein
            specified
                site NEC S85.80-
                    laceration S85.81-
                    specified type NEC S85.89-
                type NEC S85.99-
            thigh —*see* Injury, blood vessel, hip
            tibial artery —*see* Injury, blood vessel,
                tibial artery
        lesser saphenous vein (lower leg level)
            S85.40-
            laceration S85.41-
            specified type NEC S85.49-
        limb
            lower —*see* Injury, blood vessel, leg
            upper —*see* Injury, blood vessel, arm
        lower back —*see* Injury, blood vessel,
            abdomen
            specified NEC —*see* Injury, blood
                vessel, abdomen, specified, site
                NEC
        mammary (artery) (vein) —*see* Injury,
            blood vessel, thoracic, specified site
            NEC
        mesenteric (inferior) (superior)
            artery —*see* Injury, mesenteric, artery
            vein —*see* Injury, mesenteric, vein
        neck S15.9
            specified site NEC S15.8

Injury *(Continued)*
    blood vessel NEC *(Continued)*
        ovarian (artery) (vein) —*see* subcategory
            S35.8
        palmar arch (superficial) S65.20-
            deep S65.30-
                laceration S65.31-
                specified type NEC S65.39-
            laceration S65.21-
            specified type NEC S65.29-
        pelvis —*see* Injury, blood vessel, abdomen
            specified NEC —*see* Injury, blood vessel,
                abdomen, specified, site NEC
        peroneal artery S85.20-
            laceration S85.21-
            specified type NEC S85.29-
        plantar artery (deep) (foot) S95.10-
            laceration S95.11-
            specified type NEC S95.19-
        popliteal
            artery S85.00-
                laceration S85.01-
                specified type NEC S85.09-
            vein S85.50-
                laceration S85.51-
                specified type NEC S85.59-
        portal vein S35.319
            laceration S35.311
            specified type NEC S35.318
        precerebral —*see* Injury, blood vessel, neck
        pulmonary (artery) (vein) —*see* Injury,
            blood vessel, thoracic, pulmonary
        radial artery (forearm level) S55.10-
            hand and wrist (level) S65.10-
                laceration S65.11-
                specified type NEC S65.19-
            laceration S55.11-
            specified type NEC S55.19-
        renal
            artery S35.40-
                laceration S35.41-
                specified NEC S35.49-
            vein S35.40-
                laceration S35.41-
                specified NEC S35.49-
        saphenous vein (greater) (lower leg
            level) —*see* Injury, blood vessel,
            greater saphenous
            hip and thigh level —*see* Injury, blood
                vessel, greater saphenous, hip level
            lesser —*see* Injury, blood vessel, lesser
                saphenous
        shoulder
            specified NEC —*see* Injury, blood vessel,
                arm, specified site NEC
            superficial vein —*see* Injury, blood
                vessel, arm, superficial vein
        specified NEC T14.8
        splenic
            artery —*see* Injury, blood vessel, celiac
                artery, branch
            vein S35.329
                laceration S35.321
                specified NEC S35.328
        subclavian —*see* Injury, blood vessel,
            thoracic, innominate
        thigh —*see* Injury, blood vessel, hip
        thoracic S25.90
            aorta S25.00
                laceration (minor) (superficial)
                    S25.01
                    major S25.02
                specified type NEC S25.09
            azygos vein —*see* Injury, blood vessel,
                thoracic, specified, site NEC
            innominate
                artery S25.10-
                    laceration (minor) (superficial)
                        S25.11-
                        major S25.12-
                    specified type NEC S25.19-

Injury *(Continued)*
    blood vessel NEC *(Continued)*
        thoracic *(Continued)*
            innominate *(Continued)*
                vein S25.30-
                    laceration (minor) (superficial)
                        S25.31-
                        major S25.32-
                    specified type NEC S25.39-
            intercostal S25.50-
                laceration S25.51-
                specified type NEC S25.59-
            laceration S25.91
            mammary vessel —*see* Injury, blood
                vessel, thoracic, specified, site NEC
            pulmonary S25.40-
                laceration (minor) (superficial) S25.41-
                    major S25.42-
                specified type NEC S25.49-
            specified
                site NEC S25.80-
                    laceration S25.81-
                    specified type NEC S25.89-
                type NEC S25.99
            subclavian —*see* Injury, blood vessel,
                thoracic, innominate
            vena cava (superior) S25.20
                laceration (minor) (superficial) S25.21
                    major S25.22
                specified type NEC S25.29
        thumb S65.40-
            laceration S65.41-
            specified type NEC S65.49-
        tibial artery S85.10-
            anterior S85.13-
                laceration S85.14-
                specified injury NEC S85.15-
            laceration S85.11-
            posterior S85.16-
                laceration S85.17-
                specified injury NEC S85.18-
            specified injury NEC S85.12-
        ulnar artery (forearm level) S55.00-
            hand and wrist (level) S65.00-
                laceration S65.01-
                specified type NEC S65.09-
            laceration S55.01-
            specified type NEC S55.09-
        upper arm (level) —*see* Injury, blood vessel,
            arm
            superficial vein —*see* Injury, blood
                vessel, arm, superficial vein
        uterine S35.5-
            artery S35.53-
            vein S35.53-
        vena cava —*see* Injury, vena cava
        vertebral artery S15.10-
            laceration (minor) (superficial) S15.11-
                major S15.12-
            specified type NEC S15.19-
        wrist (level) —*see* Injury, blood vessel,
            hand
    brachial plexus S14.3
        newborn P14.3
    brain (traumatic) S06.9-
        diffuse (axonal) S06.2X-
        focal S06.30-
        traumatic —*see* category S06
    brainstem S06.38-
    breast NOS S29.9
    broad ligament —*see* Injury, pelvic organ,
        specified site NEC
    bronchus, bronchi —*see* Injury, intrathoracic,
        bronchus
    brow S09.90
    buttock S39.92
    canthus, eye S05.90
    cardiac plexus —*see* Injury, nerve, thorax,
        sympathetic
    cauda equina S34.3
    cavernous sinus —*see* Injury, intracranial

◀ New   ◀▦ Revised   ~~deleted~~ Deleted

Injury (*Continued*)

cecum —*see* Injury, colon
celiac ganglion or plexus —*see* Injury, nerve, lumbosacral, sympathetic
cerebellum —*see* Injury, intracranial
cerebral —*see* Injury, intracranial
cervix (uteri) —*see* Injury, uterus
cheek (wall) S09.93
chest —*see* Injury, thorax
childbirth (newborn) —*see also* Birth, injury
    maternal NEC O71.9
chin S09.93
choroid (eye) —*see* Injury, eye, specified site NEC
clitoris S39.94
coccyx —*see also* Injury, back, lower
    complicating delivery O71.6
colon —*see* Injury, intestine, large
common bile duct —*see* Injury, liver
conjunctiva (superficial) —*see* Injury, eye, conjunctiva
conus medullaris —*see* Injury, spinal, sacral cord
    spermatic (pelvic region) S37.898
        scrotal region S39.848
    spinal —*see* Injury, spinal cord, by region
cornea —*see* Injury, eye, specified site NEC
    abrasion —*see* Injury, eye, cornea, abrasion
cortex (cerebral) —*see also* Injury, intracranial
    visual —*see* Injury, nerve, optic
costal region NEC S29.9
costochondral NEC S29.9
cranial
    cavity —*see* Injury, intracranial
    nerve —*see* Injury, nerve, cranial
crushing —*see* Crush
cutaneous sensory nerve
cystic duct —*see* Injury, liver
deep tissue —*see* Contusion, by site
    meaning pressure ulcer —*see* Ulcer, pressure, unstageable, by site
delivery (newborn) P15.9
    maternal NEC O71.9
Descemet's membrane —*see* Injury, eyeball, penetrating
diaphragm —*see* Injury, intrathoracic, diaphragm
duodenum —*see* Injury, intestine, small, duodenum
ear (auricle) (external) (canal) S09.91
    abrasion —*see* Abrasion, ear
    bite —*see* Bite, ear
    blister —*see* Blister, ear
    bruise —*see* Contusion, ear
    contusion —*see* Contusion, ear
    external constriction —*see* Constriction, external, ear
    hematoma —*see* Hematoma, ear
    inner —*see* Injury, ear, middle
    laceration —*see* Laceration, ear
    middle S09.30-
        blast —*see* Injury, blast, ear
        specified NEC S09.39-
    puncture —*see* Puncture, ear
    superficial —*see* Injury, superficial, ear
eighth cranial nerve (acoustic or auditory) — *see* Injury, nerve, acoustic
elbow S59.90-
    contusion —*see* Contusion, elbow
    dislocation —*see* Dislocation, elbow
    fracture —*see* Fracture, ulna, upper end
    open —*see* Wound, open, elbow
    specified NEC S59.80-
    sprain —*see* Sprain, elbow
    superficial —*see* Injury, superficial, elbow
eleventh cranial nerve (accessory) —*see* Injury, nerve, accessory
epididymis S39.94
epigastric region S39.91
epiglottis NEC S19.89

Injury (*Continued*)

esophageal plexus —*see* Injury, nerve, thorax, sympathetic
esophagus (thoracic part) —*see also* Injury, intrathoracic, esophagus
    cervical NEC S19.85
eustachian tube S09.30-
eye S05.9-
    avulsion S05.7-
    ball —*see* Injury, eyeball
    conjunctiva S05.0-
    cornea
        abrasion S05.0-
        laceration S05.3-
            with prolapse S05.2-
    lacrimal apparatus S05.8X-
    orbit penetration S05.4-
    specified site NEC S05.8X-
eyeball S05.8X-
    contusion S05.1-
    penetrating S05.6-
        with
            foreign body S05.5-
            prolapse or loss of intraocular tissue S05.2-
        without prolapse or loss of intraocular tissue S05.3-
    specificd type NEC S05.8-
eyebrow S09.93
eyelid S09.93
    abrasion —*see* Abrasion, eyelid
    contusion —*see* Contusion, eyelid
    open —*see* Wound, open, eyelid
face S09.93
fallopian tube S37.509
    bilateral S37.502
        blast injury S37.512
        contusion S37.522
        laceration S37.532
        specified type NEC S37.592
    blast injury (primary) S37.519
        bilateral S37.512
        secondary —*see* Injury, fallopian tube, specified type NEC
        unilateral S37.511
    contusion S37.529
        bilateral S37.522
        unilateral S37.521
    laceration S37.539
        bilateral S37.532
        unilateral S37.531
    specified type NEC S37.599
        bilateral S37.592
        unilateral S37.591
    unilateral S37.501
        blast injury S37.511
        contusion S37.521
        laceration S37.531
        specified type NEC S37.591
fascia —*see* Injury, muscle
fifth cranial nerve (trigeminal) —*see* Injury, nerve, trigeminal
finger (nail) S69.9-
    blood vessel —*see* Injury, blood vessel, finger
    contusion —*see* Contusion, finger
    dislocation —*see* Dislocation, finger
    fracture —*see* Fracture, finger
    muscle —*see* Injury, muscle, finger
    nerve —*see* Injury, nerve, digital, finger
    open —*see* Wound, open, finger
    specified NEC S69.8-
    sprain —*see* Sprain, finger
    superficial —*see* Injury, superficial, finger
first cranial nerve (olfactory) —*see* Injury, nerve, olfactory
flank —*see* Injury, abdomen
foot S99.92-
    blood vessel —*see* Injury, blood vessel, foot
    contusion —*see* Contusion, foot
    dislocation —*see* Dislocation, foot

Injury (*Continued*)

foot (*Continued*)
    fracture —*see* Fracture, foot
    muscle —*see* Injury, muscle, foot
    open —*see* Wound, open, foot
    specified type NEC S99.82-
    sprain —*see* Sprain, foot
    superficial —*see* Injury, superficial, foot
forceps NOS P15.9
forearm S59.91-
    blood vessel —*see* Injury, blood vessel, forearm
    contusion —*see* Contusion, forearm
    fracture —*see* Fracture, forearm
    muscle —*see* Injury, muscle, forearm
    nerve —*see* Injury, nerve, forearm
    open —*see* Wound, open, forearm
    specified NEC S59.81-
    superficial —*see* Injury, superficial, forearm
forehead S09.90
fourth cranial nerve (trochlear) —*see* Injury, nerve, trochlear
gallbladder S36.129
    contusion S36.122
    laceration S36.123
    specified NEC S36.128
ganglion
    celiac, coeliac —*see* Injury, nerve, lumbosacral, sympathetic
    gasserian —*see* Injury, nerve, trigeminal
    stellate —*see* Injury, nerve, thorax, sympathetic
    thoracic sympathetic —*see* Injury, nerve, thorax, sympathetic
gasserian ganglion —*see* Injury, nerve, trigeminal
gastric artery —*see* Injury, blood vessel, celiac artery, branch
gastroduodenal artery —*see* Injury, blood vessel, celiac artery, branch
gastrointestinal tract —*see* Injury, intra-abdominal
    with open wound into abdominal cavity — *see* Wound, open, with penetration into peritoneal cavity
    colon —*see* Injury, intestine, large
    rectum —*see* Injury, intestine, large, rectum
        with open wound into abdominal cavity S36.61
    small intestine —*see* Injury, intestine, small
    specified site NEC —*see* Injury, intra-abdominal, specified, site NEC
    stomach —*see* Injury, stomach
genital organ (s)
    external S39.94
        specified NEC S39.848
    internal S37.90
        fallopian tube —*see* Injury, fallopian tube
        ovary —*see* Injury, ovary
        prostate —*see* Injury, prostate
        seminal vesicle —*see* Injury, pelvis, organ, specified site NEC
        uterus —*see* Injury, uterus
        vas deferens —*see* Injury, pelvis, organ, specified site NEC
    obstetrical trauma O71.9
gland
    lacrimal laceration —*see* Injury, eye, specified site NEC
    salivary S09.90
    thyroid NEC S19.84
globe (eye) S05.90
    specified NEC S05.8X-
groin —*see* Injury, abdomen
gum S09.90
hand S69.9-
    blood vessel —*see* Injury, blood vessel, hand
    contusion —*see* Contusion, hand
    fracture —*see* Fracture, hand
    muscle —*see* Injury, muscle, hand

Injury (Continued)
  hand (Continued)
    nerve —see Injury, nerve, hand
    open —see Wound, open, hand
    specified NEC S69.8-
    sprain —see Sprain, hand
    superficial —see Injury, superficial, hand
  head S09.90
    with loss of consciousness S06.9-
    specified NEC S09.8-
  heart S26.90
    with hemopericardium S26.00
      contusion S26.01
      laceration (mild) S26.020
        major S26.022
        moderate S26.021
      specified type NEC S26.09
    without hemopericardium S26.10
      contusion S26.11
      laceration S26.12
      specified type NEC S26.19
    contusion S26.91
    laceration S26.92
    specified type NEC S26.99
  heel —see Injury, foot
  hepatic
    artery —see Injury, blood vessel, celiac
        artery, branch
    duct —see Injury, liver
    vein —see Injury, vena cava, inferior
  hip S79.91-
    blood vessel —see Injury, blood vessel, hip
    contusion —see Contusion, hip
    dislocation —see Dislocation, hip
    fracture —see Fracture, femur, neck
    muscle —see Injury, muscle, hip
    nerve —see Injury, nerve, hip
    open —see Wound, open, hip
    specified NEC S79.81-
    sprain —see Sprain, hip
    superficial —see Injury, superficial, hip
  hymen S39.94
  hypogastric
    blood vessel —see Injury, blood vessel, iliac
    plexus —see Injury, nerve, lumbosacral,
        sympathetic
  ileum —see Injury, intestine, small
  iliac region S39.91
  instrumental (during surgery) —see
        Laceration, accidental complicating
        surgery
    birth injury —see Birth, injury
    nonsurgical —see Injury, by site
    obstetrical O71.9
      bladder O71.5
      cervix O71.3
      high vaginal O71.4
      perineal NOS O70.9
      urethra O71.5
      uterus O71.5
        with rupture or perforation O71.1
  internal T14.8
    aorta —see Injury, aorta
    bladder (sphincter) —see Injury, bladder
      with
        ectopic or molar pregnancy O08.6
        following ectopic or molar pregnancy
            O08.6
        obstetrical trauma O71.5
    bronchus, bronchi —see Injury,
        intrathoracic, bronchus
    cecum —see Injury, intestine, large
    cervix (uteri) —see also Injury, uterus
      with ectopic or molar pregnancy O08.6
      following ectopic or molar pregnancy
            O08.6
      obstetrical trauma O71.3
    chest —see Injury, intrathoracic
    gastrointestinal tract —see Injury,
        intra-abdominal
    heart —see Injury, heart

Injury (Continued)
  internal (Continued)
    intestine NEC —see Injury, intestine
    intrauterine —see Injury, uterus
    mesentery —see Injury, intra-abdominal,
        specified, site NEC
    pelvis, pelvic (organ) S37.90
      following ectopic or molar pregnancy
          (subsequent episode) O08.6
      obstetrical trauma NEC O71.5
        rupture or perforation O71.1
      specified NEC S39.83
    rectum —see Injury, intestine, large,
        rectum
    stomach —see Injury, stomach
    ureter —see Injury, ureter
    urethra (sphincter) following ectopic or
        molar pregnancy O08.6
    uterus —see Injury, uterus
  interscapular area —see Injury, thorax
  intestine
    large S36.509
      ascending (right) S36.500
        blast injury (primary) S36.510
          secondary S36.590
        contusion S36.520
        laceration S36.530
        specified type NEC S36.590
      blast injury (primary) S36.519
        ascending (right) S36.510
        descending (left) S36.512
        rectum S36.61
        sigmoid S36.513
        specified site NEC S36.518
        transverse S36.511
      contusion S36.529
        ascending (right) S36.520
        descending (left) S36.522
        rectum S36.62
        sigmoid S36.523
        specified site NEC S36.528
        transverse S36.521
      descending (left) S36.502
        blast injury (primary) S36.512
          secondary S36.592
        contusion S36.522
        laceration S36.532
        specified type NEC S36.592
      laceration S36.539
        ascending (right) S36.530
        descending (left) S36.532
        rectum S36.63
        sigmoid S36.533
        specified site NEC S36.538
        transverse S36.531
      rectum S36.60
        blast injury (primary) S36.61
          secondary S36.69
        contusion S36.62
        laceration S36.63
        specified type NEC S36.69
      sigmoid S36.503
        blast injury (primary) S36.513
          secondary S36.593
        contusion S36.523
        laceration S36.533
        specified type NEC S36.593
      specified
        site NEC S36.508
          blast injury (primary) S36.518
            secondary S36.598
          contusion S36.528
          laceration S36.538
          specified type NEC S36.598
        type NEC S36.599
          ascending (right) S36.590
          descending (left) S36.592
          rectum S36.69
          sigmoid S36.593
          specified site NEC S36.598
          transverse S36.591

Injury (Continued)
  intestine (Continued)
    large (Continued)
      transverse S36.501
        blast injury (primary) S36.511
          secondary S36.591
        contusion S36.521
        laceration S36.531
        specified type NEC S36.591
    small S36.409
      blast injury (primary) S36.419
        duodenum S36.410
        secondary S36.499
          duodenum S36.490
          specified site NEC S36.498
        specified site NEC S36.418
      contusion S36.429
        duodenum S36.420
        specified site NEC S36.428
      duodenum S36.400
        blast injury (primary) S36.410
          secondary S36.490
        contusion S36.420
        laceration S36.430
        specified NEC S36.490
      laceration S36.439
        duodenum S36.430
        specified site NEC S36.438
      specified
        site NEC S36.408
        type NEC S36.499
          duodenum S36.490
          specified site NEC S36.498
    intra-abdominal S36.90
      adrenal gland —see Injury, adrenal gland
      bladder —see Injury, bladder
      colon —see Injury, intestine, large
      contusion S36.92
      fallopian tube —see Injury, fallopian tube
      gallbladder —see Injury, gallbladder
      intestine —see Injury, intestine
      kidney —see Injury, kidney
      laceration S36.93
      liver —see Injury, liver
      ovary —see Injury, ovary
      pancreas —see Injury, pancreas
      pelvic NOS S37.90
      peritoneum —see Injury, intra-abdominal,
          specified, site NEC
      prostate —see Injury, prostate
      rectum —see Injury, intestine, large, rectum
      retroperitoneum —see Injury, intra-
          abdominal, specified, site NEC
      seminal vesicle —see Injury, pelvis, organ,
          specified site NEC
      small intestine —see Injury, intestine, small
      specified
        pelvic S37.90
          specified
            site NEC S37.899
              specified type NEC S37.898
            type NEC S37.99
        site NEC S36.899
          contusion S36.892
          laceration S36.893
          specified type NEC S36.898
        type NEC S36.99
      spleen —see Injury, spleen
      stomach —see Injury, stomach
      ureter —see Injury, ureter
      urethra —see Injury, urethra
      uterus —see Injury, uterus
      vas deferens —see Injury, pelvis, organ,
          specified site NEC
    intracranial (traumatic) S06.9-
      cerebellar hemorrhage, traumatic —see
          Injury, intracranial, focal
      cerebral edema, traumatic S06.1X-
        diffuse S06.1X-
        focal S06.1X-
      diffuse (axonal) S06.2X-

◀ New   ◀▥ Revised   ~~deleted~~ Deleted

Injury (*Continued*)
  intracranial (*Continued*)
    epidural hemorrhage (traumatic) S06.4X-
    focal brain injury S06.30-
      contusion —*see* Contusion, cerebral
      laceration —*see* Laceration, cerebral
    intracerebral hemorrhage, traumatic
      S06.36-
      left side S06.35-
      right side S06.34-
    subarachnoid hemorrhage, traumatic
      S06.6X-
    subdural hemorrhage, traumatic S06.5X-
  intraocular —*see* Injury, eyeball, penetrating
  intrathoracic S27.9
    bronchus S27.409
      bilateral S27.402
      blast injury (primary) S27.419
        bilateral S27.412
        secondary —*see* Injury, intrathoracic,
          bronchus, specified type NEC
        unilateral S27.411
      contusion S27.429
        bilateral S27.422
        unilateral S27.421
      laceration S27.439
        bilateral S27.432
        unilateral S27.431
      specified type NEC S27.499
        bilateral S27.492
        unilateral S27.491
      unilateral S27.401
    diaphragm S27.809
      contusion S27.802
      laceration S27.803
      specified type NEC S27.808
    esophagus (thoracic) S27.819
      contusion S27.812
      laceration S27.813
      specified type NEC S27.818
    heart —*see* Injury, heart
    hemopneumothorax S27.2
    hemothorax S27.1
    lung S27.309
      aspiration J69.0
      bilateral S27.302
      blast injury (primary) S27.319
        bilateral S27.312
        secondary —*see* Injury, intrathoracic,
          lung, specified type NEC
        unilateral S27.311
      contusion S27.329
        bilateral S27.322
        unilateral S27.321
      laceration S27.339
        bilateral S27.332
        unilateral S27.331
      specified type NEC S27.399
        bilateral S27.392
        unilateral S27.391
      unilateral S27.301
    pleura S27.60
      laceration S27.63
      specified type NEC S27.69
    pneumothorax S27.0
    specified organ NEC S27.899
      contusion S27.892
      laceration S27.893
      specified type NEC S27.898
    thoracic duct —*see* Injury, intrathoracic,
      specified organ NEC
    thymus gland —*see* Injury, intrathoracic,
      specified organ NEC
    trachea, thoracic S27.50
      blast (primary) S27.51
      contusion S27.52
      laceration S27.53
      specified type NEC S27.59
  iris —*see* Injury, eye, specified site NEC
    penetrating —*see* Injury, eyeball,
      penetrating

Injury (*Continued*)
  jaw S09.93
  jejunum —*see* Injury, intestine, small
  joint NOS T14.8
    old or residual —*see* Disorder, joint,
      specified type NEC
  kidney S37.00-
    acute (nontraumatic) N17.9
    contusion —*see* Contusion, kidney
    laceration —*see* Laceration, kidney
    specified NEC S37.09-
  knee S89.9-
    contusion —*see* Contusion, knee
    dislocation —*see* Dislocation, knee
    meniscus (lateral) (medial) —*see* Sprain,
      knee, specified site NEC
      old injury or tear —*see* Derangement,
        knee, meniscus, due to old injury
    open —*see* Wound, open, knee
    specified NEC S89.8-
    sprain —*see* Sprain, knee
    superficial —*see* Injury, superficial, knee
  labium (majus) (minus) S39.94
  labyrinth, ear S09.30-
  lacrimal apparatus, duct, gland, or sac —*see*
    Injury, eye, specified site NEC
  larynx NEC S19.81
  leg (lower) S89.9-
    blood vessel —*see* Injury, blood vessel, leg
    contusion —*see* Contusion, leg
    fracture —*see* Fracture, leg
    muscle —*see* Injury, muscle, leg
    nerve —*see* Injury, nerve, leg
    open —*see* Wound, open, leg
    specified NEC S89.8-
    superficial —*see* Injury, superficial, leg
  lens, eye —*see* Injury, eye, specified site NEC
    penetrating —*see* Injury, eyeball,
      penetrating
  limb NEC T14.8
  lip S09.93
  liver S36.119
    contusion S36.112
    laceration S36.113
      major (stellate) S36.116
      minor S36.114
      moderate S36.115
      specified NEC S36.118
  lower back S39.92
    specified NEC S39.82
  lumbar, lumbosacral (region) S39.92
    plexus —*see* Injury, lumbosacral plexus
  lumbosacral plexus S34.4
  lung —*see also* Injury, intrathoracic, lung
    aspiration J69.0
    transfusion-related (TRALI) J95.84
  lymphatic thoracic duct —*see* Injury,
    intrathoracic, specified organ NEC
  malar region S09.93
  mastoid region S09.90
  maxilla S09.93
  mediastinum —*see* Injury, intrathoracic,
    specified organ NEC
  membrane, brain —*see* Injury, intracranial
  meningeal artery —*see* Injury, intracranial,
    subdural hemorrhage
  meninges (cerebral) —*see* Injury, intracranial
  mesenteric
    artery
      branch S35.299
        laceration (minor) (superficial) S35.291
        major S35.292
        specified NEC S35.298
      inferior S35.239
        laceration (minor) (superficial) S35.231
        major S35.232
        specified NEC S35.238
      superior S35.229
        laceration (minor) (superficial) S35.221
        major S35.222
        specified NEC S35.228

Injury (*Continued*)
  mesenteric (*Continued*)
    plexus (inferior) (superior) —*see* Injury,
      nerve, lumbosacral, sympathetic
    vein
      inferior S35.349
        laceration S35.341
        specified NEC S35.348
      superior S35.339
        laceration S35.331
        specified NEC S35.338
  mesentery —*see* Injury, intra-abdominal,
    specified site NEC
  mesosalpinx —*see* Injury, pelvic organ,
    specified site NEC
  middle ear S09.30-
  midthoracic region NOS S29.9
  mouth S09.93
  multiple NOS T07
  muscle (and fascia) (and tendon)
    abdomen S39.001
      laceration S39.021
      specified type NEC S39.091
      strain S39.011
    abductor
      thumb, forearm level —*see* Injury,
        muscle, thumb, abductor
    adductor
      thigh S76.20-
        laceration S76.22-
        specified type NEC S76.29-
        strain S76.21-
    ankle —*see* Injury, muscle, foot
    anterior muscle group, at leg level (lower)
      S86.20-
      laceration S86.22-
      specified type NEC S86.29-
      strain S86.21-
    arm (upper) —*see* Injury, muscle,
      shoulder
    biceps (parts NEC) S46.20-
      laceration S46.22-
      long head S46.10-
        laceration S46.12-
        specified type NEC S46.19-
        strain S46.11-
      specified type NEC S46.29-
      strain S46.21-
    extensor
      finger (s) (other than thumb) —*see* Injury,
        muscle, finger by site, extensor
      forearm level, specified NEC —*see*
        Injury, muscle, forearm, extensor
      thumb —*see* Injury, muscle, thumb,
        extensor
      toe (large) (ankle level) (foot level) —*see*
        Injury, muscle, toe, extensor
    finger
      extensor (forearm level) S56.40-
        hand level S66.309
          laceration S66.329
          specified type NEC S66.399
          strain S66.319
        laceration S56.429
        specified type NEC S56.499
        strain S56.419
      flexor (forearm level) S56.10-
        hand level S66.109
          laceration S66.129
          specified type NEC S66.199
          strain S66.119
        laceration S56.129
        specified type NEC S56.199
        strain S56.119
      index
        extensor (forearm level)
          hand level S66.308
            laceration S66.32-
            specified type NEC S66.39-
            strain S66.31-
          specified type NEC S56.492-

Injury (Continued)
  muscle (Continued)
    finger (Continued)
      index (Continued)
        flexor (forearm level)
          hand level S66.108
            laceration S66.12-
            specified type NEC
              S66.19-
            strain S66.11-
          specified type NEC S56.19-
          strain S56.11-
        intrinsic S66.50-
          laceration S66.52-
          specified type NEC S66.59-
          strain S66.51-
      intrinsic S66.509
        laceration S66.529
        specified type NEC S66.599
        strain S66.519
      little
        extensor (forearm level)
          hand level S66.30-
            laceration S66.32-
            specified type NEC S66.39-
            strain S66.31-
          laceration S56.42-
          specified type NEC S56.49-
          strain S56.41-
        flexor (forearm level)
          hand level S66.10-
            laceration S66.12-
            specified type NEC S66.19-
            strain S66.11-
          laceration S56.12-
          specified type NEC S56.19-
          strain S56.11-
        intrinsic S66.50-
          laceration S66.52-
          specified type NEC S66.59-
          strain S66.51-
      middle
        extensor (forearm level)
          hand level S66.30-
            laceration S66.32-
            specified type NEC
              S66.39-
            strain S66.31-
          laceration S56.42-
          specified type NEC S56.49-
          strain S56.41-
        flexor (forearm level)
          hand level S66.10-
            laceration S66.12-
            specified type NEC
              S66.19-
            strain S66.11-
          laceration S56.12-
          specified type NEC S56.19-
          strain S56.11-
        intrinsic S66.50-
          laceration S66.52-
          specified type NEC S66.59-
          strain S66.51-
      ring
        extensor (forearm level)
          hand level S66.30-
            laceration S66.32-
            specified type NEC S66.39-
            strain S66.31-
          laceration S56.42-
          specified type NEC S56.49-
          strain S56.41-
        flexor (forearm level)
          hand level S66.10-
            laceration S66.12-
            specified type NEC S66.19-
            strain S66.11-
          laceration S56.12-
          specified type NEC S56.19-
          strain S56.11-

Injury (Continued)
  muscle (Continued)
    finger (Continued)
      ring (Continued)
        intrinsic S66.50-
          laceration S66.52-
          specified type NEC S66.59-
          strain S66.51-
      flexor
        finger (s) (other than thumb) — see
          Injury, muscle, finger
        forearm level, specified NEC — see
          Injury, muscle, forearm, flexor
        thumb —see Injury, muscle, thumb,
          flexor
        toe (long) (ankle level) (foot level) —see
          Injury, muscle, toe, flexor
    foot S96.90-
      intrinsic S96.20-
        laceration S96.22-
        specified type NEC S96.29-
        strain S96.21-
      laceration S96.92-
      long extensor, toe —see Injury, muscle,
        toe, extensor
      long flexor, toe —see Injury, muscle, toe,
        flexor
      specified
        site NEC S96.80-
          laceration S96.82-
          specified type NEC S96.89-
          strain S96.81-
        type NEC S96.99-
      strain S96.91-
    forearm (level) S56.90-
      extensor S56.50-
        laceration S56.52-
        specified type NEC S56.59-
        strain S56.51-
      flexor S56.20-
        laceration S56.22-
        specified type NEC S56.29-
        strain S56.21-
      laceration S56.92-
      specified S56.99-
        site NEC S56.80-
          laceration S56.82-
          strain S56.81-
        type NEC S56.89-
      strain S56.91-
    hand (level) S66.90-
      laceration S66.92-
      specified
        site NEC S66.80-
          laceration S66.82-
          specified type NEC S66.89-
          strain S66.81-
        type NEC S66.99-
      strain S66.91-
    head S09.10
      laceration S09.12
      specified type NEC S09.19
      strain S09.11
    hip NEC S76.00-
      laceration S76.02-
      specified type NEC S76.09-
      strain S76.01-
    intrinsic
      ankle and foot level —see Injury, muscle,
        foot, intrinsic
      finger (other than thumb) —see Injury,
        muscle, finger by site, intrinsic
      foot (level) —see Injury, muscle, foot,
        intrinsic
      thumb —see Injury, muscle, thumb,
        intrinsic
    leg (level) (lower) S86.90-
      Achilles tendon —see Injury, Achilles
        tendon
      anterior muscle group —see Injury,
        muscle, anterior muscle group

Injury (Continued)
  muscle (Continued)
    leg (Continued)
      laceration S86.92-
      peroneal muscle group —see Injury,
        muscle, peroneal muscle group
      posterior muscle group —see Injury,
        muscle, posterior muscle group,
        leg level
      specified
        site NEC S86.80-
          laceration S86.82-
          specified type NEC S86.89-
          strain S86.81-
        type NEC S86.99-
      strain S86.91-
    long
      extensor toe, at ankle and foot level —see
        Injury, muscle, toe, extensor
      flexor, toe, at ankle and foot level —see
        Injury, muscle, toe, flexor
      head, biceps —see Injury, muscle, biceps,
        long head
    lower back S39.002
      laceration S39.022
      specified type NEC S39.092
      strain S39.012
    neck (level) S16.9
      laceration S16.2
      specified type NEC S16.8
      strain S16.1
    pelvis S39.003
      laceration S39.023
      specified type NEC S39.093
      strain S39.013
    peroneal muscle group, at leg level (lower)
      S86.30-
      laceration S86.32-
      specified type NEC S86.39-
      strain S86.31-
    posterior muscle (group)
      leg level (lower) S86.10-
        laceration S86.12-
        specified type NEC S86.19-
        strain S86.11-
      thigh level S76.30-
        laceration S76.32-
        specified type NEC S76.39-
        strain S76.31-
    quadriceps (thigh) S76.10-
      laceration S76.12-
      specified type NEC S76.19-
      strain S76.11-
    shoulder S46.90-
      laceration S46.92-
      rotator cuff —see Injury, rotator cuff
      specified site NEC S46.80-
        laceration S46.82-
        specified type NEC S46.89-
        strain S46.81-
      specified type NEC S46.99-
      strain S46.91-
    thigh NEC (level) S76.90-
      adductor —see Injury, muscle, adductor,
        thigh
      laceration S76.92-
      posterior muscle (group) —see Injury,
        muscle, posterior muscle, thigh
        level
      quadriceps —see Injury, muscle,
        quadriceps
      specified
        site NEC S76.80-
          laceration S76.82-
          specified type NEC S76.89-
          strain S76.81-
        type NEC S76.99-
      strain S76.91-
    thorax (level) S29.009
      back wall S29.002
      front wall S29.001

◀ New ◀▥ Revised ~~deleted~~ Deleted

Injury (Continued)
  muscle (Continued)
    thorax (Continued)
      laceration S29.029
        back wall S29.022
        front wall S29.021
      specified type NEC S29.099
        back wall S29.092
        front wall S29.091
      strain S29.019
        back wall S29.012
        front wall S29.011
    thumb
      abductor (forearm level) S56.30-
        laceration S56.32-
        specified type NEC S56.39-
        strain S56.31-
      extensor (forearm level) S56.30-
        hand level S66.20-
          laceration S66.22-
          specified type NEC S66.29-
          strain S66.21-
        laceration S56.32-
        specified type NEC S56.39-
        strain S56.31-
      flexor (forearm level) S56.00-
        hand level S66.00-
          laceration S66.02-
          specified type NEC S66.09-
          strain S66.01-
        laceration S56.02-
        specified type NEC S56.09-
        strain S56.01-
        wrist level —see Injury, muscle,
          thumb, flexor, hand level
      intrinsic S66.40-
        laceration S66.42-
        specified type NEC S66.49-
        strain S66.41-
    toe —see also Injury, muscle, foot
      extensor, long S96.10-
        laceration S96.12-
        specified type NEC S96.19-
        strain S96.11-
      flexor, long S96.00-
        laceration S96.02-
        specified type NEC S96.09-
        strain S96.01-
    triceps S46.30-
      laceration S46.32-
      specified type NEC S46.39-
      strain S46.31-
    wrist (and hand) level —see Injury, muscle,
      hand
  musculocutaneous nerve —see Injury, nerve,
    musculocutaneous
  myocardium —see Injury, heart
  nape —see Injury, neck
  nasal (septum) (sinus) S09.92
  nasopharynx S09.92
  neck S19.9
    specified NEC S19.80
      specified site NEC S19.89
  nerve NEC T14.8
    abdomen S34.9
      peripheral S34.6
      specified site NEC S34.8
    abducens S04.4-
      contusion S04.4-
      laceration S04.4-
      specified type NEC S04.4-
    abducent —see Injury, nerve,
      abducens
    accessory S04.7-
      contusion S04.7-
      laceration S04.7-
      specified type NEC S04.7-
    acoustic S04.6-
      contusion S04.6-
      laceration S04.6-
      specified type NEC S04.6-

Injury (Continued)
  nerve NEC (Continued)
    ankle S94.9-
      cutaneous sensory S94.3-
      specified site NEC —see subcategory
        S94.8
    anterior crural, femoral —see Injury, nerve,
      femoral
    arm (upper) S44.9-
      axillary —see Injury, nerve, axillary
      cutaneous —see Injury, nerve, cutaneous,
        arm
      median —see Injury, nerve, median,
        upper arm
      musculocutaneous —see Injury, nerve,
        musculocutaneous
      radial —see Injury, nerve, radial, upper
        arm
      specified site NEC —see subcategory
        S44.8
      ulnar —see Injury, nerve, ulnar, arm
    auditory —see Injury, nerve, acoustic
    axillary S44.3-
    brachial plexus —see Injury, brachial plexus
    cervical sympathetic S14.5
    cranial S04.9
      contusion S04.9
      eighth (acoustic or auditory) —see Injury,
        nerve, acoustic
      eleventh (accessory) —see Injury, nerve,
        accessory
      fifth (trigeminal) —see Injury, nerve,
        trigeminal
      first (olfactory) —see Injury, nerve,
        olfactory
      fourth (trochlear) —see Injury, nerve,
        trochlear
      laceration S04.9
      ninth (glossopharyngeal) —see Injury,
        nerve, glossopharyngeal
      second (optic) —see Injury, nerve, optic
      seventh (facial) —see Injury, nerve, facial
      sixth (abducent) —see Injury, nerve,
        abducens
      specified
        nerve NEC S04.89-
          contusion S04.89-
          laceration S04.89-
          specified type NEC S04.89-
        type NEC S04.9
      tenth (pneumogastric or vagus) —see
        Injury, nerve, vagus
      third (oculomotor) —see Injury, nerve,
        oculomotor
      twelfth (hypoglossal) —see Injury, nerve,
        hypoglossal
    cutaneous sensory
      ankle (level) S94.3-
      arm (upper) (level) S44.5-
      foot (level) —see Injury, nerve, cutaneous
        sensory, ankle
      forearm (level) S54.3-
      hip (level) S74.2-
      leg (lower level) S84.2-
      shoulder (level) —see Injury, nerve,
        cutaneous sensory, arm
      thigh (level) —see Injury, nerve,
        cutaneous sensory, hip
    deep peroneal —see Injury, nerve, peroneal,
      foot
    digital
      finger S64.4-
        index S64.49-
        little S64.49-
        middle S64.49-
        ring S64.49-
        thumb S64.3-
      toe —see Injury, nerve, ankle, specified
        site NEC
    eighth cranial (acoustic or auditory) —see
      Injury, nerve, acoustic

Injury (Continued)
  nerve NEC (Continued)
    eleventh cranial (accessory) —see Injury,
      nerve, accessory
    facial S04.5-
      contusion S04.5-
      laceration S04.5-
      newborn P11.3
      specified type NEC S04.5-
    femoral (hip level) (thigh level) S74.1-
    fifth cranial (trigeminal) —see Injury, nerve,
      trigeminal
    finger (digital) —see Injury, nerve, digital,
      finger
    first cranial (olfactory) —see Injury, nerve,
      olfactory
    foot S94.9-
      cutaneous sensory S94.3-
      deep peroneal S94.2-
      lateral plantar S94.0-
      medial plantar S94.1-
      specified site NEC —see subcategory
        S94.8
    forearm (level) S54.9-
      cutaneous sensory —see Injury, nerve,
        cutaneous sensory, forearm
      median —see Injury, nerve, median
      radial —see Injury, nerve, radial
      specified site NEC —see subcategory
        S54.8
      ulnar —see Injury, nerve, ulnar
    fourth cranial (trochlear) —see Injury,
      nerve, trochlear
    glossopharyngeal S04.89-
      specified type NEC S04.89-
    hand S64.9-
      median —see Injury, nerve, median,
        hand
      radial —see Injury, nerve, radial, hand
      specified NEC —see subcategory
        S64.8
      ulnar —see Injury, nerve, ulnar, hand
    hip (level) S74.9-
      cutaneous sensory —see Injury, nerve,
        cutaneous sensory, hip
      femoral —see Injury, nerve, femoral
      sciatic —see Injury, nerve, sciatic
      specified site NEC —see subcategory
        S74.8
    hypoglossal S04.89-
      specified type NEC S04.89-
    lateral plantar S94.0-
    leg (lower) S84.9-
      cutaneous sensory —see Injury, nerve,
        cutaneous sensory, leg
      peroneal —see Injury, nerve, peroneal
      specified site NEC —see subcategory
        S84.8
      tibial —see Injury, nerve, tibial
      upper —see Injury, nerve, thigh
    lower
      back —see Injury, nerve, abdomen,
        specified site NEC
        peripheral —see Injury, nerve,
          abdomen, peripheral
      limb —see Injury, nerve, leg
    lumbar plexus —see Injury, nerve,
      lumbosacral, sympathetic
    lumbar spinal —see Injury, nerve, spinal,
      lumbar
    lumbosacral
      plexus —see Injury, nerve, lumbosacral,
        sympathetic
      sympathetic S34.5
    medial plantar S94.1-
    median (forearm level) S54.1-
      hand (level) S64.1-
      upper arm (level) S44.1-
      wrist (level) —see Injury, nerve, median,
        hand
    musculocutaneous S44.4-

Injury *(Continued)*
  nerve NEC *(Continued)*
    musculospiral (upper arm level) —*see*
      Injury, nerve, radial, upper arm
    neck S14.9
      peripheral S14.4
      specified site NEC S14.8
      sympathetic S14.5
    ninth cranial (glossopharyngeal) —*see*
      Injury, nerve, glossopharyngeal
    oculomotor S04.1-
      contusion S04.1-
      laceration S04.1-
      specified type NEC S04.1-
    olfactory S04.81-
      specified type NEC S04.81-
    optic S04.01-
      contusion S04.01-
      laceration S04.01-
      specified type NEC S04.01-
    pelvic girdle —*see* Injury, nerve, hip
    pelvis —*see* Injury, nerve, abdomen,
      specified site NEC
    peripheral —*see* Injury, nerve, abdomen,
      peripheral
    peripheral NEC T14.8
      abdomen —*see* Injury, nerve, abdomen,
        peripheral
      lower back —*see* Injury, nerve, abdomen,
        peripheral
      neck —*see* Injury, nerve, neck,
        peripheral
      pelvis —*see* Injury, nerve, abdomen,
        peripheral
      specified NEC T14.8
    peroneal (lower leg level) S84.1-
      foot S94.2-
    plexus
      brachial —*see* Injury, brachial
        plexus
      celiac, coeliac —*see* Injury, nerve,
        lumbosacral, sympathetic
      mesenteric, inferior —*see* Injury, nerve,
        lumbosacral, sympathetic
      sacral —*see* Injury, lumbosacral
        plexus
      spinal
        brachial —*see* Injury, brachial
          plexus
        lumbosacral —*see* Injury, lumbosacral
          plexus
    pneumogastric —*see* Injury, nerve,
      vagus
    radial (forearm level) S54.2-
      hand (level) S64.2-
      upper arm (level) S44.2-
      wrist (level) —*see* Injury, nerve, radial,
        hand
    root —*see* Injury, nerve, spinal, root
    sacral plexus —*see* Injury, lumbosacral
      plexus
    sacral spinal —*see* Injury, nerve, spinal,
      sacral
    sciatic (hip level) (thigh level) S74.0-
    second cranial (optic) —*see* Injury, nerve,
      optic
    seventh cranial (facial) —*see* Injury, nerve,
      facial
    shoulder —*see* Injury, nerve, arm
    sixth cranial (abducent) —*see* Injury, nerve,
      abducens
    spinal
      plexus —*see* Injury, nerve, plexus,
        spinal
      root
        cervical S14.2
        dorsal S24.2
        lumbar S34.21
        sacral S34.22
        thoracic —*see* Injury, nerve, spinal,
          root, dorsal

Injury *(Continued)*
  nerve NEC *(Continued)*
    splanchnic —*see* Injury, nerve, lumbosacral,
      sympathetic
    sympathetic NEC —*see* Injury, nerve,
      lumbosacral, sympathetic
      cervical —*see* Injury, nerve, cervical
        sympathetic
    tenth cranial (pneumogastric or vagus) —
      see Injury, nerve, vagus
    thigh (level) —*see* Injury, nerve, hip
      cutaneous sensory —*see* Injury, nerve,
        cutaneous sensory, hip
      femoral —*see* Injury, nerve, femoral
      sciatic —*see* Injury, nerve, sciatic
      specified NEC —*see* Injury, nerve, hip
    third cranial (oculomotor) —*see* Injury,
      nerve, oculomotor
    thorax S24.9
      peripheral S24.3
      specified site NEC S24.8
      sympathetic S24.4
    thumb, digital —*see* Injury, nerve, digital,
      thumb
    tibial (lower leg level) (posterior)
      S84.0-
    toe —*see* Injury, nerve, ankle
    trigeminal S04.3-
      contusion S04.3-
      laceration S04.3-
      specified type NEC S04.3-
    trochlear S04.2-
      contusion S04.2-
      laceration S04.2-
      specified type NEC S04.2-
    twelfth cranial (hypoglossal) —*see* Injury,
      nerve, hypoglossal
    ulnar (forearm level) S54.0-
      arm (upper) (level) S44.0-
      hand (level) S64.0-
      wrist (level) —*see* Injury, nerve, ulnar,
        hand
    vagus S04.89-
      specified type NEC S04.89-
    wrist (level) —*see* Injury, nerve, hand
    ninth cranial nerve (glossopharyngeal) —*see*
      Injury, nerve, glossopharyngeal
    nose (septum) S09.92
    obstetrical O71.9
      specified NEC O71.89
    occipital (region) (scalp) S09.90
      lobe —*see* Injury, intracranial
    optic chiasm S04.02
    optic radiation S04.03-
    optic tract and pathways S04.03-
    orbit, orbital (region) —*see* Injury, eye
      penetrating (with foreign body) —*see*
        Injury, eye, orbit, penetrating
      specified NEC —*see* Injury, eye, specified
        site NEC
    ovary, ovarian S37.409
      bilateral S37.402
        contusion S37.422
        laceration S37.432
        specified type NEC S37.492
      blood vessel —*see* Injury, blood vessel,
        ovarian
      contusion S37.429
        bilateral S37.422
        unilateral S37.421
      laceration S37.439
        bilateral S37.432
        unilateral S37.431
      specified type NEC S37.499
        bilateral S37.492
        unilateral S37.491
      unilateral S37.401
        contusion S37.421
        laceration S37.431
        specified type NEC S37.491
    palate (hard) (soft) S09.93

Injury *(Continued)*
  pancreas S36.209
    body S36.201
      contusion S36.221
      laceration S36.231
        major S36.261
        minor S36.241
        moderate S36.251
      specified type NEC S36.291
    contusion S36.229
    head S36.200
      contusion S36.220
      laceration S36.230
        major S36.260
        minor S36.240
        moderate S36.250
      specified type NEC S36.290
    laceration S36.239
      major S36.269
      minor S36.249
      moderate S36.259
    specified type NEC S36.299
    tail S36.202
      contusion S36.222
      laceration S36.232
        major S36.262
        minor S36.242
        moderate S36.252
      specified type NEC S36.292
  parietal (region) (scalp) S09.90
    lobe —*see* Injury, intracranial
  patellar ligament (tendon) S76.10-
    laceration S76.12-
    specified NEC S76.19-
    strain S76.11-
  pelvis, pelvic (floor) S39.93
    complicating delivery O70.1
    joint or ligament, complicating delivery
      O71.6
    organ S37.90
      with ectopic or molar pregnancy O08.6
      complication of abortion —*see* Abortion
      contusion S37.92
      following ectopic or molar pregnancy
        O08.6
      laceration S37.93
      obstetrical trauma NEC O71.5
      specified
        site NEC S37.899
          contusion S37.892
          laceration S37.893
          specified type NEC S37.898
        type NEC S37.99
    specified NEC S39.83
  penis S39.94
  perineum S39.94
  peritoneum S36.81
    laceration S36.893
  periurethral tissue —*see* Injury, urethra
    complicating delivery O71.82
  phalanges
    foot —*see* Injury, foot
    hand —*see* Injury, hand
  pharynx NEC S19.85
  pleura —*see* Injury, intrathoracic, pleura
  plexus
    brachial —*see* Injury, brachial plexus
    cardiac —*see* Injury, nerve, thorax,
      sympathetic
    celiac, coeliac —*see* Injury, nerve,
      lumbosacral, sympathetic
    esophageal —*see* Injury, nerve, thorax,
      sympathetic
    hypogastric —*see* Injury, nerve,
      lumbosacral, sympathetic
    lumbar, lumbosacral —*see* Injury,
      lumbosacral plexus
    mesenteric —*see* Injury, nerve, lumbosacral,
      sympathetic
    pulmonary —*see* Injury, nerve, thorax,
      sympathetic

◀ New   ◀▥ Revised   ~~deleted~~ Deleted

Injury *(Continued)*
 postcardiac surgery (syndrome) I97.0
 prepuce S39.94
 prostate S37.829
  contusion S37.822
  laceration S37.823
  specified type NEC S37.828
 pubic region S39.94
 pudendum S39.94
 pulmonary plexus —*see* Injury, nerve, thorax,
   sympathetic
 rectovaginal septum NEC S39.83
 rectum —*see* Injury, intestine, large, rectum
 retina —*see* Injury, eye, specified site NEC
  penetrating —*see* Injury, eyeball,
    penetrating
 retroperitoneal —*see* Injury, intra-abdominal,
   specified site NEC
 rotator cuff (muscle (s)) (tendon (s)) S46.00-
  laceration S46.02-
  specified type NEC S46.09-
  strain S46.01-
 round ligament —*see* Injury, pelvic organ,
   specified site NEC
 sacral plexus —*see* Injury, lumbosacral
   plexus
 salivary duct or gland S09.93
 scalp S09.90
  newborn (birth injury) P12.9
   due to monitoring (electrode) (sampling
    incision) P12.4
   specified NEC P12.89
    caput succedaneum P12.81
 scapular region —*see* Injury, shoulder
 sclera —*see* Injury, eye, specified site NEC
  penetrating —*see* Injury, eyeball,
    penetrating
 scrotum S39.94
 second cranial nerve (optic) —*see* Injury,
   nerve, optic
 seminal vesicle —*see* Injury, pelvic organ,
   specified site NEC
 seventh cranial nerve (facial) —*see* Injury,
   nerve, facial
 shoulder S49.9-
  blood vessel —*see* Injury, blood vessel,
    arm
  contusion —*see* Contusion, shoulder
  dislocation —*see* Dislocation, shoulder
  fracture —*see* Fracture, shoulder
  muscle —*see* Injury, muscle, shoulder
  nerve —*see* Injury, nerve, shoulder
  open —*see* Wound, open, shoulder
  specified type NEC S49.8-
  sprain —*see* Sprain, shoulder girdle
  superficial —*see* Injury, superficial,
    shoulder
 sinus
  cavernous —*see* Injury, intracranial
  nasal S09.92
 sixth cranial nerve (abducent) —*see* Injury,
   nerve, abducens
 skeleton, birth injury P13.9
  specified part NEC P13.8
 skin NEC T14.8
  surface intact —*see* Injury, superficial
 skull NEC S09.90
 specified NEC T14.8
 spermatic cord (pelvic region) S37.898
  scrotal region S39.848
 spinal (cord)
  cervical (neck) S14.109
   anterior cord syndrome S14.139
    C1 level S14.131
    C2 level S14.132
    C3 level S14.133
    C4 level S14.134
    C5 level S14.135
    C6 level S14.136
    C7 level S14.137
    C8 level S14.138

Injury *(Continued)*
 spinal *(Continued)*
  cervical *(Continued)*
   Brown-Séquard syndrome
    S14.149
    C1 level S14.141
    C2 level S14.142
    C3 level S14.143
    C4 level S14.144
    C5 level S14.145
    C6 level S14.146
    C7 level S14.147
    C8 level S14.148
   C1 level S14.101
   C2 level S14.102
   C3 level S14.103
   C4 level S14.104
   C5 level S14.105
   C6 level S14.106
   C7 level S14.107
   C8 level S14.108
   central cord syndrome S14.129
    C1 level S14.121
    C2 level S14.122
    C3 level S14.123
    C4 level S14.124
    C5 level S14.125
    C6 level S14.126
    C7 level S14.127
    C8 level S14.128
   complete lesion S14.119
    C1 level S14.111
    C2 level S14.112
    C3 level S14.113
    C4 level S14.114
    C5 level S14.115
    C6 level S14.116
    C7 level S14.117
    C8 level S14.118
   concussion S14.0
   edema S14.0
   incomplete lesion specified NEC
    S14.159
    C1 level S14.151
    C2 level S14.152
    C3 level S14.153
    C4 level S14.154
    C5 level S14.155
    C6 level S14.156
    C7 level S14.157
    C8 level S14.158
   posterior cord syndrome S14.159
    C1 level S14.151
    C2 level S14.152
    C3 level S14.153
    C4 level S14.154
    C5 level S14.155
    C6 level S14.156
    C7 level S14.157
    C8 level S14.158
  dorsal —*see* Injury, spinal, thoracic
  lumbar S34.109
   complete lesion S34.119
    L1 level S34.111
    L2 level S34.112
    L3 level S34.113
    L4 level S34.114
    L5 level S34.115
   concussion S34.01
   edema S34.01
   incomplete lesion S34.129
    L1 level S34.121
    L2 level S34.122
    L3 level S34.123
    L4 level S34.124
    L5 level S34.125
   L1 level S34.101
   L2 level S34.102
   L3 level S34.103
   L4 level S34.104
   L5 level S34.105

Injury *(Continued)*
 spinal *(Continued)*
  nerve root NEC
   cervical —*see* Injury, nerve, spinal, root,
     cervical
   dorsal —*see* Injury, nerve, spinal, root,
     dorsal
   lumbar S34.21
   sacral S34.22
   thoracic —*see* Injury, nerve, spinal, root,
     dorsal
  plexus
   brachial —*see* Injury, brachial plexus
   lumbosacral —*see* Injury, lumbosacral
     plexus
  sacral S34.139
   complete lesion S34.131
   incomplete lesion S34.132
  thoracic S24.109
   anterior cord syndrome S24.139
    T1 level S24.131
    T2-T6 level S24.132
    T7-T10 level S24.133
    T11-T12 level S24.134
   Brown-Séquard syndrome
    S24.149
    T1 level S24.141
    T2-T6 level S24.142
    T7-T10 level S24.143
    T11-T12 level S24.144
   complete lesion S24.119
    T1 level S24.111
    T2-T6 level S24.112
    T7-T10 level S24.113
    T11-T12 level S24.114
   concussion S24.0
   edema S24.0
   incomplete lesion specified NEC
    S24.159
    T1 level S24.151
    T2-T6 level S24.152
    T7-T10 level S24.153
    T11-T12 level S24.154
   posterior cord syndrome S24.159
    T1 level S24.151
    T2-T6 level S24.152
    T7-T10 level S24.153
    T11-T12 level S24.154
   T1 level S24.101
   T2-T6 level S24.102
   T7-T10 level S24.103
   T11-T12 level S24.104
  splanchnic nerve —*see* Injury, nerve,
    lumbosacral, sympathetic
  spleen S36.00
   contusion S36.029
    major S36.021
    minor S36.020
   laceration S36.039
    major (massive) (stellate) S36.032
    moderate S36.031
    superficial (capsular) (minor)
     S36.030
   specified type NEC S36.09
  splenic artery —*see* Injury, blood vessel,
    celiac artery, branch
  stellate ganglion —*see* Injury, nerve,
    thorax, sympathetic
  sternal region S29.9
  stomach S36.30
   contusion S36.32
   laceration S36.33
   specified type NEC S36.39
  subconjunctival —*see* Injury, eye,
    conjunctiva
  subcutaneous NEC T14.8
  submaxillary region S09.93
  submental region S09.93
  subungual
   fingers —*see* Injury, hand
   toes —*see* Injury, foot

Injury *(Continued)*
  superficial NEC T14.8
    abdomen, abdominal (wall) S30.92
      abrasion S30.811
      bite S30.871
        insect S30.861
      contusion S30.1
      external constriction S30.841
      foreign body S30.851
    abrasion —*see* Abrasion, by site
    adnexa, eye NEC —*see* Injury, eye,
      specified site NEC
    alveolar process —*see* Injury, superficial,
      oral cavity
    ankle S90.91-
      abrasion —*see* Abrasion, ankle
      bite —*see* Bite, ankle
      blister —*see* Blister, ankle
      contusion —*see* Contusion, ankle
      external constriction —*see* Constriction,
        external, ankle
      foreign body —*see* Foreign body,
        superficial, ankle
    anus S30.98
    arm (upper) S40.92-
      abrasion —*see* Abrasion, arm
      bite —*see* Bite, superficial, arm
      blister —*see* Blister, arm (upper)
      contusion —*see* Contusion, arm
      external constriction —*see* Constriction,
        external, arm
      foreign body —*see* Foreign body,
        superficial, arm
    auditory canal (external) (meatus) —*see*
      Injury, superficial, ear
    auricle —*see* Injury, superficial, ear
    axilla —*see* Injury, superficial, arm
    back —*see also* Injury, superficial, thorax,
      back
      lower S30.91
        abrasion S30.810
        contusion S30.0
        external constriction S30.840
        superficial
          bite NEC S30.870
            insect S30.860
          foreign body S30.850
    bite NEC —*see* Bite, superficial NEC, by
      site
    blister —*see* Blister, by site
    breast S20.10-
      abrasion —*see* Abrasion, breast
      bite —*see* Bite, superficial, breast
      contusion —*see* Contusion, breast
      external constriction —*see* Constriction,
        external, breast
      foreign body —*see* Foreign body,
        superficial, breast
    brow —*see* Injury, superficial, head,
      specified NEC
    buttock S30.91
    calf —*see* Injury, superficial, leg
    canthus, eye —*see* Injury, superficial,
      periocular area
    cheek (external) —*see* Injury, superficial,
      head, specified NEC
      internal —*see* Injury, superficial, oral
        cavity
    chest wall —*see* Injury, superficial,
      thorax
    chin —*see* Injury, superficial, head NEC
    clitoris S30.95
    conjunctiva —*see* Injury, eye, conjunctiva
      with foreign body (in conjunctival
        sac) —*see* Foreign body,
        conjunctival sac
    contusion —*see* Contusion, by site
    costal region —*see* Injury, superficial,
      thorax
    digit (s)
      hand —*see* Injury, superficial, finger

Injury *(Continued)*
  superficial NEC *(Continued)*
    ear (auricle) (canal) (external) S00.40-
      abrasion —*see* Abrasion, ear
      bite —*see* Bite, superficial, ear
      contusion —*see* Contusion, ear
      external constriction —*see* Constriction,
        external, ear
      foreign body —*see* Foreign body,
        superficial, ear
    elbow S50.90-
      abrasion —*see* Abrasion, elbow
      bite —*see* Bite, superficial, elbow
      blister —*see* Blister, elbow
      contusion —*see* Contusion, elbow
      external constriction —*see* Constriction,
        external, elbow
      foreign body —*see* Foreign body,
        superficial, elbow
    epididymis S30.94
    epigastric region S30.92
    epiglottis —*see* Injury, superficial, throat
    esophagus
      cervical —*see* Injury, superficial, throat
    external constriction —*see* Constriction,
      external, by site
    extremity NEC T14.8
    eyeball NEC —*see* Injury, eye, specified
      site NEC
    eyebrow —*see* Injury, superficial,
      periocular area
    eyelid S00.20-
      abrasion —*see* Abrasion, eyelid
      bite —*see* Bite, superficial, eyelid
      contusion —*see* Contusion, eyelid
      external constriction —*see* Constriction,
        external, eyelid
      foreign body —*see* Foreign body,
        superficial, eyelid
    face NEC —*see* Injury, superficial, head,
      specified NEC
    finger (s) S60.949
      abrasion —*see* Abrasion, finger
      bite —*see* Bite, superficial, finger
      blister —*see* Blister, finger
      contusion —*see* Contusion, finger
      external constriction —*see* Constriction,
        external, finger
      foreign body —*see* Foreign body,
        superficial, finger
      index S60.94-
      insect bite —*see* Bite, by site, superficial,
        insect
      little S60.94-
      middle S60.94-
      ring S60.94-
    flank S30.92
    foot S90.92-
      abrasion —*see* Abrasion, foot
      bite —*see* Bite, foot
      blister —*see* Blister, foot
      contusion —*see* Contusion, foot
      external constriction —*see* Constriction,
        external, foot
      foreign body —*see* Foreign body,
        superficial, foot
    forearm S50.91-
      abrasion —*see* Abrasion, forearm
      bite —*see* Bite, forearm, superficial
      blister —*see* Blister, forearm
      contusion —*see* Contusion, forearm
      elbow only —*see* Injury, superficial,
        elbow
      external constriction —*see* Constriction,
        external, forearm
      foreign body —*see* Foreign body,
        superficial, forearm
    forehead —*see* Injury, superficial, head
      NEC
    foreign body —*see* Foreign body,
      superficial

Injury *(Continued)*
  superficial NEC *(Continued)*
    genital organs, external
      female S30.97
      male S30.96
    globe (eye) —*see* Injury, eye, specified site
      NEC
    groin S30.92
    gum —*see* Injury, superficial, oral cavity
    hand S60.92-
      abrasion —*see* Abrasion, hand
      bite —*see* Bite, superficial, hand
      contusion —*see* Contusion, hand
      external constriction —*see* Constriction,
        external, hand
      foreign body —*see* Foreign body,
        superficial, hand
    head S00.90
      ear —*see* Injury, superficial, ear
      eyelid —*see* Injury, superficial, eyelid
      nose S00.30
      oral cavity S00.502
      scalp S00.00
      specified site NEC S00.80
    heel —*see* Injury, superficial, foot
    hip S70.91-
      abrasion —*see* Abrasion, hip
      bite —*see* Bite, superficial, hip
      blister —*see* Blister, hip
      contusion —*see* Contusion, hip
      external constriction —*see* Constriction,
        external, hip
      foreign body —*see* Foreign body,
        superficial, hip
    iliac region —*see* Injury, superficial,
      abdomen
    inguinal region —*see* Injury, superficial,
      abdomen
    insect bite —*see* Bite, by site, superficial,
      insect
    interscapular region —*see* Injury,
      superficial, thorax, back
    jaw —*see* Injury, superficial, head, specified
      NEC
    knee S80.91-
      abrasion —*see* Abrasion, knee
      bite —*see* Bite, superficial, knee
      blister —*see* Blister, knee
      contusion —*see* Contusion, knee
      external constriction —*see* Constriction,
        external, knee
      foreign body —*see* Foreign body,
        superficial, knee
    labium (majus) (minus) S30.95
    lacrimal (apparatus) (gland) (sac) —*see*
      Injury, eye, specified site NEC
    larynx —*see* Injury, superficial, throat
    leg (lower) S80.92-
      abrasion —*see* Abrasion, leg
      bite —*see* Bite, superficial, leg
      contusion —*see* Contusion, leg
      external constriction —*see* Constriction,
        external, leg
      foreign body —*see* Foreign body,
        superficial, leg
      knee —*see* Injury, superficial, knee
    limb NEC T14.8
    lip S00.501
    lower back S30.91
    lumbar region S30.91
    malar region —*see* Injury, superficial, head,
      specified NEC
    mammary —*see* Injury, superficial, breast
    mastoid region —*see* Injury, superficial,
      head, specified NEC
    mouth —*see* Injury, superficial, oral
      cavity
    muscle NEC T14.8
    nail NEC T14.8
      finger —*see* Injury, superficial, finger
      toe —*see* Injury, superficial, toe

◀ New   ◀▦ Revised   ~~deleted~~ Deleted

Injury *(Continued)*
superficial NEC *(Continued)*
nasal (septum) —*see* Injury, superficial,
nose
neck S10.90
specified site NEC S10.80
nose (septum) S00.30
occipital region —*see* Injury, superficial,
scalp
oral cavity S00.502
orbital region —*see* Injury, superficial,
periocular area
palate —*see* Injury, superficial, oral
cavity
palm —*see* Injury, superficial, hand
parietal region —*see* Injury, superficial,
scalp
pelvis S30.91
girdle —*see* Injury, superficial, hip
penis S30.93
perineum
female S30.95
male S30.91
periocular area S00.20-
abrasion —*see* Abrasion, eyelid
bite —*see* Bite, superficial, eyelid
contusion —*see* Contusion, eyelid
external constriction —*see* Constriction,
external, eyelid
foreign body —*see* Foreign body,
superficial, eyelid
phalanges
finger —*see* Injury, superficial, finger
toe —*see* Injury, superficial, toe
pharynx —*see* Injury, superficial, throat
pinna —*see* Injury, superficial, ear
popliteal space —*see* Injury, superficial,
knee
prepuce S30.93
pubic region S30.91
pudendum
female S30.97
male S30.96
sacral region S30.91
scalp S00.00
scapular region —*see* Injury, superficial,
shoulder
sclera —*see* Injury, eye, specified site NEC
scrotum S30.94
shin —*see* Injury, superficial, leg
shoulder S40.91-
abrasion —*see* Abrasion, shoulder
bite —*see* Bite, superficial, shoulder
blister —*see* Blister, shoulder
contusion —*see* Contusion, shoulder
external constriction —*see* Constriction,
external, shoulder
foreign body —*see* Foreign body,
superficial, shoulder
skin NEC T14.8
sternal region —*see* Injury, superficial,
thorax, front
subconjunctival —*see* Injury, eye, specified
site NEC
subcutaneous NEC T14.8
submaxillary region —*see* Injury,
superficial, head, specified NEC
submental region —*see* Injury, superficial,
head, specified NEC
subungual
finger (s) —*see* Injury, superficial, finger
toe (s) —*see* Injury, superficial, toe
supraclavicular fossa —*see* Injury,
superficial, neck
supraorbital —*see* Injury, superficial, head,
specified NEC
temple —*see* Injury, superficial, head,
specified NEC
temporal region —*see* Injury, superficial,
head, specified NEC
testis S30.94

superficial NEC *(Continued)*
thigh S70.92-
abrasion —*see* Abrasion, thigh
bite —*see* Bite, superficial, thigh
blister —*see* Blister, thigh
contusion —*see* Contusion, thigh
external constriction —*see* Constriction,
external, thigh
foreign body —*see* Foreign body,
superficial, thigh
thorax, thoracic (wall) S20.90
abrasion —*see* Abrasion, thorax
back S20.40-
bite —*see* Bite, thorax, superficial
blister —*see* Blister, thorax
contusion —*see* Contusion, thorax
external constriction —*see* Constriction,
external, thorax
foreign body —*see* Foreign body,
superficial, thorax
front S20.30-
throat S10.10
abrasion S10.11
bite S10.17
insect S10.16
blister S10.12
contusion S10.0
external constriction S10.14
foreign body S10.15
thumb S60.93-
abrasion —*see* Abrasion, thumb
bite —*see* Bite, superficial, thumb
blister —*see* Blister, thumb
contusion —*see* Contusion, thumb
external constriction —*see* Constriction,
external, thumb
foreign body —*see* Foreign body,
superficial, thumb
insect bite —*see* Bite, by site, superficial,
insect
specified type NEC S60.39-
toe (s) S90.93-
abrasion —*see* Abrasion, toe
bite —*see* Bite, toe
blister —*see* Blister, toe
contusion —*see* Contusion, toe
external constriction —*see* Constriction,
external, toe
foreign body —*see* Foreign body,
superficial, toe
great S90.93-
tongue —*see* Injury, superficial, oral
cavity
tooth, teeth —*see* Injury, superficial, oral
cavity
trachea S10.10
tunica vaginalis S30.94
tympanum, tympanic membrane —*see*
Injury, superficial, ear
uvula —*see* Injury, superficial, oral cavity
vagina S30.95
vocal cords —*see* Injury, superficial, throat
vulva S30.95
wrist S60.91-
supraclavicular region —*see* Injury, neck
supraorbital S09.93
suprarenal gland (multiple) —*see* Injury,
adrenal
surgical complication (external or internal
site) —*see* Laceration, accidental
complicating surgery
temple S09.90
temporal region S09.90
tendon —*see also* Injury, muscle, by site
abdomen —*see* Injury, muscle, abdomen
Achilles —*see* Injury, Achilles tendon
lower back —*see* Injury, muscle, lower
back
pelvic organs —*see* Injury, muscle,
pelvis

Injury *(Continued)*
tenth cranial nerve (pneumogastric or
vagus) —*see* Injury, nerve, vagus
testis S39.94
thigh S79.92-
blood vessel —*see* Injury, blood vessel,
hip
contusion —*see* Contusion, thigh
fracture —*see* Fracture, femur
muscle —*see* Injury, muscle, thigh
nerve —*see* Injury, nerve, thigh
open —*see* Wound, open, thigh
specified NEC S79.82-
superficial —*see* Injury, superficial, thigh
third cranial nerve (oculomotor) —*see* Injury,
nerve, oculomotor
thorax, thoracic S29.9
blood vessel —*see* Injury, blood vessel,
thorax
cavity —*see* Injury, intrathoracic
dislocation —*see* Dislocation, thorax
external (wall) S29.9
contusion —*see* Contusion, thorax
nerve —*see* Injury, nerve, thorax
open —*see* Wound, open, thorax
specified NEC S29.8
sprain —*see* Sprain, thorax
superficial —*see* Injury, superficial,
thorax
fracture —*see* Fracture, thorax
internal —*see* Injury, intrathoracic
intrathoracic organ —*see* Injury,
intrathoracic
sympathetic ganglion —*see* Injury, nerve,
thorax, sympathetic
throat (*see also* Injury, neck) S19.9
thumb S69.9-
blood vessel —*see* Injury, blood vessel,
thumb
contusion —*see* Contusion, thumb
dislocation —*see* Dislocation, thumb
fracture —*see* Fracture, thumb
muscle —*see* Injury, muscle, thumb
nerve —*see* Injury, nerve, digital, thumb
open —*see* Wound, open, thumb
specified NEC S69.8-
sprain —*see* Sprain, thumb
superficial —*see* Injury, superficial,
thumb
thymus (gland) —*see* Injury, intrathoracic,
specified organ NEC
thyroid (gland) NEC S19.84
toe S99.92-
contusion —*see* Contusion, toe
dislocation —*see* Dislocation, toe
fracture —*see* Fracture, toe
muscle —*see* Injury, muscle, toe
open —*see* Wound, open, toe
specified type NEC S99.82-
sprain —*see* Sprain, toe
superficial —*see* Injury, superficial, toe
tongue S09.93
tonsil S09.93
tooth S09.93
trachea (cervical) NEC S19.82
thoracic —*see* Injury, intrathoracic, trachea,
thoracic
transfusion-related acute lung (TRALI)
J95.84
tunica vaginalis S39.94
twelfth cranial nerve (hypoglossal) —*see*
Injury, nerve, hypoglossal
ureter S37.10
contusion S37.12
laceration S37.13
specified type NEC S37.19
urethra (sphincter) S37.30
at delivery O71.5
contusion S37.32
laceration S37.33
specified type NEC S37.38

Injury (Continued)
urinary organ S37.899
contusion S37.92
laceration S37.93
specified
site NEC S37.899
contusion S37.892
laceration S37.893
specified type NEC S37.898
type NEC S37.99
uterus, uterine S37.60
with ectopic or molar pregnancy O08.6
blood vessel —see Injury, blood vessel, iliac
contusion S37.62
laceration S37.63
cervix at delivery O71.3
rupture associated with obstetrics —see
Rupture, uterus
specified type NEC S37.69
uvula S09.93
vagina S39.93
abrasion S30.814
bite S31.45
insect S30.864
superficial NEC S30.874
contusion S30.23
crush S38.03
during delivery —see Laceration, vagina,
during delivery
external constriction S30.844
insect bite S30.864
laceration S31.41
with foreign body S31.42
open wound S31.40
puncture S31.43
with foreign body S31.44
superficial S30.95
foreign body S30.854
vas deferens —see Injury, pelvic organ,
specified site NEC
vascular NEC T14.8
vein —see Injury, blood vessel
vena cava (superior) S25.20
inferior S35.10
laceration (minor) (superficial) S35.11
major S35.12
specified type NEC S35.19
laceration (minor) (superficial) S25.21
major S25.22
specified type NEC S25.29
vesical (sphincter) —see Injury, bladder
visual cortex S04.04-
vitreous (humor) S05.90
specified NEC S05.8X-
vocal cord NEC S19.83
vulva S39.94
abrasion S30.814
bite S31.45
insect S30.864
superficial NEC S30.874
contusion S30.23
crush S38.03
during delivery —see Laceration,
perineum, female, during delivery
external constriction S30.844
insect bite S30.864
laceration S31.41
with foreign body S31.42
open wound S31.40
puncture S31.43
with foreign body S31.44
superficial S30.95
foreign body S30.854
whiplash (cervical spine) S13.4
wrist S69.9-
blood vessel —see Injury, blood vessel,
hand
contusion —see Contusion, wrist
dislocation —see Dislocation, wrist
fracture —see Fracture, wrist
muscle —see Injury, muscle, hand

Injury (Continued)
wrist (Continued)
nerve —see Injury, nerve, hand
open —see Wound, open, wrist
specified NEC S69.8-
sprain —see Sprain, wrist
superficial —see Injury, superficial, wrist
Inoculation —see also Vaccination
complication or reaction —see Complications,
vaccination
Insanity, insane —see also Psychosis
adolescent —see Schizophrenia
confusional F28
acute or subacute F05
delusional F22
senile F03
Insect
bite —see Bite, by site, superficial, insect
venomous, poisoning NEC (by) —see Venom,
arthropod
Insensitivity
adrenocorticotropin hormone (ACTH) E27.49
androgen E34.50
complete E34.51
partial E34.52
Insertion
cord (umbilical) lateral or velamentous
O43.12-
intrauterine contraceptive device (encounter
for) —see Intrauterine contraceptive
device
Insolation (sunstroke) T67.0
Insomnia (organic) G47.00
without objective findings F51.02
adjustment F51.02
adjustment disorder F51.02
behavioral, of childhood Z73.819
combined type Z73.812
limit setting type Z73.811
sleep-onset association type Z73.810
childhood Z73.819
chronic F51.04
somatized tension F51.04
conditioned F51.04
due to
alcohol
abuse F10.182
dependence F10.282
use F10.982
amphetamines
abuse F15.182
dependence F15.282
use F15.982
anxiety disorder F51.05
caffeine
abuse F15.182
dependence F15.282
use F15.982
cocaine
abuse F14.182
dependence F14.282
use F14.982
depression F51.05
drug NEC
abuse F19.182
dependence F19.282
use F19.982
medical condition G47.01
mental disorder NEC F51.05
opioid
abuse F11.182
dependence F11.282
use F11.982
psychoactive substance NEC
abuse F19.182
dependence F19.282
use F19.982
sedative, hypnotic, or anxiolytic
abuse F13.182
dependence F13.282
use F13.982

Insomnia (Continued)
due to (Continued)
stimulant NEC
abuse F15.182
dependence F15.282
use F15.982
fatal familial (FFI) A81.83
idiopathic F51.01
learned F51.3
nonorganic origin F51.01
not due to a substance or known
physiological condition F51.01
specified NEC F51.09
paradoxical F51.03
primary F51.01
psychiatric F51.05
psychophysiologic F51.04
related to psychopathology F51.05
short-term F51.02
specified NEC G47.09
stress-related F51.02
transient F51.02
Inspiration
food or foreign body —see Foreign body, by
site
mucus —see Asphyxia, mucus
Inspissated bile syndrome (newborn)
P59.1
Instability
emotional (excessive) F60.3
joint (post-traumatic) M25.30
ankle M25.37-
due to old ligament injury —see Disorder,
ligament
elbow M25.32-
flail —see Flail, joint
foot M25.37-
hand M25.34-
hip M25.35-
knee M25.36-
lumbosacral —see subcategory M53.2
prosthesis —see Complications, joint
prosthesis, mechanical, displacement,
by site
sacroiliac —see subcategory M53.2
secondary to
old ligament injury —see Disorder,
ligament
removal of joint prosthesis M96.89
shoulder (region) M25.31-
spine —see subcategory M53.2
wrist M25.33-
knee (chronic) M23.5-
lumbosacral —see subcategory M53.2
nervous F48.8
personality (emotional) F60.3
spine —see Instability, joint, spine
vasomotor R55
Institutional syndrome (childhood) F94.2
Institutionalization, affecting child
Z62.22
disinhibited attachment F94.2
Insufficiency, insufficient
accommodation, old age H52.4
adrenal (gland) E27.40
primary E27.1
adrenocortical E27.40
drug-induced E27.3
iatrogenic E27.3
primary E27.1
anterior (occlusal) guidance M26.54
anus K62.89
aortic (valve) I35.1
with
mitral (valve) disease I08.0
with tricuspid (valve) disease
I08.3
stenosis I35.2
tricuspid (valve) disease I08.2
with mitral (valve) disease I08.3
congenital Q23.1

◀ New   ◀▥▥ Revised   ~~deleted~~ Deleted

Insufficiency, insufficient (Continued)
  aortic (Continued)
    rheumatic I06.1
      with
        mitral (valve) disease I08.0
          with tricuspid (valve) disease I08.3
        stenosis I06.2
          with mitral (valve) disease I08.0
            with tricuspid (valve) disease I08.3
        tricuspid (valve) disease I08.2
          with mitral (valve) disease I08.3
    specified cause NEC I35.1
    syphilitic A52.03
  arterial I77.1
    basilar G45.0
    carotid (hemispheric) G45.1
    cerebral I67.81
    coronary (acute or subacute) I24.8
    mesenteric K55.1
    peripheral I73.9
    precerebral (multiple) (bilateral) G45.2
    vertebral G45.0
  arteriovenous I99.8
  biliary K83.8
  cardiac —see also Insufficiency, myocardial
    due to presence of (cardiac) prosthesis I97.11-
    postprocedural I97.11-
  cardiorenal, hypertensive I13.2
  cardiovascular —see Disease, cardiovascular
  cerebrovascular (acute) I67.81
    with transient focal neurological signs and symptoms G45.8
  circulatory NEC I99.8
    newborn P29.89
  convergence H51.11
  coronary (acute or subacute) I24.8
    chronic or with a stated duration of over 4 weeks I25.89
  corticoadrenal E27.40
    primary E27.1
  dietary E63.9
  divergence H51.8
  food T73.0
  gastroesophageal K22.8
  gonadal
    ovary E28.39
    testis E29.1
  heart —see also Insufficiency, myocardial
    newborn P29.0
    valve —see Endocarditis
  hepatic —see Failure, hepatic
  idiopathic autonomic G90.09
  interocclusal distance of fully erupted teeth (ridge) M26.36
  kidney N28.9
    acute N28.9
    chronic N18.9
  lacrimal (secretion) H04.12-
    passages —see Stenosis, lacrimal
  liver —see Failure, hepatic
  lung —see Insufficiency, pulmonary
  mental (congenital) —see Disability, intellectual
  mesenteric K55.1
  mitral (valve) I34.0
    with
      aortic valve disease I08.0
        with tricuspid (valve) disease I08.3
      obstruction or stenosis I05.2
        with aortic valve disease I08.0
      tricuspid (valve) disease I08.1
        with aortic (valve) disease I08.3
    congenital Q23.3
    rheumatic I05.1
      with
        aortic valve disease I08.0
          with tricuspid (valve) disease I08.3

Insufficiency, insufficient (Continued)
  mitral (Continued)
    rheumatic (Continued)
      with (Continued)
        obstruction or stenosis I05.2
          with aortic valve disease I08.0
            with tricuspid (valve) disease I08.3
        tricuspid (valve) disease I08.1
          with aortic (valve) disease I08.3
      active or acute I01.1
        with chorea, rheumatic (Sydenham's) I02.0
    specified cause, except rheumatic I34.0
  muscle —see also Disease, muscle
    heart —see Insufficiency, myocardial
    ocular NEC H50.9
  myocardial, myocardium (with arteriosclerosis) I50.9
    with
      rheumatic fever (conditions in I00) I09.0
        active, acute or subacute I01.2
          with chorea I02.0
        inactive or quiescent (with chorea) I09.0
    congenital Q24.8
    hypertensive —see Hypertension, heart
    newborn P29.0
    rheumatic I09.0
      active, acute, or subacute I01.2
    syphilitic A52.06
  nourishment T73.0
  pancreatic K86.8
  parathyroid (gland) E20.9
  peripheral vascular (arterial) I73.9
  pituitary E23.0
  placental (mother) O36.51-
  platelets D69.6
  prenatal care affecting management of pregnancy O09.3-
  progressive pluriglandular E31.0
  pulmonary J98.4
    acute, following surgery (nonthoracic) J95.2
      thoracic J95.1
    chronic, following surgery J95.3
    following
      shock J98.4
      trauma J98.4
    newborn P28.5
    valve I37.1
      with stenosis I37.2
      congenital Q22.2
      rheumatic I09.89
        with aortic, mitral or tricuspid (valve) disease I08.8
  pyloric K31.89
  renal (acute) N28.9
    chronic N18.9
  respiratory R06.89
    newborn P28.5
  rotation —see Malrotation
  sleep syndrome F51.12
  social insurance Z59.7
  suprarenal E27.40
    primary E27.1
  tarso-orbital fascia, congenital Q10.3
  testis E29.1
  thyroid (gland) (acquired) E03.9
    congenital E03.1
  tricuspid (valve) (rheumatic) I07.1
    with
      aortic (valve) disease I08.2
        with mitral (valve) disease I08.3
      mitral (valve) disease I08.1
        with aortic (valve) disease I08.3
      obstruction or stenosis I07.2
        with aortic (valve) disease I08.2
          with mitral (valve) disease I08.3

Insufficiency, insufficient (Continued)
  tricuspid (Continued)
    congenital Q22.8
    nonrheumatic I36.1
      with stenosis I36.2
  urethral sphincter R32
  valve, valvular (heart) —see Endocarditis
    congenital Q24.8
  vascular I99.8
    intestine K55.9
      acute K55.0
    mesenteric K55.1
    peripheral I73.9
    renal —see Hypertension, kidney
  velopharyngeal
    acquired K13.79
    congenital Q38.8
  venous (chronic) (peripheral) I87.2
  ventricular —see Insufficiency, myocardial
  welfare support Z59.7
Insufflation, fallopian Z31.41
Insular —see condition
Insulinoma
  pancreas
    benign D13.7
    malignant C25.4
    uncertain behavior D37.8
  specified site
    benign —see Neoplasm, by site, benign
    malignant —see Neoplasm, by site, malignant
    uncertain behavior —see Neoplasm, by site, uncertain behavior
  unspecified site
    benign D13.7
    malignant C25.4
    uncertain behavior D37.8
Insuloma —see Insulinoma
Interference
  balancing side M26.56
  non-working side M26.56
Intermenstrual —see condition
Intermittent —see condition
Internal —see condition
Interrogation
  cardiac defibrillator (automatic) (implantable) Z45.02
  cardiac pacemaker Z45.018
  cardiac (event) (loop) recorder Z45.09
  infusion pump (implanted) (intrathecal) Z45.1
  neurostimulator Z46.2
Interruption
  phase-shift, sleep cycle —see Disorder, sleep, circadian rhythm
  sleep phase-shift, or 24 hour sleep-wake cycle —see Disorder, sleep, circadian rhythm
Interstitial —see condition
Intertrigo L30.4
  labialis K13.0
Intervertebral disc —see condition
Intestine, intestinal —see condition
Intolerance
  carbohydrate K90.4
  disaccharide, hereditary E73.0
  fat NEC K90.4
    pancreatic K90.3
  food K90.4
    dietary counseling and surveillance Z71.3
  fructose E74.10
    hereditary E74.12
  glucose(-galactose) E74.39
  gluten K90.0
  lactose E73.9
    specified NEC E73.8
  lysine E72.3
  milk NEC K90.4
    lactose E73.9
  protein K90.4

Intolerance (Continued)
  starch NEC K90.4
  sucrose (-isomaltose) E74.31
Intoxicated NEC (without dependence) —see
    Alcohol, intoxication
Intoxication
  acid E87.2
  alcoholic (acute) (without dependence) —see
    Alcohol, intoxication
  alimentary canal K52.1
  amphetamine (without dependence) —
    see Abuse, drug, stimulant, with
    intoxication
    with dependence —see Dependence, drug,
      stimulant, with intoxication
  anxiolytic (acute) (without dependence) —see
    Abuse, drug, sedative, with intoxication
    with dependence —see Dependence, drug,
      sedative, with intoxication
  caffeine (acute) (without dependence) —
    see Abuse, drug, stimulant, with
    intoxication
    with dependence —see Dependence, drug,
      stimulant, with intoxication
  cannabinoids (acute) (without dependence) —
    see Abuse, drug, cannabis, with
    intoxication
    with dependence —see Dependence, drug,
      cannabis, with intoxication
  chemical —see Table of Drugs and
    Chemicals
    via placenta or breast milk —see -
      Absorption, chemical, through
      placenta
  cocaine (acute) (without dependence) —see
    Abuse, drug, cocaine, with intoxication
    with dependence —see Dependence, drug,
      cocaine, with intoxication
  drug
    acute (without dependence) —see Abuse,
      drug, by type with intoxication
      with dependence —see Dependence,
        drug, by type with intoxication
    addictive
      via placenta or breast milk —see
        Absorption, drug, addictive,
        through placenta
    newborn P93.8
      gray baby syndrome P93.0
    overdose or wrong substance given or
      taken —see Table of Drugs and
      Chemicals, by drug, poisoning
  enteric K52.1
  foodborne A05.9
    bacterial A05.9
    classical (Clostridium botulinum) A05.1
    due to
      Bacillus cereus A05.4
      bacterium A05.9
        specified NEC A05.8
      Clostridium
        botulinum A05.1
        perfringens A05.2
        welchii A05.2
      Salmonella A02.9
        with
          (gastro) enteritis A02.0
          localized infection (s) A02.20
            arthritis A02.23
            meningitis A02.21
            osteomyelitis A02.24
            pneumonia A02.22
            pyelonephritis A02.25
            specified NEC A02.29
          sepsis A02.1
          specified manifestation NEC A02.8
      Staphylococcus A05.0
      Vibrio
        parahaemolyticus A05.3
        vulnificus A05.5
    enterotoxin, staphylococcal A05.0
    noxious —see Poisoning, food, noxious

Intoxication (Continued)
  gastrointestinal K52.1
  hallucinogenic (without dependence) —see
    Abuse, drug, hallucinogen, with
    intoxication
    with dependence —see Dependence, drug,
      hallucinogen, with intoxication
  hypnotic (acute) (without dependence) —see
    Abuse, drug, sedative, with intoxication
    with dependence —see Dependence, drug,
      sedative, with intoxication
  inhalant (acute) (without dependence) —see
    Abuse, drug, inhalant, with intoxication
    with dependence —see Dependence, drug,
      inhalant, with intoxication
  meaning
    inebriation —see category F10
    poisoning —see Table of Drugs and
      Chemicals
  methyl alcohol (acute) (without
    dependence) —see Alcohol, intoxication
  opioid (acute) (without dependence) —see
    Abuse, drug, opioid, with intoxication
    with dependence —see Dependence, drug,
      opioid, with intoxication
  pathologic NEC (without dependence) —see
    Alcohol, intoxication
  phencyclidine (without dependence) —see
    Abuse, drug, psychoactive NEC, with
    intoxication
    with dependence —see Dependence, drug,
      psychoactive NEC, with intoxication
  potassium (K) E87.5
  psychoactive substance NEC (without
    dependence) —see Abuse, drug,
    psychoactive NEC, with intoxication
    with dependence —see Dependence, drug,
      psychoactive NEC, with intoxication
  sedative (acute) (without dependence) —see
    Abuse, drug, sedative, with intoxication
    with dependence —see Dependence, drug,
      sedative, with intoxication
  serum (see also Reaction, serum) T80.69
  uremic —see Uremia
  volatile solvents (acute) (without
    dependence) —see Abuse, drug, inhalant,
    with intoxication
    with dependence —see Dependence, drug,
      inhalant, with intoxication
  water E87.79
Intracranial —see condition
Intrahepatic gallbladder Q44.1
Intraligamentous —see condition
Intrathoracic —see also condition
  kidney Q63.2
Intrauterine contraceptive device
  checking Z30.431
  in situ Z97.5
  insertion Z30.430
    immediately following removal Z30.433
  management Z30.431
  reinsertion Z30.433
  removal Z30.432
  replacement Z30.433
  retention in pregnancy O26.3-
Intraventricular —see condition
Intrinsic deformity —see Deformity
Intubation, difficult or failed T88.4
Intumescence, lens (eye) (cataract) —see Cataract
Intussusception (bowel) (colon) (enteric)
    (ileocecal) (ileocolic) (intestine) (rectum)
    K56.1
  appendix K38.8
  congenital Q43.8
  ureter (with obstruction) N13.5
Invagination (bowel, colon, intestine or rectum)
    K56.1
Inversion
  albumin-globulin (A-G) ratio E88.09
  bladder N32.89
  cecum —see Intussusception
  cervix N88.8

Inversion (Continued)
  chromosome in normal individual Q95.1
  circadian rhythm —see Disorder, sleep,
    circadian rhythm
  nipple N64.59
    congenital Q83.8
    gestational —see Retraction, nipple
    puerperal, postpartum —see Retraction,
      nipple
  nyctohemeral rhythm —see Disorder, sleep,
    circadian rhythm
  optic papilla Q14.2
  organ or site, congenital NEC —see Anomaly,
    by site
  sleep rhythm —see Disorder, sleep, circadian
    rhythm
  testis (congenital) Q55.29
  uterus (chronic) (postinfectional) (postpartal,
    old) N85.5
    postpartum O71.2
  vagina (posthysterectomy) N99.3
  ventricular Q20.5
Investigation (see also Examination) Z04.9
  clinical research subject (control) (normal
    comparison) (participant) Z00.6
Involuntary movement, abnormal R25.9
Involution, involutional —see also condition
  breast, cystic —see Dysplasia, mammary,
    specified type NEC
  depression (single episode) F32.8
    recurrent episode F33.9
  melancholia (recurrent episode) (single
    episode) F32.8
  ovary, senile —see Atrophy, ovary
  thymus failure E32.8
I.Q.
  under 20 F73
  20-34 F72
  35-49 F71
  50-69 F70
IRDS (type I) P22.0
  type II P22.1
Irideremia Q13.1
Iridis rubeosis —see Disorder, iris, vascular
Iridochoroiditis (panuveitis) —see Panuveitis
Iridocyclitis H20.9-
  acute H20.0-
    hypopyon H20.05-
    primary H20.01-
    recurrent H20.02-
    secondary (noninfectious) H20.04-
      infectious H20.03-
  chronic H20.1-
  due to allergy —see Iridocyclitis, acute,
    secondary
  endogenous —see Iridocyclitis, acute, primary
  Fuchs' —see Cyclitis, Fuchs' heterochromic
  gonococcal A54.32
  granulomatous —see Iridocyclitis, chronic
  herpes, herpetic (simplex) B00.51
    zoster B02.32
  hypopyon —see Iridocyclitis, acute, hypopyon
  in (due to)
    ankylosing spondylitis M45.9
    gonococcal infection A54.32
    herpes (simplex) virus B00.51
      zoster B02.32
    infectious disease NOS B99
    parasitic disease NOS B89 [H22]
    sarcoidosis D86.83
    syphilis A51.43
    tuberculosis A18.54
    zoster B02.32
  lens-induced H20.2-
  nongranulomatous —see Iridocyclitis, acute
  recurrent —see Iridocyclitis, acute, recurrent
  rheumatic —see Iridocyclitis, chronic
  subacute —see Iridocyclitis, acute
  sympathetic —see Uveitis, sympathetic
  syphilitic (secondary) A51.43
  tuberculous (chronic) A18.54
  Vogt-Koyanagi H20.82-

◄ New ◄▬ Revised ~~deleted~~ Deleted

Iridocyclochoroiditis (panuveitis) —*see*
    Panuveitis
Iridodialysis H21.53-
Iridodonesis H21.89
Iridoplegia (complete) (partial) (reflex) H57.09
Iridoschisis H21.25-
Iris —*see also* condition
    bombé —*see* Membrane, pupillary
Iritis —*see also* Iridocyclitis
    chronic —*see* Iridocyclitis, chronic
    diabetic —*see* E08-E13 with .39
    due to
        herpes simplex B00.51
        leprosy A30.9 [H22]
    gonococcal A54.32
    gouty M10.9
    granulomatous —*see* Iridocyclitis, chronic
    lens induced —*see* Iridocyclitis, lens-induced
    papulosa (syphilitic) A52.71
    rheumatic —*see* Iridocyclitis, chronic
    syphilitic (secondary) A51.43
        congenital (early) A50.01
        late A52.71
    tuberculous A18.54
Iron —*see* condition
Iron-miner's lung J63.4
Irradiated enamel (tooth, teeth) K03.89
Irradiation effects, adverse T66
Irreducible, irreducibility —*see* condition
Irregular, irregularity
    action, heart I49.9
    alveolar process K08.8
    bleeding N92.6
    breathing R06.89
    contour of cornea (acquired) —*see* Deformity,
        cornea
        congenital Q13.4
    contour, reconstructed breast N65.0
    dentin (in pulp) K04.3
    eye movements H55.89
        nystagmus —*see* Nystagmus
        saccadic H55.81
    labor O62.2
    menstruation (cause unknown) N92.6
    periods N92.6
    prostate N42.9
    pupil —*see* Abnormality, pupillary
    reconstructed breast N65.0
    respiratory R06.89
    septum (nasal) J34.2
    shape, organ or site, congenital NEC —*see*
        Distortion
    sleep-wake pattern (rhythm) G47.23
Irritable, irritability R45.4
    bladder N32.89
    bowel (syndrome) K58.9
        with diarrhea K58.0
        psychogenic F45.8
    bronchial —*see* Bronchitis
    cerebral, in newborn P91.3
    colon K58.9
        with diarrhea K58.0
        psychogenic F45.8
    duodenum K59.8
    heart (psychogenic) F45.8
    hip —*see* Derangement, joint, specified type
        NEC, hip
    ileum K59.8
    infant R68.12
    jejunum K59.8
    rectum K59.8
    stomach K31.89
        psychogenic F45.8
    sympathetic G90.8
    urethra N36.8
Irritation
    anus K62.89
    axillary nerve G54.0
    bladder N32.89
    brachial plexus G54.0
    bronchial —*see* Bronchitis
    cervical plexus G54.2

Irritation (*Continued*)
    cervix —*see* Cervicitis
    choroid, sympathetic —*see* Endophthalmitis
    cranial nerve —*see* Disorder, nerve, cranial
    gastric K31.89
        psychogenic F45.8
    globe, sympathetic —*see* Uveitis, sympathetic
    labyrinth —*see* subcategory H83.2
    lumbosacral plexus G54.1
    meninges (traumatic) —*see* Injury, intracranial
        nontraumatic —*see* Meningismus
    nerve —*see* Disorder, nerve
    nervous R45.0
    penis N48.89
    perineum NEC L29.3
    peripheral autonomic nervous system G90.8
    peritoneum —*see* Peritonitis
    pharynx J39.2
    plantar nerve —*see* Lesion, nerve, plantar
    spinal (cord) (traumatic) —*see also* Injury, spinal
        cord, by region
        nerve G58.9
            root NEC —*see* Radiculopathy
        nontraumatic —*see* Myelopathy
    stomach K31.89
        psychogenic F45.8
    sympathetic nerve NEC G90.8
    ulnar nerve —*see* Lesion, nerve, ulnar
    vagina N89.8
Ischemia, ischemic I99.8
    bowel (transient)
        acute K55.0
        chronic K55.1
        due to mesenteric artery insufficiency
            K55.1
    brain —*see* Ischemia, cerebral
    cardiac (*see* Disease, heart, ischemic)
    cardiomyopathy I25.5
    cerebral (chronic) (generalized) I67.82
        arteriosclerotic I67.2
        intermittent G45.9
        newborn P91.0
        recurrent focal G45.8
        transient G45.9
    colon chronic (due to mesenteric artery
        insufficiency) K55.1
    coronary —*see* Disease, heart, ischemic
    demand (coronary) (*see also* Angina) I24.8
    heart (chronic or with a stated duration of over
        4 weeks) I25.9
        acute or with a stated duration of 4 weeks or
            less I24.9
        subacute I24.9
    infarction, muscle —*see* Infarct, muscle
    intestine (large) (small) (transient) K55.9
        acute K55.0
        chronic K55.1
        due to mesenteric artery insufficiency
            K55.1
    kidney N28.0
    mesenteric, acute K55.0
    muscle, traumatic T79.6
    myocardium, myocardial (chronic or with a
        stated duration of over 4 weeks) I25.9
        acute, without myocardial infarction I24.0
        silent (asymptomatic) I25.6
        transient of newborn P29.4
    renal N28.0
    retina, retinal —*see* Occlusion, artery, retina
    small bowel
        acute K55.0
        chronic K55.1
        due to mesenteric artery insufficiency
            K55.1
    spinal cord G95.11
    subendocardial —*see* Insufficiency, coronary
    supply (coronary) (*see also* Angina) I25.9
        due to vasospasm I20.1
Ischial spine —*see* condition
Ischialgia —*see* Sciatica
Ischiopagus Q89.4
Ischium, ischial —*see* condition

Ischuria R34
Iselin's disease or osteochondrosis —*see*
    Osteochondrosis, juvenile, metatarsus
Islands of
    parotid tissue in
        lymph nodes Q38.6
        neck structures Q38.6
    submaxillary glands in
        fascia Q38.6
        lymph nodes Q38.6
        neck muscles Q38.6
Islet cell tumor, pancreas D13.7
Isoimmunization NEC —*see also* Incompatibility
    affecting management of pregnancy (ABO)
        (with hydrops fetalis) O36.11-
        anti-A sensitization O36.11-
        anti-B sensitization O36.19-
        anti-c sensitization O36.09-
        anti-C sensitization O36.09-
        anti-e sensitization O36.09-
        anti-E sensitization O36.09-
        Rh NEC O36.09-
            anti-D antibody O36.01-
        specified NEC O36.19-
    newborn P55.9
        with
            hydrops fetalis P56.0
            kernicterus P57.0
        ABO (blood groups) P55.1
        Rhesus (Rh) factor P55.0
        specified type NEC P55.8
Isolation, isolated
    dwelling Z59.8
    family Z63.79
    social Z60.4
Isoleucinosis E71.19
Isomerism atrial appendages (with asplenia or
    polysplenia) Q20.6
Isosporiasis, isosporosis A07.3
Isovaleric acidemia E71.110
Issue of
    medical certificate Z02.79
        for disability determination Z02.71
    repeat prescription (appliance) (glasses)
        (medicinal substance, medicament,
        medicine) Z76.0
        contraception —*see* Contraception
Itch, itching —*see also* Pruritus
    baker's L23.6
    barber's B35.0
    bricklayer's L24.5
    cheese B88.0
    clam digger's B65.3
    coolie B76.9
    copra B88.0
    dew B76.9
    dhobi B35.6
    filarial —*see* Infestation, filarial
    grain B88.0
    grocer's B88.0
    ground B76.9
    harvest B88.0
    jock B35.6
    Malabar B35.5
        beard B35.0
        foot B35.3
        scalp B35.0
    meaning scabies B86
    Norwegian B86
    perianal L29.0
    poultrymen's B88.0
    sarcoptic B86
    scabies B86
    scrub B88.0
    straw B88.0
    swimmer's B65.3
    water B76.9
    winter L29.8
Ivemark's syndrome (asplenia with congenital
    heart disease) Q89.01
Ivory bones Q78.2
Ixodiasis NEC B88.8

J

Jaccoud's syndrome —*see* Arthropathy,
  postrheumatic, chronic
Jackson's
  membrane Q43.3
  paralysis or syndrome G83.89
  veil Q43.3
Jacquet's dermatitis (diaper dermatitis) L22
Jadassohn-Pellizari's disease or anetoderma
  L90.2
Jadassohn's
  blue nevus —*see* Nevus
  intraepidermal epithelioma —*see* Neoplasm,
    skin, benign
Jaffe-Lichtenstein (-Uehlinger) syndrome —*see*
  Dysplasia, fibrous, bone NEC
Jakob-Creutzfeldt disease or syndrome —*see*
  Creutzfeldt-Jakob disease or syndrome
Jaksch-Luzet disease D64.89
Jamaican
  neuropathy G92
  paraplegic tropical ataxic-spastic syndrome
    G92
Janet's disease F48.8
Janiceps Q89.4
Jansky-Bielschowsky amaurotic idiocy
  E75.4
Japanese
  B-type encephalitis A83.0
  river fever A75.3
Jaundice (yellow) R17
  acholuric (familial) (splenomegalic) —*see also*
    Spherocytosis
    acquired D59.8
  breast-milk (inhibitor) P59.3
  catarrhal (acute) B15.9
    with hepatic coma B15.0
  cholestatic (benign) R17
  due to or associated with
    delayed conjugation P59.8
      associated with (due to) preterm
        delivery P59.0
      preterm delivery P59.0
  epidemic (catarrhal) B15.9
    with hepatic coma B15.0
    leptospiral A27.0
    spirochetal A27.0
  familial nonhemolytic (congenital) (Gilbert)
    E80.4
    Crigler-Najjar E80.5
  febrile (acute) B15.9
    with hepatic coma B15.0
    leptospiral A27.0
    spirochetal A27.0
  hematogenous D59.9
  hemolytic (acquired) D59.9
    congenital —*see* Spherocytosis

Jaundice (*Continued*)
  hemorrhagic (acute) (leptospiral)
    (spirochetal) A27.0
  infectious (acute) (subacute) B15.9
    with hepatic coma B15.0
    leptospiral A27.0
    spirochetal A27.0
  leptospiral (hemorrhagic) A27.0
  malignant (without coma) K72.90
    with coma K72.91
  neonatal —*see* Jaundice, newborn
  newborn P59.9
    due to or associated with
      ABO
        antibodies P55.1
        incompatibility, maternal/fetal
          P55.1
        isoimmunization P55.1
      absence or deficiency of enzyme
        system for bilirubin conjugation
        (congenital) P59.8
      bleeding P58.1
      breast milk inhibitors to conjugation
        P59.3
        associated with preterm delivery
          P59.0
      bruising P58.0
      Crigler-Najjar syndrome E80.5
      delayed conjugation P59.8
        associated with preterm delivery
          P59.0
      drugs or toxins
        given to newborn P58.42
        transmitted from mother P58.41
      excessive hemolysis P58.9
        due to
          bleeding P58.1
          bruising P58.0
          drugs or toxins
            given to newborn P58.42
            transmitted from mother P58.41
          infection P58.2
          polycythemia P58.3
          swallowed maternal blood P58.5
        specified type NEC P58.8
      galactosemia E74.21
      Gilbert syndrome E80.4
      hemolytic disease P55.9
        ABO isoimmunization P55.1
        Rh isoimmunization P55.0
        specified NEC P55.8
      hepatocellular damage P59.20
        specified NEC P59.29
      hereditary hemolytic anemia P58.8
      hypothyroidism, congenital E03.1
      incompatibility, maternal/fetal NOS
        P55.9
      infection P58.2

Jaundice (*Continued*)
  newborn (*Continued*)
    due to or associated with (*Continued*)
      inspissated bile syndrome P59.1
      isoimmunization NOS P55.9
      mucoviscidosis E84.9
      polycythemia P58.3
      preterm delivery P59.0
      Rh
        antibodies P55.0
        incompatibility, maternal/fetal P55.0
        isoimmunization P55.0
      specified cause NEC P59.8
      swallowed maternal blood P58.5
    spherocytosis (congenital) D58.0
    nonhemolytic congenital familial (Gilbert)
      E80.4
    nuclear, newborn (*see also* Kernicterus of
      newborn) P57.9
    obstructive (*see also* Obstruction, bile duct)
      K83.1
    post-immunization —*see* Hepatitis, viral,
      type, B
    post-transfusion —*see* Hepatitis, viral, type, B
    regurgitation (*see also* Obstruction, bile duct)
      K83.1
    serum (homologous) (prophylactic)
      (therapeutic) —*see* Hepatitis, viral,
      type, B
    spirochetal (hemorrhagic) A27.0
    symptomatic R17
      newborn P59.9
Jaw —*see* condition
Jaw-winking phenomenon or syndrome Q07.8
Jealousy
  alcoholic F10.988
  childhood F93.8
  sibling F93.8
Jejunitis —*see* Enteritis
Jejunostomy status Z93.4
Jejunum, jejunal —*see* condition
Jensen's disease —*see* Inflammation,
  chorioretinal, focal, juxtapapillary
Jerks, myoclonic G25.3
Jervell-Lange-Nielsen syndrome I45.81
Jeune's disease Q77.2
Jigger disease B88.1
Job's syndrome (chronic granulomatous
  disease) D71
Joint —*see also* condition
  mice —*see* Loose, body, joint
    knee M23.4-
Jordan's anomaly or syndrome D72.0
Joseph-Diamond-Blackfan anemia (congenital
  hypoplastic) D61.01
Jungle yellow fever A95.0
Jüngling's disease —*see* Sarcoidosis
Juvenile —*see* condition

◀ New   ◀▥ Revised   ~~deleted~~ Deleted

K

Kahler's disease C90.0-
Kakke E51.11
Kala-azar B55.0
Kallmann's syndrome E23.0
Kanner's syndrome (autism) —*see* Psychosis, childhood
Kaposi's
　dermatosis (xeroderma pigmentosum) Q82.1
　lichen ruber L44.0
　　acuminatus L44.0
　sarcoma
　　colon C46.4
　　connective tissue C46.1
　　gastrointestinal organ C46.4
　　lung C46.5-
　　lymph node (multiple) C46.3
　　palate (hard) (soft) C46.2
　　rectum C46.4
　　skin (multiple sites) C46.0
　　specified site NEC C46.7
　　stomach C46.4
　　unspecified site C46.9
　varicelliform eruption B00.0
　　vaccinia T88.1
Kartagener's syndrome or triad (sinusitis, bronchiectasis, situs inversus) Q89.3
Karyotype
　with abnormality except iso (Xq) Q96.2
　45,X Q96.0
　46,X
　　iso (Xq) Q96.1
　46,XX Q98.3
　　with streak gonads Q50.32
　　hermaphrodite (true) Q99.1
　　male Q98.3
　46,XY
　　with streak gonads Q56.1
　　female Q97.3
　　hermaphrodite (true) Q99.1
　47,XXX Q97.0
　47,XXY Q98.0
　47,XYY Q98.5
Kaschin-Beck disease —*see* Disease, Kaschin-Beck
Katayama's disease or fever B65.2
Kawasaki's syndrome M30.3
Kayser-Fleischer ring (cornea) (pseudosclerosis) H18.04-
Kaznelson's syndrome (congenital hypoplastic anemia) D61.01
Kearns-Sayre syndrome H49.81-
Kedani fever A75.3
Kelis L91.0
Kelly (-Patterson) syndrome (sideropenic dysphagia) D50.1
Keloid, cheloid L91.0
　acne L73.0
　Addison's L94.0
　cornea —*see* Opacity, cornea
　Hawkin's L91.0
　scar L91.0
Keloma L91.0
Kenya fever A77.1
Keratectasia —*see also* Ectasia, cornea
　congenital Q13.4
Keratinization of alveolar ridge mucosa
　excessive K13.23
　minimal K13.22
Keratinized residual ridge mucosa
　excessive K13.23
　minimal K13.22
Keratitis (nodular) (nonulcerative) (simple) (zonular) H16.9
　with ulceration (central) (marginal) (perforated) (ring) —*see* Ulcer, cornea
　actinic —*see* Photokeratitis
　arborescens (herpes simplex) B00.52
　areolar H16.11-
　bullosa H16.8

Keratitis *(Continued)*
　deep H16.309
　　specified type NEC H16.399
　dendritic (a) (herpes simplex) B00.52
　disciform (is) (herpes simplex) B00.52
　　varicella B01.81
　filamentary H16.12-
　gonococcal (congenital or prenatal) A54.33
　herpes, herpetic (simplex) B00.52
　　zoster B02.33
　in (due to)
　　acanthamebiasis B60.13
　　adenovirus B30.0
　　exanthema (*see also* Exanthem) B09
　　herpes (simplex) virus B00.52
　　measles B05.81
　　syphilis A50.31
　　tuberculosis A18.52
　　zoster B02.33
　interstitial (nonsyphilitic) H16.30-
　　diffuse H16.32-
　　herpes, herpetic (simplex) B00.52
　　　zoster B02.33
　　sclerosing H16.33-
　　specified type NEC H16.39-
　　syphilitic (congenital) (late) A50.31
　　tuberculous A18.52
　macular H16.11-
　nummular H16.11-
　oyster shuckers' H16.8
　parenchymatous —*see* Keratitis, interstitial
　petrificans H16.8
　postmeasles B05.81
　punctata
　　leprosa A30.9 [H16.14-]
　　syphilitic (profunda) A50.31
　punctate H16.14-
　purulent H16.8
　rosacea L71.8
　sclerosing H16.33-
　specified type NEC H16.8
　stellate H16.11-
　striate H16.11-
　superficial H16.10-
　　with conjunctivitis —*see* Keratoconjunctivitis
　　due to light —*see* Photokeratitis
　suppurative H16.8
　syphilitic (congenital) (prenatal) A50.31
　trachomatous A71.1
　　sequelae B94.0
　tuberculous A18.52
　vesicular H16.8
　xerotic (*see also* Keratomalacia) H16.8
　　vitamin A deficiency E50.4
Keratoacanthoma L85.8
Keratocele —*see* Descemetocele
Keratoconjunctivitis H16.20-
　Acanthamoeba B60.13
　adenoviral B30.0
　epidemic B30.0
　exposure H16.21-
　herpes, herpetic (simplex) B00.52
　　zoster B02.33
　in exanthema (*see also* Exanthem) B09
　infectious B30.0
　lagophthalmic —*see* Keratoconjunctivitis, specified type NEC
　neurotrophic H16.23-
　phlyctenular H16.25-
　postmeasles B05.81
　shipyard B30.0
　sicca (Sjogren's) M35.0-
　　not Sjogren's H16.22-
　specified type NEC H16.29-
　tuberculous (phlyctenular) A18.52
　vernal H16.26-
Keratoconus H18.60-
　congenital Q13.4
　stable H18.61-
　unstable H18.62-

Keratocyst (dental) (odontogenic) —*see* Cyst, calcifying odontogenic
Keratoderma, keratodermia (congenital) (palmaris et plantaris) (symmetrical) Q82.8
　acquired L85.1
　　in diseases classified elsewhere L86
　climactericum L85.1
　gonococcal A54.89
　gonorrheal A54.89
　punctata L85.2
　Reiter's —*see* Reiter's disease
Keratodermatocele —*see* Descemetocele
Keratoglobus H18.79
　congenital Q15.8
　　with glaucoma Q15.0
Keratohemia —*see* Pigmentation, cornea, stromal
Keratoiritis —*see also* Iridocyclitis
　syphilitic A50.39
　tuberculous A18.54
Keratoma L57.0
　palmaris and plantaris hereditarium Q82.8
　senile L57.0
Keratomalacia H18.44-
　vitamin A deficiency E50.4
Keratomegaly Q13.4
Keratomycosis B49
　nigrans, nigricans (palmaris) B36.1
Keratopathy H18.9
　band H18.42-
　bullous H18.1-
　bullous (aphakic), following cataract surgery H59.01-
Keratoscleritis, tuberculous A18.52
Keratosis L57.0
　actinic L57.0
　arsenical L85.8
　congenital, specified NEC Q80.8
　female genital NEC N94.89
　follicularis Q82.8
　　acquired L11.0
　　congenita Q82.8
　　et parafollicularis in cutem penetrans L87.0
　　spinulosa (decalvans) Q82.8
　　vitamin A deficiency E50.8
　gonococcal A54.89
　male genital (external) N50.8
　nigricans L83
　obturans, external ear (canal) —*see* Cholesteatoma, external ear
　palmaris et plantaris (inherited) (symmetrical) Q82.8
　　acquired L85.1
　penile N48.89
　pharynx J39.2
　pilaris, acquired L85.8
　punctata (palmaris et plantaris) L85.2
　scrotal N50.8
　seborrheic L82.1
　　inflamed L82.0
　senile L57.0
　solar L57.0
　tonsillaris J35.8
　vagina N89.4
　vegetans Q82.8
　vitamin A deficiency E50.8
　vocal cord J38.3
Kerato-uveitis —*see* Iridocyclitis
Kerion (celsi) B35.0
Kernicterus of newborn (not due to isoimmunization) P57.9
　due to isoimmunization (conditions in P55.0-P55.9) P57.0
　specified type NEC P57.8
Kerunoparalysis T75.09
Keshan disease E59
Ketoacidosis E87.2
　diabetic —*see* Diabetes, by type, with ketoacidosis
Ketonuria R82.4

Ketosis NEC E88.89
   diabetic —*see* Diabetes, by type, with
      ketoacidosis
Kew Garden fever A79.1
Kidney —*see* condition
Kienböck's disease —*see also* Osteochondrosis,
      juvenile, hand, carpal lunate
   adult M93.1
Kimmelstiel (-Wilson) disease —*see* Diabetes,
      Kimmelstiel (-Wilson) disease
Kimura disease D21.9
   specified site (see Neoplasm, connective
      tissue benign)
Kink, kinking
   artery I77.1
   hair (acquired) L67.8
   ileum or intestine —*see* Obstruction,
      intestine
   Lane's —*see* Obstruction, intestine
   organ or site, congenital NEC —*see* Anomaly,
      by site
   ureter (pelvic junction) N13.5
      with
         hydronephrosis N13.1
            with infection N13.6
         pyelonephritis (chronic) N11.1
      congenital Q62.39
   vein (s) I87.8
      caval I87.1
      peripheral I87.1
Kinnier Wilson's disease (hepatolenticular
      degeneration) E83.01
Kissing spine M48.20
   cervical region M48.22
   cervicothoracic region M48.23
   lumbar region M48.26
   lumbosacral region M48.27
   occipito-atlanto-axial region M48.21
   thoracic region M48.24
   thoracolumbar region M48.25
Klatskin's tumor C24.0
Klauder's disease A26.8
Klebs' disease (*see also* Glomerulonephritis)
      N05.-
**Klebsiella (K.) pneumoniae, as cause of
      disease classified elsewhere** B96.1
Klein (e)-Levin syndrome G47.13
Kleptomania F63.2
Klinefelter's syndrome Q98.4
   karyotype 47,XXY Q98.0
   male with more than two X chromosomes
      Q98.1
Klippel-Feil deficiency, disease, or syndrome
      (brevicollis) Q76.1
Klippel's disease I67.2
Klippel-Trenaunay (-Weber) syndrome
      Q87.2
Klumpke (-Déjerine) palsy, paralysis (birth)
      (newborn) P14.1
Knee —*see* condition
Knock knee (acquired) M21.06-
   congenital Q74.1

Knot (s)
   intestinal, syndrome (volvulus) K56.2
   surfer S89.8-
   umbilical cord (true) O69.2
Knotting (of)
   hair L67.8
   intestine K56.2
Knuckle pad (Garrod's) **M72.1**
Koch's
   infection —*see* Tuberculosis
   relapsing fever A68.9
Koch-Weeks' conjunctivitis —*see*
      Conjunctivitis, acute, mucopurulent
Köebner's syndrome Q81.8
Köenig's disease (osteochondritis dissecans) —
      see Osteochondritis, dissecans
Köhler-Pellegrini-Steida disease or syndrome
      (calcification, knee joint) —*see* Bursitis,
      tibial collateral
Köhler's disease
   patellar —*see* Osteochondrosis, juvenile,
      patella
   tarsal navicular —*see* Osteochondrosis,
      juvenile, tarsus
Koilonychia L60.3
   congenital Q84.6
Kojevnikov's, epilepsy —*see* Kozhevnikof's
      epilepsy
Koplik's spots B05.9
Kopp's asthma E32.8
**Korsakoff's (Wernicke) disease, psychosis or
      syndrome** (alcoholic) F10.96
   with dependence F10.26
   drug-induced
      due to drug abuse —*see* Abuse, drug, by
         type, with amnestic disorder
      due to drug dependence —*see* Dependence,
         drug, by type, with amnestic disorder
   nonalcoholic F04
Korsakov's disease, psychosis or syndrome —
      see Korsakoff's disease
Korsakow's disease, psychosis or syndrome —
      see Korsakoff's disease
Kostmann's disease or syndrome (infantile
      genetic agranulocytosis) —*see*
      Agranulocytosis
Kozhevnikof's epilepsy G40.109
   intractable G40.119
      with status epilepticus G40.111
      without status epilepticus G40.119
   not intractable G40.109
      with status epilepticus G40.101
      without status epilepticus G40.109
Krabbe's
   disease E75.23
   syndrome, congenital muscle hypoplasia
      Q79.8
Kraepelin-Morel disease —*see* Schizophrenia
Kraft-Weber-Dimitri disease Q85.8
Kraurosis
   ani K62.89
   penis N48.0

Kraurosis (*Continued*)
   vagina N89.8
   vulva N90.4
Kreotoxism A05.9
Krukenberg's
   spindle —*see* Pigmentation, cornea, posterior
   tumor C79.6-
Kufs' disease E75.4
Kugelberg-Welander disease G12.1
Kuhnt-Junius degeneration (*see also*
      Degeneration, macula) H35.32
Kümmell's disease or spondylitis —*see*
      Spondylopathy, traumatic
Kupffer cell sarcoma C22.3
Kuru A81.81
Kussmaul's
   disease M30.0
   respiration E87.2
      in diabetic acidosis —*see* Diabetes, by type,
         with ketoacidosis
Kwashiorkor E40
   marasmic, marasmus type E42
Kyasanur Forest disease A98.2
Kyphoscoliosis, kyphoscoliotic (acquired) (*see
      also* Scoliosis) M41.9
   congenital Q67.5
   heart (disease) I27.1
   sequelae of rickets E64.3
   tuberculous A18.01
Kyphosis, kyphotic (acquired) M40.209
   cervical region M40.202
   cervicothoracic region M40.203
   congenital Q76.419
      cervical region Q76.412
      cervicothoracic region Q76.413
      occipito-atlanto-axial region Q76.411
      thoracic region Q76.414
      thoracolumbar region Q76.415
   Morquio-Brailsford type (spinal) (*see also*
      subcategory M49.8) E76.219
   postlaminectomy M96.3
   postradiation therapy M96.2
   postural (adolescent) M40.00
      cervicothoracic region M40.03
      thoracic region M40.04
      thoracolumbar region M40.05
   secondary NEC M40.10
      cervical region M40.12
      cervicothoracic region M40.13
      thoracic region M40.14
      thoracolumbar region M40.15
   sequelae of rickets E64.3
   specified type NEC M40.299
      cervical region M40.292
      cervicothoracic region M40.293
      thoracic region M40.294
      thoracolumbar region M40.295
   syphilitic, congenital A50.56
   thoracic region M40.204
   thoracolumbar region M40.205
   tuberculous A18.01
Kyrle disease L87.0

K

L

Labia, labium —*see* condition
Labile
  blood pressure R09.89
  vasomotor system I73.9
Labioglossal paralysis G12.29
Labium leporinum —*see* Cleft, lip
Labor —*see* Delivery
Labored breathing —*see* Hyperventilation
Labyrinthitis (circumscribed) (destructive)
    (diffuse) (inner ear) (latent) (purulent)
    (suppurative) (*see also* subcategory)
    H83.0
  syphilitic A52.79
Laceration
  with abortion —*see* Abortion, by type,
      complicated by laceration of pelvic
      organs
  abdomen, abdominal
    wall S31.119
      with
        foreign body S31.129
        penetration into peritoneal cavity
          S31.619
          with foreign body S31.629
      epigastric region S31.112
        with
          foreign body S31.122
          penetration into peritoneal cavity
            S31.612
            with foreign body S31.622
      left
        lower quadrant S31.114
          with
            foreign body S31.124
            penetration into peritoneal cavity
              S31.614
              with foreign body S31.624
        upper quadrant S31.111
          with
            foreign body S31.121
            penetration into peritoneal cavity
              S31.611
              with foreign body S31.621
      periumbilic region S31.115
        with
          foreign body S31.125
          penetration into peritoneal cavity
            S31.615
            with foreign body S31.625
      right
        lower quadrant S31.113
          with
            foreign body S31.123
            penetration into peritoneal cavity
              S31.613
              with foreign body S31.623
        upper quadrant S31.110
          with
            foreign body S31.120
            penetration into peritoneal cavity
              S31.610
              with foreign body S31.620
  accidental, complicating surgery —*see*
      Complications, surgical, accidental
      puncture or laceration
  Achilles tendon S86.02-
  adrenal gland S37.813
  alveolar (process) —*see* Laceration, oral cavity
  ankle S91.01-
    with
      foreign body S91.02-
  antecubital space —*see* Laceration, elbow
  anus (sphincter) S31.831
    with
      ectopic or molar pregnancy O08.6
      foreign body S31.832
    complicating delivery —*see* Delivery,
      complicated, by, laceration, anus
      (sphincter)

Laceration (*Continued*)
  anus (*Continued*)
    following ectopic or molar pregnancy
      O08.6
    nontraumatic, nonpuerperal —*see* Fissure,
      anus
  arm (upper) S41.11-
    with foreign body S41.12-
    lower —*see* Laceration, forearm
  auditory canal (external) (meatus) —*see*
    Laceration, ear
  auricle, ear —*see* Laceration, ear
  axilla —*see* Laceration, arm
  back —*see also* Laceration, thorax, back
    lower S31.010
      with
        foreign body S31.020
          with penetration into
            retroperitoneal space S31.021
        penetration into retroperitoneal space
          S31.011
  bile duct S36.13
  bladder S37.23
    with ectopic or molar pregnancy O08.6
    following ectopic or molar pregnancy
      O08.6
    obstetrical trauma O71.5
  blood vessel —*see* Injury, blood vessel
  bowel —*see also* Laceration, intestine
    with ectopic or molar pregnancy O08.6
    complicating abortion —*see* Abortion,
      by type, complicated by, specified
      condition NEC
    following ectopic or molar pregnancy
      O08.6
    obstetrical trauma O71.5
  brain (any part) (cortex) (diffuse)
    (membrane) —*see also* Injury,
    intracranial, diffuse
    during birth P10.8
      with hemorrhage P10.1
    focal —*see* Injury, intracranial, focal brain
      injury
  brainstem S06.38-
  breast S21.01-
    with foreign body S21.02-
  broad ligament S37.893
    with ectopic or molar pregnancy O08.6
    following ectopic or molar pregnancy
      O08.6
    laceration syndrome N83.8
    obstetrical trauma O71.6
    syndrome (laceration) N83.8
  buttock S31.801
    with foreign body S31.802
    left S31.821
      with foreign body S31.822
    right S31.811
      with foreign body S31.812
  calf —*see* Laceration, leg
  canaliculus lacrimalis —*see* Laceration,
    eyelid
  canthus, eye —*see* Laceration, eyelid
  capsule, joint —*see* Sprain
  causing eversion of cervix uteri (old) N86
  central (perineal), complicating delivery
    O70.9
  cerebellum, traumatic S06.37-
  cerebral S06.33-
    during birth P10.8
      with hemorrhage P10.1
    left side S06.32-
    right side S06.31-
  cervix (uteri)
    with ectopic or molar pregnancy O08.6
    following ectopic or molar pregnancy
      O08.6
    nonpuerperal, nontraumatic N88.1
    obstetrical trauma (current) O71.3
    old (postpartal) N88.1
    traumatic S37.63

Laceration (*Continued*)
  cheek (external) S01.41-
    with foreign body S01.42-
    internal —*see* Laceration, oral cavity
  chest wall —*see* Laceration, thorax
  chin —*see* Laceration, head, specified site
    NEC
  chordae tendinae NEC I51.1
    concurrent with acute myocardial
      infarction —*see* Infarct, myocardium
    following acute myocardial infarction
      (current complication) I23.4
  clitoris —*see* Laceration, vulva
  colon —*see* Laceration, intestine, large,
    colon
  common bile duct S36.13
  cortex (cerebral) —*see* Injury, intracranial,
    diffuse
  costal region —*see* Laceration, thorax
  cystic duct S36.13
  diaphragm S27.803
  digit (s)
    foot —*see* Laceration, toe
    hand —*see* Laceration, finger
  duodenum S36.430
  ear (canal) (external) S01.31-
    with foreign body S01.32-
    drum S09.2-
  elbow S51.01-
    with
      foreign body S51.02-
  epididymis —*see* Laceration, testis
  epigastric region —*see* Laceration, abdomen,
    wall, epigastric region
  esophagus K22.8
    traumatic
      cervical S11.21
        with foreign body S11.22
      thoracic S27.813
  eye (ball) S05.3-
    with prolapse or loss of intraocular tissue
      S05.2-
    penetrating S05.6-
  eyebrow —*see* Laceration, eyelid
  eyelid S01.11-
    with foreign body S01.12-
  face NEC —*see* Laceration, head, specified
    site NEC
  fallopian tube S37.539
    bilateral S37.532
    unilateral S37.531
  finger (s) S61.219
    with
      damage to nail S61.319
        with
          foreign body S61.329
      foreign body S61.229
    index S61.218
      with
        damage to nail S61.318
          with
            foreign body S61.328
        foreign body S61.228
      left S61.211
        with
          damage to nail S61.311
            with
              foreign body S61.321
          foreign body S61.221
      right S61.210
        with
          damage to nail S61.310
            with
              foreign body S61.320
          foreign body S61.220
    little S61.218
      with
        damage to nail S61.318
          with
            foreign body S61.328
        foreign body S61.228

Laceration *(Continued)*
finger *(Continued)*
little *(Continued)*
left S61.217
with
damage to nail S61.317
with
foreign body S61.327
foreign body S61.227
right S61.216
with
damage to nail S61.316
with
foreign body S61.326
foreign body S61.226
middle S61.218
with
damage to nail S61.318
with
foreign body S61.328
foreign body S61.228
left S61.213
with
damage to nail S61.313
with
foreign body S61.323
foreign body S61.223
right S61.212
with
damage to nail S61.312
with
foreign body S61.322
foreign body S61.222
ring S61.218
with
damage to nail S61.318
with
foreign body S61.328
foreign body S61.228
left S61.215
with
damage to nail S61.315
with
foreign body S61.325
foreign body S61.225
right S61.214
with
damage to nail S61.314
with
foreign body S61.324
foreign body S61.224
flank S31.119
with foreign body S31.129
foot (except toe (s) alone) S91.319
with foreign body S91.329
left S91.312
with foreign body S91.322
right S91.311
with foreign body S91.321
toe —*see* Laceration, toe
forearm S51.819
with
foreign body S51.829
elbow only —*see* Laceration,
elbow
left S51.812
with
foreign body S51.822
right S51.811
with
foreign body S51.821
forehead S01.81
with foreign body S01.82
fourchette O70.0
with ectopic or molar pregnancy
O08.6
complicating delivery O70.0
following ectopic or molar pregnancy
O08.6
gallbladder S36.123

Laceration *(Continued)*
genital organs, external
female S31.512
with foreign body S31.522
vagina —*see* Laceration, vagina
vulva —*see* Laceration, vulva
male S31.511
with foreign body S31.521
penis —*see* Laceration, penis
scrotum —*see* Laceration, scrotum
testis —*see* Laceration, testis
groin —*see* Laceration, abdomen, wall
gum —*see* Laceration, oral cavity
hand S61.419
with
foreign body S61.429
finger —*see* Laceration, finger
left S61.412
with
foreign body S61.422
right S61.411
with
foreign body S61.421
thumb —*see* Laceration, thumb
head S01.91
with foreign body S01.92
cheek —*see* Laceration, cheek
ear —*see* Laceration, ear
eyelid —*see* Laceration, eyelid
lip —*see* Laceration, lip
nose —*see* Laceration, nose
oral cavity —*see* Laceration, oral
cavity
scalp S01.01
with foreign body S01.02
specified site NEC S01.81
with foreign body S01.82
temporomandibular area —*see* Laceration,
cheek
heart —*see* Injury, heart, laceration
heel —*see* Laceration, foot
hepatic duct S36.13
hip S71.019
with foreign body S71.029
left S71.012
with foreign body S71.022
right S71.011
with foreign body S71.021
hymen —*see* Laceration, vagina
hypochondrium —*see* Laceration, abdomen,
wall
hypogastric region —*see* Laceration,
abdomen, wall
ileum S36.438
inguinal region —*see* Laceration, abdomen,
wall
instep —*see* Laceration, foot
internal organ —*see* Injury, by site
interscapular region —*see* Laceration, thorax,
back
intestine
large
colon S36.539
ascending S36.530
descending S36.532
sigmoid S36.533
specified site NEC S36.538
rectum S36.63
transverse S36.531
small S36.439
duodenum S36.430
specified site NEC S36.438
intra-abdominal organ S36.93
intestine —*see* Laceration, intestine
liver —*see* Laceration, liver
pancreas —*see* Laceration, pancreas
peritoneum S36.81
specified site NEC S36.893
spleen —*see* Laceration, spleen
stomach —*see* Laceration, stomach

Laceration *(Continued)*
intracranial NEC —*see also* Injury,
intracranial, diffuse
birth injury P10.9
jaw —*see* Laceration, head, specified site NEC
jejunum S36.438
joint capsule —*see* Sprain, by site
kidney S37.03-
major (greater than 3 cm) (massive)
(stellate) S37.06-
minor (less than 1 cm) S37.04-
moderate (1 to 3 cm) S37.05-
multiple S37.06-
knee S81.01-
with foreign body S81.02-
labium (majus) (minus) —*see* Laceration,
vulva
lacrimal duct —*see* Laceration, eyelid
large intestine —*see* Laceration, intestine,
large
larynx S11.011
with foreign body S11.012
leg (lower) S81.819
with foreign body S81.829
foot —*see* Laceration, foot
knee —*see* Laceration, knee
left S81.812
with foreign body S81.822
right S81.811
with foreign body S81.821
upper —*see* Laceration, thigh
ligament —*see* Sprain
lip S01.511
with foreign body S01.521
liver S36.113
major (stellate) S36.116
minor S36.114
moderate S36.115
loin —*see* Laceration, abdomen, wall
lower back —*see* Laceration, back, lower
lumbar region —*see* Laceration, back, lower
lung S27.339
bilateral S27.332
unilateral S27.331
malar region —*see* Laceration, head, specified
site NEC
mammary —*see* Laceration, breast
mastoid region —*see* Laceration, head,
specified site NEC
meninges —*see* Injury, intracranial, diffuse
meniscus —*see* Tear, meniscus
mesentery S36.893
mesosalpinx S37.893
mouth —*see* Laceration, oral cavity
muscle —*see* Injury, muscle, by site,
laceration
nail
finger —*see* Laceration, finger, with
damage to nail
toe —*see* Laceration, toe, with damage to
nail
nasal (septum) (sinus) —*see* Laceration,
nose
nasopharynx —*see* Laceration, head, specified
site NEC
neck S11.91
with foreign body S11.92
involving
cervical esophagus S11.21
with foreign body S11.22
larynx —*see* Laceration, larynx
pharynx —*see* Laceration, pharynx
thyroid gland —*see* Laceration, thyroid
gland
trachea —*see* Laceration, trachea
specified site NEC S11.81
with foreign body S11.82
nerve —*see* Injury, nerve
nose (septum) (sinus) S01.21
with foreign body S01.22

◀ New ◀▥▥ Revised ~~deleted~~ Deleted

Laceration *(Continued)*
  ocular NOS S05.3-
    adnexa NOS S01.11-
  oral cavity S01.512
    with foreign body S01.522
  orbit (eye) —*see* Wound, open, ocular, orbit
  ovary S37.439
    bilateral S37.432
    unilateral S37.431
  palate —*see* Laceration, oral cavity
  palm —*see* Laceration, hand
  pancreas S36.239
    body S36.231
      major S36.261
      minor S36.241
      moderate S36.251
    head S36.230
      major S36.260
      minor S36.240
      moderate S36.250
    major S36.269
    minor S36.249
    moderate S36.259
    tail S36.232
      major S36.262
      minor S36.242
      moderate S36.252
  pelvic S31.010
    with
      foreign body S31.020
        penetration into retroperitoneal cavity
          S31.021
      penetration into retroperitoneal cavity
        S31.011
    floor —*see also* Laceration, back, lower
      with ectopic or molar pregnancy O08.6
      complicating delivery O70.1
      following ectopic or molar pregnancy
        O08.6
      old (postpartal) N81.89
    organ S37.93
      with ectopic or molar pregnancy O08.6
      adrenal gland S37.813
      bladder S37.23
      fallopian tube —*see* Laceration, fallopian
        tube
      following ectopic or molar pregnancy
        O08.6
      kidney —*see* Laceration, kidney
      obstetrical trauma O71.5
      ovary —*see* Laceration, ovary
      prostate S37.823
      specified site NEC S37.893
      ureter S37.13
      urethra S37.33
      uterus S37.63
  penis S31.21
    with foreign body S31.22
  perineum
    female S31.41
      with
        ectopic or molar pregnancy O08.6
        foreign body S31.42
      during delivery O70.9
        first degree O70.0
        fourth degree O70.3
        second degree O70.1
        third degree O70.2
      old (postpartal) N81.89
      postpartal N81.89
      secondary (postpartal) O90.1
    male S31.119
      with foreign body S31.129
  periocular area (with or without lacrimal
    passages) —*see* Laceration, eyelid
  peritoneum S36.893
  periumbilic region —*see* Laceration,
    abdomen, wall, periumbilic
  periurethral tissue —*see* Laceration,
    urethra

Laceration *(Continued)*
  phalanges
    finger —*see* Laceration, finger
    toe —*see* Laceration, toe
  pharynx S11.21
    with foreign body S11.22
  pinna —*see* Laceration, ear
  popliteal space —*see* Laceration, knee
  prepuce —*see* Laceration, penis
  prostate S37.823
  pubic region S31.119
    with foreign body S31.129
  pudendum —*see* Laceration, genital organs,
    external
  rectovaginal septum —*see* Laceration, vagina
  rectum S36.63
  retroperitoneum S36.893
  round ligament S37.893
  sacral region —*see* Laceration, back, lower
  sacroiliac region —*see* Laceration, back,
    lower
  salivary gland —*see* Laceration, oral cavity
  scalp S01.01
    with foreign body S01.02
  scapular region —*see* Laceration, shoulder
  scrotum S31.31
    with foreign body S31.32
  seminal vesicle S37.893
  shin —*see* Laceration, leg
  shoulder S41.019
    with foreign body S41.029
    left S41.012
      with foreign body S41.022
    right S41.011
      with foreign body S41.021
  small intestine —*see* Laceration, intestine,
    small
  spermatic cord —*see* Laceration, testis
  spinal cord (meninges) —*see also* Injury,
    spinal cord, by region
    due to injury at birth P11.5
    newborn (birth injury) P11.5
  spleen S36.039
    major (massive) (stellate) S36.032
    moderate S36.031
    superficial (minor) S36.030
  sternal region —*see* Laceration, thorax, front
  stomach S36.33
  submaxillary region —*see* Laceration, head,
    specified site NEC
  submental region —*see* Laceration, head,
    specified site NEC
  subungual
    finger (s) —*see* Laceration, finger, with
      damage to nail
    toe (s) —*see* Laceration, toe, with damage
      to nail
  suprarenal gland —*see* Laceration, adrenal
    gland
  temple, temporal region —*see* Laceration,
    head, specified site NEC
  temporomandibular area —*see* Laceration,
    cheek
  tendon —*see* Injury, muscle, by site,
    laceration
    Achilles S86.02-
  tentorium cerebelli —*see* Injury, intracranial,
    diffuse
  testis S31.31
    with foreign body S31.32
  thigh S71.11-
    with foreign body S71.12-
  thorax, thoracic (wall) S21.91
    with foreign body S21.92
    back S21.22-
      with penetration into thoracic cavity
        S21.42-
    front S21.12-
      with penetration into thoracic cavity
        S21.32-

Laceration *(Continued)*
  thorax, thoracic *(Continued)*
    back S21.21-
      with
        foreign body S21.22-
          with penetration into thoracic
            cavity S21.42-
        penetration into thoracic cavity
          S21.41-
    breast —*see* Laceration, breast
    front S21.11-
      with
        foreign body S21.12-
          with penetration into thoracic
            cavity S21.32-
        penetration into thoracic cavity
          S21.31-
  thumb S61.019
    with
      damage to nail S61.119
        with
          foreign body S61.129
      foreign body S61.029
    left S61.012
      with
        damage to nail S61.112
          with
            foreign body S61.122
        foreign body S61.022
    right S61.011
      with
        damage to nail S61.111
          with
            foreign body S61.121
        foreign body S61.021
  thyroid gland S11.11
    with foreign body S11.12
  toe (s) S91.119
    with
      damage to nail S91.219
        with
          foreign body S91.229
      foreign body S91.129
    great S91.113
      with
        damage to nail S91.213
          with
            foreign body S91.223
        foreign body S91.123
      left S91.112
        with
          damage to nail S91.212
            with
              foreign body S91.222
          foreign body S91.122
      right S91.111
        with
          damage to nail S91.211
            with
              foreign body S91.221
          foreign body S91.121
    lesser S91.116
      with
        damage to nail S91.216
          with
            foreign body S91.226
        foreign body S91.126
      left S91.115
        with
          damage to nail S91.215
            with
              foreign body S91.225
          foreign body S91.125
      right S91.114
        with
          damage to nail S91.214
            with
              foreign body S91.224
          foreign body S91.124
  tongue —*see* Laceration, oral cavity

Laceration *(Continued)*
trachea S11.021
with foreign body S11.022
tunica vaginalis —*see* Laceration, testis
tympanum, tympanic membrane —*see* Laceration, ear, drum
umbilical region S31.115
with foreign body S31.125
ureter S37.13
urethra S37.33
with or following ectopic or molar pregnancy O08.6
obstetrical trauma O71.5
urinary organ NEC S37.893
uterus S37.63
with ectopic or molar pregnancy O08.6
following ectopic or molar pregnancy O08.6
nonpuerperal, nontraumatic N85.8
obstetrical trauma NEC O71.81
old (postpartal) N85.8
uvula —*see* Laceration, oral cavity
vagina S31.41
with
ectopic or molar pregnancy O08.6
foreign body S31.42
during delivery O71.4
with perineal laceration —*see* Laceration, perineum, female, during delivery
following ectopic or molar pregnancy O08.6
nonpuerperal, nontraumatic N89.8
old (postpartal) N89.8
vas deferens S37.893
vesical —*see* Laceration, bladder
vocal cords S11.031
with foreign body S11.032
vulva S31.41
with
ectopic or molar pregnancy O08.6
foreign body S31.42
complicating delivery O70.0
following ectopic or molar pregnancy O08.6
nonpuerperal, nontraumatic N90.89
old (postpartal) N90.89
wrist S61.519
with
foreign body S61.529
left S61.512
with
foreign body S61.522
right S61.511
with
foreign body S61.521
Lack of
achievement in school Z55.3
adequate
food Z59.4
intermaxillary vertical dimension of fully erupted teeth M26.36
sleep Z72.820
appetite (*see* Anorexia) R63.0
awareness R41.9
care
in home Z74.2
of infant (at or after birth) T76.02
confirmed T74.02
cognitive functions R41.9
coordination R27.9
ataxia R27.0
specified type NEC R27.8
development (physiological) R62.50
failure to thrive (child over 28 days old) R62.51
adult R62.7
newborn P92.6
short stature R62.52
specified type NEC R62.59
energy R53.83
financial resources Z59.6

Lack of *(Continued)*
food T73.0
growth R62.52
heating Z59.1
housing (permanent) (temporary) Z59.0
adequate Z59.1
learning experiences in childhood Z62.898
leisure time (affecting life-style) Z73.2
material resources Z59.9
memory —*see also* Amnesia
mild, following organic brain damage F06.8
ovulation N97.0
parental supervision or control of child Z62.0
person able to render necessary care Z74.2
physical exercise Z72.3
play experience in childhood Z62.898
posterior occlusal support M26.57
relaxation (affecting life-style) Z73.2
sexual
desire F52.0
enjoyment F52.1
shelter Z59.0
sleep (adequate) Z72.820
supervision of child by parent Z62.0
support, posterior occlusal M26.57
water T73.1
Lacrimal —*see* condition
Lacrimation, abnormal —*see* Epiphora
Lacrimonasal duct —*see* condition
Lactation, lactating (breast) (puerperal, postpartum)
associated
cracked nipple O92.13
retracted nipple O92.03
defective O92.4
disorder NEC O92.79
excessive O92.6
failed (complete) O92.3
partial O92.4
mastitis NEC —*see* Mastitis, obstetric
mother (care and/or examination) Z39.1
nonpuerperal N64.3
Lacticemia, excessive E87.2
Lacunar skull Q75.8
Laennec's cirrhosis K74.69
alcoholic K70.30
with ascites K70.31
Lafora's disease —*see* Epilepsy, generalized, idiopathic
Lag, lid (nervous) —*see* Retraction, lid
Lagophthalmos (eyelid) (nervous) H02.209
cicatricial H02.219
left H02.216
lower H02.215
upper H02.214
right H02.213
lower H02.212
upper H02.211
keratoconjunctivitis —*see* Keratoconjunctivitis
left H02.206
lower H02.205
upper H02.204
mechanical H02.229
left H02.226
lower H02.225
upper H02.224
right H02.223
lower H02.222
upper H02.221
paralytic H02.239
left H02.236
lower H02.235
upper H02.234
right H02.233
lower H02.232
upper H02.231
right H02.203
lower H02.202
upper H02.201

Laki-Lorand factor deficiency —*see* Defect, coagulation, specified type NEC
Lalling F80.0
Lambert-Eaton syndrome —*see* Syndrome, Lambert-Eaton
Lambliasis, lambliosis A07.1
Landau-Kleffner syndrome —*see* Epilepsy, specified NEC
Landouzy-Déjérine dystrophy or facioscapulohumeral atrophy G71.0
Landouzy's disease (icterohemorrhagic leptospirosis) A27.0
Landry-Guillain-Barré, syndrome or paralysis G61.0
Landry's disease or paralysis G61.0
Lane's
band Q43.3
kink —*see* Obstruction, intestine
syndrome K90.2
Langdon Down's syndrome —*see* Trisomy, 21
Lapsed immunization schedule status Z28.3
Large
baby (regardless of gestational age) (4000g to 4499g) P08.1
ear, congenital Q17.1
physiological cup Q14.2
stature R68.89
Large-for-dates NEC (infant) (4000g to 4499g) P08.1
affecting management of pregnancy O36.6-
exceptionally (4500g or more) P08.0
Larsen-Johansson disease orosteochondrosis —*see* Osteochondrosis, juvenile, patella
Larsen's syndrome (flattened facies and multiple congenital dislocations) Q74.8
Larva migrans
cutaneous B76.9
Ancylostoma B76.0
visceral B83.0
Laryngeal —*see* condition
Laryngismus (stridulus) J38.5
congenital P28.89
diphtheritic A36.2
Laryngitis (acute) (edematous) (fibrinous) (infective) (infiltrative) (malignant) (membranous) (phlegmonous) (pneumococcal) (pseudomembranous) (septic) (subglottic) (suppurative) (ulcerative) J04.0
with
influenza, flu, or grippe —*see* Influenza, with, laryngitis
tracheitis (acute) —*see* Laryngotracheitis
atrophic J37.0
catarrhal J37.0
chronic J37.0
with tracheitis (chronic) J37.1
diphtheritic A36.2
due to external agent —*see* Inflammation, respiratory, upper, due to
Hemophilus influenzae J04.0
H. influenzae J04.0
hypertrophic J37.0
influenzal —*see* Influenza, with, respiratory manifestations NEC
obstructive J05.0
sicca J37.0
spasmodic J05.0
acute J04.0
streptococcal J04.0
stridulous J05.0
syphilitic (late) A52.73
congenital A50.59 *[J99]*
early A50.03 *[J99]*
tuberculous A15.5
Vincent's A69.1
Laryngocele (congenital) (ventricular) Q31.3
Laryngofissure J38.7
congenital Q31.8
Laryngomalacia (congenital) Q31.5

◀ New ◀◀ Revised ~~deleted~~ Deleted

Laryngopharyngitis (acute) J06.0
 chronic J37.0
 due to external agent —*see* Inflammation,
  respiratory, upper, due to
Laryngoplegia J38.00
 bilateral J38.02
 unilateral J38.01
Laryngoptosis J38.7
Laryngospasm J38.5
Laryngostenosis J38.6
Laryngotracheitis (acute) (Infectional)
  (infective) (viral) J04.2
 atrophic J37.1
 catarrhal J37.1
 chronic J37.1
 diphtheritic A36.2
 due to external agent —*see* Inflammation,
  respiratory, upper, due to
 Hemophilus influenzae J04.2
 hypertrophic J37.1
 influenzal —*see* Influenza, with, respiratory
  manifestations NEC
 pachydermic J38.7
 sicca J37.1
 spasmodic J38.5
  acute J05.0
 streptococcal J04.2
 stridulous J38.5
 syphilitic (late) A52.73
  congenital A50.59 *[J99]*
   early A50.03 *[J99]*
 tuberculous A15.5
 Vincent's A69.1
Laryngotracheobronchitis —*see* Bronchitis
Larynx, laryngeal —*see* condition
Lassa fever A96.2
Lassitude —*see* Weakness
Late
 talker R62.0
 walker R62.0
Late effect (s) —*see* Sequelae
Latent —*see* condition
Laterocession —*see* Lateroversion
Lateroflexion —*see* Lateroversion
Lateroversion
 cervix —*see* Lateroversion, uterus
 uterus, uterine (cervix) (postinfectional)
  (postpartal, old) N85.4
  congenital Q51.818
  in pregnancy or childbirth O34.59-
Lathyrism —*see* Poisoning, food, noxious, plant
Launois' syndrome (pituitary gigantism) E22.0
Launois-Bensaude adenolipomatosis E88.89
Laurence-Moon (-Bardet)-Biedl syndrome
 Q87.89
Lax, laxity —*see also* Relaxation
 ligament (ous) —*see also* Disorder, ligament
  familial M35.7
  knee —*see* Derangement, knee
 skin (acquired) L57.4
  congenital Q82.8
Laxative habit F55.2
Lazy leukocyte syndrome D70.8
Lead miner's lung J63.6
Leak, leakage
 air NEC J93.82
  postprocedural J95.812
 amniotic fluid —*see* Rupture, membranes,
  premature
 blood (microscopic), fetal, into maternal
  circulation affecting management of
  pregnancy —*see* Pregnancy, complicated
  by
 cerebrospinal fluid G96.0
  from spinal (lumbar) puncture G97.0
 device, implant or graft —*see also*
  Complications, by site and type,
  mechanical
  arterial graft NEC —*see* Complication,
   cardiovascular device, mechanical,
   vascular

Leak, leakage *(Continued)*
 device, implant or graft *(Continued)*
  breast (implant) T85.43
  catheter NEC T85.638
   dialysis (renal) T82.43
    intraperitoneal T85.631
   infusion NEC T82.534
    spinal (epidural) (subdural) T85.630
   urinary, indwelling T83.038
    cystostomy T83.030
  gastrointestinal —*see* Complications,
   prosthetic device, mechanical,
   gastrointestinal device
  genital NEC T83.498
   penile prosthesis T83.490
  heart NEC —*see* Complication,
   cardiovascular device, mechanical
  joint prosthesis —*see* Complications, joint
   prosthesis, mechanical, specified
   NEC, by site
  ocular NEC —*see* Complications,
   prosthetic device, mechanical, ocular
   device
  orthopedic NEC —*see* Complication,
   orthopedic, device, mechanical
  persistent air J93.82
  specified NEC T85.638
  urinary NEC —*see also* Complication,
   genitourinary, device, urinary,
   mechanical
   graft T83.23
  vascular NEC —*see* Complication,
   cardiovascular device, mechanical
  ventricular intracranial shunt T85.03
 urine —*see* Incontinence
Leaky heart —*see* Endocarditis
Learning defect (specific) F81.9
Leather bottle stomach C16.9
Leber's
 congenital amaurosis H35.50
 optic atrophy (hereditary) H47.22
Lederer's anemia D59.1
Leeches (external) —*see* Hirudiniasis
Leg —*see* condition
Legg (-Calvé)-Perthes disease, syndrome or
 osteochondrosis M91.1-
Legionellosis A48.1
 nonpneumonic A48.2
Legionnaires'
 disease A48.1
  nonpneumonic A48.2
 pneumonia A48.1
Leigh's disease G31.82
Leiner's disease L21.1
Leiofibromyoma —*see* Leiomyoma
Leiomyoblastoma —*see* Neoplasm, connective
 tissue, benign
Leiomyofibroma —*see also* Neoplasm,
 connective tissue, benign
 uterus (cervix) (corpus) D25.9
Leiomyoma —*see also* Neoplasm, connective
 tissue, benign
 bizarre —*see* Neoplasm, connective tissue,
  benign
 cellular —*see* Neoplasm, connective tissue,
  benign
 epithelioid —*see* Neoplasm, connective
  tissue, benign
 uterus (cervix) (corpus) D25.9
  intramural D25.1
  submucous D25.0
  subserosal D25.2
 vascular —*see* Neoplasm, connective tissue,
  benign
Leiomyoma, leiomyomatosis (intravascular) —
 see Neoplasm, connective tissue, uncertain
 behavior
Leiomyosarcoma —*see also* Neoplasm,
 connective tissue, malignant
 epithelioid —*see* Neoplasm, connective
  tissue, malignant

Leiomyosarcoma *(Continued)*
 myxoid —*see* Neoplasm, connective tissue,
  malignant
Leishmaniasis B55.9
 American (mucocutaneous) B55.2
  cutaneous B55.1
 Asian Desert B55.1
 Brazilian B55.2
 cutaneous (any type) B55.1
 dermal —*see also* Leishmaniasis, cutaneous
  post-kala-azar B55.0
 eyelid B55.1
 infantile B55.0
 Mediterranean B55.0
 mucocutaneous (American) (New World)
  B55.2
 naso-oral B55.2
 nasopharyngeal B55.2
 old world B55.1
 tegumentaria diffusa B55.1
 visceral B55.0
Leishmanoid, dermal —*see also* Leishmaniasis,
 cutaneous
 post-kala-azar B55.0
Lenegre's disease I44.2
Lengthening, leg —*see* Deformity, limb,
 unequal length
Lennert's lymphoma —*see* Lymphoma,
 Lennert's
Lennox-Gastaut syndrome G40.812
 intractable G40.814
  with status epilepticus G40.813
  without status epilepticus G40.814
 not intractable G40.812
  with status epilepticus G40.811
  without status epilepticus G40.812
Lens —*see* condition
Lenticonus (anterior) (posterior) (congenital)
 Q12.8
Lenticular degeneration, progressive E83.01
Lentiglobus (posterior) (congenital) Q12.8
Lentigo (congenital) L81.4
 maligna —*see also* Melanoma, in situ
  melanoma —*see* Melanoma
Lentivirus, as cause of disease classified
 elsewhere B97.31
Leontiasis
 ossium M85.2
 syphilitic (late) A52.78
  congenital A50.59
Lepothrix A48.8
Lepra —*see* Leprosy
Leprechaunism E34.8
Leprosy A30.-
 with muscle disorder A30.9 *[M63.80]*
  ankle A30.9 *[M63.87-]*
  foot A30.9 *[M63.87-]*
  forearm A30.9 *[M63.83-]*
  hand A30.9 *[M63.84-]*
  lower leg A30.9 *[M63.86-]*
  multiple sites A30.9 *[M63.89]*
  pelvic region A30.9 *[M63.85-]*
  shoulder region A30.9 *[M63.81-]*
  specified site NEC A30.9 *[M63.88]*
  thigh A30.9 *[M63.85-]*
  upper arm A30.9 *[M63.82-]*
 anesthetic A30.9
 BB A30.3
 BL A30.4
 borderline (infiltrated) (neuritic) A30.3
  lepromatous A30.4
  tuberculoid A30.2
 BT A30.2
 dimorphous (infiltrated) (neuritic) A30.3
 I A30.0
 indeterminate (macular) (neuritic) A30.0
 lepromatous (diffuse) (infiltrated) (macular)
  (neuritic) (nodular) A30.5
 LL A30.5
 macular (early) (neuritic) (simple) A30.9
 maculoanesthetic A30.9

Leprosy *(Continued)*
  mixed A30.3
  neural A30.9
  nodular A30.5
  primary neuritic A30.3
  specified type NEC A30.8
  TT A30.1
  tuberculoid (major) (minor) A30.1
Leptocytosis, hereditary D56.9
Leptomeningitis (chronic) (circumscribed)
      (hemorrhagic) (nonsuppurative) —*see*
      Meningitis
Leptomeningopathy G96.19
Leptospiral —*see* condition
Leptospirochetal —*see* condition
Leptospirosis A27.9
  canicola A27.89
  due to Leptospira interrogans serovar
      icterohaemorrhagiae A27.0
  icterohemorrhagica A27.0
  pomona A27.89
  Weil's disease A27.0
Leptus dermatitis B88.0
Leriche's syndrome (aortic bifurcation
      occlusion) I74.09
Leri's pleonosteosis Q78.8
Leri-Weill syndrome Q77.8
Lermoyez' syndrome —*see* Vertigo, peripheral
      NEC
Lesch-Nyhan syndrome E79.1
Leser-Trélat disease L82.1
  inflamed L82.0
Lesion (s) (nontraumatic)
  abducens nerve —*see* Strabismus, paralytic,
      sixth nerve
  alveolar process K08.9
  angiocentric immunoproliferative D47.Z9
  anorectal K62.9
  aortic (valve) I35.9
  auditory nerve —*see* subcategory H93.3
  basal ganglion G25.9
  bile duct —*see* Disease, bile duct
  biomechanical M99.9
    specified type NEC M99.89
      abdomen M99.89
      acromioclavicular M99.87
      cervical region M99.81
      cervicothoracic M99.81
      costochondral M99.88
      costovertebral M99.88
      head region M99.80
      hip M99.85
      lower extremity M99.86
      lumbar region M99.83
      lumbosacral M99.83
      occipitocervical M99.80
      pelvic region M99.85
      pubic M99.85
      rib cage M99.88
      sacral region M99.84
      sacrococcygeal M99.84
      sacroiliac M99.84
      specified NEC M99.89
      sternochondral M99.88
      sternoclavicular M99.87
      thoracic region M99.82
      thoracolumbar M99.82
      upper extremity M99.87
  bladder N32.9
  bone —*see* Disorder, bone
  brachial plexus G54.0
  brain G93.9
    congenital Q04.9
    vascular I67.9
      degenerative I67.9
      hypertensive I67.4
  buccal cavity K13.79
  calcified —*see* Calcification
  canthus —*see* Disorder, eyelid
  carate —*see* Pinta, lesions
  cardia K22.9

Lesion *(Continued)*
  cardiac (*see also* Disease, heart) I51.9
    congenital Q24.9
    valvular —*see* Endocarditis
  cauda equina G83.4
  cecum K63.9
  cerebral —*see* Lesion, brain
  cerebrovascular I67.9
    degenerative I67.9
    hypertensive I67.4
  cervical (nerve) root NEC G54.2
  chiasmal —*see* Disorder, optic, chiasm
  chorda tympani G51.8
  coin, lung R91.1
  colon K63.9
  congenital —*see* Anomaly, by site
  conjunctiva H11.9
  conus medullaris —*see* Injury, conus
      medullaris
  coronary artery —*see* Ischemia, heart
  cranial nerve G52.9
    eighth —*see* Disorder, ear
    eleventh G52.9
    fifth G50.9
    first G52.0
    fourth —*see* Strabismus, paralytic, fourth
        nerve
    seventh G51.9
    sixth —*see* Strabismus, paralytic, sixth
        nerve
    tenth G52.2
    twelfth G52.3
  cystic —*see* Cyst
  degenerative —*see* Degeneration
  duodenum K31.9
  edentulous (alveolar) ridge, associated with
      trauma, due to traumatic occlusion
      K06.2
  en coup de sabre L94.1
  eyelid —*see* Disorder, eyelid
  gasserian ganglion G50.8
  gastric K31.9
  gastroduodenal K31.9
  gastrointestinal K63.9
  gingiva, associated with trauma K06.2
  glomerular
    focal and segmental (*see also* N00-N07 with
        fourth character .1) N05.1
    minimal change (*see also* N00-N07 with
        fourth character .0) N05.0
  heart (organic) —*see* Disease, heart
  hyperchromic, due to pinta (carate)
      A67.1
  hyperkeratotic —*see* Hyperkeratosis
  hypothalamic E23.7
  ileocecal K63.9
  ileum K63.9
  iliohypogastric nerve G57.8-
  inflammatory —*see* Inflammation
  intestine K63.9
  intracerebral —*see* Lesion, brain
  intrachiasmal (optic) —*see* Disorder, optic,
      chiasm
  intracranial, space-occupying R90.0
  joint —*see* Disorder, joint
    sacroiliac (old) M53.3
  keratotic —*see* Keratosis
  kidney —*see* Disease, renal
  laryngeal nerve (recurrent) G52.2
  lip K13.0
  liver K76.9
  lumbosacral
    plexus G54.1
    root (nerve) NEC G54.4
  lung (coin) R91.1
  maxillary sinus J32.0
  mitral I05.9
  Morel-Lavallée —*see* Hematoma,
      by site
  motor cortex NEC G93.89
  mouth K13.79

Lesion *(Continued)*
  nerve G58.9
    femoral G57.2-
    median G56.1-
      carpal tunnel syndrome —*see* Syndrome,
          carpal tunnel
    plantar G57.6-
    popliteal (lateral) G57.3-
      medial G57.4-
    radial G56.3-
    sciatic G57.0-
    spinal —*see* Injury, nerve, spinal
    ulnar G56.2-
  nervous system, congenital Q07.9
  nonallopathic —*see* Lesion, biomechanical
  nose (internal) J34.89
  obstructive —*see* Obstruction
  obturator nerve G57.8-
  oral mucosa K13.70
  organ or site NEC —*see* Disease, by site
  osteolytic —*see* Osteolysis
  peptic K27.9
  periodontal, due to traumatic occlusion
      K05.5
  pharynx J39.2
  pigment, pigmented (skin) L81.9
  pinta —*see* Pinta, lesions
  polypoid —*see* Polyp
  prechiasmal (optic) —*see* Disorder, optic,
      chiasm
  primary (*see also* Syphilis, primary) A51.0
    carate A67.0
    pinta A67.0
    yaws A66.0
  pulmonary J98.4
    valve I37.9
  pylorus K31.9
  rectosigmoid K63.9
  retina, retinal H35.9
  sacroiliac (joint) (old) M53.3
  salivary gland K11.9
    benign lymphoepithelial K11.8
  saphenous nerve G57.8-
  sciatic nerve G57.0-
  secondary —*see* Syphilis, secondary
  shoulder (region) M75.9-
    specified NEC M75.8-
  sigmoid K63.9
  sinus (accessory) (nasal) J34.89
  skin L98.9
    suppurative L08.0
  SLAP S43.43-
  spinal cord G95.9
    congenital Q06.9
  spleen D73.89
  stomach K31.9
  superior glenoid labrum S43.43-
  syphilitic —*see* Syphilis
  tertiary —*see* Syphilis, tertiary
  thoracic root (nerve) NEC G54.3
  tonsillar fossa J35.9
  tooth, teeth K08.9
    white spot
      chewing surface K02.51
      pit and fissure surface K02.51
      smooth surface K02.61
  traumatic —*see* specific type of injury
      by site
  tricuspid (valve) I07.9
    nonrheumatic I36.9
  trigeminal nerve G50.9
  ulcerated or ulcerative —*see* Ulcer, skin
  uterus N85.9
  vagus nerve G52.2
  valvular —*see* Endocarditis
  vascular I99.9
    affecting central nervous system I67.9
    following trauma NEC T14.8
    umbilical cord, complicating delivery
        O69.5
  warty —*see* Verruca

◀ New   ◀◀ Revised   ~~deleted~~ Deleted

Lesion *(Continued)*
 white spot (tooth)
  chewing surface K02.51
  pit and fissure surface K02.51
  smooth surface K02.61
Lethargic —*see* condition
Lethargy R53.83
Letterer-Siwe's disease C96.0
Leukemia, leukemic C95.9-
 acute basophilic C94.8-
 acute bilineal C95.0-
 acute erythroid C94.0-
 acute lymphoblastic C91.0-
 acute megakaryoblastic C94.2-
 acute megakaryocytic C94.2-
 acute mixed lineage C95.0-
 acute monoblastic (monoblastic/monocytic)
   C93.0-
 acute monocytic (monoblastic/monocytic)
   C93.0-
 acute myeloblastic (minimal differentiation)
   (with maturation) C92.0-
 acute myeloid
  with
   11q23-abnormality C92.6-
   dysplasia of remaining hematopoesis
     and/or myelodysplastic disease in
     its history C92.A-
   multilineage dysplasia C92.A-
   variation of MLL-gene C92.6-
  M6 (a)(b) C94.0-
  M7 C94.2-
 acute myelomonocytic C92.5-
 acute promyelocytic C92.4-
 adult T-cell (HTLV-1-associated)
   (acute variant) (chronic variant)
   (lymphomatoid variant) (smouldering
   variant) C91.5-
 aggressive NK-cell C94.8-
 AML (1/ETO) (M0) (M1) (M2) (without a
   FAB classification) C92.0-
 AML M3 C92.4-
 AML M4 (Eo with inv(16) or t(16;16))
   C92.5-
 AML M5 C93.0-
 AML M5a C93.0-
 AML M5b C93.0-
 AML Me with t (15;17) and variants C92.4-
 atypical chronic myeloid, BCR/ABL-negative
   C92.2-
 biphenotypic acute C95.0-
 blast cell C95.0-
 Burkitt-type, mature B-cell C91.A-
 chronic lymphocytic, of B-cell type C91.1-
 chronic monocytic C93.1-
 chronic myelogenous (Philadelphia
   chromosome (Ph1) positive) (t(9;22))
   (q34;q11) (with crisis of blast cells)
   C92.1-
 chronic myeloid, BCR/ABL-positive C92.1-
  atypical, BCR/ABL-negative C92.2-
 chronic myelomonocytic C93.1-
 chronic neutrophilic D47.1
 CMML (-1) (-2) (with eosinophilia) C93.1-
 granulocytic (*see also* Category C92) C92.9-
 hairy-cell C91.4-
 juvenile myelomonocytic C93.3-
 lymphoid C91.9-
  specified NEC C91.Z-
 mast cell C94.3-
 mature B-cell, Burkitt-type C91.A-
 monocytic (subacute) C93.9-
  specified NEC C93.Z-
 myelogenous (*see also* Category C92) C92.9-
 myeloid C92.9-
  specified NEC C92.Z-
 plasma cell C90.1-
 plasmacytic C90.1-
 prolymphocytic
  of B-cell type C91.3-
  of T-cell type C91.6-

Leukemia, leukemic *(Continued)*
 specified NEC C94.8-
 stem cell, of unclear lineage C95.0-
 subacute lymphocytic C91.9-
 T-cell large granular lymphocytic C91.Z-
 unspecified cell type C95.9-
  acute C95.0-
  chronic C95.1-
Leukemoid reaction (*see also* Reaction,
   leukemoid) D72.823-
Leukoaraiosis (hypertensive) I67.81
Leukoariosis —*see* Leukoaraiosis
Leukocoria —*see* Disorder, globe, degenerated
   condition, leucocoria
Leukocytopenia D72.819
Leukocytosis D72.829
 eosinophilic D72.1
Leukoderma, leukodermia NEC L81.5
 syphilitic A51.39
  late A52.79
Leukodystrophy E75.29
Leukoedema, oral epithelium K13.29
Leukoencephalitis G04.81
 acute (subacute) hemorrhagic G36.1
  postimmunization or postvaccinal G04.02
 postinfectious G04.01
 subacute sclerosing A81.1
 van Bogaert's (sclerosing) A81.1
Leukoencephalopathy (*see also*
   Encephalopathy) G93.49
 Binswanger's I67.3
 heroin vapor G92
 metachromatic E75.25
 multifocal (progressive) A81.2
 postimmunization and postvaccinal G04.02
 progressive multifocal A81.2
 reversible, posterior G93.6
 van Bogaert's (sclerosing) A81.1
 vascular, progressive I67.3
Leukoerythroblastosis D75.9
Leukokeratosis —*see also* Leukoplakia
 mouth K13.21
 nicotina palati K13.24
 oral mucosa K13.21
 tongue K13.21
 vocal cord J38.3
Leukokraurosis vulva (e) N90.4
Leukoma (cornea) —*see also* Opacity, cornea
 adherent H17.0-
 interfering with central vision —*see* Opacity,
   cornea, central
Leukomalacia, cerebral, newborn P91.2
 periventricular P91.2
Leukomelanopathy, hereditary D72.0
Leukonychia (punctata) (striata) L60.8
 congenital Q84.4
Leukopathia unguium L60.8
 congenital Q84.4
Leukopenia D72.819
 basophilic D72.818
 chemotherapy (cancer) induced D70.1
 congenital D70.0
 cyclic D70.0
 drug induced NEC D70.2
  due to cytoreductive cancer chemotherapy
    D70.1
 eosinophilic D72.818
 familial D70.0
 infantile genetic D70.0
 malignant D70.9
 periodic D70.0
 transitory neonatal P61.5
Leukopenic —*see* condition
Leukoplakia
 anus K62.89
 bladder (postinfectional) N32.89
 buccal K13.21
 cervix (uteri) N88.0
 esophagus K22.8
 gingiva K13.21
 hairy (oral mucosa) (tongue) K13.3

Leukoplakia *(Continued)*
 kidney (pelvis) N28.89
 larynx J38.7
 lip K13.21
 mouth K13.21
 oral epithelium, including tongue (mucosa)
   K13.21
 palate K13.21
 pelvis (kidney) N28.89
 penis (infectional) N48.0
 rectum K62.89
 syphilitic (late) A52.79
 tongue K13.21
 ureter (postinfectional) N28.89
 urethra (postinfectional) N36.8
 uterus N85.8
 vagina N89.4
 vocal cord J38.3
 vulva N90.4
Leukorrhea N89.8
 due to Trichomonas (vaginalis)
   A59.00
 trichomonal A59.00
Leukosarcoma C85.9
Levocardia (isolated) Q24.1
 with situs inversus Q89.3
Levotransposition Q20.5
Lev's disease or syndrome (acquired complete
   heart block) I44.2
Levulosuria —*see* Fructosuria
Levurid L30.2
Lewy body (ies) (dementia) (disease)
   G31.83
Leyden-Moebius dystrophy G71.0
Leydig cell
 carcinoma
  specified site —*see* Neoplasm, malignant,
    by site
  unspecified site
   female C56.9-
   male C62.9-
 tumor
  benign
   specified site —*see* Neoplasm, benign,
     by site
   unspecified site
    female D27.-
    male D29.2-
  malignant
   specified site —*see* Neoplasm,
     malignant, by site
   unspecified site
    female C56.-
    male C62.9-
  specified site —*see* Neoplasm, uncertain
    behavior, by site
  unspecified site
   female D39.1-
   male D40.1-
Leydig-Sertoli cell tumor
 specified site —*see* Neoplasm, benign,
   by site
 unspecified site
  female D27.-
  male D29.2-
LGSIL (Low grade squamous intraepithelial
   lesion on cytologic smear of)
 anus R85.612
 cervix R87.612
 vagina R87.622
Liar, pathologic F60.2
Libido
 decreased R68.82
Libman-Sacks disease M32.11
Lice (infestation) B85.2
 body (Pediculus corporis) B85.1
 crab B85.3
 head (Pediculus capitis) B85.0
 mixed (classifiable to more than one of the
   titles B85.0-B85.3) B85.4
 pubic (Phthirus pubis) B85.3

Lichen L28.0
  albus L90.0
    penis N48.0
    vulva N90.4
  amyloidosis E85.4 [L99]
  atrophicus L90.0
    penis N48.0
    vulva N90.4
  congenital Q82.8
  myxedematosus L98.5
  nitidus L44.1
  pilaris Q82.8
    acquired L85.8
  planopilaris L66.1
  planus (chronicus) L43.9
    annularis L43.8
    bullous L43.1
    follicular L66.1
    hypertrophic L43.0
    moniliformis L44.3
    of Wilson L43.9
    specified NEC L43.8
    subacute (active) L43.3
    tropicus L43.3
  ruber
    acuminatus L44.0
    moniliformis L44.3
    planus L43.9
  sclerosus (et atrophicus) L90.0
    penis N48.0
    vulva N90.4
  scrofulosus (primary) (tuberculous) A18.4
  simplex (chronicus) (circumscriptus) L28.0
  striatus L44.2
  urticatus L28.2
Lichenification L28.0
Lichenoides tuberculosis (primary) A18.4
Lichtheim's disease or syndrome —*see*
  Degeneration, combined
Lien migrans D73.89
Ligament —*see* condition
Light
  for gestational age —*see* Light for dates
  headedness R42
Light-for-dates (infant) P05.00
  with weight of
    499 grams or less P05.01
    500-749 grams P05.02
    750-999 grams P05.03
    1000-1249 grams P05.04
    1250-1499 grams P05.05
    1500-1749 grams P05.06
    1750-1999 grams P05.07
    2000-2499 grams P05.08
  affecting management of pregnancy O36.59-
  and small-for-dates —*see* Small for dates
Lightning (effects) (stroke) (struck by) T75.00
  burn —*see* Burn
  foot E53.8
  shock T75.01
  specified effect NEC T75.09
Lightwood-Albright syndrome N25.89
Lightwood's disease or syndrome (renal
  tubular acidosis) N25.89
Lignac (-de Toni) (-Fanconi) (-Debré) **disease or**
  syndrome E72.09
  with cystinosis E72.04
Ligneous thyroiditis E06.5
Likoff's syndrome I20.8
Limb —*see* condition
Limbic epilepsy personality syndrome F07.0
Limitation, limited
  activities due to disability Z73.6
  cardiac reserve —*see* Disease, heart
  eye muscle duction, traumatic —*see*
    Strabismus, mechanical
  mandibular range of motion M26.52
Lindau (-von Hippel) **disease** Q85.8
Line (s)
  Beau's L60.4
  Harris' —*see* Arrest, epiphyseal

Line (*Continued*)
  Hudson's (cornea) —*see* Pigmentation,
    cornea, anterior
  Stähli's (cornea) —*see* Pigmentation, cornea,
    anterior
Linea corneae senilis —*see* Change, cornea,
  senile
Lingua
  geographica K14.1
  nigra (villosa) K14.3
  plicata K14.5
  tylosis K13.29
Lingual —*see* condition
Linguatulosis B88.8
Linitis (gastric) **plastica** C16.9
Lip —*see* condition
Lipedema —*see* Edema
Lipemia —*see also* Hyperlipidemia
  retina, retinalis E78.3
Lipidosis E75.6
  cerebral (infantile) (juvenile) (late) E75.4
  cerebroretinal E75.4
  cerebroside E75.22
  cholesterol (cerebral) E75.5
  glycolipid E75.21
  hepatosplenomegalic E78.3
  sphingomyelin —*see* Niemann-Pick disease
    or syndrome
  sulfatide E75.29
Lipoadenoma —*see* Neoplasm, benign,
  by site
Lipoblastoma —*see* Lipoma
Lipoblastomatosis —*see* Lipoma
Lipochondrodystrophy E76.01
Lipochrome histiocytosis (familial) D71
Lipodermatosclerosis —*see* Varix, leg, with,
  inflammation
  ulcerated —*see* Varix, leg, with, ulcer, with
    inflammation by site
Lipodystrophia progressiva E88.1
Lipodystrophy (progressive) E88.1
  insulin E88.1
  intestinal K90.81
  mesenteric K65.4
Lipofibroma —*see* Lipoma
Lipofuscinosis, neuronal (with ceroidosis)
  E75.4
Lipogranuloma, sclerosing L92.8
Lipogranulomatosis E78.89
Lipoid —*see also* condition
  histiocytosis D76.3
    essential E75.29
  nephrosis N04.9
  proteinosis of Urbach E78.89
Lipoidemia —*see* Hyperlipidemia
Lipoidosis —*see* Lipidosis
Lipoma D17.9
  fetal D17.9
    fat cell D17.9
  infiltrating D17.9
  intramuscular D17.9
  pleomorphic D17.9
  site classification
    arms (skin) (subcutaneous) D17.2-
    connective tissue D17.30
      intra-abdominal D17.5
      intrathoracic D17.4
      peritoneum D17.79
      retroperitoneum D17.79
      specified site NEC D17.39
      spermatic cord D17.6
    face (skin) (subcutaneous) D17.0
    genitourinary organ NEC D17.72
    head (skin) (subcutaneous) D17.0
    intra-abdominal D17.5
    intrathoracic D17.4
    kidney D17.71
    legs (skin) (subcutaneous) D17.2-
    neck (skin) (subcutaneous) D17.0
    peritoneum D17.79
    retroperitoneum D17.79

Lipoma (*Continued*)
  site classification (*Continued*)
    skin D17.30
      specified site NEC D17.39
    specified site NEC D17.79
    spermatic cord D17.6
    subcutaneous D17.30
      specified site NEC D17.39
    trunk (skin) (subcutaneous) D17.1
    unspecified D17.9
  spindle cell D17.9
Lipomatosis E88.2
  dolorosa (Dercum) E88.2
  fetal —*see* Lipoma
  Launois-Bensaude E88.89
Lipomyoma —*see* Lipoma
Lipomyxoma —*see* Lipoma
Lipomyxosarcoma —*see* Neoplasm, connective
  tissue, malignant
Lipoprotein metabolism disorder E78.9
Lipoproteinemia E78.5
  broad-beta E78.2
  floating-beta E78.2
  hyper-pre-beta E78.1
Liposarcoma —*see also* Neoplasm, connective
  tissue, malignant
  dedifferentiated —*see* Neoplasm, connective
    tissue, malignant
  differentiated type —*see* Neoplasm,
    connective tissue, malignant
  embryonal —*see* Neoplasm, connective tissue,
    malignant
  mixed type —*see* Neoplasm, connective
    tissue, malignant
  myxoid —*see* Neoplasm, connective tissue,
    malignant
  pleomorphic —*see* Neoplasm, connective
    tissue, malignant
  round cell —*see* Neoplasm, connective tissue,
    malignant
  well differentiated type —*see* Neoplasm,
    connective tissue, malignant
Liposynovitis prepatellaris E88.89
Lipping, cervix N86
Lipschütz disease or ulcer N76.6
Lipuria R82.0
  schistosomiasis (bilharziasis) B65.0
Lisping F80.0
Lissauer's paralysis A52.17
Lissencephalia, lissencephaly Q04.3
Listeriosis, listerellosis A32.9
  congenital (disseminated) P37.2
  cutaneous A32.0
  neonatal, newborn (disseminated) P37.2
  oculoglandular A32.81
  specified NEC A32.89
Lithemia E79.0
Lithiasis —*see* Calculus
Lithosis J62.8
Lithuria R82.99
Litigation, anxiety concerning Z65.3
Little leaguer's elbow —*see* Epicondylitis,
  medial
Little's disease G80.9
Littre's
  gland —*see* condition
  hernia —*see* Hernia, abdomen
Littritis —*see* Urethritis
Livedo (annularis) (racemosa) (reticularis) R23.1
Liver —*see* condition
Living alone (problems with) Z60.2
  with handicapped person Z74.2
Lloyd's syndrome —*see* Adenomatosis,
  endocrine
Loa loa, loaiasis, loasis B74.3
Lobar —*see* condition
Lobomycosis B48.0
Lobo's disease B48.0
Lobotomy syndrome F07.0
Lobstein (-Ekman) **disease or syndrome** Q78.0
Lobster-claw hand Q71.6-

◄ New   ◄▐ Revised   ~~deleted~~ Deleted

Lobulation (congenital) —*see also* Anomaly, by site
  kidney, Q63.1
  liver, abnormal Q44.7
  spleen Q89.09
Lobule, lobular —*see* condition
Local, localized —*see* condition
Locked twins causing obstructed labor O66.1
Locked-in state G83.5
Locking
  joint —*see* Derangement, joint, specified type NEC
    knee —*see* Derangement, knee
Lockjaw —*see* Tetanus
Löffler's
  endocarditis I42.3
  eosinophilia J82
  pneumonia J82
  syndrome (eosinophilic pneumonitis) J82
Loiasis (with conjunctival infestation) (eyelid) B74.3
Lone Star fever A77.0
Long
  labor O63.9
    first stage O63.0
    second stage O63.1
  QT syndrome I45.81
Long-term (current) (prophylactic) drug therapy (use of)
  agents affecting estrogen receptors and estrogen levels NEC Z79.818
  anastrozole (Arimidex) Z79.811
  antibiotics Z79.2
    short-term use - omit code
  anticoagulants Z79.01
  anti-inflammatory, non-steroidal (NSAID) Z79.1
  antiplatelet Z79.02
  antithrombotics Z79.02
  aromatase inhibitors Z79.811
  aspirin Z79.82
  birth control pill or patch Z79.3
  bisphosphonates Z79.83
  contraceptive, oral Z79.3
  drug, specified NEC Z79.899
  estrogen receptor downregulators Z79.818
  Evista Z79.810
  exemestane (Aromasin) Z79.811
  Fareston Z79.810
  fulvestrant (Faslodex) Z79.818
  gonadotropin-releasing hormone (GnRH) agonist Z79.818
  goserelin acetate (Zoladex) Z79.818
  hormone replacement (postmenopausal) Z79.890
  insulin Z79.4
  letrozole (Femara) Z79.811
  leuprolide acetate (leuprorelin) (Lupron) Z79.818
  megestrol acetate (Megace) Z79.818
  methadone for pain management Z79.891
  Nolvadex Z79.810
  non-steroidal anti-inflammatories (NSAID) Z79.1
  opiate analgesic Z79.891
  oral contraceptive Z79.3
  raloxifene (Evista) Z79.810
  selective estrogen receptor modulators (SERMs) Z79.810
  steroids
    inhaled Z79.51
    systemic Z79.52
  tamoxifen (Nolvadex) Z79.810
  toremifene (Fareston) Z79.810
Longitudinal stripes or grooves, nails L60.8
  congenital Q84.6
Loop
  intestine —*see* Volvulus
  vascular on papilla (optic) Q14.2

Loose —*see also* condition
  body
    joint M24.00
      ankle M24.07-
      elbow M24.02-
      hand M24.04-
      hip M24.05-
      knee M23.4-
      shoulder (region) M24.01-
      specified site NEC M24.08
      toe M24.07-
      vertebra M24.08
      wrist M24.03-
    knee M23.4-
    sheath, tendon —*see* Disorder, tendon, specified type NEC
  cartilage —*see* Loose, body, joint
  tooth, teeth K08.8
Loosening
  aseptic
    joint prosthesis —*see* Complications, joint prosthesis, mechanical, loosening, by site
    epiphysis —*see* Osteochondropathy
  mechanical
    joint prosthesis —*see* Complications, joint prosthesis, mechanical, loosening, by site
Looser-Milkman (-Debray) **syndrome** M83.8
Lop ear (deformity) Q17.3
Lorain (-Levi) **short stature syndrome** E23.0
Lordosis M40.50
  acquired —*see* Lordosis, specified type NEC
  congenital Q76.429
    lumbar region Q76.426
    lumbosacral region Q76.427
    sacral region Q76.428
    sacrococcygeal region Q76.428
    thoracolumbar region Q76.425
  lumbar region M40.56
  lumbosacral region M40.57
  postsurgical M96.4
  postural —*see* Lordosis, specified type NEC
  rachitic (late effect) (sequelae) E64.3
  sequelae of rickets E64.3
  specified type NEC M40.40
    lumbar region M40.46
    lumbosacral region M40.47
    thoracolumbar region M40.45
  thoracolumbar region M40.55
  tuberculous A18.01
Loss (of)
  appetite (*see* Anorexia) R63.0
    hysterical F50.8
    nonorganic origin F50.8
    psychogenic F50.8
  blood —*see* Hemorrhage
  consciousness, transient R55
    traumatic —*see* Injury, intracranial
  control, sphincter, rectum R15.9
    nonorganic origin F98.1
  elasticity, skin R23.4
  family (member) in childhood Z62.898
  fluid (acute) E86.9
    with
      hypernatremia E87.0
      hyponatremia E87.1
  function of labyrinth —*see* subcategory H83.2
  hair, nonscarring —*see* Alopecia
  hearing —*see also* Deafness
    central NOS H90.5
    neural NOS H90.5
    perceptive NOS H90.5
    sensorineural NOS H90.5
    sensory NOS H90.5
  height R29.890
  limb or member, traumatic, current —*see* Amputation, traumatic
  love relationship in childhood Z62.898

Loss (*Continued*)
  memory —*see also* Amnesia
    mild, following organic brain damage F06.8
  mind —*see* Psychosis
  occlusal vertical dimension of fully erupted teeth M26.37
  organ or part —*see* Absence, by site, acquired
  ossicles, ear (partial) H74.32-
  parent in childhood Z63.4
  pregnancy, recurrent N96
    without current pregnancy N96
    care in current pregnancy O26.2-
  recurrent pregnancy —*see* Loss, pregnancy, recurrent
  self-esteem, in childhood Z62.898
  sense of
    smell —*see* Disturbance, sensation, smell
    taste —*see* Disturbance, sensation, taste
    touch R20.8
  sensory R44.9
    dissociative F44.6
  sexual desire F52.0
  sight (acquired) (complete) (congenital) —*see* Blindness
  substance of
    bone —*see* Disorder, bone, density and structure, specified NEC
    cartilage —*see* Disorder, cartilage, specified type NEC
      auricle (ear) —*see* Disorder, pinna, specified type NEC
    vitreous (humor) H15.89
  tooth, teeth —*see* Absence, teeth, acquired
  vision, visual H54.7
    both eyes H54.3
    one eye H54.60
      left (normal vision on right) H54.62
      right (normal vision on left) H54.61
    specified as blindness —*see* Blindness
    subjective
      sudden H53.13-
      transient H53.12-
  vitreous —*see* Prolapse, vitreous
  voice —*see* Aphonia
  weight (abnormal) (cause unknown) R63.4
Louis-Bar syndrome (ataxia-telangiectasia) G11.3
Louping ill (encephalitis) A84.8
Louse, lousiness —*see* Lice
Low
  achiever, school Z55.3
  back syndrome M54.5
  basal metabolic rate R94.8
  birthweight (2499 grams or less) P07.10
    with weight of
      1000-1249 grams P07.14
      1250-1499 grams P07.15
      1500-1749 grams P07.16
      1750-1999 grams P07.17
      2000-2499 grams P07.18
    extreme (999 grams or less) P07.00
      with weight of
        499 grams or less P07.01
        500-749 grams P07.02
        750-999 grams P07.03
    for gestational age —*see* Light for dates
  blood pressure —*see also* Hypotension
    reading (incidental) (isolated) (nonspecific) R03.1
  cardiac reserve —*see* Disease, heart
  function —*see also* Hypofunction
    kidney N28.9
  hematocrit D64.9
  hemoglobin D64.9
  income Z59.6
  level of literacy Z55.0
  lying
    kidney N28.89
    organ or site, congenital —*see* Malposition, congenital

◀ New   ◀▥▥ Revised   ~~deleted~~ Deleted

Low (*Continued*)
  output syndrome (cardiac) —*see* Failure,
    heart
  platelets (blood) —*see* Thrombocytopenia
  reserve, kidney N28.89
  salt syndrome E87.1
  self esteem R45.81
  set ears Q17.4
  vision H54.2
    one eye (other eye normal) H54.50
      left (normal vision on right) H54.52
        other eye blind —*see* Blindness
      right (normal vision on left) H54.51
Low-density-lipoprotein-type (LDL)
  hyperlipoproteinemia E78.0
Lowe's syndrome E72.03
Lown-Ganong-Levine syndrome I45.6
LSD reaction (acute) (without dependence)
  F16.90
  with dependence F16.20
L-shaped kidney Q63.8
Ludwig's angina or disease K12.2
Lues (venerea), **luetic** —*see* Syphilis
Luetscher's syndrome (dehydration) E86.0
Lumbago, lumbalgia M54.5
  with sciatica M54.4-
    due to intervertebral disc disorder M51.17
  due to displacement, intervertebral disc
    M51.27
    with sciatica M51.17
Lumbar —*see* condition
Lumbarization, vertebra, congenital Q76.49
Lumbermen's itch B88.0
Lump —*see* Mass
Lunacy —*see* Psychosis
Lung —*see* condition
Lupoid (miliary) **of Boeck** D86.3
Lupus
  anticoagulant D68.62
    with
      hemorrhagic disorder D68.312
      hypercoagulable state D68.62
    finding without diagnosis R76.0
  discoid (local) L93.0
  erythematosus (discoid) (local) L93.0
    disseminated —*see* Lupus, erythematosus,
      systemic
    eyelid H01.129
      left H01.126
        lower H01.125
        upper H01.124
      right H01.123
        lower H01.122
        upper H01.121
    profundus L93.2
    specified NEC L93.2
    subacute cutaneous L93.1
    systemic M32.9
      with organ or system involvement M32.10
        endocarditis M32.11
        lung M32.13
        pericarditis M32.12
        renal (glomerular) M32.14
          tubulo-interstitial M32.15
        specified organ or system NEC
          M32.19
      drug-induced M32.0
      inhibitor (presence of) D68.62
        with
          hemorrhagic disorder D68.312
          hypercoagulable state D68.62
        finding without diagnosis R76.0
      specified NEC M32.8
  exedens A18.4
  hydralazine M32.0
    correct substance properly administered —
      see Table of Drugs and Chemicals, by
      drug, adverse effect
    overdose or wrong substance given or
      taken —*see* Table of Drugs and
      Chemicals, by drug, poisoning

Lupus (*Continued*)
  nephritis (chronic) M32.14
  nontuberculous, not disseminated L93.0
  panniculitis L93.2
  pernio (Besnier) D86.3
  systemic —*see* Lupus, erythematosus,
    systemic
  tuberculous A18.4
    eyelid A18.4
  vulgaris A18.4
    eyelid A18.4
Luteinoma D27.-
Lutembacher's disease or syndrome (atrial
  septal defect with mitral stenosis) Q21.1
Luteoma D27.-
Lutz (-Splendore-de Almeida) **disease** —*see*
  Paracoccidioidomycosis
Luxation —*see also* Dislocation
  eyeball (nontraumatic) —*see* Luxation, globe
    birth injury P15.3
  globe, nontraumatic H44.82-
  lacrimal gland —*see* Dislocation, lacrimal
    gland
  lens (old) (partial) (spontaneous)
    congenital Q12.1
    syphilitic A50.39
Lycanthropy F22
Lyell's syndrome L51.2
  due to drug L51.2
    correct substance properly administered —
      see Table of Drugs and Chemicals, by
      drug, adverse effect
    overdose or wrong substance given or
      taken —*see* Table of Drugs and
      Chemicals, by drug, poisoning
Lyme disease A69.20
Lymph
  gland or node —*see* condition
  scrotum —*see* Infestation, filarial
Lymphadenitis I88.9
  with ectopic or molar pregnancy O08.0
  acute L04.9
    axilla L04.2
    face L04.0
    head L04.0
    hip L04.3
    limb
      lower L04.3
      upper L04.2
    neck L04.0
    shoulder L04.2
    specified site NEC L04.8
    trunk L04.1
  anthracosis (occupational) J60
  any site, except mesenteric I88.9
    chronic I88.1
    subacute I88.1
  breast
    gestational —*see* Mastitis, obstetric
    puerperal, postpartum (nonpurulent)
      O91.22
  chancroidal (congenital) A57
  chronic I88.1
    mesenteric I88.0
  due to
    Brugia (malayi) B74.1
      timori B74.2
    chlamydial lymphogranuloma A55
    diphtheria (toxin) A36.89
    lymphogranuloma venereum A55
    Wuchereria bancrofti B74.0
  following ectopic or molar pregnancy O08.0
  gonorrheal A54.89
  infective —*see* Lymphadenitis, acute
  mesenteric (acute) (chronic) (nonspecific)
    (subacute) I88.0
    due to Salmonella typhi A01.09
    tuberculous A18.39
  mycobacterial A31.8
  purulent —*see* Lymphadenitis, acute
  pyogenic —*see* Lymphadenitis, acute

Lymphadenitis (*Continued*)
  regional, nonbacterial I88.8
  septic —*see* Lymphadenitis, acute
  subacute, unspecified site I88.1
  suppurative —*see* Lymphadenitis, acute
  syphilitic (early) (secondary) A51.49
    late A52.79
  tuberculous —*see* Tuberculosis, lymph gland
  venereal (chlamydial) A55
Lymphadenoid goiter E06.3
Lymphadenopathy (generalized) R59.1
  angioimmunoblastic, with dysproteinemia
    (AILD) C86.5
  due to toxoplasmosis (acquired) B58.89
    congenital (acute) (subacute) (chronic)
      P37.1
  localized R59.0
  syphilitic (early) (secondary) A51.49
Lymphadenosis R59.1
Lymphangiectasis I89.0
  conjunctiva H11.89
  postinfectional I89.0
  scrotum I89.0
Lymphangiectatic elephantiasis, nonfilarial
  I89.0
Lymphangioendothelioma D18.1
  malignant —*see* Neoplasm, connective tissue,
    malignant
Lymphangioleiomyomatosis J84.81
Lymphangioma D18.1
  capillary D18.1
  cavernous D18.1
  cystic D18.1
  malignant —*see* Neoplasm, connective tissue,
    malignant
Lymphangiomyoma D18.1
Lymphangiomyomatosis J84.81
Lymphangiosarcoma —*see* Neoplasm,
  connective tissue, malignant
Lymphangitis I89.1
  with
    abscess - code by site under Abscess
    cellulitis - code by site under Cellulitis
    ectopic or molar pregnancy O08.0
  acute L03.91
    abdominal wall L03.321
    ankle —*see* Lymphangitis, acute, lower
      limb
    arm —*see* Lymphangitis, acute, upper limb
    auricle (ear) —*see* Lymphangitis, acute, ear
    axilla L03.12-
    back (any part) L03.322
    buttock L03.327
    cervical (meaning neck) L03.222
    cheek (external) L03.212
    chest wall L03.323
    digit
      finger —*see* Lymphangitis, acute, finger
      toe —*see* Lymphangitis, acute, toe
    ear (external) H60.1-
    external auditory canal —*see*
      Lymphangitis, acute, ear
    eyelid —*see* Abscess, eyelid
    face NEC L03.212
    finger (intrathecal) (periosteal)
      (subcutaneous) (subcuticular) L03.02-
    foot —*see* Lymphangitis, acute, lower limb
    gluteal (region) L03.327
    groin L03.324
    hand —*see* Lymphangitis, acute, upper
      limb
    head NEC L03.891
      face (any part, except ear, eye and nose)
        L03.212
    heel —*see* Lymphangitis, acute, lower limb
    hip —*see* Lymphangitis, acute, lower limb
    jaw (region) L03.212
    knee —*see* Lymphangitis, acute, lower limb
    leg —*see* Lymphangitis, acute, lower limb
    lower limb L03.12-
      toe —*see* Lymphangitis, acute, toe

Lymphangitis (Continued)
  acute (Continued)
    navel L03.326
    neck (region) L03.222
    orbit, orbital —see Cellulitis, orbit
    pectoral (region) L03.323
    perineal, perineum L03.325
    scalp (any part) L03.891
    shoulder —see Lymphangitis, acute, upper
      limb
    specified site NEC L03.898
    thigh —see Lymphangitis, acute, lower
      limb
    thumb (intrathecal) (periosteal)
      (subcutaneous) (subcuticular) —see
      Lymphangitis, acute, finger
    toe (intrathecal) (periosteal) (subcutaneous)
      (subcuticular) L03.04-
    trunk L03.329
      abdominal wall L03.321
      back (any part) L03.322
      buttock L03.327
      chest wall L03.323
      groin L03.324
      perineal, perineum L03.325
      umbilicus L03.326
    umbilicus L03.326
    upper limb L03.12-
      axilla —see Lymphangitis, acute, axilla
      finger —see Lymphangitis, acute, finger
      thumb —see Lymphangitis, acute, finger
      wrist —see Lymphangitis, acute, upper
        limb
  breast
    gestational —see Mastitis, obstetric
  chancroidal A57
  chronic (any site) I89.1
  due to
    Brugia (malayi) B74.1
      timori B74.2
    Wuchereria bancrofti B74.0
  following ectopic or molar pregnancy O08.89
  penis
    acute N48.29
    gonococcal (acute) (chronic) A54.09
  puerperal, postpartum, childbirth O86.89
  strumous, tuberculous A18.2
  subacute (any site) I89.1
  tuberculous —see Tuberculosis, lymph gland
Lymphatic (vessel) —see condition
Lymphatism E32.8
Lymphectasia I89.0
Lymphedema (acquired) —see also Elephantiasis
  congenital Q82.0
  hereditary (chronic) (idiopathic) Q82.0
  postmastectomy I97.2
  praecox I89.0
  secondary I89.0
  surgical NEC I97.89
    postmastectomy (syndrome) I97.2
Lymphoblastic —see condition
Lymphoblastoma (diffuse) —see Lymphoma,
  lymphoblastic (diffuse)
  giant follicular —see Lymphoma,
    lymphoblastic (diffuse)
  macrofollicular —see Lymphoma,
    lymphoblastic (diffuse)
Lymphocele I89.8
Lymphocytic
  chorioencephalitis (acute) (serous) A87.2
  choriomeningitis (acute) (serous) A87.2
  meningoencephalitis A87.2

Lymphocytoma, benign cutis L98.8
Lymphocytopenia D72.810
Lymphocytosis (symptomatic)
  D72.820
  infectious (acute) B33.8
Lymphoepithelioma —see Neoplasm,
  malignant, by site
Lymphogranuloma (malignant) —see also
  Lymphoma, Hodgkin
  chlamydial A55
  inguinale A55
  venereum (any site) (chlamydial) (with
    stricture of rectum) A55
Lymphogranulomatosis (malignant) —see also
  Lymphoma, Hodgkin
  benign (Boeck's sarcoid) (Schaumann's)
    D86.1
Lymphohistiocytosis, hemophagocytic
  (familial) D76.1
Lymphoid —see condition
Lymphoma (of) (malignant) C85.90
  adult T-cell (HTLV-1-associated)
    (acute variant) (chronic variant)
    (lymphomatoid variant) (smouldering
    variant) C91.5-
  anaplastic large cell
    ALK-negative C84.7-
    ALK-positive C84.6-
    CD30-positive C84.6-
    primary cutaneous C86.6
  angioimmunoblastic T-cell C86.5
  BALT C88.4
  B-cell C85.1-
  B-precursor C83.5-
  blastic NK-cell C86.4
  bronchial-associated lymphoid tissue
    [BALT-lymphoma] C88.4
  Burkitt (atypical) C83.7-
  Burkitt-like C83.7-
  centrocytic C83.1-
  cutaneous follicle center C82.6-
  cutaneous T-cell C84.A-
  diffuse follicle center C82.5-
  diffuse large cell C83.3-
    anaplastic C83.3-
    B-cell C83.3-
    CD30-positive C83.3-
    centroblastic C83.3-
    immunoblastic C83.3-
    plasmablastic C83.3-
    subtype not specified C83.3-
    T-cell rich C83.3-
  enteropathy-type (associated) (intestinal)
    T-cell C86.2
  extranodal marginal zone B-cell
    lymphoma of mucosa-associated
    lymphoid tissue [MALT-lymphoma]
    C88.4
  extranodal NK/T-cell, nasal type
    C86.0
  follicular C82.9-
    grade
      I C82.0-
      II C82.1-
      III C82.2-
      IIIa C82.3-
      IIIb C82.4-
    specified NEC C82.8-
  hepatosplenic T-cell (alpha-beta)
    (gamma-delta) C86.1
  histiocytic C85.9-
    true C96.A

Lymphoma (Continued)
  Hodgkin C81.9
    classical C81.7-
      lymphocyte-rich C81.4-
      lymphocytic depletion C81.3-
      mixed cellularity C81.2-
      nodular sclerosis C81.1-
      specified NEC C81.7-
    lymphocyte-rich classical C81.4-
    lymphocyte depleted classical C81.3-
    mixed cellularity classical C81.2-
    nodular
      lymphocyte predominant C81.0-
      sclerosis classical C81.1-
  intravascular large B-cell C83.8-
  Lennert's C84.4-
  lymphoblastic (diffuse) C83.5-
  lymphoblastic B-cell C83.5-
  lymphoblastic T-cell C83.5-
  lymphoepithelioid C84.4-
  lymphoplasmacytic C83.0-
    with IgM-production C88.0
  MALT C88.4
  mantle cell C83.1-
  mature T-cell NEC C84.4-
  mature T/NK-cell C84.9-
    specified NEC C84.Z-
  mediastinal (thymic) large B-cell
    C85.2-
  Mediterranean C88.3
  mucosa-associated lymphoid tissue
    [MALT-lymphoma] C88.4
  NK/T cell C84.9-
  nodal marginal zone C83.0-
  non-follicular (diffuse) C83.9-
    specified NEC C83.8-
  non-Hodgkin (see also Lymphoma, by type)
    C85.9-
    specified NEC C85.8-
  non-leukemic variant of B-CLL C83.0-
  peripheral T-cell, not classified C84.4-
  primary cutaneous
    anaplastic large cell C86.6
    CD30-positive large T-cell C86.6
  primary effusion B-cell C83.8-
  SALT C88.4
  skin-associated lymphoid tissue [SALT-
    lymphoma] C88.4
  small cell B-cell C83.0-
  splenic marginal zone C83.0-
  subcutaneous panniculitis-like T-cell
    C86.3
  T-precursor C83.5-
  true histiocytic C96.A
Lymphomatosis —see Lymphoma
Lymphopathia venerum, veneris A55
Lymphopenia D72.810
Lymphoplasmacytic leukemia —see Leukemia,
  chronic lymphocytic, B-cell type
Lymphoproliferation, X-linked disease
  D82.3
Lymphoreticulosis, benign (of inoculation)
  A28.1
Lymphorrhea I89.8
Lymphosarcoma (diffuse) (see also Lymphoma)
  C85.9-
Lymphostasis I89.8
Lypemania —see Melancholia
Lysine and hydroxylysine metabolism
  disorder E72.3
Lyssa —see Rabies

M

Macacus ear Q17.3
Maceration, wet feet, tropical (syndrome)
    T69.02-
MacLeod's syndrome J43.0
Macrocephalia, macrocephaly Q75.3
Macrocheilia, macrochilia (congenital)Q18.6
Macrocolon (*see also* Megacolon) Q43.1
Macrocornea Q15.8
    with glaucoma Q15.0
Macrocytic —*see* condition
Macrocytosis D75.89
Macrodactylia, macrodactylism (fingers)
    (thumbs) Q74.0
    toes Q74.2
Macrodontia K00.2
Macrogenia M26.05
Macrogenitosomia (adrenal) (male) (praecox)
    E25.9
    congenital E25.0
Macroglobulinemia (idiopathic) (primary)
    C88.0
    monoclonal (essential) D47.2
    Waldenström C88.0
Macroglossia (congenital) Q38.2
    acquired K14.8
Macrognathia, macrognathism (congenital)
    (mandibular) (maxillary) M26.09
Macrogyria (congenital) Q04.8
Macrohydrocephalus —*see* Hydrocephalus
Macromastia —*see* Hypertrophy, breast
Macrophthalmos Q11.3
    in congenital glaucoma Q15.0
Macropsia H53.15
Macrosigmoid K59.3
    congenital Q43.2
Macrospondylitis, acromegalic E22.0
Macrostomia (congenital) Q18.4
Macrotia (external ear) (congenital) Q17.1
Macula
    cornea, corneal —*see* Opacity, cornea
    degeneration (atrophic) (exudative)
        (senile) —*see also* Degeneration, macula
    hereditary —*see* Dystrophy, retina
Maculae ceruleae — B85.1
Maculopathy, toxic —*see* Degeneration, macula,
    toxic
Madarosis (eyelid) H02.729
    left H02.726
        lower H02.725
        upper H02.724
    right H02.723
        lower H02.722
        upper H02.721
Madelung's
    deformity (radius) Q74.0
    disease
        radial deformity Q74.0
        symmetrical lipomas, neck E88.89
Madness —*see* Psychosis
Madura
    foot B47.9
        actinomycotic B47.1
        mycotic B47.0
Maduromycosis B47.0
Maffucci's syndrome Q78.4
Magnesium metabolism disorder —*see*
    Disorder, metabolism, magnesium
Main en griffe (acquired) —*see also* Deformity,
    limb, clawhand
    congenital Q74.0
Maintenance (encounter for)
    antineoplastic chemotherapy Z51.11
    antineoplastic radiation therapy Z51.0
    methadone F11.20
Majocchi's
    disease L81.7
    granuloma B35.8
Major —*see* condition
Malabar itch (any site) B35.5

Malabsorption K90.9
    calcium K90.89
    carbohydrate K90.4
    disaccharide E73.9
    fat K90.4
    galactose E74.20
    glucose(-galactose) E74.39
    intestinal K90.9
        specified NEC K90.89
    isomaltose E74.31
    lactose E73.9
    methionine E72.19
    monosaccharide E74.39
    postgastrectomy K91.2
    postsurgical K91.2
    protein K90.4
    starch K90.4
    sucrose E74.39
    syndrome K90.9
        postsurgical K91.2
Malacia, bone (adult) M83.9
    juvenile —*see* Rickets
Malacoplakia
    bladder N32.89
    pelvis (kidney) N28.89
    ureter N28.89
    urethra N36.8
Malacosteon, juvenile —*see* Rickets
Maladaptation —*see* Maladjustment
Maladie de Roger Q21.0
Maladjustment
    conjugal Z63.0
        involving divorce or estrangement Z63.5
    educational Z55.4
    family Z63.9
    marital Z63.0
        involving divorce or estrangement Z63.5
    occupational NEC Z56.89
    simple, adult —*see* Disorder, adjustment
    situational —*see* Disorder, adjustment
    social Z60.9
        due to
            acculturation difficulty Z60.3
            discrimination and persecution
                (perceived) Z60.5
            exclusion and isolation Z60.4
            life-cycle (phase of life) transition Z60.0
            rejection Z60.4
            specified reason NEC Z60.8
Malaise R53.81
Malakoplakia —*see* Malacoplakia
Malaria, malarial (fever) B54
    with
        blackwater fever B50.8
            hemoglobinuric (bilious) B50.8
        hemoglobinuria B50.8
    accidentally induced (therapeutically) - code
        by type under Malaria
    algid B50.9
    cerebral B50.0 *[G94]*
    clinically diagnosed (without parasitological
        confirmation) B54
    congenital NEC P37.4
        falciparum P37.3
    congestion, congestive B54
    continued (fever) B50.9
    estivo-autumnal B50.9
    falciparum B50.9
        with complications NEC B50.8
            cerebral B50.0 *[G94]*
            severe B50.8
    hemorrhagic B54
    malariae B52.9
        with
            complications NEC B52.8
            glomerular disorder B52.0
    malignant (tertian) —*see* Malaria, falciparum
    mixed infections — code to first listed type
        in B50-B53
    ovale B53.0
    parasitologically confirmed NEC B53.8

Malaria, malarial (*Continued*)
    pernicious, acute —*see* Malaria, falciparum
    Plasmodium (P.)
        falciparum NEC —*see* Malaria, falciparum
        malariae NEC B52.9
            with Plasmodium
                falciparum (and or vivax) —*see*
                    Malaria, falciparum
                vivax —*see also* Malaria, vivax
                    and falciparum —*see* Malaria,
                      falciparum
        ovale B53.0
            with Plasmodium malariae —*see also*
                Malaria, malariae
            and vivax —*see also* Malaria, vivax
                and falciparum —*see* Malaria,
                    falciparum
        simian B53.1
            with Plasmodium malariae —*see also*
                Malaria, malariae
            and vivax —*see also* Malaria, vivax
                and falciparum —*see* Malaria,
                    falciparum
        vivax NEC B51.9
            with Plasmodium falciparum —*see*
                Malaria, falciparum
    quartan —*see* Malaria, malariae
    quotidian —*see* Malaria, falciparum
    recurrent B54
    remittent B54
    specified type NEC (parasitologically
        confirmed) B53.8
    spleen B54
    subtertian (fever) —*see* Malaria, falciparum
    tertian (benign) —*see also* Malaria, vivax
        malignant B50.9
    tropical B50.9
    typhoid B54
    vivax B51.9
        with
            complications NEC B51.8
            ruptured spleen B51.0
Malassez's disease (cystic) N50.8
Malassimilation K90.9
Mal de los pintos —*see* Pinta
Mal de mer T75.3
Maldescent, testis Q53.9
    bilateral Q53.20
        abdominal Q53.21
        perineal Q53.22
    unilateral Q53.10
        abdominal Q53.11
        perineal Q53.12
Maldevelopment —*see also* Anomaly
    brain Q07.9
    colon Q43.9
    hip Q74.2
        congenital dislocation Q65.2
            bilateral Q65.1
            unilateral Q65.0-
    mastoid process Q75.8
    middle ear Q16.4
        except ossicles Q16.4
        ossicles Q16.3
    ossicles Q16.3
    spine Q76.49
    toe Q74.2
Male type pelvis Q74.2
    with disproportion (fetopelvic) O33.3
        causing obstructed labor O65.3
Malformation (congenital) —*see also* Anomaly
    adrenal gland Q89.1
    affecting multiple systems with skeletal
        changes NEC Q87.5
    alimentary tract Q45.9
        specified type NEC Q45.8
        upper Q40.9
            specified type NEC Q40.8
    aorta Q25.9
        atresia Q25.2
        coarctation (preductal) (postductal) Q25.1

◀ New   ⬖ Revised   ~~deleted~~ Deleted

Malformation (Continued)
aorta (Continued)
  patent ductus arteriosus Q25.0
  specified type NEC Q25.4
  stenosis (supravalvular) Q25.3
aortic valve Q23.9
  specified NEC Q23.8
arteriovenous, aneurysmatic (congenital)
    Q27.30
  brain Q28.2
  cerebral Q28.2
  peripheral Q27.30
    digestive system Q27.33
    lower limb Q27.32
    other specified site Q27.39
    renal vessel Q27.34
    upper limb Q27.31
  precerebral vessels (nonruptured) Q28.0
auricle
  ear (congenital) Q17.3
    acquired H61.119
      left H61.112
        with right H61.113
      right H61.111
        with left H61.113
bile duct Q44.5
bladder Q64.79
  aplasia Q64.5
  diverticulum Q64.6
  exstrophy —see Exstrophy, bladder
  neck obstruction Q64.31
bone Q79.9
  face Q75.9
    specified type NEC Q75.8
  skull Q75.9
    specified type NEC Q75.8
brain (multiple) Q04.9
  arteriovenous Q28.2
  specified type NEC Q04.8
branchial cleft Q18.2
breast Q83.9
  specified type NEC Q83.8
broad ligament Q50.6
bronchus Q32.4
bursa Q79.9
cardiac
  chambers Q20.9
    specified type NEC Q20.8
  septum Q21.9
    specified type NEC Q21.8
cerebral Q04.9
  vessels Q28.3
cervix uteri Q51.9
  specified type NEC Q51.828
Chiari
  Type I G93.5
  Type II Q07.01
choroid (congenital) Q14.3
  plexus Q07.8
circulatory system Q28.9
cochlea Q16.5
cornea Q13.4
coronary vessels Q24.5
corpus callosum (congenital) Q04.0
diaphragm Q79.1
digestive system NEC, specified type NEC
    Q45.8
dura Q07.9
  brain Q04.9
  spinal Q06.9
ear Q17.9
  causing impairment of hearing Q16.9
  external Q17.9
    accessory auricle Q17.0
    causing impairment of hearing Q16.9
    absence of
      auditory canal Q16.1
      auricle Q16.0
    macrotia Q17.1
    microtia Q17.2
    misplacement Q17.4

Malformation (Continued)
ear (Continued)
  external (Continued)
    misshapen NEC Q17.3
    prominence Q17.5
    specified type NEC Q17.8
  inner Q16.5
  middle Q16.4
    absence of eustachian tube Q16.2
    ossicles (fusion) Q16.3
  ossicles Q16.3
  specified type NEC Q17.8
epididymis Q55.4
esophagus Q39.9
  specified type NEC Q39.8
eye Q15.9
  lid Q10.3
  specified NEC Q15.8
fallopian tube Q50.6
genital organ —see Anomaly, genitalia
great
  artery Q25.9
    aorta —see Malformation, aorta
    pulmonary artery —see Malformation,
        pulmonary, artery
    specified type NEC Q25.8
  vein Q26.9
    anomalous
      portal venous connection Q26.5
      pulmonary venous connection Q26.4
        partial Q26.3
        total Q26.2
    persistent left superior vena cava Q26.1
    portal vein-hepatic artery fistula Q26.6
    specified type NEC Q26.8
    vena cava stenosis, congenital Q26.0
gum Q38.6
hair Q84.2
heart Q24.9
  specified type NEC Q24.8
integument Q84.9
  specified type NEC Q84.8
internal ear Q16.5
intestine Q43.9
  specified type NEC Q43.8
iris Q13.2
joint Q74.9
  ankle Q74.2
  lumbosacral Q76.49
  sacroiliac Q74.2
  specified type NEC Q74.8
kidney Q63.9
  accessory Q63.0
  giant Q63.3
  horseshoe Q63.1
  hydronephrosis Q62.0
  malposition Q63.2
  specified type NEC Q63.8
lacrimal apparatus Q10.6
lingual Q38.3
lip Q38.0
liver Q44.7
lung Q33.9
meninges or membrane (congenital) Q07.9
  cerebral Q04.8
  spinal (cord) Q06.9
middle ear Q16.4
  ossicles Q16.3
mitral valve Q23.9
  specified NEC Q23.8
Mondini's (congenital) (malformation,
    cochlea) Q16.5
mouth (congenital) Q38.6
multiple types NEC Q89.7
musculoskeletal system Q79.9
myocardium Q24.8
nail Q84.6
nervous system (central) Q07.9
nose Q30.9
  specified type NEC Q30.8
optic disc Q14.2

Malformation (Continued)
orbit Q10.7
ovary Q50.39
palate Q38.5
parathyroid gland Q89.2
pelvic organs or tissues NEC
  in pregnancy or childbirth O34.8-
    causing obstructed labor O65.5
penis Q55.69
  aplasia Q55.5
  curvature (lateral) Q55.61
  hypoplasia Q55.62
pericardium Q24.8
peripheral vascular system Q27.9
  specified type NEC Q27.8
pharynx Q38.8
precerebral vessels Q28.1
prostate Q55.4
pulmonary
  arteriovenous Q25.72
  artery Q25.9
    atresia Q25.5
    specified type NEC Q25.79
    stenosis Q25.6
  valve Q22.3
renal artery Q27.2
respiratory system Q34.9
retina Q14.1
scrotum —see Malformation, testis and
    scrotum
seminal vesicles Q55.4
sense organs NEC Q07.9
skin Q82.9
  specified NEC Q89.8
spinal
  cord Q06.9
  nerve root Q07.8
spine Q76.49
  kyphosis —see Kyphosis, congenital
  lordosis —see Lordosis, congenital
spleen Q89.09
stomach Q40.3
  specified type NEC Q40.2
teeth, tooth K00.9
tendon Q79.9
testis and scrotum Q55.20
  aplasia Q55.0
  hypoplasia Q55.1
  polyorchism Q55.21
  retractile testis Q55.22
  scrotal transposition Q55.23
  specified NEC Q55.29
thorax, bony Q76.9
throat Q38.8
thyroid gland Q89.2
tongue (congenital) Q38.3
  hypertrophy Q38.2
  tie Q38.1
trachea Q32.1
tricuspid valve Q22.9
  specified type NEC Q22.8
umbilical cord NEC (complicating delivery)
    O69.89
umbilicus Q89.9
ureter Q62.8
  agenesis Q62.4
  duplication Q62.5
  malposition —see Malposition, congenital,
      ureter
  obstructive defect —see Defect, obstructive,
      ureter
  vesico-uretero-renal reflux Q62.7
urethra Q64.79
  aplasia Q64.5
  duplication Q64.74
  posterior valves Q64.2
  prolapse Q64.71
  stricture Q64.32
urinary system Q64.9
uterus Q51.9
  specified type NEC Q51.818

Malformation (Continued)
- vagina Q52.4
- vascular system, peripheral Q27.9
- vas deferens Q55.4
  - atresia Q55.3
- venous —see Anomaly, vein (s)
- vulva Q52.70

Malfunction —see also Dysfunction
- cardiac electronic device T82.119
  - electrode T82.110
  - pulse generator T82.111
  - specified type NEC T82.118
- catheter device NEC T85.618
  - cystostomy T83.010
  - dialysis (renal) (vascular) T82.41
    - intraperitoneal T85.611
  - infusion NEC T82.514
    - spinal (epidural) (subdural) T85.610
  - urinary, indwelling T83.018
- colostomy K94.03
  - valve K94.03
- cystostomy (stoma) N99.512
  - catheter T83.010
- enteric stoma K94.13
- enterostomy K94.13
- esophagostomy K94.33
- gastroenteric K31.89
- gastrostomy K94.23
- ileostomy K94.13
  - valve K94.13
- jejunostomy K94.13
- pacemaker —see Malfunction, cardiac electronic device
- prosthetic device, internal —see Complications, prosthetic device, by site, mechanical
- tracheostomy J95.03
- urinary device NEC —see Complication, genitourinary, device, urinary, mechanical
- valve
  - colostomy K94.03
  - heart T82.09
  - ileostomy K94.13
- vascular graft or shunt NEC —see Complication, cardiovascular device, mechanical, vascular
- ventricular (communicating shunt) T85.01

Malherbe's tumor —see Neoplasm, skin, benign
Malibu disease L98.8-
Malignancy —see also Neoplasm, malignant, by site
- unspecified site (primary) C80.1
Malignant —see condition
Malingerer, malingering Z76.5
Mallet finger (acquired) —see Deformity, finger, mallet finger
- congenital Q74.0
- sequelae of rickets E64.3
Malleus A24.0
Mallory's bodies R89.7
Mallory-Weiss syndrome K22.6
Malnutrition E46
- degree
  - first E44.1
  - mild (protein) E44.1
  - moderate (protein) E44.0
  - second E44.0
  - severe (protein-energy) E43
    - intermediate form E42
      - with
        - kwashiorkor (and marasmus) E42
        - marasmus E41
  - third E43
- following gastrointestinal surgery K91.2
- intrauterine
  - light-for-dates —see Light for dates
  - small-for-dates —see Small for dates
- lack of care, or neglect (child) (infant) T76.02
  - confirmed T74.02
- malignant E40

Malnutrition (Continued)
- protein E46
  - calorie E46
    - mild E44.1
    - moderate E44.0
    - severe E43
      - intermediate form E42
        - with
          - kwashiorkor (and marasmus) E42
          - marasmus E41
  - energy E46
    - mild E44.1
    - moderate E44.0
    - severe E43
      - intermediate form E42
        - with
          - kwashiorkor (and marasmus) E42
          - marasmus E41
  - severe (protein-energy) E43
    - with
      - kwashiorkor (and marasmus) E42
      - marasmus E41
Malocclusion (teeth) M26.4
- Angle's M26.219
  - class I M26.211
  - class II M26.212
  - class III M26.213
- due to
  - abnormal swallowing M26.59
  - mouth breathing M26.59
  - tongue, lip or finger habits M26.59
- temporomandibular (joint) M26.69
Malposition
- cervix —see Malposition, uterus
- congenital
  - adrenal (gland) Q89.1
  - alimentary tract Q45.8
    - lower Q43.8
    - upper Q40.8
  - aorta Q25.4
  - appendix Q43.8
  - arterial trunk Q20.0
  - artery (peripheral) Q27.8
    - coronary Q24.5
    - digestive system Q27.8
    - lower limb Q27.8
    - pulmonary Q25.79
    - specified site NEC Q27.8
    - upper limb Q27.8
  - auditory canal Q17.8
    - causing impairment of hearing Q16.9
  - auricle (ear) Q17.4
    - causing impairment of hearing Q16.9
    - cervical Q18.2
  - biliary duct or passage Q44.5
  - bladder (mucosa) —see Exstrophy, bladder
  - brachial plexus Q07.8
  - brain tissue Q04.8
  - breast Q83.8
  - bronchus Q32.4
  - cecum Q43.8
  - clavicle Q74.0
  - colon Q43.8
  - digestive organ or tract NEC Q45.8
    - lower Q43.8
    - upper Q40.8
  - ear (auricle) (external) Q17.4
    - ossicles Q16.3
  - endocrine (gland) NEC Q89.2
  - epiglottis Q31.8
  - eustachian tube Q17.8
  - eye Q15.8
  - facial features Q18.8
  - fallopian tube Q50.6
  - finger (s) Q68.1
    - supernumerary Q69.0
  - foot Q66.9
  - gallbladder Q44.1
  - gastrointestinal tract Q45.8

Malposition (Continued)
- congenital (Continued)
  - genitalia, genital organ (s) or tract
    - female Q52.8
      - external Q52.79
      - internal NEC Q52.8
    - male Q55.8
  - glottis Q31.8
  - hand Q68.1
  - heart Q24.8
    - dextrocardia Q24.0
      - with complete transposition of viscera Q89.3
  - hepatic duct Q44.5
  - hip (joint) Q65.89
  - intestine (large) (small) Q43.8
    - with anomalous adhesions, fixation or malrotation Q43.3
  - joint NEC Q68.8
  - kidney Q63.2
  - larynx Q31.8
  - limb Q68.8
    - lower Q68.8
    - upper Q68.8
  - liver Q44.7
  - lung (lobe) Q33.8
  - nail (s) Q84.6
  - nerve Q07.8
  - nervous system NEC Q07.8
  - nose, nasal (septum) Q30.8
  - organ or site not listed —see Anomaly, by site
  - ovary Q50.39
  - pancreas Q45.3
  - parathyroid (gland) Q89.2
  - patella Q74.1
  - peripheral vascular system Q27.8
  - pituitary (gland) Q89.2
  - respiratory organ or system NEC Q34.8
  - rib (cage) Q76.6
    - supernumerary in cervical region Q76.5
  - scapula Q74.0
  - shoulder Q74.0
  - spinal cord Q06.8
  - spleen Q89.09
  - sternum NEC Q76.7
  - stomach Q40.2
  - symphysis pubis Q74.2
  - thymus (gland) Q89.2
  - thyroid (gland) (tissue) Q89.2
    - cartilage Q31.8
  - toe (s) Q66.9
    - supernumerary Q69.2
  - tongue Q38.3
  - trachea Q32.1
  - ureter Q62.60
    - deviation Q62.61
    - displacement Q62.62
    - ectopia Q62.63
    - specified type NEC Q62.69
  - uterus Q51.818
  - vein (s) (peripheral) Q27.8
    - great Q26.8
  - vena cava (inferior) (superior) Q26.8
- device, implant or graft (see also Complications, by site and type, mechanical) T85.628
  - arterial graft NEC —see Complication, cardiovascular device, mechanical, vascular
  - breast (implant) T85.42
  - catheter NEC T85.628
    - cystostomy T83.020
    - dialysis (renal) T82.42
      - intraperitoneal T85.621
    - infusion NEC T82.524
      - spinal (epidural) (subdural) T85.620
    - urinary, indwelling T83.028

◀ New　◀▥ Revised　~~deleted~~ Deleted

Malposition (Continued)
  device, implant or graft (Continued)
    electronic (electrode) (pulse generator)
      (stimulator)
      bone T84.320
      cardiac T82.129
        electrode T82.120
        pulse generator T82.121
        specified type NEC T82.128
      nervous system —see Complication,
        prosthetic device, mechanical,
        electronic nervous system
        stimulator
      urinary —see Complication,
        genitourinary, device, urinary,
        mechanical
    fixation, internal (orthopedic) NEC —see
      Complication, fixation device,
      mechanical
    gastrointestinal —see Complications,
      prosthetic device, mechanical,
      gastrointestinal device
    genital NEC T83.428
      intrauterine contraceptive device T83.32
      penile prosthesis T83.420
    heart NEC —see Complication,
      cardiovascular device, mechanical
    joint prosthesis —see Complication, joint
      prosthesis, mechanical
    ocular NEC —see Complications, prosthetic
      device, mechanical, ocular device
    orthopedic NEC —see Complication,
      orthopedic, device, mechanical
    specified NEC T85.628
    urinary NEC —see also Complication,
      genitourinary, device, urinary,
      mechanical
      graft T83.22
    vascular NEC —see Complication,
      cardiovascular device, mechanical
    ventricular intracranial shunt T85.02
  fetus —see Pregnancy, complicated by
    (management affected by), presentation,
    fetal
  gallbladder K82.8
  gastrointestinal tract, congenital Q45.8
  heart, congenital NEC Q24.8
  joint prosthesis —see Complications, joint
    prosthesis, mechanical, displacement,
    by site
  stomach K31.89
    congenital Q40.2
  tooth, teeth, fully erupted M26.30
  uterus (acute) (acquired) (adherent)
    (asymptomatic) (postinfectional)
    (postpartal, old) N85.4
    anteflexion or anteversion N85.4
      congenital Q51.818
    flexion N85.4
      lateral —see Lateroversion, uterus
    inversion N85.5
    lateral (flexion) (version) —see
      Lateroversion, uterus
    in pregnancy or childbirth —see
      subcategory O34.5
    retroflexion or retroversion —see
      Retroversion, uterus
Malposture R29.3
Malrotation
  cecum Q43.3
  colon Q43.3
  intestine Q43.3
  kidney Q63.2
Malta fever —see Brucellosis
Maltreatment
  adult
    abandonment
      confirmed T74.01
      suspected T76.01
    confirmed T74.91
    history of Z91.419

Maltreatment (Continued)
  adult (Continued)
    neglect
      confirmed T74.01
      suspected T76.01
    physical abuse
      confirmed T74.11
      suspected T76.11
    psychological abuse
      confirmed T74.31
      history of Z91.411
      suspected T76.31
    sexual abuse
      confirmed T74.21
      suspected T76.21
    suspected T76.91
  child
    abandonment
      confirmed T74.02
      suspected T76.02
    confirmed T74.92
    history of —see History, personal (of),
      abuse
    neglect
      confirmed T74.02
      history of —see History, personal (of),
        abuse
      suspected T76.02
    physical abuse
      confirmed T74.12
      history of —see History, personal (of),
        abuse
      suspected T76.12
    psychological abuse
      confirmed T74.32
      history of —see History, personal (of),
        abuse
      suspected T76.32
    sexual abuse
      confirmed T74.22
      history of —see History, personal (of),
        abuse
      suspected T76.22
    suspected T76.92
  personal history of Z91.89
Maltworker's lung J67.4
Malunion, fracture —see Fracture, by site
Mammillitis N61
  puerperal, postpartum O91.02
Mammitis —see Mastitis
Mammogram (examination) Z12.39
  routine Z12.31
Mammoplasia N62
Management (of)
  bone conduction hearing device (implanted)
    Z45.320
  cardiac pacemaker NEC Z45.018
  cerebrospinal fluid drainage device Z45.41
  cochlear device (implanted) Z45.321
  contraceptive Z30.9
    specified NEC Z30.8
  implanted device Z45.9
    specified NEC Z45.89
  infusion pump Z45.1
  procreative Z31.9
    male factor infertility in female Z31.81
    specified NEC Z31.89
  prosthesis (external) (see also Fitting)
    Z44.9
    implanted Z45.9
      specified NEC Z45.89
  renal dialysis catheter Z49.01
  vascular access device Z45.2
Mangled —see specified injury by site
Mania (monopolar) —see also Disorder, mood,
  manic episode
  with psychotic symptoms F30.2
  without psychotic symptoms F30.10
    mild F30.11
    moderate F30.12
    severe F30.13

Mania (Continued)
  Bell's F30.8
  chronic (recurrent) F31.89
  hysterical F44.89
  puerperal F30.8
  recurrent F31.89
Manic-depressive insanity, psychosis, or
  syndrome —see Disorder, bipolar
Mannosidosis E77.1
Mansonelliasis, mansonellosis B74.4
Manson's
  disease B65.1
  schistosomiasis B65.1
Manual —see condition
Maple-bark-stripper's lung (disease) J67.6
Maple-syrup-urine disease E71.0
Marable's syndrome (celiac artery
  compression) I77.4
Marasmus E41
  due to malnutrition E41
  intestinal E41
  nutritional E41
  senile R54
  tuberculous NEC —see Tuberculosis
Marble
  bones Q78.2
  skin R23.8
Marburg virus disease A98.3
March
  fracture —see Fracture, traumatic, stress, by
    site
  hemoglobinuria D59.6
Marchesani (-Weill) syndrome Q87.0
Marchiafava (-Bignami) syndrome or disease
  G37.1
Marchiafava-Micheli syndrome D59.5
Marcus Gunn's syndrome Q07.8
Marfan's syndrome —see Syndrome, Marfan's
Marie-Bamberger disease —see
  Osteoarthropathy, hypertrophic, specified
  NEC
Marie-Charcot-Tooth neuropathic muscular
  atrophy G60.0
Marie's
  cerebellar ataxia (late-onset) G11.2
  disease or syndrome (acromegaly) E22.0
Marie-Strümpell arthritis, disease or
  spondylitis —see Spondylitis, ankylosing
Marion's disease (bladder neck obstruction)
  N32.0
Marital conflict Z63.0
Mark
  port wine Q82.5
  raspberry Q82.5
  strawberry Q82.5
  stretch L90.6
  tattoo L81.8
Marker heterochromatin —see Extra, marker
  chromosomes
Maroteaux-Lamy syndrome (mild) (severe)
  E76.29
Marrow (bone)
  arrest D61.9
  poor function D75.89
Marseilles fever A77.1
Marsh fever —see Malaria
Marshall's (hidrotic) **ectodermal dysplasia**
  Q82.4
Marsh's disease (exophthalmic goiter) E05.00
  with storm E05.01
Masculinization (female) **with adrenal**
  hyperplasia E25.9
  congenital E25.0
Masculinovoblastoma D27.-
Masochism (sexual) F65.51
Mason's lung J62.8
Mass
  abdominal R19.00
    epigastric R19.06
    generalized R19.07
    left lower quadrant R19.04

Mass *(Continued)*
  abdominal *(Continued)*
    left upper quadrant R19.02
    periumbilic R19.05
    right lower quadrant R19.03
    right upper quadrant R19.01
    specified site NEC R19.09
  breast N63
  chest R22.2
  cystic —*see* Cyst
  ear H93.8-
  head R22.0
  intra-abdominal (diffuse) (generalized) —*see*
      Mass, abdominal
  kidney N28.89
  liver R16.0
  localized (skin) R22.9
    chest R22.2
    head R22.0
    limb
      lower R22.4-
      upper R22.3-
    neck R22.1
    trunk R22.2
  lung R91.8
  malignant —*see* Neoplasm, malignant,
      by site
  neck R22.1
  pelvic (diffuse) (generalized) —*see* Mass,
      abdominal
  specified organ NEC —*see* Disease, by site
  splenic R16.1
  substernal thyroid —*see* Goiter
  superficial (localized) R22.9
  umbilical (diffuse) (generalized) R19.09
Massive —*see* condition
Mast cell
  disease, systemic tissue D47.0
  leukemia C94.3-
  sarcoma C96.2
  tumor D47.0
    malignant C96.2
Mastalgia N64.4
Masters-Allen syndrome N83.8
Mastitis (acute) (diffuse) (nonpuerperal)
    (subacute) N61
  chronic (cystic) —*see* Mastopathy, cystic
  cystic (Schimmelbusch's type) —*see*
      Mastopathy, cystic
  fibrocystic —*see* Mastopathy, cystic
  infective N61
    newborn P39.0
  interstitial, gestational or puerperal —*see*
      Mastitis, obstetric
  neonatal (noninfective) P83.4
    infective P39.0
  obstetric (interstitial) (nonpurulent)
    associated with
      lactation O91.23
      pregnancy O91.21-
      puerperium O91.22
    purulent
      associated with
        lactation O91.13
        pregnancy O91.11-
        puerperium O91.12
  periductal —*see* Ectasia, mammary duct
  phlegmonous —*see* Mastopathy, cystic
  plasma cell —*see* Ectasia, mammary duct
Mastocytoma D47.0
  malignant C96.2
Mastocytosis Q82.2
  aggressive systemic C96.2
  indolent systemic D47.0
  malignant C96.2
  systemic, associated with clonal hematopoetic
      non-mast-cell disease (SM-AHNMD)
      D47.0
Mastodynia N64.4
Mastoid —*see* condition
Mastoidalgia —*see* subcategory H92.0

Mastoiditis (coalescent) (hemorrhagic)
    (suppurative) H70.9-
  acute, subacute H70.00-
    complicated NEC H70.09-
    subperiosteal H70.01-
  chronic (necrotic) (recurrent) H70.1-
  in (due to)
    infectious disease NEC B99 *[H75.0-]*
    parasitic disease NEC B89 *[H75.0-]*
    tuberculosis A18.03
  petrositis —*see* Petrositis
  postauricular fistula —*see* Fistula,
      postauricular
  specified NEC H70.89-
  tuberculous A18.03
Mastopathy, mastopathia N64.9
  chronica cystica —*see* Mastopathy, cystic
  cystic (chronic) (diffuse) N60.1
    with epithelial proliferation N60.3-
  diffuse cystic —*see* Mastopathy, cystic
  estrogenic, oestrogenica N64.89
  ovarian origin N64.89
Mastoplasia, mastoplastia N62
Masturbation (excessive) F98.8
Maternal care (for) —*see* Pregnancy
    (complicated by) (management
    affected by)
Matheiu's disease (leptospiral jaundice)
    A27.0
Mauclaire's disease or osteochondrosis —
    see Osteochondrosis, juvenile, hand,
    metacarpal
Maxcy's disease A75.2
Maxilla, maxillary —*see* condition
May (-Hegglin) **anomaly or syndrome**
    D72.0
McArdle (-Schmid)(-Pearson) **disease**
    (glycogen storage) E74.04
McCune-Albright syndrome Q78.1
McQuarrie's syndrome (idiopathic familial
    hypoglycemia) E16.2
Meadow's syndrome Q86.1
Measles (black) (hemorrhagic) (suppressed)
    B05.9
  with
    complications NEC B05.89
    encephalitis B05.0
    intestinal complications B05.4
    keratitis (keratoconjunctivitis) B05.81
    meningitis B05.1
    otitis media B05.3
    pneumonia B05.2
  French —*see* Rubella
  German —*see* Rubella
  Liberty —*see* Rubella
Meatitis, urethral —*see* Urethritis
Meatus, meatal —*see* condition
Meat-wrappers' asthma J68.9
Meckel-Gruber syndrome Q61.9
Meckel's diverticulitis, diverticulum
    (displaced) (hypertrophic) Q43.0
Meconium
  ileus, newborn P76.0
    in cystic fibrosis E84.11
    meaning meconium plug (without cystic
        fibrosis) P76.0
  obstruction, newborn P76.0
    due to fecaliths P76.0
    in mucoviscidosis E84.11
  peritonitis P78.0
  plug syndrome (newborn) NEC P76.0
Median —*see also* condition
  arcuate ligament syndrome I77.4
  bar (prostate) (vesical orifice) —*see*
      Hyperplasia, prostate
  rhomboid glossitis K14.2
Mediastinal shift R93.8
Mediastinitis (acute) (chronic)
    J98.5
  syphilitic A52.73
  tuberculous A15.8

Mediastinopericarditis —*see also* Pericarditis
  acute I30.9
  adhesive I31.0
  chronic I31.8
  rheumatic I09.2
Mediastinum, mediastinal —*see* condition
Medicine poisoning —*see* Table of Drugs and
    Chemicals, by drug, poisoning
Mediterranean
  fever —*see* Brucellosis
    familial E85.0
    tick A77.1
  kala-azar B55.0
  leishmaniasis B55.0
  tick fever A77.1
Medulla —*see* condition
Medullary cystic kidney Q61.5
Medullated fibers
  optic (nerve) Q14.8
  retina Q14.1
Medulloblastoma
  desmoplastic C71.6
  specified site —*see* Neoplasm, malignant, by
      site
  unspecified site C71.6
Medulloepithelioma —*see also* Neoplasm,
    malignant, by site
  teratoid —*see* Neoplasm, malignant, by site
Medullomyoblastoma
  specified site —*see* Neoplasm, malignant, by
      site
  unspecified site C71.6
Meekeren-Ehlers-Danlos syndrome
    Q79.6
Megacolon (acquired) (functional) (not
    Hirschsprung's disease) (in) K59.3
  Chagas' disease B57.32
  congenital, congenitum (aganglionic)
      Q43.1
  Hirschsprung's (disease) Q43.1
  toxic NEC K59.3
    due to Clostridium difficile A04.7
Megaesophagus (functional) K22.0
  congenital Q39.5
  in (due to) Chagas' disease B57.31
Megalencephaly Q04.5
Megalerythema (epidemic) B08.3
Megaloappendix Q43.8
Megalocephalus, megalocephaly NEC Q75.3
Megalocornea Q15.8
  with glaucoma Q15.0
Megalocytic anemia D53.1
Megalodactylia (fingers) (thumbs) (congenital)
    Q74.0
  toes Q74.2
Megaloduodenum Q43.8
Megaloesophagus (functional) K22.0
  congenital Q39.5
Megalogastria (acquired) K31.89
  congenital Q40.2
Megalophthalmos Q11.3
Megalopsia H53.15
Megalosplenia —*see* Splenomegaly
Megaloureter N28.82
  congenital Q62.2
Megarectum K62.89
Megasigmoid K59.3
  congenital Q43.2
Megaureter N28.82
  congenital Q62.2
Megavitamin-B6 syndrome E67.2
Megrim —*see* Migraine
Meibomian
  cyst, infected —*see* Hordeolum
  gland —*see* condition
  sty, stye —*see* Hordeolum
Meibomitis —*see* Hordeolum
Meige-Milroy disease (chronic hereditary
    edema) Q82.0
Meige's syndrome Q82.0
Melalgia, nutritional E53.8

◀ New   ◀▥▥ Revised   ~~deleted~~ Deleted

Melancholia F32.9
- climacteric (single episode) F32.8
  - recurrent episode F33.9
- hypochondriac F45.29
- intermittent (single episode) F32.8
  - recurrent episode F33.9
- involutional (single episode) F32.8
  - recurrent episode F33.9
- menopausal (single episode) F32.8
  - recurrent episode F33.9
- puerperal F32.8
- reactive (emotional stress or trauma) F32.3
- recurrent F33.9
- senile F03
- stuporous (single episode) F32.8
  - recurrent episode F33.9

Melanemia R79.89

Melanoameloblastoma —*see* Neoplasm, bone, benign

Melanoblastoma —*see* Melanoma

Melanocarcinoma —*see* Melanoma

Melanocytoma, eyeball D31.4-

Melanocytosis, neurocutaneous Q82.8

Melanoderma, melanodermia L81.4

Melanodontia, infantile K03.89

Melanodontoclasia K03.89

Melanoepithelioma —*see* Melanoma

Melanoma (malignant) C43.9
- acral lentiginous, malignant —*see* Melanoma, skin, by site
- amelanotic —*see* Melanoma, skin, by site
- balloon cell —*see* Melanoma, skin, by site
- benign —*see* Nevus
- desmoplastic, malignant —*see* Melanoma, skin, by site
- epithelioid cell —*see* Melanoma, skin, by site
  - with spindle cell, mixed —*see* Melanoma, skin, by site
- in
  - giant pigmented nevus —*see* Melanoma, skin, by site
  - Hutchinson's melanotic freckle —*see* Melanoma, skin, by site
  - junctional nevus —*see* Melanoma, skin, by site
  - precancerous melanosis —*see* Melanoma, skin, by site
- in situ D03.9
  - abdominal wall D03.59
  - ala nasi D03.39
  - ankle D03.7-
  - anus, anal (margin) (skin) D03.51
  - arm D03.6-
  - auditory canal D03.2-
  - auricle (ear) D03.2-
  - auricular canal (external) D03.2-
  - axilla, axillary fold D03.59
  - back D03.59
  - breast D03.52
  - brow D03.39
  - buttock D03.59
  - canthus (eye) D03.1-
  - cheek (external) D03.39
  - chest wall D03.59
  - chin D03.39
  - choroid D03.8
  - conjunctiva D03.8
  - ear (external) D03.2-
  - external meatus (ear) D03.2-
  - eye D03.8
  - eyebrow D03.39
  - eyelid (lower) (upper) D03.1-
  - face D03.30
    - specified NEC D03.39
  - female genital organ (external) NEC D03.8
  - finger D03.6-
  - flank D03.59
  - foot D03.7-
  - forearm D03.6-
  - forehead D03.39
  - foreskin D03.8

Melanoma (Continued)
- in situ (Continued)
  - gluteal region D03.59
  - groin D03.59
  - hand D03.6-
  - heel D03.7-
  - helix D03.2-
  - hip D03.7-
  - interscapular region D03.59
  - iris D03.8
  - jaw D03.39
  - knee D03.7-
  - labium (majus) (minus) D03.8
  - lacrimal gland D03.8
  - leg D03.7-
  - lip (lower) (upper) D03.0
  - lower limb NEC D03.7-
  - male genital organ (external) NEC D03.8
  - nail D03.9
    - finger D03.6-
    - toe D03.7-
  - neck D03.4
  - nose (external) D03.39
  - orbit D03.8
  - penis D03.8
  - perianal skin D03.51
  - perineum D03.51
  - pinna D03.2-
  - popliteal fossa or space D03.7-
  - prepuce D03.8
  - pudendum D03.8
  - retina D03.8
  - retrobulbar D03.8
  - scalp D03.4
  - scrotum D03.8
  - shoulder D03.6-
  - specified site NEC D03.8
  - submammary fold D03.52
  - temple D03.39
  - thigh D03.7-
  - toe D03.7-
  - trunk NEC D03.59
  - umbilicus D03.59
  - upper limb NEC D03.6-
  - vulva D03.8
- juvenile —*see* Nevus
- malignant, of soft parts except skin —*see* Neoplasm, connective tissue, malignant
- metastatic
  - breast C79.81
  - genital organ C79.82
  - specified site NEC C79.89
- neurotropic, malignant —*see* Melanoma, skin, by site
- nodular —*see* Melanoma, skin, by site
- regressing, malignant —*see* Melanoma, skin, by site
- skin C43.9
  - abdominal wall C43.59
  - ala nasi C43.31
  - ankle C43.7-
  - anus, anal (skin) C43.51
  - arm C43.6-
  - auditory canal (external) C43.2-
  - auricle (ear) C43.2-
  - auricular canal (external) C43.2-
  - axilla, axillary fold C43.59
  - back C43.59
  - breast (female) (male) C43.52
  - brow C43.39
  - buttock C43.59
  - canthus (eye) C43.1-
  - cheek (external) C43.39
  - chest wall C43.59
  - chin C43.39
  - ear (external) C43.2-
  - elbow C43.6-
  - external meatus (ear) C43.2-
  - eyebrow C43.39

Melanoma (Continued)
- skin (Continued)
  - eyelid (lower) (upper) C43.1-
  - face C43.30
    - specified NEC C43.39
  - female genital organ (external) NEC C51.9
  - finger C43.6-
  - flank C43.59
  - foot C43.7-
  - forearm C43.6-
  - forehead C43.39
  - foreskin C60.0
  - glabella C43.39
  - gluteal region C43.59
  - groin C43.59
  - hand C43.6-
  - heel C43.7-
  - helix C43.2-
  - hip C43.7-
  - interscapular region C43.59
  - jaw (external) C43.39
  - knee C43.7-
  - labium C51.9
    - majus C51.0
    - minus C51.1
  - leg C43.7-
  - lip (lower) (upper) C43.0
  - lower limb NEC C43.7-
  - male genital organ (external) NEC C63.9
  - nail
    - finger C43.6-
    - toe C43.7-
  - nasolabial groove C43.39
  - nates C43.59
  - neck C43.4
  - nose (external) C43.31
  - overlapping site C43.8
  - palpebra C43.1-
  - penis C60.9
  - perianal skin C43.51
  - perineum C43.51
  - pinna C43.2-
  - popliteal fossa or space C43.7-
  - prepuce C60.0
  - pudendum C51.9
  - scalp C43.4
  - scrotum C63.2
  - shoulder C43.6-
  - skin NEC C43.9
  - submammary fold C43.52
  - temple C43.39
  - thigh C43.7-
  - toe C43.7-
  - trunk NEC C43.59
  - umbilicus C43.59
  - upper limb NEC C43.6-
  - vulva C51.9
    - overlapping sites C51.8
- spindle cell
  - with epithelioid, mixed —*see* Melanoma, skin, by site
  - type A C69.4-
  - type B C69.4-
- superficial spreading —*see* Melanoma, skin, by site

Melanosarcoma —*see also* Melanoma
- epithelioid cell —*see* Melanoma

Melanosis L81.4
- addisonian E27.1
  - tuberculous A18.7
- adrenal E27.1
- colon K63.89
- conjunctiva —*see* Pigmentation, conjunctiva
  - congenital Q13.89
- cornea (presenile) (senile) —*see also* Pigmentation, cornea
  - congenital Q13.4
- eye NEC H57.8
  - congenital Q15.8
- lenticularis progressiva Q82.1
- liver K76.89

M

Melanosis (*Continued*)
  precancerous —*see also* Melanoma, in situ
    malignant melanoma in —*see* Melanoma
  Riehl's L81.4
  sclera H15.89
    congenital Q13.89
  suprarenal E27.1
  tar L81.4
  toxic L81.4
Melanuria R82.99
MELAS syndrome E88.41
Melasma L81.1
  adrenal (gland) E27.1
  suprarenal (gland) E27.1
Melena K92.1
  with ulcer - code by site under Ulcer, with
    hemorrhage K27.4
  due to swallowed maternal blood P78.2
  newborn, neonatal P54.1
    due to swallowed maternal blood P78.2
Meleney's
  gangrene (cutaneous) —*see* Ulcer, skin
  ulcer (chronic undermining) —*see* Ulcer, skin
Melioidosis A24.9
  acute A24.1
  chronic A24.2
  fulminating A24.1
  pneumonia A24.1
  pulmonary (chronic) A24.2
    acute A24.1
    subacute A24.2
  sepsis A24.1
  specified NEC A24.3
  subacute A24.2
Melitensis, febris A23.0
Melkersson (-Rosenthal) **syndrome** G51.2
Mellitus, diabetes —*see* Diabetes
Melorheostosis (bone) —*see* Disorder, bone,
    density and structure, specified NEC
Meloschisis Q18.4
Melotia Q17.4
Membrana
  capsularis lentis posterior Q13.89
  epipapillaris Q14.2
Membranacea placenta O43.19-
Membranaceous uterus N85.8
Membrane (s), **membranous** —*see also*
    condition
  cyclitic —*see* Membrane, pupillary
  folds, congenital —*see* Web
  Jackson's Q43.3
  over face of newborn P28.9
  premature rupture —*see* Rupture,
    membranes, premature
  pupillary H21.4-
    persistent Q13.89
  retained (with hemorrhage) (complicating
    delivery) O72.2
    without hemorrhage O73.1
  secondary cataract —*see* Cataract, secondary
  unruptured (causing asphyxia) —*see*
    Asphyxia, newborn
  vitreous —*see* Opacity, vitreous, membranes
    and strands
Membranitis —*see* Chorioamnionitis
Memory disturbance, lack or loss —*see also*
    Amnesia
  mild, following organic brain damage F06.8
Menadione deficiency E56.1
Menarche
  delayed E30.0
  precocious E30.1
Mendacity, pathologic F60.2
Mendelson's syndrome (due to anesthesia)
    J95.4
  in labor and delivery O74.0
  in pregnancy O29.01-
  obstetric O74.0
  postpartum, puerperal O89.01
Ménétrier's disease or syndrome K29.60
  with bleeding K29.61

Ménière's disease, syndrome or vertigo H81.0-
Meninges, meningeal —*see* condition
Meningioma —*see also* Neoplasm, meninges,
    benign
  angioblastic —*see* Neoplasm, meninges,
    benign
  angiomatous —*see* Neoplasm, meninges,
    benign
  endotheliomatous —*see* Neoplasm, meninges,
    benign
  fibroblastic —*see* Neoplasm, meninges,
    benign
  fibrous —*see* Neoplasm, meninges, benign
  hemangioblastic —*see* Neoplasm, meninges,
    benign
  hemangiopericytic —*see* Neoplasm,
    meninges, benign
  malignant —*see* Neoplasm, meninges,
    malignant
  meningiothelial —*see* Neoplasm, meninges,
    benign
  meningotheliomatous —*see* Neoplasm,
    meninges, benign
  mixed —*see* Neoplasm, meninges, benign
  multiple —*see* Neoplasm, meninges,
    uncertain behavior
  papillary —*see* Neoplasm, meninges,
    uncertain behavior
  psammomatous —*see* Neoplasm, meninges,
    benign
  syncytial —*see* Neoplasm, meninges, benign
  transitional —*see* Neoplasm, meninges,
    benign
Meningiomatosis (diffuse) —*see* Neoplasm,
    meninges, uncertain behavior
Meningism —*see* Meningismus
Meningismus (infectional) (pneumococcal)
    R29.1
  due to serum or vaccine R29.1
  influenzal —*see* Influenza, with,
    manifestations NEC
Meningitis (basal) (basic) (brain) (cerebral)
    (cervical) (congestive) (diffuse)
    (hemorrhagic) infantile) (membranous)
    (metastatic) (nonspecific) (pontine)
    (progressive) (simple) (spinal) (subacute)
    (sympathetic) (toxic) G03.9
  abacterial G03.0
  actinomycotic A42.81
  adenoviral A87.1
  arbovirus A87.8
  aseptic (acute) G03.0
  bacterial G00.9
    Escherichia coli (E. coli) G00.8
    Friedländer (bacillus) G00.8
    gram-negative G00.9
    H. influenzae G00.0
    Klebsiella G00.8
    pneumococcal G00.1
    specified organism NEC G00.8
    staphylococcal G00.3
    streptococcal (acute) G00.2
  benign recurrent (Mollaret) G03.2
  candidal B37.5
  caseous (tuberculous) A17.0
  cerebrospinal A39.0
  chronic NEC G03.1
  clear cerebrospinal fluid NEC G03.0
  coxsackievirus A87.0
  cryptococcal B45.1
  diplococcal (gram positive) A39.0
  echovirus A87.0
  enteroviral A87.0
  eosinophilic B83.2
  epidemic NEC A39.0
  Escherichia coli (E. coli) G00.8
  fibrinopurulent G00.9
    specified organism NEC G00.8
  Friedländer (bacillus) G00.8
  gonococcal A54.81
  gram-negative cocci G00.9

Meningitis (*Continued*)
  gram-positive cocci G00.9
  Haemophilus (influenzae) G00.0
  H. influenzae G00.0
  in (due to)
    adenovirus A87.1
    African trypanosomiasis B56.9 [G02]
    anthrax A22.8
    bacterial disease NEC A48.8 [G01]
    Chagas' disease (chronic) B57.41
    chickenpox B01.0
    coccidioidomycosis B38.4
    Diplococcus pneumoniae G00.1
    enterovirus A87.0
    herpes (simplex) virus B00.3
      zoster B02.1
    infectious mononucleosis B27.92
    leptospirosis A27.81
    Listeria monocytogenes A32.11
    Lyme disease A69.21
    measles B05.1
    mumps (virus) B26.1
    neurosyphilis (late) A52.13
    parasitic disease NEC B89 [G02]
    poliovirus A80.9 [G02]
    preventive immunization, inoculation or
      vaccination G03.8
    rubella B06.02
    Salmonella infection A02.21
    specified cause NEC G03.8
    typhoid fever A01.01
    varicella B01.0
    viral disease NEC A87.8
    whooping cough A37.90
    zoster B02.1
  infectious G00.9
  influenzal (H. influenzae) G00.0
  Klebsiella G00.8
  leptospiral (aseptic) A27.81
  lymphocytic (acute) (benign) (serous)
    A87.2
  meningococcal A39.0
  Mima polymorpha G00.8
  Mollaret (benign recurrent) G03.2
  monilial B37.5
  mycotic NEC B49 [G02]
  Neisseria A39.0
  nonbacterial G03.0
  nonpyogenic NEC G03.0
  ossificans G96.19
  pneumococcal G00.1
  poliovirus A80.9 [G02]
  postmeasles B05.1
  purulent G00.9
    specified organism NEC G00.8
  pyogenic G00.9
    specified organism NEC G00.8
  Salmonella (arizonae) (Cholerae-Suis)
    (enteritidis) (typhimurium) A02.21
  septic G00.9
    specified organism NEC G00.8
  serosa circumscripta NEC G03.0
  serous NEC G93.2
  specified organism NEC G00.8
  sporotrichosis B42.81
  staphylococcal G00.3
  sterile G03.0
  streptococcal (acute) G00.2
  suppurative G00.9
    specified organism NEC G00.8
  syphilitic (late) (tertiary) A52.13
    acute A51.41
    congenital A50.41
    secondary A51.41
  Torula histolytica (cryptococcal) B45.1
  traumatic (complication of injury)
    T79.8
  tuberculous A17.0
  typhoid A01.01
  viral NEC A87.9
  Yersinia pestis A20.3

Meningocele (spinal) —*see also* Spina bifida
  with hydrocephalus —*see* Spina bifida, by
    site, with hydrocephalus
  acquired (traumatic) G96.19
  cerebral —*see* Encephalocele
Meningocerebritis —*see* Meningoencephalitis
Meningococcemia A39.4
  acute A39.2
  chronic A39.3
Meningococcus, meningococcal (*see also*
    condition) A39.9
  adrenalitis, hemorrhagic A39.1
  carrier (suspected) of Z22.31
  meningitis (cerebrospinal) A39.0
Meningoencephalitis (*see also* Encephalitis)
    G04.90
  acute NEC (*see also* Encephalitis, viral) A86
  bacterial NEC G04.2
  California A83.5
  diphasic A84.1
  eosinophilic B83.2
  epidemic A39.81
  herpesviral, herpetic B00.4
    due to herpesvirus 6 B10.01
    due to herpesvirus 7 B10.09
    specified NEC B10.09
  in (due to)
    blastomycosis NEC B40.81
    diseases classified elsewhere G05.3
    free-living amebae B60.2
    Hemophilus influenzae (H. influenzae)
      G04.2
    herpes B00.4
      due to herpesvirus 6 B10.01
      due to herpesvirus 7 B10.09
      specified NEC B10.09
    H. influenzae G00.0
    Lyme disease A69.22
    mercury —*see* subcategory T56.1
    mumps B26.2
    Naegleria (amebae) (organisms) (fowleri)
      B60.2
    Parastrongylus cantonensis B83.2
    toxoplasmosis (acquired) B58.2
      congenital P37.1
  infectious (acute) (viral) A86
  influenzal (H. influenzae) G04.2
  Listeria monocytogenes A32.12
  lymphocytic (serous) A87.2
  mumps B26.2
  parasitic NEC B89 [G05.3]
  pneumococcal G00.1
  primary amebic B60.2
  specific (syphilitic) A52.14
  specified organism NEC G04.81
  staphylococcal G04.2
  streptococcal G04.2
  syphilitic A52.14
  toxic NEC G92
    due to mercury —*see* subcategory
      T56.1
  tuberculous A17.82
  virus NEC A86
Meningoencephalocele —*see also*
    Encephalocele
  syphilitic A52.19
  congenital A50.49
Meningoencephalomyelitis —*see also*
    Meningoencephalitis
  acute NEC (viral) A86
    disseminated G04.00
      postimmunization or postvaccination
        G04.02
      postinfectious G04.01
    due to
      actinomycosis A42.82
      Torula B45.1
      Toxoplasma or toxoplasmosis (acquired)
        B58.2
        congenital P37.1
  postimmunization or postvaccination G04.02

Meningoencephalomyelopathy G96.9
Meningoencephalopathy G96.9
Meningomyelitis —*see also*
    Meningoencephalitis
  bacterial NEC G04.2
  blastomycotic NEC B40.81
  cryptococcal B45.1
  in diseases classified elsewhere G05.4
  meningococcal A39.81
  syphilitic A52.14
  tuberculous A17.82
Meningomyelocele —*see also* Spina bifida
  syphilitic A52.19
Meningomyeloneuritis —*see*
    Meningoencephalitis
Meningoradiculitis —*see* Meningitis
Meningovascular —*see* condition
Menkes' disease or syndrome E83.09
  meaning maple-syrup-urine disease E71.0
Menometrorrhagia N92.1
Menopause, menopausal (asymptomatic)
    (state) Z78.0
  arthritis (any site) NEC —*see* Arthritis,
    specified form NEC
  bleeding N92.4
  depression (single episode) F32.8
    agitated (single episode) F32.2
      recurrent episode F33.9
    psychotic (single episode) F32.8
      recurrent episode F33.9
    recurrent episode F33.9
  melancholia (single episode) F32.8
    recurrent episode F33.9
  paranoid state F22
  premature E28.319
    asymptomatic E28.319
      postirradiation E89.40
      postsurgical E89.40
    symptomatic E28.310
      postirradiation E89.41
      postsurgical E89.41
  psychosis NEC F28
  symptomatic N95.1
  toxic polyarthritis NEC —*see* Arthritis,
    specified form NEC
Menorrhagia (primary) N92.0
  climacteric N92.4
    menopausal N92.4
  menopausal N92.4
  postclimacteric N95.0
  postmenopausal N95.0
  preclimacteric or premenopausal N92.4
  pubertal (menses retained) N92.2
Menostaxis N92.0
Menses, retention N94.89
Menstrual —*see* Menstruation
Menstruation
  absent —*see* Amenorrhea
  anovulatory N97.0
  cycle, irregular N92.6
  delayed N91.0
  disorder N93.9
    psychogenic F45.8
  during pregnancy O20.8
  excessive (with regular cycle) N92.0
    with irregular cycle N92.1
    at puberty N92.2
  frequent N92.0
  infrequent —*see* Oligomenorrhea
  irregular N92.6
    specified NEC N92.5
  latent N92.5
  membranous N92.5
  painful (*see also* Dysmenorrhea) N94.6
    primary N94.4
    psychogenic F45.8
    secondary N94.5
  passage of clots N92.0
  precocious E30.1
  protracted N92.5
  rare —*see* Oligomenorrhea

Menstruation (*Continued*)
  retained N94.89
  retrograde N92.5
  scanty —*see* Oligomenorrhea
  suppression N94.89
  vicarious (nasal) N94.89
Mental —*see also* condition
  deficiency —*see* Disability, intellectual
  deterioration —*see* Psychosis
  disorder —*see* Disorder, mental
  exhaustion F48.8
  insufficiency (congenital) —*see* Disability,
    intellectual
  observation without need for further medical
    care Z03.89
  retardation —*see* Disability, intellectual
  subnormality —*see* Disability, intellectual
  upset —*see* Disorder, mental
Meralgia paresthetica G57.1-
Mercurial —*see* condition
Mercurialism —*see* subcategory T56.1
MERRF syndrome (myoclonic epilepsy
    associated with ragged-red fiber)
    E88.42
Merkel cell tumor —*see* Carcinoma,
    Merkel cell
Merocele —*see* Hernia, femoral
Meromelia
  lower limb —*see* Defect, reduction, lower
    limb
    intercalary
      femur —*see* Defect, reduction, lower
        limb, specified type NEC
      tibiofibular (complete) (incomplete) —
        see Defect, reduction, lower
        limb
  upper limb —*see* Defect, reduction, upper
    limb
    intercalary, humeral, radioulnar —*see*
      Agenesis, arm, with hand present
Merzbacher-Pelizaeus disease E75.29
Mesaortitis —*see* Aortitis
Mesarteritis —*see* Arteritis
Mesencephalitis —*see* Encephalitis
Mesenchymoma —*see also* Neoplasm,
    connective tissue, uncertain behavior
  benign —*see* Neoplasm, connective tissue,
    benign
  malignant —*see* Neoplasm, connective tissue,
    malignant
Mesenteritis
  retractile K65.4
  sclerosing K65.4
Mesentery, mesenteric —*see* condition
Mesiodens, mesiodentes K00.1
Mesio-occlusion M26.213
Mesocolon —*see* condition
Mesonephroma (malignant) —*see* Neoplasm,
    malignant, by site
  benign —*see* Neoplasm, benign, by site
Mesophlebitis —*see* Phlebitis
Mesostromal dysgenesia Q13.89
Mesothelioma (malignant) C45.9
  benign
    mesentery D19.1
    mesocolon D19.1
    omentum D19.1
    peritoneum D19.1
    pleura D19.0
    specified site NEC D19.7
    unspecified site D19.9
  biphasic C45.9
    benign
      mesentery D19.1
      mesocolon D19.1
      omentum D19.1
      peritoneum D19.1
      pleura D19.0
      specified site NEC D19.7
      unspecified site D19.9
  cystic D48.4

M

◀ New   ◀⁞⁞ Revised   ~~deleted~~ Deleted

Migraine (Continued)
basilar —see Migraine, with aura
classical —see Migraine, with aura
common —see Migraine, without aura
complicated G43.109
equivalents —see Migraine, with aura
familiar —see Migraine, hemiplegic
hemiplegic G43.409
with refractory migraine G43.419
with status migrainosus G43.411
without status migrainosus G43.419
intractable G43.419
with status migrainosus G43.411
without status migrainosus G43.419
not intractable G43.409
with status migrainosus G43.401
without status migrainosus G43.409
without refractory migraine G43.409
with status migrainosus G43.401
without status migrainosus G43.409
intractable G43.919
with status migrainosus G43.911
without status migrainosus G43.919
menstrual G43.829
with refractory migraine G43.839
with status migrainosus G43.831
without status migrainosus G43.839
intractable G43.839
with status migrainosus G43.831
without status migrainosus G43.839
not intractable G43.829
with status migrainosus G43.821
without status migrainosus G43.829
without refractory migraine G43.829
with status migrainosus G43.821
without status migrainosus G43.829
menstrually related —see Migraine, menstrual
not intractable G43.909
with status migrainosus G43.901
without status migrainosus G43.919
ophthalmoplegic G43.B0
with refractory migraine G43.B1
intractable G43.B1
not intractable G43.B0
without refractory migraine G43.B0
persistent aura (with, without) cerebral infarction —see Migraine, with aura, persistent
preceded or accompanied by transient focal neurological phenomena —see Migraine, with aura
pre-menstrual —see Migraine, menstrual
pure menstrual —see Migraine, menstrual
retinal —see Migraine, with aura
specified NEC G43.809
intractable G43.819
with status migrainosus G43.811
without status migrainosus G43.819
not intractable G43.809
with status migrainosus G43.801
without status migrainosus G43.809
sporadic —see Migraine, hemiplegic
transformed —see Migraine, without aura, chronic
triggered seizures —see Migraine, with aura
without aura G43.009
with refractory migraine G43.019
with status migrainosus G43.011
without status migrainosus G43.019
chronic G43.709
with refractory migraine G43.719
with status migrainosus G43.711
without status migrainosus G43.719
intractable
with status migrainosus G43.711
without status migrainosus G43.719
not intractable
with status migrainosus G43.701
without status migrainosus G43.709

Migraine (Continued)
without aura (Continued)
chronic (Continued)
without refractory migraine G43.709
with status migrainosus G43.701
without status migrainosus G43.709
intractable
with status migrainosus G43.011
without status migrainosus G43.019
not intractable
with status migrainosus G43.001
without status migrainosus G43.009
without mention of refractory migraine G43.009
with status migrainosus G43.001
without status migrainosus G43.009
without refractory migraine G43.909
with status migrainosus G43.901
without status migrainosus G43.919
Migrant, social Z59.0
Migration, anxiety concerning Z60.3
Migratory, migrating —see also condition
person Z59.0
testis Q55.29
Mikity-Wilson disease or syndrome P27.0
Mikulicz' disease or syndrome K11.8
Miliaria L74.3
alba L74.1
apocrine L75.2
crystallina L74.1
profunda L74.2
rubra L74.0
tropicalis L74.2
Miliary —see condition
Milium L72.0
colloid L57.8
Milk
crust L21.0
excessive secretion O92.6
poisoning —see Poisoning, food, noxious
retention O92.79
sickness —see Poisoning, food, noxious
spots I31.0
Milk-alkali disease or syndrome E83.52
Milk-leg (deep vessels) (nonpuerperal) —see Embolism, vein, lower extremity
complicating pregnancy O22.3-
puerperal, postpartum, childbirth O87.1
Milkman's disease or syndrome M83.8
Milky urine —see Chyluria
Millard-Gubler (-Foville) **paralysis or syndrome** G46.3
Millar's asthma J38.5
Miller-Fisher syndrome G61.0
Mills' disease —see Hemiplegia
Millstone maker's pneumoconiosis J62.8
Milroy's disease (chronic hereditary edema) Q82.0
Minamata disease T26.1
Miners' asthma or lung J60
Minkowski-Chauffard syndrome —see Spherocytosis
Minor —see condition
Minor's disease (hematomyelia) G95.19
Minot's disease (hemorrhagic disease), newborn P53
Minot-von Willebrand-Jurgens disease or syndrome (angiohemophilia) D68.0
Minus (and plus) **hand** (intrinsic) —see Deformity, limb, specified type NEC, forearm
Miosis (pupil) H57.03
Mirizzi's syndrome (hepatic duct stenosis) K83.1
Mirror writing F81.0
Misadventure (of) (prophylactic) (therapeutic) (see also Complications) T88.9
administration of insulin (by accident) —see subcategory T38.3
infusion —see Complications, infusion

Misadventure (Continued)
local applications (of fomentations, plasters, etc.) T88.9
burn or scald —see Burn
specified NEC T88.8
medical care (early) (late) T88.9
adverse effect of drugs or chemicals —see Table of Drugs and Chemicals
medical care (early) (late)
burn or scald —see Burn
specified NEC T88.8
specified NEC T88.8
surgical procedure (early) (late) —see Complications, surgical procedure
transfusion —see Complications, transfusion
vaccination or other immunological procedure —see Complications, vaccination
Miscarriage O03.9
Misdirection, aqueous H40.83-
Misperception, sleep state F51.02
Misplaced, misplacement
ear Q17.4
kidney (acquired) N28.89
congenital Q63.2
organ or site, congenital NEC —see Malposition, congenital
Missed
abortion O02.1
delivery O36.4
Missing —see Absence
Misuse of drugs F19.99
Mitchell's disease (erythromelalgia) I73.81
Mite (s) (infestation) B88.9
diarrhea B88.0
grain (itch) B88.0
hair follicle (itch) B88.0
in sputum B88.0
Mitral —see condition
Mittelschmerz N94.0
Mixed —see condition
MNGIE (Mitochondrial Neurogastrointestinal Encephalopathy) syndrome E88.49
Mobile, mobility
cecum Q43.3
excessive —see Hypermobility
gallbladder, congenital Q44.1
kidney N28.89
organ or site, congenital NEC —see Malposition, congenital
Mobitz heart block (atrioventricular) I44.1
Moebius, Möbius
disease (ophthalmoplegic migraine) —see Migraine, ophthalmoplegic
syndrome Q87.0
congenital oculofacial paralysis (with other anomalies) Q87.0
ophthalmoplegic migraine —see Migraine, ophthalmoplegic
Moeller's glossitis K14.0
Mohr's syndrome (Types I and II) Q87.0
Mola destruens D39.2
Molar pregnancy O02.0
Molarization of premolars K00.2
Molding, head (during birth) - omit code
Mole (pigmented) —see also Nevus
blood O02.0
Breus' O02.0
cancerous —see Melanoma
carneous O02.0
destructive D39.2
fleshy O02.0
hydatid, hydatidiform (benign) (complicating pregnancy) (delivered) (undelivered) O01.9
classical O01.0
complete O01.0
incomplete O01.1
invasive D39.2
malignant D39.2
partial O01.1

Mole *(Continued)*
  intrauterine O02.0
  invasive (hydatidiform) D39.2
  malignant
    meaning
      malignant hydatidiform mole D39.2
      melanoma —*see* Melanoma
  nonhydatidiform O02.0
  nonpigmented —*see* Nevus
  pregnancy NEC O02.0
  skin —*see* Nevus
  tubal O00.1
  vesicular —*see* Mole, hydatidiform
Molimen, molimina (menstrual) N94.3
Molluscum contagiosum (epitheliale) B08.1
Mönckeberg's arteriosclerosis, disease, or
  sclerosis —*see* Arteriosclerosis, extremities
Mondini's malformation (cochlea) Q16.5
Mondor's disease I80.8
Monge's disease T70.29
Monilethrix (congenital) Q84.1
Moniliasis (*see also* Candidiasis) B37.9
  neonatal P37.5
Monitoring (encounter for)
  therapeutic drug level Z51.81
Monkey malaria B53.1
Monkeypox B04
Monoarthritis M13.10
  ankle M13.17-
  elbow M13.12-
  foot joint M13.17-
  hand joint M13.14-
  hip M13.15-
  knee M13.16-
  shoulder M13.11-
  wrist M13.13-
Monoblastic —*see* condition
Monochromat (ism), **monochromatopsia**
  (acquired) (congenital) H53.51
Monocytic —*see* condition
Monocytopenia D72.818
Monocytosis (symptomatic) D72.821
Monomania —*see* Psychosis
Mononeuritis G58.9
  cranial nerve —*see* Disorder, nerve,
    cranial
  femoral nerve G57.2-
  lateral
    cutaneous nerve of thigh G57.1-
    popliteal nerve G57.3-
  lower limb G57.9-
    specified nerve NEC G57.8-
  medial popliteal nerve G57.4-
  median nerve G56.1-
  multiplex G58.7
  plantar nerve G57.6-
  posterior tibial nerve G57.5-
  radial nerve G56.3-
  sciatic nerve G57.0-
  specified NEC G58.8
  tibial nerve G57.4-
  ulnar nerve G56.2-
  upper limb G56.9-
    specified nerve NEC G56.8-
  vestibular —*see* subcategory H93.3
Mononeuropathy G58.9
  carpal tunnel syndrome —*see* Syndrome,
    carpal tunnel
  diabetic NEC —*see* E08-E13 with .41
  femoral nerve —*see* Lesion, nerve, femoral
  ilioinguinal nerve G57.8-
  in diseases classified elsewhere —*see* category
    G59
  intercostal G58.0
  lower limb G57.9-
    causalgia —*see* Causalgia, lower limb
    femoral nerve —*see* Lesion, nerve, femoral
    meralgia paresthetica G57.1-
    plantar nerve —*see* Lesion, nerve, plantar
    popliteal nerve —*see* Lesion, nerve,
      popliteal

Mononeuropathy *(Continued)*
  lower limb *(Continued)*
    sciatic nerve —*see* Lesion, nerve, sciatic
    specified NEC G57.8-
    tarsal tunnel syndrome —*see* Syndrome,
      tarsal tunnel
  median nerve —*see* Lesion, nerve, median
  multiplex G58.7
  obturator nerve G57.8-
  popliteal nerve —*see* Lesion, nerve, popliteal
  radial nerve —*see* Lesion, nerve, radial
  saphenous nerve G57.8-
  specified NEC G58.8
  tarsal tunnel syndrome —*see* Syndrome,
    tarsal tunnel
  tuberculous A17.83
  ulnar nerve —*see* Lesion, nerve, ulnar
  upper limb G56.9-
    carpal tunnel syndrome —*see* Syndrome,
      carpal tunnel
    causalgia —*see* Causalgia
    median nerve —*see* Lesion, nerve, median
    radial nerve —*see* Lesion, nerve, radial
    specified site NEC G56.8-
    ulnar nerve —*see* Lesion, nerve, ulnar
Mononucleosis, infectious B27.90
  with
    complication NEC B27.99
    meningitis B27.92
    polyneuropathy B27.91
  cytomegaloviral B27.10
    with
      complication NEC B27.19
      meningitis B27.12
      polyneuropathy B27.11
  Epstein-Barr (virus) B27.00
    with
      complication NEC B27.09
      meningitis B27.02
      polyneuropathy B27.01
  gammaherpesviral B27.00
    with
      complication NEC B27.09
      meningitis B27.02
      polyneuropathy B27.01
  specified NEC B27.80
    with
      complication NEC B27.89
      meningitis B27.82
      polyneuropathy B27.81
Monoplegia G83.3-
  congenital (cerebral) G80.8
    spastic G80.1
  embolic (current episode) I63.4
  following
    cerebrovascular disease
      cerebral infarction
        lower limb I69.34-
        upper limb I69.33-
      intracerebral hemorrhage
        lower limb I69.14-
        upper limb I69.13-
      lower limb I69.94-
      nontraumatic intracranial hemorrhage
        NEC
        lower limb I69.24-
        upper limb I69.23-
      specified disease NEC
        lower limb I69.84-
        upper limb I69.83-
      stroke NOS
        lower limb I69.34-
        upper limb I69.33-
      subarachnoid hemorrhage
        lower limb I69.04-
        upper limb I69.03-
      upper limb I69.93-
  hysterical (transient) F44.4
  lower limb G83.1-
  psychogenic (conversion reaction) F44.4
  thrombotic (current episode) I63.3

Monoplegia *(Continued)*
  transient R29.818
  upper limb G83.2-
Monorchism, monorchidism Q55.0
Monosomy (*see also* Deletion, chromosome)
  Q93.9
  specified NEC Q93.89
  whole chromosome
    meiotic nondisjunction Q93.0
    mitotic nondisjunction Q93.1
    mosaicism Q93.1
  X Q96.9
Monster, monstrosity (single) Q89.7
  acephalic Q00.0
  twin Q89.4
Monteggia's fracture (-dislocation) S52.27-
Mooren's ulcer (cornea) —*see* Ulcer, cornea,
  Mooren's
Moore's syndrome —*see* Epilepsy, specified
  NEC
Mooser-Neill reaction A75.2
Mooser's bodies A75.2
Morbidity not stated or unknown R69
Morbilli —*see* Measles
Morbus —*see also* Disease
  angelicus, anglorum E55.0
  Beigel B36.2
  caducus —*see* Epilepsy
  celiacus K90.0
  comitialis —*see* Epilepsy
  cordis (*see also* Disease, heart) I51.9
    valvulorum —*see* Endocarditis
  coxae senilis M16.9
    tuberculous A18.02
  hemorrhagicus neonatorum P53
  maculosus neonatorum P54.5
Morel (-Stewart)(-Morgagni) **syndrome** M85.2
Morel-Kraepelin disease —*see* Schizophrenia
Morel-Moore syndrome M85.2
Morgagni's
  cyst, organ, hydatid, or appendage
    female Q50.5
    male (epididymal) Q55.4
      testicular Q55.29
  syndrome M85.2
Morgagni-Stewart-Morel syndrome M85.2
Morgagni-Stokes-Adams syndrome I45.9
Morgagni-Turner (-Albright) **syndrome** Q96.9
Moria F07.0
Moron (I.Q. 50-69) F70
Morphea L94.0
Morphinism (without remission) F11.20
  with remission F11.21
Morphinomania (without remission) F11.20
  with remission F11.21
Morquio (-Ullrich)(-Brailsford) **disease or**
  syndrome —*see* Mucopolysaccharidosis
Mortification (dry) (moist) —*see* Gangrene
Morton's metatarsalgia (neuralgia)(neuroma)
  (syndrome) G57.6
Morvan's disease or syndrome G60.8
Mosaicism, mosaic (autosomal) (chromosomal)
  45,X/46,XX Q96.3
  45,X/other cell lines NEC with abnormal sex
    chromosome Q96.4
  sex chromosome
    female Q97.8
    lines with various numbers of X
      chromosomes Q97.2
    male Q98.7
  XY Q96.3
Moschowitz' disease M31.1
Mother yaw A66.0
Motion sickness (from travel, any vehicle)
  (from roundabouts or swings) T75.3
Mottled, mottling, teeth (enamel) (endemic)
  (nonendemic) K00.3
Mounier-Kuhn syndrome Q32.4
  with bronchiectasis J47.9
    exacerbation (acute) J47.1
    lower respiratory infection J47.0

◀ New   ◀▥ Revised   ~~deleted~~ Deleted

Mounier-Kuhn syndrome (Continued)
acquired J98.09
with bronchiectasis J47.9
with
exacerbation (acute) J47.1
lower respiratory infection J47.0
Mountain
sickness T70.29
with polycythemia , acquired (acute) D75.1
tick fever A93.2
Mouse, joint —see Loose, body, joint
knee M23.4-
Mouth —see condition
Movable
coccyx —see subcategory M53.2
kidney N28.89
congenital Q63.8
spleen D73.89
Movements, dystonic R25.8
Moyamoya disease I67.5
MRSA (Methicillin resistant Staphylococcus
aureus)
infection A49.02
as the cause of diseases classified
elsewhere B95.62
sepsis A41.02
MSSA (Methicillin susceptible Staphylococcus
aureus)
infection A49.01
as the cause of diseases classified
elsewhere B95.61
sepsis A41.01
Mucha-Habermann disease L41.0
Mucinosis (cutaneous) (focal) (papular)
(reticular erythematous) (skin) L98.5
oral K13.79
Mucocele
appendix K38.8
buccal cavity K13.79
gallbladder K82.1
lacrimal sac, chronic H04.43-
nasal sinus J34.1
nose J34.1
salivary gland (any) K11.6
sinus (accessory) (nasal) J34.1
turbinate (bone) (middle) (nasal) J34.1
uterus N85.8
Mucolipidosis
I E77.1
II, III E77.0
IV E75.11
Mucopolysaccharidosis E76.3
beta-gluduronidase deficiency E76.29
cardiopathy E76.3 [I52]
Hunter's syndrome E76.1
Hurler's syndrome E76.01
Hurler-Scheie syndrome E76.02
Maroteaux-Lamy syndrome E76.29
Morquio syndrome E76.219
A E76.210
B E76.211
classic E76.210
Sanfilippo syndrome E76.22
Scheie's syndrome E76.03
specified NEC E76.29
type
I
Hurler's syndrome E76.01
Hurler-Scheie syndrome E76.02
Scheie's syndrome E76.03
II E76.1
III E76.22
IV E76.219
IVA E76.210
IVB E76.211
VI E76.29
VII E76.29
Mucormycosis B46.5
cutaneous B46.3
disseminated B46.4
gastrointestinal B46.2

Mucormycosis (Continued)
generalized B46.4
pulmonary B46.0
rhinocerebral B46.1
skin B46.3
subcutaneous B46.3
Mucositis (ulcerative) K12.30
due to drugs NEC K12.32
gastrointestinal K92.81
mouth (oral) (oropharyngeal) K12.30
due to antineoplastic therapy K12.31
due to drugs NEC K12.32
due to radiation K12.33
specified NEC K12.39
viral K12.39
nasal J34.81
oral cavity —see Mucositis, mouth
oral soft tissues —see Mucositis, mouth
vagina and vulva N76.81
Mucositis necroticans agranulocytica —see
Agranulocytosis
Mucous —see also condition
patches (syphilitic) A51.39
congenital A50.07
Mucoviscidosis E84.9
with meconium obstruction E84.11
Mucus
asphyxia or suffocation —see Asphyxia,
mucus
in stool R19.5
plug —see Asphyxia, mucus
Muguet B37.0
Mulberry molars (congenital syphilis) A50.52
Müllerian mixed tumor
specified site —see Neoplasm, malignant, by
site
unspecified site C54.9
Multicystic kidney (development) Q61.4
Multiparity (grand) Z64.1
affecting management of pregnancy, labor
and delivery (supervision only)
O09.4-
requiring contraceptive management —see
Contraception
Multipartita placenta O43.19-
Multiple, multiplex —see also condition
digits (congenital) Q69.9
endocrine neoplasia —see Neoplasia,
endocrine, multiple [MEN]
personality F44.81
Mumps B26.9
arthritis B26.85
complication NEC B26.89
encephalitis B26.2
hepatitis B26.81
meningitis (aseptic) B26.1
meningoencephalitis B26.2
myocarditis B26.82
oophoritis B26.89
orchitis B26.0
pancreatitis B26.3
polyneuropathy B26.84
Mumu (see also Infestation, filarial) B74.9 [N51]
Münchhausen's syndrome —see Disorder,
factitious
Münchmeyer's syndrome —see Myositis,
ossificans, progressiva
Mural —see condition
Murmur (cardiac) (heart) (organic) R01.1
abdominal R19.15
aortic (valve) —see Endocarditis, aortic
benign R01.0
diastolic —see Endocarditis
Flint I35.1
functional R01.0
Graham Steell I37.1
innocent R01.0
mitral (valve) —see Insufficiency, mitral
nonorganic R01.0
presystolic, mitral —see Insufficiency, mitral
pulmonic (valve) I37.8

Murmur (Continued)
systolic (valvular) —see Endocarditis
tricuspid (valve) I07.9
valvular —see Endocarditis
Murri's disease (intermittent hemoglobinuria)
D59.6
Muscle, muscular —see also condition
carnitine (palmityltransferase) deficiency
E71.314
Musculoneuralgia —see Neuralgia
Mushroom-workers' (pickers') **disease or lung**
J67.5
Mushrooming hip —see Derangement, joint,
specified NEC, hip
Mutation (s)
factor V Leiden D68.51
surfactant, of lung J84.83
prothrombin gene D68.52
Mutism —see also Aphasia
deaf (acquired) (congenital) NEC H91.3
elective (adjustment reaction) (childhood)
F94.0
hysterical F44.4
selective (childhood) F94.0
MVD (microvillus inclusion disease) Q43.8
MVID (microvillus inclusion disease) Q43.8
Myalgia M79.1
epidemic (cervical) B33.0
traumatic NEC T14.8
Myasthenia G70.9
congenital G70.2
cordis —see Failure, heart
developmental G70.2
gravis G70.00
with exacerbation (acute) G70.01
in crisis G70.01
neonatal, transient P94.0
pseudoparalytica G70.00
with exacerbation (acute) G70.01
in crisis G70.01
stomach, psychogenic F45.8
syndrome
in
diabetes mellitus —see E08-E13 with .44
neoplastic disease (see also Neoplasm)
D49.9 [G73.3]
pernicious anemia D51.0 [G73.3]
thyrotoxicosis E05.90 [G73.3]
with thyroid storm E05.91 [G73.3]
Myasthenic M62.81
Mycelium infection B49
Mycetismus —see Poisoning, food, noxious,
mushroom
Mycetoma B47.9
actinomycotic B47.1
bone (mycotic) B47.9 [M90.80]
eumycotic B47.0
foot B47.9
actinomycotic B47.1
mycotic B47.0
madurae NEC B47.9
mycotic B47.0
maduromycotic B47.0
mycotic B47.0
nocardial B47.1
Mycobacteriosis —see Mycobacterium
Mycobacterium, mycobacterial (infection)
A31.9
anonymous A31.9
atypical A31.9
cutaneous A31.1
pulmonary A31.0
tuberculous —see Tuberculosis,
pulmonary
specified site NEC A31.8
avium (intracellulare complex) A31.0
balnei A31.1
Battey A31.0
chelonei A31.8
cutaneous A31.1
extrapulmonary systemic A31.8

Mycobacterium, mycobacterial (*Continued*)
  fortuitum A31.8
  intracellulare (Battey bacillus) A31.0
  kakaferifu A31.8
  kansasii (yellow bacillus) A31.0
  kasongo A31.8
  leprae (*see also* Leprosy) A30.9
  luciflavum A31.1
  marinum (M. balnei) A31.1
  nonspecific —*see* Mycobacterium, atypical
  pulmonary (atypical) A31.0
    tuberculous —*see* Tuberculosis, pulmonary
  scrofulaceum A31.8
  simiae A31.8
  systemic, extrapulmonary A31.8
  szulgai A31.8
  terrae A31.8
  triviale A31.8
  tuberculosis (human, bovine) —*see*
    Tuberculosis
  ulcerans A31.1
  xenopi A31.8
Mycoplasma (M.) pneumoniae, as cause of
  disease classified elsewhere B96.0
Mycosis, mycotic B49
  cutaneous NEC B36.9
  ear B36.8
  fungoides (extranodal) (solid organ)
    C84.0-
  mouth B37.0
  nails B35.1
  opportunistic B48.8
  skin NEC B36.9
  specified NEC B48.8
  stomatitis B37.0
  vagina, vaginitis (candidal) B37.3
Mydriasis (pupil) H57.04
Myelatelia Q06.1
Myelinolysis, pontine, central G37.2
Myelitis (acute) (ascending) (childhood)
  (chronic) (descending) (diffuse)
  (disseminated) (idiopathic) (pressure)
  (progressive) (spinal cord) (subacute) (*see*
  also Encephalitis) G04.91
  herpes simplex B00.82
  herpes zoster B02.24
  in diseases classified elsewhere G05.4
  necrotizing, subacute G37.4
  optic neuritis in G36.0
  postchickenpox B01.12
  postherpetic B02.24
  postimmunization G04.02
  postinfectious NEC G04.89
  postvaccinal G04.02
  specified NEC G04.89
  syphilitic (transverse) A52.14
  toxic G92
  transverse (in demyelinating diseases of
    central nervous system) G37.3
  tuberculous A17.82
  varicella B01.12
Myeloblastic —*see* condition
Myeloblastoma
  granular cell —*see also* Neoplasm, connective
    tissue
    malignant —*see* Neoplasm, connective
      tissue, malignant
    tongue D10.1
Myelocele —*see* Spina bifida
Myelocystocele —*see* Spina bifida
Myelocytic —*see* condition
Myelodysplasia D46.9
  specified NEC D46.Z
  spinal cord (congenital) Q06.1
Myelodysplastic syndrome D46.9
  with
    5q deletion D46.C
    isolated del (5q) chromosomal abnormality
      C46.C
  specified NEC D46.Z
Myeloencephalitis —*see* Encephalitis

Myelofibrosis D75.81
  with myeloid metaplasia D47.4
  acute C94.4-
  idiopathic (chronic) D47.4
  primary D47.1
  secondary D75.81
    in myeloproliferative disease D47.4
Myelogenous —*see* condition
Myeloid —*see* condition
Myelokathexis D70.9
Myeloleukodystrophy E75.29
Myelolipoma —*see* Lipoma
Myeloma (multiple) C90.0-
  monostotic C90.3
    plasma cell C90.0-
  plasma cell C90.0-
  solitary (*see also* Plasmacytoma, solitary)
    C90.3-
Myelomalacia G95.89
Myelomatosis C90.0-
Myelomeningitis —*see* Meningoencephalitis
Myelomeningocele (spinal cord) —*see* Spina
  bifida
Myelo-osteo-musculodysplasia hereditaria
  Q79.8
Myelopathic
  anemia D64.89
  muscle atrophy —*see* Atrophy, muscle, spinal
  pain syndrome G89.0
Myelopathy (spinal cord) G95.9
  drug-induced G95.89
  in (due to)
    degeneration or displacement,
      intervertebral disc NEC —*see*
      Disorder, disc, with, myelopathy
    infection —*see* Encephalitis
    intervertebral disc disorder —*see also*
      Disorder, disc, with, myelopathy
    mercury —*see* subcategory T56.1
    neoplastic disease (*see also* Neoplasm)
      D49.9 [*G99.2*]
    pernicious anemia D51.0 [*G99.2*]
    spondylosis —*see* Spondylosis, with
      myelopathy NEC
  necrotic (subacute) (vascular) G95.19
  radiation-induced G95.89
  spondylogenic NEC —*see* Spondylosis, with
    myelopathy NEC
  toxic G95.89
  transverse, acute G37.3
  vascular G95.19
  vitamin B12 E53.8 [*G32.0*]
Myelophthisis D61.82
Myeloradiculitis G04.91
Myeloradiculodysplasia (spinal) Q06.1
Myelosarcoma C92.3-
Myelosclerosis D75.89
  with myeloid metaplasia D47.4
  disseminated, of nervous system G35
  megakaryocytic D47.4
    with myeloid metaplasia D47.4
Myelosis
  acute C92.0-
  aleukemic C92.9-
  chronic D47.1
  erythremic (acute) C94.0-
  megakaryocytic C94.2-
  nonleukemic D72.828
  subacute C92.9-
Myiasis (cavernous) B87.9
  aural B87.4
  creeping B87.0
  cutaneous B87.0
  dermal B87.0
  ear (external) (middle) B87.4
  eye B87.2
  genitourinary B87.81
  intestinal B87.82
  laryngeal B87.3
  nasopharyngeal B87.3
  ocular B87.2

Myiasis (*Continued*)
  orbit B87.2
  skin B87.0
  specified site NEC B87.89
  traumatic B87.1
  wound B87.1
Myoadenoma, prostate —*see* Hyperplasia,
  prostate
Myoblastoma
  granular cell —*see also* Neoplasm, connective
    tissue, benign
    malignant —*see* Neoplasm, connective
      tissue, malignant
  tongue D10.1
Myocardial —*see* condition
Myocardiopathy (congestive) (constrictive)
  (familial) (hypertrophic nonobstructive)
  (idiopathic) (infiltrative) (obstructive)
  (primary) (restrictive) (sporadic) (*see also*
  Cardiomyopathy) I42.9
  alcoholic I42.6
  cobalt-beer I42.6
  glycogen storage E74.02 [*I43*]
  hypertrophic obstructive I42.1
  in (due to)
    beriberi E51.12
    cardiac glycogenosis E74.02 [*I43*]
    Friedreich's ataxia G11.1 [*I43*]
    myotonia atrophica G71.11 [*I43*]
    progressive muscular dystrophy G71.0
      [*I43*]
  obscure (African) I42.8
  secondary I42.9
  thyrotoxic E05.90 [*I43*]
    with storm E05.91 [*I43*]
  toxic NEC I42.7
Myocarditis (with arteriosclerosis) (chronic)
  (fibroid) (interstitial) (old) (progressive)
  (senile) I51.4
  with
    rheumatic fever (conditions in I00) I09.0
      active —*see* Myocarditis, acute,
        rheumatic
      inactive or quiescent (with chorea) I09.0
  active I40.9
    rheumatic I01.2
      with chorea (acute) (rheumatic)
        (Sydenham's) I02.0
  acute or subacute (interstitial) I40.9
    due to
      streptococcus (beta-hemolytic) I01.2
    idiopathic I40.1
    rheumatic I01.2
      with chorea (acute) (rheumatic)
        (Sydenham's) I02.0
    specified NEC I40.8
  aseptic of newborn B33.22
  bacterial (acute) I40.0
  Coxsackie (virus) B33.22
  diphtheritic A36.81
  eosinophilic I40.1
  epidemic of newborn (Coxsackie) B33.22
  Fiedler's (acute) (isolated) I40.1
  giant cell (acute) (subacute) I40.1
  gonococcal A54.83
  granulomatous (idiopathic) (isolated)
    (nonspecific) I40.1
  hypertensive —*see* Hypertension, heart
  idiopathic (granulomatous) I40.1
  in (due to)
    diphtheria A36.81
    epidemic louse-borne typhus A75.0 [*I41*]
    Lyme disease A69.29
    sarcoidosis D86.85
    scarlet fever A38.1
    toxoplasmosis (acquired) B58.81
    typhoid A01.02
    typhus NEC A75.9 [*I41*]
  infective I40.0
  influenzal —*see* Influenza, with, myocarditis
  isolated (acute) I40.1

◀ New   ◀▥ Revised   ~~deleted~~ Deleted

Myocarditis *(Continued)*
- meningococcal A39.52
- mumps B26.82
- nonrheumatic, active I40.9
- parenchymatous I40.9
- pneumococcal I40.0
- rheumatic (chronic) (inactive) (with chorea)
  - I09.0
  - active or acute I01.2
    - with chorea (acute) (rheumatic)
      - (Sydenham's) I02.0
- rheumatoid —*see* Rheumatoid, carditis
- septic I40.0
- staphylococcal I40.0
- suppurative I40.0
- syphilitic (chronic) A52.06
- toxic I40.8
  - rheumatic —*see* Myocarditis, acute,
    - rheumatic
- tuberculous A18.84
- typhoid A01.02
- valvular —*see* Endocarditis
- virus, viral I40.0
  - of newborn (Coxsackie) B33.22

Myocardium, myocardial —*see* condition
Myocardosis —*see* Cardiomyopathy
Myoclonus, myoclonic, myoclonia (familial)
(essential) (multifocal) (simplex) G25.3
- drug-induced G25.3
- epilepsy (*see also* Epilepsy, generalized,
  - specified NEC) G40.4-
  - familial (progressive) G25.3
- epileptica G40.409
  - with status epilepticus G40.401
- facial G51.3
- familial progressive G25.3
- Friedreich's G25.3
- jerks G25.3
- massive G25.3
- palatal G25.3
- pharyngeal G25.3

Myocytolysis I51.5
Myodiastasis —*see* Diastasis, muscle
Myoendocarditis —*see* Endocarditis
Myoepithelioma —*see* Neoplasm, benign, by
site
Myofasciitis (acute) —*see* Myositis
Myofibroma —*see also* Neoplasm, connective
tissue, benign
- uterus (cervix) (corpus) —*see* Leiomyoma
Myofibromatosis D48.1
- infantile Q89.8
Myofibrosis M62.89
- heart —*see* Myocarditis
- scapulohumeral —*see* Lesion, shoulder,
  - specified NEC
Myofibrositis M79.7
- scapulohumeral —*see* Lesion, shoulder,
  - specified NEC
Myoglobulinuria, myoglobinuria (primary)
R82.1
Myokymia, facial G51.4
Myolipoma —*see* Lipoma
Myoma —*see also* Neoplasm, connective tissue,
benign
- malignant —*see* Neoplasm, connective tissue,
  - malignant
- prostate D29.1
- uterus (cervix) (corpus) —*see* Leiomyoma
Myomalacia M62.89
Myometritis —*see* Endometritis
Myometrium —*see* condition
Myonecrosis, clostridial A48.0
Myopathy G72.9
- acute
  - necrotizing G72.81
  - quadriplegic G72.81
- alcoholic G72.1
- benign congenital G71.2
- central core G71.2
- centronuclear G71.2

Myopathy *(Continued)*
- congenital (benign) G71.2
- critical illness G72.81
- distal G71.0
- drug-induced G72.0
- endocrine NEC E34.9 *[G73.7]*
- extraocular muscles H05.82-
- facioscapulohumeral G71.0
- hereditary G71.9
  - specified NEC G71.8
- immune NEC G72.49
- in (due to)
  - Addison's disease E27.1 *[G73.7]*
  - alcohol G72.1
  - amyloidosis E85.0 *[G73.7]*
  - cretinism E00.9 *[G73.7]*
  - Cushing's syndrome E24.9 *[G73.7]*
  - drugs G72.0
  - endocrine disease NEC E34.9 *[G73.7]*
  - giant cell arteritis M31.6 *[G73.7]*
  - glycogen storage disease E74.00 *[G73.7]*
  - hyperadrenocorticism E24.9 *[G73.7]*
  - hyperparathyroidism NEC E21.3 *[G73.7]*
  - hypoparathyroidism E20.9 *[G73.7]*
  - hypopituitarism E23.0 *[G73.7]*
  - hypothyroidism E03.9 *[G73.7]*
  - infectious disease NEC B99 *[G73.7]*
  - lipid storage disease E75.6 *[G73.7]*
  - metabolic disease NEC E88.9 *[G73.7]*
  - myxedema E03.9 *[G73.7]*
  - parasitic disease NEC B89 *[G73.7]*
  - polyarteritis nodosa M30.0 *[G73.7]*
  - rheumatoid arthritis —*see* Rheumatoid,
    - myopathy
  - sarcoidosis D86.87
  - scleroderma M34.82
  - sicca syndrome M35.03
  - Sjögren's syndrome M35.03
  - systemic lupus erythematosus M32.19
  - thyrotoxicosis (hyperthyroidism) E05.90
    - *[G73.7]*
    - with thyroid storm E05.91 *[G73.7]*
  - toxic agent NEC G72.2
- inflammatory NEC G72.49
- intensive care (ICU) G72.81
- limb-girdle G71.0
- mitochondrial NEC G71.3
- myotubular G71.2
- myotonic, proximal (PROMM) G71.11
- nemaline G71.2
- ocular G71.0
- oculopharyngeal G71.0
- of critical illness G72.81
- primary G71.9
  - specified NEC G71.8
- progressive NEC G72.89
- proximal myotonic (PROMM) G71.11
- rod G71.2
- scapulohumeral G71.0
- specified NEC G72.89
- toxic G72.2
Myopericarditis —*see also* Pericarditis
- chronic rheumatic I09.2
Myopia (axial) (congenital) H52.1-
- degenerative (malignant) H44.2-
- malignant H44.2-
- pernicious H44.2-
- progressive high (degenerative) H44.2-
Myosarcoma —*see* Neoplasm, connective tissue,
malignant
Myosis (pupil) H57.03
- stromal (endolymphatic) D39.0
Myositis M60.9
- clostridial A48.0
- due to posture —*see* Myositis, specified type
  - NEC
- epidemic B33.0
- fibrosa or fibrous (chronic), Volkmann's
  - T79.6
- foreign body granuloma —*see* Granuloma,
  - foreign body

Myositis *(Continued)*
- in (due to)
  - bilharziasis B65.9 *[M63.8-]*
  - cysticercosis B69.81
  - leprosy A30.9 *[M63.8-]*
  - mycosis B49 *[M63.8-]*
  - sarcoidosis D86.87
  - schistosomiasis B65.9 *[M63.8-]*
  - syphilis
    - late A52.78
    - secondary A51.49
  - toxoplasmosis (acquired) B58.82
  - trichinellosis B75 *[M63.8-]*
  - tuberculosis A18.09
- inclusion body [IBM] G72.41
- infective M60.009
  - arm M60.002
    - left M60.001
    - right M60.000
  - leg M60.005
    - left M60.004
    - right M60.003
  - lower limb M60.005
    - ankle M60.07-
    - foot M60.07-
    - lower leg M60.06-
    - thigh M60.05-
    - toe M60.07-
  - multiple sites M60.09
  - specified site NEC M60.08
  - upper limb M60.002
    - finger M60.04-
    - forearm M60.03-
    - hand M60.04-
    - shoulder region M60.01-
    - upper arm M60.02-
- interstitial M60.10
  - ankle M60.17-
  - foot M60.17-
  - forearm M60.13-
  - hand M60.14-
  - lower leg M60.16-
  - multiple sites M60.19
  - shoulder region M60.11-
  - specified site NEC M60.18
  - thigh M60.15-
  - upper arm M60.12-
- mycotic B49 *[M63.8-]*
- ossificans or ossifying (circumscripta) —*see
  - also* Ossification, muscle, specified NEC
  - in (due to)
    - burns M61.30
      - ankle M61.37-
      - foot M61.37-
      - forearm M61.33-
      - hand M61.34-
      - lower leg M61.36-
      - multiple sites M61.39
      - pelvic region M61.35-
      - shoulder region M61.31-
      - specified site NEC M61.38
      - thigh M61.35-
      - upper arm M61.32-
    - quadriplegia or paraplegia M61.20
      - ankle M61.27-
      - foot M61.27-
      - forearm M61.23-
      - hand M61.24-
      - lower leg M61.26-
      - multiple sites M61.29
      - pelvic region M61.25-
      - shoulder region M61.21-
      - specified site NEC M61.28
      - thigh M61.25-
      - upper arm M61.22-
  - progressiva M61.10
    - ankle M61.17-
    - finger M61.14-
    - foot M61.17-
    - forearm M61.13-
    - hand M61.14-

Myositis *(Continued)*
  ossificans or ossifying *(Continued)*
    progressiva *(Continued)*
      lower leg M61.16-
      multiple sites M61.19
      pelvic region M61.15-
      shoulder region M61.11-
      specified site NEC M61.18
      thigh M61.15-
      toe M61.17-
      upper arm M61.12-
    traumatica M61.00
      ankle M61.07-
      foot M61.07-
      forearm M61.03-
      hand M61.04-
      lower leg M61.06-
      multiple sites M61.09
      pelvic region M61.05-
      shoulder region M61.01-
      specified site NEC M61.08
      thigh M61.05-
      upper arm M61.02-
  purulent —*see* Myositis, infective
  specified type NEC M60.80
    ankle M60.87-
    foot M60.87-
    forearm M60.83-
    hand M60.84-
    lower leg M60.86-
    multiple sites M60.89
    pelvic region M60.85-

Myositis *(Continued)*
  specified type NEC *(Continued)*
    shoulder region M60.81-
    specified site NEC M60.88
    thigh M60.85-
    upper arm M60.82-
  suppurative —*see* Myositis, infective
  traumatic (old) —*see* Myositis, specified type NEC
Myospasia impulsiva F95.2
Myotonia (acquisita) (intermittens) M62.89
  atrophica G71.11
  chondrodystrophic G71.13
  congenita (acetazolamide responsive) (dominant) (recessive) G71.12
  drug-induced G71.14
  dystrophica G71.11
  fluctuans G71.19
  levior G71.12
  permanens G71.19
  symptomatic G71.19
Myotonic pupil —*see* Anomaly, pupil, function, tonic pupil
Myriapodiasis B88.2
Myringitis H73.2-
  with otitis media —*see* Otitis, media
  acute H73.00-
    bullous H73.01-
    specified NEC H73.09-
  bullous —*see* Myringitis, acute, bullous
  chronic H73.1-
Mysophobia F40.228

Mytilotoxism —*see* Poisoning, fish
Myxadenitis labialis K13.0
Myxedema (adult) (idiocy) (infantile) (juvenile) (*see also* Hypothyroidism) E03.9
  circumscribed E05.90
    with storm E05.91
  coma E03.5
  congenital E00.1
  cutis L98.5
  localized (pretibial) E05.90
    with storm E05.91
  papular L98.5
Myxochondrosarcoma —*see* Neoplasm, cartilage, malignant
Myxofibroma —*see* Neoplasm, connective tissue, benign
  odontogenic —*see* Cyst, calcifying odontogenic
Myxofibrosarcoma —*see* Neoplasm, connective tissue, malignant
Myxolipoma D17.9
Myxoliposarcoma —*see* Neoplasm, connective tissue, malignant
Myxoma —*see also* Neoplasm, connective tissue, benign
  nerve sheath —*see* Neoplasm, nerve, benign
  odontogenic —*see* Cyst, calcifying odontogenic
Myxosarcoma —*see* Neoplasm, connective tissue, malignant

◄ New   ◄▥ Revised   ~~deleted~~ Deleted

N

Naegeli's
  disease Q82.8
  leukemia, monocytic C93.1-
Naegleriasis (with meningoencephalitis) B60.2
Naffziger's syndrome G54.0
Naga sore —*see* Ulcer, skin
Nägele's pelvis M95.5
  with disproportion (fetopelvic) O33.0
    causing obstructed labor O65.0
Nail —*see also* condition
  biting F98.8
  patella syndrome Q87.2
Nanism, nanosomia —*see* Dwarfism
Nanophyetiasis B66.8
Nanukayami A27.89
Napkin rash L22
Narcolepsy G47.419
  with cataplexy G47.411
  in conditions classified elsewhere G47.429
    with cataplexy G47.421
Narcosis R06.89
Narcotism —*see* Dependence
NARP (Neuropathy, Ataxia and Retinitis
    pigmentosa) syndrome E88.49
Narrow
  anterior chamber angle H40.03-
  pelvis —*see* Contraction, pelvis
Narrowing —*see also* Stenosis
  artery I77.1
    auditory, internal I65.8
    basilar —*see* Occlusion, artery, basilar
    carotid —*see* Occlusion, artery, carotid
    cerebellar —*see* Occlusion, artery, cerebellar
    cerebral —*see* Occlusion artery, cerebral
    choroidal —*see* Occlusion, artery, cerebral,
      specified NEC
    communicating posterior —*see* Occlusion,
      artery, cerebral, specified NEC
    coronary —*see also* Disease, heart, ischemic,
      atherosclerotic
      congenital Q24.5
      syphilitic A50.54 [152]
      due to syphilis NEC A52.06
    hypophyseal —*see* Occlusion, artery,
      cerebral, specified NEC
    pontine —*see* Occlusion, artery, cerebral,
      specified NEC
    precerebral —*see* Occlusion, artery,
      precerebral
    vertebral —*see* Occlusion, artery, vertebral
  auditory canal (external) —*see* Stenosis,
    external ear canal
  eustachian tube —*see* Obstruction, eustachian
    tube
  eyelid —*see* Disorder, eyelid function
  larynx J38.6
  mesenteric artery K55.0
  palate M26.89
  palpebral fissure —*see* Disorder, eyelid
    function
  ureter N13.5
    with infection N13.6
  urethra —*see* Stricture, urethra
Narrowness, abnormal, eyelid Q10.3
Nasal —*see* condition
Nasolachrymal, nasolacrimal —*see* condition
Nasopharyngeal —*see also* condition
  pituitary gland Q89.2
  torticollis M43.6
Nasopharyngitis (acute) (infective)
    (streptococcal) (subacute) J00
  chronic (suppurative) (ulcerative) J31.1
Nasopharynx, nasopharyngeal —*see* condition
Natal tooth, teeth K00.6
Nausea (without vomiting) R11.0
  with vomiting R11.2
  gravidarum —*see* Hyperemesis, gravidarum
  marina T75.3
  navalis T75.3

Navel —*see* condition
Neapolitan fever —*see* Brucellosis
Near drowning T75.1
Nearsightedness —*see* Myopia
Near-syncope R55
Nebula, cornea —*see* Opacity, cornea
Necator americanus infestation B76.1
Necatoriasis B76.1
Neck —*see* condition
Necrobiosis R68.89
  lipoidica NEC L92.1
    with diabetes —*see* E08-E13 with .620
Necrolysis, toxic epidermal L51.2
  due to drug
    correct substance properly administered —
      see Table of Drugs and Chemicals, by
      drug, adverse effect
    overdose or wrong substance given or
      taken —*see* Table of Drugs and
      Chemicals, by drug, poisoning
Necrophilia F65.89
Necrosis, necrotic (ischemic) —*see also*
    Gangrene
  adrenal (capsule) (gland) E27.49
  amputation stump (surgical) (late)
    T87.50
    arm T87.5-
    leg T87.5-
  antrum J32.0
  aorta (hyaline) —*see also* Aneurysm, aorta
    cystic medial —*see* Dissection, aorta
  artery I77.5
  bladder (aseptic) (sphincter) N32.89
  bone (*see also* Osteonecrosis) M87.9
    aseptic or avascular —*see* Osteonecrosis
      idiopathic M87.00
    ethmoid J32.2
    jaw M27.2
    tuberculous —*see* Tuberculosis, bone
  brain I67.89
  breast (aseptic) (fat) (segmental) N64.1
  bronchus J98.09
  central nervous system NEC I67.89
  cerebellar I67.89
  cerebral I67.89
  colon K55.0
  cornea H18.40
  cortical (acute) (renal) N17.1
  cystic medial (aorta) —*see* Dissection, aorta
  dental pulp K04.1
  esophagus K22.8
  ethmoid (bone) J32.2
  eyelid —*see* Disorder, eyelid, degenerative
  fat, fatty (generalized) —*see also* Disorder, soft
    tissue, specified type NEC
    abdominal wall K65.4
    breast (aseptic) (segmental) N64.1
    localized —*see* Degeneration, by site,
      fatty
    mesentery K65.4
    omentum K65.4
    pancreas K86.8
    peritoneum K65.4
    skin (subcutaneous), newborn P83.0
    subcutaneous, due to birth injury P15.6
  gallbladder —*see* Cholecystitis, acute
  heart —*see* Infarct, myocardium
  hip, aseptic or avascular —*see* Osteonecrosis,
    by type, femur
  intestine (acute) (hemorrhagic) (massive)
    K55.0
  jaw M27.2
  kidney (bilateral) N28.0
    acute N17.9
    cortical (acute) (bilateral) N17.1
      with ectopic or molar pregnancy
        O08.4
    medullary (bilateral) (in acute renal
      failure) (papillary) N17.2
    papillary (bilateral) (in acute renal
      failure) N17.2

Necrosis, necrotic (*Continued*)
  kidney (*Continued*)
    tubular N17.0
      with ectopic or molar pregnancy O08.4
      complicating
        abortion —*see* Abortion, by type,
          complicated by, tubular necrosis
        ectopic or molar pregnancy O08.4
        pregnancy —*see* Pregnancy,
          complicated by, diseases of,
          specified type or system NEC
      following ectopic or molar pregnancy
        O08.4
    traumatic T79.5
  larynx J38.7
  liver (with hepatic failure) (cell) —*see* Failure,
    hepatic
    hemorrhagic, central K76.2
  lung J85.0
  lymphatic gland —*see* Lymphadenitis, acute
  mammary gland (fat) (segmental) N64.1
  mastoid (chronic) —*see* Mastoiditis, chronic
  medullary (acute) (renal) N17.2
  mesentery K55.0
    fat K65.4
  mitral valve —*see* Insufficiency, mitral
  myocardium, myocardial —*see* Infarct,
    myocardium
  nose J34.0
  omentum (with mesenteric infarction)
    K55.0
    fat K65.4
  orbit, orbital —*see* Osteomyelitis, orbit
  ossicles, ear —*see* Abnormal, ear ossicles
  ovary N70.92
  pancreas (aseptic) (duct) (fat) K86.8
    acute (infective) —*see* Pancreatitis, acute
    infective —*see* Pancreatitis, acute
  papillary (acute) (renal) N17.2
  perineum N90.89
  peritoneum (with mesenteric infarction)
    K55.0
    fat K65.4
  pharynx J02.9
    in granulocytopenia —*see* Neutropenia
    Vincent's A69.1
  phosphorus —*see* subcategory T54.2
  pituitary (gland) (postpartum) (Sheehan)
    E23.0
  pressure —*see* Ulcer, pressure, by site
  pulmonary J85.0
  pulp (dental) K04.1
  radiation —*see* Necrosis, by site
  radium —*see* Necrosis, by site
  renal —*see* Necrosis, kidney
  sclera H15.89
  scrotum N50.8
  skin or subcutaneous tissue NEC I96
  spine, spinal (column) —*see also*
    Osteonecrosis, by type, vertebra
    cord G95.19
  spleen D73.5
  stomach K31.89
  stomatitis (ulcerative) A69.0
  subcutaneous fat, newborn P83.8
  subendocardial (acute) I21.4
    chronic I25.89
  suprarenal (capsule) (gland) E27.49
  testis N50.8
  thymus (gland) E32.8
  tonsil J35.8
  trachea J39.8
  tuberculous NEC —*see* Tuberculosis
  tubular (acute) (anoxic) (renal) (toxic) N17.0
    postprocedural N99.0
  vagina N89.8
  vertebra —*see also* Osteonecrosis, by type,
    vertebra
    tuberculous A18.01
  vulva N90.89
  X-ray —*see* Necrosis, by site

Necrospermia —see Infertility, male
Need (for)
  care provider because (of)
    assistance with personal care Z74.1
    continuous supervision required Z74.3
    impaired mobility Z74.09
    no other household member able to render
      care Z74.2
    specified reason NEC Z74.8
  immunization —see Vaccination
  vaccination —see Vaccination
Neglect
  adult
    confirmed T74.01
    history of Z91.412
    suspected T76.01
  child (childhood)
    confirmed T74.02
    history of Z62.812
    suspected T76.02
  emotional, in childhood Z62.898
  hemispatial R41.4
  left-sided R41.4
  sensory R41.4
  visuospatial R41.4
Neisserian infection NEC —see Gonococcus
Nelaton's syndrome G60.8
Nelson's syndrome E24.1
Nematodiasis (intestinal) B82.0
  Ancylostoma B76.0
Neonatal —see also Newborn
  acne L70.4
  bradycardia P29.12
  screening, abnormal findings on P09
  tachycardia P29.11
  tooth, teeth K00.6
Neonatorum —see condition
Neoplasia
  endocrine, multiple (MEN) E31.20
    type I E31.21
    type IIA E31.22
    type IIB E31.23
  intraepithelial (histologically confirmed)
    anal (AIN) (histologically confirmed)
      K62.82
      grade I K62.82
      grade II K62.82
      severe D01.3
    cervical glandular (histologically
      confirmed) D06.9
    cervix (uteri) (CIN) (histologically
      confirmed) N87.9
      glandular D06.9
      grade I N87.0
      grade II N87.1
      grade III (severe dysplasia) —see also
        Carcinoma, cervix uteri, in situ
        D06.9
    prostate (histologically confirmed) (PIN I)
      (PIN II) N42.3
      grade I N42.3
      grade II N42.3
      severe D07.5
    vagina (histologically confirmed) (VAIN)
      N89.3
      grade I N89.0
      grade II N89.1
      grade III (severe dysplasia) D07.2
    vulva (histologically confirmed) (VIN)
      N90.3
      grade I N90.0
      grade II N90.1
      grade III (severe dysplasia) D07.1
Neoplasm, neoplastic —see also Table of
  Neoplasms
  lipomatous, benign —see Lipoma
Neovascularization
  ciliary body —see Disorder, iris, vascular
  cornea H16.40-
    deep H16.44-
    ghost vessels —see Ghost, vessels

Neovascularization (Continued)
  cornea (Continued)
    localized H16.43-
    pannus —see Pannus
  iris —see Disorder, iris, vascular
  retina H35.05-
Nephralgia N23
Nephritis, nephritic (albuminuric) (azotemic)
  (congenital) (disseminated) (epithelial)
  (familial) (focal) (granulomatous)
  (hemorrhagic) (infantile) (nonsuppurative,
  excretory) (uremic) N05.9
  with
    dense deposit disease N05.6
    diffuse
      crescentic glomerulonephritis N05.7
      endocapillary proliferative
        glomerulonephritis N05.4
      membranous glomerulonephritis
        N05.2
      mesangial proliferative
        glomerulonephritis N05.3
      mesangiocapillary glomerulonephritis
        N05.5
    edema —see Nephrosis
    focal and segmental glomerular lesions
      N05.1
    foot process disease N04.9
    glomerular lesion
      diffuse sclerosing N05.8
      hypocomplementemic —see Nephritis,
        membranoproliferative
      IgA —see Nephropathy, IgA
      lobular, lobulonodular —see Nephritis,
        membranoproliferative
      nodular —see Nephritis,
        membranoproliferative
    lesion of
      glomerulonephritis, proliferative
        N05.8
      renal necrosis N05.9
    minor glomerular abnormality N05.0
    specified morphological changes NEC
      N05.8
  acute N00.9
    with
      dense deposit disease N00.6
      diffuse
        crescentic glomerulonephritis
          N00.7
        endocapillary proliferative
          glomerulonephritis N00.4
        membranous glomerulonephritis
          N00.2
        mesangial proliferative
          glomerulonephritis N00.3
        mesangiocapillary glomerulonephritis
          N00.5
      focal and segmental glomerular lesions
        N00.1
      minor glomerular abnormality N00.0
      specified morphological changes NEC
        N00.8
  amyloid E85.4 [N08]
  antiglomerular basement membrane (anti-
    GBM) antibody NEC
    in Goodpasture's syndrome M31.0
  antitubular basement membrane
    (tubulo-interstitial) NEC N12
    toxic —see Nephropathy, toxic
  arteriolar —see Hypertension, kidney
  arteriosclerotic —see Hypertension,
    kidney
  ascending —see Nephritis, tubulo-interstitial
  atrophic N03.9
  Balkan (endemic) N15.0
  calculous, calculus —see Calculus,
    kidney
  cardiac —see Hypertension, kidney
  cardiovascular —see Hypertension,
    kidney

Nephritis, nephritic (Continued)
  chronic N03.9
    with
      dense deposit disease N03.6
      diffuse
        crescentic glomerulonephritis
          N03.7
        endocapillary proliferative
          glomerulonephritis N03.4
        membranous glomerulonephritis
          N03.2
        mesangial proliferative
          glomerulonephritis N03.3
        mesangiocapillary glomerulonephritis
          N03.5
      focal and segmental glomerular lesions
        N03.1
      minor glomerular abnormality
        N03.0
      specified morphological changes
        NEC N03.8
  arteriosclerotic —see Hypertension,
    kidney
  cirrhotic N26.9
  complicating pregnancy O26.83-
  croupous N00.9
  degenerative —see Nephrosis
  diffuse sclerosing N05.8
  due to
    diabetes mellitus —see E08-E13 with .21
    subacute bacterial endocarditis I33.0
    systemic lupus erythematosus (chronic)
      M32.14
    typhoid fever A01.09
  gonococcal (acute) (chronic) A54.21
  hypocomplementemic —see Nephritis,
    membranoproliferative
  IgA —see Nephropathy, IgA
  immune complex (circulating) NEC N05.8
  infective —see Nephritis, tubulo-interstitial
  interstitial —see Nephritis, tubulo-interstitial
  lead N14.3
  membranoproliferative (diffuse) (type 1 or 3)
    (see also N00-N07 with fourth character
    .5) N05.5
    type 2 (see also N00-N07 with fourth
      character .6) N05.6
  minimal change N05.0
  necrotic, necrotizing NEC (see also
    N00-N07 with fourth character .8)
    N05.8
  nephrotic —see Nephrosis
  nodular —see Nephritis,
    membranoproliferative
  polycystic Q61.3
    adult type Q61.2
    autosomal
      dominant Q61.2
      recessive NEC Q61.19
    childhood type NEC Q61.19
    infantile type NEC Q61.19
  poststreptococcal N05.9
    acute N00.9
    chronic N03.9
    rapidly progressive N01.9
  proliferative NEC (see also N00-N07 with
    fourth character .8) N05.8
  purulent —see Nephritis, tubulo-interstitial
  rapidly progressive N01.9
    with
      dense deposit disease N01.6
      diffuse
        crescentic glomerulonephritis N01.7
        endocapillary proliferative
          glomerulonephritis N01.4
        membranous glomerulonephritis
          N01.2
        mesangial proliferative
          glomerulonephritis N01.3
        mesangiocapillary glomerulonephritis
          N01.5

◀ New   ◀▦ Revised   ~~deleted~~ Deleted

Nephritis, nephritic *(Continued)*
  rapidly progressive *(Continued)*
    with *(Continued)*
      focal and segmental glomerular lesions N01.1
      minor glomerular abnormality N01.0
      specified morphological changes NEC N01.8
  salt losing or wasting NEC N28.89
  saturnine N14.3
  sclerosing, diffuse N05.8
  septic —*see* Nephritis, tubulo-interstitial
  specified pathology NEC *(see also* N00-N07 with fourth character .8) N05.8
  subacute N01.9
  suppurative —*see* Nephritis, tubulo-interstitial
  syphilitic (late) A52.75
    congenital A50.59 *[N08]*
    early (secondary) A51.44
  toxic —*see* Nephropathy, toxic
  tubal, tubular —*see* Nephritis, tubulo-interstitial
  tuberculous A18.11
  tubulo-interstitial (in) N12
    acute (infectious) N10
    chronic (infectious) N11.9
      nonobstructive N11.8
        reflux-associated N11.0
      obstructive N11.1
      specified NEC N11.8
    due to
      brucellosis A23.9 *[N16]*
      cryoglobulinemia D89.1 *[N16]*
      glycogen storage disease E74.00 *[N16]*
      Sjögren's syndrome M35.04
  vascular —*see* Hypertension, kidney
  war N00.9
Nephroblastoma (epithelial) (mesenchymal) C64-
Nephrocalcinosis E83.59 *[N29]*
Nephrocystitis, pustular —*see* Nephritis, tubulo-interstitial
Nephrolithiasis (congenital) (pelvis) (recurrent) —*see also* Calculus, kidney
Nephroma C64-
  mesoblastic D41.0-
Nephronephritis —*see* Nephrosis
Nephronophthisis Q61.5
Nephropathia epidemica A98.5
Nephropathy *(see also* Nephritis) N28.9
  with
    edema —*see* Nephrosis
    glomerular lesion —*see* Glomerulonephritis
  amyloid, hereditary E85.0
  analgesic N14.0
    with medullary necrosis, acute N17.2
  Balkan (endemic) N15.0
  chemical —*see* Nephropathy, toxic
  diabetic —*see* E08-E13 with .21
  drug-induced N14.2
    specified NEC N14.1
  focal and segmental hyalinosis or sclerosis N02.1
  heavy metal-induced N14.3
  hereditary NEC N07.9
    with
      dense deposit disease N07.6
      diffuse
        crescentic glomerulonephritis N07.7
        endocapillary proliferative glomerulonephritis N07.4
        membranous glomerulonephritis N07.2
        mesangial proliferative glomerulonephritis N07.3
        mesangiocapillary glomerulonephritis N07.5

Nephropathy *(Continued)*
  hereditary NEC *(Continued)*
    with *(Continued)*
      focal and segmental glomerular lesions N07.1
      minor glomerular abnormality N07.0
      specified morphological changes NEC N07.8
  hypercalcemic N25.89
  hypertensive —*see* Hypertension, kidney
  hypokalemic (vacuolar) N25.89
  IgA N02.8
    with glomerular lesion N02.9
      focal and segmental hyalinosis or sclerosis N02.1
      membranoproliferative (diffuse) N02.5
      membranous (diffuse) N02.2
      mesangial proliferative (diffuse) N02.3
      mesangiocapillary (diffuse) N02.5
      proliferative NEC N02.8
      specified pathology NEC N02.8
  lead N14.3
  membranoproliferative (diffuse) N02.5
  membranous (diffuse) N02.2
  mesangial (IgA/IgG) —*see* Nephropathy, IgA
    proliferative (diffuse) N02.3
  mesangiocapillary (diffuse) N02.5
  obstructive N13.8
  phenacetin N17.2
  phosphate-losing N25.0
  potassium depletion N25.89
  pregnancy-related O26.83-
  proliferative NEC *(see also* N00-N07 with fourth character .8) N05.8
  protein-losing N25.89
  saturnine N14.3
  sickle-cell D57.- *[N08]*
  toxic NEC N14.4
    due to
      drugs N14.2
        analgesic N14.0
        specified NEC N14.1
      heavy metals N14.3
  vasomotor N17.0
  water-losing N25.89
Nephroptosis N28.83
Nephropyosis —*see* Abscess, kidney
Nephrorrhagia N28.89
Nephrosclerosis (arteriolar) (arteriosclerotic) (chronic) (hyaline) —*see also* Hypertension, kidney
  hyperplastic —*see* Hypertension, kidney
  senile N26.9
Nephrosis, nephrotic (Epstein's) (syndrome) (congenital) N04.9
  with
    foot process disease N04.9
    glomerular lesion N04.1
    hypocomplementemic N04.5
  acute N04.9
  anoxic —*see* Nephrosis, tubular
  chemical —*see* Nephrosis, tubular
  cholemic K76.7
  diabetic —*see* E08-E13 with .21
  Finnish type (congenital) Q89.8
  hemoglobin N10
  hemoglobinuric —*see* Nephrosis, tubular
  in
    amyloidosis E85.4 *[N08]*
    diabetes mellitus —*see* E08-E13 with .21
    epidemic hemorrhagic fever A98.5
    malaria (malariae) B52.0
  ischemic —*see* Nephrosis, tubular
  lipoid N04.9
  lower nephron —*see* Nephrosis, tubular
  malarial (malariae) B52.0
  minimal change N04.0
  myoglobin N10
  necrotizing —*see* Nephrosis, tubular
  osmotic (sucrose) N25.89
  radiation N04.9

Nephrosis, nephrotic *(Continued)*
  syphilitic (late) A52.75
  toxic —*see* Nephrosis, tubular
  tubular (acute) N17.0
    postprocedural N99.0
    radiation N04.9
Nephrosonephritis, hemorrhagic (endemic) A98.5
Nephrostomy
  attention to Z43.6
  status Z93.6
Nerve —*see also* condition
  injury —*see* Injury, nerve, by body site
Nerves R45.0
Nervous *(see also* condition) R45.0
  heart F45.8
  stomach F45.8
  tension R45.0
Nervousness R45.0
Nesidioblastoma
  pancreas D13.7
  specified site NEC —*see* Neoplasm, benign, by site
  unspecified site D13.7
Nettleship's syndrome Q82.2
Neumann's disease or syndrome L10.1
Neuralgia, neuralgic (acute) M79.2
  accessory (nerve) G52.8
  acoustic (nerve) —*see* subcategory H93.3
  auditory (nerve) —*see* subcategory H93.3
  ciliary G44.009
    intractable G44.001
    not intractable G44.009
  cranial
    nerve —*see also* Disorder, nerve, cranial
      fifth or trigeminal —*see* Neuralgia, trigeminal
    postherpetic, postzoster B02.29
  ear —*see* subcategory H92.0
  facialis vera G51.1
  Fothergill's —*see* Neuralgia, trigeminal
  glossopharyngeal (nerve) G52.1
  Horton's G44.099
    intractable G44.091
    not intractable G44.099
  Hunt's B02.21
  hypoglossal (nerve) G52.3
  infraorbital —*see* Neuralgia, trigeminal
  malarial —*see* Malaria
  migrainous G44.009
    intractable G44.001
    not intractable G44.009
  Morton's G57.6-
  nerve, cranial —*see* Disorder, nerve, cranial
  nose G52.0
  occipital M54.81
  olfactory G52.0
  penis N48.9
  perineum R10.2
  postherpetic NEC B02.29
    trigeminal B02.22
  pubic region R10.2
  scrotum R10.2
  Sluder's G44.89
  specified nerve NEC G58.8
  spermatic cord R10.2
  sphenopalatine (ganglion) G90.09
  trifacial —*see* Neuralgia, trigeminal
  trigeminal G50.0
    postherpetic, postzoster B02.22
  vagus (nerve) G52.2
  writer's F48.8
    organic G25.89
Neurapraxia —*see* Injury, nerve
Neurasthenia F48.8
  cardiac F45.8
  gastric F45.8
  heart F45.8

Neurilemmoma —see also Neoplasm, nerve, benign
  acoustic (nerve) D33.3
  malignant —see also Neoplasm, nerve, malignant
    acoustic (nerve) C72.4
Neurilemmosarcoma —see Neoplasm, nerve, malignant
Neurinoma —see Neoplasm, nerve, benign
Neurinomatosis —see Neoplasm, nerve, uncertain behavior
Neuritis (rheumatoid) M79.2
  abducens (nerve) —see Strabismus, paralytic, sixth nerve
  accessory (nerve) G52.8
  acoustic (nerve) (see also subcategory) H93.3
    in (due to)
      infectious disease NEC B99 [H94.0-]
      parasitic disease NEC B89 [H94.0-]
    syphilitic A52.15
  alcoholic G62.1
    with psychosis —see Psychosis, alcoholic
  amyloid, any site E85.4 [G63]
  auditory (nerve) —see subcategory H93.3
  brachial —see Radiculopathy
    due to displacement, intervertebral disc — see Disorder, disc, cervical, with neuritis
  cranial nerve
    due to Lyme disease A69.22
    eighth or acoustic or auditory —see subcategory H93.3
    eleventh or accessory G52.8
    fifth or trigeminal G51.0
    first or olfactory G52.0
    fourth or trochlear —see Strabismus, paralytic, fourth nerve
    second or optic —see Neuritis, optic
    seventh or facial G51.8
      newborn (birth injury) P11.3
    sixth or abducent —see Strabismus, paralytic, sixth nerve
    tenth or vagus G52.2
    third or oculomotor —see Strabismus, paralytic, third nerve
    twelfth or hypoglossal G52.3
  Déjérine-Sottas G60.0
  diabetic (mononeuropathy) —see E08-E13 with .41
    polyneuropathy —see E08-E13 with .42
  due to
    beriberi E51.11
    displacement, prolapse or rupture, intervertebral disc —see Disorder, disc, with, radiculopathy
    herniation, nucleus pulposus M51.9 [G55]
  endemic E51.11
  facial G51.8
    newborn (birth injury) P11.3
  general —see Polyneuropathy
  geniculate ganglion G51.1
    due to herpes (zoster) B02.21
  gouty M10.00 [G63]
  hypoglossal (nerve) G52.3
  ilioinguinal (nerve) G57.9-
  infectious (multiple) NEC G61.0
  interstitial hypertrophic progressive G60.0
  lumbar M54.16
  lumbosacral M54.17
  multiple —see also Polyneuropathy
    endemic E51.11
    infective, acute G61.0
  multiplex endemica E51.11
  nerve root —see Radiculopathy
  oculomotor (nerve) —see Strabismus, paralytic, third nerve
  olfactory nerve G52.0
  optic (nerve) (hereditary) (sympathetic) H46.9
    with demyelination G36.0
      in myelitis G36.0
    nutritional H46.2

Neuritis (Continued)
  optic (Continued)
    papillitis —see Papillitis, optic
    retrobulbar H46.1-
      specified type NEC H46.8
    toxic H46.3
  peripheral (nerve) G62.9
    multiple —see Polyneuropathy
    single —see Mononeuritis
  pneumogastric (nerve) G52.2
  postherpetic, postzoster B02.29
  progressive hypertrophic interstitial G60.0
  retrobulbar —see also Neuritis, optic, retrobulbar
    in (due to)
      late syphilis A52.15
      meningococcal infection A39.82
    meningococcal A39.82
    syphilitic A52.15
  sciatic (nerve) —see also Sciatica
    due to displacement of intervertebral disc —see Disorder, disc, with, radiculopathy
  serum (see also Reaction, serum) T80.69
  shoulder-girdle G54.5
  specified nerve NEC G58.8
  spinal (nerve) root —see Radiculopathy
  syphilitic A52.15
  thenar (median) G56.1-
  thoracic M54.14
  toxic NEC G62.2
  trochlear (nerve) —see Strabismus, paralytic, fourth nerve
  vagus (nerve) G52.2
Neuroastrocytoma —see Neoplasm, uncertain behavior, by site
Neuroavitaminosis E56.9 [G99.8]
Neuroblastoma
  olfactory C30.0
  specified site —see Neoplasm, malignant, by site
  unspecified site C74.90
Neurochorioretinitis —see Chorioretinitis
Neurocirculatory asthenia F45.8
Neurocysticercosis B69.0
Neurocytoma —see Neoplasm, benign, by site
Neurodermatitis (circumscribed) (circumscripta) (local) L28.0
  atopic L20.81
  diffuse (Brocq) L20.81
  disseminated L20.81
Neuroencephalomyelopathy, optic G36.0
Neuroepithelioma —see also Neoplasm, malignant, by site
  olfactory C30.0
Neurofibroma —see also Neoplasm, nerve, benign
  melanotic —see Neoplasm, nerve, benign
  multiple —see Neurofibromatosis
  plexiform —see Neoplasm, nerve, benign
Neurofibromatosis (multiple) (nonmalignant) Q85.00
  acoustic Q85.02
  malignant —see Neoplasm, nerve, malignant
  specified NEC Q85.09
  type 1 (von Recklinghausen) Q85.01
  type 2 Q85.02
Neurofibrosarcoma —see Neoplasm, nerve, malignant
Neurogenic —see also condition
  bladder (see also Dysfunction, bladder, neuromuscular) N31.9
    cauda equina syndrome G83.4
  bowel NEC K59.2
  heart F45.8
Neuroglioma —see Neoplasm, uncertain behavior, by site
Neurolabyrinthitis (of Dix and Hallpike) —see Neuronitis, vestibular
Neurolathyrism —see Poisoning, food, noxious, plant

Neuroleprosy A30.9
Neuroma —see also Neoplasm, nerve, benign
  acoustic (nerve) D33.3
  amputation (stump) (traumatic) (surgical complication) (late) T87.3-
    arm T87.3-
    leg T87.3-
  digital (toe) G57.6-
  interdigital (toe) G58.8
    lower limb G57.8-
    upper limb G56.8-
  intermetatarsal G57.8-
  Morton's G57.6-
  nonneoplastic
    arm G56.9-
    leg G57.9-
    lower extremity G57.9-
    upper extremity G56.9-
  optic (nerve) D33.3
  plantar G57.6-
  plexiform —see Neoplasm, nerve, benign
  surgical (nonneoplastic)
    arm G56.9-
    leg G57.9-
    lower extremity G57.9-
    upper extremity G56.9-
Neuromyalgia —see Neuralgia
Neuromyasthenia (epidemic) (postinfectious) G93.3
Neuromyelitis G36.9
  ascending G61.0
  optica G36.0
Neuromyopathy G70.9
  paraneoplastic D49.9 [G13.0]
Neuromyotonia (Isaacs) G71.19
Neuronevus —see Nevus
Neuronitis G58.9
  ascending (acute) G57.2-
  vestibular H81.2-
Neuroparalytic —see condition
Neuropathy, neuropathic G62.9
  acute motor G62.81
  alcoholic G62.1
    with psychosis —see Psychosis, alcoholic
  arm G56.9-
  autonomic, peripheral —see Neuropathy, peripheral, autonomic
  axillary G56.9-
  bladder N31.9
    atonic (motor) (sensory) N31.2
    autonomous N31.2
    flaccid N31.2
    nonreflex N31.2
    reflex N31.1
    uninhibited N31.0
  brachial plexus G54.0
  cervical plexus G54.2
  chronic
    progressive segmentally demyelinating G62.89
    relapsing demyelinating G62.89
  Déjérine-Sottas G60.0
  diabetic —see E08-E13 with .40
    mononeuropathy —see E08-E13 with .41
    polyneuropathy —see E08-E13 with .42
  entrapment G58.9
    iliohypogastric nerve G57.8-
    ilioinguinal nerve G57.8-
    lateral cutaneous nerve of thigh G57.1-
    median nerve G56.0-
    obturator nerve G57.8-
    peroneal nerve G57.3-
    posterior tibial nerve G57.5-
    saphenous nerve G57.8-
    ulnar nerve G56.2-
  facial nerve G51.9
  hereditary G60.9
    motor and sensory (types I-IV) G60.0
    sensory G60.8
    specified NEC G60.8

◀ New   ⬅ Revised   ~~deleted~~ Deleted

Neuropathy, neuropathic (*Continued*)
  hypertrophic G60.0
    Charcot-Marie-Tooth G60.0
    Déjérine-Sottas G60.0
    interstitial progressive G60.0
    of infancy G60.0
    Refsum G60.1
  idiopathic G60.9
    progressive G60.3
    specified NEC G60.8
  in association with hereditary ataxia G60.2
  intercostal G58.0
  ischemic —*see* Disorder, nerve
  Jamaica (ginger) G62.2
  leg NEC G57.9-
  lower extremity G57.9-
  lumbar plexus G54.1
  median nerve G56.1-
  motor and sensory —*see also* Polyneuropathy
    hereditary (types I-IV) G60.0
  multiple (acute) (chronic) —*see*
    Polyneuropathy
  optic (nerve) —*see also* Neuritis, optic
    ischemic H47.01-
  paraneoplastic (sensorial) (Denny Brown)
    D49.9 [*G13.0*]
  peripheral (nerve) (*see also* Polyneuropathy)
    G62.9
    autonomic G90.9
      idiopathic G90.09
      in (due to)
        amyloidosis E85.4 [*G99.0*]
        diabetes mellitus —*see* E08-E13 with
          .43
        endocrine disease NEC E34.9 [*G99.0*]
        gout M10.00 [*G99.0*]
        hyperthyroidism E05.90 [*G99.0*]
          with thyroid storm E05.91 [*G99.0*]
        metabolic disease NEC E88.9 [*G99.0*]
      idiopathic G60.9
        progressive G60.3
      in (due to)
        antitetanus serum G62.0
        arsenic G62.2
        drugs NEC G62.0
        lead G62.2
        organophosphate compounds G62.2
        toxic agent NEC G62.2
    plantar nerves G57.6-
  progressive
    hypertrophic interstitial G60.0
    inflammatory G62.81
  radicular NEC —*see* Radiculopathy
  sacral plexus G54.1
  sciatic G57.0-
  serum G61.1
  toxic NEC G62.2
  trigeminal sensory G50.8
  ulnar nerve G56.2-
  uremic N18.9 [*G63*]
  vitamin B12 E53.8 [*G63*]
    with anemia (pernicious) D51.0 [*G63*]
      due to dietary deficiency D51.3 [*G63*]
Neurophthisis —*see also* Disorder, nerve
  peripheral, diabetic —*see* E08-E13 with .42
Neuroretinitis —*see* Chorioretinitis
Neuroretinopathy, hereditary optic H47.22
Neurosarcoma —*see* Neoplasm, nerve,
  malignant
Neurosclerosis —*see* Disorder, nerve
Neurosis, neurotic F48.9
  anankastic F42
  anxiety (state) F41.1
    panic type F41.0
  asthenic F48.8
  bladder F45.8
  cardiac (reflex) F45.8
  cardiovascular F45.8
  character F60.9
  colon F45.8
  compensation F68.1

Neurosis, neurotic (*Continued*)
  compulsive, compulsion F42
  conversion F44.9
  craft F48.8
  cutaneous F45.8
  depersonalization F48.1
  depressive (reaction) (type) F34.1
  environmental F48.8
  excoriation L98.1
  fatigue F48.8
  functional —*see* Disorder, somatoform
  gastric F45.8
  gastrointestinal F45.8
  heart F45.8
  hypochondriacal F45.21
  hysterical F44.9
  incoordination F45.8
    larynx F45.8
    vocal cord F45.8
  intestine F45.8
  larynx (sensory) F45.8
    hysterical F44.4
  mixed NEC F48.8
  musculoskeletal F45.8
  obsessional F42
  obsessive-compulsive F42
  occupational F48.8
  ocular NEC F45.8
  organ —*see* Disorder, somatoform
  pharynx F45.8
  phobic F40.9
  posttraumatic (situational) F43.10
    acute F43.11
    chronic F43.12
  psychasthenic (type) F48.8
  railroad F48.8
  rectum F45.8
  respiratory F45.8
  rumination F45.8
  sexual F65.9
  situational F48.8
  social F40.10
    generalized F40.11
    specified type NEC F48.8
  state F48.9
    with depersonalization episode F48.1
  stomach F45.8
  traumatic F43.10
    acute F43.11
    chronic F43.12
  vasomotor F45.8
  visceral F45.8
  war F48.8
Neurospongioblastosis diffusa Q85.1
Neurosyphilis (arrested) (early) (gumma) (late)
  (latent) (recurrent) (relapse) A52.3
  with ataxia (cerebellar) (locomotor) (spastic)
    (spinal) A52.19
  aneurysm (cerebral) A52.05
  arachnoid (adhesive) A52.13
  arteritis (any artery) (cerebral) A52.04
  asymptomatic A52.2
  congenital A50.40
  dura (mater) A52.13
  general paresis A52.17
  hemorrhagic A52.05
  juvenile (asymptomatic) (meningeal)
    A50.40
  leptomeninges (aseptic) A52.13
  meningeal, meninges (adhesive) A52.13
  meningitis A52.13
  meningovascular (diffuse) A52.13
  optic atrophy A52.15
  parenchymatous (degenerative) A52.19
  paresis, paretic A52.17
    juvenile A50.45
  remission in (sustained) A52.3
  serological (without symptoms) A52.2
  specified nature or site NEC A52.19
  tabes, tabetic (dorsalis) A52.11
    juvenile A50.45

Neurosyphilis (*Continued*)
  taboparesis A52.17
    juvenile A50.45
  thrombosis (cerebral) A52.05
  vascular (cerebral) NEC A52.05
Neurothekeoma —*see* Neoplasm, nerve, benign
Neurotic —*see* Neurosis
Neurotoxemia —*see* Toxemia
Neutroclusion M26.211
Neutropenia, neutropenic (chronic) (genetic)
  (idiopathic) (immune) (infantile)
  (malignant) (pernicious) (splenic) D70.9
  congenital (primary) D70.0
  cyclic D70.4
  cytoreductive cancer chemotherapy sequela
    D70.1
  drug-induced D70.2
    due to cytoreductive cancer chemotherapy
      D70.1
  due to infection D70.3
  fever D70.9
  neonatal, transitory (isoimmune) (maternal
    transfer) P61.5
  periodic D70.4
  secondary (cyclic) (periodic) (splenic) D70.4
    drug-induced D70.2
      due to cytoreductive cancer
        chemotherapy D70.1
  toxic D70.8
Neutrophilia, hereditary giant D72.0
Nevocarcinoma —*see* Melanoma
Nevus D22.9
  achromic —*see* Neoplasm, skin, benign
  amelanotic —*see* Neoplasm, skin, benign
  angiomatous D18.00
    intra-abdominal D18.03
    intracranial D18.02
    skin D18.01
    specified site NEC D18.09
  araneus I78.1
  balloon cell —*see* Neoplasm, skin, benign
  bathing trunk D48.5
  blue —*see* Neoplasm, skin, benign
    cellular —*see* Neoplasm, skin, benign
    giant —*see* Neoplasm, skin, benign
    Jadassohn's —*see* Neoplasm, skin, benign
    malignant —*see* Melanoma
  capillary D18.00
    intra-abdominal D18.03
    intracranial D18.02
    skin D18.01
    specified site NEC D18.09
  cavernous D18.00
    intra-abdominal D18.03
    intracranial D18.02
    skin D18.01
    specified site NEC D18.09
  cellular —*see* Neoplasm, skin, benign
    blue —*see* Neoplasm, skin, benign
  choroid D31.3-
  comedonicus Q82.5
  conjunctiva D31.0-
  dermal —*see* Neoplasm, skin, benign
    with epidermal nevus —*see* Neoplasm,
      skin, benign
  dysplastic —*see* Neoplasm, skin, benign
  eye D31.9-
  flammeus Q82.5
  hemangiomatous D18.00
    intra-abdominal D18.03
    intracranial D18.02
    skin D18.01
    specified site NEC D18.09
  iris D31.4-
  lacrimal gland D31.5-
  lymphatic D18.1
  magnocellular
    specified site —*see* Neoplasm, benign, by
      site
    unspecified site D31.40
  malignant —*see* Melanoma

Nevus (*Continued*)
- meaning hemangioma D18.00
  - intra-abdominal D18.03
  - intracranial D18.02
  - skin D18.01
  - specified site NEC D18.09
- mouth (mucosa) D10.30
  - specified site NEC D10.39
  - white sponge Q38.6
- multiplex Q85.1
- non-neoplastic I78.1
- oral mucosa D10.30
  - specified site NEC D10.39
  - white sponge Q38.6
- orbit D31.6-
- pigmented
  - giant (*see also* Neoplasm, skin, uncertain behavior) D48.5
    - malignant melanoma in —*see* Melanoma
- portwine Q82.5
- retina D31.2-
- retrobulbar D31.6-
- sanguineous Q82.5
- senile I78.1
- skin D22.9
  - abdominal wall D22.5
  - ala nasi D22.39
  - ankle D22.7-
  - anus, anal D22.5
  - arm D22.6-
  - auditory canal (external) D22.2-
  - auricle (ear) D22.2-
  - auricular canal (external) D22.2-
  - axilla, axillary fold D22.5
  - back D22.5
  - breast D22.5
  - brow D22.39
  - buttock D22.5
  - canthus (eye) D22.1-
  - cheek (external) D22.39
  - chest wall D22.5
  - chin D22.39
  - ear (external) D22.2-
  - external meatus (ear) D22.2-
  - eyebrow D22.39
  - eyelid (lower) (upper) D22.1-
  - face D22.30
    - specified NEC D22.39
  - female genital organ (external) NEC D28.0
  - finger D22.6-
  - flank D22.5
  - foot D22.7-
  - forearm D22.6-
  - forehead D22.39
  - foreskin D29.0
  - genital organ (external) NEC
    - female D28.0
    - male D29.9
  - gluteal region D22.5
  - groin D22.5
  - hand D22.6-
  - heel D22.7-
  - helix D22.2-
  - hip D22.7-
  - interscapular region D22.5
  - jaw D22.39
  - knee D22.7-
  - labium (majus) (minus) D28.0
  - leg D22.7-
  - lip (lower) (upper) D22.0
  - lower limb D22.7-
  - male genital organ (external) D29.9
  - nail D22.9
    - finger D22.6-
    - toe D22.7-
  - nasolabial groove D22.39
  - nates D22.5
  - neck D22.4
  - nose (external) D22.39
  - palpebra D22.1-

Nevus (*Continued*)
- skin (*Continued*)
  - penis D29.0
  - perianal skin D22.5
  - perineum D22.5
  - pinna D22.2-
  - popliteal fossa or space D22.7-
  - prepuce D29.0
  - pudendum D28.0
  - scalp D22.4
  - scrotum D29.4
  - shoulder D22.6-
  - submammary fold D22.5
  - temple D22.39
  - thigh D22.7-
  - toe D22.7-
  - trunk NEC D22.5
  - umbilicus D22.5
  - upper limb D22.6-
  - vulva D28.0
  - specified site NEC —*see* Neoplasm, benign, by site
- spider I78.1
- stellar I78.1
- strawberry Q82.5
- Sutton's —*see* Neoplasm, skin, benign
- unius lateris Q82.5
- Unna's Q82.5
- vascular Q82.5
- verrucous Q82.5

Newborn (infant) (liveborn) (singleton) Z38.2
- abstinence syndrome P96.1
- acne L70.4
- affected by (suspected to be)
  - abnormalities of membranes P02.9
    - specified NEC P02.8
  - abruptio placenta P02.1
  - amino-acid metabolic disorder, transitory P74.8
  - amniocentesis (while in utero) P00.6
  - amnionitis P02.7
  - apparent life threatening event (ALTE) R68.13
  - bleeding (into)
    - cerebral cortex P52.22
    - germinal matrix P52.0
    - ventricles P52.1
  - breech delivery P03.0
  - cardiac arrest P29.81
  - cardiomyopathy I42.8
    - congenital I42.4
  - cerebral ischemia P91.0
  - Cesarean delivery P03.4
  - chemotherapy agents P04.1
  - chorioamnionitis P02.7
  - cocaine (crack) P04.41
  - complications of labor and delivery P03.9
    - specified NEC P03.89
  - compression of umbilical cord NEC P02.5
  - contracted pelvis P03.1
  - delivery P03.9
    - Cesarean P03.4
    - forceps P03.2
    - vacuum extractor P03.3
  - entanglement (knot) in umbilical cord P02.5
  - environmental chemicals P04.6
  - fetal (intrauterine)
    - growth retardation P05.9
    - malnutrition not light or small for gestational age P05.2
  - forceps delivery P03.2
  - heart rate abnormalities
    - bradycardia P29.12
    - intrauterine P03.819
      - before onset of labor P03.810
      - during labor P03.811
    - tachycardia P29.11

Newborn (*Continued*)
- affected by (*Continued*)
  - hemorrhage (antepartum) P02.1
    - cerebellar (nontraumatic) P52.6
    - intracerebral (nontraumatic) P52.4
    - intracranial (nontraumatic) P52.9
      - specified NEC P52.8
    - intraventricular (nontraumatic) P52.3
      - grade 1 P52.0
      - grade 2 P52.1
      - grade 3 P52.21
      - grade 4 P52.22
    - posterior fossa (nontraumatic) P52.6
    - subarachnoid (nontraumatic) P52.5
    - subependymal P52.0
      - with intracerebral extension P52.22
      - with intraventricular extension P52.1
        - with enlargment of ventricles P52.21
      - without intraventricular extension P52.0
  - hypoxic ischemic encephalopathy [HIE] P91.60
    - mild P91.61
    - moderate P91.62
    - severe P91.63
  - induction of labor P03.89
  - intestinal perforation P78.0
  - intrauterine (fetal) blood loss P50.9
    - due to (from)
      - cut end of co-twin cord P50.5
      - hemorrhage into
        - co-twin P50.3
          - maternal circulation P50.4
        - placenta P50.2
      - ruptured cord blood P50.1
      - vasa previa P50.0
    - specified NEC P50.8
  - intrauterine (fetal) hemorrhage P50.9
  - intrauterine (in utero) procedure P96.5
  - malpresentation (malposition) NEC P03.1
  - maternal (complication of) (use of)
    - alcohol P04.3
    - analgesia (maternal) P04.0
    - anesthesia (maternal) P04.0
    - blood loss P02.1
    - circulatory disease P00.3
    - condition P00.9
      - specified NEC P00.89
    - delivery P03.9
      - Cesarean P03.4
      - forceps P03.2
      - vacuum extractor P03.3
    - diabetes mellitus (pre-existing) P70.1
    - disorder P00.9
      - specified NEC P00.89
    - drugs (addictive) (illegal) NEC P04.49
    - ectopic pregnancy P01.4
    - gestational diabetes P70.0
    - hemorrhage P02.1
    - hypertensive disorder P00.0
    - incompetent cervix P01.0
    - infectious disease P00.2
    - injury P00.5
    - labor and delivery P03.9
    - malpresentation before labor P01.7
    - maternal death P01.6
    - medical procedure P00.7
    - medication P04.1
    - multiple pregnancy P01.5
    - nutritional disorder P00.4
    - oligohydramnios P01.2
    - parasitic disease P00.2
    - periodontal disease P00.81
    - placenta previa P02.0
    - polyhydramnios P01.3
    - precipitate delivery P03.5
    - pregnancy P01.9
      - specified P01.8
    - premature rupture of membranes P01.1
    - renal disease P00.1

◀ New ◀‖‖ Revised ~~deleted~~ Deleted

Newborn (Continued)
  affected by (Continued)
    maternal (Continued)
      respiratory disease P00.3
      surgical procedure P00.6
      urinary tract disease P00.1
      uterine contraction (abnormal) P03.6
    meconium peritonitis P78.0
    medication (legal) (maternal use)
      (prescribed) P04.1
    membrane abnormalities P02.9
      specified NEC P02.8
    membranitis P02.7
    methamphetamine (s) P04.49
    mixed metabolic and respiratory acidosis
      P84
    neonatal abstinence syndrome P96.1
    noxious substances transmitted via
      placenta or breast milk P04.9
      specified NEC P04.8
    nutritional supplements P04.5
    placenta previa P02.0
    placental
      abnormality (functional)
        (morphological) P02.20
        specified NEC P02.29
      dysfunction P02.29
      infarction P02.29
      insufficiency P02.29
      separation NEC P02.1
      transfusion syndromes P02.3
    placentitis P02.7
    precipitate delivery P03.5
    prolapsed cord P02.4
    respiratory arrest P28.81
    slow intrauterine growth P05.9
    tobacco P04.2
    twin to twin transplacental transfusion
      P02.3
    umbilical cord (tightly) around neck
      P02.5
    umbilical cord condition P02.60
      short cord P02.69
      specified NEC P02.69
    uterine contractions (abnormal) P03.6
    vasa previa P02.69
      from intrauterine blood loss P50.0
  apnea P28.3
    obstructive P28.4
    primary P28.3
    specified P28.4
  born in hospital Z38.00
    by cesarean Z38.01
  born outside hospital Z38.1
  breast buds P96.89
  breast engorgement P83.4
  check-up —see Newborn, examination
  convulsion P90
  dehydration P74.1
  examination
    8 to 28 days old Z00.111
    under 8 days old Z00.110
  fever P81.9
    environmentally-induced P81.0
  hyperbilirubinemia P59.9
    of prematurity P59.0
  hypernatremia P74.2
  hyponatremia P74.2
  infection P39.9
    candidal P37.5
    specified NEC P39.8
    urinary tract P39.3
  jaundice P59.8
    due to
      breast milk inhibitor P59.3
      hepatocellular damage P59.20
        specified NEC P59.29
      preterm delivery P59.0
    of prematurity P59.0
    specified NEC P59.8
  late metabolic acidosis P74.0

Newborn (Continued)
  mastitis P39.0
    infective P39.0
    noninfective P83.4
  multiple born NEC Z38.8
    born in hospital Z38.68
      by cesarean Z38.69
    born outside hospital Z38.7
  omphalitis P38.9
    with mild hemorrhage P38.1
    without hemorrhage P38.9
  post-term P08.21
  prolonged gestation (over 42 completed
    weeks) P08.22
  quadruplet Z38.8
    born in hospital Z38.63
      by ccsarean Z38.64
    born outside hospital Z38.7
  quintuplet Z38.8
    born in hospital Z38.65
      by cesarean Z38.66
    born outside hospital Z38.7
  seizure P90
  sepsis (congenital) P36.9
    due to
      anaerobes NEC P36.5
      Escherichia coli P36.4
      Staphylococcus P36.30
        aureus P36.2
        specified NEC P36.39
      Streptococcus P36.10
        group B P36.0
        specified NEC P36.19
      specified NEC P36.8
  triplet Z38.8
    born in hospital Z38.61
      by cesarean Z38.62
    born outside hospital Z38.7
  twin Z38.5
    born in hospital Z38.30
      by cesarean Z38.31
    born outside hospital Z38.4
  vomiting P92.09
    bilious P92.01
  weight check Z00.111
Newcastle conjunctivitis or disease B30.8
Nezelof's syndrome (pure alymphocytosis)
  D81.4
Niacin (amide) **deficiency** E52
Nicolas (-Durand)-**Favre disease** A55
Nicotine —see Tobacco
Nicotinic acid deficiency E52
Niemann-Pick disease or syndrome E75.249
  specified NEC E75.248
  type
    A E75.240
    B E75.241
    C E75.242
    D E75.243
Night
  blindness —see Blindness, night
  sweats R61
  terrors (child) F51.4
Nightmares (REM sleep type) F51.5
Nipple —see condition
Nisbet's chancre A57
Nishimoto (-Takeuchi) **disease** I67.5
Nitritoid crisis or reaction —see Crisis,
  nitritoid
Nitrosohemoglobinemia D74.8
Njovera A65
Nocardiosis, nocardiasis A43.9
  cutaneous A43.1
  lung A43.0
  pneumonia A43.0
  pulmonary A43.0
  specified site NEC A43.8
Nocturia R35.1
  psychogenic F45.8
Nocturnal —see condition
Nodal rhythm I49.8

Node (s) —see also Nodule
  Bouchard's (with arthropathy) M15.2
  Haygarth's M15.8
  Heberden's (with arthropathy) M15.1
  larynx J38.7
  lymph —see condition
  milker's B08.03
  Osler's I33.0
  Schmorl's —see Schmorl's disease
  singer's J38.2
  teacher's J38.2
  tuberculous —see Tuberculosis, lymph
    gland
  vocal cord J38.2
Nodule (s), **nodular**
  actinomycotic —see Actinomycosis
  breast NEC N63
  colloid (cystic), thyroid E04.1
  cutaneous —see Swelling, localized
  endometrial (stromal) D26.1
  Haygarth's M15.8
  inflammatory —see Inflammation
  juxta-articular
    syphilitic A52.77
    yaws A66.7
  larynx J38.7
  lung, solitary (subsegmental branch of the
    bronchial tree) R91.1
    multiple R91.8
  milker's B08.03
  prostate N40.2
    with lower urinary tract symptoms (LUTS)
      N40.3
    without lower urinary tract symptoms
      (LUTS) N40.2
  pulmonary, solitary (subsegmental branch of
    the bronchial tree) R91.1
  retrocardiac R09.89
  rheumatoid M06.30
    ankle M06.37-
    elbow M06.32-
    foot joint M06.37-
    hand joint M06.34-
    hip M06.35-
    knee M06.36-
    multiple site M06.39
    shoulder M06.31-
    vertebra M06.38
    wrist M06.33-
  scrotum (inflammatory) N49.2
  singer's J38.2
  solitary, lung (subsegmental branch of the
    bronchial tree) R91.1
    multiple R91.8
  subcutaneous —see Swelling, localized
  teacher's J38.2
  thyroid (cold) (gland) (nontoxic) E04.1
    with thyrotoxicosis E05.20
      with thyroid storm E05.21
    toxic or with hyperthyroidism E05.20
      with thyroid storm E05.21
  vocal cord J38.2
Noma (gangrenous) (hospital) (infective)
  A69.0
  auricle I96
  mouth A69.0
  pudendi N76.89
  vulvae N76.89
Nomad, nomadism Z59.0
Nonautoimmune hemolytic anemia D59.4
  drug-induced D59.2
Nonclosure —see also Imperfect, closure
  ductus arteriosus (Botallo's) Q25.0
  foramen
    botalli Q21.1
    ovale Q21.1
Noncompliance Z91.19
  with
    dialysis Z91.15
    dietary regimen Z91.11
    medical treatment Z91.19

Noncompliance *(Continued)*
  with *(Continued)*
    medication regimen NEC Z91.14
      underdosing *(see also* Table of Drugs and Chemicals, categories T36-T50, with final character 6) Z91.14
      intentional NEC Z91.128
        due to financial hardship of patient Z91.120
      unintentional NEC Z91.138
        due to patient's age related debility Z91.130
    renal dialysis Z91.15
Nondescent (congenital) *—see also* Malposition, congenital
  cecum Q43.3
  colon Q43.3
  testicle Q53.9
    bilateral Q53.20
      abdominal Q53.21
      perineal Q53.22
    unilateral Q53.10
      abdominal Q53.11
      perineal Q53.12
Nondevelopment
  brain Q02
    part of Q04.3
  heart Q24.8
  organ or site, congenital NEC *—see* Hypoplasia
Nonengagement
  head NEC O32.4
    in labor, causing obstructed labor O64.8
Nonexanthematous tick fever A93.2
Nonexpansion, lung (newborn) P28.0
Nonfunctioning
  cystic duct *(see also* Disease, gallbladder) K82.8
  gallbladder *(see also* Disease, gallbladder) K82.8
  kidney N28.9
  labyrinth *—see* subcategory H83.2

Non-Hodgkin lymphoma NEC *—see* Lymphoma, non-Hodgkin
Nonimplantation, ovum N97.2
Noninsufflation, fallopian tube N97.1
Non-ketotic hyperglycinemia E72.51
Nonne-Milroy syndrome Q82.0
Nonovulation N97.0
Nonpatent fallopian tube N97.1
Nonpneumatization, lung NEC P28.0
Nonrotation *—see* Malrotation
Nonsecretion, urine *—see* Anuria
Nonunion
  fracture *—see* Fracture, by site
  organ or site, congenital NEC *—see* Imperfect, closure
  symphysis pubis, congenital Q74.2
Nonvisualization, gallbladder R93.2
Nonvital, nonvitalized tooth K04.99
Non-working side interference M26.56
Noonan's syndrome Q87.1
Normocytic anemia (infectional) due to blood loss (chronic) D50.0
  acute D62
Norrie's disease (congenital) Q15.8
North American blastomycosis B40.9
Norwegian itch B86
Nose, nasal *—see* condition
Nosebleed R04.0
Nose-picking F98.8
Nosomania F45.21
Nosophobia F45.22
Nostalgia F43.20
Notch of iris Q13.2
Notching nose, congenital (tip) Q30.2
Nothnagel's
  syndrome *—see* Strabismus, paralytic, third nerve
  vasomotor acroparesthesia I73.89
Novy's relapsing fever A68.9
  louse-borne A68.0
  tick-borne A68.1

Noxious
  foodstuffs, poisoning by *—see* Poisoning, food, noxious, plant
  substances transmitted through placenta or breast milk P04.9
Nucleus pulposus *—see* condition
Numbness R20.0
Nuns' knee *—see* Bursitis, prepatellar
Nursemaid's elbow S53.03-
Nutcracker esophagus K22.4
Nutmeg liver K76.1
Nutrient element deficiency E61.9
  specified NEC E61.8
Nutrition deficient or insufficient *(see also* Malnutrition) E46
  due to
    insufficient food T73.0
    lack of
      care (child) T76.02
        adult T76.01
      food T73.0
Nutritional stunting E45
Nyctalopia (night blindness) *—see* Blindness, night
Nycturia R35.1
  psychogenic F45.8
Nymphomania F52.8
Nystagmus H55.00
  benign paroxysmal *—see* Vertigo, benign paroxysmal
  central positional H81.4-
  congenital H55.01
  dissociated H55.04
  latent H55.02
  miners' H55.09
  positional
    benign paroxysmal H81.4-
    central H81.4-
  specified form NEC H55.09
  visual deprivation H55.03

O

Obermeyer's relapsing fever (European) A68.0
Obesity E66.9
  with alveolar hyperventilation E66.2
  adrenal E27.8
  complicating
    childbirth O99.214
    pregnancy O99.21-
    puerperium O99.215
  constitutional E66.8
  dietary counseling and surveillance Z71.3
  drug-induced E66.1
  due to
    drug E66.1
    excess calories E66.09
      morbid E66.01
      severe E66.01
  endocrine E66.8
  endogenous E66.8
  familial E66.8
  glandular E66.8
  hypothyroid —see Hypothyroidism
  morbid E66.01
    with alveolar hypoventilation E66.2
    due to excess calories E66.01
  nutritional E66.09
  pituitary E23.6
  severe E66.01
  specified type NEC E66.8
Oblique —see condition
Obliteration
  appendix (lumen) K38.8
  artery I77.1
  bile duct (noncalculous) K83.1
  common duct (noncalculous) K83.1
  cystic duct —see Obstruction, gallbladder
  disease, arteriolar I77.1
  endometrium N85.8
  eye, anterior chamber —see Disorder, globe, hypotony
  fallopian tube N97.1
  lymphatic vessel I89.0
    due to mastectomy I97.2
  organ or site, congenital NEC —see Atresia, by site
  ureter N13.5
    with infection N13.6
  urethra —see Stricture, urethra
  vein I87.8
  vestibule (oral) K08.8
Observation (following) (for) (without need for further medical care) Z04.9
  accident NEC Z04.3
    at work Z04.2
    transport Z04.1
  adverse effect of drug Z03.6
  alleged rape or sexual assault (victim), ruled out
    adult Z04.41
    child Z04.42
  criminal assault Z04.8
  development state
    adolescent Z00.3
    period of rapid growth in childhood Z00.2
    puberty Z00.3
  disease, specified NEC Z03.89
  following work accident Z04.2
  growth and development state —see Observation, development state
  injuries (accidental) NEC —see also Observation, accident
  newborn (for suspected condition, ruled out) —see Newborn, affected by (suspected to be), maternal (complication of) (use of)
  postpartum
    immediately after delivery Z39.0
    routine follow-up Z39.2

Observation (Continued)
  pregnancy (normal) (without complication) Z34.9-
    high risk O09.9-
  suicide attempt, alleged NEC Z03.89
    self-poisoning Z03.6
  suspected, ruled out —see also Suspected condition, ruled out
    abuse, physical
      adult Z04.71
      child Z04.72
    accident at work Z04.2
    adult battering victim Z04.71
    child battering victim Z04.72
    condition NEC Z03.89
      newborn —see Newborn, affected by (suspected to be), maternal (complication of) (use of)
    drug poisoning or adverse effect Z03.6
    exposure (to)
      anthrax Z03.810
      biological agent NEC Z03.818
    inflicted injury NEC Z04.8
    suicide attempt, alleged Z03.89
      self-poisoning Z03.6
    toxic effects from ingested substance (drug) (poison) Z03.6
  toxic effects from ingested substance (drug) (poison) Z03.6
Obsession, obsessional state F42
Obsessive-compulsive neurosis or reaction F42
Obstetric embolism, septic —see Embolism, obstetric, septic
Obstetrical trauma (complicating delivery) O71.9
  with or following ectopic or molar pregnancy O08.6
  specified type NEC O71.89
Obstipation —see Constipation
Obstruction, obstructed, obstructive
  airway J98.8
    with
      allergic alveolitis J67.9
      asthma J45.909
        with
          exacerbation (acute) J45.901
          status asthmaticus J45.902
      bronchiectasis J47.9
        with
          exacerbation (acute) J47.1
          lower respiratory infection J47.0
      bronchitis (chronic) J44.9
      emphysema J43.9
      chronic J44.9
        with
          allergic alveolitis —see Pneumonitis, hypersensitivity
          bronchiectasis J47.9
            with
              exacerbation (acute) J47.1
              lower respiratory infection J47.0
    due to
      foreign body —see Foreign body, by site, causing asphyxia
      inhalation of fumes or vapors J68.9
      laryngospasm J38.5
  ampulla of Vater K83.1
  aortic (heart) (valve) —see Stenosis, aortic
  aortoiliac I74.09
  aqueduct of Sylvius G91.1
    congenital Q03.0
      with spina bifida —see Spina bifida, by site, with hydrocephalus
  Arnold-Chiari —see Arnold-Chiari disease
  artery (see also Embolism, artery) I74.9
    basilar (complete) (partial) —see Occlusion, artery, basilar
    carotid (complete) (partial) —see Occlusion, artery, carotid
    cerebellar —see Occlusion, artery, cerebellar

Obstruction, obstructed, obstructive (Continued)
  artery (Continued)
    cerebral (anterior) (middle) (posterior) —see Occlusion, artery, cerebral
    precerebral —see Occlusion, artery, precerebral
    renal N28.0
    retinal NEC —see Occlusion, artery, retina
    vertebral (complete) (partial) —see Occlusion, artery, vertebral
  band (intestinal) K56.69
  bile duct or passage (common) (hepatic) (noncalculous) K83.1
    with calculus K80.51
    congenital (causing jaundice) Q44.3
  biliary (duct) (tract) K83.1
    gallbladder K82.0
  bladder-neck (acquired) N32.0
    congenital Q64.31
    due to hyperplasia (hypertrophy) of prostate —see Hyperplasia, prostate
  bowel —see Obstruction, intestine
  bronchus J98.09
  canal, ear —see Stenosis, external ear canal
  cardia K22.2
  caval veins (inferior) (superior) I87.1
  cecum —see Obstruction, intestine
  circulatory I99.8
  colon —see Obstruction, intestine
  common duct (noncalculous) K83.1
  coronary (artery) —see Occlusion, coronary
  cystic duct —see also Obstruction, gallbladder
    with calculus K80.21
  device, implant or graft (see also Complications, by site and type, mechanical) T85.698
    arterial graft NEC —see Complication, cardiovascular device, mechanical, vascular
    catheter NEC T85.628
      cystostomy T83.090
      dialysis (renal) T82.49
        intraperitoneal T85.691
      infusion NEC T82.594
        spinal (epidural) (subdural) T85.690
      urinary, indwelling T83.098
    due to infection T85.79
    gastrointestinal —see Complications, prosthetic device, mechanical, gastrointestinal device
    genital NEC T83.498
      intrauterine contraceptive device T83.39
      penile prosthesis T83.490
    heart NEC —see Complication, cardiovascular device, mechanical
    joint prosthesis —see Complications, joint prosthesis, mechanical, specified NEC, by site
    orthopedic NEC —see Complication, orthopedic, device, mechanical
    specified NEC T85.628
    urinary NEC —see also Complication, genitourinary, device, urinary, mechanical
      graft T83.29
    vascular NEC —see Complication, cardiovascular device, mechanical
    ventricular intracranial shunt T85.09
  due to foreign body accidentally left in operative wound T81.529
  duodenum K31.5
  ejaculatory duct N50.8
  esophagus K22.2
  eustachian tube (complete) (partial) H68.10-
    cartilagenous (extrinsic) H68.13-
      intrinsic H68.12-
    osseous H68.11-
  fallopian tube (bilateral) N97.1

Obstruction, obstructed, obstructive
  (Continued)
  fecal K56.41
    with hernia —*see* Hernia, by site, with
      obstruction
  foramen of Monro (congenital) Q03.8
    with spina bifida —*see* Spina bifida,
      by site, with hydrocephalus
  foreign body —*see* Foreign body
  gallbladder K82.0
    with calculus, stones K80.21
    congenital Q44.1
  gastric outlet K31.1
  gastrointestinal —*see* Obstruction, intestine
  hepatic K76.89
    duct (noncalculous) K83.1
  hepatobiliary K83.1
  ileum —*see* Obstruction, intestine
  iliofemoral (artery) I74.5
  intestine K56.60
    with
      adhesions (intestinal) (peritoneal)
        K56.5
    adynamic K56.0
    by gallstone K56.3
    congenital (small) Q41.9
      large Q42.9
        specified part NEC Q42.8
    neurogenic K56.0
      Hirschsprung's disease or megacolon
        Q43.1
    newborn P76.9
      due to
        fecaliths P76.8
        inspissated milk P76.2
        meconium (plug) P76.0
          in mucoviscidosis E84.11
      specified NEC P76.8
    postoperative K91.3
    reflex K56.0
    specified NEC K56.69
    volvulus K56.2
  intracardiac ball valve prosthesis T82.09
  jejunum —*see* Obstruction, intestine
  joint prosthesis —*see* Complications, joint
    prosthesis, mechanical, specified NEC,
    by site
  kidney (calices) N28.89
  labor —*see* Delivery
  lacrimal (passages) (duct)
    by
      dacryolith —*see* Dacryolith
      stenosis —*see* Stenosis, lacrimal
    congenital Q10.5
    neonatal H04.53-
  lacrimonasal duct —*see* Obstruction,
    lacrimal
  lacteal, with steatorrhea K90.2
  laryngitis —*see* Laryngitis
  larynx NEC J38.6
    congenital Q31.8
  lung J98.4
    disease, chronic J44.9
  lymphatic I89.0
  meconium (plug)
    newborn P76.0
      due to fecaliths P76.0
      in mucoviscidosis E84.11
  mitral —*see* Stenosis, mitral
  nasal J34.89
  nasolacrimal duct —*see also* Obstruction,
    lacrimal
    congenital Q10.5
  nasopharynx J39.2
  nose J34.89
  organ or site, congenital NEC —*see* Atresia,
    by site
  pancreatic duct K86.8
  parotid duct or gland K11.8
  pelviureteral junction N13.5
    congenital Q62.39

Obstruction, obstructed, obstructive
  (Continued)
  pharynx J39.2
  portal (circulation) (vein) I81
  prostate —*see also* Hyperplasia, prostate
    valve (urinary) N32.0
  pulmonary valve (heart) I37.0
  pyelonephritis (chronic) N11.1
  pylorus
    adult K31.1
    congenital or infantile Q40.0
  rectosigmoid —*see* Obstruction,
    intestine
  rectum K62.4
  renal N28.89
    outflow N13.8
    pelvis, congenital Q62.39
  respiratory J98.8
    chronic J44.9
  retinal (vessels) H34.9
  salivary duct (any) K11.8
    with calculus K11.5
  sigmoid —*see* Obstruction, intestine
  sinus (accessory) (nasal) J34.89
  Stensen's duct K11.8
  stomach NEC K31.89
    acute K31.0
    congenital Q40.2
    due to pylorospasm K31.3
  submandibular duct K11.8
  submaxillary gland K11.8
    with calculus K11.5
  thoracic duct I89.0
  thrombotic —*see* Thrombosis
  trachea J39.8
  tracheostomy airway J95.03
  tricuspid (valve) —*see* Stenosis,
    tricuspid
  upper respiratory, congenital Q34.8
  ureter (functional) (pelvic junction) NEC
    N13.5
    with
      hydronephrosis N13.1
        with infection N13.6
      pyelonephritis (chronic) N11.1
    congenital Q62.39
    due to calculus —*see* Calculus, ureter
  urethra NEC N36.8
    congenital Q64.39
  urinary (moderate) N13.9
    due to hyperplasia (hypertrophy) of
      prostate —*see* Hyperplasia,
      prostate
    organ or tract (lower) N13.9
    prostatic valve N32.0
    specified NEC N13.8
  uropathy N13.9
  uterus N85.8
  vagina N89.5
  valvular —*see* Endocarditis
  vein, venous I87.1
    caval (inferior) (superior) I87.1
    thrombotic —*see* Thrombosis
  vena cava (inferior) (superior) I87.1
  vesical NEC N32.0
  vesicourethral orifice N32.0
    congenital Q64.31
  vessel NEC I99.8
Obturator —*see* condition
Occlusal wear, teeth K03.0
Occlusio pupillae —*see* Membrane,
  pupillary
Occlusion, occluded
  anus K62.4
    congenital Q42.3
      with fistula Q42.2
  aortoiliac (chronic) I74.09
  aqueduct of Sylvius G91.1
    congenital Q03.0
      with spina bifida —*see* Spina bifida, by
      site, with hydrocephalus

Occlusion, occluded *(Continued)*
  artery (*see also* Embolism, artery) I74.9
    auditory, internal I65.8
    basilar I65.1
      with
        infarction I63.22
        due to
          embolism I63.12
          thrombosis I63.02
    brain or cerebral I66.9
      with infarction (due to) I63.5
        embolism I63.4
        thrombosis I63.3
    carotid I65.2-
      with
        infarction I63.23-
        due to
          embolism I63.13-
          thrombosis I63.03-
    cerebellar (anterior inferior) (posterior
      inferior) (superior) I66.3
      with infarction I63.54-
        due to
          embolism I63.44-
          thrombosis I63.34-
    cerebral I66.9
      with infarction I63.50
        due to
          embolism I63.40
            specified NEC I63.49
          thrombosis I63.30
            specified NEC I63.39
      anterior I66.1-
        with infarction I63.52-
        due to
          embolism I63.42-
          thrombosis I63.32-
      middle I66.0-
        with infarction I63.51-
        due to
          embolism I63.41-
          thrombosis I63.31-
      posterior I66.2-
        with infarction I63.53-
        due to
          embolism I63.43-
          thrombosis I63.33-
      specified NEC I66.8
        with infarction I63.59
        due to
          embolism I63.4
          thrombosis I63.3
    choroidal (anterior) —*see* Occlusion,
      artery, cerebral, specified NEC
    communicating posterior —*see*
      Occlusion, artery, precerebral,
      specified NEC
    complete
      coronary I25.82
      extremities I70.92
    coronary (acute) (thrombotic) (without
      myocardial infarction) I24.0
      with myocardial infarction —*see*
        Infarction, myocardium
      chronic total I25.82
      complete I25.82
      healed or old I25.2
      total (chronic) I25.82
    hypophyseal —*see* Occlusion, artery,
      precerebral, specified NEC
    iliac I74.5
    lower extremities due to stenosis or
      stricture I77.1
    mesenteric (embolic) (thrombotic)
      K55.0
    perforating —*see* Occlusion, artery,
      cerebral, specified NEC
    peripheral I77.9
      thrombotic or embolic I74.4
    pontine —*see* Occlusion, artery, cerebral,
      specified NEC

◀ New   ◀|||| Revised   ~~deleted~~ Deleted

Occlusion, occluded (Continued)
  artery (Continued)
    precerebral I65.9
      with infarction I63.20
        due to
          embolism I63.10
            specified NEC I63.19
          thrombosis I63.00
            specified NEC I63.09
        specified NEC I63.29
      basilar —see Occlusion, artery, basilar
      carotid —see Occlusion, artery, carotid
      puerperal O88.23
      specified NEC I65.8
        with infarction I63.29
          due to
            embolism I63.19
            thrombosis I63.00
      vertebral —see Occlusion, artery,
        vertebral
    renal N28.0
    retinal
      branch H34.23-
      central H34.1-
      partial H34.21-
      transient H34.0-
    spinal —see Occlusion, artery, precerebral,
      vertebral
    total (chronic)
      coronary I25.82
      extremities I70.92
    vertebral I65.0-
      with
        infarction I63.21-
          due to
            embolism I63.11-
            thrombosis I63.01-
  basilar artery —see Occlusion, artery, basilar
  bile duct (common) (hepatic) (noncalculous)
    K83.1
  bowel —see Obstruction, intestine
  carotid (artery) (common) (internal) —see
    Occlusion, artery, carotid
  centric (of teeth) M26.59
    maximum intercuspation discrepancy
      M26.55
  cerebellar (artery) —see Occlusion, artery,
    cerebellar
  cerebral (artery) —see Occlusion, artery,
    cerebral
  cerebrovascular —see also Occlusion, artery,
    cerebral
    with infarction I63.5
  cervical canal —see Stricture, cervix
  cervix (uteri) —see Stricture, cervix
  choanal Q30.0
  choroidal (artery) —see Occlusion, artery,
    precerebral, specified NEC
  colon —see Obstruction, intestine
  communicating posterior artery —see
    Occlusion, artery, precerebral, specified
    NEC
  coronary (artery) (vein) (thrombotic) —see
    also Infarct, myocardium
    chronic total I25.82
    healed or old I25.2
    not resulting in infarction I24.0
    total (chronic) I25.82
  cystic duct —see Obstruction, gallbladder
  embolic —see Embolism
  fallopian tube N97.1
    congenital Q50.6
  gallbladder —see also Obstruction,
    gallbladder
    congenital (causing jaundice) Q44.1
  gingiva, traumatic K06.2
  hymen N89.6
    congenital Q52.3
  hypophyseal (artery) —see Occlusion, artery,
    precerebral, specified NEC
  iliac artery I74.5

Occlusion, occluded (Continued)
  intestine —see Obstruction, intestine
  lacrimal passages —see Obstruction, lacrimal
  lung J98.4
  lymph or lymphatic channel I89.0
  mammary duct N64.89
  mesenteric artery (embolic) (thrombotic)
    K55.0
  nose J34.89
    congenital Q30.0
  organ or site, congenital NEC —see Atresia,
    by site
  oviduct N97.1
    congenital Q50.6
  peripheral arteries
    due to stricture or stenosis I77.1
    upper extremity I74.2
  pontine (artery) —see Occlusion, artery,
    precerebral, specified NEC
  posterior lingual, of mandibular teeth M26.29
  precerebral artery —see Occlusion, artery,
    precerebral
  punctum lacrimale —see Obstruction,
    lacrimal
  pupil —see Membrane, pupillary
  pylorus, adult (see also Stricture, pylorus)
    K31.1
  renal artery N28.0
  retina, retinal
    artery —see Occlusion, artery, retinal
    vein (central) H34.81-
      engorgement H34.82-
      tributary H34.83-
    vessels H34.9
  spinal artery —see Occlusion, artery,
    precerebral, vertebral
  teeth (mandibular) (posterior lingual)
    M26.29
  thoracic duct I89.0
  thrombotic —see Thrombosis, artery
  traumatic
    edentulous (alveolar) ridge K06.2
    gingiva K06.2
    periodontal K05.5
  tubal N97.1
  ureter (complete) (partial) N13.5
    congenital Q62.10
  ureteropelvic junction N13.5
    congenital Q62.11
  ureterovesical orifice N13.5
    congenital Q62.12
  urethra —see Stricture, urethra
  uterus N85.8
  vagina N89.5
  vascular NEC I99.8
  vein —see Thrombosis
    retinal —see Occlusion, retinal, vein
  vena cava (inferior) (superior) —see
    Embolism, vena cava
  ventricle (brain) NEC G91.1
  vertebral (artery) —see Occlusion, artery,
    vertebral
  vessel (blood) I99.8
  vulva N90.5
Occult
  blood in feces (stools) R19.5
Occupational
  problems NEC Z56.89
Ochlophobia —see Agoraphobia
Ochronosis (endogenous) E70.29
Ocular muscle —see condition
Oculogyric crisis or disturbance H51.8
  psychogenic F45.8
Oculomotor syndrome H51.9
Oculopathy
  syphilitic NEC A52.71
    congenital
      early A50.01
      late A50.30
    early (secondary) A51.43
    late A52.71

Oddi's sphincter spasm K83.4
Odontalgia K08.8
Odontoameloblastoma —see Cyst, calcifying
  odontogenic
Odontoclasia K03.89
Odontodysplasia, regional K00.4
Odontogenesis imperfecta K00.5
Odontoma (ameloblastic) (complex)
  (compound) (fibroameloblastic) —see Cyst,
  calcifying odontogenic
Odontomyelitis (closed) (open) K04.0
Odontorrhagia K08.8
Odontosarcoma, ameloblastic C41.1
  upper jaw (bone) C41.0
Oestriasis —see Myiasis
Oguchi's disease H53.63
Ohara's disease —see Tularemia
Oidiomycosis —see Candidiasis
Oidium albicans infection —see Candidiasis
Old (previous) myocardial infarction
  I25.2
Old age (without mention of debility)
  R54-
  dementia F03
Olfactory —see condition
Oligemia —see Anemia
Oligoastrocytoma
  specified site —see Neoplasm, malignant,
    by site
  unspecified site C71.9
Oligocythemia D64.9
Oligodendroblastoma
  specified site —see Neoplasm, malignant
  unspecified site C71.9
Oligodendroglioma
  anaplastic type
    specified site —see Neoplasm, malignant,
      by site
    unspecified site C71.9
  specified site —see Neoplasm, malignant,
    by site
  unspecified site C71.9
Oligodontia —see Anodontia
Oligoencephalon Q02
Oligohidrosis L74.4
Oligohydramnios O41.0-
Oligohydrosis L74.4
Oligomenorrhea N91.5
  primary N91.3
  secondary N91.4
Oligophrenia —see also Disability, intellectual
  phenylpyruvic E70.0
Oligospermia N46.11
  due to
    drug therapy N46.121
    efferent duct obstruction N46.123
    infection N46.122
    radiation N46.124
    specified cause NEC N46.129
    systemic disease N46.125
Oligotrichia —see Alopecia
Oliguria R34
  with, complicating or following ectopic or
    molar pregnancy O08.4
  postprocedural N99.0
Ollier's disease Q78.4
Omenotocele —see Hernia, abdomen, specified
  site NEC
Omentitis —see Peritonitis
Omentum, omental —see condition
Omphalitis (congenital) (newborn) P38.9
  with mild hemorrhage P38.1
  without hemorrhage P38.9
  not of newborn L08.82
  tetanus A33
Omphalocele Q79.2
Omphalomesenteric duct, persistent
  Q43.0
Omphalorrhagia, newborn P51.9
Omsk hemorrhagic fever A98.1
Onanism (excessive) F98.8

Onchocerciasis, onchocercosis B73.1
  with
    eye disease B73.00
      endophthalmitis B73.01
      eyelid B73.09
      glaucoma B73.02
      specified NEC B73.09
    eye NEC B73.00
    eyelid B73.09
Oncocytoma —see Neoplasm, benign, by site
Oncovirus, as cause of disease classified
    elsewhere B97.32
Ondine's curse —see Apnea, sleep
Oneirophrenia F23
Onychauxis L60.2
  congenital Q84.5
Onychia —see also Cellulitis, digit
  with lymphangitis —see Lymphangitis, acute,
    digit
  candidal B37.2
  dermatophytic B35.1
Onychitis —see also Cellulitis, digit
  with lymphangitis —see Lymphangitis, acute,
    digit
Onychocryptosis L60.0
Onychodystrophy L60.3
  congenital Q84.6
Onychogryphosis, onychogryposis L60.2
Onycholysis L60.1
Onychomadesis L60.8
Onychomalacia L60.3
Onychomycosis (finger) (toe) B35.1
Onycho-osteodysplasia Q79.8
Onychophagia F98.8
Onychophosis L60.8
Onychoptosis L60.8
Onychorrhexis L60.3
  congenital Q84.6
Onychoschizia L60.3
Onyxis (finger) (toe) L60.0
Onyxitis —see also Cellulitis, digit
  with lymphangitis —see Lymphangitis, acute,
    digit
Oophoritis (cystic) (infectional) (interstitial)
    N70.92
  with salpingitis N70.93
  acute N70.02
    with salpingitis N70.03
  chronic N70.12
    with salpingitis N70.13
  complicating abortion —see Abortion, by
    type, complicated by, oophoritis
Oophorocele N83.4
Opacity, opacities
  cornea H17.-
    central H17.1-
    congenital Q13.3
    degenerative —see Degeneration, cornea
    hereditary —see Dystrophy, cornea
    inflammatory —see Keratitis
    minor H17.81-
    peripheral H17.82-
    sequelae of trachoma (healed) B94.0
    specified NEC H17.89
  enamel (teeth) (fluoride) (nonfluoride)
    K00.3
  lens —see Cataract
  snowball —see Deposit, crystalline
  vitreous (humor) NEC H43.39-
    congenital Q14.0
    membranes and strands H43.31-
Opalescent dentin (hereditary) K00.5
Open, opening
  abnormal, organ or site, congenital —see
    Imperfect, closure
  angle with
    borderline
      findings
        high risk H40.02-
        low risk H40.01-
      intraocular pressure H40.00-

Open, opening (Continued)
  angle with (Continued)
    cupping of discs H40.01-
    glaucoma (primary) —see Glaucoma, open
      angle
  bite
    anterior M26.220
    posterior M26.221
  false —see Imperfect, closure
  margin on tooth restoration K08.51
  restoration margins of tooth K08.51
  wound —see Wound, open
Operational fatigue F48.8
Operative —see condition
Operculitis —see Periodontitis
Operculum —see Break, retina
Ophiasis L63.2
Ophthalmia (see also Conjunctivitis) H10.9
  actinic rays —see Photokeratitis
  allergic (acute) —see Conjunctivitis, acute,
    atopic
  blennorrhagic (gonococcal) (neonatorum)
    A54.31
  diphtheritic A36.86
  Egyptian A71.1
  electrica —see Photokeratitis
  gonococcal (neonatorum) A54.31
  metastatic —see Endophthalmitis, purulent
  migraine —see Migraine, ophthalmoplegic
  neonatorum, newborn P39.1
    gonococcal A54.31
  nodosa H16.24-
  purulent —see Conjunctivitis, acute,
    mucopurulent
  spring —see Conjunctivitis, acute, atopic
  sympathetic —see Uveitis, sympathetic
Ophthalmitis —see Ophthalmia
Ophthalmocele (congenital) Q15.8
Ophthalmoneuromyelitis G36.0
Ophthalmoplegia —see also Strabismus,
    paralytic
  anterior internuclear —see Ophthalmoplegia,
    internuclear
  ataxia-areflexia G61.0
  diabetic —see E08-E13 with .39
  exophthalmic E05.00
    with thyroid storm E05.01
  external H49.88-
    progressive H49.4-
      with pigmentary retinopathy —see
        Kearns-Sayre syndrome
    total H49.3-
  internal (complete) (total) H52.51-
  internuclear H51.2-
  migraine —see Migraine, ophthalmoplegic
  Parinaud's H49.88-
  progressive external —see Ophthalmoplegia,
    external, progressive
  supranuclear, progressive G23.1
  total (external) —see Ophthalmoplegia,
    external, total
Opioid (s)
  abuse —see Abuse, drug, opioids
  dependence —see Dependence, drug, opioids
Opisthognathism M26.09
Opisthorchiasis (felineus) (viverrini) B66.0
Opitz' disease D73.2
Opiumism —see Dependence, drug, opioid
Oppenheim's disease G70.2
Oppenheim-Urbach disease (necrobiosis
    lipoidica diabeticorum) —see E08-E13 with
    .620
Optic nerve —see condition
Orbit —see condition
Orchioblastoma C62.9-
Orchitis (gangrenous) (nonspecific) (septic)
    (suppurative) N45.2
  blennorrhagic (gonococcal) (acute) (chronic)
    A54.23
  chlamydial A56.19
  filarial (see also Infestation, filarial) B74.9
    [N51]

Orchitis (Continued)
  gonococcal (acute) (chronic) A54.23
  mumps B26.0
  syphilitic A52.76
  tuberculous A18.15
Orf (virus disease) B08.02
Organic —see also condition
  brain syndrome F09
  heart —see Disease, heart
  mental disorder F09
  psychosis F09
Orgasm
  anejaculatory N53.13
Oriental
  bilharziasis B65.2
  schistosomiasis B65.2
Orifice —see condition
Origin of both great vessels from right
    ventricle Q20.1
Ormond's disease (with ureteral obstruction)
    N13.5
  with infection N13.6
Ornithine metabolism disorder E72.4
Ornithinemia (Type I) (Type II) E72.4
Ornithosis A70
Orotaciduria, oroticaciduria (congenital)
    (hereditary) (pyrimidine deficiency) E79.8
  anemia D53.0
Orthodontics
  adjustment Z46.4
  fitting Z46.4
Orthopnea R06.01
Orthopoxvirus B08.09
  specified NEC B08.09
Os, uterus —see condition
Osgood-Schlatter disease or
    osteochondrosis —see Osteochondrosis,
    juvenile, tibia
Osler (-Weber)-Rendu disease I78.0
Osler's nodes I33.0
Osmidrosis L75.0
Osseous —see condition
Ossification
  artery —see Arteriosclerosis
  auricle (ear) —see Disorder, pinna, specified
    type NEC
  bronchial J98.09
  cardiac —see Degeneration, myocardial
  cartilage (senile) —see Disorder, cartilage,
    specified type NEC
  coronary (artery) —see Disease, heart,
    ischemic, atherosclerotic
  diaphragm J98.6
  ear, middle —see Otosclerosis
  falx cerebri G96.19
  fontanel, premature Q75.0
  heart —see also Degeneration, myocardial
    valve —see Endocarditis
  larynx J38.7
  ligament —see Disorder, tendon, specified
    type NEC
    posterior longitudinal —see
      Spondylopathy, specified NEC
  meninges (cerebral) (spinal) G96.19
  multiple, eccentric centers —see Disorder,
    bone, development or growth
  muscle —see also Calcification, muscle
    due to burns —see Myositis, ossificans, in,
      burns
    paralytic —see Myositis, ossificans, in,
      quadriplegia
    progressive —see Myositis, ossificans,
      progressiva
    specified NEC M61.50
      ankle M61.57-
      foot M61.57-
      forearm M61.53-
      hand M61.54-
      lower leg M61.56-
      multiple sites M61.59
      pelvic region M61.55-

◀ New   ◀▦ Revised   ~~deleted~~ Deleted

Ossification (*Continued*)
  muscle (*Continued*)
    specified NEC (*Continued*)
      shoulder region M61.51-
      specified site NEC M61.58
      thigh M61.55-
      upper arm M61.52-
    traumatic —*see* Myositis, ossificans, traumatica
  myocardium, myocardial —*see* Degeneration, myocardial
  penis N48.89
  periarticular —*see* Disorder, joint, specified type NEC
  pinna —*see* Disorder, pinna, specified type NEC
  rider's bone —*see* Ossification, muscle, specified NEC
  sclera H15.89
  subperiosteal, post-traumatic M89.8X-
  tendon —*see* Disorder, tendon, specified type NEC
  trachea J39.8
  tympanic membrane —*see* Disorder, tympanic membrane, specified NEC
  vitreous (humor) —*see* Deposit, crystalline
Osteitis —*see also* Osteomyelitis
  alveolar M27.3
  condensans M85.30
    ankle M85.37-
    foot M85.37-
    forearm M85.33-
    hand M85.34-
    lower leg M85.36-
    multiple site M85.39
    neck M85.38
    rib M85.38
    shoulder M85.31-
    skull M85.38
    specified site NEC M85.38
    thigh M85.35-
    toe M85.37-
    upper arm M85.32-
    vertebra M85.38
  deformans M88.9
    in (due to)
      malignant neoplasm of bone C41.9 [M90.60]
      neoplastic disease (*see also* Neoplasm) D49.9 [M90.60]
        carpus D49.9 [M90.64-]
        clavicle D49.9 [M90.61-]
        femur D49.9 [M90.65-]
        fibula D49.9 [M90.66-]
        finger D49.9 [M90.64-]
        humerus D49.9 [M90.62-]
        ilium D49.9 [M90.65-]
        ischium D49.9 [M90.65-]
        metacarpus D49.9 [M90.64-]
        metatarsus D49.9 [M90.67-]
        multiple sites D49.9 [M90.69]
        neck D49.9 [M90.68]
        radius D49.9 [M90.63-]
        rib D49.9 [M90.68]
        scapula D49.9 [M90.61-]
        skull D49.9 [M90.68]
        tarsus D49.9 [M90.67-]
        tibia D49.9 [M90.66-]
        toe D49.9 [M90.67-]
        ulna D49.9 [M90.63-]
        vertebra D49.9 [M90.68]
    skull M88.0
    specified NEC —*see* Paget's disease, bone, by site
    vertebra M88.1
  due to yaws A66.6
  fibrosa NEC —*see* Cyst, bone, by site
    circumscripta —*see* Dysplasia, fibrous, bone NEC

Osteitis (*Continued*)
  fibrosa NEC (*Continued*)
    cystica (generalisata) E21.0
    disseminata Q78.1
    osteoplastica E21.0
  fragilitans Q78.0
  Garr's (sclerosing) —*see* Osteomyelitis, specified type NEC
  jaw (acute) (chronic) (lower) (suppurative) (upper) M27.2
  parathyroid E21.0
  petrous bone (acute) (chronic) —*see* Petrositis
  sclerotic, nonsuppurative —*see* Osteomyelitis, specified type NEC
  tuberculosa A18.09
    cystica D86.89
    multiplex cystoides D86.89
Osteoarthritis M19.90
  ankle M19.07-
  elbow M19.02-
  foot joint M19.07-
  generalized M15.9
    erosive M15.4
    primary M15.0
    specified NEC M15.8
  hand joint M19.04-
    first carpometacarpal joint M18.9-
  hip M16.1-
    bilateral M16.0
    due to hip dysplasia (unilateral) M16.3-
      bilateral M16.2
  interphalangeal
    distal (Heberden) M15.1
    proximal (Bouchard) M15.2
  knee M17.9-
    bilateral M17.0
  post-traumatic NEC M19.92
    ankle M19.17-
    elbow M19.12-
    foot joint M19.17-
    hand joint M19.14-
      first carpometacarpal joint M18.3-
        bilateral M18.2
    hip M16.5-
      bilateral M16.4
    knee M17.3-
      bilateral M17.2
    shoulder M19.11-
    wrist M19.13-
  primary M19.91
    ankle M19.07-
    elbow M19.02-
    foot joint M19.07-
    hand joint M19.04-
      first carpometacarpal joint M18.1-
        bilateral M18.0
    hip M16.1-
      bilateral M16.0
    knee M17.1-
      bilateral M17.0
    shoulder M19.01-
    spine —*see* Spondylosis
    wrist M19.03-
  secondary M19.93
    ankle M19.27-
    elbow M19.22-
    foot joint M19.27-
    hand joint M19.24-
      first carpometacarpal joint M18.5-
        bilateral M18.4
    hip M16.7
      bilateral M16.6
    knee M17.5
      bilateral M17.4
    multiple M15.3
    shoulder M19.21-
    spine —*see* Spondylosis
    wrist M19.23-
  shoulder M19.01-
  spine —*see* Spondylosis
  wrist M19.03-

Osteoarthropathy (hypertrophic) M19.90
  ankle —*see* Osteoarthritis, primary, ankle
  elbow —*see* Osteoarthritis, primary, elbow
  foot joint —*see* Osteoarthritis, primary, foot
  hand joint —*see* Osteoarthritis, primary, hand joint
  knee joint —*see* Osteoarthritis, primary, knee
  multiple site —*see* Osteoarthritis, primary, multiple joint
  pulmonary —*see also* Osteoarthropathy, specified type NEC
  hypertrophic —*see* Osteoarthropathy, hypertrophic, specified type NEC
  secondary —*see* Osteoarthropathy, specified type NEC
  secondary hypertrophic —*see* Osteoarthropathy, specified type NEC
  shoulder —*see* Osteoarthritis, primary, shoulder
  specified joint NEC —*see* Osteoarthritis, primary, specified joint NEC
  specified type NEC M89.40
    carpus M89.44-
    clavicle M89.41-
    femur M89.45-
    fibula M89.46-
    finger M89.44-
    humerus M89.42-
    ilium M89.459
    ischium M89.459
    metacarpus M89.44-
    metatarsus M89.47-
    multiple sites M89.49
    neck M89.48
    radius M89.43-
    rib M89.48
    scapula M89.41-
    skull M89.48
    tarsus M89.47-
    tibia M89.46-
    toe M89.47-
    ulna M89.43-
    vertebra M89.48
  spine —*see* Spondylosis
  wrist —*see* Osteoarthritis, primary, wrist
Osteoarthrosis (degenerative) (hypertrophic) (joint) —*see also* Osteoarthritis
  deformans alkaptonurica E70.29 [M36.8]
  erosive M15.4
  generalized M15.9
    primary M15.0
  polyarticular M15.9
  spine —*see* Spondylosis
Osteoblastoma —*see* Neoplasm, bone, benign
  aggressive —*see* Neoplasm, bone, uncertain behavior
Osteochondroarthrosis deformans endemica —*see* Disease, Kaschin-Beck
Osteochondritis —*see also* Osteochondropathy, by site
  Brailsford's —*see* Osteochondrosis, juvenile, radius
  dissecans M93.20
    ankle M93.27-
    elbow M93.22-
    foot M93.27-
    hand M93.24-
    hip M93.25-
    knee M93.26-
    multiple sites M93.29
    shoulder joint M93.21-
    specified site NEC M93.28
    wrist M93.23-
  juvenile M92.9
    patellar —*see* Osteochondrosis, juvenile, patella
  syphilitic (congenital) (early) A50.02 [M90.80]
    ankle A50.02 [M90.87-]
    elbow A50.02 [M90.82-]
    foot A50.02 [M90.87-]
    forearm A50.02 [M90.83-]

Osteochondritis *(Continued)*
  syphilitic *(Continued)*
    hand A50.02 *[M90.84-]*
    hip A50.02 *[M90.85-]*
    knee A50.02 *[M90.86-]*
    multiple sites A50.02 *[M90.89]*
    shoulder joint A50.02 *[M90.81-]*
    specified site NEC A50.02 *[M90.88]*
Osteochondrodysplasia Q78.9
  with defects of growth of tubular bones and spine Q77.9
    specified NEC Q77.8
  specified NEC Q78.8
Osteochondrodystrophy E78.9
Osteochondrolysis —*see* Osteochondritis, dissecans
Osteochondroma —*see* Neoplasm, bone, benign
Osteochondromatosis D48.0
  syndrome Q78.4
Osteochondromyxosarcoma —*see* Neoplasm, bone, malignant
Osteochondropathy M93.90
  ankle M93.97-
  elbow M93.92-
  foot M93.97-
  hand M93.94-
  hip M93.95-
  Kienböck's disease of adults M93.1
  knee M93.96-
  multiple joints M93.99
  osteochondritis dissecans —*see* Osteochondritis, dissecans
  osteochondrosis —*see* Osteochondrosis
  shoulder region M93.91-
  slipped upper femoral epiphysis —*see* Slipped, epiphysis, upper femoral
  specified joint NEC M93.98
  specified type NEC M93.80
    ankle M93.87-
    elbow M93.82-
    foot M93.87-
    hand M93.84-
    hip M93.85-
    knee M93.86-
    multiple joints M93.89
    shoulder region M93.81-
    specified joint NEC M93.88
    wrist M93.83-
  syphilitic, congenital
    early A50.02 *[M90.80]*
    late A50.56 *[M90.80]*
  wrist M93.93-
Osteochondrosarcoma —*see* Neoplasm, bone, malignant
Osteochondrosis —*see also* Osteochondropathy, by site
  acetabulum (juvenile) M91.0
  adult —*see* Osteochondropathy, specified type NEC, by site
  astragalus (juvenile) —*see* Osteochondrosis, juvenile, tarsus
  Blount's —*see* Osteochondrosis, juvenile, tibia
  Buchanan's M91.0
  Burns' —*see* Osteochondrosis, juvenile, ulna
  calcaneus (juvenile) —*see* Osteochondrosis, juvenile, tarsus
  capitular epiphysis (femur) (juvenile) —*see* Legg-Calvé-Perthes disease
  carpal (juvenile) (lunate) (scaphoid) —*see* Osteochondrosis, juvenile, hand, carpal lunate
    adult M93.1
  coxae juvenilis —*see* Legg-Calvé-Perthes disease
  deformans juvenilis, coxae —*see* Legg-Calvé-Perthes disease
  Diaz's —*see* Osteochondrosis, juvenile, tarsus
  dissecans (knee) (shoulder) —*see* Osteochondritis, dissecans
  femoral capital epiphysis (juvenile) —*see* Legg-Calvé-Perthes disease

Osteochondrosis *(Continued)*
  femur (head), juvenile —*see* Legg-Calvé-Perthes disease
  fibula (juvenile) —*see* Osteochondrosis, juvenile, fibula
  foot NEC (juvenile) M92.8
  Freiberg's —*see* Osteochondrosis, juvenile, metatarsus
  Haas' (juvenile) —*see* Osteochondrosis, juvenile, humerus
  Haglund's —*see* Osteochondrosis, juvenile, tarsus
  hip (juvenile) —*see* Legg-Calvé-Perthes disease
  humerus (capitulum) (head) (juvenile) —*see* Osteochondrosis, juvenile, humerus
  ilium, iliac crest (juvenile) M91.0
  ischiopubic synchondrosis M91.0
  Iselin's —*see* Osteochondrosis, juvenile, metatarsus
  juvenile, juvenilis M92.9
    after congenital dislocation of hip reduction —*see* Osteochondrosis, juvenile, hip, specified NEC
    arm —*see* Osteochondrosis, juvenile, upper limb NEC
    capitular epiphysis (femur) —*see* Legg-Calvé-Perthes disease
    clavicle, sternal epiphysis —*see* Osteochondrosis, juvenile, upper limb NEC
    coxae —*see* Legg-Calvé-Perthes disease
    deformans M92.9
    fibula M92.5-
    foot NEC M92.8
    hand M92.20-
      carpal lunate M92.21-
      metacarpal head M92.22-
      specified site NEC M92.29-
    head of femur —*see* Legg-Calvé-Perthes disease
    hip and pelvis M91.9-
      coxa plana —*see* Coxa, plana
      femoral head —*see* Legg-Calvé-Perthes disease
      pelvis M91.0
      pseudocoxalgia —*see* Pseudocoxalgia
      specified NEC M91.8-
    humerus M92.0-
    limb
      lower NEC M92.8
      upper NEC —*see* Osteochondrosis, juvenile, upper limb NEC
    medial cuneiform bone —*see* Osteochondrosis, juvenile, tarsus
    metatarsus M92.7-
    patella M92.4-
    radius M92.1-
    specified site NEC M92.8
    spine M42.00
      cervical region M42.02
      cervicothoracic region M42.03
      lumbar region M42.06
      lumbosacral region M42.07
      multiple sites M42.09
      occipito-atlanto-axial region M42.01
      sacrococcygeal region M42.08
      thoracic region M42.04
      thoracolumbar region M42.05
    tarsus M92.6-
    tibia M92.5-
    ulna M92.1-
    upper limb NEC M92.3-
    vertebra (body) (epiphyseal plates) (Calvé's) (Scheuermann's) —*see* Osteochondrosis, juvenile, spine
  Kienböck's —*see* Osteochondrosis, juvenile, hand, carpal lunate
    adult M93.1

Osteochondrosis *(Continued)*
  Köhler's
    patellar —*see* Osteochondrosis, juvenile, patella
    tarsal navicular —*see* Osteochondrosis, juvenile, tarsus
  Legg-Perthes (-Calvé's) (-Waldenström) —*see* Legg-Calvé-Perthes disease
  limb
    lower NEC (juvenile) M92.8
    upper NEC (juvenile) —*see* Osteochondrosis, juvenile, upper limb NEC
  lunate bone (carpal) (juvenile) —*see also* Osteochondrosis, juvenile, hand, carpal lunate
    adult M93.1
  Mauclaire's —*see* Osteochondrosis, juvenile, hand, metacarpal
  metacarpal (head) (juvenile) —*see* Osteochondrosis, juvenile, hand, metacarpal
  metatarsus (fifth) (head) (juvenile) (second) —*see* Osteochondrosis, juvenile, metatarsus
  navicular (juvenile) —*see* Osteochondrosis, juvenile, tarsus
  os
    calcis (juvenile) —*see* Osteochondrosis, juvenile, tarsus
    tibiale externum (juvenile) —*see* Osteochondrosis, juvenile, tarsus
  Osgood-Schlatter —*see* Osteochondrosis, juvenile, tibia
  Panner's —*see* Osteochondrosis, juvenile, humerus
  patellar center (juvenile) (primary) (secondary) —*see* Osteochondrosis, juvenile, patella
  pelvis (juvenile) M91.0
  Pierson's M91.0
  radius (head) (juvenile) —*see* Osteochondrosis, juvenile, radius
  Scheuermann's —*see* Osteochondrosis, juvenile, spine
  Sever's —*see* Osteochondrosis, juvenile, tarsus
  Sinding-Larsen —*see* Osteochondrosis, juvenile, patella
  spine M42.9
    adult M42.10
      cervical region M42.12
      cervicothoracic region M42.13
      lumbar region M42.16
      lumbosacral region M42.17
      multiple sites M42.19
      occipito-atlanto-axial region M42.11
      sacrococcygeal region M42.18
      thoracic region M42.14
      thoracolumbar region M42.15
    juvenile —*see* Osteochondrosis, juvenile, spine
  symphysis pubis (juvenile) M91.0
  syphilitic (congenital) A50.02
  talus (juvenile) —*see* Osteochondrosis, juvenile, tarsus
  tarsus (navicular) (juvenile) —*see* Osteochondrosis, juvenile, tarsus
  tibia (proximal) (tubercle) (juvenile) —*see* Osteochondrosis, juvenile, tibia
  tuberculous —*see* Tuberculosis, bone
  ulna (lower) (juvenile) —*see* Osteochondrosis, juvenile, ulna
  van Neck's M91.0
  vertebral —*see* Osteochondrosis, spine
Osteoclastoma D48.0
  malignant —*see* Neoplasm, bone, malignant
Osteodynia —*see* Disorder, bone, specified type NEC

◀ New   ◀▦ Revised   ~~deleted~~ Deleted

Osteodystrophy Q78.9
  azotemic N25.0
  congenital Q78.9
  parathyroid, secondary E21.1
  renal N25.0
Osteofibroma —*see* Neoplasm, bone,
    benign
Osteofibrosarcoma —*see* Neoplasm,
    bone, malignant
Osteogenesis imperfecta Q78.0
Osteogenic —*see* condition
Osteolysis M89.50
  carpus M89.54-
  clavicle M89.51-
  femur M89.55-
  fibula M89.56-
  finger M89.54-
  humerus M89.52-
  ilium M89.559
  ischium M89.559
  joint prosthesis (periprosthetic) —*see*
      Complications, joint prosthesis,
      mechanical, periprosthetic, osteolysis,
      by site
  metacarpus M89.54-
  metatarsus M89.57-
  multiple sites M89.59
  neck M89.58
  periprosthetic —*see* Complications, joint
      prosthesis, mechanical, periprosthetic,
      osteolysis, by site
  radius M89.53-
  rib M89.58
  scapula M89.51-
  skull M89.58
  tarsus M89.57-
  tibia M89.56-
  toe M89.57-
  ulna M89.53-
  vertebra M89.58
Osteoma —*see also* Neoplasm, bone, benign
  osteoid —*see also* Neoplasm, bone, benign
    giant —*see* Neoplasm, bone, benign
Osteomalacia M83.9
  adult M83.9
    drug-induced NEC M83.5
    due to
        malabsorption (postsurgical)
            M83.2
        malnutrition M83.3
      specified NEC M83.8
    aluminium-induced M83.4
  infantile —*see* Rickets
  juvenile —*see* Rickets
  oncogenic E83.89
  pelvis M83.8
  puerperal M83.0
  senile M83.1
  vitamin-D-resistant in adults E83.31
        [*M90.8-*]
    carpus E83.31 [*M90.84-*]
    clavicle E83.31 [*M90.81-*]
    femur E83.31 [*M90.85-*]
    fibula E83.31 [*M90.86-*]
    finger E83.31 [*M90.84-*]
    humerus E83.31 [*M90.82-*]
    ilium E83.31 [*M90.859*]
    ischium E83.31 [*M90.859*]
    metacarpus E83.31 [*M90.84-*]
    metatarsus E83.31 [*M90.87-*]
    multiple sites E83.31 [*M90.89*]
    neck E83.31 [*M90.88*]
    radius E83.31 [*M90.83-*]
    rib E83.31 [*M90.88*]
    scapula E83.31 [*M90.819*]
    skull E83.31 [*M90.88*]
    tarsus E83.31 [*M90.879*]
    tibia E83.31 [*M90.869*]
    toe E83.31 [*M90.879*]
    ulna E83.31 [*M90.839*]
    vertebra E83.31 [*M90.88*]

Osteomyelitis (general) (infective)
    (localized) (neonatal) (purulent)
    (septic) (staphylococcal) (streptococcal)
    (suppurative) (with periostitis) M86.9
  acute M86.10
    carpus M86.14-
    clavicle M86.11-
    femur M86.15-
    fibula M86.16-
    finger M86.14-
    hematogenous M86.00
      carpus M86.04-
      clavicle M86.01-
      femur M86.05-
      fibula M86.06-
      finger M86.04-
      humerus M86.02-
      ilium M86.059
      ischium M86.059
      mandible M27.2
      metacarpus M86.04-
      metatarsus M86.07-
      multiple sites M86.09
      neck M86.08
      orbit H05.02-
      petrous bone —*see* Petrositis
      radius M86.03-
      rib M86.08
      scapula M86.01-
      skull M86.08
      tarsus M86.07-
      tibia M86.06-
      toe M86.07-
      ulna M86.03-
      vertebra —*see* Osteomyelitis, vertebra
    humerus M86.12-
    ilium M86.159
    ischium M86.159
    mandible M27.2
    metacarpus M86.14-
    metatarsus M86.17-
    multiple sites M86.19
    neck M86.18
    orbit H05.02-
    petrous bone —*see* Petrositis
    radius M86.13-
    rib M86.18
    scapula M86.11-
    skull M86.18
    tarsus M86.17-
    tibia M86.16-
    toe M86.17-
    ulna M86.13-
    vertebra —*see* Osteomyelitis, vertebra
  chronic (or old) M86.60
    with draining sinus M86.40
      carpus M86.44-
      clavicle M86.41-
      femur M86.45-
      fibula M86.46-
      finger M86.44-
      humerus M86.42-
      ilium M86.459
      ischium M86.459
      mandible M27.2
      metacarpus M86.44-
      metatarsus M86.47-
      multiple sites M86.49
      neck M86.48
      orbit H05.02-
      petrous bone —*see* Petrositis
      radius M86.43-
      rib M86.48
      scapula M86.41-
      skull M86.48
      tarsus M86.47-
      tibia M86.46-
      toe M86.47-
      ulna M86.43-
      vertebra —*see* Osteomyelitis, vertebra
    carpus M86.64-

Osteomyelitis (*Continued*)
  chronic (*Continued*)
    clavicle M86.61-
    femur M86.65-
    fibula M86.66-
    finger M86.64-
    hematogenous NEC M86.50
      carpus M86.54-
      clavicle M86.51-
      femur M86.55-
      fibula M86.56-
      finger M86.54-
      humerus M86.52-
      ilium M86.559
      ischium M86.559
      mandible M27.2
      metacarpus M86.54-
      metatarsus M86.57-
      multifocal M86.30
        carpus M86.34-
        clavicle M86.31-
        femur M86.35-
        fibula M86.36-
        finger M86.34-
        humerus M86.32-
        ilium M86.359
        ischium M86.359
        metacarpus M86.34-
        metatarsus M86.37-
        multiple sites M86.39
        neck M86.38
        radius M86.33-
        rib M86.38
        scapula M86.31-
        skull M86.38
        tarsus M86.37-
        tibia M86.36-
        toe M86.37-
        ulna M86.33-
        vertebra —*see* Osteomyelitis, vertebra
      multiple sites M86.59
      neck M86.58
      orbit H05.02-
      petrous bone —*see* Petrositis
      radius M86.53-
      rib M86.58
      scapula M86.51-
      skull M86.58
      tarsus M86.57-
      tibia M86.56-
      toe M86.57-
      ulna M86.53-
      vertebra —*see* Osteomyelitis, vertebra
    humerus M86.62-
    ilium M86.659
    ischium M86.659
    mandible M27.2
    metacarpus M86.64-
    metatarsus M86.67-
    multifocal —*see* Osteomyelitis, chronic,
        hematogenous, multifocal
    multiple sites M86.69
    neck M86.68
    orbit H05.02-
    petrous bone —*see* Petrositis
    radius M86.63-
    rib M86.68
    scapula M86.61-
    skull M86.68
    tarsus M86.67-
    tibia M86.66-
    toe M86.67-
    ulna M86.63-
    vertebra —*see* Osteomyelitis, vertebra
  echinococcal B67.2
  Garr's —*see* Osteomyelitis, specified type
        NEC
  jaw (acute) (chronic) (lower) (neonatal)
        (suppurative) (upper) M27.2
  nonsuppurating —*see* Osteomyelitis,
        specified type NEC

Osteomyelitis (Continued)
orbit H05.02-
petrous bone —see Petrositis
Salmonella (arizonae) (cholerae-suis)
    (enteritidis) (typhimurium) A02.24
sclerosing, nonsuppurative —see
    Osteomyelitis, specified type NEC
specified type NEC (see also subcategory)
    M86.8X-
  mandible M27.2
  orbit H05.02-
  petrous bone —see Petrositis
  vertebra —see Osteomyelitis, vertebra
subacute M86.20
  carpus M86.24-
  clavicle M86.21-
  femur M86.25-
  fibula M86.26-
  finger M86.24-
  humerus M86.22-
  mandible M27.2
  metacarpus M86.24-
  metatarsus M86.27-
  multiple sites M86.29
  neck M86.28
  orbit H05.02-
  petrous bone —see Petrositis
  radius M86.23-
  rib M86.28
  scapula M86.21-
  skull M86.28
  tarsus M86.27-
  tibia M86.26-
  toe M86.27-
  ulna M86.23-
  vertebra —see Osteomyelitis, vertebra
syphilitic A52.77
  congenital (early) A50.02 [M90.80]
tuberculous —see Tuberculosis, bone
typhoid A01.05
vertebra M46.20
  cervical region M46.22
  cervicothoracic region M46.23
  lumbar region M46.26
  lumbosacral region M46.27
  occipito-atlanto-axial region M46.21
  sacrococcygeal region M46.28
  thoracic region M46.24
  thoracolumbar region M46.25
Osteomyelofibrosis D75.89
Osteomyelosclerosis D75.89
Osteonecrosis M87.9
due to
  drugs —see Osteonecrosis, secondary, due
    to, drugs
  trauma —see Osteonecrosis, secondary, due
    to, trauma
idiopathic aseptic M87.00
  ankle M87.07-
  carpus M87.03-
  clavicle M87.01-
  femur M87.05-
  fibula M87.06-
  finger M87.04-
  humerus M87.02-
  ilium M87.050
  ischium M87.050
  metacarpus M87.04-
  metatarsus M87.07-
  multiple sites M87.09
  neck M87.08
  pelvis M87.050
  radius M87.03-
  rib M87.08
  scapula M87.01-
  skull M87.08
  tarsus M87.07-
  tibia M87.06-
  toe M87.07-
  ulna M87.03-
  vertebra M87.08

Osteonecrosis (Continued)
secondary NEC M87.30
  carpus M87.33-
  clavicle M87.31-
  due to
    drugs M87.10
      carpus M87.13-
      clavicle M87.11-
      femur M87.15-
      fibula M87.16-
      finger M87.14-
      humerus M87.12-
      ilium M87.159
      ischium M87.159
      jaw M87.180
      metacarpus M87.14-
      metatarsus M87.17-
      multiple sites M87.19
      neck M87.18
      radius M87.13-
      rib M87.18
      scapula M87.11-
      skull M87.18
      tarsus M87.17-
      tibia M87.16-
      toe M87.17-
      ulna M87.13-
      vertebra M87.18
    hemoglobinopathy NEC D58.2 [M90.50]
      carpus D58.2 [M90.54-]
      clavicle D58.2 [M90.51-]
      femur D58.2 [M90.55-]
      fibula D58.2 [M90.56-]
      finger D58.2 [M90.54-]
      humerus D58.2 [M90.52-]
      ilium D58.2 [M90.55-]
      ischium D58.2 [M90.55-]
      metacarpus D58.2 [M90.54-]
      metatarsus D58.2 [M90.57-]
      multiple sites D58.2 [M90.58]
      neck D58.2 [M90.58]
      radius D58.2 [M90.53-]
      rib D58.2 [M90.58]
      scapula D58.2 [M90.51-]
      skull D58.2 [M90.58]
      tarsus D58.2 [M90.57-]
      tibia D58.2 [M90.56-]
      toe D58.2 [M90.57-]
      ulna D58.2 [M90.53-]
      vertebra D58.2 [M90.58]
    trauma (previous) M87.20
      carpus M87.23-
      clavicle M87.21-
      femur M87.25-
      fibula M87.26-
      finger M87.24-
      humerus M87.22-
      ilium M87.25-
      ischium M87.25-
      metacarpus M87.24-
      metatarsus M87.27-
      multiple sites M87.29
      neck M87.28
      radius M87.23-
      rib M87.28
      scapula M87.21-
      skull M87.28
      tarsus M87.27-
      tibia M87.26-
      toe M87.27-
      ulna M87.23-
      vertebra M87.28
  femur M87.35-
  fibula M87.36-
  finger M87.34-
  humerus M87.32
  ilium M87.350
  in
    caisson disease T70.3 [M90.50]
      carpus T70.3 [M90.54-]
      clavicle T70.3 [M90.51-]

Osteonecrosis (Continued)
secondary NEC (Continued)
  in (Continued)
    caisson disease (Continued)
      femur T70.3 [M90.55-]
      fibula T70.3 [M90.56-]
      finger T70.3 [M90.54-]
      humerus T70.3 [M90.52-]
      ilium T70.3 [M90.55-]
      ischium T70.3 [M90.55-]
      metacarpus T70.3 [M90.54-]
      metatarsus T70.3 [M90.57-]
      multiple sites T70.3 [M90.59]
      neck T70.3 [M90.58]
      radius T70.3 [M90.53-]
      rib T70.3 [M90.58]
      scapula T70.3 [M90.51-]
      skull T70.3 [M90.58]
      tarsus T70.3 [M90.57-]
      tibia T70.3 [M90.56-]
      toe T70.3 [M90.57-]
      ulna T70.3 [M90.53-]
      vertebra T70.3 [M90.58]
  ischium M87.350
  metacarpus M87.34-
  metatarsus M87.37-
  multiple site M87.39
  neck M87.38
  radius M87.33-
  rib M87.38
  scapula M87.319
  skull M87.38
  tarsus M87.379
  tibia M87.366
  toe M87.379
  ulna M87.33-
  vertebra M87.38
specified type NEC M87.80
  carpus M87.83-
  clavicle M87.81-
  femur M87.85-
  fibula M87.86-
  finger M87.84-
  humerus M87.82-
  ilium M87.85-
  ischium M87.85-
  metacarpus M87.84-
  metatarsus M87.87-
  multiple sites M87.89
  neck M87.88
  radius M87.83-
  rib M87.88-
  scapula M87.81-
  skull M87.88
  tarsus M87.87-
  tibia M87.86-
  toe M87.87-
  ulna M87.83-
  vertebra M87.88
Osteo-onycho-arthro-dysplasia Q79.8
Osteo-onychodysplasia, hereditary Q79.8
Osteopathia condensans disseminata Q78.8
Osteopathy —see also Osteomyelitis,
  Osteonecrosis, Osteoporosis
after poliomyelitis M89.60
  carpus M89.64-
  clavicle M89.61-
  femur M89.65-
  fibula M89.66-
  finger M89.64-
  humerus M89.62-
  ilium M89.659
  ischium M89.659
  metacarpus M89.64-
  metatarsus M89.67-
  multiple sites M89.69
  neck M89.68
  radius M89.63-
  rib M89.68
  scapula M89.61-
  skull M89.68

◀ New   ◀█ Revised   ~~deleted~~ Deleted

Otitis *(Continued)*
  media *(Continued)*
    chronic *(Continued)*
      catarrhal —*see* Otitis, media,
        nonsuppurative, chronic, serous
      exudative —*see* Otitis, media,
        nonsuppurative, chronic
      mucinous —*see* Otitis, media,
        nonsuppurative, chronic, mucoid
      mucoid —*see* Otitis, media,
        nonsuppurative, chronic, mucoid
      nonsuppurative NEC —*see* Otitis, media,
        nonsuppurative, chronic
      purulent —*see* Otitis, media,
        suppurative, chronic
      secretory —*see* Otitis, media,
        nonsuppurative, chronic, mucoid
      seromucinous —*see* Otitis, media,
        nonsuppurative, chronic
      serous —*see* Otitis, media,
        nonsuppurative, chronic, serous
      suppurative —*see* Otitis, media,
        suppurative, chronic
      transudative —*see* Otitis, media,
        nonsuppurative, chronic, mucoid
    exudative —*see* Otitis, media,
      nonsuppurative
    in (due to) (with)
      influenza —*see* Influenza, with, otitis
        media
      measles B05.3
      scarlet fever A38.0
      tuberculosis A18.6
      viral disease NEC B34.- *[H67.-]*
    mucoid —*see* Otitis, media,
      nonsuppurative
    nonsuppurative H65.9-
      acute or subacute NEC H65.19-
        allergic H65.11-
          recurrent H65.11-
        recurrent H65.19-
        secretory —*see* Otitis, media,
          nonsuppurative, serous
        serous H65.0-
          recurrent H65.0-
      chronic H65.49-
        allergic H65.41-
        mucoid H65.3-
        serous H65.2-
      postmeasles B05.3
    purulent —*see* Otitis, media, suppurative
    secretory —*see* Otitis, media,
      nonsuppurative
    seromucinous —*see* Otitis, media,
      nonsuppurative
    serous —*see* Otitis, media, nonsuppurative
    suppurative H66.4-
      acute H66.00-
        with rupture of ear drum H66.01-
        recurrent H66.00-
          with rupture of ear drum H66.01-
      chronic (*see also* subcategory) H66.3
        atticoantral H66.2-
        benign —*see* Otitis, media,
          suppurative, chronic,
          tubotympanic
        tubotympanic H66.1-
    transudative —*see* Otitis, media,
      nonsuppurative
    tuberculous A18.6

Otocephaly Q18.2
Otolith syndrome —*see* subcategory H81.8
Otomycosis (diffuse) NEC B36.9 *[H62.40]*
  in
    aspergillosis B44.89
    candidiasis B37.84
    moniliasis B37.84
Otoporosis —*see* Otosclerosis
Otorrhagia (nontraumatic) H92.2-
  traumatic - code by Type of injury
Otorrhea H92.1-
  cerebrospinal G96.0
Otosclerosis (general) H80.9-
  cochlear (endosteal) H80.2-
  involving
    otic capsule —*see* Otosclerosis, cochlear
    oval window
      nonobliterative H80.0-
      obliterative H80.1-
    round window —*see* Otosclerosis, cochlear
  nonobliterative —*see* Otosclerosis, involving,
    oval window, nonobliterative
  obliterative —*see* Otosclerosis, involving, oval
    window, obliterative
  specified NEC H80.8-
Otospongiosis —*see* Otosclerosis
Otto's disease or pelvis M24.7
Outcome of delivery Z37.9
  multiple births Z37.9
    all liveborn Z37.50
      quadruplets Z37.52
      quintuplets Z37.53
      sextuplets Z37.54
      specified number NEC Z37.59
      triplets Z37.51
    all stillborn Z37.7
    some liveborn Z37.60
      quadruplets Z37.62
      quintuplets Z37.63
      sextuplets Z37.64
      specified number NEC Z37.69
      triplets Z37.61
  single NEC Z37.9
    liveborn Z37.0
    stillborn Z37.1
  twins NEC Z37.9
    both liveborn Z37.2
    both stillborn Z37.4
    one liveborn, one stillborn Z37.3
Outlet —*see* condition
Ovalocytosis (congenital) (hereditary) —*see*
  Elliptocytosis
Ovarian —*see* Condition
Ovariocele N83.4
Ovaritis (cystic) —*see* Oophoritis
Ovary, ovarian —*see also* condition
  resistant syndrome E28.39
  vein syndrome N13.8
Overactive —*see also* Hyperfunction
  adrenal cortex NEC E27.0
  bladder N32.81
  hypothalamus E23.3
  thyroid —*see* Hyperthyroidism
Overactivity R46.3
  child —*see* Disorder, attention-deficit
    hyperactivity
Overbite (deep) (excessive) (horizontal)
  (vertical) M26.29
Overbreathing —*see* Hyperventilation
Overconscientious personality F60.5

Overdevelopment —*see* Hypertrophy
Overdistension —*see* Distension
Overdose, overdosage (drug) —*see* Table
  of Drugs and Chemicals, by drug,
  poisoning
Overeating R63.2
  nonorganic origin F50.8
  psychogenic F50.8
Overexertion (effects) (exhaustion) T73.3
Overexposure (effects) T73.9
  exhaustion T73.2
Overfeeding —*see* Overeating
  newborn P92.4
Overfill, endodontic M27.52
Overgrowth, bone —*see* Hypertrophy, bone
Overhanging of dental restorative material
  (unrepairable) K08.52
Overheated (places) (effects) —*see* Heat
Overjet (excessive horizontal) M26.23
Overlaid, overlying (suffocation) —*see* Asphyxia,
  traumatic, due to mechanical threat
Overlap, excessive horizontal (teeth) M26.23
Overlapping toe (acquired) —*see also*
  Deformity, toe, specified NEC
  congenital (fifth toe) Q66.89
Overload
  circulatory, due to transfusion (blood) (blood
    components) (TACO) E87.71
  fluid E87.70
    due to transfusion (blood) (blood
      components) E87.71
    specified NEC E87.79
  iron, due to repeated red blood cell
    transfusions E83.111
  potassium (K) E87.5
  sodium (Na) E87.0
Overnutrition —*see* Hyperalimentation
Overproduction —*see also* Hypersecretion
  ACTH E27.0
  catecholamine E27.5
  growth hormone E22.0
Overprotection, child by parent Z62.1
Overriding
  aorta Q25.4
  finger (acquired) —*see* Deformity, finger
    congenital Q68.1
  toe (acquired) —*see also* Deformity, toe,
    specified NEC
    congenital Q66.89
Overstrained R53.83
  heart —*see* Hypertrophy, cardiac
Overuse, muscle NEC M70.8-
Overweight E66.3
Overworked R53.83
Oviduct —*see* condition
Ovotestis Q56.0
Ovulation (cycle)
  failure or lack of N97.0
  pain N94.0
Ovum —*see* condition
Owren's disease or syndrome (parahemophilia)
  D68.2
Ox heart —*see* Hypertrophy, cardiac
Oxalosis E72.53
Oxaluria E72.53
Oxycephaly, oxycephalic Q75.0
  syphilitic, congenital A50.02
Oxyuriasis B80
Oxyuris vermicularis (infestation) B80
Ozena J31.0

◄ New   ◀▥ Revised   ~~deleted~~ Deleted

P

Pachyderma, pachydermia L85.9
  larynx (verrucosa) J38.7
Pachydermatocele (congenital) Q82.8
Pachydermoperiostosis —*see also*
    Osteoarthropathy, hypertrophic, specified
     type NEC
  clubbed nail M89.40 *[L62]*
Pachygyria Q04.3
Pachymeningitis (adhesive) (basal) (brain)
    (cervical) (chronic) (circumscribed)
    (external) (fibrous) (hemorrhagic)
    (hypertrophic) (internal) (purulent)
    (spinal) (suppurative) —*see* Meningitis
Pachyonychia (congenital) Q84.5
Pacinian tumor —*see* Neoplasm, skin, benign
Pad, knuckle or Garrod's M72.1
Paget-Schroetter syndrome I82.890
Paget's disease
  with infiltrating duct carcinoma —*see*
    Neoplasm, breast, malignant
  bone M88.9
    carpus M88.84-
    clavicle M88.81-
    femur M88.85-
    fibula M88.86-
    finger M88.84-
    humerus M88.82-
    ilium M88.85-
    in neoplastic disease —*see* Osteitis,
     deformans, in neoplastic disease
    ischium M88.85-
    metacarpus M88.84-
    metatarsus M88.87-
    multiple sites M88.89
    neck M88.88
    radius M88.83-
    rib M88.88
    scapula M88.81-
    skull M88.0
    tarsus M88.87-
    tibia M88.86-
    toe M88.87-
    ulna M88.83-
    vertebra M88.88
  breast (female) C50.01-
    male C50.02-
  extramammary —*see also* Neoplasm, skin,
    malignant
    anus C21.0
     margin C44.590
     skin C44.590
  intraductal carcinoma —*see* Neoplasm,
    breast, malignant
  malignant —*see* Neoplasm, skin, malignant
    breast (female) C50.01-
     male C50.02-
    unspecified site (female) C50.01-
     male C50.02-
  mammary —*see* Paget's disease, breast
  nipple —*see* Paget's disease, breast
  osteitis deformans —*see* Paget's disease, bone
Pain (s) (*see also* Painful) R52
  abdominal R10.9
    colic R10.83
    generalized R10.84
     with acute abdomen R10.0
    lower R10.30
     left quadrant R10.32
     pelvic or perineal R10.2
     periumbilical R10.33
     right quadrant R10.31
    rebound —*see* Tenderness, abdominal,
     rebound
    severe with abdominal rigidity R10.0
    tenderness —*see* Tenderness, abdominal
    upper R10.10
     epigastric R10.13
     left quadrant R10.12
     right quadrant R10.11

Pain (*Continued*)
  acute R52
    due to trauma G89.11
    neoplasm related G89.3
    postprocedural NEC G89.18
    post-thoracotomy G89.12
    specified by site — code to Pain, by site
  adnexa (uteri) R10.2
  anginoid —*see* Pain, precordial
  anus K62.89
  arm —*see* Pain, limb, upper
  axillary (axilla) M79.62-
  back (postural) M54.9
  bladder R39.89
    associated with micturition —*see*
     Micturition, painful
  bone —*see* Disorder, bone, specified type
    NEC
  breast N64.4
  broad ligament R10.2
  cancer associated (acute) (chronic) G89.3
  cecum —*see* Pain, abdominal
  cervicobrachial M53.1
  chest (central) R07.9
    anterior wall R07.89
    atypical R07.89
    ischemic I20.9
    musculoskeletal R07.89
    non-cardiac R07.89
    on breathing R07.1
    pleurodynia R07.81
    precordial R07.2
    wall (anterior) R07.89
  chronic G89.29
    associated with significant psychosocial
     dysfunction G89.4
    due to trauma G89.21
    neoplasm related G89.3
    postoperative NEC G89.28
    postprocedural NEC G89.28
    post-thoracotomy G89.22
    specified NEC G89.29
  coccyx M53.3
  colon —*see* Pain, abdominal
  coronary —*see* Angina
  costochondral R07.1
  diaphragm R07.1
  due to cancer G89.3
  due to device, implant or graft (*see also*
    Complications, by site and type,
     specified NEC) T85.84
    arterial graft NEC T82.848
    breast (implant) T85.84
    catheter NEC T85.84
     dialysis (renal) T82.848
      intraperitoneal T85.84
     infusion NEC T82.848
      spinal (epidural) (subdural) T85.84
     urinary (indwelling) T83.84
    electronic (electrode) (pulse generator)
     (stimulator)
     bone T84.84
     cardiac T82.847
     nervous system (brain) (peripheral
      nerve) (spinal) T85.84
     urinary T83.84
    fixation, internal (orthopedic) NEC
     T84.84
    gastrointestinal (bile duct) (esophagus)
     T85.84
    genital NEC T83.84
    heart NEC T82.847
    infusion NEC T85.84
    joint prosthesis T84.84
    ocular (corneal graft) (orbital implant)
     NEC T85.84
    orthopedic NEC T84.84
    specified NEC T85.84
    urinary NEC T83.84
    vascular NEC T82.848
    ventricular intracranial shunt T85.84

Pain (*Continued*)
  due to malignancy (primary) (secondary)
    G89.3
  ear —*see* subcategory H92.0
  epigastric, epigastrium R10.13
  eye —*see* Pain, ocular
  face, facial R51
    atypical G50.1
  female genital organs NEC N94.89
  finger —*see* Pain, limb, upper
  flank —*see* Pain, abdominal
  foot —*see* Pain, limb, lower
  gallbladder K82.9
  gas (intestinal) R14.1
  gastric —*see* Pain, abdominal
  generalized NOS R52
  genital organ
    female N94.89
    male N50.8
  groin —*see* Pain, abdominal, lower
  hand —*see* Pain, limb, upper
  head —*see* Headache
  heart —*see* Pain, precordial
  infra-orbital —*see* Neuralgia, trigeminal
  intercostal R07.82
  intermenstrual N94.0
  jaw R68.84
  joint M25.50
    ankle M25.57-
    elbow M25.52-
    finger M79.64-
    foot M25.57-
    hand M79.64-
    hip M25.55-
    knee M25.56-
    shoulder M25.51-
    toe M25.57-
    wrist M25.53-
  kidney N23
  laryngeal R07.0
  leg —*see* Pain, limb, lower
  limb M79.609
    lower M79.60-
     foot M79.67-
     lower leg M79.66-
     thigh M79.65-
     toe M79.67-
    upper M79.60-
     axilla M79.62-
     finger M79.64-
     forearm M79.63-
     hand M79.64-
     upper arm M79.62-
  loin M54.5
  low back M54.5
  lumbar region M54.5
  mandibular R68.84
  mastoid —*see* subcategory H92.0
  maxilla R68.84
  menstrual (*see also* Dysmenorrhea) N94.6
  metacarpophalangeal (joint) —*see* Pain, joint,
    hand
  metatarsophalangeal (joint) —*see* Pain, joint,
    foot
  mouth K13.79
  muscle —*see* Myalgia
  musculoskeletal (*see also* Pain, by site) M79.1
  myofascial M79.1
  nasal J34.89
  nasopharynx J39.2
  neck NEC M54.2
  nerve NEC —*see* Neuralgia
  neuromuscular —*see* Neuralgia
  nose J34.89
  ocular H57.1-
  ophthalmic —*see* Pain, ocular
  orbital region —*see* Pain, ocular
  ovary N94.89
  over heart —*see* Pain, precordial
  ovulation N94.0
  pelvic (female) R10.2

Pain *(Continued)*
  penis N48.89
  pericardial —*see* Pain, precordial
  perineal, perineum R10.2
  pharynx J39.2
  pleura, pleural, pleuritic R07.81
  postoperative NOS G89.18
  postprocedural NOS G89.18
  post-thoracotomy G89.12
  precordial (region) R07.2
  premenstrual N94.3
  psychogenic (persistent) (any site) F45.41
  radicular (spinal) —*see* Radiculopathy
  rectum K62.89
  respiration R07.1
  retrosternal R07.2
  rheumatoid, muscular —*see* Myalgia
  rib R07.81
  root (spinal) —*see* Radiculopathy
  round ligament (stretch) R10.2
  sacroiliac M53.3
  sciatic —*see* Sciatica
  scrotum N50.8
  seminal vesicle N50.8
  shoulder M25.51-
  spermatic cord N50.8
  spinal root —*see* Radiculopathy
  spine M54.9
    cervical M54.2
    low back M54.5
      with sciatica M54.4-
    thoracic M54.6
  stomach —*see* Pain, abdominal
  substernal R07.2
  temporomandibular (joint) M26.62
  testis N50.8
  thoracic spine M54.6
    with radicular and visceral pain
      M54.14
  throat R07.0
  tibia —*see* Pain, limb, lower
  toe —*see* Pain, limb, lower
  tongue K14.6
  tooth K08.8
  trigeminal —*see* Neuralgia, trigeminal
  tumor associated G89.3
  ureter N23
  urinary (organ) (system) N23
  uterus NEC N94.89
  vagina R10.2
  vertebrogenic (syndrome) M54.89
  vesical R39.89
    associated with micturition —*see*
      Micturition, painful
  vulva R10.2
Painful —*see also* Pain
  coitus
    female N94.1
    male N53.12
    psychogenic F52.6
  ejaculation (semen) N53.12
    psychogenic F52.6
  erection —*see* Priapism
  feet syndrome E53.8
  joint replacement (hip) (knee) T84.84
  menstruation —*see* Dysmenorrhea
    psychogenic F45.8
  micturition —*see* Micturition, painful
  respiration R07.1
  scar NEC L90.5
  wire sutures T81.89
Painter's colic —*see* subcategory T56.0
Palate —*see* condition
Palatoplegia K13.79
Palatoschisis —*see* Cleft, palate
Palilalia R48.8
Palliative care Z51.5
Pallor R23.1
  optic disc, temporal —*see* Atrophy, optic
Palmar —*see also* condition
  fascia —*see* condition

Palpable
  cecum K63.89
  kidney N28.89
  ovary N83.8
  prostate N42.9
  spleen —*see* Splenomegaly
Palpitations (heart) R00.2
  psychogenic F45.8
Palsy (*see also* Paralysis) G83.9
  atrophic diffuse (progressive) G12.22
  Bell's —*see also* Palsy, facial
    newborn P11.3
  brachial plexus NEC G54.0
    newborn (birth injury) P14.3
  brain —*see* Palsy, cerebral
  bulbar (progressive) (chronic) G12.22
    of childhood (Fazio-Londe) G12.1
    pseudo NEC G12.29
    supranuclear (progressive) G23.1
  cerebral (congenital) G80.9
    ataxic G80.4
    athetoid G80.3
    choreathetoid G80.3
    diplegic G80.8
      spastic G80.1
    dyskinetic G80.3
      athetoid G80.3
      choreathetoid G80.3
      distonic G80.3
    dystonic G80.3
    hemiplegic G80.8
      spastic G80.2
    mixed G80.8
    monoplegic G80.8
      spastic G80.1
    paraplegic G80.8
      spastic G80.1
    quadriplegic G80.8
      spastic G80.0
    spastic G80.1
      diplegic G80.1
      hemiplegic G80.2
      monoplegic G80.1
      quadriplegic G80.0
      specified NEC G80.1
      tetrapelgic G80.0
    specified NEC G80.8
    syphilitic A52.12
      congenital A50.49
    tetraplegic G80.8
      spastic G80.0
  cranial nerve —*see also* Disorder, nerve,
    cranial
    multiple G52.7
      in
        infectious disease B99 [G53]
        neoplastic disease (*see also* Neoplasm)
          D49.9 [G53]
        parasitic disease B89 [G53]
        sarcoidosis D86.82
  creeping G12.22
  diver's T70.3
  Erb's P14.0
  facial G51.0
    newborn (birth injury) P11.3
  glossopharyngeal G52.1
  Klumpke (-Déjérine) P14.1
  lead —*see* subcategory T56.0
  median nerve (tardy) G56.1-
  nerve G58.9
    specified NEC G58.8
  peroneal nerve (acute) (tardy) G57.3-
  progressive supranuclear G23.1
  pseudobulbar NEC G12.29
  radial nerve (acute) G56.3-
  seventh nerve —*see also* Palsy, facial
    newborn P11.3
  shaking —*see* Parkinsonism
  spastic (cerebral) (spinal) G80.1
  ulnar nerve (tardy) G56.2-
  wasting G12.29

Paludism —*see* Malaria
Panangiitis M30.0
Panaris, panaritium —*see also* Cellulitis, digit
  with lymphangitis —*see* Lymphangitis, acute,
    digit
Panarteritis nodosa M30.0
  brain or cerebral I67.7
Pancake heart R93.1
  with cor pulmonale (chronic) I27.81
Pancarditis (acute) (chronic) I51.89
  rheumatic I09.89
    active or acute I01.8
Pancoast's syndrome or tumor C34.1-
Pancolitis, ulcerative (chronic) K51.00
  with
    abscess K51.014
    complication K51.019
    fistula K51.013
    obstruction K51.012
    rectal bleeding K51.011
    specified complication NEC K51.018
Pancreas, pancreatic —*see* condition
Pancreatitis (annular) (apoplectic) (calcareous)
  (edematous) (hemorrhagic) (malignant)
  (recurrent) (subacute) (suppurative) K85.9
  acute K85.9
    alcohol induced K85.2
    biliary K85.1
    drug induced K85.3
    gallstone K85.1
    idiopathic K85.0
    specified NEC K85.8
  chronic (infectious) K86.1
    alcohol-induced K86.0
    recurrent K86.1
    relapsing K86.1
  cystic (chronic) K86.1
  cytomegaloviral B25.2
  fibrous (chronic) K86.1
  gallstone K85.1
  gangrenous K85.8
  interstitial (chronic) K86.1
    acute K85.8
  mumps B26.3
  recurrent (chronic) K86.1
  relapsing, chronic K86.1
  syphilitic A52.74
Pancreatoblastoma —*see* Neoplasm, pancreas,
  malignant
Pancreolithiasis K86.8
Pancytolysis D75.89
Pancytopenia (acquired) D61.818
  with
    malformations D61.09
    myelodysplastic syndrome —*see*
      Syndrome, myelodysplastic
  antineoplastic chemotherapy induced
    D61.810
  congenital D61.09
  drug-induced NEC D61.811
Panencephalitis, subacute, sclerosing
  A81.1
Panhematopenia D61.9
  congenital D61.09
  constitutional D61.09
  splenic, primary D73.1
Panhemocytopenia D61.9
  congenital D61.09
  constitutional D61.09
Panhypogonadism E29.1
Panhypopituitarism E23.0
  prepubertal E23.0
Panic (attack) (state) F41.0
  reaction to exceptional stress (transient)
    F43.0
Panmyelopathy, familial, constitutional
  D61.09
Panmyelophthisis D61.82
  congenital D61.09
Panmyelosis (acute) (with myelofibrosis)
  C94.4-

◀ New   ◀▥ Revised   ~~deleted~~ Deleted

Panner's disease —see Osteochondrosis,
  juvenile, humerus
Panneuritis endemica E51.11
Panniculitis (nodular) (nonsuppurative) M79.3
  back M54.00
    cervical region M54.02
    cervicothoracic region M54.03
    lumbar region M54.06
    lumbosacral region M54.07
    multiple sites M54.09
    occipito-atlanto-axial region M54.01
    sacrococcygeal region M54.08
    thoracic region M54.04
    thoracolumbar region M54.05
  lupus L93.2
  mesenteric K65.4
  neck M54.02
    cervicothoracic region M54.03
    occipito-atlanto-axial region M54.01
  relapsing M35.6
Panniculus adiposus (abdominal) E65
Pannus (allergic) (cornea) (degenerativus)
    (keratic) H16.42-
  abdominal (symptomatic) E65
  trachomatosus, trachomatous (active) A71.1
Panophthalmitis H44.01-
Pansinusitis (chronic) (hyperplastic)
    (nonpurulent) (purulent) J32.4
  acute J01.40
    recurrent J01.41
  tuberculous A15.8
Panuveitis (sympathetic) H44.11-
Panvalvular disease I08.9
  specified NEC I08.8
Papanicolaou smear, cervix Z12.4
  as part of routine gynecological examination
      Z01.419
    with abnormal findings Z01.411
  for suspected neoplasm Z12.4
  nonspecific abnormal finding R87.619
  routine Z01.419
    with abnormal findings Z01.411
Papilledema (choked disc) H47.10
  associated with
    decreased ocular pressure H47.12
    increased intracranial pressure H47.11
    retinal disorder H47.13
  Foster-Kennedy syndrome H47.14-
Papillitis H46.00
  anus K62.89
  chronic lingual K14.4
  necrotizing, kidney N17.2
  optic H46.0-
  rectum K62.89
  renal, necrotizing N17.2
  tongue K14.0
Papilloma —see also Neoplasm, benign,
    by site
  acuminatum (female) (male) (anogenital)
      A63.0
  benign pinta (primary) A67.0
  bladder (urinary) (transitional cell) D41.4
  choroid plexus (lateral ventricle) (third
      ventricle) D33.0
    anaplastic C71.5
    fourth ventricle D33.1
    malignant C71.5
  renal pelvis (transitional cell) D41.1-
    benign D30.1-
  Schneiderian
    specified site —see Neoplasm, benign, by
        site
    unspecified site D14.0
  serous surface
    borderline malignancy
      specified site —see Neoplasm, uncertain
          behavior, by site
      unspecified site D39.10
    specified site —see Neoplasm, benign, by
        site
    unspecified site D27.9

Papilloma (Continued)
  transitional (cell)
    bladder (urinary) D41.4
    inverted type —see Neoplasm, uncertain
        behavior, by site
    renal pelvis D41.1-
    ureter D41.2-
  ureter (transitional cell) D41.2-
    benign D30.2-
  urothelial —see Neoplasm, uncertain
      behavior, by site
  villous —see Neoplasm, uncertain behavior,
      by site
    adenocarcinoma in —see Neoplasm,
        malignant, by site
    in situ —see Neoplasm, in situ
  yaws, plantar or palmar A66.1
Papillomata, multiple, of yaws A66.1
Papillomatosis —see also Neoplasm, benign,
    by site
  confluent and reticulated L83
  cystic, breast —see Mastopathy, cystic
  ductal, breast —see Mastopathy, cystic
  intraductal (diffuse) —see Neoplasm, benign,
      by site
  subareolar duct D24-
Papillomavirus, as cause of disease classified
    elsewhere B97.7
Papillon-Léage and Psaume syndrome
    Q87.0
Papule (s) R23.8
  carate (primary) A67.0
  fibrous, of nose D22.39
  Gottron's L94.4
  pinta (primary) A67.0
Papulosis
  lymphomatoid C86.6
  malignant I77.89
Papyraceous fetus O31.0-
Para-albuminemia E88.09
Paracephalus Q89.7
Parachute mitral valve Q23.2
Paracoccidioidomycosis B41.9
  disseminated B41.7
  generalized B41.7
  mucocutaneous-lymphangitic B41.8
  pulmonary B41.0
  specified NEC B41.8
  visceral B41.8
Paradentosis K05.4
Paraffinoma T88.8
Paraganglioma D44.7
  adrenal D35.0-
    malignant C74.1-
  aortic body D44.7
    malignant C75.5
  carotid body D44.6
    malignant C75.4
  chromaffin —see also Neoplasm, benign, by
      site
    malignant —see Neoplasm, malignant, by
        site
  extra-adrenal D44.7
    malignant C75.5
      specified site —see Neoplasm,
          malignant, by site
      unspecified site C75.5
    specified site —see Neoplasm, uncertain
        behavior, by site
    unspecified site D44.7
  gangliocytic D13.2
    specified site —see Neoplasm, benign, by
        site
    unspecified site D13.2
  glomus jugulare D44.7
    malignant C75.5
  jugular D44.7
  malignant C75.5
    specified site —see Neoplasm, malignant,
        by site
    unspecified site C75.5

Paraganglioma (Continued)
  nonchromaffin D44.7
    malignant C75.5
      specified site —see Neoplasm,
          malignant, by site
      unspecified site C75.5
    specified site —see Neoplasm, uncertain
        behavior, by site
    unspecified site D44.7
  parasympathetic D44.7
    specified site —see Neoplasm, uncertain
        behavior, by site
    unspecified site D44.7
  specified site —see Neoplasm, uncertain
      behavior, by site
  sympathetic D44.7
    specified site —see Neoplasm, uncertain
        behavior, by site
    unspecified site D44.7
  unspecified site D44.7
Parageusia R43.2
  psychogenic F45.8
Paragonimiasis B66.4
Paragranuloma, Hodgkin —see
    Lymphoma, Hodgkin, classical,
    specified NEC
Parahemophilia (see also Defect, coagulation)
    D68.2
Parakeratosis R23.4
  variegata L41.0
Paralysis, paralytic (complete) (incomplete)
    G83.9
  with
    syphilis A52.17
  abducens, abducent (nerve) —see Strabismus,
      paralytic, sixth nerve
  abductor, lower extremity G57.9-
  accessory nerve G52.8
  accommodation —see also Paresis, of
      accommodation
    hysterical F44.89
  acoustic nerve (except Deafness) —see
      subcategory H93.3
  agitans (see also Parkinsonism) G20
    arteriosclerotic G21.4
  alternating (oculomotor) G83.89
  amyotrophic G12.21
  ankle G57.9-
  anus (sphincter) K62.89
  arm —see Monoplegia, upper limb
  ascending (spinal), acute G61.0
  association G12.29
  asthenic bulbar G70.00
    with exacerbation (acute) G70.01
    in crisis G70.01
  ataxic (hereditary) G11.9
    general (syphilitic) A52.17
  atrophic G58.9
    infantile, acute —see Poliomyelitis,
        paralytic
    progressive G12.22
    spinal (acute) —see Poliomyelitis,
        paralytic
  axillary G54.0
  Babinski-Nageotte's G83.89
  Bell's G51.0
    newborn P11.3
  Benedikt's G46.3
  birth injury P14.9
    spinal cord P11.5
  bladder (neurogenic) (sphincter)
      N31.2
  bowel, colon or intestine K56.0
  brachial plexus G54.0
    birth injury P14.3
    newborn (birth injury) P14.3
  brain G83.9
    diplegia G83.0
    triplegia G83.89
  bronchial J98.09
  Brown-Séquard G83.81

Paralysis, paralytic *(Continued)*
bulbar (chronic) (progressive) G12.22
infantile —*see* Poliomyelitis, paralytic
poliomyelitic —*see* Poliomyelitis, paralytic
pseudo G12.29
bulbospinal G70.00
with exacerbation (acute) G70.01
in crisis G70.01
cardiac (*see also* Failure, heart) I50.9
cerebrocerebellar, diplegic G80.1
cervical
plexus G54.2
sympathetic G90.09
Céstan-Chenais G46.3
Charcot-Marie-Tooth type G60.0
Clark's G80.9
colon K56.0
compressed air T70.3
compression
arm G56.9-
leg G57.9-
lower extremity G57.9-
upper extremity G56.9-
congenital (cerebral) —*see* Palsy, cerebral
conjugate movement (gaze) (of eye) H51.0
cortical (nuclear) (supranuclear) H51.0
cordis —*see* Failure, heart
cranial or cerebral nerve G52.9
creeping G12.22
crossed leg G83.89
crutch —*see* Injury, brachial plexus
deglutition R13.0
hysterical F44.4
dementia A52.17
descending (spinal) NEC G12.29
diaphragm (flaccid) J98.6
due to accidental dissection of phrenic
nerve during procedure —*see*
Puncture, accidental complicating
surgery
digestive organs NEC K59.8
diplegic —*see* Diplegia
divergence (nuclear) H51.8
diver's T70.3
Duchenne's
birth injury P14.0
due to or associated with
motor neuron disease G12.22
muscular dystrophy G71.0
due to intracranial or spinal birth injury —*see*
Palsy, cerebral
embolic (current episode) I63.4
Erb (-Duchenne) (birth) (newborn) P14.0
Erb's syphilitic spastic spinal A52.17
esophagus K22.8
eye muscle (extrinsic) H49.9
intrinsic —*see also* Paresis, of
accommodation
facial (nerve) G51.0
birth injury P11.3
congenital P11.3
following operation NEC —*see* Puncture,
accidental complicating surgery
newborn (birth injury) P11.3
familial (recurrent) (periodic) G72.3
spastic G11.4
fauces J39.2
finger G56.9-
gait R26.1
gastric nerve (nondiabetic) G52.2
gaze, conjugate H51.0
general (progressive) (syphilitic) A52.17
juvenile A50.45
glottis J38.00
bilateral J38.02
unilateral J38.01
gluteal G54.1
Gubler (-Millard) G46.3
hand —*see* Monoplegia, upper limb
heart —*see* Arrest, cardiac
hemiplegic —*see* Hemiplegia

Paralysis, paralytic *(Continued)*
hyperkalemic periodic (familial) G72.3
hypoglossal (nerve) G52.3
hypokalemic periodic G72.3
hysterical F44.4
ileus K56.0
infantile (*see also* Poliomyelitis, paralytic)
A80.30
bulbar —*see* Poliomyelitis, paralytic
cerebral —*see* Palsy, cerebral
spastic —*see* Palsy, cerebral, spastic
infective —*see* Poliomyelitis, paralytic
inferior nuclear G83.9
internuclear —*see* Ophthalmoplegia,
internuclear
intestine K56.0
iris H57.09
due to diphtheria (toxin) A36.89
ischemic, Volkmann's (complicating trauma)
T79.6
Jackson's G83.89
jake —*see* Poisoning, food, noxious, plant
Jamaica ginger (jake) G62.2
juvenile general A50.45
Klumpke (-Déjérine) (birth) (newborn) P14.1
labioglossal (laryngeal) (pharyngeal) G12.29
Landry's G61.0
laryngeal nerve (recurrent) (superior)
(unilateral) J38.00
bilateral J38.02
unilateral J38.01
larynx J38.00
bilateral J38.02
due to diphtheria (toxin) A36.2
unilateral J38.01
lateral G12.21
lead —*see* subcategory T56.0
left side —*see* Hemiplegia
leg G83.1-
both —*see* Paraplegia
crossed G83.89
hysterical F44.4
psychogenic F44.4
transient or transitory R29.818
traumatic NEC —*see* Injury, nerve, leg
levator palpebrae superioris —*see*
Blepharoptosis, paralytic
limb —*see* Monoplegia
lip K13.0
Lissauer's A52.17
lower limb —*see* Monoplegia, lower limb
both —*see* Paraplegia
lung J98.4
median nerve G56.1-
medullary (tegmental) G83.89
mesencephalic NEC G83.89
tegmental G83.89
middle alternating G83.89
Millard-Gubler-Foville G46.3
monoplegic —*see* Monoplegia
motor G83.9
muscle, muscular NEC G72.89
due to nerve lesion G58.9
eye (extrinsic) H49.9
intrinsic —*see* Paresis, of accommodation
oblique —*see* Strabismus, paralytic,
fourth nerve
iris sphincter H21.9
ischemic (Volkmann's) (complicating
trauma) T79.6
progressive G12.21
pseudohypertrophic G71.0
musculocutaneous nerve G56.9-
musculospiral G56.9-
nerve —*see also* Disorder, nerve
abducent —*see* Strabismus, paralytic, sixth
nerve
accessory G52.8
auditory (except Deafness) —*see*
subcategory H93.3
birth injury P14.9

Paralysis, paralytic *(Continued)*
nerve *(Continued)*
cranial or cerebral G52.9
facial G51.0
birth injury P11.3
congenital P11.3
newborn (birth injury) P11.3
fourth or trochlear —*see* Strabismus,
paralytic, fourth nerve
newborn (birth injury) P14.9
oculomotor —*see* Strabismus, paralytic,
third nerve
phrenic (birth injury) P14.2
radial G56.3-
seventh or facial G51.0
newborn (birth injury) P11.3
sixth or abducent —*see* Strabismus,
paralytic, sixth nerve
syphilitic A52.15
third or oculomotor —*see* Strabismus,
paralytic, third nerve
trigeminal G50.9
trochlear —*see* Strabismus, paralytic,
fourth nerve
ulnar G56.2-
normokalemic periodic G72.3
ocular H49.9
alternating G83.89
oculofacial, congenital (Moebius) Q87.0
oculomotor (external bilateral) (nerve) —*see*
Strabismus, paralytic, third nerve
palate (soft) K13.79
paratrigeminal G50.9
periodic (familial) (hyperkalemic)
(hypokalemic) (myotonic)
(normokalemic) (potassium sensitive)
(secondary) G72.3
peripheral autonomic nervous system —*see*
Neuropathy, peripheral, autonomic
peroneal (nerve) G57.3-
pharynx J39.2
phrenic nerve G56.8-
plantar nerve (s) G57.6-
pneumogastric nerve G52.2
poliomyelitis (current) —*see* Poliomyelitis,
paralytic
popliteal nerve G57.3-
postepileptic transitory G83.84
progressive (atrophic) (bulbar) (spinal)
G12.22
general A52.17
infantile acute —*see* Poliomyelitis, paralytic
supranuclear G23.1
pseudobulbar G12.29
pseudohypertrophic (muscle) G71.0
psychogenic F44.4
quadriceps G57.9-
quadriplegic —*see* Tetraplegia
radial nerve G56.3-
rectus muscle (eye) H49.9
recurrent isolated sleep G47.53
respiratory (muscle) (system) (tract) R06.81
center NEC G93.89
congenital P28.89
newborn P28.89
right side —*see* Hemiplegia
saturnine —*see* subcategory T56.0
sciatic nerve G57.0-
senile G83.9
shaking —*see* Parkinsonism
shoulder G56.9-
sleep, recurrent isolated G47.53
spastic G83.9
cerebral —*see* Palsy, cerebral, spastic
congenital (cerebral) —*see* Palsy, cerebral,
spastic
familial G11.4
hereditary G11.4
quadriplegic G80.0
syphilitic (spinal) A52.17
sphincter, bladder —*see* Paralysis, bladder

◀ New   ⬅ Revised   ~~deleted~~ Deleted

Paralysis, paralytic (Continued)
spinal (cord) G83.9
accessory nerve G52.8
acute —see Poliomyelitis, paralytic
ascending acute G61.0
atrophic (acute) —see also Poliomyelitis, paralytic
spastic, syphilitic A52.17
congenital NEC —see Palsy, cerebral
hereditary G95.89
infantile —see Poliomyelitis, paralytic
progressive G12.21
sequelae NEC G83.89
sternomastoid G52.8
stomach K31.84
diabetic —see Diabetes, by type, with gastroparesis
nerve G52.2
diabetic —see Diabetes, by type, with gastroparesis
stroke —see Infarct, brain
subcapsularis G56.8-
supranuclear (progressive) G23.1
sympathetic G90.8
cervical G90.09
nervous system —see Neuropathy, peripheral, autonomic
syndrome G83.9
specified NEC G83.89
syphilitic spastic spinal (Erb's) A52.17
thigh G57.9-
throat J39.2
diphtheritic A36.0
muscle J39.2
thrombotic (current episode) I63.3
thumb C56.9-
tick —see Toxicity, venom, arthropod, specified NEC
Todd's (postepileptic transitory paralysis) G83.84
toe G57.6-
tongue K14.8
transient R29.5
arm or leg NEC R29.818
traumatic NEC —see Injury, nerve
trapezius G52.8
traumatic, transient NEC —see Injury, nerve
trembling —see Parkinsonism
triceps brachii G56.9-
trigeminal nerve G50.9
trochlear (nerve) —see Strabismus, paralytic, fourth nerve
ulnar nerve G56.2-
upper limb —see Monoplegia, upper limb
uremic N18.9 [G99.8]
uveoparotitic D86.89
uvula K13.79
postdiphtheritic A36.0
vagus nerve G52.2
vasomotor NEC G90.8
velum palati K13.79
vesical —see Paralysis, bladder
vestibular nerve (except Vertigo) —see subcategory H93.3
vocal cords J38.00
bilateral J38.02
unilateral J38.01
Volkmann's (complicating trauma) T79.6
wasting G12.29
Weber's G46.3
wrist G56.9-
Paramedial urethrovesical orifice Q64.79
Paramenia N92.6
Parametritis (see also Disease, pelvis, inflammatory) N73.2
acute N73.0
complicating abortion —see Abortion, by type, complicated by, parametritis
Parametrium, parametric —see condition
Paramnesia —see Amnesia

Paramolar K00.1
Paramyloidosis E85.8
Paramyoclonus multiplex G25.3
Paramyotonia (congenita) G71.19
Parangi —see Yaws
Paranoia (querulans) F22
senile F03
Paranoid
dementia (senile) F03
praecox —see Schizophrenia
personality F60.0
psychosis (climacteric) (involutional) (menopausal) F22
psychogenic (acute) F23
senile F03
reaction (acute) F23
chronic F22
schizophrenia F20.0
state (climacteric) (involutional) (menopausal) (simple) F22
senile F03
tendencies F60.0
traits F60.0
trends F60.0
type, psychopathic personality F60.0
Paraparesis —see Paraplegia
Paraphasia R47.02
Paraphilia F65.9
Paraphimosis (congenital) N47.2
chancroidal A57
Paraphrenia, paraphrenic (late) F22
schizophrenia F20.0
Paraplegia (lower) G82.20
ataxic —see Degeneration, combined, spinal cord
complete G82.21
congenital (cerebral) G80.8
spastic G80.1
familial spastic G11.4
functional (hysterical) F44.4
hereditary, spastic G11.4
hysterical F44.4
incomplete G82.22
Pott's A18.01
psychogenic F44.4
spastic
Erb's spinal, syphilitic A52.17
hereditary G11.4
tropical G04.1
syphilitic (spastic) A52.17
tropical spastic G04.1
Parapoxvirus B08.60
specified NEC B08.69
Paraproteinemia D89.2
benign (familial) D89.2
monoclonal D47.2
secondary to malignant disease D47.2
Parapsoriasis L41.9
en plaques L41.4
guttata L41.1
large plaque L41.4
retiform, retiformis L41.5
small plaque L41.3
specified NEC L41.8
varioliformis (acuta) L41.0
Parasitic —see also condition
disease NEC B89
stomatitis B37.0
sycosis (beard) (scalp) B35.0
twin Q89.4
Parasitism B89
intestinal B82.9
skin B88.9
specified —see Infestation
Parasitophobia F40.218
Parasomnia G47.50
due to
alcohol
abuse F10.182
dependence F10.282
use F10.982

Parasomnia (Continued)
due to (Continued)
amphetamines
abuse F15.182
dependence F15.282
use F15.982
caffeine
abuse F15.182
dependence F15.282
use F15.982
cocaine
abuse F14.182
dependence F14.282
use F14.982
drug NEC
abuse F19.182
dependence F19.282
use F19.982
opioid
abuse F11.182
dependence F11.282
use F11.982
psychoactive substance NEC
abuse F19.182
dependence F19.282
use F19.982
sedative, hypnotic, or anxiolytic
abuse F13.182
dependence F13.282
use F13.982
stimulant NEC
abuse F15.182
dependence F15.282
use F15.982
in conditions classified elsewhere G47.54
nonorganic origin F51.8
organic G47.50
specified NEC G47.59
Paraspadias Q54.9
Paraspasmus facialis G51.8
Parasuicide (attempt)
history of (personal) Z91.5
in family Z81.8
Parathyroid gland —see condition
Parathyroid tetany E20.9
Paratrachoma A74.0
Paratyphilis —see Appendicitis
Paratyphoid (fever) —see Fever, paratyphoid
Paratyphus —see Fever, paratyphoid
Paraurethral duct Q64.79
nonorganic origin F51.5
Paraurethritis —see also Urethritis
gonococcal (acute) (chronic) (with abscess) A54.1
Paravaccinia NEC B08.04
Paravaginitis —see Vaginitis
Parencephalitis —see also Encephalitis
sequelae G09
Parent-child conflict —see Conflict, parent-child
estrangement NEC Z62.890
Paresis —see also Paralysis
accommodation —see Paresis, of accommodation
Bernhardt's G57.1-
bladder (sphincter) —see also Paralysis, bladder
tabetic A52.17
bowel, colon or intestine K56.0
extrinsic muscle, eye H49.9
general (progressive) (syphilitic) A52.17
juvenile A50.45
heart —see Failure, heart
insane (syphilitic) A52.17
juvenile (general) A50.45
of accommodation H52.52-
peripheral progressive (idiopathic) G60.3
pseudohypertrophic G71.0
senile G83.9
syphilitic (general) A52.17
congenital A50.45
vesical NEC N31.2

Paresthesia —*see also* Disturbance, sensation
  Bernhardt G57.1-
Paretic —*see* condition
Parinaud's
  conjunctivitis H10.89
  oculoglandular syndrome H10.89
  ophthalmoplegia H49.88
Parkinsonism (idiopathic) (primary) G20
  with neurogenic orthostatic hypotension
      (symptomatic) G90.3
  arteriosclerotic G21.4
  dementia G31.83 *[F02.80]*
    with behavioral disturbance G31.83
        [F02.81]
  due to
    drugs NEC G21.19
      neuroleptic G21.11
  neuroleptic induced G21.11
  postencephalitic G21.3
  secondary G21.9
    due to
      arteriosclerosis G21.4
      drugs NEC G21.19
        neuroleptic G21.11
      encephalitis G21.3
      external agents NEC G21.2
      syphilis A52.19
    specified NEC G21.8
  syphilitic A52.19
  treatment-induced NEC G21.19
  vascular G21.4
Parkinson's disease, syndrome or tremor —*see*
  Parkinsonism
Parodontitis —*see* Periodontitis
Parodontosis K05.4
Paronychia —*see also* Cellulitis, digit
  with lymphangitis —*see* Lymphangitis, acute,
      digit
  candidal (chronic) B37.2
  tuberculous (primary) A18.4
Parorexia (psychogenic) F50.8
Parosmia R43.1
  psychogenic F45.8
Parotid gland —*see* condition
Parotitis, parotiditis (allergic) (nonspecific
    toxic) (purulent) (septic) (suppurative) —
    see also Sialoadenitis
  epidemic —*see* Mumps
  infectious —*see* Mumps
  postoperative K91.89
  surgical K91.89
Parrot fever A70
Parrot's disease (early congenital syphilitic
    pseudoparalysis) A50.02
Parry-Romberg syndrome G51.8
Parry's disease or syndrome E05.00
  with thyroid storm E05.01
Pars planitis —*see* Cyclitis
Parsonage (-Aldren)-**Turner syndrome** G54.5
Parson's disease (exophthalmic goiter)
    E05.00
  with thyroid storm E05.01
Particolored infant Q82.8
Parturition —*see* Delivery
Parulis K04.7
  with sinus K04.6
Parvovirus, as cause of disease classified
    elsewhere B97.6
Pasini and Pierini's atrophoderma L90.3
Passage
  false, urethra N36.5
  meconium (newborn) during delivery
    P03.82
  of sounds or bougies —*see* Attention to,
    artificial, opening
Passive —*see* condition
  smoking Z77.22
Pasteurella septica A28.0
Pasteurellosis —*see* Infection, Pasteurella
PAT (paroxysmal atrial tachycardia) I47.1
Patau's syndrome —*see* Trisomy, 13

Patches
  mucous (syphilitic) A51.39
    congenital A50.07
  smokers' (mouth) K13.24
Patellar —*see* condition
Patent —*see also* Imperfect, closure
  canal of Nuck Q52.4
  cervix N88.3
  ductus arteriosus or Botallo's Q25.0
  foramen
    botalli Q21.1
    ovale Q21.1
  interauricular septum Q21.1
  interventricular septum Q21.0
  omphalomesenteric duct Q43.0
  os (uteri) —*see* Patent, cervix
  ostium secundum Q21.1
  urachus Q64.4
  vitelline duct Q43.0
Paterson (-Brown)(-Kelly) **syndrome or web**
    D50.1
Pathologic, pathological —*see also* condition
  asphyxia R09.01
  fire-setting F63.1
  gambling F63.0
  ovum O02.0
  resorption, tooth K03.3
  stealing F63.2
Pathology (of) —*see* Disease
  periradicular, associated with previous
      endodontic treatment NEC M27.59
Pattern, sleep-wake, irregular G47.23
Patulous —*see also* Imperfect, closure
    (congenital)
  alimentary tract Q45.8
    lower Q43.8
    upper Q40.8
  eustachian tube H69.0-
Pause, sinoatrial I49.5
Paxton's disease B36.2
Pearl (s)
  enamel K00.2
  Epstein's K09.8
Pearl-worker's disease —*see* Osteomyelitis,
    specified type NEC
Pectenosis K62.4
Pectoral —*see* condition
Pectus
  carinatum (congenital) Q67.7
    acquired M95.4
    rachitic sequelae (late effect) E64.3
  excavatum (congenital) Q67.6
    acquired M95.4
    rachitic sequelae (late effect) E64.3
  recurvatum (congenital) Q67.6
Pedatrophia E41
Pederosis F65.4
Pediculosis (infestation) B85.2
  capitis (head-louse) (any site) B85.0
  corporis (body-louse) (any site) B85.1
  eyelid B85.0
  mixed (classifiable to more than one of the
      titles B85.0-B85.3) B85.4
  pubis (pubic louse) (any site) B85.3
  vestimenti B85.1
  vulvae B85.3
Pediculus (infestation) —*see* Pediculosis
Pedophilia F65.4
Peg-shaped teeth K00.2
Pelade —*see* Alopecia, areata
Pelger-Huët anomaly or syndrome D72.0
Peliosis (rheumatica) D69.0
  hepatis K76.4
    with toxic liver disease K71.8
Pelizaeus-Merzbacher disease E75.29
Pellagra (alcoholic) (with polyneuropathy) E52
Pellagra-cerebellar-ataxia-renal aminoaciduria
    syndrome E72.02
Pellegrini (-Stieda) **disease or syndrome** —*see*
    Bursitis, tibial collateral
Pellizzi's syndrome E34.8

Pel's crisis A52.11
Pelvic —*see also* condition
  examination (periodic) (routine) Z01.419
    with abnormal findings Z01.411
  kidney, congenital Q63.2
Pelviolithiasis —*see* Calculus, kidney
Pelviperitonitis —*see also* Peritonitis, pelvic
  gonococcal A54.24
  puerperal O85
Pelvis —*see* condition or type
Pemphigoid L12.9
  benign, mucous membrane L12.1
  bullous L12.0
  cicatricial L12.1
  juvenile L12.2
  ocular L12.1
  specified NEC L12.8
Pemphigus L10.9
  benign familial (chronic) Q82.8
  Brazilian L10.3
  circinatus L13.0
  conjunctiva L12.1
  drug-induced L10.5
  erythematosus L10.4
  foliaceous L10.2
  gangrenous —*see* Gangrene
  neonatorum L01.03
  ocular L12.1
  paraneoplastic L10.81
  specified NEC L10.89
  syphilitic (congenital) A50.06
  vegetans L10.1
  vulgaris L10.0
  wildfire L10.3
Pendred's syndrome E07.1
Pendulous
  abdomen, in pregnancy —*see* Pregnancy,
      complicated by, abnormal, pelvic organs
      or tissues NEC
  breast N64.89
Penetrating wound —*see also* Puncture
  with internal injury —*see* Injury, by site
  eyeball —*see* Puncture, eyeball
  orbit (with or without foreign body) —*see*
      Puncture, orbit
  uterus by instrument with or following
      ectopic or molar pregnancy O08.6
Penicillosis B48.4
Penis —*see* condition
Penitis N48.29
Pentalogy of Fallot Q21.8
Pentasomy X syndrome Q97.1
Pentosuria (essential) E74.8
Percreta placenta O43.23-
Peregrinating patient —*see* Disorder, factitious
Perforation, perforated (nontraumatic) (of)
  accidental during procedure (blood vessel)
      (nerve) (organ) —*see* Complication,
      accidental puncture or laceration
  antrum —*see* Sinusitis, maxillary
  appendix K35.2
  atrial septum, multiple Q21.1
  attic, ear —*see* Perforation, tympanum, attic
  bile duct (common) (hepatic) K83.2
    cystic K82.2
  bladder (urinary)
    with or following ectopic or molar
        pregnancy O08.6
    obstetrical trauma O71.5
    traumatic S37.29
      at delivery O71.5
  bowel K63.1
    with or following ectopic or molar
        pregnancy O08.6
    newborn P78.0
    obstetrical trauma O71.5
    traumatic —*see* Laceration, intestine
  broad ligament N83.8
    with or following ectopic or molar
        pregnancy O08.6
    obstetrical trauma O71.6

◀ New   ◀‖‖ Revised   ~~deleted~~ Deleted

Perforation, perforated *(Continued)*
by
device, implant or graft *(see also*
Complications, by site and type,
mechanical) T85.628
arterial graft NEC —*see* Complication,
cardiovascular device, mechanical,
vascular
breast (implant) T85.49
catheter NEC T85.698
cystostomy T83.090
dialysis (renal) T82.49
intraperitoneal T85.691
infusion NEC T82.594
spinal (epidural) (subdural)
T85.690
electronic (electrode) (pulse generator)
(stimulator)
bone T84.390
cardiac T82.199
electrode T82.190
pulse generator T82.191
specified type NEC T82.198
nervous system —*see* Complication,
prosthetic device, mechanical,
electronic nervous system
stimulator
urinary —*see* Complication,
genitourinary, device, urinary,
mechanical
fixation, internal (orthopedic) NEC —*see*
Complication, fixation device,
mechanical
gastrointestinal —*see* Complications,
prosthetic device, mechanical,
gastrointestinal device
genital NEC T83.498
intrauterine contraceptive device
T83.39
penile prosthesis T83.490
heart NEC —*see* Complication,
cardiovascular device,
mechanical
joint prosthesis —*see* Complications,
joint prosthesis, mechanical,
specified NEC, by site
ocular NEC —*see* Complications,
prosthetic device, mechanical,
ocular device
orthopedic NEC —*see* Complication,
orthopedic, device, mechanical
specified NEC T85.628
urinary NEC —*see also* Complication,
genitourinary, device, urinary,
mechanical
graft T83.29
urinary, indwelling T83.098
vascular NEC —*see* Complication,
cardiovascular device,
mechanical
ventricular intracranial shunt
T85.09
foreign body left accidentally in
operative wound T81.539
instrument (any) during a procedure,
accidental —*see* Puncture, accidental
complicating surgery
cecum K35.2
cervix (uteri) N88.8
with or following ectopic or molar
pregnancy O08.6
obstetrical trauma O71.3
colon K63.1
newborn P78.0
obstetrical trauma O71.5
traumatic —*see* Laceration, intestine,
large
common duct (bile) K83.2
cornea (due to ulceration) —*see* Ulcer,
cornea, perforated
cystic duct K82.2

Perforation, perforated *(Continued)*
diverticulum (intestine) K57.80
with bleeding K57.81
large intestine K57.20
with
bleeding K57.21
small intestine K57.40
with bleeding K57.41
small intestine K57.00
with
bleeding K57.01
large intestine K57.40
with bleeding K57.41
ear drum —*see* Perforation, tympanum
esophagus K22.3
ethmoidal sinus —*see* Sinusitis, ethmoidal
frontal sinus —*see* Sinusitis, frontal
gallbladder K82.2
heart valve —*see* Endocarditis
ileum K63.1
newborn P78.0
obstetrical trauma O71.5
traumatic —*see* Laceration, intestine, small
instrumental, surgical (accidental) (blood
vessel) (nerve) (organ) —*see* Puncture,
accidental complicating surgery
intestine NEC K63.1
with ectopic or molar pregnancy O08.6
newborn P78.0
obstetrical trauma O71.5
traumatic —*see* Laceration, intestine
ulcerative NEC K63.1
newborn P78.0
jejunum, jejunal K63.1
obstetrical trauma O71.5
traumatic —*see* Laceration, intestine, small
ulcer —*see* Ulcer, gastrojejunal, with
perforation
joint prosthesis —*see* Complications, joint
prosthesis, mechanical, specified NEC,
by site
mastoid (antrum) (cell) —*see* Disorder,
mastoid, specified NEC
maxillary sinus —*see* Sinusitis, maxillary
membrana tympani —*see* Perforation,
tympanum
nasal
septum J34.89
congenital Q30.3
syphilitic A52.73
sinus J34.89
congenital Q30.8
due to sinusitis —*see* Sinusitis
palate (*see also* Cleft, palate) Q35.9
syphilitic A52.79
palatine vault (*see also* Cleft, palate, hard)
Q35.1
syphilitic A52.79
congenital A50.59
pars flaccida (ear drum) —*see* Perforation,
tympanum, attic
pelvic
floor S31.030
with
ectopic or molar pregnancy O08.6
penetration into retroperitoneal space
S31.031
retained foreign body S31.040
with penetration into
retroperitoneal space S31.041
following ectopic or molar pregnancy
O08.6
obstetrical trauma O70.1
organ S37.99
adrenal gland S37.818
bladder —*see* Perforation, bladder
fallopian tube S37.599
bilateral S37.592
unilateral S37.591
kidney S37.09-
obstetrical trauma O71.5

Perforation, perforated *(Continued)*
pelvic *(Continued)*
organ *(Continued)*
ovary S37.499
bilateral S37.492
unilateral S37.491
prostate S37.828
specified organ NEC S37.898
ureter —*see* Perforation, ureter
urethra —*see* Perforation, urethra
uterus —*see* Perforation, uterus
perineum —*see* Laceration, perineum
pharynx J39.2
rectum K63.1
newborn P78.0
obstetrical trauma O71.5
traumatic S36.63
root canal space due to endodontic treatment
M27.51
sigmoid K63.1
newborn P78.0
obstetrical trauma O71.5
traumatic S36.533
sinus (accessory) (chronic) (nasal) J34.89
sphenoidal sinus —*see* Sinusitis, sphenoidal
surgical (accidental) (by instrument) (blood
vessel) (nerve) (organ) —*see* Puncture,
accidental complicating surgery
traumatic
external —*see* Puncture
eye —*see* Puncture, eyeball
internal organ —*see* Injury, by site
tympanum, tympanic (membrane) (persistent
post-traumatic) (postinflammatory)
H72.9-
attic H72.1-
multiple —*see* Perforation, tympanum,
multiple
total —*see* Perforation, tympanum, total
central H72.0-
multiple —*see* Perforation, tympanum,
multiple
total —*see* Perforation, tympanum, total
marginal NEC —*see* subcategory H72.2
multiple H72.81-
pars flaccida —*see* Perforation, tympanum,
attic
total H72.82-
traumatic, current episode S09.2-
typhoid, gastrointestinal —*see* Typhoid
ulcer —*see* Ulcer, by site, with perforation
ureter N28.89
traumatic S37.19
urethra N36.8
with ectopic or molar pregnancy O08.6
following ectopic or molar pregnancy
O08.6
obstetrical trauma O71.5
traumatic S37.39
at delivery O71.5
uterus
with ectopic or molar pregnancy O08.6
by intrauterine contraceptive device T83.39
following ectopic or molar pregnancy
O08.6
obstetrical trauma O71.1
traumatic S37.69
obstetric O71.1
uvula K13.79
syphilitic A52.79
vagina
obstetrical trauma O71.4
other trauma - see Puncture, vagina
Periadenitis mucosa necrotica recurrens K12.0
Periappendicitis (acute) —*see* Appendicitis
Periarteritis nodosa (disseminated) (infectious)
(necrotizing) M30.0
Periarthritis (joint) —*see also* Enthesopathy
Duplay's M75.0-
gonococcal A54.42
humeroscapularis —*see* Capsulitis, adhesive

Periarthritis (Continued)
  scapulohumeral —see Capsulitis, adhesive
  shoulder —see Capsulitis, adhesive
  wrist M77.2-
Periarthrosis (angioneural) —see
    Enthesopathy
Pericapsulitis, adhesive (shoulder) —see
    Capsulitis, adhesive
Pericarditis (with decompensation) (with
    effusion) I31.9
  with rheumatic fever (conditions in I00)
    active —see Pericarditis, rheumatic
    inactive or quiescent I09.2
  acute (hemorrhagic) (nonrheumatic) (Sicca)
    I30.9
    with chorea (acute) (rheumatic)
        (Sydenham's) I02.0
    benign I30.8
    nonspecific I30.0
    rheumatic I01.0
      with chorea (acute) (Sydenham's)
          I02.0
  adhesive or adherent (chronic) (external)
      (internal) I31.0
    acute —see Pericarditis, acute
    rheumatic I09.2
  bacterial (acute) (subacute) (with serous or
      seropurulent effusion) I30.1
  calcareous I31.1
  cholesterol (chronic) I31.8
    acute I30.9
  chronic (nonrheumatic) I31.9
    rheumatic I09.2
  constrictive (chronic) I31.1
  coxsackie B33.23
  fibrinocaseous (tuberculous) A18.84
  fibrinopurulent I30.1
  fibrinous I30.8
  fibrous I31.0
  gonococcal A54.83
  idiopathic I30.0
  in systemic lupus erythematosus M32.12
  infective I30.1
  meningococcal A39.53
  neoplastic (chronic) I31.8
    acute I30.9
  obliterans, obliterating I31.0
  plastic I31.0
  pneumococcal I30.1
  postinfarction I24.1
  purulent I30.1
  rheumatic (active) (acute) (with effusion)
      (with pneumonia) I01.0
    with chorea (acute) (rheumatic)
        (Sydenham's) I02.0
    chronic or inactive (with chorea) I09.2
  rheumatoid —see Rheumatoid, carditis
  septic I30.1
  serofibrinous I30.8
  staphylococcal I30.1
  streptococcal I30.1
  suppurative I30.1
  syphilitic A52.06
  tuberculous A18.84
  uremic N18.9 [I32]
  viral I30.1
Pericardium, pericardial —see condition
Pericellulitis —see Cellulitis
Pericementitis (chronic) (suppurative) —see also
    Periodontitis
  acute K05.20
    generalized K05.22
    localized K05.21
Perichondritis
  auricle —see Perichondritis, ear
  bronchus J98.09
  ear (external) H61.00-
    acute H61.01-
    chronic H61.02-
  external auditory canal —see Perichondritis,
      ear

Perichondritis (Continued)
  larynx J38.7
    syphilitic A52.73
    typhoid A01.09
  nose J34.89
  pinna —see Perichondritis, ear
  trachea J39.8
Periclasia K05.4
Pericoronitis —see Periodontitis
Pericystitis N30.90
  with hematuria N30.91
Peridiverticulitis (intestine) K57.92
  cecum —see Diverticulitis, intestine, large
  colon —see Diverticulitis, intestine, large
  duodenum —see Diverticulitis, intestine,
      small
  intestine —see Diverticulitis, intestine
  jejunum —see Diverticulitis, intestine, small
  rectosigmoid —see Diverticulitis, intestine,
      large
  rectum —see Diverticulitis, intestine, large
  sigmoid —see Diverticulitis, intestine, large
Periendocarditis —see Endocarditis
Periepididymitis N45.1
Perifolliculitis L01.02
  abscedens, caput, scalp L66.3
  capitis, abscedens (et suffodiens) L66.3
  superficial pustular L01.02
Perihepatitis K65.8
Perilabyrinthitis (acute) —see subcategory
    H83.0
Perimeningitis —see Meningitis
Perimetritis —see Endometritis
Perimetrosalpingitis —see Salpingo-oophoritis
Perineocele N81.81
Perinephric, perinephritic —see condition
Perinephritis —see also Infection, kidney
  purulent —see Abscess, kidney
Perineum, perineal —see condition
Perineuritis NEC —see Neuralgia
Periodic —see condition
Periodontitis (chronic) (complex) (compound)
    (local) (simplex) K05.30
  acute K05.20
    generalized K05.22
    localized K05.21
  apical K04.5
    acute (pulpal origin) K04.4
  generalized K05.32
  localized K05.31
Periodontoclasia K05.4
Periodontosis (juvenile) K05.4
Periods —see also Menstruation
  heavy N92.0
  irregular N92.6
  shortened intervals (irregular) N92.1
Perionychia —see also Cellulitis, digit
  with lymphangitis —see Lymphangitis, acute,
      digit
Perioophoritis —see Salpingo-oophoritis
Periorchitis N45.2
Periosteum, periosteal —see condition
Periostitis (albuminosa) (circumscribed)
    (diffuse) (infective) (monomelic) —see also
    Osteomyelitis
  alveolar M27.3
  alveolodental M27.3
  dental M27.3
  gonorrheal A54.43
  jaw (lower) (upper) M27.2
  orbit H05.03-
  syphilitic A52.77
    congenital (early) A50.02 [M90.80]
    secondary A51.46
  tuberculous —see Tuberculosis, bone
  yaws (hypertrophic) (early) (late) A66.6
      [M90.80]
Periostosis (hyperplastic) —see also Disorder,
    bone, specified type NEC
  with osteomyelitis —see Osteomyelitis,
      specified type NEC

Peripartum
  cardiomyopathy O90.3
Periphlebitis —see Phlebitis
Periproctitis K62.89
Periprostatitis —see Prostatitis
Perirectal —see condition
Perirenal —see condition
Perisalpingitis —see Salpingo-oophoritis
Perisplenitis (infectional) D73.89
Peristalsis, visible or reversed R19.2
Peritendinitis —see Enthesopathy
Peritoneum, peritoneal —see condition
Peritonitis (adhesive) (bacterial) (fibrinous)
    (hemorrhagic) (idiopathic) (localized)
    (perforative) (primary) (with adhesions)
    (with effusion) K65.9
  with or following
    abscess K65.1
    appendicitis K35.2
      with perforation or rupture K35.2
      generalized K35.2
      localized K35.3
    diverticular disease (intestine) K57.80
      with bleeding K57.81
    ectopic or molar pregnancy O08.0
    large intestine K57.20
      with
        bleeding K57.21
        small intestine K57.40
          with bleeding K57.41
    small intestine K57.00
      with
        bleeding K57.01
        large intestine K57.40
          with bleeding K57.41
  acute (generalized) K65.0
  aseptic T81.61
  bile, biliary K65.3
  chemical T81.61
  chlamydial A74.81
  chronic proliferative K65.8
  complicating abortion —see Abortion, by
      type, complicated by, pelvic peritonitis
  congenital P78.1
  diaphragmatic K65.0
  diffuse K65.0
  diphtheritic A36.89
  disseminated K65.0
  due to
    bile K65.3
    foreign
      body or object accidentally left during
          a procedure (instrument) (sponge)
          (swab) T81.599
      substance accidentally left during a
          procedure (chemical) (powder)
          (talc) T81.61
    talc T81.61
    urine K65.8
  eosinophilic K65.8
    acute K65.0
  fibrocaseous (tuberculous) A18.31
  fibropurulent K65.0
  following ectopic or molar pregnancy O08.0
  general (ized) K65.0
  gonococcal A54.85
  meconium (newborn) P78.0
  neonatal P78.1
    meconium P78.0
  pancreatic K65.0
  paroxysmal, familial E85.0
    benign E85.0
  pelvic
    female N73.5
      acute N73.3
      chronic N73.4
        with adhesions N73.6
    male K65.0
  periodic, familial E85.0
  proliferative, chronic K65.8
  puerperal, postpartum, childbirth O85

◀ New   ◀||||| Revised   ~~deleted~~ Deleted

Peritonitis (Continued)
  purulent K65.0
  septic K65.0
  specified NEC K65.8
  spontaneous bacterial K65.2
  subdiaphragmatic K65.0
  subphrenic K65.0
  suppurative K65.0
  syphilitic A52.74
    congenital (early) A50.08 [K67]
  talc T81.61
  tuberculous A18.31
  urine K65.8
Peritonsillar —see condition
Peritonsillitis J36
Perityphlitis K37
Periureteritis N28.89
Periurethral —see condition
Periurethritis (gangrenous) —see Urethritis
Periuterine —see condition
Perivaginitis —see Vaginitis
Perivasculitis, retinal H35.06-
Perivasitis (chronic) N49.1
Perivesiculitis (seminal) —see Vesiculitis
Perlèche NEC K13.0
  due to
    candidiasis B37.83
    moniliasis B37.83
    riboflavin deficiency E53.0
    vitamin B2 (riboflavin) deficiency E53.0
Pernicious —see condition
Pernio, perniosis T69.1
Perpetrator (of abuse) —see Index to External
    Causes of Injury, Perpetrator
Persecution
  delusion F22
  social Z60.5
Perseveration (tonic) R48.8
Persistence, persistent (congenital)
  anal membrane Q42.3
    with fistula Q42.2
  arteria stapedia Q16.3
  atrioventricular canal Q21.2
  branchial cleft Q18.0
  bulbus cordis in left ventricle Q21.8
  canal of Cloquet Q14.0
  capsule (opaque) Q12.8
  cilioretinal artery or vein Q14.8
  cloaca Q43.7
  communication —see Fistula, congenital
  convolutions
    aortic arch Q25.4
    fallopian tube Q50.6
    oviduct Q50.6
    uterine tube Q50.6
  double aortic arch Q25.4
  ductus arteriosus (Botalli) Q25.0
  fetal
    circulation P29.3
    form of cervix (uteri) Q51.828
    hemoglobin, hereditary (HPFH) D56.4
  foramen
    Botalli Q21.1
    ovale Q21.1
  Gartner's duct Q52.4
  hemoglobin, fetal (hereditary) (HPFH)
    D56.4
  hyaloid
    artery (generally incomplete) Q14.0
    system Q14.8
  hymen, in pregnancy or childbirth —see
    Pregnancy, complicated by, abnormal,
    vulva
  lanugo Q84.2
  left
    posterior cardinal vein Q26.8
    root with right arch of aorta Q25.4
    superior vena cava Q26.1
  Meckel's diverticulum Q43.0
    malignant —see Table of Neoplasms, small
      intestine, malignant

Persistence, persistent (Continued)
  mucosal disease (middle ear) —see
    Otitis, media, suppurative, chronic,
    tubotympanic
  nail (s), anomalous Q84.6
  omphalomesenteric duct Q43.0
  organ or site not listed —see Anomaly, by site
  ostium
    atrioventriculare commune Q21.2
    primum Q21.2
    secundum Q21.1
  ovarian rests in fallopian tube Q50.6
  pancreatic tissue in intestinal tract Q43.8
  primary (deciduous)
    teeth K00.6
    vitreous hyperplasia Q14.0
  pupillary membrane Q13.89
  rhesus (Rh)titer —see Complication (s),
    transfusion, incompatibility reaction,
    Rh (factor)
  right aortic arch Q25.4
  sinus
    urogenitalis
      female Q52.8
      male Q55.8
    venosus with imperfect incorporation in
      right auricle Q26.8
  thymus (gland) (hyperplasia) E32.0
  thyroglossal duct Q89.2
  thyrolingual duct Q89.2
  truncus arteriosus or communis Q20.0
  tunica vasculosa lentis Q12.2
  umbilical sinus Q64.4
  urachus Q64.4
  vitelline duct Q43.0
Person (with)
  admitted for clinical research, as a control
    subject (normal comparison)
    (participant) Z00.6
  awaiting admission to adequate facility
    elsewhere Z75.1
  concern (normal) about sick person in family
    Z63.6
  consulting on behalf of another Z71.0
  feigning illness Z76.5
  living (in)
    without
      adequate housing (heating) (space) Z59.1
      housing (permanent) (temporary) Z59.0
      person able to render necessary care
        Z74.2
      shelter Z59.0
    alone Z60.2
    boarding school Z59.3
    residential institution Z59.3
  on waiting list Z75.1
  sick or handicapped in family Z63.6
Personality (disorder) F60.9
  accentuation of traits (type A pattern) Z73.1
  affective F34.0
  aggressive F60.3
  amoral F60.2
  anacastic, ananankastic F60.5
  antisocial F60.2
  anxious F60.6
  asocial F60.2
  asthenic F60.7
  avoidant F60.6
  borderline F60.3
  change due to organic condition (enduring)
    F07.0
  compulsive F60.5
  cycloid F34.0
  cyclothymic F34.0
  dependent F60.7
  depressive F34.1
  dissocial F60.2
  dual F44.81
  eccentric F60.89
  emotionally unstable F60.3
  expansive paranoid F60.0

Personality (Continued)
  explosive F60.3
  fanatic F60.0
  haltlose type F60.89
  histrionic F60.4
  hyperthymic F34.0
  hypothymic F34.1
  hysterical F60.4
  immature F60.89
  inadequate F60.7
  labile (emotional) F60.3
  mixed (nonspecific) F60.81
  morally defective F60.2
  multiple F44.81
  narcissistic F60.81
  obsessional F60.5
  obsessive (-compulsive) F60.5
  organic F07.0
  overconscientious F60.5
  paranoid F60.0
  passive (-dependent) F60.7
  passive-aggressive F60.89
  pathologic F60.9
  pattern defect or disturbance F60.9
  pseudopsychopathic (organic) F07.0
  pseudoretarded (organic) F07.0
  psychoinfantile F60.4
  psychoneurotic NEC F60.89
  psychopathic F60.2
  querulant F60.0
  sadistic F60.89
  schizoid F60.1
  self-defeating F60.7
  sensitive paranoid F60.0
  sociopathic (amoral) (antisocial) (asocial)
    (dissocial) F60.2
  specified NEC F60.89
  type A Z73.1
  unstable (emotional) F60.3
Perthes' disease —see Legg-Calvé-Perthes
    disease
Pertussis (see also Whooping cough)
    A37.90
Perversion, perverted
  appetite F50.8
    psychogenic F50.8
  function
    pituitary gland E23.2
      posterior lobe E22.2
  sense of smell and taste R43.8
    psychogenic F45.8
  sexual —see Deviation, sexual
Pervious, congenital —see also Imperfect,
    closure
  ductus arteriosus Q25.0
Pes (congenital) —see also Talipes
  acquired —see also Deformity, limb, foot,
    specified NEC
    planus —see Deformity, limb, flat foot
  adductus Q66.89
  cavus Q66.7
  deformity NEC, acquired —see Deformity,
    limb, foot, specified NEC
  planus (acquired) (any degree) —see also
    Deformity, limb, flat foot
    rachitic sequelae (late effect) E64.3
  valgus Q66.6
Pest, pestis —see Plague
Petechia, petechiae R23.3
  newborn P54.5
Petechial typhus A75.9
Peter's anomaly Q13.4
Petit mal seizure —see Epilepsy, generalized,
    specified NEC
Petit's hernia —see Hernia, abdomen, specified
    site NEC
Petrellidosis B48.2
Petrositis H70.20-
  acute H70.21-
  chronic H70.22-
Peutz-Jeghers disease or syndrome Q85.8

Peyronie's disease N48.6
Pfeiffer's disease —*see* Mononucleosis, infectious
Phagedena (dry) (moist) (sloughing) —*see also* Gangrene
  geometric L88
  penis N48.29
  tropical —*see* Ulcer, skin
  vulva N76.6
Phagedenic —*see* condition
Phakoma H35.89
Phakomatosis (*see also* specific eponymous syndromes) Q85.9
  Bourneville's Q85.1
  specified NEC Q85.8
Phantom limb syndrome (without pain) G54.7
  with pain G54.6
Pharyngeal pouch syndrome D82.1
Pharyngitis (acute) (catarrhal) (gangrenous) (infective) (malignant) (membranous) (phlegmonous) (pseudomembranous) (simple) (subacute) (suppurative) (ulcerative) (viral) J02.9
  with influenza, flu, or grippe —*see* Influenza, with, pharyngitis
  aphthous B08.5
  atrophic J31.2
  chlamydial A56.4
  chronic (atrophic) (granular) (hypertrophic) J31.2
  coxsackievirus B08.5
  diphtheritic A36.0
  enteroviral vesicular B08.5
  follicular (chronic) J31.2
  fusospirochetal A69.1
  gonococcal A54.5
  granular (chronic) J31.2
  herpesviral B00.2
  hypertrophic J31.2
  infectional, chronic J31.2
  influenzal —*see* Influenza, with, respiratory manifestations NEC
  lymphonodular, acute (enteroviral) B08.8
  pneumococcal J02.8
  purulent J02.9
  putrid J02.9
  septic J02.0
  sicca J31.2
  specified organism NEC J02.8
  staphylococcal J02.8
  streptococcal J02.0
  syphilitic, congenital (early) A50.03
  tuberculous A15.8
  vesicular, enteroviral B08.5
  viral NEC J02.8
Pharyngoconjunctivitis, viral B30.2
Pharyngolaryngitis (acute) J06.0
  chronic J37.0
Pharyngoplegia J39.2
Pharyngotonsillitis, herpesviral B00.2
Pharyngotracheitis, chronic J42
Pharynx, pharyngeal —*see* condition
Phenomenon
  Arthus' —*see* Arthus' phenomenon
  jaw-winking Q07.8
  lupus erythematosus (LE) cell M32.9
  Raynaud's (secondary) I73.00
    with gangrene I73.01
  vasomotor R55
  vasospastic I73.9
  vasovagal R55
  Wenckebach's I44.1
Phenylketonuria E70.1
  classical E70.0
  maternal E70.1
Pheochromoblastoma
  specified site —*see* Neoplasm, malignant, by site
  unspecified site C74.10

Pheochromocytoma
  malignant
    specified site —*see* Neoplasm, malignant, by site
    unspecified site C74.10
  specified site —*see* Neoplasm, benign, by site
  unspecified site D35.00
Pheohyphomycosis —*see* Chromomycosis
Pheomycosis —*see* Chromomycosis
Phimosis (congenital) (due to infection) N47.1
  chancroidal A57
Phlebectasia —*see also* Varix
  congenital Q27.4
Phlebitis (infective) (pyemic) (septic) (suppurative) I80.9
  antepartum —*see* Thrombophlebitis, antepartum
  blue —*see* Phlebitis, leg, deep
  breast, superficial I80.8
  cavernous (venous) sinus —*see* Phlebitis, intracranial (venous) sinus
  cerebral (venous) sinus —*see* Phlebitis, intracranial (venous) sinus
  chest wall, superficial I80.8
  cranial (venous) sinus —*see* Phlebitis, intracranial (venous) sinus
  deep (vessels) —*see* Phlebitis, leg, deep
  due to implanted device —*see* Complications, by site and type, specified NEC
  during or resulting from a procedure T81.72
  femoral vein (superficial) I80.1-
  femoropopliteal vein I80.0-
  gestational —*see* Phlebopathy, gestational
  hepatic veins I80.8
  iliofemoral —*see* Phlebitis, femoral vein
  intracranial (venous) sinus (any) G08
    nonpyogenic I67.6
  intraspinal venous sinuses and veins G08
    nonpyogenic G95.19
  lateral (venous) sinus —*see* Phlebitis, intracranial (venous) sinus
  leg I80.3
    antepartum —*see* Thrombophlebitis, antepartum
    deep (vessels) NEC I80.20-
      iliac I80.21-
      popliteal vein I80.22-
      specified vessel NEC I80.29-
      tibial vein I80.23-
    femoral vein (superficial) I80.1-
    superficial (vessels) I80.0-
  longitudinal sinus —*see* Phlebitis, intracranial (venous) sinus
  lower limb —*see* Phlebitis, leg
  migrans, migrating (superficial) I82.1
  pelvic
    with ectopic or molar pregnancy O08.0
    following ectopic or molar pregnancy O08.0
    puerperal, postpartum O87.1
  popliteal vein —*see* Phlebitis, leg, deep, popliteal
  portal (vein) K75.1
  postoperative T81.72
  pregnancy —*see* Thrombophlebitis, antepartum
  puerperal, postpartum, childbirth O87.0
    deep O87.1
    pelvic O87.1
    superficial O87.0
  retina —*see* Vasculitis, retina
  saphenous (accessory) (great) (long) (small) —*see* Phlebitis, leg, superficial
  sinus (meninges) —*see* Phlebitis, intracranial (venous) sinus
  specified site NEC I80.8
  syphilitic A52.09
  tibial vein —*see* Phlebitis, leg, deep, tibial
  ulcerative I80.9
    leg —*see* Phlebitis, leg
  umbilicus I80.8

Phlebitis (*Continued*)
  uterus (septic) —*see* Endometritis
  varicose (leg) (lower limb) —*see* Varix, leg, with, inflammation
Phlebofibrosis I87.8
Phleboliths I87.8
Phlebopathy
  gestational O22.9-
  puerperal O87.9
Phlebosclerosis I87.8
Phlebothrombosis —*see also* Thrombosis
  antepartum —*see* Thrombophlebitis, antepartum
  pregnancy —*see* Thrombophlebitis, antepartum
  puerperal —*see* Thrombophlebitis, puerperal
Phlebotomus fever A93.1
Phlegmasia
  alba dolens O87.1
    nonpuerperal —*see* Phlebitis, femoral vein
  cerulea dolens —*see* Phlebitis, leg, deep
Phlegmon —*see* Abscess
Phlegmonous —*see* condition
Phlyctenulosis (allergic) (keratoconjunctivitis) (nontuberculous) —*see also* Keratoconjunctivitis
  cornea —*see* Keratoconjunctivitis
  tuberculous A18.52
Phobia, phobic F40.9
  animal F40.218
    spiders F40.210
  examination F40.298
  reaction F40.9
  simple F40.298
  social F40.10
    generalized F40.11
  specific (isolated) F40.298
    animal F40.218
      spiders F40.210
    blood F40.230
    injection F40.231
    injury F40.233
    men F40.290
    natural environment F40.228
      thunderstorms F40.220
    situational F40.248
      bridges F40.242
      closed in spaces F40.240
      flying F40.243
      heights F40.241
      specified focus NEC F40.298
    transfusion F40.231
    women F40.291
  specified NEC F40.8
    medical care NEC F40.232
  state F40.9
Phocas' disease —*see* Mastopathy, cystic
Phocomelia Q73.1
  lower limb —*see* Agenesis, leg, with foot present
  upper limb —*see* Agenesis, arm, with hand present
Phoria H50.50
Phosphate-losing tubular disorder N25.0
Phosphatemia E83.39
Phosphaturia E83.39
Photodermatitis (sun) L56.8
  chronic L57.8
  due to drug L56.8
  light other than sun L59.8
Photokeratitis H16.13-
Photophobia H53.14-
Photophthalmia —*see* Photokeratitis
Photopsia H53.19
Photoretinitis —*see* Retinopathy, solar
Photosensitivity, photosensitization (sun) skin L56.8
  light other than sun L59.8
Phrenitis —*see* Encephalitis
Phrynoderma (vitamin A deficiency) E50.8

◀ New   ◀▭ Revised   ~~deleted~~ Deleted

Phthiriasis (pubis) B85.3
  with any infestation classifiable to
    B85.0-B85.2 B85.4
Phthirus infestation —see Phthiriasis
Phthisis —see also Tuberculosis
  bulbi (infectional) —see Disorder, globe,
    degenerated condition, atrophy
  eyeball (due to infection) —see Disorder,
    globe, degenerated condition, atrophy
Phycomycosis —see Zygomycosis
Physalopteriasis B81.8
Physical restraint status Z78.1
Phytobezoar T18.9
  intestine T18.3
  stomach T18.2
Pian —see Yaws
Pianoma A66.1
Pica F50.8
  in adults F50.8
  infant or child F98.3
Picking, nose F98.8
Pick-Niemann disease —see Niemann-Pick
  disease or syndrome
Pick's
  cerebral atrophy G31.01 [F02.80]
    with behavioral disturbance G31.01
      [F02.81]
  disease or syndrome (brain) G31.01 [F02.80]
    with behavioral disturbance G31.01
      [F02.81]
Pickwickian syndrome E66.2
Piebaldism E70.39
Piedra (beard) (scalp) B36.8
  black B36.3
  white B36.2
Pierre Robin deformity or syndrome Q87.0
Pierson's disease or osteochondrosis M91.0
Pig-bel A05.2
Pigeon
  breast or chest (acquired) M95.4
    congenital Q67.7
    rachitic sequelae (late effect) E64.3
  breeder's disease or lung J67.2
  fancier's disease or lung J67.2
  toe —see Deformity, toe, specified NEC
Pigmentation (abnormal) (anomaly) L81.9
  conjunctiva H11.13-
  cornea (anterior) H18.01-
    posterior H18.05-
    stromal H18.06-
  diminished melanin formation NEC L81.6
  iron L81.8
  lids, congenital Q82.8
  limbus corneae —see Pigmentation, cornea
  metals L81.8
  optic papilla, congenital Q14.2
  retina, congenital (grouped) (nevoid) Q14.1
  scrotum, congenital Q82.8
  tattoo L81.8
Piles (see also Hemorrhoids) K64.9
Pili
  annulati or torti (congenital) Q84.1
  incarnati L73.1
Pill roller hand (intrinsic) —see Parkinsonism
Pilomatrixoma —see Neoplasm, skin, benign
  malignant —see Neoplasm, skin, malignant
Pilonidal —see condition
Pimple R23.8
Pinched nerve —see Neuropathy, entrapment
Pindborg tumor —see Cyst, calcifying
  odontogenic
Pineal body or gland —see condition
Pinealoblastoma C75.3
Pinealoma D44.5
  malignant C75.3
Pineoblastoma C75.3
Pineocytoma D44.5
Pinguecula H11.15-
Pingueculitis H10.81-
Pinhole meatus (see also Stricture, urethra)
  N35.9

Pink
  disease —see subcategory T56.1
  eye —see Conjunctivitis, acute, mucopurulent
Pinkus' disease (lichen nitidus) L44.1
Pinpoint
  meatus —see Stricture, urethra
  os (uteri) —see Stricture, cervix
Pins and needles R20.2
Pinta A67.9
  cardiovascular lesions A67.2
  chancre (primary) A67.0
  erythematous plaques A67.1
  hyperchromic lesions A67.1
  hyperkeratosis A67.1
  lesions A67.9
    cardiovascular A67.2
    hyperchromic A67.1
    intermediate A67.1
    late A67.2
    mixed A67.3
    primary A67.0
    skin (achromic) (cicatricial) (dyschromic)
      A67.2
      hyperchromic A67.1
      mixed (achromic and hyperchromic)
        A67.3
  papule (primary) A67.0
  skin lesions (achromic) (cicatricial)
    (dyschromic) A67.2
    hyperchromic A67.1
    mixed (achromic and hyperchromic) A67.3
  vitiligo A67.2
Pintids A67.1
Pinworm (disease) (infection) (infestation) B80
Piroplasmosis B60.0
Pistol wound —see Gunshot wound
Pitchers' elbow —see Derangement, joint,
  specified type NEC, elbow
Pithecoid pelvis Q74.2
  with disproportion (fetopelvic) O33.0
    causing obstructed labor O65.0
Pithiatism F48.8
Pitted —see Pitting
Pitting —see also Edema R60.9
  lip R60.0
  nail L60.8
  teeth K00.4
Pituitary gland —see condition
Pituitary-snuff-taker's disease J67.8
Pityriasis (capitis) L21.0
  alba L30.5
  circinata (et maculata) L42
  furfuracea L21.0
  Hebra's L26
  lichenoides L41.0
    chronica L41.1
    et varioliformis (acuta) L41.0
  maculata (et circinata) L30.5
  nigra B36.1
  pilaris, Hebra's L44.0
  rosea L42
  rotunda L44.8
  rubra (Hebra) pilaris L44.0
  simplex L30.5
  specified type NEC L30.5
  streptogenes L30.5
  versicolor (scrotal) B36.0
Placenta, placental —see Pregnancy,
  complicated by (care of) (management
  affected by), specified condition
Placentitis O41.14-
Plagiocephaly Q67.3
Plague A20.9
  abortive A20.8
  ambulatory A20.8
  asymptomatic A20.8
  bubonic A20.0
  cellulocutaneous A20.1
  cutaneobubonic A20.1
  lymphatic gland A20.0
  meningitis A20.3

Plague (Continued)
  pharyngeal A20.8
  pneumonic (primary) (secondary) A20.2
  pulmonary, pulmonic A20.2
  septicemic A20.7
  tonsillar A20.8
    septicemic A20.7
Planning, family
  contraception Z30.9
  procreation Z31.69
Plaque (s)
  artery, arterial —see Arteriosclerosis
  calcareous —see Calcification
  coronary, lipid rich I25.83
  epicardial I31.8
  erythematous, of pinta A67.1
  Hollenhorst's —see Occlusion, artery, retina
  lipid rich, coronary I25.83
  pleural (without asbestos) J92.9
    with asbestos J92.0
  tongue K13.29
Plasmacytoma C90.3-
  extramedullary C90.2-
  medullary C90.0-
  solitary C90.3-
Plasmacytopenia D72.818
Plasmacytosis D72.822
Plaster ulcer —see Ulcer, pressure, by site
Plateau iris syndrome (post-iridectomy)
    (postprocedural) (without glaucoma)
    H21.82
  with glaucoma H40.22-
Platybasia Q75.8
Platyonychia (congenital) Q84.6
  acquired L60.8
Platypelloid pelvis M95.5
  with disproportion (fetopelvic) O33.0
    causing obstructed labor O65.0
  congenital Q74.2
Platyspondylisis Q76.49
Plaut (-Vincent) disease (see also Vincent's)
    A69.1
Plethora R23.2
  newborn P61.1
Pleura, pleural —see condition
Pleuralgia R07.81
Pleurisy (acute) (adhesive) (chronic) (costal)
    (diaphragmatic) (double) (dry) (fibrinous)
    (fibrous) (interlobar) (latent) (plastic)
    (primary) (residual) (sicca) (sterile)
    (subacute) (unresolved) R09.1
  with
    adherent pleura J86.0
    effusion J90
      chylous, chyliform J94.0
      tuberculous (non primary) A15.6
        primary (progressive) A15.7
      tuberculosis —see Pleurisy, tuberculous
        (non primary)
  encysted —see Pleurisy, with effusion
  exudative —see Pleurisy, with effusion
  fibrinopurulent, fibropurulent —see
    Pyothorax
  hemorrhagic —see Hemothorax
  pneumococcal J90
  purulent —see Pyothorax
  septic —see Pyothorax
  serofibrinous —see Pleurisy, with effusion
  seropurulent —see Pyothorax
  serous —see Pleurisy, with effusion
  staphylococcal J86.9
  streptococcal J90
  suppurative —see Pyothorax
  traumatic (post) (current) —see Injury,
    intrathoracic, pleura
  tuberculous (with effusion) (non primary)
    A15.6
    primary (progressive) A15.7
Pleuritis sicca —see Pleurisy
Pleurobronchopneumonia —see Pneumonia,
  broncho

Pleurodynia R07.81
  epidemic B33.0
  viral B33.0
Pleuropericarditis —*see also* Pericarditis
  acute I30.9
Pleuropneumonia (acute) (bilateral) (double)
  (septic) (*see also* Pneumonia) J18.8
  chronic —*see* Fibrosis, lung
Pleuro-pneumonia-like-organism (PPLO),
  as cause of disease classified elsewhere
  B96.0
Pleurorrhea —*see* Pleurisy, with effusion
Plexitis, brachial G54.0
Plica
  polonica B85.0
  syndrome, knee M67.5
  tonsil J35.8
Plicated tongue K14.5
Plug
  bronchus NEC J98.09
  meconium (newborn) NEC syndrome P76.0
  mucus —*see* Asphyxia, mucus
Plumbism —*see* subcategory T56.0
Plummer's disease E05.20
  with thyroid storm E05.21
Plummer-Vinson syndrome D50.1
Pluricarential syndrome of infancy E40
Plus (and minus) **hand** (intrinsic) —*see*
  Deformity, limb, specified type NEC,
  forearm
Pneumathemia —*see* Air, embolism
Pneumatic hammer (drill) **syndrome** T75.21
Pneumatocele (lung) J98.4
  intracranial G93.89
  tension J44.9
Pneumatosis
  cystoides intestinalis K63.89
  intestinalis K63.89
  peritonei K66.8
Pneumaturia R39.89
Pneumoblastoma —*see* Neoplasm, lung,
  malignant
Pneumocephalus G93.89
Pneumococcemia A40.3
Pneumococcus, pneumococcal —*see* condition
Pneumoconiosis (due to) (inhalation of) J64
  with tuberculosis (any type in A15) J65
  aluminum J63.0
  asbestos J61
  bagasse, bagassosis J67.1
  bauxite J63.1
  beryllium J63.2
  coal miners' (simple) J60
  coalworkers' (simple) J60
  collier's J60
  cotton dust J66.0
  diatomite (diatomaceous earth) J62.8
  dust
    inorganic NEC J63.6
    lime J62.8
    marble J62.8
    organic NEC J66.8
  fumes or vapors (from silo) J68.9
  graphite J63.3
  grinder's J62.8
  kaolin J62.8
  mica J62.8
  millstone maker's J62.8
  mineral fibers NEC J61
  miner's J60
  moldy hay J67.0
  potter's J62.8
  rheumatoid —*see* Rheumatoid, lung
  sandblaster's J62.8
  silica, silicate NEC J62.8
    with carbon J60
  stonemason's J62.8
  talc (dust) J62.0
Pneumocystis carinii pneumonia B59
Pneumocystis jiroveci (pneumonia) B59
Pneumocystosis (with pneumonia) B59

Pneumohemopericardium I31.2
Pneumohemothorax J94.2
  traumatic S27.2
Pneumohydropericardium —*see* Pericarditis
Pneumohydrothorax —*see* Hydrothorax
Pneumomediastinum J98.2
  congenital or perinatal P25.2
Pneumomycosis B49 [*J99*]
Pneumonia (acute) (double) (migratory)
  (purulent) (septic) (unresolved) J18.9
  with
    influenza —*see* Influenza, with, pneumonia
    lung abscess J85.1
      due to specified organism —*see*
        Pneumonia, in (due to)
  adenoviral J12.0
  adynamic J18.2
  alba A50.04
  allergic (eosinophilic) J82
  alveolar —*see* Pneumonia, lobar
  anaerobes J15.8
  anthrax A22.1
  apex, apical —*see* Pneumonia, lobar
  Ascaris B77.81
  aspiration J69.0
    due to
      aspiration of microorganisms
        bacterial J15.9
        viral J12.9
      food (regurgitated) J69.0
      gastric secretions J69.0
      milk (regurgitated) J69.0
      oils, essences J69.1
      solids, liquids NEC J69.8
      vomitus J69.0
    newborn P24.81
      amniotic fluid (clear) P24.11
      blood P24.21
      food (regurgitated) P24.31
      liquor (amnii) P24.11
      meconium P24.01
      milk P24.31
      mucus P24.11
      specified NEC P24.81
      stomach contents P24.31
    postprocedural J95.4
  atypical NEC J18.9
  bacillus J15.9
    specified NEC J15.8
  bacterial J15.9
    specified NEC J15.8
  Bacteroides (fragilis) (oralis)
    (melaninogenicus) J15.8
  basal, basic, basilar —*see* Pneumonia, by type
  bronchiolitis obliterans organized (BOOP)
    J84.89
  broncho-, bronchial (confluent) (croupous)
    (diffuse) (disseminated) (hemorrhagic)
    (involving lobes) (lobar) (terminal) J18.0
    allergic (eosinophilic) J82
    aspiration —*see* Pneumonia, aspiration
    bacterial J15.9
      specified NEC J15.8
    chronic —*see* Fibrosis, lung
    diplococcal J13
    Eaton's agent J15.7
    Escherichia coli (E. coli) J15.5
    Friedländer's bacillus J15.0
    Hemophilus influenzae J14
    hypostatic J18.2
    inhalation (*see also* Pneumonia, aspiration
      due to fumes or vapors (chemical) J68.0
      of oils or essences J69.1
    Klebsiella (pneumoniae) J15.0
    lipid, lipoid J69.1
      endogenous J84.89
    Mycoplasma (pneumoniae) J15.7
    pleuro-pneumonia-like-organisms (PPLO)
      J15.7
    pneumococcal J13
    Proteus J15.6

Pneumonia (*Continued*)
  broncho-, bronchial (*Continued*)
    Pseudomonas J15.1
    Serratia marcescens J15.6
    specified organism NEC J16.8
    staphylococcal —*see* Pneumonia,
      staphylococcal
    streptococcal NEC J15.4
      group B J15.3
      pneumoniae J13
    viral, virus —*see* Pneumonia, viral
  Butyrivibrio (fibriosolvens) J15.8
  Candida B37.1
  caseous —*see* Tuberculosis, pulmonary
  catarrhal —*see* Pneumonia, broncho
  chlamydial J16.0
    congenital P23.1
  cholesterol J84.89
  cirrhotic (chronic) —*see* Fibrosis, lung
  Clostridium (haemolyticum) (novyi) J15.8
  confluent —*see* Pneumonia, broncho
  congenital (infective) P23.9
    due to
      bacterium NEC P23.6
      Chlamydia P23.1
      Escherichia coli P23.4
      Haemophilus influenzae P23.6
      infective organism NEC P23.8
      Klebsiella pneumoniae P23.6
      Mycoplasma P23.6
      Pseudomonas P23.5
      Staphylococcus P23.2
      Streptococcus (except group B) P23.6
        group B P23.3
      viral agent P23.0
    specified NEC P23.8
  croupous —*see* Pneumonia, lobar
  cryptogenic organizing J84.116
  cytomegalic inclusion B25.0
  cytomegaloviral B25.0
  deglutition —*see* Pneumonia, aspiration
  desquamative interstitial J84.117
  diffuse —*see* Pneumonia, broncho
  diplococcal, diplococcus (broncho-) (lobar)
    J13
  disseminated (focal) —*see* Pneumonia,
    broncho
  Eaton's agent J15.7
  embolic, embolism —*see* Embolism,
    pulmonary
  Enterobacter J15.6
  eosinophilic J82
  Escherichia coli (E. coli) J15.5
  Eubacterium J15.8
  fibrinous —*see* Pneumonia, lobar
  fibroid, fibrous (chronic) —*see* Fibrosis, lung
  Friedländer's bacillus J15.0
  Fusobacterium (nucleatum) J15.8
  gangrenous J85.0
  giant cell (measles) B05.2
  gonococcal A54.84
  gram-negative bacteria NEC J15.6
    anaerobic J15.8
  Hemophilus influenzae (broncho) (lobar) J14
  human metapneumovirus J12.3
  hypostatic (broncho) (lobar) J18.2
  in (due to)
    actinomycosis A42.0
    adenovirus J12.0
    anthrax A22.1
    ascariasis B77.81
    aspergillosis B44.9
    Bacillus anthracis A22.1
    Bacterium anitratum J15.6
    candidiasis B37.1
    chickenpox B01.2
    Chlamydia J16.0
      neonatal P23.1
    coccidioidomycosis B38.2
      acute B38.0
      chronic B38.1

◀ New   ◀▥ Revised   ~~deleted~~ Deleted

Pneumonia (Continued)
  in (Continued)
    cytomegalovirus disease B25.0
    Diplococcus (pneumoniae) J13
    Eaton's agent J15.7
    Enterobacter J15.6
    Escherichia coli (E. coli) J15.5
    Friedländer's bacillus J15.0
    fumes and vapors (chemical) (inhalation)
      J68.0
    gonorrhea A54.84
    Hemophilus influenzae (H. influenzae)
      J14
    Herellea J15.6
    histoplasmosis B39.2
      acute B39.0
      chronic B39.1
    human metapneumovirus J12.3
    Klebsiella (pneumoniae) J15.0
    measles B05.2
    Mycoplasma (pneumoniae) J15.7
    nocardiosis, nocardiasis A43.0
    ornithosis A70
    parainfluenza virus J12.2
    pleuro-pneumonia-like-organism (PPLO)
      J15.7
    pneumococcus J13
    pneumocystosis (Pneumocystis carinii)
      (Pneumocystis jiroveci) B59
    Proteus J15.6
    Pseudomonas NEC J15.1
      pseudomallei A24.1
    psittacosis A70
    Q fever A78
    respiratory syncytial virus J12.1
    rheumatic fever I00 [J17]
    rubella B06.81
    Salmonella (infection) A02.22
      typhi A01.03
    schistosomiasis B65.9 [J17]
    Serratia marcescens J15.6
    specified
      bacterium NEC J15.8
      organism NEC J16.8
      spirochetal NEC A69.8
    Staphylococcus J15.20
      aureus (methicillin susceptible) (MSSA)
        J15.211
        methicillin resistant (MRSA)
          J15.212
      specified NEC J15.29
    Streptococcus J15.4
      group B J15.3
      pneumoniae J13
      specified NEC J15.4
    toxoplasmosis B58.3
    tularemia A21.2
    typhoid (fever) A01.03
    varicella B01.2
    virus —see Pneumonia, viral
    whooping cough A37.91
      due to
        Bordetella parapertussis
          A37.11
        Bordetella pertussis A37.01
        specified NEC A37.81
    Yersinia pestis A20.2
  inhalation of food or vomit —see Pneumonia,
    aspiration
  interstitial J84.9
    chronic J84.111
    desquamative J84.117
    due to
      collagen vascular disease J84.17
      known underlying cause J84.17
    idiopathic NOS J84.111
    in disease classified elsewhere J84.17
    lymphocytic (due to collagen vascular
      disease) (in diseases classified
      elsewhere) J84.17
    lymphoid J84.2

Pneumonia (Continued)
  interstitial (Continued)
    non-specific J84.89
      due to
        collagen vascular disease J84.17
        known underlying cause J84.17
      idiopathic (J84.113)
      in diseases classified elsewhere J84.17
    plasma cell B59
    pseudomonas J15.1
    usual J84.112
      due to collagen vascular disease J84.17
      idiopathic J84.112
      in diseases classified elsewhere J84.17
  Klebsiella (pneumoniae) J15.0
  lipid, lipoid (exogenous) J69.1
    endogenous J84.89
  lobar (disseminated) (double) (interstitial)
    J18.1
    bacterial J15.9
      specified NEC J15.8
    chronic —see Fibrosis, lung
    Escherichia coli (E. coli) J15.5
    Friedländer's bacillus J15.0
    Hemophilus influenzae J14
    hypostatic J18.2
    Klebsiella (pneumoniae) J15.0
    pneumococcal J13
    Proteus J15.6
    Pseudomonas J15.1
    specified organism NEC J16.8
    staphylococcal —see Pneumonia,
      staphylococcal
    streptococcal NEC J15.4
    Streptococcus pneumoniae J13
    viral, virus —see Pneumonia, viral
  lobular —see Pneumonia, broncho
  Löffler's J82
  lymphoid interstitial J84.2
  massive —see Pneumonia, lobar
  meconium P24.01
  MSSA (methicillin susceptible Staphylococcus
    aureus) J15.211
  multilobar —see Pneumonia, by type
  Mycoplasma (pneumoniae) J15.7
  necrotic J85.0
  neonatal P23.9
    aspiration —see Aspiration, by substance,
      with pneumonia
  nitrogen dioxide J68.9
  organizing J84.89
    due to
      collagen vascular disease J84.17
      known underlying cause J84.17
    in diseases classified elsewhere J84.17
  orthostatic J18.2
  parainfluenza virus J12.2
  parenchymatous —see Fibrosis, lung
  passive J18.2
  patchy —see Pneumonia, broncho
  Peptococcus J15.8
  Peptostreptococcus J15.8
  plasma cell (of infants) B59
  pleurolobar —see Pneumonia, lobar
  pleuro-pneumonia-like organism (PPLO)
    J15.7
  pneumococcal (broncho) (lobar) J13
  Pneumocystis (carinii) (jiroveci) B59
  postinfectional NEC B99 [J17]
  postmeasles B05.2
  Proteus J15.6
  Pseudomonas J15.1
  psittacosis A70
  radiation J70.0
  respiratory syncytial virus J12.1
  resulting from a procedure J95.89
  rheumatic I00 [J17]
  Salmonella (arizonae) (cholerae-suis)
    (enteritidis) (typhimurium) A02.22
    typhi A01.03
    typhoid fever A01.03

Pneumonia (Continued)
  SARS-associated coronavirus J12.81
  segmented, segmental —see Pneumonia,
    broncho-
  Serratia marcescens J15.6
  specified NEC J18.8
    bacterium NEC J15.8
    organism NEC J16.8
    virus NEC J12.89
  spirochetal NEC A69.8
  staphylococcal (broncho) (lobar) J15.20
    aureus (methicillin susceptible) (MSSA)
      J15.211
      methicillin resistant (MRSA) J15.212
    specified NEC J15.29
  static, stasis J18.2
  streptococcal NEC (broncho) (lobar) J15.4
    group
      A J15.4
      B J15.3
      specified NEC J15.4
  Streptococcus pneumoniae J13
  syphilitic, congenital (early) A50.04
  traumatic (complication) (early) (secondary)
    T79.8
  tuberculous (any) —see Tuberculosis,
    pulmonary
  tularemic A21.2
  varicella B01.2
  Veillonella J15.8
  ventilator associated J95.851
  viral, virus (broncho) (interstitial) (lobar) J12.9
    adenoviral J12.0
    congenital P23.0
    human metapneumovirus J12.3
    parainfluenza J12.2
    respiratory syncytial J12.1
    SARS-associated coronavirus J12.81
    specified NEC J12.89
  white (congenital) A50.04
Pneumonic —see condition
Pneumonitis (acute) (primary) —see also
  Pneumonia
  air-conditioner J67.7
  allergic (due to) J67.9
    organic dust NEC J67.8
    red cedar dust J67.8
    sequoiosis J67.8
    wood dust J67.8
  aspiration J69.0
    due to
      anesthesia J95.4
        during
          labor and delivery O74.0
            pregnancy O29.01-
            puerperium O89.01
      fumes or gases J68.0
      obstetric O74.0
  chemical (due to gases, fumes or vapors)
    (inhalation) J68.0
    due to anesthesia J95.4
  cholesterol J84.89
  chronic —see Fibrosis, lung
  congenital rubella P35.0
  crack (cocaine) J68.0
  due to
    beryllium J68.0
    cadmium J68.0
    crack (cocaine) J68.0
    detergent J69.8
    fluorocarbon-polymer J68.0
    food, vomit (aspiration) J69.0
    fumes or vapors J68.0
    gases, fumes or vapors (inhalation) J68.0
    inhalation
      blood J69.8
      essences J69.1
      food (regurgitated), milk, vomit J69.0
      oils, essences J69.1
      saliva J69.0
      solids, liquids NEC J69.8

Pneumonitis *(Continued)*
  due to *(Continued)*
    manganese J68.0
    nitrogen dioxide J68.0
    oils, essences J69.1
    solids, liquids NEC J69.8
    toxoplasmosis (acquired) B58.3
      congenital P37.1
    vanadium J68.0
    ventilator J95.851
  eosinophilic J82
  hypersensitivity J67.9
    air conditioner lung J67.7
    bagassosis J67.1
    bird fancier's lung J67.2
    farmer's lung J67.0
    maltworker's lung J67.4
    maple bark-stripper's lung J67.6
    mushroom worker's lung J67.5
    specified organic dust NEC J67.8
    suberosis J67.3
  interstitial (chronic) J84.89
    acute J84.114
    lymphoid J84.2
    non-specific J84.89
      idiopathic J84.113
  lymphoid, interstitial J84.2
  meconium P24.01
  postanesthetic J95.4
    correct substance properly administered —
      see Table of Drugs and Chemcials, by
      drug, adverse effect
    in labor and delivery O74.0
    in pregnancy O29.01-
      obstetric O74.0
    overdose or wrong substance given or
      taken (by accident) —*see* Table of
      Drugs and Chemicals, by drug,
      poisoning
    postpartum, puerperal O89.01
  postoperative J95.4
    obstetric O74.0
  radiation J70.0
  rubella, congenital P35.0
  ventilation (air-conditioning) J67.7
  ventilator associated J95.851
  wood-dust J67.8
Pneumonoconiosis —*see* Pneumoconiosis
Pneumoparotid K11.8
Pneumopathy NEC J98.4
  alveolar J84.09
  due to organic dust NEC J66.8
  parietoalveolar J84.09
Pneumopericarditis —*see also* Pericarditis
  acute I30.9
Pneumopericardium —*see also* Pericarditis
  congenital P25.3
  newborn P25.3
  traumatic (post) —*see* Injury, heart
Pneumophagia (psychogenic) F45.8
Pneumopleurisy, pneumopleuritis *(see also*
  Pneumonia) J18.8
Pneumopyopericardium I30.1
Pneumopyothorax —*see* Pyopneumothorax
  with fistula J86.0
Pneumorrhagia —*see also* Hemorrhage, lung
  tuberculous —*see* Tuberculosis, pulmonary
Pneumothorax NOS J93.9
  acute J93.83
  chronic J93.81
  congenital P25.1
  perinatal period P25.1
  postprocedural J95.811
  specified NEC J93.83
  spontaneous NOS J93.83
    newborn P25.1
    primary J93.11
    secondary J93.12
    tension J93.0
  tense valvular, infectional J93.0
  tension (spontaneous) J93.0

Pneumothorax NOS *(Continued)*
  traumatic S27.0
    with hemothorax S27.2
  tuberculous —*see* Tuberculosis, pulmonary
Podagra *(see also* Gout) M10.9
Podencephalus Q01.9
Poikilocytosis R71.8
Poikiloderma L81.6
  Civatte's L57.3
  congenital Q82.8
  vasculare atrophicans L94.5
Poikilodermatomyositis M33.10
  with
    myopathy M33.12
    respiratory involvement M33.11
    specified organ involvement NEC M33.19
Pointed ear (congenital) Q17.3
**Poison ivy, oak, sumac or other plant
  dermatitis** (allergic) (contact) L23.7
Poisoning (acute) —*see also* Table of Drugs and
  Chemicals
  algae and toxins T65.82-
  Bacillus B (aertrycke) (cholerae (suis))
    (paratyphosus) (suipestifer) A02.9
    botulinus A05.1
  bacterial toxins A05.9
  berries, noxious —*see* Poisoning, food,
    noxious, berries
  botulism A05.1
  ciguatera fish T61.0-
  Clostridium botulinum A05.1
  death-cap (Amanita phalloides) (Amanita
    verna) —*see* Poisoning, food, noxious,
    mushrooms
  drug —*see* Table of Drugs and Chemicals, by
    drug, poisoning
  epidemic, fish (noxious) —*see* Poisoning,
    seafood
    bacterial A05.9
  fava bean D55.0
  fish (noxious) T61.9-
    bacterial —*see* Intoxication, foodborne, by
      agent
    ciguatera fish —*see* Poisoning, ciguatera
      fish
    scombroid fish —*see* Poisoning, scombroid
      fish
    specified type NEC T61.77-
  food (acute) (diseased) (infected) (noxious)
    NEC T62.9-
    bacterial —*see* Intoxication, foodborne, by
      agent
    due to
      Bacillus (aertrycke) (choleraesuis)
        (paratyphosus) (suipestifer) A02.9
        botulinus A05.1
      Clostridium (perfringens) (Welchii)
        A05.2
      salmonella (aertrycke) (callinarum)
        (choleraesuis) (enteritidis)
        (paratyphi) (suipestifer) A02.9
        with
          gastroenteritis A02.0
          sepsis A02.1
      staphylococcus A05.0
      Vibrio
        parahaemolyticus A05.3
        vulnificus A05.5
    noxious or naturally toxic T62.9-
      berries —*see* subcategory T62.1-
      fish —*see* Poisoning, seafood
      mushrooms —*see* subcategory T62.0X-
      plants NEC —*see* subcategory T62.2X-
      seafood —*see* Poisoning, seafood
      specified NEC —*see* subcategory T62.8X-
    ichthyotoxism —*see* Poisoning, seafood
  kreotoxism, food A05.9
  latex T65.81-
  lead T56.0-
  mushroom —*see* Poisoning, food, noxious,
    mushroom

Poisoning *(Continued)*
  mussels —*see also* Poisoning, shellfish
    bacterial —*see* Intoxication, foodborne, by
      agent
  nicotine (tobacco) T65.2-
  noxious foodstuffs —*see* Poisoning, food,
    noxious
  plants, noxious —*see* Poisoning, food,
    noxious, plants NEC
  ptomaine —*see* Poisoning, food
  radiation J70.0
  Salmonella (arizonae) (cholerae-suis)
    (enteritidis) (typhimurium) A02.9
  scombroid fish T61.1-
  seafood (noxious) T61.9-
    bacterial —*see* Intoxication, foodborne, by
      agent
    fish —*see* Poisoning, fish
    shellfish —*see* Poisoning, shellfish
    specified NEC —*see* subcategory T61.8X-
  shellfish (amnesic) (azaspiracid) (diarrheic)
    (neurotoxic) (noxious) (paralytic)
    T61.78-
    bacterial —*see* Intoxication, foodborne, by
      agent
    ciguatera mollusk —*see* Poisoning,
      ciguatera fish
  specified substance NEC T65.891
  Staphylococcus, food A05.0
  tobacco (nicotine) T65.2-
  water E87.79
Poker spine —*see* Spondylitis, ankylosing
Poland syndrome Q79.8
Polioencephalitis (acute) (bulbar) A80.9
  inferior G12.22
  influenzal —*see* Influenza, with,
    encephalopathy
  superior hemorrhagic (acute) (Wernicke's)
    E51.2
  Wernicke's E51.2
Polioencephalomyelitis (acute) (anterior)
  A80.9
  with beriberi E51.2
Polioencephalopathy, superior hemorrhagic
  E51.2
  with
    beriberi E51.11
    pellagra E52
Poliomeningoencephalitis —*see*
  Meningoencephalitis
Poliomyelitis (acute) (anterior) (epidemic)
  A80.9
  with paralysis (bulbar) —*see* Poliomyelitis,
    paralytic
  abortive A80.4
  ascending (progressive) —*see* Poliomyelitis,
    paralytic
  bulbar (paralytic) —*see* Poliomyelitis,
    paralytic
  congenital P35.8
  nonepidemic A80.9
  nonparalytic A80.4
  paralytic A80.30
    specified NEC A80.39
    vaccine-associated A80.0
    wild virus
      imported A80.1
      indigenous A80.2
  spinal, acute A80.9
Poliosis (eyebrow) (eyelashes) L67.1
  circumscripta, acquired L67.1
Pollakiuria R35.0
  psychogenic F45.8
Pollinosis J30.1
Pollitzer's disease L73.2
Polyadenitis —*see also* Lymphadenitis
  malignant A20.0
Polyalgia M79.89
Polyangiitis M30.0
  microscopic M31.7
  overlap syndrome M30.8

◀ New   ⬅ Revised   ~~deleted~~ Deleted

Polyarteritis
  microscopic M31.7
  nodosa M30.0
    with lung involvement M30.1
    juvenile M30.2
    related condition NEC M30.8
Polyarthralgia —*see* Pain, joint
Polyarthritis, polyarthropathy (*see also* Arthritis) M13.0
  due to or associated with other specified conditions —*see* Arthritis
  epidemic (Australian) (with exanthema) B33.1
  infective —*see* Arthritis, pyogenic or pyemic
  inflammatory M06.4
  juvenile (chronic) (seronegative) M08.3
  migratory —*see* Fever, rheumatic
  rheumatic, acute —*see* Fever, rheumatic
Polyarthrosis M15.9
  post-traumatic M15.3
  primary M15.0
  specified NEC M15.8
Polycarential syndrome of infancy E40
Polychondritis (atrophic) (chronic) —*see also* Disorder, cartilage, specified type NEC
  relapsing M94.1
Polycoria Q13.2
Polycystic (disease)
  degeneration, kidney Q61.3
    autosomal dominant (adult type) Q61.2
    autosomal recessive (infantile type) NEC Q61.19
  kidney Q61.3
    autosomal
      dominant Q61.2
      recessive NEC Q61.19
    autosomal dominant (adult type) Q61.2
    autosomal recessive (childhood type) NEC Q61.19
    infantile type NEC Q61.19
  liver Q44.6
  lung J98.4
    congenital Q33.0
  ovary, ovaries E28.2
  spleen Q89.09
Polycythemia (secondary) D75.1
  acquired D75.1
  benign (familial) D75.0
  due to
    donor twin P61.1
    erythropoietin D75.1
    fall in plasma volume D75.1
    high altitude D75.1
    maternal-fetal transfusion P61.1
    stress D75.1
  emotional D75.1
  erythropoietin D75.1
  familial (benign) D75.0
  Gaisböck's (hypertonica) D75.1
  high altitude D75.1
  hypertonica D75.1
  hypoxemic D75.1
  neonatorum P61.1
  nephrogenous D75.1
  relative D75.1
  secondary D75.1
  spurious D75.1
  stress D75.1
  vera D45
Polycytosis cryptogenica D75.1
Polydactylism, polydactyly Q69.9
  toes Q69.2
Polydipsia R63.1
Polydystrophy, pseudo-Hurler E77.0
Polyembryoma —*see* Neoplasm, malignant, by site
Polyglandular
  deficiency E31.0
  dyscrasia E31.9
  dysfunction E31.9
  syndrome E31.8

Polyhydramnios O40.-
Polymastia Q83.1
Polymenorrhea N92.0
Polymyalgia M35.3
  arteritica, giant cell M31.5
  rheumatica M35.3
    with giant cell arteritis M31.5
Polymyositis (acute) (chronic) (hemorrhagic) M33.20
  with
    myopathy M33.22
    respiratory involvement M33.21
    skin involvement —*see* Dermatopolymyositis
    specified organ involvement NEC M33.29
  ossificans (generalisata) (progressiva) —*see* Myositis, ossificans, progressiva
Polyneuritis, polyneuritic —*see also* Polyneuropathy
  acute (post-)infective G61.0
  alcoholic G62.1
  cranialis G52.7
  demyelinating, chronic inflammatory (CIDP) G61.81
  diabetic —*see* Diabetes, polyneuropathy
  diphtheritic A36.83
  due to lack of vitamin NEC E56.9 *[G63]*
  endemic E51.11
  erythredema —*see* subcategory T56.1
  febrile, acute G61.0
  hereditary ataxic G60.1
  idiopathic, acute G61.0
  infective (acute) G61.0
  inflammatory, chronic demyelinating (CIDP) G61.81
  nutritional E63.9 *[G63]*
  postinfective (acute) G61.0
  specified NEC G62.89
Polyneuropathy (peripheral) G62.9
  alcoholic G62.1
  amyloid (Portuguese) E85.1 *[G63]*
  arsenical G62.2
  critical illness G62.81
  demyelinating, chronic inflammatory (CIDP) G61.81
  diabetic —*see* Diabetes, polyneuropathy
  drug-induced G62.0
  hereditary G60.9
    specified NEC G60.8
  idiopathic G60.9
    progressive G60.3
  in (due to)
    alcohol G62.1
      sequelae G65.2
    amyloidosis, familial (Portuguese) E85.1 *[G63]*
    antitetanus serum G61.1
    arsenic G62.2
      sequelae G65.2
    avitaminosis NEC E56.9 *[G63]*
    beriberi E51.11
    collagen vascular disease NEC M35.9 *[G63]*
    deficiency (of)
      B (-complex) vitamins E53.9 *[G63]*
      vitamin B6 E53.1 *[G63]*
    diabetes —*see* Diabetes, polyneuropathy
    diphtheria A36.83
    drug or medicament G62.0
      correct substance properly administered —*see* Table of Drugs and Chemicals, by drug, adverse effect
      overdose or wrong substance given or taken —*see* Table of Drugs and Chemicals, by drug, poisoning
    endocrine disease NEC E34.9 *[G63]*
    herpes zoster B02.23
    hypoglycemia E16.2 *[G63]*
    infectious
      disease NEC B99 *[G63]*
      mononucleosis B27.91

Polyneuropathy (*Continued*)
  in (*Continued*)
    lack of vitamin NEC E56.9 *[G63]*
    lead G62.2
      sequelae G65.2
    leprosy A30.9 *[G63]*
    Lyme disease A69.22
    metabolic disease NEC E88.9 *[G63]*
    microscopic polyangiitis M31.7 *[G63]*
    mumps B26.84
    neoplastic disease (*see also* Neoplasm) D49.9 *[G63]*
    nutritional deficiency NEC E63.9 *[G63]*
    organophosphate compounds G62.2
      sequelae G65.2
    parasitic disease NEC B89 *[G63]*
    pellagra E52 *[G63]*
    polyarteritis nodosa M30.0
    porphyria E80.20 *[G63]*
    radiation G62.82
    rheumatoid arthritis —*see* Rheumatoid, polyneuropathy
    sarcoidosis D86.89
    serum G61.1
    syphilis (late) A52.15
      congenital A50.43
    systemic
      connective tissue disorder M35.9 *[G63]*
      lupus erythematosus M32.19
    toxic agent NEC G62.2
      sequelae G65.2
    triorthocresyl phosphate G62.2
      sequelae G65.2
    tuberculosis A17.89
    uremia N18.9 *[G63]*
    vitamin B12 deficiency E53.8 *[G63]*
      with anemia (pernicious) D51.0 *[G63]*
      due to dietary deficiency D51.3 *[G63]*
    zoster B02.23
  inflammatory G61.9
    chronic demyelinating (CIDP) G61.81
    sequelae G65.1
    specified NEC G61.89
  lead G62.2
    sequelae G65.2
  nutritional NEC E63.9 *[G63]*
  postherpetic (zoster) B02.23
  progressive G60.3
  radiation-induced G62.82
  sensory (hereditary) (idiopathic) G60.8
  specified NEC G62.89
  syphilitic (late) A52.15
    congenital A50.43
Polyopia H53.8
Polyorchism, polyorchidism Q55.21
Polyosteoarthritis (*see also* Osteoarthritis, generalized) M15.9-
  post-traumatic M15.3
  specified NEC M15.8
Polyostotic fibrous dysplasia Q78.1
Polyotia Q17.0
Polyp, polypus
  accessory sinus J33.8
  adenocarcinoma in —*see* Neoplasm, malignant, by site
  adenocarcinoma in situ in —*see* Neoplasm, in situ, by site
  adenoid tissue J33.0
  adenomatous —*see also* Neoplasm, benign, by site
    adenocarcinoma in —*see* Neoplasm, malignant, by site
    adenocarcinoma in situ in —*see* Neoplasm, in situ, by site
    carcinoma in —*see* Neoplasm, malignant, by site
    carcinoma in situ in —*see* Neoplasm, in situ, by site

Polyp, polypus (Continued)
  adenomatous (Continued)
    multiple —see Neoplasm, benign
      adenocarcinoma in —see Neoplasm,
        malignant, by site
      adenocarcinoma in situ in —see
        Neoplasm, in situ, by site
  antrum J33.8
  anus, anal (canal) K62.0
  Bartholin's gland N84.3
  bladder D41.4
  carcinoma in —see Neoplasm, malignant, by
    site
  carcinoma in situ in —see Neoplasm, in situ,
    by site
  cecum D12.0
  cervix (uteri) N84.1
    in pregnancy or childbirth —see Pregnancy,
      complicated by, abnormal, cervix
    mucous N84.1
    nonneoplastic N84.1
  choanal J33.0
  cholesterol K82.4
  clitoris N84.3
  colon K63.5
    adenomatous D12.6
    ascending D12.2
    cecum D12.0
    descending D12.4
    inflammatory K51.40
      with
        abscess K51.414
        complication K51.419
          specified NEC K51.418
        fistula K51.413
        intestinal obstruction K51.412
        rectal bleeding K51.411
    sigmoid D12.5
    transverse D12.3
  corpus uteri N84.0
  dental K04.0
  duodenum K31.7
  ear (middle) H74.4-
  endometrium N84.0
  ethmoidal (sinus) J33.8
  fallopian tube N84.8
  female genital tract N84.9
    specified NEC N84.8
  frontal (sinus) J33.8
  gallbladder K82.4
  gingiva, gum K06.8
  labia, labium (majus) (minus) N84.3
  larynx (mucous) J38.1
    adenomatous D14.1
  malignant —see Neoplasm, malignant, by site
  maxillary (sinus) J33.8
  middle ear —see Polyp, ear (middle)
  myometrium N84.0
  nares
    anterior J33.9
    posterior J33.0
  nasal (mucous) J33.9
    cavity J33.0
    septum J33.0
  nasopharyngeal J33.0
  nose (mucous) J33.9
  oviduct N84.8
  pharynx J39.2
  placenta O90.89
  prostate —see Enlargement, enlarged,
    prostate
  pudenda, pudendum N84.3
  pulpal (dental) K04.0
  rectum (nonadenomatous) K62.1
    adenomatous —see Polyp, adenomatous
  septum (nasal) J33.0
  sinus (accessory) (ethmoidal) (frontal)
    (maxillary) (sphenoidal) J33.8
  sphenoidal (sinus) J33.8
  stomach K31.7
    adenomatous D13.1

Polyp, polypus (Continued)
  tube, fallopian N84.8
  turbinate, mucous membrane J33.8
  umbilical, newborn P83.6
  ureter N28.89
  urethra N36.2
  uterus (body) (corpus) (mucous) N84.0
    cervix N84.1
    in pregnancy or childbirth —see Pregnancy,
      complicated by, tumor, uterus
  vagina N84.2
  vocal cord (mucous) J38.1
  vulva N84.3
Polyphagia R63.2
Polyploidy Q92.7
Polypoid —see condition
Polyposis —see also Polyp
  coli (adenomatous) D12.6
    adenocarcinoma in C18.9
    adenocarcinoma in situ in —see Neoplasm,
      in situ, by site
    carcinoma in C18.9
  colon (adenomatous) D12.6
  familial D12.6
    adenocarcinoma in situ in —see Neoplasm,
      in situ, by site
  intestinal (adenomatous) D12.6
  malignant lymphomatous C83.1
  multiple, adenomatous (see also Neoplasm,
    benign) D36.9
Polyradiculitis —see Polyneuropathy
Polyradiculoneuropathy (acute) (postinfective)
  (segmentally demyelinating) G61.0
Polyserositis
  due to pericarditis I31.1
  pericardial I31.1
  periodic, familial E85.0
  tuberculous A19.9
    acute A19.1
    chronic A19.8
Polysplenia syndrome Q89.09
Polysyndactyly (see also Syndactylism,
  syndactyly) Q70.4
Polytrichia L68.3
Polyunguia Q84.6
Polyuria R35.8
  nocturnal R35.1
  psychogenic F45.8
Pompe's disease (glycogen storage) E74.02
Pompholyx L30.1
Poncet's disease (tuberculous rheumatism)
  A18.09
Pond fracture —see Fracture, skull
Ponos B55.0
Pons, pontine —see condition
Poor
  aesthetic of existing restoration of tooth
    K08.56
  contractions, labor O62.2
  gingival margin to tooth restoration K08.51
  personal hygiene R46.0
  prenatal care, affecting management of
    pregnancy —see Pregnancy, complicated
    by, insufficient, prenatal care
  sucking reflex (newborn) R29.2
  urinary stream R39.12
  vision NEC H54.7
Poradenitis, nostras inguinalis or venerea A55
Porencephaly (congenital) (developmental)
  (true) Q04.6
  acquired G93.0
  nondevelopmental G93.0
  traumatic (post) F07.89
Porocephaliasis B88.8
Porokeratosis Q82.8
Poroma, eccrine —see Neoplasm, skin, benign
Porphyria (South African) E80.20
  acquired E80.20
  acute intermittent (hepatic) (Swedish) E80.21
  cutanea tarda (hereditary) (symptomatic)
    E80.1

Porphyria (Continued)
  due to drugs E80.20
    correct substance properly administered —
      see Table of Drugs and Chemicals, by
      drug, adverse effect
    overdose or wrong substance given or
      taken —see Table of Drugs and
      Chemicals, by drug, poisoning
  erythropoietic (congenital) (hereditary)
    E80.0
  hepatocutaneous type E80.1
  secondary E80.20
  toxic NEC E80.20
  variegata E80.20
Porphyrinuria —see Porphyria
Porphyruria —see Porphyria
Portal —see condition
Port wine nevus, mark, or stain Q82.5
Posadas-Wernicke disease B38.9
Positive
  culture (nonspecific)
    blood R78.81
    bronchial washings R84.5
    cerebrospinal fluid R83.5
    cervix uteri R87.5
    nasal secretions R84.5
    nipple discharge R89.5
    nose R84.5
      staphylococcus (Methicillin susceptible)
        Z22.321
        Methicillin resistant Z22.322
    peritoneal fluid R85.5
    pleural fluid R84.5
    prostatic secretions R86.5
    saliva R85.5
    seminal fluid R86.5
    sputum R84.5
    synovial fluid R89.5
    throat scrapings R84.5
    urine R82.7
    vagina R87.5
    vulva R87.5
    wound secretions R89.5
  PPD (skin test) R76.11
  serology for syphilis A53.0
    with signs or symptoms - code as Syphilis,
      by site and stage
    false R76.8
  skin test, tuberculin (without active
    tuberculosis) R76.11
  test, human immunodeficiency virus (HIV)
    R75
  VDRL A53.0
    with signs or symptoms - code by site and
      stage under Syphilis A53.9
  Wassermann reaction A53.0
Postcardiotomy syndrome I97.0
Postcaval ureter Q62.62
Postcholecystectomy syndrome K91.5
Postclimacteric bleeding N95.0
Postcommissurotomy syndrome I97.0
Postconcussion syndrome F07.81
Postcontusional syndrome F07.81
Postcricoid region —see condition
Post-dates (40-42 weeks) (pregnancy) (mother)
  O48.0
  more than 42 weeks gestation O48.1
Postencephalitic syndrome F07.89
Posterior —see condition
Posterolateral sclerosis (spinal cord) —see
  Degeneration, combined
Postexanthematous —see condition
Postfebrile —see condition
Postgastrectomy dumping syndrome K91.1
Posthemiplegic chorea —see Monoplegia
Posthemorrhagic anemia (chronic) D50.0
  acute D62
  newborn P61.3
Postherpetic neuralgia (zoster) B02.29
  trigeminal B02.22
Posthitis N47.7

◀ New   ◀═ Revised   ~~deleted~~ Deleted

Postimmunization complication or reaction — *see* Complications, vaccination
Postinfectious —*see* condition
Postlaminectomy syndrome NEC M96.1
Postleukotomy syndrome F07.0
Postmastectomy lymphedema (syndrome) I97.2
Postmaturity, postmature (over 42 weeks)
   maternal (over 42 weeks gestation) O48.1
   newborn P08.22
Postmeasles complication NEC (*see also* condition) B05.89
Postmenopausal
   endometrium (atrophic) N95.8
      suppurative (*see also* Endometritis) N71.9
   osteoporosis —*see* Osteoporosis, postmenopausal
Postnasal drip R09.82
   due to
      allergic rhinitis —*see* Rhinitis, allergic
      common cold J00
      gastroesophageal reflux —*see* Reflux, gastroesophageal
      nasopharyngitis —*see* Nasopharyngitis
      other know condition — code to condition
      sinusitis —*see* Sinusitis
Postnatal —*see* condition
Postoperative (postprocedural) —*see* Complication, postoperative
   pneumothorax, therapeutic Z98.3
   state NEC Z98.89
Postpancreatectomy hyperglycemia E89.1
Postpartum —*see* Puerperal
Postphlebitic syndrome —*see* Syndrome, postthrombotic
Postpolio (myelitic) syndrome G14
Postpoliomyelitic —*see also* condition
   osteopathy —*see* Osteopathy, after poliomyelitis
Postprocedural —*see also* Postoperative
   hypoinsulinemia E89.1
Postschizophrenic depression F32.8
Postsurgery status —*see also* Status (post)
   pneumothorax, therapeutic Z98.3
Post-term (40-42 weeks) (pregnancy) (mother) O48.0
   infant P08.21
   more than 42 weeks gestation (mother) O48.1
Post-traumatic brain syndrome, nonpsychotic F07.81
Post-typhoid abscess A01.09
Postures, hysterical F44.2
Postvaccinal reaction or complication —*see* Complications, vaccination
Postvalvulotomy syndrome I97.0
Potain's
   disease (pulmonary edema) —*see* Edema, lung
   syndrome (gastrectasis with dyspepsia) K31.0
Potter's
   asthma J62.8
   facies Q60.6
   lung J62.8
   syndrome (with renal agenesis) Q60.6
Pott's
   curvature (spinal) A18.01
   disease or paraplegia A18.01
   spinal curvature A18.01
   tumor, puffy —*see* Osteomyelitis, specified type NEC
Pouch
   bronchus Q32.4
   Douglas' —*see* condition
   esophagus, esophageal, congenital Q39.6
      acquired K22.5
   gastric K31.4
   Hartmann's K82.8
   pharynx, pharyngeal (congenital) Q38.7
Pouchitis K91.850
Poultrymen's itch B88.0
Poverty NEC Z59.6
   extreme Z59.5

Poxvirus NEC B08.8
Prader-Willi syndrome Q87.1
Preauricular appendage or tag Q17.0
Prebetalipoproteinemia (acquired) (essential) (familial) (hereditary) (primary) (secondary) E78.1
   with chylomicronemia E78.3
Precipitate labor or delivery O62.3
Preclimacteric bleeding (menorrhagia) N92.4
Precocious
   adrenarche E30.1
   menarche E30.1
   menstruation E30.1
   pubarche E30.1
   puberty E30.1
      central E22.8
   sexual development NEC E30.1
   thelarche E30.8
Precocity, sexual (constitutional) (cryptogenic) (female) (idiopathic) (male) E30.1
   with adrenal hyperplasia E25.9
      congenital E25.0
Precordial pain R07.2
Predeciduous teeth K00.2
Prediabetes, prediabetic R73.09
   complicating
      pregnancy —*see* Pregnancy, complicated by, diseases of, specified type or system NEC
      puerperium O99.89
Predislocation status of hip at birth Q65.6
Pre-eclampsia O14.9-
   with pre-existing hypertension —*see* Hypertension, complicating pregnancy, pre-existing, with, pre-eclampsia
   mild O14.0-
   moderate O14.0-
   severe O14.1-
      with hemolysis, elevated liver enzymes and low platelet count (HELLP) O14.2-
Pre-eruptive color change, teeth, tooth K00.8
Pre-excitation atrioventricular conduction I45.6
Preglaucoma H40.00-
Pregnancy (single) (uterine) —*see also* Delivery and Puerperal

> Note: The Tabular must be reviewed for assignment of the appropriate character indicating the trimester of the pregnancy
>
> Note: The Tabular must be reviewed for assignment of appropriate seventh character for multiple gestation codes in Chapter 15

   abdominal (ectopic) O00.0
      with viable fetus O36.7-
   ampullar O00.1
   biochemical O02.81
   broad ligament O00.8
   cervical O00.8
   chemical O02.81
   complicated NOS O26.9-
   complicated by (care of) (management affected by)
      abnormal, abnormality
         cervix O34.4-
            causing obstructed labor O65.5
         cord (umbilical) O69.9
         findings on antenatal screening of mother O28.9
            biochemical O28.1
            chromosomal O28.5
            cytological O28.2
            genetic O28.5
            hematological O28.0
            radiological O28.4
            specified NEC O28.8
            ultrasonic O28.3
         glucose (tolerance) NEC O99.810

Pregnancy (*Continued*)
   complicated by (*Continued*)
      abnormal, abnormality (*Continued*)
         pelvic organs O34.9-
            specified NEC O34.8-
               causing obstructed labor O65.5
         pelvis (bony) (major) NEC O33.0
         perineum O34.7-
         position
            placenta O44.1-
               without hemorrhage O44.0-
            uterus O34.59-
         uterus O34.59-
            causing obstructed labor O65.5
            congenital O34.0-
         vagina O34.6-
            causing obstructed labor O65.5
         vulva O34.7-
            causing obstructed labor O65.5
      abruptio placentae —*see* Abruptio placentae
      abscess or cellulitis
         bladder O23.1-
         breast O91.11-
         genital organ or tract O23.9-
      abuse
         physical O9A.31-
         psychological O9A.51-
         sexual O9A.41-
      adverse effect anesthesia O29.9-
         aspiration pneumonitis O29.01-
         cardiac arrest O29.11-
         cardiac complication NEC O29.19-
         cardiac failure O29.12-
         central nervous system complication NEC O29.29-
         cerebral anoxia O29.21-
         failed or difficult intubation O29.6-
         inhalation of stomach contents or secretions NOS O29.01-
         local, toxic reaction O29.3X-
         Mendelson's syndrome O29.01-
         pressure collapse of lung O29.02-
         pulmonary complications NEC O29.09-
         specified NEC O29.8X-
         spinal and epidural type NEC O29.5X-
            induced headache O29.4-
      albuminuria O12.1-
      alcohol use O99.31-
      amnionitis O41.12-
      anaphylactoid syndrome of pregnancy O88.01-
      anemia (conditions in D50-D64) (pre-existing) O99.01-
         complicating the puerperium O99.03
      antepartum hemorrhage O46.9-
         with coagulation defect —*see* Hemorrhage, antepartum, with coagulation defect
         specified NEC O46.8X-
      appendicitis O99.61-
      atrophy (yellow) (acute) liver (subacute) O26.61-
      bariatric surgery status O99.84-
      bicornis or bicornuate uterus O34.59-
      biliary tract problems O26.61-
      breech presentation O32.1
      cardiovascular diseases (conditions in I00-I09, I20-I52, I70-I99) O99.41-
      cerebrovascular disorders (conditions in I60-I69) O99.41-
      cervical shortening O26.87-
      cervicitis O23.51-
      chloasma (gravidarum) O26.89-
      cholecystitis O99.61-
      cholestasis (intrahepatic) O26.61-
      chorioamnionitis O41.12-
      circulatory system disorder (conditions in I00-I09, I20-I99, O99.41-)
      compound presentation O32.6
      conjoined twins O30.02-

Pregnancy *(Continued)*
  complicated by *(Continued)*
    connective system disorders (conditions in M00-M99) O99.89
    contracted pelvis (general) O33.1
      inlet O33.2
      outlet O33.3
    convulsions (eclamptic) (uremic) *(see also* Eclampsia) O15.9-
    cracked nipple O92.11-
    cystitis O23.1-
    cystocele O34.8-
    death of fetus (near term) O36.4
      early pregnancy O02.1
      of one fetus or more in multiple gestation O31.2-
    deciduitis O41.14-
    decreased fetal movement O36.81-
    dental problems O99.61-
    diabetes (mellitus) O24.91-
      gestational (pregnancy induced) *—see* Diabetes, gestational
      pre-existing O24.31-
        specified NEC O24.81-
        type 1 O24.01-
        type 2 O24.11-
    digestive system disorders (conditions in K00-K93) O99.61-
    diseases of *—see* Pregnancy, complicated by, specified body system disease
      biliary tract O26.61-
      blood NEC (conditions in D65-D77) O99.11-
      liver O26.61-
      specified NEC O99.89
    disorders of *—see* Pregnancy, complicated by, specified body system disorder
      amniotic fluid and membranes O41.9-
        specified NEC O41.8X-
      biliary tract O26.61-
      ear and mastoid process (conditions in H60-H95) O99.89
      eye and adnexa (conditions in H00-H59) O99.89
      liver O26.61-
      skin (conditions in L00-L99) O99.71-
      specified NEC O99.89
    displacement, uterus NEC O34.59-
      causing obstructed labor O65.5
    disproportion (due to) O33.9
      fetal deformities NEC O33.7
      generally contracted pelvis O33.1
      hydrocephalic fetus O33.6
      inlet contraction of pelvis O33.2
      mixed maternal and fetal origin O33.4
      specified NEC O33.8
    double uterus O34.59-
      causing obstructed labor O65.5
    drug use (conditions in F11-F19) O99.32-
    eclampsia, eclamptic (coma) (convulsions) (delirium) (nephritis) (uremia) *(see also* Eclampsia) O15-
    ectopic pregnancy *—see* Pregnancy, ectopic
    edema O12.0-
      with
        gestational hypertension, mild *(see also* Pre-eclampsia) O14.0-
        proteinuria O12.2-
    effusion, amniotic fluid *—see* Pregnancy, complicated by, premature rupture of membranes
    elderly
      multigravida O09.52-
      primigravida O09.51-
    embolism *(see also* Embolism, obstetric, pregnancy) O88.-
    endocrine diseases NEC O99.28-
    endometritis O86.12
    excessive weight gain O26.0-
    exhaustion O26.81-
      during labor and delivery O75.81

Pregnancy *(Continued)*
  complicated by *(Continued)*
    face presentation O32.3
    failed induction of labor O61.9
    failed or difficult intubation for anesthesia O29.6-
      instrumental O61.1
      mechanical O61.1
      medical O61.0
      specified NEC O61.8
      surgical O61.1
    false labor (pains) O47.9
      at or after 37 completed weeks of pregnancy O47.1
      before 37 completed weeks of pregnancy O47.0-
    fatigue O26.81-
      during labor and delivery O75.81
    fatty metamorphosis of liver O26.61-
    female genital mutilation O34.8- *[N90.81-]*
    fetal (maternal care for)
      abnormality or damage O35.9
        acid-base balance O68
        specified type NEC O35.8
      acidemia O68
      acidosis O68
      alkalosis O68
      anemia and thrombocytopenia O36.82-
      anencephaly O35.0
      chromosomal abnormality (conditions in Q90-Q99) O35.1
      conjoined twins O30.02-
      damage from
        amniocentesis O35.7
        biopsy procedures O35.7
        drug addiction O35.5
        hematological investigation O35.7
        intrauterine contraceptive device O35.7
        maternal
          alcohol addiction O35.4
          cytomegalovirus infection O35.3
          disease NEC O35.8
          drug addiction O35.5
          listeriosis O35.8
          rubella O35.3
          toxoplasmosis O35.8
          viral infection O35.3
        medical procedure NEC O35.7
        radiation O35.6
      death (near term) O36.4
        early pregnancy O02.1
      decreased movement O36.81-
      disproportion due to deformity (fetal) O33.7
      excessive growth (large for dates) O36.6-
      growth retardation O36.59-
        light for dates O36.59-
        small for dates O36.59-
      heart rate irregularity (bradycardia) (decelerations) (tachycardia) O76
      hereditary disease O35.2
      hydrocephalus O35.0
      intrauterine death O36.4
      poor growth O36.59-
        light for dates O36.59-
        small for dates O36.59-
      problem O36.9-
        specified NEC O36.89-
      reduction (elective) O31.3-
      selective termination O31.3-
      spina bifida O35.0
      thrombocytopenia O36.82-
    fibroid (tumor) (uterus) O34.1-
    fissure of nipple O92.11-
    gallstones O99.61-
    gastric banding status O99.84-
    gastric bypass status O99.84-
    genital herpes (asymptomatic) (history of) (inactive) O98.51-
    genital tract infection O23.9-

Pregnancy *(Continued)*
  complicated by *(Continued)*
    glomerular diseases (conditions in N00-N07) O26.83-
      with hypertension, pre-existing *—see* Hypertension, complicating, pregnancy, pre-existing, with, renal disease
    gonorrhea O98.21-
    grand multiparity O09.4
    habitual aborter *—see* Pregnancy, complicated by, recurrent pregnancy loss
    HELLP syndrome (hemolysis, elevated liver enzymes and low platelet count) O14.2-
    hemorrhage
      antepartum *—see* Hemorrhage, antepartum
      before 20 completed weeks gestation O20.9
        specified NEC O20.8
      due to premature separation, placenta *(see also* Abruptio placentae) O45.9-
      early O20.9
        specified NEC O20.8
      threatened abortion O20.0
    hemorrhoids O22.4-
    hepatitis (viral) O98.41-
    herniation of uterus O34.59-
    high
      head at term O32.4
      risk *—see* Supervision (of) (for), high-risk
    history of in utero procedure during previous pregnancy O09.82-
    HIV O98.71-
    human immunodeficiency virus (HIV) disease O98.71-
    hydatidiform mole *(see also* Mole, hydatidiform) O01.9-
    hydramnios O40.-
    hydrocephalic fetus (disproportion) O33.6
    hydrops
      amnii O40.-
      fetalis O36.2-
        associated with isoimmunization *(see also* Pregnancy, complicated by, isoimmunization) O36.11-
    hydrorrhea O42.90
    hyperemesis (gravidarum) (mild) *(see also* Hyperemesis, gravidarum) O21.0-
    hypertension *—see* Hypertension, complicating pregnancy
    hypertensive
      heart and renal disease, pre-existing *— see* Hypertension, complicating, pregnancy, pre-existing, with, heart disease, with renal disease
      heart disease, pre-existing *—see* Hypertension, complicating, pregnancy, pre-existing, with, heart disease
      renal disease, pre-existing *—see* Hypertension, complicating, pregnancy, pre-existing, with, renal disease
    hypotension O26.5-
    immune disorders NEC (conditions in D80-D89) O99.11-
    incarceration, uterus O34.51-
    incompetent cervix O34.3-
    inconclusive fetal viability O36.80
    infection (s) O98.91-
      amniotic fluid or sac O41.10-
      bladder O23.1-
      carrier state NEC O99.830
        streptococcus B O99.820
      genital organ or tract O23.9-
        specified NEC O23.59-
      genitourinary tract O23.9-

◀ New   ◀▥ Revised   ~~deleted~~ Deleted

Pregnancy *(Continued)*
  complicated by *(Continued)*
    infection *(Continued)*
      gonorrhea O98.21-
      hepatitis (viral) O98.41-
      HIV O98.71-
      human immunodeficiency virus (HIV)
          O98.71-
      kidney O23.0-
      nipple O91.01-
      parasitic disease O98.91-
        specified NEC O98.81-
      protozoal disease O98.61-
      sexually transmitted NEC O98.31-
      specified type NEC O98.81-
      syphilis O98.11-
      tuberculosis O98.01-
      urethra O23.2-
      urinary (tract) O23.4-
        specified NEC O23.3-
      viral disease O98.51-
    injury or poisoning (conditions in S00-T88)
        O9A.21-
      due to abuse
        physical O9A.31-
        psychological O9A.51-
        sexual O9A.41-
    insufficient
      prenatal care O09.3-
      weight gain O26.1-
    insulin resistance O26.89
    intrauterine fetal death (near term) O36.4
      early pregnancy O02.1
      multiple gestation (one fetus or more)
          O31.2-
    isoimmunization O36.11-
      anti-A sensitization O36.11-
      anti-B sensitization O36.19-
      Rh O36.09-
        anti-D antibody O36.01-
      specified NEC O36.19-
    laceration of uterus NEC O71.81
    malformation
      placenta, placental (vessel) O43.10-
        specified NEC O43.19-
      uterus (congenital) O34.0-
    malnutrition (conditions in E40-E46) O25.1-
    maternal hypotension syndrome O26.5-
    mental disorders (conditions in F01-F09,
        F20-F99) O99.34-
      alcohol use O99.31-
      drug use O99.32-
      smoking O99.33-
    mentum presentation O32.3
    metabolic disorders O99.28-
    missed
      abortion O02.1
      delivery O36.4
    multiple gestations O30.9-
      conjoined twins O30.02-
      quadruplet —see Pregnancy, quadruplet
      specified complication NEC O31.8X-
      specified number of multiples NEC —see
          Pregnancy, multiple (gestation),
          specified NEC
      triplet —see Pregnancy, triplet
      twin —see Pregnancy, twin
    musculoskeletal condition (conditions is
        M00-M99) O99.89
    necrosis, liver (conditions in K72) O26.61-
    neoplasm
      benign
        cervix O34.4-
        corpus uteri O34.1-
        uterus O34.1-
      malignant O9A.11-
    nephropathy NEC O26.83-
    nervous system condition (conditions in
        G00-G99) O99.35-
    nutritional diseases NEC O99.28-
    obesity (pre-existing) O99.21-

Pregnancy *(Continued)*
  complicated by *(Continued)*
    obesity surgery status O99.84-
    oblique lie or presentation O32.2
    older mother —see Pregnancy, complicated
        by, elderly
    oligohydramnios O41.0-
      with premature rupture of membranes
          (*see also* Pregnancy, complicated by,
          premature rupture of membranes)
          O42-
    onset (spontaneous) of labor after 37
        completed weeks of gestation but
        before 39 completed weeks gestation,
        with delivery by (planned) cesarean
        section O75.82
    oophoritis O23.52-
    overdose, drug (*see also* Table of Drugs
        and Chemicals, by drug, poisoning)
        O9A.21-
    oversize fetus O33.5
    papyraceous fetus O31.0-
    pelvic inflammatory disease O99.89
    periodontal disease O99.61-
    peripheral neuritis O26.82-
    peritoneal (pelvic) adhesions O99.89
    phlebitis O22.9-
    phlebopathy O22.9-
    phlebothrombosis (superficial) O22.2-
      deep O22.3-
    placenta accreta O43.21-
    placenta increta O43.22-
    placenta percreta O43.23-
    placenta previa O44.1-
      without hemorrhage O44.0-
    placental disorder O43.9-
      specified NEC O43.89-
    placental dysfunction O43.89-
    placental infarction O43.81-
    placental insufficiency O36.51-
    placental transfusion syndromes
      fetomaternal O43.01-
      fetus to fetus O43.02-
      maternofetal O43.01-
    placentitis O41.14-
    pneumonia O99.51-
    poisoning (*see also* Table of Drugs and
        Chemicals) O9A.21-
    polyhydramnios O40-
    polymorphic eruption of pregnancy
        O26.86
    poor obstetric history NEC O09.29-
    postmaturity (post-term) (40 to 42 weeks)
        O48.0
      more than 42 completed weeks gestation
          (prolonged) O48.1
    pre-eclampsia O14.9-
      mild O14.0-
      moderate O14.0-
      severe O14.1-
        with hemolysis, elevated liver
            enzymes and low platelet count
            (HELLP) O14.2-
    premature labor —see Pregnancy,
        complicated by, preterm labor
    premature rupture of membranes O42.90
      with onset of labor
        within 24 hours O42.00
          after 37 weeks gestation O42.02
          pre-term (before 37 completed
              weeks of gestation) O42.01-
        after 24 hours O42.10
          after 37 weeks gestation O42.12
          pre-term (before 37 completed
              weeks of gestation) O42.11-
        after 37 weeks gestation O42.92
        full-term O42.92
        pre-term (before 37 completed weeks of
            gestation) O42.91-
    premature separation of placenta - (*see also*
        Abruptio placentae) O45.9-

Pregnancy *(Continued)*
  complicated by *(Continued)*
    presentation, fetal —see Delivery,
        complicated by, malposition
    preterm delivery O60.10
    preterm labor
      with delivery O60.10
        preterm O60.10
        term O60.20
      second trimester
        with preterm delivery
          second trimester O60.12
          third trimester O60.13
        with term delivery O60.22
        without delivery O60.02
      third trimester
        with term delivery O60.23
        with third trimester preterm delivery
            O60.14
        without delivery O60.03
      without delivery O60.00
        second trimester O60.02
        third trimester O60.03
    previous history of —see Pregnancy,
        supervision of, high-risk
    prolapse, uterus O34.52-
    proteinuria (gestational) O12.1-
      with edema O12.2-
    pruritic urticarial papules and plaques of
        pregnancy (PUPPP) O26.86
    pruritus (neurogenic) O26.89-
    psychosis or psychoneurosis (puerperal)
        F53
    ptyalism O26.89-
    PUPPP (pruritic urticarial papules and
        plaques of pregnancy) O26.86
    pyelitis O23.0-
    recurrent pregnancy loss O26.2-
    renal disease or failure NEC O26.83-
      with secondary hypertension,
          pre-existing —see Hypertension,
          complicating, pregnancy,
          pre-existing, secondary
      hypertensive, pre-existing —see
          Hypertension, complicating,
          pregnancy, pre-existing, with, renal
          disease
    respiratory condition (conditions in
        J00-J99) O99.51-
    retained, retention
      dead ovum O02.0
      intrauterine contraceptive device
          O26.3-
    retroversion, uterus O34.53-
    Rh immunization, incompatibility or
        sensitization NEC O36.09-
      anti-D antibody O36.01-
    rupture
      amnion (premature) (*see also* Pregnancy,
          complicated by, premature rupture
          of membranes) O42-
      membranes (premature) (*see also*
          Pregnancy, complicated by,
          premature rupture of membranes)
          O42-
      uterus (during labor) O71.1
        before onset of labor O71.0-
    salivation (excessive) O26.89-
    salpingitis O23.52-
    salpingo-oophoritis O23.52-
    sepsis (conditions in A40, A41) O98.81-
    size date discrepancy (uterine) O26.84-
    skin condition (conditions in L00-L99)
        O99.71-
    smoking (tobacco) O99.33-
    social problem O09.7-
    specified condition NEC O26.89-
    spotting O26.85-
    streptococcus B carrier state O99.820
    subluxation of symphysis (pubis) O26.71-
    syphilis (conditions in Λ50-A53) O98.11-

◀ New ◀▥▥ Revised ~~deleted~~ Deleted

Pregnancy *(Continued)*
  supervision of *(Continued)*
    high-risk *(Continued)*
      due to *(Continued)*
        in utero procedure during previous
          pregnancy O09.82-
        in vitro fertilization O09.81-
        molar pregnancy O09.1-
        multiple previous pregnancies O09.4-
        older mother —*see* Pregnancy,
          supervision of, elderly mother
        poor reproductive or obstetric history
          NEC O09.29-
        pre-term labor O09.21-
        previous
          neonatal death O09.29-
        social problems O09.7-
        specified NEC O09.89
        very young mother —*see* Pregnancy,
          supervision, young mother
      resulting from in vitro fertilization
        O09.81-
    normal Z34.9-
      first Z34.0-
      specified NEC Z34.8-
    young mother
      multigravida O09.62-
      primigravida O09.61-
  triplet O30.10-
    with
      two or more monoamniotic fetuses
        O30.12-
      two or more monochorionic fetuses
        O30.11-
    two or more monoamniotic fetuses O30.12-
    two or more monochorionic fetuses O30.11-
    unable to determine number of placenta
      and number of amniotic sacs O30.19-
    unspecified number of placenta and
      unspecified number of amniotic sacs
      O30.10-
  tubal (with abortion) (with rupture) O00.1
  twin O30.00-
    conjoined O30.02-
    dichorionic/diamniotic (two placenta, two
      amniotic sacs) O30.04-
    monochorionic/diamniotic (one placenta,
      two amniotic sacs) O30.03-
    monochorionic/monoamniotic (one
      placenta, one amniotic sac) O30.01-
    unable to determine number of placenta
      and number of amniotic sacs O30.09-
    unspecified number of placenta and
      unspecified number of amniotic sacs
      O30.00-
  unwanted Z64.0
  weeks of gestation
    8 weeks Z3A.08
    9 weeks Z3A.09
    10 weeks Z3A.10
    11 weeks Z3A.11
    12 weeks Z3A.12
    13 weeks Z3A.13
    14 weeks Z3A.14
    15 weeks Z3A.15
    16 weeks Z3A.16
    17 weeks Z3A.17
    18 weeks Z3A.18
    19 weeks Z3A.19
    20 weeks Z3A.20
    21 weeks Z3A.21
    22 weeks Z3A.22
    23 weeks Z3A.23
    24 weeks Z3A.24
    25 weeks Z3A.25
    26 weeks Z3A.26
    27 weeks Z3A.27
    28 weeks Z3A.28
    29 weeks Z3A.29
    30 weeks Z3A.30
    31 weeks Z3A.31
    32 weeks Z3A.32

Pregnancy *(Continued)*
  weeks of gestation *(Continued)*
    33 weeks Z3A.33
    34 weeks Z3A.34
    35 weeks Z3A.35
    36 weeks Z3A.36
    37 weeks Z3A.37
    38 weeks Z3A.38
    39 weeks Z3A.39
    40 weeks Z3A.40
    41 weeks Z3A.41
    42 weeks Z3A.42
    greater than 42 weeks Z3A.49
    less than 8 weeks Z3A.01
    not specified Z3A.00
Preiser's disease —*see* Osteonecrosis,
  secondary, due to, trauma, metacarpus
Pre-kwashiorkor —*see* Malnutrition, severe
Preleukemia (syndrome) D46.9
Preluxation, hip, congenital Q65.6
Premature —*see also* condition
  adrenarche E27.0
  aging E34.8
  beats I49.40
    atrial I49.1
    auricular I49.1
    supraventricular I49.1
  birth NEC —*see* Preterm, newborn
  closure, foramen ovale Q21.8
  contraction
    atrial I49.1
    atrioventricular I49.49
    auricular I49.1
    auriculoventricular I49.2
    heart (extrasystole) I49.49
    junctional I49.2
    ventricular I49.3
  delivery (*see also* Pregnancy, complicated by,
    preterm labor) O60.10
  ejaculation F52.4
  infant NEC —*see* Preterm, newborn
    light-for-dates —*see* Light for dates
  labor —*see* Pregnancy, complicated by,
    preterm labor
  lungs P28.0
  menopause E28.319
    asymptomatic E28.319
    symptomatic E28.310
  newborn
    extreme (less than 28 completed weeks) —
      see Immaturity, extreme
    less than 37 completed weeks —*see*
      Preterm, newborn
  puberty E30.1
  rupture membranes or amnion —*see*
    Pregnancy, complicated by, premature
    rupture of membranes
  senility E34.8
  thelarche E30.8
  ventricular systole I49.3
Prematurity NEC (less than 37 completed
  weeks) —*see* Preterm, newborn
  extreme (less than 28 completed weeks) —*see*
    Immaturity, extreme
Premenstrual
  dysphoric disorder (PMDD) N94.3
  tension (syndrome) N94.3
Premolarization, cuspids K00.2
Prenatal
  care, normal pregnancy —*see* Pregnancy,
    normal
  screening of mother Z36
  teeth K00.6
**Preparatory care for subsequent treatment
  NEC**
  for dialysis Z49.01
    peritoneal Z49.02
Prepartum —*see* condition
Preponderance, left or right ventricular I51.7
Prepuce —*see* condition
PRES (posterior reversible encephalopathy
  syndrome) I67.83

Presbycardia R54
Presbycusis, presbyacusia H91.1-
Presbyesophagus K22.8
Presbyophrenia F03
Presbyopia H52.4
Prescription of contraceptives (initial) Z30.019
  emergency (postcoital) Z30.012
  implantable subdermal Z30.019
  injectable Z30.013
  intrauterine contraceptive device Z30.014
  pills Z30.011
  postcoital (emergency) Z30.012
  repeat Z30.40
    implantable subdermal Z30.49
    injectable Z30.42
    pills Z30.41
    specified type NEC Z30.49
  specified type NEC Z30.018
Presence (of)
  ankle-joint implant (functional) (prosthesis)
    Z96.66-
  aortocoronary (bypass) graft Z95.1
  arterial-venous shunt (dialysis) Z99.2
  artificial
    eye (globe) Z97.0
    heart (fully implantable) (mechanical)
      Z95.812
      valve Z95.2
    larynx Z96.3
    lens (intraocular) Z96.1
    limb (complete) (partial) Z97.1-
      arm Z97.1-
        bilateral Z97.15
      leg Z97.1-
        bilateral Z97.16
  audiological implant (functional) Z96.29
  bladder implant (functional) Z96.0
  bone
    conduction hearing device Z96.29
    implant (functional) NEC Z96.7
    joint (prosthesis) —*see* Presence, joint
      implant
  cardiac
    defibrillator (functional) (with synchronous
      cardiac pacemaker) Z95.810
    implant or graft Z95.9
      specified type NEC Z95.818
    pacemaker Z95.0
  cerebrospinal fluid drainage device Z98.2
  cochlear implant (functional) Z96.21
  contact lens (es) Z97.3
  coronary artery graft or prosthesis Z95.5
  CSF shunt Z98.2
  dental prosthesis device Z97.2
  dentures Z97.2
  device (external) NEC Z97.8
    cardiac NEC Z95.818
    heart assist Z95.811
    implanted (functional) Z96.9
      specified NEC Z96.89
    prosthetic Z97.8
  ear implant Z96.20
    cochlear implant Z96.21
    myringotomy tube Z96.22
    specified type NEC Z96.29
  elbow-joint implant (functional) (prosthesis)
    Z96.62-
  endocrine implant (functional) NEC Z96.49
  eustachian tube stent or device (functional)
    Z96.29
  external hearing-aid or device Z97.4
  finger-joint implant (functional) (prosthetic)
    Z96.69-
  functional implant Z96.9
    specified NEC Z96.89
  graft
    cardiac NEC Z95.818
    vascular NEC Z95.828
  hearing-aid or device (external) Z97.4
    implant (bone) (cochlear) (functional)
      Z96.21
  heart assist device Z95.811

◀ New   ◀▥ Revised   ~~deleted~~ Deleted

Problem (Continued)
  digestive K92.9
  drug addict in family Z63.72
  ear —see Disorder, ear
  economic Z59.9
    affecting care Z59.9
    specified NEC Z59.8
  education Z55.9
    specified NEC Z55.8
  employment Z56.9
    change of job Z56.1
    discord Z56.4
    environment Z56.5
    sexual harassment Z56.81
    specified NEC Z56.89
    stress NEC Z56.6
    stressful schedule Z56.3
    threat of job loss Z56.2
    unemployment Z56.0
  enuresis, child F98.0
  eye H57.9
  failed examinations (school) Z55.2
  falling Z91.81
  family (see also Disruption, family) Z63.9-
    specified NEC Z63.8
  feeding (elderly) (infant) R63.3
    newborn P92.9
      breast P92.5
      overfeeding P92.4
      slow P92.2
      specified NEC P92.8
      underfeeding P92.3
    nonorganic F50.8
  finance Z59.9
    specified NEC Z59.8
  foreclosure on loan Z59.8
  foster child Z62.822
  frightening experience (s) in childhood
    Z62.898
  genital NEC
    female N94.9
    male N50.9
  health care Z75.9
    specified NEC Z75.8
  hearing —see Deafness
  homelessness Z59.0
  housing Z59.9
    inadequate Z59.1
    isolated Z59.8
    specified NEC Z59.8
  identity (of childhood) F93.8
  illegitimate pregnancy (unwanted) Z64.0
  illiteracy Z55.0
  impaired mobility Z74.09
  imprisonment or incarceration Z65.1
  inadequate teaching affecting education
    Z55.8
  inappropriate (excessive) parental pressure
    Z62.6
  influencing health status NEC Z78.9
  in-law Z63.1
  institutionalization, affecting child
    Z62.22
  intrafamilial communication Z63.8
  jealousy, child F93.8
  landlord Z59.2
  language (developmental) F80.9
  learning (developmental) F81.9
  legal Z65.3
    conviction without imprisonment Z65.0
    imprisonment Z65.1
    release from prison Z65.2
  life-management Z73.9
    specified NEC Z73.89
  life-style Z72.9
    gambling Z72.6
    high-risk sexual behavior (heterosexual)
      Z72.51
      bisexual Z72.53
      homosexual Z72.52
    inappropriate eating habits Z72.4

Problem (Continued)
  life-style (Continued)
    self-damaging behavior NEC Z72.89
    specified NEC Z72.89
    tobacco use Z72.0
  literacy Z55.9
    low level Z55.0
    specified NEC Z55.8
  living alone Z60.2
  lodgers Z59.2
  loss of love relationship in childhood Z62.898
  marital Z63.0
    involving
      divorce Z63.5
      estrangement Z63.5
      gender identity F66
  mastication K08.8
  medical
    care, within family Z63.6
    facilities Z75.9
      specified NEC Z75.8
  mental F48.9
  multiparity Z64.1
  negative life events in childhood Z62.9
    altered pattern of family relationships
      Z62.898
    frightening experience Z62.898
    loss of
      love relationship Z62.898
      self-esteem Z62.898
    physical abuse (alleged) —see
      Maltreatment, child
    removal from home Z62.29
    specified event NEC Z62.898
  neighbor Z59.2
  neurological NEC R29.818
  new step-parent affecting child Z62.898
  none (feared complaint unfounded) Z71.1
  occupational NEC Z56.89
  parent-child —see Conflict, parent-child
  personal hygiene Z91.89
  personality F69
  phase-of-life transition, adjustment Z60.0
  presence of sick or disabled person in family
    or household Z63.79
    needing care Z63.6
  primary support group (family) Z63.9
    specified NEC Z63.8
  probation officer Z64.4
  psychiatric F99
  psychosexual (development) F66
  psychosocial Z65.9
    specified NEC Z65.8
  relationship Z63.9
    childhood F93.8
  release from prison Z65.2
  removal from home affecting child Z62.29
  seeking and accepting known hazardous and
    harmful
    behavioral or psychological interventions
      Z65.5
    chemical, nutritional or physical
      interventions Z65.8
  sexual function (nonorganic) F52.9
  sight H54.7
  sleep disorder, child F51.9
  smell —see Disturbance, sensation, smell
  social
    environment Z60.9
      specified NEC Z60.8
    exclusion and rejection Z60.4
    worker Z64.4
  speech R47.9
    developmental F80.9
    specified NEC R47.89
  swallowing —see Dysphagia
  taste —see Disturbance, sensation, taste
  tic, child F95.0
  underachievement in school Z55.3
  unemployment Z56.0
    threatened Z56.2

Problem (Continued)
  unwanted pregnancy Z64.0
  upbringing Z62.9
    specified NEC Z62.898
  urinary N39.9
  voice production R47.89
  work schedule (stressful) Z56.3
Procedure (surgical)
  for purpose other than remedying health
    state Z41.9
    specified NEC Z41.8
  not done Z53.9
    because of
      administrative reasons Z53.8
      contraindication Z53.09
        smoking Z53.01
      patient's decision Z53.20
        for reasons of belief or group pressure
          Z53.1
        left against medical advice (AMA)
          Z53.21
        specified reason NEC Z53.29
      specified reason NEC Z53.8
Procidentia (uteri) N81.3
Proctalgia K62.89
  fugax K59.4
  spasmodic K59.4
Proctitis K62.89
  amebic (acute) A06.0
  chlamydial A56.3
  gonococcal A54.6
  granulomatous —see Enteritis, regional, large
    intestine
  herpetic A60.1
  radiation K62.7
  tuberculous A18.32
  ulcerative (chronic) K51.20
    with
      complication K51.219
        abscess K51.214
        fistula K51.213
        obstruction K51.212
        rectal bleeding K51.211
        specified NEC K51.218
Proctocele
  female (without uterine prolapse) N81.6
    with uterine prolapse N81.2
      complete N81.3
  male K62.3
Proctocolitis, mucosal —see Rectosigmoiditis,
  ulcerative
Proctoptosis K62.3
Proctorrhagia K62.5
Proctosigmoiditis K63.89
  ulcerative (chronic) —see Rectosigmoiditis,
    ulcerative
Proctospasm K59.4
  psychogenic F45.8
Profichet's disease —see Disorder, soft tissue,
  specified type NEC
Progeria E34.8
Prognathism (mandibular) (maxillary)
  M26.19
Progonoma (melanotic) —see Neoplasm,
  benign, by site
Progressive —see condition
Prolactinoma
  specified site —see Neoplasm, benign,
    by site
  unspecified site D35.2
Prolapse, prolapsed
  anus, anal (canal) (sphincter) K62.2
  arm or hand O32.2
    causing obstructed labor O64.4
  bladder (mucosa) (sphincter) (acquired)
    congenital Q79.4
    female —see Cystocele
    male N32.89
  breast implant (prosthetic) T85.49
  cecostomy K94.09
  cecum K63.4

Prolapse, prolapsed (Continued)
  cervix, cervical (hypertrophied) N81.2
    anterior lip, obstructing labor O65.5
    congenital Q51.828
    postpartal, old N81.2
    stump N81.85
  ciliary body (traumatic) —see Laceration,
      eye(ball), with prolapse or loss of
      interocular tissue
  colon (pedunculated) K63.4
  colostomy K94.09
  disc (intervertebral) —see Displacement,
      intervertebral disc
  eye implant (orbital) T85.398
    lens (ocular) —see Complications,
        intraocular lens
  fallopian tube N83.4
  gastric (mucosa) K31.89
  genital, female N81.9
    specified NEC N81.89
  globe, nontraumatic —see Luxation, globe
  ileostomy bud K94.19
  intervertebral disc —see Displacement,
      intervertebral disc
  intestine (small) K63.4
  iris (traumatic) —see Laceration, eye(ball),
      with prolapse or loss of interocular
      tissue
    nontraumatic H21.89
  kidney N28.83
    congenital Q63.2
  laryngeal muscles or ventricle J38.7
  liver K76.89
  meatus urinarius N36.8
  mitral (valve) I34.1
  ocular lens implant —see Complications,
      intraocular lens
  organ or site, congenital NEC —see
      Malposition, congenital
  ovary N83.4
  pelvic floor, female N81.89
  perineum, female N81.89
  rectum (mucosa) (sphincter) K62.3
    due to trichuris trichuria B79
  spleen D73.89
  stomach K31.89
  umbilical cord
    complicating delivery O69.0
  urachus, congenital Q64.4
  ureter N28.89
    with obstruction N13.5
      with infection N13.6
  ureterovesical orifice N28.89
  urethra (acquired) (infected) (mucosa)
      N36.8
    congenital Q64.71
  urinary meatus N36.8
    congenital Q64.72
  uterovaginal N81.4
    complete N81.3
    incomplete N81.2
  uterus (with prolapse of vagina) N81.4
    complete N81.3
    congenital Q51.818
    first degree N81.2
    in pregnancy or childbirth —see
        Pregnancy, complicated by,
        abnormal, uterus
    incomplete N81.2
    postpartal (old) N81.4
    second degree N81.2
    third degree N81.3
  uveal (traumatic) —see Laceration, eye(ball),
      with prolapse or loss of interocular
      tissue
  vagina (anterior) (wall) —see Cystocele
    with prolapse of uterus N81.4
      complete N81.3
      incomplete N81.2
    posterior wall N81.6
    posthysterectomy N99.3

Prolapse, prolapsed (Continued)
  vitreous (humor) H43.0-
    in wound —see Laceration, eye(ball), with
        prolapse or loss of interocular tissue
  womb —see Prolapse, uterus
Prolapsus, female N81.9
  specified NEC N81.89
Proliferation (s)
  primary cutaneous CD30-positive large T-cell
      C86.6
Proliferative —see condition
Prolonged, prolongation (of)
  bleeding (time) (idiopathic) R79.1
  coagulation (time) R79.1
  gestation (over 42 completed weeks)
    mother O48.1
    newborn P08.22
  interval I44.0
  labor O63.9
    first stage O63.0
    second stage O63.1
  partial thromboplastin time (PTT) R79.1
  pregnancy (more than 42 weeks gestation)
      O48.1
  prothrombin time R79.1
  QT interval I45.81
  uterine contractions in labor O62.4
Prominence, prominent
  with disproportion (fetopelvic) O33.0
    causing obstructed labor O65.0
  auricle (congenital) (ear) Q17.5
  ischial spine or sacral promontory
  nose (congenital) acquired M95.0
Promiscuity —see High, risk, sexual behavior
Pronation
  ankle —see Deformity, limb, foot, specified
      NEC
  foot —see also Deformity, limb, foot, specified
      NEC
    congenital Q74.2
Prophylactic
  administration of
    antibiotics, long-term Z79.2
      short-term use - omit code
    drug (see also Long-term (current) drug
        therapy (use of)) Z79.899-
  medication Z79.899
  organ removal (for neoplasia management)
      Z40.00
    breast Z40.01
    ovary Z40.02
    specified site NEC Z40.09
  surgery Z40.9
    for risk factors related to malignant
        neoplasm —see Prophylactic, organ
        removal
    specified NEC Z40.8
  vaccination Z23
Propionic acidemia E71.121
Proptosis (ocular) —see also Exophthalmos
  thyroid —see Hyperthyroidism, with goiter
Prosecution, anxiety concerning Z65.3
Prosopagnosia R48.3
Prostadynia N42.81
Prostate, prostatic —see condition
Prostatism —see Hyperplasia, prostate
Prostatitis (congestive) (suppurative) (with
    cystitis) N41.9
  acute N41.0
  cavitary N41.8
  chronic N41.1
  diverticular N41.8
  due to Trichomonas (vaginalis) A59.02
  fibrous N41.1
  gonococcal (acute) (chronic) A54.22
  granulomatous N41.4
  hypertrophic N41.1
  subacute N41.1
  trichomonal A59.02
  tuberculous A18.14
Prostatocystitis N41.3

Prostatorrhea N42.89
Prostatosis N42.82
Prostration R53.83
  heat —see also Heat, exhaustion
    anhydrotic T67.3
    due to
      salt (and water) depletion T67.4
      water depletion T67.3
  nervous F48.8
  senile R54
Protanomaly (anomalous trichromat) H53.54
Protanopia (complete) (incomplete) H53.54
Protection (against) (from) —see Prophylactic
Protein
  deficiency NEC —see Malnutrition
  malnutrition —see Malnutrition
  sickness (see also Reaction, serum) T80.69
Proteinemia R77.9
Proteinosis
  alveolar (pulmonary) J84.01
  lipid or lipoid (of Urbach) E78.89
Proteinuria R80.9
  Bence Jones R80.3
  complicating pregnancy —see Proteinuria,
      gestational
  gestational O12.1-
    with edema O12.2-
  idiopathic R80.0
  isolated R80.0
    with glomerular lesion N06.9
      dense deposit disease N06.6
      diffuse
        crescentic glomerulonephritis N06.7
        endocapillary proliferative
            glomerulonephritis N06.4
        mesangiocapillary glomerulonephritis
            N06.5
      focal and segmental hyalinosis or
          sclerosis N06.1
      membranous (diffuse) N06.2
      mesangial proliferative (diffuse)
          N06.3
      minimal change N06.0
      specified pathology NEC N06.8
  orthostatic R80.2
    with glomerular lesion —see Proteinuria,
        isolated, with glomerular lesion
  persistent R80.1
    with glomerular lesion —see Proteinuria,
        isolated, with glomerular lesion
  postural R80.2
    with glomerular lesion —see Proteinuria,
        isolated, with glomerular lesion
  pre-eclamptic —see Pre-eclampsia
  specified type NEC R80.8
Proteolysis, pathologic D65
Proteus (mirabilis) (morganii), as cause of
    disease classified elsewhere B96.4
Prothrombin gene mutation D68.52
Protoporphyria, erythropoietic E80.0
Protozoal —see also condition
  disease B64
    specified NEC B60.8
Protrusion, protrusio
  acetabuli M24.7
  acetabulum (into pelvis) M24.7
  device, implant or graft (see also
      Complications, by site and type,
      mechanical) T85.698
    arterial graft NEC —see Complication,
        cardiovascular device, mechanical,
        vascular
    breast (implant) T85.49
    catheter NEC T85.698
      cystostomy T83.090
      dialysis (renal) T82.49
        intraperitoneal T85.691
      infusion NEC T82.594
        spinal (epidural) (subdural)
            T85.690
      urinary, indwelling T83.098

◀ New   ◀▥ Revised   ~~deleted~~ Deleted

Protrusion, protrusio (Continued)
  device, implant or graft (Continued)
    electronic (electrode) (pulse generator)
        (stimulator)
      bone T84.390
        nervous system —see Complication,
            prosthetic device, mechanical,
            electronic nervous system
            stimulator
    fixation, internal (orthopedic) NEC —see
        Complication, fixation device,
        mechanical
    gastrointestinal —see Complications,
        prosthetic device, mechanical,
        gastrointestinal device
    genital NEC T83.498
      intrauterine contraceptive device
          T83.39
      penile prosthesis T83.490
    heart NEC —see Complication,
        cardiovascular device, mechanical
    joint prosthesis —see Complications, joint
        prosthesis, mechanical, specified
        NEC, by site
    ocular NEC —see Complications, prosthetic
        device, mechanical, ocular device
    orthopedic NEC —see Complication,
        orthopedic, device, mechanical
    specified NEC T85.628
    urinary NEC —see also Complication,
        genitourinary, device, urinary,
        mechanical
      graft T83.29
    vascular NEC —see Complication,
        cardiovascular device, mechanical
    ventricular intracranial shunt T85.09
  intervertebral disc —see Displacement,
      intervertebral disc
  joint prosthesis —see Complications, joint
      prosthesis, mechanical, specified NEC,
      by site
  nucleus pulposus —see Displacement,
      intervertebral disc
Prune belly (syndrome) Q79.4
Prurigo (ferox) (gravis) (Hebrae) (Hebra's)
    (mitis) (simplex) L28.2
  Besnier's L20.0
  estivalis L56.4
  nodularis L28.1
  psychogenic F45.8
Pruritus, pruritic (essential) L29.9
  ani, anus L29.0
    psychogenic F45.8
  anogenital L29.3
    psychogenic F45.8
  due to onchocerca volvulus B73.1
  gravidarum —see Pregnancy, complicated by,
      specified pregnancy-related condition
      NEC
  hiemalis L29.8
  neurogenic (any site) F45.8
  perianal L29.0
  psychogenic (any site) F45.8
  scroti, scrotum L29.1
    psychogenic F45.8
  senile, senilis L29.8
  specified NEC L29.8
    psychogenic F45.8
  Trichomonas A59.9
  vulva, vulvae L29.2
    psychogenic F45.8
Pseudarthrosis, pseudoarthrosis (bone) —see
    Nonunion, fracture
  clavicle, congenital Q74.0
  joint, following fusion or arthrodesis
      M96.0
Pseudoaneurysm —see Aneurysm
Pseudoangina (pectoris) —see Angina
Pseudoangioma I81
Pseudoarteriosus Q28.8
Pseudoarthrosis —see Pseudarthrosis

Pseudobulbar affect (PBA) F48.2
Pseudochromhidrosis L67.8
Pseudocirrhosis, liver, pericardial I31.1
Pseudocowpox B08.03
Pseudocoxalgia M91.3-
Pseudocroup J38.5
Pseudo-Cushing's syndrome, alcohol-induced
    E24.4
Pseudocyesis F45.8
Pseudocyst
  lung J98.4
  pancreas K86.3
  retina —see Cyst, retina
Pseudoelephantiasis neuroarthritica
    Q82.0
Pseudoexfoliation, capsule (lens) —see
    Cataract, specified NEC
Pseudofolliculitis barbae L73.1
Pseudoglioma H44.89
Pseudohemophilia (Bernuth's) (hereditary)
    (type B) D68.0
  Type A D69.8
  vascular D69.8
Pseudohermaphroditism Q56.3
  adrenal E25.8
  female Q56.2
    with adrenocortical disorder E25.8
    without adrenocortical disorder
        Q56.2
    adrenal, congenital E25.0
  male Q56.1
    with
      adrenocortical disorder E25.8
      androgen resistance E34.51
      cleft scrotum Q56.1
      feminizing testis E34.51
      5-alpha-reductase deficiency E29.1
    without gonadal disorder Q56.1
    adrenal E25.8
Pseudo-Hurler's polydystrophy E77.0
Pseudohydrocephalus G93.2
Pseudohypertrophic muscular dystrophy
    (Erb's) G71.0
Pseudohypertrophy, muscle G71.0
Pseudohypoparathyroidism E20.1
Pseudoinsomnia F51.03
Pseudoleukemia, infantile D64.89
Pseudomembranous —see condition
Pseudomeningocele (cerebral) (infective)
    (post-traumatic) G96.19
  postprocedural (spinal) G97.82
Pseudomenses (newborn) P54.6
Pseudomenstruation (newborn) P54.6
Pseudomonas
  aeruginosa, as cause of disease classified
      elsewhere B96.5
  mallei infection A24.0
    as cause of disease classified elsewhere
        B96.5
  pseudomallei, as cause of disease classified
      elsewhere B96.5
Pseudomyotonia G71.19
Pseudomyxoma peritonei C78.6
Pseudoneuritis, optic (nerve) (disc) (papilla),
    congenital Q14.2
Pseudo-obstruction intestine (acute) (chronic)
    (idiopathic) (intermittent secondary)
    (primary) K59.8
Pseudopapilledema H47.33-
  congenital Q14.2
Pseudoparalysis
  arm or leg R29.818
  atonic, congenital P94.2
Pseudopelade L66.0
Pseudophakia Z96.1
Pseudopolyarthritis, rhizomelic M35.3
Pseudopolycythemia D75.1
Pseudopseudohypoparathyroidism
    E20.1
Pseudopterygium H11.81-
Pseudoptosis (eyelid) —see Blepharochalasis

Pseudopuberty, precocious
  female heterosexual E25.8
  male isosexual E25.8
Pseudorickets (renal) N25.0
Pseudorubella B08.20
Pseudosclerema, newborn P83.8
Pseudosclerosis (brain)
  Jakob's —see Creutzfeldt-Jakob disease or
      syndrome
  of Westphal (Strüümpell) E83.01
  spastic —see Creutzfeldt-Jakob disease or
      syndrome
Pseudotetanus —see Convulsions
Pseudotetany R29.0
  hysterical F44.5
Pseudotruncus arteriosus Q25.4
Pseudotuberculosis A28.2
  enterocolitis A04.8
  pasteurella (infection) A28.0
Pseudotumor
  cerebri G93.2
  orbital H05.11-
Pseudoxanthoma elasticum Q82.8
Psilosis (sprue) (tropical) K90.1
  nontropical K90.0
Psittacosis A70
Psoitis M60.88
Psoriasis L40.9
  arthropathic L40.50
    arthritis mutilans L40.52
    distal interphalangeal L40.51
    juvenile L40.54
    other specified L40.59
    spondylitis L40.53
  buccal K13.29
  flexural L40.8
  guttate L40.4
  mouth K13.29
  nummular L40.0
  plaque L40.0
  psychogenic F54
  pustular (generalized) L40.1
    palmaris et plantaris L40.3
  specified NEC L40.8
  vulgaris L40.0
Psychasthenia F48.8
Psychiatric disorder or problem F99
Psychogenic —see also condition
  factors associated with physical conditions
      F54
Psychological and behavioral factors affecting
    medical condition F59
Psychoneurosis, psychoneurotic —see also
    Neurosis
  anxiety (state) F41.1
  depersonalization F48.1
  hypochondriacal F45.21
  hysteria F44.9
  neurasthenic F48.8
  personality NEC F60.89
Psychopathy, psychopathic
  affectionless F94.2
  autistic F84.5
  constitution, post-traumatic F07.81
  personality —see Disorder, personality
  sexual —see Deviation, sexual
  state F60.2
Psychosexual identity disorder of childhood
    F64.2
Psychosis, psychotic F29
  acute (transient) F23
    hysterical F44.9
  affective —see Disorder, mood
  alcoholic F10.959
    with
      abuse F10.159
      anxiety disorder F10.980
        with
          abuse F10.180
          dependence F10.280
      delirium tremens F10.231

Psychosis, psychotic (Continued)
  alcoholic (Continued)
    with (Continued)
      delusions F10.950
        with
          abuse F10.150
          dependence F10.250
        dementia F10.97
          with dependence F10.27
        dependence F10.259
        hallucinosis F10.951
          with
            abuse F10.151
            dependence F10.251
        mood disorder F10.94
          with
            abuse F10.14
            dependence F10.24
        paranoia F10.950
          with
            abuse F10.150
            dependence F10.250
        persisting amnesia F10.96
          with dependence F10.26
      amnestic confabulatory F10.96
        with dependence F10.26
      delirium tremens F10.231
      Korsakoff's, Korsakov's, Korsakow's F10.26
      paranoid type F10.950
        with
          abuse F10.150
          dependence F10.250
    anergastic —see Psychosis, organic
    arteriosclerotic (simple type) (uncomplicated) F01.50
      with behavioral disturbance F01.51
    childhood F84.0
      atypical F84.8
    climacteric —see Psychosis, involutional
    confusional F29
      acute or subacute F05
      reactive F23
    cycloid F23
    depressive —see Disorder, depressive
    disintegrative (childhood) F84.3
    drug-induced —see F11-F19 with .x59
      paranoid and hallucinatory states —see F11-F19 with .x50 or .x51
    due to or associated with
      addiction, drug —see F11-F19 with .X59
      dependence
        alcohol F10.259
        drug —see F11-F19 with .x59
      epilepsy F06.8
      Huntington's chorea F06.8
      ischemia, cerebrovascular (generalized) F06.8
      multiple sclerosis F06.8
      physical disease F06.8
      presenile dementia F03
      senile dementia F03
      vascular disease (arteriosclerotic) (cerebral) F01.50
        with behavioral disturbance F01.51
    epileptic F06.8
    episode F23
      due to or associated with physical condition F06.8
    exhaustive F43.0
    hallucinatory, chronic F28
    hypomanic F30.8
    hysterical (acute) F44.9
    induced F24
    infantile F84.0
      atypical F84.8
    infective (acute) (subacute) F05
    involutional F28
      depressive —see Disorder, depressive
      melancholic —see Disorder, depressive
      paranoid (state) F22

Psychosis, psychotic (Continued)
  Korsakoff's, Korsakov's, Korsakow's (nonalcoholic) F04
    alcoholic F10.96
      in dependence F10.26
    induced by other psychoactive substance —see categories F11-F19 with .x5x
  mania, manic (single episode) F30.2
    recurrent type F31.89
  manic-depressive —see Disorder, mood
  menopausal —see Psychosis, involutional
  mixed schizophrenic and affective F25.8
  multi-infarct (cerebrovascular) F01.50
    with behavioral disturbance F01.51
  nonorganic F29
    specified NEC F28
  organic F09
    due to or associated with
      arteriosclerosis (cerebral) —see Psychosis, arteriosclerotic
      cerebrovascular disease, arteriosclerotic —see Psychosis, arteriosclerotic
      childbirth —see Psychosis, puerperal
      Creutzfeldt-Jakob disease or syndrome —see Creutzfeldt-Jakob disease or syndrome
      dependence, alcohol F10.259
      disease
        alcoholic liver F10.259
        brain, arteriosclerotic —see Psychosis, arteriosclerotic
        cerebrovascular F01.50
          with behavioral disturbance F01.51
        Creutzfeldt-Jakob —see Creutzfeldt-Jakob disease or syndrome
        endocrine or metabolic F06.8
          acute or subacute F05
        liver, alcoholic F10.259
      epilepsy transient (acute) F05
      infection
        brain (intracranial) F06.8
          acute or subacute F05
      intoxication
        alcoholic (acute) F10.259
        drug F19 with .X59 F11-
      ischemia, cerebrovascular (generalized) — see Psychosis, arteriosclerotic
      puerperium —see Psychosis, puerperal
      trauma, brain (birth) (from electric current) (surgical) F06.8
        acute or subacute F05
    infective F06.8
      acute or subacute F05
    post-traumatic F06.8
      acute or subacute F05
  paranoiac F22
  paranoid (climacteric) (involutional) (menopausal) F22
    psychogenic (acute) F23
    schizophrenic F20.0
    senile F03
  postpartum F53
  presbyophrenic (type) F03
  presenile F03
  psychogenic (paranoid) F23
    depressive F32.3
  puerperal F53
    specified type —see Psychosis, by type
  reactive (brief) (transient) (emotional stress) (psychological trauma) F23
    depressive F32.3
      recurrent F33.3
    excitative type F30.8
  schizoaffective F25.9
    depressive type F25.1
    manic type F25.0
  schizophrenia, schizophrenic —see Schizophrenia

Psychosis, psychotic (Continued)
  schizophrenia-like, in epilepsy F06.2
  schizophreniform F20.81
    affective type F25.9
    brief F23
    confusional type F23
    depressive type F25.1
    manic type F25.0
    mixed type F25.0
  senile NEC F03
    depressed or paranoid type F03
    simple deterioration F03
    specified type — code to condition
  shared F24
  situational (reactive) F23
  symbiotic (childhood) F84.3
  symptomatic F09
Psychosomatic —see Disorder, psychosomatic
Psychosyndrome, organic F07.9
Psychotic episode due to or associated with physical condition F06.8
Pterygium (eye) H11.00-
  amyloid H11.01-
  central H11.02-
  colli Q18.3
  double H11.03-
  peripheral
    progressive H11.05-
    stationary H11.04-
  recurrent H11.06-
Ptilosis (eyelid) —see Madarosis
Ptomaine (poisoning) —see Poisoning, food
Ptosis —see also Blepharoptosis
  adiposa (false) —see Blepharoptosis
  breast N64.81
  cecum K63.4
  colon K63.4
  congenital (eyelid) Q10.0
    specified site NEC —see Anomaly, by site
  eyelid —see Blepharoptosis
    congenital Q10.0
  gastric K31.89
  intestine K63.4
  kidney N28.83
  liver K76.89
  renal N28.83
  splanchnic K63.4
  spleen D73.89
  stomach K31.89
  viscera K63.4
PTP D69.51
Ptyalism (periodic) K11.7
  hysterical F45.8
  pregnancy —see Pregnancy, complicated by, specified pregnancy-related condition NEC
  psychogenic F45.8
Ptyalolithiasis K11.5
Pubarche, precocious E30.1
Pubertas praecox E30.1
Puberty (development state) Z00.3
  bleeding (excessive) N92.2
  delayed E30.0
  precocious (constitutional) (cryptogenic) (idiopathic) E30.1
    central E22.8
    due to
      ovarian hyperfunction E28.1
        estrogen E28.0
      testicular hyperfunction E29.0
  premature E30.1
    due to
      adrenal cortical hyperfunction E25.8
      pineal tumor E34.8
      pituitary (anterior) hyperfunction E22.8
Puckering, macula —see Degeneration, macula, puckering
Pudenda, pudendum —see condition
Puente's disease (simple glandular cheilitis) K13.0

◄ New   ◄═ Revised   ~~deleted~~ Deleted

Puerperal, puerperium (complicated by, complications)
abnormal glucose (tolerance test) O99.815
abscess
  areola O91.02
    associated with lactation O91.03
  Bartholin's gland O86.19
  breast O91.12
    associated with lactation O91.13
  cervix (uteri) O86.11
  genital organ NEC O86.19
  kidney O86.21
  mammary O91.12
    associated with lactation O91.13
  nipple O91.02
    associated with lactation O91.03
  peritoneum O85
  subareolar O91.12
    associated with lactation O91.13
  urinary tract —*see* Puerperal, infection, urinary
  uterus O86.12
  vagina (wall) O86.13
  vaginorectal O86.13
  vulvovaginal gland O86.13
adnexitis O86.19
afibrinogenemia, or other coagulation defect O72.3
albuminuria (acute) (subacute) —*see* Proteinuria, gestational
alcohol use O99.315
anemia O90.81
  pre-existing (pre-pregnancy) O99.03
anesthetic death O89.8
apoplexy O99.43
bariatric surgery status O99.845
blood disorder NEC O99.13
blood dyscrasia O72.3
cardiomyopathy O90.3
cerebrovascular disorder (conditions in I60-I69) O99.43
cervicitis O86.11
circulatory system disorder O99.43
coagulopathy (any) O72.3
complications O90.9
  specified NEC O90.89
convulsions —*see* Eclampsia
cystitis O86.22
cystopyelitis O86.29
delirium NEC F05
diabetes O24.93
  gestational —*see* Puerperal, gestational diabetes
  pre-existing O24.33
    specified NEC O24.83
    type 1 O24.03
    type 2 O24.13
digestive system disorder O99.63
disease O90.9
  breast NEC O92.29
  cerebrovascular (acute) O99.43
  nonobstetric NEC O99.89
  tubo-ovarian O86.19
  Valsuani's O99.03
disorder O90.9
  biliary tract O26.63
  lactation O92.70
  liver O26.63
  nonobstetric NEC O99.89
disruption
  cesarean wound O90.0
  episiotomy wound O90.1
  perineal laceration wound O90.1
drug use O99.325
eclampsia (with pre-existing hypertension) O15.2
embolism (pulmonary) (blood clot) —*see* Embolism, obstetric, puerperal
endocrine, nutritional or metabolic disease NEC O99.285
endophlebitis —*see* Puerperal, phlebitis

Puerperal, puerperium *(Continued)*
endotrachelitis O86.11
failure
  lactation (complete) O92.3
    partial O92.4
  renal, acute O90.4
fever (of unknown origin) O86.4
  septic O85
fissure, nipple O92.12
  associated with lactation O92.13
fistula
  breast (due to mastitis) O91.12
    associated with lactation O91.13
  nipple O91.02
    associated with lactation O91.03
galactophoritis O91.22
  associated with lactation O91.23
galactorrhea O92.6
gastric banding status O99.845
gastric bypass status O99.845
gastrointestinal disease NEC O99.63
gestational diabetes O24.439
  diet controlled O24.430
  insulin (and diet) controlled O24.434
gonorrhea O98.23
hematoma, subdural O99.43
hemiplegia, cerebral O99.355-
  due to cerebrovascular disorder O99.43
hemorrhage O72.1
  brain O99.43
  bulbar O99.43
  cerebellar O99.43
  cerebral O99.43
  cortical O99.43
  delayed or secondary O72.2
  extradural O99.43
  internal capsule O99.43
  intracranial O99.43
  intrapontine O99.43
  meningeal O99.43
  pontine O99.43
  retained placenta O72.0
  subarachnoid O99.43
  subcortical O99.43
  subdural O99.43
  third stage O72.0
  uterine, delayed O72.2
  ventricular O99.43
hemorrhoids O87.2
hepatorenal syndrome O90.4
hypertension —*see* Hypertension, complicating, puerperium
hypertrophy, breast O92.29
induration breast (fibrous) O92.29
infection O86.4
  cervix O86.11
  generalized O85
  genital tract NEC O86.19
    obstetric surgical wound O86.0
  kidney (bacillus coli) O86.21
  maternal O98.93
    carrier state NEC O99.835
    gonorrhea O98.23
    human immunodeficiency virus (HIV) O98.73
    protozoal O98.63
    sexually transmitted NEC O98.33
    specified NEC O98.83
    streptococcus B carrier state O99.825
    syphilis O98.13
    tuberculosis O98.03
    viral hepatitis O98.43
    viral NEC O98.53
  nipple O91.02
    associated with lactation O91.03
  peritoneum O85
  renal O86.21
  specified NEC O86.89

Puerperal, puerperium *(Continued)*
infection *(Continued)*
  urinary (asymptomatic) (tract) NEC O86.20
    bladder O86.22
    kidney O86.21
    specified site NEC O86.29
    urethra O86.22
  vagina O86.13
  vein —*see* Puerperal, phlebitis
ischemia, cerebral O99.43
lymphangitis O86.89
  breast O91.22
    associated with lactation O91.23
malignancy O9A.13
malnutrition O25.3
mammillitis O91.02
  associated with lactation O91.03
mammitis O91.22
  associated with lactation O91.23
mania F30.8
mastitis O91.22
  associated with lactation O91.23
  purulent O91.12
    associated with lactation O91.13
melancholia —*see* Disorder, depressive
mental disorder NEC O99.345
metroperitonitis O85
metrorrhagia —*see* Hemorrhage, postpartum
metrosalpingitis O86.19
metrovaginitis O86.13
milk leg O87.1
monoplegia, cerebral O99.43
mood disturbance O90.6
necrosis, liver (acute) (subacute) (conditions in subcategory K72.0) O26.63
  with renal failure O90.4
nervous system disorder O99.355
neuritis O90.89
obesity (pre-existing prior to pregnancy) O99.215
obesity surgery status O99.845
occlusion, precerebral artery O99.43
paralysis
  bladder (sphincter) O90.89
  cerebral O99.43
paralytic stroke O99.43
parametritis O85
paravaginitis O86.13
pelviperitonitis O85
perimetritis O86.12
perimetrosalpingitis O86.19
perinephritis O86.21
periphlebitis —*see* Puerperal phlebitis
peritoneal infection O85
peritonitis (pelvic) O85
perivaginitis O86.13
phlebitis O87.0
  deep O87.1
  pelvic O87.1
  superficial O87.0
phlebothrombosis, deep O87.1
phlegmasia alba dolens O87.1
placental polyp O90.89
pneumonia, embolic —*see* Embolism, obstetric, puerperal
pre-eclampsia —*see* Pre-eclampsia
psychosis F53
pyelitis O86.21
pyelocystitis O86.29
pyelonephritis O86.21
pyelonephrosis O86.21
pyemia O86.21
pyocystitis O86.29
pyohemia O85
pyometra O86.12
pyonephritis O86.21
pyosalpingitis O86.19
pyrexia (of unknown origin) O86.4
renal
  disease NEC O90.89
  failure O90.4

Puerperal, puerperium (Continued)
respiratory disease NEC O99.53
retention
decidua —see Retention, decidua
placenta O72.0
secundines —see Retention,
secundines
retrated nipple O92.02
salpingo-ovaritis O86.19
salpingoperitonitis O85
secondary perineal tear O90.1
sepsis O85
sepsis (pelvic) O85
septic thrombophlebitis O86.81
skin disorder NEC O99.73
specified condition NEC O99.89
stroke O99.43
subinvolution (uterus) O90.89
subluxation of symphysis (pubis)
O26.73
suppuration —see Puerperal, abscess
tetanus A34
thelitis O91.02
associated with lactation O91.03
thrombocytopenia O72.3
thrombophlebitis (superficial) O87.0
deep O87.1
pelvic O87.1
septic O86.81
thrombosis (venous) —see Thrombosis,
puerperal
thyroiditis O90.5
toxemia (eclamptic) (pre-eclamptic)
(with convulsions) O15.2
trauma, non-obstetric O9A.23
caused by abuse (physical) (suspected)
O9A.33
confirmed O9A.33
psychological (suspected)
O9A.53
confirmed O9A.53
sexual (suspected) O9A.43
confirmed O9A.43
uremia (due to renal failure)
O90.4
urethritis O86.22
vaginitis O86.13
varicose veins (legs) O87.4
vulva or perineum O87.8
venous O87.9
vulvitis O86.19
vulvovaginitis O86.13
white leg O87.1
Puerperium —see Puerperal
Pulmolithiasis J98.4
Pulmonary —see condition
Pulpitis (acute) (anachoretic) (chronic)
(hyperplastic) (irreversible) (putrescent)
(reversible) (suppurative) (ulcerative)
K04.0
Pulpless tooth K04.99
Pulse
alternating R00.8
bigeminal R00.8
fast R00.0
feeble, rapid due to shock following injury
T79.4
rapid R00.0
weak R09.89
Pulsus alternans or trigeminus R00.8
Punch drunk F07.81
Punctum lacrimale occlusion —see Obstruction,
lacrimal
Puncture
abdomen, abdominal
wall S31.139
with
foreign body S31.149
penetration into peritoneal cavity
S31.639
with foreign body S31.649

Puncture (Continued)
abdomen, abdominal (Continued)
wall (Continued)
epigastric region S31.132
with
foreign body S31.142
penetration into peritoneal cavity
S31.632
with foreign body S31.642
left
lower quadrant S31.134
with
foreign body S31.144
penetration into peritoneal cavity
S31.634
with foreign body S31.644
upper quadrant S31.131
with
foreign body S31.141
penetration into peritoneal cavity
S31.631
with foreign body S31.641
periumbilic region S31.135
with
foreign body S31.145
penetration into peritoneal cavity
S31.635
with foreign body S31.645
right
lower quadrant S31.133
with
foreign body S31.143
penetration into peritoneal cavity
S31.633
with foreign body S31.643
upper quadrant S31.130
with
foreign body S31.140
penetration into peritoneal cavity
S31.630
with foreign body S31.640
accidental, complicating surgery —see
Complication, accidental puncture or
laceration
alveolar (process) —see Puncture, oral cavity
ankle S91.039
with
foreign body S91.049
left S91.032
with
foreign body S91.042
right S91.031
with
foreign body S91.041
anus S31.833
with foreign body S31.834
arm (upper) S41.139
with foreign body S41.149
left S41.132
with foreign body S41.142
lower —see Puncture, forearm
right S41.131
with foreign body S41.141
auditory canal (external) (meatus) —see
Puncture, ear
auricle, ear —see Puncture, ear
axilla —see Puncture, arm
back —see also Puncture, thorax, back
lower S31.030
with
foreign body S31.040
with penetration into
retroperitoneal space S31.041
penetration into retroperitoneal space
S31.031
bladder (traumatic) S37.29
nontraumatic N32.89
breast S21.039
with foreign body S21.049
left S21.032
with foreign body S21.042

Puncture (Continued)
breast (Continued)
right S21.031
with foreign body S21.041
buttock S31.803
with foreign body S31.804
left S31.823
with foreign body S31.824
right S31.813
with foreign body S31.814
by
device, implant or graft —see
Complications, by site and type,
mechanical
foreign body left accidentally in operative
wound T81.539
instrument (any) during a procedure,
accidental —see Puncture, accidental
complicating surgery
calf —see Puncture, leg
canaliculus lacrimalis —see Puncture,
eyelid
canthus, eye —see Puncture, eyelid
cervical esophagus S11.23
with foreign body S11.24
cheek (external) S01.439
with foreign body S01.449
internal —see Puncture, oral cavity
left S01.432
with foreign body S01.442
right S01.431
with foreign body S01.441
chest wall —see Puncture, thorax
chin —see Puncture, head, specified site NEC
clitoris —see Puncture, vulva
costal region —see Puncture, thorax
digit (s)
foot —see Puncture, toe
hand —see Puncture, finger
ear (canal) (external) S01.339
with foreign body S01.349
drum S09.2-
left S01.332
with foreign body S01.342
right S01.331
with foreign body S01.341
elbow S51.039
with
foreign body S51.049
left S51.032
with
foreign body S51.042
right S51.031
with
foreign body S51.041
epididymis —see Puncture, testis
epigastric region —see Puncture, abdomen,
wall, epigastric
epiglottis S11.83
with foreign body S11.84
esophagus
cervical S11.23
with foreign body S11.24
thoracic S27.818
eyeball S05.6-
with foreign body S05.5-
eyebrow —see Puncture, eyelid
eyelid S01.13-
with foreign body S01.14-
left S01.132
with foreign body S01.142
right S01.131
with foreign body S01.141
face NEC —see Puncture, head, specified site
NEC
finger (s) S61.239
with
damage to nail S61.339
with
foreign body S61.349
foreign body S61.249

◀ New   ◀▥ Revised   ~~deleted~~ Deleted

Puncture (Continued)
  finger (Continued)
    index S61.238
      with
        damage to nail S61.338
          with
            foreign body S61.348
        foreign body S61.248
      left S61.231
        with
          damage to nail S61.331
            with
              foreign body S61.341
          foreign body S61.241
      right S61.230
        with
          damage to nail S61.330
            with
              foreign body S61.340
          foreign body S61.240
    little S61.238
      with
        damage to nail S61.338
          with
            foreign body S61.348
        foreign body S61.248
      left S61.237
        with
          damage to nail S61.337
            with
              foreign body S61.347
          foreign body S61.247
      right S61.236
        with
          damage to nail S61.336
            with
              foreign body S61.346
          foreign body S61.246
    middle S61.238
      with
        damage to nail S61.338
          with
            foreign body S61.348
        foreign body S61.248
      left S61.233
        with
          damage to nail S61.333
            with
              foreign body S61.343
          foreign body S61.243
      right S61.232
        with
          damage to nail S61.332
            with
              foreign body S61.342
          foreign body S61.242
    ring S61.238
      with
        damage to nail S61.338
          with
            foreign body S61.348
        foreign body S61.248
      left S61.235
        with
          damage to nail S61.335
            with
              foreign body S61.345
          foreign body S61.245
      right S61.234
        with
          damage to nail S61.334
            with
              foreign body
                S61.344
          foreign body S61.244
  flank S31.139
    with foreign body S31.149
  foot (except toe (s) alone) S91.339
    with foreign body S91.349
    left S91.332
      with foreign body S91.342

Puncture (Continued)
  foot (Continued)
    right S91.331
      with foreign body S91.341
    toe —see Puncture, toe
  forearm S51.839
    with
      foreign body S51.849
    elbow only —see Puncture, elbow
    left S51.832
      with
        foreign body S51.842
    right S51.831
      with
        foreign body S51.841
  forehead —see Puncture, head, specified site
    NEC
  genital organs, external
    female S31.532
      with foreign body S31.542
      vagina —see Puncture, vagina
      vulva —see Puncture, vulva
    male S31.531
      with foreign body S31.541
      penis —see Puncture, penis
      scrotum —see Puncture, scrotum
      testis —see Puncture, testis
  groin —see Puncture, abdomen, wall
  gum —see Puncture, oral cavity
  hand S61.439
    with
      foreign body S61.449
    finger —see Puncture, finger
    left S61.432
      with
        foreign body S61.442
    right S61.431
      with
        foreign body S61.441
    thumb —see Puncture, thumb
  head S01.93
    with foreign body S01.94
    cheek —see Puncture, cheek
    ear —see Puncture, ear
    eyelid —see Puncture, eyelid
    lip —see Puncture, oral cavity
    nose —see Puncture, nose
    oral cavity —see Puncture, oral cavity
    scalp S01.03
      with foreign body S01.04
    specified site NEC S01.83
      with foreign body S01.84
    temporomandibular area —see Puncture,
      cheek
  heart S26.99
    with hemopericardium S26.09
    without hemopericardium S26.19
  heel —see Puncture, foot
  hip S71.039
    with foreign body S71.049
    left S71.032
      with foreign body S71.042
    right S71.031
      with foreign body S71.041
  hymen —see Puncture, vagina
  hypochondrium —see Puncture, abdomen,
    wall
  hypogastric region —see Puncture, abdomen,
    wall
  inguinal region —see Puncture, abdomen,
    wall
  instep —see Puncture, foot
  internal organs —see Injury, by site
  interscapular region —see Puncture, thorax,
    back
  intestine
    large
      colon S36.599
        ascending S36.590
        descending S36.592
        sigmoid S36.593

Puncture (Continued)
  intestine (Continued)
    large (Continued)
      colon (Continued)
        specified site NEC S36.598
        transverse S36.591
      rectum S36.69
    small S36.499
      duodenum S36.490
      specified site NEC S36.498
  intra-abdominal organ S36.99
    gallbladder S36.128
    intestine —see Puncture, intestine
    liver S36.118
    pancreas —see Puncture, pancreas
    peritoneum S36.81
    specified site NEC S36.898
    spleen S36.09
    stomach S36.39
  jaw —see Puncture, head, specified site
    NEC
  knee S81.039
    with foreign body S81.049
    left S81.032
      with foreign body S81.042
    right S81.031
      with foreign body S81.041
  labium (majus) (minus) —see Puncture,
    vulva
  lacrimal duct —see Puncture, eyelid
  larynx S11.013
    with foreign body S11.014
  leg (lower) S81.839
    with foreign body S81.849
    foot —see Puncture, foot
    knee —see Puncture, knee
    left S81.832
      with foreign body S81.842
    right S81.831
      with foreign body S81.841
    upper —see Puncture, thigh
  lip S01.531
    with foreign body S01.541
  loin —see Puncture, abdomen, wall
  lower back —see Puncture, back, lower
  lumbar region —see Puncture, back, lower
  malar region —see Puncture, head, specified
    site NEC
  mammary —see Puncture, breast
  mastoid region —see Puncture, head,
    specified site NEC
  mouth —see Puncture, oral cavity
  nail
    finger —see Puncture, finger, with damage
      to nail
    toe —see Puncture, toe, with damage to
      nail
  nasal (septum) (sinus) —see Puncture,
    nose
  nasopharynx —see Puncture, head, specified
    site NEC
  neck S11.93
    with foreign body S11.94
    involving
      cervical esophagus —see Puncture,
        cervical esophagus
      larynx —see Puncture, larynx
      pharynx —see Puncture, pharynx
      thyroid gland —see Puncture, thyroid
        gland
      trachea —see Puncture, trachea
    specified site NEC S11.83
      with foreign body S11.84
  nose (septum) (sinus) S01.23
    with foreign body S01.24
  ocular —see Puncture, eyeball - oral cavity
    S01.532
    with foreign body S01.542
  orbit S05.4-
  palate —see Puncture, oral cavity
  palm —see Puncture, hand

Puncture (Continued)
- pancreas S36.299
  - body S36.291
  - head S36.290
  - tail S36.292
- pelvis —see Puncture, back, lower
- penis S31.23
  - with foreign body S31.24
- perineum
  - female S31.43
    - with foreign body S31.44
  - male S31.139
    - with foreign body S31.149
- periocular area (with or without lacrimal passages) —see Puncture, eyelid
- phalanges
  - finger —see Puncture, finger
  - toe —see Puncture, toe
- pharynx S11.23
  - with foreign body S11.24
- pinna —see Puncture, ear
- popliteal space —see Puncture, knee
- prepuce —see Puncture, penis
- pubic region S31.139
  - with foreign body S31.149
- pudendum —see Puncture, genital organs, external
- rectovaginal septum —see Puncture, vagina
- sacral region —see Puncture, back, lower
- sacroiliac region —see Puncture, back, lower
- salivary gland —see Puncture, oral cavity
- scalp S01.03
  - with foreign body S01.04
- scapular region —see Puncture, shoulder
- scrotum S31.33
  - with foreign body S31.34
- shin —see Puncture, leg
- shoulder S41.039
  - with foreign body S41.049
  - left S41.032
    - with foreign body S41.042
  - right S41.031
    - with foreign body S41.041
- spermatic cord —see Puncture, testis
- sternal region —see Puncture, thorax, front
- submaxillary region —see Puncture, head, specified site NEC
- submental region —see Puncture, head, specified site NEC
- subungual
  - finger (s) —see Puncture, finger, with damage to nail
  - toe —see Puncture, toe, with damage to nail
- supraclavicular fossa —see Puncture, neck, specified site NEC
- temple, temporal region —see Puncture, head, specified site NEC
- temporomandibular area —see Puncture, cheek
- testis S31.33
  - with foreign body S31.34
- thigh S71.139
  - with foreign body S71.149
  - left S71.132
    - with foreign body S71.142
  - right S71.131
    - with foreign body S71.141
- thorax, thoracic (wall) S21.93
  - with foreign body S21.94
  - back S21.23-
    - with
      - foreign body S21.24-
        - with penetration S21.44
      - penetration S21.43
    - breast —see Puncture, breast

Puncture (Continued)
- thorax, thoracic (Continued)
  - front S21.13-
    - with
      - foreign body S21.14-
        - with penetration S21.34
      - penetration S21.33
  - throat —see Puncture, neck
- thumb S61.039
  - with
    - damage to nail S61.139
      - with
        - foreign body S61.149
    - foreign body S61.049
  - left S61.032
    - with
      - damage to nail S61.132
        - with
          - foreign body S61.142
      - foreign body S61.042
  - right S61.031
    - with
      - damage to nail S61.131
        - with
          - foreign body S61.141
      - foreign body S61.041
- thyroid gland S11.13
  - with foreign body S11.14
- toe (s) S91.139
  - with
    - damage to nail S91.239
      - with
        - foreign body S91.249
    - foreign body S91.149
  - great S91.133
    - with
      - damage to nail S91.233
        - with
          - foreign body S91.243
      - foreign body S91.143
    - left S91.132
      - with
        - damage to nail S91.232
          - with
            - foreign body S91.242
        - foreign body S91.142
    - right S91.131
      - with
        - damage to nail S91.231
          - with
            - foreign body S91.241
        - foreign body S91.141
  - lesser S91.136
    - with
      - damage to nail S91.236
        - with
          - foreign body S91.246
      - foreign body S91.146
    - left S91.135
      - with
        - damage to nail S91.235
          - with
            - foreign body S91.245
        - foreign body S91.145
    - right S91.134
      - with
        - damage to nail S91.234
          - with
            - foreign body S91.244
        - foreign body S91.144
- tongue —see Puncture, oral cavity
- trachea S11.023
  - with foreign body S11.024
- tunica vaginalis —see Puncture, testis
- tympanum, tympanic membrane S09.2-
- umbilical region S31.135
  - with foreign body S31.145
- uvula —see Puncture, oral cavity
- vagina S31.43
  - with foreign body S31.44

Puncture (Continued)
- vocal cords S11.033
  - with foreign body S11.034
- vulva S31.43
  - with foreign body S31.44
- wrist S61.539
  - with
    - foreign body S61.549
  - left S61.532
    - with
      - foreign body S61.542
  - right S61.531
    - with
      - foreign body S61.541

PUO (pyrexia of unknown origin) R50.9

Pupillary membrane (persistent) Q13.89

Pupillotonia —see Anomaly, pupil, function, tonic pupil

Purpura D69.2
- abdominal D69.0
- allergic D69.0
- anaphylactoid D69.0
- annularis telangiectodes L81.7
- arthritic D69.0
- autoerythrocyte sensitization D69.2
- autoimmune D69.0
- bacterial D69.0
- Bateman's (senile) D69.2
- capillary fragility (hereditary) (idiopathic) D69.8
- cryoglobulinemic D89.1
- Devil's pinches D69.2
- fibrinolytic —see Fibrinolysis
- fulminans, fulminous D65
- gangrenous D65
- hemorrhagic, hemorrhagica D69.3
  - not due to thrombocytopenia D69.0
- Henoch (-Schönlein) (allergic) D69.0
- hypergammaglobulinemic (benign) (Waldenström's) D89.0
- idiopathic (thrombocytopenic) D69.3
  - nonthrombocytopenic D69.0
- immune thrombocytopenic D69.3
- infectious D69.0
- malignant D69.0
- neonatorum P54.5
- nervosa D69.0
- newborn P54.5
- nonthrombocytopenic D69.2
  - hemorrhagic D69.0
  - idiopathic D69.0
- nonthrombopenic D69.2
- peliosis rheumatica D69.0
- posttransfusion (post-transfusion) (from (fresh) whole blood or blood products) D69.51
- primary D69.49
- red cell membrane sensitivity D69.2
- rheumatica D69.0
- Schönlein (-Henoch) (allergic) D69.0
- scorbutic E54 [D77]
- senile D69.2
- simplex D69.2
- symptomatica D69.0
- telangiectasia annularis L81.7
- thrombocytopenic D69.49
  - congenital D69.42
  - hemorrhagic D69.3
  - hereditary D69.42
  - idiopathic D69.3
  - immune D69.3
  - neonatal, transitory P61.0
  - thrombotic M31.1
- thrombohemolytic —see Fibrinolysis
- thrombolytic —see Fibrinolysis
- thrombopenic D69.49
- thrombotic, thrombocytopenic M31.1
- toxic D69.0
- vascular D69.0
- visceral symptoms D69.0

Purpuric spots R23.3

◀ New   ◀▥ Revised   ~~deleted~~ Deleted

Purulent —*see* condition
Pus
  in
    stool R19.5
    urine N39.0
  tube (rupture) —*see* Salpingo-oophoritis
Pustular rash L08.0
Pustule (nonmalignant) L08.9
  malignant A22.0
Pustulosis palmaris et plantaris L40.3
Putnam (-Dana) **disease or syndrome** —*see*
  Degeneration, combined
Putrescent pulp (dental) K04.1
Pyarthritis, pyarthrosis —*see* Arthritis,
  pyogenic or pyemic
  tuberculous —*see* Tuberculosis, joint
Pyelectasis —*see* Hydronephrosis
Pyelitis (congenital) (uremic) —*see also*
  Pyelonephritis
  with
    calculus — *see* category N20
      with hydronephrosis N13.2
    contracted kidney N11.9
  acute N10
  chronic N11.9
    with calculus —*see* category N20
      with hydronephrosis N13.2
  cystica N28.84
  puerperal (postpartum) O86.21
  tuberculous A18.11
Pyelocystitis —*see* Pyelonephritis
Pyelonephritis —*see also* Nephritis,
  tubulo-interstitial
  with
    calculus —*see* category N20
      with hydronephrosis N13.2
    contracted kidney N11.9
  acute N10
  calculous —*see* category N20
    with hydronephrosis N13.2
  chronic N11.9
    with calculus —*see* category N20
      with hydronephrosis N13.2
    associated with ureteral obstruction or
      stricture N11.1
    nonobstructive N11.8
      with reflux (vesicoureteral) N11.0
    obstructive N11.1
    specified NEC N11.8
  in (due to)
    brucellosis A23.9 *[N16]*
    cryoglobulinemia (mixed) D89.1 *[N16]*
    cystinosis E72.04
    diphtheria A36.84

Pyelonephritis (*Continued*)
  in (*Continued*)
    glycogen storage disease E74.09 *[N16]*
    leukemia NEC C95.9- *[N16]*
    lymphoma NEC C85.90 *[N16]*
    multiple myeloma C90.0- *[N16]*
    obstruction N11.1
    Salmonella infection A02.25
    sarcoidosis D86.84
    sepsis A41.9 *[N16]*
    Sjögren's disease M35.04
    toxoplasmosis B58.83
    transplant rejection T86.91 *[N16]*
    Wilson's disease E83.01 *[N16]*
    nonobstructive N12
      with reflux (vesicoureteral) N11.0
      chronic N11.8
    syphilitic A52.75
Pyelonephrosis (obstructive) N11.1
  chronic N11.9
Pyelophlebitis I80.8
Pyeloureteritis cystica N28.85
Pyemia, pyemic (fever) (infection) (purulent) —
  see also Sepsis
  joint —*see* Arthritis, pyogenic or pyemic
  liver K75.1
  pneumococcal A40.3
  portal K75.1
  postvaccinal T88.0
  puerperal, postpartum, childbirth O85
  specified organism NEC A41.89
  tuberculous —*see* Tuberculosis, miliary
Pygopagus Q89.4
Pyknoepilepsy (idiopathic) —*see* Pyknolepsy
Pyknolepsy G40.A09
  intractable G40.A19
    with status epilepticus G40.A11
    without status epilepticus G40.A19
  not intractable G40.A09
    with status epilepticus G40.A01
    without status epilepticus G40.A09
Pylephlebitis K75.1
Pyle's syndrome Q78.5
Pylethrombophlebitis K75.1
Pylethrombosis K75.1
Pyloritis K29.90
  with bleeding K29.91
Pylorospasm (reflex) NEC K31.3
  congenital or infantile Q40.0
  neurotic F45.8
  newborn Q40.0
  psychogenic F45.8
Pylorus, pyloric —*see* condition

Pyoarthrosis —*see* Arthritis, pyogenic or
  pyemic
Pyocele
  mastoid —*see* Mastoiditis, acute
  sinus (accessory) —*see* Sinusitis
  turbinate (bone) J32.9
  urethra (*see also* Urethritis) N34.0
Pyocolpos —*see* Vaginitis
Pyocystitis N30.80
  with hematuria N30.81
Pyoderma, pyodermia L08.0
  gangrenosum L88
  newborn P39.4
  phagedenic L88
  vegetans L08.81
Pyodermatitis L08.0
  vegetans L08.81
Pyogenic —*see* condition
Pyohydronephrosis N13.6
Pyometra, pyometrium, pyometritis —*see*
  Endometritis
Pyomyositis (tropical) —*see* Myositis, infective
Pyonephritis N12
Pyonephrosis N13.6
  tuberculous A18.11
Pyo-oophoritis —*see* Salpingo-oophoritis
Pyo-ovarium —*see* Salpingo-oophoritis
Pyopericarditis, pyopericardium I30.1
Pyophlebitis —*see* Phlebitis
Pyopneumopericardium I30.1
Pyopneumothorax (infective) J86.9
  with fistula J86.0
  tuberculous NEC A15.6
Pyosalpinx, pyosalpingitis —*see also*
  Salpingo-oophoritis
Pyothorax J86.9
  with fistula J86.0
  tuberculous NEC A15.6
Pyoureter N28.89
  tuberculous A18.11
Pyramidopallidonigral syndrome G20
Pyrexia (of unknown origin) R50.9
  atmospheric T67.0
  during labor NEC O75.2
  heat T67.0
  newborn P81.9
    environmentally-induced P81.0
  persistent R50.9
  puerperal O86.4
Pyroglobulinemia NEC E88.09
Pyromania F63.1
Pyrosis R12
Pyuria (bacterial) N39.0

Q

Q fever A78
with pneumonia A78
Quadricuspid aortic valve Q23.8
Quadrilateral fever A78
Quadriparesis —*see* Quadriplegia
meaning muscle weakness M62.81
Quadriplegia G82.50-
complete
C1-C4 level G82.51
C5-C7 level G82.53
congenital (cerebral) (spinal) G80.8
spastic G80.0

Quadriplegia (*Continued*)
embolic (current episode) I63.4
functional R53.2
incomplete
C1-C4 level G82.52
C5-C7 level G82.54
thrombotic (current episode) I63.3
traumatic — code to injury with seventh
character S
current episode —*see* Injury, spinal (cord),
cervical
Quadruplet, pregnancy —*see* Pregnancy,
quadruplet
Quarrelsomeness F60.3

Queensland fever A77.3
Quervain's disease M65.4
thyroid E06.1
Queyrat's erythroplasia D07.4
penis D07.4
specified site —*see* Neoplasm, skin,
in situ
unspecified site D07.4
Quincke's disease or edema T78.3
hereditary D84.1
Quinsy (gangrenous) J36
Quintan fever A79.0
Quintuplet, pregnancy —*see* Pregnancy,
quintuplet

◀ New ◀▮▮ Revised ~~deleted~~ Deleted

R

Rabbit fever —*see* Tularemia
Rabies A82.9
  contact Z20.3
  exposure to Z20.3
  inoculation reaction —*see* Complications,
    vaccination
  sylvatic A82.0
  urban A82.1
Rachischisis —*see* Spina bifida
Rachitic —*see also* condition
  deformities of spine (late effect) (sequelae)
    E64.3
  pelvis (late effect) (sequelae) E64.3
    with disproportion (fetopelvic)
      O33.0
      causing obstructed labor O65.0
Rachitis, rachitism (acute) (tarda) —*see also*
    Rickets
  renalis N25.0
  sequelae E64.3
Radial nerve —*see* condition
Radiation
  burn —*see* Burn
  effects NOS T66
  sickness NOS T66
  therapy, encounter for Z51.0
Radiculitis (pressure) (vertebrogenic) —*see*
    Radiculopathy
Radiculomyelitis —*see also* Encephalitis
  toxic, due to
    Clostridium tetani A35
    Corynebacterium diphtheriae
      A36.82
Radiculopathy M54.10
  cervical region M54.12
  cervicothoracic region M54.13
  due to
    disc disorder
      C3 M50.11
      C4 M50.11
      C5 M50.12
      C6 M50.12
      C7 M50.12
      C8 M50.13
    displacement of intervertebral disc —*see*
      Disorder, disc, with, radiculopathy
  leg M54.1-
  lumbar region M54.16
  lumbosacral region M54.17
  occipito-atlanto-axial region M54.11
  postherpetic B02.29
  sacrococcygeal region M54.18
  syphilitic A52.11
  thoracic region (with visceral pain)
    M54.14
  thoracolumbar region M54.15
Radiodermal burns (acute, chronic, or
    occupational) —*see* Burn
Radiodermatitis L58.9
  acute L58.0
  chronic L58.1
Radiotherapy session Z51.0
Rage, meaning rabies —*see* Rabies
Ragpicker's disease A22.1
Ragsorter's disease A22.1
Raillietiniasis B71.8
Railroad neurosis F48.8
Railway spine F48.8
Raised —*see also* Elevated
  antibody titer R76.0
Rake teeth, tooth M26.39
Rales R09.89
Ramifying renal pelvis Q63.8
Ramsay-Hunt disease or syndrome (*see also*
    Hunt's disease) B02.21
  meaning dyssynergia cerebellaris myoclonica
    G11.1
Ranula K11.6
  congenital Q38.4

Rape
  adult
    confirmed T74.21
    suspected T76.21
  alleged, observation or examination, ruled out
    adult Z04.41
    child Z04.42
  child
    confirmed T74.22
    suspected T76.22
Rapid
  feeble pulse, due to shock, following injury
    T79.4
  heart (beat) R00.0
    psychogenic F45.8
  second stage (delivery) O62.3
  time-zone change syndrome —*see* Disorder,
    sleep, circadian rhythm, psychogenic
Rarefaction, bone —*see* Disorder, bone, density
    and structure, specified NEC
Rash (toxic) R21
  canker A38.9
  diaper L22
  drug (internal use) L27.0
    contact (*see also* Dermatitis, due to, drugs,
      external) L25.1
  following immunization T88.1
  food —*see* Dermatitis, due to, food
  heat L74.0
  napkin (psoriasiform) L22
  nettle —*see* Urticaria
  pustular L08.0
  rose R21
    epidemic B06.9
  scarlet A38.9
  serum (*see also* Reaction, serum) T80.69
  wandering tongue K14.1
Rasmussen aneurysm —*see* Tuberculosis,
    pulmonary
Rasmussen encephalitis G04.81
Rat-bite fever A25.9
  due to Streptobacillus moniliformis A25.1
  spirochetal (morsus muris) A25.0
Rathke's pouch tumor D44.3
Raymond (-Céstan) syndrome I65.8
Raynaud's disease, phenomenon or syndrome
    (secondary) I73.00
  with gangrene (symmetric) I73.01
RDS (newborn) (type I) P22.0
  type II P22.1
Reaction —*see also* Disorder
  adaptation —*see* Disorder, adjustment
  adjustment (anxiety) (conduct disorder)
    (depressiveness) (distress) —*see*
    Disorder, adjustment
    with
      mutism, elective (child) (adolescent) F94.0
  adverse
    food (any) (ingested) NEC T78.1
      anaphylactic —*see* Shock, anaphylactic,
        due to food
  anaphylactoid —*see* Shock, anaphylactic
  affective —*see* Disorder, mood
  allergic —*see* Allergy
  anaphylactic —*see* Shock, anaphylactic
  anesthesia —*see* Anesthesia, complication
  antitoxin (prophylactic) (therapeutic) —*see*
    Complications, vaccination
  anxiety F41.1
  Arthus —*see* Arthus' phenomenon
  asthenic F48.8
  combat and operational stress F43.0
  compulsive F42
  conversion F44.9
  crisis, acute F43.0
  deoxyribonuclease (DNA) (DNase)
    hypersensitivity D69.2
  depressive (single episode) F32.9
    affective (single episode) F31.4
      recurrent episode F33.9
    neurotic F34.1
    psychoneurotic F34.1

Reaction (Continued)
  depressive (Continued)
    psychotic F32.3
    recurrent —*see* Disorder, depressive,
      recurrent
  dissociative F44.9
  drug NEC T88.7
    addictive —*see* Dependence, drug
      transmitted via placenta or breast
        milk —*see* Absorption, drug,
        addictive, through placenta
    allergic —*see* Allergy, drug
    lichenoid L43.2
    newborn P93.8
      gray baby syndrome P93.0
    overdose or poisoning (by accident) —*see*
      Table of Drugs and Chemicals, by
      drug, poisoning
    photoallergic L56.1
    phototoxic L56.0
    withdrawal —*see* Dependence, by drug,
      with, withdrawal
      infant of dependent mother P96.1
      newborn P96.1
    wrong substance given or taken (by
      accident) —*see* Table of Drugs and
      Chemicals, by drug, poisoning
  fear F40.9
    child (abnormal) F93.8
  febrile nonhemolytic transfusion (FNHTR)
    R50.84
  fluid loss, cerebrospinal G97.1
  foreign
    body NEC —*see* Granuloma, foreign body
      in operative wound (inadvertently
        left) —*see* Foreign body,
        accidentally left during a
        procedure
    substance accidentally left during a
      procedure (chemical) (powder) (talc)
      T81.60
      aseptic peritonitis T81.61
      body or object (instrument) (sponge)
        (swab) —*see* Foreign body,
        accidentally left during a
        procedure
      specified reaction NEC T81.69
  grief —*see* Disorder, adjustment
  Herxheimer's R68.89
  hyperkinetic —*see* Hyperkinesia
  hypochondriacal F45.20
  hypoglycemic, due to insulin E16.0
    with coma (diabetic) —*see* Diabetes, coma
      nondiabetic E15
    therapeutic misadventure —*see*
      subcategory T38.3
  hypomanic F30.8
  hysterical F44.9
  immunization —*see* Complications, vaccination
  incompatibility
    ABO blood group (infusion) (transfusion) —
      see Complication (s), transfusion,
      incompatibility reaction, ABO
      delayed serologic T80.39
    minor blood group (Duffy) (E) (K(ell))
      (Kidd) (Lewis) (M) (N) (P) (S) T80.89
    Rh (factor) (infusion) (transfusion) —*see*
      Complication (s), transfusion,
      incompatibility reaction, Rh (factor)
  inflammatory —*see* Infection
  infusion —*see* Complications, infusion
  inoculation (immune serum) —*see*
    Complications, vaccination
  insulin T38.3-
  involutional psychotic —*see* Disorder,
    depressive
  leukemoid D72.823
    basophilic D72.823
    lymphocytic D72.823
    monocytic D72.823
    myelocytic D72.823
    neutrophilic D72.823

Reaction *(Continued)*
  LSD (acute)
    due to drug abuse —*see* Abuse, drug, hallucinogen
    due to drug dependence —*see* Dependence, drug, hallucinogen
  lumbar puncture G97.1
  manic-depressive —*see* Disorder, bipolar
  neurasthenic F48.8
  neurogenic —*see* Neurosis
  neurotic F48.9
  neurotic-depressive F34.1
  nitritoid —*see* Crisis, nitritoid - obsessive-compulsive F42
  nonspecific
    to
      cell mediated immunity measurement of gamma interferon antigen response without active tuberculosis R76.12
      QuantiFERON-TB test (QFT) without active tuberculosis R76.12
      tuberculin test *(see also* Reaction, tuberculin skin test) R76.11
  obsessive-compulsive F42
  organic, acute or subacute —*see* Delirium
  paranoid (acute) F23
    chronic F22
    senile F03
  passive dependency F60.7
  phobic F40.9
  post-traumatic stress, uncomplicated Z73.3
  psychogenic F99
  psychoneurotic —*see also* Neurosis
    compulsive F42
    depersonalization F48.1
    depressive F34.1
    hypochondriacal F45.20
    neurasthenic F48.8
    obsessive F42
  psychophysiologic —*see* Disorder, somatoform
  psychosomatic —*see* Disorder, somatoform
  psychotic —*see* Psychosis
  scarlet fever toxin —*see* Complications, vaccination
  schizophrenic F23
    acute (brief) (undifferentiated) F23
    latent F21
    undifferentiated (acute) (brief) F23
  serological for syphilis —*see* Serology for syphilis
  serum T80.69
    anaphylactic (immediate) *(see also* Shock, anaphylactic) T80.59
    specified reaction NEC
      due to
        administration of blood and blood products T80.61
        immunization T80.62
        serum specified NEC T80.69
        vaccination T80.62
  situational —*see* Disorder, adjustment
  somatization —*see* Disorder, somatoform
  spinal puncture G97.1
  stress (severe) F43.9
    acute (agitation) ("daze") (disorientation) (disturbance of consciousness) (flight reaction) (fugue) F43.0
    specified NEC F43.8
  surgical procedure —*see* Complications, surgical procedure
  tetanus antitoxin —*see* Complications, vaccination
  toxic, to local anesthesia T81.89
    in labor and delivery O74.4
    in pregnancy O29.3X-
    postpartum, puerperal O89.3
  toxin-antitoxin —*see* Complications, vaccination

Reaction *(Continued)*
  transfusion (blood) (bone marrow) (lymphocytes) (allergic) —*see* Complications, transfusion
  tuberculin skin test, abnormal R76.11
  vaccination (any) —*see* Complications, vaccination
  withdrawing, child or adolescent F93.8
Reactive airway disease —*see* Asthma
Reactive depression —*see* Reaction, depressive
Rearrangement
  chromosomal
    balanced (in) Q95.9
      abnormal individual (autosomal) Q95.2
      non-sex (autosomal) chromosomes Q95.2
      sex/non-sex chromosomes Q95.3
      specified NEC Q95.8
Recalcitrant patient —*see* Noncompliance
Recanalization, thrombus —*see* Thrombosis
Recession, receding
  chamber angle (eye) H21.55-
  chin M26.09
  gingival (generalized) (localized) (postinfective) (postoperative) K06.0
Recklinghausen's disease Q85.01
  bones E21.0
Reclus' disease (cystic) —*see* Mastopathy, cystic
Recrudescent typhus (fever) A75.1
Recruitment, auditory H93.21-
Rectalgia K62.89
Rectitis K62.89
Rectocele
  female (without uterine prolapse) N81.6
    with uterine prolapse N81.4
      incomplete N81.2
  in pregnancy —*see* Pregnancy, complicated by, abnormal, pelvic organs or tissues NEC
  male K62.3
Rectosigmoid junction —*see* condition
Rectosigmoiditis K63.89
  ulcerative (chronic) K51.30
    with
      complication K51.319
        abscess K51.314
        fistula K51.313
        obstruction K51.312
        rectal bleeding K51.311
        specified NEC K51.318
Rectourethral —*see* condition
Rectovaginal —*see* condition
Rectovesical —*see* condition
Rectum, rectal —*see* condition
Recurrent —*see* condition
  pregnancy loss —*see* Loss (of), pregnancy, recurrent
Red bugs B88.0
Red-cedar lung or pneumonitis J67.8
Red tide *(see also* Table of Drugs and Chemicals) T65.82-
Reduced
  mobility Z74.09
  ventilatory or vital capacity R94.2
Redundant, redundancy
  anus (congenital) Q43.8
  clitoris N90.89
  colon (congenital) Q43.8
  foreskin (congenital) N47.8
  intestine (congenital) Q43.8
  labia N90.6
  organ or site, congenital NEC —*see* Accessory
  panniculus (abdominal) E65
  prepuce (congenital) N47.8
  pylorus K31.89
  rectum (congenital) Q43.8
  scrotum N50.8
  sigmoid (congenital) Q43.8
  skin (of face) L57.4
    eyelids —*see* Blepharochalasis
  stomach K31.89

Reduplication —*see* Duplication
Reflex R29.2
  hyperactive gag J39.2
  pupillary, abnormal —*see* Anomaly, pupil, function
  vasoconstriction I73.9
  vasovagal R55
Reflux K21.9
  acid K21.9
  esophageal K21.9
    with esophagitis K21.0
    newborn P78.83
  gastroesophageal K21.9
    with esophagitis K21.0
  mitral —*see* Insufficiency, mitral
  ureteral —*see* Reflux, vesicoureteral
  vesicoureteral (with scarring) N13.70
    with
      nephropathy N13.729
        with hydroureter N13.739
          bilateral N13.732
          unilateral N13.731
        without hydroureter N13.729
          bilateral N13.722
          unilateral N13.721
      bilateral N13.722
      unilateral N13.721
      pyelonephritis (chronic) N11.0
    without nephropathy N13.71
    congenital Q62.7
Reforming, artificial openings —*see* Attention to, artificial, opening
Refractive error —*see* Disorder, refraction
Refsum's disease or syndrome G60.1
Refusal of
  food, psychogenic F50.8
  treatment (because of) Z53.20
    left against medical advice (AMA) Z53.21
    patient's decision NEC Z53.29
    reasons of belief or group pressure Z53.1
Regional —*see* condition
Regurgitation R11.10
  aortic (valve) —*see* Insufficiency, aortic
  food —*see also* Vomiting
    with reswallowing —*see* Rumination
    newborn P92.1
  gastric contents —*see* Vomiting
  heart —*see* Endocarditis
  mitral (valve) —*see* Insufficiency, mitral
    congenital Q23.3
  myocardial —*see* Endocarditis
  pulmonary (valve) (heart) I37.1
    congenital Q22.2
    syphilitic A52.03
  tricuspid —*see* Insufficiency, tricuspid
  valve, valvular —*see* Endocarditis
    congenital Q24.8
  vesicoureteral —*see* Reflux, vesicoureteral
Reichmann's disease or syndrome K31.89
Reifenstein syndrome E34.52
Reinsertion, contraceptive device Z30.433
Reiter's disease, syndrome, or urethritis M02.30
  ankle M02.37-
  elbow M02.32-
  foot joint M02.37-
  hand joint M02.34-
  hip M02.35-
  knee M02.36-
  multiple site M02.39
  shoulder M02.31-
  vertebra M02.38
  wrist M02.33-
Rejection
  food, psychogenic F50.8
  transplant T86.91
    bone T86.830
      marrow T86.01
    cornea T86.840
    heart T86.21
      with lung (s) T86.31

◀ New   ⬤▮ Revised   ~~deleted~~ Deleted

Rejection (Continued)
   transplant (Continued)
      intestine T86.850
      kidney T86.11
      liver T86.41
      lung (s) T86.810
         with heart T86.31
      organ (immune or nonimmune cause)
         T86.91
      pancreas T86.890
      skin (allograft) (autograft) T86.820
      specified NEC T86.890
      stem cell (peripheral blood) (umbilical
         cord) T86.5
Relapsing fever A68.9
   Carter's (Asiatic) A68.1
   Dutton's (West African) A68.1
   Koch's A68.9
   louse-borne (epidemic) A68.0
   Novy's (American) A68.1
   Obermeyers's (European) A68.0
   Spirillum A68.9
   tick-borne (endemic) A68.1
Relationship
   occlusal
      open anterior M26.220
      open posterior M26.221
Relaxation
   anus (sphincter) K62.89
      psychogenic F45.8
   arch (foot) —see also Deformity, limb, flat
      foot
   back ligaments —see Instability, joint, spine
   bladder (sphincter) N31.2
   cardioesophageal K21.9
   cervix —see Incompetency, cervix
   diaphragm J98.6
   joint (capsule) (ligament) (paralytic) —see
      Flail, joint
      congenital NEC Q74.8
   lumbosacral (joint) —see subcategory M53.2
   pelvic floor N81.89
   perineum N81.89
   posture R29.3
   rectum (sphincter) K62.89
   sacroiliac (joint) —see subcategory M53.2
   scrotum N50.8
   urethra (sphincter) N36.44
   vesical N31.2
Release from prison, anxiety concerning
   Z65.2
Remains
   canal of Cloquet Q14.0
   capsule (opaque) Q14.8
Remittent fever (malarial) B54
Remnant
   canal of Cloquet Q14.0
   capsule (opaque) Q14.8
   cervix, cervical stump (acquired)
      (postoperative) N88.8
   cystic duct, postcholecystectomy K91.5
   fingernail L60.8
      congenital Q84.6
   meniscus, knee —see Derangement, knee,
      meniscus, specified NEC
   thyroglossal duct Q89.2
   tonsil J35.8
      infected (chronic) J35.01
   urachus Q64.4
Removal (from) (of)
   artificial
      arm Z44.00-
         complete Z44.01-
         partial Z44.02-
      eye Z44.2-
      leg Z44.10-
         complete Z44.11-
         partial Z44.12-
   breast implant Z45.81
   cardiac pulse generator (battery) (end-of-life)
      Z45.010

Removal (Continued)
   catheter (urinary) (indwelling) Z46.6
      from artificial opening —see Attention to,
         artificial, opening
      non-vascular Z46.82
      vascular NEC Z45.2
   device Z46.9
      contraceptive Z30.432
      implanted NEC Z45.89
      specified NEC Z46.89
   drains Z48.03
   dressing (nonsurgical) Z48.00
      surgical Z48.01
   external
      fixation device — code to fracture with
         seventh character D
      prosthesis, prosthetic device Z44.9
         breast Z44.3-
         specified NEC Z44.8
   home in childhood (to foster home or
      institution) Z62.29
   ileostomy Z43.2
   insulin pump Z46.81
   myringotomy device (stent) (tube) Z45.82
   nervous system device NEC Z46.2
      brain neuropacemaker Z46.2
      visual substitution device Z46.2
         implanted Z45.31
   non-vascular catheter Z46.82
   organ, prophylactic (for neoplasia
      management) —see Prophylactic, organ
      removal
   orthodontic device Z46.4
   staples Z48.02
   stent
      ureteral Z46.6
   suture Z48.02
   urinary device Z46.6
   vascular access device or catheter Z45.2
Ren
   arcuatus Q63.1
   mobile, mobilis N28.89
      congenital Q63.8
   unguliformis Q63.1
Renal —see condition
Rendu-Osler-Weber disease or syndrome I78.0
Reninoma D41.0-
Renon-Delille syndrome E23.3
Reovirus, as cause of disease classified
   elsewhere B97.5
Repeated falls NEC R29.6
Replaced chromosome by dicentric ring Q93.2
Replacement by artificial or mechanical device
   or prosthesis of
   bladder Z96.0
   blood vessel NEC Z95.828
   bone NEC Z96.7
   cochlea Z96.21
   coronary artery Z95.5
   eustachian tube Z96.29
   eye globe Z97.0
   heart Z95.812
      valve Z95.2
         prosthetic Z95.2
         specified NEC Z95.4
         xenogenic Z95.3
   intestine Z96.89
   joint Z96.60
      hip —see Presence, hip joint implant
      knee —see Presence, knee joint implant
      specified site NEC Z96.698
   larynx Z96.3
   lens Z96.1
   limb (s) —see Presence, artificial, limb
   mandible NEC (for tooth root implant (s))
      Z96.5
   organ NEC Z96.89
   peripheral vessel NEC Z95.828
   stapes Z96.29
   teeth Z97.2
   tendon Z96.7

Replacement by artificial or mechanical device
   or prosthesis of (Continued)
   tissue NEC Z96.89
   tooth root (s) Z96.5
   vessel NEC Z95.828
      coronary (artery) Z95.5
Request for expert evidence Z04.8
Reserve, decreased or low
   cardiac —see Disease, heart
   kidney N28.89
Residual —see also condition
   ovary syndrome N99.83
   state, schizophrenic F20.5
   urine R39.19
Resistance, resistant (to)
   activated protein C D68.51
   complicating pregnancy O26.89
   insulin E88.81
   organism (s)
      to
         drug
            aminoglycosides Z16.29
            amoxicillin Z16.11
            ampicillin Z16.11
            antibiotic (s) Z16.20
               multiple Z16.24
               specified NEC Z16.29
            antifungal Z16.32
            antimicrobial (single) Z16.30
               multiple Z16.35
               specified NEC Z16.39
            antimycbacterial (single) Z16.341
               multiple Z16.342
            antiparasitic Z16.31
            antiviral Z16.33
            beta lactam antibiotics Z16.10
               specified NEC Z16.19
            cephalosporins Z16.19
            extended beta lactamase (ESBL)
               Z16.12
            fluoroquinolones Z16.23
            macrolides Z16.29
            methicillin —see MRSA
            multiple drugs (MDRO)
               antibiotics Z16.24
            penicillins Z16.11
            quinine (and related compounds)
               Z16.31
            quinolones Z16.23
            sulfonamides Z16.29
            tetracyclines Z16.29
            tuberculostatics (single) Z16.341
               multiple Z16.342
            vancomycin Z16.21
            related antibiotics Z16.22
   thyroid hormone E07.89
Resorption
   dental (roots) K03.3
      alveoli M26.79
   teeth (external) (internal) (pathological)
      (roots) K03.3
Respiration
   Cheyne-Stokes R06.3
   decreased due to shock, following injury
      T79.4
   disorder of, psychogenic F45.8
   insufficient, or poor R06.89
      newborn P28.5
   painful R07.1
   sighing, psychogenic F45.8
Respiratory —see also condition
   distress syndrome (newborn) (type I)
      P22.0
      type II P22.1
   syncytial virus, as cause of disease classified
      elsewhere B97.4
Respite care Z75.5
Response (drug)
   photoallergic L56.1
   phototoxic L56.0
Restless legs (syndrome) G25.81

Restlessness R45.1
Restoration (of)
  dental
    aesthetically inadequate or displeasing
      K08.56
    defective K08.50
      specified NEC K08.59
    failure of marginal integrity K08.51
    failure of periodontal anatomical intergrity
      K08.54
  organ continuity from previous sterilization
    (tuboplasty) (vasoplasty) Z31.0
    aftercare Z31.42
  tooth (existing)
    contours biologically incompatible with
      oral health K08.54
    open margins K08.51
    overhanging K08.52
    poor aesthetic K08.56
    poor gingival margins K08.51
    unsatisfactory, of tooth K08.50
      specified NEC K08.59
Restorative material (dental)
  allergy to K08.55
  fractured K08.539
    with loss of material K08.531
    without loss of material K08.530
  unrepairable overhanging of K08.52
Restriction of housing space Z59.1
Rests, ovarian, in fallopian tube Q50.6
Restzustand (schizophrenic) F20.5
Retained —see also Retention
  cholelithiasis following cholecystectomy
    K91.86
  foreign body fragments (type of) Z18.9
    acrylics Z18.2
    animal quill (s) or spines Z18.31
    cement Z18.83
    concrete Z18.83
    crystalline Z18.83
    depleted isotope Z18.09
    depleted uranium Z18.01
    diethylhexylphthalates Z18.2
    glass Z18.81
    isocyanate Z18.2
    magnetic metal Z18.11
    metal Z18.10
    nonmagnetic metal Z18.12
    nontherapeutic radioactive Z18.09
    organic NEC Z18.39
    plastic Z18.2
    quill (s) (animal) Z18.31
    radioactive (nontherapeutic) NEC
      Z18.09
    specified NEC Z18.89
    spine (s) (animal) Z18.31
    stone Z18.83
    tooth (teeth) Z18.32
    wood Z18.33
  fragments (type of) Z18.9
    acrylics Z18.2
    animal quill (s) or spines Z18.31
    cement Z18.83
    concrete Z18.83
    crystalline Z18.83
    depleted isotope Z18.09
    depleted uranium Z18.01
    diethylhexylphthalates Z18.2
    glass Z18.81
    isocyanate Z18.2
    magnetic metal Z18.11
    metal Z18.10
    nonmagnectic metal Z18.12
    nontherapeutic radioactive Z18.09
    organic NEC Z18.39
    plastic Z18.2
    quill (s) (animal) Z18.31
    radioactive (nontherapeutic) NEC
      Z18.09
    specified NEC Z18.89
    spine (s) (animal) Z18.31

Retained (Continued)
  fragments (Continued)
    stone Z18.83
    tooth (teeth) Z18.32
    wood Z18.33
  gallstones, following cholecystectomy K91.86
Retardation
  development, developmental, specific —see
    Disorder, developmental
  endochondral bone growth —see Disorder,
    bone, development or growth
  growth R62.50
    due to malnutrition E45
  mental —see Disability, intellectual
  motor function, specific F82
  physical (child) R62.52
    due to malnutrition E45
  reading (specific) F81.0
  spelling (specific) (without reading disorder)
    F81.81
Retching —see Vomiting
Retention —see also Retained
  bladder —see Retention, urine
  carbon dioxide E87.2
  cholelithiasis following cholecystectomy
    K91.86
  cyst —see Cyst
  dead
    fetus (at or near term) (mother) O36.4
      early fetal death O02.1
    ovum O02.0
  decidua (fragments) (following delivery)
    (with hemorrhage) O72.2
    without hemorrhage O73.1
  deciduous tooth K00.6
  dental root K08.3
  fecal —see Constipation
  fetus
    dead O36.4
    early O02.1
  fluid R60.9
  foreign body —see also Foreign body, retained
    current trauma - code as Foreign body, by
      site or type
  gallstones, following cholecystectomy
    K91.86
  gastric K31.89
  intrauterine contraceptive device, in
    pregnancy —see Pregnancy, complicated
    by, retention, intrauterine device
  membranes (complicating delivery) (with
    hemorrhage) O72.2
    with abortion —see Abortion, by type
    without hemorrhage O73.1
  meniscus —see Derangement, meniscus
  menses N94.89
  milk (puerperal, postpartum) O92.79
  nitrogen, extrarenal R39.2
  ovary syndrome N99.83
  placenta (total) (with hemorrhage) O72.0
    without hemorrhage O73.0
    portions or fragments (with hemorrhage)
      O72.2
      without hemorrhage O73.1
  products of conception
    early pregnancy (dead fetus) O02.1
    following
      delivery (with hemorrhage) O72.2
        without hemorrhage O73.1
  secundines (following delivery) (with
    hemorrhage) O72.0
    without hemorrhage O73.0
    complicating puerperium (delayed
      hemorrhage) O72.2
    partial O72.2
      without hemorrhage O73.1
  smegma, clitoris N90.89
  urine R33.9
    drug-induced R33.0
    due to hyperplasia (hypertrophy) of
      prostate —see Hyperplasia, prostate

Retention (Continued)
  urine (Continued)
    organic R33.8
      drug-induced R33.0
    psychogenic F45.8
    specified NEC R33.8
  water (in tissues) —see Edema
Reticular erythematous mucinosis L98.5
Reticulation, dust —see Pneumoconiosis
Reticulocytosis R70.1
Reticuloendotheliosis
  acute infantile C96.0
  leukemic C91.4-
  malignant C96.9
  nonlipid C96.0
Reticulohistiocytoma (giant-cell) D76.3
Reticuloid, actinic L57.1
Reticulosis (skin)
  acute of infancy C96.0
  hemophagocytic, familial D76.1
  histiocytic medullary C96.9
  lipomelanotic I89.8
  malignant (midline) C86.0
  nonlipid C96.0
  polymorphic C86.0
  Sézary —see Sézary disease
Retina, retinal —see also condition
  dark area D49.81
Retinitis —see also Inflammation, chorioretinal
  albuminurica N18.9 [H32]
  diabetic —see Diabetes, retinitis
  disciformis —see Degeneration, macula
  focal —see Inflammation, chorioretinal,
    focal
  gravidarum —see Pregnancy, complicated by,
    specified pregnancy-related condition
    NEC
  juxtapapillaris —see Inflammation,
    chorioretinal, focal, juxtapapillary
  luetic —see Retinitis, syphilitic
  pigmentosa H35.52
  proliferans —see Disorder, globe,
    degenerative, specified type NEC
  proliferating —see Disorder, globe,
    degenerative, specified type NEC
  renal N18.9 [H32]
  syphilitic (early) (secondary) A51.43
    central, recurrent A52.71
    congenital (early) A50.01 [H32]
    late A52.71
  tuberculous A18.53
Retinoblastoma C69.2-
  differentiated C69.2-
  undifferentiated C69.2-
Retinochoroiditis —see also Inflammation,
  chorioretinal
  disseminated —see Inflammation,
    chorioretinal, disseminated
  syphilitic A52.71
  focal —see Inflammation, chorioretinal
  juxtapapillaris —see Inflammation,
    chorioretinal, focal, juxtapapillary
Retinopathy (background) H35.00
  arteriosclerotic I70.8 [H35.0-]
  atherosclerotic I70.8 [H35.0-]
  central serous —see Chorioretinopathy,
    central serous
  Coats H35.02-
  diabetic —see Diabetes, retinopathy
  exudative H35.02-
  hypertensive H35.03-
  in (due to)
    diabetes —see Diabetes, retinopathy
  sickle-cell disorders D57.- [H36]
  of prematurity H35.10-
    stage 0 H35.11-
    stage 1 H35.12-
    stage 2 H35.13-
    stage 3 H35.14-
    stage 4 H35.15-
    stage 5 H35.16-

◀ New   ◀|||| Revised   ~~deleted~~ Deleted

Retinopathy *(Continued)*
 pigmentary, congenital —*see* Dystrophy,
  retina
 proliferative NEC H35.2-
  diabetic —*see* Diabetes, retinopathy,
   proliferative
  sickle-cell D57.- *[H36]*
 solar H31.02-
Retinoschisis H33.10-
 congenital Q14.1
 specified type NEC H33.19-
Retortamoniasis A07.8
Retractile testis Q55.22
Retraction
 cervix —*see* Retroversion, uterus
 drum (membrane) —*see* Disorder, tympanic
  membrane, specified NEC
 finger —*see* Deformity, finger
 lid H02.539
  left H02.536
   lower H02.535
   upper H02.534
  right H02.533
   lower H02.532
   upper H02.531
 lung J98.4
 mediastinum J98.5
 nipple N64.53
  associated with
   lactation O92.03
   pregnancy O92.01-
   puerperium O92.02
  congenital Q83.8
 palmar fascia M72.0
 pleura —*see* Pleurisy
 ring, uterus (Bandl's) (pathological) O62.4
 sternum (congenital) Q76.7
  acquired M95.4
 uterus —*see* Retroversion, uterus
 valve (heart) —*see* Endocarditis
Retrobulbar —*see* condition
Retrocecal —*see* condition
Retrocession —*see* Retroversion
Retrodisplacement —*see* Retroversion
Retroflection, retroflexion —*see* Retroversion
Retrognathia, retrognathism (mandibular)
  (maxillary) M26.19
Retrograde menstruation N92.5
Retroperineal —*see* condition
Retroperitoneal —*see* condition
Retroperitonitis K68.9
Retropharyngeal —*see* condition
Retroplacental —*see* condition
Retroposition —*see* Retroversion
Retroprosthetic membrane T85.398
Retrosternal thyroid (congenital) Q89.2
Retroversion, retroverted
 cervix —*see* Retroversion, uterus
 female NEC —*see* Retroversion, uterus
 iris H21.89
 testis (congenital) Q55.29
 uterus (acquired) (acute) (any
   degree) (asymptomatic) (cervix)
   (postinfectional) (postpartal, old)
   N85.4
  congenital Q51.818
  in pregnancy O34.53-
Retrovirus, as cause of disease classified
  elsewhere B97.30
 human
  immunodeficiency, type 2 (HIV 2) B97.35
  T-cell lymphotropic
   type I (HTLV-I) B97.33
   type II (HTLV-II) B97.34
 lentivirus B97.31
 oncovirus B97.32
 specified NEC B97.39
Retrusion, premaxilla (developmental)
  M26.09
Rett's disease or syndrome F84.2
Reverse peristalsis R19.2

Reye's syndrome G93.7
Rh (factor)
 hemolytic disease (newborn) P55.0
 incompatibility, immunization or
  sensitization
  affecting management of pregnancy NEC
   O36.09-
   anti-D antibody O36.01-
  newborn P55.0
  transfusion reaction —*see* Complication (s),
   transfusion, incompatibility reaction,
   Rh (factor)
 negative mother affecting newborn P55.0
 titer elevated —*see* Complication (s),
  transfusion, incompatibility reaction,
  Rh (factor)
 transfusion reaction —*see* Complication (s),
  transfusion, incompatibility reaction,
  Rh (factor)
Rhabdomyolysis (idiopathic) **NEC** M62.82
 traumatic T79.6
Rhabdomyoma —*see also* Neoplasm, connective
  tissue, benign
 adult —*see* Neoplasm, connective tissue,
  benign
 fetal —*see* Neoplasm, connective tissue, benign
 glycogenic —*see* Neoplasm, connective tissue,
  benign
Rhabdomyosarcoma (any type) —*see*
  Neoplasm, connective tissue, malignant
Rhabdosarcoma —*see* Rhabdomyosarcoma
Rhesus (factor) **incompatibility** —*see* Rh,
  incompatibility
Rheumatic (acute) (subacute) (chronic)
 adherent pericardium I09.2
 coronary arteritis I01.9
 degeneration, myocardium I09.0
 fever (acute) —*see* Fever, rheumatic
 heart —*see* Disease, heart, rheumatic
 myocardial degeneration —*see* Degeneration,
  myocardium
 myocarditis (chronic) (inactive) (with chorea)
  I09.0
  with chorea (acute) (rheumatic)
   (Sydenham's) I02.0
  active or acute I01.2
 pancarditis, acute I01.8
  with chorea (acute (rheumatic)
   Sydenham's) I02.0
 pericarditis (active) (acute) (with effusion)
   (with pneumonia) I01.0
  with chorea (acute) (rheumatic)
   (Sydenham's) I02.0
  chronic or inactive I09.2
 pneumonia I00 *[J17]*
 torticollis M43.6
 typhoid fever A01.09
Rheumatism (articular) (neuralgic)
  (nonarticular) M79.0
 gout —*see* Arthritis, rheumatoid
 intercostal, meaning Tietze's disease M94.0
 palindromic (any site) M12.30
  ankle M12.37-
  elbow M12.32-
  foot joint M12.37-
  hand joint M12.34-
  hip M12.35-
  knee M12.36-
  multiple site M12.39
  shoulder M12.31-
  specified joint NEC M12.38
  vertebrae M12.38
  wrist M12.33-
 sciatic M54.4-
Rheumatoid —*see also* condition
 arthritis —*see also* Arthritis, rheumatoid
  with involvement of organs NEC M05.60
   ankle M05.67-
   elbow M05.62-
   foot joint M05.67-
   hand joint M05.64-

Rheumatoid *(Continued)*
 arthritis *(Continued)*
  with involvement of organs NEC
   (Continued)
   hip M05.65-
   knee M05.66-
   multiple site M05.69
   shoulder M05.61-
   vertebra —*see* Spondylitis, ankylosing
   wrist M05.63-
  seronegative —*see* Arthritis, rheumatoid,
   seronegative
  seropositive —*see* Arthritis, rheumatoid,
   seropositive
 carditis M05.30
  ankle M05.37-
  elbow M05.32-
  foot joint M05.37-
  hand joint M05.34-
  hip M05.35-
  knee M05.36-
  multiple site M05.39
  shoulder M05.31-
  vertebra —*see* Spondylitis, ankylosing
  wrist M05.33-
 endocarditis —*see* Rheumatoid, carditis
 lung (disease) M05.10
  ankle M05.17-
  elbow M05.12-
  foot joint M05.17-
  hand joint M05.14-
  hip M05.15-
  knee M05.16-
  multiple site M05.19
  shoulder M05.11-
  vertebra —*see* Spondylitis, ankylosing
  wrist M05.13-
 myocarditis —*see* Rheumatoid, carditis
 myopathy M05.40
  ankle M05.47-
  elbow M05.42-
  foot joint M05.47-
  hand joint M05.44-
  hip M05.45-
  knee M05.46-
  multiple site M05.49
  shoulder M05.41-
  vertebra —*see* Spondylitis, ankylosing
  wrist M05.43-
 pericarditis —*see* Rheumatoid, carditis
 polyarthritis —*see* Arthritis, rheumatoid
 polyneuropathy M05.50
  ankle M05.57-
  elbow M05.52-
  foot joint M05.57-
  hand joint M05.54-
  hip M05.55-
  knee M05.56-
  multiple site M05.59
  shoulder M05.51-
  vertebra —*see* Spondylitis, ankylosing
  wrist M05.53-
 vasculitis M05.20
  ankle M05.27-
  elbow M05.22-
  foot joint M05.27-
  hand joint M05.24-
  hip M05.25-
  knee M05.26-
  multiple site M05.29
  shoulder M05.21-
  vertebra —*see* Spondylitis, ankylosing
  wrist M05.23-
Rhinitis (atrophic) (catarrhal) (chronic)
  (croupous) (fibrinous) (granulomatous)
  (hyperplastic) (hypertrophic)
  (membranous) (obstructive) (purulent)
  (suppurative) (ulcerative) J31.0
 with
  sore throat —*see* Nasopharyngitis,
 acute J00

Rhinitis *(Continued)*
  allergic J30.9
    with asthma J45.909
      with
        exacerbation (acute) J45.901
        status asthmaticus J45.902
      due to
        food J30.5
        pollen J30.1
    nonseasonal J30.89
    perennial J30.89
    seasonal NEC J30.2
    specified NEC J30.89
  infective J00
  pneumococcal J00
  syphilitic A52.73
    congenital A50.05 *[J99]*
  tuberculous A15.8
  vasomotor J30.0
Rhinoantritis (chronic) —*see* Sinusitis,
    maxillary
Rhinodacryolith —*see* Dacryolith
Rhinolith (nasal sinus) J34.89
Rhinomegaly J34.89
Rhinopharyngitis (acute) (subacute) —*see also*
    Nasopharyngitis
  chronic J31.1
  destructive ulcerating A66.5
  mutilans A66.5
Rhinophyma L71.1
Rhinorrhea J34.89
  cerebrospinal (fluid) G96.0
  paroxysmal —*see* Rhinitis, allergic
  spasmodic —*see* Rhinitis, allergic
Rhinosalpingitis —*see* Salpingitis,
    eustachian
Rhinoscleroma A48.8
Rhinosporidiosis B48.1
Rhinovirus infection NEC B34.8
Rhizomelic chondrodysplasia punctata
    E71.540
Rhythm
  atrioventricular nodal I49.8
  disorder I49.9
    coronary sinus I49.8
    ectopic I49.8
    nodal I49.8
  escape I49.9
  heart, abnormal I49.9
  idioventricular I44.2
  nodal I49.8
  sleep, inversion G47.2-
    nonorganic origin —*see* Disorder, sleep,
      circadian rhythm, psychogenic
Rhytidosis facialis L98.8
Rib —*see also* condition
  cervical Q76.5
Riboflavin deficiency E53.0
Rice bodies —*see also* Loose, body, joint
  knee M23.4-
Richter syndrome —*see* Leukemia, chronic
    lymphocytic, B-cell type
Richter's hernia —*see* Hernia, abdomen, with
    obstruction
Ricinism —*see* Poisoning, food, noxious,
    plant
Rickets (active) (acute) (adolescent) (chest
    wall) (congenital) (current) (infantile)
    (intestinal) E55.0
  adult —*see* Osteomalacia
  celiac K90.0
  hypophosphatemic with nephrotic-glycosuric
    dwarfism E72.09
  inactive E64.3
  kidney N25.0
  renal N25.0
  sequelae, any E64.3
  vitamin-D-resistant E83.31 *[M90.80]*
Rickettsial disease A79.9
  specified type NEC A79.89
Rickettsialpox (Rickettsia akari) A79.1

Rickettsiosis A79.9
  due to
    Ehrlichia sennetsu A79.81
    Rickettsia akari (rickettsialpox) A79.1
  specified type NEC A79.89
  tick-borne A77.9
  vesicular A79.1
Rider's bone —*see* Ossification, muscle,
    specified NEC
Ridge, alveolus —*see also* condition
  flabby K06.8
Ridged ear, congenital Q17.3
Riedel's
  lobe, liver Q44.7
  struma, thyroiditis or disease E06.5
Rieger's anomaly or syndrome Q13.81
Riehl's melanosis L81.4
Rietti-Greppi-Micheli anemia D56.9
Rieux's hernia —*see* Hernia, abdomen, specified
    site NEC
Riga (-Fede) **disease** K14.0
Riggs' disease —*see* Periodontitis
Right middle lobe syndrome J98.11
Rigid, rigidity —*see also* condition
  abdominal R19.30
    with severe abdominal pain R10.0
      epigastric R19.36
      generalized R19.37
      left lower quadrant R19.34
      left upper quadrant R19.32
      periumbilic R19.35
      right lower quadrant R19.33
      right upper quadrant R19.31
  articular, multiple, congenital Q68.8
  cervix (uteri) in pregnancy —*see* Pregnancy,
    complicated by, abnormal, cervix
  hymen (acquired) (congenital) N89.6
  nuchal R29.1
  pelvic floor in pregnancy —*see* Pregnancy,
    complicated by, abnormal, pelvic organs
    or tissues NEC
  perineum or vulva in pregnancy —*see*
    Pregnancy, complicated by, abnormal,
    vulva
  spine —*see* Dorsopathy, specified NEC
  vagina in pregnancy —*see* Pregnancy,
    complicated by, abnormal, vagina
Rigors R68.89
  with fever R50.9
Riley-Day syndrome G90.1
RIND (reversible ischemic neurologic deficit)
    I63.9
Ring (s)
  aorta (vascular) Q25.4
  Bandl's O62.4
  contraction, complicating delivery O62.4
  esophageal, lower (muscular) K22.2
  Fleischer's (cornea) H18.04-
  hymenal, tight (acquired) (congenital)
    N89.6
  Kayser-Fleischer (cornea) H18.04-
  retraction, uterus, pathological O62.4
  Schatzki's (esophagus) (lower) K22.2
    congenital Q39.3
  Soemmerring's —*see* Cataract, secondary
  vascular (congenital) Q25.8
    aorta Q25.4
Ringed hair (congenital) Q84.1
Ringworm B35.9
  beard B35.0
  black dot B35.0
  body B35.4
  Burmese B35.5
  corporeal B35.4
  foot B35.3
  groin B35.6
  hand B35.2
  honeycomb B35.0
  nails B35.1
  perianal (area) B35.6
  scalp B35.0

Ringworm *(Continued)*
  specified NEC B35.8
  Tokelau B35.5
Rise, venous pressure I87.8
Risk, suicidal
  meaning personal history of attempted
    suicide Z91.5
  meaning suicidal ideation —*see* Ideation,
    suicidal
Ritter's disease L00
Rivalry, sibling Z62.891
Rivalta's disease A42.2
River blindness B73.01
Robert's pelvis Q74.2
  with disproportion (fetopelvic) O33.0
    causing obstructed labor O65.0
Robin (-Pierre) **syndrome** Q87.0
Robinow-Silvermann-Smith syndrome Q87.1
Robinson's (hidrotic) **ectodermal dysplasia or**
    syndrome Q82.4
Robles' disease B73.01
Rocky Mountain (spotted) **fever** A77.0
Roetheln —*see* Rubella
Roger's disease Q21.0
Rokitansky-Aschoff sinuses (gallbladder)
    K82.8
Rolando's fracture (displaced) S62.22-
  nondisplaced S62.22-
Romano-Ward (prolonged QT interval)
    syndrome I45.81
Romberg's disease or syndrome G51.8
Roof, mouth —*see* condition
Rosacea L71.9
  acne L71.9
  keratitis L71.8
  specified NEC L71.8
Rosary, rachitic E55.0
Rose
  cold J30.1
  fever J30.1
  rash R21
    epidemic B06.9
Rosenbach's erysipeloid A26.0
Rosenthal's disease or syndrome D68.1
Roseola B09
  infantum B08.20
    due to human herpesvirus 6 B08.21
    due to human herpesvirus 7 B08.22
Ross River disease or fever B33.1
Rossbach's disease K31.89
  psychogenic F45.8
Rostan's asthma (cardiac) —*see* Failure,
    ventricular, left
Rotation
  anomalous, incomplete or insufficient,
    intestine Q43.3
  cecum (congenital) Q43.3
  colon (congenital) Q43.3
  spine, incomplete or insufficient —*see*
    Dorsopathy, deforming, specified NEC
  tooth, teeth, fully erupted M26.35
  vertebra, incomplete or insufficient —*see*
    Dorsopathy, deforming, specified NEC
Rotes Quérol disease or syndrome —*see*
    Hyperostosis, ankylosing
Roth (-Bernhardt) **disease or syndrome** —*see*
    Meralgia paraesthetica
Rothmund (-Thomson) **syndrome** Q82.8
Rotor's disease or syndrome E80.6
Round
  back (with wedging of vertebrae) —*see*
    Kyphosis
  sequelae (late effect) of rickets E64.3
  worms (large) (infestation) NEC B82.0
    Ascariasis (*see also* Ascariasis) B77.9
Roussy-Lévy syndrome G60.0
Rubella (German measles) B06.9
  complication NEC B06.09
    neurological B06.00
  congenital P35.0
  contact Z20.4

◄ New   ◄▥ Revised   ~~deleted~~ Deleted

Rubella (Continued)
exposure to Z20.4
maternal
care for (suspected) damage to fetus O35.3
manifest rubella in infant P35.0
suspected damage to fetus affecting
management of pregnancy O35.3
specified complications NEC B06.89
Rubeola (meaning measles) —see Measles
meaning rubella —see Rubella
Rubeosis, iris —see Disorder, iris, vascular
Rubinstein-Taybi syndrome Q87.2
Rudimentary (congenital) —see also Agenesis
arm —see Defect, reduction, upper limb
bone Q79.9
cervix uteri Q51.828
eye Q11.2
lobule of ear Q17.3
patella Q74.1
respiratory organs in thoracopagus Q89.4
tracheal bronchus Q32.4
uterus Q51.818
in male Q56.1
vagina Q52.0
Ruled out condition —see Observation,
suspected
Rumination R11.10
with nausea R11.2
disorder of infancy F98.21
neurotic F42
newborn P92.1
obsessional F42
psychogenic F42
Runeberg's disease D51.0
Runny nose R09.89
Rupia (syphilitic) A51.39
congenital A50.06
tertiary A52.79
Rupture, ruptured
abscess (spontaneous) - code by site under
Abscess
aneurysm —see Aneurysm
anus (sphincter) —see Laceration, anus
aorta, aortic I71.8
abdominal I71.3
arch I71.1
ascending I71.1
descending I71.8
abdominal I71.3
thoracic I71.1
syphilitic A52.01
thoracoabdominal I71.5
thorax, thoracic I71.1
transverse I71.1
traumatic —see Injury, aorta, laceration,
major
valve or cusp (see also Endocarditis, aortic)
I35.8
appendix (with peritonitis) K35.2
arteriovenous fistula, brain I60.8
artery I77.2
brain —see Hemorrhage, intracranial,
intracerebral
coronary —see Infarct, myocardium
heart —see Infarct, myocardium
pulmonary I28.8
traumatic (complication) —see Injury,
blood vessel
bile duct (common) (hepatic) K83.2
cystic K82.2
bladder (sphincter) (nontraumatic)
(spontaneous) N32.89
following ectopic or molar pregnancy
O08.6
obstetrical trauma O71.5
traumatic S37.29
blood vessel —see also Hemorrhage
brain —see Hemorrhage, intracranial,
intracerebral
heart —see Infarct, myocardium
traumatic (complication) —see Injury,
blood vessel, laceration, major, by site

Rupture, ruptured (Continued)
bone —see Fracture
bowel (nontraumatic) K63.1
brain
aneurysm (congenital) —see also
Hemorrhage, intracranial,
subarachnoid
syphilitic A52.05
hemorrhagic —see Hemorrhage,
intracranial, intracerebral
capillaries I78.8
cardiac (auricle) (ventricle) (wall) I23.3
with hemopericardium I23.0
infectional I40.9
traumatic —see Injury, heart
cartilage (articular) (current) —see also Sprain
knee S83.3-
semilunar —see Tear, meniscus
cecum (with peritonitis) K65.0
with peritoneal abscess K35.3
traumatic S36.598
celiac artery, traumatic —see Injury, blood
vessel, celiac artery, laceration, major
cerebral aneurysm (congenital) (see
Hemorrhage, intracranial,
subarachnoid)
cervix (uteri)
with ectopic or molar pregnancy O08.6
following ectopic or molar pregnancy
O08.6
obstetrical trauma O71.3
traumatic S37.69
chordae tendineae NEC I51.1
concurrent with acute myocardial
infarction —see Infarct, myocardium
following acute myocardial infarction
(current complication) I23.4
choroid (direct) (indirect) (traumatic) H31.32-
circle of Willis I60.6
colon (nontraumatic) K63.1
traumatic —see Injury, intestine, large
cornea (traumatic) —see Injury, eye, laceration
coronary (artery) (thrombotic) —see Infarct,
myocardium
corpus luteum (infected) (ovary) N83.1
cyst —see Cyst
cystic duct K82.2
Descemet's membrane —see Change, corneal
membrane, Descemet's, rupture
traumatic —see Injury, eye, laceration
diaphragm, traumatic —see Injury,
intrathoracic, diaphragm
disc —see Rupture, intervertebral disc
diverticulum (intestine) K57.80
with bleeding K57.81
bladder N32.3
large intestine K57.20
with
bleeding K57.21
small intestine K57.40
with bleeding K57.41
small intestine K57.00
with
bleeding K57.01
large intestine K57.40
with bleeding K57.41
duodenal stump K31.89
ear drum (nontraumatic) —see also
Perforation, tympanum
traumatic S09.2-
due to blast injury —see Injury, blast, ear
esophagus K22.3
eye (without prolapse or loss of intraocular
tissue) —see Injury, eye, laceration
fallopian tube NEC (nonobstetric)
(nontraumatic) N83.8
due to pregnancy O00.1
fontanel P13.1
gallbladder K82.2
traumatic S36.128
gastric —see also Rupture, stomach
vessel K92.2

Rupture, ruptured (Continued)
globe (eye) (traumatic) —see Injury, eye,
laceration
graafian follicle (hematoma) N83.0
heart —see Rupture, cardiac
hymen (nontraumatic) (nonintentional)
N89.8
internal organ, traumatic —see Injury, by site
intervertebral disc —see Displacement,
intervertebral disc
traumatic —see Rupture, traumatic,
intervertebral disc
intestine NEC (nontraumatic) K63.1
traumatic —see Injury, intestine
iris —see also Abnormality, pupillary
traumatic —see Injury, eye, laceration
joint capsule, traumatic —see Sprain
kidney (traumatic) S37.06-
birth injury P15.8
nontraumatic N28.89
lacrimal duct (traumatic) —see Injury, eye,
specified site NEC
lens (cataract) (traumatic) —see Cataract,
traumatic
ligament, traumatic —see Rupture, traumatic,
ligament, by site
liver S36.116
birth injury P15.0
lymphatic vessel I89.8
marginal sinus (placental) (with
hemorrhage) —see Hemorrhage,
antepartum, specified cause NEC
membrana tympani (nontraumatic) —see
Perforation, tympanum
membranes (spontaneous)
artificial
delayed delivery following O75.5
delayed delivery following —see
Pregnancy, complicated by,
premature rupture of membranes
meningeal artery I60.8
meniscus (knee) —see also Tear, meniscus
old —see Derangement, meniscus
site other than knee - code as Sprain
mesenteric artery, traumatic —see Injury,
mesenteric, artery, laceration, major
mesentery (nontraumatic) K66.8
traumatic —see Injury, intra-abdominal,
specified, site NEC
mitral (valve) I34.8
muscle (traumatic) —see also Strain
diastasis —see Diastasis, muscle
nontraumatic M62.10
ankle M62.17-
foot M62.17-
forearm M62.13-
hand M62.14-
lower leg M62.16-
pelvic region M62.15-
shoulder region M62.11-
specified site NEC M62.18
thigh M62.15-
upper arm M62.12-
traumatic —see Strain, by site
musculotendinous junction NEC,
nontraumatic —see Rupture, tendon,
spontaneous
mycotic aneurysm causing cerebral
hemorrhage —see Hemorrhage,
intracranial, subarachnoid
myocardium, myocardial —see Rupture,
cardiac
traumatic —see Injury, heart
nontraumatic, meaning hernia —see Hernia
obstructed —see Hernia, by site, obstructed
operation wound —see Disruption, wound,
operation
ovary, ovarian N83.8
corpus luteum cyst N83.1
follicle (graafian) N83.0
oviduct (nonobstetric) (nontraumatic) N83.8
due to pregnancy O00.1

Rupture, ruptured *(Continued)*
  pancreas (nontraumatic) K86.8
    traumatic S36.299
  papillary muscle NEC I51.2
    following acute myocardial infarction
      (current complication) I23.5
  pelvic
    floor, complicating delivery O70.1
    organ NEC, obstetrical trauma O71.5
  perineum (nonobstetric) (nontraumatic)
    N90.89
    complicating delivery —*see* Delivery,
      complicated, by, laceration, anus
      (sphincter)
  postoperative wound —*see* Disruption,
    wound, operation
  prostate (traumatic) S37.828
  pulmonary
    artery I28.8
    valve (heart) I37.8
    vein I28.8
    vessel I28.8
  pus tube —*see* Salpingitis
  pyosalpinx —*see* Salpingitis
  rectum (nontraumatic) K63.1
    traumatic S36.69
  retina, retinal (traumatic) (without
      detachment) —*see also* Break, retina
    with detachment —*see* Detachment, retina,
      with retinal, break
  rotator cuff (nontraumatic) M75.10-
    complete M75.12-
    incomplete M75.11-
  sclera —*see* Injury, eye, laceration
  sigmoid (nontraumatic) K63.1
    traumatic S36.593
  spinal cord —*see also* Injury, spinal cord, by
      region
    due to injury at birth P11.5
    newborn (birth injury) P11.5
  spleen (traumatic) S36.09
    birth injury P15.1
    congenital (birth injury) P15.1
    due to P. vivax malaria B51.0
    nontraumatic D73.5
    spontaneous D73.5
  splenic vein R58
    traumatic —*see* Injury, blood vessel,
      splenic vein
  stomach (nontraumatic) (spontaneous)
      K31.89
    traumatic S36.39
  supraspinatus (complete) (incomplete)
      (nontraumatic) —*see* Tear, rotator
      cuff
  symphysis pubis
    obstetric O71.6
    traumatic S33.4
  synovium (cyst) M66.10
    ankle M66.17-
    elbow M66.12-
    finger M66.14-
    foot M66.17-
    forearm M66.13-
    hand M66.14-
    pelvic region M66.15-
    shoulder region M66.11-
    specified site NEC M66.18
    thigh M66.15-
    toe M66.17-
    upper arm M66.12-
    wrist M66.13-
  tendon (traumatic) —*see* Strain
    nontraumatic (spontaneous) M66.9
      ankle M66.87-
      extensor M66.20
        ankle M66.27-
        foot M66.27-
        forearm M66.23-
        hand M66.24-
        lower leg M66.26-
        multiple sites M66.29

Rupture, ruptured *(Continued)*
  tendon *(Continued)*
    nontraumatic *(Continued)*
      extensor *(Continued)*
        pelvic region M66.25-
        shoulder region M66.21-
        specified site NEC M66.28
        thigh M66.25-
        upper arm M66.22-
      flexor M66.30
        ankle M66.37-
        foot M66.37-
        forearm M66.33-
        hand M66.34-
        lower leg M66.36-
        multiple sites M66.39
        pelvic region M66.35-
        shoulder region M66.31-
        specified site NEC M66.38
        thigh M66.35-
        upper arm M66.32-
      foot M66.87-
      forearm M66.83-
      hand M66.84-
      lower leg M66.86-
      multiple sites M66.89
      pelvic region M66.85-
      shoulder region M66.81-
      specified
        site NEC M66.88
        tendon M66.80
      thigh M66.85-
      upper arm M66.82-
  thoracic duct I89.8
  tonsil J35.8
  traumatic
    aorta —*see* Injury, aorta, laceration, major
    diaphragm —*see* Injury, intrathoracic,
      diaphragm
    external site —*see* Wound, open, by site
    eye —*see* Injury, eye, laceration
    internal organ —*see* Injury, by site
    intervertebral disc
      cervical S13.0
      lumbar S33.0
      thoracic S23.0
    kidney S37.06-
    ligament —*see also* Sprain
      ankle —*see* Sprain, ankle
      carpus —*see* Rupture, traumatic,
        ligament, wrist
      collateral (hand) —*see* Rupture,
        traumatic, ligament, finger,
        collateral
      finger (metacarpophalangeal)
        (interphalangeal) S63.40-
        collateral S63.41-
          index S63.41-
          little S63.41-
          middle S63.41-
          ring S63.41-
        index S63.40-
        little S63.40-
        middle S63.40-
        palmar S63.42-
          index S63.42-
          little S63.42-
          middle S63.42-
          ring S63.42-
        ring S63.40-
        specified site NEC S63.499
          index S63.49-
          little S63.49-
          middle S63.49-
          ring S63.49-
        volar plate S63.43-
          index S63.43-
          little S63.43-
          middle S63.43-
          ring S63.43-
      foot —*see* Sprain, foot
      radial collateral S53.2-

Rupture, ruptured *(Continued)*
  traumatic *(Continued)*
    ligament *(Continued)*
      radiocarpal —*see* Rupture, traumatic,
        ligament, wrist, radiocarpal
      ulnar collateral S53.3-
      ulnocarpal —*see* Rupture, traumatic,
        ligament, wrist, ulnocarpal
      wrist S63.30-
        collateral S63.31-
        radiocarpal S63.32-
        specified site NEC S63.39-
        ulnocarpal (palmar) S63.33-
    liver S36.116
    membrana tympani —*see* Rupture, ear
      drum, traumatic
    muscle or tendon —*see* Strain
    myocardium —*see* Injury, heart
    pancreas S36.299
    rectum S36.69
    sigmoid S36.593
    spleen S36.09
    stomach S36.39
    symphysis pubis S33.4
    tympanum, tympanic (membrane) —*see*
      Rupture, ear drum, traumatic
    ureter S37.19
    uterus S37.69
    vagina —*see* Injury, vagina
    vena cava —*see* Injury, vena cava,
      laceration, major
  tricuspid (heart) (valve) I07.8
  tube, tubal (nonobstetric) (nontraumatic)
    N83.8
    abscess —*see* Salpingitis
    due to pregnancy O00.1
  tympanum, tympanic (membrane)
    (nontraumatic) (*see also* Perforation,
    tympanic membrane) H72.9-
    traumatic —*see* Rupture, ear drum,
      traumatic
  umbilical cord, complicating delivery
    O69.89
  ureter (traumatic) S37.19
    nontraumatic N28.89
  urethra (nontraumatic) N36.8
    with ectopic or molar pregnancy
      O08.6
    following ectopic or molar pregnancy
      O08.6
    obstetrical trauma O71.5
    traumatic S37.39
  uterosacral ligament (nonobstetric)
    (nontraumatic) N83.8
  uterus (traumatic) S37.69
    before labor O71.0-
    during or after labor O71.1
    nonpuerperal, nontraumatic N85.8
    pregnant (during labor) O71.1
      before labor O71.0-
  vagina —*see* Injury, vagina
  valve, valvular (heart) —*see* Endocarditis
  varicose vein —*see* Varix
  varix —*see* Varix
  vena cava R58
    traumatic —*see* Injury, vena cava,
      laceration, major
  vesical (urinary) N32.89
  vessel (blood) R58
    pulmonary I28.8
    traumatic —*see* Injury, blood vessel
  viscus R19.8
  vulva complicating delivery O70.0
Russell-Silver syndrome Q87.1
Russian spring-summer type encephalitis
  A84.0
Rust's disease (tuberculous cervical spondylitis)
  A18.01
Ruvalcaba-Myhre-Smith syndrome
  E71.440
Rytand-Lipsitch syndrome I44.2

◀ New ◀▦ Revised ~~deleted~~ Deleted

S

Saber, sabre shin or tibia (syphilitic) A50.56
  [M90.8-]
Sac lacrimal —*see* condition
Saccharomyces infection B37.9
Saccharopinuria E72.3
Saccular —*see* condition
Sacculation
  aorta (nonsyphilitic) —*see* Aneurysm,
    aorta
  bladder N32.3
  intralaryngeal (congenital) (ventricular)
    Q31.3
  larynx (congenital) (ventricular) Q31.3
  organ or site, congenital —*see* Distortion
  pregnant uterus —*see* Pregnancy, complicated
    by, abnormal, uterus
  ureter N28.89
  urethra N36.1
  vesical N32.3
Sachs' amaurotic familial idiocy or disease
  E75.02
Sachs-Tay disease E75.02
Sacks-Libman disease M32.11
Sacralgia M53.3
Sacralization Q76.49
Sacrodynia M53.3
Sacroiliac joint —*see* condition
Sacroiliitis NEC M46.1
Sacrum —*see* condition
Saddle
  back —*see* Lordosis
  embolus
    abdominal aorta I74.01
    pulmonary artery I26.92
      with acute cor pulmonale I26.02
  injury — code to condition
  nose M95.0
    due to syphilis A50.57
Sadism (sexual) F65.52
Sadness, postpartal O90.6
Sadomasochism F65.50
Saemisch's ulcer (cornea) —*see* Ulcer, cornea,
  central
Sahib disease B55.0
Sailors' skin L57.8
Saint
  Anthony's fire —*see* Erysipelas
  triad —*see* Hernia, diaphragm
  Vitus' dance —*see* Chorea, Sydenham's
Salaam
  attack (s) —*see* Epilepsy, spasms
  tic R25.8
Salicylism
  abuse F55.8
  overdose or wrong substance given —*see*
    Table of Drugs and Chemicals, by drug,
    poisoning
Salivary duct or gland —*see* condition
Salivation, excessive K11.7
Salmonella —*see* Infection, Salmonella
Salmonellosis A02.0
Salpingitis (catarrhal) (fallopian tube) (nodular)
  (pseudofollicular) (purulent) (septic)
  N70.91
  with oophoritis N70.93
  acute N70.01
    with oophoritis N70.03
  chlamydial A56.11
  chronic N70.11
    with oophoritis N70.13
  complicating abortion —*see* Abortion, by
    type, complicated by, salpingitis
  ear —*see* Salpingitis, eustachian
  eustachian (tube) H68.00-
    acute H68.01-
    chronic H68.02-
  follicularis N70.11
    with oophoritis N70.13
  gonococcal (acute) (chronic) A54.24

Salpingitis *(Continued)*
  interstitial, chronic N70.11
    with oophoritis N70.13
  isthmica nodosa N70.11
    with oophoritis N70.13
  specific (gonococcal) (acute) (chronic) A54.24
  tuberculous (acute) (chronic) A18.17
  venereal (gonococcal) (acute) (chronic) A54.24
Salpingocele N83.4
Salpingo-oophoritis (catarrhal) (purulent)
  (ruptured) (septic) (suppurative) N70.93
  acute N70.03
    with ectopic or molar pregnancy O08.0
    following ectopic or molar pregnancy
      O08.0
    gonococcal A54.24
  chronic N70.13
  following ectopic or molar pregnancy O08.0
  gonococcal (acute) (chronic) A54.24
  puerperal O86.19
  specific (gonococcal) (acute) (chronic) A54.24
  subacute N70.03
  tuberculous (acute) (chronic) A18.17
  venereal (gonococcal) (acute) (chronic)
    A54.24
Salpingo-ovaritis —*see* Salpingo-oophoritis
Salpingoperitonitis —*see* Salpingo-oophoritis
Salzmann's nodular dystrophy —*see*
  Degeneration, cornea, nodular
Sampson's cyst or tumor N80.1
San Joaquin (Valley) **fever** B38.0
Sandblaster's asthma, lung or pneumoconiosis
  J62.8
Sander's disease (paranoia) F22
Sandfly fever A93.1
Sandhoff's disease E75.01
Sanfilippo (Type B) (Type C) (Type D)
  syndrome E76.22
Sanger-Brown ataxia G11.2
Sao Paulo fever or typhus A77.0
Saponification, mesenteric K65.8
Sarcocele (benign)
  syphilitic A52.76
    congenital A50.59
Sarcocystosis A07.8
Sarcoepiplocele —*see* Hernia
Sarcoepiplomphalocele Q79.2
Sarcoid —*see also* Sarcoidosis
  arthropathy D86.86
  Boeck's D86.9
  Darier-Roussy D86.3
  iridocyclitis D86.83
  meningitis D86.81
  myocarditis D86.85
  myositis D86.87
  pyelonephritis D86.84
  Spiegler-Fendt L08.89
Sarcoidosis D86.9
  with
    cranial nerve palsies D86.82
    hepatic granuloma D86.89
    polyarthritis D86.86
    tubulo-interstitial nephropathy D86.84
  combined sites NEC D86.89
  lung D86.0
    and lymph nodes D86.2
  lymph nodes D86.1
    and lung D86.2
  meninges D86.81
  skin D86.3
  specified type NEC D86.89
Sarcoma (of) —*see also* Neoplasm, connective
  tissue, malignant
  alveolar soft part —*see* Neoplasm, connective
    tissue, malignant
  ameloblastic C41.1
    upper jaw (bone) C41.0
  botryoid —*see* Neoplasm, connective tissue,
    malignant
  botryoides —*see* Neoplasm, connective tissue,
    malignant

Sarcoma *(Continued)*
  cerebellar C71.6
    circumscribed (arachnoidal) C71.6
  circumscribed (arachnoidal) cerebellar
    C71.6
  clear cell —*see also* Neoplasm, connective
    tissue, malignant
    kidney C64.-
  dendritic cells (accessory cells) C96.4
  embryonal —*see* Neoplasm, connective tissue,
    malignant
  endometrial (stromal) C54.1
    isthmus C54.0
  epithelioid (cell) —*see* Neoplasm, connective
    tissue, malignant
  Ewing's —*see* Neoplasm, bone, malignant
  follicular dendritic cell C96.4
  germinoblastic (diffuse) —*see* Lymphoma,
    diffuse, large cell
    follicular —*see* Lymphoma, follicular,
      specified NEC
  giant cell (except of bone) —*see also* Neoplasm,
    connective tissue, malignant
    bone —*see* Neoplasm, bone, malignant
  glomoid —*see* Neoplasm, connective tissue,
    malignant
  granulocytic C92.3-
  hemangioendothelial —*see* Neoplasm,
    connective tissue, malignant
  hemorrhagic, multiple —*see* Sarcoma,
    Kaposi's
  histiocytic C96.A
  Hodgkin —*see* Lymphoma, Hodgkin
  immunoblastic (diffuse) —*see* Lymphoma,
    diffuse large cell
  interdigitating dendritic cell C96.4
  Kaposi's
    colon C46.4
    connective tissue C46.1
    gastrointestinal organ C46.4
    lung C46.5-
    lymph node (s) C46.3
    palate (hard) (soft) C46.2
    rectum C46.4
    skin C46.0
    specified site NEC C46.7
    stomach C46.4
    unspecified site C46.9
  Kupffer cell C22.3
  Langerhans cell C96.4
  leptomeningeal —*see* Neoplasm, meninges,
    malignant
  liver NEC C22.4
  lymphangioendothelial —*see* Neoplasm,
    connective tissue, malignant
  lymphoblastic —*see* Lymphoma,
    lymphoblastic (diffuse)
  lymphocytic —*see* Lymphoma, small cell
    B-cell
  mast cell C96.2
  melanotic —*see* Melanoma
  meningeal —*see* Neoplasm, meninges,
    malignant
  meningothelial —*see* Neoplasm, meninges,
    malignant
  mesenchymal —*see also* Neoplasm,
    connective tissue, malignant
    mixed —*see* Neoplasm, connective tissue,
      malignant
  mesothelial —*see* Mesothelioma
  monstrocellular
    specified site —*see* Neoplasm, malignant,
      by site
    unspecified site C71.9
  myeloid C92.3-
  neurogenic —*see* Neoplasm, nerve,
    malignant
  odontogenic C41.1
    upper jaw (bone) C41.0
  osteoblastic —*see* Neoplasm, bone,
    malignant

Sarcoma *(Continued)*
- osteogenic —*see also* Neoplasm, bone, malignant
  - juxtacortical —*see* Neoplasm, bone, malignant
  - periosteal —*see* Neoplasm, bone, malignant
- periosteal —*see also* Neoplasm, bone, malignant
  - osteogenic —*see* Neoplasm, bone, malignant
- pleomorphic cell —*see* Neoplasm, connective tissue, malignant
- reticulum cell (diffuse) —*see* Lymphoma, diffuse large cell
  - nodular —*see* Lymphoma, follicular
  - pleomorphic cell type —*see* Lymphoma, diffuse large cell
- rhabdoid —*see* Neoplasm, malignant, by site
- round cell —*see* Neoplasm, connective tissue, malignant
- small cell —*see* Neoplasm, connective tissue, malignant
- soft tissue —*see* Neoplasm, connective tissue, malignant
- spindle cell —*see* Neoplasm, connective tissue, malignant
- stromal (endometrial) C54.1
  - isthmus C54.0
- synovial —*see also* Neoplasm, connective tissue, malignant
  - biphasic —*see* Neoplasm, connective tissue, malignant
  - epithelioid cell —*see* Neoplasm, connective tissue, malignant
  - spindle cell —*see* Neoplasm, connective tissue, malignant

Sarcomatosis
- meningeal —*see* Neoplasm, meninges, malignant
- specified site NEC —*see* Neoplasm, connective tissue, malignant
- unspecified site C80.1

Sarcosinemia E72.59
Sarcosporidiosis (intestinal) A07.8
Satiety, early R68.81
Saturnine —*see* condition
Saturnism
- overdose or wrong substance given or taken —*see* Table of Drugs and Chemicals, by drug, poisoning

Satyriasis F52.8
Sauriasis —*see* Ichthyosis
SBE (subacute bacterial endocarditis) I33.0
Scabies (any site) B86
Scabs R23.4
Scaglietti-Dagnini syndrome E22.0
Scald —*see* Burn
Scalenus anticus (anterior) **syndrome** G54.0
Scales R23.4
Scaling, skin R23.4
Scalp —*see* condition
Scapegoating affecting child Z62.3
Scaphocephaly Q75.0
Scapulalgia M89.8X1
Scapulohumeral myopathy G71.0
Scar, scarring (*see also* Cicatrix) L90.5
- adherent L90.5
- atrophic L90.5
- cervix
  - in pregnancy or childbirth —*see* Pregnancy, complicated by, abnormal cervix
- cheloid L91.0
- chorioretinal H31.00-
  - posterior pole macula H31.01-
  - postsurgical H59.81-
  - solar retinopathy H31.02-
  - specified type NEC H31.09-
- choroid —*see* Scar, chorioretinal
- conjunctiva H11.24-

Scar, scarring *(Continued)*
- cornea H17.9
  - xerophthalmic —*see also* Opacity, cornea
    - vitamin A deficiency E50.6
- duodenum, obstructive K31.5
- hypertrophic L91.0
- keloid L91.0
- labia N90.89
- lung (base) J98.4
- macula —*see* Scar, chorioretinal, posterior pole
- muscle M62.89
- myocardium, myocardial I25.2
- painful L90.5
- posterior pole (eye) —*see* Scar, chorioretinal, posterior pole
- retina —*see* Scar, chorioretinal
- trachea J39.8
- uterus N85.8
  - in pregnancy O34.29
- vagina N89.8
  - postoperative N99.2
- vulva N90.89

Scarabiasis B88.2
Scarlatina (anginosa) (maligna) (ulcerosa) A38.9
- myocarditis (acute) A38.1
  - old —*see* Myocarditis
- otitis media A38.0

Scarlet fever (albuminuria) (angina) A38.9
Schamberg's disease (progressive pigmentary dermatosis) L81.7
Schatzki's ring (acquired) (esophagus) (lower) K22.2
- congenital Q39.3

Schaufenster krankheit I20.8
Schaumann's
- benign lymphogranulomatosis D86.1
- disease or syndrome —*see* Sarcoidosis

Scheie's syndrome E76.03
Schenck's disease B42.1
Scheuermann's disease or osteochondrosis —*see* Osteochondrosis, juvenile, spine
Schilder (-Flatau) disease G37.0
Schilling-type monocytic leukemia C93.0-
Schimmelbusch's disease, cystic mastitis, or hyperplasia —*see* Mastopathy, cystic
Schistosoma infestation —*see* Infestation, Schistosoma
Schistosomiasis B65.9
- with muscle disorder B65.9 *[M63.80]*
  - ankle B65.9 *[M63.87-]*
  - foot B65.9 *[M63.87-]*
  - forearm B65.9 *[M63.83-]*
  - hand B65.9 *[M63.84-]*
  - lower leg B65.9 *[M63.86-]*
  - multiple sites B65.9 *[M63.89]*
  - pelvic region B65.9 *[M63.85-]*
  - shoulder region B65.9 *[M63.81-]*
  - specified site NEC B65.9 *[M63.88]*
  - thigh B65.9 *[M63.85-]*
  - upper arm B65.9 *[M63.82-]*
- Asiatic B65.2
- bladder B65.0
- chestermani B65.8
- colon B65.1
- cutaneous B65.3
- due to
  - S. haematobium B65.0
  - S. japonicum B65.2
  - S. mansoni B65.1
  - S. mattheii B65.8
- Eastern B65.2
- genitourinary tract B65.0
- intestinal B65.1
- lung NEC B65.9 *[J99]*
  - pneumonia B65.9 *[J17]*
- Manson's (intestinal) B65.1
- oriental B65.2
- pulmonary NEC B65.9 *[J99]*
  - pneumonia B65.9

Schistosomiasis *(Continued)*
- Schistosoma
  - haematobium B65.0
  - japonicum B65.2
  - mansoni B65.1
- specified type NEC B65.8
- urinary B65.0
- vesical B65.0

Schizencephaly Q04.6
Schizoaffective psychosis F25.9
Schizodontia K00.2
Schizoid personality F60.1
Schizophrenia, schizophrenic F20.9
- acute (brief) (undifferentiated) F23
- atypical (form) F20.3
- borderline F21
- catalepsy F20.2
- catatonic (type) (excited) (withdrawn) F20.2
- cenesthopathic, cenesthesiopathic F20.89
- childhood type F84.5
- chronic undifferentiated F20.5
- cyclic (type) F25.0
- disorganized (type) F20.1
- flexibilitas cerea F20.2
- hebephrenic (type) F20.1
- incipient F21
- latent F21
- negative type F20.5
- paranoid (type) F20.0
- paraphrenic F20.0
- post-psychotic depression F32.8
- prepsychotic F21
- prodromal F21
- pseudoneurotic F21
- pseudopsychopathic F21
- reaction F23
- residual (state) (type) F20.5
- restzustand F20.5
- schizoaffective (type) —*see* Psychosis, schizoaffective
- simple (type) F20.89
- simplex F20.89
- specified type NEC F20.89
- stupor F20.2
- syndrome of childhood F84.5
- undifferentiated (type) F20.3
  - chronic F20.5

Schizothymia (persistent) F60.1
Schlatter-Osgood disease or osteochondrosis —*see* Osteochondrosis, juvenile, tibia
Schlatter's tibia —*see* Osteochondrosis, juvenile, tibia
Schmidt's syndrome (polyglandular, autoimmune) E31.0
Schmincke's carcinoma or tumor —*see* Neoplasm, nasopharynx, malignant
Schmitz (-Stutzer) dysentery A03.0
Schmorl's disease or nodes
- lumbar region M51.46
- lumbosacral region M51.47
- sacrococcygeal region M53.3
- thoracic region M51.44
- thoracolumbar region M51.45

Schneiderian
- papilloma —*see* Neoplasm, nasopharynx, benign
  - specified site —*see* Neoplasm, benign, by site
  - unspecified site D14.0
- specified site —*see* Neoplasm, malignant, by site
- unspecified site C30.0

Scholte's syndrome (malignant carcinoid) E34.0
Scholz (-Bielchowsky-Henneberg) disease or syndrome E75.25
Schönlein (-Henoch) disease or purpura (primary) (rheumatic) D69.0
Schottmuller's disease A01.4
Schroeder's syndrome (endocrine hypertensive) E27.0

◄ New ◄≡ Revised ~~deleted~~ Deleted

Schüller-Christian disease or syndrome C96.5
Schultze's type acroparesthesia, simple I73.89
Schultz's disease or syndrome —see
  Agranulocytosis
Schwalbe-Ziehen-Oppenheim disease G24.1
Schwannoma —see also Neoplasm, nerve,
    benign
  malignant —see also Neoplasm, nerve,
      malignant
    with rhabdomyoblastic differentiation —
        see Neoplasm, nerve, malignant
  melanocytic —see Neoplasm, nerve, benign
  pigmented —see Neoplasm, nerve, benign
Schwannomatosis Q85.03
Schwartz (-Jampel) syndrome G71.13
Schwartz-Bartter syndrome E22.2
Schweniger-Buzzi anetoderma L90.1
Sciatic —see condition
Sciatica (infective)
  with lumbago M54.4-
    due to intervertebral disc disorder —see
        Disorder, disc, with, radiculopathy
  due to displacement of intervertebral disc
      (with lumbago) —see Disorder, disc,
      with, radiculopathy
  wallet M54.3-
Scimitar syndrome Q26.8
Sclera —see condition
Sclerectasia H15.84-
Scleredema
  adultorum —see Sclerosis, systemic
  Buschke's —see Sclerosis, systemic
  newborn P83.0
Sclerema (adiposum) (edematosum)
    (neonatorum) (newborn) P83.0
  adultorum —see Sclerosis, systemic
Scleriasis —see Scleroderma
Scleritis H15.00-
  with corneal involvement H15.04-
  anterior H15.01-
  brawny H15.02-
  in (due to) zoster B02.34
  posterior H15.03-
  specified type NEC H15.09-
  syphilitic A52.71
  tuberculous (nodular) A18.51
Sclerochoroiditis H31.8
Scleroconjunctivitis —see Scleritis
Sclerocystic ovary syndrome E28.2
Sclerodactyly, sclerodactylia L94.3
Scleroderma, sclerodermia (acrosclerotic)
    (diffuse) (generalized) (progressive)
    (pulmonary) (see also Sclerosis, systemic)
    M34.9-
  circumscribed L94.0
  linear L94.1
  localized L94.0
  newborn P83.8
  systemic M34.9
Sclerokeratitis H16.8
  tuberculous A18.52
Scleroma nasi A48.8
Scleromalacia (perforans) H15.05-
Scleromyxedema L98.5
Sclérose en plaques G35
Sclerosis, sclerotic
  adrenal (gland) E27.8
  Alzheimer's —see Disease, Alzheimer's
  amyotrophic (lateral) G12.21
  aorta, aortic I70.0
    valve —see Endocarditis, aortic
  artery, arterial, arteriolar, arteriovascular —
      see Arteriosclerosis
  ascending multiple G35
  brain (generalized) (lobular) G37.9
    artery, arterial I67.2
    diffuse G37.0
    disseminated G35
    insular G35
    Krabbe's E75.23
    miliary G35

Sclerosis, sclerotic (Continued)
  brain (Continued)
    multiple G35
    presenile (Alzheimer's) —see Disease,
        Alzheimer's, early onset
    senile (arteriosclerotic) I67.2
    stem, multiple G35
    tuberous Q85.1
  bulbar, multiple G35
  bundle of I Iis I44.39
  cardiac —see Disease, heart, ischemic,
      atherosclerotic
  cardiorenal —see Hypertension, cardiorenal
  cardiovascular —see also Disease,
      cardiovascular
    renal —see Hypertension, cardiorenal
  cerebellar —see Sclerosis, brain
  cerebral —see Sclerosis, brain
  cerebrospinal (disseminated) (multiple) G35
  cerebrovascular I67.2
  choroid —see Degeneration, choroid
  combined (spinal cord) —see also
      Degeneration, combined
    multiple G35
  concentric (Balo) G37.5
  cornea —see Opacity, cornea
  coronary (artery) I25.10
    with angina pectoris —see Arteriosclerosis,
        coronary (artery),
  corpus cavernosum
    female N90.89
    male N48.6
  diffuse (brain) (spinal cord) G37.0
  disseminated G35
  dorsal G35
  dorsolateral (spinal cord) —see Degeneration,
      combined
  endometrium N85.5
  extrapyramidal G25.9
  eye, nuclear (senile) —see Cataract, senile,
      nuclear
  focal and segmental (glomerular) (see also
      N00-N07 with fourth character .1)
      N05.1
  Friedreich's (spinal cord) G11.1
  funicular (spermatic cord) N50.8
  general (vascular) —see Arteriosclerosis
  gland (lymphatic) I89.8
  hepatic K74.1
    alcoholic K70.2
  hereditary
    cerebellar G11.9
    spinal (Friedreich's ataxia) G11.1
  hippocampal G93.81
  insular G35
  kidney —see Sclerosis, renal
  larynx J38.7
  lateral (amyotrophic) (descending) (primary)
      (spinal) G12.21
  lens, senile nuclear —see Cataract, senile,
      nuclear
  liver K74.1
    with fibrosis K74.2
      alcoholic K70.2
    alcoholic K70.2
    cardiac K76.1
  lung —see Fibrosis, lung
  mastoid —see Mastoiditis, chronic
  mesial temporal G93.81
  mitral I05.8
  Mönckeberg's (medial) —see Arteriosclerosis,
      extremities
  multiple (brain stem) (cerebral) (generalized)
      (spinal cord) G35
  myocardium, myocardial —see Disease, heart,
      ischemic, atherosclerotic
  nuclear (senile), eye —see Cataract, senile,
      nuclear
  ovary N83.8
  pancreas K86.8
  penis N48.6

Sclerosis, sclerotic (Continued)
  peripheral arteries —see Arteriosclerosis,
      extremities
  plaques G35
  pluriglandular E31.8
  polyglandular E31.8
  posterolateral (spinal cord) —see
      Degeneration, combined
  presenile (Alzheimer's) —see Disease,
      Alzheimer's, early onset
  primary, lateral G12.29
  progressive, systemic M34.0
  pulmonary —see Fibrosis, lung
    artery I27.0
    valve (heart) —see Endocarditis,
        pulmonary
  renal N26.9
    with
      cystine storage disease E72.09
      hypertensive heart disease (conditions
          in I11) —see Hypertension,
          cardiorenal
      arteriolar (hyaline) (hyperplastic) —see
          Hypertension, kidney
  retina (senile) (vascular) H35.00
  senile (vascular) —see Arteriosclerosis
  spinal (cord) (progressive) G95.89
    ascending G61.0
    combined —see also Degeneration,
        combined
      multiple G35
      syphilitic A52.11
    disseminated G35
    dorsolateral —see Degeneration, combined
    hereditary (Friedreich's) (mixed form)
        G11.1
    lateral (amyotrophic) G12.21
    multiple G35
    posterior (syphilitic) A52.11
  stomach K31.89
  subendocardial, congenital I42.4
  systemic M34.9
    with
      lung involvement M34.81
      myopathy M34.82
      polyneuropathy M34.83
    drug-induced M34.2
    due to chemicals NEC M34.2
    progressive M34.0
    specified NEC M34.89
  temporal (mesial) G93.81
  tricuspid (heart) (valve) I07.8
  tuberous (brain) Q85.1
  tympanic membrane —see Disorder,
      tympanic membrane, specified NEC
  valve, valvular (heart) —see Endocarditis
  vascular —see Arteriosclerosis
  vein I87.8
Scoliosis (acquired) (postural) M41.9
  adolescent (idiopathic) —see Scoliosis,
      idiopathic, juvenile
  congenital Q67.5
    due to bony malformation Q76.3
    failure of segmentation (hemivertebra)
        Q76.3
    hemivertebra fusion Q76.3
    postural Q67.5
  idiopathic M41.20
    adolescent M41.129
      cervical region M41.122
      cervicothoracic region M41.123
      lumbar region M41.126
      lumbosacral region M41.127
      thoracic region M41.124
      thoracolumbar region M41.125
    cervical region M41.22
    cervicothoracic region M41.23
    infantile M41.00
      cervical region M41.02
      cervicothoracic region M41.03
      lumbar region M41.06

Scoliosis (Continued)
  idiopathic (Continued)
    infantile (Continued)
      lumbosacral region M41.07
      sacrococcygeal region M41.08
      thoracic region M41.04
      thoracolumbar region M41.05
    juvenile M41.119
      cervical region M41.112
      cervicothoracic region M41.113
      lumbar region M41.116
      lumbosacral region M41.117
      thoracic region M41.114
      thoracolumbar region M41.115
    lumbar region M41.26
    lumbosacral region M41.27
    thoracic region M41.24
    thoracolumbar region M41.25
  neuromuscular M41.40
    cervical region M41.42
    cervicothoracic region M41.43
    lumbar region M41.46
    lumbosacral region M41.47
    occipito-atlanto-axial region M41.41
    thoracic region M41.44
    thoracolumbar region M41.45
  paralytic —see Scoliosis, neuromuscular
  postradiation therapy M96.5
  rachitic (late effect or sequelae) E64.3
      [M49.80]
    cervical region E64.3 [M49.82]
    cervicothoracic region E64.3 [M49.83]
    lumbar region E64.3 [M49.86]
    lumbosacral region E64.3 [M49.87]
    multiple sites E64.3 [M49.89]
    occipito-atlanto-axial region E64.3 [M49.81]
    sacrococcygeal region E64.3 [M49.88]
    thoracic region E64.3 [M49.84]
    thoracolumbar region E64.3 [M49.85]
  sciatic M54.4-
  secondary (to) NEC M41.50
    cerebral palsy, Friedreich's ataxia,
        poliomyelitis, neuromuscular
        disorders —see Scoliosis,
        neuromuscular
    cervical region M41.52
    cervicothoracic region M41.53
    lumbar region M41.56
    lumbosacral region M41.57
    thoracic region M41.54
    thoracolumbar region M41.55
  specified form NEC M41.80
    cervical region M41.82
    cervicothoracic region M41.83
    lumbar region M41.86
    lumbosacral region M41.87
    thoracic region M41.84
    thoracolumbar region M41.85
  thoracogenic M41.30
    thoracic region M41.34
    thoracolumbar region M41.35
  tuberculous A18.01
Scoliotic pelvis
  with disproportion (fetopelvic) O33.0
    causing obstructed labor O65.0
Scorbutus, scorbutic —see also Scurvy
  anemia D53.2
Scotoma (arcuate) (Bjerrum) (central) (ring) —
    see also Defect, visual field, localized,
    scotoma
  scintillating H53.19
Scratch —see Abrasion
Scratchy throat R09.89
Screening (for) Z13.9
  alcoholism Z13.89
  anemia Z13.0
  anomaly, congenital Z13.89
  antenatal, of mother Z36
  arterial hypertension Z13.6
  arthropod-borne viral disease NEC Z11.59
  bacteriuria, asymptomatic Z13.89

Screening (Continued)
  behavioral disorder Z13.89
  brain injury, traumatic Z13.850
  bronchitis, chronic Z13.83
  brucellosis Z11.2
  cardiovascular disorder Z13.6
  cataract Z13.5
  chlamydial diseases Z11.8
  cholera Z11.0
  chromosomal abnormalities (nonprocreative)
      NEC Z13.79
  colonoscopy Z12.11
  congenital
    dislocation of hip Z13.89
    eye disorder Z13.5
    malformation or deformation Z13.89
  contamination NEC Z13.88
  cystic fibrosis Z13.228
  dengue fever Z11.59
  dental disorder Z13.84
  depression Z13.89
  developmental handicap Z13.4
    in early childhood Z13.4
  diabetes mellitus Z13.1
  diphtheria Z11.2
  disability, intellectual Z13.4
  disease or disorder Z13.9
    bacterial NEC Z11.2
      intestinal infectious Z11.0
      respiratory tuberculosis Z11.1
    blood or blood-forming organ Z13.0
    cardiovascular Z13.6
    Chagas' Z11.6
    chlamydial Z11.8
    dental Z13.89
    developmental Z13.4
    digestive tract NEC Z13.818
      lower GI Z13.811
      upper GI Z13.810
    ear Z13.5
    endocrine Z13.29
    eye Z13.5
    genitourinary Z13.89
    heart Z13.6
    human immunodeficiency virus (HIV)
        infection Z11.4
    immunity Z13.0
    infection
      intestinal Z11.0
      specified NEC Z11.6
    infectious Z11.9
    mental Z13.89
    metabolic Z13.228
    neurological Z13.89
    nutritional Z13.21
      metabolic Z13.228
        lipoid disorders Z13.220
    protozoal Z11.6
      intestinal Z11.0
    respiratory Z13.83
    rheumatic Z13.828
    rickettsial Z11.8
    sexually-transmitted NEC Z11.3
      human immunodeficiency virus (HIV)
          Z11.4
    sickle-cell (trait) Z13.0
    skin Z13.89
    specified NEC Z13.89
    spirochetal Z11.8
    thyroid Z13.29
    vascular Z13.6
    venereal Z11.3
    viral NEC Z11.59
      human immunodeficiency virus (HIV)
          Z11.4
      intestinal Z11.0
  elevated titer Z13.89
  emphysema Z13.83
  encephalitis, viral (mosquito- or tick-borne)
      Z11.59
  exposure to contaminants (toxic) Z13.88

Screening (Continued)
  fever
    dengue Z11.59
      hemorrhagic Z11.59
      yellow Z11.59
  filariasis Z11.6
  galactosemia Z13.228
  gastrointestinal condition Z13.818
  genetic (nonprocreative)- for procreative
      management —see Testing, genetic, for
      procreative management
    disease carrier status (nonprocreative)
        Z13.71
    specified NEC (nonprocreative) Z13.79
  genitourinary condition Z13.89
  glaucoma Z13.5
  gonorrhea Z11.3
  gout Z13.89
  helminthiasis (intestinal) Z11.6
  hematopoietic malignancy Z12.89
  hemoglobinopathies NEC Z13.0
  hemorrhagic fever Z11.59
  Hodgkin disease Z12.89
  human immunodeficiency virus (HIV)
      Z11.4
  human papillomavirus Z11.51
  hypertension Z13.6
  immunity disorders Z13.0
  infection
    mycotic Z11.8
    parasitic Z11.8
  ingestion of radioactive substance Z13.88
  intellectual disability Z13.4
  intestinal
    helminthiasis Z11.6
    infectious disease Z11.0
  leishmaniasis Z11.6
  leprosy Z11.2
  leptospirosis Z11.8
  leukemia Z12.89
  lymphoma Z12.89
  malaria Z11.6
  malnutrition Z13.29
    metabolic Z13.228
    nutritional Z13.21
  measles Z11.59
  mental disorder Z13.89
  metabolic errors, inborn Z13.228
  multiphasic Z13.89
  musculoskeletal disorder Z13.828
    osteoporosis Z13.820
  mycoses Z11.8
  myocardial infarction (acute) Z13.6
  neoplasm (malignant) (of) Z12.9
    bladder Z12.6
    blood Z12.89
    breast Z12.39
      routine mammogram Z12.31
    cervix Z12.4
    colon Z12.11
    genitourinary organs NEC Z12.79
      bladder Z12.6
      cervix Z12.4
      ovary Z12.73
      prostate Z12.5
      testis Z12.71
      vagina Z12.72
    hematopoietic system Z12.89
    intestinal tract Z12.10
      colon Z12.11
      rectum Z12.12
      small intestine Z12.13
    lung Z12.2
    lymph (glands) Z12.89
    nervous system Z12.82
    oral cavity Z12.81
    prostate Z12.5
    rectum Z12.12
    respiratory organs Z12.2
    skin Z12.83
    small intestine Z12.13

◀ New   ◀▥ Revised   ~~deleted~~ Deleted

Screening *(Continued)*
  neoplasm *(Continued)*
    specified site NEC Z12.89
    stomach Z12.0
  nephropathy Z13.89
  nervous system disorders NEC Z13.858
  neurological condition Z13.89
  osteoporosis Z13.820
  parasitic infestation Z11.9
    specified NEC Z11.8
  phenylketonuria Z13.228
  plague Z11.2
  poisoning (chemical) (heavy metal)
      Z13.88
  poliomyelitis Z11.59
  postnatal, chromosomal abnormalities
      Z13.89
  prenatal, of mother Z36
  protozoal disease Z11.6
    intestinal Z11.0
  pulmonary tuberculosis Z11.1
  radiation exposure Z13.88
  respiratory condition Z13.83
  respiratory tuberculosis Z11.1
  rheumatoid arthritis Z13.828
  rubella Z11.59
  schistosomiasis Z11.6
  sexually-transmitted disease NEC Z11.3
    human immunodeficiency virus (HIV)
        Z11.4
  sickle-cell disease or trait Z13.0
  skin condition Z13.89
  sleeping sickness Z11.6
  special Z13.9
    specified NEC Z13.89
  syphilis Z11.3
  tetanus Z11.2
  trachoma Z11.8
  traumatic brain injury Z13.850
  trypanosomiasis Z11.6
  tuberculosis, respiratory Z11.1
  venereal disease Z11.3
  viral encephalitis (mosquito- or tick-borne)
      Z11.59
  whooping cough Z11.2
  worms, intestinal Z11.6
  yaws Z11.8
  yellow fever Z11.59
Scrofula, scrofulosis (tuberculosis of cervical
    lymph glands) A18.2
Scrofulide (primary) (tuberculous) A18.4
Scrofuloderma, scrofulodermia (any site)
    (primary) A18.4
Scrofulosus lichen (primary) (tuberculous)
    A18.4
Scrofulous —*see* condition
Scrotal tongue K14.5
Scrotum —*see* condition
Scurvy, scorbutic E54
  anemia D53.2
  gum E54
  infantile E54
  rickets E55.0 *[M90.80]*
Sealpox B08.62
Seasickness T75.3
Seatworm (infection) (infestation) B80
Sebaceous —*see also* condition
  cyst —*see* Cyst, sebaceous
Seborrhea, seborrheic L21.9
  capillitii R23.8
  capitis L21.0
  dermatitis L21.9
    infantile L21.1
  eczema L21.9
    infantile L21.1
  sicca L21.0
Seckel's syndrome Q87.1
Seclusion, pupil —*see* Membrane, pupillary
Second hand tobacco smoke exposure (acute)
    (chronic) Z77.22
  in the perinatal period P96.81

Secondary
  dentin (in pulp) K04.3
  neoplasm, secondaries —*see* Table of
      Neoplasms, secondary
Secretion
  antidiuretic hormone, inappropriate E22.2
  catecholamine, by pheochromocytoma
      E27.5
  hormone
    antidiuretic, inappropriate (syndrome)
        E22.2
    by
      carcinoid tumor E34.0
      pheochromocytoma E27.5
    ectopic NEC E34.2
  urinary
    excessive R35.8
    suppression R34
Section
  nerve, traumatic —*see* Injury, nerve
Segmentation, incomplete (congenital) —*see
    also* Fusion
  bone NEC Q78.8
  lumbosacral (joint) (vertebra) Q76.49
Seitelberger's syndrome (infantile neuraxonal
    dystrophy) G31.89
Seizure (s) (*see also* Convulsions) R56.9
  akinetic —*see* Epilepsy, generalized, specified
      NEC
  atonic —*see* Epilepsy, generalized, specified
      NEC
  autonomic (hysterical) F44.5
  convulsive —*see* Convulsions
  cortical (focal) (motor) —*see* Epilepsy,
      localization-related, symptomatic, with
      simple partial seizures
  disorder (*see also* Epilepsy) G40.909
  due to stroke —*see* Sequelae (of), disease,
      cerebrovascular, by type, specified
      NEC
  epileptic —*see* Epilepsy
  febrile (simple) R56.00
    with status epilepticus G40.901
    complex (atypical) (complicated)
        R56.01
      with status epilepticus G40.901
  grand mal G40.409
    intractable G40.419
      with status epilepticus G40.411
      without status epilepticus G40.419
    not intractable G40.409
      with status epilepticus G40.401
      without status epilepticus G40.409
  heart —*see* Disease, heart
  hysterical F44.5
  intractable G40.919
    with status epilepticus G40.911
  Jacksonian (focal) (motor type) (sensory
      type) —*see* Epilepsy, localization-
      related, symptomatic, with simple
      partial seizures
  newborn P90
  nonspecific epileptic
    atonic —*see* Epilepsy, generalized, specified
        NEC
    clonic —*see* Epilepsy, generalized, specified
        NEC
    myoclonic —*see* Epilepsy, generalized,
        specified NEC
    tonic —*see* Epilepsy, generalized, specified
        NEC
    tonic-clonic —*see* Epilepsy, generalized,
        specified NEC
  partial, developing into secondarily
      generalized seizures
    complex —*see* Epilepsy, localization-
        related, symptomatic, with complex
        partial seizures
    simple —*see* Epilepsy, localization-related,
        symptomatic, with simple partial
        seizures

Seizure *(Continued)*
  petit mal G40.409
    intractable G40.419
      with status epilepticus G40.411
      without status epilepticus G40.419
    not intractable G40.409
      with status epilepticus G40.401
      without status epilepticus G40.409
  post traumatic R56.1
  recurrent G40.909
  specified NEC G40.89
  uncinate —*see* Epilepsy, localization-related,
      symptomatic, with complex partial
      seizures
Selenium deficiency, dietary E59
Self-damaging behavior (life-style) Z72.89
Self-harm (attempted)
  history (personal) Z91.5
    in family Z81.8
Self-mutilation (attempted)
  history (personal) Z91.5
    in family Z81.8
Self-poisoning
  history (personal) Z91.5
    in family Z81.8
  observation following (alleged) attempt Z03.6
Semicoma R40.1
Seminal vesiculitis N49.0
Seminoma C62.9-
  specified site —*see* Neoplasm, malignant, by
      site
Senear-Usher disease or syndrome L10.4
Senectus R54
Senescence (without mention of psychosis) R54
Senile, senility (*see also* condition) R41.81
  with
    acute confusional state F05
    mental changes NOS F03
    psychosis NEC —*see* Psychosis, senile
  asthenia R54
  cervix (atrophic) N88.8
  debility R54
  endometrium (atrophic) N85.8
  fallopian tube (atrophic) —*see* Atrophy,
      fallopian tube
  heart (failure) R54
  ovary (atrophic) —*see* Atrophy, ovary
  premature E34.8
  vagina, vaginitis (atrophic) N95.2
  wart L82.1
Sensation
  burning (skin) R20.8
    tongue K14.6
  loss of R20.8
  prickling (skin) R20.2
  tingling (skin) R20.2
Sense loss
  smell —*see* Disturbance, sensation, smell
  taste —*see* Disturbance, sensation, taste
  touch R20.8
Sensibility disturbance (cortical) (deep)
    (vibratory) R20.9
Sensitive, sensitivity —*see also* Allergy
  carotid sinus G90.01
  child (excessive) F93.8
  cold, autoimmune D59.1
  dentin K03.89
  latex Z91.040
  methemoglobin D74.8
  tuberculin, without clinical or radiological
      symptoms R76.11
  visual
    glare H53.71
    impaired contrast H53.72
Sensitiver Beziehungswahn F22
Sensitization, auto-erythrocytic D69.2
Separation
  anxiety, abnormal (of childhood) F93.0
  apophysis, traumatic - code as Fracture, by
      site
  choroid —*see* Detachment, choroid

Separation (Continued)
  epiphysis, epiphyseal
    nontraumatic —see also
        Osteochondropathy, specified type
        NEC
      upper femoral —see Slipped, epiphysis,
        upper femoral
    traumatic - code as Fracture, by site
  fracture —see Fracture
  infundibulum cardiac from right ventricle by
    a partition Q24.3
  joint (traumatic) (current) - code by site under
    Dislocation
  pubic bone, obstetrical trauma O71.6
  retina, retinal —see Detachment, retina
  symphysis pubis, obstetrical trauma O71.6
  tracheal ring, incomplete, congenital Q32.1
Sepsis (generalized) (unspecified organism)
    A41.9
  with
    organ dysfunction (acute) (multiple) R65.20
      with septic shock R65.21
  actinomycotic A42.7
  adrenal hemorrhage syndrome
    (meningococcal) A39.1
  anaerobic A41.4
  Bacillus anthracis A22.7
  Brucella (see also Brucellosis) A23.9
  candidal B37.7
  cryptogenic A41.9
  due to device, implant or graft T85.79
    arterial graft NEC T82.7
    breast (implant) T85.79
    catheter NEC T85.79
      dialysis (renal) T82.7
        intraperitoneal T85.71
      infusion NEC T82.7
        spinal (epidural) (subdural) T85.79
      urinary (indwelling) T83.51
    ectopic or molar pregnancy O08.82
    electronic (electrode) (pulse generator)
      (stimulator)
      bone T84.7
      cardiac T82.7
      nervous system (brain) (peripheral
        nerve) (spinal) T85.79
      urinary T83.59
    fixation, internal (orthopedic) —see
        Complication, fixation device,
        infection
    gastrointestinal (bile duct) (esophagus)
      T85.79
    genital T83.6
    heart NEC T82.7
      valve (prosthesis) T82.6
        graft T82.7
    joint prosthesis —see Complication, joint
        prosthesis, infection
    ocular (corneal graft) (orbital implant)
      T85.79
    orthopedic NEC T84.7
      fixation device, internal —see
          Complication, fixation device,
          infection
    specified NEC T85.79
    vascular T82.7
    ventricular intracranial shunt T85.79
  during labor O75.3
  Enterococcus A41.81
  Erysipelothrix (rhusiopathiae) (erysipeloid)
    A26.7
  Escherichia coli (E. coli) A41.5
  extraintestinal yersiniosis A28.2
  following
    abortion (subsequent episode) O08.0
      current episode —see Abortion
    ectopic or molar pregnancy O08.82
    immunization T88.0
    infusion, therapeutic injection or
      transfusion NEC T80.29
  gangrenous A41.9

Sepsis (Continued)
  gonococcal A54.86
  Gram-negative (organism) A41.5
    anaerobic A41.4
  Haemophilus influenzae A41.3
  herpesviral B00.7
  intra-abdominal K65.1
  intraocular —see Endophthalmitis, purulent
  Listeria monocytogenes A32.7
  localized — code to specific localized
      infection
    in operation wound T81.4
    skin —see Abscess
  malleus A24.0
  melioidosis A24.1
  meningeal —see Meningitis
  meningococcal A39.4
    acute A39.2
    chronic A39.3
  MSSA (Methicillin susceptible
      Staphylococcus aureus) A41.01
  newborn P36.9
    due to
      anaerobes NEC P36.5
      Escherichia coli P36.4
      Staphylococcus P36.30
        aureus P36.2
        specified NEC P36.39
      Streptococcus P36.10
        group B P36.0
        specified NEC P36.19
    specified NEC P36.8
  Pasteurella multocida A28.0
  pelvic, puerperal, postpartum, childbirth O85
  pneumococcal A40.3
  postprocedural T81.4
  puerperal, postpartum, childbirth (pelvic)
    O85
  Salmonella (arizonae) (cholerae-suis)
      (enteritidis) (typhimurium) A02.1
  severe R65.20
    with septic shock R65.21
  Shigella (see also Dysentery, bacillary) A03.9
  skin, localized —see Abscess
  specified organism NEC A41.89
  Staphylococcus, staphylococcal A41.2
    aureus (methicillin susceptible) (MSSA)
      A41.01
      methicillin resistant (MRSA) A41.02
    coagulase-negative A41.1
    specified NEC A41.1
  Streptococcus, streptococcal A40.9
    agalactiae A40.1
    group
      A A40.0
      B A40.1
      D A41.81
    neonatal P36.10
      group B P36.0
      specified NEC P36.19
    pneumoniae A40.3
    pyogenes A40.0
    specified NEC A40.8
  tracheostomy stoma J95.02
  tularemic A21.7
  umbilical, umbilical cord (newborn) —see
    Sepsis, newborn
  Yersinia pestis A20.7
Septate —see Septum
Septic —see condition
  arm —see Cellulitis, upper limb
    with lymphangitis —see Lymphangitis,
      acute, upper limb
  embolus —see Embolism
  finger —see Cellulitis, digit
    with lymphangitis —see Lymphangitis,
      acute, digit
  foot —see Cellulitis, lower limb
    with lymphangitis —see Lymphangitis,
      acute, lower limb
  gallbladder (acute) K81.0

Septic (Continued)
  hand —see Cellulitis, upper limb
    with lymphangitis —see Lymphangitis,
      acute, upper limb
  joint —see Arthritis, pyogenic or pyemic
  leg —see Cellulitis, lower limb
    with lymphangitis —see Lymphangitis,
      acute, lower limb
  nail —see also Cellulitis, digit
    with lymphangitis —see Lymphangitis,
      acute, digit
  sore —see also Abscess
    throat J02.0
      streptococcal J02.0
  spleen (acute) D73.89
  teeth, tooth (pulpal origin) K04.4
  throat —see Pharyngitis
  thrombus —see Thrombosis
  toe —see Cellulitis, digit
    with lymphangitis —see Lymphangitis,
      acute, digit
  tonsils, chronic J35.01
    with adenoiditis J35.03
  uterus —see Endometritis
Septicemia A41.9
  meaning sepsis —see Sepsis
Septum, septate (congenital) —see also
    Anomaly, by site
  anal Q42.3
    with fistula Q42.2
  aqueduct of Sylvius Q03.0
    with spina bifida —see Spina bifida, by site,
      with hydrocephalus
  uterus (complete) (partial) Q51.2
  vagina Q52.10
    in pregnancy —see Pregnancy, complicated
      by, abnormal vagina
    causing obstructed labor O65.5
    longitudinal (with or without obstruction)
      Q52.12
    transverse Q52.11
Sequelae (of) —see also condition
  abscess, intracranial or intraspinal (conditions
    in G06) G09
  amputation — code to injury with seventh
    character S
  burn and corrosion — code to injury with
    seventh character S
  calcium deficiency E64.8
  cerebrovascular disease —see Sequelae,
    disease, cerebrovascular
  childbirth O94
  contusion — code to injury with seventh
    character S
  corrosion —see Sequelae, burn and
    corrosion
  crushing injury — code to injury with
    seventh character S
  disease
    cerebrovascular I69.90
      alteration of sensation I69.998
      aphasia I69.920
      apraxia I69.990
      ataxia I69.993
      cognitive deficits I69.91
      disturbance of vision I69.998
      dysarthria I69.922
      dysphagia I69.991
      dysphasia I69.921
      facial droop I69.992
      facial weakness I69.992
      fluency disorder I69.923
      hemiplegia I69.95-
      hemorrhage
        intracerebral —see Sequelae,
            hemorrhage, intracerebral
        intracranial, nontraumatic NEC —
            see Sequelae, hemorrhage,
            intracranial, nontraumatic
        subarachnoid —see Sequelae,
            hemorrhage, subarachnoid

◀ New   ◀▥ Revised   ~~deleted~~ Deleted

Sequelae (Continued)
  disease (Continued)
    cerebrovascular (Continued)
      language deficit I69.928
      monoplegia
        lower limb I69.84-
        upper limb I69.93-
      paralytic syndrome I69.96-
      specified effect NEC I69.998
      specified type NEC I69.80
        alteration of sensation I69.898
        aphasia I69.820
        apraxia I69.890
        ataxia I69.893
        cognitive deficits I69.81
        disturbance of vision I69.898
        dysarthria I69.822
        dysphagia I69.891
        dysphasia I69.821
        facial droop I69.892
        facial weakness I69.892
        fluency disorder I69.823
        hemiplegia I69.85-
        language deficit I69.828
        monoplegia
          lower limb I69.84-
          upper limb I69.83-
        paralytic syndrome I69.86-
        specified effect NEC I69.898
      speech deficit I69.928
        speech deficit I69.828
      stroke NOS —see Sequelae, stroke
          NOS
  dislocation — code to injury with seventh
      character S
  encephalitis or encephalomyelitis (conditions
      in G04) G09
    in infectious disease NEC B94.8
    viral B94.1
  external cause — code to injury with seventh
      character S
  foreign body entering natural orifice — code
      to injury with seventh character S
  fracture — code to injury with seventh
      character S
  frostbite — code to injury with seventh
      character S
  Hansen's disease B92
  hemorrhage
    intracerebral I69.10
      alteration of sensation I69.198
      aphasia I69.120
      apraxia I69.190
      ataxia I69.193
      cognitive deficits I69.11
      disturbance of vision I69.198
      dysarthria I69.122
      dysphagia I69.191
      dysphasia I69.121
      facial droop I69.192
      facial weakness I69.192
      fluency disorder I69.123
      hemiplegia I69.15-
      language deficit NEC I69.128
      monoplegia
        lower limb I69.14-
        upper limb I69.13-
      paralytic syndrome I69.16-
      specified effect NEC I69.198
      speech deficit NEC I69.128
    intracranial, nontraumatic NEC I69.20
      alteration of sensation I69.298
      aphasia I69.220
      apraxia I69.290
      ataxia I69.293
      cognitive deficits I69.21
      disturbance of vision I69.298
      dysarthria I69.222
      dysphagia I69.291
      dysphasia I69.221
      facial droop I69.292

Sequelae (Continued)
  hemorrhage (Continued)
    intracranial, nontraumatic NEC
        (Continued)
      facial weakness I69.292
      fluency disorder I69.223
      hemiplegia I69.25-
      language deficit NEC I69.228
      monoplegia
        lower limb I69.24-
        upper limb I69.23-
      paralytic syndrome I69.26-
      specified effect NEC I69.298
      speech deficit NEC I69.228
    subarachnoid I69.00
      alteration of sensation I69.098
      aphasia I69.020
      apraxia I69.090
      ataxia I69.093
      cognitive deficits I69.01
      disturbance of vision I69.098
      dysarthria I69.022
      dysphagia I69.091
      dysphasia I69.021
      facial droop I69.092
      facial weakness I69.092
      fluency disorder I69.023
      hemiplegia I69.05-
      language deficit NEC I69.028
      monoplegia
        lower limb I69.04-
        upper limb I69.03-
      paralytic syndrome I69.06-
      specified effect NEC I69.098
      speech deficit NEC I69.028
  hepatitis, viral B94.2
  hyperalimentation E68
  infarction
    cerebral I69.30
      alteration of sensation I69.398
      aphasia I69.320
      apraxia I69.390
      ataxia I69.393
      cognitive deficits I69.31
      disturbance of vision I69.398
      dysarthria I69.322
      dysphagia I69.391
      dysphasia I69.321
      facial droop I69.392
      facial weakness I69.392
      fluency disorder I69.323
      hemiplegia I69.35-
      language deficit NEC I69.328
      monoplegia
        lower limb I69.34-
        upper limb I69.33-
      paralytic syndrome I69.36-
      specified effect NEC I69.398
      speech deficit NEC I69.328
  infection, pyogenic, intracranial or intraspinal
      G09
  infectious disease B94.9
    specified NEC B94.8
  injury — code to injury with seventh
      character S
  leprosy B92
  meningitis
    bacterial (conditions in G00) G09
    other or unspecified cause (conditions in
        G03) G09
  muscle (and tendon) injury — code to injury
      with seventh character S
  myelitis —see Sequelae, encephalitis
  niacin deficiency E64.8
  nutritional deficiency E64.9
    specified NEC E64.8
  obstetrical condition O94
  parasitic disease B94.9
  phlebitis or thrombophlebitis of intracranial
      or intraspinal venous sinuses and veins
      (conditions in G08) G09

Sequelae (Continued)
  poisoning — code to poisoning with seventh
      character S
    nonmedicinal substance —see Sequelae,
        toxic effect, nonmedicinal substance
  poliomyelitis (acute) B91
  pregnancy O94
  protein-energy malnutrition E64.0
  puerperium O94
  rickets E64.3
  selenium deficiency E64.8
  sprain and strain — code to injury with
      seventh character S
  stroke NOS I69.30
    alteration in sensation I69.398
    aphasia I69.320
    apraxia I69.390
    ataxia I69.393
    cognitive deficits I69.31
    disturbance of vision I69.398
    dysarthria I69.322
    dysphagia I69.391
    dysphasia I69.321
    facial droop I69.392
    facial weakness I69.392
    hemiplegia I69.35-
    language deficit NEC I69.328
    monoplegia
      lower limb I69.34-
      upper limb I69.33-
    paralytic syndrome I69.36-
    specified effect NEC I69.398
    speech deficit NEC I69.328
  tendon and muscle injury — code to injury
      with seventh character S
  thiamine deficiency E64.8
  trachoma B94.0
  tuberculosis B90.9
    bones and joints B90.2
    central nervous system B90.0
    genitourinary B90.1
    pulmonary (respiratory) B90.9
    specified organs NEC B90.8
  viral
    encephalitis B94.1
    hepatitis B94.2
  vitamin deficiency NEC E64.8
    A E64.1
    B E64.8
    C E64.2
  wound, open — code to injury with seventh
      character S
Sequestration —see also Sequestrum
  lung, congenital Q33.2
Sequestrum
  bone —see Osteomyelitis, chronic
  dental M27.2
  jaw bone M27.2
  orbit —see Osteomyelitis, orbit
  sinus (accessory) (nasal) —see Sinusitis
Sequoiosis lung or pneumonitis J67.8
Serology for syphilis
  doubtful
    with signs or symptoms - code by site and
        stage under Syphilis
    follow-up of latent syphilis —see Syphilis,
        latent
  negative, with signs or symptoms — code by
      site and stage under Syphilis
  positive A53.0
    with signs or symptoms - code by site and
        stage under Syphilis
  reactivated A53.0
Seroma —see also Hematoma
  traumatic, secondary and recurrent
      T79.2
Seropurulent —see condition
Serositis, multiple K65.8
  pericardial I31.1
  peritoneal K65.8
Serous —see condition

S

Sertoli cell
  adenoma
    specified site —*see* Neoplasm, benign, by
      site
    unspecified site
      female D27.9
      male D29.20
  carcinoma
    specified site —*see* Neoplasm, malignant,
      by site
    unspecified site (male) C62.9-
      female C56.9
  tumor
    with lipid storage
      specified site —*see* Neoplasm, benign,
        by site
      unspecified site
        female D27.9
        male D29.20
    specified site —*see* Neoplasm, benign, by
      site
    unspecified site
      female D27.9
      male D29.20
Sertoli-Leydig cell tumor —*see* Neoplasm,
    benign, by site
  specified site —*see* Neoplasm, benign,
    by site
  unspecified site
    female D27.9
    male D29.20
Serum
  allergy, allergic reaction (*see also* Reaction,
    serum) T80.69
    shock (*see also* Shock, anaphylactic) T80.59
  arthritis (*see also* Reaction, serum) T80.69
  complication or reaction NEC (*see also*
    Reaction, serum) T80.69
  disease NEC (*see also* Reaction, serum) T80.69
  hepatitis —*see also* Hepatitis, viral, type B
    carrier (suspected) of Z22.51
  intoxication (*see also* Reaction, serum) T80.69
  neuritis (*see also* Reaction, serum) T80.69
  neuropathy G61.1
  poisoning NEC (*see also* Reaction, serum)
    T80.69
  rash NEC (*see also* Reaction, serum) T80.69
  reaction NEC (*see also* Reaction, serum)
    T80.69
  sickness NEC (*see also* Reaction, serum)
    T80.69
  urticaria (*see also* Reaction, serum) T80.69
Sesamoiditis M25.8-
Sever's disease or osteochondrosis —*see*
    Osteochondrosis, juvenile, tarsus
Severe sepsis R65.20
  with septic shock R65.21
Sex
  chromosome mosaics Q97.8
    lines with various numbers of
      X chromosomes Q97.2
  education Z70.8
  reassignment surgery status Z87.890
Sextuplet pregnancy —*see* Pregnancy,
    sextuplet
Sexual
  function, disorder of (psychogenic) F52.9
  immaturity (female) (male) E30.0
  impotence (psychogenic) organic origin
    NEC —*see* Dysfunction, sexual, male
  precocity (constitutional) (cryptogenic)
    (female) (idiopathic) (male) E30.1
Sexuality, pathologic —*see* Deviation, sexual
Sézary disease C84.1-
Shadow, lung R91.8
Shaking palsy or paralysis —*see* Parkinsonism
Shallowness, acetabulum —*see* Derangement,
    joint, specified type NEC, hip
Shaver's disease J63.1
Sheath (tendon) —*see* condition
Sheathing, retinal vessels H35.01-

Shedding
  nail L60.8
  premature, primary (deciduous) teeth K00.6
Sheehan's disease or syndrome E23.0
Shelf, rectal K62.89
Shell teeth K00.5
Shellshock (current) F43.0
  lasting state —*see* Disorder, post-traumatic
    stress
Shield kidney Q63.1
Shift
  auditory threshold (temporary) H93.24-
  mediastinal R93.8
Shifting sleep-work schedule (affecting sleep)
    G47.26
Shiga (-Kruse) dysentery A03.0
Shiga's bacillus A03.0
Shigella (dysentery) —*see* Dysentery, bacillary
Shigellosis A03.9
  Group A A03.0
  Group B A03.1
  Group C A03.2
  Group D A03.3
Shin splints S86.89
Shingles —*see* Herpes, zoster
Shipyard disease or eye B30.0
Shirodkar suture, in pregnancy —*see*
    Pregnancy, complicated by, incompetent
    cervix
Shock R57.9
  with ectopic or molar pregnancy O08.3
  adrenal (cortical) (Addisonian) E27.2
  adverse food reaction (anaphylactic) —*see*
    Shock, anaphylactic, due to food
  allergic —*see* Shock, anaphylactic
  anaphylactic T78.2
    chemical —*see* Table of Drugs and
      Chemicals
    due to drug or medicinal substance
      correct substance properly administered
        T88.6
      overdose or wrong substance given or
        taken (by accident) —*see* Table of
        Drugs and Chemicals, by drug,
        poisoning
    due to food (nonpoisonous) T78.00
      additives T78.06
      dairy products T78.07
      eggs T78.08
      fish T78.03
        shellfish T78.02
      fruit T78.04
      milk T78.07
      nuts T78.05
        peanuts T78.01
      peanuts T78.01
      seeds T78.05
      specified type NEC T78.09
      vegetable T78.04
    following sting (s) —*see* Venom
    immunization T80.52
    serum T80.59
      blood and blood products T80.51
      immunization T80.52
      specified NEC T80.59
      vaccination T80.52
  anaphylactoid —*see* Shock, anaphylactic
  anesthetic
    correct substance properly administered
      T88.2
    overdose or wrong substance given or
      taken —*see* Table of Drugs and
      Chemicals, by drug, poisoning
    specified anesthetic —*see* Table of
      Drugs and Chemicals, by drug,
      poisoning
  cardiogenic R57.0
  chemical substance —*see* Table of Drugs and
    Chemicals
  complicating ectopic or molar pregnancy O08.3
  culture —*see* Disorder, adjustment

Shock (*Continued*)
  drug
    due to correct substance properly
      administered T88.6
    overdose or wrong substance given or
      taken (by accident) —*see* Table of
      Drugs and Chemicals, by drug,
      poisoning
  during or after labor and delivery O75.1
  electric T75.4
    (taser) T75.4
  endotoxic R65.21
    postprocedural (during or resulting from a
      procedure, not elsewhere classified)
      T81.12
  following
    ectopic or molar pregnancy O08.3
    injury (immediate) (delayed) T79.4
    labor and delivery O75.1
  food (anaphylactic) —*see* Shock, anaphylactic,
    due to food
  from electroshock gun (taser) T75.4
  gram-negative R65.21
    postprocedural (during or resulting from a
      procedure, not elsewhere classified)
      T81.12
  hematologic R57.8
  hemorrhagic
    surgery (intraoperative) (postoperative)
      T81.19
    trauma T79.4
  hypovolemic R57.1
    surgical T81.19
    traumatic T79.4
  insulin E15
    therapeutic misadventure —*see*
      subcategory T38.3
  kidney N17.0
    traumatic (following crushing) T79.5
  lightning T75.01
  lung J80
  obstetric O75.1
    with ectopic or molar pregnancy O08.3
    following ectopic or molar pregnancy
      O08.3
  pleural (surgical) T81.19
    due to trauma T79.4
  postprocedural (postoperative) T81.10
    with ectopic or molar pregnancy O08.3
    cardiogenic T81.11
    endotoxic T81.12
    following ectopic or molar pregnancy
      O08.3
    gram-negative T81.12
    hypovolemic T81.19
    septic T81.12
    specified type NEC T81.19
  psychic F43.0
  septic (due to severe sepsis) R65.21
  specified NEC R57.8
  surgical T81.10
  taser gun (taser) T75.4
  therapeutic misadventure NEC T81.10
  thyroxin
    overdose or wrong substance given or
      taken —*see* Table of Drugs and
      Chemicals, by drug, poisoning
  toxic, syndrome A48.3
  transfusion —*see* Complications, transfusion
  traumatic (immediate) (delayed) T79.4
Shoemaker's chest M95.4
Short, shortening, shortness
  arm (acquired) —*see also* Deformity, limb,
    unequal length
    congenital Q71.81-
    forearm —*see* Deformity, limb, unequal
      length
  bowel syndrome K91.2
  breath R06.02
  cervical (complicating pregnancy) O26.87-
    non-gravid uterus N88.3

◀ New ◀▥ Revised ~~deleted~~ Deleted

Short, shortening, shortness *(Continued)*
  common bile duct, congenital Q44.5
  cord (umbilical), complicating delivery O69.3
  cystic duct, congenital Q44.5
  esophagus (congenital) Q39.8
  femur (acquired) —*see* Deformity, limb,
      unequal length, femur
    congenital —*see* Defect, reduction, lower
        limb, longitudinal, femur
  frenum, frenulum, linguae (congenital) Q38.1
  hip (acquired) —*see also* Deformity, limb,
      unequal length
    congenital Q65.89
  leg (acquired) —*see also* Deformity, limb,
      unequal length
    congenital Q72.81-
      lower leg —*see also* Deformity, limb,
          unequal length
  limbed stature, with immunodeficiency D82.2
  lower limb (acquired) —*see also* Deformity,
      limb, unequal length
    congenital Q72.81-
  organ or site, congenital NEC —*see* Distortion
  palate, congenital Q38.5
  radius (acquired) —*see also* Deformity, limb,
      unequal length
    congenital —*see* Defect, reduction, upper
        limb, longitudinal, radius
  rib syndrome Q77.2
  stature (child) (hereditary) (idiopathic) NEC
      R62.52
    constitutional E34.3
    due to endocrine disorder E34.3
    Laron-type E34.3
  tendon —*see also* Contraction, tendon
    with contracture of joint —*see* Contraction,
        joint
    Achilles (acquired) M67.0-
      congenital Q66.89
    congenital Q79.8
  thigh (acquired) —*see also* Deformity, limb,
      unequal length, femur
    congenital —*see* Defect, reduction, lower
        limb, longitudinal, femur
  tibialis anterior (tendon) —*see* Contraction,
      tendon
  umbilical cord
    complicating delivery O69.3
  upper limb, congenital —*see* Defect,
      reduction, upper limb, specified type
      NEC
  urethra N36.8
  uvula, congenital Q38.5
  vagina (congenital) Q52.4
Shortsightedness —*see* Myopia
Shoshin (acute fulminating beriberi) E51.11
Shoulder —*see* condition
Shovel-shaped incisors K00.2
Shower, thromboembolic —*see* Embolism
Shunt
  arterial-venous (dialysis) Z99.2
  arteriovenous, pulmonary (acquired) I28.0
    congenital Q25.72
  cerebral ventricle (communicating) in situ
      Z98.2
  surgical, prosthetic, with complications —*see*
      Complications, cardiovascular, device
      or implant Shutdown, renal N28.9
Shutdown, renal N28.9
Shy-Drager syndrome G90.3
Sialadenitis, sialadenosis (any gland) (chronic)
    (periodic) (suppurative) —*see* Sialoadenitis
Sialectasia K11.8
Sialidosis E77.1
Sialitis, silitis (any gland) (chronic)
    (suppurative) —*see* Sialoadenitis
Sialoadenitis (any gland) (periodic)
      (suppurative) K11.20
    acute K11.21
      recurrent K11.22
    chronic K11.23

Sialoadenopathy K11.9
Sialoangitis —*see* Sialoadenitis
Sialodochitis (fibrinosa) —*see* Sialoadenitis
Sialodocholithiasis K11.5
Sialolithiasis K11.5
Sialometaplasia, necrotizing K11.8
Sialorrhea —*see also* Ptyalism
    periodic —*see* Sialoadenitis
Sialosis K11.7
Siamese twin Q89.4
Sibling rivalry Z62.891
Sicard's syndrome G52.7
Sicca syndrome M35.00
    with
      keratoconjunctivitis M35.01
      lung involvement M35.02
      myopathy M35.03
      renal tubulo-interstitial disorders M35.04
    specified organ involvement NEC M35.09
Sick R69
    or handicapped person in family Z63.79
      needing care at home Z63.6
    sinus (syndrome) I49.5
Sick-euthyroid syndrome E07.81
Sickle-cell
    anemia —*see* Disease, sickle-cell
    trait D57.3
Sicklemia —*see also* Disease, sickle-cell
    trait D57.3
Sickness
    air (travel) T75.3
    airplane T75.3
    alpine T70.29
    altitude T70.20
    Andes T70.29
    aviator's T70.29
    balloon T70.29
    car T75.3
    compressed air T70.3
    decompression T70.3
    green D50.8
    milk —*see* Poisoning, food, noxious
    motion T75.3
    mountain T70.29
      acute D75.1
    protein (*see also* Reaction, serum) T80.69
    radiation T66
    roundabout (motion) T75.3
    sea T75.3
    serum NEC (*see also* Reaction, serum) T80.69
    sleeping (African) B56.9
      by Trypanosoma B56.9
        brucei
          gambiense B56.0
          rhodesiense B56.1
        East African B56.1
        Gambian B56.0
        Rhodesian B56.1
        West African B56.0
    swing (motion) T75.3
    train (railway) (travel) T75.3
    travel (any vehicle) T75.3
Sideropenia —*see* Anemia, iron deficiency
Siderosilicosis J62.8
Siderosis (lung) J63.4
    eye (globe) —*see* Disorder, globe,
        degenerative, siderosis
Siemens' syndrome (ectodermal dysplasia) Q82.8
Sighing R06.89
    psychogenic F45.8
Sigmoid —*see also* condition
    flexure —*see* condition
    kidney Q63.1
Sigmoiditis (*see also* Enteritis) K52.9
    infectious A09
    noninfectious K52.9
Silfversköld's syndrome Q78.9
Silicosiderosis J62.8
Silicosis, silicotic (simple) (complicated) J62.8
    with tuberculosis J65
Silicotuberculosis J65

Silo-fillers' disease J68.8
    bronchitis J68.0
    pneumonitis J68.0
    pulmonary edema J68.1
Silver's syndrome Q87.1
Simian malaria B53.1
Simmonds' cachexia or disease E23.0
Simons' disease or syndrome (progressive
      lipodystrophy) E88.1
Simple, simplex —*see* condition
Simulation, conscious (of illness) Z76.5
Simultanagnosia (asimultagnosia) R48.3
Sin Nombre virus disease (Hantavirus)
      (cardio)-pulmonary syndrome) B33.4
Sinding-Larsen disease or osteochondrosis —
      see Osteochondrosis, juvenile, patella
Singapore hemorrhagic fever A91
Singer's node or nodule J38.2
Single
    atrium Q21.2
    coronary artery Q24.5
    umbilical artery Q27.0
    ventricle Q20.4
Singultus R06.6
    epidemicus B33.0
Sinus —*see also* Fistula
    abdominal K63.89
    arrest I45.5
    arrhythmia I49.8
    bradycardia R00.1
    branchial cleft (internal) (external) Q18.0
    coccygeal —*see* Sinus, pilonidal
    dental K04.6
    dermal (congenital) Q06.8
      with abscess Q06.8
      coccygeal, pilonidal —*see* Sinus,
          coccygeal
    infected, skin NEC L08.89
    marginal, ruptured or bleeding —*see*
        Hemorrhage, antepartum, specified
        cause NEC
    medial, face and neck Q18.8
    pause I45.5
    pericranii Q01.9
    pilonidal (infected) (rectum) L05.92
      with abscess L05.02
    preauricular Q18.1
    rectovaginal N82.3
    Rokitansky-Aschoff (gallbladder) K82.8
    sacrococcygeal (dermoid) (infected) —*see*
        Sinus, pilonidal
    tachycardia R00.0
      paroxysmal I47.1
    tarsi syndrome M25.57-
    testis N50.8
    tract (postinfective) —*see* Fistula
    urachus Q64.4
Sinusitis (accessory) (chronic) (hyperplastic)
      (nasal) (nonpurulent) (purulent) J32.9
    acute J01.90
      ethmoidal J01.20
        recurrent J01.21
      frontal J01.10
        recurrent J01.11
      involving more than one sinus, other than
          pansinusitis J01.80
        recurrent J01.81
      maxillary J01.00
        recurrent J01.01
      pansinusitis J01.40
        recurrent J01.41
      recurrent J01.91
      specified NEC J01.80
        recurrent J01.81
      sphenoidal J01.30
        recurrent J01.31
    allergic —*see* Rhinitis, allergic
    due to high altitude T70.1
    ethmoidal J32.2
      acute J01.20
        recurrent J01.21

S

Sinusitis *(Continued)*
  frontal J32.1
    acute J01.10
      recurrent J01.11
  influenzal —*see* Influenza, with, respiratory
    manifestations NEC
  involving more than one sinus but not
    pansinusitis J32.8
    acute J01.80
      recurrent J01.81
  maxillary J32.0
    acute J01.00
      recurrent J01.01
  sphenoidal J32.3
    acute J01.30
      recurrent J01.31
  tuberculous, any sinus A15.8
Sinusitis-bronchiectasis-situs inversus
  (syndrome) (triad) Q89.3
Sipple's syndrome E31.22
Sirenomelia (syndrome) Q87.2
Siriasis T67.0
Sirkari's disease B55.0
Siti A65
Situation, psychiatric F99
Situational
  disturbance (transient) —*see* Disorder,
    adjustment
    acute F43.0
  maladjustment —*see* Disorder, adjustment
  reaction —*see* Disorder, adjustment
    acute F43.0
Situs inversus or transversus (abdominalis)
  (thoracis) Q89.3
Sixth disease B08.20
  due to human herpesvirus 6 B08.21
  due to human herpesvirus 7 B08.22
Sjögren-Larsson syndrome Q87.1
Sjögren's syndrome or disease —*see* Sicca
  syndrome
Skeletal —*see* condition
Skene's gland —*see* condition
Skenitis —*see* Urethritis
Skerljevo A65
Skevas-Zerfus disease —*see* Toxicity, venom,
  marine animal, sea anemone
Skin —*see also* condition
  clammy R23.1
  donor —*see* Donor, skin
  hidebound M35.9
Slate-dressers' or slate-miners' lung J62.8
Sleep
  apnea —*see* Apnea, sleep
  deprivation Z72.820
  disorder or disturbance G47.9
    child F51.9
    nonorganic origin F51.9
    specified NEC G47.8
  disturbance G47.9
    nonorganic origin F51.9
  drunkenness F51.9
  rhythm inversion G47.2-
  terrors F51.4
  walking F51.3
    hysterical F44.89
Sleep hygiene
  abuse Z72.821
  inadequate Z72.821
  poor Z72.821
Sleeping sickness —*see* Sickness, sleeping
Sleeplessness —*see* Insomnia
  menopausal N95.11
Sleep-wake schedule disorder G47.20
Slim disease (in HIV infection) B20
Slipped, slipping
  epiphysis (traumatic) —*see also*
    Osteochondropathy, specified type
    NEC
    capital femoral (traumatic)
      acute (on chronic) S79.01-
    current traumatic - code as Fracture, by site

Slipped, slipping *(Continued)*
  epiphysis *(Continued)*
    upper femoral (nontraumatic) M93.00-
      acute M93.01-
      on chronic M93.03-
      chronic M93.02-
  intervertebral disc —*see* Displacement,
    intervertebral disc
  ligature, umbilical P51.8
  patella —*see* Disorder, patella, derangement
    NEC
  rib M89.8X8
  sacroiliac joint —*see* subcategory M53.2
  tendon —*see* Disorder, tendon
  ulnar nerve, nontraumatic —*see* Lesion,
    nerve, ulnar
  vertebra NEC —*see* Spondylolisthesis
Slocumb's syndrome E27.0
Sloughing (multiple) (phagedena) (skin) —*see
  also* Gangrene
  abscess —*see* Abscess
  appendix K38.8
  fascia —*see* Disorder, soft tissue, specified
    type NEC
  scrotum N50.8
  tendon —*see* Disorder, tendon
  transplanted organ —*see* Rejection, transplant
  ulcer —*see* Ulcer, skin
Slow
  feeding, newborn P92.2
  flow syndrome, coronary I20.8
  heart(beat) R00.1
Slowing, urinary stream R39.19
Sluder's neuralgia (syndrome) G44.89
Slurred, slurring speech R47.81
Small (ness)
  for gestational age —*see* Small for dates
  introitus, vagina N89.6
  kidney (unknown cause) N27.9
    bilateral N27.1
    unilateral N27.0
  ovary (congenital) Q50.39
  pelvis
    with disproportion (fetopelvic) O33.1
      causing obstructed labor O65.1
  uterus N85.8
  white kidney N03.9
Small-and-light-for-dates —*see* Small for
  dates
Small-for-dates (infant) P05.10
  with weight of
    499 grams or less P05.11
    500-749 grams P05.12
    750-999 grams P05.13
    1000-1249 grams P05.14
    1250-1499 grams P05.15
    1500-1749 grams P05.16
    1750-1999 grams P05.17
    2000-2499 grams P05.18
Smallpox B03
Smearing, fecal R15.1
Smith-Lemli-Opitz syndrome E78.72
Smith's fracture S52.54-
Smoker —*see* Dependence, drug, nicotine
Smoker's
  bronchitis J41.0
  cough J41.0
  palate K13.24
  throat J31.2
  tongue K13.24
Smoking
  passive Z77.22
Smothering spells R06.81
Snaggle teeth, tooth M26.39
Snapping
  finger —*see* Trigger finger
  hip —*see* Derangement, joint, specified type
    NEC, hip
    involving the iliotiblial band M76.3-
  knee —*see* Derangement, knee
    involving the iliotiblial band M76.3-

Sneddon-Wilkinson disease or syndrome (subcorneal pustular dermatosis) L13.1
Sneezing (intractable) R06.7
Sniffing
  cocaine
    abuse —*see* Abuse, drug, cocaine
    dependence —*see* Dependence, drug,
      cocaine
  gasoline
    abuse —*see* Abuse, drug, inhalant
    dependence —*see* Dependence, drug,
      inhalant
  glue (airplane)
    abuse —*see* Abuse, drug, inhalant
    drug dependence —*see* Dependence, drug,
      inhalant
Sniffles (non-syphilitic) R06.5
  newborn P28.89
Snoring R06.83
Snow blindness —*see* Photokeratitis
Snuffles (non-syphilitic) R06.5
  newborn P28.89
  syphilitic (infant) A50.05 *[J99]*
Social
  exclusion Z60.4
    due to discrimination or persecution
      (perceived) Z60.5
  migrant Z59.0
    acculturation difficulty Z60.3
  rejection Z60.4
    due to discrimination or persecution
      Z60.5
  role conflict NEC Z73.5
  skills inadequacy NEC Z73.4
  transplantation Z60.3
Sodoku A25.0
Soemmerring's ring —*see* Cataract, secondary
Soft —*see also* condition
  nails L60.3
Softening
  bone —*see* Osteomalacia
  brain (necrotic) (progressive) G93.89
    congenital Q04.8
    embolic I63.4
    hemorrhagic —*see* Hemorrhage,
      intracranial, intracerebral
    occlusive I63.5
    thrombotic I63.3
  cartilage M94.2-
    patella M22.4-
  cerebellar —*see* Softening, brain
  cerebral —*see* Softening, brain
  cerebrospinal —*see* Softening, brain
  myocardial, heart —*see* Degeneration,
    myocardial
  spinal cord G95.89
  stomach K31.89
Soldier's
  heart F45.8
  patches I31.0
Solitary
  cyst, kidney N28.1
  kidney, congenital Q60.0
Solvent abuse —*see* Abuse, drug, inhalant
  dependence —*see* Dependence, drug,
    inhalant
Somatization reaction, somatic reaction —*see*
  Disorder, somatoform
Somnambulism F51.3
  hysterical F44.89
Somnolence R40.0
  nonorganic origin F51.11
Sonne dysentery A03.3
Soor B37.0
Sore
  bed —*see* Ulcer, pressure, by site
  chiclero B55.1
  Delhi B55.1
  desert —*see* Ulcer, skin
  eye H57.1-
  Lahore B55.1

◀ New   ◀═ Revised   ~~deleted~~ Deleted

Sore *(Continued)*
  mouth K13.79
    canker K12.0
  muscle M79.1
  Naga —*see* Ulcer, skin
  of skin —*see* Ulcer, skin - oriental B55.1
  pressure —*see* Ulcer, pressure, by site
  skin L98.9
  soft A57
  throat (acute) —*see also* Pharyngitis
    with influenza, flu, or grippe —*see*
      Influenza, with, respiratory
      manifestations NEC
    chronic J31.2
    coxsackie (virus) B08.5
    diphtheritic A36.0
    herpesviral B00.2
    influenzal —*see* Influenza, with, respiratory
      manifestations NEC
    septic J02.0
    streptococcal (ulcerative) J02.0
    viral NEC J02.8
      coxsackie B08.5
    tropical —*see* Ulcer, skin
    veldt —*see* Ulcer, skin
Soto's syndrome (cerebral gigantism) Q87.3
South African cardiomyopathy syndrome I42.8
Southeast Asian hemorrhagic fever A91
Spacing
  abnormal, tooth, teeth, fully erupted M26.30
  excessive, tooth, fully erupted M26.32
Spade-like hand (congenital) Q68.1
Spading nail L60.8
  congenital Q84.6
Spanish collar N47.1
Sparganosis B70.1
Spasm (s), spastic, spasticity (*see also* condition)
  R25.2
  accommodation —*see* Spasm, of
    accommodation
  ampulla of Vater K83.4
  anus, ani (sphincter) (reflex) K59.4
    psychogenic F45.8
  artery I73.9
    cerebral G45.9
  Bell's G51.3
  bladder (sphincter, external or internal)
    N32.89
    psychogenic F45.8
  bronchus, bronchiole J98.01
  cardia K22.0
  cardiac I20.1
  carpopedal —*see* Tetany
  cerebral (arteries) (vascular) G45.9
  cervix, complicating delivery O62.4
  ciliary body (of accommodation) —*see* Spasm,
    of accommodation
  colon K58.9
    with diarrhea K58.0
    psychogenic F45.8
  common duct K83.8
  compulsive —*see* Tic
  conjugate H51.8
  coronary (artery) I20.1
  diaphragm (reflex) R06.6
    epidemic B33.0
    psychogenic F45.8
  duodenum K59.8
  epidemic diaphragmatic (transient) B33.0
  esophagus (diffuse) K22.4
    psychogenic F45.8
  facial G51.3
  fallopian tube N83.8
  gastrointestinal (tract) K31.89
    psychogenic F45.8
  glottis J38.5
    hysterical F44.4
    psychogenic F45.8
      conversion reaction F44.4
    reflex through recurrent laryngeal nerve
      J38.5

Spasm (s), spastic, spasticity *(Continued)*
  habit —*see* Tic
  heart I20.1
  hemifacial (clonic) G51.3
  hourglass —*see* Contraction, hourglass
  hysterical F44.4
  infantile —*see* Epilepsy, spasms
  inferior oblique, eye H51.8
  intestinal (*see also* Syndrome, irritable bowel)
    K58.9
    psychogenic F45.8
  larynx, laryngeal J38.5
    hysterical F44.4
    psychogenic F45.8
      conversion reaction F44.4
  levator palpebrae superioris —*see* Disorder,
    eyelid function
  muscle NEC M62.838
    back M62.830
  nerve, trigeminal G51.0
  nervous F45.8
  nodding F98.4
  occupational F48.8
  oculogyric H51.8
    psychogenic F45.8
  of accommodation H52.53-
  ophthalmic artery —*see* Occlusion, artery,
    retina
  perineal, female N94.89
  peroneo-extensor —*see also* Deformity, limb,
    flat foot
  pharynx (reflex) J39.2
    hysterical F45.8
    psychogenic F45.8
  psychogenic F45.8
  pylorus NEC K31.3
    adult hypertrophic K31.89
    congenital or infantile Q40.0
    psychogenic F45.8
  rectum (sphincter) K59.4
    psychogenic F45.8
  retinal (artery) —*see* Occlusion, artery, retina
  sigmoid (*see also* Syndrome, irritable bowel)
    K58.9
    psychogenic F45.8
  sphincter of Oddi K83.4
  stomach K31.89
    neurotic F45.8
  throat J39.2
    hysterical F45.8
    psychogenic F45.8
  tic F95.9
    chronic F95.1
    transient of childhood F95.0
  tongue K14.8
  torsion (progressive) G24.1
  trigeminal nerve —*see* Neuralgia, trigeminal
  ureter N13.5
  urethra (sphincter) N35.9
  uterus N85.8
    complicating labor O62.4
  vagina N94.2
    psychogenic F52.5
  vascular I73.9
  vasomotor I73.9
  vein NEC I87.8
  viscera —*see* Pain, abdominal
Spasmodic —*see* condition
Spasmophilia —*see* Tetany
Spasmus nutans F98.4
Spastic, spasticity —*see also* Spasm
  child (cerebral) (congenital) (paralysis) G80.1
Speaker's throat R49.8
Specific, specified —*see* condition
Speech
  defect, disorder, disturbance, impediment
    R47.9
    psychogenic, in childhood and adolescence
      F98.8
    slurring R47.81
    specified NEC R47.89

Spencer's disease A08.19
Spens' syndrome (syncope with heart block)
  I45.9
Sperm counts (fertility testing) Z31.41
  postvasectomy Z30.8
  reversal Z31.42
Spermatic cord —*see* condition
Spermatocele N43.40
  congenital Q55.4
  multiple N43.42
  single N43.41
Spermatocystitis N49.0
Spermatocytoma C62.9-
  specified site —*see* Neoplasm, malignant, by
    site
Spermatorrhea N50.8
Sphacelus —*see* Gangrene
Sphenoidal —*see* condition
Sphenoiditis (chronic) —*see* Sinusitis,
  sphenoidal
Sphenopalatine ganglion neuralgia
  G90.09
Sphericity, increased, lens (congenital)
  Q12.4
Spherocytosis (congenital) (familial)
  (hereditary) D58.0
  hemoglobin disease D58.0
  sickle-cell (disease) D57.8-
Spherophakia Q12.4
Sphincter —*see* condition
Sphincteritis, sphincter of Oddi —*see*
  Cholangitis
Sphingolipidosis E75.3
  specified NEC E75.29
Sphingomyelinosis E75.3
Spicule tooth K00.2
Spider
  bite —*see* Toxicity, venom, spider
  fingers —*see* Syndrome, Marfan's
  nevus I78.1
  toes —*see* Syndrome, Marfan's
  vascular I78.1
Spiegler-Fendt
  benign lymphocytoma L98.8
  sarcoid L08.89
Spielmeyer-Vogt disease E75.4
Spina bifida (aperta) Q05.9
  with hydrocephalus NEC Q05.4
  cervical Q05.5
    with hydrocephalus Q05.0
  dorsal Q05.6
    with hydrocephalus Q05.1
  lumbar Q05.7
    with hydrocephalus Q05.2
  lumbosacral Q05.7
    with hydrocephalus Q05.2
  occulta Q76.0
  sacral Q05.8
    with hydrocephalus Q05.3
  thoracic Q05.6
    with hydrocephalus Q05.1
  thoracolumbar Q05.6
    with hydrocephalus Q05.1
Spindle, Krukenberg's —*see* Pigmentation,
  cornea, posterior
Spine, spinal —*see* condition
Spiradenoma (eccrine) —*see* Neoplasm, skin,
  benign
Spirillosis A25.0
Spirillum
  minus A25.0
  obermeieri infection A68.0
Spirochetal —*see* condition
Spirochetosis A69.9
  arthritic, arthritica A69.9
  bronchopulmonary A69.8
  icterohemorrhagic A27.0
  lung A69.8
Spirometrosis B70.1
Spitting blood —*see* Hemoptysis
Splanchnoptosis K63.4

Spleen, splenic —see condition
Splenectasis —see Splenomegaly
Splenitis (interstitial) (malignant) (nonspecific)
    D73.89
    malarial (see also Malaria) B54 [D77]
    tuberculous A18.85
Splenocele D73.89
Splenomegaly, splenomegalia (Bengal)
        (cryptogenic) (idiopathic) (tropical) R16.1
    with hepatomegaly R16.2
    cirrhotic D73.2
    congenital Q89.09
    congestive, chronic D73.2
    Egyptian B65.1
    Gaucher's E75.22
    malarial (see also Malaria) B54 [D77]
    neutropenic D73.81
    Niemann-Pick —see Niemann-Pick disease or
        syndrome
    siderotic D73.2
    syphilitic A52.79
        congenital (early) A50.08 [D77]
Splenopathy D73.9
Splenoptosis D73.89
Splenosis D73.89
Splinter —see Foreign body, superficial, by site
Split, splitting
    foot Q72.7-
    heart sounds R01.2
    lip, congenital —see Cleft, lip
    nails L60.3
    urinary stream R39.13
Spondylarthrosis —see Spondylosis
Spondylitis (chronic) —see also Spondylopathy,
        inflammatory
    ankylopoietica —see Spondylitis, ankylosing
    ankylosing (chronic) M45.9
        with lung involvement M45.9 [J99]
        cervical region M45.2
        cervicothoracic region M45.3
        juvenile M08.1
        lumbar region M45.6
        lumbosacral region M45.7
        multiple sites M45.0
        occipito-atlanto-axial region M45.1
        sacrococcygeal region M45.8
        thoracic region M45.4
        thoracolumbar region M45.5
    atrophic (ligamentous) —see Spondylitis,
        ankylosing
    deformans (chronic) —see Spondylosis
    gonococcal A54.41
    gouty M10.08
    in (due to)
        brucellosis A23.9 [M49.80]
            cervical region A23.9 [M49.82]
            cervicothoracic region A23.9 [M49.83]
            lumbar region A23.9 [M49.86]
            lumbosacral region A23.9 [M49.87]
            multiple sites A23.9 [M49.89]
            occipito-atlanto-axial region A23.9
                [M49.81]
            sacrococcygeal region A23.9 [M49.88]
            thoracic region A23.9 [M49.84]
            thoracolumbar region A23.9 [M49.85]
        enterobacteria (see also subcategory M49.8)
            A04.9
        tuberculosis A18.01
    infectious NEC —see Spondylopathy,
        infective
    juvenile ankylosing (chronic) M08.1
    Kümmell's —see Spondylopathy, traumatic
    Marie-Strümpell —see Spondylitis,
        ankylosing
    muscularis —see Spondylopathy, specified
        NEC
    psoriatic L40.53
    rheumatoid —see Spondylitis, ankylosing
    rhizomelica —see Spondylitis, ankylosing
    sacroiliac NEC M46.1
    senescent, senile —see Spondylosis

Spondylitis (Continued)
    traumatic (chronic) or post-traumatic —see
        Spondylopathy, traumatic
    tuberculous A18.01
    typhosa A01.05
Spondylolisthesis (acquired) (degenerative)
        M43.10
    with disproportion (fetopelvic) O33.0
        causing obstructed labor O65.0
    cervical region M43.12
    cervicothoracic region M43.13
    congenital Q76.2
    lumbar region M43.16
    lumbosacral region M43.17
    multiple sites M43.19
    occipito-atlanto-axial region M43.11
    sacrococcygeal region M43.18
    thoracic region M43.14
    thoracolumbar region M43.15
    traumatic (old) M43.10
        acute
            fifth cervical (displaced) S12.430
                nondisplaced S12.431
                specified type NEC (displaced)
                    S12.450
                    nondisplaced S12.451
                type III S12.44
            fourth cervical (displaced) S12.330
                nondisplaced S12.331
                specified type NEC (displaced)
                    S12.350
                    nondisplaced S12.351
                type III S12.34
            second cervical (displaced) S12.130
                nondisplaced S12.131
                specified type NEC (displaced)
                    S12.150
                    nondisplaced S12.151
                type III S12.14
            seventh cervical (displaced) S12.630
                nondisplaced S12.631
                specified type NEC (displaced)
                    S12.650
                    nondisplaced S12.651
                type III S12.64
            sixth cervical (displaced) S12.530
                nondisplaced S12.531
                specified type NEC (displaced)
                    S12.550
                    nondisplaced S12.551
                type III S12.54
            third cervical (displaced) S12.230
                nondisplaced S12.231
                specified type NEC (displaced)
                    S12.250
                    nondisplaced S12.251
                type III S12.24
Spondylolysis (acquired) M43.00
    cervical region M43.02
    cervicothoracic region M43.03
    congenital Q76.2
    lumbar region M43.06
    lumbosacral region M43.07
        with disproportion (fetopelvic) O33.0
            causing obstructed labor O65.8
    multiple sites M43.09
    occipito-atlanto-axial region M43.01
    sacrococcygeal region M43.08
    thoracic region M43.04
    thoracolumbar region M43.05
Spondylopathy M48.9
    infective NEC M46.50
        cervical region M46.52
        cervicothoracic region M46.53
        lumbar region M46.56
        lumbosacral region M46.57
        multiple sites M46.59
        occipito-atlanto-axial region M46.51
        sacrococcygeal region M46.58
        thoracic region M46.54
        thoracolumbar region M46.55

Spondylopathy (Continued)
    inflammatory M46.90
        cervical region M46.92
        cervicothoracic region M46.93
        lumbar region M46.96
        lumbosacral region M46.97
        multiple sites M46.99
        occipito-atlanto-axial region M46.91
        sacrococcygeal region M46.98
        specified type NEC M46.80
            cervical region M46.82
            cervicothoracic region M46.83
            lumbar region M46.86
            lumbosacral region M46.87
            multiple sites M46.89
            occipito-atlanto-axial region M46.81
            sacrococcygeal region M46.88
            thoracic region M46.84
            thoracolumbar region M46.85
        thoracic region M46.94
        thoracolumbar region M46.95
    neuropathic, in
        syringomyelia and syringobulbia G95.0
        tabes dorsalis A52.11
    specified NEC —see subcategory M48.8
    traumatic M48.30
        cervical region M48.32
        cervicothoracic region M48.33
        lumbar region M48.36
        lumbosacral region M48.37
        occipito-atlanto-axial region M48.31
        sacrococcygeal region M48.38
        thoracic region M48.34
        thoracolumbar region M48.35
Spondylosis M47.9
    with
        disproportion (fetopelvic) O33.0
            causing obstructed labor O65.0
        myelopathy NEC M47.10
            cervical region M47.12
            cervicothoracic region M47.13
            lumbar region M47.16
            occipito-atlanto-axial region
                M47.11
            thoracic region M47.14
            thoracolumbar region M47.15
        radiculopathy M47.20
            cervical region M47.22
            cervicothoracic region M47.23
            lumbar region M47.26
            lumbosacral region M47.27
            occipito-atlanto-axial region
                M47.21
            sacrococcygeal region M47.28
            thoracic region M47.24
            thoracolumbar region M47.25
    without myelopathy or radiculopathy
        M47.819
        cervical region M47.812
        cervicothoracic region M47.813
        lumbar region M47.816
        lumbosacral region M47.817
        occipito-atlanto-axial region M47.811
        sacrococcygeal region M47.818
        thoracic region M47.814
        thoracolumbar region M47.815
    specified NEC M47.899
        cervical region M47.892
        cervicothoracic region M47.893
        lumbar region M47.896
        lumbosacral region M47.897
        occipito-atlanto-axial region M47.891
        sacrococcygeal region M47.898
        thoracic region M47.894
        thoracolumbar region M47.895
    traumatic —see Spondylopathy, traumatic
Sponge
    inadvertently left in operation wound —see
        Foreign body, accidentally left during a
        procedure
    kidney (medullary) Q61.5

◀ New   ◀▥ Revised   ~~deleted~~ Deleted

Sprain *(Continued)*
  sternum S23.429
    chondrosternal joint S23.421
    specified site NEC S23.428
    sternoclavicular (joint) (ligament) S23.420
  symphysis
    jaw S03.4
      old M26.69
    mandibular S03.4
      old M26.69
  talofibular —*see* Sprain, ankle
  tarsal —*see* Sprain, foot, specified site NEC
  tarsometatarsal —*see* Sprain, foot, specified site NEC
  temporomandibular S03.4
    old M26.69
  thorax S23.9
    ribs S23.41
    specified site NEC S23.8
    spine S23.3
    sternum —*see* Sprain, sternum
  thumb S63.60-
    interphalangeal (joint) S63.62-
    metacarpophalangeal (joint) S63.64-
    specified site NEC S63.68-
  thyroid cartilage or region S13.5
  tibia (proximal end) —*see* Sprain, knee, specified site NEC
  tibial collateral, knee —*see* Sprain, knee, collateral
  tibiofibular
    distal —*see* Sprain, ankle
    superior —*see* Sprain, knee, specified site NEC
  toe (s) S93.50-
    great S93.50-
    interphalangeal joint S93.51-
      great S93.51-
      lesser S93.51-
    lesser S93.50-
    metatarsophalangeal joint S93.52-
      great S93.52-
      lesser S93.52-
  ulna, collateral —*see* Rupture, traumatic, ligament, ulnar collateral
  ulnohumeral —*see* Sprain, elbow
  wrist S63.50-
    carpal S63.51-
    radiocarpal S63.52-
    specified site NEC S63.59-
  xiphoid cartilage —*see* Sprain, sternum
Sprengel's deformity (congenital) Q74.0
Sprue (tropical) K90.1
  celiac K90.0
  idiopathic K90.0
  meaning thrush B37.0
  nontropical K90.0
Spur, bone —*see also* Enthesopathy
  calcaneal M77.3-
  iliac crest M76.2-
  nose (septum) J34.89
Spurway's syndrome Q78.0
Sputum
  abnormal (amount) (color) (odor) (purulent) R09.3
  blood-stained R04.2
  excessive (cause unknown) R09.3
Squamous —*see also* condition
  epithelium N19
    cervical canal (congenital) Q51.828
    uterine mucosa (congenital) Q51.818
Squashed nose M95.0
  congenital Q67.4
Squeeze, diver's T70.3
Squint —*see also* Strabismus
  accommodative —*see* Strabismus, convergent concomitant
St. Hubert's disease A82.9
Stab —*see also* Laceration
  internal organs —*see* Injury, by site

Stafne's cyst or cavity M27.0
Staggering gait R26.0
  hysterical F44.4
Staghorn calculus —*see* Calculus, kidney
Stähli's line (cornea) (pigment) —*see* Pigmentation, cornea, anterior
Stain, staining
  meconium (newborn) P96.83
  port wine Q82.5
  tooth, teeth (hard tissues) (extrinsic) K03.6
    due to
      accretions K03.6
      deposits (betel) (black) (green) (materia alba) (orange) (soft) (tobacco) K03.6
      metals (copper) (silver) K03.7
      nicotine K03.6
      pulpal bleeding K03.7
      tobacco K03.6
    intrinsic K00.8
Stammering (*see also* Disorder, fluency) F80.81
Standstill
  auricular I45.5
  cardiac —*see* Arrest, cardiac
  sinoatrial I45.5
  ventricular —*see* Arrest, cardiac
Stannosis J63.5
Stanton's disease —*see* Melioidosis
Staphylitis (acute) (catarrhal) (chronic) (gangrenous) (membranous) (suppurative) (ulcerative) K12.2
Staphylococcal scalded skin syndrome L00
Staphylococcemia A41.2
Staphylococcus, staphylococcal —*see also* condition
  as cause of disease classified elsewhere B95.8
    aureus (methicillin susceptible) (MSSA) B95.61
      methicillin resistant (MRSA) B95.62
    specified NEC, as cause of disease classified elsewhere B95.7
Staphyloma (sclera)
  cornea H18.72-
  equatorial H15.81-
  localized (anterior) H15.82-
  posticum H15.83-
  ring H15.85-
Stargardt's disease —*see* Dystrophy, retina
Starvation (inanition) (due to lack of food) T73.0
  edema —*see* Malnutrition, severe
Stasis
  bile (noncalculous) K83.1
  bronchus J98.09
    with infection —*see* Bronchitis
  cardiac —*see* Failure, heart, congestive
  cecum K59.8
  colon K59.8
  dermatitis —*see* Varix, leg, with, inflammation
  duodenal K31.5
  eczema —*see* Varix, leg, with, inflammation
  edema —*see* Hypertension, venous (chronic), idiopathic
  foot T69.0-
  ileocecal coil K59.8
  ileum K59.8
  intestinal K59.8
  jejunum K59.8
  kidney N19
  liver (cirrhotic) K76.1
  lymphatic I89.8
  pneumonia J18.2
  pulmonary —*see* Edema, lung
  rectal K59.8
  renal N19
    tubular N17.0
  ulcer —*see* Varix, leg, with, ulcer
    without varicose veins I87.2
  urine —*see* Retention, urine
  venous I87.8

State (of)
  affective and paranoid, mixed, organic psychotic F06.8
  agitated R45.1
    acute reaction to stress F43.0
  anxiety (neurotic) F41.1
  apprehension F41.1
  burn-out Z73.0
  climacteric, female Z78.0
    symptomatic N95.1
  compulsive F42
    mixed with obsessional thoughts F42
  confusional (psychogenic) F44.89
    acute —*see also* Delirium
      with
        arteriosclerotic dementia F01.50
          with behavioral disturbance F01.51
        senility or dementia F05
      alcoholic F10.231
      epileptic F05
    reactive (from emotional stress, psychological trauma) F44.89
    subacute —*see* Delirium
  convulsive —*see* Convulsions
  crisis F43.0
  depressive F32.9
    neurotic F34.1
  dissociative F44.9
  emotional shock (stress) R45.7
  hypercoagulation —*see* Hypercoagulable
  locked-in G83.5
  menopausal Z78.0
    symptomatic N95.1
  neurotic F48.9
    with depersonalization F48.1
  obsessional F42
  oneiroid (schizophrenia-like) F23
  organic
    hallucinatory (nonalcoholic) F06.0
    paranoid (-hallucinatory) F06.2
  panic F41.0
  paranoid F22
    climacteric F22
    involutional F22
    menopausal F22
    organic F06.2
    senile F03
    simple F22
  persistent vegetative R40.3
  phobic F40.9
  postleukotomy F07.0
  pregnant, incidental Z33.1
  psychogenic, twilight F44.89
  psychopathic (constitutional) F60.2
  psychotic, organic —*see also* Psychosis, organic
    mixed paranoid and affective F06.8
    senile or presenile F03
    transient NEC F06.8
      with
        depression F06.31
        hallucinations F06.0
  residual schizophrenic F20.5
  restlessness R45.1
  stress (emotional) R45.7
  tension (mental) F48.9
    specified NEC F48.8
  transient organic psychotic NEC F06.8
    depressive type F06.31
    hallucinatory type F06.30
  twilight
    epileptic F05
    psychogenic F44.89
  vegetative, persistent R40.3
  vital exhaustion Z73.0
  withdrawal —*see* Withdrawal, state
Status (post) —*see also* Presence (of)
  absence, epileptic —*see* Epilepsy, by type, with status epilepticus

◀ New   ⬅ Revised   ~~deleted~~ Deleted

Status (*Continued*)

administration of tPA (rtPA) in a different facility within the last 24 hours prior to admission to the current facility Z92.82
adrenalectomy (unilateral) (bilateral) E89.6
anastomosis Z98.0
anginosus I20.9
angioplasty (peripheral) Z98.62
  with implant Z95.820
    coronary artery Z98.61
      with implant Z95.5
aortocoronary bypass Z95.1
arthrodesis Z98.1
artificial opening (of) Z93.9
  gastrointestinal tract Z93.4
  specified NEC Z93.8
  urinary tract Z93.6
  vagina Z93.8
asthmaticus —*see* Asthma, by type, with status asthmaticus
awaiting organ transplant Z76.82
bariatric surgery Z98.84
bed confinement Z74.01
bleb, filtering (vitreous), after glaucoma surgery Z98.83
breast implant Z98.82
  removal Z98.86
cataract extraction Z98.4-
cholecystectomy Z90.49
clitorectomy N90.811
  with excision of labia minora N90.812
colectomy (complete) (partial) Z90.49
colonization —*see* Carrier (suspected) of
colostomy Z93.3
convulsivus idiopathicus —*see* Epilepsy, by type, with status epilepticus
coronary artery angioplasty —*see* Status, angioplasty, coronary artery
cystectomy (urinary bladder) Z90.6
cystostomy Z93.50
  appendico-vesicostomy Z93.52
  cutaneous Z93.51
  specified NEC Z93.59
delinquent immunization Z28.3
dental Z98.818
  crown Z98.811
  fillings Z98.811
  restoration Z98.811
  sealant Z98.810
  specified NEC Z98.818
deployment (current) (military) Z56.82
dialysis (hemodialysis) (peritoneal) Z99.2
do not resuscitate (DNR) Z66
donor —*see* Donor
embedded fragments —*see* Retained, foreign body fragments (type of)
embedded splinter —*see* Retained, foreign body fragments (type of)
enterostomy Z93.4
epileptic, epilepticus (*see also* Epilepsy, by type, with status epilepticus) G40.901
estrogen receptor
  negative Z17.1
  positive Z17.0
female genital cutting —*see* Female genital mutilation status
female genital mutilation —*see* Female genital mutilation status
filtering (vitreous) bleb after glaucoma surgery Z98.83
gastrectomy (complete) (partial) Z90.3
gastric banding Z98.84
gastric bypass for obesity Z98.84
gastrostomy Z93.1
human immunodeficiency virus (HIV) infection, asymptomatic Z21
hysterectomy (complete) (total) Z90.710
  partial (with remaining cervical stump) Z90.711
ileostomy Z93.2

Status (*Continued*)

implant
  breast Z98.82
infibulation N90.813
intestinal bypass Z98.0
jejunostomy Z93.4
lapsed immunization schedule Z28.3
laryngectomy Z90.02
lymphaticus E32.8
marmoratus G80.3
mastectomy (unilateral) (bilateral) Z90.1-
military deployment status (current) Z56.82
  in theater or in support of military war, peacekeeping and humanitarian operations Z56.82
nephrectomy (unilateral) (bilateral) Z90.5
nephrostomy Z93.6
obesity surgery Z98.84
oophorectomy
  bilateral Z90.722
  unilateral Z90.721
organ replacement
  by artificial or mechanical device or prosthesis of
    artery Z95.828
    bladder Z96.0
    blood vessel Z95.828
    breast Z97.8
    eye globe Z97.0
    heart Z95.812
      valve Z95.2
    intestine Z97.8
    joint Z96.60
      hip —*see* Presence, hip joint implant
      knee —*see* Presence, knee joint implant
      specified site NEC Z96.698
    kidney Z97.8
    larynx Z96.3
    lens Z96.1
    limbs —*see* Presence, artificial, limb
    liver Z97.8
    lung Z97.8
    pancreas Z97.8
  by organ transplant (heterologous) (homologous) —*see* Transplant
pacemaker
  brain Z96.89
  cardiac Z95.0
  specified NEC Z96.89
pancreatectomy Z90.410
  complete Z90.410
  partial Z90.411
  total Z90.410
pneumonectomy (complete) (partial) Z90.2
pneumothorax, therapeutic Z98.3
postcommotio cerebri F07.81
postoperative (postprocedural) NEC Z98.89
  breast implant Z98.82
  dental Z98.818
    crown Z98.811
    fillings Z98.811
    restoration Z98.811
    sealant Z98.810
    specified NEC Z98.818
  pneumothorax, therapeutic Z98.3
postpartum (routine follow-up) Z39.2
  care immediately after delivery Z39.0
postsurgical (postprocedural) NEC Z98.89
  pneumothorax, therapeutic Z98.3
pregnancy, incidental Z33.1
prosthesis coronary angioplasty Z95.5
pseudophakia Z96.1
renal dialysis (hemodialysis) (peritoneal) Z99.2
retained foreign body —*see* Retained, foreign body fragments (type of)
reversed jejunal transposition (for bypass) Z98.0

Status (*Continued*)

salpingo-oophorectomy
  bilateral Z90.722
  unilateral Z90.721
sex reassignment surgery status Z87.890
shunt
  arteriovenous (for dialysis) Z99.2
  cerebrospinal fluid Z98.2
  ventricular (communicating) (for drainage) Z98.2
splenectomy Z90.81
thymicolymphaticus E32.8
thymicus E32.8
thymolymphaticus E32.8
thyroidectomy (hypothyroidism) E89.0
tooth (teeth) extraction (*see also* Absence, teeth, acquired) K08.409
tPA (rtPA) administration in a different facility within the last 24 hours prior to admission to current facility Z92.82
tracheostomy Z93.0
transplant —*see* Transplant
  organ removed Z98.85
tubal ligation Z98.51
underimmunization Z28.3
ureterostomy Z93.6
urethrostomy Z93.6
vagina, artificial Z93.8
vasectomy Z98.52
wheelchair confinement Z99.3

Stealing
child problem F91.8
in company with others Z72.810
pathological (compulsive) F63.2

Steam burn —*see* Burn
Steatocystoma multiplex L72.2
Steatohepatitis (nonalcoholic) (NASH) K75.81
Steatoma L72.3
eyelid (cystic) —*see* Dermatosis, eyelid
infected —*see* Hordeolum
Steatorrhea (chronic) K90.4
with lacteal obstruction K90.2
idiopathic (adult) (infantile) K90.0
pancreatic K90.3
primary K90.0
tropical K90.1
Steatosis E88.89
heart —*see* Degeneration, myocardial
kidney N28.89
liver NEC K76.0
Steele-Richardson-Olszewski disease or syndrome G23.1
Steinbrocker's syndrome G90.8
Steinert's disease G71.11
Stein-Leventhal syndrome E28.2
Stein's syndrome E28.2
STEMI (*see also* - Infarct, myocardium, ST elevation) I21.3
Stenocardia I20.8
Stenocephaly Q75.8
Stenosis, stenotic (cicatricial) —*see also* Stricture
ampulla of Vater K83.1
anus, anal (canal) (sphincter) K62.4
  and rectum K62.4
  congenital Q42.3
    with fistula Q42.2
aorta (ascending) (supraventricular) (congenital) Q25.3
  arteriosclerotic I70.0
  calcified I70.0
aortic (valve) I35.0
  with insufficiency I35.2
  congenital Q23.0
  rheumatic I06.0
    with
      incompetency, insufficiency or regurgitation I06.2
      with mitral (valve) disease I08.0
        with tricuspid (valve) disease I08.3

Stenosis, stenotic *(Continued)*
  aortic *(Continued)*
    rheumatic *(Continued)*
      with *(Continued)*
        mitral (valve) disease I08.0
          with tricuspid (valve) disease
            I08.3
        tricuspid (valve) disease I08.2
          with mitral (valve) disease I08.3
    specified cause NEC I35.0
    syphilitic A52.03
  aqueduct of Sylvius (congenital) Q03.0
    with spina bifida —*see* Spina bifida,
      by site, with hydrocephalus
    acquired G91.1
  artery NEC (*see also* Arteriosclerosis)
    I77.1
    celiac I77.4
    cerebral —*see* Occlusion, artery, cerebral
    extremities —*see* Arteriosclerosis,
      extremities
    precerebral —*see* Occlusion, artery,
      precerebral
    pulmonary (congenital) Q25.6
      acquired I28.8
    renal I70.1
  bile duct (common) (hepatic) K83.1
    congenital Q44.3
  bladder-neck (acquired) N32.0
    congenital Q64.31
  brain G93.89
  bronchus J98.09
    congenital Q32.3
    syphilitic A52.72
  cardia (stomach) K22.2
    congenital Q39.3
  cardiovascular —*see* Disease, cardiovascular
  caudal M48.08
  cervix, cervical (canal) N88.2
    congenital Q51.828
    in pregnancy or childbirth —*see* Pregnancy,
      complicated by, abnormal cervix
  colon —*see also* Obstruction, intestine
    congenital Q42.9
      specified NEC Q42.8
  colostomy K94.03
  common (bile) duct K83.1
    congenital Q44.3
  coronary (artery) —*see* Disease, heart,
    ischemic, atherosclerotic
  cystic duct —*see* Obstruction, gallbladder
  due to presence of device, implant or graft
    (*see also* Complications, by site and type,
      specified NEC) T85.85
    arterial graft NEC T82.858
    breast (implant) T85.85
    catheter T85.85
      dialysis (renal) T82.858
        intraperitoneal T85.85
      infusion NEC T82.858
        spinal (epidural) (subdural) T85.85
      urinary (indwelling) T83.85
    fixation, internal (orthopedic) NEC
      T84.85
    gastrointestinal (bile duct) (esophagus)
      T85.85
    genital NEC T83.85
    heart NEC T82.857
    joint prosthesis T84.85
    ocular (corneal graft) (orbital implant)
      NEC T85.85
    orthopedic NEC T84.85
    specified NEC T85.85
    urinary NEC T83.85
    vascular NEC T82.858
    ventricular intracranial shunt T85.85
  duodenum K31.5
    congenital Q41.0
  ejaculatory duct NEC N50.8
  endocervical os —*see* Stenosis, cervix
  enterostomy K94.13

Stenosis, stenotic *(Continued)*
  esophagus K22.2
    congenital Q39.3
    syphilitic A52.79
      congenital A50.59 *[K23]*
  eustachian tube —*see* Obstruction, eustachian
    tube
  external ear canal (acquired) H61.30-
    congenital Q16.1
    due to
      inflammation H61.32-
      trauma H61.31-
    postprocedural H95.81-
    specified cause NEC H61.39-
  gallbladder —*see* Obstruction, gallbladder
  glottis J38.6
  heart valve (congenital) Q24.8
    aortic Q23.0
    mitral Q23.2
    pulmonary Q22.1
    tricuspid Q22.4
  hepatic duct K83.1
  hymen N89.6
  hypertrophic subaortic (idiopathic) I42.1
  ileum K56.69
    congenital Q41.2
  infundibulum cardia Q24.3
  intervertebral foramina —*see also* Lesion,
    biomechanical, specified NEC
    connective tissue M99.79
      abdomen M99.79
      cervical region M99.71
      cervicothoracic M99.71
      head region M99.70
      lumbar region M99.73
      lumbosacral M99.73
      occipitocervical M99.70
      sacral region M99.74
      sacrococcygeal M99.74
      sacroiliac M99.74
      specified NEC M99.79
      thoracic region M99.72
      thoracolumbar M99.72
    disc M99.79
      abdomen M99.79
      cervical region M99.71
      cervicothoracic M99.71
      head region M99.70
      lower extremity M99.76
      lumbar region M99.73
      lumbosacral M99.73
      occipitocervical M99.70
      pelvic M99.75
      rib cage M99.78
      sacral region M99.74
      sacrococcygeal M99.74
      sacroiliac M99.74
      specified NEC M99.79
      thoracic region M99.72
      thoracolumbar M99.72
      upper extremity M99.77
    osseous M99.69
      abdomen M99.69
      cervical region M99.61
      cervicothoracic M99.61
      head region M99.60
      lower extremity M99.66
      lumbar region M99.63
      lumbosacral M99.63
      occipitocervical M99.60
      pelvic M99.65
      rib cage M99.68
      sacral region M99.64
      sacrococcygeal M99.64
      sacroiliac M99.64
      specified NEC M99.69
      thoracic region M99.62
      thoracolumbar M99.62
      upper extremity M99.67
    subluxation —*see* Stenosis, intervertebral
      foramina, osseous

Stenosis, stenotic *(Continued)*
  intestine —*see also* Obstruction, intestine
    congenital (small) Q41.9
      large Q42.9
        specified NEC Q42.8
      specified NEC Q41.8
  jejunum K56.69
    congenital Q41.1
  lacrimal (passage)
    canaliculi H04.54-
    congenital Q10.5
    duct H04.55-
    punctum H04.56-
    sac H04.57-
  lacrimonasal duct —*see* Stenosis, lacrimal,
    duct
    congenital Q10.5
  larynx J38.6
    congenital NEC Q31.8
      subglottic Q31.1
    syphilitic A52.73
      congenital A50.59 *[J99]*
  mitral (chronic) (inactive) (valve) I05.0
    with
      aortic valve disease I08.0
      incompetency, insufficiency or
        regurgitation I05.2
    active or acute I01.1
      with rheumatic or Sydenham's chorea
        I02.0
    congenital Q23.2
    specified cause, except rheumatic I34.2
    syphilitic A52.03
  myocardium, myocardial —*see also*
    Degeneration, myocardial
    hypertrophic subaortic (idiopathic) I42.1
  nares (anterior) (posterior) J34.89
    congenital Q30.0
  nasal duct —*see also* Stenosis, lacrimal, duct
    congenital Q10.5
  nasolacrimal duct —*see also* Stenosis, lacrimal,
    duct
    congenital Q10.5
  neural canal —*see also* Lesion, biomechanical,
    specified NEC
    connective tissue M99.49
      abdomen M99.49
      cervical region M99.41
      cervicothoracic M99.41
      head region M99.40
      lower extremity M99.46
      lumbar region M99.43
      lumbosacral M99.43
      occipitocervical M99.40
      pelvic M99.45
      rib cage M99.48
      sacral region M99.44
      sacrococcygeal M99.44
      sacroiliac M99.44
      specified NEC M99.49
      thoracic region M99.42
      thoracolumbar M99.42
      upper extremity M99.47
    intervertebral disc M99.59
      abdomen M99.59
      cervical region M99.51
      cervicothoracic M99.51
      head region M99.50
      lower extremity M99.56
      lumbar region M99.53
      lumbosacral M99.53
      occipitocervical M99.50
      pelvic M99.55
      rib cage M99.58
      sacral region M99.54
      sacrococcygeal M99.54
      sacroiliac M99.54
      specified NEC M99.59
      thoracic region M99.52
      thoracolumbar M99.52
      upper extremity M99.57

◀ New   ◀◀ Revised   ~~deleted~~ Deleted

Stenosis, stenotic *(Continued)*
  neural canal *(Continued)*
    osseous M99.39
      abdomen M99.39
      cervical region M99.31
      cervicothoracic M99.31
      head region M99.30
      lower extremity M99.36
      lumbar region M99.33
      lumbosacral M99.33
      occipitocervical M99.30
      pelvic M99.35
      rib cage M99.38
      sacral region M99.34
      sacrococcygeal M99.34
      sacroiliac M99.34
      specified NEC M99.39
      thoracic region M99.32
      thoracolumbar M99.32
      upper extremity M99.37
    subluxation M99.29
      cervical region M99.21
      cervicothoracic M99.21
      head region M99.20
      lower extremity M99.26
      lumbar region M99.23
      lumbosacral M99.23
      occipitocervical M99.20
      pelvic M99.25
      rib cage M99.28
      sacral region M99.24
      sacrococcygeal M99.24
      sacroiliac M99.24
      specified NEC M99.29
      thoracic region M99.22
      thoracolumbar M99.22
      upper extremity M99.27
  organ or site, congenital NEC —*see* Atresia, by site
  papilla of Vater K83.1
  pulmonary (artery) (congenital) Q25.6
    with ventricular septal defect, transposition of aorta, and hypertrophy of right ventricle Q21.3
    acquired I28.8
    in tetralogy of Fallot Q21.3
    infundibular Q24.3
    subvalvular Q24.3
    supravalvular Q25.6
    valve I37.0
      with insufficiency I37.2
      congenital Q22.1
      rheumatic I09.89
        with aortic, mitral or tricuspid (valve) disease I08.8
    vein, acquired I28.8
    vessel NEC I28.8
  pulmonic (congenital) Q22.1
    infundibular Q24.3
    subvalvular Q24.3
  pylorus (hypertrophic) (acquired) K31.1
    adult K31.1
    congenital Q40.0
    infantile Q40.0
  rectum (sphincter) —*see* Stricture, rectum
  renal artery I70.1
    congenital Q27.1
  salivary duct (any) K11.8
  sphincter of Oddi K83.1
  spinal M48.00
    cervical region M48.02
    cervicothoracic region M48.03
    lumbar region M48.06
    lumbosacral region M48.07
    occipito-atlanto-axial region M48.01
    sacrococcygeal region M48.08
    thoracic region M48.04
    thoracolumbar region M48.05
  stomach, hourglass K31.2

Stenosis, stenotic *(Continued)*
  subaortic (congenital) Q24.4
    hypertrophic (idiopathic) I42.1
  subglottic J38.6
    congenital Q31.1
    postprocedural J95.5
  trachea J39.8
    congenital Q32.1
    syphilitic A52.73
    tuberculous NEC A15.5
  tracheostomy J95.03
  tricuspid (valve) I07.0
    with
      aortic (valve) disease I08.2
      incompetency, insufficiency or regurgitation I07.2
        with aortic (valve) disease I08.2
          with mitral (valve) disease I08.3
      mitral (valve) disease I08.1
        with aortic (valve) disease I08.3
    congenital Q22.4
    nonrheumatic I36.0
      with insufficiency I36.2
  tubal N97.1
  ureter —*see* Atresia, ureter
  ureteropelvic junction, congenital Q62.11
  ureterovesical orifice, congenital Q62.12
  urethra (valve) —*see also* Stricture, urethra
    congenital Q64.32
  urinary meatus, congenital Q64.33
  vagina N89.5
    congenital Q52.4
    in pregnancy —*see* Pregnancy, complicated by, abnormal vagina
      causing obstructed labor O65.5
  valve (cardiac) (heart) (*see also* Endocarditis) I38
    congenital Q24.8
      aortic Q23.0
      mitral Q23.2
      pulmonary Q22.1
      tricuspid Q22.4
  vena cava (inferior) (superior) I87.1
    congenital Q26.0
  vesicourethral orifice Q64.31
  vulva N90.5
Stent jail T82.897
Stercolith (impaction) K56.41
  appendix K38.1
Stercoraceous, stercoral ulcer K63.3
  anus or rectum K62.6
Stereotypies NEC F98.4
Sterility —*see* Infertility
Sterilization —*see* Encounter (for), sterilization
Sternalgia —*see* Angina
Sternopagus Q89.4
Sternum bifidum Q76.7
Steroid
  effects (adverse) (adrenocortical) (iatrogenic)
    cushingoid E24.2
      correct substance properly administered —*see* Table of Drugs and Chemicals, by drug, adverse effect
      overdose or wrong substance given or taken —*see* Table of Drugs and Chemicals, by drug, poisoning
    diabetes —*see* category E09
      correct substance properly administered —*see* Table of Drugs and Chemicals, by drug, adverse effect
      overdose or wrong substance given or taken —*see* Table of Drugs and Chemicals, by drug, poisoning
    fever R50.2
    insufficiency E27.3
      correct substance properly administered —*see* Table of Drugs and Chemicals, by drug, adverse effect

Steroid *(Continued)*
  effects *(Continued)*
    insufficiency *(Continued)*
      overdose or wrong substance given or taken —*see* Table of Drugs and Chemicals, by drug, poisoning
    responder H40.04-
Stevens-Johnson disease or syndrome L51.1
  toxic epidermal necrolysis overlap L51.3
Stewart-Morel syndrome M85.2
Sticker's disease B08.3
Sticky eye —*see* Conjunctivitis, acute, mucopurulent
Stieda's disease —*see* Bursitis, tibial collateral
Stiff neck —*see* Torticollis
Stiff-man syndrome G25.82
Stiffness, joint NEC M25.60-
  ankle M25.67-
  ankylosis —*see* Ankylosis, joint
  contracture —*see* Contraction, joint
  elbow M25.62-
  foot M25.67-
  hand M25.64-
  hip M25.65-
  knee M25.66-
  shoulder M25.61-
  wrist M25.63-
Stigmata congenital syphilis A50.59
Stillbirth P95
Still-Felty syndrome —*see* Felty's syndrome
Still's disease or syndrome (juvenile) M08.20
  adult-onset M06.1
  ankle M08.27-
  elbow M08.22-
  foot joint M08.27-
  hand joint M08.24-
  hip M08.25-
  knee M08.26-
  multiple site M08.29
  shoulder M08.21-
  vertebra M08.28
  wrist M08.23-
Stimulation, ovary E28.1
Sting (venomous) (with allergic or anaphylactic shock) —*see* Table of Drugs and Chemicals, by animal or substance, poisoning
Stippled epiphyses Q78.8
Stitch
  abscess T81.4
  burst (in operation wound) —*see* Disruption, wound, operation
Stokes-Adams disease or syndrome I45.9
Stokes' disease E05.00
  with thyroid storm E05.01
Stokvis (-Talma) disease D74.8
Stoma malfunction
  colostomy K94.03
  enterostomy K94.13
  gastrostomy K94.23
  ileostomy K94.13
  tracheostomy J95.03
Stomach —*see* condition
Stomatitis (denture) (ulcerative) K12.1
  angular K13.0
    due to dietary or vitamin deficiency E53.0
  aphthous K12.0
  bovine B08.61
  candidal B37.0
  catarrhal K12.1
  diphtheritic A36.89
  due to
    dietary deficiency E53.0
    thrush B37.0
    vitamin deficiency
      B group NEC E53.9
      B2 (riboflavin) E53.0
  epidemic B08.8
  epizootic B08.8
  follicular K12.1
  gangrenous A69.0
  Geotrichum B48.3

Stomatitis (Continued)
  herpesviral, herpetic B00.2
  herpetiformis K12.0
  malignant K12.1
  membranous acute K12.1
  monilial B37.0
  mycotic B37.0
  necrotizing ulcerative A69.0
  parasitic B37.0
  septic K12.1
  spirochetal A69.1
  suppurative (acute) K12.2
  ulceromembranous A69.1
  vesicular K12.1
    with exanthem (enteroviral) B08.4
    virus disease A93.8
  Vincent's A69.1
Stomatocytosis D58.8
Stomatomycosis B37.0
Stomatorrhagia K13.79
Stone (s) —see also Calculus
  bladder (diverticulum) N21.0
  cystine E72.09
  heart syndrome I50.1
  kidney N20.0
  prostate N42.0
  pulpal (dental) K04.2
  renal N20.0
  salivary gland or duct (any) K11.5
  urethra (impacted) N21.1
  urinary (duct) (impacted) (passage) N20.9
    bladder (diverticulum) N21.0
    lower tract N21.9
    specified NEC N21.8
  xanthine E79.8 [N22]
Stonecutter's lung J62.8
Stonemason's asthma, disease, lung or pneumoconiosis J62.8
Stoppage
  heart —see Arrest, cardiac
  urine —see Retention, urine
Storm, thyroid —see Thyrotoxicosis
Strabismus (congenital) (nonparalytic) H50.9
  concomitant H50.40
    convergent —see Strabismus, convergent concomitant
    divergent —see Strabismus, divergent concomitant
  convergent concomitant H50.00
    accommodative component H50.43
    alternating H50.05
      with
        A pattern H50.06
        specified nonconcomitances NEC H50.08
        V pattern H50.07
    monocular H50.01-
      with
        A pattern H50.02-
        specified nonconcomitances NEC H50.04-
        V pattern H50.03-
      intermittent H50.31-
        alternating H50.32
  cyclotropia H50.1-
  divergent concomitant H50.10
    alternating H50.15
      with
        A pattern H50.16
        specified nonconcomitances NEC H50.18
        V pattern H50.17
    monocular H50.11-
      with
        A pattern H50.12-
        specified nonconcomitances NEC H50.14-
        V pattern H50.13-
      intermittent H50.33-
        alternating H50.34
  Duane's syndrome H50.81-

Strabismus (Continued)
  due to adhesions, scars H50.69
  heterophoria H50.50
    alternating H50.55
    cyclophoria H50.54
    esophoria H50.51
    exophoria H50.52
    vertical H50.53
  heterotropia H50.40
    intermittent H50.30
  hypertropia H50.2-
  hypotropia —see Hypertropia
  latent H50.50
  mechanical H50.60
    Brown's sheath syndrome H50.61-
    specified type NEC H50.69
  monofixation syndrome H50.42
  paralytic H49.9
    abducens nerve H49.2-
    fourth nerve H49.1-
    Kearns-Sayre syndrome H49.81-
    ophthalmoplegia (external)
      progressive H49.4-
        with pigmentary retinopathy H49.81-
      total H49.3-
    sixth nerve H49.2-
    specified type NEC H49.88-
    third nerve H49.0-
    trochlear nerve H49.1-
  specified type NEC H50.89
  vertical H50.2-
Strain
  back S39.012
  cervical S16.1
  eye NEC —see Disturbance, vision, subjective
  heart —see Disease, heart
  low back S39.012
  mental NOS Z73.3
    work-related Z56.6
  muscle (tendon) —see Injury, muscle, by site, strain
  neck S16.1
  physical NOS Z73.3
    work-related Z56.6
  postural —see also Disorder, soft tissue, due to use
  psychological NEC Z73.3
  tendon —see Injury, muscle, by site, strain
Straining, on urination R39.16
Strand, vitreous —see Opacity, vitreous, membranes and strands
Strangulation, strangulated —see also Asphyxia, traumatic
  appendix K38.8
  bladder-neck N32.0
  bowel or colon K56.2
  food or foreign body —see Foreign body, by site
  hemorrhoids —see Hemorrhoids, with complication
  hernia —see also Hernia, by site, with obstruction
    with gangrene —see Hernia, by site, with gangrene
  intestine (large) (small) K56.2
    with hernia —see also Hernia, by site, with obstruction
      with gangrene —see Hernia, by site, with gangrene
  mesentery K56.2
  mucus —see Asphyxia, mucus
  omentum K56.2
  organ or site, congenital NEC —see Atresia, by site
  ovary —see Torsion, ovary
  penis N48.89
    foreign body T19.4
  rupture —see Hernia, by site, with obstruction

Strangulation, strangulated (Continued)
  stomach due to hernia —see also Hernia, by site, with obstruction
    with gangrene —see Hernia, by site, with gangrene
  vesicourethral orifice N32.0
Strangury R30.0
Straw itch B88.0
Strawberry
  gallbladder K82.4
  mark Q82.5
  tongue (red) (white) K14.3
Streak (s)
  macula, angioid H35.33
  ovarian Q50.32
Strephosymbolia F81.0
  secondary to organic lesion R48.8
Streptobacillary fever A25.1
Streptobacillosis A25.1
Streptobacillus moniliformis A25.1
Streptococcus, streptococcal —see also condition
  as cause of disease classified elsewhere B95.5
  group
    A, as cause of disease classified elsewhere B95.0
    B, as cause of disease classified elsewhere B95.1
    D, as cause of disease classified elsewhere B95.2
  pneumoniae, as cause of disease classified elsewhere B95.3
  specified NEC, as cause of disease classified elsewhere B95.4
Streptomycosis B47.1
Streptotrichosis A48.8
Stress F43.9
  family —see Disruption, family
  fetal P84
    complicating pregnancy O77.9
      due to drug administration O77.1
  mental NEC Z73.3
    work-related Z56.6
  physical NEC Z73.3
    work-related Z56.6
  polycythemia D75.1
  reaction (see also Reaction, stress) F43.9
  work schedule Z56.3
Stretching, nerve —see Injury, nerve
Striae albicantes, atrophicae or distensae (cutis) L90.6
Stricture —see also Stenosis
  ampulla of Vater K83.1
  anus (sphincter) K62.4
    congenital Q42.3
      with fistula Q42.2
    infantile Q42.3
      with fistula Q42.2
  aorta (ascending) (congenital) Q25.3
    arteriosclerotic I70.0
    calcified I70.0
    supravalvular, congenital Q25.3
  aortic (valve) —see Stenosis, aortic
  aqueduct of Sylvius (congenital) Q03.0
    with spina bifida —see Spina bifida, by site, with hydrocephalus
    acquired G91.1
  artery I77.1
    basilar —see Occlusion, artery, basilar
    carotid —see Occlusion, artery, carotid
    celiac I77.4
    congenital (peripheral) Q27.8
      cerebral Q28.3
      coronary Q24.5
      digestive system Q27.8
      lower limb Q27.8
      retinal Q14.1
      specified site NEC Q27.8
      umbilical Q27.0
      upper limb Q27.8

◀ New   ◀◀ Revised   ~~deleted~~ Deleted

Stricture *(Continued)*
  artery *(Continued)*
    coronary —*see* Disease, heart, ischemic,
      atherosclerotic
      congenital Q24.5
    precerebral —*see* Occlusion, artery,
      precerebral
    pulmonary (congenital) Q25.6
      acquired I28.8
    renal I70.1
    vertebral —*see* Occlusion, artery, vertebral
  auditory canal (external) (congenital)
    acquired —*see* Stenosis, external ear canal
  bile duct (common) (hepatic) K83.1
    congenital Q44.3
    postoperative K91.89
  bladder N32.89
    neck N32.0
  bowel —*see* Obstruction, intestine
  brain G93.89
  bronchus J98.09
    congenital Q32.3
    syphilitic A52.72
  cardia (stomach) K22.2
    congenital Q39.3
  cardiac —*see also* Disease, heart
    orifice (stomach) K22.2
  cecum —*see* Obstruction, intestine
  cervix, cervical (canal) N88.2
    congenital Q51.828
    in pregnancy —*see* Pregnancy, complicated
      by, abnormal cervix
      causing obstructed labor O65.5
  colon —*see also* Obstruction, intestine
    congenital Q42.9
      specified NEC Q42.8
  colostomy K94.03
  common (bile) duct K83.1
  coronary (artery) —*see* Disease, heart,
    ischemic, atherosclerotic
  cystic duct —*see* Obstruction, gallbladder
  digestive organs NEC, congenital Q45.8
  duodenum K31.5
    congenital Q41.0
  ear canal (external) (congenital) Q16.1
    acquired —*see* Stricture, auditory canal,
      acquired
  ejaculatory duct N50.8
  enterostomy K94.13
  esophagus K22.2
    congenital Q39.3
    syphilitic A52.79
      congenital A50.59 *[K23]*
  eustachian tube —*see also* Obstruction,
    eustachian tube
    congenital Q17.8
  fallopian tube N97.1
    gonococcal A54.24
    tuberculous A18.17
  gallbladder —*see* Obstruction, gallbladder
  glottis J38.6
  heart —*see also* Disease, heart
    valve *(see also* Endocarditis) I38
      aortic Q23.0
      mitral Q23.4
      pulmonary Q22.1
      tricuspid Q22.4
  hepatic duct K83.1
  hourglass, of stomach K31.2
  hymen N89.6
  hypopharynx J39.2
  ileum K56.69
    congenital Q41.2
  intestine —*see also* Obstruction, intestine
    congenital (small) Q41.9
      large Q42.9
        specified NEC Q42.8
      specified NEC Q41.8
    ischemic K55.1
  jejunum K56.69
    congenital Q41.1

Stricture *(Continued)*
  lacrimal passages —*see also* Stenosis, lacrimal
    congenital Q10.5
  larynx J38.6
    congenital NEC Q31.8
      subglottic Q31.1
    syphilitic A52.73
      congenital A50.59 *[J99]*
  meatus
    ear (congenital) Q16.1
      acquired —*see* Stricture, auditory canal,
        acquired
    osseous (ear) (congenital) Q16.1
      acquired —*see* Stricture, auditory canal,
        acquired
    urinarius —*see also* Stricture, urethra
      congenital Q64.33
  mitral (valve) —*see* Stenosis, mitral
  myocardium, myocardial I51.5
    hypertrophic subaortic (idiopathic)
      I42.1
  nares (anterior) (posterior) J34.89
    congenital Q30.0
  nasal duct —*see also* Stenosis, lacrimal, duct
    congenital Q10.5
  nasolacrimal duct —*see also* Stenosis, lacrimal,
    duct
    congenital Q10.5
  nasopharynx J39.2
    syphilitic A52.73
  nose J34.89
    congenital Q30.0
  nostril (anterior) (posterior) J34.89
    congenital Q30.0
    syphilitic A52.73
      congenital A50.59 *[J99]*
  organ or site, congenital NEC —*see* Atresia,
    by site
  os uteri —*see* Stricture, cervix
  osseous meatus (ear) (congenital) Q16.1
    acquired —*see* Stricture, auditory canal,
      acquired
  oviduct —*see* Stricture, fallopian tube
  pelviureteric junction (congenital)
    Q62.11
  penis, by foreign body T19.4
  pharynx J39.2
  prostate N42.89
  pulmonary, pulmonic
    artery (congenital) Q25.6
      acquired I28.8
      noncongenital I28.8
    infundibulum (congenital) Q24.3
    valve I37.0
      congenital Q22.1
    vein, acquired I28.8
    vessel NEC I28.8
  punctum lacrimale —*see also* Stenosis,
    lacrimal, punctum
    congenital Q10.5
  pylorus (hypertrophic) K31.1
    adult K31.1
    congenital Q40.0
    infantile Q40.0
  rectosigmoid K56.69
  rectum (sphincter) K62.4
    congenital Q42.1
      with fistula Q42.0
    due to
      chlamydial lymphogranuloma A55
      irradiation K91.89
      lymphogranuloma venereum A55
    gonococcal A54.6
    inflammatory (chlamydial) A55
    syphilitic A52.74
    tuberculous A18.32
  renal artery I70.1
    congenital Q27.1
  salivary duct or gland (any) K11.8
  sigmoid (flexure) —*see* Obstruction, intestine
  spermatic cord N50.8

Stricture *(Continued)*
  stoma (following) (of)
    colostomy K94.03
    enterostomy K94.13
    gastrostomy K94.23
    ileostomy K94.13
    tracheostomy J95.03
  stomach K31.89
    congenital Q40.2
    hourglass K31.2
  subaortic Q24.4
    hypertrophic (acquired) (idiopathic) I42.1
  subglottic J38.6
  syphilitic NEC A52.79
  trachea J39.8
    congenital Q32.1
    syphilitic A52.73
    tuberculous NEC A15.5
  tracheostomy J95.03
  tricuspid (valve) —*see* Stenosis, tricuspid
  tunica vaginalis N50.8
  ureter (postoperative) N13.5
    with
      hydronephrosis N13.1
        with infection N13.6
      pyelonephritis (chronic) N11.1
    congenital —*see* Atresia, ureter
    tuberculous A18.11
  ureteropelvic junction (congenital) Q62.11
  ureterovesical orifice N13.5
    with infection N13.6
  urethra (organic) (spasmodic) N35.9
    associated with schistosomiasis B65.0 *[N37]*
    congenital Q64.39
      valvular (posterior) Q64.2
    due to
      infection —*see* Stricture, urethra,
        postinfective
      trauma —*see* Stricture, urethra,
        post-traumatic
    gonococcal, gonorrheal A54.01
    infective NEC —*see* Stricture, urethra,
      postinfective
    late effect (sequelae) of injury —*see*
      Stricture, urethra, post-traumatic
    postcatheterization —*see* Stricture, urethra,
      postprocedural
    postinfective NEC
      female N35.12
      male N35.119
        anterior urethra N35.114
        bulbous urethra N35.112
        meatal N35.111
        membranous urethra N35.113
    postobstetric N35.021
    postoperative —*see* Stricture, urethra,
      postprocedural
    postprocedural
      female N99.12
      male N99.114
        anterior urethra N99.113
        bulbous urethra N99.111
        meatal N99.110
        membranous urethra N99.112
    post-traumatic
      female N35.028
        due to childbirth N35.021
      male N35.014
        anterior urethra N35.013
        bulbous urethra N35.011
        meatal N35.010
        membranous urethra N35.012
    sequela (late effect) of
      childbirth N35.021
      injury —*see* Stricture, urethra,
        post-traumatic
    specified cause NEC N35.8
    syphilitic A52.76
    traumatic —*see* Stricture, urethra,
      post-traumatic
    valvular (posterior), congenital Q64.2

Stricture (*Continued*)
  urinary meatus —*see* Stricture, urethra
  uterus, uterine (synechiae) N85.6
    os (external) (internal) —*see* Stricture,
      cervix
  vagina (outlet) —*see* Stenosis, vagina
  valve (cardiac) (heart) —*see also* Endocarditis
    congenital
      aortic Q23.0
      mitral Q23.2
      pulmonary Q22.1
      tricuspid Q22.4
  vas deferens N50.8
    congenital Q55.4
  vein I87.1
  vena cava (inferior) (superior) NEC I87.1
    congenital Q26.0
  vesicourethral orifice N32.0
    congenital Q64.31
  vulva (acquired) N90.5
Stridor R06.1
  congenital (larynx) P28.89
Stridulous —*see* condition
Stroke (apoplectic) (brain) (embolic) (ischemic)
    (paralytic) (thrombotic) I63.9
  epileptic —*see* Epilepsy
  heat T67.0
  in evolution I63.9
  intraoperative
    during cardiac surgery I97.810
    during other surgery I97.811
  lightning —*see* Lightning
  meaning
    cerebral hemorrhage — code to
      Hemorrhage, intracranial
    cerebral infarction — code to Infarction,
      cerebral
  postprocedural
    following cardiac surgery I97.820
    following other surgery I97.821
  unspecified (NOS) I63.9
Stromatosis, endometrial D39.0
Strongyloidiasis, strongyloidosis B78.9
  cutaneous B78.1
  disseminated B78.7
  intestinal B78.0
Strophulus pruriginosus L28.2
Struck by lightning —*see* Lightning
Struma —*see also* Goiter
  Hashimoto E06.3
  lymphomatosa E06.3
  nodosa (simplex) E04.9
    endemic E01.2
      multinodular E01.1
    multinodular E04.2
      iodine-deficiency related E01.1
    toxic or with hyperthyroidism E05.20
      with thyroid storm E05.21
      multinodular E05.20
        with thyroid storm E05.21
      uninodular E05.10
        with thyroid storm E05.11
    toxicosa E05.20
      with thyroid storm E05.21
      multinodular E05.20
        with thyroid storm E05.21
      uninodular E05.10
        with thyroid storm E05.11
    uninodular E04.1
  ovarii D27.-
  Riedel's E06.5
Strumipriva cachexia E03.4
Strümpell-Marie spine —*see* Spondylitis,
    ankylosing
Strümpell-Westphal pseudosclerosis E83.01
Stuart deficiency disease (factor X) D68.2
Stuart-Prower factor deficiency (factor X)
    D68.2
Student's elbow —*see* Bursitis, elbow,
    olecranon
Stump —*see* Amputation

Stunting, nutritional E45
Stupor (catatonic) R40.1
  depressive F32.8
  dissociative F44.2
  manic F30.2
  manic-depressive F31.89
  psychogenic (anergic) F44.2
  reaction to exceptional stress (transient)
    F43.0
Sturge (-Weber) (-Dimitri) (-Kalischer) **disease
    or syndrome** Q85.8
Stuttering F80.81
  adult onset F98.5
  childhood onset F80.81
  following cerebrovascular disease —
    see Disorder, fluency, following
      cerebrovascular disease
  in conditions classified elsewhere R47.82
Sty, stye (external) (internal) (meibomian)
    (zeisian) —*see* Hordeolum
Subacidity, gastric K31.89
  psychogenic F45.8
Subacute —*see* condition
Subarachnoid —*see* condition
Subcortical —*see* condition
Subcostal syndrome, nerve compression —*see*
    Mononeuropathy, upper limb, specified
    site NEC
Subcutaneous, subcuticular —*see* condition
Subdural —*see* condition
Subendocardium —*see* condition
Subependymoma
  specified site —*see* Neoplasm, uncertain
    behavior, by site
  unspecified site D43.2
Suberosis J67.3
Subglossitis —*see* Glossitis
Subhemophilia D66
Subinvolution
  breast (postlactational) (postpuerperal)
    N64.89
  puerperal O90.89
  uterus (chronic) (nonpuerperal) N85.3
    puerperal O90.89
Sublingual —*see* condition
Sublinguitis —*see* Sialoadenitis
Subluxatable hip Q65.6
Subluxation —*see also* Dislocation
  acromioclavicular S43.11-
  ankle S93.0-
  atlantoaxial, recurrent M43.4
    with myelopathy M43.3
  carpometacarpal (joint) NEC S63.05-
    thumb S63.04-
  complex, vertebral —*see* Complex,
    subluxation
  congenital —*see also* Malposition,
    congenital
    hip —*see* Dislocation, hip, congenital,
      partial
    joint (excluding hip)
      lower limb Q68.8
      shoulder Q68.8
      upper limb Q68.8
  elbow (traumatic) S53.10-
    anterior S53.11-
    lateral S53.14-
    medial S53.13-
    posterior S53.12-
    specified type NEC S53.19-
  finger S63.20-
    index S63.20-
    interphalangeal S63.22-
      distal S63.24-
        index S63.24-
        little S63.24-
        middle S63.24-
        ring S63.24-
      index S63.22-
      little S63.22-
      middle S63.22-

Subluxation (*Continued*)
  finger (*Continued*)
    interphalangeal (*Continued*)
      proximal S63.23-
        index S63.23-
        little S63.23-
        middle S63.23-
        ring S63.23-
      ring S63.22-
    little S63.20-
    metacarpophalangeal S63.21-
      index S63.21-
      little S63.21-
      middle S63.21-
      ring S63.21-
    middle S63.20-
    ring S63.20-
  foot S93.30-
    specified site NEC S93.33-
    tarsal joint S93.31-
    tarsometatarsal joint S93.32-
    toe —*see* Subluxation, toe
  hip S73.00-
    anterior S73.03-
      obturator S73.02-
    central S73.04-
    posterior S73.01-
  interphalangeal (joint)
    finger S63.22-
      distal joint S63.24-
        index S63.24-
        little S63.24-
        middle S63.24-
        ring S63.24-
      index S63.22-
      little S63.22-
      middle S63.22-
      proximal joint S63.23-
        index S63.23-
        little S63.23-
        middle S63.23-
        ring S63.23-
      ring S63.22-
    thumb S63.12-
      distal joint S63.14-
      proximal joint S63.13-
    toe S93.13-
      great S93.13-
      lesser S93.13-
  joint prosthesis —*see* Complications, joint
    prosthesis, mechanical, displacement,
    by site
  knee S83.10-
    cap —*see* Subluxation, patella
    patella —*see* Subluxation, patella
    proximal tibia
      anteriorly S83.11-
      laterally S83.14-
      medially S83.13-
      posteriorly S83.12-
    specified type NEC S83.19-
  lens —*see* Dislocation, lens, partial
  ligament, traumatic —*see* Sprain, by site
  metacarpal (bone)
    proximal end S63.06-
  metacarpophalangeal (joint)
    finger S63.21-
      index S63.21-
      little S63.21-
      middle S63.21-
      ring S63.21-
    thumb S63.11-
  metatarsophalangeal joint S93.14-
    great toe S93.14-
    lesser toe S93.14-
  midcarpal (joint) S63.03-
  patella S83.00-
    lateral S83.01-
    recurrent (nontraumatic) —*see* Dislocation,
      patella, recurrent, incomplete
    specified type NEC S83.09-

◀ New   ◀▦ Revised   ~~deleted~~ Deleted

Subluxation *(Continued)*
 pathological —*see* Dislocation, pathological
 radial head S53.00-
  anterior S53.01-
  nursemaid's elbow S53.03-
  posterior S53.02-
  specified type NEC S53.09-
 radiocarpal (joint) S63.02-
 radioulnar (joint)
  distal S63.01-
  proximal —*see* Subluxation, elbow
 shoulder
  congenital Q68.8
  girdle S43.30-
   scapula S43.31-
   specified site NEC S43.39-
  traumatic S43.00-
   anterior S43.01-
   inferior S43.03-
   posterior S43.02-
   specified type NEC S43.08-
 sternoclavicular (joint) S43.20-
  anterior S43.21-
  posterior S43.22-
 symphysis (pubis)
 thumb S63.103
  interphalangeal joint —*see* Subluxation,
   interphalangeal (joint), thumb
  metacarpophalangeal joint —*see*
   Subluxation, metacarpophalangeal
   (joint), thumb
 toe (s) S93.10-
  great S93.10-
   interphalangeal joint S93.13-
   metatarsophalangeal joint S93.14-
  interphalangeal joint S93.13-
  lesser S93.10-
   interphalangeal joint S93.13-
   metatarsophalangeal joint S93.14-
  metatarsophalangeal joint S93.149
 ulnohumeral joint —*see* Subluxation, elbow
 vertebral
  recurrent NEC —*see* subcategory M43.5
  traumatic
   cervical S13.100
    atlantoaxial joint S13.120
    atlantooccipital joint S13.110
    atloidooccipital joint S13.110
    joint between
     C0 and C1 S13.110
     C1 and C2 S13.120
     C2 and C3 S13.130
     C3 and C4 S13.140
     C4 and C5 S13.150
     C5 and C6 S13.160
     C6 and C7 S13.170
     C7 and T1 S13.180
    occipitoatloid joint S13.110
   lumbar S33.100
    joint between
     L1 and L2 S33.110
     L2 and L3 S33.120
     L3 and L4 S33.130
     L4 and L5 S33.140
   thoracic S23.100
    joint between
     T1 and T2 S23.110
     T2 and T3 S23.120
     T3 and T4 S23.122
     T4 and T5 S23.130
     T5 and T6 S23.132
     T6 and T7 S23.140
     T7 and T8 S23.142
     T8 and T9 S23.150
     T9 and T10 S23.152
     T10 and T11 S23.160
     T11 and T12 S23.162
     T12 and L1 S23.170
 ulna
  distal end S63.07-
  proximal end —*see* Subluxation, elbow

Subluxation *(Continued)*
 wrist (carpal bone) S63.00-
  carpometacarpal joint —*see* Subluxation,
   carpometacarpal (joint)
  distal radioulnar joint —*see* Subluxation,
   radioulnar (joint), distal
  metacarpal bone, proximal —*see*
   Subluxation, metacarpal (bone),
   proximal end
  midcarpal —*see* Subluxation, midcarpal
   (joint)
  radiocarpal joint —*see* Subluxation,
   radiocarpal (joint)
  recurrent —*see* Dislocation, recurrent, wrist
  specified site NEC S63.09-
  ulna —*see* Subluxation, ulna, distal end
Submaxillary —*see* condition
Submersion (fatal) (nonfatal) T75.1
Submucous —*see* condition
Subnormal, subnormality
 accommodation (old age) H52.4
 mental —*see* Disability, intellectual
 temperature (accidental) T68
Subphrenic —*see* condition
Subscapular nerve —*see* condition
Subseptus uterus Q51.2
Subsiding appendicitis K36
Substernal thyroid E04.9
 congenital Q89.2
Substitution disorder F44.9
Subtentorial —*see* condition
Subthyroidism (acquired) —*see also*
  Hypothyroidism
 congenital E03.1
Succenturiate placenta O43.19-
Sucking thumb, child (excessive) F98.8
Sudamen, sudamina L74.1
Sudanese kala-azar B55.0
Sudden
 hearing loss —*see* Deafness, sudden
 heart failure —*see* Failure, heart
Sudeck's atrophy, disease, or syndrome —*see*
  Algoneurodystrophy
Suffocation —*see* Asphyxia, traumatic
Sugar
 blood
  high (transient) R73.9
  low (transient) E16.2
 in urine R81
Suicide, suicidal (attempted) T14.91
 by poisoning —*see* Table of Drugs and
  Chemicals
 history of (personal) Z91.5
  in family Z81.8
 ideation —*see* Ideation, suicidal
 risk
  meaning personal history of attempted
   suicide Z91.5
  meaning suicidal ideation —*see* Ideation,
   suicidal
 tendencies
  meaning personal history of attempted
   suicide Z91.5
  meaning suicidal ideation —*see* Ideation,
   suicidal
 trauma —*see* nature of injury by site
Suipestifer infection —*see* Infection, salmonella
Sulfhemoglobinemia, sulphemoglobinemia
  (acquired) (with methemoglobinemia)
  D74.8
Sumatran mite fever A75.3
Summer —*see* condition
Sunburn L55.9
 first degree L55.0
 second degree L55.1
 third degree L55.2
SUNCT (short lasting unilateral neuralgiform
  headache with conjunctival injection and
  tearing) G44.059
 intractable G44.051
 not intractable G44.059

Sunken acetabulum —*see* Derangement, joint,
  specified type NEC, hip
Sunstroke T67.0
Superfecundation —*see* Pregnancy,
  multiple
Superfetation —*see* Pregnancy, multiple
Superinvolution (uterus) N85.8
Supernumerary (congenital)
 aortic cusps Q23.8
 auditory ossicles Q16.3
 bone Q79.8
 breast Q83.1
 carpal bones Q74.0
 cusps, heart valve NEC Q24.8
  aortic Q23.8
  mitral Q23.2
  pulmonary Q22.3
 digit (s) Q69.9
 ear (lobule) Q17.0
 fallopian tube Q50.6
 finger Q69.0
 hymen Q52.4
 kidney Q63.0
 lacrimonasal duct Q10.6
 lobule (ear) Q17.0
 mitral cusps Q23.2
 muscle Q79.8
 nipple (s) Q83.3
 organ or site not listed —*see* Accessory
 ossicles, auditory Q16.3
 ovary Q50.31
 oviduct Q50.6
 pulmonary, pulmonic cusps Q22.3
 rib Q76.6
  cervical or first (syndrome) Q76.5
 roots (of teeth) K00.2
 spleen Q89.09
 tarsal bones Q74.2
 teeth K00.1
 testis Q55.29
 thumb Q69.1
 toe Q69.2
 uterus Q51.2
 vagina Q52.1
 vertebra Q76.49
Supervision (of)
 contraceptive —*see* Prescription,
  contraceptives
 dietary (for) Z71.3
  allergy (food) Z71.3
  colitis Z71.3
  diabetes mellitus Z71.3
  food allergy or intolerance Z71.3
  gastritis Z71.3
  hypercholesterolemia Z71.3
  hypoglycemia Z71.3
  intolerance (food) Z71.3
  obesity Z71.3
  specified NEC Z71.3
 healthy infant or child Z76.2
  foundling Z76.1
 high-risk pregnancy —*see* Pregnancy,
  complicated by, high, risk
 lactation Z39.1
 pregnancy —*see* Pregnancy, supervision of
Supplemental teeth K00.1
Suppression
 binocular vision H53.34
 lactation O92.5
 menstruation N94.89
 ovarian secretion E28.39
 renal N28.9
 urine, urinary secretion R34
Suppuration, suppurative —*see also* condition
 accessory sinus (chronic) —*see* Sinusitis
 adrenal gland
 antrum (chronic) —*see* Sinusitis,
  maxillary
 bladder —*see* Cystitis
 brain G06.0
  sequelae G09

Suppuration, suppurative (Continued)
  breast N61
    puerperal, postpartum or gestational —see
        Mastitis, obstetric, purulent
  dental periosteum M27.3
  ear (middle) —see also Otitis, media
    external NEC —see Otitis, externa,
        infective
    internal —see subcategory H83.0
  ethmoidal (chronic) (sinus) —see Sinusitis,
        ethmoidal
  fallopian tube —see Salpingo-oophoritis
  frontal (chronic) (sinus) —see Sinusitis,
        frontal
  gallbladder (acute) K81.0
  gum K05.20
    generalized K05.22
    localized K05.21
  intracranial G06.0
  joint —see Arthritis, pyogenic or pyemic
  labyrinthine —see subcategory H83.0
  lung —see Abscess, lung
  mammary gland N61
    puerperal, postpartum O91.12
      associated with lactation O91.13
  maxilla, maxillary M27.2
    sinus (chronic) —see Sinusitis, maxillary
  muscle —see Myositis, infective
  nasal sinus (chronic) —see Sinusitis
  pancreas, acute K85.8
  parotid gland —see Sialoadenitis
  pelvis, pelvic
    female —see Disease, pelvis, inflammatory
    male K65.0
  pericranial —see Osteomyelitis
  salivary duct or gland (any) —see
        Sialoadenitis
  sinus (accessory) (chronic) (nasal) —see
        Sinusitis
  sphenoidal sinus (chronic) —see Sinusitis,
        sphenoidal
  thymus (gland) E32.1
  thyroid (gland) E06.0
  tonsil —see Tonsillitis
  uterus —see Endometritis
Supraeruption of tooth (teeth) M26.34
Supraglottitis J04.30
  with obstruction J04.31
Suprarenal (gland) —see condition
Suprascapular nerve —see condition
Suprasellar —see condition
Surfer's knots or nodules S89.8-
Surgical
  emphysema T81.82
  procedures, complication or misadventure —
      see Complications, surgical procedures
  shock T81.10
Surveillance (of) (for) —see also Observation
  alcohol abuse Z71.41
  contraceptive —see Prescription,
        contraceptives
  dietary Z71.3
  drug abuse Z71.51
Susceptibility to disease, genetic Z15.89
  malignant neoplasm Z15.09
    breast Z15.01
    endometrium Z15.04
    ovary Z15.02
    prostate Z15.03
    specified NEC Z15.09
  multiple endocrine neoplasia Z15.81
Suspected condition, ruled out —see also
      Observation, suspected
  amniotic cavity and membrane Z03.71
  cervical shortening Z03.75
  fetal anomaly Z03.73
  fetal growth Z03.74
  maternal and fetal conditions NEC Z03.79
  oligohydramnios Z03.71
  placental problem Z03.72
  polyhydramnios Z03.71

Suspended uterus
  in pregnancy or childbirth —see Pregnancy,
      complicated by, abnormal uterus
Sutton's nevus D22.9
Suture
  burst (in operation wound) T81.31
    external operation wound T81.31
    internal operation wound T81.32
  inadvertently left in operation wound —see
      Foreign body, accidentally left during a
      procedure
  removal Z48.02
Swab inadvertently left in operation wound —
    see Foreign body, accidentally left during
    a procedure
Swallowed, swallowing
  difficulty —see Dysphagia
  foreign body —see Foreign body, alimentary
      tract
Swan-neck deformity (finger) —see Deformity,
    finger, swan-neck
Swearing, compulsive F42
  in Gilles de la Tourette's syndrome F95.2
Sweat, sweats
  fetid L75.0
  night R61
Sweating, excessive R61
Sweeley-Klionsky disease E75.21
Sweet's disease or dermatosis L98.2
Swelling (of) R60.9
  abdomen, abdominal (not referable to any
        particular organ) —see Mass,
        abdominal
  ankle —see Effusion, joint, ankle
  arm M79.89
    forearm M79.89
  breast N63
  Calabar B74.3
  cervical gland R59.0
  chest, localized R22.2
  ear H93.8-
  extremity (lower) (upper) —see Disorder, soft
      tissue, specified type NEC
  finger M79.89
  foot M79.89
  glands R59.9
    generalized R59.1
    localized R59.0
  hand M79.89
  head (localized) R22.0
  inflammatory —see Inflammation
  intra-abdominal —see Mass, abdominal
  joint —see Effusion, joint
  leg M79.89
    lower M79.89
  limb —see Disorder, soft tissue, specified type
      NEC
  localized (skin) R22.9
    chest R22.2
    head R22.0
    limb
      lower —see Mass, localized, limb,
          lower
      upper —see Mass, localized, limb,
          upper
    neck R22.1
    trunk R22.2
  neck (localized) R22.1
  pelvic —see Mass, abdominal
  scrotum N50.8
  splenic —see Splenomegaly
  testis N50.8
  toe M79.89
  umbilical R19.09
  wandering, due to Gnathostoma
        (spinigerum) B83.1
  white —see Tuberculosis, arthritis
Swift (-Feer) disease
  overdose or wrong substance given or
      taken —see Table of Drugs and
      Chemicals, by drug, poisoning

Swimmer's
  cramp T75.1
  ear H60.33-
  itch B65.3
Swimming in the head R42
Swollen —see Swelling
Swyer syndrome Q99.1
Sycosis L73.8
  barbae (not parasitic) L73.8
  contagiosa (mycotic) B35.0
  lupoides L73.8
  mycotic B35.0
  parasitic B35.0
  vulgaris L73.8
Sydenham's chorea —see Chorea, Sydenham's
Sylvatic yellow fever A95.0
Sylvest's disease B33.0
Symblepharon H11.23-
  congenital Q10.3
Symond's syndrome G93.2
Sympathetic —see condition
Sympatheticotonia G90.8
Sympathicoblastoma
  specified site —see Neoplasm, malignant, by
      site
  unspecified site C74.90
Sympathogonioma —see Sympathicoblastoma
Symphalangy (fingers) (toes) Q70.9
Symptoms NEC R68.89
  breast NEC N64.59
  development NEC R63.8
  factitious, self-induced —see Disorder,
      factitious
  genital organs, female R10.2
  involving
    abdomen NEC R19.8
    appearance NEC R46.89
    awareness R41.9
      altered mental status R41.82
      amnesia —see Amnesia
      borderline intellectual functioning
          R41.83
      coma —see Coma
      disorientation R41.0
      neurologic neglect syndrome R41.4
      senile cognitive decline R41.81
      specified symptom NEC R41.89
    behavior NEC R46.89
    cardiovascular system NEC R09.89
    chest NEC R09.89
    circulatory system NEC R09.89
    cognitive functions R41.9
      altered mental status R41.82
      amnesia —see Amnesia
      borderline intellectual functioning
          R41.83
      coma —see Coma
      disorientation R41.0
      neurologic neglect syndrome R41.4
      senile cognitive decline R41.81
      specified symptom NEC R41.89
    development NEC R62.50
    digestive system NEC R19.8
    emotional state NEC R45.89
      emotional lability R45.86
    food and fluid intake R63.8
    general perceptions and sensations
        R44.9
      specified NEC R44.8
    musculoskeletal system R29.91
      specified NEC R29.898
    nervous system R29.90
      specified NEC R29.818
    pelvis NEC R19.8
    respiratory system NEC R09.89
    skin and integument R23.9
    urinary system R39.9
  menopausal N95.1
  metabolism NEC R63.8
  neurotic F48.8
  of infancy R68.19

◀ New   ◀▥ Revised   ~~deleted~~ Deleted

Symptoms NEC *(Continued)*
pelvis NEC, female R10.2
skin and integument NEC R23.9
subcutaneous tissue NEC R23.9
Sympus Q74.2
Syncephalus Q89.4
Synchondrosis
abnormal (congenital) Q78.8
ischiopubic M91.0
Synchysis (scintillans) (senile) (vitreous body)
H43.89
Syncope (near) (pre-) R55
anginosa I20.8
bradycardia R00.1
cardiac R55
carotid sinus G90.01
due to spinal (lumbar) puncture G97.1
heart R55
heat T67.1
laryngeal R05
psychogenic F48.8
tussive R05
vasoconstriction R55
vasodepressor R55
vasomotor R55
vasovagal R55
Syndactylism, syndactyly Q70.9
complex (with synostosis)
fingers Q70.0-
toes Q70.2-
simple (without synostosis)
fingers Q70.1-
toes Q70.3-
Syndrome —*see also* Disease
5q minus NOS D46.C
48,XXXX Q97.1
49,XXXXX Q97.1
abdominal
acute R10.0
muscle deficiency Q79.4
abnormal innervation H02.519
left H02.516
lower H02.515
upper H02.514
right H02.513
lower H02.512
upper H02.511
abstinence, neonatal P96.1
acid pulmonary aspiration, obstetric O74.0
acquired immunodeficiency —*see* Human,
immunodeficiency virus (HIV)
disease
acute abdominal R10.0
acute respiratory distress (adult) (child) J80
Adair-Dighton Q78.0
Adams-Stokes (-Morgagni) I45.9
adiposogenital E23.6
adrenal
hemorrhage (meningococcal) A39.1
meningococcic A39.1
adrenocortical —*see* Cushing's, syndrome
adrenogenital E25.9
congenital, associated with enzyme
deficiency E25.0
afferent loop NEC K91.89
Alagille's Q44.7
alcohol withdrawal (without convulsions) —
see Dependence, alcohol, with,
withdrawal
Alder's D72.0
Aldrich (-Wiskott) D82.0
alien hand R41.4
Alport Q87.81
alveolar hypoventilation E66.2
alveolocapillary block J84.10
amnesic, amnestic (confabulatory) (due to) —
see Disorder, amnesic
amyostatic (Wilson's disease) E83.01
androgen insensitivity E34.50
complete E34.51
partial E34.52

Syndrome *(Continued)*
androgen resistance (*see also* Syndrome,
androgen insensitivity) E34.50
Angelman Q93.5
anginal —*see* Angina
ankyloglossia superior Q38.1
anterior
chest wall R07.89
cord G83.82
spinal artery G95.19
compression M47.019
cervical region M47.012
cervicothoracic region M47.013
lumbar region M47.016
occipito-atlanto-axial region M47.011
thoracic region M47.014
thoracolumbar region M47.015
tibial M76.81-
antibody deficiency D80.9
agammaglobulinemic D80.1
hereditary D80.0
congenital D80.0
hypogammaglobulinemic D80.1
hereditary D80.0
anticardiolipin (-antibody) D68.61
antiphospholipid (-antibody) D68.61
aortic
arch M31.4
bifurcation I74.09
aortomesenteric duodenum occlusion K31.5
apical ballooning (transient left ventricular)
I51.81
arcuate ligament I77.4
argentaffin, argintaffinoma E34.0
Arnold-Chiari —*see* Arnold-Chiari disease
Arrillaga-Ayerza I27.0
Asherman's N85.6
aspiration, of newborn —*see* Aspiration, by
substance, with pneumonia
meconium P24.01
ataxia-telangiectasia G11.3
auriculotemporal G50.8
autoerythrocyte sensitization (Gardner-
Diamond) D69.2
autoimmune lymphoproliferative [ALPS]
D89.82
autoimmune polyglandular E31.0
autosomal —*see* Abnormal, autosomes
Avellis' G46.8
Ayerza (-Arrillaga) I27.0
Babinski-Nageotte G83.89
Bakwin-Krida Q79.8
bare lymphocyte D81.6
Barré-Guillain G61.0
Barré-Liéou M53.0
Barrett's —*see* Barrett's, esophagus
Barsony-Polgar K22.4
Barsony-Teschendorf K22.4
Barth E78.71
Bartter's E26.81
basal cell nevus Q87.89
Basedow's E05.00
with thyroid storm E05.01
basilar artery G45.0
Batten-Steinert G71.11
battered
baby or child —*see* Maltreatment, child,
physical abuse
spouse —*see* Maltreatment, adult, physical
abuse
Beals Q87.40
Beau's I51.5
Beck's I65.8
Benedikt's G46.3
Béquez César (-Steinbrinck-Chédiak-Higashi)
D70.330
Bernhardt-Roth —*see* Meralgia paresthetica
Bernheim's I50.9
big spleen D73.1
bilateral polycystic ovarian E28.2
Bing-Horton's —*see* Horton's headache

Syndrome *(Continued)*
Birt-Hogg-Dube syndrome Q87.89
Björck (-Thorsen) E34.0
black
lung J60
widow spider bite —*see* Toxicity, venom,
spider, black widow
Blackfan-Diamond D61.01
blind loop K90.2
congenital Q43.8
postsurgical K91.2
blue sclera Q78.0
blue toe I75.02-
Boder-Sedgewick G11.3
Boerhaave's K22.3
Borjeson Forssman Lehmann Q89.8
Bouillaud's I01.9
Bourneville (-Pringle) Q85.1
Bouveret (-Hoffman) I47.9
brachial plexus G54.0
bradycardia-tachycardia I49.5
brain (nonpsychotic) F09
with psychosis, psychotic reaction F09
acute or subacute —*see* Delirium
congenital —*see* Disability, intellectual
organic F09
post-traumatic (nonpsychotic) F07.81
psychotic F09
personality change F07.0
postcontusional F07.81
post-traumatic, nonpsychotic F07.81
psycho-organic F09
psychotic F06.8
brain stem stroke G46.3
Brandt's (acrodermatitis enteropathica) E83.2
broad ligament laceration N83.8
Brock's J98.11
bronze baby P83.8
Brown-Sequard G83.81
bubbly lung P27.0
Buchem's M85.2
Budd-Chiari I82.0
bulbar (progressive) G12.22
Bürger-Grütz E78.3
Burke's K86.8
Burnett's (milk-alkali) E83.52
burning feet E53.9
Bywaters' T79.5
Call-Fleming I67.841
carbohydrate-deficient glycoprotein (CDGS)
E77.8
carcinogenic thrombophlebitis I82.1
carcinoid E34.0
cardiac asthma I50.1
cardiacos negros I27.0
cardiofaciocutaneous Q87.89
cardiopulmonary-obesity E66.2
cardiorenal —*see* Hypertension, cardiorenal
cardiorespiratory distress (idiopathic),
newborn P22.0
cardiovascular renal —*see* Hypertension,
cardiorenal
carotid
artery (hemispheric) (internal) G45.1
body G90.01
sinus G90.01
carpal tunnel G56.0-
Cassidy (-Scholte) E34.0
cat-cry Q93.4
cat eye Q92.8
cauda equina G83.4
causalgia —*see* Causalgia
celiac K90.0
artery compression I77.4
axis I77.4
central pain G89.0
cerebellar
hereditary G11.9
stroke G46.4
cerebellomedullary malformation —*see* Spina
bifida

S

Syndrome (*Continued*)
cerebral
  artery
    anterior G46.1
    middle G46.0
    posterior G46.2
  gigantism E22.0
cervical (root) M53.1
  disc —*see* Disorder, disc, cervical, with
    neuritis
  fusion Q76.1
  posterior, sympathicus M53.0
  rib Q76.5
  sympathetic paralysis G90.2
cervicobrachial (diffuse) M53.1
cervicocranial M53.0
cervicodorsal outlet G54.2
cervicothoracic outlet G54.0
Céstan (-Raymond) I65.8
Charcot's (angina cruris) (intermittent
  claudication) I73.9
Charcot-Weiss-Baker G90.09
CHARGE Q89.8
Chédiak-Higashi (-Steinbrinck) E70.330
chest wall R07.1
Chiari's (hepatic vein thrombosis) I82.0
Chilaiditi's Q43.3
child maltreatment —*see* Maltreatment,
  child
chondrocostal junction M94.0
chondroectodermal dysplasia Q77.6
chromosome 4 short arm deletion Q93.3
chromosome 5 short arm deletion Q93.4
chronic
  pain G89.4
    personality F68.8
Clarke-Hadfield K86.8
Clerambault's automatism G93.89
Clouston's (hidrotic ectodermal dysplasia)
  Q82.4
clumsiness, clumsy child F82
cluster headache G44.009
  intractable G44.001
  not intractable G44.009
Coffin-Lowry Q89.8
cold injury (newborn) P80.0
combined immunity deficiency D81.9
compartment (deep) (posterior) (traumatic)
  T79.A0
  abdomen T79.A3
  lower extremity (hip, buttock, thigh, leg,
    foot, toes) T79.A2
  nontraumatic
    abdomen M79.A3
    lower extremity (hip, buttock, thigh, leg,
      foot, toes) M79.A2-
    specified site NEC M79.A9
    upper extremity (shoulder, arm, forearm,
      wrist, hand, fingers) M79.A1-
  postprocedural —*see* Syndrome
    compartment, nontraumatic
  specified site NEC T79.A9
  upper extremity (shoulder, arm, forearm,
    wrist, hand, fingers) T79.A1
complex regional pain —*see* Syndrome, pain,
  complex regional
compression T79.5
  anterior spinal —*see* Syndrome, anterior,
    spinal artery, compression
  cauda equina G83.4
  celiac artery I77.4
  vertebral artery M47.029
    cervical region M47.022
    occipito-atlanto-axial region M47.021
concussion F07.81
congenital
  affecting multiple systems NEC Q87.89
  central alveolar hypoventilation G47.35
  facial diplegia Q87.0
  muscular hypertrophy-cerebral Q87.89
  oculo-auriculovertebral Q87.0

Syndrome (*Continued*)
congenital (*Continued*)
  oculofacial diplegia (Moebius) Q87.0
  rubella (manifest) P35.0
congestion-fibrosis (pelvic), female N94.89
congestive dysmenorrhea N94.6
Conn's E26.01
connective tissue M35.9
  overlap NEC M35.1
conus medullaris G95.81
cord
  anterior G83.82
  posterior G83.83
coronary
  acute NEC I24.9
  insufficiency or intermediate I20.0
  slow flow I20.8
Costen's (complex) M26.69
costochondral junction M94.0
costoclavicular G54.0
costovertebral E22.0
Cowden Q85.8
craniovertebral M53.0
Creutzfeldt-Jakob —*see* Creutzfeldt-Jakob
  disease or syndrome
cri-du-chat Q93.4
crib death R99
cricopharyngeal —*see* Dysphagia
croup J05.0
CRPS I —*see* Syndrome, pain, complex
  regional I
crush T79.5
cryptophthalmos Q87.0
cubital tunnel —*see* Lesion, nerve, ulnar
Curschmann (-Batten) (-Steinert) G71.11
Cushing's E24.9
  alcohol-induced E24.4
  drug-induced E24.2
  due to
    alcohol
    drugs E24.2
    ectopic ACTH E24.3
    overproduction of pituitary ACTH E24.0
  overdose or wrong substance given or
    taken —*see* Table of Drugs and
    Chemicals, by drug, poisoning
  pituitary-dependent E24.0
  specified type NEC E24.8
cystic duct stump K91.5
Dana-Putnam D51.0
Danbolt (-Cross) (acrodermatitis
  enteropathica) E83.2
Dandy-Walker Q03.1
  with spina bifida Q07.01
Danlos' Q79.8
defibrination —*see also* Fibrinolysis
  with
    antepartum hemorrhage —*see*
      Hemorrhage, antepartum, with
      coagulation defect
    intrapartum hemorrhage —*see*
      Hemorrhage, complicating,
      delivery
  newborn P60
  postpartum O72.3
Degos' I77.8
Déjérine-Roussy G89.0
delayed sleep phase G47.21
demyelinating G37.9
dependence —*see* F10-F19 with fourth
  character .2
depersonalization (-derealization) F48.1
De Quervain E34.51
de Toni-Fanconi (-Debré) E72.09
  with cystinosis E72.04
diabetes mellitus-hypertension-nephrosis —
  see Diabetes, nephrosis
diabetes mellitus in newborn infant P70.2
diabetes-nephrosis —*see* Diabetes, nephrosis
diabetic amyotrophy —*see* Diabetes,
  amyotrophy

Syndrome (*Continued*)
Diamond-Blackfan D61.01
Diamond-Gardener D69.2
DIC (diffuse or disseminated intravascular
  coagulopathy) D65
di George's D82.1
Dighton's Q78.0
disequilibrium E87.8
Döhle body-panmyelopathic D72.0
dorsolateral medullary G46.4
double athetosis G80.3
Down (*see also* Down syndrome) Q90.9
Dresbach's (elliptocytosis) D58.1
Dressler's (postmyocardial infarction)
  I24.1
  postcardiotomy I97.0
drug withdrawal, infant of dependent mother
  P96.1
dry eye H04.12-
due to abnormality
  chromosomal Q99.9
    sex
      female phenotype Q97.9
      male phenotype Q98.9
    specified NEC Q99.8
dumping (postgastrectomy) K91.1
  nonsurgical K31.89
Dupré's (meningism) R29.1
dysmetabolic X E88.81
dyspraxia, developmental F82
Eagle-Barrett Q79.4
Eaton-Lambert —*see* Syndrome,
  Lambert-Eaton
Ebstein's Q22.5
ectopic ACTH E24.3
eczema-thrombocytopenia D82.0
Eddowes' Q78.0
effort (psychogenic) F45.8
Ehlers-Danlos Q79.6
Eisenmenger's I27.89
Ekman's Q78.0
electric feet E53.8
Ellis-van Creveld Q77.6
empty nest Z60.0
endocrine-hypertensive E27.0
entrapment —*see* Neuropathy,
  entrapment
eosinophilia-myalgia M35.8
epileptic —*see also* Epilepsy, by type
  absence G40.A09
    intractable G40.A19
      with status epilepticus G40.A11
      without status epilepticus G40.A19
    not intractable G40.A09
      with status epilepticus G40.A01
      without status epilepticus G40.A09
Erdheim-Chester (ECD) E88.89
Erdheim's E22.0
erythrocyte fragmentation D59.4
Evans D69.41
exhaustion F48.8
extrapyramidal G25.9
  specified NEC G25.89
eye retraction —*see* Strabismus
eyelid-malar-mandible Q87.0
Faber's D50.9
facial pain, paroxysmal G50.0
Fallot's Q21.3
familial eczema-thrombocytopenia
  (Wiskott-Aldrich) D82.0
Fanconi (-de Toni) (-Debré) E72.09
  with cystinosis E72.04
Fanconi's (anemia) (congenital pancytopenia)
  D61.09
fatigue
  chronic R53.82
  psychogenic F48.8
faulty bowel habit K59.3
Feil-Klippel (brevicollis) Q76.1
Felty's —*see* Felty's syndrome
fertile eunuch E23.0

◀ New   ◀◀◀ Revised   ~~deleted~~ Deleted

Syndrome *(Continued)*
  fetal
    alcohol (dysmorphic) Q86.0
    hydantoin Q86.1
  Fiedler's I40.1
  first arch Q87.0
  fish odor E72.8
  Fisher's G61.0
  Fitzhugh-Curtis
    due to
      Chlamydia trachomatis A74.81
      Neisseria gonorrhorea (gonococcal
        peritonitis) A54.85
  Fitz's K85.8
  Flajani (-Basedow) E05.00
    with thyroid storm E05.01
  flatback —*see* Flatback syndrome
  floppy
    baby P94.2
    iris (intraoeprative) (IFIS) H21.81
    mitral valve I34.1
  flush E34.0
  Foix-Alajouanine G95.19
  Fong's Q79.8
  foramen magnum G93.5
  Foster-Kennedy H47.14-
  Foville's (peduncular) G46.3
  fragile X Q99.2
  Franceschetti Q75.4
  Frey's
    auriculotemporal G50.8
    hyperhidrosis L74.52
  Friderichsen-Waterhouse A39.1
  Froin's G95.89
  frontal lobe F07.0
  Fukuhara E88.49
  functional
    bowel K59.9
    prepubertal castrate E29.1
  Gaisböck's D75.1
  ganglion (basal ganglia brain) G25.9
    geniculi G51.1
  Gardner-Diamond D69.2
  gastroesophageal
    junction K22.0
    laceration-hemorrhage K22.6
  gastrojejunal loop obstruction K91.89
  Gee-Herter-Heubner K90.0
  Gelineau's G47.419
    with cataplexy G47.411
  genito-anorectal A55
  Gerstmann-Sträussler-Scheinker (GSS)
    A81.82
  Gianotti-Crosti L44.4
  giant platelet (Bernard-Soulier) D69.1
  Gilles de la Tourette's F95.2
  goiter-deafness E07.1
  Goldberg Q89.8
  Goldberg-Maxwell E34.51
  Good's D83.8
  Gopalan' (burning feet) E53.8
  Gorlin's Q87.89
  Gougerot-Blum L81.7
  Gouley's I31.1
  Gower's R55
  gray or grey (newborn) P93.0
    platelet D69.1
  Gubler-Millard G46.3
  Guillain-Barré (-Strohl) G61.0
  gustatory sweating G50.8
  Hadfield-Clarke K86.8
  hair tourniquet —*see* Constriction, external,
    by site
  Hamman's J98.19
  hand-foot L27.1
  hand-shoulder G90.8
  hantavirus (cardio)-pulmonary (HPS) (HCPS)
    B33.4
  happy puppet Q93.5
  Harada's H30.81-
  Hayem-Faber D50.9

Syndrome *(Continued)*
  headache NEC G44.89
    complicated NEC G44.59
  Heberden's I20.8
  Hedinger's E34.0
  Hegglin's D72.0
  HELLP (hemolysis, elevated liver enzymes
    and low platelet count) O14.2-
  hemolytic-uremic D59.3
  hemophagocytic, infection-associated
    D76.2
  Henoch-Schönlein D69.0
  hepatic flexure K59.8
  hepatopulmonary K76.81
  hepatorenal K76.7
    following delivery O90.4
    postoperative or postprocedural K91.83
    postpartum, puerperal O90.4
  hepatourologic K76.7
  Herter (-Gee) (nontropical sprue) K90.0
  Heubner-Herter K90.0
  Heyd's K76.7
  Hilger's G90.09
  histamine-like (fish poisoning) —*see*
    Poisoning, fish
  histiocytic D76.3
  histiocytosis NEC D76.3
  HIV infection, acute B20
  Hoffmann-Werdnig G12.0
  Hollander-Simons E88.1
  Hoppe-Goldflam G70.00
    with exacerbation (acute) G70.01
    in crisis G70.01
  Horner's G90.2
  hungry bone E83.81
  hunterian glossitis D51.0
  Hutchinson's triad A50.53
  hyperabduction G54.0
  hyperammonemia-hyperornithinemia-
    homocitrullinemia E72.4
  hypereosinophilic (idiopathic) D72.1
  hyperimmunoglobulin E (IgE) D82.4
  hyperkalemic E87.5
  hyperkinetic —*see* Hyperkinesia
  hypermobility M35.7
  hypernatremia E87.0
  hyperosmolarity E87.0
  hyperperfusion G97.82
  hypersplenic D73.1
  hypertransfusion, newborn P61.1
  hyperventilation F45.8
  hyperviscosity (of serum)
    polycythemic D75.1
    sclerothymic D58.8
  hypoglycemic (familial) (neonatal) E16.2
  hypokalemic E87.6
  hyponatremic E87.1
  hypopituitarism E23.0
  hypoplastic left-heart Q23.4
  hypopotassemia E87.6
  hyposmolality E87.1
  hypotension, maternal O26.5-
  hypothenar hammer I73.89
  ICF (intravascular coagulation-fibrinolysis)
    D65
  idiopathic
    cardiorespiratory distress, newborn P22.0
    nephrotic (infantile) N04.9
  iliotibial band M76.3-
  immobility, immobilization (paraplegic)
    M62.3
  immune reconstitution D89.3
  immune reconstitution inflammatory [IRIS]
    D89.3
  immunity deficiency, combined D81.9
  immunodeficiency
    acquired —*see* Human, immunodeficiency
      virus (HIV) disease
    combined D81.9
  impending coronary I20.0
  impingement, shoulder M75.4-

Syndrome *(Continued)*
  inappropriate secretion of antidiuretic
    hormone E22.2
  infant
    gestational diabetes P70.0
    of diabetic mother P70.1
  infantilism (pituitary) E23.0
  inferior vena cava I87.1
  inspissated bile (newborn) P59.1
  institutional (childhood) F94.2
  insufficient sleep F51.12
  intermediate coronary (artery) I20.0
  interspinous ligament —*see* Spondylopathy,
    specified NEC
  intestinal
    carcinoid E34.0
    knot K56.2
  intravascular coagulation-fibrinolysis (ICF)
    D65
  iodine-deficiency, congenital E00.9
    type
      mixed E00.2
      myxedematous E00.1
      neurological E00.0
  IRDS (idiopathic respiratory distress,
    newborn) P22.0
  irritable
    bowel K58.9
      with diarrhea K58.0
      psychogenic F45.8
    heart (psychogenic) F45.8
    weakness F48.8
  ischemic bowel (transient) K55.9
    chronic K55.1
    due to mesenteric artery insufficiency
      K55.1
  IVC (intravascular coagulopathy) D65
  Ivemark's Q89.01
  Jaccoud's —*see* Arthropathy, postrheumatic,
    chronic
  Jackson's G83.89
  Jakob-Creutzfeldt —*see* Creutzfeldt-Jakob
    disease or syndrome
  jaw-winking Q07.8
  Jervell-Lange-Nielsen I45.81
  jet lag G47.25
  Job's D71
  Joseph-Diamond-Blackfan D61.01
  jugular foramen G52.7
  Kabuki Q89.8
  Kanner's (autism) F84.0
  Kartagener's Q89.3
  Kelly's D50.1
  Kimmelstiel-Wilson —*see* Diabetes, specified
    type, with Kimmelstiel-Wilson disease
  Klein (e)-Levine G47.13
  Klippel-Feil (brevicollis) Q76.1
  Köhler-Pellegrini-Steida —*see* Bursitis, tibial
    collateral
  König's K59.8
  Korsakoff (-Wernicke) (nonalcoholic) F04
    alcoholic F10.26
  Kostmann's D70.0
  Krabbe's congenital muscle hypoplasia Q79.8
  labyrinthine —*see* subcategory H83.2
  lacunar NEC G46.7
  Lambert-Eaton G70.80
    in
      neoplastic disease G73.1
      specified disease NEC G70.81
  Landau-Kleffner —*see* Epilepsy, specified
    NEC
  Larsen's Q74.8
  lateral
    cutaneous nerve of thigh G57.1-
    medullary G46.4
  Launois' E22.0
  lazy
    leukocyte D70.8
    posture M62.3
  Lemiere I80.8

Syndrome (Continued)
Lennox-Gastaut G40.812
  intractable G40.814
    with status epilepticus G40.813
    without status epilepticus G40.814
  not intractable G40.812
    with status epilepticus G40.811
    without status epilepticus G40.812
lenticular, progressive E83.01
Leopold-Levi's E05.90
Lev's I44.2
Li-Fraumeni Z15.01
Lichtheim's D51.0
Lightwood's N25.89
Lignac (de Toni) (-Fanconi) (-Debré) E72.09
  with cystinosis E72.04
Likoff's I20.8
limbic epilepsy personality F07.0
liver-kidney K76.7
lobotomy F07.0
Loffler's J82
long arm 18 or 21 deletion Q93.89
long QT I45.81
Louis-Barré G11.3
low
  atmospheric pressure T70.29
  back M54.5
  output (cardiac) I50.9
lower radicular, newborn (birth injury) P14.8
Luetscher's (dehydration) E86.0
Lupus anticoagulant D68.62
Lutembacher's Q21.1
macrophage activation D76.1
  due to infection D76.2
magnesium-deficiency R29.0
Mal de Debarquement R42
malabsorption K90.9
  postsurgical K91.2
malformation, congenital, due to
  alcohol Q86.0
  exogenous cause NEC Q86.8
  hydantoin Q86.1
  warfarin Q86.2
malignant
  carcinoid E34.0
  neuroleptic G21.0
Mallory-Weiss K22.6
mandibulofacial dysostosis Q75.4
manic-depressive —see Disorder, bipolar,
  affective
maple-syrup-urine E71.0
Marable's I77.4
Marfan's Q87.40
  with
    cardiovascular manifestations Q87.418
      aortic dilation Q87.410
    ocular manifestations Q87.42
    skeletal manifestations Q87.43
Marie's (acromegaly) E22.0
maternal hypotension —see Syndrome,
  hypotension, maternal
May (-Hegglin) D72.0
McArdle (-Schmidt) (-Pearson) E74.04
McQuarrie's E16.2
meconium plug (newborn) P76.0
median arcuate ligament I77.4
Meekeren-Ehlers-Danlos Q79.6
megavitamin-B6 E67.2
Meige G24.4
MELAS E88.41
Mendelson's O74.0
MERRF (myoclonic epilepsy associated with
  ragged-red fibers) E88.42
mesenteric
  artery (superior) K55.1
  vascular insufficiency K55.1
metabolic E88.81
metastatic carcinoid E34.0
micrognathia-glossoptosis Q87.0
midbrain NEC G93.89
middle lobe (lung) J98.19

Syndrome (Continued)
middle radicular G54.0
migraine (see also Migraine) G43.909-
Mikulicz' K11.8
milk-alkali E83.52
Millard-Gubler G46.3
Miller-Dieker Q93.88
Miller-Fisher G61.0
Minkowski-Chauffard D58.0
Mirizzi's K83.1
MNGIE (Mitochondrial Neurogastrointestinal
  Encephalopathy) E88.49
Möbius, ophthalmoplegic migraine —see
  Migraine, ophthalmoplegic
monofixation H50.42
Morel-Moore M85.2
Morel-Morgagni M85.2
Morgagni (-Morel) (-Stewart) M85.2
Morgagni-Adams-Stokes I45.9
Mounier-Kuhn Q32.4
  with bronchiectasis J47.9
    with
      exacerbation (acute) J47.1
      lower respiratory infection J47.0
  acquired J98.09
    with bronchiectasis J47.9
      with
        exacerbation (acute) J47.1
        lower respiratory infection J47.0
mucocutaneous lymph node (acute febrile)
  (MCLS) M30.3
multiple endocrine neoplasia (MEN) —see
  Neoplasia, endocrine, multiple (MEN}
multiple operations —see Disorder, factitious
myasthenic G70.9
  in
    diabetes mellitus —see Diabetes,
      amyotrophy
    endocrine disease NEC E34.9 [G73.3]
    neoplastic disease (see also Neoplasm)
      D49.9 [G73.3]
    thyrotoxicosis (hyperthyroidism) E05.90
      [G73.3]
      with thyroid storm E05.91 [G73.3]
myelodysplastic D46.9
  with
    5q deletion D46.C
    isolated del (5q) chromosomal
      abnormality D46.C
  lesions, low grade D46.20
  specified NEC D46.Z
myelopathic pain G89.0
myeloproliferative (chronic) D47.1
myofascial pain M79.1
Naffziger's G54.0
nail patella Q87.2
NARP (Neuropathy, Ataxia and Retinitis
  pigmentosa) E88.49
neonatal abstinence P96.1
nephritic —see also Nephritis
  with edema —see Nephrosis
  acute N00.9
  chronic N03.9
  rapidly progressive N01.9
nephrotic (congenital) (see also Nephrosis)
  N04.9
  with
    dense deposit disease N04.6
    diffuse
      crescentic glomerulonephritis
        N04.7
      endocapillary proliferative
        glomerulonephritis N04.4
      membranous glomerulonephritis
        N04.2
      mesangial proliferative
        glomerulonephritis N04.3
      mesangiocapillary glomerulonephritis
        N04.5
    focal and segmental glomerular lesions
      N04.1

Syndrome (Continued)
nephrotic (Continued)
  with (Continued)
    minor glomerular abnormality N04.0
    specified morphological changes NEC
      N04.8
  diabetic —see Diabetes, nephrosis
neurologic neglect R41.4
Nezelof's D81.4
Nonne-Milroy-Meige Q82.0
Nothnagel's vasomotor acroparesthesia
  I73.89
oculomotor H51.9
ophthalmoplegia-cerebellar ataxia —see
  Strabismus, paralytic, third nerve
oral-facial-digital Q87.0
organic
  affective F06.30
  amnesic (not alcohol- or drug-induced) F04
  brain F09
  depressive F06.31
  hallucinosis F06.0
  personality F07.0
Ormond's N13.5
oro-facial-digital Q87.0
os trigonum Q68.8
Osler-Weber-Rendu I78.0
osteoporosis-osteomalacia M83.8
Osterreicher-Turner Q79.8
otolith —see subcategory H81.8
oto-palatal-digital Q87.0
outlet (thoracic) G54.0
ovary
  polycystic E28.2
  resistant E28.39
  sclerocystic E28.2
Owren's D68.2
Paget-Schroetter I82.890
pain —see also Pain
  complex regional I G90.50
    lower limb G90.52-
      specified site NEC G90.59
      upper limb G90.51-
  complex regional II —see Causalgia
painful
  bruising D69.2
  feet E53.8
  prostate N42.81
paralysis agitans —see Parkinsonism
paralytic G83.9
  specified NEC G83.89
Parinaud's H51.0
parkinsonian —see Parkinsonism
Parkinson's —see Parkinsonism
paroxysmal facial pain G50.0
Parry's E05.00
  with thyroid storm E05.01
Parsonage (-Aldren)-Turner G54.5
patella clunk M25.86-
Paterson (-Brown) (-Kelly) D50.1
pectoral girdle I77.89
pectoralis minor I77.89
Pelger-Huet D72.0
pellagra-cerebellar ataxia-renal
  aminoaciduria E72.02
pellagroid E52
Pellegrini-Stieda —see Bursitis, tibial
  collateral
pelvic congestion-fibrosis, female N94.89
penta X Q97.1
peptic ulcer —see Ulcer, peptic
perabduction I77.89
periodic headache, in adults and children —
  see Headache, periodic syndromes in
  adults and children
periurethral fibrosis N13.5
phantom limb (without pain) G54.7
  with pain G54.6
pharyngeal pouch D82.1
Pick's (heart) (liver) I31.1
Pickwickian E66.2

◀ New   ◀▥ Revised   ~~deleted~~ Deleted

Syndrome *(Continued)*
PIE (pulmonary infiltration with eosinophilia) J82
pigmentary pallidal degeneration (progressive) G23.0
pineal E34.8
pituitary E22.0
placental transfusion —*see* Pregnancy, complicated by, placental transfusion syndromes
plantar fascia M72.2
plateau iris (post-iridectomy) (postprocedural) H21.82
Plummer-Vinson D50.1
pluricarential of infancy E40
plurideficiency E40
pluriglandular (compensatory) E31.8
  autoimmune E31.0
pneumatic hammer T75.21
polyangiitis overlap M30.8
polycarential of infancy E40
polyglandular E31.8
  autoimmune E31.0
polysplenia Q89.09
pontine NEC G93.89
popliteal
  artery entrapment I77.89
  web Q87.89
postcardiac injury
  postcardiotomy I97.0
  postmyocardial infarction I24.1
postcardiotomy I97.0
post chemoembolization — code to associated conditions
postcholecystectomy K91.5
postcommissurotomy I97.0
postconcussional F07.81
postcontusional F07.81
postencephalitic F07.89
posterior
  cervical sympathetic M53.0
  cord G83.83
  fossa compression G93.5
  reversible encephalopathy (PRES) I67.83
postgastrectomy (dumping) K91.1
postgastric surgery K91.1
postinfarction I24.1
postlaminectomy NEC M96.1
postleukotomy F07.0
postmastectomy lymphedema I97.2
postmyocardial infarction I24.1
postoperative NEC T81.9
  blind loop K90.2
postpartum panhypopituitary (Sheehan) E23.0
postpolio (myelitic) G14
postthrombotic I87.009
  with
    inflammation I87.02-
      with ulcer I87.03-
    specified complication NEC I87.09-
    ulcer I87.01-
      with inflammation I87.03-
  asymptomatic I87.00-
postvagotomy K91.1
postvalvulotomy I97.0
postviral NEC G93.3
  fatigue G93.3
Potain's K31.0
potassium intoxication E87.5
precerebral artery (multiple) (bilateral) G45.2
preinfarction I20.0
preleukemic D46.9
premature senility E34.8
premenstrual dysphoric N94.3
premenstrual tension N94.3
Prinzmetal-Massumi R07.1
prune belly Q79.4
pseudocarpal tunnel (sublimis) —*see* Syndrome, carpal tunnel

Syndrome *(Continued)*
pseudoparalytica G70.00
  with exacerbation (acute) G70.01
  in crisis G70.01
pseudo -Turner's Q87.1
psycho-organic (nonpsychotic severity) F07.9
  acute or subacute F05
  depressive type F06.31
  hallucinatory type F06.0
  nonpsychotic severity F07.0
  specified NEC F07.89
pulmonary
  arteriosclerosis I27.0
  dysmaturity (Wilson-Mikity) P27.0
  hypoperfusion (idiopathic) P22.0
  renal (hemorrhagic) (Goodpasture's) M31.0
pure
  motor lacunar G46.5
  sensory lacunar G46.6
Putnam-Dana D51.0
pyramidopallidonigral G20
pyriformis —*see* Lesion, nerve, sciatic
QT interval prolongation I45.81
radicular NEC —*see* Radiculopathy
  upper limbs, newborn (birth injury) P14.3
rapid time-zone change G47.25
Rasmussen G04.81
Raymond (-Céstan) I65.8
Raynaud's I73.00
  with gangrene I73.01
RDS (respiratory distress syndrome, newborn) P22.0
reactive airways dysfunction J68.3
Refsum's G60.1
Reifenstein E34.52
renal glomerulohyalinosis-diabetic —*see* Diabetes, nephrosis
Rendu-Osler-Weber I78.0
residual ovary N99.83
resistant ovary E28.39
respiratory
  distress
    acute J80
      adult J80
      child J80
    newborn (idiopathic) (type I) P22.0
      type II P22.1
restless legs G25.81
retinoblastoma (familial) C69.2
retroperitoneal fibrosis N13.5
retroviral seroconversion (acute) Z21
Reye's G93.7
Richter —*see* Leukemia, chronic lymphocytic, B-cell type
Ridley's I50.1
right
  heart, hypoplastic Q22.6
  ventricular obstruction —*see* Failure, heart, congestive
Romano-Ward (prolonged QT interval) I45.81
rotator cuff, shoulder (*see also* Tear, rotator cuff) M75.10-
Rotes Quérol —*see* Hyperostosis, ankylosing
Roth —*see* Meralgia paresthetica
rubella (congenital) P35.0
Ruvalcaba-Myhre-Smith E71.440
Rytand-Lipsitch I44.2
salt
  depletion E87.1
    due to heat NEC T67.8
      causing heat exhaustion or prostration T67.4
  low E87.1
salt-losing N28.89
Scaglietti-Dagnini E22.0
scalenus anticus (anterior) G54.0
scapulocostal —*see* Mononeuropathy, upper limb, specified site NEC
scapuloperoneal G71.0
schizophrenic, of childhood NEC F84.5
Schnitzler D47.2

Syndrome *(Continued)*
Scholte's E34.0
Schroeder's E27.0
Schüller-Christian C96.5
Schwachman's —*see* Syndrome, Shwachman's
Schwartz (-Jampel) G71.13
Schwartz-Bartter E22.2
scimitar Q26.8
sclerocystic ovary E28.2
Seitelberger's G31.89
septicemic adrenal hemorrhage A39.1
seroconversion, retroviral (acute) Z21
serous meningitis G93.2
severe acute respiratory (SARS) J12.81
shaken infant T74.4
shock (traumatic) T79.4
  kidney N17.0
    following crush injury T79.5
  toxic A48.3
shock-lung J80
Shone's — code to specific anomalies
short
  bowel K91.2
  rib Q77.2
shoulder-hand —*see* Algoneurodystrophy
Shwachman's D70.4
sicca —*see* Sicca syndrome
sick
  cell E87.1
  sinus I49.5
sick-euthyroid E07.81
sideropenic D50.1
Siemens' ectodermal dysplasia Q82.4
Silfversköld's Q78.9
Simons' E88.1
sinus tarsi M25.57-
sinusitis-bronchiectasis-situs inversus Q89.3
Sipple's E31.22
sirenomelia Q87.2
Slocumb's E27.0
slow flow, coronary I20.8
Sluder's G44.89
Smith-Magenis Q93.88
Sneddon-Wilkinson L13.1
Sotos' E22.0
South African cardiomyopathy I42.8
spasmodic
  upward movement, eyes H51.8
  winking F95.8
Spen's I45.9
splenic
  agenesis Q89.01
  flexure K59.8
  neutropenia D73.81
Spurway's Q78.0
staphylococcal scalded skin L00
Stein-Leventhal E28.2
Stein's E28.2
Stevens-Johnson syndrome L51.1
  toxic epidermal necrolysis overlap L51.3
Stewart-Morel M85.2
Stickler Q89.8
stiff baby Q89.8
stiff man G25.82
Still-Felty —*see* Felty's syndrome
Stokes (-Adams) I45.9
stone heart I50.1
straight back, congenital Q76.49
subclavian steal G45.8
subcoracoid-pectoralis minor G54.0
subcostal nerve compression I77.89
subphrenic interposition Q43.3
superior
  cerebellar artery I63.8
  mesenteric artery K55.1
  semi-circular canal dehiscence H83.8X-
  vena cava I87.1
supine hypotensive (maternal) —*see* Syndrome, hypotension, maternal

S

Syndrome (*Continued*)
suprarenal cortical E27.0
supraspinatus (*see also* Tear, rotator cuff)
  M75.10-
Susac G93.49
swallowed blood P78.2
sweat retention L74.0
Swyer Q99.1
Symond's G93.2
sympathetic
  cervical paralysis G90.2
  pelvic, female N94.89
systemic inflammatory response (SIRS), of
  non-infectious origin (without organ
  dysfunction) R65.10
  with acute organ dysfunction R65.11
tachycardia-bradycardia I49.5
takotsubo I51.81
TAR (thrombocytopenia with absent radius)
  Q87.2
tarsal tunnel G57.5-
teething K00.7
tegmental G93.89
telangiectasic-pigmentation-cataract
  Q82.8
temporal pyramidal apex —*see* Otitis,
  media, suppurative, acute
temporomandibular joint-pain-dysfunction
  M26.62
Terry's H44.2-
testicular feminization (*see also* Syndrome,
  androgen insensitivity) E34.51
thalamic pain (hyperesthetic) G89.0
thoracic outlet (compression) G54.0
Thorson-Björck E34.0
thrombocytopenia with absent radius (TAR)
  Q87.2
thyroid-adrenocortical insufficiency E31.0
tibial
  anterior M76.81-
  posterior M76.82-
Tietze's M94.0
time-zone (rapid) G47.25
Toni-Fanconi E72.09
  with cystinosis E72.04
Touraine's Q79.8
tourniquet —*see* Constriction, external,
  by site
toxic shock A48.3
transient left ventricular apical ballooning
  I51.81
traumatic vasospastic T75.22
Treacher Collins Q75.4
triple X, female Q97.0
trisomy Q92.9
  13 Q91.7
    meiotic nondisjunction Q91.4
    mitotic nondisjunction Q91.5
    mosaicism Q91.5
    translocation Q91.6
  18 Q91.3
    meiotic nondisjunction Q91.0
    mitotic nondisjunction Q91.1
    mosaicism Q91.1
    translocation Q91.2
  20 (q)(p) Q92.8
  21 Q90.9
    meiotic nondisjunction Q90.0
    mitotic nondisjunction Q90.1
    mosaicism Q90.1
    translocation Q90.2
  22 Q92.8
tropical wet feet T69.0-
Trousseau's I82.1
tumor lysis (following antineoplastic
  chemotherapy) (spontaneous) NEC
  E88.3
Twiddler's (due to)
  automatic implantable defibrillator
    T82.198
  cardiac pacemaker T82.198

Syndrome (*Continued*)
Unverricht (-Lundborg) —*see* Epilepsy,
  generalized, idiopathic
upward gaze H51.8
uremia, chronic (*see also* Disease, kidney,
  chronic) N18.9
urethral N34.3
urethro-oculo-articular —*see* Reiter's disease
urohepatic K76.7
vago-hypoglossal G52.7
van Buchem's M85.2
van der Hoeve's Q78.0
vascular NEC in cerebrovascular disease
  G46.8
vasoconstriction, reversible cerebrovascular
  I67.841
vasomotor I73.9
vasospastic (traumatic) T75.22
vasovagal R55
VATER Q87.2
velo-cardio-facial Q93.81
vena cava (inferior) (superior) (obstruction)
  I87.1
vertebral
  artery G45.0
    compression —*see* Syndrome, anterior,
      spinal artery, compression
  steal G45.0
vertebro-basilar artery G45.0
vertebrogenic (pain) M54.89
vertiginous —*see* Disorder, vestibular
  function
Vinson-Plummer D50.1
virus B34.9
visceral larva migrans B83.0
visual disorientation H53.8
vitamin B6 deficiency E53.1
vitreal corneal H59.01-
vitreous (touch) H59.01-
Vogt-Koyanagi H20.82-
Volkmann's T79.6
von Schroetter's I82.890
von Willebrand (-Jürgen) D68.0
Waldenström-Kjellberg D50.1
Wallenberg's G46.3
water retention E87.79
Waterhouse (-Friderichsen) A39.1
Weber-Gubler G46.3
Weber-Leyden G46.3
Weber's G46.3
Wegener's M31.30
  with
    kidney involvement M31.31
    lung involvement M31.30
      with kidney involvement M31.31
Weingarten's (tropical eosinophilia) J82
Weiss-Baker G90.09
Werdnig-Hoffman G12.0
Wermer's E31.21
Werner's E34.8
Wernicke-Korsakoff (nonalcoholic) F04
  alcoholic F10.26
West's —*see* Epilepsy, spasms
Westphal-Strümpell E83.01
wet
  feet (maceration) (tropical) T69.0-
  lung, newborn P22.1
whiplash S13.4
whistling face Q87.0
Wilkie's K55.1
Wilkinson-Sneddon L13.1
Willebrand (-Jürgens) D68.0
Wilson's (hepatolenticular degeneration)
  E83.01
Wiskott-Aldrich D82.0
withdrawal —*see* Withdrawal, state
  drug
    infant of dependent mother P96.1
    therapeutic use, newborn P96.2
Woakes' (ethmoiditis) J33.1
Wright's (hyperabduction) I77.89

Syndrome (*Continued*)
X I20.9
XXXX Q97.1
XXXXX Q97.1
XXXXY Q98.1
XXY Q98.0
yellow nail L60.5
Zahorsky's B08.5
Zellweger syndrome E71.510
Zellweger-like syndrome E71.541
Synechia (anterior) (iris) (posterior) (pupil) —
  see also Adhesions, iris
  intra-uterine (traumatic) N85.6
Synesthesia R20.8
Syngamiasis, syngamosis B83.3
Synodontia K00.2
Synorchidism, synorchism Q55.1
Synostosis (congenital) Q78.8
  astragalo-scaphoid Q74.2
  radioulnar Q74.0
Synovial sarcoma —*see* Neoplasm, connective
  tissue, malignant
Synovioma (malignant) —*see also* Neoplasm,
  connective tissue, malignant
  benign —*see* Neoplasm, connective tissue,
    benign
Synoviosarcoma —*see* Neoplasm, connective
  tissue, malignant
Synovitis —*see also* Tenosynovitis
  crepitant
    hand M70.0-
    wrist M70.03-
  gonococcal A54.49
  gouty —*see* Gout, idiopathic
  in (due to)
    crystals M65.8-
    gonorrhea A54.49
    syphilis (late) A52.78
    use, overuse, pressure —*see* Disorder, soft
      tissue, due to use
  infective NEC —*see* Tenosynovitis, infective
    NEC
  specified NEC —*see* Tenosynovitis, specified
    type NEC
  syphilitic A52.78
    congenital (early) A50.02
  toxic —*see* Synovitis, transient
  transient M67.3-
    ankle M67.37-
    elbow M67.32-
    foot joint M67.37-
    hand joint M67.34-
    hip M67.35-
    knee M67.36-
    multiple site M67.39
    pelvic region M67.35-
    shoulder M67.31-
    specified joint NEC M67.38
    wrist M67.33-
  traumatic, current —*see* Sprain
  tuberculous —*see* Tuberculosis, synovitis
  villonodular (pigmented) M12.2-
    ankle M12.27-
    elbow M12.22-
    foot joint M12.27-
    hand joint M12.24-
    hip M12.25-
    knee M12.26-
    multiple site M12.29
    pelvic region M12.25-
    shoulder M12.21-
    specified joint NEC M12.28
    vertebrae M12.28
    wrist M12.23-
Syphilid A51.39
  congenital A50.06
  newborn A50.06
  tubercular (late) A52.79
Syphilis, syphilitic (acquired) A53.9
  abdomen (late) A52.79
  acoustic nerve A52.15

◀ New   ◀▦ Revised   ~~deleted~~ Deleted

Syphilis, syphilitic *(Continued)*
  adenopathy (secondary) A51.49
  adrenal (gland) (with cortical hypofunction)
    A52.79
  age under 2 years NOS —*see also* Syphilis,
      congenital, early
    acquired A51.9
  alopecia (secondary) A51.32
  anemia (late) A52.79 *[D63.8]*
  aneurysm (aorta) (ruptured) A52.01
    central nervous system A52.05
    congenital A50.54 *[I79.0]*
  anus (late) A52.74
    primary A51.1
    secondary A51.39
  aorta (arch) (abdominal) (thoracic) A52.02
    aneurysm A52.01
  aortic (insufficiency) (regurgitation)
        (stenosis) A52.03
    aneurysm A52.01
  arachnoid (adhesive) (cerebral) (spinal)
      A52.13
  asymptomatic —*see* Syphilis, latent
  ataxia (locomotor) A52.11
  atrophoderma maculatum A51.39
  auricular fibrillation A52.06
  bladder (late) A52.76
  bone A52.77
    secondary A51.46
  brain A52.17
  breast (late) A52.79
  bronchus (late) A52.72
  bubo (primary) A51.0
  bulbar palsy A52.19
  bursa (late) A52.78
  cardiac decompensation A52.06
  cardiovascular A52.00
  central nervous system (late) (recurrent)
        (relapse) (tertiary) A52.3
    with
      ataxia A52.11
      general paralysis A52.17
        juvenile A50.45
      paresis (general) A52.17
        juvenile A50.45
      tabes (dorsalis) A52.11
        juvenile A50.45
      taboparesis A52.17
        juvenile A50.45
    aneurysm A52.05
    congenital A50.40
    juvenile A50.40
    remission in (sustained) A52.3
    serology doubtful, negative, or positive
      A52.3
    specified nature or site NEC A52.19
    vascular A52.05
  cerebral A52.17
    meningovascular A52.13
    nerves (multiple palsies) A52.15
    sclerosis A52.17
    thrombosis A52.05
  cerebrospinal (tabetic type) A52.12
  cerebrovascular A52.05
  cervix (late) A52.76
  chancre (multiple) A51.0
    extragenital A51.2
    Rollet's A51.0
  Charcot's joint A52.16
  chorioretinitis A51.43
    congenital A50.01
    late A52.71
    prenatal A50.01
  choroiditis —*see* Syphilitic chorioretinitis
  choroidoretinitis —*see* Syphilitic
      chorioretinitis
  ciliary body (secondary) A51.43
    late A52.71
  colon (late) A52.74
  combined spinal sclerosis A52.11
  condyloma (latum) A51.31

Syphilis, syphilitic *(Continued)*
  congenital A50.9
    with
      paresis (general) A50.45
      tabes (dorsalis) A50.45
      taboparesis A50.45
    chorioretinitis, choroiditis A50.01 *[H32]*
    early, or less than 2 years after birth NEC
        A50.2
      with manifestations —*see* Syphilis,
          congenital, early, symptomatic
      latent (without manifestations) A50.1
        negative spinal fluid test A50.1
        serology positive A50.1
      symptomatic A50.09
        cutaneous A50.06
        mucocutaneous A50.07
        oculopathy A50.01
        osteochondropathy A50.02
        pharyngitis A50.03
        pneumonia A50.04
        rhinitis A50.05
        visceral A50.08
    interstitial keratitis A50.31
    juvenile neurosyphilis A50.45
    late, or 2 years or more after birth NEC
        A50.7
      chorioretinitis, choroiditis A50.32
      interstitial keratitis A50.31
      juvenile neurosyphilis A50.45
      latent (without manifestations) A50.6
        negative spinal fluid test A50.6
        serology positive A50.6
      symptomatic or with manifestations
          NEC A50.59
        arthropathy A50.55
        cardiovascular A50.54
        Clutton's joints A50.51
        Hutchinson's teeth A50.52
        Hutchinson's triad A50.53
        osteochondropathy A50.56
        saddle nose A50.57
  conjugal A53.9
    tabes A52.11
  conjunctiva (late) A52.71
  contact Z20.2
  cord bladder A52.19
  cornea, late A52.71
  coronary (artery) (sclerosis) A52.06
  coryza, congenital A50.05
  cranial nerve A52.15
    multiple palsies A52.15
  cutaneous —*see* Syphilis, skin
  dacryocystitis (late) A52.71
  degeneration, spinal cord A52.12
  dementia paralytica A52.17
    juvenilis A50.45
  destruction of bone A52.77
  dilatation, aorta A52.01
  due to blood transfusion A53.9
  dura mater A52.13
  ear A52.79
    inner A52.79
      nerve (eighth) A52.15
      neurorecurrence A52.15
  early A51.9
    cardiovascular A52.00
    central nervous system A52.3
    latent (without manifestations) (less
        than 2 years after infection)
        A51.5
      negative spinal fluid test A51.5
      serological relapse after treatment
        A51.5
      serology positive A51.5
    relapse (treated, untreated) A51.9
    skin A51.39
    symptomatic A51.9
      extragenital chancre A51.2
      primary, except extragenital chancre
        A51.0

Syphilis, syphilitic *(Continued)*
  early *(Continued)*
    symptomatic *(Continued)*
      secondary (*see also* Syphilis, secondary)
          A51.39
        relapse (treated, untreated) A51.49
      ulcer A51.39
  eighth nerve (neuritis) A52.15
  endemic A65
  endocarditis A52.03
    aortic A52.03
    pulmonary A52.03
  epididymis (late) A52.76
  epiglottis (late) A52.73
  epiphysitis (congenital) (early) A50.02
  episcleritis (late) A52.71
  esophagus A52.79
  eustachian tube A52.73
  exposure to Z20.2
  eye A52.71
  eyelid (late) (with gumma) A52.71
  fallopian tube (late) A52.76
  fracture A52.77
  gallbladder (late) A52.74
  gastric (polyposis) (late) A52.74
  general A53.9
    paralysis A52.17
      juvenile A50.45
  genital (primary) A51.0
  glaucoma A52.71
  gumma NEC A52.79
    cardiovascular system A52.00
    central nervous system A52.3
    congenital A50.59
  heart (block) (decompensation) (disease)
      (failure) A52.06 *[I52]*
    valve NEC A52.03
  hemianesthesia A52.19
  hemianopsia A52.71
  hemiparesis A52.17
  hemiplegia A52.17
  hepatic artery A52.09
  hepatis A52.74
  hepatomegaly, congenital A50.08
  hereditaria tarda —*see* Syphilis, congenital,
      late
  hereditary —*see* Syphilis, congenital
  Hutchinson's teeth A50.52
  hyalitis A52.71
  inactive —*see* Syphilis, latent
  infantum —*see* Syphilis, congenital
  inherited —*see* Syphilis, congenital
  internal ear A52.79
  intestine (late) A52.74
  iris, iritis (secondary) A51.43
    late A52.71
  joint (late) A52.77
  keratitis (congenital) (interstitial) (late)
      A50.31
  kidney (late) A52.75
  lacrimal passages (late) A52.71
  larynx (late) A52.73
  late A52.9
    cardiovascular A52.00
    central nervous system A52.3
    kidney A52.75
    latent or 2 years or more after infection
        (without manifestations) A52.8
      negative spinal fluid test A52.8
      serology positive A52.8
    paresis A52.17
    specified site NEC A52.79
    symptomatic or with manifestations A52.79
    tabes A52.11
  latent A53.0
    with signs or symptoms - code by site and
        stage under Syphilis
    central nervous system A52.2
    date of infection unspecified A53.0
    early, or less than 2 years after infection
        A51.5

Syphilis, syphilitic *(Continued)*
  latent *(Continued)*
    follow-up of latent syphilis A53.0
      date of infection unspecified A53.0
      late, or 2 years or more after infection
        A52.8
      late, or 2 years or more after infection
        A52.8
      positive serology (only finding) A53.0
        date of infection unspecified A53.0
        early, or less than 2 years after infection
          A51.5
        late, or 2 years or more after infection
          A52.8
  lens (late) A52.71
  leukoderma A51.39
    late A52.79
  lienitis A52.79
  lip A51.39
    chancre (primary) A51.2
    late A52.79
  Lissauer's paralysis A52.17
  liver A52.74
  locomotor ataxia A52.11
  lung A52.72
  lymph gland (early) (secondary) A51.49
    late A52.79
  lymphadenitis (secondary) A51.49
  macular atrophy of skin A51.39
    striated A52.79
  mediastinum (late) A52.73
  meninges (adhesive) (brain) (spinal cord)
    A52.13
  meningitis A52.13
    acute (secondary) A51.41
    congenital A50.41
  meningoencephalitis A52.14
  meningovascular A52.13
    congenital A50.41
  mesarteritis A52.09
    brain A52.04
  middle ear A52.77
  mitral stenosis A52.03
  monoplegia A52.17
  mouth (secondary) A51.39
    late A52.79
  mucocutaneous (secondary) A51.39
    late A52.79
  mucous
    membrane (secondary) A51.39
      late A52.79
    patches A51.39
      congenital A50.07
  mulberry molars A50.52
  muscle A52.78
  myocardium A52.06
  nasal sinus (late) A52.73
  neonatorum —*see* Syphilis, congenital
  nephrotic syndrome (secondary)
    A51.44
  nerve palsy (any cranial nerve)
    A52.15
    multiple A52.15
  nervous system, central A52.3
  neuritis A52.15
    acoustic A52.15
  neurorecidive of retina A52.19
  neuroretinitis A52.19
  newborn —*see* Syphilis, congenital
  nodular superficial (late) A52.79
  nonvenereal A65
  nose (late) A52.73
    saddle back deformity A50.57
  occlusive arterial disease A52.09
  oculopathy A52.71
  ophthalmic (late) A52.71
  optic nerve (atrophy) (neuritis) (papilla)
    A52.15
  orbit (late) A52.71
  organic A53.9
  osseous (late) A52.77

Syphilis, syphilitic *(Continued)*
  osteochondritis (congenital) (early) A50.02
    [M90.80]
  osteoporosis A52.77
  ovary (late) A52.76
  oviduct (late) A52.76
  palate (late) A52.79
  pancreas (late) A52.74
  paralysis A52.17
    general A52.17
      juvenile A50.45
  paresis (general) A52.17
    juvenile A50.45
  paresthesia A52.19
  Parkinson's disease or syndrome A52.19
  paroxysmal tachycardia A52.06
  pemphigus (congenital) A50.06
  penis (chancre) A51.0
    late A52.76
  pericardium A52.06
  perichondritis, larynx (late) A52.73
  periosteum (late) A52.77
    congenital (early) A50.02 [M90.80]
    early (secondary) A51.46
  peripheral nerve A52.79
  petrous bone (late) A52.77
  pharynx (late) A52.73
    secondary A51.39
  pituitary (gland) A52.79
  pleura (late) A52.73
  pneumonia, white A50.04
  pontine lesion A52.17
  portal vein A52.09
  primary A51.0
    anal A51.1
    and secondary —*see* Syphilis, secondary
    central nervous system A52.3
    extragenital chancre NEC A51.2
    fingers A51.2
    genital A51.0
    lip A51.2
    specified site NEC A51.2
    tonsils A51.2
  prostate (late) A52.76
  ptosis (eyelid) A52.71
  pulmonary (late) A52.72
    artery A52.09
  pyelonephritis (late) A52.75
  recently acquired, symptomatic A51.9
  rectum (late) A52.74
  respiratory tract (late) A52.73
  retina, late A52.71
  retrobulbar neuritis A52.15
  salpingitis A52.76
  sclera (late) A52.71
  sclerosis
    cerebral A52.17
    coronary A52.06
    multiple A52.11
  scotoma (central) A52.71
  scrotum (late) A52.76
  secondary (and primary) A51.49
    adenopathy A51.49
    anus A51.39
    bone A51.46
    chorioretinitis, choroiditis A51.43
    hepatitis A51.45
    liver A51.45
    lymphadenitis A51.49
    meningitis (acute) A51.41
    mouth A51.39
    mucous membranes A51.39
    periosteum, periostitis A51.46
    pharynx A51.39
    relapse (treated, untreated) A51.49
    skin A51.39
    specified form NEC A51.49
    tonsil A51.39
    ulcer A51.39
    viscera NEC A51.49
    vulva A51.39

Syphilis, syphilitic *(Continued)*
  seminal vesicle (late) A52.76
  seronegative with signs or symptoms -
    code by site and stage under
    Syphilis
  seropositive
    with signs or symptoms - code
      by site and stage under
      Syphilis
    follow-up of latent syphilis —*see* Syphilis,
      latent
    only finding —*see* Syphilis, latent
  seventh nerve (paralysis) A52.15
  sinus, sinusitis (late) A52.73
  skeletal system A52.77
  skin (with ulceration) (early) (secondary)
    A51.39
    late or tertiary A52.79
  small intestine A52.74
  spastic spinal paralysis A52.17
  spermatic cord (late) A52.76
  spinal (cord) A52.12
  spleen A52.79
  splenomegaly A52.79
  spondylitis A52.77
  staphyloma A52.71
  stigmata (congenital) A50.59
  stomach A52.74
  synovium A52.78
  tabes dorsalis (late) A52.11
    juvenile A50.45
  tabetic type A52.11
    juvenile A50.45
  taboparesis A52.17
    juvenile A50.45
  tachycardia A52.06
  tendon (late) A52.78
  tertiary A52.9
    with symptoms NEC A52.79
    cardiovascular A52.00
    central nervous system A52.3
    multiple NEC A52.79
    specified site NEC A52.79
  testis A52.76
  thorax A52.73
  throat A52.73
  thymus (gland) (late) A52.79
  thyroid (late) A52.79
  tongue (late) A52.79
  tonsil (lingual) (late) A52.73
    primary A51.2
    secondary A51.39
  trachea (late) A52.73
  tunica vaginalis (late) A52.76
  ulcer (any site) (early) (secondary)
    A51.39
    late A52.79
    perforating A52.79
      foot A52.11
  urethra (late) A52.76
  urogenital (late) A52.76
  uterus (late) A52.76
  uveal tract (secondary) A51.43
    late A52.71
  uveitis (secondary) A51.43
    late A52.71
  uvula (late) (perforated) A52.79
  vagina A51.0
    late A52.76
  valvulitis NEC A52.03
  vascular A52.00
    brain (cerebral) A52.05
  ventriculi A52.74
  vesicae urinariae (late) A52.76
  viscera (abdominal) (late) A52.74
    secondary A51.49
  vitreous (opacities) (late) A52.71
    hemorrhage A52.71
  vulva A51.0
    late A52.76
    secondary A51.39

◀ New   ◀|||| Revised   ~~deleted~~ Deleted

Syphiloma A52.79
cardiovascular system A52.00
central nervous system A52.3
circulatory system A52.00
congenital A50.59
Syphilophobia F45.29
Syringadenoma —*see also* Neoplasm, skin, benign
papillary —*see* Neoplasm, skin, benign
Syringobulbia G95.0

Syringocystadenoma —*see* Neoplasm, skin, benign
papillary —*see* Neoplasm, skin, benign
Syringoma —*see also* Neoplasm, skin, benign
chondroid —*see* Neoplasm, skin, benign
Syringomyelia G95.0
Syringomyelitis —*see* Encephalitis
Syringomyelocele —*see* Spina bifida
Syringopontia G95.0

System, systemic —*see also* condition
disease, combined —*see* Degeneration, combined
inflammatory response syndrome (SIRS) of non-infectious origin (without organ dysfunction) R65.10
with acute organ dysfunction R65.11
lupus erythematosus M32.9
inhibitor present D68.62

T

Tabacism, tabacosis, tabagism —*see also*
  Poisoning, tobacco
  meaning dependence (without remission)
    F17.200
  with
    disorder F17.299
      remission F17.211
      specified disorder NEC F17.298
    withdrawal F17.203
Tabardillo A75.9
  flea-borne A75.2
  louse-borne A75.0
Tabes, tabetic A52.10
  with
    central nervous system syphilis A52.10
    Charcot's joint A52.16
    cord bladder A52.19
    crisis, viscera (any) A52.19
    paralysis, general A52.17
    paresis (general) A52.17
    perforating ulcer (foot) A52.19
  arthropathy (Charcot) A52.16
  bladder A52.19
  bone A52.11
  cerebrospinal A52.12
  congenital A50.45
  conjugal A52.10
  dorsalis A52.11
    juvenile A50.49
  juvenile A50.49
  latent A52.19
  mesenterica A18.39
  paralysis, insane, general A52.17
  spasmodic A52.17
  syphilis (cerebrospinal) A52.12
Taboparalysis A52.17
Taboparesis (remission) A52.17
  juvenile A50.45
TAC (trigeminal autonomic cephalgia) NEC
    G44.099
  intractable G44.091
  not intractable G44.099
Tache noir S60.22-
Tachyalimentation K91.2
Tachyarrhythmia, tachyrhythmia —*see*
    Tachycardia
Tachycardia R00.0
  atrial (paroxysmal) I47.1
  auricular I47.1
  AV nodal re-entry (re-entrant) I47.1
  junctional (paroxysmal) I47.1
  newborn P29.11
  nodal (paroxysmal) I47.1
  non-paroxysmal AV nodal I45.89
  paroxysmal (sustained) (nonsustained)
    I47.9
    with sinus bradycardia I49.5
    atrial (PAT) I47.1
    atrioventricular (AV) (re-entrant) I47.1
      psychogenic F54
    junctional I47.1
      ectopic I47.1
    nodal I47.1
    psychogenic (atrial) (supraventricular)
      (ventricular) F54
    supraventricular (sustained) I47.1
      psychogenic F54
    ventricular I47.2
      psychogenic F54
  psychogenic F45.8
  sick sinus I49.5
  sinoauricular NOS R00.0
    paroxysmal I47.1
  sinus [sinusal] NOS R00.0
    paroxysmal I47.1
  supraventricular I47.1
  ventricular (paroxysmal) (sustained) I47.2
    psychogenic F54
Tachygastria K31.89

Tachypnea R06.82
  hysterical F45.8
  newborn (idiopathic) (transitory) P22.1
  psychogenic F45.8
  transitory, of newborn P22.1
TACO (transfusion associated circulatory
    overload) E87.71
Taenia (infection) (infestation) B68.9
  diminuta B71.0
  echinococcal infestation B67.90
  mediocanellata B68.1
  nana B71.0
  saginata B68.1
  solium (intestinal form) B68.0
    larval form —*see* Cysticercosis
Taeniasis (intestine) —*see* Taenia
Tag (hypertrophied skin) (infected) L91.8
  adenoid J35.8
  anus K64.4
  hemorrhoidal K64.4
  hymen N89.8
  perineal N90.89
  preauricular Q17.0
  sentinel K64.4
  skin L91.8
    accessory (congenital) Q82.8
    anus K64.4
    congenital Q82.8
    preauricular Q17.0
  tonsil J35.8
  urethra, urethral N36.8
  vulva N90.89
Tahyna fever B33.8
Takahara's disease E80.3
Takayasu's disease or syndrome M31.4
Talcosis (pulmonary) J62.0
Talipes (congenital) Q66.89
  acquired, planus —*see* Deformity, limb, flat
    foot
  asymmetric Q66.89
  calcaneovalgus Q66.4
  calcaneovarus Q66.1
  calcaneus Q66.89
  cavus Q66.7
  equinovalgus Q66.6
  equinovarus Q66.0
  equinus Q66.89
  percavus Q66.7
  planovalgus Q66.6
  planus (acquired) (any degree) —*see also*
    Deformity, limb, flat foot
    congenital Q66.5-
    due to rickets (sequelae) E64.3
  valgus Q66.6
  varus Q66.3
Tall stature, constitutional E34.4
Talma's disease M62.89
Talon noir S90.3-
  hand S60.22-
  heel S90.3-
  toe S90.1-
Tamponade, heart I31.4
Tanapox (virus disease) B08.71
Tangier disease E78.6
Tantrum, child problem F91.8
Tapeworm (infection) (infestation) —*see*
    Infestation, tapeworm
Tapia's syndrome G52.7
TAR (thrombocytopenia with absent radius)
    syndrome Q87.2
Tarral-Besnier disease L44.0
Tarsal tunnel syndrome —*see* Syndrome, tarsal
    tunnel
Tarsalgia —*see* Pain, limb, lower
Tarsitis (eyelid) H01.8
  syphilitic A52.71
  tuberculous A18.4
Tartar (teeth) (dental calculus) K03.6
Tattoo (mark) L81.8
Tauri's disease E74.09
Taurodontism K00.2

Taussig-Bing syndrome Q20.1
Taybi's syndrome Q87.2
Tay-Sachs amaurotic familial idiocy or disease
    E75.02
TBI (traumatic brain injury) —*see* category
    S06
Teacher's node or nodule J38.2
Tear, torn (traumatic) —*see also* Laceration
  with abortion —*see* Abortion
  annular fibrosis M51.35
  anus, anal (sphincter) S31.831
    complicating delivery
      with third degree perineal laceration
        O70.2
        with mucosa O70.3
      without third degree perineal laceration
        O70.4
    nontraumatic (healed) (old) K62.81
  articular cartilage, old —*see* Derangement,
    joint, articular cartilage, by site
  bladder
    with ectopic or molar pregnancy O08.6
    following ectopic or molar pregnancy
      O08.6
    obstetrical O71.5
    traumatic —*see* Injury, bladder
  bowel
    with ectopic or molar pregnancy O08.6
    following ectopic or molar pregnancy
      O08.6
    obstetrical trauma O71.5
  broad ligament
    with ectopic or molar pregnancy O08.6
    following ectopic or molar pregnancy
      O08.6
    obstetrical trauma O71.6
  bucket handle (knee) (meniscus) —*see* Tear,
    meniscus
  capsule, joint —*see* Sprain
  cartilage —*see also* Sprain
    articular, old —*see* Derangement, joint,
      articular cartilage, by site
  cervix
    with ectopic or molar pregnancy O08.6
    following ectopic or molar pregnancy
      O08.6
    obstetrical trauma (current) O71.3
    old N88.1
    traumatic —*see* Injury, uterus
  dural G97.41
    nontraumatic G96.11
  internal organ —*see* Injury, by site
  knee cartilage
    articular (current) S83.3-
    old —*see* Derangement, knee, meniscus,
      due to old tear
  ligament —*see* Sprain
  meniscus (knee) (current injury) S83.209
    bucket-handle S83.20-
    lateral
      bucket-handle S83.25-
      complex S83.27-
      peripheral S83.26-
      specified type NEC S83.28-
    medial
      bucket-handle S83.21-
      complex S83.23-
      peripheral S83.22-
      specified type NEC S83.24-
    old —*see* Derangement, knee, meniscus,
      due to old tear
    site other than knee - code as Sprain
    specified type NEC S83.20-
  muscle —*see* Strain
  pelvic
    floor, complicating delivery O70.1
    organ NEC, obstetrical trauma O71.5
      with ectopic or molar pregnancy O08.6
      following ectopic or molar pregnancy
        O08.6
  perineal, secondary O90.1

◀ New   ◀ Revised   ~~deleted~~ Deleted

Tear, torn *(Continued)*
  periurethral tissue, obstetrical trauma O71.82
    with ectopic or molar pregnancy O08.6
    following ectopic or molar pregnancy
      O08.6
  rectovaginal septum —*see* Laceration, vagina
  retina, retinal (without detachment)
      (horseshoe) —*see also* Break, retina,
      horseshoe
    with detachment —*see* Detachment, retina,
      with retinal, break
  rotator cuff (nontraumatic) M75.10-
    complete M75.12-
    incomplete M75.11-
    traumatic S46.01-
      capsule S43.42-
  semilunar cartilage, knee —*see* Tear, meniscus
  supraspinatus (complete) (incomplete)
      (nontraumatic) (*see also* Tear, rotator
      cuff) M75.10-
  tendon —*see* Strain
  tentorial, at birth P10.4
  umbilical cord
    complicating delivery O69.89
  urethra
    with ectopic or molar pregnancy O08.6
    following ectopic or molar pregnancy
      O08.6
    obstetrical trauma O71.5
  uterus —*see* Injury, uterus
  vagina —*see* Laceration, vagina
  vessel, from catheter —*see* Puncture,
      accidental complicating surgery
  vulva, complicating delivery O70.0
Tear-stone —*see* Dacryolith
Teeth —*see also* condition
  grinding
    psychogenic F45.8
    sleep related G47.63
Teething (syndrome) K00.7
Telangiectasia, telangiectasis (verrucous)
      I78.1
  ataxic (cerebellar) (Louis-Bar) G11.3
  familial I78.0
  hemorrhagic, hereditary (congenital) (senile)
      I78.0
  hereditary, hemorrhagic (congenital) (senile)
      I78.0
  juxtafoveal H35.07-
  macular H35.07-
  parafoveal H35.07-
  retinal (idiopathic) (juxtafoveal) (macular)
      (parafoveal) H35.07-
  spider I78.1
Telephone scatologia F65.89
Telescoped bowel or intestine K56.1
  congenital Q43.8
Temperature
  body, high (of unknown origin) R50.9
  cold, trauma from T69.9
    newborn P80.0
    specified effect NEC T69.8
Temple —*see* condition
Temporal —*see* condition
Temporomandibular joint pain-dysfunction
      syndrome M26.62
Temporosphenoidal —*see* condition
Tendency
  bleeding —*see* Defect, coagulation
  suicide
    meaning personal history of attempted
      suicide Z91.5
    meaning suicidal ideation —*see* Ideation,
      suicidal
  to fall R29.6
Tenderness, abdominal R10.819
  epigastric R10.816
  generalized R10.817
  left lower quadrant R10.814
  left upper quadrant R10.812
  periumbic R10.815

Tenderness, abdominal *(Continued)*
  rebound R10.829
    epigastric R10.826
    generalized R10.827
    left lower quadrant R10.824
    left upper quadrant R10.822
    periumbic R10.825
    right lower quadrant R10.823
    right upper quadrant R10.821
  right lower quadrant R10.813
  right upper quadrant R10.811
Tendinitis, tendonitis —*see also* Enthesopathy
  Achilles M76.6-
  adhesive —*see* Tenosynovitis, specified type
      NEC
    shoulder —*see* Capsulitis, adhesive
  bicipital M75.2-
  calcific M65.2-
    ankle M65.27-
    foot M65.27-
    forearm M65.23-
    hand M65.24-
    lower leg M65.26-
    multiple sites M65.29
    pelvic region M65.25-
    shoulder M75.3-
    specified site NEC M65.28
    thigh M65.25-
    upper arm M65.22-
  due to use, overuse, pressure —*see also*
      Disorder, soft tissue, due to use
    specified NEC —*see* Disorder, soft tissue,
      due to use, specified NEC
  gluteal M76.0-
  patellar M76.5-
  peroneal M76.7-
  psoas M76.1-
  tibial (posterior) M76.82-
    anterior M76.81-
  trochanteric —*see* Bursitis, hip, trochanteric
Tendon —*see* condition
Tendosynovitis —*see* Tenosynovitis
Tenesmus (rectal) R19.8
  vesical R30.1
Tennis elbow —*see* Epicondylitis, lateral
Tenonitis —*see also* Tenosynovitis
  eye (capsule) H05.04-
Tenontosynovitis —*see* Tenosynovitis
Tenontothecitis —*see* Tenosynovitis
Tenophyte —*see* Disorder, synovium, specified
      type NEC
Tenosynovitis (*see also* Synovitis) M65.9
  adhesive —*see* Tenosynovitis, specified type
      NEC
    shoulder —*see* Capsulitis, adhesive
  bicipital (calcifying) —*see* Tendinitis,
      bicipital
  gonococcal A54.49
  in (due to)
    crystals M65.8-
    gonorrhea A54.49
    syphilis (late) A52.78
    use, overuse, pressure —*see also* Disorder,
      soft tissue, due to use
    specified NEC —*see* Disorder, soft tissue,
      due to use, specified NEC
  infective NEC M65.1-
    ankle M65.17-
    foot M65.17-
    forearm M65.13-
    hand M65.14-
    lower leg M65.16-
    multiple sites M65.19
    pelvic region M65.15-
    shoulder region M65.11-
    specified site NEC M65.18
    thigh M65.15-
    upper arm M65.12-
  radial styloid M65.4
  shoulder region M65.81-
    adhesive —*see* Capsulitis, adhesive

Tenosynovitis *(Continued)*
  specified type NEC M65.88-
    ankle M65.87-
    foot M65.87-
    forearm M65.83-
    hand M65.84-
    lower leg M65.86-
    multiple sites M65.89
    pelvic region M65.85-
    shoulder region M65.81-
    specified site NEC M65.88
    thigh M65.85-
    upper arm M65.82-
  tuberculous —*see* Tuberculosis, tenosynovitis
Tenovaginitis —*see* Tenosynovitis
Tension
  arterial, high —*see also* Hypertension
    without diagnosis of hypertension R03.0
  headache G44.209
    intractable G44.201
    not intractable G44.209
  nervous R45.0
  pneumothorax J93.0
  premenstrual N94.3
  state (mental) F48.9
Tentorium —*see* condition
Teratencephalus Q89.8
Teratism Q89.7
Teratoblastoma (malignant) —*see* Neoplasm,
      malignant, by site
Teratocarcinoma —*see also* Neoplasm,
      malignant, by site
  liver C22.7
Teratoma (solid) —*see also* Neoplasm, uncertain
      behavior, by site
  with embryonal carcinoma, mixed —*see*
      Neoplasm, malignant, by site
  with malignant transformation —*see*
      Neoplasm, malignant, by site
  adult (cystic) —*see* Neoplasm, benign, by site
  benign —*see* Neoplasm, benign, by site
  combined with choriocarcinoma —*see*
      Neoplasm, malignant, by site
  cystic (adult) —*see* Neoplasm, benign, by site
  differentiated —*see* Neoplasm, benign, by site
  embryonal —*see also* Neoplasm, malignant,
      by site
    liver C22.7
  immature —*see* Neoplasm, malignant, by site
  liver C22.7
    adult, benign, cystic, differentiated type or
      mature D13.4
  malignant —*see also* Neoplasm, malignant,
      by site
    anaplastic —*see* Neoplasm, malignant, by
      site
    intermediate —*see* Neoplasm, malignant,
      by site
    specified site —*see* Neoplasm,
      malignant, by site
    unspecified site C62.90
    undifferentiated —*see* Neoplasm,
      malignant, by site
  mature —*see* Neoplasm, uncertain behavior,
      by site
    malignant —*see* Neoplasm, by site,
      malignant, by site
  ovary D27.-
    embryonal, immature or malignant C56-
  solid —*see* Neoplasm, uncertain behavior,
      by site
  testis C62.9-
    adult, benign, cystic, differentiated type or
      mature D29.2-
    scrotal C62.1-
    undescended C62.0-
Termination
  anomalous —*see also* Malposition,
      congenital
    right pulmonary vein Q26.3
  pregnancy, elective Z33.2

Ternidens diminutus infestation B81.8
Ternidensiasis B81.8
Terror (s) night (child) F51.4
Terrorism, victim of Z65.4
Terry's syndrome H44.2-
Tertiary —see condition
Test, tests, testing (for)
  adequacy (for dialysis)
    hemodialysis Z49.31
    peritoneal Z49.32
  blood pressure Z01.30
    abnormal reading —see Blood, pressure
  blood typing Z01.83
    Rh typing Z01.83
  blood-alcohol Z04.8
    positive —see Findings, abnormal, in
      blood
  blood-drug Z04.8
    positive —see Findings, abnormal, in
      blood
  cardiac pulse generator (battery) Z45.010
  fertility Z31.41
  genetic
    disease carrier status for procreative
      management
      female Z31.430
      male Z31.440
    male partner of patient with recurrent
      pregnancy loss Z31.441
    procreative management NEC
      female Z31.438
      male Z31.448
  hearing Z01.10
    with abnormal findings NEC Z01.118
  HIV (human immunodeficiency virus)
    nonconclusive (in infants) R75
    positive Z21
    seropositive Z21
  immunity status Z01.84
  intelligence NEC Z01.89
  laboratory (as part of a general medical
    examination) Z00.00
    with abnormal finding Z00.01
    for medicolegal reason NEC Z04.8
  male partner of patient with recurrent
    pregnancy loss Z31.441
  Mantoux (for tuberculosis) Z11.1
    abnormal result R76.11
  pregnancy, positive first pregnancy —see
    Pregnancy, normal, first
  procreative Z31.49
    fertility Z31.41
  skin, diagnostic
    allergy Z01.82
      special screening examination —see
        Screening, by name of disease
    Mantoux Z11.1
    tuberculin Z11.1
  specified NEC Z01.89
  tuberculin Z11.1
    abnormal result R76.11
  vision Z01.00
    with abnormal findings Z01.01
  Wassermann Z11.3
    positive —see Serology for syphilis,
      positive
Testicle, testicular, testis —see also condition
  feminization syndrome (see also Syndrome,
    androgen insensitivity) E34.51
  migrans Q55.29
Tetanus, tetanic (cephalic) (convulsions) A35
  with
    abortion A34
    ectopic or molar pregnancy O08.0
  following ectopic or molar pregnancy
    O08.0
  inoculation reaction (due to serum) —see
    Complications, vaccination
  neonatorum A33
  obstetrical A34
  puerperal, postpartum, childbirth A34

Tetany (due to) R29.0
  alkalosis E87.3
  associated with rickets E55.0
  convulsions R29.0
    hysterical F44.5
  functional (hysterical) F44.5
  hyperkinetic R29.0
    hysterical F44.5
  hyperpnea R06.4
    hysterical F44.5
    psychogenic F45.8
  hyperventilation (see also Hyperventilation)
    R06.4
    hysterical F44.5
  neonatal (without calcium or magnesium
    deficiency) P71.3
  parathyroid (gland) E20.9
  parathyroprival E89.2
  post- (para)thyroidectomy E89.2
  postoperative E89.2
  pseudotetany R29.0
  psychogenic (conversion reaction) F44.5
Tetralogy of Fallot Q21.3
Tetraplegia (chronic) (see also Quadriplegia)
  G82.50-
Thailand hemorrhagic fever A91
Thalassanemia —see Thalassemia
Thalassemia (anemia) (disease) D56.9
  with other hemoglobinopathy D56.8
  alpha (major) (severe) (triple gene defect)
    D56.0
    minor D56.3
    silent carrier D56.3
    trait D56.3
  beta (severe) D56.1
    homozygous D56.1
    major D56.1
    minor D56.3
    trait D56.3
  delta-beta (homozygous) D56.2
    minor D56.3
    trait D56.3
  dominant D56.8
  hemoglobin
    C D56.8
    E-beta D56.5
  intermedia D56.1
  major D56.1
  minor D56.3
  mixed D56.8
  sickle-cell —see Disease, sickle-cell,
    thalassemia
  specified type NEC D56.8
  trait D56.3
  variants D56.8
Thanatophoric dwarfism or short stature Q77.1
Thaysen-Gee disease (nontropical sprue) K90.0
Thaysen's disease K90.0
Thecoma D27-
  luteinized D27-
  malignant C56-
Thelarche, premature E30.8
Thelaziasis B83.8
Thelitis N61
  puerperal, postpartum or gestational —see
    Infection, nipple
Therapeutic —see condition
Therapy
  drug, long-term (current) (prophylactic)
    agents affecting estrogen receptors and
      estrogen levels NEC Z79.818
    anastrozole (Arimidex) Z79.811
    antibiotics Z79.2
      short-term use - omit code
    anticoagulants Z79.01
    anti-inflammatory Z79.1
    antiplatelet Z79.02
    antithrombotics Z79.02
    aromatase inhibitors Z79.811
    aspirin Z79.82
    birth control pill or patch Z79.3

Therapy (Continued)
  drug, long-term (Continued)
    bisphosphonates Z79.83
    contraceptive, oral Z79.3
    drug, specified NEC Z79.899
    estrogen receptor downregulators
      Z79.818
    Evista Z79.810
    exemestane (Aromasin) Z79.811
    Fareston Z79.810
    fulvestrant (Faslodex) Z79.818
    gonadotropin-releasing hormone (GnRH)
      agonist Z79.818
    goserelin acetate (Zoladex) Z79.818
    hormone replacement (postmenopausal)
      Z79.890
    insulin Z79.4
    letrozole (Femara) Z79.811
    leuprolide acetate (leuprorelin) (Lupron)
      Z79.818
    megestrol acetate (Megace) Z79.818
    methadone
      for pain management Z79.891
      maintenance therapy F11.20
    Nolvadex Z79.810
    opiate analgesic Z79.891
    oral contraceptive Z79.3
    raloxifene (Evista) Z79.810
    selective estrogen receptor modulators
      (SERMs) Z79.810
    short term - omit code
    steroids
      inhaled Z79.51
      systemic Z79.52
    tamoxifen (Nolvadex) Z79.810
    toremifene (Fareston) Z79.810
Thermic —see condition
Thermography (abnormal) (see also Abnormal,
    diagnostic imaging) R93.8
  breast R92.8
Thermoplegia T67.0
Thesaurismosis, glycogen —see Disease,
    glycogen storage
Thiamin deficiency E51.9
  specified NEC E51.8
Thiaminic deficiency with beriberi E51.11
Thibierge-Weissenbach syndrome —see
    Sclerosis, systemic
Thickening
  bone —see Hypertrophy, bone
  breast N64.59
  endometrium R93.8
  epidermal L85.9
    specified NEC L85.8
  hymen N89.6
  larynx J38.7
  nail L60.2
    congenital Q84.5
  periosteal —see Hypertrophy, bone
  pleura J92.9
    with asbestos J92.0
  skin R23.4
  subepiglottic J38.7
  tongue K14.8
  valve, heart —see Endocarditis
Thigh —see condition
Thinning vertebra —see Spondylopathy,
    specified NEC
Thirst, excessive R63.1
  due to deprivation of water T73.1
Thomsen disease G71.12
Thoracic —see also condition
  kidney Q63.2
  outlet syndrome G54.0
Thoracogastroschisis (congenital) Q79.8
Thoracopagus Q89.4
Thorax —see condition
Thorn's syndrome N28.89
Thorson-Björck syndrome E34.0
Threadworm (infection) (infestation)
  B80

◀ New   ◀▥ Revised   ~~deleted~~ Deleted

Threatened
abortion O20.0
with subsequent abortion O03.9
job loss, anxiety concerning Z56.2
labor (without delivery) O47.9
after 37 completed weeks of gestation O47.1
before 37 completed weeks of gestation O47.0-
loss of job, anxiety concerning Z56.2
miscarriage O20.0
unemployment, anxiety concerning Z56.2
Three-day fever A93.1
Threshers' lung J67.0
Thrix annulata (congenital) Q84.1
Throat —see condition
Thrombasthenia (Glanzmann) (hemorrhagic) (hereditary) D69.1
Thromboangiitis I73.1
obliterans (general) I73.1
cerebral I67.89
vessels
brain I67.89
spinal cord I67.89
Thromboarteritis —see Arteritis
Thromboasthenia (Glanzmann) (hemorrhagic) (hereditary) D69.1
Thrombocytasthenia (Glanzmann) D69.1
Thrombocythemia (essential) (hemorrhagic) (idiopathic) (primary) D47.3
Thrombocytopathy (dystrophic) (granulopenic) D69.1
Thrombocytopenia, thrombocytopenic D69.6
with absent radius (TAR) Q87.2
congenital D69.42
dilutional D69.59
due to
drugs D69.59
extracorporeal circulation of blood D69.59
(massive)blood transfusion D69.59
platelet alloimmunization D69.59
essential D69.3
heparin induced (HIT) D75.82
hereditary D69.42
idiopathic D69.3
neonatal, transitory P61.0
due to
exchange transfusion P61.0
idiopathic maternal thrombocytopenia P61.0
isoimmunization P61.0
primary NEC D69.49
idiopathic D69.3
puerperal, postpartum O72.3
secondary D69.59
transient neonatal P61.0
Thrombocytosis, essential D47.3
primary D47.3
Thromboembolism —see Embolism
Thrombopathy (Bernard-Soulier) D69.1
constitutional D68.0
Willebrand-Jurgens D68.0
Thrombopenia —see Thrombocytopenia
Thrombophilia D68.59
primary NEC D68.59
secondary NEC D68.69
specified NEC D68.69
Thrombophlebitis I80.9
antepartum O22.2-
deep O22.3-
superficial O22.2-
cavernous (venous) sinus G08
complicating pregnancy O22.5-
nonpyogenic I67.6
cerebral (sinus) (vein) G08
nonpyogenic I67.6
sequelae G09
due to implanted device —see Complications, by site and type, specified NEC
during or resulting from a procedure NEC T81.72

Thrombophlebitis (Continued)
femoral vein (superficial) I80.1-
femoropopliteal vein I80.0-
hepatic (vein) I80.8
idiopathic, recurrent I82.1
iliofemoral I80.1-
intracranial venous sinus (any) G08
nonpyogenic I67.6
sequelae G09
intraspinal venous sinuses and veins G08
nonpyogenic G95.19
lateral (venous) sinus G08
nonpyogenic I67.6
leg I80.299
superficial I80.0-
longitudinal (venous) sinus G08
nonpyogenic I67.6
lower extremity I80.299
migrans, migrating I82.1
pelvic
with ectopic or molar pregnancy O08.0
following ectopic or molar pregnancy O08.0
puerperal O87.1
popliteal vein —see Phlebitis, leg, deep, popliteal
portal (vein) K75.1
postoperative T81.72
pregnancy —see Thrombophlebitis, antepartum
puerperal, postpartum, childbirth O87.0
deep O87.1
pelvic O87.1
septic O86.81
superficial O87.0
saphenous (greater) (lesser) I80.0-
sinus (intracranial) G08
nonpyogenic I67.6
specified site NEC I80.8
tibial vein I80.23-
Thrombosis, thrombotic (bland) (multiple) (progressive) (silent) (vessel) I82.90
anal K64.5
antepartum —see Thrombophlebitis, antepartum
aorta, aortic I74.10
abdominal I74.09
saddle I74.01
bifurcation I74.09
saddle I74.01
specified site NEC I74.19
terminal I74.09
thoracic I74.11
valve —see Endocarditis, aortic
apoplexy I63.3
artery, arteries (postinfectional) I74.9
auditory, internal —see Occlusion, artery, precerebral, specified NEC
basilar —see Occlusion, artery, basilar
carotid (common) (internal) —see Occlusion, artery, carotid
cerebellar (anterior inferior) (posterior inferior) (superior) —see Occlusion, artery, cerebellar
cerebral —see Occlusion, artery, cerebral
choroidal (anterior) —see Occlusion, artery, cerebral, specified NEC
communicating, posterior —see Occlusion, artery, cerebral, specified NEC
coronary —see also Infarct, myocardium
not resulting in infarction I24.0
hepatic I74.8
hypophyseal —see Occlusion, artery, cerebral, specified NEC
iliac I74.5
limb I74.4
lower I74.3
upper I74.2
meningeal, anterior or posterior —see Occlusion, artery, cerebral, specified NEC

Thrombosis, thrombotic (Continued)
artery, arteries (Continued)
mesenteric (with gangrene) K55.0
ophthalmic —see Occlusion, artery, retina
pontine —see Occlusion, artery, cerebral, specified NEC
precerebral —see Occlusion, artery, precerebral
pulmonary (iatrogenic) —see Embolism, pulmonary
renal N28.0
retinal —see Occlusion, artery, retina
spinal, anterior or posterior G95.11
traumatic NEC T14.8
vertebral —see Occlusion, artery, vertebral
atrium, auricular —see also Infarct, myocardium
following acute myocardial infarction (current complication) I23.6
not resulting in infarction I24.0
basilar (artery) —see Occlusion, artery, basilar
brain (artery) (stem) —see also Occlusion, artery, cerebral
due to syphilis A52.05
puerperal O99.43
sinus —see Thrombosis, intracranial venous sinus
capillary I78.8
cardiac —see also Infarct, myocardium
not resulting in infarction I24.0
valve —see Endocarditis
carotid (artery) (common) (internal) —see Occlusion, artery, carotid
cavernous (venous) sinus —see Thrombosis, intracranial venous sinus
cerebellar artery (anterior inferior) (posterior inferior) (superior) I66.3
cerebral (artery) —see Occlusion, artery, cerebral
cerebrovenous sinus —see also Thrombosis, intracranial venous sinus
puerperium O87.3
chronic I82.91
coronary (artery) (vein) —see also Infarct, myocardium
not resulting in infarction I24.0
corpus cavernosum N48.89
cortical I66.9
deep —see Embolism, vein, lower extremity
due to device, implant or graft (see also Complications, by site and type, specified NEC) T85.86
arterial graft NEC T82.868
breast (implant) T85.86
catheter NEC T85.86
dialysis (renal) T82.868
intraperitoneal T85.86
infusion NEC T82.868
spinal (epidural) (subdural) T85.86
urinary (indwelling) T83.86
electronic (electrode) (pulse generator) (stimulator)
bone T84.86
cardiac T82.867
nervous system (brain) (peripheral nerve) (spinal) T85.86
urinary T83.86
fixation, internal (orthopedic) NEC T84.86
gastrointestinal (bile duct) (esophagus) T85.86
genital NEC T83.86
heart T82.867
joint prosthesis T84.86
ocular (corneal graft) (orbital implant) NEC T85.86
orthopedic NEC T84.86
specified NEC T85.86
urinary NEC T83.86
vascular NEC T82.868
ventricular intracranial shunt T85.86

Thrombosis, thrombotic (Continued)
during the puerperium —see Thrombosis, puerperal
endocardial —see also Infarct, myocardium
  not resulting in infarction I24.0
eye —see Occlusion, retina
genital organ
  female NEC N94.89
    pregnancy —see Thrombophlebitis, antepartum
  male N50.1
gestational —see Phlebopathy, gestational
heart (chamber) —see also Infarct, myocardium
  not resulting in infarction I24.0
hepatic (vein) I82.0
  artery I74.8
history (of) Z86.718
intestine (with gangrene) K55.0
intracardiac NEC (apical) (atrial) (auricular) (ventricular) (old) I51.3
intracranial (arterial) I66.9
  venous sinus (any) G08
    nonpyogenic origin I67.6
    puerperium O87.3
intramural —see also Infarct, myocardium
  not resulting in infarction I24.0
intraspinal venous sinuses and veins G08
  nonpyogenic G95.19
kidney (artery) N28.0
lateral (venous) sinus —see Thrombosis, intracranial venous sinus
leg —see Thrombosis, vein, lower extremity
  arterial I74.3
liver (venous) I82.0
  artery I74.8
  portal vein I81
longitudinal (venous) sinus —see Thrombosis, intracranial venous sinus
lower limb —see Thrombosis, vein, lower extremity
lung (iatrogenic) (postoperative) —see Embolism, pulmonary
meninges (brain) (arterial) I66.8
mesenteric (artery) (with gangrene) K55.0
  vein (inferior) (superior) I81
mitral I34.8
mural —see also Infarct, myocardium
  due to syphilis A52.06
  not resulting in infarction I24.0
omentum (with gangrene) K55.0
ophthalmic —see Occlusion, retina
pampiniform plexus (male) N50.1
parietal —see also Infarct, myocardium
  not resulting in infarction I24.0
penis, superficial vein N48.81
perianal venous K64.5
peripheral arteries I74.4
  upper I74.2
personal history (of) Z86.718
portal I81
  due to syphilis A52.09
precerebral artery —see Occlusion, artery, precerebral
puerperal, postpartum O87.0
  brain (artery) O99.43
    venous (sinus) O87.3
  cardiac O99.43
  cerebral (artery) O99.43
    venous (sinus) O87.3
  superficial O87.0
pulmonary (artery) (iatrogenic) (postoperative) (vein) —see Embolism, pulmonary
renal (artery) N28.0
  vein I82.3
resulting from presence of device, implant or graft —see Complications, by site and type, specified NEC
retina, retinal —see Occlusion, retina

Thrombosis, thrombotic (Continued)
scrotum N50.1
seminal vesicle N50.1
sigmoid (venous) sinus —see Thrombosis, intracranial venous sinus
sinus, intracranial (any) —see Thrombosis, intracranial venous sinus
specified site NEC I82.890
  chronic I82.891
spermatic cord N50.1
spinal cord (arterial) G95.11
  due to syphilis A52.09
  pyogenic origin G06.1
spleen, splenic D73.5
  artery I74.8
testis N50.1
traumatic NEC T14.8
tricuspid I07.8
tumor —see Neoplasm, by site
tunica vaginalis N50.1
umbilical cord (vessels), complicating delivery O69.5
vas deferens N50.1
vein (acute) I82.90
  antecubital I82.61-
    chronic I82.71-
  axillary I82.A1-
    chronic I82.A2-
  basilic I82.61-
    chronic I82.71-
  brachial I82.62-
    chronic I82.72-
  brachiocephalic (innominate) I82.290
    chronic I82.291
  cerebral, nonpyogenic I67.6
  cephalic I82.61-
    chronic I82.71-
  chronic I82.91
  deep (DVT) I82.40-
    calf I82.4Z-
      chronic I82.5Z-
    lower leg I82.4Z-
      chronic I82.5Z-
    thigh I82.4Y-
      chronic I82.5Y-
    upper leg I82.4Y
      chronic I82.5y-
  femoral I82.41-
    chronic I82.51-
  iliac (iliofemoral) I82.42-
    chronic I82.52-
  innominate I82.290
    chronic I82.291
  internal jugular I82.C1-
    chronic I82.C2-
  lower extremity
    deep I82.40-
      chronic I82.50-
        specified NEC I82.49-
          chronic NEC I82.59-
      distal
        deep I82.4Z-
      proximal
        deep I82.4Y-
          chronic I82.5Y-
    superficial I82.81-
  perianal K64.5
  popliteal I82.43-
    chronic I82.53-
  radial I82.62-
    chronic I82.72-
  renal I82.3
  saphenous (greater) (lesser) I82.81-
  specified NEC I82.890
    chronic NEC I82.891
  subclavian I82.B1-
    chronic I82.B2-
  thoracic NEC I82.290
    chronic I82.291
  tibial I82.44-
    chronic I82.54-

Thrombosis, thrombotic (Continued)
vein (Continued)
  ulnar I82.62-
    chronic I82.72-
  upper extremity I82.60-
    chronic I82.70-
    deep I82.62-
      chronic I82.72-
    superficial I82.61-
      chronic I82.71-
  vena cava
    inferior I82.220
      chronic I82.221
    superior I82.210
      chronic I82.211
  venous, perianal K64.5
ventricle —see also Infarct, myocardium
  following acute myocardial infarction (current complication) I23.6
  not resulting in infarction I24.0
Thrombus —see Thrombosis
Thrush —see also Candidiasis
newborn P37.5
oral B37.0
vaginal B37.3
Thumb —see also condition
sucking (child problem) F98.8
Thymitis E32.8
Thymoma (benign) D15.0
malignant C37
Thymus, thymic (gland) —see condition
Thyrocele —see Goiter
Thyroglossal —see also condition
cyst Q89.2
duct, persistent Q89.2
Thyroid (gland) (body) —see also condition
hormone resistance E07.89
lingual Q89.2
nodule (cystic) (nontoxic) (single) E04.1
Thyroiditis E06.9
acute (nonsuppurative) (pyogenic) (suppurative) E06.0
autoimmune E06.3
chronic (nonspecific) (sclerosing) E06.5
  with thyrotoxicosis, transient E06.2
  fibrous E06.5
  lymphadenoid E06.3
  lymphocytic E06.3
  lymphoid E06.3
de Quervain's E06.1
drug-induced E06.4
fibrous (chronic) E06.5
giant-cell (follicular) E06.1
granulomatous (de Quervain) (subacute) E06.1
Hashimoto's (struma lymphomatosa) E06.3
iatrogenic E06.4
ligneous E06.5
lymphocytic (chronic) E06.3
lymphoid E06.3
lymphomatous E06.3
nonsuppurative E06.1
postpartum, puerperal O90.5
pseudotuberculous E06.1
pyogenic E06.0
radiation E06.4
Riedel's E06.5
subacute (granulomatous) E06.1
suppurative E06.0
tuberculous A18.81
viral E06.1
woody E06.5
Thyrolingual duct, persistent Q89.2
Thyromegaly E01.0
Thyrotoxic
crisis —see Thyrotoxicosis
heart disease or failure (see also Thyrotoxicosis) E05.90 [I43]
  with thyroid storm E05.91 [I43]
storm —see Thyrotoxicosis

◀ New   ⬅ Revised   ~~deleted~~ Deleted

Thyrotoxicosis (recurrent) E05.90
  with
    goiter (diffuse) E05.00
      with thyroid storm E05.01
      adenomatous uninodular E05.10
        with thyroid storm E05.11
      multinodular E05.20
        with thyroid storm E05.21
      nodular E05.20
        with thyroid storm E05.21
      uninodular E05.10
        with thyroid storm E05.11
    infiltrative
      dermopathy E05.00
        with thyroid storm E05.01
      ophthalmopathy E05.00
        with thyroid storm E05.01
    single thyroid nodule E05.10
      with thyroid storm E05.11
    thyroid storm E05.91
  due to
    ectopic thyroid nodule or tissue E05.30
      with thyroid storm E05.31
    ingestion of (excessive) thyroid material
      E05.40
      with thyroid storm E05.41
    overproduction of thyroid-stimulating
      hormone E05.80
      with thyroid storm E05.81
    specified cause NEC E05.80
      with thyroid storm E05.81
  factitia E05.40
    with thyroid storm E05.41
  heart E05.90 *[I43]*
    with thyroid storm E05.91 *[I43]*
    failure E05.90 *[I43]*
  neonatal (transient) P72.1
  transient with chronic thyroiditis E06.2
Tibia vara —*see* Osteochondrosis, juvenile, tibia
Tic (disorder) F95.9
  breathing F95.8
  child problem F95.0
  compulsive F95.1
  de la Tourette F95.2
  degenerative (generalized) (localized) G25.69
    facial G25.69
  disorder
    chronic
      motor F95.1
      vocal F95.1
    combined vocal and multiple motor F95.2
    transient F95.0
  douloureux G50.0
    atypical G50.1
    postherpetic, postzoster B02.22
  drug-induced G25.61
  eyelid F95.8
  habit F95.9
    chronic F95.1
    transient of childhood F95.0
  lid, transient of childhood F95.0
  motor-verbal F95.2
  occupational F48.8
  orbicularis F95.8
    transient of childhood F95.0
  organic origin G25.69
  postchoreic G25.69
  psychogenic, compulsive F95.1
  salaam R25.8
  spasm (motor or vocal) F95.9
    chronic F95.1
    transient of childhood F95.0
  specified NEC F95.8
Tick-borne —*see* condition
Tietze's disease or syndrome M94.0
Tight, tightness
  anus K62.89
  chest R07.89
  fascia (lata) M62.89
  foreskin (congenital) N47.1
  hymen, hymenal ring N89.6

Tight, tightness *(Continued)*
  introitus (acquired) (congenital) N89.6
  rectal sphincter K62.89
  tendon —*see* Short, tendon
  urethral sphincter N35.9
Tilting vertebra —*see* Dorsopathy, deforming,
  specified NEC
Timidity, child F93.8
Tin-miner's lung J63.5
Tinea (intersecta) (tarsi) B35.9
  amiantacea L44.8
  asbestina B35.0
  barbae B35.0
  beard B35.0
  black dot B35.0
  blanca B36.2
  capitis B35.0
  corporis B35.4
  cruris B35.6
  flava B36.0
  foot B35.3
  furfuracea B36.0
  imbricata (Tokelau) B35.5
  kerion B35.0
  manuum B35.2
  microsporic —*see* Dermatophytosis
  nigra B36.1
  nodosa —*see* Piedra
  pedis B35.3
  scalp B35.0
  specified site NEC B35.8
  sycosis B35.0
  tonsurans B35.0
  trichophytic —*see* Dermatophytosis
  unguium B35.1
  versicolor B36.0
Tingling sensation (skin) R20.2
Tinnitus (audible) (aurium) (subjective) —*see*
  subcategory H93.1
Tipped tooth (teeth) M26.33
Tipping
  pelvis M95.5
    with disproportion (fetopelvic) O33.0
      causing obstructed labor O65.0
  tooth (teeth), fully erupted M26.33
Tiredness R53.83
Tissue —*see* condition
Tobacco (nicotine)
  dependence —*see* Dependence, drug, nicotine
  harmful use Z72.0
  heart —*see* Tobacco, toxic effect
  maternal use, affecting newborn P04.2
  toxic effect —*see* Table of Drugs and
    Chemicals, by substance, poisoning
    chewing tobacco —*see* Table of Drugs
      and Chemicals, by substance,
      poisoning
    cigarettes —*see* Table of Drugs and
      Chemicals, by substance,
      poisoning
  use Z72.0
    complicating
      childbirth O99.334
      pregnancy O99.33-
      puerperium O99.335
    counseling and surveillance Z71.6
  withdrawal state —*see* Dependence, drug,
    nicotine
Tocopherol deficiency E56.0
Todd's
  cirrhosis K74.3
  paralysis (postepileptic) (transitory) G83.84
Toe —*see* condition
Toilet, artificial opening —*see* Attention to,
  artificial, opening
Tokelau (ringworm) B35.5
Tollwut —*see* Rabies
Tommaselli's disease R31.9
  correct substance properly administered —*see*
    Table of Drugs and Chemicals, by drug,
    adverse effect

Tommaselli's disease *(Continued)*
  overdose or wrong substance given or
    taken —*see* Table of Drugs and
    Chemicals, by drug, poisoning
Tongue —*see also* condition
  tie Q38.1
Tonic pupil —*see* Anomaly, pupil, function,
  tonic pupil
Toni-Fanconi syndrome (cystinosis) E72.09
  with cystinosis E72.04
Tonsil —*see* condition
Tonsillitis (acute) (catarrhal) (croupous)
    (follicular) (gangrenous) (infective)
    (lacunar) (lingual) (malignant)
    (membranous) (parenchymatous)
    (phlegmonous) (pseudomembranous)
    (purulent) (septic) (subacute)
    (suppurative) (toxic) (ulcerative)
    (vesicular) (viral) J03.90
  chronic J35.01
    with adenoiditis J35.03
  diphtheritic A36.0
  hypertrophic J35.01
    with adenoiditis J35.03
  recurrent J03.91
  specified organism NEC J03.80
    recurrent J03.81
  staphylococcal J03.80
    recurrent J03.81
  streptococcal J03.00
    recurrent J03.01
  tuberculous A15.8
  Vincent's A69.1
Tooth, teeth —*see* condition
Toothache K08.8
Topagnosis R20.8
Tophi —*see* Gout, chronic
TORCH infection —*see* Infection, congenital
  without active infection P00.2
Torn —*see* Tear
Tornwaldt's cyst or disease J39.2
Torsion
  accessory tube —*see* Torsion, fallopian tube
  adnexa (female) —*see* Torsion, fallopian tube
  aorta, acquired I77.1
  appendix epididymis N44.04
  appendix testis N44.03
  bile duct (common) (hepatic) K83.8
    congenital Q44.5
  bowel, colon or intestine K56.2
  cervix —*see* Malposition, uterus
  cystic duct K82.8
  dystonia —*see* Dystonia, torsion
  epididymis (appendix) N44.04
  fallopian tube N83.52
    with ovary N83.53
  gallbladder K82.8
    congenital Q44.1
  hydatid of Morgagni
    female N83.52
    male N44.03
  kidney (pedicle) (leading to infarction)
    N28.0
  Meckel's diverticulum (congenital) Q43.0
    malignant —*see* Table of Neoplasms, small
      intestine, malignant
  mesentery K56.2
  omentum K56.2
  organ or site, congenital NEC —*see* Anomaly,
    by site
  ovary (pedicle) N83.51
    with fallopian tube N83.53
    congenital Q50.2
  oviduct —*see* Torsion, fallopian tube
  penis (acquired) N48.82
    congenital Q55.63
  spasm —*see* Dystonia, torsion
  spermatic cord N44.02
    extravaginal N44.01
    intravaginal N44.02
  spleen D73.5

Torsion (Continued)
testis, testicle N44.00
  appendix N44.03
tibia —see Deformity, limb, specified type
  NEC, lower leg
uterus —see Malposition, uterus
Torticollis (intermittent) (spastic) M43.6
congenital (sternomastoid) Q68.0
due to birth injury P15.8
hysterical F44.4
ocular R29.891
psychogenic F45.8
  conversion reaction F44.4
rheumatic M43.6
rheumatoid M06.88
spasmodic G24.3
traumatic, current S13.4
Tortipelvis G24.1
Tortuous
artery I77.1
organ or site, congenital NEC —see Distortion
retinal vessel, congenital Q14.1
ureter N13.8
urethra N36.8
vein —see Varix
Torture, victim of Z65.4
Torula, torular (histolytica) (infection) —see
  Cryptococcosis
Torulosis —see Cryptococcosis
Torus (mandibularis) (palatinus) M27.0
fracture —see Fracture, by site, torus
Touraine's syndrome Q79.8
Tourette's syndrome F95.2
Tourniquet syndrome —see Constriction,
  external, by site
Tower skull Q75.0
with exophthalmos Q87.0
Toxemia R68.89
bacterial —see Sepsis
burn —see Burn
eclamptic (with pre-existing hypertension) —
  see Eclampsia
erysipelatous —see Erysipelas
fatigue R68.89
food —see Poisoning, food
gastrointestinal K52.1
intestinal K52.1
kidney —see Uremia
malarial —see Malaria
myocardial —see Myocarditis, toxic
of pregnancy —see Pre-eclampsia
pre-eclamptic —see Pre-eclampsia
small intestine K52.1
staphylococcal, due to food A05.0
stasis R68.89
uremic —see Uremia
urinary —see Uremia
Toxemica cerebropathia psychica
  (nonalcoholic) F04
alcoholic —see Alcohol, amnestic disorder
Toxic (poisoning) —see also condition T65.91
effect —see Table of Drugs and Chemicals, by
  substance, poisoning
shock syndrome A48.3
thyroid (gland) —see Thyrotoxicosis
Toxicemia —see Toxemia
Toxicity —see Table of Drugs and Chemicals, by
  substance, poisoning
fava bean D55.0
food, noxious —see Poisoning, food
from drug or nonmedicinal substance —see
  Table of Drugs and Chemicals, by
  drug
Toxicosis —see also Toxemia
capillary, hemorrhagic D69.0
Toxinfection, gastrointestinal K52.1
Toxocariasis B83.0
Toxoplasma, toxoplasmosis (acquired) B58.9
with
  hepatitis B58.1
  meningoencephalitis B58.2
  ocular involvement B58.00

Toxoplasma, toxoplasmosis (Continued)
with (Continued)
  other organ involvement B58.89
  pneumonia, pneumonitis B58.3
congenital (acute) (subacute) (chronic) P37.1
maternal, manifest toxoplasmosis in infant
  (acute) (subacute) (chronic) P37.1
tPA (rtPA) administation in a different facility
  within the last 24 hours prior to admission
  to current facility Z92.82
Trabeculation, bladder N32.89
Trachea —see condition
Tracheitis (catarrhal) (infantile) (membranous)
  (plastic) (septal) (suppurative) (viral)
  J04.10
with
  bronchitis (15 years of age and above) J40
   acute or subacute —see Bronchitis,
    acute
   chronic J42
   tuberculous NEC A15.5
   under 15 years of age J20.9
  laryngitis (acute) J04.2
   chronic J37.1
   tuberculous NEC A15.5
acute J04.10
  with obstruction J04.11
chronic J42
  with
   bronchitis (chronic) J42
   laryngitis (chronic) J37.1
diphtheritic (membranous) A36.89
due to external agent —see Inflammation,
  respiratory, upper, due to
syphilitic A52.73
tuberculous A15.5
Trachelitis (nonvenereal) —see Cervicitis
Tracheobronchial —see condition
Tracheobronchitis (15 years of age and
  above) —see also Bronchitis
due to
  Bordetella bronchiseptica A37.80
   with pneumonia A37.81
  Francisella tularensis A21.8
Tracheobronchomegaly Q32.4
with bronchiectasis J47.9
  with
   exacerbation (acute) J47.1
   lower respiratory infection J47.0
acquired J98.09
  with bronchiectasis J47.9
   with
    exacerbation (acute) J47.1
    lower respiratory infection J47.0
Tracheobronchopneumonitis —see Pneumonia,
  broncho-
Tracheocele (external) (internal) J39.8
congenital Q32.1
Tracheomalacia J39.8
congenital Q32.0
Tracheopharyngitis (acute) J06.9
chronic J42
due to external agent —see Inflammation,
  respiratory, upper, due to
Tracheostenosis J39.8
Tracheostomy
complication —see Complication,
  tracheostomy
status Z93.0
  attention to Z43.0
  malfunctioning J95.03
Trachoma, trachomatous A71.9
active (stage) A71.1
contraction of conjunctiva A71.1
dubium A71.0
healed or sequelae B94.0
initial (stage) A71.0
pannus A71.1
Türck's J37.0
Traction, vitreomacular H43.82-
Train sickness T75.3

Trait (s)
Hb-S D57.3
hemoglobin
  abnormal NEC D58.2
   with thalassemia D56.3
  C —see Disease, hemoglobin C
  S (Hb-S) D57.3
Lepore D56.3
personality, accentuated Z73.1
sickle-cell D57.3
  with elliptocytosis or spherocytosis
   D57.3
type A personality Z73.1
Tramp Z59.0
Trance R41.89
hysterical F44.89
Transaminasemia R74.0
Transection
abdomen (partial) S38.3
aorta (incomplete) —see also Injury, aorta
  complete —see Injury, aorta, laceration,
   major
carotid artery (incomplete) —see also Injury,
  blood vessel, carotid, laceration
  complete —see Injury, blood vessel, carotid,
   laceration, major
celiac artery (incomplete) S35.211
  branch (incomplete) S35.291
   complete S35.292
  complete S35.212
innominate
  artery (incomplete) —see also Injury, blood
   vessel, thoracic, innominate, artery,
   laceration
   complete —see Injury, blood vessel,
    thoracic, innominate, artery,
    laceration, major
  vein (incomplete) —see also Injury, blood
   vessel, thoracic, innominate, vein,
   laceration
   complete —see Injury, blood vessel,
    thoracic, innominate, vein,
    laceration, major
jugular vein (external) (incomplete) —see
  also Injury, blood vessel, jugular vein,
  laceration
  complete —see Injury, blood vessel, jugular
   vein, laceration, major
  internal (incomplete) —see also Injury,
   blood vessel, jugular vein, internal,
   laceration
   complete —see Injury, blood vessel,
    jugular vein, internal, laceration,
    major
mesenteric artery (incomplete) —see also
  Injury, mesenteric, artery, laceration
  complete —see Injury, mesenteric artery,
   laceration, major
pulmonary vessel (incomplete) —see
  also Injury, blood vessel, thoracic,
  pulmonary, laceration
  complete —see Injury, blood vessel,
   thoracic, pulmonary, laceration,
   major
subclavian —see Transection, innominate
vena cava (incomplete) —see also Injury, vena
  cava
  complete —see Injury, vena cava,
   laceration, major
vertebral artery (incomplete) —see also
  Injury, blood vessel, vertebral,
  laceration
  complete —see Injury, blood vessel,
   vertebral, laceration, major
Transfusion
associated (red blood cell) hemochromatosis
  E83.111
blood
  ABO incompatible —see Complication (s),
   transfusion, incompatibility reaction,
   ABO

◀ New   ⬅ Revised   ~~deleted~~ Deleted

Transfusion *(Continued)*
  blood *(Continued)*
    minor blood group (Duffy) (E) (K(ell))
      (Kidd) (Lewis) (M) (N) (P) (S) T80.89
    reaction or complication —*see*
      Complications, transfusion
    fetomaternal (mother) —*see* Pregnancy,
      complicated by, placenta, transfusion
      syndrome
    maternofetal (mother) —*see* Pregnancy,
      complicated by, placenta, transfusion
      syndrome
    placental (syndrome) (mother) —*see*
      Pregnancy, complicated by, placenta,
      transfusion syndrome
    reaction (adverse) —*see* Complications,
      transfusion
    related acute lung injury (TRALI) J95.84
    twin-to-twin —*see* Pregnancy, complicated by,
      placenta, transfusion syndrome, fetus
      to fetus
Transient (meaning homeless) *(see also*
  condition) Z59.0
Translocation
  balanced autosomal Q95.9
    in normal individual Q95.0
  chromosomes NEC Q99.8
    balanced and insertion in normal
      individual Q95.0
  Down's syndrome Q90.2
  trisomy
    13 Q91.6
    18 Q91.2
    21 Q90.2
Translucency, iris —*see* Degeneration, iris
**Transmission of chemical substances through
  the placenta** —*see* Absorption, chemical,
  through placenta
Transparency, lung, unilateral J43.0
Transplant (ed) (status) Z94.9
  awaiting organ Z76.82
  bone Z94.6
    marrow Z94.81
  candidate Z76.82
  complication —*see* Complication, transplant
  cornea Z94.7
  heart Z94.1
    and lung (s) Z94.3
    valve Z95.2
      prosthetic Z95.2
      specified NEC Z95.4
      xenogenic Z95.3
  intestine Z94.82
  kidney Z94.0
  liver Z94.4
  lung (s) Z94.2
    and heart Z94.3
  organ (failure) (infection) (rejection)Z94.9
    removal status Z98.85
  pancreas Z94.83
  skin Z94.5
  social Z60.3
  specified organ or tissue NEC Z94.89
  stem cells Z94.84
  tissue Z94.9
Transplants, ovarian, endometrial N80.1
Transposed —*see* Transposition
Transposition (congenital) —*see also*
  Malposition, congenital
  abdominal viscera Q89.3
  aorta (dextra) Q20.3
  appendix Q43.8
  colon Q43.8
  corrected Q20.5
  great vessels (complete) (partial) Q20.3
  heart Q24.0
    with complete transposition of viscera
      Q89.3
  intestine (large) (small) Q43.8
  reversed jejunal (for bypass) (status) Z98.0
  scrotum Q55.23

Transposition *(Continued)*
  stomach Q40.2
    with general transposition of viscera Q89.3
  tooth, teeth, fully erupted M26.30
  vessels, great (complete) (partial) Q20.3
  viscera (abdominal) (thoracic) Q89.3
Transsexualism F64.1
Transverse —*see also* condition
  arrest (deep), in labor O64.0
  lie (mother) O32.2
    causing obstructed labor O64.8
Transvestism, transvestitism (dual-role) F64.1
  fetishistic F65.1
Trapped placenta (with hemorrhage) O72.0
  without hemorrhage O73.0
Trauma, traumatism —*see also* Injury
  acoustic —*see* subcategory H83.3
  birth —*see* Birth, injury
  complicating ectopic or molar pregnancy
    O08.6
  during delivery O71.9
  following ectopic or molar pregnancy O08.6
  obstetric O71.9
    specified NEC O71.89
Traumatic —*see also* condition
  brain injury —*see* category S06
Treacher Collins syndrome Q75.4
Treitz's hernia —*see* Hernia, abdomen, specified
  site NEC
Trematode infestation —*see* Infestation, fluke
Trematodiasis —*see* Infestation, fluke
Trembling paralysis —*see* Parkinsonism
Tremor (s) R25.1
  drug induced G25.1
  essential (benign) G25.0
  familial G25.0
  hereditary G25.0
  hysterical F44.4
  intention G25.2
  medication induced postural G25.1
  mercurial —*see* subcategory T56.1
  Parkinson's —*see* Parkinsonism
  psychogenic (conversion reaction) F44.4
  senilis R54
  specified type NEC G25.2
Trench
  fever A79.0
  foot —*see* Immersion, foot
  mouth A69.1
Treponema pallidum infection —*see* Syphilis
Treponematosis
  due to
    T. pallidum —*see* Syphilis
    T. pertenue —*see* Yaws
Triad
  Hutchinson's (congenital syphilis) A50.53
  Kartagener's Q89.3
  Saint's —*see* Hernia, diaphragm
Trichiasis (eyelid) H02.059
  with entropion —*see* Entropion
  left H02.056
    lower H02.055
    upper H02.054
  right H02.053
    lower H02.052
    upper H02.051
Trichinella spiralis (infection) (infestation) B75
**Trichinellosis, trichiniasis, trichinelliasis,
  trichinosis** B75
  with muscle disorder B75 *[M63.80]*
    ankle B75 *[M63.87-]*
    foot B75 *[M63.87-]*
    forearm B75 *[M63.83-]*
    hand B75 *[M63.84-]*
    lower leg B75 *[M63.86-]*
    multiple sites B75 *[M63.89]*
    pelvic region B75 *[M63.85-]*
    shoulder region B75 *[M63.81-]*
    specified site NEC B75 *[M63.88]*
    thigh B75 *[M63.85-]*
    upper arm B75 *[M63.82-]*

Trichobezoar T18.9
  intestine T18.3
  stomach T18.2
Trichocephaliasis, trichocephalosis B79
Trichocephalus infestation B79
Trichoclasis L67.8
Trichoepithelioma —*see also* Neoplasm, skin,
  benign
  malignant —*see* Neoplasm, skin, malignant
Trichofolliculoma —*see* Neoplasm, skin,
  benign
Tricholemmoma —*see* Neoplasm, skin,
  benign
Trichomoniasis A59.9
  bladder A59.03
  cervix A59.09
  intestinal A07.8
  prostate A59.02
  seminal vesicles A59.09
  specified site NEC A59.8
  urethra A59.03
  urogenitalis A59.00
  vagina A59.01
  vulva A59.01
Trichomycosis
  axillaris A48.8
  nodosa, nodularis B36.8
Trichonodosis L67.8
Trichophytid, trichophyton infection —*see*
  Dermatophytosis
Trichophytobezoar T18.9
  intestine T18.3
  stomach T18.2
Trichophytosis —*see* Dermatophytosis
Trichoptilosis L67.8
Trichorrhexis (nodosa) (invaginata) L67.0
Trichosis axillaris A48.8
Trichosporosis nodosa B36.2
Trichostasis spinulosa (congenital) Q84.1
Trichostrongyliasis, trichostrongylosis (small
  intestine) B81.2
Trichostrongylus infection B81.2
Trichotillomania F63.3
Trichromat, trichromatopsia, anomalous
  (congenital) H53.55
Trichuriasis B79
Trichuris trichiura (infection) (infestation) (any
  site) B79
Tricuspid (valve) —*see* condition
Trifid —*see also* Accessory
  kidney (pelvis) Q63.8
  tongue Q38.3
Trigeminal neuralgia —*see* Neuralgia,
  trigeminal
Trigeminy R00.8
Trigger finger (acquired) M65.30
  congenital Q74.0
  index finger M65.32-
  little finger M65.35-
  middle finger M65.33-
  ring finger M65.34-
  thumb M65.31-
Trigonitis (bladder) (chronic)
  (pseudomembranous) N30.30
  with hematuria N30.31
Trigonocephaly Q75.0
Trilocular heart —*see* Cor triloculare
Trimethylaminuria E72.52
Tripartite placenta O43.19-
Triphalangeal thumb Q74.0
Triple —*see also* Accessory
  kidneys Q63.0
  uteri Q51.818
  X, female Q97.0
Triplegia G83.89
  congenital G80.8
Triplet (newborn) —*see also* Newborn, triplet
  complicating pregnancy —*see* Pregnancy,
  triplet
Triplication —*see* Accessory
Triploidy Q92.7

Trismus R25.2
  neonatorum A33
  newborn A33
Trisomy (syndrome) Q92.9
  13 (partial) Q91.7
    meiotic nondisjunction Q91.4
    mitotic nondisjunction Q91.5
    mosaicism Q91.5
    translocation Q91.6
  18 (partial) Q91.3
    meiotic nondisjunction Q91.0
    mitotic nondisjunction Q91.1
    mosaicism Q91.1
    translocation Q91.2
  20 Q92.8
  21 (partial) Q90.9
    meiotic nondisjunction Q90.0
    mitotic nondisjunction Q90.1
    mosaicism Q90.1
    translocation Q90.2
  22 Q92.8
  autosomes Q92.9
  chromosome specified NEC Q92.8
    partial Q92.2
      due to unbalanced translocation Q92.5
    specified NEC Q92.8
    whole (nonsex chromosome)
      meiotic nondisjunction Q92.0
      mitotic nondisjunction Q92.1
      mosaicism Q92.1
  due to
    dicentrics —*see* Extra, marker
        chromosomes
    extra rings —*see* Extra, marker
        chromosomes
    isochromosomes —*see* Extra, marker
        chromosomes
  specified NEC Q92.8
  whole chromosome Q92.9
    meiotic nondisjunction Q92.0
    mitotic nondisjunction Q92.1
    mosaicism Q92.1
    partial Q92.9
    specified NEC Q92.8
Tritanomaly, tritanopia H53.55
Trombiculosis, trombiculiasis, trombidiosis
    B88.0
Trophedema (congenital) (hereditary) Q82.0
Trophoblastic disease (*see also* Mole,
    hydatidiform) O01.9
Tropholymphedema Q82.0
Trophoneurosis NEC G96.8
  disseminated M34.9
Tropical —*see* condition
Trouble —*see also* Disease
  heart —*see* Disease, heart
  kidney —*see* Disease, renal
  nervous R45.0
  sinus —*see* Sinusitis
Trousseau's syndrome (thrombophlebitis
    migrans) I82.1
Truancy, childhood
  from school Z72.810
Truncus
  arteriosus (persistent) Q20.0
  communis Q20.0
Trunk —*see* condition
Trypanosomiasis
  African B56.9
    by Trypanosoma brucei
      gambiense B56.0
      rhodesiense B56.1
  American —*see* Chagas' disease
  Brazilian —*see* Chagas' disease
  by Trypanosoma
    brucei gambiense B56.0
    brucei rhodesiense B56.1
    cruzi —*see* Chagas' disease
  gambiensis, Gambian B56.0
  rhodesiensis, Rhodesian B56.1
  South American —*see* Chagas' disease

Trypanosomiasis (*Continued*)
  where
    African trypanosomiasis is prevalent B56.9
    Chagas' disease is prevalent B57.2
T-shaped incisors K00.2
Tsutsugamushi (disease) (fever) A75.3
Tube, tubal, tubular —*see* condition
Tubercle —*see also* Tuberculosis
  brain, solitary A17.81
  Darwin's Q17.8
  Ghon, primary infection A15.7
Tuberculid, tuberculide (indurating,
    subcutaneous) (lichenoid) (miliary)
    (papulonecrotic) (primary) (skin) A18.4
Tuberculoma —*see also* Tuberculosis
  brain A17.81
  meninges (cerebral) (spinal) A17.1
  spinal cord A17.81
Tuberculosis, tubercular, tuberculous
    (calcification) (calcified) (caseous)
    (chromogenic acid-fast bacilli)
    (degeneration) (fibrocaseous) (fistula)
    (interstitial) (isolated circumscribed
    lesions) (necrosis) (parenchymatous)
    (ulcerative) A15.9
  with pneumoconiosis (any condition in
    J60-J64) J65
  abdomen (lymph gland) A18.39
  abscess (respiratory) A15.9
    bone A18.03
      hip A18.02
      knee A18.02
      sacrum A18.01
      specified site NEC A18.03
      spinal A18.01
      vertebra A18.01
    brain A17.81
    breast A18.89
    Cowper's gland A18.15
    dura (mater) (cerebral) (spinal) A17.81
    epidural (cerebral) (spinal) A17.81
    female pelvis A18.17
    frontal sinus A15.8
    genital organs NEC A18.10
    genitourinary A18.10
    gland (lymphatic) —*see* Tuberculosis,
        lymph gland
    hip A18.02
    intestine A18.32
    ischiorectal A18.32
    joint NEC A18.02
      hip A18.02
      knee A18.02
      specified NEC A18.02
      vertebral A18.01
    kidney A18.11
    knee A18.02
    latent R76.11
    lumbar (spine) A18.01
    lung —*see* Tuberculosis, pulmonary
    meninges (cerebral) (spinal) A17.0
    muscle A18.09
    perianal (fistula) A18.32
    perinephritic A18.11
    perirectal A18.32
    rectum A18.32
    retropharyngeal A15.8
    sacrum A18.01
    scrofulous A18.2
    scrotum A18.15
    skin (primary) A18.4
    spinal cord A17.81
    spine or vertebra (column) A18.01
    subdiaphragmatic A18.31
    testis A18.15
    urinary A18.13
    uterus A18.17
  accessory sinus —*see* Tuberculosis, sinus
  Addison's disease A18.7
  adenitis —*see* Tuberculosis, lymph gland
  adenoids A15.8

Tuberculosis, tubercular, tuberculous
    (*Continued*)
  adenopathy —*see* Tuberculosis, lymph gland
  adherent pericardium A18.84
  adnexa (uteri) A18.17
  adrenal (capsule) (gland) A18.7
  alimentary canal A18.32
  anemia A18.89
  ankle (joint) (bone) A18.02
  anus A18.32
  apex, apical —*see* Tuberculosis, pulmonary
  appendicitis, appendix A18.32
  arachnoid A17.0
  artery, arteritis A18.89
    cerebral A18.89
  arthritis (chronic) (synovial) A18.02
    spine or vertebra (column) A18.01
  articular —*see* Tuberculosis, joint
  ascites A18.31
  asthma —*see* Tuberculosis, pulmonary
  axilla, axillary (gland) A18.2
  bladder A18.12
  bone A18.03
    hip A18.02
    knee A18.02
    limb NEC A18.03
    sacrum A18.01
    spine or vertebral column A18.01
  bowel (miliary) A18.32
  brain A17.81
  breast A18.89
  broad ligament A18.17
  bronchi, bronchial, bronchus A15.5
    ectasia, ectasis (bronchiectasis) —*see*
        Tuberculosis, pulmonary
    fistula A15.5
      primary (progressive) A15.7
    gland or node A15.4
      primary (progressive) A15.7
    lymph gland or node A15.4
      primary (progressive) A15.7
  bronchiectasis —*see* Tuberculosis, pulmonary
  bronchitis A15.5
  bronchopleural A15.6
  bronchopneumonia, bronchopneumonic —*see*
        Tuberculosis, pulmonary
  bronchorrhagia A15.5
  bronchotracheal A15.5
  bronze disease A18.7
  buccal cavity A18.83
  bulbourethral gland A18.15
  bursa A18.09
  cachexia A15.9
  cardiomyopathy A18.84
  caries —*see* Tuberculosis, bone
  cartilage A18.02
    intervertebral A18.01
  catarrhal —*see* Tuberculosis, respiratory
  cecum A18.32
  cellulitis (primary) A18.4
  cerebellum A17.81
  cerebral, cerebrum A17.81
  cerebrospinal A17.81
    meninges A17.0
  cervical (lymph gland or node) A18.2
  cervicitis, cervix (uteri) A18.16
  chest —*see* Tuberculosis, respiratory
  chorioretinitis A18.53
  choroid, choroiditis A18.53
  ciliary body A18.54
  colitis A18.32
  collier's J65
  colliquativa (primary) A18.4
  colon A18.32
  complex, primary A15.7
  congenital P37.0
  conjunctiva A18.59
  connective tissue (systemic) A18.89
  contact Z20.1
  cornea (ulcer) A18.52
  Cowper's gland A18.15

◀ New   ◀|||| Revised   ~~deleted~~ Deleted

Tuberculosis, tubercular, tuberculous
(Continued)
coxae A18.02
coxalgia A18.02
cul-de-sac of Douglas A18.17
curvature, spine A18.01
cutis (colliquativa) (primary) A18.4
cyst, ovary A18.18
cystitis A18.12
dactylitis A18.03
diarrhea A18.32
diffuse —*see* Tuberculosis, miliary
digestive tract A18.32
disseminated —*see* Tuberculosis, miliary
duodenum A18.32
dura (mater) (cerebral) (spinal) A17.0
   abscess (cerebral) (spinal) A17.81
dysentery A18.32
ear (inner) (middle) A18.6
   bone A18.03
   external (primary) A18.4
   skin (primary) A18.4
elbow A18.02
emphysema —*see* Tuberculosis, pulmonary
empyema A15.6
encephalitis A17.82
endarteritis A18.89
endocarditis A18.84
   aortic A18.84
   mitral A18.84
   pulmonary A18.84
   tricuspid A18.84
endocrine glands NEC A18.82
endometrium A18.17
enteric, enterica, enteritis A18.32
enterocolitis A18.32
epididymis, epididymitis A18.15
epidural abscess (cerebral) (spinal) A17.81
epiglottis A15.5
episcleritis A18.51
erythema (induratum) (nodosum) (primary)
   A18.4
esophagus A18.83
eustachian tube A18.6
exposure (to) Z20.1
exudative —*see* Tuberculosis, pulmonary
eye A18.50
eyelid (primary) (lupus) A18.4
fallopian tube (acute) (chronic) A18.17
fascia A18.09
fauces A15.8
female pelvic inflammatory disease A18.17
finger A18.03
first infection A15.7
gallbladder A18.83
ganglion A18.09
gastritis A18.83
gastrocolic fistula A18.32
gastroenteritis A18.32
gastrointestinal tract A18.32
general, generalized —*see* Tuberculosis,
   miliary
genital organs A18.10
genitourinary A18.10
genu A18.02
glandula suprarenalis A18.7
glandular, general A18.2
glottis A15.5
grinder's J65
gum A18.83
hand A18.03
heart A18.84
hematogenous —*see* Tuberculosis, miliary
hemoptysis —*see* Tuberculosis, pulmonary
hemorrhage NEC —*see* Tuberculosis,
   pulmonary
hemothorax A15.6
hepatitis A18.83
hilar lymph nodes A15.4
   primary (progressive) A15.7
hip (joint) (disease) (bone) A18.02

Tuberculosis, tubercular, tuberculous
(Continued)
hydropneumothorax A15.6
hydrothorax A15.6
hypoadrenalism A18.7
hypopharynx A15.8
ileocecal (hyperplastic) A18.32
ileocolitis A18.32
ileum A18.32
iliac spine (superior) A18.03
immunological findings only A15.7
indurativa (primary) A18.4
infantile A15.7
infection A15.9
   without clinical manifestations A15.7
infraclavicular gland A18.2
inguinal gland A18.2
inguinalis A18.2
intestine (any part) A18.32
iridocyclitis A18.54
iris, iritis A18.54
ischiorectal A18.32
jaw A18.03
jejunum A18.32
joint A18.02
   vertebral A18.01
keratitis (interstitial) A18.52
keratoconjunctivitis A18.52
kidney A18.11
knee (joint) A18.02
kyphosis, kyphoscoliosis A18.01
laryngitis A15.5
larynx A15.5
latent R76.11
leptomeninges, leptomeningitis (cerebral)
   (spinal) A17.0
lichenoides (primary) A18.4
linguae A18.83
lip A18.83
liver A18.83
lordosis A18.01
lung —*see* Tuberculosis, pulmonary
lupus vulgaris A18.4
lymph gland or node (peripheral) A18.2
   abdomen A18.39
   bronchial A15.4
      primary (progressive) A15.7
   cervical A18.2
   hilar A15.4
      primary (progressive) A15.7
   intrathoracic A15.4
      primary (progressive) A15.7
   mediastinal A15.4
      primary (progressive) A15.7
   mesenteric A18.39
   retroperitoneal A18.39
   tracheobronchial A15.4
      primary (progressive) A15.7
lymphadenitis —*see* Tuberculosis, lymph
   gland
lymphangitis —*see* Tuberculosis, lymph
   gland
lymphatic (gland) (vessel) —*see* Tuberculosis,
   lymph gland
mammary gland A18.89
marasmus A15.9
mastoiditis A18.03
mediastinal lymph gland or node
   A15.4
   primary (progressive) A15.7
mediastinitis A15.8
   primary (progressive) A15.7
mediastinum A15.8
   primary (progressive) A15.7
medulla A17.81
melanosis, Addisonian A18.7
meninges, meningitis (basilar) (cerebral)
   (cerebrospinal) (spinal) A17.0
meningoencephalitis A17.82
mesentery, mesenteric (gland or node)
   A18.39

Tuberculosis, tubercular, tuberculous
(Continued)
miliary A19.9
   acute A19.2
      multiple sites A19.1
      single specified site A19.0
   chronic A19.8
   specified NEC A19.8
millstone makers' J65
miner's J65
molder's J65
mouth A18.83
multiple A19.9
   acute A19.1
   chronic A19.8
muscle A18.09
myelitis A17.82
myocardium, myocarditis A18.84
nasal (passage) (sinus) A15.8
nasopharynx A15.8
neck gland A18.2
nephritis A18.11
nerve (mononeuropathy) A17.83
nervous system A17.9
nose (septum) A15.8
ocular A18.50
omentum A18.31
oophoritis (acute) (chronic) A18.17
optic (nerve trunk) (papilla) A18.59
orbit A18.59
orchitis A18.15
organ, specified NEC A18.89
osseous —*see* Tuberculosis, bone
osteitis —*see* Tuberculosis, bone
osteomyelitis —*see* Tuberculosis, bone
otitis media A18.6
ovary, ovaritis (acute) (chronic) A18.17
oviduct (acute) (chronic) A18.17
pachymeningitis A17.0
palate (soft) A18.83
pancreas A18.83
papulonecrotic (a) (primary) A18.4
parathyroid glands A18.82
paronychia (primary) A18.4
parotid gland or region A18.83
pelvis (bony) A18.03
penis A18.15
peribronchitis A15.5
pericardium, pericarditis A18.84
perichondritis, larynx A15.5
periostitis —*see* Tuberculosis, bone
perirectal fistula A18.32
peritoneum NEC A18.31
peritonitis A18.31
pharynx, pharyngitis A15.8
phlyctenulosis (keratoconjunctivitis) A18.52
phthisis NEC —*see* Tuberculosis, pulmonary
pituitary gland A18.82
pleura, pleural, pleurisy, pleuritis (fibrinous)
   (obliterative) (purulent) (simple plastic)
   (with effusion) A15.6
   primary (progressive) A15.7
pneumonia, pneumonic —*see* Tuberculosis,
   pulmonary
pneumothorax (spontaneous) (tense
   valvular) —*see* Tuberculosis, pulmonary
polyneuropathy A17.89
polyserositis A19.9
   acute A19.1
   chronic A19.8
potter's J65
prepuce A18.15
primary (complex) A15.7
proctitis A18.32
prostate, prostatitis A18.14
pulmonalis —*see* Tuberculosis, pulmonary
pulmonary (cavitated) (fibrotic) (infiltrative)
   (nodular) A15.0
   childhood type or first infection A15.7
   primary (complex) A15.7
pyelitis A18.11

Tuberculosis, tubercular, tuberculous
(Continued)
pyelonephritis A18.11
pyemia —see Tuberculosis, miliary
pyonephrosis A18.11
pyopneumothorax A15.6
pyothorax A15.6
rectum (fistula) (with abscess) A18.32
reinfection stage —see Tuberculosis,
pulmonary
renal A18.11
renis A18.11
respiratory A15.9
primary A15.7
specified site NEC A15.8
retina, retinitis A18.53
retroperitoneal (lymph gland or node)
A18.39
rheumatism NEC A18.09
rhinitis A15.8
sacroiliac (joint) A18.01
sacrum A18.01
salivary gland A18.83
salpingitis (acute) (chronic) A18.17
sandblaster's J65
sclera A18.51
scoliosis A18.01
scrofulous A18.2
scrotum A18.15
seminal tract or vesicle A18.15
senile A15.9
septic —see Tuberculosis, miliary
shoulder (joint) A18.02
blade A18.03
sigmoid A18.32
sinus (any nasal) A15.8
bone A18.03
epididymis A18.15
skeletal NEC A18.03
skin (any site) (primary) A18.4
small intestine A18.32
soft palate A18.83
spermatic cord A18.15
spine, spinal (column) A18.01
cord A17.81
medulla A17.81
membrane A17.0
meninges A17.0
spleen, splenitis A18.85
spondylitis A18.01
sternoclavicular joint A18.02
stomach A18.83
stonemason's J65
subcutaneous tissue (cellular) (primary)
A18.4
subcutis (primary) A18.4
subdeltoid bursa A18.83
submaxillary (region) A18.83
supraclavicular gland A18.2
suprarenal (capsule) (gland) A18.7
swelling, joint (see also category M01) (see also
Tuberculosis, joint) A18.02
symphysis pubis A18.02
synovitis A18.09
articular A18.02
spine or vertebra A18.01
systemic —see Tuberculosis, miliary
tarsitis A18.4
tendon (sheath) —see Tuberculosis,
tenosynovitis
tenosynovitis A18.09
spine or vertebra A18.01
testis A18.15
throat A15.8
thymus gland A18.82
thyroid gland A18.81
tongue A18.83
tonsil, tonsillitis A15.8
trachea, tracheal A15.5
lymph gland or node A15.4
primary (progressive) A15.7

Tuberculosis, tubercular, tuberculous
(Continued)
tracheobronchial A15.5
lymph gland or node A15.4
primary (progressive) A15.7
tubal (acute) (chronic) A18.17
tunica vaginalis A18.15
ulcer (skin) (primary) A18.4
bowel or intestine A18.32
specified NEC - code under Tuberculosis,
by site
unspecified site A15.9
ureter A18.11
urethra, urethral (gland) A18.13
urinary organ or tract A18.13
uterus A18.17
uveal tract A18.54
uvula A18.83
vagina A18.18
vas deferens A18.15
verruca, verrucosa (cutis) (primary)
A18.4
vertebra (column) A18.01
vesiculitis A18.15
vulva A18.18
wrist (joint) A18.02
Tuberculum
Carabelli (see Note at) K00.2
occlusal (see Note at) K00.2
paramolare K00.2
Tuberosity, enitre maxillary M26.07
Tuberous sclerosis (brain) Q85.1
Tubo-ovarian —see condition
Tuboplasty, after previous sterilization
Z31.0
aftercare Z31.42
Tubotympanitis, catarrhal (chronic) —see
Otitis, media, nonsuppurative, chronic,
serous
Tularemia A21.9
with
conjunctivitis A21.1
pneumonia A21.2
abdominal A21.3
bronchopneumonic A21.2
conjunctivitis A21.1
cryptogenic A21.3
enteric A21.3
gastrointestinal A21.3
generalized A21.7
ingestion A21.3
intestinal A21.3
oculoglandular A21.1
ophthalmic A21.1
pneumonia (any), pneumonic A21.2
pulmonary A21.2
sepsis A21.7
specified NEC A21.8
typhoidal A21.7
ulceroglandular A21.0
Tularensis conjunctivitis A21.1
Tumefaction —see also Swelling
liver —see Hypertrophy, liver
Tumor —see also Neoplasm, unspecified
behavior, by site
acinar cell —see Neoplasm, uncertain
behavior, by site
acinic cell —see Neoplasm, uncertain
behavior, by site
adenocarcinoid —see Neoplasm, malignant,
by site
adenomatoid —see also Neoplasm, benign,
by site
odontogenic —see Cyst, calcifying
odontogenic
adnexal (skin) —see Neoplasm, skin, benign,
by site
adrenal
cortical (benign) D35.0-
malignant C74.0-
rest —see Neoplasm, benign, by site

Tumor (Continued)
alpha-cell
malignant
pancreas C25.4
specified site NEC —see Neoplasm,
malignant, by site
unspecified site C25.4
pancreas D13.7
specified site NEC —see Neoplasm, benign,
by site
unspecified site D13.7
aneurysmal —see Aneurysm
aortic body D44.7
malignant C75.5
Askin's —see Neoplasm, connective tissue,
malignant
basal cell (see also Neoplasm, skin, uncertain
behavior) D48.5
Bednar —see Neoplasm, skin, malignant
benign (unclassified) —see Neoplasm, benign,
by site
beta-cell
malignant
pancreas C25.4
specified site NEC —see Neoplasm,
malignant, by site
unspecified site C25.4
pancreas D13.7
specified site NEC —see Neoplasm, benign,
by site
unspecified site D13.7
Brenner D27.9
borderline malignancy D39.1-
malignant C56-
proliferating D39.1
bronchial alveolar, intravascular D38.1
Brooke's —see Neoplasm, skin, benign
brown fat —see Lipoma
Burkitt —see Lymphoma, Burkitt
calcifying epithelial odontogenic —see Cyst,
calcifying odontogenic
carcinoid
benign D3A.00
appendix D3A.020
ascending colon D3A.022
bronchus (lung) D3A.090
cecum D3A.021
colon D3A.029
descending colon D3A.024
duodenum D3A.010
foregut NOS D3A.094
hindgut NOS D3A.096
ileum D3A.012
jejunum D3A.011
kidney D3A.093
large intestine D3A.029
lung (bronchus) D3A.090
midgut NOS D3A.095
rectum D3A.026
sigmoid colon D3A.025
small intestine D3A.019
specified NEC D3A.098
stomach D3A.092
thymus D3A.091
transverse colon D3A.023
malignant C7A.00
appendix C7A.020
ascending colon C7A.022
bronchus (lung) C7A.090
cecum C7A.021
colon C7A.029
descending colon C7A.024
duodenum C7A.010
foregut NOS C7A.094
hindgut NOS C7A.096
ileum C7A.012
jejunum C7A.011
kidney C7A.093
large intestine C7A.029
lung (bronchus) C7A.090
midgut NOS C7A.095

◀ New   ◀▥ Revised   ~~deleted~~ Deleted

Tumor *(Continued)*
  carcinoid *(Continued)*
    malignant *(Continued)*
      rectum C7A.026
      sigmoid colon C7A.025
      small intestine C7A.019
      specified NEC C7A.098
      stomach C7A.092
      thymus C7A.091
      transverse colon C7A.023
    mesentary metastasis C7B.04
    secondary C7B.00
      bone C7B.03
      distant lymph nodes C7B.01
      liver C7B.02
      peritoneum C7B.04
      specified NEC C7B.09
  carotid body D44.6
    malignant C75.4
  cells —*see also* Neoplasm, unspecified behavior, by site
    benign —*see* Neoplasm, benign, by site
    malignant —*see* Neoplasm, malignant, by site
    uncertain whether benign or malignant —*see* Neoplasm, uncertain behavior, by site
  cervix, in pregnancy or childbirth —*see* Pregnancy, complicated by, tumor, cervix
  chondromatous giant cell —*see* Neoplasm, bone, benign
  chromaffin —*see also* Neoplasm, benign, by site
    malignant —*see* Neoplasm, malignant, by site
  Cock's peculiar L72.3
  Codman's —*see* Neoplasm, bone, benign
  dentigerous, mixed —*see* Cyst, calcifying odontogenic
  dermoid —*see* Neoplasm, benign, by site
    with malignant transformation C56-
  desmoid (extra-abdominal) —*see also* Neoplasm, connective tissue, uncertain behavior
    abdominal —*see* Neoplasm, connective tissue, uncertain behavior
  embolus —*see* Neoplasm, secondary, by site
  embryonal (mixed) —*see also* Neoplasm, uncertain behavior, by site
    liver C22.7
  endodermal sinus
    specified site —*see* Neoplasm, malignant, by site
    unspecified site
      female C56.-
      male C62.90
  epithelial
    benign —*see* Neoplasm, benign, by site
    malignant —*see* Neoplasm, malignant, by site
  Ewing's —*see* Neoplasm, bone, malignant, by site
  fatty —*see* Lipoma
  fibroid —*see* Leiomyoma
  G cell
    malignant
      pancreas C25.4
      specified site NEC —*see* Neoplasm, malignant, by site
      unspecified site C25.4
    specified site —*see* Neoplasm, uncertain behavior, by site
    unspecified site D37.8
  germ cell —*see also* Neoplasm, malignant, by site
    mixed —*see* Neoplasm, malignant, by site
  ghost cell, odontogenic —*see* Cyst, calcifying odontogenic

Tumor *(Continued)*
  giant cell —*see also* Neoplasm, uncertain behavior, by site
    bone D48.0
      malignant —*see* Neoplasm, bone, malignant
    chondromatous —*see* Neoplasm, bone, benign
    malignant —*see* Neoplasm, malignant, by site
    soft parts —*see* Neoplasm, connective tissue, uncertain behavior
      malignant —*see* Neoplasm, connective tissue, malignant
  glomus D18.00
    intra-abdominal D18.03
    intracranial D18.02
    jugulare D44.7
      malignant C75.5
    skin D18.01
    specified site NEC D18.09
  gonadal stromal —*see* Neoplasm, uncertain behavior, by site
  granular cell —*see also* Neoplasm, connective tissue, benign
    malignant —*see* Neoplasm, connective tissue, malignant
  granulosa cell D39.1-
    juvenile D39.1-
    malignant C56-
  granulosa cell-theca cell D39.1-
    malignant C56-
  Grawitz's C64-
  hemorrhoidal —*see* Hemorrhoids
  hilar cell D27-
  hilus cell D27-
  Hurthle cell (benign) D34
    malignant C73
  hydatid —*see* Echinococcus
  hypernephroid —*see also* Neoplasm, uncertain behavior, by site
  interstitial cell —*see also* Neoplasm, uncertain behavior, by site
    benign —*see* Neoplasm, benign, by site
    malignant —*see* Neoplasm, malignant, by site
  intravascular bronchial alveolar D38.1
  islet cell —*see* Neoplasm, benign, by site
    malignant —*see* Neoplasm, malignant, by site
      pancreas C25.4
      specified site NEC —*see* Neoplasm, malignant, by site
      unspecified site C25.4
    pancreas D13.7
    specified site NEC —*see* Neoplasm, benign, by site
    unspecified site D13.7
  juxtaglomerular D41.0-
  Klatskin's C24.0
  Krukenberg's C79.6-
  Leydig cell —*see* Neoplasm, uncertain behavior, by site
    benign —*see* Neoplasm, benign, by site
      specified site —*see* Neoplasm, benign, by site
      unspecified site
        female D27.9
        male D29.20
    malignant —*see* Neoplasm, malignant, by site
      specified site —*see* Neoplasm, malignant, by site
      unspecified site
        female C56.9
        male C62.90
    specified site —*see* Neoplasm, uncertain behavior, by site
    unspecified site
      female D39.10
      male D40.10

Tumor *(Continued)*
  lipid cell, ovary D27-
  lipoid cell, ovary D27-
  malignant (*see also* Neoplasm, malignant, by site) C80.1
    fusiform cell (type) C80.1
    giant cell (type) C80.1
    localized, plasma cell —*see* Plasmacytoma, solitary
    mixed NEC C80.1
    small cell (type) C80.1
    spindle cell (type) C80.1
    unclassified C80.1
  mast cell D47.0
    malignant C96.2
  melanotic, neuroectodermal —*see* Neoplasm, benign, by site
  Merkel cell —*see* Carcinoma, Merkel cell
  mesenchymal
    malignant —*see* Neoplasm, connective tissue, malignant
    mixed —*see* Neoplasm, connective tissue, uncertain behavior
  mesodermal, mixed —*see also* Neoplasm, malignant, by site
    liver C22.4
  mesonephric —*see also* Neoplasm, uncertain behavior, by site
    malignant —*see* Neoplasm, malignant, by site
  metastatic
    from specified site —*see* Neoplasm, malignant, by site
    of specified site —*see* Neoplasm, malignant, by site
    to specified site —*see* Neoplasm, secondary, by site
  mixed NEC —*see also* Neoplasm, benign, by site
    malignant —*see* Neoplasm, malignant, by site
  mucinous of low malignant potential
    specified site —*see* Neoplasm, malignant, by site
    unspecified site C56.9
  mucocarcinoid
    specified site —*see* Neoplasm, malignant, by site
    unspecified site C18.1
  mucoepidermoid —*see* Neoplasm, uncertain behavior, by site
  Müllerian, mixed
    specified site —*see* Neoplasm, malignant, by site
    unspecified site C54.9
  myoepithelial —*see* Neoplasm, benign, by site
  neuroectodermal (peripheral) —*see* Neoplasm, malignant, by site
    primitive
      specified site —*see* Neoplasm, malignant, by site
      unspecified site C71.9
  neuroendocrine D3A.8
    malignant poorly differentiated C7A.1
    secondary NEC C7B.8
    specified NEC C7A.8
  neurogenic olfactory C30.0
  nonencapsulated sclerosing C73
  odontogenic (adenomatoid) (benign) (calcifying epithelial) (keratocystic) (squamous) —*see* Cyst, calcifying odontogenic
    malignant C41.1
      upper jaw (bone) C41.0
  ovarian stromal D39.1-
  ovary, in pregnancy —*see* Pregnancy, complicated by
  pacinian —*see* Neoplasm, skin, benign
  Pancoast's —*see* Pancoast's syndrome

Tumor (Continued)
- papillary —*see also* Papilloma
  - cystic D37.9
  - mucinous of low malignant potential C56-
    - specified site —*see* Neoplasm, malignant, by site
    - unspecified site C56.9
  - serous of low malignant potential
    - specified site —*see* Neoplasm, malignant, by site
    - unspecified site C56.9
- pelvic, in pregnancy or childbirth —*see* Pregnancy, complicated by
- phantom F45.8
- phyllodes D48.6-
  - benign D24-
  - malignant —*see* Neoplasm, breast, malignant
- Pindborg —*see* Cyst, calcifying odontogenic
- placental site trophoblastic D39.2
- plasma cell (malignant) (localized) —*see* Plasmacytoma, solitary
- polyvesicular vitelline
  - specified site —*see* Neoplasm, malignant, by site
  - unspecified site
    - female C56.9
    - male C62.90
- Pott's puffy —*see* Osteomyelitis, specified NEC
- Rathke's pouch D44.3
- retinal anlage —*see* Neoplasm, benign, by site
- salivary gland type, mixed —*see* Neoplasm, salivary gland, benign
  - malignant —*see* Neoplasm, salivary gland, malignant
- Sampson's N80.1
- Schmincke's —*see* Neoplasm, nasopharynx, malignant
- sclerosing stromal D27-
- sebaceous —*see* Cyst, sebaceous
- secondary —*see* Neoplasm, secondary, by site
  - carcinoid C7B.00
    - bone C7B.03
    - distant lymph nodes C7B.01
    - liver C7B.02
    - peritoneum C7B.04
    - specified NEC C7B.09
  - neuroendocrine NEC C7B.8
- serous of low malignant potential
  - specified site —*see* Neoplasm, malignant, by site
  - unspecified site C56.9
- Sertoli cell —*see* Neoplasm, benign, by site
  - with lipid storage
    - specified site —*see* Neoplasm, benign, by site
    - unspecified site
      - female D27.9
      - male D29.20
  - specified site —*see* Neoplasm, benign, by site
  - unspecified site
    - female D27.9
    - male D29.20
- Sertoli-Leydig cell —*see* Neoplasm, benign, by site
  - specified site —*see* Neoplasm, benign, by site
  - unspecified site
    - female D27.9
    - male D29.20
- sex cord(-stromal) —*see* Neoplasm, uncertain behavior, by site
  - with annular tubules D39.1-
- skin appendage —*see* Neoplasm, skin, benign
- smooth muscle —*see* Neoplasm, connective tissue, uncertain behavior

Tumor (Continued)
- soft tissue
  - benign —*see* Neoplasm, connective tissue, benign
  - malignant —*see* Neoplasm, connective tissue, malignant
- sternomastoid (congenital) Q68.0
- stromal
  - endometrial D39.0
  - gastric D48.1
    - benign D21.4
    - malignant C16.9
    - uncertain behavior D48.1
  - gastrointestinal
    - benign D21.4
    - malignant C49.4
    - uncertain behavior D48.1
  - intestine
    - benign D21.4
    - malignant C49.4
    - uncertain behavior D48.1
  - ovarian D39.1-
  - stomach
    - benign D21.4
    - malignant C16.9
    - uncertain behavior D48.1
- sweat gland —*see also* Neoplasm, skin, uncertain behavior
  - benign —*see* Neoplasm, skin, benign
  - malignant —*see* Neoplasm, skin, malignant
- syphilitic, brain A52.17
- testicular D40.10
- testicular stromal D40.1-
- theca cell D27.-
- theca cell-granulosa cell D39.1-
- Triton, malignant —*see* Neoplasm, nerve, malignant
- trophoblastic, placental site D39.2
- turban D23.4
- uterus (body), in pregnancy or childbirth — *see* Pregnancy, complicated by, tumor, uterus
- vagina, in pregnancy or childbirth —*see* Pregnancy, complicated by
- varicose —*see* Varix
- von Recklinghausen's —*see* Neurofibromatosis
- vulva or perineum, in pregnancy or childbirth —*see* Pregnancy, complicated by
  - causing obstructed labor O65.5
- Warthin's —*see* Neoplasm, salivary gland, benign
- Wilms' C64-
- yolk sac —*see* Neoplasm, malignant, by site
  - specified site —*see* Neoplasm, malignant, by site
  - unspecified site
    - female C56.9
    - male C62.90
Tumor lysis syndrome (following antineoplastic chemotherapy) (spontaneous) NEC E88.3
Tumorlet —*see* Neoplasm, uncertain behavior, by site
Tungiasis B88.1
Tunica vasculosa lentis Q12.2
Turban tumor D23.4
Türck's trachoma J37.0
Turner-Kieser syndrome Q79.8
Turner-like syndrome Q87.1
Turner's
- hypoplasia (tooth) K00.4
- syndrome Q96.9
  - specified NEC Q96.8
- tooth K00.4
Turner-Ullrich syndrome Q96.9
Tussis convulsiva —*see* Whooping cough
Twiddler's syndrome (due to)
- automatic implantable defibrillator T82.198
- cardiac pacemaker T82.198

Twilight state
- epileptic F05
- psychogenic F44.89
Twin (newborn) —*see also* Newborn, twin
- conjoined Q89.4
- pregnancy —*see* Pregnancy, twin, conjoined
Twinning, teeth K00.2
Twist, twisted
- bowel, colon or intestine K56.2
- hair (congenital) Q84.1
- mesentery K56.2
- omentum K56.2
- organ or site, congenital NEC —*see* Anomaly, by site
- ovarian pedicle —*see* Torsion, ovary
Twitching R25.3
Tylosis (acquired) L84
- buccalis K13.29
- linguae K13.29
- palmaris et plantaris (congenital) (inherited) Q82.8
- acquired L85.1
Tympanism R14.0
Tympanites (abdominal) (intestinal) R14.0
Tympanitis —*see* Myringitis
Tympanosclerosis —*see* subcategory H74.0
Tympanum —*see* condition
Tympany
- abdomen R14.0
- chest R09.89
Type A behavior pattern Z73.1
Typhlitis —*see* Appendicitis
Typhoenteritis —*see* Typhoid
Typhoid (abortive) (ambulant) (any site) (clinical) (fever) (hemorrhagic) (infection) (intermittent) (malignant) (rheumatic) (Widal negative) A01.00
- with pneumonia A01.03
- abdominal A01.09
- arthritis A01.04
- carrier (suspected) of Z22.0
- cholecystitis (current) A01.09
- endocarditis A01.02
- heart involvement A01.02
- inoculation reaction —*see* Complications, vaccination
- meningitis A01.01
- mesenteric lymph nodes A01.09
- myocarditis A01.02
- osteomyelitis A01.05
- perichondritis, larynx A01.09
- pneumonia A01.03
- specified NEC A01.09
- spine A01.05
- ulcer (perforating) A01.09
Typhomalaria (fever) —*see* Malaria
Typhomania A01.00
Typhoperitonitis A01.09
Typhus (fever) A75.9
- abdominal, abdominalis —*see* Typhoid
- African tick A77.1
- amarillic A95.9
- brain A75.9 [G94]
- cerebral A75.9 [G94]
- classical A75.0
- due to Rickettsia
  - prowazekii A75.0
    - recrudescent A75.1
  - tsutsugamushi A75.3
  - typhi A75.2
- endemic (flea-borne) A75.2
- epidemic (louse-borne) A75.0
- exanthematic NEC A75.0
- exanthematicus SAI A75.0
  - brillii SAI A75.1
  - mexicanus SAI A75.2
  - typhus murinus A75.2
- flea-borne A75.2
- India tick A77.1
- Kenya (tick) A77.1
- louse-borne A75.0

◄ New ◄▥ Revised ~~deleted~~ Deleted

Typhus *(Continued)*
  Mexican A75.2
  mite-borne A75.3
  murine A75.2
  North Asian tick-borne A77.2
  petechial A75.9
  Queensland tick A77.3
  rat A75.2

Typhus *(Continued)*
  recrudescent A75.1
  recurrens —*see* Fever, relapsing
  Sao Paulo A77.0
  scrub (China) (India) (Malaysia) (New
    Guinea) A75.3
  shop (of Malaysia) A75.2
  Siberian tick A77.2

Typhus *(Continued)*
  tick-borne A77.9
  tropical (mite-borne) A75.3
Tyrosinemia E70.21
  newborn, transitory P74.5
Tyrosinosis E70.21
Tyrosinuria E70.29

U

Uhl's anomaly or disease Q24.8
Ulcer, ulcerated, ulcerating, ulceration, ulcerative
  alveolar process M27.3
  amebic (intestine) A06.1
    skin A06.7
  anastomotic —*see* Ulcer, gastrojejunal
  anorectal K62.6
  antral —*see* Ulcer, stomach
  anus (sphincter) (solitary) K62.6
  aorta —*see* Aneurysm
  aphthous (oral) (recurrent) K12.0
    genital organ (s)
      female N76.6
      male N50.8
  artery I77.2
  atrophic —*see* Ulcer, skin
    decubitus —*see* Ulcer, pressure, by site
  back L98.429
    with
      bone necrosis L98.424
      exposed fat layer L98.422
      muscle necrosis L98.423
      skin breakdown only L98.421
  Barrett's (esophagus) K22.10
    with bleeding K22.11
  bile duct (common) (hepatic) K83.8
  bladder (solitary) (sphincter) NEC N32.89
    bilharzial B65.9 [N33]
    in schistosomiasis (bilharzial) B65.9 [N33]
    submucosal —*see* Cystitis, interstitial
    tuberculous A18.12
  bleeding K27.4
  bone —*see* Osteomyelitis, specified type NEC
  bowel —*see* Ulcer, intestine
  breast N61
  bronchus J98.09
  buccal (cavity) (traumatic) K12.1
  Buruli A31.1
  buttock L98.419
    with
      bone necrosis L98.414
      exposed fat layer L98.412
      muscle necrosis L98.413
      skin breakdown only L98.411
  cancerous —*see* Neoplasm, malignant, by site
  cardia K22.10
    with bleeding K22.11
  cardioesophageal (peptic) K22.10
    with bleeding K22.11
  cecum —*see* Ulcer, intestine
  cervix (uteri) (decubitus) (trophic) N86
    with cervicitis N72
  chancroidal A57
  chiclero B55.1
  chronic (cause unknown) —*see* Ulcer, skin
  Cochin-China B55.1
  colon —*see* Ulcer, intestine
  conjunctiva H10.89
  cornea H16.00-
    with hypopyon H16.03-
    central H16.01-
    dendritic (herpes simplex) B00.52
    marginal H16.04-
    Mooren's H16.05-
    mycotic H16.06-
    perforated H16.07-
    ring H16.02-
    tuberculous (phlyctenular) A18.52
  corpus cavernosum (chronic) N48.5
  crural —*see* Ulcer, lower limb
  Curling's —*see* Ulcer, peptic, acute
  Cushing's —*see* Ulcer, peptic, acute
  cystic duct K82.8
  cystitis (interstitial) —*see* Cystitis, interstitial
  decubitus —*see* Ulcer, pressure, by site
  dendritic, cornea (herpes simplex) B00.52
  diabetes, diabetic —*see* Diabetes, ulcer
  Dieulafoy's K25.0

Ulcer, ulcerated, ulcerating, ulceration, ulcerative (Continued)
  due to
    infection NEC —*see* Ulcer, skin
    radiation NEC L59.8
    trophic disturbance (any region) —*see* Ulcer, skin
    X-ray L58.1
  duodenum, duodenal (eroded) (peptic) K26.9
    with
      hemorrhage K26.4
        and perforation K26.6
      perforation K26.5
    acute K26.3
      with
        hemorrhage K26.0
          and perforation K26.2
        perforation K26.1
    chronic K26.7
      with
        hemorrhage K26.4
          and perforation K26.6
        perforation K26.5
  dysenteric A09
  elusive —*see* Cystitis, interstitial
  endocarditis (acute) (chronic) (subacute) I28.8
  epiglottis J38.7
  esophagus (peptic) K22.10
    with bleeding K22.11
    due to
      aspirin K22.10
        with bleeding K22.11
      gastrointestinal reflux disease K21.0
      ingestion of chemical or medicament K22.10
        with bleeding K22.11
    fungal K22.10
      with bleeding K22.11
    infective K22.10
      with bleeding K22.11
    varicose —*see* Varix, esophagus
  eyelid (region) H01.8
  fauces J39.2
  Fenwick (-Hunner) (solitary) —*see* Cystitis, interstitial
  fistulous —*see* Ulcer, skin
  foot (indolent) (trophic) —*see* Ulcer, lower limb
  frambesial, initial A66.0
  frenum (tongue) K14.0
  gallbladder or duct K82.8
  gangrenous —*see* Gangrene
  gastric —*see* Ulcer, stomach
  gastrocolic —*see* Ulcer, gastrojejunal
  gastroduodenal —*see* Ulcer, peptic
  gastroesophageal —*see* Ulcer, stomach
  gastrointestinal —*see* Ulcer, gastrojejunal
  gastrojejunal (peptic) K28.9
    with
      hemorrhage K28.4
        and perforation K28.6
      perforation K28.5
    acute K28.3
      with
        hemorrhage K28.0
          and perforation K28.2
        perforation K28.1
    chronic K28.7
      with
        hemorrhage K28.4
          and perforation K28.6
        perforation K28.5
  gastrojejunocolic —*see* Ulcer, gastrojejunal
  gingiva K06.8
  gingivitis K05.10
    nonplaque induced K05.11
    plaque induced K05.10
  glottis J38.7
  granuloma of pudenda A58
  gum K06.8
  gumma, due to yaws A66.4

Ulcer, ulcerated, ulcerating, ulceration, ulcerative (Continued)
  heel —*see* Ulcer, lower limb
  hemorrhoid (*see also* Hemorrhoids, by degree) K64.8
  Hunner's —*see* Cystitis, interstitial
  hypopharynx J39.2
  hypopyon (chronic) (subacute) —*see* Ulcer, cornea, with hypopyon
  hypostaticum —*see* Ulcer, varicose
  ileum —*see* Ulcer, intestine
  intestine, intestinal K63.3
    with perforation K63.1
    amebic A06.1
    duodenal —*see* Ulcer, duodenum
    granulocytopenic (with hemorrhage) —*see* Neutropenia
    marginal —*see* Ulcer, gastrojejunal
    perforating K63.1
      newborn P78.0
    primary, small intestine K63.3
    rectum K62.6
    stercoraceous, stercoral K63.3
    tuberculous A18.32
    typhoid (fever) —*see* Typhoid
    varicose I86.8
  jejunum, jejunal —*see* Ulcer, gastrojejunal
  keratitis —*see* Ulcer, cornea
  knee —*see* Ulcer, lower limb
  labium (majus) (minus) N76.6
  laryngitis —*see* Laryngitis
  larynx (aphthous) (contact) J38.7
    diphtheritic A36.2
  leg —*see* Ulcer, lower limb
  lip K13.0
  Lipschütz's N76.6
  lower limb (atrophic) (chronic) (neurogenic) (perforating) (pyogenic) (trophic) (tropical) L97.909
    with
      bone necrosis L97.904
      exposed fat layer L97.902
      muscle necrosis L97.903
      skin breakdown only L97.901
    ankle L97.309
      with
        bone necrosis L97.304
        exposed fat layer L97.302
        muscle necrosis L97.303
        skin breakdown only L97.301
      left L97.329
        with
          bone necrosis L97.324
          exposed fat layer L97.322
          muscle necrosis L97.323
          skin breakdown only L97.321
      right L97.319
        with
          bone necrosis L97.314
          exposed fat layer L97.312
          muscle necrosis L97.313
          skin breakdown only L97.311
    calf L97.209
      with
        bone necrosis L97.204
        exposed fat layer L97.202
        muscle necrosis L97.203
        skin breakdown only L97.201
      left L97.229
        with
          bone necrosis L97.224
          exposed fat layer L97.222
          muscle necrosis L97.223
          skin breakdown only L97.221
      right L97.219
        with
          bone necrosis L97.214
          exposed fat layer L97.212
          muscle necrosis L97.213
          skin breakdown only L97.211
    decubitus —*see* Ulcer, pressure, by site

◀ New   ◀▥ Revised   ~~deleted~~ Deleted

Ulcer, ulcerated, ulcerating, ulceration, ulcerative (Continued)
lower limb (Continued)
foot specified NEC L97.509
with
bone necrosis L97.504
exposed fat layer L97.502
muscle necrosis L97.503
skin breakdown only L97.501
left L97.529
with
bone necrosis L97.524
exposed fat layer L97.522
muscle necrosis L97.523
skin breakdown only L97.521
right L97.519
with
bone necrosis L97.514
exposed fat layer L97.512
muscle necrosis L97.513
skin breakdown only L97.511
heel L97.409
with
bone necrosis L97.404
exposed fat layer L97.402
muscle necrosis L97.403
skin breakdown only L97.401
left L97.429
with
bone necrosis L97.424
exposed fat layer L97.422
muscle necrosis L97.423
skin breakdown only L97.421
right L97.419
with
bone necrosis L97.414
exposed fat layer L97.412
muscle necrosis L97.413
skin breakdown only L97.411
left L97.929
with
bone necrosis L97.924
exposed fat layer L97.922
muscle necrosis L97.923
skin breakdown only L97.921
lower leg NOS L97.909
with
bone necrosis L97.904
exposed fat layer L97.902
muscle necrosis L97.903
skin breakdown only L97.901
left L97.929
with
bone necrosis L97.924
exposed fat layer L97.922
muscle necrosis L97.923
skin breakdown only L97.921
right L97.919
with
bone necrosis L97.914
exposed fat layer L97.912
muscle necrosis L97.913
skin breakdown only L97.911
specified site NEC L97.809
with
bone necrosis L97.804
exposed fat layer L97.802
muscle necrosis L97.803
skin breakdown only L97.801
left L97.829
with
bone necrosis L97.824
exposed fat layer L97.822
muscle necrosis L97.823
skin breakdown only L97.821
right L97.819
with
bone necrosis L97.814
exposed fat layer L97.812
muscle necrosis L97.813
skin breakdown only L97.811

Ulcer, ulcerated, ulcerating, ulceration, ulcerative (Continued)
lower limb (Continued)
midfoot L97.409
with
bone necrosis L97.404
exposed fat layer L97.402
muscle necrosis L97.403
skin breakdown only L97.401
left L97.429
with
bone necrosis L97.424
exposed fat layer L97.422
muscle necrosis L97.423
skin breakdown only L97.421
right L97.419
with
bone necrosis L97.414
exposed fat layer L97.412
muscle necrosis L97.413
skin breakdown only L97.411
right L97.919
with
bone necrosis L97.914
exposed fat layer L97.912
muscle necrosis L97.913
skin breakdown only L97.911
thigh L97.109
with
bone necrosis L97.104
exposed fat layer L97.102
muscle necrosis L97.103
skin breakdown only L97.101
left L97.129
with
bone necrosis L97.124
exposed fat layer L97.122
muscle necrosis L97.123
skin breakdown only L97.121
right L97.119
with
bone necrosis L97.114
exposed fat layer L97.112
muscle necrosis L97.113
skin breakdown only L97.111
toe L97.509
with
bone necrosis L97.504
exposed fat layer L97.502
muscle necrosis L97.503
skin breakdown only L97.501
left L97.529
with
bone necrosis L97.524
exposed fat layer L97.522
muscle necrosis L97.523
skin breakdown only L97.521
right L97.519
with
bone necrosis L97.514
exposed fat layer L97.512
muscle necrosis L97.513
skin breakdown only L97.511
leprous A30.1
syphilitic A52.19
varicose —see Varix, leg, with, ulcer
luetic —see Ulcer, syphilitic
lung J98.4
tuberculous —see Tuberculosis, pulmonary
malignant —see Neoplasm, malignant, by site
marginal NEC —see Ulcer, gastrojejunal
meatus (urinarius) N34.2
Meckel's diverticulum Q43.0
malignant —see Table of Neoplasms, small intestine, malignant
Meleney's (chronic undermining) —see Ulcer, skin
Mooren's (cornea) —see Ulcer, cornea, Mooren's
mycobacterial (skin) A31.1
nasopharynx J39.2

Ulcer, ulcerated, ulcerating, ulceration, ulcerative (Continued)
neck, uterus N86
neurogenic NEC —see Ulcer, skin
nose, nasal (passage) (infective) (septum) J34.0
skin —see Ulcer, skin
spirochetal A69.8
varicose (bleeding) I86.8
oral mucosa (traumatic) K12.1
palate (soft) K12.1
penis (chronic) N48.5
peptic (site unspecified) K27.9
with
hemorrhage K27.4
and perforation K27.6
perforation K27.5
acute K27.3
with
hemorrhage K27.0
and perforation K27.2
perforation K27.1
chronic K27.7
with
hemorrhage K27.4
and perforation K27.6
perforation K27.5
esophagus K22.10
with bleeding K22.11
newborn P78.82
perforating K27.5
skin —see Ulcer, skin
peritonsillar J35.8
phagedenic (tropical) —see Ulcer, skin
pharynx J39.2
phlebitis —see Phlebitis
plaster —see Ulcer, pressure, by site
popliteal space —see Ulcer, lower limb
postpyloric —see Ulcer, duodenum
prepuce N47.7
prepyloric —see Ulcer, stomach
pressure (pressure area) L89.9-
ankle L89.5-
back L89.1-
buttock L89.3-
coccyx L89.15-
contiguous site of back, buttock, hip L89.4-
elbow L89.0-
face L89.81-
head L89.81-
heel L89.6-
hip L89.2-
sacral region (tailbone) L89.15-
specified site NEC L89.89-
stage 1 (healing) (pre-ulcer skin changes limited to persistent focal edema)
ankle L89.5-
back L89.1-
buttock L89.3-
coccyx L89.15-
contiguous site of back, buttock, hip L89.4-
elbow L89.0-
face L89.81-
head L89.81-
heel L89.6-
hip L89.2-
sacral region (tailbone) L89.15-
specified site NEC L89.89-
stage 2 (healing) (abrasion, blister, partial thickness skin loss involving epidermis and/or dermis)
ankle L89.5-
back L89.1-
buttock L89.3-
coccyx L89.15-
contiguous site of back, buttock, hip L89.4-
elbow L89.0-
face L89.81-
head L89.81-

◀ New ◀▦▦ Revised ~~deleted~~ Deleted

Underdosing (*see also* Table of Drugs and Chemicals, categories T36-T50, with final character 6) Z91.14
  intentional NEC Z91.128
    due to financial hardship of patient Z91.120
  unintentional NEC Z91.138
    due to patient's age related debility Z91.130
Underfeeding, newborn P92.3
Underfill, endodontic M27.53
Underimmunization status Z28.3
Undernourishment —*see* Malnutrition
Undernutrition —*see* Malnutrition
Under observation —*see* Observation
Underweight R63.6
  for gestational age —*see* Light for dates
Underwood's disease P83.0
Undescended —*see also* Malposition, congenital
  cecum Q43.3
  colon Q43.3
  testicle —*see* Cryptorchid
Undeveloped, undevelopment —*see also* Hypoplasia
  brain (congenital) Q02
  cerebral (congenital) Q02
  heart Q24.8
  lung Q33.6
  testis E29.1
  uterus E30.0
Undiagnosed (disease) R69
Undulant fever —*see* Brucellosis
Unemployment, anxiety concerning Z56.0
  threatened Z56.2
Unequal length (acquired) (limb) —*see also* Deformity, limb, unequal length
  leg —*see also* Deformity, limb, unequal length
    congenital Q72.9-
Unextracted dental root K08.3
Unguis incarnatus L60.0
Unhappiness R45.2
Unicornate uterus Q51.4
Unilateral —*see also* condition
  development, breast N64.89
  organ or site, congenital NEC —*see* Agenesis, by site
Unilocular heart Q20.8
Union, abnormal —*see also* Fusion
  larynx and trachea Q34.8
Universal mesentery Q43.3
Unrepairable overhanging of dental restorative materials K08.52
Unsatisfactory
  restoration of tooth K08.50
    specified NEC K08.59
  sample of cytologic smear
    anus R85.615
    cervix R87.615
    vagina R87.625
  surroundings Z59.1
  work Z56.5
Unsoundness of mind —*see* Psychosis
Unstable
  back NEC —*see* Instability, joint, spine
  hip (congenital) Q65.6
    acquired —*see* Derangement, joint, specified type NEC, hip
  joint —*see* Instability, joint
    secondary to removal of joint prosthesis M96.89
  lie (mother) O32.0
  lumbosacral joint (congenital)
    acquired —*see* subcategory M53.2
  sacroiliac —*see* subcategory M53.2
  spine NEC —*see* Instability, joint, spine
Unsteadiness on feet R26.81
Untruthfulness, child problem F91.8
Unverricht(-Lundborg) **disease or epilepsy** — *see* Epilepsy, generalized, idiopathic
Unwanted pregnancy Z64.0

Upbringing, institutional Z62.22
  away from parents NEC Z62.29
  in care of non-parental family member Z62.21
  in foster care Z62.21
  in orphanage or group home Z62.22
  in welfare custody Z62.21
Upper respiratory —*see* condition
Upset
  gastric K30
  gastrointestinal K30
    psychogenic F45.8
  intestinal (large) (small) K59.9
    psychogenic F45.8
  menstruation N93.9
  mental F48.9
  stomach K30
    psychogenic F45.8
Urachus —*see also* condition
  patent or persistent Q64.4
Urbach-Oppenheim disease (necrobiosis lipoidica diabeticorum) —*see* E08-E13 with .620
Urbach's lipoid proteinosis E78.89
Urbach-Wiethe disease E78.89
Urban yellow fever A95.1
Urea
  blood, high —*see* Uremia
  cycle metabolism disorder —*see* Disorder, urea cycle metabolism
Uremia, uremic N19
  with
    ectopic or molar pregnancy O08.4
    polyneuropathy N18.9 *[G63]*
  chronic (*see also* Disease, kidney, chronic) N18.9
    due to hypertension —*see* Hypertensive, kidney
  complicating
    ectopic or molar pregnancy O08.4
  congenital P96.0
  extrarenal R39.2
  following ectopic or molar pregnancy O08.4
  newborn P96.0
  prerenal R39.2
Ureter, ureteral —*see* condition
Ureteralgia N23
Ureterectasis —*see* Hydroureter
Ureteritis N28.89
  cystica N28.86
  due to calculus N20.1
    with calculus, kidney N20.2
      with hydronephrosis N13.2
  gonococcal (acute) (chronic) A54.21
  nonspecific N28.89
Ureterocele N28.89
  congenital (orthotopic) Q62.31
  ectopic Q62.32
Ureterolith, ureterolithiasis —*see* Calculus, ureter
Ureterostomy
  attention to Z43.6
  status Z93.6
Urethra, urethral —*see* condition
Urethralgia R39.89
Urethritis (anterior) (posterior) N34.2
  calculous N21.1
  candidal B37.41
  chlamydial A56.01
  diplococcal (gonococcal) A54.01
    with abscess (accessory gland) (periurethral) A54.1
  gonococcal A54.01
    with abscess (accessory gland) (periurethral) A54.1
  nongonococcal N34.1
    Reiter's —*see* Reiter's disease
  nonspecific N34.1
  nonvenereal N34.1
  postmenopausal N34.2
  puerperal O86.22
  Reiter's —*see* Reiter's disease

Urethritis (*Continued*)
  specified NEC N34.2
  trichomonal or due to Trichomonas (vaginalis) A59.03
Urethrocele N81.0
  with
    cystocele —*see* Cystocele
    prolapse of uterus —*see* Prolapse, uterus
Urethrolithiasis (with colic or infection) N21.1
Urethrorectal —*see* condition
Urethrorrhagia N36.8
Urethrorrhea R36.9
Urethrostomy
  attention to Z43.6
  status Z93.6
Urethrotrigonitis —*see* Trigonitis
Urethrovaginal —*see* condition
Urgency
  fecal R15.2
  hypertensive —*see* Hypertension
  urinary N39.41
Urhidrosis, uridrosis L74.8
Uric acid in blood (increased) E79.0
Uricacidemia (asymptomatic) E79.0
Uricemia (asymptomatic) E79.0
Uricosuria R82.99
Urinary —*see* condition
Urination
  frequent R35.0
  painful R30.9
Urine
  blood in —*see* Hematuria
  discharge, excessive R35.8
  enuresis, nonorganic origin F98.0
  extravasation R39.0
  frequency R35.0
  incontinence R32
    nonorganic origin F98.0
  intermittent stream R39.19
  pus in N39.0
  retention or stasis R33.9
    organic R33.8
      drug-induced R33.0
    psychogenic F45.8
  secretion
    deficient R34
    excessive R35.8
    frequency R35.0
  stream
    intermittent R39.19
    slowing R39.19
    splitting R39.13
    weak R39.12
Urinemia —*see* Uremia
Urinoma, urethra N36.8
Uroarthritis, infectious (Reiter's) —*see* Reiter's disease
Urodialysis R34
Urolithiasis —*see* Calculus, urinary
Uronephrosis —*see* Hydronephrosis
Uropathy N39.9
  obstructive N13.9
    specified NEC N13.8
  reflux N13.9
    specified NEC N13.8
  vesicoureteral reflux-associated —*see* Reflux, vesicoureteral
Urosepsis — code to condition
Urticaria L50.9
  with angioneurotic edema T78.3
    hereditary D84.1
  allergic L50.0
  cholinergic L50.5
  chronic L50.8
  cold, familial L50.2
  contact L50.6
  dermatographic L50.3
  due to
    cold or heat L50.2
    drugs L50.0
    food L50.0

Urticaria (Continued)
 due to (Continued)
  inhalants L50.0
  plants L50.6
  serum (see also Reaction, serum) T80.69
 factitial L50.3
 giant T78.3
  hereditary D84.1
 gigantea T78.3
 idiopathic L50.1
 larynx T78.3
  hereditary D84.1
 neonatorum P83.8
 nonallergic L50.1
 papulosa (Hebra) L28.2
 pigmentosa Q82.2
 recurrent periodic L50.8
 serum (see also Reaction, serum) T80.69
 solar L56.3
 specified type NEC L50.8
 thermal (cold) (heat) L50.2
 vibratory L50.4
 xanthelasmoidea Q82.2
Use (of)
 alcohol F10.99
  with sleep disorder F10.982
  harmful —see Abuse, alcohol
 amphetamines —see Use, stimulant NEC
 caffeine —see Use, stimulant NEC
 cannabis F12.90
  with
   anxiety disorder F12.980
   intoxication F12.929
    with
     delirium F12.921
     perceptual disturbance F12.922
    uncomplicated F12.920
   other specified disorder F12.988
   psychosis F12.959
    delusions F12.950
    hallucinations F12.951
   unspecified disorder F12.99
 cocaine F14.90
  with
   anxiety disorder F14.980
   intoxication F14.929
    with
     delirium F14.921
     perceptual disturbance F14.922
    uncomplicated F14.920
   other specified disorder F14.988
   psychosis F14.959
    delusions F14.950
    hallucinations F14.951
   sexual dysfunction F14.981
   sleep disorder F14.982
   unspecified disorder F14.99
  harmful —see Abuse, drug, cocaine
 drug (s) NEC F19.90
  with sleep disorder F19.982
  harmful —see Abuse, drug, by type
 hallucinogen NEC F16.90
  with
   anxiety disorder F16.980
   intoxication F16.929
    with
     delirium F16.921
    uncomplicated F16.920
   mood disorder F16.94
   other specified disorder F16.988
   perception disorder (flashbacks)
    F16.983

Use (Continued)
 hallucinogen NEC (Continued)
  with (Continued)
   psychosis F16.959
    delusions F16.950
    hallucinations F16.951
   unspecified disorder F16.99
  harmful —see Abuse, drug, hallucinogen
   NEC
 inhalants F18.90
  with
   anxiety disorder F18.980
   intoxication F18.929
    with delirium F18.921
    uncomplicated F18.920
   mood disorder F18.94
   other specified disorder F18.988
   persisting dementia F18.97
   psychosis F18.959
    delusions F18.950
    hallucinations F18.951
   unspecified disorder F18.99
  harmful —see Abuse, drug, inhalant
 methadone F11.20
 nonprescribed drugs F19.90
  harmful —see Abuse, non-psychoactive
   substance
 opioid F11.90
  with
   disorder F11.99
    mood F11.94
    sleep F11.982
    specified type NEC F11.988
   intoxication F11.929
    with
     delirium F11.921
     perceptual disturbance
      F11.922
    uncomplicated F11.920
   withdrawal F11.93
  harmful —see Abuse, drug, opioid
 patent medicines F19.90
  harmful —see Abuse, non-psychoactive
   substance
 psychoactive drug NEC F19.90
  with
   anxiety disorder F19.980
   intoxication F19.929
    with
     delirium F19.921
     perceptual disturbance
      F19.922
    uncomplicated F19.920
   mood disorder F19.94
   other specified disorder F19.988
   persisting
    amnestic disorder F19.96
    dementia F19.97
   psychosis F19.959
    delusions F19.950
    hallucinations F19.951
   sexual dysfunction F19.981
   sleep disorder F19.982
   unspecified disorder F19.99
   withdrawal F19.939
    with
     delirium F19.931
     perceptual disturbance
      F19.932
    uncomplicated F19.930
  harmful —see Abuse, drug NEC,
   psychoactive NEC

Use (Continued)
 sedative, hypnotic, or anxiolytic F13.90
  with
   anxiety disorder F13.980
   intoxication F13.929
    with
     delirium F13.921
    uncomplicated F13.920
   other specified disorder F13.988
   persisting
    amnestic disorder F13.96
    dementia F13.97
   psychosis F13.959
    delusions F13.950
    hallucinations F13.951
   sexual dysfunction F13.981
   sleep disorder F13.982
   unspecified disorder F13.99
  harmful —see Abuse, drug, sedative,
   hypnotic, or anxiolytic
 stimulant NEC F15.90
  with
   anxiety disorder F15.980
   intoxication F15.929
    with
     delirium F15.921
     perceptual disturbance F15.922
    uncomplicated F15.920
   mood disorder F15.94
   other specified disorder F15.988
   psychosis F15.959
    delusions F15.950
    hallucinations F15.951
   sexual dysfunction F15.981
   sleep disorder F15.982
   unspecified disorder F15.99
   withdrawal F15.93
  harmful —see Abuse, drug, stimulant NEC
 tobacco Z72.0
  with dependence —see Dependence, drug,
   nicotine
 volatile solvents (see also Use, inhalant) F18.90
  harmful —see Abuse, drug, inhalant
Usher-Senear disease or syndrome L10.4
Uta B55.1
Uteromegaly N85.2
Uterovaginal —see condition
Uterovesical —see condition
Uveal —see condition
Uveitis (anterior) —see also Iridocyclitis
 acute —see Iridocyclitis, acute
 chronic —see Iridocyclitis, chronic
 due to toxoplasmosis (acquired) B58.09
  congenital P37.1
 granulomatous —see Iridocyclitis, chronic
 heterochromic —see Cyclitis, Fuchs'
  heterochromic
 lens-induced —see Iridocyclitis, lens-induced
 posterior —see Chorioretinitis
 sympathetic H44.13-
 syphilitic (secondary) A51.43
  congenital (early) A50.01
  late A52.71
 tuberculous A18.54
Uveoencephalitis —see Inflammation,
 chorioretinal
Uveokeratitis —see Iridocyclitis
Uveoparotitis D86.89
Uvula —see condition
Uvulitis (acute) (catarrhal) (chronic)
 (membranous) (suppurative) (ulcerative)
 K12.2

◀ New   ◀▨ Revised   ~~deleted~~ Deleted

V

Vaccination (prophylactic)
　complication or reaction —*see* Complications, vaccination
　delayed Z28.9
　encounter for Z23
　not done —*see* Immunization, not done, because (of)
Vaccinia (generalized) (localized) T88.1
　without vaccination B08.011
　congenital P35.8
Vacuum, in sinus (accessory) (nasal) J34.89
Vagabond, vagabondage Z59.0
Vagabond's disease B85.1
Vagina, vaginal —*see* condition
Vaginalitis (tunica) (testis) N49.1
Vaginismus (reflex) N94.2
　functional F52.5
　nonorganic F52.5
　psychogenic F52.5
　secondary N94.2
Vaginitis (acute) (circumscribed) (diffuse) (emphysematous) (nonvenereal) (ulcerative) N76.0
　with ectopic or molar pregnancy O08.0
　amebic A06.82
　atrophic, postmenopausal N95.2
　bacterial N76.0
　blennorrhagic (gonococcal) A54.02
　candidal B37.3
　chlamydial A56.02
　chronic N76.1
　due to Trichomonas (vaginalis) A59.01
　following ectopic or molar pregnancy O08.0
　gonococcal A54.02
　　with abscess (accessory gland) (periurethral) A54.1
　granuloma A58
　in (due to)
　　candidiasis B37.3
　　herpesviral (herpes simplex) infection A60.04
　　pinworm infection B80 [N77.1]
　monilial B37.3
　mycotic (candidal) B37.3
　postmenopausal atrophic N95.2
　puerperal (postpartum) O86.13
　senile (atrophic) N95.2
　subacute or chronic N76.1
　syphilitic (early) A51.0
　　late A52.76
　trichomonal A59.01
　tuberculous A18.18
Vaginosis —*see* Vaginitis
Vagotonia G52.2
Vagrancy Z59.0
VAIN —*see* Neoplasia, intraepithelial, vagina
Vallecula —*see* condition
Valley fever B38.0
Valsuani's disease —*see* Anemia, obstetric
Valve, valvular (formation) —*see also* condition
　cerebral ventricle (communicating) in situ Z98.2
　cervix, internal os Q51.828
　congenital NEC —*see* Atresia, by site
　ureter (pelvic junction) (vesical orifice) Q62.39
　urethra (congenital) (posterior) Q64.2
Valvulitis (chronic) —*see* Endocarditis
Valvulopathy —*see* Endocarditis
Van Bogaert's leukoencephalopathy (sclerosing) (subacute) A81.1
Van Bogaert-Scherer-Epstein disease or syndrome E75.5
Van Buchem's syndrome M85.2
Van Creveld-von Gierke disease E74.01
Van der Hoeve (-de Kleyn) **syndrome** Q78.0
Van der Woude's syndrome Q38.0
Van Neck's disease or osteochondrosis M91.0
Vanishing lung J44.9

Vapor asphyxia or suffocation T59.9
　specified agent —*see* Table of Drugs and Chemicals
Variance, lethal ball, prosthetic heart valve T82.09
Variants, thalassemic D56.8
Variations in hair color L67.1
Varicella B01.9
　with
　　complications NEC B01.89
　　encephalitis B01.11
　　encephalomyelitis B01.11
　　meningitis B01.0
　　myelitis B01.12
　　pneumonia B01.2
　congenital P35.8
Varices —*see* Varix
Varicocele (scrotum) (thrombosed) I86.1
　ovary I86.2
　perineum I86.3
　spermatic cord (ulcerated) I86.1
Varicose
　aneurysm (ruptured) I77.0
　dermatitis —*see* Varix, leg, with, inflammation
　eczema —*see* Varix, leg, with, inflammation
　phlebitis —*see* Varix, with, inflammation
　tumor —*see* Varix
　ulcer (lower limb, any part) —*see also* Varix, leg, with, ulcer
　　anus (*see also* Hemorrhoids) K64.8
　　esophagus —*see* Varix, esophagus
　　inflamed or infected —*see* Varix, leg, with ulcer, with inflammation
　　nasal septum I86.8
　　perineum I86.3
　　scrotum I86.1
　　specified site NEC I86.8
　vein —*see* Varix
　vessel —*see* Varix, leg
Varicosis, varicosities, varicosity —*see* Varix
Variola (major) (minor) B03
Varioloid B03
Varix (lower limb) (ruptured) I83.90
　with
　　edema I83.899
　　inflammation I83.10
　　　with ulcer (venous) I83.209
　　pain I83.819
　　specified complication NEC I83.899
　　stasis dermatitis I83.10
　　　with ulcer (venous) I83.209
　　swelling I83.899
　　ulcer I83.009
　　　with inflammation I83.209
　aneurysmal I77.0
　asymptomatic I83.9-
　bladder I86.2
　broad ligament I86.2
　complicating
　　childbirth (lower extremity) O87.4
　　　anus or rectum O87.2
　　　genital (vagina, vulva or perineum) O87.8
　　pregnancy (lower extremity) O22.0-
　　　anus or rectum O22.4-
　　　genital (vagina, vulva or perineum) O22.1-
　　puerperium (lower extremity) O87.4
　　　anus or rectum O87.2
　　　genital (vagina, vulva, perineum) O87.8
　congenital (any site) Q27.8
　esophagus (idiopathic) (primary) (ulcerated) I85.00
　　bleeding I85.01
　　congenital Q27.8
　　in (due to)
　　　alcoholic liver disease I85.10
　　　　bleeding I85.11
　　　cirrhosis of liver I85.10
　　　　bleeding I85.11

Varix (*Continued*)
　esophagus (*Continued*)
　　in (*Continued*)
　　　portal hypertension I85.10
　　　　bleeding I85.11
　　　schistosomiasis I85.10
　　　　bleeding I85.11
　　　toxic liver disease I85.10
　　　　bleeding I85.11
　　secondary I85.10
　　　bleeding I85.11
　gastric I86.4
　inflamed or infected I83.10
　　ulcerated I83.209
　labia (majora) I86.3
　leg (asymptomatic) I83.90
　　with
　　　edema I83.899
　　　inflammation I83.10
　　　　with ulcer —*see* Varix, leg, with, ulcer, with inflammation by site
　　　pain I83.819
　　　specified complication NEC I83.899
　　　swelling I83.899
　　　ulcer I83.009
　　　　with inflammation I83.209
　　　　ankle I83.003
　　　　　with inflammation I83.203
　　　　calf I83.002
　　　　　with inflammation I83.202
　　　　foot NEC I83.005
　　　　　with inflammation I83.205
　　　　heel I83.004
　　　　　with inflammation I83.204
　　　　lower leg NEC I83.008
　　　　　with inflammation I83.208
　　　　midfoot I83.004
　　　　　with inflammation I83.204
　　　　thigh I83.001
　　　　　with inflammation I83.201
　　bilateral (asymptomatic) I83.93
　　　with
　　　　edema I83.893
　　　　pain I83.813
　　　　specified complication NEC I83.893
　　　　swelling I83.893
　　　　ulcer I83.009
　　　　　with inflammation I83.209
　　left (asymptomatic) I83.92
　　　with
　　　　edema I83.892
　　　　inflammation I83.12
　　　　　with ulcer —*see* Varix, leg, with, ulcer, with inflammation by site
　　　　pain I83.812
　　　　specified complication NEC I83.892
　　　　swelling I83.892
　　　　ulcer I83.029
　　　　　with inflammation I83.229
　　　　ankle I83.023
　　　　　with inflammation I83.223
　　　　calf I83.022
　　　　　with inflammation I83.222
　　　　foot NEC I83.025
　　　　　with inflammation I83.225
　　　　heel I83.024
　　　　　with inflammation I83.224
　　　　lower leg NEC I83.028
　　　　　with inflammation I83.228
　　　　midfoot I83.024
　　　　　with inflammation I83.224
　　　　thigh I83.021
　　　　　with inflammation I83.221
　　right (asymptomatic) I83.91
　　　with
　　　　edema I83.891
　　　　inflammation I83.11
　　　　　with ulcer —*see* Varix, leg, with, ulcer, with inflammation by site

◄ New   ◄▥ Revised   ~~deleted~~ Deleted

Virilization (female) (suprarenal) E25.9
  congenital E25.0
  isosexual E28.2
Virulent bubo A57
Virus, viral —*see also* condition
  as cause of disease classified elsewhere
    B97.89
  cytomegalovirus B25.9
  human immunodeficiency (HIV) —*see*
    Human, immunodeficiency virus (HIV)
    disease
  infection —*see* Infection, virus
  specified NEC B34.8
  swine influenza (viruses that normally cause
    infections in pigs) (*see also* Influenza,
    due to, identified novel influenza A
    virus) J09.X2
  West Nile (fever) A92.30
    with
      complications NEC A92.39
      cranial nerve disorders A92.32
      encephalitis A92.31
      encephalomyelitis A92.31
      neurologic manifestation NEC A92.32
      optic neuritis A92.32
      polyradiculitis A92.32
Viscera, visceral —*see* condition
Visceroptosis K63.4
Visible peristalsis R19.2
Vision, visual
  binocular, suppression H53.34
  blurred, blurring H53.8
    hysterical F44.6
  defect, defective NEC H54.7
  disorientation (syndrome) H53.8
  disturbance H53.9
    hysterical F44.6
  double H53.2
  examination Z01.00
    with abnormal findings Z01.01
  field, limitation (defect) —*see* Defect, visual
    field
  hallucinations R44.1
  halos H53.19
  loss —*see* Loss, vision
    sudden —*see* Disturbance, vision,
      subjective, loss, sudden
  low (both eyes) —*see* Low, vision
  perception, simultaneous without fusion
    H53.33
Vitality, lack or want of R53.83
  newborn P96.89
Vitamin deficiency —*see* Deficiency, vitamin
Vitelline duct, persistent Q43.0
Vitiligo L80
  eyelid H02.739
    left H02.736
      lower H02.735
      upper H02.734

Vitiligo (*Continued*)
  eyelid (*Continued*)
    right H02.733
      lower H02.732
      upper H02.731
  pinta A67.2
  vulva N90.89
Vitreal corneal syndrome H59.01-
Vitreoretinopathy, proliferative —*see also*
  Retinopathy, proliferative
  with retinal detachment —*see* Detachment,
    retina, traction
Vitreous —*see also* condition
  touch syndrome —*see* Complication,
    postprocedural, following cataract
    surgery
Vocal cord —*see* condition
Vogt-Koyanagi syndrome H20.82-
Vogt's disease or syndrome G80.3
Vogt-Spielmeyer amaurotic idiocy or disease
  E75.4
Voice
  change R49.9
    specified NEC R49.8
  loss —*see* Aphonia
Volhynian fever A79.0
Volkmann's ischemic contracture or paralysis
  (complicating trauma) T79.6
Volvulus (bowel) (colon) (duodenum)
  (intestine) K56.2
  with perforation K56.2
  congenital Q43.8
  fallopian tube —*see* Torsion, fallopian
    tube
  oviduct —*see* Torsion, fallopian tube
  stomach (due to absence of gastrocolic
    ligament) K31.89
Vomiting R11.10
  with nausea R11.2
  without nausea R11.11
  asphyxia —*see* Foreign body, by site, causing
    asphyxia, gastric contents
  bilious (cause unknown) R11.14
    following gastro-intestinal surgery
      K91.0
    in newborn P92.01
  blood —*see* Hematemesis
  causing asphyxia, choking, or suffocation —
    see Foreign body, by site
  cyclical G43.A0
    with refractory migraine G43.A1
    intractable G43.A1
    not intractable G43.A0
    psychogenic F50.8
    without refractory migraine G43.A0
  fecal mater R11.13
  following gastrointestinal surgery
    K91.0
  psychogenic F50.8

Vomiting (*Continued*)
  functional K31.89
  hysterical F50.8
  nervous F50.8
  neurotic F50.8
  newborn NEC P92.09
    bilious P92.01
  periodic R11.10
    psychogenic F50.8
  projectile R11.12
  psychogenic F50.8
  uremic —*see* Uremia
Vomito negro —*see* Fever, yellow
Von Bezold's abscess —*see* Mastoiditis,
  acute
Von Economo-Cruchet disease A85.8
Von Eulenburg's disease G71.19
Von Gierke's disease E74.01
Von Hippel (-Lindau) **disease or syndrome**
  Q85.8
Von Jaksch's anemia or disease D64.89
Von Recklinghausen
  disease (neurofibromatosis) Q85.01
  bones E21.0
Von Schroetter's syndrome I82.890
Von Willebrand (-Jurgens)(-Minot) **disease or**
  syndrome D68.0
Von Zumbusch's disease L40.1
Voyeurism F65.3
Vrolik's disease Q78.0
Vulva —*see* condition
Vulvismus N94.2
Vulvitis (acute) (allergic) (atrophic)
  (hypertrophic) (intertriginous) (senile)
  N76.3
  with ectopic or molar pregnancy O08.0
  adhesive, congenital Q52.79
  blennorrhagic (gonococcal) A54.02
  candidal B37.3
  chlamydial A56.02
  due to Haemophilus ducreyi A57
  following ectopic or molar pregnancy
    O08.0
  gonococcal A54.02
    with abscess (accessory gland)
      (periurethral) A54.1
  herpesviral A60.04
  leukoplakic N90.4
  monilial B37.3
  puerperal (postpartum) O86.19
  subacute or chronic N76.3
  syphilitic (early) A51.0
    late A52.76
  trichomonal A59.01
  tuberculous A18.18
Vulvodynia N94.819
  specified NEC N94.818
Vulvorectal —*see* condition
Vulvovaginitis (acute) —*see* Vaginitis

W

Waiting list, person on Z75.1
  for organ transplant Z76.82
  undergoing social agency investigation Z75.2
Waldenström
  hypergammaglobulinemia D89.0
  syndrome or macroglobulinemia C88.0
Waldenström-Kjellberg syndrome D50.1
Walking
  difficulty R26.2
    psychogenic F44.4
  sleep F51.3
    hysterical F44.89
Wall, abdominal —*see* condition
Wallenberg's disease or syndrome G46.3
Wallgren's disease I87.8
Wandering
  gallbladder, congenital Q44.1
  in diseases classified elsewhere Z91.83
  kidney, congenital Q63.8
  organ or site, congenital NEC —*see*
    Malposition, congenital, by site
  pacemaker (heart) I49.8
  spleen D73.89
War neurosis F48.8
Wart (due to HPV) (filiform) (infectious) (viral)
  B07.9
  anogenital region (venereal) A63.0
  common B07.8
  external genital organs (venereal) A63.0
  flat B07.8
  Hassal-Henle's (of cornea) H18.49
  Peruvian A44.1
  plantar B07.0
  prosector (tuberculous) A18.4
  seborrheic L82.1
    inflamed L82.0
  senile (seborrheic) L82.1
    inflamed L82.0
  tuberculous A18.4
  venereal A63.0
Warthin's tumor —*see* Neoplasm, salivary
  gland, benign
Wassilieff's disease A27.0
Wasting
  disease R64
    due to malnutrition E41
  extreme (due to malnutrition) E41
  muscle NEC —*see* Atrophy, muscle
Water
  clefts (senile cataract) —*see* Cataract, senile,
    incipient
  deprivation of T73.1
  intoxication E87.79
  itch B76.9
  lack of T73.1
  loading E87.70
  on
    brain —*see* Hydrocephalus
    chest J94.8
  poisoning E87.79
Waterbrash R12
Waterhouse(-Friderichsen) **syndrome or**
  disease (meningococcal) A39.1
Water-losing nephritis N25.89
Watermelon stomach K31.819
  with hemorrhage K31.811
  without hemorrhage K31.819
Watsoniasis B66.8
Wax in ear —*see* Impaction, cerumen
Weak, weakening, weakness (generalized)
  R53.1
  arches (acquired) —*see also* Deformity, limb,
    flat foot
  bladder (sphincter) R32
  facial R29.810
    following
      cerebrovascular disease I69.992
        cerebral infarction I69.392
        intracerebral hemorrhage I69.192

Weak, weakening, weakness *(Continued)*
  facial *(Continued)*
    following *(Continued)*
      cerebrovascular disease *(Continued)*
        nontraumatic intracranial hemorrhage
          NEC I69.292
        specified disease NEC I69.892
        stroke I69.392
        subarachnoid hemorrhage I69.092
  foot (double) —*see* Weak, arches
  heart, cardiac —*see* Failure, heart
  mind F70
  muscle M62.81
  myocardium —*see* Failure, heart
  newborn P96.89
  pelvic fundus N81.89
  pubocervical tissue N81.82
  rectovaginal tissue N81.83
  senile R54
  urinary stream R39.12
  valvular —*see* Endocarditis
Wear, worn (with normal or routine use)
  articular bearing surface of internal joint
    prosthesis —*see* Complications, joint
    prosthesis, mechanical, wear of articular
    bearing surfaces, by site
  device, implant or graft —*see* Complications,
    by site, mechanical complication
  tooth, teeth (approximal) (hard tissues)
    (interproximal) (occlusal) K03.0
Weather, weathered
  effects of
    cold T69.9
      specified effect NEC T69.8
    hot —*see* Heat
  skin L57.8
Weaver's syndrome Q87.3
Web, webbed (congenital)
  duodenal Q43.8
  esophagus Q39.4
  fingers Q70.1
  larynx (glottic) (subglottic) Q31.0
  neck (pterygium colli) Q18.3
  Paterson-Kelly D50.1
  popliteal syndrome Q87.89
  toes Q70.3
Weber-Christian disease M35.6
Weber-Cockayne syndrome (epidermolysis
  bullosa) Q81.8
Weber-Gubler syndrome G46.3
Weber-Leyden syndrome G46.3
Weber-Osler syndrome I78.0
Weber's paralysis or syndrome G46.3
Wedge-shaped or wedging vertebra —*see*
  Collapse, vertebra NEC
Wegener's granulomatosis or syndrome
  M31.30
  with
    kidney involvement M31.31
    lung involvement M31.30
      with kidney involvement M31.31
Wegner's disease A50.02
Weight
  1000-2499 grams at birth (low) —*see* Low,
    birthweight
  999 grams or less at birth (extremely low) —
    see Low, birthweight, extreme
  gain (abnormal) (excessive) R63.5
    in pregnancy —*see* Pregnancy, complicated
      by, excessive weight gain
      low —*see* Pregnancy, complicated by,
        insufficient, weight gain
  loss (abnormal) (cause unknown) R63.4
Weightlessness (effect of) T75.82
Weil (l)-**Marchesani syndrome** Q87.1
Weil's disease A27.0
Weingarten's syndrome J82
Weir Mitchell's disease I73.81
Weiss-Baker syndrome G90.09
Wells' disease L98.3
Wen —*see* Cyst, sebaceous

Wenckebach's block or phenomenon I44.1
Werdnig-Hoffmann syndrome (muscular
  atrophy) G12.0
Werlhof's disease D69.3
Werner-His disease A79.0
Werner's disease or syndrome E31.21
Werner's disease or syndrome E34.8
Wernicke-Korsakoff's syndrome or psychosis
  (alcoholic) F10.96
  with dependence F10.26
  drug-induced
    due to drug abuse —*see* Abuse, drug, by
      type, with amnestic disorder
    due to drug dependence —*see* Dependence,
      drug, by type, with amnestic disorder
  nonalcoholic F04
Wernicke-Posadas disease B38.9
Wernicke's
  developmental aphasia F80.2
  disease or syndrome E51.2
  encephalopathy E51.2
  polioencephalitis, superior E51.2
West African fever B50.8
Westphal-Strümpell syndrome E83.01
West's syndrome —*see* Epilepsy, spasms
Wet
  feet, tropical (maceration) (syndrome) —*see*
    Immersion, foot
  lung (syndrome), newborn P22.1
Wharton's duct —*see* condition
Wheal —*see* Urticaria
Wheezing R06.2
Whiplash injury S13.4
Whipple's disease (see also subcategory M14.8-)
  K90.81
Whipworm (disease) (infection) (infestation)
  B79
Whistling face Q87.0
White —*see also* condition
  kidney, small N03.9
  leg, puerperal, postpartum, childbirth O87.1
  mouth B37.0
  patches of mouth K13.29
  spot lesions, teeth
    chewing surface K02.51
    pit and fissure surface K02.51
    smooth surface K02.61
Whitehead L70.0
Whitlow —*see also* Cellulitis, digit
  with lymphangitis —*see* Lymphangitis, acute,
    digit
  herpesviral B00.89
Whitmore's disease or fever —*see* Melioidosis
Whooping cough A37.90
  with pneumonia A37.91
    due to Bordetella
      bronchiseptica A37.81
      parapertussis A37.11
      pertussis A37.01
      specified organism NEC A37.81
  due to
    Bordetella
      bronchiseptica A37.80
        with pneumonia A37.81
      parapertussis A37.10
        with pneumonia A37.11
      pertussis A37.00
        with pneumonia A37.01
      specified NEC A37.80
        with pneumonia A37.81
Wichman's asthma J38.5
Wide cranial sutures, newborn P96.3
Widening aorta —*see* Ectasia, aorta
  with aneurysm —*see* Aneurysm, aorta
Wilkie's disease or syndrome K55.1
Wilkinson-Sneddon disease or syndrome
  L13.1
Willebrand (-Jürgens) **thrombopathy** D68.0
Willige-Hunt disease or syndrome G23.1
Wilms' tumor C64-
Wilson-Mikity syndrome P27.0

◀ New   ◀||| Revised   ~~deleted~~ Deleted

Wilson's
  disease or syndrome E83.01
  hepatolenticular degeneration E83.01
  lichen ruber L43.9
Window —*see also* Imperfect, closure
  aorticopulmonary Q21.4
Winter —*see* condition
Wiskott-Aldrich syndrome D82.0
Withdrawal state —*see also* Dependence, drug
    by type, with withdrawal
  newborn
    correct therapeutic substance properly
      administered P96.2
    infant of dependent mother P96.1
    therapeutic substance, neonatal P96.2
Witts' anemia D50.8
Witzelsucht F07.0
Woakes' ethmoiditis or syndrome J33.1
Wolff-Hirschorn syndrome Q93.3
Wolff-Parkinson-White syndrome I45.6
Wolhynian fever A79.0
Wolman's disease E75.5
Wood lung or pneumonitis J67.8
Woolly, wooly hair (congenital) (nevus)
    Q84.1
Woolsorter's disease A22.1
Word
  blindness (congenital) (developmental)
    F81.0
  deafness (congenital) (developmental)
    H93.25
Worm (s) (infection) (infestation) —*see also*
    Infestation, helminth
  guinea B72
  in intestine NEC B82.0
Worm-eaten soles A66.3
Worn out —*see* Exhaustion
  cardiac
    defibrillator (with synchronous cardiac
      pacemaker) Z45.02
    pacemaker
      battery Z45.010
      lead Z45.018
  device, implant or graft —*see* Complications,
    by site, mechanical
Worried well Z71.1
Worries R45.82
Wound, open
  abdomen, abdominal
    wall S31.109
      with penetration into peritoneal cavity
        S31.609
      bite —*see* Bite, abdomen, wall
      epigastric region S31.102
        with penetration into peritoneal cavity
          S31.602
        bite —*see* Bite, abdomen, wall,
          epigastric region
        laceration —*see* Laceration, abdomen,
          wall, epigastric region
        puncture —*see* Puncture, abdomen,
          wall, epigastric region
      laceration —*see* Laceration, abdomen,
        wall
      left
        lower quadrant S31.104
          with penetration into peritoneal
            cavity S31.604
          bite —*see* Bite, abdomen, wall, left,
            lower quadrant
          laceration —*see* Laceration,
            abdomen, wall, left, lower
            quadrant
          puncture —*see* Puncture,
            abdomen, wall, left, lower
            quadrant
        upper quadrant S31.101
          with penetration into peritoneal
            cavity S31.601
          bite —*see* Bite, abdomen, wall, left,
            upper quadrant

Wound, open *(Continued)*
  abdomen, abdominal *(Continued)*
    wall *(Continued)*
      left *(Continued)*
        upper quadrant *(Continued)*
          laceration —*see* Laceration,
            abdomen, wall, left, upper
            quadrant
          puncture —*see* Puncture, abdomen,
            wall, left, upper quadrant
      periumbilic region S31.105
        with penetration into peritoneal cavity
          S31.605
        bite —*see* Bite, abdomen, wall,
          periumbilic region
        laceration —*see* Laceration, abdomen,
          wall, periumbilic region
        puncture —*see* Puncture, abdomen,
          wall, periumbilic region
      puncture —*see* Puncture, abdomen, wall
      right
        lower quadrant S31.103
          with penetration into peritoneal
            cavity S31.603
          bite —*see* Bite, abdomen, wall, right,
            lower quadrant
          laceration —*see* Laceration,
            abdomen, wall, right, lower
            quadrant
          puncture —*see* Puncture, abdomen,
            wall, right, lower quadrant
        upper quadrant S31.100
          with penetration into peritoneal
            cavity S31.600
          bite —*see* Bite, abdomen, wall, right,
            upper quadrant
          laceration —*see* Laceration,
            abdomen, wall, right, upper
            quadrant
          puncture —*see* Puncture, abdomen,
            wall, right, upper quadrant
    alveolar (process) —*see* Wound, open, oral
      cavity
    ankle S91.00-
      bite —*see* Bite, ankle
      laceration —*see* Laceration, ankle
      puncture —*see* Puncture, ankle
    antecubital space —*see* Wound, open, elbow
    anterior chamber, eye —*see* Wound, open,
      ocular
    anus S31.839
      bite S31.835
      laceration —*see* Laceration, anus
      puncture —*see* Puncture, anus
    arm (upper) S41.10-
      with amputation —*see* Amputation,
        traumatic, arm
      bite —*see* Bite, arm
      forearm —*see* Wound, open, forearm
      laceration —*see* Laceration, arm
      puncture —*see* Puncture, arm
    auditory canal (external) (meatus) —*see*
      Wound, open, ear
    auricle, ear —*see* Wound, open, ear
    axilla —*see* Wound, open, arm
    back —*see also* Wound, open, thorax, back
      lower S31.000
        with penetration into retroperitoneal
          space S31.001
        bite —*see* Bite, back, lower
        laceration —*see* Laceration, back,
          lower
        puncture —*see* Puncture, back, lower
    bite —*see* Bite
    blood vessel —*see* Injury, blood vessel
    breast S21.00-
      with amputation —*see* Amputation,
        traumatic, breast
      bite —*see* Bite, breast
      laceration —*see* Laceration, breast
      puncture —*see* Puncture, breast

Wound, open *(Continued)*
  buttock S31.809
    bite —*see* Bite, buttock
    laceration —*see* Laceration, buttock
    left S31.829
    puncture —*see* Puncture, buttock
    right S31.819
  calf —*see* Wound, open, leg
  canaliculus lacrimalis —*see* Wound,
    open, eyelid
  canthus, eye —*see* Wound, open,
    eyelid
  cervical esophagus S11.20
    bite S11.25
    laceration —*see* Laceration, esophagus,
      traumatic, cervical
    puncture —*see* Puncture, cervical
      esophagus
  cheek (external) S01.40-
    bite —*see* Bite, cheek
    internal —*see* Wound, open, oral
      cavity
    laceration —*see* Laceration, cheek
    puncture —*see* Puncture, cheek
  chest wall —*see* Wound, open, thorax
  chin —*see* Wound, open, head, specified site
    NEC
  choroid —*see* Wound, open, ocular
  ciliary body (eye) —*see* Wound, open,
    ocular
  clitoris S31.40
    with amputation —*see* Amputation,
      traumatic, clitoris
    bite S31.45
    laceration —*see* Laceration, vulva
    puncture —*see* Puncture, vulva
  conjunctiva —*see* Wound, open, ocular
  cornea —*see* Wound, open, ocular
  costal region —*see* Wound, open, thorax
  Descemet's membrane —*see* Wound, open,
    ocular
  digit (s)
    foot —*see* Wound, open, toe
    hand —*see* Wound, open, finger
  ear (canal) (external) S01.30-
    with amputation —*see* Amputation,
      traumatic, ear
    bite —*see* Bite, ear
    drum S09.2-
    laceration —*see* Laceration, ear
    puncture —*see* Puncture, ear
  elbow S51.00-
    bite —*see* Bite, elbow
    laceration —*see* Laceration, elbow
    puncture —*see* Puncture, elbow
  epididymis —*see* Wound, open, testis
  epigastric region S31.102
    with penetration into peritoneal cavity
      S31.602
    bite —*see* Bite, abdomen, wall, epigastric
      region
    laceration —*see* Laceration, abdomen, wall,
      epigastric region
    puncture —*see* Puncture, abdomen, wall,
      epigastric region
  epiglottis —*see* Wound, open, neck, specified
    site NEC
  esophagus (thoracic) S27.819
    cervical —*see* Wound, open, cervical
      esophagus
    laceration S27.813
    specified type NEC S27.818
  eye —*see* Wound, open, ocular
  eyeball —*see* Wound, open, ocular
  eyebrow —*see* Wound, open, eyelid
  eyelid S01.10-
    bite —*see* Bite, eyelid
    laceration —*see* Laceration, eyelid
    puncture —*see* Puncture, eyelid
  face NEC —*see* Wound, open, head, specified
    site NEC

W

Wound, open *(Continued)*
  finger (s) S61.209
    with
      amputation —*see* Amputation,
        traumatic, finger
      damage to nail S61.309
    bite —*see* Bite, finger
    index S61.208
      with
        damage to nail S61.308
      left S61.201
        with
          damage to nail S61.301
      right S61.200
        with
          damage to nail S61.300
    laceration —*see* Laceration, finger
    little S61.208
      with
        damage to nail S61.308
      left S61.207
        with damage to nail S61.307
      right S61.206
        with damage to nail S61.306
    middle S61.208
      with
        damage to nail S61.308
      left S61.203
        with damage to nail S61.303
      right S61.202
        with damage to nail S61.302
    puncture —*see* Puncture, finger
    ring S61.208
      with
        damage to nail S61.308
      left S61.205
        with damage to nail S61.305
      right S61.204
        with damage to nail S61.304
  flank —*see* Wound, open, abdomen, wall
  foot (except toe (s) alone) S91.30-
    with amputation —*see* Amputation,
      traumatic, foot
    bite —*see* Bite, foot
    laceration —*see* Laceration, foot
    puncture —*see* Puncture, foot
    toe —*see* Wound, open, toe
  forearm S51.80-
    with
      amputation —*see* Amputation,
        traumatic, forearm
    bite —*see* Bite, forearm
    elbow only —*see* Wound, open, elbow
    laceration —*see* Laceration, forearm
    puncture —*see* Puncture, forearm
  forehead —*see* Wound, open, head, specified
    site NEC
  genital organs, external
    with amputation —*see* Amputation,
      traumatic, genital organs
    bite —*see* Bite, genital organ
    female S31.502
      vagina S31.40
      vulva S31.40
      laceration —*see* Laceration, genital
        organ
    male S31.501
      penis S31.20
      scrotum S31.30
      testes S31.30
    puncture —*see* Puncture, genital organ
  globe (eye) —*see* Wound, open, ocular
  groin —*see* Wound, open, abdomen, wall
  gum —*see* Wound, open, oral cavity
  hand S61.40-
    with
      amputation —*see* Amputation,
        traumatic, hand
    bite —*see* Bite, hand
    finger (s) —*see* Wound, open, finger
    laceration —*see* Laceration, hand

Wound, open *(Continued)*
  hand *(Continued)*
      puncture —*see* Puncture, hand
      thumb —*see* Wound, open, thumb
  head S01.90
    bite —*see* Bite, head
    cheek —*see* Wound, open, cheek
    ear —*see* Wound, open, ear
    eyelid —*see* Wound, open, eyelid
    laceration —*see* Laceration, head
    lip —*see* Wound, open, lip
    nose S01.20
    oral cavity —*see* Wound, open, oral cavity
    puncture —*see* Puncture, head
    scalp —*see* Wound, open, scalp
    specified site NEC S01.80
    temporomandibular area —*see* Wound,
      open, cheek
  heel —*see* Wound, open, foot
  hip S71.00-
    with amputation —*see* Amputation,
      traumatic, hip
    bite —*see* Bite, hip
    laceration —*see* Laceration, hip
    puncture —*see* Puncture, hip
  hymen S31.40
    bite —*see* Bite, vulva
    laceration —*see* Laceration, vagina
    puncture —*see* Puncture, vagina
  hypochondrium S31.109
    bite —*see* Bite, hypochondrium
    laceration —*see* Laceration,
      hypochondrium
    puncture —*see* Puncture, hypochondrium
  hypogastric region S31.109
    bite —*see* Bite, hypogastric region
    laceration —*see* Laceration, hypogastric
      region
    puncture —*see* Puncture, hypogastric
      region
  iliac (region) —*see* Wound, open, inguinal
    region
  inguinal region S31.109
    bite —*see* Bite, abdomen, wall, lower
      quadrant
    laceration —*see* Laceration, inguinal region
    puncture —*see* Puncture, inguinal region
  instep —*see* Wound, open, foot
  interscapular region —*see* Wound, open,
    thorax, back
  intraocular —*see* Wound, open, ocular
  iris —*see* Wound, open, ocular
  jaw —*see* Wound, open, head, specified site
    NEC
  knee S81.00-
    bite —*see* Bite, knee
    laceration —*see* Laceration, knee
    puncture —*see* Puncture, knee
  labium (majus) (minus) —*see* Wound, open,
    vulva
  laceration —*see* Laceration, by site
  lacrimal duct —*see* Wound, open, eyelid
  larynx S11.019
    bite —*see* Bite, larynx
    laceration —*see* Laceration, larynx
    puncture —*see* Puncture, larynx
  left
    lower quadrant S31.104
      with penetration into peritoneal cavity
        S31.604
      bite —*see* Bite, abdomen, wall, left, lower
        quadrant
      laceration —*see* Laceration, abdomen,
        wall, left, lower quadrant
      puncture —*see* Puncture, abdomen, wall,
        left, lower quadrant
    upper quadrant S31.101
      with penetration into peritoneal cavity
        S31.601
      bite —*see* Bite, abdomen, wall, left,
        upper quadrant

Wound, open *(Continued)*
  left *(Continued)*
    upper quadrant *(Continued)*
      laceration —*see* Laceration, abdomen,
        wall, left, upper quadrant
      puncture —*see* Puncture, abdomen, wall,
        left, upper quadrant
  leg (lower) S81.80-
    with amputation —*see* Amputation,
      traumatic, leg
    ankle —*see* Wound, open, ankle
    bite —*see* Bite, leg
    foot —*see* Wound, open, foot
    knee —*see* Wound, open, knee
    laceration —*see* Laceration, leg
    puncture —*see* Puncture, leg
    toe —*see* Wound, open, toe
    upper —*see* Wound, open, thigh
  lip S01.501
    bite —*see* Bite, lip
    laceration —*see* Laceration, lip
    puncture —*see* Puncture, lip
  loin S31.109
    bite —*see* Bite, abdomen, wall
    laceration —*see* Laceration, loin
    puncture —*see* Puncture, loin
  lower back —*see* Wound, open, back,
    lower
  lumbar region —*see* Wound, open, back,
    lower
  malar region —*see* Wound, open, head,
    specified site NEC
  mammary —*see* Wound, open, breast
  mastoid region —*see* Wound, open, head,
    specified site NEC
  mouth —*see* Wound, open, oral cavity
  nail
    finger —*see* Wound, open, finger, with
      damage to nail
    toe —*see* Wound, open, toe, with damage
      to nail
  nape (neck) —*see* Wound, open, neck
  nasal (septum) (sinus) —*see* Wound, open,
    nose
  nasopharynx —*see* Wound, open, head,
    specified site NEC
  neck S11.90
    bite —*see* Bite, neck
    involving
      cervical esophagus S11.20
      larynx —*see* Wound, open, larynx
      pharynx S11.20
      thyroid S11.10
      trachea (cervical) S11.029
        bite —*see* Bite, trachea
        laceration S11.021
          with foreign body S11.022
        puncture S11.023
          with foreign body S11.024
    laceration —*see* Laceration, neck
    puncture —*see* Puncture, neck
    specified site NEC S11.80
      specified type NEC S11.89
  nose (septum) (sinus) S01.20
    with amputation —*see* Amputation,
      traumatic, nose
    bite —*see* Bite, nose
    laceration —*see* Laceration, nose
    puncture —*see* Puncture, nose
  ocular S05.90
    avulsion (traumatic enucleation) S05.7-
    eyeball S05.6-
      with foreign body S05.5-
    eyelid —*see* Wound, open, eyelid
    laceration and rupture S05.3-
      with prolapse or loss of intraocular
        tissue S05.2-
    orbit (penetrating) (with or without foreign
      body) S05.4-
    periocular area —*see* Wound, open, eyelid
    specified NEC S05.8X-

W

X

Xanthelasma (eyelid) (palpebrarum) H02.60
  left H02.66
    lower H02.65
    upper H02.64
  right H02.63
    lower H02.62
    upper H02.61
Xanthelasmatosis (essential) E78.2
Xanthinuria, hereditary E79.8
Xanthoastrocytoma
  specified site —*see* Neoplasm, malignant, by
      site
  unspecified site C71.9
Xanthofibroma —*see* Neoplasm, connective
      tissue, benign
Xanthogranuloma D76.3
Xanthoma (s), **xanthomatosis** (primary)
      (familial) (hereditary) E75.5
  with
    hyperlipoproteinemia
      Type I E78.3
      Type III E78.2
      Type IV E78.1
      Type V E78.3
  bone (generalisata) C96.5
  cerebrotendinous E75.5
  cutaneotendinous E75.5

Xanthoma (s), **xanthomatosis** (*Continued*)
  disseminatum (skin) E78.2
  eruptive E78.2
  hypercholesterinemic E78.0
  hypercholesterolemic E78.0
  hyperlipidemic E78.5
  joint E75.5
  multiple (skin) E78.2
  tendon (sheath) E75.5
  tuberosum E78.2
  tuberous E78.2
  tubo-eruptive E78.2
  verrucous, oral mucosa K13.4
Xanthosis R23.8
Xenophobia F40.10
Xeroderma —*see also* Ichthyosis
  acquired L85.0
    eyelid H01.149
      left H01.146
        lower H01.145
        upper H01.144
      right H01.143
        lower H01.142
        upper H01.141
  pigmentosum Q82.1
  vitamin A deficiency E50.8
Xerophthalmia (vitamin A deficiency) E50.7
  unrelated to vitamin A deficiency —*see*
      Keratoconjunctivitis

Xerosis
  conjunctiva H11.14-
    with Bitot's spots —*see also* Pigmentation,
        conjunctiva
      vitamin A deficiency E50.1
    vitamin A deficiency E50.0
  cornea H18.89-
    with ulceration —*see* Ulcer, cornea
      vitamin A deficiency E50.3
    vitamin A deficiency E50.2
  cutis L85.3
  skin L85.3
Xerostomia K11.7
Xiphopagus Q89.4
XO syndrome Q96.9
X-ray (of)
  abnormal findings —*see* Abnormal,
      diagnostic imaging
  breast (mammogram) (routine) Z12.31
  chest
    routine (as part of a general medical
        examination) Z00.00
      with abnormal findings Z00.01
    routine (as part of a general medical
        examination) Z00.00
      with abnormal findings Z00.01
XXXXY syndrome Q98.1
XXY syndrome Q98.0

◀ New   ◀▦ Revised   ~~deleted~~ Deleted

Y

Yaba pox virus disease B08.72
Yatapoxvirus B08.70
  specified NEC B08.79
Yawning R06.89
  psychogenic F45.8
Yaws A66.9
  bone lesions A66.6
  butter A66.1
  chancre A66.0
  cutaneous, less than five years after infection
    A66.2
  early (cutaneous) (macular) (maculopapular)
    (micropapular) (papular) A66.2
    frambeside A66.2
    skin lesions NEC A66.2
  eyelid A66.2
  ganglion A66.6
  gangosis, gangosa A66.5
  gumma, gummata A66.4
    bone A66.6
  gummatous
    frambeside A66.4
    osteitis A66.6
    periostitis A66.6
  hydrarthrosis (*see also* subcategory M14.8-)
    A66.6
  hyperkeratosis (early) (late) A66.3

Yaws (*Continued*)
  initial lesions A66.0
  joint lesions (*see also* subcategory M14.8-)
    A66.6
  juxta-articular nodules A66.7
  late nodular (ulcerated) A66.4
  latent (without clinical manifestations) (with
    positive serology) A66.8
  mother A66.0
  mucosal A66.7
  multiple papillomata A66.1
  nodular, late (ulcerated) A66.4
  osteitis A66.6
  papilloma, plantar or palmar A66.1
  periostitis (hypertrophic) A66.6
  specified NEC A66.7
  ulcers A66.4
  wet crab A66.1
Yeast infection (*see also* Candidiasis) B37.9
Yellow
  atrophy (liver) —*see* Failure, hepatic
  fever —*see* Fever, yellow
  jack —*see* Fever, yellow
  jaundice —*see* Jaundice
  nail syndrome L60.5
Yersiniosis —*see also* Infection, Yersinia
  extraintestinal A28.2
  intestinal A04.6

Z

Zahorsky's syndrome (herpangina) B08.5
Zellweger's syndrome Q87.89
Zenker's diverticulum (esophagus) K22.5
Ziehen-Oppenheim disease G24.1
Zieve's syndrome K70.0
Zinc
  deficiency, dietary E60
  metabolism disorder E83.2
Zollinger-Ellison syndrome E16.4
Zona —*see* Herpes, zoster
Zoophobia F40.218
Zoster (herpes) —*see* Herpes, zoster
Zygomycosis B46.9
  specified NEC B46.8
Zymotic —*see* condition

Y & Z

ICD-10-CM
Table of Neoplasms

ICD-10-CM
Table of Neoplasms

	Malignant Primary	Malignant Secondary	Ca in situ	Benign	Uncertain Behavior	Unspecified Behavior
The list below gives the code numbers for neoplasms by anatomical site. For each site there are six possible code numbers according to whether the neoplasm in question is malignant, benign, in situ, of uncertain behavior, or of unspecified nature. The description of the neoplasm will often indicate which of the six columns is appropriate; e.g., malignant melanoma of skin, benign fibroadenoma of breast, carcinoma in situ of cervix uteri.						
Where such descriptors are not present, the remainder of the Index should be consulted where guidance is given to the appropriate column for each morphological (histological) variety listed; e.g., Mesonephroma—*see Neoplasm, malignant;* Embryoma—*see also Neoplasm, uncertain behavior;* Disease, Bowen's—*see Neoplasm, skin, in situ.* However, the guidance in the Index can be overridden if one of the descriptors mentioned above is present; e.g., malignant adenoma of colon is coded to C18.9 and not to D12.6 as the adjective "malignant" overrides the Index entry "Adenoma—*see also Neoplasm, benign.*"						
Codes listed with a dash -, following the code have a required additional character for laterality. The tablular must be reviewed for the complete code.						
Neoplasm, neoplastic	C80.1	C79.9	D09.9	D36.9	D48.9	D49.9
abdomen, abdominal	C76.2	C79.8-	D09.8	D36.7	D48.7	D49.89
cavity	C76.2	C79.8-	D09.8	D36.7	D48.7	D49.89
organ	C76.2	C79.8-	D09.8	D36.7	D48.7	D49.89
viscera	C76.2	C79.8-	D09.8	D36.7	D48.7	D49.89
wall—*see also Neoplasm, abdomen, wall, skin*	C44.509	C79.2-	D04.5	D23.5	D48.5	D49.2
connective tissue	C49.4	C79.8-	—	D21.4	D48.1	D49.2
skin	C44.509					
basal cell carcinoma	C44.519	—	—	—	—	—
specified type NEC	C44.599	—	—	—	—	—
squamous cell carcinoma	C44.529	—	—	—	—	—
abdominopelvic	C76.8	C79.8-	—	D36.7	D48.7	D49.89
accessory sinus—*see Neoplasm, sinus*						
acoustic nerve	C72.4-	C79.49	—	D33.3	D43.3	D49.7
adenoid (pharynx) (tissue)	C11.1	C79.89	D00.08	D10.6	D37.05	D49.0
adipose tissue—*see also Neoplasm, connective tissue*	C49.4	C79.89	—	D21.9	D48.1	D49.2
adnexa (uterine)	C57.4	C79.89	D07.39	D28.7	D39.8	D49.5
adrenal	C74.9-	C79.7-	D09.3	D35.0-	D44.1-	D49.7
capsule	C74.9-	C79.7-	D09.3	D35.0-	D44.1-	D49.7
cortex	C74.0-	C79.7-	D09.3	D35.0-	D44.1-	D49.7
gland	C74.9-	C79.7-	D09.3	D35.0-	D44.1-	D49.7
medulla	C74.1-	C79.7-	D09.3	D35.0-	D44.1-	D49.7
ala nasi (external)—*see also Neoplasm, skin, nose*	C44.301	C79.2	D04.39	D23.39	D48.5	D49.2
alimentary canal or tract NEC	C26.9	C78.80	D01.9	D13.9	D37.9	D49.0
alveolar	C03.9	C79.89	D00.03	D10.39	D37.09	D49.0
mucosa	C03.9	C79.89	D00.03	D10.39	D37.09	D49.0
lower	C03.1	C79.89	D00.03	D10.39	D37.09	D49.0
upper	C03.0	C79.89	D00.03	D10.39	D37.09	D49.0
ridge or process	C41.1	C79.51	—	D16.5-	D48.0	D49.2
carcinoma	C03.9	C79.8-	—	—	—	—
lower	C03.1	C79.8-	—	—	—	—
upper	C03.0	C79.8-	—	—	—	—

TABLE OF NEOPLASMS

	Malignant Primary	Malignant Secondary	Ca in situ	Benign	Uncertain Behavior	Unspecified Behavior
alveolar *(Continued)*						
ridge or process *(Continued)*						
lower	C41.1	C79.51	—	D16.5-	D48.0	D49.2
mucosa	C03.9	C79.89	D00.03	D10.39	D37.09	D49.0
lower	C03.1	C79.89	D00.03	D10.39	D37.09	D49.0
upper	C03.0	C79.89	D00.03	D10.39	D37.09	D49.0
upper	C41.0	C79.51	—	D16.4-	D48.0	D49.2
sulcus	C06.1	C79.89	D00.02	D10.39	D37.09	D49.0
alveolus	C03.9	C79.89	D00.03	D10.39	D37.09	D49.0
lower	C03.1	C79.89	D00.03	D10.39	D37.09	D49.0
upper	C03.0	C79.89	D00.03	D10.39	D37.09	D49.0
ampulla of Vater	C24.1	C78.89	D01.5	D13.5	D37.6	D49.0
ankle NEC	C76.5-	C79.89	D04.7-	D36.7	D48.7	D49.89
anorectum, anorectal (junction)	C21.8	C78.5	D01.3	D12.9	D37.8	D49.0
antecubital fossa or space	C76.4-	C79.89	D04.6-	D36.7	D48.7	D49.89
antrum (Highmore) (maxillary)	C31.0	C78.39	D02.3	D14.0	D38.5	D49.1
pyloric	C16.3	C78.89	D00.2	D13.1	D37.1	D49.0
tympanicum	C30.1	C78.39	D02.3	D14.0	D38.5	D49.1
anus, anal	C21.0	C78.5	D01.3	D12.9	D37.8	D49.0
canal	C21.1	C78.5	D01.3	D12.9	D37.8	D49.0
cloacogenic zone	C21.2	C78.5	D01.3	D12.9	D37.8	D49.0
margin — *see also Neoplasm, anus, skin*	C44.500	C79.2	D04.5	D23.5	D48.5	D49.2
overlapping lesion with rectosigmoid junction or rectum	C21.8	—	—	—	—	—
skin	C44.500	C79.2	D04.5	D23.5	D48.5	D49.2
basal cell carcinoma	C44.510	—	—	—	—	—
specified type NEC	C44.590	—	—	—	—	—
squamous cell carcinoma	C44.520	—	—	—	—	—
sphincter	C21.1	C78.5	D01.3	D12.9	D37.8	D49.0
aorta (thoracic)	C49.3	C79.89	—	D21.3	D48.1	D49.2
abdominal	C49.4	C79.89	—	D21.4	D48.1	D49.2
aortic body	C75.5	C79.89	—	D35.6	D44.7	D49.7
aponeurosis	C49.9	C79.89	—	D21.9	D48.1	D49.2
palmar	C49.1-	C79.89	—	D21.1-	D48.1	D49.2
plantar	C49.2-	C79.89	—	D21.2-	D48.1	D49.2
appendix	C18.1	C78.5	D01.0	D12.1	D37.3	D49.0
arachnoid	C70.9	C79.49	—	D32.9	D42.9	D49.7
cerebral	C70.0	C79.32	—	D32.0	D42.0	D49.7
spinal	C70.1	C79.49	—	D32.1	D42.1	D49.7
areola	C50.0-	C79.81	D05.-	D24.-	D48.6-	D49.3
arm NEC	C76.4-	C79.89	D04.6-	D36.7	D48.7	D49.89
artery — *see Neoplasm, connective tissue*						

	Malignant Primary	Malignant Secondary	Ca in situ	Benign	Uncertain Behavior	Unspecified Behavior
aryepiglottic fold	C13.1	C79.89	D00.08	D10.7	D37.05	D49.0
hypopharyngeal aspect	C13.1	C79.89	D00.08	D10.7	D37.05	D49.0
laryngeal aspect	C32.1	C78.39	D02.0	D14.1	D38.0	D49.1
marginal zone	C13.1	C79.89	D00.08	D10.7	D37.05	D49.0
arytenoid (cartilage)	C32.3	C78.39	D02.0	D14.1	D38.0	D49.1
fold — *see Neoplasm, aryepiglottic*						
associated with transplanted organ	C80.2	—	—	—	—	—
atlas	C41.2	C79.51	—	D16.6	D48.0	D49.2
atrium, cardiac	C38.0	C79.89	—	D15.1	D48.7	D49.89
auditory						
canal (external) (skin) A81	C44.20-	C79.2	D04.2-	D23.2-	D48.5	D49.2
internal	C30.1	C78.39	D02.3	D14.0	D38.5	D49.1
nerve	C72.4-	C79.49	—	D33.3	D43.3	D49.7
tube	C30.1	C78.39	D02.3	D14.0	D38.5	D49.1
opening	C11.2	C79.89	D00.08	D10.6	D37.05	D49.0
auricle, ear — *see also Neoplasm, skin, ear*	C44.20-	C79.2	D04.2-	D23.2-	D48.5	D49.2
auricular canal (external) — *see also Neoplasm, skin, ear*	C44.20-	C79.2	D04.2-	D23.2-	D48.5	D49.2
internal	C30.1	C78.39	D02.3	D14.0	D38.5	D49.2
autonomic nerve or nervous system NEC *(see Neoplasm, nerve, peripheral)*						
axilla, axillary	C76.1	C79.89	D09.8	D36.7	D48.7	D49.89
fold — *see also Neoplasm, skin, trunk*	C44.509	C79.2	D04.5	D23.5	D48.5	D49.2
back NEC	C76.8	C79.89	D04.5	D36.7	D48.7	D49.89
Bartholin's gland	C51.0	C79.82	D07.1	D28.0	D39.8	D49.5
basal ganglia	C71.0	C79.31	—	D33.0	D43.0	D49.6
basis pedunculi	C71.7	C79.31	—	D33.1	D43.1	D49.6
bile or biliary (tract)	C24.9	C78.89	D01.5	D13.5	D37.6	D49.0
canaliculi (biliferi) (intrahepatic)	C22.1	C78.7	D01.5	D13.4	D37.6	D49.0
canals, interlobular	C22.1	C78.89	D01.5	D13.4	D37.6	D49.0
duct or passage (common) (cystic) (extrahepatic)	C24.0	C78.89	D01.5	D13.5	D37.6	D49.0
interlobular	C22.1	C78.89	D01.5	D13.4	D37.6	D49.0
intrahepatic	C22.1	C78.7	D01.5	D13.4	D37.6	D49.0
and extrahepatic	C24.8	C78.89	D01.5	D13.5	D37.6	D49.0
bladder (urinary)	C67.9	C79.11	D09.0	D30.3	D41.4	D49.4
dome	C67.1	C79.11	D09.0	D30.3	D41.4	D49.4
neck	C67.5	C79.11	D09.0	D30.3	D41.4	D49.4
orifice	C67.9	C79.11	D09.0	D30.3	D41.4	D49.4
ureteric	C67.6	C79.11	D09.0	D30.3	D41.4	D49.4
urethral	C67.5	C79.11	D09.0	D30.3	D41.4	D49.4
overlapping lesion	C67.8	—	—	—	—	—
sphincter	C67.8	C79.11	D09.0	D30.3	D41.4	D49.4
trigone	C67.0	C79.11	D09.0	D30.3	D41.4	D49.4
urachus	C67.7	C79.11	D09.0	D30.3	D41.4	D49.4

◀ New   ◀▦ Revised   ~~deleted~~ Deleted

TABLE OF NEOPLASMS

	Malignant Primary	Malignant Secondary	Ca in situ	Benign	Uncertain Behavior	Unspecified Behavior
bladder (urinary) *(Continued)*						
wall	C67.9	C79.11	D09.0	D30.3	D41.4	D49.4
anterior	C67.3	C79.11	D09.0	D30.3	D41.4	D49.4
lateral	C67.2	C79.11	D09.0	D30.3	D41.4	D49.4
posterior	C67.4	C79.11	D09.0	D30.3	D41.4	D49.4
blood vessel — *see Neoplasm, connective tissue*						
bone (periosteum)	C41.9	C79.51	—	D16.9-	D48.0	D49.2
acetabulum	C41.4	C79.51	—	D16.8-	D48.0	D49.2
ankle	C40.3-	C79.51	—	D16.3-	—	—
arm NEC	C40.0-	C79.51	—	D16.0-	—	—
astragalus	C40.3-	C79.51	—	D16.3-	—	—
atlas	C41.2	C79.51	—	D16.6-	D48.0	D49.2
axis	C41.2	C79.51	—	D16.6-	D48.0	D49.2
back NEC	C41.2	C79.51	—	D16.6-	D48.0	D49.2
calcaneus	C40.3-	C79.51	—	D16.3-	—	—
calvarium	C41.0	C79.51	—	D16.4-	D48.0	D49.2
carpus (any)	C40.1-	C79.51	—	D16.1-	—	—
cartilage NEC	C41.9	C79.51	—	D16.9-	D48.0	D49.2
clavicle	C41.3	C79.51	—	D16.7-	D48.0	D49.2
clivus	C41.0	C79.51	—	D16.4-	D48.0	D49.2
coccygeal vertebra	C41.4	C79.51	—	D16.8-	D48.0	D49.2
coccyx	C41.4	C79.51	—	D16.8-	D48.0	D49.2
costal cartilage	C41.3	C79.51	—	D16.7-	D48.0	D49.2
costovertebral joint	C41.3	C79.51	—	D16.7-	D48.0	D49.2
cranial	C41.0	C79.51	—	D16.4-	D48.0	D49.2
cuboid	C40.3-	C79.51	—	D16.3-	—	—
cuneiform	C41.9	C79.51	—	D16.9-	D48.0	D49.2
elbow	C40.0-	C79.51	—	D16.0-	—	—
ethmoid (labyrinth)	C41.0	C79.51	—	D16.4-	D48.0	D49.2
face	C41.0	C79.51	—	D16.4-	D48.0	D49.2
femur (any part)	C40.2-	C79.51	—	D16.2-	—	—
fibula (any part)	C40.2-	C79.51	—	D16.2-	—	—
finger (any)	C40.1-	C79.51	—	D16.1-	—	—
foot	C40.3-	C79.51	—	D16.3-	—	—
forearm	C40.0-	C79.51	—	D16.0-	—	—
frontal	C41.0	C79.51	—	D16.4-	D48.0	D49.2
hand	C40.1-	C79.51	—	D16.1-	—	—
heel	C40.3-	C79.51	—	D16.3-	—	—
hip	C41.4	C79.51	—	D16.8-	D48.0	D49.2
humerus (any part)	C40.0-	C79.51	—	D16.0-	—	—
hyoid	C41.0	C79.51	—	D16.4-	D48.0	D49.2
ilium	C41.4	C79.51	—	D16.8-	D48.0	D49.2
innominate	C41.4	C79.51	—	D16.8-	D48.0	D49.2

◀ New ◀══ Revised ~~deleted~~ Deleted

	Malignant Primary	Malignant Secondary	Ca in situ	Benign	Uncertain Behavior	Unspecified Behavior
bone *(Continued)*						
intervertebral cartilage or disc	C41.2	C79.51	—	D16.6-	D48.0	D49.2
ischium	C41.4	C79.51	—	D16.8-	D48.0	D49.2
jaw (lower)	C41.1	C79.51	—	D16.5-	D48.0	D49.2
knee	C40.2-	C79.51	—	D16.2-	—	—
leg NEC	C40.2-	C79.51	—	D16.2-	—	—
limb NEC	C40.9-	C79.51	—	D16.9-	—	—
lower (long bones)	C40.2-	C79.51	—	D16.2-	—	—
short bones	C40.3-	C79.51	—	D16.3-	—	—
upper (long bones)	C40.0-	C79.51	—	D16.0-	—	—
short bones	C40.1-	C79.51	—	D16.1-	—	—
malar	C41.0	C79.51	—	D16.4-	D48.0	D49.2
mandible	C41.1	C79.51	—	D16.5-	D48.0	D49.2
marrow NEC (any bone)	C96.9	C79.52	—	—	D47.9	D49.89
mastoid	C41.0	C79.51	—	D16.4-	D48.0	D49.2
maxilla, maxillary (superior)	C41.0	C79.51	—	D16.4-	D48.0	D49.2
inferior	C41.1	C79.51	—	D16.5-	D48.0	D49.2
metacarpus (any)	C40.1-	C79.51	—	D16.1-	—	—
metatarsus (any)	C40.3-	C79.51	—	D16.3-	—	—
overlapping sites	C40.8-	—	—	—	—	—
navicular						
ankle	C40.3-	C79.51	—	—	—	—
hand	C40.1-	C79.51	—	—	—	—
nose, nasal	C41.0	C79.51	—	D16.4-	D48.0	D49.2
occipital	C41.0	C79.51	—	D16.4-	D48.0	D49.2
orbit	C41.0	C79.51	—	D16.4-	D48.0	D49.2
parietal	C41.0	C79.51	—	D16.4-	D48.0	D49.2
patella	C40.2-	C79.51	—	—	—	—
pelvic	C41.4	C79.51	—	D16.8	D48.0	D49.2
phalanges						
foot	C40.3-	C79.51	—	—	—	—
hand	C40.1-	C79.51	—	—	—	—
pubic	C41.4	C79.51	—	D16.8	D48.0	D49.2
radius (any part)	C40.0-	C79.51	—	D16.0-	—	—
rib	C41.3	C79.51	—	D16.7	D48.0	D49.2
sacral vertebra	C41.4	C79.51	—	D16.8	D48.0	D49.2
sacrum	C41.4	C79.51	—	D16.8	D48.0	D49.2
scaphoid					—	—
of ankle	C40.3-	C79.51	—	—	—	—
of hand	C40.1-	C79.51	—	—	—	—
scapula (any part)	C40.0-	C79.51	—	D16.0-	—	—
sella turcica	C41.0	C79.51	—	D16.4-	D48.0	D49.2
shoulder	C40.0-	C79.51	—	D16.0-	—	—

	Malignant Primary	Malignant Secondary	Ca in situ	Benign	Uncertain Behavior	Unspecified Behavior
bone *(Continued)*						
skull	C41.0	C79.51	—	D16.4-	D48.0	D49.2
sphenoid	C41.0	C79.51	—	D16.4-	D48.0	D49.2
spine, spinal (column)	C41.2	C79.51	—	D16.6	D48.0	D49.2
coccyx	C41.4	C79.51	—	D16.8	D48.0	D49.2
sacrum	C41.4	C79.51	—	D16.8	D48.0	D49.2
sternum	C41.3	C79.51	—	D16.7	D48.0	D49.2
tarsus (any)	C40.3-	C79.51	—	—	—	—
temporal	C41.0	C79.51	—	D16.4-	D48.0	D49.2
thumb	C40.1-	C79.51	—	—	—	—
tibia (any part)	C40.2-	C79.51	—	—	—	—
toe (any)	C40.3-	C79.51	—	—	—	—
trapezium	C40.1-	C79.51	—	—	—	—
trapezoid	C40.1-	C79.51	—	—	—	—
turbinate	C41.0	C79.51	—	D16.4-	D48.0	D49.2
ulna (any part)	C40.0-	C79.51	—	D16.0-	—	—
unciform	C40.1-	C79.51	—	—	—	—
vertebra (column)	C41.2	C79.51	—	D16.6	D48.0	D49.2
coccyx	C41.4	C79.51	—	D16.8	D48.0	D49.2
sacrum	C41.4	C79.51	—	D16.8	D48.0	D49.2
vomer	C41.0	C79.51	—	D16.4-	D48.0	D49.2
wrist	C40.1-	C79.51	—	—	—	—
xiphoid process	C41.3	C79.51	—	D16.7	D48.0	D49.2
zygomatic	C41.0	C79.51	—	D16.4-	D48.0	D49.2
book-leaf (mouth)	C06.89	C79.89	D00.00	D10.39	D37.09	D49.0
bowel — *see* Neoplasm, intestine						
brachial plexus	C47.1-	C79.89	—	D36.12	D48.2	D49.2
brain NEC	C71.9	C79.31	—	D33.2	D43.2	D49.6
basal ganglia	C71.0	C79.31	—	D33.0	D43.0	D49.6
cerebellopontine angle	C71.6	C79.31	—	D33.1	D43.1	D49.6
cerebellum NOS	C71.6	C79.31	—	D33.1	D43.1	D49.6
cerebrum	C71.0	C79.31	—	D33.0	D43.0	D49.6
choroid plexus	C71.7	C79.31	—	D33.1	D43.1	D49.6
corpus callosum	C71.8	C79.31	—	D33.2	D43.2	D49.6
corpus striatum	C71.0	C79.31	—	D33.0	D43.0	D49.6
cortex (cerebral)	C71.0	C79.31	—	D33.0	D43.0	D49.6
frontal lobe	C71.1	C79.31	—	D33.0	D43.0	D49.6
globus pallidus	C71.0	C79.31	—	D33.0	D43.0	D49.6
hippocampus	C71.2	C79.31	—	D33.0	D43.0	D49.6
hypothalamus	C71.0	C79.31	—	D33.0	D43.0	D49.6
internal capsule	C71.0	C79.31	—	D33.0	D43.0	D49.6
medulla oblongata	C71.7	C79.31	—	D33.1	D43.1	D49.6
meninges	C70.0	C79.32	—	D32.0	D42.0	D49.7

◀ New   ◀▥ Revised   ~~deleted~~ Deleted

	Malignant Primary	Malignant Secondary	Ca in situ	Benign	Uncertain Behavior	Unspecified Behavior
brain NEC *(Continued)*						
midbrain	C71.7	C79.31	—	D33.1	D43.1	D49.6
occipital lobe	C71.4	C79.31	—	D33.0	D43.0	D49.6
overlapping lesion	C71.8	C79.31	—	—	—	—
parietal lobe	C71.3	C79.31	—	D33.0	D43.0	D49.6
peduncle	C71.7	C79.31	—	D33.1	D43.1	D49.6
pons	C71.7	C79.31	—	D33.1	D43.1	D49.6
stem	C71.7	C79.31	—	D33.1	D43.1	D49.6
tapetum	C71.8	C79.31	—	D33.2	D43.2	D49.6
temporal lobe	C71.2	C79.31	—	D33.0	D43.0	D49.6
thalamus	C71.0	C79.31	—	D33.0	D43.0	D49.6
uncus	C71.2	C79.31	—	D33.0	D43.0	D49.6
ventricle (floor)	C71.5	C79.31	—	D33.0	D43.0	D49.6
fourth	C71.7	C79.31	—	D33.1	D43.1	D49.6
branchial (cleft) (cyst) (vestiges)	C10.4	C79.89	D00.08	D10.5	D37.05	D49.0
breast (connective tissue) (glandular tissue) (soft parts)	C50.9-	C79.81	D05.-	D24.-	D48.6-	D49.3
areola	C50.0-	C79.81	D05.-	D24.-	D48.6-	D49.3
axillary tail	C50.6-	C79.81	D05.-	D24.-	D48.6-	D49.3
central portion	C50.1-	C79.81	D05.-	D24.-	D48.6-	D49.3
inner	C50.8-	C79.81	D05.-	D24.-	D48.6-	D49.3
lower	C50.8-	C79.81	D05.-	D24.-	D48.6-	D49.3
lower-inner quadrant	C50.3-	C79.81	D05.-	D24.-	D48.6-	D49.3
lower-outer quadrant	C50.5-	C79.81	D05.-	D24.-	D48.6-	D49.3
mastectomy site (skin) — *see also* Neoplasm, breast, skin	C44.501	C79.2	—	—	—	—
specified as breast tissue	C50.8-	C79.81	—	—	—	—
midline	C50.8-	C79.81	D05.-	D24.-	D48.6-	D49.3
nipple	C50.0-	C79.81	D05.-	D24.-	D48.6-	D49.3
outer	C50.8-	C79.81	D05.-	D24.-	D48.6-	D49.3
overlapping lesion	C50.8-	—	—	—	—	—
skin	C44.501	C79.2	D04.5	D23.5	D48.5	D49.2
basal cell carcinoma	C44.511	—	—	—	—	—
specified type NEC	C44.591	—	—	—	—	—
squamous cell carcinoma	C44.521	—	—	—	—	—
tail (axillary)	C50.6-	C79.81	D05.-	D24.-	D48.6-	D49.3
upper	C50.8-	C79.81	D05.-	D24.-	D48.6-	D49.3
upper-inner quadrant	C50.2-	C79.81	D05.-	D24.-	D48.6-	D49.3
upper-outer quadrant	C50.4-	C79.81	D05.-	D24.-	D48.6-	D49.3
broad ligament	C57.1	C79.82	D07.39	D28.2	D39.8	D49.5
bronchiogenic, bronchogenic (lung)	C34.9-	C78.0-	D02.2-	D14.3-	D38.1	D49.1
bronchiole	C34.9-	C78.0-	D02.2-	D14.3-	D38.1	D49.1
bronchus	C34.9-	C78.0-	D02.2-	D14.3-	D38.1	D49.1
carina	C34.0-	C78.0-	D02.2-	D14.3-	D38.1	D49.1
lower lobe of lung	C34.3-	C78.0-	D02.2-	D14.3-	D38.1	D49.1

TABLE OF NEOPLASMS

TABLE OF NEOPLASMS

	Malignant Primary	Malignant Secondary	Ca in situ	Benign	Uncertain Behavior	Unspecified Behavior
bronchus *(Continued)*						
main	C34.0-	C78.0-	D02.2-	D14.3-	D38.1	D49.1
middle lobe of lung	C34.2	C78.0-	D02.21	D14.31	D38.1	D49.1
overlapping lesion	C34.8-	—	—	—	—	—
upper lobe of lung	C34.1-	C78.0-	D02.2-	D14.3-	D38.1	D49.1
brow	C44.309	C79.2	D04.39	D23.39	D48.5	D49.2
basal cell carcinoma	C44.319	—	—	—	—	—
specified type NEC	C44.399	—	—	—	—	—
squamous cell carcinoma	C44.329	—	—	—	—	—
buccal (cavity)	C06.9	C79.89	D00.00	D10.39	D37.09	D49.0
commissure	C06.0	C79.89	D00.02	D10.39	D37.09	D49.0
groove (lower) (upper)	C06.1	C79.89	D00.02	D10.39	D37.09	D49.0
mucosa	C06.0	C79.89	D00.02	D10.39	D37.09	D49.0
sulcus (lower) (upper)	C06.1	C79.89	D00.02	D10.39	D37.09	D49.0
bulbourethral gland	C68.0	C79.19	D09.19	D30.4	D41.3	D49.5
bursa — *see Neoplasm, connective tissue*						
buttock NEC	C76.3	C79.89	D04.5	D36.7	D48.7	D49.89
calf	C76.5-	C79.89	D04.7-	D36.7	D48.7	D49.89
calvarium	C41.0	C79.51	—	D16.4-	D48.0	D49.2
calyx, renal	C65.-	C79.0-	D09.19	D30.1-	D41.1-	D49.5
canal						
anal	C21.1	C78.5	D01.3	D12.9	D37.8	D49.0
auditory (external) — *see also Neoplasm, skin, ear*	C44.20-	C79.2	D04.2-	D23.2-	D48.5	D49.2
auricular (external) — *see also Neoplasm, skin, ear*	C44.20-	C79.2	D04.2-	D23.2-	D48.5	D49.2
canaliculi, biliary (biliferi) (intrahepatic)	C22.1	C78.7	D01.5	D13.4	D37.6	D49.0
canthus (eye) (inner) (outer)	C44.10-	C79.2	D04.1-	D23.1-	D48.5	D49.2
basal cell carcinoma	C44.11-	—	—	—	—	—
specified type NEC	C44.19-	—	—	—	—	—
squamous cell carcinoma	C44.12-	—	—	—	—	—
capillary — *see Neoplasm, connective tissue*						
caput coli	C18.0	C78.5	D01.0	D12.0	D37.4	D49.0
carcinoid — *see Tumor, carcinoid*						
cardia (gastric)	C16.0	C78.89	D00.2	D13.1	D37.1	D49.0
cardiac orifice (stomach)	C16.0	C78.89	D00.2	D13.1	D37.1	D49.0
cardio-esophageal junction	C16.0	C78.89	D00.2	D13.1	D37.1	D49.0
cardio-esophagus	C16.0	C78.89	D00.2	D13.1	D37.1	D49.0
carina (bronchus)	C34.0-	C78.0-	D02.2-	D14.3-	D38.1	D49.1
carotid (artery)	C49.0	C79.89	—	D21.0	D48.1	D49.2
body	C75.4	C79.89	—	D35.5	D44.6	D49.7
carpus (any bone)	C40.1-	C79.51	—	D16.1-	—	—
cartilage (articular) (joint) NEC — *see also Neoplasm, bone*	C41.9	C79.51	—	D16.9-	D48.0	D49.2
arytenoid	C32.3	C78.39	D02.0	D14.1	D38.0	D49.1
auricular	C49.0	C79.89	—	D21.0	D48.1	D49.2

◀ New ◀▥▥ Revised ~~deleted~~ Deleted

	Malignant Primary	Malignant Secondary	Ca in situ	Benign	Uncertain Behavior	Unspecified Behavior
cartilage NEC *(Continued)*						
bronchi	C34.0-	C78.39	—	D14.3-	D38.1	D49.1
costal	C41.3	C79.51	—	D16.7	D48.0	D49.2
cricoid	C32.3	C78.39	D02.0	D14.1	D38.0	D49.1
cuneiform	C32.3	C78.39	D02.0	D14.1	D38.0	D49.1
ear (external)	C49.0	C79.89	—	D21.0	D48.1	D49.2
ensiform	C41.3	C79.51	—	D16.7	D48.0	D49.2
epiglottis	C32.1	C78.39	D02.0	D14.1	D38.0	D49.1
anterior surface	C10.1	C79.89	D00.08	D10.5	D37.05	D49.0
eyelid	C49.0	C79.89	—	D21.0	D48.1	D49.2
intervertebral	C41.2	C79.51	—	D16.6	D48.0	D49.2
larynx, laryngeal	C32.3	C78.39	D02.0	D14.1	D38.0	D49.1
nose, nasal	C30.0	C78.39	D02.3	D14.0	D38.5	D49.1
pinna	C49.0	C79.89	—	D21.0	D48.1	D49.2
rib	C41.3	C79.51	—	D16.7	D48.0	D49.2
semilunar (knee)	C40.2-	C79.51	—	D16.2-	D48.0	D49.2
thyroid	C32.3	C78.39	D02.0	D14.1	D38.0	D49.1
trachea	C33	C78.39	D02.1	D14.2	D38.1	D49.1
cauda equina	C72.1	C79.49	—	D33.4	D43.4	D49.7
cavity						
buccal	C06.9	C79.89	D00.00	D10.30	D37.09	D49.0
nasal	C30.0	C78.39	D02.3	D14.0	D38.5	D49.1
oral	C06.9	C79.89	D00.00	D10.30	D37.09	D49.0
peritoneal	C48.2	C78.6	—	D20.1	D48.4	D49.0
tympanic	C30.1	C78.39	D02.3	D14.0	D38.5	D49.1
cecum	C18.0	C78.5	D01.0	D12.0	D37.4	D49.0
central nervous system	C72.9	C79.40	—	—	—	—
cerebellopontine (angle)	C71.6	C79.31	—	D33.1	D43.1	D49.6
cerebellum, cerebellar	C71.6	C79.31	—	D33.1	D43.1	D49.6
cerebrum, cerebral (cortex) (hemisphere) (white matter)	C71.0	C79.31	—	D33.0	D43.0	D49.6
meninges	C70.0	C79.32	—	D32.0	D42.0	D49.7
peduncle	C71.7	C79.31	—	D33.1	D43.1	D49.6
ventricle	C71.5	C79.31	—	D33.0	D43.0	D49.6
fourth	C71.7	C79.31	—	D33.1	D43.1	D49.6
cervical region	C76.0	C79.89	D09.8	D36.7	D48.7	D49.89
cervix (cervical) (uteri) (uterus)	C53.9	C79.82	D06.9	D26.0	D39.0	D49.5
canal	C53.0	C79.82	D06.0	D26.0	D39.0	D49.5
endocervix (canal) (gland)	C53.0	C79.82	D06.0	D26.0	D39.0	D49.5
exocervix	C53.1	C79.82	D06.1	D26.0	D39.0	D49.5
external os	C53.1	C79.82	D06.1	D26.0	D39.0	D49.5
internal os	C53.0	C79.82	D06.0	D26.0	D39.0	D49.5
nabothian gland	C53.0	C79.82	D06.0	D26.0	D39.0	D49.5
overlapping lesion	C53.8	—	—	—	—	—

TABLE OF NEOPLASMS

	Malignant Primary	Malignant Secondary	Ca in situ	Benign	Uncertain Behavior	Unspecified Behavior
cervix *(Continued)*						
squamocolumnar junction	C53.8	C79.82	D06.7	D26.0	D39.0	D49.5
stump	C53.8	C79.82	D06.7	D26.0	D39.0	D49.5
cheek	C76.0	C79.89	D09.8	D36.7	D48.7	D49.89
external	C44.309	C79.2	D04.39	D23.39	D48.5	D49.2
basal cell carcinoma	C44.319	—	—	—	—	—
specified type NEC	C44.399	—	—	—	—	—
squamous cell carcinoma	C44.329	—	—	—	—	—
inner aspect	C06.0	C79.89	D00.02	D10.39	D37.09	D49.0
internal	C06.0	C79.89	D00.02	D10.39	D37.09	D49.0
mucosa	C06.0	C79.89	D00.02	D10.39	D37.09	D49.0
chest (wall) NEC	C76.1	C79.89	D09.8	D36.7	D48.7	D49.89
chiasma opticum	C72.3-	C79.49	—	D33.3	D43.3	D49.7
chin	C44.309	C79.2	D04.39	D23.39	D48.5	D49.2
basal cell carcinoma	C44.319	—	—	—	—	—
specified type NEC	C44.399	—	—	—	—	—
squamous cell carcinoma	C44.329	—	—	—	—	—
choana	C11.3	C79.89	D00.08	D10.6	D37.05	D49.0
cholangiole	C22.1	C78.89	D01.5	D13.4	D37.6	D49.0
choledochal duct	C24.0	C78.89	D01.5	D13.5	D37.6	D49.0
choroid	C69.3-	C79.49	D09.2-	D31.3-	D48.7	D49.81
plexus	C71.5	C79.31	—	D33.0	D43.0	D49.6
ciliary body	C69.4-	C79.49	D09.2-	D31.4-	D48.7	D49.89
clavicle	C41.3	C79.51	—	D16.7	D48.0	D49.2
clitoris	C51.2	C79.82	D07.1	D28.0	D39.8	D49.5
clivus	C41.0	C79.51	—	D16.4-	D48.0	D49.2
cloacogenic zone	C21.2	C78.5	D01.3	D12.9	D37.8	D49.0
coccygeal						
body or glomus	C49.5	C79.89	—	D21.5	D48.1	D49.2
vertebra	C41.4	C79.51	—	D16.8	D48.0	D49.2
coccyx	C41.4	C79.51	—	D16.8	D48.0	D49.2
colon — *see also Neoplasm, intestine, large*	C18.9	C78.5	—	—	—	—
with rectum	C19	C78.5	D01.1	D12.7	D37.5	D49.0
column, spinal — *see Neoplasm, spine*						
columnella — *see also Neoplasm, skin, face*	C44.390	C79.2	D04.39	D23.39	D48.5	D49.2
commissure						
labial, lip	C00.6	C79.89	D00.01	D10.39	D37.01	D49.0
laryngeal	C32.0	C78.39	D02.0	D14.1	D38.0	D49.1
common (bile) duct	C24.0	C78.89	D01.5	D13.5	D37.6	D49.0
concha — *see also Neoplasm, skin, ear*	C44.20-	C79.2	D04.2-	D23.2-	D48.5	D49.2
nose	C30.0	C78.39	D02.3	D14.0	D38.5	D49.1
conjunctiva	C69.0-	C79.49	D09.2-	D31.0-	D48.7	D49.89

◀ New ◀▥ Revised ~~deleted~~ Deleted

	Malignant Primary	Malignant Secondary	Ca in situ	Benign	Uncertain Behavior	Unspecified Behavior
connective tissue NEC	C49.9	C79.89	—	D21.9	D48.1	D49.2

Note: For neoplasms of connective tissue (blood vessel, bursa, fascia, ligament, muscle, peripheral nerves, sympathetic and parasympathetic nerves and ganglia, synovia, tendon, etc.) or of morphological types that indicate connective tissue, code according to the list under "Neoplasm, connective tissue". For sites that do not appear in this list, code to neoplasm of that site; e.g., fibrosarcoma, pancreas (C25.9)

Note: Morphological types that indicate connective tissue appear in their proper place in the alphabetic index with the instruction "*see Neoplasm, connective tissue ....*"

	Malignant Primary	Malignant Secondary	Ca in situ	Benign	Uncertain Behavior	Unspecified Behavior
abdomen	C49.4	C79.89	—	D21.4	D48.1	D49.2
abdominal wall	C49.4	C79.89	—	D21.4	D48.1	D49.2
ankle	C49.2-	C79.89	—	D21.2-	D48.1	D49.2
antecubital fossa or space	C49.1-	C79.89	—	D21.1-	D48.1	D49.2
arm	C49.1-	C79.89	—	D21.1-	D48.1	D49.2
auricle (ear)	C49.0	C79.89	—	D21.0	D48.1	D49.2
axilla	C49.3	C79.89	—	D21.3	D48.1	D49.2
back	C49.6	C79.89	—	D21.6	D48.1	D49.2
breast — *see Neoplasm, breast*						
buttock	C49.5	C79.89	—	D21.5	D48.1	D49.2
calf	C49.2-	C79.89	—	D21.2-	D48.1	D49.2
cervical region	C49.0	C79.89	—	D21.0	D48.1	D49.2
cheek	C49.0	C79.89	—	D21.0	D48.1	D49.2
chest (wall)	C49.3	C79.89	—	D21.3	D48.1	D49.2
chin	C49.0	C79.89	—	D21.0	D48.1	D49.2
diaphragm	C49.3	C79.89	—	D21.3	D48.1	D49.2
ear (external)	C49.0	C79.89	—	D21.0	D48.1	D49.2
elbow	C49.1-	C79.89	—	D21.1-	D48.1	D49.2
extrarectal	C49.5	C79.89	—	D21.5	D48.1	D49.2
extremity	C49.9	C79.89	—	D21.9	D48.1	D49.2
lower	C49.2-	C79.89	—	D21.2-	D48.1	D49.2
upper	C49.1-	C79.89	—	D21.1-	D48.1	D49.2
eyelid	C49.0	C79.89	—	D21.0	D48.1	D49.2
face	C49.0	C79.89	—	D21.0	D48.1	D49.2
finger	C49.1-	C79.89	—	D21.1-	D48.1	D49.2
flank	C49.6	C79.89	—	D21.6	D48.1	D49.2
foot	C49.2-	C79.89	—	D21.2-	D48.1	D49.2
forearm	C49.1-	C79.89	—	D21.1-	D48.1	D49.2
forehead	C49.0	C79.89	—	D21.0	D48.1	D49.2
gastric	C49.4	C79.89	—	D21.4	D48.1	D49.2
gastrointestinal	C49.4	C79.89	—	D21.4	D48.1	D49.2
gluteal region	C49.5	C79.89	—	D21.5	D48.1	D49.2
great vessels NEC	C49.3	C79.89	—	D21.3	D48.1	D49.2
groin	C49.5	C79.89	—	D21.5	D48.1	D49.2
hand	C49.1-	C79.89	—	D21.1-	D48.1	D49.2

connective tissue NEC *(Continued)*	Malignant Primary	Malignant Secondary	Ca in situ	Benign	Uncertain Behavior	Unspecified Behavior
head	C49.0	C79.89	—	D21.0	D48.1	D49.2
heel	C49.2-	C79.89	—	D21.2-	D48.1	D49.2
hip	C49.2-	C79.89	—	D21.2-	D48.1	D49.2
hypochondrium	C49.4	C79.89	—	D21.4	D48.1	D49.2
iliopsoas muscle	C49.5	C79.89	—	D21.5	D48.1	D49.2
infraclavicular region	C49.3	C79.89	—	D21.3	D48.1	D49.2
inguinal (canal) (region)	C49.5	C79.89	—	D21.5	D48.1	D49.2
intestinal	C49.4	C79.89	—	D21.4	D48.1	D49.2
intrathoracic	C49.3	C79.89	—	D21.3	D48.1	D49.2
ischiorectal fossa	C49.5	C79.89	—	D21.5	D48.1	D49.2
jaw	C03.9	C79.89	D00.03	D10.39	D48.1	D49.0
knee	C49.2-	C79.89	—	D21.2-	D48.1	D49.2
leg	C49.2-	C79.89	—	D21.2-	D48.1	D49.2
limb NEC	C49.9	C79.89	—	D21.9	D48.1	D49.2
lower	C49.2-	C79.89	—	D21.2-	D48.1	D49.2
upper	C49.1-	C79.89	—	D21.1-	D48.1	D49.2
nates	C49.5	C79.89	—	D21.5	D48.1	D49.2
neck	C49.0	C79.89	—	D21.0	D48.1	D49.2
orbit	C69.6-	C79.49	D09.2-	D31.6-	D48.1	D49.89
overlapping lesion	C49.8	—	—	—	—	—
pararectal	C49.5	C79.89	—	D21.5	D48.1	D49.2
para-urethral	C49.5	C79.89	—	D21.5	D48.1	D49.2
paravaginal	C49.5	C79.89	—	D21.5	D48.1	D49.2
pelvis (floor)	C49.5	C79.89	—	D21.5	D48.1	D49.2
pelvo-abdominal	C49.8	C79.89	—	D21.6	D48.1	D49.2
perineum	C49.5	C79.89	—	D21.5	D48.1	D49.2
perirectal (tissue)	C49.5	C79.89	—	D21.5	D48.1	D49.2
periurethral (tissue)	C49.5	C79.89	—	D21.5	D48.1	D49.2
popliteal fossa or space	C49.2-	C79.89	—	D21.2-	D48.1	D49.2
presacral	C49.5	C79.89	—	D21.5	D48.1	D49.2
psoas muscle	C49.4	C79.89	—	D21.4	D48.1	D49.2
pterygoid fossa	C49.0	C79.89	—	D21.0	D48.1	D49.2
rectovaginal septum or wall	C49.5	C79.89	—	D21.5	D48.1	D49.2
rectovesical	C49.5	C79.89	—	D21.5	D48.1	D49.2
retroperitoneum	C48.0	C78.6	—	D20.0	D48.3	D49.0
sacrococcygeal region	C49.5	C79.89	—	D21.5	D48.1	D49.2
scalp	C49.0	C79.89	—	D21.0	D48.1	D49.2
scapular region	C49.3	C79.89	—	D21.3	D48.1	D49.2
shoulder	C49.1-	C79.89	—	D21.1-	D48.1	D49.2
skin (dermis) NEC — *see also Neoplasm, skin, by site*	C44.90	C79.2	D04.9	D23.9	D48.5	D49.2
stomach	C49.4	C79.89	—	D21.4	D48.1	D49.2
submental	C49.0	C79.89	—	D21.0	D48.1	D49.2

◀ New ◀ Revised ~~deleted~~ Deleted

	Malignant Primary	Malignant Secondary	Ca in situ	Benign	Uncertain Behavior	Unspecified Behavior
connective tissue NEC *(Continued)*						
supraclavicular region	C49.0	C79.89	—	D21.0	D48.1	D49.2
temple	C49.0	C79.89	—	D21.0	D48.1	D49.2
temporal region	C49.0	C79.89	—	D21.0	D48.1	D49.2
thigh	C49.2-	C79.89	—	D21.2-	D48.1	D49.2
thoracic (duct) (wall)	C49.3	C79.89	—	D21.3	D48.1	D49.2
thorax	C49.3	C79.89	—	D21.3	D48.1	D49.2
thumb	C49.1-	C79.89	—	D21.1-	D48.1	D49.2
toe	C49.2-	C79.89	—	D21.2-	D48.1	D49.2
trunk	C49.6	C79.89	—	D21.6	D48.1	D49.2
umbilicus	C49.4	C79.89	—	D21.4	D48.1	D49.2
vesicorectal	C49.5	C79.89	—	D21.5	D48.1	D49.2
wrist	C49.1-	C79.89	—	D21.1-	D48.1	D49.2
conus medullaris	C72.0	C79.49	—	D33.4	D43.4	D49.7
cord (true) (vocal)	C32.0	C78.39	D02.0	D14.1	D38.0	D49.1
false	C32.1	C78.39	D02.0	D14.1	D38.0	D49.1
spermatic	C63.1-	C79.82	D07.69	D29.8	D40.8	D49.5
spinal (cervical) (lumbar) (thoracic)	C72.0	C79.49	—	D33.4	D43.4	D49.7
cornea (limbus)	C69.1-	C79.49	D09.2-	D31.1-	D48.7	D49.89
corpus						
albicans	C56.-	C79.6-	D07.39	D27.-	D39.1-	D49.5
callosum, brain	C71.0	C79.31	—	D33.2	D43.2	D49.6
cavernosum	C60.2	C79.82	D07.4	D29.0	D40.8	D49.5
gastric	C16.2	C78.89	D00.2	D13.1	D37.1	D49.0
overlapping sites	C54.8	—	—	—	—	—
penis	C60.2	C79.82	D07.4	D29.0	D40.8	D49.5
striatum, cerebrum	C71.0	C79.31	—	D33.0	D43.0	D49.6
uteri	C54.9	C79.82	D07.0	D26.1	D39.0	D49.5
isthmus	C54.0	C79.82	D07.0	D26.1	D39.0	D49.5
cortex						
adrenal	C74.0-	C79.7-	D09.3	D35.0-	D44.1-	D49.7
cerebral	C71.0	C79.31	—	D33.0	D43.0	D49.6
costal cartilage	C41.3	C79.51	—	D16.7	D48.0	D49.2
costovertebral joint	C41.3	C79.51	—	D16.7	D48.0	D49.2
Cowper's gland	C68.0	C79.19	D09.19	D30.4	D41.3	D49.5
cranial (fossa, any)	C71.9	C79.31	—	D33.2	D43.2	D49.6
meninges	C70.0	C79.32	—	D32.0	D42.0	D49.7
nerve	C72.50	C79.49	—	D33.3	D43.3	D49.7
specified NEC	C72.59	C79.49	—	D33.3	D43.3	D49.7
craniobuccal pouch	C75.2	C79.89	D09.3	D35.2	D44.3	D49.7
craniopharyngeal (duct) (pouch)	C75.2	C79.89	D09.3	D35.3	D44.4	D49.7
cricoid	C13.0	C79.89	D00.08	D10.7	D37.05	D49.0
cartilage	C32.3	C78.39	D02.0	D14.1	D38.0	D49.1

TABLE OF NEOPLASMS

TABLE OF NEOPLASMS

	Malignant Primary	Malignant Secondary	Ca in situ	Benign	Uncertain Behavior	Unspecified Behavior
cricopharynx	C13.0	C79.89	D00.08	D10.7	D37.05	D49.0
crypt of Morgagni	C21.8	C78.5	D01.3	D12.9	D37.8	D49.0
crystalline lens	C69.4-	C79.49	D09.2-	D31.4-	D48.7	D49.89
cul-de-sac (Douglas')	C48.1	C78.6	—	D20.1	D48.4	D49.0
cuneiform cartilage	C32.3	C78.39	D02.0	D14.1	D38.0	D49.1
cutaneous — see Neoplasm, skin						
cutis — see Neoplasm, skin						
cystic (bile) duct (common)	C24.0	C78.89	D01.5	D13.5	D37.6	D49.0
dermis — see Neoplasm, skin						
diaphragm	C49.3	C79.89	—	D21.3	D48.1	D49.2
digestive organs, system, tube, or tract NEC	C26.9	C78.89	D01.9	D13.9	D37.9	D49.0
disc, intervertebral	C41.2	C79.51		D16.6	D48.0	D49.2
disease, generalized	C80.0	—	—	—	—	—
disseminated	C80.0	—	—	—	—	—
Douglas' cul-de-sac or pouch	C48.1	C78.6	—	D20.1	D48.4	D49.0
duodenojejunal junction	C17.8	C78.4	D01.49	D13.39	D37.2	D49.0
duodenum	C17.0	C78.4	D01.49	D13.2	D37.2	D49.0
dura (cranial) (mater)	C70.9	C79.49	—	D32.9	D42.9	D49.7
cerebral	C70.0	C79.32	—	D32.0	D42.0	D49.7
spinal	C70.1	C79.49	—	D32.1	D42.1	D49.7
ear (external) — see also Neoplasm, skin, ear	C44.20-	C79.2	D04.2-	D23.2-	D48.5	D49.2
auricle or auris — see also Neoplasm, skin, ear	C44.20-	C79.2	D04.2-	D23.2-	D48.5	D49.2
canal, external — see also Neoplasm, skin, ear	C44.20-	C79.2	D04.2-	D23.2-	D48.5	D49.2
cartilage	C49.0	C79.89	—	D21.0	D48.1	D49.2
external meatus — see also Neoplasm, skin, ear	C44.20-	C79.2	D04.2-	D23.2-	D48.5	D49.2
inner	C30.1	C78.39	D02.3	D14.0	D38.5	D49.1
lobule — see also Neoplasm, skin, ear	C44.20-	C79.2	D04.2-	D23.2-	D48.5	D49.2
middle	C30.1	C78.39	D02.3	D14.0	D38.5	D49.1
overlapping lesion with accessory sinuses	C31.8	—	—	—	—	—
skin	C44.20-	C79.2	D04.2-	D23.2-	D48.5	D49.2
basal cell carcinoma	C44.21-	—	—	—	—	—
specified type NEC	C44.29-	—	—	—	—	—
squamous cell carcinoma	C44.22-	—	—	—	—	—
earlobe	C44.20-	C79.2	D04.2-	D23.2-	D48.5	D49.2
basal cell carcinoma	C44.21-	—	—	—	—	—
specified type NEC	C44.29-	—	—	—	—	—
squamous cell carcinoma	C44.22-	—	—	—	—	—
ejaculatory duct	C63.7	C79.82	D07.69	D29.8	D40.8	D49.5
elbow NEC	C76.4-	C79.89	D04.6-	D36.7	D48.7	D49.89
endocardium	C38.0	C79.89	—	D15.1	D48.7	D49.89
endocervix (canal) (gland)	C53.0	C79.82	D06.0	D26.0	D39.0	D49.5
endocrine gland NEC	C75.9	C79.89	D09.3	D35.9	D44.9	D49.7
pluriglandular	C75.8	C79.89	D09.3	D35.7	D44.9	D49.7

◀ New ◀▥ Revised ~~deleted~~ Deleted

	Malignant Primary	Malignant Secondary	Ca in situ	Benign	Uncertain Behavior	Unspecified Behavior
endometrium (gland) (stroma)	C54.1	C79.82	D07.0	D26.1	D39.0	D49.5
ensiform cartilage	C41.3	C79.51	—	D16.7	D48.0	D49.2
enteric — see Neoplasm, intestine						
ependyma (brain)	C71.5	C79.31	—	D33.0	D43.0	D49.6
fourth ventricle	C71.7	C79.31	—	D33.1	D43.1	D49.6
epicardium	C38.0	C79.89	—	D15.1	D48.7	D49.89
epididymis	C63.0-	C79.82	D07.69	D29.3-	D40.8	D49.5
epidural	C72.9	C79.49	—	D33.9	D43.9	D49.7
epiglottis	C32.1	C78.39	D02.0	D14.1	D38.0	D49.1
anterior aspect or surface	C10.1	C79.89	D00.08	D10.5	D37.05	D49.0
cartilage	C32.3	C78.39	D02.0	D14.1	D38.0	D49.1
free border (margin)	C10.1	C79.89	D00.08	D10.5	D37.05	D49.0
junctional region	C10.8	C79.89	D00.08	D10.5	D37.05	D49.0
posterior (laryngeal) surface	C32.1	C78.39	D02.0	D14.1	D38.0	D49.1
suprahyoid portion	C32.1	C78.39	D02.0	D14.1	D38.0	D49.1
esophagogastric junction	C16.0	C78.89	D00.2	D13.1	D37.1	D49.0
esophagus	C15.9	C78.89	D00.1	D13.0	D37.8	D49.0
abdominal	C15.5	C78.89	D00.1	D13.0	D37.8	D49.0
cervical	C15.3	C78.89	D00.1	D13.0	D37.8	D49.0
distal (third)	C15.5	C78.89	D00.1	D13.0	D37.8	D49.0
lower (third)	C15.5	C78.89	D00.1	D13.0	D37.8	D49.0
middle (third)	C15.4	C78.89	D00.1	D13.0	D37.8	D49.0
overlapping lesion	C15.8	—	—	—	—	—
proximal (third)	C15.3	C78.89	D00.1	D13.0	D37.8	D49.0
thoracic	C15.4	C78.89	D00.1	D13.0	D37.8	D49.0
upper (third)	C15.3	C78.89	D00.1	D13.0	D37.8	D49.0
ethmoid (sinus)	C31.1	C78.39	D02.3	D14.0	D38.5	D49.1
bone or labyrinth	C41.0	C79.51	—	D16.4-	D48.0	D49.2
eustachian tube	C30.1	C78.39	D02.3	D14.0	D38.5	D49.1
exocervix	C53.1	C79.82	D06.1	D26.0	D39.0	D49.5
external						
meatus (ear) — see also Neoplasm, skin, ear	C44.20-	C79.2	D04.2-	D23.2-	D48.5	D49.2
os, cervix uteri	C53.1	C79.82	D06.1	D26.0	D39.0	D49.5
extradural	C72.9	C79.49	—	D33.9	D43.9	D49.7
extrahepatic (bile) duct	C24.0	C78.89	D01.5	D13.5	D37.6	D49.0
overlapping lesion with gallbladder	C24.8	—	—	—	—	—
extraocular muscle	C69.6-	C79.49	D09.2-	D31.6-	D48.7	D49.89
extrarectal	C76.3	C79.89	D09.8	D36.7	D48.7	D49.89
extremity	C76.8	C79.89	D04.8	D36.7	D48.7	D49.89
lower	C76.5-	C79.89	D04.7-	D36.7	D48.7	D49.89
upper	C76.4-	C79.89	D04.6-	D36.7	D48.7	D49.89
eye NEC	C69.9-	C79.49	D09.2	D31.9	D48.7	D49.89
overlapping sites	C69.8	—	—	—	—	—
eyeball	C69.9-	C79.49	D09.2-	D31.9-	D48.7	D49.89

◀ New ◀▤ Revised ~~deleted~~ Deleted

TABLE OF NEOPLASMS

	Malignant Primary	Malignant Secondary	Ca in situ	Benign	Uncertain Behavior	Unspecified Behavior
eyebrow	C44.309	C79.2	D04.39	D23.39	D48.5	D49.2
basal cell carcinoma	C44.319	—	—	—	—	—
specified type NEC	C44.399	—	—	—	—	—
squamous cell carcinoma	C44.329	—	—	—	—	—
eyelid (lower) (skin) (upper)	C44.10-	—	—	—	—	—
basal cell carcinoma	C44.11-	—	—	—	—	—
cartilage	C49.0	C79.89	—	D21.0	D48.1	D49.2
specified type NEC	C44.19-	—	—	—	—	—
squamous cell carcinoma	C44.12-	—	—	—	—	—
face NEC	C76.0	C79.89	D04.39	D36.7	D48.7	D49.89
fallopian tube (accessory)	C57.0-	C79.82	D07.39	D28.2	D39.8	D49.5
falx (cerebella) (cerebri)	C70.0	C79.32	—	D32.0	D42.0	D49.7
fascia — see also Neoplasm, connective tissue						
palmar	C49.1-	C79.89	—	D21.1-	D48.1	D49.2
plantar	C49.2-	C79.89	—	D21.2-	D48.1	D49.2
fatty tissue — see Neoplasm, connective tissue						
fauces, faucial NEC	C10.9	C79.89	D00.08	D10.5	D37.05	D49.0
pillars	C09.1	C79.89	D00.08	D10.5	D37.05	D49.0
tonsil	C09.9	C79.89	D00.08	D10.4	D37.05	D49.0
femur (any part)	C40.2-	—	—	D16.2-	—	—
fetal membrane	C58	C79.82	D07.0	D26.7	D39.2	D49.5
fibrous tissue — see Neoplasm, connective tissue						
fibula (any part)	C40.2-	C79.51	—	D16.2-	—	—
filum terminale	C72.0	C79.49	—	D33.4	D43.4	D49.7
finger NEC	C76.4-	C79.89	D04.6-	D36.7	D48.7	D49.89
flank NEC	C76.8	C79.89	D04.5	D36.7	D48.7	D49.89
follicle, nabothian	C53.0	C79.82	D06.0	D26.0	D39.0	D49.5
foot NEC	C76.5-	C79.89	D04.7-	D36.7	D48.7	D49.89
forearm NEC	C76.4-	C79.89	D04.6-	D36.7	D48.7	D49.89
forehead (skin)	C44.309	C79.2	D04.39	D23.39	D48.5	D49.2
basal cell carcinoma	C44.319	—	—	—	—	—
specified type NEC	C44.399	—	—	—	—	—
squamous cell carcinoma	C44.329	—	—	—	—	—
foreskin	C60.0	C79.82	D07.4	D29.0	D40.8	D49.5
fornix						
pharyngeal	C11.3	C79.89	D00.08	D10.6	D37.05	D49.0
vagina	C52	C79.82	D07.2	D28.1	D39.8	D49.5
fossa (of)						
anterior (cranial)	C71.9	C79.31	—	D33.2	D43.2	D49.6
cranial	C71.9	C79.31	—	D33.2	D43.2	D49.6
ischiorectal	C76.3	C79.89	D09.8	D36.7	D48.7	D49.89
middle (cranial)	C71.9	C79.31	—	D33.2	D43.2	D49.6
piriform	C12	C79.89	D00.08	D10.7	D37.05	D49.0

◄ New ◄ Revised ~~deleted~~ Deleted

TABLE OF NEOPLASMS

	Malignant Primary	Malignant Secondary	Ca in situ	Benign	Uncertain Behavior	Unspecified Behavior
fossa *(Continued)*						
pituitary	C75.1	C79.89	D09.3	D35.2	D44.3	D49.7
posterior (cranial)	C71.9	C79.31	—	D33.2	D43.2	D49.6
pterygoid	C49.0	C79.89	—	D21.0	D48.1	D49.2
pyriform	C12	C79.89	D00.08	D10.7	D37.05	D49.0
Rosenmuller	C11.2	C79.89	D00.08	D10.6	D37.05	D49.0
tonsillar	C09.0	C79.89	D00.08	D10.5	D37.05	D49.0
fourchette	C51.9	C79.82	D07.1	D28.0	D39.8	D49.5
frenulum						
labii — *see Neoplasm, lip, internal*						
linguae	C02.2	C79.89	D00.07	D10.1	D37.02	D49.0
frontal						
bone	C41.0	C79.51	—	D16.4-	D48.0	D49.2
lobe, brain	C71.1	C79.31	—	D33.0	D43.0	D49.6
pole	C71.1	C79.31	—	D33.0	D43.0	D49.6
sinus	C31.2	C78.39	D02.3	D14.0	D38.5	D49.1
fundus						
stomach	C16.1	C78.89	D00.2	D13.1	D37.1	D49.0
uterus	C54.3	C79.82	D07.0	D26.1	D39.0	D49.5
gall duct (extrahepatic)	C24.0	C78.89	D01.5	D13.5	D37.6	D49.0
intrahepatic	C22.1	C78.7	D01.5	D13.4	D37.6	D49.0
gallbladder	C23	C78.89	D01.5	D13.5	D37.6	D49.0
overlapping lesion with extrahepatic bile ducts	C24.8	—	—	—	—	—
ganglia — *see also Neoplasm, nerve, peripheral*	C47.9	C79.89	—	D36.10	D48.2	D49.2
basal	C71.0	C79.31	—	D33.0	D43.0	D49.6
cranial nerve	C72.50	C79.49	—	D33.3	D43.3	D49.7
Gartner's duct	C52	C79.82	D07.2	D28.1	D39.8	D49.5
gastric — *see Neoplasm, stomach*						
gastrocolic	C26.9	C78.89	D01.9	D13.9	D37.9	D49.0
gastroesophageal junction	C16.0	C78.89	D00.2	D13.1	D37.1	D49.0
gastrointestinal (tract) NEC	C26.9	C78.89	D01.9	D13.9	D37.9	D49.0
generalized	C80.0	—	—	—	—	—
genital organ or tract						
female NEC	C57.9	C79.82	D07.30	D28.9	D39.9	D49.5
overlapping lesion	C57.8	—	—	—	—	—
specified site NEC	C57.7	C79.82	D07.39	D28.7	D39.8	D49.5
male NEC	C63.9	C79.82	D07.60	D29.9	D40.9	D49.5
overlapping lesion	C63.8	—	—	—	—	—
specified site NEC	C63.7	C79.82	D07.69	D29.8	D40.8	D49.5
genitourinary tract						
female	C57.9	C79.82	D07.30	D28.9	D39.9	D49.5
male	C63.9	C79.82	D07.60	D29.9	D40.9	D49.5

	Malignant Primary	Malignant Secondary	Ca in situ	Benign	Uncertain Behavior	Unspecified Behavior
gingiva (alveolar) (marginal)	C03.9	C79.89	D00.03	D10.39	D37.09	D49.0
lower	C03.1	C79.89	D00.03	D10.39	D37.09	D49.0
mandibular	C03.1	C79.89	D00.03	D10.39	D37.09	D49.0
maxillary	C03.0	C79.89	D00.03	D10.39	D37.09	D49.0
upper	C03.0	C79.89	D00.03	D10.39	D37.09	D49.0
gland, glandular (lymphatic) (system) — see also Neoplasm, lymph gland						
endocrine NEC	C75.9	C79.89	D09.3	D35.9	D44.9	D49.7
salivary — see Neoplasm, salivary gland						
glans penis	C60.1	C79.82	D07.4	D29.0	D40.8	D49.5
globus pallidus	C71.0	C79.31	—	D33.0	D43.0	D49.6
glomus						
coccygeal	C49.5	C79.89	—	D21.5	D48.1	D49.2
jugularis	C75.5	C79.89	—	D35.6	D44.7	D49.7
glosso-epiglottic fold(s)	C10.1	C79.89	D00.08	D10.5	D37.05	D49.0
glossopalatine fold	C09.1	C79.89	D00.08	D10.5	D37.05	D49.0
glossopharyngeal sulcus	C09.0	C79.89	D00.08	D10.5	D37.05	D49.0
glottis	C32.0	C78.39	D02.0	D14.1	D38.0	D49.1
gluteal region	C76.3	C79.89	D04.5	D36.7	D48.7	D49.89
great vessels NEC	C49.3	C79.89	—	D21.3	D48.1	D49.2
groin NEC	C76.3	C79.89	D04.5	D36.7	D48.7	D49.89
gum	C03.9	C79.89	D00.03	D10.39	D37.09	D49.0
lower	C03.1	C79.89	D00.03	D10.39	D37.09	D49.0
upper	C03.0	C79.89	D00.03	D10.39	D37.09	D49.0
hand NEC	C76.4-	C79.89	D04.6-	D36.7	D48.7	D49.89
head NEC	C76.0	C79.89	D04.4	D36.7	D48.7	D49.89
heart	C38.0	C79.89	—	D15.1	D48.7	D49.89
heel NEC	C76.5-	C79.89	D04.7-	D36.7	D48.7	D49.89
helix — see also Neoplasm, skin, ear	C44.20-	C79.2	D04.2-	D23.2-	D48.5	D49.2
hematopoietic, hemopoietic tissue NEC	C96.9	—	—	—	—	—
specified NEC	C96.Z	—	—	—	—	—
hemisphere, cerebral	C71.0	C79.31	—	D33.0	D43.0	D49.6
hemorrhoidal zone	C21.1	C78.5	D01.3	D12.9	D37.8	D49.0
hepatic — see also Index to disease, by histology	C22.9	C78.7	D01.5	D13.4	D37.6	D49.0
duct (bile)	C24.0	C78.89	D01.5	D13.5	D37.6	D49.0
flexure (colon)	C18.3	C78.5	D01.0	D12.3	D37.4	D49.0
primary	C22.8	C78.7	D01.5	D13.4	D37.6	D49.0
hepatobiliary	C24.9	C79.89	D01.5	D13.5	D37.6	D49.0
hepatoblastoma	C22.2	C78.7	D01.5	D13.4	D37.6	D49.0
hepatoma	C22.0	C78.7	D01.5	D13.4	D37.6	D49.0
hilus of lung	C34.0-	C78.0-	D02.2-	D14.3-	D38.1	D49.1
hip NEC	C76.5-	C79.89	D04.7-	D36.7	D48.7	D49.89
hippocampus, brain	C71.2	C79.31	—	D33.0	D43.0	D49.6
humerus (any part)	C40.0-	C79.51	—	D16.0-	—	—
hymen	C52	C79.82	D07.2	D28.1	D39.8	D49.5

◄ New   ◄ Revised   ~~deleted~~ Deleted

	Malignant Primary	Malignant Secondary	Ca in situ	Benign	Uncertain Behavior	Unspecified Behavior
hypopharynx, hypopharyngeal NEC	C13.9	C79.89	D00.08	D10.7	D37.05	D49.0
overlapping lesion	C13.8	—	—	—	—	—
postcricoid region	C13.0	C79.89	D00.08	D10.7	D37.05	D49.0
posterior wall	C13.2	C79.89	D00.08	D10.7	D37.05	D49.0
pyriform fossa (sinus)	C12	C79.89	D00.08	D10.7	D37.05	D49.0
hypophysis	C75.1	C79.89	D09.3	D35.2	D44.3	D49.7
hypothalamus	C71.0	C79.31	—	D33.0	D43.0	D49.6
ileocecum, ileocecal (coil) (junction) (valve)	C18.0	C78.5	D01.0	D12.0	D37.4	D49.0
ileum	C17.2	C78.4	D01.49	D13.39	D37.2	D49.0
ilium	C41.4	C79.51	—	D16.8	D48.0	D49.2
immunoproliferative NEC	C88.9	—	—	—	—	—
infraclavicular (region)	C76.1	C79.89	D04.5	D36.7	D48.7	D49.89
inguinal (region)	C76.3	C79.89	D04.5	D36.7	D48.7	D49.89
insula	C71.0	C79.31	—	D33.0	D43.0	D49.6
insular tissue (pancreas)	C25.4	C78.89	D01.7	D13.7	D37.8	D49.0
brain	C71.0	C79.31	—	D33.0	D43.0	D49.6
interarytenoid fold	C13.1	C79.89	D00.08	D10.7	D37.05	D49.0
hypopharyngeal aspect	C13.1	C79.89	D00.08	D10.7	D37.05	D49.0
laryngeal aspect	C32.1	C78.39	D02.0	D14.1	D38.0	D49.1
marginal zone	C13.1	C79.89	D00.08	D10.7	D37.05	D49.0
interdental papillae	C03.9	C79.89	D00.03	D10.39	D37.09	D49.0
lower	C03.1	C79.89	D00.03	D10.39	D37.09	D49.0
upper	C03.0	C79.89	D00.03	D10.39	D37.09	D49.0
internal						
capsule	C71.0	C79.31	—	D33.0	D43.0	D49.6
os (cervix)	C53.0	C79.82	D06.0	D26.0	D39.0	D49.5
intervertebral cartilage or disc	C41.2	C79.51	—	D16.6	D48.0	D49.2
intestine, intestinal	C26.0	C78.80	D01.40	D13.9	D37.8	D49.0
large	C18.9	C78.5	D01.0	D12.6	D37.4	D49.0
appendix	C18.1	C78.5	D01.0	D12.1	D37.3	D49.0
caput coli	C18.0	C78.5	D01.0	D12.0	D37.4	D49.0
cecum	C18.0	C78.5	D01.0	D12.0	D37.4	D49.0
colon	C18.9	C78.5	D01.0	D12.6	D37.4	D49.0
and rectum	C19	C78.5	D01.1	D12.7	D37.5	D49.0
ascending	C18.2	C78.5	D01.0	D12.2	D37.4	D49.0
caput	C18.0	C78.5	D01.0	D12.0	D37.4	D49.0
descending	C18.6	C78.5	D01.0	D12.4	D37.4	D49.0
distal	C18.6	C78.5	D01.0	D12.4	D37.4	D49.0
left	C18.6	C78.5	D01.0	D12.4	D37.4	D49.0
overlapping lesion	C18.8	—	—	—	—	—
pelvic	C18.7	C78.5	D01.0	D12.5	D37.4	D49.0
right	C18.2	C78.5	D01.0	D12.2	D37.4	D49.0
sigmoid (flexure)	C18.7	C78.5	D01.0	D12.5	D37.4	D49.0
transverse	C18.4	C78.5	D01.0	D12.3	D37.4	D49.0

	Malignant Primary	Malignant Secondary	Ca in situ	Benign	Uncertain Behavior	Unspecified Behavior
intestine, intestinal *(Continued)*						
large *(Continued)*						
hepatic flexure	C18.3	C78.5	D01.0	D12.3	D37.4	D49.0
ileocecum, ileocecal (coil) (valve)	C18.0	C78.5	D01.0	D12.0	D37.4	D49.0
overlapping lesion	C18.8	—	—	—	—	—
sigmoid flexure (lower) (upper)	C18.7	C78.5	D01.0	D12.5	D37.4	D49.0
splenic flexure	C18.5	C78.5	D01.0	D12.3	D37.4	D49.0
small	C17.9	C78.4	D01.40	D13.30	D37.2	D49.0
duodenum	C17.0	C78.4	D01.49	D13.2	D37.2	D49.0
ileum	C17.2	C78.4	D01.49	D13.39	D37.2	D49.0
jejunum	C17.1	C78.4	D01.49	D13.39	D37.2	D49.0
overlapping lesion	C17.8	—	—	—	—	—
tract NEC	C26.0	C78.89	D01.40	D13.9	D37.8	D49.0
intra-abdominal	C76.2	C79.89	D09.8	D36.7	D48.7	D49.89
intracranial NEC	C71.9	C79.31	—	D33.2	D43.2	D49.6
intrahepatic (bile) duct	C22.1	C78.7	D01.5	D13.4	D37.6	D49.0
intraocular	C69.9-	C79.49	D09.2-	D31.9-	D48.7	D49.89
intraorbital	C69.6-	C79.49	D09.2-	D31.6-	D48.7	D49.89
intrasellar	C75.1	C79.89	D09.3	D35.2	D44.3	D49.7
intrathoracic (cavity) (organs)	C76.1	C79.89	D09.8	D15.9	D48.7	D49.89
specified NEC	C76.1	C79.89	D09.8	D15.7	—	—
iris	C69.4-	C79.49	D09.2-	D31.4-	D48.7	D49.89
ischiorectal (fossa)	C76.3	C79.89	D09.8	D36.7	D48.7	D49.89
ischium	C41.4	C79.51	—	D16.8	D48.0	D49.2
island of Reil	C71.0	C79.31	—	D33.0	D43.0	D49.6
islands or islets of Langerhans	C25.4	C78.89	D01.7	D13.7	D37.8	D49.0
isthmus uteri	C54.0	C79.82	D07.0	D26.1	D39.0	D49.5
jaw	C76.0	C79.89	D09.8	D36.7	D48.7	D49.89
bone	C41.1	C79.51	—	D16.5-	D48.0	D49.2
lower	C41.1	C79.51	—	D16.5-	—	—
upper	C41.0	C79.51	—	D16.4-	—	—
carcinoma (any type) (lower) (upper)	C76.0	C79.89	—	—	—	—
skin — *see also Neoplasm, skin, face*	C44.309	C79.2	D04.39	D23.39	D48.5	D49.2
soft tissues	C03.9	C79.89	D00.03	D10.39	D37.09	D49.0
lower	C03.1	C79.89	D00.03	D10.39	D37.09	D49.0
upper	C03.0	C79.89	D00.03	D10.39	D37.09	D49.0
jejunum	C17.1	C78.4	D01.49	D13.39	D37.2	D49.0
joint NEC — *see also Neoplasm, bone*	C41.9	C79.51	—	D16.9-	D48.0	D49.2
acromioclavicular	C40.0-	C79.51	—	D16.0-	—	—
bursa or synovial membrane — *see Neoplasm, connective tissue*						
costovertebral	C41.3	C79.51	—	D16.7	D48.0	D49.2
sternocostal	C41.3	C79.51	—	D16.7	D48.0	D49.2
temporomandibular	C41.1	C79.51	—	D16.5-	D48.0	D49.2

◄ New ◄▒ Revised ~~deleted~~ Deleted

TABLE OF NEOPLASMS

	Malignant Primary	Malignant Secondary	Ca in situ	Benign	Uncertain Behavior	Unspecified Behavior
junction						
anorectal	C21.8	C78.5	D01.3	D12.9	D37.8	D49.0
cardioesophageal	C16.0	C78.89	D00.2	D13.1	D37.1	D49.0
esophagogastric	C16.0	C78.89	D00.2	D13.1	D37.1	D49.0
gastroesophageal	C16.0	C78.89	D00.2	D13.1	D37.1	D49.0
hard and soft palate	C05.9	C79.89	D00.00	D10.39	D37.09	D49.0
ileocecal	C18.0	C78.5	D01.0	D12.0	D37.4	D49.0
pelvirectal	C19	C78.5	D01.1	D12.7	D37.5	D49.0
pelviureteric	C65.-	C79.0-	D09.19	D30.1-	D41.1-	D49.5
rectosigmoid	C19	C78.5	D01.1	D12.7	D37.5	D49.0
squamocolumnar, of cervix	C53.8	C79.82	D06.7	D26.0	D39.0	D49.5
Kaposi's sarcoma — *see Kaposi's, sarcoma*						
kidney (parenchymal)	C64.-	C79.0-	D09.19	D30.0-	D41.0-	D49.5
calyx	C65.-	C79.0-	D09.19	D30.1-	D41.1-	D49.5
hilus	C65.-	C79.0-	D09.19	D30.1-	D41.1-	D49.5
pelvis	C65.-	C79.0-	D09.19	D30.1-	D41.1-	D49.5
knee NEC	C76.5-	C79.89	D04.7-	D36.7	D48.7	D49.89
labia (skin)	C51.9	C79.82	D07.1	D28.0	D39.8	D49.5
majora	C51.0	C79.82	D07.1	D28.0	D39.8	D49.5
minora	C51.1	C79.82	D07.1	D28.0	D39.8	D49.5
labial — *see also Neoplasm, lip*	C00.9	C79.89	D00.01	D10.0	D37.01	D49.0
sulcus (lower) (upper)	C06.1	C79.89	D00.02	D10.39	D37.09	D49.0
labium (skin)	C51.9	C79.82	D07.1	D28.0	D39.8	D49.5
majus	C51.0	C79.82	D07.1	D28.0	D39.8	D49.5
minus	C51.1	C79.82	D07.1	D28.0	D39.8	D49.5
lacrimal						
canaliculi	C69.5-	C79.49	D09.2-	D31.5-	D48.7	D49.89
duct (nasal)	C69.5-	C79.49	D09.2-	D31.5-	D48.7	D49.89
gland	C69.5-	C79.49	D09.2-	D31.5-	D48.7	D49.89
punctum	C69.5-	C79.49	D09.2-	D31.5-	D48.7	D49.89
sac	C69.5-	C79.49	D09.2-	D31.5-	D48.7	D49.89
Langerhans, islands or islets	C25.4	C78.89	D01.7	D13.7	D37.8	D49.0
laryngopharynx	C13.9	C79.89	D00.08	D10.7	D37.05	D49.0
larynx, laryngeal NEC	C32.9	C78.39	D02.0	D14.1	D38.0	D49.1
aryepiglottic fold	C32.1	C78.39	D02.0	D14.1	D38.0	D49.1
cartilage (arytenoid) (cricoid) (cuneiform) (thyroid)	C32.3	C78.39	D02.0	D14.1	D38.0	D49.1
commissure (anterior) (posterior)	C32.0	C78.39	D02.0	D14.1	D38.0	D49.1
extrinsic NEC	C32.1	C78.39	D02.0	D14.1	D38.0	D49.1
meaning hypopharynx	C13.9	C79.89	D00.08	D10.7	D37.05	D49.0
interarytenoid fold	C32.1	C78.39	D02.0	D14.1	D38.0	D49.1
intrinsic	C32.0	C78.39	D02.0	D14.1	D38.0	D49.1
overlapping lesion	C32.8	—	—	—	—	—
ventricular band	C32.1	C78.39	D02.0	D14.1	D38.0	D49.1
leg NEC	C76.5-	C79.89	D04.7-	D36.7	D48.7	D49.89

TABLE OF NEOPLASMS

TABLE OF NEOPLASMS

	Malignant Primary	Malignant Secondary	Ca in situ	Benign	Uncertain Behavior	Unspecified Behavior
lens, crystalline	C69.4-	C79.49	D09.2-	D31.4-	D48.7	D49.89
lid (lower) (upper)	C44.10-	C79.2	D04.1-	D23.1-	D48.5	D49.2
basal cell carcinoma	C44.11-	—	—	—	—	—
specified type NEC	C44.19-	—	—	—	—	—
squamous cell carcinoma	C44.12-	—	—	—	—	—
ligament — *see also Neoplasm, connective tissue*						
broad	C57.1	C79.82	D07.39	D28.2	D39.8	D49.5
Mackenrodt's	C57.7	C79.82	D07.39	D28.7	D39.8	D49.5
non-uterine — *see Neoplasm, connective tissue*						
round	C57.2	C79.82	—	D28.2	D39.8	D49.5
sacro-uterine	C57.3	C79.82	—	D28.2	D39.8	D49.5
uterine	C57.3	C79.82	—	D28.2	D39.8	D49.5
utero-ovarian	C57.7	C79.82	D07.39	D28.2	D39.8	D49.5
uterosacral	C57.3	C79.82	—	D28.2	D39.8	D49.5
limb	C76.8	C79.89	D04.8	D36.7	D48.7	D49.89
lower	C76.5-	C79.89	D04.7-	D36.7	D48.7	D49.89
upper	C76.4-	C79.89	D04.6-	D36.7	D48.7	D49.89
limbus of cornea	C69.1-	C79.49	D09.2-	D31.1-	D48.7	D49.89
lingual NEC — *see also Neoplasm, tongue*	C02.9	C79.89	D00.07	D10.1	D37.02	D49.0
lingula, lung	C34.1-	C78.0-	D02.2-	D14.3-	D38.1	D49.1
lip	C00.9	C79.89	D00.01	D10.0	D37.01	D49.0
buccal aspect — *see Neoplasm, lip, internal*						
commissure	C00.6	C79.89	D00.01	D10.0	D37.01	D49.0
external	C00.2	C79.89	D00.01	D10.0	D37.01	D49.0
lower	C00.1	C79.89	D00.01	D10.0	D37.01	D49.0
upper	C00.0	C79.89	D00.01	D10.0	D37.01	D49.0
frenulum — *see Neoplasm, lip, internal*						
inner aspect — *see Neoplasm, lip, internal*						
internal	C00.5	C79.89	D00.01	D10.0	D37.01	D49.0
lower	C00.4	C79.89	D00.01	D10.0	D37.01	D49.0
upper	C00.3	C79.89	D00.01	D10.0	D37.01	D49.0
lipstick area	C00.2	C79.89	D00.01	D10.0	D37.01	D49.0
lower	C00.1	C79.89	D00.01	D10.0	D37.01	D49.0
upper	C00.0	C79.89	D00.01	D10.0	D37.01	D49.0
lower	C00.1	C79.89	D00.01	D10.0	D37.01	D49.0
internal	C00.4	C79.89	D00.01	D10.0	D37.01	D49.0
mucosa — *see Neoplasm, lip, internal*						
oral aspect — *see Neoplasm, lip, internal*						
overlapping lesion	C00.8	—	—	—	—	—
with oral cavity or pharynx	C14.8	—	—	—	—	—
skin (commissure) (lower) (upper)	C44.00	C79.2	D04.0	D23.0	D48.5	D49.2
basal cell carcinoma	C44.01	—	—	—	—	—
specified type NEC	C44.09	—	—	—	—	—
squamous cell carcinoma	C44.02	—	—	—	—	—

◀ New   ◀▥ Revised   ~~deleted~~ Deleted

	Malignant Primary	Malignant Secondary	Ca in situ	Benign	Uncertain Behavior	Unspecified Behavior
lip *(Continued)*						
upper	C00.0	C79.89	D00.01	D10.0	D37.01	D49.0
internal	C00.3	C79.89	D00.01	D10.0	D37.01	D49.0
vermilion border	C00.2	C79.89	D00.01	D10.0	D37.01	D49.0
lower	C00.1	C79.89	D00.01	D10.0	D37.01	D49.0
upper	C00.0	C79.89	D00.01	D10.0	D37.01	D49.0
lipomatous — *see Lipoma, by site*						
liver — *see also Index to disease, by histology*	C22.9	C78.7	D01.5	D13.4	D37.6	D49.0
primary	C22.8	C78.7	D01.5	D13.4	D37.6	D49.0
lumbosacral plexus	C47.5	C79.89	—	D36.16	D48.2	D49.2
lung	C34.9-	C78.0-	D02.2-	D14.3-	D38.1	D49.1
azygos lobe	C34.1-	C78.0-	D02.2-	D14.3-	D38.1	D49.1
carina	C34.0-	C78.0-	D02.2-	D14.3-	D38.1	D49.1
hilus	C34.0-	C78.0-	D02.2-	D14.3-	D38.1	D49.1
lingula	C34.1-	C78.0-	D02.2-	D14.3-	D38.1	D49.1
lobe NEC	C34.9-	C78.0-	D02.2-	D14.3-	D38.1	D49.1
lower lobe	C34.3-	C78.0-	D02.2-	D14.3-	D38.1	D49.1
main bronchus	C34.0-	C78.0-	D02.2-	D14.3-	D38.1	D49.1
mesothelioma — *see Mesothelioma*						
middle lobe	C34.2	C78.0-	D02.21	D14.31	D38.1	D49.1
overlapping lesion	C34.8-	—	—	—	—	—
upper lobe	C34.1-	C78.0-	D02.2-	D14.3-	D38.1	D49.1
lymph, lymphatic channel NEC	C49.9	C79.89	—	D21.9	D48.1	D49.2
gland (secondary)	—	C77.9	—	D36.0	D48.7	D49.89
abdominal	—	C77.2	—	D36.0	D48.7	D49.89
aortic	—	C77.2	—	D36.0	D48.7	D49.89
arm	—	C77.3	—	D36.0	D48.7	D49.89
auricular (anterior) (posterior)	—	C77.0	—	D36.0	D48.7	D49.89
axilla, axillary	—	C77.3	—	D36.0	D48.7	D49.89
brachial	—	C77.3	—	D36.0	D48.7	D49.89
bronchial	—	C77.1	—	D36.0	D48.7	D49.89
bronchopulmonary	—	C77.1	—	D36.0	D48.7	D49.89
celiac	—	C77.2	—	D36.0	D48.7	D49.89
cervical	—	C77.0	—	D36.0	D48.7	D49.89
cervicofacial	—	C77.0	—	D36.0	D48.7	D49.89
Cloquet	—	C77.4	—	D36.0	D48.7	D49.89
colic	—	C77.2	—	D36.0	D48.7	D49.89
common duct	—	C77.2	—	D36.0	D48.7	D49.89
cubital	—	C77.3	—	D36.0	D48.7	D49.89
diaphragmatic	—	C77.1	—	D36.0	D48.7	D49.89
epigastric, inferior	—	C77.1	—	D36.0	D48.7	D49.89
epitrochlear	—	C77.3	—	D36.0	D48.7	D49.89
esophageal	—	C77.1	—	D36.0	D48.7	D49.89
face	—	C77.0	—	D36.0	D48.7	D49.89

	Malignant Primary	Malignant Secondary	Ca in situ	Benign	Uncertain Behavior	Unspecified Behavior
lymph, lymphatic channel NEC *(Continued)*						
gland *(Continued)*						
femoral	—	C77.4	—	D36.0	D48.7	D49.89
gastric	—	C77.2	—	D36.0	D48.7	D49.89
groin	—	C77.4	—	D36.0	D48.7	D49.89
head	—	C77.0	—	D36.0	D48.7	D49.89
hepatic	—	C77.2	—	D36.0	D48.7	D49.89
hilar (pulmonary)	—	C77.1	—	D36.0	D48.7	D49.89
splenic	—	C77.2	—	D36.0	D48.7	D49.89
hypogastric	—	C77.5	—	D36.0	D48.7	D49.89
ileocolic	—	C77.2	—	D36.0	D48.7	D49.89
iliac	—	C77.5	—	D36.0	D48.7	D49.89
infraclavicular	—	C77.3	—	D36.0	D48.7	D49.89
inguina, inguinal	—	C77.4	—	D36.0	D48.7	D49.89
innominate	—	C77.1	—	D36.0	D48.7	D49.89
intercostal	—	C77.1	—	D36.0	D48.7	D49.89
intestinal	—	C77.2	—	D36.0	D48.7	D49.89
intrabdominal	—	C77.2	—	D36.0	D48.7	D49.89
intrapelvic	—	C77.5	—	D36.0	D48.7	D49.89
intrathoracic	—	C77.1	—	D36.0	D48.7	D49.89
jugular	—	C77.0	—	D36.0	D48.7	D49.89
leg	—	C77.4	—	D36.0	D48.7	D49.89
limb						
lower	—	C77.4	—	D36.0	D48.7	D49.89
upper	—	C77.3	—	D36.0	D48.7	D49.89
lower limb	—	C77.4	—	D36.0	D48.7	D49.89
lumbar	—	C77.2	—	D36.0	D48.7	D49.89
mandibular	—	C77.0	—	D36.0	D48.7	D49.89
mediastinal	—	C77.1	—	D36.0	D48.7	D49.89
mesenteric (inferior) (superior)	—	C77.2	—	D36.0	D48.7	D49.89
midcolic	—	C77.2	—	D36.0	D48.7	D49.89
multiple sites in categories C77.0 - C77.5	—	C77.8	—	D36.0	D48.7	D49.89
neck	—	C77.0	—	D36.0	D48.7	D49.89
obturator	—	C77.5	—	D36.0	D48.7	D49.89
occipital	—	C77.0	—	D36.0	D48.7	D49.89
pancreatic	—	C77.2	—	D36.0	D48.7	D49.89
para-aortic	—	C77.2	—	D36.0	D48.7	D49.89
paracervical	—	C77.5	—	D36.0	D48.7	D49.89
parametrial	—	C77.5	—	D36.0	D48.7	D49.89
parasternal	—	C77.1	—	D36.0	D48.7	D49.89
parotid	—	C77.0	—	D36.0	D48.7	D49.89
pectoral	—	C77.3	—	D36.0	D48.7	D49.89
pelvic	—	C77.5	—	D36.0	D48.7	D49.89

TABLE OF NEOPLASMS

◀ New ◀ Revised ~~deleted~~ Deleted

	Malignant Primary	Malignant Secondary	Ca in situ	Benign	Uncertain Behavior	Unspecified Behavior
lymph, lymphatic channel NEC *(Continued)*						
gland *(Continued)*						
peri-aortic	—	C77.2	—	D36.0	D48.7	D49.89
peripancreatic	—	C77.2	—	D36.0	D48.7	D49.89
popliteal	—	C77.4	—	D36.0	D48.7	D49.89
porta hepatis	—	C77.2	—	D36.0	D48.7	D49.89
portal	—	C77.2	—	D36.0	D48.7	D49.89
preauricular	—	C77.0	—	D36.0	D48.7	D49.89
prelaryngeal	—	C77.0	—	D36.0	D48.7	D49.89
presymphysial	—	C77.5	—	D36.0	D48.7	D49.89
pretracheal	—	C77.0	—	D36.0	D48.7	D49.89
primary (any site) NEC	C96.9	—	—	—	—	—
pulmonary (hiler)	—	C77.1	—	D36.0	D48.7	D49.89
pyloric	—	C77.2	—	D36.0	D48.7	D49.89
retroperitoneal	—	C77.2	—	D36.0	D48.7	D49.89
retropharyngeal	—	C77.0	—	D36.0	D48.7	D49.89
Rosenmuller's	—	C77.4	—	D36.0	D48.7	D49.89
sacral	—	C77.5	—	D36.0	D48.7	D49.89
scalene	—	C77.0	—	D36.0	D48.7	D49.89
site NEC	—	C77.9	—	D36.0	D48.7	D49.89
splenic (hilar)	—	C77.2	—	D36.0	D48.7	D49.89
subclavicular	—	C77.3	—	D36.0	D48.7	D49.89
subinguinal	—	C77.4	—	D36.0	D48.7	D49.89
sublingual	—	C77.0	—	D36.0	D48.7	D49.89
submandibular	—	C77.0	—	D36.0	D48.7	D49.89
submaxillary	—	C77.0	—	D36.0	D48.7	D49.89
submental	—	C77.0	—	D36.0	D48.7	D49.89
subscapular	—	C77.3	—	D36.0	D48.7	D49.89
supraclavicular	—	C77.0	—	D36.0	D48.7	D49.89
thoracic	—	C77.1	—	D36.0	D48.7	D49.89
tibial	—	C77.4	—	D36.0	D48.7	D49.89
tracheal	—	C77.1	—	D36.0	D48.7	D49.89
tracheobronchial	—	C77.1	—	D36.0	D48.7	D49.89
upper limb	—	C77.3	—	D36.0	D48.7	D49.89
Virchow's	—	C77.0	—	D36.0	D48.7	D49.89
node — *see also Neoplasm, lymph gland*						
primary NEC	C96.9	—	—	—	—	—
vessel — *see also Neoplasm, connective tissue*	C49.9	C79.89	—	D21.9	D48.1	D49.2
Mackenrodt's ligament	C57.7	C79.82	D07.39	D28.7	D39.8	D49.5
malar	C41.0	C79.51	—	D16.4-	D48.0	D49.2
region — *see Neoplasm, cheek*						
mammary gland — *see Neoplasm, breast*						

TABLE OF NEOPLASMS

	Malignant Primary	Malignant Secondary	Ca in situ	Benign	Uncertain Behavior	Unspecified Behavior
mandible	C41.1	C79.51	—	D16.5-	D48.0	D49.2
alveolar						
mucosa (carcinoma)	C03.1	C79.89	D00.03	D10.39	D37.09	D49.0
ridge or process	C41.1	C79.51	—	D16.5-	D48.0	D49.2
marrow (bone) NEC	C96.9	C79.52	—	—	D47.9	D49.89
mastectomy site (skin) — see also Neoplasm, breast, skin	C44.501	C79.2	—	—	—	—
specified as breast tissue	C50.8-	C79.81	—	—	—	—
mastoid (air cells) (antrum) (cavity)	C30.1	C78.39	D02.3	D14.0	D38.5	D49.1
bone or process	C41.0	C79.51	—	D16.4-	D48.0	D49.2
maxilla, maxillary (superior)	C41.0	C79.51	—	D16.4-	D48.0	D49.2
alveolar						
mucosa	C03.0	C79.89	D00.03	D10.39	D37.09	D49.0
ridge or process (carcinoma)	C41.0	C79.51	—	D16.4-	D48.0	D49.2
antrum	C31.0	C78.39	D02.3	D14.0	D38.5	D49.1
carcinoma	C03.0	C79.51	—	—	—	—
inferior — see Neoplasm, mandible						
sinus	C31.0	C78.39	D02.3	D14.0	D38.5	D49.1
meatus external (ear) — see also Neoplasm, skin, ear	C44.20-	C79.2	D04.2-	D23.2-	D48.5	D49.2
Meckel diverticulum, malignant	C17.3	C78.4	D01.49	D13.39	D37.2	D49.0
mediastinum, mediastinal	C38.3	C78.1	—	D15.2	D38.3	D49.89
anterior	C38.1	C78.1	—	D15.2	D38.3	D49.89
posterior	C38.2	C78.1	—	D15.2	D38.3	D49.89
medulla						
adrenal	C74.1-	C79.7-	D09.3	D35.0-	D44.1-	D49.7
oblongata	C71.7	C79.31	—	D33.1	D43.1	D49.6
meibomian gland	C44.10-	C79.2	D04.1-	D23.1-	D48.5	D49.2
basal cell carcinoma	C44.11-	—	—	—	—	—
specified type NEC	C44.19-	—	—	—	—	—
squamous cell carcinoma	C44.12-	—	—	—	—	—
melanoma — see Melanoma						
meninges	C70.9	C79.49	—	D32.9	D42.9	D49.7
brain	C70.0	C79.32	—	D32.0	D42.0	D49.7
cerebral	C70.0	C79.32	—	D32.0	D42.0	D49.7
crainial	C70.0	C79.32	—	D32.0	D42.0	D49.7
intracranial	C70.0	C79.32	—	D32.0	D42.0	D49.7
spinal (cord)	C70.1	C79.49	—	D32.1	D42.1	D49.7
meniscus, knee joint (lateral) (medial)	C40.2-	C79.51	—	D16.2-	D48.0	D49.2
Merkel cell — see Carcinoma, Merkel cell						
mesentery, mesenteric	C48.1	C78.6	—	D20.1	D48.4	D49.0
mesoappendix	C48.1	C78.6	—	D20.1	D48.4	D49.0
mesocolon	C48.1	C78.6	—	D20.1	D48.4	D49.0
mesopharynx — see Neoplasm, oropharynx						
mesosalpinx	C57.1	C79.82	D07.39	D28.2	D39.8	D49.5

◄ New   ◄⫶⫶ Revised   ~~deleted~~ Deleted

	Malignant Primary	Malignant Secondary	Ca in situ	Benign	Uncertain Behavior	Unspecified Behavior
mesothelial tissue — *see Mesothelioma*						
mesothelioma — *see Mesothelioma*						
mesovarium	C57.1	C79.82	D07.39	D28.2	D39.8	D49.5
metacarpus (any bone)	C40.1-	C79.51	—	D16.1-	—	—
metastatic NEC — *see also Neoplasm, by site, secondary*	—	C79.9	—	—	—	—
metatarsus (any bone)	C40.3-	C79.51	—	D16.3-	—	—
midbrain	C71.7	C79.31	—	D33.1	D43.1	D49.6
milk duct — *see Neoplasm, breast*						
mons						
pubis	C51.9	C79.82	D07.1	D28.0	D39.8	D49.5
veneris	C51.9	C79.82	D07.1	D28.0	D39.8	D49.5
motor tract	C72.9	C79.49	—	D33.9	D43.9	D49.7
brain	C71.9	C79.31	—	D33.2	D43.2	D49.6
cauda equina	C72.1	C79.49	—	D33.4	D43.4	D49.7
spinal	C72.0	C79.49	—	D33.4	D43.4	D49.7
mouth	C06.9	C79.89	D00.00	D10.30	D37.09	D49.0
book-leaf	C06.89	C79.89	—	—	—	—
floor	C04.9	C79.89	D00.06	D10.2	D37.09	D49.0
anterior portion	C04.0	C79.89	D00.06	D10.2	D37.09	D49.0
lateral portion	C04.1	C79.89	D00.06	D10.2	D37.09	D49.0
overlapping lesion	C04.8	—	—	—	—	—
overlapping NEC	C06.80	—	—	—	—	—
roof	C05.9	C79.89	D00.00	D10.39	D37.09	D49.0
specified part NEC	C06.89	C79.89	D00.00	D10.39	D37.09	D49.0
vestibule	C06.1	C79.89	D00.00	D10.39	D37.09	D49.0
mucosa						
alveolar (ridge or process)	C03.9	C79.89	D00.03	D10.39	D37.09	D49.0
lower	C03.1	C79.89	D00.03	D10.39	D37.09	D49.0
upper	C03.0	C79.89	D00.03	D10.39	D37.09	D49.0
buccal	C06.0	C79.89	D00.02	D10.39	D37.09	D49.0
cheek	C06.0	C79.89	D00.02	D10.39	D37.09	D49.0
lip — *see Neoplasm, lip, internal*						
nasal	C30.0	C78.39	D02.3	D14.0	D38.5	D49.1
oral	C06.0	C79.89	D00.02	D10.39	D37.09	D49.0
Mullerian duct						
female	C57.7	C79.82	D07.39	D28.7	D39.8	D49.5
male	C63.7	C79.82	D07.69	D29.8	D40.8	D49.5
muscle — *see also Neoplasm, connective tissue*						
extraocular	C69.6-	C79.49	D09.2-	D31.6-	D48.7	D49.89
myocardium	C38.0	C79.89	—	D15.1	D48.7	D49.89
myometrium	C54.2	C79.82	D07.0	D26.1	D39.0	D49.5
myopericardium	C38.0	C79.89	—	D15.1	D48.7	D49.89
nabothian gland (follicle)	C53.0	C79.82	D06.0	D26.0	D39.0	D49.5

TABLE OF NEOPLASMS

	Malignant Primary	Malignant Secondary	Ca in situ	Benign	Uncertain Behavior	Unspecified Behavior
nail — see also Neoplasm, skin, limb	C44.90	C79.2	D04.9	D23.9	D48.5	D49.2
finger — see also Neoplasm, skin, limb, upper	C44.60-	C79.2	D04.6-	D23.6-	D48.5	D49.2
toe — see also Neoplasm, skin, limb, lower	C44.70-	C79.2	D04.7-	D23.7-	D48.5	D49.2
nares, naris (anterior) (posterior)	C30.0	C78.39	D02.3	D14.0	D38.5	D49.1
nasal — see Neoplasm, nose						
nasolabial groove — see also Neoplasm, skin, face	C44.309	C79.2	D04.39	D23.39	D48.5	D49.2
nasolacrimal duct	C69.5-	C79.49	D09.2-	D31.5-	D48.7	D49.89
nasopharynx, nasopharyngeal	C11.9	C79.89	D00.08	D10.6	D37.05	D49.0
floor	C11.3	C79.89	D00.08	D10.6	D37.05	D49.0
overlapping lesion	C11.8	—	—	—	—	—
roof	C11.0	C79.89	D00.08	D10.6	D37.05	D49.0
wall	C11.9	C79.89	D00.08	D10.6	D37.05	D49.0
anterior	C11.3	C79.89	D00.08	D10.6	D37.05	D49.0
lateral	C11.2	C79.89	D00.08	D10.6	D37.05	D49.0
posterior	C11.1	C79.89	D00.08	D10.6	D37.05	D49.0
superior	C11.0	C79.89	D00.08	D10.6	D37.05	D49.0
nates — see also Neoplasm, skin, trunk	C44.509	C79.2	D04.5	D23.5	D48.5	D49.2
neck NEC	C76.0	C79.89	D09.8	D36.7	D48.7	D49.89
skin	C44.40	—	—	—	—	—
basal cell carcinoma	C44.41	—	—	—	—	—
specified type NEC	C44.49	—	—	—	—	—
squamous cell carcinoma	C44.42	—	—	—	—	—
nerve (ganglion)	C47.9	C79.89	—	D36.10	D48.2	D49.2
abducens	C72.59	C79.49	—	D33.3	D43.3	D49.7
accessory (spinal)	C72.59	C79.49	—	D33.3	D43.3	D49.7
acoustic	C72.4-	C79.49	—	D33.3	D43.3	D49.7
auditory	C72.4-	C79.49	—	D33.3	D43.3	D49.7
autonomic NEC — see also Neoplasm, nerve, peripheral	C47.9	C79.89	—	D36.10	D48.2	D49.2
brachial	C47.1-	C79.89	—	D36.12	D48.2	D49.2
cranial	C72.50	C79.49	—	D33.3	D43.3	D49.7
specified NEC	C72.59	C79.49	—	D33.3	D43.3	D49.7
facial	C72.59	C79.49	—	D33.3	D43.3	D49.7
femoral	C47.2-	C79.89	—	D36.13	D48.2	D49.2
ganglion NEC — see also Neoplasm, nerve, peripheral	C47.9	C79.89	—	D36.10	D48.2	D49.2
glossopharyngeal	C72.59	C79.49	—	D33.3	D43.3	D49.7
hypoglossal	C72.59	C79.49	—	D33.3	D43.3	D49.7
intercostal	C47.3	C79.89	—	D36.14	D48.2	D49.2
lumbar	C47.6	C79.89	—	D36.17	D48.2	D49.2
median	C47.1-	C79.89	—	D36.12	D48.2	D49.2
obturator	C47.2-	C79.89	—	D36.13	D48.2	D49.2
oculomotor	C72.59	C79.49	—	D33.3	D43.3	D49.7
olfactory	C47.2-	C79.49	—	D33.3	D43.3	D49.7
optic	C72.3-	C79.49	—	D33.3	D43.3	D49.7
parasympathetic NEC	C47.9	C79.89	—	D36.10	D48.2	D49.2

◀ New ◀▬ Revised ~~deleted~~ Deleted

	Malignant Primary	Malignant Secondary	Ca in situ	Benign	Uncertain Behavior	Unspecified Behavior
nerve *(Continued)*						
peripheral NEC	C47.9	C79.89	—	D36.10	D48.2	D49.2
abdomen	C47.4	C79.89	—	D36.15	D48.2	D49.2
abdominal wall	C47.4	C79.89	—	D36.15	D48.2	D49.2
ankle	C47.2-	C79.89	—	D36.13	D48.2	D49.2
antecubital fossa or space	C47.1-	C79.89	—	D36.12	D48.2	D49.2
arm	C47.1-	C79.89	—	D36.12	D48.2	D49.2
auricle (ear)	C47.0	C79.89	—	D36.11	D48.2	D49.2
axilla	C47.3	C79.89	—	D36.12	D48.2	D49.2
back	C47.6	C79.89	—	D36.17	D48.2	D49.2
buttock	C47.5	C79.89	—	D36.16	D48.2	D49.2
calf	C47.2-	C79.89	—	D36.13	D48.2	D49.2
cervical region	C47.0	C79.89	—	D36.11	D48.2	D49.2
cheek	C47.0	C79.89	—	D36.11	D48.2	D49.2
chest (wall)	C47.3	C79.89	—	D36.14	D48.2	D49.2
chin	C47.0	C79.89	—	D36.11	D48.2	D49.2
ear (external)	C47.0	C79.89	—	D36.11	D48.2	D49.2
elbow	C47.1-	C79.89	—	D36.12	D48.2	D49.2
extrarectal	C47.5	C79.89	—	D36.16	D48.2	D49.2
extremity	C47.9	C79.89	—	D36.10	D48.2	D49.2
lower	C47.2-	C79.89	—	D36.13	D48.2	D49.2
upper	C47.1-	C79.89	—	D36.12	D48.2	D49.2
eyelid	C47.0	C79.89	—	D36.11	D48.2	D49.2
face	C47.0	C79.89	—	D36.11	D48.2	D49.2
finger	C47.1-	C79.89	—	D36.12	D48.2	D49.2
flank	C47.6	C79.89	—	D36.17	D48.2	D49.2
foot	C47.2-	C79.89	—	D36.13	D48.2	D49.2
forearm	C47.1-	C79.89	—	D36.12	D48.2	D49.2
forehead	C47.0	C79.89	—	D36.11	D48.2	D49.2
gluteal region	C47.5	C79.89	—	D36.16	D48.2	D49.2
groin	C47.5	C79.89	—	D36.16	D48.2	D49.2
hand	C47.1-	C79.89	—	D36.12	D48.2	D49.2
head	C47.0	C79.89	—	D36.11	D48.2	D49.2
heel	C47.2-	C79.89	—	D36.13	D48.2	D49.2
hip	C47.2-	C79.89	—	D36.13	D48.2	D49.2
infraclavicular region	C47.3	C79.89	—	D36.14	D48.2	D49.2
inguinal (canal) (region)	C47.5	C79.89	—	D36.16	D48.2	D49.2
intrathoracic	C47.3	C79.89	—	D36.14	D48.2	D49.2
ischiorectal fossa	C47.5	C79.89	—	D36.16	D48.2	D49.2
knee	C47.2-	C79.89	—	D36.13	D48.2	D49.2
leg	C47.2-	C79.89	—	D36.13	D48.2	D49.2
limb NEC	C47.9	C79.89	—	D36.10	D48.2	D49.2
lower	C47.2-	C79.89	—	D36.13	D48.2	D49.2
upper	C47.1-	C79.89	—	D36.12	D48.2	D49.2

TABLE OF NEOPLASMS

	Malignant Primary	Malignant Secondary	Ca in situ	Benign	Uncertain Behavior	Unspecified Behavior
nerve *(Continued)*						
peripheral NEC *(Continued)*						
nates	C47.5	C79.89	—	D36.16	D48.2	D49.2
neck	C47.0	C79.89	—	D36.11	D48.2	D49.2
orbit	C69.6-	C79.49	—	D31.6-	D48.7	D49.2
pararectal	C47.5	C79.89	—	D36.16	D48.2	D49.2
paraurethral	C47.5	C79.89	—	D36.16	D48.2	D49.2
paravaginal	C47.5	C79.89	—	D36.16	D48.2	D49.2
pelvis (floor)	C47.5	C79.89	—	D36.16	D48.2	D49.2
pelvoabdominal	C47.8	C79.89	—	D36.17	D48.2	D49.2
perineum	C47.5	C79.89	—	D36.16	D48.2	D49.2
perirectal (tissue)	C47.5	C79.89	—	D36.16	D48.2	D49.2
periurethral (tissue)	C47.5	C79.89	—	D36.16	D48.2	D49.2
popliteal fossa or space	C47.2-	C79.89	—	D36.13	D48.2	D49.2
presacral	C47.5	C79.89	—	D36.16	D48.2	D49.2
pterygoid fossa	C47.0	C79.89	—	D36.11	D48.2	D49.2
rectovaginal septum or wall	C47.5	C79.89	—	D36.16	D48.2	D49.2
rectovesical	C47.5	C79.89	—	D36.16	D48.2	D49.2
sacrococcygeal region	C47.5	C79.89	—	D36.16	D48.2	D49.2
scalp	C47.0	C79.89	—	D36.11	D48.2	D49.2
scapular region	C47.3	C79.89	—	D36.14	D48.2	D49.2
shoulder	C47.1-	C79.89	—	D36.12	D48.2	D49.2
submental	C47.0	C79.89	—	D36.11	D48.2	D49.2
supraclavicular region	C47.0	C79.89	—	D36.11	D48.2	D49.2
temple	C47.0	C79.89	—	D36.11	D48.2	D49.2
temporal region	C47.0	C79.89	—	D36.11	D48.2	D49.2
thigh	C47.2-	C79.89	—	D36.13	D48.2	D49.2
thoracic (duct) (wall)	C47.3	C79.89	—	D36.14	D48.2	D49.2
thorax	C47.3	C79.89	—	D36.14	D48.2	D49.2
thumb	C47.1-	C79.89	—	D36.12	D48.2	D49.2
toe	C47.2-	C79.89	—	D36.13	D48.2	D49.2
trunk	C47.6	C79.89	—	D36.17	D48.2	D49.2
umbilicus	C47.4	C79.89	—	D36.15	D48.2	D49.2
vesicorectal	C47.5	C79.89	—	D36.16	D48.2	D49.2
wrist	C47.1-	C79.89	—	D36.12	D48.2	D49.2
radial	C47.1-	C79.89	—	D36.12	D48.2	D49.2
sacral	C47.5	C79.89	—	D36.16	D48.2	D49.2
sciatic	C47.2-	C79.89	—	D36.13	D48.2	D49.2
spinal NEC	C47.9	C79.89	—	D36.10	D48.2	D49.2
accessory	C72.59	C79.49	—	D33.3	D43.3	D49.7
sympathetic NEC — *see also* Neoplasm, nerve, peripheral	C47.9	C79.89	—	D36.10	D48.2	D49.2
trigeminal	C72.59	C79.49	—	D33.3	D43.3	D49.7
trochlear	C72.59	C79.49	—	D33.3	D43.3	D49.7

◀ New   ◀◀ Revised   ~~deleted~~ Deleted

	Malignant Primary	Malignant Secondary	Ca in situ	Benign	Uncertain Behavior	Unspecified Behavior
nerve *(Continued)*						
ulnar	C47.1-	C79.89	—	D36.12	D48.2	D49.2
vagus	C72.59	C79.49	—	D33.3	D43.3	D49.7
nervous system (central)	C72.9	C79.40	—	D33.9	D43.9	D49.7
autonomic — *see Neoplasm, nerve, peripheral*						
parasympathetic — *see Neoplasm, nerve, peripheral*						
specified site NEC	—	C79.49	—	D33.7	D43.8	—
sympathetic — *see Neoplasm, nerve, peripheral*						
nevus — *see Nevus*						
nipple	C50.0-	C79.81	D05.-	D24.-	—	—
nose, nasal	C76.0	C79.89	D09.8	D36.7	D48.7	D49.89
ala (external) (nasi) — *see also Neoplasm, nose, skin*	C44.301	C79.2	D04.39	D23.39	D48.5	D49.2
bone	C41.0	C79.51	—	D16.4-	D48.0	D49.2
cartilage	C30.0	C78.39	D02.3	D14.0	D38.5	D49.1
cavity	C30.0	C78.39	D02.3	D14.0	D38.5	D49.1
choana	C11.3	C79.89	D00.08	D10.6	D37.05	D49.0
external (skin) — *see also Neoplasm, nose, skin*	C44.301	C79.2	D04.39	D23.39	D48.5	D49.2
fossa	C30.0	C78.39	D02.3	D14.0	D38.5	D49.1
internal	C30.0	C78.39	D02.3	D14.0	D38.5	D49.1
mucosa	C30.0	C78.39	D02.3	D14.0	D38.5	D49.1
septum	C30.0	C78.39	D02.3	D14.0	D38.5	D49.1
posterior margin	C11.3	C79.89	D00.08	D10.6	D37.05	D49.0
sinus — *see Neoplasm, sinus*						
skin	C44.301	C79.2	D04.39	D23.39	D48.5	D49.2
basal cell carcinoma	C44.311	—	—	—	—	—
specified type NEC	C44.391	—	—	—	—	—
squamous cell carcinoma	C44.321	—	—	—	—	—
turbinate (mucosa)	C30.0	C78.39	D02.3	D14.0	D38.5	D49.1
bone	C41.0	C79.51	—	D16.4-	D48.0	D49.2
vestibule	C30.0	C78.39	D02.3	D14.0	D38.5	D49.1
nostril	C30.0	C78.39	D02.3	D14.0	D38.5	D49.1
nucleus pulposus	C41.2	C79.51	—	D16.6	D48.0	D49.2
occipital						
bone	C41.0	C79.51	—	D16.4-	D48.0	D49.2
lobe or pole, brain	C71.4	C79.31	—	D33.0	D43.0	D49.6
odontogenic — *see Neoplasm, jaw bone*						
olfactory nerve or bulb	C72.2-	C79.49	—	D33.3	D43.3	D49.7
olive (brain)	C71.7	C79.31	—	D33.1	D43.1	D49.6
omentum	C48.1	C78.6	—	D20.1	D48.4	D49.0
operculum (brain)	C71.0	C79.31	—	D33.0	D43.0	D49.6
optic nerve, chiasm, or tract	C72.3-	C79.49	—	D33.3	D43.3	D49.7
oral (cavity)	C06.9	C79.89	D00.00	D10.30	D37.09	D49.0
ill-defined	C14.8	C79.89	D00.00	D10.30	D37.09	D49.0
mucosa	C06.0	C79.89	D00.02	D10.39	D37.09	D49.0

◀ New   ◀═ Revised   ~~deleted~~ Deleted

TABLE OF NEOPLASMS

	Malignant Primary	Malignant Secondary	Ca in situ	Benign	Uncertain Behavior	Unspecified Behavior
orbit	C69.6-	C79.49	D09.2-	D31.6-	D48.7	D49.89
autonomic nerve	C69.6-	C79.49	—	D31.6-	D48.7	D49.2
bone	C41.0	C79.51	—	D16.4-	D48.0	D49.2
eye	C69.6-	C79.49	D09.2-	D31.6-	D48.7	D49.89
peripheral nerves	C69.6-	C79.49	—	D31.6-	D48.7	D49.2
soft parts	C69.6-	C79.49	D09.2-	D31.6-	D48.7	D49.89
organ of Zuckerkandl	C75.5	C79.89	—	D35.6	D44.7	D49.7
oropharynx	C10.9	C79.89	D00.08	D10.5	D37.05	D49.0
branchial cleft (vestige)	C10.4	C79.89	D00.08	D10.5	D37.05	D49.0
junctional region	C10.8	C79.89	D00.08	D10.5	D37.05	D49.0
lateral wall	C10.2	C79.89	D00.08	D10.5	D37.05	D49.0
overlapping lesion	C10.8	—	—	—	—	—
pillars or fauces	C09.1	C79.89	D00.08	D10.5	D37.05	D49.0
posterior wall	C10.3	C79.89	D00.08	D10.5	D37.05	D49.0
vallecula	C10.0	C79.89	D00.08	D10.5	D37.05	D49.0
os						
external	C53.1	C79.82	D06.1	D26.0	D39.0	D49.5
internal	C53.0	C79.82	D06.0	D26.0	D39.0	D49.5
ovary	C56.-	C79.6-	D07.39	D27.-	D39.1-	D49.5
oviduct	C57.0-	C79.82	D07.39	D28.2	D39.8	D49.5
palate	C05.9	C79.89	D00.00	D10.39	D37.09	D49.0
hard	C05.0	C79.89	D00.05	D10.39	D37.09	D49.0
junction of hard and soft palate	C05.9	C79.89	D00.00	D10.39	D37.09	D49.0
overlapping lesions	C05.8	—	—	—	—	—
soft	C05.1	C79.89	D00.04	D10.39	D37.09	D49.0
nasopharyngeal surface	C11.3	C79.89	D00.08	D10.6	D37.05	D49.0
posterior surface	C11.3	C79.89	D00.08	D10.6	D37.05	D49.0
superior surface	C11.3	C79.89	D00.08	D10.6	D37.05	D49.0
palatoglossal arch	C09.1	C79.89	D00.00	D10.5	D37.09	D49.0
palatopharyngeal arch	C09.1	C79.89	D00.00	D10.5	D37.09	D49.0
pallium	C71.0	C79.31	—	D33.0	D43.0	D49.6
palpebra	C44.10-	C79.2	D04.1-	D23.1-	D48.5	D49.2
basal cell carcinoma	C44.11-	—	—	—	—	—
specified type NEC	C44.19-	—	—	—	—	—
squamous cell carcinoma	C44.12-	—	—	—	—	—
pancreas	C25.9	C78.89	D01.7	D13.6	D37.8	D49.0
body	C25.1	C78.89	D01.7	D13.6	D37.8	D49.0
duct (of Santorini) (of Wirsung)	C25.3	C78.89	D01.7	D13.6	D37.8	D49.0
ectopic tissue	C25.7	C78.89	—	D13.6	D37.8	D49.0
head	C25.0	C78.89	D01.7	D13.6	D37.8	D49.0
islet cells	C25.4	C78.89	D01.7	D13.7	D37.8	D49.0
neck	C25.7	C78.89	D01.7	D13.6	D37.8	D49.0
overlapping lesion	C25.8	—	—	—	—	—
tail	C25.2	C78.89	D01.7	D13.6	D37.8	D49.0

◀ New   ◀▥ Revised   ~~deleted~~ Deleted

	Malignant Primary	Malignant Secondary	Ca in situ	Benign	Uncertain Behavior	Unspecified Behavior
para-aortic body	C75.5	C79.89	—	D35.6	D44.7	D49.7
paraganglion NEC	C75.5	C79.89	—	D35.6	D44.7	D49.7
parametrium	C57.3	C79.82	—	D28.2	D39.8	D49.5
paranephric	C48.0	C78.6	—	D20.0	D48.3	D49.0
pararectal	C76.3	C79.89	—	D36.7	D48.7	D49.89
parasagittal (region)	C76.0	C79.89	D09.8	D36.7	D48.7	D49.89
parasellar	C72.9	C79.49	—	D33.9	D43.8	D49.7
parathyroid (gland)	C75.0	C79.89	D09.3	D35.1	D44.2	D49.7
paraurethral	C76.3	C79.89	—	D36.7	D48.7	D49.89
gland	C68.1	C79.19	D09.19	D30.8	D41.8	D49.5
paravaginal	C76.3	C79.89	—	D36.7	D48.7	D49.89
parenchyma, kidney	C64.-	C79.0-	D09.19	D30.0-	D41.0-	D49.5
parietal						
bone	C41.0	C79.51	—	D16.4-	D48.0	D49.2
lobe, brain	C71.3	C79.31	—	D33.0	D43.0	D49.6
paroophoron	C57.1	C79.82	D07.39	D28.2	D39.8	D49.5
parotid (duct) (gland)	C07	C79.89	D00.00	D11.0	D37.030	D49.0
parovarium	C57.1	C79.82	D07.39	D28.2	D39.8	D49.5
patella	C40.20	C79.51	—	—	—	—
peduncle, cerebral	C71.7	C79.31	—	D33.1	D43.1	D49.6
pelvirectal junction	C19	C78.5	D01.1	D12.7	D37.5	D49.0
pelvis, pelvic	C76.3	C79.89	D09.8	D36.7	D48.7	D49.89
bone	C41.4	C79.51	—	D16.8	D48.0	D49.2
floor	C76.3	C79.89	D09.8	D36.7	D48.7	D49.89
renal	C65.-	C79.0-	D09.19	D30.1-	D41.1-	D49.5
viscera	C76.3	C79.89	D09.8	D36.7	D48.7	D49.89
wall	C76.3	C79.89	D09.8	D36.7	D48.7	D49.89
pelvo-abdominal	C76.8	C79.89	D09.8	D36.7	D48.7	D49.89
penis	C60.9	C79.82	D07.4	D29.0	D40.8	D49.5
body	C60.2	C79.82	D07.4	D29.0	D40.8	D49.5
corpus (cavernosum)	C60.2	C79.82	D07.4	D29.0	D40.8	D49.5
glans	C60.1	C79.82	D07.4	D29.0	D40.8	D49.5
overlapping sites	C60.8	—	—	—	—	—
skin NEC	C60.9	C79.82	D07.4	D29.0	D40.8	D49.5
periadrenal (tissue)	C48.0	C78.6	—	D20.0	D48.3	D49.0
perianal (skin) — see also Neoplasm, anus, skin	C44.500	C79.2	D04.5	D23.5	D48.5	D49.2
pericardium	C38.0	C79.89	—	D15.1	D48.7	D49.89
perinephric	C48.0	C78.6	—	D20.0	D48.3	D49.0
perineum	C76.3	C79.89	D09.8	D36.7	D48.7	D49.89
periodontal tissue NEC	C03.9	C79.89	D00.03	D10.39	D37.09	D49.0
periosteum — see Neoplasm, bone						
peripancreatic	C48.0	C78.6	—	D20.0	D48.3	D49.0
peripheral nerve NEC	C47.9	C79.89	—	D36.10	D48.2	D49.2
perirectal (tissue)	C76.3	C79.89	—	D36.7	D48.7	D49.89

TABLE OF NEOPLASMS

	Malignant Primary	Malignant Secondary	Ca in situ	Benign	Uncertain Behavior	Unspecified Behavior
perirenal (tissue)	C48.0	C78.6	—	D20.0	D48.3	D49.0
peritoneum, peritoneal (cavity)	C48.2	C78.6	—	D20.1	D48.4	D49.0
benign mesothelial tissue — see Mesothelioma, benign						
overlapping lesion	C48.8	—	—	—	—	—
with digestive organs	C26.9	—	—	—	—	—
parietal	C48.1	C78.6	—	D20.1	D48.4	D49.0
pelvic	C48.1	C78.6	—	D20.1	D48.4	D49.0
specified part NEC	C48.1	C78.6	—	D20.1	D48.4	D49.0
peritonsillar (tissue)	C76.0	C79.89	D09.8	D36.7	D48.7	D49.89
periurethral tissue	C76.3	C79.89	—	D36.7	D48.7	D49.89
phalanges						
foot	C40.3-	C79.51	—	D16.3-	—	—
hand	C40.1-	C79.51	—	D16.1-	—	—
pharynx, pharyngeal	C14.0	C79.89	D00.08	D10.9	D37.05	D49.0
bursa	C11.1	C79.89	D00.08	D10.6	D37.05	D49.0
fornix	C11.3	C79.89	D00.08	D10.6	D37.05	D49.0
recess	C11.2	C79.89	D00.08	D10.6	D37.05	D49.0
region	C14.0	C79.89	D00.08	D10.9	D37.05	D49.0
tonsil	C11.1	C79.89	D00.08	D10.6	D37.05	D49.0
wall (lateral) (posterior)	C14.0	C79.89	D00.08	D10.9	D37.05	D49.0
pia mater	C70.9	C79.40	—	D32.9	D42.9	D49.7
cerebral	C70.0	C79.32	—	D32.0	D42.0	D49.7
cranial	C70.0	C79.32	—	D32.0	D42.0	D49.7
spinal	C70.1	C79.49	—	D32.1	D42.1	D49.7
pillars of fauces	C09.1	C79.89	D00.08	D10.5	D37.05	D49.0
pineal (body) (gland)	C75.3	C79.89	D09.3	D35.4	D44.5	D49.7
pinna (ear) NEC — see also Neoplasm, skin, ear	C44.20-	C79.2	D04.2-	D23.2-	D48.5	D49.2
piriform fossa or sinus	C12	C79.89	D00.08	D10.7	D37.05	D49.0
pituitary (body) (fossa) (gland) (lobe)	C75.1	C79.89	D09.3	D35.2	D44.3	D49.7
placenta	C58	C79.82	D07.0	D26.7	D39.2	D49.5
pleura, pleural (cavity)	C38.4	C78.2	—	D19.0	D38.2	D49.1
overlapping lesion with heart or mediastinum	C38.8	—	—	—	—	—
parietal	C38.4	C78.2	—	D19.0	D38.2	D49.1
visceral	C38.4	C78.2	—	D19.0	D38.2	D49.1
plexus						
brachial	C47.1-	C79.89	—	D36.12	D48.2	D49.2
cervical	C47.0	C79.89	—	D36.11	D48.2	D49.2
choroid	C71.5	C79.31	—	D33.0	D43.0	D49.6
lumbosacral	C47.5	C79.89	—	D36.16	D48.2	D49.2
sacral	C47.5	C79.89	—	D36.16	D48.2	D49.2
pluriendocrine	C75.8	C79.89	D09.3	D35.7	D44.9	D49.7
pole						
frontal	C71.1	C79.31	—	D33.0	D43.0	D49.6
occipital	C71.4	C79.31	—	D33.0	D43.0	D49.6

◀ New ◀▥ Revised ~~deleted~~ Deleted

	Malignant Primary	Malignant Secondary	Ca in situ	Benign	Uncertain Behavior	Unspecified Behavior
pons (varolii)	C71.7	C79.31	—	D33.1	D43.1	D49.6
popliteal fossa or space	C76.5-	C79.89	D04.7-	D36.7	D48.7	D49.89
postcricoid (region)	C13.0	C79.89	D00.08	D10.7	D37.05	D49.0
posterior fossa (cranial)	C71.9	C79.31	—	D33.2	D43.2	D49.6
postnasal space	C11.9	C79.89	D00.08	D10.6	D37.05	D49.0
prepuce	C60.0	C79.82	D07.4	D29.0	D40.8	D49.5
prepylorus	C16.4	C78.89	D00.2	D13.1	D37.1	D49.0
presacral (region)	C76.3	C79.89	—	D36.7	D48.7	D49.89
prostate (gland)	C61	C79.82	D07.5	D29.1	D40.0	D49.5
utricle	C68.0	C79.19	D09.19	D30.4	D41.3	D49.5
pterygoid fossa	C49.0	C79.89	—	D21.0	D48.1	D49.2
pubic bone	C41.4	C79.51	—	D16.8	D48.0	D49.2
pudenda, pudendum (female)	C51.9	C79.82	D07.1	D28.0	D39.8	D49.5
pulmonary — *see also Neoplasm, lung*	C34.9-	C78.0-	D02.2-	D14.3-	D38.1	D49.1
putamen	C71.0	C79.31	—	D33.0	D43.0	D49.6
pyloric						
antrum	C16.3	C78.89	D00.2	D13.1	D37.1	D49.0
canal	C16.4	C78.89	D00.2	D13.1	D37.1	D49.0
pylorus	C16.4	C78.89	D00.2	D13.1	D37.1	D49.0
pyramid (brain)	C71.7	C79.31	—	D33.1	D43.1	D49.6
pyriform fossa or sinus	C12	C79.89	D00.08	D10.7	D37.05	D49.0
radius (any part)	C40.0-	C79.51	—	D16.0-	—	—
Rathke's pouch	C75.1	C79.89	D09.3	D35.2	D44.3	D49.7
rectosigmoid (junction)	C19	C78.5	D01.1	D12.7	D37.5	D49.0
overlapping lesion with anus or rectum	C21.8	—	—	—	—	—
rectouterine pouch	C48.1	C78.6	—	D20.1	D48.4	D49.0
rectovaginal septum or wall	C76.3	C79.89	D09.8	D36.7	D48.7	D49.89
rectovesical septum	C76.3	C79.89	D09.8	D36.7	D48.7	D49.89
rectum (ampulla)	C20	C78.5	D01.2	D12.8	D37.5	D49.0
and colon	C19	C78.5	D01.1	D12.7	D37.5	D49.0
overlapping lesion with anus or rectosigmoid junction	C21.8	—	—	—	—	—
renal	C64.-	C79.0-	D09.19	D30.0-	D41.0-	D49.5
calyx	C65.-	C79.0-	D09.19	D30.1-	D41.1-	D49.5
hilus	C65.-	C79.0-	D09.19	D30.1-	D41.1-	D49.5
parenchyma	C64.-	C79.0-	D09.19	D30.0-	D41.0-	D49.5
pelvis	C65.-	C79.0-	D09.19	D30.1-	D41.1-	D49.5
respiratory						
organs or system NEC	C39.9	C78.30	D02.4	D14.4	D38.6	D49.1
tract NEC	C39.9	C78.30	D02.4	D14.4	D38.5	D49.1
upper	C39.0	C78.30	D02.4	D14.4	D38.5	D49.1
retina	C69.2-	C79.49	D09.2-	D31.2-	D48.7	D49.81
retrobulbar	C69.6-	C79.49	—	D31.6-	D48.7	D49.89
retrocecal	C48.0	C78.6	—	D20.0	D48.3	D49.0
retromolar (area) (triangle) (trigone)	C06.2	C79.89	D00.00	D10.39	D37.09	D49.0

TABLE OF NEOPLASMS

	Malignant Primary	Malignant Secondary	Ca in situ	Benign	Uncertain Behavior	Unspecified Behavior
retro-orbital	C76.0	C79.89	D09.8	D36.7	D48.7	D49.89
retroperitoneal (space) (tissue)	C48.0	C78.6	—	D20.0	D48.3	D49.0
retroperitoneum	C48.0	C78.6	—	D20.0	D48.3	D49.0
retropharyngeal	C14.0	C79.89	D00.08	D10.9	D37.05	D49.0
retrovesical (septum)	C76.3	C79.89	D09.8	D36.7	D48.7	D49.89
rhinencephalon	C71.0	C79.31	—	D33.0	D43.0	D49.6
rib	C41.3	C79.51	—	D16.7	D48.0	D49.2
Rosenmuller's fossa	C11.2	C79.89	D00.08	D10.6	D37.05	D49.0
round ligament	C57.2	C79.82	—	D28.2	D39.8	D49.5
sacrococcyx, sacrococcygeal	C41.4	C79.51	—	D16.8	D48.0	D49.2
region	C76.3	C79.89	D09.8	D36.7	D48.7	D49.89
sacrouterine ligament	C57.3	C79.82	—	D28.2	D39.8	D49.5
sacrum, sacral (vertebra)	C41.4	C79.51	—	D16.8	D48.0	D49.2
salivary gland or duct (major)	C08.9	C79.89	D00.00	D11.9	D37.039	D49.0
minor NEC	C06.9	C79.89	D00.00	D10.39	D37.04	D49.0
overlapping lesion	C08.9	—	—	—	—	—
parotid	C07	C79.89	D00.00	D11.0	D37.030	D49.0
pluriglandular	C08.9	C79.89	D00.00	D11.9	D37.039	D49.0
sublingual	C08.1	C79.89	D00.00	D11.7	D37.031	D49.0
submandibular	C08.0	C79.89	D00.00	D11.7	D37.032	D49.0
submaxillary	C08.0	C79.89	D00.00	D11.7	D37.032	D49.0
salpinx (uterine)	C57.0-	C79.82	D07.39	D28.2	D39.8	D49.5
Santorini's duct	C25.3	C78.89	D01.7	D13.6	D37.8	D49.0
scalp	C44.40	C79.2	D04.4	D23.4	D48.5	D49.2
basal cell carcinoma	C44.41	—	—	—	—	—
specified type NEC	C44.49	—	—	—	—	—
squamous cell carcinoma	C44.42	—	—	—	—	—
scapula (any part)	C40.0-	C79.51	—	D16.0-	—	—
scapular region	C76.1	C79.89	D09.8	D36.7	D48.7	D49.89
scar NEC — see also Neoplasm, skin, by site	C44.90	C79.2	D04.9	D23.9	D48.5	D49.2
sciatic nerve	C47.2-	C79.89	—	D36.13	D48.2	D49.2
sclera	C69.4-	C79.49	D09.2-	D31.4-	D48.7	D49.89
scrotum (skin)	C63.2	C79.82	D07.61	D29.4	D40.8	D49.5
sebaceous gland — see Neoplasm, skin						
sella turcica	C75.1	C79.89	D09.3	D35.2	D44.3	D49.7
bone	C41.0	C79.51	—	D16.4-	D48.0	D49.2
semilunar cartilage (knee)	C40.2-	C79.51	—	D16.2-	D48.0	D49.2
seminal vesicle	C63.7	C79.82	D07.69	D29.8	D40.8	D49.5
septum						
nasal	C30.0	C78.39	D02.3	D14.0	D38.5	D49.1
posterior margin	C11.3	C79.89	D00.08	D10.6	D37.05	D49.0
rectovaginal	C76.3	C79.89	D09.8	D36.7	D48.7	D49.89
rectovesical	C76.3	C79.89	D09.8	D36.7	D48.7	D49.89

◀ New　◀▥ Revised　~~deleted~~ Deleted

	Malignant Primary	Malignant Secondary	Ca in situ	Benign	Uncertain Behavior	Unspecified Behavior
septum *(Continued)*						
urethrovaginal	C57.9	C79.82	D07.30	D28.9	D39.9	D49.5
vesicovaginal	C57.9	C79.82	D07.30	D28.9	D39.9	D49.5
shoulder NEC	C76.4-	C79.89	D04.6-	D36.7	D48.7	D49.89
sigmoid flexure (lower) (upper)	C18.7	C78.5	D01.0	D12.5	D37.4	D49.0
sinus (accessory)	C31.9	C78.39	D02.3	D14.0	D38.5	D49.1
bone (any)	C41.0	C79.51	—	D16.4-	D48.0	D49.2
ethmoidal	C31.1	C78.39	D02.3	D14.0	D38.5	D49.1
frontal	C31.2	C78.39	D02.3	D14.0	D38.5	D49.1
maxillary	C31.0	C78.39	D02.3	D14.0	D38.5	D49.1
nasal, paranasal NEC	C31.9	C78.39	D02.3	D14.0	D38.5	D49.1
overlapping lesion	C31.8	—	—	—	—	—
pyriform	C12	C79.89	D00.08	D10.7	D37.05	D49.0
sphenoid	C31.3	C78.39	D02.3	D14.0	D38.5	D49.1
skeleton, skeletal NEC	C41.9	C79.51	—	D16.9-	D48.0	D49.2
Skene's gland	C68.1	C79.19	D09.19	D30.8	D41.8	D49.5
skin NOS	C44.90	C79.2	D04.9	D23.9	D48.5	D49.2
abdominal wall	C44.509	C79.2	D04.5	D23.5	D48.5	D49.2
basal cell carcinoma	C44.519	—	—	—	—	—
specified type NEC	C44.599	—	—	—	—	—
squamous cell carcinoma	C44.529	—	—	—	—	—
ala nasi — *see also Neoplasm, nose, skin*	C44.301	C79.2	D04.39	D23.39	D48.5	D49.2
ankle — *see also Neoplasm, skin, limb, lower*	C44.70-	C79.2	D04.7-	D23.7-	D48.5	D49.2
antecubital space — *see also Neoplasm, skin, limb, upper*	C44.60-	C79.2	D04.6-	D23.6-	D48.5	D49.2
anus	C44.500	C79.2	D04.5	D23.5	D48.5	D49.2
basal cell carcinoma	C44.510	—	—	—	—	—
specified type NEC	C44.590	—	—	—	—	—
squamous cell carcinoma	C44.520	—	—	—	—	—
arm — *see also Neoplasm, skin, limb, upper*	C44.60-	C79.2	D04.6-	D23.6-	D48.5	D49.2
auditory canal (external) — *see also Neoplasm, skin, ear*	C44.20-	C79.2	D04.2-	D23.2-	D48.5	D49.2
auricle (ear) — *see also Neoplasm, skin, ear*	C44.20-	C79.2	D04.2-	D23.2-	D48.5	D49.2
auricular canal (external) — *see also Neoplasm, skin, ear*	C44.20-	C79.2	D04.2-	D23.2-	D48.5	D49.2
axilla, axillary fold — *see also Neoplasm, skin, trunk*	C44.509	C79.2	D04.5	D23.5	D48.5	D49.2
back — *see also Neoplasm, skin, trunk*	C44.509	C79.2	D04.5	D23.5	D48.5	D49.2
basal cell carcinoma	C44.91					
breast	C44.501	C79.2	D04.5	D23.5	D48.5	D49.2
basal cell carcinoma	C44.511	—	—	—	—	—
specified type NEC	C44.591	—	—	—	—	—
squamous cell carcinoma	C44.521	—	—	—	—	—
brow — *see also Neoplasm, skin, face*	C44.309	C79.2	D04.39	D23.39	D48.5	D49.2
buttock — *see also Neoplasm, skin, trunk*	C44.509	C79.2	D04.5	D23.5	D48.5	D49.2
calf — *see also Neoplasm, skin, limb, lower*	C44.70-	C79.2	D04.7-	D23.7-	D48.5	D49.2

	Malignant Primary	Malignant Secondary	Ca in situ	Benign	Uncertain Behavior	Unspecified Behavior
skin NOS *(Continued)*						
canthus (eye) (inner) (outer)	C44.10-	C79.2	D04.1-	D23.1-	D48.5	D49.2
basal cell carcinoma	C44.11-	—	—	—	—	—
specified type NEC	C44.19-	—	—	—	—	—
squamous cell carcinoma	C44.12-	—	—	—	—	—
cervical region — *see also Neoplasm, skin, neck*	C44.40	C79.2	D04.4	D23.4	D48.5	D49.2
cheek (external) — *see also Neoplasm, skin, face*	C44.309	C79.2	D04.39	D23.39	D48.5	D49.2
chest (wall) — *see also Neoplasm, skin, trunk*	C44.509	C79.2	D04.5	D23.5	D48.5	D49.2
chin — *see also Neoplasm, skin, face*	C44.309	C79.2	D04.39	D23.39	D48.5	D49.2
clavicular area — *see also Neoplasm, skin, trunk*	C44.509	C79.2	D04.5	D23.5	D48.5	D49.2
clitoris	C51.2	C79.82	D07.1	D28.0	D39.8	D49.5
columnella — *see also Neoplasm, skin, face*	C44.309	C79.2	D04.39	D23.39	D48.5	D49.2
concha — *see also Neoplasm, skin, ear*	C44.20-	C79.2	D04.2-	D23.2-	D48.5	D49.2
ear (external)	C44.20-	C79.2	D04.2-	D23.2-	D48.5	D49.2
basal cell carcinoma	C44.21-	—	—	—	—	—
specified type NEC	C44.29-	—	—	—	—	—
squamous cell carcinoma	C44.22-	—	—	—	—	—
elbow — *see also Neoplasm, skin, limb, upper*	C44.60-	C79.2	D04.6-	D23.6-	D48.5	D49.2
eyebrow — *see also Neoplasm, skin, face*	C44.309	C79.2	D04.39	D23.39	D48.5	D49.2
eyelid	C44.10-	C79.2	D04.1-	D23.1-	D48.5	D49.2
basal cell carcinoma	C44.11-	—	—	—	—	—
specified type NEC	C44.19-	—	—	—	—	—
squamous cell carcinoma	C44.12-	—	—	—	—	—
face NOS	C44.300	C79.2	D04.30	D23.30	D48.5	D49.2
basal cell carcinoma	C44.310	—	—	—	—	—
specified type NEC	C44.390	—	—	—	—	—
squamous cell carcinoma	C44.320	—	—	—	—	—
female genital organs (external)	C51.9	C79.82	D07.1	D28.0	D39.8	D49.5
clitoris	C51.2	C79.82	D07.1	D28.0	D39.8	D49.5
labium NEC	C51.9	C79.82	D07.1	D28.0	D39.8	D49.5
majus	C51.0	C79.82	D07.1	D28.0	D39.8	D49.5
minus	C51.1	C79.82	D07.1	D28.0	D39.8	D49.5
pudendum	C51.9	C79.82	D07.1	D28.0	D39.8	D49.5
vulva	C51.9	C79.82	D07.1	D28.0	D39.8	D49.5
finger — *see also Neoplasm, skin, limb, upper*	C44.60-	C79.2	D04.6-	D23.6-	D48.5	D49.2
flank — *see also Neoplasm, skin, trunk*	C44.509	C79.2	D04.5	D23.5	D48.5	D49.2
foot — *see also Neoplasm, skin, limb, lower*	C44.70-	C79.2	D04.7-	D23.7-	D48.5	D49.2
forearm — *see also Neoplasm, skin, limb, upper*	C44.60-	C79.2	D04.6-	D23.6-	D48.5	D49.2
forehead — *see also Neoplasm, skin, face*	C44.309	C79.2	D04.39	D23.39	D48.5	D49.2
glabella — *see also Neoplasm, skin, face*	C44.309	C79.2	D04.39	D23.39	D48.5	D49.2
gluteal region — *see also Neoplasm, skin, trunk*	C44.509	C79.2	D04.5	D23.5	D48.5	D49.2
groin — *see also Neoplasm, skin, trunk*	C44.509	C79.2	D04.5	D23.5	D48.5	D49.2
hand — *see also Neoplasm, skin, limb, upper*	C44.60-	C79.2	D04.6-	D23.6-	D48.5	D49.2

◀ New   ⇐ Revised   ~~deleted~~ Deleted

	Malignant Primary	Malignant Secondary	Ca in situ	Benign	Uncertain Behavior	Unspecified Behavior
skin NOS *(Continued)*						
head NEC — *see also Neoplasm, skin, scalp*	C44.40	C79.2	D04.4	D23.4	D48.5	D49.2
heel — *see also Neoplasm, skin, limb, lower*	C44.70-	C79.2	D04.7-	D23.7-	D48.5	D49.2
helix — *see also Neoplasm, skin, ear*	C44.20-	C79.2	D04.2-	D23.2-	D48.5	D49.2
hip — *see also Neoplasm, skin, limb, lower*	C44.70-	C79.2	D04.7-	D23.7-	D48.5	D49.2
infraclavicular region — *see also Neoplasm, skin, trunk*	C44.509	C79.2	D04.5	D23.5	D48.5	D49.2
inguinal region — *see also Neoplasm, skin, trunk*	C44.509	C79.2	D04.5	D23.5	D48.5	D49.2
jaw — *see also Neoplasm, skin, face*	C44.309	C79.2	D04.39	D23.39	D48.5	D49.2
Kaposi's sarcoma — *see Kaposi's, sarcoma, skin*						
knee — *see also Neoplasm, skin, limb, lower*	C44.70-	C79.2	D04.7-	D23.7-	D48.5	D49.2
labia						
majora	C51.0	C79.82	D07.1	D28.0	D39.8	D49.5
minora	C51.1	C79.82	D07.1	D28.0	D39.8	D49.5
leg — *see also Neoplasm, skin, limb, lower*	C44.70-	C79.2	D04.7-	D23.7-	D48.5	D49.2
lid (lower) (upper)	C44.10-	C79.2	D04.1-	D23.1-	D48.5	D49.2
basal cell carcinoma	C44.11-	—	—	—	—	—
specified type NEC	C44.19-	—	—	—	—	—
squamous cell carcinoma	C44.12-	—	—	—	—	—
limb NEC	C44.90	C79.2	D04.9	D23.9	D48.5	D49.2
basal cell carcinoma	C44.91					
lower	C44.70-	C79.2	D04.7-	D23.7-	D48.5	D49.2
basal cell carcinoma	C44.71-	—	—	—	—	—
specified type NEC	C44.79-	—	—	—	—	—
squamous cell carcinoma	C44.72-	—	—	—	—	—
upper	C44.60-	C79.2	D04.6-	D23.6-	D48.5	D49.2
basal cell carcinoma	C44.61-	—	—	—	—	—
specified type NEC	C44.69-	—	—	—	—	—
squamous cell carcinoma	C44.62-	—	—	—	—	—
lip (lower) (upper)	C44.00	C79.2	D04.0	D23.0	D48.5	D49.2
basal cell carcinoma	C44.01	—	—	—	—	—
specified type NEC	C44.09	—	—	—	—	—
squamous cell carcinoma	C44.02	—	—	—	—	—
male genital organs	C63.9	C79.82	D07.60	D29.9	D40.8	D49.5
penis	C60.9	C79.82	D07.4	D29.0	D40.8	D49.5
prepuce	C60.0	C79.82	D07.4	D29.0	D40.8	D49.5
scrotum	C63.2	C79.82	D07.61	D29.4	D40.8	D49.5
mastectomy site (skin) — *see also Neoplasm, skin, breast*	C44.501	C79.2	—	—	—	—
specified as breast tissue	C50.8-	C79.81	—	—	—	—
meatus, acoustic (external) — *see also Neoplasm, skin, ear*	C44.20-	C79.2	D04.2-	D23.2-	D48.5	D49.2
melanotic — *see Melanoma*						
Merkel cell — *see Carcinoma, Merkel cell*						
nates — *see also Neoplasm, skin, trunk*	C44.509	C79.2	D04.5	D23.5	D48.5	D49.2

	Malignant Primary	Malignant Secondary	Ca in situ	Benign	Uncertain Behavior	Unspecified Behavior
skin NOS *(Continued)*						
neck	C44.40	C79.2	D04.4	D23.4	D48.5	D49.2
basal cell carcinoma	C44.41	—	—	—	—	—
specified type NEC	C44.49	—	—	—	—	—
squamous cell carcinoma	C44.42	—	—	—	—	—
nevus — *see Nevus, skin*						
nose (external) — *see also Neoplasm, nose, skin*	C44.301	C79.2	D04.39	D23.39	D48.5	D49.2
overlapping lesion	C44.80	—	—	—	—	—
basal cell carcinoma	C44.81	—	—	—	—	—
specified type NEC	C44.89	—	—	—	—	—
squamous cell carcinoma	C44.82	—	—	—	—	—
palm — *see also Neoplasm, skin, limb, upper*	C44.60-	C79.2	D04.6-	D23.6-	D48.5	D49.2
palpebra	C44.10-	C79.2	D04.1-	D23.1-	D48.5	D49.2
basal cell carcinoma	C44.11-	—	—	—	—	—
specified type NEC	C44.19-	—	—	—	—	—
squamous cell carcinoma	C44.12-	—	—	—	—	—
penis NEC	C60.9	C79.82	D07.4	D29.0	D40.8	D49.5
perianal — *see also Neoplasm, skin, anus*	C44.500	C79.2	D04.5	D23.5	D48.5	D49.2
perineum — *see also Neoplasm, skin, anus*	C44.500	C79.2	D04.5	D23.5	D48.5	D49.2
pinna — *see also Neoplasm, skin, ear*	C44.20-	C79.2	D04.2-	D23.2-	D48.5	D49.2
plantar — *see also Neoplasm, skin, limb, lower*	C44.70-	C79.2	D04.7-	D23.7-	D48.5	D49.2
popliteal fossa or space — *see also Neoplasm, skin, limb, lower*	C44.70-	C79.2	D04.7-	D23.7-	D48.5	D49.2
prepuce	C60.0	C79.82	D07.4	D29.0	D40.8	D49.5
pubes — *see also Neoplasm, skin, trunk*	C44.509	C79.2	D04.5	D23.5	D48.5	D49.2
sacrococcygeal region — *see also Neoplasm, skin, trunk*	C44.509	C79.2	D04.5	D23.5	D48.5	D49.2
scalp	C44.40	C79.2	D04.4	D23.4	D48.5	D49.2
basal cell carcinoma	C44.41	—	—	—	—	—
specified type NEC	C44.49	—	—	—	—	—
squamous cell carcinoma	C44.42	—	—	—	—	—
scapular region — *see also Neoplasm, skin, trunk*	C44.509	C79.2	D04.5	D23.5	D48.5	D49.2
scrotum	C63.2	C79.82	D07.61	D29.4	D40.8	D49.5
shoulder — *see also Neoplasm, skin, limb, upper*	C44.60-	C79.2	D04.6-	D23.6-	D48.5	D49.2
sole (foot) — *see also Neoplasm, skin, limb, lower*	C44.70-	C79.2	D04.7-	D23.7-	D48.5	D49.2
specified sites NEC	C44.80	C79.2	D04.8	D23.9	D48.5	D49.2
basal cell carcinoma	C44.81	—	—	—	—	—
specified type NEC	C44.89	—	—	—	—	—
squamous cell carcinoma	C44.82	—	—	—	—	—
specified type NEC	C44.99					
squamous cell carcinoma	C44.92	—	—	—	—	—
submammary fold — *see also Neoplasm, skin, trunk*	C44.509	C79.2	D04.5	D23.5	D48.5	D49.2
supraclavicular region — *see also Neoplasm, skin, neck*	C44.40	C79.2	D04.4	D23.4	D48.5	D49.2
temple — *see also Neoplasm, skin, face*	C44.309	C79.2	D04.39	D23.39	D48.5	D49.2
thigh — *see also Neoplasm, skin, limb, lower*	C44.70-	C79.2	D04.7-	D23.7-	D48.5	D49.2
thoracic wall — *see also Neoplasm, skin, trunk*	C44.509	C79.2	D04.5	D23.5	D48.5	D49.2

◀ New   ◀▬ Revised   ~~deleted~~ Deleted

	Malignant Primary	Malignant Secondary	Ca in situ	Benign	Uncertain Behavior	Unspecified Behavior
skin NOS *(Continued)*						
thumb — *see also Neoplasm, skin, limb, upper*	C44.60-	C79.2	D04.6-	D23.6-	D48.5	D49.2
toe — *see also Neoplasm, skin, limb, lower*	C44.70-	C79.2	D04.7-	D23.7-	D48.5	D49.2
tragus — *see also Neoplasm, skin, ear*	C44.20-	C79.2	D04.2-	D23.2-	D48.5	D49.2
trunk	C44.509	C79.2	D04.5	D23.5	D48.5	D49.2
basal cell carcinoma	C44.519	—	—	—	—	—
specified type NEC	C44.599	—	—	—	—	—
squamous cell carcinoma	C44.529	—	—	—	—	—
umbilicus — *see also Neoplasm, skin, trunk*	C44.509	C79.2	D04.5	D23.5	D48.5	D49.2
vulva	C51.9	C79.82	D07.1	D28.0	D39.8	D49.5
overlapping lesion	C51.8	—	—	—	—	—
wrist — *see also Neoplasm, skin, limb, upper*	C44.60-	C79.2	D04.6-	D23.6-	D48.5	D49.2
skull	C41.0	C79.51	—	D16.4-	D48.0	D49.2
soft parts or tissues — *see Neoplasm, connective tissue*						
specified site NEC	C76.8	C79.89	D09.8	D36.7	D48.7	D49.89
spermatic cord	C63.1-	C79.82	D07.69	D29.8	D40.8	D49.5
sphenoid	C31.3	C78.39	D02.3	D14.0	D38.5	D49.1
bone	C41.0	C79.51	—	D16.4-	D48.0	D49.2
sinus	C31.3	C78.39	D02.3	D14.0	D38.5	D49.1
sphincter						
anal	C21.1	C78.5	D01.3	D12.9	D37.8	D49.0
of Oddi	C24.0	C78.89	D01.5	D13.5	D37.6	D49.0
spine, spinal (column)	C41.2	C79.51	—	D16.6	D48.0	D49.2
bulb	C71.7	C79.31	—	D33.1	D43.1	D49.6
coccyx	C41.4	C79.51	—	D16.8	D48.0	D49.2
cord (cervical) (lumbar) (sacral) (thoracic)	C72.0	C79.49	—	D33.4	D43.4	D49.7
dura mater	C70.1	C79.49	—	D32.1	D42.1	D49.7
lumbosacral	C41.2	C79.51	—	D16.6	D48.0	D49.2
marrow NEC	C96.9	C79.52	—	—	D47.9	D49.89
membrane	C70.1	C79.49	—	D32.1	D42.1	D49.7
meninges	C70.1	C79.49	—	D32.1	D42.1	D49.7
nerve (root)	C47.9	C79.89	—	D36.10	D48.2	D49.2
pia mater	C70.1	C79.49	—	D32.1	D42.1	D49.7
root	C47.9	C79.89	—	D36.10	D48.2	D49.2
sacrum	C41.4	C79.51	—	D16.8	D48.0	D49.2
spleen, splenic NEC	C26.1	C78.89	D01.7	D13.9	D37.8	D49.0
flexure (colon)	C18.5	C78.5	D01.0	D12.3	D37.4	D49.0
stem, brain	C71.7	C79.31	—	D33.1	D43.1	D49.6
Stensen's duct	C07	C79.89	D00.00	D11.0	D37.030	D49.0
sternum	C41.3	C79.51	—	D16.7	D48.0	D49.2
stomach	C16.9	C78.89	D00.2	D13.1	D37.1	D49.0
antrum (pyloric)	C16.3	C78.89	D00.2	D13.1	D37.1	D49.0
body	C16.2	C78.89	D00.2	D13.1	D37.1	D49.0
cardia	C16.0	C78.89	D00.2	D13.1	D37.1	D49.0

	Malignant Primary	Malignant Secondary	Ca in situ	Benign	Uncertain Behavior	Unspecified Behavior
stomach *(Continued)*						
cardiac orifice	C16.0	C78.89	D00.2	D13.1	D37.1	D49.0
corpus	C16.2	C78.89	D00.2	D13.1	D37.1	D49.0
fundus	C16.1	C78.89	D00.2	D13.1	D37.1	D49.0
greater curvature NEC	C16.6	C78.89	D00.2	D13.1	D37.1	D49.0
lesser curvature NEC	C16.5	C78.89	D00.2	D13.1	D37.1	D49.0
overlapping lesion	C16.8	—	—	—	—	—
prepylorus	C16.4	C78.89	D00.2	D13.1	D37.1	D49.0
pylorus	C16.4	C78.89	D00.2	D13.1	D37.1	D49.0
wall NEC	C16.9	C78.89	D00.2	D13.1	D37.1	D49.0
anterior NEC	C16.8	C78.89	D00.2	D13.1	D37.1	D49.0
posterior NEC	C16.8	C78.89	D00.2	D13.1	D37.1	D49.0
stroma, endometrial	C54.1	C79.82	D07.0	D26.1	D39.0	D49.5
stump, cervical	C53.8	C79.82	D06.7	D26.0	D39.0	D49.5
subcutaneous (nodule) (tissue) NEC — *see Neoplasm, connective tissue*						
subdural	C70.9	C79.32	—	D32.9	D42.9	D49.7
subglottis, subglottic	C32.2	C78.39	D02.0	D14.1	D38.0	D49.1
sublingual	C04.9	C79.89	D00.06	D10.2	D37.09	D49.0
gland or duct	C08.1	C79.89	D00.00	D11.7	D37.031	D49.0
submandibular gland	C08.0	C79.89	D00.00	D11.7	D37.032	D49.0
submaxillary gland or duct	C08.0	C79.89	D00.00	D11.7	D37.032	D49.0
submental	C76.0	C79.89	D09.8	D36.7	D48.7	D49.89
subpleural	C34.9-	C78.0-	D02.2-	D14.3-	D38.1	D49.1
substernal	C38.1	C78.1	—	D15.2	D38.3	D49.89
sudoriferous, sudoriparous gland, site unspecified	C44.90	C79.2	D04.9	D23.9	D48.5	D49.2
specified site — *see Neoplasm, skin*						
supraclavicular region	C76.0	C79.89	D09.8	D36.7	D48.7	D49.89
supraglottis	C32.1	C78.39	D02.0	D14.1	D38.0	D49.1
suprarenal	C74.9-	C79.7-	D09.3	D35.0-	D44.1-	D49.7
capsule	C74.9-	C79.7-	D09.3	D35.0-	D44.1-	D49.7
cortex	C74.0-	C79.7-	D09.3	D35.0-	D44.1-	D49.7
gland	C74.9-	C79.7-	D09.3	D35.0-	D44.1-	D49.7
medulla	C74.1-	C79.7-	D09.3	D35.0-	D44.1-	D49.7
suprasellar (region)	C71.9	C79.31	—	D33.2	D43.2	D49.6
supratentorial (brain) NEC	C71.0	C79.31	—	D33.0	D43.0	D49.6
sweat gland (apocrine) (eccrine), site unspecified	C44.90	C79.2	D04.9	D23.9	D48.5	D49.2
specified site — *see Neoplasm, skin*						
sympathetic nerve or nervous system NEC	C47.9	C79.89	—	D36.10	D48.2	D49.2
symphysis pubis	C41.4	C79.51	—	D16.8	D48.0	D49.2
synovial membrane — *see Neoplasm, connective tissue*						
tapetum, brain	C71.8	C79.31	—	D33.2	D43.2	D49.6
tarsus (any bone)	C40.3-	C79.51	—	D16.3-	—	—
temple (skin) — *see also Neoplasm, skin, face*	C44.309	C79.2	D04.39	D23.39	D48.5	D49.2

◀ New ◀▥ Revised ~~deleted~~ Deleted

	Malignant Primary	Malignant Secondary	Ca in situ	Benign	Uncertain Behavior	Unspecified Behavior
temporal						
bone	C41.0	C79.51	—	D16.4-	D48.0	D49.2
lobe or pole	C71.2	C79.31	—	D33.0	D43.0	D49.6
region	C76.0	C79.89	D09.8	D36.7	D48.7	D49.89
skin — *see also Neoplasm, skin, face*	C44.309	C79.2	D04.39	D23.39	D48.5	D49.2
tendon (sheath) — *see Neoplasm, connective tissue*						
tentorium (cerebelli)	C70.0	C79.32	—	D32.0	D42.0	D49.7
testis, testes	C62.9-	C79.82	D07.69	D29.2-	D40.1-	D49.5
descended	C62.1-	C79.82	D07.69	D29.2-	D40.1-	D49.5
ectopic	C62.0-	C79.82	D07.69	D29.2-	D40.1-	D49.5
retained	C62.0-	C79.82	D07.69	D29.2-	D40.1-	D49.5
scrotal	C62.1-	C79.82	D07.69	D29.2-	D40.1-	D49.5
undescended	C62.0-	C79.82	D07.69	D29.2-	D40.1-	D49.5
unspecified whether descended or undescended	C62.9-	C79.82	D07.69	D29.2-	D40.1-	D49.5
thalamus	C71.0	C79.31	—	D33.0	D43.0	D49.6
thigh NEC	C76.5-	C79.89	D04.7-	D36.7	D48.7	D49.89
thorax, thoracic (cavity) (organs NEC)	C76.1	C79.89	D09.8	D36.7	D48.7	D49.89
duct	C49.3	C79.89	—	D21.3	D48.1	D49.2
wall NEC	C76.1	C79.89	D09.8	D36.7	D48.7	D49.89
throat	C14.0	C79.89	D00.08	D10.9	D37.05	D49.0
thumb NEC	C76.4-	C79.89	D04.6-	D36.7	D48.7	D49.89
thymus (gland)	C37	C79.89	D09.3	D15.0	D38.4	D49.89
thyroglossal duct	C73	C79.89	D09.3	D34	D44.0	D49.7
thyroid (gland)	C73	C79.89	D09.3	D34	D44.0	D49.7
cartilage	C32.3	C78.39	D02.0	D14.1	D38.0	D49.1
tibia (any part)	C40.2-	C79.51	—	D16.2-	—	—
toe NEC	C76.5-	C79.89	D04.7-	D36.7	D48.7	D49.89
tongue	C02.9	C79.89	D00.07	D10.1	D37.02	D49.0
anterior (two-thirds) NEC	C02.3	C79.89	D00.07	D10.1	D37.02	D49.0
dorsal surface	C02.0	C79.89	D00.07	D10.1	D37.02	D49.0
ventral surface	C02.2	C79.89	D00.07	D10.1	D37.02	D49.0
base (dorsal surface)	C01	C79.89	D00.07	D10.1	D37.02	D49.0
border (lateral)	C02.1	C79.89	D00.07	D10.1	D37.02	D49.0
dorsal surface NEC	C02.0	C79.89	D00.07	D10.1	D37.02	D49.0
fixed part NEC	C01	C79.89	D00.07	D10.1	D37.02	D49.0
foreamen cecum	C02.0	C79.89	D00.07	D10.1	D37.02	D49.0
frenulum linguae	C02.2	C79.89	D00.07	D10.1	D37.02	D49.0
junctional zone	C02.8	C79.89	D00.07	D10.1	D37.02	D49.0
margin (lateral)	C02.1	C79.89	D00.07	D10.1	D37.02	D49.0
midline NEC	C02.0	C79.89	D00.07	D10.1	D37.02	D49.0
mobile part NEC	C02.3	C79.89	D00.07	D10.1	D37.02	D49.0
overlapping lesion	C02.8	—	—	—	—	—
posterior (third)	C01	C79.89	D00.07	D10.1	D37.02	D49.0

◀ New   ◀▥ Revised   ~~deleted~~ Deleted

	Malignant Primary	Malignant Secondary	Ca in situ	Benign	Uncertain Behavior	Unspecified Behavior
tongue *(Continued)*						
root	C01	C79.89	D00.07	D10.1	D37.02	D49.0
surface (dorsal)	C02.0	C79.89	D00.07	D10.1	D37.02	D49.0
base	C01	C79.89	D00.07	D10.1	D37.02	D49.0
ventral	C02.2	C79.89	D00.07	D10.1	D37.02	D49.0
tip	C02.1	C79.89	D00.07	D10.1	D37.02	D49.0
tonsil	C02.4	C79.89	D00.07	D10.1	D37.02	D49.0
tonsil	C09.9	C79.89	D00.08	D10.4	D37.05	D49.0
fauces, faucial	C09.9	C79.89	D00.08	D10.4	D37.05	D49.0
lingual	C02.4	C79.89	D00.07	D10.1	D37.02	D49.0
overlapping sites	C09.8	—	—	—	—	—
palatine	C09.9	C79.89	D00.08	D10.4	D37.05	D49.0
pharyngeal	C11.1	C79.89	D00.08	D10.6	D37.05	D49.0
pillar (anterior) (posterior)	C09.1	C79.89	D00.08	D10.5	D37.05	D49.0
tonsillar fossa	C09.0	C79.89	D00.08	D10.5	D37.05	D49.0
tooth socket NEC	C03.9	C79.89	D00.03	D10.39	D37.09	D49.0
trachea (cartilage) (mucosa)	C33	C78.39	D02.1	D14.2	D38.1	D49.1
overlapping lesion with bronchus or lung	C34.8-	—	—	—	—	—
tracheobronchial	C34.8-	C78.39	D02.1	D14.2	D38.1	D49.1
overlapping lesion with lung	C34.8-	—	—	—	—	—
tragus — *see also Neoplasm, skin, ear*	C44.20-	C79.2	D04.2-	D23.2-	D48.5	D49.2
trunk NEC	C76.8	C79.89	D04.5	D36.7	D48.7	D49.89
tubo-ovarian	C57.8	C79.82	D07.39	D28.7	D39.8	D49.5
tunica vaginalis	C63.7	C79.82	D07.69	D29.8	D40.8	D49.5
turbinate (bone)	C41.0	C79.51	—	D16.4-	D48.0	D49.2
nasal	C30.0	C78.39	D02.3	D14.0	D38.5	D49.1
tympanic cavity	C30.1	C78.39	D02.3	D14.0	D38.5	D49.1
ulna (any part)	C40.0-	C79.51	—	D16.0-	—	—
umbilicus, umbilical — *see also Neoplasm, skin, trunk*	C44.509	C79.2	D04.5	D23.5	D48.5	D49.2
uncus, brain	C71.2	C79.31	—	D33.0	D43.0	D49.6
unknown site or unspecified	C80.1	C79.9	D09.9	D36.9	D48.9	D49.9
urachus	C67.7	C79.11	D09.0	D30.3	D41.4	D49.4
ureter, ureteral	C66.-	C79.19	D09.19	D30.2-	D41.2-	D49.5
orifice (bladder)	C67.6	C79.11	D09.0	D30.3	D41.4	D49.4
ureter-bladder (junction)	C67.6	C79.11	D09.0	D30.3	D41.4	D49.4
urethra, urethral (gland)	C68.0	C79.19	D09.19	D30.4	D41.3	D49.5
orifice, internal	C67.5	C79.11	D09.0	D30.3	D41.4	D49.4
urethrovaginal (septum)	C57.9	C79.82	D07.30	D28.9	D39.8	D49.5
urinary organ or system	C68.9	C79.10	D09.10	D30.9	D41.9	D49.5
bladder — *see Neoplasm, bladder*						
overlapping lesion	C68.8	—	—	—	—	—
specified sites NEC	C68.8	C79.19	D09.19	D30.8	D41.8	D49.5

◀ New ◀ Revised ~~deleted~~ Deleted

	Malignant Primary	Malignant Secondary	Ca in situ	Benign	Uncertain Behavior	Unspecified Behavior
utero-ovarian	C57.8	C79.82	D07.39	D28.7	D39.8	D49.5
ligament	C57.1	C79.82	D07.39	D28.2	D39.8	D49.5
uterosacral ligament	C57.3	C79.82	—	D28.2	D39.8	D49.5
uterus, uteri, uterine	C55	C79.82	D07.0	D26.9	D39.0	D49.5
adnexa NEC	C57.4	C79.82	D07.39	D28.7	D39.8	D49.5
body	C54.9	C79.82	D07.0	D26.1	D39.0	D49.5
cervix	C53.9	C79.82	D06.9	D26.0	D39.0	D49.5
cornu	C54.9	C79.82	D07.0	D26.1	D39.0	D49.5
corpus	C54.9	C79.82	D07.0	D26.1	D39.0	D49.5
endocervix (canal) (gland)	C53.0	C79.82	D06.0	D26.0	D39.0	D49.5
endometrium	C54.1	C79.82	D07.0	D26.1	D39.0	D49.5
exocervix	C53.1	C79.82	D06.1	D26.0	D39.0	D49.5
external os	C53.1	C79.82	D06.1	D26.0	D39.0	D49.5
fundus	C54.3	C79.82	D07.0	D26.1	D39.0	D49.5
internal os	C53.0	C79.82	D06.0	D26.0	D39.0	D49.5
isthmus	C54.0	C79.82	D07.0	D26.1	D39.0	D49.5
ligament	C57.3	C79.82	—	D28.2	D39.8	D49.5
broad	C57.1	C79.82	D07.39	D28.2	D39.8	D49.5
round	C57.2	C79.82	—	D28.2	D39.8	D49.5
lower segment	C54.0	C79.82	D07.0	D26.1	D39.0	D49.5
myometrium	C54.2	C79.82	D07.0	D26.1	D39.0	D49.5
overlapping sites	C54.8	—	—	—	—	—
squamocolumnar junction	C53.8	C79.82	D06.7	D26.0	D39.0	D49.5
tube	C57.0-	C79.82	D07.39	D28.2	D39.8	D49.5
utricle, prostatic	C68.0	C79.19	D09.19	D30.4	D41.3	D49.5
uveal tract	C69.4-	C79.49	D09.2-	D31.4-	D48.7	D49.89
uvula	C05.2	C79.89	D00.04	D10.39	D37.09	D49.0
vagina, vaginal (fornix) (vault) (wall)	C52	C79.82	D07.2	D28.1	D39.8	D49.5
vaginovesical	C57.9	C79.82	D07.30	D28.9	D39.9	D49.5
septum	C57.9	C79.82	D07.30	D28.9	D39.9	D49.5
vallecula (epigiottis)	C10.0	C79.89	D00.08	D10.5	D37.05	D49.0
vas deferens	C63.1-	C79.82	D07.69	D29.8	D40.8	D49.5
vascular — see Neoplasm, connective tissue						
Vater's ampulla	C24.1	C78.89	D01.5	D13.5	D37.6	D49.0
vein, venous — see Neoplasm, connective tissue						
vena cava (abdominal) (inferior)	C49.4	C79.89	—	D21.4	D48.1	D49.2
superior	C49.3	C79.89	—	D21.3	D48.1	D49.2
ventricle (cerebral) (floor) (lateral) (third)	C71.5	C79.31	—	D33.0	D43.0	D49.6
cardiac (left) (right)	C38.0	C79.89	—	D15.1	D48.7	D49.89
fourth	C71.7	C79.31	—	D33.1	D43.1	D49.6
ventricular band of larynx	C32.1	C78.39	D02.0	D14.1	D38.0	D49.1
ventriculus — see Neoplasm, stomach						

TABLE OF NEOPLASMS

	Malignant Primary	Malignant Secondary	Ca in situ	Benign	Uncertain Behavior	Unspecified Behavior
vermillion border — *see Neoplasm, lip*						
vermis, cerebellum	C71.6	C79.31	—	D33.1	D43.1	D49.6
vertebra (column)	C41.2	C79.51	—	D16.6	D48.0	D49.2
coccyx	C41.4	C79.51	—	D16.8-	D48.0	D49.2
marrow NEC	C96.9	C79.52	—	—	D47.9	D49.89
sacrum	C41.4	C79.51	—	D16.8-	D48.0	D49.2
vesical — *see Neoplasm, bladder*						
vesicle, seminal	C63.7	C79.82	D07.69	D29.8	D40.8	D49.5
vesicocervical tissue	C57.9	C79.82	D07.30	D28.9	D39.9	D49.5
vesicorectal	C76.3	C79.82	D09.8	D36.7	D48.7	D49.89
vesicovaginal	C57.9	C79.82	D07.30	D28.9	D39.9	D49.5
septum	C57.9	C79.82	D07.30	D28.9	D39.8	D49.5
vessel (blood) — *see Neoplasm, connective tissue*						
vestibular gland, greater	C51.0	C79.82	D07.1	D28.0	D39.8	D49.5
vestibule						
mouth	C06.1	C79.89	D00.00	D10.39	D37.09	D49.0
nose	C30.0	C78.39	D02.3	D14.0	D38.5	D49.1
Virchow's gland	C77.0	C77.0	—	D36.0	D48.7	D49.89
viscera NEC	C76.8	C79.89	D09.8	D36.7	D48.7	D49.89
vocal cords (true)	C32.0	C78.39	D02.0	D14.1	D38.0	D49.1
false	C32.1	C78.39	D02.0	D14.1	D38.0	D49.1
vomer	C41.0	C79.51	—	D16.4-	D48.0	D49.2
vulva	C51.9	C79.82	D07.1	D28.0	D39.8	D49.5
vulvovaginal gland	C51.0	C79.82	D07.1	D28.0	D39.8	D49.5
Waldeyer's ring	C14.2	C79.89	D00.08	D10.9	D37.05	D49.0
Wharton's duct	C08.0	C79.89	D00.00	D11.7	D37.032	D49.0
white matter (central) (cerebral)	C71.0	C79.31	—	D33.0	D43.0	D49.6
windpipe	C33	C78.39	D02.1	D14.2	D38.1	D49.1
Wirsung's duct	C25.3	C78.89	D01.7	D13.6	D37.8	D49.0
wolffian (body) (duct)						
female	C57.7	C79.82	D07.39	D28.7	D39.8	D49.5
male	C63.7	C79.82	D07.69	D29.8	D40.8	D49.5
womb — *see Neoplasm, uterus*						
wrist NEC	C76.4-	C79.89	D04.6-	D36.7	D48.7	D49.89
xiphoid process	C41.3	C79.51	—	D16.7	D48.0	D49.2
Zuckerkandl organ	C75.5	C79.89	—	D35.6	D44.7	D49.7

◄ New ◄ Revised ~~deleted~~ Deleted

ICD-10-CM
Table of Drugs and Chemicals

ICD-10-CM

Table of Drugs and Chemicals

Substance	External Cause (T-Code)					
	Poisoning, Accidental (Unintentional)	Poisoning, Intentional Self-Harm	Poisoning, Assault	Poisoning, Undetermined	Adverse Effect	Underdosing
#						
1-propanol	T51.3X1	T51.3X2	T51.3X3	T51.3X4	—	—
2-propanol	T51.2X1	T51.2X2	T51.2X3	T51.2X4	—	—
2,4-D (dichlorophen-oxyacetic acid)	T60.3X1	T60.3X2	T60.3X3	T60.3X4	—	—
2,4-toluene diisocyanate	T65.0X1	T65.0X2	T65.0X3	T65.0X4	—	—
2,4,5-T (trichloro-phenoxyacetic acid)	T60.1X1	T60.1X2	T60.1X3	T60.1X4	—	—
14-hydroxydihydro-morphinone	T40.2X1	T40.2X2	T40.2X3	T40.2X4	T40.2X5	T40.2X6
A						
ABOB	T37.5X1	T37.5X2	T37.5X3	T37.5X4	T37.5X5	T37.5X6
Abrine	T62.2X1	T62.2X2	T62.2X3	T62.2X4	—	—
Abrus (seed)	T62.2X1	T62.2X2	T62.2X3	T62.2X4	—	—
Absinthe	T51.0X1	T51.0X2	T51.0X3	T51.0X4	—	—
beverage	T51.0X1	T51.0X2	T51.0X3	T51.0X4	—	—
Acaricide	T60.8X1	T60.8X2	T60.8X3	T60.8X4	—	—
Acebutolol	T44.7X1	T44.7X2	T44.7X3	T44.7X4	T44.7X5	T44.7X6
Acecarbromal	T42.6X1	T42.6X2	T42.6X3	T42.6X4	T42.6X5	T42.6X6
Aceclidine	T44.1X1	T44.1X2	T44.1X3	T44.1X4	T44.1X5	T44.1X6
Acedapsone	T37.0X1	T37.0X2	T37.0X3	T37.0X4	T37.0X5	T37.0X6
Acefylline piperazine	T48.6X1	T48.6X2	T48.6X3	T48.6X4	T48.6X5	T48.6X6
Acemorphan	T40.2X1	T40.2X2	T40.2X3	T40.2X4	T40.2X5	T40.2X6
Acenocoumarin	T45.511	T45.512	T45.513	T45.514	T45.515	T45.516
Acenocoumarol	T45.511	T45.512	T45.513	T45.514	T45.515	T45.516
Acepifylline	T48.6X1	T48.6X2	T48.6X3	T48.6X4	T48.6X5	T48.6X6
Acepromazine	T43.3X1	T43.3X2	T43.3X3	T43.3X4	T43.3X5	T43.3X6
Acesulfamethoxypyridazine	T37.0X1	T37.0X2	T37.0X3	T37.0X4	T37.0X5	T37.0X6
Acetal	T52.8X1	T52.8X2	T52.8X3	T52.8X4	—	—
Acetaldehyde (vapor)	T52.8X1	T52.8X2	T52.8X3	T52.8X4	—	—
liquid	T65.891	T65.892	T65.893	T65.894	—	—
P-Acetamidophenol	T39.1X1	T39.1X2	T39.1X3	T39.1X4	T39.1X5	T39.1X6
Acetaminophen	T39.1X1	T39.1X2	T39.1X3	T39.1X4	T39.1X5	T39.1X6
Acetaminosalol	T39.1X1	T39.1X2	T39.1X3	T39.1X4	T39.1X5	T39.1X6
Acetanilide	T39.1X1	T39.1X2	T39.1X3	T39.1X4	T39.1X5	T39.1X6
Acetarsol	T37.3X1	T37.3X2	T37.3X3	T37.3X4	T37.3X5	T37.3X6
Acetazolamide	T50.2X1	T50.2X2	T50.2X3	T50.2X4	T50.2X5	T50.2X6
Acetiamine	T45.2X1	T45.2X2	T45.2X3	T45.2X4	T45.2X5	T45.2X6
Acetic						
acid	T54.2X1	T54.2X2	T54.2X3	T54.2X4	—	—
with sodium acetate (ointment)	T49.3X1	T49.3X2	T49.3X3	T49.3X4	T49.3X5	T49.3X6
ester (solvent) (vapor)	T52.8X1	T52.8X2	T52.8X3	T52.8X4	—	—

◀ New   ◀▦ Revised   ~~deleted~~ Deleted

TABLE OF DRUGS AND CHEMICALS

Substance	External Cause (T-Code)					
	Poisoning, Accidental (Unintentional)	Poisoning, Intentional Self-Harm	Poisoning, Assault	Poisoning, Undetermined	Adverse Effect	Underdosing
Acetic *(Continued)*						
acid *(Continued)*						
irrigating solution	T50.3X1	T50.3X2	T50.3X3	T50.3X4	T50.3X5	T50.3X6
medicinal (lotion)	T49.2X1	T49.2X2	T49.2X3	T49.2X4	T49.2X5	T49.2X6
anhydride	T65.891	T65.892	T65.893	T65.894	—	—
ether (vapor)	T52.8X1	T52.8X2	T52.8X3	T52.8X4	—	—
Acetohexamide	T38.3X1	T38.3X2	T38.3X3	T38.3X4	T38.3X5	T38.3X6
Acetohydroxamic acid	T50.991	T50.992	T50.993	T50.994	T50.995	T50.996
Acetomenaphthone	T45.7X1	T45.7X2	T45.7X3	T45.7X4	T45.7X5	T45.7X6
Acetomorphine	T40.1X1	T40.1X2	T40.1X3	T40.1X4	—	—
Acetone (oils)	T52.4X1	T52.4X2	T52.4X3	T52.4X4	—	—
chlorinated	T52.4X1	T52.4X2	T52.4X3	T52.4X4	—	—
vapor	T52.4X1	T52.4X2	T52.4X3	T52.4X4	—	—
Acetonitrile	T52.8X1	T52.8X2	T52.8X3	T52.8X4	—	—
Acetophenazine	T43.3X1	T43.3X2	T43.3X3	T43.3X4	T43.3X5	T43.3X6
Acetophenetedin	T39.1X1	T39.1X2	T39.1X3	T39.1X4	T39.1X5	T39.1X6
Acetophenone	T52.4X1	T52.4X2	T52.4X3	T52.4X4	—	—
Acetorphine	T40.2X1	T40.2X2	T40.2X3	T40.2X4	—	—
Acetosulfone (sodium)	T37.1X1	T37.1X2	T37.1X3	T37.1X4	T37.1X5	T37.1X6
Acetrizoate (sodium)	T50.8X1	T50.8X2	T50.8X3	T50.8X4	T50.8X5	T50.8X6
Acetylcarbromal	T42.6X1	T42.6X2	T42.6X3	T42.6X4	T42.6X5	T42.6X6
Acetrizoic acid	T50.8X1	T50.8X2	T50.8X3	T50.8X4	T50.8X5	T50.8X6
Acetyl						
bromide	T53.6X1	T53.6X2	T53.6X3	T53.6X4	—	—
chloride	T53.6X1	T53.6X2	T53.6X3	T53.6X4	—	—
Acetylcholine						
chloride	T44.1X1	T44.1X2	T44.1X3	T44.1X4	T44.1X5	T44.1X6
derivative	T44.1X1	T44.1X2	T44.1X3	T44.1X4	T44.1X5	T44.1X6
Acetylcysteine	T48.4X1	T48.4X2	T48.4X3	T48.4X4	T48.4X5	T48.4X6
Acetyldigitoxin	T46.0X1	T46.0X2	T46.0X3	T46.0X4	T46.0X5	T46.0X6
Acetyldigoxin	T46.0X1	T46.0X2	T46.0X3	T46.0X4	T46.0X5	T46.0X6
Acetyldihydrocodeine	T40.2X1	T40.2X2	T40.2X3	T40.2X4	—	—
Acetyldihydrocodeinone	T40.2X1	T40.2X2	T40.2X3	T40.2X4	—	—
Acetylene (gas)	T59.891	T59.892	T59.893	T59.894	—	—
dichloride	T53.6X1	T53.6X2	T53.6X3	T53.6X4	—	—
incomplete combustion of	T58.11	T58.12	T58.13	T58.14		
industrial	T59.891	T59.892	T59.893	T59.894	—	—
tetrachloride	T53.6X1	T53.6X2	T53.6X3	T53.6X4	—	—
vapor	T53.6X1	T53.6X2	T53.6X3	T53.6X4	—	—
Acetylphenylhydrazine	T39.8X1	T39.8X2	T39.8X3	T39.8X4	T39.8X5	T39.8X6

◀ New   ◀▥ Revised   ~~deleted~~ Deleted

Substance	External Cause (T-Code)					
	Poisoning, Accidental (Unintentional)	Poisoning, Intentional Self-Harm	Poisoning, Assault	Poisoning, Undetermined	Adverse Effect	Underdosing
Acetylpheneturide	T42.6X1	T42.6X2	T42.6X3	T42.6X4	T42.6X5	T42.6X6
Acetylsalicylic acid (salts)	T39.011	T39.012	T39.013	T39.014	T39.015	T39.016
enteric coated	T39.011	T39.012	T39.013	T39.014	T39.015	T39.016
Acetylsulfamethoxypyridazine	T37.0X1	T37.0X2	T37.0X3	T37.0X4	T37.0X5	T37.0X6
Achromycin	T36.4X1	T36.4X2	T36.4X3	T36.4X4	T36.4X5	T36.4X6
ophthalmic preparation	T49.5X1	T49.5X2	T49.5X3	T49.5X4	T49.5X5	T49.5X6
topical NEC	T49.0X1	T49.0X2	T49.0X3	T49.0X4	T49.0X5	T49.0X6
Aciclovir	T37.5X1	T37.5X2	T37.5X3	T37.5X4	T37.5X5	T37.5X6
Acid (corrosive) NEC	T54.2X1	T54.2X2	T54.2X3	T54.2X4	—	—
Acidifying agent NEC	T50.901	T50.902	T50.903	T50.904	T50.905	T50.906
Acipimox	T46.6X1	T46.6X2	T46.6X3	T46.6X4	T46.6X5	T46.6X6
Acitretin	T50.991	T50.992	T50.993	T50.994	T50.995	T50.996
Aclarubicin	T45.1X1	T45.1X2	T45.1X3	T45.1X4	T45.1X5	T45.1X6
Aclatonium napadisilate	T48.1X1	T48.1X2	T48.1X3	T48.1X4	T48.1X5	T48.1X6
Aconite (wild)	T46.991	T46.992	T46.993	T46.994	T46.995	T46.996
Aconitine	T46.991	T46.992	T46.993	T46.994	T46.995	T46.996
Aconitum ferox	T46.991	T46.992	T46.993	T46.994	T46.995	T46.996
Acridine	T65.6X1	T65.6X2	T65.6X3	T65.6X4	—	—
vapor	T59.891	T59.892	T59.893	T59.894	—	—
Acriflavine	T37.91	T37.92	T37.93	T37.94	T37.95	T37.96
Acriflavinium chloride	T49.0X1	T49.0X2	T49.0X3	T49.0X4	T49.0X5	T49.0X6
Acrinol	T49.0X1	T49.0X2	T49.0X3	T49.0X4	T49.0X5	T49.0X6
Acrisorcin	T49.0X1	T49.0X2	T49.0X3	T49.0X4	T49.0X5	T49.0X6
Acrivastine	T45.0X1	T45.0X2	T45.0X3	T45.0X4	T45.0X5	T45.0X6
Acrolein (gas)	T59.891	T59.892	T59.893	T59.894	—	—
liquid	T54.1X1	T54.1X2	T54.1X3	T54.1X4	—	—
Acrylamide	T65.891	T65.892	T65.893	T65.894	—	—
Acrylic resin	T49.3X1	T49.3X2	T49.3X3	T49.3X4	T49.3X5	T49.3X6
Acrylonitrile	T65.891	T65.892	T65.893	T65.894	—	—
Actaea spicata	T62.2X1	T62.2X2	T62.2X3	T62.2X4	—	—
berry	T62.1X1	T62.1X2	T62.1X3	T62.1X4	—	—
Acterol	T37.3X1	T37.3X2	T37.3X3	T37.3X4	T37.3X5	T37.3X6
ACTH	T38.811	T38.812	T38.813	T38.814	T38.815	T38.816
Actinomycin C	T45.1X1	T45.1X2	T45.1X3	T45.1X4	T45.1X5	T45.1X6
Actinomycin D	T45.1X1	T45.1X2	T45.1X3	T45.1X4	T45.1X5	T45.1X6
Activated charcoal — see also Charcoal, medicinal	T47.6X1	T47.6X2	T47.6X3	T47.6X4	T47.6X5	T47.6X6
Acyclovir	T37.5X1	T37.5X2	T37.5X3	T37.5X4	T37.5X5	T37.5X6
Adenine	T45.2X1	T45.2X2	T45.2X3	T45.2X4	T45.2X5	T45.2X6
arabinoside	T37.5X1	T37.5X2	T37.5X3	T37.5X4	T37.5X5	T37.5X6
Adenosine (phosphate)	T46.2X1	T46.2X2	T46.2X3	T46.2X4	T46.2X5	T46.2X6

◀ New   ◀ Revised   ~~deleted~~ Deleted

TABLE OF DRUGS AND CHEMICALS

TABLE OF DRUGS AND CHEMICALS

Substance	Poisoning, Accidental (Unintentional)	Poisoning, Intentional Self-Harm	Poisoning, Assault	Poisoning, Undetermined	Adverse Effect	Underdosing
	External Cause (T-Code)					
ADH	T38.891	T38.892	T38.893	T38.894	T38.895	T38.896
Adhesive NEC	T65.891	T65.892	T65.893	T65.894	—	—
Adicillin	T36.0X1	T36.0X2	T36.0X3	T36.0X4	T36.0X5	T36.0X6
Adiphenine	T44.3X1	T44.3X2	T44.3X3	T44.3X4	T44.3X5	T44.3X6
Adipiodone	T50.8X1	T50.8X2	T50.8X3	T50.8X4	T50.8X5	T50.8X6
Adjunct, pharmaceutical	T50.901	T50.902	T50.903	T50.904	T50.905	T50.906
Adrenal (extract, cortex or medulla) (glucocorticoids) (hormones) (mineralocorticoids)	T38.0X1	T38.0X2	T38.0X3	T38.0X4	T38.0X5	T38.0X6
ENT agent	T49.6X1	T49.6X2	T49.6X3	T49.6X4	T49.6X5	T49.6X6
ophthalmic preparation	T49.5X1	T49.5X2	T49.5X3	T49.5X4	T49.5X5	T49.5X6
topical NEC	T49.0X1	T49.0X2	T49.0X3	T49.0X4	T49.0X5	T49.0X6
Adrenaline	T44.5X1	T44.5X2	T44.5X3	T44.5X4	T44.5X5	T44.5X6
Adrenalin — see Adrenaline						
Adrenergic NEC	T44.901	T44.902	T44.903	T44.904	T44.905	T44.906
blocking agent NEC	T44.8X1	T44.8X2	T44.8X3	T44.8X4	T44.8X5	T44.8X6
beta, heart	T44.7X1	T44.7X2	T44.7X3	T44.7X4	T44.7X5	T44.7X6
specified NEC	T44.991	T44.992	T44.993	T44.994	T44.995	T44.996
Adrenochrome						
(mono) semicarbazone	T46.991	T46.992	T46.993	T46.994	T46.995	T46.996
derivative	T46.991	T46.992	T46.993	T46.994	T46.995	T46.996
Adrenocorticotrophic hormone	T38.811	T38.812	T38.813	T38.814	T38.815	T38.816
Adrenocorticotrophin	T38.811	T38.812	T38.813	T38.814	T38.815	T38.816
Adriamycin	T45.1X1	T45.1X2	T45.1X3	T45.1X4	T45.1X5	T45.1X6
Aerosol spray NEC	T65.91	T65.92	T65.93	T65.94	—	—
Aerosporin	T36.8X1	T36.8X2	T36.8X3	T36.8X4	T36.8X5	T36.8X6
ENT agent	T49.6X1	T49.6X2	T49.6X3	T49.6X4	T49.6X5	T49.6X6
ophthalmic preparation	T49.5X1	T49.5X2	T49.5X3	T49.5X4	T49.5X5	T49.5X6
topical NEC	T49.0X1	T49.0X2	T49.0X3	T49.0X4	T49.0X5	T49.0X6
Aethusa cynapium	T62.2X1	T62.2X2	T62.2X3	T62.2X4	—	—
Afghanistan black	T40.7X1	T40.7X2	T40.7X3	T40.7X4	T40.7X5	T40.7X6
Aflatoxin	T64.01	T64.02	T64.03	T64.04	—	—
Afloqualone	T42.8X1	T42.8X2	T42.8X3	T42.8X4	T42.8X5	T42.8X6
African boxwood	T62.2X1	T62.2X2	T62.2X3	T62.2X4	—	—
Agar	T47.4X1	T47.4X2	T47.4X3	T47.4X4	T47.4X5	T47.4X6
Agonist						
predominantly						
alpha-adrenoreceptor	T44.4X1	T44.4X2	T44.4X3	T44.4X4	T44.4X5	T44.4X6
beta-adrenoreceptor	T44.5X1	T44.5X2	T44.5X3	T44.5X4	T44.5X5	T44.5X6
Agricultural agent NEC	T65.91	T65.92	T65.93	T65.94	—	—
Agrypnal	T42.3X1	T42.3X2	T42.3X3	T42.3X4	T42.3X5	T42.3X6

◀ New　◀▥ Revised　~~deleted~~ Deleted

Substance	Poisoning, Accidental (Unintentional)	Poisoning, Intentional Self-Harm	Poisoning, Assault	Poisoning, Undetermined	Adverse Effect	Underdosing
AHLG	T50.Z11	T50.Z12	T50.Z13	T50.Z14	T50.Z15	T50.Z16
Air contaminant(s), source/type NOS	T65.91	T65.92	T65.93	T65.94	—	—
Ajmaline	T46.2X1	T46.2X2	T46.2X3	T46.2X4	T46.2X5	T46.2X6
Akritoin	T37.8X1	T37.8X2	T37.8X3	T37.8X4	T37.8X5	T37.8X6
Akee	T62.1X1	T62.1X2	T62.1X3	T62.1X4	—	—
Akrinol	T49.0X1	T49.0X2	T49.0X3	T49.0X4	T49.0X5	T49.0X6
Alacepril	T46.4X1	T46.4X2	T46.4X3	T46.4X4	T46.4X5	T46.4X6
Alantolactone	T37.4X1	T37.4X2	T37.4X3	T37.4X4	T37.4X5	T37.4X6
Albamycin	T36.8X1	T36.8X2	T36.8X3	T36.8X4	T36.8X5	T36.8X6
Albendazole	T37.4X1	T37.4X2	T37.4X3	T37.4X4	T37.4X5	T37.4X6
Albumin						
bovine	T45.8X1	T45.8X2	T45.8X3	T45.8X4	T45.8X5	T45.8X6
human serum	T45.8X1	T45.8X2	T45.8X3	T45.8X4	T45.8X5	T45.8X6
salt-poor	T45.8X1	T45.8X2	T45.8X3	T45.8X4	T45.8X5	T45.8X6
normal human serum	T45.8X1	T45.8X2	T45.8X3	T45.8X4	T45.8X5	T45.8X6
Albuterol	T48.6X1	T48.6X2	T48.6X3	T48.6X4	T48.6X5	T48.6X6
Albutoin	T42.0X1	T42.0X2	T42.0X3	T42.0X4	T42.0X5	T42.0X6
Alclometasone	T49.0X1	T49.0X2	T49.0X3	T49.0X4	T49.0X5	T49.0X6
Alcohol	T51.91	T51.92	T51.93	T51.94	—	—
absolute	T51.0X1	T51.0X2	T51.0X3	T51.0X4	—	—
beverage	T51.0X1	T51.0X2	T51.0X3	T51.0X4	—	—
allyl	T51.8X1	T51.8X2	T51.8X3	T51.8X4	—	—
amyl	T51.3X1	T51.3X2	T51.3X3	T51.3X4	—	—
antifreeze	T51.1X1	T51.1X2	T51.1X3	T51.1X4	—	—
beverage	T51.0X1	T51.0X2	T51.0X3	T51.0X4	—	—
butyl	T51.3X1	T51.3X2	T51.3X3	T51.3X4	—	—
dehydrated	T51.0X1	T51.0X2	T51.0X3	T51.0X4	—	—
beverage	T51.0X1	T51.0X2	T51.0X3	T51.0X4	—	—
denatured	T51.0X1	T51.0X2	T51.0X3	T51.0X4	—	—
deterrent NEC	T50.6X1	T50.6X2	T50.6X3	T50.6X4	T50.6X5	T50.6X6
diagnostic (gastric function)	T50.8X1	T50.8X2	T50.8X3	T50.8X4	T50.8X5	T50.8X6
ethyl	T51.0X1	T51.0X2	T51.0X3	T51.0X4	—	—
beverage	T51.0X1	T51.0X2	T51.0X3	T51.0X4	—	—
grain	T51.0X1	T51.0X2	T51.0X3	T51.0X4	—	—
beverage	T51.0X1	T51.0X2	T51.0X3	T51.0X4	—	—
industrial	T51.0X1	T51.0X2	T51.0X3	T51.0X4	—	—
isopropyl	T51.2X1	T51.2X2	T51.2X3	T51.2X4	—	—
methyl	T51.1X1	T51.1X2	T51.1X3	T51.1X4	—	—
preparation for consumption	T51.0X1	T51.0X2	T51.0X3	T51.0X4	—	—

TABLE OF DRUGS AND CHEMICALS

Substance	External Cause (T-Code)					
	Poisoning, Accidental (Unintentional)	Poisoning, Intentional Self-Harm	Poisoning, Assault	Poisoning, Undetermined	Adverse Effect	Underdosing
Alcohol (Continued)						
propyl	T51.3X1	T51.3X2	T51.3X3	T51.3X4	—	—
secondary	T51.2X1	T51.2X2	T51.2X3	T51.2X4	—	—
radiator	T51.1X1	T51.1X2	T51.1X3	T51.1X4	—	—
rubbing	T51.2X1	T51.2X2	T51.2X3	T51.2X4	—	—
specified type NEC	T51.8X1	T51.8X2	T51.8X3	T51.8X4	—	—
surgical	T51.0X1	T51.0X2	T51.0X3	T51.0X4	—	—
vapor (from any type of Alcohol)	T59.891	T59.892	T59.893	T59.894	—	—
wood	T51.1X1	T51.1X2	T51.1X3	T51.1X4	—	—
Alcuronium (chloride)	T48.1X1	T48.1X2	T48.1X3	T48.1X4	T48.1X5	T48.1X6
Aldactone	T50.0X1	T50.0X2	T50.0X3	T50.0X4	T50.0X5	T50.0X6
Aldesulfone sodium	T37.1X1	T37.1X2	T37.1X3	T37.1X4	T37.1X5	T37.1X6
Aldicarb	T60.0X1	T60.0X2	T60.0X3	T60.0X4	—	—
Aldomet	T46.5X1	T46.5X2	T46.5X3	T46.5X4	T46.5X5	T46.5X6
Aldosterone	T50.0X1	T50.0X2	T50.0X3	T50.0X4	T50.0X5	T50.0X6
Aldrin (dust)	T60.1X1	T60.1X2	T60.1X3	T60.1X4	—	—
Aleve — see Naproxen						
Alexitol sodium	T47.1X1	T47.1X2	T47.1X3	T47.1X4	T47.1X5	T47.1X6
Alfacalcidol	T45.2X1	T45.2X2	T45.2X3	T45.2X4	T45.2X5	T45.2X6
Alfadolone	T41.1X1	T41.1X2	T41.1X3	T41.1X4	T41.1X5	T41.1X6
Alfaxalone	T41.1X1	T41.1X2	T41.1X3	T41.1X4	T41.1X5	T41.1X6
Alfentanil	T40.4X1	T40.4X2	T40.4X3	T40.4X4	T40.4X5	T40.4X6
Alfuzosin (hydrochloride)	T44.8X1	T44.8X2	T44.8X3	T44.8X4	T44.8X5	T44.8X6
Algae (harmful) (toxin)	T65.821	T65.822	T65.823	T65.824	—	—
Algeldrate	T47.1X1	T47.1X2	T47.1X3	T47.1X4	T47.1X5	T47.1X6
Algin	T47.8X1	T47.8X2	T47.8X3	T47.8X4	T47.8X5	T47.8X6
Alglucerase	T45.3X1	T45.3X2	T45.3X3	T45.3X4	T45.3X5	T45.3X6
Alidase	T45.3X1	T45.3X2	T45.3X3	T45.3X4	T45.3X5	T45.3X6
Alimemazine	T43.3X1	T43.3X2	T43.3X3	T43.3X4	T43.3X5	T43.3X6
Aliphatic thiocyanates	T65.0X1	T65.0X2	T65.0X3	T65.0X4	—	—
Alizapride	T45.0X1	T45.0X2	T45.0X3	T45.0X4	T45.0X5	T45.0X6
Alkali (caustic)	T54.3X1	T54.3X2	T54.3X3	T54.3X4	—	—
Alkalizing agent NEC	T50.901	T50.902	T50.903	T50.904	T50.905	T50.906
Alkaline antiseptic solution (aromatic)	T49.6X1	T49.6X2	T49.6X3	T49.6X4	T49.6X5	T49.6X6
Alkalinizing agents (medicinal)	T50.901	T50.902	T50.903	T50.904	T50.905	T50.906
Alka-seltzer	T39.011	T39.012	T39.013	T39.014	T39.015	T39.016
Alkavervir	T46.5X1	T46.5X2	T46.5X3	T46.5X4	T46.5X5	T46.5X6
Alkonium (bromide)	T49.0X1	T49.0X2	T49.0X3	T49.0X4	T49.0X5	T49.0X6
Alkylating drug NEC	T45.1X1	T45.1X2	T45.1X3	T45.1X4	T45.1X5	T45.1X6
antimyeloproliferative	T45.1X1	T45.1X2	T45.1X3	T45.1X4	T45.1X5	T45.1X6
lymphatic	T45.1X1	T45.1X2	T45.1X3	T45.1X4	T45.1X5	T45.1X6

◀ New ◀ Revised ~~deleted~~ Deleted

Substance	External Cause (T-Code)					
	Poisoning, Accidental (Unintentional)	Poisoning, Intentional Self-Harm	Poisoning, Assault	Poisoning, Undetermined	Adverse Effect	Underdosing
Alkylisocyanate	T65.0X1	T65.0X2	T65.0X3	T65.0X4	—	—
Allantoin	T49.411	T49.412	T49.413	T49.414	T49.415	T49.416
Allegron	T43.0X1	T43.0X2	T43.0X3	T43.0X4	T43.0X5	T43.0X6
Allethrin	T49.0X1	T49.0X2	T49.0X3	T49.0X4	T49.0X5	T49.0X6
Allobarbital	T42.3X1	T42.3X2	T42.3X3	T42.3X4	T42.3X5	T42.3X6
Allopurinol	T50.4X1	T50.4X2	T50.4X3	T50.4X4	T50.4X5	T50.4X6
Allyl						
alcohol	T51.8X1	T51.8X2	T51.8X3	T51.8X4	—	—
disulfide	T46.6X1	T46.6X2	T46.6X3	T46.6X4	T46.6X5	T46.6X6
Allylestrenol	T38.5X1	T38.5X2	T38.5X3	T38.5X4	T38.5X5	T38.5X6
Allylisopropylacetylurea	T42.6X1	T42.6X2	T42.6X3	T42.6X4	T42.6X5	T42.6X6
Allylisopropylmalonylurea	T42.3X1	T42.3X2	T42.3X3	T42.3X4	T42.3X5	T42.3X6
Allylthiourea	T49.3X1	T49.3X2	T49.3X3	T49.3X4	T49.3X5	T49.3X6
Allyltribromide	T42.6X1	T42.6X2	T42.6X3	T42.6X4	T42.6X5	T42.6X6
Allypropymal	T42.3X1	T42.3X2	T42.3X3	T42.3X4	T42.3X5	T42.3X6
Almagate	T47.1X1	T47.1X2	T47.1X3	T47.1X4	T47.1X5	T47.1X6
Almasilate	T47.1X1	T47.1X2	T47.1X3	T47.1X4	T47.1X5	T47.1X6
Almitrine	T50.7X1	T50.7X2	T50.7X3	T50.7X4	T50.7X5	T50.7X6
Aloes	T47.2X1	T47.2X2	T47.2X3	T47.2X4	T47.2X5	T47.2X6
Aloglutamol	T47.1X1	T47.1X2	T47.1X3	T47.1X4	T47.1X5	T47.1X6
Aloin	T47.2X1	T47.2X2	T47.2X3	T47.2X4	T47.2X5	T47.2X6
Aloxidone	T42.2X1	T42.2X2	T42.2X3	T42.2X4	T42.2X5	T42.2X6
Alpha						
acetyldigoxin	T46.0X1	T46.0X2	T46.0X3	T46.0X4	T46.0X5	T46.0X6
adrenergic blocking drug	T44.6X1	T44.6X2	T44.6X3	T44.6X4	T44.6X5	T44.6X6
amylase	T45.3X1	T45.3X2	T45.3X3	T45.3X4	T45.3X5	T45.3X6
tocoferol (acetate)	T45.2X1	T45.2X2	T45.2X3	T45.2X4	T45.2X5	T45.2X6
tocopherol	T45.2X1	T45.2X2	T45.2X3	T45.2X4	T45.2X5	T45.2X6
Alphadolone	T41.1X1	T41.1X2	T41.1X3	T41.1X4	T41.1X5	T41.1X6
Alphaprodine	T40.4X1	T40.4X2	T40.4X3	T40.4X4	T40.4X5	T40.4X6
Alphaxalone	T41.1X1	T41.1X2	T41.1X3	T41.1X4	T41.1X5	T41.1X6
Alprazolam	T42.4X1	T42.4X2	T42.4X3	T42.4X4	T42.4X5	T42.4X6
Alprenolol	T44.7X1	T44.7X2	T44.7X3	T44.7X4	T44.7X5	T44.7X6
Alprostadil	T46.7X1	T46.7X2	T46.7X3	T46.7X4	T46.7X5	T46.7X6
Alsactide	T38.811	T38.812	T38.813	T38.814	T38.815	T38.816
Alseroxylon	T46.5X1	T46.5X2	T46.5X3	T46.5X4	T46.5X5	T46.5X6
Alteplase	T45.611	T45.612	T45.613	T45.614	T45.615	T45.616
Altizide	T50.2X1	T50.2X2	T50.2X3	T50.2X4	T50.2X5	T50.2X6
Altretamine	T45.1X1	T45.1X2	T45.1X3	T45.1X4	T45.1X5	T45.1X6

◀ New   ◀▥ Revised   ~~deleted~~ Deleted

TABLE OF DRUGS AND CHEMICALS

Substance	External Cause (T-Code)					
	Poisoning, Accidental (Unintentional)	Poisoning, Intentional Self-Harm	Poisoning, Assault	Poisoning, Undetermined	Adverse Effect	Underdosing
Alum (medicinal)	T49.4X1	T49.4X2	T49.4X3	T49.4X4	T49.4X5	T49.4X6
nonmedicinal (ammonium) (potassium)	T56.891	T56.892	T56.893	T56.894	—	—
Aluminium, aluminum						
acetate	T49.2X1	T49.2X2	T49.2X3	T49.2X4	T49.2X5	T49.2X6
solution	T49.0X1	T49.0X2	T49.0X3	T49.0X4	T49.0X5	T49.0X6
aspirin	T39.011	T39.012	T39.013	T39.014	T39.015	T39.016
bis (acetylsalicylate)	T39.011	T39.012	T39.013	T39.014	T39.015	T39.016
carbonate (gel, basic)	T47.1X1	T47.1X2	T47.1X3	T47.1X4	T47.1X5	T47.1X6
chlorhydroxide-complex	T47.1X1	T47.1X2	T47.1X3	T47.1X4	T47.1X5	T47.1X6
chloride	T49.2X1	T49.2X2	T49.2X3	T49.2X4	T49.2X5	T49.2X6
clofibrate	T46.6X1	T46.6X2	T46.6X3	T46.6X4	T46.6X5	T46.6X6
diacetate	T49.2X1	T49.2X2	T49.2X3	T49.2X4	T49.2X5	T49.2X6
glycinate	T47.1X1	T47.1X2	T47.1X3	T47.1X4	T47.1X5	T47.1X6
hydroxide (gel)	T47.1X1	T47.1X2	T47.1X3	T47.1X4	T47.1X5	T47.1X6
hydroxide-magnesium carb. gel	T47.1X1	T47.1X2	T47.1X3	T47.1X4	T47.1X5	T47.1X6
magnesium silicate	T47.1X1	T47.1X2	T47.1X3	T47.1X4	T47.1X5	T47.1X6
nicotinate	T46.7X1	T46.7X2	T46.7X3	T46.7X4	T46.7X5	T46.7X6
ointment (surgical) (topical)	T49.3X1	T49.3X2	T49.3X3	T49.3X4	T49.3X5	T49.3X6
phosphate	T47.1X1	T47.1X2	T47.1X3	T47.1X4	T47.1X5	T47.1X6
salicylate	T39.091	T39.092	T39.093	T39.094	T39.095	T39.096
silicate	T47.1X1	T47.1X2	T47.1X3	T47.1X4	T47.1X5	T47.1X6
sodium silicate	T47.1X1	T47.1X2	T47.1X3	T47.1X4	T47.1X5	T47.1X6
subacetate	T49.2X1	T49.2X2	T49.2X3	T49.2X4	T49.2X5	T49.2X6
sulfate	T49.0X1	T49.0X2	T49.0X3	T49.0X4	T49.0X5	T49.0X6
tannate	T47.6X1	T47.6X2	T47.6X3	T47.6X4	T47.6X5	T47.6X6
topical NEC	T49.3X1	T49.3X2	T49.3X3	T49.3X4	T49.3X5	T49.3X6
Alurate	T42.3X1	T42.3X2	T42.3X3	T42.3X4	T42.3X5	T42.3X6
Alverine	T44.3X1	T44.3X2	T44.3X3	T44.3X4	T44.3X5	T44.3X6
Alvodine	T40.2X1	T40.2X2	T40.2X3	T40.2X4	T40.2X5	T40.2X6
Amanita phalloides	T62.0X1	T62.0X2	T62.0X3	T62.0X4	—	—
Amanitine	T62.0X1	T62.0X2	T62.0X3	T62.0X4	—	—
Amantadine	T42.8X1	T42.8X2	T42.8X3	T42.8X4	T42.8X5	T42.8X6
Ambazone	T49.6X1	T49.6X2	T49.6X3	T49.6X4	T49.6X5	T49.6X6
Ambenonium (chloride)	T44.0X1	T44.0X2	T44.0X3	T44.0X4	T44.0X5	T44.0X6
Ambroxol	T48.4X1	T48.4X2	T48.4X3	T48.4X4	T48.4X5	T48.4X6
Ambuphylline	T48.6X1	T48.6X2	T48.6X3	T48.6X4	T48.6X5	T48.6X6
Ambutonium bromide	T44.3X1	T44.3X2	T44.3X3	T44.3X4	T44.3X5	T44.3X6
Amcinonide	T49.0X1	T49.0X2	T49.0X3	T49.0X4	T49.0X5	T49.0X6
Amdinocilline	T36.0X1	T36.0X2	T36.0X3	T36.0X4	T36.0X5	T36.0X6

◀ New   ◀▦ Revised   ~~deleted~~ Deleted

Substance	External Cause (T-Code)					
	Poisoning, Accidental (Unintentional)	Poisoning, Intentional Self-Harm	Poisoning, Assault	Poisoning, Undetermined	Adverse Effect	Underdosing
Ametazole	T50.8X1	T50.8X2	T50.8X3	T50.8X4	T50.8X5	T50.8X6
Amethocaine	T41.3X1	T41.3X2	T41.3X3	T41.3X4	T41.3X5	T41.3X6
regional	T41.3X1	T41.3X2	T41.3X3	T41.3X4	T41.3X5	T41.3X6
spinal	T41.3X1	T41.3X2	T41.3X3	T41.3X4	T41.3X5	T41.3X6
Amethopterin	T45.1X1	T45.1X2	T45.1X3	T45.1X4	T45.1X5	T45.1X6
Amezinium metilsulfate	T44.991	T44.992	T44.993	T44.994	T44.995	T44.996
Amfebutamone	T43.291	T43.292	T43.293	T43.294	T43.295	T43.296
Amfepramone	T50.5X1	T50.5X2	T50.5X3	T50.5X4	T50.5X5	T50.5X6
Amfetamine	T43.621	T43.622	T43.623	T43.624	T43.625	T43.626
Amfetaminil	T43.621	T43.622	T43.623	T43.624	T43.625	T43.626
Amfomycin	T36.8X1	T36.8X2	T36.8X3	T36.8X4	T36.8X5	T36.8X6
Amidefrine mesilate	T48.5X1	T48.5X2	T48.5X3	T48.5X4	T48.5X5	T48.5X6
Amidone	T40.3X1	T40.3X2	T40.3X3	T40.3X4	T40.3X5	T40.3X6
Amidopyrine	T39.2X1	T39.2X2	T39.2X3	T39.2X4	T39.2X5	T39.2X6
Amidotrizoate	T50.8X1	T50.8X2	T50.8X3	T50.8X4	T50.8X5	T50.8X6
Amiflamine	T43.1X1	T43.1X2	T43.1X3	T43.1X4	T43.1X5	T43.1X6
Amikacin	T36.5X1	T36.5X2	T36.5X3	T36.5X4	T36.5X5	T36.5X6
Amikhelline	T46.3X1	T46.3X2	T46.3X3	T46.3X4	T46.3X5	T46.3X6
Amiloride	T50.2X1	T50.2X2	T50.2X3	T50.2X4	T50.2X5	T50.2X6
Aminacrine	T49.0X1	T49.0X2	T49.0X3	T49.0X4	T49.0X5	T49.0X6
Amineptine	T43.011	T43.012	T43.013	T43.014	T43.015	T43.016
Aminitrozole	T37.3X1	T37.3X2	T37.3X3	T37.3X4	T37.3X5	T37.3X6
Aminoacetic acid (derivatives)	T50.3X1	T50.3X2	T50.3X3	T50.3X4	T50.3X5	T50.3X6
Amino acids	T50.3X1	T50.3X2	T50.3X3	T50.3X4	T50.3X5	T50.3X6
Aminoacridine	T49.0X1	T49.0X2	T49.0X3	T49.0X4	T49.0X5	T49.0X6
Aminobenzoic acid (-p)	T49.3X1	T49.3X2	T49.3X3	T49.3X4	T49.3X5	T49.3X6
4-Aminobutyric acid	T43.8X1	T43.8X2	T43.8X3	T43.8X4	T43.8X5	T43.8X6
Aminocaproic acid	T45.621	T45.622	T45.623	T45.624	T45.625	T45.626
Aminofenazone	T39.2X1	T39.2X2	T39.2X3	T39.2X4	T39.2X5	T39.2X6
Aminoethylisothiourium	T45.8X1	T45.8X2	T45.8X3	T45.8X4	T45.8X5	T45.8X6
Aminoglutethimide	T45.1X1	T45.1X2	T45.1X3	T45.1X4	T45.1X5	T45.1X6
Aminohippuric acid	T50.8X1	T50.8X2	T50.8X3	T50.8X4	T50.8X5	T50.8X6
Aminomethylbenzoic acid	T45.691	T45.692	T45.693	T45.694	T45.695	T45.696
Aminometradine	T50.2X1	T50.2X2	T50.2X3	T50.2X4	T50.2X5	T50.2X6
Aminopentamide	T44.3X1	T44.3X2	T44.3X3	T44.3X4	T44.3X5	T44.3X6
Aminophenazone	T39.2X1	T39.2X2	T39.2X3	T39.2X4	T39.2X5	T39.2X6
Aminophenol	T54.0X1	T54.0X2	T54.0X3	T54.0X4	—	—
4-Aminophenol derivatives	T39.1X1	T39.1X2	T39.1X3	T39.1X4	T39.1X5	T39.1X6
Aminophenylpyridone	T43.591	T43.592	T43.593	T43.594	T43.595	T43.596

TABLE OF DRUGS AND CHEMICALS

Substance	External Cause (T-Code)					
	Poisoning, Accidental (Unintentional)	Poisoning, Intentional Self-Harm	Poisoning, Assault	Poisoning, Undetermined	Adverse Effect	Underdosing
Aminophylline	T48.6X1	T48.6X2	T48.6X3	T48.6X4	T48.6X5	T48.6X6
Aminopterin sodium	T45.1X1	T45.1X2	T45.1X3	T45.1X4	T45.1X5	T45.1X6
Aminopyrine	T39.2X1	T39.2X2	T39.2X3	T39.2X4	T39.2X5	T39.2X6
8-Aminoquinoline drugs	T37.2X1	T37.2X2	T37.2X3	T37.2X4	T37.2X5	T37.2X6
Aminorex	T50.5X1	T50.5X2	T50.5X3	T50.5X4	T50.5X5	T50.5X6
Aminosalicylic acid	T37.1X1	T37.1X2	T37.1X3	T37.1X4	T37.1X5	T37.1X6
Aminosalylum	T37.1X1	T37.1X2	T37.1X3	T37.1X4	T37.1X5	T37.1X6
Amiodarone	T46.2X1	T46.2X2	T46.2X3	T46.2X4	T46.2X5	T46.2X6
Amiphenazole	T50.7X1	T50.7X2	T50.7X3	T50.7X4	T50.7X5	T50.7X6
Amiquinsin	T46.5X1	T46.5X2	T46.5X3	T46.5X4	T46.5X5	T46.5X6
Amisometradine	T50.2X1	T50.2X2	T50.2X3	T50.2X4	T50.2X5	T50.2X6
Amisulpride	T43.591	T43.592	T43.593	T43.594	T43.595	T43.596
Amitriptyline	T43.021	T43.022	T43.023	T43.024	T43.025	T43.026
Amitriptylinoxide	T43.021	T43.022	T43.023	T43.024	T43.025	T43.026
Amlexanox	T48.6X1	T48.6X2	T48.6X3	T48.6X4	T48.6X5	T48.6X6
Ammonia (fumes) (gas) (vapor)	T59.891	T59.892	T59.893	T59.894	—	—
aromatic spirit	T48.991	T48.992	T48.993	T48.994	T48.995	T48.996
liquid (household)	T54.3X1	T54.3X2	T54.3X3	T54.3X4	—	—
Ammoniated mercury	T49.0X1	T49.0X2	T49.0X3	T49.0X4	T49.0X5	T49.0X6
Ammonium						
acid tartrate	T49.5X1	T49.5X2	T49.5X3	T49.5X4	T49.5X5	T49.5X6
bromide	T42.6X1	T42.6X2	T42.6X3	T42.6X4	T42.6X5	T42.6X6
carbonate	T54.3X1	T54.3X2	T54.3X3	T54.3X4	—	—
chloride	T50.991	T50.992	T50.993	T50.994	T50.995	T50.996
expectorant	T48.4X1	T48.4X2	T48.4X3	T48.4X4	T48.4X5	T48.4X6
compounds (household) NEC	T54.3X1	T54.3X2	T54.3X3	T54.3X4	—	—
fumes (any usage)	T59.891	T59.892	T59.893	T59.894	—	—
industrial	T54.3X1	T54.3X2	T54.3X3	T54.3X4	—	—
ichthyosulronate	T49.4X1	T49.4X2	T49.4X3	T49.4X4	T49.4X5	T49.4X6
mandelate	T37.91	T37.92	T37.93	T37.94	T37.95	T37.96
sulfamate	T60.3X1	T60.3X2	T60.3X3	T60.3X4	—	—
sulfonate resin	T47.8X1	T47.8X2	T47.8X3	T47.8X4	T47.8X5	T47.8X6
Amobarbital (sodium)	T42.3X1	T42.3X2	T42.3X3	T42.3X4	T42.3X5	T42.3X6
Amodiaquine	T37.2X1	T37.2X2	T37.2X3	T37.2X4	T37.2X5	T37.2X6
Amopyroquin(e)	T37.2X1	T37.2X2	T37.2X3	T37.2X4	T37.2X5	T37.2X6
Amoxapine	T43.011	T43.012	T43.013	T43.014	T43.015	T43.016
Amoxicillin	T36.0X1	T36.0X2	T36.0X3	T36.0X4	T36.0X5	T36.0X6
Amperozide	T43.591	T43.592	T43.593	T43.594	T43.595	T43.596
Amphenidone	T43.591	T43.592	T43.593	T43.594	T43.595	T43.596
Amphetamine NEC	T43.621	T43.622	T43.623	T43.624	T43.625	T43.626

◀ New   ◀ Revised   ~~deleted~~ Deleted

Substance	External Cause (T-Code)					
	Poisoning, Accidental (Unintentional)	Poisoning, Intentional Self-Harm	Poisoning, Assault	Poisoning, Undetermined	Adverse Effect	Underdosing
Amphomycin	T36.8X1	T36.8X2	T36.8X3	T36.8X4	T36.8X5	T36.8X6
Amphotalide	T37.4X1	T37.4X2	T37.4X3	T37.4X4	T37.4X5	T37.4X6
Amphotericin B	T36.7X1	T36.7X2	T36.7X3	T36.7X4	T36.7X5	T36.7X6
topical	T49.0X1	T49.0X2	T49.0X3	T49.0X4	T49.0X5	T49.0X6
Ampicillin	T36.0X1	T36.0X2	T36.0X3	T36.0X4	T36.0X5	T36.0X6
Amprotropine	T44.3X1	T44.3X2	T44.3X3	T44.3X4	T44.3X5	T44.3X6
Amsacrine	T45.1X1	T45.1X2	T45.1X3	T45.1X4	T45.1X5	T45.1X6
Amygdaline	T62.2X1	T62.2X2	T62.2X3	T62.2X4	—	—
Amyl						
acetate	T52.8X1	T52.8X2	T52.8X3	T52.8X4	—	—
vapor	T59.891	T59.892	T59.893	T59.894	—	—
alcohol	T51.3X1	T51.3X2	T51.3X3	T51.3X4	—	—
chloride	T53.6X1	T53.6X2	T53.6X3	T53.6X4	—	—
formate	T52.8X1	T52.8X2	T52.8X3	T52.8X4	—	—
nitrite	T46.3X1	T46.3X2	T46.3X3	T46.3X4	T46.3X5	T46.3X6
propionate	T65.891	T65.892	T65.893	T65.894	—	—
Amylase	T47.5X1	T47.5X2	T47.5X3	T47.5X4	T47.5X5	T47.5X6
Amyleine, regional	T41.3X1	T41.3X2	T41.3X3	T41.3X4	T41.3X5	T41.3X6
Amylene						
dichloride	T53.6X1	T53.6X2	T53.6X3	T53.6X4	—	—
hydrate	T51.3X1	T51.3X2	T51.3X3	T51.3X4	—	—
Amylmetacresol	T49.6X1	T49.6X2	T49.6X3	T49.6X4	T49.6X5	T49.6X6
Amylobarbitone	T42.3X1	T42.3X2	T42.3X3	T42.3X4	T42.3X5	T42.3X6
Amylocaine, regional	T41.3X1	T41.3X2	T41.3X3	T41.3X4	T41.3X5	T41.3X6
infiltration (subcutaneous)	T41.3X1	T41.3X2	T41.3X3	T41.3X4	T41.3X5	T41.3X6
nerve block (peripheral) (plexus)	T41.3X1	T41.3X2	T41.3X3	T41.3X4	T41.3X5	T41.3X6
spinal	T41.3X1	T41.3X2	T41.3X3	T41.3X4	T41.3X5	T41.3X6
topical (surface)	T41.3X1	T41.3X2	T41.3X3	T41.3X4	T41.3X5	T41.3X6
Amylopectin	T47.6X1	T47.6X2	T47.6X3	T47.6X4	T47.6X5	T47.6X6
Amytal (sodium)	T42.3X1	T42.3X2	T42.3X3	T42.3X4	T42.3X5	T42.3X6
Anabolic steroid	T38.7X1	T38.7X2	T38.7X3	T38.7X4	T38.7X5	T38.7X6
Analeptic NEC	T50.7X1	T50.7X2	T50.7X3	T50.7X4	T50.7X5	T50.7X6
Analgesic	T39.91	T39.92	T39.93	T39.94	T39.95	T39.96
anti-inflammatory NEC	T39.91	T39.92	T39.93	T39.94	T39.95	T39.96
propionic acid derivative	T39.311	T39.312	T39.313	T39.314	T39.315	T39.316
antirheumatic NEC	T39.4X1	T39.4X2	T39.4X3	T39.4X4	T39.4X5	T39.4X6
aromatic NEC	T39.1X1	T39.1X2	T39.1X3	T39.1X4	T39.1X5	T39.1X6
narcotic NEC	T40.601	T40.602	T40.603	T40.604	T40.605	T40.606
combination	T40.601	T40.602	T40.603	T40.604	T40.605	T40.606
obstetric	T40.601	T40.602	T40.603	T40.604	T40.605	T40.606

◄ New ◄▥ Revised ~~deleted~~ Deleted

Substance	External Cause (T-Code)					
	Poisoning, Accidental (Unintentional)	Poisoning, Intentional Self-Harm	Poisoning, Assault	Poisoning, Undetermined	Adverse Effect	Underdosing
Analgesic *(Continued)*						
non-narcotic NEC	T39.91	T39.92	T39.93	T39.94	T39.95	T39.96
combination	T39.91	T39.92	T39.93	T39.94	T39.95	T39.96
pyrazole	T39.2X1	T39.2X2	T39.2X3	T39.2X4	T39.2X5	T39.2X6
specified NEC	T39.8X1	T39.8X2	T39.8X3	T39.8X4	T39.8X5	T39.8X6
Analgin	T39.2X1	T39.2X2	T39.2X3	T39.2X4	T39.2X5	T39.2X6
Anamirta cocculus	T62.1X1	T62.1X2	T62.1X3	T62.1X4	—	—
Ancillin	T36.0X1	T36.0X2	T36.0X3	T36.0X4	T36.0X5	T36.0X6
Ancrod	T45.691	T45.692	T45.693	T45.694	T45.695	T45.696
Androgen	T38.7X1	T38.7X2	T38.7X3	T38.7X4	T38.7X5	T38.7X6
Androgen-estrogen mixture	T38.7X1	T38.7X2	T38.7X3	T38.7X4	T38.7X5	T38.7X6
Androstalone	T38.7X1	T38.7X2	T38.7X3	T38.7X4	T38.7X5	T38.7X6
Androstanolone	T38.7X1	T38.7X2	T38.7X3	T38.7X4	T38.7X5	T38.7X6
Androsterone	T38.7X1	T38.7X2	T38.7X3	T38.7X4	T38.7X5	T38.7X6
Anemone pulsatilla	T62.2X1	T62.2X2	T62.2X3	T62.2X4	—	—
Anesthesia						
caudal	T41.3X1	T41.3X2	T41.3X3	T41.3X4	T41.3X5	T41.3X6
endotracheal	T41.0X1	T41.0X2	T41.0X3	T41.0X4	T41.0X5	T41.0X6
epidural	T41.3X1	T41.3X2	T41.3X3	T41.3X4	T41.3X5	T41.3X6
inhalation	T41.0X1	T41.0X2	T41.0X3	T41.0X4	T41.0X5	T41.0X6
local	T41.3X1	T41.3X2	T41.3X3	T41.3X4	T41.3X5	T41.3X6
mucosal	T41.3X1	T41.3X2	T41.3X3	T41.3X4	T41.3X5	T41.3X6
muscle relaxation	T48.1X1	T48.1X2	T48.1X3	T48.1X4	T48.1X5	T48.1X6
nerve blocking	T41.3X1	T41.3X2	T41.3X3	T41.3X4	T41.3X5	T41.3X6
plexus blocking	T41.3X1	T41.3X2	T41.3X3	T41.3X4	T41.3X5	T41.3X6
potentiated	T41.201	T41.202	T41.203	T41.204	T41.205	T41.206
rectal	T41.201	T41.202	T41.203	T41.204	T41.205	T41.206
general	T41.201	T41.202	T41.203	T41.204	T41.205	T41.206
local	T41.3X1	T41.3X2	T41.3X3	T41.3X4	T41.3X5	T41.3X6
regional	T41.3X1	T41.3X2	T41.3X3	T41.3X4	T41.3X5	T41.3X6
surface	T41.3X1	T41.3X2	T41.3X3	T41.3X4	T41.3X5	T41.3X6
Anesthetic NEC—*see also Anesthesia*	T41.41	T41.42	T41.43	T41.44	T41.45	T41.46
with muscle relaxant	T41.201	T41.202	T41.203	T41.204	T41.205	T41.206
general	T41.201	T41.202	T41.203	T41.204	T41.205	T41.206
local	T41.3X1	T41.3X2	T41.3X3	T41.3X4	T41.3X5	T41.3X6
gaseous NEC	T41.0X1	T41.0X2	T41.0X3	T41.0X4	T41.0X5	T41.0X6
general NEC	T41.201	T41.202	T41.203	T41.204	T41.205	T41.206
halogenated hydrocarbon derivatives NEC	T41.0X1	T41.0X2	T41.0X3	T41.0X4	T41.0X5	T41.0X6
infiltration NEC	T41.3X1	T41.3X2	T41.3X3	T41.3X4	T41.3X5	T41.3X6
intravenous NEC	T41.1X1	T41.1X2	T41.1X3	T41.1X4	T41.1X5	T41.1X6

◀ New ◀ Revised ~~deleted~~ Deleted

Substance	External Cause (T-Code)					
	Poisoning, Accidental (Unintentional)	Poisoning, Intentional Self-Harm	Poisoning, Assault	Poisoning, Undetermined	Adverse Effect	Underdosing
Anesthetic NEC *(Continued)*						
local NEC	T41.3X1	T41.3X2	T41.3X3	T41.3X4	T41.3X5	T41.3X6
rectal	T41.201	T41.202	T41.203	T41.204	T41.205	T41.206
general	T41.201	T41.202	T41.203	T41.204	T41.205	T41.206
local	T41.3X1	T41.3X2	T41.3X3	T41.3X4	T41.3X5	T41.3X6
regional NEC	T41.3X1	T41.3X2	T41.3X3	T41.3X4	T41.3X5	T41.3X6
spinal NEC	T41.3X1	T41.3X2	T41.3X3	T41.3X4	T41.3X5	T41.3X6
thiobarbiturate	T41.1X1	T41.1X2	T41.1X3	T41.1X4	T41.1X5	T41.1X6
topical	T41.3X1	T41.3X2	T41.3X3	T41.3X4	T41.3X5	T41.3X6
Aneurine	T45.2X1	T45.2X2	T45.2X3	T45.2X4	T45.2X5	T45.2X6
Angio-Conray	T50.8X1	T50.8X2	T50.8X3	T50.8X4	T50.8X5	T50.8X6
Angiotensin	T44.5X1	T44.5X2	T44.5X3	T44.5X4	T44.5X5	T44.5X6
Angiotensinamide	T44.991	T44.992	T44.993	T44.994	T44.995	T44.996
Anhydrohydroxy-progesterone	T38.5X1	T38.5X2	T38.5X3	T38.5X4	T38.5X5	T38.5X6
Anhydron	T50.2X1	T50.2X2	T50.2X3	T50.2X4	T50.2X5	T50.2X6
Anileridine	T40.4X1	T40.4X2	T40.4X3	T40.4X4	T40.4X5	T40.4X6
Aniline (dye) (liquid)	T65.3X1	T65.3X2	T65.3X3	T65.3X4	—	—
analgesic	T39.1X1	T39.1X2	T39.1X3	T39.1X4	T39.1X5	T39.1X6
derivatives, therapeutic NEC	T39.1X1	T39.1X2	T39.1X3	T39.1X4	T39.1X5	T39.1X6
vapor	T65.3X1	T65.3X2	T65.3X3	T65.3X4	—	—
Anise oil	T47.5X1	T47.5X2	T47.5X3	T47.5X4	T47.5X5	T47.5X6
Aniscoropine	T44.3X1	T44.3X2	T44.3X3	T44.3X4	T44.3X5	T44.3X6
Anisidine	T65.3X1	T65.3X2	T65.3X3	T65.3X4	—	—
Anisindione	T45.511	T45.512	T45.513	T45.514	T45.515	T45.516
Anisotropine methyl-bromide	T44.3X1	T44.3X2	T44.3X3	T44.3X4	T44.3X5	T44.3X6
Anistreplase	T45.611	T45.612	T45.613	T45.614	T45.615	T45.616
Anorexiant (central)	T50.5X1	T50.5X2	T50.5X3	T50.5X4	T50.5X5	T50.5X6
Anorexic agents	T50.5X1	T50.5X2	T50.5X3	T50.5X4	T50.5X5	T50.5X6
Ansamycin	T36.6X1	T36.6X2	T36.6X3	T36.6X4	T36.6X5	T36.6X6
Ant (bite) (sting)	T63.421	T63.422	T63.423	T63.424	—	—
Antabuse	T50.6X1	T50.6X2	T50.6X3	T50.6X4	T50.6X5	T50.6X6
Ant poison — *see Insecticide*						
Antacid NEC	T47.1X1	T47.1X2	T47.1X3	T47.1X4	T47.1X5	T47.1X6
Antagonist						
Aldosterone	T50.0X1	T50.0X2	T50.0X3	T50.0X4	T50.0X5	T50.0X6
alpha-adrenoreceptor	T44.6X1	T44.6X2	T44.6X3	T44.6X4	T44.6X5	T44.6X6
anticoagulant	T45.7X1	T45.7X2	T45.7X3	T45.7X4	T45.7X5	T45.7X6
beta-adrenoreceptor	T44.7X1	T44.7X2	T44.7X3	T44.7X4	T44.7X5	T44.7X6
extrapyramidal NEC	T44.3X1	T44.3X2	T44.3X3	T44.3X4	T44.3X5	T44.3X6
folic acid	T45.1X1	T45.1X2	T45.1X3	T45.1X4	T45.1X5	T45.1X6

◀ New   ◀— Revised   ~~deleted~~ Deleted

TABLE OF DRUGS AND CHEMICALS

Substance	External Cause (T-Code)					
	Poisoning, Accidental (Unintentional)	Poisoning, Intentional Self-Harm	Poisoning, Assault	Poisoning, Undetermined	Adverse Effect	Underdosing
Antagonist *(Continued)*						
H2 receptor	T47.0X1	T47.0X2	T47.0X3	T47.0X4	T47.0X5	T47.0X6
heavy metal	T45.8X1	T45.8X2	T45.8X3	T45.8X4	T45.8X5	T45.8X6
narcotic analgesic	T50.7X1	T50.7X2	T50.7X3	T50.7X4	T50.7X5	T50.7X6
opiate	T50.7X1	T50.7X2	T50.7X3	T50.7X4	T50.7X5	T50.7X6
pyrimidine	T45.1X1	T45.1X2	T45.1X3	T45.1X4	T45.1X5	T45.1X6
serotonin	T46.5X1	T46.5X2	T46.5X3	T46.5X4	T46.5X5	T46.5X6
Antazolin(e)	T45.0X1	T45.0X2	T45.0X3	T45.0X4	T45.0X5	T45.0X6
Anterior pituitary hormone NEC	T38.811	T38.812	T38.813	T38.814	T38.815	T38.816
Anthelmintic NEC	T37.4X1	T37.4X2	T37.4X3	T37.4X4	T37.4X5	T37.4X6
Anthiolimine	T37.4X1	T37.4X2	T37.4X3	T37.4X4	T37.4X5	T37.4X6
Anthralin	T49.4X1	T49.4X2	T49.4X3	T49.4X4	T49.4X5	T49.4X6
Anthramycin	T45.1X1	T45.1X2	T45.1X3	T45.1X4	T45.1X5	T45.1X6
Antiadrenergic NEC	T44.8X1	T44.8X2	T44.8X3	T44.8X4	T44.8X5	T44.8X6
Antiallergic NEC	T45.0X1	T45.0X2	T45.0X3	T45.0X4	T45.0X5	T45.0X6
Anti-anemic (drug) (preparation)	T45.8X1	T45.8X2	T45.8X3	T45.8X4	T45.8X5	T45.8X6
Antiandrogen NEC	T38.6X1	T38.6X2	T38.6X3	T38.6X4	T38.6X5	T38.6X6
Antianxiety drug NEC	T43.501	T43.502	T43.503	T43.504	T43.505	T43.506
Antiaris toxicaria	T65.891	T65.892	T65.893	T65.894	—	—
Antiarteriosclerotic drug	T46.6X1	T46.6X2	T46.6X3	T46.6X4	T46.6X5	T46.6X6
Antiasthmatic drug NEC	T48.6X1	T48.6X2	T48.6X3	T48.6X4	T48.6X5	T48.6X6
Antibiotic NEC	T36.91	T36.92	T36.93	T36.94	T36.95	T36.96
aminoglycoside	T36.5X1	T36.5X2	T36.5X3	T36.5X4	T36.5X5	T36.5X6
anticancer	T45.1X1	T45.1X2	T45.1X3	T45.1X4	T45.1X5	T45.1X6
antifungal	T36.7X1	T36.7X2	T36.7X3	T36.7X4	T36.7X5	T36.7X6
antimycobacterial	T36.5X1	T36.5X2	T36.5X3	T36.5X4	T36.5X5	T36.5X6
antineoplastic	T45.1X1	T45.1X2	T45.1X3	T45.1X4	T45.1X5	T45.1X6
cephalosporin (group)	T36.1X1	T36.1X2	T36.1X3	T36.1X4	T36.1X5	T36.1X6
chloramphenicol (group)	T36.2X1	T36.2X2	T36.2X3	T36.2X4	T36.2X5	T36.2X6
ENT	T49.6X1	T49.6X2	T49.6X3	T49.6X4	T49.6X5	T49.6X6
eye	T49.5X1	T49.5X2	T49.5X3	T49.5X4	T49.5X5	T49.5X6
fungicidal (local)	T49.0X1	T49.0X2	T49.0X3	T49.0X4	T49.0X5	T49.0X6
intestinal	T36.8X1	T36.8X2	T36.8X3	T36.8X4	T36.8X5	T36.8X6
b-lactam NEC	T36.1X1	T36.1X2	T36.1X3	T36.1X4	T36.1X5	T36.1X6
local	T49.0X1	T49.0X2	T49.0X3	T49.0X4	T49.0X5	T49.0X6
macrolides	T36.3X1	T36.3X2	T36.3X3	T36.3X4	T36.3X5	T36.3X6
polypeptide	T36.8X1	T36.8X2	T36.8X3	T36.8X4	T36.8X5	T36.8X6
specified NEC	T36.8X1	T36.8X2	T36.8X3	T36.8X4	T36.8X5	T36.8X6
tetracycline (group)	T36.4X1	T36.4X2	T36.4X3	T36.4X4	T36.4X5	T36.4X6
throat	T49.6X1	T49.6X2	T49.6X3	T49.6X4	T49.6X5	T49.6X6

◄ New ◀ Revised ~~deleted~~ Deleted

Substance	External Cause (T-Code)					
	Poisoning, Accidental (Unintentional)	Poisoning, Intentional Self-Harm	Poisoning, Assault	Poisoning, Undetermined	Adverse Effect	Underdosing
Anticancer agents NEC	T45.1X1	T45.1X2	T45.1X3	T45.1X4	T45.1X5	T45.1X6
Anticholesterolemic drug NEC	T46.6X1	T46.6X2	T46.6X3	T46.6X4	T46.6X5	T46.6X6
Anticholinergic NEC	T44.3X1	T44.3X2	T44.3X3	T44.3X4	T44.3X5	T44.3X6
Anticholinesterase	T44.0X1	T44.0X2	T44.0X3	T44.0X4	T44.0X5	T44.0X6
organophosphorus	T44.0X1	T44.0X2	T44.0X3	T44.0X4	T44.0X5	T44.0X6
insecticide	T60.0X1	T60.0X2	T60.0X3	T60.0X4	—	—
nerve gas	T59.891	T59.892	T59.893	T59.894	—	—
reversible	T44.0X1	T44.0X2	T44.0X3	T44.0X4	T44.0X5	T44.0X6
ophthalmological	T49.5X1	T49.5X2	T49.5X3	T49.5X4	T49.5X5	T49.5X6
Anticoagulant NEC	T45.511	T45.512	T45.513	T45.514	T45.515	T45.516
Antagonist	T45.7X1	T45.7X2	T45.7X3	T45.7X4	T45.7X5	T45.7X6
Anti-common-cold drug NEC	T48.5X1	T48.5X2	T48.5X3	T48.5X4	T48.5X5	T48.5X6
Anticonvulsant	T42.71	T42.72	T42.73	T42.74	T42.75	T42.76
barbiturate	T42.3X1	T42.3X2	T42.3X3	T42.3X4	T42.3X5	T42.3X6
combination (with barbiturate)	T42.3X1	T42.3X2	T42.3X3	T42.3X4	T42.3X5	T42.3X6
hydantoin	T42.0X1	T42.0X2	T42.0X3	T42.0X4	T42.0X5	T42.0X6
hypnotic NEC	T42.6X1	T42.6X2	T42.6X3	T42.6X4	T42.6X5	T42.6X6
oxazolidinedione	T42.2X1	T42.2X2	T42.2X3	T42.2X4	T42.2X5	T42.2X6
pyrimidinedione	T42.6X1	T42.6X2	T42.6X3	T42.6X4	T42.6X5	T42.6X6
specified NEC	T42.6X1	T42.6X2	T42.6X3	T42.6X4	T42.6X5	T42.6X6
succinimide	T42.2X1	T42.2X2	T42.2X3	T42.2X4	T42.2X5	T42.2X6
Anti-D immunoglobulin (human)	T50.Z11	T50.Z12	T50.Z13	T50.Z14	T50.Z15	T50.Z16
Antidepressant NEC	T43.201	T43.202	T43.203	T43.204	T43.205	T43.206
monoamine oxidase inhibitor	T43.1X1	T43.1X2	T43.1X3	T43.1X4	T43.1X5	T43.1X6
selective serotonin norepinephrine reuptake inhibitor	T43.211	T43.212	T43.213	T43.214	T43.215	T43.216
selective serotonin reuptake inhibitor	T43.221	T43.222	T43.223	T43.224	T43.225	T43.226
specified NEC	T43.291	T43.292	T43.293	T43.294	T43.295	T43.296
tetracyclic	T43.021	T43.022	T43.023	T43.024	T43.025	T43.026
triazolopyridine	T43.221	T43.222	T43.223	T43.224	T43.225	T43.226
tricyclic	T43.011	T43.012	T43.013	T43.014	T43.015	T43.016
Antidiabetic NEC	T38.3X1	T38.3X2	T38.3X3	T38.3X4	T38.3X5	T38.3X6
biguanide	T38.3X1	T38.3X2	T38.3X3	T38.3X4	T38.3X5	T38.3X6
and sulfonyl combined	T38.3X1	T38.3X2	T38.3X3	T38.3X4	T38.3X5	T38.3X6
combined	T38.3X1	T38.3X2	T38.3X3	T38.3X4	T38.3X5	T38.3X6
sulfonylurea	T38.3X1	T38.3X2	T38.3X3	T38.3X4	T38.3X5	T38.3X6
Antidiarrheal drug NEC	T47.6X1	T47.6X2	T47.6X3	T47.6X4	T47.6X5	T47.6X6
absorbent	T47.6X1	T47.6X2	T47.6X3	T47.6X4	T47.6X5	T47.6X6
Antidiphtheria serum	T50.Z11	T50.Z12	T50.Z13	T50.Z14	T50.Z15	T50.Z16
Antidiuretic hormone	T38.891	T38.892	T38.893	T38.894	T38.895	T38.896

TABLE OF DRUGS AND CHEMICALS

TABLE OF DRUGS AND CHEMICALS

Substance	External Cause (T-Code)					
	Poisoning, Accidental (Unintentional)	Poisoning, Intentional Self-Harm	Poisoning, Assault	Poisoning, Undetermined	Adverse Effect	Underdosing
Antidote NEC	T50.6X1	T50.6X2	T50.6X3	T50.6X4	T50.6X5	T50.6X6
heavy metal	T45.8X1	T45.8X2	T45.8X3	T45.8X4	T45.8X5	T45.8X6
Antidysrhythmic NEC	T46.2X1	T46.2X2	T46.2X3	T46.2X4	T46.2X5	T46.2X6
Antiemetic drug	T45.0X1	T45.0X2	T45.0X3	T45.0X4	T45.0X5	T45.0X6
Antiepilepsy agent	T42.71	T42.72	T42.73	T42.74	T42.75	T42.76
combination	T42.5X1	T42.5X2	T42.5X2	T42.5X4	T42.5X5	T42.5X6
mixed	T42.5X1	T42.5X2	T42.5X3	T42.5X4	T42.5X5	T42.5X6
specified, NEC	T42.6X1	T42.6X2	T42.6X3	T42.6X4	T42.6X5	T42.6X6
Antiestrogen NEC	T38.6X1	T38.6X2	T38.6X3	T38.6X4	T38.6X5	T38.6X6
Antifertility pill	T38.4X1	T38.4X2	T38.4X3	T38.4X4	T38.4X5	T38.4X6
Antifibrinolytic drug	T45.621	T45.622	T45.623	T45.624	T45.625	T45.626
Antifilarial drug	T37.4X1	T37.4X2	T37.4X3	T37.4X4	T37.4X5	T37.4X6
Antiflatulent	T47.5X1	T47.5X2	T47.5X3	T47.5X4	T47.5X5	T47.5X6
Antifreeze	T65.91	T65.92	T65.93	T65.94	—	—
alcohol	T51.1X1	T51.1X2	T51.1X3	T51.1X4	—	—
ethylene glycol	T51.8X1	T51.8X2	T51.8X3	T51.8X4	—	—
Antifungal						
antibiotic (systemic)	T36.7X1	T36.7X2	T36.7X3	T36.7X4	T36.7X5	T36.7X6
anti-infective NEC	T37.91	T37.92	T37.93	T37.94	T37.95	T37.96
disinfectant, local	T49.0X1	T49.0X2	T49.0X3	T49.0X4	T49.0X5	T49.0X6
nonmedicinal (spray)	T60.3X1	T60.3X2	T60.3X3	T60.3X4	—	—
topical	T49.0X1	T49.0X2	T49.0X3	T49.0X4	T49.0X5	T49.0X6
Anti-gastric-secretion drug NEC	T47.1X1	T47.1X2	T47.1X3	T47.1X4	T47.1X5	T47.1X6
Antigonadotrophin NEC	T38.6X1	T38.6X2	T38.6X3	T38.6X4	T38.6X5	T38.6X6
Antihallucinogen	T43.501	T43.502	T43.503	T43.504	T43.505	T43.506
Antihelmintics	T37.4X1	T37.4X2	T37.4X3	T37.4X4	T37.4X5	T37.4X6
Antihemophilic						
factor	T45.8X1	T45.8X2	T45.8X3	T45.8X4	T45.8X5	T45.8X6
fraction	T45.8X1	T45.8X2	T45.8X3	T45.8X4	T45.8X5	T45.8X6
globulin concentrate	T45.7X1	T45.7X2	T45.7X3	T45.7X4	T45.7X5	T45.7X6
human plasma	T45.8X1	T45.8X2	T45.8X3	T45.8X4	T45.8X5	T45.8X6
plasma, dried	T45.7X1	T45.7X2	T45.7X3	T45.7X4	T45.7X5	T45.7X6
Antihemorrhoidal preparation	T49.2X1	T49.2X2	T49.2X3	T49.2X4	T49.2X5	T49.2X6
Antiheparin drug	T45.7X1	T45.7X2	T45.7X3	T45.7X4	T45.7X5	T45.7X6
Antihistamine	T45.0X1	T45.0X2	T45.0X3	T45.0X4	T45.0X5	T45.0X6
Antihookworm drug	T37.4X1	T37.4X2	T37.4X3	T37.4X4	T37.4X5	T37.4X6
Anti-human lymphocytic globulin	T50.Z11	T50.Z12	T50.Z13	T50.Z14	T50.Z15	T50.Z16
Antihyperlipidemic drug	T46.6X1	T46.6X2	T46.6X3	T46.6X4	T46.6X5	T46.6X6
Antihypertensive drug NEC	T46.5X1	T46.5X2	T46.5X3	T46.5X4	T46.5X5	T46.5X6

◀ New ◀▥ Revised ~~deleted~~ Deleted

	External Cause (T-Code)					
Substance	Poisoning, Accidental (Unintentional)	Poisoning, Intentional Self-Harm	Poisoning, Assault	Poisoning, Undetermined	Adverse Effect	Underdosing
Anti-infective NEC	T37.91	T37.92	T37.93	T37.94	T37.95	T37.96
anthelmintic	T37.4X1	T37.4X2	T37.4X3	T37.4X4	T37.4X5	T37.4X6
antibiotics	T36.91	T36.92	T36.93	T36.94	T36.95	T36.96
specified NEC	T36.8X1	T36.8X2	T36.8X3	T36.8X4	T36.8X5	T36.8X6
antimalarial	T37.2X1	T37.2X2	T37.2X3	T37.2X4	T37.2X5	T37.2X6
antimycobacterial NEC	T37.1X1	T37.1X2	T37.1X3	T37.1X4	T37.1X5	T37.1X6
antibiotics	T36.5X1	T36.5X2	T36.5X3	T36.5X4	T36.5X5	T36.5X6
antiprotozoal NEC	T37.3X1	T37.3X2	T37.3X3	T37.3X4	T37.3X5	T37.3X6
blood	T37.2X1	T37.2X2	T37.2X3	T37.2X4	T37.2X5	T37.2X6
antiviral	T37.5X1	T37.5X2	T37.5X3	T37.5X4	T37.5X5	T37.5X6
arsenical	T37.8X1	T37.8X2	T37.8X3	T37.8X4	T37.8X5	T37.8X6
bismuth, local	T49.0X1	T49.0X2	T49.0X3	T49.0X4	T49.0X5	T49.0X6
ENT	T49.6X1	T49.6X2	T49.6X3	T49.6X4	T49.6X5	T49.6X6
eye NEC	T49.5X1	T49.5X2	T49.5X3	T49.5X4	T49.5X5	T49.5X6
heavy metals NEC	T37.8X1	T37.8X2	T37.8X3	T37.8X4	T37.8X5	T37.8X6
local NEC	T49.0X1	T49.0X2	T49.0X3	T49.0X4	T49.0X5	T49.0X6
specified NEC	T49.0X1	T49.0X2	T49.0X3	T49.0X4	T49.0X5	T49.0X6
mixed	T37.91	T37.92	T37.93	T37.94	T37.95	T37.96
ophthalmic preparation	T49.5X1	T49.5X2	T49.5X3	T49.5X4	T49.5X5	T49.5X6
topical NEC	T49.0X1	T49.0X2	T49.0X3	T49.0X4	T49.0X5	T49.0X6
Anti-inflammatory drug NEC	T49.0X1	T49.0X2	T49.0X3	T49.0X4	T49.0X5	T49.0X6
local	T49.0X1	T49.0X2	T49.0X3	T49.0X4	T49.0X5	T49.0X6
nonsteroidal NEC	T39.391	T39.392	T39.393	T39.394	T39.395	T39.396
propionic acid derivative	T39.311	T39.312	T39.313	T39.314	T39.315	T39.316
specified NEC	T39.391	T39.392	T39.393	T39.394	T39.395	T39.396
Antikaluretic	T50.3X1	T50.3X2	T50.3X3	T50.3X4	T50.3X5	T50.3X6
Antiknock (tetraethyl lead)	T56.0X1	T56.0X2	T56.0X3	T56.0X4	—	—
Antilipemic drug NEC	T46.6X1	T46.6X2	T46.6X3	T46.6X4	T46.6X5	T46.6X6
Antimalarial	T37.2X1	T37.2X2	T37.2X3	T37.2X4	T37.2X5	T37.2X6
prophylactic NEC	T37.2X1	T37.2X2	T37.2X3	T37.2X4	T37.2X5	T37.2X6
pyrimidine derivative	T37.2X1	T37.2X2	T37.2X3	T37.2X4	T37.2X5	T37.2X6
Antimetabolite	T45.1X1	T45.1X2	T45.1X3	T45.1X4	T45.1X5	T45.1X6
Antimitotic agent	T45.1X1	T45.1X2	T45.1X3	T45.1X4	T45.1X5	T45.1X6
Antimony (compounds) (vapor) NEC	T56.891	T56.892	T56.893	T56.894	—	—
anti-infectives	T37.8X1	T37.8X2	T37.8X3	T37.8X4	T37.8X5	T37.8X6
dimercaptosuccinate	T37.3X1	T37.3X2	T37.3X3	T37.3X4	T37.3X5	T37.3X6
hydride	T56.891	T56.892	T56.893	T56.894	—	—
pesticide (vapor)	T60.8X1	T60.8X2	T60.8X3	T60.8X4	—	—
potassium (sodium) tartrate	T37.8X1	T37.8X2	T37.8X3	T37.8X4	T37.8X5	T37.8X6

Substance	External Cause (T-Code)					
	Poisoning, Accidental (Unintentional)	Poisoning, Intentional Self-Harm	Poisoning, Assault	Poisoning, Undetermined	Adverse Effect	Underdosing
Antimony NEC *(Continued)*						
sodium dimercaptosuccinate	T37.3X1	T37.3X2	T37.3X3	T37.3X4	T37.3X5	T37.3X6
tartrated	T37.8X1	T37.8X2	T37.8X3	T37.8X4	T37.8X5	T37.8X6
Antimuscarinic NEC	T44.3X1	T44.3X2	T44.3X3	T44.3X4	T44.3X5	T44.3X6
Antimycobacterial drug NEC	T37.1X1	T37.1X2	T37.1X3	T37.1X4	T37.1X5	T37.1X6
antibiotics	T36.5X1	T36.5X2	T36.5X3	T36.5X4	T36.5X5	T36.5X6
combination	T37.1X1	T37.1X2	T37.1X3	T37.1X4	T37.1X5	T37.1X6
Antinausea drug	T45.0X1	T45.0X2	T45.0X3	T45.0X4	T45.0X5	T45.0X6
Antinematode drug	T37.4X1	T37.4X2	T37.4X3	T37.4X4	T37.4X5	T37.4X6
Antineoplastic NEC	T45.1X1	T45.1X2	T45.1X3	T45.1X4	T45.1X5	T45.1X6
alkaloidal	T45.1X1	T45.1X2	T45.1X3	T45.1X4	T45.1X5	T45.1X6
antibiotics	T45.1X1	T45.1X2	T45.1X3	T45.1X4	T45.1X5	T45.1X6
combination	T45.1X1	T45.1X2	T45.1X3	T45.1X4	T45.1X5	T45.1X6
estrogen	T38.5X1	T38.5X2	T38.5X3	T38.5X4	T38.5X5	T38.5X6
steroid	T38.7X1	T38.7X2	T38.7X3	T38.7X4	T38.7X5	T38.7X6
Antiparasitic drug (systemic)	T37.91	T37.92	T37.93	T37.94	T37.95	T37.96
local	T49.0X1	T49.0X2	T49.0X3	T49.0X4	T49.0X5	T49.0X6
specified NEC	T37.8X1	T37.8X2	T37.8X3	T37.8X4	T37.8X5	T37.8X6
Antiparkinsonism drug NEC	T42.8X1	T42.8X2	T42.8X3	T42.8X4	T42.8X5	T42.8X6
Antiperspirant NEC	T49.2X1	T49.2X2	T49.2X3	T49.2X4	T49.2X5	T49.2X6
Antiphlogistic NEC	T39.4X1	T39.4X2	T39.4X3	T39.4X4	T39.4X5	T39.4X6
Antiplatyhelmintic drug	T37.4X1	T37.4X2	T37.4X3	T37.4X4	T37.4X5	T37.4X6
Antiprotozoal drug NEC	T37.3X1	T37.3X2	T37.3X3	T37.3X4	T37.3X5	T37.3X6
blood	T37.2X1	T37.2X2	T37.2X3	T37.2X4	T37.2X5	T37.2X6
local	T49.0X1	T49.0X2	T49.0X3	T49.0X4	T49.0X5	T49.0X6
Antipruritic drug NEC	T49.1X1	T49.1X2	T49.1X3	T49.1X4	T49.1X5	T49.1X6
Antipsychotic drug	T43.501	T43.502	T43.503	T43.504	T43.505	T43.506
specified NEC	T43.591	T43.592	T43.593	T43.594	T43.595	T43.596
Antipyretic	T39.91	T39.92	T39.93	T39.94	T39.95	T39.96
specified NEC	T39.8X1	T39.8X2	T39.8X3	T39.8X4	T39.8X5	T39.8X6
Antipyrine	T39.2X1	T39.2X2	T39.2X3	T39.2X4	T39.2X5	T39.2X6
Antirabies hyperimmune serum	T50.Z11	T50.Z12	T50.Z13	T50.Z14	T50.Z15	T50.Z16
Antirheumatic NEC	T39.4X1	T39.4X2	T39.4X3	T39.4X4	T39.4X5	T39.4X6
Antirigidity drug NEC	T42.8X1	T42.8X2	T42.8X3	T42.8X4	T42.8X5	T42.8X6
Antischistosomal drug	T37.4X1	T37.4X2	T37.4X3	T37.4X4	T37.4X5	T37.4X6
Antiscorpion sera	T50.Z11	T50.Z12	T50.Z13	T50.Z14	T50.Z15	T50.Z16
Antiseborrheics	T49.4X1	T49.4X2	T49.4X3	T49.4X4	T49.4X5	T49.4X6
Antiseptics (external) (medicinal)	T49.0X1	T49.0X2	T49.0X3	T49.0X4	T49.0X5	T49.0X6
Antistine	T45.0X1	T45.0X2	T45.0X3	T45.0X4	T45.0X5	T45.0X6
Antitapeworm drug	T37.4X1	T37.4X2	T37.4X3	T37.4X4	T37.4X5	T37.4X6

◀ New   ◀▥ Revised   ~~deleted~~ Deleted

Substance	External Cause (T-Code)					
	Poisoning, Accidental (Unintentional)	Poisoning, Intentional Self-Harm	Poisoning, Assault	Poisoning, Undetermined	Adverse Effect	Underdosing
Antitetanus immunoglobulin	T50.Z11	T50.Z12	T50.Z13	T50.Z14	T50.Z15	T50.Z16
Antithyroid drug NEC	T38.2X1	T38.2X2	T38.2X3	T38.2X4	T38.2X5	T38.2X6
Antitoxin	T50.Z11	T50.Z12	T50.Z13	T50.Z14	T50.Z15	T50.Z16
diphtheria	T50.Z11	T50.Z12	T50.Z13	T50.Z14	T50.Z15	T50.Z16
gas gangrene	T50.Z11	T50.Z12	T50.Z13	T50.Z14	T50.Z15	T50.Z16
tetanus	T50.Z11	T50.Z12	T50.Z13	T50.Z14	T50.Z15	T50.Z16
Antitoxin, any	T50.901	T50.902	T50.903	T50.904	T50.905	T50.906
Antitrichomonal drug	T37.3X1	T37.3X2	T37.3X3	T37.3X4	T37.3X5	T37.3X6
Antituberculars	T37.1X1	T37.1X2	T37.1X3	T37.1X4	T37.1X5	T37.1X6
antibiotics	T36.5X1	T36.5X2	T36.5X3	T36.5X4	T36.5X5	T36.5X6
Antitussive NEC	T48.3X1	T48.3X2	T48.3X3	T48.3X4	T48.3X5	T48.3X6
codeine mixture	T40.2X1	T40.2X2	T40.2X3	T40.2X4	T40.2X5	T40.2X6
opiate	T40.2X1	T40.2X2	T40.2X3	T40.2X4	T40.2X5	T40.2X6
Antivaricose drug	T46.8X1	T46.8X2	T46.8X3	T46.8X4	T46.8X5	T46.8X6
Antivenin, antivenom (sera)	T50.Z11	T50.Z12	T50.Z13	T50.Z14	T50.Z15	T50.Z16
crotaline	T50.Z11	T50.Z12	T50.Z13	T50.Z14	T50.Z15	T50.Z16
spider bite	T50.Z11	T50.Z12	T50.Z13	T50.Z14	T50.Z15	T50.Z16
Antivertigo drug	T45.0X1	T45.0X2	T45.0X3	T45.0X4	T45.0X5	T45.0X6
Antiviral drug NEC	T37.5X1	T37.5X2	T37.5X3	T37.5X4	T37.5X5	T37.5X6
eye	T49.5X1	T49.5X2	T49.5X3	T49.5X4	T49.5X5	T49.5X6
Antiwhipworm drug	T37.4X1	T37.4X2	T37.4X3	T37.4X4	T37.4X5	T37.4X6
Ant poisons — see Pesticides						
Antrol — see also by specific chemical substance	T60.91	T60.92	T60.93	T60.94	—	—
fungicide	T60.91	T60.92	T60.93	T60.94	—	—
ANTU (alpha naphthylthiourea)	T60.4X1	T60.4X2	T60.4X3	T60.4X4	—	—
Apalcillin	T36.0X1	T36.0X2	T36.0X3	T36.0X4	T36.0X5	T36.0X6
APC	T48.5X1	T48.5X2	T48.5X3	T48.5X4	T48.5X5	T48.5X6
Aplonidine	T44.4X1	T44.4X2	T44.4X3	T44.4X4	T44.4X5	T44.4X6
Apomorphine	T47.7X1	T47.7X2	T47.7X3	T47.7X4	T47.7X5	T47.7X6
Appetite depressants, central	T50.5X1	T50.5X2	T50.5X3	T50.5X4	T50.5X5	T50.5X6
Apraclonidine (hydrochloride)	T44.4X1	T44.4X2	T44.4X3	T44.4X4	T44.4X5	T44.4X6
Apresoline	T46.5X1	T46.5X2	T46.5X3	T46.5X4	T46.5X5	T46.5X6
Aprindine	T46.2X1	T46.2X2	T46.2X3	T46.2X4	T46.2X5	T46.2X6
Aprobarbital	T42.3X1	T42.3X2	T42.3X3	T42.3X4	T42.3X5	T42.3X6
Apronalide	T42.6X1	T42.6X2	T42.6X3	T42.6X4	T42.6X5	T42.6X6
Aprotinin	T45.621	T45.622	T45.623	T45.624	T45.625	T45.626
Aptocaine	T41.3X1	T41.3X2	T41.3X3	T41.3X4	T41.3X5	T41.3X6
Aqua fortis	T54.2X1	T54.2X2	T54.2X3	T54.2X4	—	—
Ara-A	T37.5X1	T37.5X2	T37.5X3	T37.5X4	T37.5X5	T37.5X6
Ara-C	T45.1X1	T45.1X2	T45.1X3	T45.1X4	T45.1X5	T45.1X6

◀ New ◀▥ Revised ~~deleted~~ Deleted

Substance	Poisoning, Accidental (Unintentional)	Poisoning, Intentional Self-Harm	Poisoning, Assault	Poisoning, Undetermined	Adverse Effect	Underdosing
Arachis oil	T49.3X1	T49.3X2	T49.3X3	T49.3X4	T49.3X5	T49.3X6
cathartic	T47.4X1	T47.4X2	T47.4X3	T47.4X4	T47.4X5	T47.4X6
Aralen	T37.2X1	T37.2X2	T37.2X3	T37.2X4	T37.2X5	T37.2X6
Arecoline	T44.1X1	T44.1X2	T44.1X3	T44.1X4	T44.1X5	T44.1X6
Arginine	T50.991	T50.992	T50.993	T50.994	T50.995	T50.996
glutamate	T50.991	T50.992	T50.993	T50.994	T50.995	T50.996
Argyrol	T49.0X1	T49.0X2	T49.0X3	T49.0X4	T49.0X5	T49.0X6
ENT agent	T49.6X1	T49.6X2	T49.6X3	T49.6X4	T49.6X5	T49.6X6
ophthalmic preparation	T49.5X1	T49.5X2	T49.5X3	T49.5X4	T49.5X5	T49.5X6
Aristocort	T38.0X1	T38.0X2	T38.0X3	T38.0X4	T38.0X5	T38.0X6
ENT agent	T49.6X1	T49.6X2	T49.6X3	T49.6X4	T49.6X5	T49.6X6
ophthalmic preparation	T49.5X1	T49.5X2	T49.5X3	T49.5X4	T49.5X5	T49.5X6
topical NEC	T49.0X1	T49.0X2	T49.0X3	T49.0X4	T49.0X5	T49.0X6
Aromatics, corrosive	T54.1X1	T54.1X2	T54.1X3	T54.1X4	—	—
disinfectants	T54.1X1	T54.1X2	T54.1X3	T54.1X4	—	—
Arsenate of lead	T57.0X1	T57.0X2	T57.0X3	T57.0X4	—	—
herbicide	T57.0X1	T57.0X2	T57.0X3	T57.0X4	—	—
Arsenic, arsenicals (compounds) (dust) (vapor) NEC	T57.0X1	T57.0X2	T57.0X3	T57.0X4	—	—
anti-infectives	T37.8X1	T37.8X2	T37.8X3	T37.8X4	T37.8X5	T37.8X6
pesticide (dust) (fumes)	T57.0X1	T57.0X2	T57.0X3	T57.0X4	—	—
Arsine (gas)	T57.0X1	T57.0X2	T57.0X3	T57.0X4	—	—
Arsphenamine (silver)	T37.8X1	T37.8X2	T37.8X3	T37.8X4	T37.8X5	T37.8X6
Arsthinol	T37.3X1	T37.3X2	T37.3X3	T37.3X4	T37.3X5	T37.3X6
Artane	T44.3X1	T44.3X2	T44.3X3	T44.3X4	T44.3X5	T44.3X6
Arthropod (venomous) NEC	T63.481	T63.482	T63.483	T63.484	—	—
Articaine	T41.3X1	T41.3X2	T41.3X3	T41.3X4	T41.3X5	T41.3X6
Asbestos	T57.8X1	T57.8X2	T57.8X3	T57.8X4	—	—
Ascaridole	T37.4X1	T37.4X2	T37.4X3	T37.4X4	T37.4X5	T37.4X6
Ascorbic acid	T45.2X1	T45.2X2	T45.2X3	T45.2X4	T45.2X5	T45.2X6
Asiaticoside	T49.0X1	T49.0X2	T49.0X3	T49.0X4	T49.0X5	T49.0X6
Asparaginase	T45.1X1	T45.1X2	T45.1X3	T45.1X4	T45.1X5	T45.1X6
Aspidium (oleoresin)	T37.4X1	T37.4X2	T37.4X3	T37.4X4	T37.4X5	T37.4X6
Aspirin (aluminum) (soluble)	T39.011	T39.012	T39.013	T39.014	T39.015	T39.016
Aspoxicillin	T36.0X1	T36.0X2	T36.0X3	T36.0X4	T36.0X5	T36.0X6
Astemizole	T45.0X1	T45.0X2	T45.0X3	T45.0X4	T45.0X5	T45.0X6
Astringent (local)	T49.2X1	T49.2X2	T49.2X3	T49.2X4	T49.2X5	T49.2X6
specified NEC	T49.2X1	T49.2X2	T49.2X3	T49.2X4	T49.2X5	T49.2X6
Astromicin	T36.5X1	T36.5X2	T36.5X3	T36.5X4	T36.5X5	T36.5X6
Ataractic drug NEC	T43.501	T43.502	T43.503	T43.504	T43.505	T43.506

◀ New   ◀= Revised   ~~deleted~~ Deleted

Substance	External Cause (T-Code)					
	Poisoning, Accidental (Unintentional)	Poisoning, Intentional Self-Harm	Poisoning, Assault	Poisoning, Undetermined	Adverse Effect	Underdosing
Atenolol	T44.7X1	T44.7X2	T44.7X3	T44.7X4	T44.7X5	T44.7X6
Atonia drug, intestinal	T47.4X1	T47.4X2	T47.4X3	T47.4X4	T47.4X5	T47.4X6
Atophan	T50.4X1	T50.4X2	T50.4X3	T50.4X4	T50.4X5	T50.4X6
Atracurium besilate	T48.1X1	T48.1X2	T48.1X3	T48.1X4	T48.1X5	T48.1X6
Atropine	T44.3X1	T44.3X2	T44.3X3	T44.3X4	T44.3X5	T44.3X6
derivative	T44.3X1	T44.3X2	T44.3X3	T44.3X4	T44.3X5	T44.3X6
methonitrate	T44.3X1	T44.3X2	T44.3X3	T44.3X4	T44.3X5	T44.3X6
Attapulgite	T47.6X1	T47.6X2	T47.6X3	T47.6X4	T47.6X5	T47.6X6
Attenuvax	T50.991	T50.992	T50.993	T50.994	T50.995	T50.996
Auramine	T65.891	T65.892	T65.893	T65.894	—	—
dye	T65.6X1	T65.6X2	T65.6X3	T65.6X4	—	—
fungicide	T60.3X1	T60.3X2	T60.3X3	T60.3X4	—	—
Auranofin	T39.4X1	T39.4X2	T39.4X3	T39.4X4	T39.4X5	T39.4X6
Aurantiin	T46.991	T46.992	T46.993	T46.994	T46.995	T46.996
Aureomycin	T36.4X1	T36.4X2	T36.4X3	T36.4X4	T36.4X5	T36.4X6
ophthalmic preparation	T49.5X1	T49.5X2	T49.5X3	T49.5X4	T49.5X5	T49.5X6
topical NEC	T49.0X1	T49.0X2	T49.0X3	T49.0X4	T49.0X5	T49.0X6
Aurothioglucose	T39.4X1	T39.4X2	T39.4X3	T39.4X4	T39.4X5	T39.4X6
Aurothioglycanide	T39.4X1	T39.4X2	T39.4X3	T39.4X4	T39.4X5	T39.4X6
Aurothiomalate sodium	T39.4X1	T39.4X2	T39.4X3	T39.4X4	T39.4X5	T39.4X6
Aurotioprol	T39.4X1	T39.4X2	T39.4X3	T39.4X4	T39.4X5	T39.4X6
Automobile fuel	T52.0X1	T52.0X2	T52.0X3	T52.0X4	—	—
Autonomic nervous system agent NEC	T44.901	T44.902	T44.903	T44.904	T44.905	T44.906
Avlosulfon	T37.1X1	T37.1X2	T37.1X3	T37.1X4	T37.1X5	T37.1X6
Avomine	T42.6X1	T42.6X2	T42.6X3	T42.6X4	T42.6X5	T42.6X6
Axerophthol	T45.2X1	T45.2X2	T45.2X3	T45.2X4	T45.2X5	T45.2X6
Azacitidine	T45.1X1	T45.1X2	T45.1X3	T45.1X4	T45.1X5	T45.1X6
Azacyclonol	T43.591	T43.592	T43.593	T43.594	T43.595	T43.596
Azadirachta	T60.2X1	T60.2X2	T60.2X3	T60.2X4	—	—
Azanidazole	T37.3X1	T37.3X2	T37.3X3	T37.3X4	T37.3X5	T37.3X6
Azapetine	T46.7X1	T46.7X2	T46.7X3	T46.7X4	T46.7X5	T46.7X6
Azapropazone	T39.2X1	T39.2X2	T39.2X3	T39.2X4	T39.2X5	T39.2X6
Azaribine	T45.1X1	T45.1X2	T45.1X3	T45.1X4	T45.1X5	T45.1X6
Azaserine	T45.1X1	T45.1X2	T45.1X3	T45.1X4	T45.1X5	T45.1X6
Azatadine	T45.0X1	T45.0X2	T45.0X3	T45.0X4	T45.0X5	T45.0X6
Azatepa	T45.1X1	T45.1X2	T45.1X3	T45.1X4	T45.1X5	T45.1X6
Azathioprine	T45.1X1	T45.1X2	T45.1X3	T45.1X4	T45.1X5	T45.1X6
Azelaic acid	T49.0X1	T49.0X2	T49.0X3	T49.0X4	T49.0X5	T49.0X6
Azelastine	T45.0X1	T45.0X2	T45.0X3	T45.0X4	T45.0X5	T45.0X6

◄ New   ◄◄ Revised   ~~deleted~~ Deleted

Substance	External Cause (T-Code)					
	Poisoning, Accidental (Unintentional)	Poisoning, Intentional Self-Harm	Poisoning, Assault	Poisoning, Undetermined	Adverse Effect	Underdosing
Azidocillin	T36.0X1	T36.0X2	T36.0X3	T36.0X4	T36.0X5	T36.0X6
Azidothymidine	T37.5X1	T37.5X2	T37.5X3	T37.5X4	T37.5X5	T37.5X6
Azinphos (ethyl) (methyl)	T60.0X1	T60.0X2	T60.0X3	T60.0X4	—	—
Aziridine (chelating)	T54.1X1	T54.1X2	T54.1X3	T54.1X4	—	—
Azithromycin	T36.3X1	T36.3X2	T36.3X3	T36.3X4	T36.3X5	T36.3X6
Azlocillin	T36.01	T36.02	T36.03	T36.04	T36.05	T36.06
Azobenzene smoke	T65.3X1	T65.3X2	T65.3X3	T65.3X4	—	—
acaricide	T60.8X1	T60.8X2	T60.8X3	T60.8X4	—	—
Azosulfamide	T37.0X1	T37.0X2	T37.0X3	T37.0X4	T37.0X5	T37.0X6
AZT	T37.5X1	T37.5X2	T37.5X3	T37.5X4	T37.5X5	T37.5X6
Aztreonam	T36.1X1	T36.1X2	T36.1X3	T36.1X4	T36.1X5	T36.1X6
Azulfidine	T37.0X1	T37.0X2	T37.0X3	T37.0X4	T37.0X5	T37.0X6
Azuresin	T50.8X1	T50.8X2	T50.8X3	T50.8X4	T50.8X5	T50.8X6
B						
Bacampicillin	T36.0X1	T36.0X2	T36.0X3	T36.0X4	T36.0X5	T36.0X6
Bacillus						
lactobacillus	T47.8X1	T47.8X2	T47.8X3	T47.8X4	T47.8X5	T47.8X6
subtilis	T47.6X1	T47.6X2	T47.6X3	T47.6X4	T47.6X5	T47.6X6
Bacimycin	T49.0X1	T49.0X2	T49.0X3	T49.0X4	T49.0X5	T49.0X6
ophthalmic preparation	T49.5X1	T49.5X2	T49.5X3	T49.5X4	T49.5X5	T49.5X6
Bacitracin zinc	T49.0X1	T49.0X2	T49.0X3	T49.0X4	T49.0X5	T49.0X6
with neomycin	T49.0X1	T49.0X2	T49.0X3	T49.0X4	T49.0X5	T49.0X6
ENT agent	T49.6X1	T49.6X2	T49.6X3	T49.6X4	T49.6X5	T49.6X6
ophthalmic preparation	T49.5X1	T49.5X2	T49.5X3	T49.5X4	T49.5X5	T49.5X6
topical NEC	T49.0X1	T49.0X2	T49.0X3	T49.0X4	T49.0X5	T49.0X6
Baclofen	T42.8X1	T42.8X2	T42.8X3	T42.8X4	T42.8X5	T42.8X6
Baking soda	T50.991	T50.992	T50.993	T50.994	T50.995	T50.996
BAL	T45.8X1	T45.8X2	T45.8X3	T45.8X4	T45.8X5	T45.8X6
Bambuterol	T48.6X1	T48.6X2	T48.6X3	T48.6X4	T48.6X5	T48.6X6
Bamethan (sulfate)	T46.7X1	T46.7X2	T46.7X3	T46.7X4	T46.7X5	T46.7X6
Bamifylline	T48.6X1	T48.6X2	T48.6X3	T48.6X4	T48.6X5	T48.6X6
Bamipine	T45.0X1	T45.0X2	T45.0X3	T45.0X4	T45.0X5	T45.0X6
Baneberry — see Actaea spicata						
Banewort — see Belladonna						
Barbenyl	T42.3X1	T42.3X2	T42.3X3	T42.3X4	T42.3X5	T42.3X6
Barbexaclone	T42.6X1	T42.6X2	T42.6X3	T42.6X4	T42.6X5	T42.6X6
Barbital	T42.3X1	T42.3X2	T42.3X3	T42.3X4	T42.3X5	T42.3X6
sodium	T42.3X1	T42.3X2	T42.3X3	T42.3X4	T42.3X5	T42.3X6
Barbitone	T42.3X1	T42.3X2	T42.3X3	T42.3X4	T42.3X5	T42.3X6

TABLE OF DRUGS AND CHEMICALS

◄ New   ◄⁐ Revised   ~~deleted~~ Deleted

Substance	Poisoning, Accidental (Unintentional)	Poisoning, Intentional Self-Harm	Poisoning, Assault	Poisoning, Undetermined	Adverse Effect	Underdosing
Barbiturate NEC	T42.3X1	T42.3X2	T42.3X3	T42.3X4	T42.3X5	T42.3X6
with tranquilizer	T42.3X1	T42.3X2	T42.3X3	T42.3X4	T42.3X5	T42.3X6
anesthetic (intravenous)	T41.1X1	T41.1X2	T41.1X3	T41.1X4	T41.1X5	T41.1X6
Barium (carbonate) (chloride) (sulfite)	T57.8X1	T57.8X2	T57.8X3	T57.8X4	—	—
diagnostic agent	T50.8X1	T50.8X2	T50.8X3	T50.8X4	T50.8X5	T50.8X6
pesticide	T60.4X1	T60.4X2	T60.4X3	T60.4X4	—	—
rodenticide	T60.4X1	T60.4X2	T60.4X3	T60.4X4	—	—
sulfate (medicinal)	T50.8X1	T50.8X2	T50.8X3	T50.8X4	T50.8X5	T50.8X6
Barrier cream	T49.3X1	T49.3X2	T49.3X3	T49.3X4	T49.3X5	T49.3X6
Basic fuchsin	T49.0X1	T49.0X2	T49.0X3	T49.0X4	T49.0X5	T49.0X6
Battery acid or fluid	T54.2X1	T54.2X2	T54.2X3	T54.2X4	—	—
Bay rum	T51.8X1	T51.8X2	T51.8X3	T51.8X4	—	—
BCG (vaccine)	T50.A91	T50.A92	T50.A93	T50.A94	T50.A95	T50.A96
BCNU	T45.1X1	T45.1X2	T45.1X3	T45.1X4	T45.1X5	T45.1X6
Bearsfoot	T62.2X1	T62.2X2	T62.2X3	T62.2X4	—	—
Beclamide	T42.6X1	T42.6X2	T42.6X3	T42.6X4	T42.6X5	T42.6X6
Beclomethasone	T44.5X1	T44.5X2	T44.5X3	T44.5X4	T44.5X5	T44.5X6
Bee (sting) (venom)	T63.441	T63.442	T63.443	T63.444	—	—
Befunolol	T49.5X1	T49.5X2	T49.5X3	T49.5X4	T49.5X5	T49.5X6
Bekanamycin	T36.5X1	T36.5X2	T36.5X3	T36.5X4	T36.5X5	T36.5X6
Belladonna—see also Nightshade						
alkaloids	T44.3X1	T44.3X2	T44.3X3	T44.3X4	T44.3X5	T44.3X6
extract	T44.3X1	T44.3X2	T44.3X3	T44.3X4	T44.3X5	T44.3X6
herb	T44.3X1	T44.3X2	T44.3X3	T44.3X4	T44.3X5	T44.3X6
Bemegride	T50.7X1	T50.7X2	T50.7X3	T50.7X4	T50.7X5	T50.7X6
Benactyzine	T44.3X1	T44.3X2	T44.3X3	T44.3X4	T44.3X5	T44.3X6
Benadryl	T45.0X1	T45.0X2	T45.0X3	T45.0X4	T45.0X5	T45.0X6
Benaprizine	T44.3X1	T44.3X2	T44.3X3	T44.3X4	T44.3X5	T44.3X6
Benazepril	T46.4X1	T46.4X2	T46.4X3	T46.4X4	T46.4X5	T46.4X6
Bencyclane	T46.7X1	T46.7X2	T46.7X3	T46.7X4	T46.7X5	T46.7X6
Bendazol	T46.3X1	T46.3X2	T46.3X3	T46.3X4	T46.3X5	T46.3X6
Bendrofluazide	T50.2X1	T50.2X2	T50.2X3	T50.2X4	T50.2X5	T50.2X6
Bendroflumethiazide	T50.2X1	T50.2X2	T50.2X3	T50.2X4	T50.2X5	T50.2X6
Benemid	T50.4X1	T50.4X2	T50.4X3	T50.4X4	T50.4X5	T50.4X6
Benethamine penicillin	T36.0X1	T36.0X2	T36.0X3	T36.0X4	T36.0X5	T36.0X6
Benisone	T49.0X1	T49.0X2	T49.0X3	T49.0X4	T49.0X5	T49.0X6
Benexate	T47.1X1	T47.1X2	T47.1X3	T47.1X4	T47.1X5	T47.1X6
Benfluorex	T46.6X1	T46.6X2	T46.6X3	T46.6X4	T46.6X5	T46.6X6
Benfotiamine	T45.2X1	T45.2X2	T45.2X3	T45.2X4	T45.2X5	T45.2X6
Benomyl	T60.0X1	T60.0X2	T60.0X3	T60.0X4	—	—

◄ New   ◄▥ Revised   ~~deleted~~ Deleted

TABLE OF DRUGS AND CHEMICALS

	External Cause (T-Code)					
Substance	Poisoning, Accidental (Unintentional)	Poisoning, Intentional Self-Harm	Poisoning, Assault	Poisoning, Undetermined	Adverse Effect	Underdosing
Benoquin	T49.8X1	T49.8X2	T49.8X3	T49.8X4	T49.8X5	T49.8X6
Benoxinate	T41.3X1	T41.3X2	T41.3X3	T41.3X4	T41.3X5	T41.3X6
Benperidol	T43.4X1	T43.4X2	T43.4X3	T43.4X4	T43.4X5	T43.4X6
Benproperine	T48.3X1	T48.3X2	T48.3X3	T48.3X4	T48.3X5	T48.3X6
Benserazide	T42.8X1	T42.8X2	T42.8X3	T42.8X4	T42.8X5	T42.8X6
Bentazepam	T42.4X1	T42.4X2	T42.4X3	T42.4X4	T42.4X5	T42.4X6
Bentiromide	T50.8X1	T50.8X2	T50.8X3	T50.8X4	T50.8X5	T50.8X6
Bentonite	T49.3X1	T49.3X2	T49.3X3	T49.3X4	T49.3X5	T49.3X6
Benzalbutyramide	T46.6X1	T46.6X2	T46.6X3	T46.6X4	T46.6X5	T46.6X6
Benzalkonium (chloride)	T49.0X1	T49.0X2	T49.0X3	T49.0X4	T49.0X5	T49.0X6
ophthalmic preparation	T49.5X1	T49.5X2	T49.5X3	T49.5X4	T49.5X5	T49.5X6
Benzamine	T41.3X1	T41.3X2	T41.3X3	T41.3X4	T41.3X5	T41.3X6
lactate	T49.1X1	T49.1X2	T49.1X3	T49.1X4	T49.1X5	T49.1X6
Benzamidosalicylate (calcium)	T37.1X1	T37.1X2	T37.1X3	T37.1X4	T37.1X5	T37.1X6
Benzamphetamine	T50.5X1	T50.5X2	T50.5X3	T50.5X4	T50.5X5	T50.5X6
Benzapril hydrochloride	T46.5X1	T46.5X2	T46.5X3	T46.5X4	T46.5X5	T46.5X6
Benzathine benzylpenicillin	T36.0X1	T36.0X2	T36.0X3	T36.0X4	T36.0X5	T36.0X6
Benzathine penicillin	T36.0X1	T36.0X2	T36.0X3	T36.0X4	T36.0X5	T36.0X6
Benzatropine	T42.8X1	T42.8X2	T42.8X3	T42.8X4	T42.8X5	T42.8X6
Benzbromarone	T50.4X1	T50.4X2	T50.4X3	T50.4X4	T50.4X5	T50.4X6
Benzcarbimine	T45.1X1	T45.1X2	T45.1X3	T45.1X4	T45.1X5	T45.1X6
Benzedrex	T44.991	T44.992	T44.993	T44.994	T44.995	T44.996
Benzedrine (amphetamine)	T43.621	T43.622	T43.623	T43.624	T43.625	T43.626
Benzenamine	T65.3X1	T65.3X2	T65.3X3	T65.3X4	—	—
Benzene	T52.1X1	T52.1X2	T52.1X3	T52.1X4	—	—
homologues (acetyl) (dimethyl) (methyl) (solvent)	T52.2X1	T52.2X2	T52.2X3	T52.2X4	—	—
Benzethonium (chloride)	T49.0X1	T49.0X2	T49.0X3	T49.0X4	T49.0X5	T49.0X6
Benzfetamine	T50.5X1	T50.5X2	T50.5X3	T50.5X4	T50.5X5	T50.5X6
Benzhexol	T44.3X1	T44.3X2	T44.3X3	T44.3X4	T44.3X5	T44.3X6
Benzhydramine (chloride)	T45.0X1	T45.0X2	T45.0X3	T45.0X4	T45.0X5	T45.0X6
Benzidine	T65.891	T65.892	T65.893	T65.894	—	—
Benzilonium bromide	T44.3X1	T44.3X2	T44.3X3	T44.3X4	T44.3X5	T44.3X6
Benzimidazole	T60.3X1	T60.3X2	T60.3X3	T60.3X4	—	—
Benzin(e) — see Ligroin						
Benziodarone	T46.3X1	T46.3X2	T46.3X3	T46.3X4	T46.3X5	T46.3X6
Benznidazole	T37.3X1	T37.3X2	T37.3X3	T37.3X4	T37.3X5	T37.3X6
Benzocaine	T41.3X1	T41.3X2	T41.3X3	T41.3X4	T41.3X5	T41.3X6
Benzoctamine	T43.0X1	T43.0X2	T43.0X3	T43.0X4	T43.0X5	T43.0X6
Benzodiapin	T42.4X1	T42.4X2	T42.4X3	T42.4X4	T42.4X5	T42.4X6
Benzodiazepine NEC	T42.4X1	T42.4X2	T42.4X3	T42.4X4	T42.4X5	T42.4X6

◀ New   ◀ Revised   ~~deleted~~ Deleted

Substance	External Cause (T-Code)					
	Poisoning, Accidental (Unintentional)	Poisoning, Intentional Self-Harm	Poisoning, Assault	Poisoning, Undetermined	Adverse Effect	Underdosing
Benzoic acid	T49.0X1	T49.0X2	T49.0X3	T49.0X4	T49.0X5	T49.0X6
with salicylic acid	T49.0X1	T49.0X2	T49.0X3	T49.0X4	T49.0X5	T49.0X6
Benzoin (tincture)	T48.5X1	T48.5X2	T48.5X3	T48.5X4	T48.5X5	T48.5X6
Benzol (benzene)	T52.1X1	T52.1X2	T52.1X3	T52.1X4	—	—
vapor	T52.0X1	T52.0X2	T52.0X3	T52.0X4	—	—
Benzomorphan	T40.2X1	T40.2X2	T40.2X3	T40.2X4	T40.2X5	T40.2X6
Benzonatate	T48.3X1	T48.3X2	T48.3X3	T48.3X4	T48.3X5	T48.3X6
Benzophenones	T49.3X1	T49.3X2	T49.3X3	T49.3X4	T49.3X5	T49.3X6
Benzopyrone	T46.991	T46.992	T46.993	T46.994	T46.995	T46.996
Benzothiadiazides	T50.2X1	T50.2X2	T50.2X3	T50.2X4	T50.2X5	T50.2X6
Benzoxonium chloride	T49.0X1	T49.0X2	T49.0X3	T49.0X4	T49.0X5	T49.0X6
Benzoyl peroxide	T49.0X1	T49.0X2	T49.0X3	T49.0X4	T49.0X5	T49.0X6
Benzoylpas calcium	T37.1X1	T37.1X2	T37.1X3	T37.1X4	T37.1X5	T37.1X6
Benzperidin	T43.591	T43.592	T43.593	T43.594	T43.595	T43.596
Benzperidol	T43.591	T43.592	T43.593	T43.594	T43.595	T43.596
Benzphetamine	T50.5X1	T50.5X2	T50.5X3	T50.5X4	T50.5X5	T50.5X6
Benzpyrinium bromide	T44.1X1	T44.1X2	T44.1X3	T44.1X4	T44.1X5	T44.1X6
Benzquinamide	T45.0X1	T45.0X2	T45.0X3	T45.0X4	T45.0X5	T45.0X6
Benzthiazide	T50.2X1	T50.2X2	T50.2X3	T50.2X4	T50.2X5	T50.2X6
Benztropine						
anticholinergic	T44.3X1	T44.3X2	T44.3X3	T44.3X4	T44.3X5	T44.3X6
antiparkinson	T42.8X1	T42.8X2	T42.8X3	T42.8X4	T42.8X5	T42.8X6
Benzydamine	T49.0X1	T49.0X2	T49.0X3	T49.0X4	T49.0X5	T49.0X6
Benzyl						
acetate	T52.8X1	T52.8X2	T52.8X3	T52.8X4	—	—
alcohol	T49.0X1	T49.0X2	T49.0X3	T49.0X4	T49.0X5	T49.0X6
benzoate	T49.0X1	T49.0X2	T49.0X3	T49.0X4	T49.0X5	T49.0X6
Benzoic acid	T49.0X1	T49.0X2	T49.0X3	T49.0X4	T49.0X5	T49.0X6
morphine	T40.2X1	T40.2X2	T40.2X3	T40.2X4	—	—
nicotinate	T46.6X1	T46.6X2	T46.6X3	T46.6X4	T46.6X5	T46.6X6
penicillin	T36.0X1	T36.0X2	T36.0X3	T36.0X4	T36.0X5	T36.0X6
Benzylhydrochlorthia-zide	T50.2X1	T50.2X2	T50.2X3	T50.2X4	T50.2X5	T50.2X6
Benzylpenicillin	T36.0X1	T36.0X2	T36.0X3	T36.0X4	T36.0X5	T36.0X6
Benzylthiouracil	T38.2X1	T38.2X2	T38.2X3	T38.2X4	T38.2X5	T38.2X6
Bephenium hydroxy-naphthoate	T37.4X1	T37.4X2	T37.4X3	T37.4X4	T37.4X5	T37.4X6
Bepridil	T46.1X1	T46.1X2	T46.1X3	T46.1X4	T46.1X5	T46.1X6
Bergamot oil	T65.891	T65.892	T65.893	T65.894	—	—
Bergapten	T50.991	T50.992	T50.993	T50.994	T50.995	T50.996
Berries, poisonous	T62.1X1	T62.1X2	T62.1X3	T62.1X4	—	—
Beryllium (compounds)	T56.7X1	T56.7X2	T56.7X3	T56.7X4	—	—

◀ New ◀ Revised ~~deleted~~ Deleted

TABLE OF DRUGS AND CHEMICALS

Substance	External Cause (T-Code)					
	Poisoning, Accidental (Unintentional)	Poisoning, Intentional Self-Harm	Poisoning, Assault	Poisoning, Undetermined	Adverse Effect	Underdosing
b-acetyldigoxin	T46.0X1	T46.0X2	T46.0X3	T46.0X4	T46.0X5	T46.0X6
beta adrenergic blocking agent, heart	T44.7X1	T44.7X2	T44.7X3	T44.7X4	T44.7X5	T44.7X6
b-benzalbutyramide	T46.6X1	T46.6X2	T46.6X3	T46.6X4	T46.6X5	T46.6X6
Betacarotene	T45.2X1	T45.2X2	T45.2X3	T45.2X4	T45.2X5	T45.2X6
b-eucaine	T49.1X1	T49.1X2	T49.1X3	T49.1X4	T49.1X5	T49.1X6
Beta-Chlor	T42.6X1	T42.6X2	T42.6X3	T42.6X4	T42.6X5	T42.6X6
b-galactosidase	T47.5X1	T47.5X2	T47.5X3	T47.5X4	T47.5X5	T47.5X6
Betahistine	T46.7X1	T46.7X2	T46.7X3	T46.7X4	T46.7X5	T46.7X6
Betaine	T47.5X1	T47.5X2	T47.5X3	T47.5X4	T47.5X5	T47.5X6
Betamethasone	T49.0X1	T49.0X2	T49.0X3	T49.0X4	T49.0X5	T49.0X6
topical	T49.0X1	T49.0X2	T49.0X3	T49.0X4	T49.0X5	T49.0X6
Betamicin	T36.8X1	T36.8X2	T36.8X3	T36.8X4	T36.8X5	T36.8X6
Betanidine	T46.5X1	T46.5X2	T46.5X3	T46.5X4	T46.5X5	T46.5X6
b-sitosterol(s)	T46.6X1	T46.6X2	T46.6X3	T46.6X4	T46.6X5	T46.6X6
Betaxolol	T44.7X1	T44.7X2	T44.7X3	T44.7X4	T44.7X5	T44.7X6
Betazole	T50.8X1	T50.8X2	T50.8X3	T50.8X4	T50.8X5	T50.8X6
Bethanechol	T44.1X1	T44.1X2	T44.1X3	T44.1X4	T44.1X5	T44.1X6
chloride	T44.1X1	T44.1X2	T44.1X3	T44.1X4	T44.1X5	T44.1X6
Bethanidine	T46.5X1	T46.5X2	T46.5X3	T46.5X4	T46.5X5	T46.5X6
Betoxycaine	T41.3X1	T41.3X2	T41.3X3	T41.3X4	T41.3X5	T41.3X6
Betula oil	T49.3X1	T49.3X2	T49.3X3	T49.3X4	T49.3X5	T49.3X6
Bevantolol	T44.7X1	T44.7X2	T44.7X3	T44.7X4	T44.7X5	T44.7X6
Bevonium metilsulfate	T44.3X1	T44.3X2	T44.3X3	T44.3X4	T44.3X5	T44.3X6
Bezafibrate	T46.6X1	T46.6X2	T46.6X3	T46.6X4	T46.6X5	T46.6X6
Bezitramide	T40.4X1	T40.4X2	T40.4X3	T40.4X4	T40.4X5	T40.4X6
BHA	T50.991	T50.992	T50.993	T50.994	T50.995	T50.996
Bhang	T40.7X1	T40.7X2	T40.7X3	T40.7X4	T40.7X5	T40.7X6
BHC (medicinal)	T49.0X1	T49.0X2	T49.0X3	T49.0X4	T49.0X5	T49.0X6
nonmedicinal (vapor)	T53.6X1	T53.6X2	T53.6X3	T53.6X4	—	—
Bialamicol	T37.3X1	T37.3X2	T37.3X3	T37.3X4	T37.3X5	T37.3X6
Bibenzonium bromide	T48.3X1	T48.3X2	T48.3X3	T48.3X4	T48.3X5	T48.3X6
Bibrocathol	T49.5X1	T49.5X2	T49.5X3	T49.5X4	T49.5X5	T49.5X6
Bichloride of mercury — see Mercury, chloride						
Bichromates (calcium) (potassium) (sodium) (crystals)	T57.8X1	T57.8X2	T57.8X3	T57.8X4	—	—
fumes	T56.2X1	T56.2X2	T56.2X3	T56.2X4	—	—
Biclotymol	T49.6X1	T49.6X2	T49.6X3	T49.6X4	T49.6X5	T49.6X6
Bicucculine	T50.7X1	T50.7X2	T50.7X3	T50.7X4	T50.7X5	T50.7X6
Bifemelane	T43.291	T43.292	T43.293	T43.294	T43.295	T43.296
Biguanide derivatives, oral	T38.3X1	T38.3X2	T38.3X3	T38.3X4	T38.3X5	T38.3X6

◄ New ◄◄ Revised ~~deleted~~ Deleted

Substance	External Cause (T-Code)					
	Poisoning, Accidental (Unintentional)	Poisoning, Intentional Self-Harm	Poisoning, Assault	Poisoning, Undetermined	Adverse Effect	Underdosing
Biligrafin	T50.8X1	T50.8X2	T50.8X3	T50.8X4	T50.8X5	T50.8X6
Bile salts	T47.5X1	T47.5X2	T47.5X3	T47.5X4	T47.5X5	T47.5X6
Bilopaque	T50.8X1	T50.8X2	T50.8X3	T50.8X4	T50.8X5	T50.8X6
Binifibrate	T46.6X1	T46.6X2	T46.6X3	T46.6X4	T46.6X5	T46.6X6
Binitrobenzol	T65.3X1	T65.3X2	T65.3X3	T65.3X4	—	—
Bioflavonoid(s)	T46.991	T46.992	T46.993	T46.994	T46.995	T46.996
Biological substance NEC	T50.901	T50.902	T50.903	T50.904	T50.905	T50.906
Biotin	T45.2X1	T45.2X2	T45.2X3	T45.2X4	T45.2X5	T45.2X6
Biperiden	T44.3X1	T44.3X2	T44.3X3	T44.3X4	T44.3X5	T44.3X6
Bisacodyl	T47.2X1	T47.2X2	T47.2X3	T47.2X4	T47.2X5	T47.2X6
Bisbentiamine	T45.2X1	T45.2X2	T45.2X3	T45.2X4	T45.2X5	T45.2X6
Bisbutiamine	T45.2X1	T45.2X2	T45.2X3	T45.2X4	T45.2X5	T45.2X6
Bisdequalinium (salts) (diacetate)	T49.6X1	T49.6X2	T49.6X3	T49.6X4	T49.6X5	T49.6X6
Bishydroxycoumarin	T45.511	T45.512	T45.513	T45.514	T45.515	T45.516
Bismarsen	T37.8X1	T37.8X2	T37.8X3	T37.8X4	T37.8X5	T37.8X6
Bismuth salts	T47.6X1	T47.6X2	T47.6X3	T47.6X4	T47.6X5	T47.6X6
aluminate	T47.1X1	T47.1X2	T47.1X3	T47.1X4	T47.1X5	T47.1X6
anti-infectives	T37.8X1	T37.8X2	T37.8X3	T37.8X4	T37.8X5	T37.8X6
formic iodide	T49.0X1	T49.0X2	T49.0X3	T49.0X4	T49.0X5	T49.0X6
glycolylarsenate	T49.0X1	T49.0X2	T49.0X3	T49.0X4	T49.0X5	T49.0X6
nonmedicinal (compounds) NEC	T65.91	T65.92	T65.93	T65.94	—	—
subcarbonate	T47.6X1	T47.6X2	T47.6X3	T47.6X4	T47.6X5	T47.6X6
subsalicylate	T37.8X1	T37.8X2	T37.8X3	T37.8X4	T37.8X5	T37.8X6
sulfarsphenamine	T37.8X1	T37.8X2	T37.8X3	T37.8X4	T37.8X5	T37.8X6
Bisoprolol	T44.7X1	T44.7X2	T44.7X3	T44.7X4	T44.7X5	T44.7X6
Bisoxatin	T47.2X1	T47.2X2	T47.2X3	T47.2X4	T47.2X5	T47.2X6
Bisulepin (hydrochloride)	T45.0X1	T45.0X2	T45.0X3	T45.0X4	T45.0X5	T45.0X6
Bithionol	T37.8X1	T37.8X2	T37.8X3	T37.8X4	T37.8X5	T37.8X6
anthelminthic	T37.4X1	T37.4X2	T37.4X3	T37.4X4	T37.4X5	T37.4X6
Bitolterol	T48.6X1	T48.6X2	T48.6X3	T48.6X4	T48.6X5	T48.6X6
Bitoscanate	T37.4X1	T37.4X2	T37.4X3	T37.4X4	T37.4X5	T37.4X6
Bitter almond oil	T62.8X1	T62.8X2	T62.8X3	T62.8X4	—	—
Bittersweet	T62.2X1	T62.2X2	T62.2X3	T62.2X4	—	—
Black						
flag	T60.91	T60.92	T60.93	T60.94	—	—
henbane	T62.2X1	T62.2X2	T62.2X3	T62.2X4	—	—
leaf (40)	T60.91	T60.92	T60.93	T60.94	—	—
widow spider (bite)	T63.311	T63.312	T63.313	T63.314	—	—
antivenin	T50.Z11	T50.Z12	T50.Z13	T50.Z14	T50.Z15	T50.Z16
Blast furnace gas (carbon monoxide from)	T58.8X1	T58.8X2	T58.8X3	T58.8X4		

Substance	External Cause (T-Code)					
	Poisoning, Accidental (Unintentional)	Poisoning, Intentional Self-Harm	Poisoning, Assault	Poisoning, Undetermined	Adverse Effect	Underdosing
Bleach	T54.91	T54.92	T54.93	T54.94	—	—
Bleaching agent (medicinal)	T49.4X1	T49.4X2	T49.4X3	T49.4X4	T49.4X5	T49.4X6
Bleomycin	T45.1X1	T45.1X2	T45.1X3	T45.1X4	T45.1X5	T45.1X6
Blockain	T41.3X1	T41.3X2	T41.3X3	T41.3X4	T41.3X5	T41.3X6
infiltration (subcutaneous)	T41.3X1	T41.3X2	T41.3X3	T41.3X4	T41.3X5	T41.3X6
nerve block (peripheral) (plexus)	T41.3X1	T41.3X2	T41.3X3	T41.3X4	T41.3X5	T41.3X6
topical (surface)	T41.3X1	T41.3X2	T41.3X3	T41.3X4	T41.3X5	T41.3X6
Blockers, calcium channel	T46.1X1	T46.1X2	T46.1X3	T46.1X4	T46.1X5	T46.1X6
Blood (derivatives) (natural) (plasma) (whole)	T45.8X1	T45.8X2	T45.8X3	T45.8X4	T45.8X5	T45.8X6
dried	T45.8X1	T45.8X2	T45.8X3	T45.8X4	T45.8X5	T45.8X6
drug affecting NEC	T45.91	T45.92	T45.93	T45.94	T45.95	T45.96
expander NEC	T45.8X1	T45.8X2	T45.8X3	T45.8X4	T45.8X5	T45.8X6
fraction NEC	T45.8X1	T45.8X2	T45.8X3	T45.8X4	T45.8X5	T45.8X6
substitute (macromolecular)	T45.8X1	T45.8X2	T45.8X3	T45.8X4	T45.8X5	T45.8X6
Blue velvet	T40.2X1	T40.2X2	T40.2X3	T40.2X4	—	—
Bone meal	T62.8X1	T62.8X2	T62.8X3	T62.8X4	—	—
Bonine	T45.0X1	T45.0X2	T45.0X3	T45.0X4	T45.0X5	T45.0X6
Bopindolol	T44.7X1	T44.7X2	T44.7X3	T44.7X4	T44.7X5	T44.7X6
Boracic acid	T49.0X1	T49.0X2	T49.0X3	T49.0X4	T49.0X5	T49.0X6
ENT agent	T49.6X1	T49.6X2	T49.6X3	T49.6X4	T49.6X5	T49.6X6
ophthalmic preparation	T49.5X1	T49.5X2	T49.5X3	T49.5X4	T49.5X5	T49.5X6
Borane complex	T57.8X1	T57.8X2	T57.8X3	T57.8X4	—	—
Borate(s)	T57.8X1	T57.8X2	T57.8X3	T57.8X4	—	—
buffer	T50.991	T50.992	T50.993	T50.994	T50.995	T50.996
cleanser	T54.91	T54.92	T54.93	T54.94	—	—
sodium	T57.8X1	T57.8X2	T57.8X3	T57.8X4	—	—
Borax (cleanser)	T54.91	T54.92	T54.93	T54.94	—	—
Bordeaux mixture	T60.3X1	T60.3X2	T60.3X3	T60.3X4	—	—
Boric acid	T49.0X1	T49.0X2	T49.0X3	T49.0X4	T49.0X5	T49.0X6
ENT agent	T49.6X1	T49.6X2	T49.6X3	T49.6X4	T49.6X5	T49.6X6
ophthalmic preparation	T49.5X1	T49.5X2	T49.5X3	T49.5X4	T49.5X5	T49.5X6
Bornaprine	T44.3X1	T44.3X2	T44.3X3	T44.3X4	T44.3X5	T44.3X6
Boron	T57.8X1	T57.8X2	T57.8X3	T57.8X4	—	—
hydride NEC	T57.8X1	T57.8X2	T57.8X3	T57.8X4	—	—
fumes or gas	T57.8X1	T57.8X2	T57.8X3	T57.8X4	—	—
trifluoride	T59.891	T59.892	T59.893	T59.894	—	—
Botox	T48.291	T48.292	T48.293	T48.294	T48.295	T48.296
Botulinus anti-toxin (type A, B)	T50.Z11	T50.Z12	T50.Z13	T50.Z14	T50.Z15	T50.Z16
Brake fluid vapor	T59.891	T59.892	T59.893	T59.894	—	—
Brallobarbital	T42.3X1	T42.3X2	T42.3X3	T42.3X4	T42.3X5	T42.3X6

◀ New ◀▮ Revised ~~deleted~~ Deleted

Substance	External Cause (T-Code)					
	Poisoning, Accidental (Unintentional)	Poisoning, Intentional Self-Harm	Poisoning, Assault	Poisoning, Undetermined	Adverse Effect	Underdosing
Bran (wheat)	T47.4X1	T47.4X2	T47.4X3	T47.4X4	T47.4X5	T47.4X6
Brass (fumes)	T56.891	T56.892	T56.893	T56.894	—	—
Brasso	T52.0X1	T52.0X2	T52.0X3	T52.0X4	—	—
Bretylium tosilate	T46.2X1	T46.2X2	T46.2X3	T46.2X4	T46.2X5	T46.2X6
Brevital (sodium)	T41.1X1	T41.1X2	T41.1X3	T41.1X4	T41.1X5	T41.1X6
Brinase	T45.3X1	T45.3X2	T45.3X3	T45.3X4	T45.3X5	T45.3X6
British antilewisite	T45.8X1	T45.8X2	T45.8X3	T45.8X4	T45.8X5	T45.8X6
Brodifacoum	T60.4X1	T60.4X2	T60.4X3	T60.4X4	—	—
Bromal (hydrate)	T42.6X1	T42.6X2	T42.6X3	T42.6X4	T42.6X5	T42.6X6
Bromazepam	T42.4X1	T42.4X2	T42.4X3	T42.4X4	T42.4X5	T42.4X6
Bromazine	T45.0X1	T45.0X2	T45.0X3	T45.0X4	T45.0X5	T45.0X6
Brombenzylcyanide	T59.3X1	T59.3X2	T59.3X3	T59.3X4	—	—
Bromelains	T45.3X1	T45.3X2	T45.3X3	T45.3X4	T45.3X5	T45.3X6
Bromethalin	T60.4X1	T60.4X2	T60.4X3	T60.4X4	—	—
Bromhexine	T48.4X1	T48.4X2	T48.4X3	T48.4X4	T48.4X5	T48.4X6
Bromide salts	T42.6X1	T42.6X2	T42.6X3	T42.6X4	T42.6X5	T42.6X6
Bromindione	T45.511	T45.512	T45.513	T45.514	T45.515	T45.516
Bromine						
compounds (medicinal)	T42.6X1	T42.6X2	T42.6X3	T42.6X4	T42.6X5	T42.6X6
sedative	T42.6X1	T42.6X2	T42.6X3	T42.6X4	T42.6X5	T42.6X6
vapor	T59.891	T59.892	T59.893	T59.894	—	—
Bromisovalum	T42.6X1	T42.6X2	T42.6X3	T42.6X4	T42.6X5	T42.6X6
Bromisoval	T42.6X1	T42.6X2	T42.6X3	T42.6X4	T42.6X5	T42.6X6
Bromobenzylcyanide	T59.3X1	T59.3X2	T59.3X3	T59.3X4	—	—
Bromochlorosalicylani-lide	T49.0X1	T49.0X2	T49.0X3	T49.0X4	T49.0X5	T49.0X6
Bromocriptine	T42.8X1	T42.8X2	T42.8X3	T42.8X4	T42.8X5	T42.8X6
Bromodiphenhydramine	T45.0X1	T45.0X2	T45.0X3	T45.0X4	T45.0X5	T45.0X6
Bromoform	T42.6X1	T42.6X2	T42.6X3	T42.6X4	T42.6X5	T42.6X6
Bromophenol blue reagent	T50.991	T50.992	T50.993	T50.994	T50.995	T50.996
Bromopride	T47.8X1	T47.8X2	T47.8X3	T47.8X4	T47.8X5	T47.8X6
Bromosalicylchloranitide	T49.0X1	T49.0X2	T49.0X3	T49.0X4	T49.0X5	T49.0X6
Bromosalicylhydroxamic acid	T37.1X1	T37.1X2	T37.1X3	T37.1X4	T37.1X5	T37.1X6
Bromo-seltzer	T39.1X1	T39.1X2	T39.1X3	T39.1X4	T39.1X5	T39.1X6
Bromoxynil	T60.3X1	T60.3X2	T60.3X3	T60.3X4	—	—
Bromperidol	T43.4X1	T43.4X2	T43.4X3	T43.4X4	T43.4X5	T43.4X6
Brompheniramine	T45.0X1	T45.0X2	T45.0X3	T45.0X4	T45.0X5	T45.0X6
Bromsulfophthalein	T50.8X1	T50.8X2	T50.8X3	T50.8X4	T50.8X5	T50.8X6
Bromural	T42.6X1	T42.6X2	T42.6X3	T42.6X4	T42.6X5	T42.6X6
Bromvaletone	T42.6X1	T42.6X2	T42.6X3	T42.6X4	T42.6X5	T42.6X6
Bronchodilator NEC	T48.6X1	T48.6X2	T48.6X3	T48.6X4	T48.6X5	T48.6X6

◀ New   ◀⫴ Revised   ~~deleted~~ Deleted

TABLE OF DRUGS AND CHEMICALS

Substance	External Cause (T-Code)					
	Poisoning, Accidental (Unintentional)	Poisoning, Intentional Self-Harm	Poisoning, Assault	Poisoning, Undetermined	Adverse Effect	Underdosing
Brotizolam	T42.4X1	T42.4X2	T42.4X3	T42.4X4	T42.4X5	T42.4X6
Brovincamine	T46.7X1	T46.7X2	T46.7X3	T46.7X4	T46.7X5	T46.7X6
Brown spider (bite) (venom)	T63.391	T63.392	T63.393	T63.394	—	—
Brown recluse spider (bite) (venom)	T63.331	T63.332	T63.333	T63.334	—	—
Broxaterol	T48.6X1	T48.6X2	T48.6X3	T48.6X4	T48.6X5	T48.6X6
Broxuridine	T45.1X1	T45.1X2	T45.1X3	T45.1X4	T45.1X5	T45.1X6
Broxyquinoline	T37.8X1	T37.8X2	T37.8X3	T37.8X4	T37.8X5	T37.8X6
Bruceine	T48.291	T48.292	T48.293	T48.294	T48.295	T48.296
Brucia	T62.2X1	T62.2X2	T62.2X3	T62.2X4	—	—
Brucine	T65.1X1	T65.1X2	T65.1X3	T65.1X4	—	—
Brunswick green — see Copper						
Bruten — see Ibuprofen						
Bryonia	T47.2X1	T47.2X2	T47.2X3	T47.2X4	T47.2X5	T47.2X6
Buclizine	T45.0X1	T45.0X2	T45.0X3	T45.0X4	T45.0X5	T45.0X6
Buclosamide	T49.0X1	T49.0X2	T49.0X3	T49.0X4	T49.0X5	T49.0X6
Budesonide	T44.5X1	T44.5X2	T44.5X3	T44.5X4	T44.5X5	T44.5X6
Budralazine	T46.5X1	T46.5X2	T46.5X3	T46.5X4	T46.5X5	T46.5X6
Bufferin	T39.011	T39.012	T39.013	T39.014	T39.015	T39.016
Buflomedil	T46.7X1	T46.7X2	T46.7X3	T46.7X4	T46.7X5	T46.7X6
Buformin	T38.3X1	T38.3X2	T38.3X3	T38.3X4	T38.3X5	T38.3X6
Bufotenine	T40.991	T40.992	T40.993	T40.994	—	—
Bufrolin	T48.6X1	T48.6X2	T48.6X3	T48.6X4	T48.6X5	T48.6X6
Bufylline	T48.6X1	T48.6X2	T48.6X3	T48.6X4	T48.6X5	T48.6X6
Bulk filler	T50.5X1	T50.5X2	T50.5X3	T50.5X4	T50.5X5	T50.5X6
cathartic	T47.4X1	T47.4X2	T47.4X3	T47.4X4	T47.4X5	T47.4X6
Bumetanide	T50.1X1	T50.1X2	T50.1X3	T50.1X4	T50.1X5	T50.1X6
Bunaftine	T46.2X1	T46.2X2	T46.2X3	T46.2X4	T46.2X5	T46.2X6
Bunamiodyl	T50.8X1	T50.8X2	T50.8X3	T50.8X4	T50.8X5	T50.8X6
Bunazosin	T44.6X1	T44.6X2	T44.6X3	T44.6X4	T44.6X5	T44.6X6
Bunitrolol	T44.7X1	T44.7X2	T44.7X3	T44.7X4	T44.7X5	T44.7X6
Buphenine	T46.7X1	T46.7X2	T46.7X3	T46.7X4	T46.7X5	T46.7X6
Bupivacaine	T41.3X1	T41.3X2	T41.3X3	T41.3X4	T41.3X5	T41.3X6
infiltration (subcutaneous)	T41.3X1	T41.3X2	T41.3X3	T41.3X4	T41.3X5	T41.3X6
nerve block (peripheral) (plexus)	T41.3X1	T41.3X2	T41.3X3	T41.3X4	T41.3X5	T41.3X6
spinal	T41.3X1	T41.3X2	T41.3X3	T41.3X4	T41.3X5	T41.3X6
Bupranolol	T44.7X1	T44.7X2	T44.7X3	T44.7X4	T44.7X5	T44.7X6
Buprenorphine	T40.4X1	T40.4X2	T40.4X3	T40.4X4	T40.4X5	T40.4X6
Bupropion	T43.291	T43.292	T43.293	T43.294	T43.295	T43.296
Burimamide	T47.1X1	T47.1X2	T47.1X3	T47.1X4	T47.1X5	T47.1X6
Buserelin	T38.891	T38.892	T38.893	T38.894	T38.895	T38.896

◄ New ◄▦ Revised ~~deleted~~ Deleted

Substance	External Cause (T-Code)					
	Poisoning, Accidental (Unintentional)	Poisoning, Intentional Self-Harm	Poisoning, Assault	Poisoning, Undetermined	Adverse Effect	Underdosing
Buspirone	T43.591	T43.592	T43.593	T43.594	T43.595	T43.596
Busulfan, busulphan	T45.1X1	T45.1X2	T45.1X3	T45.1X4	T45.1X5	T45.1X6
Butabarbital (sodium)	T42.3X1	T42.3X2	T42.3X3	T42.3X4	T42.3X5	T42.3X6
Butabarbitone	T42.3X1	T42.3X2	T42.3X3	T42.3X4	T42.3X5	T42.3X6
Butabarpal	T42.3X1	T42.3X2	T42.3X3	T42.3X4	T42.3X5	T42.3X6
Butacaine	T41.3X1	T41.3X2	T41.3X3	T41.3X4	T41.3X5	T41.3X6
Butalamine	T46.7X1	T46.7X2	T46.7X3	T46.7X4	T46.7X5	T46.7X6
Butalbital	T42.3X1	T42.3X2	T42.3X3	T42.3X4	T42.3X5	T42.3X6
Butallylonal	T42.3X1	T42.3X2	T42.3X3	T42.3X4	T42.3X5	T42.3X6
Butamben	T41.3X1	T41.3X2	T41.3X3	T41.3X4	T41.3X5	T41.3X6
Butamirate	T48.3X1	T48.3X2	T48.3X3	T48.3X4	T48.3X5	T48.3X6
Butane (distributed in mobile container)	T59.891	T59.892	T59.893	T59.894	—	—
distributed through pipes	T59.891	T59.892	T59.893	T59.894	—	—
incomplete combustion	T58.11	T58.12	T58.13	T58.14	—	—
Butanilicaine	T41.3X1	T41.3X2	T41.3X3	T41.3X4	T41.3X5	T41.3X6
Butanol	T51.3X1	T51.3X2	T51.3X3	T51.3X4	—	—
Butanone, 2-butanone	T52.4X1	T52.4X2	T52.4X3	T52.4X4	—	—
Butantrone	T49.4X1	T49.4X2	T49.4X3	T49.4X4	T49.4X5	T49.4X6
Butaperazine	T43.3X1	T43.3X2	T43.3X3	T43.3X4	T43.3X5	T43.3X6
Butazolidin	T39.2X1	T39.2X2	T39.2X3	T39.2X4	T39.2X5	T39.2X6
Butetamate	T48.6X1	T48.6X2	T48.6X3	T48.6X4	T48.6X5	T48.6X6
Butethal	T42.3X1	T42.3X2	T42.3X3	T42.3X4	T42.3X5	T42.3X6
Butethamate	T44.3X1	T44.3X2	T44.3X3	T44.3X4	T44.3X5	T44.3X6
Buthalitone (sodium)	T41.1X1	T41.1X2	T41.1X3	T41.1X4	T41.1X5	T41.1X6
Butisol (sodium)	T42.3X1	T42.3X2	T42.3X3	T42.3X4	T42.3X5	T42.3X6
Butizide	T50.2X1	T50.2X2	T50.2X3	T50.2X4	T50.2X5	T50.2X6
Butobarbital	T42.3X1	T42.3X2	T42.3X3	T42.3X4	T42.3X5	T42.3X6
sodium	T42.3X1	T42.3X2	T42.3X3	T42.3X4	T42.3X5	T42.3X6
Butobarbitone	T42.3X1	T42.3X2	T42.3X3	T42.3X4	T42.3X5	T42.3X6
Butoconazole (nitrate)	T49.0X1	T49.0X2	T49.0X3	T49.0X4	T49.0X5	T49.0X6
Butorphanol	T40.4X1	T40.4X2	T40.4X3	T40.4X4	T40.4X5	T40.4X6
Butriptyline	T43.011	T43.012	T43.013	T43.014	T43.015	T43.016
Butropium bromide	T44.3X1	T44.3X2	T44.3X3	T44.3X4	T44.3X5	T44.3X6
Buttercups	T62.2X1	T62.2X2	T62.2X3	T62.2X4	—	—
Butter of antimony — see Antimony						
Butyl						
acetate (secondary)	T52.8X1	T52.8X2	T52.8X3	T52.8X4	—	—
alcohol	T51.3X1	T51.3X2	T51.3X3	T51.3X4	—	—
aminobenzoate	T41.3X1	T41.3X2	T41.3X3	T41.3X4	T41.3X5	T41.3X6
butyrate	T52.8X1	T52.8X2	T52.8X3	T52.8X4	—	—

TABLE OF DRUGS AND CHEMICALS

Substance	External Cause (T-Code)					
	Poisoning, Accidental (Unintentional)	Poisoning, Intentional Self-Harm	Poisoning, Assault	Poisoning, Undetermined	Adverse Effect	Underdosing
Butyl *(Continued)*						
carbinol	T51.3X1	T51.3X2	T51.3X3	T51.3X4	—	—
carbitol	T52.3X1	T52.3X2	T52.3X3	T52.3X4	—	—
cellosolve	T52.3X1	T52.3X2	T52.3X3	T52.3X4	—	—
chloral (hydrate)	T42.6X1	T42.6X2	T42.6X3	T42.6X4	T42.6X5	T42.6X6
formate	T52.8X1	T52.8X2	T52.8X3	T52.8X4	—	—
lactate	T52.8X1	T52.8X2	T52.8X3	T52.8X4	—	—
propionate	T52.8X1	T52.8X2	T52.8X3	T52.8X4	—	—
scopolamine bromide	T44.3X1	T44.3X2	T44.3X3	T44.3X4	T44.3X5	T44.3X6
thiobarbital sodium	T41.1X1	T41.1X2	T41.1X3	T41.1X4	T41.1X5	T41.1X6
Butylated hydroxy-anisole	T50.991	T50.992	T50.993	T50.994	T50.995	T50.996
Butylchloral hydrate	T42.6X1	T42.6X2	T42.6X3	T42.6X4	T42.6X5	T42.6X6
Butyltoluene	T52.2X1	T52.2X2	T52.2X3	T52.2X4	—	—
Butyn	T41.3X1	T41.3X2	T41.3X3	T41.3X4	T41.3X5	T41.3X6
Butyrophenone (-based tranquilizers)	T43.4X1	T43.4X2	T43.4X3	T43.4X4	T43.4X5	T43.4X6
C						
Cabergoline	T42.8X1	T42.8X2	T42.8X3	T42.8X4	T42.8X5	T42.8X6
Cacodyl, cacodylic acid	T57.0X1	T57.0X2	T57.0X3	T57.0X4	—	—
Cactinomycin	T45.1X1	T45.1X2	T45.1X3	T45.1X4	T45.1X5	T45.1X6
Cade oil	T49.4X1	T49.4X2	T49.4X3	T49.4X4	T49.4X5	T49.4X6
Cadexomer iodine	T49.0X1	T49.0X2	T49.0X3	T49.0X4	T49.0X5	T49.0X6
Cadmium (chloride) (fumes) (oxide)	T56.3X1	T56.3X2	T56.3X3	T56.3X4	—	—
sulfide (medicinal) NEC	T49.4X1	T49.4X2	T49.4X3	T49.4X4	T49.4X5	T49.4X6
Cadralazine	T46.5X1	T46.5X2	T46.5X3	T46.5X4	T46.5X5	T46.5X6
Caffeine	T43.611	T43.612	T43.613	T43.614	T43.615	T43.616
Calabar bean	T62.2X1	T62.2X2	T62.2X3	T62.2X4	—	—
Caladium seguinum	T62.2X1	T62.2X2	T62.2X3	T62.2X4	—	—
Calamine (lotion)	T49.3X1	T49.3X2	T49.3X3	T49.3X4	T49.3X5	T49.3X6
Calcifediol	T45.2X1	T45.2X2	T45.2X3	T45.2X4	T45.2X5	T45.2X6
Calciferol	T45.2X1	T45.2X2	T45.2X3	T45.2X4	T45.2X5	T45.2X6
Calcitonin	T50.991	T50.992	T50.993	T50.994	T50.995	T50.996
Calcitriol	T45.2X1	T45.2X2	T45.2X3	T45.2X4	T45.2X5	T45.2X6
Calcium	T50.3X1	T50.3X2	T50.3X3	T50.3X4	T50.3X5	T50.3X6
actylsalicylate	T39.011	T39.012	T39.013	T39.014	T39.015	T39.016
benzamidosalicylate	T37.1X1	T37.1X2	T37.1X3	T37.1X4	T37.1X5	T37.1X6
bromide	T42.6X1	T42.6X2	T42.6X3	T42.6X4	T42.6X5	T42.6X6
bromolactobionate	T42.6X1	T42.6X2	T42.6X3	T42.6X4	T42.6X5	T42.6X6
carbaspirin	T39.011	T39.012	T39.013	T39.014	T39.015	T39.016
carbimide	T50.6X1	T50.6X2	T50.6X3	T50.6X4	T50.6X5	T50.6X6

◀ New ◀▥ Revised ~~deleted~~ Deleted

	External Cause (T-Code)					
Substance	Poisoning, Accidental (Unintentional)	Poisoning, Intentional Self-Harm	Poisoning, Assault	Poisoning, Undetermined	Adverse Effect	Underdosing
Calcium *(Continued)*						
carbonate	T47.1X1	T47.1X2	T47.1X3	T47.1X4	T47.1X5	T47.1X6
chloride	T50.991	T50.992	T50.993	T50.994	T50.995	T50.996
anhydrous	T50.991	T50.992	T50.993	T50.994	T50.995	T50.996
cyanide	T57.8X1	T57.8X2	T57.8X3	T57.8X4	—	—
dioctyl sulfosuccinate	T47.4X1	T47.4X2	T47.4X3	T47.4X4	T47.4X5	T47.4X6
disodium edathamil	T45.8X1	T45.8X2	T45.8X3	T45.8X4	T45.8X5	T45.8X6
disodium edetate	T45.8X1	T45.8X2	T45.8X3	T45.8X4	T45.8X5	T45.8X6
dobesilate	T46.991	T46.992	T46.993	T46.994	T46.995	T46.996
EDTA	T45.8X1	T45.8X2	T45.8X3	T45.8X4	T45.8X5	T45.8X6
ferrous citrate	T45.4X1	T45.4X2	T45.4X3	T45.4X4	T45.4X5	T45.4X6
folinate	T45.8X1	T45.8X2	T45.8X3	T45.8X4	T45.8X5	T45.8X6
glubionate	T50.3X1	T50.3X2	T50.3X3	T50.3X4	T50.3X5	T50.3X6
gluconate	T50.3X1	T50.3X2	T50.3X3	T50.3X4	T50.3X5	T50.3X6
gluconogalactogluconate	T50.3X1	T50.3X2	T50.3X3	T50.3X4	T50.3X5	T50.3X6
hydrate, hydroxide	T54.3X1	T54.3X2	T54.3X3	T54.3X4	—	—
hypochlorite	T54.3X1	T54.3X2	T54.3X3	T54.3X4	—	—
iodide	T48.4X1	T48.4X2	T48.4X3	T48.4X4	T48.4X5	T48.4X6
ipodate	T50.8X1	T50.8X2	T50.8X3	T50.8X4	T50.8X5	T50.8X6
lactate	T50.3X1	T50.3X2	T50.3X3	T50.3X4	T50.3X5	T50.3X6
leucovorin	T45.8X1	T45.8X2	T45.8X3	T45.8X4	T45.8X5	T45.8X6
mandelate	T37.91	T37.92	T37.93	T37.94	T37.95	T37.96
oxide	T54.3X1	T54.3X2	T54.3X3	T54.3X4	—	—
pantothenate	T45.2X1	T45.2X2	T45.2X3	T45.2X4	T45.2X5	T45.2X6
phosphate	T50.3X1	T50.3X2	T50.3X3	T50.3X4	T50.3X5	T50.3X6
salicylate	T39.091	T39.092	T39.093	T39.094	T39.095	T39.096
salts	T50.3X1	T50.3X2	T50.3X3	T50.3X4	T50.3X5	T50.3X6
Calculus-dissolving drug	T50.991	T50.992	T50.993	T50.994	T50.995	T50.996
Calomel	T49.0X1	T49.0X2	T49.0X3	T49.0X4	T49.0X5	T49.0X6
Caloric agent	T50.3X1	T50.3X2	T50.3X3	T50.3X4	T50.3X5	T50.3X6
Calusterone	T38.7X1	T38.7X2	T38.7X3	T38.7X4	T38.7X5	T38.7X6
Camazepam	T42.4X1	T42.4X2	T42.4X3	T42.4X4	T42.4X5	T42.4X6
Camomile	T49.0X1	T49.0X2	T49.0X3	T49.0X4	T49.0X5	T49.0X6
Camoquin	T37.2X1	T37.2X2	T37.2X3	T37.2X4	T37.2X5	T37.2X6
Camphor						
insecticide	T60.2X1	T60.2X2	T60.2X3	T60.2X4	—	—
medicinal	T49.8X1	T49.8X2	T49.8X3	T49.8X4	T49.8X5	T49.8X6
Camylofin	T44.3X1	T44.3X2	T44.3X3	T44.3X4	T44.3X5	T44.3X6
Cancer chemotherapy drug regimen	T45.1X1	T45.1X2	T45.1X3	T45.1X4	T45.1X5	T45.1X6
Candeptin	T49.0X1	T49.0X2	T49.0X3	T49.0X4	T49.0X5	T49.0X6

TABLE OF DRUGS AND CHEMICALS

TABLE OF DRUGS AND CHEMICALS

Substance	External Cause (T-Code)					
	Poisoning, Accidental (Unintentional)	Poisoning, Intentional Self-Harm	Poisoning, Assault	Poisoning, Undetermined	Adverse Effect	Underdosing
Candicidin	T49.0X1	T49.0X2	T49.0X3	T49.0X4	T49.0X5	T49.0X6
Cannabinol	T40.7X1	T40.7X2	T40.7X3	T40.7X4	T40.7X5	T40.7X6
Cannabis (derivatives)	T40.7X1	T40.7X2	T40.7X3	T40.7X4	T40.7X5	T40.7X6
Canned heat	T51.1X1	T51.1X2	T51.1X3	T51.1X4	—	—
Canrenoic acid	T50.0X1	T50.0X2	T50.0X3	T50.0X4	T50.0X5	T50.0X6
Canrenone	T50.0X1	T50.0X2	T50.0X3	T50.0X4	T50.0X5	T50.0X6
Cantharides, cantharidin, cantharis	T49.8X1	T49.8X2	T49.8X3	T49.8X4	T49.8X5	T49.8X6
Canthaxanthin	T50.991	T50.992	T50.993	T50.994	T50.995	T50.996
Capillary-active drug NEC	T46.901	T46.902	T46.903	T46.904	T46.905	T46.906
Capreomycin	T36.8X1	T36.8X2	T36.8X3	T36.8X4	T36.8X5	T36.8X6
Capsicum	T49.4X1	T49.4X2	T49.4X3	T49.4X4	T49.4X5	T49.4X6
Captafol	T60.3X1	T60.3X2	T60.3X3	T60.3X4	—	—
Captan	T60.3X1	T60.3X2	T60.3X3	T60.3X4	—	—
Captodiame, captodiamine	T43.591	T43.592	T43.593	T43.594	T43.595	T43.596
Captopril	T46.4X1	T46.4X2	T46.4X3	T46.4X4	T46.4X5	T46.4X6
Caramiphen	T44.3X1	T44.3X2	T44.3X3	T44.3X4	T44.3X5	T44.3X6
Carazolol	T44.7X1	T44.7X2	T44.7X3	T44.7X4	T44.7X5	T44.7X6
Carbachol	T44.1X1	T44.1X2	T44.1X3	T44.1X4	T44.1X5	T44.1X6
Carbacrylamine (resin)	T50.3X1	T50.3X2	T50.3X3	T50.3X4	T50.3X5	T50.3X6
Carbamate (insecticide)	T60.0X1	T60.0X2	T60.0X3	T60.0X4	—	—
Carbamate (sedative)	T42.6X1	T42.6X2	T42.6X3	T42.6X4	T42.6X5	T42.6X6
herbicide	T60.0X1	T60.0X2	T60.0X3	T60.0X4	—	—
insecticide	T60.0X1	T60.0X2	T60.0X3	T60.0X4	—	—
Carbamazepine	T42.1X1	T42.1X2	T42.1X3	T42.1X4	T42.1X5	T42.1X6
Carbamide	T47.3X1	T47.3X2	T47.3X3	T47.3X4	T47.3X5	T47.3X6
peroxide	T49.0X1	T49.0X2	T49.0X3	T49.0X4	T49.0X5	T49.0X6
topical	T49.8X1	T49.8X2	T49.8X3	T49.8X4	T49.8X5	T49.8X6
Carbamylcholine chloride	T44.1X1	T44.1X2	T44.1X3	T44.1X4	T44.1X5	T44.1X6
Carbaril	T60.0X1	T60.0X2	T60.0X3	T60.0X4	—	—
Carbarsone	T37.3X1	T37.3X2	T37.3X3	T37.3X4	T37.3X5	T37.3X6
Carbaryl	T60.0X1	T60.0X2	T60.0X3	T60.0X4	—	—
Carbaspirin	T39.011	T39.012	T39.013	T39.014	T39.015	T39.016
Carbazochrome (salicylate) (sodium sulfonate)	T49.4X1	T49.4X2	T49.4X3	T49.4X4	T49.4X5	T49.4X6
Carbenicillin	T36.0X1	T36.0X2	T36.0X3	T36.0X4	T36.0X5	T36.0X6
Carbenoxolone	T47.1X1	T47.1X2	T47.1X3	T47.1X4	T47.1X5	T47.1X6
Carbetapentane	T48.3X1	T48.3X2	T48.3X3	T48.3X4	T48.3X5	T48.3X6
Carbethyl salicylate	T39.091	T39.092	T39.093	T39.094	T39.095	T39.096
Carbidopa (with levodopa)	T42.8X1	T42.8X2	T42.8X3	T42.8X4	T42.8X5	T42.8X6
Carbimazole	T38.2X1	T38.2X2	T38.2X3	T38.2X4	T38.2X5	T38.2X6

◀ New   ◀||| Revised   ~~deleted~~ Deleted

Substance	External Cause (T-Code)					
	Poisoning, Accidental (Unintentional)	Poisoning, Intentional Self-Harm	Poisoning, Assault	Poisoning, Undetermined	Adverse Effect	Underdosing
Carbinol	T51.1X1	T51.1X2	T51.1X3	T51.1X4	—	—
Carbinoxamine	T45.0X1	T45.0X2	T45.0X3	T45.0X4	T45.0X5	T45.0X6
Carbiphene	T39.8X1	T39.8X2	T39.8X3	T39.8X4	T39.8X5	T39.8X6
Carbitol	T52.3X1	T52.3X2	T52.3X3	T52.3X4	—	—
Carbocaine	T41.3X1	T41.3X2	T41.3X3	T41.3X4	T41.3X5	T41.3X6
infiltration (subcutaneous)	T41.3X1	T41.3X2	T41.3X3	T41.3X4	T41.3X5	T41.3X6
nerve block (peripheral) (plexus)	T41.3X1	T41.3X2	T41.3X3	T41.3X4	T41.3X5	T41.3X6
topical (surface)	T41.3X1	T41.3X2	T41.3X3	T41.3X4	T41.3X5	T41.3X6
Carbo medicinalis	T47.6X1	T47.6X2	T47.6X3	T47.6X4	T47.6X5	T47.6X6
Carbomycin	T36.8X1	T36.8X2	T36.8X3	T36.8X4	T36.8X5	T36.8X6
Carbocisteine	T48.4X1	T48.4X2	T48.4X3	T48.4X4	T48.4X5	T48.4X6
Carbocromen	T46.3X1	T46.3X2	T46.3X3	T46.3X4	T46.3X5	T46.3X6
Carbol fuchsin	T49.0X1	T49.0X2	T49.0X3	T49.0X4	T49.0X5	T49.0X6
Carbolic acid — see also Phenol	T54.0X1	T54.0X2	T54.0X3	T54.0X4	—	—
Carbolonium (bromide)	T48.1X1	T48.1X2	T48.1X3	T48.1X4	T48.1X5	T48.1X6
Carbon						
bisulfide (liquid)	T65.4X1	T65.4X2	T65.4X3	T65.4X4	—	—
vapor	T65.4X1	T65.4X2	T65.4X3	T65.4X4	—	—
dioxide (gas)	T59.7X1	T59.7X2	T59.7X3	T59.7X4	—	—
medicinal	T41.5X1	T41.5X2	T41.5X3	T41.5X4	T41.5X5	T41.5X6
nonmedicinal	T59.7X1	T59.7X2	T59.7X3	T59.7X4	—	—
snow	T49.4X1	T49.4X2	T49.4X3	T49.4X4	T49.4X5	T49.4X6
disulfide (liquid)	T65.4X1	T65.4X2	T65.4X3	T65.4X4	—	—
vapor	T65.4X1	T65.4X2	T65.4X3	T65.4X4	—	—
monoxide (from incomplete combustion)	T58.91	T58.92	T58.93	T58.94	—	—
blast furnace gas	T58.8X1	T58.8X2	T58.8X3	T58.8X4	—	—
butane (distributed in mobile container)	T58.11	T58.12	T58.13	T58.14	—	—
distributed through pipes	T58.11	T58.12	T58.13	T58.14	—	—
charcoal fumes	T58.2X1	T58.2X2	T58.2X3	T58.2X4	—	—
coal	T58.2X1	T58.2X2	T58.2X3	T58.2X4		
coke (in domestic stoves, fireplaces)	T58.2X1	T58.2X2	T58.2X3	T58.2X4	—	—
gas (piped)	T58.11	T58.12	T58.13	T58.14	—	—
solid (in domestic stoves, fireplaces)	T58.2X1	T58.2X2	T58.2X3	T58.2X4	—	—
exhaust gas (motor) not in transit	T58.01	T58.02	T58.03	T58.04	—	—
combustion engine, any not in watercraft	T58.01	T58.02	T58.03	T58.04	—	—
farm tractor, not in transit	T58.01	T58.02	T58.03	T58.04	—	—
gas engine	T58.01	T58.02	T58.03	T58.04	—	—
motor pump	T58.01	T58.02	T58.03	T58.04	—	—
motor vehicle, not in transit	T58.01	T58.02	T58.03	T58.04	—	—

TABLE OF DRUGS AND CHEMICALS

Substance	External Cause (T-Code)					
	Poisoning, Accidental (Unintentional)	Poisoning, Intentional Self-Harm	Poisoning, Assault	Poisoning, Undetermined	Adverse Effect	Underdosing
Carbon *(Continued)*						
monoxide *(Continued)*						
fuel (in domestic use)	T58.2X1	T58.2X2	T58.2X3	T58.2X4	—	—
gas (piped)	T58.11	T58.12	T58.13	T58.14	—	—
in mobile container	T58.11	T58.12	T58.13	T58.14	—	—
utility	T58.11	T58.12	T58.13	T58.14	—	—
in mobile container	T58.11	T58.12	T58.13	T58.14	—	—
piped (natural)	T58.11	T58.12	T58.13	T58.14	—	—
illuminating gas	T58.11	T58.12	T58.13	T58.14	—	—
industrial fuels or gases, any	T58.8X1	T58.8X2	T58.8X3	T58.8X4	—	—
kerosene (in domestic stoves, fireplaces)	T58.2X1	T58.2X2	T58.2X3	T58.2X4	—	—
kiln gas or vapor	T58.8X1	T58.8X2	T58.8X3	T58.8X4	—	—
motor exhaust gas, not in transit	T58.01	T58.02	T58.03	T58.04	—	—
piped gas (manufactured) (natural)	T58.11	T58.12	T58.13	T58.14	—	—
producer gas	T58.8X1	T58.8X2	T58.8X3	T58.8X4	—	—
propane (distributed in mobile container)	T58.11	T58.12	T58.13	T58.14	—	—
distributed through pipes	T58.11	T58.12	T58.13	T58.14	—	—
specified source NEC	T58.8X1	T58.8X2	T58.8X3	T58.8X4	—	—
stove gas	T58.11	T58.12	T58.13	T58.14	—	—
piped	T58.11	T58.12	T58.13	T58.14	—	—
utility gas	T58.11	T58.12	T58.13	T58.14	—	—
piped	T58.11	T58.12	T58.13	T58.14	—	—
water gas	T58.11	T58.12	T58.13	T58.14	—	—
wood (in domestic stoves, fireplaces)	T58.2X1	T58.2X2	T58.2X3	T58.2X4	—	—
tetrachloride (vapor) NEC	T53.0X1	T53.0X2	T53.0X3	T53.0X4	—	—
liquid (cleansing agent) NEC	T53.0X1	T53.0X2	T53.0X3	T53.0X4	—	—
solvent	T53.0X1	T53.0X2	T53.0X3	T53.0X4	—	—
Carbonic acid gas	T59.7X1	T59.7X2	T59.7X3	T59.7X4	—	—
anhydrase inhibitor NEC	T50.2X1	T50.2X2	T50.2X3	T50.2X4	T50.2X5	T50.2X6
Carbophenothion	T60.0X1	T60.0X2	T60.0X3	T60.0X4	—	—
Carboplatin	T45.1X1	T45.1X2	T45.1X3	T45.1X4	T45.1X5	T45.1X6
Carboprost	T48.0X1	T48.0X2	T48.0X3	T48.0X4	T48.0X5	T48.0X6
Carboquone	T45.1X1	T45.1X2	T45.1X3	T45.1X4	T45.1X5	T45.1X6
Carbowax	T49.3X1	T49.3X2	T49.3X3	T49.3X4	T49.3X5	T49.3X6
Carboxymethyl-cellulose	T47.4X1	T47.4X2	T47.4X3	T47.4X4	T47.4X5	T47.4X6
S-Carboxymethyl-cysteine	T48.4X1	T48.4X2	T48.4X3	T48.4X4	T48.4X5	T48.4X6
Carbrital	T42.3X1	T42.3X2	T42.3X3	T42.3X4	T42.3X5	T42.3X6
Carbromal	T42.6X1	T42.6X2	T42.6X3	T42.6X4	T42.6X5	T42.6X6
Carbutamide	T38.3X1	T38.3X2	T38.3X3	T38.3X4	T38.3X5	T38.3X6
Carbuterol	T48.6X1	T48.6X2	T48.6X3	T48.6X4	T48.6X5	T48.6X6

◀ New   ◀▥ Revised   ~~deleted~~ Deleted

	External Cause (T-Code)					
Substance	Poisoning, Accidental (Unintentional)	Poisoning, Intentional Self-Harm	Poisoning, Assault	Poisoning, Undetermined	Adverse Effect	Underdosing
Cardiac						
depressants	T46.2X1	T46.2X2	T46.2X3	T46.2X4	T46.2X5	T46.2X6
rhythm regulator	T46.2X1	T46.2X2	T46.2X3	T46.2X4	T46.2X5	T46.2X6
specified NEC	T46.2X1	T46.2X2	T46.2X3	T46.2X4	T46.2X5	T46.2X6
Cardiografin	T50.8X1	T50.8X2	T50.8X3	T50.8X4	T50.8X5	T50.8X6
Cardio-green	T50.8X1	T50.8X2	T50.8X3	T50.8X4	T50.8X5	T50.8X6
Cardiotonic (glycoside) NEC	T46.0X1	T46.0X2	T46.0X3	T46.0X4	T46.0X5	T46.0X6
Cardiovascular drug NEC	T46.901	T46.902	T46.903	T46.904	T46.905	T46.906
Cardrase	T50.2X1	T50.2X2	T50.2X3	T50.2X4	T50.2X5	T50.2X6
Carfusin	T49.0X1	T49.0X2	T49.0X3	T49.0X4	T49.0X5	T49.0X6
Carfecillin	T36.0X1	T36.0X2	T36.0X3	T36.0X4	T36.0X5	T36.0X6
Carfenazine	T43.3X1	T43.3X2	T43.3X3	T43.3X4	T43.3X5	T43.3X6
Carindacillin	T36.0X1	T36.0X2	T36.0X3	T36.0X4	T36.0X5	T36.0X6
Carisoprodol	T42.8X1	T42.8X2	T42.8X3	T42.8X4	T42.8X5	T42.8X6
Carmellose	T47.4X1	T47.4X2	T47.4X3	T47.4X4	T47.4X5	T47.4X6
Carminative	T47.5X1	T47.5X2	T47.5X3	T47.5X4	T47.5X5	T47.5X6
Carmofur	T45.1X1	T45.1X2	T45.1X3	T45.1X4	T45.1X5	T45.1X6
Carmustine	T45.1X1	T45.1X2	T45.1X3	T45.1X4	T45.1X5	T45.1X6
Carotene	T45.2X1	T45.2X2	T45.2X3	T45.2X4	T45.2X5	T45.2X6
Carphenazine	T43.3X1	T43.3X2	T43.3X3	T43.3X4	T43.3X5	T43.3X6
Carpipramine	T42.4X1	T42.4X2	T42.4X3	T42.4X4	T42.4X5	T42.4X6
Carprofen	T39.311	T39.312	T39.313	T39.314	T39.315	T39.316
Carpronium chloride	T44.3X1	T44.3X2	T44.3X3	T44.3X4	T44.3X5	T44.3X6
Carrageenan	T47.8X1	T47.8X2	T47.8X3	T47.8X4	T47.8X5	T47.8X6
Carteolol	T44.7X1	T44.7X2	T44.7X3	T44.7X4	T44.7X5	T44.7X6
Carter's Little Pills	T47.2X1	T47.2X2	T47.2X3	T47.2X4	T47.2X5	T47.2X6
Cascara (sagrada)	T47.2X1	T47.2X2	T47.2X3	T47.2X4	T47.2X5	T47.2X6
Cassava	T62.2X1	T62.2X2	T62.2X3	T62.2X4	—	—
Castellani's paint	T49.0X1	T49.0X2	T49.0X3	T49.0X4	T49.0X5	T49.0X6
Castor						
bean	T62.2X1	T62.2X2	T62.2X3	T62.2X4	—	—
oil	T47.2X1	T47.2X2	T47.2X3	T47.2X4	T47.2X5	T47.2X6
Catalase	T45.3X1	T45.3X2	T45.3X3	T45.3X4	T45.3X5	T45.3X6
Caterpillar (sting)	T63.431	T63.432	T63.433	T63.434	—	—
Catha (edulis) (tea)	T43.691	T43.692	T43.693	T43.694	—	—
Cathartic NEC	T47.4X1	T47.4X2	T47.4X3	T47.4X4	T47.4X5	T47.4X6
anthacene derivative	T47.2X1	T47.2X2	T47.2X3	T47.2X4	T47.2X5	T47.2X6
bulk	T47.4X1	T47.4X2	T47.4X3	T47.4X4	T47.4X5	T47.4X6
contact	T47.2X1	T47.2X2	T47.2X3	T47.2X4	T47.2X5	T47.2X6
emollient NEC	T47.4X1	T47.4X2	T47.4X3	T47.4X4	T47.4X5	T47.4X6

◀ New   ◀▥ Revised   ~~deleted~~ Deleted

TABLE OF DRUGS AND CHEMICALS

Substance	Poisoning, Accidental (Unintentional)	Poisoning, Intentional Self-Harm	Poisoning, Assault	Poisoning, Undetermined	Adverse Effect	Underdosing
			External Cause (T-Code)			
Cathartic NEC *(Continued)*						
irritant NEC	T47.2X1	T47.2X2	T47.2X3	T47.2X4	T47.2X5	T47.2X6
mucilage	T47.4X1	T47.4X2	T47.4X3	T47.4X4	T47.4X5	T47.4X6
saline	T47.3X1	T47.3X2	T47.3X3	T47.3X4	T47.3X5	T47.3X6
vegetable	T47.2X1	T47.2X2	T47.2X3	T47.2X4	T47.2X5	T47.2X6
Cathine	T50.5X1	T50.5X2	T50.5X3	T50.5X4	T50.5X5	T50.5X6
Cathomycin	T36.8X1	T36.8X2	T36.8X3	T36.8X4	T36.8X5	T36.8X6
Cation exchange resin	T50.3X1	T50.3X2	T50.3X3	T50.3X4	T50.3X5	T50.3X6
Caustic(s) NEC	T54.91	T54.92	T54.93	T54.94	—	—
alkali	T54.3X1	T54.3X2	T54.3X3	T54.3X4	—	—
hydroxide	T54.3X1	T54.3X2	T54.3X3	T54.3X4	—	—
potash	T54.3X1	T54.3X2	T54.3X3	T54.3X4	—	—
soda	T54.3X1	T54.3X2	T54.3X3	T54.3X4	—	—
specified NEC	T54.91	T54.92	T54.93	T54.94	—	—
Ceepryn	T49.0X1	T49.0X2	T49.0X3	T49.0X4	T49.0X5	T49.0X6
ENT agent	T49.6X1	T49.6X2	T49.6X3	T49.6X4	T49.6X5	T49.6X6
lozenges	T49.6X1	T49.6X2	T49.6X3	T49.6X4	T49.6X5	T49.6X6
Cefacetrile	T36.1X1	T36.1X2	T36.1X3	T36.1X4	T36.1X5	T36.1X6
Cefaclor	T36.1X1	T36.1X2	T36.1X3	T36.1X4	T36.1X5	T36.1X6
Cefadroxil	T36.1X1	T36.1X2	T36.1X3	T36.1X4	T36.1X5	T36.1X6
Cefalexin	T36.1X1	T36.1X2	T36.1X3	T36.1X4	T36.1X5	T36.1X6
Cefaloglycin	T36.1X1	T36.1X2	T36.1X3	T36.1X4	T36.1X5	T36.1X6
Cefaloridine	T36.1X1	T36.1X2	T36.1X3	T36.1X4	T36.1X5	T36.1X6
Cefalosporins	T36.1X1	T36.1X2	T36.1X3	T36.1X4	T36.1X5	T36.1X6
Cefalotin	T36.1X1	T36.1X2	T36.1X3	T36.1X4	T36.1X5	T36.1X6
Cefamandole	T36.1X1	T36.1X2	T36.1X3	T36.1X4	T36.1X5	T36.1X6
Cefamycin antibiotic	T36.1X1	T36.1X2	T36.1X3	T36.1X4	T36.1X5	T36.1X6
Cefapirin	T36.1X1	T36.1X2	T36.1X3	T36.1X4	T36.1X5	T36.1X6
Cefatrizine	T36.1X1	T36.1X2	T36.1X3	T36.1X4	T36.1X5	T36.1X6
Cefazedone	T36.1X1	T36.1X2	T36.1X3	T36.1X4	T36.1X5	T36.1X6
Cefazolin	T36.1X1	T36.1X2	T36.1X3	T36.1X4	T36.1X5	T36.1X6
Cefbuperazone	T36.1X1	T36.1X2	T36.1X3	T36.1X4	T36.1X5	T36.1X6
Cefetamet	T36.1X1	T36.1X2	T36.1X3	T36.1X4	T36.1X5	T36.1X6
Cefixime	T36.1X1	T36.1X2	T36.1X3	T36.1X4	T36.1X5	T36.1X6
Cefmenoxime	T36.1X1	T36.1X2	T36.1X3	T36.1X4	T36.1X5	T36.1X6
Cefmetazole	T36.1X1	T36.1X2	T36.1X3	T36.1X4	T36.1X5	T36.1X6
Cefminox	T36.1X1	T36.1X2	T36.1X3	T36.1X4	T36.1X5	T36.1X6
Cefonicid	T36.1X1	T36.1X2	T36.1X3	T36.1X4	T36.1X5	T36.1X6
Cefoperazone	T36.1X1	T36.1X2	T36.1X3	T36.1X4	T36.1X5	T36.1X6

◀ New　◀▥ Revised　~~deleted~~ Deleted

Substance	External Cause (T-Code)					
	Poisoning, Accidental (Unintentional)	Poisoning, Intentional Self-Harm	Poisoning, Assault	Poisoning, Undetermined	Adverse Effect	Underdosing
Ceforanide	T36.1X1	T36.1X2	T36.1X3	T36.1X4	T36.1X5	T36.1X6
Cefotaxime	T36.1X1	T36.1X2	T36.1X3	T36.1X4	T36.1X5	T36.1X6
Cefotetan	T36.1X1	T36.1X2	T36.1X3	T36.1X4	T36.1X5	T36.1X6
Cefotiam	T36.1X1	T36.1X2	T36.1X3	T36.1X4	T36.1X5	T36.1X6
Cefoxitin	T36.1X1	T36.1X2	T36.1X3	T36.1X4	T36.1X5	T36.1X6
Cefpimizole	T36.1X1	T36.1X2	T36.1X3	T36.1X4	T36.1X5	T36.1X6
Cefpiramide	T36.1X1	T36.1X2	T36.1X3	T36.1X4	T36.1X5	T36.1X6
Cefradine	T36.1X1	T36.1X2	T36.1X3	T36.1X4	T36.1X5	T36.1X6
Cefroxadine	T36.1X1	T36.1X2	T36.1X3	T36.1X4	T36.1X5	T36.1X6
Cefsulodin	T36.1X1	T36.1X2	T36.1X3	T36.1X4	T36.1X5	T36.1X6
Ceftazidime	T36.1X1	T36.1X2	T36.1X3	T36.1X4	T36.1X5	T36.1X6
Cefteram	T36.1X1	T36.1X2	T36.1X3	T36.1X4	T36.1X5	T36.1X6
Ceftezole	T36.1X1	T36.1X2	T36.1X3	T36.1X4	T36.1X5	T36.1X6
Ceftizoxime	T36.1X1	T36.1X2	T36.1X3	T36.1X4	T36.1X5	T36.1X6
Ceftriaxone	T36.1X1	T36.1X2	T36.1X3	T36.1X4	T36.1X5	T36.1X6
Cefuroxime	T36.1X1	T36.1X2	T36.1X3	T36.1X4	T36.1X5	T36.1X6
Cefuzonam	T36.1X1	T36.1X2	T36.1X3	T36.1X4	T36.1X5	T36.1X6
Celestone	T38.0X1	T38.0X2	T38.0X3	T38.0X4	T38.0X5	T38.0X6
topical	T49.0X1	T49.0X2	T49.0X3	T49.0X4	T49.0X5	T49.0X6
Celiprolol	T44.7X1	T44.7X2	T44.7X3	T44.7X4	T44.7X5	T44.7X6
Cellosolve	T52.91	T52.92	T52.93	T52.94	—	—
Cell stimulants and proliferants	T49.8X1	T49.8X2	T49.8X3	T49.8X4	T49.8X5	T49.8X6
Cellulose						
cathartic	T47.4X1	T47.4X2	T47.4X3	T47.4X4	T47.4X5	T47.4X6
hydroxyethyl	T47.4X1	T47.4X2	T47.4X3	T47.4X4	T47.4X5	T47.4X6
nitrates (topical)	T49.3X1	T49.3X2	T49.3X3	T49.3X4	T49.3X5	T49.3X6
oxidized	T49.4X1	T49.4X2	T49.4X3	T49.4X4	T49.4X5	T49.4X6
Centipede (bite)	T63.411	T63.412	T63.413	T63.414	—	—
Central nervous system						
depressants	T42.71	T42.72	T42.73	T42.74	T42.75	T42.76
anesthetic (general) NEC	T41.201	T41.202	T41.203	T41.204	T41.205	T41.206
gases NEC	T41.0X1	T41.0X2	T41.0X3	T41.0X4	T41.0X5	T41.0X6
intravenous	T41.1X1	T41.1X2	T41.1X3	T41.1X4	T41.1X5	T41.1X6
barbiturates	T42.3X1	T42.3X2	T42.3X3	T42.3X4	T42.3X5	T42.3X6
benzodiazepines	T42.4X1	T42.4X2	T42.4X3	T42.4X4	T42.4X5	T42.4X6
bromides	T42.6X1	T42.6X2	T42.6X3	T42.6X4	T42.6X5	T42.6X6
cannabis sativa	T40.7X1	T40.7X2	T40.7X3	T40.7X4	T40.7X5	T40.7X6
chloral hydrate	T42.6X1	T42.6X2	T42.6X3	T42.6X4	T42.6X5	T42.6X6
ethanol	T51.0X1	T51.0X2	T51.0X3	T51.0X4	—	—

TABLE OF DRUGS AND CHEMICALS

Substance	Poisoning, Accidental (Unintentional)	Poisoning, Intentional Self-Harm	Poisoning, Assault	Poisoning, Undetermined	Adverse Effect	Underdosing
				External Cause (T-Code)		
Central nervous system *(Continued)*						
depressants *(Continued)*						
hallucinogenics	T40.901	T40.902	T40.903	T40.904	T40.905	T40.906
hypnotics	T42.71	T42.72	T42.73	T42.74	T42.75	T42.76
specified NEC	T42.6X1	T42.6X2	T42.6X3	T42.6X4	T42.6X5	T42.6X6
muscle relaxants	T42.8X1	T42.8X2	T42.8X3	T42.8X4	T42.8X5	T42.8X6
paraldehyde	T42.6X1	T42.6X2	T42.6X3	T42.6X4	T42.6X5	T42.6X6
sedatives; sedative-hypnotics	T42.71	T42.72	T42.73	T42.74	T42.75	T42.76
mixed NEC	T42.6X1	T42.6X2	T42.6X3	T42.6X4	T42.6X5	T42.6X6
specified NEC	T42.6X1	T42.6X2	T42.6X3	T42.6X4	T42.6X5	T42.6X6
muscle-tone depressants	T42.8X1	T42.8X2	T42.8X3	T42.8X4	T42.8X5	T42.8X6
stimulants	T43.601	T43.602	T43.603	T43.604	T43.605	T43.606
amphetamines	T43.621	T43.622	T43.623	T43.624	T43.625	T43.626
analeptics	T50.7X1	T50.7X2	T50.7X3	T50.7X4	T50.7X5	T50.7X6
antidepressants	T43.201	T43.202	T43.203	T43.204	T43.205	T43.206
opiate antagonists	T50.7X1	T50.7X2	T50.7X3	T50.7X4	T50.7X5	T50.7X6
specified NEC	T43.691	T43.692	T43.693	T43.694	T43.695	T43.696
Cephalexin	T36.1X1	T36.1X2	T36.1X3	T36.1X4	T36.1X5	T36.1X6
Cephaloglycin	T36.1X1	T36.1X2	T36.1X3	T36.1X4	T36.1X5	T36.1X6
Cephaloridine	T36.1X1	T36.1X2	T36.1X3	T36.1X4	T36.1X5	T36.1X6
Cephalosporins	T36.1X1	T36.1X2	T36.1X3	T36.1X4	T36.1X5	T36.1X6
N (adicillin)	T36.0X1	T36.0X2	T36.0X3	T36.0X4	T36.0X5	T36.0X6
Cephalothin	T36.1X1	T36.1X2	T36.1X3	T36.1X4	T36.1X5	T36.1X6
Cephalotin	T36.1X1	T36.1X2	T36.1X3	T36.1X4	T36.1X5	T36.1X6
Cephradine	T36.1X1	T36.1X2	T36.1X3	T36.1X4	T36.1X5	T36.1X6
Cerbera (odallam)	T62.2X1	T62.2X2	T62.2X3	T62.2X4	—	—
Cerberin	T46.0X1	T46.0X2	T46.0X3	T46.0X4	T46.0X5	T46.0X6
Cerebral stimulants	T43.601	T43.602	T43.603	T43.604	T43.605	T43.606
psychotherapeutic	T43.601	T43.602	T43.603	T43.604	T43.605	T43.606
specified NEC	T43.691	T43.692	T43.693	T43.694	T43.695	T43.696
Cerium oxalate	T45.0X1	T45.0X2	T45.0X3	T45.0X4	T45.0X5	T45.0X6
Cerous oxalate	T45.0X1	T45.0X2	T45.0X3	T45.0X4	T45.0X5	T45.0X6
Ceruletide	T50.8X1	T50.8X2	T50.8X3	T50.8X4	T50.8X5	T50.8X6
Cetalkonium (chloride)	T49.0X1	T49.0X2	T49.0X3	T49.0X4	T49.0X5	T49.0X6
Cethexonium chloride	T49.0X1	T49.0X2	T49.0X3	T49.0X4	T49.0X5	T49.0X6
Cetiedil	T46.7X1	T46.7X2	T46.7X3	T46.7X4	T46.7X5	T46.7X6
Cetirizine	T45.0X1	T45.0X2	T45.0X3	T45.0X4	T45.0X5	T45.0X6
Cetomacrogol	T50.991	T50.992	T50.993	T50.994	T50.995	T50.996
Cetotiamine	T45.2X1	T45.2X2	T45.2X3	T45.2X4	T45.2X5	T45.2X6

◀ New ◀◀ Revised ~~deleted~~ Deleted

Substance	External Cause (T-Code)					
	Poisoning, Accidental (Unintentional)	Poisoning, Intentional Self-Harm	Poisoning, Assault	Poisoning, Undetermined	Adverse Effect	Underdosing
Cetoxime	T45.0X1	T45.0X2	T45.0X3	T45.0X4	T45.0X5	T45.0X6
Cetraxate	T47.1X1	T47.1X2	T47.1X3	T47.1X4	T47.1X5	T47.1X6
Cetrimide	T49.0X1	T49.0X2	T49.0X3	T49.0X4	T49.0X5	T49.0X6
Cetrimonium (bromide)	T49.0X1	T49.0X2	T49.0X3	T49.0X4	T49.0X5	T49.0X6
Cetylpyridinium chloride	T49.0X1	T49.0X2	T49.0X3	T49.0X4	T49.0X5	T49.0X6
ENT agent	T49.6X1	T49.6X2	T49.6X3	T49.6X4	T49.6X5	T49.6X6
lozenges	T49.6X1	T49.6X2	T49.6X3	T49.6X4	T49.6X5	T49.6X6
Cevadillasee Sabadilla						
Cevitamic acid	T45.2X1	T45.2X2	T45.2X3	T45.2X4	T45.2X5	T45.2X6
Chalk, precipitated	T47.1X1	T47.1X2	T47.1X3	T47.1X4	T47.1X5	T47.1X6
Chamomile	T49.0X1	T49.0X2	T49.0X3	T49.0X4	T49.0X5	T49.0X6
Ch'an su	T46.0X1	T46.0X2	T46.0X3	T46.0X4	T46.0X5	T46.0X6
Charcoal	T47.6X1	T47.6X2	T47.6X3	T47.6X4	T47.6X5	T47.6X6
activated — see also Charcoal, medicinal	T47.6X1	T47.6X2	T47.6X3	T47.6X4	T47.6X5	T47.6X6
fumes (Carbon monoxide)	T58.2X1	T58.2X2	T58.2X3	T58.2X4	—	—
industrial	T58.8X1	T58.8X2	T58.8X3	T58.8X4	—	—
medicinal (activated)	T47.6X1	T47.6X2	T47.6X3	T47.6X4	T47.6X5	T47.6X6
antidiarrheal	T47.6X1	T47.6X2	T47.6X3	T47.6X4	T47.6X5	T47.6X6
poison control	T47.8X1	T47.8X2	T47.8X3	T47.8X4	T47.8X5	T47.8X6
specified use other than for diarrhea	T47.8X1	T47.8X2	T47.8X3	T47.8X4	T47.8X5	T47.8X6
topical	T49.8X1	T49.8X2	T49.8X3	T49.8X4	T49.8X5	T49.8X6
Chaulmosulfone	T37.1X1	T37.1X2	T37.1X3	T37.1X4	T37.1X5	T37.1X6
Chelating agent NEC	T50.6X1	T50.6X2	T50.6X3	T50.6X4	T50.6X5	T50.6X6
Chelidonium majus	T62.2X1	T62.2X2	T62.2X3	T62.2X4	—	—
Chemical substance NEC	T65.91	T65.92	T65.93	T65.94	—	—
Chenodeoxycholic acid	T47.5X1	T47.5X2	T47.5X3	T47.5X4	T47.5X5	T47.5X6
Chenodiol	T47.5X1	T47.5X2	T47.5X3	T47.5X4	T47.5X5	T47.5X6
Chenopodium	T37.4X1	T37.4X2	T37.4X3	T37.4X4	T37.4X5	T37.4X6
Cherry laurel	T62.2X1	T62.2X2	T62.2X3	T62.2X4	—	—
Chinidin(e)	T46.2X1	T46.2X2	T46.2X3	T46.2X4	T46.2X5	T46.2X6
Chiniofon	T37.8X1	T37.8X2	T37.8X3	T37.8X4	T37.8X5	T37.8X6
Chlophedianol	T48.3X1	T48.3X2	T48.3X3	T48.3X4	T48.3X5	T48.3X6
Chloral	T42.6X1	T42.6X2	T42.6X3	T42.6X4	T42.6X5	T42.6X6
derivative	T42.6X1	T42.6X2	T42.6X3	T42.6X4	T42.6X5	T42.6X6
hydrate	T42.6X1	T42.6X2	T42.6X3	T42.6X4	T42.6X5	T42.6X6
Chloralamide	T42.6X1	T42.6X2	T42.6X3	T42.6X4	T42.6X5	T42.6X6
Chloralodol	T42.6X1	T42.6X2	T42.6X3	T42.6X4	T42.6X5	T42.6X6
Chloralose	T60.4X1	T60.4X2	T60.4X3	T60.4X4	—	—
Chlorambucil	T45.1X1	T45.1X2	T45.1X3	T45.1X4	T45.1X5	T45.1X6

◀ New ◀ Revised ~~deleted~~ Deleted

Substance	External Cause (T-Code)					
	Poisoning, Accidental (Unintentional)	Poisoning, Intentional Self-Harm	Poisoning, Assault	Poisoning, Undetermined	Adverse Effect	Underdosing
Chloramine	T57.8X1	T57.8X2	T57.8X3	T57.8X4	—	—
T	T49.0X1	T49.0X2	T49.0X3	T49.0X4	T49.0X5	T49.0X6
topical	T49.0X1	T49.0X2	T49.0X3	T49.0X4	T49.0X5	T49.0X6
Chloramphenicol	T36.2X1	T36.2X2	T36.2X3	T36.2X4	T36.2X5	T36.2X6
ENT agent	T49.6X1	T49.6X2	T49.6X3	T49.6X4	T49.6X5	T49.6X6
ophthalmic preparation	T49.5X1	T49.5X2	T49.5X3	T49.5X4	T49.5X5	T49.5X6
topical NEC	T49.0X1	T49.0X2	T49.0X3	T49.0X4	T49.0X5	T49.0X6
Chlorate (potassium) (sodium) NEC	T60.3X1	T60.3X2	T60.3X3	T60.3X4	—	—
herbicide	T60.3X1	T60.3X2	T60.3X3	T60.3X4	—	—
Chlorazanil	T50.2X1	T50.2X2	T50.2X3	T50.2X4	T50.2X5	T50.2X6
Chlorbenzene, chlorbenzol	T53.7X1	T53.7X2	T53.7X3	T53.7X4	—	—
Chlorbenzoxamine	T44.3X1	T44.3X2	T44.3X3	T44.3X4	T44.3X5	T44.3X6
Chlorbutol	T42.6X1	T42.6X2	T42.6X3	T42.6X4	T42.6X5	T42.6X6
Chlorcyclizine	T45.0X1	T45.0X2	T45.0X3	T45.0X4	T45.0X5	T45.0X6
Chlordan(e) (dust)	T60.1X1	T60.1X2	T60.1X3	T60.1X4	—	—
Chlordantoin	T49.0X1	T49.0X2	T49.0X3	T49.0X4	T49.0X5	T49.0X6
Chlordiazepoxide	T42.4X1	T42.4X2	T42.4X3	T42.4X4	T42.4X5	T42.4X6
Chlordiethyl benzamide	T49.3X1	T49.3X2	T49.3X3	T49.3X4	T49.3X5	T49.3X6
Chloresium	T49.8X1	T49.8X2	T49.8X3	T49.8X4	T49.8X5	T49.8X6
Chlorethiazol	T42.6X1	T42.6X2	T42.6X3	T42.6X4	T42.6X5	T42.6X6
Chlorethyl — see Ethyl chloride						
Chloretone	T42.6X1	T42.6X2	T42.6X3	T42.6X4	T42.6X5	T42.6X6
Chlorex	T53.6X1	T53.6X2	T53.6X3	T53.6X4	—	—
insecticide	T60.1X1	T60.1X2	T60.1X3	T60.1X4	—	—
Chlorfenvinphos	T60.0X1	T60.0X2	T60.0X3	T60.0X4	—	—
Chlorhexadol	T42.6X1	T42.6X2	T42.6X3	T42.6X4	T42.6X5	T42.6X6
Chlorhexamide	T45.1X1	T45.1X2	T45.1X3	T45.1X4	T45.1X5	T45.1X6
Chlorhexidine	T49.0X1	T49.0X2	T49.0X3	T49.0X4	T49.0X5	T49.0X6
Chlorhydroxyquinolin	T49.0X1	T49.0X2	T49.0X3	T49.0X4	T49.0X5	T49.0X6
Chloride of lime (bleach)	T54.3X1	T54.3X2	T54.3X3	T54.3X4	—	—
Chlorimipramine	T43.011	T43.012	T43.013	T43.014	T43.015	T43.016
Chlorinated						
camphene	T53.6X1	T53.6X2	T53.6X3	T53.6X4	—	—
diphenyl	T53.7X1	T53.7X2	T53.7X3	T53.7X4	—	—
hydrocarbons NEC	T53.91	T53.92	T53.93	T53.94	—	—
solvents	T53.91	T53.92	T53.93	T53.94	—	—
lime (bleach)	T54.3X1	T54.3X2	T54.3X3	T54.3X4	—	—
and boric acid solution	T49.0X1	T49.0X2	T49.0X3	T49.0X4	T49.0X5	T49.0X6
naphthalene (insecticide)	T60.1X1	T60.1X2	T60.1X3	T60.1X4		
industrial (non-pesticide)	T53.7X1	T53.7X2	T53.7X3	T53.7X4	—	—

◀ New ◀◀ Revised ~~deleted~~ Deleted

Substance	External Cause (T-Code)					
	Poisoning, Accidental (Unintentional)	Poisoning, Intentional Self-Harm	Poisoning, Assault	Poisoning, Undetermined	Adverse Effect	Underdosing
Chlorinated *(Continued)*						
pesticide NEC	T60.8X1	T60.8X2	T60.8X3	T60.8X4	—	—
soda — *see also sodium hypochlorite*						
solution	T49.0X1	T49.0X2	T49.0X3	T49.0X4	T49.0X5	T49.0X6
Chlorine (fumes) (gas)	T59.4X1	T59.4X2	T59.4X3	T59.4X4	—	—
bleach	T54.3X1	T54.3X2	T54.3X3	T54.3X4	—	—
compound gas NEC	T59.4X1	T59.4X2	T59.4X3	T59.4X4	—	—
disinfectant	T59.4X1	T59.4X2	T59.4X3	T59.4X4	—	—
releasing agents NEC	T59.4X1	T59.4X2	T59.4X3	T59.4X4	—	—
Chlorisondamine chloride	T46.991	T46.992	T46.993	T46.994	T46.995	T46.996
Chlormadinone	T38.5X1	T38.5X2	T38.5X3	T38.5X4	T38.5X5	T38.5X6
Chlormephos	T60.0X1	T60.0X2	T60.0X3	T60.0X4	—	—
Chlormerodrin	T50.2X1	T50.2X2	T50.2X3	T50.2X4	T50.2X5	T50.2X6
Chlormethiazole	T42.6X1	T42.6X2	T42.6X3	T42.6X4	T42.6X5	T42.6X6
Chlormethine	T45.1X1	T45.1X2	T45.1X3	T45.1X4	T45.1X5	T45.1X6
Chlormethylenecycline	T36.4X1	T36.4X2	T36.4X3	T36.4X4	T36.4X5	T36.4X6
Chlormezanone	T42.6X1	T42.6X2	T42.6X3	T42.6X4	T42.6X5	T42.6X6
Chloroacetic acid	T60.3X1	T60.3X2	T60.3X3	T60.3X4	—	—
Chloroacetone	T59.3X1	T59.3X2	T59.3X3	T59.3X4	—	—
Chloroacetophenone	T59.3X1	T59.3X2	T59.3X3	T59.3X4	—	—
Chloroaniline	T53.7X1	T53.7X2	T53.7X3	T53.7X4	—	—
Chlorobenzene, chlorobenzol	T53.7X1	T53.7X2	T53.7X3	T53.7X4	—	—
Chlorobromomethane (fire extinguisher)	T53.6X1	T53.6X2	T53.6X3	T53.6X4	—	—
Chlorobutanol	T49.0X1	T49.0X2	T49.0X3	T49.0X4	T49.0X5	T49.0X6
Chlorocresol	T49.0X1	T49.0X2	T49.0X3	T49.0X4	T49.0X5	T49.0X6
Chlorodehydro-methyltestosterone	T38.7X1	T38.7X2	T38.7X3	T38.7X4	T38.7X5	T38.7X6
Chlorodinitrobenzene	T53.7X1	T53.7X2	T53.7X3	T53.7X4	—	—
dust or vapor	T53.7X1	T53.7X2	T53.7X3	T53.7X4	—	—
Chlorodiphenyl	T53.7X1	T53.7X2	T53.7X3	T53.7X4	—	—
Chloroethane — *see Ethyl chloride*						
Chloroethylene	T53.6X1	T53.6X2	T53.6X3	T53.6X4	—	—
Chlorofluorocarbons	T53.5X1	T53.5X2	T53.5X3	T53.5X4	—	—
Chloroform (fumes) (vapor)	T53.1X1	T53.1X2	T53.1X3	T53.1X4	—	—
anesthetic	T41.0X1	T41.0X2	T41.0X3	T41.0X4	T41.0X5	T41.0X6
solvent	T53.1X1	T53.1X2	T53.1X3	T53.1X4	—	—
water, concentrated	T41.0X1	T41.0X2	T41.0X3	T41.0X4	T41.0X5	T41.0X6
Chloroguanide	T37.2X1	T37.2X2	T37.2X3	T37.2X4	T37.2X5	T37.2X6
Chloromycetin	T36.2X1	T36.2X2	T36.2X3	T36.2X4	T36.2X5	T36.2X6
ENT agent	T49.6X1	T49.6X2	T49.6X3	T49.6X4	T49.6X5	T49.6X6
ophthalmic preparation	T49.5X1	T49.5X2	T49.5X3	T49.5X4	T49.5X5	T49.5X6

TABLE OF DRUGS AND CHEMICALS

Substance	External Cause (T-Code)					
	Poisoning, Accidental (Unintentional)	Poisoning, Intentional Self-Harm	Poisoning, Assault	Poisoning, Undetermined	Adverse Effect	Underdosing
Chloromycetin *(Continued)*						
otic solution	T49.6X1	T49.6X2	T49.6X3	T49.6X4	T49.6X5	T49.6X6
topical NEC	T49.0X1	T49.0X2	T49.0X3	T49.0X4	T49.0X5	T49.0X6
Chloronitrobenzene	T53.7X1	T53.7X2	T53.7X3	T53.7X4	—	—
dust or vapor	T53.7X1	T53.7X2	T53.7X3	T53.7X4	—	—
Chlorophacinone	T60.4X1	T60.4X2	T60.4X3	T60.4X4	—	—
Chlorophenol	T53.7X1	T53.7X2	T53.7X3	T53.7X4	—	—
Chlorophenothane	T60.1X1	T60.1X2	T60.1X3	T60.1X4		
Chlorophyll	T50.991	T50.992	T50.993	T50.994	T50.995	T50.996
Chloropicrin (fumes)	T53.6X1	T53.6X2	T53.6X3	T53.6X4	—	—
fumigant	T60.8X1	T60.8X2	T60.8X3	T60.8X4	—	—
fungicide	T60.3X1	T60.3X2	T60.3X3	T60.3X4	—	—
pesticide	T60.8X1	T60.8X2	T60.8X3	T60.8X4	—	—
Chloroprocaine	T41.3X1	T41.3X2	T41.3X3	T41.3X4	T41.3X5	T41.3X6
infiltration (subcutaneous)	T41.3X1	T41.3X2	T41.3X3	T41.3X4	T41.3X5	T41.3X6
nerve block (peripheral) (plexus)	T41.3X1	T41.3X2	T41.3X3	T41.3X4	T41.3X5	T41.3X6
spinal	T41.3X1	T41.3X2	T41.3X3	T41.3X4	T41.3X5	T41.3X6
Chloroptic	T49.5X1	T49.5X2	T49.5X3	T49.5X4	T49.5X5	T49.5X6
Chloropurine	T45.1X1	T45.1X2	T45.1X3	T45.1X4	T45.1X5	T45.1X6
Chloropyramine	T45.0X1	T45.0X2	T45.0X3	T45.0X4	T45.0X5	T45.0X6
Chloropyrifos	T60.0X1	T60.0X2	T60.0X3	T60.0X4	—	—
Chloropyrilene	T45.0X1	T45.0X2	T45.0X3	T45.0X4	T45.0X5	T45.0X6
Chloroquine	T37.2X1	T37.2X2	T37.2X3	T37.2X4	T37.2X5	T37.2X6
Chlorothalonil	T60.3X1	T60.3X2	T60.3X3	T60.3X4	—	—
Chlorothen	T45.0X1	T45.0X2	T45.0X3	T45.0X4	T45.0X5	T45.0X6
Chlorothiazide	T50.2X1	T50.2X2	T50.2X3	T50.2X4	T50.2X5	T50.2X6
Chlorothymol	T49.4X1	T49.4X2	T49.4X3	T49.4X4	T49.4X5	T49.4X6
Chlorotrianisene	T38.5X1	T38.5X2	T38.5X3	T38.5X4	T38.5X5	T38.5X6
Chlorovinyldichloro-arsine, not in war	T57.0X1	T57.0X2	T57.0X3	T57.0X4	—	—
Chloroxine	T49.4X1	T49.4X2	T49.4X3	T49.4X4	T49.4X5	T49.4X6
Chloroxylenol	T49.0X1	T49.0X2	T49.0X3	T49.0X4	T49.0X5	T49.0X6
Chlorphenamine	T45.0X1	T45.0X2	T45.0X3	T45.0X4	T45.0X5	T45.0X6
Chlorphenesin	T42.8X1	T42.8X2	T42.8X3	T42.8X4	T42.8X5	T42.8X6
topical (antifungal)	T49.0X1	T49.0X2	T49.0X3	T49.0X4	T49.0X5	T49.0X6
Chlorpheniramine	T45.0X1	T45.0X2	T45.0X3	T45.0X4	T45.0X5	T45.0X6
Chlorphenoxamine	T45.0X1	T45.0X2	T45.0X3	T45.0X4	T45.0X5	T45.0X6
Chlorphentermine	T50.5X1	T50.5X2	T50.5X3	T50.5X4	T50.5X5	T50.5X6
Chlorprocaine — *see Chloroprocaine*						
Chlorproguanil	T37.2X1	T37.2X2	T37.2X3	T37.2X4	T37.2X5	T37.2X6
Chlorpromazine	T43.3X1	T43.3X2	T43.3X3	T43.3X4	T43.3X5	T43.3X6

◄ New ◀ Revised ~~deleted~~ Deleted

Substance	External Cause (T-Code)					
	Poisoning, Accidental (Unintentional)	Poisoning, Intentional Self-Harm	Poisoning, Assault	Poisoning, Undetermined	Adverse Effect	Underdosing
Chlorpropamide	T38.3X1	T38.3X2	T38.3X3	T38.3X4	T38.3X5	T38.3X6
Chlorprothixene	T43.4X1	T43.4X2	T43.4X3	T43.4X4	T43.4X5	T43.4X6
Chlorquinaldol	T49.0X1	T49.0X2	T49.0X3	T49.0X4	T49.0X5	T49.0X6
Chlorquinol	T49.0X1	T49.0X2	T49.0X3	T49.0X4	T49.0X5	T49.0X6
Chlortalidone	T50.2X1	T50.2X2	T50.2X3	T50.2X4	T50.2X5	T50.2X6
Chlortetracycline	T36.4X1	T36.4X2	T36.4X3	T36.4X4	T36.4X5	T36.4X6
Chlorthalidone	T50.2X1	T50.2X2	T50.2X3	T50.2X4	T50.2X5	T50.2X6
Chlorthiophos	T60.0X1	T60.0X2	T60.0X3	T60.0X4	—	—
Chlorotrianisene	T38.5X1	T38.5X2	T38.5X3	T38.5X4	T38.5X5	T38.5X6
Chlor-Trimeton	T45.0X1	T45.0X2	T45.0X3	T45.0X4	T45.0X5	T45.0X6
Chlorthion	T60.0X1	T60.0X2	T60.0X3	T60.0X4	—	—
Chlorzoxazone	T42.8X1	T42.8X2	T42.8X3	T42.8X4	T42.8X5	T42.8X6
Choke damp	T59.7X1	T59.7X2	T59.7X3	T59.7X4	—	—
Cholagogues	T47.5X1	T47.5X2	T47.5X3	T47.5X4	T47.5X5	T47.5X6
Cholebrine	T50.8X1	T50.8X2	T50.8X3	T50.8X4	T50.8X5	T50.8X6
Cholecalciferol	T45.2X1	T45.2X2	T45.2X3	T45.2X4	T45.2X5	T45.2X6
Cholecystokinin	T50.8X1	T50.8X2	T50.8X3	T50.8X4	T50.8X5	T50.8X6
Cholera vaccine	T50.A91	T50.A92	T50.A93	T50.A94	T50.A95	T50.A96
Choleretic	T47.5X1	T47.5X2	T47.5X3	T47.5X4	T47.5X5	T47.5X6
Cholesterol-lowering agents	T46.6X1	T46.6X2	T46.6X3	T46.6X4	T46.6X5	T46.6X6
Cholestyramine (resin)	T46.6X1	T46.6X2	T46.6X3	T46.6X4	T46.6X5	T46.6X6
Cholic acid	T47.5X1	T47.5X2	T47.5X3	T47.5X4	T47.5X5	T47.5X6
Choline	T48.6X1	T48.6X2	T48.6X3	T48.6X4	T48.6X5	T48.6X6
chloride	T50.991	T50.992	T50.993	T50.994	T50.995	T50.996
dihydrogen citrate	T50.991	T50.992	T50.993	T50.994	T50.995	T50.996
salicylate	T39.091	T39.092	T39.093	T39.094	T39.095	T39.096
theophyllinate	T48.6X1	T48.6X2	T48.6X3	T48.6X4	T48.6X5	T48.6X6
Cholinergic (drug) NEC	T44.1X1	T44.1X2	T44.1X3	T44.1X4	T44.1X5	T44.1X6
muscle tone enhancer	T44.1X1	T44.1X2	T44.1X3	T44.1X4	T44.1X5	T44.1X6
organophosphorus	T44.0X1	T44.0X2	T44.0X3	T44.0X4	T44.0X5	T44.0X6
insecticide	T60.0X1	T60.0X2	T60.0X3	T60.0X4	—	—
nerve gas	T59.891	T59.892	T59.893	T59.894	—	—
trimethyl ammonium propanediol	T44.1X1	T44.1X2	T44.1X3	T44.1X4	T44.1X5	T44.1X6
Cholinesterase reactivator	T50.6X1	T50.6X2	T50.6X3	T50.6X4	T50.6X5	T50.6X6
Cholografin	T50.8X1	T50.8X2	T50.8X3	T50.8X4	T50.8X5	T50.8X6
Chorionic gonadotropin	T38.891	T38.892	T38.893	T38.894	T38.895	T38.896
Chromate	T56.2X1	T56.2X2	T56.2X3	T56.2X4	—	—
dust or mist	T56.2X1	T56.2X2	T56.2X3	T56.2X4	—	—
lead — *see also lead*	T56.0X1	T56.0X2	T56.0X3	T56.0X4	—	—
paint	T56.0X1	T56.0X2	T56.0X3	T56.0X4	—	—

◀ New ◀▥ Revised ~~deleted~~ Deleted

Substance	Poisoning, Accidental (Unintentional)	Poisoning, Intentional Self-Harm	Poisoning, Assault	Poisoning, Undetermined	Adverse Effect	Underdosing
			External Cause (T-Code)			
Chromic						
acid	T56.2X1	T56.2X2	T56.2X3	T56.2X4	—	—
dust or mist	T56.2X1	T56.2X2	T56.2X3	T56.2X4	—	—
phosphate 32P	T45.1X1	T45.1X2	T45.1X3	T45.1X4	T45.1X5	T45.1X6
Chromium	T56.2X1	T56.2X2	T56.2X3	T56.2X4	—	—
compounds — see Chromate						
sesquioxide	T50.8X1	T50.8X2	T50.8X3	T50.8X4	T50.8X5	T50.8X6
Chromomycin A3	T45.1X1	T45.1X2	T45.1X3	T45.1X4	T45.1X5	T45.1X6
Chromonar	T46.3X1	T46.3X2	T46.3X3	T46.3X4	T46.3X5	T46.3X6
Chromyl chloride	T56.2X1	T56.2X2	T56.2X3	T56.2X4	—	—
Chrysarobin	T49.4X1	T49.4X2	T49.4X3	T49.4X4	T49.4X5	T49.4X6
Chrysazin	T47.2X1	T47.2X2	T47.2X3	T47.2X4	T47.2X5	T47.2X6
Chymar	T45.3X1	T45.3X2	T45.3X3	T45.3X4	T45.3X5	T45.3X6
ophthalmic preparation	T49.5X1	T49.5X2	T49.5X3	T49.5X4	T49.5X5	T49.5X6
Chymopapain	T45.3X1	T45.3X2	T45.3X3	T45.3X4	T45.3X5	T45.3X6
Chymotrypsin	T45.3X1	T45.3X2	T45.3X3	T45.3X4	T45.3X5	T45.3X6
ophthalmic preparation	T49.5X1	T49.5X2	T49.5X3	T49.5X4	T49.5X5	T49.5X6
Cianidanol	T50.991	T50.992	T50.993	T50.994	T50.995	T50.996
Cianopramine	T43.011	T43.012	T43.013	T43.014	T43.015	T43.016
Cibenzoline	T46.2X1	T46.2X2	T46.2X3	T46.2X4	T46.2X5	T46.2X6
Ciclacillin	T36.0X1	T36.0X2	T36.0X3	T36.0X4	T36.0X5	T36.0X6
Ciclobarbital — see Hexobarbital						
Ciclonicate	T46.7X1	T46.7X2	T46.7X3	T46.7X4	T46.7X5	T46.7X6
Ciclopirox (olamine)	T49.0X1	T49.0X2	T49.0X3	T49.0X4	T49.0X5	T49.0X6
Ciclosporin	T45.1X1	T45.1X2	T45.1X3	T45.1X4	T45.1X5	T45.1X6
Cicuta maculata or virosa	T62.2X1	T62.2X2	T62.2X3	T62.2X4	—	—
Cicutoxin	T62.2X1	T62.2X2	T62.2X3	T62.2X4	—	—
Cigarette lighter fluid	T52.0X1	T52.0X2	T52.0X3	T52.0X4	—	—
Cigarettes (tobacco)	T65.221	T65.222	T65.223	T65.224		
Ciguatoxin	T61.01	T61.02	T61.03	T61.04	—	—
Cilazapril	T46.4X1	T46.4X2	T46.4X3	T46.4X4	T46.4X5	T46.4X6
Cimetidine	T47.0X1	T47.0X2	T47.0X3	T47.0X4	T47.0X5	T47.0X6
Cimetropium bromide	T44.3X1	T44.3X2	T44.3X3	T44.3X4	T44.3X5	T44.3X6
Cinchocaine	T41.3X1	T41.3X2	T41.3X3	T41.3X4	T41.3X5	T41.3X6
topical (surface)	T41.3X1	T41.3X2	T41.3X3	T41.3X4	T41.3X5	T41.3X6
Cinchona	T37.2X1	T37.2X2	T37.2X3	T37.2X4	T37.2X5	T37.2X6
Cinchonine alkaloids	T37.2X1	T37.2X2	T37.2X3	T37.2X4	T37.2X5	T37.2X6
Cinchophen	T50.4X1	T50.4X2	T50.4X3	T50.4X4	T50.4X5	T50.4X6
Cinepazide	T46.7X1	T46.7X2	T46.7X3	T46.7X4	T46.7X5	T46.7X6
Cinnamedrine	T48.5X1	T48.5X2	T48.5X3	T48.5X4	T48.5X5	T48.5X6

◀ New   ◀▥ Revised   ~~deleted~~ Deleted

Substance	Poisoning, Accidental (Unintentional)	Poisoning, Intentional Self-Harm	Poisoning, Assault	Poisoning, Undetermined	Adverse Effect	Underdosing
		External Cause (T-Code)				
Cinnarizine	T45.0X1	T45.0X2	T45.0X3	T45.0X4	T45.0X5	T45.0X6
Cinoxacin	T37.8X1	T37.8X2	T37.8X3	T37.8X4	T37.8X5	T37.8X6
Ciprofibrate	T46.6X1	T46.6X2	T46.6X3	T46.6X4	T46.6X5	T46.6X6
Ciprofloxacin	T36.8X1	T36.8X2	T36.8X3	T36.8X4	T36.8X5	T36.8X6
Cisapride	T47.8X1	T47.8X2	T47.8X3	T47.8X4	T47.8X5	T47.8X6
Cisplatin	T45.1X1	T45.1X2	T45.1X3	T45.1X4	T45.1X5	T45.1X6
Citalopram	T43.221	T43.222	T43.223	T43.224	T43.225	T43.226
Citanest	T41.3X1	T41.3X2	T41.3X3	T41.3X4	T41.3X5	T41.3X6
infiltration (subcutaneous)	T41.3X1	T41.3X2	T41.3X3	T41.3X4	T41.3X5	T41.3X6
nerve block (peripheral) (plexus)	T41.3X1	T41.3X2	T41.3X3	T41.3X4	T41.3X5	T41.3X6
Citric acid	T47.5X1	T47.5X2	T47.5X3	T47.5X4	T47.5X5	T47.5X6
Citrovorum (factor)	T45.8X1	T45.8X2	T45.8X3	T45.8X4	T45.8X5	T45.8X6
Claviceps purpurea	T62.2X1	T62.2X2	T62.2X3	T62.2X4	—	—
Clavulanic acid	T36.1X1	T36.1X2	T36.1X3	T36.1X4	T36.1X5	T36.1X6
Cleaner, cleansing agent, type not specified	T65.891	T65.892	T65.893	T65.894	—	—
of paint or varnish	T52.91	T52.92	T52.93	T52.94	—	—
specified type NEC	T65.891	T65.892	T65.893	T65.894	—	—
Clebopride	T47.8X1	T47.8X2	T47.8X3	T47.8X4	T47.8X5	T47.8X6
Clefamide	T37.3X1	T37.3X2	T37.3X3	T37.3X4	T37.3X5	T37.3X6
Clemastine	T45.0X1	T45.0X2	T45.0X3	T45.0X4	T45.0X5	T45.0X6
Clematis vitalba	T62.2X1	T62.2X2	T62.2X3	T62.2X4	—	—
Clemizole	T45.0X1	T45.0X2	T45.0X3	T45.0X4	T45.0X5	T45.0X6
penicillin	T36.0X1	T36.0X2	T36.0X3	T36.0X4	T36.0X5	T36.0X6
Clenbuterol	T48.6X1	T48.6X2	T48.6X3	T48.6X4	T48.6X5	T48.6X6
Clidinium bromide	T44.3X1	T44.3X2	T44.3X3	T44.3X4	T44.3X5	T44.3X6
Clindamycin	T36.8X1	T36.8X2	T36.8X3	T36.8X4	T36.8X5	T36.8X6
Clinofibrate	T46.6X1	T46.6X2	T46.6X3	T46.6X4	T46.6X5	T46.6X6
Clioquinol	T37.8X1	T37.8X2	T37.8X3	T37.8X4	T37.8X5	T37.8X6
Cliradon	T40.2X1	T40.2X2	T40.2X3	T40.2X4	—	—
Clobazam	T42.4X1	T42.4X2	T42.4X3	T42.4X4	T42.4X5	T42.4X6
Clobenzorex	T50.5X1	T50.5X2	T50.5X3	T50.5X4	T50.5X5	T50.5X6
Clobetasol	T49.0X1	T49.0X2	T49.0X3	T49.0X4	T49.0X5	T49.0X6
Clobetasone	T49.0X1	T49.0X2	T49.0X3	T49.0X4	T49.0X5	T49.0X6
Clobutinol	T48.3X1	T48.3X2	T48.3X3	T48.3X4	T48.3X5	T48.3X6
Clocapramine	T43.0X1	T43.0X2	T43.0X3	T43.0X4	T43.0X5	T43.0X6
Clocortolone	T38.0X1	T38.0X2	T38.0X3	T38.0X4	T38.0X5	T38.0X6
Clodantoin	T49.0X1	T49.0X2	T49.0X3	T49.0X4	T49.0X5	T49.0X6
Clodronic acid	T50.991	T50.992	T50.993	T50.994	T50.995	T50.996
Clofazimine	T37.1X1	T37.1X2	T37.1X3	T37.1X4	T37.1X5	T37.1X6
Clofedanol	T48.3X1	T48.3X2	T48.3X3	T48.3X4	T48.3X5	T48.3X6

◀ New ◀ Revised ~~deleted~~ Deleted

Substance	Poisoning, Accidental (Unintentional)	Poisoning, Intentional Self-Harm	Poisoning, Assault	Poisoning, Undetermined	Adverse Effect	Underdosing
			External Cause (T-Code)			
Clofenamide	T50.2X1	T50.2X2	T50.2X3	T50.2X4	T50.2X5	T50.2X6
Clofenotane	T49.0X1	T49.0X2	T49.0X3	T49.0X4	T49.0X5	T49.0X6
Clofezone	T39.2X1	T39.2X2	T39.2X3	T39.2X4	T39.2X5	T39.2X6
Clofibrate	T46.6X1	T46.6X2	T46.6X3	T46.6X4	T46.6X5	T46.6X6
Clofibride	T46.6X1	T46.6X2	T46.6X3	T46.6X4	T46.6X5	T46.6X6
Cloforex	T50.5X1	T50.5X2	T50.5X3	T50.5X4	T50.5X5	T50.5X6
Clomacran	T43.0X1	T43.0X2	T43.0X3	T43.0X4	T43.0X5	T43.0X6
Clomethiazole	T42.6X1	T42.6X2	T42.6X3	T42.6X4	T42.6X5	T42.6X6
Clometocillin	T36.0X1	T36.0X2	T36.0X3	T36.0X4	T36.0X5	T36.0X6
Clomifene	T38.5X1	T38.5X2	T38.5X3	T38.5X4	T38.5X5	T38.5X6
Clomiphene	T38.5X1	T38.5X2	T38.5X3	T38.5X4	T38.5X5	T38.5X6
Clomipramine	T43.011	T43.012	T43.013	T43.014	T43.015	T43.016
Clomocycline	T36.4X1	T36.4X2	T36.4X3	T36.4X4	T36.4X5	T36.4X6
Clonazepam	T42.4X1	T42.4X2	T42.4X3	T42.4X4	T42.4X5	T42.4X6
Clonidine	T46.5X1	T46.5X2	T46.5X3	T46.5X4	T46.5X5	T46.5X6
Clonixin	T39.8X1	T39.8X2	T39.8X3	T39.8X4	T39.8X5	T39.8X6
Clopamide	T50.2X1	T50.2X2	T50.2X3	T50.2X4	T50.2X5	T50.2X6
Clopenthixol	T43.4X1	T43.4X2	T43.4X3	T43.4X4	T43.4X5	T43.4X6
Cloperastine	T48.3X1	T48.3X2	T48.3X3	T48.3X4	T48.3X5	T48.3X6
Clophedianol	T48.3X1	T48.3X2	T48.3X3	T48.3X4	T48.3X5	T48.3X6
Cloponone	T36.2X1	T36.2X2	T36.2X3	T36.2X4	T36.2X5	T36.2X6
Cloprednol	T38.0X1	T38.0X2	T38.0X3	T38.0X4	T38.0X5	T38.0X6
Cloral betaine	T42.6X1	T42.6X2	T42.6X3	T42.6X4	T42.6X5	T42.6X6
Cloramfenicol	T36.2X1	T36.2X2	T36.2X3	T36.2X4	T36.2X5	T36.2X6
Clorazepate (dipotassium)	T42.4X1	T42.4X2	T42.4X3	T42.4X4	T42.4X5	T42.4X6
Clorexolone	T50.2X1	T50.2X2	T50.2X3	T50.2X4	T50.2X5	T50.2X6
Clorox (bleach)	T54.91	T54.92	T54.93	T54.94	—	—
Clorfenamine	T45.0X1	T45.0X2	T45.0X3	T45.0X4	T45.0X5	T45.0X6
Clorgiline	T43.1X1	T43.1X2	T43.1X3	T43.1X4	T43.1X5	T43.1X6
Clorotepine	T44.3X1	T44.3X2	T44.3X3	T44.3X4	T44.3X5	T44.3X6
Clorprenaline	T48.6X1	T48.6X2	T48.6X3	T48.6X4	T48.6X5	T48.6X6
Clortermine	T50.5X1	T50.5X2	T50.5X3	T50.5X4	T50.5X5	T50.5X6
Clotiapine	T43.591	T43.592	T43.593	T43.594	T43.595	T43.596
Clotiazepam	T42.4X1	T42.4X2	T42.4X3	T42.4X4	T42.4X5	T42.4X6
Clotibric acid	T46.6X1	T46.6X2	T46.6X3	T46.6X4	T46.6X5	T46.6X6
Clotrimazole	T49.0X1	T49.0X2	T49.0X3	T49.0X4	T49.0X5	T49.0X6
Cloxacillin	T36.0X1	T36.0X2	T36.0X3	T36.0X4	T36.0X5	T36.0X6
Cloxazolam	T42.4X1	T42.4X2	T42.4X3	T42.4X4	T42.4X5	T42.4X6
Cloxiquine	T49.0X1	T49.0X2	T49.0X3	T49.0X4	T49.0X5	T49.0X6
Clozapine	T42.4X1	T42.4X2	T42.4X3	T42.4X4	T42.4X5	T42.4X6

TABLE OF DRUGS AND CHEMICALS

◄ New ◄▥ Revised ~~deleted~~ Deleted

Substance	External Cause (T-Code)					
	Poisoning, Accidental (Unintentional)	Poisoning, Intentional Self-Harm	Poisoning, Assault	Poisoning, Undetermined	Adverse Effect	Underdosing
Coagulant NEC	T45.7X1	T45.7X2	T45.7X3	T45.7X4	T45.7X5	T45.7X6
Coal (carbon monoxide from)—*see also Carbon, monoxide, coal*	T58.2X1	T58.2X2	T58.2X3	T58.2X4	—	—
oil—*see Kerosene*						
tar	T49.1X1	T49.1X2	T49.1X3	T49.1X4	T49.1X5	T49.1X6
fumes	T59.891	T59.892	T59.893	T59.894	—	—
medicinal (ointment)	T49.4X1	T49.4X2	T49.4X3	T49.4X4	T49.4X5	T49.4X6
analgesics NEC	T39.2X1	T39.2X2	T39.2X3	T39.2X4	T39.2X5	T39.2X6
naphtha (solvent)	T52.0X1	T52.0X2	T52.0X3	T52.0X4		
Cobalamine	T45.2X1	T45.2X2	T45.2X3	T45.2X4	T45.2X5	T45.2X6
Cobalt (nonmedicinal) (fumes) (industrial)	T56.891	T56.892	T56.893	T56.894		
medicinal (trace) (chloride)	T45.8X1	T45.8X2	T45.8X3	T45.8X4	T45.8X5	T45.8X6
Cobra (venom)	T63.041	T63.042	T63.043	T63.044		
Coca (leaf)	T40.5X1	T40.5X2	T40.5X3	T40.5X4	T40.5X5	T40.5X6
Cocaine	T40.5X1	T40.5X2	T40.5X3	T40.5X4	T40.5X5	T40.5X6
topical anesthetic	T41.3X1	T41.3X2	T41.3X3	T41.3X4	T41.3X5	T41.3X6
Cocarboxylase	T45.3X1	T45.3X2	T45.3X3	T45.3X4	T45.3X5	T45.3X6
Coccidioidin	T50.8X1	T50.8X2	T50.8X3	T50.8X4	T50.8X5	T50.8X6
Cocculus indicus	T62.1X1	T62.1X2	T62.1X3	T62.1X4		
Cochineal	T65.6X1	T65.6X2	T65.6X3	T65.6X4		
medicinal products	T50.991	T50.992	T50.993	T50.994	T50.995	T50.996
Codeine	T40.2X1	T40.2X2	T40.2X3	T40.2X4	T40.2X5	T40.2X6
Cod-liver oil	T45.2X1	T45.2X2	T45.2X3	T45.2X4	T45.2X5	T45.2X6
Coenzyme A	T50.991	T50.992	T50.993	T50.994	T50.995	T50.996
Coffee	T62.8X1	T62.8X2	T62.8X3	T62.8X4	—	—
Cogalactoisomerase	T50.991	T50.992	T50.993	T50.994	T50.995	T50.996
Cogentin	T44.3X1	T44.3X2	T44.3X3	T44.3X4	T44.3X5	T44.3X6
Coke fumes or gas (carbon monoxide)	T58.2X1	T58.2X2	T58.2X3	T58.2X4	—	—
industrial use	T58.8X1	T58.8X2	T58.8X3	T58.8X4	—	—
Colace	T47.4X1	T47.4X2	T47.4X3	T47.4X4	T47.4X5	T47.4X6
Colaspase	T45.1X1	T45.1X2	T45.1X3	T45.1X4	T45.1X5	T45.1X6
Colchicine	T50.4X1	T50.4X2	T50.4X3	T50.4X4	T50.4X5	T50.4X6
Colchicum	T62.2X1	T62.2X2	T62.2X3	T62.2X4	—	—
Cold cream	T49.3X1	T49.3X2	T49.3X3	T49.3X4	T49.3X5	T49.3X6
Colecalciferol	T45.2X1	T45.2X2	T45.2X3	T45.2X4	T45.2X5	T45.2X6
Colestipol	T46.6X1	T46.6X2	T46.6X3	T46.6X4	T46.6X5	T46.6X6
Colestyramine	T46.6X1	T46.6X2	T46.6X3	T46.6X4	T46.6X5	T46.6X6
Colimycin	T36.8X1	T36.8X2	T36.8X3	T36.8X4	T36.8X5	T36.8X6
Colistimethate	T36.8X1	T36.8X2	T36.8X3	T36.8X4	T36.8X5	T36.8X6
Colistin	T36.8X1	T36.8X2	T36.8X3	T36.8X4	T36.8X5	T36.8X6
sulfate (eye preparation)	T49.5X1	T49.5X2	T49.5X3	T49.5X4	T49.5X5	T49.5X6

TABLE OF DRUGS AND CHEMICALS

Substance	External Cause (T-Code)					
	Poisoning, Accidental (Unintentional)	Poisoning, Intentional Self-Harm	Poisoning, Assault	Poisoning, Undetermined	Adverse Effect	Underdosing
Collagen	T50.991	T50.992	T50.993	T50.994	T50.995	T50.996
Collagenase	T49.4X1	T49.4X2	T49.4X3	T49.4X4	T49.4X5	T49.4X6
Collodion	T49.3X1	T49.3X2	T49.3X3	T49.3X4	T49.3X5	T49.3X6
Colocynth	T47.2X1	T47.2X2	T47.2X3	T47.2X4	T47.2X5	T47.2X6
Colophony adhesive	T49.3X1	T49.3X2	T49.3X3	T49.3X4	T49.3X5	T49.3X6
Colorant — *see also Dye*	T50.991	T50.992	T50.993	T50.994	T50.995	T50.996
Coloring matter — *see Dye(s)*						
Combustion gas (after combustion) — *see Carbon, monoxide*						
prior to combustion	T59.891	T59.892	T59.893	T59.894	—	—
Compazine	T43.3X1	T43.3X2	T43.3X3	T43.3X4	T43.3X5	T43.3X6
Compound						
42 (warfarin)	T60.4X1	T60.4X2	T60.4X3	T60.4X4	—	—
269 (endrin)	T60.1X1	T60.1X2	T60.1X3	T60.1X4	—	—
497 (dieldrin)	T60.1X1	T60.1X2	T60.1X3	T60.1X4	—	—
1080 (sodium fluoroacetate)	T60.4X1	T60.4X2	T60.4X3	T60.4X4	—	—
3422 (parathion)	T60.0X1	T60.0X2	T60.0X3	T60.0X4	—	—
3911 (phorate)	T60.0X1	T60.0X2	T60.0X3	T60.0X4	—	—
3956 (toxaphene)	T60.1X1	T60.1X2	T60.1X3	T60.1X4	—	—
4049 (malathion)	T60.0X1	T60.0X2	T60.0X3	T60.0X4	—	—
4069 (malathion)	T60.0X1	T60.0X2	T60.0X3	T60.0X4	—	—
4124 (dicapthon)	T60.0X1	T60.0X2	T60.0X3	T60.0X4	—	—
E (cortisone)	T38.0X1	T38.0X2	T38.0X3	T38.0X4	T38.0X5	T38.0X6
F (hydrocortisone)	T38.0X1	T38.0X2	T38.0X3	T38.0X4	T38.0X5	T38.0X6
Congener, anabolic	T38.7X1	T38.7X2	T38.7X3	T38.7X4	T38.7X5	T38.7X6
Congo red	T50.8X1	T50.8X2	T50.8X3	T50.8X4	T50.8X5	T50.8X6
Coniine, conine	T62.2X1	T62.2X2	T62.2X3	T62.2X4	—	—
Conium (maculatum)	T62.2X1	T62.2X2	T62.2X3	T62.2X4	—	—
Conjugated estrogenic substances	T38.5X1	T38.5X2	T38.5X3	T38.5X4	T38.5X5	T38.5X6
Contac	T48.5X1	T48.5X2	T48.5X3	T48.5X4	T48.5X5	T48.5X6
Contact lens solution	T49.5X1	T49.5X2	T49.5X3	T49.5X4	T49.5X5	T49.5X6
Contraceptive (oral)	T38.4X1	T38.4X2	T38.4X3	T38.4X4	T38.4X5	T38.4X6
vaginal	T49.8X1	T49.8X2	T49.8X3	T49.8X4	T49.8X5	T49.8X6
Contrast medium, radiography	T50.8X1	T50.8X2	T50.8X3	T50.8X4	T50.8X5	T50.8X6
Convallaria glycosides	T46.0X1	T46.0X2	T46.0X3	T46.0X4	T46.0X5	T46.0X6
Convallaria majalis	T62.2X1	T62.2X2	T62.2X3	T62.2X4	—	—
berry	T62.1X1	T62.1X2	T62.1X3	T62.1X4	—	—
Copper (dust) (fumes) (nonmedicinal) NEC	T56.4X1	T56.4X2	T56.4X3	T56.4X4	—	—
arsenate, arsenite	T57.0X1	T57.0X2	T57.0X3	T57.0X4	—	—
insecticide	T60.2X1	T60.2X2	T60.2X3	T60.2X4	—	—

◀ New   ◀◀ Revised   ~~deleted~~ Deleted

Substance	External Cause (T-Code)					
	Poisoning, Accidental (Unintentional)	Poisoning, Intentional Self-Harm	Poisoning, Assault	Poisoning, Undetermined	Adverse Effect	Underdosing
Copper NEC *(Continued)*						
emetic	T47.7X1	T47.7X2	T47.7X3	T47.7X4	T47.7X5	T47.7X6
fungicide	T60.3X1	T60.3X2	T60.3X3	T60.3X4	—	—
gluconate	T49.0X1	T49.0X2	T49.0X3	T49.0X4	T49.0X5	T49.0X6
insecticide	T60.2X1	T60.2X2	T60.2X3	T60.2X4	—	—
medicinal (trace)	T45.8X1	T45.8X2	T45.8X3	T45.8X4	T45.8X5	T45.8X6
oleate	T49.0X1	T49.0X2	T49.0X3	T49.0X4	T49.0X5	T49.0X6
sulfate	T56.4X1	T56.4X2	T56.4X3	T56.4X4		
cupric	T56.4X1	T56.4X2	T56.4X3	T56.4X4	—	—
fungicide	T60.3X1	T60.3X2	T60.3X3	T60.3X4	—	—
medicinal						
ear	T49.6X1	T49.6X2	T49.6X3	T49.6X4	T49.6X5	T49.6X6
emetic	T47.7X1	T47.7X2	T47.7X3	T47.7X4	T47.7X5	T47.7X6
eye	T49.5X1	T49.5X2	T49.5X3	T49.5X4	T49.5X5	T49.5X6
cuprous	T56.4X1	T56.4X2	T56.4X3	T56.4X4	—	—
fungicide	T60.3X1	T60.3X2	T60.3X3	T60.3X4	—	—
medicinal						
ear	T49.6X1	T49.6X2	T49.6X3	T49.6X4	T49.6X5	T49.6X6
emetic	T47.7X1	T47.7X2	T47.7X3	T47.7X4	T47.7X5	T47.7X6
eye	T49.5X1	T49.5X2	T49.5X3	T49.5X4	T49.5X5	T49.5X6
Copperhead snake (bite) (venom)	T63.061	T63.062	T63.063	T63.064	—	—
Coral (sting)	T63.691	T63.692	T63.693	T63.694	—	—
snake (bite) (venom)	T63.021	T63.022	T63.023	T63.024	—	—
Corbadrine	T49.6X1	T49.6X2	T49.6X3	T49.6X4	T49.6X5	T49.6X6
Cordran	T49.0X1	T49.0X2	T49.0X3	T49.0X4	T49.0X5	T49.0X6
Cordite	T65.891	T65.892	T65.893	T65.894	—	—
vapor	T59.891	T59.892	T59.893	T59.894	—	—
Corn cures	T49.4X1	T49.4X2	T49.4X3	T49.4X4	T49.4X5	T49.4X6
Cornhusker's lotion	T49.3X1	T49.3X2	T49.3X3	T49.3X4	T49.3X5	T49.3X6
Corn starch	T49.3X1	T49.3X2	T49.3X3	T49.3X4	T49.3X5	T49.3X6
Coronary vasodilator NEC	T46.3X1	T46.3X2	T46.3X3	T46.3X4	T46.3X5	T46.3X6
Corrosive NEC	T54.91	T54.92	T54.93	T54.94	—	—
acid NEC	T54.2X1	T54.2X2	T54.2X3	T54.2X4	—	—
aromatics	T54.1X1	T54.1X2	T54.1X3	T54.1X4	—	—
disinfectant	T54.1X1	T54.1X2	T54.1X3	T54.1X4	—	—
fumes NEC	T54.91	T54.92	T54.93	T54.94	—	—
specified NEC	T54.91	T54.92	T54.93	T54.94	—	—
sublimate	T56.1X1	T56.1X2	T56.1X3	T56.1X4	—	—
Cortate	T38.0X1	T38.0X2	T38.0X3	T38.0X4	T38.0X5	T38.0X6

◄ New   ◄▥ Revised   ~~deleted~~ Deleted

Substance	External Cause (T-Code)					
	Poisoning, Accidental (Unintentional)	Poisoning, Intentional Self-Harm	Poisoning, Assault	Poisoning, Undetermined	Adverse Effect	Underdosing
Cort-Dome	T38.0X1	T38.0X2	T38.0X3	T38.0X4	T38.0X5	T38.0X6
ENT agent	T49.6X1	T49.6X2	T49.6X3	T49.6X4	T49.6X5	T49.6X6
ophthalmic preparation	T49.5X1	T49.5X2	T49.5X3	T49.5X4	T49.5X5	T49.5X6
topical NEC	T49.0X1	T49.0X2	T49.0X3	T49.0X4	T49.0X5	T49.0X6
Cortef	T38.0X1	T38.0X2	T38.0X3	T38.0X4	T38.0X5	T38.0X6
ENT agent	T49.6X1	T49.6X2	T49.6X3	T49.6X4	T49.6X5	T49.6X6
ophthalmic preparation	T49.5X1	T49.5X2	T49.5X3	T49.5X4	T49.5X5	T49.5X6
topical NEC	T49.0X1	T49.0X2	T49.0X3	T49.0X4	T49.0X5	T49.0X6
Corticosteroid	T38.0X1	T38.0X2	T38.0X3	T38.0X4	T38.0X5	T38.0X6
ENT agent	T49.6X1	T49.6X2	T49.6X3	T49.6X4	T49.6X5	T49.6X6
mineral	T50.0X1	T50.0X2	T50.0X3	T50.0X4	T50.0X5	T50.0X6
ophthalmic	T49.5X1	T49.5X2	T49.5X3	T49.5X4	T49.5X5	T49.5X6
topical NEC	T49.0X1	T49.0X2	T49.0X3	T49.0X4	T49.0X5	T49.0X6
Corticotropin	T38.811	T38.812	T38.813	T38.814	T38.815	T38.816
Cortisol	T49.0X1	T49.0X2	T49.0X3	T49.0X4	T49.0X5	T49.0X6
ENT agent	T49.6X1	T49.6X2	T49.6X3	T49.6X4	T49.6X5	T49.6X6
ophthalmic preparation	T49.5X1	T49.5X2	T49.5X3	T49.5X4	T49.5X5	T49.5X6
topical NEC	T49.0X1	T49.0X2	T49.0X3	T49.0X4	T49.0X5	T49.0X6
Cortisone (acetate)	T38.0X1	T38.0X2	T38.0X3	T38.0X4	T38.0X5	T38.0X6
ENT agent	T49.6X1	T49.6X2	T49.6X3	T49.6X4	T49.6X5	T49.6X6
ophthalmic preparation	T49.5X1	T49.5X2	T49.5X3	T49.5X4	T49.5X5	T49.5X6
topical NEC	T49.0X1	T49.0X2	T49.0X3	T49.0X4	T49.0X5	T49.0X6
Cortivazol	T38.0X1	T38.0X2	T38.0X3	T38.0X4	T38.0X5	T38.0X6
Cortogen	T38.0X1	T38.0X2	T38.0X3	T38.0X4	T38.0X5	T38.0X6
ENT agent	T49.6X1	T49.6X2	T49.6X3	T49.6X4	T49.6X5	T49.6X6
ophthalmic preparation	T49.5X1	T49.5X2	T49.5X3	T49.5X4	T49.5X5	T49.5X6
Cortone	T38.0X1	T38.0X2	T38.0X3	T38.0X4	T38.0X5	T38.0X6
ENT agent	T49.6X1	T49.6X2	T49.6X3	T49.6X4	T49.6X5	T49.6X6
ophthalmic preparation	T49.5X1	T49.5X2	T49.5X3	T49.5X4	T49.5X5	T49.5X6
Cortril	T38.0X1	T38.0X2	T38.0X3	T38.0X4	T38.0X5	T38.0X6
ENT agent	T49.6X1	T49.6X2	T49.6X3	T49.6X4	T49.6X5	T49.6X6
ophthalmic preparation	T49.5X1	T49.5X2	T49.5X3	T49.5X4	T49.5X5	T49.5X6
topical NEC	T49.0X1	T49.0X2	T49.0X3	T49.0X4	T49.0X5	T49.0X6
Corynebacterium parvum	T45.1X1	T45.1X2	T45.1X3	T45.1X4	T45.1X5	T45.1X6
Cosmetic preparation	T49.8X1	T49.8X2	T49.8X3	T49.8X4	T49.8X5	T49.8X6
Cosmetics	T49.8X1	T49.8X2	T49.8X3	T49.8X4	T49.8X5	T49.8X6
Cosyntropin	T38.811	T38.812	T38.813	T38.814	T38.815	T38.816
Cotarnine	T45.7X1	T45.7X2	T45.7X3	T45.7X4	T45.7X5	T45.7X6
Co-trimoxazole	T36.8X1	T36.8X2	T36.8X3	T36.8X4	T36.8X5	T36.8X6
Cottonseed oil	T49.3X1	T49.3X2	T49.3X3	T49.3X4	T49.3X5	T49.3X6

◀ New   ◀▥ Revised   ~~deleted~~ Deleted

Substance	Poisoning, Accidental (Unintentional)	Poisoning, Intentional Self-Harm	Poisoning, Assault	Poisoning, Undetermined	Adverse Effect	Underdosing
			External Cause (T-Code)			
Cough mixture (syrup)	T48.4X1	T48.4X2	T48.4X3	T48.4X4	T48.4X5	T48.4X6
containing opiates	T40.2X1	T40.2X2	T40.2X3	T40.2X4	T40.2X5	T40.2X6
expectorants	T48.4X1	T48.4X2	T48.4X3	T48.4X4	T48.4X5	T48.4X6
Coumadin	T45.511	T45.512	T45.513	T45.514	T45.515	T45.516
rodenticide	T60.4X1	T60.4X2	T60.4X3	T60.4X4	—	—
Coumaphos	T60.0X1	T60.0X2	T60.0X3	T60.0X4	—	—
Coumarin	T45.511	T45.512	T45.513	T45.514	T45.515	T45.516
Coumetarol	T45.511	T45.512	T45.513	T45.514	T45.515	T45.516
Cowbane	T62.2X1	T62.2X2	T62.2X3	T62.2X4	—	—
Cozyme	T45.2X1	T45.2X2	T45.2X3	T45.2X4	T45.2X5	T45.2X6
Crack	T40.5X1	T40.5X2	T40.5X3	T40.5X4	—	—
Crataegus extract	T46.0X1	T46.0X2	T46.0X3	T46.0X4	T46.0X5	T46.0X6
Creolin	T54.1X1	T54.1X2	T54.1X3	T54.1X4	—	—
disinfectant	T54.1X1	T54.1X2	T54.1X3	T54.1X4	—	—
Creosol (compound)	T49.0X1	T49.0X2	T49.0X3	T49.0X4	T49.0X5	T49.0X6
Creosote (coal tar) (beechwood)	T49.0X1	T49.0X2	T49.0X3	T49.0X4	T49.0X5	T49.0X6
medicinal (expectorant)	T48.4X1	T48.4X2	T48.4X3	T48.4X4	T48.4X5	T48.4X6
syrup	T48.4X1	T48.4X2	T48.4X3	T48.4X4	T48.4X5	T48.4X6
Cresol(s)	T49.0X1	T49.0X2	T49.0X3	T49.0X4	T49.0X5	T49.0X6
and soap solution	T49.0X1	T49.0X2	T49.0X3	T49.0X4	T49.0X5	T49.0X6
Cresyl acetate	T49.0X1	T49.0X2	T49.0X3	T49.0X4	T49.0X5	T49.0X6
Cresylic acid	T49.0X1	T49.0X2	T49.0X3	T49.0X4	T49.0X5	T49.0X6
Crimidine	T60.4X1	T60.4X2	T60.4X3	T60.4X4	—	—
Croconazole	T37.8X1	T37.8X2	T37.8X3	T37.8X4	T37.8X5	T37.8X6
Cromoglicic acid	T48.6X1	T48.6X2	T48.6X3	T48.6X4	T48.6X5	T48.6X6
Cromolyn	T48.6X1	T48.6X2	T48.6X3	T48.6X4	T48.6X5	T48.6X6
Cromonar	T46.3X1	T46.3X2	T46.3X3	T46.3X4	T46.3X5	T46.3X6
Cropropamide	T39.8X1	T39.8X2	T39.8X3	T39.8X4	T39.8X5	T39.8X6
with crotethamide	T50.7X1	T50.7X2	T50.7X3	T50.7X4	T50.7X5	T50.7X6
Crotamiton	T49.0X1	T49.0X2	T49.0X3	T49.0X4	T49.0X5	T49.0X6
Crotethamide	T39.8X1	T39.8X2	T39.8X3	T39.8X4	T39.8X5	T39.8X6
with cropropamide	T50.7X1	T50.7X2	T50.7X3	T50.7X4	T50.7X5	T50.7X6
Croton (oil)	T47.2X1	T47.2X2	T47.2X3	T47.2X4	T47.2X5	T47.2X6
chloral	T42.6X1	T42.6X2	T42.6X3	T42.6X4	T42.6X5	T42.6X6
Crude oil	T52.0X1	T52.0X2	T52.0X3	T52.0X4	—	—
Cryogenine	T39.8X1	T39.8X2	T39.8X3	T39.8X4	T39.8X5	T39.8X6
Cryolite (vapor)	T60.1X1	T60.1X2	T60.1X3	T60.1X4	—	—
insecticide	T60.1X1	T60.1X2	T60.1X3	T60.1X4	—	—
Cryptenamine (tannates)	T46.5X1	T46.5X2	T46.5X3	T46.5X4	T46.5X5	T46.5X6
Crystal violet	T49.0X1	T49.0X2	T49.0X3	T49.0X4	T49.0X5	T49.0X6

TABLE OF DRUGS AND CHEMICALS

◀ New ◀ Revised ~~deleted~~ Deleted

Substance	External Cause (T-Code)					
	Poisoning, Accidental (Unintentional)	Poisoning, Intentional Self-Harm	Poisoning, Assault	Poisoning, Undetermined	Adverse Effect	Underdosing
Cuckoopint	T62.2X1	T62.2X2	T62.2X3	T62.2X4	—	—
Cumetharol	T45.511	T45.512	T45.513	T45.514	T45.515	T45.516
Cupric						
acetate	T60.3X1	T60.3X2	T60.3X3	T60.3X4	—	—
acetoarsenite	T57.0X1	T57.0X2	T57.0X3	T57.0X4	—	—
arsenate	T57.0X1	T57.0X2	T57.0X3	T57.0X4	—	—
gluconate	T49.0X1	T49.0X2	T49.0X3	T49.0X4	T49.0X5	T49.0X6
oleate	T49.0X1	T49.0X2	T49.0X3	T49.0X4	T49.0X5	T49.0X6
sulfate	T56.4X1	T56.4X2	T56.4X3	T56.4X4	—	—
Cuprous sulfate — see also Copper sulfate	T56.4X1	T56.4X2	T56.4X3	T56.4X4	—	—
Curare, curarine	T48.1X1	T48.1X2	T48.1X3	T48.1X4	T48.1X5	T48.1X6
Cyamemazine	T43.3X1	T43.3X2	T43.3X3	T43.3X4	T43.3X5	T43.3X6
Cyamopsis tetragono-loba	T46.6X1	T46.6X2	T46.6X3	T46.6X4	T46.6X5	T46.6X6
Cyanacetyl hydrazide	T37.1X1	T37.1X2	T37.1X3	T37.1X4	T37.1X5	T37.1X6
Cyanic acid (gas)	T59.891	T59.892	T59.893	T59.894	—	—
Cyanide(s) (compounds) (potassium) (sodium) NEC	T65.0X1	T65.0X2	T65.0X3	T65.0X4	—	—
dust or gas (inhalation) NEC	T57.3X1	T57.3X2	T57.3X3	T57.3X4	—	—
fumigant	T65.0X1	T65.0X2	T65.0X3	T65.0X4	—	—
hydrogen	T57.3X1	T57.3X2	T57.3X3	T57.3X4	—	—
mercuric — see Mercury						
pesticide (dust) (fumes)	T65.0X1	T65.0X2	T65.0X3	T65.0X4	—	—
Cyanoacrylate adhesive	T49.3X1	T49.3X2	T49.3X3	T49.3X4	T49.3X5	T49.3X6
Cyanocobalamin	T45.8X1	T45.8X2	T45.8X3	T45.8X4	T45.8X5	T45.8X6
Cyanogen (chloride) (gas) NEC	T59.891	T59.892	T59.893	T59.894	—	—
Cyclacillin	T36.0X1	T36.0X2	T36.0X3	T36.0X4	T36.0X5	T36.0X6
Cyclaine	T41.3X1	T41.3X2	T41.3X3	T41.3X4	T41.3X5	T41.3X6
Cyclamate	T50.991	T50.992	T50.993	T50.994	T50.995	T50.996
Cyclamen europaeum	T62.2X1	T62.2X2	T62.2X3	T62.2X4	—	—
Cyclandelate	T46.7X1	T46.7X2	T46.7X3	T46.7X4	T46.7X5	T46.7X6
Cyclazocine	T50.7X1	T50.7X2	T50.7X3	T50.7X4	T50.7X5	T50.7X6
Cyclizine	T45.0X1	T45.0X2	T45.0X3	T45.0X4	T45.0X5	T45.0X6
Cyclobarbital	T42.3X1	T42.3X2	T42.3X3	T42.3X4	T42.3X5	T42.3X6
Cyclobarbitone	T42.3X1	T42.3X2	T42.3X3	T42.3X4	T42.3X5	T42.3X6
Cyclobenzaprine	T48.1X1	T48.1X2	T48.1X3	T48.1X4	T48.1X5	T48.1X6
Cyclodrine	T44.3X1	T44.3X2	T44.3X3	T44.3X4	T44.3X5	T44.3X6
Cycloguanil embonate	T37.2X1	T37.2X2	T37.2X3	T37.2X4	T37.2X5	T37.2X6
Cycloheptadiene	T43.291	T43.292	T43.293	T43.294	T43.295	T43.296
Cyclohexane	T52.8X1	T52.8X2	T52.8X3	T52.8X4	—	—
Cyclohexanol	T51.8X1	T51.8X2	T51.8X3	T51.8X4	—	—
Cyclohexanone	T52.4X1	T52.4X2	T52.4X3	T52.4X4	—	—

◀ New ◀▥ Revised ~~deleted~~ Deleted

Substance	External Cause (T-Code)					
	Poisoning, Accidental (Unintentional)	Poisoning, Intentional Self-Harm	Poisoning, Assault	Poisoning, Undetermined	Adverse Effect	Underdosing
Cycloheximide	T60.3X1	T60.3X2	T60.3X3	T60.3X4	—	—
Cyclohexyl acetate	T52.8X1	T52.8X2	T52.8X3	T52.8X4	—	—
Cycloleucin	T45.1X1	T45.1X2	T45.1X3	T45.1X4	T45.1X5	T45.1X6
Cyclomethycaine	T41.3X1	T41.3X2	T41.3X3	T41.3X4	T41.3X5	T41.3X6
Cyclopentamine	T44.4X1	T44.4X2	T44.4X3	T44.4X4	T44.4X5	T44.4X6
Cyclopenthiazide	T50.2X1	T50.2X2	T50.2X3	T50.2X4	T50.2X5	T50.2X6
Cyclopentolate	T44.3X1	T44.3X2	T44.3X3	T44.3X4	T44.3X5	T44.3X6
Cyclophosphamide	T45.1X1	T45.1X2	T45.1X3	T45.1X4	T45.1X5	T45.1X6
Cycloplegic drug	T49.5X1	T49.5X2	T49.5X3	T49.5X4	T49.5X5	T49.5X6
Cyclopropane	T41.291	T41.292	T41.293	T41.294	T41.295	T41.296
Cyclopyrabital	T39.8X1	T39.8X2	T39.8X3	T39.8X4	T39.8X5	T39.8X6
Cycloserine	T37.1X1	T37.1X2	T37.1X3	T37.1X4	T37.1X5	T37.1X6
Cyclosporin	T45.1X1	T45.1X2	T45.1X3	T45.1X4	T45.1X5	T45.1X6
Cyclothiazide	T50.2X1	T50.2X2	T50.2X3	T50.2X4	T50.2X5	T50.2X6
Cycrimine	T44.3X1	T44.3X2	T44.3X3	T44.3X4	T44.3X5	T44.3X6
Cyhalothrin	T60.1X1	T60.1X2	T60.1X3	T60.1X4	—	—
Cymarin	T46.0X1	T46.0X2	T46.0X3	T46.0X4	T46.0X5	T46.0X6
Cypermethrin	T60.1X1	T60.1X2	T60.1X3	T60.1X4	—	—
Cyphenothrin	T60.2X1	T60.2X2	T60.2X3	T60.2X4	—	—
Cyproheptadine	T45.0X1	T45.0X2	T45.0X3	T45.0X4	T45.0X5	T45.0X6
Cyprolidol	T43.291	T43.292	T43.293	T43.294	T43.295	T43.296
Cyproterone	T38.6X1	T38.6X2	T38.6X3	T38.6X4	T38.6X5	T38.6X6
Cysteamine	T50.6X1	T50.6X2	T50.6X3	T50.6X4	T50.6X5	T50.6X6
Cytarabine	T45.1X1	T45.1X2	T45.1X3	T45.1X4	T45.1X5	T45.1X6
Cytisus						
laburnum	T62.2X1	T62.2X2	T62.2X3	T62.2X4	—	—
scoparius	T62.2X1	T62.2X2	T62.2X3	T62.2X4	—	—
Cytochrome C	T47.5X1	T47.5X2	T47.5X3	T47.5X4	T47.5X5	T47.5X6
Cytomel	T38.1X1	T38.1X2	T38.1X3	T38.1X4	T38.1X5	T38.1X6
Cytosine arabinoside	T45.1X1	T45.1X2	T45.1X3	T45.1X4	T45.1X5	T45.1X6
Cytoxan	T45.1X1	T45.1X2	T45.1X3	T45.1X4	T45.1X5	T45.1X6
Cytozyme	T45.7X1	T45.7X2	T45.7X3	T45.7X4	T45.7X5	T45.7X6
2,4-D	T60.3X1	T60.3X2	T60.3X3	T60.3X4	—	—
D						
Dacarbazine	T45.1X1	T45.1X2	T45.1X3	T45.1X4	T45.1X5	T45.1X6
Dactinomycin	T45.1X1	T45.1X2	T45.1X3	T45.1X4	T45.1X5	T45.1X6
DADPS	T37.1X1	T37.1X2	T37.1X3	T37.1X4	T37.1X5	T37.1X6
Dakin's solution	T49.0X1	T49.0X2	T49.0X3	T49.0X4	T49.0X5	T49.0X6
Dalapon (sodium)	T60.3X1	T60.3X2	T60.3X3	T60.3X4	—	—

◀ New ◀▥ Revised ~~deleted~~ Deleted

Substance	External Cause (T-Code)					
	Poisoning, Accidental (Unintentional)	Poisoning, Intentional Self-Harm	Poisoning, Assault	Poisoning, Undetermined	Adverse Effect	Underdosing
Dalmane	T42.4X1	T42.4X2	T42.4X3	T42.4X4	T42.4X5	T42.4X6
Danazol	T38.6X1	T38.6X2	T38.6X3	T38.6X4	T38.6X5	T38.6X6
Danilone	T45.511	T45.512	T45.513	T45.514	T45.515	T45.516
Danthron	T47.2X1	T47.2X2	T47.2X3	T47.2X4	T47.2X5	T47.2X6
Dantrolene	T42.8X1	T42.8X2	T42.8X3	T42.8X4	T42.8X5	T42.8X6
Dantron	T47.2X1	T47.2X2	T47.2X3	T47.2X4	T47.2X5	T47.2X6
Daphne (gnidium) (mezereum)	T62.2X1	T62.2X2	T62.2X3	T62.2X4	—	—
berry	T62.1X1	T62.1X2	T62.1X3	T62.1X4	—	—
Dapsone	T37.1X1	T37.1X2	T37.1X3	T37.1X4	T37.1X5	T37.1X6
Daraprim	T37.2X1	T37.2X2	T37.2X3	T37.2X4	T37.2X5	T37.2X6
Darnel	T62.2X1	T62.2X2	T62.2X3	T62.2X4	—	—
Darvon	T39.8X1	T39.8X2	T39.8X3	T39.8X4	T39.8X5	T39.8X6
Daunomycin	T45.1X1	T45.1X2	T45.1X3	T45.1X4	T45.1X5	T45.1X6
Daunorubicin	T45.1X1	T45.1X2	T45.1X3	T45.1X4	T45.1X5	T45.1X6
DBI	T38.3X1	T38.3X2	T38.3X3	T38.3X4	T38.3X5	T38.3X6
D-Con	T60.91	T60.92	T60.93	T60.94	—	—
insecticide	T60.2X1	T60.2X2	T60.2X3	T60.2X4	—	—
rodenticide	T60.4X1	T60.4X2	T60.4X3	T60.4X4	—	—
DDAVP	T38.891	T38.892	T38.893	T38.894	T38.895	T38.896
DDE (bis(chlorophenyl)-dichloroethylene)	T60.2X1	T60.2X2	T60.2X3	T60.2X4	—	—
DDS	T37.1X1	T37.1X2	T37.1X3	T37.1X4	T37.1X5	T37.1X6
DDT (dust)	T60.1X1	T60.1X2	T60.1X3	T60.1X4	—	—
Deadly nightshade — see also Belladonna	T62.2X1	T62.2X2	T62.2X3	T62.2X4	—	—
berry	T62.1X1	T62.1X2	T62.1X3	T62.1X4	—	—
Deamino-D-arginine vasopressin	T38.891	T38.892	T38.893	T38.894	T38.895	T38.896
Deanol (aceglumate)	T50.991	T50.992	T50.993	T50.994	T50.995	T50.996
Debrisoquine	T46.5X1	T46.5X2	T46.5X3	T46.5X4	T46.5X5	T46.5X6
Decaborane	T57.8X1	T57.8X2	T57.8X3	T57.8X4	—	—
fumes	T59.891	T59.892	T59.893	T59.894	—	—
Decadron	T38.0X1	T38.0X2	T38.0X3	T38.0X4	T38.0X5	T38.0X6
ENT agent	T49.6X1	T49.6X2	T49.6X3	T49.6X4	T49.6X5	T49.6X6
ophthalmic preparation	T49.5X1	T49.5X2	T49.5X3	T49.5X4	T49.5X5	T49.5X6
topical NEC	T49.0X1	T49.0X2	T49.0X3	T49.0X4	T49.0X5	T49.0X6
Decahydronaphthalene	T52.8X1	T52.8X2	T52.8X3	T52.8X4	—	—
Decalin	T52.8X1	T52.8X2	T52.8X3	T52.8X4	—	—
Decamethonium (bromide)	T48.1X1	T48.1X2	T48.1X3	T48.1X4	T48.1X5	T48.1X6
Decholin	T47.5X1	T47.5X2	T47.5X3	T47.5X4	T47.5X5	T47.5X6
Declomycin	T36.4X1	T36.4X2	T36.4X3	T36.4X4	T36.4X5	T36.4X6
Decongestant, nasal (mucosa)	T48.5X1	T48.5X2	T48.5X3	T48.5X4	T48.5X5	T48.5X6
combination	T48.5X1	T48.5X2	T48.5X3	T48.5X4	T48.5X5	T48.5X6

◀ New ◀ Revised ~~deleted~~ Deleted

Substance	External Cause (T-Code)					
	Poisoning, Accidental (Unintentional)	Poisoning, Intentional Self-Harm	Poisoning, Assault	Poisoning, Undetermined	Adverse Effect	Underdosing
Deet	T60.8X1	T60.8X2	T60.8X3	T60.8X4	—	—
Deferoxamine	T45.8X1	T45.8X2	T45.8X3	T45.8X4	T45.8X5	T45.8X6
Deflazacort	T38.0X1	T38.0X2	T38.0X3	T38.0X4	T38.0X5	T38.0X6
Deglycyrrhizinized extract of licorice	T48.4X1	T48.4X2	T48.4X3	T48.4X4	T48.4X5	T48.4X6
Dehydrocholic acid	T47.5X1	T47.5X2	T47.5X3	T47.5X4	T47.5X5	T47.5X6
Dehydroemetine	T37.3X1	T37.3X2	T37.3X3	T37.3X4	T37.3X5	T37.3X6
Dekalin	T52.8X1	T52.8X2	T52.8X3	T52.8X4	—	—
Delalutin	T38.5X1	T38.5X2	T38.5X3	T38.5X4	T38.5X5	T38.5X6
Delphinium	T62.2X1	T62.2X2	T62.2X3	T62.2X4	—	—
Deltasone	T38.0X1	T38.0X2	T38.0X3	T38.0X4	T38.0X5	T38.0X6
Deltra	T38.0X1	T38.0X2	T38.0X3	T38.0X4	T38.0X5	T38.0X6
Delvinal	T42.3X1	T42.3X2	T42.3X3	T42.3X4	T42.3X5	T42.3X6
Delorazepam	T42.4X1	T42.4X2	T42.4X3	T42.4X4	T42.4X5	T42.4X6
Deltamethrin	T60.1X1	T60.1X2	T60.1X3	T60.1X4	—	—
Demecarium (bromide)	T49.5X1	T49.5X2	T49.5X3	T49.5X4	T49.5X5	T49.5X6
Demeclocycline	T36.4X1	T36.4X2	T36.4X3	T36.4X4	T36.4X5	T36.4X6
Demecolcine	T45.1X1	T45.1X2	T45.1X3	T45.1X4	T45.1X5	T45.1X6
Demegestone	T38.5X1	T38.5X2	T38.5X3	T38.5X4	T38.5X5	T38.5X6
Demelanizing agents	T49.8X1	T49.8X2	T49.8X3	T49.8X4	T49.8X5	T49.8X6
Demephion -O and -S	T60.0X1	T60.0X2	T60.0X3	T60.0X4	—	—
Demerol	T40.2X1	T40.2X2	T40.2X3	T40.2X4	T40.2X5	T40.2X6
Demethylchlortetracycline	T36.4X1	T36.4X2	T36.4X3	T36.4X4	T36.4X5	T36.4X6
Demethyltetracycline	T36.4X1	T36.4X2	T36.4X3	T36.4X4	T36.4X5	T36.4X6
Demeton -O and -S	T60.0X1	T60.0X2	T60.0X3	T60.0X4	—	—
Demulcent (external)	T49.3X1	T49.3X2	T49.3X3	T49.3X4	T49.3X5	T49.3X6
specified NEC	T49.3X1	T49.3X2	T49.3X3	T49.3X4	T49.3X5	T49.3X6
Demulen	T38.4X1	T38.4X2	T38.4X3	T38.4X4	T38.4X5	T38.4X6
Denatured alcohol	T51.0X1	T51.0X2	T51.0X3	T51.0X4	—	—
Dendrid	T49.5X1	T49.5X2	T49.5X3	T49.5X4	T49.5X5	T49.5X6
Dental drug, topical application NEC	T49.7X1	T49.7X2	T49.7X3	T49.7X4	T49.7X5	T49.7X6
Dentifrice	T49.7X1	T49.7X2	T49.7X3	T49.7X4	T49.7X5	T49.7X6
Deodorant spray (feminine hygiene)	T49.8X1	T49.8X2	T49.8X3	T49.8X4	T49.8X5	T49.8X6
Deoxycortone	T50.0X1	T50.0X2	T50.0X3	T50.0X4	T50.0X5	T50.0X6
2-Deoxy-5-fluorouridine	T45.1X1	T45.1X2	T45.1X3	T45.1X4	T45.1X5	T45.1X6
5-Deoxy-5-fluorouridine	T45.1X1	T45.1X2	T45.1X3	T45.1X4	T45.1X5	T45.1X6
Deoxyribonuclease (pancreatic)	T45.3X1	T45.3X2	T45.3X3	T45.3X4	T45.3X5	T45.3X6
Depilatory	T49.4X1	T49.4X2	T49.4X3	T49.4X4	T49.4X5	T49.4X6
Deprenalin	T42.8X1	T42.8X2	T42.8X3	T42.8X4	T42.8X5	T42.8X6
Deprenyl	T42.8X1	T42.8X2	T42.8X3	T42.8X4	T42.8X5	T42.8X6

◀ New   ◀═ Revised   ~~deleted~~ Deleted

TABLE OF DRUGS AND CHEMICALS

Substance	External Cause (T-Code)					
	Poisoning, Accidental (Unintentional)	Poisoning, Intentional Self-Harm	Poisoning, Assault	Poisoning, Undetermined	Adverse Effect	Underdosing
Depressant, appetite	T50.5X1	T50.5X2	T50.5X3	T50.5X4	T50.5X5	T50.5X6
Depressant						
appetite, central	T50.5X1	T50.5X2	T50.5X3	T50.5X4	T50.5X5	T50.5X6
cardiac	T46.2X1	T46.2X2	T46.2X3	T46.2X4	T46.2X5	T46.2X6
central nervous system (anesthetic) — *see also Central nervous system, depressants*	T42.71	T42.72	T42.73	T42.74	T42.75	T42.76
general anesthetic	T41.201	T41.202	T41.203	T41.204	T41.205	T41.206
muscle tone	T42.8X1	T42.8X2	T42.8X3	T42.8X4	T42.8X5	T42.8X6
muscle tone, central	T42.8X1	T42.8X2	T42.8X3	T42.8X4	T42.8X5	T42.8X6
psychotherapeutic	T43.501	T43.502	T43.503	T43.504	T43.505	T43.506
Deptropine	T45.0X1	T45.0X2	T45.0X3	T45.0X4	T45.0X5	T45.0X6
Dequalinium (chloride)	T49.0X1	T49.0X2	T49.0X3	T49.0X4	T49.0X5	T49.0X6
Derris root	T60.2X1	T60.2X2	T60.2X3	T60.2X4	—	—
Deserpidine	T43.011	T43.012	T43.013	T43.014	T43.015	T43.016
Desferrioxamine	T45.8X1	T45.8X2	T45.8X3	T45.8X4	T45.8X5	T45.8X6
Desipramine	T43.0X1	T43.0X2	T43.0X3	T43.0X4	T43.0X5	T43.0X6
Deslanoside	T46.0X1	T46.0X2	T46.0X3	T46.0X4	T46.0X5	T46.0X6
Desloughing agent	T49.4X1	T49.4X2	T49.4X3	T49.4X4	T49.4X5	T49.4X6
Desmethylimipramine	T43.011	T43.012	T43.013	T43.014	T43.015	T43.016
Desmopressin	T38.891	T38.892	T38.893	T38.894	T38.895	T38.896
Desocodeine	T40.2X1	T40.2X2	T40.2X3	T40.2X4	T40.2X5	T40.2X6
Desogestrel	T38.5X1	T38.5X2	T38.5X3	T38.5X4	T38.5X5	T38.5X6
Desomorphine	T40.2X1	T40.2X2	T40.2X3	T40.2X4	—	—
Desonide	T49.0X1	T49.0X2	T49.0X3	T49.0X4	T49.0X5	T49.0X6
Desoximetasone	T49.0X1	T49.0X2	T49.0X3	T49.0X4	T49.0X5	T49.0X6
Desoxycorticosteroid	T50.0X1	T50.0X2	T50.0X3	T50.0X4	T50.0X5	T50.0X6
Desoxycortone	T50.0X1	T50.0X2	T50.0X3	T50.0X4	T50.0X5	T50.0X6
Desoxyephedrine	T43.621	T43.622	T43.623	T43.624	T43.625	T43.626
Detaxtran	T46.6X1	T46.6X2	T46.6X3	T46.6X4	T46.6X5	T46.6X6
Detergent	T49.2X1	T49.2X2	T49.2X3	T49.2X4	T49.2X5	T49.2X6
external medication	T49.2X1	T49.2X2	T49.2X3	T49.2X4	T49.2X5	T49.2X6
local	T49.2X1	T49.2X2	T49.2X3	T49.2X4	T49.2X5	T49.2X6
medicinal	T49.2X1	T49.2X2	T49.2X3	T49.2X4	T49.2X5	T49.2X6
nonmedicinal	T55.1X1	T55.1X2	T55.1X3	T55.1X4	—	—
specified NEC	T55.1X1	T55.1X2	T55.1X3	T55.1X4	T55.1X5	T55.1X6
Deterrent, alcohol	T50.6X1	T50.6X2	T50.6X3	T50.6X4	T50.6X5	T50.6X6
Detoxifying agent	T50.6X1	T50.6X2	T50.6X3	T50.6X4	T50.6X5	T50.6X6
Detrothyronine	T38.1X1	T38.1X2	T38.1X3	T38.1X4	T38.1X5	T38.1X6
Dettol (external medication)	T49.0X1	T49.0X2	T49.0X3	T49.0X4	T49.0X5	T49.0X6

◀ New   ◀ Revised   ~~deleted~~ Deleted

TABLE OF DRUGS AND CHEMICALS

Substance	External Cause (T-Code)					
	Poisoning, Accidental (Unintentional)	Poisoning, Intentional Self-Harm	Poisoning, Assault	Poisoning, Undetermined	Adverse Effect	Underdosing
Dexamethasone	T38.0X1	T38.0X2	T38.0X3	T38.0X4	T38.0X5	T38.0X6
ENT agent	T49.6X1	T49.6X2	T49.6X3	T49.6X4	T49.6X5	T49.6X6
ophthalmic preparation	T49.5X1	T49.5X2	T49.5X3	T49.5X4	T49.5X5	T49.5X6
topical NEC	T49.0X1	T49.0X2	T49.0X3	T49.0X4	T49.0X5	T49.0X6
Dexamfetamine	T43.621	T43.622	T43.623	T43.624	T43.625	T43.626
Dexamphetamine	T43.621	T43.622	T43.623	T43.624	T43.625	T43.626
Dexbrompheniramine	T45.0X1	T45.0X2	T45.0X3	T45.0X4	T45.0X5	T45.0X6
Dexchlorpheniramine	T45.0X1	T45.0X2	T45.0X3	T45.0X4	T45.0X5	T45.0X6
Dexedrine	T43.621	T43.622	T43.623	T43.624	T43.625	T43.626
Dexetimide	T44.3X1	T44.3X2	T44.3X3	T44.3X4	T44.3X5	T44.3X6
Dexfenfluramine	T50.5X1	T50.5X2	T50.5X3	T50.5X4	T50.5X5	T50.5X6
Dexpanthenol	T45.2X1	T45.2X2	T45.2X3	T45.2X4	T45.2X5	T45.2X6
Dextran (40) (70) (150)	T45.8X1	T45.8X2	T45.8X3	T45.8X4	T45.8X5	T45.8X6
Dextriferron	T45.4X1	T45.4X2	T45.4X3	T45.4X4	T45.4X5	T45.4X6
Dextroamphetamine	T43.621	T43.622	T43.623	T43.624	T43.625	T43.626
Dextro calcium pantothenate	T45.2X1	T45.2X2	T45.2X3	T45.2X4	T45.2X5	T45.2X6
Dextromethorphan	T48.3X1	T48.3X2	T48.3X3	T48.3X4	T48.3X5	T48.3X6
Dextromoramide	T40.4X1	T40.4X2	T40.4X3	T40.4X4	—	—
topical	T49.8X1	T49.8X2	T49.8X3	T49.8X4	T49.8X5	T49.8X6
Dextro pantothenyl alcohol	T45.2X1	T45.2X2	T45.2X3	T45.2X4	T45.2X5	T45.2X6
Dextropropoxyphene	T40.4X1	T40.4X2	T40.4X3	T40.4X4	T40.4X5	T40.4X6
Dextrorphan	T40.2X1	T40.2X2	T40.2X3	T40.2X4	T40.2X5	T40.2X6
Dextrose	T50.3X1	T50.3X2	T50.3X3	T50.3X4	T50.3X5	T50.3X6
concentrated solution, intravenous	T46.8X1	T46.8X2	T46.8X3	T46.8X4	T46.8X5	T46.8X6
Dextrothyroxin	T38.1X1	T38.1X2	T38.1X3	T38.1X4	T38.1X5	T38.1X6
Dextrothyroxine sodium	T38.1X1	T38.1X2	T38.1X3	T38.1X4	T38.1X5	T38.1X6
DFP	T44.0X1	T44.0X2	T44.0X3	T44.0X4	T44.0X5	T44.0X6
DHE	T37.3X1	T37.3X2	T37.3X3	T37.3X4	T37.3X5	T37.3X6
45	T46.5X1	T46.5X2	T46.5X3	T46.5X4	T46.5X5	T46.5X6
Diabinese	T38.3X1	T38.3X2	T38.3X3	T38.3X4	T38.3X5	T38.3X6
Diacetone alcohol	T52.4X1	T52.4X2	T52.4X3	T52.4X4	—	—
Diacetyl monoxime	T50.991	T50.992	T50.993	T50.994	—	—
Diacetylmorphine	T40.1X1	T40.1X2	T40.1X3	T40.1X4	—	—
Diachylon plaster	T49.4X1	T49.4X2	T49.4X3	T49.4X4	T49.4X5	T49.4X6
Diaethylstilboestrolum	T38.5X1	T38.5X2	T38.5X3	T38.5X4	T38.5X5	T38.5X6
Diagnostic agent NEC	T50.8X1	T50.8X2	T50.8X3	T50.8X4	T50.8X5	T50.8X6
Dial (soap)	T49.2X1	T49.2X2	T49.2X3	T49.2X4	T49.2X5	T49.2X6
sedative	T42.3X1	T42.3X2	T42.3X3	T42.3X4	T42.3X5	T42.3X6
Dialkyl carbonate	T52.91	T52.92	T52.93	T52.94	—	—

◀ New ◀ Revised ~~deleted~~ Deleted

Substance	External Cause (T-Code)					
	Poisoning, Accidental (Unintentional)	Poisoning, Intentional Self-Harm	Poisoning, Assault	Poisoning, Undetermined	Adverse Effect	Underdosing
Diallylbarbituric acid	T42.3X1	T42.3X2	T42.3X3	T42.3X4	T42.3X5	T42.3X6
Diallymal	T42.3X1	T42.3X2	T42.3X3	T42.3X4	T42.3X5	T42.3X6
Dialysis solution (intraperitoneal)	T50.3X1	T50.3X2	T50.3X3	T50.3X4	T50.3X5	T50.3X6
Diaminodiphenylsulfone	T37.1X1	T37.1X2	T37.1X3	T37.1X4	T37.1X5	T37.1X6
Diamorphine	T40.1X1	T40.1X2	T40.1X3	T40.1X4	—	—
Diamox	T50.2X1	T50.2X2	T50.2X3	T50.2X4	T50.2X5	T50.2X6
Diamthazole	T49.0X1	T49.0X2	T49.0X3	T49.0X4	T49.0X5	T49.0X6
Dianthone	T47.2X1	T47.2X2	T47.2X3	T47.2X4	T47.2X5	T47.2X6
Diaphenylsulfone	T37.0X1	T37.0X2	T37.0X3	T37.0X4	T37.0X5	T37.0X6
Diasone (sodium)	T37.1X1	T37.1X2	T37.1X3	T37.1X4	T37.1X5	T37.1X6
Diastase	T47.5X1	T47.5X2	T47.5X3	T47.5X4	T47.5X5	T47.5X6
Diatrizoate	T50.8X1	T50.8X2	T50.8X3	T50.8X4	T50.8X5	T50.8X6
Diazepam	T42.4X1	T42.4X2	T42.4X3	T42.4X4	T42.4X5	T42.4X6
Diazinon	T60.0X1	T60.0X2	T60.0X3	T60.0X4	—	—
Diazomethane (gas)	T59.891	T59.892	T59.893	T59.894	—	—
Diazoxide	T46.5X1	T46.5X2	T46.5X3	T46.5X4	T46.5X5	T46.5X6
Dibekacin	T36.5X1	T36.5X2	T36.5X3	T36.5X4	T36.5X5	T36.5X6
Dibenamine	T44.6X1	T44.6X2	T44.6X3	T44.6X4	T44.6X5	T44.6X6
Dibenzepin	T43.011	T43.012	T43.013	T43.014	T43.015	T43.016
Dibenzheptropine	T45.0X1	T45.0X2	T45.0X3	T45.0X4	T45.0X5	T45.0X6
Dibenzyline	T44.6X1	T44.6X2	T44.6X3	T44.6X4	T44.6X5	T44.6X6
Diborane (gas)	T59.891	T59.892	T59.893	T59.894	—	—
Dibromochloropropane	T60.8X1	T60.8X2	T60.8X3	T60.8X4	—	—
Dibromodulcitol	T45.1X1	T45.1X2	T45.1X3	T45.1X4	T45.1X5	T45.1X6
Dibromoethane	T53.6X1	T53.6X2	T53.6X3	T53.6X4	—	—
Dibromomannitol	T45.1X1	T45.1X2	T45.1X3	T45.1X4	T45.1X5	T45.1X6
Dibromopropamidine isethionate	T49.0X1	T49.0X2	T49.0X3	T49.0X4	T49.0X5	T49.0X6
Dibrompropamidine	T49.0X1	T49.0X2	T49.0X3	T49.0X4	T49.0X5	T49.0X6
Dibucaine	T41.3X1	T41.3X2	T41.3X3	T41.3X4	T41.3X5	T41.3X6
topical (surface)	T41.3X1	T41.3X2	T41.3X3	T41.3X4	T41.3X5	T41.3X6
Dibunate sodium	T48.3X1	T48.3X2	T48.3X3	T48.3X4	T48.3X5	T48.3X6
Dibutoline sulfate	T44.3X1	T44.3X2	T44.3X3	T44.3X4	T44.3X5	T44.3X6
Dicamba	T60.3X1	T60.3X2	T60.3X3	T60.3X4	—	—
Dicapthon	T60.0X1	T60.0X2	T60.0X3	T60.0X4	—	—
Dichlobenil	T60.3X1	T60.3X2	T60.3X3	T60.3X4	—	—
Dichlone	T60.3X1	T60.3X2	T60.3X3	T60.3X4	—	—
Dichloralphenozone	T42.6X1	T42.6X2	T42.6X3	T42.6X4	T42.6X5	T42.6X6
Dichlorbenzidine	T65.3X1	T65.3X2	T65.3X3	T65.3X4	—	—
Dichlorhydrin	T52.8X1	T52.8X2	T52.8X3	T52.8X4	—	—
Dichlorhydroxyquinoline	T37.8X1	T37.8X2	T37.8X3	T37.8X4	T37.8X5	T37.8X6

◀ New   ◀▦ Revised   ~~deleted~~ Deleted

Substance	Poisoning, Accidental (Unintentional)	Poisoning, Intentional Self-Harm	Poisoning, Assault	Poisoning, Undetermined	Adverse Effect	Underdosing
			External Cause (T-Code)			
Dichlorobenzene	T53.7X1	T53.7X2	T53.7X3	T53.7X4	—	—
Dichlorobenzyl alcohol	T49.6X1	T49.6X2	T49.6X3	T49.6X4	T49.6X5	T49.6X6
Dichlorodifluoromethane	T53.5X1	T53.5X2	T53.5X3	T53.5X4	—	—
Dichloroethane	T52.8X1	T52.8X2	T52.8X3	T52.8X4	—	—
Sym-Dichloroethyl ether	T53.6X1	T53.6X2	T53.6X3	T53.6X4	—	—
Dichloroethyl sulfide, not in war	T59.891	T59.892	T59.893	T59.894	—	—
Dichloroethylene	T53.6X1	T53.6X2	T53.6X3	T53.6X4	—	—
Dichloroformoxine, not in war	T59.891	T59.892	T59.893	T59.894	—	—
Dichlorohydrin, alpha-dichlorohydrin	T52.8X1	T52.8X2	T52.8X3	T52.8X4	—	—
Dichloromethane (solvent)	T53.4X1	T53.4X2	T53.4X3	T53.4X4	—	—
vapor	T53.4X1	T53.4X2	T53.4X3	T53.4X4	—	—
Dichloronaphthoquinone	T60.3X1	T60.3X2	T60.3X3	T60.3X4	—	—
Dichlorophen	T37.4X1	T37.4X2	T37.4X3	T37.4X4	T37.4X5	T37.4X6
2,4-Dichlorophenoxy-acetic acid	T60.3X1	T60.3X2	T60.3X3	T60.3X4	—	—
Dichloropropene	T60.3X1	T60.3X2	T60.3X3	T60.3X4	—	—
Dichloropropionic acid	T60.3X1	T60.3X2	T60.3X3	T60.3X4	—	—
Dichlorphenamide	T50.2X1	T50.2X2	T50.2X3	T50.2X4	T50.2X5	T50.2X6
Dichlorvos	T60.0X1	T60.0X2	T60.0X3	T60.0X4	—	—
Diclofenac	T39.391	T39.392	T39.393	T39.394	T39.395	T39.396
Diclofenamide	T50.2X1	T50.2X2	T50.2X3	T50.2X4	T50.2X5	T50.2X6
Diclofensine	T43.291	T43.292	T43.293	T43.294	T43.295	T43.296
Diclonixine	T39.8X1	T39.8X2	T39.8X3	T39.8X4	T39.8X5	T39.8X6
Dicloxacillin	T36.0X1	T36.0X2	T36.0X3	T36.0X4	T36.0X5	T36.0X6
Dicophane	T49.0X1	T49.0X2	T49.0X3	T49.0X4	T49.0X5	T49.0X6
Dicoumarol, dicoumarin, dicumarol	T45.511	T45.512	T45.513	T45.514	T45.515	T45.516
Dicrotophos	T60.0X1	T60.0X2	T60.0X3	T60.0X4	—	—
Dicyanogen (gas)	T65.0X1	T65.0X2	T65.0X3	T65.0X4	—	—
Dicyclomine	T44.3X1	T44.3X2	T44.3X3	T44.3X4	T44.3X5	T44.3X6
Dicycloverine	T44.3X1	T44.3X2	T44.3X3	T44.3X4	T44.3X5	T44.3X6
Dideoxycytidine	T37.5X1	T37.5X2	T37.5X3	T37.5X4	T37.5X5	T37.5X6
Dideoxyinosine	T37.5X1	T37.5X2	T37.5X3	T37.5X4	T37.5X5	T37.5X6
Dieldrin (vapor)	T60.1X1	T60.1X2	T60.1X3	T60.1X4	—	—
Diemal	T42.3X1	T42.3X2	T42.3X3	T42.3X4	T42.3X5	T42.3X6
Dienestrol	T38.5X1	T38.5X2	T38.5X3	T38.5X4	T38.5X5	T38.5X6
Dienoestrol	T38.5X1	T38.5X2	T38.5X3	T38.5X4	T38.5X5	T38.5X6
Dietetic drug NEC	T50.901	T50.902	T50.903	T50.904	T50.905	T50.906
Diethazine	T42.8X1	T42.8X2	T42.8X3	T42.8X4	T42.8X5	T42.8X6
Diethyl						
barbituric acid	T42.3X1	T42.3X2	T42.3X3	T42.3X4	T42.3X5	T42.3X6
carbamazine	T37.4X1	T37.4X2	T37.4X3	T37.4X4	T37.4X5	T37.4X6

TABLE OF DRUGS AND CHEMICALS

TABLE OF DRUGS AND CHEMICALS

Substance	External Cause (T-Code)					
	Poisoning, Accidental (Unintentional)	Poisoning, Intentional Self-Harm	Poisoning, Assault	Poisoning, Undetermined	Adverse Effect	Underdosing
Diethyl *(Continued)*						
carbinol	T51.3X1	T51.3X2	T51.3X3	T51.3X4	—	—
carbonate	T52.8X1	T52.8X2	T52.8X3	T52.8X4	—	—
ether (vapor) — *see also ether*	T41.0X1	T41.0X2	T41.0X3	T41.0X4	T41.0X5	T41.0X6
oxide	T52.8X1	T52.8X2	T52.8X3	T52.8X4	—	—
propion	T50.5X1	T50.5X2	T50.5X3	T50.5X4	T50.5X5	T50.5X6
stilbestrol	T38.5X1	T38.5X2	T38.5X3	T38.5X4	T38.5X5	T38.5X6
toluamide (nonmedicinal)	T60.8X1	T60.8X2	T60.8X3	T60.8X4	—	—
medicinal	T49.3X1	T49.3X2	T49.3X3	T49.3X4	T49.3X5	T49.3X6
Diethylcarbamazine	T37.4X1	T37.4X2	T37.4X3	T37.4X4	T37.4X5	T37.4X6
Diethylene						
dioxide	T52.8X1	T52.8X2	T52.8X3	T52.8X4	—	—
glycol (monoacetate) (monobutyl ether) (monoethyl ether)	T52.3X1	T52.3X2	T52.3X3	T52.3X4	—	—
Diethylhexylphthalate	T65.891	T65.892	T65.893	T65.894	—	—
Diethylpropion	T50.5X1	T50.5X2	T50.5X3	T50.5X4	T50.5X5	T50.5X6
Diethylstilbestrol	T38.5X1	T38.5X2	T38.5X3	T38.5X4	T38.5X5	T38.5X6
Diethylstilboestrol	T38.5X1	T38.5X2	T38.5X3	T38.5X4	T38.5X5	T38.5X6
Diethylsulfone-diethylmethane	T42.6X1	T42.6X2	T42.6X3	T42.6X4	T42.6X5	T42.6X6
Diethyltoluamide	T49.0X1	T49.0X2	T49.0X3	T49.0X4	T49.0X5	T49.0X6
Diethyltryptamine (DET)	T40.991	T40.992	T40.993	T40.994	—	—
Difebarbamate	T42.3X1	T42.3X2	T42.3X3	T42.3X4	T42.3X5	T42.3X6
Difencloxazine	T40.2X1	T40.2X2	T40.2X3	T40.2X4	T40.2X5	T40.2X6
Difenidol	T45.0X1	T45.0X2	T45.0X3	T45.0X4	T45.0X5	T45.0X6
Difenoxin	T47.6X1	T47.6X2	T47.6X3	T47.6X4	T47.6X5	T47.6X6
Difetarsone	T37.3X1	T37.3X2	T37.3X3	T37.3X4	T37.3X5	T37.3X6
Diffusin	T45.3X1	T45.3X2	T45.3X3	T45.3X4	T45.3X5	T45.3X6
Diflorasone	T49.0X1	T49.0X2	T49.0X3	T49.0X4	T49.0X5	T49.0X6
Diflubenzuron	T60.1X1	T60.1X2	T60.1X3	T60.1X4	—	—
Diflos	T44.0X1	T44.0X2	T44.0X3	T44.0X4	T44.0X5	T44.0X6
Diflucortolone	T49.0X1	T49.0X2	T49.0X3	T49.0X4	T49.0X5	T49.0X6
Diflunisal	T39.091	T39.092	T39.093	T39.094	T39.095	T39.096
Difluoromethyldopa	T42.8X1	T42.8X2	T42.8X3	T42.8X4	T42.8X5	T42.8X6
Difluorophate	T44.0X1	T44.0X2	T44.0X3	T44.0X4	T44.0X5	T44.0X6
Digestant NEC	T47.5X1	T47.5X2	T47.5X3	T47.5X4	T47.5X5	T47.5X6
Digitalin(e)	T46.0X1	T46.0X2	T46.0X3	T46.0X4	T46.0X5	T46.0X6
Digitalis (leaf) (glycoside)	T46.0X1	T46.0X2	T46.0X3	T46.0X4	T46.0X5	T46.0X6
lanata	T46.0X1	T46.0X2	T46.0X3	T46.0X4	T46.0X5	T46.0X6
purpurea	T46.0X1	T46.0X2	T46.0X3	T46.0X4	T46.0X5	T46.0X6
Digitoxin	T46.0X1	T46.0X2	T46.0X3	T46.0X4	T46.0X5	T46.0X6

◄ New ◄▥ Revised ~~deleted~~ Deleted

Substance	External Cause (T-Code)					
	Poisoning, Accidental (Unintentional)	Poisoning, Intentional Self-Harm	Poisoning, Assault	Poisoning, Undetermined	Adverse Effect	Underdosing
Digitoxose	T46.0X1	T46.0X2	T46.0X3	T46.0X4	T46.0X5	T46.0X6
Digoxin	T46.0X1	T46.0X2	T46.0X3	T46.0X4	T46.0X5	T46.0X6
Digoxine	T46.0X1	T46.0X2	T46.0X3	T46.0X4	T46.0X5	T46.0X6
Dihydralazine	T46.5X1	T46.5X2	T46.5X3	T46.5X4	T46.5X5	T46.5X6
Dihydrazine	T46.5X1	T46.5X2	T46.5X3	T46.5X4	T46.5X5	T46.5X6
Dihydrocodeinone	T40.2X1	T40.2X2	T40.2X3	T40.2X4	T40.2X5	T40.2X6
Dihydroergocornine	T46.7X1	T46.7X2	T46.7X3	T46.7X4	T46.7X5	T46.7X6
Dihydroergocristine (mesilate)	T46.7X1	T46.7X2	T46.7X3	T46.7X4	T46.7X5	T46.7X6
Dihydroergokryptine	T46.7X1	T46.7X2	T46.7X3	T46.7X4	T46.7X5	T46.7X6
Dihydroergotamine	T46.5X1	T46.5X2	T46.5X3	T46.5X4	T46.5X5	T46.5X6
Dihydroergotoxine	T46.7X1	T46.7X2	T46.7X3	T46.7X4	T46.7X5	T46.7X6
mesilate	T46.7X1	T46.7X2	T46.7X3	T46.7X4	T46.7X5	T46.7X6
Dihydrohydroxycodein-one	T40.2X1	T40.2X2	T40.2X3	T40.2X4	T40.2X5	T40.2X6
Dihydrohydroxymorphinone	T40.2X1	T40.2X2	T40.2X3	T40.2X4	T40.2X5	T40.2X6
Dihydroisocodeine	T40.2X1	T40.2X2	T40.2X3	T40.2X4	T40.2X5	T40.2X6
Dihydromorphine	T40.2X1	T40.2X2	T40.2X3	T40.2X4	—	—
Dihydromorphinone	T40.2X1	T40.2X2	T40.2X3	T40.2X4	T40.2X5	T40.2X6
Dihydrostreptomycin	T36.5X1	T36.5X2	T36.5X3	T36.5X4	T36.5X5	T36.5X6
Dihydrotachysterol	T45.2X1	T45.2X2	T45.2X3	T45.2X4	T45.2X5	T45.2X6
Dihydroxyaluminum aminoacetate	T47.1X1	T47.1X2	T47.1X3	T47.1X4	T47.1X5	T47.1X6
Dihydroxyaluminum sodium carbonate	T47.1X1	T47.1X2	T47.1X3	T47.1X4	T47.1X5	T47.1X6
Dihydroxyanthraquinone	T47.2X1	T47.2X2	T47.2X3	T47.2X4	T47.2X5	T47.2X6
Dihydroxycodeinone	T40.2X1	T40.2X2	T40.2X3	T40.2X4	T40.2X5	T40.2X6
Dihydroxypropyl theophylline	T50.2X1	T50.2X2	T50.2X3	T50.2X4	T50.2X5	T50.2X6
Diiodohydroxyquin	T37.8X1	T37.8X2	T37.8X3	T37.8X4	T37.8X5	T37.8X6
topical	T49.0X1	T49.0X2	T49.0X3	T49.0X4	T49.0X5	T49.0X6
Diiodohydroxyquinoline	T37.8X1	T37.8X2	T37.8X3	T37.8X4	T37.8X5	T37.8X6
Diiodotyrosine	T38.2X1	T38.2X2	T38.2X3	T38.2X4	T38.2X5	T38.2X6
Diisopromine	T44.3X1	T44.3X2	T44.3X3	T44.3X4	T44.3X5	T44.3X6
Diisopropylamine	T46.3X1	T46.3X2	T46.3X3	T46.3X4	T46.3X5	T46.3X6
Diisopropylfluorophosphonate	T44.0X1	T44.0X2	T44.0X3	T44.0X4	T44.0X5	T44.0X6
Dilantin	T42.0X1	T42.0X2	T42.0X3	T42.0X4	T42.0X5	T42.0X6
Dilaudid	T40.2X1	T40.2X2	T40.2X3	T40.2X4	T40.2X5	T40.2X6
Dilazep	T46.3X1	T46.3X2	T46.3X3	T46.3X4	T46.3X5	T46.3X6
Dill	T47.5X1	T47.5X2	T47.5X3	T47.5X4	T47.5X5	T47.5X6
Diloxanide	T37.3X1	T37.3X2	T37.3X3	T37.3X4	T37.3X5	T37.3X6
Diltiazem	T46.1X1	T46.1X2	T46.1X3	T46.1X4	T46.1X5	T46.1X6
Dimazole	T49.0X1	T49.0X2	T49.0X3	T49.0X4	T49.0X5	T49.0X6
Dimefline	T50.7X1	T50.7X2	T50.7X3	T50.7X4	T50.7X5	T50.7X6

TABLE OF DRUGS AND CHEMICALS

◄ New ◄‖‖ Revised ~~deleted~~ Deleted

TABLE OF DRUGS AND CHEMICALS

Substance	Poisoning, Accidental (Unintentional)	Poisoning, Intentional Self-Harm	Poisoning, Assault	Poisoning, Undetermined	Adverse Effect	Underdosing
	External Cause (T-Code)					
Dimefox	T60.0X1	T60.0X2	T60.0X3	T60.0X4	—	—
Dimemorfan	T48.3X1	T48.3X2	T48.3X3	T48.3X4	T48.3X5	T48.3X6
Dimenhydrinate	T45.0X1	T45.0X2	T45.0X3	T45.0X4	T45.0X5	T45.0X6
Dimercaprol (British anti-lewisite)	T45.8X1	T45.8X2	T45.8X3	T45.8X4	T45.8X5	T45.8X6
Dimercaptopropanol	T45.8X1	T45.8X2	T45.8X3	T45.8X4	T45.8X5	T45.8X6
Dimestrol	T38.5X1	T38.5X2	T38.5X3	T38.5X4	T38.5X5	T38.5X6
Dimetane	T45.0X1	T45.0X2	T45.0X3	T45.0X4	T45.0X5	T45.0X6
Dimethicone	T47.1X1	T47.1X2	T47.1X3	T47.1X4	T47.1X5	T47.1X6
Dimethindene	T45.0X1	T45.0X2	T45.0X3	T45.0X4	T45.0X5	T45.0X6
Dimethisoquin	T49.1X1	T49.1X2	T49.1X3	T49.1X4	T49.1X5	T49.1X6
Dimethisterone	T38.5X1	T38.5X2	T38.5X3	T38.5X4	T38.5X5	T38.5X6
Dimethoate	T60.0X1	T60.0X2	T60.0X3	T60.0X4	—	—
Dimethocaine	T41.3X1	T41.3X2	T41.3X3	T41.3X4	T41.3X5	T41.3X6
Dimethoxanate	T48.3X1	T48.3X2	T48.3X3	T48.3X4	T48.3X5	T48.3X6
Dimethyl						
arsine, arsinic acid	T57.0X1	T57.0X2	T57.0X3	T57.0X4	—	—
carbinol	T51.2X1	T51.2X2	T51.2X3	T51.2X4	—	—
carbonate	T52.8X1	T52.8X2	T52.8X3	T52.8X4	—	—
diguanide	T38.3X1	T38.3X2	T38.3X3	T38.3X4	T38.3X5	T38.3X6
ketone	T52.4X1	T52.4X2	T52.4X3	T52.4X4	—	—
vapor	T52.4X1	T52.4X2	T52.4X3	T52.4X4	—	—
meperidine	T40.2X1	T40.2X2	T40.2X3	T40.2X4	T40.2X5	T40.2X6
parathion	T60.0X1	T60.0X2	T60.0X3	T60.0X4	—	—
phthlate	T49.3X1	T49.3X2	T49.3X3	T49.3X4	T49.3X5	T49.3X6
polysiloxane	T47.8X1	T47.8X2	T47.8X3	T47.8X4	T47.8X5	T47.8X6
sulfate (fumes)	T59.891	T59.892	T59.893	T59.894	—	—
liquid	T65.891	T65.892	T65.893	T65.894	—	—
sulfoxide (nonmedicinal)	T52.8X1	T52.8X2	T52.8X3	T52.8X4	—	—
medicinal	T49.4X1	T49.4X2	T49.4X3	T49.4X4	T49.4X5	T49.4X6
tryptamine	T40.991	T40.992	T40.993	T40.994	—	—
tubocurarine	T48.1X1	T48.1X2	T48.1X3	T48.1X4	T48.1X5	T48.1X6
Dimethylamine sulfate	T49.4X1	T49.4X2	T49.4X3	T49.4X4	T49.4X5	T49.4X6
Dimethylformamide	T52.8X1	T52.8X2	T52.8X3	T52.8X4	—	—
Dimethyltubocurarinium chloride	T48.1X1	T48.1X2	T48.1X3	T48.1X4	T48.1X5	T48.1X6
Dimeticone	T47.1X1	T47.1X2	T47.1X3	T47.1X4	T47.1X5	T47.1X6
Dimetilan	T60.0X1	T60.0X2	T60.0X3	T60.0X4	—	—
Dimetindene	T45.0X1	T45.0X2	T45.0X3	T45.0X4	T45.0X5	T45.0X6
Dimetotiazine	T43.3X1	T43.3X2	T43.3X3	T43.3X4	T43.3X5	T43.3X6

◄ New   ◄▦ Revised   ~~deleted~~ Deleted

Substance	External Cause (T-Code)					
	Poisoning, Accidental (Unintentional)	Poisoning, Intentional Self-Harm	Poisoning, Assault	Poisoning, Undetermined	Adverse Effect	Underdosing
Dimorpholamine	T50.7X1	T50.7X2	T50.7X3	T50.7X4	T50.7X5	T50.7X6
Dimoxyline	T46.3X1	T46.3X2	T46.3X3	T46.3X4	T46.3X5	T46.3X6
Dinitrobenzene	T65.3X1	T65.3X2	T65.3X3	T65.3X4	—	—
vapor	T59.891	T59.892	T59.893	T59.894	—	—
Dinitrobenzol	T65.3X1	T65.3X2	T65.3X3	T65.3X4	—	—
vapor	T59.891	T59.892	T59.893	T59.894	—	—
Dinitrobutylphenol	T65.3X1	T65.3X2	T65.3X3	T65.3X4	—	—
Dinitro (-ortho-)cresol (pesticide) (spray)	T65.3X1	T65.3X2	T65.3X3	T65.3X4	—	—
Dinitrocyclohexylphenol	T65.3X1	T65.3X2	T65.3X3	T65.3X4	—	—
Dinitrophenol	T65.3X1	T65.3X2	T65.3X3	T65.3X4	—	—
Dinoprost	T48.0X1	T48.0X2	T48.0X3	T48.0X4	T48.0X5	T48.0X6
Dinoprostone	T48.0X1	T48.0X2	T48.0X3	T48.0X4	T48.0X5	T48.0X6
Dinoseb	T60.3X1	T60.3X2	T60.3X3	T60.3X4	—	—
Dioctyl sulfosuccinate (calcium) (sodium)	T47.4X1	T47.4X2	T47.4X3	T47.4X4	T47.4X5	T47.4X6
Diodone	T50.8X1	T50.8X2	T50.8X3	T50.8X4	T50.8X5	T50.8X6
Diodoquin	T37.8X1	T37.8X2	T37.8X3	T37.8X4	T37.8X5	T37.8X6
Dionin	T40.2X1	T40.2X2	T40.2X3	T40.2X4	T40.2X5	T40.2X6
Diosmin	T46.991	T46.992	T46.993	T46.994	T46.995	T46.996
Dioxane	T52.8X1	T52.8X2	T52.8X3	T52.8X4	—	—
Dioxathion	T60.0X1	T60.0X2	T60.0X3	T60.0X4	—	—
Dioxin	T53.7X1	T53.7X2	T53.7X3	T53.7X4	—	—
Dioxopromethazine	T43.3X1	T43.3X2	T43.3X3	T43.3X4	T43.3X5	T43.3X6
Dioxyline	T46.3X1	T46.3X2	T46.3X3	T46.3X4	T46.3X5	T46.3X6
Dipentene	T52.8X1	T52.8X2	T52.8X3	T52.8X4	—	—
Diperodon	T41.3X1	T41.3X2	T41.3X3	T41.3X4	T41.3X5	T41.3X6
Diphacinone	T60.4X1	T60.4X2	T60.4X3	T60.4X4	—	—
Diphemanil	T44.3X1	T44.3X2	T44.3X3	T44.3X4	T44.3X5	T44.3X6
metilsulfate	T44.3X1	T44.3X2	T44.3X3	T44.3X4	T44.3X5	T44.3X6
Diphenadione	T45.511	T45.512	T45.513	T45.514	T45.515	T45.516
rodenticide	T60.4X1	T60.4X2	T60.4X3	T60.4X4	—	—
Diphenhydramine	T45.0X1	T45.0X2	T45.0X3	T45.0X4	T45.0X5	T45.0X6
Diphenidol	T45.0X1	T45.0X2	T45.0X3	T45.0X4	T45.0X5	T45.0X6
Diphenoxylate	T47.6X1	T47.6X2	T47.6X3	T47.6X4	T47.6X5	T47.6X6
Diphenylamine	T65.3X1	T65.3X2	T65.3X3	T65.3X4	—	—
Diphenylbutazone	T39.2X1	T39.2X2	T39.2X3	T39.2X4	T39.2X5	T39.2X6
Diphenylchloroarsine, not in war	T57.0X1	T57.0X2	T57.0X3	T57.0X4	—	—
Diphenylhydantoin	T42.0X1	T42.0X2	T42.0X3	T42.0X4	T42.0X5	T42.0X6
Diphenylmethane dye	T52.1X1	T52.1X2	T52.1X3	T52.1X4	—	—

◀ New   ◀▥ Revised   ~~deleted~~ Deleted

TABLE OF DRUGS AND CHEMICALS

TABLE OF DRUGS AND CHEMICALS

Substance	External Cause (T-Code)					
	Poisoning, Accidental (Unintentional)	Poisoning, Intentional Self-Harm	Poisoning, Assault	Poisoning, Undetermined	Adverse Effect	Underdosing
Diphenylpyraline	T45.0X1	T45.0X2	T45.0X3	T45.0X4	T45.0X5	T45.0X6
Diphtheria						
antitoxin	T50.Z11	T50.Z12	T50.Z13	T50.Z14	T50.Z15	T50.Z16
toxoid	T50.A91	T50.A92	T50.A93	T50.A94	T50.A95	T50.A96
with tetanus toxoid	T50.A21	T50.A22	T50.A23	T50.A24	T50.A25	T50.A26
with pertussis component	T50.A11	T50.A12	T50.A13	T50.A14	T50.A15	T50.A16
vaccine (combination)	T50.A91	T50.A92	T50.A93	T50.A94	T50.A95	T50.A96
combination						
including pertussis	T50.A11	T50.A12	T50.A13	T50.A14	T50.A15	T50.A16
without pertussis	T50.A21	T50.A22	T50.A23	T50.A24	T50.A25	T50.A26
Diphylline	T50.2X1	T50.2X2	T50.2X3	T50.2X4	T50.2X5	T50.2X6
Dipipanone	T40.4X1	T40.4X2	T40.4X3	T40.4X4	—	—
Dipivefrine	T49.5X1	T49.5X2	T49.5X3	T49.5X4	T49.5X5	T49.5X6
Diplovax	T50.B91	T50.B92	T50.B93	T50.B94	T50.B95	T50.B96
Diprophylline	T50.2X1	T50.2X2	T50.2X3	T50.2X4	T50.2X5	T50.2X6
Dipropyline	T48.291	T48.292	T48.293	T48.294	T48.295	T48.296
Dipyridamole	T46.3X1	T46.3X2	T46.3X3	T46.3X4	T46.3X5	T46.3X6
Dipyrone	T39.2X1	T39.2X2	T39.2X3	T39.2X4	T39.2X5	T39.2X6
Diquat (dibromide)	T60.3X1	T60.3X2	T60.3X3	T60.3X4	—	—
Disinfectant	T65.891	T65.892	T65.893	T65.894	—	—
alkaline	T54.3X1	T54.3X2	T54.3X3	T54.3X4	—	—
aromatic	T54.1X1	T54.1X2	T54.1X3	T54.1X4	—	—
intestinal	T37.8X1	T37.8X2	T37.8X3	T37.8X4	T37.8X5	T37.8X6
Disipal	T42.8X1	T42.8X2	T42.8X3	T42.8X4	T42.8X5	T42.8X6
Disodium edetate	T50.6X1	T50.6X2	T50.6X3	T50.6X4	T50.6X5	T50.6X6
Disoprofol	T41.291	T41.292	T41.293	T41.294	T41.295	T41.296
Disopyramide	T46.2X1	T46.2X2	T46.2X3	T46.2X4	T46.2X5	T46.2X6
Distigmine (bromide)	T44.0X1	T44.0X2	T44.0X3	T44.0X4	T44.0X5	T44.0X6
Disulfamide	T50.2X1	T50.2X2	T50.2X3	T50.2X4	T50.2X5	T50.2X6
Disulfanilamide	T37.0X1	T37.0X2	T37.0X3	T37.0X4	T37.0X5	T37.0X6
Disulfiram	T50.6X1	T50.6X2	T50.6X3	T50.6X4	T50.6X5	T50.6X6
Disulfoton	T60.0X1	T60.0X2	T60.0X3	T60.0X4	—	—
Dithiazanine iodide	T37.4X1	T37.4X2	T37.4X3	T37.4X4	T37.4X5	T37.4X6
Dithiocarbamate	T60.0X1	T60.0X2	T60.0X3	T60.0X4	—	—
Dithranol	T49.4X1	T49.4X2	T49.4X3	T49.4X4	T49.4X5	T49.4X6
Diucardin	T50.2X1	T50.2X2	T50.2X3	T50.2X4	T50.2X5	T50.2X6
Diupres	T50.2X1	T50.2X2	T50.2X3	T50.2X4	T50.2X5	T50.2X6
Diuretic NEC	T50.2X1	T50.2X2	T50.2X3	T50.2X4	T50.2X5	T50.2X6
benzothiadiazine	T50.2X1	T50.2X2	T50.2X3	T50.2X4	T50.2X5	T50.2X6
carbonic acid anhydrase inhibitors	T50.2X1	T50.2X2	T50.2X3	T50.2X4	T50.2X5	T50.2X6

◀ New   ◀ Revised   ~~deleted~~ Deleted

Substance	External Cause (T-Code)					
	Poisoning, Accidental (Unintentional)	Poisoning, Intentional Self-Harm	Poisoning, Assault	Poisoning, Undetermined	Adverse Effect	Underdosing
Diuretic NEC *(Continued)*						
furfuryl NEC	T50.2X1	T50.2X2	T50.2X3	T50.2X4	T50.2X5	T50.2X6
loop (high-ceiling)	T50.1X1	T50.1X2	T50.1X3	T50.1X4	T50.1X5	T50.1X6
mercurial NEC	T50.2X1	T50.2X2	T50.2X3	T50.2X4	T50.2X5	T50.2X6
osmotic	T50.2X1	T50.2X2	T50.2X3	T50.2X4	T50.2X5	T50.2X6
purine NEC	T50.2X1	T50.2X2	T50.2X3	T50.2X4	T50.2X5	T50.2X6
saluretic NEC	T50.2X1	T50.2X2	T50.2X3	T50.2X4	T50.2X5	T50.2X6
sulfonamide	T50.2X1	T50.2X2	T50.2X3	T50.2X4	T50.2X5	T50.2X6
thiazide NEC	T50.2X1	T50.2X2	T50.2X3	T50.2X4	T50.2X5	T50.2X6
xanthine	T50.2X1	T50.2X2	T50.2X3	T50.2X4	T50.2X5	T50.2X6
Diurgin	T50.2X1	T50.2X2	T50.2X3	T50.2X4	T50.2X5	T50.2X6
Diuril	T50.2X1	T50.2X2	T50.2X3	T50.2X4	T50.2X5	T50.2X6
Diuron	T60.3X1	T60.3X2	T60.3X3	T60.3X4	—	—
Divalproex	T42.6X1	T42.6X2	T42.6X3	T42.6X4	T42.6X5	T42.6X6
Divinyl ether	T41.0X1	T41.0X2	T41.0X3	T41.0X4	T41.0X5	T41.0X6
Dixanthogen	T49.0X1	T49.0X2	T49.0X3	T49.0X4	T49.0X5	T49.0X6
Dixyrazine	T43.3X1	T43.3X2	T43.3X3	T43.3X4	T43.3X5	T43.3X6
D-lysergic acid diethylamide	T40.8X1	T40.8X2	T40.8X3	T40.8X4	—	—
DMCT	T36.4X1	T36.4X2	T36.4X3	T36.4X4	T36.4X5	T36.4X6
DMSO — *see Dimethyl sulfoxide*						
DNBP	T60.3X1	T60.3X2	T60.3X3	T60.3X4	—	—
DNOC	T65.3X1	T65.3X2	T65.3X3	T65.3X4	—	—
DOCA	T38.0X1	T38.0X2	T38.0X3	T38.0X4	T38.0X5	T38.0X6
Dobutamine	T44.5X1	T44.5X2	T44.5X3	T44.5X4	T44.5X5	T44.5X6
Docusate sodium	T47.4X1	T47.4X2	T47.4X3	T47.4X4	T47.4X5	T47.4X6
Dodicin	T49.0X1	T49.0X2	T49.0X3	T49.0X4	T49.0X5	T49.0X6
Dofamium chloride	T49.0X1	T49.0X2	T49.0X3	T49.0X4	T49.0X5	T49.0X6
Dolophine	T40.3X1	T40.3X2	T40.3X3	T40.3X4	T40.3X5	T40.3X6
Doloxene	T39.8X1	T39.8X2	T39.8X3	T39.8X4	T39.8X5	T39.8X6
Domestic gas (after combustion) — *see Gas, utility*						
prior to combustion	T59.891	T59.892	T59.893	T59.894	—	—
Domiodol	T48.4X1	T48.4X2	T48.4X3	T48.4X4	T48.4X5	T48.4X6
Domiphen (bromide)	T49.0X1	T49.0X2	T49.0X3	T49.0X4	T49.0X5	T49.0X6
Domperidone	T45.0X1	T45.0X2	T45.0X3	T45.0X4	T45.0X5	T45.0X6
Dopa	T42.8X1	T42.8X2	T42.8X3	T42.8X4	T42.8X5	T42.8X6
Dopamine	T44.991	T44.992	T44.993	T44.994	T44.995	T44.996
Doriden	T42.6X1	T42.6X2	T42.6X3	T42.6X4	T42.6X5	T42.6X6
Dormiral	T42.3X1	T42.3X2	T42.3X3	T42.3X4	T42.3X5	T42.3X6
Dormison	T42.6X1	T42.6X2	T42.6X3	T42.6X4	T42.6X5	T42.6X6
Dornase	T48.4X1	T48.4X2	T48.4X3	T48.4X4	T48.4X5	T48.4X6

TABLE OF DRUGS AND CHEMICALS

Substance	External Cause (T-Code)					
	Poisoning, Accidental (Unintentional)	Poisoning, Intentional Self-Harm	Poisoning, Assault	Poisoning, Undetermined	Adverse Effect	Underdosing
Dorsacaine	T41.3X1	T41.3X2	T41.3X3	T41.3X4	T41.3X5	T41.3X6
Dosulepin	T43.011	T43.012	T43.013	T43.014	T43.015	T43.016
Dothiepin	T43.011	T43.012	T43.013	T43.014	T43.015	T43.016
Doxantrazole	T48.6X1	T48.6X2	T48.6X3	T48.6X4	T48.6X5	T48.6X6
Doxapram	T50.7X1	T50.7X2	T50.7X3	T50.7X4	T50.7X5	T50.7X6
Doxazosin	T44.6X1	T44.6X2	T44.6X3	T44.6X4	T44.6X5	T44.6X6
Doxepin	T43.011	T43.012	T43.013	T43.014	T43.015	T43.016
Doxifluridine	T45.1X1	T45.1X2	T45.1X3	T45.1X4	T45.1X5	T45.1X6
Doxorubicin	T45.1X1	T45.1X2	T45.1X3	T45.1X4	T45.1X5	T45.1X6
Doxycycline	T36.4X1	T36.4X2	T36.4X3	T36.4X4	T36.4X5	T36.4X6
Doxylamine	T45.0X1	T45.0X2	T45.0X3	T45.0X4	T45.0X5	T45.0X6
Dramamine	T45.0X1	T45.0X2	T45.0X3	T45.0X4	T45.0X5	T45.0X6
Drano (drain cleaner)	T54.3X1	T54.3X2	T54.3X3	T54.3X4	—	—
Dressing, live pulp	T49.7X1	T49.7X2	T49.7X3	T49.7X4	T49.7X5	T49.7X6
Drocode	T40.2X1	T40.2X2	T40.2X3	T40.2X4	T40.2X5	T40.2X6
Dromoran	T40.2X1	T40.2X2	T40.2X3	T40.2X4	T40.2X5	T40.2X6
Dromostanolone	T38.7X1	T38.7X2	T38.7X3	T38.7X4	T38.7X5	T38.7X6
Dronabinol	T40.7X1	T40.7X2	T40.7X3	T40.7X4	T40.7X5	T40.7X6
Droperidol	T43.591	T43.592	T43.593	T43.594	T43.595	T43.596
Dropropizine	T48.3X1	T48.3X2	T48.3X3	T48.3X4	T48.3X5	T48.3X6
Drostanolone	T38.7X1	T38.7X2	T38.7X3	T38.7X4	T38.7X5	T38.7X6
Drotaverine	T44.3X1	T44.3X2	T44.3X3	T44.3X4	T44.3X5	T44.3X6
Drotrecogin alfa	T45.511	T45.512	T45.513	T45.514	T45.515	T45.516
Drug NEC	T50.901	T50.902	T50.903	T50.904	T50.905	T50.906
specified NEC	T50.991	T50.992	T50.993	T50.994	T50.995	T50.996
DTIC	T45.1X1	T45.1X2	T45.1X3	T45.1X4	T45.1X5	T45.1X6
Duboisine	T44.3X1	T44.3X2	T44.3X3	T44.3X4	T44.3X5	T44.3X6
Dulcolax	T47.2X1	T47.2X2	T47.2X3	T47.2X4	T47.2X5	T47.2X6
Duponol (C) (EP)	T49.2X1	T49.2X2	T49.2X3	T49.2X4	T49.2X5	T49.2X6
Durabolin	T38.7X1	T38.7X2	T38.7X3	T38.7X4	T38.7X5	T38.7X6
Dyclone	T41.3X1	T41.3X2	T41.3X3	T41.3X4	T41.3X5	T41.3X6
Dyclonine	T41.3X1	T41.3X2	T41.3X3	T41.3X4	T41.3X5	T41.3X6
Dydrogesterone	T38.5X1	T38.5X2	T38.5X3	T38.5X4	T38.5X5	T38.5X6
Dye NEC	T65.6X1	T65.6X2	T65.6X3	T65.6X4	—	—
antiseptic	T49.0X1	T49.0X2	T49.0X3	T49.0X4	T49.0X5	T49.0X6
diagnostic agents	T50.8X1	T50.8X2	T50.8X3	T50.8X4	T50.8X5	T50.8X6
pharmaceutical NEC	T50.901	T50.902	T50.903	T50.904	T50.905	T50.906
Dyflos	T44.0X1	T44.0X2	T44.0X3	T44.0X4	T44.0X5	T44.0X6
Dymelor	T38.3X1	T38.3X2	T38.3X3	T38.3X4	T38.3X5	T38.3X6

◀ New   ◀▥ Revised   ~~deleted~~ Deleted

Substance	External Cause (T-Code)					
	Poisoning, Accidental (Unintentional)	Poisoning, Intentional Self-Harm	Poisoning, Assault	Poisoning, Undetermined	Adverse Effect	Underdosing
Dynamite	T65.3X1	T65.3X2	T65.3X3	T65.3X4	—	—
fumes	T59.891	T59.892	T59.893	T59.894	—	—
Dyphylline	T44.3X1	T44.3X2	T44.3X3	T44.3X4	T44.3X5	T44.3X6
E						
Ear drug NEC	T49.6X1	T49.6X2	T49.6X3	T49.6X4	T49.6X5	T49.6X6
Ear preparations	T49.6X1	T49.6X2	T49.6X3	T49.6X4	T49.6X5	T49.6X6
Econazole	T49.0X1	T49.0X2	T49.0X3	T49.0X4	T49.0X5	T49.0X6
Ecothiopate iodide	T49.5X1	T49.5X2	T49.5X3	T49.5X4	T49.5X5	T49.5X6
Echothiophate, echothiopate, ecothiopate	T49.5X1	T49.5X2	T49.5X3	T49.5X4	T49.5X5	T49.5X6
Ecstasy	T43.621	T43.622	T43.623	T43.624	T43.625	T43.626
Ectylurea	T42.6X1	T42.6X2	T42.6X3	T42.6X4	T42.6X5	T42.6X6
Edathamil disodium	T45.8X1	T45.8X2	T45.8X3	T45.8X4	T45.8X5	T45.8X6
Edecrin	T50.1X1	T50.1X2	T50.1X3	T50.1X4	T50.1X5	T50.1X6
Edetate, disodium (calcium)	T45.8X1	T45.8X2	T45.8X3	T45.8X4	T45.8X5	T45.8X6
Edoxudine	T49.5X1	T49.5X2	T49.5X3	T49.5X4	T49.5X5	T49.5X6
Edrophonium	T44.0X1	T44.0X2	T44.0X3	T44.0X4	T44.0X5	T44.0X6
chloride	T44.0X1	T44.0X2	T44.0X3	T44.0X4	T44.0X5	T44.0X6
EDTA	T50.6X1	T50.6X2	T50.6X3	T50.6X4	T50.6X5	T50.6X6
Eflornithine	T37.2X1	T37.2X2	T37.2X3	T37.2X4	T37.2X5	T37.2X6
Efloxate	T46.3X1	T46.3X2	T46.3X3	T46.3X4	T46.3X5	T46.3X6
Elase	T49.8X1	T49.8X2	T49.8X3	T49.8X4	T49.8X5	T49.8X6
Elastase	T47.5X1	T47.5X2	T47.5X3	T47.5X4	T47.5X5	T47.5X6
Elaterium	T47.2X1	T47.2X2	T47.2X3	T47.2X4	T47.2X5	T47.2X6
Elcatonin	T50.991	T50.992	T50.993	T50.994	T50.995	T50.996
Elder	T62.2X1	T62.2X2	T62.2X3	T62.2X4	—	—
berry (unripe)	T62.1X1	T62.1X2	T62.1X3	T62.1X4	—	—
Electrolyte balance drug	T50.3X1	T50.3X2	T50.3X3	T50.3X4	T50.3X5	T50.3X6
Electrolytes NEC	T50.3X1	T50.3X2	T50.3X3	T50.3X4	T50.3X5	T50.3X6
Electrolytic agent NEC	T50.3X1	T50.3X2	T50.3X3	T50.3X4	T50.3X5	T50.3X6
Elemental diet	T50.901	T50.902	T50.903	T50.904	T50.905	T50.906
Elliptinium acetate	T45.1X1	T45.1X2	T45.1X3	T45.1X4	T45.1X5	T45.1X6
Embramine	T45.0X1	T45.0X2	T45.0X3	T45.0X4	T45.0X5	T45.0X6
Emepronium (salts)	T44.3X1	T44.3X2	T44.3X3	T44.3X4	T44.3X5	T44.3X6
bromide	T44.3X1	T44.3X2	T44.3X3	T44.3X4	T44.3X5	T44.3X6
Emetic NEC	T47.7X1	T47.7X2	T47.7X3	T47.7X4	T47.7X5	T47.7X6
Emetine	T37.3X1	T37.3X2	T37.3X3	T37.3X4	T37.3X5	T37.3X6
Emollient NEC	T49.3X1	T49.3X2	T49.3X3	T49.3X4	T49.3X5	T49.3X6
Emorfazone	T39.8X1	T39.8X2	T39.8X3	T39.8X4	T39.8X5	T39.8X6

◀ New ◀◀ Revised ~~deleted~~ Deleted

TABLE OF DRUGS AND CHEMICALS

Substance	Poisoning, Accidental (Unintentional)	Poisoning, Intentional Self-Harm	Poisoning, Assault	Poisoning, Undetermined	Adverse Effect	Underdosing
			External Cause (T-Code)			
Emylcamate	T43.591	T43.592	T43.593	T43.594	T43.595	T43.596
Enalapril	T46.4X1	T46.4X2	T46.4X3	T46.4X4	T46.4X5	T46.4X6
Enalaprilat	T46.4X1	T46.4X2	T46.4X3	T46.4X4	T46.4X5	T46.4X6
Encainide	T46.2X1	T46.2X2	T46.2X3	T46.2X4	T46.2X5	T46.2X6
Endocaine	T41.3X1	T41.3X2	T41.3X3	T41.3X4	T41.3X5	T41.3X6
Endosulfan	T60.2X1	T60.2X2	T60.2X3	T60.2X4	—	—
Endothall	T60.3X1	T60.3X2	T60.3X3	T60.3X4	—	—
Endralazine	T46.5X1	T46.5X2	T46.5X3	T46.5X4	T46.5X5	T46.5X6
Endrin	T60.1X1	T60.1X2	T60.1X3	T60.1X4	—	—
Enflurane	T41.0X1	T41.0X2	T41.0X3	T41.0X4	T41.0X5	T41.0X6
Enhexymal	T42.3X1	T42.3X2	T42.3X3	T42.3X4	T42.3X5	T42.3X6
Enocitabine	T45.1X1	T45.1X2	T45.1X3	T45.1X4	T45.1X5	T45.1X6
Enovid	T38.4X1	T38.4X2	T38.4X3	T38.4X4	T38.4X5	T38.4X6
Enoxacin	T36.8X1	T36.8X2	T36.8X3	T36.8X4	T36.8X5	T36.8X6
Enoxaparin (sodium)	T45.511	T45.512	T45.513	T45.514	T45.515	T45.516
Enpiprazole	T43.591	T43.592	T43.593	T43.594	T43.595	T43.596
Enprofylline	T48.6X1	T48.6X2	T48.6X3	T48.6X4	T48.6X5	T48.6X6
Enprostil	T47.1X1	T47.1X2	T47.1X3	T47.1X4	T47.1X5	T47.1X6
ENT preparations (anti-infectives)	T49.6X1	T49.6X2	T49.6X3	T49.6X4	T49.6X5	T49.6X6
Enviomycin	T36.8X1	T36.8X2	T36.8X3	T36.8X4	T36.8X5	T36.8X6
Enzodase	T45.3X1	T45.3X2	T45.3X3	T45.3X4	T45.3X5	T45.3X6
Enzyme NEC	T45.3X1	T45.3X2	T45.3X3	T45.3X4	T45.3X5	T45.3X6
depolymerizing	T49.8X1	T49.8X2	T49.8X3	T49.8X4	T49.8X5	T49.8X6
fibrolytic	T45.3X1	T45.3X2	T45.3X3	T45.3X4	T45.3X5	T45.3X6
gastric	T47.5X1	T47.5X2	T47.5X3	T47.5X4	T47.5X5	T47.5X6
intestinal	T47.5X1	T47.5X2	T47.5X3	T47.5X4	T47.5X5	T47.5X6
local action	T49.4X1	T49.4X2	T49.4X3	T49.4X4	T49.4X5	T49.4X6
proteolytic	T49.4X1	T49.4X2	T49.4X3	T49.4X4	T49.4X5	T49.4X6
thrombolytic	T45.3X1	T45.3X2	T45.3X3	T45.3X4	T45.3X5	T45.3X6
EPAB	T41.3X1	T41.3X2	T41.3X3	T41.3X4	T41.3X5	T41.3X6
Epanutin	T42.0X1	T42.0X2	T42.0X3	T42.0X4	T42.0X5	T42.0X6
Ephedra	T44.991	T44.992	T44.993	T44.994	T44.995	T44.996
Ephedrine	T44.991	T44.992	T44.993	T44.994	T44.995	T44.996
Epichlorhydrin, epichlorohydrin	T52.8X1	T52.8X2	T52.8X3	T52.8X4	—	—
Epicillin	T36.0X1	T36.0X2	T36.0X3	T36.0X4	T36.0X5	T36.0X6
Epiestriol	T38.5X1	T38.5X2	T38.5X3	T38.5X4	T38.5X5	T38.5X6
Epilim — see Sodium valproate						
Epimestrol	T38.5X1	T38.5X2	T38.5X3	T38.5X4	T38.5X5	T38.5X6
Epinephrine	T44.5X1	T44.5X2	T44.5X3	T44.5X4	T44.5X5	T44.5X6

◄ New ◄ Revised ~~deleted~~ Deleted

Substance	Poisoning, Accidental (Unintentional)	Poisoning, Intentional Self-Harm	Poisoning, Assault	Poisoning, Undetermined	Adverse Effect	Underdosing
Epirubicin	T45.1X1	T45.1X2	T45.1X3	T45.1X4	T45.1X5	T45.1X6
Epitiostanol	T38.7X1	T38.7X2	T38.7X3	T38.7X4	T38.7X5	T38.7X6
Epitizide	T50.2X1	T50.2X2	T50.2X3	T50.2X4	T50.2X5	T50.2X6
EPN	T60.0X1	T60.0X2	T60.0X3	T60.0X4	—	—
EPO	T45.8X1	T45.8X2	T45.8X3	T45.8X4	T45.8X5	T45.8X6
Epoetin alpha	T45.8X1	T45.8X2	T45.8X3	T45.8X4	T45.8X5	T45.8X6
Epomediol	T50.991	T50.992	T50.993	T50.994	T50.995	T50.996
Epoprostenol	T45.521	T45.522	T45.523	T45.524	T45.525	T45.526
Epoxy resin	T65.891	T65.892	T65.893	T65.894	—	—
Eprazinone	T48.4X1	T48.4X2	T48.4X3	T48.4X4	T48.4X5	T48.4X6
Epsilon amino-caproic acid	T45.621	T45.622	T45.623	T45.624	T45.625	T45.626
Epsom salt	T47.3X1	T47.3X2	T47.3X3	T47.3X4	T47.3X5	T47.3X6
Eptazocine	T40.4X1	T40.4X2	T40.4X3	T40.4X4	T40.4X5	T40.4X6
Equanil	T43.591	T43.592	T43.593	T43.594	T43.595	T43.596
Equisetum	T62.2X1	T62.2X2	T62.2X3	T62.2X4	—	—
diuretic	T50.2X1	T50.2X2	T50.2X3	T50.2X4	T50.2X5	T50.2X6
Ergobasine	T48.0X1	T48.0X2	T48.0X3	T48.0X4	T48.0X5	T48.0X6
Ergocalciferol	T45.2X1	T45.2X2	T45.2X3	T45.2X4	T45.2X5	T45.2X6
Ergoloid mesylates	T46.7X1	T46.7X2	T46.7X3	T46.7X4	T46.7X5	T46.7X6
Ergometrine	T48.0X1	T48.0X2	T48.0X3	T48.0X4	T48.0X5	T48.0X6
Ergonovine	T48.0X1	T48.0X2	T48.0X3	T48.0X4	T48.0X5	T48.0X6
Ergot NEC	T64.81	T64.82	T64.83	T64.84	—	—
derivative	T48.0X1	T48.0X2	T48.0X3	T48.0X4	T48.0X5	T48.0X6
medicinal (alkaloids)	T48.0X1	T48.0X2	T48.0X3	T48.0X4	T48.0X5	T48.0X6
prepared	T48.0X1	T48.0X2	T48.0X3	T48.0X4	T48.0X5	T48.0X6
Ergotamine	T46.5X1	T46.5X2	T46.5X3	T46.5X4	T46.5X5	T46.5X6
Ergotocine	T48.0X1	T48.0X2	T48.0X3	T48.0X4	T48.0X5	T48.0X6
Ergotrate	T48.0X1	T48.0X2	T48.0X3	T48.0X4	T48.0X5	T48.0X6
Eritrityl tetranitrate	T46.3X1	T46.3X2	T46.3X3	T46.3X4	T46.3X5	T46.3X6
Erythrityl tetranitrate	T46.3X1	T46.3X2	T46.3X3	T46.3X4	T46.3X5	T46.3X6
Erythrol tetranitrate	T46.3X1	T46.3X2	T46.3X3	T46.3X4	T46.3X5	T46.3X6
Erythromycin (salts)	T36.3X1	T36.3X2	T36.3X3	T36.3X4	T36.3X5	T36.3X6
ophthalmic preparation	T49.5X1	T49.5X2	T49.5X3	T49.5X4	T49.5X5	T49.5X6
topical NEC	T49.0X1	T49.0X2	T49.0X3	T49.0X4	T49.0X5	T49.0X6
Erythropoietin	T45.8X1	T45.8X2	T45.8X3	T45.8X4	T45.8X5	T45.8X6
human	T45.8X1	T45.8X2	T45.8X3	T45.8X4	T45.8X5	T45.8X6
Escin	T46.991	T46.992	T46.993	T46.994	T46.995	T46.996
Esculin	T45.2X1	T45.2X2	T45.2X3	T45.2X4	T45.2X5	T45.2X6
Esculoside	T45.2X1	T45.2X2	T45.2X3	T45.2X4	T45.2X5	T45.2X6

◀ New   ◀▦ Revised   ~~deleted~~ Deleted

TABLE OF DRUGS AND CHEMICALS

Substance	External Cause (T-Code)					
	Poisoning, Accidental (Unintentional)	Poisoning, Intentional Self-Harm	Poisoning, Assault	Poisoning, Undetermined	Adverse Effect	Underdosing
ESDT (ether-soluble tar distillate)	T49.1X1	T49.1X2	T49.1X3	T49.1X4	T49.1X5	T49.1X6
Eserine	T49.5X1	T49.5X2	T49.5X3	T49.5X4	T49.5X5	T49.5X6
Esflurbiprofen	T39.311	T39.312	T39.313	T39.314	T39.315	T39.316
Eskabarb	T42.3X1	T42.3X2	T42.3X3	T42.3X4	T42.3X5	T42.3X6
Eskalith	T43.8X1	T43.8X2	T43.8X3	T43.8X4	T43.8X5	T43.8X6
Esmolol	T44.7X1	T44.7X2	T44.7X3	T44.7X4	T44.7X5	T44.7X6
Estanozolol	T38.7X1	T38.7X2	T38.7X3	T38.7X4	T38.7X5	T38.7X6
Estazolam	T42.4X1	T42.4X2	T42.4X3	T42.4X4	T42.4X5	T42.4X6
Estradiol	T38.5X1	T38.5X2	T38.5X3	T38.5X4	T38.5X5	T38.5X6
with testosterone	T38.7X1	T38.7X2	T38.7X3	T38.7X4	T38.7X5	T38.7X6
benzoate	T38.5X1	T38.5X2	T38.5X3	T38.5X4	T38.5X5	T38.5X6
Estramustine	T45.1X1	T45.1X2	T45.1X3	T45.1X4	T45.1X5	T45.1X6
Estriol	T38.5X1	T38.5X2	T38.5X3	T38.5X4	T38.5X5	T38.5X6
Estrogen	T38.5X1	T38.5X2	T38.5X3	T38.5X4	T38.5X5	T38.5X6
with progesterone	T38.5X1	T38.5X2	T38.5X3	T38.5X4	T38.5X5	T38.5X6
conjugated	T38.5X1	T38.5X2	T38.5X3	T38.5X4	T38.5X5	T38.5X6
Estrone	T38.5X1	T38.5X2	T38.5X3	T38.5X4	T38.5X5	T38.5X6
Estropipate	T38.5X1	T38.5X2	T38.5X3	T38.5X4	T38.5X5	T38.5X6
Etacrynate sodium	T50.1X1	T50.1X2	T50.1X3	T50.1X4	T50.1X5	T50.1X6
Etacrynic acid	T50.1X1	T50.1X2	T50.1X3	T50.1X4	T50.1X5	T50.1X6
Etafedrine	T48.6X1	T48.6X2	T48.6X3	T48.6X4	T48.6X5	T48.6X6
Etafenone	T46.3X1	T46.3X2	T46.3X3	T46.3X4	T46.3X5	T46.3X6
Etambutol	T37.1X1	T37.1X2	T37.1X3	T37.1X4	T37.1X5	T37.1X6
Etamiphyllin	T48.6X1	T48.6X2	T48.6X3	T48.6X4	T48.6X5	T48.6X6
Etamivan	T50.7X1	T50.7X2	T50.7X3	T50.7X4	T50.7X5	T50.7X6
Etamsylate	T45.7X1	T45.7X2	T45.7X3	T45.7X4	T45.7X5	T45.7X6
Etebenecid	T50.4X1	T50.4X2	T50.4X3	T50.4X4	T50.4X5	T50.4X6
Ethacridine	T49.0X1	T49.0X2	T49.0X3	T49.0X4	T49.0X5	T49.0X6
Ethacrynic acid	T50.1X1	T50.1X2	T50.1X3	T50.1X4	T50.1X5	T50.1X6
Ethadione	T42.2X1	T42.2X2	T42.2X3	T42.2X4	T42.2X5	T42.2X6
Ethambutol	T37.1X1	T37.1X2	T37.1X3	T37.1X4	T37.1X5	T37.1X6
Ethamide	T50.2X1	T50.2X2	T50.2X3	T50.2X4	T50.2X5	T50.2X6
Ethamivan	T50.7X1	T50.7X2	T50.7X3	T50.7X4	T50.7X5	T50.7X6
Ethamsylate	T45.7X1	T45.7X2	T45.7X3	T45.7X4	T45.7X5	T45.7X6
Ethanol	T51.0X1	T51.0X2	T51.0X3	T51.0X4	—	—
beverage	T51.0X1	T51.0X2	T51.0X3	T51.0X4	—	—
Ethanolamine oleate	T46.8X1	T46.8X2	T46.8X3	T46.8X4	T46.8X5	T46.8X6
Ethaverine	T44.3X1	T44.3X2	T44.3X3	T44.3X4	T44.3X5	T44.3X6
Ethchlorvynol	T42.6X1	T42.6X2	T42.6X3	T42.6X4	T42.6X5	T42.6X6
Ethebenecid	T50.4X1	T50.4X2	T50.4X3	T50.4X4	T50.4X5	T50.4X6

◀ New ◀Ⅲ Revised ~~deleted~~ Deleted

TABLE OF DRUGS AND CHEMICALS

Substance	External Cause (T-Code)					
	Poisoning, Accidental (Unintentional)	Poisoning, Intentional Self-Harm	Poisoning, Assault	Poisoning, Undetermined	Adverse Effect	Underdosing
Ether (vapor)	T41.0X1	T41.0X2	T41.0X3	T41.0X4	T41.0X5	T41.0X6
anesthetic	T41.0X1	T41.0X2	T41.0X3	T41.0X4	T41.0X5	T41.0X6
divinyl	T41.0X1	T41.0X2	T41.0X3	T41.0X4	T41.0X5	T41.0X6
ethyl (medicinal)	T41.0X1	T41.0X2	T41.0X3	T41.0X4	T41.0X5	T41.0X6
nonmedicinal	T52.8X1	T52.8X2	T52.8X3	T52.8X4	—	—
petroleum — see Ligroin						
solvent	T52.8X1	T52.8X2	T52.8X3	T52.8X4	—	—
Ethiazide	T50.2X1	T50.2X2	T50.2X3	T50.2X4	T50.2X5	T50.2X6
Ethidium chloride (vapor)	T59.891	T59.892	T59.893	T59.894	—	—
Ethinamate	T42.6X1	T42.6X2	T42.6X3	T42.6X4	T42.6X5	T42.6X6
Ethinylestradiol, ethinyloestradiol	T38.5X1	T38.5X2	T38.5X3	T38.5X4	T38.5X5	T38.5X6
with						
levonorgestrel	T38.4X1	T38.4X2	T38.4X3	T38.4X4	T38.4X5	T38.4X6
norethisterone	T38.4X1	T38.4X2	T38.4X3	T38.4X4	T38.4X5	T38.4X6
Ethiodized oil (131 I)	T50.8X1	T50.8X2	T50.8X3	T50.8X4	T50.8X5	T50.8X6
Ethion	T60.0X1	T60.0X2	T60.0X3	T60.0X4	—	—
Ethionamide	T37.1X1	T37.1X2	T37.1X3	T37.1X4	T37.1X5	T37.1X6
Ethioniamide	T37.1X1	T37.1X2	T37.1X3	T37.1X4	T37.1X5	T37.1X6
Ethisterone	T38.5X1	T38.5X2	T38.5X3	T38.5X4	T38.5X5	T38.5X6
Ethobral	T42.3X1	T42.3X2	T42.3X3	T42.3X4	T42.3X5	T42.3X6
Ethocaine (infiltration) (topical)	T41.3X1	T41.3X2	T41.3X3	T41.3X4	T41.3X5	T41.3X6
nerve block (peripheral) (plexus)	T41.3X1	T41.3X2	T41.3X3	T41.3X4	T41.3X5	T41.3X6
spinal	T41.3X1	T41.3X2	T41.3X3	T41.3X4	T41.3X5	T41.3X6
Ethoheptazine	T40.4X1	T40.4X2	T40.4X3	T40.4X4	T40.4X5	T40.4X6
Ethopropazine	T44.3X1	T44.3X2	T44.3X3	T44.3X4	T44.3X5	T44.3X6
Ethosuximide	T42.2X1	T42.2X2	T42.2X3	T42.2X4	T42.2X5	T42.2X6
Ethotoin	T42.0X1	T42.0X2	T42.0X3	T42.0X4	T42.0X5	T42.0X6
Ethoxazene	T37.91	T37.92	T37.93	T37.94	T37.95	T37.96
Ethoxazorutoside	T46.991	T46.992	T46.993	T46.994	T46.995	T46.996
2-Ethoxyethanol	T52.3X1	T52.3X2	T52.3X3	T52.3X4	—	—
Ethoxzolamide	T50.2X1	T50.2X2	T50.2X3	T50.2X4	T50.2X5	T50.2X6
Ethyl						
acetate	T52.8X1	T52.8X2	T52.8X3	T52.8X4	—	—
alcohol	T51.0X1	T51.0X2	T51.0X3	T51.0X4	—	—
beverage	T51.0X1	T51.0X2	T51.0X3	T51.0X4	—	—
aldehyde (vapor)	T59.891	T59.892	T59.893	T59.894	—	—
liquid	T52.8X1	T52.8X2	T52.8X3	T52.8X4	—	—
aminobenzoate	T41.3X1	T41.3X2	T41.3X3	T41.3X4	T41.3X5	T41.3X6
aminophenothiazine	T43.3X1	T43.3X2	T43.3X3	T43.3X4	T43.3X5	T43.3X6
benzoate	T52.8X1	T52.8X2	T52.8X3	T52.8X4		

TABLE OF DRUGS AND CHEMICALS

Substance	Poisoning, Accidental (Unintentional)	Poisoning, Intentional Self-Harm	Poisoning, Assault	Poisoning, Undetermined	Adverse Effect	Underdosing
External Cause (T-Code)						
Ethyl *(Continued)*						
biscoumacetate	T45.511	T45.512	T45.513	T45.514	T45.515	T45.516
bromide (anesthetic)	T41.0X1	T41.0X2	T41.0X3	T41.0X4	T41.0X5	T41.0X6
carbamate	T45.1X1	T45.1X2	T45.1X3	T45.1X4	T45.1X5	T45.1X6
carbinol	T51.3X1	T51.3X2	T51.3X3	T51.3X4	—	—
carbonate	T52.8X1	T52.8X2	T52.8X3	T52.8X4	—	—
chaulmoograte	T37.1X1	T37.1X2	T37.1X3	T37.1X4	T37.1X5	T37.1X6
chloride (anesthetic)	T41.0X1	T41.0X2	T41.0X3	T41.0X4	T41.0X5	T41.0X6
anesthetic (local)	T41.3X1	T41.3X2	T41.3X3	T41.3X4	T41.3X5	T41.3X6
inhaled	T41.0X1	T41.0X2	T41.0X3	T41.0X4	T41.0X5	T41.0X6
local	T49.4X1	T49.4X2	T49.4X3	T49.4X4	T49.4X5	T49.4X6
solvent	T53.6X1	T53.6X2	T53.6X3	T53.6X4	—	—
dibunate	T48.3X1	T48.3X2	T48.3X3	T48.3X4	T48.3X5	T48.3X6
dichloroarsine (vapor)	T57.0X1	T57.0X2	T57.0X3	T57.0X4	—	—
estranol	T38.7X1	T38.7X2	T38.7X3	T38.7X4	T38.7X5	T38.7X6
ether — *see also ether*	T52.8X1	T52.8X2	T52.8X3	T52.8X4	—	—
formate NEC (solvent)	T52.0X1	T52.0X2	T52.0X3	T52.0X4	—	—
fumarate	T49.4X1	T49.4X2	T49.4X3	T49.4X4	T49.4X5	T49.4X6
hydroxyisobutyrate NEC (solvent)	T52.8X1	T52.8X2	T52.8X3	T52.8X4	—	—
iodoacetate	T59.3X1	T59.3X2	T59.3X3	T59.3X4	—	—
lactate NEC (solvent)	T52.8X1	T52.8X2	T52.8X3	T52.8X4	—	—
loflazepate	T42.4X1	T42.4X2	T42.4X3	T42.4X4	T42.4X5	T42.4X6
mercuric chloride	T56.1X1	T56.1X2	T56.1X3	T56.1X4	—	—
methylcarbinol	T51.8X1	T51.8X2	T51.8X3	T51.8X4	—	—
morphine	T40.2X1	T40.2X2	T40.2X3	T40.2X4	T40.2X5	T40.2X6
noradrenaline	T48.6X1	T48.6X2	T48.6X3	T48.6X4	T48.6X5	T48.6X6
oxybutyrate NEC (solvent)	T52.8X1	T52.8X2	T52.8X3	T52.8X4	—	—
Ethylene (gas)	T59.891	T59.892	T59.893	T59.894	—	—
anesthetic (general)	T41.0X1	T41.0X2	T41.0X3	T41.0X4	T41.0X5	T41.0X6
chlorohydrin	T52.8X1	T52.8X2	T52.8X3	T52.8X4	—	—
vapor	T53.6X1	T53.6X2	T53.6X3	T53.6X4	—	—
dichloride	T52.8X1	T52.8X2	T52.8X3	T52.8X4	—	—
vapor	T53.6X1	T53.6X2	T53.6X3	T53.6X4	—	—
dinitrate	T52.3X1	T52.3X2	T52.3X3	T52.3X4	—	—
glycol(s)	T52.8X1	T52.8X2	T52.8X3	T52.8X4	—	—
dinitrate	T52.3X1	T52.3X2	T52.3X3	T52.3X4	—	—
monobutyl ether	T52.3X1	T52.3X2	T52.3X3	T52.3X4	—	—
imine	T54.1X1	T54.1X2	T54.1X3	T54.1X4	—	—
oxide (fumigant) (nonmedicinal)	T59.891	T59.892	T59.893	T59.894	—	—
medicinal	T49.0X1	T49.0X2	T49.0X3	T49.0X4	T49.0X5	T49.0X6

◀ New　◀ Revised　~~deleted~~ Deleted

Substance	External Cause (T-Code)					
	Poisoning, Accidental (Unintentional)	Poisoning, Intentional Self-Harm	Poisoning, Assault	Poisoning, Undetermined	Adverse Effect	Underdosing
Ethylenediamine theophylline	T48.6X1	T48.6X2	T48.6X3	T48.6X4	T48.6X5	T48.6X6
Ethylenediaminetetra-acetic acid	T50.6X1	T50.6X2	T50.6X3	T50.6X4	T50.6X5	T50.6X6
Ethylenedinitrilotetra-acetate	T50.6X1	T50.6X2	T50.6X3	T50.6X4	T50.6X5	T50.6X6
Ethylestrenol	T38.7X1	T38.7X2	T38.7X3	T38.7X4	T38.7X5	T38.7X6
Ethylhydroxycellulose	T47.4X1	T47.4X2	T47.4X3	T47.4X4	T47.4X5	T47.4X6
Ethylidene						
chloride NEC	T53.6X1	T53.6X2	T53.6X3	T53.6X4	—	—
diacetate	T60.3X1	T60.3X2	T60.3X3	T60.3X4	—	—
dicoumarin	T45.511	T45.512	T45.513	T45.514	T45.515	T45.516
dicoumarol	T45.511	T45.512	T45.513	T45.514	T45.515	T45.516
diethyl ether	T52.0X1	T52.0X2	T52.0X3	T52.0X4	—	—
Ethylmorphine	T40.2X1	T40.2X2	T40.2X3	T40.2X4	T40.2X5	T40.2X6
Ethylnorepinephrine	T48.6X1	T48.6X2	T48.6X3	T48.6X4	T48.6X5	T48.6X6
Ethylparachlorophen-oxyisobutyrate	T46.6X1	T46.6X2	T46.6X3	T46.6X4	T46.6X5	T46.6X6
Ethynodiol	T38.4X1	T38.4X2	T38.4X3	T38.4X4	T38.4X5	T38.4X6
with mestranol diacetate	T38.4X1	T38.4X2	T38.4X3	T38.4X4	T38.4X5	T38.4X6
Etidocaine	T41.3X1	T41.3X2	T41.3X3	T41.3X4	T41.3X5	T41.3X6
infiltration (subcutaneous)	T41.3X1	T41.3X2	T41.3X3	T41.3X4	T41.3X5	T41.3X6
nerve (peripheral) (plexus)	T41.3X1	T41.3X2	T41.3X3	T41.3X4	T41.3X5	T41.3X6
Etidronate	T50.991	T50.992	T50.993	T50.994	T50.995	T50.996
Etidronic acid (disodium salt)	T50.991	T50.992	T50.993	T50.994	T50.995	T50.996
Etifoxine	T42.6X1	T42.6X2	T42.6X3	T42.6X4	T42.6X5	T42.6X6
Etilefrine	T44.4X1	T44.4X2	T44.4X3	T44.4X4	T44.4X5	T44.4X6
Etilfen	T42.3X1	T42.3X2	T42.3X3	T42.3X4	T42.3X5	T42.3X6
Etinodiol	T38.4X1	T38.4X2	T38.4X3	T38.4X4	T38.4X5	T38.4X6
Etiroxate	T46.6X1	T46.6X2	T46.6X3	T46.6X4	T46.6X5	T46.6X6
Etizolam	T42.4X1	T42.4X2	T42.4X3	T42.4X4	T42.4X5	T42.4X6
Etodolac	T39.391	T39.392	T39.393	T39.394	T39.395	T39.396
Etofamide	T37.3X1	T37.3X2	T37.3X3	T37.3X4	T37.3X5	T37.3X6
Etofibrate	T46.6X1	T46.6X2	T46.6X3	T46.6X4	T46.6X5	T46.6X6
Etofylline	T46.7X1	T46.7X2	T46.7X3	T46.7X4	T46.7X5	T46.7X6
clofibrate	T46.6X1	T46.6X2	T46.6X3	T46.6X4	T46.6X5	T46.6X6
Etoglucid	T45.1X1	T45.1X2	T45.1X3	T45.1X4	T45.1X5	T45.1X6
Etomidate	T41.1X1	T41.1X2	T41.1X3	T41.1X4	T41.1X5	T41.1X6
Etomide	T39.8X1	T39.8X2	T39.8X3	T39.8X4	T39.8X5	T39.8X6
Etomidoline	T44.3X1	T44.3X2	T44.3X3	T44.3X4	T44.3X5	T44.3X6
Etoposide	T45.1X1	T45.1X2	T45.1X3	T45.1X4	T45.1X5	T45.1X6
Etorphine	T40.2X1	T40.2X2	T40.2X3	T40.2X4	T40.2X5	T40.2X6
Etoval	T42.3X1	T42.3X2	T42.3X3	T42.3X4	T42.3X5	T42.3X6
Etozolin	T50.1X1	T50.1X2	T50.1X3	T50.1X4	T50.1X5	T50.1X6

◀ New　◀▥ Revised　~~deleted~~ Deleted

Substance	External Cause (T-Code)					
	Poisoning, Accidental (Unintentional)	Poisoning, Intentional Self-Harm	Poisoning, Assault	Poisoning, Undetermined	Adverse Effect	Underdosing
Etretinate	T50.991	T50.992	T50.993	T50.994	T50.995	T50.996
Etryptamine	T43.691	T43.692	T43.693	T43.694	T43.695	T43.696
Etybenzatropine	T44.3X1	T44.3X2	T44.3X3	T44.3X4	T44.3X5	T44.3X6
Etynodiol	T38.4X1	T38.4X2	T38.4X3	T38.4X4	T38.4X5	T38.4X6
Eucaine	T41.3X1	T41.3X2	T41.3X3	T41.3X4	T41.3X5	T41.3X6
Eucalyptus oil	T49.7X1	T49.7X2	T49.7X3	T49.7X4	T49.7X5	T49.7X6
Eucatropine	T49.5X1	T49.5X2	T49.5X3	T49.5X4	T49.5X5	T49.5X6
Eucodal	T40.2X1	T40.2X2	T40.2X3	T40.2X4	T40.2X5	T40.2X6
Euneryl	T42.3X1	T42.3X2	T42.3X3	T42.3X4	T42.3X5	T42.3X6
Euphthalmine	T44.3X1	T44.3X2	T44.3X3	T44.3X4	T44.3X5	T44.3X6
Eurax	T49.0X1	T49.0X2	T49.0X3	T49.0X4	T49.0X5	T49.0X6
Euresol	T49.4X1	T49.4X2	T49.4X3	T49.4X4	T49.4X5	T49.4X6
Euthroid	T38.1X1	T38.1X2	T38.1X3	T38.1X4	T38.1X5	T38.1X6
Evans blue	T50.8X1	T50.8X2	T50.8X3	T50.8X4	T50.8X5	T50.8X6
Evipal	T42.3X1	T42.3X2	T42.3X3	T42.3X4	T42.3X5	T42.3X6
sodium	T41.1X1	T41.1X2	T41.1X3	T41.1X4	T41.1X5	T41.1X6
Evipan	T42.3X1	T42.3X2	T42.3X3	T42.3X4	T42.3X5	T42.3X6
sodium	T41.1X1	T41.1X2	T41.1X3	T41.1X4	T41.1X5	T41.1X6
Exalamide	T49.0X1	T49.0X2	T49.0X3	T49.0X4	T49.0X5	T49.0X6
Exalgin	T39.1X1	T39.1X2	T39.1X3	T39.1X4	T39.1X5	T39.1X6
Excipients, pharmaceutical	T50.901	T50.902	T50.903	T50.904	T50.905	T50.906
Exhaust gas (engine) (motor vehicle)	T58.01	T58.02	T58.03	T58.04	—	—
Ex-Lax (phenolphthalein)	T47.2X1	T47.2X2	T47.2X3	T47.2X4	T47.2X5	T47.2X6
Expectorant NEC	T48.4X1	T48.4X2	T48.4X3	T48.4X4	T48.4X5	T48.4X6
Extended insulin zinc suspension	T38.3X1	T38.3X2	T38.3X3	T38.3X4	T38.3X5	T38.3X6
External medications (skin) (mucous membrane)	T49.91	T49.92	T49.93	T49.94	T49.95	T49.96
dental agent	T49.7X1	T49.7X2	T49.7X3	T49.7X4	T49.7X5	T49.7X6
ENT agent	T49.6X1	T49.6X2	T49.6X3	T49.6X4	T49.6X5	T49.6X6
ophthalmic preparation	T49.5X1	T49.5X2	T49.5X3	T49.5X4	T49.5X5	T49.5X6
specified NEC	T49.8X1	T49.8X2	T49.8X3	T49.8X4	T49.8X5	T49.8X6
Extrapyramidal antagonist NEC	T44.3X1	T44.3X2	T44.3X3	T44.3X4	T44.3X5	T44.3X6
Eye agents (anti-infective)	T49.5X1	T49.5X2	T49.5X3	T49.5X4	T49.5X5	T49.5X6
Eye drug NEC	T49.5X1	T49.5X2	T49.5X3	T49.5X4	T49.5X5	T49.5X6
F						
FAC (fluorouracil + doxorubicin + cyclophosphamide)	T45.1X1	T45.1X2	T45.1X3	T45.1X4	T45.1X5	T45.1X6
Factor						
I (fibrinogen)	T45.8X1	T45.8X2	T45.8X3	T45.8X4	T45.8X5	T45.8X6
III (thromboplastin)	T45.8X1	T45.8X2	T45.8X3	T45.8X4	T45.8X5	T45.8X6
VIII (antihemophilic Factor) (Concentrate)	T45.8X1	T45.8X2	T45.8X3	T45.8X4	T45.8X5	T45.8X6

◀ New　◀▥ Revised　~~deleted~~ Deleted

Substance	Poisoning, Accidental (Unintentional)	Poisoning, Intentional Self-Harm	Poisoning, Assault	Poisoning, Undetermined	Adverse Effect	Underdosing
Factor *(Continued)*						
IX complex	T45.7X1	T45.7X2	T45.7X3	T45.7X4	T45.7X5	T45.7X6
human	T45.8X1	T45.8X2	T45.8X3	T45.8X4	T45.8X5	T45.8X6
Famotidine	T47.0X1	T47.0X2	T47.0X3	T47.0X4	T47.0X5	T47.0X6
Fat suspension, intravenous	T50.991	T50.992	T50.993	T50.994	T50.995	T50.996
Fazadinium bromide	T48.1X1	T48.1X2	T48.1X3	T48.1X4	T48.1X5	T48.1X6
Febarbamate	T42.3X1	T42.3X2	T42.3X3	T42.3X4	T42.3X5	T42.3X6
Fecal softener	T47.4X1	T47.4X2	T47.4X3	T47.4X4	T47.4X5	T47.4X6
Fedrilate	T48.3X1	T48.3X2	T48.3X3	T48.3X4	T48.3X5	T48.3X6
Felodipine	T46.1X1	T46.1X2	T46.1X3	T46.1X4	T46.1X5	T46.1X6
Felypressin	T38.891	T38.892	T38.893	T38.894	T38.895	T38.896
Femoxetine	T43.221	T43.222	T43.223	T43.224	T43.225	T43.226
Fenalcomine	T46.3X1	T46.3X2	T46.3X3	T46.3X4	T46.3X5	T46.3X6
Fenamisal	T37.1X1	T37.1X2	T37.1X3	T37.1X4	T37.1X5	T37.1X6
Fenazone	T39.2X1	T39.2X2	T39.2X3	T39.2X4	T39.2X5	T39.2X6
Fenbendazole	T37.4X1	T37.4X2	T37.4X3	T37.4X4	T37.4X5	T37.4X6
Fenbutrazate	T50.5X1	T50.5X2	T50.5X3	T50.5X4	T50.5X5	T50.5X6
Fencamfamine	T43.691	T43.692	T43.693	T43.694	T43.695	T43.696
Fendiline	T46.1X1	T46.1X2	T46.1X3	T46.1X4	T46.1X5	T46.1X6
Fenetylline	T43.691	T43.692	T43.693	T43.694	T43.695	T43.696
Fenflumizole	T39.391	T39.392	T39.393	T39.394	T39.395	T39.396
Fenfluramine	T50.5X1	T50.5X2	T50.5X3	T50.5X4	T50.5X5	T50.5X6
Fenobarbital	T42.3X1	T42.3X2	T42.3X3	T42.3X4	T42.3X5	T42.3X6
Fenofibrate	T46.6X1	T46.6X2	T46.6X3	T46.6X4	T46.6X5	T46.6X6
Fenoprofen	T39.311	T39.312	T39.313	T39.314	T39.315	T39.316
Fenoterol	T48.6X1	T48.6X2	T48.6X3	T48.6X4	T48.6X5	T48.6X6
Fenoverine	T44.3X1	T44.3X2	T44.3X3	T44.3X4	T44.3X5	T44.3X6
Fenoxazoline	T48.5X1	T48.5X2	T48.5X3	T48.5X4	T48.5X5	T48.5X6
Fenproporex	T50.5X1	T50.5X2	T50.5X3	T50.5X4	T50.5X5	T50.5X6
Fenquizone	T50.2X1	T50.2X2	T50.2X3	T50.2X4	T50.2X5	T50.2X6
Fentanyl	T40.4X1	T40.4X2	T40.4X3	T40.4X4	T40.4X5	T40.4X6
Fentazin	T43.3X1	T43.3X2	T43.3X3	T43.3X4	T43.3X5	T43.3X6
Fenthion	T60.0X1	T60.0X2	T60.0X3	T60.0X4	—	—
Fenticlor	T49.0X1	T49.0X2	T49.0X3	T49.0X4	T49.0X5	T49.0X6
Fenylbutazone	T39.2X1	T39.2X2	T39.2X3	T39.2X4	T39.2X5	T39.2X6
Feprazone	T39.2X1	T39.2X2	T39.2X3	T39.2X4	T39.2X5	T39.2X6
Fer de lance (bite) (venom)	T63.061	T63.062	T63.063	T63.064	—	—
Ferric — *see also Iron*						
chloride	T45.4X1	T45.4X2	T45.4X3	T45.4X4	T45.4X5	T45.4X6
citrate	T45.4X1	T45.4X2	T45.4X3	T45.4X4	T45.4X5	T45.4X6

Substance	External Cause (T-Code)					
	Poisoning, Accidental (Unintentional)	Poisoning, Intentional Self-Harm	Poisoning, Assault	Poisoning, Undetermined	Adverse Effect	Underdosing
Ferric *(Continued)*						
hydroxide						
colloidal	T45.4X1	T45.4X2	T45.4X3	T45.4X4	T45.4X5	T45.4X6
polymaltose	T45.4X1	T45.4X2	T45.4X3	T45.4X4	T45.4X5	T45.4X6
pyrophosphate	T45.4X1	T45.4X2	T45.4X3	T45.4X4	T45.4X5	T45.4X6
Ferritin	T45.4X1	T45.4X2	T45.4X3	T45.4X4	T45.4X5	T45.4X6
Ferrocholinate	T45.4X1	T45.4X2	T45.4X3	T45.4X4	T45.4X5	T45.4X6
Ferrodextrane	T45.4X1	T45.4X2	T45.4X3	T45.4X4	T45.4X5	T45.4X6
Ferropolimaler	T45.4X1	T45.4X2	T45.4X3	T45.4X4	T45.4X5	T45.4X6
Ferrous— *see also Iron*						
phosphate	T45.4X1	T45.4X2	T45.4X3	T45.4X4	T45.4X5	T45.4X6
salt	T45.4X1	T45.4X2	T45.4X3	T45.4X4	T45.4X5	T45.4X6
with folic acid	T45.4X1	T45.4X2	T45.4X3	T45.4X4	T45.4X5	T45.4X6
Ferrous fumerate, gluconate, lactate, salt NEC, sulfate (medicinal)	T45.4X1	T45.4X2	T45.4X3	T45.4X4	T45.4X5	T45.4X6
Ferrovanadium (fumes)	T59.891	T59.892	T59.893	T59.894	—	—
Ferrum— *see Iron*						
Fertilizers NEC	T65.891	T65.892	T65.893	T65.894	—	—
with herbicide mixture	T60.3X1	T60.3X2	T60.3X3	T60.3X4	—	—
Fetoxilate	T47.6X1	T47.6X2	T47.6X3	T47.6X4	T47.6X5	T47.6X6
Fiber, dietary	T47.4X1	T47.4X2	T47.4X3	T47.4X4	T47.4X5	T47.4X6
Fibrinogen (human)	T45.8X1	T45.8X2	T45.8X3	T45.8X4	T45.8X5	T45.8X6
Fibrinolysin (human)	T45.691	T45.692	T45.693	T45.694	T45.695	T45.696
Fibrinolysis						
affecting drug	T45.601	T45.602	T45.603	T45.604	T45.605	T45.606
inhibitor NEC	T45.621	T45.622	T45.623	T45.624	T45.625	T45.626
Fibrinolytic drug	T45.611	T45.612	T45.613	T45.614	T45.615	T45.616
Filix mas	T37.4X1	T37.4X2	T37.4X3	T37.4X4	T37.4X5	T37.4X6
Filtering cream	T49.3X1	T49.3X2	T49.3X3	T49.3X4	T49.3X5	T49.3X6
Fiorinal	T39.011	T39.012	T39.013	T39.014	T39.015	T39.016
Firedamp	T59.891	T59.892	T59.893	T59.894	—	—
Fish, noxious, nonbacterial	T61.91	T61.92	T61.93	T61.94	—	—
ciguatera	T61.01	T61.02	T61.03	T61.04	—	—
scombroid	T61.11	T61.12	T61.13	T61.14	—	—
shell	T61.781	T61.782	T61.783	T61.784	—	—
specified NEC	T61.771	T61.772	T61.773	T61.774	—	—
Flagyl	T37.3X1	T37.3X2	T37.3X3	T37.3X4	T37.3X5	T37.3X6
Flavine adenine dinucleotide	T45.2X1	T45.2X2	T45.2X3	T45.2X4	T45.2X5	T45.2X6
Flavodic acid	T46.991	T46.992	T46.993	T46.994	T46.995	T46.996
Flavoxate	T44.3X1	T44.3X2	T44.3X3	T44.3X4	T44.3X5	T44.3X6

◀ New   ◀▥ Revised   ~~deleted~~ Deleted

Substance	External Cause (T-Code)					
	Poisoning, Accidental (Unintentional)	Poisoning, Intentional Self-Harm	Poisoning, Assault	Poisoning, Undetermined	Adverse Effect	Underdosing
Flaxedil	T48.1X1	T48.1X2	T48.1X3	T48.1X4	T48.1X5	T48.1X6
Flaxseed (medicinal)	T49.3X1	T49.3X2	T49.3X3	T49.3X4	T49.3X5	T49.3X6
Flecainide	T46.2X1	T46.2X2	T46.2X3	T46.2X4	T46.2X5	T46.2X6
Fleroxacin	T36.8X1	T36.8X2	T36.8X3	T36.8X4	T36.8X5	T36.8X6
Floctafenine	T39.8X1	T39.8X2	T39.8X3	T39.8X4	T39.8X5	T39.8X6
Flomax	T44.6X1	T44.6X2	T44.6X3	T44.6X4	T44.6X5	T44.6X6
Flomoxef	T36.1X1	T36.1X2	T36.1X3	T36.1X4	T36.1X5	T36.1X6
Flopropione	T44.3X1	T44.3X2	T44.3X3	T44.3X4	T44.3X5	T44.3X6
Florantyrone	T47.5X1	T47.5X2	T47.5X3	T47.5X4	T47.5X5	T47.5X6
Floraquin	T37.8X1	T37.8X2	T37.8X3	T37.8X4	T37.8X5	T37.8X6
Florinef	T38.0X1	T38.0X2	T38.0X3	T38.0X4	T38.0X5	T38.0X6
ENT agent	T49.6X1	T49.6X2	T49.6X3	T49.6X4	T49.6X5	T49.6X6
ophthalmic preparation	T49.5X1	T49.5X2	T49.5X3	T49.5X4	T49.5X5	T49.5X6
topical NEC	T49.0X1	T49.0X2	T49.0X3	T49.0X4	T49.0X5	T49.0X6
Flowers of sulfur	T49.4X1	T49.4X2	T49.4X3	T49.4X4	T49.4X5	T49.4X6
Floxuridine	T45.1X1	T45.1X2	T45.1X3	T45.1X4	T45.1X5	T45.1X6
Fluanisone	T43.4X1	T43.4X2	T43.4X3	T43.4X4	T43.4X5	T43.4X6
Flubendazole	T37.4X1	T37.4X2	T37.4X3	T37.4X4	T37.4X5	T37.4X6
Fluclorolone acetonide	T49.0X1	T49.0X2	T49.0X3	T49.0X4	T49.0X5	T49.0X6
Flucloxacillin	T36.0X1	T36.0X2	T36.0X3	T36.0X4	T36.0X5	T36.0X6
Fluconazole	T37.8X1	T37.8X2	T37.8X3	T37.8X4	T37.8X5	T37.8X6
Flucytosine	T37.8X1	T37.8X2	T37.8X3	T37.8X4	T37.8X5	T37.8X6
Fludeoxyglucose (18F)	T50.8X1	T50.8X2	T50.8X3	T50.8X4	T50.8X5	T50.8X6
Fludiazepam	T42.4X1	T42.4X2	T42.4X3	T42.4X4	T42.4X5	T42.4X6
Fludrocortisone	T50.0X1	T50.0X2	T50.0X3	T50.0X4	T50.0X5	T50.0X6
ENT agent	T49.6X1	T49.6X2	T49.6X3	T49.6X4	T49.6X5	T49.6X6
ophthalmic preparation	T49.5X1	T49.5X2	T49.5X3	T49.5X4	T49.5X5	T49.5X6
topical NEC	T49.0X1	T49.0X2	T49.0X3	T49.0X4	T49.0X5	T49.0X6
Fludroxycortide	T49.0X1	T49.0X2	T49.0X3	T49.0X4	T49.0X5	T49.0X6
Flufenamic acid	T39.391	T39.392	T39.393	T39.394	T39.395	T39.396
Fluindione	T45.511	T45.512	T45.513	T45.514	T45.515	T45.516
Flumequine	T37.8X1	T37.8X2	T37.8X3	T37.8X4	T37.8X5	T37.8X6
Flumethasone	T49.0X1	T49.0X2	T49.0X3	T49.0X4	T49.0X5	T49.0X6
Flumethiazide	T50.2X1	T50.2X2	T50.2X3	T50.2X4	T50.2X5	T50.2X6
Flumidin	T37.5X1	T37.5X2	T37.5X3	T37.5X4	T37.5X5	T37.5X6
Flunarizine	T46.7X1	T46.7X2	T46.7X3	T46.7X4	T46.7X5	T46.7X6
Flunidazole	T37.8X1	T37.8X2	T37.8X3	T37.8X4	T37.8X5	T37.8X6
Flunisolide	T48.6X1	T48.6X2	T48.6X3	T48.6X4	T48.6X5	T48.6X6
Flunitrazepam	T42.4X1	T42.4X2	T42.4X3	T42.4X4	T42.4X5	T42.4X6

Substance	External Cause (T-Code)					
	Poisoning, Accidental (Unintentional)	Poisoning, Intentional Self-Harm	Poisoning, Assault	Poisoning, Undetermined	Adverse Effect	Underdosing
Fluocinolone (acetonide)	T49.0X1	T49.0X2	T49.0X3	T49.0X4	T49.0X5	T49.0X6
Fluocinonide	T49.0X1	T49.0X2	T49.0X3	T49.0X4	T49.0X5	T49.0X6
Fluocortin (butyl)	T49.0X1	T49.0X2	T49.0X3	T49.0X4	T49.0X5	T49.0X6
Fluocortolone	T49.0X1	T49.0X2	T49.0X3	T49.0X4	T49.0X5	T49.0X6
Fluohydrocortisone	T38.0X1	T38.0X2	T38.0X3	T38.0X4	T38.0X5	T38.0X6
ENT agent	T49.6X1	T49.6X2	T49.6X3	T49.6X4	T49.6X5	T49.6X6
ophthalmic preparation	T49.5X1	T49.5X2	T49.5X3	T49.5X4	T49.5X5	T49.5X6
topical NEC	T49.0X1	T49.0X2	T49.0X3	T49.0X4	T49.0X5	T49.0X6
Fluonid	T49.0X1	T49.0X2	T49.0X3	T49.0X4	T49.0X5	T49.0X6
Fluopromazine	T43.3X1	T43.3X2	T43.3X3	T43.3X4	T43.3X5	T43.3X6
Fluoroacetate	T60.8X1	T60.8X2	T60.8X3	T60.8X4	—	—
Fluorescein	T50.8X1	T50.8X2	T50.8X3	T50.8X4	T50.8X5	T50.8X6
Fluorhydrocortisone	T50.0X1	T50.0X2	T50.0X3	T50.0X4	T50.0X5	T50.0X6
Fluoride (nonmedicinal) (pesticide) (sodium) NEC	T60.8X1	T60.8X2	T60.8X3	T60.8X4	—	—
hydrogen — see Hydrofluoric acid						
medicinal NEC	T50.991	T50.992	T50.993	T50.994	T50.995	T50.996
dental use	T49.7X1	T49.7X2	T49.7X3	T49.7X4	T49.7X5	T49.7X6
not pesticide NEC	T54.91	T54.92	T54.93	T54.94	—	—
stannous	T49.7X1	T49.7X2	T49.7X3	T49.7X4	T49.7X5	T49.7X6
Fluorinated corticosteroids	T38.0X1	T38.0X2	T38.0X3	T38.0X4	T38.0X5	T38.0X6
Fluorine (gas)	T59.5X1	T59.5X2	T59.5X3	T59.5X4	—	—
salt — see Fluoride(s)						
Fluoristan	T49.7X1	T49.7X2	T49.7X3	T49.7X4	T49.7X5	T49.7X6
Fluormetholone	T49.0X1	T49.0X2	T49.0X3	T49.0X4	T49.0X5	T49.0X6
Fluoroacetate	T60.8X1	T60.8X2	T60.8X3	T60.8X4	—	—
Fluorocarbon monomer	T53.6X1	T53.6X2	T53.6X3	T53.6X4	—	—
Fluorocytosine	T37.8X1	T37.8X2	T37.8X3	T37.8X4	T37.8X5	T37.8X6
Fluorodeoxyuridine	T45.1X1	T45.1X2	T45.1X3	T45.1X4	T45.1X5	T45.1X6
Fluorometholone	T49.0X1	T49.0X2	T49.0X3	T49.0X4	T49.0X5	T49.0X6
ophthalmic preparation	T49.5X1	T49.5X2	T49.5X3	T49.5X4	T49.5X5	T49.5X6
Fluorophosphate insecticide	T60.0X1	T60.0X2	T60.0X3	T60.0X4	—	—
Fluorosol	T46.3X1	T46.3X2	T46.3X3	T46.3X4	T46.3X5	T46.3X6
Fluorouracil	T45.1X1	T45.1X2	T45.1X3	T45.1X4	T45.1X5	T45.1X6
Fluorphenylalanine	T49.5X1	T49.5X2	T49.5X3	T49.5X4	T49.5X5	T49.5X6
Fluothane	T41.0X1	T41.0X2	T41.0X3	T41.0X4	T41.0X5	T41.0X6
Fluoxetine	T43.221	T43.222	T43.223	T43.224	T43.225	T43.226
Fluoxymesterone	T38.7X1	T38.7X2	T38.7X3	T38.7X4	T38.7X5	T38.7X6
Flupenthixol	T43.4X1	T43.4X2	T43.4X3	T43.4X4	T43.4X5	T43.4X6
Flupentixol	T43.4X1	T43.4X2	T43.4X3	T43.4X4	T43.4X5	T43.4X6
Fluphenazine	T43.3X1	T43.3X2	T43.3X3	T43.3X4	T43.3X5	T43.3X6

◀ New   ◀ Revised   ~~deleted~~ Deleted

Substance	External Cause (T-Code)					
	Poisoning, Accidental (Unintentional)	Poisoning, Intentional Self-Harm	Poisoning, Assault	Poisoning, Undetermined	Adverse Effect	Underdosing
Fluprednidene	T49.0X1	T49.0X2	T49.0X3	T49.0X4	T49.0X5	T49.0X6
Fluprednisolone	T38.0X1	T38.0X2	T38.0X3	T38.0X4	T38.0X5	T38.0X6
Fluradoline	T39.8X1	T39.8X2	T39.8X3	T39.8X4	T39.8X5	T39.8X6
Flurandrenolide	T49.0X1	T49.0X2	T49.0X3	T49.0X4	T49.0X5	T49.0X6
Flurandrenolone	T49.0X1	T49.0X2	T49.0X3	T49.0X4	T49.0X5	T49.0X6
Flurazepam	T42.4X1	T42.4X2	T42.4X3	T42.4X4	T42.4X5	T42.4X6
Flurbiprofen	T39.311	T39.312	T39.313	T39.314	T39.315	T39.316
Flurobate	T49.0X1	T49.0X2	T49.0X3	T49.0X4	T49.0X5	T49.0X6
Flurotyl	T43.291	T43.292	T43.293	T43.294	T43.295	T43.296
Fluroxene	T41.0X1	T41.0X2	T41.0X3	T41.0X4	T41.0X5	T41.0X6
Fluspirilene	T43.591	T43.592	T43.593	T43.594	T43.595	T43.596
Flutamide	T38.6X1	T38.6X2	T38.6X3	T38.6X4	T38.6X5	T38.6X6
Flutazolam	T42.4X1	T42.4X2	T42.4X3	T42.4X4	T42.4X5	T42.4X6
Fluticasone propionate	T49.1X1	T49.1X2	T49.1X3	T49.1X4	T49.1X5	T49.1X6
Flutoprazepam	T42.4X1	T42.4X2	T42.4X3	T42.4X4	T42.4X5	T42.4X6
Flutropium bromide	T48.6X1	T48.6X2	T48.6X3	T48.6X4	T48.6X5	T48.6X6
Fluvoxamine	T43.221	T43.222	T43.223	T43.224	T43.225	T43.226
Folacin	T45.8X1	T45.8X2	T45.8X3	T45.8X4	T45.8X5	T45.8X6
Folic acid	T45.8X1	T45.8X2	T45.8X3	T45.8X4	T45.8X5	T45.8X6
with ferrous salt	T45.2X1	T45.2X2	T45.2X3	T45.2X4	T45.2X5	T45.2X6
antagonist	T45.1X1	T45.1X2	T45.1X3	T45.1X4	T45.1X5	T45.1X6
Folinic acid	T45.8X1	T45.8X2	T45.8X3	T45.8X4	T45.8X5	T45.8X6
Folium stramoniae	T48.6X1	T48.6X2	T48.6X3	T48.6X4	T48.6X5	T48.6X6
Follicle-stimulating hormone, human	T38.811	T38.812	T38.813	T38.814	T38.815	T38.816
Folpet	T60.3X1	T60.3X2	T60.3X3	T60.3X4	—	—
Fominoben	T48.3X1	T48.3X2	T48.3X3	T48.3X4	T48.3X5	T48.3X6
Food, foodstuffs, noxious, nonbacterial, NEC	T62.91	T62.92	T62.93	T62.94	—	—
berries	T62.1X1	T62.1X2	T62.1X3	T62.1X4	—	—
fish—see also Fish	T61.91	T61.92	T61.93	T61.94	—	—
mushrooms	T62.0X1	T62.0X2	T62.0X3	T62.0X4	—	—
plants	T62.2X1	T62.2X2	T62.2X3	T62.2X4	—	—
seafood	T61.91	T61.92	T61.93	T61.94	—	—
specified NEC	T61.8X1	T61.8X2	T61.8X3	T61.8X4	—	—
seeds	T62.2X1	T62.2X2	T62.2X3	T62.2X4	—	—
shellfish	T61.781	T61.782	T61.783	T61.784	—	—
specified NEC	T62.8X1	T62.8X2	T62.8X3	T62.8X4	—	—
Fool's parsley	T62.2X1	T62.2X2	T62.2X3	T62.2X4	—	—
Formaldehyde (solution), gas or vapor	T59.2X1	T59.2X2	T59.2X3	T59.2X4	—	—
fungicide	T60.3X1	T60.3X2	T60.3X3	T60.3X4	—	—

TABLE OF DRUGS AND CHEMICALS

Substance	External Cause (T-Code)					
	Poisoning, Accidental (Unintentional)	Poisoning, Intentional Self-Harm	Poisoning, Assault	Poisoning, Undetermined	Adverse Effect	Underdosing
Formalin	T59.2X1	T59.2X2	T59.2X3	T59.2X4	—	—
fungicide	T60.3X1	T60.3X2	T60.3X3	T60.3X4	—	—
vapor	T59.2X1	T59.2X2	T59.2X3	T59.2X4	—	—
Formic acid	T54.2X1	T54.2X2	T54.2X3	T54.2X4	—	—
vapor	T59.891	T59.892	T59.893	T59.894	—	—
Foscarnet sodium	T37.5X1	T37.5X2	T37.5X3	T37.5X4	T37.5X5	T37.5X6
Fosfestrol	T38.5X1	T38.5X2	T38.5X3	T38.5X4	T38.5X5	T38.5X6
Fosfomycin	T36.8X1	T36.8X2	T36.8X3	T36.8X4	T36.8X5	T36.8X6
Fosfonet sodium	T37.5X1	T37.5X2	T37.5X3	T37.5X4	T37.5X5	T37.5X6
Fosinopril	T46.4X1	T46.4X2	T46.4X3	T46.4X4	T46.4X5	T46.4X6
sodium	T46.4X1	T46.4X2	T46.4X3	T46.4X4	T46.4X5	T46.4X6
Fowler's solution	T57.0X1	T57.0X2	T57.0X3	T57.0X4	—	—
Foxglove	T62.2X1	T62.2X2	T62.2X3	T62.2X4	—	—
Framycetin	T36.5X1	T36.5X2	T36.5X3	T36.5X4	T36.5X5	T36.5X6
Frangula	T47.2X1	T47.2X2	T47.2X3	T47.2X4	T47.2X5	T47.2X6
extract	T47.2X1	T47.2X2	T47.2X3	T47.2X4	T47.2X5	T47.2X6
Frei antigen	T50.8X1	T50.8X2	T50.8X3	T50.8X4	T50.8X5	T50.8X6
Freon	T53.5X1	T53.5X2	T53.5X3	T53.5X4	—	—
Fructose	T50.3X1	T50.3X2	T50.3X3	T50.3X4	T50.3X5	T50.3X6
Frusemide	T50.1X1	T50.1X2	T50.1X3	T50.1X4	T50.1X5	T50.1X6
FSH	T38.811	T38.812	T38.813	T38.814	T38.815	T38.816
Ftorafur	T45.1X1	T45.1X2	T45.1X3	T45.1X4	T45.1X5	T45.1X6
Fuel						
automobile	T52.0X1	T52.0X2	T52.0X3	T52.0X4	—	—
exhaust gas, not in transit	T58.01	T58.02	T58.03	T58.04	—	—
vapor NEC	T52.0X1	T52.0X2	T52.0X3	T52.0X4	—	—
gas (domestic use) — see also Carbon, monoxide, fuel, utility	T59.891	T59.892	T59.893	T59.894	—	—
utility	T59.891	T59.892	T59.893	T59.894	—	—
in mobile container	T59.891	T59.892	T59.893	T59.894	—	—
incomplete combustion of — see Carbon, monoxide, fuel, utility						
piped (natural)	T59.891	T59.892	T59.893	T59.894	—	—
industrial, incomplete combustion	T58.8X1	T58.8X2	T58.8X3	T58.8X4	—	—
Fugillin	T36.8X1	T36.8X2	T36.8X3	T36.8X4	T36.8X5	T36.8X6
Fulminate of mercury	T56.1X1	T56.1X2	T56.1X3	T56.1X4	—	—
Fulvicin	T36.7X1	T36.7X2	T36.7X3	T36.7X4	T36.7X5	T36.7X6
Fumadil	T36.8X1	T36.8X2	T36.8X3	T36.8X4	T36.8X5	T36.8X6
Fumagillin	T36.8X1	T36.8X2	T36.8X3	T36.8X4	T36.8X5	T36.8X6
Fumaric acid	T49.4X1	T49.4X2	T49.4X3	T49.4X4	T49.4X5	T49.4X6
Fumes (from)	T59.91	T59.92	T59.93	T59.94	—	—
carbon monoxide — see Carbon, monoxide						
charcoal (domestic use) — see Charcoal, fumes						

◀ New   ◀━ Revised   ~~deleted~~ Deleted

Substance	External Cause (T-Code)					
	Poisoning, Accidental (Unintentional)	Poisoning, Intentional Self-Harm	Poisoning, Assault	Poisoning, Undetermined	Adverse Effect	Underdosing
Fumes *(Continued)*						
chloroform — *see Chloroform*						
coke (in domestic stoves, fireplaces) — *see Coke, fumes*						
corrosive NEC	T54.91	T54.92	T54.93	T54.94	—	—
ether — *see ether*						
freons	T53.5X1	T53.5X2	T53.5X3	T53.5X4	—	—
hydrocarbons	T59.891	T59.892	T59.893	T59.894	—	—
petroleum (liquefied)	T59.891	T59.892	T59.893	T59.894	—	—
distributed through pipes (pure or mixed with air)	T59.891	T59.892	T59.893	T59.894	—	—
lead — *see lead*						
metal — *see Metals, or the specified metal*						
nitrogen dioxide	T59.0X1	T59.0X2	T59.0X3	T59.0X4	—	—
pesticides — *see Pesticides*						
petroleum (liquefied)	T59.891	T59.892	T59.893	T59.894	—	—
distributed through pipes (pure or mixed with air)	T59.891	T59.892	T59.893	T59.894	—	—
polyester	T59.891	T59.892	T59.893	T59.894	—	—
specified source NEC — *see also substance specified*	T59.891	T59.892	T59.893	T59.894	—	—
sulfur dioxide	T59.1X1	T59.1X2	T59.1X3	T59.1X4	—	—
Fumigant NEC	T60.91	T60.92	T60.93	T60.94	—	—
Fungi, noxious, used as food	T62.0X1	T62.0X2	T62.0X3	T62.0X4	—	—
Fungicide NEC (nonmedicinal)	T60.3X1	T60.3X2	T60.3X3	T60.3X4	—	—
Fungizone	T36.7X1	T36.7X2	T36.7X3	T36.7X4	T36.7X5	T36.7X6
topical	T49.0X1	T49.0X2	T49.0X3	T49.0X4	T49.0X5	T49.0X6
Furacin	T49.0X1	T49.0X2	T49.0X3	T49.0X4	T49.0X5	T49.0X6
Furadantin	T37.91	T37.92	T37.93	T37.94	T37.95	T37.96
Furazolidone	T37.8X1	T37.8X2	T37.8X3	T37.8X4	T37.8X5	T37.8X6
Furazolium chloride	T49.0X1	T49.0X2	T49.0X3	T49.0X4	T49.0X5	T49.0X6
Furfural	T52.8X1	T52.8X2	T52.8X3	T52.8X4	—	—
Furnace (coal burning) (domestic), gas from industrial	T58.2X1	T58.2X2	T58.2X3	T58.2X4	—	—
industrial	T58.8X1	T58.8X2	T58.8X3	T58.8X4	—	—
Furniture polish	T65.891	T65.892	T65.893	T65.894	—	—
Furosemide	T50.1X1	T50.1X2	T50.1X3	T50.1X4	T50.1X5	T50.1X6
Furoxone	T37.91	T37.92	T37.93	T37.94	T37.95	T37.96
Fursultiamine	T45.2X1	T45.2X2	T45.2X3	T45.2X4	T45.2X5	T45.2X6
Fusafungine	T36.8X1	T36.8X2	T36.8X3	T36.8X4	T36.8X5	T36.8X6
Fusel oil (any) (amyl) (butyl) (propyl), vapor	T51.3X1	T51.3X2	T51.3X3	T51.3X4	—	—
Fusidate (ethanolamine) (sodium)	T36.8X1	T36.8X2	T36.8X3	T36.8X4	T36.8X5	T36.8X6
Fusidic acid	T36.8X1	T36.8X2	T36.8X3	T36.8X4	T36.8X5	T36.8X6
Fytic acid, nonasodium	T50.6X1	T50.6X2	T50.6X3	T50.6X4	T50.6X5	T50.6X6

◀ New ◀⁞⁞⁞ Revised ~~deleted~~ Deleted

TABLE OF DRUGS AND CHEMICALS

Substance	External Cause (T-Code)					
	Poisoning, Accidental (Unintentional)	Poisoning, Intentional Self-Harm	Poisoning, Assault	Poisoning, Undetermined	Adverse Effect	Underdosing
G						
GABA	T43.8X1	T43.8X2	T43.8X3	T43.8X4	T43.8X5	T43.8X6
Gadopentetic acid	T50.8X1	T50.8X2	T50.8X3	T50.8X4	T50.8X5	T50.8X6
Galactose	T50.3X1	T50.3X2	T50.3X3	T50.3X4	T50.3X5	T50.3X6
b-Galactosidase	T47.5X1	T47.5X2	T47.5X3	T47.5X4	T47.5X5	T47.5X6
Galantamine	T44.0X1	T44.0X2	T44.0X3	T44.0X4	T44.0X5	T44.0X6
Gallamine (triethiodide)	T48.1X1	T48.1X2	T48.1X3	T48.1X4	T48.1X5	T48.1X6
Gallium citrate	T50.991	T50.992	T50.993	T50.994	T50.995	T50.996
Gallopamil	T46.1X1	T46.1X2	T46.1X3	T46.1X4	T46.1X5	T46.1X6
Gamboge	T47.2X1	T47.2X2	T47.2X3	T47.2X4	T47.2X5	T47.2X6
Gamimune	T50.Z11	T50.Z12	T50.Z13	T50.Z14	T50.Z15	T50.Z16
Gamma-aminobutyric acid	T43.8X1	T43.8X2	T43.8X3	T43.8X4	T43.8X5	T43.8X6
Gamma-benzene hexachloride (medicinal)	T49.0X1	T49.0X2	T49.0X3	T49.0X4	T49.0X5	T49.0X6
nonmedicinal, vapor	T53.6X1	T53.6X2	T53.6X3	T53.6X4	—	—
Gamma-BHC (medicinal) — see also Gamma-benzene hexachloride	T49.0X1	T49.0X2	T49.0X3	T49.0X4	T49.0X5	T49.0X6
Gamma globulin	T50.Z11	T50.Z12	T50.Z13	T50.Z14	T50.Z15	T50.Z16
Gamulin	T50.Z11	T50.Z12	T50.Z13	T50.Z14	T50.Z15	T50.Z16
Ganciclovir (sodium)	T37.5X1	T37.5X2	T37.5X3	T37.5X4	T37.5X5	T37.5X6
Ganglionic blocking drug NEC	T44.2X1	T44.2X2	T44.2X3	T44.2X4	T44.2X5	T44.2X6
specified NEC	T44.2X1	T44.2X2	T44.2X3	T44.2X4	T44.2X5	T44.2X6
Ganja	T40.7X1	T40.7X2	T40.7X3	T40.7X4	T40.7X5	T40.7X6
Garamycin	T36.5X1	T36.5X2	T36.5X3	T36.5X4	T36.5X5	T36.5X6
ophthalmic preparation	T49.5X1	T49.5X2	T49.5X3	T49.5X4	T49.5X5	T49.5X6
topical NEC	T49.0X1	T49.0X2	T49.0X3	T49.0X4	T49.0X5	T49.0X6
Gardenal	T42.3X1	T42.3X2	T42.3X3	T42.3X4	T42.3X5	T42.3X6
Gardepanyl	T42.3X1	T42.3X2	T42.3X3	T42.3X4	T42.3X5	T42.3X6
Gas	T59.91	T59.92	T59.93	T59.94	—	—
acetylene	T59.891	T59.892	T59.893	T59.894	—	—
incomplete combustion of	T58.11	T58.12	T58.13	T58.14	—	—
air contaminants, source or type not specified	T59.91	T59.92	T59.93	T59.94	—	—
anesthetic	T41.0X1	T41.0X2	T41.0X3	T41.0X4	T41.0X5	T41.0X6
blast furnace	T58.8X1	T58.8X2	T58.8X3	T58.8X4	—	—
butane — see butane						
carbon monoxide — see Carbon, monoxide						
chlorine	T59.4X1	T59.4X2	T59.4X3	T59.4X4	—	—
coal	T58.2X1	T58.2X2	T58.2X3	T58.2X4	—	—
cyanide	T57.3X1	T57.3X2	T57.3X3	T57.3X4	—	—
dicyanogen	T65.0X1	T65.0X2	T65.0X3	T65.0X4	—	—
domestic — see Domestic gas	T57.91	T57.92	T57.93	T57.94	—	—

◀ New   ◀▥ Revised   ~~deleted~~ Deleted

Substance	External Cause (T-Code)					
	Poisoning, Accidental (Unintentional)	Poisoning, Intentional Self-Harm	Poisoning, Assault	Poisoning, Undetermined	Adverse Effect	Underdosing
Gas *(Continued)*						
exhaust	T57.91	T57.92	T57.93	T57.94	—	—
from utility (for cooking, heating, or lighting) (after combustion) — *see Carbon, monoxide, fuel, utility*						
prior to combustion	T59.891	T59.892	T59.893	T59.894	—	—
from wood or coal-burning stove or fireplace	T57.91	T57.92	T57.93	T57.94	—	—
fuel (domestic use) (after combustion) — *see also Carbon, monoxide, fuel*	T57.91	T57.92	T57.93	T57.94	—	—
industrial use	T58.8X1	T58.8X2	T58.8X3	T58.8X4	—	—
prior to combustion	T59.891	T59.892	T59.893	T59.894	—	—
utility	T59.891	T59.892	T59.893	T59.894	—	—
in mobile container	T59.891	T59.892	T59.893	T59.894	—	—
incomplete combustion of — *see Carbon, monoxide, fuel, utility*						
piped (natural)	T59.891	T59.892	T59.893	T59.894	—	—
garage	T58.01	T58.02	T58.03	T58.04	—	—
hydrocarbon NEC	T59.891	T59.892	T59.893	T59.894	—	—
incomplete combustion of — *see Carbon, monoxide, fuel, utility*						
liquefied — *see butane*						
piped	T59.891	T59.892	T59.893	T59.894	—	—
hydrocyanic acid	T65.0X1	T65.0X2	T65.0X3	T65.0X4	—	—
illuminating (after combustion)	T58.11	T58.12	T58.13	T58.14	—	—
prior to combustion	T59.891	T59.892	T59.893	T59.894	—	—
incomplete combustion, any — *see Carbon, monoxide*						
kiln	T58.8X1	T58.8X2	T58.8X3	T58.8X4	—	—
lacrimogenic	T59.3X1	T59.3X2	T59.3X3	T59.3X4	—	—
liquefied petroleum — *see butane*						
marsh	T59.891	T59.892	T59.893	T59.894	—	—
motor exhaust, not in transit	T58.01	T58.02	T58.03	T58.04	—	—
mustard, not in war	T59.891	T59.892	T59.893	T59.894	—	—
natural	T59.891	T59.892	T59.893	T59.894	—	—
nerve, not in war	T59.91	T59.92	T59.93	T59.94	—	—
oil	T52.0X1	T52.0X2	T52.0X3	T52.0X4	—	—
petroleum (liquefied) (distributed in mobile containers)	T59.891	T59.892	T59.893	T59.894	—	—
piped (pure or mixed with air)	T59.891	T59.892	T59.893	T59.894	—	—
piped (manufactured) (natural) NEC	T59.891	T59.892	T59.893	T59.894	—	—
producer	T58.8X1	T58.8X2	T58.8X3	T58.8X4	—	—
propane — *see propane*						
refrigerant (chlorofluoro-carbon)	T53.5X1	T53.5X2	T53.5X3	T53.5X4	—	—
not chlorofluoro-carbon	T59.891	T59.892	T59.893	T59.894	—	—
sewer	T59.91	T59.92	T59.93	T59.94	—	—
specified source NEC	T59.91	T59.92	T59.93	T59.94	—	—

◀ New   ◀▦ Revised   ~~deleted~~ Deleted

Substance	External Cause (T-Code)					
	Poisoning, Accidental (Unintentional)	Poisoning, Intentional Self-Harm	Poisoning, Assault	Poisoning, Undetermined	Adverse Effect	Underdosing
Gas (Continued)						
stove (after combustion)	T58.11	T58.12	T58.13	T58.14	—	—
tear	T59.3X1	T59.3X2	T59.3X3	T59.3X4	—	—
therapeutic	T41.5X1	T41.5X2	T41.5X3	T41.5X4	T41.5X5	T41.5X6
utility (for cooking, heating, or lighting) (piped) NEC	T59.891	T59.892	T59.893	T59.894	—	—
in mobile container	T59.891	T59.892	T59.893	T59.894	—	—
incomplete combustion of — see Carbon, monoxide, fuel, utilty						
piped (natural)	T59.891	T59.892	T59.893	T59.894	—	—
water	T58.11	T58.12	T58.13	T58.14	—	—
incomplete combustion of — see Carbon, monoxide, fuel, utility						
Gaseous substance — see Gas						
Gasoline	T52.0X1	T52.0X2	T52.0X3	T52.0X4	—	—
vapor	T52.0X1	T52.0X2	T52.0X3	T52.0X4	—	—
Gastric enzymes	T47.5X1	T47.5X2	T47.5X3	T47.5X4	T47.5X5	T47.5X6
Gastrografin	T50.8X1	T50.8X2	T50.8X3	T50.8X4	T50.8X5	T50.8X6
Gastrointestinal drug	T47.91	T47.92	T47.93	T47.94	T47.95	T47.96
biological	T47.8X1	T47.8X2	T47.8X3	T47.8X4	T47.8X5	T47.8X6
specified NEC	T47.8X1	T47.8X2	T47.8X3	T47.8X4	T47.8X5	T47.8X6
Gaultheria procumbens	T62.2X1	T62.2X2	T62.2X3	T62.2X4	—	—
Gelatin (intravenous)	T45.8X1	T45.8X2	T45.8X3	T45.8X4	T45.8X5	T45.8X6
absorbable (sponge)	T45.7X1	T45.7X2	T45.7X3	T45.7X4	T45.7X5	T45.7X6
Gefarnate	T44.3X1	T44.3X2	T44.3X3	T44.3X4	T44.3X5	T44.3X6
Gelfilm	T49.8X1	T49.8X2	T49.8X3	T49.8X4	T49.8X5	T49.8X6
Gelfoam	T45.7X1	T45.7X2	T45.7X3	T45.7X4	T45.7X5	T45.7X6
Gelsemine	T50.991	T50.992	T50.993	T50.994	T50.995	T50.996
Gelsemium (sempervirens)	T62.2X1	T62.2X2	T62.2X3	T62.2X4	—	—
Gemeprost	T48.0X1	T48.0X2	T48.0X3	T48.0X4	T48.0X5	T48.0X6
Gemfibrozil	T46.6X1	T46.6X2	T46.6X3	T46.6X4	T46.6X5	T46.6X6
Gemonil	T42.3X1	T42.3X2	T42.3X3	T42.3X4	T42.3X5	T42.3X6
Gentamicin	T36.5X1	T36.5X2	T36.5X3	T36.5X4	T36.5X5	T36.5X6
ophthalmic preparation	T49.5X1	T49.5X2	T49.5X3	T49.5X4	T49.5X5	T49.5X6
topical NEC	T49.0X1	T49.0X2	T49.0X3	T49.0X4	T49.0X5	T49.0X6
Gentian	T47.5X1	T47.5X2	T47.5X3	T47.5X4	T47.5X5	T47.5X6
violet	T49.0X1	T49.0X2	T49.0X3	T49.0X4	T49.0X5	T49.0X6
Gepefrine	T44.4X1	T44.4X2	T44.4X3	T44.4X4	T44.4X5	T44.4X6
Gestonorone caproate	T38.5X1	T38.5X2	T38.5X3	T38.5X4	T38.5X5	T38.5X6
Gexane	T49.0X1	T49.0X2	T49.0X3	T49.0X4	T49.0X5	T49.0X6
Gila monster (venom)	T63.111	T63.112	T63.113	T63.114	—	—
Ginger	T47.5X1	T47.5X2	T47.5X3	T47.5X4	T47.5X5	T47.5X6
Jamaica — see Jamaica, ginger						

TABLE OF DRUGS AND CHEMICALS

◄ New   ◄ Revised   deleted Deleted

Substance	Poisoning, Accidental (Unintentional)	Poisoning, Intentional Self-Harm	Poisoning, Assault	Poisoning, Undetermined	Adverse Effect	Underdosing
	External Cause (T-Code)					
Gitalin	T46.0X1	T46.0X2	T46.0X3	T46.0X4	T46.0X5	T46.0X6
amorphous	T46.0X1	T46.0X2	T46.0X3	T46.0X4	T46.0X5	T46.0X6
Gitaloxin	T46.0X1	T46.0X2	T46.0X3	T46.0X4	T46.0X5	T46.0X6
Gitoxin	T46.0X1	T46.0X2	T46.0X3	T46.0X4	T46.0X5	T46.0X6
Glafenine	T39.8X1	T39.8X2	T39.8X3	T39.8X4	T39.8X5	T39.8X6
Glandular extract (medicinal) NEC	T50.Z91	T50.Z92	T50.Z93	T50.Z94	T50.Z95	T50.Z96
Glaucarubin	T37.3X1	T37.3X2	T37.3X3	T37.3X4	T37.3X5	T37.3X6
Glibenclamide	T38.3X1	T38.3X2	T38.3X3	T38.3X4	T38.3X5	T38.3X6
Glibornuride	T38.3X1	T38.3X2	T38.3X3	T38.3X4	T38.3X5	T38.3X6
Gliclazide	T38.3X1	T38.3X2	T38.3X3	T38.3X4	T38.3X5	T38.3X6
Glimidine	T38.3X1	T38.3X2	T38.3X3	T38.3X4	T38.3X5	T38.3X6
Glipizide	T38.3X1	T38.3X2	T38.3X3	T38.3X4	T38.3X5	T38.3X6
Gliquidone	T38.3X1	T38.3X2	T38.3X3	T38.3X4	T38.3X5	T38.3X6
Glisolamide	T38.3X1	T38.3X2	T38.3X3	T38.3X4	T38.3X5	T38.3X6
Glisoxepide	T38.3X1	T38.3X2	T38.3X3	T38.3X4	T38.3X5	T38.3X6
Globin zinc insulin	T38.3X1	T38.3X2	T38.3X3	T38.3X4	T38.3X5	T38.3X6
Globulin						
antilymphocytic	T50.Z11	T50.Z12	T50.Z13	T50.Z14	T50.Z15	T50.Z16
antirhesus	T50.Z11	T50.Z12	T50.Z13	T50.Z14	T50.Z15	T50.Z16
antivenin	T50.Z11	T50.Z12	T50.Z13	T50.Z14	T50.Z15	T50.Z16
antiviral	T50.Z11	T50.Z12	T50.Z13	T50.Z14	T50.Z15	T50.Z16
Glucagon	T38.3X1	T38.3X2	T38.3X3	T38.3X4	T38.3X5	T38.3X6
Glucocorticoids	T38.0X1	T38.0X2	T38.0X3	T38.0X4	T38.0X5	T38.0X6
Glucocorticosteroid	T38.0X1	T38.0X2	T38.0X3	T38.0X4	T38.0X5	T38.0X6
Gluconic acid	T50.991	T50.992	T50.993	T50.994	T50.995	T50.996
Glucosamine sulfate	T39.4X1	T39.4X2	T39.4X3	T39.4X4	T39.4X5	T39.4X6
Glucose	T50.3X1	T50.3X2	T50.3X3	T50.3X4	T50.3X5	T50.3X6
with sodium chloride	T50.3X1	T50.3X2	T50.3X3	T50.3X4	T50.3X5	T50.3X6
Glucosulfone sodium	T37.1X1	T37.1X2	T37.1X3	T37.1X4	T37.1X5	T37.1X6
Glucurolactone	T47.8X1	T47.8X2	T47.8X3	T47.8X4	T47.8X5	T47.8X6
Glue NEC	T52.8X1	T52.8X2	T52.8X3	T52.8X4	—	—
Glutamic acid	T47.5X1	T47.5X2	T47.5X3	T47.5X4	T47.5X5	T47.5X6
Glutaral (medicinal)	T49.0X1	T49.0X2	T49.0X3	T49.0X4	T49.0X5	T49.0X6
nonmedicinal	T65.891	T65.892	T65.893	T65.894	—	—
Glutaraldehyde (nonmedicinal)	T65.891	T65.892	T65.893	T65.894	—	—
medicinal	T49.0X1	T49.0X2	T49.0X3	T49.0X4	T49.0X5	T49.0X6
Glutathione	T50.6X1	T50.6X2	T50.6X3	T50.6X4	T50.6X5	T50.6X6
Glutethimide	T42.6X1	T42.6X2	T42.6X3	T42.6X4	T42.6X5	T42.6X6
Glyburide	T38.3X1	T38.3X2	T38.3X3	T38.3X4	T38.3X5	T38.3X6

◀ New ◀▥ Revised ~~deleted~~ Deleted

TABLE OF DRUGS AND CHEMICALS

Substance	Poisoning, Accidental (Unintentional)	Poisoning, Intentional Self-Harm	Poisoning, Assault	Poisoning, Undetermined	Adverse Effect	Underdosing
			External Cause (T-Code)			
Glycerin	T47.4X1	T47.4X2	T47.4X3	T47.4X4	T47.4X5	T47.4X6
Glycerol	T47.4X1	T47.4X2	T47.4X3	T47.4X4	T47.4X5	T47.4X6
borax	T49.6X1	T49.6X2	T49.6X3	T49.6X4	T49.6X5	T49.6X6
intravenous	T50.3X1	T50.3X2	T50.3X3	T50.3X4	T50.3X5	T50.3X6
iodinated	T48.4X1	T48.4X2	T48.4X3	T48.4X4	T48.4X5	T48.4X6
Glycerophosphate	T50.991	T50.992	T50.993	T50.994	T50.995	T50.996
Glyceryl						
gualacolate	T48.4X1	T48.4X2	T48.4X3	T48.4X4	T48.4X5	T48.4X6
nitrate	T46.3X1	T46.3X2	T46.3X3	T46.3X4	T46.3X5	T46.3X6
triacetate (topical)	T49.0X1	T49.0X2	T49.0X3	T49.0X4	T49.0X5	T49.0X6
trinitrate	T46.3X1	T46.3X2	T46.3X3	T46.3X4	T46.3X5	T46.3X6
Glycine	T50.3X1	T50.3X2	T50.3X3	T50.3X4	T50.3X5	T50.3X6
Glyclopyramide	T38.3X1	T38.3X2	T38.3X3	T38.3X4	T38.3X5	T38.3X6
Glycobiarsol	T37.3X1	T37.3X2	T37.3X3	T37.3X4	T37.3X5	T37.3X6
Glycols (ether)	T52.3X1	T52.3X2	T52.3X3	T52.3X4	—	—
Glyconiazide	T37.1X1	T37.1X2	T37.1X3	T37.1X4	T37.1X5	T37.1X6
Glycopyrrolate	T44.3X1	T44.3X2	T44.3X3	T44.3X4	T44.3X5	T44.3X6
Glycopyrronium	T44.3X1	T44.3X2	T44.3X3	T44.3X4	T44.3X5	T44.3X6
bromide	T44.3X1	T44.3X2	T44.3X3	T44.3X4	T44.3X5	T44.3X6
Glycoside, cardiac (stimulant)	T46.0X1	T46.0X2	T46.0X3	T46.0X4	T46.0X5	T46.0X6
Glycyclamide	T38.3X1	T38.3X2	T38.3X3	T38.3X4	T38.3X5	T38.3X6
Glycyrrhiza extract	T48.4X1	T48.4X2	T48.4X3	T48.4X4	T48.4X5	T48.4X6
Glycyrrhizic acid	T48.4X1	T48.4X2	T48.4X3	T48.4X4	T48.4X5	T48.4X6
Glycyrrhizinate potassium	T48.4X1	T48.4X2	T48.4X3	T48.4X4	T48.4X5	T48.4X6
Glymidine sodium	T38.3X1	T38.3X2	T38.3X3	T38.3X4	T38.3X5	T38.3X6
Glyphosate	T60.3X1	T60.3X2	T60.3X3	T60.3X4	—	—
Glyphylline	T48.6X1	T48.6X2	T48.6X3	T48.6X4	T48.6X5	T48.6X6
Gold						
colloidal (l98Au)	T45.1X1	T45.1X2	T45.1X3	T45.1X4	T45.1X5	T45.1X6
salts	T39.4X1	T39.4X2	T39.4X3	T39.4X4	T39.4X5	T39.4X6
Golden sulfide of antimony	T56.891	T56.892	T56.893	T56.894	—	—
Goldylocks	T62.2X1	T62.2X2	T62.2X3	T62.2X4	—	—
Gonadal tissue extract	T38.901	T38.902	T38.903	T38.904	T38.905	T38.906
female	T38.5X1	T38.5X2	T38.5X3	T38.5X4	T38.5X5	T38.5X6
male	T38.7X1	T38.7X2	T38.7X3	T38.7X4	T38.7X5	T38.7X6
Gonadorelin	T38.891	T38.892	T38.893	T38.894	T38.895	T38.896
Gonadotropin	T38.891	T38.892	T38.893	T38.894	T38.895	T38.896
chorionic	T38.891	T38.892	T38.893	T38.894	T38.895	T38.896
pituitary	T38.811	T38.812	T38.813	T38.814	T38.815	T38.816
Goserelin	T45.1X1	T45.1X2	T45.1X3	T45.1X4	T45.1X5	T45.1X6

◀ New ◀▦ Revised ~~deleted~~ Deleted

Substance	External Cause (T-Code)					
	Poisoning, Accidental (Unintentional)	Poisoning, Intentional Self-Harm	Poisoning, Assault	Poisoning, Undetermined	Adverse Effect	Underdosing
Grain alcohol	T51.0X1	T51.0X2	T51.0X3	T51.0X4	—	—
Gramicidin	T49.0X1	T49.0X2	T49.0X3	T49.0X4	T49.0X5	T49.0X6
Granisetron	T45.0X1	T45.0X2	T45.0X3	T45.0X4	T45.0X5	T45.0X6
Gratiola officinalis	T62.2X1	T62.2X2	T62.2X3	T62.2X4	—	—
Grease	T65.891	T65.892	T65.893	T65.894	—	—
Green hellebore	T62.2X1	T62.2X2	T62.2X3	T62.2X4	—	—
Green soap	T49.2X1	T49.2X2	T49.2X3	T49.2X4	T49.2X5	T49.2X6
Grifulvin	T36.7X1	T36.7X2	T36.7X3	T36.7X4	T36.7X5	T36.7X6
Griseofulvin	T36.7X1	T36.7X2	T36.7X3	T36.7X4	T36.7X5	T36.7X6
Growth hormone	T38.811	T38.812	T38.813	T38.814	T38.815	T38.816
Guaiacol derivatives	T48.4X1	T48.4X2	T48.4X3	T48.4X4	T48.4X5	T48.4X6
Guaiac reagent	T50.991	T50.992	T50.993	T50.994	T50.995	T50.996
Guaifenesin	T48.4X1	T48.4X2	T48.4X3	T48.4X4	T48.4X5	T48.4X6
Guaimesal	T48.4X1	T48.4X2	T48.4X3	T48.4X4	T48.4X5	T48.4X6
Guaiphenesin	T48.4X1	T48.4X2	T48.4X3	T48.4X4	T48.4X5	T48.4X6
Guamecycline	T36.4X1	T36.4X2	T36.4X3	T36.4X4	T36.4X5	T36.4X6
Guanabenz	T46.5X1	T46.5X2	T46.5X3	T46.5X4	T46.5X5	T46.5X6
Guanacline	T46.5X1	T46.5X2	T46.5X3	T46.5X4	T46.5X5	T46.5X6
Guanadrel	T46.5X1	T46.5X2	T46.5X3	T46.5X4	T46.5X5	T46.5X6
Guanatol	T37.2X1	T37.2X2	T37.2X3	T37.2X4	T37.2X5	T37.2X6
Guanethidine	T46.5X1	T46.5X2	T46.5X3	T46.5X4	T46.5X5	T46.5X6
Guanfacine	T46.5X1	T46.5X2	T46.5X3	T46.5X4	T46.5X5	T46.5X6
Guano	T65.891	T65.892	T65.893	T65.894	—	—
Guanochlor	T46.5X1	T46.5X2	T46.5X3	T46.5X4	T46.5X5	T46.5X6
Guanoclor	T46.5X1	T46.5X2	T46.5X3	T46.5X4	T46.5X5	T46.5X6
Guanoctine	T46.5X1	T46.5X2	T46.5X3	T46.5X4	T46.5X5	T46.5X6
Guanoxabenz	T46.5X1	T46.5X2	T46.5X3	T46.5X4	T46.5X5	T46.5X6
Guanoxan	T46.5X1	T46.5X2	T46.5X3	T46.5X4	T46.5X5	T46.5X6
Guar gum (medicinal)	T46.6X1	T46.6X2	T46.6X3	T46.6X4	T46.6X5	T46.6X6
H						
Hachimycin	T36.7X1	T36.7X2	T36.7X3	T36.7X4	T36.7X5	T36.7X6
Hair						
dye	T49.4X1	T49.4X2	T49.4X3	T49.4X4	T49.4X5	T49.4X6
preparation NEC	T49.4X1	T49.4X2	T49.4X3	T49.4X4	T49.4X5	T49.4X6
Halazepam	T42.4X1	T42.4X2	T42.4X3	T42.4X4	T42.4X5	T42.4X6
Halcinolone	T49.0X1	T49.0X2	T49.0X3	T49.0X4	T49.0X5	T49.0X6
Halcinonide	T49.0X1	T49.0X2	T49.0X3	T49.0X4	T49.0X5	T49.0X6
Halethazole	T49.0X1	T49.0X2	T49.0X3	T49.0X4	T49.0X5	T49.0X6
Hallucinogen NEC	T40.901	T40.902	T40.903	T40.904	T40.905	T40.906

◀ New ◀▥ Revised ~~deleted~~ Deleted

TABLE OF DRUGS AND CHEMICALS

Substance	Poisoning, Accidental (Unintentional)	Poisoning, Intentional Self-Harm	Poisoning, Assault	Poisoning, Undetermined	Adverse Effect	Underdosing
Halofantrine	T37.2X1	T37.2X2	T37.2X3	T37.2X4	T37.2X5	T37.2X6
Halofenate	T46.6X1	T46.6X2	T46.6X3	T46.6X4	T46.6X5	T46.6X6
Halometasone	T49.0X1	T49.0X2	T49.0X3	T49.0X4	T49.0X5	T49.0X6
Haloperidol	T43.4X1	T43.4X2	T43.4X3	T43.4X4	T43.4X5	T43.4X6
Haloprogin	T49.0X1	T49.0X2	T49.0X3	T49.0X4	T49.0X5	T49.0X6
Halotex	T49.0X1	T49.0X2	T49.0X3	T49.0X4	T49.0X5	T49.0X6
Halothane	T41.0X1	T41.0X2	T41.0X3	T41.0X4	T41.0X5	T41.0X6
Haloxazolam	T42.4X1	T42.4X2	T42.4X3	T42.4X4	T42.4X5	T42.4X6
Halquinols	T49.0X1	T49.0X2	T49.0X3	T49.0X4	T49.0X5	T49.0X6
Hamamelis	T49.2X1	T49.2X2	T49.2X3	T49.2X4	T49.2X5	T49.2X6
Haptendextran	T45.8X1	T45.8X2	T45.8X3	T45.8X4	T45.8X5	T45.8X6
Harmonyl	T46.5X1	T46.5X2	T46.5X3	T46.5X4	T46.5X5	T46.5X6
Hartmann's solution	T50.3X1	T50.3X2	T50.3X3	T50.3X4	T50.3X5	T50.3X6
Hashish	T40.7X1	T40.7X2	T40.7X3	T40.7X4	T40.7X5	T40.7X6
Hawaiian Woodrose seeds	T40.991	T40.992	T40.993	T40.994	—	—
HCB	T60.3X1	T60.3X2	T60.3X3	T60.3X4	—	—
HCH	T53.6X1	T53.6X2	T53.6X3	T53.6X4	—	—
medicinal	T49.0X1	T49.0X2	T49.0X3	T49.0X4	T49.0X5	T49.0X6
HCN	T57.3X1	T57.3X2	T57.3X3	T57.3X4	—	—
Headache cures, drugs, powders NEC	T50.901	T50.902	T50.903	T50.904	T50.905	T50.906
Heavenly Blue (morning glory)	T40.991	T40.992	T40.993	T40.994	—	—
Heavy metal antidote	T45.8X1	T45.8X2	T45.8X3	T45.8X4	T45.8X5	T45.8X6
Hedaquinium	T49.0X1	T49.0X2	T49.0X3	T49.0X4	T49.0X5	T49.0X6
Hedge hyssop	T62.2X1	T62.2X2	T62.2X3	T62.2X4	—	—
Heet	T49.8X1	T49.8X2	T49.8X3	T49.8X4	T49.8X5	T49.8X6
Helium	T48.991	T48.992	T48.993	T48.994	T48.995	T48.996
Helenin	T37.4X1	T37.4X2	T37.4X3	T37.4X4	T37.4X5	T37.4X6
Hellebore (black) (green) (white)	T62.2X1	T62.2X2	T62.2X3	T62.2X4	—	—
Helium (nonmedicinal) NEC	T59.891	T59.892	T59.893	T59.894	—	—
medicinal	T48.991	T48.992	T48.993	T48.994	T48.995	T48.996
Hematin	T45.8X1	T45.8X2	T45.8X3	T45.8X4	T45.8X5	T45.8X6
Hematinic preparation	T45.8X1	T45.8X2	T45.8X3	T45.8X4	T45.8X5	T45.8X6
Hemlock	T62.2X1	T62.2X2	T62.2X3	T62.2X4	—	—
Hemostatic	T45.621	T45.622	T45.623	T45.624	T45.625	T45.626
drug, systemic	T45.621	T45.622	T45.623	T45.624	T45.625	T45.626
Hemostyptic	T49.4X1	T49.4X2	T49.4X3	T49.4X4	T49.4X5	T49.4X6
Henbane	T62.2X1	T62.2X2	T62.2X3	T62.2X4	—	—
Heparin (sodium)	T45.511	T45.512	T45.513	T45.514	T45.515	T45.516
action reverser	T45.7X1	T45.7X2	T45.7X3	T45.7X4	T45.7X5	T45.7X6
Heparin-fraction	T45.511	T45.512	T45.513	T45.514	T45.515	T45.516

◀ New ◀▐ Revised ~~deleted~~ Deleted

Substance	External Cause (T-Code)					
	Poisoning, Accidental (Unintentional)	Poisoning, Intentional Self-Harm	Poisoning, Assault	Poisoning, Undetermined	Adverse Effect	Underdosing
Heparinoid (systemic)	T45.511	T45.512	T45.513	T45.514	T45.515	T45.516
Hepatic secretion stimulant	T47.8X1	T47.8X2	T47.8X3	T47.8X4	T47.8X5	T47.8X6
Hepatitis B						
immune globulin	T50.Z11	T50.Z12	T50.Z13	T50.Z14	T50.Z15	T50.Z16
vaccine	T50.B91	T50.B92	T50.B93	T50.B94	T50.B95	T50.B96
Hepronicate	T46.7X1	T46.7X2	T46.7X3	T46.7X4	T46.7X5	T46.7X6
Heptabarb	T42.3X1	T42.3X2	T42.3X3	T42.3X4	T42.3X5	T42.3X6
Heptabarbitone	T42.3X1	T42.3X2	T42.3X3	T42.3X4	T42.3X5	T42.3X6
Heptabarbital	T42.3X1	T42.3X2	T42.3X3	T42.3X4	T42.3X5	T42.3X6
Heptachlor	T60.1X1	T60.1X2	T60.1X3	T60.1X4	—	—
Heptalgin	T40.2X1	T40.2X2	T40.2X3	T40.2X4	T40.2X5	T40.2X6
Heptaminol	T46.3X1	T46.3X2	T46.3X3	T46.3X4	T46.3X5	T46.3X6
Herbicide NEC	T60.3X1	T60.3X2	T60.3X3	T60.3X4	—	—
Heroin	T40.1X1	T40.1X2	T40.1X3	T40.1X4	—	—
Herplex	T49.5X1	T49.5X2	T49.5X3	T49.5X4	T49.5X5	T49.5X6
HES	T45.8X1	T45.8X2	T45.8X3	T45.8X4	T45.8X5	T45.8X6
Hesperidin	T46.991	T46.992	T46.993	T46.994	T46.995	T46.996
Hetacillin	T36.0X1	T36.0X2	T36.0X3	T36.0X4	T36.0X5	T36.0X6
Hetastarch	T45.8X1	T45.8X2	T45.8X3	T45.8X4	T45.8X5	T45.8X6
HETP	T60.0X1	T60.0X2	T60.0X3	T60.0X4	—	—
Hexachlorobenzene (vapor)	T60.3X1	T60.3X2	T60.3X3	T60.3X4	—	—
Hexachlorocyclohexane	T53.6X1	T53.6X2	T53.6X3	T53.6X4	—	—
Hexachlorophene	T49.0X1	T49.0X2	T49.0X3	T49.0X4	T49.0X5	T49.0X6
Hexadiline	T46.3X1	T46.3X2	T46.3X3	T46.3X4	T46.3X5	T46.3X6
Hexadimethrine (bromide)	T45.7X1	T45.7X2	T45.7X3	T45.7X4	T45.7X5	T45.7X6
Hexadylamine	T46.3X1	T46.3X2	T46.3X3	T46.3X4	T46.3X5	T46.3X6
Hexaethyl tetraphosphate	T60.0X1	T60.0X2	T60.0X3	T60.0X4	—	—
Hexafluorenium bromide	T48.1X1	T48.1X2	T48.1X3	T48.1X4	T48.1X5	T48.1X6
Hexafluorodiethyl ether	T43.291	T43.292	T43.293	T43.294	T43.295	T43.296
Hexafluronium (bromide)	T48.1X1	T48.1X2	T48.1X3	T48.1X4	T48.1X5	T48.1X6
Hexahydrobenzol	T52.8X1	T52.8X2	T52.8X3	T52.8X4	—	—
Hexahydrocresol(s)	T51.8X1	T51.8X2	T51.8X3	T51.8X4	—	—
arsenide	T57.0X1	T57.0X2	T57.0X3	T57.0X4	—	—
arseniurated	T57.0X1	T57.0X2	T57.0X3	T57.0X4	—	—
cyanide	T57.3X1	T57.3X2	T57.3X3	T57.3X4	—	—
gas	T59.891	T59.892	T59.893	T59.894	—	—
Fluoride (liquid)	T57.8X1	T57.8X2	T57.8X3	T57.8X4	—	—
vapor	T59.891	T59.892	T59.893	T59.894	—	—
phophorated	T60.0X1	T60.0X2	T60.0X3	T60.0X4	—	—
sulfate	T57.8X1	T57.8X2	T57.8X3	T57.8X4	—	—

TABLE OF DRUGS AND CHEMICALS

Substance	External Cause (T-Code)					
	Poisoning, Accidental (Unintentional)	Poisoning, Intentional Self-Harm	Poisoning, Assault	Poisoning, Undetermined	Adverse Effect	Underdosing
Hexahydrocresol(s) *(Continued)*						
sulfide (gas)	T59.6X1	T59.6X2	T59.6X3	T59.6X4	—	—
arseniurated	T57.0X1	T57.0X2	T57.0X3	T57.0X4	—	—
sulfurated	T57.8X1	T57.8X2	T57.8X3	T57.8X4	—	—
Hexahydrophenol	T51.8X1	T51.8X2	T51.8X3	T51.8X4	—	—
Hexa-germ	T49.2X1	T49.2X2	T49.2X3	T49.2X4	T49.2X5	T49.2X6
Hexalen	T51.8X1	T51.8X2	T51.8X3	T51.8X4	—	—
Hexamethonium bromide	T44.2X1	T44.2X2	T44.2X3	T44.2X4	T44.2X5	T44.2X6
Hexamethylene	T52.8X1	T52.8X2	T52.8X3	T52.8X4	—	—
Hexamethylmelamine	T45.1X1	T45.1X2	T45.1X3	T45.1X4	T45.1X5	T45.1X6
Hexamidine	T49.0X1	T49.0X2	T49.0X3	T49.0X4	T49.0X5	T49.0X6
Hexamine (mandelate)	T37.8X1	T37.8X2	T37.8X3	T37.8X4	T37.8X5	T37.8X6
Hexanone, 2-hexanone	T52.4X1	T52.4X2	T52.4X3	T52.4X4	—	—
Hexanuorenium	T48.1X1	T48.1X2	T48.1X3	T48.1X4	T48.1X5	T48.1X6
Hexapropymate	T42.6X1	T42.6X2	T42.6X3	T42.6X4	T42.6X5	T42.6X6
Hexasonium iodide	T44.3X1	T44.3X2	T44.3X3	T44.3X4	T44.3X5	T44.3X6
Hexcarbacholine bromide	T48.1X1	T48.1X2	T48.1X3	T48.1X4	T48.1X5	T48.1X6
Hexemal	T42.3X1	T42.3X2	T42.3X3	T42.3X4	T42.3X5	T42.3X6
Hexestrol	T38.5X1	T38.5X2	T38.5X3	T38.5X4	T38.5X5	T38.5X6
Hexethal (sodium)	T42.3X1	T42.3X2	T42.3X3	T42.3X4	T42.3X5	T42.3X6
Hexetidine	T37.8X1	T37.8X2	T37.8X3	T37.8X4	T37.8X5	T37.8X6
Hexobarbital	T42.3X1	T42.3X2	T42.3X3	T42.3X4	T42.3X5	T42.3X6
rectal	T41.291	T41.292	T41.293	T41.294	T41.295	T41.296
sodium	T41.1X1	T41.1X2	T41.1X3	T41.1X4	T41.1X5	T41.1X6
Hexobendine	T46.3X1	T46.3X2	T46.3X3	T46.3X4	T46.3X5	T46.3X6
Hexocyclium	T44.3X1	T44.3X2	T44.3X3	T44.3X4	T44.3X5	T44.3X6
metilsulfate	T44.3X1	T44.3X2	T44.3X3	T44.3X4	T44.3X5	T44.3X6
Hexoestrol	T38.5X1	T38.5X2	T38.5X3	T38.5X4	T38.5X5	T38.5X6
Hexone	T52.4X1	T52.4X2	T52.4X3	T52.4X4	—	—
Hexoprenaline	T48.6X1	T48.6X2	T48.6X3	T48.6X4	T48.6X5	T48.6X6
Hexylcaine	T41.3X1	T41.3X2	T41.3X3	T41.3X4	T41.3X5	T41.3X6
Hexylresorcinol	T52.2X1	T52.2X2	T52.2X3	T52.2X4	—	—
HGH (human growth hormone)	T38.811	T38.812	T38.813	T38.814	T38.815	T38.816
Hinkle's pills	T47.2X1	T47.2X2	T47.2X3	T47.2X4	T47.2X5	T47.2X6
Histalog	T50.8X1	T50.8X2	T50.8X3	T50.8X4	T50.8X5	T50.8X6
Histamine (phosphate)	T50.8X1	T50.8X2	T50.8X3	T50.8X4	T50.8X5	T50.8X6
Histoplasmin	T50.8X1	T50.8X2	T50.8X3	T50.8X4	T50.8X5	T50.8X6
Holly berries	T62.2X1	T62.2X2	T62.2X3	T62.2X4	—	—
Homatropine	T44.3X1	T44.3X2	T44.3X3	T44.3X4	T44.3X5	T44.3X6
methylbromide	T44.3X1	T44.3X2	T44.3X3	T44.3X4	T44.3X5	T44.3X6

◀ New ◀▥ Revised ~~deleted~~ Deleted

Substance	Poisoning, Accidental (Unintentional)	Poisoning, Intentional Self-Harm	Poisoning, Assault	Poisoning, Undetermined	Adverse Effect	Underdosing
Homochlorcyclizine	T45.0X1	T45.0X2	T45.0X3	T45.0X4	T45.0X5	T45.0X6
Homosalate	T49.3X1	T49.3X2	T49.3X3	T49.3X4	T49.3X5	T49.3X6
Homo-tet	T50.Z11	T50.Z12	T50.Z13	T50.Z14	T50.Z15	T50.Z16
Hormone	T38.801	T38.802	T38.803	T38.804	T38.805	T38.806
adrenal cortical steroids	T38.0X1	T38.0X2	T38.0X3	T38.0X4	T38.0X5	T38.0X6
androgenic	T38.7X1	T38.7X2	T38.7X3	T38.7X4	T38.7X5	T38.7X6
anterior pituitary NEC	T38.811	T38.812	T38.813	T38.814	T38.815	T38.816
antidiabetic agents	T38.3X1	T38.3X2	T38.3X3	T38.3X4	T38.3X5	T38.3X6
antidiuretic	T38.891	T38.892	T38.893	T38.894	T38.895	T38.896
cancer therapy	T45.1X1	T45.1X2	T45.1X3	T45.1X4	T45.1X5	T45.1X6
follicle stimulating	T38.811	T38.812	T38.813	T38.814	T38.815	T38.816
gonadotropic	T38.891	T38.892	T38.893	T38.894	T38.895	T38.896
pituitary	T38.811	T38.812	T38.813	T38.814	T38.815	T38.816
growth	T38.811	T38.812	T38.813	T38.814	T38.815	T38.816
luteinizing	T38.811	T38.812	T38.813	T38.814	T38.815	T38.816
ovarian	T38.5X1	T38.5X2	T38.5X3	T38.5X4	T38.5X5	T38.5X6
oxytocic	T48.0X1	T48.0X2	T48.0X3	T48.0X4	T48.0X5	T48.0X6
parathyroid (derivatives)	T50.991	T50.992	T50.993	T50.994	T50.995	T50.996
pituitary (posterior) NEC	T38.891	T38.892	T38.893	T38.894	T38.895	T38.896
anterior	T38.811	T38.812	T38.813	T38.814	T38.815	T38.816
specified, NEC	T38.891	T38.892	T38.893	T38.894	T38.895	T38.896
thyroid	T38.1X1	T38.1X2	T38.1X3	T38.1X4	T38.1X5	T38.1X6
Hornet (sting)	T63.451	T63.452	T63.453	T63.454	—	—
Horse anti-human lymphocytic serum	T50.Z11	T50.Z12	T50.Z13	T50.Z14	T50.Z15	T50.Z16
Horticulture agent NEC	T65.91	T65.92	T65.93	T65.94	—	—
with pesticide	T60.91	T60.92	T60.93	T60.94	—	—
Human						
albumin	T45.8X1	T45.8X2	T45.8X3	T45.8X4	T45.8X5	T45.8X6
growth hormone (HGH)	T38.811	T38.812	T38.813	T38.814	T38.815	T38.816
immune serum	T50.Z11	T50.Z12	T50.Z13	T50.Z14	T50.Z15	T50.Z16
Hyaluronidase	T45.3X1	T45.3X2	T45.3X3	T45.3X4	T45.3X5	T45.3X6
Hyazyme	T45.3X1	T45.3X2	T45.3X3	T45.3X4	T45.3X5	T45.3X6
Hycodan	T40.2X1	T40.2X2	T40.2X3	T40.2X4	T40.2X5	T40.2X6
Hydantoin derivative NEC	T42.0X1	T42.0X2	T42.0X3	T42.0X4	T42.0X5	T42.0X6
Hydeltra	T38.0X1	T38.0X2	T38.0X3	T38.0X4	T38.0X5	T38.0X6
Hydergine	T44.6X1	T44.6X2	T44.6X3	T44.6X4	T44.6X5	T44.6X6
Hydrabamine penicillin	T36.0X1	T36.0X2	T36.0X3	T36.0X4	T36.0X5	T36.0X6
Hydralazine	T46.5X1	T46.5X2	T46.5X3	T46.5X4	T46.5X5	T46.5X6
Hydrargaphen	T49.0X1	T49.0X2	T49.0X3	T49.0X4	T49.0X5	T49.0X6

◀ New ◀▥ Revised deleted Deleted

Substance	External Cause (T-Code)					
	Poisoning, Accidental (Unintentional)	Poisoning, Intentional Self-Harm	Poisoning, Assault	Poisoning, Undetermined	Adverse Effect	Underdosing
Hydrargyri amino-chloridum	T49.0X1	T49.0X2	T49.0X3	T49.0X4	T49.0X5	T49.0X6
Hydrastine	T48.291	T48.292	T48.293	T48.294	T48.295	T48.296
Hydrazine	T54.1X1	T54.1X2	T54.1X3	T54.1X4	—	—
monoamine oxidase inhibitors	T43.1X1	T43.1X2	T43.1X3	T43.1X4	T43.1X5	T43.1X6
Hydrazoic acid, azides	T54.2X1	T54.2X2	T54.2X3	T54.2X4		
Hydriodic acid	T48.4X1	T48.4X2	T48.4X3	T48.4X4	T48.4X5	T48.4X6
Hydrocarbon gas	T59.891	T59.892	T59.893	T59.894	—	—
incomplete combustion of — see Carbon, monoxide, fuel, utility						
liquefied (mobile container)	T59.891	T59.892	T59.893	T59.894	—	—
piped (natural)	T59.891	T59.892	T59.893	T59.894	—	—
Hydrochloric acid (liquid)	T54.2X1	T54.2X2	T54.2X3	T54.2X4		—
medicinal (digestant)	T47.5X1	T47.5X2	T47.5X3	T47.5X4	T47.5X5	T47.5X6
vapor	T59.891	T59.892	T59.893	T59.894	—	—
Hydrochlorothiazide	T50.2X1	T50.2X2	T50.2X3	T50.2X4	T50.2X5	T50.2X6
Hydrocodone	T40.2X1	T40.2X2	T40.2X3	T40.2X4	T40.2X5	T40.2X6
Hydrocortisone (derivatives)	T49.0X1	T49.0X2	T49.0X3	T49.0X4	T49.0X5	T49.0X6
aceponate	T49.0X1	T49.0X2	T49.0X3	T49.0X4	T49.0X5	T49.0X6
ENT agent	T49.6X1	T49.6X2	T49.6X3	T49.6X4	T49.6X5	T49.6X6
ophthalmic preparation	T49.5X1	T49.5X2	T49.5X3	T49.5X4	T49.5X5	T49.5X6
topical NEC	T49.0X1	T49.0X2	T49.0X3	T49.0X4	T49.0X5	T49.0X6
Hydrocortone	T38.0X1	T38.0X2	T38.0X3	T38.0X4	T38.0X5	T38.0X6
ENT agent	T49.6X1	T49.6X2	T49.6X3	T49.6X4	T49.6X5	T49.6X6
ophthalmic preparation	T49.5X1	T49.5X2	T49.5X3	T49.5X4	T49.5X5	T49.5X6
topical NEC	T49.0X1	T49.0X2	T49.0X3	T49.0X4	T49.0X5	T49.0X6
Hydrocyanic acid (liquid)	T57.3X1	T57.3X2	T57.3X3	T57.3X4	—	—
gas	T65.0X1	T65.0X2	T65.0X3	T65.0X4	—	—
Hydroflumethiazide	T50.2X1	T50.2X2	T50.2X3	T50.2X4	T50.2X5	T50.2X6
Hydrofluoric acid (liquid)	T54.2X1	T54.2X2	T54.2X3	T54.2X4	—	—
vapor	T59.891	T59.892	T59.893	T59.894	—	—
Hydrogen	T59.891	T59.892	T59.893	T59.894	—	—
arsenide	T57.0X1	T57.0X2	T57.0X3	T57.0X4	—	—
arseniureted	T57.0X1	T57.0X2	T57.0X3	T57.0X4	—	—
chloride	T57.8X1	T57.8X2	T57.8X3	T57.8X4	—	—
cyanide (salts)	T57.3X1	T57.3X2	T57.3X3	T57.3X4	—	—
gas	T57.3X1	T57.3X2	T57.3X3	T57.3X4	—	—
Fluoride	T59.5X1	T59.5X2	T59.5X3	T59.5X4	—	—
vapor	T59.5X1	T59.5X2	T59.5X3	T59.5X4	—	—
peroxide	T49.0X1	T49.0X2	T49.0X3	T49.0X4	T49.0X5	T49.0X6
phosphureted	T57.1X1	T57.1X2	T57.1X3	T57.1X4	—	—

◀ New ◀ Revised ~~deleted~~ Deleted

Substance	External Cause (T-Code)					
	Poisoning, Accidental (Unintentional)	Poisoning, Intentional Self-Harm	Poisoning, Assault	Poisoning, Undetermined	Adverse Effect	Underdosing
Hydrogen *(Continued)*						
sulfide	T59.6X1	T59.6X2	T59.6X3	T59.6X4	—	—
arseniureted	T57.0X1	T57.0X2	T57.0X3	T57.0X4	—	—
sulfureted	T59.6X1	T59.6X2	T59.6X3	T59.6X4	—	—
Hydromethylpyridine	T46.7X1	T46.7X2	T46.7X3	T46.7X4	T46.7X5	T46.7X6
Hydromorphinol	T40.2X1	T40.2X2	T40.2X3	T40.2X4	—	—
Hydromorphinone	T40.2X1	T40.2X2	T40.2X3	T40.2X4	T40.2X5	T40.2X6
Hydromorphone	T40.2X1	T40.2X2	T40.2X3	T40.2X4	T40.2X5	T40.2X6
Hydromox	T50.2X1	T50.2X2	T50.2X3	T50.2X4	T50.2X5	T50.2X6
Hydrophilic lotion	T49.3X1	T49.3X2	T49.3X3	T49.3X4	T49.3X5	T49.3X6
Hydroquinidine	T46.2X1	T46.2X2	T46.2X3	T46.2X4	T46.2X5	T46.2X6
Hydroquinone	T52.2X1	T52.2X2	T52.2X3	T52.2X4	—	—
vapor	T59.891	T59.892	T59.893	T59.894	—	—
Hydrosulfuric acid (gas)	T59.6X1	T59.6X2	T59.6X3	T59.6X4	—	—
Hydrotalcite	T47.1X1	T47.1X2	T47.1X3	T47.1X4	T47.1X5	T47.1X6
Hydrous wool fat	T49.3X1	T49.3X2	T49.3X3	T49.3X4	T49.3X5	T49.3X6
Hydroxide, caustic	T54.3X1	T54.3X2	T54.3X3	T54.3X4	—	—
Hydroxocobalamin	T45.8X1	T45.8X2	T45.8X3	T45.8X4	T45.8X5	T45.8X6
Hydroxyamphetamine	T49.5X1	T49.5X2	T49.5X3	T49.5X4	T49.5X5	T49.5X6
Hydroxycarbamide	T45.1X1	T45.1X2	T45.1X3	T45.1X4	T45.1X5	T45.1X6
Hydroxychloroquine	T37.8X1	T37.8X2	T37.8X3	T37.8X4	T37.8X5	T37.8X6
Hydroxydihydrocodeinone	T40.2X1	T40.2X2	T40.2X3	T40.2X4	T40.2X5	T40.2X6
Hydroxyestrone	T38.5X1	T38.5X2	T38.5X3	T38.5X4	T38.5X5	T38.5X6
Hydroxyethyl starch	T45.8X1	T45.8X2	T45.8X3	T45.8X4	T45.8X5	T45.8X6
Hydroxymethylpentanone	T52.4X1	T52.4X2	T52.4X3	T52.4X4	—	—
Hydroxyphenamate	T43.591	T43.592	T43.593	T43.594	T43.595	T43.596
Hydroxyphenylbutazone	T39.2X1	T39.2X2	T39.2X3	T39.2X4	T39.2X5	T39.2X6
Hydroxyprogesterone	T38.5X1	T38.5X2	T38.5X3	T38.5X4	T38.5X5	T38.5X6
caproate	T38.5X1	T38.5X2	T38.5X3	T38.5X4	T38.5X5	T38.5X6
Hydroxyquinoline (derivatives) NEC	T37.8X1	T37.8X2	T37.8X3	T37.8X4	T37.8X5	T37.8X6
Hydroxystilbamidine	T37.3X1	T37.3X2	T37.3X3	T37.3X4	T37.3X5	T37.3X6
Hydroxytoluene (nonmedicinal)	T54.0X1	T54.0X2	T54.0X3	T54.0X4	—	—
medicinal	T49.0X1	T49.0X2	T49.0X3	T49.0X4	T49.0X5	T49.0X6
Hydroxyurea	T45.1X1	T45.1X2	T45.1X3	T45.1X4	T45.1X5	T45.1X6
Hydroxyzine	T43.591	T43.592	T43.593	T43.594	T43.595	T43.596
Hyoscine	T44.3X1	T44.3X2	T44.3X3	T44.3X4	T44.3X5	T44.3X6
Hyoscyamine	T44.3X1	T44.3X2	T44.3X3	T44.3X4	T44.3X5	T44.3X6
Hyoscyamus	T44.3X1	T44.3X2	T44.3X3	T44.3X4	T44.3X5	T44.3X6
dry extract	T44.3X1	T44.3X2	T44.3X3	T44.3X4	T44.3X5	T44.3X6

◀ New ◀═ Revised ~~deleted~~ Deleted

TABLE OF DRUGS AND CHEMICALS

Substance	External Cause (T-Code)					
	Poisoning, Accidental (Unintentional)	Poisoning, Intentional Self-Harm	Poisoning, Assault	Poisoning, Undetermined	Adverse Effect	Underdosing
Hypaque	T50.8X1	T50.8X2	T50.8X3	T50.8X4	T50.8X5	T50.8X6
Hypertussis	T50.Z11	T50.Z12	T50.Z13	T50.Z14	T50.Z15	T50.Z16
Hypnotic	T42.71	T42.72	T42.73	T42.74	T42.75	T42.76
anticonvulsant	T42.71	T42.72	T42.73	T42.74	T42.75	T42.76
specified NEC	T42.6X1	T42.6X2	T42.6X3	T42.6X4	T42.6X5	T42.6X6
Hypochlorite	T49.0X1	T49.0X2	T49.0X3	T49.0X4	T49.0X5	T49.0X6
Hypophysis, posterior	T38.891	T38.892	T38.893	T38.894	T38.895	T38.896
Hypotensive NEC	T46.5X1	T46.5X2	T46.5X3	T46.5X4	T46.5X5	T46.5X6
Hypromellose	T49.5X1	T49.5X2	T49.5X3	T49.5X4	T49.5X5	T49.5X6
I						
Ibacitabine	T37.5X1	T37.5X2	T37.5X3	T37.5X4	T37.5X5	T37.5X6
Ibopamine	T44.991	T44.992	T44.993	T44.994	T44.995	T44.996
Ibufenac	T39.311	T39.312	T39.313	T39.314	T39.315	T39.316
Ibuprofen	T39.311	T39.312	T39.313	T39.314	T39.315	T39.316
Ibuproxam	T39.311	T39.312	T39.313	T39.314	T39.315	T39.316
Ibuterol	T48.6X1	T48.6X2	T48.6X3	T48.6X4	T48.6X5	T48.6X6
Ichthammol	T49.0X1	T49.0X2	T49.0X3	T49.0X4	T49.0X5	T49.0X6
Ichthyol	T49.4X1	T49.4X2	T49.4X3	T49.4X4	T49.4X5	T49.4X6
Idarubicin	T45.1X1	T45.1X2	T45.1X3	T45.1X4	T45.1X5	T45.1X6
Idrocilamide	T42.8X1	T42.8X2	T42.8X3	T42.8X4	T42.8X5	T42.8X6
Ifenprodil	T46.7X1	T46.7X2	T46.7X3	T46.7X4	T46.7X5	T46.7X6
Ifosfamide	T45.1X1	T45.1X2	T45.1X3	T45.1X4	T45.1X5	T45.1X6
Iletin	T38.3X1	T38.3X2	T38.3X3	T38.3X4	T38.3X5	T38.3X6
Ilex	T62.2X1	T62.2X2	T62.2X3	T62.2X4	—	—
Illuminating gas (after combustion)	T58.11	T58.12	T58.13	T58.14	—	—
prior to combustion	T59.891	T59.892	T59.893	T59.894	—	—
Ilopan	T45.2X1	T45.2X2	T45.2X3	T45.2X4	T45.2X5	T45.2X6
Iloprost	T46.7X1	T46.7X2	T46.7X3	T46.7X4	T46.7X5	T46.7X6
Ilotycin	T36.3X1	T36.3X2	T36.3X3	T36.3X4	T36.3X5	T36.3X6
ophthalmic preparation	T49.5X1	T49.5X2	T49.5X3	T49.5X4	T49.5X5	T49.5X6
topical NEC	T49.0X1	T49.0X2	T49.0X3	T49.0X4	T49.0X5	T49.0X6
Imidazole-4-carboxamide	T45.1X1	T45.1X2	T45.1X3	T45.1X4	T45.1X5	T45.1X6
Imipenem	T36.0X1	T36.0X2	T36.0X3	T36.0X4	T36.0X5	T36.0X6
Imipramine	T43.011	T43.012	T43.013	T43.014	T43.015	T43.016
Iminostilbene	T42.1X1	T42.1X2	T42.1X3	T42.1X4	T42.1X5	T42.1X6
Immu-G	T50.Z11	T50.Z12	T50.Z13	T50.Z14	T50.Z15	T50.Z16
Immuglobin	T50.Z11	T50.Z12	T50.Z13	T50.Z14	T50.Z15	T50.Z16
Immune						
globulin	T50.Z11	T50.Z12	T50.Z13	T50.Z14	T50.Z15	T50.Z16
serum globulin	T50.Z11	T50.Z12	T50.Z13	T50.Z14	T50.Z15	T50.Z16

◀ New   ◀||| Revised   ~~deleted~~ Deleted

| | External Cause (T-Code) | | | | | |
Substance	Poisoning, Accidental (Unintentional)	Poisoning, Intentional Self-Harm	Poisoning, Assault	Poisoning, Undetermined	Adverse Effect	Underdosing
Immunoglobin human (intravenous) (normal)	T50.Z11	T50.Z12	T50.Z13	T50.Z14	T50.Z15	T50.Z16
unmodified	T50.Z11	T50.Z12	T50.Z13	T50.Z14	T50.Z15	T50.Z16
Immunosuppressive drug	T45.1X1	T45.1X2	T45.1X3	T45.1X4	T45.1X5	T45.1X6
Immu-tetanus	T50.Z11	T50.Z12	T50.Z13	T50.Z14	T50.Z15	T50.Z16
Indalpine	T43.221	T43.222	T43.223	T43.224	T43.225	T43.226
Indanazoline	T48.5X1	T48.5X2	T48.5X3	T48.5X4	T48.5X5	T48.5X6
Indandione (derivatives)	T45.511	T45.512	T45.513	T45.514	T45.515	T45.516
Indapamide	T46.5X1	T46.5X2	T46.5X3	T46.5X4	T46.5X5	T46.5X6
Indendione (derivatives)	T45.511	T45.512	T45.513	T45.514	T45.515	T45.516
Indenolol	T44.7X1	T44.7X2	T44.7X3	T44.7X4	T44.7X5	T44.7X6
Inderal	T44.7X1	T44.7X2	T44.7X3	T44.7X4	T44.7X5	T44.7X6
Indian						
hemp	T40.7X1	T40.7X2	T40.7X3	T40.7X4	T40.7X5	T40.7X6
tobacco	T62.2X1	T62.2X2	T62.2X3	T62.2X4	—	—
Indigo carmine	T50.8X1	T50.8X2	T50.8X3	T50.8X4	T50.8X5	T50.8X6
Indobufen	T45.521	T45.522	T45.523	T45.524	T45.525	T45.526
Indocin	T39.2X1	T39.2X2	T39.2X3	T39.2X4	T39.2X5	T39.2X6
Indocyanine green	T50.8X1	T50.8X2	T50.8X3	T50.8X4	T50.8X5	T50.8X6
Indometacin	T39.391	T39.392	T39.393	T39.394	T39.395	T39.396
Indomethacin	T39.391	T39.392	T39.393	T39.394	T39.395	T39.396
farnesil	T39.4X1	T39.4X2	T39.4X3	T39.4X4	T39.4X5	T39.4X6
Indoramin	T44.6X1	T44.6X2	T44.6X3	T44.6X4	T44.6X5	T44.6X6
Industrial						
alcohol	T51.0X1	T51.0X2	T51.0X3	T51.0X4	—	—
fumes	T59.891	T59.892	T59.893	T59.894	—	—
solvents (fumes) (vapors)	T52.91	T52.92	T52.93	T52.94	—	—
Influenza vaccine	T50.B91	T50.B92	T50.B93	T50.B94	T50.B95	T50.B96
Ingested substance NEC	T65.91	T65.92	T65.93	T65.94		
INH	T37.1X1	T37.1X2	T37.1X3	T37.1X4	T37.1X5	T37.1X6
Inhalation, gas (noxious) — see Gas						
Inhibitor						
angiotensin-converting enzyme	T46.4X1	T46.4X2	T46.4X3	T46.4X4	T46.4X5	T46.4X6
carbonic anhydrase	T50.2X1	T50.2X2	T50.2X3	T50.2X4	T50.2X5	T50.2X6
fibrinolysis	T45.621	T45.622	T45.623	T45.624	T45.625	T45.626
monoamine oxidase NEC	T43.1X1	T43.1X2	T43.1X3	T43.1X4	T43.1X5	T43.1X6
hydrazine	T43.1X1	T43.1X2	T43.1X3	T43.1X4	T43.1X5	T43.1X6
postsynaptic	T43.8X1	T43.8X2	T43.8X3	T43.8X4	T43.8X5	T43.8X6
prothrombin synthesis	T45.511	T45.512	T45.513	T45.514	T45.515	T45.516
Ink	T65.891	T65.892	T65.893	T65.894	—	—
Inorganic substance NEC	T57.91	T57.92	T57.93	T57.94	—	—

Substance	External Cause (T-Code)					
	Poisoning, Accidental (Unintentional)	Poisoning, Intentional Self-Harm	Poisoning, Assault	Poisoning, Undetermined	Adverse Effect	Underdosing
Inosine pranobex	T37.5X1	T37.5X2	T37.5X3	T37.5X4	T37.5X5	T37.5X6
Inositol	T50.991	T50.992	T50.993	T50.994	T50.995	T50.996
nicotinate	T46.7X1	T46.7X2	T46.7X3	T46.7X4	T46.7X5	T46.7X6
Inproquone	T45.1X1	T45.1X2	T45.1X3	T45.1X4	T45.1X5	T45.1X6
Insect (sting), venomous	T63.481	T63.482	T63.483	T63.484	—	—
ant	T63.421	T63.422	T63.423	T63.424	—	—
bee	T63.441	T63.442	T63.443	T63.444	—	—
caterpillar	T63.431	T63.432	T63.433	T63.434	—	—
hornet	T63.451	T63.452	T63.453	T63.454	—	—
wasp	T63.461	T63.462	T63.463	T63.464	—	—
Insecticide NEC	T60.91	T60.92	T60.93	T60.94	—	—
carbamate	T60.0X1	T60.0X2	T60.0X3	T60.0X4	—	—
chlorinated	T60.1X1	T60.1X2	T60.1X3	T60.1X4	—	—
mixed	T60.91	T60.92	T60.93	T60.94	—	—
organochlorine	T60.1X1	T60.1X2	T60.1X3	T60.1X4	—	—
organophosphorus	T60.0X1	T60.0X2	T60.0X3	T60.0X4	—	—
Insular tissue extract	T38.3X1	T38.3X2	T38.3X3	T38.3X4	T38.3X5	T38.3X6
Insulin (amorphous) (globin) (isophane) (Lente) (NPH) (Semilente) (Ultralente)	T38.3X1	T38.3X2	T38.3X3	T38.3X4	T38.3X5	T38.3X6
defalan	T38.3X1	T38.3X2	T38.3X3	T38.3X4	T38.3X5	T38.3X6
human	T38.3X1	T38.3X2	T38.3X3	T38.3X4	T38.3X5	T38.3X6
injection, soluble	T38.3X1	T38.3X2	T38.3X3	T38.3X4	T38.3X5	T38.3X6
biphasic	T38.3X1	T38.3X2	T38.3X3	T38.3X4	T38.3X5	T38.3X6
intermediate acting	T38.3X1	T38.3X2	T38.3X3	T38.3X4	T38.3X5	T38.3X6
protamine zinc	T38.3X1	T38.3X2	T38.3X3	T38.3X4	T38.3X5	T38.3X6
slow acting	T38.3X1	T38.3X2	T38.3X3	T38.3X4	T38.3X5	T38.3X6
zinc						
protamine injection	T38.3X1	T38.3X2	T38.3X3	T38.3X4	T38.3X5	T38.3X6
suspension (amorphous) (crystalline)	T38.3X1	T38.3X2	T38.3X3	T38.3X4	T38.3X5	T38.3X6
Interferon (alpha) (beta) (gamma)	T37.5X1	T37.5X2	T37.5X3	T37.5X4	T37.5X5	T37.5X6
Intestinal motility control drug	T47.6X1	T47.6X2	T47.6X3	T47.6X4	T47.6X5	T47.6X6
biological	T47.8X1	T47.8X2	T47.8X3	T47.8X4	T47.8X5	T47.8X6
Intranarcon	T41.1X1	T41.1X2	T41.1X3	T41.1X4	T41.1X5	T41.1X6
Intravenous						
amino acids	T50.991	T50.992	T50.993	T50.994	T50.995	T50.996
fat suspension	T50.991	T50.992	T50.993	T50.994	T50.995	T50.996
Inulin	T50.8X1	T50.8X2	T50.8X3	T50.8X4	T50.8X5	T50.8X6
Invert sugar	T50.3X1	T50.3X2	T50.3X3	T50.3X4	T50.3X5	T50.3X6
Inza — *see Naproxen*						
Iobenzamic acid	T50.8X1	T50.8X2	T50.8X3	T50.8X4	T50.8X5	T50.8X6
Iocarmic acid	T50.8X1	T50.8X2	T50.8X3	T50.8X4	T50.8X5	T50.8X6

◀ New ◀▪▪ Revised ~~deleted~~ Deleted

Substance	External Cause (T-Code)					
	Poisoning, Accidental (Unintentional)	Poisoning, Intentional Self-Harm	Poisoning, Assault	Poisoning, Undetermined	Adverse Effect	Underdosing
Iocetamic acid	T50.8X1	T50.8X2	T50.8X3	T50.8X4	T50.8X5	T50.8X6
Iodamide	T50.8X1	T50.8X2	T50.8X3	T50.8X4	T50.8X5	T50.8X6
Iodide NEC—see also Iodine	T49.0X1	T49.0X2	T49.0X3	T49.0X4	T49.0X5	T49.0X6
mercury (ointment)	T49.0X1	T49.0X2	T49.0X3	T49.0X4	T49.0X5	T49.0X6
methylate	T49.0X1	T49.0X2	T49.0X3	T49.0X4	T49.0X5	T49.0X6
potassium (expectorant) NEC	T48.4X1	T48.4X2	T48.4X3	T48.4X4	T48.4X5	T48.4X6
Iodinated						
contrast medium	T50.8X1	T50.8X2	T50.8X3	T50.8X4	T50.8X5	T50.8X6
glycerol	T48.4X1	T48.4X2	T48.4X3	T48.4X4	T48.4X5	T48.4X6
human serum albumin (131I)	T50.8X1	T50.8X2	T50.8X3	T50.8X4	T50.8X5	T50.8X6
Iodine (antiseptic, external) (tincture) NEC	T49.0X1	T49.0X2	T49.0X3	T49.0X4	T49.0X5	T49.0X6
125—see also Radiation sickness, and Exposure to radioactivce isotopes	T50.8X1	T50.8X2	T50.8X3	T50.8X4	T50.8X5	T50.8X6
therapeutic	T50.991	T50.992	T50.993	T50.994	T50.995	T50.996
131—see also Radiation sickness, and Exposure to radioactivce isotopes	T50.8X1	T50.8X2	T50.8X3	T50.8X4	T50.8X5	T50.8X6
therapeutic	T38.2X1	T38.2X2	T38.2X3	T38.2X4	T38.2X5	T38.2X6
diagnostic	T50.8X1	T50.8X2	T50.8X3	T50.8X4	T50.8X5	T50.8X6
for thyroid conditions (antithyroid)	T38.2X1	T38.2X2	T38.2X3	T38.2X4	T38.2X5	T38.2X6
solution	T49.0X1	T49.0X2	T49.0X3	T49.0X4	T49.0X5	T49.0X6
vapor	T59.891	T59.892	T59.893	T59.894	—	—
Iodipamide	T50.8X1	T50.8X2	T50.8X3	T50.8X4	T50.8X5	T50.8X6
Iodized (poppy seed) oil	T50.8X1	T50.8X2	T50.8X3	T50.8X4	T50.8X5	T50.8X6
Iodobismitol	T37.8X1	T37.8X2	T37.8X3	T37.8X4	T37.8X5	T37.8X6
Iodochlorhydroxyquin	T37.8X1	T37.8X2	T37.8X3	T37.8X4	T37.8X5	T37.8X6
topical	T49.0X1	T49.0X2	T49.0X3	T49.0X4	T49.0X5	T49.0X6
Iodochlorhydroxyquino-line	T37.8X1	T37.8X2	T37.8X3	T37.8X4	T37.8X5	T37.8X6
Iodocholesterol (131I)	T50.8X1	T50.8X2	T50.8X3	T50.8X4	T50.8X5	T50.8X6
Iodoform	T49.0X1	T49.0X2	T49.0X3	T49.0X4	T49.0X5	T49.0X6
Iodohippuric acid	T50.8X1	T50.8X2	T50.8X3	T50.8X4	T50.8X5	T50.8X6
Iodopanoic acid	T50.8X1	T50.8X2	T50.8X3	T50.8X4	T50.8X5	T50.8X6
Iodophthalein (sodium)	T50.8X1	T50.8X2	T50.8X3	T50.8X4	T50.8X5	T50.8X6
Iodopyracet	T50.8X1	T50.8X2	T50.8X3	T50.8X4	T50.8X5	T50.8X6
Iodoquinol	T37.8X1	T37.8X2	T37.8X3	T37.8X4	T37.8X5	T37.8X6
Iodoxamic acid	T50.8X1	T50.8X2	T50.8X3	T50.8X4	T50.8X5	T50.8X6
Iofendylate	T50.8X1	T50.8X2	T50.8X3	T50.8X4	T50.8X5	T50.8X6
Ioglycamic acid	T50.8X1	T50.8X2	T50.8X3	T50.8X4	T50.8X5	T50.8X6
Iohexol	T50.8X1	T50.8X2	T50.8X3	T50.8X4	T50.8X5	T50.8X6
Ion exchange resin						
anion	T47.8X1	T47.8X2	T47.8X3	T47.8X4	T47.8X5	T47.8X6
cation	T50.3X1	T50.3X2	T50.3X3	T50.3X4	T50.3X5	T50.3X6

◀ New ◀|||| Revised ~~deleted~~ Deleted

Substance	External Cause (T-Code)					
	Poisoning, Accidental (Unintentional)	Poisoning, Intentional Self-Harm	Poisoning, Assault	Poisoning, Undetermined	Adverse Effect	Underdosing
Ion exchange resin *(Continued)*						
cholestyramine	T46.6X1	T46.6X2	T46.6X3	T46.6X4	T46.6X5	T46.6X6
intestinal	T47.8X1	T47.8X2	T47.8X3	T47.8X4	T47.8X5	T47.8X6
Iopamidol	T50.8X1	T50.8X2	T50.8X3	T50.8X4	T50.8X5	T50.8X6
Iopanoic acid	T50.8X1	T50.8X2	T50.8X3	T50.8X4	T50.8X5	T50.8X6
Iophenoic acid	T50.8X1	T50.8X2	T50.8X3	T50.8X4	T50.8X5	T50.8X6
Iopodate, sodium	T50.8X1	T50.8X2	T50.8X3	T50.8X4	T50.8X5	T50.8X6
Iopodic acid	T50.8X1	T50.8X2	T50.8X3	T50.8X4	T50.8X5	T50.8X6
Iopromide	T50.8X1	T50.8X2	T50.8X3	T50.8X4	T50.8X5	T50.8X6
Iopydol	T50.8X1	T50.8X2	T50.8X3	T50.8X4	T50.8X5	T50.8X6
Iotalamic acid	T50.8X1	T50.8X2	T50.8X3	T50.8X4	T50.8X5	T50.8X6
Iothalamate	T50.8X1	T50.8X2	T50.8X3	T50.8X4	T50.8X5	T50.8X6
Iothiouracil	T38.2X1	T38.2X2	T38.2X3	T38.2X4	T38.2X5	T38.2X6
Iotrol	T50.8X1	T50.8X2	T50.8X3	T50.8X4	T50.8X5	T50.8X6
Iotrolan	T50.8X1	T50.8X2	T50.8X3	T50.8X4	T50.8X5	T50.8X6
Iotroxate	T50.8X1	T50.8X2	T50.8X3	T50.8X4	T50.8X5	T50.8X6
Iotroxic acid	T50.8X1	T50.8X2	T50.8X3	T50.8X4	T50.8X5	T50.8X6
Ioversol	T50.8X1	T50.8X2	T50.8X3	T50.8X4	T50.8X5	T50.8X6
Ioxaglate	T50.8X1	T50.8X2	T50.8X3	T50.8X4	T50.8X5	T50.8X6
Ioxaglic acid	T50.8X1	T50.8X2	T50.8X3	T50.8X4	T50.8X5	T50.8X6
Ioxitalamic acid	T50.8X1	T50.8X2	T50.8X3	T50.8X4	T50.8X5	T50.8X6
Ipecac	T47.7X1	T47.7X2	T47.7X3	T47.7X4	T47.7X5	T47.7X6
Ipecacuanha	T48.4X1	T48.4X2	T48.4X3	T48.4X4	T48.4X5	T48.4X6
Ipodate, calcium	T50.8X1	T50.8X2	T50.8X3	T50.8X4	T50.8X5	T50.8X6
Ipral	T42.3X1	T42.3X2	T42.3X3	T42.3X4	T42.3X5	T42.3X6
Ipratropium (bromide)	T48.6X1	T48.6X2	T48.6X3	T48.6X4	T48.6X5	T48.6X6
Ipriflavone	T46.3X1	T46.3X2	T46.3X3	T46.3X4	T46.3X5	T46.3X6
Iprindole	T43.011	T43.012	T43.013	T43.014	T43.015	T43.016
Iproclozide	T43.1X1	T43.1X2	T43.1X3	T43.1X4	T43.1X5	T43.1X6
Iprofenin	T50.8X1	T50.8X2	T50.8X3	T50.8X4	T50.8X5	T50.8X6
Iproheptine	T49.2X1	T49.2X2	T49.2X3	T49.2X4	T49.2X5	T49.2X6
Iproniazid	T43.1X1	T43.1X2	T43.1X3	T43.1X4	T43.1X5	T43.1X6
Iproplatin	T45.1X1	T45.1X2	T45.1X3	T45.1X4	T45.1X5	T45.1X6
Iproveratril	T46.1X1	T46.1X2	T46.1X3	T46.1X4	T46.1X5	T46.1X6
Iron (compounds) (medicinal) NEC	T45.4X1	T45.4X2	T45.4X3	T45.4X4	T45.4X5	T45.4X6
ammonium	T45.4X1	T45.4X2	T45.4X3	T45.4X4	T45.4X5	T45.4X6
dextran injection	T45.4X1	T45.4X2	T45.4X3	T45.4X4	T45.4X5	T45.4X6
nonmedicinal	T56.891	T56.892	T56.893	T56.894	—	—

◀ New   ◀▥▥ Revised   ~~deleted~~ Deleted

Substance	External Cause (T-Code)					
	Poisoning, Accidental (Unintentional)	Poisoning, Intentional Self-Harm	Poisoning, Assault	Poisoning, Undetermined	Adverse Effect	Underdosing
Iron NEC *(Continued)*						
salts	T45.4X1	T45.4X2	T45.4X3	T45.4X4	T45.4X5	T45.4X6
sorbitex	T45.4X1	T45.4X2	T45.4X3	T45.4X4	T45.4X5	T45.4X6
sorbitol citric acid complex	T45.4X1	T45.4X2	T45.4X3	T45.4X4	T45.4X5	T45.4X6
Irrigating fluid (vaginal)	T49.8X1	T49.8X2	T49.8X3	T49.8X4	T49.8X5	T49.8X6
eye	T49.5X1	T49.5X2	T49.5X3	T49.5X4	T49.5X5	T49.5X6
Isepamicin	T36.5X1	T36.5X2	T36.5X3	T36.5X4	T36.5X5	T36.5X6
Isoaminile (citrate)	T48.3X1	T48.3X2	T48.3X3	T48.3X4	T48.3X5	T48.3X6
Isoamyl nitrite	T46.3X1	T46.3X2	T46.3X3	T46.3X4	T46.3X5	T46.3X6
Isobenzan	T60.1X1	T60.1X2	T60.1X3	T60.1X4	—	—
Isobutyl acetate	T52.8X1	T52.8X2	T52.8X3	T52.8X4	—	—
Isocarboxazid	T43.1X1	T43.1X2	T43.1X3	T43.1X4	T43.1X5	T43.1X6
Isoconazole	T49.0X1	T49.0X2	T49.0X3	T49.0X4	T49.0X5	T49.0X6
Isocyanate	T65.0X1	T65.0X2	T65.0X3	T65.0X4	—	—
Isoephedrine	T44.991	T44.992	T44.993	T44.994	T44.995	T44.996
Isoetarine	T48.6X1	T48.6X2	T48.6X3	T48.6X4	T48.6X5	T48.6X6
Isoethadione	T42.2X1	T42.2X2	T42.2X3	T42.2X4	T42.2X5	T42.2X6
Isoetharine	T44.5X1	T44.5X2	T44.5X3	T44.5X4	T44.5X5	T44.5X6
Isoflurane	T41.0X1	T41.0X2	T41.0X3	T41.0X4	T41.0X5	T41.0X6
Isoflurophate	T44.0X1	T44.0X2	T44.0X3	T44.0X4	T44.0X5	T44.0X6
Isomaltose, ferric complex	T45.4X1	T45.4X2	T45.4X3	T45.4X4	T45.4X5	T45.4X6
Isometheptene	T44.3X1	T44.3X2	T44.3X3	T44.3X4	T44.3X5	T44.3X6
Isoniazid	T37.1X1	T37.1X2	T37.1X3	T37.1X4	T37.1X5	T37.1X6
with						
rifampicin	T36.6X1	T36.6X2	T36.6X3	T36.6X4	T36.6X5	T36.6X6
thioacetazone	T37.1X1	T37.1X2	T37.1X3	T37.1X4	T37.1X5	T37.1X6
Isonicotinic acid hydrazide	T37.1X1	T37.1X2	T37.1X3	T37.1X4	T37.1X5	T37.1X6
Isonipecaine	T40.4X1	T40.4X2	T40.4X3	T40.4X4	T40.4X5	T40.4X6
Isopentaquine	T37.2X1	T37.2X2	T37.2X3	T37.2X4	T37.2X5	T37.2X6
Isophane insulin	T38.3X1	T38.3X2	T38.3X3	T38.3X4	T38.3X5	T38.3X6
Isophorone	T65.891	T65.892	T65.893	T65.894	—	—
Isophosphamide	T45.1X1	T45.1X2	T45.1X3	T45.1X4	T45.1X5	T45.1X6
Isopregnenone	T38.5X1	T38.5X2	T38.5X3	T38.5X4	T38.5X5	T38.5X6
Isoprenaline	T48.6X1	T48.6X2	T48.6X3	T48.6X4	T48.6X5	T48.6X6
Isopromethazine	T43.3X1	T43.3X2	T43.3X3	T43.3X4	T43.3X5	T43.3X6
Isopropamide	T44.3X1	T44.3X2	T44.3X3	T44.3X4	T44.3X5	T44.3X6
iodide	T44.3X1	T44.3X2	T44.3X3	T44.3X4	T44.3X5	T44.3X6
Isopropanol	T51.2X1	T51.2X2	T51.2X3	T51.2X4	—	—

◄ New ◄⦚ Revised ~~deleted~~ Deleted

TABLE OF DRUGS AND CHEMICALS

Substance	Poisoning, Accidental (Unintentional)	Poisoning, Intentional Self-Harm	Poisoning, Assault	Poisoning, Undetermined	Adverse Effect	Underdosing
			External Cause (T-Code)			
Isopropyl						
acetate	T52.8X1	T52.8X2	T52.8X3	T52.8X4	—	—
alcohol	T51.2X1	T51.2X2	T51.2X3	T51.2X4	—	—
medicinal	T49.4X1	T49.4X2	T49.4X3	T49.4X4	T49.4X5	T49.4X6
ether	T52.8X1	T52.8X2	T52.8X3	T52.8X4	—	—
Isopropylaminophena-zone	T39.2X1	T39.2X2	T39.2X3	T39.2X4	T39.2X5	T39.2X6
Isoproterenol	T48.6X1	T48.6X2	T48.6X3	T48.6X4	T48.6X5	T48.6X6
Isosorbide dinitrate	T46.3X1	T46.3X2	T46.3X3	T46.3X4	T46.3X5	T46.3X6
Isothipendyl	T45.0X1	T45.0X2	T45.0X3	T45.0X4	T45.0X5	T45.0X6
Isotretinoin	T50.991	T50.992	T50.993	T50.994	T50.995	T50.996
Isoxazolyl penicillin	T36.0X1	T36.0X2	T36.0X3	T36.0X4	T36.0X5	T36.0X6
Isoxicam	T39.391	T39.392	T39.393	T39.394	T39.395	T39.396
Isoxsuprine	T46.7X1	T46.7X2	T46.7X3	T46.7X4	T46.7X5	T46.7X6
Ispagula	T47.4X1	T47.4X2	T47.4X3	T47.4X4	T47.4X5	T47.4X6
husk	T47.4X1	T47.4X2	T47.4X3	T47.4X4	T47.4X5	T47.4X6
Isradipine	T46.1X1	T46.1X2	T46.1X3	T46.1X4	T46.1X5	T46.1X6
I-thyroxine sodium	T38.1X1	T38.1X2	T38.1X3	T38.1X4	T38.1X5	T38.1X6
Itraconazole	T37.8X1	T37.8X2	T37.8X3	T37.8X4	T37.8X5	T37.8X6
Itramin tosilate	T46.3X1	T46.3X2	T46.3X3	T46.3X4	T46.3X5	T46.3X6
Ivermectin	T37.4X1	T37.4X2	T37.4X3	T37.4X4	T37.4X5	T37.4X6
Izoniazid	T37.1X1	T37.1X2	T37.1X3	T37.1X4	T37.1X5	T37.1X6
with thioacetazone	T37.1X1	T37.1X2	T37.1X3	T37.1X4	T37.1X5	T37.1X6
J						
Jalap	T47.2X1	T47.2X2	T47.2X3	T47.2X4	T47.2X5	T47.2X6
Jamaica						
dogwood (bark)	T39.8X1	T39.8X2	T39.8X3	T39.8X4	T39.8X5	T39.8X6
ginger	T65.891	T65.892	T65.893	T65.894	—	—
root	T62.2X1	T62.2X2	T62.2X3	T62.2X4	—	—
Jatropha	T62.2X1	T62.2X2	T62.2X3	T62.2X4	—	—
curcas	T62.2X1	T62.2X2	T62.2X3	T62.2X4	—	—
Jectofer	T45.4X1	T45.4X2	T45.4X3	T45.4X4	T45.4X5	T45.4X6
Jellyfish (sting)	T63.621	T63.622	T63.623	T63.624	—	—
Jequirity (bean)	T62.2X1	T62.2X2	T62.2X3	T62.2X4	—	—
Jimson weed (stramonium)	T62.2X1	T62.2X2	T62.2X3	T62.2X4	—	—
seeds	T62.2X1	T62.2X2	T62.2X3	T62.2X4	—	—
Josamycin	T36.3X1	T36.3X2	T36.3X3	T36.3X4	T36.3X5	T36.3X6
Juniper tar	T49.1X1	T49.1X2	T49.1X3	T49.1X4	T49.1X5	T49.1X6

◀ New   ◀▌ Revised   ~~deleted~~ Deleted

Substance	External Cause (T-Code)					
	Poisoning, Accidental (Unintentional)	Poisoning, Intentional Self-Harm	Poisoning, Assault	Poisoning, Undetermined	Adverse Effect	Underdosing
K						
Kallidinogenase	T46.7X1	T46.7X2	T46.7X3	T46.7X4	T46.7X5	T46.7X6
Kallikrein	T46.7X1	T46.7X2	T46.7X3	T46.7X4	T46.7X5	T46.7X6
Kanamycin	T36.5X1	T36.5X2	T36.5X3	T36.5X4	T36.5X5	T36.5X6
Kantrex	T36.5X1	T36.5X2	T36.5X3	T36.5X4	T36.5X5	T36.5X6
Kaolin	T47.6X1	T47.6X2	T47.6X3	T47.6X4	T47.6X5	T47.6X6
light	T47.6X1	T47.6X2	T47.6X3	T47.6X4	T47.6X5	T47.6X6
Karaya (gum)	T47.4X1	T47.4X2	T47.4X3	T47.4X4	T47.4X5	T47.4X6
Kebuzone	T39.2X1	T39.2X2	T39.2X3	T39.2X4	T39.2X5	T39.2X6
Kelevan	T60.1X1	T60.1X2	T60.1X3	T60.1X4	—	—
Kemithal	T41.1X1	T41.1X2	T41.1X3	T41.1X4	T41.1X5	T41.1X6
Kenacort	T38.0X1	T38.0X2	T38.0X3	T38.0X4	T38.0X5	T38.0X6
Keratolytic drug NEC	T49.4X1	T49.4X2	T49.4X3	T49.4X4	T49.4X5	T49.4X6
anthracene	T49.4X1	T49.4X2	T49.4X3	T49.4X4	T49.4X5	T49.4X6
Keratoplastic NEC	T49.4X1	T49.4X2	T49.4X3	T49.4X4	T49.4X5	T49.4X6
Kerosene, kerosine (fuel) (solvent) NEC	T52.0X1	T52.0X2	T52.0X3	T52.0X4	—	—
insecticide	T52.0X1	T52.0X2	T52.0X3	T52.0X4	—	—
vapor	T52.0X1	T52.0X2	T52.0X3	T52.0X4	—	—
Ketamine	T41.291	T41.292	T41.293	T41.294	T41.295	T41.296
Ketazolam	T42.4X1	T42.4X2	T42.4X3	T42.4X4	T42.4X5	T42.4X6
Ketazon	T39.2X1	T39.2X2	T39.2X3	T39.2X4	T39.2X5	T39.2X6
Ketobemidone	T40.4X1	T40.4X2	T40.4X3	T40.4X4	—	—
Ketoconazole	T49.0X1	T49.0X2	T49.0X3	T49.0X4	T49.0X5	T49.0X6
Ketols	T52.4X1	T52.4X2	T52.4X3	T52.4X4	—	—
Ketone oils	T52.4X1	T52.4X2	T52.4X3	T52.4X4	—	—
Ketoprofen	T39.311	T39.312	T39.313	T39.314	T39.315	T39.316
Ketorolac	T39.8X1	T39.8X2	T39.8X3	T39.8X4	T39.8X5	T39.8X6
Ketotifen	T45.0X1	T45.0X2	T45.0X3	T45.0X4	T45.0X5	T45.0X6
Khat	T43.691	T43.692	T43.693	T43.694	—	—
Khellin	T46.3X1	T46.3X2	T46.3X3	T46.3X4	T46.3X5	T46.3X6
Khelloside	T46.3X1	T46.3X2	T46.3X3	T46.3X4	T46.3X5	T46.3X6
Kiln gas or vapor (carbon monoxide)	T58.8X1	T58.8X2	T58.8X3	T58.8X4	—	—
Kitasamycin	T36.3X1	T36.3X2	T36.3X3	T36.3X4	T36.3X5	T36.3X6
Konsyl	T47.4X1	T47.4X2	T47.4X3	T47.4X4	T47.4X5	T47.4X6
Kosam seed	T62.2X1	T62.2X2	T62.2X3	T62.2X4	—	—
Krait (venom)	T63.091	T63.092	T63.093	T63.094	—	—
Kwell (insecticide)	T60.1X1	T60.1X2	T60.1X3	T60.1X4	—	—
anti-infective (topical)	T49.0X1	T49.0X2	T49.0X3	T49.0X4	T49.0X5	T49.0X6

Substance	Poisoning, Accidental (Unintentional)	External Cause (T-Code)			Adverse Effect	Underdosing
		Poisoning, Intentional Self-Harm	Poisoning, Assault	Poisoning, Undetermined		

L

Substance	Poisoning, Accidental (Unintentional)	Poisoning, Intentional Self-Harm	Poisoning, Assault	Poisoning, Undetermined	Adverse Effect	Underdosing
Labetalol	T44.8X1	T44.8X2	T44.8X3	T44.8X4	T44.8X5	T44.8X6
Laburnum (seeds)	T62.2X1	T62.2X2	T62.2X3	T62.2X4	—	—
leaves	T62.2X1	T62.2X2	T62.2X3	T62.2X4	—	—
Lachesine	T49.5X1	T49.5X2	T49.5X3	T49.5X4	T49.5X5	T49.5X6
Lacidipine	T46.5X1	T46.5X2	T46.5X3	T46.5X4	T46.5X5	T46.5X6
Lacquer	T65.6X1	T65.6X2	T65.6X3	T65.6X4	—	—
Lacrimogenic gas	T59.3X1	T59.3X2	T59.3X3	T59.3X4	—	—
Lactated potassic saline	T50.3X1	T50.3X2	T50.3X3	T50.3X4	T50.3X5	T50.3X6
Lactic acid	T49.8X1	T49.8X2	T49.8X3	T49.8X4	T49.8X5	T49.8X6
Lactobacillus						
acidophilus	T47.6X1	T47.6X2	T47.6X3	T47.6X4	T47.6X5	T47.6X6
compound	T47.6X1	T47.6X2	T47.6X3	T47.6X4	T47.6X5	T47.6X6
bifidus, lyophilized	T47.6X1	T47.6X2	T47.6X3	T47.6X4	T47.6X5	T47.6X6
bulgaricus	T47.6X1	T47.6X2	T47.6X3	T47.6X4	T47.6X5	T47.6X6
sporogenes	T47.6X1	T47.6X2	T47.6X3	T47.6X4	T47.6X5	T47.6X6
Lactoflavin	T45.2X1	T45.2X2	T45.2X3	T45.2X4	T45.2X5	T45.2X6
Lactose (as excipient)	T50.901	T50.902	T50.903	T50.904	T50.905	T50.906
Lactuca (virosa) (extract)	T42.6X1	T42.6X2	T42.6X3	T42.6X4	T42.6X5	T42.6X6
Lactucarium	T42.6X1	T42.6X2	T42.6X3	T42.6X4	T42.6X5	T42.6X6
Lactulose	T47.3X1	T47.3X2	T47.3X3	T47.3X4	T47.3X5	T47.3X6
Laevo—see Levo-						
Lanatosides	T46.0X1	T46.0X2	T46.0X3	T46.0X4	T46.0X5	T46.0X6
Lanolin	T49.3X1	T49.3X2	T49.3X3	T49.3X4	T49.3X5	T49.3X6
Largactil	T43.3X1	T43.3X2	T43.3X3	T43.3X4	T43.3X5	T43.3X6
Larkspur	T62.2X1	T62.2X2	T62.2X3	T62.2X4	—	—
Laroxyl	T43.011	T43.012	T43.013	T43.014	T43.015	T43.016
Lassar's paste	T49.4X1	T49.4X2	T49.4X3	T49.4X4	T49.4X5	T49.4X6
Lasix	T50.1X1	T50.1X2	T50.1X3	T50.1X4	T50.1X5	T50.1X6
Latamoxef	T36.1X1	T36.1X2	T36.1X3	T36.1X4	T36.1X5	T36.1X6
Latex	T65.811	T65.812	T65.813	T65.814	—	—
Lathyrus (seed)	T62.2X1	T62.2X2	T62.2X3	T62.2X4	—	—
Laudanum	T40.0X1	T40.0X2	T40.0X3	T40.0X4	T40.0X5	T40.0X6
Laudexium	T48.1X1	T48.1X2	T48.1X3	T48.1X4	T48.1X5	T48.1X6
Laughing gas	T41.0X1	T41.0X2	T41.0X3	T41.0X4	T41.0X5	T41.0X6
Laurel, black or cherry	T62.2X1	T62.2X2	T62.2X3	T62.2X4	—	—
Laurolinium	T49.0X1	T49.0X2	T49.0X3	T49.0X4	T49.0X5	T49.0X6
Lauryl sulfoacetate	T49.2X1	T49.2X2	T49.2X3	T49.2X4	T49.2X5	T49.2X6

◀ New   ◀ Revised   ~~deleted~~ Deleted

Substance	External Cause (T-Code)					
	Poisoning, Accidental (Unintentional)	Poisoning, Intentional Self-Harm	Poisoning, Assault	Poisoning, Undetermined	Adverse Effect	Underdosing
Laxative NEC	T47.4X1	T47.4X2	T47.4X3	T47.4X4	T47.4X5	T47.4X6
osmotic	T47.3X1	T47.3X2	T47.3X3	T47.3X4	T47.3X5	T47.3X6
saline	T47.3X1	T47.3X2	T47.3X3	T47.3X4	T47.3X5	T47.3X6
stimulant	T47.2X1	T47.2X2	T47.2X3	T47.2X4	T47.2X5	T47.2X6
L-dopa	T42.8X1	T42.8X2	T42.8X3	T42.8X4	T42.8X5	T42.8X6
Lead (dust) (fumes) (vapor) NEC	T56.0X1	T56.0X2	T56.0X3	T56.0X4	—	—
acetate	T49.2X1	T49.2X2	T49.2X3	T49.2X4	T49.2X5	T49.2X6
alkyl (fuel additive)	T56.0X1	T56.0X2	T56.0X3	T56.0X4	—	—
anti-infectives	T37.8X1	T37.8X2	T37.8X3	T37.8X4	T37.8X5	T37.8X6
antiknock compound (tetraethyl)	T56.0X1	T56.0X2	T56.0X3	T56.0X4	—	—
arsenate, arsenite (dust) (herbicide) (insecticide) (vapor)	T57.0X1	T57.0X2	T57.0X3	T57.0X4	—	—
carbonate	T56.0X1	T56.0X2	T56.0X3	T56.0X4	—	—
paint	T56.0X1	T56.0X2	T56.0X3	T56.0X4	—	—
chromate	T56.0X1	T56.0X2	T56.0X3	T56.0X4	—	—
paint	T56.0X1	T56.0X2	T56.0X3	T56.0X4	—	—
dioxide	T56.0X1	T56.0X2	T56.0X3	T56.0X4	—	—
inorganic	T56.0X1	T56.0X2	T56.0X3	T56.0X4	—	—
iodide	T56.0X1	T56.0X2	T56.0X3	T56.0X4	—	—
pigment (paint)	T56.0X1	T56.0X2	T56.0X3	T56.0X4	—	—
monoxide (dust)	T56.0X1	T56.0X2	T56.0X3	T56.0X4	—	—
paint	T56.0X1	T56.0X2	T56.0X3	T56.0X4	—	—
organic	T56.0X1	T56.0X2	T56.0X3	T56.0X4	—	—
oxide	T56.0X1	T56.0X2	T56.0X3	T56.0X4	—	—
paint	T56.0X1	T56.0X2	T56.0X3	T56.0X4	—	—
paint	T56.0X1	T56.0X2	T56.0X3	T56.0X4	—	—
salts	T56.0X1	T56.0X2	T56.0X3	T56.0X4	—	—
specified compound NEC	T56.0X1	T56.0X2	T56.0X3	T56.0X4	—	—
tetra-ethyl	T56.0X1	T56.0X2	T56.0X3	T56.0X4	—	—
Lebanese red	T40.7X1	T40.7X2	T40.7X3	T40.7X4	T40.7X5	T40.7X6
Lefetamine	T39.8X1	T39.8X2	T39.8X3	T39.8X4	T39.8X5	T39.8X6
Lenperone	T43.4X1	T43.4X2	T43.4X3	T43.4X4	T43.4X5	T43.4X6
Lente lietin (insulin)	T38.3X1	T38.3X2	T38.3X3	T38.3X4	T38.3X5	T38.3X6
Leptazol	T50.7X1	T50.7X2	T50.7X3	T50.7X4	T50.7X5	T50.7X6
Leptophos	T60.0X1	T60.0X2	T60.0X3	T60.0X4	—	—
Leritine	T40.2X1	T40.2X2	T40.2X3	T40.2X4	T40.2X5	T40.2X6
Letosteine	T48.4X1	T48.4X2	T48.4X3	T48.4X4	T48.4X5	T48.4X6
Letter	T38.1X1	T38.1X2	T38.1X3	T38.1X4	T38.1X5	T38.1X6
Lettuce opium	T42.6X1	T42.6X2	T42.6X3	T42.6X4	T42.6X5	T42.6X6
Leucinocaine	T41.3X1	T41.3X2	T41.3X3	T41.3X4	T41.3X5	T41.3X6

TABLE OF DRUGS AND CHEMICALS

TABLE OF DRUGS AND CHEMICALS

Substance	External Cause (T-Code)					
	Poisoning, Accidental (Unintentional)	Poisoning, Intentional Self-Harm	Poisoning, Assault	Poisoning, Undetermined	Adverse Effect	Underdosing
Leucocianidol	T46.991	T46.992	T46.993	T46.994	T46.995	T46.996
Leucovorin (factor)	T45.8X1	T45.8X2	T45.8X3	T45.8X4	T45.8X5	T45.8X6
Leukeran	T45.1X1	T45.1X2	T45.1X3	T45.1X4	T45.1X5	T45.1X6
Leuprolide	T38.891	T38.892	T38.893	T38.894	T38.895	T38.896
Levalbuterol	T48.6X1	T48.6X2	T48.6X3	T48.6X4	T48.6X5	T48.6X6
Levallorphan	T50.7X1	T50.7X2	T50.7X3	T50.7X4	T50.7X5	T50.7X6
Levamisole	T37.4X1	T37.4X2	T37.4X3	T37.4X4	T37.4X5	T37.4X6
Levanil	T42.6X1	T42.6X2	T42.6X3	T42.6X4	T42.6X5	T42.6X6
Levarterenol	T44.4X1	T44.4X2	T44.4X3	T44.4X4	T44.4X5	T44.4X6
Levdropropizine	T48.3X1	T48.3X2	T48.3X3	T48.3X4	T48.3X5	T48.3X6
Levobunolol	T49.5X1	T49.5X2	T49.5X3	T49.5X4	T49.5X5	T49.5X6
Levocabastine (hydrochloride)	T45.0X1	T45.0X2	T45.0X3	T45.0X4	T45.0X5	T45.0X6
Levocarnitine	T50.991	T50.992	T50.993	T50.994	T50.995	T50.996
Levodopa	T42.8X1	T42.8X2	T42.8X3	T42.8X4	T42.8X5	T42.8X6
with carbidopa	T42.8X1	T42.8X2	T42.8X3	T42.8X4	T42.8X5	T42.8X6
Levo-dromoran	T40.2X1	T40.2X2	T40.2X3	T40.2X4	T40.2X5	T40.2X6
Levoglutamide	T50.991	T50.992	T50.993	T50.994	T50.995	T50.996
Levoid	T38.1X1	T38.1X2	T38.1X3	T38.1X4	T38.1X5	T38.1X6
Levo-iso-methadone	T40.3X1	T40.3X2	T40.3X3	T40.3X4	T40.3X5	T40.3X6
Levomepromazine	T43.3X1	T43.3X2	T43.3X3	T43.3X4	T43.3X5	T43.3X6
Levonordefrin	T49.6X1	T49.6X2	T49.6X3	T49.6X4	T49.6X5	T49.6X6
Levonorgestrel	T38.4X1	T38.4X2	T38.4X3	T38.4X4	T38.4X5	T38.4X6
with ethinylestradiol	T38.5X1	T38.5X2	T38.5X3	T38.5X4	T38.5X5	T38.5X6
Levopromazine	T43.3X1	T43.3X2	T43.3X3	T43.3X4	T43.3X5	T43.3X6
Levoprome	T42.6X1	T42.6X2	T42.6X3	T42.6X4	T42.6X5	T42.6X6
Levopropoxyphene	T40.4X1	T40.4X2	T40.4X3	T40.4X4	T40.4X5	T40.4X6
Levopropylhexedrine	T50.5X1	T50.5X2	T50.5X3	T50.5X4	T50.5X5	T50.5X6
Levoproxyphylline	T48.6X1	T48.6X2	T48.6X3	T48.6X4	T48.6X5	T48.6X6
Levorphanol	T40.4X1	T40.4X2	T40.4X3	T40.4X4	T40.4X5	T40.4X6
Levothyroxine	T38.1X1	T38.1X2	T38.1X3	T38.1X4	T38.1X5	T38.1X6
sodium	T38.1X1	T38.1X2	T38.1X3	T38.1X4	T38.1X5	T38.1X6
Levsin	T44.3X1	T44.3X2	T44.3X3	T44.3X4	T44.3X5	T44.3X6
Levulose	T50.3X1	T50.3X2	T50.3X3	T50.3X4	T50.3X5	T50.3X6
Lewisite (gas), not in war	T57.0X1	T57.0X2	T57.0X3	T57.0X4	—	—
Librium	T42.4X1	T42.4X2	T42.4X3	T42.4X4	T42.4X5	T42.4X6
Lidex	T49.0X1	T49.0X2	T49.0X3	T49.0X4	T49.0X5	T49.0X6
Lidocaine	T41.3X1	T41.3X2	T41.3X3	T41.3X4	T41.3X5	T41.3X6
regional	T41.3X1	T41.3X2	T41.3X3	T41.3X4	T41.3X5	T41.3X6
spinal	T41.3X1	T41.3X2	T41.3X3	T41.3X4	T41.3X5	T41.3X6
Lidofenin	T50.8X1	T50.8X2	T50.8X3	T50.8X4	T50.8X5	T50.8X6

◄ New ◄▦ Revised ~~deleted~~ Deleted

Substance	External Cause (T-Code)					
	Poisoning, Accidental (Unintentional)	Poisoning, Intentional Self-Harm	Poisoning, Assault	Poisoning, Undetermined	Adverse Effect	Underdosing
Lidoflazine	T46.1X1	T46.1X2	T46.1X3	T46.1X4	T46.1X5	T46.1X6
Lighter fluid	T52.0X1	T52.0X2	T52.0X3	T52.0X4	—	—
Lignin hemicellulose	T47.6X1	T47.6X2	T47.6X3	T47.6X4	T47.6X5	T47.6X6
Lignocaine	T41.3X1	T41.3X2	T41.3X3	T41.3X4	T41.3X5	T41.3X6
regional	T41.3X1	T41.3X2	T41.3X3	T41.3X4	T41.3X5	T41.3X6
spinal	T41.3X1	T41.3X2	T41.3X3	T41.3X4	T41.3X5	T41.3X6
Ligroin(e) (solvent)	T52.0X1	T52.0X2	T52.0X3	T52.0X4	—	—
vapor	T59.891	T59.892	T59.893	T59.894	—	—
Ligustrum vulgare	T62.2X1	T62.2X2	T62.2X3	T62.2X4	—	—
Lily of the valley	T62.2X1	T62.2X2	T62.2X3	T62.2X4	—	—
Lime (chloride)	T54.3X1	T54.3X2	T54.3X3	T54.3X4	—	—
Limonene	T52.8X1	T52.8X2	T52.8X3	T52.8X4	—	—
Lincomycin	T36.8X1	T36.8X2	T36.8X3	T36.8X4	T36.8X5	T36.8X6
Lindane (insecticide) (nonmedicinal) (vapor)	T53.6X1	T53.6X2	T53.6X3	T53.6X4	—	—
medicinal	T49.0X1	T49.0X2	T49.0X3	T49.0X4	T49.0X5	T49.0X6
Liniments NEC	T49.91	T49.92	T49.93	T49.94	T49.95	T49.96
Linoleic acid	T46.6X1	T46.6X2	T46.6X3	T46.6X4	T46.6X5	T46.6X6
Linolenic acid	T46.6X1	T46.6X2	T46.6X3	T46.6X4	T46.6X5	T46.6X6
Linseed	T47.4X1	T47.4X2	T47.4X3	T47.4X4	T47.4X5	T47.4X6
Liothyronine	T38.1X1	T38.1X2	T38.1X3	T38.1X4	T38.1X5	T38.1X6
Liotrix	T38.1X1	T38.1X2	T38.1X3	T38.1X4	T38.1X5	T38.1X6
Lipancreatin	T47.5X1	T47.5X2	T47.5X3	T47.5X4	T47.5X5	T47.5X6
Lipo-alprostadil	T46.7X1	T46.7X2	T46.7X3	T46.7X4	T46.7X5	T46.7X6
Lipo-Lutin	T38.5X1	T38.5X2	T38.5X3	T38.5X4	T38.5X5	T38.5X6
Lipotropic drug NEC	T50.901	T50.902	T50.903	T50.904	T50.905	T50.906
Liquefied petroleum gases	T59.891	T59.892	T59.893	T59.894	—	—
piped (pure or mixed with air)	T59.891	T59.892	T59.893	T59.894	—	—
Liquid						
paraffin	T47.4X1	T47.4X2	T47.4X3	T47.4X4	T47.4X5	T47.4X6
petrolatum	T47.4X1	T47.4X2	T47.4X3	T47.4X4	T47.4X5	T47.4X6
topical	T49.3X1	T49.3X2	T49.3X3	T49.3X4	T49.3X5	T49.3X6
specified NEC	T65.891	T65.892	T65.893	T65.894	—	—
substance	T65.91	T65.92	T65.93	T65.94	—	—
Liquor creosolis compositus	T65.891	T65.892	T65.893	T65.894	—	—
Liquorice	T48.4X1	T48.4X2	T48.4X3	T48.4X4	T48.4X5	T48.4X6
extract	T47.8X1	T47.8X2	T47.8X3	T47.8X4	T47.8X5	T47.8X6
Lirugen	T50.991	T50.992	T50.993	T50.994	T50.995	T50.996
Lisinopril	T46.4X1	T46.4X2	T46.4X3	T46.4X4	T46.4X5	T46.4X6
Lisuride	T42.8X1	T42.8X2	T42.8X3	T42.8X4	T42.8X5	T42.8X6
Lithane	T43.8X1	T43.8X2	T43.8X3	T43.8X4	T43.8X5	T43.8X6

◀ New ◀◁ Revised ~~deleted~~ Deleted

TABLE OF DRUGS AND CHEMICALS

Substance	Poisoning, Accidental (Unintentional)	Poisoning, Intentional Self-Harm	Poisoning, Assault	Poisoning, Undetermined	Adverse Effect	Underdosing
External Cause (T-Code)						
Lithium	T56.891	T56.892	T56.893	T56.894	—	—
gluconate	T43.591	T43.592	T43.593	T43.594	T43.595	T43.596
salts (carbonate)	T43.591	T43.592	T43.593	T43.594	T43.595	T43.596
Lithonate	T43.8X1	T43.8X2	T43.8X3	T43.8X4	T43.8X5	T43.8X6
Liver						
extract	T45.8X1	T45.8X2	T45.8X3	T45.8X4	T45.8X5	T45.8X6
for parenteral use	T45.8X1	T45.8X2	T45.8X3	T45.8X4	T45.8X5	T45.8X6
fraction 1	T45.8X1	T45.8X2	T45.8X3	T45.8X4	T45.8X5	T45.8X6
hydrolysate	T45.8X1	T45.8X2	T45.8X3	T45.8X4	T45.8X5	T45.8X6
Lizard (bite) (venom)	T63.121	T63.122	T63.123	T63.124	—	—
LMD	T45.8X1	T45.8X2	T45.8X3	T45.8X4	T45.8X5	T45.8X6
Lobelia	T62.2X1	T62.2X2	T62.2X3	T62.2X4	—	—
Lobeline	T50.7X1	T50.7X2	T50.7X3	T50.7X4	T50.7X5	T50.7X6
Local action drug NEC	T49.8X1	T49.8X2	T49.8X3	T49.8X4	T49.8X5	T49.8X6
Locorten	T49.0X1	T49.0X2	T49.0X3	T49.0X4	T49.0X5	T49.0X6
Lofepramine	T43.011	T43.012	T43.013	T43.014	T43.015	T43.016
Lolium temulentum	T62.2X1	T62.2X2	T62.2X3	T62.2X4	—	—
Lomotil	T47.6X1	T47.6X2	T47.6X3	T47.6X4	T47.6X5	T47.6X6
Lomustine	T45.1X1	T45.1X2	T45.1X3	T45.1X4	T45.1X5	T45.1X6
Lonidamine	T45.1X1	T45.1X2	T45.1X3	T45.1X4	T45.1X5	T45.1X6
Loperamide	T47.6X1	T47.6X2	T47.6X3	T47.6X4	T47.6X5	T47.6X6
Loprazolam	T42.4X1	T42.4X2	T42.4X3	T42.4X4	T42.4X5	T42.4X6
Lorajmine	T46.2X1	T46.2X2	T46.2X3	T46.2X4	T46.2X5	T46.2X6
Loratidine	T45.0X1	T45.0X2	T45.0X3	T45.0X4	T45.0X5	T45.0X6
Lorazepam	T42.4X1	T42.4X2	T42.4X3	T42.4X4	T42.4X5	T42.4X6
Lorcainide	T46.2X1	T46.2X2	T46.2X3	T46.2X4	T46.2X5	T46.2X6
Lormetazepam	T42.4X1	T42.4X2	T42.4X3	T42.4X4	T42.4X5	T42.4X6
Lotions NEC	T49.91	T49.92	T49.93	T49.94	T49.95	T49.96
Lotusate	T42.3X1	T42.3X2	T42.3X3	T42.3X4	T42.3X5	T42.3X6
Lovastatin	T46.6X1	T46.6X2	T46.6X3	T46.6X4	T46.6X5	T46.6X6
Loxapine	T43.591	T43.592	T43.593	T43.594	T43.595	T43.596
Lowila	T49.2X1	T49.2X2	T49.2X3	T49.2X4	T49.2X5	T49.2X6
Lozenges (throat)	T49.6X1	T49.6X2	T49.6X3	T49.6X4	T49.6X5	T49.6X6
LSD	T40.8X1	T40.8X2	T40.8X3	T40.8X4	—	—
L-Tryptophan—see amino acid						
Lubricant, eye	T49.5X1	T49.5X2	T49.5X3	T49.5X4	T49.5X5	T49.5X6
Lubricating oil NEC	T52.0X1	T52.0X2	T52.0X3	T52.0X4	—	—
Lucanthone	T37.4X1	T37.4X2	T37.4X3	T37.4X4	T37.4X5	T37.4X6
Luminal	T42.3X1	T42.3X2	T42.3X3	T42.3X4	T42.3X5	T42.3X6
Lung irritant (gas) NEC	T59.91	T59.92	T59.93	T59.94	—	—

◀ New ◀║ Revised ~~deleted~~ Deleted

Substance	External Cause (T-Code)					
	Poisoning, Accidental (Unintentional)	Poisoning, Intentional Self-Harm	Poisoning, Assault	Poisoning, Undetermined	Adverse Effect	Underdosing
Luteinizing hormone	T38.811	T38.812	T38.813	T38.814	T38.815	T38.816
Lutocylol	T38.5X1	T38.5X2	T38.5X3	T38.5X4	T38.5X5	T38.5X6
Lutromone	T38.5X1	T38.5X2	T38.5X3	T38.5X4	T38.5X5	T38.5X6
Lututrin	T48.291	T48.292	T48.293	T48.294	T48.295	T48.296
Lye (Concentrated)	T54.3X1	T54.3X2	T54.3X3	T54.3X4	—	—
Lygranum (skin test)	T50.8X1	T50.8X2	T50.8X3	T50.8X4	T50.8X5	T50.8X6
Lymecycline	T36.4X1	T36.4X2	T36.4X3	T36.4X4	T36.4X5	T36.4X6
Lymphogranuloma venereum antigen	T50.8X1	T50.8X2	T50.8X3	T50.8X4	T50.8X5	T50.8X6
Lynestrenol	T38.4X1	T38.4X2	T38.4X3	T38.4X4	T38.4X5	T38.4X6
Lypressin	T38.891	T38.892	T38.893	T38.894	T38.895	T38.896
Lyovac Sodium Edecrin	T50.1X1	T50.1X2	T50.1X3	T50.1X4	T50.1X5	T50.1X6
Lysergic acid diethylamide	T40.8X1	T40.8X2	T40.8X3	T40.8X4	—	—
Lysergide	T40.8X1	T40.8X2	T40.8X3	T40.8X4	—	—
Lysine vasopressin	T38.891	T38.892	T38.893	T38.894	T38.895	T38.896
Lysol	T54.1X1	T54.1X2	T54.1X3	T54.1X4	—	—
Lysozyme	T49.0X1	T49.0X2	T49.0X3	T49.0X4	T49.0X5	T49.0X6
Lytta (vitatta)	T49.8X1	T49.8X2	T49.8X3	T49.8X4	T49.8X5	T49.8X6
M						
Mace	T59.3X1	T59.3X2	T59.3X3	T59.3X4	—	—
Macrogol	T50.991	T50.992	T50.993	T50.994	T50.995	T50.996
Macrolide						
anabolic drug	T38.7X1	T38.7X2	T38.7X3	T38.7X4	T38.7X5	T38.7X6
antibiotic	T36.3X1	T36.3X2	T36.3X3	T36.3X4	T36.3X5	T36.3X6
Mafenide	T49.0X1	T49.0X2	T49.0X3	T49.0X4	T49.0X5	T49.0X6
Magaldrate	T47.1X1	T47.1X2	T47.1X3	T47.1X4	T47.1X5	T47.1X6
Magic mushroom	T40.991	T40.992	T40.993	T40.994	—	—
Magnamycin	T36.8X1	T36.8X2	T36.8X3	T36.8X4	T36.8X5	T36.8X6
Magnesia magma	T47.1X1	T47.1X2	T47.1X3	T47.1X4	T47.1X5	T47.1X6
Magnesium NEC	T56.891	T56.892	T56.893	T56.894	—	—
carbonate	T47.1X1	T47.1X2	T47.1X3	T47.1X4	T47.1X5	T47.1X6
citrate	T47.4X1	T47.4X2	T47.4X3	T47.4X4	T47.4X5	T47.4X6
hydroxide	T47.1X1	T47.1X2	T47.1X3	T47.1X4	T47.1X5	T47.1X6
oxide	T47.1X1	T47.1X2	T47.1X3	T47.1X4	T47.1X5	T47.1X6
peroxide	T49.0X1	T49.0X2	T49.0X3	T49.0X4	T49.0X5	T49.0X6
salicylate	T39.091	T39.092	T39.093	T39.094	T39.095	T39.096
silicofluoride	T50.3X1	T50.3X2	T50.3X3	T50.3X4	T50.3X5	T50.3X6
sulfate	T47.4X1	T47.4X2	T47.4X3	T47.4X4	T47.4X5	T47.4X6
thiosulfate	T45.0X1	T45.0X2	T45.0X3	T45.0X4	T45.0X5	T45.0X6
trisilicate	T47.1X1	T47.1X2	T47.1X3	T47.1X4	T47.1X5	T47.1X6

TABLE OF DRUGS AND CHEMICALS

Substance	External Cause (T-Code)					
	Poisoning, Accidental (Unintentional)	Poisoning, Intentional Self-Harm	Poisoning, Assault	Poisoning, Undetermined	Adverse Effect	Underdosing
Malathion (medicinal)	T49.0X1	T49.0X2	T49.0X3	T49.0X4	T49.0X5	T49.0X6
insecticide	T60.0X1	T60.0X2	T60.0X3	T60.0X4	—	—
Male fern extract	T37.4X1	T37.4X2	T37.4X3	T37.4X4	T37.4X5	T37.4X6
M-AMSA	T45.1X1	T45.1X2	T45.1X3	T45.1X4	T45.1X5	T45.1X6
Mandelic acid	T37.8X1	T37.8X2	T37.8X3	T37.8X4	T37.8X5	T37.8X6
Manganese (dioxide) (salts)	T57.2X1	T57.2X2	T57.2X3	T57.2X4	—	—
medicinal	T50.991	T50.992	T50.993	T50.994	T50.995	T50.996
Mannitol	T47.3X1	T47.3X2	T47.3X3	T47.3X4	T47.3X5	T47.3X6
hexanitrate	T46.3X1	T46.3X2	T46.3X3	T46.3X4	T46.3X5	T46.3X6
Mannomustine	T45.1X1	T45.1X2	T45.1X3	T45.1X4	T45.1X5	T45.1X6
MAO inhibitors	T43.1X1	T43.1X2	T43.1X3	T43.1X4	T43.1X5	T43.1X6
Mapharsen	T37.8X1	T37.8X2	T37.8X3	T37.8X4	T37.8X5	T37.8X6
Maphenide	T49.0X1	T49.0X2	T49.0X3	T49.0X4	T49.0X5	T49.0X6
Maprotiline	T43.021	T43.022	T43.023	T43.024	T43.025	T43.026
Marcaine	T41.3X1	T41.3X2	T41.3X3	T41.3X4	T41.3X5	T41.3X6
infiltration (subcutaneous)	T41.3X1	T41.3X2	T41.3X3	T41.3X4	T41.3X5	T41.3X6
nerve block (peripheral) (plexus)	T41.3X1	T41.3X2	T41.3X3	T41.3X4	T41.3X5	T41.3X6
Marezine	T45.0X1	T45.0X2	T45.0X3	T45.0X4	T45.0X5	T45.0X6
Marihuana	T40.7X1	T40.7X2	T40.7X3	T40.7X4	T40.7X5	T40.7X6
Marijuana	T40.7X1	T40.7X2	T40.7X3	T40.7X4	T40.7X5	T40.7X6
Marine (sting)	T63.691	T63.692	T63.693	T63.694	—	—
animals (sting)	T63.691	T63.692	T63.693	T63.694	—	—
plants (sting)	T63.711	T63.712	T63.713	T63.714	—	—
Marplan	T43.1X1	T43.1X2	T43.1X3	T43.1X4	T43.1X5	T43.1X6
Marsh gas	T59.891	T59.892	T59.893	T59.894	—	—
Marsilid	T43.1X1	T43.1X2	T43.1X3	T43.1X4	T43.1X5	T43.1X6
Matulane	T45.1X1	T45.1X2	T45.1X3	T45.1X4	T45.1X5	T45.1X6
Mazindol	T50.5X1	T50.5X2	T50.5X3	T50.5X4	T50.5X5	T50.5X6
MCPA	T60.3X1	T60.3X2	T60.3X3	T60.3X4	—	—
MDMA	T43.621	T43.622	T43.623	T43.624	T43.625	T43.626
Meadow saffron	T62.2X1	T62.2X2	T62.2X3	T62.2X4	—	—
Measles virus vaccine (attenuated)	T50.B91	T50.B92	T50.B93	T50.B94	T50.B95	T50.B96
Meat, noxious	T62.8X1	T62.8X2	T62.8X3	T62.8X4	—	—
Meballymal	T42.3X1	T42.3X2	T42.3X3	T42.3X4	T42.3X5	T42.3X6
Mebanazine	T43.1X1	T43.1X2	T43.1X3	T43.1X4	T43.1X5	T43.1X6
Mebaral	T42.3X1	T42.3X2	T42.3X3	T42.3X4	T42.3X5	T42.3X6
Mebendazole	T37.4X1	T37.4X2	T37.4X3	T37.4X4	T37.4X5	T37.4X6
Mebeverine	T44.3X1	T44.3X2	T44.3X3	T44.3X4	T44.3X5	T44.3X6
Mebhydrolin	T45.0X1	T45.0X2	T45.0X3	T45.0X4	T45.0X5	T45.0X6
Mebumal	T42.3X1	T42.3X2	T42.3X3	T42.3X4	T42.3X5	T42.3X6

◀ New ◀▬ Revised ~~deleted~~ Deleted

	External Cause (T-Code)					
Substance	Poisoning, Accidental (Unintentional)	Poisoning, Intentional Self-Harm	Poisoning, Assault	Poisoning, Undetermined	Adverse Effect	Underdosing
Mebutamate	T43.591	T43.592	T43.593	T43.594	T43.595	T43.596
Mecamylamine	T44.2X1	T44.2X2	T44.2X3	T44.2X4	T44.2X5	T44.2X6
Mechlorethamine	T45.1X1	T45.1X2	T45.1X3	T45.1X4	T45.1X5	T45.1X6
Mecillinam	T36.0X1	T36.0X2	T36.0X3	T36.0X4	T36.0X5	T36.0X6
Meclizine (hydrochloride)	T45.0X1	T45.0X2	T45.0X3	T45.0X4	T45.0X5	T45.0X6
Meclocycline	T36.4X1	T36.4X2	T36.4X3	T36.4X4	T36.4X5	T36.4X6
Meclofenamate	T39.391	T39.392	T39.393	T39.394	T39.395	T39.396
Meclofenamic acid	T39.391	T39.392	T39.393	T39.394	T39.395	T39.396
Meclofenoxate	T43.691	T43.692	T43.693	T43.694	T43.695	T43.696
Meclozine	T45.0X1	T45.0X2	T45.0X3	T45.0X4	T45.0X5	T45.0X6
Mecobalamin	T45.8X1	T45.8X2	T45.8X3	T45.8X4	T45.8X5	T45.8X6
Mecoprop	T60.3X1	T60.3X2	T60.3X3	T60.3X4	—	—
Mecrilate	T49.3X1	T49.3X2	T49.3X3	T49.3X4	T49.3X5	T49.3X6
Mecysteine	T48.4X1	T48.4X2	T48.4X3	T48.4X4	T48.4X5	T48.4X6
Medazepam	T42.4X1	T42.4X2	T42.4X3	T42.4X4	T42.4X5	T42.4X6
Medicament NEC	T50.901	T50.902	T50.903	T50.904	T50.905	T50.906
Medinal	T42.3X1	T42.3X2	T42.3X3	T42.3X4	T42.3X5	T42.3X6
Medomin	T42.3X1	T42.3X2	T42.3X3	T42.3X4	T42.3X5	T42.3X6
Medrogestone	T38.5X1	T38.5X2	T38.5X3	T38.5X4	T38.5X5	T38.5X6
Medroxalol	T44.8X1	T44.8X2	T44.8X3	T44.8X4	T44.8X5	T44.8X6
Medroxyprogesterone acetate (depot)	T38.5X1	T38.5X2	T38.5X3	T38.5X4	T38.5X5	T38.5X6
Medrysone	T49.0X1	T49.0X2	T49.0X3	T49.0X4	T49.0X5	T49.0X6
Mefenamic acid	T39.391	T39.392	T39.393	T39.394	T39.395	T39.396
Mefenorex	T50.5X1	T50.5X2	T50.5X3	T50.5X4	T50.5X5	T50.5X6
Mefloquine	T37.2X1	T37.2X2	T37.2X3	T37.2X4	T37.2X5	T37.2X6
Mefruside	T50.2X1	T50.2X2	T50.2X3	T50.2X4	T50.2X5	T50.2X6
Megahallucinogen	T40.901	T40.902	T40.903	T40.904	T40.905	T40.906
Megestrol	T38.5X1	T38.5X2	T38.5X3	T38.5X4	T38.5X5	T38.5X6
Meglumine						
antimoniate	T37.8X1	T37.8X2	T37.8X3	T37.8X4	T37.8X5	T37.8X6
diatrizoate	T50.8X1	T50.8X2	T50.8X3	T50.8X4	T50.8X5	T50.8X6
iodipamide	T50.8X1	T50.8X2	T50.8X3	T50.8X4	T50.8X5	T50.8X6
iotroxate	T50.8X1	T50.8X2	T50.8X3	T50.8X4	T50.8X5	T50.8X6
MEK (methyl ethyl ketone)	T52.4X1	T52.4X2	T52.4X3	T52.4X4	—	—
Meladrazine	T44.3X1	T44.3X2	T44.3X3	T44.3X4	T44.3X5	T44.3X6
Meladinin	T49.3X1	T49.3X2	T49.3X3	T49.3X4	T49.3X5	T49.3X6
Melaleuca alternifolia oil	T49.0X1	T49.0X2	T49.0X3	T49.0X4	T49.0X5	T49.0X6
Melanizing agents	T49.3X1	T49.3X2	T49.3X3	T49.3X4	T49.3X5	T49.3X6
Melanocyte-stimulating hormone	T38.891	T38.892	T38.893	T38.894	T38.895	T38.896
Melarsonyl potassium	T37.3X1	T37.3X2	T37.3X3	T37.3X4	T37.3X5	T37.3X6

◀ New ◀ Revised deleted Deleted

Substance	External Cause (T-Code)					
	Poisoning, Accidental (Unintentional)	Poisoning, Intentional Self-Harm	Poisoning, Assault	Poisoning, Undetermined	Adverse Effect	Underdosing
Melarsoprol	T37.3X1	T37.3X2	T37.3X3	T37.3X4	T37.3X5	T37.3X6
Melia azedarach	T62.2X1	T62.2X2	T62.2X3	T62.2X4	—	—
Melitracen	T43.011	T43.012	T43.013	T43.014	T43.015	T43.016
Mellaril	T43.3X1	T43.3X2	T43.3X3	T43.3X4	T43.3X5	T43.3X6
Meloxine	T49.3X1	T49.3X2	T49.3X3	T49.3X4	T49.3X5	T49.3X6
Melperone	T43.4X1	T43.4X2	T43.4X3	T43.4X4	T43.4X5	T43.4X6
Melphalan	T45.1X1	T45.1X2	T45.1X3	T45.1X4	T45.1X5	T45.1X6
Memantine	T43.8X1	T43.8X2	T43.8X3	T43.8X4	T43.8X5	T43.8X6
Menadiol	T45.7X1	T45.7X2	T45.7X3	T45.7X4	T45.7X5	T45.7X6
sodium sulfate	T45.7X1	T45.7X2	T45.7X3	T45.7X4	T45.7X5	T45.7X6
Menadione	T45.7X1	T45.7X2	T45.7X3	T45.7X4	T45.7X5	T45.7X6
sodium bisulfite	T45.7X1	T45.7X2	T45.7X3	T45.7X4	T45.7X5	T45.7X6
Menaphthone	T45.7X1	T45.7X2	T45.7X3	T45.7X4	T45.7X5	T45.7X6
Menaquinone	T45.7X1	T45.7X2	T45.7X3	T45.7X4	T45.7X5	T45.7X6
Menatetrenone	T45.7X1	T45.7X2	T45.7X3	T45.7X4	T45.7X5	T45.7X6
Meningococcal vaccine	T50.A91	T50.A92	T50.A93	T50.A94	T50.A95	T50.A96
Menningovax (-AC) (-C)	T50.A91	T50.A92	T50.A93	T50.A94	T50.A95	T50.A96
Menotropins	T38.811	T38.812	T38.813	T38.814	T38.815	T38.816
Menthol	T48.5X1	T48.5X2	T48.5X3	T48.5X4	T48.5X5	T48.5X6
Mepacrine	T37.2X1	T37.2X2	T37.2X3	T37.2X4	T37.2X5	T37.2X6
Meparfynol	T42.6X1	T42.6X2	T42.6X3	T42.6X4	T42.6X5	T42.6X6
Mepartricin	T36.7X1	T36.7X2	T36.7X3	T36.7X4	T36.7X5	T36.7X6
Mepazine	T43.3X1	T43.3X2	T43.3X3	T43.3X4	T43.3X5	T43.3X6
Mepenzolate	T44.3X1	T44.3X2	T44.3X3	T44.3X4	T44.3X5	T44.3X6
bromide	T44.3X1	T44.3X2	T44.3X3	T44.3X4	T44.3X5	T44.3X6
Meperidine	T40.4X1	T40.4X2	T40.4X3	T40.4X4	T40.4X5	T40.4X6
Mephebarbital	T42.3X1	T42.3X2	T42.3X3	T42.3X4	T42.3X5	T42.3X6
Mephenamin(e)	T42.8X1	T42.8X2	T42.8X3	T42.8X4	T42.8X5	T42.8X6
Mephenesin	T42.8X1	T42.8X2	T42.8X3	T42.8X4	T42.8X5	T42.8X6
Mephenhydramine	T45.0X1	T45.0X2	T45.0X3	T45.0X4	T45.0X5	T45.0X6
Mephenoxalone	T42.8X1	T42.8X2	T42.8X3	T42.8X4	T42.8X5	T42.8X6
Mephentermine	T44.991	T44.992	T44.993	T44.994	T44.995	T44.996
Mephenytoin	T42.0X1	T42.0X2	T42.0X3	T42.0X4	T42.0X5	T42.0X6
with phenobarbital	T42.3X1	T42.3X2	T42.3X3	T42.3X4	T42.3X5	T42.3X6
Mephobarbital	T42.3X1	T42.3X2	T42.3X3	T42.3X4	T42.3X5	T42.3X6
Mephosfolan	T60.0X1	T60.0X2	T60.0X3	T60.0X4	—	—
Mepindolol	T44.7X1	T44.7X2	T44.7X3	T44.7X4	T44.7X5	T44.7X6
Mepiperphenidol	T44.3X1	T44.3X2	T44.3X3	T44.3X4	T44.3X5	T44.3X6
Mepitiostane	T38.7X1	T38.7X2	T38.7X3	T38.7X4	T38.7X5	T38.7X6

TABLE OF DRUGS AND CHEMICALS

◄ New   ◄ Revised   ~~deleted~~ Deleted

Substance	Poisoning, Accidental (Unintentional)	Poisoning, Intentional Self-Harm	Poisoning, Assault	Poisoning, Undetermined	Adverse Effect	Underdosing
	External Cause (T-Code)					
Mepivacaine	T41.3X1	T41.3X2	T41.3X3	T41.3X4	T41.3X5	T41.3X6
epidural	T41.3X1	T41.3X2	T41.3X3	T41.3X4	T41.3X5	T41.3X6
Meprednisone	T38.0X1	T38.0X2	T38.0X3	T38.0X4	T38.0X5	T38.0X6
Meprobam	T43.591	T43.592	T43.593	T43.594	T43.595	T43.596
Meprobamate	T43.591	T43.592	T43.593	T43.594	T43.595	T43.596
Meproscillarin	T46.0X1	T46.0X2	T46.0X3	T46.0X4	T46.0X5	T46.0X6
Meprylcaine	T41.3X1	T41.3X2	T41.3X3	T41.3X4	T41.3X5	T41.3X6
Meptazinol	T39.8X1	T39.8X2	T39.8X3	T39.8X4	T39.8X5	T39.8X6
Mepyramine	T45.0X1	T45.0X2	T45.0X3	T45.0X4	T45.0X5	T45.0X6
Mequitazine	T43.3X1	T43.3X2	T43.3X3	T43.3X4	T43.3X5	T43.3X6
Meralluride	T50.2X1	T50.2X2	T50.2X3	T50.2X4	T50.2X5	T50.2X6
Merbaphen	T50.2X1	T50.2X2	T50.2X3	T50.2X4	T50.2X5	T50.2X6
Merbromin	T49.0X1	T49.0X2	T49.0X3	T49.0X4	T49.0X5	T49.0X6
Mercaptobenzothiazole salts	T49.0X1	T49.0X2	T49.0X3	T49.0X4	T49.0X5	T49.0X6
Mercaptomerin	T50.2X1	T50.2X2	T50.2X3	T50.2X4	T50.2X5	T50.2X6
Mercaptopurine	T45.1X1	T45.1X2	T45.1X3	T45.1X4	T45.1X5	T45.1X6
Mercumatilin	T50.2X1	T50.2X2	T50.2X3	T50.2X4	T50.2X5	T50.2X6
Mercuramide	T50.2X1	T50.2X2	T50.2X3	T50.2X4	T50.2X5	T50.2X6
Mercurochrome	T49.0X1	T49.0X2	T49.0X3	T49.0X4	T49.0X5	T49.0X6
Mercurophylline	T50.2X1	T50.2X2	T50.2X3	T50.2X4	T50.2X5	T50.2X6
Mercury, mercurial, mercuric, mercurous (compounds) (cyanide) (fumes) (nonmedicinal) (vapor) NEC	T56.1X1	T56.1X2	T56.1X3	T56.1X4	—	—
ammoniated	T49.0X1	T49.0X2	T49.0X3	T49.0X4	T49.0X5	T49.0X6
anti-infective						
local	T49.0X1	T49.0X2	T49.0X3	T49.0X4	T49.0X5	T49.0X6
systemic	T37.8X1	T37.8X2	T37.8X3	T37.8X4	T37.8X5	T37.8X6
topical	T49.0X1	T49.0X2	T49.0X3	T49.0X4	T49.0X5	T49.0X6
chloride (ammoniated)	T49.0X1	T49.0X2	T49.0X3	T49.0X4	T49.0X5	T49.0X6
fungicide	T56.1X1	T56.1X2	T56.1X3	T56.1X4	—	—
diuretic NEC	T50.2X1	T50.2X2	T50.2X3	T50.2X4	T50.2X5	T50.2X6
fungicide	T56.1X1	T56.1X2	T56.1X3	T56.1X4	—	—
organic (fungicide)	T56.1X1	T56.1X2	T56.1X3	T56.1X4	—	—
oxide, yellow	T49.0X1	T49.0X2	T49.0X3	T49.0X4	T49.0X5	T49.0X6
Mersalyl	T50.2X1	T50.2X2	T50.2X3	T50.2X4	T50.2X5	T50.2X6
Merthiolate	T49.0X1	T49.0X2	T49.0X3	T49.0X4	T49.0X5	T49.0X6
ophthalmic preparation	T49.5X1	T49.5X2	T49.5X3	T49.5X4	T49.5X5	T49.5X6
Meruvax	T50.B91	T50.B92	T50.B93	T50.B94	T50.B95	T50.B96
Mesalazine	T47.8X1	T47.8X2	T47.8X3	T47.8X4	T47.8X5	T47.8X6
Mescal buttons	T40.991	T40.992	T40.993	T40.994	—	—

◀ New　◀▥ Revised　~~deleted~~ Deleted

Substance	External Cause (T-Code)					
	Poisoning, Accidental (Unintentional)	Poisoning, Intentional Self-Harm	Poisoning, Assault	Poisoning, Undetermined	Adverse Effect	Underdosing
Mescaline	T40.991	T40.992	T40.993	T40.994	—	—
Mesna	T48.4X1	T48.4X2	T48.4X3	T48.4X4	T48.4X5	T48.4X6
Mesoglycan	T46.6X1	T46.6X2	T46.6X3	T46.6X4	T46.6X5	T46.6X6
Mesoridazine	T43.3X1	T43.3X2	T43.3X3	T43.3X4	T43.3X5	T43.3X6
Mestanolone	T38.7X1	T38.7X2	T38.7X3	T38.7X4	T38.7X5	T38.7X6
Mesterolone	T38.7X1	T38.7X2	T38.7X3	T38.7X4	T38.7X5	T38.7X6
Mestranol	T38.5X1	T38.5X2	T38.5X3	T38.5X4	T38.5X5	T38.5X6
Mesulergine	T42.8X1	T42.8X2	T42.8X3	T42.8X4	T42.8X5	T42.8X6
Mesulfen	T49.0X1	T49.0X2	T49.0X3	T49.0X4	T49.0X5	T49.0X6
Mesuximide	T42.2X1	T42.2X2	T42.2X3	T42.2X4	T42.2X5	T42.2X6
Metabutethamine	T41.3X1	T41.3X2	T41.3X3	T41.3X4	T41.3X5	T41.3X6
Metactesylacetate	T49.0X1	T49.0X2	T49.0X3	T49.0X4	T49.0X5	T49.0X6
Metacycline	T36.4X1	T36.4X2	T36.4X3	T36.4X4	T36.4X5	T36.4X6
Metaldehyde (snail killer) NEC	T60.8X1	T60.8X2	T60.8X3	T60.8X4	—	—
Metals (heavy) (nonmedicinal)	T56.91	T56.92	T56.93	T56.94	—	—
dust, fumes, or vapor NEC	T56.91	T56.92	T56.93	T56.94	—	—
light NEC	T56.91	T56.92	T56.93	T56.94	—	—
dust, fumes, or vapor NEC	T56.91	T56.92	T56.93	T56.94	—	—
specified NEC	T56.891	T56.892	T56.893	T56.894	—	—
thallium	T56.811	T56.812	T56.813	T56.814	—	—
Metamfetamine	T43.621	T43.622	T43.623	T43.624	T43.625	T43.626
Metamizole sodium	T39.2X1	T39.2X2	T39.2X3	T39.2X4	T39.2X5	T39.2X6
Metampicillin	T36.0X1	T36.0X2	T36.0X3	T36.0X4	T36.0X5	T36.0X6
Metamucil	T47.4X1	T47.4X2	T47.4X3	T47.4X4	T47.4X5	T47.4X6
Metaphen	T49.0X1	T49.0X2	T49.0X3	T49.0X4	T49.0X5	T49.0X6
Metandienone	T38.7X1	T38.7X2	T38.7X3	T38.7X4	T38.7X5	T38.7X6
Metandrostenolone	T38.7X1	T38.7X2	T38.7X3	T38.7X4	T38.7X5	T38.7X6
Metaphos	T60.0X1	T60.0X2	T60.0X3	T60.0X4	—	—
Metapramine	T43.011	T43.012	T43.013	T43.014	T43.015	T43.016
Metaproterenol	T48.291	T48.292	T48.293	T48.294	T48.295	T48.296
Metaraminol	T44.4X1	T44.4X2	T44.4X3	T44.4X4	T44.4X5	T44.4X6
Metaxalone	T42.8X1	T42.8X2	T42.8X3	T42.8X4	T42.8X5	T42.8X6
Metenolone	T38.7X1	T38.7X2	T38.7X3	T38.7X4	T38.7X5	T38.7X6
Metergoline	T42.8X1	T42.8X2	T42.8X3	T42.8X4	T42.8X5	T42.8X6
Metescufylline	T46.991	T46.992	T46.993	T46.994	T46.995	T46.996
Metetoin	T42.0X1	T42.0X2	T42.0X3	T42.0X4	T42.0X5	T42.0X6
Metformin	T38.3X1	T38.3X2	T38.3X3	T38.3X4	T38.3X5	T38.3X6
Methacholine	T44.1X1	T44.1X2	T44.1X3	T44.1X4	T44.1X5	T44.1X6
Methacycline	T36.4X1	T36.4X2	T36.4X3	T36.4X4	T36.4X5	T36.4X6
Methadone	T40.3X1	T40.3X2	T40.3X3	T40.3X4	T40.3X5	T40.3X6

◀ New   ◀▥ Revised   ~~deleted~~ Deleted

Substance	External Cause (T-Code)					
	Poisoning, Accidental (Unintentional)	Poisoning, Intentional Self-Harm	Poisoning, Assault	Poisoning, Undetermined	Adverse Effect	Underdosing
Methallenestril	T38.5X1	T38.5X2	T38.5X3	T38.5X4	T38.5X5	T38.5X6
Methallenoestril	T38.5X1	T38.5X2	T38.5X3	T38.5X4	T38.5X5	T38.5X6
Methamphetamine	T43.621	T43.622	T43.623	T43.624	T43.625	T43.626
Methampyrone	T39.2X1	T39.2X2	T39.2X3	T39.2X4	T39.2X5	T39.2X6
Methandienone	T38.7X1	T38.7X2	T38.7X3	T38.7X4	T38.7X5	T38.7X6
Methandriol	T38.7X1	T38.7X2	T38.7X3	T38.7X4	T38.7X5	T38.7X6
Methandrostenolone	T38.7X1	T38.7X2	T38.7X3	T38.7X4	T38.7X5	T38.7X6
Methane	T59.891	T59.892	T59.893	T59.894	—	—
Methanethiol	T59.891	T59.892	T59.893	T59.894	—	—
Methaniazide	T37.1X1	T37.1X2	T37.1X3	T37.1X4	T37.1X5	T37.1X6
Methanol (vapor)	T51.1X1	T51.1X2	T51.1X3	T51.1X4	—	—
Methantheline	T44.3X1	T44.3X2	T44.3X3	T44.3X4	T44.3X5	T44.3X6
Methanthelinium bromide	T44.3X1	T44.3X2	T44.3X3	T44.3X4	T44.3X5	T44.3X6
Methaphenilene	T45.0X1	T45.0X2	T45.0X3	T45.0X4	T45.0X5	T45.0X6
Methapyrilene	T45.0X1	T45.0X2	T45.0X3	T45.0X4	T45.0X5	T45.0X6
Methaqualone (compound)	T42.6X1	T42.6X2	T42.6X3	T42.6X4	T42.6X5	T42.6X6
Metharbital	T42.3X1	T42.3X2	T42.3X3	T42.3X4	T42.3X5	T42.3X6
Methazolamide	T50.2X1	T50.2X2	T50.2X3	T50.2X4	T50.2X5	T50.2X6
Methdilazine	T43.3X1	T43.3X2	T43.3X3	T43.3X4	T43.3X5	T43.3X6
Methedrine	T43.621	T43.622	T43.623	T43.624	T43.625	T43.626
Methenamine (mandelate)	T37.8X1	T37.8X2	T37.8X3	T37.8X4	T37.8X5	T37.8X6
Methenolone	T38.7X1	T38.7X2	T38.7X3	T38.7X4	T38.7X5	T38.7X6
Methergine	T48.0X1	T48.0X2	T48.0X3	T48.0X4	T48.0X5	T48.0X6
Methetoin	T42.0X1	T42.0X2	T42.0X3	T42.0X4	T42.0X5	T42.0X6
Methiacil	T38.2X1	T38.2X2	T38.2X3	T38.2X4	T38.2X5	T38.2X6
Methicillin	T36.0X1	T36.0X2	T36.0X3	T36.0X4	T36.0X5	T36.0X6
Methimazole	T38.2X1	T38.2X2	T38.2X3	T38.2X4	T38.2X5	T38.2X6
Methiodal sodium	T50.8X1	T50.8X2	T50.8X3	T50.8X4	T50.8X5	T50.8X6
Methionine	T50.991	T50.992	T50.993	T50.994	T50.995	T50.996
Methisazone	T37.5X1	T37.5X2	T37.5X3	T37.5X4	T37.5X5	T37.5X6
Methisoprinol	T37.5X1	T37.5X2	T37.5X3	T37.5X4	T37.5X5	T37.5X6
Methitural	T42.3X1	T42.3X2	T42.3X3	T42.3X4	T42.3X5	T42.3X6
Methixene	T44.3X1	T44.3X2	T44.3X3	T44.3X4	T44.3X5	T44.3X6
Methobarbital, methobarbitone	T42.3X1	T42.3X2	T42.3X3	T42.3X4	T42.3X5	T42.3X6
Methocarbamol	T42.8X1	T42.8X2	T42.8X3	T42.8X4	T42.8X5	T42.8X6
skeletal muscle relaxant	T48.1X1	T48.1X2	T48.1X3	T48.1X4	T48.1X5	T48.1X6
Methohexital	T41.1X1	T41.1X2	T41.1X3	T41.1X4	T41.1X5	T41.1X6
Methohexitone	T41.1X1	T41.1X2	T41.1X3	T41.1X4	T41.1X5	T41.1X6
Methoin	T42.0X1	T42.0X2	T42.0X3	T42.0X4	T42.0X5	T42.0X6
Methopholine	T39.8X1	T39.8X2	T39.8X3	T39.8X4	T39.8X5	T39.8X6

TABLE OF DRUGS AND CHEMICALS

◄ New   ◄ⅲ Revised   ~~deleted~~ Deleted

TABLE OF DRUGS AND CHEMICALS

Substance	External Cause (T-Code)					
	Poisoning, Accidental (Unintentional)	Poisoning, Intentional Self-Harm	Poisoning, Assault	Poisoning, Undetermined	Adverse Effect	Underdosing
Methopromazine	T43.3X1	T43.3X2	T43.3X3	T43.3X4	T43.3X5	T43.3X6
Methorate	T48.3X1	T48.3X2	T48.3X3	T48.3X4	T48.3X5	T48.3X6
Methoserpidine	T46.5X1	T46.5X2	T46.5X3	T46.5X4	T46.5X5	T46.5X6
Methotrexate	T45.1X1	T45.1X2	T45.1X3	T45.1X4	T45.1X5	T45.1X6
Methotrimeprazine	T43.3X1	T43.3X2	T43.3X3	T43.3X4	T43.3X5	T43.3X6
Methoxa-Dome	T49.3X1	T49.3X2	T49.3X3	T49.3X4	T49.3X5	T49.3X6
Methoxamine	T44.4X1	T44.4X2	T44.4X3	T44.4X4	T44.4X5	T44.4X6
Methoxsalen	T50.991	T50.992	T50.993	T50.994	T50.995	T50.996
Methoxyaniline	T65.3X1	T65.3X2	T65.3X3	T65.3X4	—	—
Methoxybenzyl penicillin	T36.0X1	T36.0X2	T36.0X3	T36.0X4	T36.0X5	T36.0X6
Methoxychlor	T53.7X1	T53.7X2	T53.7X3	T53.7X4	—	—
Methoxy-DDT	T53.7X1	T53.7X2	T53.7X3	T53.7X4	—	—
2-Methoxyethanol	T52.3X1	T52.3X2	T52.3X3	T52.3X4	—	—
Methoxyflurane	T41.0X1	T41.0X2	T41.0X3	T41.0X4	T41.0X5	T41.0X6
Methoxyphenamine	T48.6X1	T48.6X2	T48.6X3	T48.6X4	T48.6X5	T48.6X6
Methoxypromazine	T43.3X1	T43.3X2	T43.3X3	T43.3X4	T43.3X5	T43.3X6
5-Methoxypsoralen (5-MOP)	T50.991	T50.992	T50.993	T50.994	T50.995	T50.996
8-Methoxypsoralen (8-MOP)	T50.991	T50.992	T50.993	T50.994	T50.995	T50.996
Methscopolamine bromide	T44.3X1	T44.3X2	T44.3X3	T44.3X4	T44.3X5	T44.3X6
Methsuximide	T42.2X1	T42.2X2	T42.2X3	T42.2X4	T42.2X5	T42.2X6
Methyclothiazide	T50.2X1	T50.2X2	T50.2X3	T50.2X4	T50.2X5	T50.2X6
Methyl						
acetate	T52.4X1	T52.4X2	T52.4X3	T52.4X4	—	—
acetone	T52.4X1	T52.4X2	T52.4X3	T52.4X4	—	—
acrylate	T65.891	T65.892	T65.893	T65.894	—	—
alcohol	T51.1X1	T51.1X2	T51.1X3	T51.1X4	—	—
aminophenol	T65.3X1	T65.3X2	T65.3X3	T65.3X4	—	—
amphetamine	T43.621	T43.622	T43.623	T43.624	T43.625	T43.626
androstanolone	T38.7X1	T38.7X2	T38.7X3	T38.7X4	T38.7X5	T38.7X6
atropine	T44.3X1	T44.3X2	T44.3X3	T44.3X4	T44.3X5	T44.3X6
benzene	T52.2X1	T52.2X2	T52.2X3	T52.2X4	—	—
benzoate	T52.8X1	T52.8X2	T52.8X3	T52.8X4	—	—
benzol	T52.2X1	T52.2X2	T52.2X3	T52.2X4	—	—
bromide (gas)	T59.891	T59.892	T59.893	T59.894	—	—
fumigant	T60.8X1	T60.8X2	T60.8X3	T60.8X4	—	—
butanol	T51.3X1	T51.3X2	T51.3X3	T51.3X4	—	—
carbinol	T51.1X1	T51.1X2	T51.1X3	T51.1X4	—	—
carbonate	T52.8X1	T52.8X2	T52.8X3	T52.8X4	—	—
CCNU	T45.1X1	T45.1X2	T45.1X3	T45.1X4	T45.1X5	T45.1X6
cellosolve	T52.91	T52.92	T52.93	T52.94	—	—

◀ New ◀▥ Revised ~~deleted~~ Deleted

Substance	External Cause (T-Code)					
	Poisoning, Accidental (Unintentional)	Poisoning, Intentional Self-Harm	Poisoning, Assault	Poisoning, Undetermined	Adverse Effect	Underdosing
Methyl *(Continued)*						
cellulose	T47.4X1	T47.4X2	T47.4X3	T47.4X4	T47.4X5	T47.4X6
chloride (gas)	T59.891	T59.892	T59.893	T59.894	—	—
chloroformate	T59.3X1	T59.3X2	T59.3X3	T59.3X4	—	—
cyclohexane	T52.8X1	T52.8X2	T52.8X3	T52.8X4	—	—
cyclohexanol	T51.8X1	T51.8X2	T51.8X3	T51.8X4	—	—
cyclohexanone	T52.8X1	T52.8X2	T52.8X3	T52.8X4	—	—
cyclohexyl acetate	T52.8X1	T52.8X2	T52.8X3	T52.8X4	—	—
demeton	T60.0X1	T60.0X2	T60.0X3	T60.0X4		
dihydromorphinone	T40.2X1	T40.2X2	T40.2X3	T40.2X4	T40.2X5	T40.2X6
ergometrine	T48.0X1	T48.0X2	T48.0X3	T48.0X4	T48.0X5	T48.0X6
ergonovine	T48.0X1	T48.0X2	T48.0X3	T48.0X4	T48.0X5	T48.0X6
ethyl ketone	T52.4X1	T52.4X2	T52.4X3	T52.4X4	—	—
glucamine antimonate	T37.8X1	T37.8X2	T37.8X3	T37.8X4	T37.8X5	T37.8X6
hydrazine	T65.891	T65.892	T65.893	T65.894	—	—
iodide	T65.891	T65.892	T65.893	T65.894	—	—
isobutyl ketone	T52.4X1	T52.4X2	T52.4X3	T52.4X4	—	—
isothiocyanate	T60.3X1	T60.3X2	T60.3X3	T60.3X4	—	—
mercaptan	T59.891	T59.892	T59.893	T59.894	—	—
morphine NEC	T40.2X1	T40.2X2	T40.2X3	T40.2X4	T40.2X5	T40.2X6
nicotinate	T49.4X1	T49.4X2	T49.4X3	T49.4X4	T49.4X5	T49.4X6
paraben	T49.0X1	T49.0X2	T49.0X3	T49.0X4	T49.0X5	T49.0X6
parafynol	T42.6X1	T42.6X2	T42.6X3	T42.6X4	T42.6X5	T42.6X6
parathion	T60.0X1	T60.0X2	T60.0X3	T60.0X4	—	—
peridol	T43.4X1	T43.4X2	T43.4X3	T43.4X4	T43.4X5	T43.4X6
phenidate	T43.631	T43.632	T43.633	T43.634	T43.635	T43.636
prednisolone	T38.0X1	T38.0X2	T38.0X3	T38.0X4	T38.0X5	T38.0X6
ENT agent	T49.6X1	T49.6X2	T49.6X3	T49.6X4	T49.6X5	T49.6X6
ophthalmic preparation	T49.5X1	T49.5X2	T49.5X3	T49.5X4	T49.5X5	T49.5X6
topical NEC	T49.0X1	T49.0X2	T49.0X3	T49.0X4	T49.0X5	T49.0X6
propylcarbinol	T51.3X1	T51.3X2	T51.3X3	T51.3X4	—	—
rosaniline NEC	T49.0X1	T49.0X2	T49.0X3	T49.0X4	T49.0X5	T49.0X6
salicylate	T49.2X1	T49.2X2	T49.2X3	T49.2X4	T49.2X5	T49.2X6
sulfate (fumes)	T59.891	T59.892	T59.893	T59.894	—	—
liquid	T52.8X1	T52.8X2	T52.8X3	T52.8X4	—	—
sulfonal	T42.6X1	T42.6X2	T42.6X3	T42.6X4	T42.6X5	T42.6X6
testosterone	T38.7X1	T38.7X2	T38.7X3	T38.7X4	T38.7X5	T38.7X6
thiouracil	T38.2X1	T38.2X2	T38.2X3	T38.2X4	T38.2X5	T38.2X6
Methylamphetamine	T43.621	T43.622	T43.623	T43.624	T43.625	T43.626
Methylated spirit	T51.1X1	T51.1X2	T51.1X3	T51.1X4	—	—

TABLE OF DRUGS AND CHEMICALS

Substance	External Cause (T-Code)					
	Poisoning, Accidental (Unintentional)	Poisoning, Intentional Self-Harm	Poisoning, Assault	Poisoning, Undetermined	Adverse Effect	Underdosing
Methylatropine nitrate	T44.3X1	T44.3X2	T44.3X3	T44.3X4	T44.3X5	T44.3X6
Methylbenactyzium bromide	T44.3X1	T44.3X2	T44.3X3	T44.3X4	T44.3X5	T44.3X6
Methylbenzethonium chloride	T49.0X1	T49.0X2	T49.0X3	T49.0X4	T49.0X5	T49.0X6
Methylcellulose	T47.4X1	T47.4X2	T47.4X3	T47.4X4	T47.4X5	T47.4X6
laxative	T47.4X1	T47.4X2	T47.4X3	T47.4X4	T47.4X5	T47.4X6
Methylchlorophenoxy-acetic acid	T60.3X1	T60.3X2	T60.3X3	T60.3X4	—	—
Methyldopa	T46.5X1	T46.5X2	T46.5X3	T46.5X4	T46.5X5	T46.5X6
Methyldopate	T46.5X1	T46.5X2	T46.5X3	T46.5X4	T46.5X5	T46.5X6
Methylene						
blue	T50.6X1	T50.6X2	T50.6X3	T50.6X4	T50.6X5	T50.6X6
chloride or dichloride (solvent) NEC	T53.4X1	T53.4X2	T53.4X3	T53.4X4	—	—
Methylenedioxyamphet-amine	T43.621	T43.622	T43.623	T43.624	T43.625	T43.626
Methylenedioxymethamphetamine	T43.621	T43.622	T43.623	T43.624	T43.625	T43.626
Methylergometrine	T48.0X1	T48.0X2	T48.0X3	T48.0X4	T48.0X5	T48.0X6
Methylergonovine	T48.0X1	T48.0X2	T48.0X3	T48.0X4	T48.0X5	T48.0X6
Methylestrenolone	T38.5X1	T38.5X2	T38.5X3	T38.5X4	T38.5X5	T38.5X6
Methylethyl cellulose	T50.991	T50.992	T50.993	T50.994	T50.995	T50.996
Methylhexabital	T42.3X1	T42.3X2	T42.3X3	T42.3X4	T42.3X5	T42.3X6
Methylmorphine	T40.2X1	T40.2X2	T40.2X3	T40.2X4	T40.2X5	T40.2X6
Methylparaben (ophthalmic)	T49.5X1	T49.5X2	T49.5X3	T49.5X4	T49.5X5	T49.5X6
Methylparafynol	T42.6X1	T42.6X2	T42.6X3	T42.6X4	T42.6X5	T42.6X6
Methylpentynol, methylpenthynol	T42.6X1	T42.6X2	T42.6X3	T42.6X4	T42.6X5	T42.6X6
Methylphenidate	T43.631	T43.632	T43.633	T43.634	T43.635	T43.636
Methylphenobarbital	T42.3X1	T42.3X2	T42.3X3	T42.3X4	T42.3X5	T42.3X6
Methylpolysiloxane	T47.1X1	T47.1X2	T47.1X3	T47.1X4	T47.1X5	T47.1X6
Methylprednisolone — see Methyl, prednisolone						
Methylrosaniline	T49.0X1	T49.0X2	T49.0X3	T49.0X4	T49.0X5	T49.0X6
Methylrosanilinium chloride	T49.0X1	T49.0X2	T49.0X3	T49.0X4	T49.0X5	T49.0X6
Methyltestosterone	T38.7X1	T38.7X2	T38.7X3	T38.7X4	T38.7X5	T38.7X6
Methylthionine chloride	T50.6X1	T50.6X2	T50.6X3	T50.6X4	T50.6X5	T50.6X6
Methylthioninium chloride	T50.6X1	T50.6X2	T50.6X3	T50.6X4	T50.6X5	T50.6X6
Methylthiouracil	T38.2X1	T38.2X2	T38.2X3	T38.2X4	T38.2X5	T38.2X6
Methyprylon	T42.6X1	T42.6X2	T42.6X3	T42.6X4	T42.6X5	T42.6X6
Methysergide	T46.5X1	T46.5X2	T46.5X3	T46.5X4	T46.5X5	T46.5X6
Metiamide	T47.1X1	T47.1X2	T47.1X3	T47.1X4	T47.1X5	T47.1X6
Meticillin	T36.0X1	T36.0X2	T36.0X3	T36.0X4	T36.0X5	T36.0X6
Meticrane	T50.2X1	T50.2X2	T50.2X3	T50.2X4	T50.2X5	T50.2X6
Metildigoxin	T46.0X1	T46.0X2	T46.0X3	T46.0X4	T46.0X5	T46.0X6
Metipranolol	T49.5X1	T49.5X2	T49.5X3	T49.5X4	T49.5X5	T49.5X6

◄ New ◄ⅲ Revised ~~deleted~~ Deleted

Substance	Poisoning, Accidental (Unintentional)	Poisoning, Intentional Self-Harm	Poisoning, Assault	Poisoning, Undetermined	Adverse Effect	Underdosing
	External Cause (T-Code)					
Metirosine	T46.5X1	T46.5X2	T46.5X3	T46.5X4	T46.5X5	T46.5X6
Metisazone	T37.5X1	T37.5X2	T37.5X3	T37.5X4	T37.5X5	T37.5X6
Metixene	T44.3X1	T44.3X2	T44.3X3	T44.3X4	T44.3X5	T44.3X6
Metizoline	T48.5X1	T48.5X2	T48.5X3	T48.5X4	T48.5X5	T48.5X6
Metoclopramide	T45.0X1	T45.0X2	T45.0X3	T45.0X4	T45.0X5	T45.0X6
Metofenazate	T43.3X1	T43.3X2	T43.3X3	T43.3X4	T43.3X5	T43.3X6
Metofoline	T39.8X1	T39.8X2	T39.8X3	T39.8X4	T39.8X5	T39.8X6
Metolazone	T50.2X1	T50.2X2	T50.2X3	T50.2X4	T50.2X5	T50.2X6
Metopon	T40.2X1	T40.2X2	T40.2X3	T40.2X4	T40.2X5	T40.2X6
Metoprine	T45.1X1	T45.1X2	T45.1X3	T45.1X4	T45.1X5	T45.1X6
Metoprolol	T44.7X1	T44.7X2	T44.7X3	T44.7X4	T44.7X5	T44.7X6
Metrifonate	T60.0X1	T60.0X2	T60.0X3	T60.0X4	—	—
Metrizamide	T50.8X1	T50.8X2	T50.8X3	T50.8X4	T50.8X5	T50.8X6
Metrizoic acid	T50.8X1	T50.8X2	T50.8X3	T50.8X4	T50.8X5	T50.8X6
Metronidazole	T37.8X1	T37.8X2	T37.8X3	T37.8X4	T37.8X5	T37.8X6
Metycaine	T41.3X1	T41.3X2	T41.3X3	T41.3X4	T41.3X5	T41.3X6
infiltration (subcutaneous)	T41.3X1	T41.3X2	T41.3X3	T41.3X4	T41.3X5	T41.3X6
nerve block (peripheral) (plexus)	T41.3X1	T41.3X2	T41.3X3	T41.3X4	T41.3X5	T41.3X6
topical (surface)	T41.3X1	T41.3X2	T41.3X3	T41.3X4	T41.3X5	T41.3X6
Metyrapone	T50.8X1	T50.8X2	T50.8X3	T50.8X4	T50.8X5	T50.8X6
Mevinphos	T60.0X1	T60.0X2	T60.0X3	T60.0X4	—	—
Mexazolam	T42.4X1	T42.4X2	T42.4X3	T42.4X4	T42.4X5	T42.4X6
Mexenone	T49.3X1	T49.3X2	T49.3X3	T49.3X4	T49.3X5	T49.3X6
Mexiletine	T46.2X1	T46.2X2	T46.2X3	T46.2X4	T46.2X5	T46.2X6
Mezereon	T62.2X1	T62.2X2	T62.2X3	T62.2X4	—	—
berries	T62.1X1	T62.1X2	T62.1X3	T62.1X4	—	—
Mezlocillin	T36.0X1	T36.0X2	T36.0X3	T36.0X4	T36.0X5	T36.0X6
Mianserin	T43.021	T43.022	T43.023	T43.024	T43.025	T43.026
Micatin	T49.0X1	T49.0X2	T49.0X3	T49.0X4	T49.0X5	T49.0X6
Miconazole	T49.0X1	T49.0X2	T49.0X3	T49.0X4	T49.0X5	T49.0X6
Micronomicin	T36.5X1	T36.5X2	T36.5X3	T36.5X4	T36.5X5	T36.5X6
Midazolam	T42.4X1	T42.4X2	T42.4X3	T42.4X4	T42.4X5	T42.4X6
Midecamycin	T36.3X1	T36.3X2	T36.3X3	T36.3X4	T36.3X5	T36.3X6
Mifepristone	T38.6X1	T38.6X2	T38.6X3	T38.6X4	T38.6X5	T38.6X6
Milk of magnesia	T47.1X1	T47.1X2	T47.1X3	T47.1X4	T47.1X5	T47.1X6
Millipede (tropical) (venomous)	T63.411	T63.412	T63.413	T63.414	—	—
Miltown	T43.591	T43.592	T43.593	T43.594	T43.595	T43.596
Milverine	T44.3X1	T44.3X2	T44.3X3	T44.3X4	T44.3X5	T44.3X6
Minaprine	T43.291	T43.292	T43.293	T43.294	T43.295	T43.296

◀ New ◀▥ Revised ~~deleted~~ Deleted

Substance	Poisoning, Accidental (Unintentional)	Poisoning, Intentional Self-Harm	Poisoning, Assault	Poisoning, Undetermined	Adverse Effect	Underdosing
			External Cause (T-Code)			
Minaxolone	T41.291	T41.292	T41.293	T41.294	T41.295	T41.296
Mineral						
acids	T54.2X1	T54.2X2	T54.2X3	T54.2X4	—	—
oil (laxative) (medicinal)	T47.4X1	T47.4X2	T47.4X3	T47.4X4	T47.4X5	T47.4X6
emulsion	T47.2X1	T47.2X2	T47.2X3	T47.2X4	T47.2X5	T47.2X6
nonmedicinal	T52.0X1	T52.0X2	T52.0X3	T52.0X4	—	—
topical	T49.3X1	T49.3X2	T49.3X3	T49.3X4	T49.3X5	T49.3X6
salt NEC	T50.3X1	T50.3X2	T50.3X3	T50.3X4	T50.3X5	T50.3X6
spirits	T52.0X1	T52.0X2	T52.0X3	T52.0X4	—	—
Mineralocorticosteroid	T50.0X1	T50.0X2	T50.0X3	T50.0X4	T50.0X5	T50.0X6
Minocycline	T36.4X1	T36.4X2	T36.4X3	T36.4X4	T36.4X5	T36.4X6
Minoxidil	T46.7X1	T46.7X2	T46.7X3	T46.7X4	T46.7X5	T46.7X6
Miokamycin	T36.3X1	T36.3X2	T36.3X3	T36.3X4	T36.3X5	T36.3X6
Miotic drug	T49.5X1	T49.5X2	T49.5X3	T49.5X4	T49.5X5	T49.5X6
Mipafox	T60.0X1	T60.0X2	T60.0X3	T60.0X4	—	—
Mirex	T60.1X1	T60.1X2	T60.1X3	T60.1X4	—	—
Mirtazapine	T43.021	T43.022	T43.023	T43.024	T43.025	T43.026
Misonidazole	T37.3X1	T37.3X2	T37.3X3	T37.3X4	T37.3X5	T37.3X6
Misoprostol	T47.1X1	T47.1X2	T47.1X3	T47.1X4	T47.1X5	T47.1X6
Mithramycin	T45.1X1	T45.1X2	T45.1X3	T45.1X4	T45.1X5	T45.1X6
Mitobronitol	T45.1X1	T45.1X2	T45.1X3	T45.1X4	T45.1X5	T45.1X6
Mitoguazone	T45.1X1	T45.1X2	T45.1X3	T45.1X4	T45.1X5	T45.1X6
Mitolactol	T45.1X1	T45.1X2	T45.1X3	T45.1X4	T45.1X5	T45.1X6
Mitomycin	T45.1X1	T45.1X2	T45.1X3	T45.1X4	T45.1X5	T45.1X6
Mitopodozide	T45.1X1	T45.1X2	T45.1X3	T45.1X4	T45.1X5	T45.1X6
Mitotane	T45.1X1	T45.1X2	T45.1X3	T45.1X4	T45.1X5	T45.1X6
Mitoxantrone	T45.1X1	T45.1X2	T45.1X3	T45.1X4	T45.1X5	T45.1X6
Mivacurium chloride	T48.1X1	T48.1X2	T48.1X3	T48.1X4	T48.1X5	T48.1X6
Miyari bacteria	T47.6X1	T47.6X2	T47.6X3	T47.6X4	T47.6X5	T47.6X6
Moclobemide	T43.1X1	T43.1X2	T43.1X3	T43.1X4	T43.1X5	T43.1X6
Moderil	T46.5X1	T46.5X2	T46.5X3	T46.5X4	T46.5X5	T46.5X6
Mofebutazone	T39.2X1	T39.2X2	T39.2X3	T39.2X4	T39.2X5	T39.2X6
Mogadon — see Nitrazepam						
Molindone	T43.591	T43.592	T43.593	T43.594	T43.595	T43.596
Molsidomine	T46.3X1	T46.3X2	T46.3X3	T46.3X4	T46.3X5	T46.3X6
Mometasone	T49.0X1	T49.0X2	T49.0X3	T49.0X4	T49.0X5	T49.0X6
Monistat	T49.0X1	T49.0X2	T49.0X3	T49.0X4	T49.0X5	T49.0X6
Monkshood	T62.2X1	T62.2X2	T62.2X3	T62.2X4	—	—
Monoamine oxidase inhibitor NEC	T43.1X1	T43.1X2	T43.1X3	T43.1X4	T43.1X5	T43.1X6
hydrazine	T43.1X1	T43.1X2	T43.1X3	T43.1X4	T43.1X5	T43.1X6

◀ New   ◀▬ Revised   ~~deleted~~ Deleted

Substance	External Cause (T-Code)					
	Poisoning, Accidental (Unintentional)	Poisoning, Intentional Self-Harm	Poisoning, Assault	Poisoning, Undetermined	Adverse Effect	Underdosing
Monobenzone	T49.4X1	T49.4X2	T49.4X3	T49.4X4	T49.4X5	T49.4X6
Monochloroacetic acid	T60.3X1	T60.3X2	T60.3X3	T60.3X4	—	—
Monochlorobenzene	T53.7X1	T53.7X2	T53.7X3	T53.7X4	—	—
Monoethanolamine	T46.8X1	T46.8X2	T46.8X3	T46.8X4	T46.8X5	T46.8X6
oleate	T46.8X1	T46.8X2	T46.8X3	T46.8X4	T46.8X5	T46.8X6
Monooctanoin	T50.991	T50.992	T50.993	T50.994	T50.995	T50.996
Monophenylbutazone	T39.2X1	T39.2X2	T39.2X3	T39.2X4	T39.2X5	T39.2X6
Monosodium glutamate	T65.891	T65.892	T65.893	T65.894	—	—
Monosulfiram	T49.0X1	T49.0X2	T49.0X3	T49.0X4	T49.0X5	T49.0X6
Monoxide, carbon — see Carbon, monoxide	T57.91	T57.92	T57.93	T57.94	—	—
Monoxidine hydrochloride	T46.1X1	T46.1X2	T46.1X3	T46.1X4	T46.1X5	T46.1X6
Monuron	T60.3X1	T60.3X2	T60.3X3	T60.3X4	—	—
Moperone	T43.4X1	T43.4X2	T43.4X3	T43.4X4	T43.4X5	T43.4X6
Mopidamol	T45.1X1	T45.1X2	T45.1X3	T45.1X4	T45.1X5	T45.1X6
MOPP (mechlorethamine + vincristine + prednisone + procarbazine)	T45.1X1	T45.1X2	T45.1X3	T45.1X4	T45.1X5	T45.1X6
Morfin	T40.2X1	T40.2X2	T40.2X3	T40.2X4	T40.2X5	T40.2X6
Morinamide	T37.1X1	T37.1X2	T37.1X3	T37.1X4	T37.1X5	T37.1X6
Morning glory seeds	T40.991	T40.992	T40.993	T40.994	—	—
Moroxydine	T37.5X1	T37.5X2	T37.5X3	T37.5X4	T37.5X5	T37.5X6
Morphazinamide	T37.1X1	T37.1X2	T37.1X3	T37.1X4	T37.1X5	T37.1X6
Morphine	T40.2X1	T40.2X2	T40.2X3	T40.2X4	T40.2X5	T40.2X6
antagonist	T50.7X1	T50.7X2	T50.7X3	T50.7X4	T50.7X5	T50.7X6
Morpholinylethylmorphine	T40.2X1	T40.2X2	T40.2X3	T40.2X4	—	—
Morsuximide	T42.2X1	T42.2X2	T42.2X3	T42.2X4	T42.2X5	T42.2X6
Mosapramine	T43.591	T43.592	T43.593	T43.594	T43.595	T43.596
Moth balls — see also Pesticides	T60.2X1	T60.2X2	T60.2X3	T60.2X4	—	—
naphthalene	T60.2X1	T60.2X2	T60.2X3	T60.2X4	—	—
paradichlorobenzene	T60.1X1	T60.1X2	T60.1X3	T60.1X4	—	—
Motor exhaust gas	T58.01	T58.02	T58.03	T58.04	—	—
Mouthwash (antiseptic) (zinc chloride)	T49.6X1	T49.6X2	T49.6X3	T49.6X4	T49.6X5	T49.6X6
Moxastine	T45.0X1	T45.0X2	T45.0X3	T45.0X4	T45.0X5	T45.0X6
Moxaverine	T44.3X1	T44.3X2	T44.3X3	T44.3X4	T44.3X5	T44.3X6
Moxifensine	T43.291	T43.292	T43.293	T43.294	T43.295	T43.296
Moxisylyte	T46.7X1	T46.7X2	T46.7X3	T46.7X4	T46.7X5	T46.7X6
Mucilage, plant	T47.4X1	T47.4X2	T47.4X3	T47.4X4	T47.4X5	T47.4X6
Mucolytic drug	T48.4X1	T48.4X2	T48.4X3	T48.4X4	T48.4X5	T48.4X6
Mucomyst	T48.4X1	T48.4X2	T48.4X3	T48.4X4	T48.4X5	T48.4X6
Mucous membrane agents (external)	T49.91	T49.92	T49.93	T49.94	T49.95	T49.96
specified NEC	T49.8X1	T49.8X2	T49.8X3	T49.8X4	T49.8X5	T49.8X6

TABLE OF DRUGS AND CHEMICALS

Substance	External Cause (T-Code)					
	Poisoning, Accidental (Unintentional)	Poisoning, Intentional Self-Harm	Poisoning, Assault	Poisoning, Undetermined	Adverse Effect	Underdosing
Mumps						
immune globulin (human)	T50.Z11	T50.Z12	T50.Z13	T50.Z14	T50.Z15	T50.Z16
skin test antigen	T50.8X1	T50.8X2	T50.8X3	T50.8X4	T50.8X5	T50.8X6
vaccine	T50.B91	T50.B92	T50.B93	T50.B94	T50.B95	T50.B96
Mumpsvax	T50.B91	T50.B92	T50.B93	T50.B94	T50.B95	T50.B96
Mupirocin	T49.0X1	T49.0X2	T49.0X3	T49.0X4	T49.0X5	T49.0X6
Muriatic acid — *see Hydrochloric acid*						
Muromonab-CD3	T45.1X1	T45.1X2	T45.1X3	T45.1X4	T45.1X5	T45.1X6
Muscle relaxant — *see Relaxant, muscle*						
Muscle-action drug NEC	T48.201	T48.202	T48.203	T48.204	T48.205	T48.206
Muscle affecting agents NEC	T48.201	T48.202	T48.203	T48.204	T48.205	T48.206
oxytocic	T48.0X1	T48.0X2	T48.0X3	T48.0X4	T48.0X5	T48.0X6
relaxants	T48.201	T48.202	T48.203	T48.204	T48.205	T48.206
central nervous system	T42.8X1	T42.8X2	T42.8X3	T42.8X4	T42.8X5	T42.8X6
skeletal	T48.1X1	T48.1X2	T48.1X3	T48.1X4	T48.1X5	T48.1X6
smooth	T44.3X1	T44.3X2	T44.3X3	T44.3X4	T44.3X5	T44.3X6
Muscle-tone depressant, central NEC	T42.8X1	T42.8X2	T42.8X3	T42.8X4	T42.8X5	T42.8X6
specified NEC	T42.8X1	T42.8X2	T42.8X3	T42.8X4	T42.8X5	T42.8X6
Mushroom, noxious	T62.0X1	T62.0X2	T62.0X3	T62.0X4	—	—
Mussel, noxious	T61.781	T61.782	T61.783	T61.784	—	—
Mustard (emetic)	T47.7X1	T47.7X2	T47.7X3	T47.7X4	T47.7X5	T47.7X6
black	T47.7X1	T47.7X2	T47.7X3	T47.7X4	T47.7X5	T47.7X6
gas, not in war	T59.91	T59.92	T59.93	T59.94	—	—
nitrogen	T45.1X1	T45.1X2	T45.1X3	T45.1X4	T45.1X5	T45.1X6
Mustine	T45.1X1	T45.1X2	T45.1X3	T45.1X4	T45.1X5	T45.1X6
M-vac	T45.1X1	T45.1X2	T45.1X3	T45.1X4	T45.1X5	T45.1X6
Mycifradin	T36.5X1	T36.5X2	T36.5X3	T36.5X4	T36.5X5	T36.5X6
topical	T49.0X1	T49.0X2	T49.0X3	T49.0X4	T49.0X5	T49.0X6
Mycitracin	T36.8X1	T36.8X2	T36.8X3	T36.8X4	T36.8X5	T36.8X6
ophthalmic preparation	T49.5X1	T49.5X2	T49.5X3	T49.5X4	T49.5X5	T49.5X6
Mycostatin	T36.7X1	T36.7X2	T36.7X3	T36.7X4	T36.7X5	T36.7X6
topical	T49.0X1	T49.0X2	T49.0X3	T49.0X4	T49.0X5	T49.0X6
Mycotoxins	T64.81	T64.82	T64.83	T64.84	—	—
aflatoxin	T64.01	T64.02	T64.03	T64.04	—	—
specified NEC	T64.81	T64.82	T64.83	T64.84	—	—
Mydriacyl	T44.3X1	T44.3X2	T44.3X3	T44.3X4	T44.3X5	T44.3X6
Mydriatic drug	T49.5X1	T49.5X2	T49.5X3	T49.5X4	T49.5X5	T49.5X6
Myelobromal	T45.1X1	T45.1X2	T45.1X3	T45.1X4	T45.1X5	T45.1X6
Myleran	T45.1X1	T45.1X2	T45.1X3	T45.1X4	T45.1X5	T45.1X6
Myochrysin(e)	T39.2X1	T39.2X2	T39.2X3	T39.2X4	T39.2X5	T39.2X6

◄ New   ◄▥ Revised   ~~deleted~~ Deleted

TABLE OF DRUGS AND CHEMICALS

Substance	External Cause (T-Code)					
	Poisoning, Accidental (Unintentional)	Poisoning, Intentional Self-Harm	Poisoning, Assault	Poisoning, Undetermined	Adverse Effect	Underdosing
Myoneural blocking agents	T48.1X1	T48.1X2	T48.1X3	T48.1X4	T48.1X5	T48.1X6
Myralact	T49.0X1	T49.0X2	T49.0X3	T49.0X4	T49.0X5	T49.0X6
Myristica fragrans	T62.2X1	T62.2X2	T62.2X3	T62.2X4	—	—
Myristicin	T65.891	T65.892	T65.893	T65.894	—	—
Mysoline	T42.3X1	T42.3X2	T42.3X3	T42.3X4	T42.3X5	T42.3X6
			N			
Nabilone	T40.7X1	T40.7X2	T40.7X3	T40.7X4	T40.7X5	T40.7X6
Nabumetone	T39.391	T39.392	T39.393	T39.394	T39.395	T39.396
Nadolol	T44.7X1	T44.7X2	T44.7X3	T44.7X4	T44.7X5	T44.7X6
Nafcillin	T36.0X1	T36.0X2	T36.0X3	T36.0X4	T36.0X5	T36.0X6
Nafoxidine	T38.6X1	T38.6X2	T38.6X3	T38.6X4	T38.6X5	T38.6X6
Naftazone	T46.991	T46.992	T46.993	T46.994	T46.995	T46.996
Naftidrofuryl (oxalate)	T46.7X1	T46.7X2	T46.7X3	T46.7X4	T46.7X5	T46.7X6
Naftifine	T49.0X1	T49.0X2	T49.0X3	T49.0X4	T49.0X5	T49.0X6
Nail polish remover	T52.91	T52.92	T52.93	T52.94	—	—
Nalbuphine	T40.4X1	T40.4X2	T40.4X3	T40.4X4	T40.4X5	T40.4X6
Naled	T60.0X1	T60.0X2	T60.0X3	T60.0X4	—	—
Nalidixic acid	T37.8X1	T37.8X2	T37.8X3	T37.8X4	T37.8X5	T37.8X6
Nalorphine	T50.7X1	T50.7X2	T50.7X3	T50.7X4	T50.7X5	T50.7X6
Naloxone	T50.7X1	T50.7X2	T50.7X3	T50.7X4	T50.7X5	T50.7X6
Naltrexone	T50.7X1	T50.7X2	T50.7X3	T50.7X4	T50.7X5	T50.7X6
Namenda	T43.8X1	T43.8X2	T43.8X3	T43.8X4	T43.8X5	T43.8X6
Nandrolone	T38.7X1	T38.7X2	T38.7X3	T38.7X4	T38.7X5	T38.7X6
Naphazoline	T48.5X1	T48.5X2	T48.5X3	T48.5X4	T48.5X5	T48.5X6
Naphtha (painters') (petroleum)	T52.0X1	T52.0X2	T52.0X3	T52.0X4	—	—
solvent	T52.0X1	T52.0X2	T52.0X3	T52.0X4	—	—
vapor	T52.0X1	T52.0X2	T52.0X3	T52.0X4	—	—
Naphthalene (non-chlorinated)	T60.2X1	T60.2X2	T60.2X3	T60.2X4	—	—
chlorinated	T60.1X1	T60.1X2	T60.1X3	T60.1X4	—	—
vapor	T60.1X1	T60.1X2	T60.1X3	T60.1X4	—	—
insecticide or moth repellent	T60.2X1	T60.2X2	T60.2X3	T60.2X4	—	—
chlorinated	T60.1X1	T60.1X2	T60.1X3	T60.1X4	—	—
vapor	T60.2X1	T60.2X2	T60.2X3	T60.2X4	—	—
chlorinated	T60.1X1	T60.1X2	T60.1X3	T60.1X4	—	—
Naphthol	T65.891	T65.892	T65.893	T65.894	—	—
Naphthylamine	T65.891	T65.892	T65.893	T65.894	—	—
Naphthylthiourea (ANTU)	T60.4X1	T60.4X2	T60.4X3	T60.4X4	—	—
Naprosyn — see Naproxen						
Naproxen	T39.311	T39.312	T39.313	T39.314	T39.315	T39.316

TABLE OF DRUGS AND CHEMICALS

Substance	External Cause (T-Code)					
	Poisoning, Accidental (Unintentional)	Poisoning, Intentional Self-Harm	Poisoning, Assault	Poisoning, Undetermined	Adverse Effect	Underdosing
Narcotic (drug)	T40.601	T40.602	T40.603	T40.604	T40.605	T40.606
analgesic NEC	T40.601	T40.602	T40.603	T40.604	T40.605	T40.606
antagonist	T50.7X1	T50.7X2	T50.7X3	T50.7X4	T50.7X5	T50.7X6
specified NEC	T40.691	T40.692	T40.693	T40.694	T40.695	T40.696
synthetic	T40.4X1	T40.4X2	T40.4X3	T40.4X4	T40.4X5	T40.4X6
Narcotine	T48.3X1	T48.3X2	T48.3X3	T48.3X4	T48.3X5	T48.3X6
Nardil	T43.1X1	T43.1X2	T43.1X3	T43.1X4	T43.1X5	T43.1X6
Nasal drug NEC	T49.6X1	T49.6X2	T49.6X3	T49.6X4	T49.6X5	T49.6X6
Natamycin	T49.0X1	T49.0X2	T49.0X3	T49.0X4	T49.0X5	T49.0X6
Natrium cyanide — see Cyanide(s)						
Natural gas	T59.891	T59.892	T59.893	T59.894	—	—
incomplete combustion	T57.91	T57.92	T57.93	T57.94	—	—
Natural						
blood (product)	T45.8X1	T45.8X2	T45.8X3	T45.8X4	T45.8X5	T45.8X6
gas (piped)	T59.891	T59.892	T59.893	T59.894	—	—
incomplete combustion	T58.11	T58.12	T58.13	T58.14	—	—
Nealbarbital	T42.3X1	T42.3X2	T42.3X3	T42.3X4	T42.3X5	T42.3X6
Nectadon	T48.3X1	T48.3X2	T48.3X3	T48.3X4	T48.3X5	T48.3X6
Nedocromil	T48.6X1	T48.6X2	T48.6X3	T48.6X4	T48.6X5	T48.6X6
Nefopam	T39.8X1	T39.8X2	T39.8X3	T39.8X4	T39.8X5	T39.8X6
Nematocyst (sting)	T63.691	T63.692	T63.693	T63.694	—	—
Nembutal	T42.3X1	T42.3X2	T42.3X3	T42.3X4	T42.3X5	T42.3X6
Nemonapride	T43.591	T43.592	T43.593	T43.594	T43.595	T43.596
Neoarsphenamine	T37.8X1	T37.8X2	T37.8X3	T37.8X4	T37.8X5	T37.8X6
Neocinchophen	T50.4X1	T50.4X2	T50.4X3	T50.4X4	T50.4X5	T50.4X6
Neomycin (derivatives)	T36.5X1	T36.5X2	T36.5X3	T36.5X4	T36.5X5	T36.5X6
with						
bacitracin	T49.0X1	T49.0X2	T49.0X3	T49.0X4	T49.0X5	T49.0X6
neostigmine	T44.0X1	T44.0X2	T44.0X3	T44.0X4	T44.0X5	T44.0X6
ENT agent	T49.6X1	T49.6X2	T49.6X3	T49.6X4	T49.6X5	T49.6X6
ophthalmic preparation	T49.5X1	T49.5X2	T49.5X3	T49.5X4	T49.5X5	T49.5X6
topical NEC	T49.0X1	T49.0X2	T49.0X3	T49.0X4	T49.0X5	T49.0X6
Neonal	T42.3X1	T42.3X2	T42.3X3	T42.3X4	T42.3X5	T42.3X6
Neoprontosil	T37.0X1	T37.0X2	T37.0X3	T37.0X4	T37.0X5	T37.0X6
Neosalvarsan	T37.8X1	T37.8X2	T37.8X4	T37.8X4	T37.8X5	T37.8X6
Neosilversalvarsan	T37.8X1	T37.8X2	T37.8X3	T37.8X4	T37.8X5	T37.8X6
Neosporin	T36.8X1	T36.8X2	T36.8X3	T36.8X4	T36.8X5	T36.8X6
ENT agent	T49.6X1	T49.6X2	T49.6X3	T49.6X4	T49.6X5	T49.6X6
opthalmic preparation	T49.5X1	T49.5X2	T49.5X3	T49.5X4	T49.5X5	T49.5X6
topical NEC	T49.0X1	T49.0X2	T49.0X3	T49.0X4	T49.0X5	T49.0X6

◀ New   ⇐ Revised   ~~deleted~~ Deleted

TABLE OF DRUGS AND CHEMICALS

Substance	External Cause (T-Code)					
	Poisoning, Accidental (Unintentional)	Poisoning, Intentional Self-Harm	Poisoning, Assault	Poisoning, Undetermined	Adverse Effect	Underdosing
Neostigmine bromide	T44.0X1	T44.0X2	T44.0X3	T44.0X4	T44.0X5	T44.0X6
Neraval	T42.3X1	T42.3X2	T42.3X3	T42.3X4	T42.3X5	T42.3X6
Neravan	T42.3X1	T42.3X2	T42.3X3	T42.3X4	T42.3X5	T42.3X6
Nerium oleander	T62.2X1	T62.2X2	T62.2X3	T62.2X4	—	—
Nerve gas, not in war	T59.91	T59.92	T59.93	T59.94	—	—
Nesacaine	T41.3X1	T41.3X2	T41.3X3	T41.3X4	T41.3X5	T41.3X6
infiltration (subcutaneous)	T41.3X1	T41.3X2	T41.3X3	T41.3X4	T41.3X5	T41.3X6
nerve block (peripheral) (plexus)	T41.3X1	T41.3X2	T41.3X3	T41.3X4	T41.3X5	T41.3X6
Netilmicin	T36.5X1	T36.5X2	T36.5X3	T36.5X4	T36.5X5	T36.5X6
Neurobarb	T42.3X1	T42.3X2	T42.3X3	T42.3X4	T42.3X5	T42.3X6
Neuroleptic drug NEC	T43.501	T43.502	T43.503	T43.504	T43.505	T43.506
Neuromuscular blocking drug	T48.1X1	T48.1X2	T48.1X3	T48.1X4	T48.1X5	T48.1X6
Neutral insulin injection	T38.3X1	T38.3X2	T38.3X3	T38.3X4	T38.3X5	T38.3X6
Neutral spirits	T51.0X1	T51.0X2	T51.0X3	T51.0X4	—	—
beverage	T51.0X1	T51.0X2	T51.0X3	T51.0X4	—	—
Niacin	T46.7X1	T46.7X2	T46.7X3	T46.7X4	T46.7X5	T46.7X6
Niacinamide	T45.2X1	T45.2X2	T45.2X3	T45.2X4	T45.2X5	T45.2X6
Nialamide	T43.1X1	T43.1X2	T43.1X3	T43.1X4	T43.1X5	T43.1X6
Niaprazine	T42.6X1	T42.6X2	T42.6X3	T42.6X4	T42.6X5	T42.6X6
Nicametate	T46.7X1	T46.7X2	T46.7X3	T46.7X4	T46.7X5	T46.7X6
Nicardipine	T46.1X1	T46.1X2	T46.1X3	T46.1X4	T46.1X5	T46.1X6
Nicergoline	T46.7X1	T46.7X2	T46.7X3	T46.7X4	T46.7X5	T46.7X6
Nickel (carbonyl) (tetra-carbonyl) (fumes) (vapor)	T56.891	T56.892	T56.893	T56.894	—	—
Nickelocene	T56.891	T56.892	T56.893	T56.894	—	—
Niclosamide	T37.4X1	T37.4X2	T37.4X3	T37.4X4	T37.4X5	T37.4X6
Nicofuranose	T46.7X1	T46.7X2	T46.7X3	T46.7X4	T46.7X5	T46.7X6
Nicomorphine	T40.2X1	T40.2X2	T40.2X3	T40.2X4	—	—
Nicorandil	T46.3X1	T46.3X2	T46.3X3	T46.3X4	T46.3X5	T46.3X6
Nicotiana (plant)	T62.2X1	T62.2X2	T62.2X3	T62.2X4	—	—
Nicotinamide	T45.2X1	T45.2X2	T45.2X3	T45.2X4	T45.2X5	T45.2X6
Nicotine (insecticide) (spray) (sulfate) NEC	T60.2X1	T60.2X2	T60.2X3	T60.2X4	—	—
from tobacco	T65.291	T65.292	T65.293	T65.294	—	—
cigarettes	T65.221	T65.222	T65.223	T65.224	—	—
not insecticide	T65.291	T65.292	T65.293	T65.294	—	—
Nicotinic acid	T46.7X1	T46.7X2	T46.7X3	T46.7X4	T46.7X5	T46.7X6
Nicotinyl alcohol	T46.7X1	T46.7X2	T46.7X3	T46.7X4	T46.7X5	T46.7X6
Nicoumalone	T45.511	T45.512	T45.513	T45.514	T45.515	T45.516
Nifedipine	T46.1X1	T46.1X2	T46.1X3	T46.1X4	T46.1X5	T46.1X6
Nifenazone	T39.2X1	T39.2X2	T39.2X3	T39.2X4	T39.2X5	T39.2X6
Nifuraldezone	T37.91	T37.92	T37.93	T37.94	T37.95	T37.96

TABLE OF DRUGS AND CHEMICALS

TABLE OF DRUGS AND CHEMICALS

Substance	External Cause (T-Code)					
	Poisoning, Accidental (Unintentional)	Poisoning, Intentional Self-Harm	Poisoning, Assault	Poisoning, Undetermined	Adverse Effect	Underdosing
Nifuratel	T37.8X1	T37.8X2	T37.8X3	T37.8X4	T37.8X5	T37.8X6
Nifurtimox	T37.3X1	T37.3X2	T37.3X3	T37.3X4	T37.3X5	T37.3X6
Nifurtoinol	T37.8X1	T37.8X2	T37.8X3	T37.8X4	T37.8X5	T37.8X6
Nightshade, deadly (solanum) — see also Belladonna	T62.2X1	T62.2X2	T62.2X3	T62.2X4	—	—
berry	T62.1X1	T62.1X2	T62.1X3	T62.1X4	—	—
Nikethamide	T50.7X1	T50.7X2	T50.7X3	T50.7X4	T50.7X5	T50.7X6
Nilstat	T36.7X1	T36.7X2	T36.7X3	T36.7X4	T36.7X5	T36.7X6
topical	T49.0X1	T49.0X2	T49.0X3	T49.0X4	T49.0X5	T49.0X6
Nilutamide	T38.6X1	T38.6X2	T38.6X3	T38.6X4	T38.6X5	T38.6X6
Nimesulide	T39.391	T39.392	T39.393	T39.394	T39.395	T39.396
Nimetazepam	T42.4X1	T42.4X2	T42.4X3	T42.4X4	T42.4X5	T42.4X6
Nimodipine	T46.1X1	T46.1X2	T46.1X3	T46.1X4	T46.1X5	T46.1X6
Nimorazole	T37.3X1	T37.3X2	T37.3X3	T37.3X4	T37.3X5	T37.3X6
Nimustine	T45.1X1	T45.1X2	T45.1X3	T45.1X4	T45.1X5	T45.1X6
Niridazole	T37.4X1	T37.4X2	T37.4X3	T37.4X4	T37.4X5	T37.4X6
Nisentil	T40.2X1	T40.2X2	T40.2X3	T40.2X4	T40.2X5	T40.2X6
Nisoldipine	T46.1X1	T46.1X2	T46.1X3	T46.1X4	T46.1X5	T46.1X6
Nitramine	T65.3X1	T65.3X2	T65.3X3	T65.3X4	—	—
Nitrate, organic	T46.3X1	T46.3X2	T46.3X3	T46.3X4	T46.3X5	T46.3X6
Nitrazepam	T42.4X1	T42.4X2	T42.4X3	T42.4X4	T42.4X5	T42.4X6
Nitrefazole	T50.6X1	T50.6X2	T50.6X3	T50.6X4	T50.6X5	T50.6X6
Nitrendipine	T46.1X1	T46.1X2	T46.1X3	T46.1X4	T46.1X5	T46.1X6
Nitric						
acid (liquid)	T54.2X1	T54.2X2	T54.2X3	T54.2X4	—	—
vapor	T59.891	T59.892	T59.893	T59.894	—	—
oxide (gas)	T59.0X1	T59.0X2	T59.0X3	T59.0X4	—	—
Nitrimidazine	T37.3X1	T37.3X2	T37.3X3	T37.3X4	T37.3X5	T37.3X6
Nitrite, amyl (medicinal) (vapor)	T46.3X1	T46.3X2	T46.3X3	T46.3X4	T46.3X5	T46.3X6
Nitroaniline	T65.3X1	T65.3X2	T65.3X3	T65.3X4	—	—
vapor	T59.891	T59.892	T59.893	T59.894	—	—
Nitrobenzene, nitrobenzol	T65.3X1	T65.3X2	T65.3X3	T65.3X4	—	—
vapor	T65.3X1	T65.3X2	T65.3X3	T65.3X4	—	—
Nitrocellulose	T65.891	T65.892	T65.893	T65.894	—	—
lacquer	T65.891	T65.892	T65.893	T65.894	—	—
Nitrodiphenyl	T65.3X1	T65.3X2	T65.3X3	T65.3X4	—	—
Nitrofural	T49.0X1	T49.0X2	T49.0X3	T49.0X4	T49.0X5	T49.0X6
Nitrofurantoin	T37.8X1	T37.8X2	T37.8X3	T37.8X4	T37.8X5	T37.8X6
Nitrofurazone	T49.0X1	T49.0X2	T49.0X3	T49.0X4	T49.0X5	T49.0X6
Nitrogen	T59.0X1	T59.0X2	T59.0X3	T59.0X4	—	—
mustard	T45.1X1	T45.1X2	T45.1X3	T45.1X4	T45.1X5	T45.1X6

◀ New ◀▥ Revised ~~deleted~~ Deleted

Substance	External Cause (T-Code)					
	Poisoning, Accidental (Unintentional)	Poisoning, Intentional Self-Harm	Poisoning, Assault	Poisoning, Undetermined	Adverse Effect	Underdosing
Nitroglycerin, nitro-glycerol (medicinal)	T46.3X1	T46.3X2	T46.3X3	T46.3X4	T46.3X5	T46.3X6
nonmedicinal	T65.5X1	T65.5X2	T65.5X3	T65.5X4	—	—
fumes	T65.5X1	T65.5X2	T65.5X3	T65.5X4	—	—
Nitroglycol	T52.3X1	T52.3X2	T52.3X3	T52.3X4	—	—
Nitrohydrochloric acid	T54.2X1	T54.2X2	T54.2X3	T54.2X4	—	—
Nitromersol	T49.0X1	T49.0X2	T49.0X3	T49.0X4	T49.0X5	T49.0X6
Nitronaphthalene	T65.891	T65.892	T65.893	T65.894	—	—
Nitrophenol	T54.0X1	T54.0X2	T54.0X3	T54.0X4	—	—
Nitropropane	T52.8X1	T52.8X2	T52.8X3	T52.8X4	—	—
Nitroprusside	T46.5X1	T46.5X2	T46.5X3	T46.5X4	T46.5X5	T46.5X6
Nitrosodimethylamine	T65.3X1	T65.3X2	T65.3X3	T65.3X4	—	—
Nitrothiazol	T37.4X1	T37.4X2	T37.4X3	T37.4X4	T37.4X5	T37.4X6
Nitrotoluene, nitrotoluol	T65.3X1	T65.3X2	T65.3X3	T65.3X4	—	—
vapor	T65.3X1	T65.3X2	T65.3X3	T65.3X4	—	—
Nitrous						
acid (liquid)	T54.2X1	T54.2X2	T54.2X3	T54.2X4	—	—
fumes	T59.891	T59.892	T59.893	T59.894	—	—
ether spirit	T46.3X1	T46.3X2	T46.3X3	T46.3X4	T46.3X5	T46.3X6
oxide	T41.0X1	T41.0X2	T41.0X3	T41.0X4	T41.0X5	T41.0X6
Nitroxoline	T37.8X1	T37.8X2	T37.8X3	T37.8X4	T37.8X5	T37.8X6
Nitrozone	T49.0X1	T49.0X2	T49.0X3	T49.0X4	T49.0X5	T49.0X6
Nizatidine	T47.0X1	T47.0X2	T47.0X3	T47.0X4	T47.0X5	T47.0X6
Nizofenone	T43.8X1	T43.8X2	T43.8X3	T43.8X4	T43.8X5	T43.8X6
Noctec	T42.6X1	T42.6X2	T42.6X3	T42.6X4	T42.6X5	T42.6X6
Noludar	T42.6X1	T42.6X2	T42.6X3	T42.6X4	T42.6X5	T42.6X6
Noptil	T42.3X1	T42.3X2	T42.3X3	T42.3X4	T42.3X5	T42.3X6
Nomegestrol	T38.5X1	T38.5X2	T38.5X3	T38.5X4	T38.5X5	T38.5X6
Nomifensine	T43.291	T43.292	T43.293	T43.294	T43.295	T43.296
Nonoxinol	T49.8X1	T49.8X2	T49.8X3	T49.8X4	T49.8X5	T49.8X6
Nonylphenoxy (polyethoxy-ethanol)	T49.8X1	T49.8X2	T49.8X3	T49.8X4	T49.8X5	T49.8X6
Noptil	T42.3X1	T42.3X2	T42.3X3	T42.3X4	T42.3X5	T42.3X6
Noradrenaline	T44.4X1	T44.4X2	T44.4X3	T44.4X4	T44.4X5	T44.4X6
Noramidopyrine	T39.2X1	T39.2X2	T39.2X3	T39.2X4	T39.2X5	T39.2X6
methanesulfonate sodium	T39.2X1	T39.2X2	T39.2X3	T39.2X4	T39.2X5	T39.2X6
Norbormide	T60.4X1	T60.4X2	T60.4X3	T60.4X4	—	—
Nordazepam	T42.4X1	T42.4X2	T42.4X3	T42.4X4	T42.4X5	T42.4X6
Norepinephrine	T44.4X1	T44.4X2	T44.4X3	T44.4X4	T44.4X5	T44.4X6
Norethandrolone	T38.7X1	T38.7X2	T38.7X3	T38.7X4	T38.7X5	T38.7X6
Norethindrone	T38.4X1	T38.4X2	T38.4X3	T38.4X4	T38.4X5	T38.4X6

◀ New   ◀ Revised   ~~deleted~~ Deleted

TABLE OF DRUGS AND CHEMICALS

Substance	Poisoning, Accidental (Unintentional)	Poisoning, Intentional Self-Harm	Poisoning, Assault	Poisoning, Undetermined	Adverse Effect	Underdosing
			External Cause (T-Code)			
Norethisterone (acetate) (enantate)	T38.4X1	T38.4X2	T38.4X3	T38.4X4	T38.4X5	T38.4X6
with ethinylestradiol	T38.5X1	T38.5X2	T38.5X3	T38.5X4	T38.5X5	T38.5X6
Noretynodrel	T38.5X1	T38.5X2	T38.5X3	T38.5X4	T38.5X5	T38.5X6
Norfenefrine	T44.4X1	T44.4X2	T44.4X3	T44.4X4	T44.4X5	T44.4X6
Norfloxacin	T36.8X1	T36.8X2	T36.8X3	T36.8X4	T36.8X5	T36.8X6
Norgestrel	T38.4X1	T38.4X2	T38.4X3	T38.4X4	T38.4X5	T38.4X6
Norgestrienone	T38.4X1	T38.4X2	T38.4X3	T38.4X4	T38.4X5	T38.4X6
Norlestrin	T38.4X1	T38.4X2	T38.4X3	T38.4X4	T38.4X5	T38.4X6
Norlutin	T38.4X1	T38.4X2	T38.4X3	T38.4X4	T38.4X5	T38.4X6
Normal serum albumin (human), salt-poor	T45.8X1	T45.8X2	T45.8X3	T45.8X4	T45.8X5	T45.8X6
Normethandrone	T38.5X1	T38.5X2	T38.5X3	T38.5X4	T38.5X5	T38.5X6
Normison — see Benzodiazepines						
Normorphine	T40.2X1	T40.2X2	T40.2X3	T40.2X4	—	—
Norpseudoephedrine	T50.5X1	T50.5X2	T50.5X3	T50.5X4	T50.5X5	T50.5X6
Nortestosterone (furanpropionate)	T38.7X1	T38.7X2	T38.7X3	T38.7X4	T38.7X5	T38.7X6
Nortriptyline	T43.011	T43.012	T43.013	T43.014	T43.015	T43.016
Noscapine	T48.3X1	T48.3X2	T48.3X3	T48.3X4	T48.3X5	T48.3X6
Nose preparations	T49.6X1	T49.6X2	T49.6X3	T49.6X4	T49.6X5	T49.6X6
Novobiocin	T36.5X1	T36.5X2	T36.5X3	T36.5X4	T36.5X5	T36.5X6
Novocain (infiltration) (topical)	T41.3X1	T41.3X2	T41.3X3	T41.3X4	T41.3X5	T41.3X6
nerve block (peripheral) (plexus)	T41.3X1	T41.3X2	T41.3X3	T41.3X4	T41.3X5	T41.3X6
spinal	T41.3X1	T41.3X2	T41.3X3	T41.3X4	T41.3X5	T41.3X6
Noxious foodstuff	T62.91	T62.92	T62.93	T62.94	—	—
specified NEC	T62.8X1	T62.8X2	T62.8X3	T62.8X4	—	—
Noxiptiline	T43.011	T43.012	T43.013	T43.014	T43.015	T43.016
Noxytiolin	T49.0X1	T49.0X2	T49.0X3	T49.0X4	T49.0X5	T49.0X6
NPH Iletin (insulin)	T38.3X1	T38.3X2	T38.3X3	T38.3X4	T38.3X5	T38.3X6
Numorphan	T40.2X1	T40.2X2	T40.2X3	T40.2X4	T40.2X5	T40.2X6
Nunol	T42.3X1	T42.3X2	T42.3X3	T42.3X4	T42.3X5	T42.3X6
Nupercaine (spinal anesthetic)	T41.3X1	T41.3X2	T41.3X3	T41.3X4	T41.3X5	T41.3X6
topical (surface)	T41.3X1	T41.3X2	T41.3X3	T41.3X4	T41.3X5	T41.3X6
Nutmeg oil (liniment)	T49.3X1	T49.3X2	T49.3X3	T49.3X4	T49.3X5	T49.3X6
Nutritional supplement	T50.901	T50.902	T50.903	T50.904	T50.905	T50.906
Nux vomica	T65.1X1	T65.1X2	T65.1X3	T65.1X4	—	—
Nydrazid	T37.1X1	T37.1X2	T37.1X3	T37.1X4	T37.1X5	T37.1X6
Nylidrin	T46.7X1	T46.7X2	T46.7X3	T46.7X4	T46.7X5	T46.7X6
Nystatin	T36.7X1	T36.7X2	T36.7X3	T36.7X4	T36.7X5	T36.7X6
topical	T49.0X1	T49.0X2	T49.0X3	T49.0X4	T49.0X5	T49.0X6
Nytol	T45.0X1	T45.0X2	T45.0X3	T45.0X4	T45.0X5	T45.0X6

◀ New   ⬅ Revised   ~~deleted~~ Deleted

Substance	External Cause (T-Code)					
	Poisoning, Accidental (Unintentional)	Poisoning, Intentional Self-Harm	Poisoning, Assault	Poisoning, Undetermined	Adverse Effect	Underdosing
O						
Obidoxime chloride	T50.6X1	T50.6X2	T50.6X3	T50.6X4	T50.6X5	T50.6X6
Octafonium (chloride)	T49.3X1	T49.3X2	T49.3X3	T49.3X4	T49.3X5	T49.3X6
Octamethyl pyrophos-phoramide	T60.0X1	T60.0X2	T60.0X3	T60.0X4	—	—
Octanoin	T50.991	T50.992	T50.993	T50.994	T50.995	T50.996
Octatropine methyl-bromide	T44.3X1	T44.3X2	T44.3X3	T44.3X4	T44.3X5	T44.3X6
Octotiamine	T45.2X1	T45.2X2	T45.2X3	T45.2X4	T45.2X5	T45.2X6
Octoxinol (9)	T49.8X1	T49.8X2	T49.8X3	T49.8X4	T49.8X5	T49.8X6
Octreotide	T38.991	T38.992	T38.993	T38.994	T38.995	T38.996
Octyl nitrite	T46.3X1	T46.3X2	T46.3X3	T46.3X4	T46.3X5	T46.3X6
Oestradiol	T38.5X1	T38.5X2	T38.5X3	T38.5X4	T38.5X5	T38.5X6
Oestriol	T38.5X1	T38.5X2	T38.5X3	T38.5X4	T38.5X5	T38.5X6
Oestrogen	T38.5X1	T38.5X2	T38.5X3	T38.5X4	T38.5X5	T38.5X6
Oestrone	T38.5X1	T38.5X2	T38.5X3	T38.5X4	T38.5X5	T38.5X6
Ofloxacin	T36.8X1	T36.8X2	T36.8X3	T36.8X4	T36.8X5	T36.8X6
Oil (of)	T65.891	T65.892	T65.893	T65.894	—	—
bitter almond	T62.8X1	T62.8X2	T62.8X3	T62.8X4	—	—
cloves	T49.7X1	T49.7X2	T49.7X3	T49.7X4	T49.7X5	T49.7X6
colors	T65.6X1	T65.6X2	T65.6X3	T65.6X4	—	—
fumes	T59.891	T59.892	T59.893	T59.894	—	—
lubricating	T52.0X1	T52.0X2	T52.0X3	T52.0X4	—	—
Niobe	T52.8X1	T52.8X2	T52.8X3	T52.8X4	—	—
vitriol (liquid)	T54.2X1	T54.2X2	T54.2X3	T54.2X4	—	—
fumes	T54.2X1	T54.2X2	T54.2X3	T54.2X4	—	—
wintergreen (bitter) NEC	T49.3X1	T49.3X2	T49.3X3	T49.3X4	T49.3X5	T49.3X6
Oily preparation (for skin)	T49.3X1	T49.3X2	T49.3X3	T49.3X4	T49.3X5	T49.3X6
Ointment NEC	T49.3X1	T49.3X2	T49.3X3	T49.3X4	T49.3X5	T49.3X6
Olanzapine	T43.591	T43.592	T43.593	T43.594	T43.595	T43.596
Oleander	T62.2X1	T62.2X2	T62.2X3	T62.2X4	—	—
Oleandomycin	T36.3X1	T36.3X2	T36.3X3	T36.3X4	T36.3X5	T36.3X6
Oleandrin	T46.0X1	T46.0X2	T46.0X3	T46.0X4	T46.0X5	T46.0X6
Oleic acid	T46.6X1	T46.6X2	T46.6X3	T46.6X4	T46.6X5	T46.6X6
Oleovitamin A	T45.2X1	T45.2X2	T45.2X3	T45.2X4	T45.2X5	T45.2X6
Oleum ricini	T47.2X1	T47.2X2	T47.2X3	T47.2X4	T47.2X5	T47.2X6
Olive oil (medicinal) NEC	T47.4X1	T47.4X2	T47.4X3	T47.4X4	T47.4X5	T47.4X6
Olivomycin	T45.1X1	T45.1X2	T45.1X3	T45.1X4	T45.1X5	T45.1X6
Olsalazine	T47.8X1	T47.8X2	T47.8X3	T47.8X4	T47.8X5	T47.8X6
Omeprazole	T47.1X1	T47.1X2	T47.1X3	T47.1X4	T47.1X5	T47.1X6

TABLE OF DRUGS AND CHEMICALS

Substance	Poisoning, Accidental (Unintentional)	Poisoning, Intentional Self-Harm	Poisoning, Assault	Poisoning, Undetermined	Adverse Effect	Underdosing
OMPA	T60.0X1	T60.0X2	T60.0X3	T60.0X4	—	—
Ondansetron	T45.0X1	T45.0X2	T45.0X3	T45.0X4	T45.0X5	T45.0X6
Oncovin	T45.1X1	T45.1X2	T45.1X3	T45.1X4	T45.1X5	T45.1X6
Ophthaine	T41.3X1	T41.3X2	T41.3X3	T41.3X4	T41.3X5	T41.3X6
Ophthetic	T41.3X1	T41.3X2	T41.3X3	T41.3X4	T41.3X5	T41.3X6
Opiate NEC	T40.601	T40.602	T40.603	T40.604	T40.605	T40.606
antagonists	T50.7X1	T50.7X2	T50.7X3	T50.7X4	T50.7X5	T50.7X6
Opioid NEC	T40.2X1	T40.2X2	T40.2X3	T40.2X4	T40.2X5	T40.2X6
Opipramol	T43.011	T43.012	T43.013	T43.014	T43.015	T43.016
Opium alkaloids (total)	T40.0X1	T40.0X2	T40.0X3	T40.0X4	T40.0X5	T40.0X6
standardized powdered	T40.0X1	T40.0X2	T40.0X3	T40.0X4	T40.0X5	T40.0X6
tincture (camphorated)	T40.0X1	T40.0X2	T40.0X3	T40.0X4	T40.0X5	T40.0X6
Oracon	T38.4X1	T38.4X2	T38.4X3	T38.4X4	T38.4X5	T38.4X6
Oragrafin	T50.8X1	T50.8X2	T50.8X3	T50.8X4	T50.8X5	T50.8X6
Oral contraceptives	T38.4X1	T38.4X2	T38.4X3	T38.4X4	T38.4X5	T38.4X6
Oral rehydration salts	T50.3X1	T50.3X2	T50.3X3	T50.3X4	T50.3X5	T50.3X6
Orazamide	T50.991	T50.992	T50.993	T50.994	T50.995	T50.996
Orciprenaline	T48.291	T48.292	T48.293	T48.294	T48.295	T48.296
Organidin	T48.4X1	T48.4X2	T48.4X3	T48.4X4	T48.4X5	T48.4X6
Organonitrate NEC	T46.3X1	T46.3X2	T46.3X3	T46.3X4	T46.3X5	T46.3X6
Organophosphates	T60.0X1	T60.0X2	T60.0X3	T60.0X4	—	—
Orimune	T50.B91	T50.B92	T50.B93	T50.B94	T50.B95	T50.B96
Orinase	T38.3X1	T38.3X2	T38.3X3	T38.3X4	T38.3X5	T38.3X6
Ormeloxifene	T38.6X1	T38.6X2	T38.6X3	T38.6X4	T38.6X5	T38.6X6
Ornidazole	T37.3X1	T37.3X2	T37.3X3	T37.3X4	T37.3X5	T37.3X6
Ornithine aspartate	T50.991	T50.992	T50.993	T50.994	T50.995	T50.996
Ornoprostil	T47.1X1	T47.1X2	T47.1X3	T47.1X4	T47.1X5	T47.1X6
Orphenadrine (hydrochloride)	T42.8X1	T42.8X2	T42.8X3	T42.8X4	T42.8X5	T42.8X6
Ortal (sodium)	T42.3X1	T42.3X2	T42.3X3	T42.3X4	T42.3X5	T42.3X6
Orthoboric acid	T49.0X1	T49.0X2	T49.0X3	T49.0X4	T49.0X5	T49.0X6
ENT agent	T49.6X1	T49.6X2	T49.6X3	T49.6X4	T49.6X5	T49.6X6
ophthalmic preparation	T49.5X1	T49.5X2	T49.5X3	T49.5X4	T49.5X5	T49.5X6
Orthocaine	T41.3X1	T41.3X2	T41.3X3	T41.3X4	T41.3X5	T41.3X6
Orthodichlorobenzene	T53.7X1	T53.7X2	T53.7X3	T53.7X4	—	—
Ortho-Novum	T38.4X1	T38.4X2	T38.4X3	T38.4X4	T38.4X5	T38.4X6
Orthotolidine (reagent)	T54.2X1	T54.2X2	T54.2X3	T54.2X4	—	—
Osmic acid (liquid)	T54.2X1	T54.2X2	T54.2X3	T54.2X4	—	—
fumes	T54.2X1	T54.2X2	T54.2X3	T54.2X4	—	—
Osmotic diuretics	T50.2X1	T50.2X2	T50.2X3	T50.2X4	T50.2X5	T50.2X6
Otilonium bromide	T44.3X1	T44.3X2	T44.3X3	T44.3X4	T44.3X5	T44.3X6

◀ New   ◀▦ Revised   ~~deleted~~ Deleted

Substance	External Cause (T-Code)					
	Poisoning, Accidental (Unintentional)	Poisoning, Intentional Self-Harm	Poisoning, Assault	Poisoning, Undetermined	Adverse Effect	Underdosing
Otorhinolaryngological drug NEC	T49.6X1	T49.6X2	T49.6X3	T49.6X4	T49.6X5	T49.6X6
Ouabain(e)	T46.0X1	T46.0X2	T46.0X3	T46.0X4	T46.0X5	T46.0X6
Ovarian						
hormone	T38.5X1	T38.5X2	T38.5X3	T38.5X4	T38.5X5	T38.5X6
stimulant	T38.5X1	T38.5X2	T38.5X3	T38.5X4	T38.5X5	T38.5X6
Ovral	T38.4X1	T38.4X2	T38.4X3	T38.4X4	T38.4X5	T38.4X6
Ovulen	T38.4X1	T38.4X2	T38.4X3	T38.4X4	T38.4X5	T38.4X6
Oxacillin	T36.0X1	T36.0X2	T36.0X3	T36.0X4	T36.0X5	T36.0X6
Oxalic acid	T54.2X1	T54.2X2	T54.2X3	T54.2X4	—	—
ammonium salt	T50.991	T50.992	T50.993	T50.994	T50.995	T50.996
Oxamniquine	T37.4X1	T37.4X2	T37.4X3	T37.4X4	T37.4X5	T37.4X6
Oxanamide	T43.591	T43.592	T43.593	T43.594	T43.595	T43.596
Oxandrolone	T38.7X1	T38.7X2	T38.7X3	T38.7X4	T38.7X5	T38.7X6
Oxantel	T37.4X1	T37.4X2	T37.4X3	T37.4X4	T37.4X5	T37.4X6
Oxapium iodide	T44.3X1	T44.3X2	T44.3X3	T44.3X4	T44.3X5	T44.3X6
Oxaprotiline	T43.021	T43.022	T43.023	T43.024	T43.025	T43.026
Oxaprozin	T39.311	T39.312	T39.313	T39.314	T39.315	T39.316
Oxatomide	T45.0X1	T45.0X2	T45.0X3	T45.0X4	T45.0X5	T45.0X6
Oxazepam	T42.4X1	T42.4X2	T42.4X3	T42.4X4	T42.4X5	T42.4X6
Oxazimedrine	T50.5X1	T50.5X2	T50.5X3	T50.5X4	T50.5X5	T50.5X6
Oxazolam	T42.4X1	T42.4X2	T42.4X3	T42.4X4	T42.4X5	T42.4X6
Oxazolidine derivatives	T42.2X1	T42.2X2	T42.2X3	T42.2X4	T42.2X5	T42.2X6
Oxazolidinedione (derivative)	T42.2X1	T42.2X2	T42.2X3	T42.2X4	T42.2X5	T42.2X6
Ox bile extract	T47.5X1	T47.5X2	T47.5X3	T47.5X4	T47.5X5	T47.5X6
Oxcarbazepine	T42.1X1	T42.1X2	T42.1X3	T42.1X4	T42.1X5	T42.1X6
Oxedrine	T44.4X1	T44.4X2	T44.4X3	T44.4X4	T44.4X5	T44.4X6
Oxeladin (citrate)	T48.3X1	T48.3X2	T48.3X3	T48.3X4	T48.3X5	T48.3X6
Oxendolone	T38.5X1	T38.5X2	T38.5X3	T38.5X4	T38.5X5	T38.5X6
Oxetacaine	T41.3X1	T41.3X2	T41.3X3	T41.3X4	T41.3X5	T41.3X6
Oxethazine	T41.3X1	T41.3X2	T41.3X3	T41.3X4	T41.3X5	T41.3X6
Oxetorone	T39.8X1	T39.8X2	T39.8X3	T39.8X4	T39.8X5	T39.8X6
Oxiconazole	T49.0X1	T49.0X2	T49.0X3	T49.0X4	T49.0X5	T49.0X6
Oxidizing agent NEC	T54.91	T54.92	T54.93	T54.94	—	—
Oxipurinol	T50.4X1	T50.4X2	T50.4X3	T50.4X4	T50.4X5	T50.4X6
Oxitriptan	T43.291	T43.292	T43.293	T43.294	T43.295	T43.296
Oxitropium bromide	T48.6X1	T48.6X2	T48.6X3	T48.6X4	T48.6X5	T48.6X6
Oxodipine	T46.1X1	T46.1X2	T46.1X3	T46.1X4	T46.1X5	T46.1X6
Oxolamine	T48.3X1	T48.3X2	T48.3X3	T48.3X4	T48.3X5	T48.3X6
Oxolinic acid	T37.8X1	T37.8X2	T37.8X3	T37.8X4	T37.8X5	T37.8X6
Oxomemazine	T43.3X1	T43.3X2	T43.3X3	T43.3X4	T43.3X5	T43.3X6

TABLE OF DRUGS AND CHEMICALS

◄ New ◄▥ Revised ~~deleted~~ Deleted

Substance	Poisoning, Accidental (Unintentional)	Poisoning, Intentional Self-Harm	Poisoning, Assault	Poisoning, Undetermined	Adverse Effect	Underdosing
Oxophenarsine	T37.3X1	T37.3X2	T37.3X3	T37.3X4	T37.3X5	T37.3X6
Oxprenolol	T44.7X1	T44.7X2	T44.7X3	T44.7X4	T44.7X5	T44.7X6
Oxsoralen	T49.3X1	T49.3X2	T49.3X3	T49.3X4	T49.3X5	T49.3X6
Oxtriphylline	T48.6X1	T48.6X2	T48.6X3	T48.6X4	T48.6X5	T48.6X6
Oxybate sodium	T41.291	T41.292	T41.293	T41.294	T41.295	T41.296
Oxybuprocaine	T41.3X1	T41.3X2	T41.3X3	T41.3X4	T41.3X5	T41.3X6
Oxybutynin	T44.3X1	T44.3X2	T44.3X3	T44.3X4	T44.3X5	T44.3X6
Oxychlorosene	T49.0X1	T49.0X2	T49.0X3	T49.0X4	T49.0X5	T49.0X6
Oxycodone	T40.2X1	T40.2X2	T40.2X3	T40.2X4	T40.2X5	T40.2X6
Oxyfedrine	T46.3X1	T46.3X2	T46.3X3	T46.3X4	T46.3X5	T46.3X6
Oxygen	T41.5X1	T41.5X2	T41.5X3	T41.5X4	T41.5X5	T41.5X6
Oxylone	T49.0X1	T49.0X2	T49.0X3	T49.0X4	T49.0X5	T49.0X6
ophthalmic preparation	T49.5X1	T49.5X2	T49.5X3	T49.5X4	T49.5X5	T49.5X6
Oxymesterone	T38.7X1	T38.7X2	T38.7X3	T38.7X4	T38.7X5	T38.7X6
Oxymetazoline	T48.5X1	T48.5X2	T48.5X3	T48.5X4	T48.5X5	T48.5X6
Oxymetholone	T38.7X1	T38.7X2	T38.7X3	T38.7X4	T38.7X5	T38.7X6
Oxymorphone	T40.2X1	T40.2X2	T40.2X3	T40.2X4	T40.2X5	T40.2X6
Oxypertine	T43.591	T43.592	T43.593	T43.594	T43.595	T43.596
Oxyphenbutazone	T39.2X1	T39.2X2	T39.2X3	T39.2X4	T39.2X5	T39.2X6
Oxyphencyclimine	T44.3X1	T44.3X2	T44.3X3	T44.3X4	T44.3X5	T44.3X6
Oxyphenisatine	T47.2X1	T47.2X2	T47.2X3	T47.2X4	T47.2X5	T47.2X6
Oxyphenonium bromide	T44.3X1	T44.3X2	T44.3X3	T44.3X4	T44.3X5	T44.3X6
Oxypolygelatin	T45.8X1	T45.8X2	T45.8X3	T45.8X4	T45.8X5	T45.8X6
Oxyquinoline (derivatives)	T37.8X1	T37.8X2	T37.8X3	T37.8X4	T37.8X5	T37.8X6
Oxytetracycline	T36.4X1	T36.4X2	T36.4X3	T36.4X4	T36.4X5	T36.4X6
Oxytocic drug NEC	T48.0X1	T48.0X2	T48.0X3	T48.0X4	T48.0X5	T48.0X6
Oxytocin (synthetic)	T48.0X1	T48.0X2	T48.0X3	T48.0X4	T48.0X5	T48.0X6
Ozone	T59.891	T59.892	T59.893	T59.894	—	—

P

Substance	Poisoning, Accidental (Unintentional)	Poisoning, Intentional Self-Harm	Poisoning, Assault	Poisoning, Undetermined	Adverse Effect	Underdosing
PABA	T49.3X1	T49.3X2	T49.3X3	T49.3X4	T49.3X5	T49.3X6
Packed red cells	T45.8X1	T45.8X2	T45.8X3	T45.8X4	T45.8X5	T45.8X6
Padimate	T49.3X1	T49.3X2	T49.3X3	T49.3X4	T49.3X5	T49.3X6
Paint NEC	T65.6X1	T65.6X2	T65.6X3	T65.6X4	—	—
cleaner	T52.91	T52.92	T52.93	T52.94	—	—
fumes NEC	T59.891	T59.892	T59.893	T59.894	—	—
lead (fumes)	T56.0X1	T56.0X2	T56.0X3	T56.0X4	—	—
solvent NEC	T52.8X1	T52.8X2	T52.8X3	T52.8X4	—	—
stripper	T52.8X1	T52.8X2	T52.8X3	T52.8X4	—	—
Palfium	T40.2X1	T40.2X2	T40.2X3	T40.2X4	—	—

◀ New   ◀▥ Revised   ~~deleted~~ Deleted

Substance	External Cause (T-Code)					
	Poisoning, Accidental (Unintentional)	Poisoning, Intentional Self-Harm	Poisoning, Assault	Poisoning, Undetermined	Adverse Effect	Underdosing
Palm kernel oil	T50.991	T50.992	T50.993	T50.994	T50.995	T50.996
Paludrine	T37.2X1	T37.2X2	T37.2X3	T37.2X4	T37.2X5	T37.2X6
PAM (pralidoxime)	T50.6X1	T50.6X2	T50.6X3	T50.6X4	T50.6X5	T50.6X6
Pamaquine (naphthoute)	T37.2X1	T37.2X2	T37.2X3	T37.2X4	T37.2X5	T37.2X6
Panadol	T39.1X1	T39.1X2	T39.1X3	T39.1X4	T39.1X5	T39.1X6
Pancreatic						
digestive secretion stimulant	T47.8X1	T47.8X2	T47.8X3	T47.8X4	T47.8X5	T47.8X6
dornase	T45.3X1	T45.3X2	T45.3X3	T45.3X4	T45.3X5	T45.3X6
Pancreatin	T47.5X1	T47.5X2	T47.5X3	T47.5X4	T47.5X5	T47.5X6
Pancrelipase	T47.5X1	T47.5X2	T47.5X3	T47.5X4	T47.5X5	T47.5X6
Pancuronium (bromide)	T48.1X1	T48.1X2	T48.1X3	T48.1X4	T48.1X5	T48.1X6
Pangamic acid	T45.2X1	T45.2X2	T45.2X3	T45.2X4	T45.2X5	T45.2X6
Panthenol	T45.2X1	T45.2X2	T45.2X3	T45.2X4	T45.2X5	T45.2X6
topical	T49.8X1	T49.8X2	T49.8X3	T49.8X4	T49.8X5	T49.8X6
Pantopon	T40.0X1	T40.0X2	T40.0X3	T40.0X4	T40.0X5	T40.0X6
Pantothenic acid	T45.2X1	T45.2X2	T45.2X3	T45.2X4	T45.2X5	T45.2X6
Panwarfin	T45.511	T45.512	T45.513	T45.514	T45.515	T45.516
Papain	T47.5X1	T47.5X2	T47.5X3	T47.5X4	T47.5X5	T47.5X6
digestant	T47.5X1	T47.5X2	T47.5X3	T47.5X4	T47.5X5	T47.5X6
Papaveretum	T40.0X1	T40.0X2	T40.0X3	T40.0X4	T40.0X5	T40.0X6
Papaverine	T44.3X1	T44.3X2	T44.3X3	T44.3X4	T44.3X5	T44.3X6
Para-acetamidophenol	T39.1X1	T39.1X2	T39.1X3	T39.1X4	T39.1X5	T39.1X6
Para-aminobenzoic acid	T49.3X1	T49.3X2	T49.3X3	T49.3X4	T49.3X5	T49.3X6
Para-aminophenol derivatives	T39.1X1	T39.1X2	T39.1X3	T39.1X4	T39.1X5	T39.1X6
Para-aminosalicylic acid	T37.1X1	T37.1X2	T37.1X3	T37.1X4	T37.1X5	T37.1X6
Paracetaldehyde	T42.6X1	T42.6X2	T42.6X3	T42.6X4	T42.6X5	T42.6X6
Paracetamol	T39.1X1	T39.1X2	T39.1X3	T39.1X4	T39.1X5	T39.1X6
Parachlorophenol (camphorated)	T49.0X1	T49.0X2	T49.0X3	T49.0X4	T49.0X5	T49.0X6
Paracodin	T40.2X1	T40.2X2	T40.2X3	T40.2X4	T40.2X5	T40.2X6
Paradione	T42.2X1	T42.2X2	T42.2X3	T42.2X4	T42.2X5	T42.2X6
Paraffin(s) (wax)	T52.0X1	T52.0X2	T52.0X3	T52.0X4	—	—
liquid (medicinal)	T47.4X1	T47.4X2	T47.4X3	T47.4X4	T47.4X5	T47.4X6
nonmedicinal	T52.0X1	T52.0X2	T52.0X3	T52.0X4	—	—
Paraformaldehyde	T60.3X1	T60.3X2	T60.3X3	T60.3X4	—	—
Paraldehyde	T42.6X1	T42.6X2	T42.6X3	T42.6X4	T42.6X5	T42.6X6
Paramethadione	T42.2X1	T42.2X2	T42.2X3	T42.2X4	T42.2X5	T42.2X6
Paramethasone	T38.0X1	T38.0X2	T38.0X3	T38.0X4	T38.0X5	T38.0X6
acetate	T49.0X1	T49.0X2	T49.0X3	T49.0X4	T49.0X5	T49.0X6
Paraoxon	T60.0X1	T60.0X2	T60.0X3	T60.0X4	—	—
Paraquat	T60.3X1	T60.3X2	T60.3X3	T60.3X4	—	—

◀ New   ◀▥ Revised   ~~deleted~~ Deleted

	External Cause (T-Code)					
Substance	Poisoning, Accidental (Unintentional)	Poisoning, Intentional Self-Harm	Poisoning, Assault	Poisoning, Undetermined	Adverse Effect	Underdosing
Parasympatholytic NEC	T44.3X1	T44.3X2	T44.3X3	T44.3X4	T44.3X5	T44.3X6
Parasympathomimetic drug NEC	T44.1X1	T44.1X2	T44.1X3	T44.1X4	T44.1X5	T44.1X6
Parathion	T60.0X1	T60.0X2	T60.0X3	T60.0X4	—	—
Parathormone	T50.991	T50.992	T50.993	T50.994	T50.995	T50.996
Parathyroid extract	T50.991	T50.992	T50.993	T50.994	T50.995	T50.996
Paratyphoid vaccine	T50.A91	T50.A92	T50.A93	T50.A94	T50.A95	T50.A96
Paredrine	T44.4X1	T44.4X2	T44.4X3	T44.4X4	T44.4X5	T44.4X6
Paregoric	T40.0X1	T40.0X2	T40.0X3	T40.0X4	T40.0X5	T40.0X6
Pargyline	T46.5X1	T46.5X2	T46.5X3	T46.5X4	T46.5X5	T46.5X6
Paris green	T57.0X1	T57.0X2	T57.0X3	T57.0X4	—	—
insecticide	T57.0X1	T57.0X2	T57.0X3	T57.0X4	—	—
Parnate	T43.1X1	T43.1X2	T43.1X3	T43.1X4	T43.1X5	T43.1X6
Paromomycin	T36.5X1	T36.5X2	T36.5X3	T36.5X4	T36.5X5	T36.5X6
Paroxypropione	T45.1X1	T45.1X2	T45.1X3	T45.1X4	T45.1X5	T45.1X6
Parzone	T40.2X1	T40.2X2	T40.2X3	T40.2X4	T40.2X5	T40.2X6
PAS	T37.1X1	T37.1X2	T37.1X3	T37.1X4	T37.1X5	T37.1X6
Pasiniazid	T37.1X1	T37.1X2	T37.1X3	T37.1X4	T37.1X5	T37.1X6
PBB (polybrominated biphenyls)	T65.891	T65.892	T65.893	T65.894	—	—
PCB	T65.891	T65.892	T65.893	T65.894	—	—
PCP						
meaning pentachlorophenol	T60.1X1	T60.1X2	T60.1X3	T60.1X4	—	—
fungicide	T60.3X1	T60.3X2	T60.3X3	T60.3X4	—	—
herbicide	T60.3X1	T60.3X2	T60.3X3	T60.3X4	—	—
insecticide	T60.1X1	T60.1X2	T60.1X3	T60.1X4	—	—
meaning phencyclidine	T40.991	T40.992	T40.993	T40.994	—	—
Peach kernel oil (emulsion)	T47.4X1	T47.4X2	T47.4X3	T47.4X4	T47.4X5	T47.4X6
Peanut oil (emulsion) NEC	T47.4X1	T47.4X2	T47.4X3	T47.4X4	T47.4X5	T47.4X6
topical	T49.3X1	T49.3X2	T49.3X3	T49.3X4	T49.3X5	T49.3X6
Pearly Gates (morning glory seeds)	T40.991	T40.992	T40.993	T40.994	—	—
Pecazine	T43.3X1	T43.3X2	T43.3X3	T43.3X4	T43.3X5	T43.3X6
Pectin	T47.6X1	T47.6X2	T47.6X3	T47.6X4	T47.6X5	T47.6X6
Pefloxacin	T37.8X1	T37.8X2	T37.8X3	T37.8X4	T37.8X5	T37.8X6
Pegademase, bovine	T50.Z91	T50.Z92	T50.Z93	T50.Z94	T50.Z95	T50.Z96
Pelletierine tannate	T37.4X1	T37.4X2	T37.4X3	T37.4X4	T37.4X5	T37.4X6
Pemirolast (potassium)	T48.6X1	T48.6X2	T48.6X3	T48.6X4	T48.6X5	T48.6X6
Pemoline	T50.7X1	T50.7X2	T50.7X3	T50.7X4	T50.7X5	T50.7X6
Pempidine	T44.2X1	T44.2X2	T44.2X3	T44.2X4	T44.2X5	T44.2X6
Penamecillin	T36.0X1	T36.0X2	T36.0X3	T36.0X4	T36.0X5	T36.0X6
Penbutolol	T44.7X1	T44.7X2	T44.7X3	T44.7X4	T44.7X5	T44.7X6
Penethamate	T36.0X1	T36.0X2	T36.0X3	T36.0X4	T36.0X5	T36.0X6

◀ New ◀◀ Revised ~~deleted~~ Deleted

Substance	Poisoning, Accidental (Unintentional)	Poisoning, Intentional Self-Harm	Poisoning, Assault	Poisoning, Undetermined	Adverse Effect	Underdosing
			External Cause (T-Code)			
Penfluridol	T43.591	T43.592	T43.593	T43.594	T43.595	T43.596
Penflutizide	T50.2X1	T50.2X2	T50.2X3	T50.2X4	T50.2X5	T50.2X6
Pengitoxin	T46.0X1	T46.0X2	T46.0X3	T46.0X4	T46.0X5	T46.0X6
Penicillamine	T50.6X1	T50.6X2	T50.6X3	T50.6X4	T50.6X5	T50.6X6
Penicillin (any)	T36.0X1	T36.0X2	T36.0X3	T36.0X4	T36.0X5	T36.0X6
Penicillinase	T45.3X1	T45.3X2	T45.3X3	T45.3X4	T45.3X5	T45.3X6
Penicilloyl polylysine	T50.8X1	T50.8X2	T50.8X3	T50.8X4	T50.8X5	T50.8X6
Penimepicycline	T36.4X1	T36.4X2	T36.4X3	T36.4X4	T36.4X5	T36.4X6
Pentachloroethane	T53.6X1	T53.6X2	T53.6X3	T53.6X4	—	—
Pentachloronaphthalene	T53.7X1	T53.7X2	T53.7X3	T53.7X4	—	—
Pentachlorophenol (pesticide)	T60.1X1	T60.1X2	T60.1X3	T60.1X4	—	—
fungicide	T60.3X1	T60.3X2	T60.3X3	T60.3X4	—	—
herbicide	T60.3X1	T60.3X2	T60.3X3	T60.3X4	—	—
insecticide	T60.1X1	T60.1X2	T60.1X3	T60.1X4	—	—
Pentaerythritol tetranitrate	T46.3X1	T46.3X2	T46.3X3	T46.3X4	T46.3X5	T46.3X6
Pentaerythritol	T46.3X1	T46.3X2	T46.3X3	T46.3X4	T46.3X5	T46.3X6
chloral	T42.6X1	T42.6X2	T42.6X3	T42.6X4	T42.6X5	T42.6X6
tetranitrate NEC	T46.3X1	T46.3X2	T46.3X3	T46.3X4	T46.3X5	T46.3X6
Pentagastrin	T50.8X1	T50.8X2	T50.8X3	T50.8X4	T50.8X5	T50.8X6
Pentalin	T53.6X1	T53.6X2	T53.6X3	T53.6X4	—	—
Pentamethonium bromide	T44.2X1	T44.2X2	T44.2X3	T44.2X4	T44.2X5	T44.2X6
Pentamidine	T37.3X1	T37.3X2	T37.3X3	T37.3X4	T37.3X5	T37.3X6
Pentanol	T51.3X1	T51.3X2	T51.3X3	T51.3X4	—	—
Pentapyrrolinium (bitartrate)	T44.2X1	T44.2X2	T44.2X3	T44.2X4	T44.2X5	T44.2X6
Pentaquine	T37.2X1	T37.2X2	T37.2X3	T37.2X4	T37.2X5	T37.2X6
Pentazocine	T40.4X1	T40.4X2	T40.4X3	T40.4X4	T40.4X5	T40.4X6
Pentetrazole	T50.7X1	T50.7X2	T50.7X3	T50.7X4	T50.7X5	T50.7X6
Penthienate bromide	T44.3X1	T44.3X2	T44.3X3	T44.3X4	T44.3X5	T44.3X6
Pentifylline	T46.7X1	T46.7X2	T46.7X3	T46.7X4	T46.7X5	T46.7X6
Pentobarbital	T42.3X1	T42.3X2	T42.3X3	T42.3X4	T42.3X5	T42.3X6
sodium	T42.3X1	T42.3X2	T42.3X3	T42.3X4	T42.3X5	T42.3X6
Pentobarbitone	T42.3X1	T42.3X2	T42.3X3	T42.3X4	T42.3X5	T42.3X6
Pentolonium tartrate	T44.2X1	T44.2X2	T44.2X3	T44.2X4	T44.2X5	T44.2X6
Pentosan polysulfate (sodium)	T39.8X1	T39.8X2	T39.8X3	T39.8X4	T39.8X5	T39.8X6
Pentostatin	T45.1X1	T45.1X2	T45.1X3	T45.1X4	T45.1X5	T45.1X6
Pentothal	T41.1X1	T41.1X2	T41.1X3	T41.1X4	T41.1X5	T41.1X6
Pentoxifylline	T46.7X1	T46.7X2	T46.7X3	T46.7X4	T46.7X5	T46.7X6
Pentoxyverine	T48.3X1	T48.3X2	T48.3X3	T48.3X4	T48.3X5	T48.3X6
Pentrinat	T46.3X1	T46.3X2	T46.3X3	T46.3X4	T46.3X5	T46.3X6
Pentylenetetrazole	T50.7X1	T50.7X2	T50.7X3	T50.7X4	T50.7X5	T50.7X6

◀ New ◀▥ Revised ~~deleted~~ Deleted

Substance	External Cause (T-Code)					
	Poisoning, Accidental (Unintentional)	Poisoning, Intentional Self-Harm	Poisoning, Assault	Poisoning, Undetermined	Adverse Effect	Underdosing
Pentylsalicylamide	T37.1X1	T37.1X2	T37.1X3	T37.1X4	T37.1X5	T37.1X6
Pentymal	T42.3X1	T42.3X2	T42.3X3	T42.3X4	T42.3X5	T42.3X6
Peplomycin	T45.1X1	T45.1X2	T45.1X3	T45.1X4	T45.1X5	T45.1X6
Peppermint (oil)	T47.5X1	T47.5X2	T47.5X3	T47.5X4	T47.5X5	T47.5X6
Pepsin	T47.5X1	T47.5X2	T47.5X3	T47.5X4	T47.5X5	T47.5X6
digestant	T47.5X1	T47.5X2	T47.5X3	T47.5X4	T47.5X5	T47.5X6
Pepstatin	T47.1X1	T47.1X2	T47.1X3	T47.1X4	T47.1X5	T47.1X6
Peptavlon	T50.8X1	T50.8X2	T50.8X3	T50.8X4	T50.8X5	T50.8X6
Perazine	T43.3X1	T43.3X2	T43.3X3	T43.3X4	T43.3X5	T43.3X6
Percaine (spinal)	T41.3X1	T41.3X2	T41.3X3	T41.3X4	T41.3X5	T41.3X6
topical (surface)	T41.3X1	T41.3X2	T41.3X3	T41.3X4	T41.3X5	T41.3X6
Perchloroethylene	T53.3X1	T53.3X2	T53.3X3	T53.3X4	—	—
medicinal	T37.4X1	T37.4X2	T37.4X3	T37.4X4	T37.4X5	T37.4X6
vapor	T53.3X1	T53.3X2	T53.3X3	T53.3X4	—	—
Percodan	T40.2X1	T40.2X2	T40.2X3	T40.2X4	T40.2X5	T40.2X6
Percogesic — *see also acetaminophen*	T45.0X1	T45.0X2	T45.0X3	T45.0X4	T45.0X5	T45.0X6
Percorten	T38.0X1	T38.0X2	T38.0X3	T38.0X4	T38.0X5	T38.0X6
Pergolide	T42.8X1	T42.8X2	T42.8X3	T42.8X4	T42.8X5	T42.8X6
Pergonal	T38.811	T38.812	T38.813	T38.814	T38.815	T38.816
Perhexilene	T46.3X1	T46.3X2	T46.3X3	T46.3X4	T46.3X5	T46.3X6
Perhexiline (maleate)	T46.3X1	T46.3X2	T46.3X3	T46.3X4	T46.3X5	T46.3X6
Periactin	T45.0X1	T45.0X2	T45.0X3	T45.0X4	T45.0X5	T45.0X6
Periciazine	T43.3X1	T43.3X2	T43.3X3	T43.3X4	T43.3X5	T43.3X6
Periclor	T42.6X1	T42.6X2	T42.6X3	T42.6X4	T42.6X5	T42.6X6
Perindopril	T46.4X1	T46.4X2	T46.4X3	T46.4X4	T46.4X5	T46.4X6
Perisoxal	T39.8X1	T39.8X2	T39.8X3	T39.8X4	T39.8X5	T39.8X6
Peritrate	T46.3X1	T46.3X2	T46.3X3	T46.3X4	T46.3X5	T46.3X6
Peritoneal dialysis solution	T50.3X1	T50.3X2	T50.3X3	T50.3X4	T50.3X5	T50.3X6
Perlapine	T42.4X1	T42.4X2	T42.4X3	T42.4X4	T42.4X5	T42.4X6
Permanganate	T65.891	T65.892	T65.893	T65.894	—	—
Permethrin	T60.1X1	T60.1X2	T60.1X3	T60.1X4	—	—
Pernocton	T42.3X1	T42.3X2	T42.3X3	T42.3X4	T42.3X5	T42.3X6
Pernoston	T42.3X1	T42.3X2	T42.3X3	T42.3X4	T42.3X5	T42.3X6
Peronine	T40.2X1	T40.2X2	T40.2X3	T40.2X4	—	—
Perphenazine	T43.3X1	T43.3X2	T43.3X3	T43.3X4	T43.3X5	T43.3X6
Pertofrane	T43.011	T43.012	T43.013	T43.014	T43.015	T43.016
Pertussis						
immune serum (human)	T50.Z11	T50.Z12	T50.Z13	T50.Z14	T50.Z15	T50.Z16
vaccine (with diphtheria toxoid) (with tetanus toxoid)	T50.A11	T50.A12	T50.A13	T50.A14	T50.A15	T50.A16
Peruvian balsam	T49.0X1	T49.0X2	T49.0X3	T49.0X4	T49.0X5	T49.0X6

◀ New   ◀◀ Revised   ~~deleted~~ Deleted

Substance	Poisoning, Accidental (Unintentional)	Poisoning, Intentional Self-Harm	Poisoning, Assault	Poisoning, Undetermined	Adverse Effect	Underdosing
	External Cause (T-Code)					
Peruvoside	T46.0X1	T46.0X2	T46.0X3	T46.0X4	T46.0X5	T46.0X6
Pesticide (dust) (fumes) (vapor) NEC	T60.91	T60.92	T60.93	T60.94	—	—
arsenic	T57.0X1	T57.0X2	T57.0X3	T57.0X4	—	—
chlorinated	T60.1X1	T60.1X2	T60.1X3	T60.1X4	—	—
cyanide	T65.0X1	T65.0X2	T65.0X3	T65.0X4	—	—
kerosene	T52.0X1	T52.0X2	T52.0X3	T52.0X4	—	—
mixture (of compounds)	T60.91	T60.92	T60.93	T60.94	—	—
naphthalene	T60.2X1	T60.2X2	T60.2X3	T60.2X4	—	—
organochlorine (compounds)	T60.1X1	T60.1X2	T60.1X3	T60.1X4	—	—
petroleum (distillate) (products) NEC	T60.8X1	T60.8X2	T60.8X3	T60.8X4	—	—
specified ingredient NEC	T60.8X1	T60.8X2	T60.8X3	T60.8X4	—	—
strychnine	T65.1X1	T65.1X2	T65.1X3	T65.1X4	—	—
thallium	T60.4X1	T60.4X2	T60.4X3	T60.4X4	—	—
Pethidine	T40.4X1	T40.4X2	T40.4X3	T40.4X4	T40.4X5	T40.4X6
Petrichloral	T42.6X1	T42.6X2	T42.6X3	T42.6X4	T42.6X5	T42.6X6
Petrol	T52.0X1	T52.0X2	T52.0X3	T52.0X4	—	—
vapor	T52.0X1	T52.0X2	T52.0X3	T52.0X4	—	—
Petrolatum	T49.3X1	T49.3X2	T49.3X3	T49.3X4	T49.3X5	T49.3X6
hydrophilic	T49.3X1	T49.3X2	T49.3X3	T49.3X4	T49.3X5	T49.3X6
liquid	T47.4X1	T47.4X2	T47.4X3	T47.4X4	T47.4X5	T47.4X6
topical	T49.3X1	T49.3X2	T49.3X3	T49.3X4	T49.3X5	T49.3X6
nonmedicinal	T52.0X1	T52.0X2	T52.0X3	T52.0X4	—	—
red veterinary	T49.3X1	T49.3X2	T49.3X3	T49.3X4	T49.3X5	T49.3X6
white	T49.3X1	T49.3X2	T49.3X3	T49.3X4	T49.3X5	T49.3X6
Petroleum (products) NEC	T52.0X1	T52.0X2	T52.0X3	T52.0X4	—	—
benzine(s) — *see Ligroin*						
ether — *see Ligroin*						
jelly — *see Petrolatum*						
naphtha — *see Ligroin*						
pesticide	T60.8X1	T60.8X2	T60.8X3	T60.8X4	—	—
solids	T52.0X1	T52.0X2	T52.0X3	T52.0X4	—	—
solvents	T52.0X1	T52.0X2	T52.0X3	T52.0X4	—	—
vapor	T52.0X1	T52.0X2	T52.0X3	T52.0X4	—	—
Peyote	T40.991	T40.992	T40.993	T40.994	—	—
Phanodorm, phanodorn	T42.3X1	T42.3X2	T42.3X3	T42.3X4	T42.3X5	T42.3X6
Phanquinone	T37.3X1	T37.3X2	T37.3X3	T37.3X4	T37.3X5	T37.3X6
Phanquone	T37.3X1	T37.3X2	T37.3X3	T37.3X4	T37.3X5	T37.3X6
Pharmaceutical						
adjunct NEC	T50.901	T50.902	T50.903	T50.904	T50.905	T50.906
excipient NEC	T50.901	T50.902	T50.903	T50.904	T50.905	T50.906

	External Cause (T-Code)					
Substance	Poisoning, Accidental (Unintentional)	Poisoning, Intentional Self-Harm	Poisoning, Assault	Poisoning, Undetermined	Adverse Effect	Underdosing
Pharmaceutical *(Continued)*						
sweetener	T50.901	T50.902	T50.903	T50.904	T50.905	T50.906
viscous agent	T50.901	T50.902	T50.903	T50.904	T50.905	T50.906
Phemitone	T42.3X1	T42.3X2	T42.3X3	T42.3X4	T42.3X5	T42.3X6
Phenacaine	T41.3X1	T41.3X2	T41.3X3	T41.3X4	T41.3X5	T41.3X6
Phenacemide	T42.6X1	T42.6X2	T42.6X3	T42.6X4	T42.6X5	T42.6X6
Phenacetin	T39.1X1	T39.1X2	T39.1X3	T39.1X4	T39.1X5	T39.1X6
Phenadoxone	T40.2X1	T40.2X2	T40.2X3	T40.2X4	—	—
Phenaglycodol	T43.591	T43.592	T43.593	T43.594	T43.595	T43.596
Phenantoin	T42.0X1	T42.0X2	T42.0X3	T42.0X4	T42.0X5	T42.0X6
Phenaphthazine reagent	T50.991	T50.992	T50.993	T50.994	T50.995	T50.996
Phenazocine	T40.4X1	T40.4X2	T40.4X3	T40.4X4	T40.4X5	T40.4X6
Phenazone	T39.2X1	T39.2X2	T39.2X3	T39.2X4	T39.2X5	T39.2X6
Phenazopyridine	T39.8X1	T39.8X2	T39.8X3	T39.8X4	T39.8X5	T39.8X6
Phenbenicillin	T36.0X1	T36.0X2	T36.0X3	T36.0X4	T36.0X5	T36.0X6
Phenbutrazate	T50.5X1	T50.5X2	T50.5X3	T50.5X4	T50.5X5	T50.5X6
Phencyclidine	T40.991	T40.992	T40.993	T40.994	T40.995	T40.996
Phendimetrazine	T50.5X1	T50.5X2	T50.5X3	T50.5X4	T50.5X5	T50.5X6
Phenelzine	T43.1X1	T43.1X2	T43.1X3	T43.1X4	T43.1X5	T43.1X6
Phenemal	T42.3X1	T42.3X2	T42.3X3	T42.3X4	T42.3X5	T42.3X6
Phenergan	T42.6X1	T42.6X2	T42.6X3	T42.6X4	T42.6X5	T42.6X6
Pheneticillin	T36.0X1	T36.0X2	T36.0X3	T36.0X4	T36.0X5	T36.0X6
Pheneturide	T42.6X1	T42.6X2	T42.6X3	T42.6X4	T42.6X5	T42.6X6
Phenformin	T38.3X1	T38.3X2	T38.3X3	T38.3X4	T38.3X5	T38.3X6
Phenglutarimide	T44.3X1	T44.3X2	T44.3X3	T44.3X4	T44.3X5	T44.3X6
Phenicarbazide	T39.8X1	T39.8X2	T39.8X3	T39.8X4	T39.8X5	T39.8X6
Phenindamine	T45.0X1	T45.0X2	T45.0X3	T45.0X4	T45.0X5	T45.0X6
Phenindione	T45.511	T45.512	T45.513	T45.514	T45.515	T45.516
Pheniprazine	T43.1X1	T43.1X2	T43.1X3	T43.1X4	T43.1X5	T43.1X6
Pheniramine	T45.0X1	T45.0X2	T45.0X3	T45.0X4	T45.0X5	T45.0X6
Phenisatin	T47.2X1	T47.2X2	T47.2X3	T47.2X4	T47.2X5	T47.2X6
Phenmetrazine	T50.5X1	T50.5X2	T50.5X3	T50.5X4	T50.5X5	T50.5X6
Phenobal	T42.3X1	T42.3X2	T42.3X3	T42.3X4	T42.3X5	T42.3X6
Phenobarbital	T42.3X1	T42.3X2	T42.3X3	T42.3X4	T42.3X5	T42.3X6
with						
mephenytoin	T42.3X1	T42.3X2	T42.3X3	T42.3X4	T42.3X5	T42.3X6
phenytoin	T42.3X1	T42.3X2	T42.3X3	T42.3X4	T42.3X5	T42.3X6
sodium	T42.3X1	T42.3X2	T42.3X3	T42.3X4	T42.3X5	T42.3X6
Phenobarbitone	T42.3X1	T42.3X2	T42.3X3	T42.3X4	T42.3X5	T42.3X6

◀ New ◀‖‖ Revised ~~deleted~~ Deleted

TABLE OF DRUGS AND CHEMICALS

Substance	Poisoning, Accidental (Unintentional)	Poisoning, Intentional Self-Harm	Poisoning, Assault	Poisoning, Undetermined	Adverse Effect	Underdosing
			External Cause (T-Code)			
Phenobutiodil	T50.8X1	T50.8X2	T50.8X3	T50.8X4	T50.8X5	T50.8X6
Phenoctide	T49.0X1	T49.0X2	T49.0X3	T49.0X4	T49.0X5	T49.0X6
Phenol	T49.0X1	T49.0X2	T49.0X3	T49.0X4	T49.0X5	T49.0X6
disinfectant	T54.0X1	T54.0X2	T54.0X3	T54.0X4	—	—
in oil injection	T46.8X1	T46.8X2	T46.8X3	T46.8X4	T46.8X5	T46.8X6
medicinal	T49.1X1	T49.1X2	T49.1X3	T49.1X4	T49.1X5	T49.1X6
nonmedicinal NEC	T54.0X1	T54.0X2	T54.0X3	T54.0X4	—	—
pesticide	T60.8X1	T60.8X2	T60.8X3	T60.8X4	—	—
red	T50.8X1	T50.8X2	T50.8X3	T50.8X4	T50.8X5	T50.8X6
Phenolic preparation	T49.1X1	T49.1X2	T49.1X3	T49.1X4	T49.1X5	T49.1X6
Phenolphthalein	T47.2X1	T47.2X2	T47.2X3	T47.2X4	T47.2X5	T47.2X6
Phenolsulfonphthalein	T50.8X1	T50.8X2	T50.8X3	T50.8X4	T50.8X5	T50.8X6
Phenomorphan	T40.2X1	T40.2X2	T40.2X3	T40.2X4	—	—
Phenonyl	T42.3X1	T42.3X2	T42.3X3	T42.3X4	T42.3X5	T42.3X6
Phenoperidine	T40.4X1	T40.4X2	T40.4X3	T40.4X4	—	—
Phenopyrazone	T46.991	T46.992	T46.993	T46.994	T46.995	T46.996
Phenoquin	T50.4X1	T50.4X2	T50.4X3	T50.4X4	T50.4X5	T50.4X6
Phenothiazine (psychotropic) NEC	T43.3X1	T43.3X2	T43.3X3	T43.3X4	T43.3X5	T43.3X6
insecticide	T60.2X1	T60.2X2	T60.2X3	T60.2X4	—	—
Phenothrin	T49.0X1	T49.0X2	T49.0X3	T49.0X4	T49.0X5	T49.0X6
Phenoxybenzamine	T46.7X1	T46.7X2	T46.7X3	T46.7X4	T46.7X5	T46.7X6
Phenoxyethanol	T49.0X1	T49.0X2	T49.0X3	T49.0X4	T49.0X5	T49.0X6
Phenoxymethyl penicillin	T36.0X1	T36.0X2	T36.0X3	T36.0X4	T36.0X5	T36.0X6
Phenprobamate	T42.8X1	T42.8X2	T42.8X3	T42.8X4	T42.8X5	T42.8X6
Phenprocoumon	T45.511	T45.512	T45.513	T45.514	T45.515	T45.516
Phensuximide	T42.2X1	T42.2X2	T42.2X3	T42.2X4	T42.2X5	T42.2X6
Phentermine	T50.5X1	T50.5X2	T50.5X3	T50.5X4	T50.5X5	T50.5X6
Phenthicillin	T36.0X1	T36.0X2	T36.0X3	T36.0X4	T36.0X5	T36.0X6
Phentolamine	T46.7X1	T46.7X2	T46.7X3	T46.7X4	T46.7X5	T46.7X6
Phenyl						
butazone	T39.2X1	T39.2X2	T39.2X3	T39.2X4	T39.2X5	T39.2X6
enediamine	T65.3X1	T65.3X2	T65.3X3	T65.3X4	—	—
hydrazine	T65.3X1	T65.3X2	T65.3X3	T65.3X4	—	—
antineoplastic	T45.1X1	T45.1X2	T45.1X3	T45.1X4	T45.1X5	T45.1X6
mercuric compounds — *see Mercury*						
salicylate	T49.3X1	T49.3X2	T49.3X3	T49.3X4	T49.3X5	T49.3X6
Phenylalanine mustard	T45.1X1	T45.1X2	T45.1X3	T45.1X4	T45.1X5	T45.1X6
Phenylbutazone	T39.2X1	T39.2X2	T39.2X3	T39.2X4	T39.2X5	T39.2X6
Phenylenediamine	T65.3X1	T65.3X2	T65.3X3	T65.3X4	—	—

◀ New   ◀ Revised   ~~deleted~~ Deleted

Substance	External Cause (T-Code)					
	Poisoning, Accidental (Unintentional)	Poisoning, Intentional Self-Harm	Poisoning, Assault	Poisoning, Undetermined	Adverse Effect	Underdosing
Phenylephrine	T44.4X1	T44.4X2	T44.4X3	T44.4X4	T44.4X5	T44.4X6
Phenylethylbiguanide	T38.3X1	T38.3X2	T38.3X3	T38.3X4	T38.3X5	T38.3X6
Phenylmercuric						
acetate	T49.0X1	T49.0X2	T49.0X3	T49.0X4	T49.0X5	T49.0X6
borate	T49.0X1	T49.0X2	T49.0X3	T49.0X4	T49.0X5	T49.0X6
nitrate	T49.0X1	T49.0X2	T49.0X3	T49.0X4	T49.0X5	T49.0X6
Phenylmethylbarbitone	T42.3X1	T42.3X2	T42.3X3	T42.3X4	T42.3X5	T42.3X6
Phenylpropanol	T47.5X1	T47.5X2	T47.5X3	T47.5X4	T47.5X5	T47.5X6
Phenylpropanolamine	T44.991	T44.992	T44.993	T44.994	T44.995	T44.996
Phenylsulfthion	T60.0X1	T60.0X2	T60.0X3	T60.0X4	—	—
Phenyltoloxamine	T45.0X1	T45.0X2	T45.0X3	T45.0X4	T45.0X5	T45.0X6
Phenyramidol, phenyramidon	T39.8X1	T39.8X2	T39.8X3	T39.8X4	T39.8X5	T39.8X6
Phenytoin	T42.0X1	T42.0X2	T42.0X3	T42.0X4	T42.0X5	T42.0X6
with Phenobarbital	T42.3X1	T42.3X2	T42.3X3	T42.3X4	T42.3X5	T42.3X6
pHisoHex	T49.2X1	T49.2X2	T49.2X3	T49.2X4	T49.2X5	T49.2X6
Pholcodine	T48.3X1	T48.3X2	T48.3X3	T48.3X4	T48.3X5	T48.3X6
Pholedrine	T46.991	T46.992	T46.993	T46.994	T46.995	T46.996
Phorate	T60.0X1	T60.0X2	T60.0X3	T60.0X4	—	—
Phosdrin	T60.0X1	T60.0X2	T60.0X3	T60.0X4	—	—
Phosfolan	T60.0X1	T60.0X2	T60.0X3	T60.0X4	—	—
Phosgene (gas)	T59.891	T59.892	T59.893	T59.894	—	—
Phosphamidon	T60.0X1	T60.0X2	T60.0X3	T60.0X4	—	—
Phosphate	T65.891	T65.892	T65.893	T65.894	—	—
laxative	T47.4X1	T47.4X2	T47.4X3	T47.4X4	T47.4X5	T47.4X6
organic	T60.0X1	T60.0X2	T60.0X3	T60.0X4	—	—
solvent	T52.91	T52.92	T52.93	T52.94	—	—
tricresyl	T65.891	T65.892	T65.893	T65.894	—	—
Phosphine	T57.1X1	T57.1X2	T57.1X3	T57.1X4	—	—
fumigant	T57.1X1	T57.1X2	T57.1X3	T57.1X4	—	—
Phospholine	T49.5X1	T49.5X2	T49.5X3	T49.5X4	T49.5X5	T49.5X6
Phosphoric acid	T54.2X1	T54.2X2	T54.2X3	T54.2X4	—	—
Phosphorus (compound) NEC	T57.1X1	T57.1X2	T57.1X3	T57.1X4	—	—
pesticide	T60.0X1	T60.0X2	T60.0X3	T60.0X4	—	—
Phthalates	T65.891	T65.892	T65.893	T65.894	—	—
Phthalic anhydride	T65.891	T65.892	T65.893	T65.894	—	—
Phthalimidoglutarimide	T42.6X1	T42.6X2	T42.6X3	T42.6X4	T42.6X5	T42.6X6
Phthalylsulfathiazole	T37.0X1	T37.0X2	T37.0X3	T37.0X4	T37.0X5	T37.0X6
Phylloquinone	T45.7X1	T45.7X2	T45.7X3	T45.7X4	T45.7X5	T45.7X6
Physeptone	T40.3X1	T40.3X2	T40.3X3	T40.3X4	T40.3X5	T40.3X6

TABLE OF DRUGS AND CHEMICALS

◀ New ◀ Revised ~~deleted~~ Deleted

Substance	External Cause (T-Code)					
	Poisoning, Accidental (Unintentional)	Poisoning, Intentional Self-Harm	Poisoning, Assault	Poisoning, Undetermined	Adverse Effect	Underdosing
Physostigma venenosum	T62.2X1	T62.2X2	T62.2X3	T62.2X4	—	—
Physostigmine	T49.5X1	T49.5X2	T49.5X3	T49.5X4	T49.5X5	T49.5X6
Phytolacca decandra	T62.2X1	T62.2X2	T62.2X3	T62.2X4		—
berries	T62.1X1	T62.1X2	T62.1X3	T62.1X4	—	—
Phytomenadione	T45.7X1	T45.7X2	T45.7X3	T45.7X4	T45.7X5	T45.7X6
Phytonadione	T45.7X1	T45.7X2	T45.7X3	T45.7X4	T45.7X5	T45.7X6
Picoperine	T48.3X1	T48.3X2	T48.3X3	T48.3X4	T48.3X5	T48.3X6
Picosulfate (sodium)	T47.2X1	T47.2X2	T47.2X3	T47.2X4	T47.2X5	T47.2X6
Picric (acid)	T54.2X1	T54.2X2	T54.2X3	T54.2X4	—	—
Picrotoxin	T50.7X1	T50.7X2	T50.7X3	T50.7X4	T50.7X5	T50.7X6
Piketoprofen	T49.0X1	T49.0X2	T49.0X3	T49.0X4	T49.0X5	T49.0X6
Pilocarpine	T44.1X1	T44.1X2	T44.1X3	T44.1X4	T44.1X5	T44.1X6
Pilocarpus (jaborandi) extract	T44.1X1	T44.1X2	T44.1X3	T44.1X4	T44.1X5	T44.1X6
Pilsicainide (hydrochloride)	T46.2X1	T46.2X2	T46.2X3	T46.2X4	T46.2X5	T46.2X6
Pimaricin	T36.7X1	T36.7X2	T36.7X3	T36.7X4	T36.7X5	T36.7X6
Pimeclone	T50.7X1	T50.7X2	T50.7X3	T50.7X4	T50.7X5	T50.7X6
Pimelic ketone	T52.8X1	T52.8X2	T52.8X3	T52.8X4	—	—
Pimethixene	T45.0X1	T45.0X2	T45.0X3	T45.0X4	T45.0X5	T45.0X6
Piminodine	T40.2X1	T40.2X2	T40.2X3	T40.2X4	T40.2X5	T40.2X6
Pimozide	T43.591	T43.592	T43.593	T43.594	T43.595	T43.596
Pinacidil	T46.5X1	T46.5X2	T46.5X3	T46.5X4	T46.5X5	T46.5X6
Pinaverium bromide	T44.3X1	T44.3X2	T44.3X3	T44.3X4	T44.3X5	T44.3X6
Pinazepam	T42.4X1	T42.4X2	T42.4X3	T42.4X4	T42.4X5	T42.4X6
Pindolol	T44.7X1	T44.7X2	T44.7X3	T44.7X4	T44.7X5	T44.7X6
Pindone	T60.4X1	T60.4X2	T60.4X3	T60.4X4	—	—
Pine oil (disinfectant)	T65.891	T65.892	T65.893	T65.894	—	—
Pinkroot	T37.4X1	T37.4X2	T37.4X3	T37.4X4	T37.4X5	T37.4X6
Pipadone	T40.2X1	T40.2X2	T40.2X3	T40.2X4		
Pipamazine	T45.0X1	T45.0X2	T45.0X3	T45.0X4	T45.0X5	T45.0X6
Pipamperone	T43.4X1	T43.4X2	T43.4X3	T43.4X4	T43.4X5	T43.4X6
Pipazetate	T48.3X1	T48.3X2	T48.3X3	T48.3X4	T48.3X5	T48.3X6
Pipemidic acid	T37.8X1	T37.8X2	T37.8X3	T37.8X4	T37.8X5	T37.8X6
Pipenzolate bromide	T44.3X1	T44.3X2	T44.3X3	T44.3X4	T44.3X5	T44.3X6
Piperacetazine	T43.3X1	T43.3X2	T43.3X3	T43.3X4	T43.3X5	T43.3X6
Piperacillin	T36.0X1	T36.0X2	T36.0X3	T36.0X4	T36.0X5	T36.0X6
Piperazine	T37.4X1	T37.4X2	T37.4X3	T37.4X4	T37.4X5	T37.4X6
estrone sulfate	T38.5X1	T38.5X2	T38.5X3	T38.5X4	T38.5X5	T38.5X6
Piper cubeba	T62.2X1	T62.2X2	T62.2X3	T62.2X4	—	—
Piperidione	T48.3X1	T48.3X2	T48.3X3	T48.3X4	—	—

◀ New   ◀||| Revised   ~~deleted~~ Deleted

Substance	External Cause (T-Code)					
	Poisoning, Accidental (Unintentional)	Poisoning, Intentional Self-Harm	Poisoning, Assault	Poisoning, Undetermined	Adverse Effect	Underdosing
Piperidolate	T44.3X1	T44.3X2	T44.3X3	T44.3X4	T44.3X5	T44.3X6
Piperocaine	T41.3X1	T41.3X2	T41.3X3	T41.3X4	T41.3X5	T41.3X6
infiltration (subcutaneous)	T41.3X1	T41.3X2	T41.3X3	T41.3X4	T41.3X5	T41.3X6
nerve block (peripheral) (plexus)	T41.3X1	T41.3X2	T41.3X3	T41.3X4	T41.3X5	T41.3X6
topical (surface)	T41.3X1	T41.3X2	T41.3X3	T41.3X4	T41.3X5	T41.3X6
Piperonyl butoxide	T60.8X1	T60.8X2	T60.8X3	T60.8X4	—	—
Pipethanate	T44.3X1	T44.3X2	T44.3X3	T44.3X4	T44.3X5	T44.3X6
Pipobroman	T45.1X1	T45.1X2	T45.1X3	T45.1X4	T45.1X5	T45.1X6
Pipofezine	T43.0X1	T43.0X2	T43.0X3	T43.0X4	T43.0X5	T43.0X6
Pipotiazine	T43.3X1	T43.3X2	T43.3X3	T43.3X4	T43.3X5	T43.3X6
Pipoxizine	T45.0X1	T45.0X2	T45.0X3	T45.0X4	T45.0X5	T45.0X6
Pipradrol	T43.691	T43.692	T43.693	T43.694	T43.695	T43.696
Piprinhydrinate	T45.0X1	T45.0X2	T45.0X3	T45.0X4	T45.0X5	T45.0X6
Pirarubicin	T45.1X1	T45.1X2	T45.1X3	T45.1X4	T45.1X5	T45.1X6
Pirazinamide	T37.1X1	T37.1X2	T37.1X3	T37.1X4	T37.1X5	T37.1X6
Pirbuterol	T48.6X1	T48.6X2	T48.6X3	T48.6X4	T48.6X5	T48.6X6
Pirenzepine	T47.1X1	T47.1X2	T47.1X3	T47.1X4	T47.1X5	T47.1X6
Piretanide	T50.1X1	T50.1X2	T50.1X3	T50.1X4	T50.1X5	T50.1X6
Piribedil	T42.8X1	T42.8X2	T42.8X3	T42.8X4	T42.8X5	T42.8X6
Piridoxilate	T46.3X1	T46.3X2	T46.3X3	T46.3X4	T46.3X5	T46.3X6
Piritramide	T40.4X1	T40.4X2	T40.4X3	T40.4X4	—	—
Pirlindole	T43.0X1	T43.0X2	T43.0X3	T43.0X4	T43.0X5	T43.0X6
Piromidic acid	T37.8X1	T37.8X2	T37.8X3	T37.8X4	T37.8X5	T37.8X6
Piroxicam	T39.391	T39.392	T39.393	T39.394	T39.395	T39.396
beta-cyclodextrin complex	T39.8X1	T39.8X2	T39.8X3	T39.8X4	T39.8X5	T39.8X6
Pirozadil	T46.6X1	T46.6X2	T46.6X3	T46.6X4	T46.6X5	T46.6X6
Piscidia (bark) (erythrina)	T39.8X1	T39.8X2	T39.8X3	T39.8X4	T39.8X5	T39.8X6
Pitch	T65.891	T65.892	T65.893	T65.894	—	—
Pitkin's solution	T41.3X1	T41.3X2	T41.3X3	T41.3X4	T41.3X5	T41.3X6
Pitocin	T48.0X1	T48.0X2	T48.0X3	T48.0X4	T48.0X5	T48.0X6
Pitressin (tannate)	T38.891	T38.892	T38.893	T38.894	T38.895	T38.896
Pituitary extracts (posterior)	T38.891	T38.892	T38.893	T38.894	T38.895	T38.896
anterior	T38.811	T38.812	T38.813	T38.814	T38.815	T38.816
Pituitrin	T38.891	T38.892	T38.893	T38.894	T38.895	T38.896
Pivampicillin	T36.0X1	T36.0X2	T36.0X3	T36.0X4	T36.0X5	T36.0X6
Pivmecillinam	T36.0X1	T36.0X2	T36.0X3	T36.0X4	T36.0X5	T36.0X6
Placental hormone	T38.891	T38.892	T38.893	T38.894	T38.895	T38.896
Placidyl	T42.6X1	T42.6X2	T42.6X3	T42.6X4	T42.6X5	T42.6X6
Plague vaccine	T50.A91	T50.A92	T50.A93	T50.A94	T50.A95	T50.A96

◄ New ◄|||| Revised ~~deleted~~ Deleted

Substance	Poisoning, Accidental (Unintentional)	Poisoning, Intentional Self-Harm	Poisoning, Assault	Poisoning, Undetermined	Adverse Effect	Underdosing
Plant						
food or fertilizer NEC	T65.891	T65.892	T65.893	T65.894	—	—
containing herbicide	T60.3X1	T60.3X2	T60.3X3	T60.3X4	—	—
noxious, used as food	T62.2X1	T62.2X2	T62.2X3	T62.2X4	—	—
berries	T62.1X1	T62.1X2	T62.1X3	T62.1X4	—	—
seeds	T62.2X1	T62.2X2	T62.2X3	T62.2X4	—	—
specified type NEC	T62.2X1	T62.2X2	T62.2X3	T62.2X4	—	—
Plasma	T45.8X1	T45.8X2	T45.8X3	T45.8X4	T45.8X5	T45.8X6
expander NEC	T45.8X1	T45.8X2	T45.8X3	T45.8X4	T45.8X5	T45.8X6
protein fraction (human)	T45.8X1	T45.8X2	T45.8X3	T45.8X4	T45.8X5	T45.8X6
Plasmanate	T45.8X1	T45.8X2	T45.8X3	T45.8X4	T45.8X5	T45.8X6
Plasminogen (tissue) activator	T45.611	T45.612	T45.613	T45.614	T45.615	T45.616
Plaster dressing	T49.3X1	T49.3X2	T49.3X3	T49.3X4	T49.3X5	T49.3X6
Plastic dressing	T49.3X1	T49.3X2	T49.3X3	T49.3X4	T49.3X5	T49.3X6
Plegicil	T43.3X1	T43.3X2	T43.3X3	T43.3X4	T43.3X5	T43.3X6
Plicamycin	T45.1X1	T45.1X2	T45.1X3	T45.1X4	T45.1X5	T45.1X6
Podophyllotoxin	T49.8X1	T49.8X2	T49.8X3	T49.8X4	T49.8X5	T49.8X6
Podophyllum (resin)	T49.4X1	T49.4X2	T49.4X3	T49.4X4	T49.4X5	T49.4X6
Poison NEC	T65.91	T65.92	T65.93	T65.94	—	—
Poisonous berries	T62.1X1	T62.1X2	T62.1X3	T62.1X4	—	—
Pokeweed (any part)	T62.2X1	T62.2X2	T62.2X3	T62.2X4	—	—
Poldine metilsulfate	T44.3X1	T44.3X2	T44.3X3	T44.3X4	T44.3X5	T44.3X6
Polidexide (sulfate)	T46.6X1	T46.6X2	T46.6X3	T46.6X4	T46.6X5	T46.6X6
Polidocanol	T46.8X1	T46.8X2	T46.8X3	T46.8X4	T46.8X5	T46.8X6
Poliomyelitis vaccine	T50.B91	T50.B92	T50.B93	T50.B94	T50.B95	T50.B96
Polish (car) (floor) (furniture) (metal) (porcelain) (silver)	T65.891	T65.892	T65.893	T65.894	—	—
abrasive	T65.891	T65.892	T65.893	T65.894	—	—
porcelain	T65.891	T65.892	T65.893	T65.894	—	—
Poloxalkol	T47.4X1	T47.4X2	T47.4X3	T47.4X4	T47.4X5	T47.4X6
Poloxamer	T47.4X1	T47.4X2	T47.4X3	T47.4X4	T47.4X5	T47.4X6
Polyaminostyrene resins	T50.3X1	T50.3X2	T50.3X3	T50.3X4	T50.3X5	T50.3X6
Polycarbophil	T47.4X1	T47.4X2	T47.4X3	T47.4X4	T47.4X5	T47.4X6
Polychlorinated biphenyl	T65.891	T65.892	T65.893	T65.894	—	—
Polycycline	T36.4X1	T36.4X2	T36.4X3	T36.4X4	T36.4X5	T36.4X6
Polyester fumes	T59.891	T59.892	T59.893	T59.894	—	—
Polyester resin hardener	T52.91	T52.92	T52.93	T52.94	—	—
fumes	T59.891	T59.892	T59.893	T59.894	—	—
Polyestradiol phosphate	T38.5X1	T38.5X2	T38.5X3	T38.5X4	T38.5X5	T38.5X6
Polyethanolamine alkyl sulfate	T49.2X1	T49.2X2	T49.2X3	T49.2X4	T49.2X5	T49.2X6

TABLE OF DRUGS AND CHEMICALS

Substance	Poisoning, Accidental (Unintentional)	Poisoning, Intentional Self-Harm	Poisoning, Assault	Poisoning, Undetermined	Adverse Effect	Underdosing
				External Cause (T-Code)		
Polyethylene adhesive	T49.3X1	T49.3X2	T49.3X3	T49.3X4	T49.3X5	T49.3X6
Polyferose	T45.4X1	T45.4X2	T45.4X3	T45.4X4	T45.4X5	T45.4X6
Polygeline	T45.8X1	T45.8X2	T45.8X3	T45.8X4	T45.8X5	T45.8X6
Polymyxin	T36.8X1	T36.8X2	T36.8X3	T36.8X4	T36.8X5	T36.8X6
B	T36.8X1	T36.8X2	T36.8X3	T36.8X4	T36.8X5	T36.8X6
ENT agent	T49.6X1	T49.6X2	T49.6X3	T49.6X4	T49.6X5	T49.6X6
ophthalmic preparation	T49.5X1	T49.5X2	T49.5X3	T49.5X4	T49.5X5	T49.5X6
topical NEC	T49.0X1	T49.0X2	T49.0X3	T49.0X4	T49.0X5	T49.0X6
E sulfate (eye preparation)	T49.5X1	T49.5X2	T49.5X3	T49.5X4	T49.5X5	T49.5X6
Polynoxylin	T49.0X1	T49.0X2	T49.0X3	T49.0X4	T49.0X5	T49.0X6
Polyoestradiol phosphate	T38.5X1	T38.5X2	T38.5X3	T38.5X4	T38.5X5	T38.5X6
Polyoxymethyleneurea	T49.0X1	T49.0X2	T49.0X3	T49.0X4	T49.0X5	T49.0X6
Polysilane	T47.8X1	T47.8X2	T47.8X3	T47.8X4	T47.8X5	T47.8X6
Polytetrafluoroethylene (inhaled)	T59.891	T59.892	T59.893	T59.894	—	—
Polythiazide	T50.2X1	T50.2X2	T50.2X3	T50.2X4	T50.2X5	T50.2X6
Polyvidone	T45.8X1	T45.8X2	T45.8X3	T45.8X4	T45.8X5	T45.8X6
Polyvinylpyrrolidone	T45.8X1	T45.8X2	T45.8X3	T45.8X4	T45.8X5	T45.8X6
Pontocaine (hydrochloride) (infiltration) (topical)	T41.3X1	T41.3X2	T41.3X3	T41.3X4	T41.3X5	T41.3X6
nerve block (peripheral) (plexus)	T41.3X1	T41.3X2	T41.3X3	T41.3X4	T41.3X5	T41.3X6
spinal	T41.3X1	T41.3X2	T41.3X3	T41.3X4	T41.3X5	T41.3X6
Porfiromycin	T45.1X1	T45.1X2	T45.1X3	T45.1X4	T45.1X5	T45.1X6
Posterior pituitary hormone NEC	T38.891	T38.892	T38.893	T38.894	T38.895	T38.896
Pot	T40.7X1	T40.7X2	T40.7X3	T40.7X4	T40.7X5	T40.7X6
Potash (caustic)	T54.3X1	T54.3X2	T54.3X3	T54.3X4	—	—
Potassic saline injection (lactated)	T50.3X1	T50.3X2	T50.3X3	T50.3X4	T50.3X5	T50.3X6
Potassium (salts) NEC	T50.3X1	T50.3X2	T50.3X3	T50.3X4	T50.3X5	T50.3X6
aminobenzoate	T45.8X1	T45.8X2	T45.8X3	T45.8X4	T45.8X5	T45.8X6
aminosalicylate	T37.1X1	T37.1X2	T37.1X3	T37.1X4	T37.1X5	T37.1X6
antimony 'tartrate'	T37.8X1	T37.8X2	T37.8X3	T37.8X4	T37.8X5	T37.8X6
arsenite (solution)	T57.0X1	T57.0X2	T57.0X3	T57.0X4	—	—
bichromate	T56.2X1	T56.2X2	T56.2X3	T56.2X4	—	—
bisulfate	T47.3X1	T47.3X2	T47.3X3	T47.3X4	T47.3X5	T47.3X6
bromide	T42.6X1	T42.6X2	T42.6X3	T42.6X4	T42.6X5	T42.6X6
canrenoate	T50.0X1	T50.0X2	T50.0X3	T50.0X4	T50.0X5	T50.0X6
carbonate	T54.3X1	T54.3X2	T54.3X3	T54.3X4	—	—
chlorate NEC	T65.891	T65.892	T65.893	T65.894	—	—
chloride	T50.3X1	T50.3X2	T50.3X3	T50.3X4	T50.3X5	T50.3X6
citrate	T50.991	T50.992	T50.993	T50.994	T50.995	T50.996
cyanide	T65.0X1	T65.0X2	T65.0X3	T65.0X4	—	—

◀ New   ◀◀ Revised   ~~deleted~~ Deleted

Substance	Poisoning, Accidental (Unintentional)	Poisoning, Intentional Self-Harm	Poisoning, Assault	Poisoning, Undetermined	Adverse Effect	Underdosing
Potassium NEC *(Continued)*						
ferric hexacyanoferrate (medicinal)	T50.6X1	T50.6X2	T50.6X3	T50.6X4	T50.6X5	T50.6X6
nonmedicinal	T65.891	T65.892	T65.893	T65.894	—	—
Fluoride	T57.8X1	T57.8X2	T57.8X3	T57.8X4	—	—
glucaldrate	T47.1X1	T47.1X2	T47.1X3	T47.1X4	T47.1X5	T47.1X6
hydroxide	T54.3X1	T54.3X2	T54.3X3	T54.3X4	—	—
iodate	T49.0X1	T49.0X2	T49.0X3	T49.0X4	T49.0X5	T49.0X6
iodide	T48.4X1	T48.4X2	T48.4X3	T48.4X4	T48.4X5	T48.4X6
nitrate	T57.8X1	T57.8X2	T57.8X3	T57.8X4	—	—
oxalate	T65.891	T65.892	T65.893	T65.894	—	—
perchlorate (nonmedicinal) NEC	T65.891	T65.892	T65.893	T65.894	—	—
antithyroid	T38.2X1	T38.2X2	T38.2X3	T38.2X4	T38.2X5	T38.2X6
medicinal	T38.2X1	T38.2X2	T38.2X3	T38.2X4	T38.2X5	T38.2X6
Permanganate (nonmedicinal)	T65.891	T65.892	T65.893	T65.894	—	—
medicinal	T49.0X1	T49.0X2	T49.0X3	T49.0X4	T49.0X5	T49.0X6
sulfate	T47.2X1	T47.2X2	T47.2X3	T47.2X4	T47.2X5	T47.2X6
Potassium-removing resin	T50.3X1	T50.3X2	T50.3X3	T50.3X4	T50.3X5	T50.3X6
Potassium-retaining drug	T50.3X1	T50.3X2	T50.3X3	T50.3X4	T50.3X5	T50.3X6
Povidone	T45.8X1	T45.8X2	T45.8X3	T45.8X4	T45.8X5	T45.8X6
iodine	T49.0X1	T49.0X2	T49.0X3	T49.0X4	T49.0X5	T49.0X6
Practolol	T44.7X1	T44.7X2	T44.7X3	T44.7X4	T44.7X5	T44.7X6
Prajmalium bitartrate	T46.2X1	T46.2X2	T46.2X3	T46.2X4	T46.2X5	T46.2X6
Pralidoxime (iodide)	T50.6X1	T50.6X2	T50.6X3	T50.6X4	T50.6X5	T50.6X6
chloride	T50.6X1	T50.6X2	T50.6X3	T50.6X4	T50.6X5	T50.6X6
Pramiverine	T44.3X1	T44.3X2	T44.3X3	T44.3X4	T44.3X5	T44.3X6
Pramocaine	T49.1X1	T49.1X2	T49.1X3	T49.1X4	T49.1X5	T49.1X6
Pramoxine	T49.1X1	T49.1X2	T49.1X3	T49.1X4	T49.1X5	T49.1X6
Prasterone	T38.7X1	T38.7X2	T38.7X3	T38.7X4	T38.7X5	T38.7X6
Pravastatin	T46.6X1	T46.6X2	T46.6X3	T46.6X4	T46.6X5	T46.6X6
Prazepam	T42.4X1	T42.4X2	T42.4X3	T42.4X4	T42.4X5	T42.4X6
Praziquantel	T37.4X1	T37.4X2	T37.4X3	T37.4X4	T37.4X5	T37.4X6
Prazitone	T43.291	T43.292	T43.293	T43.294	T43.295	T43.296
Prazosin	T44.6X1	T44.6X2	T44.6X3	T44.6X4	T44.6X5	T44.6X6
Prednicarbate	T49.0X1	T49.0X2	T49.0X3	T49.0X4	T49.0X5	T49.0X6
Prednimustine	T45.1X1	T45.1X2	T45.1X3	T45.1X4	T45.1X5	T45.1X6
Prednisolone	T38.0X1	T38.0X2	T38.0X3	T38.0X4	T38.0X5	T38.0X6
ENT agent	T49.6X1	T49.6X2	T49.6X3	T49.6X4	T49.6X5	T49.6X6
ophthalmic preparation	T49.5X1	T49.5X2	T49.5X3	T49.5X4	T49.5X5	T49.5X6
steaglate	T49.0X1	T49.0X2	T49.0X3	T49.0X4	T49.0X5	T49.0X6
topical NEC	T49.0X1	T49.0X2	T49.0X3	T49.0X4	T49.0X5	T49.0X6

Substance	External Cause (T-Code)					
	Poisoning, Accidental (Unintentional)	Poisoning, Intentional Self-Harm	Poisoning, Assault	Poisoning, Undetermined	Adverse Effect	Underdosing
Prednisone	T38.0X1	T38.0X2	T38.0X3	T38.0X4	T38.0X5	T38.0X6
Prednylidene	T38.0X1	T38.0X2	T38.0X3	T38.0X4	T38.0X5	T38.0X6
Pregnandiol	T38.5X1	T38.5X2	T38.5X3	T38.5X4	T38.5X5	T38.5X6
Pregneninolone	T38.5X1	T38.5X2	T38.5X3	T38.5X4	T38.5X5	T38.5X6
Preludin	T43.691	T43.692	T43.693	T43.694	T43.695	T43.696
Premarin	T38.5X1	T38.5X2	T38.5X3	T38.5X4	T38.5X5	T38.5X6
Premedication anesthetic	T41.201	T41.202	T41.203	T41.204	T41.205	T41.206
Prenalterol	T44.5X1	T44.5X2	T44.5X3	T44.5X4	T44.5X5	T44.5X6
Prenoxdiazine	T48.3X1	T48.3X2	T48.3X3	T48.3X4	T48.3X5	T48.3X6
Prenylamine	T46.3X1	T46.3X2	T46.3X3	T46.3X4	T46.3X5	T46.3X6
Preparation, local	T49.4X1	T49.4X2	T49.4X3	T49.4X4	T49.4X5	T49.4X6
Preparation H	T49.8X1	T49.8X2	T49.8X3	T49.8X4	T49.8X5	T49.8X6
Preservative (nonmedicinal)	T65.891	T65.892	T65.893	T65.894	—	—
medicinal	T50.901	T50.902	T50.903	T50.904	T50.905	T50.906
wood	T60.91	T60.92	T60.93	T60.94	—	—
Prethcamide	T50.7X1	T50.7X2	T50.7X3	T50.7X4	T50.7X5	T50.7X6
Pride of China	T62.2X1	T62.2X2	T62.2X3	T62.2X4	—	—
Pridinol	T44.3X1	T44.3X2	T44.3X3	T44.3X4	T44.3X5	T44.3X6
Prifinium bromide	T44.3X1	T44.3X2	T44.3X3	T44.3X4	T44.3X5	T44.3X6
Prilocaine	T41.3X1	T41.3X2	T41.3X3	T41.3X4	T41.3X5	T41.3X6
infiltration (subcutaneous)	T41.3X1	T41.3X2	T41.3X3	T41.3X4	T41.3X5	T41.3X6
nerve block (peripheral) (plexus)	T41.3X1	T41.3X2	T41.3X3	T41.3X4	T41.3X5	T41.3X6
regional	T41.3X1	T41.3X2	T41.3X3	T41.3X4	T41.3X5	T41.3X6
Primaquine	T37.2X1	T37.2X2	T37.2X3	T37.2X4	T37.2X5	T37.2X6
Primidone	T42.6X1	T42.6X2	T42.6X3	T42.6X4	T42.6X5	T42.6X6
Primula (veris)	T62.2X1	T62.2X2	T62.2X3	T62.2X4	—	—
Prinadol	T40.2X1	T40.2X2	T40.2X3	T40.2X4	T40.2X5	T40.2X6
Priscol, Priscoline	T44.6X1	T44.6X2	T44.6X3	T44.6X4	T44.6X5	T44.6X6
Pristinamycin	T36.3X1	T36.3X2	T36.3X3	T36.3X4	T36.3X5	T36.3X6
Privet	T62.2X1	T62.2X2	T62.2X3	T62.2X4	—	—
berries	T62.1X1	T62.1X2	T62.1X3	T62.1X4	—	—
Privine	T44.4X1	T44.4X2	T44.4X3	T44.4X4	T44.4X5	T44.4X6
Pro-Banthine	T44.3X1	T44.3X2	T44.3X3	T44.3X4	T44.3X5	T44.3X6
Probarbital	T42.3X1	T42.3X2	T42.3X3	T42.3X4	T42.3X5	T42.3X6
Probenecid	T50.4X1	T50.4X2	T50.4X3	T50.4X4	T50.4X5	T50.4X6
Probucol	T46.6X1	T46.6X2	T46.6X3	T46.6X4	T46.6X5	T46.6X6
Procainamide	T46.2X1	T46.2X2	T46.2X3	T46.2X4	T46.2X5	T46.2X6
Procaine	T41.3X1	T41.3X2	T41.3X3	T41.3X4	T41.3X5	T41.3X6
benzylpenicillin	T36.0X1	T36.0X2	T36.0X3	T36.0X4	T36.0X5	T36.0X6
nerve block (periphreal) (plexus)	T41.3X1	T41.3X2	T41.3X3	T41.3X4	T41.3X5	T41.3X6

◀ New   ◀ Revised   ~~deleted~~ Deleted

Substance	External Cause (T-Code)					
	Poisoning, Accidental (Unintentional)	Poisoning, Intentional Self-Harm	Poisoning, Assault	Poisoning, Undetermined	Adverse Effect	Underdosing
Procaine *(Continued)*						
penicillin G	T36.0X1	T36.0X2	T36.0X3	T36.0X4	T36.0X5	T36.0X6
regional	T41.3X1	T41.3X2	T41.3X3	T41.3X4	T41.3X5	T41.3X6
spinal	T41.3X1	T41.3X2	T41.3X3	T41.3X4	T41.3X5	T41.3X6
Procalmidol	T43.591	T43.592	T43.593	T43.594	T43.595	T43.596
Procarbazine	T45.1X1	T45.1X2	T45.1X3	T45.1X4	T45.1X5	T45.1X6
Procaterol	T44.5X1	T44.5X2	T44.5X3	T44.5X4	T44.5X5	T44.5X6
Prochlorperazine	T43.3X1	T43.3X2	T43.3X3	T43.3X4	T43.3X5	T43.3X6
Procyclidine	T44.3X1	T44.3X2	T44.3X3	T44.3X4	T44.3X5	T44.3X6
Producer gas	T58.8X1	T58.8X2	T58.8X3	T58.8X4	—	—
Profadol	T40.4X1	T40.4X2	T40.4X3	T40.4X4	T40.4X5	T40.4X6
Profenamine	T44.3X1	T44.3X2	T44.3X3	T44.3X4	T44.3X5	T44.3X6
Profenil	T44.3X1	T44.3X2	T44.3X3	T44.3X4	T44.3X5	T44.3X6
Proflavine	T49.0X1	T49.0X2	T49.0X3	T49.0X4	T49.0X5	T49.0X6
Progabide	T42.6X1	T42.6X2	T42.6X3	T42.6X4	T42.6X5	T42.6X6
Progestin	T38.5X1	T38.5X2	T38.5X3	T38.5X4	T38.5X5	T38.5X6
oral contraceptive	T38.4X1	T38.4X2	T38.4X3	T38.4X4	T38.4X5	T38.4X6
Progesterone	T38.5X1	T38.5X2	T38.5X3	T38.5X4	T38.5X5	T38.5X6
Progestogen NEC	T38.5X1	T38.5X2	T38.5X3	T38.5X4	T38.5X5	T38.5X6
Progestone	T38.5X1	T38.5X2	T38.5X3	T38.5X4	T38.5X5	T38.5X6
Proglumide	T47.1X1	T47.1X2	T47.1X3	T47.1X4	T47.1X5	T47.1X6
Proguanil	T37.2X1	T37.2X2	T37.2X3	T37.2X4	T37.2X5	T37.2X6
Prolactin	T38.811	T38.812	T38.813	T38.814	T38.815	T38.816
Prolintane	T43.691	T43.692	T43.693	T43.694	T43.695	T43.696
Proloid	T38.1X1	T38.1X2	T38.1X3	T38.1X4	T38.1X5	T38.1X6
Proluton	T38.5X1	T38.5X2	T38.5X3	T38.5X4	T38.5X5	T38.5X6
Promacetin	T37.1X1	T37.1X2	T37.1X3	T37.1X4	T37.1X5	T37.1X6
Promazine	T43.3X1	T43.3X2	T43.3X3	T43.3X4	T43.3X5	T43.3X6
Promedol	T40.2X1	T40.2X2	T40.2X3	T40.2X4	—	—
Promegestone	T38.5X1	T38.5X2	T38.5X3	T38.5X4	T38.5X5	T38.5X6
Promethazine (teoclate)	T43.3X1	T43.3X2	T43.3X3	T43.3X4	T43.3X5	T43.3X6
Promin	T37.1X1	T37.1X2	T37.1X3	T37.1X4	T37.1X5	T37.1X6
Pronase	T45.3X1	T45.3X2	T45.3X3	T45.3X4	T45.3X5	T45.3X6
Pronestyl (hydrochloride)	T46.2X1	T46.2X2	T46.2X3	T46.2X4	T46.2X5	T46.2X6
Pronetalol	T44.7X1	T44.7X2	T44.7X3	T44.7X4	T44.7X5	T44.7X6
Prontosil	T37.0X1	T37.0X2	T37.0X3	T37.0X4	T37.0X5	T37.0X6
Propachlor	T60.3X1	T60.3X2	T60.3X3	T60.3X4	—	—
Propafenone	T46.2X1	T46.2X2	T46.2X3	T46.2X4	T46.2X5	T46.2X6
Propallylonal	T42.3X1	T42.3X2	T42.3X3	T42.3X4	T42.3X5	T42.3X6
Propamidine	T49.0X1	T49.0X2	T49.0X3	T49.0X4	T49.0X5	T49.0X6

TABLE OF DRUGS AND CHEMICALS

Substance	External Cause (T-Code)					
	Poisoning, Accidental (Unintentional)	Poisoning, Intentional Self-Harm	Poisoning, Assault	Poisoning, Undetermined	Adverse Effect	Underdosing
Propane (distributed in mobile container)	T59.891	T59.892	T59.893	T59.894	—	—
distributed through pipes	T59.891	T59.892	T59.893	T59.894	—	—
incomplete combustion	T57.11	T57.12	T57.13	T57.14	—	—
Propanidid	T41.291	T41.292	T41.293	T41.294	T41.295	T41.296
Propanil	T60.3X1	T60.3X2	T60.3X3	T60.3X4		
1-Propanol	T51.3X1	T51.3X2	T51.3X3	T51.3X4	—	—
2-Propanol	T51.2X1	T51.2X2	T51.2X3	T51.2X4	—	—
Propantheline	T44.3X1	T44.3X2	T44.3X3	T44.3X4	T44.3X5	T44.3X6
bromide	T44.3X1	T44.3X2	T44.3X3	T44.3X4	T44.3X5	T44.3X6
Proparacaine	T41.3X1	T41.3X2	T41.3X3	T41.3X4	T41.3X5	T41.3X6
Propatylnitrate	T46.3X1	T46.3X2	T46.3X3	T46.3X4	T46.3X5	T46.3X6
Propicillin	T36.0X1	T36.0X2	T36.0X3	T36.0X4	T36.0X5	T36.0X6
Propiolactone	T49.0X1	T49.0X2	T49.0X3	T49.0X4	T49.0X5	T49.0X6
Propiomazine	T45.0X1	T45.0X2	T45.0X3	T45.0X4	T45.0X5	T45.0X6
Propionaidehyde (medicinal)	T42.6X1	T42.6X2	T42.6X3	T42.6X4	T42.6X5	T42.6X6
Propionate (calcium) (sodium)	T49.0X1	T49.0X2	T49.0X3	T49.0X4	T49.0X5	T49.0X6
Propion gel	T49.0X1	T49.0X2	T49.0X3	T49.0X4	T49.0X5	T49.0X6
Propitocaine	T41.3X1	T41.3X2	T41.3X3	T41.3X4	T41.3X5	T41.3X6
infiltration (subcutaneous)	T41.3X1	T41.3X2	T41.3X3	T41.3X4	T41.3X5	T41.3X6
nerve block (peripheral) (plexus)	T41.3X1	T41.3X2	T41.3X3	T41.3X4	T41.3X5	T41.3X6
Propofol	T41.291	T41.292	T41.293	T41.294	T41.295	T41.296
Propoxur	T60.0X1	T60.0X2	T60.0X3	T60.0X4	—	—
Propoxycaine	T41.3X1	T41.3X2	T41.3X3	T41.3X4	T41.3X5	T41.3X6
infiltration (subcutaneous)	T41.3X1	T41.3X2	T41.3X3	T41.3X4	T41.3X5	T41.3X6
nerve block (peripheral) (plexus)	T41.3X1	T41.3X2	T41.3X3	T41.3X4	T41.3X5	T41.3X6
topical (surface)	T41.3X1	T41.3X2	T41.3X3	T41.3X4	T41.3X5	T41.3X6
Propoxyphene	T40.4X1	T40.4X2	T40.4X3	T40.4X4	T40.4X5	T40.4X6
Propranolol	T44.7X1	T44.7X2	T44.7X3	T44.7X4	T44.7X5	T44.7X6
Propyl						
alcohol	T51.3X1	T51.3X2	T51.3X3	T51.3X4	—	—
carbinol	T51.3X1	T51.3X2	T51.3X3	T51.3X4	—	—
hexadrine	T44.4X1	T44.4X2	T44.4X3	T44.4X4	T44.4X5	T44.4X6
iodone	T50.8X1	T50.8X2	T50.8X3	T50.8X4	T50.8X5	T50.8X6
thiouracil	T38.2X1	T38.2X2	T38.2X3	T38.2X4	T38.2X5	T38.2X6
Propylaminophenothiazine	T43.3X1	T43.3X2	T43.3X3	T43.3X4	T43.3X5	T43.3X6
Propylene	T59.891	T59.892	T59.893	T59.894	—	—
Propylhexedrine	T48.5X1	T48.5X2	T48.5X3	T48.5X4	T48.5X5	T48.5X6
Propyliodone	T50.8X1	T50.8X2	T50.8X3	T50.8X4	T50.8X5	T50.8X6
Propylthiouracil	T38.2X1	T38.2X2	T38.2X3	T38.2X4	T38.2X5	T38.2X6
Propylparaben (ophthalmic)	T49.5X1	T49.5X2	T49.5X3	T49.5X4	T49.5X5	T49.5X6

◀ New   ◀⁗ Revised   ~~deleted~~ Deleted

Substance	External Cause (T-Code)					
	Poisoning, Accidental (Unintentional)	Poisoning, Intentional Self-Harm	Poisoning, Assault	Poisoning, Undetermined	Adverse Effect	Underdosing
Propyphenazone	T39.2X1	T39.2X2	T39.2X3	T39.2X4	T39.2X5	T39.2X6
Proquazone	T39.391	T39.392	T39.393	T39.394	T39.395	T39.396
Proscillaridin	T46.0X1	T46.0X2	T46.0X3	T46.0X4	T46.0X5	T46.0X6
Prostacyclin	T45.521	T45.522	T45.523	T45.524	T45.525	T45.526
Prostaglandin (I2)	T45.521	T45.522	T45.523	T45.524	T45.525	T45.526
E1	T46.7X1	T46.7X2	T46.7X3	T46.7X4	T46.7X5	T46.7X6
E2	T48.0X1	T48.0X2	T48.0X3	T48.0X4	T48.0X5	T48.0X6
F2 alpha	T48.0X1	T48.0X2	T48.0X3	T48.0X4	T48.0X5	T48.0X6
Prostigmin	T44.0X1	T44.0X2	T44.0X3	T44.0X4	T44.0X5	T44.0X6
Prosultiamine	T45.2X1	T45.2X2	T45.2X3	T45.2X4	T45.2X5	T45.2X6
Protamine sulfate	T45.7X1	T45.7X2	T45.7X3	T45.7X4	T45.7X5	T45.7X6
zinc insulin	T38.3X1	T38.3X2	T38.3X3	T38.3X4	T38.3X5	T38.3X6
Protease	T47.5X1	T47.5X2	T47.5X3	T47.5X4	T47.5X5	T47.5X6
Protectant, skin NEC	T49.3X1	T49.3X2	T49.3X3	T49.3X4	T49.3X5	T49.3X6
Protein hydrolysate	T50.991	T50.992	T50.993	T50.994	T50.995	T50.996
Prothiaden — *see Dothiepin hydrochloride*						
Prothionamide	T37.1X1	T37.1X2	T37.1X3	T37.1X4	T37.1X5	T37.1X6
Prothipendyl	T43.591	T43.592	T43.593	T43.594	T43.595	T43.596
Prothoate	T60.0X1	T60.0X2	T60.0X3	T60.0X4	—	—
Prothrombin						
activator	T45.7X1	T45.7X2	T45.7X3	T45.7X4	T45.7X5	T45.7X6
synthesis inhibitor	T45.511	T45.512	T45.513	T45.514	T45.515	T45.516
Protionamide	T37.1X1	T37.1X2	T37.1X3	T37.1X4	T37.1X5	T37.1X6
Protirelin	T38.891	T38.892	T38.893	T38.894	T38.895	T38.896
Protokylol	T48.6X1	T48.6X2	T48.6X3	T48.6X4	T48.6X5	T48.6X6
Protopam	T50.6X1	T50.6X2	T50.6X3	T50.6X4	T50.6X5	T50.6X6
Protoveratrine(s) (A) (B)	T46.5X1	T46.5X2	T46.5X3	T46.5X4	T46.5X5	T46.5X6
Protriptyline	T43.011	T43.012	T43.013	T43.014	T43.015	T43.016
Provera	T38.5X1	T38.5X2	T38.5X3	T38.5X4	T38.5X5	T38.5X6
Provitamin A	T45.2X1	T45.2X2	T45.2X3	T45.2X4	T45.2X5	T45.2X6
Proxibarbal	T42.3X1	T42.3X2	T42.3X3	T42.3X4	T42.3X5	T42.3X6
Proxymetacaine	T41.3X1	T41.3X2	T41.3X3	T41.3X4	T41.3X5	T41.3X6
Proxyphylline	T48.6X1	T48.6X2	T48.6X3	T48.6X4	T48.6X5	T48.6X6
Prozac — *see Fluoxetine hydrochloride*						
Prunus						
laurocerasus	T62.2X1	T62.2X2	T62.2X3	T62.2X4	—	—
virginiana	T62.2X1	T62.2X2	T62.2X3	T62.2X4	—	—
Prussian blue						
commercial	T65.891	T65.892	T65.893	T65.894	—	—
therapeutic	T50.6X1	T50.6X2	T50.6X3	T50.6X4	T50.6X5	T50.6X6

TABLE OF DRUGS AND CHEMICALS

Substance	External Cause (T-Code)					
	Poisoning, Accidental (Unintentional)	Poisoning, Intentional Self-Harm	Poisoning, Assault	Poisoning, Undetermined	Adverse Effect	Underdosing
Prussic acid	T65.0X1	T65.0X2	T65.0X3	T65.0X4	—	—
vapor	T57.3X1	T57.3X2	T57.3X3	T57.3X4	—	—
Pseudoephedrine	T44.991	T44.992	T44.993	T44.994	T44.995	T44.996
Psilocin	T40.991	T40.992	T40.993	T40.994	—	—
Psilocybin	T40.991	T40.992	T40.993	T40.994	—	—
Psilocybine	T40.991	T40.992	T40.993	T40.994	—	—
Psoralene (nonmedicinal)	T65.891	T65.892	T65.893	T65.894	—	—
Psoralens (medicinal)	T50.991	T50.992	T50.993	T50.994	T50.995	T50.996
PSP (phenolsulfonphthalein)	T50.8X1	T50.8X2	T50.8X3	T50.8X4	T50.8X5	T50.8X6
Psychodysleptic drug NEC	T40.901	T40.902	T40.903	T40.904	T40.905	T40.906
Psychostimulant	T43.601	T43.602	T43.603	T43.604	T43.605	T43.606
amphetamine	T43.621	T43.622	T43.623	T43.624	T43.625	T43.626
caffeine	T43.611	T43.612	T43.613	T43.614	T43.615	T43.616
methylphenidate	T43.631	T43.632	T43.633	T43.634	T43.635	T43.636
specified NEC	T43.691	T43.692	T43.693	T43.694	T43.695	T43.696
Psychotherapeutic drug NEC	T43.91	T43.92	T43.93	T43.94	T43.95	T43.96
antidepressants— see also Antidepressant	T43.201	T43.202	T43.203	T43.204	T43.205	T43.206
specified NEC	T43.8X1	T43.8X2	T43.8X3	T43.8X4	T43.8X5	T43.8X6
tranquilizers NEC	T43.501	T43.502	T43.503	T43.504	T43.505	T43.506
Psychotomimetic agents	T40.901	T40.902	T40.903	T40.904	T40.905	T40.906
Psychotropic drug NEC	T43.91	T43.92	T43.93	T43.94	T43.95	T43.96
specified NEC	T43.8X1	T43.8X2	T43.8X3	T43.8X4	T43.8X5	T43.8X6
Psyllium hydrophilic mucilloid	T47.4X1	T47.4X2	T47.4X3	T47.4X4	T47.4X5	T47.4X6
Pteroylglutamic acid	T45.8X1	T45.8X2	T45.8X3	T45.8X4	T45.8X5	T45.8X6
Pteroyltriglutamate	T45.1X1	T45.1X2	T45.1X3	T45.1X4	T45.1X5	T45.1X6
PTFE— see Polytetrafluoroethylene						
Pulp						
devitalizing paste	T49.7X1	T49.7X2	T49.7X3	T49.7X4	T49.7X5	T49.7X6
dressing	T49.7X1	T49.7X2	T49.7X3	T49.7X4	T49.7X5	T49.7X6
Pulsatilla	T62.2X1	T62.2X2	T62.2X3	T62.2X4	—	—
Pumpkin seed extract	T37.4X1	T37.4X2	T37.4X3	T37.4X4	T37.4X5	T37.4X6
Purex (bleach)	T54.91	T54.92	T54.93	T54.94	—	—
Purgative NEC— see also Cathartic	T47.4X1	T47.4X2	T47.4X3	T47.4X4	T47.4X5	T47.4X6
Purine analogue (antineoplastic)	T45.1X1	T45.1X2	T45.1X3	T45.1X4	T45.1X5	T45.1X6
Purine diuretics	T50.2X1	T50.2X2	T50.2X3	T50.2X4	T50.2X5	T50.2X6
Purinethol	T45.1X1	T45.1X2	T45.1X3	T45.1X4	T45.1X5	T45.1X6
PVP	T45.8X1	T45.8X2	T45.8X3	T45.8X4	T45.8X5	T45.8X6
Pyrabital	T39.8X1	T39.8X2	T39.8X3	T39.8X4	T39.8X5	T39.8X6
Pyramidon	T39.2X1	T39.2X2	T39.2X3	T39.2X4	T39.2X5	T39.2X6
Pyrantel	T37.4X1	T37.4X2	T37.4X3	T37.4X4	T37.4X5	T37.4X6

◄ New ◄ Revised ~~deleted~~ Deleted

Substance	External Cause (T-Code)					
	Poisoning, Accidental (Unintentional)	Poisoning, Intentional Self-Harm	Poisoning, Assault	Poisoning, Undetermined	Adverse Effect	Underdosing
Pyrathiazine	T45.0X1	T45.0X2	T45.0X3	T45.0X4	T45.0X5	T45.0X6
Pyrazinamide	T37.1X1	T37.1X2	T37.1X3	T37.1X4	T37.1X5	T37.1X6
Pyrazinoic acid (amide)	T37.1X1	T37.1X2	T37.1X3	T37.1X4	T37.1X5	T37.1X6
Pyrazole (derivatives)	T39.2X1	T39.2X2	T39.2X3	T39.2X4	T39.2X5	T39.2X6
Pyrazolone analgesic NEC	T39.2X1	T39.2X2	T39.2X3	T39.2X4	T39.2X5	T39.2X6
Pyrethrin, pyrethrum (nonmedicinal)	T60.2X1	T60.2X2	T60.2X3	T60.2X4	—	—
Pyrethrum extract	T49.0X1	T49.0X2	T49.0X3	T49.0X4	T49.0X5	T49.0X6
Pyribenzamine	T45.0X1	T45.0X2	T45.0X3	T45.0X4	T45.0X5	T45.0X6
Pyridine	T52.8X1	T52.8X2	T52.8X3	T52.8X4	—	—
aldoxime methiodide	T50.6X1	T50.6X2	T50.6X3	T50.6X4	T50.6X5	T50.6X6
aldoxime methyl chloride	T50.6X1	T50.6X2	T50.6X3	T50.6X4	T50.6X5	T50.6X6
vapor	T59.891	T59.892	T59.893	T59.894	—	—
Pyridium	T39.8X1	T39.8X2	T39.8X3	T39.8X4	T39.8X5	T39.8X6
Pyridostigmine bromide	T44.0X1	T44.0X2	T44.0X3	T44.0X4	T44.0X5	T44.0X6
Pyridoxal phosphate	T45.2X1	T45.2X2	T45.2X3	T45.2X4	T45.2X5	T45.2X6
Pyridoxine	T45.2X1	T45.2X2	T45.2X3	T45.2X4	T45.2X5	T45.2X6
Pyrilamine	T45.0X1	T45.0X2	T45.0X3	T45.0X4	T45.0X5	T45.0X6
Pyrimethamine	T37.2X1	T37.2X2	T37.2X3	T37.2X4	T37.2X5	T37.2X6
with sulfadoxine	T37.2X1	T37.2X2	T37.2X3	T37.2X4	T37.2X5	T37.2X6
Pyrimidine antagonist	T45.1X1	T45.1X2	T45.1X3	T45.1X4	T45.1X5	T45.1X6
Pyriminil	T60.4X1	T60.4X2	T60.4X3	T60.4X4	—	—
Pyrithione zinc	T49.4X1	T49.4X2	T49.4X3	T49.4X4	T49.4X5	T49.4X6
Pyrithyldione	T42.6X1	T42.6X2	T42.6X3	T42.6X4	T42.6X5	T42.6X6
Pyrogallic acid	T49.0X1	T49.0X2	T49.0X3	T49.0X4	T49.0X5	T49.0X6
Pyrogallol	T49.0X1	T49.0X2	T49.0X3	T49.0X4	T49.0X5	T49.0X6
Pyroxylin	T49.3X1	T49.3X2	T49.3X3	T49.3X4	T49.3X5	T49.3X6
Pyrrobutamine	T45.0X1	T45.0X2	T45.0X3	T45.0X4	T45.0X5	T45.0X6
Pyrrolizidine alkaloids	T62.8X1	T62.8X2	T62.8X3	T62.8X4	—	—
Pyrvinium chloride	T37.4X1	T37.4X2	T37.4X3	T37.4X4	T37.4X5	T37.4X6
PZI	T38.3X1	T38.3X2	T38.3X3	T38.3X4	T38.3X5	T38.3X6
Q						
Quaalude	T42.6X1	T42.6X2	T42.6X3	T42.6X4	T42.6X5	T42.6X6
Quarternary ammonium						
anti-infective	T49.0X1	T49.0X2	T49.0X3	T49.0X4	T49.0X5	T49.0X6
ganglion blocking	T44.2X1	T44.2X2	T44.2X3	T44.2X4	T44.2X5	T44.2X6
parasympatholytic	T44.3X1	T44.3X2	T44.3X3	T44.3X4	T44.3X5	T44.3X6
Quazepam	T42.4X1	T42.4X2	T42.4X3	T42.4X4	T42.4X5	T42.4X6
Quicklime	T54.3X1	T54.3X2	T54.3X3	T54.3X4	—	—
Quillaja extract	T48.4X1	T48.4X2	T48.4X3	T48.4X4	T48.4X5	T48.4X6

TABLE OF DRUGS AND CHEMICALS

◀ New   ◀▦ Revised   ~~deleted~~ Deleted

TABLE OF DRUGS AND CHEMICALS

Substance	Poisoning, Accidental (Unintentional)	Poisoning, Intentional Self-Harm	Poisoning, Assault	Poisoning, Undetermined	Adverse Effect	Underdosing
			External Cause (T-Code)			
Quinacrine	T37.2X1	T37.2X2	T37.2X3	T37.2X4	T37.2X5	T37.2X6
Quinaglute	T46.2X1	T46.2X2	T46.2X3	T46.2X4	T46.2X5	T46.2X6
Quinalbarbital	T42.3X1	T42.3X2	T42.3X3	T42.3X4	T42.3X5	T42.3X6
Quinalbarbitone sodium	T42.3X1	T42.3X2	T42.3X3	T42.3X4	T42.3X5	T42.3X6
Quinalphos	T60.0X1	T60.0X2	T60.0X3	T60.0X4	—	—
Quinapril	T46.4X1	T46.4X2	T46.4X3	T46.4X4	T46.4X5	T46.4X6
Quinestradiol	T38.5X1	T38.5X2	T38.5X3	T38.5X4	T38.5X5	T38.5X6
Quinestradol	T38.5X1	T38.5X2	T38.5X3	T38.5X4	T38.5X5	T38.5X6
Quinestrol	T38.5X1	T38.5X2	T38.5X3	T38.5X4	T38.5X5	T38.5X6
Quinethazone	T50.2X1	T50.2X2	T50.2X3	T50.2X4	T50.2X5	T50.2X6
Quingestanol	T38.4X1	T38.4X2	T38.4X3	T38.4X4	T38.4X5	T38.4X6
Quinidine	T46.2X1	T46.2X2	T46.2X3	T46.2X4	T46.2X5	T46.2X6
Quinine	T37.2X1	T37.2X2	T37.2X3	T37.2X4	T37.2X5	T37.2X6
Quiniobine	T37.8X1	T37.8X2	T37.8X3	T37.8X4	T37.8X5	T37.8X6
Quinisocaine	T49.1X1	T49.1X2	T49.1X3	T49.1X4	T49.1X5	T49.1X6
Quinocide	T37.2X1	T37.2X2	T37.2X3	T37.2X4	T37.2X5	T37.2X6
Quinoline (derivatives) NEC	T37.8X1	T37.8X2	T37.8X3	T37.8X4	T37.8X5	T37.8X6
Quinupramine	T43.011	T43.012	T43.013	T43.014	T43.015	T43.016
Quotane	T41.3X1	T41.3X2	T41.3X3	T41.3X4	T41.3X5	T41.3X6
R						
Rabies						
immune globulin (human)	T50.Z11	T50.Z12	T50.Z13	T50.Z14	T50.Z15	T50.Z16
vaccine	T50.B91	T50.B92	T50.B93	T50.B94	T50.B95	T50.B96
Racemoramide	T40.2X1	T40.2X2	T40.2X3	T40.2X4	—	—
Racemorphan	T40.2X1	T40.2X2	T40.2X3	T40.2X4	T40.2X5	T40.2X6
Racepinefrin	T44.5X1	T44.5X2	T44.5X3	T44.5X4	T44.5X5	T44.5X6
Raclopride	T43.591	T43.592	T43.593	T43.594	T43.595	T43.596
Radiator alcohol	T51.1X1	T51.1X2	T51.1X3	T51.1X4	—	—
Radioactive drug NEC	T50.8X1	T50.8X2	T50.8X3	T50.8X4	T50.8X5	T50.8X6
Radio-opaque (drugs) (materials)	T50.8X1	T50.8X2	T50.8X3	T50.8X4	T50.8X5	T50.8X6
Ramifenazone	T39.2X1	T39.2X2	T39.2X3	T39.2X4	T39.2X5	T39.2X6
Ramipril	T46.4X1	T46.4X2	T46.4X3	T46.4X4	T46.4X5	T46.4X6
Ranitidine	T47.0X1	T47.0X2	T47.0X3	T47.0X4	T47.0X5	T47.0X6
Ranunculus	T62.2X1	T62.2X2	T62.2X3	T62.2X4	—	—
Rat poison NEC	T60.4X1	T60.4X2	T60.4X3	T60.4X4	—	—
Rattlesnake (venom)	T63.011	T63.012	T63.013	T63.014	—	—
Raubasine	T46.7X1	T46.7X2	T46.7X3	T46.7X4	T46.7X5	T46.7X6
Raudixin	T46.5X1	T46.5X2	T46.5X3	T46.5X4	T46.5X5	T46.5X6
Rautensin	T46.5X1	T46.5X2	T46.5X3	T46.5X4	T46.5X5	T46.5X6

◀ New   ◀▥ Revised   ~~deleted~~ Deleted

Substance	External Cause (T-Code)					
	Poisoning, Accidental (Unintentional)	Poisoning, Intentional Self-Harm	Poisoning, Assault	Poisoning, Undetermined	Adverse Effect	Underdosing
Rautina	T46.5X1	T46.5X2	T46.5X3	T46.5X4	T46.5X5	T46.5X6
Rautotal	T46.5X1	T46.5X2	T46.5X3	T46.5X4	T46.5X5	T46.5X6
Rauwiloid	T46.5X1	T46.5X2	T46.5X3	T46.5X4	T46.5X5	T46.5X6
Rauwoldin	T46.5X1	T46.5X2	T46.5X3	T46.5X4	T46.5X5	T46.5X6
Rauwolfia (alkaloids)	T46.5X1	T46.5X2	T46.5X3	T46.5X4	T46.5X5	T46.5X6
Razoxane	T45.1X1	T45.1X2	T45.1X3	T45.1X4	T45.1X5	T45.1X6
Realgar	T57.0X1	T57.0X2	T57.0X3	T57.0X4	—	—
Recombinant (R) — see specific protein						
Red blood cells, packed	T45.8X1	T45.8X2	T45.8X3	T45.8X4	T45.8X5	T45.8X6
Red squill (scilliroside)	T60.4X1	T60.4X2	T60.4X3	T60.4X4	—	—
Reducing agent, industrial NEC	T65.891	T65.892	T65.893	T65.894	—	—
Refrigerant gas (chlorofluoro-carbon)	T53.5X1	T53.5X2	T53.5X3	T53.5X4	—	—
not chlorofluoro-carbon	T59.891	T59.892	T59.893	T59.894	—	—
Regroton	T50.2X1	T50.2X2	T50.2X3	T50.2X4	T50.2X5	T50.2X6
Rehydration salts (oral)	T50.3X1	T50.3X2	T50.3X3	T50.3X4	T50.3X5	T50.3X6
Rela	T42.8X1	T42.8X2	T42.8X3	T42.8X4	T42.8X5	T42.8X6
Relaxant, muscle						
anesthetic	T48.1X1	T48.1X2	T48.1X3	T48.1X4	T48.1X5	T48.1X6
central nervous system	T42.8X1	T42.8X2	T42.8X3	T42.8X4	T42.8X5	T42.8X6
skeletal NEC	T48.1X1	T48.1X2	T48.1X3	T48.1X4	T48.1X5	T48.1X6
smooth NEC	T44.3X1	T44.3X2	T44.3X3	T44.3X4	T44.3X5	T44.3X6
Remoxipride	T43.591	T43.592	T43.593	T43.594	T43.595	T43.596
Renese	T50.2X1	T50.2X2	T50.2X3	T50.2X4	T50.2X5	T50.2X6
Renografin	T50.8X1	T50.8X2	T50.8X3	T50.8X4	T50.8X5	T50.8X6
Replacement solution	T50.3X1	T50.3X2	T50.3X3	T50.3X4	T50.3X5	T50.3X6
Reproterol	T48.6X1	T48.6X2	T48.6X3	T48.6X4	T48.6X5	T48.6X6
Rescinnamine	T46.5X1	T46.5X2	T46.5X3	T46.5X4	T46.5X5	T46.5X6
Reserpin(e)	T46.5X1	T46.5X2	T46.5X3	T46.5X4	T46.5X5	T46.5X6
Resorcin, resorcinol (nonmedicinal)	T65.891	T65.892	T65.893	T65.894	—	—
medicinal	T49.4X1	T49.4X2	T49.4X3	T49.4X4	T49.4X5	T49.4X6
Respaire	T48.4X1	T48.4X2	T48.4X3	T48.4X4	T48.4X5	T48.4X6
Respiratory drug NEC	T48.901	T48.902	T48.903	T48.904	T48.905	T48.906
antiasthmatic NEC	T48.6X1	T48.6X2	T48.6X3	T48.6X4	T48.6X5	T48.6X6
anti-common-cold NEC	T48.5X1	T48.5X2	T48.5X3	T48.5X4	T48.5X5	T48.5X6
expectorant NEC	T48.4X1	T48.4X2	T48.4X3	T48.4X4	T48.4X5	T48.4X6
stimulant	T48.901	T48.902	T48.903	T48.904	T48.905	T48.906
Retinoic acid	T49.0X1	T49.0X2	T49.0X3	T49.0X4	T49.0X5	T49.0X6
Retinol	T45.2X1	T45.2X2	T45.2X3	T45.2X4	T45.2X5	T45.2X6
Rh (D) immune globulin (human)	T50.Z11	T50.Z12	T50.Z13	T50.Z14	T50.Z15	T50.Z16
Rhodine	T39.011	T39.012	T39.013	T39.014	T39.015	T39.016

◀ New ◀ Revised ~~deleted~~ Deleted

TABLE OF DRUGS AND CHEMICALS

Substance	External Cause (T-Code)					
	Poisoning, Accidental (Unintentional)	Poisoning, Intentional Self-Harm	Poisoning, Assault	Poisoning, Undetermined	Adverse Effect	Underdosing
RhoGAM	T50.Z11	T50.Z12	T50.Z13	T50.Z14	T50.Z15	T50.Z16
Rhubarb						
dry extract	T47.2X1	T47.2X2	T47.2X3	T47.2X4	T47.2X5	T47.2X6
tincture, compound	T47.2X1	T47.2X2	T47.2X3	T47.2X4	T47.2X5	T47.2X6
Ribavirin	T37.5X1	T37.5X2	T37.5X3	T37.5X4	T37.5X5	T37.5X6
Riboflavin	T45.2X1	T45.2X2	T45.2X3	T45.2X4	T45.2X5	T45.2X6
Ribostamycin	T36.5X1	T36.5X2	T36.5X3	T36.5X4	T36.5X5	T36.5X6
Ricin	T62.2X1	T62.2X2	T62.2X3	T62.2X4	—	—
Ricinus communis	T62.2X1	T62.2X2	T62.2X3	T62.2X4	—	—
Rickettsial vaccine NEC	T50.A91	T50.A92	T50.A93	T50.A94	T50.A95	T50.A96
Rifabutin	T36.6X1	T36.6X2	T36.6X3	T36.6X4	T36.6X5	T36.6X6
Rifamide	T36.6X1	T36.6X2	T36.6X3	T36.6X4	T36.6X5	T36.6X6
Rifampicin	T36.6X1	T36.6X2	T36.6X3	T36.6X4	T36.6X5	T36.6X6
with isoniazid	T37.1X1	T37.1X2	T37.1X3	T37.1X4	T37.1X5	T37.1X6
Rifampin	T36.6X1	T36.6X2	T36.6X3	T36.6X4	T36.6X5	T36.6X6
Rifamycin	T36.6X1	T36.6X2	T36.6X3	T36.6X4	T36.6X5	T36.6X6
Rifaximin	T36.6X1	T36.6X2	T36.6X3	T36.6X4	T36.6X5	T36.6X6
Rimantadine	T37.5X1	T37.5X2	T37.5X3	T37.5X4	T37.5X5	T37.5X6
Rimazolium metilsulfate	T39.8X1	T39.8X2	T39.8X3	T39.8X4	T39.8X5	T39.8X6
Rimifon	T37.1X1	T37.1X2	T37.1X3	T37.1X4	T37.1X5	T37.1X6
Rimiterol	T48.6X1	T48.6X2	T48.6X3	T48.6X4	T48.6X5	T48.6X6
Ringer (lactate) solution	T50.3X1	T50.3X2	T50.3X3	T50.3X4	T50.3X5	T50.3X6
Ristocetin	T36.8X1	T36.8X2	T36.8X3	T36.8X4	T36.8X5	T36.8X6
Ritalin	T43.631	T43.632	T43.633	T43.634	T43.635	T43.636
Ritodrine	T44.5X1	T44.5X2	T44.5X3	T44.5X4	T44.5X5	T44.5X6
Roach killer — see Insecticide						
Rociverine	T44.3X1	T44.3X2	T44.3X3	T44.3X4	T44.3X5	T44.3X6
Rocky Mountain spotted fever vaccine	T50.A91	T50.A92	T50.A93	T50.A94	T50.A95	T50.A96
Rodenticide NEC	T60.4X1	T60.4X2	T60.4X3	T60.4X4	—	—
Rohypnol	T42.4X1	T42.4X2	T42.4X3	T42.4X4	T42.4X5	T42.4X6
Rokitamycin	T36.3X1	T36.3X2	T36.3X3	T36.3X4	T36.3X5	T36.3X6
Rolaids	T47.1X1	T47.1X2	T47.1X3	T47.1X4	T47.1X5	T47.1X6
Rolitetracycline	T36.4X1	T36.4X2	T36.4X3	T36.4X4	T36.4X5	T36.4X6
Romilar	T48.3X1	T48.3X2	T48.3X3	T48.3X4	T48.3X5	T48.3X6
Ronifibrate	T46.6X1	T46.6X2	T46.6X3	T46.6X4	T46.6X5	T46.6X6
Rosaprostol	T47.1X1	T47.1X2	T47.1X3	T47.1X4	T47.1X5	T47.1X6
Rose bengal sodium (131I)	T50.8X1	T50.8X2	T50.8X3	T50.8X4	T50.8X5	T50.8X6
Rose water ointment	T49.3X1	T49.3X2	T49.3X3	T49.3X4	T49.3X5	T49.3X6
Rosoxacin	T37.8X1	T37.8X2	T37.8X3	T37.8X4	T37.8X5	T37.8X6
Rotenone	T60.2X1	T60.2X2	T60.2X3	T60.2X4	—	—

◀ New   ◀▪▪ Revised   ~~deleted~~ Deleted

Substance	External Cause (T-Code)					
	Poisoning, Accidental (Unintentional)	Poisoning, Intentional Self-Harm	Poisoning, Assault	Poisoning, Undetermined	Adverse Effect	Underdosing
Rotoxamine	T45.0X1	T45.0X2	T45.0X3	T45.0X4	T45.0X5	T45.0X6
Rough-on-rats	T60.4X1	T60.4X2	T60.4X3	T60.4X4	—	—
Roxatidine	T47.0X1	T47.0X2	T47.0X3	T47.0X4	T47.0X5	T47.0X6
Roxithromycin	T36.3X1	T36.3X2	T36.3X3	T36.3X4	T36.3X5	T36.3X6
Rt-PA	T45.611	T45.612	T45.613	T45.614	T45.615	T45.616
Rubbing alcohol	T51.2X1	T51.2X2	T51.2X3	T51.2X4	—	—
Rubefacient	T49.4X1	T49.4X2	T49.4X3	T49.4X4	T49.4X5	T49.4X6
Rubella vaccine	T50.B91	T50.B92	T50.B93	T50.B94	T50.B95	T50.B96
Rubelogen	T50.B91	T50.B92	T50.B93	T50.B94	T50.B95	T50.B96
Rubeovax	T50.991	T50.992	T50.993	T50.994	T50.995	T50.996
Rubidium chloride Rb82	T50.8X1	T50.8X2	T50.8X3	T50.8X4	T50.8X5	T50.8X6
Rubidomycin	T45.1X1	T45.1X2	T45.1X3	T45.1X4	T45.1X5	T45.1X6
Rue	T62.2X1	T62.2X2	T62.2X3	T62.2X4	—	—
Rufocromomycin	T45.1X1	T45.1X2	T45.1X3	T45.1X4	T45.1X5	T45.1X6
Russel's viper venin	T45.7X1	T45.7X2	T45.7X3	T45.7X4	T45.7X5	T45.7X6
Ruta (graveolens)	T62.2X1	T62.2X2	T62.2X3	T62.2X4	—	—
Rutinum	T46.991	T46.992	T46.993	T46.994	T46.995	T46.996
Rutoside	T46.991	T46.992	T46.993	T46.994	T46.995	T46.996
S						
Sabadilla (plant)	T62.2X1	T62.2X2	T62.2X3	T62.2X4	—	—
pesticide	T60.2X1	T60.2X2	T60.2X3	T60.2X4	—	—
Saccharated iron oxide	T45.8X1	T45.8X2	T45.8X3	T45.8X4	T45.8X5	T45.8X6
Saccharin	T50.901	T50.902	T50.903	T50.904	T50.905	T50.906
Saccharomyces boulardii	T47.6X1	T47.6X2	T47.6X3	T47.6X4	T47.6X5	T47.6X6
Safflower oil	T46.6X1	T46.6X2	T46.6X3	T46.6X4	T46.6X5	T46.6X6
Safrazine	T43.1X1	T43.1X2	T43.1X3	T43.1X4	T43.1X5	T43.1X6
Salazosulfapyridine	T37.0X1	T37.0X2	T37.0X3	T37.0X4	T37.0X5	T37.0X6
Salbutamol	T48.6X1	T48.6X2	T48.6X3	T48.6X4	T48.6X5	T48.6X6
Salicylamide	T39.091	T39.092	T39.093	T39.094	T39.095	T39.096
Salicylate NEC	T39.091	T39.092	T39.093	T39.094	T39.095	T39.096
methyl	T49.3X1	T49.3X2	T49.3X3	T49.3X4	T49.3X5	T49.3X6
theobromine calcium	T50.2X1	T50.2X2	T50.2X3	T50.2X4	T50.2X5	T50.2X6
Salicylazosulfapyridine	T37.0X1	T37.0X2	T37.0X3	T37.0X4	T37.0X5	T37.0X6
Salicylhydroxamic acid	T49.0X1	T49.0X2	T49.0X3	T49.0X4	T49.0X5	T49.0X6
Salicylic acid	T49.4X1	T49.4X2	T49.4X3	T49.4X4	T49.4X5	T49.4X6
with benzoic acid	T49.4X1	T49.4X2	T49.4X3	T49.4X4	T49.4X5	T49.4X6
congeners	T39.091	T39.092	T39.093	T39.094	T39.095	T39.096
derivative	T39.091	T39.092	T39.093	T39.094	T39.095	T39.096
salts	T39.091	T39.092	T39.093	T39.094	T39.095	T39.096

TABLE OF DRUGS AND CHEMICALS

Substance	Poisoning, Accidental (Unintentional)	Poisoning, Intentional Self-Harm	Poisoning, Assault	Poisoning, Undetermined	Adverse Effect	Underdosing
Salinazid	T37.1X1	T37.1X2	T37.1X3	T37.1X4	T37.1X5	T37.1X6
Salmeterol	T48.6X1	T48.6X2	T48.6X3	T48.6X4	T48.6X5	T48.6X6
Salol	T49.3X1	T49.3X2	T49.3X3	T49.3X4	T49.3X5	T49.3X6
Salsalate	T39.091	T39.092	T39.093	T39.094	T39.095	T39.096
Salt substitute	T50.901	T50.902	T50.903	T50.904	T50.905	T50.906
Salt-replacing drug	T50.901	T50.902	T50.903	T50.904	T50.905	T50.906
Salt-retaining mineralocorticoid	T50.0X1	T50.0X2	T50.0X3	T50.0X4	T50.0X5	T50.0X6
Saluretic NEC	T50.2X1	T50.2X2	T50.2X3	T50.2X4	T50.2X5	T50.2X6
Saluron	T50.2X1	T50.2X2	T50.2X3	T50.2X4	T50.2X5	T50.2X6
Salvarsan 606 (neosilver) (silver)	T37.8X1	T37.8X2	T37.8X3	T37.8X4	T37.8X5	T37.8X6
Sambucus canadensis	T62.2X1	T62.2X2	T62.2X3	T62.2X4	—	—
berry	T62.1X1	T62.1X2	T62.1X3	T62.1X4	—	—
Sandril	T46.5X1	T46.5X2	T46.5X3	T46.5X4	T46.5X5	T46.5X6
Sanguinaria canadensis	T62.2X1	T62.2X2	T62.2X3	T62.2X4	—	—
Saniflush (cleaner)	T54.2X1	T54.2X2	T54.2X3	T54.2X4	—	—
Santonin	T37.4X1	T37.4X2	T37.4X3	T37.4X4	T37.4X5	T37.4X6
Santyl	T49.8X1	T49.8X2	T49.8X3	T49.8X4	T49.8X5	T49.8X6
Saralasin	T46.5X1	T46.5X2	T46.5X3	T46.5X4	T46.5X5	T46.5X6
Sarcolysin	T45.1X1	T45.1X2	T45.1X3	T45.1X4	T45.1X5	T45.1X6
Sarkomycin	T45.1X1	T45.1X2	T45.1X3	T45.1X4	T45.1X5	T45.1X6
Saroten	T43.011	T43.012	T43.013	T43.014	T43.015	T43.016
Saturnine—see Lead						
Savin (oil)	T49.4X1	T49.4X2	T49.4X3	T49.4X4	T49.4X5	T49.4X6
Scammony	T47.2X1	T47.2X2	T47.2X3	T47.2X4	T47.2X5	T47.2X6
Scarlet red	T49.8X1	T49.8X2	T49.8X3	T49.8X4	T49.8X5	T49.8X6
Scheele's green	T57.0X1	T57.0X2	T57.0X3	T57.0X4	—	—
insecticide	T57.0X1	T57.0X2	T57.0X3	T57.0X4	—	—
Schizontozide (blood) (tissue)	T37.2X1	T37.2X2	T37.2X3	T37.2X4	T37.2X5	T37.2X6
Schradan	T60.0X1	T60.0X2	T60.0X3	T60.0X4		
Schweinfurth green	T57.0X1	T57.0X2	T57.0X3	T57.0X4	—	—
insecticide	T57.0X1	T57.0X2	T57.0X3	T57.0X4	—	—
Scilla, rat poison	T60.4X1	T60.4X2	T60.4X3	T60.4X4	—	—
Scillaren	T60.4X1	T60.4X2	T60.4X3	T60.4X4	—	—
Sclerosing agent	T46.8X1	T46.8X2	T46.8X3	T46.8X4	T46.8X5	T46.8X6
Scombrotoxin	T61.11	T61.12	T61.13	T61.14	—	—
Scopolamine	T44.3X1	T44.3X2	T44.3X3	T44.3X4	T44.3X5	T44.3X6
Scopolia extract	T44.3X1	T44.3X2	T44.3X3	T44.3X4	T44.3X5	T44.3X6
Scouring powder	T65.891	T65.892	T65.893	T65.894	—	—

◀ New ◀▥ Revised ~~deleted~~ Deleted

Substance	External Cause (T-Code)					
	Poisoning, Accidental (Unintentional)	Poisoning, Intentional Self-Harm	Poisoning, Assault	Poisoning, Undetermined	Adverse Effect	Underdosing
Sea						
anemone (sting)	T63.631	T63.632	T63.633	T63.634	—	—
cucumber (sting)	T63.691	T63.692	T63.693	T63.694	—	—
snake (bite) (venom)	T63.091	T63.092	T63.093	T63.094	—	—
urchin spine (puncture)	T63.691	T63.692	T63.693	T63.694	—	—
Seafood	T61.91	T61.92	T61.93	T61.94	—	—
specified NEC	T61.8X1	T61.8X2	T61.8X3	T61.8X4	—	—
Secbutabarbital	T42.3X1	T42.3X2	T42.3X3	T42.3X4	T42.3X5	T42.3X6
Secbutabarbitone	T42.3X1	T42.3X2	T42.3X3	T42.3X4	T42.3X5	T42.3X6
Secnidazole	T37.3X1	T37.3X2	T37.3X3	T37.3X4	T37.3X5	T37.3X6
Secobarbital	T42.3X1	T42.3X2	T42.3X3	T42.3X4	T42.3X5	T42.3X6
Seconal	T42.3X1	T42.3X2	T42.3X3	T42.3X4	T42.3X5	T42.3X6
Secretin	T50.8X1	T50.8X2	T50.8X3	T50.8X4	T50.8X5	T50.8X6
Sedative NEC	T42.71	T42.72	T42.73	T42.74	T42.75	T42.76
mixed NEC	T42.6X1	T42.6X2	T42.6X3	T42.6X4	T42.6X5	T42.6X6
Sedormid	T42.6X1	T42.6X2	T42.6X3	T42.6X4	T42.6X5	T42.6X6
Seed disinfectant or dressing	T60.8X1	T60.8X2	T60.8X3	T60.8X4	—	—
Seeds (poisonous)	T62.2X1	T62.2X2	T62.2X3	T62.2X4	—	—
Selegiline	T42.8X1	T42.8X2	T42.8X3	T42.8X4	T42.8X5	T42.8X6
Selenium NEC	T56.891	T56.892	T56.893	T56.894	—	—
disulfide or sulfide	T49.4X1	T49.4X2	T49.4X3	T49.4X4	T49.4X5	T49.4X6
fumes	T59.891	T59.892	T59.893	T59.894	—	—
sulfide	T49.4X1	T49.4X2	T49.4X3	T49.4X4	T49.4X5	T49.4X6
Selenomethionine (75Se)	T50.8X1	T50.8X2	T50.8X3	T50.8X4	T50.8X5	T50.8X6
Selsun	T49.4X1	T49.4X2	T49.4X3	T49.4X4	T49.4X5	T49.4X6
Semustine	T45.1X1	T45.1X2	T45.1X3	T45.1X4	T45.1X5	T45.1X6
Senega syrup	T48.4X1	T48.4X2	T48.4X3	T48.4X4	T48.4X5	T48.4X6
Senna	T47.2X1	T47.2X2	T47.2X3	T47.2X4	T47.2X5	T47.2X6
Sennoside A+B	T47.2X1	T47.2X2	T47.2X3	T47.2X4	T47.2X5	T47.2X6
Septisol	T49.2X1	T49.2X2	T49.2X3	T49.2X4	T49.2X5	T49.2X6
Seractide	T38.811	T38.812	T38.813	T38.814	T38.815	T38.816
Serax	T42.4X1	T42.4X2	T42.4X3	T42.4X4	T42.4X5	T42.4X6
Serenesil	T42.6X1	T42.6X2	T42.6X3	T42.6X4	T42.6X5	T42.6X6
Serenium (hydrochloride)	T37.91	T37.92	T37.93	T37.94	T37.95	T37.96
Serepax — see Oxazepam						
Sermorelin	T38.891	T38.892	T38.893	T38.894	T38.895	T38.896
Sernyl	T41.1X1	T41.1X2	T41.1X3	T41.1X4	T41.1X5	T41.1X6
Serotonin	T50.991	T50.992	T50.993	T50.994	T50.995	T50.996

TABLE OF DRUGS AND CHEMICALS

◀ New   ◀▥ Revised   ~~deleted~~ Deleted

TABLE OF DRUGS AND CHEMICALS

Substance	Poisoning, Accidental (Unintentional)	Poisoning, Intentional Self-Harm	Poisoning, Assault	Poisoning, Undetermined	Adverse Effect	Underdosing
			External Cause (T-Code)			
Serpasil	T46.5X1	T46.5X2	T46.5X3	T46.5X4	T46.5X5	T46.5X6
Serrapeptase	T45.3X1	T45.3X2	T45.3X3	T45.3X4	T45.3X5	T45.3X6
Serum						
antibotulinus	T50.Z11	T50.Z12	T50.Z13	T50.Z14	T50.Z15	T50.Z16
anticytotoxic	T50.Z11	T50.Z12	T50.Z13	T50.Z14	T50.Z15	T50.Z16
antidiphtheria	T50.Z11	T50.Z12	T50.Z13	T50.Z14	T50.Z15	T50.Z16
antimeningococcus	T50.Z11	T50.Z12	T50.Z13	T50.Z14	T50.Z15	T50.Z16
anti-Rh	T50.Z11	T50.Z12	T50.Z13	T50.Z14	T50.Z15	T50.Z16
anti-snake-bite	T50.Z11	T50.Z12	T50.Z13	T50.Z14	T50.Z15	T50.Z16
antitetanic	T50.Z11	T50.Z12	T50.Z13	T50.Z14	T50.Z15	T50.Z16
antitoxic	T50.Z11	T50.Z12	T50.Z13	T50.Z14	T50.Z15	T50.Z16
complement (inhibitor)	T45.8X1	T45.8X2	T45.8X3	T45.8X4	T45.8X5	T45.8X6
convalescent	T50.Z11	T50.Z12	T50.Z13	T50.Z14	T50.Z15	T50.Z16
hemolytic complement	T45.8X1	T45.8X2	T45.8X3	T45.8X4	T45.8X5	T45.8X6
immune (human)	T50.Z11	T50.Z12	T50.Z13	T50.Z14	T50.Z15	T50.Z16
protective NEC	T50.Z11	T50.Z12	T50.Z13	T50.Z14	T50.Z15	T50.Z16
Setastine	T45.0X1	T45.0X2	T45.0X3	T45.0X4	T45.0X5	T45.0X6
Setoperone	T43.591	T43.592	T43.593	T43.594	T43.595	T43.596
Sewer gas	T59.91	T59.92	T59.93	T59.94	—	—
Shampoo	T55.0X1	T55.0X2	T55.0X3	T55.0X4	—	—
Shellfish, noxious, nonbacterial	T61.781	T61.782	T61.783	T61.784	—	—
Sildenafil	T46.7X1	T46.7X2	T46.7X3	T46.7X4	T46.7X5	T46.7X6
Silibinin	T50.991	T50.992	T50.993	T50.994	T50.995	T50.996
Silicone NEC	T65.891	T65.892	T65.893	T65.894	—	—
medicinal	T49.3X1	T49.3X2	T49.3X3	T49.3X4	T49.3X5	T49.3X6
Silvadene	T49.0X1	T49.0X2	T49.0X3	T49.0X4	T49.0X5	T49.0X6
Silver	T49.0X1	T49.0X2	T49.0X3	T49.0X4	T49.0X5	T49.0X6
anti-infectives	T49.0X1	T49.0X2	T49.0X3	T49.0X4	T49.0X5	T49.0X6
arsphenamine	T37.8X1	T37.8X2	T37.8X3	T37.8X4	T37.8X5	T37.8X6
colloidal	T49.0X1	T49.0X2	T49.0X3	T49.0X4	T49.0X5	T49.0X6
nitrate	T49.0X1	T49.0X2	T49.0X3	T49.0X4	T49.0X5	T49.0X6
ophthalmic preparation	T49.5X1	T49.5X2	T49.5X3	T49.5X4	T49.5X5	T49.5X6
toughened (keratolytic)	T49.4X1	T49.4X2	T49.4X3	T49.4X4	T49.4X5	T49.4X6
nonmedicinal (dust)	T56.891	T56.892	T56.893	T56.894	—	—
protein	T49.5X1	T49.5X2	T49.5X3	T49.5X4	T49.5X5	T49.5X6
salvarsan	T37.8X1	T37.8X2	T37.8X3	T37.8X4	T37.8X5	T37.8X6
sulfadiazine	T49.4X1	T49.4X2	T49.4X3	T49.4X4	T49.4X5	T49.4X6
Silymarin	T50.991	T50.992	T50.993	T50.994	T50.995	T50.996
Simaldrate	T47.1X1	T47.1X2	T47.1X3	T47.1X4	T47.1X5	T47.1X6
Simazine	T60.3X1	T60.3X2	T60.3X3	T60.3X4	—	—

◄ New   ◄▦ Revised   ~~deleted~~ Deleted

Substance	Poisoning, Accidental (Unintentional)	Poisoning, Intentional Self-Harm	Poisoning, Assault	Poisoning, Undetermined	Adverse Effect	Underdosing
	External Cause (T-Code)					
Simethicone	T47.1X1	T47.1X2	T47.1X3	T47.1X4	T47.1X5	T47.1X6
Simfibrate	T46.6X1	T46.6X2	T46.6X3	T46.6X4	T46.6X5	T46.6X6
Simvastatin	T46.6X1	T46.6X2	T46.6X3	T46.6X4	T46.6X5	T46.6X6
Sincalide	T50.8X1	T50.8X2	T50.8X3	T50.8X4	T50.8X5	T50.8X6
Sinequan	T43.011	T43.012	T43.013	T43.014	T43.015	T43.016
Singoserp	T46.5X1	T46.5X2	T46.5X3	T46.5X4	T46.5X5	T46.5X6
Sintrom	T45.511	T45.512	T45.513	T45.514	T45.515	T45.516
Sisomicin	T36.5X1	T36.5X2	T36.5X3	T36.5X4	T36.5X5	T36.5X6
Sitosterols	T46.6X1	T46.6X2	T46.6X3	T46.6X4	T46.6X5	T46.6X6
Skeletal muscle relaxants	T48.1X1	T48.1X2	T48.1X3	T48.1X4	T48.1X5	T48.1X6
Skin						
agents (external)	T49.91	T49.92	T49.93	T49.94	T49.95	T49.96
specified NEC	T49.8X1	T49.8X2	T49.8X3	T49.8X4	T49.8X5	T49.8X6
test antigen	T50.8X1	T50.8X2	T50.8X3	T50.8X4	T50.8X5	T50.8X6
Sleep-eze	T45.0X1	T45.0X2	T45.0X3	T45.0X4	T45.0X5	T45.0X6
Sleeping draught, pill	T42.71	T42.72	T42.73	T42.74	T42.75	T42.76
Smallpox vaccine	T50.B11	T50.B12	T50.B13	T50.B14	T50.B15	T50.B16
Smelter fumes NEC	T56.91	T56.92	T56.93	T56.94	—	—
Smog	T59.1X1	T59.1X2	T59.1X3	T59.1X4	—	—
Smoke NEC	T59.811	T59.812	T59.813	T59.814	—	—
Smooth muscle relaxant	T44.3X1	T44.3X2	T44.3X3	T44.3X4	T44.3X5	T44.3X6
Snail killer NEC	T60.8X1	T60.8X2	T60.8X3	T60.8X4	—	—
Snake venom or bite	T63.001	T63.002	T63.003	T63.004	—	—
hemocoagulase	T45.7X1	T45.7X2	T45.7X3	T45.7X4	T45.7X5	T45.7X6
Snuff	T65.211	T65.212	T65.213	T65.214	—	—
Soap (powder) (product)	T55.0X1	T55.0X2	T55.0X3	T55.0X4	—	—
enema	T47.4X1	T47.4X2	T47.4X3	T47.4X4	T47.4X5	T47.4X6
medicinal, soft	T49.2X1	T49.2X2	T49.2X3	T49.2X4	T49.2X5	T49.2X6
superfatted	T49.2X1	T49.2X2	T49.2X3	T49.2X4	T49.2X5	T49.2X6
Sobrerol	T48.4X1	T48.4X2	T48.4X3	T48.4X4	T48.4X5	T48.4X6
Soda (caustic)	T54.3X1	T54.3X2	T54.3X3	T54.3X4	—	—
bicarb	T47.1X1	T47.1X2	T47.1X3	T47.1X4	T47.1X5	T47.1X6
chlorinated — *see Sodium, hypochlorite*						
Sodium						
acetosulfone	T37.1X1	T37.1X2	T37.1X3	T37.1X4	T37.1X5	T37.1X6
acetrizoate	T50.8X1	T50.8X2	T50.8X3	T50.8X4	T50.8X5	T50.8X6
acid phosphate	T50.3X1	T50.3X2	T50.3X3	T50.3X4	T50.3X5	T50.3X6
alginate	T47.8X1	T47.8X2	T47.8X3	T47.8X4	T47.8X5	T47.8X6
amidotrizoate	T50.8X1	T50.8X2	T50.8X3	T50.8X4	T50.8X5	T50.8X6
aminopterin	T45.1X1	T45.1X2	T45.1X3	T45.1X4	T45.1X5	T45.1X6

Substance	Poisoning, Accidental (Unintentional)	Poisoning, Intentional Self-Harm	Poisoning, Assault	Poisoning, Undetermined	Adverse Effect	Underdosing
Sodium *(Continued)*						
amylosulfate	T47.8X1	T47.8X2	T47.8X3	T47.8X4	T47.8X5	T47.8X6
amytal	T42.3X1	T42.3X2	T42.3X3	T42.3X4	T42.3X5	T42.3X6
antimony gluconate	T37.3X1	T37.3X2	T37.3X3	T37.3X4	T37.3X5	T37.3X6
arsenate	T57.0X1	T57.0X2	T57.0X3	T57.0X4	—	—
aurothiomalate	T39.4X1	T39.4X2	T39.4X3	T39.4X4	T39.4X5	T39.4X6
aurothiosulfate	T39.4X1	T39.4X2	T39.4X3	T39.4X4	T39.4X5	T39.4X6
barbiturate	T42.3X1	T42.3X2	T42.3X3	T42.3X4	T42.3X5	T42.3X6
basic phosphate	T47.4X1	T47.4X2	T47.4X3	T47.4X4	T47.4X5	T47.4X6
bicarbonate	T47.1X1	T47.1X2	T47.1X3	T47.1X4	T47.1X5	T47.1X6
bichromate	T57.8X1	T57.8X2	T57.8X3	T57.8X4	—	—
biphosphate	T50.3X1	T50.3X2	T50.3X3	T50.3X4	T50.3X5	T50.3X6
bisulfate	T65.891	T65.892	T65.893	T65.894	—	—
borate						
cleanser	T57.8X1	T57.8X2	T57.8X3	T57.8X4	—	—
eye	T49.5X1	T49.5X2	T49.5X3	T49.5X4	T49.5X5	T49.5X6
therapeutic	T49.8X1	T49.8X2	T49.8X3	T49.8X4	T49.8X5	T49.8X6
bromide	T42.6X1	T42.6X2	T42.6X3	T42.6X4	T42.6X5	T42.6X6
cacodylate (nonmedicinal) NEC	T50.8X1	T50.8X2	T50.8X3	T50.8X4	T50.8X5	T50.8X6
anti-infective	T37.8X1	T37.8X2	T37.8X3	T37.8X4	T37.8X5	T37.8X6
herbicide	T60.3X1	T60.3X2	T60.3X3	T60.3X4	—	—
calcium edetate	T45.8X1	T45.8X2	T45.8X3	T45.8X4	T45.8X5	T45.8X6
carbonate NEC	T54.3X1	T54.3X2	T54.3X3	T54.3X4	—	—
chlorate NEC	T65.891	T65.892	T65.893	T65.894	—	—
herbicide	T54.91	T54.92	T54.93	T54.94	—	—
chloride	T50.3X1	T50.3X2	T50.3X3	T50.3X4	T50.3X5	T50.3X6
with glucose	T50.3X1	T50.3X2	T50.3X3	T50.3X4	T50.3X5	T50.3X6
chromate	T65.891	T65.892	T65.893	T65.894	—	—
citrate	T50.991	T50.992	T50.993	T50.994	T50.995	T50.996
cromoglicate	T48.6X1	T48.6X2	T48.6X3	T48.6X4	T48.6X5	T48.6X6
cyanide	T65.0X1	T65.0X2	T65.0X3	T65.0X4	—	—
cyclamate	T50.3X1	T50.3X2	T50.3X3	T50.3X4	T50.3X5	T50.3X6
dehydrocholate	T45.8X1	T45.8X2	T45.8X3	T45.8X4	T45.8X5	T45.8X6
diatrizoate	T50.8X1	T50.8X2	T50.8X3	T50.8X4	T50.8X5	T50.8X6
dibunate	T48.4X1	T48.4X2	T48.4X3	T48.4X4	T48.4X5	T48.4X6
dioctyl sulfosuccinate	T47.4X1	T47.4X2	T47.4X3	T47.4X4	T47.4X5	T47.4X6
dipantoyl ferrate	T45.8X1	T45.8X2	T45.8X3	T45.8X4	T45.8X5	T45.8X6
edetate	T45.8X1	T45.8X2	T45.8X3	T45.8X4	T45.8X5	T45.8X6
ethacrynate	T50.1X1	T50.1X2	T50.1X3	T50.1X4	T50.1X5	T50.1X6
feredetate	T45.8X1	T45.8X2	T45.8X3	T45.8X4	T45.8X5	T45.8X6

◀ New   ◀▥ Revised   ~~deleted~~ Deleted

Substance	External Cause (T-Code)					
	Poisoning, Accidental (Unintentional)	Poisoning, Intentional Self-Harm	Poisoning, Assault	Poisoning, Undetermined	Adverse Effect	Underdosing
Sodium *(Continued)*						
Fluoride — *see Fluoride*						
fluoroacetate (dust) (pesticide)	T60.4X1	T60.4X2	T60.4X3	T60.4X4	—	—
free salt	T50.3X1	T50.3X2	T50.3X3	T50.3X4	T50.3X5	T50.3X6
fusidate	T36.8X1	T36.8X2	T36.8X3	T36.8X4	T36.8X5	T36.8X6
glucaldrate	T47.1X1	T47.1X2	T47.1X3	T47.1X4	T47.1X5	T47.1X6
glucosulfone	T37.1X1	T37.1X2	T37.1X3	T37.1X4	T37.1X5	T37.1X6
glutamate	T45.8X1	T45.8X2	T45.8X3	T45.8X4	T45.8X5	T45.8X6
hydrogen carbonate	T50.3X1	T50.3X2	T50.3X3	T50.3X4	T50.3X5	T50.3X6
hydroxide	T54.3X1	T54.3X2	T54.3X3	T54.3X4	—	—
hypochlorite (bleach) NEC	T54.3X1	T54.3X2	T54.3X3	T54.3X4	—	—
disinfectant	T54.3X1	T54.3X2	T54.3X3	T54.3X4	—	—
medicinal (anti-infective) (external)	T49.0X1	T49.0X2	T49.0X3	T49.0X4	T49.0X5	T49.0X6
vapor	T54.3X1	T54.3X2	T54.3X3	T54.3X4	—	—
hyposulfite	T49.0X1	T49.0X2	T49.0X3	T49.0X4	T49.0X5	T49.0X6
indigotin disulfonate	T50.8X1	T50.8X2	T50.8X3	T50.8X4	T50.8X5	T50.8X6
iodide	T50.991	T50.992	T50.993	T50.994	T50.995	T50.996
I-131	T50.8X1	T50.8X2	T50.8X3	T50.8X4	T50.8X5	T50.8X6
therapeutic	T38.2X1	T38.2X2	T38.2X3	T38.2X4	T38.2X5	T38.2X6
iodohippurate (131I)	T50.8X1	T50.8X2	T50.8X3	T50.8X4	T50.8X5	T50.8X6
iopodate	T50.8X1	T50.8X2	T50.8X3	T50.8X4	T50.8X5	T50.8X6
iothalamate	T50.8X1	T50.8X2	T50.8X3	T50.8X4	T50.8X5	T50.8X6
iron edetate	T45.4X1	T45.4X2	T45.4X3	T45.4X4	T45.4X5	T45.4X6
lactate (compound solution)	T45.8X1	T45.8X2	T45.8X3	T45.8X4	T45.8X5	T45.8X6
lauryl (sulfate)	T49.2X1	T49.2X2	T49.2X3	T49.2X4	T49.2X5	T49.2X6
(L)-triiodothyronine	T38.1X1	T38.1X2	T38.1X3	T38.1X4	T38.1X5	T38.1X6
magnesium citrate	T50.991	T50.992	T50.993	T50.994	T50.995	T50.996
mersalate	T50.2X1	T50.2X2	T50.2X3	T50.2X4	T50.2X5	T50.2X6
metasilicate	T65.891	T65.892	T65.893	T65.894	—	—
metrizoate	T50.8X1	T50.8X2	T50.8X3	T50.8X4	T50.8X5	T50.8X6
monofluoroacetate (pesticide)	T60.1X1	T60.1X2	T60.1X3	T60.1X4	—	—
morrhuate	T46.8X1	T46.8X2	T46.8X3	T46.8X4	T46.8X5	T46.8X6
nafcillin	T36.0X1	T36.0X2	T36.0X3	T36.0X4	T36.0X5	T36.0X6
nitrate (oxidizing agent)	T65.891	T65.892	T65.893	T65.894	—	—
nitrite	T50.6X1	T50.6X2	T50.6X3	T50.6X4	T50.6X5	T50.6X6
nitroferricyanide	T46.5X1	T46.5X2	T46.5X3	T46.5X4	T46.5X5	T46.5X6
nitroprusside	T46.5X1	T46.5X2	T46.5X3	T46.5X4	T46.5X5	T46.5X6
oxalate	T65.891	T65.892	T65.893	T65.894	—	—
oxide/peroxide	T65.891	T65.892	T65.893	T65.894	—	—
oxybate	T41.291	T41.292	T41.293	T41.294	T41.295	T41.296

Substance	External Cause (T-Code)					
	Poisoning, Accidental (Unintentional)	Poisoning, Intentional Self-Harm	Poisoning, Assault	Poisoning, Undetermined	Adverse Effect	Underdosing
Sodium (Continued)						
para-aminohippurate	T50.8X1	T50.8X2	T50.8X3	T50.8X4	T50.8X5	T50.8X6
perborate (nonmedicinal) NEC	T65.891	T65.892	T65.893	T65.894	—	—
medicinal	T49.0X1	T49.0X2	T49.0X3	T49.0X4	T49.0X5	T49.0X6
soap	T55.0X1	T55.0X2	T55.0X3	T55.0X4	—	
percarbonate — see Sodium, perborate						
pertechnetate Tc99m	T50.8X1	T50.8X2	T50.8X3	T50.8X4	T50.8X5	T50.8X6
phosphate						
cellulose	T45.8X1	T45.8X2	T45.8X3	T45.8X4	T45.8X5	T45.8X6
dibasic	T47.2X1	T47.2X2	T47.2X3	T47.2X4	T47.2X5	T47.2X6
monobasic	T47.2X1	T47.2X2	T47.2X3	T47.2X4	T47.2X5	T47.2X6
phytate	T50.6X1	T50.6X2	T50.6X3	T50.6X4	T50.6X5	T50.6X6
picosulfate	T47.2X1	T47.2X2	T47.2X3	T47.2X4	T47.2X5	T47.2X6
polyhydroxyaluminium monocarbonate	T47.1X1	T47.1X2	T47.1X3	T47.1X4	T47.1X5	T47.1X6
polystyrene sulfonate	T50.3X1	T50.3X2	T50.3X3	T50.3X4	T50.3X5	T50.3X6
propionate	T49.0X1	T49.0X2	T49.0X3	T49.0X4	T49.0X5	T49.0X6
propyl hydroxybenzoate	T50.991	T50.992	T50.993	T50.994	T50.995	T50.996
psylliate	T46.8X1	T46.8X2	T46.8X3	T46.8X4	T46.8X5	T46.8X6
removing resins	T50.3X1	T50.3X2	T50.3X3	T50.3X4	T50.3X5	T50.3X6
salicylate	T39.091	T39.092	T39.093	T39.094	T39.095	T39.096
salt NEC	T50.3X1	T50.3X2	T50.3X3	T50.3X4	T50.3X5	T50.3X6
selenate	T60.2X1	T60.2X2	T60.2X3	T60.2X4	—	—
stibogluconate	T37.3X1	T37.3X2	T37.3X3	T37.3X4	T37.3X5	T37.3X6
sulfate	T47.4X1	T47.4X2	T47.4X3	T47.4X4	T47.4X5	T47.4X6
sulfoxone	T37.1X1	T37.1X2	T37.1X3	T37.1X4	T37.1X5	T37.1X6
tetradecyl sulfate	T46.8X1	T46.8X2	T46.8X3	T46.8X4	T46.8X5	T46.8X6
thiopental	T41.1X1	T41.1X2	T41.1X3	T41.1X4	T41.1X5	T41.1X6
thiosalicylate	T39.091	T39.092	T39.093	T39.094	T39.095	T39.096
thiosulfate	T50.6X1	T50.6X2	T50.6X3	T50.6X4	T50.6X5	T50.6X6
tolbutamide	T38.3X1	T38.3X2	T38.3X3	T38.3X4	T38.3X5	T38.3X6
l-triiodothyronine	T38.1X1	T38.1X2	T38.1X3	T38.1X4	T38.1X5	T38.1X6
tyropanoate	T50.8X1	T50.8X2	T50.8X3	T50.8X4	T50.8X5	T50.8X6
valproate	T42.6X1	T42.6X2	T42.6X3	T42.6X4	T42.6X5	T42.6X6
versenate	T50.6X1	T50.6X2	T50.6X3	T50.6X4	T50.6X5	T50.6X6
Sodium-free salt	T50.901	T50.902	T50.903	T50.904	T50.905	T50.906
Sodium-removing resin	T50.3X1	T50.3X2	T50.3X3	T50.3X4	T50.3X5	T50.3X6
Soft soap	T55.0X1	T55.0X2	T55.0X3	T55.0X4	—	—
Solanine	T62.2X1	T62.2X2	T62.2X3	T62.2X4	—	—
berries	T62.1X1	T62.1X2	T62.1X3	T62.1X4	—	—

◀ New ◀◍ Revised ~~deleted~~ Deleted

Substance	External Cause (T-Code)					
	Poisoning, Accidental (Unintentional)	Poisoning, Intentional Self-Harm	Poisoning, Assault	Poisoning, Undetermined	Adverse Effect	Underdosing
Solanum dulcamara	T62.2X1	T62.2X2	T62.2X3	T62.2X4	—	—
berries	T62.1X1	T62.1X2	T62.1X3	T62.1X4	—	—
Solapsone	T37.1X1	T37.1X2	T37.1X3	T37.1X4	T37.1X5	T37.1X6
Solar lotion	T49.3X1	T49.3X2	T49.3X3	T49.3X4	T49.3X5	T49.3X6
Solasulfone	T37.1X1	T37.1X2	T37.1X3	T37.1X4	T37.1X5	T37.1X6
Soldering fluid	T65.891	T65.892	T65.893	T65.894	—	—
Solid substance	T65.91	T65.92	T65.93	T65.94	—	—
specified NEC	T65.891	T65.892	T65.893	T65.894	—	—
Solvent, industrial NEC	T52.91	T52.92	T52.93	T52.94	—	—
naphtha	T52.0X1	T52.0X2	T52.0X3	T52.0X4	—	—
petroleum	T52.0X1	T52.0X2	T52.0X3	T52.0X4	—	—
specified NEC	T52.8X1	T52.8X2	T52.8X3	T52.8X4	—	—
Soma	T42.8X1	T42.8X2	T42.8X3	T42.8X4	T42.8X5	T42.8X6
Somatorelin	T38.891	T38.892	T38.893	T38.894	T38.895	T38.896
Somatostatin	T38.991	T38.992	T38.993	T38.994	T38.995	T38.996
Somatotropin	T38.811	T38.812	T38.813	T38.814	T38.815	T38.816
Somatrem	T38.811	T38.812	T38.813	T38.814	T38.815	T38.816
Somatropin	T38.811	T38.812	T38.813	T38.814	T38.815	T38.816
Sominex	T45.0X1	T45.0X2	T45.0X3	T45.0X4	T45.0X5	T45.0X6
Somnos	T42.6X1	T42.6X2	T42.6X3	T42.6X4	T42.6X5	T42.6X6
Somonal	T42.3X1	T42.3X2	T42.3X3	T42.3X4	T42.3X5	T42.3X6
Soneryl	T42.3X1	T42.3X2	T42.3X3	T42.3X4	T42.3X5	T42.3X6
Soothing syrup	T50.901	T50.902	T50.903	T50.904	T50.905	T50.906
Sopor	T42.6X1	T42.6X2	T42.6X3	T42.6X4	T42.6X5	T42.6X6
Soporific	T42.71	T42.72	T42.73	T42.74	T42.75	T42.76
Soporific drug	T42.71	T42.72	T42.73	T42.74	T42.75	T42.76
specified type NEC	T42.6X1	T42.6X2	T42.6X3	T42.6X4	T42.6X5	T42.6X6
Sorbide nitrate	T46.3X1	T46.3X2	T46.3X3	T46.3X4	T46.3X5	T46.3X6
Sorbitol	T47.4X1	T47.4X2	T47.4X3	T47.4X4	T47.4X5	T47.4X6
Sotalol	T44.7X1	T44.7X2	T44.7X3	T44.7X4	T44.7X5	T44.7X6
Sotradecol	T46.8X1	T46.8X2	T46.8X3	T46.8X4	T46.8X5	T46.8X6
Soysterol	T46.6X1	T46.6X2	T46.6X3	T46.6X4	T46.6X5	T46.6X6
Spacoline	T44.3X1	T44.3X2	T44.3X3	T44.3X4	T44.3X5	T44.3X6
Spanish fly	T49.8X1	T49.8X2	T49.8X3	T49.8X4	T49.8X5	T49.8X6
Sparine	T43.3X1	T43.3X2	T43.3X3	T43.3X4	T43.3X5	T43.3X6
Sparteine	T48.0X1	T48.0X2	T48.0X3	T48.0X4	T48.0X5	T48.0X6
Spasmolytic						
anticholinergics	T44.3X1	T44.3X2	T44.3X3	T44.3X4	T44.3X5	T44.3X6
autonomic	T44.3X1	T44.3X2	T44.3X3	T44.3X4	T44.3X5	T44.3X6

TABLE OF DRUGS AND CHEMICALS

TABLE OF DRUGS AND CHEMICALS

Substance	Poisoning, Accidental (Unintentional)	Poisoning, Intentional Self-Harm	Poisoning, Assault	Poisoning, Undetermined	Adverse Effect	Underdosing
External Cause (T-Code)						
Spasmolytic *(Continued)*						
bronchial NEC	T48.6X1	T48.6X2	T48.6X3	T48.6X4	T48.6X5	T48.6X6
quaternary ammonium	T44.3X1	T44.3X2	T44.3X3	T44.3X4	T44.3X5	T44.3X6
skeletal muscle NEC	T48.1X1	T48.1X2	T48.1X3	T48.1X4	T48.1X5	T48.1X6
Spectinomycin	T36.5X1	T36.5X2	T36.5X3	T36.5X4	T36.5X5	T36.5X6
Speed	T43.621	T43.622	T43.623	T43.624	T43.625	T43.626
Spermicide	T49.8X1	T49.8X2	T49.8X3	T49.8X4	T49.8X5	T49.8X6
Spider (bite) (venom)	T63.391	T63.392	T63.393	T63.394	—	—
antivenin	T50.Z11	T50.Z12	T50.Z13	T50.Z14	T50.Z15	T50.Z16
Spigelia (root)	T37.4X1	T37.4X2	T37.4X3	T37.4X4	T37.4X5	T37.4X6
Spindle inactivator	T50.4X1	T50.4X2	T50.4X3	T50.4X4	T50.4X5	T50.4X6
Spiperone	T43.4X1	T43.4X2	T43.4X3	T43.4X4	T43.4X5	T43.4X6
Spiramycin	T36.3X1	T36.3X2	T36.3X3	T36.3X4	T36.3X5	T36.3X6
Spirapril	T46.4X1	T46.4X2	T46.4X3	T46.4X4	T46.4X5	T46.4X6
Spirilene	T43.591	T43.592	T43.593	T43.594	T43.595	T43.596
Spirit(s) (neutral) NEC	T51.0X1	T51.0X2	T51.0X3	T51.0X4	—	—
beverage	T51.0X1	T51.0X2	T51.0X3	T51.0X4	—	—
industrial	T51.0X1	T51.0X2	T51.0X3	T51.0X4	—	—
mineral	T52.0X1	T52.0X2	T52.0X3	T52.0X4	—	—
of salt — *see Hydrochloric acid*						
surgical	T51.0X1	T51.0X2	T51.0X3	T51.0X4	—	—
Spironolactone	T50.0X1	T50.0X2	T50.0X3	T50.0X4	T50.0X5	T50.0X6
Spiroperidol	T43.4X1	T43.4X2	T43.4X3	T43.4X4	T43.4X5	T43.4X6
Sponge, absorbable (gelatin)	T45.7X1	T45.7X2	T45.7X3	T45.7X4	T45.7X5	T45.7X6
Sporostacin	T49.0X1	T49.0X2	T49.0X3	T49.0X4	T49.0X5	T49.0X6
Spray (aerosol)	T65.91	T65.92	T65.93	T65.94	—	—
cosmetic	T65.891	T65.892	T65.893	T65.894	—	—
medicinal NEC	T50.901	T50.902	T50.903	T50.904	T50.905	T50.906
pesticides — *see Pesticides*						
specified content — *see specific substance*						
Spurge flax	T62.2X1	T62.2X2	T62.2X3	T62.2X4	—	—
Spurges	T62.2X1	T62.2X2	T62.2X3	T62.2X4	—	—
Sputum viscosity-lowering drug	T48.4X1	T48.4X2	T48.4X3	T48.4X4	T48.4X5	T48.4X6
Squill	T46.0X1	T46.0X2	T46.0X3	T46.0X4	T46.0X5	T46.0X6
rat poison	T60.4X1	T60.4X2	T60.4X3	T60.4X4	—	—
Squirting cucumber (cathartic)	T47.2X1	T47.2X2	T47.2X3	T47.2X4	T47.2X5	T47.2X6
Stains	T65.6X1	T65.6X2	T65.6X3	T65.6X4	—	—
Stannous fluoride	T49.7X1	T49.7X2	T49.7X3	T49.7X4	T49.7X5	T49.7X6
Stanolone	T38.7X1	T38.7X2	T38.7X3	T38.7X4	T38.7X5	T38.7X6
Stanozolol	T38.7X1	T38.7X2	T38.7X3	T38.7X4	T38.7X5	T38.7X6

◄ New   ◄◄ Revised   ~~deleted~~ Deleted

Substance	External Cause (T-Code)					
	Poisoning, Accidental (Unintentional)	Poisoning, Intentional Self-Harm	Poisoning, Assault	Poisoning, Undetermined	Adverse Effect	Underdosing
Staphisagria or stavesacre (pediculicide)	T49.0X1	T49.0X2	T49.0X3	T49.0X4	T49.0X5	T49.0X6
Starch	T50.901	T50.902	T50.903	T50.904	T50.905	T50.906
Stelazine	T43.3X1	T43.3X2	I43.3X3	T43.3X4	T43.3X5	T43.3X6
Stemetil	T43.3X1	T43.3X2	T43.3X3	T43.3X4	T43.3X5	T43.3X6
Stepronin	T48.4X1	T48.4X2	T48.4X3	T48.4X4	T48.4X5	T48.4X6
Sterculia	T47.4X1	T47.4X2	T47.4X3	T47.4X4	T47.4X5	T47.4X6
Sternutator gas	T59.891	T59.892	T59.893	T59.894	—	—
Steroid	T38.0X1	T38.0X2	T38.0X3	T38.0X4	T38.0X5	T38.0X6
anabolic	T38.7X1	T38.7X2	T38.7X3	T38.7X4	T38.7X5	T38.7X6
androgenic	T38.7X1	T38.7X2	T38.7X3	T38.7X4	T38.7X5	T38.7X6
antineoplastic, hormone	T38.7X1	T38.7X2	T38.7X3	T38.7X4	T38.7X5	T38.7X6
estrogen	T38.5X1	T38.5X2	T38.5X3	T38.5X4	T38.5X5	T38.5X6
ENT agent	T49.6X1	T49.6X2	T49.6X3	T49.6X4	T49.6X5	T49.6X6
ophthalmic preparation	T49.5X1	T49.5X2	T49.5X3	T49.5X4	T49.5X5	T49.5X6
topical NEC	T49.0X1	T49.0X2	T49.0X3	T49.0X4	T49.0X5	T49.0X6
Stibine	T56.891	T56.892	T56.893	T56.894	—	—
Stibogluconate	T37.3X1	T37.3X2	T37.3X3	T37.3X4	T37.3X5	T37.3X6
Stibophen	T37.4X1	T37.4X2	T37.4X3	T37.4X4	T37.4X5	T37.4X6
Stilbamidine (isetionate)	T37.3X1	T37.3X2	T37.3X3	T37.3X4	T37.3X5	T37.3X6
Stilbestrol	T38.5X1	T38.5X2	T38.5X3	T38.5X4	T38.5X5	T38.5X6
Stilboestrol	T38.5X1	T38.5X2	T38.5X3	T38.5X4	T38.5X5	T38.5X6
Stimulant						
central nervous system — *see also Psychostimulant*	T43.601	T43.602	T43.603	T43.604	T43.605	T43.606
analeptics	T50.7X1	T50.7X2	T50.7X3	T50.7X4	T50.7X5	T50.7X6
opiate antagonist	T50.7X1	T50.7X2	T50.7X3	T50.7X4	T50.7X5	T50.7X6
psychotherapeutic NEC — *see also Psychotherapeutic drug*	T43.601	T43.602	T43.603	T43.604	T43.605	T43.606
specified NEC	T43.691	T43.692	T43.693	T43.694	T43.695	T43.696
respiratory	T48.901	T48.902	T48.903	T48.904	T48.905	T48.906
Stone-dissolving drug	T50.901	T50.902	T50.903	T50.904	T50.905	T50.906
Storage battery (cells) (acid)	T54.2X1	T54.2X2	T54.2X3	T54.2X4	—	—
Stovaine	T41.3X1	T41.3X2	T41.3X3	T41.3X4	T41.3X5	T41.3X6
infiltration (subcutaneous)	T41.3X1	T41.3X2	T41.3X3	T41.3X4	T41.3X5	T41.3X6
nerve block (peripheral) (plexus)	T41.3X1	T41.3X2	T41.3X3	T41.3X4	T41.3X5	T41.3X6
spinal	T41.3X1	T41.3X2	T41.3X3	T41.3X4	T41.3X5	T41.3X6
topical (surface)	T41.3X1	T41.3X2	T41.3X3	T41.3X4	T41.3X5	T41.3X6
Stovarsal	T37.8X1	T37.8X2	T37.8X3	T37.8X4	T37.8X5	T37.8X6
Stove gas — *see Gas, stove*	T57.91	T57.92	T57.93	T57.94	—	—
Stoxil	T49.5X1	T49.5X2	T49.5X3	T49.5X4	T49.5X5	T49.5X6
Stramonium	T48.6X1	T48.6X2	T48.6X3	T48.6X4	T48.6X5	T48.6X6
natural state	T62.2X1	T62.2X2	T62.2X3	T62.2X4	—	—

◀ New ◀▥ Revised ~~deleted~~ Deleted

TABLE OF DRUGS AND CHEMICALS

TABLE OF DRUGS AND CHEMICALS

Substance	External Cause (T-Code)					
	Poisoning, Accidental (Unintentional)	Poisoning, Intentional Self-Harm	Poisoning, Assault	Poisoning, Undetermined	Adverse Effect	Underdosing
Streptodornase	T45.3X1	T45.3X2	T45.3X3	T45.3X4	T45.3X5	T45.3X6
Streptoduocin	T36.5X1	T36.5X2	T36.5X3	T36.5X4	T36.5X5	T36.5X6
Streptokinase	T45.611	T45.612	T45.613	T45.614	T45.615	T45.616
Streptomycin (derivative)	T36.5X1	T36.5X2	T36.5X3	T36.5X4	T36.5X5	T36.5X6
Streptonivicin	T36.5X1	T36.5X2	T36.5X3	T36.5X4	T36.5X5	T36.5X6
Streptovarycin	T36.5X1	T36.5X2	T36.5X3	T36.5X4	T36.5X5	T36.5X6
Streptozocin	T45.1X1	T45.1X2	T45.1X3	T45.1X4	T45.1X5	T45.1X6
Streptozotocin	T45.1X1	T45.1X2	T45.1X3	T45.1X4	T45.1X5	T45.1X6
Stripper (paint) (solvent)	T52.8X1	T52.8X2	T52.8X3	T52.8X4	—	—
Strobane	T60.1X1	T60.1X2	T60.1X3	T60.1X4	—	—
Strofantina	T46.0X1	T46.0X2	T46.0X3	T46.0X4	T46.0X5	T46.0X6
Strophanthin (g) (k)	T46.0X1	T46.0X2	T46.0X3	T46.0X4	T46.0X5	T46.0X6
Strophanthus	T46.0X1	T46.0X2	T46.0X3	T46.0X4	T46.0X5	T46.0X6
Strophantin	T46.0X1	T46.0X2	T46.0X3	T46.0X4	T46.0X5	T46.0X6
Strophantin-g	T46.0X1	T46.0X2	T46.0X3	T46.0X4	T46.0X5	T46.0X6
Strychnine (nonmedicinal) (pesticide) (salts)	T65.1X1	T65.1X2	T65.1X3	T65.1X4	—	—
medicinal	T48.291	T48.292	T48.293	T48.294	T48.295	T48.296
Strychnos (ignatii) — see Strychnine						
Styramate	T42.8X1	T42.8X2	T42.8X3	T42.8X4	T42.8X5	T42.8X6
Styrene	T65.891	T65.892	T65.893	T65.894	—	—
Succinimide, antiepileptic or anticonvulsant	T42.2X1	T42.2X2	T42.2X3	T42.2X4	T42.2X5	T42.2X6
mercuric — see Mercury						
Succinylcholine	T48.1X1	T48.1X2	T48.1X3	T48.1X4	T48.1X5	T48.1X6
Succinylsulfathiazole	T37.0X1	T37.0X2	T37.0X3	T37.0X4	T37.0X5	T37.0X6
Sucralfate	T47.1X1	T47.1X2	T47.1X3	T47.1X4	T47.1X5	T47.1X6
Sucrose	T50.3X1	T50.3X2	T50.3X3	T50.3X4	T50.3X5	T50.3X6
Sufentanil	T40.4X1	T40.4X2	T40.4X3	T40.4X4	T40.4X5	T40.4X6
Sulbactam	T36.0X1	T36.0X2	T36.0X3	T36.0X4	T36.0X5	T36.0X6
Sulbenicillin	T36.0X1	T36.0X2	T36.0X3	T36.0X4	T36.0X5	T36.0X6
Sulbentine	T49.0X1	T49.0X2	T49.0X3	T49.0X4	T49.0X5	T49.0X6
Sulfacetamide	T49.0X1	T49.0X2	T49.0X3	T49.0X4	T49.0X5	T49.0X6
ophthalmic preparation	T49.5X1	T49.5X2	T49.5X3	T49.5X4	T49.5X5	T49.5X6
Sulfachlorpyridazine	T37.0X1	T37.0X2	T37.0X3	T37.0X4	T37.0X5	T37.0X6
Sulfacitine	T37.0X1	T37.0X2	T37.0X3	T37.0X4	T37.0X5	T37.0X6
Sulfadiasulfone sodium	T37.0X1	T37.0X2	T37.0X3	T37.0X4	T37.0X5	T37.0X6
Sulfadiazine	T37.0X1	T37.0X2	T37.0X3	T37.0X4	T37.0X5	T37.0X6
silver (topical)	T49.0X1	T49.0X2	T49.0X3	T49.0X4	T49.0X5	T49.0X6
Sulfadimethoxine	T37.0X1	T37.0X2	T37.0X3	T37.0X4	T37.0X5	T37.0X6
Sulfadimidine	T37.0X1	T37.0X2	T37.0X3	T37.0X4	T37.0X5	T37.0X6

◀ New ◀ Revised ~~deleted~~ Deleted

Substance	External Cause (T-Code)					
	Poisoning, Accidental (Unintentional)	Poisoning, Intentional Self-Harm	Poisoning, Assault	Poisoning, Undetermined	Adverse Effect	Underdosing
Sulfadoxine	T37.0X1	T37.0X2	T37.0X3	T37.0X4	T37.0X5	T37.0X6
with pyrimethamine	T37.2X1	T37.2X2	T37.2X3	T37.2X4	T37.2X5	T37.2X6
Sulfaethidole	T37.0X1	T37.0X2	T37.0X3	T37.0X4	T37.0X5	T37.0X6
Sulfafurazole	T37.0X1	T37.0X2	T37.0X3	T37.0X4	T37.0X5	T37.0X6
Sulfaguanidine	T37.0X1	T37.0X2	T37.0X3	T37.0X4	T37.0X5	T37.0X6
Sulfalene	T37.0X1	T37.0X2	T37.0X3	T37.0X4	T37.0X5	T37.0X6
Sulfaloxate	T37.0X1	T37.0X2	T37.0X3	T37.0X4	T37.0X5	T37.0X6
Sulfaloxic acid	T37.0X1	T37.0X2	T37.0X3	T37.0X4	T37.0X5	T37.0X6
Sulfamazone	T39.2X1	T39.2X2	T39.2X3	T39.2X4	T39.2X5	T39.2X6
Sulfamerazine	T37.0X1	T37.0X2	T37.0X3	T37.0X4	T37.0X5	T37.0X6
Sulfameter	T37.0X1	T37.0X2	T37.0X3	T37.0X4	T37.0X5	T37.0X6
Sulfamethazine	T37.0X1	T37.0X2	T37.0X3	T37.0X4	T37.0X5	T37.0X6
Sulfamethizole	T37.0X1	T37.0X2	T37.0X3	T37.0X4	T37.0X5	T37.0X6
Sulfamethoxazole	T37.0X1	T37.0X2	T37.0X3	T37.0X4	T37.0X5	T37.0X6
with trimethoprim	T36.8X1	T36.8X2	T36.8X3	T36.8X4	T36.8X5	T36.8X6
Sulfamethoxydiazine	T37.0X1	T37.0X2	T37.0X3	T37.0X4	T37.0X5	T37.0X6
Sulfamethoxypyridazine	T37.0X1	T37.0X2	T37.0X3	T37.0X4	T37.0X5	T37.0X6
Sulfamethylthiazole	T37.0X1	T37.0X2	T37.0X3	T37.0X4	T37.0X5	T37.0X6
Sulfametoxydiazine	T37.0X1	T37.0X2	T37.0X3	T37.0X4	T37.0X5	T37.0X6
Sulfamidopyrine	T39.2X1	T39.2X2	T39.2X3	T39.2X4	T39.2X5	T39.2X6
Sulfamonomethoxine	T37.0X1	T37.0X2	T37.0X3	T37.0X4	T37.0X5	T37.0X6
Sulfamoxole	T37.0X1	T37.0X2	T37.0X3	T37.0X4	T37.0X5	T37.0X6
Sulfamylon	T49.0X1	T49.0X2	T49.0X3	T49.0X4	T49.0X5	T49.0X6
Sulfan blue (diagnostic dye)	T50.8X1	T50.8X2	T50.8X3	T50.8X4	T50.8X5	T50.8X6
Sulfanilamide	T37.0X1	T37.0X2	T37.0X3	T37.0X4	T37.0X5	T37.0X6
Sulfanilylguanidine	T37.0X1	T37.0X2	T37.0X3	T37.0X4	T37.0X5	T37.0X6
Sulfaperin	T37.0X1	T37.0X2	T37.0X3	T37.0X4	T37.0X5	T37.0X6
Sulfaphenazole	T37.0X1	T37.0X2	T37.0X3	T37.0X4	T37.0X5	T37.0X6
Sulfaphenylthiazole	T37.0X1	T37.0X2	T37.0X3	T37.0X4	T37.0X5	T37.0X6
Sulfaproxyline	T37.0X1	T37.0X2	T37.0X3	T37.0X4	T37.0X5	T37.0X6
Sulfapyridine	T37.0X1	T37.0X2	T37.0X3	T37.0X4	T37.0X5	T37.0X6
Sulfapyrimidine	T37.0X1	T37.0X2	T37.0X3	T37.0X4	T37.0X5	T37.0X6
Sulfarsphenamine	T37.8X1	T37.8X2	T37.8X3	T37.8X4	T37.8X5	T37.8X6
Sulfasalazine	T37.0X1	T37.0X2	T37.0X3	T37.0X4	T37.0X5	T37.0X6
Sulfasuxidine	T37.0X1	T37.0X2	T37.0X3	T37.0X4	T37.0X5	T37.0X6
Sulfasymazine	T37.0X1	T37.0X2	T37.0X3	T37.0X4	T37.0X5	T37.0X6
Sulfated amylopectin	T47.8X1	T47.8X2	T47.8X3	T47.8X4	T47.8X5	T47.8X6
Sulfathiazole	T37.0X1	T37.0X2	T37.0X3	T37.0X4	T37.0X5	T37.0X6
Sulfatostearate	T49.2X1	T49.2X2	T49.2X3	T49.2X4	T49.2X5	T49.2X6

◀ New   ◀▥ Revised   ~~deleted~~ Deleted

TABLE OF DRUGS AND CHEMICALS

Substance	External Cause (T-Code)					
	Poisoning, Accidental (Unintentional)	Poisoning, Intentional Self-Harm	Poisoning, Assault	Poisoning, Undetermined	Adverse Effect	Underdosing
Sulfinpyrazone	T50.4X1	T50.4X2	T50.4X3	T50.4X4	T50.4X5	T50.4X6
Sulfiram	T49.0X1	T49.0X2	T49.0X3	T49.0X4	T49.0X5	T49.0X6
Sulfisomidine	T37.0X1	T37.0X2	T37.0X3	T37.0X4	T37.0X5	T37.0X6
Sulfisoxazole	T37.0X1	T37.0X2	T37.0X3	T37.0X4	T37.0X5	T37.0X6
ophthalmic preparation	T49.5X1	T49.5X2	T49.5X3	T49.5X4	T49.5X5	T49.5X6
Sulfobromophthalein (sodium)	T50.8X1	T50.8X2	T50.8X3	T50.8X4	T50.8X5	T50.8X6
Sulfobromphthalein	T50.8X1	T50.8X2	T50.8X3	T50.8X4	T50.8X5	T50.8X6
Sulfogaiacol	T48.4X1	T48.4X2	T48.4X3	T48.4X4	T48.4X5	T48.4X6
Sulfomyxin	T36.8X1	T36.8X2	T36.8X3	T36.8X4	T36.8X5	T36.8X6
Sulfonal	T42.6X1	T42.6X2	T42.6X3	T42.6X4	T42.6X5	T42.6X6
Sulfonamide NEC	T37.0X1	T37.0X2	T37.0X3	T37.0X4	T37.0X5	T37.0X6
eye	T49.5X1	T49.5X2	T49.5X3	T49.5X4	T49.5X5	T49.5X6
Sulfonazide	T37.1X1	T37.1X2	T37.1X3	T37.1X4	T37.1X5	T37.1X6
Sulfones	T37.1X1	T37.1X2	T37.1X3	T37.1X4	T37.1X5	T37.1X6
Sulfonethylmethane	T42.6X1	T42.6X2	T42.6X3	T42.6X4	T42.6X5	T42.6X6
Sulfonmethane	T42.6X1	T42.6X2	T42.6X3	T42.6X4	T42.6X5	T42.6X6
Sulfonphthal, sulfonphthol	T50.8X1	T50.8X2	T50.8X3	T50.8X4	T50.8X5	T50.8X6
Sulfonylurea derivatives, oral	T38.3X1	T38.3X2	T38.3X3	T38.3X4	T38.3X5	T38.3X6
Sulforidazine	T43.3X1	T43.3X2	T43.3X3	T43.3X4	T43.3X5	T43.3X6
Sulfoxone	T37.1X1	T37.1X2	T37.1X3	T37.1X4	T37.1X5	T37.1X6
Sulfur, sulfurated, sulfuric, sulfurous, sulfuryl (compounds NEC) (medicinal)	T49.4X1	T49.4X2	T49.4X3	T49.4X4	T49.4X5	T49.4X6
acid	T54.2X1	T54.2X2	T54.2X3	T54.2X4	—	—
dioxide (gas)	T59.1X1	T59.1X2	T59.1X3	T59.1X4	—	—
ether — see Ether(s)						
hydrogen	T59.6X1	T59.6X2	T59.6X3	T59.6X4	—	—
medicinal (keratolytic) (ointment) NEC	T49.4X1	T49.4X2	T49.4X3	T49.4X4	T49.4X5	T49.4X6
ointment	T49.0X1	T49.0X2	T49.0X3	T49.0X4	T49.0X5	T49.0X6
pesticide (vapor)	T60.91	T60.92	T60.93	T60.94	—	—
vapor NEC	T59.891	T59.892	T59.893	T59.894	—	—
Sulfuric acid	T54.2X1	T54.2X2	T54.2X3	T54.2X4	—	—
Sulglicotide	T47.1X1	T47.1X2	T47.1X3	T47.1X4	T47.1X5	T47.1X6
Sulindac	T39.391	T39.392	T39.393	T39.394	T39.395	T39.396
Sulisatin	T47.2X1	T47.2X2	T47.2X3	T47.2X4	T47.2X5	T47.2X6
Sulisobenzone	T49.3X1	T49.3X2	T49.3X3	T49.3X4	T49.3X5	T49.3X6
Sulkowitch's reagent	T50.8X1	T50.8X2	T50.8X3	T50.8X4	T50.8X5	T50.8X6
Sulmetozine	T44.3X1	T44.3X2	T44.3X3	T44.3X4	T44.3X5	T44.3X6
Suloctidil	T46.7X1	T46.7X2	T46.7X3	T46.7X4	T46.7X5	T46.7X6
Sulph — see also Sulf-						
Sulphadiazine	T37.0X1	T37.0X2	T37.0X3	T37.0X4	T37.0X5	T37.0X6
Sulphadimethoxine	T37.0X1	T37.0X2	T37.0X3	T37.0X4	T37.0X5	T37.0X6

◀ New   ◀═ Revised   ~~deleted~~ Deleted

Substance	External Cause (T-Code)					
	Poisoning, Accidental (Unintentional)	Poisoning, Intentional Self-Harm	Poisoning, Assault	Poisoning, Undetermined	Adverse Effect	Underdosing
Sulphadimidine	T37.0X1	T37.0X2	T37.0X3	T37.0X4	T37.0X5	T37.0X6
Sulphadione	T37.1X1	T37.1X2	T37.1X3	T37.1X4	T37.1X5	T37.1X6
Sulphafurazole	T37.0X1	T37.0X2	T37.0X3	T37.0X4	T37.0X5	T37.0X6
Sulphamethizole	T37.0X1	T37.0X2	T37.0X3	T37.0X4	T37.0X5	T37.0X6
Sulphamethoxazole	T37.0X1	T37.0X2	T37.0X3	T37.0X4	T37.0X5	T37.0X6
Sulphan blue	T50.8X1	T50.8X2	T50.8X3	T50.8X4	T50.8X5	T50.8X6
Sulphaphenazole	T37.0X1	T37.0X2	T37.0X3	T37.0X4	T37.0X5	T37.0X6
Sulphapyridine	T37.0X1	T37.0X2	T37.0X3	T37.0X4	T37.0X5	T37.0X6
Sulphasalazine	T37.0X1	T37.0X2	T37.0X3	T37.0X4	T37.0X5	T37.0X6
Sulphinpyrazone	T50.4X1	T50.4X2	T50.4X3	T50.4X4	T50.4X5	T50.4X6
Sulpiride	T43.591	T43.592	T43.593	T43.594	T43.595	T43.596
Sulprostone	T48.0X1	T48.0X2	T48.0X3	T48.0X4	T48.0X5	T48.0X6
Sulpyrine	T39.2X1	T39.2X2	T39.2X3	T39.2X4	T39.2X5	T39.2X6
Sultamicillin	T36.0X1	T36.0X2	T36.0X3	T36.0X4	T36.0X5	T36.0X6
Sulthiame	T42.6X1	T42.6X2	T42.6X3	T42.6X4	T42.6X5	T42.6X6
Sultiame	T42.6X1	T42.6X2	T42.6X3	T42.6X4	T42.6X5	T42.6X6
Sultopride	T43.591	T43.592	T43.593	T43.594	T43.595	T43.596
Sumatriptan	T39.8X1	T39.8X2	T39.8X3	T39.8X4	T39.8X5	T39.8X6
Sunflower seed oil	T46.6X1	T46.6X2	T46.6X3	T46.6X4	T46.6X5	T46.6X6
Superinone	T48.4X1	T48.4X2	T48.4X3	T48.4X4	T48.4X5	T48.4X6
Suprofen	T39.311	T39.312	T39.313	T39.314	T39.315	T39.316
Suramin (sodium)	T37.4X1	T37.4X2	T37.4X3	T37.4X4	T37.4X5	T37.4X6
Surfacaine	T41.3X1	T41.3X2	T41.3X3	T41.3X4	T41.3X5	T41.3X6
Surital	T41.1X1	T41.1X2	T41.1X3	T41.1X4	T41.1X5	T41.1X6
Sutilains	T45.3X1	T45.3X2	T45.3X3	T45.3X4	T45.3X5	T45.3X6
Suxamethonium (chloride)	T48.1X1	T48.1X2	T48.1X3	T48.1X4	T48.1X5	T48.1X6
Suxethonium (chloride)	T48.1X1	T48.1X2	T48.1X3	T48.1X4	T48.1X5	T48.1X6
Suxibuzone	T39.2X1	T39.2X2	T39.2X3	T39.2X4	T39.2X5	T39.2X6
Sweet oil (birch)	T49.3X1	T49.3X2	T49.3X3	T49.3X4	T49.3X5	T49.3X6
Sweet niter spirit	T46.3X1	T46.3X2	T46.3X3	T46.3X4	T46.3X5	T46.3X6
Sweetener	T50.901	T50.902	T50.903	T50.904	T50.905	T50.906
Sym-dichloroethyl ether	T53.6X1	T53.6X2	T53.6X3	T53.6X4	—	—
Sympatholytic NEC	T44.8X1	T44.8X2	T44.8X3	T44.8X4	T44.8X5	T44.8X6
haloalkylamine	T44.8X1	T44.8X2	T44.8X3	T44.8X4	T44.8X5	T44.8X6
Sympathomimetic NEC	T44.901	T44.902	T44.903	T44.904	T44.905	T44.906
anti-common-cold	T48.5X1	T48.5X2	T48.5X3	T48.5X4	T48.5X5	T48.5X6
bronchodilator	T48.6X1	T48.6X2	T48.6X3	T48.6X4	T48.6X5	T48.6X6
specified NEC	T44.991	T44.992	T44.993	T44.994	T44.995	T44.996
Synagis	T50.B91	T50.B92	T50.B93	T50.B94	T50.B95	T50.B96
Synalar	T49.0X1	T49.0X2	T49.0X3	T49.0X4	T49.0X5	T49.0X6

TABLE OF DRUGS AND CHEMICALS

	External Cause (T-Code)					
Substance	Poisoning, Accidental (Unintentional)	Poisoning, Intentional Self-Harm	Poisoning, Assault	Poisoning, Undetermined	Adverse Effect	Underdosing
Synthroid	T38.1X1	T38.1X2	T38.1X3	T38.1X4	T38.1X5	T38.1X6
Syntocinon	T48.0X1	T48.0X2	T48.0X3	T48.0X4	T48.0X5	T48.0X6
Syrosingopine	T46.5X1	T46.5X2	T46.5X3	T46.5X4	T46.5X5	T46.5X6
Systemic drug	T45.91	T45.92	T45.93	T45.94	T45.95	T45.96
specified NEC	T45.8X1	T45.8X2	T45.8X3	T45.8X4	T45.8X5	T45.8X6
2,4,5-T	T60.3X1	T60.3X2	T60.3X3	T60.3X4	—	—
T						
Tablets — see also specified substance	T50.901	T50.902	T50.903	T50.904	T50.905	T50.906
Tace	T38.5X1	T38.5X2	T38.5X3	T38.5X4	T38.5X5	T38.5X6
Tacrine	T44.0X1	T44.0X2	T44.0X3	T44.0X4	T44.0X5	T44.0X6
Tadalafil	T46.7X1	T46.7X2	T46.7X3	T46.7X4	T46.7X5	T46.7X6
Talampicillin	T36.0X1	T36.0X2	T36.0X3	T36.0X4	T36.0X5	T36.0X6
Talbutal	T42.3X1	T42.3X2	T42.3X3	T42.3X4	T42.3X5	T42.3X6
Talc powder	T49.3X1	T49.3X2	T49.3X3	T49.3X4	T49.3X5	T49.3X6
Talcum	T49.3X1	T49.3X2	T49.3X3	T49.3X4	T49.3X5	T49.3X6
Taleranol	T38.6X1	T38.6X2	T38.6X3	T38.6X4	T38.6X5	T38.6X6
Tamoxifen	T38.6X1	T38.6X2	T38.6X3	T38.6X4	T38.6X5	T38.6X6
Tamsulosin	T44.6X1	T44.6X2	T44.6X3	T44.6X4	T44.6X5	T44.6X6
Tandearil, tanderil	T39.2X1	T39.2X2	T39.2X3	T39.2X4	T39.2X5	T39.2X6
Tannic acid	T49.2X1	T49.2X2	T49.2X3	T49.2X4	T49.2X5	T49.2X6
medicinal (astringent)	T49.2X1	T49.2X2	T49.2X3	T49.2X4	T49.2X5	T49.2X6
Tannin — see Tannic acid						
Tansy	T62.2X1	T62.2X2	T62.2X3	T62.2X4	—	—
TAO	T36.3X1	T36.3X2	T36.3X3	T36.3X4	T36.3X5	T36.3X6
Tapazole	T38.2X1	T38.2X2	T38.2X3	T38.2X4	T38.2X5	T38.2X6
Tar NEC	T52.0X1	T52.0X2	T52.0X3	T52.0X4	—	—
camphor	T60.1X1	T60.1X2	T60.1X3	T60.1X4	—	—
distillate	T49.1X1	T49.1X2	T49.1X3	T49.1X4	T49.1X5	T49.1X6
fumes	T59.891	T59.892	T59.893	T59.894	—	—
medicinal	T49.1X1	T49.1X2	T49.1X3	T49.1X4	T49.1X5	T49.1X6
ointment	T49.1X1	T49.1X2	T49.1X3	T49.1X4	T49.1X5	T49.1X6
Taractan	T43.591	T43.592	T43.593	T43.594	T43.595	T43.596
Tarantula (venomous)	T63.321	T63.322	T63.323	T63.324	—	—
Tartar emetic	T37.8X1	T37.8X2	T37.8X3	T37.8X4	T37.8X5	T37.8X6
Tartaric acid	T65.891	T65.892	T65.893	T65.894	—	—
Tartrated antimony (anti-infective)	T37.8X1	T37.8X2	T37.8X3	T37.8X4	T37.8X5	T37.8X6
Tartrate, laxative	T47.4X1	T47.4X2	T47.4X3	T47.4X4	T47.4X5	T47.4X6
Tauromustine	T45.1X1	T45.1X2	T45.1X3	T45.1X4	T45.1X5	T45.1X6
TCA — see Trichloroacetic acid						

◄ New ◄ Revised ~~deleted~~ Deleted

Substance	External Cause (T-Code)					
	Poisoning, Accidental (Unintentional)	Poisoning, Intentional Self-Harm	Poisoning, Assault	Poisoning, Undetermined	Adverse Effect	Underdosing
TCDD	T53.7X1	T53.7X2	T53.7X3	T53.7X4	—	—
TDI (vapor)	T65.0X1	T65.0X2	T65.0X3	T65.0X4	—	—
Tear						
gas	T59.3X1	T59.3X2	T59.3X3	T59.3X4	—	—
solution	T49.5X1	T49.5X2	T49.5X3	T49.5X4	T49.5X5	T49.5X6
Teclothiazide	T50.2X1	T50.2X2	T50.2X3	T50.2X4	T50.2X5	T50.2X6
Teclozan	T37.3X1	T37.3X2	T37.3X3	T37.3X4	T37.3X5	T37.3X6
Tegafur	T45.1X1	T45.1X2	T45.1X3	T45.1X4	T45.1X5	T45.1X6
Tegretol	T42.1X1	T42.1X2	T42.1X3	T42.1X4	T42.1X5	T42.1X6
Teicoplanin	T36.8X1	T36.8X2	T36.8X3	T36.8X4	T36.8X5	T36.8X6
Telepaque	T50.8X1	T50.8X2	T50.8X3	T50.8X4	T50.8X5	T50.8X6
Tellurium	T56.891	T56.892	T56.893	T56.894	—	—
fumes	T56.891	T56.892	T56.893	T56.894	—	—
TEM	T45.1X1	T45.1X2	T45.1X3	T45.1X4	T45.1X5	T45.1X6
Temazepam	T42.4X1	T42.4X2	T42.4X3	T42.4X4	T42.4X5	T42.4X6
Temocillin	T36.0X1	T36.0X2	T36.0X3	T36.0X4	T36.0X5	T36.0X6
Tenamfetamine	T43.621	T43.622	T43.623	T43.624	T43.625	T43.626
Teniposide	T45.1X1	T45.1X2	T45.1X3	T45.1X4	T45.1X5	T45.1X6
Tenitramine	T46.3X1	T46.3X2	T46.3X3	T46.3X4	T46.3X5	T46.3X6
Tenoglicin	T48.4X1	T48.4X2	T48.4X3	T48.4X4	T48.4X5	T48.4X6
Tenonitrozole	T37.3X1	T37.3X2	T37.3X3	T37.3X4	T37.3X5	T37.3X6
Tenoxicam	T39.391	T39.392	T39.393	T39.394	T39.395	T39.396
TEPA	T45.1X1	T45.1X2	T45.1X3	T45.1X4	T45.1X5	T45.1X6
TEPP	T60.0X1	T60.0X2	T60.0X3	T60.0X4	—	—
Teprotide	T46.5X1	T46.5X2	T46.5X3	T46.5X4	T46.5X5	T46.5X6
Terazosin	T44.6X1	T44.6X2	T44.6X3	T44.6X4	T44.6X5	T44.6X6
Terbufos	T60.0X1	T60.0X2	T60.0X3	T60.0X4	—	—
Terbutaline	T48.6X1	T48.6X2	T48.6X3	T48.6X4	T48.6X5	T48.6X6
Terconazole	T49.0X1	T49.0X2	T49.0X3	T49.0X4	T49.0X5	T49.0X6
Terfenadine	T45.0X1	T45.0X2	T45.0X3	T45.0X4	T45.0X5	T45.0X6
Teriparatide (acetate)	T50.991	T50.992	T50.993	T50.994	T50.995	T50.996
Terizidone	T37.1X1	T37.1X2	T37.1X3	T37.1X4	T37.1X5	T37.1X6
Terlipressin	T38.891	T38.892	T38.893	T38.894	T38.895	T38.896
Terodiline	T46.3X1	T46.3X2	T46.3X3	T46.3X4	T46.3X5	T46.3X6
Teroxalene	T37.4X1	T37.4X2	T37.4X3	T37.4X4	T37.4X5	T37.4X6
Terpin(cis) hydrate	T48.4X1	T48.4X2	T48.4X3	T48.4X4	T48.4X5	T48.4X6
Terramycin	T36.4X1	T36.4X2	T36.4X3	T36.4X4	T36.4X5	T36.4X6
Tertatolol	T44.7X1	T44.7X2	T44.7X3	T44.7X4	T44.7X5	T44.7X6
Tessalon	T48.3X1	T48.3X2	T48.3X3	T48.3X4	T48.3X5	T48.3X6
Testolactone	T38.7X1	T38.7X2	T38.7X3	T38.7X4	T38.7X5	T38.7X6

◀ New   ◀▥ Revised   ~~deleted~~ Deleted

TABLE OF DRUGS AND CHEMICALS

Substance	Poisoning, Accidental (Unintentional)	Poisoning, Intentional Self-Harm	Poisoning, Assault	Poisoning, Undetermined	Adverse Effect	Underdosing
	External Cause (T-Code)					
Testosterone	T38.7X1	T38.7X2	T38.7X3	T38.7X4	T38.7X5	T38.7X6
Tetanus toxoid or vaccine	T50.A91	T50.A92	T50.A93	T50.A94	T50.A95	T50.A96
antitoxin	T50.Z11	T50.Z12	T50.Z13	T50.Z14	T50.Z15	T50.Z16
immune globulin (human)	T50.Z11	T50.Z12	T50.Z13	T50.Z14	T50.Z15	T50.Z16
toxoid	T50.A91	T50.A92	T50.A93	T50.A94	T50.A95	T50.A96
with diphtheria toxoid	T50.A21	T50.A22	T50.A23	T50.A24	T50.A25	T50.A26
with pertussis	T50.A11	T50.A12	T50.A13	T50.A14	T50.A15	T50.A16
Tetrabenazine	T43.591	T43.592	T43.593	T43.594	T43.595	T43.596
Tetracaine	T41.3X1	T41.3X2	T41.3X3	T41.3X4	T41.3X5	T41.3X6
nerve block (peripheral) (plexus)	T41.3X1	T41.3X2	T41.3X3	T41.3X4	T41.3X5	T41.3X6
regional	T41.3X1	T41.3X2	T41.3X3	T41.3X4	T41.3X5	T41.3X6
spinal	T41.3X1	T41.3X2	T41.3X3	T41.3X4	T41.3X5	T41.3X6
Tetrachlorethylene — see Tetrachloroethylene						
Tetrachlormethiazide	T50.2X1	T50.2X2	T50.2X3	T50.2X4	T50.2X5	T50.2X6
2,3,7,8-Tetrachlorodibenzo-p-dioxin	T53.7X1	T53.7X2	T53.7X3	T53.7X4	—	—
Tetrachloroethane	T53.6X1	T53.6X2	T53.6X3	T53.6X4	—	—
vapor	T53.6X1	T53.6X2	T53.6X3	T53.6X4	—	—
paint or varnish	T53.6X1	T53.6X2	T53.6X3	T53.6X4	—	—
Tetrachloroethylene (liquid)	T53.3X1	T53.3X2	T53.3X3	T53.3X4		
medicinal	T37.4X1	T37.4X2	T37.4X3	T37.4X4	T37.4X5	T37.4X6
vapor	T53.3X1	T53.3X2	T53.3X3	T53.3X4	—	—
Tetrachloromethane — see Carbon tetrachloride						
Tetracosactide	T38.811	T38.812	T38.813	T38.814	T38.815	T38.816
Tetracosactrin	T38.811	T38.812	T38.813	T38.814	T38.815	T38.816
Tetracycline	T36.4X1	T36.4X2	T36.4X3	T36.4X4	T36.4X5	T36.4X6
ophthalmic preparation	T49.5X1	T49.5X2	T49.5X3	T49.5X4	T49.5X5	T49.5X6
topical NEC	T49.0X1	T49.0X2	T49.0X3	T49.0X4	T49.0X5	T49.0X6
Tetradifon	T60.8X1	T60.8X2	T60.8X3	T60.8X4	—	—
Tetradotoxin	T61.771	T61.772	T61.773	T61.774	—	—
Tetraethyl						
lead	T56.0X1	T56.0X2	T56.0X3	T56.0X4	—	—
pyrophosphate	T60.0X1	T60.0X2	T60.0X3	T60.0X4	—	—
Tetraethylammonium chloride	T44.2X1	T44.2X2	T44.2X3	T44.2X4	T44.2X5	T44.2X6
Tetraethylthiuram disulfide	T50.6X1	T50.6X2	T50.6X3	T50.6X4	T50.6X5	T50.6X6
Tetrahydroaminoacridine	T44.0X1	T44.0X2	T44.0X3	T44.0X4	T44.0X5	T44.0X6
Tetrahydrocannabinol	T40.7X1	T40.7X2	T40.7X3	T40.7X4	T40.7X5	T40.7X6
Tetrahydrofuran	T52.8X1	T52.8X2	T52.8X3	T52.8X4	—	—
Tetrahydronaphthalene	T52.8X1	T52.8X2	T52.8X3	T52.8X4	—	—
Tetrahydrozoline	T49.5X1	T49.5X2	T49.5X3	T49.5X4	T49.5X5	T49.5X6
Tetralin	T52.8X1	T52.8X2	T52.8X3	T52.8X4	—	—

◀ New   ◀ Revised   ~~deleted~~ Deleted

Substance	Poisoning, Accidental (Unintentional)	Poisoning, Intentional Self-Harm	Poisoning, Assault	Poisoning, Undetermined	Adverse Effect	Underdosing
	External Cause (T-Code)					
Tetramethrin	T60.2X1	T60.2X2	T60.2X3	T60.2X4	—	—
Tetramethylthiuram (disulfide) NEC	T60.3X1	T60.3X2	T60.3X3	T60.3X4	—	—
medicinal	T49.0X1	T49.0X2	T49.0X3	T49.0X4	T49.0X5	T49.0X6
Tetramisole	T37.4X1	T37.4X2	T37.4X3	T37.4X4	T37.4X5	T37.4X6
Tetranicotinoyl fructose	T46.7X1	T46.7X2	T46.7X3	T46.7X4	T46.7X5	T46.7X6
Tetronal	T42.6X1	T42.6X2	T42.6X3	T42.6X4	T42.6X5	T42.6X6
Tetrazepam	T42.4X1	T42.4X2	T42.4X3	T42.4X4	T42.4X5	T42.4X6
Tetryl	T65.3X1	T65.3X2	T65.3X3	T65.3X4	—	—
Tetrylammonium chloride	T44.2X1	T44.2X2	T44.2X3	T44.2X4	T44.2X5	T44.2X6
Tetryzoline	T49.5X1	T49.5X2	T49.5X3	T49.5X4	T49.5X5	T49.5X6
Thalidomide	T45.1X1	T45.1X2	T45.1X3	T45.1X4	T45.1X5	T45.1X6
Thallium (compounds) (dust) NEC	T56.811	T56.812	T56.813	T56.814	—	—
pesticide	T60.4X1	T60.4X2	T60.4X3	T60.4X4	—	—
THC	T40.7X1	T40.7X2	T40.7X3	T40.7X4	T40.7X5	T40.7X6
Thebacon	T48.3X1	T48.3X2	T48.3X3	T48.3X4	T48.3X5	T48.3X6
Thebaine	T40.2X1	T40.2X2	T40.2X3	T40.2X4	T40.2X5	T40.2X6
Thenoic acid	T49.6X1	T49.6X2	T49.6X3	T49.6X4	T49.6X5	T49.6X6
Thenyldiamine	T45.0X1	T45.0X2	T45.0X3	T45.0X4	T45.0X5	T45.0X6
Theobromine (calcium salicylate)	T48.6X1	T48.6X2	T48.6X3	T48.6X4	T48.6X5	T48.6X6
sodium salicylate	T48.6X1	T48.6X2	T48.6X3	T48.6X4	T48.6X5	T48.6X6
Theophyllamine	T48.6X1	T48.6X2	T48.6X3	T48.6X4	T48.6X5	T48.6X6
Theophylline	T48.6X1	T48.6X2	T48.6X3	T48.6X4	T48.6X5	T48.6X6
aminobenzoic acid	T48.6X1	T48.6X2	T48.6X3	T48.6X4	T48.6X5	T48.6X6
ethylenediamine	T48.6X1	T48.6X2	T48.6X3	T48.6X4	T48.6X5	T48.6X6
piperazine p-amino-benzoate	T48.6X1	T48.6X2	T48.6X3	T48.6X4	T48.6X5	T48.6X6
Thiabendazole	T37.4X1	T37.4X2	T37.4X3	T37.4X4	T37.4X5	T37.4X6
Thialbarbital	T41.1X1	T41.1X2	T41.1X3	T41.1X4	T41.1X5	T41.1X6
Thiamazole	T38.2X1	T38.2X2	T38.2X3	T38.2X4	T38.2X5	T38.2X6
Thiambutosine	T37.1X1	T37.1X2	T37.1X3	T37.1X4	T37.1X5	T37.1X6
Thiamine	T45.2X1	T45.2X2	T45.2X3	T45.2X4	T45.2X5	T45.2X6
Thiamphenicol	T36.2X1	T36.2X2	T36.2X3	T36.2X4	T36.2X5	T36.2X6
Thiamylal	T41.1X1	T41.1X2	T41.1X3	T41.1X4	T41.1X5	T41.1X6
sodium	T41.1X1	T41.1X2	T41.1X3	T41.1X4	T41.1X5	T41.1X6
Thiazesim	T43.291	T43.292	T43.293	T43.294	T43.295	T43.296
Thiazides (diuretics)	T50.2X1	T50.2X2	T50.2X3	T50.2X4	T50.2X5	T50.2X6
Thiazinamium metilsulfate	T43.3X1	T43.3X2	T43.3X3	T43.3X4	T43.3X5	T43.3X6
Thiethylperazine	T43.3X1	T43.3X2	T43.3X3	T43.3X4	T43.3X5	T43.3X6
Thimerosal	T49.0X1	T49.0X2	T49.0X3	T49.0X4	T49.0X5	T49.0X6
ophthalmic preparation	T49.5X1	T49.5X2	T49.5X3	T49.5X4	T49.5X5	T49.5X6

◀ New   ◀▥ Revised   ~~deleted~~ Deleted

TABLE OF DRUGS AND CHEMICALS

Substance	External Cause (T-Code)					
	Poisoning, Accidental (Unintentional)	Poisoning, Intentional Self-Harm	Poisoning, Assault	Poisoning, Undetermined	Adverse Effect	Underdosing
Thioacetazone	T37.1X1	T37.1X2	T37.1X3	T37.1X4	T37.1X5	T37.1X6
with isoniazid	T37.1X1	T37.1X2	T37.1X3	T37.1X4	T37.1X5	T37.1X6
Thiobarbital sodium	T41.1X1	T41.1X2	T41.1X3	T41.1X4	T41.1X5	T41.1X6
Thiobarbiturate anesthetic	T41.1X1	T41.1X2	T41.1X3	T41.1X4	T41.1X5	T41.1X6
Thiobismol	T37.8X1	T37.8X2	T37.8X3	T37.8X4	T37.8X5	T37.8X6
Thiobutabarbital sodium	T41.1X1	T41.1X2	T41.1X3	T41.1X4	T41.1X5	T41.1X6
Thiocarbamate (insecticide)	T60.0X1	T60.0X2	T60.0X3	T60.0X4	—	—
Thiocarbamide	T38.2X1	T38.2X2	T38.2X3	T38.2X4	T38.2X5	T38.2X6
Thiocarbarsone	T37.8X1	T37.8X2	T37.8X3	T37.8X4	T37.8X5	T37.8X6
Thiocarlide	T37.1X1	T37.1X2	T37.1X3	T37.1X4	T37.1X5	T37.1X6
Thioctamide	T50.991	T50.992	T50.993	T50.994	T50.995	T50.996
Thioctic acid	T50.991	T50.992	T50.993	T50.994	T50.995	T50.996
Thiofos	T60.0X1	T60.0X2	T60.0X3	T60.0X4	—	—
Thioglycolate	T49.4X1	T49.4X2	T49.4X3	T49.4X4	T49.4X5	T49.4X6
Thioglycolic acid	T65.891	T65.892	T65.893	T65.894	—	—
Thioguanine	T45.1X1	T45.1X2	T45.1X3	T45.1X4	T45.1X5	T45.1X6
Thiomercaptomerin	T50.2X1	T50.2X2	T50.2X3	T50.2X4	T50.2X5	T50.2X6
Thiomerin	T50.2X1	T50.2X2	T50.2X3	T50.2X4	T50.2X5	T50.2X6
Thiomersal	T49.0X1	T49.0X2	T49.0X3	T49.0X4	T49.0X5	T49.0X6
Thionazin	T60.0X1	T60.0X2	T60.0X3	T60.0X4	—	—
Thiopental (sodium)	T41.1X1	T41.1X2	T41.1X3	T41.1X4	T41.1X5	T41.1X6
Thiopentone (sodium)	T41.1X1	T41.1X2	T41.1X3	T41.1X4	T41.1X5	T41.1X6
Thiopropazate	T43.3X1	T43.3X2	T43.3X3	T43.3X4	T43.3X5	T43.3X6
Thioproperazine	T43.3X1	T43.3X2	T43.3X3	T43.3X4	T43.3X5	T43.3X6
Thioridazine	T43.3X1	T43.3X2	T43.3X3	T43.3X4	T43.3X5	T43.3X6
Thiosinamine	T49.3X1	T49.3X2	T49.3X3	T49.3X4	T49.3X5	T49.3X6
Thiotepa	T45.1X1	T45.1X2	T45.1X3	T45.1X4	T45.1X5	T45.1X6
Thiothixene	T43.4X1	T43.4X2	T43.4X3	T43.4X4	T43.4X5	T43.4X6
Thiouracil (benzyl) (methyl) (propyl)	T38.2X1	T38.2X2	T38.2X3	T38.2X4	T38.2X5	T38.2X6
Thiourea	T38.2X1	T38.2X2	T38.2X3	T38.2X4	T38.2X5	T38.2X6
Thiphenamil	T44.3X1	T44.3X2	T44.3X3	T44.3X4	T44.3X5	T44.3X6
Thiram	T60.3X1	T60.3X2	T60.3X3	T60.3X4	—	—
medicinal	T49.2X1	T49.2X2	T49.2X3	T49.2X4	T49.2X5	T49.2X6
Thonzylamine (systemic)	T45.0X1	T45.0X2	T45.0X3	T45.0X4	T45.0X5	T45.0X6
mucosal decongestant	T48.5X1	T48.5X2	T48.5X3	T48.5X4	T48.5X5	T48.5X6
Thorazine	T43.3X1	T43.3X2	T43.3X3	T43.3X4	T43.3X5	T43.3X6
Thorium dioxide suspension	T50.8X1	T50.8X2	T50.8X3	T50.8X4	T50.8X5	T50.8X6
Thornapple	T62.2X1	T62.2X2	T62.2X3	T62.2X4	—	—
Throat drug NEC	T49.6X1	T49.6X2	T49.6X3	T49.6X4	T49.6X5	T49.6X6
Thrombin	T45.7X1	T45.7X2	T45.7X3	T45.7X4	T45.7X5	T45.7X6

TABLE OF DRUGS AND CHEMICALS

◄ New ◄▬ Revised ~~deleted~~ Deleted

Substance	External Cause (T-Code)					
	Poisoning, Accidental (Unintentional)	Poisoning, Intentional Self-Harm	Poisoning, Assault	Poisoning, Undetermined	Adverse Effect	Underdosing
Thrombolysin	T45.611	T45.612	T45.613	T45.614	T45.615	T45.616
Thromboplastin	T45.7X1	T45.7X2	T45.7X3	T45.7X4	T45.7X5	T45.7X6
Thurfyl nicotinate	T46.7X1	T46.7X2	T46.7X3	T46.7X4	T46.7X5	T46.7X6
Thymol	T49.0X1	T49.0X2	T49.0X3	T49.0X4	T49.0X5	T49.0X6
Thymopentin	T37.5X1	T37.5X2	T37.5X3	T37.5X4	T37.5X5	T37.5X6
Thymoxamine	T46.7X1	T46.7X2	T46.7X3	T46.7X4	T46.7X5	T46.7X6
Thymus extract	T38.891	T38.892	T38.893	T38.894	T38.895	T38.896
Thyreotrophic hormone	T38.811	T38.812	T38.813	T38.814	T38.815	T38.816
Thyroglobulin	T38.1X1	T38.1X2	T38.1X3	T38.1X4	T38.1X5	T38.1X6
Thyroid (hormone)	T38.1X1	T38.1X2	T38.1X3	T38.1X4	T38.1X5	T38.1X6
Thyrolar	T38.1X1	T38.1X2	T38.1X3	T38.1X4	T38.1X5	T38.1X6
Thyrotrophin	T38.811	T38.812	T38.813	T38.814	T38.815	T38.816
Thyrotropic hormone	T38.811	T38.812	T38.813	T38.814	T38.815	T38.816
Thyroxine	T38.1X1	T38.1X2	T38.1X3	T38.1X4	T38.1X5	T38.1X6
Tiabendazole	T37.4X1	T37.4X2	T37.4X3	T37.4X4	T37.4X5	T37.4X6
Tiamizide	T50.2X1	T50.2X2	T50.2X3	T50.2X4	T50.2X5	T50.2X6
Tianeptine	T43.291	T43.292	T43.293	T43.294	T43.295	T43.296
Tiapamil	T46.1X1	T46.1X2	T46.1X3	T46.1X4	T46.1X5	T46.1X6
Tiapride	T43.591	T43.592	T43.593	T43.594	T43.595	T43.596
Tiaprofenic acid	T39.311	T39.312	T39.313	T39.314	T39.315	T39.316
Tiaramide	T39.8X1	T39.8X2	T39.8X3	T39.8X4	T39.8X5	T39.8X6
Ticarcillin	T36.0X1	T36.0X2	T36.0X3	T36.0X4	T36.0X5	T36.0X6
Ticlatone	T49.0X1	T49.0X2	T49.0X3	T49.0X4	T49.0X5	T49.0X6
Ticlopidine	T45.521	T45.522	T45.523	T45.524	T45.525	T45.526
Ticrynafen	T50.1X1	T50.1X2	T50.1X3	T50.1X4	T50.1X5	T50.1X6
Tidiacic	T50.991	T50.992	T50.993	T50.994	T50.995	T50.996
Tiemonium	T44.3X1	T44.3X2	T44.3X3	T44.3X4	T44.3X5	T44.3X6
iodide	T44.3X1	T44.3X2	T44.3X3	T44.3X4	T44.3X5	T44.3X6
Tienilic acid	T50.1X1	T50.1X2	T50.1X3	T50.1X4	T50.1X5	T50.1X6
Tifenamil	T44.3X1	T44.3X2	T44.3X3	T44.3X4	T44.3X5	T44.3X6
Tigan	T45.0X1	T45.0X2	T45.0X3	T45.0X4	T45.0X5	T45.0X6
Tigloidine	T44.3X1	T44.3X2	T44.3X3	T44.3X4	T44.3X5	T44.3X6
Tilactase	T47.5X1	T47.5X2	T47.5X3	T47.5X4	T47.5X5	T47.5X6
Tiletamine	T41.291	T41.292	T41.293	T41.294	T41.295	T41.296
Tilidine	T40.4X1	T40.4X2	T40.4X3	T40.4X4	—	—
Timepidium bromide	T44.3X1	T44.3X2	T44.3X3	T44.3X4	T44.3X5	T44.3X6
Timiperone	T43.4X1	T43.4X2	T43.4X3	T43.4X4	T43.4X5	T43.4X6
Timolol	T44.7X1	T44.7X2	T44.7X3	T44.7X4	T44.7X5	T44.7X6
Tin (chloride) (dust) (oxide) NEC	T56.6X1	T56.6X2	T56.6X3	T56.6X4	—	—
anti-infectives	T37.8X1	T37.8X2	T37.8X3	T37.8X4	T37.8X5	T37.8X6

◀ New ◀▥ Revised ~~deleted~~ Deleted

TABLE OF DRUGS AND CHEMICALS

	External Cause (T-Code)					
Substance	Poisoning, Accidental (Unintentional)	Poisoning, Intentional Self-Harm	Poisoning, Assault	Poisoning, Undetermined	Adverse Effect	Underdosing
Tincture, iodine—see Iodine						
Tindal	T43.3X1	T43.3X2	T43.3X3	T43.3X4	T43.3X5	T43.3X6
Tinidazole	T37.3X1	T37.3X2	T37.3X3	T37.3X4	T37.3X5	T37.3X6
Tinoridine	T39.8X1	T39.8X2	T39.8X3	T39.8X4	T39.8X5	T39.8X6
Tiocarlide	T37.1X1	T37.1X2	T37.1X3	T37.1X4	T37.1X5	T37.1X6
Tioclomarol	T45.511	T45.512	T45.513	T45.514	T45.515	T45.516
Tioconazole	T49.0X1	T49.0X2	T49.0X3	T49.0X4	T49.0X5	T49.0X6
Tioguanine	T45.1X1	T45.1X2	T45.1X3	T45.1X4	T45.1X5	T45.1X6
Tiopronin	T50.991	T50.992	T50.993	T50.994	T50.995	T50.996
Tiotixene	T43.4X1	T43.4X2	T43.4X3	T43.4X4	T43.4X5	T43.4X6
Tioxolone	T49.4X1	T49.4X2	T49.4X3	T49.4X4	T49.4X5	T49.4X6
Tipepidine	T48.3X1	T48.3X2	T48.3X3	T48.3X4	T48.3X5	T48.3X6
Tiquizium bromide	T44.3X1	T44.3X2	T44.3X3	T44.3X4	T44.3X5	T44.3X6
Tiratricol	T38.1X1	T38.1X2	T38.1X3	T38.1X4	T38.1X5	T38.1X6
Tisopurine	T50.4X1	T50.4X2	T50.4X3	T50.4X4	T50.4X5	T50.4X6
Titanium (compounds) (vapor)	T56.891	T56.892	T56.893	T56.894	—	—
dioxide	T49.3X1	T49.3X2	T49.3X3	T49.3X4	T49.3X5	T49.3X6
ointment	T49.3X1	T49.3X2	T49.3X3	T49.3X4	T49.3X5	T49.3X6
oxide	T49.3X1	T49.3X2	T49.3X3	T49.3X4	T49.3X5	T49.3X6
tetrachloride	T56.891	T56.892	T56.893	T56.894	—	—
Titanocene	T56.891	T56.892	T56.893	T56.894	—	—
Titroid	T38.1X1	T38.1X2	T38.1X3	T38.1X4	T38.1X5	T38.1X6
Tizanidine	T42.8X1	T42.8X2	T42.8X3	T42.8X4	T42.8X5	T42.8X6
TMTD	T60.3X1	T60.3X2	T60.3X3	T60.3X4	—	—
TNT (fumes)	T65.3X1	T65.3X2	T65.3X3	T65.3X4	—	—
Toadstool	T62.0X1	T62.0X2	T62.0X3	T62.0X4	—	—
Tobacco NEC	T65.291	T65.292	T65.293	T65.294	—	—
cigarettes	T65.221	T65.222	T65.223	T65.224	—	—
Indian	T62.2X1	T62.2X2	T62.2X3	T62.2X4	—	—
smoke, second-hand	T65.221	T65.222	T65.223	T65.224	—	—
Tobramycin	T36.5X1	T36.5X2	T36.5X3	T36.5X4	T36.5X5	T36.5X6
Tocainide	T46.2X1	T46.2X2	T46.2X3	T46.2X4	T46.2X5	T46.2X6
Tocoferol	T45.2X1	T45.2X2	T45.2X3	T45.2X4	T45.2X5	T45.2X6
Tocopherol	T45.2X1	T45.2X2	T45.2X3	T45.2X4	T45.2X5	T45.2X6
acetate	T45.2X1	T45.2X2	T45.2X3	T45.2X4	T45.2X5	T45.2X6
Tocosamine	T48.0X1	T48.0X2	T48.0X3	T48.0X4	T48.0X5	T48.0X6
Todralazine	T46.5X1	T46.5X2	T46.5X3	T46.5X4	T46.5X5	T46.5X6
Tofisopam	T42.4X1	T42.4X2	T42.4X3	T42.4X4	T42.4X5	T42.4X6
Tofranil	T43.011	T43.012	T43.013	T43.014	T43.015	T43.016
Toilet deodorizer	T65.891	T65.892	T65.893	T65.894	—	—

◀ New ◀▥ Revised ~~deleted~~ Deleted

Substance	Poisoning, Accidental (Unintentional)	Poisoning, Intentional Self-Harm	Poisoning, Assault	Poisoning, Undetermined	Adverse Effect	Underdosing
			External Cause (T-Code)			
Tolamolol	T44.7X1	T44.7X2	T44.7X3	T44.7X4	T44.7X5	T44.7X6
Tolazamide	T38.3X1	T38.3X2	T38.3X3	T38.3X4	T38.3X5	T38.3X6
Tolazoline	T46.7X1	T46.7X2	T46.7X3	T46.7X4	T46.7X5	T46.7X6
Tolbutamide (sodium)	T38.3X1	T38.3X2	T38.3X3	T38.3X4	T38.3X5	T38.3X6
Tolciclate	T49.0X1	T49.0X2	T49.0X3	T49.0X4	T49.0X5	T49.0X6
Tolmetin	T39.391	T39.392	T39.393	T39.394	T39.395	T39.396
Tolnaftate	T49.0X1	T49.0X2	T49.0X3	T49.0X4	T49.0X5	T49.0X6
Tolonidine	T46.5X1	T46.5X2	T46.5X3	T46.5X4	T46.5X5	T46.5X6
Toloxatone	T42.6X1	T42.6X2	T42.6X3	T42.6X4	T42.6X5	T42.6X6
Tolperisone	T44.3X1	T44.3X2	T44.3X3	T44.3X4	T44.3X5	T44.3X6
Tolserol	T42.8X1	T42.8X2	T42.8X3	T42.8X4	T42.8X5	T42.8X6
Toluene (liquid)	T52.2X1	T52.2X2	T52.2X3	T52.2X4	—	—
diisocyanate	T65.0X1	T65.0X2	T65.0X3	T65.0X4	—	—
Toluidine	T65.891	T65.892	T65.893	T65.894	—	—
vapor	T59.891	T59.892	T59.893	T59.894	—	—
Toluol (liquid)	T52.2X1	T52.2X2	T52.2X3	T52.2X4	—	—
vapor	T52.2X1	T52.2X2	T52.2X3	T52.2X4	—	—
Toluylenediamine	T65.3X1	T65.3X2	T65.3X3	T65.3X4	—	—
Tolylene-2,4-diisocyanate	T65.0X1	T65.0X2	T65.0X3	T65.0X4	—	—
Tonic NEC	T50.901	T50.902	T50.903	T50.904	T50.905	T50.906
Topical action drug NEC	T49.91	T49.92	T49.93	T49.94	T49.95	T49.96
ear, nose or throat	T49.6X1	T49.6X2	T49.6X3	T49.6X4	T49.6X5	T49.6X6
eye	T49.5X1	T49.5X2	T49.5X3	T49.5X4	T49.5X5	T49.5X6
skin	T49.91	T49.92	T49.93	T49.94	T49.95	T49.96
specified NEC	T49.8X1	T49.8X2	T49.8X3	T49.8X4	T49.8X5	T49.8X6
Toquizine	T44.3X1	T44.3X2	T44.3X3	T44.3X4	T44.3X5	T44.3X6
Toremifene	T38.6X1	T38.6X2	T38.6X3	T38.6X4	T38.6X5	T38.6X6
Tosylchloramide sodium	T49.8X1	T49.8X2	T49.8X3	T49.8X4	T49.8X5	T49.8X6
Toxaphene (dust) (spray)	T60.1X1	T60.1X2	T60.1X3	T60.1X4	—	—
Toxin, diphtheria (Schick Test)	T50.8X1	T50.8X2	T50.8X3	T50.8X4	T50.8X5	T50.8X6
Toxoid						
combined	T50.A21	T50.A22	T50.A23	T50.A24	T50.A25	T50.A26
diphtheria	T50.A91	T50.A92	T50.A93	T50.A94	T50.A95	T50.A96
tetanus	T50.A91	T50.A92	T50.A93	T50.A94	T50.A95	T50.A96
Trace element NEC	T45.8X1	T45.8X2	T45.8X3	T45.8X4	T45.8X5	T45.8X6
Tractor fuel NEC	T52.0X1	T52.0X2	T52.0X3	T52.0X4	—	—
Tragacanth	T50.991	T50.992	T50.993	T50.994	T50.995	T50.996
Tramadol	T40.4X1	T40.4X2	T40.4X3	T40.4X4	T40.4X5	T40.4X6
Tramazoline	T48.5X1	T48.5X2	T48.5X3	T48.5X4	T48.5X5	T48.5X6
Tranexamic acid	T45.621	T45.622	T45.623	T45.624	T45.625	T45.626

◄ New ◄ Revised ~~deleted~~ Deleted

TABLE OF DRUGS AND CHEMICALS

Substance	Poisoning, Accidental (Unintentional)	Poisoning, Intentional Self-Harm	Poisoning, Assault	Poisoning, Undetermined	Adverse Effect	Underdosing
	External Cause (T-Code)					
Tranilast	T45.0X1	T45.0X2	T45.0X3	T45.0X4	T45.0X5	T45.0X6
Tranquilizer NEC	T43.501	T43.502	T43.503	T43.504	T43.505	T43.506
with hypnotic or sedative	T42.6X1	T42.6X2	T42.6X3	T42.6X4	T42.6X5	T42.6X6
benzodiazepine NEC	T42.4X1	T42.4X2	T42.4X3	T42.4X4	T42.4X5	T42.4X6
butyrophenone NEC	T43.4X1	T43.4X2	T43.4X3	T43.4X4	T43.4X5	T43.4X6
carbamate	T43.591	T43.592	T43.593	T43.594	T43.595	T43.596
dimethylamine	T43.3X1	T43.3X2	T43.3X3	T43.3X4	T43.3X5	T43.3X6
ethylamine	T43.3X1	T43.3X2	T43.3X3	T43.3X4	T43.3X5	T43.3X6
hydroxyzine	T43.591	T43.592	T43.593	T43.594	T43.595	T43.596
major NEC	T43.501	T43.502	T43.503	T43.504	T43.505	T43.506
penothiazine NEC	T43.3X1	T43.3X2	T43.3X3	T43.3X4	T43.3X5	T43.3X6
phenothiazine-based	T43.3X1	T43.3X2	T43.3X3	T43.3X4	T43.3X5	T43.3X6
piperazine NEC	T43.3X1	T43.3X2	T43.3X3	T43.3X4	T43.3X5	T43.3X6
piperidine	T43.3X1	T43.3X2	T43.3X3	T43.3X4	T43.3X5	T43.3X6
propylamine	T43.3X1	T43.3X2	T43.3X3	T43.3X4	T43.3X5	T43.3X6
specified NEC	T43.591	T43.592	T43.593	T43.594	T43.595	T43.596
thioxanthene NEC	T43.591	T43.592	T43.593	T43.594	T43.595	T43.596
Tranxene	T42.4X1	T42.4X2	T42.4X3	T42.4X4	T42.4X5	T42.4X6
Tranylcypromine	T43.1X1	T43.1X2	T43.1X3	T43.1X4	T43.1X5	T43.1X6
Trapidil	T46.3X1	T46.3X2	T46.3X3	T46.3X4	T46.3X5	T46.3X6
Trasentine	T44.3X1	T44.3X2	T44.3X3	T44.3X4	T44.3X5	T44.3X6
Travert	T50.3X1	T50.3X2	T50.3X3	T50.3X4	T50.3X5	T50.3X6
Trazodone	T43.211	T43.212	T43.213	T43.214	T43.215	T43.216
Trecator	T37.1X1	T37.1X2	T37.1X3	T37.1X4	T37.1X5	T37.1X6
Treosulfan	T45.1X1	T45.1X2	T45.1X3	T45.1X4	T45.1X5	T45.1X6
Tretamine	T45.1X1	T45.1X2	T45.1X3	T45.1X4	T45.1X5	T45.1X6
Tretinoin	T49.0X1	T49.0X2	T49.0X3	T49.0X4	T49.0X5	T49.0X6
Tretoquinol	T48.6X1	T48.6X2	T48.6X3	T48.6X4	T48.6X5	T48.6X6
Triacetin	T49.0X1	T49.0X2	T49.0X3	T49.0X4	T49.0X5	T49.0X6
Triacetoxyanthracene	T49.4X1	T49.4X2	T49.4X3	T49.4X4	T49.4X5	T49.4X6
Triacetyloleandomycin	T36.3X1	T36.3X2	T36.3X3	T36.3X4	T36.3X5	T36.3X6
Triamcinolone	T49.0X1	T49.0X2	T49.0X3	T49.0X4	T49.0X5	T49.0X6
ENT agent	T49.6X1	T49.6X2	T49.6X3	T49.6X4	T49.6X5	T49.6X6
hexacetonide	T49.0X1	T49.0X2	T49.0X3	T49.0X4	T49.0X5	T49.0X6
ophthalmic preparation	T49.5X1	T49.5X2	T49.5X3	T49.5X4	T49.5X5	T49.5X6
topical NEC	T49.0X1	T49.0X2	T49.0X3	T49.0X4	T49.0X5	T49.0X6
Triampyzine	T44.3X1	T44.3X2	T44.3X3	T44.3X4	T44.3X5	T44.3X6
Triamterene	T50.2X1	T50.2X2	T50.2X3	T50.2X4	T50.2X5	T50.2X6
Triazine (herbicide)	T60.3X1	T60.3X2	T60.3X3	T60.3X4	—	—
Triaziquone	T45.1X1	T45.1X2	T45.1X3	T45.1X4	T45.1X5	T45.1X6

◀ New ◀▥ Revised ~~deleted~~ Deleted

Substance	External Cause (T-Code)					
	Poisoning, Accidental (Unintentional)	Poisoning, Intentional Self-Harm	Poisoning, Assault	Poisoning, Undetermined	Adverse Effect	Underdosing
Triazolam	T42.4X1	T42.4X2	T42.4X3	T42.4X4	T42.4X5	T42.4X6
Triazole (herbicide)	T60.3X1	T60.3X2	T60.3X3	T60.3X4	—	—
Tribenoside	T46.991	T46.992	T46.993	T46.994	T46.995	T46.996
Tribromacetaldehyde	T42.6X1	T42.6X2	T42.6X3	T42.6X4	T42.6X5	T42.6X6
Tribromoethanol, rectal	T41.291	T41.292	T41.293	T41.294	T41.295	T41.296
Tribromomethane	T42.6X1	T42.6X2	T42.6X3	T42.6X4	T42.6X5	T42.6X6
Trichlorethane	T53.2X1	T53.2X2	T53.2X3	T53.2X4	—	—
Trichlorethylene	T53.2X1	T53.2X2	T53.2X3	T53.2X4	—	—
Trichlorfon	T60.0X1	T60.0X2	T60.0X3	T60.0X4	—	—
Trichlormethiazide	T50.2X1	T50.2X2	T50.2X3	T50.2X4	T50.2X5	T50.2X6
Trichlormethine	T45.1X1	T45.1X2	T45.1X3	T45.1X4	T45.1X5	T45.1X6
Trichloroacetic acid, Trichloracetic acid	T54.2X1	T54.2X2	T54.2X3	T54.2X4	—	—
medicinal	T49.4X1	T49.4X2	T49.4X3	T49.4X4	T49.4X5	T49.4X6
Trichloroethane	T53.2X1	T53.2X2	T53.2X3	T53.2X4	—	—
Trichloroethanol	T42.6X1	T42.6X2	T42.6X3	T42.6X4	T42.6X5	T42.6X6
Trichloroethylene (liquid) (vapor)	T53.2X1	T53.2X2	T53.2X3	T53.2X4	—	—
anesthetic (gas)	T41.0X1	T41.0X2	T41.0X3	T41.0X4	T41.0X5	T41.0X6
vapor NEC	T53.2X1	T53.2X2	T53.2X3	T53.2X4	—	—
Trichloroethyl phosphate	T42.6X1	T42.6X2	T42.6X3	T42.6X4	T42.6X5	T42.6X6
Trichlorofluoromethane NEC	T53.5X1	T53.5X2	T53.5X3	T53.5X4	—	—
Trichloronate	T60.0X1	T60.0X2	T60.0X3	T60.0X4	—	—
2,4,5-Trichlorophen-oxyacetic acid	T60.3X1	T60.3X2	T60.3X3	T60.3X4	—	—
Trichloropropane	T53.6X1	T53.6X2	T53.6X3	T53.6X4	—	—
Trichlorotriethylamine	T45.1X1	T45.1X2	T45.1X3	T45.1X4	T45.1X5	T45.1X6
Trichomonacides NEC	T37.3X1	T37.3X2	T37.3X3	T37.3X4	T37.3X5	T37.3X6
Trichomycin	T36.7X1	T36.7X2	T36.7X3	T36.7X4	T36.7X5	T36.7X6
Triclobisonium chloride	T49.0X1	T49.0X2	T49.0X3	T49.0X4	T49.0X5	T49.0X6
Triclocarban	T49.0X1	T49.0X2	T49.0X3	T49.0X4	T49.0X5	T49.0X6
Triclofos	T42.6X1	T42.6X2	T42.6X3	T42.6X4	T42.6X5	T42.6X6
Triclosan	T49.0X1	T49.0X2	T49.0X3	T49.0X4	T49.0X5	T49.0X6
Tricresyl phosphate	T65.891	T65.892	T65.893	T65.894	—	—
solvent	T52.91	T52.92	T52.93	T52.94	—	—
Tricyclamol chloride	T44.3X1	T44.3X2	T44.3X3	T44.3X4	T44.3X5	T44.3X6
Tridesilon	T49.0X1	T49.0X2	T49.0X3	T49.0X4	T49.0X5	T49.0X6
Tridihexethyl iodide	T44.3X1	T44.3X2	T44.3X3	T44.3X4	T44.3X5	T44.3X6
Tridione	T42.2X1	T42.2X2	T42.2X3	T42.2X4	T42.2X5	T42.2X6
Trientine	T45.8X1	T45.8X2	T45.8X3	T45.8X4	T45.8X5	T45.8X6
Triethanolamine NEC	T54.3X1	T54.3X2	T54.3X3	T54.3X4	—	—
detergent	T54.3X1	T54.3X2	T54.3X3	T54.3X4	—	—
trinitrate (biphosphate)	T46.3X1	T46.3X2	T46.3X3	T46.3X4	T46.3X5	T46.3X6

TABLE OF DRUGS AND CHEMICALS

TABLE OF DRUGS AND CHEMICALS

Substance	Poisoning, Accidental (Unintentional)	Poisoning, Intentional Self-Harm	Poisoning, Assault	Poisoning, Undetermined	Adverse Effect	Underdosing
Triethanomelamine	T45.1X1	T45.1X2	T45.1X3	T45.1X4	T45.1X5	T45.1X6
Triethylenemelamine	T45.1X1	T45.1X2	T45.1X3	T45.1X4	T45.1X5	T45.1X6
Triethylenephosphoramide	T45.1X1	T45.1X2	T45.1X3	T45.1X4	T45.1X5	T45.1X6
Triethylenethiophosphoramide	T45.1X1	T45.1X2	T45.1X3	T45.1X4	T45.1X5	T45.1X6
Trifluoperazine	T43.3X1	T43.3X2	T43.3X3	T43.3X4	T43.3X5	T43.3X6
Trifluoroethyl vinyl ether	T41.0X1	T41.0X2	T41.0X3	T41.0X4	T41.0X5	T41.0X6
Trifluperidol	T43.4X1	T43.4X2	T43.4X3	T43.4X4	T43.4X5	T43.4X6
Triflupromazine	T43.3X1	T43.3X2	T43.3X3	T43.3X4	T43.3X5	T43.3X6
Trifluridine	T37.5X1	T37.5X2	T37.5X3	T37.5X4	T37.5X5	T37.5X6
Triflusal	T45.521	T45.522	T45.523	T45.524	T45.525	T45.526
Trihexyphenidyl	T44.3X1	T44.3X2	T44.3X3	T44.3X4	T44.3X5	T44.3X6
Triiodothyronine	T38.1X1	T38.1X2	T38.1X3	T38.1X4	T38.1X5	T38.1X6
Trilene	T41.0X1	T41.0X2	T41.0X3	T41.0X4	T41.0X5	T41.0X6
Trilostane	T38.991	T38.992	T38.993	T38.994	T38.995	T38.996
Trimebutine	T44.3X1	T44.3X2	T44.3X3	T44.3X4	T44.3X5	T44.3X6
Trimecaine	T41.3X1	T41.3X2	T41.3X3	T41.3X4	T41.3X5	T41.3X6
Trimeprazine (tartrate)	T44.3X1	T44.3X2	T44.3X3	T44.3X4	T44.3X5	T44.3X6
Trimetaphan camsilate	T44.2X1	T44.2X2	T44.2X3	T44.2X4	T44.2X5	T44.2X6
Trimetazidine	T46.7X1	T46.7X2	T46.7X3	T46.7X4	T46.7X5	T46.7X6
Trimethadione	T42.2X1	T42.2X2	T42.2X3	T42.2X4	T42.2X5	T42.2X6
Trimethaphan	T44.2X1	T44.2X2	T44.2X3	T44.2X4	T44.2X5	T44.2X6
Trimethidinium	T44.2X1	T44.2X2	T44.2X3	T44.2X4	T44.2X5	T44.2X6
Trimethobenzamide	T45.0X1	T45.0X2	T45.0X3	T45.0X4	T45.0X5	T45.0X6
Trimethoprim	T37.8X1	T37.8X2	T37.8X3	T37.8X4	T37.8X5	T37.8X6
with sulfamethoxazole	T36.8X1	T36.8X2	T36.8X3	T36.8X4	T36.8X5	T36.8X6
Trimethylcarbinol	T51.3X1	T51.3X2	T51.3X3	T51.3X4	—	—
Trimethylpsoralen	T49.3X1	T49.3X2	T49.3X3	T49.3X4	T49.3X5	T49.3X6
Trimeton	T45.0X1	T45.0X2	T45.0X3	T45.0X4	T45.0X5	T45.0X6
Trimetrexate	T45.1X1	T45.1X2	T45.1X3	T45.1X4	T45.1X5	T45.1X6
Trimipramine	T43.011	T43.012	T43.013	T43.014	T43.015	T43.016
Trimustine	T45.1X1	T45.1X2	T45.1X3	T45.1X4	T45.1X5	T45.1X6
Trinitrine	T46.3X1	T46.3X2	T46.3X3	T46.3X4	T46.3X5	T46.3X6
Trinitrobenzol	T65.3X1	T65.3X2	T65.3X3	T65.3X4	—	—
Trinitrophenol	T65.3X1	T65.3X2	T65.3X3	T65.3X4	—	—
Trinitrotoluene (fumes)	T65.3X1	T65.3X2	T65.3X3	T65.3X4	—	—
Trional	T42.6X1	T42.6X2	T42.6X3	T42.6X4	T42.6X5	T42.6X6
Triorthocresyl phosphate	T65.891	T65.892	T65.893	T65.894	—	—
Trioxide of arsenic	T57.0X1	T57.0X2	T57.0X3	T57.0X4	—	—
Trioxysalen	T49.4X1	T49.4X2	T49.4X3	T49.4X4	T49.4X5	T49.4X6
Tripamide	T50.2X1	T50.2X2	T50.2X3	T50.2X4	T50.2X5	T50.2X6

◀ New ◀ Revised ~~deleted~~ Deleted

Substance	Poisoning, Accidental (Unintentional)	Poisoning, Intentional Self-Harm	Poisoning, Assault	Poisoning, Undetermined	Adverse Effect	Underdosing
	External Cause (T-Code)					
Triparanol	T46.6X1	T46.6X2	T46.6X3	T46.6X4	T46.6X5	T46.6X6
Tripelennamine	T45.0X1	T45.0X2	T45.0X3	T45.0X4	T45.0X5	T45.0X6
Triperiden	I44.3X1	T44.3X2	T44.3X3	T44.3X4	T44.3X5	T44.3X6
Triperidol	T43.4X1	T43.4X2	T43.4X3	T43.4X4	T43.4X5	T43.4X6
Triphenylphosphate	T65.891	T65.892	T65.893	T65.894	—	—
Triple						
bromides	T42.6X1	T42.6X2	T42.6X3	T42.6X4	T42.6X5	T42.6X6
carbonate	T47.1X1	T47.1X2	T47.1X3	T47.1X4	T47.1X5	T47.1X6
vaccine						
DPT	T50.A11	T50.A12	T50.A13	T50.A14	T50.A15	T50.A16
including pertussis	T50.A11	T50.A12	T50.A13	T50.A14	T50.A15	T50.A16
MMR	T50.B91	T50.B92	—	—	—	—
Triprolidine	T45.0X1	T45.0X2	T45.0X3	T45.0X4	T45.0X5	T45.0X6
Trisodium hydrogen edetate	T50.6X1	T50.6X2	T50.6X3	T50.6X4	T50.6X5	T50.6X6
Trisoralen	T49.3X1	T49.3X2	T49.3X3	T49.3X4	T49.3X5	T49.3X6
Trisulfapyrimidines	T37.0X1	T37.0X2	T37.0X3	T37.0X4	T37.0X5	T37.0X6
Trithiozine	T44.3X1	T44.3X2	T44.3X3	T44.3X4	T44.3X5	T44.3X6
Tritiozine	T44.3X1	T44.3X2	T44.3X3	T44.3X4	T44.3X5	T44.3X6
Tritoqualine	T45.0X1	T45.0X2	T45.0X3	T45.0X4	T45.0X5	T45.0X6
Trofosfamide	T45.1X1	T45.1X2	T45.1X3	T45.1X4	T45.1X5	T45.1X6
Troleandomycin	T36.3X1	T36.3X2	T36.3X3	T36.3X4	T36.3X5	T36.3X6
Trolnitrate (phosphate)	T46.3X1	T46.3X2	T46.3X3	T46.3X4	T46.3X5	T46.3X6
Tromantadine	T37.5X1	T37.5X2	T37.5X3	T37.5X4	T37.5X5	T37.5X6
Trometamol	T50.2X1	T50.2X2	T50.2X3	T50.2X4	T50.2X5	T50.2X6
Tromethamine	T50.2X1	T50.2X2	T50.2X3	T50.2X4	T50.2X5	T50.2X6
Tronothane	T41.3X1	T41.3X2	T41.3X3	T41.3X4	T41.3X5	T41.3X6
Tropacine	T44.3X1	T44.3X2	T44.3X3	T44.3X4	T44.3X5	T44.3X6
Tropatepine	T44.3X1	T44.3X2	T44.3X3	T44.3X4	T44.3X5	T44.3X6
Tropicamide	T44.3X1	T44.3X2	T44.3X3	T44.3X4	T44.3X5	T44.3X6
Trospium chloride	T44.3X1	T44.3X2	T44.3X3	T44.3X4	T44.3X5	T44.3X6
Troxerutin	T46.991	T46.992	T46.993	T46.994	T46.995	T46.996
Troxidone	T42.2X1	T42.2X2	T42.2X3	T42.2X4	T42.2X5	T42.2X6
Tryparsamide	T37.3X1	T37.3X2	T37.3X3	T37.3X4	T37.3X5	T37.3X6
Trypsin	T45.3X1	T45.3X2	T45.3X3	T45.3X4	T45.3X5	T45.3X6
Tryptizol	T43.011	T43.012	T43.013	T43.014	T43.015	T43.016
TSH	T38.811	T38.812	T38.813	T38.814	T38.815	T38.816
Tuaminoheptane	T48.5X1	T48.5X2	T48.5X3	T48.5X4	T48.5X5	T48.5X6
Tuberculin, purified protein derivative (PPD)	T50.8X1	T50.8X2	T50.8X3	T50.8X4	T50.8X5	T50.8X6
Tubocurare	T48.1X1	T48.1X2	T48.1X3	T48.1X4	T48.1X5	T48.1X6
Tubocurarine (chloride)	T48.1X1	T48.1X2	T48.1X3	T48.1X4	T48.1X5	T48.1X6

TABLE OF DRUGS AND CHEMICALS

TABLE OF DRUGS AND CHEMICALS

Substance	External Cause (T-Code)					
	Poisoning, Accidental (Unintentional)	Poisoning, Intentional Self-Harm	Poisoning, Assault	Poisoning, Undetermined	Adverse Effect	Underdosing
Tulobuterol	T48.6X1	T48.6X2	T48.6X3	T48.6X4	T48.6X5	T48.6X6
Turpentine (spirits of)	T52.8X1	T52.8X2	T52.8X3	T52.8X4	—	—
vapor	T52.8X1	T52.8X2	T52.8X3	T52.8X4	—	—
Tybamate	T43.591	T43.592	T43.593	T43.594	T43.595	T43.596
Tyloxapol	T48.4X1	T48.4X2	T48.4X3	T48.4X4	T48.4X5	T48.4X6
Tymazoline	T48.5X1	T48.5X2	T48.5X3	T48.5X4	T48.5X5	T48.5X6
Typhoid-paratyphoid vaccine	T50.A91	T50.A92	T50.A93	T50.A94	T50.A95	T50.A96
Typhus vaccine	T50.A91	T50.A92	T50.A93	T50.A94	T50.A95	T50.A96
Tyropanoate	T50.8X1	T50.8X2	T50.8X3	T50.8X4	T50.8X5	T50.8X6
Tyrothricin	T49.6X1	T49.6X2	T49.6X3	T49.6X4	T49.6X5	T49.6X6
ENT agent	T49.6X1	T49.6X2	T49.6X3	T49.6X4	T49.6X5	T49.6X6
ophthalmic preparation	T49.5X1	T49.5X2	T49.5X3	T49.5X4	T49.5X5	T49.5X6
U						
Ufenamate	T39.391	T39.392	T39.393	T39.394	T39.395	T39.396
Ultraviolet light protectant	T49.3X1	T49.3X2	T49.3X3	T49.3X4	T49.3X5	T49.3X6
Undecenoic acid	T49.0X1	T49.0X2	T49.0X3	T49.0X4	T49.0X5	T49.0X6
Undecoylium	T49.0X1	T49.0X2	T49.0X3	T49.0X4	T49.0X5	T49.0X6
Undecylenic acid (derivatives)	T49.0X1	T49.0X2	T49.0X3	T49.0X4	T49.0X5	T49.0X6
Unna's boot	T49.3X1	T49.3X2	T49.3X3	T49.3X4	T49.3X5	T49.3X6
Unsaturated fatty acid	T46.6X1	T46.6X2	T46.6X3	T46.6X4	T46.6X5	T46.6X6
Uracil mustard	T45.1X1	T45.1X2	T45.1X3	T45.1X4	T45.1X5	T45.1X6
Uramustine	T45.1X1	T45.1X2	T45.1X3	T45.1X4	T45.1X5	T45.1X6
Urapidil	T46.5X1	T46.5X2	T46.5X3	T46.5X4	T46.5X5	T46.5X6
Urari	T48.1X1	T48.1X2	T48.1X3	T48.1X4	T48.1X5	T48.1X6
Urate oxidase	T50.4X1	T50.4X2	T50.4X3	T50.4X4	T50.4X5	T50.4X6
Urea	T47.3X1	T47.3X2	T47.3X3	T47.3X4	T47.3X5	T47.3X6
peroxide	T49.0X1	T49.0X2	T49.0X3	T49.0X4	T49.0X5	T49.0X6
stibamine	T37.4X1	T37.4X2	T37.4X3	T37.4X4	T37.4X5	T37.4X6
topical	T49.8X1	T49.8X2	T49.8X3	T49.8X4	T49.8X5	T49.8X6
Urethane	T45.1X1	T45.1X2	T45.1X3	T45.1X4	T45.1X5	T45.1X6
Urginea (maritima) (scilla) — see Squill						
Uric acid metabolism drug NEC	T50.4X1	T50.4X2	T50.4X3	T50.4X4	T50.4X5	T50.4X6
Uricosuric agent	T50.4X1	T50.4X2	T50.4X3	T50.4X4	T50.4X5	T50.4X6
Urinary anti-infective	T37.8X1	T37.8X2	T37.8X3	T37.8X4	T37.8X5	T37.8X6
Urofollitropin	T38.811	T38.812	T38.813	T38.814	T38.815	T38.816
Urokinase	T45.611	T45.612	T45.613	T45.614	T45.615	T45.616
Urokon	T50.8X1	T50.8X2	T50.8X3	T50.8X4	T50.8X5	T50.8X6
Ursodeoxycholic acid	T50.991	T50.992	T50.993	T50.994	T50.995	T50.996
Ursodiol	T50.991	T50.992	T50.993	T50.994	T50.995	T50.996

◀ New ◀▥ Revised ~~deleted~~ Deleted

	External Cause (T-Code)					
Substance	Poisoning, Accidental (Unintentional)	Poisoning, Intentional Self-Harm	Poisoning, Assault	Poisoning, Undetermined	Adverse Effect	Underdosing
Urtica	T62.2X1	T62.2X2	T62.2X3	T62.2X4	—	—
Utility gas—*see Gas, utility*						
V						
Vaccine NEC	T50.Z91	T50.Z92	T50.Z93	T50.Z94	T50.Z95	T50.Z96
antineoplastic	T50.Z91	T50.Z92	T50.Z93	T50.Z94	T50.Z95	T50.Z96
bacterial NEC	T50.A91	T50.A92	T50.A93	T50.A94	T50.A95	T50.A96
with						
other bacterial component	T50.A91	T50.A92	T50.A93	T50.A94	T50.A95	T50.A96
pertussis component	T50.A91	T50.A92	T50.A93	T50.A94	T50.A95	T50.A96
viral-rickettsial component	T50.A91	T50.A92	T50.A93	T50.A94	T50.A95	T50.A96
mixed NEC	T50.A91	T50.A92	T50.A93	T50.A94	T50.A95	T50.A96
BCG	T50.A91	T50.A92	T50.A93	T50.A94	T50.A95	T50.A96
cholera	T50.A91	T50.A92	T50.A93	T50.A94	T50.A95	T50.A96
diphtheria	T50.A91	T50.A92	T50.A93	T50.A94	T50.A95	T50.A96
with tetanus	T50.A21	T50.A22	T50.A23	T50.A24	T50.A25	T50.A26
and pertussis	T50.A11	T50.A12	T50.A13	T50.A14	T50.A15	T50.A16
influenza	T50.B91	T50.B92	T50.B93	T50.B94	T50.B95	T50.B96
measles	T50.B91	T50.B92	T50.B93	T50.B94	T50.B95	T50.B96
with mumps and rubella	T50.B91	T50.B92	T50.B93	T50.B94	T50.B95	T50.B96
meningococcal	T50.A91	T50.A92	T50.A93	T50.A94	T50.A95	T50.A96
mumps	T50.B91	T50.B92	T50.B93	T50.B94	T50.B95	T50.B96
paratyphoid	T50.A91	T50.A92	T50.A93	T50.A94	T50.A95	T50.A96
pertussis	T50.A11	T50.A12	T50.A13	T50.A14	T50.A15	T50.A16
with diphtheria	T50.A11	T50.A12	T50.A13	T50.A14	T50.A15	T50.A16
and tetanus	T50.A11	T50.A12	T50.A13	T50.A14	T50.A15	T50.A16
plague	T50.A91	T50.A92	T50.A93	T50.A94	T50.A95	T50.A96
poliomyelitis	T50.B91	T50.B92	T50.B93	T50.B94	T50.B95	T50.B96
poliovirus	T50.B91	T50.B92	T50.B93	T50.B94	T50.B95	T50.B96
rabies	T50.B91	T50.B92	T50.B93	T50.B94	T50.B95	T50.B96
respiratory syncytial virus	T50.B91	T50.B92	T50.B93	T50.B94	T50.B95	T50.B96
rickettsial NEC	T50.A91	T50.A92	T50.A93	T50.A94	T50.A95	T50.A96
with						
bacterial component	T50.A21	T50.A22	T50.A23	T50.A24	T50.A25	T50.A26
Rocky Mountain spotted fever	T50.A91	T50.A92	T50.A93	T50.A94	T50.A95	T50.A96
rubella	T50.B91	T50.B92	T50.B93	T50.B94	T50.B95	T50.B96
sabin oral	T50.B91	T50.B92	T50.B93	T50.B94	T50.B95	T50.B96
smallpox	T50.B11	T50.B12	T50.B13	T50.B14	T50.B15	T50.B16
TAB	T50.A91	T50.A92	T50.A93	T50.A94	T50.A95	T50.A96
tetanus	T50.A91	T50.A92	T50.A93	T50.A94	T50.A95	T50.A96

TABLE OF DRUGS AND CHEMICALS

◀ New　◀▥ Revised　~~deleted~~ Deleted

TABLE OF DRUGS AND CHEMICALS

Substance	External Cause (T-Code)					
	Poisoning, Accidental (Unintentional)	Poisoning, Intentional Self-Harm	Poisoning, Assault	Poisoning, Undetermined	Adverse Effect	Underdosing
Vaccine NEC *(Continued)*						
typhoid	T50.A91	T50.A92	T50.A93	T50.A94	T50.A95	T50.A96
typhus	T50.A91	T50.A92	T50.A93	T50.A94	T50.A95	T50.A96
viral NEC	T50.B91	T50.B92	T50.B93	T50.B94	T50.B95	T50.B96
yellow fever	T50.B91	T50.B92	T50.B93	T50.B94	T50.B95	T50.B96
Vaccinia immune globulin	T50.Z11	T50.Z12	T50.Z13	T50.Z14	T50.Z15	T50.Z16
Vaginal contraceptives	T49.8X1	T49.8X2	T49.8X3	T49.8X4	T49.8X5	T49.8X6
Valerian						
root	T42.6X1	T42.6X2	T42.6X3	T42.6X4	T42.6X5	T42.6X6
tincture	T42.6X1	T42.6X2	T42.6X3	T42.6X4	T42.6X5	T42.6X6
Valethamate bromide	T44.3X1	T44.3X2	T44.3X3	T44.3X4	T44.3X5	T44.3X6
Valisone	T49.0X1	T49.0X2	T49.0X3	T49.0X4	T49.0X5	T49.0X6
Valium	T42.4X1	T42.4X2	T42.4X3	T42.4X4	T42.4X5	T42.4X6
Valmid	T42.6X1	T42.6X2	T42.6X3	T42.6X4	T42.6X5	T42.6X6
Valnoctamide	T42.6X1	T42.6X2	T42.6X3	T42.6X4	T42.6X5	T42.6X6
Valproate (sodium)	T42.6X1	T42.6X2	T42.6X3	T42.6X4	T42.6X5	T42.6X6
Valproic acid	T42.6X1	T42.6X2	T42.6X3	T42.6X4	T42.6X5	T42.6X6
Valpromide	T42.6X1	T42.6X2	T42.6X3	T42.6X4	T42.6X5	T42.6X6
Vanadium	T56.891	T56.892	T56.893	T56.894	—	—
Vancomycin	T36.8X1	T36.8X2	T36.8X3	T36.8X4	T36.8X5	T36.8X6
Vapor — *see also Gas*	T59.91	T59.92	T59.93	T59.94	—	—
kiln (carbon monoxide)	T58.8X1	T58.8X2	T58.8X3	T58.8X4	—	—
lead — *see lead*						
specified source NEC	T59.891	T59.892	T59.893	T59.894	—	—
Vardenafil	T46.7X1	T46.7X2	T46.7X3	T46.7X4	T46.7X5	T46.7X6
Varicose reduction drug	T46.8X1	T46.8X2	T46.8X3	T46.8X4	T46.8X5	T46.8X6
Varnish	T65.4X1	T65.4X2	T65.4X3	T65.4X4	—	—
cleaner	T52.91	T52.92	T52.93	T52.94	—	—
Vaseline	T49.3X1	T49.3X2	T49.3X3	T49.3X4	T49.3X5	T49.3X6
Vasodilan	T46.7X1	T46.7X2	T46.7X3	T46.7X4	T46.7X5	T46.7X6
Vasodilator						
coronary NEC	T46.3X1	T46.3X2	T46.3X3	T46.3X4	T46.3X5	T46.3X6
peripheral NEC	T46.7X1	T46.7X2	T46.7X3	T46.7X4	T46.7X5	T46.7X6
Vasopressin	T38.891	T38.892	T38.893	T38.894	T38.895	T38.896
Vasopressor drugs	T38.891	T38.892	T38.893	T38.894	T38.895	T38.896
Vecuronium bromide	T48.1X1	T48.1X2	T48.1X3	T48.1X4	T48.1X5	T48.1X6
Vegetable extract, astringent	T49.2X1	T49.2X2	T49.2X3	T49.2X4	T49.2X5	T49.2X6
Venlafaxine	T43.211	T43.212	T43.213	T43.214	T43.215	T43.216

◀ New   ◀ Revised   ~~deleted~~ Deleted

Substance	External Cause (T-Code)					
	Poisoning, Accidental (Unintentional)	Poisoning, Intentional Self-Harm	Poisoning, Assault	Poisoning, Undetermined	Adverse Effect	Underdosing
Venom, venomous (bite) (sting)	T63.91	T63.92	T63.93	T63.94	—	—
amphibian NEC	T63.831	T63.832	T63.833	T63.834	—	—
animal NEC	T63.891	T63.892	T63.893	T63.894	—	—
ant	T63.421	T63.422	T63.423	T63.424	—	—
arthropod NEC	T63.481	T63.482	T63.483	T63.484	—	—
bee	T63.441	T63.442	T63.443	T63.444	—	—
centipede	T63.411	T63.412	T63.413	T63.414	—	—
fish	T63.591	T63.592	T63.593	T63.594	—	—
frog	T63.811	T63.812	T63.813	T63.814	—	—
hornet	T63.451	T63.452	T63.453	T63.454	—	—
insect NEC	T63.481	T63.482	T63.483	T63.484	—	—
lizard	T63.121	T63.122	T63.123	T63.124	—	—
marine						
animals	T63.691	T63.692	T63.693	T63.694	—	—
bluebottle	T63.611	T63.612	T63.613	T63.614	—	—
jellyfish NEC	T63.621	T63.622	T63.623	T63.624	—	—
Portugese Man-o-war	T63.611	T63.612	T63.613	T63.614	—	—
sea anemone	T63.631	T63.632	T63.633	T63.634	—	—
specified NEC	T63.691	T63.692	T63.693	T63.694	—	—
fish	T63.591	T63.592	T63.593	T63.594	—	—
plants	T63.711	T63.712	T63.713	T63.714	—	—
sting ray	T63.511	T63.512	T63.513	T63.514	—	—
millipede (tropical)	T63.411	T63.412	T63.413	T63.414	—	—
plant NEC	T63.791	T63.792	T63.793	T63.794	—	—
marine	T63.711	T63.712	T63.713	T63.714	—	—
reptile	T63.191	T63.192	T63.193	T63.194	—	—
gila monster	T63.111	T63.112	T63.113	T63.114	—	—
lizard NEC	T63.121	T63.122	T63.123	T63.124	—	—
scorpion	T63.2X1	T63.2X2	T63.2X3	T63.2X4	—	—
snake	T63.001	T63.002	T63.003	T63.004	—	—
African NEC	T63.081	T63.082	T63.083	T63.084	—	—
American (North) (South) NEC	T63.061	T63.062	T63.063	T63.064	—	—
Asian	T63.081	T63.082	T63.083	T63.084	—	—
Australian	T63.071	T63.072	T63.073	T63.074	—	—
cobra	T63.041	T63.042	T63.043	T63.044	—	—
coral snake	T63.021	T63.022	T63.023	T63.024	—	—
rattlesnake	T63.011	T63.012	T63.013	T63.014	—	—
specified NEC	T63.091	T63.092	T63.093	T63.094	—	—
taipan	◀ T63.031	T63.032	T63.033	T63.034	—	—

TABLE OF DRUGS AND CHEMICALS

Substance	External Cause (T-Code)					
	Poisoning, Accidental (Unintentional)	Poisoning, Intentional Self-Harm	Poisoning, Assault	Poisoning, Undetermined	Adverse Effect	Underdosing
Venom, venomous *(Continued)*						
specified NEC	T63.891	T63.892	T63.893	T63.894	—	—
spider	T63.301	T63.302	T63.303	T63.304	—	—
black widow	T63.311	T63.312	T63.313	T63.314	—	—
brown recluse	T63.331	T63.332	T63.333	T63.334	—	—
specified NEC	T63.391	T63.392	T63.393	T63.394	—	—
tarantula	T63.321	T63.322	T63.323	T63.324	—	—
sting ray	T63.511	T63.512	T63.513	T63.514	—	—
toad	T63.821	T63.822	T63.823	T63.824	—	—
wasp	T63.461	T63.462	T63.463	T63.464	—	—
Venous sclerosing drug NEC	T46.8X1	T46.8X2	T46.8X3	T46.8X4	T46.8X5	T46.8X6
Ventolin — *see Albuterol*						
Verapamil	T46.1X1	T46.1X2	T46.1X3	T46.1X4	T46.1X5	T46.1X6
Veramon	T42.3X1	T42.3X2	T42.3X3	T42.3X4	T42.3X5	T42.3X6
Veratrine	T46.5X1	T46.5X2	T46.5X3	T46.5X4	T46.5X5	T46.5X6
Veratrum						
album	T62.2X1	T62.2X2	T62.2X3	T62.2X4	—	—
alkaloids	T46.5X1	T46.5X2	T46.5X3	T46.5X4	T46.5X5	T46.5X6
viride	T62.2X1	T62.2X2	T62.2X3	T62.2X4	—	—
Verdigris	T60.3X1	T60.3X2	T60.3X3	T60.3X4	—	—
Veronal	T42.3X1	T42.3X2	T42.3X3	T42.3X4	T42.3X5	T42.3X6
Veroxil	T37.4X1	T37.4X2	T37.4X3	T37.4X4	T37.4X5	T37.4X6
Versenate	T50.6X1	T50.6X2	T50.6X3	T50.6X4	T50.6X5	T50.6X6
Versidyne	T39.8X1	T39.8X2	T39.8X3	T39.8X4	T39.8X5	T39.8X6
Vetrabutine	T48.0X1	T48.0X2	T48.0X3	T48.0X4	T48.0X5	T48.0X6
Vidarabine	T37.5X1	T37.5X2	T37.5X3	T37.5X4	T37.5X5	T37.5X6
Vienna						
green	T57.0X1	T57.0X2	T57.0X3	T57.0X4	—	—
insecticide	T60.2X1	T60.2X2	T60.2X3	T60.2X4	—	—
red	T57.0X1	T57.0X2	T57.0X3	T57.0X4	—	—
pharmaceutical dye	T50.991	T50.992	T50.993	T50.994	T50.995	T50.996
Vigabatrin	T42.6X1	T42.6X2	T42.6X3	T42.6X4	T42.6X5	T42.6X6
Viloxazine	T43.291	T43.292	T43.293	T43.294	T43.295	T43.296
Viminol	T39.8X1	T39.8X2	T39.8X3	T39.8X4	T39.8X5	T39.8X6
Vinbarbital, vinbarbitone	T42.3X1	T42.3X2	T42.3X3	T42.3X4	T42.3X5	T42.3X6
Vinblastine	T45.1X1	T45.1X2	T45.1X3	T45.1X4	T45.1X5	T45.1X6
Vinburnine	T46.7X1	T46.7X2	T46.7X3	T46.7X4	T46.7X5	T46.7X6
Vincamine	T45.1X1	T45.1X2	T45.1X3	T45.1X4	T45.1X5	T45.1X6
Vincristine	T45.1X1	T45.1X2	T45.1X3	T45.1X4	T45.1X5	T45.1X6
Vindesine	T45.1X1	T45.1X2	T45.1X3	T45.1X4	T45.1X5	T45.1X6

◄ New ◀▦ Revised ~~deleted~~ Deleted

Substance	Poisoning, Accidental (Unintentional)	Poisoning, Intentional Self-Harm	Poisoning, Assault	Poisoning, Undetermined	Adverse Effect	Underdosing
			External Cause (T-Code)			
Vinesthene, vinethene	T41.0X1	T41.0X2	T41.0X3	T41.0X4	T41.0X5	T41.0X6
Vinorelbine tartrate	T45.1X1	T45.1X2	T45.1X3	T45.1X4	T45.1X5	T45.1X6
Vinpocetine	T46.7X1	T46.7X2	T46.7X3	T46.7X4	T46.7X5	T46.7X6
Vinyl						
acetate	T65.891	T65.892	T65.893	T65.894	—	—
bital	T42.3X1	T42.3X2	T42.3X3	T42.3X4	T42.3X5	T42.3X6
bromide	T65.891	T65.892	T65.893	T65.894	—	—
chloride	T59.891	T59.892	T59.893	T59.894	—	—
ether	T41.0X1	T41.0X2	T41.0X3	T41.0X4	T41.0X5	T41.0X6
Vinylbital	T42.3X1	T42.3X2	T42.3X3	T42.3X4	T42.3X5	T42.3X6
Vinylidene chloride	T65.891	T65.892	T65.893	T65.894	—	—
Vioform	T37.8X1	T37.8X2	T37.8X3	T37.8X4	T37.8X5	T37.8X6
topical	T49.0X1	T49.0X2	T49.0X3	T49.0X4	T49.0X5	T49.0X6
Viomycin	T36.8X1	T36.8X2	T36.8X3	T36.8X4	T36.8X5	T36.8X6
Viosterol	T45.2X1	T45.2X2	T45.2X3	T45.2X4	T45.2X5	T45.2X6
Viper (venom)	T63.091	T63.092	T63.093	T63.094	—	—
Viprynium	T37.4X1	T37.4X2	T37.4X3	T37.4X4	T37.4X5	T37.4X6
Viquidil	T46.7X1	T46.7X2	T46.7X3	T46.7X4	T46.7X5	T46.7X6
Viral vaccine NEC	T50.B91	T50.B92	T50.B93	T50.B94	T50.B95	T50.B96
Virginiamycin	T36.8X1	T36.8X2	T36.8X3	T36.8X4	T36.8X5	T36.8X6
Virugon	T37.5X1	T37.5X2	T37.5X3	T37.5X4	T37.5X5	T37.5X6
Viscous agent	T50.901	T50.902	T50.903	T50.904	T50.905	T50.906
Visine	T49.5X1	T49.5X2	T49.5X3	T49.5X4	T49.5X5	T49.5X6
Visnadine	T46.3X1	T46.3X2	T46.3X3	T46.3X4	T46.3X5	T46.3X6
Vitamin NEC	T45.2X1	T45.2X2	T45.2X3	T45.2X4	T45.2X5	T45.2X6
A	T45.2X1	T45.2X2	T45.2X3	T45.2X4	T45.2X5	T45.2X6
B NEC	T45.2X1	T45.2X2	T45.2X3	T45.2X4	T45.2X5	T45.2X6
nicotinic acid	T46.7X1	T46.7X2	T46.7X3	T46.7X4	T46.7X5	T46.7X6
B1	T45.2X1	T45.2X2	T45.2X3	T45.2X4	T45.2X5	T45.2X6
B2	T45.2X1	T45.2X2	T45.2X3	T45.2X4	T45.2X5	T45.2X6
B6	T45.2X1	T45.2X2	T45.2X3	T45.2X4	T45.2X5	T45.2X6
B12	T45.2X1	T45.2X2	T45.2X3	T45.2X4	T45.2X5	T45.2X6
B15	T45.2X1	T45.2X2	T45.2X3	T45.2X4	T45.2X5	T45.2X6
C	T45.2X1	T45.2X2	T45.2X3	T45.2X4	T45.2X5	T45.2X6
D	T45.2X1	T45.2X2	T45.2X3	T45.2X4	T45.2X5	T45.2X6
D2	T45.2X1	T45.2X2	T45.2X3	T45.2X4	T45.2X5	T45.2X6
D3	T45.2X1	T45.2X2	T45.2X3	T45.2X4	T45.2X5	T45.2X6
E	T45.2X1	T45.2X2	T45.2X3	T45.2X4	T45.2X5	T45.2X6
E acetate	T45.2X1	T45.2X2	T45.2X3	T45.2X4	T45.2X5	T45.2X6
hematopoietic	T45.8X1	T45.8X2	T45.8X3	T45.8X4	T45.8X5	T45.8X6

TABLE OF DRUGS AND CHEMICALS

Substance	External Cause (T-Code)					
	Poisoning, Accidental (Unintentional)	Poisoning, Intentional Self-Harm	Poisoning, Assault	Poisoning, Undetermined	Adverse Effect	Underdosing
Vitamin NEC *(Continued)*						
K NEC	T45.7X1	T45.7X2	T45.7X3	T45.7X4	T45.7X5	T45.7X6
K1	T45.7X1	T45.7X2	T45.7X3	T45.7X4	T45.7X5	T45.7X6
K2	T45.7X1	T45.7X2	T45.7X3	T45.7X4	T45.7X5	T45.7X6
PP	T45.2X1	T45.2X2	T45.2X3	T45.2X4	T45.2X5	T45.2X6
ulceroprotectant	T47.1X1	T47.1X2	T47.1X3	T47.1X4	T47.1X5	T47.1X6
Vleminckx's solution	T49.4X1	T49.4X2	T49.4X3	T49.4X4	T49.4X5	T49.4X6
Voltaren — *see Diclofenac sodium*						
W						
Warfarin	T45.511	T45.512	T45.513	T45.514	T45.515	T45.516
rodenticide	T60.4X1	T60.4X2	T60.4X3	T60.4X4	—	—
sodium	T60.4X1	T60.4X2	T60.4X3	T60.4X4	—	—
Wasp (sting)	T63.461	T63.462	T63.463	T63.464	—	—
Water						
balance drug	T50.3X1	T50.3X2	T50.3X3	T50.3X4	T50.3X5	T50.3X6
distilled	T50.3X1	T50.3X2	T50.3X3	T50.3X4	T50.3X5	T50.3X6
gas — *see Gas, water*						
incomplete combustion of — *see Carbon, monoxide, fuel, utility*						
hemlock	T62.2X1	T62.2X2	T62.2X3	T62.2X4	—	—
moccasin (venom)	T63.061	T63.062	T63.063	T63.064	—	—
purified	T50.3X1	T50.3X2	T50.3X3	T50.3X4	T50.3X5	T50.3X6
Wax (paraffin) (petroleum)	T52.0X1	T52.0X2	T52.0X3	T52.0X4	—	—
automobile	T65.891	T65.892	T65.893	T65.894	—	—
floor	T52.0X1	T52.0X2	T52.0X3	T52.0X4	—	—
Weed killers NEC	T60.3X1	T60.3X2	T60.3X3	T60.3X4	—	—
Welldorm	T42.6X1	T42.6X2	T42.6X3	T42.6X4	T42.6X5	T42.6X6
White						
arsenic	T57.0X1	T57.0X2	T57.0X3	T57.0X4	—	—
hellebore	T62.2X1	T62.2X2	T62.2X3	T62.2X4	—	—
lotion (keratolytic)	T49.4X1	T49.4X2	T49.4X3	T49.4X4	T49.4X5	T49.4X6
spirit	T52.0X1	T52.0X2	T52.0X3	T52.0X4	—	—
Whitewash	T65.891	T65.892	T65.893	T65.894	—	—
Whole blood (human)	T45.8X1	T45.8X2	T45.8X3	T45.8X4	T45.8X5	T45.8X6
Wild						
black cherry	T62.2X1	T62.2X2	T62.2X3	T62.2X4	—	—
poisonous plants NEC	T62.2X1	T62.2X2	T62.2X3	T62.2X4	—	—
Window cleaning fluid	T65.891	T65.892	T65.893	T65.894	—	—
Wintergreen (oil)	T49.3X1	T49.3X2	T49.3X3	T49.3X4	T49.3X5	T49.3X6

◀ New   ◀║ Revised   ~~deleted~~ Deleted

Substance	External Cause (T-Code)					
	Poisoning, Accidental (Unintentional)	Poisoning, Intentional Self-Harm	Poisoning, Assault	Poisoning, Undetermined	Adverse Effect	Underdosing
Wisterine	T62.2X1	T62.2X2	T62.2X3	T62.2X4	—	—
Witch hazel	T49.2X1	T49.2X2	T49.2X3	T49.2X4	T49.2X5	T49.2X6
Wood alcohol or spirit	T51.1X1	T51.1X2	T51.1X3	T51.1X4	—	—
Wool fat (hydrous)	T49.3X1	T49.3X2	T49.3X3	T49.3X4	T49.3X5	T49.3X6
Woorali	T48.1X1	T48.1X2	T48.1X3	T48.1X4	T48.1X5	T48.1X6
Wormseed, American	T37.4X1	T37.4X2	T37.4X3	T37.4X4	T37.4X5	T37.4X6
X						
Xamoterol	T44.5X1	T44.5X2	T44.5X3	T44.5X4	T44.5X5	T44.5X6
Xanthine diuretics	T50.2X1	T50.2X2	T50.2X3	T50.2X4	T50.2X5	T50.2X6
Xanthinol nicotinate	T46.7X1	T46.7X2	T46.7X3	T46.7X4	T46.7X5	T46.7X6
Xanthotoxin	T49.3X1	T49.3X2	T49.3X3	T49.3X4	T49.3X5	T49.3X6
Xantinol nicotinate	T46.7X1	T46.7X2	T46.7X3	T46.7X4	T46.7X5	T46.7X6
Xantocillin	T36.0X1	T36.0X2	T36.0X3	T36.0X4	T36.0X5	T36.0X6
Xenon (127Xe) (133Xe)	T50.8X1	T50.8X2	T50.8X3	T50.8X4	T50.8X5	T50.8X6
Xenysalate	T49.4X1	T49.4X2	T49.4X3	T49.4X4	T49.4X5	T49.4X6
Xibornol	T37.8X1	T37.8X2	T37.8X3	T37.8X4	T37.8X5	T37.8X6
Xigris	T45.511	T45.512	T45.513	T45.514	T45.515	T45.516
Xipamide	T50.2X1	T50.2X2	T50.2X3	T50.2X4	T50.2X5	T50.2X6
Xylene (vapor)	T52.2X1	T52.2X2	T52.2X3	T52.2X4	—	—
Xylocaine (infiltration) (topical)	T41.3X1	T41.3X2	T41.3X3	T41.3X4	T41.3X5	T41.3X6
nerve block (peripheral) (plexus)	T41.3X1	T41.3X2	T41.3X3	T41.3X4	T41.3X5	T41.3X6
spinal	T41.3X1	T41.3X2	T41.3X3	T41.3X4	T41.3X5	T41.3X6
Xylol (vapor)	T52.2X1	T52.2X2	T52.2X3	T52.2X4	—	—
Xylometazoline	T48.5X1	T48.5X2	T48.5X3	T48.5X4	T48.5X5	T48.5X6
Y						
Yeast	T45.2X1	T45.2X2	T45.2X3	T45.2X4	T45.2X5	T45.2X6
dried	T45.2X1	T45.2X2	T45.2X3	T45.2X4	T45.2X5	T45.2X6
Yellow						
fever vaccine	T50.B91	T50.B92	T50.B93	T50.B94	T50.B95	T50.B96
jasmine	T62.2X1	T62.2X2	T62.2X3	T62.2X4	—	—
phenolphthalein	T47.2X1	T47.2X2	T47.2X3	T47.2X4	T47.2X5	T47.2X6
Yew	T62.2X1	T62.2X2	T62.2X3	T62.2X4	—	—
Yohimbic acid	T40.991	T40.992	T40.993	T40.994	T40.995	T40.996
Z						
Zactane	T39.8X1	T39.8X2	T39.8X3	T39.8X4	T39.8X5	T39.8X6
Zalcitabine	T37.5X1	T37.5X2	T37.5X3	T37.5X4	T37.5X5	T37.5X6
Zaroxolyn	T50.2X1	T50.2X2	T50.2X3	T50.2X4	T50.2X5	T50.2X6

◀ New ◀▥ Revised ~~deleted~~ Deleted

TABLE OF DRUGS AND CHEMICALS

TABLE OF DRUGS AND CHEMICALS

	External Cause (T-Code)					
Substance	Poisoning, Accidental (Unintentional)	Poisoning, Intentional Self-Harm	Poisoning, Assault	Poisoning, Undetermined	Adverse Effect	Underdosing
Zephiran (topical)	T49.0X1	T49.0X2	T49.0X3	T49.0X4	T49.0X5	T49.0X6
ophthalmic preparation	T49.5X1	T49.5X2	T49.5X3	T49.5X4	T49.5X5	T49.5X6
Zeranol	T38.7X1	T38.7X2	T38.7X3	T38.7X4	T38.7X5	T38.7X6
Zerone	T51.1X1	T51.1X2	T51.1X3	T51.1X4	—	—
Zidovudine	T37.5X1	T37.5X2	T37.5X3	T37.5X4	T37.5X5	T37.5X6
Zimeldine	T43.221	T43.222	T43.223	T43.224	T43.225	T43.226
Zinc (compounds) (fumes) (vapor) NEC	T56.5X1	T56.5X2	T56.5X3	T56.5X4	—	—
anti-infectives	T49.0X1	T49.0X2	T49.0X3	T49.0X4	T49.0X5	T49.0X6
antivaricose	T46.8X1	T46.8X2	T46.8X3	T46.8X4	T46.8X5	T46.8X6
bacitracin	T49.0X1	T49.0X2	T49.0X3	T49.0X4	T49.0X5	T49.0X6
chloride (mouthwash)	T49.6X1	T49.6X2	T49.6X3	T49.6X4	T49.6X5	T49.6X6
chromate	T56.5X1	T56.5X2	T56.5X3	T56.5X4	—	—
gelatin	T49.3X1	T49.3X2	T49.3X3	T49.3X4	T49.3X5	T49.3X6
oxide	T49.3X1	T49.3X2	T49.3X3	T49.3X4	T49.3X5	T49.3X6
plaster	T49.3X1	T49.3X2	T49.3X3	T49.3X4	T49.3X5	T49.3X6
peroxide	T49.0X1	T49.0X2	T49.0X3	T49.0X4	T49.0X5	T49.0X6
pesticides	T56.5X1	T56.5X2	T56.5X3	T56.5X4	—	—
phosphide	T60.4X1	T60.4X2	T60.4X3	T60.4X4	—	—
pyrithionate	T49.4X1	T49.4X2	T49.4X3	T49.4X4	T49.4X5	T49.4X6
stearate	T49.3X1	T49.3X2	T49.3X3	T49.3X4	T49.3X5	T49.3X6
sulfate	T49.5X1	T49.5X2	T49.5X3	T49.5X4	T49.5X5	T49.5X6
ENT agent	T49.6X1	T49.6X2	T49.6X3	T49.6X4	T49.6X5	T49.6X6
ophthalmic solution	T49.5X1	T49.5X2	T49.5X3	T49.5X4	T49.5X5	T49.5X6
topical NEC	T49.0X1	T49.0X2	T49.0X3	T49.0X4	T49.0X5	T49.0X6
undecylenate	T49.0X1	T49.0X2	T49.0X3	T49.0X4	T49.0X5	T49.0X6
Zineb	T60.0X1	T60.0X2	T60.0X3	T60.0X4	—	—
Zinostatin	T45.1X1	T45.1X2	T45.1X3	T45.1X4	T45.1X5	T45.1X6
Zipeprol	T48.3X1	T48.3X2	T48.3X3	T48.3X4	T48.3X5	T48.3X6
Zofenopril	T46.4X1	T46.4X2	T46.4X3	T46.4X4	T46.4X5	T46.4X6
Zolpidem	T42.6X1	T42.6X2	T42.6X3	T42.6X4	T42.6X5	T42.6X6
Zomepirac	T39.391	T39.392	T39.393	T39.394	T39.395	T39.396
Zopiclone	T42.6X1	T42.6X2	T42.6X3	T42.6X4	T42.6X5	T42.6X6
Zorubicin	T45.1X1	T45.1X2	T45.1X3	T45.1X4	T45.1X5	T45.1X6
Zotepine	T43.591	T43.592	T43.593	T43.594	T43.595	T43.596
Zovant	T45.511	T45.512	T45.513	T45.514	T45.515	T45.516
Zoxazolamine	T42.8X1	T42.8X2	T42.8X3	T42.8X4	T42.8X5	T42.8X6
Zuclopenthixol	T43.4X1	T43.4X2	T43.4X3	T43.4X4	T43.4X5	T43.4X6
Zygadenus (venenosus)	T62.2X1	T62.2X2	T62.2X3	T62.2X4	—	—
Zyprexa	T43.591	T43.592	T43.593	T43.594	T43.595	T43.596

◀ New   ◀▥ Revised   ~~deleted~~ Deleted

External Cause
of Injuries Index

A

Abandonment (causing exposure to weather conditions) (with intent to injure or kill) NEC X58

Abuse (adult) (child) (mental) (physical) (sexual) X58

Accident (to) X58
  aircraft (in transit) (powered) —*see also* Accident, transport, aircraft
    due to, caused by cataclysm —*see* Forces of nature, by type
  animal-drawn vehicle —*see* Accident, transport, animal-drawn vehicle occupant
  animal-rider —*see* Accident, transport, animal-rider
  automobile —*see* Accident, transport, car occupant
  bare foot water skiier V94.4
  boat, boating —*see also* Accident, watercraft
    striking swimmer
      powered V94.11
      unpowered V94.12
  bus —*see* Accident, transport, bus occupant
  cable car, not on rails V98.0
    on rails —*see* Accident, transport, streetcar occupant
  car —*see* Accident, transport, car occupant
  caused by, due to
    animal NEC W64
    chain hoist W24.0
    cold (excessive) —*see* Exposure, cold
    corrosive liquid, substance —*see* Table of Drugs and Chemicals
    cutting or piercing instrument —*see* Contact, with, by type of instrument
    drive belt W24.0
    electric
      current —*see* Exposure, electric current
        motor (*see also* Contact, with, by type of machine) W31.3
        current (of) W86.8
    environmental factor NEC X58
    explosive material —*see* Explosion
    fire, flames —*see* Exposure, fire
    firearm missile —*see* Discharge, firearm by type
    heat (excessive) —*see* Heat
    hot —*see* Contact, with, hot
    ignition —*see* Ignition
    lifting device W24.0
    lightning —*see* subcategory T75.0
      causing fire —*see* Exposure, fire
    machine, machinery —*see* Contact, with, by type of machine
    natural factor NEC X58
    pulley (block) W24.0
    radiation —*see* Radiation
    steam X13.1
      inhalation X13.0
      pipe X16
    thunderbolt —*see* subcategory T75.0
      causing fire —*see* Exposure, fire
    transmission device W24.1
  coach —*see* Accident, transport, bus occupant
  coal car —*see* Accident, transport, industrial vehicle occupant
  diving —*see also* Fall, into, water
    with
      drowning or submersion —*see* Drowning
  forklift —*see* Accident, transport, industrial vehicle occupant
  heavy transport vehicle NOS —*see* Accident, transport, truck occupant
  ice yacht V98.2

Accident (*Continued*)
  in
    medical, surgical procedure
      as, or due to misadventure —*see* Misadventure
      causing an abnormal reaction or later complication without mention of misadventure (*see also* Complication of or following, by type of procedure) Y84.9
  land yacht V98.1
  late effect of —*see* W00-X58 with 7th character S
  logging car —*see* Accident, transport, industrial vehicle occupant
  machine, machinery —*see also* Contact, with, by type of machine
    on board watercraft V93.69
      explosion —*see* Explosion, in, watercraft
      fire —*see* Burn, on board watercraft
      powered craft V93.63
        ferry boat V93.61
        fishing boat V93.62
        jetskis V93.63
        liner V93.61
        merchant ship V93.60
        passenger ship V93.61
        sailboat V93.64
  mine tram —*see* Accident, transport, industrial vehicle occupant
  mobility scooter (motorized) —*see* Accident, transport, pedestrian, conveyance, specified type NEC
  motor scooter —*see* Accident, transport, motorcyclist
  motor vehicle NOS (traffic) (*see also* Accident, transport) V89.2
    nontraffic V89.0
    three-wheeled NOS —*see* Accident, transport, three-wheeled motor vehicle occupant
  motorcycle NOS —*see* Accident, transport, motorcyclist
  nonmotor vehicle NOS (nontraffic) (*see also* Accident, transport) V89.1
    traffic NOS V89.3
  nontraffic (victim's mode of transport NOS) V88.9
    collision (between) V88.7
      bus and truck V88.5
      car and:
        bus V88.3
        pickup V88.2
        three-wheeled motor vehicle V88.0
        train V88.6
        truck V88.4
        two-wheeled motor vehicle V88.0
        van V88.2
      specified vehicle NEC and:
        three-wheeled motor vehicle V88.1
        two-wheeled motor vehicle V88.1
    known mode of transport —*see* Accident, transport, by type of vehicle
    noncollision V88.8
  on board watercraft V93.89
    powered craft V93.83
      ferry boat V93.81
      fishing boat V93.82
      jetskis V93.83
      liner V93.81
      merchant ship V93.80
      passenger ship V93.81
    unpowered craft V93.88
      canoe V93.85
      inflatable V93.86
        in tow
          recreational V94.31
          specified NEC V94.32
      kayak V93.85

Accident (*Continued*)
  on board watercraft (*Continued*)
    unpowered craft (*Continued*)
      sailboat V93.84
      surf-board V93.88
      water skis V93.87
      windsurfer V93.88
  parachutist V97.29
    entangled in object V97.21
    injured on landing V97.22
  pedal cycle —*see* Accident, transport, pedal cyclist
  pedestrian (on foot)
    with
      another pedestrian W51
        with fall W03
          due to ice or snow W00.0
          on pedestrian conveyance NEC V00.09
      roller skater (in-line) V00.01
      skate boarder V00.02
      transport vehicle —*see* Accident, transport
    on pedestrian conveyance —*see* Accident, transport, pedestrian, conveyance
  pick-up truck or van —*see* Accident, transport, pickup truck occupant
  quarry truck —*see* Accident, transport, industrial vehicle occupant
  railway vehicle (any) (in motion) —*see* Accident, transport, railway vehicle occupant
    due to cataclysm —*see* Forces of nature, by type
  scooter (non-motorized) —*see* Accident, transport, pedestrian, conveyance, scooter
  sequelae of —*see* W00-X58 with 7th character S
  skateboard —*see* Accident, transport, pedestrian, conveyance, skateboard
  ski (ing) —*see* Accident, transport, pedestrian, conveyance
    lift V98.3
  specified cause NEC X58
  streetcar —*see* Accident, transport, streetcar occupant
  traffic (victim's mode of transport NOS) V87.9
    collision (between) V87.7
      bus and truck V87.5
      car and:
        bus V87.3
        pickup V87.2
        three-wheeled motor vehicle V87.0
        train V87.6
        truck V87.4
        two-wheeled motor vehicle V87.0
        van V87.2
      specified vehicle NEC and:
        three-wheeled motor vehicle V87.1
        two-wheeled motor vehicle V87.1
    known mode of transport —*see* Accident, transport, by type of vehicle
    noncollision V87.8
  transport (involving injury to) V99
    18 wheeler —*see* Accident, transport, truck occupant
    agricultural vehicle occupant (nontraffic) V84.9
      driver V84.5
      hanger-on V84.7
      passenger V84.6
      traffic V84.3
        driver V84.0
        hanger-on V84.2
        passenger V84.1
      while boarding or alighting V84.4

Accident (Continued)
  transport (Continued)
    aircraft NEC V97.89
      military NEC V97.818
        with civilian aircraft V97.810
        civilian injured by V97.811
      occupant injured (in)
        nonpowered craft accident
          V96.9
          balloon V96.00
            collision V96.03
            crash V96.01
            explosion V96.05
            fire V96.04
            forced landing V96.02
            specified type NEC V96.09
          glider V96.20
            collision V96.23
            crash V96.21
            explosion V96.25
            fire V96.24
            forced landing V96.22
            specified type NEC V96.29
          hang glider V96.10
            collision V96.13
            crash V96.11
            explosion V96.15
            fire V96.14
            forced landing V96.12
            specified type NEC V96.19
         specified craft NEC V96.8
        powered craft accident V95.9
          fixed wing NEC
            commercial V95.30
              collision V95.33
              crash V95.31
              explosion V95.35
              fire V95.34
              forced landing V95.32
              specified type NEC
                V95.39
            private V95.20
              collision V95.23
              crash V95.21
              explosion V95.25
              fire V95.24
              forced landing V95.22
              specified type NEC
                V95.29
          glider V95.10
            collision V95.13
            crash V95.11
            explosion V95.15
            fire V95.14
            forced landing V95.12
            specified type NEC V95.19
          helicopter V95.00
            collision V95.03
            crash V95.01
            explosion V95.05
            fire V95.04
            forced landing V95.02
            specified type NEC V95.09
          spacecraft V95.40
            collision V95.43
            crash V95.41
            explosion V95.45
            fire V95.44
            forced landing V95.42
            specified type NEC V95.49
         specified craft NEC V95.8
        ultralight V95.10
          collision V95.13
          crash V95.11
          explosion V95.15
          fire V95.14
          forced landing V95.12
          specified type NEC V95.19
      specified accident NEC V97.0
      while boarding or alighting
        V97.1

Accident (Continued)
  transport (Continued)
    aircraft NEC (Continued)
      person (injured by)
        falling from, in or on aircraft V97.0
        machinery on aircraft V97.89
        on ground with aircraft involvement
          V97.39
        rotating propeller V97.32
        struck by object falling from aircraft
          V97.31
        sucked into aircraft jet V97.33
        while boarding or alighting aircraft
          V97.1
    airport (battery-powered) passenger
      vehicle —see Accident, transport,
      industrial vehicle occupant
    all-terrain vehicle occupant (nontraffic)
      V86.99
      driver V86.59
      dune buggy —see Accident, transport,
        dune buggy occupant
      hanger-on V86.79
      passenger V86.69
      snowmobile —see Accident, transport,
        snowmobile occupant
      traffic V86.39
        driver V86.09
        hanger-on V86.29
        passenger V86.19
      while boarding or alighting V86.49
    ambulance occupant (traffic) V86.31
      driver V86.01
      hanger-on V86.21
      nontraffic V86.91
        driver V86.51
        hanger-on V86.71
        passenger V86.61
      passenger V86.11
      while boarding or alighting V86.41
    animal-drawn vehicle occupant (in)
      V80.929
      collision (with)
        animal V80.12
          being ridden V80.711
        animal-drawn vehicle V80.721
        bus V80.42
        car V80.42
        fixed or stationary object V80.82
        military vehicle V80.920
        nonmotor vehicle V80.791
        pedal cycle V80.22
        pedestrian V80.12
        pickup V80.42
        railway train or vehicle V80.62
        specified motor vehicle NEC V80.52
        streetcar V80.731
        truck V80.42
        two-or three-wheeled motor vehicle
          V80.32
        van V80.42
      noncollision V80.02
      specified circumstance NEC V80. 928
    animal-rider V80.919
      collision (with)
        animal V80.11
          being ridden V80.710
        animal-drawn vehicle V80.720
        bus V80.41
        car V80.41
        fixed or stationary object V80.81
        military vehicle V80.910
        nonmotor vehicle V80.790
        pedal cycle V80.21
        pedestrian V80.11
        pickup V80.41
        railway train or vehicle V80.61
        specified motor vehicle NEC
          V80.51
        streetcar V80.730
        truck V80.41

Accident (Continued)
  transport (Continued)
    animal-rider (Continued)
      collision (Continued)
        two- or three-wheeled motor vehicle
          V80.31
        van V80.41
      noncollision V80.018
        specified as horse rider V80.010
      specified circumstance NEC V80.918
    armored car —see Accident, transport,
      truck occupant
    battery-powered truck (baggage) (mail) —
      see Accident, transport, industrial
      vehicle occupant
    bus occupant V79.9
      collision (with)
        animal (traffic) V70.9
          being ridden (traffic) V76.9
            nontraffic V76.3
            while boarding or alighting V76.4
          nontraffic V70.3
          while boarding or alighting V70.4
        animal-drawn vehicle (traffic) V76.9
          nontraffic V76.3
          while boarding or alighting V76.4
        bus (traffic) V74.9
          nontraffic V74.3
          while boarding or alighting V74.4
        car (traffic) V73.9
          nontraffic V73.3
          while boarding or alighting V73.4
        motor vehicle NOS (traffic) V79.60
          nontraffic V79.20
          specified type NEC (traffic) V79.69
            nontraffic V79.29
        pedal cycle (traffic) V71.9
          nontraffic V71.3
          while boarding or alighting V71.4
        pickup truck (traffic) V73.9
          nontraffic V73.3
          while boarding or alighting V73.4
        railway vehicle (traffic) V75.9
          nontraffic V75.3
          while boarding or alighting V75.4
        specified vehicle NEC (traffic) V76.9
          nontraffic V76.3
          while boarding or alighting V76.4
        stationary object (traffic) V77.9
          nontraffic V77.3
          while boarding or alighting V77.4
        streetcar (traffic) V76.9
          nontraffic V76.3
          while boarding or alighting V76.4
        three wheeled motor vehicle (traffic)
          V72.9
          nontraffic V72.3
          while boarding or alighting V72.4
        truck (traffic) V74.9
          nontraffic V74.3
          while boarding or alighting V74.4
        two wheeled motor vehicle (traffic)
          V72.9
          nontraffic V72.3
          while boarding or alighting V72.4
        van (traffic) V73.9
          nontraffic V73.3
          while boarding or alighting V73.4
      driver
        collision (with)
          animal (traffic) V70.5
            being ridden (traffic) V76.5
              nontraffic V76.0
            nontraffic V70.0
          animal-drawn vehicle (traffic)
            V76.5
            nontraffic V76.0
          bus (traffic) V74.5
            nontraffic V74.0
          car (traffic) V73.5
            nontraffic V73.0

Accident (Continued)
 transport (Continued)
  bus occupant (Continued)
   driver (Continued)
    collision (Continued)
     motor vehicle NOS (traffic) V79.40
      nontraffic V79.00
     specified type NEC (traffic)
       V79.49
      nontraffic V79.09
     pedal cycle (traffic) V71.5
      nontraffic V71.0
     pickup truck (traffic) V73.5
      nontraffic V73.0
     railway vehicle (traffic) V75.5
      nontraffic V75.0
     specified vehicle NEC (traffic)
       V76.5
      nontraffic V76.0
     stationary object (traffic) V77.5
      nontraffic V77.0
     streetcar (traffic) V76.5
      nontraffic V76.0
     three wheeled motor vehicle
       (traffic) V72.5
      nontraffic V72.0
     truck (traffic) V74.5
      nontraffic V74.0
     two wheeled motor vehicle (traffic)
       V72.5
      nontraffic V72.0
     van (traffic) V73.5
      nontraffic V73.0
    noncollision accident (traffic) V78.5
     nontraffic V78.0
   hanger-on
    collision (with)
     animal (traffic) V70.7
      being ridden (traffic) V76.7
       nontraffic V76.2
      nontraffic V70.2
     animal-drawn vehicle (traffic) V76.7
      nontraffic V76.2
     bus (traffic) V74.7
      nontraffic V74.2
     car (traffic) V73.7
      nontraffic V73.2
     pedal cycle (traffic) V71.7
      nontraffic V71.2
     pickup truck (traffic) V73.7
      nontraffic V73.2
     railway vehicle (traffic) V75.7
      nontraffic V75.2
     specified vehicle NEC (traffic) V76.7
      nontraffic V76.2
     stationary object (traffic) V77.7
      nontraffic V77.2
     streetcar (traffic) V76.7
      nontraffic V76.2
     three wheeled motor vehicle
       (traffic) V72.7
      nontraffic V72.2
     truck (traffic) V74.7
      nontraffic V74.2
     two wheeled motor vehicle (traffic)
       V72.7
      nontraffic V72.2
     van (traffic) V73.7
      nontraffic V73.2
    noncollision accident (traffic) V78.7
     nontraffic V78.2
   noncollision accident (traffic) V78.9
    nontraffic V78.3
    while boarding or alighting V78.4
   nontraffic V79.3
   passenger
    collision (with)
     animal (traffic) V70.6
      being ridden (traffic) V76.6
       nontraffic V76.1
      nontraffic V70.1

Accident (Continued)
 transport (Continued)
  bus occupant (Continued)
   passenger (Continued)
    collision (Continued)
     animal-drawn vehicle (traffic) V76.6
      nontraffic V76.1
     bus (traffic) V74.6
      nontraffic V74.1
     car (traffic) V73.6
      nontraffic V73.1
     motor vehicle NOS (traffic) V79.50
      nontraffic V79.10
     specified type NEC (traffic)
       V79.59
      nontraffic V79.19
     pedal cycle (traffic) V71.6
      nontraffic V71.1
     pickup truck (traffic) V73.6
      nontraffic V73.1
     railway vehicle (traffic) V75.6
      nontraffic V75.1
     specified vehicle NEC (traffic) V76.6
      nontraffic V76.1
     stationary object (traffic) V77.6
      nontraffic V77.1
     streetcar (traffic) V76.6
      nontraffic V76.1
     three wheeled motor vehicle
       (traffic) V72.6
      nontraffic V72.1
     truck (traffic) V74.6
      nontraffic V74.1
     two wheeled motor vehicle (traffic)
       V72.6
      nontraffic V72.1
     van (traffic) V73.6
      nontraffic V73.1
    noncollision accident (traffic) V78.6
     nontraffic V78.1
    specified type NEC V79.88
    military vehicle V79.81
  cable car, not on rails V98.0
   on rails —see Accident, transport,
     streetcar occupant
  car occupant V49.9
   ambulance occupant —see Accident,
     transport, ambulance occupant
   collision (with)
    animal (traffic) V40.9
     being ridden (traffic) V46.9
      nontraffic V46.3
      while boarding or alighting
        V46.4
     nontraffic V40.3
     while boarding or alighting V40.4
    animal-drawn vehicle (traffic) V46.9
     nontraffic V46.3
     while boarding or alighting V46.4
    bus (traffic) V44.9
     nontraffic V44.3
     while boarding or alighting V44.4
    car (traffic) V43.92
     nontraffic V43.32
     while boarding or alighting V43.42
    motor vehicle NOS (traffic) V49.60
     nontraffic V49.20
     specified type NEC (traffic) V49.69
      nontraffic V49.29
    pedal cycle (traffic) V41.9
     nontraffic V41.3
     while boarding or alighting V41.4
    pickup truck (traffic) V43.93
     nontraffic V43.33
     while boarding or alighting V43.43
    railway vehicle (traffic) V45.9
     nontraffic V45.3
     while boarding or alighting V45.4
    specified vehicle NEC (traffic) V46.9
     nontraffic V46.3
     while boarding or alighting V46.4

Accident (Continued)
 transport (Continued)
  car occupant (Continued)
   collision (Continued)
    sport utility vehicle (traffic) V43.91
     nontraffic V43.31
     while boarding or alighting V43.41
    stationary object (traffic) V47.92
     nontraffic V47.32
     while boarding or alighting V47.4
    streetcar (traffic) V46.9
     nontraffic V46.3
     while boarding or alighting V46.4
    three wheeled motor vehicle (traffic)
       V42.9
     nontraffic V42.3
     while boarding or alighting V42.4
    truck (traffic) V44.9
     nontraffic V44.3
     while boarding or alighting V44.4
    two wheeled motor vehicle (traffic)
       V42.9
     nontraffic V42.3
     while boarding or alighting V42.4
    van (traffic) V43.94
     nontraffic V43.34
     while boarding or alighting V43.44
   driver
    collision (with)
     animal (traffic) V40.5
      being ridden (traffic) V46.5
       nontraffic V46.0
      nontraffic V40.0
     animal-drawn vehicle (traffic) V46.5
      nontraffic V46.0
     bus (traffic) V44.5
      nontraffic V44.0
     car (traffic) V43.52
      nontraffic V43.02
     motor vehicle NOS (traffic) V49.40
      nontraffic V49.00
      specified type NEC (traffic)
        V49.49
       nontraffic V49.09
     pedal cycle (traffic) V41.5
      nontraffic V41.0
     pickup truck (traffic) V43.53
      nontraffic V43.03
     railway vehicle (traffic) V45.5
      nontraffic V45.0
     specified vehicle NEC (traffic) V46.5
      nontraffic V46.0
     sport utility vehicle (traffic) V43.51
      nontraffic V43.01
     stationary object (traffic) V47.52
      nontraffic V47.02
     streetcar (traffic) V46.5
      nontraffic V46.0
     three wheeled motor vehicle
       (traffic) V42.5
      nontraffic V42.0
     truck (traffic) V44.5
      nontraffic V44.0
     two wheeled motor vehicle (traffic)
       V42.5
      nontraffic V42.0
     van (traffic) V43.54
      nontraffic V43.04
    noncollision accident (traffic) V48.5
     nontraffic V48.0
   hanger-on
    collision (with)
     animal (traffic) V40.7
      being ridden (traffic) V46.7
       nontraffic V46.2
      nontraffic V40.2
     animal-drawn vehicle (traffic)
       V46.7
      nontraffic V46.2
     bus (traffic) V44.7
      nontraffic V44.2

◀ New   ◀▥ Revised   ~~deleted~~ Deleted

Accident *(Continued)*
transport *(Continued)*
car occupant *(Continued)*
hanger-on *(Continued)*
collision *(Continued)*
car (traffic) V43.72
nontraffic V43.22
pedal cycle (traffic) V41.7
nontraffic V41.2
pickup truck (traffic) V43.73
nontraffic V43.23
railway vehicle (traffic) V45.7
nontraffic V45.2
specified vehicle NEC (traffic) V46.7
nontraffic V46.2
sport utility vehicle (traffic) V43.71
nontraffic V43.21
stationary object (traffic) V47.7
nontraffic V47.2
streetcar (traffic) V46.7
nontraffic V46.2
three wheeled motor vehicle
(traffic) V42.7
nontraffic V42.2
truck (traffic) V44.7
nontraffic V44.2
two wheeled motor vehicle (traffic)
V42.7
nontraffic V42.2
van (traffic) V43.74
nontraffic V43.24
noncollision accident (traffic) V48.7
nontraffic V48.2
noncollision accident (traffic) V48.9
nontraffic V48.3
while boarding or alighting V48.4
nontraffic V49.3
passenger
collision (with)
animal (traffic) V40.6
being ridden (traffic) V46.6
nontraffic V46.1
nontraffic V40.1
animal-drawn vehicle (traffic) V46.6
nontraffic V46.1
bus (traffic) V44.6
nontraffic V44.1
car (traffic) V43.62
nontraffic V43.12
motor vehicle NOS (traffic) V49.50
nontraffic V49.10
specified type NEC (traffic) V49.59
nontraffic V49.19
pedal cycle (traffic) V41.6
nontraffic V41.1
pickup truck (traffic) V43.63
nontraffic V43.13
railway vehicle (traffic) V45.6
nontraffic V45.1
specified vehicle NEC (traffic) V46.6
nontraffic V46.1
sport utility vehicle (traffic) V43.61
nontraffic V43.11
stationary object (traffic) V47.62
nontraffic V47.12
streetcar (traffic) V46.6
nontraffic V46.1
three wheeled motor vehicle
(traffic) V42.6
nontraffic V42.1
truck (traffic) V44.6
nontraffic V44.1
two wheeled motor vehicle (traffic)
V42.6
nontraffic V42.1
van (traffic) V43.64
nontraffic V43.14
noncollision accident (traffic) V48.6
nontraffic V48.1
specified type NEC V49.88
military vehicle V49.81

Accident *(Continued)*
transport *(Continued)*
coal car —*see* Accident, transport,
industrial vehicle occupant
construction vehicle occupant (nontraffic)
V85.9
driver V85.5
hanger-on V85.7
passenger V85.6
traffic V85.3
driver V85.0
hanger-on V85.2
passenger V85.1
while boarding or alighting V85.4
dirt bike rider —*see* Accident, transport,
all-terrain vehicle occupant
due to cataclysm —*see* Forces of nature,
by type
dune buggy occupant (nontraffic) V86.93
driver V86.53
hanger-on V86.73
passenger V86.63
traffic V86.33
driver V86.03
hanger-on V86.23
passenger V86.13
while boarding or alighting V86.43
forklift —*see* Accident, transport, industrial
vehicle occupant
go cart —*see* Accident, transport, all-terrain
vehicle occupant
golf cart —*see* Accident, transport, all-
terrain vehicle occupant
heavy transport vehicle occupant —*see*
Accident, transport, truck occupant
ice yacht V98.2
industrial vehicle occupant (nontraffic)
V83.9
driver V83.5
hanger-on V83.7
passenger V83.6
traffic V83.3
driver V83.0
hanger-on V83.2
passenger V83.1
while boarding or alighting V83.4
interurban electric car —*see* Accident,
transport, streetcar
land yacht V98.1
logging car —*see* Accident, transport,
industrial vehicle occupant
military vehicle occupant (traffic) V86.34
driver V86.04
hanger-on V86.24
nontraffic V86.94
driver V86.54
hanger-on V86.74
passenger V86.64
passenger V86.14
while boarding or alighting V86.44
mine tram —*see* Accident, transport,
industrial vehicle occupant
motor vehicle NEC occupant (traffic) V86.39
driver V86.09
hanger-on V86.29
nontraffic V86.99
driver V86.59
hanger-on V86.79
passenger V86.69
passenger V86.19
while boarding or alighting V86.49
motorcoach —*see* Accident, transport, bus
occupant
motorcyclist V29.9
collision (with)
animal (traffic) V20.9
being ridden (traffic) V26.9
nontraffic V26.2
while boarding or alighting V26.3
nontraffic V20.2
while boarding or alighting V20.3

Accident *(Continued)*
transport *(Continued)*
motorcyclist *(Continued)*
collision *(Continued)*
animal-drawn vehicle (traffic) V26.9
nontraffic V26.2
while boarding or alighting V26.3
bus (traffic) V24.9
nontraffic V24.2
while boarding or alighting V24.3
car (traffic) V23.9
nontraffic V23.2
while boarding or alighting V23.3
motor vehicle NOS (traffic) V29.60
nontraffic V29.20
specified type NEC (traffic) V29.69
nontraffic V29.29
pedal cycle (traffic) V21.9
nontraffic V21.2
while boarding or alighting V21.3
pickup truck (traffic) V23.9
nontraffic V23.2
while boarding or alighting V23.3
railway vehicle (traffic) V25.9
nontraffic V25.2
while boarding or alighting V25.3
specified vehicle NEC (traffic) V26.9
nontraffic V26.2
while boarding or alighting V26.3
stationary object (traffic) V27.9
nontraffic V27.2
while boarding or alighting V27.3
streetcar (traffic) V26.9
nontraffic V26.2
while boarding or alighting V26.3
three wheeled motor vehicle (traffic)
V22.9
nontraffic V22.2
while boarding or alighting V22.3
truck (traffic) V24.9
nontraffic V24.2
while boarding or alighting V24.3
two wheeled motor vehicle (traffic)
V22.9
nontraffic V22.2
while boarding or alighting V22.3
van (traffic) V23.9
nontraffic V23.2
while boarding or alighting V23.3
driver
collision (with)
animal (traffic) V20.4
being ridden (traffic) V26.4
nontraffic V26.0
nontraffic V20.0
animal-drawn vehicle (traffic) V26.4
nontraffic V26.0
bus (traffic) V24.4
nontraffic V24.0
car (traffic) V23.4
nontraffic V23.0
motor vehicle NOS (traffic) V29.40
nontraffic V29.00
specified type NEC (traffic)
V29.49
nontraffic V29.09
pedal cycle (traffic) V21.4
nontraffic V21.0
pickup truck (traffic) V23.4
nontraffic V23.0
railway vehicle (traffic) V25.4
nontraffic V25.0
specified vehicle NEC (traffic) V26.4
nontraffic V26.0
stationary object (traffic) V27.4
nontraffic V27.0
streetcar (traffic) V26.4
nontraffic V26.0
three wheeled motor vehicle
(traffic) V22.4
nontraffic V22.0

Accident (*Continued*)
  transport (*Continued*)
    motorcyclist (*Continued*)
      driver (*Continued*)
        collision (*Continued*)
          truck (traffic) V24.4
            nontraffic V24.0
          two wheeled motor vehicle (traffic) V22.4
            nontraffic V22.0
          van (traffic) V23.4
            nontraffic V23.0
        noncollision accident (traffic) V28.4
          nontraffic V28.0
      noncollision accident (traffic) V28.9
        nontraffic V28.2
        while boarding or alighting V28.3
      nontraffic V29.3
      passenger
        collision (with)
          animal (traffic) V20.5
            being ridden (traffic) V26.5
              nontraffic V26.1
            nontraffic V20.1
          animal-drawn vehicle (traffic) V26.5
            nontraffic V26.1
          bus (traffic) V24.5
            nontraffic V24.1
          car (traffic) V23.5
            nontraffic V23.1
          motor vehicle NOS (traffic) V29.50
            nontraffic V29.10
            specified type NEC (traffic) V29.59
              nontraffic V29.19
          pedal cycle (traffic) V21.5
            nontraffic V21.1
          pickup truck (traffic) V23.5
            nontraffic V23.1
          railway vehicle (traffic) V25.5
            nontraffic V25.1
          specified vehicle NEC (traffic) V26.5
            nontraffic V26.1
          stationary object (traffic) V27.5
            nontraffic V27.1
          streetcar (traffic) V26.5
            nontraffic V26.1
          three wheeled motor vehicle (traffic) V22.5
            nontraffic V22.1
          truck (traffic) V24.5
            nontraffic V24.1
          two wheeled motor vehicle (traffic) V22.5
            nontraffic V22.1
          van (traffic) V23.5
            nontraffic V23.1
        noncollision accident (traffic) V28.5
          nontraffic V28.1
      specified type NEC V29.88
      military vehicle V29.81
    occupant (of)
      aircraft (powered) V95.9
        fixed wing
          commercial —*see* Accident, transport, aircraft, occupant, powered, fixed wing, commercial
          private —*see* Accident, transport, aircraft, occupant, powered, fixed wing, private
        nonpowered V96.9
        specified NEC V95.8
      airport battery-powered vehicle —*see* Accident, transport, industrial vehicle occupant
      all-terrain vehicle (ATV) —*see* Accident, transport, all-terrain vehicle occupant

Accident (*Continued*)
  transport (*Continued*)
    occupant (*Continued*)
      animal-drawn vehicle —*see* Accident, transport, animal-drawn vehicle occupant
      automobile —*see* Accident, transport, car occupant
      balloon V96.00
      battery-powered vehicle —*see* Accident, transport, industrial vehicle occupant
      bicycle —*see* Accident, transport, pedal cyclist
        motorized —*see* Accident, transport, motorcycle rider
      boat NEC —*see* Accident, watercraft
      bulldozer —*see* Accident, transport, construction vehicle occupant
      bus —*see* Accident, transport, bus occupant
      cable car (on rails) —*see also* Accident, transport, streetcar occupant
        not on rails V98.0
      car —*see also* Accident, transport, car occupant
        cable (on rails) —*see also* Accident, transport, streetcar occupant
          not on rails V98.0
      coach —*see* Accident, transport, bus occupant
      coal-car —*see* Accident, transport, industrial vehicle occupant
      digger —*see* Accident, transport, construction vehicle occupant
      dump truck —*see* Accident, transport, construction vehicle occupant
      earth-leveler —*see* Accident, transport, construction vehicle occupant
      farm machinery (self-propelled) —*see* Accident, transport, agricultural vehicle occupant
      forklift —*see* Accident, transport, industrial vehicle occupant
      glider (unpowered) V96.20
        hang V96.10
        powered (microlight) (ultralight) —*see* Accident, transport, aircraft, occupant, powered, glider
      glider (unpowered) NEC V96.20
      hang-glider V96.10
      harvester —*see* Accident, transport, agricultural vehicle occupant
      heavy (transport) vehicle —*see* Accident, transport, truck occupant
      helicopter —*see* Accident, transport, aircraft, occupant, helicopter
      ice-yacht V98.2
      kite (carrying person) V96.8
      land-yacht V98.1
      logging car —*see* Accident, transport, industrial vehicle occupant
      mechanical shovel —*see* Accident, transport, construction vehicle occupant
      microlight —*see* Accident, transport, aircraft, occupant, powered, glider
      minibus —*see* Accident, transport, car occupant
      minivan —*see* Accident, transport, car occupant
      moped —*see* Accident, transport, motorcycle
      motor scooter —*see* Accident, transport, motorcycle
      motorcycle (with sidecar) —*see* Accident, transport, motorcycle
      pedal cycle —*see also* Accident, transport, pedal cyclist
      pick-up (truck) —*see* Accident, transport, pickup truck occupant

Accident (*Continued*)
  transport (*Continued*)
    occupant (*Continued*)
      railway (train) (vehicle) (subterranean) (elevated) —*see* Accident, transport, railway vehicle occupant
      rickshaw —*see* Accident, transport, pedal cycle
        pedal driven —*see* Accident, transport, pedal cyclist
      road-roller —*see* Accident, transport, construction vehicle occupant
      ship NOS V94.9
      ski-lift (chair) (gondola) V98.3
      snowmobile —*see* Accident, transport, snowmobile occupant
      spacecraft, spaceship —*see* Accident, transport, aircraft, occupant, spacecraft
      sport utility vehicle —*see* Accident, transport, car occupant
      streetcar (interurban) (operating on public street or highway) —*see* Accident, transport, streetcar occupant
      SUV —*see* Accident, transport, car occupant
      téléférique V98.0
      three-wheeled vehicle (motorized) —*see also* Accident, transport, three-wheeled motor vehicle occupant
        nonmotorized —*see* Accident, transport, pedal cycle
      tractor (farm) (and trailer) —*see* Accident, transport, agricultural vehicle occupant
      train —*see* Accident, transport, railway vehicle occupant
      tram —*see* Accident, transport, streetcar occupant
        in mine or quarry —*see* Accident, transport, industrial vehicle occupant
      tricycle —*see* Accident, transport, pedal cycle
        motorized —*see* Accident, transport, three-wheeled motor vehicle
      trolley —*see* Accident, transport, streetcar occupant
        in mine or quarry —*see* Accident, transport, industrial vehicle occupant
      tub, in mine or quarry —*see* Accident, transport, industrial vehicle occupant
      ultralight —*see* Accident, transport, aircraft, occupant, powered, glider
      van —*see* Accident, transport, van occupant
      vehicle NEC V89.9
        heavy transport —*see* Accident, transport, truck occupant
        motor (traffic) NEC V89.2
          nontraffic NEC V89.0
      watercraft NOS V94.9
        causing drowning —*see* Drowning, resulting from accident to boat
    parachutist V97.29
      after accident to aircraft —*see* Accident, transport, aircraft
      entangled in object V97.21
      injured on landing V97.22
    pedal cyclist V19.9
      collision (with)
        animal (traffic) V10.9
          being ridden (traffic) V16.9
            nontraffic V16.2
            while boarding or alighting V16.3
          nontraffic V10.2
          while boarding or alighting V10.3

Accident *(Continued)*
transport *(Continued)*
pedal cyclist *(Continued)*
collision *(Continued)*
animal-drawn vehicle (traffic) V16.9
nontraffic V16.2
while boarding or alighting V16.3
bus (traffic) V14.9
nontraffic V14.2
while boarding or alighting V14.3
car (traffic) V13.9
nontraffic V13.2
while boarding or alighting V13.3
motor vehicle NOS (traffic) V19.60
nontraffic V19.20
specified type NEC (traffic) V19.69
nontraffic V19.29
pedal cycle (traffic) V11.9
nontraffic V11.2
while boarding or alighting V11.3
pickup truck (traffic) V13.9
nontraffic V13.2
while boarding or alighting V13.3
railway vehicle (traffic) V15.9
nontraffic V15.2
while boarding or alighting V15.3
specified vehicle NEC (traffic) V16.9
nontraffic V16.2
while boarding or alighting V16.3
stationary object (traffic) V17.9
nontraffic V17.2
while boarding or alighting V17.3
streetcar (traffic) V16.9
nontraffic V16.2
while boarding or alighting V16.3
three wheeled motor vehicle (traffic)
V12.9
nontraffic V12.2
while boarding or alighting V12.3
truck (traffic) V14.9
nontraffic V14.2
while boarding or alighting V14.3
two wheeled motor vehicle (traffic)
V12.9
nontraffic V12.2
while boarding or alighting V12.3
van (traffic) V13.9
nontraffic V13.2
while boarding or alighting V13.3
driver
collision (with)
animal (traffic) V10.4
being ridden (traffic) V16.4
nontraffic V16.0
nontraffic V10.0
animal-drawn vehicle (traffic) V16.4
nontraffic V16.0
bus (traffic) V14.4
nontraffic V14.0
car (traffic) V13.4
nontraffic V13.0
motor vehicle NOS (traffic) V19.40
nontraffic V19.00
specified type NEC (traffic)
V19.49
nontraffic V19.09
pedal cycle (traffic) V11.4
nontraffic V11.0
pickup truck (traffic) V13.4
nontraffic V13.0
railway vehicle (traffic) V15.4
nontraffic V15.0
specified vehicle NEC (traffic) V16.4
nontraffic V16.0
stationary object (traffic) V17.4
nontraffic V17.0
streetcar (traffic) V16.4
nontraffic V16.0
three wheeled motor vehicle
(traffic) V12.4
nontraffic V12.0

Accident *(Continued)*
transport *(Continued)*
pedal cyclist *(Continued)*
driver *(Continued)*
collision *(Continued)*
truck (traffic) V14.4
nontraffic V14.0
two wheeled motor vehicle (traffic)
V12.4
nontraffic V12.0
van (traffic) V13.4
nontraffic V13.0
noncollision accident (traffic) V18.4
nontraffic V18.0
noncollision accident (traffic) V18.9
nontraffic V18.2
while boarding or alighting V18.3
nontraffic V19.3
passenger
collision (with)
animal (traffic) V10.5
being ridden (traffic) V16.5
nontraffic V16.1
nontraffic V10.1
animal-drawn vehicle (traffic) V16.5
nontraffic V16.1
bus (traffic) V14.5
nontraffic V14.1
car (traffic) V13.5
nontraffic V13.1
motor vehicle NOS (traffic) V19.50
nontraffic V19.10
specified type NEC (traffic)
V19.59
nontraffic V19.19
pedal cycle (traffic) V11.5
nontraffic V11.1
pickup truck (traffic) V13.5
nontraffic V13.1
railway vehicle (traffic) V15.5
nontraffic V15.1
specified vehicle NEC (traffic) V16.5
nontraffic V16.1
stationary object (traffic) V17.5
nontraffic V17.1
streetcar (traffic) V16.5
nontraffic V16.1
three wheeled motor vehicle
(traffic) V12.5
nontraffic V12.1
truck (traffic) V14.5
nontraffic V14.1
two wheeled motor vehicle (traffic)
V12.5
nontraffic V12.1
van (traffic) V13.5
nontraffic V13.1
noncollision accident (traffic) V18.5
nontraffic V18.1
specified type NEC V19.88
military vehicle V19.81
pedestrian
conveyance (occupant) V09.9
babystroller V00.828
collision (with) V09.9
animal being ridden or animal
drawn vehicle V06.99
nontraffic V06.09
traffic V06.19
bus or heavy transport V04.99
nontraffic V04.09
traffic V04.19
car V03.99
nontraffic V03.09
traffic V03.19
pedal cycle V01.99
nontraffic V01.09
traffic V01.19
pick-up truck or van V03.99
nontraffic V03.09
traffic V03.19

Accident *(Continued)*
transport *(Continued)*
pedestrian *(Continued)*
conveyance *(Continued)*
babystroller *(Continued)*
collision *(Continued)*
railway (train) (vehicle) V05.99
nontraffic V05.09
traffic V05.19
stationary object V00.822
streetcar V06.99
nontraffic V06.09
traffic V06.19
two- or three-wheeled motor
vehicle V02.99
nontraffic V02.09
traffic V02.19
vehicle V09.9
animal-drawn V06.99
nontraffic V06.09
traffic V06.19
motor
nontraffic V09.00
traffic V09.20
fall V00.821
nontraffic V09.1
involving motor vehicle NEC
V09.00
traffic V09.3
involving motor vehicle NEC
V09.20
flat-bottomed NEC V00.388
collision (with) V09.9
animal being ridden or animal
drawn vehicle V06.99
nontraffic V06.09
traffic V06.19
bus or heavy transport V04.99
nontraffic V04.09
traffic V04.19
car V03.99
nontraffic V03.09
traffic V03.19
pedal cycle V01.99
nontraffic V01.09
traffic V01.19
pick-up truck or van V03.99
nontraffic V03.09
traffic V03.19
railway (train) (vehicle) V05.99
nontraffic V05.09
traffic V05.19
stationary object V00.382
streetcar V06.99
nontraffic V06.09
traffic V06.19
two-or three-wheeled motor
vehicle V02.99
nontraffic V02.09
traffic V02.19
vehicle V09.9
animal-drawn V06.99
nontraffic V06.09
traffic V06.19
motor
nontraffic V09.00
traffic V09.20
fall V00.381
nontraffic V09.1
involving motor vehicle NEC
V09.00
snow
board —*see* Accident, transport,
pedestrian, conveyance,
snow board
ski —*see* Accident, transport,
pedestrian, conveyance, skis
(snow)
traffic V09.3
involving motor vehicle NEC
V09.20

Accident (Continued)
  transport (Continued)
    pedestrian (Continued)
      conveyance (Continued)
        gliding type NEC V00.288
          collision (with) V09.9
            animal being ridden or animal
                drawn vehicle V06.99
              nontraffic V06.09
              traffic V06.19
            bus or heavy transport
                V04.99
              nontraffic V04.09
              traffic V04.19
            car V03.99
              nontraffic V03.09
              traffic V03.19
            pedal cycle V01.99
              nontraffic V01.09
              traffic V01.19
            pick-up truck or van V03.99
              nontraffic V03.09
              traffic V03.19
            railway (train) (vehicle) V05.99
              nontraffic V05.09
              traffic V05.19
            stationary object V00.282
            streetcar V06.99
              nontraffic V06.09
              traffic V06.19
            two- or three-wheeled motor
                vehicle V02.99
              nontraffic V02.09
              traffic V02.19
            vehicle V09.9
              animal-drawn V06.99
                nontraffic V06.09
                traffic V06.19
              motor
                nontraffic V09.00
                traffic V09.20
          fall V00.281
          heelies —see Accident, transport,
              pedestrian, conveyance,
              heelies
          ice skate —see Accident, transport,
              pedestrian, conveyance, ice
              skate
          nontraffic V09.1
            involving motor vehicle NEC
                V09.00
          sled —see Accident, transport,
              pedestrian, conveyance, sled
          traffic V09.3
            involving motor vehicle NEC
                V09.20
          wheelies —see Accident,
              transport, pedestrian,
              conveyance, heelies
        heelies V00.158
          colliding with stationary object
              V00.152
          fall V00.151
        ice skates V00.218
          collision (with) V09.9
            animal being ridden or animal
                drawn vehicle V06.99
              nontraffic V06.09
              traffic V06.19
            bus or heavy transport V04.99
              nontraffic V04.09
              traffic V04.19
            car V03.99
              nontraffic V03.09
              traffic V03.19
            pedal cycle V01.99
              nontraffic V01.09
              traffic V01.19
            pick-up truck or van V03.99
              nontraffic V03.09
              traffic V03.19

Accident (Continued)
  transport (Continued)
    pedestrian (Continued)
      conveyance (Continued)
        ice skates (Continued)
          collision (Continued)
            railway (train) (vehicle)
                V05.99
              nontraffic V05.09
              traffic V05.19
            stationary object V00.212
            streetcar V06.99
              nontraffic V06.09
              traffic V06.19
            two- or three-wheeled motor
                vehicle V02.99
              nontraffic V02.09
              traffic V02.19
            vehicle V09.9
              animal-drawn V06.99
                nontraffic V06.09
                traffic V06.19
              motor
                nontraffic V09.00
                traffic V09.20
          fall V00.211
          nontraffic V09.1
            involving motor vehicle NEC
                V09.00
          traffic V09.3
            involving motor vehicle NEC
                V09.20
        motorized mobility scooter
            V00.838
          collision with stationary object
              V00.832
          fall from V00.831
        nontraffic V09.1
          involving motor vehicle
              V09.00
            military V09.01
            specified type NEC V09.09
        roller skates (non in-line) V00.128
          collision (with) V09.9
            animal being ridden or animal
                drawn vehicle V06.91
              nontraffic V06.01
              traffic V06.11
            bus or heavy transport
                V04.91
              nontraffic V04.01
              traffic V04.11
            car V03.91
              nontraffic V03.01
              traffic V03.11
            pedal cycle V01.91
              nontraffic V01.01
              traffic V01.11
            pick-up truck or van V03.91
              nontraffic V03.01
              traffic V03.11
            railway (train) (vehicle)
                V05.91
              nontraffic V05.01
              traffic V05.11
            stationary object V00.122
            streetcar V06.91
              nontraffic V06.01
              traffic V06.11
            two- or three-wheeled motor
                vehicle V02.91
              nontraffic V02.01
              traffic V02.11
            vehicle V09.9
              animal-drawn V06.91
                nontraffic V06.01
                traffic V06.11
              motor
                nontraffic V09.00
                traffic V09.20
          fall V00.121

Accident (Continued)
  transport (Continued)
    pedestrian (Continued)
      conveyance (Continued)
        roller skates (Continued)
          in-line V00.118
            collision —see also Accident,
                transport, pedestrian,
                conveyance occupant, roller
                skates, collision
              with stationary object
                  V00.112
            fall V00.111
            nontraffic V09.1
              involving motor vehicle NEC
                  V09.00
            traffic V09.3
              involving motor vehicle NEC
                  V09.20
        rolling shoes V00.158
          colliding with stationary object
              V00.152
          fall V00.151
        rolling type NEC V00.188
          collision (with) V09.9
            animal being ridden or animal
                drawn vehicle V06.99
              nontraffic V06.09
              traffic V06.19
            bus or heavy transport V04.99
              nontraffic V04.09
              traffic V04.19
            car V03.99
              nontraffic V03.09
              traffic V03.19
            pedal cycle V01.99
              nontraffic V01.09
              traffic V01.19
            pick-up truck or van V03.99
              nontraffic V03.09
              traffic V03.19
            railway (train) (vehicle)
                V05.99
              nontraffic V05.09
              traffic V05.19
            stationary object V00.182
            streetcar V06.99
              nontraffic V06.09
              traffic V06.19
            two- or three-wheeled motor
                vehicle V02.99
              nontraffic V02.09
              traffic V02.19
            vehicle V09.9
              animal-drawn V06.99
                nontraffic V06.09
                traffic V06.19
              motor
                nontraffic V09.00
                traffic V09.20
          fall V00.181
          in-line roller skate —see Accident,
              transport, pedestrian,
              conveyance, roller skate,
              in-line
          nontraffic V09.1
            involving motor vehicle NEC
                V09.00
          roller skate —see Accident,
              transport, pedestrian,
              conveyance, roller skate
          scooter (non-motorized) —
              see Accident, transport,
              pedestrian, conveyance,
              scooter
          skateboard —see Accident,
              transport, pedestrian,
              conveyance, skateboard
          traffic V09.3
            involving motor vehicle NEC
                V09.20

◀ New   ◀║║ Revised   ~~deleted~~ Deleted

Accident *(Continued)*
  transport *(Continued)*
    pedestrian *(Continued)*
      conveyance *(Continued)*
        scooter (non-motorized) V00.148
          collision (with) V09.9
            animal being ridden or animal
              drawn vehicle V06.99
              nontraffic V06.09
              traffic V06.19
            bus or heavy transport
              V04.99
              nontraffic V04.09
              traffic V04.19
            car V03.99
              nontraffic V03.09
              traffic V03.19
            pedal cycle V01.99
              nontraffic V01.09
              traffic V01.19
            pick-up truck or van V03.99
              nontraffic V03.09
              traffic V03.19
            railway (train) (vehicle)
              V05.99
              nontraffic V05.09
              traffic V05.19
            stationary object V00.142
            streetcar V06.99
              nontraffic V06.09
              traffic V06.19
            two- or three-wheeled motor
              vehicle V02.99
              nontraffic V02.09
              traffic V02.19
            vehicle V09.9
              animal-drawn V06.99
                nontraffic V06.09
                traffic V06.19
              motor
                nontraffic V09.00
                traffic V09.20
          fall V00.141
          nontraffic V09.1
            involving motor vehicle NEC
              V09.00
          traffic V09.3
            involving motor vehicle NEC
              V09.20
        skate board V00.138
          collision (with) V09.9
            animal being ridden or
              animal drawn vehicle
              V06.92
              nontraffic V06.02
              traffic V06.12
            bus or heavy transport
              V04.92
              nontraffic V04.02
              traffic V04.12
            car V03.92
              nontraffic V03.02
              traffic V03.12
            pedal cycle V01.92
              nontraffic V01.02
              traffic V01.12
            pick-up truck or van V03.92
              nontraffic V03.02
              traffic V03.12
            railway (train) (vehicle)
              V05.92
              nontraffic V05.02
              traffic V05.12
            stationary object V00.132
            streetcar V06.92
              nontraffic V06.02
              traffic V06.12
            two- or three-wheeled motor
              vehicle V02.92
              nontraffic V02.02
              traffic V02.12

Accident *(Continued)*
  transport *(Continued)*
    pedestrian *(Continued)*
      conveyance *(Continued)*
        skate board *(Continued)*
          collision *(Continued)*
            vehicle V09.9
              animal-drawn V06.92
                nontraffic V06.02
                traffic V06.12
              motor
                nontraffic V09.00
                traffic V09.20
          fall V00.131
          nontraffic V09.1
            involving motor vehicle NEC
              V09.00
          traffic V09.3
            involving motor vehicle NEC
              V09.20
        skis (snow) V00.328
          collision (with) V09.9
            animal being ridden or animal
              drawn vehicle V06.99
              nontraffic V06.09
              traffic V06.19
            bus or heavy transport V04.99
              nontraffic V04.09
              traffic V04.19
            car V03.99
              nontraffic V03.09
              traffic V03.19
            pedal cycle V01.99
              nontraffic V01.09
              traffic V01.19
            pick-up truck or van V03.99
              nontraffic V03.09
              traffic V03.19
            railway (train) (vehicle) V05.99
              nontraffic V05.09
              traffic V05.19
            stationary object V00.322
            streetcar V06.99
              nontraffic V06.09
              traffic V06.19
            two- or three-wheeled motor
              vehicle V02.99
              nontraffic V02.09
              traffic V02.19
            vehicle V09.9
              animal-drawn V06.99
                nontraffic V06.09
                traffic V06.19
              motor
                nontraffic V09.00
                traffic V09.20
          fall V00.321
          nontraffic V09.1
            involving motor vehicle NEC
              V09.00
          traffic V09.3
            involving motor vehicle NEC
              V09.20
        sled V00.228
          collision (with) V09.9
            animal being ridden or animal
              drawn vehicle V06.99
              nontraffic V06.09
              traffic V06.19
            bus or heavy transport V04.99
              nontraffic V04.09
              traffic V04.19
            car V03.99
              nontraffic V03.09
              traffic V03.19
            pedal cycle V01.99
              nontraffic V01.09
              traffic V01.19
            pick-up truck or van V03.99
              nontraffic V03.09
              traffic V03.19

Accident *(Continued)*
  transport *(Continued)*
    pedestrian *(Continued)*
      conveyance *(Continued)*
        sled *(Continued)*
          collision *(Continued)*
            railway (train) (vehicle)
              V05.99
              nontraffic V05.09
              traffic V05.19
            stationary object V00.222
            streetcar V06.99
              nontraffic V06.09
              traffic V06.19
            two- or three-wheeled motor
              vehicle V02.99
              nontraffic V02.09
              traffic V02.19
            vehicle V09.9
              animal-drawn V06.99
                nontraffic V06.09
                traffic V06.19
              motor
                nontraffic V09.00
                traffic V09.20
          fall V00.221
          nontraffic V09.1
            involving motor vehicle NEC
              V09.00
          traffic V09.3
            involving motor vehicle NEC
              V09.20
        snow board V00.318
          collision (with) V09.9
            animal being ridden or animal
              drawn vehicle V06.99
              nontraffic V06.09
              traffic V06.19
            bus or heavy transport V04.99
              nontraffic V04.09
              traffic V04.19
            car V03.99
              nontraffic V03.09
              traffic V03.19
            pedal cycle V01.99
              nontraffic V01.09
              traffic V01.19
            pick-up truck or van V03.99
              nontraffic V03.09
              traffic V03.19
            railway (train) (vehicle) V05.99
              nontraffic V05.09
              traffic V05.19
            stationary object V00.312
            streetcar V06.99
              nontraffic V06.09
              traffic V06.19
            two- or three-wheeled motor
              vehicle V02.99
              nontraffic V02.09
              traffic V02.19
            vehicle V09.9
              animal-drawn V06.99
                nontraffic V06.09
                traffic V06.19
              motor
                nontraffic V09.00
                traffic V09.20
          fall V00.311
          nontraffic V09.1
            involving motor vehicle NEC
              V09.00
          traffic V09.3
            involving motor vehicle NEC
              V09.20
        specified type NEC V00.898
          collision (with) V09.9
            animal being ridden or animal
              drawn vehicle V06.99
              nontraffic V06.09
              traffic V06.19

Accident (Continued)
  transport (Continued)
    pedestrian (Continued)
      conveyance (Continued)
        specified type NEC (Continued)
          collision (Continued)
            bus or heavy transport
                V04.99
              nontraffic V04.09
              traffic V04.19
            car V03.99
              nontraffic V03.09
              traffic V03.19
            pedal cycle V01.99
              nontraffic V01.09
              traffic V01.19
            pick-up truck or van V03.99
              nontraffic V03.09
              traffic V03.19
            railway (train) (vehicle)
                V05.99
              nontraffic V05.09
              traffic V05.19
            stationary object V00.892
            streetcar V06.99
              nontraffic V06.09
              traffic V06.19
            two- or three-wheeled motor
                vehicle V02.99
              nontraffic V02.09
              traffic V02.19
            vehicle V09.9
              animal-drawn V06.99
                nontraffic V06.09
                traffic V06.19
              motor
                nontraffic V09.00
                traffic V09.20
          fall V00.891
          nontraffic V09.1
            involving motor vehicle NEC
                V09.00
          traffic V09.3
            involving motor vehicle NEC
                V09.20
        traffic V09.3
          involving motor vehicle V09.20
            military V09.21
            specified type NEC V09.29
      wheelchair (powered) V00.818
        collision (with) V09.9
          animal being ridden or
              animal drawn vehicle
              V06.99
            nontraffic V06.09
            traffic V06.19
          bus or heavy transport
              V04.99
            nontraffic V04.09
            traffic V04.19
          car V03.99
            nontraffic V03.09
            traffic V03.19
          pedal cycle V01.99
            nontraffic V01.09
            traffic V01.19
          pick-up truck or van V03.99
            nontraffic V03.09
            traffic V03.19
          railway (train) (vehicle)
              V05.99
            nontraffic V05.09
            traffic V05.19
          stationary object V00.812
          streetcar V06.99
            nontraffic V06.09
            traffic V06.19
          two- or three-wheeled motor
              vehicle V02.99
            nontraffic V02.09
            traffic V02.19

Accident (Continued)
  transport (Continued)
    pedestrian (Continued)
      conveyance (Continued)
        wheelchair (Continued)
          collision (Continued)
            vehicle V09.9
              animal-drawn V06.99
                nontraffic V06.09
                traffic V06.19
              motor
                nontraffic V09.00
                traffic V09.20
          fall V00.811
          nontraffic V09.1
            involving motor vehicle NEC
                V09.00
          traffic V09.3
            involving motor vehicle NEC
                V09.20
        wheeled shoe V00.158
          colliding with stationary object
              V00.152
          fall V00.151
    on foot —see also Accident, pedestrian
      collision (with)
        animal being ridden or animal
            drawn vehicle V06.90
          nontraffic V06.00
          traffic V06.10
        bus or heavy transport V04.90
          nontraffic V04.00
          traffic V04.10
        car V03.90
          nontraffic V03.00
          traffic V03.10
        pedal cycle V01.90
          nontraffic V01.00
          traffic V01.10
        pick-up truck or van V03.90
          nontraffic V03.00
          traffic V03.10
        railway (train) (vehicle) V05.90
          nontraffic V05.00
          traffic V05.10
        streetcar V06.90
          nontraffic V06.00
          traffic V06.10
        two- or three-wheeled motor
            vehicle V02.90
          nontraffic V02.00
          traffic V02.10
        vehicle V09.9
          animal-drawn V06.90
            nontraffic V06.00
            traffic V06.10
          motor
            nontraffic V09.00
            traffic V09.20
        nontraffic V09.1
          involving motor vehicle V09.00
            military V09.01
            specified type NEC V09.09
        traffic V09.3
          involving motor vehicle V09.20
            military V09.21
            specified type NEC V09.29
    person NEC (unknown way or
        transportation) V99
      collision (between)
        bus (with)
          heavy transport vehicle (traffic)
              V87.5
          nontraffic V88.5
        car (with)
          nontraffic V88.5
          bus (traffic) V87.3
            nontraffic V88.3
          heavy transport vehicle (traffic)
              V87.4
            nontraffic V88.4

Accident (Continued)
  transport (Continued)
    person NEC (Continued)
      collision (Continued)
        car (Continued)
          pick-up truck or van (traffic) V87.2
            nontraffic V88.2
          train or railway vehicle (traffic)
              V87.6
            nontraffic V88.6
          two- or three-wheeled motor
              vehicle (traffic) V87.0
            nontraffic V88.0
          motor vehicle (traffic) NEC V87.7
            nontraffic V88.7
          two- or three-wheeled vehicle (with)
              (traffic)
            motor vehicle NEC V87.1
              nontraffic V88.1
          nonmotor vehicle (collision)
              (noncollision) (traffic) V87.9
            nontraffic V88.9
      pickup truck occupant V59.9
        collision (with)
          animal (traffic) V50.9
            being ridden (traffic) V56.9
              nontraffic V56.3
              while boarding or alighting V56.4
            nontraffic V50.3
            while boarding or alighting V50.4
          animal-drawn vehicle (traffic) V56.9
            nontraffic V56.3
            while boarding or alighting V56.4
          bus (traffic) V54.9
            nontraffic V54.3
            while boarding or alighting V54.4
          car (traffic) V53.9
            nontraffic V53.3
            while boarding or alighting V53.4
          motor vehicle NOS (traffic) V59.60
            nontraffic V59.20
            specified type NEC (traffic) V59.69
              nontraffic V59.29
          pedal cycle (traffic) V51.9
            nontraffic V51.3
            while boarding or alighting V51.4
          pickup truck (traffic) V53.9
            nontraffic V53.3
            while boarding or alighting V53.4
          railway vehicle (traffic) V55.9
            nontraffic V55.3
            while boarding or alighting V55.4
          specified vehicle NEC (traffic) V56.9
            nontraffic V56.3
            while boarding or alighting V56.4
          stationary object (traffic) V57.9
            nontraffic V57.3
            while boarding or alighting V57.4
          streetcar (traffic) V56.9
            nontraffic V56.3
            while boarding or alighting V56.4
          three wheeled motor vehicle (traffic)
              V52.9
            nontraffic V52.3
            while boarding or alighting V52.4
          truck (traffic) V54.9
            nontraffic V54.3
            while boarding or alighting V54.4
          two wheeled motor vehicle (traffic)
              V52.9
            nontraffic V52.3
            while boarding or alighting V52.4
          van (traffic) V53.9
            nontraffic V53.3
            while boarding or alighting V53.4
        driver
          collision (with)
            animal (traffic) V50.5
              being ridden (traffic) V56.5
                nontraffic V56.0
              nontraffic V50.0

◀ New   ⬅▥ Revised   ~~deleted~~ Deleted

Accident (*Continued*)
  transport (*Continued*)
    pickup truck occupant (*Continued*)
      driver (*Continued*)
        collision (*Continued*)
          animal-drawn vehicle (traffic)
            V56.5
            nontraffic V56.0
          bus (traffic) V54.5
            nontraffic V54.0
          car (traffic) V53.5
            nontraffic V53.0
          motor vehicle NOS (traffic) V59.40
            nontraffic V59.00
            specified type NEC (traffic)
              V59.49
              nontraffic V59.09
          pedal cycle (traffic) V51.5
            nontraffic V51.0
          pickup truck (traffic) V53.5
            nontraffic V53.0
          railway vehicle (traffic) V55.5
            nontraffic V55.0
          specified vehicle NEC (traffic) V56.5
            nontraffic V56.0
          stationary object (traffic) V57.5
            nontraffic V57.0
          streetcar (traffic) V56.5
            nontraffic V56.0
          three wheeled motor vehicle
            (traffic) V52.5
            nontraffic V52.0
          truck (traffic) V54.5
            nontraffic V54.0
          two wheeled motor vehicle (traffic)
            V52.5
            nontraffic V52.0
          van (traffic) V53.5
            nontraffic V53.0
        noncollision accident (traffic) V58.5
          nontraffic V58.0
      hanger-on
        collision (with)
          animal (traffic) V50.7
            being ridden (traffic) V56.7
              nontraffic V56.2
            nontraffic V50.2
          animal-drawn vehicle (traffic) V56.7
            nontraffic V56.2
          bus (traffic) V54.7
            nontraffic V54.2
          car (traffic) V53.7
            nontraffic V53.2
          pedal cycle (traffic) V51.7
            nontraffic V51.2
          pickup truck (traffic) V53.7
            nontraffic V53.2
          railway vehicle (traffic) V55.7
            nontraffic V55.2
          specified vehicle NEC (traffic) V56.7
            nontraffic V56.2
          stationary object (traffic) V57.7
            nontraffic V57.2
          streetcar (traffic) V56.7
            nontraffic V56.2
          three wheeled motor vehicle
            (traffic) V52.7
            nontraffic V52.2
          truck (traffic) V54.7
            nontraffic V54.2
          two wheeled motor vehicle (traffic)
            V52.7
            nontraffic V52.2
          van (traffic) V53.7
            nontraffic V53.2
        noncollision accident (traffic) V58.7
          nontraffic V58.2
      noncollision accident (traffic) V58.9
        nontraffic V58.3
        while boarding or alighting V58.4
      nontraffic V59.3

Accident (*Continued*)
  transport (*Continued*)
    pickup truck occupant (*Continued*)
      passenger
        collision (with)
          animal (traffic) V50.6
            being ridden (traffic) V56.6
              nontraffic V56.1
            nontraffic V50.1
          animal-drawn vehicle (traffic)
            V56.6
            nontraffic V56.1
          bus (traffic) V54.6
            nontraffic V54.1
          car (traffic) V53.6
            nontraffic V53.1
          motor vehicle NOS (traffic) V59.50
            nontraffic V59.10
            specified type NEC (traffic)
              V59.59
              nontraffic V59.19
          pedal cycle (traffic) V51.6
            nontraffic V51.1
          pickup truck (traffic) V53.6
            nontraffic V53.1
          railway vehicle (traffic) V55.6
            nontraffic V55.1
          specified vehicle NEC (traffic)
            V56.6
            nontraffic V56.1
          stationary object (traffic) V57.6
            nontraffic V57.1
          streetcar (traffic) V56.6
            nontraffic V56.1
          three wheeled motor vehicle
            (traffic) V52.6
            nontraffic V52.1
          truck (traffic) V54.6
            nontraffic V54.1
          two wheeled motor vehicle (traffic)
            V52.6
            nontraffic V52.1
          van (traffic) V53.6
            nontraffic V53.1
        noncollision accident (traffic) V58.6
          nontraffic V58.1
    specified type NEC V59.88
    military vehicle V59.81
  quarry truck —*see* Accident, transport,
    industrial vehicle occupant
  race car —*see* Accident, transport, motor
    vehicle NEC occupant
  railway vehicle occupant V81.9
    collision (with) V81.3
      motor vehicle (non-military) (traffic)
        V81.1
        military V81.83
        nontraffic V81.0
      rolling stock V81.2
      specified object NEC V81.3
    during derailment V81.7
      with antecedent collision —*see*
        Accident, transport, railway
        vehicle occupant, collision
    explosion V81.81
    fall (in railway vehicle) V81.5
      during derailment V81.7
        with antecedent collision —*see*
          Accident, transport, railway
          vehicle occupant, collision
      from railway vehicle V81.6
        during derailment V81.7
          with antecedent collision —*see*
            Accident, transport, railway
            vehicle occupant, collision
      while boarding or alighting V81.4
    fire V81.81
    object falling onto train V81.82
    specified type NEC V81.89
    while boarding or alighting V81.4
  ski lift V98.3

Accident (*Continued*)
  transport (*Continued*)
    snowmobile occupant (nontraffic)
      V86.92
      driver V86.52
      hanger-on V86.72
      passenger V86.62
      traffic V86.32
        driver V86.02
        hanger-on V86.22
        passenger V86.12
      while boarding or alighting V86.42
    specified NEC V98.8
    sport utility vehicle occupant —*see also*
      Accident, transport, car occupant
      collision (with)
        stationary object (traffic) V47.91
          nontraffic V47.31
      driver
        collision (with)
          stationary object (traffic) V47.51
            nontraffic V47.01
      passenger
        collision (with)
          stationary object (traffic) V47.61
            nontraffic V47.11
    streetcar occupant V82.9
      collision (with) V82.3
        motor vehicle (traffic) V82.1
          nontraffic V82.0
        rolling stock V82.2
      during derailment V82.7
        with antecedent collision —*see*
          Accident, transport, streetcar
          occupant, collision
      fall (in streetcar) V82.5
        during derailment V82.7
          with antecedent collision —*see*
            Accident, transport, streetcar
            occupant, collision
        from streetcar V82.6
          during derailment V82.7
            with antecedent collision —*see*
              Accident, transport, streetcar
              occupant, collision
          while boarding or alighting V82.4
      while boarding or alighting V82.4
      specified type NEC V82.8
      while boarding or alighting V82.4
    three-wheeled motor vehicle occupant
      V39.9
      collision (with)
        animal (traffic) V30.9
          being ridden (traffic) V36.9
            nontraffic V36.3
            while boarding or alighting
              V36.4
          nontraffic V30.3
          while boarding or alighting V30.4
        animal-drawn vehicle (traffic) V36.9
          nontraffic V36.3
          while boarding or alighting V36.4
        bus (traffic) V34.9
          nontraffic V34.3
          while boarding or alighting V34.4
        car (traffic) V33.9
          nontraffic V33.3
          while boarding or alighting V33.4
        motor vehicle NOS (traffic) V39.60
          nontraffic V39.20
          specified type NEC (traffic) V39.69
            nontraffic V39.29
        pedal cycle (traffic) V31.9
          nontraffic V31.3
          while boarding or alighting V31.4
        pickup truck (traffic) V33.9
          nontraffic V33.3
          while boarding or alighting V33.4
        railway vehicle (traffic) V35.9
          nontraffic V35.3
          while boarding or alighting V35.4

◀ New   ◀|||| Revised   ~~deleted~~ Deleted

Accident *(Continued)*
  transport *(Continued)*
    three-wheeled motor vehicle occupant
    (Continued)
      collision *(Continued)*
        specified vehicle NEC (traffic) V36.9
          nontraffic V36.3
          while boarding or alighting V36.4
        stationary object (traffic) V37.9
          nontraffic V37.3
          while boarding or alighting V37.4
        streetcar (traffic) V36.9
          nontraffic V36.3
          while boarding or alighting V36.4
        three wheeled motor vehicle (traffic)
          V32.9
          nontraffic V32.3
          while boarding or alighting V32.4
        truck (traffic) V34.9
          nontraffic V34.3
          while boarding or alighting V34.4
        two wheeled motor vehicle (traffic)
          V32.9
          nontraffic V32.3
          while boarding or alighting V32.4
        van (traffic) V33.9
          nontraffic V33.3
          while boarding or alighting V33.4
      driver
        collision (with)
          animal (traffic) V30.5
            being ridden (traffic) V36.5
              nontraffic V36.0
            nontraffic V30.0
          animal-drawn vehicle (traffic) V36.5
            nontraffic V36.0
          bus (traffic) V34.5
            nontraffic V34.0
          car (traffic) V33.5
            nontraffic V33.0
          motor vehicle NOS (traffic) V39.40
            nontraffic V39.00
            specified type NEC (traffic)
              V39.49
              nontraffic V39.09
          pedal cycle (traffic) V31.5
            nontraffic V31.0
          pickup truck (traffic) V33.5
            nontraffic V33.0
          railway vehicle (traffic) V35.5
            nontraffic V35.0
          specified vehicle NEC (traffic) V36.5
            nontraffic V36.0
          stationary object (traffic) V37.5
            nontraffic V37.0
          streetcar (traffic) V36.5
            nontraffic V36.0
          three wheeled motor vehicle
            (traffic) V32.5
            nontraffic V32.0
          truck (traffic) V34.5
            nontraffic V34.0
          two wheeled motor vehicle (traffic)
            V32.5
            nontraffic V32.0
          van (traffic) V33.5
            nontraffic V33.0
        noncollision accident (traffic) V38.5
          nontraffic V38.0
      hanger-on
        collision (with)
          animal (traffic) V30.7
            being ridden (traffic) V36.7
              nontraffic V36.2
            nontraffic V30.2
          animal-drawn vehicle (traffic) V36.7
            nontraffic V36.2
          bus (traffic) V34.7
            nontraffic V34.2
          car (traffic) V33.7
            nontraffic V33.2

Accident *(Continued)*
  transport *(Continued)*
    three-wheeled motor vehicle occupant
    (Continued)
      hanger-on *(Continued)*
        collision *(Continued)*
          pedal cycle (traffic) V31.7
            nontraffic V31.2
          pickup truck (traffic) V33.7
            nontraffic V33.2
          railway vehicle (traffic) V35.7
            nontraffic V35.2
          specified vehicle NEC (traffic) V36.7
            nontraffic V36.2
          stationary object (traffic) V37.7
            nontraffic V37.2
          streetcar (traffic) V36.7
            nontraffic V36.2
          three wheeled motor vehicle
            (traffic) V32.7
            nontraffic V32.2
          truck (traffic) V34.7
            nontraffic V34.2
          two wheeled motor vehicle (traffic)
            V32.7
            nontraffic V32.2
          van (traffic) V33.7
            nontraffic V33.2
        noncollision accident (traffic) V38.7
          nontraffic V38.2
      noncollision accident (traffic) V38.9
        nontraffic V38.3
        while boarding or alighting V38.4
      nontraffic V39.3
      passenger
        collision (with)
          animal (traffic) V30.6
            being ridden (traffic) V36.6
              nontraffic V36.1
            nontraffic V30.1
          animal-drawn vehicle (traffic) V36.6
            nontraffic V36.1
          bus (traffic) V34.6
            nontraffic V34.1
          car (traffic) V33.6
            nontraffic V33.1
          motor vehicle NOS (traffic) V39.50
            nontraffic V39.10
            specified type NEC (traffic)
              V39.59
              nontraffic V39.19
          pedal cycle (traffic) V31.6
            nontraffic V31.1
          pickup truck (traffic) V33.6
            nontraffic V33.1
          railway vehicle (traffic) V35.6
            nontraffic V35.1
          specified vehicle NEC (traffic)
            V36.6
            nontraffic V36.1
          stationary object (traffic) V37.6
            nontraffic V37.1
          streetcar (traffic) V36.6
            nontraffic V36.1
          three wheeled motor vehicle
            (traffic) V32.6
            nontraffic V32.1
          truck (traffic) V34.6
            nontraffic V34.1
          two wheeled motor vehicle (traffic)
            V32.6
            nontraffic V32.1
          van (traffic) V33.6
            nontraffic V33.1
        noncollision accident (traffic) V38.6
          nontraffic V38.1
      specified type NEC V39.89
      military vehicle V39.81
      tractor (farm) (and trailer) —*see* Accident,
        transport, agricultural vehicle
        occupant

Accident *(Continued)*
  transport *(Continued)*
    tram —*see* Accident, transport, streetcar
      in mine or quarry —*see* Accident,
        transport, industrial vehicle
        occupant
    trolley —*see* Accident, transport, streetcar
      in mine or quarry —*see* Accident,
        transport, industrial vehicle
        occupant
    truck (heavy) occupant V69.9
      collision (with)
        animal (traffic) V60.9
          being ridden (traffic) V66.9
            nontraffic V66.3
            while boarding or alighting V66.4
          nontraffic V60.3
          while boarding or alighting V60.4
        animal-drawn vehicle (traffic) V66.9
          nontraffic V66.3
          while boarding or alighting V66.4
        bus (traffic) V64.9
          nontraffic V64.3
          while boarding or alighting V64.4
        car (traffic) V63.9
          nontraffic V63.3
          while boarding or alighting V63.4
        motor vehicle NOS (traffic) V69.60
          nontraffic V69.20
          specified type NEC (traffic) V69.69
            nontraffic V69.29
        pedal cycle (traffic) V61.9
          nontraffic V61.3
          while boarding or alighting V61.4
        pickup truck (traffic) V63.9
          nontraffic V63.3
          while boarding or alighting V63.4
        railway vehicle (traffic) V65.9
          nontraffic V65.3
          while boarding or alighting V65.4
        specified vehicle NEC (traffic) V66.9
          nontraffic V66.3
          while boarding or alighting V66.4
        stationary object (traffic) V67.9
          nontraffic V67.3
          while boarding or alighting V67.4
        streetcar (traffic) V66.9
          nontraffic V66.3
          while boarding or alighting V66.4
        three wheeled motor vehicle (traffic)
          V62.9
          nontraffic V62.3
          while boarding or alighting V62.4
        truck (traffic) V64.9
          nontraffic V64.3
          while boarding or alighting V64.4
        two wheeled motor vehicle (traffic)
          V62.9
          nontraffic V62.3
          while boarding or alighting V62.4
        van (traffic) V63.9
          nontraffic V63.3
          while boarding or alighting V63.4
      driver
        collision (with)
          animal (traffic) V60.5
            being ridden (traffic) V66.5
              nontraffic V66.0
            nontraffic V60.0
          animal-drawn vehicle (traffic)
            V66.5
            nontraffic V66.0
          bus (traffic) V64.5
            nontraffic V64.0
          car (traffic) V63.5
            nontraffic V63.0
          motor vehicle NOS (traffic) V69.40
            nontraffic V69.00
            specified type NEC (traffic)
              V69.49
              nontraffic V69.09

◀ New   ◀▥ Revised   ~~deleted~~ Deleted

Accident (Continued)
  transport (Continued)
    truck occupant (Continued)
      driver (Continued)
        collision (Continued)
          pedal cycle (traffic) V61.5
            nontraffic V61.0
          pickup truck (traffic) V63.5
            nontraffic V63.0
          railway vehicle (traffic) V65.5
            nontraffic V65.0
          specified vehicle NEC (traffic) V66.5
            nontraffic V66.0
          stationary object (traffic) V67.5
            nontraffic V67.0
          streetcar (traffic) V66.5
            nontraffic V66.0
          three wheeled motor vehicle
              (traffic) V62.5
            nontraffic V62.0
          truck (traffic) V64.5
            nontraffic V64.0
          two wheeled motor vehicle (traffic)
              V62.5
            nontraffic V62.0
          van (traffic) V63.5
            nontraffic V63.0
        noncollision accident (traffic) V68.5
          nontraffic V68.0
      dump —see Accident, transport,
          construction vehicle occupant
      hanger-on
        collision (with)
          animal (traffic) V60.7
            being ridden (traffic) V66.7
              nontraffic V66.2
            nontraffic V60.2
          animal-drawn vehicle (traffic) V66.7
            nontraffic V66.2
          bus (traffic) V64.7
            nontraffic V64.2
          car (traffic) V63.7
            nontraffic V63.2
          pedal cycle (traffic) V61.7
            nontraffic V61.2
          pickup truck (traffic) V63.7
            nontraffic V63.2
          railway vehicle (traffic) V65.7
            nontraffic V65.2
          specified vehicle NEC (traffic) V66.7
            nontraffic V66.2
          stationary object (traffic) V67.7
            nontraffic V67.2
          streetcar (traffic) V66.7
            nontraffic V66.2
          three wheeled motor vehicle
              (traffic) V62.7
            nontraffic V62.2
          truck (traffic) V64.7
            nontraffic V64.2
          two wheeled motor vehicle (traffic)
              V62.7
            nontraffic V62.2
          van (traffic) V63.7
            nontraffic V63.2
        noncollision accident (traffic) V68.7
          nontraffic V68.2
      noncollision accident (traffic) V68.9
        nontraffic V68.3
        while boarding or alighting V68.4
      nontraffic V69.3
      passenger
        collision (with)
          animal (traffic) V60.6
            being ridden (traffic) V66.6
              nontraffic V66.1
            nontraffic V60.1
          animal-drawn vehicle (traffic) V66.6
            nontraffic V66.1
          bus (traffic) V64.6
            nontraffic V64.1

Accident (Continued)
  transport (Continued)
    truck occupant (Continued)
      passenger (Continued)
        collision (Continued)
          car (traffic) V63.6
            nontraffic V63.1
          motor vehicle NOS (traffic) V69.50
            nontraffic V69.10
            specified type NEC (traffic)
                V69.59
              nontraffic V69.19
          pedal cycle (traffic) V61.6
            nontraffic V61.1
          pickup truck (traffic) V63.6
            nontraffic V63.1
          railway vehicle (traffic) V65.6
            nontraffic V65.1
          specified vehicle NEC (traffic)
              V66.6
            nontraffic V66.1
          stationary object (traffic) V67.6
            nontraffic V67.1
          streetcar (traffic) V66.6
            nontraffic V66.1
          three wheeled motor vehicle
              (traffic) V62.6
            nontraffic V62.1
          truck (traffic) V64.6
            nontraffic V64.1
          two wheeled motor vehicle (traffic)
              V62.6
            nontraffic V62.1
          van (traffic) V63.6
            nontraffic V63.1
        noncollision accident (traffic) V68.6
          nontraffic V68.1
    pickup —see Accident, transport, pickup
        truck occupant
    specified type NEC V69.88
      military vehicle V69.81
    van occupant V59.9
      collision (with)
        animal (traffic) V50.9
          being ridden (traffic) V56.9
            nontraffic V56.3
            while boarding or alighting
                V56.4
          nontraffic V50.3
          while boarding or alighting V50.4
        animal-drawn vehicle (traffic) V56.9
          nontraffic V56.3
          while boarding or alighting V56.4
        bus (traffic) V54.9
          nontraffic V54.3
          while boarding or alighting V54.4
        car (traffic) V53.9
          nontraffic V53.3
          while boarding or alighting V53.4
        motor vehicle NOS (traffic) V59.60
          nontraffic V59.20
          specified type NEC (traffic) V59.69
            nontraffic V59.29
        pedal cycle (traffic) V51.9
          nontraffic V51.3
          while boarding or alighting V51.4
        pickup truck (traffic) V53.9
          nontraffic V53.3
          while boarding or alighting V53.4
        railway vehicle (traffic) V55.9
          nontraffic V55.3
          while boarding or alighting V55.4
        specified vehicle NEC (traffic) V56.9
          nontraffic V56.3
          while boarding or alighting V56.4
        stationary object (traffic) V57.9
          nontraffic V57.3
          while boarding or alighting V57.4
        streetcar (traffic) V56.9
          nontraffic V56.3
          while boarding or alighting V56.4

Accident (Continued)
  transport (Continued)
    van occupant (Continued)
      collision (Continued)
        three wheeled motor vehicle (traffic)
            V52.9
          nontraffic V52.3
          while boarding or alighting V52.4
        truck (traffic) V54.9
          nontraffic V54.3
          while boarding or alighting V54.4
        two wheeled motor vehicle (traffic)
            V52.9
          nontraffic V52.3
          while boarding or alighting V52.4
        van (traffic) V53.9
          nontraffic V53.3
          while boarding or alighting V53.4
      driver
        collision (with)
          animal (traffic) V50.5
            being ridden (traffic) V56.5
              nontraffic V56.0
            nontraffic V50.0
          animal-drawn vehicle (traffic) V56.5
            nontraffic V56.0
          bus (traffic) V54.5
            nontraffic V54.0
          car (traffic) V53.5
            nontraffic V53.0
          motor vehicle NOS (traffic) V59.40
            nontraffic V59.00
            specified type NEC (traffic)
                V59.49
              nontraffic V59.09
          pedal cycle (traffic) V51.5
            nontraffic V51.0
          pickup truck (traffic) V53.5
            nontraffic V53.0
          railway vehicle (traffic) V55.5
            nontraffic V55.0
          specified vehicle NEC (traffic) V56.5
            nontraffic V56.0
          stationary object (traffic) V57.5
            nontraffic V57.0
          streetcar (traffic) V56.5
            nontraffic V56.0
          three wheeled motor vehicle
              (traffic) V52.5
            nontraffic V52.0
          truck (traffic) V54.5
            nontraffic V54.0
          two wheeled motor vehicle (traffic)
              V52.5
            nontraffic V52.0
          van (traffic) V53.5
            nontraffic V53.0
        noncollision accident (traffic) V58.5
          nontraffic V58.0
      hanger-on
        collision (with)
          animal (traffic) V50.7
            being ridden (traffic) V56.7
              nontraffic V56.2
            nontraffic V50.2
          animal-drawn vehicle (traffic) V56.7
            nontraffic V56.2
          bus (traffic) V54.7
            nontraffic V54.2
          car (traffic) V53.7
            nontraffic V53.2
          pedal cycle (traffic) V51.7
            nontraffic V51.2
          pickup truck (traffic) V53.7
            nontraffic V53.2
          railway vehicle (traffic) V55.7
            nontraffic V55.2
          specified vehicle NEC (traffic) V56.7
            nontraffic V56.2
          stationary object (traffic) V57.7
            nontraffic V57.2

A

Accident *(Continued)*
  transport *(Continued)*
    van occupant *(Continued)*
      hanger-on *(Continued)*
        collision *(Continued)*
          streetcar (traffic) V56.7
            nontraffic V56.2
          three wheeled motor vehicle
            (traffic) V52.7
            nontraffic V52.2
          truck (traffic) V54.7
            nontraffic V54.2
          two wheeled motor vehicle (traffic)
            V52.7
            nontraffic V52.2
          van (traffic) V53.7
            nontraffic V53.2
        noncollision accident (traffic) V58.7
          nontraffic V58.2
        noncollision accident (traffic) V58.9
          nontraffic V58.3
          while boarding or alighting V58.4
        nontraffic V59.3
      passenger
        collision (with)
          animal (traffic) V50.6
            being ridden (traffic) V56.6
              nontraffic V56.1
            nontraffic V50.1
          animal-drawn vehicle (traffic) V56.6
            nontraffic V56.1
          bus (traffic) V54.6
            nontraffic V54.1
          car (traffic) V53.6
            nontraffic V53.1
          motor vehicle NOS (traffic) V59.50
            nontraffic V59.10
            specified type NEC (traffic) V59.59
              nontraffic V59.19
          pedal cycle (traffic) V51.6
            nontraffic V51.1
          pickup truck (traffic) V53.6
            nontraffic V53.1
          railway vehicle (traffic) V55.6
            nontraffic V55.1
          specified vehicle NEC (traffic) V56.6
            nontraffic V56.1
          stationary object (traffic) V57.6
            nontraffic V57.1
          streetcar (traffic) V56.6
            nontraffic V56.1
          three wheeled motor vehicle
            (traffic) V52.6
            nontraffic V52.1
          truck (traffic) V54.6
            nontraffic V54.1
          two wheeled motor vehicle (traffic)
            V52.6
            nontraffic V52.1
          van (traffic) V53.6
            nontraffic V53.1
        noncollision accident (traffic) V58.6
          nontraffic V58.1
      specified type NEC V59.88
      military vehicle V59.81
    watercraft occupant —*see* Accident,
      watercraft
    vehicle NEC V89.9
      animal-drawn NEC —*see* Accident,
        transport, animal-drawn vehicle
        occupant
      special
        agricultural —*see* Accident, transport,
          agricultural vehicle occupant
        construction —*see* Accident, transport,
          construction vehicle occupant
        industrial —*see* Accident, transport,
          industrial vehicle occupant
        three-wheeled NEC (motorized) —*see*
          Accident, transport, three-wheeled
          motor vehicle occupant

Accident *(Continued)*
  watercraft V94.9
    causing
      drowning —*see* Drowning, due to,
        accident to, watercraft
      injury NEC V91.89
        crushed between craft and object
          V91.19
          powered craft V91.13
            ferry boat V91.11
            fishing boat V91.12
            jetskis V91.13
            liner V91.11
            merchant ship V91.10
            passenger ship V91.11
          unpowered craft V91.18
            canoe V91.15
            inflatable V91.16
            kayak V91.15
            sailboat V91.14
            surf-board V91.18
            windsurfer V91.18
        fall on board V91.29
          powered craft V91.23
            ferry boat V91.21
            fishing boat V91.22
            jetskis V91.23
            liner V91.21
            merchant ship V91.20
            passenger ship V91.21
          unpowered craft
            canoe V91.25
            inflatable V91.26
            kayak V91.25
            sailboat V91.24
        fire on board causing burn V91.09
          powered craft V91.03
            ferry boat V91.01
            fishing boat V91.02
            jetskis V91.03
            liner V91.01
            merchant ship V91.00
            passenger ship V91.01
          unpowered craft V91.08
            canoe V91.05
            inflatable V91.06
            kayak V91.05
            sailboat V91.04
            surf-board V91.08
            water skis V91.07
            windsurfer V91.08
        hit by falling object V91.39
          powered craft V91.33
            ferry boat V91.31
            fishing boat V91.32
            jetskis V91.33
            liner V91.31
            merchant ship V91.30
            passenger ship V91.31
          unpowered craft V91.38
            canoe V91.35
            inflatable V91.36
            kayak V91.35
            sailboat V91.34
            surf-board V91.38
            water skis V91.37
            windsurfer V91.38
        specified type NEC V91.89
          powered craft V91.83
            ferry boat V91.81
            fishing boat V91.82
            jetskis V91.83
            liner V91.81
            merchant ship V91.80
            passenger ship V91.81
          unpowered craft V91.88
            canoe V91.85
            inflatable V91.86
            kayak V91.85
            sailboat V91.84
            surf-board V91.88

Accident *(Continued)*
  watercraft *(Continued)*
    causing *(Continued)*
      injury NEC *(Continued)*
        specified type NEC *(Continued)*
          unpowered craft *(Continued)*
            water skis V91.87
            windsurfer V91.88
      due to, caused by cataclysm —*see* Forces of
        nature, by type
      military NEC V94.818
        with civilian watercraft V94.810
        civilian in water injured by V94.811
      nonpowered, struck by
        nonpowered vessel V94.22
        powered vessel V94.21
      specified type NEC V94.89
      striking swimmer
        powered V94.11
        unpowered V94.12
Acid throwing (assault) Y08.89
Activity (involving) (of victim at time of event)
  Y93.9
  aerobic and step exercise (class) Y93.A3
  alpine skiing Y93.23
  animal care NEC Y93.K9
  arts and handcrafts NEC Y93.D9
  athletics NEC Y93.79
  athletics played as a team or group NEC
    Y93.69
  athletics played individually NEC Y93.59
  baking Y93.G3
  ballet Y93.41
  barbells Y93.B3
  BASE (Building, Antenna, Span, Earth)
    jumping Y93.33
  baseball Y93.64
  basketball Y93.67
  bathing (personal) Y93.E1
  beach volleyball Y93.68
  bike riding Y93.55
  boogie boarding Y93.18
  bowling Y93.54
  boxing Y93.71
  brass instrument playing Y93.J4
  building construction Y93.H3
  bungee jumping Y93.34
  calisthenics Y93.A2
  canoeing (in calm and turbulent water)
    Y93.16
  capture the flag Y93.6A
  cardiorespiratory exercise NEC Y93.A9
  caregiving (providing) NEC Y93.F9
    bathing Y93.F1
    lifting Y93.F2
  cellular
    communication device Y93.C2
    telephone Y93.C2
  challenge course Y93.A5
  cheerleading Y93.45
  circuit training Y93.A4
  cleaning
    floor Y93.E5
  climbing NEC Y93.39
    mountain Y93.31
    rock Y93.31
    wall Y93.31
  clothing care and maintenance NEC
    Y93.E9
  combatives Y93.75
  computer
    keyboarding Y93.C1
    technology NEC Y93.C9
  confidence course Y93.A5
  construction (building) Y93.H3
  cooking and baking Y93.G3
  cool down exercises Y93.A2
  cricket Y93.69
  crocheting Y93.D1
  cross country skiing Y93.24
  dancing (all types) Y93.41

◀ New   ⬅ Revised   ~~deleted~~ Deleted

Activity *(Continued)*
  digging
    dirt Y93.H1
  dirt digging Y93.H1
  dishwashing Y93.G1
  diving (platform) (springboard) Y93.12
    underwater Y93.15
  dodge ball Y93.6A
  downhill skiing Y93.23
  drum playing Y93.J2
  dumbbells Y93.B3
  electronic
    devices NEC Y93.C9
      hand held interactive Y93.C2
    game playing (using) (with)
      interactive device Y93.C2
      keyboard or other stationary device
        Y93.C1
  elliptical machine Y93.A1
  exercise (s)
    machines ((primarily) for)
      cardiorespiratory conditioning Y93.A1
      muscle strengthening Y93.B1
    muscle strengthening (non-machine) NEC
      Y93.B9
  external motion NEC Y93.I9
    rollercoaster Y93.I1
  field hockey Y93.65
  figure skating (pairs) (singles) Y93.21
  flag football Y93.62
  floor mopping and cleaning Y93.E5
  food preparation and clean up Y93.G1
  football (American) NOS Y93.61
    flag Y93.62
    tackle Y93.61
    touch Y93.62
  four square Y93.6A
  free weights Y93.B3
  frisbee (ultimate) Y93.74
  furniture
    building Y93.D3
    finishing Y93.D3
    repair Y93.D3
  game playing (electronic)
    using interactive device Y93.C2
    using keyboard or other stationary device
      Y93.C1
  gardening Y93.H2
  golf Y93.53
  grass drills Y93.A6
  grilling and smoking food Y93.G2
  grooming and shearing an animal Y93.K3
  guerilla drills Y93.A6
  gymnastics (rhythmic) Y93.43
  hand held interactive electronic device Y93.
    C2
  handball Y93.73
  handcrafts NEC Y93.D9
  hang gliding Y93.35
  hiking (on level or elevated terrain) Y93.01
  hockey (ice) Y93.22
    field Y93.65
  horseback riding Y93.52
  household (interior) maintenance NEC Y93.
    E9
  ice NEC Y93.29
    dancing Y93.21
    hockey Y93.22
    skating Y93.21
  inline roller skating Y93.51
  ironing Y93.E4
  judo Y93.75
  jumping (off) NEC Y93.39
    BASE (Building, Antenna, Span, Earth)
      Y93.33
    bungee Y93.34
    jacks Y93.A2
    rope Y93.56
  jumping jacks Y93.A2
  jumping rope Y93.56
  karate Y93.75

Activity *(Continued)*
  kayaking (in calm and turbulent water)
    Y93.16
  keyboarding (computer) Y93.C1
  kickball Y93.6A
  knitting Y93.D1
  lacrosse Y93.65
  land maintenance NEC Y93.H9
  landscaping Y93.H2
  laundry Y93.E2
  machines (exercise)
    primarily for cardiorespiratory
      conditioning Y93.A1
    primarily for muscle strengthening Y93.B1
  maintenance
    exterior building NEC Y93.H9
    household (interior) NEC Y93.E9
    land Y93.H9
    property Y93.H9
  marching (on level or elevated terrain) Y93.01
  martial arts Y93.75
  microwave oven Y93.G3
  milking an animal Y93.K2
  mopping (floor) Y93.E5
  mountain climbing Y93.31
  muscle strengthening
    exercises (non-machine) NEC Y93.B9
    machines Y93.B1
  musical keyboard (electronic) playing Y93.J1
  nordic skiing Y93.24
  obstacle course Y93.A5
  oven (microwave) Y93.G3
  packing up and unpacking in moving to a
    new residence Y93.E6
  parasailing Y93.19
  percussion instrument playing NEC Y93.J2
  personal
    bathing and showering Y93.E1
    hygiene NEC Y93.E8
    showering Y93.E1
  physical games generally associated with
    school recess, summer camp and
    children Y93.6A
  physical training NEC Y93.A9
  piano playing Y93.J1
  pilates Y93.B4
  platform diving Y93.12
  playing musical instrument
    brass instrument Y93.J4
    drum Y93.J2
    musical keyboard (electronic) Y93.J1
    percussion instrument NEC Y93.J2
    piano Y93.J1
    string instrument Y93.J3
    winds instrument Y93.J4
  property maintenance
    exterior NEC Y93.H9
    interior NEC Y93.E9
  pruning (garden and lawn) Y93.H2
  pull-ups Y93.B2
  push-ups Y93.B2
  racquetball Y93.73
  rafting (in calm and turbulent water) Y93.16
  raking (leaves) Y93.H1
  rappelling Y93.32
  refereeing a sports activity Y93.81
  residential relocation Y93.E6
  rhythmic gymnastics Y93.43
  rhythmic movement NEC Y93.49
  riding
    horseback Y93.52
    rollercoaster Y93.I1
  rock climbing Y93.31
  roller skating (inline) Y93.51
  rollercoaster riding Y93.I1
  rough housing and horseplay Y93.83
  rowing (in calm and turbulent water)
    Y93.16
  rugby Y93.63
  SCUBA diving Y93.15
  sewing Y93.D2

Activity *(Continued)*
  shoveling Y93.H1
    dirt Y93.H1
    snow Y93.H1
  showering (personal) Y93.E1
  sit-ups Y93.B2
  skateboarding Y93.51
  skating (ice) Y93.21
    roller Y93.51
  skiing (alpine) (downhill) Y93.23
    cross country Y93.24
    nordic Y93.24
    water Y93.17
  sledding (snow) Y93.23
  sleeping (sleep) Y93.84
  smoking and grilling food Y93.G2
  snorkeling Y93.15
  snow NEC Y93.29
    boarding Y93.23
    shoveling Y93.H1
    sledding Y93.23
    tubing Y93.23
  soccer Y93.66
  softball Y93.64
  specified NEC Y93.89
  spectator at an event Y93.82
  sports NEC Y93.79
    sports played as a team or group NEC
      Y93.69
    sports played individually NEC Y93.59
  springboard diving Y93.12
  squash Y93.73
  stationary bike Y93.A1
  step (stepping) exercise (class) Y93.A3
  stepper machine Y93.A1
  stove Y93.G3
  string instrument playing Y93.J3
  surfing Y93.18
    wind Y93.18
  swimming Y93.11
  tackle football Y93.61
  tap dancing Y93.41
  tennis Y93.73
  tobogganing Y93.23
  touch football Y93.62
  track and field events (non-running) Y93.57
    running Y93.02
  trampoline Y93.44
  treadmill Y93.A1
  trimming shrubs Y93.H2
  tubing (in calm and turbulent water) Y93.16
    snow Y93.23
  ultimate frisbee Y93.74
  underwater diving Y93.15
  unpacking in moving to a new residence
    Y93.E6
  use of stove, oven and microwave oven Y93.
    G3
  vacuuming Y93.E3
  volleyball (beach) (court) Y93.68
  wake boarding Y93.17
  walking (on level or elevated terrain) Y93.01
    an animal Y93.K1
  walking an animal Y93.K1
  wall climbing Y93.31
  warm up and cool down exercises Y93.A2
  water NEC Y93.19
    aerobics Y93.14
    craft NEC Y93.19
    exercise Y93.14
    polo Y93.13
    skiing Y93.17
    sliding Y93.18
    survival training and testing Y93.19
  weeding (garden and lawn) Y93.H2
  wind instrument playing Y93.J4
  windsurfing Y93.18
  wrestling Y93.72
  yoga Y93.42
Adverse effect of drugs —*see* Table of Drugs
  and Chemicals

Aerosinusitis —*see* Air, pressure
After-effect, late —*see* Sequelae
Air
  blast in war operations —*see* War operations,
    air blast
  pressure
    change, rapid
      during
        ascent W94.29
          while (in) (surfacing from)
            aircraft W94.23
            deep water diving W94.21
            underground W94.22
        descent W94.39
          in
            aircraft W94.31
            water W94.32
    high, prolonged W94.0
    low, prolonged W94.12
      due to residence or long visit at high
        altitude W94.11
Alpine sickness W94.11
Altitude sickness W94.11
Anaphylactic shock, anaphylaxis —*see* Table of
  Drugs and Chemicals
Andes disease W94.11
Arachnidism, arachnoidism X58
Arson (with intent to injure or kill) X97
Asphyxia, asphyxiation
  by
    food (bone) (seed) —*see* categories T17
      and T18
    gas —*see also* Table of Drugs and Chemicals
      legal
        execution —*see* Legal, intervention,
          gas
        intervention —*see* Legal, intervention,
          gas
  from
    fire —*see also* Exposure, fire
      in war operations —*see* War operations,
        fire
    ignition —*see* Ignition
    vomitus T17.81
  in war operations —*see* War operations,
    restriction of airway
Aspiration
  food (any type) (into respiratory tract) (with
    asphyxia, obstruction respiratory tract,
    suffocation) —*see* categories T17 and T18
  foreign body —*see* Foreign body, aspiration
  vomitus (with asphyxia, obstruction
    respiratory tract, suffocation) T17.81
Assassination (attempt) —*see* Assault
Assault (homicidal) (by) (in) Y09
  arson X97
  bite (of human being) Y04.1
  bodily force Y04.8
    bite Y04.1
    bumping into Y04.2
    sexual —*see* subcategories T74.0, T76.0
    unarmed fight Y04.0

Assault *(Continued)*
  bomb X96.9
    antipersonnel X96.0
    fertilizer X96.3
    gasoline X96.1
    letter X96.2
    petrol X96.1
    pipe X96.3
    specified NEC X96.8
  brawl (hand) (fists) (foot) (unarmed) Y04.0
  burning, burns (by fire) NEC X97
    acid Y08.89
    caustic, corrosive substance Y08.89
    chemical from swallowing caustic,
      corrosive substance —*see* Table of
      Drugs and Chemicals
    cigarette (s) X97
    hot object X98.9
      fluid NEC X98.2
      household appliance X98.3
      specified NEC X98.8
      steam X98.0
      tap water X98.1
      vapors X98.0
    scalding —*see* Assault, burning
    steam X98.0
    vitriol Y08.89
  caustic, corrosive substance (gas) Y08.89
  crashing of
    aircraft Y08.81
    motor vehicle Y03.8
      pushed in front of Y02.0
      run over Y03.0
      specified NEC Y03.8
  cutting or piercing instrument X99.9
    dagger X99.2
    glass X99.0
    knife X99.1
    specified NEC X99.8
    sword X99.2
  dagger X99.2
  drowning (in) X92.9
    bathtub X92.0
    natural water X92.3
    specified NEC X92.8
    swimming pool X92.1
      following fall X92.2
  dynamite X96.8
  explosive (s) (material) X96.9
  fight (hand) (fists) (foot) (unarmed) Y04.0
    with weapon —*see* Assault, by type of
      weapon
  fire X97
  firearm X95.9
    airgun X95.01
    handgun X93
    hunting rifle X94.1
    larger X94.9
      specified NEC X94.8
    machine gun X94.2
    shotgun X94.0
    specified NEC X95.8

Assault *(Continued)*
  from high place Y01
  gunshot (wound) NEC —*see* Assault, firearm,
    by type
  incendiary device X97
  injury Y09
    to child due to criminal abortion attempt
      NEC Y08.89
  knife X99.1
  late effect of —*see* X92-Y08 with 7th character
    S
  placing before moving object NEC Y02.8
    motor vehicle Y02.0
  poisoning —*see* categories T36-T65 with 7th
    character S
  puncture, any part of body —*see* Assault,
    cutting or piercing instrument
  pushing
    before moving object NEC Y02.8
      motor vehicle Y02.0
      subway train Y02.1
      train Y02.1
  rape T74.2-
  scalding —*see* Assault, burning
  sequelae of —*see* X92-Y08 with 7th character
    S
  sexual (by bodily force) T74.2-
  shooting —*see* Assault, firearm
  specified means NEC Y08.89
  stab, any part of body —*see* Assault, cutting
    or piercing instrument
  steam X98.0
  striking against
    other person Y04.2
    sports equipment Y08.09
      baseball bat Y08.02
      hockey stick Y08.01
  struck by
    sports equipment Y08.09
      baseball bat Y08.02
      hockey stick Y08.01
  submersion —*see* Assault, drowning
  violence Y09
  weapon Y09
    blunt Y00
    cutting or piercing —*see* Assault, cutting or
      piercing instrument
    firearm —*see* Assault, firearm
  wound Y09
    cutting —*see* Assault, cutting or piercing
      instrument
    gunshot —*see* Assault, firearm
    knife X99.1
    piercing —*see* Assault, cutting or piercing
      instrument
    puncture —*see* Assault, cutting or piercing
      instrument
    stab —*see* Assault, cutting or piercing
      instrument
Attack by mammals NEC W55.89
Avalanche —*see* Landslide
Aviator's disease —*see* Air, pressure

◀ New   ◀≡ Revised   ~~deleted~~ Deleted

B

Barotitis, barodontalgia, barosinusitis, barotrauma (otitic) (sinus) —*see* Air, pressure
Battered (baby) (child) (person) (syndrome) X58
Bayonet wound W26.1
  in
    legal intervention —*see* Legal, intervention, sharp object, bayonet
    war operations —*see* War operations, combat
  stated as undetermined whether accidental or intentional Y28.8
  suicide (attempt) X78.2
Bean in nose —*see* categories T17 and T18
Bed set on fire NEC —*see* Exposure, fire, uncontrolled, building, bed
Beheading (by guillotine)
  homicide X99.9
  legal execution —*see* Legal, intervention
Bending, injury in —*see* category Y93
Bends —*See* Air, pressure, change
Bite, bitten by
  alligator W58.01
  arthropod (nonvenomous) NEC W57
  bull W55.21
  cat W55.01
  cow W55.21
  crocodile W58.11
  dog W54.0
  goat W55.31
  hoof stock NEC W55.31
  horse W55.11
  human being (accidentally) W50.3
    with intent to injure or kill Y04.1
    as, or caused by, a crowd or human stampede (with fall) W52
    assault Y04.1
    homicide (attempt) Y04.1
    in
      fight Y04.1
  insect (nonvenomous) W57
  lizard (nonvenomous) W59.01
  mammal NEC W55.81
    marine W56.31
  marine animal (nonvenomous) W56.81
  millipede W57
  moray eel W56.51
  mouse W53.01
  person (s) (accidentally) W50.3
    with intent to injure or kill Y04.1
    as, or caused by, a crowd or human stampede (with fall) W52
    assault Y04.1
    homicide (attempt) Y04.1
    in
      fight Y04.1
  pig W55.41
  raccoon W55.51
  rat W53.11
  reptile W59.81
    lizard W59.01
    snake W59.11
    turtle W59.21
      terrestrial W59.81
  rodent W53.81
    mouse W53.01
    rat W53.11
    specified NEC W53.81
    squirrel W53.21
  shark W56.41
  sheep W55.31
  snake (nonvenomous) W59.11
  spider (nonvenomous) W57
  squirrel W53.21
Blast (air) **in war operations** —*see* War operations, blast
Blizzard X37.2

Blood alcohol level Y90.9
  20-39mg/100ml Y90.1
  40-59mg/100ml Y90.2
  60-79mg/100ml Y90.3
  80-99mg/100ml Y90.4
  100-119mg/100ml Y90.5
  120-199mg/100ml Y90.6
  200-239mg/100ml Y90.7
  less than 20mg/100ml Y90.0
  presence in blood, level not specified Y90.9
Blow X58
  by law-enforcing agent, police (on duty) —*see* Legal, intervention, manhandling
    blunt object —*see* Legal, intervention, blunt object
Blowing up —*see* Explosion
Brawl (hand) (fists) (foot) Y04.0
Breakage (accidental) (part of)
  ladder (causing fall) W11
  scaffolding (causing fall) W12
Broken
  glass, contact with —*see* Contact, with, glass
  power line (causing electric shock) W85
Bumping against, into (accidentally)
  object NEC W22.8
    with fall —*see* Fall, due to, bumping against, object
    caused by crowd or human stampede (with fall) W52
    sports equipment W21.9
  person (s) W51
    with fall W03
      due to ice or snow W00.0
    assault Y04.2
    caused by, a crowd or human stampede (with fall) W52
    homicide (attempt) Y04.2
  sports equipment W21.9
Burn, burned, burning (accidental) (by) (from) (on)
  acid NEC —*see* Table of Drugs and Chemicals
  bed linen —*see* Exposure, fire, uncontrolled, in building, bed
  blowtorch X08.8
    with ignition of clothing NEC X06.2
      nightwear X05
  bonfire, campfire (controlled) —*see also* Exposure, fire, controlled, not in building
    uncontrolled —*see* Exposure, fire, uncontrolled, not in building
  candle X08.8
    with ignition of clothing NEC X06.2
      nightwear X05
  caustic liquid, substance (external) (internal) NEC —*see* Table of Drugs and Chemicals
  chemical (external) (internal) —*see also* Table of Drugs and Chemicals
    in war operations —*see* War operations, fire
  cigar (s) or cigarette (s) X08.8
    with ignition of clothing NEC X06.2
      nightwear X05
  clothes, clothing NEC (from controlled fire) X06.2
    with conflagration —*see* Exposure, fire, uncontrolled, building
      not in building or structure —*see* Exposure, fire, uncontrolled, not in building
  cooker (hot) X15.8
    stated as undetermined whether accidental or intentional Y27.3
    suicide (attempt) X77.3
  electric blanket X16
  engine (hot) X17
  fire, flames —*see* Exposure, fire
  flare, Very pistol —*see* Discharge, firearm NEC

Burn, burned, burning (Continued)
  heat
    from appliance (electrical) (household) X15.8
      cooker X15.8
      hotplate X15.2
      kettle X15.8
      light bulb X15.8
      saucepan X15.3
      skillet X15.3
      stated as undetermined whether accidental or intentional Y27.3
      stove X15.0
      suicide (attempt) X77.3
      toaster X15.1
    in local application or packing during medical or surgical procedure Y63.5
  heating
    appliance, radiator or pipe X16
  homicide (attempt) —*see* Assault, burning
  hot
    air X14.1
    cooker X15.8
    drink X10.0
    engine X17
    fat X10.2
    fluid NEC X12
    food X10.1
    gases X14.1
    heating appliance X16
    household appliance NEC X15.8
    kettle X15.8
    liquid NEC X12
    machinery X17
    metal (molten) (liquid) NEC X18
    object (not producing fire or flames) NEC X19
    oil (cooking) X10.2
    pipe (s) X16
    radiator X16
    saucepan (glass) (metal) X15.3
    stove (kitchen) X15.0
    substance NEC X19
      caustic or corrosive NEC —*see* Table of Drugs and Chemicals
    toaster X15.1
    tool X17
    vapor X13.1
    water (tap) —*see* Contact, with, hot, tap water
  hotplate X15.2
    suicide (attempt) X77.3
  ignition —*see* Ignition
  in war operations —*see* War operations, fire
  inflicted by other person X97
    by hot objects, hot vapor, and steam —*see* Assault, burning, hot object
  internal, from swallowed caustic, corrosive liquid, substance —*see* Table of Drugs and Chemicals
  iron (hot) X15.8
    stated as undetermined whether accidental or intentional Y27.3
    suicide (attempt) X77.3
  kettle (hot) X15.8
    stated as undetermined whether accidental or intentional Y27.3
    suicide (attempt) X77.3
  lamp (flame) X08.8
    with ignition of clothing NEC X06.2
      nightwear X05
  lighter (cigar) (cigarette) X08.8
    with ignition of clothing NEC X06.2
      nightwear X05
  lightning —*see* subcategory T75.0
    causing fire —*see* Exposure, fire
  liquid (boiling) (hot) NEC X12
    stated as undetermined whether accidental or intentional Y27.2
    suicide (attempt) X77.2

Burn, burned, burning (*Continued*)
  local application of externally applied
      substance in medical or surgical care
      Y63.5
  machinery (hot) X17
  matches X08.8
    with ignition of clothing NEC X06.2
      nightwear X05
  mattress —*see* Exposure, fire, uncontrolled,
    building, bed
  medicament, externally applied Y63.5
  metal (hot) (liquid) (molten) NEC X18
  nightwear (nightclothes, nightdress, gown,
    pajamas, robe) X05
  object (hot) NEC X19
  on board watercraft
    due to
      accident to watercraft V91.09
        powered craft V91.03
          ferry boat V91.01
          fishing boat V91.02
          jetskis V91.03
          liner V91.01
          merchant ship V91.00
          passenger ship V91.01
        unpowered craft V91.08
          canoe V91.05
          inflatable V91.06
          kayak V91.05
          sailboat V91.04
          surf-board V91.08
          water skis V91.07
          windsurfer V91.08
      fire on board V93.09
        ferry boat V93.01
        fishing boat V93.02
        jetskis V93.03
        liner V93.01
        merchant ship V93.00
        passenger ship V93.01
        powered craft NEC V93.03
        sailboat V93.04

Burn, burned, burning (*Continued*)
  on board watercraft (*Continued*)
    due to (*Continued*)
      specified heat source NEC on board
        V93.19
        ferry boat V93.11
        fishing boat V93.12
        jetskis V93.13
        liner V93.11
        merchant ship V93.10
        passenger ship V93.11
        powered craft NEC V93.13
        sailboat V93.14
  pipe (hot) X16
    smoking X08.8
      with ignition of clothing NEC X06.2
        nightwear X05
  powder —*see* Powder burn
  radiator (hot) X16
  saucepan (hot) (glass) (metal) X15.3
    stated as undetermined whether
      accidental or intentional
      Y27.3
    suicide (attempt) X77.3
  self-inflicted X76
    stated as undetermined whether
      accidental or intentional
      Y26
  stated as undetermined whether
    accidental or intentional Y27.0
  steam X13.1
    pipe X16
      stated as undetermined whether
        accidental or intentional
        Y27.8
    stated as undetermined whether
      accidental or intentional Y27.0
    suicide (attempt) X77.0
  stove (hot) (kitchen) X15.0
    stated as undetermined whether
      accidental or intentional Y27.3
    suicide (attempt) X77.3

Burn, burned, burning (*Continued*)
  substance (hot) NEC X19
    boiling X12
      stated as undetermined whether
        accidental or intentional Y27.2
      suicide (attempt) X77.2
    molten (metal) X18
  suicide (attempt) NEC X76
    hot
      household appliance X77.3
      object X77.9
  stated as undetermined whether accidental or
    intentional Y27.0
  therapeutic misadventure
    heat in local application or packing during
      medical or surgical procedure Y63.5
    overdose of radiation Y63.2
  toaster (hot) X15.1
    stated as undetermined whether accidental
      or intentional Y27.3
    suicide (attempt) X77.3
  tool (hot) X17
  torch, welding X08.8
    with ignition of clothing NEC X06.2
      nightwear X05
  trash fire (controlled) —*see* Exposure, fire,
    controlled, not in building
    uncontrolled —*see* Exposure, fire,
      uncontrolled, not in building
  vapor (hot) X13.1
    stated as undetermined whether accidental
      or intentional Y27.0
    suicide (attempt) X77.0
  Very pistol —*see* Discharge, firearm NEC
Butted by animal W55.82
  bull W55.22
  cow W55.22
  goat W55.32
  horse W55.12
  pig W55.42
  sheep W55.32

◄ New   ⬅ Revised   ~~deleted~~ Deleted

C

Caisson disease —*see* Air, pressure, change
Campfire (exposure to) (controlled) —*see also* Exposure, fire, controlled, not in building
  uncontrolled —*see* Exposure, fire, uncontrolled, not in building
Capital punishment (any means) —*see* Legal, intervention
Car sickness T75.3
Casualty (not due to war) NEC X58
  war —*see* War operations
Cat
  bite W55.01
  scratch W55.03
Cataclysm, cataclysmic (any injury) NEC —*see* Forces of nature
Catching fire —*see* Exposure, fire
Caught
  between
    folding object W23.0
    objects (moving) (stationary and moving) W23.0
      and machinery —*see* Contact, with, by type of machine
      stationary W23.1
    sliding door and door frame W23.0
  by, in
    machinery (moving parts of) —*see* Contact, with, by type of machine
    washing-machine wringer W23.0
  under packing crate (due to losing grip) W23.1
Cave-in caused by cataclysmic earth surface movement or eruption —*see* Landslide
Change (s) **in air pressure** —*see* Air, pressure, change
Choked, choking (on) (any object except food or vomitus)
  food (bone) (seed) —*see* categories T17 and T18
  vomitus T17.81-
Civil insurrection —*see* War operations
Cloudburst (any injury) X37.8
Cold, exposure to (accidental) (excessive) (extreme) (natural) (place) **NEC** —*see* Exposure, cold
Collapse
  building W20.1
    burning (uncontrolled fire) X00.2
  dam or man-made structure (causing earth movement) X36.0
  machinery —*see* Contact, with, by type of machine
  structure W20.1
    burning (uncontrolled fire) X00.2
Collision (accidental) **NEC** (*see also* Accident, transport) V89.9
  pedestrian W51
    with fall W03
      due to ice or snow W00.0
      involving pedestrian conveyance —*see* Accident, transport, pedestrian, conveyance
    and
      crowd or human stampede (with fall) W52
      object W22.8
        with fall —*see* Fall, due to, bumping against, object
    person (s) —*see* Collision, pedestrian
  transport vehicle NEC V89.9
    and
      avalanche, fallen or not moving —*see* Accident, transport
        falling or moving —*see* Landslide
      landslide, fallen or not moving —*see* Accident, transport
        falling or moving —*see* Landslide

Collision NEC (*Continued*)
  transport vehicle NEC (*Continued*)
    due to cataclysm —*see* Forces of nature, by type
      intentional, purposeful suicide (attempt) —*see* Suicide, collision
Combustion, spontaneous —*see* Ignition
Complication (delayed) **of or following**
  (medical or surgical procedure) Y84.9
  with misadventure —*see* Misadventure
  amputation of limb (s) Y83.5
  anastomosis (arteriovenous) (blood vessel) (gastrojejunal) (tendon) (natural or artificial material) Y83.2
  aspiration (of fluid) Y84.4
    tissue Y84.8
  biopsy Y84.8
  blood
    sampling Y84.7
    transfusion
      procedure Y84.8
  bypass Y83.2
  catheterization (urinary) Y84.6
    cardiac Y84.0
  colostomy Y83.3
  cystostomy Y83.3
  dialysis (kidney) Y84.1
  drug —*see* Table of Drugs and Chemicals
  due to misadventure —*see* Misadventure
  duodenostomy Y83.3
  electroshock therapy Y84.3
  external stoma, creation of Y83.3
  formation of external stoma Y83.3
  gastrostomy Y83.3
  graft Y83.2
  hypothermia (medically-induced) Y84.8
  implant, implantation (of)
    artificial
      internal device (cardiac pacemaker) (electrodes in brain) (heart valve prosthesis) (orthopedic) Y83.1
      material or tissue (for anastomosis or bypass) Y83.2
        with creation of external stoma Y83.3
      natural tissues (for anastomosis or bypass) Y83.2
        with creation of external stoma Y83.3
  infusion
    procedure Y84.8
  injection —*see* Table of Drugs and Chemicals
    procedure Y84.8
  insertion of gastric or duodenal sound Y84.5
  insulin-shock therapy Y84.3
  paracentesis (abdominal) (thoracic) (aspirative) Y84.4
  procedures other than surgical operation —*see* Complication of or following, by type of procedure
  radiological procedure or therapy Y84.2
  removal of organ (partial) (total) NEC Y83.6
  sampling
    blood Y84.7
    fluid NEC Y84.4
    tissue Y84.8
  shock therapy Y84.3
  surgical operation NEC (*see also* Complication of or following, by type of operation) Y83.9
    reconstructive NEC Y83.4
      with
        anastomosis, bypass or graft Y83.2
        formation of external stoma Y83.3
    specified NEC Y83.8
  transfusion —*see also* Table of Drugs and Chemicals
    procedure Y84.8
  transplant, transplantation (heart) (kidney) (liver) (whole organ, any) Y83.0
    partial organ Y83.4
  ureterostomy Y83.3

Complication of or following (*Continued*)
  vaccination —*see also* Table of Drugs and Chemicals
    procedure Y84.8
Compression
  divers' squeeze —*see* Air, pressure, change
  trachea by
    food (lodged in esophagus) —*see* categories T17 and T18
    vomitus (lodged in esophagus) T17.81-
Conflagration —*see* Exposure, fire, uncontrolled
Constriction (external)
  hair W49.01
  jewelry W49.04
  ring W49.04
  rubber band W49.03
  specified item NEC W49.09
  string W49.02
  thread W49.02
Contact (accidental)
  with
    abrasive wheel (metalworking) W31.1
    alligator W58.09
      bite W58.01
      crushing W58.03
      strike W58.02
    amphibian W62.9
      frog W62.0
      toad W62.1
    animal (nonvenomous) NEC W64
      marine W56.89
        bite W56.81
        dolphin —*see* Contact, with, dolphin
        fish NEC —*see* Contact, with, fish
        mammal —*see* Contact, with, mammal, marine
        orca —*see* Contact, with, orca
        sea lion —*see* Contact, with, sea lion
        shark —*see* Contact, with, shark
        strike W56.82
    animate mechanical force NEC W64
    arrow W21.89
      not thrown, projected or falling W45.8
    arthropods (nonvenomous) W57
    axe W27.0
    band-saw (industrial) W31.2
    bayonet —*see* Bayonet wound
    bee (s) X58
    bench-saw (industrial) W31.2
    bird W61.99
      bite W61.91
      chicken —*see* Contact, with, chicken
      duck —*see* Contact, with, duck
      goose —*see* Contact, with, goose
      macaw —*see* Contact, with, macaw
      parrot —*see* Contact, with, parrot
      psittacine —*see* Contact, with, psittacine
      strike W61.92
      turkey —*see* Contact, with, turkey
    blender W29.0
    boiling water X12
      stated as undetermined whether accidental or intentional Y27.2
      suicide (attempt) X77.2
    bore, earth-drilling or mining (land) (seabed) W31.0
    buffalo —*see* Contact, with, hoof stock NEC
    bull W55.29
      bite W55.21
      gored W55.22
      strike W55.22
    bumper cars W31.81
    camel —*see* Contact, with, hoof stock NEC
    can
      lid W45.2
      opener W27.4
        powered W29.0
    cat W55.09
      bite W55.01
      scratch W55.03
    caterpillar (venomous) X58

Contact (*Continued*)
  with (*Continued*)
    centipede (venomous) X58
    chain
      hoist W24.0
        agricultural operations W30.89
      saw W29.3
    chicken W61.39
      peck W61.33
      strike W61.32
    chisel W27.0
    circular saw W31.2
    cobra X58
    combine (harvester) W30.0
    conveyer belt W24.1
    cooker (hot) X15.8
      stated as undetermined whether
        accidental or intentional Y27.3
      suicide (attempt) X77.3
    coral X58
    cotton gin W31.82
    cow W55.29
      bite W55.21
      strike W55.22
    crane W24.0
      agricultural operations W30.89
    crocodile W58.19
      bite W58.11
      crushing W58.13
      strike W58.12
    dagger W26.1
      stated as undetermined whether
        accidental or intentional Y28.2
      suicide (attempt) X78.2
    dairy equipment W31.82
    dart W21.89
      not thrown, projected or falling W45.8
    deer —*see* Contact, with, hoof stock
      NEC
    derrick W24.0
      agricultural operations W30.89
        hay W30.2
    dog W54.8
      bite W54.0
      strike W54.1
    dolphin W56.09
      bite W56.01
      strike W56.02
    donkey —*see* Contact, with, hoof stock
      NEC
    drill (powered) W29.8
      earth (land) (seabed) W31.0
      nonpowered W27.8
    drive belt W24.0
      agricultural operations W30.89
    dry ice —*see* Exposure, cold, man-made
    dryer (clothes) (powered) (spin) W29.2
    duck W61.69
      bite W61.61
      strike W61.62
    earth(-)
      drilling machine (industrial) W31.0
      scraping machine in stationary use
        W31.83
    edge of stiff paper W45.1
    electric
      beater W29.0
      blanket X16
      fan W29.2
        commercial W31.82
      knife W29.1
      mixer W29.0
    elevator (building) W24.0
      agricultural operations W30.89
        grain W30.3
    engine (s), hot NEC X17
    excavating machine W31.0
    farm machine W30.9
    feces —*see* Contact, with, by type of
      animal
    fer de lance X58

Contact (*Continued*)
  with (*Continued*)
    fish W56.59
      bite W56.51
      shark —*see* Contact, with, shark
      strike W56.52
    flying horses W31.81
    forging (metalworking) machine
      W31.1
    fork W27.4
    forklift (truck) W24.0
      agricultural operations W30.89
    frog W62.0
    garden
      cultivator (powered) W29.3
        riding W30.89
      fork W27.1
    gas turbine W31.3
    Gila monster X58
    giraffe —*see* Contact, with, hoof stock
      NEC
    glass (sharp) (broken) W25
      with subsequent fall W18.02
      assault X99.0
      due to fall —*see* Fall, by type
      stated as undetermined whether
        accidental or intentional Y28. 0
      suicide (attempt) X78.0
    goat W55.39
      bite W55.31
      strike W55.32
    goose W61.59
      bite W61.51
      strike W61.52
    hand
      saw W27.0
      tool (not powered) NEC W27.8
        powered W29.8
    harvester W30.0
    hay-derrick W30.2
    heat NEC X19
      from appliance (electrical)
        (household) —*see* Contact, with,
        hot, household appliance
        heating appliance X16
    heating
      appliance (hot) X16
      pad (electric) X16
    hedge-trimmer (powered) W29.3
    hoe W27.1
    hoist (chain) (shaft) NEC W24.0
      agricultural W30.89
    hoof stock NEC W55.39
      bite W55.31
      strike W55.32
    hornet (s) X58
    horse W55.19
      bite W55.11
      strike W55.12
    hot
      air X14.1
        inhalation X14.0
      cooker X15.8
      drinks X10.0
      engine X17
      fats X10.2
      fluids NEC X12
        assault X98.2
        suicide (attempt) X77.2
        undetermined whether accidental or
          intentional Y27.2
      food X10.1
      gases X14.1
        inhalation X14.0
      heating appliance X16
      household appliance X15.8
        assault X98.3
        cooker X15.8
        hotplate X15.2
        kettle X15.8
        light bulb X15.8

Contact (*Continued*)
  with (*Continued*)
    hot (*Continued*)
      household appliance (*Continued*)
        object NEC X19
          assault X98.8
          stated as undetermined whether
            accidental or intentional Y27.9
          suicide (attempt) X77.8
        saucepan X15.3
        skillet X15.3
        stated as undetermined whether
          accidental or intentional Y27.3
        stove X15.0
        suicide (attempt) X77.3
        toaster X15.1
      kettle X15.8
      light bulb X15.8
      liquid NEC (*see also* Burn) X12
        drinks X10.0
        stated as undetermined whether
          accidental or intentional Y27.2
        suicide (attempt) X77.2
        tap water X11.8
          stated as undetermined whether
            accidental or intentional Y27.1
          suicide (attempt) X77.1
      machinery X17
      metal (molten) (liquid) NEC X18
      object (not producing fire or flames)
        NEC X19
      oil (cooking) X10.2
      pipe X16
      plate X15.2
      radiator X16
      saucepan (glass) (metal) X15.3
      skillet X15.3
      stove (kitchen) X15.0
      substance NEC X19
      tap-water X11.8
        assault X98.1
        heated on stove X12
          stated as undetermined whether
            accidental or intentional Y27.2
          suicide (attempt) X77.2
        in bathtub X11.0
        running X11.1
        stated as undetermined whether
          accidental or intentional Y27.1
        suicide (attempt) X77.1
      toaster X15.1
      tool X17
      vapors X13.1
        inhalation X13.0
      water (tap) X11.8
        boiling X12
          stated as undetermined whether
            accidental or intentional Y27.2
          suicide (attempt) X77.2
        heated on stove X12
          stated as undetermined whether
            accidental or intentional Y27.2
          suicide (attempt) X77.2
        in bathtub X11.0
        running X11.1
        stated as undetermined whether
          accidental or intentional Y27.1
        suicide (attempt) X77.1
    hotplate X15.2
    ice-pick W27.4
    insect (nonvenomous) NEC W57
    kettle (hot) X15.8
    knife W26.0
      assault X99.1
      electric W29.1
      stated as undetermined whether
        accidental or intentional Y28.1
      suicide (attempt) X78.1
    lathe (metalworking) W31.1
      turnings W45.8
      woodworking W31.2

◀ New   ◀▥ Revised   ~~deleted~~ Deleted

Contact *(Continued)*
  with *(Continued)*
    lawnmower (powered) (ridden) W28
      causing electrocution W86.8
        suicide (attempt) X83.1
      unpowered W27.1
    lift, lifting (devices) W24.0
      agricultural operations W30.89
      shaft W24.0
    liquefied gas —*see* Exposure, cold,
        man-made
    liquid air, hydrogen, nitrogen —*see*
        Exposure, cold, man-made
    lizard (nonvenomous) W59.09
      bite W59.01
      strike W59.02
    llama —*see* Contact, with, hoof stock NEC
    macaw W61.19
      bite W61.11
      strike W61.12
    machine, machinery W31.9
      abrasive wheel W31.1
      agricultural including animal-powered
          W30.9
        combine harvester W30.0
        grain storage elevator W30.3
        hay derrick W30.2
        power take-off device W30.1
        reaper W30.0
        specified NEC W30.89
        thresher W30.0
        transport vehicle, stationary W30.81
      band saw W31.2
      bench saw W31.2
      circular saw W31.2
      commercial NEC W31.82
      drilling, metal (industrial) W31.1
      earth-drilling W31.0
      earthmoving or scraping W31.89
      excavating W31.89
      forging machine W31.1
      gas turbine W31.3
      hot X17
      internal combustion engine W31.3
      land drill W31.0
      lathe W31.1
      lifting (devices) W24.0
      metal drill W31.1
      metalworking (industrial) W31.1
      milling, metal W31.1
      mining W31.0
      molding W31.2
      overhead plane W31.2
      power press, metal W31.1
      prime mover W31.3
      printing W31.89
      radial saw W31.2
      recreational W31.81
      roller-coaster W31.81
      rolling mill, metal W31.1
      sander W31.2
      seabed drill W31.0
      shaft
        hoist W31.0
        lift W31.0
      specified NEC W31.89
      spinning W31.89
      steam engine W31.3
      transmission W24.1
      undercutter W31.0
      water driven turbine W31.3
      weaving W31.89
      woodworking or forming (industrial)
          W31.2
    mammal (feces) (urine) W55.89
      bull —*see* Contact, with, bull
      cat —*see* Contact, with, cat
      cow —*see* Contact, with, cow
      goat —*see* Contact, with, goat
      hoof stock —*see* Contact, with, hoof
          stock

Contact *(Continued)*
  with *(Continued)*
    mammal *(Continued)*
      horse —*see* Contact, with, horse
      marine W56.39
        dolphin —*see* Contact, with, dolphin
        orca —*see* Contact, with, orca
        sea lion —*see* Contact, with, sea lion
        specified NEC W56.39
          bite W56.31
          strike W56.32
      pig —*see* Contact, with, pig
      raccoon —*see* Contact, with, raccoon
      rodent —*see* Contact, with, rodent
      sheep —*see* Contact, with, sheep
      specified NEC W55.89
        bite W55.81
        strike W55.82
    marine
      animal W56.89
        bite W56.81
        dolphin —*see* Contact, with, dolphin
        fish NEC —*see* Contact, with, fish
        mammal —*see* Contact, with,
            mammal, marine
        orca —*see* Contact, with, orca
        sea lion —*see* Contact, with, sea lion
        shark —*see* Contact, with, shark
        strike W56.82
    meat
      grinder (domestic) W29.0
        industrial W31.82
        nonpowered W27.4
      slicer (domestic) W29.0
        industrial W31.82
    merry go round W31.81
    metal, (hot) (liquid) (molten) NEC X18
    millipede W57
    nail W45.0
      gun W29.4
    needle (sewing) W27.3
      hypodermic W46.0
        contaminated W46.1
    object (blunt) NEC
      hot NEC X19
      legal intervention —*see* Legal,
          intervention, blunt object
      sharp NEC W45.8
        inflicted by other person NEC W45.8
          stated as
            intentional homicide (attempt) —
                see Assault, cutting or
                piercing instrument
          legal intervention —*see* Legal,
              intervention, sharp object
          self-inflicted X78.9
    orca W56.29
      bite W56.21
      strike W56.22
    overhead plane W31.2
    paper (as sharp object) W45.1
    paper-cutter W27.5
    parrot W61.09
      bite W61.01
      strike W61.02
    pig W55.49
      bite W55.41
      strike W55.42
    pipe, hot X16
    pitchfork W27.1
    plane (metal) (wood) W27.0
      overhead W31.2
    plant thorns, spines, sharp leaves or other
        mechanisms W60
    powered
      garden cultivator W29.3
      household appliance, implement, or
          machine W29.8
      saw (industrial) W31.2
        hand W29.8
    printing machine W31.89

Contact *(Continued)*
  with *(Continued)*
    psittacine bird W61.29
      bite W61.21
      macaw —*see* Contact, with, macaw
      parrot —*see* Contact, with, parrot
      strike W61.22
    pulley (block) (transmission) W24.0
      agricultural operations W30.89
    raccoon W55.59
      bite W55.51
      strike W55.52
    radial-saw (industrial) W31.2
    radiator (hot) X16
    rake W27.1
    rattlesnake X58
    reaper W30.0
    reptile W59.89
      lizard —*see* Contact, with, lizard
      snake —*see* Contact, with, snake
      specified NEC W59.89
        bite W59.81
        crushing W59.83
        strike W59.82
      turtle —*see* Contact, with, turtle
    rivet gun (powered) W29.4
    road scraper —*see* Accident, transport,
        construction vehicle
    rodent (feces) (urine) W53.89
      bite W53.81
      mouse W53.09
        bite W53.01
      rat W53.19
        bite W53.11
      specified NEC W53.89
        bite W53.81
      squirrel W53.29
        bite W53.21
    roller coaster W31.81
    rope NEC W24.0
      agricultural operations W30.89
    saliva —*see* Contact, with, by type of
        animal
    sander W29.8
      industrial W31.2
    saucepan (hot) (glass) (metal) X15.3
    saw W27.0
      band (industrial) W31.2
      bench (industrial) W31.2
      chain W29.3
      hand W27.0
    sawing machine, metal W31.1
    scissors W27.2
    scorpion X58
    screwdriver W27.0
      powered W29.8
    sea
      anemone, cucumber or urchin (spine)
          X58
      lion W56.19
        bite W56.11
        strike W56.12
    serpent —*see* Contact, with, snake, by type
    sewing-machine (electric) (powered)
        W29.2
      not powered W27.8
    shaft (hoist) (lift) (transmission) NEC
        W24.0
      agricultural W30.89
    shark W56.49
      bite W56.41
      strike W56.42
    shears (hand) W27.2
      powered (industrial) W31.1
        domestic W29.2
    sheep W55.39
      bite W55.31
      strike W55.32
    shovel W27.8
      steam —*see* Accident, transport,
          construction vehicle

Contact *(Continued)*
  with *(Continued)*
    snake (nonvenomous) W59.19
      bite W59.11
      crushing W59.13
      strike W59.12
    spade W27.1
    spider (venomous) X58
    spin-drier W29.2
    spinning machine W31.89
    splinter W45.8
    sports equipment W21.9
    staple gun (powered) W29.8
    steam X13.1
      engine W31.3
      inhalation X13.0
      pipe X16
      shovel W31.89
    stove (hot) (kitchen) X15.0
    substance, hot NEC X19
      molten (metal) X18
    sword W26.1
      assault X99.2
      stated as undetermined whether
        accidental or intentional
        Y28.2
      suicide (attempt) X78.2
    tarantula X58
    thresher W30.0
    tin can lid W45.2
    toad W62.1
    toaster (hot) X15.1
    tool W27.8
      hand (not powered) W27.8
        auger W27.0
        axe W27.0
        can opener W27.4
        chisel W27.0
        fork W27.4
        garden W27.1
        handsaw W27.0
        hoe W27.1
        ice-pick W27.4
        kitchen utensil W27.4
        manual
          lawn mower W27.1
          sewing machine W27.8
        meat grinder W27.4
        needle (sewing) W27.3
          hypodermic W46.0
            contaminated W46.1
        paper cutter W27.5
        pitchfork W27.1
        rake W27.1
        scissors W27.2
        screwdriver W27.0
        specified NEC W27.8
        workbench W27.0
      hot X17
      powered W29.8
        blender W29.0
          commercial W31.82
        can opener W29.0
          commercial W31.82
        chainsaw W29.3
        clothes dryer W29.2
          commercial W31.82
        dishwasher W29.2
          commercial W31.82
        edger W29.3
        electric fan W29.2
          commercial W31.82
        electric knife W29.1
        food processor W29.0
          commercial W31.82
        garbage disposal W29.0
          commercial W31.82

Contact *(Continued)*
  with *(Continued)*
    tool *(Continued)*
      powered *(Continued)*
        garden tool W29.3
        hedge trimmer W29.3
        ice maker W29.0
          commercial W31.82
        kitchen appliance W29.0
          commercial W31.82
        lawn mower W28
        meat grinder W29.0
          commercial W31.82
        mixer W29.0
          commercial W31.82
        rototiller W29.3
        sewing machine W29.2
          commercial W31.82
        washing machine W29.2
          commercial W31.82
      transmission device (belt, cable, chain,
        gear, pinion, shaft) W24.1
        agricultural operations W30.89
      turbine (gas) (water-driven) W31.3
      turkey W61.49
        peck W61.43
        strike W61.42
      turtle (nonvenomous) W59.29
        bite W59.21
        strike W59.22
        terrestrial W59.89
          bite W59.81
          crushing W59.83
          strike W59.82
      under-cutter W31.0
      urine —*see* Contact, with, by type of
        animal
      vehicle
        agricultural use (transport) —*see*
          Accident, transport, agricultural
          vehicle
          not on public highway W30.81
        industrial use (transport) —*see*
          Accident, transport, industrial
          vehicle
          not on public highway W31.83
        off-road use (transport) —*see* Accident,
          transport, all-terrain or off-road
          vehicle
          not on public highway W31.83
        special construction use (transport) —*see*
          Accident, transport, construction
          vehicle
          not on public highway W31.83
      venomous
        animal X58
        arthropods X58
        lizard X58
        marine animal NEC X58
        marine plant NEC X58
        millipedes (tropical) X58
        plant (s) X58
        snake X58
        spider X58
      viper X58
      washing-machine (powered) W29.2
      wasp X58
      weaving-machine W31.89
      winch W24.0
        agricultural operations W30.89
      wire NEC W24.0
        agricultural operations W30.89
      wood slivers W45.8
      yellow jacket X58
      zebra —*see* Contact, with, hoof stock
        NEC
Coup de soleil X32

Crash
  aircraft (in transit) (powered) V95.9
    balloon V96.01
    fixed wing NEC (private) V95.21
      commercial V95.31
    glider V96.21
      hang V96.11
      powered V95.11
    helicopter V95.01
    in war operations —*see* War operations,
      destruction of aircraft
    microlight V95.11
    nonpowered V96.9
      specified NEC V96.8
    powered NEC V95.8
    stated as
      homicide (attempt) Y08.81
      suicide (attempt) X83.0
    ultralight V95.11
  spacecraft V95.41
  transport vehicle NEC (*see also* Accident,
    transport) V89.9
    homicide (attempt) Y03.8
    motor NEC (traffic) V89.2
      homicide (attempt) Y03.8
    suicide (attempt) —*see* Suicide, collision
Cruelty (mental) (physical) (sexual) X58
Crushed (accidentally) X58
  between objects (moving) (stationary and
    moving) W23.0
    stationary W23.1
  by
    alligator W58.03
    avalanche NEC —*see* Landslide
    cave-in W20.0
      caused by cataclysmic earth surface
        movement —*see* Landslide
    crocodile W58.13
    crowd or human stampede W52
    falling
      aircraft V97.39
        in war operations —*see* War
          operations, destruction of aircraft
      earth, material W20.0
        caused by cataclysmic earth surface
          movement —*see* Landslide
      object NEC W20.8
    landslide NEC —*see* Landslide
    lizard (nonvenomous) W59.09
    machinery —*see* Contact, with, by type of
      machine
    reptile NEC W59.89
    snake (nonvenomous) W59.13
  in
    machinery —*see* Contact, with, by type of
      machine
Cut, cutting (any part of body) (accidental) —
  see also Contact, with, by object or machine
  during medical or surgical treatment as
    misadventure —*see* Index to Diseases
    and Injuries, Complications
  homicide (attempt) —*see* Assault, cutting or
    piercing instrument
  inflicted by other person —*see* Assault,
    cutting or piercing instrument
  legal
    execution —*see* Legal, intervention
    intervention —*see* Legal, intervention,
      sharp object
  machine NEC (*see also* Contact, with, by type
    of machine) W31.9
  self-inflicted —*see* Suicide, cutting or piercing
    instrument
  suicide (attempt) —*see* Suicide, cutting or
    piercing instrument
Cyclone (any injury) X37.1

◀ New   ◀▥ Revised   ~~deleted~~ Deleted

D

Decapitation (accidental circumstances)
NEC X58
homicide X99.9
legal execution —*see* Legal, intervention
Dehydration from lack of water X58
Deprivation X58
Derailment (accidental)
railway (rolling stock) (train) (vehicle)
(without antecedent collision) V81.7
with antecedent collision —*see* Accident,
transport, railway vehicle occupant
streetcar (without antecedent collision)
V82.7
with antecedent collision —*see* Accident,
transport, streetcar occupant
Descent
parachute (voluntary) (without accident to
aircraft) V97.29
due to accident to aircraft —*see* Accident,
transport, aircraft
Desertion X58
Destitution X58
Disability, late effect or sequela of injury —*see*
Sequelae
Discharge (accidental)
airgun W34.010
assault X95.01
homicide (attempt) X95.01
stated as undetermined whether accidental
or intentional Y24.0
suicide (attempt) X74.01
BB gun —*see* Discharge, airgun
firearm (accidental) W34.00
assault X95.9
handgun (pistol) (revolver) W32.0
assault X93
homicide (attempt) X93
legal intervention —*see* Legal,
intervention, firearm, handgun
stated as undetermined whether
accidental or intentional Y22
suicide (attempt) X72
homicide (attempt) X95.9
hunting rifle W33.02
assault X94.1
homicide (attempt) X94.1
legal intervention
injuring
bystander Y35.032
law enforcement personnel
Y35.031
suspect Y35.033
stated as undetermined whether
accidental or intentional Y23.1
suicide (attempt) X73.1
larger W33.00
assault X94.9
homicide (attempt) X94.9
hunting rifle —*see* Discharge, firearm,
hunting rifle
legal intervention —*see* Legal,
intervention, firearm by type of
firearm
machine gun —*see* Discharge, firearm,
machine gun
shotgun —*see* Discharge, firearm,
shotgun
specified NEC W33.09
assault X94.8
homicide (attempt) X94.8
legal intervention
injuring
bystander Y35.092
law enforcement personnel
Y35.091
suspect Y35.093
stated as undetermined whether
accidental or intentional Y23.8
suicide (attempt) X73.8

Discharge (Continued)
firearm (Continued)
larger (Continued)
stated as undetermined whether
accidental or intentional Y23.9
suicide (attempt) X73.9
legal intervention
injuring
bystander Y35.002
law enforcement personnel Y35.001
suspect Y35.03
using rubber bullet
injuring
bystander Y35.042
law enforcement personnel
Y35.041
suspect Y35.043
machine gun W33.03
assault X94.2
homicide (attempt) X94.2
legal intervention —*see* Legal,
intervention, firearm, machine gun
stated as undetermined whether
accidental or intentional Y23.3
suicide (attempt) X73.2
pellet gun —*see* Discharge, airgun
shotgun W33.01
assault X94.0
homicide (attempt) X94.0
legal intervention —*see* Legal,
intervention, firearm, specified NEC
stated as undetermined whether
accidental or intentional Y23.0
suicide (attempt) X73.0
specified NEC W34.09
assault X95.8
homicide (attempt) X95.8
legal intervention —*see* Legal,
intervention, firearm, specified NEC
stated as undetermined whether
accidental or intentional Y24.8
suicide (attempt) X74.8
stated as undetermined whether accidental
or intentional Y24.9
suicide (attempt) X74.9
Very pistol W34.09
assault X95.8
homicide (attempt) X95.8
stated as undetermined whether
accidental or intentional Y24.8
suicide (attempt) X74.8
firework (s) W39
stated as undetermined whether accidental
or intentional Y25
gas-operated gun NEC W34.018
airgun —*see* Discharge, airgun
assault X95.09
homicide (attempt) X95.09
paintball gun —*see* Discharge, paintball
gun
stated as undetermined whether accidental
or intentional Y24.8
suicide (attempt) X74.09
gun NEC —*see also* Discharge, firearm NEC
air —*see* Discharge, airgun
BB —*see* Discharge, airgun
for single hand use —*see* Discharge,
firearm, handgun
hand —*see* Discharge, firearm, handgun
machine —*see* Discharge, firearm, machine
gun
other specified —*see* Discharge, firearm
NEC
paintball —*see* Discharge, paintball gun
pellet —*see* Discharge, airgun
handgun —*see* Discharge, firearm, handgun
machine gun —*see* Discharge, firearm,
machine gun
paintball gun W34.011
assault X95.02
homicide (attempt) X95.02

Discharge (Continued)
paintball gun (Continued)
stated as undetermined whether accidental
or intentional Y24.8
suicide (attempt) X74.02
pistol —*see* Discharge, firearm, handgun
flare —*see* Discharge, firearm, Very pistol
pellet —*see* Discharge, airgun
Very —*see* Discharge, firearm, Very pistol
revolver —*see* Discharge, firearm, handgun
rifle (hunting) —*see* Discharge, firearm,
hunting rifle
shotgun —*see* Discharge, firearm, shotgun
spring-operated gun NEC W34.018
assault X95.09
homicide (attempt) X95.09
stated as undetermined whether accidental
or intentional Y24.8
suicide (attempt) X74.09
Disease
Andes W94.11
aviator's —*see* Air, pressure
range W94.11
Diver's disease, palsy, paralysis, squeeze —*see*
Air, pressure
Diving (into water) —*see* Accident, diving
Dog bite W54.0
Dragged by transport vehicle NEC (*see also*
Accident, transport) V09.9
Drinking poison (accidental) —*see* Table of
Drugs and Chemicals
Dropped (accidentally) **while being carried or
supported by other person** W04
Drowning (accidental) W74
assault X92.9
due to
accident (to)
machinery —*see* Contact, with, by type
of machine
watercraft V90.89
burning V90.29
powered V90.23
fishing boat V90.22
jetskis V90.23
merchant ship V90.20
passenger ship V90.21
unpowered V90.28
canoe V90.25
inflatable V90.26
kayak V90.25
sailboat V90.24
water skis V90.27
crushed V90.39
powered V90.33
fishing boat V90.32
jetskis V90.33
merchant ship V90.30
passenger ship V90.31
unpowered V90.38
canoe V90.35
inflatable V90.36
kayak V90.35
sailboat V90.34
water skis V90.37
overturning V90.09
powered V90.03
fishing boat V90.02
jetskis V90.03
merchant ship V90.00
passenger ship V90.01
unpowered V90.08
canoe V90.05
inflatable V90.06
kayak V90.05
sailboat V90.04
sinking V90.19
powered V90.13
fishing boat V90.12
jetskis V90.13
merchant ship V90.10
passenger ship V90.11

Drowning (Continued)
  due to (Continued)
    accident (Continued)
      watercraft (Continued)
        sinking (Continued)
          unpowered V90.18
            canoe V90.15
            inflatable V90.16
            kayak V90.15
            sailboat V90.14
          specified type NEC V90.89
          powered V90.83
            fishing boat V90.82
            jetskis V90.83
            merchant ship V90.80
            passenger ship V90.81
          unpowered V90.88
            canoe V90.85
            inflatable V90.86
            kayak V90.85
            sailboat V90.84
            water skis V90.87
    avalanche —see Landslide
    cataclysmic
      earth surface movement NEC —see
        Forces of nature, earth movement
      storm —see Forces of nature, cataclysmic
        storm
    cloudburst X37.8
    cyclone X37.1
    fall overboard (from) V92.09
      powered craft V92.03
        ferry boat V92.01
        fishing boat V92.02
        jetskis V92.03
        liner V92.01
        merchant ship V92.00
        passenger ship V92.01
      resulting from
        accident to watercraft —see Drowning,
          due to, accident to, watercraft
        being washed overboard (from)
          V92.29
          powered craft V92.23
            ferry boat V92.21
            fishing boat V92.22
            jetskis V92.23
            liner V92.21
            merchant ship V92.20
            passenger ship V92.21
          unpowered craft V92.28
            canoe V92.25
            inflatable V92.26
            kayak V92.25
            sailboat V92.24
            surf-board V92.28
            water skis V92.27
            windsurfer V92.28
        motion of watercraft V92.19
          powered craft V92.13
            ferry boat V92.11
            fishing boat V92.12
            jetskis V92.13
            liner V92.11
            merchant ship V92.10
            passenger ship V92.11
          unpowered craft
            canoe V92.15
            inflatable V92.16
            kayak V92.15
            sailboat V92.14
      unpowered craft V92.08
        canoe V92.05
        inflatable V92.06
        kayak V92.05

Drowning (Continued)
  due to (Continued)
    fall overboard (Continued)
      unpowered craft (Continued)
        sailboat V92.04
        surf-board V92.08
        water skis V92.07
        windsurfer V92.08
    hurricane X37.0
    jumping into water from watercraft
      (involved in accident) —see also
      Drowning, due to, accident to,
      watercraft
      without accident to or on watercraft
        W16.711
    tidal wave NEC —see Forces of nature,
      tidal wave
    torrential rain X37.8
  following
    fall
      into
        bathtub W16.211
        bucket W16.221
        fountain —see Drowning, following,
          fall, into, water, specified NEC
        quarry —see Drowning, following,
          fall, into, water, specified NEC
        reservoir —see Drowning, following,
          fall, into, water, specified NEC
        swimming-pool W16.011
          stated as undetermined whether
            accidental or intentional
            Y21.3
          striking
            bottom W16.021
            wall W16.031
          suicide (attempt) X71.2
        water NOS W16.41
          natural (lake) (open sea) (river)
            (stream) (pond) W16.111
            striking
              bottom W16.121
              side W16.131
          specified NEC W16.311
            striking
              bottom W16.321
              wall W16.331
      overboard NEC —see Drowning, due to,
        fall overboard
    jump or dive
      from boat W16.711
        striking bottom W16.721
      into
        fountain —see Drowning, following,
          jump or dive, into, water,
          specified NEC
        quarry —see Drowning, following,
          jump or dive, into, water,
          specified NEC
        reservoir —see Drowning, following,
          jump or dive, into, water,
          specified NEC
        swimming-pool W16.511
          striking
            bottom W16.521
            wall W16.531
          suicide (attempt) X71.2
        water NOS W16.91
          natural (lake) (open sea) (river)
            (stream) (pond) W16.611
          specified NEC W16.811
            striking
              bottom W16.821
              wall W16.831
          striking bottom W16.621

Drowning (Continued)
  homicide (attempt) X92.9
  in
    bathtub (accidental) W65
      assault X92.0
      following fall W16.211
        stated as undetermined whether
          accidental or intentional
          Y21.1
      stated as undetermined whether
        accidental or intentional Y21.0
      suicide (attempt) X71.0
    lake —see Drowning, in, natural water
    natural water (lake) (open sea) (river)
      (stream) (pond) W69
      assault X92.3
      following
        dive or jump W16.611
          striking bottom W16.621
        fall W16.111
          striking
            bottom W16.121
            side W16.131
      stated as undetermined whether
        accidental or intentional Y21.4
      suicide (attempt) X71.3
    quarry —see Drowning, in, specified place
      NEC
    quenching tank —see Drowning, in,
      specified place NEC
    reservoir —see Drowning, in, specified
      place NEC
    river —see Drowning, in, natural water
    sea —see Drowning, in, natural water
    specified place NEC W73
      assault X92.8
      following
        dive or jump W16.811
          striking
            bottom W16.821
            wall W16.831
        fall W16.311
          striking
            bottom W16.321
            wall W16.331
      stated as undetermined whether
        accidental or intentional Y21.8
      suicide (attempt) X71.8
    stream —see Drowning, in, natural water
    swimming-pool W67
      assault X92.1
        following fall X92.2
      following
        dive or jump W16.511
          striking
            bottom W16.521
            wall W16.531
        fall W16.011
          striking
            bottom W16.021
            wall W16.031
      stated as undetermined whether
        accidental or intentional Y21.2
        following fall Y21.3
      suicide (attempt) X71.1
        following fall X71.2
    war operations —see War operations,
      restriction of airway
  resulting from accident to watercraft —see
    Drowning, due to, accident, watercraft
  self-inflicted X71.9
  stated as undetermined whether accidental or
    intentional Y21.9
  suicide (attempt) X71.9

◀ New   ◀⁞⁞ Revised   ~~deleted~~ Deleted

E

Earth (surface) movement NEC —*see* Forces of
nature, earth movement
Earth falling (on) W20.0
caused by cataclysmic earth surface
movement or eruption —*see* Landslide
Earthquake (any injury) X34
Effect (s) (adverse) of
air pressure (any) —*see* Air, pressure
cold, excessive (exposure to) —*see* Exposure,
cold
heat (excessive) —*see* Heat
hot place (weather) —*see* Heat
insolation X30
late —*see* Sequelae
motion —*see* Motion
nuclear explosion or weapon in war
operations —*see* War operations, nuclear
weapon
radiation —*see* Radiation
travel —*see* Travel
Electric shock (accidental) (by) (in) —*see*
Exposure, electric current
Electrocution (accidental) —*see* Exposure,
electric current
Endotracheal tube wrongly placed during
anesthetic procedure Y65.3
Entanglement
in
bed linen, causing suffocation —*see*
category T71
wheel of pedal cycle V19.88
Entry of foreign body or material —*see* Foreign
body
Environmental pollution related condition —
see Z57
Execution, legal (any method) —*see* Legal,
intervention
Exhaustion
cold —*see* Exposure, cold
due to excessive exertion —*see* category Y93
heat —*see* Heat
Explosion (accidental) (of) (with secondary fire)
W40.9
acetylene W40.1
aerosol can W36.1
air tank (compressed) (in machinery) W36.2
aircraft (in transit) (powered) NEC V95.9
balloon V96.05
fixed wing NEC (private) V95.25
commercial V95.35
glider V96.25
hang V96.15
powered V95.15
helicopter V95.05
in war operations —*see* War operations,
destruction of aircraft
microlight V95.15
nonpowered V96.9
specified NEC V96.8
powered NEC V95.8
stated as
homicide (attempt) Y03.8
suicide (attempt) X83.0
ultralight V95.15
anesthetic gas in operating room W40.1
antipersonnel bomb W40.8
assault X96.0
homicide (attempt) X96.0
suicide (attempt) X75
assault X96.9
bicycle tire W37.0
blasting (cap) (materials) W40.0
boiler (machinery), not on transport vehicle
W35
on watercraft —*see* Explosion, in,
watercraft
butane W40.1
caused by other person X96.9
coal gas W40.1

Explosion (*Continued*)
detonator W40.0
dump (munitions) W40.8
dynamite W40.0
in
assault X96.8
homicide (attempt) X96.8
legal intervention
injuring
bystander Y35.112
law enforcement personnel Y35.111
suspect Y35.113
suicide (attempt) X75
explosive (material) W40.9
gas W40.1
in blasting operation W40.0
specified NEC W40.8
in
assault X96.8
homicide (attempt) X96.8
legal intervention
injuring
bystander Y35.192
law enforcement personnel
Y35.191
suspect Y35.193
suicide (attempt) X75
factory (munitions) W40.8
fertilizer bomb W40.8
assault X96.3
homicide (attempt) X96.3
suicide (attempt) X75
fire-damp W40.1
firearm (parts) NEC W34.19
airgun W34.110
BB gun W34.110
gas, air or spring-operated gun NEC
W34.118
handgun W32.1
hunting rifle W33.12
larger firearm W33.10
specified NEC W33.19
machine gun W33.13
paintball gun W34.111
pellet gun W34.110
shotgun W33.11
Very pistol [flare] W34.19
fireworks W39
gas (coal) (explosive) W40.1
cylinder W36.9
aerosol can W36.1
air tank W36.2
pressurized W36.3
specified NEC W36.8
gasoline (fumes) (tank) not in moving motor
vehicle W40.1
bomb W40.8
assault X96.1
homicide (attempt) X96.1
suicide (attempt) X75
in motor vehicle —*see* Accident, transport,
by type of vehicle
grain store W40.8
grenade W40.8
in
assault X96.8
homicide (attempt) X96.8
legal intervention
injuring
bystander Y35.192
law enforcement personnel
Y35.191
suspect Y35.193
suicide (attempt) X75
handgun (parts) —*see* Explosion, firearm,
handgun (parts)
homicide (attempt) X96.9
antipersonnel bomb —*see* Explosion,
antipersonnel bomb
fertilizer bomb —*see* Explosion, fertilizer
bomb

Explosion (*Continued*)
homicide (*Continued*)
gasoline bomb —*see* Explosion, gasoline
bomb
letter bomb —*see* Explosion, letter bomb
pipe bomb —*see* Explosion, pipe bomb
specified NEC X96.8
hose, pressurized W37.8
hot water heater, tank (in machinery) W35
on watercraft —*see* Explosion, in,
watercraft
in, on
dump W40.8
factory W40.8
mine (of explosive gases) NEC W40.1
watercraft V93.59
powered craft V93.53
ferry boat V93.51
fishing boat V93.52
jetskis V93.53
liner V93.51
merchant ship V93.50
passenger ship V93.51
sailboat V93.54
letter bomb W40.8
assault X96.2
homicide (attempt) X96.2
suicide (attempt) X75
machinery —*see also* Contact, with, by type
of machine
on board watercraft —*see* Explosion, in,
watercraft
pressure vessel —*see* Explosion, by type
of vessel
methane W40.1
mine W40.1
missile NEC W40.8
mortar bomb W40.8
in
assault X96.8
homicide (attempt) X96.8
legal intervention
injuring
bystander Y35.192
law enforcement personnel
Y35.191
suspect Y35.193
suicide (attempt) X75
munitions (dump) (factory) W40.8
pipe, pressurized W37.8
bomb W40.8
assault X96.4
homicide (attempt) X96.4
suicide (attempt) X75
pressure, pressurized
cooker W38
gas tank (in machinery) W36.3
hose W37.8
pipe W37.8
specified device NEC W38
tire W37.8
bicycle W37.0
vessel (in machinery) W38
propane W40.1
self-inflicted X75
shell (artillery) NEC W40.8
during war operations —*see* War
operations, explosion
in
legal intervention
injuring
bystander Y35.122
law enforcement personnel Y35.121
suspect Y35.123
war —*see* War operations, explosion
spacecraft V95.45
stated as undetermined whether accidental or
intentional Y25
steam or water lines (in machinery) W37.8
stove W40.9
suicide (attempt) X75

Explosion (Continued)
  tire, pressurized W37.8
    bicycle W37.0
  undetermined whether accidental or
      intentional Y25
  vehicle tire NEC W37.8
    bicycle W37.0
  war operations —see War operations,
      explosion
Exposure (to) X58
  air pressure change —see Air, pressure
  cold (accidental) (excessive) (extreme)
      (natural) (place) X31
    assault Y08.89
    due to
      man-made conditions W93.8
        dry ice (contact) W93.01
          inhalation W93.02
        liquid air (contact) (hydrogen)
            (nitrogen) W93.11
          inhalation W93.12
        refrigeration unit (deep freeze)
            W93.2
      suicide (attempt) X83.2
      weather (conditions) X31
    homicide (attempt) Y08.89
    self-inflicted X83.2
  due to abandonment or neglect X58
  electric current W86.8
    appliance (faulty) W86.8
      domestic W86.0
    caused by other person Y08.89
    conductor (faulty) W86.1
    control apparatus (faulty) W86.1
    electric power generating plant,
        distribution station W86.1
    electroshock gun —see Exposure, electric
        current, taser
    high-voltage cable W85
    homicide (attempt) Y08.89
    legal execution —see Legal, intervention,
        specified means NEC
    lightning —see subcategory T75.0
    live rail W86.8
    misadventure in medical or surgical
        procedure in electroshock therapy
        Y63.4
    motor (electric) (faulty) W86.8
      domestic W86.0
    self-inflicted X83.1
    specified NEC W86.8
      domestic W86.0
    stun gun —see Exposure, electric current,
        taser
    suicide (attempt) X83.1
    taser W86.8
      assault Y08.89
      legal intervention —see category Y35
      self-harm (intentional) X83.8
      undetermined intent Y33
    third rail W86.8
    transformer (faulty) W86.1
    transmission lines W85
  environmental tobacco smoke X58
  excessive
    cold —see Exposure, cold
    heat (natural) NEC X30
      man-made W92
  factor (s) NOS X58
    environmental NEC X58
      man-made NEC W99
    natural NEC —see Forces of nature
    specified NEC X58
  fire, flames (accidental) X08.8
    assault X97
    campfire —see Exposure, fire, controlled,
        not in building
    controlled (in)
      with ignition (of) clothing (see also
          Ignition, clothes) X06.2
        nightwear X05

Exposure (Continued)
  fire, flames (Continued)
    controlled (Continued)
      bonfire —see Exposure, fire, controlled,
          not in building
      brazier (in building or structure) —see
          also Exposure, fire, controlled,
          building
        not in building or structure —see
            Exposure, fire, controlled, not in
            building
      building or structure X02.0
        with
          fall from building X02.3
          from building X02.5
          injury due to building collapse
              X02.2
          smoke inhalation X02.1
        hit by object from building X02.4
        specified mode of injury NEC X02.8
      fireplace, furnace or stove —see
          Exposure, fire, controlled, building
      not in building or structure X03.0
        with
          fall X03.3
          smoke inhalation X03.1
        hit by object X03.4
        specified mode of injury NEC X03.8
      trash —see Exposure, fire, controlled, not
          in building
    fireplace —see Exposure, fire, controlled,
        building
    fittings or furniture (in building or
        structure) (uncontrolled) —see
        Exposure, fire, uncontrolled, building
    forest (uncontrolled) —see Exposure, fire,
        uncontrolled, not in building
    grass (uncontrolled) —see Exposure, fire,
        uncontrolled, not in building
    hay (uncontrolled) —see Exposure, fire,
        uncontrolled, not in building
    homicide (attempt) X97
    ignition of highly flammable material X04
    in, of, on, starting in
      machinery —see Contact, with, by type
          of machine
      motor vehicle (in motion) (see also
          Accident, transport, occupant by
          type of vehicle) V87.8
        with collision —see Collision
      railway rolling stock, train, vehicle
          V81.81
        with collision —see Accident,
            transport, railway vehicle
            occupant
      street car (in motion) V82.8
        with collision —see Accident,
            transport, streetcar occupant
      transport vehicle NEC —see also
          Accident, transport
        with collision —see Collision
      war operations —see also War operations,
          fire
        from nuclear explosion —see War
            operations, nuclear weapons
      watercraft (in transit) (not in transit)
          V91.09
        localized —see Burn, on board
            watercraft, due to, fire on board
        powered craft V91.03
          ferry boat V91.01
          fishing boat V91.02
          jet skis V91.03
          liner V91.01
          merchant ship V91.00
          passenger ship V91.01
        unpowered craft V91.08
          canoe V91.05
          inflatable V91.06
          kayak V91.05
          sailboat V91.04

Exposure (Continued)
  fire, flames (Continued)
    in, of, on, starting in (Continued)
      watercraft (Continued)
        unpowered craft (Continued)
          surf-board V91.08
          waterskis V91.07
          windsurfer V91.08
    lumber (uncontrolled) —see Exposure, fire,
        uncontrolled, not in building
    mine (uncontrolled) —see Exposure, fire,
        uncontrolled, not in building
    prairie (uncontrolled) —see Exposure, fire,
        uncontrolled, not in building
    resulting from
      explosion —see Explosion
      lightning X08.8
    self-inflicted X76
    specified NEC X08.8
    started by other person X97
    stated as undetermined whether accidental
        or intentional Y26
    stove —see Exposure, fire, controlled,
        building
    suicide (attempt) X76
    tunnel (uncontrolled) —see Exposure, fire,
        uncontrolled, not in building
    uncontrolled
      in building or structure X00.0
        with
          fall from building X00.3
          injury due to building collapse
              X00.2
          jump from building X00.5
          smoke inhalation X00.1
        bed X08.00
          due to
            cigarette X08.01
            specified material NEC X08.09
        furniture NEC X08.20
          due to
            cigarette X08.21
            specified material NEC X08.29
        hit by object from building X00.4
        sofa X08.10
          due to
            cigarette X08.11
            specified material NEC
                X08.19
        specified mode of injury NEC
            X00.8
      not in building or structure (any)
          X01.0
        with
          fall X01.3
          smoke inhalation X01.1
        hit by object X01.4
        specified mode of injury NEC
            X01.8
    undetermined whether accidental or
        intentional Y26
  forces of nature NEC —see Forces of nature
  G-forces (abnormal) W49.9
  gravitational forces (abnormal) W49.9
  heat (natural) NEC —see Heat
  high-pressure jet (hydraulic) (pneumatic)
      W49.9
  hydraulic jet W49.9
  inanimate mechanical force W49.9
  jet, high-pressure (hydraulic) (pneumatic)
      W49.9
  lightning —see subcategory T75.0
    causing fire —see Exposure, fire
  mechanical forces NEC W49.9
    animate NEC W64
    inanimate NEC W49.9
  noise W42.9
    supersonic W42.0
  noxious substance —see Table of Drugs and
      Chemical
  pneumatic jet W49.9

Exposure *(Continued)*
  prolonged in deep-freeze unit or refrigerator
    W93.2
  radiation —*see* Radiation
  smoke —*see also* Exposure, fire
    tobacco, second hand Z77.22
  specified factors NEC X58
  sunlight X32
    man-made (sun lamp) W89.8
      tanning bed W89.1
  supersonic waves W42.0
  transmission line (s), electric W85
  vibration W49.9

Exposure *(Continued)*
  waves
    infrasound W49.9
    sound W42.9
    supersonic W42.0
  weather NEC —*see* Forces of nature
External cause status Y99.9
  child assisting in compensated work for
    family Y99.8
  civilian activity done for financial or other
    compensation Y99.0
  civilian activity done for income or pay
    Y99.0

External cause status *(Continued)*
  family member assisting in compensated
    work for other family member Y99.8
  hobby not done for income Y99.8
  leisure activity Y99.8
  military activity Y99.1
  off-duty activity of military personnel Y99.8
  recreation or sport not for income or while a
    student Y99.8
  specified NEC Y99.8
  student activity Y99.8
  volunteer activity Y99.2

F

Factors, supplemental
  alcohol
    blood level
      less than 20mg/100ml Y90.0
      presence in blood, level not specified
          Y90.9
      20-39mg/100ml Y90.1
      40-59mg/100ml Y90.2
      60-79mg/100ml Y90.3
      80-99mg/100ml Y90.4
      100-119mg/100ml Y90.5
      120-199mg/100ml Y90.6
      200-239mg/100ml Y90.7
      240mg/100ml or more Y90.8
      presence in blood, but level not specified
          Y90.9
    environmental-pollution-related condition —
        see Z57
    nosocomial condition Y95
    work-related condition Y99.0
Failure
  in suture or ligature during surgical
      procedure Y65.2
  mechanical, of instrument or apparatus
      (any) (during any medical or surgical
      procedure) Y65.8
  sterile precautions (during medical and
      surgical care) —see Misadventure,
      failure, sterile precautions, by type of
      procedure
  to
    introduce tube or instrument Y65.4
      endotracheal tube during anesthesia Y65.3
    make curve (transport vehicle) NEC —see
        Accident, transport
    remove tube or instrument Y65.4
Fall, falling (accidental) W19
  building W20.1
    burning (uncontrolled fire) X00.3
  down
    embankment W17.81
    escalator W10.0
    hill W17.81
    ladder W11
    ramp W10.2
    stairs, steps W10.9
  due to
    bumping against
      object W18.00
        sharp glass W18.02
        specified NEC W18.09
        sports equipment W18.01
      person W03
        due to ice or snow W00.0
        on pedestrian conveyance —see
            Accident, transport, pedestrian,
            conveyance
    collision with another person W03
      due to ice or snow W00.0
      involving pedestrian conveyance —see
          Accident, transport, pedestrian,
          conveyance
    grocery cart tipping over W17.82
    ice or snow W00.9
      from one level to another W00.2
        on stairs or steps W00.1
      involving pedestrian conveyance —see
          Accident, transport, pedestrian,
          conveyance
      on same level W00.0
    slipping (on moving sidewalk) W01.0
      with subsequent striking against object
          W01.10
        furniture W01.190
        sharp object W01.119
          glass W01.110
          power tool or machine W01.111
          specified NEC W01.118
        specified NEC W01.198

Fall, falling (Continued)
  due to (Continued)
    striking against
      object W18.00
        sharp glass W18.02
        specified NEC W18.09
        sports equipment W18.01
      person W03
        due to ice or snow W00.0
        on pedestrian conveyance —see
            Accident, transport, pedestrian,
            conveyance
  earth (with asphyxia or suffocation (by
      pressure)) —see Earth, falling
  from, off, out of
    aircraft NEC (with accident to aircraft
        NEC) V97.0
      while boarding or alighting V97.1
    balcony W13.0
    bed W06
    boat, ship, watercraft NEC (with
        drowning or submersion) —
        see Drowning, due to, fall
        overboard
      with hitting bottom or object V94.0
    bridge W13.1
    building W13.9
      burning (uncontrolled fire) X00.3
    cavity W17.2
    chair W07
    cherry picker W17.89
    cliff W15
    dock W17.4
    embankment W17.81
    escalator W10.0
    flagpole W13.8
    furniture NEC W08
    grocery cart W17.82
    haystack W17.89
    high place NEC W17.89
      stated as undetermined whether
          accidental or intentional Y30
    hole W17.2
    incline W10.2
    ladder W11
    lifting device W17.89
    machine, machinery —see also Contact,
        with, by type of machine
      not in operation W17.89
    manhole W17.1
    mobile elevated work platform [MEWP]
        W17.89
    motorized mobility scooter W05.2
    one level to another NEC W17.89
      intentional, purposeful, suicide
          (attempt) X80
      stated as undetermined whether
          accidental or intentional Y30
    pit W17.2
    playground equipment W09.8
      jungle gym W09.2
      slide W09.0
      swing W09.1
    quarry W17.89
    railing W13.9
    ramp W10.2
    roof W13.2
    scaffolding W12
    scooter (nonmotorized) W05.1
      motorized mobility W05.2
    sky lift W17.89
    stairs, steps W10.9
      curb W10.1
      due to ice or snow W00.1
      escalator W10.0
      incline W10.2
      ramp W10.2
      sidewalk curb W10.1
      specified NEC W10.8
    stepladder W11
    storm drain W17.1

Fall, falling (Continued)
  from, off, out of (Continued)
    streetcar NEC V82.6
      with antecedent collision —see
          Accident, transport, streetcar
          occupant
      while boarding or alighting V82.4
    structure NEC W13.8
      burning (uncontrolled fire) X00.3
    table W08
    toilet W18.11
      with subsequent striking against object
          W18.12
    train NEC V81.6
      during derailment (without antecedent
          collision) V81.7
      with antecedent collision —see
          Accident, transport, railway
          vehicle occupant
      while boarding or alighting V81.4
    transport vehicle after collision —see
        Accident, transport, by type of
        vehicle, collision
    tree W14
    vehicle (in motion) NEC (see also Accident,
        transport) V89.9
      motor NEC (see also Accident, transport,
          occupant, by type of vehicle)
          V87.8
      stationary W17.89
        while boarding or alighting —see
            Accident, transport, by type
            of vehicle, while boarding or
            alighting
    viaduct W13.8
    wall W13.8
    watercraft —see also Drowning, due to, fall
        overboard
      with hitting bottom or object V94.0
    well W17.0
    wheelchair, non-moving W05.0
      powered —see Accident, transport,
          pedestrian, conveyance occupant,
          specified type NEC
    window W13.4
  in, on
    aircraft NEC V97.0
      with accident to aircraft V97.0
      while boarding or alighting
          V97.1
    bathtub (empty) W18.2
      filled W16.212
        causing drowning W16.211
    escalator W10.0
    incline W10.2
    ladder W11
    machine, machinery —see Contact, with,
        by type of machine
    object, edged, pointed or sharp (with
        cut) —see Fall, by type
    playground equipment W09.8
      jungle gym W09.2
      slide W09.0
      swing W09.1
    ramp W10.2
    scaffolding W12
    shower W18.2
      causing drowning W16.211
    staircase, stairs, steps W10.9
      curb W10.1
      due to ice or snow W00.1
      escalator W10.0
      incline W10.2
      specified NEC W10.8
    streetcar (without antecedent collision)
        V82.5
      with antecedent collision —see
          Accident, transport, streetcar
          occupant
      while boarding or alighting
          V82.4

◄ New   ◄▥ Revised   ~~deleted~~ Deleted

Fall, falling (Continued)
  in, on (Continued)
    train (without antecedent collision) V81.5
      with antecedent collision —see Accident, transport, railway vehicle occupant
      during derailment (without antecedent collision) V81.7
        with antecedent collision —see Accident, transport, railway vehicle occupant
      while boarding or alighting V81.4
    transport vehicle after collision —see Accident, transport, by type of vehicle, collision
    watercraft V93.39
      due to
        accident to craft V91.29
          powered craft V91.23
            ferry boat V91.21
            fishing boat V91.22
            jetskis V91.23
            liner V91.21
            merchant ship V91.20
            passenger ship V91.21
          unpowered craft
            canoe V91.25
            inflatable V91.26
            kayak V91.25
            sailboat V91.24
      powered craft V93.33
        ferry boat V93.31
        fishing boat V93.32
        jetskis V93.33
        liner V93.31
        merchant ship V93.30
        passenger ship V93.31
      unpowered craft V93.38
        canoe V93.35
        inflatable V93.36
        kayak V93.35
        sailboat V93.34
        surf-board V93.38
        windsurfer V93.38
  into
    cavity W17.2
    dock W17.4
    fire —see Exposure, fire, by type
    haystack W17.89
    hole W17.2
    lake —see Fall, into, water
    manhole W17.1
    moving part of machinery —see Contact, with, by type of machine
    ocean —see Fall, into, water
    opening in surface NEC W17.89
    pit W17.2
    pond —see Fall, into, water
    quarry W17.89
    river —see Fall, into, water
    shaft W17.89
    storm drain W17.1
    stream —see Fall, into, water
    swimming pool —see also Fall, into, water, in, swimming pool
      empty W17.3
    tank W17.89
    water W16.42
      causing drowning W16.41
      from watercraft —see Drowning, due to, fall overboard
      hitting diving board W21.4
      in
        bathtub W16.212
          causing drowning W16.211
        bucket W16.222
          causing drowning W16.221
        natural body of water W16.112
          causing drowning W16.111
          striking
            bottom W16.122
              causing drowning W16.121

Fall, falling (Continued)
  into (Continued)
    water (Continued)
      in (Continued)
        natural body of water (Continued)
          striking (Continued)
            side W16.132
              causing drowning W16.131
        specified water NEC W16.312
          causing drowning W16.311
          striking
            bottom W16.322
              causing drowning W16.321
            wall W16.332
              causing drowning W16.331
        swimming pool W16.012
          causing drowning W16.011
          striking
            bottom W16.022
              causing drowning W16.021
            wall W16.032
              causing drowning W16.031
        utility bucket W16.222
          causing drowning W16.221
    well W17.0
  involving
    bed W06
    chair W07
    furniture NEC W08
    glass —see Fall, by type
    playground equipment W09.8
      jungle gym W09.2
      slide W09.0
      swing W09.1
    roller blades —see Accident, transport, pedestrian, conveyance
    skateboard (s) —see Accident, transport, pedestrian, conveyance
    skates (ice) (in line) (roller) —see Accident, transport, pedestrian, conveyance
    skis —see Accident, transport, pedestrian, conveyance
    table W08
    wheelchair, non-moving W05.0
      powered —see Accident, transport, pedestrian, conveyance, specified type NEC
  object —see Struck by, object, falling
  off
    toilet W18.11
      with subsequent striking against object W18.12
  on same level W18.30
    due to
      specified NEC W18.39
      stepping on an object W18.31
  out of
    bed W06
    building NEC W13.8
    chair W07
    furniture NEC W08
    wheelchair, non-moving W05.0
      powered —see Accident, transport, pedestrian, conveyance, specified type NEC
    window W13.4
  over
    animal W01.0
    cliff W15
    embankment W17.81
    small object W01.0
  rock W20.8
  same level W18.30
    from
      being crushed, pushed, or stepped on by a crowd or human stampede W52
      collision, pushing, shoving, by or with other person W03
      slipping, stumbling, tripping W01.0

Fall, falling (Continued)
  same level (Continued)
    involving ice or snow W00.0
      involving skates (ice) (roller), skateboard, skis —see Accident, transport, pedestrian, conveyance
  snowslide (avalanche) —see Landslide
  stone W20.8
  structure W20.1
    burning (uncontrolled fire) X00.3
  through
    bridge W13.1
    floor W13.3
    roof W13.2
    wall W13.8
    window W13.4
  timber W20.8
  tree (caused by lightning) W20.8
  while being carried or supported by other person (s) W04
Fallen on by
  animal (not being ridden) NEC W55.89
Felo-de-se —see Suicide
Fight (hand) (fists) (foot) —see Assault, fight
Fire (accidental) —see Exposure, fire
Firearm discharge —see Discharge, firearm
Fireball effects from nuclear explosion in war operations —see War operations, nuclear weapons
Fireworks (explosion) W39
Flash burns from explosion —see Explosion
Flood (any injury) (caused by) X38
  collapse of man-made structure causing earth movement X36.0
  tidal wave —see Forces of nature, tidal wave
Food (any type) in
  air passages (with asphyxia, obstruction, or suffocation) —see categories T17 and T18
  alimentary tract causing asphyxia (due to compression of trachea) —see categories T17 and T18
Forces of nature X39.8
  avalanche X36.1
    causing transport accident —see Accident, transport, by type of vehicle
  blizzard X37.2
  cataclysmic storm X37.9
    with flood X38
    blizzard X37.2
    cloudburst X37.8
    cyclone X37.1
    dust storm X37.3
    hurricane X37.0
    specified storm NEC X37.8
    storm surge X37.0
    tornado X37.1
    twister X37.1
    typhoon X37.0
  cloudburst X37.8
  cold (natural) X31
  cyclone X37.1
  dam collapse causing earth movement X36.0
  dust storm X37.3
  earth movement X36.1
    caused by dam or structure collapse X36.0
    earthquake X34
  earthquake X34
  flood (caused by) X38
    dam collapse X36.0
    tidal wave —see Forces of nature, tidal wave
  heat (natural) X30
  hurricane X37.0
  landslide X36.1
    causing transport accident —see Accident, transport, by type of vehicle
  lightning —see subcategory T75.0
    causing fire —see Exposure, fire
  mudslide X36.1
    causing transport accident —see Accident, transport, by type of vehicle

Forces of nature (*Continued*)
 radiation (natural) X39.08
  radon X39.01
 radon X39.01
 specified force NEC X39.8
 storm surge X37.0
 structure collapse causing
   earth movement
   X36.0
 sunlight X32
 tidal wave X37.41
  due to
   earthquake X37.41
   landslide X37.43
   storm X37.42
   volcanic eruption X37.41
 tornado X37.1

Forces of nature (*Continued*)
 tsunami X37.41
 twister X37.1
 typhoon X37.0
 volcanic eruption X35
Foreign body
 aspiration - *see* Index to Diseases and
   Injuries. Foreign body, respitory
   tract
 entering through skin
   W45.8
  can lid W45.2
  nail W45.0
  paper W45.1
  specified NEC 45.8
  splinter W45.8

Forest fire (exposure to) —*see* Exposure, fire,
  uncontrolled, not in building
Found injured X58
 from exposure (to) —*see* Exposure
 on
   highway, road(way), street V89.9
   railway right of way V81.9
Fracture (circumstances unknown or
  unspecified) X58
 due to specified cause NEC X58
Freezing —*see* Exposure, cold
Frostbite X31
 due to man-made conditions —*see* Exposure,
   cold, man-made
Frozen —*see* Exposure, cold

G

Gored by bull W55.22
Gunshot wound W34.00

H

Hailstones, injured by X39.8
Hanged herself or himself —*see* Hanging,
  self-inflicted
Hanging (accidental) (*see also* category T71)
 legal execution —*see* Legal, intervention,
   specified means NEC
Heat (effects of) (excessive) X30
 due to
   man-made conditions W92
    on board watercraft V93.29
     fishing boat V93.22
     merchant ship V93.20
     passenger ship V93.21
     sailboat V93.24
     specified powered craft NEC V93.23
   weather (conditions) X30

Heat (*Continued*)
 from
   electric heating apparatus causing
    burning X16
   nuclear explosion in war operations —
    see War operations, nuclear
    weapons
 inappropriate in local application or
   packing in medical or surgical
   procedure Y63.5
Hemorrhage
 delayed following medical or surgical
   treatment without mention of
   misadventure —*see* Index to Diseases
   and Injuries, Complication(s)
 during medical or surgical treatment as
   misadventure —*see* Index to Diseases
   and Injuries, Complication(s)

High
 altitude (effects) —*see* Air, pressure, low
 level of radioactivity, effects —*see* Radiation
 pressure (effects) —*see* Air, pressure, high
 temperature, effects —*see* Heat
Hit, hitting (accidental) by —*see* Struck by
Hitting against —*see* Striking against
Homicide (attempt) (justifiable) —*see* Assault
Hot
 place, effects —*see also* Heat
 weather, effects X30
House fire (uncontrolled) —*see* Exposure, fire,
  uncontrolled, building
Humidity, causing problem X39.8
Hunger X58
Hurricane (any injury) X37.0
Hypobarism, hypobaropathy —*see* Air,
  pressure, low

◀ New   ◀▥ Revised   ~~deleted~~ Deleted

F, G, & H

I

Ictus
- caloris —*see also* Heat
- solaris X30

Ignition (accidental) (*see also* Exposure, fire) X08.8
- anesthetic gas in operating room W40.1
- apparel X06.2
  - from highly flammable material X04
  - nightwear X05
- bed linen (sheets) (spreads) (pillows) (mattress) —*see* Exposure, fire, uncontrolled, building, bed
- benzine X04
- clothes, clothing NEC (from controlled fire) X06.2
  - from
    - highly flammable material X04
- ether X04
  - in operating room W40.1
- explosive material —*see* Explosion
- gasoline X04
- jewelry (plastic) (any) X06.0
- kerosene X04
- material
  - explosive —*see* Explosion
  - highly flammable with secondary explosion X04
- nightwear X05
- paraffin X04
- petrol X04

Immersion (accidental) —*see also* Drowning
- hand or foot due to cold (excessive) X31

Implantation of quills of porcupine W55.89

Inanition (from) (hunger) X58
- thirst X58.8

Inappropriate operation performed
- correct operation on wrong side or body part (wrong side) (wrong site) Y65.53
- operation intended for another patient done on wrong patient Y65.52
- wrong operation performed on correct patient Y65.51

Inattention after, at birth (homicidal intent) (infanticidal intent) X58

Incident, adverse
- device
  - anesthesiology Y70.8
    - accessory Y70.2
    - diagnostic Y70.0
    - miscellaneous Y70.8
    - monitoring Y70.0
    - prosthetic Y70.2
    - rehabilitative Y70.1
    - surgical Y70.3
    - therapeutic Y70.1
  - cardiovascular Y71.8
    - accessory Y71.2
    - diagnostic Y71.0
    - miscellaneous Y71.8
    - monitoring Y71.0
    - prosthetic Y71.2
    - rehabilitative Y71.1
    - surgical Y71.3
    - therapeutic Y71.1
  - gastroenterology Y73.8
    - accessory Y73.2
    - diagnostic Y73.0
    - miscellaneous Y73.8
    - monitoring Y73.0
    - prosthetic Y73.2
    - rehabilitative Y73.1
    - surgical Y73.3
    - therapeutic Y73.1
  - general
    - hospital Y74.8
      - accessory Y74.2
      - diagnostic Y74.0

Incident, adverse (*Continued*)
- device (*Continued*)
  - general (*Continued*)
    - hospital (*Continued*)
      - miscellaneous Y74.8
      - monitoring Y74.0
      - prosthetic Y74.2
      - rehabilitative Y74.1
      - surgical Y74.3
      - therapeutic Y74.1
    - surgical Y81.8
      - accessory Y81.2
      - diagnostic Y81.0
      - miscellaneous Y81.8
      - monitoring Y81.0
      - prosthetic Y81.2
      - rehabilitative Y81.1
      - surgical Y81.3
      - therapeutic Y81.1
  - gynecological Y76.8
    - accessory Y76.2
    - diagnostic Y76.0
    - miscellaneous Y76.8
    - monitoring Y76.0
    - prosthetic Y76.2
    - rehabilitative Y76.1
    - surgical Y76.3
    - therapeutic Y76.1
  - medical Y82.9
    - specified type NEC Y82.8
  - neurological Y75.8
    - accessory Y75.2
    - diagnostic Y75.0
    - miscellaneous Y75.8
    - monitoring Y75.0
    - prosthetic Y75.2
    - rehabilitative Y75.1
    - surgical Y75.3
    - therapeutic Y75.1
  - obstetrical Y76.8
    - accessory Y76.2
    - diagnostic Y76.0
    - miscellaneous Y76.8
    - monitoring Y76.0
    - prosthetic Y76.2
    - rehabilitative Y76.1
    - surgical Y76.3
    - therapeutic Y76.1
  - ophthalmic Y77.8
    - accessory Y77.2
    - diagnostic Y77.0
    - miscellaneous Y77.8
    - monitoring Y77.0
    - prosthetic Y77.2
    - rehabilitative Y77.1
    - surgical Y77.3
    - therapeutic Y77.1
  - orthopedic Y79.8
    - accessory Y79.2
    - diagnostic Y79.0
    - miscellaneous Y79.8
    - monitoring Y79.0
    - prosthetic Y79.2
    - rehabilitative Y79.1
    - surgical Y79.3
    - therapeutic Y79.1
  - otorhinolaryngological Y72.8
    - accessory Y72.2
    - diagnostic Y72.0
    - miscellaneous Y72.8
    - monitoring Y72.0
    - prosthetic Y72.2
    - rehabilitative Y72.1
    - surgical Y72.3
    - therapeutic Y72.1
  - personal use Y74.8
    - accessory Y74.2
    - diagnostic Y74.0
    - miscellaneous Y74.8
    - monitoring Y74.0
    - prosthetic Y74.2

Incident, adverse (*Continued*)
- device (*Continued*)
  - personal use (*Continued*)
    - rehabilitative Y74.1
    - surgical Y74.3
    - therapeutic Y74.1
  - physical medicine Y80.8
    - accessory Y80.2
    - diagnostic Y80.0
    - miscellaneous Y80.8
    - monitoring Y80.0
    - prosthetic Y80.2
    - rehabilitative Y80.1
    - surgical Y80.3
    - therapeutic Y80.1
  - plastic surgical Y81.8
    - accessory Y81.2
    - diagnostic Y81.0
    - miscellaneous Y81.8
    - monitoring Y81.0
    - prosthetic Y81.2
    - rehabilitative Y81.1
    - surgical Y81.3
    - therapeutic Y81.1
  - radiological Y78.8
    - accessory Y78.2
    - diagnostic Y78.0
    - miscellaneous Y78.8
    - monitoring Y78.0
    - prosthetic Y78.2
    - rehabilitative Y78.1
    - surgical Y78.3
    - therapeutic Y78.1
  - urology Y73.8
    - accessory Y73.2
    - diagnostic Y73.0
    - miscellaneous Y73.8
    - monitoring Y73.0
    - prosthetic Y73.2
    - rehabilitative Y73.1
    - surgical Y73.3
    - therapeutic Y73.1

Incineration (accidental) —*see* Exposure, fire

Infanticide —*see* Assault

Infrasound waves (causing injury) W49.9

Ingestion
- foreign body (causing injury) (with obstruction) —*see* Foreign body, alimentary canal
- poisonous
  - plant (s) X58
  - substance NEC —*see* Table of Drugs and Chemicals

Inhalation
- excessively cold substance, man-made —*see* Exposure, cold, man-made
- food (any type) (into respiratory tract) (with asphyxia, obstruction respiratory tract, suffocation) —*see* categories T17 and T18
- foreign body —*see* Foreign body, aspiration
- gastric contents (with asphyxia, obstruction respiratory passage, suffocation) T17.81-
- hot air or gases X14.0
- liquid air, hydrogen, nitrogen W93.12
  - suicide (attempt) X83.2
- steam X13.0
  - assault X98.0
  - stated as undetermined whether accidental or intentional Y27.0
  - suicide (attempt) X77.0
- toxic gas —*see* Table of Drugs and Chemicals
- vomitus (with asphyxia, obstruction respiratory passage, suffocation) T17.81-

Injury, injured (accidental(ly)) **NOS** X58
- by, caused by, from
  - assault —*see* Assault
  - law-enforcing agent, police, in course of legal intervention —*see* Legal intervention
  - suicide (attempt) X83.8

Injury, injured NOS (*Continued*)
due to, in
civil insurrection —*see* War
operations
fight (*see also* Assault, fight)
Y04.0
war operations —*see* War
operations
homicide (*see also* Assault) Y09
inflicted (by)
in course of arrest (attempted), suppression
of disturbance, maintenance of order,
by law-enforcing agents —*see* Legal
intervention

Injury, injured NOS (*Continued*)
inflicted (*Continued*)
other person
stated as
accidental X58
intentional, homicide (attempt) —*see*
Assault
undetermined whether accidental or
intentional Y33
purposely (inflicted) by other person (s) —*see*
Assault
self-inflicted X83.8
stated as accidental X58
specified cause NEC X58

Injury, injured NOS (*Continued*)
undetermined whether accidental or
intentional Y33
Insolation, effects X30
Insufficient nourishment X58
Interruption of respiration (by)
food (lodged in esophagus) —*see* categories
T17 and T18
vomitus (lodged in esophagus) T17.81-
Intervention, legal —*see* Legal intervention
Intoxication
drug —*see* Table of Drugs and Chemicals
poison —*see* Table of Drugs and
Chemicals

J

Jammed (accidentally)
between objects (moving) (stationary and
moving) W23.0
stationary W23.1
Jumped, jumping
before moving object NEC X81.8
motor vehicle X81.0
subway train X81.1
train X81.1
undetermined whether accidental or
intentional Y31
from
boat (into water) voluntarily,
without accident (to or on boat)
W16.712
with
accident to or on boat —*see* Accident,
watercraft
drowning or submersion W16.711
suicide (attempt) X71.3

Jumped, jumping (*Continued*)
from (*Continued*)
boat voluntarily, without accident
(*Continued*)
striking bottom W16.722
causing drowning W16.721
building (*see also* Jumped, from,
high place) W13.9
burning (uncontrolled fire)
X00.5
high place NEC W17.89
suicide (attempt) X80
undetermined whether accidental or
intentional Y30
structure (*see also* Jumped, from, high
place) W13.9
burning (uncontrolled fire)
X00.5
into water W16.92
causing drowning W16.91
from, off watercraft —*see* Jumped, from,
boat

Jumped, jumping (*Continued*)
into water (*Continued*)
in
natural body W16.612
causing drowning W16.611
striking bottom W16.622
causing drowning W16.621
specified place NEC W16.812
causing drowning W16.811
striking
bottom W16.822
causing drowning W16.821
wall W16.832
causing drowning W16.831
swimming pool W16.512
causing drowning W16.511
striking
bottom W16.522
causing drowning W16.521
wall W16.532
causing drowning W16.531
suicide (attempt) X71.3

K

Kicked by
animal NEC W55.82
person (s) (accidentally) W50.1
with intent to injure or kill Y04.0
as, or caused by, a crowd or human
stampede (with fall) W52
assault Y04.0
homicide (attempt) Y04.0
in
fight Y04.0
legal intervention
injuring
bystander Y35.812
law enforcement personnel Y35.811
suspect Y35.813

Kicking against
object W22.8
sports equipment W21.9
stationary W22.09
sports equipment W21.89
person —*see* Striking against, person
sports equipment W21.9
Killed, killing (accidentally) **NOS** (*see also*
Injury) X58
in
action —*see* War operations
brawl, fight (hand) (fists) (foot) Y04.0
by weapon —*see also* Assault
cutting, piercing —*see* Assault, cutting
or piercing instrument
firearm —*see* Discharge, firearm, by
type, homicide

Killed, killing NOS (*Continued*)
self
stated as
accident NOS X58
suicide —*see* Suicide
undetermined whether accidental or
intentional Y33
Knocked down (accidentally) (by) **NOS** X58
animal (not being ridden) NEC —*see also*
Struck by, by type of animal
crowd or human stampede W52
person W51
in brawl, fight Y04.0
transport vehicle NEC (*see also* Accident,
transport) V09.9

◀ New   ◀▥ Revised   ~~deleted~~ Deleted

L

Laceration NEC —*see* Injury
Lack of
  care (helpless person) (infant) (newborn) X58
  food except as result of abandonment or
    neglect X58
    due to abandonment or neglect X58
  water except as result of transport accident X58
    due to transport accident —*see* Accident,
      transport, by type
  helpless person, infant, newborn X58
Landslide (falling on transport vehicle) X36.1
  caused by collapse of man-made structure
    X36.0
Late effect —*see* Sequelae
Legal
  execution (any method) —*see* Legal,
    intervention
  intervention (by)
    baton —*see* Legal, intervention, blunt
      object, baton
    bayonet —*see* Legal, intervention, sharp
      object, bayonet
    blow —*see* Legal, intervention,
      manhandling
    blunt object
      baton
        injuring
          bystander Y35.312
          law enforcement personnel Y35.311
          suspect Y35.313
      injuring
        bystander Y35.302
        law enforcement personnel Y35.301
        suspect Y35.303
      specified NEC
        injuring
          bystander Y35.392
          law enforcement personnel Y35.391
          suspect Y35.393
      stave
        injuring
          bystander Y35.392
          law enforcement personnel Y35.391
          suspect Y35.393
    bomb —*see* Legal, intervention, explosive
    cutting or piercing instrument —*see* Legal,
      intervention, sharp object
    dynamite —*see* Legal, intervention,
      explosive, dynamite
    explosive (s)
      dynamite
        injuring
          bystander Y35.112
          law enforcement personnel Y35.111
          suspect Y35.113
      grenade
        injuring
          bystander Y35.192
          law enforcement personnel Y35.191
          suspect Y35.193
      injuring
        bystander Y35.102
        law enforcement personnel Y35.101
        suspect Y35.103

Legal (*Continued*)
  intervention (*Continued*)
    explosive (*Continued*)
      mortar bomb
        injuring
          bystander Y35.192
          law enforcement personnel
            Y35.191
          suspect Y35.193
      shell
        injuring
          bystander Y35.122
          law enforcement personnel Y35.121
          suspect Y35.123
      specified NEC
        injuring
          bystander Y35.192
          law enforcement personnel Y35.191
          suspect Y35.193
    firearm (s) (discharge)
      handgun
        injuring
          bystander Y35.022
          law enforcement personnel Y35.021
          suspect Y35.023
      injuring
        bystander Y35.002
        law enforcement personnel Y35.001
        suspect Y35.003
      machine gun
        injuring
          bystander Y35.012
          law enforcement personnel Y35.011
          suspect Y35.013
      rifle pellet
        injuring
          bystander Y35.032
          law enforcement personnel Y35.031
          suspect Y35.033
      rubber bullet
        injuring
          bystander Y35.042
          law enforcement personnel Y35.041
          suspect Y35.043
      shotgun —*see* Legal, intervention,
        firearm, specified NEC
      specified NEC
        injuring
          bystander Y35.092
          law enforcement personnel Y35.091
          suspect Y35.093
    gas (asphyxiation) (poisoning)
      injuring
        bystander Y35.202
        law enforcement personnel Y35.201
        suspect Y35.203
      specified NEC
        injuring
          bystander Y35.292
          law enforcement personnel Y35.291
          suspect Y35.293
      tear gas
        injuring
          bystander Y35.212
          law enforcement personnel Y35.211
          suspect Y35.213

Legal (*Continued*)
  intervention (*Continued*)
    grenade —*see* Legal, intervention,
      explosive, grenade
    injuring
      bystander Y35.92
      law enforcement personnel Y35.91
      suspect Y35.93
    late effect (of) (*see* with 7th character S)
      Y35
    manhandling
      injuring
        bystander Y35.812
        law enforcement personnel Y35.811
        suspect Y35.813
    sequelae (of) (*see* with 7th character S)
      Y35
    sharp objects
      bayonet
        injuring
          bystander Y35.412
          law enforcement personnel
            Y35.411
          suspect Y35.413
      injuring
        bystander Y35.402
        law enforcement personnel Y35.401
        suspect Y35.403
      specified NEC
        injuring
          bystander Y35.492
          law enforcement personnel
            Y35.491
          suspect Y35.493
    specified means NEC
      injuring
        bystander Y35.892
        law enforcement personnel Y35.891
        suspect Y35.893
    stabbing —*see* Legal, intervention, sharp
      object
    stave —*see* Legal, intervention, blunt
      object, stave
    tear gas —*see* Legal, intervention, gas, tear
      gas
    truncheon —*see* Legal, intervention, blunt
      object, stave
Lightning (shock) (stroke) (struck by) —*see*
  subcategory T75.0
  causing fire —*see* Exposure, fire
Loss of control (transport vehicle) **NEC** —*see*
  Accident, transport
Lost at sea NOS —*see* Drowning, due to, fall
  overboard
Low
  pressure (effects) —*see* Air, pressure, low
  temperature (effects) —*see* Exposure, cold
**Lying before train, vehicle or other moving
  object** X81.8
  subway train X81.1
  train X81.1
  undetermined whether accidental or
    intentional Y31
Lynching —*see* Assault

M

Malfunction (mechanism or component) (of)
  firearm
    airgun W34.10
    BB gun W34.110
    gas, air or spring-operated gun NEC
      W34.118
    handgun W32.1
    hunting rifle W33.12
    larger firearm W33.10
      specified NEC W33.19
    machine gun W33.13
    paintball gun W34.111
    pellet gun W34.110
    shotgun W33.11
    specified NEC W34.19
    Very pistol [flare] W34.19
  handgun —*see* Malfunction, firearm,
    handgun
Maltreatment —*see* Perpetrator
Mangled (accidentally) **NOS** X58
Manhandling (in brawl, fight) Y04.0
  legal intervention —*see* Legal, intervention,
    manhandling
Manslaughter (nonaccidental) —*see* Assault
Mauled by animal NEC W55.89
Medical procedure, complication of
  (delayed or as an abnormal reaction
    without mention of misadventure) —*see*
    Complication of or following, by specified
    type of procedure
  due to or as a result of misadventure —*see*
    Misadventure
Melting (due to fire) —*see also* Exposure, fire
  apparel NEC X06.3
  clothes, clothing NEC X06.3
    nightwear X05
  fittings or furniture (burning building)
    (uncontrolled fire) X00.8
  nightwear X05
  plastic jewelry X06.1
Mental cruelty X58
Military operations (injuries to military and
    civilians occuring during peacetime on
    military property and during routine
    military exercises and operations) (by)
    (from) (involving) Y37.90-
  air blast Y37.20-
  aircraft
    destruction —*see* Military operations,
      destruction of aircraft
    airway restriction —*see* Military operations,
      restriction of airways
    asphyxiation —*see* Military operations,
      restriction of airways
  biological weapons Y37.6X-
  blast Y37.20-
  blast fragments Y37.20-
  blast wave Y37.20-
  blast wind Y37.20-
  bomb Y37.20-
    dirty Y37.50-
    gasoline Y37.31-
    incendiary Y37.31-
    petrol Y37.31-
  bullet Y37.43-
    incendiary Y37.32-
    rubber Y37.41-
  chemical weapons Y37.7X-
  combat
    hand to hand (unarmed) combat
      Y37.44-
    using blunt or piercing object Y37.45-
  conflagration —*see* Military operations, fire
  conventional warfare NEC Y37.49-
  depth-charge Y37.01-
  destruction of aircraft Y37.10-
    due to
      air to air missile Y37.11-
      collision with other aircraft Y37.12-

Military operations (*Continued*)
  destruction of aircraft (*Continued*)
    due to (*Continued*)
      detonation (accidental) of onboard
        munitions and explosives Y37.14-
      enemy fire or explosives Y37.11-
      explosive placed on aircraft Y37.11-
      onboard fire Y37.13-
      rocket propelled grenade [RPG] Y37.11-
      small arms fire Y37.11-
      surface to air missile Y37.11-
    specified NEC Y37.19-
  detonation (accidental) of
    onboard marine weapons Y37.05-
    own munitions or munitions launch device
      Y37.24-
  dirty bomb Y37.50-
  explosion (of) Y37.20-
    aerial bomb Y37.21-
    bomb NOS (*see also* Military operations,
      bomb (s)) Y37.20-
    fragments Y37.20-
    grenade Y37.29-
    guided missile Y37.22-
    improvised explosive device [IED] (person-
      borne) (roadside) (vehicle-borne)
      Y37.23-
    land mine Y37.29-
    marine mine (at sea) (in harbor) Y37.02-
    marine weapon Y37.00-
      specified NEC Y37.09-
    own munitions or munitions launch device
      (accidental) Y37.24-
    sea-based artillery shell Y37.03-
    specified NEC Y37.29-
    torpedo Y37.04-
  fire Y37.30-
    specified NEC Y37.39-
  firearms
    discharge Y37.43-
    pellets Y37.42-
  flamethrower Y37.33-
  fragments (from) (of)
    improvised explosive device [IED] (person-
      borne) (roadside) (vehicle-borne)
      Y37.26-
    munitions Y37.25-
    specified NEC Y37.29-
    weapons Y37.27-
  friendly fire Y37.92-
  hand to hand (unarmed) combat Y37.44-
  hot substances —*see* Military operations, fire
  incendiary bullet Y37.32-
  nuclear weapon (effects of) Y37.50-
    acute radiation exposure Y37.54-
    blast pressure Y37.51-
    direct blast Y37.51-
    direct heat Y37.53-
    fallout exposure Y37.54-
    fireball Y37.53-
    indirect blast (struck or crushed by blast
      debris) (being thrown by blast)
      Y37.52-
    ionizing radiation (immediate exposure)
      Y37.54-
    nuclear radiation Y37.54-
    radiation
      ionizing (immediate exposure) Y37.54-
      nuclear Y37.54-
      thermal Y37.53-
    secondary effects Y37.54-
    specified NEC Y37.59-
    thermal radiation Y37.53-
  restriction of air (airway)
    intentional Y37.46-
    unintentional Y37.47-
  rubber bullets Y37.41-
  shrapnel NOS Y37.29-
  suffocation —*see* Military operations,
    restriction of airways
  unconventional warfare NEC Y37.7X-

Military operations (*Continued*)
  underwater blast NOS Y37.00-
  warfare
    conventional NEC Y37.49-
    unconventional NEC Y37.7X-
  weapon of mass destruction [WMD] Y37.91-
  weapons
    biological weapons Y37.6X-
    chemical Y37.7X-
    nuclear (effects of) Y37.50-
      acute radiation exposure Y37.54-
      blast pressure Y37.51-
      direct blast Y37.51-
      direct heat Y37.53-
      fallout exposure Y37.54-
      fireball Y37.53-
      indirect blast (struck or crushed by blast
        debris) (being thrown by blast)
        Y37.52-
      radiation
        ionizing (immediate exposure) Y37.54-
        nuclear Y37.54-
        thermal Y37.53-
      secondary effects Y37.54-
      specified NEC Y37.59-
    of mass destruction [WMD] Y37.91-
**Misadventure (s) to patient (s) during surgical
  or medical care** Y69
  contaminated medical or biological substance
    (blood, drug, fluid) Y64.9
    administered (by) NEC Y64.9
      immunization Y64.1
      infusion Y64.0
      injection Y64.1
      specified means NEC Y64.8
      transfusion Y64.0
      vaccination Y64.1
  excessive amount of blood or other fluid
    during transfusion or infusion Y63.0
  failure
    in dosage Y63.9
      electroshock therapy Y63.4
      inappropriate temperature (too hot or
        too cold) in local application and
        packing Y63.5
      infusion
        excessive amount of fluid Y63.0
        incorrect dilution of fluid Y63.1
      insulin-shock therapy Y63.4
      nonadministration of necessary drug or
        biological substance Y63.6
      overdose —*see* Table of Drugs and
        Chemicals
      radiation, in therapy Y63.2
      radiation
        overdose Y63.2
      specified procedure NEC Y63.8
      transfusion
        excessive amount of blood Y63.0
    mechanical, of instrument or apparatus
      (any) (during any procedure) Y65.8
    sterile precautions (during procedure)
      Y62.9
      aspiration of fluid or tissue (by puncture
        or catheterization, except heart)
        Y62.6
      biopsy (except needle aspiration) Y62.8
        needle (aspirating) Y62.6
      blood sampling Y62.6
      catheterization Y62.6
        heart Y62.5
      dialysis (kidney) Y62.2
      endoscopic examination Y62.4
      enema Y62.8
      immunization Y62.3
      infusion Y62.1
      injection Y62.3
      needle biopsy Y62.6
      paracentesis (abdominal) (thoracic)
        Y62.6
      perfusion Y62.2

Misadventure (s) to patient (s) during surgical or medical care *(Continued)*
failure *(Continued)*
sterile precautions *(Continued)*
puncture (lumbar) Y62.6
removal of catheter or packing Y62.8
specified procedure NEC Y62.8
surgical operation Y62.0
transfusion Y62.1
vaccination Y62.3
suture or ligature during surgical procedure Y65.2
to introduce or to remove tube or instrument —*see* Failure, to
hemorrhage —*see* Index to Diseases and Injuries, Complication(s)
inadvertent exposure of patient to radiation Y63.3
inappropriate
operation performed —*see* Inappropriate operation performed
temperature (too hot or too cold) in local application or packing Y63.5

Misadventure (s) to patient (s) during surgical or medical care *(Continued)*
infusion (*see also* Misadventure, by type, infusion) Y69
excessive amount of fluid Y63.0
incorrect dilution of fluid Y63.1
wrong fluid Y65.1
mismatched blood in transfusion Y65.0
nonadministration of necessary drug or biological substance Y63.6
overdose —*see* Table of Drugs and Chemicals
radiation (in therapy) Y63.2
perforation —*see* Index to Diseases and Injuries, Complication(s)
performance of inappropriate operation — *see* Inappropriate operation performed
puncture —*see* Index to Diseases and Injuries, Complication(s)
specified type NEC Y65.8
failure
suture or ligature during surgical operation Y65.2
to introduce or to remove tube or instrument —*see* Failure, to
infusion of wrong fluid Y65.1

Misadventure (s) to patient (s) during surgical or medical care *(Continued)*
specified type NEC *(Continued)*
performance of inappropriate operation — *see* Inappropriate operation performed
transfusion of mismatched blood Y65.0
wrong
fluid in infusion Y65.1
placement of endotracheal tube during anesthetic procedure Y65.3
transfusion —*see* Misadventure, by type, transfusion
excessive amount of blood Y63.0
mismatched blood Y65.0
wrong
drug given in error —*see* Table of Drugs and Chemicals
fluid in infusion Y65.1
placement of endotracheal tube during anesthetic procedure Y65.3
Mismatched blood in transfusion Y65.0
Motion sickness T75.3
Mountain sickness W94.11
Mudslide (of cataclysmic nature) —*see* Landslide
Murder (attempt) —*see* Assault

N

Nail, contact with W45.0
gun W29.4
Neglect (criminal) (homicidal intent) X58
Noise (causing injury) (pollution) W42.9
supersonic W42.0

Nonadministration (of)
drug or biological substance (necessary) Y63.6
surgical and medical care Y66
Nosocomial condition Y95

O

Object
falling
from, in, on, hitting
machinery —*see* Contact, with, by type of machine
set in motion by
accidental explosion or rupture of pressure vessel W38
firearm —*see* Discharge, firearm, by type
machine (ry) —*see* Contact, with, by type of machine

Overdose (drug) —*see* Table of Drugs and Chemicals
radiation Y63.2
Overexertion —*see* category Y93
Overexposure (accidental) (to)
cold (*see also* Exposure, cold) X31
due to man-made conditions —*see* Exposure, cold, man-made
heat (*see also* Heat) X30
radiation —*see* Radiation
radioactivity W88.0
sun (sunburn) X32
weather NEC —*see* Forces of nature
wind NEC —*see* Forces of nature

Overheated —*see* Heat
Overturning (accidental)
machinery —*see* Contact, with, by type of machine
transport vehicle NEC (*see also* Accident, transport) V89.9
watercraft (causing drowning, submersion) —*see also* Drowning, due to, accident to, watercraft, overturning
causing injury except drowning or submersion —*see* Accident, watercraft, causing, injury NEC

P

Parachute descent (voluntary) (without
    accident to aircraft) V97.29
  due to accident to aircraft —*see* Accident,
    transport, aircraft
Pecked by bird W61.99
Perforation during medical or surgical
    treatment as misadventure —*see* Index to
    Diseases and Injuries, Complication(s)
Perpetrator, perpetration, of assault,
    maltreatment and neglect (by)
    Y07.9
  boyfriend Y07.03
  brother Y07.410
    stepbrother Y07.435
  coach Y07.53
  cousin
    female Y07.491
    male Y07.490
  daycare provider Y07.519
    at-home
      adult care Y07.512
      childcare Y07.510
    care center
      adult care Y07.513
      childcare Y07.511
  family member NEC Y07.499
  father Y07.11
    adoptive Y07.13
    foster Y07.420
    stepfather Y07.430
  foster father Y07.420
  foster mother Y07.421
  girl friend Y07.04
  healthcare provider Y07.529
    mental health Y07.521
    specified NEC Y07.528
  husband Y07.01
  instructor Y07.53
  mother Y07.12
    adoptive Y07.14
    foster Y07.421
    stepmother Y07.433
  nonfamily member Y07.50
    specified NEC Y07.59
  nurse Y07.528
  occupational therapist Y07.528
  partner of parent
    female Y07.434
    male Y07.432
  physical therapist Y07.528
  sister Y07.411
  speech therapist Y07.528
  stepbrother Y07.435
  stepfather Y07.430
  stepmother Y07.433
  stepsister Y07.436
  teacher Y07.53
  wife Y07.02
Piercing —*see* Contact, with, by type of object
    or machine
Pinched
  between objects (moving) (stationary and
    moving) W23.0
    stationary W23.1
Pinned under machine (ry) —*see* Contact, with,
    by type of machine
Place of occurrence Y92.9
  abandoned house Y92.89
  airplane Y92.813
  airport Y92.520
  ambulatory health services establishment
    NEC Y92.538
  ambulatory surgery center Y92.530
  amusement park Y92.831
  apartment (co-op) —*see* Place of occurrence,
    residence, apartment
  assembly hall Y92.29
  bank Y92.510
  barn Y92.71
  baseball field Y92.320

Place of occurrence (*Continued*)
  basketball court Y92.310
  beach Y92.832
  boarding house —*see* Place of occurrence,
    residence, boarding house
  boat Y92.814
  bowling alley Y92.39
  bridge Y92.89
  building under construction Y92.61
  bus Y92.811
    station Y92.521
  cafe Y92.511
  campsite Y92.833
  campus —*see* Place of occurrence, school
  canal Y92.89
  car Y92.810
  casino Y92.59
  children's home —*see* Place of occurrence,
    residence, institutional, orphanage
  church Y92.22
  cinema Y92.26
  clubhouse Y92.29
  coal pit Y92.64
  college (community) Y92.214
  condominium —*see* Place of occurrence,
    residence, apartment
  construction area —*see* Place of occurrence,
    industrial and construction area
  convalescent home —*see* Place of occurrence,
    residence, institutional, nursing home
  court-house Y92.240
  cricket ground Y92.328
  cultural building Y92.258
    art gallery Y92.250
    museum Y92.251
    music hall Y92.252
    opera house Y92.253
    specified NEC Y92.258
    theater Y92.254
  dancehall Y92.252
  day nursery Y92.210
  dentist office Y92.531
  derelict house Y92.89
  desert Y92.820
  dock NOS Y92.89
  dockyard Y92.62
  doctor's office Y92.531
  dormitory —*see* Place of occurrence,
    residence, institutional, school dormitory
  dry dock Y92.62
  factory (building) (premises) Y92.63
  farm (land under cultivation) (outbuildings)
    Y92.79
    barn Y92.71
    chicken coop Y92.72
    field Y92.73
    hen house Y92.72
    house —*see* Place of occurrence, residence,
      house
    orchard Y92.74
    specified NEC Y92.79
  football field Y92.321
  forest Y92.821
  freeway Y92.411
  gallery Y92.250
  garage (commercial) Y92.59
    boarding house Y92.044
    military base Y92.135
    mobile home Y92.025
    nursing home Y92.124
    orphanage Y92.114
    private house Y92.015
    reform school Y92.155
  gas station Y92.524
  gasworks Y92.69
  golf course Y92.39
  gravel pit Y92.64
  grocery Y92.512
  gymnasium Y92.39
  handball court Y92.318
  harbor Y92.89

Place of occurrence (*Continued*)
  harness racing course Y92.39
  healthcare provider office Y92.531
  highway (interstate) Y92.411
  hill Y92.828
  hockey rink Y92.330
  home —*see* Place of occurrence, residence
  hospice —*see* Place of occurrence, residence,
    institutional, nursing home
  hospital Y92.239
    cafeteria Y92.233
    corridor Y92.232
    operating room Y92.234
    patient
      bathroom Y92.231
      room Y92.230
    specified NEC Y92.238
  hotel Y92.59
  house —*see also* Place of occurrence, residence
    abandoned Y92.89
    under construction Y92.61
  industrial and construction area (yard)
    Y92.69
    building under construction Y92.61
    dock Y92.62
    dry dock Y92.62
    factory Y92.63
    gasworks Y92.69
    mine Y92.64
    oil rig Y92.65
    pit Y92.64
    power station Y92.69
    shipyard Y92.62
    specified NEC Y92.69
    tunnel under construction Y92.69
    workshop Y92.69
  kindergarten Y92.211
  lacrosse field Y92.328
  lake Y92.828
  library Y92.241
  mall Y92.59
  market Y92.512
  marsh Y92.828
  military
    base —*see* Place of occurrence, residence,
      institutional, military base
    training ground Y92.84
  mine Y92.64
  mosque Y92.22
  motel Y92.59
  motorway (interstate) Y92.411
  mountain Y92.828
  movie-house Y92.26
  museum Y92.251
  music-hall Y92.252
  not applicable Y92.9
  nuclear power station Y92.69
  nursing home —*see* Place of occurrence,
    residence, institutional, nursing home
  office building Y92.59
  offshore installation Y92.65
  oil rig Y92.65
  old people's home —*see* Place of occurrence,
    residence, institutional, specified NEC
  opera-house Y92.253
  orphanage —*see* Place of occurrence,
    residence, institutional, orphanage
  outpatient surgery center Y92.530
  park (public) Y92.830
    amusement Y92.831
  parking garage Y92.89
    lot Y92.481
  pavement Y92.480
  physician office Y92.531
  polo field Y92.328
  pond Y92.828
  post office Y92.242
  power station Y92.69
  prairie Y92.828
  prison —*see* Place of occurrence, residence,
    institutional, prison

◀ New   ◀ Revised   ~~deleted~~ Deleted

Place of occurrence *(Continued)*
  public
    administration building Y92.248
      city hall Y92.243
      courthouse Y92.240
      library Y92.241
      post office Y92.242
      specified NEC Y92.248
    building NEC Y92.29
    hall Y92.29
    place NOS Y92.89
  race course Y92.39
  radio station Y92.59
  railway line (bridge) Y92.85
  ranch (outbuildings) —*see* Place of
    occurrence, farm
  recreation area Y92.838
    amusement park Y92.831
    beach Y92.832
    campsite Y92.833
    park (public) Y92.830
    seashore Y92.832
    specified NEC Y92.838
  reform school —*see* Place of occurrence,
    residence, institutional, reform school
  religious institution Y92.22
  residence (non-institutional) (private) Y92.009
    apartment Y92.039
      bathroom Y92.031
      bedroom Y92.032
      kitchen Y92.030
      specified NEC Y92.038
    bathroom Y92.002
    bedroom Y92.003
    boarding house Y92.049
      bathroom Y92.041
      bedroom Y92.042
      driveway Y92.043
      garage Y92.044
      garden Y92.046
      kitchen Y92.040
      specified NEC Y92.048
      swimming pool Y92.045
      yard Y92.046
    dining room Y92.001
    garden Y92.007
    home Y92.009
    house, single family Y92.019
      bathroom Y92.012
      bedroom Y92.013
      dining room Y92.011
      driveway Y92.014
      garage Y92.015
      garden Y92.017
      kitchen Y92.010
      specified NEC Y92.018
      swimming pool Y92.016
      yard Y92.017
    institutional Y92.10
      children's home —*see* Place of
        occurrence, residence, institutional,
        orphanage
      hospice —*see* Place of occurrence,
        residence, institutional, nursing
        home
      military base Y92.139
        barracks Y92.133
        garage Y92.135
        garden Y92.137
        kitchen Y92.130
        mess hall Y92.131
        specified NEC Y92.138
        swimming pool Y92.136
        yard Y92.137
      nursing home Y92.129
        bathroom Y92.121
        bedroom Y92.122
        driveway Y92.123
        garage Y92.124
        garden Y92.126
        kitchen Y92.120

Place of occurrence *(Continued)*
  residence *(Continued)*
    institutional *(Continued)*
      nursing home *(Continued)*
        specified NEC Y92.128
        swimming pool Y92.125
        yard Y92.126
      orphanage Y92.119
        bathroom Y92.111
        bedroom Y92.112
        driveway Y92.113
        garage Y92.114
        garden Y92.116
        kitchen Y92.110
        specified NEC Y92.118
        swimming pool Y92.115
        yard Y92.116
      prison Y92.149
        bathroom Y92.142
        cell Y92.143
        courtyard Y92.147
        dining room Y92.141
        kitchen Y92.140
        specified NEC Y92.148
        swimming pool Y92.146
      reform school Y92.159
        bathroom Y92.152
        bedroom Y92.153
        dining room Y92.151
        driveway Y92.154
        garage Y92.155
        garden Y92.157
        kitchen Y92.150
        specified NEC Y92.158
        swimming pool Y92.156
        yard Y92.157
      school dormitory Y92.169
        bathroom Y92.162
        bedroom Y92.163
        dining room Y92.161
        kitchen Y92.160
        specified NEC Y92.168
      specified NEC Y92.199
        bathroom Y92.192
        bedroom Y92.193
        dining room Y92.191
        driveway Y92.194
        garage Y92.195
        garden Y92.197
        kitchen Y92.190
        specified NEC Y92.198
        swimming pool Y92.196
        yard Y92.197
    kitchen Y92.000
    mobile home Y92.029
      bathroom Y92.022
      bedroom Y92.023
      dining room Y92.021
      driveway Y92.024
      garage Y92.025
      garden Y92.027
      kitchen Y92.020
      specified NEC Y92.028
      swimming pool Y92.026
      yard Y92.027
    specified place in residence NEC Y92.008
    specified residence type NEC Y92.099
      bathroom Y92.091
      bedroom Y92.092
      driveway Y92.093
      garage Y92.094
      garden Y92.096
      kitchen Y92.090
      specified NEC Y92.098
      swimming pool Y92.095
      yard Y92.096
  restaurant Y92.511
  riding school Y92.39
  river Y92.828
  road Y92.488
  rodeo ring Y92.39

Place of occurrence *(Continued)*
  rugby field Y92.328
  same day surgery center Y92.530
  sand pit Y92.64
  school (private) (public) (state) Y92.219
    college Y92.214
    daycare center Y92.210
    elementary school Y92.211
    high school Y92.213
    kindergarten Y92.211
    middle school Y92.212
    specified NEC Y92.218
    trace school Y92.215
    university Y92.214
    vocational school Y92.215
  sea (shore) Y92.832
  senior citizen center Y92.29
  service area
    airport Y92.520
    bus station Y92.521
    gas station Y92.524
    highway rest stop Y92.523
    railway station Y92.522
  shipyard Y92.62
  shop(commercial) Y92.513
  sidewalk Y92.480
  silo Y92.79
  skating rink (roller) Y92.331
    ice Y92.330
  slaughter house Y92.86
  soccer field Y92.322
  specified place NEC Y92.89
  sports area Y92.39
    athletic
      court Y92.318
        basketball Y92.310
        specified NEC Y92.318
        squash Y92.311
        tennis Y92.312
      field Y92.328
        baseball Y92.320
        cricket ground Y92.328
        football Y92.321
        hockey Y92.328
        soccer Y92.322
        specified NEC Y92.328
    golf course Y92.39
    gymnasium Y92.39
    riding school Y92.39
    skating rink (roller) Y92.331
      ice Y92.330
    stadium Y92.39
    swimming pool Y92.34
  squash court Y92.311
  stadium Y92.39
  steeplechasing course Y92.39
  store Y92.512
  stream Y92.828
  street and highway Y92.410
    bike path Y92.482
    freeway Y92.411
    highway ramp Y92.415
    interstate highway Y92.411
    local residential or business street
      Y92.414
    motorway Y92.411
    parking lot Y92.481
    parkway Y92.412
    sidewalk Y92.480
    specified NEC Y92.488
    state road Y92.413
  subway car Y92.816
  supermarket Y92.512
  swamp Y92.828
  swimming pool (public) Y92.34
    private (at) Y92.095
      boarding house Y92.045
      military base Y92.136
      mobile home Y92.026
      nursing home Y92.125
      orphanage Y92.115

Place of occurrence (Continued)
  swimming pool (Continued)
    private (Continued)
      prison Y92.146
      reform school Y92.156
      single family residence
        Y92.016
  synagogue Y92.22
  television station Y92.59
  tennis court Y92.312
  theater Y92.254
  trade area Y92.59
    bank Y92.510
    cafe Y92.511
    casino Y92.59
    garage Y92.59
    hotel Y92.59
    market Y92.512
    office building Y92.59
    radio station Y92.59
    restaurant Y92.511
    shop Y92.513
    shopping mall Y92.59
    store Y92.512
    supermarket Y92.512
    television station Y92.59
    warehouse Y92.59
  trailer park, residential —see Place of
    occurrence, residence, mobile
    home
  trailer site NOS Y92.89
  train Y92.815
    station Y92.522
  truck Y92.812
  tunnel under construction Y92. 69
  university Y92.214
  urgent (health) care center Y92.532
  vehicle (transport) Y92.818
    airplane Y92.813
    boat Y92.814
    bus Y92.811
    car Y92.810
    specified NEC Y92.818
    subway car Y92.816
    train Y92.815
    truck Y92.812
  warehouse Y92.59
  water reservoir Y92.89
  wilderness area Y92.828
    desert Y92.820
    forest Y92.821
    marsh Y92.828
    mountain Y92.828
    prairie Y92.828
    specified NEC Y92.828
    swamp Y92.828
  workshop Y92.69
  yard, private Y92.096
    boarding house Y92.046
    mobile home Y92.027
    single family house Y92.017

Place of occurrence (Continued)
  youth center Y92.29
  zoo (zoological garden) Y92.834
Plumbism —see Table of Drugs and Chemicals,
  lead
Poisoning (accidental) (by) —see also Table of
  Drugs and Chemicals
  by plant, thorns, spines, sharp leaves or other
    mechanisms NEC X58
  carbon monoxide
    generated by
      motor vehicle —see Accident, transport
      watercraft (in transit) (not in transit)
        V93.89
        ferry boat V93.81
        fishing boat V93.82
        jet skis V93.83
        liner V93.81
        merchant ship V93.80
        passenger ship V93.81
        powered craft NEC V93.83
  caused by injection of poisons into skin by
    plant thorns, spines, sharp leaves X58
  marine or sea plants (venomous) X58
  exhaust gas
    generated by
      motor vehicle —see Accident, transport
      watercraft (in transit) (not in transit)
        V93.89
        ferry boat V93.81
        fishing boat V93.82
        jet skis V93.83
        liner V93.81
        merchant ship V93.80
        passenger ship V93.81
        powered craft NEC V93.83
  fumes or smoke due to
    explosion (see also Explosion) W40.9
    fire —see Exposure, fire
    ignition —see Ignition
  gas
    in legal intervention —see Legal,
      intervention, gas
    legal execution —see Legal, intervention,
      gas
  in war operations —see War operations
  legal
    execution —see Legal, intervention, gas
    intervention
      by gas —see Legal, intervention, gas
      other specified means —see Legal,
        intervention, specified means
        NEC
Powder burn (by) (from)
  airgun W34.110
  BB gun W34.110
  firearm NEC W34.19
  gas, air or spring-operated gun NEC
    W34.118
  handgun W32.1
  hunting rifle W33.12

Powder burn (Continued)
  larger firearm W33.10
    specified NEC W33.19
  machine gun W33.13
  paintball gun W34.111
  pellet gun W34.110
  shotgun W33.11
  Very pistol [flare] W34.19
Premature cessation (of) **surgical and medical**
  care Y66
Privation (food) (water) X58
Procedure (operation)
  correct, on wrong side or body part (wrong
    side) (wrong site) Y65.53
  intended for another patient done on wrong
    patient Y65.52
  performed on patient not scheduled for
    surgery Y65.52
  performed on wrong patient Y65.52
  wrong, performed on correct patient Y65.51
Prolonged
  sitting in transport vehicle —see Travel, by
    type of vehicle
  stay in
    high altitude as cause of anoxia,
      barodontalgia, barotitis or hypoxia
      W94.11
    weightless environment X52
Pulling, excessive —see category Y93
Puncture, puncturing —see also Contact, with,
  by type of object or machine
  by
    plant thorns, spines, sharp leaves or other
      mechanisms NEC W60
  during medical or surgical treatment as
    misadventure —see Index to Diseases
    and Injuries, Complication(s)
Pushed, pushing (accidental) (injury in)
  (overexertion) —see also category Y93
  by other person (s) (accidental) W51
    with fall W03
      due to ice or snow W00.0
    as, or caused by, a crowd or human
      stampede (with fall) W52
    before moving object NEC Y02.8
      motor vehicle Y02.0
      subway train Y02.1
      train Y02.1
    from
      high place NEC
        in accidental circumstances W17.89
        stated as
          intentional, homicide (attempt) Y01
          undetermined whether accidental
            or intentional Y30
      transport vehicle NEC (see also Accident,
        transport) V89.9
        stated as
          intentional, homicide (attempt)
            Y08.89

P

R

Radiation (exposure to)
  arc lamps W89.0
  atomic power plant (malfunction) NEC
    W88.1
  complication of or abnormal reaction to
    medical radiotherapy Y84.2
  electromagnetic, ionizing W88.0
  gamma rays W88.1
  in
    war operations (from or following
      nuclear explosion) —*see also* War
      operations
  inadvertent exposure of patient (receiving
    test or therapy) Y63.3
  infrared (heaters and lamps) W90.1
    excessive heat from W92
  ionized, ionizing (particles, artificially
    accelerated)
    radioisotopes W88.1
    specified NEC W88.8
    x-rays W88.0
  isotopes, radioactive —*see* Radiation,
    radioactive isotopes
  laser (s) W90.2
    in war operations —*see* War operations
    misadventure in medical care Y63.2
  light sources (man-made visible and
    ultraviolet) W89.9
    natural X32
    specified NEC W89.8
    tanning bed W89.1
    welding light W89.0
  man-made visible light W89.9
    specified NEC W89.8
    tanning bed W89.1
    welding light W89.0
  microwave W90.8
  misadventure in medical or surgical
    procedure Y63.2

Radiation *(Continued)*
  natural NEC X39.08
    radon X39.01
  overdose (in medical or surgical procedure)
    Y63.2
  radar W90.0
  radioactive isotopes (any) W88.1
    atomic power plant malfunction W88.1
    misadventure in medical or surgical
      treatment Y63.2
  radiofrequency W90.0
  radium NEC W88.1
  sun X32
  ultraviolet (light) (man-made) W89.9
    natural X32
    specified NEC W89.8
    tanning bed W89.1
    welding light W89.0
  welding arc, torch, or light W89.0
    excessive heat from W92
  x-rays (hard) (soft) W88.0
Range disease W94.11
Rape (attempted) T74.2-
Rat bite W53.11
Reaction, abnormal to medical procedure *(see
  also* Complication of or following, by type
  of procedure) Y84.9
  with misadventure —*see* Misadventure
  biologicals —*see* Table of Drugs and
    Chemicals
  drugs —*see* Table of Drugs and
    Chemicals
  vaccine —*see* Table of Drugs and
    Chemicals
Recoil
  airgun W34.110
  BB gun W34.110
  firearm NEC W34.19
  gas, air or spring-operated gun NEC
    W34.118

Recoil *(Continued)*
  handgun W32.1
  hunting rifle W33.12
  larger firearm W33.10
    specified NEC W33.19
  machine gun W33.13
  paintball gun W34.111
  pellet W34.110
  shotgun W33.11
  Very pistol [flare] W34.19
Reduction in
  atmospheric pressure —*see* Air, pressure,
    change
Rock falling on or hitting (accidentally)
  (person) W20.8
  in cave-in W20.0
Run over (accidentally) (by)
  animal (not being ridden) NEC W55.89
  machinery —*see* Contact, with, by specified
    type of machine
  transport vehicle NEC (*see also* Accident,
    transport) V09.9
    intentional homicide (attempt) Y03.0
    motor NEC V09.20
      intentional homicide (attempt)
        Y03.0
Running
  before moving object X81.8
  motor vehicle X81.0
Running off, away
  animal (being ridden) (*see also* Accident,
    transport) V80.918
    not being ridden W55.89
  animal-drawn vehicle NEC (*see also* Accident,
    transport) V80.928
  highway, road(way), street
    transport vehicle NEC (*see also* Accident,
      transport) V89.9
Rupture pressurized devices —*see* Explosion,
  by type of device

S

Saturnism —*see* Table of Drugs and Chemicals, lead
Scald, scalding (accidental) (by) (from) (in) X19
  air (hot) X14.1
  gases (hot) X14.1
  homicide (attempt) —*see* Assault, burning, hot object
  inflicted by other person
    stated as intentional, homicide (attempt) —*see* Assault, burning, hot object
  liquid (boiling) (hot) NEC X12
    stated as undetermined whether accidental or intentional Y27.2
    suicide (attempt) X77.2
  local application of externally applied substance in medical or surgical care Y63.5
  metal (molten) (liquid) (hot) NEC X18
  self-inflicted X77.9
  stated as undetermined whether accidental or intentional Y27.8
  steam X13.1
    assault X98.0
    stated as undetermined whether accidental or intentional Y27.0
    suicide (attempt) X77.0
  suicide (attempt) X77.9
  vapor (hot) X13.1
    assault X98.0
    stated as undetermined whether accidental or intentional Y27.0
    suicide (attempt) X77.0
Scratched by
  cat W55.03
  person (s) (accidentally) W50.4
    with intent to injure or kill Y04.0
    as, or caused by, a crowd or human stampede (with fall) W52
    assault Y04.0
    homicide (attempt) Y04.0
    in
      fight Y04.0
      legal intervention
        injuring
          bystander Y35.892
          law enforcement personnel Y35.891
          suspect Y35.893
Seasickness T75.3
Self-harm NEC —*see also* External cause by type, undetermined whether accidental or intentional
  intentional —*see* Suicide
  poisoning NEC —*see* Table of drugs and biologicals, accident
Self-inflicted (injury) **NEC** —*see also* External cause by type, undetermined whether accidental or intentional
  intentional —*see* Suicide
  poisoning NEC —*see* Table of drugs and biologicals, accident
Sequelae (of)
  accident NEC —*see* W00-X58 with 7th character S
  assault (homicidal) (any means) —*see* X92-Y08 with 7th character S
  homicide, attempt (any means) —*see* X92-Y08 with 7th character S
  injury undetermined whether accidentally or purposely inflicted —*see* Y21-Y33 with 7th character S
  intentional self-harm (classifiable to X71-X83) —*see* X71-X83 with 7th character S
  legal intervention (*see* with 7th character S Y35)
  motor vehicle accident —*see* V00-V99 with 7th character S
  suicide, attempt (any means) —*see* X71-X83 with 7th character S

Sequelae (*Continued*)
  transport accident —*see* V00-V99 with 7th character S
  war operations —*see* War operations
Shock
  electric —*see* Exposure, electric current
  from electric appliance (any) (faulty) W86.8
    domestic W86.0
    suicide (attempt) X83.1
Shooting, shot (accidental (ly)) —*see also* Discharge, firearm, by type
  herself or himself —*see* Discharge, firearm by type, self-inflicted
  homicide (attempt) —*see* Discharge, firearm by type, homicide
  in war operations —*see* War operations
  inflicted by other person —*see* Discharge, firearm by type, homicide
    accidental —*see* Discharge, firearm, by type of firearm
  legal
    execution —*see* Legal, intervention, firearm
    intervention —*see* Legal, intervention, firearm
  self-inflicted —*see* Discharge, firearm by type, suicide
    accidental —*see* Discharge, firearm, by type of firearm
  suicide (attempt) —*see* Discharge, firearm by type, suicide
Shoving (accidentally) **by other person** —*see* Pushed, by other person
Sickness
  alpine W94.11
  motion —*see* Motion
  mountain W94.11
Sinking (accidental)
  watercraft (causing drowning, submersion) —*see also* Drowning, due to, accident to, watercraft, sinking
    causing injury except drowning or submersion —*see* Accident, watercraft, causing, injury NEC
Siriasis X32
Slashed wrists —*see* Cut, self-inflicted
Slipping (accidental) (on same level) (with fall) W01.0
  without fall W18.40
    due to
      specified NEC W18.49
      stepping from one level to another W18.43
      stepping into hole or opening W18.42
      stepping on object W18.41
  on
    ice W00.0
      with skates —*see* Accident, transport, pedestrian, conveyance
    mud W01.0
    oil W01.0
    snow W00.0
      with skis —*see* Accident, transport, pedestrian, conveyance
    surface (slippery) (wet) NEC W01.0
Sliver, wood, contact with W45.8
Smoldering (due to fire) —*see* Exposure, fire
Sodomy (attempted) **by force** T74.2-
Sound waves (causing injury) W42.9
  supersonic W42.0
Splinter, contact with W45.8
Stab, stabbing —*see* Cut
Starvation X58
Status of external cause Y99.9
  child assisting in compensated work for family Y99.8
  civilian activity done for financial or other compensation Y99.0
  civilian activity done for income or pay Y99.0
  family member assisting in compensated work for other family member Y99.8
  hobby not done for income Y99.8

Status of external cause (*Continued*)
  leisure activity Y99.8
  military activity Y99.1
  off-duty activity of military personnel Y99.8
  recreation or sport not for income or while a student Y99.8
  specified NEC Y99.8
  student activity Y99.8
  volunteer activity Y99.2
Stepped on
  by
    animal (not being ridden) NEC W55.89
    crowd or human stampede W52
    person W50.0
Stepping on
  object W22.8
    with fall W18.31
    sports equipment W21.9
    stationary W22.09
      sports equipment W21.89
  person W51
    by crowd or human stampede W52
    sports equipment W21.9
Sting
  arthropod, nonvenomous W57
  insect, nonvenomous W57
Storm (cataclysmic) —*see* Forces of nature, cataclysmic storm
Straining, excessive —*see* category Y93
Strangling —*see* Strangulation
Strangulation (accidental) —*see* category T71
Strenuous movements —*see* category Y93
Striking against
  airbag (automobile) W22.10
    driver side W22.11
    front passenger side W22.12
    specified NEC W22.19
  bottom when
    diving or jumping into water (in) W16.822
      causing drowning W16.821
      from boat W16.722
        causing drowning W16.721
      natural body W16.622
        causing drowning W16.821
      swimming pool W16.522
        causing drowning W16.521
    falling into water (in) W16.322
      causing drowning W16.321
      fountain —*see* Striking against, bottom when, falling into water, specified NEC
      natural body W16.122
        causing drowning W16.121
      reservoir —*see* Striking against, bottom when, falling into water, specified NEC
      specified NEC W16.322
        causing drowning W16.321
      swimming pool W16.022
        causing drowning W16.021
  diving board (swimming-pool) W21.4
  object W22.8
    with
      drowning or submersion —*see* Drowning
      fall —*see* Fall, due to, bumping against, object
    caused by crowd or human stampede (with fall) W52
    furniture W22.03
    lamppost W22.02
    sports equipment W21.9
    stationary W22.09
      sports equipment W21.89
    wall W22.01
  person (s) W51
    with fall W03
      due to ice or snow W00.0
    as, or caused by, a crowd or human stampede (with fall) W52

◀ New   ⬱ Revised   ~~deleted~~ Deleted

Striking against (Continued)
  person (Continued)
    assault Y04.2
    homicide (attempt) Y04.2
  sports equipment W21.9
  wall (when) W22.01
    diving or jumping into water (in) W16.832
      causing drowning W16.831
      swimming pool W16.532
        causing drowning W16.531
    falling into water (in) W16.332
      causing drowning W16.331
      fountain —see Striking against, wall
        when, falling into water, specified
        NEC
      natural body W16.132
        causing drowning W16.131
      reservoir —see Striking against, wall
        when, falling into water, specified
        NEC
      specified NEC W16.332
        causing drowning W16.331
      swimming pool W16.032
        causing drowning W16.031
    swimming pool (when) W22.042
      causing drowning W22.041
      diving or jumping into water W16.532
        causing drowning W16.531
      falling into water W16.032
        causing drowning W16.031

Struck (accidentally) by
  airbag (automobile) W22.10
    driver side W22.11
    front passenger side W22.12
    specified NEC W22.19
  alligator W58.02
  animal (not being ridden) NEC W55.89
  avalanche —see Landslide
  ball (hit) (thrown) W21.00
    assault Y08.09
    baseball W21.03
    basketball W21.05
    football W21.01
    golf ball W21.04
    football W21.01
    soccer W21.02
    softball W21.07
    specified NEC W21.09
    volleyball W21.06
  bat or racquet
    baseball bat W21.11
      assault Y08.02
    golf club W21.13
      assault Y08.09
    specified NEC W21.19
      assault Y08.09
    tennis racquet W21.12
      assault Y08.09
  bullet —see also Discharge, firearm by type
    in war operations —see War operations
  crocodile W58.12
  dog W54.1
  flare, Very pistol —see Discharge, firearm
    NEC
  hailstones X39.8
  hockey (ice)
    field
      puck W21.221
      stick W21.211
    puck W21.220
    stick W21.210
      assault Y08.01
  landslide —see Landslide
  law-enforcement agent (on duty) —see Legal,
    intervention, manhandling
    with blunt object —see Legal, intervention,
      blunt object
  lightning —see subcategory T75.0
    causing fire —see Exposure, fire
  machine —see Contact, with, by type of
    machine

Struck by (Continued)
  mammal NEC W55.89
    marine W56.32
  marine animal W56.82
  missile
    firearm —see Discharge, firearm by type
    in war operations —see War operations,
      missile
  object W22.8
    blunt W22.8
      assault Y00
      suicide (attempt) X79
      undetermined whether accidental or
        intentional Y29
    falling W20.8
      from, in, on
        building W20.1
          burning (uncontrolled fire) X00.4
        cataclysmic
          earth surface movement NEC —see
            Landslide
          storm —see Forces of nature,
            cataclysmic storm
        cave-in W20.0
        earthquake X34
        machine (in operation) —see Contact,
          with, by type of machine
        structure W20.1
          burning X00.4
        transport vehicle (in motion) —see
          Accident, transport, by type of
          vehicle
        watercraft V93.49
          due to
            accident to craft V91.39
              powered craft V91.33
                ferry boat V91.31
                fishing boat V91.32
                jetskis V91.33
                liner V91.31
                merchant ship V91.30
                passenger ship V91.31
              unpowered craft V91.38
                canoe V91.35
                inflatable V91.36
                kayak V91.35
                sailboat V91.34
                surf-board V91.38
                windsurfer V91.38
            powered craft V93.43
              ferry boat V93.41
              fishing boat V93.42
              jetskis V93.43
              liner V93.41
              merchant ship V93.40
              passenger ship V93.41
            unpowered craft V93.48
              sailboat V93.44
              surf-board V93.48
              windsurfer V93.48
    moving NEC W20.8
    projected W20.8
      assault Y00
      in sports W21.9
        assault Y08.09
        ball W21.00
          baseball W21.03
          basketball W21.05
          football W21.01
          golf ball W21.04
          soccer W21.02
          softball W21.07
          specified NEC W21.09
          volleyball W21.06
        bat or racquet
          baseball bat W21.11
            assault Y08.02
          golf club W21.13
            assault Y08.09-
          specified NEC W21.19
            assault Y08.09

Struck by (Continued)
  object (Continued)
    projected (Continued)
      in sports (Continued)
        bat or racquet (Continued)
          tennis racquet W21.12
            assault Y08.09
        hockey (ice)
          field
            puck W21.221
            stick W21.211
          puck W21.220
          stick W21.210
            assault Y08.01
        specified NEC W21.89
      set in motion by explosion —see
        Explosion
    thrown W20.8
      assault Y00
      in sports W21.9
        assault Y08.09
        ball W21.00
          baseball W21.03
          basketball W21.05
          football W21.01
          golf ball W21.04
          soccer W21.02
          soft ball W21.07
          specified NEC W21.09
          volleyball W21.06
        bat or racquet
          baseball bat W21.11
            assault Y08.02
          golf club W21.13
            assault Y08.09
          specified NEC W21.19
            assault Y08.09
          tennis racquet W21.12
            assault Y08.09
        hockey (ice)
          field
            puck W21.221
            stick W21.211
          puck W21.220
          stick W21.210
            assault Y08.01
        specified NEC W21.89
  other person (s) W50.0
    with
      blunt object W22.8
        intentional, homicide (attempt) Y00
        sports equipment W21.9
        undetermined whether accidental or
          intentional Y29
      fall W03
        due to ice or snow W00.0
      as, or caused by, a crowd or human
        stampede (with fall) W52
    assault Y04.2
    homicide (attempt) Y04.2
    in legal intervention
      injuring
        bystander Y35.812
        law enforcement personnel Y35.811
        suspect Y35.813
    sports equipment W21.9
  police (on duty) —see Legal, intervention,
    manhandling
    with blunt object —see Legal, intervention,
      blunt object
  sports equipment W21.9
    assault Y08.09
    ball W21.00
      baseball W21.03
      basketball W21.05
      football W21.01
      golf ball W21.04
      soccer W21.02
      soft ball W21.07
      specified NEC W21.09
      volleyball W21.06

Struck by (Continued)
  sports equipment (Continued)
    bat or racquet
      baseball bat W21.11
        assault Y08.02
      golf club W21.13
        assault Y08.09
      specified NEC W21.19
      tennis racquet W21.12
        assault Y08.09
    cleats (shoe) W21.31
    foot wear NEC W21.39
    football helmet W21.81
    hockey (ice)
      field
        puck W21.221
        stick W21.211
      puck W21.220
      stick W21.210
        assault Y08.01
    skate blades W21.32
    specified NEC W21.89
      assault Y08.09
  thunderbolt —see subcategory
    T75.0
  causing fire —see Exposure, fire
  transport vehicle NEC (see also Accident,
    transport) V09.9
  intentional, homicide (attempt) Y03.0
  motor NEC (see also Accident, transport)
    V09.20
  homicide Y03.0
  vehicle (transport) NEC —see Accident,
    transport, by type of vehicle
  stationary (falling from jack,
    hydraulic lift, ramp)
    W20.8
Stumbling
  without fall W18.40
    due to
      specified NEC W18.49
      stepping from one level to another
        W18.43
      stepping into hole or opening
        W18.42
      stepping on object W18.41
  over
    animal NEC W01.0
      with fall W18.09
    carpet, rug or (small) object
      W22.8
      with fall W18.09
    person W51
      with fall W03
        due to ice or snow W00.0
Submersion (accidental) —see Drowning

Suffocation (accidental) (by external means) (by
  pressure) (mechanical) —see also category
  T71
  due to, by
    avalanche —see Landslide
    explosion —see Explosion
    fire —see Exposure, fire
    food, any type (aspiration) (ingestion)
      (inhalation) —see categories T17 and
      T18
    ignition —see Ignition
    landslide —see Landslide
    machine (ry) —see Contact, with, by type
      of machine
    vomitus (aspiration) (inhalation)
      T17.81-
  in
    burning building X00.8
Suicide, suicidal (attempted) (by) X83.8
  blunt object X79
  burning, burns X76
    hot object X77.9
      fluid NEC X77.2
      household appliance X77.3
      specified NEC X77.8
      steam X77.0
      tap water X77.1
      vapors X77.0
  caustic substance —see Table of Drugs and
    Chemicals
  cold, extreme X83.2
  collision of motor vehicle with
    motor vehicle X82.0
    specified NEC X82.8
    train X82.1
    tree X82.2
  crashing of aircraft X83.0
  cut (any part of body) X78.9
  cutting or piercing instrument X78.9
    dagger X78.2
    glass X78.0
    knife X78.1
    specified NEC X78.8
    sword X78.2
  drowning (in) X71.9
    bathtub X71.0
    natural water X71.3
    specified NEC X71.8
    swimming pool X71.1
      following fall X71.2
  electrocution X83.1
  explosive (s) (material) X75
  fire, flames X76
  firearm X74.9
    airgun X74.01
    handgun X72

Suicide, suicidal (Continued)
  firearm (Continued)
    hunting rifle X73.1
    larger X73.9
      specified NEC X73.8
    machine gun X73.2
    shotgun X73.0
    specified NEC X74.8
  hanging X83.8
  hot object —see Suicide, burning, hot object
  jumping
    before moving object X81.8
      motor vehicle X81.0
      subway train X81.1
      train X81.1
    from high place X80
  late effect of attempt —see X71-X83 with 7th
    character S
  lying before moving object, train, vehicle X81.8
  poisoning —see Table of Drugs and
    Chemicals
  puncture (any part of body) —see Suicide,
    cutting or piercing instrument
  scald —see Suicide, burning, hot object
  sequelae of attempt —see X71-X83 with 7th
    character S
  sharp object (any) —see Suicide, cutting or
    piercing instrument
  shooting —see Suicide, firearm
  specified means NEC X83.8
  stab (any part of body) —see Suicide, cutting
    or piercing instrument
  steam, hot vapors X77.0
  strangulation X83.8
  submersion —see Suicide, drowning
  suffocation X83.8
  wound NEC X83.8
Sunstroke X32
Supersonic waves (causing injury) W42.0
Surgical procedure, complication of (delayed
  or as an abnormal reaction without
  mention of misadventure) —see also
  Complication of or following, by type of
  procedure
  due to or as a result of misadventure —see
    Misadventure
Swallowed, swallowing
  foreign body —see Foreign body, alimentary
    canal
  poison —see Table of Drugs and Chemicals
  substance
    caustic or corrosive —see Table of Drugs
      and Chemicals
    poisonous —see Table of Drugs and
      Chemicals

T

Tackle in sport W03
Terrorism (involving) Y38.80
  biological weapons Y38.6X-
  chemical weapons Y38.7X-
  conflagration Y38.3X-
  drowning and submersion Y38.89-
  explosion Y38.2X-
    destruction of aircraft Y38.1X-
    marine weapons Y38.0X-
  fire Y38.3X-
  firearms Y38.4X-
  hot substances Y38.5X-
  lasers Y38.89-
  nuclear weapons Y38.5X-
  piercing or stabbing instruments
    Y38.89-
  secondary effects Y38.9X-
  specified method NEC Y38.89-
  suicide bomber Y38.81-
Thirst X58
Threat to breathing
  aspiration —see Aspiration
  due to cave-in, falling earth or substance
    NEC —see category T71
Thrown (accidentally)
  against part (any) of or object in transport
    vehicle (in motion) NEC (see also
    Accident, transport)

Thrown (Continued)
  from
    high place, homicide (attempt) Y01
    machinery —see Contact, with, by type of
      machine
    transport vehicle NEC (see also Accident,
      transport) V89.9
  off —see Thrown, from
Thunderbolt —see subcategory T75.0
  causing fire —see Exposure, fire
Tidal wave (any injury) **NEC** —see Forces of
    nature, tidal wave
Took
  overdose (drug) —see Table of Drugs and
    Chemicals
  poison —see Table of Drugs and
    Chemicals
Tornado (any injury) X37.1
Torrential rain (any injury) X37.8
Torture X58
Trampled by animal NEC W55.89
Trapped (accidentally)
  between objects (moving) (stationary and
    moving) —see Caught
  by part (any) of
    motorcycle V29.88
    pedal cycle V19.88
    transport vehicle NEC (see also Accident,
      transport) V89.9
Travel (effects) (sickness) T75.3

Tree falling on or hitting (accidentally)
    (person) W20.8
Tripping
  without fall W18.40
    due to
      specified NEC W18.49
      stepping from one level to another
        W18.43
      stepping into hole or opening
        W18.42
      stepping on object W18.41
    over
      animal W01.0
        with fall W01.0
      carpet, rug or (small) object W22.8
        with fall W18.09
      person W51
        with fall W03
          due to ice or snow W00.0
Twisted by person (s) (accidentally) W50.2
  with intent to injure or kill Y04.0
  as, or caused by, a crowd or human stampede
    (with fall) W52
  assault Y04.0
  homicide (attempt) Y04.0
  in
    fight Y04.0
    legal intervention —see Legal, intervention,
      manhandling
Twisting, excessive —see category Y93

U

Underdosing of necessary drugs, medicaments
  or biological substances Y63.6
Undetermined intent (contact) (exposure)
  automobile collision Y32
  blunt object Y29
  drowning (submersion) (in) Y21.9
    bathtub Y21.0
      after fall Y21.1
    natural water (lake) (ocean) (pond) (river)
      (stream) Y21.4
    specified place NEC Y21.8
    swimming pool Y21.2
      after fall Y21.3
  explosive material Y25
  fall, jump or push from high place Y30
  falling, lying or running before moving object
    Y31
  fire Y26

Undetermined intent (Continued)
  firearm discharge Y24.9
    airgun (BB) (pellet) Y24.0
    handgun (pistol) (revolver) Y22
    hunting rifle Y23.1
    larger Y23.9
      hunting rifle Y23.1
      machine gun Y23.3
      military Y23.2
      shotgun Y23.0
      specified type NEC Y23.8
    machine gun Y23.3
    military Y23.2
    shotgun Y23.0
    specified type NEC Y24.8
    Very pistol Y24.8
  hot object Y27.9
    fluid NEC Y27.2
    household appliance Y27.3
    specified object NEC Y27.8

Undetermined intent (Continued)
  hot object (Continued)
    steam Y27.0
    tap water Y27.1
    vapor Y27.0
  jump, fall or push from high place Y30
  lying, falling or running before moving object
    Y31
  motor vehicle crash Y32
  push, fall or jump from high place Y30
  running, falling or lying before moving object
    Y31
  sharp object Y28.9
    dagger Y28.2
    glass Y28.0
    knife Y28.1
    specified object NEC Y28.8
    sword Y28.2
  smoke Y26
  specified event NEC Y33

V

Vibration (causing injury) W49.9
Victim (of)
  avalanche —see Landslide
  earth movements NEC —see Forces of nature,
    earth movement
  earthquake X34

Victim (Continued)
  flood —see Flood
  landslide —see Landslide
  lightning —see subcategory T75.0
    causing fire —see Exposure, fire
  storm (cataclysmic) NEC —see Forces of
    nature, cataclysmic storm
  volcanic eruption X35

Volcanic eruption (any injury) X35
Vomitus, gastric contents in air passages
    (with asphyxia, obstruction or
    suffocation) T17.81-

W

Walked into stationary object (any) W22.09
  furniture W22.03
  lamppost W22.02
  wall W22.01
War operations (injuries to military personnel
  and civilians during war, civil insurrection
  and peacekeeping missions) (by) (from)
  (involving) Y36.90-
  after cessation of hostilities Y36.89-
    explosion (of)
      bomb placed during war operations
        Y36.82-
      mine placed during war operations
        Y36.81-
    specified NEC Y36.88-
  air blast Y36.20-
  aircraft
    destruction —*see* War operations,
      destruction of aircraft
    airway restriction —*see* War operations,
      restriction of airways
  asphyxiation —*see* War operations, restriction
    of airways
  biological weapons Y36.6X-
  blast Y36.20-
  blast fragments Y36.20-
  blast wave Y36.20-
  blast wind Y36.20-
  bomb Y36.20-
    dirty Y36.50-
    gasoline Y36.31-
    incendiary Y36.31-
    petrol Y36.31-
  bullet Y36.43-
    incendiary Y36.32-
    rubber Y36.41-
  chemical weapons Y36.7X-
  combat
    hand to hand (unarmed) combat Y36.44-
    using blunt or piercing object Y36.45-
  conflagration —*see* War operations, fire
  conventional warfare NEC Y36.49-
  depth-charge Y36.01-
  destruction of aircraft Y36.10-
    due to
      air to air missile Y36.11-
      collision with other aircraft Y36.12-
      detonation (accidental) of onboard
        munitions and explosives Y36.14-
      enemy fire or explosives Y36.11-
      explosive placed on aircraft Y36.11-
      onboard fire Y36.13-
      rocket propelled grenade [RPG] Y36.11-
      small arms fire Y36.11-
      surface to air missile Y36.11-
    specified NEC Y36.19-
  detonation (accidental) of
    onboard marine weapons Y36.05-
    own munitions or munitions launch device
      Y36.24-

War operations (*Continued*)
  dirty bomb Y36.50-
  explosion (of) Y36.20-
    aerial bomb Y36.21-
    after cessation of hostilities
      bomb placed during war operations
        Y36.82-
      mine placed during war operations
        Y36.81-
    bomb NOS (*see also* War operations,
      bomb (s)) Y36.20-
    fragments Y36.20-
    grenade Y36.29-
    guided missile Y36.22-
    improvised explosive device [IED]
      (person-borne) (roadside)
      (vehicle-borne) Y36.23-
    land mine Y36.29-
    marine mine (at sea) (in harbor)
      Y36.02-
    marine weapon Y36.00-
      specified NEC Y36.09-
    own munitions or munitions launch
      device (accidental) Y36.24-
    sea-based artillery shell Y36.03-
    specified NEC Y36.29-
    torpedo Y36.04-
  fire Y36.30-
    specified NEC Y36.39-
  firearms
    discharge Y36.43-
    pellets Y36.42-
  flamethrower Y36.33-
  fragments (from) (of)
    improvised explosive device [IED]
      (person-borne) (roadside)
      (vehicle-borne) Y36.26-
    munitions Y36.25-
    specified NEC Y36.29-
    weapons Y36.27-
  friendly fire Y36.92
  hand to hand (unarmed) combat
    Y36.44-
  hot substances —*see* War operations,
    fire
  incendiary bullet Y36.32-
  nuclear weapon (effects of) Y36.50-
    acute radiation exposure Y36.54-
    blast pressure Y36.51-
    direct blast Y36.51-
    direct heat Y36.53-
    fallout exposure Y36.54-
    fireball Y36.53-
    indirect blast (struck or crushed by blast
      debris) (being thrown by blast)
      Y36.52-
    ionizing radiation (immediate exposure)
      Y36.54-
    nuclear radiation Y36.54-
    radiation
      ionizing (immediate exposure)
        Y36.54-

War operations (*Continued*)
  nuclear weapon (*Continued*)
    radiation (*Continued*)
      nuclear Y36.54-
      thermal Y36.53-
    secondary effects Y36.54-
    specified NEC Y36.59-
    thermal radiation Y36.53-
  restriction of air (airway)
    intentional Y36.46-
    unintentional Y36.47-
  rubber bullets Y36.41-
  shrapnel NOS Y36.29-
  suffocation —*see* War operations, restriction
    of airways
  unconventional warfare NEC Y36.7X-
  underwater blast NOS Y36.00-
  warfare
    conventional NEC Y36.49-
    unconventional NEC Y36.7X-
  weapon of mass destruction [WMD] Y36.91
  weapons
    biological weapons Y36.6X-
    chemical Y36.7X-
    nuclear (effects of) Y36.50-
      acute radiation exposure Y36.54-
      blast pressure Y36.51-
      direct blast Y36.51-
      direct heat Y36.53-
      fallout exposure Y36.54-
      fireball Y36.53-
      indirect blast (struck or crushed by blast
        debris) (being thrown by blast)
        Y36.52-
      radiation
        ionizing (immediate exposure) Y36.54-
        nuclear Y36.54-
        thermal Y36.53-
      secondary effects Y36.54-
      specified NEC Y36.59-
    of mass destruction [WMD] Y36.91-
Washed
  away by flood —*see* Flood
  off road by storm (transport vehicle) —*see*
    Forces of nature, cataclysmic storm
Weather exposure NEC —*see* Forces of nature
Weightlessness (causing injury) (effects of) (in
  spacecraft, real or simulated) X52
Work related condition Y99.0
Wound (accidental) **NEC** (*see also* Injury) X58
  battle (*see also* War operations) Y36.90
  gunshot —*see* Discharge, firearm by type
Wreck transport vehicle NEC (*see also* Accident,
  transport) V89.9
Wrong
  device implanted into correct surgical site
    Y65.51
  fluid in infusion Y65.1
  patient, procedure performed on Y65.52
  procedure (operation) on correct patient
    Y65.51

◀ New   ◀▥ Revised   ~~deleted~~ Deleted

PART III

ICD-10-CM Tabular List of Diseases and Injuries

CHAPTER 1

CERTAIN INFECTIOUS AND PARASITIC DISEASES (A00-B99)

Includes diseases generally recognized as communicable or transmissible

Use additional code to identify resistance to antimicrobial drugs (Z16.-)

Excludes1 certain localized infections - see body system-related chapters

Excludes2 carrier or suspected carrier of infectious disease (Z22.-)

infectious and parasitic diseases complicating pregnancy, childbirth and the puerperium (O98.-)

infectious and parasitic diseases specific to the perinatal period (P35-P39)

influenza and other acute respiratory infections (J00-J22)

This chapter contains the following blocks:

A00-A09	Intestinal infectious diseases
A15-A19	Tuberculosis
A20-A28	Certain zoonotic bacterial diseases
A30-A49	Other bacterial diseases
A50-A64	Infections with a predominantly sexual mode of transmission
A65-A69	Other spirochetal diseases
A70-A74	Other diseases caused by chlamydiae
A75-A79	Rickettsioses
A80-A89	Viral and prion infections of the central nervous system
A90-A99	Arthropod-borne viral fevers and viral hemorrhagic fevers
B00-B09	Viral infections characterized by skin and mucous membrane lesions
B10	Other human herpesviruses
B15-B19	Viral hepatitis
B20	Human immunodeficiency virus [HIV] disease
B25-B34	Other viral diseases
B35-B49	Mycoses
B50-B64	Protozoal diseases
B65-B83	Helminthiases
B85-B89	Pediculosis, acariasis and other infestations
B90-B94	Sequelae of infectious and parasitic diseases
B95-B97	Bacterial and viral infectious agents
B99	Other infectious diseases

INTESTINAL INFECTIOUS DISEASES (A00-A09)

● **A00 Cholera**
A serious, often deadly, infectious disease of the small intestine

     A00.0 Cholera due to Vibrio cholerae 01, biovar cholerae
        Classical cholera

     A00.1 Cholera due to Vibrio cholerae 01, biovar eltor
        Cholera eltor

     A00.9 Cholera, unspecified

● **A01 Typhoid and paratyphoid fevers**
Caused by Salmonella typhi and Salmonella paratyphi A, B, and C bacteria

    ● **A01.0 Typhoid fever**
        Infection due to Salmonella typhi

        A01.00 Typhoid fever, unspecified

        A01.01 Typhoid meningitis

        A01.02 Typhoid fever with heart involvement
           Typhoid endocarditis
           Typhoid myocarditis

        A01.03 Typhoid pneumonia

        A01.04 Typhoid arthritis

        A01.05 Typhoid osteomyelitis

        A01.09 Typhoid fever with other complications

     A01.1 Paratyphoid fever A

     A01.2 Paratyphoid fever B

Item 1–1 Salmonella is a bacterium that lives in the intestines of fowl and mammals and can spread to humans through improper food preparation and cooking. Salmonellosis is an infection with the bacterium. Symptoms include diarrhea, fever, and abdominal cramps 12 to 72 hours after infection. The illness usually lasts 4 to 7 days, and most persons recover without treatment. The diarrhea may be so severe that the patient needs to be hospitalized. Patients with immunocompromised systems in chronic, ill health are more likely to have the infection invade their bloodstream with life-threatening results. For example, patients with sickle cell disease are more prone to salmonella osteomyelitis than others.

     A01.3 Paratyphoid fever C

     A01.4 Paratyphoid fever, unspecified
        Infection due to Salmonella paratyphi NOS

● **A02 Other salmonella infections**

     Includes infection or foodborne intoxication due to any Salmonella species other than S. typhi and S. paratyphi

     A02.0 Salmonella enteritis
        Salmonellosis

     A02.1 Salmonella sepsis

    ● **A02.2 Localized salmonella infections**

        A02.20 Localized salmonella infection, unspecified
           Specified in the documentation as localized, but unspecified as to type

        A02.21 Salmonella meningitis
           Specified as localized in the meninges

        A02.22 Salmonella pneumonia
           Specified as localized in the lungs

        A02.23 Salmonella arthritis
           Specified as localized in the joints

        A02.24 Salmonella osteomyelitis
           Specified as localized in bone

        A02.25 Salmonella pyelonephritis
           Salmonella tubulo-interstitial nephropathy

        A02.29 Salmonella with other localized infection
           Specified as localized (because it is still under localized heading) but does not assign into any of the above codes

     A02.8 Other specified salmonella infections
        Any specified salmonella infection which does NOT assign into any of the above codes (not specified as localized)

     A02.9 Salmonella infection, unspecified
        Unspecified in the documentation as to specific type of salmonella

● **A03 Shigellosis**
An infectious disease caused by bacteria (Shigella)

     A03.0 Shigellosis due to Shigella dysenteriae
        Group A shigellosis [Shiga-Kruse dysentery]

     A03.1 Shigellosis due to Shigella flexneri
        Group B shigellosis

     A03.2 Shigellosis due to Shigella boydii
        Group C shigellosis

     A03.3 Shigellosis due to Shigella sonnei
        Group D shigellosis

     A03.8 Other shigellosis

     A03.9 Shigellosis, unspecified
        Bacillary dysentery NOS

● **A04 Other bacterial intestinal infections**

     Excludes1 bacterial foodborne intoxications, NEC (A05.-)
        tuberculous enteritis (A18.32)

     A04.0 Enteropathogenic Escherichia coli infection
        Pertaining to or producing intestinal disease

     A04.1 Enterotoxigenic Escherichia coli infection
        Producing or containing intestinal toxin

     A04.2 Enteroinvasive Escherichia coli infection
        Capable of penetrating and spreading through intestinal mucosal epithelium

     A04.3 Enterohemorrhagic Escherichia coli infection
        Causing bloody diarrhea, resulting from microorganisms

---

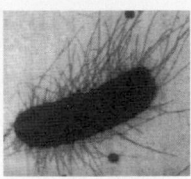

Figure 1-1 Electron micrograph of escherichia coli (E. coli) expressing P fimbriae. (From Mandell, Bennett, & Dolin: Principles and Practice of Infectious Diseases, ed 7, Churchill Livingstone, An Imprint of Elsevier, 2009)

Item 1–2 *Escherichia coli [E. coli]* is a gram-negative bacterium found in the intestinal tracts of humans and animals and is usually nonpathogenic. Pathogenic strains can cause diarrhea or pyogenic (pus-producing) infections. Can be a threat to food safety.

A04.4 Other intestinal Escherichia coli infections
Escherichia coli enteritis NOS

A04.5 Campylobacter enteritis
Spiral shaped bacterium

A04.6 Enteritis due to Yersinia enterocolitica
> **Excludes1** extraintestinal yersiniosis (A28.2)

Transmitted by infected food /water and person-to-person contact, affecting intestinal tract

A04.7 Enterocolitis due to Clostridium difficile
Foodborne intoxication by Clostridium difficile
Pseudomembraneous colitis
Marked by fibrinous deposit (false membrane) with enmeshed necrotic cells

A04.8 Other specified bacterial intestinal infections

A04.9 Bacterial intestinal infection, unspecified
Bacterial enteritis NOS

● **A05 Other bacterial foodborne intoxications, not elsewhere classified**
> **Excludes1** Clostridium difficile foodborne intoxication and infection (A04.7)
> Escherichia coli infection (A04.0-A04.4)
> listeriosis (A32.-)
> salmonella foodborne intoxication and infection (A02.-)
> toxic effect of noxious foodstuffs (T61-T62)

A05.0 Foodborne staphylococcal intoxication

A05.1 Botulism food poisoning
Botulism NOS
Classical foodborne intoxication due to Clostridium botulinum
> **Excludes1** infant botulism (A48.51)
> wound botulism (A48.52)

A05.2 Foodborne Clostridium perfringens [Clostridium welchii] intoxication
Type A causes gas gangrene and necrotizing colitis; major cause of food poisoning in humans
Enteritis necroticans
Pig-bel

A05.3 Foodborne Vibrio parahaemolyticus intoxication
Organism that survives only in high salt environment (halophilic), major cause of gastroenteritis due to consumption of raw or improperly cooked fish/seafood

A05.4 Foodborne Bacillus cereus intoxication
Spore-forming species commonly found in soil, causes food poisoning from formation of intestinal toxins in contaminated foods

A05.5 Foodborne Vibrio vulnificus intoxication
Species that survives in high salt environment (halophilic) with infection by eating raw seafood causes septicemia and cellulitis

A05.8 Other specified bacterial foodborne intoxications

A05.9 Bacterial foodborne intoxication, unspecified

● **A06 Amebiasis**
An intestinal illness caused by the microscopic parasite Entamoeba histolytica
> **Includes**   infection due to Entamoeba histolytica
> **Excludes1** other protozoal intestinal diseases (A07.-)
> **Excludes2** acanthamebiasis (B60.1-)
> Naegleriasis (B60.2)

A06.0 Acute amebic dysentery
Acute amebiasis
Intestinal amebiasis NOS

A06.1 Chronic intestinal amebiasis

A06.2 Amebic nondysenteric colitis
Pertaining to single cell microorganism

A06.3 Ameboma of intestine
Tumorlike mass produced by localized inflammation often in intestine
Ameboma NOS

A06.4 Amebic liver abscess
Hepatic amebiasis

A06.5 Amebic lung abscess
Amebic abscess of lung (and liver)

A06.6 Amebic brain abscess
Amebic abscess of brain (and liver) (and lung)

A06.7 Cutaneous amebiasis

● **A06.8 Amebic infection of other sites**

    A06.81 Amebic cystitis

    A06.82 Other amebic genitourinary infections
    Amebic balanitis
    Amebic vesiculitis
    Amebic vulvovaginitis

    A06.89 Other amebic infections
    Amebic appendicitis
    Amebic splenic abscess

A06.9 Amebiasis, unspecified

● **A07 Other protozoal intestinal diseases**

A07.0 Balantidiasis
Balantidial dysentery
Infection by protozoa that may cause diarrhea and dysentery, with ulceration of colonic mucous membranes

A07.1 Giardiasis [lambliasis]
Common infection in small intestine spread by contaminated food, water, or direct person-to-person contact

A07.2 Cryptosporidiosis
Human infection with protozoa usually seen as self-limited diarrhea in those who work with cattle

A07.3 Isosporiasis
Human intestinal disease caused by protozoa
Infection due to Isospora belli and Isospora hominis
Intestinal coccidiosis
Isosporosis

A07.4 Cyclosporiasis
Infection by protozoa with most common species infecting humans being C cayetanensis

A07.8 Other specified protozoal intestinal diseases
Intestinal microsporidiosis
Intestinal trichomoniasis
Sarcocystosis
Sarcosporidiosis

A07.9 Protozoal intestinal disease, unspecified
Flagellate diarrhea
Protozoal colitis
Protozoal diarrhea
Protozoal dysentery

CHAPTER 1 (A00-B99)

CHAPTER 1 (A00-B99)

● **A08**   **Viral and other specified intestinal infections**

> **Excludes1**   influenza with involvement of gastrointestinal tract (J09.X3, J10.2, J11.2)

    A08.0   **Rotaviral enteritis**

● **A08.1**   **Acute gastroenteropathy due to Norwalk agent and other small round viruses**

        A08.11   **Acute gastroenteropathy due to Norwalk agent**
            Acute gastroenteropathy due to Norovirus
            Acute gastroenteropathy due to Norwalk-like agent

        A08.19   **Acute gastroenteropathy due to other small round viruses**
            Acute gastroenteropathy due to small round virus [SRV] NOS

    A08.2   **Adenoviral enteritis**

● **A08.3**   **Other viral enteritis**

        A08.31   **Calicivirus enteritis**

        A08.32   **Astrovirus enteritis**

        A08.39   **Other viral enteritis**
            Coxsackie virus enteritis
            Echovirus enteritis
            Enterovirus enteritis NEC
            Torovirus enteritis

    A08.4   **Viral intestinal infection, unspecified**
        Viral enteritis NOS
        Viral gastroenteritis NOS
        Viral gastroenteropathy NOS

    A08.8   **Other specified intestinal infections**

A09   **Infectious gastroenteritis and colitis, unspecified**
    Infectious colitis NOS
    Infectious enteritis NOS
    Infectious gastroenteritis NOS

> **Excludes1**   colitis NOS (K52.9)
>   diarrhea NOS (R19.7)
>   enteritis NOS (K52.9)
>   gastroenteritis NOS (K52.9)
>   noninfective gastroenteritis and colitis, unspecified (K52.9)

TUBERCULOSIS (A15-A19)

> **Includes**   infections due to Mycobacterium tuberculosis and Mycobacterium bovis

> **Excludes1**   congenital tuberculosis (P37.0)
>   nonspecific reaction to test for tuberculosis without active tuberculosis (R76.1-)
>   pneumoconiosis associated with tuberculosis, any type in A15 (J65)
>   positive PPD (R76.11)
>   positive tuberculin skin test without active tuberculosis (R76.11)
>   sequelae of tuberculosis (B90.-)
>   silicotuberculosis (J65)

● **A15**   **Respiratory tuberculosis**

    A15.0   **Tuberculosis of lung**
        Tuberculous bronchiectasis
        Chronic dilatation of bronchi
        Tuberculous fibrosis of lung
        Tuberculous pneumonia
        Tuberculous pneumothorax

    A15.4   **Tuberculosis of intrathoracic lymph nodes**
        Tuberculosis of hilar lymph nodes
        Tuberculosis of mediastinal lymph nodes
        Tuberculosis of tracheobronchial lymph nodes

> **Excludes1**   tuberculosis specified as primary (A15.7)

    A15.5   **Tuberculosis of larynx, trachea and bronchus**
        Tuberculosis of bronchus
        Tuberculosis of glottis
        Tuberculosis of larynx
        Tuberculosis of trachea

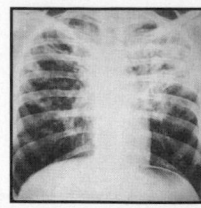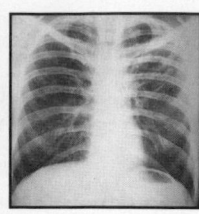

Figure 1-2   Far advanced bilateral pulmonary tuberculosis before and after 8 months of treatment with streptomycin, PAS, and isoniazid. (From Hinshaw HC, Garland LH: Diseases of the Chest, ed 4, Philadelphia, WB Saunders, 1980)

Item 1–3 **Tuberculosis** is a common and deadly infectious disease caused by the *Mycobacterium tuberculosis* organism. The first tuberculosis infection is called the **primary infection** and most commonly attacks the lungs but can affect the central nervous system, lymphatic system, circulatory system, genitourinary system, bones, joints, and even the skin. A **Ghon** lesion is the **initial lesion.** A **secondary lesion** occurs when the tubercle bacilli are carried to other areas.

Item 1–4 **Although** it primarily affects the lungs, the bacteria ***Mycobacterium tuberculosis*** can travel from the pulmonary circulation to virtually any organ in the body, much as a cancer metastasizes to a secondary site. If the immune system becomes compromised by age or disease, what would otherwise be a self-limiting primary tuberculosis in the lungs will develop in other organs. These are known as extrapulmonary sites.

    A15.6   **Tuberculous pleurisy**
        Tuberculosis of pleura
        Tuberculous empyema

> **Excludes1**   primary respiratory tuberculosis (A15.7)

    A15.7   **Primary respiratory tuberculosis**

    A15.8   **Other respiratory tuberculosis**
        Mediastinal tuberculosis
        Nasopharyngeal tuberculosis
        Tuberculosis of nose
        Tuberculosis of sinus [any nasal]

    A15.9   **Respiratory tuberculosis unspecified**

● **A17**   **Tuberculosis of nervous system**

    A17.0   **Tuberculous meningitis**
        Tuberculosis of meninges (cerebral) (spinal)
        Tuberculous leptomeningitis

> **Excludes1**   tuberculous meningoencephalitis (A17.82)

    A17.1   **Meningeal tuberculoma**
        Tuberculoma of meninges (cerebral) (spinal)

> **Excludes2**   tuberculoma of brain and spinal cord (A17.81)

● **A17.8**   **Other tuberculosis of nervous system**

        A17.81   **Tuberculoma of brain and spinal cord**
            Tuberculous abscess of brain and spinal cord

        A17.82   **Tuberculous meningoencephalitis**
            Inflammation of brain and meninges; AKA cerebromeningitis and encephalomeningitis
            Tuberculous myelitis

        A17.83   **Tuberculous neuritis**
            Tuberculous mononeuropathy

        A17.89   **Other tuberculosis of nervous system**
            Tuberculous polyneuropathy

    A17.9   **Tuberculosis of nervous system, unspecified**

◀ New   ⬅ Revised   ~~deleted~~ Deleted   Excludes 1   Excludes 2   Includes   Use additional   Code first   Code also   Unspecified

OGCR Official Guidelines   **X** Assign placeholder X   ● Use Additional Character(s)   ▶ Manifestation Code   **Coding Clinic**

● **A18 Tuberculosis of other organs**
  ● **A18.0 Tuberculosis of bones and joints**
      A18.01 Tuberculosis of spine
        Pott's disease or curvature of spine
        Tuberculous arthritis
        Tuberculous osteomyelitis of spine
        Tuberculous spondylitis
      A18.02 Tuberculous arthritis of other joints
        Tuberculosis of hip (joint)
        Tuberculosis of knee (joint)
      A18.03 Tuberculosis of other bones
        Tuberculous mastoiditis
        Tuberculous osteomyelitis
      A18.09 Other musculoskeletal tuberculosis
        Tuberculous myositis
        Tuberculous synovitis
        Tuberculous tenosynovitis
  ● **A18.1 Tuberculosis of genitourinary system**
      A18.10 Tuberculosis of genitourinary system, unspecified
      A18.11 Tuberculosis of kidney and ureter
      A18.12 Tuberculosis of bladder
      A18.13 Tuberculosis of other urinary organs
        Tuberculous urethritis
      A18.14 Tuberculosis of prostate ♂   A
      A18.15 Tuberculosis of other male genital organs ♂
      A18.16 Tuberculosis of cervix ♀
      A18.17 Tuberculous female pelvic inflammatory disease ♀
        Tuberculous endometritis
        Tuberculous oophoritis and salpingitis
          Oophoritis = inflammation of ovary
          Salpingitis = inflammation of fallopian tube
      A18.18 Tuberculosis of other female genital organs ♀
        Tuberculous ulceration of vulva
    A18.2 Tuberculous peripheral lymphadenopathy
      Tuberculous adenitis
      Excludes2 tuberculosis of bronchial and mediastinal lymph nodes (A15.4)
        tuberculosis of mesenteric and retroperitoneal lymph nodes (A18.39)
        tuberculous tracheobronchial adenopathy (A15.4)
  ● **A18.3 Tuberculosis of intestines, peritoneum and mesenteric glands**
      A18.31 Tuberculous peritonitis
        Tuberculous ascites
      A18.32 Tuberculous enteritis
        Tuberculosis of anus and rectum
        Tuberculosis of intestine (large) (small)
      A18.39 Retroperitoneal tuberculosis
        Tuberculosis of mesenteric glands
        Tuberculosis of retroperitoneal (lymph glands)
    A18.4 Tuberculosis of skin and subcutaneous tissue
      Erythema induratum, tuberculous
      Lupus excedens
      Lupus vulgaris NOS
      Lupus vulgaris of eyelid
        Cutaneous tuberculosis characterized by reddish brown plaque on skin surrounded by papules and nodules
      Scrofuloderma
        Type of cutaneous tuberculosis, with direct extension of tuberculosis into skin from underlying structures; AKA tuberculosis colliquativa
      Tuberculosis of external ear
      Excludes2 lupus erythematosus (L93.-)
        lupus NOS (M32.9)
        systemic (M32.-)

  ● **A18.5 Tuberculosis of eye**
      Excludes2 lupus vulgaris of eyelid (A18.4)
      A18.50 Tuberculosis of eye, unspecified
      A18.51 Tuberculous episcleritis
        Inflammation of episclera and adjacent tissues
      A18.52 Tuberculous keratitis
        Tuberculous interstitial keratitis
        Tuberculous keratoconjunctivitis (interstitial) (phlyctenular)
        Inflammation of cornea and conjunctiva
      A18.53 Tuberculous chorioretinitis
        Inflammation of choroid and retina; retinochoroiditis
      A18.54 Tuberculous iridocyclitis
        Inflammation of iris and ciliary body
      A18.59 Other tuberculosis of eye
        Tuberculous conjunctivitis
    A18.6 Tuberculosis of (inner) (middle) ear
      Tuberculous otitis media
      Excludes2 tuberculosis of external ear (A18.4)
        tuberculous mastoiditis (A18.03)
    A18.7 Tuberculosis of adrenal glands
      Tuberculous Addison's disease
  ● **A18.8 Tuberculosis of other specified organs**
      A18.81 Tuberculosis of thyroid gland
      A18.82 Tuberculosis of other endocrine glands
        Tuberculosis of pituitary gland
        Tuberculosis of thymus gland
      A18.83 Tuberculosis of digestive tract organs, not elsewhere classified
        Excludes1 tuberculosis of intestine (A18.32)
      A18.84 Tuberculosis of heart
        Tuberculous cardiomyopathy
        Tuberculous endocarditis
        Tuberculous myocarditis
        Tuberculous pericarditis
      A18.85 Tuberculosis of spleen
      A18.89 Tuberculosis of other sites
        Tuberculosis of muscle
        Tuberculous cerebral arteritis

● **A19 Miliary tuberculosis**
    Includes disseminated tuberculosis
      generalized tuberculosis
      tuberculous polyserositis
    A19.0 Acute miliary tuberculosis of a single specified site
    A19.1 Acute miliary tuberculosis of multiple sites
    A19.2 Acute miliary tuberculosis, unspecified
    A19.8 Other miliary tuberculosis
    A19.9 Miliary tuberculosis, unspecified

Item 1–5 Miliary tuberculosis can be a life-threatening condition. If a tuberculous lesion enters a blood vessel, immense dissemination of tuberculous organisms can occur if the immune system is weak. High-risk populations—children under 4 years of age, the elderly, or the immunocompromised—are particularly prone to this type of infection. The lesions will have a millet seedlike appearance on chest x-ray. Bronchial washings and biopsy may aid in diagnosis.

CHAPTER 1 (A00-B99)

CERTAIN ZOONOTIC BACTERIAL DISEASES (A20-A28)

● **A20 Plague**
Infectious disease caused by a Yersinia pestis bacterium, transmitted by a rodent flea bite or handling of infected animal

Includes infection due to Yersinia pestis

A20.0 Bubonic plague

A20.1 Cellulocutaneous plague
Skin and subcutaneous tissue plague

A20.2 Pneumonic plague

A20.3 Plague meningitis

A20.7 Septicemic plague

A20.8 Other forms of plague
Abortive plague
Asymptomatic plague
Pestis minor
Systemic bacterial disease

A20.9 Plague, unspecified

● **A21 Tularemia**
Caused by Francisella tularensis bacterium found in rodents, rabbits, and hares and transmitted to humans by contact with infected animal tissues or by ticks, biting flies, or mosquitoes

Includes deer-fly fever
infection due to Francisella tularensis
rabbit fever

A21.0 Ulceroglandular tularemia
Most common form of tularemia in humans is painful, swollen, erythematous papule at point of inoculation that ruptures to form shallow ulcer

A21.1 Oculoglandular tularemia
Primary site of entry is conjunctival sac, results in granulomatous corneal lesions
Ophthalmic tularemia

A21.2 Pulmonary tularemia

A21.3 Gastrointestinal tularemia
Abdominal tularemia

A21.7 Generalized tularemia

A21.8 Other forms of tularemia

A21.9 Tularemia, unspecified

● **A22 Anthrax**
An acute infectious disease caused by the spore-forming Bacillus anthracis; occurs in humans exposed to infected animals or tissue from infected animals

Includes infection due to Bacillus anthracis

A22.0 Cutaneous anthrax
Malignant carbuncle
Malignant pustule

A22.1 Pulmonary anthrax
Inhalation anthrax
Ragpicker's disease
Woolsorter's disease

A22.2 Gastrointestinal anthrax

A22.7 Anthrax sepsis
Infectious bacterial disease

A22.8 Other forms of anthrax
Anthrax meningitis

A22.9 Anthrax, unspecified

Item 1-6 Brucellosis: An infectious disease caused by the bacterium Brucella. Humans are infected by contact with contaminated animals or animal products. In humans brucellosis symptoms that are similar to the flu include fever, sweats, headaches, back pains, and physical weakness. Severe infections of the central nervous system or lining of the heart may occur. Brucellosis can also cause chronic symptoms that include recurrent fevers, joint pain, and fatigue.

● **A23 Brucellosis**

Includes Malta fever
Mediterranean fever
undulant fever

A23.0 Brucellosis due to Brucella melitensis
Resulting in flu-like symptoms that may lead to chronic symptoms that include recurrent fevers, joint pain, and fatigue

A23.1 Brucellosis due to Brucella abortus
Most common cause of brucellosis in humans; AKA Bang bacillus

A23.2 Brucellosis due to Brucella suis
Species found primarily in pigs, rabbits, and reindeer

A23.3 Brucellosis due to Brucella canis
Species that causes respiratory tract infection in humans

A23.8 Other brucellosis

A23.9 Brucellosis, unspecified

● **A24 Glanders and melioidosis**
Infection, usually of rodents, which spreads to other animals and humans, caused by Burkholderia pseudomallei through break in skin contaminated with infested soil or water

A24.0 Glanders
Infection due to Pseudomonas mallei
Malleus

A24.1 Acute and fulminating melioidosis
Melioidosis pneumonia
Melioidosis sepsis

A24.2 Subacute and chronic melioidosis

A24.3 Other melioidosis

A24.9 Melioidosis, unspecified
Infection due to Pseudomonas pseudomallei NOS
Whitmore's disease

● **A25 Rat-bite fevers**
RBF, infectious disease caused by Streptobacillus moniliformis or Spirillum minus.

A25.0 Spirillosis
Any disease condition caused by spirilla
Sodoku

A25.1 Streptobacillosis
Acute, febrile human illness caused by bacteria transmitted by rats in most cases, passed from rodent to human via rodent's urine or mucous secretions; AKA rat fever
Epidemic arthritic erythema
Haverhill fever
Streptobacillary rat-bite fever

A25.9 Rat-bite fever, unspecified

● **A26 Erysipeloid**
Infection with Erysipelothrix rhusiopathiae, occurring often as occupational disease resulting from handling infected fish, shellfish, meat, or poultry

A26.0 Cutaneous erysipeloid
Erythema migrans

A26.7 Erysipelothrix sepsis

A26.8 Other forms of erysipeloid

A26.9 Erysipeloid, unspecified

◀ New   ⬅ Revised   ~~deleted~~ Deleted   Excludes 1   Excludes 2   Includes   Use additional   Code first   Code also   Unspecified

OGCR Official Guidelines   X Assign placeholder X   ● Use Additional Character(s)   ▶ Manifestation Code   **Coding Clinic**

● **A27**   **Leptospirosis**
          Occurs most commonly in the tropics
     A27.0   **Leptospirosis icterohemorrhagica**
            Leptospiral or spirochetal jaundice (hemorrhagic)
            Weil's disease
   ● **A27.8**   **Other forms of leptospirosis**
         A27.81   **Aseptic meningitis in leptospirosis**
         A27.89   **Other forms of leptospirosis**
     A27.9   **Leptospirosis,** `unspecified`

● **A28**   **Other zoonotic bacterial diseases, not elsewhere classified**
     A28.0   **Pasteurellosis**
            Infection of humans or other animals by species of
               Pasteurella
     A28.1   **Cat-scratch disease**
            Cat-scratch fever
     A28.2   **Extraintestinal yersiniosis**
            Infection from Yersinia enterocolitica; AKA enteric
               yersiniosis, intestinal yersiniosis, Yersinia enteritis
         `Excludes1`   enteritis due to Yersinia enterocolitica
                       (A04.6)
                       plague (A20.-)
     A28.8   **Other specified zoonotic bacterial diseases, not elsewhere classified**
     A28.9   **Zoonotic bacterial disease,** `unspecified`

─────── **OTHER BACTERIAL DISEASES (A30-A49)** ───────

● **A30**   **Leprosy [Hansen's disease]**
          Chronic infectious disease attacking the skin, peripheral nerves, and
            mucous membranes
       `Includes`   infection due to Mycobacterium leprae
       `Excludes1`   sequelae of leprosy (B92)
     A30.0   **Indeterminate leprosy**
            I leprosy
     A30.1   **Tuberculoid leprosy**
            TT leprosy
     A30.2   **Borderline tuberculoid leprosy**
            BT leprosy
     A30.3   **Borderline leprosy**
            BB leprosy
     A30.4   **Borderline lepromatous leprosy**
            BL leprosy
     A30.5   **Lepromatous leprosy**
            LL leprosy
     A30.8   **Other forms of leprosy**
     A30.9   **Leprosy,** `unspecified`

● **A31**   **Infection due to other mycobacteria**
       `Excludes2`   leprosy (A30.-)
                 tuberculosis (A15-A19)
     A31.0   **Pulmonary mycobacterial infection**
            Infection due to Mycobacterium avium
            Infection due to Mycobacterium intracellulare [Battey
               bacillus]
            Infection due to Mycobacterium kansasii
     A31.1   **Cutaneous mycobacterial infection**
            Buruli ulcer
            Infection due to Mycobacterium marinum
            Infection due to Mycobacterium ulcerans
     A31.2   **Disseminated mycobacterium avium-intracellulare complex (DMAC)**
            MAC sepsis
     A31.8   **Other mycobacterial infections**
     A31.9   **Mycobacterial infection,** `unspecified`
            Atypical mycobacterial infection NOS
            Mycobacteriosis NOS

● **A32**   **Listeriosis**
          Infection caused by Listeria monocytogenes
       `Includes`   listerial foodborne infection
       `Excludes1`   neonatal (disseminated) listeriosis (P37.2)
     A32.0   **Cutaneous listeriosis**
   ● **A32.1**   **Listerial meningitis and meningoencephalitis**
         A32.11   **Listerial meningitis**
         A32.12   **Listerial meningoencephalitis**
     A32.7   **Listerial sepsis**
   ● **A32.8**   **Other forms of listeriosis**
         A32.81   **Oculoglandular listeriosis**
               Primary infection site is conjunctival sac, which if
                  untreated may result in perforation of cornea
                  and optic atrophy
         A32.82   **Listerial endocarditis**
               Exudative and proliferative inflammatory condition
                  of endocardium caused by listeria bacteria
         A32.89   **Other forms of listeriosis**
               Listerial cerebral arteritis
     A32.9   **Listeriosis,** `unspecified`

A33   **Tetanus neonatorum**   **N**
          Neonate = newborn

A34   **Obstetrical tetanus** ♀   **M**

A35   **Other tetanus**
          Tetanus NOS
       `Excludes1`   tetanus neonatorum (A33)
                 obstetrical tetanus (A34)

● **A36**   **Diphtheria**
     A36.0   **Pharyngeal diphtheria**
            Diphtheritic membranous angina
            Tonsillar diphtheria
     A36.1   **Nasopharyngeal diphtheria**
     A36.2   **Laryngeal diphtheria**
            Diphtheritic laryngotracheitis
     A36.3   **Cutaneous diphtheria**
         `Excludes2`   erythrasma (L08.1)
   ● **A36.8**   **Other diphtheria**
         A36.81   **Diphtheritic cardiomyopathy**
               Diphtheritic myocarditis
         A36.82   **Diphtheritic radiculomyelitis**
         A36.83   **Diphtheritic polyneuritis**
         A36.84   **Diphtheritic tubulo-interstitial nephropathy**
         A36.85   **Diphtheritic cystitis**
         A36.86   **Diphtheritic conjunctivitis**
         A36.89   **Other diphtheritic complications**
               Diphtheritic peritonitis
     A36.9   **Diphtheria,** `unspecified`

Item 1-7 Diptheria: A highly contagious bacterial disease that results in the formation of an adherent membrane in the throat that may lead to suffocation. In its most poisonous form, it attacks the heart and lungs. It is spread by direct physical contact or breathing the aerosolized secretions of infected individuals. The exact location is specified in the codes.

CHAPTER 1 (A00-B99)

● **A37   Whooping cough**
Pertussis is a highly contagious disease caused by the bacterium Bordetella pertussis and results in a whooping sounding cough.

  ● **A37.0   Whooping cough due to Bordetella pertussis**

     A37.00   Whooping cough due to Bordetella pertussis without pneumonia

     A37.01   Whooping cough due to Bordetella pertussis with pneumonia

  ● **A37.1   Whooping cough due to Bordetella parapertussis**

     A37.10   Whooping cough due to Bordetella parapertussis without pneumonia

     A37.11   Whooping cough due to Bordetella parapertussis with pneumonia

  ● **A37.8   Whooping cough due to other Bordetella species**

     A37.80   Whooping cough due to other Bordetella species without pneumonia

     A37.81   Whooping cough due to other Bordetella species with pneumonia

  ● **A37.9   Whooping cough, unspecified species**

     A37.90   Whooping cough, unspecified species without pneumonia

     A37.91   Whooping cough, unspecified species with pneumonia

● **A38   Scarlet fever**
Most commonly caused by the bacteria Streptococcus pneumoniae and Neisseria meningitides

   Includes   scarlatina

   Excludes2   streptococcal sore throat (J02.0)

   A38.0   Scarlet fever with otitis media

   A38.1   Scarlet fever with myocarditis

   A38.8   Scarlet fever with other complications

   A38.9   Scarlet fever, uncomplicated
     Scarlet fever, NOS

● **A39   Meningococcal infection**
Most commonly caused by the bacteria Streptococcus pneumoniae and Neisseria meningitides

   A39.0   Meningococcal meningitis

   A39.1   Waterhouse-Friderichsen syndrome
     Fulminating complication of meningococcemia
     Meningococcal hemorrhagic adrenalitis
     Meningococcic adrenal syndrome

   A39.2   Acute meningococcemia

   A39.3   Chronic meningococcemia

   A39.4   Meningococcemia, unspecified

  ● **A39.5   Meningococcal heart disease**

     A39.50   Meningococcal carditis, unspecified

     A39.51   Meningococcal endocarditis

     A39.52   Meningococcal myocarditis

     A39.53   Meningococcal pericarditis

  ● **A39.8   Other meningococcal infections**

     A39.81   Meningococcal encephalitis

     A39.82   Meningococcal retrobulbar neuritis
       Optic neuritis in portion of optic nerve posterior to eyeball; AKA postocular optic neuritis

     A39.83   Meningococcal arthritis

     A39.84   Postmeningococcal arthritis

     A39.89   Other meningococcal infections
       Meningococcal conjunctivitis

   A39.9   Meningococcal infection, unspecified
     Meningococcal disease NOS

● **A40   Streptococcal sepsis**
   Code first
     postprocedural streptococcal sepsis (T81.4)
     streptococcal sepsis during labor (O75.3)
     streptococcal sepsis following abortion or ectopic or molar pregnancy (O03-O07, O08.0)
     streptococcal sepsis following immunization (T88.0)
     streptococcal sepsis following infusion, transfusion or therapeutic injection (T80.2-)

   Excludes1   neonatal (P36.0-P36.1)
       puerperal sepsis (O85)
       sepsis due to Streptococcus, group D (A41.81)

   A40.0   Sepsis due to streptococcus, group A

   A40.1   Sepsis due to streptococcus, group B

   A40.3   Sepsis due to Streptococcus pneumoniae
     Pneumococcal sepsis

   A40.8   Other streptococcal sepsis

   A40.9   Streptococcal sepsis, unspecified

● **A41   Other sepsis**
   Code first
     postprocedural sepsis (T81.4)
     sepsis during labor (O75.3)
     sepsis following abortion, ectopic or molar pregnancy (O03-O07, O08.0)
     sepsis following immunization (T88.0)
     sepsis following infusion, transfusion or therapeutic injection (T80.2-)

   Excludes1   bacteremia NOS (R78.81)
       neonatal (P36.-)
       puerperal sepsis (O85)
       sepsis NOS (A41.9)
       streptococcal sepsis (A40.-)

   Excludes2   sepsis (due to) (in) actinomycotic (A42.7)
       sepsis (due to) (in) anthrax (A22.7)
       sepsis (due to) (in) candidal (B37.7)
       sepsis (due to) (in) Erysipelothrix (A26.7)
       sepsis (due to) (in) extraintestinal yersiniosis (A28.2)
       sepsis (due to) (in) gonococcal (A54.86)
       sepsis (due to) (in) herpesviral (B00.7)
       sepsis (due to) (in) listerial (A32.7)
       sepsis (due to) (in) melioidosis (A24.1)
       sepsis (due to) (in) meningococcal (A39.2-A39.4)
       sepsis (due to) (in) plague (A20.7)
       sepsis (due to) (in) tularemia (A21.7)
       toxic shock syndrome (A48.3)

  ● **A41.0   Sepsis due to Staphylococcus aureus**

     A41.01   Sepsis due to Methicillin susceptible Staphylococcus aureus
       MSSA sepsis
       Staphylococcus aureus sepsis NOS

     A41.02   Sepsis due to Methicillin resistant Staphylococcus aureus

   A41.1   Sepsis due to other specified staphylococcus
     Coagulase negative staphylococcus sepsis

   A41.2   Sepsis due to unspecified staphylococcus

   A41.3   Sepsis due to Hemophilus influenzae

   A41.4   Sepsis due to anaerobes

     Excludes1   gas gangrene (A48.0)

  ● **A41.5   Sepsis due to other Gram-negative organisms**

     A41.50   Gram-negative sepsis, unspecified
       Gram-negative sepsis NOS

     A41.51   Sepsis due to Escherichia coli [E. coli]

     A41.52   Sepsis due to Pseudomonas
       Pseudomonas aeroginosa

     A41.53   Sepsis due to Serratia

     A41.59   Other Gram-negative sepsis

◄ New   ◄▬ Revised   ~~deleted~~ Deleted   Excludes 1   Excludes 2   Includes   Use additional   Code first   Code also   Unspecified

OGCR Official Guidelines   **X** Assign placeholder X   ● Use Additional Character(s)   ▶ Manifestation Code   **Coding Clinic**

Item 1–8 Gas gangrene is a necrotizing subcutaneous infection that will cause tissue death. Patients with poor circulation (e.g., diabetes, peripheral nephropathy) will have low oxygen content in their tissues (hypoxia), which allows the Clostridium bacteria to flourish. Gas gangrene often occurs at the site of a surgical wound or trauma. Onset is sudden and dramatic. Treatment can include debridement, amputation, and/or hyperbaric oxygen treatments.

● **A41.8   Other specified sepsis**
    A41.81   Sepsis due to Enterococcus
    A41.89   Other specified sepsis
  A41.9   Sepsis, unspecified organism
    Septicemia NOS

● **A42   Actinomycosis**
    Excludes1   actinomycetoma (B47.1)
  A42.0   Pulmonary actinomycosis
  A42.1   Abdominal actinomycosis
  A42.2   Cervicofacial actinomycosis
  A42.7   Actinomycotic sepsis
● **A42.8   Other forms of actinomycosis**
    A42.81   Actinomycotic meningitis
    A42.82   Actinomycotic encephalitis
    A42.89   Other forms of actinomycosis
  A42.9   Actinomycosis, unspecified

● **A43   Nocardiosis**
  A43.0   Pulmonary nocardiosis
  A43.1   Cutaneous nocardiosis
  A43.8   Other forms of nocardiosis
  A43.9   Nocardiosis, unspecified

● **A44   Bartonellosis**
  A44.0   Systemic bartonellosis
    Oroya fever
  A44.1   Cutaneous and mucocutaneous bartonellosis
    Verruga peruana
  A44.8   Other forms of bartonellosis
  A44.9   Bartonellosis, unspecified

  A46   Erysipelas
    Excludes1   postpartum or puerperal erysipelas (O86.89)

● **A48   Other bacterial diseases, not elsewhere classified**
    Excludes1   actinomycetoma (B47.1)
  A48.0   Gas gangrene
    Clostridial cellulitis
    Clostridial myonecrosis
  A48.1   Legionnaires' disease
  A48.2   Nonpneumonic Legionnaires' disease [Pontiac fever]
  A48.3   Toxic shock syndrome
    Use additional code to identify the organism (B95, B96)
    Excludes1   endotoxic shock NOS (R57.8)
        sepsis NOS (A41.9)
  A48.4   Brazilian purpuric fever
    Systemic Hemophilus aegyptius infection
● **A48.5   Other specified botulism**
    Non-foodborne intoxication due to toxins of Clostridium botulinum [C. botulinum]
    Excludes1   food poisoning due to toxins of Clostridium botulinum (A05.1)
    A48.51   Infant botulism   P
    A48.52   Wound botulism
        Non-foodborne botulism NOS
        Use additional code for associated wound
  A48.8   Other specified bacterial diseases

● **A49   Bacterial infection of unspecified site**
    Excludes1   bacterial agents as the cause of diseases classified elsewhere (B95-B96)
        chlamydial infection NOS (A74.9)
        meningococcal infection NOS (A39.9)
        rickettsial infection NOS (A79.9)
        spirochetal infection NOS (A69.9)
● **A49.0   Staphylococcal infection, unspecified site**
    A49.01   Methicillin susceptible Staphylococcus aureus infection, unspecified site
        Methicillin susceptible Staphylococcus aureus (MSSA) infection
        Staphylococcus aureus infection NOS
    A49.02   Methicillin resistant Staphylococcus aureus infection, unspecified site
        Methicillin resistant Staphylococcus aureus (MRSA) infection
  A49.1   Streptococcal infection, unspecified site
  A49.2   Hemophilus influenzae infection, unspecified site
    Any of seven bacterium of genus Haemophilus
  A49.3   Mycoplasma infection, unspecified site
    Bacterium of class Mollicutes, unusual group of bacteria distinguished by absence of cell wall
  A49.8   Other bacterial infections of unspecified site
  A49.9   Bacterial infection, unspecified
    Excludes1   bacteremia NOS (R78.81)

INFECTIONS WITH A PREDOMINANTLY SEXUAL MODE OF TRANSMISSION (A50-A64)

    Excludes1   human immunodeficiency virus [HIV] disease (B20)
        nonspecific and nongonococcal urethritis (N34.1)
        Reiter's disease (M02.3-)

● **A50   Congenital syphilis**
● **A50.0   Early congenital syphilis, symptomatic**
    Any congenital syphilitic condition specified as early or manifest less than two years after birth
    A50.01   Early congenital syphilitic oculopathy
    A50.02   Early congenital syphilitic osteochondropathy
    A50.03   Early congenital syphilitic pharyngitis
        Early congenital syphilitic laryngitis
    A50.04   Early congenital syphilitic pneumonia
    A50.05   Early congenital syphilitic rhinitis
    A50.06   Early cutaneous congenital syphilis
    A50.07   Early mucocutaneous congenital syphilis
    A50.08   Early visceral congenital syphilis
    A50.09   Other early congenital syphilis, symptomatic
  A50.1   Early congenital syphilis, latent
    Congenital syphilis without clinical manifestations, with positive serological reaction and negative spinal fluid test, less than two years after birth
  A50.2   Early congenital syphilis, unspecified
    Congenital syphilis NOS less than two years after birth
● **A50.3   Late congenital syphilitic oculopathy**
    Excludes1   Hutchinson's triad (A50.53)
    A50.30   Late congenital syphilitic oculopathy, unspecified
    A50.31   Late congenital syphilitic interstitial keratitis
    A50.32   Late congenital syphilitic chorioretinitis
    A50.39   Other late congenital syphilitic oculopathy

CHAPTER 1 (A00-B99)

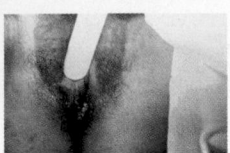

Figure 1-3 Chancre of primary syphilis. (From Mandell, Bennett, & Dolin: Principles and Practice of Infectious Diseases, ed 7, Churchill Livingstone, An Imprint of Elsevier, 2009)

Item 1–9 Syphilis, also known as lues, is the most serious of the venereal diseases caused by *Treponema pallidum.* The **primary** stage is characterized by an ulceration known as **chancre,** which usually appears on the genitals but can also develop on the anus, lips, tonsils, breasts, or fingers. Syphilis is easy to cure in its early stages. A single intramuscular injection of penicillin will usually cure a person who has had syphilis for less than a year.

The **secondary** stage is characterized by a rash that can affect any area of the body. **Latent** syphilis is divided into **early,** which is diagnosed within two years of infection, and **late,** which is diagnosed two years or more after infection. Additional doses of penicillin or another antibiotic are needed to treat someone who has had syphilis for longer than a year. For those allergic to penicillin, there are other antibiotic treatments. **Congenital** syphilis is also labeled **early** or **late** based on the time of diagnosis.

- **A50.4 Late congenital neurosyphilis [juvenile neurosyphilis]**

    Use additional code to identify any associated mental disorder

    Excludes1 Hutchinson's triad (A50.53)

    A50.40 Late congenital neurosyphilis, unspecified
    Juvenile neurosyphilis NOS

    A50.41 Late congenital syphilitic meningitis

    A50.42 Late congenital syphilitic encephalitis

    A50.43 Late congenital syphilitic polyneuropathy

    A50.44 Late congenital syphilitic optic nerve atrophy

    A50.45 Juvenile general paresis
    Dementia paralytica juvenilis
    Juvenile tabetoparetic neurosyphilis

    A50.49 Other late congenital neurosyphilis
    Juvenile tabes dorsalis

- **A50.5 Other late congenital syphilis, symptomatic**
    Any congenital syphilitic condition specified as late or manifest two years or more after birth

    A50.51 Clutton's joints

    A50.52 Hutchinson's teeth

    A50.53 Hutchinson's triad

    A50.54 Late congenital cardiovascular syphilis

    A50.55 Late congenital syphilitic arthropathy

    A50.56 Late congenital syphilitic osteochondropathy

    A50.57 Syphilitic saddle nose

    A50.59 Other late congenital syphilis, symptomatic

    A50.6 Late congenital syphilis, latent
    Congenital syphilis without clinical manifestations, with positive serological reaction and negative spinal fluid test, two years or more after birth.

    A50.7 Late congenital syphilis, unspecified
    Congenital syphilis NOS two years or more after birth.

    A50.9 Congenital syphilis, unspecified

- **A51 Early syphilis**

    A51.0 Primary genital syphilis
    Syphilitic chancre NOS

    A51.1 Primary anal syphilis

    A51.2 Primary syphilis of other sites

- **A51.3 Secondary syphilis of skin and mucous membranes**

    A51.31 Condyloma latum

    A51.32 Syphilitic alopecia

    A51.39 Other secondary syphilis of skin
    Syphilitic leukoderma
    Syphilitic mucous patch

    Excludes1 late syphilitic leukoderma (A52.79)

A51.4 Other secondary syphilis

    A51.41 Secondary syphilitic meningitis

    A51.42 Secondary syphilitic female pelvic disease ♀

    A51.43 Secondary syphilitic oculopathy
    Secondary syphilitic chorioretinitis
    Secondary syphilitic iridocyclitis, iritis
    Secondary syphilitic uveitis

    A51.44 Secondary syphilitic nephritis

    A51.45 Secondary syphilitic hepatitis

    A51.46 Secondary syphilitic osteopathy

    A51.49 Other secondary syphilitic conditions
    Secondary syphilitic lymphadenopathy
    Secondary syphilitic myositis

    A51.5 Early syphilis, latent
    Syphilis (acquired) without clinical manifestations, with positive serological reaction and negative spinal fluid test, less than two years after infection.

    A51.9 Early syphilis, unspecified

- **A52 Late syphilis**

- **A52.0 Cardiovascular and cerebrovascular syphilis**

    A52.00 Cardiovascular syphilis, unspecified

    A52.01 Syphilitic aneurysm of aorta

    A52.02 Syphilitic aortitis

    A52.03 Syphilitic endocarditis
    Syphilitic aortic valve incompetence or stenosis
    Syphilitic mitral valve stenosis
    Syphilitic pulmonary valve regurgitation

    A52.04 Syphilitic cerebral arteritis

    A52.05 Other cerebrovascular syphilis
    Syphilitic cerebral aneurysm (ruptured) (non-ruptured)
    Syphilitic cerebral thrombosis

    A52.06 Other syphilitic heart involvement
    Syphilitic coronary artery disease
    Syphilitic myocarditis
    Syphilitic pericarditis

    A52.09 Other cardiovascular syphilis

- **A52.1 Symptomatic neurosyphilis**

    A52.10 Symptomatic neurosyphilis, unspecified

    A52.11 Tabes dorsalis
    Cognitive decline with progressive degeneration of posterior columns, roots, and ganglia of spinal cord, occur 15-20 years after initial infection of syphilis; AKA Duchenne disease
    Locomotor ataxia (progressive)
    Tabetic neurosyphilis

    A52.12 Other cerebrospinal syphilis

    A52.13 Late syphilitic meningitis

    A52.14 Late syphilitic encephalitis

    A52.15 Late syphilitic neuropathy
    Late syphilitic acoustic neuritis
    Late syphilitic optic (nerve) atrophy
    Late syphilitic polyneuropathy
    Late syphilitic retrobulbar neuritis

    A52.16 Charcôt's arthropathy (tabetic)
    Progressive musculoskeletal condition characterized by joint dislocation, fractures, and deformities, results in progressive destruction of bone and soft tissue of weight-bearing joints

    A52.17 General paresis
    Chronic meningoencephalitis results in loss of cortical function, or progressive dementia and generalized paralysis, occurring 10-20 years after initial infection of syphilis; AKA Bayle disease, dementia paralytica, paralytic dementiaparetic neurosyphilis, syphilitic meningoencephalitis
    Dementia paralytica

    A52.19 Other symptomatic neurosyphilis
    Syphilitic parkinsonism

A52.2   **Asymptomatic neurosyphilis**

A52.3   **Neurosyphilis, unspecified**
Gumma (syphilitic)
Destructive lesions of syphilis
Syphilis (late)
Syphiloma

● **A52.7**   **Other symptomatic late syphilis**

     A52.71   **Late syphilitic oculopathy**
Late syphilitic chorioretinitis
Late syphilitic episcleritis

     A52.72   **Syphilis of lung and bronchus**

     A52.73   **Symptomatic late syphilis of other respiratory organs**

     A52.74   **Syphilis of liver and other viscera**
Late syphilitic peritonitis

     A52.75   **Syphilis of kidney and ureter**
Syphilitic glomerular disease

     A52.76   **Other genitourinary symptomatic late syphilis**
Late syphilitic female pelvic inflammatory disease

     A52.77   **Syphilis of bone and joint**

     A52.78   **Syphilis of other musculoskeletal tissue**
Late syphilitic bursitis
Syphilis [stage unspecified] of bursa
Syphilis [stage unspecified] of muscle
Syphilis [stage unspecified] of synovium
Syphilis [stage unspecified] of tendon

     A52.79   **Other symptomatic late syphilis**
Late syphilitic leukoderma
Syphilis of adrenal gland
Syphilis of pituitary gland
Syphilis of thyroid gland
Syphilitic splenomegaly

         Excludes1   syphilitic leukoderma (secondary) (A51.39)

A52.8   **Late syphilis, latent**
Syphilis (acquired) without clinical manifestations, with positive serological reaction and negative spinal fluid test, two years or more after infection

A52.9   **Late syphilis, unspecified**

● **A53**   **Other and unspecified syphilis**

     A53.0   **Latent syphilis, unspecified as early or late**
Latent syphilis NOS
Positive serological reaction for syphilis

     A53.9   **Syphilis, unspecified**
Infection due to Treponema pallidum NOS
Syphilis (acquired) NOS

         Excludes1   syphilis NOS under two years of age (A50.2)

● **A54**   **Gonococcal infection**

  ● **A54.0**   **Gonococcal infection of lower genitourinary tract without periurethral or accessory gland abscess**

         Excludes1   gonococcal infection with genitourinary gland abscess (A54.1)
gonococcal infection with periurethral abscess (A54.1)

     A54.00   **Gonococcal infection of lower genitourinary tract, unspecified**

     A54.01   **Gonococcal cystitis and urethritis, unspecified**

     A54.02   **Gonococcal vulvovaginitis, unspecified** ♀

     A54.03   **Gonococcal cervicitis, unspecified** ♀

     A54.09   **Other gonococcal infection of lower genitourinary tract**

     A54.1   **Gonococcal infection of lower genitourinary tract with periurethral and accessory gland abscess**
Gonococcal Bartholin's gland abscess

Item 1-10 An STD (sexually transmitted disease) caused by **Neisseria gonorrhoeae** that flourishes in the warm, moist areas of the reproductive tract. Untreated gonorrhea spreads to other parts of the body, causing inflammation of the testes or prostate or pelvic inflammatory disease (PID).

  ● **A54.2**   **Gonococcal pelviperitonitis and other gonococcal genitourinary infection**

     A54.21   **Gonococcal infection of kidney and ureter**

     A54.22   **Gonococcal prostatitis** ♂

     A54.23   **Gonococcal infection of other male genital organs** ♂
Gonococcal epididymitis
Gonococcal orchitis

     A54.24   **Gonococcal female pelvic inflammatory disease** ♀
Gonococcal pelviperitonitis

         Excludes1   gonococcal peritonitis (A54.85)

     A54.29   **Other gonococcal genitourinary infections**

  ● **A54.3**   **Gonococcal infection of eye**

     A54.30   **Gonococcal infection of eye, unspecified**

     A54.31   **Gonococcal conjunctivitis**
Form of bacterial conjunctivitis contracted by newborns during delivery; AKA neonatal conjunctivitis
Ophthalmia neonatorum due to gonococcus

     A54.32   **Gonococcal iridocyclitis**
Inflammation of iris and of ciliary body due to gonococcal infection

     A54.33   **Gonococcal keratitis**
Inflammation of cornea due to gonococcal infection; AKA keratoconjunctivitis, keratopathy

     A54.39   **Other gonococcal eye infection**
Gonococcal endophthalmia

  ● **A54.4**   **Gonococcal infection of musculoskeletal system**

     A54.40   **Gonococcal infection of musculoskeletal system, unspecified**

     A54.41   **Gonococcal spondylopathy**
Disorder of vertebrae due to gonococcal infection; AKA rachiopathy

     A54.42   **Gonococcal arthritis**

         Excludes2   gonococcal infection of spine (A54.41)

     A54.43   **Gonococcal osteomyelitis**

         Excludes2   gonococcal infection of spine (A54.41)

     A54.49   **Gonococcal infection of other musculoskeletal tissue**
Gonococcal bursitis
Gonococcal myositis
Gonococcal synovitis
Gonococcal tenosynovitis

     A54.5   **Gonococcal pharyngitis**

     A54.6   **Gonococcal infection of anus and rectum**

  ● **A54.8**   **Other gonococcal infections**

     A54.81   **Gonococcal meningitis**

     A54.82   **Gonococcal brain abscess**

     A54.83   **Gonococcal heart infection**
Gonococcal endocarditis
Gonococcal myocarditis
Gonococcal pericarditis

     A54.84   **Gonococcal pneumonia**

     A54.85   **Gonococcal peritonitis**

         Excludes1   gonococcal pelviperitonitis (A54.24)

     A54.86   **Gonococcal sepsis**

     A54.89   **Other gonococcal infections**
Gonococcal keratoderma
Gonococcal lymphadenitis

     A54.9   **Gonococcal infection, unspecified**

CHAPTER 1 (A00-B99)

A55   Chlamydial lymphogranuloma (venereum)
    Climatic or tropical bubo
    Durand-Nicolas-Favre disease
    Esthiomene
    Lymphogranuloma inguinale

● **A56   Other sexually transmitted chlamydial diseases**

    Includes   sexually transmitted diseases due to Chlamydia trachomatis

    Excludes1   neonatal chlamydial conjunctivitis (P39.1)
                  neonatal chlamydial pneumonia (P23.1)

    Excludes2   chlamydial lymphogranuloma (A55)
                  conditions classified to A74.-

   ● **A56.0   Chlamydial infection of lower genitourinary tract**

       A56.00   Chlamydial infection of lower genitourinary tract, unspecified

       A56.01   Chlamydial cystitis and urethritis

       A56.02   Chlamydial vulvovaginitis ♀

       A56.09   Other chlamydial infection of lower genitourinary tract
             Chlamydial cervicitis

   ● **A56.1   Chlamydial infection of pelviperitoneum and other genitourinary organs**

       A56.11   Chlamydial female pelvic inflammatory disease ♀

       A56.19   Other chlamydial genitourinary infection
             Chlamydial epididymitis
             Chlamydial orchitis

    A56.2   Chlamydial infection of genitourinary tract, unspecified

    A56.3   Chlamydial infection of anus and rectum

    A56.4   Chlamydial infection of pharynx

    A56.8   Sexually transmitted chlamydial infection of other sites

A57   Chancroid
    Ulcus molle
    Sexually transmitted infection caused by bacteria, Haemophilus ducreyi

A58   Granuloma inguinale
    Chronic, progressive, ulcerative granulomatous disease
    Donovanosis

● **A59   Trichomoniasis**

    Excludes2   intestinal trichomoniasis (A07.8)

    A common STD caused by a parasite, Trichomonas vaginalis

   ● **A59.0   Urogenital trichomoniasis**

       A59.00   Urogenital trichomoniasis, unspecified
             Fluor (vaginalis) due to Trichomonas
             Leukorrhea (vaginalis) due to Trichomonas

       A59.01   Trichomonal vulvovaginitis ♀

       A59.02   Trichomonal prostatitis ♂

       A59.03   Trichomonal cystitis and urethritis

       A59.09   Other urogenital trichomoniasis
             Common sexually transmitted disease (STD) caused by single-celled protozoan parasite; AKA trich
             Trichomonas cervicitis

    A59.8   Trichomoniasis of other sites

    A59.9   Trichomoniasis, unspecified

● **A60   Anogenital herpesviral [herpes simplex] infections**

   ● **A60.0   Herpesviral infection of genitalia and urogenital tract**

       A60.00   Herpesviral infection of urogenital system, unspecified

       A60.01   Herpesviral infection of penis ♂

       A60.02   Herpesviral infection of other male genital organs ♂

       A60.03   Herpesviral cervicitis ♀

       A60.04   Herpesviral vulvovaginitis ♀
             Herpesviral [herpes simplex] ulceration
             Herpesviral [herpes simplex] vaginitis
             Herpesviral [herpes simplex] vulvitis

       A60.09   Herpesviral infection of other urogenital tract

    A60.1   Herpesviral infection of perianal skin and rectum

    A60.9   Anogenital herpesviral infection, unspecified

● **A63   Other predominantly sexually transmitted diseases, not elsewhere classified**

    Excludes2   molluscum contagiosum (B08.1)
                  papilloma of cervix (D26.0)

    A63.0   Anogenital (venereal) warts
       Anogenital warts due to (human) papillomavirus [HPV]
       Condyloma acuminatum

    A63.8   Other specified predominantly sexually transmitted diseases

A64   Unspecified sexually transmitted disease

OTHER SPIROCHETAL DISEASES (A65-A69)

    Excludes2   leptospirosis (A27.-)
                  syphilis (A50-A53)

A65   Nonvenereal syphilis
    Bejel
    Endemic syphilis
    Njovera

● **A66   Yaws**
    Endemic, infectious, tropical disease caused by spirochete, spread by direct contact; AKA frambesia, framboesia, frambesia tropica

    Includes   bouba
                frambesia (tropica)
                pian

    A66.0   Initial lesions of yaws
       Chancre of yaws
       Frambesia, initial or primary
       Initial frambesial ulcer
       Mother yaw

    A66.1   Multiple papillomata and wet crab yaws
       Frambesioma
       Pianoma
       Plantar or palmar papilloma of yaws

    A66.2   Other early skin lesions of yaws
       Cutaneous yaws, less than five years after infection
       Early yaws (cutaneous)(macular)(maculopapular) (micropapular)(papular)
       Frambeside of early yaws

    A66.3   Hyperkeratosis of yaws
       Hypertrophy of stratum corneum of skin in which there are small, hard, verrucous scales
       Ghoul hand
       Hyperkeratosis, palmar or plantar (early) (late) due to yaws
       Worm-eaten soles

◀ New   ◀▥ Revised   ~~deleted~~ Deleted   Excludes 1   Excludes 2   Includes   Use additional   Code first   Code also   Unspecified

750   **OGCR** Official Guidelines   **X** Assign placeholder X   ● Use Additional Character(s)   ▶ Manifestation Code   **Coding Clinic**

A66.4 Gummata and ulcers of yaws
Small, rubbery granuloma with necrotic center and inflamed characteristic of advanced stage of syphilis; AKA syphiloma
Gummatous frambeside
Nodular late yaws (ulcerated)

A66.5 Gangosa
Manifestation of yaws that develops in the soft palate and spreads eroding bone, cartilage, and soft tissue
Rhinopharyngitis mutilans

A66.6 Bone and joint lesions of yaws
Yaws ganglion
Yaws goundou
Yaws gumma, bone
Yaws gummatous osteitis or periostitis
Yaws hydrarthrosis
Yaws osteitis
Yaws periostitis (hypertrophic)

A66.7 Other manifestations of yaws
Juxta-articular nodules of yaws
Mucosal yaws

A66.8 Latent yaws
Yaws without clinical manifestations, with positive serology

A66.9 Yaws, unspecified

● **A67 Pinta [carate]**
Group of nonvenereal diseases caused by Treponema species

A67.0 Primary lesions of pinta
Chancre (primary) of pinta
Papule (primary) of pinta

A67.1 Intermediate lesions of pinta
Erythematous plaques of pinta
Hyperchromic lesions of pinta
Hyperkeratosis of pinta
Pintids

A67.2 Late lesions of pinta
Achromic skin lesions of pinta
Cicatricial skin lesions of pinta
Dyschromic skin lesions of pinta

A67.3 Mixed lesions of pinta
Achromic with hyperchromic skin lesions of pinta [carate]

A67.9 Pinta, unspecified

● **A68 Relapsing fevers**
Includes recurrent fever
Excludes2 Lyme disease (A69.2-)

A68.0 Louse-borne relapsing fever
Relapsing fever due to Borrelia recurrentis

A68.1 Tick-borne relapsing fever
Relapsing fever due to any Borrelia species other than Borrelia recurrentis

A68.9 Relapsing fever, unspecified

● **A69 Other spirochetal infections**

A69.0 Necrotizing ulcerative stomatitis
Cancrum oris
Fusospirochetal gangrene
Noma
Stomatitis gangrenosa

A69.1 Other Vincent's infections
Fusospirochetal pharyngitis
Necrotizing ulcerative (acute) gingivitis
Necrotizing ulcerative (acute) gingivostomatitis
Spirochetal stomatitis
Trench mouth
Vincent's angina
Vincent's gingivitis

Item 1-11 Cancrum oris, also known as **noma** or **gangrenous stomatitis,** begins as an ulcer of the gingiva and results in a progressive gangrenous process.

● **A69.2 Lyme disease**
Erythema chronicum migrans due to Borrelia burgdorferi

A69.20 Lyme disease, unspecified

A69.21 Meningitis due to Lyme disease

A69.22 Other neurologic disorders in Lyme disease
Cranial neuritis
Meningoencephalitis
Polyneuropathy

A69.23 Arthritis due to Lyme disease

A69.29 Other conditions associated with Lyme disease
Myopericarditis due to Lyme disease

A69.8 Other specified spirochetal infections

A69.9 Spirochetal infection, unspecified

OTHER DISEASES CAUSED BY CHLAMYDIAE (A70-A74)

Excludes1 sexually transmitted chlamydial diseases (A55-A56)

A70 Chlamydia psittaci infections
Ornithosis
Parrot fever
Psittacosis

● **A71 Trachoma**
Excludes1 sequelae of trachoma (B94.0)

A71.0 Initial stage of trachoma
Trachoma dubium

A71.1 Active stage of trachoma
Granular conjunctivitis (trachomatous)
Trachomatous follicular conjunctivitis
Trachomatous pannus

A71.9 Trachoma, unspecified

● **A74 Other diseases caused by chlamydiae**
Excludes1 neonatal chlamydial conjunctivitis (P39.1)
neonatal chlamydial pneumonia (P23.1)
Reiter's disease (M02.3-)
sexually transmitted chlamydial diseases (A55-A56)

Excludes2 chlamydial pneumonia (J16.0)

A74.0 Chlamydial conjunctivitis
Paratrachoma

● **A74.8 Other chlamydial diseases**

A74.81 Chlamydial peritonitis

A74.89 Other chlamydial diseases

A74.9 Chlamydial infection, unspecified
Chlamydiosis NOS

RICKETTSIOSES (A75-A79)

● **A75 Typhus fever**
Excludes1 rickettsiosis due to Ehrlichia sennetsu (A79.81)

A75.0 Epidemic louse-borne typhus fever due to Rickettsia prowazekii
Organisms transmitted between humans via louse
Classical typhus (fever)
Epidemic (louse-borne) typhus

A75.1 Recrudescent typhus [Brill's disease]
Brill-Zinsser disease

A75.2 Typhus fever due to Rickettsia typhi
Murine (flea-borne) typhus

A75.3 Typhus fever due to Rickettsia tsutsugamushi
Scrub (mite-borne) typhus
Tsutsugamushi fever

A75.9 Typhus fever, unspecified
Typhus (fever) NOS

Item 1–12 Rickettsioses are diseases spread from ticks, lice, fleas, or mites to humans.

Typhus is spread to humans chiefly by the fleas of rats.

Endemic identifies a disease as being present in low numbers of humans at all times, whereas **epidemic** identifies a disease as being present in high numbers of humans at a specific time. Morbidity (death) is higher in epidemic diseases.

Brill's disease, also known as **Brill-Zinsser disease,** is spread from human to human by body lice and also from the lice of flying squirrels. **Scrub typhus** is spread in the same ways as Brill's disease.

Malaria is spread to humans by mosquitoes.

● **A77   Spotted fever [tick-borne rickettsioses]**
   A77.0   Spotted fever due to Rickettsia rickettsii
         Rocky Mountain spotted fever
         Sao Paulo fever

   A77.1   Spotted fever due to Rickettsia conorii
         African tick typhus
         Boutonneuse fever
         India tick typhus
         Kenya tick typhus
         Marseilles fever
         Mediterranean tick fever

   A77.2   Spotted fever due to Rickettsia siberica
         North Asian tick fever
         Siberian tick typhus

   A77.3   Spotted fever due to Rickettsia australis
         Queensland tick typhus

● **A77.4   Ehrlichiosis**
         Type of tick-borne fever caused by bacteria infection
         `Excludes1`   Rickettsiosis due to Ehrlichia sennetsu
                       (A79.81)

         A77.40   Ehrlichiosis, `unspecified`
         A77.41   Ehrlichiosis chafeensis [E. chafeensis]
         A77.49   Other ehrlichiosis

   A77.8   Other spotted fevers
   A77.9   Spotted fever, `unspecified`
         Tick-borne typhus NOS

  A78   Q fever
         Infection due to Coxiella burnetii
         Nine Mile fever
         Quadrilateral fever

● **A79   Other rickettsioses**
   A79.0   Trench fever
         Quintan fever
         Wolhynian fever

   A79.1   Rickettsialpox due to Rickettsia akari
         Kew Garden fever
         Vesicular rickettsiosis

● **A79.8   Other specified rickettsioses**
         A79.81   Rickettsiosis due to Ehrlichia sennetsu
         A79.89   Other specified rickettsioses

   A79.9   Rickettsiosis, `unspecified`
         Rickettsial infection NOS

VIRAL AND PRION INFECTIONS OF THE CENTRAL NERVOUS SYSTEM (A80-A89)

         `Excludes1`   postpolio syndrome (G14)
                       sequelae of poliomyelitis (B91)
                       sequelae of viral encephalitis (B94.1)

● **A80   Acute poliomyelitis**
   A80.0   Acute paralytic poliomyelitis, vaccine-associated
   A80.1   Acute paralytic poliomyelitis, wild virus, imported
   A80.2   Acute paralytic poliomyelitis, wild virus, indigenous
● **A80.3   Acute paralytic poliomyelitis, other and unspecified**
         A80.30   Acute paralytic poliomyelitis, `unspecified`
         A80.39   Other acute paralytic poliomyelitis
   A80.4   Acute nonparalytic poliomyelitis
   A80.9   Acute poliomyelitis, `unspecified`

Item 1–13 Acute Poliomyelitis: Also called infantile paralysis and is caused by the poliovirus, which enters the body orally and infects the intestinal wall and then enters the blood stream and central nervous system, causing muscle weakness and paralysis. This disease has been nearly eradicated with the polio vaccine.

● **A81   Atypical virus infections of central nervous system**
         `Includes`   diseases of the central nervous system caused by
                      prions
         Use additional code to identify:
            dementia with behavioral disturbance (F02.81)
            dementia without behavioral disturbance (F02.80)
● **A81.0   Creutzfeldt-Jakob disease**
         A81.00   Creutzfeldt-Jakob disease, `unspecified`
                     Jakob-Creutzfeldt disease, unspecified
         A81.01   Variant Creutzfeldt-Jakob disease
                     vCJD
         A81.09   Other Creutzfeldt-Jakob disease
                     CJD
                     Familial Creutzfeldt-Jakob disease
                     Iatrogenic Creutzfeldt-Jakob disease
                     Sporadic Creutzfeldt-Jakob disease
                     Subacute spongiform encephalopathy (with
                       dementia)

   A81.1   Subacute sclerosing panencephalitis
         *Type of viral encephalitis that causes parenchymatous lesions
            in gray and white matter of brain*
         Dawson's inclusion body encephalitis
         Van Bogaert's sclerosing leukoencephalopathy

   A81.2   Progressive multifocal leukoencephalopathy
         Group of diseases affecting white matter of brain
         Multifocal leukoencephalopathy NOS

● **A81.8   Other atypical virus infections of central nervous system**
         A81.81   Kuru
         A81.82   Gerstmann-Sträussler-Scheinker syndrome
                     GSS syndrome
         A81.83   Fatal familial insomnia
                     FFI
         **A81.89   Other atypical virus infections of central
                     nervous system**

   **A81.9   Atypical virus infection of central nervous system,
              `unspecified`**
         Prion diseases of the central nervous system NOS

● **A82   Rabies**
         *Viral disease affecting the central nervous system and transmitted
            from infected mammals to man.*
   A82.0   Sylvatic rabies
   A82.1   Urban rabies
   A82.9   Rabies, `unspecified`

● **A83   Mosquito-borne viral encephalitis**
         *Inflammation of the brain caused most commonly by Herpes Simplex
            virus.*
         `Includes`   mosquito-borne viral meningoencephalitis
         `Excludes2`   Venezuelan equine encephalitis (A92.2)
                       West Nile fever (A92.3-)
                       West Nile virus (A92.3-)

   A83.0   Japanese encephalitis
   A83.1   Western equine encephalitis
   A83.2   Eastern equine encephalitis
   A83.3   St. Louis encephalitis
   A83.4   Australian encephalitis
         Kunjin virus disease
   A83.5   California encephalitis
         California meningoencephalitis
         La Crosse encephalitis

◀ New   ◀▬ Revised   ~~deleted~~ Deleted   `Excludes 1`   `Excludes 2`   `Includes`   `Use additional`   `Code first`   `Code also`   `Unspecified`

OGCR Official Guidelines   **X** Assign placeholder X   ● Use Additional Character(s)   ▶ Manifestation Code   **Coding Clinic**

Item 1-14 **Encephalitis** is an inflammation of the brain most often caused by a virus but may also be caused by a bacteria and most commonly transmitted by a mosquito. **Myelitis** is an inflammation of the spinal cord that may disrupt CNS function. Untreated myelitis may rapidly lead to permanent damage to the spinal cord. **Encephalomyelitis** is a general term for an inflammation of the brain and spinal cord.

A83.6   **Rocio virus disease**
    Mosquito-borne virus

A83.8   **Other mosquito-borne viral encephalitis**

A83.9   **Mosquito-borne viral encephalitis, unspecified**

● **A84**   **Tick-borne viral encephalitis**
> **Includes**   tick-borne viral meningoencephalitis

A84.0   **Far Eastern tick-borne encephalitis [Russian spring-summer encephalitis]**

A84.1   **Central European tick-borne encephalitis**

A84.8   **Other tick-borne viral encephalitis**
    Louping ill
    Powassan virus disease

A84.9   **Tick-borne viral encephalitis, unspecified**

● **A85**   **Other viral encephalitis, not elsewhere classified**
> **Includes**   specified viral encephalomyelitis NEC
>   specified viral meningoencephalitis NEC
>
> **Excludes1**   benign myalgic encephalomyelitis (G93.3)
>   encephalitis due to cytomegalovirus (B25.8)
>   encephalitis due to herpesvirus NEC (B10.0-)
>   encephalitis due to herpesvirus [herpes simplex] (B00.4)
>   encephalitis due to measles virus (B05.0)
>   encephalitis due to mumps virus (B26.2)
>   encephalitis due to poliomyelitis virus (A80.-)
>   encephalitis due to zoster (B02.0)
>   lymphocytic choriomeningitis (A87.2)

A85.0   **Enteroviral encephalitis**
    Enteroviral encephalomyelitis

A85.1   **Adenoviral encephalitis**
    Adenoviral meningoencephalitis

A85.2   **Arthropod-borne viral encephalitis, unspecified**
> **Excludes1**   West nile virus with encephalitis (A92.31)

A85.8   **Other specified viral encephalitis**
    Encephalitis lethargica
    Von Economo-Cruchet disease

A86   **Unspecified viral encephalitis**
    Viral encephalomyelitis NOS
    Viral meningoencephalitis NOS

● **A87**   **Viral meningitis**
> **Excludes1**   meningitis due to herpesvirus [herpes simplex] (B00.3)
>   meningitis due to measles virus (B05.1)
>   meningitis due to mumps virus (B26.1)
>   meningitis due to poliomyelitis virus (A80.-)
>   meningitis due to zoster (B02.1)

A87.0   **Enteroviral meningitis**
    Group of common viruses responsible for the majority of viral meningitis
    Coxsackievirus meningitis
    Echovirus meningitis

A87.1   **Adenoviral meningitis**

A87.2   **Lymphocytic choriomeningitis**
    Lymphocytic meningoencephalitis

A87.8   **Other viral meningitis**

A87.9   **Viral meningitis, unspecified**

● **A88**   **Other viral infections of central nervous system, not elsewhere classified**
> **Excludes1**   viral encephalitis NOS (A86)
>   viral meningitis NOS (A87.9)

A88.0   **Enteroviral exanthematous fever [Boston exanthem]**
    Infectious skin eruption

A88.1   **Epidemic vertigo**

A88.8   **Other specified viral infections of central nervous system**

● **A89**   **Unspecified viral infection of central nervous system**

ARTHROPOD-BORNE VIRAL FEVERS AND VIRAL HEMORRHAGIC FEVERS (A90-A99)

A90   **Dengue fever [classical dengue]**
    Acute, self-limited disease, characterized by fever, prostration, severe muscle pains, headache, rash, lymphadenopathy, and leukopenia, caused by dengue virus; AKA breakbone, dandy
> **Excludes1**   dengue hemorrhagic fever (A91)

A91   **Dengue hemorrhagic fever**
    Serious follow-up to regular dengue, with symptoms of hemorrhage

● **A92**   **Other mosquito-borne viral fevers**
> **Excludes1**   Ross River disease (B33.1)

A92.0   **Chikungunya virus disease**
    Transmitted by mosquitoes
    Chikungunya (hemorrhagic) fever

A92.1   **O'nyong-nyong fever**
    Acute, nonfatal febrile disease transmitted by mosquitoes, which clinically resembles dengue and chikungunya

A92.2   **Venezuelan equine fever**
    Venezuelan equine encephalitis
    Venezuelan equine encephalomyelitis virus disease

● **A92.3**   **West Nile virus infection**
    West Nile fever

    A92.30   **West Nile virus infection, unspecified**
       West Nile fever NOS
       West Nile fever without complications
       West Nile virus NOS

    A92.31   **West Nile virus infection with encephalitis**
       West Nile encephalitis
       West Nile encephalomyelitis

    A92.32   **West Nile virus infection with other neurologic manifestation**
       Use additional code to specify the neurologic manifestation

    A92.39   **West Nile virus infection with other complications**
       Use additional code to specify the other conditions

A92.4   **Rift Valley fever**

A92.8   **Other specified mosquito-borne viral fevers**

A92.9   **Mosquito-borne viral fever, unspecified**

● **A93**   **Other arthropod-borne viral fevers, not elsewhere classified**

A93.0   **Oropouche virus disease**
    Tropical viral infection
    Oropouche fever

A93.1   **Sandfly fever**
    Pappataci fever
    Phlebotomus fever

A93.2   **Colorado tick fever**

A93.8   **Other specified arthropod-borne viral fevers**
    Piry virus disease
    Vesicular stomatitis virus disease [Indiana fever]

A94   **Unspecified arthropod-borne viral fever**
    Arboviral fever NOS
    Arbovirus infection NOS

● **A95   Yellow fever**
Acute infectious disease transmitted by mosquitoes

    A95.0   Sylvatic yellow fever
          Jungle yellow fever

    A95.1   Urban yellow fever

    A95.9   Yellow fever, unspecified

● **A96   Arenaviral hemorrhagic fever**
Virus that causes various hemorrhagic fevers

    A96.0   Junin hemorrhagic fever
          Argentinian hemorrhagic fever

    A96.1   Machupo hemorrhagic fever
          Transmitted by contact with infected rodents
          Bolivian hemorrhagic fever

    A96.2   Lassa fever
          Acute type of hemorrhagic fever caused by contact with
            disease carrying mouse or person

    A96.8   Other arenaviral hemorrhagic fevers

    A96.9   Arenaviral hemorrhagic fever, unspecified

● **A98   Other viral hemorrhagic fevers, not elsewhere classified**
    Excludes1   chikungunya hemorrhagic fever (A92.0)
                dengue hemorrhagic fever (A91)

    A98.0   Crimean-Congo hemorrhagic fever
          Virus transmitted by ticks and contact with blood, secretions,
            or fluids from infected humans or animals
          Central Asian hemorrhagic fever

    A98.1   Omsk hemorrhagic fever
          Transmitted to humans by bites of infected ticks or contact
            with infected muskrats

    A98.2   Kyasanur Forest disease
          Transmitted via infected monkeys, voles, ticks

    A98.3   Marburg virus disease
          Rare, acute, often fatal type of hemorrhagic fever

    A98.4   Ebola virus disease

    A98.5   Hemorrhagic fever with renal syndrome
          Epidemic hemorrhagic fever
          Korean hemorrhagic fever
          Russian hemorrhagic fever
          Hantaan virus disease
          Hantavirus disease with renal manifestations
          Nephropathia epidemica
          Songo fever
          Excludes1   hantavirus (cardio)-pulmonary syndrome
                   (B33.4)

    A98.8   Other specified viral hemorrhagic fevers

A99   Unspecified viral hemorrhagic fever

◀ New   ◀▥ Revised   ~~deleted~~ Deleted   Excludes 1   Excludes 2   Includes   Use additional   Code first   Code also   Unspecified
OGCR Official Guidelines   **X** Assign placeholder X   ● Use Additional Character(s)   ▌ Manifestation Code   **Coding Clinic**
754

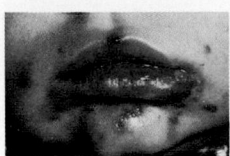

Figure 1-4 Primary herpes simplex in and around the mouth. The infection is usually acquired from siblings or parents and is readily transmitted to other direct contacts. (From Forbes, Jackson: Colour Atlas and Text of Clinical Medicine, International Edition, Mosby, 2002)

Item 1–15   Herpes is a viral disease for which there is no cure. There are two types of the herpes simplex virus: **Type I** causes **cold sores** or **fever blisters,** and **Type II** causes **genital herpes.** The virus can be spread from a sore on the lips to the genitals or from the genitals to the lips.

VIRAL INFECTIONS CHARACTERIZED BY SKIN AND MUCOUS MEMBRANE LESIONS (B00-B09)

● **B00   Herpesviral [herpes simplex] infections**
    Excludes1   congenital herpesviral infections (P35.2)
    Excludes2   anogenital herpesviral infection (A60.-)
                 gammaherpesviral mononucleosis (B27.0-)
                 herpangina (B08.5)

  B00.0   Eczema herpeticum
      Cutaneous eruption caused by herpes simplex virus (HSV) type 1, HSV-2, coxsackievirus A16, or vaccinia virus
      Kaposi's varicelliform eruption

  B00.1   Herpesviral vesicular dermatitis
      Vesicle formation; characteristics include formation of blisters and scabs on feet and legs
      Herpes simplex facialis
      Herpes simplex labialis
      Herpes simplex otitis externa
      Vesicular dermatitis of ear
      Vesicular dermatitis of lip

  B00.2   Herpesviral gingivostomatitis and pharyngotonsillitis
      Inflammation involving both gingivae and oral mucosa
      Herpesviral pharyngitis
        Inflammation of pharynx and tonsils; AKA tonsillopharyngitis

  B00.3   Herpesviral meningitis

  B00.4   Herpesviral encephalitis
      Herpesviral meningoencephalitis
      Simian B disease
      Excludes1   herpesviral encephalitis due to herpesvirus 6 and 7 (B10.01, B10.09)
                  non-simplex herpesviral encephalitis (B10.0-)

● **B00.5   Herpesviral ocular disease**
    B00.50   Herpesviral ocular disease, unspecified
    B00.51   Herpesviral iridocyclitis
        Herpesviral iritis
        Herpesviral uveitis, anterior
    B00.52   Herpesviral keratitis
        Herpesviral keratoconjunctivitis
    B00.53   Herpesviral conjunctivitis
    B00.59   Other herpesviral disease of eye
        Herpesviral dermatitis of eyelid

  B00.7   Disseminated herpesviral disease
      Herpesviral sepsis

● **B00.8   Other forms of herpesviral infections**
    B00.81   Herpesviral hepatitis
    B00.82   Herpes simplex myelitis
    B00.89   Other herpesviral infection
        Herpesviral whitlow

  B00.9   Herpesviral infection, unspecified
      Herpes simplex infection NOS

Item 1-16 Zoster: Also known as **shingles** and is caused by the same virus as chickenpox. After exposure, the virus lies dormant in nerve tissue and is activated by factors including aging, stress, suppression of the immune system, and certain medication. It begins as a unilateral rash that leads to blisters and sores on the skin. It may involve the nerve pathways of the eye, forehead, nose, and eyelids and may be very painful with long term systemic effects.

● **B01   Varicella [chickenpox]**
      Very contagious disease caused by the varicella zoster virus that results in an itchy outbreak of skin blisters (varicella). The same virus causes shingles (zoster).

  B01.0   Varicella meningitis

● **B01.1   Varicella encephalitis, myelitis and encephalomyelitis**
      Postchickenpox encephalitis, myelitis and encephalomyelitis
    B01.11 Varicella encephalitis and encephalomyelitis
        Postchickenpox encephalitis and encephalomyelitis
    B01.12 Varicella myelitis
        Postchickenpox myelitis

  B01.2   Varicella pneumonia

● **B01.8   Varicella with other complications**
    B01.81   Varicella keratitis
    B01.89   Other varicella complications

  B01.9   Varicella without complication
      Varicella NOS

● **B02   Zoster [herpes zoster]**
    Includes   shingles
            zona

  B02.0   Zoster encephalitis
      Zoster meningoencephalitis

  B02.1   Zoster meningitis

● **B02.2   Zoster with other nervous system involvement**
    B02.21   Postherpetic geniculate ganglionitis
    B02.22   Postherpetic trigeminal neuralgia
    B02.23   Postherpetic polyneuropathy
    B02.24   Postherpetic myelitis
        Herpes zoster myelitis
    B02.29   Other postherpetic nervous system involvement
        Postherpetic radiculopathy

● **B02.3   Zoster ocular disease**
    B02.30   Zoster ocular disease, unspecified
    B02.31   Zoster conjunctivitis
    B02.32   Zoster iridocyclitis
    B02.33   Zoster keratitis
        Herpes zoster keratoconjunctivitis
    B02.34   Zoster scleritis
    B02.39   Other herpes zoster eye disease
        Zoster blepharitis

  B02.7   Disseminated zoster

  B02.8   Zoster with other complications
      Herpes zoster otitis externa

  B02.9   Zoster without complications
      Zoster NOS

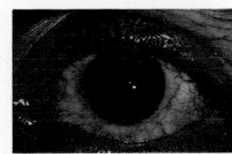

Figure 1-5 Photograph of eyelids with marginal blepharitis. (From Mandell, Bennett, & Dolin: Principles and Practice of Infectious Diseases, ed 7, Churchill Livingstone, An Imprint of Elsevier, 2009)

Item 1–17 Blepharitis is a common condition in which the eyelid is swollen and yellow scaling and conjunctivitis develop. Usually the hair on the scalp and brow is involved.

CHAPTER 1 (A00-B99)

B03   Smallpox
Note: In 1980 the 33rd World Health Assembly declared that smallpox had been eradicated. The classification is maintained for surveillance purposes.

B04   Monkeypox
Disease occurring in captive monkeys and other mammals that may be transmitted to humans, clinically similar to smallpox

● **B05   Measles**
Includes   morbilli
Excludes1   subacute sclerosing panencephalitis (A81.1)

B05.0   Measles complicated by encephalitis
Postmeasles encephalitis

B05.1   Measles complicated by meningitis
Postmeasles meningitis

B05.2   Measles complicated by pneumonia
Postmeasles pneumonia

B05.3   Measles complicated by otitis media
Postmeasles otitis media

B05.4   Measles with intestinal complications

● B05.8   Measles with other complications
B05.81   Measles keratitis and keratoconjunctivitis
B05.89   Other measles complications

B05.9   Measles without complication
Measles NOS

● **B06   Rubella [German measles]**
Excludes1   congenital rubella (P35.0)

● B06.0   Rubella with neurological complications
B06.00   Rubella with neurological complication, unspecified
B06.01   Rubella encephalitis
Rubella meningoencephalitis
B06.02   Rubella meningitis
B06.09   Other neurological complications of rubella

● B06.8   Rubella with other complications
B06.81   Rubella pneumonia
B06.82   Rubella arthritis
B06.89   Other rubella complications

B06.9   Rubella without complication
Rubella NOS

● **B07   Viral warts**
Includes   verruca simplex
verruca vulgaris
viral warts due to human papillomavirus

Excludes2   anogenital (venereal) warts (A63.0)
papilloma of bladder (D41.4)
papilloma of cervix (D26.0)
papilloma larynx (D14.1)

B07.0   Plantar wart
Verruca plantaris

B07.8   Other viral warts
Common wart
Flat wart
Verruca plana

B07.9   Viral wart, unspecified

● **B08   Other viral infections characterized by skin and mucous membrane lesions, not elsewhere classified**
Excludes1   vesicular stomatitis virus disease (A93.8)

● B08.0   Other orthopoxvirus infections
Excludes2   monkeypox (B04)

● B08.01   Cowpox and vaccinia not from vaccine
B08.010   Cowpox
B08.011   Vaccinia not from vaccine
Excludes1   vaccinia (from vaccination) (generalized) (T88.1)

B08.02   Orf virus disease
Contagious pustular dermatitis
Ecthyma contagiosum

B08.03   Pseudocowpox [milker's node]

B08.04   Paravaccinia, unspecified

B08.09   Other orthopoxvirus infections
Orthopoxvirus infection NOS

B08.1   Molluscum contagiosum
Various skin diseases characterized by soft, rounded, cutaneous lesions

● B08.2   Exanthema subitum [sixth disease] Roseola infantum
Acute, short-lived high fever in infants and young children followed by a rash mainly on the trunk, caused by human herpesvirus 6

B08.20   Exanthema subitum [sixth disease], unspecified Roseola infantum, unspecified   P

B08.21   Exanthema subitum [sixth disease] due to human herpesvirus 6 Roseola infantum due to human herpesvirus 6   P
Virus results in sudden rash; infection results in lifelong persistence

B08.22   Exanthema subitum [sixth disease] due to human herpesvirus 7 Roseola infantum due to human herpesvirus 7   P

B08.3   Erythema infectiosum [fifth disease]
Moderately contagious, epidemic disease in children caused by B19 virus; onset of rash that begins as redness of cheeks, later there is rash on trunk and limbs; when this fades, there may be central clearing that leaves lacelike pattern

B08.4   Enteroviral vesicular stomatitis with exanthem
Hand, foot and mouth disease
Check your documentation—this code is HAND, foot, and mouth disease. Code B08.8 is foot and mouth disease.

B08.5   Enteroviral vesicular pharyngitis
Herpangina

● B08.6   Parapoxvirus infections
B08.60   Parapoxvirus infection, unspecified
B08.61   Bovine stomatitis
B08.62   Sealpox
B08.69   Other parapoxvirus infections

● B08.7   Yatapoxvirus infections
B08.70   Yatapoxvirus infection, unspecified
B08.71   Tanapox virus disease
B08.72   Yaba pox virus disease
Yaba monkey tumor disease
B08.79   Other yatapoxvirus infections

B08.8   Other specified viral infections characterized by skin and mucous membrane lesions
Enteroviral lymphonodular pharyngitis
Foot-and-mouth disease
Check your documentation. Code B08.4 is for HAND, foot, and mouth disease.
Poxvirus NEC

B09   Unspecified viral infection characterized by skin and mucous membrane lesions
Viral enanthema NOS
Viral exanthema NOS

◀ New   ◀▥ Revised   d̶e̶l̶e̶t̶e̶d̶ Deleted   Excludes 1   Excludes 2   Includes   Use additional   Code first   Code also   Unspecified
OGCR Official Guidelines   X Assign placeholder X   ● Use Additional Character(s)   ▶ Manifestation Code   **Coding Clinic**

OTHER HUMAN HERPESVIRUSES (B10)

● **B10** **Other human herpesviruses**

    Excludes2 cytomegalovirus (B25.9)
                Epstein-Barr virus (B27.0-)
                herpes NOS (B00.9)
                herpes simplex (B00.-)
                herpes zoster (B02.-)
                human herpesvirus NOS (B00.-)
                human herpesvirus 1 and 2 (B00.-)
                human herpesvirus 3 (B01.-, B02.-)
                human herpesvirus 4 (B27.0-)
                human herpesvirus 5 (B25.-)
                varicella (B01.-)
                zoster (B02.-)

● **B10.0** **Other human herpesvirus encephalitis**

    Excludes2 herpes encephalitis NOS (B00.4)
                herpes simplex encephalitis (B00.4)
                human herpesvirus encephalitis (B00.4)
                simian B herpes virus encephalitis (B00.4)

    B10.01 **Human herpesvirus 6 encephalitis**
            Sudden rash or roseola

    B10.09 **Other human herpesvirus encephalitis**
            Human herpesvirus 7 encephalitis
            Virus closely related to human herpesvirus 6, but
               not known to cause any disease

● **B10.8** **Other human herpesvirus infection**

    B10.81 **Human herpesvirus 6 infection**
            Causative agent of exanthema subitum that results
               in sudden rash

    B10.82 **Human herpesvirus 7 infection**
            Closely related to human herpesvirus 6, but not
               known cause any disease

    B10.89 **Other human herpesvirus infection**
            Human herpesvirus 8 infection
            May be the cause of Kaposi sarcoma, a malignant
               tumor
            Kaposi's sarcoma-associated herpesvirus
               infection

VIRAL HEPATITIS (B15-B19)

    Excludes1 sequelae of viral hepatitis (B94.2)
    Excludes2 cytomegaloviral hepatitis (B25.1)
                herpesviral [herpes simplex] hepatitis (B00.81)

● **B15** **Acute hepatitis A**
    B15.0 **Hepatitis A with hepatic coma**
    B15.9 **Hepatitis A without hepatic coma**
            Hepatitis A (acute) (viral) NOS

● **B16** **Acute hepatitis B**
    B16.0 **Acute hepatitis B with delta-agent with hepatic coma**
    B16.1 **Acute hepatitis B with delta-agent without hepatic coma**
    B16.2 **Acute hepatitis B without delta-agent with hepatic coma**
    B16.9 **Acute hepatitis B without delta-agent and without**
            hepatic coma
            Hepatitis B (acute) (viral) NOS

● **B17** **Other acute viral hepatitis**
    B17.0 **Acute delta-(super) infection of hepatitis B carrier**
  ● **B17.1** **Acute hepatitis C**
      B17.10 **Acute hepatitis C without hepatic coma**
              Acute hepatitis C NOS
      B17.11 **Acute hepatitis C with hepatic coma**
    B17.2 **Acute hepatitis E**
    B17.8 **Other specified acute viral hepatitis**
            Hepatitis non-A non-B (acute) (viral) NEC
    B17.9 **Acute viral hepatitis, unspecified**
            Acute hepatitis NOS

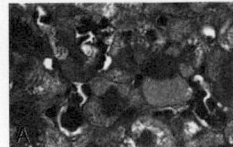 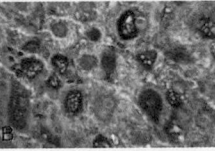

Figure 1-6 Hepatitis B viral infection. **A.** Liver parenchyma showing hepatocytes with diffuse granular cytoplasm, so-called ground glass hepatocytes (H&E). **B.** Immunoperoxidase stains from the same case, showing cytoplasmic inclusions of viral particles. (From Kumar: Robbins and Cotran: Pathologic Basis of Disease, ed 8, Saunders, An Imprint of Elsevier, 2009)

Item 1-18 Hepatitis A (HAV) was formerly called epidemic, infectious, short-incubation, or acute catarrhal jaundice hepatitis. The primary transmission mode is the oral–fecal route. **Hepatitis B (HBV)** was formerly called long-incubation period, serum, or homologous serum hepatitis. Transmission modes are through blood from infected persons and from body fluids of infected mother to neonate. **Hepatitis C (HCV),** caused by the hepatitis C virus, is primarily transfusion associated. **Hepatitis D (HDV),** also called delta hepatitis, is caused by the hepatitis D virus in patients formerly or currently infected with hepatitis B. **Hepatitis E (HEV)** is also called enterically transmitted non-A, non-B hepatitis. The primary transmission mode is the oral–fecal route, usually through contaminated water.

● **B18** **Chronic viral hepatitis**
    B18.0 **Chronic viral hepatitis B with delta-agent**
    B18.1 **Chronic viral hepatitis B without delta-agent**
            Chronic (viral) hepatitis B
    B18.2 **Chronic viral hepatitis C**
    B18.8 **Other chronic viral hepatitis**
    B18.9 **Chronic viral hepatitis, unspecified**

● **B19** **Unspecified viral hepatitis**
    B19.0 **Unspecified viral hepatitis with hepatic coma**
  ● **B19.1** **Unspecified viral hepatitis B**
      B19.10 **Unspecified viral hepatitis B without hepatic**
            coma
            Unspecified viral hepatitis B NOS
      B19.11 **Unspecified viral hepatitis B with hepatic coma**
  ● **B19.2** **Unspecified viral hepatitis C**
      B19.20 **Unspecified viral hepatitis C without hepatic**
            coma
            Viral hepatitis C NOS
      B19.21 **Unspecified viral hepatitis C with hepatic coma**
    B19.9 **Unspecified viral hepatitis without hepatic coma**
            Viral hepatitis NOS

CHAPTER 1 (A00-B99)

CHAPTER 1 (A00-B99)

OGCR Section I. C.1.a

Certain Infectious and Parasitic Diseases (A00-B99)

a. Human Immunodeficiency Virus (HIV) Infections

1) Code only confirmed cases

Code only confirmed cases of HIV infection illness. This is an exception to the hospital inpatient guideline Section II, H.

In this context, "confirmation" does not require documentation of positive serology or culture for HIV; the provider's diagnostic statement that the patient is HIV positive, or has an HIV-related illness is sufficient.

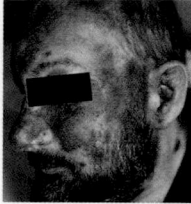

Figure 1-7 Kaposi's sarcoma. There are large confluent hyperpigmented patch-stage lesions with lymphedema. (From Cohen & Powderly: Infectious Diseases, ed 3, Mosby, An Imprint of Elsevier, 2010)

Item 1–19 AIDS (acquired immune deficiency syndrome) is caused by **HIV** (human immunodeficiency virus). HIV affects certain white blood cells (T-4 lymphocytes) and destroys the ability of the cells to fight infections, making patients susceptible to a host of infectious diseases (e.g., **Pneumocystis carinii pneumonia (PCP)**, **Kaposi's sarcoma,** and **lymphoma**). **AIDS-related complex (ARC)** is an early stage of AIDS in which tests for HIV are positive but the symptoms are mild.

HUMAN IMMUNODEFICIENCY VIRUS [HIV] DISEASE (B20)

B20   Human immunodeficiency virus [HIV] disease

> **Includes**   acquired immune deficiency syndrome [AIDS]
> AIDS-related complex [ARC]
> HIV infection, symptomatic

> *Code first* Human immunodeficiency virus [HIV] disease complicating pregnancy, childbirth and the puerperium, if applicable (O98.7-)

> Use additional code(s) to identify all manifestations of HIV infection

> **Excludes1**   asymptomatic human immunodeficiency virus [HIV] infection status (Z21)
> exposure to HIV virus (Z20.6)
> inconclusive serologic evidence of HIV (R75)

OTHER VIRAL DISEASES (B25-B34)

● **B25   Cytomegaloviral disease**
> *AKA: HCMV or Human Herpesvirus 5 (HHV-5)*
> **Excludes1**   congenital cytomegalovirus infection (P35.1)
> cytomegaloviral mononucleosis (B27.1-)

   B25.0   **Cytomegaloviral pneumonitis**

   B25.1   **Cytomegaloviral hepatitis**

   B25.2   **Cytomegaloviral pancreatitis**

   B25.8   **Other cytomegaloviral diseases**
     Cytomegaloviral encephalitis

   B25.9   **Cytomegaloviral disease, unspecified**

● **B26   Mumps**
> **Includes**   epidemic parotitis
> infectious parotitis
> *Acute, contagious, viral disease*

   B26.0   **Mumps orchitis ♂**

   B26.1   **Mumps meningitis**

   B26.2   **Mumps encephalitis**

   B26.3   **Mumps pancreatitis**

●   B26.8   **Mumps with other complications**

     B26.81   **Mumps hepatitis**

     B26.82   **Mumps myocarditis**

     B26.83   **Mumps nephritis**

     B26.84   **Mumps polyneuropathy**

     B26.85   **Mumps arthritis**

     B26.89   **Other mumps complications**

   B26.9   **Mumps without complication**
     Mumps NOS
     Mumps parotitis NOS

● **B27   Infectious mononucleosis**
> **Includes**   glandular fever
> monocytic angina
> Pfeiffer's disease

● **B27.0   Gammaherpesviral mononucleosis**
> *AKA: Pfeiffer's disease, infective mononucleosis*
> Mononucleosis due to Epstein-Barr virus

     B27.00   **Gammaherpesviral mononucleosis without complication**
       Infective mononucleosis

     B27.01   **Gammaherpesviral mononucleosis with polyneuropathy**

     B27.02   **Gammaherpesviral mononucleosis with meningitis**

     B27.09   **Gammaherpesviral mononucleosis with other complications**
       Hepatomegaly in gammaherpesviral mononucleosis

● **B27.1   Cytomegaloviral mononucleosis**
> *Infectious disease resembling infectious mononucleosis*

     B27.10   **Cytomegaloviral mononucleosis without complications**

     B27.11   **Cytomegaloviral mononucleosis with polyneuropathy**

     B27.12   **Cytomegaloviral mononucleosis with meningitis**

     B27.19   **Cytomegaloviral mononucleosis with other complication**
       Hepatomegaly in cytomegaloviral mononucleosis

● **B27.8   Other infectious mononucleosis**

     B27.80   **Other infectious mononucleosis without complication**

     B27.81   **Other infectious mononucleosis with polyneuropathy**

     B27.82   **Other infectious mononucleosis with meningitis**

     B27.89   **Other infectious mononucleosis with other complication**
       Hepatomegaly in other infectious mononucleosis

● **B27.9   Infectious mononucleosis, unspecified**

     B27.90   **Infectious mononucleosis, unspecified without complication**

     B27.91   **Infectious mononucleosis, unspecified with polyneuropathy**

     B27.92   **Infectious mononucleosis, unspecified with meningitis**

     B27.99   **Infectious mononucleosis, unspecified with other complication**
       Hepatomegaly in unspecified infectious mononucleosis

● **B30   Viral conjunctivitis**
> **Excludes1**   herpesviral [herpes simplex] ocular disease (B00.5)
> ocular zoster (B02.3)

   B30.0   **Keratoconjunctivitis due to adenovirus**
     Epidemic keratoconjunctivitis
     Shipyard eye

   B30.1   **Conjunctivitis due to adenovirus**
     Acute adenoviral follicular conjunctivitis
     Swimming-pool conjunctivitis

◀ New   ◀▥ Revised   ~~deleted~~ Deleted   Excludes 1   Excludes 2   Includes   Use additional   Code first   Code also   Unspecified

OGCR Official Guidelines   X Assign placeholder X   ● Use Additional Character(s)   ▶ Manifestation Code   **Coding Clinic**

B30.2   **Viral pharyngoconjunctivitis**

B30.3   **Acute epidemic hemorrhagic conjunctivitis (enteroviral)**
Conjunctivitis due to coxsackievirus 24
Conjunctivitis due to enterovirus 70
Hemorrhagic conjunctivitis (acute)(epidemic)

B30.8   **Other viral conjunctivitis**
Newcastle conjunctivitis

B30.9   **Viral conjunctivitis, unspecified**

● **B33**   **Other viral diseases, not elsewhere classified**

B33.0   **Epidemic myalgia**
Acute infectious disease, caused by group A coxsackie viruses or other enteroviruses with symptoms that include sudden pain in chest or upper abdomen with fever
Bornholm disease

B33.1   **Ross River disease**
Epidemic polyarthritis and exanthema
Ross River fever

● **B33.2**   **Viral carditis**
Coxsackie (virus) carditis

    B33.20   **Viral carditis, unspecified**

    B33.21   **Viral endocarditis**

    B33.22   **Viral myocarditis**

    B33.23   **Viral pericarditis**

    B33.24   **Viral cardiomyopathy**

B33.3   **Retrovirus infections, not elsewhere classified**
Retrovirus infection NOS

B33.4   **Hantavirus (cardio)-pulmonary syndrome [HPS] [HCPS]**
Hantavirus disease with pulmonary manifestations
Sin nombre virus disease

    Use additional code to identify any associated acute kidney failure (N17.9)

    Excludes1   hantavirus disease with renal manifestations (A98.5)
hemorrhagic fever with renal manifestations (A98.5)

B33.8   **Other specified viral diseases**

    Excludes1   anogenital human papillomavirus infection (A63.0)
viral warts due to human papillomavirus infection (B07)

● **B34**   **Viral infection of unspecified site**

    Excludes1   anogenital human papillomavirus infection (A63.0)
cytomegaloviral disease NOS (B25.9)
herpesvirus [herpes simplex] infection NOS (B00.9)
retrovirus infection NOS (B33.3)
viral agents as the cause of diseases classified elsewhere (B97.-)
viral warts due to human papillomavirus infection (B07)

B34.0   **Adenovirus infection, unspecified**

B34.1   **Enterovirus infection, unspecified**
Intestinal tract infection
Coxsackievirus infection NOS
Echovirus infection NOS

B34.2   **Coronavirus infection, unspecified**

    Excludes1   pneumonia due to SARS-associated coronavirus (J12.81)

B34.3   **Parvovirus infection, unspecified**

B34.4   **Papovavirus infection, unspecified**

B34.8   **Other viral infections of unspecified site**

B34.9   **Viral infection, unspecified**
Viremia NOS

MYCOSES (B35-B49)

    Excludes2   hypersensitivity pneumonitis due to organic dust (J67.-)
mycosis fungoides (C84.0-)

● **B35**   **Dermatophytosis**
AKA tinea or ringworm

    Includes   favus
infections due to species of Epidermophyton, Micro-sporum and Trichophyton
tinea, any type except those in B36.-

B35.0   **Tinea barbae and tinea capitis**
Beard ringworm
Kerion
Scalp ringworm
Sycosis, mycotic

B35.1   **Tinea unguium**
White patches or pits on surface or edges of nails, followed by infection under nail plate
Dermatophytic onychia
Dermatophytosis of nail
Onychomycosis
Ringworm of nails

B35.2   **Tinea manuum**
Tinea of hands
Dermatophytosis of hand
Hand ringworm

B35.3   **Tinea pedis**
Tinea affecting feet
Athlete's foot
Dermatophytosis of foot
Foot ringworm

B35.4   **Tinea corporis**
Infecting skin areas other than hands
Ringworm of the body

B35.5   **Tinea imbricata**
Chronic tropical tinea corporis; AKA Oriental ringworm, tinea inguinalis, tinea cruris
Tokelau

B35.6   **Tinea cruris**
In groin or perineal area, spreading to adjacent regions; AKA jock itch, eczema marginatum, ringworm of groin, or t inguinalis
Dhobi itch
Groin ringworm
Jock itch

B35.8   **Other dermatophytoses**
Disseminated dermatophytosis
Granulomatous dermatophytosis

B35.9   **Dermatophytosis, unspecified**
Ringworm NOS

● **B36**   **Other superficial mycoses**

B36.0   **Pityriasis versicolor**
Common, chronic, symptomless disorder that includes macular patches of various sizes and shapes; AKA liver spots
Tinea flava
Tinea versicolor

B36.1   **Tinea nigra**
Minor fungal infection, with dark lesions, usually on skin of hands
Keratomycosis nigricans palmaris
Microsporosis nigra
Pityriasis nigra

B36.2   **White piedra**
White to light brown nodules on hair of beard, axilla, or groin; AKA trichosporosis
Tinea blanca

B36.3   **Black piedra**
Characterized by small black or brown nodules on shafts of scalp hair

B36.8   **Other specified superficial mycoses**

B36.9   **Superficial mycosis, unspecified**

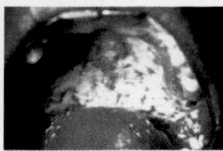

Figure 1-8   Oral candidiasis (thrush). *(Courtesy of Stephen Raffanti, MD, MPH.)* (From Mandell, Bennett, & Dolin: Principles and Practice of Infectious Diseases, ed 7, Churchill Livingstone, An Imprint of Elsevier, 2009)

Item 1–20   Candidiasis, also called oidiomycosis or moniliasis, is a fungal infection. It most often appears on moist cutaneous areas of the body but can also be responsible for a variety of systemic infections such as endocarditis, meningitis, arthritis, and myositis. Antifungal medications cure most yeast infections.

● **B37   Candidiasis**

> **Includes**   candidosis
>   moniliasis
>
> **Excludes1**   neonatal candidiasis (P37.5)

    B37.0   Candidal stomatitis
           Oral thrush

    B37.1   Pulmonary candidiasis
           Candidal bronchitis
           Candidal pneumonia

    B37.2   Candidiasis of skin and nail
           Candidal onychia
           Candidal paronychia

>   **Excludes2**   diaper dermatitis (L22)

    B37.3   Candidiasis of vulva and vagina ♀
           Candidal vulvovaginitis
           Monilial vulvovaginitis
           Vaginal thrush

   ● **B37.4   Candidiasis of other urogenital sites**

       B37.41   Candidal cystitis and urethritis

       B37.42   Candidal balanitis
               Male condition only

       B37.49   Other urogenital candidiasis
               Candidal pyelonephritis

    B37.5   Candidal meningitis

    B37.6   Candidal endocarditis

    B37.7   Candidal sepsis
           Disseminated candidiasis systemic candidiasis

   ● **B37.8   Candidiasis of other sites**

       B37.81   Candidal esophagitis

       B37.82   Candidal enteritis
               Candidal proctitis

       B37.83   Candidal cheilitis
               Inflammation affecting lip

       B37.84   Candidal otitis externa
               Inflammation of external auditory canal

       B37.89   Other sites of candidiasis
               Infection manifested by invasive candidiasis
               Candidal osteomyelitis

    B37.9   Candidiasis, unspecified
           Thrush NOS

● **B38   Coccidioidomycosis**
     Fungal disease; AKA coccidioidosis, coccidioidal granuloma, Posadas, or Posadas-Wernicke disease

    B38.0   Acute pulmonary coccidioidomycosis

    B38.1   Chronic pulmonary coccidioidomycosis

    B38.2   Pulmonary coccidioidomycosis, unspecified

    B38.3   Cutaneous coccidioidomycosis

    B38.4   Coccidioidomycosis meningitis

    B38.7   Disseminated coccidioidomycosis
           Generalized coccidioidomycosis

   ● **B38.8   Other forms of coccidioidomycosis**

       B38.81   Prostatic coccidioidomycosis ♂

       B38.89   Other forms of coccidioidomycosis

    B38.9   Coccidioidomycosis, unspecified

Item 1–21   Bird and bat droppings that fall into the soil give rise to a fungus that can spread airborne spores. When inhaled into the lungs, these spores divide and multiply into lesions. Histoplasmosis capsulatum takes three forms: primary (lodged in the lungs only), chronic (resembles TB), and disseminated (infection has moved to other organs). This is an opportunistic infection in immunosuppressed patients.

● **B39   Histoplasmosis**
     Infection resulting from inhalation or ingestion of spores; AKA Darling disease

> Code first associated AIDS (B20)

> Use additional code for any associated manifestations, such as:
>   endocarditis (I39)
>   meningitis (G02)
>   pericarditis (I32)
>   retinititis (H32)

    B39.0   Acute pulmonary histoplasmosis capsulati

    B39.1   Chronic pulmonary histoplasmosis capsulati

    B39.2   Pulmonary histoplasmosis capsulati, unspecified

    B39.3   Disseminated histoplasmosis capsulati
           Generalized histoplasmosis capsulati

    B39.4   Histoplasmosis capsulati, unspecified
           American histoplasmosis

    B39.5   Histoplasmosis duboisii
           African histoplasmosis

    B39.9   Histoplasmosis, unspecified

● **B40   Blastomycosis**
     Rare and potentially fatal infection caused by inhaling fungus found in moist soil in temperate climates.

> **Excludes1**   Brazilian blastomycosis (B41.-)
>   keloidal blastomycosis (B48.0)

    B40.0   Acute pulmonary blastomycosis

    B40.1   Chronic pulmonary blastomycosis

    B40.2   Pulmonary blastomycosis, unspecified

    B40.3   Cutaneous blastomycosis

    B40.7   Disseminated blastomycosis
           Generalized blastomycosis

   ● **B40.8   Other forms of blastomycosis**

       B40.81   Blastomycotic meningoencephalitis
               Meningomyelitis due to blastomycosis

       B40.89   Other forms of blastomycosis

    B40.9   Blastomycosis, unspecified

● **B41   Paracoccidioidomycosis**
     Fungal infection usually chronic that begins in lungs, spreads to mucocutaneous areas which may extend to skin, tonsils, gastrointestinal lymphatics, liver, and spleen; AKA Almeida or Lutz-Splendore-Almeida disease, Brazilian or South American blastomycosis, or paracoccidioidal granuloma

> **Includes**   Brazilian blastomycosis
>   Lutz' disease

    B41.0   Pulmonary paracoccidioidomycosis

    B41.7   Disseminated paracoccidioidomycosis
           Generalized paracoccidioidomycosis

    B41.8   Other forms of paracoccidioidomycosis

    B41.9   Paracoccidioidomycosis, unspecified

● **B42   Sporotrichosis**
     Chronic fungal infection with nodular lesions

    B42.0   Pulmonary sporotrichosis

    B42.1   Lymphocutaneous sporotrichosis

    B42.7   Disseminated sporotrichosis
           Generalized sporotrichosis

   ● **B42.8   Other forms of sporotrichosis**

       B42.81   Cerebral sporotrichosis
               Meningitis due to sporotrichosis

       B42.82   Sporotrichosis arthritis

       B42.89   Other forms of sporotrichosis

    B42.9   Sporotrichosis, unspecified

◀ New   ◀ Revised   ~~deleted~~ Deleted   Excludes 1   Excludes 2   Includes   Use additional   Code first   Code also   Unspecified

OGCR Official Guidelines   X Assign placeholder X   ● Use Additional Character(s)   ▶ Manifestation Code   **Coding Clinic**

● **B43**   **Chromomycosis and pheomycotic abscess**
Chronic fungal infection of skin, initiated at site of puncture affecting lower limb or foot (mossy foot)

    B43.0   **Cutaneous chromomycosis**
       Dermatitis verrucosa

    B43.1   **Pheomycotic brain abscess**
       Cerebral chromomycosis

    B43.2   **Subcutaneous pheomycotic abscess and cyst**

    B43.8   **Other forms of chromomycosis**

    B43.9   **Chromomycosis, `unspecified`**

● **B44**   **Aspergillosis**
Infection marked by inflammatory lesions in skin, ear, orbit, nasal sinuses, lungs, and occasionally bones and meninges

    `Includes`   aspergilloma

    B44.0   **Invasive pulmonary aspergillosis**

    B44.1   **Other pulmonary aspergillosis**

    B44.2   **Tonsillar aspergillosis**

    B44.7   **Disseminated aspergillosis**
       Generalized aspergillosis

   ● **B44.8**   **Other forms of aspergillosis**

       B44.81   **Allergic bronchopulmonary aspergillosis**

       B44.89   **Other forms of aspergillosis**

    B44.9   **Aspergillosis, `unspecified`**

● **B45**   **Cryptococcosis**
Infection in the immunocompromised and fatal if left untreated; AKA torulosis, Buschke, or Busse-Buschke disease

    B45.0   **Pulmonary cryptococcosis**

    B45.1   **Cerebral cryptococcosis**
       Cryptococcal meningitis
       Cryptococcosis meningocerebralis

    B45.2   **Cutaneous cryptococcosis**

    B45.3   **Osseous cryptococcosis**

    B45.7   **Disseminated cryptococcosis**
       Generalized cryptococcosis

    B45.8   **Other forms of cryptococcosis**

    B45.9   **Cryptococcosis, `unspecified`**

● **B46**   **Zygomycosis**
Fungal infections including subcutaneous lesions and infection of sinuses, brain, or lungs

    B46.0   **Pulmonary mucormycosis**
       Fungal infection affecting lung

    B46.1   **Rhinocerebral mucormycosis**

    B46.2   **Gastrointestinal mucormycosis**

    B46.3   **Cutaneous mucormycosis**
       Subcutaneous mucormycosis

    B46.4   **Disseminated mucormycosis**
       Generalized mucormycosis

    B46.5   **Mucormycosis, `unspecified`**

    B46.8   **Other zygomycoses**
       Entomophthoromycosis

    B46.9   **Zygomycosis, `unspecified`**
       Phycomycosis NOS

● **B47**   **Mycetoma**
Slow progressive, destructive fungal infection of cutaneous and subcutaneous tissues, fascia, and bone, primarily seen in foot (Madura foot) or leg

    B47.0   **Eumycetoma**
       Madura foot, mycotic Maduromycosis

    B47.1   **Actinomycetoma**

    B47.9   **Mycetoma, `unspecified`**
       Madura foot NOS

● **B48**   **Other mycoses, not elsewhere classified**

    B48.0   **Lobomycosis**
Infection with symptoms of red, smooth, hard cutaneous nodules resembling keloids
       Keloidal blastomycosis
       Lobo's disease

    B48.1   **Rhinosporidiosis**
Chronic, localized granulomatous fungal infection, affecting mucocutaneous tissues, usually of nose characterized by polyps, papillomas, and wartlike lesions

    B48.2   **Allescheriasis**
Fungal infection
       Infection due to Pseudallescheria boydii
       `Excludes1`   eumycetoma (B47.0)

    B48.3   **Geotrichosis**
Fungal infection usually of bronchi, lungs, mouth, or intestinal tract
       Geotrichum stomatitis

    B48.4   **Penicillosis**
Fungal infection

    B48.8   **Other specified mycoses**
       Adiaspiromycosis
       Infection of tissue and organs by Alternaria
       Infection of tissue and organs by Drechslera
       Infection of tissue and organs by Fusarium
       Infection of tissue and organs by saprophytic fungi NEC

● **B49**   **`Unspecified` mycosis**
     Fungemia NOS

PROTOZOAL DISEASES (B50-B64)

    `Excludes1`   amebiasis (A06.-)
                 other protozoal intestinal diseases (A07.-)

● **B50**   **Plasmodium falciparum malaria**
Severe form of malaria that can be fatal
    `Includes`   mixed infections of Plasmodium falciparum with any other Plasmodium species

    B50.0   **Plasmodium falciparum malaria with cerebral complications**
       Cerebral malaria NOS

    B50.8   **Other severe and complicated Plasmodium falciparum malaria**
       Severe or complicated Plasmodium falciparum malaria NOS

    B50.9   **Plasmodium falciparum malaria, `unspecified`**

● **B51**   **Plasmodium vivax malaria**
    `Includes`   mixed infections of Plasmodium vivax with other Plasmodium species, except Plasmodium falciparum

    `Excludes1`   plasmodium vivav with Plasmodium falciparum (B50.-)

    B51.0   **Plasmodium vivax malaria with rupture of spleen**

    B51.8   **Plasmodium vivax malaria with other complications**

    B51.9   **Plasmodium vivax malaria without complication**
       Plasmodium vivax malaria NOS

● **B52**   **Plasmodium malariae malaria**
Causes fever that recurs at approximately three-day intervals (quartan fever), longer than two-day (tertian) intervals of other malarial parasites
    `Includes`   mixed infections of Plasmodium malariae with other Plasmodium species, except Plasmodium falciparum and Plasmodium vivax

    `Excludes1`   plasmodium falciparum (B50.-)
                plasmodium vivax (B51.-)

    B52.0   **Plasmodium malariae malaria with nephropathy**

    B52.8   **Plasmodium malariae malaria with other complications**

    B52.9   **Plasmodium malariae malaria without complication**
       Plasmodium malariae malaria NOS

CHAPTER 1 (A00-B99)

● **B53　Other specified malaria**

B53.0　Plasmodium ovale malaria
Least diagnosed type of malaria spread by female mosquitoes of rare species

> **Excludes1**　plasmodium ovale with Plasmodium falciparum (B50.-)
> plasmodium ovale with Plasmodium malariae (B52.-)
> plasmodium ovale with Plasmodium vivax (B51.-)

B53.1　Malaria due to simian plasmodia
Malaria-like disease (parasite infection)

> **Excludes1**　malaria due to simian plasmodia with Plasmodium falciparum (B50.-)
> malaria due to simian plasmodia with Plasmodium malariae (B52.-)
> malaria due to simian plasmodia with Plasmodium ovale (B53.0)
> malaria due to simian plasmodia with Plasmodium vivax (B51.-)

B53.8　Other malaria, not elsewhere classified

B54　Unspecified malaria

● **B55　Leishmaniasis**
Protozoal infection

B55.0　Visceral leishmaniasis
Kala-azar
Post-kala-azar dermal leishmaniasis

B55.1　Cutaneous leishmaniasis

B55.2　Mucocutaneous leishmaniasis

B55.9　Leishmaniasis, unspecified

● **B56　African trypanosomiasis**
Human African trypanosomiasis (HAT) is transmitted by fly bites

B56.0　Gambiense trypanosomiasis
Infection due to Trypanosoma brucei gambiense
West African sleeping sickness

B56.1　Rhodesiense trypanosomiasis
East African sleeping sickness
Infection due to Trypanosoma brucei rhodesiense

B56.9　African trypanosomiasis, unspecified
Sleeping sickness NOS

● **B57　Chagas' disease**
Tropical parasitic disease

> **Includes**　American trypanosomiasis
> infection due to Trypanosoma cruzi

B57.0　Acute Chagas' disease with heart involvement
Acute Chagas' disease with myocarditis

B57.1　Acute Chagas' disease without heart involvement
Acute Chagas' disease NOS

B57.2　Chagas' disease (chronic) with heart involvement
American trypanosomiasis NOS
Chagas' disease (chronic) NOS
Chagas' disease (chronic) with myocarditis
Trypanosomiasis NOS

● **B57.3　Chagas' disease (chronic) with digestive system involvement**

B57.30　Chagas' disease with digestive system involvement, unspecified

B57.31　Megaesophagus in Chagas' disease

B57.32　Megacolon in Chagas' disease

B57.39　Other digestive system involvement in Chagas' disease

● **B57.4　Chagas' disease (chronic) with nervous system involvement**

B57.40　Chagas' disease with nervous system involvement, unspecified

B57.41　Meningitis in Chagas' disease

B57.42　Meningoencephalitis in Chagas' disease

B57.49　Other nervous system involvement in Chagas' disease

B57.5　Chagas' disease (chronic) with other organ involvement

Item 1–22　Toxoplasmosis is caused by the protozoa **Toxoplasma gondii,** of which the house cat can be a host. Human infection occurs when contact is made with materials containing the pathogen, such as feces, contaminated soil, or ingestion of infected lamb, goat, or pork. Of the infected, very few have symptoms because a healthy person's immune system keeps the parasite from causing illness. When the immune system is compromised, symptoms may occur. Clinical symptoms include flu-like symptoms, but the disease progresses to include the eyes and the brain in babies.

● **B58　Toxoplasmosis**
Infection by protozoon transmitted in cysts in feces of cats

> **Includes**　infection due to Toxoplasma gondii
> **Excludes1**　congenital toxoplasmosis (P37.1)

● **B58.0　Toxoplasma oculopathy**

B58.00　Toxoplasma oculopathy, unspecified

B58.01　Toxoplasma chorioretinitis

B58.09　Other toxoplasma oculopathy
Toxoplasma uveitis

B58.1　Toxoplasma hepatitis

B58.2　Toxoplasma meningoencephalitis

B58.3　Pulmonary toxoplasmosis

● **B58.8　Toxoplasmosis with other organ involvement**

B58.81　Toxoplasma myocarditis

B58.82　Toxoplasma myositis

B58.83　Toxoplasma tubulo-interstitial nephropathy
Toxoplasma pyelonephritis

B58.89　Toxoplasmosis with other organ involvement

B58.9　Toxoplasmosis, unspecified

B59　Pneumocystosis
Caused by fungus
Pneumonia due to Pneumocystis carinii
Pneumonia due to Pneumocystis jiroveci

● **B60　Other protozoal diseases, not elsewhere classified**

> **Excludes1**　cryptosporidiosis (A07.2)
> intestinal microsporidiosis (A07.8)
> isosporiasis (A07.3)

B60.0　Babesiosis
Tickborne disease caused by microscopic organisms
Piroplasmosis

● **B60.1　Acanthamebiasis**

B60.10　Acanthamebiasis, unspecified

B60.11　Meningoencephalitis due to Acanthamoeba (culbertsoni)

B60.12　Conjunctivitis due to Acanthamoeba

B60.13　Keratoconjunctivitis due to Acanthamoeba

B60.19　Other acanthamebic disease

B60.2　Naegleriasis
Infection with microscopic organisms
Primary amebic meningoencephalitis

B60.8　Other specified protozoal diseases
Microsporidiosis

B64　Unspecified protozoal disease

HELMINTHIASES (B65-B83)

Diseases or infestations caused by parasitic worms

● **B65　Schistosomiasis [bilharziasis]**
Infection with flukes (flat parasitic worms)

> **Includes**　snail fever

B65.0　Schistosomiasis due to Schistosoma haematobium [urinary schistosomiasis]

B65.1　Schistosomiasis due to Schistosoma mansoni [intestinal schistosomiasis]

B65.2　Schistosomiasis due to Schistosoma japonicum
Asiatic schistosomiasis

B65.3　Cercarial dermatitis
Swimmer's itch

◀ New　　◀▬ Revised　　~~deleted~~ Deleted　　Excludes 1　　Excludes 2　　Includes　　Use additional　　Code first　　Code also　　Unspecified

OGCR Official Guidelines　　X Assign placeholder X　　● Use Additional Character(s)　　▶ Manifestation Code　　**Coding Clinic**

B65.8   **Other schistosomiasis**
     Infection due to Schistosoma intercalatum
     Infection due to Schistosoma mattheei
     Infection due to Schistosoma mekongi

B65.9   **Schistosomiasis, unspecified**

● **B66**   **Other fluke infections**
     Trematode (parasitic worms)

B66.0   **Opisthorchiasis**
     Infection due to cat liver fluke
     Infection due to Opisthorchis (felineus)(viverrini)

B66.1   **Clonorchiasis**
     Chinese liver fluke disease
     Infection due to Clonorchis sinensis
     Oriental liver fluke disease

B66.2   **Dicroceliasis**
     Liver fluke
     Infection due to Dicrocoelium dendriticum
     Lancet fluke infection

B66.3   **Fascioliasis**
     Infection due to Fasciola gigantica
     Infection due to Fasciola hepatica
     Infection due to Fasciola indica
     Sheep liver fluke disease

B66.4   **Paragonimiasis**
     Infection due to Paragonimus species
     Lung fluke disease
     Pulmonary distomiasis

B66.5   **Fasciolopsiasis**
     Largest intestinal fluke in humans
     Infection due to Fasciolopsis buski
     Intestinal distomiasis

B66.8   **Other specified fluke infections**
     Echinostomiasis
     Heterophyiasis
     Metagonimiasis
     Nanophyetiasis
     Watsoniasis

B66.9   **Fluke infection, unspecified**

● **B67**   **Echinococcosis**
     Larval forms of tapeworms usually of liver or lungs
     Includes   hydatidosis

B67.0   **Echinococcus granulosus infection of liver**

B67.1   **Echinococcus granulosus infection of lung**

B67.2   **Echinococcus granulosus infection of bone**

● **B67.3**   **Echinococcus granulosus infection, other and multiple sites**

     B67.31   **Echinococcus granulosus infection, thyroid gland**

     B67.32   **Echinococcus granulosus infection, multiple sites**

     B67.39   **Echinococcus granulosus infection, other sites**

B67.4   **Echinococcus granulosus infection, unspecified**
     Dog tapeworm (infection)

B67.5   **Echinococcus multilocularis infection of liver**

● **B67.6**   **Echinococcus multilocularis infection, other and multiple sites**

     B67.61   **Echinococcus multilocularis infection, multiple sites**

     B67.69   **Echinococcus multilocularis infection, other sites**

B67.7   **Echinococcus multilocularis infection, unspecified**

B67.8   **Echinococcosis, unspecified, of liver**

● **B67.9**   **Echinococcosis, other and unspecified**

     B67.90   **Echinococcosis, unspecified**
         Echinococcosis NOS

     B67.99   **Other echinococcosis**

Item 1-23 Echinococcosis: Also known as hydatid disease; is caused by Echinococcus granulosus, E. multilocularis, and E. vogeli tapeworms; and is contracted from infected food. Found in southern South America, the Mediterranean, the Middle East, central Asia, and Africa and uncommon in the United States but has been reported in California, New Mexico, Arizona and Utah. The disease is treated with medication over a long course as it is resistive.

● **B68**   **Taeniasis**
     Intestinal tapeworm (cestode) infection from raw or undercooked meat of infected animal
     Excludes1   cysticercosis (B69.-)

B68.0   **Taenia solium taeniasis**
     Pork tapeworm (infection)

B68.1   **Taenia saginata taeniasis**
     Beef tapeworm (infection)
     Infection due to adult tapeworm Taenia saginata

B68.9   **Taeniasis, unspecified**

● **B69**   **Cysticercosis**
     Systemic illness caused by the larvae of pork tapeworm
     Includes   cysticerciasis infection due to larval form of Taenia solium

B69.0   **Cysticercosis of central nervous system**

B69.1   **Cysticercosis of eye**

● **B69.8**   **Cysticercosis of other sites**

     B69.81   **Myositis in cysticercosis**

     B69.89   **Cysticercosis of other sites**

B69.9   **Cysticercosis, unspecified**

● **B70**   **Diphyllobothriasis and sparganosis**
     Infection with tapeworms seen most often from inadequately cooked fish

B70.0   **Diphyllobothriasis**
     Diphyllobothrium (adult) (latum) (pacificum) infection
     Fish tapeworm (infection)
     Excludes2   larval diphyllobothriasis (B70.1)

B70.1   **Sparganosis**
     Infection with migrating tapeworm larvae, which invade subcutaneous tissues, causing inflammation and fibrosis that resembles cellulitis
     Infection due to Sparganum (mansoni) (proliferum)
     Infection due to Spirometra larva
     Larval diphyllobothriasis
     Spirometrosis

● **B71**   **Other cestode infections**

B71.0   **Hymenolepiasis**
     Intestinal infestation with tapeworms
     Dwarf tapeworm infection
     Rat tapeworm (infection)

B71.1   **Dipylidiasis**
     Infection with tapeworm common to dogs and cats and seen in children having close contact with infected pets

B71.8   **Other specified cestode infections**
     Infection by the larval stage of a tapeworm, usually through fruit or vegetables
     Coenurosis

B71.9   **Cestode infection, unspecified**
     Tapeworm (infection) NOS

B72   **Dracunculiasis**
     Infection with roundworms
     Includes   guinea worm infection
         infection due to Dracunculus medinensis

● **B73**   **Onchocerciasis**
     Infection with parasitic worm
     Includes   onchocerca volvulus infection
         onchocercosis
         river blindness

● **B73.0**   **Onchocerciasis with eye disease**

     B73.00   **Onchocerciasis with eye involvement, unspecified**

     B73.01   **Onchocerciasis with endophthalmitis**

     B73.02   **Onchocerciasis with glaucoma**

     B73.09   **Onchocerciasis with other eye involvement**
         Infestation of eyelid due to onchocerciasis

B73.1   **Onchocerciasis without eye disease**

CHAPTER 1 (A00-B99)

● **B74** **Filariasis**
Infestation with slender threadlike worms

> **Excludes2**   onchocerciasis (B73)
>   tropical (pulmonary) eosinophilia NOS (J82)

   B74.0 **Filariasis due to Wuchereria bancrofti**
       Bancroftian elephantiasis
       Bancroftian filariasis

   B74.1 **Filariasis due to Brugia malayi**

   B74.2 **Filariasis due to Brugia timori**

   B74.3 **Loiasis**
       Infection with round worms growing in subcutaneous
           connective tissue
       Calabar swelling
       Eyeworm disease of Africa
       Loa loa infection

   B74.4 **Mansonelliasis**
       Infection with filarial parasite
       Infection due to Mansonella ozzardi
       Infection due to Mansonella perstans
       Infection due to Mansonella streptocerca

   B74.8 **Other filariases**
       Dirofilariasis

   B74.9 **Filariasis, unspecified**

B75 **Trichinellosis**
Infestation with parasitic roundworms ingested in undercooked
     contaminated meat

> **Includes**   infection due to Trichinella species trichiniasis

● **B76** **Hookworm diseases**
Occurs in hot, humid parts of world where larvae are soil borne, enter
     digestive tract through skin of feet/legs or in contaminated food/
     water; AKA ground itch

> **Includes**   uncinariasis

   B76.0 **Ancylostomiasis**
       Infection due to Ancylostoma species

   B76.1 **Necatoriasis**
       Infection due to Necator americanus

   B76.8 **Other hookworm diseases**

   B76.9 **Hookworm disease, unspecified**
       Cutaneous larva migrans NOS

● **B77** **Ascariasis**
Infection by roundworm in small intestine

> **Includes**   ascaridiasis
>   roundworm infection

   B77.0 **Ascariasis with intestinal complications**

   ● **B77.8** **Ascariasis with other complications**
       B77.81 **Ascariasis pneumonia**
       B77.89 **Ascariasis with other complications**

   B77.9 **Ascariasis, unspecified**

● **B78** **Strongyloidiasis**
Infection with adult female roundworms

> **Excludes1**   trichostrongyliasis (B81.2)

   B78.0 **Intestinal strongyloidiasis**

   B78.1 **Cutaneous strongyloidiasis**

   B78.7 **Disseminated strongyloidiasis**

   B78.9 **Strongyloidiasis, unspecified**

B79 **Trichuriasis**
Intestinal infection with roundworms

> **Includes**   trichocephaliasis
>   whipworm (disease)(infection)

B80 **Enterobiasis**
Intestinal infection with pinworms

> **Includes**   oxyuriasis
>   pinworm infection
>   threadworm infection

● **B81** **Other intestinal helminthiases, not elsewhere classified**
Diseases or infestations caused by parasitic worms

> **Excludes1**   angiostrongyliasis due to Parastrongylus
>   cantonensis (B83.2)

   B81.0 **Anisakiasis**
       Roundworm infection via contaminated undercooked infected
           fish or marine mammals
       Infection due to Anisakis larva

   B81.1 **Intestinal capillariasis**
       Infestation with of parasites (nematodes)
       Capillariasis NOS
       Infection due to Capillaria philippinensis

>   **Excludes2**   hepatic capillariasis (B83.8)

   B81.2 **Trichostrongyliasis**

   B81.3 **Intestinal angiostrongyliasis**
       Angiostrongyliasis due to Parastrongylus costaricensis

   B81.4 **Mixed intestinal helminthiases**
       Infection due to intestinal helminths classified to more
          than one of the categories B65.0-B81.3 and B81.8
       Mixed helminthiasis NOS

   B81.8 **Other specified intestinal helminthiases**
       Infection due to Oesophagostomum species
          [esophagostomiasis]
       Infection due to Ternidens diminutus [ternidensiasis]

● **B82** **Unspecified intestinal parasitism**

   B82.0 **Intestinal helminthiasis, unspecified**
       Infected with worms

   B82.9 **Intestinal parasitism, unspecified**

● **B83** **Other helminthiases**
Caused by parasitic worms

> **Excludes1**   capillariasis NOS (B81.1)
> **Excludes2**   intestinal capillariasis (B81.1)

   B83.0 **Visceral larva migrans**
       Prolonged migration of nematode larvae
       Toxocariasis

   B83.1 **Gnathostomiasis**
       Infection with nematode occurring from ingested undercooked
          fish contaminated with larvae; larvae migrate to
          subcutaneous tissue or deeper tissues, results are
          abscesses
       Wandering swelling

   B83.2 **Angiostrongyliasis due to Parastrongylus cantonensis**
       Nematode infection caused by eating contaminated raw
          snails, slugs, or paratenic hosts such as prawns or
          crabs; larval worms migrate to central nervous system
          resulting in eosinophilic meningitis
       Eosinophilic meningoencephalitis due to
          Parastrongylus cantonensis

>   **Excludes2**   intestinal angiostrongyliasis (B81.3)

   B83.3 **Syngamiasis**
       Infestation with gapeworm from turkey, pheasant, guinea fowl,
          goose, and wild birds
       Syngamosis

   B83.4 **Internal hirudiniasis**
       Infestation by leeches

>   **Excludes2**   external hirudiniasis (B88.3)

   B83.8 **Other specified helminthiases**
       Parasitic worm infestation
       Acanthocephaliasis
       Gongylonemiasis
       Hepatic capillariasis
       Metastrongyliasis
       Thelaziasis

   B83.9 **Helminthiasis, unspecified**
       Worms NOS

>   **Excludes1**   intestinal helminthiasis NOS (B82.0)

◄ New   ◄■ Revised   ~~deleted~~ Deleted   Excludes 1   Excludes 2   Includes   Use additional   Code first   Code also   Unspecified

OGCR Official Guidelines   **X** Assign placeholder X   ● Use Additional Character(s)   ▶ Manifestation Code   **Coding Clinic**

PEDICULOSIS, ACARIASIS AND OTHER INFESTATIONS (B85-B89)

Infestation of lice

● **B85   Pediculosis and phthiriasis**

    B85.0   Pediculosis due to Pediculus humanus capitis
        Head-louse infestation

    B85.1   Pediculosis due to Pediculus humanus corporis
        Body-louse infestation

    B85.2   Pediculosis, unspecified

    B85.3   Phthiriasis
        Crab or pubic lice
        Infestation by crab-louse
        Infestation by Phthirus pubis

    B85.4   Mixed pediculosis and phthiriasis
        Infestation classifiable to more than one of the
        categories B85.0-B85.3

  B86   Scabies
      Sarcoptic itch
      Contagious dermatitis caused by mites

● **B87   Myiasis**
    Infestation by fly maggots
    Includes   infestation by larva of flies

    B87.0   Cutaneous myiasis
        Creeping myiasis

    B87.1   Wound myiasis
        Traumatic myiasis

    B87.2   Ocular myiasis

    B87.3   Nasopharyngeal myiasis
        Laryngeal myiasis

    B87.4   Aural myiasis

  ● **B87.8   Myiasis of other sites**

      B87.81   Genitourinary myiasis

      B87.82   Intestinal myiasis

      B87.89   Myiasis of other sites

    B87.9   Myiasis, unspecified

● **B88   Other infestations**

    B88.0   Other acariasis
        Acarine dermatitis
        Dermatitis due to Demodex species
        Dermatitis due to Dermanyssus gallinae
        Dermatitis due to Liponyssoides sanguineus
        Trombiculosis
        Excludes2   scabies (B86)

    B88.1   Tungiasis [sandflea infestation]
        Inflammatory skin disease caused by infestation of fleas

    B88.2   Other arthropod infestations
        Scarabiasis

    B88.3   External hirudiniasis
        Leech infestation NOS
        Excludes2   internal hirudiniasis (B83.4)

    B88.8   Other specified infestations
        Infection of topical fresh water fish parasite
        Ichthyoparasitism due to Vandellia cirrhosa
        Linguatulosis
        Porocephaliasis

    B88.9   Infestation, unspecified
        Infestation (skin) NOS
        Infestation by mites NOS
        Skin parasites NOS

  B89   Unspecified parasitic disease

SEQUELAE OF INFECTIOUS AND PARASITIC DISEASES (B90-B94)

Note: Categories B90-B94 are to be used to indicate conditions
in categories A00-B89 as the cause of sequelae, which are
themselves classified elsewhere. The 'sequelae' include
conditions specified as such; they also include residuals
of diseases classifiable to the above categories if there
is evidence that the disease itself is no longer present.
Codes from these categories are not to be used for chronic
infections. Code chronic current infections to active infectious
disease as appropriate.

*Code first condition resulting from (sequela) the infectious or parasitic
disease*

● **B90   Sequelae of tuberculosis**
    Condition resulting from tuberculosis

    B90.0   Sequelae of central nervous system tuberculosis

    B90.1   Sequelae of genitourinary tuberculosis

    B90.2   Sequelae of tuberculosis of bones and joints

    B90.8   Sequelae of tuberculosis of other organs
        Excludes2   sequelae of respiratory tuberculosis
            (B90.9)

    B90.9   Sequelae of respiratory and unspecified tuberculosis
        Sequelae of tuberculosis NOS

  B91   Sequelae of poliomyelitis
    Excludes1   postpolio syndrome (G14)

  B92   Sequelae of leprosy

● **B94   Sequelae of other and unspecified infectious and parasitic
diseases**

    B94.0   Sequelae of trachoma

    B94.1   Sequelae of viral encephalitis

    B94.2   Sequelae of viral hepatitis

    **B94.8   Sequelae of other specified infectious and parasitic
diseases**

    B94.9   Sequelae of unspecified infectious and parasitic disease

    OGCR Section I.C.1.b

> Certain infectious and parasitic diseases
>
> Infectious agents as the cause of diseases classified to other
> chapters
>
> Certain infections are classified in chapters other than Chapter
> 1 and no organism is identified as part of the infection code. In
> these instances, it is necessary to use an additional code from
> Chapter 1 to identify the organism. A code from category B95,
> Streptococcus, Staphylococcus, and Enterococcus as the cause
> of diseases classified to other chapters, B96, Other bacterial
> agents as the cause of diseases classified to other chapters, or
> B97, Viral agents as the cause of diseases classified to other
> chapters, is to be used as an additional code to identify the
> organism. An instructional note will be found at the infection
> code advising that an additional organism code is required.

BACTERIAL AND VIRAL INFECTIOUS AGENTS (B95-B97)

Note: These categories are provided for use as supplementary or
additional codes to identify the infectious agent(s) in diseases
classified elsewhere.
*Code the disease first, then the bacterium. Do not report codes from
B95-B97 for sepsis.*

● **B95   Streptococcus, Staphylococcus, and Enterococcus as the cause of
diseases classified elsewhere**

    **B95.0   Streptococcus, group A, as the cause of diseases
classified elsewhere**

    **B95.1   Streptococcus, group B, as the cause of diseases
classified elsewhere**

    **B95.2   Enterococcus as the cause of diseases classified
elsewhere**

    **B95.3   Streptococcus pneumoniae as the cause of diseases
classified elsewhere**

    **B95.4   Other streptococcus as the cause of diseases classified
elsewhere**

CHAPTER 1 (A00-B99)

B95.5   Unspecified streptococcus as the cause of diseases classified elsewhere

● **B95.6**   Staphylococcus aureus as the cause of diseases classified elsewhere

     B95.61   Methicillin susceptible Staphylococcus aureus infection as the cause of diseases classified elsewhere
         Methicillin susceptible Staphylococcus aureus (MSSA) infection as the cause of diseases classified elsewhere
         Staphylococcus aureus infection NOS as the cause of diseases classified elsewhere

     B95.62   Methicillin resistant Staphylococcus aureus infection as the cause of diseases classified elsewhere
         Methicillin resistant staphylococcus aureus (MRSA) infection as the cause of diseases classified elsewhere

B95.7   Other staphylococcus as the cause of diseases classified elsewhere

B95.8   Unspecified staphylococcus as the cause of diseases classified elsewhere

● **B96**   Other bacterial agents as the cause of diseases classified elsewhere

     B96.0   Mycoplasma pneumoniae [M. pneumoniae] as the cause of diseases classified elsewhere
         Pleuro-pneumonia-like-organism [PPLO]

     B96.1   Klebsiella pneumoniae [K. pneumoniae] as the cause of diseases classified elsewhere

●   **B96.2**   Escherichia coli [E. coli] as the cause of diseases classified elsewhere

     B96.20   Unspecified Escherichia coli [E. coli] as the cause of diseases classified elsewhere
         Escherichia coli [E. coli] NOS

     B96.21   Shiga toxin-producing Escherichia coli [E. coli] (STEC) O157 as the cause of diseases classified elsewhere
         E. coli O157:H- (nonmotile) with confirmation of Shiga toxin
         E. coli O157 with confirmation of Shiga toxin when H antigen is unknown, or is not H7
         O157:H7 Escherichia coli [E.coli] with or without confirmation of Shiga toxin-production
         Shiga toxin-producing Escherichia coli [E.coli] O157:H7 with or without confirmation of Shiga toxin-production
         STEC O157:H7 with or without confirmation of Shiga toxin-production

     B96.22   Other specified Shiga toxin-producing Escherichia coli [E. coli] (STEC) as the cause of diseases classified elsewhere
         Non-O157 Shiga toxin-producing Escherichia coli [E.coli]
         Non-O157 Shiga toxin-producing Escherichia coli [E.coli] with known O group

     B96.23   Unspecified Shiga toxin-producing Escherichia coli [E. coli] (STEC) as the cause of diseases classified elsewhere
         Shiga toxin-producing Escherichia coli [E. coli] with unspecified O group
         STEC NOS

     B96.29   Other Escherichia coli [E. coli] as the cause of diseases classified elsewhere
         Non-Shiga toxin-producing E. coli

     B96.3   Hemophilus influenzae [H. influenzae] as the cause of diseases classified elsewhere

     B96.4   Proteus (mirabilis) (morganii) as the cause of diseases classified elsewhere

     B96.5   Pseudomonas (aeruginosa) (mallei) (pseudomallei) as the cause of diseases classified elsewhere
         Coding Clinic: 2015, Q1, P18

B96.6   Bacteroides fragilis [B. fragilis] as the cause of diseases classified elsewhere

B96.7   Clostridium perfringens [C. perfringens] as the cause of diseases classified elsewhere

● **B96.8**   Other specified bacterial agents as the cause of diseases classified elsewhere

     B96.81   Helicobacter pylori [H. pylori] as the cause of diseases classified elsewhere

     B96.82   Vibrio vulnificus as the cause of diseases classified elsewhere

     B96.89   Other specified bacterial agents as the cause of diseases classified elsewhere

● **B97**   Viral agents as the cause of diseases classified elsewhere

     B97.0   Adenovirus as the cause of diseases classified elsewhere

●   **B97.1**   Enterovirus as the cause of diseases classified elsewhere

     B97.10   Unspecified enterovirus as the cause of diseases classified elsewhere

     B97.11   Coxsackievirus as the cause of diseases classified elsewhere

     B97.12   Echovirus as the cause of diseases classified elsewhere

     B97.19   Other enterovirus as the cause of diseases classified elsewhere

●   **B97.2**   Coronavirus as the cause of diseases classified elsewhere

     B97.21   SARS-associated coronavirus as the cause of diseases classified elsewhere
         Excludes1   pneumonia due to SARS-associated coronavirus (J12.81)

     B97.29   Other coronavirus as the cause of diseases classified elsewhere

●   **B97.3**   Retrovirus as the cause of diseases classified elsewhere
     Excludes1   human immunodeficiency virus [HIV] disease (B20)

     B97.30   Unspecified retrovirus as the cause of diseases classified elsewhere

     B97.31   Lentivirus as the cause of diseases classified elsewhere

     B97.32   Oncovirus as the cause of diseases classified elsewhere

     B97.33   Human T-cell lymphotrophic virus, type I [HTLV-I] as the cause of diseases classified elsewhere

     B97.34   Human T-cell lymphotrophic virus, type II [HTLV-II] as the cause of diseases classified elsewhere

     B97.35   Human immunodeficiency virus, type 2 [HIV 2] as the cause of diseases classified elsewhere

     B97.39   Other retrovirus as the cause of diseases classified elsewhere

     B97.4   Respiratory syncytial virus as the cause of diseases classified elsewhere

     B97.5   Reovirus as the cause of diseases classified elsewhere

     B97.6   Parvovirus as the cause of diseases classified elsewhere

     B97.7   Papillomavirus as the cause of diseases classified elsewhere

Item 1–24   **Retrovirus** develops by copying its RNA, genetic materials, into the DNA, which then produces new virus particles. It is from the Retroviridae virus family. **Human T-cell lymphotropic virus, Type I (HTLV-I)** is also called human T-cell leukemia virus, Type I, and is a retrovirus thought to cause T-cell leukemia/lymphoma. **Human T-cell lymphotropic virus, Type II (HTLV-II),** is also called human T-cell leukemia virus, Type II, and is a retrovirus associated with hematologic disorders.

     HIV-2 is one of the serotypes of HIV and is usually confined to West Africa, whereas HIV-1 is found worldwide.

◀ New   ◀▬ Revised   ~~deleted~~ Deleted   Excludes 1   Excludes 2   Includes   Use additional   Code first   Code also   Unspecified

OGCR Official Guidelines   **X** Assign placeholder X   ● Use Additional Character(s)   ▶ Manifestation Code   **Coding Clinic**

● B97.8   Other viral agents as the cause of diseases classified elsewhere

    B97.81   Human metapneumovirus as the cause of diseases classified elsewhere

    B97.89   Other viral agents as the cause of diseases classified elsewhere

OTHER INFECTIOUS DISEASES (B99)

● B99   Other and unspecified infectious diseases

    B99.8   Other infectious disease

    B99.9   Unspecified infectious disease

CHAPTER 1 (A00-B99)

Item 2–1 Neoplasm: Neo = new, plasm = growth, development, formation. This new growth (mass, tumor) can be malignant or benign, which is confirmed by the pathology report. Do not assign a code to a neoplasm until you review the pathology report. Certain CPT codes will specify benign or malignant lesion, so be certain the diagnosis code supports the procedure code.

OGCR Section I.C.2

General Guidelines

Chapter 2 of the ICD-10-CM contains the codes for the most benign and all malignant neoplasms. Certain benign neoplasms, such as prostatic adenomas, may be found in the specific body system chapters. To properly code a neoplasm, it is necessary to determine from the record if the neoplasm is benign, in-situ, malignant, or, of uncertain histologic behavior. If malignant, any secondary (metastatic) sites should also be determined.

CHAPTER 2

NEOPLASMS (C00-D49)

This chapter contains the following blocks:

C00-C14	Malignant neoplasms of lip, oral cavity and pharynx
C15-C26	Malignant neoplasms of digestive organs
C30-C39	Malignant neoplasms of respiratory and intrathoracic organs
C40-C41	Malignant neoplasms of bone and articular cartilage
C43-C44	Melanoma and other malignant neoplasms of skin
C45-C49	Malignant neoplasms of mesothelial and soft tissue
C50	Malignant neoplasms of breast
C51-C58	Malignant neoplasms of female genital organs
C60-C63	Malignant neoplasms of male genital organs
C64-C68	Malignant neoplasms of urinary tract
C69-C72	Malignant neoplasms of eye, brain and other parts of central nervous system
C73-C75	Malignant neoplasms of thyroid and other endocrine glands
C7A	Malignant neuroendocrine tumors
C7B	Secondary neuroendocrine tumors
C76-C80	Malignant neoplasms of ill-defined, other secondary and unspecified sites
C81-C96	Malignant neoplasms of lymphoid, hematopoietic and related tissue
D00-D09	In situ neoplasms
D10-D36	Benign neoplasms, except benign neuroendocrine tumors
D3A	Benign neuroendocrine tumors
D37-D48	Neoplasms of uncertain behavior, polycythemia vera and myelodysplastic syndromes
D49	Neoplasms of unspecified behavior

Notes: Functional activity

All neoplasms are classified in this chapter, whether they are functionally active or not. An additional code from Chapter 4 may be used, to identify functional activity associated with any neoplasm.

Morphology [Histology]

Chapter 2 classifies neoplasms primarily by site (topography), with broad groupings for behavior, malignant, in situ, benign, etc. The Table of Neoplasms should be used to identify the correct topography code. In a few cases, such as for malignant melanoma and certain neuroendocrine tumors, the morphology (histologic type) is included in the category and codes.

Primary malignant neoplasms overlapping site boundaries

A primary malignant neoplasm that overlaps two or more contiguous (next to each other) sites should be classified to the subcategory/code .8 ('overlapping lesion'), unless the combination is specifically indexed elsewhere. For multiple neoplasms of the same site that are not contiguous, such as tumors in different quadrants of the same breast, codes for each site should be assigned.

Malignant neoplasm of ectopic tissue

Malignant neoplasms of ectopic tissue are to be coded to the site mentioned, e.g., ectopic pancreatic malignant neoplasms are coded to pancreas, unspecified (C25.9).

MALIGNANT NEOPLASMS (C00-C96)

MALIGNANT NEOPLASMS, STATED OR PRESUMED TO BE PRIMARY (OF SPECIFIED SITES), AND CERTAIN SPECIFIED HISTOLOGIES, EXCEPT NEUROENDOCRINE, AND OF LYMPHOID, HEMATOPOIETIC AND RELATED TISSUE (C00-C75)

MALIGNANT NEOPLASMS OF LIP, ORAL CAVITY AND PHARYNX (C00-C14)

● **C00**   **Malignant neoplasm of lip**

     Use additional code to identify:
       alcohol abuse and dependence (F10.-)
       history of tobacco use (Z87.891)
       tobacco dependence (F17.-)
       tobacco use (Z72.0)

     Excludes1   malignant melanoma of lip (C43.0)
                    Merkel cell carcinoma of lip (C4A.0)
                    other and unspecified malignant neoplasm of skin of lip (C44.0-)

   C00.0   **Malignant neoplasm of external upper lip**
       Malignant neoplasm of lipstick area of upper lip
       Malignant neoplasm of upper lip NOS
       Malignant neoplasm of vermilion border of upper lip

   C00.1   **Malignant neoplasm of external lower lip**
       Malignant neoplasm of lower lip NOS
       Malignant neoplasm of lipstick area of lower lip
       Malignant neoplasm of vermilion border of lower lip

   C00.2   **Malignant neoplasm of external lip, unspecified**
       Malignant neoplasm of vermilion border of lip NOS

   C00.3   **Malignant neoplasm of upper lip, inner aspect**
       Malignant neoplasm of buccal aspect of upper lip
       Malignant neoplasm of frenulum of upper lip
       Malignant neoplasm of mucosa of upper lip
       Malignant neoplasm of oral aspect of upper lip

   C00.4   **Malignant neoplasm of lower lip, inner aspect**
       Malignant neoplasm of buccal aspect of lower lip
       Malignant neoplasm of frenulum of lower lip
       Malignant neoplasm of mucosa of lower lip
       Malignant neoplasm of oral aspect of lower lip

   C00.5   **Malignant neoplasm of lip, unspecified, inner aspect**
       Malignant neoplasm of buccal aspect of lip, unspecified
       Malignant neoplasm of frenulum of lip, unspecified
       Malignant neoplasm of mucosa of lip, unspecified
       Malignant neoplasm of oral aspect of lip, unspecified

   C00.6   **Malignant neoplasm of commissure of lip, unspecified**
       Commissure: Site of union of corresponding parts

   C00.8   **Malignant neoplasm of overlapping sites of lip**

   C00.9   **Malignant neoplasm of lip, unspecified**

◀ New   ◀┅ Revised   ~~deleted~~ Deleted   Excludes 1   Excludes 2   Includes   Use additional   Code first   Code also   Unspecified

OGCR Official Guidelines   **X** Assign placeholder X   ● Use Additional Character(s)   ▶ Manifestation Code   **Coding Clinic**

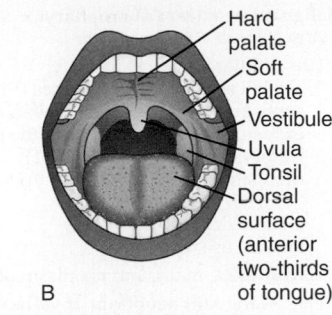

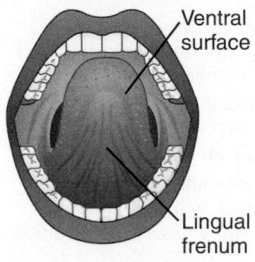

Transitional or vermilion surfaces

Lips are connected to
A   the gums by frenulum

Hard palate
Soft palate
Vestibule
Uvula
Tonsil
Dorsal surface (anterior two-thirds of tongue)

B

Ventral surface

Lingual frenum

C

Figure 2-1   Anatomical structures of the mouth and lips. **A.** Transitional or vermilion borders. Lips are connected to the gums by frenulum. **B.** Dorsal surface. **C.** Ventral surface.

C01   **Malignant neoplasm of base of tongue**
     Malignant neoplasm of dorsal surface of base of tongue
     Malignant neoplasm of fixed part of tongue NOS
     Malignant neoplasm of posterior third of tongue
     Use additional code to identify:
         alcohol abuse and dependence (F10.-)
         history of tobacco use (Z87.891)
         tobacco dependence (F17.-)
         tobacco use (Z72.0)

●**C02**   **Malignant neoplasm of other and unspecified parts of tongue**
     Use additional code to identify:
         alcohol abuse and dependence (F10.-)
         history of tobacco use (Z87.891)
         tobacco dependence (F17.-)
         tobacco use (Z72.0)

     C02.0   **Malignant neoplasm of dorsal surface of tongue**
         Malignant neoplasm of anterior two-thirds of tongue, dorsal surface
         Excludes2   malignant neoplasm of dorsal surface of base of tongue (C01)

     C02.1   **Malignant neoplasm of border of tongue**
         Malignant neoplasm of tip of tongue

     C02.2   **Malignant neoplasm of ventral surface of tongue**
         Malignant neoplasm of anterior two-thirds of tongue, ventral surface
         Malignant neoplasm of frenulum linguae

     C02.3   **Malignant neoplasm of anterior two-thirds of tongue, part unspecified**
         Malignant neoplasm of middle third of tongue NOS
         Malignant neoplasm of mobile part of tongue NOS

     C02.4   **Malignant neoplasm of lingual tonsil**
         Lingual tonsil: Aggregation of lymph follicles at root of tongue
         Excludes2   malignant neoplasm of tonsil NOS (C09.9)

     C02.8   **Malignant neoplasm of overlapping sites of tongue**
         Malignant neoplasm of two or more contiguous sites of tongue

     C02.9   **Malignant neoplasm of tongue, unspecified**

●**C03**   **Malignant neoplasm of gum**
     Includes   malignant neoplasm of alveolar (ridge) mucosa
                     malignant neoplasm of gingiva
     Use additional code to identify:
         alcohol abuse and dependence (F10.-)
         history of tobacco use (Z87.891)
         tobacco dependence (F17.-)
         tobacco use (Z72.0)
     Excludes2   malignant odontogenic neoplasms (C41.0-C41.1)

     C03.0   **Malignant neoplasm of upper gum**

     C03.1   **Malignant neoplasm of lower gum**

     C03.9   **Malignant neoplasm of gum, unspecified**

●**C04**   **Malignant neoplasm of floor of mouth**
     Use additional code to identify:
         alcohol abuse and dependence (F10.-)
         history of tobacco use (Z87.891)
         tobacco dependence (F17.-)
         tobacco use (Z72.0)

     C04.0   **Malignant neoplasm of anterior floor of mouth**
         Malignant neoplasm of anterior to the premolar-canine junction

     C04.1   **Malignant neoplasm of lateral floor of mouth**

     C04.8   **Malignant neoplasm of overlapping sites of floor of mouth**

     C04.9   **Malignant neoplasm of floor of mouth, unspecified**

●**C05**   **Malignant neoplasm of palate**
     Use additional code to identify:
         alcohol abuse and dependence (F10.-)
         history of tobacco use (Z87.891)
         tobacco dependence (F17.-)
         tobacco use (Z72.0)
     Excludes1   Kaposi's sarcoma of palate (C46.2)

     C05.0   **Malignant neoplasm of hard palate**

     C05.1   **Malignant neoplasm of soft palate**
         Excludes2   malignant neoplasm of nasopharyngeal surface of soft palate (C11.3)

     C05.2   **Malignant neoplasm of uvula**

     C05.8   **Malignant neoplasm of overlapping sites of palate**

     C05.9   **Malignant neoplasm of palate, unspecified**
         Malignant neoplasm of roof of mouth

●**C06**   **Malignant neoplasm of other and unspecified parts of mouth**
     Use additional code to identify:
         alcohol abuse and dependence (F10.-)
         history of tobacco use (Z87.891)
         tobacco dependence (F17.-)
         tobacco use (Z72.0)

     C06.0   **Malignant neoplasm of cheek mucosa**
         Malignant neoplasm of buccal mucosa NOS
         Malignant neoplasm of internal cheek

     C06.1   **Malignant neoplasm of vestibule of mouth**
         Malignant neoplasm of buccal sulcus (upper) (lower)
         Malignant neoplasm of labial sulcus (upper) (lower)

     C06.2   **Malignant neoplasm of retromolar area**

● **C06.8**   **Malignant neoplasm of overlapping sites of other and unspecified parts of mouth**

         C06.80   **Malignant neoplasm of overlapping sites of unspecified parts of mouth**

         C06.89   **Malignant neoplasm of overlapping sites of other parts of mouth 'book leaf' neoplasm [ventral surface of tongue and floor of mouth]**

     C06.9   **Malignant neoplasm of mouth, unspecified**
         Malignant neoplasm of minor salivary gland, unspecified site
         Malignant neoplasm of oral cavity NOS

CHAPTER 2 (C00-D49)

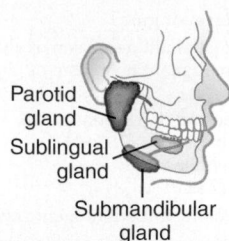

Parotid gland
Sublingual gland
Submandibular gland

Figure 2-2   Major salivary glands.

C07   **Malignant neoplasm of parotid gland**
     Use additional code to identify:
         alcohol abuse and dependence (F10.-)
         exposure to environmental tobacco smoke (Z77.22)
         exposure to tobacco smoke in the perinatal period (P96.81)
         history of tobacco use (Z87.891)
         occupational exposure to environmental tobacco smoke
            (Z57.31)
         tobacco dependence (F17.-)
         tobacco use (Z72.0)

● **C08**   **Malignant neoplasm of other and unspecified major salivary glands**
     Includes   malignant neoplasm of salivary ducts
     Use additional code to identify:
         alcohol abuse and dependence (F10.-)
         exposure to environmental tobacco smoke (Z77.22)
         exposure to tobacco smoke in the perinatal period (P96.81)
         history of tobacco use (Z87.891)
         occupational exposure to environmental tobacco smoke
            (Z57.31)
         tobacco dependence (F17.-)
         tobacco use (Z72.0)
     Excludes1   malignant neoplasms of specified minor salivary glands which are classified according to their anatomical location
     Excludes2   malignant neoplasms of minor salivary glands NOS (C06.9)
                  malignant neoplasm of parotid gland (C07)

   C08.0   **Malignant neoplasm of submandibular gland**
         Malignant neoplasm of submaxillary gland
   C08.1   **Malignant neoplasm of sublingual gland**
   C08.9   **Malignant neoplasm of major salivary gland, unspecified**
         Malignant neoplasm of salivary gland (major) NOS

(See Plate 61 on page 73.)

● **C09**   **Malignant neoplasm of tonsil**
     Use additional code to identify:
         alcohol abuse and dependence (F10.-)
         exposure to environmental tobacco smoke (Z77.22)
         exposure to tobacco smoke in the perinatal period (P96.81)
         history of tobacco use (Z87.891)
         occupational exposure to environmental tobacco smoke
            (Z57.31)
         tobacco dependence (F17.-)
         tobacco use (Z72.0)
     Excludes2   malignant neoplasm of lingual tonsil (C02.4)
                  malignant neoplasm of pharyngeal tonsil (C11.1)

   C09.0   **Malignant neoplasm of tonsillar fossa**
         Surface of palatine (two masses of lymphatic tissue on sides of throat) tonsils
   C09.1   **Malignant neoplasm of tonsillar pillar (anterior) (posterior)**
         Extension from palatine (two masses of lymphatic tissue on sides of throat) tonsils
   C09.8   **Malignant neoplasm of overlapping sites of tonsil**
   C09.9   **Malignant neoplasm of tonsil, unspecified**
         Malignant neoplasm of tonsil NOS
         Malignant neoplasm of faucial tonsils
         Malignant neoplasm of palatine tonsils

● **C10**   **Malignant neoplasm of oropharynx**
     Area of throat at back of mouth
     Use additional code to identify:
         alcohol abuse and dependence (F10.-)
         exposure to environmental tobacco smoke (Z77.22)
         exposure to tobacco smoke in the perinatal period (P96.81)
         history of tobacco use (Z87.891)
         occupational exposure to environmental tobacco smoke
            (Z57.31)
         tobacco dependence (F17.-)
         tobacco use (Z72.0)
     Excludes2   malignant neoplasm of tonsil (C09.-)

   C10.0   **Malignant neoplasm of vallecula**
         Vallecula, depression or furrow
   C10.1   **Malignant neoplasm of anterior surface of epiglottis**
         Malignant neoplasm of epiglottis, free border [margin]
         Malignant neoplasm of glossoepiglottic fold(s)
       Excludes2   malignant neoplasm of epiglottis (suprahyoid portion) NOS (C32.1)
   C10.2   **Malignant neoplasm of lateral wall of oropharynx**
   C10.3   **Malignant neoplasm of posterior wall of oropharynx**
   C10.4   **Malignant neoplasm of branchial cleft**
         Congenital slitlike openings formed between branchial arches pharyngeal groove
         Malignant neoplasm of branchial cyst [site of neoplasm]
   C10.8   **Malignant neoplasm of overlapping sites of oropharynx**
         Malignant neoplasm of junctional region of oropharynx
   C10.9   **Malignant neoplasm of oropharynx, unspecified**

● **C11**   **Malignant neoplasm of nasopharynx**
     Use additional code to identify:
         exposure to environmental tobacco smoke (Z77.22)
         exposure to tobacco smoke in the perinatal period (P96.81)
         history of tobacco use (Z87.891)
         occupational exposure to environmental tobacco smoke
            (Z57.31)
         tobacco dependence (F17.-)
         tobacco use (Z72.0)

   C11.0   **Malignant neoplasm of superior wall of nasopharynx**
         Part of pharynx that lies above soft palate
         Malignant neoplasm of roof of nasopharynx
   C11.1   **Malignant neoplasm of posterior wall of nasopharynx**
         Malignant neoplasm of adenoid
         Malignant neoplasm of pharyngeal tonsil
   C11.2   **Malignant neoplasm of lateral wall of nasopharynx**
         Malignant neoplasm of fossa of Rosenmüller
         Malignant neoplasm of opening of auditory tube
         Malignant neoplasm of pharyngeal recess
   C11.3   **Malignant neoplasm of anterior wall of nasopharynx**
         Malignant neoplasm of floor of nasopharynx
         Malignant neoplasm of nasopharyngeal (anterior) (posterior) surface of soft palate
         Malignant neoplasm of posterior margin of nasal choana
         Malignant neoplasm of posterior margin of nasal septum
   C11.8   **Malignant neoplasm of overlapping sites of nasopharynx**
   C11.9   **Malignant neoplasm of nasopharynx, unspecified**
         Malignant neoplasm of nasopharyngeal wall NOS

   C12   **Malignant neoplasm of pyriform sinus**
     Malignant neoplasm of pyriform fossa
     Use additional code to identify:
         exposure to environmental tobacco smoke (Z77.22)
         exposure to tobacco smoke in the perinatal period (P96.81)
         history of tobacco use (Z87.891)
         occupational exposure to environmental tobacco smoke
            (Z57.31)
         tobacco dependence (F17.-)
         tobacco use (Z72.0)

CHAPTER 2 (C00-D49)

◀ New   ⬅ Revised   ~~deleted~~ Deleted   Excludes 1   Excludes 2   Includes   Use additional   Code first   Code also   Unspecified

OGCR Official Guidelines   X Assign placeholder X   ● Use Additional Character(s)   ▶ Manifestation Code   **Coding Clinic**

● **C13**   **Malignant neoplasm of hypopharynx**

> Use additional code to identify:
> > exposure to environmental tobacco smoke (Z77.22)
> > exposure to tobacco smoke in the perinatal period (P96.81)
> > history of tobacco use (Z87.891)
> > occupational exposure to environmental tobacco smoke (Z57.31)
> > tobacco dependence (F17.-)
> > tobacco use (Z72.0)
>
> **Excludes2**   malignant neoplasm of pyriform sinus (C12)

C13.0   **Malignant neoplasm of postcricoid region**
> *Behind the cricoid cartilage of neck*

C13.1   **Malignant neoplasm of aryepiglottic fold, hypopharyngeal aspect**
> *Arytenoepiglottic fold, triangular opening between side of epiglottis and apex of arytenoid cartilage*
> Malignant neoplasm of aryepiglottic fold, marginal zone
> Malignant neoplasm of aryepiglottic fold NOS
> Malignant neoplasm of interarytenoid fold, marginal zone
> Malignant neoplasm of interarytenoid fold NOS
>
> > **Excludes2**   malignant neoplasm of aryepiglottic fold or interarytenoid fold, laryngeal aspect (C32.1)

C13.2   **Malignant neoplasm of posterior wall of hypopharynx**

C13.8   **Malignant neoplasm of overlapping sites of hypopharynx**

C13.9   **Malignant neoplasm of hypopharynx, unspecified**
> Malignant neoplasm of hypopharyngeal wall NOS

● **C14**   **Malignant neoplasm of other and ill-defined sites in the lip, oral cavity and pharynx**

> Use additional code to identify:
> > alcohol abuse and dependence (F10.-)
> > exposure to environmental tobacco smoke (Z77.22)
> > exposure to tobacco smoke in the perinatal period (P96.81)
> > history of tobacco use (Z87.891)
> > occupational exposure to environmental tobacco smoke (Z57.31)
> > tobacco dependence (F17.-)
> > tobacco use (Z72.0)
>
> **Excludes1**   malignant neoplasm of oral cavity NOS (C06.9)

C14.0   **Malignant neoplasm of pharynx, unspecified**

C14.2   **Malignant neoplasm of Waldeyer's ring**

C14.8   **Malignant neoplasm of overlapping sites of lip, oral cavity and pharynx**
> Primary malignant neoplasm of two or more contiguous sites of lip, oral cavity and pharynx
>
> > **Excludes1**   'book leaf' neoplasm [ventral surface of tongue and floor of mouth] (C06.89)

MALIGNANT NEOPLASM OF DIGESTIVE ORGANS (C15-C26)

> **Excludes1**   Kaposi's sarcoma of gastrointestinal sites (C46.4)

● **C15**   **Malignant neoplasms of esophagus**

> Use additional code to identify:
> > alcohol abuse and dependence (F10.-)

C15.3   **Malignant neoplasm of upper third of esophagus**

C15.4   **Malignant neoplasm of middle third of esophagus**

C15.5   **Malignant neoplasm of lower third of esophagus**
> > **Excludes1**   malignant neoplasm of cardio-esophageal junction (C16.0)

C15.8   **Malignant neoplasm of overlapping sites of esophagus**

C15.9   **Malignant neoplasm of esophagus, unspecified**

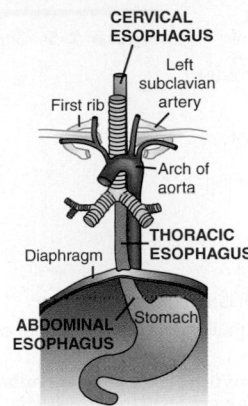

Figure 2-3   The esophagus is the muscular tube that connects the pharynx and the stomach. The 10 inch (25 cm) long esophagus is divided into three parts: **cervical, thoracic,** and **abdominal.**

● **C16**   **Malignant neoplasm of stomach**

> Use additional code to identify:
> > alcohol abuse and dependence (F10.-)
>
> **Excludes2**   malignant carcinoid tumor of the stomach (C7A.092)

C16.0   **Malignant neoplasm of cardia**
> Malignant neoplasm of cardiac orifice
> Malignant neoplasm of cardio-esophageal junction
> Malignant neoplasm of esophagus and stomach
> Malignant neoplasm of gastro-esophageal junction

C16.1   **Malignant neoplasm of fundus of stomach**

C16.2   **Malignant neoplasm of body of stomach**

C16.3   **Malignant neoplasm of pyloric antrum**
> Malignant neoplasm of gastric antrum

C16.4   **Malignant neoplasm of pylorus**
> Malignant neoplasm of prepylorus
> Malignant neoplasm of pyloric canal

C16.5   **Malignant neoplasm of lesser curvature of stomach, unspecified**
> Malignant neoplasm of lesser curvature of stomach, not classifiable to C16.1-C16.4

C16.6   **Malignant neoplasm of greater curvature of stomach, unspecified**
> Malignant neoplasm of greater curvature of stomach, not classifiable to C16.0-C16.4

C16.8   **Malignant neoplasm of overlapping sites of stomach**

C16.9   **Malignant neoplasm of stomach, unspecified**
> Gastric cancer NOS

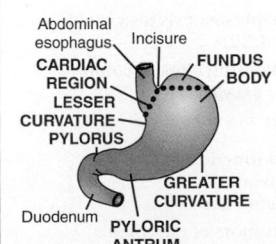

Figure 2-4   Parts of the stomach.

Item 2–2   The esophagus opens into the stomach through the **cardiac orifice,** also called the **cardioesophageal junction.** The **cardia** is adjacent to the cardiac orifice. The stomach widens into the **greater** and **lesser curvatures.** The **pyloric antrum** precedes the **pylorus,** which opens to the duodenum.

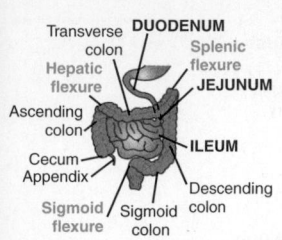

Figure 2-5 Small intestine and colon.

CHAPTER 2 (C00-D49)

● **C17 Malignant neoplasm of small intestine**

  Excludes1   malignant carcinoid tumor of the small intestine
              (C7A.01)

  C17.0   Malignant neoplasm of duodenum
          First or proximal portion of small intestine, extending from
          pylorus to jejunum

  C17.1   Malignant neoplasm of jejunum
          Second section of small intestine, extending from duodenum
          to ileum

  C17.2   Malignant neoplasm of ileum
          Distal and longest portion of small intestine, extending from
          jejunum to cecum

          Excludes1   malignant neoplasm of ileocecal valve
                      (C18.0)

  C17.3   Meckel's diverticulum, malignant
          Appendage of ileum

          Excludes1   Meckel's diverticulum, congenital (Q43.0)

  C17.8   Malignant neoplasm of overlapping sites of small
          intestine

  C17.9   Malignant neoplasm of small intestine, unspecified

● **C18 Malignant neoplasm of colon**

  Excludes1   malignant carcinoid tumors of the colon (C7A.02)

  C18.0   Malignant neoplasm of cecum
          First section of large intestine
          Malignant neoplasm of ileocecal valve

  C18.1   Malignant neoplasm of appendix
          Blind ended tube connected to the cecum; AKA vermiform
          appendix

  C18.2   Malignant neoplasm of ascending colon
          Ascending colon is between cecum and right colic flexure

  C18.3   Malignant neoplasm of hepatic flexure
          A flexure is a bending in a structure or organ. Note the three
          flexures illustrated in Figure 2–5.

  C18.4   Malignant neoplasm of transverse colon
          Portion of colon that runs transversely across upper part of
          abdomen, between right and left colic flexures

  C18.5   Malignant neoplasm of splenic flexure
          Bend at junction of transverse and descending colon

  C18.6   Malignant neoplasm of descending colon
          Portion between left colic flexure and sigmoid colon at pelvic
          brim; AKA iliac colon

  C18.7   Malignant neoplasm of sigmoid colon
          S-shaped part of colon extending from pelvic brim to third
          segment of sacrum
          Malignant neoplasm of sigmoid (flexure)

          Excludes1   malignant neoplasm of rectosigmoid
                      junction (C19)

  C18.8   Malignant neoplasm of overlapping sites of colon

  C18.9   Malignant neoplasm of colon, unspecified
          Malignant neoplasm of large intestine NOS

  C19 Malignant neoplasm of rectosigmoid junction
          Malignant neoplasm of colon with rectum
          Malignant neoplasm of rectosigmoid (colon)

          Excludes1   malignant carcinoid tumors of the colon
                      (C7A.02-)

C20 Malignant neoplasm of rectum
      Malignant neoplasm of rectal ampulla

      Excludes1   malignant carcinoid tumor of the rectum
                  (C7A.026)

● **C21 Malignant neoplasm of anus and anal canal**

      Excludes2   malignant carcinoid tumors of the colon
                  (C7A.02-)
                  malignant melanoma of anal margin (C43.51)
                  malignant melanoma of anal skin (C43.51)
                  malignant melanoma of perianal skin (C43.51)
                  other and unspecified malignant neoplasm of
                      anal margin (C44.500, C44.510, C44.520,
                      C44.590)
                  other and unspecified malignant neoplasm
                      of anal skin (C44.500, C44.510, C44.520,
                      C44.590)
                  other and unspecified malignant neoplasm of
                      perianal skin (C44.500, C44.510, C44.520,
                      C44.590)

  C21.0   Malignant neoplasm of anus, unspecified

  C21.1   Malignant neoplasm of anal canal
          Terminal part of large intestine
          Malignant neoplasm of anal sphincter

  C21.2   Malignant neoplasm of cloacogenic zone

  C21.8   Malignant neoplasm of overlapping sites of rectum,
          anus and anal canal
          Malignant neoplasm of anorectal junction
          Malignant neoplasm of anorectum
          Primary malignant neoplasm of two or more
              contiguous sites of rectum, anus and anal canal

● **C22 Malignant neoplasm of liver and intrahepatic bile ducts**
      Intrahepatic: Within liver

      Use additional code to identify:
          alcohol abuse and dependence (F10.-)
          hepatitis B (B16.-, B18.0-B18.1) hepatitis C (B17.1-, B18.2)

      Excludes1   malignant neoplasm of biliary tract NOS (C24.9)
                  secondary malignant neoplasm of liver and
                      intrahepatic bile duct (C78.7)

  C22.0   Liver cell carcinoma
          Hepatocellular carcinoma
          Hepatoma

  C22.1   Intrahepatic bile duct carcinoma
          Cholangiocarcinoma
          Adenocarcinoma (cancer that originates in glandular tissue)
          arising from epithelium of intrahepatic bile ducts

          Excludes1   malignant neoplasm of hepatic duct
                      (C24.0)

  C22.2   Hepatoblastoma
          Malignant intrahepatic tumor

  C22.3   Angiosarcoma of liver
          Kupffer cell sarcoma

  C22.4   Other sarcomas of liver

  C22.7   Other specified carcinomas of liver

  C22.8   Malignant neoplasm of liver, primary, unspecified as to
          type

  C22.9   Malignant neoplasm of liver, not specified as primary or
          secondary

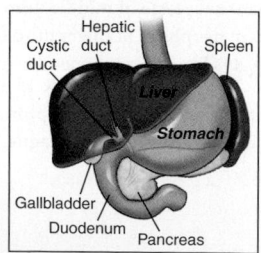

Figure 2-6 Diagram of liver, gallbladder, hepatic duct, pancreas, and
spleen. (From Thibodeau and Patton: Anatomy and Physiology, ed 7,
Mosby, 2010)

◄ New   ◄▬ Revised   ~~deleted~~ Deleted   Excludes 1   Excludes 2   Includes   Use additional   Code first   Code also   Unspecified

OGCR Official Guidelines   X Assign placeholder X   ● Use Additional Character(s)   ▶ Manifestation Code   **Coding Clinic**

C23 **Malignant neoplasm of gallbladder**

● C24 **Malignant neoplasm of other and unspecified parts of biliary tract**

> **Excludes1** malignant neoplasm of intrahepatic bile duct (C22.1)

C24.0 **Malignant neoplasm of extrahepatic bile duct**
Extrahepatic = outside the liver
Malignant neoplasm of biliary duct or passage NOS
Malignant neoplasm of common bile duct
Malignant neoplasm of cystic duct
Malignant neoplasm of hepatic duct

C24.1 **Malignant neoplasm of ampulla of Vater**
Union of pancreatic duct and common bile duct

C24.8 **Malignant neoplasm of overlapping sites of biliary tract**
Malignant neoplasm involving both intrahepatic and extrahepatic bile ducts
Primary malignant neoplasm of two or more contiguous sites of biliary tract

C24.9 **Malignant neoplasm of biliary tract, unspecified**

● C25 **Malignant neoplasm of pancreas**
Check documentation for specific site.
Use additional code to identify:
alcohol abuse and dependence (F10.-)

C25.0 **Malignant neoplasm of head of pancreas**

C25.1 **Malignant neoplasm of body of pancreas**

C25.2 **Malignant neoplasm of tail of pancreas**

C25.3 **Malignant neoplasm of pancreatic duct**

C25.4 **Malignant neoplasm of endocrine pancreas**
Malignant neoplasm of islets of Langerhans
That part of the pancreas that acts as endocrine gland and consists of islets of Langerhans
Use additional code to identify any functional activity.

C25.7 **Malignant neoplasm of other parts of pancreas**
Malignant neoplasm of neck of pancreas

C25.8 **Malignant neoplasm of overlapping sites of pancreas**

C25.9 **Malignant neoplasm of pancreas, unspecified**

● C26 **Malignant neoplasm of other and ill-defined digestive organs**

> **Excludes1** malignant neoplasm of peritoneum and retroperitoneum (C48.-)

C26.0 **Malignant neoplasm of intestinal tract, part unspecified**
Malignant neoplasm of intestine NOS

C26.1 **Malignant neoplasm of spleen**

> **Excludes1** Hodgkin lymphoma (C81.-)
> non-Hodgkin lymphoma (C82-C85)

C26.9 **Malignant neoplasm of ill-defined sites within the digestive system**
Malignant neoplasm of alimentary canal or tract NOS
Malignant neoplasm of gastrointestinal tract NOS

> **Excludes1** malignant neoplasm of abdominal NOS (C76.2)
> malignant neoplasm of intra-abdominal NOS (C76.2)

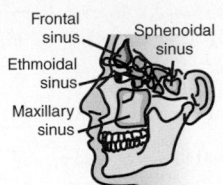

Figure 2-7 Paranasal sinuses. (From Buck CJ: Step-by-Step Medical Coding, ed 2011, Philadelphia, WB Saunders, 2011)

MALIGNANT NEOPLASMS OF RESPIRATORY AND INTRATHORACIC ORGANS (C30-C39)

> **Includes** malignant neoplasm of middle ear
> **Excludes1** mesothelioma (C45.-)

● C30 **Malignant neoplasm of nasal cavity and middle ear**

C30.0 **Malignant neoplasm of nasal cavity**
Malignant neoplasm of cartilage of nose
Malignant neoplasm of nasal concha
Malignant neoplasm of internal nose
Malignant neoplasm of septum of nose
Malignant neoplasm of vestibule of nose
Anterior part of nasal cavity

> **Excludes1** malignant neoplasm of nasal bone (C41.0)
> malignant neoplasm of nose NOS (C76.0)
> malignant neoplasm of olfactory bulb (C72.2-)
> malignant neoplasm of posterior margin of nasal septum and choana (C11.3)
> malignant melanoma of skin of nose (C43.31)
> malignant neoplasm of turbinates (C41.0)
> other and unspecified malignant neoplasm of skin of nose C44.301, C44.311, C44.321, C44.391)

C30.1 **Malignant neoplasm of middle ear**
Malignant neoplasm of antrum tympanicum
Boney cavity or chamber
Malignant neoplasm of auditory tube
Malignant neoplasm of eustachian tube
Malignant neoplasm of inner ear
Malignant neoplasm of mastoid air cells
Malignant neoplasm of tympanic cavity

> **Excludes1** malignant neoplasm of auricular canal (external) (C43.2-, C44.2-)
> malignant neoplasm of bone of ear (meatus) (C41.0)
> malignant neoplasm of cartilage of ear (C49.0)
> malignant melanoma of skin of (external) ear (C43.2-)
> other and unspecified malignant neoplasm of skin of (external) ear (C44.2-)

● C31 **Malignant neoplasm of accessory sinuses**
Paired sinuses in bones of face

C31.0 **Malignant neoplasm of maxillary sinus**
Malignant neoplasm of antrum (Highmore) (maxillary)

C31.1 **Malignant neoplasm of ethmoidal sinus**

C31.2 **Malignant neoplasm of frontal sinus**

C31.3 **Malignant neoplasm of sphenoid sinus**

C31.8 **Malignant neoplasm of overlapping sites of accessory sinuses**

C31.9 **Malignant neoplasm of accessory sinus, unspecified**

Item 2–3 Islets of Langerhans (endocrine producing cells comprising 1% to 2% of the pancreatic mass) make and secrete hormones that regulate the body's production of insulin, glucagon, and stomach acid. Breakdown of the insulin-producing cells can cause diabetes mellitus. Islet cell tumors can be benign or malignant and include glucagonomas, insulinomas, gastrinomas, and neuroendocrine tumor. The neoplasm table must be consulted for the correct neoplasm code.

N Newborn Age: 0   **P** Pediatric Age: 0–17   **M** Maternity DX: 12–55   **A** Adult Age: 15–124   ♀ Females Only   ♂ Males Only

773

CHAPTER 2 (C00-D49)

CHAPTER 2 (C00-D49)

● **C32   Malignant neoplasm of larynx**
    Use additional code to identify:
      alcohol abuse and dependence (F10.-)
      exposure to environmental tobacco smoke (Z77.22)
      exposure to tobacco smoke in the perinatal period (P96.81)
      history of tobacco use (Z87.891)
      occupational exposure to environmental tobacco smoke
        (Z57.31)
      tobacco dependence (F17.-)
      tobacco use (Z72.0)

    C32.0   Malignant neoplasm of glottis
      Vocal apparatus of larynx, consisting of true vocal cords
        (plicae vocales) and opening between them (rima
        glottidis)
      Malignant neoplasm of intrinsic larynx
      Malignant neoplasm of laryngeal commissure (anterior)
        (posterior)
      Malignant neoplasm of vocal cord (true) NOS
        True *vocal cords ("lower vocal folds") produce vocalization*
        when air from the lungs passes between them. Check
        your documentation. Code C32.1 is for malignant
        *neoplasm of the **false** vocal cords.*

    C32.1   Malignant neoplasm of supraglottis
      Area of pharynx above glottis
      Malignant neoplasm of aryepiglottic fold or
        interarytenoid fold, laryngeal aspect
      Malignant neoplasm of epiglottis (suprahyoid portion)
        NOS
      Malignant neoplasm of extrinsic larynx
      Malignant neoplasm of false vocal cord
        False *vocal cords ("upper vocal folds") are not involved in*
        vocalization. Check your documentation. Code C32.0 is
        for true vocal cords.
      Malignant neoplasm of posterior (laryngeal) surface of
        epiglottis
      Malignant neoplasm of ventricular bands

      Excludes2   malignant neoplasm of anterior surface of
            epiglottis (C10.1)
            malignant neoplasm of aryepiglottic
              fold or interarytenoid fold,
              hypopharyngeal aspect (C13.1)
            malignant neoplasm of aryepiglottic fold
              or interarytenoid fold, marginal zone
              (C13.1)
            malignant neoplasm of aryepiglottic fold
              or interarytenoid fold NOS (C13.1)

    C32.2   Malignant neoplasm of subglottis
      Lowest part of larynx from just below vocal cords down to top
        of trachea

    C32.3   Malignant neoplasm of laryngeal cartilage
      Cartilages of larynx, including cricoid, thyroid, and
        epiglottic, and two each of arytenoid, corniculate, and
        cuneiform

    C32.8   Malignant neoplasm of overlapping sites of larynx

    C32.9   Malignant neoplasm of larynx, unspecified

C33   Malignant neoplasm of trachea
    Use additional code to identify:
      exposure to environmental tobacco smoke (Z77.22)
      exposure to tobacco smoke in the perinatal period (P96.81)
      history of tobacco use (Z87.891)
      occupational exposure to environmental tobacco smoke
        (Z57.31)
      tobacco dependence (F17.-)
      tobacco use (Z72.0)

● **C34   Malignant neoplasm of bronchus and lung**
    Use additional code to identify:
      exposure to environmental tobacco smoke (Z77.22)
      exposure to tobacco smoke in the perinatal period (P96.81)
      history of tobacco use (Z87.891)
      occupational exposure to environmental tobacco smoke
        (Z57.31)
      tobacco dependence (F17.-)
      tobacco use (Z72.0)

    Excludes1   Kaposi's sarcoma of lung (C46.5-)
         malignant carcinoid tumor of the bronchus and
          lung (C7A.090)

● **C34.0   Malignant neoplasm of main bronchus**
      Malignant neoplasm of carina
        Ridgelike structure
      Malignant neoplasm of hilus (of lung)
        Anatomic depression or pit

      C34.00   Malignant neoplasm of unspecified main
            bronchus

      C34.01   Malignant neoplasm of right main bronchus

      C34.02   Malignant neoplasm of left main bronchus

● **C34.1   Malignant neoplasm of upper lobe, bronchus or lung**

      C34.10   Malignant neoplasm of unspecified bronchus
            or lung

      C34.11   Malignant neoplasm of upper lobe, right
            bronchus or lung

      C34.12   Malignant neoplasm of upper lobe, left
            bronchus or lung

    C34.2   Malignant neoplasm of middle lobe, bronchus or lung

● **C34.3   Malignant neoplasm of lower lobe, bronchus or lung**

      C34.30   Malignant neoplasm of lower lobe, unspecified
            bronchus or lung

      C34.31   Malignant neoplasm of lower lobe, right
            bronchus or lung

      C34.32   Malignant neoplasm of lower lobe, left
            bronchus or lung

● **C34.8   Malignant neoplasm of overlapping sites of bronchus
and lung**

      C34.80   Malignant neoplasm of overlapping sites
            of unspecified bronchus and lung

      C34.81   Malignant neoplasm of overlapping sites of
            right bronchus and lung

      C34.82   Malignant neoplasm of overlapping sites of left
            bronchus and lung

● **C34.9   Malignant neoplasm of unspecified part of bronchus or
lung**

      C34.90   Malignant neoplasm of unspecified part of
            unspecified bronchus or lung
             Lung cancer NOS

      C34.91   Malignant neoplasm of unspecified part of
            right bronchus or lung

      C34.92   Malignant neoplasm of unspecified part of left
            bronchus or lung

C37   Malignant neoplasm of thymus
    Excludes1   malignant carcinoid tumor of the thymus
         (C7A.091)

◀ New   ◀≡ Revised   ~~deleted~~ Deleted   Excludes 1   Excludes 2   Includes   Use additional   Code first   Code also   Unspecified

OGCR Official Guidelines   X Assign placeholder X   ● Use Additional Character(s)   ▶ Manifestation Code   **Coding Clinic**

● **C38** **Malignant neoplasm of heart, mediastinum and pleura**
  > **Excludes1**   mesothelioma (C45.-)

  C38.0 **Malignant neoplasm of heart**
  Malignant neoplasm of pericardium
  > **Excludes1**   malignant neoplasm of great vessels (C49.3)

  C38.1 **Malignant neoplasm of anterior mediastinum**

  C38.2 **Malignant neoplasm of posterior mediastinum**

  C38.3 **Malignant neoplasm of mediastinum, part unspecified**

  C38.4 **Malignant neoplasm of pleura**

  C38.8 **Malignant neoplasm of overlapping sites of heart, mediastinum and pleura**
  Pleura are comprised of serous membrane that lines the thoracic cavity (parietal) and covers the lungs (visceral).

● **C39** **Malignant neoplasm of other and ill-defined sites in the respiratory system and intrathoracic organs**
  Intrathoracic: within thorax/chest
  Use additional code to identify:
  exposure to environmental tobacco smoke (Z77.22)
  exposure to tobacco smoke in the perinatal period (P96.81)
  history of tobacco use (Z87.891)
  occupational exposure to environmental tobacco smoke (Z57.31)
  tobacco dependence (F17.-)
  tobacco use (Z72.0)
  > **Excludes1**   intrathoracic malignant neoplasm NOS (C76.1)
  > thoracic malignant neoplasm NOS (C76.1)

  C39.0 **Malignant neoplasm of upper respiratory tract, part unspecified**

  C39.9 **Malignant neoplasm of lower respiratory tract, part unspecified**
  Malignant neoplasm of respiratory tract NOS

MALIGNANT NEOPLASMS OF BONE AND ARTICULAR CARTILAGE (C40-C41)

  > **Includes**   malignant neoplasm of cartilage (articular) (joint)
  > malignant neoplasm of periosteum
  > **Excludes1**   malignant neoplasm of bone marrow NOS (C96.9)
  > malignant neoplasm of synovia (C49.-)

● **C40** **Malignant neoplasm of bone and articular cartilage of limbs**
  Use additional code to identify major osseous defect, if applicable (M89.7-)

  ● **C40.0** **Malignant neoplasm of scapula and long bones of upper limb**

    C40.00 **Malignant neoplasm of scapula and long bones of unspecified upper limb**

    C40.01 **Malignant neoplasm of scapula and long bones of right upper limb**

    C40.02 **Malignant neoplasm of scapula and long bones of left upper limb**

  ● **C40.1** **Malignant neoplasm of short bones of upper limb**

    C40.10 **Malignant neoplasm of short bones of unspecified upper limb**

    C40.11 **Malignant neoplasm of short bones of right upper limb**

    C40.12 **Malignant neoplasm of short bones of left upper limb**

  ● **C40.2** **Malignant neoplasm of long bones of lower limb**

    C40.20 **Malignant neoplasm of long bones of unspecified lower limb**

    C40.21 **Malignant neoplasm of long bones of right lower limb**

    C40.22 **Malignant neoplasm of long bones of left lower limb**

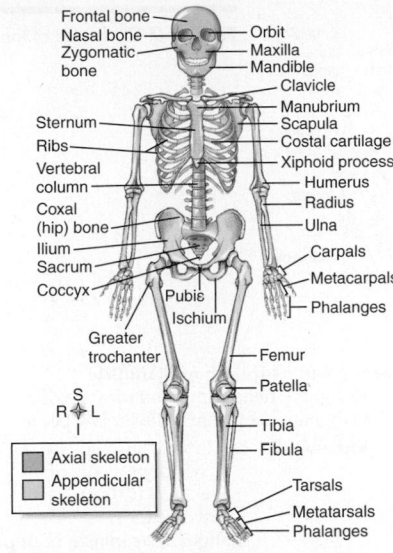

Figure 2-8   Diagram of skeleton of trunk and limbs with bones labeled. (From Thibodeau and Patton: Anatomy and Physiology, ed 7, Mosby, 2010)

● **C40.3** **Malignant neoplasm of short bones of lower limb**

  C40.30 **Malignant neoplasm of short bones of unspecified lower limb**

  C40.31 **Malignant neoplasm of short bones of right lower limb**

  C40.32 **Malignant neoplasm of short bones of left lower limb**

● **C40.8** **Malignant neoplasm of overlapping sites of bone and articular cartilage of limb**

  C40.80 **Malignant neoplasm of overlapping sites of bone and articular cartilage of unspecified limb**

  C40.81 **Malignant neoplasm of overlapping sites of bone and articular cartilage of right limb**

  C40.82 **Malignant neoplasm of overlapping sites of bone and articular cartilage of left limb**

● **C40.9** **Malignant neoplasm of unspecified bones and articular cartilage of limb**

  C40.90 **Malignant neoplasm of unspecified bones and articular cartilage of unspecified limb**

  C40.91 **Malignant neoplasm of unspecified bones and articular cartilage of right limb**

  C40.92 **Malignant neoplasm of unspecified bones and articular cartilage of left limb**

● **C41** **Malignant neoplasm of bone and articular cartilage of other and unspecified sites**
  > **Excludes1**   malignant neoplasm of bones of limbs (C40.-)
  > malignant neoplasm of cartilage of ear (C49.0)
  > malignant neoplasm of cartilage of eyelid (C49.0)
  > malignant neoplasm of cartilage of larynx (C32.3)
  > malignant neoplasm of cartilage of limbs (C40.-)
  > malignant neoplasm of cartilage of nose (C30.0)

  C41.0 **Malignant neoplasm of bones of skull and face**
  Malignant neoplasm of maxilla (superior)
  Malignant neoplasm of orbital bone
  > **Excludes2**   carcinoma, any type except intraosseous or odontogenic of:
  > maxillary sinus (C31.0)
  > upper jaw (C03.0)
  > malignant neoplasm of jaw bone (lower) (C41.1)

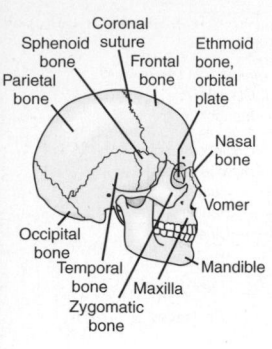

Figure 2-9 Bones of the skull.

(Labels on skull diagram: Coronal suture, Sphenoid bone, Frontal bone, Parietal bone, Ethmoid bone, orbital plate, Nasal bone, Vomer, Occipital bone, Temporal bone, Maxilla, Zygomatic bone, Mandible)

C41.1 **Malignant neoplasm of mandible**
    Malignant neoplasm of inferior maxilla
    Malignant neoplasm of lower jaw bone
    Excludes2 carcinoma, any type except intraosseous or odontogenic of:
        jaw NOS (C03.9)
        lower (C03.1)
        malignant neoplasm of upper jaw bone (C41.0)

C41.2 **Malignant neoplasm of vertebral column**
    Excludes1 malignant neoplasm of sacrum and coccyx (C41.4)

C41.3 **Malignant neoplasm of ribs, sternum and clavicle**

C41.4 **Malignant neoplasm of pelvic bones, sacrum and coccyx**

C41.9 **Malignant neoplasm of bone and articular cartilage, unspecified**

MELANOMA AND OTHER MALIGNANT NEOPLASMS OF SKIN (C43-C44)

● **C43** **Malignant melanoma of skin**
    Excludes1 melanoma in situ (D03.-)
    Excludes2 malignant melanoma of skin of genital organs (C51-C52, C60.-, C63.-)
        Merkel cell carcinoma (C4A.-)
        sites other than skin-code to malignant neoplasm of the site

C43.0 **Malignant melanoma of lip**
    Excludes1 malignant neoplasm of vermilion border of lip (C00.0-C00.2)

● **C43.1** **Malignant melanoma of eyelid, including canthus**
    Canthus: Either corner of eye where upper and lower eyelids meet
    C43.10 **Malignant melanoma of unspecified eyelid, including canthus**
    C43.11 **Malignant melanoma of right eyelid, including canthus**
    C43.12 **Malignant melanoma of left eyelid, including canthus**

● **C43.2** **Malignant melanoma of ear and external auricular canal**
    C43.20 **Malignant melanoma of unspecified ear and external auricular canal**
    C43.21 **Malignant melanoma of right ear and external auricular canal**
    C43.22 **Malignant melanoma of left ear and external auricular canal**

● **C43.3** **Malignant melanoma of other and unspecified parts of face**
    C43.30 **Malignant melanoma of unspecified part of face**
    C43.31 **Malignant melanoma of nose**
    C43.39 **Malignant melanoma of other parts of face**

C43.4 **Malignant melanoma of scalp and neck**

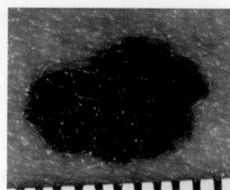

Figure 2-10 Malignant melanoma of skin. (From Goldman: Cecil Textbook of Medicine, ed 22, Saunders, 2004)

Item 2–4 **Malignant melanoma** is a serious form of skin cancer that affects the melanocytes (pigment-forming cells) and is caused by ultraviolet (UV) rays from the sun that damage skin. It is most commonly seen in the 40- to 60-year-olds with fair skin, blue or green eyes, and red or blond hair who sunburn easily.

Melanoma can spread very rapidly and is the most deadly form of skin cancer. It is less common than other types of skin cancer. The rate of melanoma is increasing and currently is the leading cause of death from skin disease.

● **C43.5** **Malignant melanoma of trunk**
    Excludes2 malignant neoplasm of anus NOS (C21.0)
        malignant neoplasm of scrotum (C63.2)
    C43.51 **Malignant melanoma of anal skin**
        Malignant melanoma of anal margin
        Malignant melanoma of perianal skin
    C43.52 **Malignant melanoma of skin of breast**
    C43.59 **Malignant melanoma of other part of trunk**

● **C43.6** **Malignant melanoma of upper limb, including shoulder**
    C43.60 **Malignant melanoma of upper limb, including shoulder, unspecified side**
    C43.61 **Malignant melanoma of right upper limb, including shoulder**
    C43.62 **Malignant melanoma of left upper limb, including shoulder**

● **C43.7** **Malignant melanoma of lower limb, including hip**
    C43.70 **Malignant melanoma of unspecified lower limb, including hip**
    C43.71 **Malignant melanoma of right lower limb, including hip**
    C43.72 **Malignant melanoma of left lower limb, including hip**

C43.8 **Malignant melanoma of overlapping sites of skin**

C43.9 **Malignant melanoma of skin, unspecified**
    Malignant melanoma of unspecified site of skin
    Melanoma (malignant) NOS

C4A **Merkel cell carcinoma**
    C4A.0 **Merkel cell carcinoma of lip**
        Excludes1 malignant neoplasm of vermilion border of lip (C00.0-C00.2)

● **C4A.1** **Merkel cell carcinoma of eyelid, including canthus**
    C4A.10 **Merkel cell carcinoma of unspecified eyelid, including canthus**
    C4A.11 **Merkel cell carcinoma of right eyelid, including canthus**
    C4A.12 **Merkel cell carcinoma of left eyelid, including canthus**

● **C4A.2** **Merkel cell carcinoma of ear and external auricular canal**
    C4A.20 **Merkel cell carcinoma of unspecified ear and external auricular canal**
    C4A.21 **Merkel cell carcinoma of right ear and external auricular canal**
    C4A.22 **Merkel cell carcinoma of left ear and external auricular canal**

◀ New   ◀▦ Revised   ~~deleted~~ Deleted   Excludes 1   Excludes 2   Includes   Use additional   Code first   Code also   Unspecified

OGCR Official Guidelines   X Assign placeholder X   ● Use Additional Character(s)   ▶ Manifestation Code   **Coding Clinic**

● **C4A.3** Merkel cell carcinoma of other and unspecified parts of face
　　　C4A.30 Merkel cell carcinoma of unspecified part of face
　　　C4A.31 Merkel cell carcinoma of nose
　　　C4A.39 Merkel cell carcinoma of other parts of face
　C4A.4 Merkel cell carcinoma of scalp and neck
● **C4A.5** Merkel cell carcinoma of trunk
　　　Excludes2　malignant neoplasm of anus NOS (C21.0)
　　　　　　　　　　malignant neoplasm of scrotum (C63.2)
　　　C4A.51 Merkel cell carcinoma of anal skin
　　　　　　Merkel cell carcinoma of anal margin
　　　　　　Merkel cell carcinoma of perianal skin
　　　C4A.52 Merkel cell carcinoma of skin of breast
　　　C4A.59 Merkel cell carcinoma of other part of trunk
● **C4A.6** Merkel cell carcinoma of upper limb, including shoulder
　　　C4A.60 Merkel cell carcinoma of unspecified upper limb, including shoulder
　　　C4A.61 Merkel cell carcinoma of right upper limb, including shoulder
　　　C4A.62 Merkel cell carcinoma of left upper limb, including shoulder
● **C4A.7** Merkel cell carcinoma of lower limb, including hip
　　　C4A.70 Merkel cell carcinoma of unspecified lower limb, including hip
　　　C4A.71 Merkel cell carcinoma of right lower limb, including hip
　　　C4A.72 Merkel cell carcinoma of left lower limb, including hip
　C4A.8 Merkel cell carcinoma of overlapping sites
　C4A.9 Merkel cell carcinoma, unspecified
　　　　Merkel cell carcinoma of unspecified site
　　　　Merkel cell carcinoma NOS

● **C44** Other and unspecified malignant neoplasm of skin
　　　Includes　malignant neoplasm of sebaceous glands
　　　　　　　　malignant neoplasm of sweat glands
　　　Excludes1　Kaposi's sarcoma of skin (C46.0)
　　　　　　　　　malignant melanoma of skin (C43.-)
　　　　　　　　　malignant neoplasm of skin of genital organs
　　　　　　　　　　(C51-C52, C60.-, C63.2)
　　　　　　　　　Merkel cell carcinoma (C4A.-)
● **C44.0** Other and unspecified malignant neoplasm of skin of lip
　　　Excludes1　malignant neoplasm of lip (C00.-)
　　　C44.00 Unspecified malignant neoplasm of skin of lip
　　　C44.01 Basal cell carcinoma of skin of lip
　　　C44.02 Squamous cell carcinoma of skin of lip
　　　C44.09 Other specified malignant neoplasm of skin of lip
● **C44.1** Other and unspecified malignant neoplasm of skin of eyelid, including canthus
　　　Excludes1　connective tissue of eyelid (C49.0)
　　● **C44.10** Unspecified malignant neoplasm of skin of eyelid, including canthus
　　　　　C44.101 Unspecified malignant neoplasm of skin of unspecified eyelid, including canthus
　　　　　C44.102 Unspecified malignant neoplasm of skin of right eyelid, including canthus
　　　　　C44.109 Unspecified malignant neoplasm of skin of left eyelid, including canthus

● **C44.11** Basal cell carcinoma of skin of eyelid, including canthus
　　　C44.111 Basal cell carcinoma of skin of unspecified eyelid, including canthus
　　　C44.112 Basal cell carcinoma of skin of right eyelid, including canthus
　　　C44.119 Basal cell carcinoma of skin of left eyelid, including canthus
● **C44.12** Squamous cell carcinoma of skin of eyelid, including canthus
　　　C44.121 Squamous cell carcinoma of skin of unspecified eyelid, including canthus
　　　C44.122 Squamous cell carcinoma of skin of right eyelid, including canthus
　　　C44.129 Squamous cell carcinoma of skin of left eyelid, including canthus
● **C44.19** Other specified malignant neoplasm of skin of eyelid, including canthus
　　　C44.191 Other specified malignant neoplasm of skin of unspecified eyelid, including canthus
　　　C44.192 Other specified malignant neoplasm of skin of right eyelid, including canthus
　　　C44.199 Other specified malignant neoplasm of skin of left eyelid, including canthus
● **C44.2** Other and unspecified malignant neoplasm of skin of ear and external auricular canal
　　　Excludes1　connective tissue of ear (C49.0)
● **C44.20** Unspecified malignant neoplasm of skin of ear and external auricular canal
　　　C44.201 Unspecified malignant neoplasm of skin of unspecified ear and external auricular canal
　　　C44.202 Unspecified malignant neoplasm of skin of right ear and external auricular canal
　　　C44.209 Unspecified malignant neoplasm of skin of left ear and external auricular canal
● **C44.21** Basal cell carcinoma of skin of ear and external auricular canal
　　　C44.211 Basal cell carcinoma of skin of unspecified ear and external auricular canal
　　　C44.212 Basal cell carcinoma of skin of right ear and external auricular canal
　　　C44.219 Basal cell carcinoma of skin of left ear and external auricular canal
● **C44.22** Squamous cell carcinoma of skin of ear and external auricular canal
　　　C44.221 Squamous cell carcinoma of skin of unspecified ear and external auricular canal
　　　C44.222 Squamous cell carcinoma of skin of right ear and external auricular canal
　　　C44.229 Squamous cell carcinoma of skin of left ear and external auricular canal

CHAPTER 2 (C00-D49)

● **C44.29** Other specified malignant neoplasm of skin of ear and external auricular canal

    C44.291 Other specified malignant neoplasm of skin of <mark>unspecified</mark> ear and external auricular canal

    C44.292 Other specified malignant neoplasm of skin of right ear and external auricular canal

    C44.299 Other specified malignant neoplasm of skin of left ear and external auricular canal

● **C44.3** Other and unspecified malignant neoplasm of skin of other and unspecified parts of face

  ● **C44.30** Unspecified malignant neoplasm of skin of other and unspecified parts of face

    C44.300 <mark>Unspecified</mark> malignant neoplasm of skin of unspecified part of face

    C44.301 <mark>Unspecified</mark> malignant neoplasm of skin of nose

    C44.309 <mark>Unspecified</mark> malignant neoplasm of skin of other parts of face

  ● **C44.31** Basal cell carcinoma of skin of other and unspecified parts of face

    C44.310 Basal cell carcinoma of skin of <mark>unspecified</mark> parts of face

    C44.311 Basal cell carcinoma of skin of nose

    C44.319 Basal cell carcinoma of skin of other parts of face

  ● **C44.32** Squamous cell carcinoma of skin of other and unspecified parts of face

    C44.320 Squamous cell carcinoma of skin of <mark>unspecified</mark> parts of face

    C44.321 Squamous cell carcinoma of skin of nose

    C44.329 Squamous cell carcinoma of skin of other parts of face

  ● **C44.39** Other specified malignant neoplasm of skin of other and unspecified parts of face

    C44.390 Other specified malignant neoplasm of skin of <mark>unspecified</mark> parts of face

    C44.391 Other specified malignant neoplasm of skin of nose

    C44.399 Other specified malignant neoplasm of skin of other parts of face

● **C44.4** Other and unspecified malignant neoplasm of skin of scalp and neck

    C44.40 <mark>Unspecified</mark> malignant neoplasm of skin of scalp and neck

    C44.41 Basal cell carcinoma of skin of scalp and neck

    C44.42 Squamous cell carcinoma of skin of scalp and neck

    C44.49 Other specified malignant neoplasm of skin of scalp and neck

● **C44.5** Other and unspecified malignant neoplasm of skin of trunk

    Excludes1 anus NOS (C21.0)
              scrotum (C63.2)

  ● **C44.50** Unspecified malignant neoplasm of skin of trunk

    C44.500 <mark>Unspecified</mark> malignant neoplasm of anal skin
        Unspecified malignant neoplasm of anal margin
        Unspecified malignant neoplasm of perianal skin

    C44.501 <mark>Unspecified</mark> malignant neoplasm of skin of breast

    C44.509 <mark>Unspecified</mark> malignant neoplasm of skin of other part of trunk

● **C44.51** Basal cell carcinoma of skin of trunk

    C44.510 Basal cell carcinoma of anal skin
        Basal cell carcinoma of anal margin
        Basal cell carcinoma of perianal skin

    C44.511 Basal cell carcinoma of skin of breast

    C44.519 Basal cell carcinoma of skin of other part of trunk

● **C44.52** Squamous cell carcinoma of skin of trunk

    C44.520 Squamous cell carcinoma of anal skin
        Squamous cell carcinoma of anal margin
        Squamous cell carcinoma of perianal skin

    C44.521 Squamous cell carcinoma of skin of breast

    C44.529 Squamous cell carcinoma of skin of other part of trunk

● **C44.59** Other specified malignant neoplasm of skin of trunk

    C44.590 Other specified malignant neoplasm of anal skin
        Other specified malignant neoplasm of anal margin
        Other specified malignant neoplasm of perianal skin

    C44.591 Other specified malignant neoplasm of skin of breast

    C44.599 Other specified malignant neoplasm of skin of other part of trunk

● **C44.6** Other and unspecified malignant neoplasm of skin of upper limb, including shoulder

  ● **C44.60** Unspecified malignant neoplasm of skin of upper limb, including shoulder

    C44.601 <mark>Unspecified</mark> malignant neoplasm of skin of unspecified upper limb, including shoulder

    C44.602 <mark>Unspecified</mark> malignant neoplasm of skin of right upper limb, including shoulder

    C44.609 <mark>Unspecified</mark> malignant neoplasm of skin of left upper limb, including shoulder

  ● **C44.61** Basal cell carcinoma of skin of upper limb, including shoulder

    C44.611 Basal cell carcinoma of skin of <mark>unspecified</mark> upper limb, including shoulder

    C44.612 Basal cell carcinoma of skin of right upper limb, including shoulder

    C44.619 Basal cell carcinoma of skin of left upper limb, including shoulder

  ● **C44.62** Squamous cell carcinoma of skin of upper limb, including shoulder

    C44.621 Squamous cell carcinoma of skin of <mark>unspecified</mark> upper limb, including shoulder

    C44.622 Squamous cell carcinoma of skin of right upper limb, including shoulder

    C44.629 Squamous cell carcinoma of skin of left upper limb, including shoulder

◄ New ⏴ Revised ~~deleted~~ Deleted | Excludes 1 | Excludes 2 | Includes | Use additional | Code first | Code also | Unspecified

OGCR Official Guidelines X Assign placeholder X ● Use Additional Character(s) ▶ Manifestation Code **Coding Clinic**

● C44.69   Other specified malignant neoplasm of skin of upper limb, including shoulder

     C44.691   Other specified malignant neoplasm of skin of unspecified upper limb, including shoulder

     C44.692   Other specified malignant neoplasm of skin of right upper limb, including shoulder

     C44.699   Other specified malignant neoplasm of skin of left upper limb, including shoulder

● C44.7   Other and unspecified malignant neoplasm of skin of lower limb, including hip

   ● C44.70   Unspecified malignant neoplasm of skin of lower limb, including hip

     C44.701   Unspecified malignant neoplasm of skin of unspecified lower limb, including hip

     C44.702   Unspecified malignant neoplasm of skin of right lower limb, including hip

     C44.709   Unspecified malignant neoplasm of skin of left lower limb, including hip

   ● C44.71   Basal cell carcinoma of skin of lower limb, including hip

     C44.711   Basal cell carcinoma of skin of unspecified lower limb, including hip

     C44.712   Basal cell carcinoma of skin of right lower limb, including hip

     C44.719   Basal cell carcinoma of skin of left lower limb, including hip

   ● C44.72   Squamous cell carcinoma of skin of lower limb, including hip

     C44.721   Squamous cell carcinoma of skin of unspecified lower limb, including hip

     C44.722   Squamous cell carcinoma of skin of right lower limb, including hip

     C44.729   Squamous cell carcinoma of skin of left lower limb, including hip

   ● C44.79   Other specified malignant neoplasm of skin of lower limb, including hip

     C44.791   Other specified malignant neoplasm of skin of unspecified lower limb, including hip

     C44.792   Other specified malignant neoplasm of skin of right lower limb, including hip

     C44.799   Other specified malignant neoplasm of skin of left lower limb, including hip

● C44.8   Other and unspecified malignant neoplasm of overlapping sites of skin

     C44.80   Unspecified malignant neoplasm of overlapping sites of skin

     C44.81   Basal cell carcinoma of overlapping sites of skin

     C44.82   Squamous cell carcinoma of overlapping sites of skin

     C44.89   Other specified malignant neoplasm of overlapping sites of skin

● C44.9   Other and unspecified malignant neoplasm of skin, unspecified

     C44.90   Unspecified malignant neoplasm of skin, unspecified

        Malignant neoplasm of unspecified site of skin

     C44.91   Basal cell carcinoma of skin, unspecified

     C44.92   Squamous cell carcinoma of skin, unspecified

     C44.99   Other specified malignant neoplasm of skin, unspecified

MALIGNANT NEOPLASMS OF MESOTHELIAL AND SOFT TISSUE (C45-C49)

● C45   Mesothelioma

Malignant cells develop in protective lining that covers internal organs (mesothelium) caused by exposure to asbestos

     C45.0   Mesothelioma of pleura

        Excludes1   other malignant neoplasm of pleura (C38.4)

     C45.1   Mesothelioma of peritoneum

        Mesothelioma of cul-de-sac
        Mesothelioma of mesentery
        Mesothelioma of mesocolon
        Mesothelioma of omentum
        Mesothelioma of peritoneum (parietal) (pelvic)

        Excludes1   other malignant neoplasm of soft tissue of peritoneum (C48.-)

     C45.2   Mesothelioma of pericardium

        Excludes1   other malignant neoplasm of pericardium (C38.0)

     C45.7   Mesothelioma of other sites

     C45.9   Mesothelioma, unspecified

● C46   Kaposi's sarcoma

Code first any human immunodeficiency virus [HIV] disease (B20)

     C46.0   Kaposi's sarcoma of skin

     C46.1   Kaposi's sarcoma of soft tissue

        Kaposi's sarcoma of blood vessel
        Kaposi's sarcoma of connective tissue
        Kaposi's sarcoma of fascia
        Kaposi's sarcoma of ligament
        Kaposi's sarcoma of lymphatic(s) NEC
        Kaposi's sarcoma of muscle

        Excludes2   Kaposi's sarcoma of lymph glands and nodes (C46.3)

     C46.2   Kaposi's sarcoma of palate

     C46.3   Kaposi's sarcoma of lymph nodes

     C46.4   Kaposi's sarcoma of gastrointestinal sites

   ● C46.5   Kaposi's sarcoma of lung

     C46.50   Kaposi's sarcoma of unspecified lung

     C46.51   Kaposi's sarcoma of right lung

     C46.52   Kaposi's sarcoma of left lung

     C46.7   Kaposi's sarcoma of other sites

     C46.9   Kaposi's sarcoma, unspecified

        Kaposi's sarcoma of unspecified site

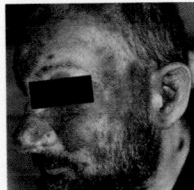

Figure 2-11   Kaposi's sarcoma. There are large confluent hyperpigmented patch-stage lesions with lymphedema. (From Cohen & Powderly: Infectious Diseases, ed 3, Mosby, An Imprint of Elsevier, 2010)

Item 2-5   Kaposi's sarcoma is a cancer that causes patches of abnormal tissue to grow under the skin; in the lining of the mouth, nose, and throat; or in other organs, often beginning and spreading to other organs. Patients who have had organ transplants or patients with AIDS are at high risk for this malignancy.

CHAPTER 2 (C00-D49)

● **C47   Malignant neoplasm of peripheral nerves and autonomic nervous system**

> **Includes**   malignant neoplasm of sympathetic and parasympathetic nerves and ganglia
>
> **Excludes1**   Kaposi's sarcoma of soft tissue (C46.1)

C47.0   Malignant neoplasm of peripheral nerves of head, face and neck

> **Excludes1**   malignant neoplasm of peripheral nerves of orbit (C69.6-)

● **C47.1   Malignant neoplasm of peripheral nerves of upper limb, including shoulder**

> **C47.10   Malignant neoplasm of peripheral nerves of unspecified upper limb, including shoulder**
>
> **C47.11   Malignant neoplasm of peripheral nerves of right upper limb, including shoulder**
>
> **C47.12   Malignant neoplasm of peripheral nerves of left upper limb, including shoulder**

● **C47.2   Malignant neoplasm of peripheral nerves of lower limb, including hip**

> **C47.20   Malignant neoplasm of peripheral nerves of unspecified lower limb, including hip**
>
> **C47.21   Malignant neoplasm of peripheral nerves of right lower limb, including hip**
>
> **C47.22   Malignant neoplasm of peripheral nerves of left lower limb, including hip**

C47.3   Malignant neoplasm of peripheral nerves of thorax

C47.4   Malignant neoplasm of peripheral nerves of abdomen

C47.5   Malignant neoplasm of peripheral nerves of pelvis

C47.6   Malignant neoplasm of peripheral nerves of trunk, unspecified

> Malignant neoplasm of peripheral nerves of unspecified part of trunk

C47.8   Malignant neoplasm of overlapping sites of peripheral nerves and autonomic nervous system

C47.9   Malignant neoplasm of peripheral nerves and autonomic nervous system, unspecified

> Malignant neoplasm of unspecified site of peripheral nerves and autonomic nervous system

● **C48   Malignant neoplasm of retroperitoneum and peritoneum**

> **Excludes1**   Kaposi's sarcoma of connective tissue (C46.1)
> mesothelioma (C45.-)

C48.0   Malignant neoplasm of retroperitoneum

> *Behind/outside of peritoneum*

C48.1   Malignant neoplasm of specified parts of peritoneum

> *Serous membrane lining abdominopelvic walls and covering viscera*
> Malignant neoplasm of cul-de-sac
> Malignant neoplasm of mesentery
> Malignant neoplasm of mesocolon
> Malignant neoplasm of omentum
> Malignant neoplasm of parietal peritoneum
> Malignant neoplasm of pelvic peritoneum

C48.2   Malignant neoplasm of peritoneum, unspecified

C48.8   Malignant neoplasm of overlapping sites of retroperitoneum and peritoneum

● **C49   Malignant neoplasm of other connective and soft tissue**

> **Includes**   malignant neoplasm of blood vessel
> malignant neoplasm of bursa
> malignant neoplasm of cartilage
> malignant neoplasm of fascia
> malignant neoplasm of fat
> malignant neoplasm of ligament, except uterine
> malignant neoplasm of lymphatic vessel
> malignant neoplasm of muscle
> malignant neoplasm of synovia
> malignant neoplasm of tendon (sheath)
>
> **Excludes1**   malignant neoplasm of cartilage (of):
> articular (C40-C41)
> larynx (C32.3)
> nose (C30.0)
> malignant neoplasm of connective tissue of breast (C50.-)
>
> **Excludes2**   Kaposi's sarcoma of soft tissue (C46.1)
> malignant neoplasm of heart (C38.0)
> malignant neoplasm of peripheral nerves and autonomic nervous system (C47.-)
> malignant neoplasm of peritoneum (C48.2)
> malignant neoplasm of retroperitoneum (C48.0)
> malignant neoplasm of uterine ligament (C57.3)
> mesothelioma (C45.-)

C49.0   Malignant neoplasm of connective and soft tissue of head, face and neck

> Malignant neoplasm of connective tissue of ear
> Malignant neoplasm of connective tissue of eyelid
>
> **Excludes1**   connective tissue of orbit (C69.6-)

● **C49.1   Malignant neoplasm of connective and soft tissue of upper limb, including shoulder**

> **C49.10   Malignant neoplasm of connective and soft tissue of unspecified upper limb, including shoulder**
>
> **C49.11   Malignant neoplasm of connective and soft tissue of right upper limb, including shoulder**
>
> **C49.12   Malignant neoplasm of connective and soft tissue of left upper limb, including shoulder**

● **C49.2   Malignant neoplasm of connective and soft tissue of lower limb, including hip**

> **C49.20   Malignant neoplasm of connective and soft tissue of unspecified lower limb, including hip**
>
> **C49.21   Malignant neoplasm of connective and soft tissue of right lower limb, including hip**
>
> **C49.22   Malignant neoplasm of connective and soft tissue of left lower limb, including hip**

C49.3   Malignant neoplasm of connective and soft tissue of thorax

> Malignant neoplasm of axilla
> Malignant neoplasm of diaphragm
> Malignant neoplasm of great vessels
>
> **Excludes1**   malignant neoplasm of breast (C50.-)
> malignant neoplasm of heart (C38.0)
> malignant neoplasm of mediastinum (C38.1-C38.3)
> malignant neoplasm of thymus (C37)

C49.4   Malignant neoplasm of connective and soft tissue of abdomen

> Malignant neoplasm of abdominal wall
> Malignant neoplasm of hypochondrium

C49.5   Malignant neoplasm of connective and soft tissue of pelvis

> Malignant neoplasm of buttock
> Malignant neoplasm of groin
> Malignant neoplasm of perineum

◀ New   ◀▦ Revised   ~~deleted~~ Deleted   Excludes 1   Excludes 2   Includes   Use additional   Code first   Code also   Unspecified

OGCR Official Guidelines   X Assign placeholder X   ● Use Additional Character(s)   ▶ Manifestation Code   **Coding Clinic**

C49.6   **Malignant neoplasm of connective and soft tissue of trunk, unspecified**
  Malignant neoplasm of back NOS

C49.8   **Malignant neoplasm of overlapping sites of connective and soft tissue**
  Primary malignant neoplasm of two or more contiguous sites of connective and soft tissue

C49.9   **Malignant neoplasm of connective and soft tissue, unspecified**

MALIGNANT NEOPLASMS OF BREAST (C50)

● **C50** **Malignant neoplasm of breast**

  Includes connective tissue of breast
      Paget's disease of breast
      Paget's disease of nipple
       Intraductal carcinoma of breast characterized by eczema-like inflammatory skin changes

  Use additional code to identify estrogen receptor status (Z17.0, Z17.1)

  Excludes1 skin of breast (C44.501, C44.511, C44.521, C44.591)

● C50.0 **Malignant neoplasm of nipple and areola**

 ● C50.01 **Malignant neoplasm of nipple and areola, female**

  C50.011 Malignant neoplasm of nipple and areola, right female breast ♀

  C50.012 Malignant neoplasm of nipple and areola, left female breast ♀

  C50.019 Malignant neoplasm of nipple and areola, unspecified female breast ♀

 ● C50.02 **Malignant neoplasm of nipple and areola, male**

  C50.021 Malignant neoplasm of nipple and areola, right male breast ♂

  C50.022 Malignant neoplasm of nipple and areola, left male breast ♂

  C50.029 Malignant neoplasm of nipple and areola, unspecified male breast ♂

● C50.1 **Malignant neoplasm of central portion of breast**

 ● C50.11 **Malignant neoplasm of central portion of breast, female**

  C50.111 Malignant neoplasm of central portion of right female breast ♀

  C50.112 Malignant neoplasm of central portion of left female breast ♀

  C50.119 Malignant neoplasm of central portion of unspecified female breast ♀

 ● C50.12 **Malignant neoplasm of central portion of breast, male**

  C50.121 Malignant neoplasm of central portion of right male breast ♂

  C50.122 Malignant neoplasm of central portion of left male breast ♂

  C50.129 Malignant neoplasm of central portion of unspecified male breast ♂

● C50.2 **Malignant neoplasm of upper-inner quadrant of breast**

 ● C50.21 **Malignant neoplasm of upper-inner quadrant of breast, female**

  C50.211 Malignant neoplasm of upper-inner quadrant of right female breast ♀

  C50.212 Malignant neoplasm of upper-inner quadrant of left female breast ♀

  C50.219 Malignant neoplasm of upper-inner quadrant of unspecified female breast ♀

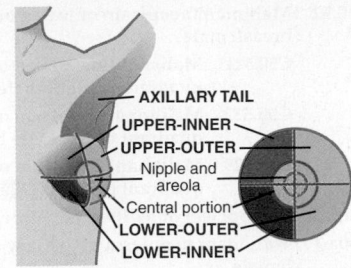

Figure 2-12 Female breast quadrants and axillary tail.

 ● C50.22 **Malignant neoplasm of upper-inner quadrant of breast, male**

  C50.221 Malignant neoplasm of upper-inner quadrant of right male breast ♂

  C50.222 Malignant neoplasm of upper-inner quadrant of left male breast ♂

  C50.229 Malignant neoplasm of upper-inner quadrant of unspecified male breast ♂

● C50.3 **Malignant neoplasm of lower-inner quadrant of breast**

 ● C50.31 **Malignant neoplasm of lower-inner quadrant of breast, female**

  C50.311 Malignant neoplasm of lower-inner quadrant of right female breast ♀

  C50.312 Malignant neoplasm of lower-inner quadrant of left female breast ♀

  C50.319 Malignant neoplasm of lower-inner quadrant of unspecified female breast ♀

 ● C50.32 **Malignant neoplasm of lower-inner quadrant of breast, male**

  C50.321 Malignant neoplasm of lower-inner quadrant of right male breast ♂

  C50.322 Malignant neoplasm of lower-inner quadrant of left male breast ♂

  C50.329 Malignant neoplasm of lower-inner quadrant of unspecified male breast ♂

● C50.4 **Malignant neoplasm of upper-outer quadrant of breast**

 ● C50.41 **Malignant neoplasm of upper-outer quadrant of breast, female**

  C50.411 Malignant neoplasm of upper-outer quadrant of right female breast ♀

  C50.412 Malignant neoplasm of upper-outer quadrant of left female breast ♀

  C50.419 Malignant neoplasm of upper-outer quadrant of unspecified female breast ♀

 ● C50.42 **Malignant neoplasm of upper-outer quadrant of breast, male**

  C50.421 Malignant neoplasm of upper-outer quadrant of right male breast ♂

  C50.422 Malignant neoplasm of upper-outer quadrant of left male breast ♂

  C50.429 Malignant neoplasm of upper-outer quadrant of unspecified male breast ♂

● C50.5 **Malignant neoplasm of lower-outer quadrant of breast**

 ● C50.51 **Malignant neoplasm of lower-outer quadrant of breast, female**

  C50.511 Malignant neoplasm of lower-outer quadrant of right female breast ♀

  C50.512 Malignant neoplasm of lower-outer quadrant of left female breast ♀

  C50.519 Malignant neoplasm of lower-outer quadrant of unspecified female breast ♀

N Newborn Age: 0 **P** Pediatric Age: 0–17 **M** Maternity DX: 12–55 **A** Adult Age: 15–124 ♀ Females Only ♂ Males Only

781

- C50.52 **Malignant neoplasm of lower-outer quadrant of breast, male**
  - C50.521 Malignant neoplasm of lower-outer quadrant of right male breast ♂
  - C50.522 Malignant neoplasm of lower-outer quadrant of left male breast ♂
  - C50.529 Malignant neoplasm of lower-outer quadrant of unspecified male breast ♂
- C50.6 **Malignant neoplasm of axillary tail of breast**
  - C50.61 **Malignant neoplasm of axillary tail of breast, female**
    - C50.611 Malignant neoplasm of axillary tail of right female breast ♀
    - C50.612 Malignant neoplasm of axillary tail of left female breast ♀
    - C50.619 Malignant neoplasm of axillary tail of unspecified female breast ♀
  - C50.62 **Malignant neoplasm of axillary tail of breast, male**
    - C50.621 Malignant neoplasm of axillary tail of right male breast ♂
    - C50.622 Malignant neoplasm of axillary tail of left male breast ♂
    - C50.629 Malignant neoplasm of axillary tail of unspecified male breast ♂
- C50.8 **Malignant neoplasm of overlapping sites of breast**
  - C50.81 **Malignant neoplasm of overlapping sites of breast, female**
    - C50.811 Malignant neoplasm of overlapping sites of right female breast ♀
    - C50.812 Malignant neoplasm of overlapping sites of left female breast ♀
    - C50.819 Malignant neoplasm of overlapping sites of unspecified female breast ♀
  - C50.82 **Malignant neoplasm of overlapping sites of breast, male**
    - C50.821 Malignant neoplasm of overlapping sites of right male breast ♂
    - C50.822 Malignant neoplasm of overlapping sites of left male breast ♂
    - C50.829 Malignant neoplasm of overlapping sites of unspecified male breast ♂
- C50.9 **Malignant neoplasm of breast of unspecified site**
  - C50.91 **Malignant neoplasm of breast of unspecified site, female**
    - C50.911 Malignant neoplasm of unspecified site of right female breast ♀
    - C50.912 Malignant neoplasm of unspecified site of left female breast ♀
    - C50.919 Malignant neoplasm of unspecified site of unspecified female breast ♀
  - C50.92 **Malignant neoplasm of breast of unspecified site, male**
    - C50.921 Malignant neoplasm of unspecified site of right male breast ♂
    - C50.922 Malignant neoplasm of unspecified site of left male breast ♂
    - C50.929 Malignant neoplasm of unspecified site of unspecified male breast ♂

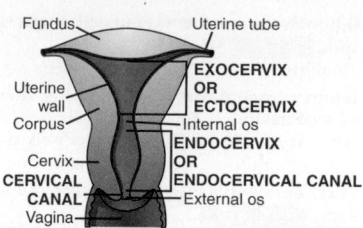

Figure 2-13 Cervix uteri.

MALIGNANT NEOPLASMS OF FEMALE GENITAL ORGANS (C51-C58)

> **Includes**   malignant neoplasm of skin of female genital organs

- C51 **Malignant neoplasm of vulva**
  > **Excludes1**   carcinoma in situ of vulva (D07.1)
  - C51.0 **Malignant neoplasm of labium majus** ♀
    Outer folds of skin external female genitalia
    Malignant neoplasm of Bartholin's [greater vestibular] gland
  - C51.1 **Malignant neoplasm of labium minus** ♀
    Two inner folds surrounding vulva in female genitalia
  - C51.2 **Malignant neoplasm of clitoris** ♀
  - C51.8 **Malignant neoplasm of overlapping sites of vulva** ♀
  - C51.9 **Malignant neoplasm of vulva, unspecified** ♀
    Malignant neoplasm of external female genitalia NOS
    Malignant neoplasm of pudendum

- C52 **Malignant neoplasm of vagina** ♀
  > **Excludes1**   carcinoma in situ of vagina (D07.2)

- C53 **Malignant neoplasm of cervix uteri**
  > **Excludes1**   carcinoma in situ of cervix uteri (D06.-)
  - C53.0 **Malignant neoplasm of endocervix** ♀
    Inside the cervix
  - C53.1 **Malignant neoplasm of exocervix** ♀
    Outside the cervix
  - C53.8 **Malignant neoplasm of overlapping sites of cervix uteri** ♀
  - C53.9 **Malignant neoplasm of cervix uteri, unspecified** ♀

- C54 **Malignant neoplasm of corpus uteri**
  - C54.0 **Malignant neoplasm of isthmus uteri** ♀
    Constricted part of uterus between cervix and body
    Malignant neoplasm of lower uterine segment
  - C54.1 **Malignant neoplasm of endometrium** ♀
    Lining of uterus
  - C54.2 **Malignant neoplasm of myometrium** ♀
    Middle layer of uterine wall consisting of smooth muscle supporting stromal and vascular tissue
  - C54.3 **Malignant neoplasm of fundus uteri** ♀
    Top rounded portion of uterus
  - C54.8 **Malignant neoplasm of overlapping sites of corpus uteri** ♀
    Main body of uterus
  - C54.9 **Malignant neoplasm of corpus uteri, unspecified** ♀

- C55 **Malignant neoplasm of uterus, part unspecified** ♀

- C56 **Malignant neoplasm of ovary**
  Use additional code to identify any functional activity
  - C56.1 **Malignant neoplasm of right ovary** ♀
  - C56.2 **Malignant neoplasm of left ovary** ♀
  - C56.9 **Malignant neoplasm of unspecified ovary** ♀

◄ New   ◄ Revised   ~~deleted~~ Deleted   Excludes 1   Excludes 2   Includes   Use additional   Code first   Code also   Unspecified

OGCR Official Guidelines   X Assign placeholder X   ● Use Additional Character(s)   ▶ Manifestation Code   **Coding Clinic**

● C57   Malignant neoplasm of other and unspecified female genital
organs
   ● C57.0   Malignant neoplasm of fallopian tube
         Malignant neoplasm of oviduct
         Malignant neoplasm of uterine tube
         C57.00   Malignant neoplasm of unspecified fallopian
                   tube ♀
         C57.01   Malignant neoplasm of right fallopian tube ♀
         C57.02   Malignant neoplasm of left fallopian tube ♀
   ● C57.1   Malignant neoplasm of broad ligament
         C57.10   Malignant neoplasm of unspecified broad
                   ligament ♀
         C57.11   Malignant neoplasm of right broad ligament ♀
         C57.12   Malignant neoplasm of left broad ligament ♀
   ● C57.2   Malignant neoplasm of round ligament
         C57.20   Malignant neoplasm of unspecified round
                   ligament ♀
         C57.21   Malignant neoplasm of right round ligament ♀
         C57.22   Malignant neoplasm of left round ligament ♀
      C57.3   Malignant neoplasm of parametrium ♀
               Malignant neoplasm of uterine ligament NOS
      C57.4   Malignant neoplasm of uterine adnexa, unspecified ♀
      C57.7   Malignant neoplasm of other specified female genital
               organs ♀
               Malignant neoplasm of wolffian body or duct
      C57.8   Malignant neoplasm of overlapping sites of female
               genital organs ♀
               Primary malignant neoplasm of two or more
                   contiguous sites of the female genital organs whose
                   point of origin cannot be determined
               Primary tubo-ovarian malignant neoplasm whose point
                   of origin cannot be determined
               Primary utero-ovarian malignant neoplasm whose
                   point of origin cannot be determined
      C57.9   Malignant neoplasm of female genital
               organ, unspecified ♀
               Malignant neoplasm of female genitourinary tract NOS

   C58   Malignant neoplasm of placenta ♀
      Includes   choriocarcinoma NOS
                      chorionepithelioma NOS
      Excludes1   chorioadenoma (destruens) (D39.2)
                      hydatidiform mole NOS (O01.9)
                      invasive hydatidiform mole (D39.2)
                      male choriocarcinoma NOS (C62.9-)
                      malignant hydatidiform mole (D39.2)

MALIGNANT NEOPLASMS OF MALE GENITAL ORGANS (C60-C63)
   Includes   malignant neoplasm of skin of male genital
                   organs

● C60   Malignant neoplasm of penis
      C60.0   Malignant neoplasm of prepuce ♂
               Malignant neoplasm of foreskin
      C60.1   Malignant neoplasm of glans penis ♂
      C60.2   Malignant neoplasm of body of penis ♂
               Malignant neoplasm of corpus cavernosum
      C60.8   Malignant neoplasm of overlapping sites of penis ♂
      C60.9   Malignant neoplasm of penis, unspecified ♂
               Malignant neoplasm of skin of penis NOS

   C61   Malignant neoplasm of prostate ♂
      Excludes1   malignant neoplasm of seminal vesicle (C63.7)

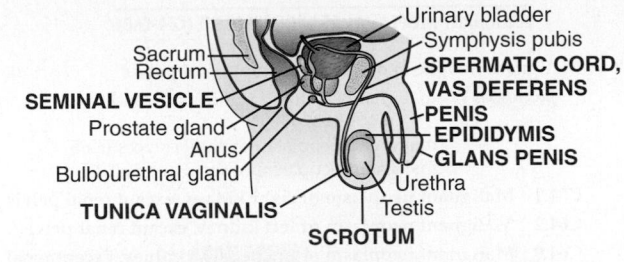

Figure 2-14   Penis and other male genital organs.

● C62   Malignant neoplasm of testis
         Use additional code to identify any functional activity.
   ● C62.0   Malignant neoplasm of undescended testis
               Malignant neoplasm of ectopic testis
               Malignant neoplasm of retained testis
         C62.00   Malignant neoplasm of unspecified
                   undescended testis ♂
         C62.01   Malignant neoplasm of undescended right
                   testis ♂
         C62.02   Malignant neoplasm of undescended left
                   testis ♂
   ● C62.1   Malignant neoplasm of descended testis
               Malignant neoplasm of scrotal testis
         C62.10   Malignant neoplasm of unspecified descended
                   testis, unspecified side ♂
         C62.11   Malignant neoplasm of descended right testis ♂
         C62.12   Malignant neoplasm of descended left testis ♂
   ● C62.9   Malignant neoplasm of testis, unspecified whether
               descended or undescended
         C62.90   Malignant neoplasm of unspecified
                   testis, unspecified whether descended or
                   undescended ♂
                   Malignant neoplasm of testis NOS
         C62.91   Malignant neoplasm of right testis, unspecified
                   whether descended or undescended ♂
         C62.92   Malignant neoplasm of left testis, unspecified
                   whether descended or undescended ♂

● C63   Malignant neoplasm of other and unspecified male genital
organs
   ● C63.0   Malignant neoplasm of epididymis
         C63.00   Malignant neoplasm of unspecified
                   epididymis ♂
         C63.01   Malignant neoplasm of right epididymis ♂
         C63.02   Malignant neoplasm of left epididymis ♂
   ● C63.1   Malignant neoplasm of spermatic cord
         C63.10   Malignant neoplasm of unspecified spermatic
                   cord ♂
         C63.11   Malignant neoplasm of right spermatic cord ♂
         C63.12   Malignant neoplasm of left spermatic cord ♂
      C63.2   Malignant neoplasm of scrotum ♂
               Malignant neoplasm of skin of scrotum
      C63.7   Malignant neoplasm of other specified male genital
               organs ♂
               Malignant neoplasm of seminal vesicle
               Malignant neoplasm of tunica vaginalis
      C63.8   Malignant neoplasm of overlapping sites of male genital
               organs ♂
               Primary malignant neoplasm of two or more
                   contiguous sites of male genital organs whose
                   point of origin cannot be determined
      C63.9   Malignant neoplasm of male genital
               organ, unspecified ♂
               Malignant neoplasm of male genitourinary tract NOS

CHAPTER 2 (C00-D49)

MALIGNANT NEOPLASMS OF URINARY TRACT (C64-C68)

● **C64**   **Malignant neoplasm of kidney, except renal pelvis**
> **Excludes1**   malignant carcinoid tumor of the kidney (C7A.093)
> malignant neoplasm of renal calyces (C65.-)
> malignant neoplasm of renal pelvis (C65.-)

    C64.1   **Malignant neoplasm of right kidney, except renal pelvis**

    C64.2   **Malignant neoplasm of left kidney, except renal pelvis**

    C64.9   **Malignant neoplasm of unspecified kidney, except renal pelvis**

● **C65**   **Malignant neoplasm of renal pelvis**
> **Includes**   malignant neoplasm of pelviureteric junction
> malignant neoplasm of renal calyces

    C65.1   **Malignant neoplasm of right renal pelvis**

    C65.2   **Malignant neoplasm of left renal pelvis**

    C65.9   **Malignant neoplasm of unspecified renal pelvis**

● **C66**   **Malignant neoplasm of ureter**
> **Excludes1**   malignant neoplasm of ureteric orifice of bladder (C67.6)

    C66.1   **Malignant neoplasm of right ureter**

    C66.2   **Malignant neoplasm of left ureter**

    C66.9   **Malignant neoplasm of unspecified ureter**

● **C67**   **Malignant neoplasm of bladder**

    C67.0   **Malignant neoplasm of trigone of bladder**
> *Triangular area formed by three openings in the floor of urinary bladder*

    C67.1   **Malignant neoplasm of dome of bladder**
> *Vaulted roof*

    C67.2   **Malignant neoplasm of lateral wall of bladder**
> *Side walls*

    C67.3   **Malignant neoplasm of anterior wall of bladder**
> *Front wall*

    C67.4   **Malignant neoplasm of posterior wall of bladder**
> *Back wall*

    C67.5   **Malignant neoplasm of bladder neck**
> *Joining of bladder and urethra*
> Malignant neoplasm of internal urethral orifice

    C67.6   **Malignant neoplasm of ureteric orifice**
> *Opening from bladder to ureters*

    C67.7   **Malignant neoplasm of urachus**
> *Embryonic canal that connects the urinary bladder with the structure that forms the umbilical cord (allantois)*

    C67.8   **Malignant neoplasm of overlapping sites of bladder**

    C67.9   **Malignant neoplasm of bladder, unspecified**

● **C68**   **Malignant neoplasm of other and unspecified urinary organs**
> **Excludes1**   malignant neoplasm of female genitourinary tract NOS (C57.9)
> malignant neoplasm of male genitourinary tract NOS (C63.9)

    C68.0   **Malignant neoplasm of urethra**
> > **Excludes1**   malignant neoplasm of urethral orifice of bladder (C67.5)

    C68.1   **Malignant neoplasm of paraurethral glands**
> *Group of glands of female urethra drained by paraurethral ducts; AKA Skene glands, female prostate*

    C68.8   **Malignant neoplasm of overlapping sites of urinary organs**
> *Primary malignant neoplasm of two or more contiguous sites of urinary organs whose point of origin cannot be determined*

    C68.9   **Malignant neoplasm of urinary organ, unspecified**
> Malignant neoplasm of urinary system NOS

MALIGNANT NEOPLASMS OF EYE, BRAIN AND OTHER PARTS OF CENTRAL NERVOUS SYSTEM (C69-C72)

● **C69**   **Malignant neoplasm of eye and adnexa**
> **Excludes1**   malignant neoplasm of connective tissue of eyelid (C49.0)
> malignant neoplasm of eyelid (skin) (C43.1-, C44.1-)
> malignant neoplasm of optic nerve (C72.3-)

● **C69.0**   **Malignant neoplasm of conjunctiva**

    C69.00   **Malignant neoplasm of unspecified conjunctiva**

    C69.01   **Malignant neoplasm of right conjunctiva**

    C69.02   **Malignant neoplasm of left conjunctiva**

● **C69.1**   **Malignant neoplasm of cornea**

    C69.10   **Malignant neoplasm of unspecified cornea**

    C69.11   **Malignant neoplasm of right cornea**

    C69.12   **Malignant neoplasm of left cornea**

● **C69.2**   **Malignant neoplasm of retina**
> **Excludes1**   dark area on retina (D49.81)
> neoplasm of unspecified behavior of retina and choroid (D49.81)
> retinal freckle (D49.81)

    C69.20   **Malignant neoplasm of unspecified retina**

    C69.21   **Malignant neoplasm of right retina**

    C69.22   **Malignant neoplasm of left retina**

● **C69.3**   **Malignant neoplasm of choroid**

    C69.30   **Malignant neoplasm of unspecified choroid**

    C69.31   **Malignant neoplasm of right choroid**

    C69.32   **Malignant neoplasm of left choroid**

● **C69.4**   **Malignant neoplasm of ciliary body**

    C69.40   **Malignant neoplasm of unspecified ciliary body**

    C69.41   **Malignant neoplasm of right ciliary body**

    C69.42   **Malignant neoplasm of left ciliary body**

● **C69.5**   **Malignant neoplasm of lacrimal gland and duct**
> Malignant neoplasm of lacrimal sac
> Malignant neoplasm of nasolacrimal duct

    C69.50   **Malignant neoplasm of unspecified lacrimal gland and duct**

    C69.51   **Malignant neoplasm of right lacrimal gland and duct**

    C69.52   **Malignant neoplasm of left lacrimal gland and duct**

● **C69.6**   **Malignant neoplasm of orbit**
> Malignant neoplasm of connective tissue of orbit
> Malignant neoplasm of extraocular muscle
> Malignant neoplasm of peripheral nerves of orbit
> Malignant neoplasm of retrobulbar tissue
> Malignant neoplasm of retro-ocular tissue
> > **Excludes1**   malignant neoplasm of orbital bone (C41.0)

    C69.60   **Malignant neoplasm of unspecified orbit**

    C69.61   **Malignant neoplasm of right orbit**

    C69.62   **Malignant neoplasm of left orbit**

● **C69.8**   **Malignant neoplasm of overlapping sites of eye and adnexa**

    C69.80   **Malignant neoplasm of overlapping sites of unspecified eye and adnexa**

    C69.81   **Malignant neoplasm of overlapping sites of right eye and adnexa**

    C69.82   **Malignant neoplasm of overlapping sites of left eye and adnexa**

● **C69.9**   **Malignant neoplasm of unspecified site of eye**
> Malignant neoplasm of eyeball

    C69.90   **Malignant neoplasm of unspecified site of unspecified eye**

    C69.91   **Malignant neoplasm of unspecified site of right eye**

    C69.92   **Malignant neoplasm of unspecified site of left eye**

◀ New   ◀▥ Revised   ~~deleted~~ Deleted   Excludes 1   Excludes 2   Includes   Use additional   Code first   Code also   Unspecified
OGCR Official Guidelines   X Assign placeholder X   ● Use Additional Character(s)   ▶ Manifestation Code   **Coding Clinic**

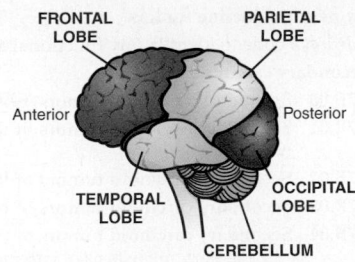

Figure 2-15 The brain.

● **C70 Malignant neoplasm of meninges**
  C70.0   Malignant neoplasm of cerebral meninges
  C70.1   Malignant neoplasm of spinal meninges
  C70.9   Malignant neoplasm of meninges, unspecified

● **C71 Malignant neoplasm of brain**
  Excludes1   malignant neoplasm of cranial nerves
                (C72.2-C72.5)
              retrobulbar malignant neoplasm (C69.6-)
  C71.0   Malignant neoplasm of cerebrum, except lobes and
          ventricles
          Malignant neoplasm of supratentorial NOS
  C71.1   Malignant neoplasm of frontal lobe
  C71.2   Malignant neoplasm of temporal lobe
  C71.3   Malignant neoplasm of parietal lobe
  C71.4   Malignant neoplasm of occipital lobe
  C71.5   Malignant neoplasm of cerebral ventricle
          Excludes1   malignant neoplasm of fourth cerebral
                        ventricle (C71.7)
  C71.6   Malignant neoplasm of cerebellum
  C71.7   Malignant neoplasm of brain stem
          Malignant neoplasm of fourth cerebral ventricle
          Infratentorial malignant neoplasm NOS
  C71.8   Malignant neoplasm of overlapping sites of brain
  C71.9   Malignant neoplasm of brain, unspecified

● **C72 Malignant neoplasm of spinal cord, cranial nerves and other**
  parts of central nervous system
  Excludes1   malignant neoplasm of meninges (C70.-)
              malignant neoplasm of peripheral nerves and
                autonomic nervous system (C47.-)
  C72.0   Malignant neoplasm of spinal cord
  C72.1   Malignant neoplasm of cauda equina
          Lower end of spinal column
  ● C72.2   **Malignant neoplasm of olfactory nerve**
            Malignant neoplasm of olfactory bulb
    C72.20   Malignant neoplasm of unspecified olfactory
             nerve
    C72.21   Malignant neoplasm of right olfactory nerve
    C72.22   Malignant neoplasm of left olfactory nerve
  ● C72.3   **Malignant neoplasm of optic nerve**
    C72.30   Malignant neoplasm of unspecified optic nerve
    C72.31   Malignant neoplasm of right optic nerve
    C72.32   Malignant neoplasm of left optic nerve
  ● C72.4   **Malignant neoplasm of acoustic nerve**
    C72.40   Malignant neoplasm of unspecified acoustic
             nerve
    C72.41   Malignant neoplasm of right acoustic nerve
    C72.42   Malignant neoplasm of left acoustic nerve

● C72.5   **Malignant neoplasm of other and unspecified cranial**
          nerves
    C72.50   Malignant neoplasm of unspecified cranial
             nerve
             Malignant neoplasm of cranial nerve NOS
    C72.59   Malignant neoplasm of other cranial nerves
  C72.9   Malignant neoplasm of central nervous
          system, unspecified
          Malignant neoplasm of unspecified site of central
            nervous system
          Malignant neoplasm of nervous system NOS

MALIGNANT NEOPLASMS OF THYROID AND OTHER ENDOCRINE GLANDS (C73-C75)

  C73   **Malignant neoplasm of thyroid gland**
        Use additional code to identify any functional activity

● **C74 Malignant neoplasm of adrenal gland**
  ● C74.0   **Malignant neoplasm of cortex of adrenal gland**
    C74.00   Malignant neoplasm of cortex of unspecified
             adrenal gland
    C74.01   Malignant neoplasm of cortex of right adrenal
             gland
    C74.02   Malignant neoplasm of cortex of left adrenal
             gland
  ● C74.1   **Malignant neoplasm of medulla of adrenal gland**
            Pair of glands situated on top of or above each kidney
            ("suprarenal")
    C74.10   Malignant neoplasm of medulla of unspecified
             adrenal gland
    C74.11   Malignant neoplasm of medulla of right
             adrenal gland
    C74.12   Malignant neoplasm of medulla of left adrenal
             gland
  ● C74.9   **Malignant neoplasm of unspecified part of adrenal**
            gland
    C74.90   Malignant neoplasm of unspecified part of
             unspecified adrenal gland
    C74.91   Malignant neoplasm of unspecified part of right
             adrenal gland
    C74.92   Malignant neoplasm of unspecified part of left
             adrenal gland

● **C75 Malignant neoplasm of other endocrine glands and related**
  structures
  Excludes1   malignant carcinoid tumors (C7A.0-)
              malignant neoplasm of adrenal gland (C74.-)
              malignant neoplasm of endocrine pancreas
                (C25.4)
              malignant neoplasm of islets of Langerhans
                (C25.4)
              malignant neoplasm of ovary (C56.-)
              malignant neoplasm of testis (C62.-)
              malignant neoplasm of thymus (C37)
              malignant neoplasm of thyroid gland (C73)
              malignant neuroendocrine tumors (C7A.-)
  C75.0   Malignant neoplasm of parathyroid gland
  C75.1   Malignant neoplasm of pituitary gland
  C75.2   Malignant neoplasm of craniopharyngeal duct
  C75.3   Malignant neoplasm of pineal gland
  C75.4   Malignant neoplasm of carotid body
  C75.5   Malignant neoplasm of aortic body and other
          paraganglia
  C75.8   Malignant neoplasm with pluriglandular
          involvement, unspecified
  C75.9   Malignant neoplasm of endocrine gland, unspecified

CHAPTER 2 (C00-D49)

CHAPTER 2 (C00-D49)

MALIGNANT NEUROENDOCRINE TUMORS (C7A)

● **C7A Malignant neuroendocrine tumors**

> Code also any associated multiple endocrine neoplasia [MEN] syndromes (E31.2-)
>
> Use additional code to identify any associated endocrine syndrome, such as:
> carcinoid syndrome (E34.0)
>
> **Excludes2**   malignant pancreatic islet cell tumors (C25.4)
> Merkel cell carcinoma (C4A.-)

   ● **C7A.0 Malignant carcinoid tumors**

     C7A.00   **Malignant carcinoid tumor of unspecified site**

     ● C7A.01   **Malignant carcinoid tumors of the small intestine**

       C7A.010   **Malignant carcinoid tumor of the duodenum**

       C7A.011   **Malignant carcinoid tumor of the jejunum**

       C7A.012   **Malignant carcinoid tumor of the ileum**

       C7A.019   **Malignant carcinoid tumor of the small intestine, unspecified portion**

     ● C7A.02   **Malignant carcinoid tumors of the appendix, large intestine, and rectum**

       C7A.020   **Malignant carcinoid tumor of the appendix**

       C7A.021   **Malignant carcinoid tumor of the cecum**

       C7A.022   **Malignant carcinoid tumor of the ascending colon**

       C7A.023   **Malignant carcinoid tumor of the transverse colon**

       C7A.024   **Malignant carcinoid tumor of the descending colon**

       C7A.025   **Malignant carcinoid tumor of the sigmoid colon**

       C7A.026   **Malignant carcinoid tumor of the rectum**

       C7A.029   **Malignant carcinoid tumor of the large intestine, unspecified portion**
> Malignant carcinoid tumor of the colon NOS

     ● C7A.09   **Malignant carcinoid tumors of other sites**

       C7A.090   **Malignant carcinoid tumor of the bronchus and lung**

       C7A.091   **Malignant carcinoid tumor of the thymus**

       C7A.092   **Malignant carcinoid tumor of the stomach**

       C7A.093   **Malignant carcinoid tumor of the kidney**

       C7A.094   **Malignant carcinoid tumor of the foregut NOS**

       C7A.095   **Malignant carcinoid tumor of the midgut NOS**

       C7A.096   **Malignant carcinoid tumor of the hindgut NOS**

       C7A.098   **Malignant carcinoid tumors of other sites**

   C7A.1   **Malignant poorly differentiated neuroendocrine tumors**
> Malignant poorly differentiated neuroendocrine tumor NOS
> Malignant poorly differentiated neuroendocrine carcinoma, any site
> High grade neuroendocrine carcinoma, any site

   C7A.8   **Other malignant neuroendocrine tumors**
> Secondary neuroendocrine tumors (C7B)

● **C7B Secondary neuroendocrine tumors**
> Use additional code to identify any functional activity

   ● **C7B.0 Secondary carcinoid tumors**

     C7B.00   **Secondary carcinoid tumors, unspecified site**

     C7B.01   **Secondary carcinoid tumors of distant lymph nodes**

     C7B.02   **Secondary carcinoid tumors of liver**

     C7B.03   **Secondary carcinoid tumors of bone**

     C7B.04   **Secondary carcinoid tumors of peritoneum**
> Mesentery metastasis of carcinoid tumor

     C7B.09   **Secondary carcinoid tumors of other sites**

   C7B.1   **Secondary Merkel cell carcinoma**
> Merkel cell carcinoma nodal presentation
> Merkel cell carcinoma visceral metastatic presentation

   C7B.8   **Other secondary neuroendocrine tumors**

MALIGNANT NEOPLASMS OF ILL-DEFINED, OTHER SECONDARY AND UNSPECIFIED SITES (C76-C80)

● **C76 Malignant neoplasm of other and ill-defined sites**

> **Excludes1**   malignant neoplasm of female genitourinary tract NOS (C57.9)
> malignant neoplasm of male genitourinary tract NOS (C63.9)
> malignant neoplasm of lymphoid, hematopoietic and related tissue (C81-C96)
> malignant neoplasm of skin (C44.-)
> malignant neoplasm of unspecified site NOS (C80.1)

   C76.0   **Malignant neoplasm of head, face and neck**
> Malignant neoplasm of cheek NOS
> Malignant neoplasm of nose NOS

   C76.1   **Malignant neoplasm of thorax**
> Intrathoracic malignant neoplasm NOS
> Malignant neoplasm of axilla NOS
> Thoracic malignant neoplasm NOS

   C76.2   **Malignant neoplasm of abdomen**

   C76.3   **Malignant neoplasm of pelvis**
> Malignant neoplasm of groin NOS
> Malignant neoplasm of sites overlapping systems within the pelvis
> Rectovaginal (septum) malignant neoplasm
> *Between rectum and vagina*
> Rectovesical (septum) malignant neoplasm
> *Between rectum and urinary bladder; AKA vesicorectal*

   ● C76.4   **Malignant neoplasm of upper limb**

     C76.40   **Malignant neoplasm of unspecified upper limb**

     C76.41   **Malignant neoplasm of right upper limb**

     C76.42   **Malignant neoplasm of left upper limb**

   ● C76.5   **Malignant neoplasm of lower limb**

     C76.50   **Malignant neoplasm of unspecified lower limb**

     C76.51   **Malignant neoplasm of right lower limb**

     C76.52   **Malignant neoplasm of left lower limb**

   C76.8   **Malignant neoplasm of other specified ill-defined sites**
> Malignant neoplasm of overlapping ill-defined sites

● **C77 Secondary and unspecified malignant neoplasm of lymph nodes**

> **Excludes1**   malignant neoplasm of lymph nodes, specified as primary (C81-C86, C88, C96.-)
> mesentary metastasis of carcinoid tumor (C7B.04)
> secondary carcinoid tumors of distant lymph nodes (C7B.01)

   C77.0   **Secondary and unspecified malignant neoplasm of lymph nodes of head, face and neck**
> Secondary and unspecified malignant neoplasm of supraclavicular lymph nodes

   C77.1   **Secondary and unspecified malignant neoplasm of intrathoracic lymph nodes**

◄ New   ◀▥ Revised   ~~deleted~~ Deleted   Excludes 1   Excludes 2   Includes   Use additional   Code first   Code also   Unspecified

OGCR Official Guidelines   X Assign placeholder X   ● Use Additional Character(s)   ▶ Manifestation Code   **Coding Clinic**

C77.2 Secondary and unspecified malignant neoplasm of intra-abdominal lymph nodes

C77.3 Secondary and unspecified malignant neoplasm of axilla and upper limb lymph nodes
> Secondary and unspecified malignant neoplasm of pectoral lymph nodes

C77.4 Secondary and unspecified malignant neoplasm of inguinal and lower limb lymph nodes

C77.5 Secondary and unspecified malignant neoplasm of intrapelvic lymph nodes

C77.8 Secondary and unspecified malignant neoplasm of lymph nodes of multiple regions

C77.9 Secondary and unspecified malignant neoplasm of lymph node, unspecified

● **C78** Secondary malignant neoplasm of respiratory and digestive organs
> **Excludes1**   lymph node metastases (C77.0)
> secondary carcinoid tumors of liver (C7B.02)
> secondary carcinoid tumors of peritoneum (C7B.04)

● **C78.0** Secondary malignant neoplasm of lung
     C78.00 Secondary malignant neoplasm of unspecified lung
     C78.01 Secondary malignant neoplasm of right lung
     C78.02 Secondary malignant neoplasm of left lung

C78.1 Secondary malignant neoplasm of mediastinum
> *Thoracic cavity between pleural cavities*

C78.2 Secondary malignant neoplasm of pleura
> *Serous membrane covering lungs and lining thoracic cavity*

● **C78.3** Secondary malignant neoplasm of other and unspecified respiratory organs
     C78.30 Secondary malignant neoplasm of unspecified respiratory organ
     C78.39 Secondary malignant neoplasm of other respiratory organs

C78.4 Secondary malignant neoplasm of small intestine

C78.5 Secondary malignant neoplasm of large intestine and rectum

C78.6 Secondary malignant neoplasm of retroperitoneum and peritoneum

C78.7 Secondary malignant neoplasm of liver and intrahepatic bile duct

● **C78.8** Secondary malignant neoplasm of other and unspecified digestive organs
     C78.80 Secondary malignant neoplasm of unspecified digestive organ
     C78.89 Secondary malignant neoplasm of other digestive organs

● **C79** Secondary malignant neoplasm of other and unspecified sites
> **Excludes1**   lymph node metastases (C77.0)
> secondary carcinoid tumors (C7B.-)
> secondary neuroendocrine tumors (C7B.-)

● **C79.0** Secondary malignant neoplasm of kidney and renal pelvis
     C79.00 Secondary malignant neoplasm of unspecified kidney and renal pelvis
     C79.01 Secondary malignant neoplasm of right kidney and renal pelvis
     C79.02 Secondary malignant neoplasm of left kidney and renal pelvis

Item 2-6 The adrenal glands are a pair of glands situated on top of or above each kidney ("suprarenal") and chiefly responsible for regulating the stress response through the synthesis of corticosteroids and catecholamines, including cortisol and adrenaline.

● **C79.1** Secondary malignant neoplasm of bladder and other and unspecified urinary organs
     C79.10 Secondary malignant neoplasm of unspecified urinary organs
     C79.11 Secondary malignant neoplasm of bladder
     C79.19 Secondary malignant neoplasm of other urinary organs

C79.2 Secondary malignant neoplasm of skin
> **Excludes1**   secondary Merkel cell carcinoma (C7B.1)

● **C79.3** Secondary malignant neoplasm of brain and cerebral meninges
     C79.31 Secondary malignant neoplasm of brain
     C79.32 Secondary malignant neoplasm of cerebral meninges

● **C79.4** Secondary malignant neoplasm of other and unspecified parts of nervous system
     C79.40 Secondary malignant neoplasm of unspecified part of nervous system
     C79.49 Secondary malignant neoplasm of other parts of nervous system

● **C79.5** Secondary malignant neoplasm of bone and bone marrow
> **Excludes1**   secondary carcinoid tumors of bone (C7B.03)
     C79.51 Secondary malignant neoplasm of bone
     C79.52 Secondary malignant neoplasm of bone marrow

● **C79.6** Secondary malignant neoplasm of ovary
     C79.60 Secondary malignant neoplasm of unspecified ovary ♀
     C79.61 Secondary malignant neoplasm of right ovary ♀
     C79.62 Secondary malignant neoplasm of left ovary ♀

● **C79.7** Secondary malignant neoplasm of adrenal gland
     C79.70 Secondary malignant neoplasm of unspecified adrenal gland
     C79.71 Secondary malignant neoplasm of right adrenal gland
     C79.72 Secondary malignant neoplasm of left adrenal gland

● **C79.8** Secondary malignant neoplasm of other specified sites
     C79.81 Secondary malignant neoplasm of breast
     C79.82 Secondary malignant neoplasm of genital organs
     C79.89 Secondary malignant neoplasm of other specified sites

C79.9 Secondary malignant neoplasm of unspecified site
> Metastatic cancer NOS
> Metastatic disease NOS
> **Excludes1**   carcinomatosis NOS (C80.0)
> generalized cancer NOS (C80.0)
> malignant (primary) neoplasm of unspecified site (C80.1)

CHAPTER 2 (C00-D49)

OGCR Section I.C.2.j and k

Disseminated malignant neoplasm, unspecified

j. Code C80.0, Disseminated malignant neoplasm, unspecified, is for use only in those cases where the patient has advanced metastatic disease and no known primary or secondary sites are specified. It should not be used in place of assigning codes for the primary site and all known secondary sites.

Malignant neoplasm without specification of site

k. Code C80.1, Malignant (primary) neoplasm, unspecified, equates to Cancer, unspecified. This code should only be used when no determination can be made as to the primary site of a malignancy. This code should rarely be used in the inpatient setting.

● C80   Malignant neoplasm without specification of site
        Excludes1   malignant carcinoid tumor of unspecified site
                    (C7A.00)
                    malignant neoplasm of specified multiple sites-
                    code to each site

   C80.0   Disseminated malignant neoplasm, unspecified
           Carcinomatosis NOS
           Generalized cancer, unspecified site (primary)
           (secondary)
           Generalized malignancy, unspecified site (primary)
           (secondary)

   C80.1   Malignant (primary) neoplasm, unspecified
           Cancer NOS
           Cancer unspecified site (primary)
           Carcinoma unspecified site (primary)
           Malignancy unspecified site (primary)
           Excludes1   secondary malignant neoplasm of
                       unspecified site (C79.9)

   C80.2   Malignant neoplasm associated with transplanted organ
           Code first complication of transplanted organ (T86.-)
           Use additional code to identify the specific malignancy

   (See Plate 315 on page 49.)

   ### MALIGNANT NEOPLASMS OF LYMPHOID, HEMATOPOIETIC AND RELATED TISSUE (C81-C96)

        Excludes2   Kaposi's sarcoma of lymph nodes (C46.3)
                    secondary and unspecified neoplasm of lymph
                    nodes (C77.-)
                    secondary neoplasm of bone marrow (C79.52)
                    secondary neoplasm of spleen (C78.89)

● C81   Hodgkin lymphoma
        *Form of malignant lymphoma with four types, nodular sclerosis,
        mixed cellularity, lymphocyte depleted, and lymphocyte
        predominant*
        Excludes1   personal history of Hodgkin lymphoma (Z85.71)

   ● C81.0   Nodular lymphocyte predominant Hodgkin lymphoma
             Least aggressive, least common, typically no symptoms
             Lymphocytic-histiocytic predominance Hodgkin's
             disease

      C81.00   Nodular lymphocyte predominant Hodgkin
               lymphoma, unspecified site
      C81.01   Nodular lymphocyte predominant Hodgkin
               lymphoma, lymph nodes of head, face, and
               neck
      C81.02   Nodular lymphocyte predominant Hodgkin
               lymphoma, intrathoracic lymph nodes
      C81.03   Nodular lymphocyte predominant Hodgkin
               lymphoma, intra-abdominal lymph nodes
      C81.04   Nodular lymphocyte predominant Hodgkin
               lymphoma, lymph nodes of axilla and upper
               limb

      C81.05   Nodular lymphocyte predominant Hodgkin
               lymphoma, lymph nodes of inguinal region and
               lower limb
      C81.06   Nodular lymphocyte predominant Hodgkin
               lymphoma, intrapelvic lymph nodes
      C81.07   Nodular lymphocyte predominant Hodgkin
               lymphoma, spleen
      C81.08   Nodular lymphocyte predominant Hodgkin
               lymphoma, lymph nodes of multiple sites
      C81.09   Nodular lymphocyte predominant Hodgkin
               lymphoma, extranodal and solid organ sites

   ● C81.1   Nodular sclerosis classical Hodgkin lymphoma
             Moderately aggressive; most common in young adults

      C81.10   Nodular sclerosis classical Hodgkin
               lymphoma, unspecified site
      C81.11   Nodular sclerosis classical Hodgkin lymphoma,
               lymph nodes of head, face, and neck
      C81.12   Nodular sclerosis classical Hodgkin lymphoma,
               intrathoracic lymph nodes
      C81.13   Nodular sclerosis classical Hodgkin lymphoma,
               intra-abdominal lymph nodes
      C81.14   Nodular sclerosis classical Hodgkin lymphoma,
               lymph nodes of axilla and upper limb
      C81.15   Nodular sclerosis classical Hodgkin lymphoma,
               lymph nodes of inguinal region and lower limb
      C81.16   Nodular sclerosis classical Hodgkin lymphoma,
               intrapelvic lymph nodes
      C81.17   Nodular sclerosis classical Hodgkin lymphoma,
               spleen
      C81.18   Nodular sclerosis classical Hodgkin lymphoma,
               lymph nodes of multiple sites
      C81.19   Nodular sclerosis classical Hodgkin lymphoma,
               extranodal and solid organ sites

   ● C81.2   Mixed cellularity classical Hodgkin lymphoma
             *A type of Hodgkin's that is moderately aggressive with mixed
             cell types*

      C81.20   Mixed cellularity classical Hodgkin
               lymphoma, unspecified site
      C81.21   Mixed cellularity classical Hodgkin lymphoma,
               lymph nodes of head, face, and neck
      C81.22   Mixed cellularity classical Hodgkin lymphoma,
               intrathoracic lymph nodes
      C81.23   Mixed cellularity classical Hodgkin lymphoma,
               intra-abdominal lymph nodes
      C81.24   Mixed cellularity classical Hodgkin lymphoma,
               lymph nodes of axilla and upper limb
      C81.25   Mixed cellularity classical Hodgkin lymphoma,
               lymph nodes of inguinal region and lower limb
      C81.26   Mixed cellularity classical Hodgkin lymphoma,
               intrapelvic lymph nodes
      C81.27   Mixed cellularity classical Hodgkin lymphoma,
               spleen
      C81.28   Mixed cellularity classical Hodgkin lymphoma,
               lymph nodes of multiple sites
      C81.29   Mixed cellularity classical Hodgkin lymphoma,
               extranodal and solid organ sites

   ● C81.3   Lymphocyte depleted classical Hodgkin lymphoma
             Most aggressive type with poor prognosis

      C81.30   Lymphocyte depleted classical Hodgkin
               lymphoma, unspecified site
      C81.31   Lymphocyte depleted classical Hodgkin
               lymphoma, lymph nodes of head, face, and
               neck
      C81.32   Lymphocyte depleted classical Hodgkin
               lymphoma, intrathoracic lymph nodes

◀ New   ◀▥ Revised   ~~deleted~~ Deleted   Excludes 1   Excludes 2   Includes   Use additional   Code first   Code also   Unspecified

OGCR Official Guidelines   X Assign placeholder X   ● Use Additional Character(s)   ▶ Manifestation Code   **Coding Clinic**

C81.33   Lymphocyte depleted classical Hodgkin lymphoma, intra-abdominal lymph nodes

C81.34   Lymphocyte depleted classical Hodgkin lymphoma, lymph nodes of axilla and upper limb

C81.35   Lymphocyte depleted classical Hodgkin lymphoma, lymph nodes of inguinal region and lower limb

C81.36   Lymphocyte depleted classical Hodgkin lymphoma, intrapelvic lymph nodes

C81.37   Lymphocyte depleted classical Hodgkin lymphoma, spleen

C81.38   Lymphocyte depleted classical Hodgkin lymphoma, lymph nodes of multiple sites

C81.39   Lymphocyte depleted classical Hodgkin lymphoma, extranodal and solid organ sites

● C81.4   Lymphocyte-rich classical Hodgkin lymphoma

    Excludes1   nodular lymphocyte predominant Hodgkin lymphoma (C81.0-)

C81.40   Lymphocyte-rich classical Hodgkin lymphoma, unspecified site

C81.41   Lymphocyte-rich classical Hodgkin lymphoma, lymph nodes of head, face, and neck

C81.42   Lymphocyte-rich classical Hodgkin lymphoma, intrathoracic lymph nodes

C81.43   Lymphocyte-rich classical Hodgkin lymphoma, intra-abdominal lymph nodes

C81.44   Lymphocyte-rich classical Hodgkin lymphoma, lymph nodes of axilla and upper limb

C81.45   Lymphocyte-rich classical Hodgkin lymphoma, lymph nodes of inguinal region and lower limb

C81.46   Lymphocyte-rich classical Hodgkin lymphoma, intrapelvic lymph nodes

C81.47   Lymphocyte-rich classical Hodgkin lymphoma, spleen

C81.48   Lymphocyte-rich classical Hodgkin lymphoma, lymph nodes of multiple sites

C81.49   Lymphocyte-rich classical Hodgkin lymphoma, extranodal and solid organ sites

● C81.7   Other classical Hodgkin lymphoma
    Classical Hodgkin lymphoma NOS

C81.70   Other classical Hodgkin lymphoma, unspecified site

C81.71   Other classical Hodgkin lymphoma, lymph nodes of head, face, and neck

C81.72   Other classical Hodgkin lymphoma, intrathoracic lymph nodes

C81.73   Other classical Hodgkin lymphoma, intra-abdominal lymph nodes

C81.74   Other classical Hodgkin lymphoma, lymph nodes of axilla and upper limb

C81.75   Other classical Hodgkin lymphoma, lymph nodes of inguinal region and lower limb

C81.76   Other classical Hodgkin lymphoma, intrapelvic lymph nodes

C81.77   Other classical Hodgkin lymphoma, spleen

C81.78   Other classical Hodgkin lymphoma, lymph nodes of multiple sites

C81.79   Other classical Hodgkin lymphoma, extranodal and solid organ sites

● C81.9   Hodgkin lymphoma, unspecified

C81.90   Hodgkin lymphoma, unspecified, unspecified site

C81.91   Hodgkin lymphoma, unspecified, lymph nodes of head, face, and neck

C81.92   Hodgkin lymphoma, unspecified, intrathoracic lymph nodes

C81.93   Hodgkin lymphoma, unspecified, intra-abdominal lymph nodes

C81.94   Hodgkin lymphoma, unspecified, lymph nodes of axilla and upper limb

C81.95   Hodgkin lymphoma, unspecified, lymph nodes of inguinal region and lower limb

C81.96   Hodgkin lymphoma, unspecified, intrapelvic lymph nodes

C81.97   Hodgkin lymphoma, unspecified, spleen

C81.98   Hodgkin lymphoma, unspecified, lymph nodes of multiple sites

C81.99   Hodgkin lymphoma, unspecified, extranodal and solid organ sites

● C82   Follicular lymphoma
    Group of malignant lymphomas

    Includes   follicular lymphoma with or without diffuse areas

    Excludes1   mature T/NK-cell lymphomas (C84.-) personal history of non-Hodgkin lymphoma (Z85.72)

● C82.0   Follicular lymphoma grade I

C82.00   Follicular lymphoma grade I, unspecified site

C82.01   Follicular lymphoma grade I, lymph nodes of head, face, and neck

C82.02   Follicular lymphoma grade I, intrathoracic lymph nodes

C82.03   Follicular lymphoma grade I, intra-abdominal lymph nodes

C82.04   Follicular lymphoma grade I, lymph nodes of axilla and upper limb

C82.05   Follicular lymphoma grade I, lymph nodes of inguinal region and lower limb

C82.06   Follicular lymphoma grade I, intrapelvic lymph nodes

C82.07   Follicular lymphoma grade I, spleen

C82.08   Follicular lymphoma grade I, lymph nodes of multiple sites

C82.09   Follicular lymphoma grade I, extranodal and solid organ sites

● C82.1   Follicular lymphoma grade II

C82.10   Follicular lymphoma grade II, unspecified site

C82.11   Follicular lymphoma grade II, lymph nodes of head, face, and neck

C82.12   Follicular lymphoma grade II, intrathoracic lymph nodes

C82.13   Follicular lymphoma grade II, intra-abdominal lymph nodes

C82.14   Follicular lymphoma grade II, lymph nodes of axilla and upper limb

C82.15   Follicular lymphoma grade II, lymph nodes of inguinal region and lower limb

C82.16   Follicular lymphoma grade II, intrapelvic lymph nodes

C82.17   Follicular lymphoma grade II, spleen

C82.18   Follicular lymphoma grade II, lymph nodes of multiple sites

C82.19   Follicular lymphoma grade II, extranodal and solid organ sites

● C82.2   Follicular lymphoma grade III, unspecified

C82.20   Follicular lymphoma grade III, unspecified, unspecified site

C82.21   Follicular lymphoma grade III, unspecified, lymph nodes of head, face, and neck

C82.22   Follicular lymphoma grade III, unspecified, intrathoracic lymph nodes

C82.23   Follicular lymphoma grade III, unspecified, intra-abdominal lymph nodes

CHAPTER 2 (C00-D49)

C82.24   Follicular lymphoma grade III, unspecified, lymph nodes of axilla and upper limb

C82.25   Follicular lymphoma grade III, unspecified, lymph nodes of inguinal region and lower limb

C82.26   Follicular lymphoma grade III, unspecified, intrapelvic lymph nodes

C82.27   Follicular lymphoma grade III, unspecified, spleen

C82.28   Follicular lymphoma grade III, unspecified, lymph nodes of multiple sites

C82.29   Follicular lymphoma grade III, unspecified, extranodal and solid organ sites

● C82.3   Follicular lymphoma grade IIIa

C82.30   Follicular lymphoma grade IIIa, unspecified site

C82.31   Follicular lymphoma grade IIIa, lymph nodes of head, face, and neck

C82.32   Follicular lymphoma grade IIIa, intrathoracic lymph nodes

C82.33   Follicular lymphoma grade IIIa, intra-abdominal lymph nodes

C82.34   Follicular lymphoma grade IIIa, lymph nodes of axilla and upper limb

C82.35   Follicular lymphoma grade IIIa, lymph nodes of inguinal region and lower limb

C82.36   Follicular lymphoma grade IIIa, intrapelvic lymph nodes

C82.37   Follicular lymphoma grade IIIa, spleen

C82.38   Follicular lymphoma grade IIIa, lymph nodes of multiple sites

C82.39   Follicular lymphoma grade IIIa, extranodal and solid organ sites

● C82.4   Follicular lymphoma grade IIIb

C82.40   Follicular lymphoma grade IIIb, unspecified site

C82.41   Follicular lymphoma grade IIIb, lymph nodes of head, face, and neck

C82.42   Follicular lymphoma grade IIIb, intrathoracic lymph nodes

C82.43   Follicular lymphoma grade IIIb, intra-abdominal lymph nodes

C82.44   Follicular lymphoma grade IIIb, lymph nodes of axilla and upper limb

C82.45   Follicular lymphoma grade IIIb, lymph nodes of inguinal region and lower limb

C82.46   Follicular lymphoma grade IIIb, intrapelvic lymph nodes

C82.47   Follicular lymphoma grade IIIb, spleen

C82.48   Follicular lymphoma grade IIIb, lymph nodes of multiple sites

C82.49   Follicular lymphoma grade IIIb, extranodal and solid organ sites

● C82.5   Diffuse follicle center lymphoma

C82.50   Diffuse follicle center lymphoma, unspecified site

C82.51   Diffuse follicle center lymphoma, lymph nodes of head, face, and neck

C82.52   Diffuse follicle center lymphoma, intrathoracic lymph nodes

C82.53   Diffuse follicle center lymphoma, intra-abdominal lymph nodes

C82.54   Diffuse follicle center lymphoma, lymph nodes of axilla and upper limb

C82.55   Diffuse follicle center lymphoma, lymph nodes of inguinal region and lower limb

C82.56   Diffuse follicle center lymphoma, intrapelvic lymph nodes

C82.57   Diffuse follicle center lymphoma, spleen

C82.58   Diffuse follicle center lymphoma, lymph nodes of multiple sites

C82.59   Diffuse follicle center lymphoma, extranodal and solid organ sites

● C82.6   Cutaneous follicle center lymphoma

C82.60   Cutaneous follicle center lymphoma, unspecified site

C82.61   Cutaneous follicle center lymphoma, lymph nodes of head, face, and neck

C82.62   Cutaneous follicle center lymphoma, intrathoracic lymph nodes

C82.63   Cutaneous follicle center lymphoma, intra-abdominal lymph nodes

C82.64   Cutaneous follicle center lymphoma, lymph nodes of axilla and upper limb

C82.65   Cutaneous follicle center lymphoma, lymph nodes of inguinal region and lower limb

C82.66   Cutaneous follicle center lymphoma, intrapelvic lymph nodes

C82.67   Cutaneous follicle center lymphoma, spleen

C82.68   Cutaneous follicle center lymphoma, lymph nodes of multiple sites

C82.69   Cutaneous follicle center lymphoma, extranodal and solid organ sites

● C82.8   Other types of follicular lymphoma

C82.80   Other types of follicular lymphoma, unspecified site

C82.81   Other types of follicular lymphoma, lymph nodes of head, face, and neck

C82.82   Other types of follicular lymphoma, intrathoracic lymph nodes

C82.83   Other types of follicular lymphoma, intra-abdominal lymph nodes

C82.84   Other types of follicular lymphoma, lymph nodes of axilla and upper limb

C82.85   Other types of follicular lymphoma, lymph nodes of inguinal region and lower limb

C82.86   Other types of follicular lymphoma, intrapelvic lymph nodes

C82.87   Other types of follicular lymphoma, spleen

C82.88   Other types of follicular lymphoma, lymph nodes of multiple sites

C82.89   Other types of follicular lymphoma, extranodal and solid organ sites

● C82.9   Follicular lymphoma, unspecified

C82.90   Follicular lymphoma, unspecified, unspecified site

C82.91   Follicular lymphoma, unspecified, lymph nodes of head, face, and neck

C82.92   Follicular lymphoma, unspecified, intrathoracic lymph nodes

C82.93   Follicular lymphoma, unspecified, intra-abdominal lymph nodes

C82.94   Follicular lymphoma, unspecified, lymph nodes of axilla and upper limb

C82.95   Follicular lymphoma, unspecified, lymph nodes of inguinal region and lower limb

C82.96   Follicular lymphoma, unspecified, intrapelvic lymph nodes

C82.97   Follicular lymphoma, unspecified, spleen

C82.98   Follicular lymphoma, unspecified, lymph nodes of multiple sites

C82.99   Follicular lymphoma, unspecified, extranodal and solid organ sites

◀ New   ◀▥ Revised   ~~deleted~~ Deleted   Excludes 1   Excludes 2   Includes   Use additional   Code first   Code also   Unspecified

OGCR Official Guidelines   X Assign placeholder X   ● Use Additional Character(s)   ▶ Manifestation Code   **Coding Clinic**

● **C83**   **Non-follicular lymphoma**

> **Excludes1**   personal history of non-Hodgkin lymphoma
> (Z85.72)

● **C83.0**   **Small cell B-cell lymphoma**
Lymphoplasmacytic lymphoma
Nodal marginal zone lymphoma
Non-leukemic variant of B-CLL
Splenic marginal zone lymphoma

> **Excludes1**   chronic lymphocytic leukemia (C91.1)
> mature T/NK-cell lymphomas (C84.-)
> Waldenström macroglobulinemia (C88.0)

C83.00   Small cell B-cell lymphoma, unspecified site

C83.01   Small cell B-cell lymphoma, lymph nodes of head, face, and neck

C83.02   Small cell B-cell lymphoma, intrathoracic lymph nodes

C83.03   Small cell B-cell lymphoma, intra-abdominal lymph nodes

C83.04   Small cell B-cell lymphoma, lymph nodes of axilla and upper limb

C83.05   Small cell B-cell lymphoma, lymph nodes of inguinal region and lower limb

C83.06   Small cell B-cell lymphoma, intrapelvic lymph nodes

C83.07   Small cell B-cell lymphoma, spleen

C83.08   Small cell B-cell lymphoma, lymph nodes of multiple sites

C83.09   Small cell B-cell lymphoma, extranodal and solid organ sites

● **C83.1**   **Mantle cell lymphoma**
Centrocytic lymphoma
Malignant lymphomatous polyposis

C83.10   Mantle cell lymphoma, unspecified site

C83.11   Mantle cell lymphoma, lymph nodes of head, face, and neck

C83.12   Mantle cell lymphoma, intrathoracic lymph nodes

C83.13   Mantle cell lymphoma, intra-abdominal lymph nodes

C83.14   Mantle cell lymphoma, lymph nodes of axilla and upper limb

C83.15   Mantle cell lymphoma, lymph nodes of inguinal region and lower limb

C83.16   Mantle cell lymphoma, intrapelvic lymph nodes

C83.17   Mantle cell lymphoma, spleen

C83.18   Mantle cell lymphoma, lymph nodes of multiple sites

C83.19   Mantle cell lymphoma, extranodal and solid organ sites

● **C83.3**   **Diffuse large B-cell lymphoma**
Anaplastic diffuse large B-cell lymphoma
CD30-positive diffuse large B-cell lymphoma
Centroblastic diffuse large B-cell lymphoma
Diffuse large B-cell lymphoma, subtype not specified
Immunoblastic diffuse large B-cell lymphoma
Plasmablastic diffuse large B-cell lymphoma
Diffuse large B-cell lymphoma, subtype not specified
T-cell rich diffuse large B-cell lymphoma

> **Excludes1**   mediastinal (thymic) large B-cell
> lymphoma (C85.2-)
> mature T/NK-cell lymphomas (C84.-)

C83.30   Diffuse large B-cell lymphoma, unspecified site

C83.31   Diffuse large B-cell lymphoma, lymph nodes of head, face, and neck

C83.32   Diffuse large B-cell lymphoma, intrathoracic lymph nodes

C83.33   Diffuse large B-cell lymphoma, intra-abdominal lymph nodes

C83.34   Diffuse large B-cell lymphoma, lymph nodes of axilla and upper limb

C83.35   Diffuse large B-cell lymphoma, lymph nodes of inguinal region and lower limb

C83.36   Diffuse large B-cell lymphoma, intrapelvic lymph nodes

C83.37   Diffuse large B-cell lymphoma, spleen

C83.38   Diffuse large B-cell lymphoma, lymph nodes of multiple sites

C83.39   Diffuse large B-cell lymphoma, extranodal and solid organ sites

● **C83.5**   **Lymphoblastic (diffuse) lymphoma**
Highly malignant type of non-Hodgkin lymphoma with diffuse infiltration
B-precursor lymphoma
Lymphoblastic B-cell lymphoma
Lymphoblastic lymphoma NOS
Lymphoblastic T-cell lymphoma
T-precursor lymphoma

C83.50   Lymphoblastic (diffuse) lymphoma, unspecified site

C83.51   Lymphoblastic (diffuse) lymphoma, lymph nodes of head, face, and neck

C83.52   Lymphoblastic (diffuse) lymphoma, intrathoracic lymph nodes

C83.53   Lymphoblastic (diffuse) lymphoma, intra-abdominal lymph nodes

C83.54   Lymphoblastic (diffuse) lymphoma, lymph nodes of axilla and upper limb

C83.55   Lymphoblastic (diffuse) lymphoma, lymph nodes of inguinal region and lower limb

C83.56   Lymphoblastic (diffuse) lymphoma, intrapelvic lymph nodes

C83.57   Lymphoblastic (diffuse) lymphoma, spleen

C83.58   Lymphoblastic (diffuse) lymphoma, lymph nodes of multiple sites

C83.59   Lymphoblastic (diffuse) lymphoma, extranodal and solid organ sites

● **C83.7**   **Burkitt lymphoma**
Form of small cell lymphoma
Atypical Burkitt lymphoma
Burkitt-like lymphoma

> **Excludes1**   mature B-cell leukemia Burkitt type
> (C91.A-)

C83.70   Burkitt lymphoma, unspecified site

C83.71   Burkitt lymphoma, lymph nodes of head, face, and neck

C83.72   Burkitt lymphoma, intrathoracic lymph nodes

C83.73   Burkitt lymphoma, intra-abdominal lymph nodes

C83.74   Burkitt lymphoma, lymph nodes of axilla and upper limb

C83.75   Burkitt lymphoma, lymph nodes of inguinal region and lower limb

C83.76   Burkitt lymphoma, intrapelvic lymph nodes

C83.77   Burkitt lymphoma, spleen

C83.78   Burkitt lymphoma, lymph nodes of multiple sites

C83.79   Burkitt lymphoma, extranodal and solid organ sites

● **C83.8**   **Other non-follicular lymphoma**
Intravascular large B-cell lymphoma
Lymphoid granulomatosis
Primary effusion B-cell lymphoma

     Excludes1   mediastinal (thymic) large B-cell
         lymphoma (C85.2-)
         T-cell rich B-cell lymphoma (C83.3-)

   C83.80   Other non-follicular lymphoma, unspecified site

   C83.81   Other non-follicular lymphoma, lymph nodes of head, face, and neck

   C83.82   Other non-follicular lymphoma, intrathoracic lymph nodes

   C83.83   Other non-follicular lymphoma, intra-abdominal lymph nodes

   C83.84   Other non-follicular lymphoma, lymph nodes of axilla and upper limb

   C83.85   Other non-follicular lymphoma, lymph nodes of inguinal region and lower limb

   C83.86   Other non-follicular lymphoma, intrapelvic lymph nodes

   C83.87   Other non-follicular lymphoma, spleen

   C83.88   Other non-follicular lymphoma, lymph nodes of multiple sites

   C83.89   Other non-follicular lymphoma, extranodal and solid organ sites

● **C83.9**   Non-follicular (diffuse) lymphoma, unspecified

   C83.90   Non-follicular (diffuse) lymphoma, unspecified, unspecified site

   C83.91   Non-follicular (diffuse) lymphoma, unspecified, lymph nodes of head, face, and neck

   C83.92   Non-follicular (diffuse) lymphoma, unspecified, intrathoracic lymph nodes

   C83.93   Non-follicular (diffuse) lymphoma, unspecified, intra-abdominal lymph nodes

   C83.94   Non-follicular (diffuse) lymphoma, unspecified, lymph nodes of axilla and upper limb

   C83.95   Non-follicular (diffuse) lymphoma, unspecified, lymph nodes of inguinal region and lower limb

   C83.96   Non-follicular (diffuse) lymphoma, unspecified, intrapelvic lymph nodes

   C83.97   Non-follicular (diffuse) lymphoma, unspecified, spleen

   C83.98   Non-follicular (diffuse) lymphoma, unspecified, lymph nodes of multiple sites

   C83.99   Non-follicular (diffuse) lymphoma, unspecified, extranodal and solid organ sites

● **C84**   **Mature T/NK-cell lymphomas**

     Excludes1   personal history of non-Hodgkin lymphoma (Z85.72)

● **C84.0**   **Mycosis fungoides**
Chronic or rapidly progressive form of cutaneous T-cell lymphoma; AKA granuloma fungoides

     Excludes1   peripheral T-cell lymphoma, not classified (C84.4-)

   C84.00   Mycosis fungoides, unspecified site

   C84.01   Mycosis fungoides, lymph nodes of head, face, and neck

   C84.02   Mycosis fungoides, intrathoracic lymph nodes

   C84.03   Mycosis fungoides, intra-abdominal lymph nodes

   C84.04   Mycosis fungoides, lymph nodes of axilla and upper limb

   C84.05   Mycosis fungoides, lymph nodes of inguinal region and lower limb

   C84.06   Mycosis fungoides, intrapelvic lymph nodes

   C84.07   Mycosis fungoides, spleen

   C84.08   Mycosis fungoides, lymph nodes of multiple sites

   C84.09   Mycosis fungoides, extranodal and solid organ sites

● **C84.1**   **Sézary disease**
Type of cutaneous lymphoma affecting T-cells

   C84.10   Sézary disease, unspecified site

   C84.11   Sézary disease, lymph nodes of head, face, and neck

   C84.12   Sézary disease, intrathoracic lymph nodes

   C84.13   Sézary disease, intra-abdominal lymph nodes

   C84.14   Sézary disease, lymph nodes of axilla and upper limb

   C84.15   Sézary disease, lymph nodes of inguinal region and lower limb

   C84.16   Sézary disease, intrapelvic lymph nodes

   C84.17   Sézary disease, spleen

   C84.18   Sézary disease, lymph nodes of multiple sites

   C84.19   Sézary disease, extranodal and solid organ sites

● **C84.4**   **Peripheral T-cell lymphoma, not classified**
Diverse group of blood carcinomas originating from T-cells, requiring aggressive chemotherapy
Lennert's lymphoma
Lymphoepithelioid lymphoma
Mature T-cell lymphoma, not elsewhere classified

   C84.40   Peripheral T-cell lymphoma, not classified, unspecified site

   C84.41   Peripheral T-cell lymphoma, not classified, lymph nodes of head, face, and neck

   C84.42   Peripheral T-cell lymphoma, not classified, intrathoracic lymph nodes

   C84.43   Peripheral T-cell lymphoma, not classified, intra-abdominal lymph nodes

   C84.44   Peripheral T-cell lymphoma, not classified, lymph nodes of axilla and upper limb

   C84.45   Peripheral T-cell lymphoma, not classified, lymph nodes of inguinal region and lower limb

   C84.46   Peripheral T-cell lymphoma, not classified, intrapelvic lymph nodes

   C84.47   Peripheral T-cell lymphoma, not classified, spleen

   C84.48   Peripheral T-cell lymphoma, not classified, lymph nodes of multiple sites

   C84.49   Peripheral T-cell lymphoma, not classified, extranodal and solid organ sites

● **C84.6**   **Anaplastic large cell lymphoma, ALK-positive**
Anaplastic large cell lymphoma, CD30-positive

   C84.60   Anaplastic large cell lymphoma, ALK-positive, unspecified site

   C84.61   Anaplastic large cell lymphoma, ALK-positive, lymph nodes of head, face, and neck

   C84.62   Anaplastic large cell lymphoma, ALK-positive, intrathoracic lymph nodes

   C84.63   Anaplastic large cell lymphoma, ALK-positive, intra-abdominal lymph nodes

◄ New   ◄ Revised   ~~deleted~~ Deleted   Excludes 1   Excludes 2   Includes   Use additional   Code first   Code also   Unspecified

OGCR Official Guidelines   **X** Assign placeholder X   ● Use Additional Character(s)   ▶ Manifestation Code   **Coding Clinic**

Item 2-7 Lymphosarcoma, also known as malignant lymphoma, is a cancer of the lymph system exhibiting abnormal cells encompassing an entire lymph node creating a diffuse pattern without any definite organization. Diffuse pattern lymphoma has a more unfavorable survival outlook than those with a follicular or nodular pattern. Reticulosarcoma is the most common aggressive form of non-Hodgkin's lymphoma.

C84.64 Anaplastic large cell lymphoma, ALK-positive, lymph nodes of axilla and upper limb

C84.65 Anaplastic large cell lymphoma, ALK-positive, lymph nodes of inguinal region and lower limb

C84.66 Anaplastic large cell lymphoma, ALK-positive, intrapelvic lymph nodes

C84.67 Anaplastic large cell lymphoma, ALK-positive, spleen

C84.68 Anaplastic large cell lymphoma, ALK-positive, lymph nodes of multiple sites

C84.69 Anaplastic large cell lymphoma, ALK-positive, extranodal and solid organ sites

● C84.7 Anaplastic large cell lymphoma, ALK-negative

Excludes1 primary cutaneous CD30-positive T-cell proliferations (C86.6-)

C84.70 Anaplastic large cell lymphoma, ALK-negative, unspecified site

C84.71 Anaplastic large cell lymphoma, ALK-negative, lymph nodes of head, face, and neck

C84.72 Anaplastic large cell lymphoma, ALK-negative, intrathoracic lymph nodes

C84.73 Anaplastic large cell lymphoma, ALK-negative, intra-abdominal lymph nodes

C84.74 Anaplastic large cell lymphoma, ALK-negative, lymph nodes of axilla and upper limb

C84.75 Anaplastic large cell lymphoma, ALK-negative, lymph nodes of inguinal region and lower limb

C84.76 Anaplastic large cell lymphoma, ALK-negative, intrapelvic lymph nodes

C84.77 Anaplastic large cell lymphoma, ALK-negative, spleen

C84.78 Anaplastic large cell lymphoma, ALK-negative, lymph nodes of multiple sites

C84.79 Anaplastic large cell lymphoma, ALK-negative, extranodal and solid organ sites

● C84.A Cutaneous T-cell lymphoma, unspecified

C84.A0 Cutaneous T-cell lymphoma, unspecified, unspecified site

C84.A1 Cutaneous T-cell lymphoma, unspecified lymph nodes of head, face, and neck

C84.A2 Cutaneous T-cell lymphoma, unspecified, intrathoracic lymph nodes

C84.A3 Cutaneous T-cell lymphoma, unspecified, intra-abdominal lymph nodes

C84.A4 Cutaneous T-cell lymphoma, unspecified, lymph nodes of axilla and upper limb

C84.A5 Cutaneous T-cell lymphoma, unspecified, lymph nodes of inguinal region and lower limb

C84.A6 Cutaneous T-cell lymphoma, unspecified, intrapelvic lymph nodes

C84.A7 Cutaneous T-cell lymphoma, unspecified, spleen

C84.A8 Cutaneous T-cell lymphoma, unspecified, lymph nodes of multiple sites

C84.A9 Cutaneous T-cell lymphoma, unspecified, extranodal and solid organ sites

● C84.Z Other mature T/NK-cell lymphomas

Note: If T-cell lineage or involvement is mentioned in conjunction with a specific lymphoma, code to the more specific description.

Excludes1 angioimmunoblastic T-cell lymphoma (C86.5)
blastic NK-cell lymphoma (C86.4)
enteropathy-type T-cell lymphoma (C86.2)
extranodal NK-cell lymphoma, nasal type (C86.0)
hepatosplenic T-cell lymphoma (C86.1)
primary cutaneous CD30-positive T-cell proliferations (C86.6)
subcutaneous panniculitis-like T-cell lymphoma (C86.3)
T-cell leukemia (C91.1-)

C84.Z0 Other mature T/NK-cell lymphomas, unspecified site

C84.Z1 Other mature T/NK-cell lymphomas, lymph nodes of head, face, and neck

C84.Z2 Other mature T/NK-cell lymphomas, intrathoracic lymph nodes

C84.Z3 Other mature T/NK-cell lymphomas, intra-abdominal lymph nodes

C84.Z4 Other mature T/NK-cell lymphomas, lymph nodes of axilla and upper limb

C84.Z5 Other mature T/NK-cell lymphomas, lymph nodes of inguinal region and lower limb

C84.Z6 Other mature T/NK-cell lymphomas, intrapelvic lymph nodes

C84.Z7 Other mature T/NK-cell lymphomas, spleen

C84.Z8 Other mature T/NK-cell lymphomas, lymph nodes of multiple sites

C84.Z9 Other mature T/NK-cell lymphomas, extranodal and solid organ sites

● C84.9 Mature T/NK-cell lymphomas, unspecified
NK/T cell lymphoma NOS

Excludes1 mature T-cell lymphoma, not elsewhere classified (C84.4-)

C84.90 Mature T/NK-cell lymphomas, unspecified, unspecified site

C84.91 Mature T/NK-cell lymphomas, unspecified, lymph nodes of head, face, and neck

C84.92 Mature T/NK-cell lymphomas, unspecified, intrathoracic lymph nodes

C84.93 Mature T/NK-cell lymphomas, unspecified, intra-abdominal lymph nodes

C84.94 Mature T/NK-cell lymphomas, unspecified, lymph nodes of axilla and upper limb

C84.95 Mature T/NK-cell lymphomas, unspecified, lymph nodes of inguinal region and lower limb

C84.96 Mature T/NK-cell lymphomas, unspecified, intrapelvic lymph nodes

C84.97 Mature T/NK-cell lymphomas, unspecified, spleen

C84.98 Mature T/NK-cell lymphomas, unspecified, lymph nodes of multiple sites

C84.99 Mature T/NK-cell lymphomas, unspecified, extranodal and solid organ sites

● **C85   Other specified and unspecified types of non-Hodgkin lymphoma**

> **Excludes1**   other specified types of T/NK-cell lymphoma (C86.-)
> personal history of non-Hodgkin lymphoma (Z85.72)

● **C85.1   Unspecified B-cell lymphoma**

> **Note:** If B-cell lineage or involvement is mentioned in conjunction with a specific lymphoma, code to the more specific description.

    C85.10   **Unspecified** B-cell lymphoma, unspecified site

    C85.11   **Unspecified** B-cell lymphoma, lymph nodes of head, face, and neck

    C85.12   **Unspecified** B-cell lymphoma, intrathoracic lymph nodes

    C85.13   **Unspecified** B-cell lymphoma, intra-abdominal lymph nodes

    C85.14   **Unspecified** B-cell lymphoma, lymph nodes of axilla and upper limb

    C85.15   **Unspecified** B-cell lymphoma, lymph nodes of inguinal region and lower limb

    C85.16   **Unspecified** B-cell lymphoma, intrapelvic lymph nodes

    C85.17   **Unspecified** B-cell lymphoma, spleen

    C85.18   **Unspecified** B-cell lymphoma, lymph nodes of multiple sites

    C85.19   **Unspecified** B-cell lymphoma, extranodal and solid organ sites

● **C85.2   Mediastinal (thymic) large B-cell lymphoma**

    C85.20   Mediastinal (thymic) large B-cell lymphoma, **unspecified** site

    C85.21   Mediastinal (thymic) large B-cell lymphoma, lymph nodes of head, face, and neck

    C85.22   Mediastinal (thymic) large B-cell lymphoma, intrathoracic lymph nodes

    C85.23   Mediastinal (thymic) large B-cell lymphoma, intra-abdominal lymph nodes

    C85.24   Mediastinal (thymic) large B-cell lymphoma, lymph nodes of axilla and upper limb

    C85.25   Mediastinal (thymic) large B-cell lymphoma, lymph nodes of inguinal region and lower limb

    C85.26   Mediastinal (thymic) large B-cell lymphoma, intrapelvic lymph nodes

    C85.27   Mediastinal (thymic) large B-cell lymphoma, spleen

    C85.28   Mediastinal (thymic) large B-cell lymphoma, lymph nodes of multiple sites

    C85.29   Mediastinal (thymic) large B-cell lymphoma, extranodal and solid organ sites

● **C85.8   Other specified types of non-Hodgkin lymphoma**

    C85.80   Other specified types of non-Hodgkin lymphoma, **unspecified** site

    C85.81   Other specified types of non-Hodgkin lymphoma, lymph nodes of head, face, and neck

    C85.82   Other specified types of non-Hodgkin lymphoma, intrathoracic lymph nodes

    C85.83   Other specified types of non-Hodgkin lymphoma, intra-abdominal lymph nodes

    C85.84   Other specified types of non-Hodgkin lymphoma, lymph nodes of axilla and upper limb

    C85.85   Other specified types of non-Hodgkin lymphoma, lymph nodes of inguinal region and lower limb

    C85.86   Other specified types of non-Hodgkin lymphoma, intrapelvic lymph nodes

    C85.87   Other specified types of non-Hodgkin lymphoma, spleen

    C85.88   Other specified types of non-Hodgkin lymphoma, lymph nodes of multiple sites

    C85.89   Other specified types of non-Hodgkin lymphoma, extranodal and solid organ sites

● **C85.9   Non-Hodgkin lymphoma, unspecified**

> Lymphoma NOS
> Malignant lymphoma NOS
> Non-Hodgkin lymphoma NOS

    C85.90   Non-Hodgkin lymphoma, **unspecified**, unspecified site

    C85.91   Non-Hodgkin lymphoma, **unspecified**, lymph nodes of head, face, and neck

    C85.92   Non-Hodgkin lymphoma, **unspecified**, intrathoracic lymph nodes

    C85.93   Non-Hodgkin lymphoma, **unspecified**, intra-abdominal lymph nodes

    C85.94   Non-Hodgkin lymphoma, **unspecified**, lymph nodes of axilla and upper limb

    C85.95   Non-Hodgkin lymphoma, **unspecified**, lymph nodes of inguinal region and lower limb

    C85.96   Non-Hodgkin lymphoma, **unspecified**, intrapelvic lymph nodes

    C85.97   Non-Hodgkin lymphoma, **unspecified**, spleen

    C85.98   Non-Hodgkin lymphoma, **unspecified**, lymph nodes of multiple sites

    C85.99   Non-Hodgkin lymphoma, **unspecified**, extranodal and solid organ sites

● **C86   Other specified types of T/NK-cell lymphoma**

> **Excludes1**   anaplastic large cell lymphoma, ALK negative (C84.7-)
> anaplastic large cell lymphoma, ALK positive (C84.6-)
> mature T/NK-cell lymphomas (C84.-)
> other specified types of non-Hodgkin lymphoma (C85.8-)

C86.0   Extranodal NK/T-cell lymphoma, nasal type

C86.1   Hepatosplenic T-cell lymphoma
> Alpha-beta and gamma delta types

C86.2   Enteropathy-type (intestinal) T-cell lymphoma
> Enteropathy associated T-cell lymphoma

C86.3   Subcutaneous panniculitis-like T-cell lymphoma

C86.4   Blastic NK-cell lymphoma

C86.5   Angioimmunoblastic T-cell lymphoma
> Angioimmunoblastic lymphadenopathy with dysproteinemia (AILD)

C86.6   Primary cutaneous CD30-positive T-cell proliferations
> Lymphomatoid papulosis
> Primary cutaneous anaplastic large cell lymphoma
> Primary cutaneous CD30-positive large T-cell lymphoma

● **C88   Malignant immunoproliferative diseases and certain other B-cell lymphomas**

> *Diseases involving immune system*

> **Excludes1**   B-cell lymphoma, unspecified (C85.1-)
> personal history of other malignant neoplasms of lymphoid, hematopoietic and related tissues (Z85.79)

C88.0   Waldenström's macroglobulinemia
> Lymphoplasmacytic lymphoma with IgM-production
> Macroglobulinemia (idiopathic) (primary)
>
> > **Excludes1**   small cell B-cell lymphoma (C83.0)

C88.2   Heavy chain disease
> Franklin disease
> Gamma heavy chain disease
> Mu heavy chain disease

C88.3   **Immunoproliferative small intestinal disease**
     Alpha heavy chain disease
     Mediterranean lymphoma

C88.4   **Extranodal marginal zone B-cell lymphoma of mucosa-associated lymphoid tissue [MALT-lymphoma]**
     Lymphoma of skin-associated lymphoid tissue [SALT-lymphoma]
     Lymphoma of bronchial-associated lymphoid tissue [BALT-lymphoma]
     Excludes1   high malignant (diffuse large B-cell) lymphoma (C83.3-)

C88.8   **Other malignant immunoproliferative diseases**

C88.9   **Malignant immunoproliferative disease, unspecified**
     Immunoproliferative disease NOS

● **C90**   **Multiple myeloma and malignant plasma cell neoplasms**
     Excludes1   personal history of other malignant neoplasms of lymphoid, hematopoietic and related tissues (Z85.79)

● **C90.0**   **Multiple myeloma**
     Kahler's disease
     Medullary plasmacytoma
     Myelomatosis
     Plasma cell myeloma
     Excludes1   solitary myeloma (C90.3-)
                 solitary plasmacytoma (C90.3-)

     C90.00   **Multiple myeloma not having achieved remission**
         Multiple myeloma with failed remission
         Multiple myeloma NOS

     C90.01   **Multiple myeloma in remission**

     C90.02   **Multiple myeloma in relapse**

● **C90.1**   **Plasma cell leukemia**
     Rare type of acute leukemia
     Plasmacytic leukemia

     C90.10   **Plasma cell leukemia not having achieved remission**
         Plasma cell leukemia with failed remission
         Plasma cell leukemia NOS

     C90.11   **Plasma cell leukemia in remission**

     C90.12   **Plasma cell leukemia in relapse**

● **C90.2**   **Extramedullary plasmacytoma**
     Malignant monoclonal plasma cell tumor growing in soft tissue; AKA plasma cell dyscrasias

     C90.20   **Extramedullary plasmacytoma not having achieved remission**
         Extramedullary plasmacytoma with failed remission
         Extramedullary plasmacytoma NOS

     C90.21   **Extramedullary plasmacytoma in remission**

     C90.22   **Extramedullary plasmacytoma in relapse**

● **C90.3**   **Solitary plasmacytoma**
     Localized malignant plasma cell tumor NOS
     Plasmacytoma NOS
     Solitary myeloma

     C90.30   **Solitary plasmacytoma not having achieved remission**
         Solitary plasmacytoma with failed remission
         Solitary plasmacytoma NOS

     C90.31   **Solitary plasmacytoma in remission**

     C90.32   **Solitary plasmacytoma in relapse**

Item 2–9   Leukemia is a cancer (acute or chronic) of the blood-forming tissues of the bone marrow. Blood cells all start out as stem cells. They mature and become red cells, white cells, or platelets. There are three main types of leukocytes (white cells that fight infection): monocytes, lymphocytes, and granulocytes. **Acute monocytic leukemia** (AML) affects monocytes. **Acute lymphoid leukemia** (ALL) affects lymphocytes, and **acute myeloid leukemia** (AML) affects cells that typically develop into white blood cells (not lymphocytes), though it may develop in other blood cells.

● **C91**   **Lymphoid leukemia**
     Type of leukemia affecting circulating cells of lymphoid origin
     Excludes1   personal history of leukemia (Z85.6)

● **C91.0**   **Acute lymphoblastic leukemia [ALL]**
     Note: Code C91.0 should only be used for T-cell and B-cell precursor leukemia

     C91.00   **Acute lymphoblastic leukemia not having achieved remission**
         Acute lymphoblastic leukemia with failed remission
         Acute lymphoblastic leukemia NOS

     C91.01   **Acute lymphoblastic leukemia, in remission**

     C91.02   **Acute lymphoblastic leukemia, in relapse**

● **C91.1**   **Chronic lymphocytic leukemia of B-cell type**
     Lymphoplasmacytic leukemia
     Richter syndrome
     Excludes1   lymphoplasmacytic lymphoma (C83.0-)

     C91.10   **Chronic lymphocytic leukemia of B-cell type not having achieved remission**
         Chronic lymphocytic leukemia of B-cell type with failed remission
         Chronic lymphocytic leukemia of B-cell type NOS

     C91.11   **Chronic lymphocytic leukemia of B-cell type in remission**

     C91.12   **Chronic lymphocytic leukemia of B-cell type in relapse**

● **C91.3**   **Prolymphocytic leukemia of B-cell type**
     Chronic leukemia with symptoms of large number of circulating lymphocytes

     C91.30   **Prolymphocytic leukemia of B-cell type not having achieved remission**
         Prolymphocytic leukemia of B-cell type with failed remission
         Prolymphocytic leukemia of B-cell type NOS

     C91.31   **Prolymphocytic leukemia of B-cell type, in remission**

     C91.32   **Prolymphocytic leukemia of B-cell type, in relapse**

● **C91.4**   **Hairy cell leukemia**
     Chronic leukemia with splenomegaly and excessive number of abnormal large mononuclear cells covered by hairlike villi
     Leukemic reticuloendotheliosis

     C91.40   **Hairy cell leukemia not having achieved remission**
         Hairy cell leukemia with failed remission
         Hairy cell leukemia NOS

     C91.41   **Hairy cell leukemia, in remission**

     C91.42   **Hairy cell leukemia, in relapse**

CHAPTER 2 (C00-D49)

Item 2–8 Multiple myeloma is a cancer of a plasma cell (a type of white blood cell) and is an incurable but treatable disease. Immunoproliferative neoplasm is a term for diseases (mostly cancers) in which the immune system cells proliferate.

● **C91.5** **Adult T-cell lymphoma/leukemia (HTLV-1-associated)**
    Acute variant of adult T-cell lymphoma/leukemia (HTLV-1-associated)
    Chronic variant of adult T-cell lymphoma/leukemia (HTLV-1-associated)
    Lymphomatoid variant of adult T-cell lymphoma/leukemia (HTLV-1-associated)
    Smouldering variant of adult T-cell lymphoma/leukemia (HTLV-1-associated)

    C91.50 **Adult T-cell lymphoma/leukemia (HTLV-1-associated) not having achieved remission**   **A**
        Adult T-cell lymphoma/leukemia (HTLV-1-associated) with failed remission
        Adult T-cell lymphoma/leukemia (HTLV-1-associated) NOS

    C91.51 **Adult T-cell lymphoma/leukemia (HTLV-1-associated), in remission**   **A**

    C91.52 **Adult T-cell lymphoma/leukemia (HTLV-1-associated), in relapse**   **A**

● **C91.6** **Prolymphocytic leukemia of T-cell type**

    C91.60 **Prolymphocytic leukemia of T-cell type not having achieved remission**
        Prolymphocytic leukemia of T-cell type with failed remission
        Prolymphocytic leukemia of T-cell type NOS

    C91.61 **Prolymphocytic leukemia of T-cell type, in remission**

    C91.62 **Prolymphocytic leukemia of T-cell type, in relapse**

● **C91.A** **Mature B-cell leukemia Burkitt-type**

    Excludes1   Burkitt lymphoma (C83.7-)

    C91.A0 **Mature B-cell leukemia Burkitt-type not having achieved remission**
        Mature B-cell leukemia Burkitt-type with failed remission
        Mature B-cell leukemia Burkitt-type NOS

    C91.A1 **Mature B-cell leukemia Burkitt-type, in remission**

    C91.A2 **Mature B-cell leukemia Burkitt-type, in relapse**

● **C91.Z** **Other lymphoid leukemia**
    T-cell large granular lymphocytic leukemia (associated with rheumatoid arthritis)

    C91.Z0 **Other lymphoid leukemia not having achieved remission**
        Other lymphoid leukemia with failed remission
        Other lymphoid leukemia NOS

    C91.Z1 **Other lymphoid leukemia, in remission**

    C91.Z2 **Other lymphoid leukemia, in relapse**

● **C91.9** **Lymphoid leukemia, unspecified**

    C91.90 **Lymphoid leukemia, unspecified not having achieved remission**
        Lymphoid leukemia with failed remission
        Lymphoid leukemia NOS

    C91.91 **Lymphoid leukemia, unspecified, in remission**

    C91.92 **Lymphoid leukemia, unspecified, in relapse**

● **C92** **Myeloid leukemia**

    Includes   granulocytic leukemia
          myelogenous leukemia

    Excludes1   personal history of leukemia (Z85.6)

● **C92.0** **Acute myeloblastic leukemia**
    Acute myeloblastic leukemia, minimal differentiation
    Acute myeloblastic leukemia (with maturation)
    Acute myeloblastic leukemia 1/ETO
    Acute myeloblastic leukemia M0
    Acute myeloblastic leukemia M1
    Acute myeloblastic leukemia M2
    Acute myeloblastic leukemia with t(8;21)
    Acute myeloblastic leukemia (without a FAB classification) NOS
    Refractory anemia with excess blasts in transformation [RAEB T]

    Excludes1   acute exacerbation of chronic myeloid leukemia (C92.10)
          refractory anemia with excess of blasts not in transformation (D46.2-)

    C92.00 **Acute myeloblastic leukemia, not having achieved remission**
        Acute myeloblastic leukemia with failed remission
        Acute myeloblastic leukemia NOS

    C92.01 **Acute myeloblastic leukemia, in remission**

    C92.02 **Acute myeloblastic leukemia, in relapse**

● **C92.1** **Chronic myeloid leukemia, BCR/ABL-positive**
    Chronic myelogenous leukemia, Philadelphia chromosome (Ph1) positive
    Chronic myelogenous leukemia, t(9;22) (q34;q11)
    Chronic myelogenous leukemia with crisis of blast cells

    Excludes1   atypical chronic myeloid leukemia BCR/ABL-negative (C92.2-)
          chronic myelomonocytic leukemia (C93.1-)
          chronic myeloproliferative disease (D47.1)

    C92.10 **Chronic myeloid leukemia, BCR/ABL-positive, not having achieved remission**
        Chronic myeloid leukemia, BCR/ABL-positive with failed remission
        Chronic myeloid leukemia, BCR/ABL-positive NOS

    C92.11 **Chronic myeloid leukemia, BCR/ABL-positive, in remission**

    C92.12 **Chronic myeloid leukemia, BCR/ABL-positive, in relapse**

● **C92.2** **Atypical chronic myeloid leukemia, BCR/ABL-negative**

    C92.20 **Atypical chronic myeloid leukemia, BCR/ABL-negative, not having achieved remission**
        Atypical chronic myeloid leukemia, BCR/ABL-negative with failed remission
        Atypical chronic myeloid leukemia, BCR/ABL-negative NOS

    C92.21 **Atypical chronic myeloid leukemia, BCR/ABL-negative, in remission**

    C92.22 **Atypical chronic myeloid leukemia, BCR/ABL-negative, in relapse**

● **C92.3** **Myeloid sarcoma**
    A malignant tumor of immature myeloid cells
    Chloroma
    Granulocytic sarcoma

    C92.30 **Myeloid sarcoma, not having achieved remission**
        Myeloid sarcoma with failed remission
        Myeloid sarcoma NOS

    C92.31 **Myeloid sarcoma, in remission**

    C92.32 **Myeloid sarcoma, in relapse**

◄ New   ◄ Revised   ~~deleted~~ Deleted   Excludes 1   Excludes 2   Includes   Use additional   Code first   Code also   Unspecified
OGCR Official Guidelines   **X** Assign placeholder X   ● Use Additional Character(s)   ▶ Manifestation Code   **Coding Clinic**

● **C92.4**   **Acute promyelocytic leukemia**
AML M3
AML Me with t(15;17) and variants

     C92.40   **Acute promyelocytic leukemia, not having achieved remission**
Acute promyelocytic leukemia with failed remission
Acute promyelocytic leukemia NOS

     C92.41   **Acute promyelocytic leukemia, in remission**

     C92.42   **Acute promyelocytic leukemia, in relapse**

● **C92.5**   **Acute myelomonocytic leukemia**
AML M4
AML M4 Eo with inv(16) or t(16;16)

     C92.50   **Acute myelomonocytic leukemia, not having achieved remission**
Acute myelomonocytic leukemia with failed remission
Acute myelomonocytic leukemia NOS

     C92.51   **Acute myelomonocytic leukemia, in remission**

     C92.52   **Acute myelomonocytic leukemia, in relapse**

● **C92.6**   **Acute myeloid leukemia with 11q23-abnormality**
Acute myeloid leukemia with variation of MLL-gene

     C92.60   **Acute myeloid leukemia with 11q23-abnormality not having achieved remission**
Acute myeloid leukemia with 11q23-abnormality with failed remission
Acute myeloid leukemia with 11q23-abnormality NOS

     C92.61   **Acute myeloid leukemia with 11q23-abnormality in remission**

     C92.62   **Acute myeloid leukemia with 11q23-abnormality in relapse**

● **C92.A**   **Acute myeloid leukemia with multilineage dysplasia**
Acute myeloid leukemia with dysplasia of remaining hematopoesis and/or myelodysplastic disease in its history

     C92.A0   **Acute myeloid leukemia with multilineage dysplasia, not having achieved remission**
Acute myeloid leukemia with multilineage dysplasia with failed remission
Acute myeloid leukemia with multilineage dysplasia NOS

     C92.A1   **Acute myeloid leukemia with multilineage dysplasia, in remission**

     C92.A2   **Acute myeloid leukemia with multilineage dysplasia, in relapse**

● **C92.Z**   **Other myeloid leukemia**

     C92.Z0   **Other myeloid leukemia not having achieved remission**
Myeloid leukemia NEC with failed remission
Myeloid leukemia NEC

     C92.Z1   **Other myeloid leukemia, in remission**

     C92.Z2   **Other myeloid leukemia, in relapse**

● **C92.9**   **Myeloid leukemia, unspecified**

     C92.90   **Myeloid leukemia, unspecified, not having achieved remission**
Myeloid leukemia, unspecified with failed remission
Myeloid leukemia, unspecified NOS

     C92.91   **Myeloid leukemia, unspecified in remission**

     C92.92   **Myeloid leukemia, unspecified in relapse**

● **C93**   **Monocytic leukemia**
    Includes   monocytoid leukemia
    Excludes1   personal history of leukemia (Z85.6)

● **C93.0**   **Acute monoblastic/monocytic leukemia**
AML M5
AML M5a
AML M5b

     C93.00   **Acute monoblastic/monocytic leukemia, not having achieved remission**
Acute monoblastic/monocytic leukemia with failed remission
Acute monoblastic/monocytic leukemia NOS

     C93.01   **Acute monoblastic/monocytic leukemia, in remission**

     C93.02   **Acute monoblastic/monocytic leukemia, in relapse**

● **C93.1**   **Chronic myelomonocytic leukemia**
Chronic monocytic leukemia
CMML-1
CMML-2
CMML with eosinophilia

     C93.10   **Chronic myelomonocytic leukemia not having achieved remission**
Chronic myelomonocytic leukemia with failed remission
Chronic myelomonocytic leukemia NOS

     C93.11   **Chronic myelomonocytic leukemia, in remission**

     C93.12   **Chronic myelomonocytic leukemia, in relapse**

● **C93.3**   **Juvenile myelomonocytic leukemia**

     C93.30   **Juvenile myelomonocytic leukemia, not having achieved remission**   **P**
Juvenile myelomonocytic leukemia with failed remission
Juvenile myelomonocytic leukemia NOS

     C93.31   **Juvenile myelomonocytic leukemia, in remission**   **P**

     C93.32   **Juvenile myelomonocytic leukemia, in relapse** **P**

● **C93.Z**   **Other monocytic leukemia**

     C93.Z0   **Other monocytic leukemia, not having achieved remission**
Other monocytic leukemia NOS

     C93.Z1   **Other monocytic leukemia, in remission**

     C93.Z2   **Other monocytic leukemia, in relapse**

● **C93.9**   **Monocytic leukemia, unspecified**

     C93.90   **Monocytic leukemia, unspecified, not having achieved remission**
Monocytic leukemia, unspecified with failed remission
Monocytic leukemia, unspecified NOS

     C93.91   **Monocytic leukemia, unspecified in remission**

     C93.92   **Monocytic leukemia, unspecified in relapse**

● **C94**   **Other leukemias of specified cell type**
    Excludes1   leukemic reticuloendotheliosis (C91.4-)
                 myelodysplastic syndromes (D46.-)
                 personal history of leukemia (Z85.6)
                 plasma cell leukemia (C90.1-)

● **C94.0**   **Acute erythroid leukemia**
Acute myeloid leukemia M6(a)(b)
Erythroleukemia

     C94.00   **Acute erythroid leukemia, not having achieved remission**
Acute erythroid leukemia with failed remission
Acute erythroid leukemia NOS

     C94.01   **Acute erythroid leukemia, in remission**

     C94.02   **Acute erythroid leukemia, in relapse**

● **C94.2** **Acute megakaryoblastic leukemia**
Acute myeloid leukemia M7
Acute megakaryocytic leukemia

    C94.20 **Acute megakaryoblastic leukemia not having achieved remission**
Acute megakaryoblastic leukemia with failed remission
Acute megakaryoblastic leukemia NOS

    C94.21 **Acute megakaryoblastic leukemia, in remission**

    C94.22 **Acute megakaryoblastic leukemia, in relapse**

● **C94.3** **Mast cell leukemia**

    C94.30 **Mast cell leukemia not having achieved remission**
Mast cell leukemia with failed remission
Mast cell leukemia NOS

    C94.31 **Mast cell leukemia, in remission**

    C94.32 **Mast cell leukemia, in relapse**

● **C94.4** **Acute panmyelosis with myelofibrosis**
Acute myelofibrosis

    Excludes1   myelofibrosis NOS (D75.81)
secondary myelofibrosis NOS (D75.81)

    C94.40 **Acute panmyelosis with myelofibrosis not having achieved remission**
Acute myelofibrosis NOS
Acute panmyelosis with myelofibrosis with failed remission
Acute panmyelosis NOS

    C94.41 **Acute panmyelosis with myelofibrosis, in remission**

    C94.42 **Acute panmyelosis with myelofibrosis, in relapse**

C94.6 **Myelodysplastic disease, not classified**
Myeloproliferative disease, not classified

● **C94.8** **Other specified leukemias**
Aggressive NK-cell leukemia
Acute basophilic leukemia

    C94.80 **Other specified leukemias not having achieved remission**
Other specified leukemia with failed remission
Other specified leukemias NOS

    C94.81 **Other specified leukemias, in remission**

    C94.82 **Other specified leukemias, in relapse**

● **C95** **Leukemia of unspecified cell type**

    Excludes1   personal history of leukemia (Z85.6)

● **C95.0** **Acute leukemia of unspecified cell type**
Acute bilineal leukemia
Acute mixed lineage leukemia
Biphenotypic acute leukemia
Stem cell leukemia of unclear lineage

    Excludes1   acute exacerbation of unspecified chronic leukemia (C95.10)

    C95.00 **Acute leukemia of unspecified cell type not having achieved remission**
Acute leukemia of unspecified cell type with failed remission
Acute leukemia NOS

    C95.01 **Acute leukemia of unspecified cell type, in remission**

    C95.02 **Acute leukemia of unspecified cell type, in relapse**

● **C95.1** **Chronic leukemia of unspecified cell type**

    C95.10 **Chronic leukemia of unspecified cell type not having achieved remission**
Chronic leukemia of unspecified cell type with failed remission
Chronic leukemia NOS

    C95.11 **Chronic leukemia of unspecified cell type, in remission**

    C95.12 **Chronic leukemia of unspecified cell type, in relapse**

● **C95.9** **Leukemia, unspecified**

    C95.90 **Leukemia, unspecified not having achieved remission**
Leukemia, unspecified with failed remission
Leukemia NOS

    C95.91 **Leukemia, unspecified, in remission**

    C95.92 **Leukemia, unspecified, in relapse**

● **C96** **Other and unspecified malignant neoplasms of lymphoid, hematopoietic and related tissue**

    Excludes1   personal history of other malignant neoplasms of lymphoid, hematopoietic and related tissues (Z85.79)

C96.0 **Multifocal and multisystemic (disseminated) Langerhans-cell histiocytosis**
Histiocytosis X, multisystemic
Letterer-Siwe disease

    Excludes1   adult pulmonary Langerhans cell histiocytosis (J84.82)
multifocal and unisystemic Langerhans-cell histiocytosis (C96.5)
unifocal Langerhans-cell histiocytosis (C96.6)

C96.2 **Malignant mast cell tumor**
Aggressive systemic mastocytosis
Mast cell sarcoma

    Excludes1   indolent mastocytosis (D47.0)
mast cell leukemia (C94.30)
mastocytosis (congenital) (cutaneous) (Q82.2)

C96.4 **Sarcoma of dendritic cells (accessory cells)**
Follicular dendritic cell sarcoma
Interdigitating dendritic cell sarcoma
Langerhans cell sarcoma

C96.5 **Multifocal and unisystemic Langerhans-cell histiocytosis**
Hand-Schüller-Christian disease
Histiocytosis X, multifocal

    Excludes1   multifocal and multisystemic (disseminated) Langerhans-cell histiocytosis (C96.0)
unifocal Langerhans-cell histiocytosis (C96.6)

C96.6 **Unifocal Langerhans-cell histiocytosis**
Eosinophilic granuloma
Histiocytosis X, unifocal
Histiocytosis X NOS
Langerhans-cell histiocytosis NOS

    Excludes1   multifocal and multisysemic (disseminated) Langerhans-cell histiocytosis (C96.0)
multifocal and unisystemic Langerhans-cell histiocytosis (C96.5)

C96.A **Histiocytic sarcoma**
Malignant histiocytosis

C96.Z **Other specified malignant neoplasms of lymphoid, hematopoietic and related tissue**

C96.9 **Malignant neoplasm of lymphoid, hematopoietic and related tissue, unspecified**

◀ New   ◀◀ Revised   ~~deleted~~ Deleted   Excludes 1   Excludes 2   Includes   Use additional   Code first   Code also   Unspecified

OGCR Official Guidelines   X Assign placeholder X   ● Use Additional Character(s)   ▶ Manifestation Code   **Coding Clinic**

In situ is carcinoma involving cells in localized tissues that has not spread to nearby tissues

IN SITU NEOPLASMS (D00-D09)

Includes   Bowen's disease
erythroplasia
grade III intraepithelial neoplasia
Queyrat's erythroplasia

● **D00   Carcinoma in situ of oral cavity, esophagus and stomach**
    Excludes1   melanoma in situ (D03.-)

   ● **D00.0   Carcinoma in situ of lip, oral cavity and pharynx**
     Use additional code to identify:
     exposure to environmental tobacco smoke (Z77.22)
     exposure to tobacco smoke in the perinatal period (P96.81)
     history of tobacco use (Z87.891)
     occupational exposure to environmental tobacco smoke (Z57.31)
     tobacco dependence (F17.-)
     tobacco use (Z72.0)

     Excludes1   carcinoma in situ of aryepiglottic fold or interarytenoid fold, laryngeal aspect (D02.0)
       carcinoma in situ of epiglottis NOS (D02.0)
       carcinoma in situ of epiglottis suprahyoid portion (D02.0)
       carcinoma in situ of skin of lip (D03.0, D04.0)

     D00.00   Carcinoma in situ of oral cavity, unspecified site
     D00.01   Carcinoma in situ of labial mucosa and vermilion border
     D00.02   Carcinoma in situ of buccal mucosa
     D00.03   Carcinoma in situ of gingiva and edentulous alveolar ridge
     D00.04   Carcinoma in situ of soft palate
     D00.05   Carcinoma in situ of hard palate
     D00.06   Carcinoma in situ of floor of mouth
     D00.07   Carcinoma in situ of tongue
     D00.08   Carcinoma in situ of pharynx
       Carcinoma in situ of aryepiglottic fold NOS
       Carcinoma in situ of hypopharyngeal aspect of aryepiglottic fold
       Carcinoma in situ of marginal zone of aryepiglottic fold

   D00.1   Carcinoma in situ of esophagus
   D00.2   Carcinoma in situ of stomach

● **D01   Carcinoma in situ of other and unspecified digestive organs**
    Excludes1   melanoma in situ (D03.-)

   D01.0   Carcinoma in situ of colon
     Excludes1   carcinoma in situ of rectosigmoid junction (D01.1)

   D01.1   Carcinoma in situ of rectosigmoid junction
   D01.2   Carcinoma in situ of rectum
   D01.3   Carcinoma in situ of anus and anal canal
     Excludes1   carcinoma in situ of anal margin (D04.5)
       carcinoma in situ of anal skin (D04.5)
       carcinoma in situ of perianal skin (D04.5)

   ● **D01.4   Carcinoma in situ of other and unspecified parts of intestine**
     Excludes1   carcinoma in situ of ampulla of Vater (D01.5)

     D01.40   Carcinoma in situ of unspecified part of intestine
     D01.49   Carcinoma in situ of other parts of intestine

   D01.5   Carcinoma in situ of liver, gallbladder and bile ducts
     Carcinoma in situ of ampulla of Vater

   D01.7   Carcinoma in situ of other specified digestive organs
     Carcinoma in situ of pancreas

   D01.9   Carcinoma in situ of digestive organ, unspecified

● **D02   Carcinoma in situ of middle ear and respiratory system**
    Use additional code to identify:
    exposure to environmental tobacco smoke (Z77.22)
    exposure to tobacco smoke in the perinatal period (P96.81)
    history of tobacco use (Z87.891)
    occupational exposure to environmental tobacco smoke (Z57.31)
    tobacco dependence (F17.-)
    tobacco use (Z72.0)

    Excludes1   melanoma in situ (D03.-)

   D02.0   Carcinoma in situ of larynx
     Carcinoma in situ of aryepiglottic fold or interarytenoid fold, laryngeal aspect
     Carcinoma in situ of epiglottis (suprahyoid portion)
     Excludes1   carcinoma in situ of aryepiglottic fold or interarytenoid fold NOS (D00.08)
       carcinoma in situ of hypopharyngeal aspect (D00.08)
       carcinoma in situ of marginal zone (D00.08)

   D02.1   Carcinoma in situ of trachea
   ● **D02.2   Carcinoma in situ of bronchus and lung**
     D02.20   Carcinoma in situ of unspecified bronchus and lung
     D02.21   Carcinoma in situ of right bronchus and lung
     D02.22   Carcinoma in situ of left bronchus and lung

   D02.3   Carcinoma in situ of other parts of respiratory system
     Carcinoma in situ of accessory sinuses
     Carcinoma in situ of middle ear
     Carcinoma in situ of nasal cavities
     Excludes1   carcinoma in situ of ear (external) (skin) (D04.2-)
       carcinoma in situ of nose NOS (D09.8)
       carcinoma in situ of skin of nose (D04.3)

   D02.4   Carcinoma in situ of respiratory system, unspecified

● **D03   Melanoma in situ**
   D03.0   Melanoma in situ of lip
   ● **D03.1   Melanoma in situ of eyelid, including canthus**
     D03.10   Melanoma in situ of unspecified eyelid, including canthus
     D03.11   Melanoma in situ of right eyelid, including canthus
     D03.12   Melanoma in situ of left eyelid, including canthus

   ● **D03.2   Melanoma in situ of ear and external auricular canal**
     D03.20   Melanoma in situ of unspecified ear and external auricular canal
     D03.21   Melanoma in situ of right ear and external auricular canal
     D03.22   Melanoma in situ of left ear and external auricular canal

   ● **D03.3   Melanoma in situ of other and unspecified parts of face**
     D03.30   Melanoma in situ of unspecified part of face
     D03.39   Melanoma in situ of other parts of face

   D03.4   Melanoma in situ of scalp and neck
   ● **D03.5   Melanoma in situ of trunk**
     D03.51   Melanoma in situ of anal skin
       Melanoma in situ of anal margin
       Melanoma in situ of perianal skin
     D03.52   Melanoma in situ of breast (skin) (soft tissue)
     D03.59   Melanoma in situ of other part of trunk

   ● **D03.6   Melanoma in situ of upper limb, including shoulder**
     D03.60   Melanoma in situ of unspecified upper limb, including shoulder
     D03.61   Melanoma in situ of right upper limb, including shoulder
     D03.62   Melanoma in situ of left upper limb, including shoulder

●D03.7   Melanoma in situ of lower limb, including hip
  D03.70 Melanoma in situ of unspecified lower limb, including hip
  D03.71 Melanoma in situ of right lower limb, including hip
  D03.72 Melanoma in situ of left lower limb, including hip

D03.8 Melanoma in situ of other sites
  Melanoma in situ of scrotum
  Excludes1 carcinoma in situ of scrotum (D07.61)

D03.9 Melanoma in situ, unspecified

●D04 Carcinoma in situ of skin
  Excludes1 erythroplasia of Queyrat (penis) NOS (D07.4)
    melanoma in situ (D03.-)

D04.0 Carcinoma in situ of skin of lip
  Excludes1 carcinoma in situ of vermilion border of lip (D00.01)

●D04.1 Carcinoma in situ of skin of eyelid, including canthus
  D04.10 Carcinoma in situ of skin of unspecified eyelid, including canthus
  D04.11 Carcinoma in situ of skin of right eyelid, including canthus
  D04.12 Carcinoma in situ of skin of left eyelid, including canthus

●D04.2 Carcinoma in situ of skin of ear and external auricular canal
  D04.20 Carcinoma in situ of skin of unspecified ear and external auricular canal
  D04.21 Carcinoma in situ of skin of right ear and external auricular canal
  D04.22 Carcinoma in situ of skin of left ear and external auricular canal

●D04.3 Carcinoma in situ of skin of other and unspecified parts of face
  D04.30 Carcinoma in situ of skin of unspecified part of face
  D04.39 Carcinoma in situ of skin of other parts of face

D04.4 Carcinoma in situ of skin of scalp and neck

D04.5 Carcinoma in situ of skin of trunk
  Carcinoma in situ of anal margin
  Carcinoma in situ of anal skin
  Carcinoma in situ of perianal skin
  Carcinoma in situ of skin of breast
  Excludes1 carcinoma in situ of anus NOS (D01.3)
    carcinoma in situ of scrotum (D07.61)
    carcinoma in situ of skin of genital organs (D07.-)

●D04.6 Carcinoma in situ of skin of upper limb, including shoulder
  D04.60 Carcinoma in situ of skin of unspecified upper limb, including shoulder
  D04.61 Carcinoma in situ of skin of right upper limb, including shoulder
  D04.62 Carcinoma in situ of skin of left upper limb, including shoulder

●D04.7 Carcinoma in situ of skin of lower limb, including hip
  D04.70 Carcinoma in situ of skin of unspecified lower limb, including hip
  D04.71 Carcinoma in situ of skin of right lower limb, including hip
  D04.72 Carcinoma in situ of skin of left lower limb, including hip

D04.8 Carcinoma in situ of skin of other sites

D04.9 Carcinoma in situ of skin, unspecified

●D05 Carcinoma in situ of breast
  Excludes1 carcinoma in situ of skin of breast (D04.5)
    melanoma in situ of breast (skin) (D03.5)
    Paget's disease of breast or nipple (C50.-)

●D05.0 Lobular carcinoma in situ of breast
  D05.00 Lobular carcinoma in situ of unspecified breast
  D05.01 Lobular carcinoma in situ of right breast
  D05.02 Lobular carcinoma in situ of left breast

●D05.1 Intraductal carcinoma in situ of breast
  D05.10 Intraductal carcinoma in situ of unspecified breast
  D05.11 Intraductal carcinoma in situ of right breast
  D05.12 Intraductal carcinoma in situ of left breast

●D05.8 Other specified type of carcinoma in situ of breast
  D05.80 Other specified type of carcinoma in situ of unspecified breast
  D05.81 Other specified type of carcinoma in situ of right breast
  D05.82 Other specified type of carcinoma in situ of left breast

●D05.9 Unspecified type of carcinoma in situ of breast
  D05.90 Unspecified type of carcinoma in situ of unspecified breast
  D05.91 Unspecified type of carcinoma in situ of right breast
  D05.92 Unspecified type of carcinoma in situ of left breast

●D06 Carcinoma in situ of cervix uteri
  Includes cervical adenocarcinoma in situ
    cervical intraepithelial glandular neoplasia
    cervical intraepithelial neoplasia III [CIN III]
    severe dysplasia of cervix uteri
  Excludes1 cervical intraepithelial neoplasia II [CIN II] (N87.1)
    cytologic evidence of malignancy of cervix without histologic confirmation (R87.614)
    high grade squamous intraepithelial lesion (HGSIL) of cervix (R87.613)
    melanoma in situ of cervix (D03.5)
    moderate cervical dysplasia (N87.1)

 D06.0 Carcinoma in situ of endocervix ♀
 D06.1 Carcinoma in situ of exocervix ♀
 D06.7 Carcinoma in situ of other parts of cervix ♀
 D06.9 Carcinoma in situ of cervix, unspecified ♀

●D07 Carcinoma in situ of other and unspecified genital organs
  Excludes1 melanoma in situ of trunk (D03.5)

 D07.0 Carcinoma in situ of endometrium ♀
 D07.1 Carcinoma in situ of vulva ♀
  Severe dysplasia of vulva
  Vulvar intraepithelial neoplasia III [VIN III]
  Excludes1 moderate dysplasia of vulva (N90.1)
    vulvar intraepithelial neoplasia II [VIN II] (N90.1)

 D07.2 Carcinoma in situ of vagina ♀
  Severe dysplasia of vagina
  Vaginal intraepithelial neoplasia III [VIN III]
  Excludes1 moderate dysplasia of vagina (N89.1)
    vaginal intraepithelial neoplasia II [VIN II] (N89.1)

●D07.3 Carcinoma in situ of other and unspecified female genital organs
  D07.30 Carcinoma in situ of unspecified female genital organs ♀
  D07.39 Carcinoma in situ of other female genital organs ♀

◀ New ⬅ Revised ~~deleted~~ Deleted Excludes 1 Excludes 2 Includes Use additional Code first Code also Unspecified
OGCR Official Guidelines X Assign placeholder X ● Use Additional Character(s) 〗 Manifestation Code **Coding Clinic**

CHAPTER 2 (C00-D49)

D07.4 **Carcinoma in situ of penis** ♂
　　　　Erythroplasia of Queyrat NOS

D07.5 **Carcinoma in situ of prostate** ♂
　　　　Prostatic intraepithelial neoplasia III (PIN III)
　　　　Severe dysplasia of prostate
　　　　　Excludes1　dysplasia (mild) (moderate) of prostate
　　　　　　　　　　(N42.3)

● **D07.6** **Carcinoma in situ of other and unspecified male genital organs**

　　D07.60 **Carcinoma in situ of unspecified male genital organs** ♂

　　D07.61 **Carcinoma in situ of scrotum** ♂

　　D07.69 **Carcinoma in situ of other male genital organs** ♂

● **D09** **Carcinoma in situ of other and unspecified sites**
　　　Excludes1　melanoma in situ (D03.-)

　D09.0 **Carcinoma in situ of bladder**

● **D09.1** **Carcinoma in situ of other and unspecified urinary organs**

　　D09.10 **Carcinoma in situ of unspecified urinary organ**

　　D09.19 **Carcinoma in situ of other urinary organs**

● **D09.2** **Carcinoma in situ of eye**
　　　Excludes1　carcinoma in situ of skin of eyelid
　　　　　　　　　(D04.1-)

　　D09.20 **Carcinoma in situ of unspecified eye**

　　D09.21 **Carcinoma in situ of right eye**

　　D09.22 **Carcinoma in situ of left eye**

　D09.3 **Carcinoma in situ of thyroid and other endocrine glands**
　　　Excludes1　carcinoma in situ of endocrine pancreas
　　　　　　　　　(D01.7)
　　　　　　　　carcinoma in situ of ovary (D07.39)
　　　　　　　　carcinoma in situ of testis (D07.69)

　D09.8 **Carcinoma in situ of other specified sites**

　D09.9 **Carcinoma in situ, unspecified**

BENIGN NEOPLASMS, EXCEPT BENIGN NEUROENDOCRINE TUMORS (D10-D36)

● **D10** **Benign neoplasm of mouth and pharynx**

　D10.0 **Benign neoplasm of lip**
　　　Benign neoplasm of lip (frenulum) (inner aspect)
　　　　(mucosa) (vermilion border)
　　　Excludes1　benign neoplasm of skin of lip (D22.0,
　　　　　　　　　D23.0)

　D10.1 **Benign neoplasm of tongue**
　　　Benign neoplasm of lingual tonsil

　D10.2 **Benign neoplasm of floor of mouth**

● **D10.3** **Other and unspecified parts of mouth**

　　D10.30 **Benign neoplasm of unspecified part of mouth**

　　D10.39 **Benign neoplasm of other parts of mouth**
　　　　Benign neoplasm of minor salivary gland NOS
　　　　　Excludes1　benign odontogenic neoplasms
　　　　　　　　　　(D16.4-D16.5)
　　　　　　　　　benign neoplasm of mucosa of
　　　　　　　　　　lip (D10.0)
　　　　　　　　　benign neoplasm of
　　　　　　　　　　nasopharyngeal surface of
　　　　　　　　　　soft palate (D10.6)

　D10.4 **Benign neoplasm of tonsil**
　　　Benign neoplasm of tonsil (faucial) (palatine)
　　　Excludes1　benign neoplasm of lingual tonsil
　　　　　　　　　(D10.1)
　　　　　　　　benign neoplasm of pharyngeal tonsil
　　　　　　　　　(D10.6)
　　　　　　　　benign neoplasm of tonsillar fossa (D10.5)
　　　　　　　　benign neoplasm of tonsillar pillars
　　　　　　　　　(D10.5)

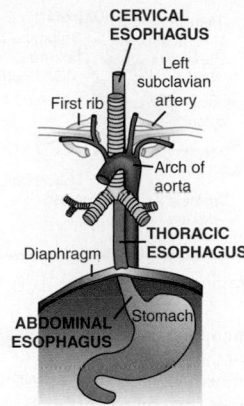

Figure 2-16 The esophagus is the muscular tube that connects the pharynx and the stomach. The 10 inch (25 cm) long esophagus is divided into three parts: **cervical, thoracic,** and **abdominal.**

　D10.5 **Benign neoplasm of other parts of oropharynx**
　　　Division of pharynx lying between soft palate and upper edge of epiglottis
　　　Benign neoplasm of epiglottis, anterior aspect
　　　Benign neoplasm of tonsillar fossa
　　　Benign neoplasm of tonsillar pillars
　　　Benign neoplasm of vallecula
　　　Excludes1　benign neoplasm of epiglottis NOS
　　　　　　　　　(D14.1)
　　　　　　　　benign neoplasm of epiglottis,
　　　　　　　　　suprahyoid portion (D14.1)

　D10.6 **Benign neoplasm of nasopharynx**
　　　Segment of pharynx that lies above soft palate
　　　Benign neoplasm of pharyngeal tonsil
　　　Benign neoplasm of posterior margin of septum and
　　　　choanae

　D10.7 **Benign neoplasm of hypopharynx**
　　　*Segment of pharynx that lies below upper edge of epiglottis
　　　and opens into larynx and esophagus*

　D10.9 **Benign neoplasm of pharynx, unspecified**

● **D11** **Benign neoplasm of major salivary glands**
　　　Excludes1　benign neoplasms of specified minor salivary
　　　　　　　　　glands which are classified according to their
　　　　　　　　　anatomical location
　　　　　　　　benign neoplasms of minor salivary glands NOS
　　　　　　　　　(D10.39)

　D11.0 **Benign neoplasm of parotid gland**

　D11.7 **Benign neoplasm of other major salivary glands**
　　　Benign neoplasm of sublingual salivary gland
　　　Benign neoplasm of submandibular salivary gland

　D11.9 **Benign neoplasm of major salivary gland, unspecified**

● **D12** **Benign neoplasm of colon, rectum, anus and anal canal**
　　　Excludes1　benign carcinoid tumors of the large intestine,
　　　　　　　　　and rectum (D3A.02-)

　D12.0 **Benign neoplasm of cecum**
　　　Benign neoplasm of ileocecal valve

　D12.1 **Benign neoplasm of appendix**
　　　Excludes1　benign carcinoid tumor of the appendix
　　　　　　　　　(D3A.020)

　D12.2 **Benign neoplasm of ascending colon**

　D12.3 **Benign neoplasm of transverse colon**
　　　Benign neoplasm of hepatic flexure
　　　Benign neoplasm of splenic flexure
　　　　*Flexure is a bending in a structure or organ. Note the
　　　　three flexures illustrated in Figure 2–17. Hepatic =
　　　　liver, sigmoid = colon, splenic = spleen.*

　D12.4 **Benign neoplasm of descending colon**

　D12.5 **Benign neoplasm of sigmoid colon**

N Newborn Age: 0　　**P** Pediatric Age: 0–17　　**M** Maternity DX: 12–55　　**A** Adult Age: 15–124　　♀ Females Only　　♂ Males Only

801

CHAPTER 2 (C00-D49)

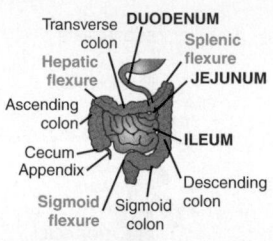

Transverse colon   **DUODENUM**   Splenic flexure
Hepatic flexure   **JEJUNUM**
Ascending colon
Cecum   **ILEUM**
Appendix   Descending colon
Sigmoid flexure   Sigmoid colon

Figure 2-17   Small intestine and colon.

D12.6   **Benign neoplasm of colon, unspecified**
Adenomatosis of colon
Benign neoplasm of large intestine NOS
Polyposis (hereditary) of colon
> **Excludes1**   inflammatory polyp of colon (K51.4-)
> polyp of colon NOS (K63.5)

D12.7   **Benign neoplasm of rectosigmoid junction**
Angle where sigmoid colon becomes rectum

D12.8   **Benign neoplasm of rectum**
> **Excludes1**   benign carcinoid tumor of the rectum (D3A.026)

D12.9   **Benign neoplasm of anus and anal canal**
Benign neoplasm of anus NOS
> **Excludes1**   benign neoplasm of anal margin (D22.5, D23.5)
> benign neoplasm of anal skin (D22.5, D23.5)
> benign neoplasm of perianal skin (D22.5, D23.5)

● **D13**   **Benign neoplasm of other and ill-defined parts of digestive system**
> **Excludes1**   benign stromal tumors of digestive system (D21.4)

D13.0   **Benign neoplasm of esophagus**

D13.1   **Benign neoplasm of stomach**
> **Excludes1**   benign carcinoid tumor of the stomach (D3A.092)

D13.2   **Benign neoplasm of duodenum**
> **Excludes1**   benign carcinoid tumor of the duodenum (D3A.010)

● **D13.3**   **Benign neoplasm of other and unspecified parts of small intestine**
> **Excludes1**   benign carcinoid tumors of the small intestine (D3A.01-)
> benign neoplasm of ileocecal valve (D12.0)

    D13.30   **Benign neoplasm of unspecified part of small intestine**

    D13.39   **Benign neoplasm of other parts of small intestine**

D13.4   **Benign neoplasm of liver**
Benign neoplasm of intrahepatic bile ducts

D13.5   **Benign neoplasm of extrahepatic bile ducts**
Extensions of common hepatic bile duct (tube that collects bile from liver)

D13.6   **Benign neoplasm of pancreas**
> **Excludes1**   benign neoplasm of endocrine pancreas (D13.7)

D13.7   **Benign neoplasm of endocrine pancreas**
Pancreatic islets: Cells scattered throughout pancreas
Islet cell tumor
Benign neoplasm of islets of Langerhans
Use additional code to identify any functional activity.

D13.9   **Benign neoplasm of ill-defined sites within the digestive system**
Benign neoplasm of digestive system NOS
Benign neoplasm of intestine NOS
Benign neoplasm of spleen

● **D14**   **Benign neoplasm of middle ear and respiratory system**

D14.0   **Benign neoplasm of middle ear, nasal cavity and accessory sinuses**
Benign neoplasm of cartilage of nose
> **Excludes1**   benign neoplasm of auricular canal (external) (D22.2-, D23.2-)
> benign neoplasm of bone of ear (D16.4)
> benign neoplasm of bone of nose (D16.4)
> benign neoplasm of cartilage of ear (D21.0)
> benign neoplasm of ear (external) (skin) (D22.2-, D23.2-)
> benign neoplasm of nose NOS (D36.7)
> benign neoplasm of skin of nose (D22.39, D23.39)
> benign neoplasm of olfactory bulb (D33.3)
> benign neoplasm of posterior margin of septum and choanae (D10.6)
> polyp of accessory sinus (J33.8)
> polyp of ear (middle) (H74.4)
> polyp of nasal (cavity) (J33.-)

D14.1   **Benign neoplasm of larynx**
Adenomatous polyp of larynx
Benign neoplasm of epiglottis (suprahyoid portion)
Horseshoe shaped bone in anterior midline of neck between chin and thyroid cartilage
> **Excludes1**   benign neoplasm of epiglottis, anterior aspect (D10.5)
> polyp (nonadenomatous) of vocal cord or larynx (J38.1)

D14.2   **Benign neoplasm of trachea**

● **D14.3**   **Benign neoplasm of bronchus and lung**
> **Excludes1**   benign carcinoid tumor of the bronchus and lung (D3A.090)

    D14.30   **Benign neoplasm of unspecified bronchus and lung**

    D14.31   **Benign neoplasm of right bronchus and lung**

    D14.32   **Benign neoplasm of left bronchus and lung**

D14.4   **Benign neoplasm of respiratory system, unspecified**

● **D15**   **Benign neoplasm of other and unspecified intrathoracic organs**
> **Excludes1**   benign neoplasm of mesothelial tissue (D19.-)

D15.0   **Benign neoplasm of thymus**
> **Excludes1**   benign carcinoid tumor of the thymus (D3A.091)

D15.1   **Benign neoplasm of heart**
> **Excludes1**   benign neoplasm of great vessels (D21.3)

D15.2   **Benign neoplasm of mediastinum**

D15.7   **Benign neoplasm of other specified intrathoracic organs**

D15.9   **Benign neoplasm of intrathoracic organ, unspecified**

● **D16**   **Benign neoplasm of bone and articular cartilage**
> **Excludes1**   benign neoplasm of connective tissue of ear (D21.0)
> benign neoplasm of connective tissue of eyelid (D21.0)
> benign neoplasm of connective tissue of larynx (D14.1)
> benign neoplasm of connective tissue of nose (D14.0)
> benign neoplasm of synovia (D21.-)

● **D16.0**   **Benign neoplasm of scapula and long bones of upper limb**

    D16.00   **Benign neoplasm of scapula and long bones of unspecified upper limb**

    D16.01   **Benign neoplasm of scapula and long bones of right upper limb**

    D16.02   **Benign neoplasm of scapula and long bones of left upper limb**

CHAPTER 2 (C00-D49)

◄ New   ◀▦ Revised   ~~deleted~~ Deleted   Excludes 1   Excludes 2   Includes   Use additional   Code first   Code also   Unspecified
OGCR Official Guidelines   **X** Assign placeholder X   ● Use Additional Character(s)   ▶ Manifestation Code   **Coding Clinic**

● D16.1   Benign neoplasm of short bones of upper limb

     D16.10   Benign neoplasm of short bones of unspecified upper limb

     D16.11   Benign neoplasm of short bones of right upper limb

     D16.12   Benign neoplasm of short bones of left upper limb

● D16.2   Benign neoplasm of long bones of lower limb

     D16.20   Benign neoplasm of long bones of unspecified lower limb

     D16.21   Benign neoplasm of long bones of right lower limb

     D16.22   Benign neoplasm of long bones of left lower limb

● D16.3   Benign neoplasm of short bones of lower limb

     D16.30   Benign neoplasm of short bones of unspecified lower limb

     D16.31   Benign neoplasm of short bones of right lower limb

     D16.32   Benign neoplasm of short bones of left lower limb

D16.4   Benign neoplasm of bones of skull and face

     Benign neoplasm of maxilla (superior)
     Benign neoplasm of orbital bone
       Cavity or socket of skull in which eye and its appendages are located
     Keratocyst of maxilla
     Keratocystic odontogenic tumor of maxilla

     Excludes1   benign neoplasm of lower jaw bone (D16.5)

D16.5   Benign neoplasm of lower jaw bone

     Keratocyst of mandible
     Keratocystic odontogenic tumor of mandible

D16.6   Benign neoplasm of vertebral column

     Excludes1   benign neoplasm of sacrum and coccyx (D16.8)

D16.7   Benign neoplasm of ribs, sternum and clavicle

D16.8   Benign neoplasm of pelvic bones, sacrum and coccyx

D16.9   Benign neoplasm of bone and articular cartilage, unspecified

● D17   Benign lipomatous neoplasm

     Slow growing benign tumors (rubbery masses) of mature fat cells enclosed in a thin fibrous capsule

D17.0   Benign lipomatous neoplasm of skin and subcutaneous tissue of head, face and neck

D17.1   Benign lipomatous neoplasm of skin and subcutaneous tissue of trunk

● D17.2   Benign lipomatous neoplasm of skin and subcutaneous tissue of limb

     D17.20   Benign lipomatous neoplasm of skin and subcutaneous tissue of unspecified limb

     D17.21   Benign lipomatous neoplasm of skin and subcutaneous tissue of right arm

     D17.22   Benign lipomatous neoplasm of skin and subcutaneous tissue of left arm

     D17.23   Benign lipomatous neoplasm of skin and subcutaneous tissue of right leg

     D17.24   Benign lipomatous neoplasm of skin and subcutaneous tissue of left leg

● D17.3   Benign lipomatous neoplasm of skin and subcutaneous tissue of other and unspecified sites

     D17.30   Benign lipomatous neoplasm of skin and subcutaneous tissue of unspecified sites

     D17.39   Benign lipomatous neoplasm of skin and subcutaneous tissue of other sites

D17.4   Benign lipomatous neoplasm of intrathoracic organs

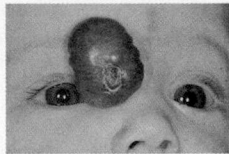

Figure 2-18   Hemangioma of skin and subcutaneous tissue. (From Yanoff: Ophthalmology, ed 3, Mosby, Inc., 2008)

Item 2–10   **Hemangiomas** are abnormally dense collections of dilated capillaries that occur on the skin or in internal organs. Hemangiomas are both deep and superficial and undergo a rapid growth phase when the size increases rapidly, followed by a rest phase, in which the tumor changes very little, followed by an involutional phase in which the tumor begins to and can disappear altogether. **Lymphangiomas** or cystic hygroma are benign collections of overgrown lymph vessels and, although rare, may occur anywhere but most commonly on the head and neck of children and infants. Visceral organs, lungs, and gastrointestinal tract may also be involved.

D17.5   Benign lipomatous neoplasm of intra-abdominal organs

     Excludes1   benign lipomatous neoplasm of peritoneum and retroperitoneum (D17.79)

D17.6   Benign lipomatous neoplasm of spermatic cord ♂

● D17.7   Benign lipomatous neoplasm of other sites

     D17.71   Benign lipomatous neoplasm of kidney

     D17.72   Benign lipomatous neoplasm of other genitourinary organ

     D17.79   Benign lipomatous neoplasm of other sites
       Benign lipomatous neoplasm of peritoneum
       Benign lipomatous neoplasm of retroperitoneum

D17.9   Benign lipomatous neoplasm, unspecified

     Lipoma NOS

● D18   Hemangioma and lymphangioma, any site

     Excludes1   benign neoplasm of glomus jugulare (D35.6)
       blue or pigmented nevus (D22.-)
       nevus NOS (D22.-)
       vascular nevus (Q82.5)

● D18.0   Hemangioma

     Common type of vascular malformation
     Angioma NOS
     Cavernous nevus

     D18.00   Hemangioma unspecified site

     D18.01   Hemangioma of skin and subcutaneous tissue

     D18.02   Hemangioma of intracranial structures

     D18.03   Hemangioma of intra-abdominal structures

     D18.09   Hemangioma of other sites

     D18.1   Lymphangioma, any site

● D19   Benign neoplasm of mesothelial tissue

     Mesothelial tissue is the membrane lining several body cavities

D19.0   Benign neoplasm of mesothelial tissue of pleura

D19.1   Benign neoplasm of mesothelial tissue of peritoneum

D19.7   Benign neoplasm of mesothelial tissue of other sites

D19.9   Benign neoplasm of mesothelial tissue, unspecified

     Benign mesothelioma NOS

● D20   Benign neoplasm of soft tissue of retroperitoneum and peritoneum

     Excludes1   benign lipomatous neoplasm of peritoneum and retroperitoneum (D17.79)
       benign neoplasm of mesothelial tissue (D19.-)

D20.0   Benign neoplasm of soft tissue of retroperitoneum

D20.1   Benign neoplasm of soft tissue of peritoneum

CHAPTER 2 (C00-D49)

● **D21 Other benign neoplasms of connective and other soft tissue**
> **Includes** benign neoplasm of blood vessel
> benign neoplasm of bursa
> benign neoplasm of cartilage
> benign neoplasm of fascia
> benign neoplasm of fat
> benign neoplasm of ligament, except uterine
> benign neoplasm of lymphatic channel
> benign neoplasm of muscle
> benign neoplasm of synovia
> benign neoplasm of tendon (sheath)
> benign stromal tumors
>
> **Excludes1** benign neoplasm of articular cartilage (D16.-)
> benign neoplasm of cartilage of larynx (D14.1)
> benign neoplasm of cartilage of nose (D14.0)
> benign neoplasm of connective tissue of breast (D24.-)
> benign neoplasm of peripheral nerves and autonomic nervous system (D36.1-)
> benign neoplasm of peritoneum (D20.1)
> benign neoplasm of retroperitoneum (D20.0)
> benign neoplasm of uterine ligament, any (D28.2)
> benign neoplasm of vascular tissue (D18.-)
> hemangioma (D18.0-)
> lipomatous neoplasm (D17.-)
> lymphangioma (D18.1)
> uterine leiomyoma (D25.-)

D21.0 Benign neoplasm of connective and other soft tissue of head, face and neck
> Benign neoplasm of connective tissue of ear
> Benign neoplasm of connective tissue of eyelid
> **Excludes1** benign neoplasm of connective tissue of orbit (D31.6-)

● **D21.1 Benign neoplasm of connective and other soft tissue of upper limb, including shoulder**
> **D21.10** Benign neoplasm of connective and other soft tissue of unspecified upper limb, including shoulder
> **D21.11** Benign neoplasm of connective and other soft tissue of right upper limb, including shoulder
> **D21.12** Benign neoplasm of connective and other soft tissue of left upper limb, including shoulder

● **D21.2 Benign neoplasm of connective and other soft tissue of lower limb, including hip**
> **D21.20** Benign neoplasm of connective and other soft tissue of unspecified lower limb, including hip
> **D21.21** Benign neoplasm of connective and other soft tissue of right lower limb, including hip
> **D21.22** Benign neoplasm of connective and other soft tissue of left lower limb, including hip

D21.3 Benign neoplasm of connective and other soft tissue of thorax
> Benign neoplasm of axilla
> Benign neoplasm of diaphragm
> Benign neoplasm of great vessels
> **Excludes1** benign neoplasm of heart (D15.1)
> benign neoplasm of mediastinum (D15.2)
> benign neoplasm of thymus (D15.0)

D21.4 Benign neoplasm of connective and other soft tissue of abdomen Benign stromal tumors of abdomen

D21.5 Benign neoplasm of connective and other soft tissue of pelvis
> **Excludes1** benign neoplasm of any uterine ligament (D28.2)
> uterine leiomyoma (D25.-)

D21.6 Benign neoplasm of connective and other soft tissue of trunk, unspecified
> Benign neoplasm of back NOS

D21.9 Benign neoplasm of connective and other soft tissue, unspecified

● **D22 Melanocytic nevi**
> **Includes** atypical nevus
> blue hairy pigmented nevus
> nevus NOS

D22.0 Melanocytic nevi of lip
> *Skin lesions composed of nests of nevus cells with macules/papules*

● **D22.1 Melanocytic nevi of eyelid, including canthus**
> **D22.10** Melanocytic nevi of unspecified eyelid, including canthus
> **D22.11** Melanocytic nevi of right eyelid, including canthus
> **D22.12** Melanocytic nevi of left eyelid, including canthus

● **D22.2 Melanocytic nevi of ear and external auricular canal**
> **D22.20** Melanocytic nevi of unspecified ear and external auricular canal
> **D22.21** Melanocytic nevi of right ear and external auricular canal
> **D22.22** Melanocytic nevi of left ear and external auricular canal

● **D22.3 Melanocytic nevi of other and unspecified parts of face**
> **D22.30** Melanocytic nevi of unspecified part of face
> **D22.39** Melanocytic nevi of other parts of face

D22.4 Melanocytic nevi of scalp and neck

D22.5 Melanocytic nevi of trunk
> Melanocytic nevi of anal margin
> Melanocytic nevi of anal skin
> Melanocytic nevi of perianal skin
> Melanocytic nevi of skin of breast

● **D22.6 Melanocytic nevi of upper limb, including shoulder**
> **D22.60** Melanocytic nevi of unspecified upper limb, including shoulder
> **D22.61** Melanocytic nevi of right upper limb, including shoulder
> **D22.62** Melanocytic nevi of left upper limb, including shoulder

● **D22.7 Melanocytic nevi of lower limb, including hip**
> **D22.70** Melanocytic nevi of unspecified lower limb, including hip
> **D22.71** Melanocytic nevi of right lower limb, including hip
> **D22.72** Melanocytic nevi of left lower limb, including hip

D22.9 Melanocytic nevi, unspecified

● **D23 Other benign neoplasms of skin**
> **Includes** benign neoplasm of hair follicles
> benign neoplasm of sebaceous glands
> benign neoplasm of sweat glands
> **Excludes1** benign lipomatous neoplasms of skin (D17.0-D17.3)
> melanocytic nevi (D22.-)

D23.0 Other benign neoplasm of skin of lip
> **Excludes1** benign neoplasm of vermilion border of lip (D10.0)

● **D23.1 Other benign neoplasm of skin of eyelid, including canthus**
> **D23.10** Other benign neoplasm of skin unspecified of eyelid, including canthus
> **D23.11** Other benign neoplasm of skin of right eyelid, including canthus
> **D23.12** Other benign neoplasm of skin of left eyelid, including canthus

◄ New   ◄▦ Revised   ~~deleted~~ Deleted   Excludes 1   Excludes 2   Includes   Use additional   Code first   Code also   Unspecified
OGCR Official Guidelines   **X** Assign placeholder X   ● Use Additional Character(s)   ▶ Manifestation Code   **Coding Clinic**

- **D23.2** Other benign neoplasm of skin of ear and external auricular canal
    - **D23.20** Other benign neoplasm of skin of unspecified ear and external auricular canal
    - **D23.21** Other benign neoplasm of skin of right ear and external auricular canal
    - **D23.22** Other benign neoplasm of skin of left ear and external auricular canal
- **D23.3** Other benign neoplasm of skin of other and unspecified parts of face
    - **D23.30** Other benign neoplasm of skin of unspecified part of face
    - **D23.39** Other benign neoplasm of skin of other parts of face
- **D23.4** Other benign neoplasm of skin of scalp and neck
- **D23.5** Other benign neoplasm of skin of trunk
    Other benign neoplasm of anal margin
    Other benign neoplasm of anal skin
    Other benign neoplasm of perianal skin
    Other benign neoplasm of skin of breast
    Excludes1   benign neoplasm of anus NOS (D12.9)
- **D23.6** Other benign neoplasm of skin of upper limb, including shoulder
    - **D23.60** Other benign neoplasm of skin of unspecified upper limb, including shoulder
    - **D23.61** Other benign neoplasm of skin of right upper limb, including shoulder
    - **D23.62** Other benign neoplasm of skin of left upper limb, including shoulder
- **D23.7** Other benign neoplasm of skin of lower limb, including hip
    - **D23.70** Other benign neoplasm of skin of unspecified lower limb, including hip
    - **D23.71** Other benign neoplasm of skin of right lower limb, including hip
    - **D23.72** Other benign neoplasm of skin of left lower limb, including hip
- **D23.9** Other benign neoplasm of skin, unspecified

- **D24** **Benign neoplasm of breast**
    Includes   benign neoplasm of connective tissue of breast
    benign neoplasm of soft parts of breast
    fibroadenoma of breast
    Excludes2   adenofibrosis of breast (N60.2)
    benign cyst of breast (N60.-)
    benign mammary dysplasia (N60.-)
    benign neoplasm of skin of breast (D22.5, D23.5)
    fibrocystic disease of breast (N60.-)
    - **D24.1** Benign neoplasm of right breast
    - **D24.2** Benign neoplasm of left breast
    - **D24.9** Benign neoplasm of unspecified breast

- **D25** **Leiomyoma of uterus**
    Benign tumors or nodules of the uterine wall
    Includes   uterine fibroid
    uterine fibromyoma
    uterine myoma
    - **D25.0** Submucous leiomyoma of uterus ♀
    - **D25.1** Intramural leiomyoma of uterus ♀
        Interstitial leiomyoma of uterus
    - **D25.2** Subserosal leiomyoma of uterus ♀
        Subperitoneal leiomyoma of uterus
    - **D25.9** Leiomyoma of uterus, unspecified ♀

- **D26** **Other benign neoplasms of uterus**
    - **D26.0** Other benign neoplasm of cervix uteri ♀
    - **D26.1** Other benign neoplasm of corpus uteri ♀
    - **D26.7** Other benign neoplasm of other parts of uterus ♀
    - **D26.9** Other benign neoplasm of uterus, unspecified ♀

Item 2–11 Teratoma: terat = monster, oma = mass, tumor. Alternate terms: dermoid cyst of the ovary, ovarian teratoma. Teratomas are neoplasms and arise from germ cells (ovaries in female and testes in male) and can be benign or malignant. Teratomas have been known to contain hair, nails, and teeth, giving them a bizarre ("monster") appearance.

- **D27** **Benign neoplasm of ovary**
    Use additional code to identify any functional activity.
    Excludes2   corpus albicans cyst (N83.2)
    corpus luteum cyst (N83.1)
    endometrial cyst (N80.1)
    follicular (atretic) cyst (N83.0)
    graafian follicle cyst (N83.0)
    ovarian cyst NEC (N83.2)
    ovarian retention cyst (N83.2)
    - **D27.0** Benign neoplasm of right ovary ♀
    - **D27.1** Benign neoplasm of left ovary ♀
    - **D27.9** Benign neoplasm of unspecified ovary ♀

- **D28** **Benign neoplasm of other and unspecified female genital organs**
    Includes   adenomatous polyp
    benign neoplasm of skin of female genital organs
    benign teratoma
    Excludes1   epoophoron cyst (Q50.5)
    fimbrial cyst (Q50.4)
    Gartner's duct cyst (Q52.4)
    parovarian cyst (Q50.5)
    - **D28.0** Benign neoplasm of vulva ♀
    - **D28.1** Benign neoplasm of vagina ♀
    - **D28.2** Benign neoplasm of uterine tubes and ligaments ♀
        Benign neoplasm of fallopian tube
        Benign neoplasm of uterine ligament (broad) (round)
    - **D28.7** Benign neoplasm of other specified female genital organs ♀
    - **D28.9** Benign neoplasm of female genital organ, unspecified ♀

- **D29** **Benign neoplasm of male genital organs**
    Includes   benign neoplasm of skin of male genital organs
    - **D29.0** Benign neoplasm of penis ♂
    - **D29.1** Benign neoplasm of prostate ♂
        Excludes1   enlarged prostate (N40.-)
    - **D29.2** Benign neoplasm of testis ♂
        Use additional code to identify any functional activity.
        - **D29.20** Benign neoplasm of unspecified testis ♂
        - **D29.21** Benign neoplasm of right testis ♂
        - **D29.22** Benign neoplasm of left testis ♂
    - **D29.3** Benign neoplasm of epididymis
        - **D29.30** Benign neoplasm of unspecified epididymis ♂
        - **D29.31** Benign neoplasm of right epididymis ♂
        - **D29.32** Benign neoplasm of left epididymis ♂
    - **D29.4** Benign neoplasm of scrotum ♂
        Benign neoplasm of skin of scrotum
    - **D29.8** Benign neoplasm of other specified male genital organs ♂
        Benign neoplasm of seminal vesicle
        Benign neoplasm of spermatic cord
        Benign neoplasm of tunica vaginalis
    - **D29.9** Benign neoplasm of male genital organ, unspecified ♂

- **D30** **Benign neoplasm of urinary organs**
    - **D30.0** Benign neoplasm of kidney
        Excludes1   benign carcinoid tumor of the kidney (D3A.093)
        benign neoplasm of renal calyces (D30.1-)
        benign neoplasm of renal pelvis (D30.1-)
        - **D30.00** Benign neoplasm of unspecified kidney
        - **D30.01** Benign neoplasm of right kidney
        - **D30.02** Benign neoplasm of left kidney

CHAPTER 2 (C00–D49)

● **D30.1**   Benign neoplasm of renal pelvis
     D30.10   Benign neoplasm of unspecified renal pelvis
     D30.11   Benign neoplasm of right renal pelvis
     D30.12   Benign neoplasm of left renal pelvis

● **D30.2**   Benign neoplasm of ureter
     Excludes1   benign neoplasm of ureteric orifice of bladder (D30.3)
     D30.20   Benign neoplasm of unspecified ureter
     D30.21   Benign neoplasm of right ureter
     D30.22   Benign neoplasm of left ureter

   D30.3   Benign neoplasm of bladder
     Benign neoplasm of ureteric orifice of bladder
     Benign neoplasm of urethral orifice of bladder

   D30.4   Benign neoplasm of urethra
     Excludes1   benign neoplasm of urethral orifice of bladder (D30.3)

   D30.8   Benign neoplasm of other specified urinary organs
     Benign neoplasm of paraurethral glands

   D30.9   Benign neoplasm of urinary organ, unspecified
     Benign neoplasm of urinary system NOS

● **D31**   Benign neoplasm of eye and adnexa
     Excludes1   benign neoplasm of connective tissue of eyelid (D21.0)
               benign neoplasm of optic nerve (D33.3)
               benign neoplasm of skin of eyelid (D22.1-, D23.1-)

● **D31.0**   Benign neoplasm of conjunctiva
     D31.00   Benign neoplasm of unspecified conjunctiva
     D31.01   Benign neoplasm of right conjunctiva
     D31.02   Benign neoplasm of left conjunctiva

● **D31.1**   Benign neoplasm of cornea
     D31.10   Benign neoplasm of unspecified cornea
     D31.11   Benign neoplasm of right cornea
     D31.12   Benign neoplasm of left cornea

● **D31.2**   Benign neoplasm of retina
     Excludes1   dark area on retina (D49.81)
               hemangioma of retina (D49.81)
               neoplasm of unspecified behavior of retina and choroid (D49.81)
               retinal freckle (D49.81)
     D31.20   Benign neoplasm of unspecified retina
     D31.21   Benign neoplasm of right retina
     D31.22   Benign neoplasm of left retina

● **D31.3**   Benign neoplasm of choroid
     D31.30   Benign neoplasm of unspecified choroid
     D31.31   Benign neoplasm of right choroid
     D31.32   Benign neoplasm of left choroid

● **D31.4**   Benign neoplasm of ciliary body
     D31.40   Benign neoplasm of unspecified ciliary body
     D31.41   Benign neoplasm of right ciliary body
     D31.42   Benign neoplasm of left ciliary body

● **D31.5**   Benign neoplasm of lacrimal gland and duct
     Benign neoplasm of lacrimal sac
     Benign neoplasm of nasolacrimal duct
     D31.50   Benign neoplasm of unspecified lacrimal gland and duct
     D31.51   Benign neoplasm of right lacrimal gland and duct
     D31.52   Benign neoplasm of left lacrimal gland and duct

● **D31.6**   Benign neoplasm of unspecified site of orbit
     Benign neoplasm of connective tissue of orbit
     Benign neoplasm of extraocular muscle
     Benign neoplasm of peripheral nerves of orbit
     Benign neoplasm of retrobulbar tissue
     Benign neoplasm of retro-ocular tissue
     Excludes1   benign neoplasm of orbital bone (D16.4)
     D31.60   Benign neoplasm of unspecified site of unspecified orbit
     D31.61   Benign neoplasm of unspecified site of right orbit
     D31.62   Benign neoplasm of unspecified site of left orbit

● **D31.9**   Benign neoplasm of unspecified part of eye
     Benign neoplasm of eyeball
     D31.90   Benign neoplasm of unspecified part of unspecified eye
     D31.91   Benign neoplasm of unspecified part of right eye
     D31.92   Benign neoplasm of unspecified part of left eye

● **D32**   Benign neoplasm of meninges
     D32.0   Benign neoplasm of cerebral meninges
     D32.1   Benign neoplasm of spinal meninges
     D32.9   Benign neoplasm of meninges, unspecified
         Meningioma NOS

● **D33**   Benign neoplasm of brain and other parts of central nervous system
     Excludes1   angioma (D18.0-)
               benign neoplasm of meninges (D32.-)
               benign neoplasm of peripheral nerves and autonomic nervous system (D36.1-)
               hemangioma (D18.0-)
               neurofibromatosis (Q85.0-)
               retro-ocular benign neoplasm (D31.6-)

     D33.0   Benign neoplasm of brain, supratentorial
         Benign neoplasm of cerebral ventricle
         Benign neoplasm of cerebrum
         Benign neoplasm of frontal lobe
         Benign neoplasm of occipital lobe
         Benign neoplasm of parietal lobe
         Benign neoplasm of temporal lobe
         Excludes1   benign neoplasm of fourth ventricle (D33.1)

     D33.1   Benign neoplasm of brain, infratentorial
         Benign neoplasm of brain stem
         Benign neoplasm of cerebellum
         Benign neoplasm of fourth ventricle

     D33.2   Benign neoplasm of brain, unspecified

     D33.3   Benign neoplasm of cranial nerves
         Benign neoplasm of olfactory bulb

     D33.4   Benign neoplasm of spinal cord

     D33.7   Benign neoplasm of other specified parts of central nervous system

     D33.9   Benign neoplasm of central nervous system, unspecified
         Benign neoplasm of nervous system (central) NOS

  D34   Benign neoplasm of thyroid gland
     Use additional code to identify any functional activity.

◄ New   ◄▪▪▪ Revised   ~~deleted~~ Deleted   Excludes 1   Excludes 2   Includes   Use additional   Code first   Code also   Unspecified

OGCR Official Guidelines   X Assign placeholder X   ● Use Additional Character(s)   ▶ Manifestation Code   **Coding Clinic**

● **D35**   **Benign neoplasm of other and unspecified endocrine glands**
Use additional code to identify any functional activity.
> **Excludes1**   benign neoplasm of endocrine pancreas (D13.7)
> benign neoplasm of ovary (D27.-)
> benign neoplasm of testis (D29.2.-)
> benign neoplasm of thymus (D15.0)

  ● **D35.0**   Benign neoplasm of adrenal gland
     D35.00   Benign neoplasm of unspecified adrenal gland
     D35.01   Benign neoplasm of right adrenal gland
     D35.02   Benign neoplasm of left adrenal gland
  D35.1   Benign neoplasm of parathyroid gland
  D35.2   Benign neoplasm of pituitary gland
  D35.3   Benign neoplasm of craniopharyngeal duct
  D35.4   Benign neoplasm of pineal gland
  D35.5   Benign neoplasm of carotid body
  D35.6   Benign neoplasm of aortic body and other paraganglia
     Benign tumor of glomus jugulare
  D35.7   Benign neoplasm of other specified endocrine glands
  D35.9   Benign neoplasm of endocrine gland, unspecified
     Benign neoplasm of unspecified endocrine gland

● **D36**   **Benign neoplasm of other and unspecified sites**
  D36.0   Benign neoplasm of lymph nodes
> **Excludes1**   lymphangioma (D18.1)

  ● **D36.1**   Benign neoplasm of peripheral nerves and autonomic nervous system
> **Excludes1**   benign neoplasm of peripheral nerves of orbit (D31.6-)
> neurofibromatosis (Q85.0-)

     D36.10   Benign neoplasm of peripheral nerves and autonomic nervous system, unspecified
     D36.11   Benign neoplasm of peripheral nerves and autonomic nervous system of face, head, and neck
     D36.12   Benign neoplasm of peripheral nerves and autonomic nervous system, upper limb, including shoulder
     D36.13   Benign neoplasm of peripheral nerves and autonomic nervous system of lower limb, including hip
     D36.14   Benign neoplasm of peripheral nerves and autonomic nervous system of thorax
     D36.15   Benign neoplasm of peripheral nerves and autonomic nervous system of abdomen
     D36.16   Benign neoplasm of peripheral nerves and autonomic nervous system of pelvis
     D36.17   Benign neoplasm of peripheral nerves and autonomic nervous system of trunk, unspecified
  D36.7   Benign neoplasm of other specified sites
     Benign neoplasm of nose NOS
  D36.9   Benign neoplasm, unspecified site

BENIGN NEUROENDOCRINE TUMORS (D3A)

● **D3A**   **Benign neuroendocrine tumors**
Code also any associated multiple endocrine neoplasia [MEN] syndromes (E31.2-)
Use additional code to identify any associated endocrine syndrome, such as:
carcinoid syndrome (E34.0)
> **Excludes2**   benign pancreatic islet cell tumors (D13.7)

  ● **D3A.0**   Benign carcinoid tumors
     D3A.00   Benign carcinoid tumor of unspecified site
       Carcinoid tumor NOS
     ● **D3A.01**   Benign carcinoid tumors of the small intestine
       D3A.010   Benign carcinoid tumor of the duodenum
       D3A.011   Benign carcinoid tumor of the jejunum

       D3A.012   Benign carcinoid tumor of the ileum
       D3A.019   Benign carcinoid tumor of the small intestine, unspecified portion
     ● **D3A.02**   Benign carcinoid tumors of the appendix, large intestine, and rectum
       D3A.020   Benign carcinoid tumor of the appendix
       D3A.021   Benign carcinoid tumor of the cecum
       D3A.022   Benign carcinoid tumor of the ascending colon
       D3A.023   Benign carcinoid tumor of the transverse colon
       D3A.024   Benign carcinoid tumor of the descending colon
       D3A.025   Benign carcinoid tumor of the sigmoid colon
       D3A.026   Benign carcinoid tumor of the rectum
       D3A.029   Benign carcinoid tumor of the large intestine, unspecified portion
        Benign carcinoid tumor of the colon NOS
     ● **D3A.09**   Benign carcinoid tumors of other sites
       D3A.090   Benign carcinoid tumor of the bronchus and lung
       D3A.091   Benign carcinoid tumor of the thymus
       D3A.092   Benign carcinoid tumor of the stomach
       D3A.093   Benign carcinoid tumor of the kidney
       D3A.094   Benign carcinoid tumor of the foregut NOS
       D3A.095   Benign carcinoid tumor of the midgut NOS
       D3A.096   Benign carcinoid tumor of the hindgut NOS
       D3A.098   Benign carcinoid tumors of other sites
  D3A.8   Other benign neuroendocrine tumors
     Neuroendocrine tumor NOS

NEOPLASMS OF UNCERTAIN BEHAVIOR, POLYCYTHEMIA VERA AND MYELODYSPLASTIC SYNDROMES (D37-D48)

Note: Categories D37-D44, and D48 classify by site neoplasms of uncertain behavior, i.e., histologic confirmation whether the neoplasm is malignant or benign cannot be made.
> **Excludes1**   neoplasms of unspecified behavior (D49.-)

● **D37**   **Neoplasm of uncertain behavior of oral cavity and digestive organs**
> **Excludes1**   stromal tumors of uncertain behavior of digestive system (D48.1)

  ● **D37.0**   Neoplasm of uncertain behavior of lip, oral cavity and pharynx
> **Excludes1**   neoplasm of uncertain behavior of aryepiglottic fold or interarytenoid fold, laryngeal aspect (D38.0)
> neoplasm of uncertain behavior of epiglottis NOS (D38.0)
> neoplasm of uncertain behavior of skin of lip (D48.5)
> neoplasm of uncertain behavior of suprahyoid portion of epiglottis (D38.0)

     D37.01   Neoplasm of uncertain behavior of lip
       Neoplasm of uncertain behavior of vermilion border of lip
     D37.02   Neoplasm of uncertain behavior of tongue

CHAPTER 2 (C00-D49)

CHAPTER 2 (C00–D49)

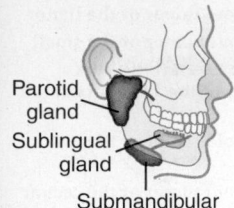

Figure 2-19   Major salivary glands.

Parotid gland
Sublingual gland
Submandibular gland

● **D37.03**   **Neoplasm of uncertain behavior of the major salivary glands**
     D37.030   **Neoplasm of uncertain behavior of the parotid salivary glands**
     D37.031   **Neoplasm of uncertain behavior of the sublingual salivary glands**
     D37.032   **Neoplasm of uncertain behavior of the submandibular salivary glands**
     D37.039   **Neoplasm of uncertain behavior of the major salivary glands, <mark>unspecified</mark>**
   D37.04   **Neoplasm of uncertain behavior of the minor salivary glands**
     Neoplasm of uncertain behavior of submucosal salivary glands of lip
     Neoplasm of uncertain behavior of submucosal salivary glands of cheek
     Neoplasm of uncertain behavior of submucosal salivary glands of hard palate
     Neoplasm of uncertain behavior of submucosal salivary glands of soft palate
   D37.05   **Neoplasm of uncertain behavior of pharynx**
     Neoplasm of uncertain behavior of aryepiglottic fold of pharynx NOS
     Neoplasm of uncertain behavior of hypopharyngeal aspect of aryepiglottic fold of pharynx
     Neoplasm of uncertain behavior of marginal zone of aryepiglottic fold of pharynx
   D37.09   **Neoplasm of uncertain behavior of other specified sites of the oral cavity**
  D37.1   **Neoplasm of uncertain behavior of stomach**
  D37.2   **Neoplasm of uncertain behavior of small intestine**
  D37.3   **Neoplasm of uncertain behavior of appendix**
  D37.4   **Neoplasm of uncertain behavior of colon**
  D37.5   **Neoplasm of uncertain behavior of rectum**
     Neoplasm of uncertain behavior of rectosigmoid junction
     Rectosigmoid junction: Angle where sigmoid colon becomes rectum
  D37.6   **Neoplasm of uncertain behavior of liver, gallbladder and bile ducts**
     Neoplasm of uncertain behavior of ampulla of Vater
     Ampulla of Vater: Enlarged segment of ducts from liver and pancreas at entry point to small intestine
  D37.8   **Neoplasm of uncertain behavior of other specified digestive organs**
     Neoplasm of uncertain behavior of anal canal
     Neoplasm of uncertain behavior of anal sphincter
     Neoplasm of uncertain behavior of anus NOS
     Neoplasm of uncertain behavior of esophagus
     Neoplasm of uncertain behavior of intestine NOS
     Neoplasm of uncertain behavior of pancreas
     Excludes1   neoplasm of uncertain behavior of anal margin (D48.5)
       neoplasm of uncertain behavior of anal skin (D48.5)
       neoplasm of uncertain behavior of perianal skin (D48.5)
  D37.9   **Neoplasm of uncertain behavior of digestive organ, <mark>unspecified</mark>**

● **D38**   **Neoplasm of uncertain behavior of middle ear and respiratory and intrathoracic organs**
     Excludes1   neoplasm of uncertain behavior of heart (D48.7)
   D38.0   **Neoplasm of uncertain behavior of larynx**
     Neoplasm of uncertain behavior of aryepiglottic fold or interarytenoid fold, laryngeal aspect
     Neoplasm of uncertain behavior of epiglottis (suprahyoid portion)
     Excludes1   neoplasm of uncertain behavior of aryepiglottic fold or interarytenoid fold NOS (D37.05)
       neoplasm of uncertain behavior of hypopharyngeal aspect of aryepiglottic fold (D37.05)
       neoplasm of uncertain behavior of marginal zone of aryepiglottic fold (D37.05)
   D38.1   **Neoplasm of uncertain behavior of trachea, bronchus and lung**
   D38.2   **Neoplasm of uncertain behavior of pleura**
   D38.3   **Neoplasm of uncertain behavior of mediastinum**
   D38.4   **Neoplasm of uncertain behavior of thymus**
   D38.5   **Neoplasm of uncertain behavior of other respiratory organs**
     Neoplasm of uncertain behavior of accessory sinuses
     Neoplasm of uncertain behavior of cartilage of nose
     Neoplasm of uncertain behavior of middle ear
     Neoplasm of uncertain behavior of nasal cavities
     Excludes1   neoplasm of uncertain behavior of ear (external) (skin) (D48.5)
       neoplasm of uncertain behavior of nose NOS (D48.7)
       neoplasm of uncertain behavior of skin of nose (D48.5)
   D38.6   **Neoplasm of uncertain behavior of respiratory organ, <mark>unspecified</mark>**

● **D39**   **Neoplasm of uncertain behavior of female genital organs**
   D39.0   **Neoplasm of uncertain behavior of uterus ♀**
  ● **D39.1**   **Neoplasm of uncertain behavior of ovary**
     Use additional code to identify any functional activity.
     D39.10   **Neoplasm of uncertain behavior of <mark>unspecified</mark> ovary ♀**
     D39.11   **Neoplasm of uncertain behavior of right ovary ♀**
     D39.12   **Neoplasm of uncertain behavior of left ovary ♀**
   D39.2   **Neoplasm of uncertain behavior of placenta ♀**
     Chorioadenoma destruens
     Invasive hydatidiform mole
     Malignant hydatidiform mole
     Excludes1   hydatidiform mole NOS (O01.9)
   D39.8   **Neoplasm of uncertain behavior of other specified female genital organs ♀**
     Neoplasm of uncertain behavior of skin of female genital organs
   D39.9   **Neoplasm of uncertain behavior of female genital organ, <mark>unspecified</mark> ♀**

● **D40**   **Neoplasm of uncertain behavior of male genital organs**
   D40.0   **Neoplasm of uncertain behavior of prostate ♂**
  ● **D40.1**   **Neoplasm of uncertain behavior of testis**
     D40.10   **Neoplasm of uncertain behavior of <mark>unspecified</mark> testis ♂**
     D40.11   **Neoplasm of uncertain behavior of right testis ♂**
     D40.12   **Neoplasm of uncertain behavior of left testis ♂**
   D40.8   **Neoplasm of uncertain behavior of other specified male genital organs ♂**
     Neoplasm of uncertain behavior of skin of male genital organs
   D40.9   **Neoplasm of uncertain behavior of male genital organ, <mark>unspecified</mark> ♂**

◀ New   ⏴ Revised   ~~deleted~~ Deleted   Excludes 1   Excludes 2   Includes   Use additional   Code first   Code also   Unspecified

808   **OGCR** Official Guidelines   **X** Assign placeholder X   ● Use Additional Character(s)   ▶ Manifestation Code   **Coding Clinic**

● **D41　Neoplasm of uncertain behavior of urinary organs**
　● **D41.0　Neoplasm of uncertain behavior of kidney**
　　　Excludes1　neoplasm of uncertain behavior of renal pelvis (D41.1-)
　　　D41.00　Neoplasm of uncertain behavior of unspecified **kidney**
　　　D41.01　Neoplasm of uncertain behavior of right kidney
　　　D41.02　Neoplasm of uncertain behavior of left kidney
　● **D41.1　Neoplasm of uncertain behavior of renal pelvis**
　　　D41.10　Neoplasm of uncertain behavior of unspecified **renal pelvis**
　　　D41.11　Neoplasm of uncertain behavior of right renal pelvis
　　　D41.12　Neoplasm of uncertain behavior of left renal pelvis
　● **D41.2　Neoplasm of uncertain behavior of ureter**
　　　D41.20　Neoplasm of uncertain behavior of unspecified **ureter**
　　　D41.21　Neoplasm of uncertain behavior of right ureter
　　　D41.22　Neoplasm of uncertain behavior of left ureter
　　D41.3　Neoplasm of uncertain behavior of urethra
　　D41.4　Neoplasm of uncertain behavior of bladder
　　D41.8　Neoplasm of uncertain behavior of other specified urinary organs
　　D41.9　Neoplasm of uncertain behavior of unspecified **urinary organ**

● **D42　Neoplasm of uncertain behavior of meninges**
　　D42.0　Neoplasm of uncertain behavior of cerebral meninges
　　D42.1　Neoplasm of uncertain behavior of spinal meninges
　　D42.9　Neoplasm of uncertain behavior of meninges, unspecified

● **D43　Neoplasm of uncertain behavior of brain and central nervous system**
　　　Excludes1　neoplasm of uncertain behavior of peripheral nerves and autonomic nervous system (D48.2)
　　D43.0　Neoplasm of uncertain behavior of brain, supratentorial
　　　Superior to tentorium of cerebellum
　　　Neoplasm of uncertain behavior of cerebral ventricle
　　　Neoplasm of uncertain behavior of cerebrum
　　　Neoplasm of uncertain behavior of frontal lobe
　　　Neoplasm of uncertain behavior of occipital lobe
　　　Neoplasm of uncertain behavior of parietal lobe
　　　Neoplasm of uncertain behavior of temporal lobe
　　　　Excludes1　neoplasm of uncertain behavior of fourth ventricle (D43.1)
　　D43.1　Neoplasm of uncertain behavior of brain, infratentorial
　　　Beneath the tentorium of cerebellum
　　　Neoplasm of uncertain behavior of brain stem
　　　Neoplasm of uncertain behavior of cerebellum
　　　Neoplasm of uncertain behavior of fourth ventricle
　　D43.2　Neoplasm of uncertain behavior of brain, unspecified
　　D43.3　Neoplasm of uncertain behavior of cranial nerves
　　D43.4　Neoplasm of uncertain behavior of spinal cord
　　D43.8　Neoplasm of uncertain behavior of other specified parts of central nervous system
　　D43.9　Neoplasm of uncertain behavior of central nervous system, unspecified
　　　Neoplasm of uncertain behavior of nervous system (central) NOS

● **D44　Neoplasm of uncertain behavior of endocrine glands**
　　　Excludes1　multiple endocrine adenomatosis (E31.2-)
　　　　　　　　multiple endocrine neoplasia (E31.2-)
　　　　　　　　neoplasm of uncertain behavior of endocrine pancreas (D37.8)
　　　　　　　　neoplasm of uncertain behavior of ovary (D39.1-)
　　　　　　　　neoplasm of uncertain behavior of testis (D40.1-)
　　　　　　　　neoplasm of uncertain behavior of thymus (D38.4)
　　D44.0　Neoplasm of uncertain behavior of thyroid gland
　● **D44.1　Neoplasm of uncertain behavior of adrenal gland**
　　　Use additional code to identify any functional activity.
　　　D44.10　Neoplasm of uncertain behavior of unspecified **adrenal gland**
　　　D44.11　Neoplasm of uncertain behavior of right adrenal gland
　　　D44.12　Neoplasm of uncertain behavior of left adrenal gland
　　D44.2　Neoplasm of uncertain behavior of parathyroid gland
　　D44.3　Neoplasm of uncertain behavior of pituitary gland
　　　Use additional code to identify any functional activity.
　　D44.4　Neoplasm of uncertain behavior of craniopharyngeal duct
　　D44.5　Neoplasm of uncertain behavior of pineal gland
　　D44.6　Neoplasm of uncertain behavior of carotid body
　　D44.7　Neoplasm of uncertain behavior of aortic body and other paraganglia
　　D44.9　Neoplasm of uncertain behavior of unspecified **endocrine gland**

　D45　Polycythemia vera
　　　Excludes1　familial polycythemia (D75.0)
　　　　　　　　secondary polycythemia (D75.1)
　　　Primary polycythemia. Secondary polycythemia is D75.1. Check your documentation. Polycythemia is caused by too many red blood cells, which increase the thickness of blood (viscosity). This can cause engorgement of the spleen (splenomegaly) with extra RBCs and potential clot formation.

● **D46　Myelodysplastic syndromes**
　　　Use additional code for adverse effect, if applicable, to identify drug (T36-T50 with fifth or sixth character 5)
　　　Excludes2　drug-induced aplastic anemia (D61.1)
　　D46.0　Refractory anemia without ring sideroblasts, so stated
　　　Refractory anemia without sideroblasts, without excess of blasts
　　D46.1　Refractory anemia with ring sideroblasts RARS
　● **D46.2　Refractory anemia with excess of blasts**
　　　Form of myelodysplasia with increased immature white blood cells (blasts) in bone marrow
　　　D46.20　Refractory anemia with excess of blasts, unspecified **RAEB NOS**
　　　D46.21　Refractory anemia with excess of blasts 1 RAEB 1
　　　　Bone marrow disease which results in insufficient RBCs (anemia) in which level of blasts is less than 10%
　　　D46.22　Refractory anemia with excess of blasts 2 RAEB 2
　　　　Bone marrow disease manifested by insufficient numbers of RBCs (anemia) with level of blasts 10-20%

CHAPTER 2 (C00-D49)

CHAPTER 2 (C00-D49)

D46.A **Refractory cytopenia with multilineage dysplasia**

D46.B **Refractory cytopenia with multilineage dysplasia and ring sideroblasts**
RCMD RS

D46.C **Myelodysplastic syndrome with isolated del(5q) chromosomal abnormality**
Myelodysplastic syndrome with 5q deletion
5q minus syndrome NOS

D46.4 **Refractory anemia, unspecified**

D46.Z **Other myelodysplastic syndromes**
Excludes1 chronic myelomonocytic leukemia (C93.1-)

D46.9 **Myelodysplastic syndrome, unspecified**
Myelodysplasia NOS

● D47 **Other neoplasms of uncertain behavior of lymphoid, hematopoietic and related tissue**

D47.0 **Histiocytic and mast cell tumors of uncertain behavior**
Indolent systemic mastocytosis
Mast cell tumor NOS
Mastocytoma NOS
Excludes1 malignant mast cell tumor (C96.2)
mastocytosis (congenital) (cutaneous) (Q82.2)

D47.1 **Chronic myeloproliferative disease**
Chronic neutrophilic leukemia
Myeloproliferative disease, unspecified
Excludes1 atypical chronic myeloid leukemia BCR/ABL-negative (C92.2-)
chronic myeloid leukemia BCR/ABL-positive (C92.1-)
myelofibrosis NOS (D75.81)
myelophthisic anemia (D61.82)
myelophthisis (D61.82)
secondary myelofibrosis NOS (D75.81)

D47.2 **Monoclonal gammopathy**
Monoclonal gammopathy of undetermined significance [MGUS]

D47.3 **Essential (hemorrhagic) thrombocythemia**
Essential thrombocytosis
Idiopathic hemorrhagic thrombocythemia

D47.4 **Osteomyelofibrosis**
Chronic idiopathic myelofibrosis
Myelofibrosis (idiopathic) (with myeloid metaplasia)
Myelosclerosis (megakaryocytic) with myeloid metaplasia
Secondary myelofibrosis in myeloproliferative disease
Excludes1 acute myelofibrosis (C94.4-)

● D47.Z **Other specified neoplasms of uncertain behavior of lymphoid, hematopoietic and related tissue**

D47.Z1 **Post-transplant lymphoproliferative disorder (PTLD)**
Code first complications of transplanted organs and tissue (T86.-)

D47.Z9 **Other specified neoplasms of uncertain behavior of lymphoid, hematopoietic and related tissue**
Histiocytic tumors of uncertain behavior

D47.9 **Neoplasm of uncertain behavior of lymphoid, hematopoietic and related tissue, unspecified**
Lymphoproliferative disease NOS

● D48 **Neoplasm of uncertain behavior of other and unspecified sites**
Excludes1 neurofibromatosis (nonmalignant) (Q85.0-)

D48.0 **Neoplasm of uncertain behavior of bone and articular cartilage**
Excludes1 neoplasm of uncertain behavior of cartilage of ear (D48.1)
neoplasm of uncertain behavior of cartilage of larynx (D38.0)
neoplasm of uncertain behavior of cartilage of nose (D38.5)
neoplasm of uncertain behavior of connective tissue of eyelid (D48.1)
neoplasm of uncertain behavior of synovia (D48.1)

D48.1 **Neoplasm of uncertain behavior of connective and other soft tissue**
Neoplasm of uncertain behavior of connective tissue of ear
Neoplasm of uncertain behavior of connective tissue of eyelid
Stromal tumors of uncertain behavior of digestive system
Excludes1 neoplasm of uncertain behavior of articular cartilage (D48.0)
neoplasm of uncertain behavior of cartilage of larynx (D38.0)
neoplasm of uncertain behavior of cartilage of nose (D38.5)
neoplasm of uncertain behavior of connective tissue of breast (D48.6-)

D48.2 **Neoplasm of uncertain behavior of peripheral nerves and autonomic nervous system**
Excludes1 neoplasm of uncertain behavior of peripheral nerves of orbit (D48.7)

D48.3 **Neoplasm of uncertain behavior of retroperitoneum**

D48.4 **Neoplasm of uncertain behavior of peritoneum**

D48.5 **Neoplasm of uncertain behavior of skin**
Neoplasm of uncertain behavior of anal margin
Neoplasm of uncertain behavior of anal skin
Neoplasm of uncertain behavior of perianal skin
Neoplasm of uncertain behavior of skin of breast
Excludes1 neoplasm of uncertain behavior of anus NOS (D37.8)
neoplasm of uncertain behavior of skin of genital organs (D39.8, D40.8)
neoplasm of uncertain behavior of vermilion border of lip (D37.0)

● D48.6 **Neoplasm of uncertain behavior of breast**
Neoplasm of uncertain behavior of connective tissue of breast
Cystosarcoma phyllodes
Excludes1 neoplasm of uncertain behavior of skin of breast (D48.5)

D48.60 **Neoplasm of uncertain behavior of unspecified breast**

D48.61 **Neoplasm of uncertain behavior of right breast**

D48.62 **Neoplasm of uncertain behavior of left breast**

D48.7 **Neoplasm of uncertain behavior of other specified sites**
Neoplasm of uncertain behavior of eye
Neoplasm of uncertain behavior of heart
Neoplasm of uncertain behavior of peripheral nerves of orbit
Excludes1 neoplasm of uncertain behavior of connective tissue (D48.1)
neoplasm of uncertain behavior of skin of eyelid (D48.5)

D48.9 **Neoplasm of uncertain behavior, unspecified**

◀ New ◀══ Revised ~~deleted~~ Deleted Excludes 1 Excludes 2 Includes Use additional Code first Code also Unspecified
OGCR Official Guidelines X Assign placeholder X ● Use Additional Character(s) ▶ Manifestation Code **Coding Clinic**

● **D49   Neoplasms of unspecified behavior**

> **Note:** Category D49 classifies by site neoplasms of unspecified morphology and behavior. The term 'mass,' unless otherwise stated, is not to be regarded as a neoplastic growth.

> | **Includes** | 'growth' NOS |
> | --- | --- |
> | | neoplasm NOS |
> | | new growth NOS |
> | | tumor NOS |

> | **Excludes1** | neoplasms of uncertain behavior (D37-D44, D48) |
> | --- | --- |

D49.0   Neoplasm of unspecified behavior of digestive system

> | **Excludes1** | neoplasm of unspecified behavior of margin of anus (D49.2) |
> | --- | --- |
> | | neoplasm of unspecified behavior of perianal skin (D49.2) |
> | | neoplasm of unspecified behavior of skin of anus (D49.2) |

D49.1   Neoplasm of unspecified behavior of respiratory system

D49.2   Neoplasm of unspecified behavior of bone, soft tissue, and skin

> | **Excludes1** | neoplasm of unspecified behavior of anal canal (D49.0) |
> | --- | --- |
> | | neoplasm of unspecified behavior of anus NOS (D49.0) |
> | | neoplasm of unspecified behavior of bone marrow (D49.89) |
> | | neoplasm of unspecified behavior of cartilage of larynx (D49.1) |
> | | neoplasm of unspecified behavior of cartilage of nose (D49.1) |
> | | neoplasm of unspecified behavior of connective tissue of breast (D49.3) |
> | | neoplasm of unspecified behavior of skin of genital organs (D49.5) |
> | | neoplasm of unspecified behavior of vermilion border of lip (D49.0) |

D49.3   Neoplasm of unspecified behavior of breast

> | **Excludes1** | neoplasm of unspecified behavior of skin of breast (D49.2) |
> | --- | --- |

D49.4   Neoplasm of unspecified behavior of bladder

D49.5   Neoplasm of unspecified behavior of other genitourinary organs

D49.6   Neoplasm of unspecified behavior of brain

> | **Excludes1** | neoplasm of unspecified behavior of cerebral meninges (D49.7) |
> | --- | --- |
> | | neoplasm of unspecified behavior of cranial nerves (D49.7) |

D49.7   Neoplasm of unspecified behavior of endocrine glands and other parts of nervous system

> | **Excludes1** | neoplasm of unspecified behavior of peripheral, sympathetic, and parasympathetic nerves and ganglia (D49.2) |
> | --- | --- |

● **D49.8   Neoplasm of unspecified behavior of other specified sites**

> | **Excludes1** | neoplasm of unspecified behavior of eyelid (skin) (D49.2) |
> | --- | --- |
> | | neoplasm of unspecified behavior of eyelid cartilage (D49.2) |
> | | neoplasm of unspecified behavior of great vessels (D49.2) |
> | | neoplasm of unspecified behavior of optic nerve (D49.7) |

D49.81   Neoplasm of unspecified behavior of retina and choroid
> Dark area on retina
> Retinal freckle

D49.89   Neoplasm of unspecified behavior of other specified sites

D49.9   Neoplasm of unspecified behavior of unspecified site

CHAPTER 2 (C00-D49)

CHAPTER 3

DISEASES OF THE BLOOD AND BLOOD-FORMING ORGANS AND CERTAIN DISORDERS INVOLVING THE IMMUNE MECHANISM (D50-D89)

> **Excludes2** autoimmune disease (systemic) NOS (M35.9)
> certain conditions originating in the perinatal period (P00-P96)
> complications of pregnancy, childbirth and the puerperium (O00-O9A)
> congenital malformations, deformations and chromosomal abnormalities (Q00-Q99)
> endocrine, nutritional and metabolic diseases (E00-E88)
> human immunodeficiency virus [HIV] disease (B20)
> injury, poisoning and certain other consequences of external causes (S00-T88)
> neoplasms (C00-D49)
> symptoms, signs and abnormal clinical and laboratory findings, not elsewhere classified (R00-R94)

This chapter contains the following blocks:

D50-D53	Nutritional anemias
D55-D59	Hemolytic anemias
D60-D64	Aplastic and other anemias and other bone marrow failure syndromes
D65-D69	Coagulation defects, purpura and other hemorrhagic conditions
D70-D77	Other disorders of blood and blood-forming organs
D78	Intraoperative and postprocedural complications of the spleen
D80-D89	Certain disorders involving the immune mechanism

NUTRITIONAL ANEMIAS (D50-D53)

● **D50 Iron deficiency anemia**
A disease characterized by a decrease in the number of red cells (hemoglobin) in the blood.

> **Includes** asiderotic anemia
> hypochromic anemia

D50.0 Iron deficiency anemia secondary to blood loss (chronic)
Posthemorrhagic anemia (chronic)

> **Excludes1** acute posthemorrhagic anemia (D62)
> congenital anemia from fetal blood loss (P61.3)

D50.1 Sideropenic dysphagia
Web-like growth of membranes in throat that makes swallowing difficult
Kelly-Paterson syndrome
Plummer-Vinson syndrome

D50.8 Other iron deficiency anemias
Iron deficiency anemia due to inadequate dietary iron intake

D50.9 Iron deficiency anemia, unspecified

● **D51 Vitamin B12 deficiency anemia**

> **Excludes1** vitamin B12 deficiency (E53.8)

D51.0 Vitamin B12 deficiency anemia due to intrinsic factor deficiency
Addison anemia
Biermer anemia
Pernicious (congenital) anemia
Congenital intrinsic factor deficiency

D51.1 Vitamin B12 deficiency anemia due to selective vitamin B12 malabsorption with proteinuria
Imerslund (Gräsbeck) syndrome
Megaloblastic hereditary anemia

D51.2 Transcobalamin II deficiency
D51.3 Other dietary vitamin B12 deficiency anemia
Vegan anemia
D51.8 Other vitamin B12 deficiency anemias
D51.9 Vitamin B12 deficiency anemia, unspecified

● **D52 Folate deficiency anemia**

> **Excludes1** folate deficiency without anemia (E53.8)

D52.0 Dietary folate deficiency anemia
Nutritional megaloblastic anemia

D52.1 Drug-induced folate deficiency anemia

> Use additional code for adverse effect, if applicable, to identify drug (T36-T50 with fifth or sixth character 5)

D52.8 Other folate deficiency anemias
D52.9 Folate deficiency anemia, unspecified
Folic acid deficiency anemia NOS

● **D53 Other nutritional anemias**

> **Includes** megaloblastic anemia unresponsive to vitamin B12 or folate therapy

D53.0 Protein deficiency anemia
Amino-acid deficiency anemia
Orotaciduric anemia

> **Excludes1** Lesch-Nyhan syndrome (E79.1)

D53.1 Other megaloblastic anemias, not elsewhere classified
Megaloblastic anemia NOS

> **Excludes1** Di Guglielmo's disease (C94.0)

D53.2 Scorbutic anemia
Anemia resulting from deficiency of ascorbic acid (vitamin C)

> **Excludes1** scurvy (E54)

D53.8 Other specified nutritional anemias
Anemia associated with deficiency of copper
Anemia associated with deficiency of molybdenum
Anemia associated with deficiency of zinc

> **Excludes1** nutritional deficiencies without anemia, such as:
> copper deficiency NOS (E61.0)
> molybdenum deficiency NOS (E61.5)
> zinc deficiency NOS (E60)

D53.9 Nutritional anemia, unspecified
Simple chronic anemia

> **Excludes1** anemia NOS (D64.9)

HEMOLYTIC ANEMIAS (D55-D59)

● **D55 Anemia due to enzyme disorders**

> **Excludes1** drug-induced enzyme deficiency anemia (D59.2)

D55.0 Anemia due to glucose-6-phosphate dehydrogenase [G6PD] deficiency
Favism
G6PD deficiency anemia

D55.1 Anemia due to other disorders of glutathione metabolism
Anemia (due to) enzyme deficiencies, except G6PD, related to the hexose monophosphate [HMP] shunt pathway
Anemia (due to) hemolytic nonspherocytic (hereditary), type I

D55.2 Anemia due to disorders of glycolytic enzymes
Hemolytic nonspherocytic (hereditary) anemia, type II
Hexokinase deficiency anemia
Pyruvate kinase [PK] deficiency anemia
Triose-phosphate isomerase deficiency anemia

> **Excludes1** disorders of glycolysis not associated with anemia (E74.8)

D55.3 Anemia due to disorders of nucleotide metabolism
D55.8 Other anemias due to enzyme disorders
D55.9 Anemia due to enzyme disorder, unspecified

◀ New ◀▬ Revised ~~deleted~~ Deleted Excludes 1 Excludes 2 Includes Use additional Code first Code also Unspecified
OGCR Official Guidelines X Assign placeholder X ● Use Additional Character(s) ▶ Manifestation Code **Coding Clinic**

● **D56**   **Thalassemia**
Hereditary disorders characterized by low production of hemoglobin or excessive destruction of red blood cells

> **Excludes1**   sickle-cell thalassemia (D57.4-)

D56.0   **Alpha thalassemia**
Alpha thalassemia major
Hemoglobin H Constant Spring
Hemoglobin H disease
Hydrops fetalis due to alpha thalassemia
Severe alpha thalassemia
Triple gene defect alpha thalassemia

Use additional code, if applicable, for hydrops fetalis due to alpha thalassemia (P56.99)

> **Excludes1**   alpha thalassemia trait or minor (D56.3)
> asymptomatic alpha thalassemia (D56.3)
> hydrops fetalis due to isoimmunization (P56.0)
> hydrops fetalis not due to immune hemolysis (P83.2)

D56.1   **Beta thalassemia**
Beta thalassemia major
Cooley's anemia
Homozygous beta thalassemia
Severe beta thalassemia
Thalassemia intermedia
Thalassemia major

> **Excludes1**   beta thalassemia minor (D56.3)
> beta thalassemia trait (D56.3)
> delta-beta thalassemia (D56.2)
> hemoglobin E-beta thalassemia (D56.5)
> sickle-cell beta thalassemia (D57.4-)

D56.2   **Delta-beta thalassemia**
Homozygous delta-beta thalassemia

> **Excludes1**   delta-beta thalassemia minor (D56.3)
> delta-beta thalassemia trait (D56.3)

D56.3   **Thalassemia minor**
Genetic disorders that have in common defective production of hemoglobin
Alpha thalassemia minor
Alpha thalassemia silent carrier
Alpha thalassemia trait
Beta thalassemia minor
Beta thalassemia trait
Delta-beta thalassemia minor
Delta-beta thalassemia trait
Thalassemia trait NOS

> **Excludes1**   alpha thalassemia (D56.0)
> beta thalassemia (D56.1)
> delta-beta thalassemia (D56.2)
> hemoglobin E-beta thalassemia (D56.5)
> sickle-cell trait (D57.3)

D56.4   **Hereditary persistence of fetal hemoglobin [HPFH]**
Persistent production of hemoglobin

D56.5   **Hemoglobin E-beta thalassemia**

> **Excludes1**   beta thalassemia (D56.1)
> beta thalassemia minor (D56.3)
> beta thalassemia trait (D56.3)
> delta-beta thalassemia (D56.2)
> delta-beta thalassemia trait (D56.3)
> hemoglobin E disease (D58.2)
> other hemoglobinopathies (D58.2)
> sickle-cell beta thalassemia (D57.4-)

D56.8   **Other thalassemias**
Dominant thalassemia
Hemoglobin C thalassemia
Mixed thalassemia
Thalassemia with other hemoglobinopathy

> **Excludes1**   hemoglobin C disease (D58.2)
> hemoglobin E disease (D58.2)
> other hemoglobinopathies (D58.2)
> sickle cell anemia (D57.-)
> sickle-cell thalassemia (D57.4)

D56.9   **Thalassemia, unspecified**
Mediterranean anemia (with other hemoglobinopathy)

● **D57**   **Sickle-cell disorders**
Inherited disease in which red blood cells, normally disc-shaped, become crescent shaped.

Use additional code for any associated fever (R50.81)

> **Excludes1**   other hemoglobinopathies (D58.-)

● **D57.0**   **Hb-SS disease with crisis**
Sickle-cell disease NOS with crisis
Hb-SS disease with vasoocclusive pain

D57.00   **Hb-SS disease with crisis, unspecified**

D57.01   **Hb-SS disease with acute chest syndrome**

D57.02   **Hb-SS disease with splenic sequestration**

D57.1   **Sickle-cell disease without crisis Hb-SS disease without crisis**
Sickle-cell anemia NOS
Sickle-cell disease NOS
Sickle-cell disorder NOS

● **D57.2**   **Sickle-cell/Hb-C disease**
Hb-SC disease
Hb-S/Hb-C disease

D57.20   **Sickle-cell/Hb-C disease without crisis**

● **D57.21**   **Sickle-cell/Hb-C disease with crisis**

D57.211   **Sickle-cell/Hb-C disease with acute chest syndrome**

D57.212   **Sickle-cell/Hb-C disease with splenic sequestration**

D57.219   **Sickle-cell/Hb-C disease with crisis, unspecified**
Sickle-cell/Hb-C disease with crisis NOS

D57.3   **Sickle-cell trait**
Hb-S trait
Heterozygous hemoglobin S

● **D57.4**   **Sickle-cell thalassemia**
Sickle-cell beta thalassemia
Thalassemia Hb-S disease

D57.40   **Sickle-cell thalassemia without crisis**
Microdrepanocytosis
Sickle-cell thalassemia NOS

● **D57.41**   **Sickle-cell thalassemia with crisis**
Sickle-cell "crisis" is precipitated when abnormally crescent-shaped red blood cells form clots and interrupt blood flow to major organs, causing severe pain and organ damage.
Sickle-cell thalassemia with vasoocclusive pain

D57.411   **Sickle-cell thalassemia with acute chest syndrome**

D57.412   **Sickle-cell thalassemia with splenic sequestration**

D57.419   **Sickle-cell thalassemia with crisis, unspecified**
Sickle-cell thalassemia with crisis NOS

● **D57.8**   **Other sickle-cell disorders**
Hb-SD disease
Hb-SE disease

D57.80   **Other sickle-cell disorders without crisis**

● **D57.81**   **Other sickle-cell disorders with crisis**

D57.811   **Other sickle-cell disorders with acute chest syndrome**

D57.812   **Other sickle-cell disorders with splenic sequestration**

D57.819   **Other sickle-cell disorders with crisis, unspecified**
Other sickle-cell disorders with crisis NOS

CHAPTER 3 (D50-D89)

● **D58 Other hereditary hemolytic anemias**
Genetic condition in which bone marrow is unable to compensate for premature destruction of red blood cells

> **Excludes1**   hemolytic anemia of the newborn (P55.-)

D58.0 Hereditary spherocytosis
Presence of spherocytes (spherically shaped red blood cells)
Acholuric (familial) jaundice
Congenital (spherocytic) hemolytic icterus
Minkowski-Chauffard syndrome

D58.1 Hereditary elliptocytosis
Presence of large numbers of elliptocytes in blood
Elliptocytosis (congenital)
Ovalocytosis (congenital) (hereditary)

D58.2 Other hemoglobinopathies
Abnormal hemoglobin NOS
Congenital Heinz body anemia
Hb-C disease
Hb-D disease
Hb-E disease
Hemoglobinopathy NOS
Unstable hemoglobin hemolytic disease

> **Excludes1**   familial polycythemia (D75.0)
> Hb-M disease (D74.0)
> hemoglobin E-beta thalassemia (D56.5)
> hereditary persistence of fetal hemoglobin [HPFH] (D56.4)
> high-altitude polycythemia (D75.1)
> methemoglobinemia (D74.-)
> other hemoglobinopathies with thalassemia (D56.8)

D58.8 Other specified hereditary hemolytic anemias
Stomatocytosis

D58.9 Hereditary hemolytic anemia, unspecified

● **D59 Acquired hemolytic anemia**

D59.0 Drug-induced autoimmune hemolytic anemia

> Use additional code for adverse effect, if applicable, to identify drug (T36-T50 with fifth or sixth character 5)

D59.1 Other autoimmune hemolytic anemias
Autoimmune hemolytic disease (cold type) (warm type)
Chronic cold hemagglutinin disease
Cold agglutinin disease
Cold agglutinin hemoglobinuria
Cold type (secondary) (symptomatic) hemolytic anemia
Warm type (secondary) (symptomatic) hemolytic anemia

> **Excludes1**   Evans syndrome (D69.41)
> hemolytic disease of newborn (P55.-)
> paroxysmal cold hemoglobinuria (D59.6)

D59.2 Drug-induced nonautoimmune hemolytic anemia
Drug-induced enzyme deficiency anemia

> Use additional code for adverse effect, if applicable, to identify drug (T36-T50 with fifth or sixth character 5)

D59.3 Hemolytic-uremic syndrome

> Use additional code to identify associated:
> E. coli infection (B96.2-)
> Pneumococcal pneumonia (J13)
> Shigella dysenteriae (A03.9)

D59.4 Other nonautoimmune hemolytic anemias
Mechanical hemolytic anemia
Microangiopathic hemolytic anemia
Toxic hemolytic anemia

D59.5 Paroxysmal nocturnal hemoglobinuria [Marchiafava-Micheli]

> **Excludes1**   hemoglobinuria NOS (R82.3)

D59.6 Hemoglobinuria due to hemolysis from other external causes
Hemoglobinuria from exertion
March hemoglobinuria
Paroxysmal cold hemoglobinuria

> Use additional code (Chapter 20) to identify external cause

> **Excludes1**   hemoglobinuria NOS (R82.3)

D59.8 Other acquired hemolytic anemias

D59.9 Acquired hemolytic anemia, unspecified
Idiopathic hemolytic anemia, chronic

APLASTIC AND OTHER ANEMIAS AND OTHER BONE MARROW FAILURE SYNDROMES (D60-D64)

● **D60 Acquired pure red cell aplasia [erythroblastopenia]**
Deficiency of erythroblasts

> **Includes**   red cell aplasia (acquired) (adult) (with thymoma)
> **Excludes1**   congenital red cell aplasia (D61.01)

D60.0 Chronic acquired pure red cell aplasia
Lack of development of blood cell

D60.1 Transient acquired pure red cell aplasia

D60.8 Other acquired pure red cell aplasias

D60.9 Acquired pure red cell aplasia, unspecified

● **D61 Other aplastic anemias and other bone marrow failure syndromes**

> **Excludes1**   neutropenia (D70.-)

● **D61.0 Constitutional aplastic anemia**
Condition where bone marrow is unable to produce blood cells

D61.01 Constitutional (pure) red blood cell aplasia
Blackfan-Diamond syndrome
Congenital (pure) red cell aplasia
Familial hypoplastic anemia
Primary (pure) red cell aplasia
Red cell (pure) aplasia of infants

> **Excludes1**   acquired red cell aplasia (D60.9)

D61.09 Other constitutional aplastic anemia
Fanconi's anemia
Pancytopenia with malformations

D61.1 Drug-induced aplastic anemia

> Use additional code for adverse effect, if applicable, to identify drug (T36-T50 with fifth or sixth character 5)

D61.2 Aplastic anemia due to other external agents

> Code first , if applicable, toxic effects of substances chiefly nonmedicinal as to source (T51-T65)

D61.3 Idiopathic aplastic anemia

◀ New   ◀▆ Revised   ~~deleted~~ Deleted   Excludes 1   Excludes 2   Includes   Use additional   Code first   Code also   Unspecified

OGCR Official Guidelines   **X** Assign placeholder X   ● Use Additional Character(s)   ▶ Manifestation Code   **Coding Clinic**

● **D61.8   Other specified aplastic anemias and other bone marrow failure syndromes**

  ● **D61.81   Pancytopenia**

    Marked deficiency of all the blood elements: Red blood cells (erythrocytes), white blood cells (leukocytes), and platelets (thrombocytes). Check laboratory results.

    Excludes1   pancytopenia (due to) (with) aplastic anemia (D61.9)

               pancytopenia (due to) (with) bone marrow infiltration (D61.82)

               pancytopenia (due to) (with) congenital (pure) red cell aplasia (D61.01)

               pancytopenia (due to) (with) hairy cell leukemia (C91.4-)

               pancytopenia (due to) (with) human immunodeficiency virus disease (B20.-)

               pancytopenia (due to) (with) leukoerythroblastic anemia (D61.82)

               pancytopenia (due to) (with) myelodysplastic syndromes (D46.-)

               pancytopenia (due to) (with) myeloproliferative disease (D47.1)

    D61.810   Antineoplastic chemotherapy induced pancytopenia

      Excludes2   aplastic anemia due to antineoplastic chemotherapy (D61.1)

    D61.811   Other drug-induced pancytopenia

      Excludes2   aplastic anemia due to drugs (D61.1)

    D61.818   Other pancytopenia

  D61.82   Myelophthisis

    Leukoerythroblastic anemia
    Myelophthisic anemia
    Panmyelophthisis

    Code also the underlying disorder, such as:
      malignant neoplasm of breast (C50.-)
      tuberculosis (A15.-)

    Excludes1   idiopathic myelofibrosis (D47.1)

             myelofibrosis NOS (D75.81)

             myelofibrosis with myeloid metaplasia (D47.4)

             primary myelofibrosis (D47.1)

             secondary myelofibrosis (D75.81)

  D61.89   Other specified aplastic anemias and other bone marrow failure syndromes

● **D61.9   Aplastic anemia, unspecified**

  Hypoplastic anemia NOS
  Medullary hypoplasia

● **D62   Acute posthemorrhagic anemia**

  Excludes1   anemia due to chronic blood loss (D50.0)
             blood loss anemia NOS (D50.0)
             congenital anemia from fetal blood loss (P61.3)

● **D63   Anemia in chronic diseases classified elsewhere**

  ▶ **D63.0   *Anemia in neoplastic disease***

    Code first neoplasm (C00-D49)

    Excludes1   anemia due to antineoplastic chemotherapy (D64.81)
             aplastic anemia due to antineoplastic chemotherapy (D61.1)

    OGCR Section I.C.2.e.2.

    2) Anemia associated with chemotherapy, immunotherapy and radiation therapy

    When the admission/encounter is for management of an anemia associated with an adverse effect of the administration of chemotherapy or immunotherapy and the only treatment is for the anemia, the anemia code is sequenced first followed by the appropriate codes for the neoplasm and the adverse effect (T45.1X5, Adverse effect of antineoplastic and immunosuppressive drugs).

  ▶ **D63.1   *Anemia in chronic kidney disease***

    Erythropoietin resistant anemia (EPO resistant anemia)

    Code first underlying chronic kidney disease (CKD) (N18.-)

  ▶ **D63.8   *Anemia in other chronic diseases classified elsewhere***

    Code first underlying disease, such as:
      diphyllobothriasis (B70.0)
      hookworm disease (B76.0-B76.9)
      hypothyroidism (E00.0-E03.9)
      malaria (B50.0-B54)
      symptomatic late syphilis (A52.79)
      tuberculosis (A18.89)

● **D64   Other anemias**

  Excludes1   refractory anemia (D46.-)
             refractory anemia with excess blasts in transformation [RAEB T] (C92.0-)

  D64.0   Hereditary sideroblastic anemia

    Abnormal production RBCs (erythrocytes)
    Sex-linked hypochromic sideroblastic anemia

  ▶ **D64.1   *Secondary sideroblastic anemia due to disease***

    Code first underlying disease

  D64.2   Secondary sideroblastic anemia due to drugs and toxins

    Code first poisoning due to drug or toxin, if applicable (T36-T65 with fifth or sixth character 1-4 or 6)

    Use additional code for adverse effect, if applicable, to identify drug (T36-T50 with fifth or sixth character 5)

  D64.3   Other sideroblastic anemias

    Sideroblastic anemia NOS
    Pyridoxine-responsive sideroblastic anemia NEC

  D64.4   Congenital dyserythropoietic anemia

    Any of several rare hereditary anemias, mostly types of macrocytic anemia
    Dyshematopoietic anemia (congenital)

    Excludes1   Blackfan-Diamond syndrome (D61.01)
             Di Guglielmo's disease (C94.0)

● **D64.8   Other specified anemias**

  D64.81   Anemia due to antineoplastic chemotherapy

    Antineoplastic chemotherapy induced anemia

    Excludes1   anemia in neoplastic disease (D63.0)
             aplastic anemia due to antineoplastic chemotherapy (D61.1)

  D64.89   Other specified anemias

    Infantile pseudoleukemia

  D64.9   Anemia, unspecified

CHAPTER 3 (D50-D89)

COAGULATION DEFECTS, PURPURA AND OTHER HEMORRHAGIC CONDITIONS (D65-D69)

D65   Disseminated intravascular coagulation [defibrination syndrome]
Blood clots form and consume all coagulation proteins and platelets and disrupt normal coagulation, resulting in abnormal bleeding
Afibrinogenemia, acquired
Consumption coagulopathy
Diffuse or disseminated intravascular coagulation [DIC]
Fibrinolytic hemorrhage, acquired
Fibrinolytic purpura
Purpura fulminans

> **Excludes1**   disseminated intravascular coagulation (complicating):
>   abortion or ectopic or molar pregnancy (O00-O07, O08.1)
>   in newborn (P60)
>   pregnancy, childbirth and the puerperium (O45.0, O46.0, O67.0, O72.3)

D66   Hereditary factor VIII deficiency
Inherited coagulation disorder carried by females but most often affecting males
Classical hemophilia
Deficiency factor VIII (with functional defect)
Hemophilia NOS
Hemophilia A

> **Excludes1**   factor VIII deficiency with vascular defect (D68.0)

D67   Hereditary factor IX deficiency
Christmas disease
Factor IX deficiency (with functional defect)
Hemophilia B
Plasma thromboplastin component [PTC] deficiency

● D68   Other coagulation defects

> **Excludes1**   abnormal coagulation profile (R79.1)
>   coagulation defects complicating abortion or ectopic or molar pregnancy (O00-O07, O08.1)
>   coagulation defects complicating pregnancy, childbirth and the puerperium (O45.0, O46.0, O67.0, O72.3)

D68.0   Von Willebrand's disease
Congenital bleeding disorder
Angiohemophilia
Factor VIII deficiency with vascular defect
Vascular hemophilia

> **Excludes1**   capillary fragility (hereditary) (D69.8)
>   factor VIII deficiency NOS (D66)
>   factor VIII deficiency with functional defect (D66)

D68.1   Hereditary factor XI deficiency
Deficiency of blood coagulation resulting in systemic blood-clotting defect
Hemophilia C
Plasma thromboplastin antecedent [PTA] deficiency
Rosenthal's disease

D68.2   Hereditary deficiency of other clotting factors
Blood clotting disorders caused by hereditary deficiencies of one or more clotting factors
AC globulin deficiency
Congenital afibrinogenemia
Deficiency of factor I [fibrinogen]
Deficiency of factor II [prothrombin]
Deficiency of factor V [labile]
Deficiency of factor VII [stable]
Deficiency of factor X [Stuart-Prower]
Deficiency of factor XII [Hageman]
Deficiency of factor XIII [fibrin stabilizing]
Dysfibrinogenemia (congenital)
Hypoproconvertinemia
Owren's disease
Proaccelerin deficiency

● D68.3   Hemorrhagic disorder due to circulating anticoagulants
Blood clotting disorders caused by anticoagulants (warfarin and heparin)

● D68.31   Hemorrhagic disorder due to intrinsic circulating anticoagulants, antibodies, or inhibitors

    D68.311   Acquired hemophilia
      Autoimmune hemophilia
      Autoimmune inhibitors to clotting factors
      Secondary hemophilia

    D68.312   Antiphospholipid antibody with hemorrhagic disorder
      Lupus anticoagulant (LAC) with hemorrhagic disorder
      Systemic lupus erythematosus [SLE] inhibitor with hemorrhagic disorder

> **Excludes1**   antiphospholipid antibody, finding without diagnosis (R76.0)
>   antiphospholipid antibody syndrome (D68.61)
>   antiphospholipid antibody with hypercoagulable state (D68.61)
>   lupus anticoagulant (LAC) finding without diagnosis (R76.0)
>   lupus anticoagulant (LAC) with hypercoagulable state (D68.62)
>   systemic lupus erythematosus [SLE] inhibitor finding without diagnosis (R76.0)
>   systemic lupus erythematosus [SLE] inhibitor with hypercoagulable state (D68.62)

    D68.318   Other hemorrhagic disorder due to intrinsic circulating anticoagulants, antibodies, or inhibitors
      Antithromboplastinemia
      Antithromboplastinogenemia
      Hemorrhagic disorder due to intrinsic increase in antithrombin
      Hemorrhagic disorder due to intrinsic increase in anti-VIIIa
      Hemorrhagic disorder due to intrinsic increase in anti-IXa
      Hemorrhagic disorder due to intrinsic increase in anti-XIa

D68.32   Hemorrhagic disorder due to extrinsic circulating anticoagulants
Drug-induced hemorrhagic disorder
Hemorrhagic disorder due to increase in anti-IIa
Hemorrhagic disorder due to increase in anti-Xa
Hyperheparinemia

> Use additional code for adverse effect, if applicable, to identify drug (T45.515, T45.525)

D68.4   **Acquired coagulation factor deficiency**
Deficiency of coagulation factor due to liver disease
Deficiency of coagulation factor due to vitamin K deficiency

> **Excludes1**   vitamin K deficiency of newborn (P53)

● **D68.5**   **Primary thrombophilia**
AKA idiopathic thrombocytopenia, may be acquired or congenital and is a common cause of coagulation disorders.
Primary hypercoagulable states

> **Excludes1**   antiphospholipid syndrome (D68.61)
> lupus anticoagulant (D68.62)
> secondary activated protein C resistance (D68.69)
> secondary antiphospholipid antibody syndrome (D68.69)
> secondary lupus anticoagulant with hypercoagulable state (D68.69)
> secondary systemic lupus erythematosus [SLE] inhibitor with hypercoagulable state (D68.69)
> systemic lupus erythematosus [SLE] inhibitor finding without diagnosis (R76.0)
> systemic lupus erythematosus [SLE] inhibitor with hemorrhagic disorder (D68.312)
> thrombotic thrombocytopenic purpura (M31.1)

     D68.51   **Activated protein C resistance**
Factor V Leiden mutation

     D68.52   **Prothrombin gene mutation**

     D68.59   **Other primary thrombophilia**
Antithrombin III deficiency
Hypercoagulable state NOS
Primary hypercoagulable state NEC
Primary thrombophilia NEC
Protein C deficiency
Protein S deficiency
Thrombophilia NOS

● **D68.6**   **Other thrombophilia**
Other hypercoagulable states

> **Excludes1**   diffuse or disseminated intravascular coagulation [DIC] (D65)
> heparin induced thrombocytopenia (HIT) (D75.82)
> hyperhomocysteinemia (E72.11)

     D68.61   **Antiphospholipid syndrome**
Anticardiolipin syndrome
Antiphospholipid antibody syndrome

> **Excludes1**   anti-phospholipid antibody, finding without diagnosis (R76.0)
> anti-phospholipid antibody with hemorrhagic disorder (D68.312)
> lupus anticoagulant syndrome (D68.62)

     D68.62   **Lupus anticoagulant syndrome**
Lupus anticoagulant
Presence of systemic lupus erythematosus [SLE] inhibitor

> **Excludes1**   anticardiolipin syndrome (D68.61)
> antiphospholipid syndrome (D68.61)
> lupus anticoagulant (LAC) finding without diagnosis (R79.0)
> lupus anticoagulant (LAC) with hemorrhagic disorder (D68.312)

     D68.69   **Other thrombophilia**
Hypercoagulable states NEC
Secondary hypercoagulable state NOS

D68.8   **Other specified coagulation defects**

> **Excludes1**   hemorrhagic disease of newborn (P53)

D68.9   **Coagulation defect, unspecified**

● **D69**   **Purpura and other hemorrhagic conditions**
Group of conditions characterized by small hemorrhages in skin, mucous membranes, or serosal surfaces

> **Excludes1**   benign hypergammaglobulinemic purpura (D89.0)
> cryoglobulinemic purpura (D89.1)
> essential (hemorrhagic) thrombocythemia (D47.3)
> hemorrhagic thrombocythemia (D47.3)
> purpura fulminans (D65)
> thrombotic thrombocytopenic purpura (M31.1)
> Waldenström hypergammaglobulinemic purpura (D89.0)

D69.0   **Allergic purpura**
Allergic vasculitis
Nonthrombocytopenic hemorrhagic purpura
Nonthrombocytopenic idiopathic purpura
Purpura anaphylactoid
Purpura Henoch(-Schönlein)
Purpura rheumatica
Vascular purpura

> **Excludes1**   thrombocytopenic hemorrhagic purpura (D69.3)

D69.1   **Qualitative platelet defects**
Bernard-Soulier [giant platelet] syndrome
Glanzmann's disease
Grey platelet syndrome
Thrombasthenia (hemorrhagic) (hereditary)
Thrombocytopathy

> **Excludes1**   von Willebrand's disease (D68.0)

D69.2   **Other nonthrombocytopenic purpura**
Purpura NOS
Purpura simplex
Senile purpura

D69.3   **Immune thrombocytopenic purpura**
Hemorrhagic (thrombocytopenic) purpura
Idiopathic thrombocytopenic purpura
Tidal platelet dysgenesis

● **D69.4**   **Other primary thrombocytopenia**

> **Excludes1**   transient neonatal thrombocytopenia (P61.0)
> Wiskott-Aldrich syndrome (D82.0)

     D69.41   **Evans syndrome**
Acquired hemolytic anemia and thrombocytopenia

     D69.42   **Congenital and hereditary thrombocytopenia purpura**
Congenital thrombocytopenia
Hereditary thrombocytopenia

       Code first congenital or hereditary disorder, such as:
thrombocytopenia with absent radius (TAR syndrome) (Q87.2)

     D69.49   **Other primary thrombocytopenia**
Megakaryocytic hypoplasia
Primary thrombocytopenia NOS

● **D69.5**   **Secondary thrombocytopenia**
Acquired reduction of number of platelets required for blood clotting

> **Excludes1**   heparin induced thrombocytopenia (HIT) (D75.82)
> transient thrombocytopenia of newborn (P61.0)

     D69.51   **Posttransfusion purpura**
Posttransfusion purpura from whole blood (fresh) or blood products PTP

     D69.59   **Other secondary thrombocytopenia**

D69.6   **Thrombocytopenia, unspecified**

D69.8   **Other specified hemorrhagic conditions**
Capillary fragility (hereditary)
Vascular pseudohemophilia

D69.9   **Hemorrhagic condition, unspecified**

CHAPTER 3 (D50-D89)

CHAPTER 3 (D50-D89)

OTHER DISORDERS OF BLOOD AND BLOOD-FORMING ORGANS (D70-D77)

● **D70 Neutropenia**
Decrease in number of neutrophils (type of white blood cell)

> **Includes** agranulocytosis
> decreased absolute neurophile count (ANC)

Use additional code for any associated:
fever (R50.81)
mucositis (J34.81, K12.3-, K92.81, N76.81)

> **Excludes1** neutropenic splenomegaly (D73.81)
> transient neonatal neutropenia (P61.5)

D70.0 Congenital agranulocytosis
Reduced numbers of neutrophils (type of white blood cell)
Congenital neutropenia
Infantile genetic agranulocytosis
Kostmann's disease

D70.1 Agranulocytosis secondary to cancer chemotherapy
Decreased numbers of granulocytes (type of white blood cell)
Code also *underlying neoplasm*
Use additional code for adverse effect, if applicable, to identify drug (T45.1X5)

D70.2 Other drug-induced agranulocytosis
Use additional code for adverse effect, if applicable, to identify drug (T36-T50 with fifth or sixth character 5)

D70.3 Neutropenia due to infection

D70.4 Cyclic neutropenia
Chronic neutropenia (low number of type of white blood cell)
Cyclic hematopoiesis
Periodic neutropenia

D70.8 Other neutropenia

D70.9 Neutropenia, unspecified

D71 Functional disorders of polymorphonuclear neutrophils
Polymorphonuclear: varying shapes of nucleus; AKA PMNs
Cell membrane receptor complex [CR3] defect
Chronic (childhood) granulomatous disease
Congenital dysphagocytosis
Progressive septic granulomatosis

● **D72 Other disorders of white blood cells**

> **Excludes1** basophilia (D72.824)
> immunity disorders (D80-D89)
> neutropenia (D70)
> preleukemia (syndrome) (D46.9)

D72.0 Genetic anomalies of leukocytes
Alder (granulation) (granulocyte) anomaly
Alder syndrome
Hereditary leukocytic hypersegmentation
Hereditary leukocytic hyposegmentation
Hereditary leukomelanopathy
May.-Hegglin (granulation) (granulocyte) anomaly
May-Hegglin syndrome
Pelger-Huët (granulation) (granulocyte) anomaly
Pelger-Huët syndrome

> **Excludes1** Chédiak (-Steinbrinck)-Higashi syndrome (E70.330)

D72.1 Eosinophilia
Formation and accumulation of high number of white cells in blood/tissue
Allergic eosinophilia
Hereditary eosinophilia

> **Excludes1** Löffler's syndrome (J82)
> pulmonary eosinophilia (J82)

● **D72.8 Other specified disorders of white blood cells**

> **Excludes1** leukemia (C91-C95)

● **D72.81 Decreased white blood cell count**

> **Excludes1** neutropenia (D70.-)

D72.810 Lymphocytopenia
Decreased lymphocytes
Reduction in number of lympho cytes in blood

D72.818 Other decreased white blood cell count
Basophilic leukopenia
Eosinophilic leukopenia
Monocytopenia
Other decreased leukocytes
Plasmacytopenia

D72.819 Decreased white blood cell count, unspecified
Decreased leukocytes, unspecified
Leukocytopenia, unspecified
Leukopenia

> **Excludes1** malignant leukopenia (D70.9)

● **D72.82 Elevated white blood cell count**

> **Excludes1** eosinophilia (D72.1)

D72.820 Lymphocytosis (symptomatic)
Elevated lymphocytes
Excess of normal lymphocytes

D72.821 Monocytosis (symptomatic)

> **Excludes1** infectious mononucleosis (B27.-)

D72.822 Plasmacytosis
Presence of excess plasma cells

D72.823 Leukemoid reaction
Basophilic leukemoid reaction
Leukemoid reaction NOS
Lymphocytic leukemoid reaction
Monocytic leukemoid reaction
Myelocytic leukemoid reaction
Neutrophilic leukemoid reaction

D72.824 Basophilia
Increase of basophils in blood

D72.825 Bandemia
Bandemia without diagnosis of specific infection
Excess number of band cells (immature white blood cells) released by bone marrow

> **Excludes1** confirmed infection
> -code to infection
> leukemia (C91.-, C92.-, C93.-, C94.-, C95.-)

D72.828 Other elevated white blood cell count

D72.829 Elevated white blood cell count, unspecified
Elevated leukocytes, unspecified
Leukocytosis, unspecified

D72.89 Other specified disorders of white blood cells
Abnormality of white blood cells NEC

D72.9 Disorder of white blood cells, unspecified
Abnormal leukocyte differential NOS

◀ New ◀▬ Revised ~~deleted~~ Deleted | Excludes 1 | Excludes 2 | Includes | Use additional | Code first | Code also | Unspecified |
OGCR Official Guidelines X Assign placeholder X ● Use Additional Character(s) ▶ Manifestation Code **Coding Clinic**

● **D73 Diseases of spleen**

    D73.0 Hyposplenism
        Diminished functioning of spleen
        Atrophy of spleen

> **Excludes1**   asplenia (congenital) (Q89.01)
>   postsurgical absence of spleen (Z90.81)

    D73.1 Hypersplenism
        Accelerated function of spleen

> **Excludes1**   neutropenic splenomegaly (D73.81)
>   primary splenic neutropenia (D73.81)
>   splenitis, splenomegaly in late syphilis
>   (A52.79)
>   splenitis, splenomegaly in tuberculosis
>   (A18.85)
>   splenomegaly NOS (R16.1)
>   splenomegaly congenital (Q89.0)

    D73.2 Chronic congestive splenomegaly
        Enlargement of spleen

    D73.3 Abscess of spleen

    D73.4 Cyst of spleen

    D73.5 Infarction of spleen
        Splenic rupture, nontraumatic
        Torsion of spleen

> **Excludes1**   rupture of spleen due to Plasmodium
>   vivax malaria (B51.0)
>   traumatic rupture of spleen (S36.03-)

●   **D73.8 Other diseases of spleen**

        D73.81 Neutropenic splenomegaly
            Werner-Schultz disease
            Enlarged spleen responding to inadequate number
            of neutrophils

        D73.89 Other diseases of spleen
            Fibrosis of spleen NOS
            Perisplenitis
            Splenitis NOS

    D73.9 Disease of spleen, unspecified

● **D74 Methemoglobinemia**
    Excessive methemoglobin (form of hemoglobin)

    D74.0 Congenital methemoglobinemia
        Congenital NADH-methemoglobin reductase
            deficiency
        Hemoglobin-M [Hb-M] disease
        Methemoglobinemia, hereditary

    D74.8 Other methemoglobinemias
        Acquired methemoglobinemia (with
            sulfhemoglobinemia)
        Toxic methemoglobinemia

    D74.9 Methemoglobinemia, unspecified

● **D75 Other and unspecified diseases of blood and blood-forming organs**

> **Excludes2**   acute lymphadenitis (L04.-)
>   chronic lymphadenitis (I88.1)
>   enlarged lymph nodes (R59.-)
>   hypergammaglobulinemia NOS (D89.2)
>   lymphadenitis NOS (I88.9)
>   mesenteric lymphadenitis (acute) (chronic) (I88.0)

    D75.0 Familial erythrocytosis
        Genetic mutation of gene that results in increased circulating
        RBCs
        Benign polycythemia
        Familial polycythemia

> **Excludes1**   hereditary ovalocytosis (D58.1)

    D75.1 Secondary polycythemia
        Increase in total red cell mass
        Acquired polycythemia
        Emotional polycythemia
        Erythrocytosis NOS
        Hypoxemic polycythemia
        Nephrogenous polycythemia
        Polycythemia due to erythropoietin
        Polycythemia due to fall in plasma volume
        Polycythemia due to high altitude
        Polycythemia due to stress
        Polycythemia NOS
        Relative polycythemia

> **Excludes1**   polycythemia neonatorum (P61.1)
>   polycythemia vera (D45)

●   **D75.8 Other specified diseases of blood and blood-forming organs**

        D75.81 Myelofibrosis
            Replacing bone marrow by fibrous tissue
            Myelofibrosis NOS
            Secondary myelofibrosis NOS

> *Code first the underlying disorder, such as:*
>   malignant neoplasm of breast (C50.-)

> Use additional code, if applicable,
>   for associated therapy-related
>   myelodysplastic syndrome (D46.-)

> Use additional code for adverse effect, if
>   applicable, to identify drug (T45.1X5)

> **Excludes1**   acute myelofibrosis (C94.4-)
>   idiopathic myelofibrosis (D47.1)
>   leukoerythroblastic anemia
>   (D61.82)
>   myelofibrosis with myeloid
>   metaplasia (D47.4)
>   myelophthisic anemia (D61.82)
>   myelophthisis (D61.82)
>   primary myelofibrosis (D47.1)

        D75.82 Heparin induced thrombocytopenia (HIT)

        D75.89 Other specified diseases of blood and blood-forming organs

    D75.9 Disease of blood and blood-forming organs, unspecified

● **D76 Other specified diseases with participation of lymphoreticular and reticulohistiocytic tissue**

> **Excludes1**   (Abt-) Letterer-Siwe disease (C96.0)
>   eosinophilic granuloma (C96.6)
>   Hand-Schüller-Christian disease (C96.5)
>   histiocytic sarcoma (C96.A)
>   histiocytosis X, multifocal (C96.5)
>   histiocytosis X, unifocal (C96.6)
>   malignant histiocytosis (C96.A)
>   Langerhans-cell histiocytosis, multifocal (C96.5)
>   Langerhans-cell histiocytosis NOS (C96.6)
>   Langerhans-cell histiocytosis, unifocal (C96.6)

> **Excludes1**   leukemic reticuloendotheliosis or reticulosis
>   (C91.4-)
>   lipomelanotic reticuloendotheliosis or reticulosis
>   (I89.8)

    D76.1 Hemophagocytic lymphohistiocytosis
        Familial hemophagocytic reticulosis
        Histiocytoses of mononuclear phagocytes

    D76.2 Hemophagocytic syndrome, infection-associated
        Use additional code to identify infectious agent or
            disease.

    D76.3 Other histiocytosis syndromes
        Reticulohistiocytoma (giant-cell)
        Sinus histiocytosis with massive lymphadenopathy
        Xanthogranuloma

CHAPTER 3 (D50-D89)

▷ **D77 Other disorders of blood and blood-forming organs in diseases classified elsewhere**

Code first underlying disease, such as:
amyloidosis (E85.-)
congenital early syphilis (A50.0)
echinococcosis (B67.0-B67.9)
malaria (B50.0-B54)
schistosomiasis [bilharziasis] (B65.0-B65.9)
vitamin C deficiency (E54)

> **Excludes1** rupture of spleen due to Plasmodium vivax malaria (B51.0)
> splenitis, splenomegaly in late syphilis (A52.79)
> splenitis, splenomegaly in tuberculosis (A18.85)

INTRAOPERATIVE AND POSTPROCEDURAL COMPLICATIONS OF THE SPLEEN (D78)

● **D78 Intraoperative and postprocedural complications of the spleen**

● **D78.0 Intraoperative hemorrhage and hematoma of the spleen complicating a procedure**

> **Excludes1** intraoperative hemorrhage and hematoma of the spleen due to accidental puncture or laceration during a procedure (D78.1-)

D78.01 Intraoperative hemorrhage and hematoma of the spleen complicating a procedure on the spleen

D78.02 Intraoperative hemorrhage and hematoma of the spleen complicating other procedure

● **D78.1 Accidental puncture and laceration of the spleen during a procedure**

D78.11 Accidental puncture and laceration of the spleen during a procedure on the spleen

D78.12 Accidental puncture and laceration of the spleen during other procedure

● **D78.2 Postprocedural hemorrhage and hematoma of the spleen following a procedure**

D78.21 Postprocedural hemorrhage and hematoma of the spleen following a procedure on the spleen

D78.22 Postprocedural hemorrhage and hematoma of the spleen following other procedure

● **D78.8 Other intraoperative and postprocedural complications of the spleen**

Use additional code, if applicable, to further specify disorder

D78.81 Other intraoperative complications of the spleen

D78.89 Other postprocedural complications of the spleen

CERTAIN DISORDERS INVOLVING THE IMMUNE MECHANISM (D80-D89)

> **Includes** defects in the complement system
> immunodeficiency disorders, except human immunodeficiency virus [HIV] disease
> sarcoidosis

> **Excludes1** autoimmune disease (systemic) NOS (M35.9)
> functional disorders of polymorphonuclear neutrophils (D71)
> human immunodeficiency virus [HIV] disease (B20)

● **D80 Immunodeficiency with predominantly antibody defects**

D80.0 Hereditary hypogammaglobulinemia
Autosomal recessive agammaglobulinemia (Swiss type)
X-linked agammaglobulinemia [Bruton] (with growth hormone deficiency)

D80.1 Nonfamilial hypogammaglobulinemia
Abnormally low levels of all classes of immunoglobulins
Agammaglobulinemia with immunoglobulin-bearing B-lymphocytes
Common variable agammaglobulinemia [CVAgamma]
Hypogammaglobulinemia NOS

D80.2 Selective deficiency of immunoglobulin A [IgA]

D80.3 Selective deficiency of immunoglobulin G [IgG] subclasses

D80.4 Selective deficiency of immunoglobulin M [IgM]

D80.5 Immunodeficiency with increased immunoglobulin M [IgM]

D80.6 Antibody deficiency with near-normal immunoglobulins or with hyperimmunoglobulinemia
Abnormally high levels of immunoglobulins in serum

D80.7 Transient hypogammaglobulinemia of infancy N

D80.8 Other immunodeficiencies with predominantly antibody defects
Kappa light chain deficiency

D80.9 Immunodeficiency with predominantly antibody defects, unspecified

● **D81 Combined immunodeficiencies**

> **Excludes1** autosomal recessive agammaglobulinemia (Swiss type) (D80.0)

D81.0 Severe combined immunodeficiency [SCID] with reticular dysgenesis

D81.1 Severe combined immunodeficiency [SCID] with low T- and B-cell numbers

D81.2 Severe combined immunodeficiency [SCID] with low or normal B-cell numbers

D81.3 Adenosine deaminase [ADA] deficiency

D81.4 Nezelof's syndrome

D81.5 Purine nucleoside phosphorylase [PNP] deficiency

D81.6 Major histocompatibility complex class I deficiency
Bare lymphocyte syndrome

D81.7 Major histocompatibility complex class II deficiency

● **D81.8 Other combined immunodeficiencies**

● **D81.81 Biotin-dependent carboxylase deficiency**
Multiple carboxylase deficiency

> **Excludes1** biotin-dependent carboxylase deficiency due to dietary deficiency of biotin (E53.8)

D81.810 Biotinidase deficiency

D81.818 Other biotin-dependent carboxylase deficiency
Holocarboxylase synthetase deficiency
Other multiple carboxylase deficiency

D81.819 Biotin-dependent carboxylase deficiency, unspecified
Multiple carboxylase deficiency, unspecified

D81.89 Other combined immunodeficiencies

D81.9 Combined immunodeficiency, unspecified
Severe combined immunodeficiency disorder [SCID] NOS

● **D82 Immunodeficiency associated with other major defects**

> **Excludes1** ataxia telangiectasia [Louis-Bar] (G11.3)

D82.0 Wiskott-Aldrich syndrome
X-linked immunodeficiency
Immunodeficiency with thrombocytopenia and eczema

D82.1 Di George's syndrome
Congenital disorder with defective development of third and fourth pharyngeal pouches
Pharyngeal pouch syndrome
Thymic alymphoplasia
Thymic aplasia or hypoplasia with immunodeficiency

D82.2 Immunodeficiency with short-limbed stature

D82.3 Immunodeficiency following hereditary defective response to Epstein-Barr virus
X-linked lymphoproliferative disease

◀ New ◀━ Revised ~~deleted~~ Deleted Excludes 1 Excludes 2 Includes Use additional Code first Code also Unspecified

OGCR Official Guidelines X Assign placeholder X ● Use Additional Character(s) ▷ Manifestation Code **Coding Clinic**

D82.4   Hyperimmunoglobulin E [IgE] syndrome
Suspected genetic defect that produces high levels of antibody immunoglobulin (IgE) that causes skin and lung infections and eczema

D82.8   Immunodeficiency associated with other specified major defects

D82.9   Immunodeficiency associated with major defect, unspecified

● **D83   Common variable immunodeficiency**

D83.0   Common variable immunodeficiency with predominant abnormalities of B-cell numbers and function

D83.1   Common variable immunodeficiency with predominant immunoregulatory T-cell disorders

D83.2   Common variable immunodeficiency with autoantibodies to B- or T-cells

D83.8   Other common variable immunodeficiencies

D83.9   Common variable immunodeficiency, unspecified

● **D84   Other immunodeficiencies**

D84.0   Lymphocyte function antigen-1 [LFA-1] defect

D84.1   Defects in the complement system
C1 esterase inhibitor [C1-INH] deficiency

D84.8   Other specified immunodeficiencies

D84.9   Immunodeficiency, unspecified

● **D86   Sarcoidosis**

D86.0   Sarcoidosis of lung

D86.1   Sarcoidosis of lymph nodes

D86.2   Sarcoidosis of lung with sarcoidosis of lymph nodes

D86.3   Sarcoidosis of skin

● **D86.8   Sarcoidosis of other sites**

D86.81   Sarcoid meningitis

D86.82   Multiple cranial nerve palsies in sarcoidosis

D86.83   Sarcoid iridocyclitis
Rare large tumor with irregular surface of iris

D86.84   Sarcoid pyelonephritis
Systemic disease of unknown etiology characterized by chronic granulomatous inflammation with tissue destruction of pelvis kidney
Tubulo-interstitial nephropathy in sarcoidosis

D86.85   Sarcoid myocarditis

D86.86   Sarcoid arthropathy
Polyarthritis in sarcoidosis

D86.87   Sarcoid myositis
Granumloma of muscle

D86.89   Sarcoidosis of other sites
Hepatic granuloma
Uveoparotid fever [Heerfordt]

D86.9   Sarcoidosis, unspecified

Item 3-1 Sarcoidosis: A symptom of an inflammation producing tiny lumps of cells (granulomas) in various organs, most commonly the lungs and lymph nodes, that affect organ function. Cause is unknown occurring primarily in 20- to 40-year-olds, African-American, especially women, and those of Asian, German, Irish, Scandinavian, and Puerto Rican heritage.

● **D89   Other disorders involving the immune mechanism, not elsewhere classified**

Excludes1   hyperglobulinemia NOS (R77.1)
monoclonal gammopathy (of undetermined significance) (D47.2)

Excludes2   transplant failure and rejection (T86.-)

D89.0   Polyclonal hypergammaglobulinemia
Benign hypergammaglobulinemic purpura
Polyclonal gammopathy NOS

D89.1   Cryoglobulinemia
Cryoglobulin (proteins) in blood that precipitate temperatures below 98.6° F; usually symptomatic of underlying disease
Cryoglobulinemic purpura
Cryoglobulinemic vasculitis
Essential cryoglobulinemia
Idiopathic cryoglobulinemia
Mixed cryoglobulinemia
Primary cryoglobulinemia
Secondary cryoglobulinemia

D89.2   Hypergammaglobulinemia, unspecified

D89.3   Immune reconstitution syndrome
Immune reconstitution inflammatory syndrome [IRIS]

Use additional code for adverse effect, if applicable, to identify drug (T36-T50 with fifth or sixth character 5)

● **D89.8   Other specified disorders involving the immune mechanism, not elsewhere classified**

● **D89.81   Graft-versus-host disease**

Code first underlying cause, such as:
complications of transplanted organs and tissue (T86.-)
complications of blood transfusion (T80.89)

Use additional code to identify associated manifestations, such as:
desquamative dermatitis (L30.8)
diarrhea (R19.7)
elevated bilirubin (R17)
hair loss (L65.9)

D89.810   Acute graft-versus-host disease

D89.811   Chronic graft-versus-host disease

D89.812   Acute on chronic graft-versus-host disease

D89.813   Graft-versus-host disease, unspecified

D89.82   Autoimmune lymphoproliferative syndrome [ALPS]

D89.89   Other specified disorders involving the immune mechanism, not elsewhere classified

Excludes1   human immunodeficiency virus disease (B20)

D89.9   Disorder involving the immune mechanism, unspecified
Immune disease NOS

CHAPTER 3 (D50-D89)

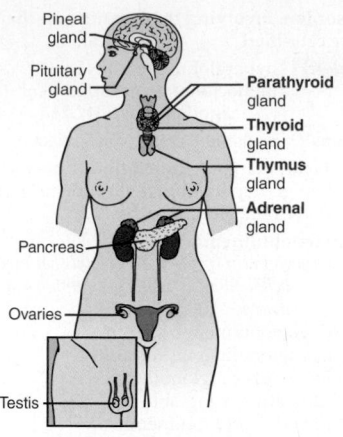

Figure 4-1 The endocrine system. (From Buck CJ: Step-by-Step Medical Coding, ed 2011, Philadelphia, WB Saunders, 2011)

CHAPTER 4

ENDOCRINE, NUTRITIONAL AND METABOLIC DISEASES (E00-E89)

All neoplasms, whether functionally active or not, are classified in Chapter 2. Appropriate codes in this chapter (i.e., E05.8, E07.0, E16-E31, E34.-) may be used as additional codes to indicate either functional activity by neoplasms and ectopic endocrine tissue or hyperfunction and hypofunction of endocrine glands associated with neoplasms and other conditions classified elsewhere.

Excludes1 transitory endocrine and metabolic disorders specific to newborn (P70-P74)

This chapter contains the following blocks:

E00-E07	Disorders of thyroid gland
E08-E13	Diabetes mellitus
E15-E16	Other disorders of glucose regulation and pancreatic internal secretion
E20-E35	Disorders of other endocrine glands
E36	Intraoperative complications of endocrine system
E40-E46	Malnutrition
E50-E64	Other nutritional deficiencies
E65-E68	Overweight, obesity and other hyperalimentation
E70-E88	Metabolic disorders
E89	Postprocedural endocrine and metabolic complications and disorders, not elsewhere classified

DISORDERS OF THYROID GLAND (E00-E07)

● **E00   Congenital iodine-deficiency syndrome**
Use additional code (F70-F79) to identify associated intellectual disabilities.
Excludes1 subclinical iodine-deficiency hypothyroidism (E02)

E00.0   Congenital iodine-deficiency syndrome, neurological type
Endemic cretinism, neurological type

E00.1   Congenital iodine-deficiency syndrome, myxedematous type
Dry, waxy type of swelling (nonpitting edema) with abnormal deposits of mucin in skin (mucinosis) and other tissues
Endemic hypothyroid cretinism
Endemic cretinism, myxedematous type

E00.2   Congenital iodine-deficiency syndrome, mixed type
Endemic cretinism, mixed type

E00.9   Congenital iodine-deficiency syndrome, unspecified
Congenital iodine-deficiency hypothyroidism NOS
Endemic cretinism NOS

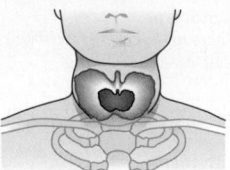

Figure 4-2   Goiter is an enlargement of the thyroid gland.

Item 4–1   Simple goiter indicates no nodules are present. The most common type of goiter is a **diffuse colloidal,** also called a **nontoxic** or **endemic** goiter.

● **E01   Iodine-deficiency related thyroid disorders and allied conditions**
Excludes1 congenital iodine-deficiency syndrome (E00.-)
subclinical iodine-deficiency hypothyroidism (E02)

E01.0   Iodine-deficiency related diffuse (endemic) goiter
Thyroid gland is enlarged

E01.1   Iodine-deficiency related multinodular (endemic) goiter
Iodine-deficiency related nodular goiter

E01.2   Iodine-deficiency related (endemic) goiter, unspecified
Endemic goiter NOS

E01.8   Other iodine-deficiency related thyroid disorders and allied conditions
Acquired iodine-deficiency hypothyroidism NOS

E02   Subclinical iodine-deficiency hypothyroidism

● **E03   Other hypothyroidism**
Excludes1 iodine-deficiency related hypothyroidism (E00-E02)
postprocedural hypothyroidism (E89.0)

E03.0   Congenital hypothyroidism with diffuse goiter
Congenital parenchymatous goiter (nontoxic)
Congenital goiter (nontoxic) NOS
Excludes1 transitory congenital goiter with normal function (P72.0)

E03.1   Congenital hypothyroidism without goiter
Aplasia of thyroid (with myxedema)
Congenital atrophy of thyroid
Congenital hypothyroidism NOS

E03.2   Hypothyroidism due to medicaments and other exogenous substances
Code first poisoning due to drug or toxin, if applicable (T36-T65 with fifth or sixth character 1-4 or 6)
Use additional code for adverse effect, if applicable, to identify drug (T36-T50 with fifth or sixth character 5)

E03.3   Postinfectious hypothyroidism

E03.4   Atrophy of thyroid (acquired)
Excludes1 congenital atrophy of thyroid (E03.1)

E03.5   Myxedema coma
Often fatal complication of long-term hypothyroidism

E03.8   Other specified hypothyroidism

E03.9   Hypothyroidism, unspecified
Myxedema NOS

Item 4–2   Hypothyroidism is a condition in which there are insufficient levels of thyroxine. **Cretinism** is congenital hypothyroidism, which can result in mental and physical retardation.

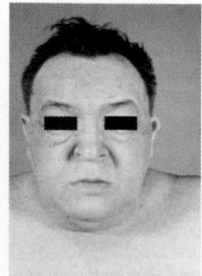

Figure 4-3 Typical appearance of patients with moderately severe primary hypothyroidism or myxedema. (From Larsen: Williams Textbook of Endocrinology, ed 10, Saunders, An Imprint of Elsevier, 2003)

● **E04**   **Other nontoxic goiter**
     Excludes1   congenital goiter (NOS) (diffuse)
                    (parenchymatous) (E03.0)
                    iodine-deficiency related goiter (E00-E02)

     E04.0   **Nontoxic diffuse goiter**
           Thyroid gland is enlarged
           Diffuse (colloid) nontoxic goiter
           Simple nontoxic goiter

     E04.1   **Nontoxic single thyroid nodule**
           Colloid nodule (cystic) (thyroid)
           Nontoxic uninodular goiter
           Thyroid (cystic) nodule NOS

     E04.2   **Nontoxic multinodular goiter**
           Enlarged thyroid gland with multiple nodules
           Cystic goiter NOS
           Multinodular (cystic) goiter NOS

     E04.8   **Other specified nontoxic goiter**

     E04.9   **Nontoxic goiter, unspecified**
           Goiter NOS
           Nodular goiter (nontoxic) NOS

● **E05**   **Thyrotoxicosis [hyperthyroidism]**
       Enlarged thyroid gland with multiple nodules
     Excludes1   chronic thyroiditis with transient thyrotoxicosis
                    (E06.2)
                    neonatal thyrotoxicosis (P72.1)

     ● **E05.0**   **Thyrotoxicosis with diffuse goiter**
           Exophthalmic or toxic goiter NOS
           Graves' disease
           Toxic diffuse goiter

         E05.00   **Thyrotoxicosis with diffuse goiter without**
                  thyrotoxic crisis or storm

         E05.01   **Thyrotoxicosis with diffuse goiter with**
                  thyrotoxic crisis or storm

     ● **E05.1**   **Thyrotoxicosis with toxic single thyroid nodule**
           Thyrotoxicosis with toxic uninodular goiter

         E05.10   **Thyrotoxicosis with toxic single thyroid nodule**
                  without thyrotoxic crisis or storm

         E05.11   **Thyrotoxicosis with toxic single thyroid nodule**
                  with thyrotoxic crisis or storm

     ● **E05.2**   **Thyrotoxicosis with toxic multinodular goiter**
           Toxic nodular goiter NOS

         E05.20   **Thyrotoxicosis with toxic multinodular goiter**
                  without thyrotoxic crisis or storm

         E05.21   **Thyrotoxicosis with toxic multinodular goiter**
                  with thyrotoxic crisis or storm

     ● **E05.3**   **Thyrotoxicosis from ectopic thyroid tissue**

         E05.30   **Thyrotoxicosis from ectopic thyroid tissue**
                  without thyrotoxic crisis or storm

         E05.31   **Thyrotoxicosis from ectopic thyroid tissue with**
                  thyrotoxic crisis or storm

     ● **E05.4**   **Thyrotoxicosis factitia**

         E05.40   **Thyrotoxicosis factitia without thyrotoxic crisis**
                  or storm

         E05.41   **Thyrotoxicosis factitia with thyrotoxic crisis or**
                  storm

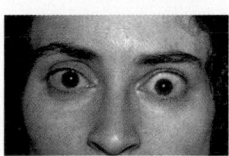

Figure 4-4   Graves' disease. In Graves' disease, exophthalmos often looks more pronounced than it actually is because of the extreme lid retraction that may occur. This patient, for instance, had minimal proptosis of the left eye but marked lid retraction.
(Courtesy Dr. HG Scheie. From Yanoff M, Fine BS: Ocular Pathology, ed 6, St. Louis, Mosby, 2008)

Item 4-3   Thyrotoxicosis is a condition caused by excessive amounts of the thyroid hormone thyroxine production or hyperthyroidism. **Graves' disease is associated with hyperthyroidism** (known as **Basedow's disease** in Europe).

● **E05.8**   **Other thyrotoxicosis**
           Overproduction of thyroid-stimulating hormone

         E05.80   **Other thyrotoxicosis without thyrotoxic crisis or**
                  storm

         E05.81   **Other thyrotoxicosis with thyrotoxic crisis or**
                  storm

● **E05.9**   **Thyrotoxicosis, unspecified**
           Hyperthyroidism NOS

         E05.90   **Thyrotoxicosis, unspecified without thyrotoxic**
                  crisis or storm

         E05.91   **Thyrotoxicosis, unspecified with thyrotoxic**
                  crisis or storm

● **E06**   **Thyroiditis**
       An inflammation of the thyroid gland which results in an inability to
       convert iodine into thyroid hormone
     Excludes1   postpartum thyroiditis (O90.5)

     E06.0   **Acute thyroiditis**
           Abscess of thyroid
           Pyogenic thyroiditis
           Suppurative thyroiditis
           Use additional code (B95-B97) to identify infectious
               agent.

     E06.1   **Subacute thyroiditis**
           Inflammation of thyroid gland following viral upper
               respiratory infection
           de Quervain thyroiditis
           Giant-cell thyroiditis
           Granulomatous thyroiditis
           Nonsuppurative thyroiditis
           Viral thyroiditis
         Excludes1   autoimmune thyroiditis (E06.3)

     E06.2   **Chronic thyroiditis with transient thyrotoxicosis**
           Chronic inflammation of thyroid gland with intermittent
               overproduction of thyroid hormone
         Excludes1   autoimmune thyroiditis (E06.3)

     E06.3   **Autoimmune thyroiditis**
           Hashimoto's thyroiditis
           Hashitoxicosis (transient)
           Lymphadenoid goiter
           Lymphocytic thyroiditis
           Struma lymphomatosa

     E06.4   **Drug-induced thyroiditis**
           Use additional code for adverse effect, if applicable,
               to identify drug (T36-T50 with fifth or sixth
               character 5)

     E06.5   **Other chronic thyroiditis**
           Chronic fibrous thyroiditis
           Chronic thyroiditis NOS
           Ligneous thyroiditis
           Riedel thyroiditis

     E06.9   **Thyroiditis, unspecified**

● **E07**   **Other disorders of thyroid**
     E07.0   **Hypersecretion of calcitonin**
           C-cell hyperplasia of thyroid
           Hypersecretion of thyrocalcitonin

     E07.1   **Dyshormogenetic goiter**
           Group of several types of goiter resulting from enzyme defects
               in hormone synthesis
           Familial dyshormogenetic goiter
           Pendred's syndrome
         Excludes1   transitory congenital goiter with normal
                    function (P72.0)

● **E07.8**   **Other specified disorders of thyroid**
         E07.81   **Sick-euthyroid syndrome**
                  Euthyroid sick-syndrome

         E07.89   **Other specified disorders of thyroid**
                  Abnormality of thyroid-binding globulin
                  Hemorrhage of thyroid
                  Infarction of thyroid

     E07.9   **Disorder of thyroid, unspecified**

CHAPTER 4 (E00-E90)

OGCR Section I.C.4.a

4.1 Diabetes mellitus

The diabetes mellitus codes are combination codes that include the type of diabetes mellitus, body system affected, and the complications affecting that body system. As many codes within a particular category as are necessary to describe all of the complications of the disease may be used. They should be sequenced based on the reason for a particular visit. Assign as many codes from categories E08–E13 as needed to identify all of the associated conditions that the patient has.

DIABETES MELLITUS (E08-E13)

A metabolic disease that results in persistent hyperglycemia.

● **E08**   **Diabetes mellitus due to underlying condition**

Code first the underlying condition, such as:
congenital rubella (P35.0)
Cushing's syndrome (E24.-)
cystic fibrosis (E84.-)
malignant neoplasm (C00-C96)
malnutrition (E40-E46)
pancreatitis and other diseases of the pancreas (K85-K86.-)

Use additional code to identify any insulin use (Z79.4)

Excludes1   drug or chemical induced diabetes mellitus (E09.-)
gestational diabetes (O24.4-)
neonatal diabetes mellitus (P70.2)
postpancreatectomy diabetes mellitus (E13.-)
postprocedural diabetes mellitus (E13.-)
secondary diabetes mellitus NEC (E13.-)
type 1 diabetes mellitus (E10.-)
type 2 diabetes mellitus (E11.-)

● **E08.0**   **Diabetes mellitus due to underlying condition with hyperosmolarity**

E08.00   **Diabetes mellitus due to underlying condition with hyperosmolarity without nonketotic hyperglycemic-hyperosmolar coma (NKHHC)**

E08.01   **Diabetes mellitus due to underlying condition with hyperosmolarity with coma**

● **E08.1**   **Diabetes mellitus due to underlying condition with ketoacidosis**

E08.10   **Diabetes mellitus due to underlying condition with ketoacidosis without coma**

E08.11   **Diabetes mellitus due to underlying condition with ketoacidosis with coma**

● **E08.2**   **Diabetes mellitus due to underlying condition with kidney complications**

E08.21   **Diabetes mellitus due to underlying condition with diabetic nephropathy**
Diabetes mellitus due to underlying condition with intercapillary glomerulosclerosis
Diabetes mellitus due to underlying condition with intracapillary glomerulonephrosis
Diabetes mellitus due to underlying condition with Kimmelstiel-Wilson disease

E08.22   **Diabetes mellitus due to underlying condition with diabetic chronic kidney disease**
Use additional code to identify stage of chronic kidney disease (N18.1-N18.6)

E08.29   **Diabetes mellitus due to underlying condition with other diabetic kidney complication**
Renal tubular degeneration in diabetes mellitus due to underlying condition

● **E08.3**   **Diabetes mellitus due to underlying condition with ophthalmic complications**
Changes in blood vessels of retina in which blood vessels swell and leak fluid into retinal surface.

● **E08.31**   **Diabetes mellitus due to underlying condition with unspecified diabetic retinopathy**

E08.311   **Diabetes mellitus due to underlying condition with unspecified diabetic retinopathy with macular edema**

E08.319   **Diabetes mellitus due to underlying condition with unspecified diabetic retinopathy without macular edema**

● **E08.32**   **Diabetes mellitus due to underlying condition with mild nonproliferative diabetic retinopathy**
Diabetes mellitus due to underlying condition with nonproliferative diabetic retinopathy NOS

E08.321   **Diabetes mellitus due to underlying condition with mild nonproliferative diabetic retinopathy with macular edema**

E08.329   **Diabetes mellitus due to underlying condition with mild nonproliferative diabetic retinopathy without macular edema**

● **E08.33**   **Diabetes mellitus due to underlying condition with moderate nonproliferative diabetic retinopathy**

E08.331   **Diabetes mellitus due to underlying condition with moderate nonproliferative diabetic retinopathy with macular edema**

E08.339   **Diabetes mellitus due to underlying condition with moderate nonproliferative diabetic retinopathy without macular edema**

● **E08.34**   **Diabetes mellitus due to underlying condition with severe nonproliferative diabetic retinopathy**

E08.341   **Diabetes mellitus due to underlying condition with severe nonproliferative diabetic retinopathy with macular edema**

E08.349   **Diabetes mellitus due to underlying condition with severe nonproliferative diabetic retinopathy without macular edema**

● **E08.35**   **Diabetes mellitus due to underlying condition with proliferative diabetic retinopathy**

E08.351   **Diabetes mellitus due to underlying condition with proliferative diabetic retinopathy with macular edema**

E08.359   **Diabetes mellitus due to underlying condition with proliferative diabetic retinopathy without macular edema**

E08.36   **Diabetes mellitus due to underlying condition with diabetic cataract**

E08.39   **Diabetes mellitus due to underlying condition with other diabetic ophthalmic complication**
Use additional code to identify manifestation, such as:
diabetic glaucoma (H40-H42)

◀ New   ◀▬ Revised   ~~deleted~~ Deleted   Excludes 1   Excludes 2   Includes   Use additional   Code first   Code also   Unspecified
OGCR Official Guidelines   X Assign placeholder X   ● Use Additional Character(s)   ❱ Manifestation Code   **Coding Clinic**

● **E08.4**   Diabetes mellitus due to underlying condition with neurological complications

     E08.40   Diabetes mellitus due to underlying condition with diabetic neuropathy, unspecified

     E08.41   Diabetes mellitus due to underlying condition with diabetic mononeuropathy

     E08.42   Diabetes mellitus due to underlying condition with diabetic polyneuropathy
         Diabetes mellitus due to underlying condition with diabetic neuralgia

     E08.43   Diabetes mellitus due to underlying condition with diabetic autonomic (poly)neuropathy
         Diabetes mellitus due to underlying condition with diabetic gastroparesis

     E08.44   Diabetes mellitus due to underlying condition with diabetic amyotrophy

     E08.49   Diabetes mellitus due to underlying condition with other diabetic neurological complication

● **E08.5**   Diabetes mellitus due to underlying condition with circulatory complications

     E08.51   Diabetes mellitus due to underlying condition with diabetic peripheral angiopathy without gangrene

     E08.52   Diabetes mellitus due to underlying condition with diabetic peripheral angiopathy with gangrene
         Diabetes mellitus due to underlying condition with diabetic gangrene

     E08.59   Diabetes mellitus due to underlying condition with other circulatory complications

● **E08.6**   Diabetes mellitus due to underlying condition with other specified complications

   ● E08.61   Diabetes mellitus due to underlying condition with diabetic arthropathy

     E08.610   Diabetes mellitus due to underlying condition with diabetic neuropathic arthropathy
         Diabetes mellitus due to underlying condition with Charcôt's joints

     E08.618   Diabetes mellitus due to underlying condition with other diabetic arthropathy

   ● E08.62   Diabetes mellitus due to underlying condition with skin complications

     E08.620   Diabetes mellitus due to underlying condition with diabetic dermatitis
         Diabetes mellitus due to underlying condition with diabetic necrobiosis lipoidica

     E08.621   Diabetes mellitus due to underlying condition with foot ulcer
         Use additional code to identify site of ulcer (L97.4-, L97.5-)

     E08.622   Diabetes mellitus due to underlying condition with other skin ulcer
         Use additional code to identify site of ulcer (L97.1-L97.9, L98.41-L98.49)

     E08.628   Diabetes mellitus due to underlying condition with other skin complications

   ● E08.63   Diabetes mellitus due to underlying condition with oral complications

     E08.630   Diabetes mellitus due to underlying condition with periodontal disease

     E08.638   Diabetes mellitus due to underlying condition with other oral complications

● **E08.64**   Diabetes mellitus due to underlying condition with hypoglycemia

     E08.641   Diabetes mellitus due to underlying condition with hypoglycemia with coma

     E08.649   Diabetes mellitus due to underlying condition with hypoglycemia without coma

     E08.65   Diabetes mellitus due to underlying condition with hyperglycemia

     E08.69   Diabetes mellitus due to underlying condition with other specified complication
         Use additional code to identify complication

   E08.8   Diabetes mellitus due to underlying condition with unspecified complications

   E08.9   Diabetes mellitus due to underlying condition without complications

● E09   **Drug or chemical induced diabetes mellitus**

     Code first poisoning due to drug or toxin, if applicable (T36-T65 with fifth or sixth character 1-4 or 6)

     Use additional code for adverse effect, if applicable, to identify drug (T36-T50 with fifth or sixth character 5)

     Use additional code to identify any insulin use (Z79.4)

     Excludes1   diabetes mellitus due to underlying condition (E08.-)
         gestational diabetes (O24.4-)
         neonatal diabetes mellitus (P70.2)
         postpancreatectomy diabetes mellitus (E13.-)
         postprocedural diabetes mellitus (E13.-)
         secondary diabetes mellitus NEC (E13.-)
         type 1 diabetes mellitus (E10.-)
         type 2 diabetes mellitus (E11.-)

● **E09.0**   Drug or chemical induced diabetes mellitus with hyperosmolarity

     E09.00   Drug or chemical induced diabetes mellitus with hyperosmolarity without nonketotic hyperglycemic-hyperosmolar coma (NKHHC)

     E09.01   Drug or chemical induced diabetes mellitus with hyperosmolarity with coma

● **E09.1**   Drug or chemical induced diabetes mellitus with ketoacidosis

     E09.10   Drug or chemical induced diabetes mellitus with ketoacidosis without coma

     E09.11   Drug or chemical induced diabetes mellitus with ketoacidosis with coma

● **E09.2**   Drug or chemical induced diabetes mellitus with kidney complications

     E09.21   Drug or chemical induced diabetes mellitus with diabetic nephropathy
         Drug or chemical induced diabetes mellitus with intercapillary glomerulosclerosis
         Drug or chemical induced diabetes mellitus with intracapillary glomerulonephrosis
         Drug or chemical induced diabetes mellitus with Kimmelstiel-Wilson disease

     E09.22   Drug or chemical induced diabetes mellitus with diabetic chronic kidney disease
         Use additional code to identify stage of chronic kidney disease (N18.1-N18.6)

     E09.29   Drug or chemical induced diabetes mellitus with other diabetic kidney complication
         Drug or chemical induced diabetes mellitus with renal tubular degeneration

● **E09.3**   **Drug or chemical induced diabetes mellitus with ophthalmic complications**

     ● **E09.31**   **Drug or chemical induced diabetes mellitus with unspecified diabetic retinopathy**

         E09.311   **Drug or chemical induced diabetes mellitus with unspecified diabetic retinopathy with macular edema**

         E09.319   **Drug or chemical induced diabetes mellitus with unspecified diabetic retinopathy without macular edema**

     ● **E09.32**   **Drug or chemical induced diabetes mellitus with mild nonproliferative diabetic retinopathy**

         Drug or chemical induced diabetes mellitus with nonproliferative diabetic retinopathy NOS

         E09.321   **Drug or chemical induced diabetes mellitus with mild nonproliferative diabetic retinopathy with macular edema**

         E09.329   **Drug or chemical induced diabetes mellitus with mild nonproliferative diabetic retinopathy without macular edema**

     ● **E09.33**   **Drug or chemical induced diabetes mellitus with moderate nonproliferative diabetic retinopathy**

         E09.331   **Drug or chemical induced diabetes mellitus with moderate nonproliferative diabetic retinopathy with macular edema**

         E09.339   **Drug or chemical induced diabetes mellitus with moderate nonproliferative diabetic retinopathy without macular edema**

     ● **E09.34**   **Drug or chemical induced diabetes mellitus with severe nonproliferative diabetic retinopathy**

         E09.341   **Drug or chemical induced diabetes mellitus with severe nonproliferative diabetic retinopathy with macular edema**

         E09.349   **Drug or chemical induced diabetes mellitus with severe nonproliferative diabetic retinopathy without macular edema**

     ● **E09.35**   **Drug or chemical induced diabetes mellitus with proliferative diabetic retinopathy**

         E09.351   **Drug or chemical induced diabetes mellitus with proliferative diabetic retinopathy with macular edema**

         E09.359   **Drug or chemical induced diabetes mellitus with proliferative diabetic retinopathy without macular edema**

     E09.36   **Drug or chemical induced diabetes mellitus with diabetic cataract**

     E09.39   **Drug or chemical induced diabetes mellitus with other diabetic ophthalmic complication**

         Use additional code to identify manifestation, such as:

           diabetic glaucoma (H40-H42)

● **E09.4**   **Drug or chemical induced diabetes mellitus with neurological complications**

     E09.40   **Drug or chemical induced diabetes mellitus with neurological complications with diabetic neuropathy, unspecified**

     E09.41   **Drug or chemical induced diabetes mellitus with neurological complications with diabetic mononeuropathy**

     E09.42   **Drug or chemical induced diabetes mellitus with neurological complications with diabetic polyneuropathy**

         Drug or chemical induced diabetes mellitus with diabetic neuralgia

     E09.43   **Drug or chemical induced diabetes mellitus with neurological complications with diabetic autonomic (poly)neuropathy**

         Drug or chemical induced diabetes mellitus with diabetic gastroparesis

     E09.44   **Drug or chemical induced diabetes mellitus with neurological complications with diabetic amyotrophy**

     E09.49   **Drug or chemical induced diabetes mellitus with neurological complications with other diabetic neurological complication**

● **E09.5**   **Drug or chemical induced diabetes mellitus with circulatory complications**

     E09.51   **Drug or chemical induced diabetes mellitus with diabetic peripheral angiopathy without gangrene**

     E09.52   **Drug or chemical induced diabetes mellitus with diabetic peripheral angiopathy with gangrene**

         Drug or chemical induced diabetes mellitus with diabetic gangrene

     E09.59   **Drug or chemical induced diabetes mellitus with other circulatory complications**

● **E09.6**   **Drug or chemical induced diabetes mellitus with other specified complications**

     ● **E09.61**   **Drug or chemical induced diabetes mellitus with diabetic arthropathy**

         E09.610   **Drug or chemical induced diabetes mellitus with diabetic neuropathic arthropathy**

           Drug or chemical induced diabetes mellitus with Charcôt's joints

           Progressive degeneration of weight bearing joint

         E09.618   **Drug or chemical induced diabetes mellitus with other diabetic arthropathy**

     ● **E09.62**   **Drug or chemical induced diabetes mellitus with skin complications**

         E09.620   **Drug or chemical induced diabetes mellitus with diabetic dermatitis**

           Drug or chemical induced diabetes mellitus with diabetic necrobiosis lipoidica

           Necrotizing skin condition

         E09.621   **Drug or chemical induced diabetes mellitus with foot ulcer**

           Use additional code to identify site of ulcer (L97.4-, L97.5-)

         E09.622   **Drug or chemical induced diabetes mellitus with other skin ulcer**

           Use additional code to identify site of ulcer (L97.1-L97.9, L98.41-L98.49)

         E09.628   **Drug or chemical induced diabetes mellitus with other skin complications**

     ● **E09.63**   **Drug or chemical induced diabetes mellitus with oral complications**

         E09.630   **Drug or chemical induced diabetes mellitus with periodontal disease**

         E09.638   **Drug or chemical induced diabetes mellitus with other oral complications**

◀ New   ◀▦ Revised   ~~deleted~~ Deleted   Excludes 1   Excludes 2   Includes   Use additional   Code first   Code also   Unspecified

OGCR Official Guidelines   **X** Assign placeholder X   ● Use Additional Character(s)   ▶ Manifestation Code   **Coding Clinic**

● **E09.64** Drug or chemical induced diabetes mellitus with hypoglycemia

    E09.641 Drug or chemical induced diabetes mellitus with hypoglycemia with coma

    E09.649 Drug or chemical induced diabetes mellitus with hypoglycemia without coma

E09.65 Drug or chemical induced diabetes mellitus with hyperglycemia

E09.69 Drug or chemical induced diabetes mellitus with other specified complication

    Use additional code to identify complication

E09.8 Drug or chemical induced diabetes mellitus with unspecified complications

E09.9 Drug or chemical induced diabetes mellitus without complications

● **E10** Type 1 diabetes mellitus

    Includes   brittle diabetes (mellitus)
                diabetes (mellitus) due to autoimmune process
                diabetes (mellitus) due to immune mediated pancreatic islet beta-cell destruction
                idiopathic diabetes (mellitus)
                juvenile onset diabetes (mellitus)
                ketosis-prone diabetes (mellitus)

    Excludes1   diabetes mellitus due to underlying condition (E08.-)
                drug or chemical induced diabetes mellitus (E09.-)
                gestational diabetes (O24.4-)
                hyperglycemia NOS (R73.9)
                neonatal diabetes mellitus (P70.2)
                postpancreatectomy diabetes mellitus (E13.-)
                postprocedural diabetes mellitus (E13.-)
                secondary diabetes mellitus NEC (E13.-)
                type 2 diabetes mellitus (E11.-)

● **E10.1** Type 1 diabetes mellitus with ketoacidosis

    Acidosis accompanied by accumulation of ketone bodies (ketosis) in body tissues and fluids

    E10.10 Type 1 diabetes mellitus with ketoacidosis without coma
          Coding Clinic: 2013, Q3, P20

    E10.11 Type 1 diabetes mellitus with ketoacidosis with coma

● **E10.2** Type 1 diabetes mellitus with kidney complications

    E10.21 Type 1 diabetes mellitus with diabetic nephropathy
        Type 1 diabetes mellitus with intercapillary glomerulosclerosis
        Type 1 diabetes mellitus with intracapillary glomerulonephrosis
        Type 1 diabetes mellitus with Kimmelstiel-Wilson disease

    E10.22 Type 1 diabetes mellitus with diabetic chronic kidney disease
        Use additional code to identify stage of chronic kidney disease (N18.1-N18.6)

    E10.29 Type 1 diabetes mellitus with other diabetic kidney complication
        Type 1 diabetes mellitus with renal tubular degeneration

● **E10.3** Type 1 diabetes mellitus with ophthalmic complications

    ● **E10.31** Type 1 diabetes mellitus with unspecified diabetic retinopathy

        E10.311 Type 1 diabetes mellitus with unspecified diabetic retinopathy with macular edema

        E10.319 Type 1 diabetes mellitus with unspecified diabetic retinopathy without macular edema

● **E10.32** Type 1 diabetes mellitus with mild nonproliferative diabetic retinopathy

    Type 1 diabetes mellitus with nonproliferative diabetic retinopathy NOS

    E10.321 Type 1 diabetes mellitus with mild nonproliferative diabetic retinopathy with macular edema

    E10.329 Type 1 diabetes mellitus with mild nonproliferative diabetic retinopathy without macular edema

● **E10.33** Type 1 diabetes mellitus with moderate nonproliferative diabetic retinopathy

    E10.331 Type 1 diabetes mellitus with moderate nonproliferative diabetic retinopathy with macular edema

    E10.339 Type 1 diabetes mellitus with moderate nonproliferative diabetic retinopathy without macular edema

● **E10.34** Type 1 diabetes mellitus with severe nonproliferative diabetic retinopathy

    E10.341 Type 1 diabetes mellitus with severe nonproliferative diabetic retinopathy with macular edema

    E10.349 Type 1 diabetes mellitus with severe nonproliferative diabetic retinopathy without macular edema

● **E10.35** Type 1 diabetes mellitus with proliferative diabetic retinopathy

    E10.351 Type 1 diabetes mellitus with proliferative diabetic retinopathy with macular edema

    E10.359 Type 1 diabetes mellitus with proliferative diabetic retinopathy without macular edema

E10.36 Type 1 diabetes mellitus with diabetic cataract

E10.39 Type 1 diabetes mellitus with other diabetic ophthalmic complication

    Use additional code to identify manifestation, such as:
    diabetic glaucoma (H40-H42)

● **E10.4** Type 1 diabetes mellitus with neurological complications

    E10.40 Type 1 diabetes mellitus with diabetic neuropathy, unspecified

    E10.41 Type 1 diabetes mellitus with diabetic mononeuropathy

    E10.42 Type 1 diabetes mellitus with diabetic polyneuropathy
        Type 1 diabetes mellitus with diabetic neuralgia

    E10.43 Type 1 diabetes mellitus with diabetic autonomic (poly)neuropathy
        Type 1 diabetes mellitus with diabetic gastroparesis

    E10.44 Type 1 diabetes mellitus with diabetic amyotrophy

    E10.49 Type 1 diabetes mellitus with other diabetic neurological complication

● **E10.5** Type 1 diabetes mellitus with circulatory complications

    E10.51 Type 1 diabetes mellitus with diabetic peripheral angiopathy without gangrene

    E10.52 Type 1 diabetes mellitus with diabetic peripheral angiopathy with gangrene
        Type 1 diabetes mellitus with diabetic gangrene

    E10.59 Type 1 diabetes mellitus with other circulatory complications

CHAPTER 4 (E00-E90)

● **E10.6**   **Type 1 diabetes mellitus with other specified complications**

     ● **E10.61**   **Type 1 diabetes mellitus with diabetic arthropathy**

         E10.610   **Type 1 diabetes mellitus with diabetic neuropathic arthropathy**
           Type 1 diabetes mellitus with Charcôt's joints

         E10.618   **Type 1 diabetes mellitus with other diabetic arthropathy**

     ● **E10.62**   **Type 1 diabetes mellitus with skin complications**

         E10.620   **Type 1 diabetes mellitus with diabetic dermatitis**
           Type 1 diabetes mellitus with diabetic necrobiosis lipoidica

         E10.621   **Type 1 diabetes mellitus with foot ulcer**
           Use additional code to identify site of ulcer (L97.4-, L97.5-)

         E10.622   **Type 1 diabetes mellitus with other skin ulcer**
           Use additional code to identify site of ulcer (L97.1-L97.9, L98.41-L98.49)

         E10.628   **Type 1 diabetes mellitus with other skin complications**

     ● **E10.63**   **Type 1 diabetes mellitus with oral complications**

         E10.630   **Type 1 diabetes mellitus with periodontal disease**

         E10.638   **Type 1 diabetes mellitus with other oral complications**

     ● **E10.64**   **Type 1 diabetes with hypoglycemia**

         E10.641   **Type 1 diabetes mellitus with hypoglycemia with coma**

         E10.649   **Type 1 diabetes mellitus with hypoglycemia without coma**

       E10.65   **Type 1 diabetes mellitus with hyperglycemia**
         Coding Clinic: 2013, Q3, P20

       E10.69   **Type 1 diabetes mellitus with other specified complication**
         Use additional code to identify complication
         Use this code with E10.65 to report hyperosmolarity in a Type 1 patient

   E10.8   Type 1 diabetes mellitus with unspecified complications

   E10.9   Type 1 diabetes mellitus without complications

● **E11**   **Type 2 diabetes mellitus**

     Includes   diabetes (mellitus) due to insulin secretory defect
              diabetes NOS
              insulin resistant diabetes (mellitus)

     Use additional code to identify any insulin use (Z79.4)

     Excludes1   diabetes mellitus due to underlying condition (E08.-)
              drug or chemical induced diabetes mellitus (E09.-)
              gestational diabetes (O24.4-)
              neonatal diabetes mellitus (P70.2)
              postpancreatectomy diabetes mellitus (E13.-)
              postprocedural diabetes mellitus (E13.-)
              secondary diabetes mellitus NEC (E13.-)
              type 1 diabetes mellitus (E10.-)

     ● **E11.0**   **Type 2 diabetes mellitus with hyperosmolarity**

       E11.00   **Type 2 diabetes mellitus with hyperosmolarity without nonketotic hyperglycemic-hyperosmolar coma (NKHHC)**

       E11.01   **Type 2 diabetes mellitus with hyperosmolarity with coma**

   ● **E11.2**   **Type 2 diabetes mellitus with kidney complications**

       E11.21   **Type 2 diabetes mellitus with diabetic nephropathy**
         Type 2 diabetes mellitus with intercapillary glomerulosclerosis
         Type 2 diabetes mellitus with intracapillary glomerulonephrosis
         Type 2 diabetes mellitus with Kimmelstiel-Wilson disease

       E11.22   **Type 2 diabetes mellitus with diabetic chronic kidney disease**
         Use additional code to identify stage of chronic kidney disease (N18.1-N18.6)

       E11.29   **Type 2 diabetes mellitus with other diabetic kidney complication**
         Type 2 diabetes mellitus with renal tubular degeneration

   ● **E11.3**   **Type 2 diabetes mellitus with ophthalmic complications**

     ● **E11.31**   **Type 2 diabetes mellitus with unspecified diabetic retinopathy**

       E11.311   **Type 2 diabetes mellitus with unspecified diabetic retinopathy with macular edema**

       E11.319   **Type 2 diabetes mellitus with unspecified diabetic retinopathy without macular edema**
         Coding Clinic: 2013, Q3, P20

     ● **E11.32**   **Type 2 diabetes mellitus with mild nonproliferative diabetic retinopathy**
         Type 2 diabetes mellitus with nonproliferative diabetic retinopathy NOS

       E11.321   **Type 2 diabetes mellitus with mild nonproliferative diabetic retinopathy with macular edema**

       E11.329   **Type 2 diabetes mellitus with mild nonproliferative diabetic retinopathy without macular edema**

     ● **E11.33**   **Type 2 diabetes mellitus with moderate nonproliferative diabetic retinopathy**

       E11.331   **Type 2 diabetes mellitus with moderate nonproliferative diabetic retinopathy with macular edema**

       E11.339   **Type 2 diabetes mellitus with moderate nonproliferative diabetic retinopathy without macular edema**

     ● **E11.34**   **Type 2 diabetes mellitus with severe nonproliferative diabetic retinopathy**

       E11.341   **Type 2 diabetes mellitus with severe nonproliferative diabetic retinopathy with macular edema**

       E11.349   **Type 2 diabetes mellitus with severe nonproliferative diabetic retinopathy without macular edema**

     ● **E11.35**   **Type 2 diabetes mellitus with proliferative diabetic retinopathy**

       E11.351   **Type 2 diabetes mellitus with proliferative diabetic retinopathy with macular edema**

       E11.359   **Type 2 diabetes mellitus with proliferative diabetic retinopathy without macular edema**

       E11.36   **Type 2 diabetes mellitus with diabetic cataract**

       E11.39   **Type 2 diabetes mellitus with other diabetic ophthalmic complication**
         Use additional code to identify manifestation, such as:
           diabetic glaucoma (H40-H42)

◀ New   ◀▦ Revised   ~~deleted~~ Deleted | Excludes 1 | | Excludes 2 | | Includes | | Use additional | | Code first | Code also | Unspecified |

OGCR Official Guidelines   **X** Assign placeholder X   ● Use Additional Character(s)   ▶ Manifestation Code   **Coding Clinic**

● **E11.4** **Type 2 diabetes mellitus with neurological complications**

　E11.40 **Type 2 diabetes mellitus with diabetic neuropathy, unspecified**

　E11.41 **Type 2 diabetes mellitus with diabetic mononeuropathy**

　E11.42 **Type 2 diabetes mellitus with diabetic polyneuropathy**
　　Type 2 diabetes mellitus with diabetic neuralgia

　E11.43 **Type 2 diabetes mellitus with diabetic autonomic (poly)neuropathy**
　　Type 2 diabetes mellitus with diabetic gastroparesis

　E11.44 **Type 2 diabetes mellitus with diabetic amyotrophy**

　E11.49 **Type 2 diabetes mellitus with other diabetic neurological complication**

● **E11.5** **Type 2 diabetes mellitus with circulatory complications**

　E11.51 **Type 2 diabetes mellitus with diabetic peripheral angiopathy without gangrene**

　E11.52 **Type 2 diabetes mellitus with diabetic peripheral angiopathy with gangrene**
　　Type 2 diabetes mellitus with diabetic gangrene

　E11.59 **Type 2 diabetes mellitus with other circulatory complications**

● **E11.6** **Type 2 diabetes mellitus with other specified complications**

　● **E11.61** **Type 2 diabetes mellitus with diabetic arthropathy**

　　E11.610 **Type 2 diabetes mellitus with diabetic neuropathic arthropathy**
　　　Type 2 diabetes mellitus with Charcôt's joints

　　E11.618 **Type 2 diabetes mellitus with other diabetic arthropathy**

　● **E11.62** **Type 2 diabetes mellitus with skin complications**

　　E11.620 **Type 2 diabetes mellitus with diabetic dermatitis**
　　　Type 2 diabetes mellitus with diabetic necrobiosis lipoidica

　　E11.621 **Type 2 diabetes mellitus with foot ulcer**
　　　Use additional code to identify site of ulcer (L97.4-, L97.5-)

　　E11.622 **Type 2 diabetes mellitus with other skin ulcer**
　　　Use additional code to identify site of ulcer (L97.1-L97.9, L98.41-L98.49)

　　E11.628 **Type 2 diabetes mellitus with other skin complications**

　● **E11.63** **Type 2 diabetes mellitus with oral complications**

　　E11.630 **Type 2 diabetes mellitus with periodontal disease**

　　E11.638 **Type 2 diabetes mellitus with other oral complications**

　● **E11.64** **Type 2 diabetes mellitus with hypoglycemia**

　　E11.641 **Type 2 diabetes mellitus with hypoglycemia with coma**

　　E11.649 **Type 2 diabetes mellitus with hypoglycemia without coma**

　E11.65 **Type 2 diabetes mellitus with hyperglycemia**
　　Coding Clinic: 2013, Q3, P20

　E11.69 **Type 2 diabetes mellitus with other specified complication**
　　Use additional code to identify complication
　　Use this code with E11.65 to report DKA in a Type 2 patient

E11.8 **Type 2 diabetes mellitus with unspecified complications**

E11.9 **Type 2 diabetes mellitus without complications**

● **E13** **Other specified diabetes mellitus**

　Includes diabetes mellitus due to genetic defects of beta-cell function
　　diabetes mellitus due to genetic defects in insulin action
　　postpancreatectomy diabetes mellitus
　　postprocedural diabetes mellitus
　　secondary diabetes mellitus NEC

　Use additional code to identify any insulin use (Z79.4)

　Excludes1 diabetes (mellitus) due to autoimmune process (E10.-)
　　diabetes (mellitus) due to immune mediated pancreatic islet beta-cell destruction (E10.-)
　　diabetes mellitus due to underlying condition (E08.-)
　　drug or chemical induced diabetes mellitus (E09.-)
　　gestational diabetes (O24.4-)
　　neonatal diabetes mellitus (P70.2)
　　type 2 diabetes mellitus (E11.-)

● **E13.0** **Other specified diabetes mellitus with hyperosmolarity**

　E13.00 **Other specified diabetes mellitus with hyperosmolarity without nonketotic hyperglycemic-hyperosmolar coma (NKHHC)**

　E13.01 **Other specified diabetes mellitus with hyperosmolarity with coma**

● **E13.1** **Other specified diabetes mellitus with ketoacidosis**

　E13.10 **Other specified diabetes mellitus with ketoacidosis without coma**
　　Coding Clinic: 2013, Q1, P26

　E13.11 **Other specified diabetes mellitus with ketoacidosis with coma**

● **E13.2** **Other specified diabetes mellitus with kidney complications**

　E13.21 **Other specified diabetes mellitus with diabetic nephropathy**
　　Other specified diabetes mellitus with intercapillary glomerulosclerosis
　　Other specified diabetes mellitus with intracapillary glomerulonephrosis
　　Other specified diabetes mellitus with Kimmelstiel-Wilson disease

　E13.22 **Other specified diabetes mellitus with diabetic chronic kidney disease**
　　Use additional code to identify stage of chronic kidney disease (N18.1-N18.6)

　E13.29 **Other specified diabetes mellitus with other diabetic kidney complication**
　　Other specified diabetes mellitus with renal tubular degeneration

● **E13.3** **Other specified diabetes mellitus with ophthalmic complications**

　● **E13.31** **Other specified diabetes mellitus with unspecified diabetic retinopathy**

　　E13.311 **Other specified diabetes mellitus with unspecified diabetic retinopathy with macular edema**

　　E13.319 **Other specified diabetes mellitus with unspecified diabetic retinopathy without macular edema**

　● **E13.32** **Other specified diabetes mellitus with mild nonproliferative diabetic retinopathy**
　　Other specified diabetes mellitus with nonproliferative diabetic retinopathy NOS

　　E13.321 **Other specified diabetes mellitus with mild nonproliferative diabetic retinopathy with macular edema**

　　E13.329 **Other specified diabetes mellitus with mild nonproliferative diabetic retinopathy without macular edema**

CHAPTER 4 (E00-E90)

● E13.33　Other specified diabetes mellitus with moderate nonproliferative diabetic retinopathy

　　E13.331　Other specified diabetes mellitus with moderate nonproliferative diabetic retinopathy with macular edema

　　E13.339　Other specified diabetes mellitus with moderate nonproliferative diabetic retinopathy without macular edema

● E13.34　Other specified diabetes mellitus with severe nonproliferative diabetic retinopathy

　　E13.341　Other specified diabetes mellitus with severe nonproliferative diabetic retinopathy with macular edema

　　E13.349　Other specified diabetes mellitus with severe nonproliferative diabetic retinopathy without macular edema

● E13.35　Other specified diabetes mellitus with proliferative diabetic retinopathy

　　E13.351　Other specified diabetes mellitus with proliferative diabetic retinopathy with macular edema

　　E13.359　Other specified diabetes mellitus with proliferative diabetic retinopathy without macular edema

　E13.36　Other specified diabetes mellitus with diabetic cataract

　E13.39　Other specified diabetes mellitus with other diabetic ophthalmic complication

　　　Use additional code to identify manifestation, such as:
　　　　diabetic glaucoma (H40-H42)

● E13.4　Other specified diabetes mellitus with neurological complications

　E13.40　Other specified diabetes mellitus with diabetic neuropathy, unspecified

　E13.41　Other specified diabetes mellitus with diabetic mononeuropathy

　E13.42　Other specified diabetes mellitus with diabetic polyneuropathy

　　　Other specified diabetes mellitus with diabetic neuralgia

　E13.43　Other specified diabetes mellitus with diabetic autonomic (poly)neuropathy

　　　Other specified diabetes mellitus with diabetic gastroparesis

　E13.44　Other specified diabetes mellitus with diabetic amyotrophy

　E13.49　Other specified diabetes mellitus with other diabetic neurological complication

● E13.5　Other specified diabetes mellitus with circulatory complications

　E13.51　Other specified diabetes mellitus with diabetic peripheral angiopathy without gangrene

　E13.52　Other specified diabetes mellitus with diabetic peripheral angiopathy with gangrene

　　　Other specified diabetes mellitus with diabetic gangrene

　E13.59　Other specified diabetes mellitus with other circulatory complications

● E13.6　Other specified diabetes mellitus with other specified complications

● E13.61　Other specified diabetes mellitus with diabetic arthropathy

　　E13.610　Other specified diabetes mellitus with diabetic neuropathic arthropathy

　　　　Other specified diabetes mellitus with Charcôt's joints

　　E13.618　Other specified diabetes mellitus with other diabetic arthropathy

● E13.62　Other specified diabetes mellitus with skin complications

　　E13.620　Other specified diabetes mellitus with diabetic dermatitis

　　　　Other specified diabetes mellitus with diabetic necrobiosis lipoidica

　　E13.621　Other specified diabetes mellitus with foot ulcer

　　　　Use additional code to identify site of ulcer (L97.4-, L97.5-)

　　E13.622　Other specified diabetes mellitus with other skin ulcer

　　　　Use additional code to identify site of ulcer (L97.1-L97.9, L98.41-L98.49)

　　E13.628　Other specified diabetes mellitus with other skin complications

● E13.63　Other specified diabetes mellitus with oral complications

　　E13.630　Other specified diabetes mellitus with periodontal disease

　　E13.638　Other specified diabetes mellitus with other oral complications

● E13.64　Other specified diabetes mellitus with hypoglycemia

　　E13.641　Other specified diabetes mellitus with hypoglycemia with coma

　　E13.649　Other specified diabetes mellitus with hypoglycemia without coma

　E13.65　Other specified diabetes mellitus with hyperglycemia

　E13.69　Other specified diabetes mellitus with other specified complication

　　　Use additional code to identify complication

E13.8　Other specified diabetes mellitus with unspecified complications

E13.9　Other specified diabetes mellitus without complications

---

OTHER DISORDERS OF GLUCOSE REGULATION AND PANCREATIC INTERNAL SECRETION (E15-E16)

E15　Nondiabetic hypoglycemic coma

　　Includes　drug-induced insulin coma in nondiabetic hyperinsulinism with hypoglycemic coma
　　　hypoglycemic coma NOS

● E16　Other disorders of pancreatic internal secretion

　E16.0　Drug-induced hypoglycemia without coma

　　　Use additional code for adverse effect, if applicable, to identify drug (T36-T50 with fifth or sixth character 5)

　E16.1　Other hypoglycemia

　　　Functional hyperinsulinism
　　　Functional nonhyperinsulinemic hypoglycemia
　　　Hyperinsulinism NOS
　　　Hyperplasia of pancreatic islet beta cells NOS

　　　Excludes1　hypoglycemia in infant of diabetic mother (P70.1)
　　　　neonatal hypoglycemia (P70.4)

　E16.2　Hypoglycemia, unspecified

　E16.3　Increased secretion of glucagon

　　　Hyperplasia of pancreatic endocrine cells with glucagon excess

　E16.4　Increased secretion of gastrin

　　　Hypergastrinemia
　　　Hyperplasia of pancreatic endocrine cells with gastrin excess
　　　Zollinger-Ellison syndrome

◀ New　◀▥ Revised　deleted Deleted　Excludes 1　Excludes 2　Includes　Use additional　Code first　Code also　Unspecified

OGCR Official Guidelines　X Assign placeholder X　● Use Additional Character(s)　▶ Manifestation Code　Coding Clinic

E16.8   Other specified disorders of pancreatic internal secretion
     Increased secretion from endocrine pancreas of growth hormone-releasing hormone
     Increased secretion from endocrine pancreas of pancreatic polypeptide
     Increased secretion from endocrine pancreas of somatostatin
     Increased secretion from endocrine pancreas of vasoactive-intestinal polypeptide

E16.9   Disorder of pancreatic internal secretion, unspecified
     Islet-cell hyperplasia NOS
     Pancreatic endocrine cell hyperplasia NOS

DISORDERS OF OTHER ENDOCRINE GLANDS (E20-E35)

   Excludes1   galactorrhea (N64.3)
                   gynecomastia (N62)

● **E20   Hypoparathyroidism**
     Greatly reduced function of parathyroid glands; AKA parathyroid insufficiency

   Excludes1   Di George's syndrome (D82.1)
                   postprocedural hypoparathyroidism (E89.2)
                   tetany NOS (R29.0)
                   transitory neonatal hypoparathyroidism (P71.4)

E20.0   Idiopathic hypoparathyroidism
     Rare condition, unknown cause; short dwarf-like with round face

E20.1   Pseudohypoparathyroidism
     Hereditary condition resembling hypoparathyroidism, but caused by inability to respond to parathyroid hormone

E20.8   Other hypoparathyroidism

E20.9   Hypoparathyroidism, unspecified
     Parathyroid tetany

● **E21   Hyperparathyroidism and other disorders of parathyroid gland**
   Excludes1   adult osteomalacia (M83.-)
                   ectopic hyperparathyroidism (E34.2)
                   familial hypocalciuric hypercalcemia (E83.52)
                   hungry bone syndrome (E83.81)
                   infantile and juvenile osteomalacia (E55.0)

E21.0   Primary hyperparathyroidism
     Hyperplasia of parathyroid
     Osteitis fibrosa cystica generalisata [von Recklinghausen's disease of bone]

E21.1   Secondary hyperparathyroidism, not elsewhere classified
   Excludes1   secondary hyperparathyroidism of renal origin (N25.81)

E21.2   Other hyperparathyroidism
     Tertiary hyperparathyroidism
   Excludes1   familial hypocalciuric hypercalcemia (E83.52)

E21.3   Hyperparathyroidism, unspecified
E21.4   Other specified disorders of parathyroid gland
E21.5   Disorder of parathyroid gland, unspecified

● **E22   Hyperfunction of pituitary gland**
   Excludes1   Cushing's syndrome (E24.-)
                   Nelson's syndrome (E24.1)
                   overproduction of ACTH not associated with Cushing's disease (E27.0)
                   overproduction of pituitary ACTH (E24.0)
                   overproduction of thyroid-stimulating hormone (E05.8-)

E22.0   Acromegaly and pituitary gigantism
     Chronic disease caused by hypersecretion of growth hormone
     Overproduction of growth hormone
   Excludes1   constitutional gigantism (E34.4)
                   constitutional tall stature (E34.4)
                   increased secretion from endocrine pancreas of growth hormone-releasing hormone (E16.8)

E22.1   Hyperprolactinemia
     Increased levels of prolactin
     Use additional code for adverse effect, if applicable, to identify drug (T36-T50 with fifth or sixth character 5)

E22.2   Syndrome of inappropriate secretion of antidiuretic hormone

E22.8   Other hyperfunction of pituitary gland
     Central precocious puberty

E22.9   Hyperfunction of pituitary gland, unspecified

● **E23   Hypofunction and other disorders of the pituitary gland**
   Includes   the listed conditions whether the disorder is in the pituitary or the hypothalamus
   Excludes1   postprocedural hypopituitarism (E89.3)

E23.0   Hypopituitarism
     Fertile eunuch syndrome
     Hypogonadotropic hypogonadism
     Idiopathic growth hormone deficiency
     Isolated deficiency of gonadotropin
     Isolated deficiency of growth hormone
     Isolated deficiency of pituitary hormone
     Kallmann's syndrome
     Lorain-Levi short stature
     Necrosis of pituitary gland (postpartum)
     Panhypopituitarism
     Pituitary cachexia
     Pituitary insufficiency NOS
     Pituitary short stature
     Sheehan's syndrome
     Simmonds' disease

E23.1   Drug-induced hypopituitarism
     Use additional code for adverse effect, if applicable, to identify drug (T36-T50 with fifth or sixth character 5)

E23.2   Diabetes insipidus
   Excludes1   nephrogenic diabetes insipidus (N25.1)

Item 4–4   Hyperparathyroidism is an overactive parathyroid gland that secretes excessive parathormone, causing increased levels of circulating calcium. This results in a loss of calcium in the bone (osteoporosis).

     Hypoparathyroidism is an underactive parathyroid gland that results in decreased levels of circulating calcium. The primary manifestation is **tetany,** a continuous muscle spasm.

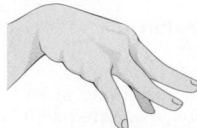

Figure 4-5   Tetany caused by hypoparathyroidism.

Item 4–5   Hyperadrenalism is overactivity of the adrenal cortex, which secretes corticosteroid hormones. Excessive glucocorticoid hormone results in hyperglycemia **(Cushing's syndrome),** and excessive aldosterone results in **Conn's syndrome. Adrenogenital syndrome** is the result of excessive secretion of androgens, male hormones, which stimulates premature sexual development. **Hypoadrenalism, Addison's disease,** is a condition in which the adrenal glands atrophy.

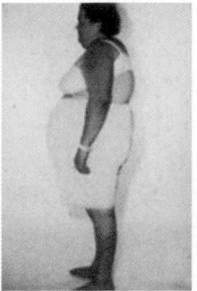

Figure 4-6   Centripetal and generalized obesity and dorsal kyphosis in a 30-year-old woman with Cushing's disease. (From Larsen: Williams Textbook of Endocrinology, ed 10, Saunders, An Imprint of Elsevier, 2003)

CHAPTER 4 (E00-E90)

E23.3   **Hypothalamic dysfunction, not elsewhere classified**
> **Excludes1**   Prader-Willi syndrome (Q87.1)
> Russell-Silver syndrome (Q87.1)

E23.6   **Other disorders of pituitary gland**
> Abscess of pituitary
> Adiposogenital dystrophy

E23.7   **Disorder of pituitary gland, unspecified**

● **E24**   **Cushing's syndrome**
> **Excludes1**   congenital adrenal hyperplasia (E25.0)

E24.0   **Pituitary-dependent Cushing's disease**
> Overproduction of pituitary ACTH
> Pituitary-dependent hypercorticalism

E24.1   **Nelson's syndrome**

E24.2   **Drug-induced Cushing's syndrome**
> Use additional code for adverse effect, if applicable, to identify drug (T36-T50 with fifth or sixth character 5)

E24.3   **Ectopic ACTH syndrome**

E24.4   **Alcohol-induced pseudo-Cushing's syndrome**

E24.8   **Other Cushing's syndrome**

E24.9   **Cushing's syndrome, unspecified**

● **E25**   **Adrenogenital disorders**
> *Disorder of production of steroid hormone in adrenal gland*
> **Includes**   adrenogenital syndromes, virilizing or feminizing, whether acquired or due to adrenal hyperplasia consequent on inborn enzyme defects in hormone synthesis
> female adrenal pseudohermaphroditism
> female heterosexual precocious pseudopuberty
> male isosexual precocious pseudopuberty
> male macrogenitosomia praecox
> male sexual precocity with adrenal hyperplasia
> male virilization (female)
>
> **Excludes1**   indeterminate sex and pseudohermaphroditism (Q56)
> chromosomal abnormalities (Q90-Q99)

E25.0   **Congenital adrenogenital disorders associated with enzyme deficiency**
> Congenital adrenal hyperplasia
> 21-Hydroxylase deficiency
> Salt-losing congenital adrenal hyperplasia

E25.8   **Other adrenogenital disorders**
> Idiopathic adrenogenital disorder
> Use additional code for adverse effect, if applicable, to identify drug (T36-T50 with fifth or sixth character 5)

E25.9   **Adrenogenital disorder, unspecified**
> Adrenogenital syndrome NOS

● **E26**   **Hyperaldosteronism**
> *Abnormality of electrolyte metabolism caused by excessive secretion of aldosterone*

● **E26.0**   **Primary hyperaldosteronism**

E26.01   **Conn's syndrome**
> Code also adrenal adenoma (D35.0-)

E26.02   **Glucocorticoid-remediable aldosteronism**
> Familial aldosteronism type I

E26.09   **Other primary hyperaldosteronism**
> Primary aldosteronism due to adrenal hyperplasia (bilateral)

E26.1   **Secondary hyperaldosteronism**

● **E26.8**   **Other hyperaldosteronism**

E26.81   **Bartter's syndrome**

E26.89   **Other hyperaldosteronism**

E26.9   **Hyperaldosteronism, unspecified**
> Aldosteronism NOS
> Hyperaldosteronism NOS

● **E27**   **Other disorders of adrenal gland**

E27.0   **Other adrenocortical overactivity**
> Overproduction of ACTH, not associated with Cushing's disease
> Premature adrenarche
> **Excludes1**   Cushing's syndrome (E24.-)

E27.1   **Primary adrenocortical insufficiency**
> Addison's disease
> Autoimmune adrenalitis
> **Excludes1**   Addison only phenotype adrenoleukodystrophy (E71.528)
> amyloidosis (E85.-)
> tuberculous Addison's disease (A18.7)
> Waterhouse-Friderichsen syndrome (A39.1)

E27.2   **Addisonian crisis**
> *Acute onset of adrenocortical insufficiency*
> Adrenal crisis
> Adrenocortical crisis

E27.3   **Drug-induced adrenocortical insufficiency**
> Use additional code for adverse effect, if applicable, to identify drug (T36-T50 with fifth or sixth character 5)

● **E27.4**   **Other and unspecified adrenocortical insufficiency**
> **Excludes1**   adrenoleukodystrophy [Addison-Schilder] (E71.528)
> Waterhouse-Friderichsen syndrome (A39.1)

E27.40   **Unspecified adrenocortical insufficiency**
> Adrenocortical insufficiency NOS
> Hypoaldosteronism

E27.49   **Other adrenocortical insufficiency**
> Adrenal hemorrhage
> Adrenal infarction

E27.5   **Adrenomedullary hyperfunction**
> Adrenomedullary hyperplasia
> Catecholamine hypersecretion

E27.8   **Other specified disorders of adrenal gland**
> Abnormality of cortisol-binding globulin

E27.9   **Disorder of adrenal gland, unspecified**

● **E28**   **Ovarian dysfunction**
> **Excludes1**   isolated gonadotropin deficiency (E23.0)
> postprocedural ovarian failure (E89.4-)

E28.0   **Estrogen excess ♀**
> Use additional code for adverse effect, if applicable, to identify drug (T36-T50 with fifth or sixth character 5)

E28.1   **Androgen excess ♀**
> Hypersecretion of ovarian androgens
> Use additional code for adverse effect, if applicable, to identify drug (T36-T50 with fifth or sixth character 5)

E28.2   **Polycystic ovarian syndrome ♀**
> Sclerocystic ovary syndrome
> Stein-Leventhal syndrome

● **E28.3**   **Primary ovarian failure**
> **Excludes1**   pure gonadal dysgenesis (Q99.1)
> Turner's syndrome (Q96.-)

● **E28.31**   **Premature menopause**

E28.310   **Symptomatic premature menopause ♀**   A
> Symptoms such as flushing, sleeplessness, headache, lack of concentration, associated with premature menopause

E28.319   **Asymptomatic premature menopause ♀**   A
> Premature menopause NOS

E28.39   **Other primary ovarian failure ♀**
> Decreased estrogen
> Resistant ovary syndrome

◀ New   ◀▬ Revised   ~~deleted~~ Deleted   Excludes 1   Excludes 2   Includes   Use additional   Code first   Code also   Unspecified
OGCR Official Guidelines   X Assign placeholder X   ● Use Additional Character(s)   ▶ Manifestation Code   **Coding Clinic**

E28.8   Other ovarian dysfunction ♀
Ovarian hyperfunction NOS
Excludes1   postprocedural ovarian failure (E89.4-)
E28.9   Ovarian dysfunction, unspecified ♀

● **E29   Testicular dysfunction**
Excludes1   androgen insensitivity syndrome (E34.5-)
azoospermia or oligospermia NOS (N46.0-N46.1)
isolated gonadotropin deficiency (E23.0)
Klinefelter's syndrome (Q98.0-Q98.2, Q98.4)
E29.0   Testicular hyperfunction ♂
Hypersecretion of testicular hormones
E29.1   Testicular hypofunction ♂
Defective biosynthesis of testicular androgen NOS
5-delta-Reductase deficiency (with male pseudohermaphroditism)
Testicular hypogonadism NOS
Use additional code for adverse effect, if applicable, to identify drug (T36-T50 with fifth or sixth character 5)
Excludes1   postprocedural testicular hypofunction (E89.5)
E29.8   Other testicular dysfunction ♂
E29.9   Testicular dysfunction, unspecified ♂

● **E30   Disorders of puberty, not elsewhere classified**
E30.0   Delayed puberty
Constitutional delay of puberty
Delayed sexual development
E30.1   Precocious puberty   P
Sexual maturation at earlier age than normal, or before age 8 in girls and 9 in boys, usually hormonal; AKA sexual precocity or pubertas praecox
Precocious menstruation
Excludes1   Albright (-McCune) (-Sternberg) syndrome (Q78.1)
central precocious puberty (E22.8)
congenital adrenal hyperplasia (E25.0)
female heterosexual precocious pseudopuberty (E25.-)
male isosexual precocious pseudopuberty (E25.-)
E30.8   Other disorders of puberty   P
Premature thelarche
E30.9   Disorder of puberty, unspecified

● **E31   Polyglandular dysfunction**
Excludes1   ataxia telangiectasia [Louis-Bar] (G11.3)
dystrophia myotonica [Steinert] (G71.11)
pseudohypoparathyroidism (E20.1)
E31.0   Autoimmune polyglandular failure
Schmidt's syndrome
E31.1   Polyglandular hyperfunction
Excludes1   multiple endocrine adenomatosis (E31.2-)
multiple endocrine neoplasia (E31.2-)
● **E31.2   Multiple endocrine neoplasia [MEN] syndromes**
Adenomatous hyperplasia and malignant tumors in endocrine glands
Multiple endocrine adenomatosis
Code also any associated malignancies and other conditions associated with the syndromes
E31.20   Multiple endocrine neoplasia [MEN] syndrome, unspecified
Multiple endocrine adenomatosis NOS
Multiple endocrine neoplasia [MEN] syndrome NOS
E31.21   Multiple endocrine neoplasia [MEN] type I
Wermer's syndrome
E31.22   Multiple endocrine neoplasia [MEN] type IIA
Sipple's syndrome
E31.23   Multiple endocrine neoplasia [MEN] type IIB
E31.8   Other polyglandular dysfunction
E31.9   Polyglandular dysfunction, unspecified

● **E32   Diseases of thymus**
Excludes1   aplasia or hypoplasia of thymus with immunodeficiency (D82.1)
myasthenia gravis (G70.0)
E32.0   Persistent hyperplasia of thymus
Hypertrophy of thymus
E32.1   Abscess of thymus
E32.8   Other diseases of thymus
Excludes1   aplasia or hypoplasia with immunodeficiency (D82.1)
thymoma (D15.0)
E32.9   Disease of thymus, unspecified

● **E34   Other endocrine disorders**
Excludes1   pseudohypoparathyroidism (E20.1)
E34.0   Carcinoid syndrome
Note: May be used as an additional code to identify functional activity associated with a carcinoid tumor.
E34.1   Other hypersecretion of intestinal hormones
E34.2   Ectopic hormone secretion, not elsewhere classified
Excludes1   ectopic ACTH syndrome (E24.3)
E34.3   Short stature due to endocrine disorder
Constitutional short stature
Laron-type short stature
Excludes1   achondroplastic short stature (Q77.4)
hypochondroplastic short stature (Q77.4)
nutritional short stature (E45)
pituitary short stature (E23.0)
progeria (E34.8)
renal short stature (N25.0)
Russell-Silver syndrome (Q87.1)
short-limbed stature with immunodeficiency (D82.2)
short stature in specific dysmorphic syndromes - code to syndrome - see Alphabetical Index
short stature NOS (R62.52)
E34.4   Constitutional tall stature
Constitutional gigantism
● **E34.5   Androgen insensitivity syndrome**
E34.50   Androgen insensitivity syndrome, unspecified
Androgen insensitivity NOS
E34.51   Complete androgen insensitivity syndrome
Complete androgen insensitivity
de Quervain syndrome
Goldberg-Maxwell syndrome
E34.52   Partial androgen insensitivity syndrome
Partial androgen insensitivity
Reifenstein syndrome
E34.8   Other specified endocrine disorders
Pineal gland dysfunction
Progeria
Excludes2   pseudohypoparathyroidism (E20.1)
E34.9   Endocrine disorder, unspecified
Endocrine disturbance NOS
Hormone disturbance NOS

▶ *E35   Disorders of endocrine glands in diseases classified elsewhere*
Code first underlying disease, such as:
late congenital syphilis of thymus gland [Dubois disease] (A50.5)
Use additional code, if applicable, to identify:
sequelae of tuberculosis of other organs (B90.8)
Excludes1   Echinococcus granulosus infection of thyroid gland (B67.3)
meningococcal hemorrhagic adrenalitis (A39.1)
syphilis of endocrine gland (A52.79)
tuberculosis of adrenal gland, except calcification (A18.7)
tuberculosis of endocrine gland NEC (A18.82)
tuberculosis of thyroid gland (A18.81)
Waterhouse-Friderichsen syndrome (A39.1)

INTRAOPERATIVE COMPLICATIONS OF ENDOCRINE SYSTEM (E36)

● **E36**   **Intraoperative complications of endocrine system**
> **Excludes2**   postprocedural endocrine and metabolic complications and disorders, not elsewhere classified (E89.-)

● **E36.0**   **Intraoperative hemorrhage and hematoma of an endocrine system organ or structure complicating a procedure**
> **Excludes1**   intraoperative hemorrhage and hematoma of an endocrine system organ or structure due to accidental puncture or laceration during a procedure (E36.1-)

     E36.01   **Intraoperative hemorrhage and hematoma of an endocrine system organ or structure complicating an endocrine system procedure**

     E36.02   **Intraoperative hemorrhage and hematoma of an endocrine system organ or structure complicating other procedure**

● **E36.1**   **Accidental puncture and laceration of an endocrine system organ or structure during a procedure**

     E36.11   **Accidental puncture and laceration of an endocrine system organ or structure during an endocrine system procedure**

     E36.12   **Accidental puncture and laceration of an endocrine system organ or structure during other procedure**

     E36.8   **Other intraoperative complications of endocrine system**
> Use additional code, if applicable, to further specify disorder

MALNUTRITION (E40-E46)

> **Excludes1**   intestinal malabsorption (K90.-)
> sequelae of protein-calorie malnutrition (E64.0)
> **Excludes2**   nutritional anemias (D50-D53)
> starvation (T73.0)

E40   **Kwashiorkor**
Malnutrition produced by severe protein deficiency
Severe malnutrition with nutritional edema with dyspigmentation of skin and hair
> **Excludes1**   marasmic kwashiorkor (E42)

E41   **Nutritional marasmus**
Severe malnutrition with marasmus
> **Excludes1**   marasmic kwashiorkor (E42)

E42   **Marasmic kwashiorkor**
Severe protein malnutrition
Intermediate form severe protein-calorie malnutrition
Severe protein-calorie malnutrition with signs of both kwashiorkor and marasmus

E43   **Unspecified severe protein-calorie malnutrition**
Starvation edema

● **E44**   **Protein-calorie malnutrition of moderate and mild degree**
     E44.0   **Moderate protein-calorie malnutrition**
     E44.1   **Mild protein-calorie malnutrition**

E45   **Retarded development following protein-calorie malnutrition**
Nutritional short stature
Nutritional stunting
Physical retardation due to malnutrition

E46   **Unspecified protein-calorie malnutrition**
Malnutrition NOS
Protein-calorie imbalance NOS
> **Excludes1**   nutritional deficiency NOS (E63.9)

Item 4–6   **Bitot's spots** are the result of a buildup of keratin debris found on the superficial surface the conjunctiva; oval, triangular, or irregular in shape; and a sign of vitamin A deficiency and associated with night blindness. The disease may progress to **keratomalacia,** which can result in eventual prolapse of the iris and loss of the lens.

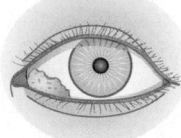

Figure 4-7   Bitot's spot on the conjunctiva.

OTHER NUTRITIONAL DEFICIENCIES (E50-E64)

> **Excludes2**   nutritional anemias (D50-D53)

● **E50**   **Vitamin A deficiency**
> **Excludes1**   sequelae of vitamin A deficiency (E64.1)

     E50.0   **Vitamin A deficiency with conjunctival xerosis**

     E50.1   **Vitamin A deficiency with Bitot's spot and conjunctival xerosis**
Bitot's spot in the young child

     E50.2   **Vitamin A deficiency with corneal xerosis**

     E50.3   **Vitamin A deficiency with corneal ulceration and xerosis**

     E50.4   **Vitamin A deficiency with keratomalacia**
Eye disorder that results in dry cornea caused by vitamin A deficiency

     E50.5   **Vitamin A deficiency with night blindness**

     E50.6   **Vitamin A deficiency with xerophthalmic scars of cornea**
Abnormal dryness and thickening of conjunctiva and cornea due to vitamin A deficiency

     E50.7   **Other ocular manifestations of vitamin A deficiency**
Xerophthalmia NOS

     E50.8   **Other manifestations of vitamin A deficiency**
Follicular keratosis
Xeroderma

     E50.9   **Vitamin A deficiency, unspecified**
Hypovitaminosis A NOS

● **E51**   **Thiamine deficiency**
> **Excludes1**   sequelae of thiamine deficiency (E64.8)

● **E51.1**   **Beriberi**

     E51.11   **Dry beriberi**
Thiamine deficiency with nervous system manifestation most often caused by excessive alcohol consumption
Beriberi NOS
Beriberi with polyneuropathy

     E51.12   **Wet beriberi**
Thiamine deficiency with cardiovascular manifestation most often caused by excessive alcohol consumption
Beriberi with cardiovascular manifestations
Cardiovascular beriberi
Shoshin disease

     E51.2   **Wernicke's encephalopathy**
Acute disease of brain due to thiamine deficiency most often associated with excessive alcohol consumption

     E51.8   **Other manifestations of thiamine deficiency**

     E51.9   **Thiamine deficiency, unspecified**

◀ New   ◀◀ Revised   ~~deleted~~ Deleted   Excludes 1   Excludes 2   Includes   Use additional   Code first   Code also   Unspecified
OGCR Official Guidelines   **X** Assign placeholder X   ● Use Additional Character(s)   ▶ Manifestation Code   **Coding Clinic**

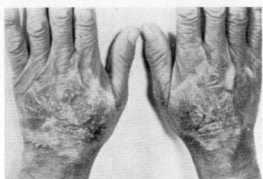

Figure 4-8 The sharply demarcated, characteristic scaling dermatitis of pellagra. (From Kumar: Robbins and Cotran: Pathologic Basis of Disease, ed 8, Saunders, An Imprint of Elsevier, 2009)

Item 4–7 Pellagra is associated with a deficiency of niacin and its precursor, **tryptophan.** Characteristics of the condition include diarrhea, dermatitis on exposed skin surfaces, dementia, and death. It is prevalent in developing countries where nutrition is inadequate. **Beriberi** is associated with thiamine deficiency.

E52   Niacin deficiency [pellagra]
Niacin (-tryptophan) deficiency
Nicotinamide deficiency
Pellagra (alcoholic)
Excludes1   sequelae of niacin deficiency (E64.8)

● **E53   Deficiency of other B group vitamins**
Excludes1   sequelae of vitamin B deficiency (E64.8)

E53.0   Riboflavin deficiency
Ariboflavinosis
Vitamin B2 deficiency

E53.1   Pyridoxine deficiency
Vitamin B6 deficiency
Excludes1   pyridoxine-responsive sideroblastic anemia (D64.3)

E53.8   Deficiency of other specified B group vitamins
Biotin deficiency
Cyanocobalamin deficiency
Folate deficiency
Folic acid deficiency
Pantothenic acid deficiency
Vitamin B12 deficiency
Excludes1   folate deficiency anemia (D52.-)
vitamin B12 deficiency anemia (D51.-)

E53.9   Vitamin B deficiency, unspecified

E54   Ascorbic acid deficiency
Deficiency of vitamin C
Scurvy
Excludes1   scorbutic anemia (D53.2)
sequelae of vitamin C deficiency (E64.2)

● **E55   Vitamin D deficiency**
Excludes1   adult osteomalacia (M83.-)
osteoporosis (M80.-)
sequelae of rickets (E64.3)

E55.0   Rickets, active
Infantile osteomalacia
Juvenile osteomalacia
Softening of bone
Excludes1   celiac rickets (K90.0)
Crohn's rickets (K50.-)
hereditary vitamin D-dependent rickets (E83.32)
inactive rickets (E64.3)
renal rickets (N25.0)
sequelae of rickets (E64.3)
vitamin D-resistant rickets (E83.31)

E55.9   Vitamin D deficiency, unspecified
Avitaminosis D

● **E56   Other vitamin deficiencies**
Excludes1   sequelae of other vitamin deficiencies (E64.8)

E56.0   Deficiency of vitamin E
E56.1   Deficiency of vitamin K
Excludes1   deficiency of coagulation factor due to vitamin K deficiency (D68.4)
vitamin K deficiency of newborn (P53)

E56.8   Deficiency of other vitamins
E56.9   Vitamin deficiency, unspecified

E58   Dietary calcium deficiency
Excludes1   disorders of calcium metabolism (E83.5-)
sequelae of calcium deficiency (E64.8)

E59   Dietary selenium deficiency
Keshan disease
Excludes1   sequelae of selenium deficiency (E64.8)

E60   Dietary zinc deficiency

● **E61   Deficiency of other nutrient elements**
Use additional code for adverse effect, if applicable, to identify drug (T36-T50 with fifth or sixth character 5)
Excludes1   disorders of mineral metabolism (E83.-)
iodine deficiency related thyroid disorders (E00-E02)
sequelae of malnutrition and other nutritional deficiencies (E64.-)

E61.0   Copper deficiency
E61.1   Iron deficiency
Excludes1   iron deficiency anemia (D50.-)

E61.2   Magnesium deficiency
E61.3   Manganese deficiency
E61.4   Chromium deficiency
E61.5   Molybdenum deficiency
E61.6   Vanadium deficiency
E61.7   Deficiency of multiple nutrient elements
E61.8   Deficiency of other specified nutrient elements
E61.9   Deficiency of nutrient element, unspecified

● **E63   Other nutritional deficiencies**
Excludes1   dehydration (E86.0)
failure to thrive, adult (R62.7)
failure to thrive, child (R62.51)
feeding problems in newborn (P92.-)
sequelae of malnutrition and other nutritional deficiencies (E64.-)

E63.0   Essential fatty acid [EFA] deficiency
E63.1   Imbalance of constituents of food intake
E63.8   Other specified nutritional deficiencies
E63.9   Nutritional deficiency, unspecified

● **E64   Sequelae of malnutrition and other nutritional deficiencies**
Pathological condition resulting from disease, injury, or other trauma
Note: This category is to be used to indicate conditions in categories E43, E44, E46, E50-E63 as the cause of sequelae, which are themselves classified elsewhere. The 'sequelae' include conditions specified as such; they also include the late effects of diseases classifiable to the above categories if the disease itself is no longer present
Code first condition resulting from (sequela) of malnutrition and other nutritional deficiencies

E64.0   Sequelae of protein-calorie malnutrition
Excludes2   retarded development following protein-calorie malnutrition (E45)

E64.1   Sequelae of vitamin A deficiency
E64.2   Sequelae of vitamin C deficiency
E64.3   Sequelae of rickets
E64.8   Sequelae of other nutritional deficiencies
E64.9   Sequelae of unspecified nutritional deficiency

CHAPTER 4 (E00-E90)

OVERWEIGHT, OBESITY AND OTHER HYPERALIMENTATION (E65-E68)

E65   **Localized adiposity**
     Fat pad

● **E66**   **Overweight and obesity**
     Code first obesity complicating pregnancy, childbirth and the puerperium, if applicable (O99.21-)
     Use additional code to identify body mass index (BMI), if known (Z68.-)

     Excludes1   adiposogenital dystrophy (E23.6)
                 lipomatosis NOS (E88.2)
                 lipomatosis dolorosa [Dercum] (E88.2)
                 Prader-Willi syndrome (Q87.1)

   ● **E66.0**   **Obesity due to excess calories**

       E66.01   **Morbid (severe) obesity due to excess calories**

          Excludes1   morbid (severe) obesity with alveolar hypoventilation (E66.2)

       E66.09   **Other obesity due to excess calories**

     E66.1   **Drug-induced obesity**

         Use additional code for adverse effect, if applicable, to identify drug (T36-T50 with fifth or sixth character 5)

     E66.2   **Morbid (severe) obesity with alveolar hypoventilation**
         Uncommon condition of unknown cause leading to inadequate ventilation in lungs, even though lungs and airways are normal
         Pickwickian syndrome

     E66.3   **Overweight**

     E66.8   **Other obesity**

     E66.9   **Obesity, unspecified**
         Obesity NOS

● **E67**   **Other hyperalimentation**
     Ingestion of more than optimal amount of nutrients

     Excludes1   hyperalimentation NOS (R63.2)
                 sequelae of hyperalimentation (E68)

     E67.0   **Hypervitaminosis A**

     E67.1   **Hypercarotinemia**

     E67.2   **Megavitamin-B6 syndrome**

     E67.3   **Hypervitaminosis D**

     E67.8   **Other specified hyperalimentation**

E68   **Sequelae of hyperalimentation**
     Code first condition resulting from (sequela) of hyperalimentation

METABOLIC DISORDERS (E70-E88)

     Excludes1   androgen insensitivity syndrome (E34.5-)
                 congenital adrenal hyperplasia (E25.0)
                 Ehlers-Danlos syndrome (Q79.6)
                 hemolytic anemias attributable to enzyme disorders (D55.-)
                 Marfan's syndrome (Q87.4)
                 5-alpha-reductase deficiency (E29.1)

● **E70**   **Disorders of aromatic amino-acid metabolism**

     E70.0   **Classical phenylketonuria**
         Inherited disorder that increases to harmful levels amino acid phenylalanine

     E70.1   **Other hyperphenylalaninemias**

   ● **E70.2**   **Disorders of tyrosine metabolism**

       Excludes1   transitory tyrosinemia of newborn (P74.5)

       E70.20   **Disorder of tyrosine metabolism, unspecified**
          Tyrosine: Nonessential amino acid occurring in most proteins

       E70.21   **Tyrosinemia**
          Congenital amino acid metabolism
          Hypertyrosinemia

       E70.29   **Other disorders of tyrosine metabolism**
          Alkaptonuria
          Ochronosis

● **E70.3**   **Albinism**
     Congenital condition of reduced or absent pigment in eyes, skin, and hair

     E70.30   **Albinism, unspecified**

   ● **E70.31**   **Ocular albinism**

       E70.310   **X-linked ocular albinism**

       E70.311   **Autosomal recessive ocular albinism**

       E70.318   **Other ocular albinism**

       E70.319   **Ocular albinism, unspecified**

   ● **E70.32**   **Oculocutaneous albinism**
       Partial or total lack of melanin pigment in eyes

       Excludes1   Chediak-Higashi syndrome (E70.330)
                 Hermansky-Pudlak syndrome (E70.331)

       E70.320   **Tyrosinase negative oculocutaneous albinism**
          Albinism I
          Oculocutaneous albinism ty-neg

       E70.321   **Tyrosinase positive oculocutaneous albinism**
          Albinism II
          Oculocutaneous albinism ty-pos

       E70.328   **Other oculocutaneous albinism**
          Cross syndrome

       E70.329   **Oculocutaneous albinism, unspecified**

   ● **E70.33**   **Albinism with hematologic abnormality**

       E70.330   **Chediak-Higashi syndrome**

       E70.331   **Hermansky-Pudlak syndrome**

       E70.338   **Other albinism with hematologic abnormality**

       E70.339   **Albinism with hematologic abnormality, unspecified**

     E70.39   **Other specified albinism**
         Piebaldism

   ● **E70.4**   **Disorders of histidine metabolism**

       E70.40   **Disorders of histidine metabolism, unspecified**

       E70.41   **Histidinemia**

       E70.49   **Other disorders of histidine metabolism**

     E70.5   **Disorders of tryptophan metabolism**

     E70.8   **Other disorders of aromatic amino-acid metabolism**

     E70.9   **Disorder of aromatic amino-acid metabolism, unspecified**

● **E71**   **Disorders of branched-chain amino-acid metabolism and fatty-acid metabolism**

     E71.0   **Maple-syrup-urine disease**
         Due to defect in amino acid catabolism, causing severe ketoacidosis with smell of maple syrup in urine and on body

● **E71.1**   **Other disorders of branched-chain amino-acid metabolism**

   ● **E71.11**   **Branched-chain organic acidurias**

       E71.110   **Isovaleric acidemia**

       E71.111   **3-methylglutaconic aciduria**

       E71.118   **Other branched-chain organic acidurias**

   ● **E71.12**   **Disorders of propionate metabolism**

       E71.120   **Methylmalonic acidemia**

       E71.121   **Propionic acidemia**

       E71.128   **Other disorders of propionate metabolism**

     E71.19   **Other disorders of branched-chain amino-acid metabolism**
         Hyperleucine-isoleucinemia
         Hypervalinemia

◄ New   ⬱ Revised   ~~deleted~~ Deleted   Excludes 1   Excludes 2   Includes   Use additional   Code first   Code also   Unspecified

OGCR Official Guidelines   X Assign placeholder X   ● Use Additional Character(s)   ▶ Manifestation Code   **Coding Clinic**

E71.2   Disorder of branched-chain amino-acid metabolism, unspecified

● **E71.3**   Disorders of fatty-acid metabolism

     Excludes1   peroxisomal disorders (E71.5)
                       Refsum's disease (G60.1)
                       Schilder's disease (G37.0)

     Excludes2   carnitine deficiency due to inborn error of metabolism (E71.42)

     E71.30   Disorder of fatty-acid metabolism, unspecified

●   **E71.31**   Disorders of fatty-acid oxidation

         E71.310   Long chain/very long chain acyl CoA dehydrogenase deficiency
                     LCAD
                     VLCAD

         E71.311   Medium chain acyl CoA dehydrogenase deficiency
                     MCAD

         E71.312   Short chain acyl CoA dehydrogenase deficiency
                     SCAD

         E71.313   Glutaric aciduria type II
                     Glutaric aciduria type II A
                     Glutaric aciduria type II B
                     Glutaric aciduria type II C

                 Excludes1   glutaric aciduria (type 1) NOS (E72.3)

         E71.314   Muscle carnitine palmitoyltransferase deficiency

         E71.318   Other disorders of fatty-acid oxidation

     E71.32   Disorders of ketone metabolism

     E71.39   Other disorders of fatty-acid metabolism

● **E71.4**   Disorders of carnitine metabolism

     Excludes1   muscle carnitine palmitoyltransferase deficiency (E71.314)

     E71.40   Disorder of carnitine metabolism, unspecified

     E71.41   Primary carnitine deficiency

     E71.42   Carnitine deficiency due to inborn errors of metabolism

         Code also associated inborn error or metabolism

     E71.43   Iatrogenic carnitine deficiency
         Iatrogenic: Outcomes from activity of physicians
         Carnitine deficiency due to hemodialysis
         Carnitine deficiency due to Valproic acid therapy

●   **E71.44**   Other secondary carnitine deficiency

         E71.440   Ruvalcaba-Myhre-Smith syndrome

         E71.448   Other secondary carnitine deficiency

● **E71.5**   Peroxisomal disorders

     Class of conditions which lead to disorders of lipid metabolism

     Excludes1   Schilder's disease (G37.0)

     E71.50   Peroxisomal disorder, unspecified

●   **E71.51**   Disorders of peroxisome biogenesis
         Group 1 peroxisomal disorders

         Excludes1   Refsum's disease (G60.1)

         E71.510   Zellweger syndrome

         E71.511   Neonatal adrenoleukodystrophy   **N**

                 Excludes1   X-linked adrenoleuko-dystrophy (E71.42-)

         E71.518   Other disorders of peroxisome biogenesis

●   **E71.52**   X-linked adrenoleukodystrophy

         E71.520   Childhood cerebral X-linked adrenoleukodystrophy

         E71.521   Adolescent X-linked adrenoleukodystrophy

         E71.522   Adrenomyeloneuropathy

         E71.528   Other X-linked adrenoleukodystrophy
                     Addison only phenotype adrenoleukodystrophy
                     Addison-Schilder adrenoleukodystrophy

         E71.529   X-linked adrenoleukodystrophy, unspecified type

     E71.53   Other group 2 peroxisomal disorders

●   **E71.54**   Other peroxisomal disorders

         E71.540   Rhizomelic chondrodysplasia punctata
                     Rare, severe, inherited disorder with limb shortening, bone and cartilage abnormalities, abnormal facial appearance, severe mental retardation, psychomotor retardation, and cataracts

                 Excludes1   chondrodysplasia punctata NOS (Q77.3)

         E71.541   Zellweger-like syndrome

         E71.542   Other group 3 peroxisomal disorders

         E71.548   Other peroxisomal disorders

● **E72**   Other disorders of amino-acid metabolism

     Excludes1   disorders of:
                     aromatic amino-acid metabolism (E70.-)
                     branched-chain amino-acid metabolism (E71.0-E71.2)
                     fatty-acid metabolism (E71.3)
                     purine and pyrimidine metabolism (E79.-)
                     gout (M1A.-, M10.-)

●   **E72.0**   Disorders of amino-acid transport

     Excludes1   disorders of tryptophan metabolism (E70.5)

     E72.00   Disorders of amino-acid transport, unspecified

     E72.01   Cystinuria
         Hereditary aminoaciduria due to impairment of renal transport with predominant symptom of urinary cystine calculi

     E72.02   Hartnup's disease
         Inborn error of metabolism

     E72.03   Lowe's syndrome
         X-linked disorder with rickets, hydrophthalmia, congenital glaucoma, cataracts, mental retardation, and renal tubule dysfunction

         Use additional code for associated glaucoma (H42)

     E72.04   Cystinosis
         Genetic disease with excessive depostits of amino acid cystine in cells
         Fanconi (-de Toni) (-Debré) syndrome with cystinosis

         Excludes1   Fanconi (-de Toni) (-Debré) syndrome without cystinosis (E72.09)

     E72.09   Other disorders of amino-acid transport
         Fanconi (-de Toni) (-Debré) syndrome, unspecified

CHAPTER 4 (E00-E90)

CHAPTER 4 (E00-E90)

● **E72.1** **Disorders of sulfur-bearing amino-acid metabolism**
     Excludes1   cystinosis (E72.04)
                      cystinuria (E72.01)
                      transcobalamin II deficiency (D51.2)

     E72.10   **Disorders of sulfur-bearing amino-acid metabolism, unspecified**

     E72.11   **Homocystinuria**
            Cystathionine synthase deficiency

     E72.12   **Methylenetetrahydrofolate reductase deficiency**

     E72.19   **Other disorders of sulfur-bearing amino-acid metabolism**
            Cystathioninuria
            Methioninemia
            Sulfite oxidase deficiency

● **E72.2** **Disorders of urea cycle metabolism**
     Excludes1   disorders of ornithine metabolism (E72.4)

     E72.20   **Disorder of urea cycle metabolism, unspecified**
            Hyperammonemia
            Elevated levels of ammonia

         Excludes1   hyperammonemia-
                       hyperornithinemia-
                       homocitrullinemia
                       syndrome E72.4
                       transient hyperammonemia of
                       newborn (P74.6)

     E72.21   **Argininemia**
            Disorder in which deficiency of enzyme arginase causes build up of arginine and ammonia in blood

     E72.22   **Arginosuccinic aciduria**
            Gene disorder of urea cycle resulting accumulation of ammonia

     E72.23   **Citrullinemia**
            Urea cycle disorder that causes ammonia and other toxic substances to accumulate in blood

     E72.29   **Other disorders of urea cycle metabolism**

E72.3 **Disorders of lysine and hydroxylysine metabolism**
     Glutaric aciduria NOS
     Glutaric aciduria (type I)
     Hydroxylysinemia
     Hyperlysinemia
     Excludes1   glutaric aciduria type II (E71.313)
                      Refsum's disease (G60.1)
                      Zellweger syndrome (E71.510)

E72.4 **Disorders of ornithine metabolism**
     Hyperammonemia-Hyperornithinemia-
         Homocitrullinemia syndrome
     Ornithinemia (types I, II)
     Ornithine transcarbamylase deficiency
     Excludes1   hereditary choroidal dystrophy (H31.2-)

● **E72.5** **Disorders of glycine metabolism**
     E72.50   **Disorder of glycine metabolism, unspecified**
     E72.51   **Non-ketotic hyperglycinemia**
     E72.52   **Trimethylaminuria**
     E72.53   **Hyperoxaluria**
            Oxalosis
            Oxaluria
     E72.59   **Other disorders of glycine metabolism**
            D-glycericacidemia
            Hyperhydroxyprolinemia
            Hyperprolinemia (types I, II)
            Sarcosinemia

E72.8 **Other specified disorders of amino-acid metabolism**
     Disorders of beta-amino-acid metabolism
     Disorders of gamma-glutamyl cycle

E72.9 **Disorder of amino-acid metabolism, unspecified**

● **E73** **Lactose intolerance**
     Intolerance for lactose, due to inherited deficiency of lactase activity in intestinal mucosa

     E73.0   **Congenital lactase deficiency**

     E73.1   **Secondary lactase deficiency**

     E73.8   **Other lactose intolerance**

     E73.9   **Lactose intolerance, unspecified**

● **E74** **Other disorders of carbohydrate metabolism**
     Excludes1   diabetes mellitus (E08-E13)
                    hypoglycemia NOS (E16.2)
                    increased secretion of glucagon (E16.3)
                    mucopolysaccharidosis (E76.0-E76.3)

   ● **E74.0** **Glycogen storage disease**
     E74.00   **Glycogen storage disease, unspecified**
     E74.01   **von Gierke's disease**
            Type I glycogen storage disease
     E74.02   **Pompe disease**
            Cardiac glycogenosis
            Type II glycogen storage disease
     E74.03   **Cori disease**
            Forbes' disease
            Type III glycogen storage disease
     E74.04   **McArdle disease**
            Type V glycogen storage disease
     E74.09   **Other glycogen storage disease**
            Andersen disease
            Hers disease
            Tauri disease
            Glycogen storage disease, types 0, IV, VI-XI
            Liver phosphorylase deficiency
            Muscle phosphofructokinase deficiency

   ● **E74.1** **Disorders of fructose metabolism**
     Excludes1   muscle phosphofructokinase deficiency (E74.09)
     E74.10   **Disorder of fructose metabolism, unspecified**
     E74.11   **Essential fructosuria**
            Fructokinase deficiency
     E74.12   **Hereditary fructose intolerance**
            Fructosemia
     E74.19   **Other disorders of fructose metabolism**
            Fructose-1, 6-diphosphatase deficiency

   ● **E74.2** **Disorders of galactose metabolism**
     E74.20   **Disorders of galactose metabolism, unspecified**
     E74.21   **Galactosemia**
            Genetic disorders resulting from defective simple sugar (galactose) metabolism
     E74.29   **Other disorders of galactose metabolism**
            Galactokinase deficiency

   ● **E74.3** **Other disorders of intestinal carbohydrate absorption**
     Excludes2   lactose intolerance (E73.-)
     E74.31   **Sucrase-isomaltase deficiency**
            Deficiency in metabolism in intestinal mucosa results in malabsorption of sucrose and starch
     E74.39   **Other disorders of intestinal carbohydrate absorption**
            Disorder of intestinal carbohydrate absorption NOS
            Glucose-galactose malabsorption
            Sucrase deficiency

   E74.4 **Disorders of pyruvate metabolism and gluconeogenesis**
     Deficiency of phosphoenolpyruvate carboxykinase
     Deficiency of pyruvate carboxylase
     Deficiency of pyruvate dehydrogenase
     Excludes1   disorders of pyruvate metabolism and gluconeogenesis with anemia (D55.-)
                    Leigh's syndrome (G31.82)

   E74.8 **Other specified disorders of carbohydrate metabolism**
     Essential pentosuria
     Renal glycosuria

   E74.9 **Disorder of carbohydrate metabolism, unspecified**

◄ New   ⬅ Revised   ~~deleted~~ Deleted   Excludes 1   Excludes 2   Includes   Use additional   Code first   Code also   Unspecified

OGCR Official Guidelines   X Assign placeholder X   ● Use Additional Character(s)   ▶ Manifestation Code   **Coding Clinic**

Item 4–8 Leukodystrophy is characterized by degeneration and/or failure of the myelin formation of the central nervous system and sometimes of the peripheral nervous system. The disease is inherited and progressive.

● **E75 Disorders of sphingolipid metabolism and other lipid storage disorders**
      Excludes1 mucolipidosis, types I-III (E77.0-E77.1)
              Refsum's disease (G60.1)

● **E75.0 GM2 gangliosidosis**
    Rare metabolic disorder that causes destruction of nerve cells of brain and spinal cord

    E75.00 GM2 gangliosidosis, unspecified

    E75.01 Sandhoff disease

    E75.02 Tay-Sachs disease

    E75.09 Other GM2 gangliosidosis
          Adult GM2 gangliosidosis
          Juvenile GM2 gangliosidosis

● **E75.1 Other and unspecified gangliosidosis**

    E75.10 Unspecified gangliosidosis
          Gangliosidosis NOS

    E75.11 Mucolipidosis IV
        Disorder with symptoms of psychomotor retardation and severe visual impairment

    E75.19 Other gangliosidosis
          GM1 gangliosidosis
          GM3 gangliosidosis

● **E75.2 Other sphingolipidosis**
    Lysosomal (a particle in a cytoplasm cell that contains digestive enzymes) storage diseases with symptoms of abnormal storage of amino acids

      Excludes1 adrenoleukodystrophy [Addison-Schilder] (E71.528)

    E75.21 Fabry (-Anderson) disease

    E75.22 Gaucher disease

    E75.23 Krabbe disease

  ● **E75.24 Niemann-Pick disease**

        E75.240 Niemann-Pick disease type A

        E75.241 Niemann-Pick disease type B

        E75.242 Niemann-Pick disease type C

        E75.243 Niemann-Pick disease type D

        E75.248 Other Niemann-Pick disease

        E75.249 Niemann-Pick disease, unspecified

    E75.25 Metachromatic leukodystrophy

    E75.29 Other sphingolipidosis
          Farber's syndrome
          Sulfatase deficiency
          Sulfatide lipidosis

  E75.3 Sphingolipidosis, unspecified

  E75.4 Neuronal ceroid lipofuscinosis
        Batten disease
        Bielschowsky-Jansky disease
        Kufs disease
        Spielmeyer-Vogt disease

  E75.5 Other lipid storage disorders
        Cerebrotendinous cholesterosis [van Bogaert-Scherer-Epstein]
        Wolman's disease

  E75.6 Lipid storage disorder, unspecified

● **E76 Disorders of glycosaminoglycan metabolism**

  ● **E76.0 Mucopolysaccharidosis, type I**
      Inborn metabolic disorder of enzymes that break down carbohydrates

    E76.01 Hurler's syndrome

    E76.02 Hurler-Scheie syndrome

    E76.03 Scheie's syndrome

  E76.1 Mucopolysaccharidosis, type II
      Inborn metabolic disorder of enzymes that break down carbohydrates occurs in 2-4 year old males
      Hunter's syndrome

● **E76.2 Other mucopolysaccharidoses**

  ● **E76.21 Morquio mucopolysaccharidoses**

    E76.210 Morquio A mucopolysaccharidoses
        Classic Morquio syndrome
        Morquio syndrome A
        Mucopolysaccharidosis, type IVA

    E76.211 Morquio B mucopolysaccharidoses
        Morquio-like mucopolysaccharidoses
        Morquio-like syndrome
        Morquio syndrome B
        Mucopolysaccharidosis, type IVB

    E76.219 Morquio mucopolysaccharidoses, unspecified
        Morquio syndrome
        Mucopolysaccharidosis, type IV

  E76.22 Sanfilippo mucopolysaccharidoses
      Mucopolysaccharidosis, type III (A) (B) (C) (D)
      Sanfilippo A syndrome
      Sanfilippo B syndrome
      Sanfilippo C syndrome
      Sanfilippo D syndrome

  E76.29 Other mucopolysaccharidoses
      beta-Glucuronidase deficiency
      Maroteaux-Lamy (mild) (severe) syndrome
      Mucopolysaccharidosis, types VI, VII

  E76.3 Mucopolysaccharidosis, unspecified

  E76.8 Other disorders of glucosaminoglycan metabolism

  E76.9 Glucosaminoglycan metabolism disorder, unspecified

● **E77 Disorders of glycoprotein metabolism**

  E77.0 Defects in post-translational modification of lysosomal enzymes
      Mucolipidosis II [I-cell disease]
      Mucolipidosis III [pseudo-Hurler polydystrophy]

  E77.1 Defects in glycoprotein degradation
      Aspartylglucosaminuria
      Fucosidosis
      Mannosidosis
      Sialidosis [mucolipidosis I]

  E77.8 Other disorders of glycoprotein metabolism

  E77.9 Disorder of glycoprotein metabolism, unspecified

● **E78 Disorders of lipoprotein metabolism and other lipidemias**
      Excludes1 sphingolipidosis (E75.0-E75.3)

  E78.0 Pure hypercholesterolemia
      Familial hypercholesterolemia
      Fredrickson's hyperlipoproteinemia, type IIa
      Hyperbetalipoproteinemia
      Hyperlipidemia, Group A
      Low-density-lipoprotein-type [LDL] hyperlipoproteinemia

  E78.1 Pure hyperglyceridemia
      Elevated fasting triglycerides
      Endogenous hyperglyceridemia
      Fredrickson's hyperlipoproteinemia, type IV
      Hyperlipidemia, group B
      Hyperprebetalipoproteinemia
      Very-low-density-lipoprotein-type [VLDL] hyperlipoproteinemia

  E78.2 Mixed hyperlipidemia
      Broad- or floating-betalipoproteinemia
      Combined hyperlipidemia NOS
      Elevated cholesterol with elevated triglycerides NEC
      Fredrickson's hyperlipoproteinemia, type IIb or III
      Hyperbetalipoproteinemia with prebetalipoproteinemia
      Hypercholesteremia with endogenous hyperglyceridemia
      Hyperlipidemia, group C
      Tubo-eruptive xanthoma
      Xanthoma tuberosum

      Excludes1 cerebrotendinous cholesterosis [van Bogaert-Scherer-Epstein] (E75.5)
              familial combined hyperlipidemia (E78.4)

CHAPTER 4 (E00-E90)

E78.3 **Hyperchylomicronemia**
Chylomicron retention disease
Fredrickson's hyperlipoproteinemia, type I or V
Hyperlipidemia, group D
Mixed hyperglyceridemia

E78.4 **Other hyperlipidemia**
Familial combined hyperlipidemia

E78.5 **Hyperlipidemia, unspecified**

E78.6 **Lipoprotein deficiency**
Abetalipoproteinemia
Depressed HDL cholesterol
High-density lipoprotein deficiency
Hypoalphalipoproteinemia
Hypobetalipoproteinemia (familial)
Lecithin cholesterol acyltransferase deficiency
Tangier disease

● **E78.7** **Disorders of bile acid and cholesterol metabolism**
   Excludes1   Niemann-Pick disease type C (E75.242)

   E78.70 **Disorder of bile acid and cholesterol metabolism, unspecified**

   E78.71 **Barth syndrome**

   E78.72 **Smith-Lemli-Opitz syndrome**

   E78.79 **Other disorders of bile acid and cholesterol metabolism**

● **E78.8** **Other disorders of lipoprotein metabolism**

   E78.81 **Lipoid dermatoarthritis**

   E78.89 **Other lipoprotein metabolism disorders**

E78.9 **Disorder of lipoprotein metabolism, unspecified**

● **E79** **Disorders of purine and pyrimidine metabolism**
Purines, along with pyrimidines, signal RNA and DNA production
   Excludes1   Ataxia-telangiectasia (Q87.1)
                   Bloom's syndrome (Q82.8)
                   Cockayne's syndrome (Q87.1)
                   calculus of kidney (N20.0)
                   combined immunodeficiency disorders (D81.-)
                   Fanconi's anemia (D61.09)
                   gout (M1A.-, M10.-)
                   orotaciduric anemia (D53.0)
                   progeria (E34.8)
                   Werner's syndrome (E34.8)
                   xeroderma pigmentosum (Q82.1)

E79.0 **Hyperuricemia without signs of inflammatory arthritis and tophaceous disease**
Asymptomatic hyperuricemia

E79.1 **Lesch-Nyhan syndrome**
HGPRT deficiency

E79.2 **Myoadenylate deaminase deficiency**

E79.8 **Other disorders of purine and pyrimidine metabolism**
Hereditary xanthinuria

E79.9 **Disorder of purine and pyrimidine metabolism, unspecified**

● **E80** **Disorders of porphyrin and bilirubin metabolism**
Group of chemical compounds in RBC's that combine with iron to form heme
   Includes   defects of catalase and peroxidase

E80.0 **Hereditary erythropoietic porphyria**
Congenital erythropoietic porphyria
Erythropoietic protoporphyria

E80.1 **Porphyria cutanea tarda**

● **E80.2** **Other and unspecified porphyria**
   E80.20 **Unspecified porphyria**
         Porphyria NOS

   E80.21 **Acute intermittent (hepatic) porphyria**

   E80.29 **Other porphyria**
         Hereditary coproporphyria

E80.3 **Defects of catalase and peroxidase**
Acatalasia [Takahara]

E80.4 **Gilbert syndrome**

E80.5 **Crigler-Najjar syndrome**

E80.6 **Other disorders of bilirubin metabolism**
Dubin-Johnson syndrome
Rotor's syndrome

E80.7 **Disorder of bilirubin metabolism, unspecified**

● **E83** **Disorders of mineral metabolism**
   Excludes1   dietary mineral deficiency (E58-E61)
                   parathyroid disorders (E20-E21)
                   vitamin D deficiency (E55.-)

● **E83.0** **Disorders of copper metabolism**

   E83.00 **Disorder of copper metabolism, unspecified**

   E83.01 **Wilson's disease**

         Code also associated Kayser Fleischer ring (H18.04-)

   E83.09 **Other disorders of copper metabolism**
         Menkes' (kinky hair) (steely hair) disease

● **E83.1** **Disorders of iron metabolism**
   Excludes1   iron deficiency anemia (D50.-)
                   sideroblastic anemia (D64.0-D64.3)

   E83.10 **Disorder of iron metabolism, unspecified**

  ● **E83.11** **Hemochromatosis**

     E83.110 **Hereditary hemochromatosis**
         Bronzed diabetes
         Pigmentary cirrhosis (of liver)
         Primary (hereditary) hemochromatosis

     E83.111 **Hemochromatosis due to repeated red blood cell transfusions**
         Iron overload due to repeated red blood cell transfusions
         Transfusion (red blood cell) associated hemochromatosis

     E83.118 **Other hemochromatosis**

     E83.119 **Hemochromatosis, unspecified**

   E83.19 **Other disorders of iron metabolism**
         Use additional code, if applicable, for idiopathic pulmonary hemosiderosis (J84.03)

E83.2 **Disorders of zinc metabolism**
Acrodermatitis enteropathica

● **E83.3** **Disorders of phosphorus metabolism and phosphatases**
   Excludes1   adult osteomalacia (M83.-)
                   osteoporosis (M80.-)

   E83.30 **Disorder of phosphorus metabolism, unspecified**

   E83.31 **Familial hypophosphatemia**
         Vitamin D-resistant osteomalacia
         Vitamin D-resistant rickets
      Excludes1   vitamin D-deficiency rickets (E55.0)

   E83.32 **Hereditary vitamin D-dependent rickets (type 1) (type 2)**
         25-hydroxyvitamin D 1-alpha-hydroxylase deficiency
         Pseudovitamin D deficiency
         Vitamin D receptor defect

   E83.39 **Other disorders of phosphorus metabolism**
         Acid phosphatase deficiency
         Hypophosphatasia

● **E83.4** **Disorders of magnesium metabolism**

   E83.40 **Disorders of magnesium metabolism, unspecified**

   E83.41 **Hypermagnesemia**

   E83.42 **Hypomagnesemia**

   E83.49 **Other disorders of magnesium metabolism**

CHAPTER 4 (E00-E90)

◀ New   ◀▥ Revised   ~~deleted~~ Deleted   Excludes 1   Excludes 2   Includes   Use additional   Code first   Code also   Unspecified

OGCR Official Guidelines   **X** Assign placeholder X   ● Use Additional Character(s)   ▶ Manifestation Code   **Coding Clinic**

● **E83.5**   **Disorders of calcium metabolism**
> **Excludes1**   chondrocalcinosis (M11.1-M11.2)
> hungry bone syndrome (E83.81)
> hyperparathyroidism (E21.0-E21.3)

     E83.50   Unspecified **disorder of calcium metabolism**

     E83.51   **Hypocalcemia**

     E83.52   **Hypercalcemia**
> Familial hypocalciuric hypercalcemia

     E83.59   **Other disorders of calcium metabolism**
> Idiopathic hypercalciuria

● **E83.8**   **Other disorders of mineral metabolism**

     E83.81   **Hungry bone syndrome**

     E83.89   **Other disorders of mineral metabolism**

     E83.9   **Disorder of mineral metabolism,** unspecified

● **E84**   **Cystic fibrosis**
> **Includes**   mucoviscidosis

     E84.0   **Cystic fibrosis with pulmonary manifestations**
> Use additional code to identify any infectious organism
> present, such as:
> Pseudomonas (B96.5)

● **E84.1**   **Cystic fibrosis with intestinal manifestations**

     E84.11   **Meconium ileus in cystic fibrosis**   **N**
> **Excludes1**   meconium ileus not due to cystic
> fibrosis (P76.0)

     E84.19   **Cystic fibrosis with other intestinal manifestations**
> Distal intestinal obstruction syndrome

     E84.8   **Cystic fibrosis with other manifestations**

     E84.9   **Cystic fibrosis,** unspecified

● **E85**   **Amyloidosis**
> *A disorder resulting from the abnormal deposition of a particular protein (amyloid) into tissues of the body.*
> **Excludes1**   Alzheimer's disease (G30.0-)

     E85.0   **Non-neuropathic heredofamilial amyloidosis**
> Familial Mediterranean fever
> Hereditary amyloid nephropathy

     E85.1   **Neuropathic heredofamilial amyloidosis**
> Amyloid polyneuropathy (Portuguese)
> **Coding Clinic: 2012, Q4, P100**

     E85.2   **Heredofamilial amyloidosis,** unspecified

     E85.3   **Secondary systemic amyloidosis**
> Hemodialysis-associated amyloidosis

     E85.4   **Organ-limited amyloidosis**
> Localized amyloidosis

     E85.8   **Other amyloidosis**

     E85.9   **Amyloidosis,** unspecified

● **E86**   **Volume depletion**
> **Excludes1**   dehydration of newborn (P74.1)
> hypovolemic shock NOS (R57.1)
> postprocedural hypovolemic shock (T81.19)
> traumatic hypovolemic shock (T79.4)

     E86.0   **Dehydration**
> *Excessive loss of body water*

     E86.1   **Hypovolemia**
> *Diminished volume of circulating blood*
> Depletion of volume of plasma

     E86.9   **Volume depletion,** unspecified

● **E87**   **Other disorders of fluid, electrolyte and acid-base balance**
> **Excludes1**   diabetes insipidus (E23.2)
> electrolyte imbalance associated with
> hyperemesis gravidarum (O21.1)
> electrolyte imbalance following ectopic or molar
> pregnancy (O08.5)
> familial periodic paralysis (G72.3)

     E87.0   **Hyperosmolality and hypernatremia**
> Sodium [Na] excess
> Sodium [Na] overload

     E87.1   **Hypo-osmolality and hyponatremia**
> Sodium [Na] deficiency
> **Excludes1**   syndrome of inappropriate secretion of
> antidiuretic hormone (E22.2)

     E87.2   **Acidosis**
> Acidosis NOS
> Lactic acidosis
> Metabolic acidosis
> Respiratory acidosis
> **Excludes1**   diabetic acidosis - see categories E08-E10,
> E13 with ketoacidosis

     E87.3   **Alkalosis**
> Alkalosis NOS
> Metabolic alkalosis
> Respiratory alkalosis

     E87.4   **Mixed disorder of acid-base balance**

     E87.5   **Hyperkalemia**
> Potassium [K] excess
> Potassium [K] overload

     E87.6   **Hypokalemia**
> Potassium [K] deficiency

● **E87.7**   **Fluid overload**
> **Excludes1**   edema NOS (R60.9)
> fluid retention (R60.9)

     E87.70   **Fluid overload,** unspecified

     E87.71   **Transfusion associated circulatory overload**
> Fluid overload due to transfusion (blood)
> (blood components) TACO

     E87.79   **Other fluid overload**

     E87.8   **Other disorders of electrolyte and fluid balance, not elsewhere classified**
> Electrolyte imbalance NOS
> Hyperchloremia
> Hypochloremia

● **E88**   **Other and unspecified metabolic disorders**
> Use additional codes for associated conditions
> **Excludes1**   histiocytosis X (chronic) (C96.6)

● **E88.0**   **Disorders of plasma-protein metabolism, not elsewhere classified**
> **Excludes1**   disorder of lipoprotein metabolism (E78.-)
> monoclonal gammopathy (of
> undetermined significance) (D47.2)
> polyclonal hypergammaglobulinemia
> (D89.0)
> Waldenström macroglobulinemia (C88.0)

     E88.01   **Alpha-1-antitrypsin deficiency AAT deficiency**

     E88.09   **Other disorders of plasma-protein metabolism, not elsewhere classified**
> Bisalbuminemia

     E88.1   **Lipodystrophy, not elsewhere classified**
> *Defective fat metabolism resulting in absence of subcutaneous fat*
> Lipodystrophy NOS
> **Excludes1**   Whipple's disease (K90.81)

     E88.2   **Lipomatosis, not elsewhere classified**
> *Abnormal tumorlike accumulations of fat in tissue*
> Lipomatosis NOS
> Lipomatosis (Check) dolorosa [Dercum]

Item 4-9   Circulating fluid volume is regulated by the amount of water and sodium ingested, excreted by the kidneys into the urine, and lost through the gastrointestinal tract, lungs, and skin. To maintain blood volume within a normal range, the kidneys regulate the amount of water and sodium lost into the urine. Too much **(fluid overload)** or too little fluid volume **(volume depletion)** will affect blood pressure. Severe cases of vomiting, diarrhea, bleeding, and burns (fluid loss through exposed burn surface area) can contribute to fluid loss. Internal body environment must maintain a precise balance (homeostasis) between too much fluid and too little fluid. This complex balancing mechanism is critical to good health.

CHAPTER 4 (E00-E90)

E88.3 **Tumor lysis syndrome**
Tumor lysis syndrome (spontaneous)
Tumor lysis syndrome following antineoplastic drug
chemotherapy
*Use additional code for adverse effect, if applicable, to
identify drug (T45.1X5)*

● E88.4 **Mitochondrial metabolism disorders**
Congenital disorder of metabolism
Excludes1   disorders of pyruvate metabolism (E74.4)
Kearns-Sayre syndrome (H49.81)
Leber's disease (H47.22)
Leigh's encephalopathy (G31.82)
Mitochondrial myopathy, NEC (G71.3)
Reye's syndrome (G93.7)

E88.40 **Mitochondrial metabolism disorder,
unspecified**

E88.41 **MELAS syndrome**
Mitochondrial myopathy, encephalopathy,
lactic acidosis and stroke-like episodes

E88.42 **MERRF syndrome**
Myoclonic epilepsy associated with ragged-red
fibers
Code also myoclonic epilepsy (G40.3-)

E88.49 **Other mitochondrial metabolism disorders**

● E88.8 **Other specified metabolic disorders**
E88.81 **Metabolic syndrome**
Dysmetabolic syndrome X
*Use additional codes for associated
manifestations, such as:*
obesity (E66.-)

E88.89 **Other specified metabolic disorders**
Launois-Bensaude adenolipomatosis
Excludes1   adult pulmonary Langerhans cell
histiocytosis (J84.82)

E88.9 **Metabolic disorder, unspecified**

POSTPROCEDURAL ENDOCRINE AND METABOLIC COMPLICATIONS
AND DISORDERS, NOT ELSEWHERE CLASSIFIED (E89)

● E89 **Postprocedural endocrine and metabolic complications and
disorders, not elsewhere classified**
Excludes2   intraoperative complications of endocrine system
organ or structure (E36.0-, E36.1-, E36.8)

E89.0 **Postprocedural hypothyroidism**
Postirradiation hypothyroidism
Postsurgical hypothyroidism

E89.1 **Postprocedural hypoinsulinemia**
Postpancreatectomy hyperglycemia
Postsurgical hypoinsulinemia
Use additional code, if applicable, to identify:
acquired absence of pancreas (Z90.41-)
diabetes mellitus (postpancreatectomy)
(postprocedural) (E13.-)
insulin use (Z79.4)
Excludes1   transient postprocedural hyperglycemia
(R73.9)
transient postprocedural hypoglycemia
(E16.2)

E89.2 **Postprocedural hypoparathyroidism**
Parathyroprival tetany

E89.3 **Postprocedural hypopituitarism**
Postirradiation hypopituitarism

● E89.4 **Postprocedural ovarian failure**
E89.40 **Asymptomatic postprocedural ovarian failure** ♀
Postprocedural ovarian failure NOS

E89.41 **Symptomatic postprocedural ovarian failure** ♀
Symptoms such as flushing, sleeplessness,
headache, lack of concentration,
associated with postprocedural
menopause

E89.5 **Postprocedural testicular hypofunction** ♂

E89.6 **Postprocedural adrenocortical (-medullary)
hypofunction**

● E89.8 **Other postprocedural endocrine and metabolic
complications and disorders**
● E89.81 **Postprocedural hemorrhage and hematoma
of an endocrine system organ or structure
following a procedure**
E89.810 **Postprocedural hemorrhage and
hematoma of an endocrine system
organ or structure following an
endocrine system procedure**

E89.811 **Postprocedural hemorrhage and
hematoma of an endocrine system
organ or structure following other
procedure**

E89.89 **Other postprocedural endocrine and metabolic
complications and disorders**
*Use additional code, if applicable, to further
specify disorder*

CHAPTER 4 (E00-E90)

CHAPTER 5

MENTAL, BEHAVIORAL AND NEURODEVELOPMENTAL DISORDERS (F01–F99)

Includes	disorders of psychological development
Excludes2	symptoms, signs and abnormal clinical laboratory findings, not elsewhere classified (R00-R99)

This chapter contains the following blocks:

F01-F09	Mental disorders due to known physiological conditions
F10-F19	Mental and behavioral disorders due to psychoactive substance use
F20-F29	Schizophrenia, schizotypal, delusional, and other non-mood psychotic disorders
F30-F39	Mood [affective] disorders
F40-F48	Anxiety, dissociative, stress-related, somatoform and other nonpsychotic mental disorders
F50-F59	Behavioral syndromes associated with physiological disturbances and physical factors
F60-F69	Disorders of adult personality and behavior
F70-F79	Intellectual disabilities
F80-F89	Pervasive and specific developmental disorders
F90-F98	Behavioral and emotional disorders with onset usually occurring in childhood and adolescence
F99	Unspecified mental disorder

MENTAL DISORDERS DUE TO KNOWN PHYSIOLOGICAL CONDITIONS (F01-F09)

This block comprises a range of mental disorders grouped together on the basis of their having in common a demonstrable etiology in cerebral disease, brain injury, or other insult leading to cerebral dysfunction. The dysfunction may be primary, as in diseases, injuries, and insults that affect the brain directly and selectively; or secondary, as in systemic diseases and disorders that attack the brain only as one of the multiple organs or systems of the body that are involved.

● **F01   Vascular dementia**

Vascular dementia as a result of infarction of the brain due to vascular disease, including hypertensive cerebrovascular disease.

Includes	arteriosclerotic dementia

Code first the underlying physiological condition or sequelae of cerebrovascular disease.

● **F01.5   Vascular dementia**

F01.50   Vascular dementia without behavioral disturbance   **A**

F01.51   Vascular dementia with behavioral disturbance   **A**

Vascular dementia with aggressive behavior
Vascular dementia with combative behavior
Vascular dementia with violent behavior

Use additional code, if applicable, to identify wandering in vascular dementia (Z91.83)

● **F02   Dementia in other diseases classified elsewhere**

Code first the underlying physiological condition, such as:
Alzheimer's (G30.-)
cerebral lipidosis (E75.4)
Creutzfeldt-Jakob disease (A81.0-)
dementia with Lewy bodies (G31.83)
epilepsy and recurrent seizures (G40.-)
frontotemporal dementia (G31.09)
hepatolenticular degeneration (E83.0)
human immunodeficiency virus [HIV] disease (B20)
hypercalcemia (E83.52)
hypothyroidism, acquired (E00-E03.-)
intoxications (T36-T65)
Jakob-Creutzfeldt disease (A81.0-)
multiple sclerosis (G35)
neurosyphilis (A52.17)
niacin deficiency [pellagra] (E52)
Parkinson's disease (G20)
Pick's disease (G31.01)
polyarteritis nodosa (M30.0)
systemic lupus erythematosus (M32.-)
trypanosomiasis (B56.-, B57.-)
vitamin B deficiency (E53.8)

Excludes1	dementia with Parkinsonism (G31.83)
Excludes2	dementia in alcohol and psychoactive substance disorders (F10-F19, with .17, .27, .97) vascular dementia (F01.5-)

● **F02.8   Dementia in other diseases classified elsewhere**

▸ **F02.80   *Dementia in other diseases classified elsewhere without behavioral disturbance***

Dementia in other diseases classified elsewhere NOS

▸ **F02.81   *Dementia in other diseases classified elsewhere with behavioral disturbance***

Dementia in other diseases classified elsewhere with aggressive behavior
Dementia in other diseases classified elsewhere with combative behavior
Dementia in other diseases classified elsewhere with violent behavior

Use additional code, if applicable, to identify wandering in dementia in conditions classified elsewhere (Z91.83)

● **F03   Unspecified dementia**

Presenile dementia NOS
Presenile psychosis NOS
Primary degenerative dementia NOS
Senile dementia NOS
Senile dementia depressed or paranoid type
Senile psychosis NOS

Excludes1	senility NOS (R41.81)
Excludes2	mild memory disturbance due to known physiological condition (F06.8) senile dementia with delirium or acute confusional state (F05)

● **F03.9   Unspecified dementia**

F03.90   Unspecified dementia without behavioral disturbance   **A**

Dementia NOS
Coding Clinic: 2012, Q4, P92

F03.91   Unspecified dementia with behavioral disturbance   **A**

Unspecified dementia with aggressive behavior
Unspecified dementia with combative behavior
Unspecified dementia with violent behavior

Use additional code, if applicable, to identify wandering in unspecified dementia (Z91.83)

Item 5-1 Psychosis was a term formerly applied to any mental disorder but is now restricted to disturbances of a great magnitude in which there is a personality disintegration and loss of contact with reality.

F04   Amnestic disorder due to known physiological condition
Korsakov's psychosis or syndrome, nonalcoholic

Code first the underlying physiological condition

Excludes1   amnesia NOS (R41.3)
anterograde amnesia (R41.1)
dissociative amnesia (F44.0)
retrograde amnesia (R41.2)

Excludes2   alcohol-induced or unspecified Korsakov's
syndrome (F10.26, F10.96)
Korsakov's syndrome induced by other
psychoactive substances (F13.26, F13.96,
F19.16, F19.26, F19.96)

F05   Delirium due to known physiological condition
Acute or subacute brain syndrome
Acute or subacute confusional state (nonalcoholic)
Acute or subacute infective psychosis
Acute or subacute organic reaction
Acute or subacute psycho-organic syndrome
Delirium of mixed etiology
Delirium superimposed on dementia
Sundowning

Code first the underlying physiological condition

Excludes1   delirium NOS (R41.0)

Excludes2   delirium tremens alcohol-induced or unspecified
(F10.231, F10.921)

● **F06   Other mental disorders due to known physiological condition**

Includes   mental disorders due to endocrine disorder
mental disorders due to exogenous hormone
mental disorders due to exogenous toxic
substance
mental disorders due to primary cerebral disease
mental disorders due to somatic illness
mental disorders due to systemic disease
affecting the brain

Code first the underlying physiological condition

Excludes1   unspecified dementia (F03)

Excludes2   delirium due to known physiological condition
(F05)
dementia as classified in F01-F02
other mental disorders associated with alcohol
and other psychoactive substances (F10-F19)

**F06.0   Psychotic disorder with hallucinations due to known
physiological condition**
Organic hallucinatory state (nonalcoholic)

Excludes2   hallucinations and perceptual disturbance
induced by alcohol and other
psychoactive substances (F10-F19
with .151, .251, .951)
schizophrenia (F20.-)

**F06.1   Catatonic disorder due to known physiological
condition**

Excludes1   catatonic stupor (R40.1)
stupor NOS (R40.1)

Excludes2   catatonic schizophrenia (F20.2)
dissociative stupor (F44.2)

**F06.2   Psychotic disorder with delusions due to known
physiological condition**
Paranoid and paranoid-hallucinatory organic states
Schizophrenia-like psychosis in epilepsy

Excludes2   alcohol and drug-induced psychotic
disorder (F10-F19 with .150, .250,
.950)
brief psychotic disorder (F23)
delusional disorder (F22)
schizophrenia (F20.-)

● **F06.3   Mood disorder due to known physiological condition**

Excludes2   mood disorders due to alcohol and other
psychoactive
substances (F10-F19 with .14, .24, .94)
mood disorders, not due to known
physiological condition or
unspecified (F30-F39)

**F06.30   Mood disorder due to known physiological
condition, unspecified**

**F06.31   Mood disorder due to known physiological
condition with depressive features**

**F06.32   Mood disorder due to known physiological
condition with major depressive-like episode**

**F06.33   Mood disorder due to known physiological
condition with manic features**

**F06.34   Mood disorder due to known physiological
condition with mixed features**

F06.4   Anxiety disorder due to known physiological condition

Excludes2   anxiety disorders due to alcohol and
other psychoactive substances
(F10-F19 with .180, .280, .980)
anxiety disorders, not due to known
physiological condition or
unspecified (F40.-, F41.-)

**F06.8   Other specified mental disorders due to known
physiological condition**
Epileptic psychosis NOS
Organic dissociative disorder
Organic emotionally labile [asthenic] disorder

● **F07   Personality and behavioral disorders due to known
physiological condition**

Code first the underlying physiological condition

**F07.0   Personality change due to known physiological
condition**
Frontal lobe syndrome
Limbic epilepsy personality syndrome
Lobotomy syndrome
Organic personality disorder
Organic pseudopsychopathic personality
Organic pseudoretarded personality
Postleucotomy syndrome

Code first underlying physiological condition

Excludes1   mild cognitive impairment (G31.84)
postconcussional syndrome (F07.81)
postencephalitic syndrome (F07.89)
signs and symptoms involving emotional
state (R45.-)

Excludes2   specific personality disorder (F60.-)

● **F07.8   Other personality and behavioral disorders due to
known physiological condition**

F07.81   Postconcussional syndrome
Postcontusional syndrome (encephalopathy)
Post-traumatic brain syndrome, nonpsychotic

Use additional code to identify associated
post-traumatic headache, if applicable
(G44.3-)

Excludes1   current concussion (brain)
(S06.0-)
postencephalitic syndrome
(F07.89)

**F07.89   Other personality and behavioral disorders due
to known physiological condition**
Postencephalitic syndrome
*Damage to temporal brain lobes with memory
loss and abnormal behavior*
Right hemispheric organic affective disorder

**F07.9   Unspecified personality and behavioral disorder due to
known physiological condition**
Organic psychosyndrome
Due to exposure to organic solvents

◀ New   ◀▬ Revised   ~~deleted~~ Deleted   Excludes 1   Excludes 2   Includes   Use additional   Code first   Code also   Unspecified

OGCR Official Guidelines   X Assign placeholder X   ● Use Additional Character(s)   ▶ Manifestation Code   **Coding Clinic**

F09   **Unspecified mental disorder due to known physiological condition**
      Mental disorder NOS due to known physiological condition
      Organic brain syndrome NOS
      Organic mental disorder NOS
      Organic psychosis NOS
      Symptomatic psychosis NOS
      Code first the underlying physiological condition
      Excludes1   psychosis NOS (F29)

MENTAL AND BEHAVIORAL DISORDERS DUE TO PSYCHOACTIVE SUBSTANCE USE (F10-F19)

● **F10**   **Alcohol related disorders**
      Use additional code for blood alcohol level, if applicable (Y90.-)

● **F10.1**   **Alcohol abuse**
      Excludes1   alcohol dependence (F10.2-)
                   alcohol use, unspecified (F10.9-)
      F10.10   Alcohol abuse, uncomplicated
    ● F10.12   Alcohol abuse with intoxication
          F10.120   Alcohol abuse with intoxication, uncomplicated
          F10.121   Alcohol abuse with intoxication, delirium
          F10.129   Alcohol abuse with intoxication, unspecified
      F10.14   Alcohol abuse with alcohol-induced mood disorder
    ● F10.15   Alcohol abuse with alcohol-induced psychotic disorder
          F10.150   Alcohol abuse with alcohol-induced psychotic disorder with delusions
          F10.151   Alcohol abuse with alcohol-induced psychotic disorder with hallucinations
          F10.159   Alcohol abuse with alcohol-induced psychotic disorder, unspecified
    ● F10.18   Alcohol abuse with other alcohol-induced disorders
          F10.180   Alcohol abuse with alcohol-induced anxiety disorder
          F10.181   Alcohol abuse with alcohol-induced sexual dysfunction
          F10.182   Alcohol abuse with alcohol-induced sleep disorder
          F10.188   Alcohol abuse with other alcohol-induced disorder
      F10.19   Alcohol abuse with unspecified alcohol-induced disorder

● **F10.2**   **Alcohol dependence**
      Excludes1   alcohol abuse (F10.1-)
                   alcohol use, unspecified (F10.9-)
      Excludes2   toxic effect of alcohol (T51.0-)
      F10.20   Alcohol dependence, uncomplicated
      F10.21   Alcohol dependence, in remission
    ● F10.22   Alcohol dependence with intoxication
          Acute drunkenness (in alcoholism)
          Excludes1   alcohol dependence with withdrawal (F10.23-)
          F10.220   Alcohol dependence with intoxication, uncomplicated
          F10.221   Alcohol dependence with intoxication delirium
          F10.229   Alcohol dependence with intoxication, unspecified

● **F10.23**   **Alcohol dependence with withdrawal**
      Excludes1   alcohol dependence with intoxication (F10.22-)
      F10.230   Alcohol dependence with withdrawal, uncomplicated
      F10.231   Alcohol dependence with withdrawal delirium
      F10.232   Alcohol dependence with withdrawal with perceptual disturbance
      F10.239   Alcohol dependence with withdrawal, unspecified
    F10.24   Alcohol dependence with alcohol-induced mood disorder

● **F10.25**   Alcohol dependence with alcohol-induced psychotic disorder
      F10.250   Alcohol dependence with alcohol-induced psychotic disorder with delusions
      F10.251   Alcohol dependence with alcohol-induced psychotic disorder with hallucinations
      F10.259   Alcohol dependence with alcohol-induced psychotic disorder, unspecified
    F10.26   Alcohol dependence with alcohol-induced persisting amnestic disorder
    F10.27   Alcohol dependence with alcohol-induced persisting dementia

● **F10.28**   Alcohol dependence with other alcohol-induced disorders
      F10.280   Alcohol dependence with alcohol-induced anxiety disorder
      F10.281   Alcohol dependence with alcohol-induced sexual dysfunction
      F10.282   Alcohol dependence with alcohol-induced sleep disorder
      F10.288   Alcohol dependence with other alcohol-induced disorder
    F10.29   Alcohol dependence with unspecified alcohol-induced disorder

● **F10.9**   **Alcohol use, unspecified**
      Excludes1   alcohol abuse (F10.1-)
                   alcohol dependence (F10.2-)
    ● F10.92   Alcohol use, unspecified with intoxication
          F10.920   Alcohol use, unspecified with intoxication, uncomplicated
          F10.921   Alcohol use, unspecified with intoxication delirium
          F10.929   Alcohol use, unspecified with intoxication, unspecified
    F10.94   Alcohol use, unspecified with alcohol-induced mood disorder
    ● F10.95   Alcohol use, unspecified with alcohol-induced psychotic disorder
          F10.950   Alcohol use, unspecified with alcohol-induced psychotic disorder with delusions
          F10.951   Alcohol use, unspecified with alcohol-induced psychotic disorder with hallucinations
          F10.959   Alcohol use, unspecified with alcohol-induced psychotic disorder, unspecified
    F10.96   Alcohol use, unspecified with alcohol-induced persisting amnestic disorder
    F10.97   Alcohol use, unspecified with alcohol-induced persisting dementia

CHAPTER 5 (F01-F99)

● F10.98 Alcohol use, unspecified with other alcohol-induced disorders

    F10.980 Alcohol use, unspecified with alcohol-induced anxiety disorder

    F10.981 Alcohol use, unspecified with alcohol-induced sexual dysfunction

    F10.982 Alcohol use, unspecified with alcohol-induced sleep disorder

    F10.988 Alcohol use, unspecified with other alcohol-induced disorder

F10.99 Alcohol use, unspecified with unspecified alcohol-induced disorder

● F11 Opioid related disorders

  ● F11.1 Opioid abuse

    Excludes1 opioid dependence (F11.2-)
               opioid use, unspecified (F11.9-)

    F11.10 Opioid abuse, uncomplicated

  ● F11.12 Opioid abuse with intoxication

    F11.120 Opioid abuse with intoxication, uncomplicated

    F11.121 Opioid abuse with intoxication delirium

    F11.122 Opioid abuse with intoxication with perceptual disturbance

    F11.129 Opioid abuse with intoxication, unspecified

    F11.14 Opioid abuse with opioid-induced mood disorder

  ● F11.15 Opioid abuse with opioid-induced psychotic disorder

    F11.150 Opioid abuse with opioid-induced psychotic disorder with delusions

    F11.151 Opioid abuse with opioid-induced psychotic disorder with hallucinations

    F11.159 Opioid abuse with opioid-induced psychotic disorder, unspecified

  ● F11.18 Opioid abuse with other opioid-induced disorder

    F11.181 Opioid abuse with opioid-induced sexual dysfunction

    F11.182 Opioid abuse with opioid-induced sleep disorder

    F11.188 Opioid abuse with other opioid-induced disorder

    F11.19 Opioid abuse with unspecified opioid-induced disorder

  ● F11.2 Opioid dependence

    Excludes1 opioid abuse (F11.1-)
               opioid use, unspecified (F11.9-)

    Excludes2 opioid poisoning (T40.0--T40.2-)

    F11.20 Opioid dependence, uncomplicated

    F11.21 Opioid dependence, in remission

  ● F11.22 Opioid dependence with intoxication

    Excludes1 opioid dependence with withdrawal (F11.23)

    F11.220 Opioid dependence with intoxication, uncomplicated

    F11.221 Opioid dependence with intoxication delirium

    F11.222 Opioid dependence with intoxication with perceptual disturbance

    F11.229 Opioid dependence with intoxication, unspecified

    F11.23 Opioid dependence with withdrawal

    Excludes1 opioid dependence with intoxication (F11.22-)

F11.24 Opioid dependence with opioid-induced mood disorder

● F11.25 Opioid dependence with opioid-induced psychotic disorder

    F11.250 Opioid dependence with opioid-induced psychotic disorder with delusions

    F11.251 Opioid dependence with opioid-induced psychotic disorder with hallucinations

    F11.259 Opioid dependence with opioid-induced psychotic disorder, unspecified

● F11.28 Opioid dependence with other opioid-induced disorder

    F11.281 Opioid dependence with opioid-induced sexual dysfunction

    F11.282 Opioid dependence with opioid-induced sleep disorder

    F11.288 Opioid dependence with other opioid-induced disorder

F11.29 Opioid dependence with unspecified opioid-induced disorder

● F11.9 Opioid use, unspecified

    Excludes1 opioid abuse (F11.1-)
               opioid dependence (F11.2-)

F11.90 Opioid use, unspecified, uncomplicated

● F11.92 Opioid use, unspecified with intoxication

    Excludes1 opioid use, unspecified with withdrawal (F11.93)

    F11.920 Opioid use, unspecified with intoxication, uncomplicated

    F11.921 Opioid use, unspecified with intoxication delirium

    F11.922 Opioid use, unspecified with intoxication with perceptual disturbance

    F11.929 Opioid use, unspecified with intoxication, unspecified

F11.93 Opioid use, unspecified with withdrawal

    Excludes1 opioid use, unspecified with intoxication (F11.92-)

F11.94 Opioid use, unspecified with opioid-induced mood disorder

● F11.95 Opioid use, unspecified with opioid-induced psychotic disorder

    F11.950 Opioid use, unspecified with opioid-induced psychotic disorder with delusions

    F11.951 Opioid use, unspecified with opioid-induced psychotic disorder with hallucinations

    F11.959 Opioid use, unspecified with opioid-induced psychotic disorder, unspecified

● F11.98 Opioid use, unspecified with other specified opioid-induced disorder

    F11.981 Opioid use, unspecified with opioid-induced sexual dysfunction

    F11.982 Opioid use, unspecified with opioid-induced sleep disorder

    F11.988 Opioid use, unspecified with other opioid-induced disorder

F11.99 Opioid use, unspecified with unspecified opioid-induced disorder

◀ New   ◀◀◀ Revised   ~~deleted~~ Deleted   Excludes 1   Excludes 2   Includes   Use additional   Code first   Code also   Unspecified

OGCR Official Guidelines   X Assign placeholder X   ● Use Additional Character(s)   ❱ Manifestation Code   **Coding Clinic**

● F12   Cannabis related disorders
>   **Includes**   marijuana

● F12.1   Cannabis abuse
>   **Excludes1**   cannabis dependence (F12.2-)
>   cannabis use, unspecified (F12.9-)

>   F12.10   Cannabis abuse, uncomplicated

● F12.12   Cannabis abuse with intoxication

>   F12.120   Cannabis abuse with intoxication, uncomplicated

>   F12.121   Cannabis abuse with intoxication delirium

>   F12.122   Cannabis abuse with intoxication with perceptual disturbance

>   F12.129   Cannabis abuse with intoxication, unspecified

● F12.15   Cannabis abuse with psychotic disorder

>   F12.150   Cannabis abuse with psychotic disorder with delusions

>   F12.151   Cannabis abuse with psychotic disorder with hallucinations

>   F12.159   Cannabis abuse with psychotic disorder, unspecified

● F12.18   Cannabis abuse with other cannabis-induced disorder

>   F12.180   Cannabis abuse with cannabis-induced anxiety disorder

>   F12.188   Cannabis abuse with other cannabis-induced disorder

>   F12.19   Cannabis abuse with unspecified cannabis-induced disorder

● F12.2   Cannabis dependence
>   **Excludes1**   cannabis abuse (F12.1-)
>   cannabis use, unspecified (F12.9-)
>
>   **Excludes2**   cannabis poisoning (T40.7-)

>   F12.20   Cannabis dependence, uncomplicated

>   F12.21   Cannabis dependence, in remission

● F12.22   Cannabis dependence with intoxication

>   F12.220   Cannabis dependence with intoxication, uncomplicated

>   F12.221   Cannabis dependence with intoxication delirium

>   F12.222   Cannabis dependence with intoxication with perceptual disturbance

>   F12.229   Cannabis dependence with intoxication, unspecified

● F12.25   Cannabis dependence with psychotic disorder

>   F12.250   Cannabis dependence with psychotic disorder with delusions

>   F12.251   Cannabis dependence with psychotic disorder with hallucinations

>   F12.259   Cannabis dependence with psychotic disorder, unspecified

● F12.28   Cannabis dependence with other cannabis-induced disorder

>   F12.280   Cannabis dependence with cannabis-induced anxiety disorder

>   F12.288   Cannabis dependence with other cannabis-induced disorder

>   F12.29   Cannabis dependence with unspecified cannabis-induced disorder

● F12.9   Cannabis use, unspecified
>   **Excludes1**   cannabis abuse (F12.1-)
>   cannabis dependence (F12.2-)

>   F12.90   Cannabis use, unspecified, uncomplicated

● F12.92   Cannabis use, unspecified with intoxication

>   F12.920   Cannabis use, unspecified with intoxication, uncomplicated

>   F12.921   Cannabis use, unspecified with intoxication delirium

>   F12.922   Cannabis use, unspecified with intoxication with perceptual disturbance

>   F12.929   Cannabis use, unspecified with intoxication, unspecified

● F12.95   Cannabis use, unspecified with psychotic disorder

>   F12.950   Cannabis use, unspecified with psychotic disorder with delusions

>   F12.951   Cannabis use, unspecified with psychotic disorder with hallucinations

>   F12.959   Cannabis use, unspecified with psychotic disorder, unspecified

● F12.98   Cannabis use, unspecified with other cannabis-induced disorder

>   F12.980   Cannabis use, unspecified with anxiety disorder

>   F12.988   Cannabis use, unspecified with other cannabis-induced disorder

>   F12.99   Cannabis use, unspecified with unspecified cannabis-induced disorder

● F13   Sedative, hypnotic, or anxiolytic related disorders

● F13.1   Sedative, hypnotic or anxiolytic-related abuse
>   **Excludes1**   sedative, hypnotic or anxiolytic-related dependence (F13.2-)
>   sedative, hypnotic, or anxiolytic use, unspecified (F13.9-)

>   F13.10   Sedative, hypnotic or anxiolytic abuse, uncomplicated

● F13.12   Sedative, hypnotic or anxiolytic abuse with intoxication

>   F13.120   Sedative, hypnotic or anxiolytic abuse with intoxication, uncomplicated

>   F13.121   Sedative, hypnotic or anxiolytic abuse with intoxication delirium

>   F13.129   Sedative, hypnotic or anxiolytic abuse with intoxication, unspecified

>   F13.14   Sedative, hypnotic or anxiolytic abuse with sedative, hypnotic or anxiolytic-induced mood disorder

● F13.15   Sedative, hypnotic or anxiolytic abuse with sedative, hypnotic or anxiolyticinduced psychotic disorder

>   F13.150   Sedative, hypnotic or anxiolytic abuse with sedative, hypnotic or anxiolytic-induced psychotic disorder with delusions

>   F13.151   Sedative, hypnotic or anxiolytic abuse with sedative, hypnotic or anxiolytic-induced psychotic disorder with hallucinations

>   F13.159   Sedative, hypnotic or anxiolytic abuse with sedative, hypnotic or anxiolytic-induced psychotic disorder, unspecified

CHAPTER 5 (F01-F99)

N Newborn Age: 0   **P** Pediatric Age: 0–17   **M** Maternity DX: 12–55   **A** Adult Age: 15–124   ♀ Females Only   ♂ Males Only

847

CHAPTER 5 (F01-F99)

● **F13.18**   Sedative, hypnotic or anxiolytic abuse with other sedative, hypnotic or anxiolytic-induced disorders

     F13.180   Sedative, hypnotic or anxiolytic abuse with sedative, hypnotic or anxiolytic-induced anxiety disorder

     F13.181   Sedative, hypnotic or anxiolytic abuse with sedative, hypnotic or anxiolytic-induced sexual dysfunction

     F13.182   Sedative, hypnotic or anxiolytic abuse with sedative, hypnotic or anxiolytic-induced sleep disorder

     F13.188   Sedative, hypnotic or anxiolytic abuse with other sedative, hypnotic or anxiolytic-induced disorder

   F13.19   Sedative, hypnotic or anxiolytic abuse with unspecified sedative, hypnotic or anxiolytic-induced disorder

● **F13.2**   Sedative, hypnotic or anxiolytic-related dependence

     Excludes1   sedative, hypnotic or anxiolytic-related abuse (F13.1-)

               sedative, hypnotic, or anxiolytic use, unspecified (F13.9-)

     Excludes2   sedative, hypnotic, or anxiolytic poisoning (T42.-)

   F13.20   Sedative, hypnotic or anxiolytic dependence, uncomplicated

   F13.21   Sedative, hypnotic or anxiolytic dependence, in remission

● **F13.22**   Sedative, hypnotic or anxiolytic dependence with intoxication

     Excludes1   sedative, hypnotic or anxiolytic dependence with withdrawal (F13.23-)

     F13.220   Sedative, hypnotic or anxiolytic dependence with intoxication, uncomplicated

     F13.221   Sedative, hypnotic or anxiolytic dependence with intoxication delirium

     F13.229   Sedative, hypnotic or anxiolytic dependence with intoxication, unspecified

● **F13.23**   Sedative, hypnotic or anxiolytic dependence with withdrawal

     Excludes1   sedative, hypnotic or anxiolytic dependence with intoxication (F13.22-)

     F13.230   Sedative, hypnotic or anxiolytic dependence with withdrawal, uncomplicated

     F13.231   Sedative, hypnotic or anxiolytic dependence with withdrawal delirium

     F13.232   Sedative, hypnotic or anxiolytic dependence with withdrawal with perceptual disturbance

     F13.239   Sedative, hypnotic or anxiolytic dependence with withdrawal, unspecified

   F13.24   Sedative, hypnotic or anxiolytic dependence with sedative, hypnotic or anxiolytic-induced mood disorder

● **F13.25**   Sedative, hypnotic or anxiolytic dependence with sedative, hypnotic or anxiolytic-induced psychotic disorder

     F13.250   Sedative, hypnotic or anxiolytic dependence with sedative, hypnotic or anxiolytic-induced psychotic disorder with delusions

     F13.251   Sedative, hypnotic or anxiolytic dependence with sedative, hypnotic or anxiolytic-induced psychotic disorder with hallucinations

     F13.259   Sedative, hypnotic or anxiolytic dependence with sedative, hypnotic or anxiolytic-induced psychotic disorder, unspecified

   F13.26   Sedative, hypnotic or anxiolytic dependence with sedative, hypnotic or anxiolytic-induced persisting amnestic disorder

   F13.27   Sedative, hypnotic or anxiolytic dependence with sedative, hypnotic or anxiolytic-induced persisting dementia

● **F13.28**   Sedative, hypnotic or anxiolytic dependence with other sedative, hypnotic or anxiolytic-induced disorders

     F13.280   Sedative, hypnotic or anxiolytic dependence with sedative, hypnotic or anxiolytic-induced anxiety disorder

     F13.281   Sedative, hypnotic or anxiolytic dependence with sedative, hypnotic or anxiolytic-induced sexual dysfunction

     F13.282   Sedative, hypnotic or anxiolytic dependence with sedative, hypnotic or anxiolytic-induced sleep disorder

     F13.288   Sedative, hypnotic or anxiolytic dependence with other sedative, hypnotic or anxiolytic-induced disorder

   F13.29   Sedative, hypnotic or anxiolytic dependence with unspecified sedative, hypnotic or anxiolytic-induced disorder

● **F13.9**   Sedative, hypnotic or anxiolytic-related use, unspecified

     Excludes1   sedative, hypnotic or anxiolytic-related abuse (F13.1-)

               sedative, hypnotic or anxiolytic-related dependence (F13.2-)

   F13.90   Sedative, hypnotic, or anxiolytic use, unspecified, uncomplicated

● **F13.92**   Sedative, hypnotic or anxiolytic use, unspecified with intoxication

     Excludes1   sedative, hypnotic or anxiolytic use, unspecified with withdrawal (F13.93-)

     F13.920   Sedative, hypnotic or anxiolytic use, unspecified with intoxication, uncomplicated

     F13.921   Sedative, hypnotic or anxiolytic use, unspecified with intoxication delirium

     F13.929   Sedative, hypnotic or anxiolytic use, unspecified with intoxication, unspecified

◀ New   ◀ Revised   ~~deleted~~ Deleted   Excludes 1   Excludes 2   Includes   Use additional   Code first   Code also   Unspecified

OGCR Official Guidelines   X Assign placeholder X   ● Use Additional Character(s)   ▌ Manifestation Code   **Coding Clinic**

● **F13.93** Sedative, hypnotic or anxiolytic use, unspecified with withdrawal

> **Excludes1**   sedative, hypnotic or anxiolytic use, unspecified with intoxication (F13.92-)

F13.930   Sedative, hypnotic or anxiolytic use, unspecified with withdrawal, uncomplicated

F13.931   Sedative, hypnotic or anxiolytic use, unspecified with withdrawal delirium

F13.932   Sedative, hypnotic or anxiolytic use, unspecified with withdrawal with perceptual disturbances

F13.939   Sedative, hypnotic or anxiolytic use, unspecified with withdrawal, unspecified

F13.94 Sedative, hypnotic or anxiolytic use, unspecified with sedative, hypnotic or anxiolytic-induced mood disorder

● **F13.95** Sedative, hypnotic or anxiolytic use, unspecified with sedative, hypnotic or anxiolytic-induced psychotic disorder

F13.950   Sedative, hypnotic or anxiolytic use, unspecified with sedative, hypnotic or anxiolytic-induced psychotic disorder with delusions

F13.951   Sedative, hypnotic or anxiolytic use, unspecified with sedative, hypnotic or anxiolytic-induced psychotic disorder with hallucinations

F13.959   Sedative, hypnotic or anxiolytic use, unspecified with sedative, hypnotic or anxiolytic-induced psychotic disorder, unspecified

F13.96 Sedative, hypnotic or anxiolytic use, unspecified with sedative, hypnotic or anxiolytic-induced persisting amnestic disorder

F13.97 Sedative, hypnotic or anxiolytic use, unspecified with sedative, hypnotic or anxiolytic-induced persisting dementia

● **F13.98** Sedative, hypnotic or anxiolytic use, unspecified with other sedative, hypnotic or anxiolytic-induced disorders

F13.980   Sedative, hypnotic or anxiolytic use, unspecified with sedative, hypnotic or anxiolytic-induced anxiety disorder

F13.981   Sedative, hypnotic or anxiolytic use, unspecified with sedative, hypnotic or anxiolytic-induced sexual dysfunction

F13.982   Sedative, hypnotic or anxiolytic use, unspecified with sedative, hypnotic or anxiolytic-induced sleep disorder

F13.988   Sedative, hypnotic or anxiolytic use, unspecified with other sedative, hypnotic or anxiolytic-induced disorder

F13.99 Sedative, hypnotic or anxiolytic use, unspecified with unspecified sedative, hypnotic or anxiolytic-induced disorder

● **F14**   Cocaine related disorders

> **Excludes2**   other stimulant-related disorders (F15.-)

● **F14.1**   Cocaine abuse

> **Excludes1**   cocaine dependence (F14.2-)
> cocaine use, unspecified (F14.9-)

F14.10   Cocaine abuse, uncomplicated

● **F14.12**   Cocaine abuse with intoxication

F14.120   Cocaine abuse with intoxication, uncomplicated

F14.121   Cocaine abuse with intoxication with delirium

F14.122   Cocaine abuse with intoxication with perceptual disturbance

F14.129   Cocaine abuse with intoxication, unspecified

F14.14   Cocaine abuse with cocaine-induced mood disorder

● **F14.15**   Cocaine abuse with cocaine-induced psychotic disorder

F14.150   Cocaine abuse with cocaine-induced psychotic disorder with delusions

F14.151   Cocaine abuse with cocaine-induced psychotic disorder with hallucinations

F14.159   Cocaine abuse with cocaine-induced psychotic disorder, unspecified

● **F14.18**   Cocaine abuse with other cocaine-induced disorder

F14.180   Cocaine abuse with cocaine-induced anxiety disorder

F14.181   Cocaine abuse with cocaine-induced sexual dysfunction

F14.182   Cocaine abuse with cocaine-induced sleep disorder

F14.188   Cocaine abuse with other cocaine-induced disorder

F14.19   Cocaine abuse with unspecified cocaine-induced disorder

● **F14.2**   Cocaine dependence

> **Excludes1**   cocaine abuse (F14.1-)
> cocaine use, unspecified (F14.9-)

> **Excludes2**   cocaine poisoning (T40.5-)

F14.20   Cocaine dependence, uncomplicated

F14.21   Cocaine dependence, in remission

● **F14.22**   Cocaine dependence with intoxication

> **Excludes1**   cocaine dependence with withdrawal (F14.23)

F14.220   Cocaine dependence with intoxication, uncomplicated

F14.221   Cocaine dependence with intoxication delirium

F14.222   Cocaine dependence with intoxication with perceptual disturbance

F14.229   Cocaine dependence with intoxication, unspecified

F14.23   Cocaine dependence with withdrawal

> **Excludes1**   cocaine dependence with intoxication (F14.22-)

F14.24   Cocaine dependence with cocaine-induced mood disorder

● F14.25   Cocaine dependence with cocaine-induced psychotic disorder

     F14.250   Cocaine dependence with cocaine-induced psychotic disorder with delusions

     F14.251   Cocaine dependence with cocaine-induced psychotic disorder with hallucinations

     F14.259   Cocaine dependence with cocaine-induced psychotic disorder, unspecified

● F14.28   Cocaine dependence with other cocaine-induced disorder

     F14.280   Cocaine dependence with cocaine-induced anxiety disorder

     F14.281   Cocaine dependence with cocaine-induced sexual dysfunction

     F14.282   Cocaine dependence with cocaine-induced sleep disorder

     F14.288   Cocaine dependence with other cocaine-induced disorder

   F14.29   Cocaine dependence with unspecified cocaine-induced disorder

● F14.9   Cocaine use, unspecified

    Excludes1   cocaine abuse (F14.1-)
                 cocaine dependence (F14.2-)

   F14.90   Cocaine use, unspecified, uncomplicated

● F14.92   Cocaine use, unspecified with intoxication

     F14.920   Cocaine use, unspecified with intoxication, uncomplicated

     F14.921   Cocaine use, unspecified with intoxication delirium

     F14.922   Cocaine use, unspecified with intoxication with perceptual disturbance

     F14.929   Cocaine use, unspecified with intoxication, unspecified

   F14.94   Cocaine use, unspecified with cocaine-induced mood disorder

● F14.95   Cocaine use, unspecified with cocaine-induced psychotic disorder

     F14.950   Cocaine use, unspecified with cocaine-induced psychotic disorder with delusions

     F14.951   Cocaine use, unspecified with cocaine-induced psychotic disorder with hallucinations

     F14.959   Cocaine use, unspecified with cocaine-induced psychotic disorder, unspecified

● F14.98   Cocaine use, unspecified with other specified cocaine-induced disorder

     F14.980   Cocaine use, unspecified with cocaine-induced anxiety disorder

     F14.981   Cocaine use, unspecified with cocaine-induced sexual dysfunction

     F14.982   Cocaine use, unspecified with cocaine-induced sleep disorder

     F14.988   Cocaine use, unspecified with other cocaine-induced disorder

   F14.99   Cocaine use, unspecified with unspecified cocaine-induced disorder

● F15   Other stimulant related disorders

    Includes   amphetamine-related disorders
                 caffeine

    Excludes2   cocaine-related disorders (F14.-)

● F15.1   Other stimulant abuse

    Excludes1   other stimulant dependence (F15.2-)
                 other stimulant use, unspecified (F15.9-)

   F15.10   Other stimulant abuse, uncomplicated

● F15.12   Other stimulant abuse with intoxication

     F15.120   Other stimulant abuse with intoxication, uncomplicated

     F15.121   Other stimulant abuse with intoxication delirium

     F15.122   Other stimulant abuse with intoxication with perceptual disturbance

     F15.129   Other stimulant abuse with intoxication, unspecified

   F15.14   Other stimulant abuse with stimulant-induced mood disorder

● F15.15   Other stimulant abuse with stimulant-induced psychotic disorder

     F15.150   Other stimulant abuse with stimulant-induced psychotic disorder with delusions

     F15.151   Other stimulant abuse with stimulant-induced psychotic disorder with hallucinations

     F15.159   Other stimulant abuse with stimulant-induced psychotic disorder, unspecified

● F15.18   Other stimulant abuse with other stimulant-induced disorder

     F15.180   Other stimulant abuse with stimulant-induced anxiety disorder

     F15.181   Other stimulant abuse with stimulant-induced sexual dysfunction

     F15.182   Other stimulant abuse with stimulant-induced sleep disorder

     F15.188   Other stimulant abuse with other stimulant-induced disorder

   F15.19   Other stimulant abuse with unspecified stimulant-induced disorder

● F15.2   Other stimulant dependence

    Excludes1   other stimulant abuse (F15.1-)
                 other stimulant use, unspecified (F15.9-)

   F15.20   Other stimulant dependence, uncomplicated

   F15.21   Other stimulant dependence, in remission

● F15.22   Other stimulant dependence with intoxication

    Excludes1   other stimulant dependence with withdrawal (F15.23)

     F15.220   Other stimulant dependence with intoxication, uncomplicated

     F15.221   Other stimulant dependence with intoxication delirium

     F15.222   Other stimulant dependence with intoxication with perceptual disturbance

     F15.229   Other stimulant dependence with intoxication, unspecified

   F15.23   Other stimulant dependence with withdrawal

    Excludes1   other stimulant dependence with intoxication (F15.22-)

◀ New   ◀▦ Revised   ~~deleted~~ Deleted   Excludes 1   Excludes 2   Includes   Use additional   Code first   Code also   Unspecified

OGCR Official Guidelines   X Assign placeholder X   ● Use Additional Character(s)   ▶ Manifestation Code   **Coding Clinic**

F15.24   Other stimulant dependence with stimulant-induced mood disorder

● F15.25   Other stimulant dependence with stimulant-induced psychotic disorder

     F15.250   Other stimulant dependence with stimulant-induced psychotic disorder with delusions

     F15.251   Other stimulant dependence with stimulant-induced psychotic disorder with hallucinations

     F15.259   Other stimulant dependence with stimulant-induced psychotic disorder, unspecified

● F15.28   Other stimulant dependence with other stimulant-induced disorder

     F15.280   Other stimulant dependence with stimulant-induced anxiety disorder

     F15.281   Other stimulant dependence with stimulant-induced sexual dysfunction

     F15.282   Other stimulant dependence with stimulant-induced sleep disorder

     F15.288   Other stimulant dependence with other stimulant-induced disorder

F15.29   Other stimulant dependence with unspecified stimulant-induced disorder

● F15.9   Other stimulant use, unspecified

     Excludes1   other stimulant abuse (F15.1-)
               other stimulant dependence (F15.2-)

F15.90   Other stimulant use, unspecified, uncomplicated

● F15.92   Other stimulant use, unspecified with intoxication

     Excludes1   other stimulant use, unspecified with withdrawal (F15.93)

     F15.920   Other stimulant use, unspecified with intoxication, uncomplicated

     F15.921   Other stimulant use, unspecified with intoxication delirium

     F15.922   Other stimulant use, unspecified with intoxication with perceptual disturbance

     F15.929   Other stimulant use, unspecified with intoxication, unspecified

F15.93   Other stimulant use, unspecified with withdrawal

     Excludes1   other stimulant use, unspecified with intoxication (F15.92-)

F15.94   Other stimulant use, unspecified with stimulant-induced mood disorder

● F15.95   Other stimulant use, unspecified with stimulant-induced psychotic disorder

     F15.950   Other stimulant use, unspecified with stimulant-induced psychotic disorder with delusions

     F15.951   Other stimulant use, unspecified with stimulant-induced psychotic disorder with hallucinations

     F15.959   Other stimulant use, unspecified with stimulant-induced psychotic disorder, unspecified

● F15.98   Other stimulant use, unspecified with other stimulant-induced disorder

     F15.980   Other stimulant use, unspecified with stimulant-induced anxiety disorder

     F15.981   Other stimulant use, unspecified with stimulant-induced sexual dysfunction

     F15.982   Other stimulant use, unspecified with stimulant-induced sleep disorder

     F15.988   Other stimulant use, unspecified with other stimulant-induced disorder

F15.99   Other stimulant use, unspecified with unspecified stimulant-induced disorder

● **F16**   **Hallucinogen related disorders**

     Includes   ecstasy
               PCP
               phencyclidine

● F16.1   Hallucinogen abuse

     Excludes1   hallucinogen dependence (F16.2-)
               hallucinogen use, unspecified (F16.9-)

F16.10   Hallucinogen abuse, uncomplicated

● F16.12   Hallucinogen abuse with intoxication

     F16.120   Hallucinogen abuse with intoxication, uncomplicated

     F16.121   Hallucinogen abuse with intoxication with delirium

     F16.122   Hallucinogen abuse with intoxication with perceptual disturbance

     F16.129   Hallucinogen abuse with intoxication, unspecified

F16.14   Hallucinogen abuse with hallucinogen-induced mood disorder

● F16.15   Hallucinogen abuse with hallucinogen-induced psychotic disorder

     F16.150   Hallucinogen abuse with hallucinogen-induced psychotic disorder with delusions

     F16.151   Hallucinogen abuse with hallucinogen-induced psychotic disorder with hallucinations

     F16.159   Hallucinogen abuse with hallucinogen-induced psychotic disorder, unspecified

● F16.18   Hallucinogen abuse with other hallucinogen-induced disorder

     F16.180   Hallucinogen abuse with hallucinogen-induced anxiety disorder

     F16.183   Hallucinogen abuse with hallucinogen persisting perception disorder (flashbacks)

     F16.188   Hallucinogen abuse with other hallucinogen-induced disorder

F16.19   Hallucinogen abuse with unspecified hallucinogen-induced disorder

● F16.2   Hallucinogen dependence

     Excludes1   hallucinogen abuse (F16.1-)
               hallucinogen use, unspecified (F16.9-)

F16.20   Hallucinogen dependence, uncomplicated

F16.21   Hallucinogen dependence, in remission

● F16.22   Hallucinogen dependence with intoxication

     F16.220   Hallucinogen dependence with intoxication, uncomplicated

     F16.221   Hallucinogen dependence with intoxication with delirium

     F16.229   Hallucinogen dependence with intoxication, unspecified

F16.24   Hallucinogen dependence with hallucinogen-induced mood disorder

● F16.25   Hallucinogen dependence with hallucinogen-induced psychotic disorder

     F16.250   Hallucinogen dependence with hallucinogen-induced psychotic disorder with delusions

     F16.251   Hallucinogen dependence with hallucinogen-induced psychotic disorder with hallucinations

     F16.259   Hallucinogen dependence with hallucinogen-induced psychotic disorder, unspecified

CHAPTER 5 (F01-F99)

- **F16.28** Hallucinogen dependence with other hallucinogen-induced disorder
  - F16.280 Hallucinogen dependence with hallucinogen-induced anxiety disorder
  - F16.283 Hallucinogen dependence with hallucinogen persisting perception disorder (flashbacks)
  - F16.288 Hallucinogen dependence with other hallucinogen-induced disorder
  - F16.29 Hallucinogen dependence with unspecified hallucinogen-induced disorder
- **F16.9** Hallucinogen use, unspecified
  - **Excludes1** hallucinogen abuse (F16.1-)
    hallucinogen dependence (F16.2-)
  - F16.90 Hallucinogen use, unspecified, uncomplicated
- **F16.92** Hallucinogen use, unspecified with intoxication
  - F16.920 Hallucinogen use, unspecified with intoxication, uncomplicated
  - F16.921 Hallucinogen use, unspecified with intoxication with delirium
  - F16.929 Hallucinogen use, unspecified with intoxication, unspecified
  - F16.94 Hallucinogen use, unspecified with hallucinogen-induced mood disorder
- **F16.95** Hallucinogen use, unspecified with hallucinogen-induced psychotic disorder
  - F16.950 Hallucinogen use, unspecified with hallucinogen-induced psychotic disorder with delusions
  - F16.951 Hallucinogen use, unspecified with hallucinogen-induced psychotic disorder with hallucinations
  - F16.959 Hallucinogen use, unspecified with hallucinogen-induced psychotic disorder, unspecified
- **F16.98** Hallucinogen use, unspecified with other specified hallucinogen-induced disorder
  - F16.980 Hallucinogen use, unspecified with hallucinogen-induced anxiety disorder
  - F16.983 Hallucinogen use, unspecified with hallucinogen persisting perception disorder (flashbacks)
  - F16.988 Hallucinogen use, unspecified with other hallucinogen-induced disorder
  - F16.99 Hallucinogen use, unspecified with unspecified hallucinogen-induced disorder

- **F17** Nicotine dependence
  - **Excludes1** history of tobacco dependence (Z87.891)
    tobacco use NOS (Z72.0)
  - **Excludes2** tobacco use (smoking) during pregnancy, childbirth and the puerperium (O99.33-)
    toxic effect of nicotine (T65.2-)
- **F17.2** Nicotine dependence
  - **F17.20** Nicotine dependence, unspecified
    - F17.200 Nicotine dependence, unspecified, uncomplicated
    - F17.201 Nicotine dependence, unspecified, in remission
    - F17.203 Nicotine dependence unspecified, with withdrawal
    - F17.208 Nicotine dependence, unspecified, with other nicotine-induced disorders
    - F17.209 Nicotine dependence, unspecified, with unspecified nicotine-induced disorders

- **F17.21** Nicotine dependence, cigarettes
  - F17.210 Nicotine dependence, cigarettes, uncomplicated
  - F17.211 Nicotine dependence, cigarettes, in remission
  - F17.213 Nicotine dependence, cigarettes, with withdrawal
  - F17.218 Nicotine dependence, cigarettes, with other nicotine-induced disorders
  - F17.219 Nicotine dependence, cigarettes, with unspecified nicotine-induced disorders
- **F17.22** Nicotine dependence, chewing tobacco
  - F17.220 Nicotine dependence, chewing tobacco, uncomplicated
  - F17.221 Nicotine dependence, chewing tobacco, in remission
  - F17.223 Nicotine dependence, chewing tobacco, with withdrawal
  - F17.228 Nicotine dependence, chewing tobacco, with other nicotine-induced disorders
  - F17.229 Nicotine dependence, chewing tobacco, with unspecified nicotine-induced disorders
- **F17.29** Nicotine dependence, other tobacco product
  - F17.290 Nicotine dependence, other tobacco product, uncomplicated
  - F17.291 Nicotine dependence, other tobacco product, in remission
  - F17.293 Nicotine dependence, other tobacco product, with withdrawal
  - F17.298 Nicotine dependence, other tobacco product, with other nicotine-induced disorders
  - F17.299 Nicotine dependence, other tobacco product, with unspecified nicotine-induced disorders

- **F18** Inhalant related disorders
  - **Includes** volatile solvents
- **F18.1** Inhalant abuse
  - **Excludes1** inhalant dependence (F18.2-)
    inhalant use, unspecified (F18.9-)
  - F18.10 Inhalant abuse, uncomplicated
- **F18.12** Inhalant abuse with intoxication
  - F18.120 Inhalant abuse with intoxication, uncomplicated
  - F18.121 Inhalant abuse with intoxication delirium
  - F18.129 Inhalant abuse with intoxication, unspecified
  - F18.14 Inhalant abuse with inhalant-induced mood disorder
- **F18.15** Inhalant abuse with inhalant-induced psychotic disorder
  - F18.150 Inhalant abuse with inhalant-induced psychotic disorder with delusions
  - F18.151 Inhalant abuse with inhalant-induced psychotic disorder with hallucinations
  - F18.159 Inhalant abuse with inhalant-induced psychotic disorder, unspecified
  - F18.17 Inhalant abuse with inhalant-induced dementia

◀ New　◀▦ Revised　~~deleted~~ Deleted　| Excludes 1 |　| Excludes 2 |　| Includes |　| Use additional |　| Code first |　| Code also |　| Unspecified |

OGCR Official Guidelines　X Assign placeholder X　● Use Additional Character(s)　▶ Manifestation Code　**Coding Clinic**

● F18.18   Inhalant abuse with other inhalant-induced disorders
  F18.180   Inhalant abuse with inhalant-induced anxiety disorder
  F18.188   Inhalant abuse with other inhalant-induced disorder
  F18.19   Inhalant abuse with unspecified inhalant-induced disorder
● F18.2   Inhalant dependence
  Excludes1   inhalant abuse (F18.1-)
  inhalant use, unspecified (F18.9-)
  F18.20   Inhalant dependence, uncomplicated
  F18.21   Inhalant dependence, in remission
● F18.22   Inhalant dependence with intoxication
  F18.220   Inhalant dependence with intoxication, uncomplicated
  F18.221   Inhalant dependence with intoxication delirium
  F18.229   Inhalant dependence with intoxication, unspecified
  F18.24   Inhalant dependence with inhalant-induced mood disorder
● F18.25   Inhalant dependence with inhalant-induced psychotic disorder
  F18.250   Inhalant dependence with inhalant-induced psychotic disorder with delusions
  F18.251   Inhalant dependence with inhalant-induced psychotic disorder with hallucinations
  F18.259   Inhalant dependence with inhalant-induced psychotic disorder, unspecified
  F18.27   Inhalant dependence with inhalant-induced dementia
● F18.28   Inhalant dependence with other inhalant-induced disorders
  F18.280   Inhalant dependence with inhalant-induced anxiety disorder
  F18.288   Inhalant dependence with other inhalant-induced disorder
  F18.29   Inhalant dependence with unspecified inhalant-induced disorder
● F18.9   Inhalant use, unspecified
  Excludes1   inhalant abuse (F18.1-)
  inhalant dependence (F18.2-)
  F18.90   Inhalant use, unspecified, uncomplicated
● F18.92   Inhalant use, unspecified with intoxication
  F18.920   Inhalant use, unspecified with intoxication, uncomplicated
  F18.921   Inhalant use, unspecified with intoxication with delirium
  F18.929   Inhalant use, unspecified with intoxication, unspecified
  F18.94   Inhalant use, unspecified with inhalant-induced mood disorder
● F18.95   Inhalant use, unspecified with inhalant-induced psychotic disorder
  F18.950   Inhalant use, unspecified with inhalant-induced psychotic disorder with delusions
  F18.951   Inhalant use, unspecified with inhalant-induced psychotic disorder with hallucinations
  F18.959   Inhalant use, unspecified with inhalant-induced psychotic disorder, unspecified

  F18.97   Inhalant use, unspecified with inhalant-induced persisting dementia
● F18.98   Inhalant use, unspecified with other inhalant-induced disorders
  F18.980   Inhalant use, unspecified with inhalant-induced anxiety disorder
  F18.988   Inhalant use, unspecified with other inhalant-induced disorder
  F18.99   Inhalant use, unspecified with unspecified inhalant-induced disorder
● F19   Other psychoactive substance related disorders
  Includes   polysubstance drug use (indiscriminate drug use)
● F19.1   Other psychoactive substance abuse
  Excludes1   other psychoactive substance dependence (F19.2-)
  other psychoactive substance use, unspecified (F19.9-)
  F19.10   Other psychoactive substance abuse, uncomplicated
● F19.12   Other psychoactive substance abuse with intoxication
  F19.120   Other psychoactive substance abuse with intoxication, uncomplicated
  F19.121   Other psychoactive substance abuse with intoxication delirium
  F19.122   Other psychoactive substance abuse with intoxication with perceptual disturbances
  F19.129   Other psychoactive substance abuse with intoxication, unspecified
  F19.14   Other psychoactive substance abuse with psychoactive substance-induced mood disorder
● F19.15   Other psychoactive substance abuse with psychoactive substance-induced psychotic disorder
  F19.150   Other psychoactive substance abuse with psychoactive substance-induced psychotic disorder with delusions
  F19.151   Other psychoactive substance abuse with psychoactive substance-induced psychotic disorder with hallucinations
  F19.159   Other psychoactive substance abuse with psychoactive substance-induced psychotic disorder, unspecified
  F19.16   Other psychoactive substance abuse with psychoactive substance-induced persisting amnestic disorder
  F19.17   Other psychoactive substance abuse with psychoactive substance-induced persisting dementia
● F19.18   Other psychoactive substance abuse with other psychoactive substance-induced disorders
  F19.180   Other psychoactive substance abuse with psychoactive substance-induced anxiety disorder
  F19.181   Other psychoactive substance abuse with psychoactive substance-induced sexual dysfunction
  F19.182   Other psychoactive substance abuse with psychoactive substance-induced sleep disorder
  F19.188   Other psychoactive substance abuse with other psychoactive substance-induced disorder
  F19.19   Other psychoactive substance abuse with unspecified psychoactive substance-induced disorder

CHAPTER 5 (F01-F99)

● **F19.2**   **Other psychoactive substance dependence**

> **Excludes1**   other psychoactive substance abuse (F19.1-)
>
> other psychoactive substance use, unspecified (F19.9-)

F19.20   Other psychoactive substance dependence, uncomplicated

F19.21   Other psychoactive substance dependence, in remission

● F19.22   Other psychoactive substance dependence with intoxication

> **Excludes1**   other psychoactive substance dependence with withdrawal (F19.23-)

F19.220   Other psychoactive substance dependence with intoxication, uncomplicated

F19.221   Other psychoactive substance dependence with intoxication delirium

F19.222   Other psychoactive substance dependence with intoxication with perceptual disturbance

F19.229   Other psychoactive substance dependence with intoxication, unspecified

● F19.23   Other psychoactive substance dependence with withdrawal

> **Excludes1**   other psychoactive substance dependence with intoxication (F19.22-)

F19.230   Other psychoactive substance dependence with withdrawal, uncomplicated

F19.231   Other psychoactive substance dependence with withdrawal delirium

F19.232   Other psychoactive substance dependence with withdrawal with perceptual disturbance

F19.239   Other psychoactive substance dependence with withdrawal, unspecified

F19.24   Other psychoactive substance dependence with psychoactive substance-induced mood disorder

● F19.25   Other psychoactive substance dependence with psychoactive substance-induced psychotic disorder

F19.250   Other psychoactive substance dependence with psychoactive substance-induced psychotic disorder with delusions

F19.251   Other psychoactive substance dependence with psychoactive substance-induced psychotic disorder with hallucinations

F19.259   Other psychoactive substance dependence with psychoactive substance-induced psychotic disorder, unspecified

F19.26   Other psychoactive substance dependence with psychoactive substance-induced persisting amnestic disorder

F19.27   Other psychoactive substance dependence with psychoactive substance-induced persisting dementia

● F19.28   Other psychoactive substance dependence with other psychoactive substance-induced disorders

F19.280   Other psychoactive substance dependence with psychoactive substance-induced anxiety disorder

F19.281   Other psychoactive substance dependence with psychoactive substance-induced sexual dysfunction

F19.282   Other psychoactive substance dependence with psychoactive substance-induced sleep disorder

F19.288   Other psychoactive substance dependence with other psychoactive substance-induced disorder

F19.29   Other psychoactive substance dependence with unspecified psychoactive substance-induced disorder

● **F19.9**   **Other psychoactive substance use, unspecified**

> **Excludes1**   other psychoactive substance abuse (F19.1-)
>
> other psychoactive substance dependence (F19.2-)

F19.90   Other psychoactive substance use, unspecified, uncomplicated

● F19.92   Other psychoactive substance use, unspecified with intoxication

> **Excludes1**   other psychoactive substance use, unspecified with withdrawal (F19.93)

F19.920   Other psychoactive substance use, unspecified with intoxication, uncomplicated

F19.921   Other psychoactive substance use, unspecified with intoxication with delirium

F19.922   Other psychoactive substance use, unspecified with intoxication with perceptual disturbance

F19.929   Other psychoactive substance use, unspecified with intoxication, unspecified

● F19.93   Other psychoactive substance use, unspecified with withdrawal

> **Excludes1**   other psychoactive substance use, unspecified with intoxication (F19.92-)

F19.930   Other psychoactive substance use, unspecified with withdrawal, uncomplicated

F19.931   Other psychoactive substance use, unspecified with withdrawal delirium

F19.932   Other psychoactive substance use, unspecified with withdrawal with perceptual disturbance

F19.939   Other psychoactive substance use, unspecified with withdrawal, unspecified

F19.94   Other psychoactive substance use, unspecified with psychoactive substance-induced mood disorder

● F19.95   Other psychoactive substance use, unspecified with psychoactive substance-induced psychotic disorder

F19.950   Other psychoactive substance use, unspecified with psychoactive substance-induced psychotic disorder with delusions

F19.951   Other psychoactive substance use, unspecified with psychoactive substance-induced psychotic disorder with hallucinations

F19.959   Other psychoactive substance use, unspecified with psychoactive substance-induced psychotic disorder, unspecified

◀ New   ◀◀ Revised   ~~deleted~~ Deleted   Excludes 1   Excludes 2   Includes   Use additional   Code first   Code also   Unspecified

OGCR Official Guidelines   X Assign placeholder X   ● Use Additional Character(s)   ▷ Manifestation Code   **Coding Clinic**

F19.96   Other psychoactive substance use, unspecified with psychoactive substance-induced persisting amnestic disorder

F19.97   Other psychoactive substance use, unspecified with psychoactive substance-induced persisting dementia

● F19.98   Other psychoactive substance use, unspecified with other psychoactive substance-induced disorders

     F19.980   Other psychoactive substance use, unspecified with psychoactive substance-induced anxiety disorder

     F19.981   Other psychoactive substance use, unspecified with psychoactive substance-induced sexual dysfunction

     F19.982   Other psychoactive substance use, unspecified with psychoactive substance-induced sleep disorder

     F19.988   Other psychoactive substance use, unspecified with other psychoactive substance-induced disorder

F19.99   Other psychoactive substance use, unspecified with unspecified psychoactive substance-induced disorder

---

SCHIZOPHRENIA, SCHIZOTYPAL, DELUSIONAL, AND OTHER NON-MOOD PSYCHOTIC DISORDERS (F20-F29)

● **F20**   **Schizophrenia**
Personality disorders characterized by multiple mental and behavioral irregularities (may exhibit disorganized thinking, delusions, and auditory hallucinations).

   Excludes1   brief psychotic disorder (F23)
              cyclic schizophrenia (F25.0)
              mood [affective] disorders with psychotic symptoms (F30.2, F31.2, F31.5, F31.64, F32.3, F33.3)
              schizoaffective disorder (F25.-)
              schizophrenic reaction NOS (F23)

   Excludes2   schizophrenic reaction in:
              alcoholism (F10.15-, F10.25-, F10.95-)
              brain disease (F06.2)
              epilepsy (F06.2)
              psychoactive drug use (F11-F19 with .15, .25, .95)
              schizotypal disorder (F21)

F20.0   **Paranoid schizophrenia**
Paraphrenic schizophrenia

   Excludes1   involutional paranoid state (F22)
              paranoia (F22)

F20.1   **Disorganized schizophrenia**
Hebephrenic schizophrenia
Hebephrenia

F20.2   **Catatonic schizophrenia**
Schizophrenic catalepsy
Schizophrenic catatonia
Schizophrenic flexibilitas cerea

   Excludes1   catatonic stupor (R40.1)

F20.3   **Undifferentiated schizophrenia**
Atypical schizophrenia

   Excludes1   acute schizophrenia-like psychotic disorder (F23)

   Excludes2   post-schizophrenic depression (F32.8)

F20.5   **Residual schizophrenia**
Restzustand (schizophrenic)
Schizophrenic residual state

● **F20.8**   **Other schizophrenia**

     F20.81   **Schizophreniform disorder**
Schizophreniform psychosis NOS

     F20.89   **Other schizophrenia**
Cenesthopathic schizophrenia
Simple schizophrenia

F20.9   **Schizophrenia, unspecified**

F21   **Schizotypal disorder**
Personality disorder characterized by need for social isolation, odd behavior and thinking, and often unconventional beliefs
Borderline schizophrenia
Latent schizophrenia
Latent schizophrenic reaction
Prepsychotic schizophrenia
Prodromal schizophrenia
Pseudoneurotic schizophrenia
Pseudopsychopathic schizophrenia
Schizotypal personality disorder

   Excludes2   Asperger's syndrome (F84.5)
              schizoid personality disorder (F60.1)

F22   **Delusional disorders**
Delusional dysmorphophobia
Involutional paranoid state
Paranoia
Paranoia querulans
Paranoid psychosis
Paranoid state
Paraphrenia (late)
Sensitiver Beziehungswahn

   Excludes1   mood [affective] disorders with psychotic symptoms (F30.2, F31.2, F31.5, F31.64, F32.3, F33.3)
              paranoid schizophrenia (F20.0)

   Excludes2   paranoid personality disorder (F60.0)
              paranoid psychosis, psychogenic (F23)
              paranoid reaction (F23)

F23   **Brief psychotic disorder**
Paranoid reaction
Psychogenic paranoid psychosis

   Excludes2   mood [affective] disorders with psychotic symptoms (F30.2, F31.2, F31.5, F31.64, F32.3, F33.3)

F24   **Shared psychotic disorder**
Folie à deux
Induced paranoid disorder
Induced psychotic disorder

● **F25**   **Schizoaffective disorders**
Mental disorder exhibiting major depressive episode, manic episode, or mixed episode occurs with symptoms of schizophrenia, and mood disorder

   Excludes1   mood [affective] disorders with psychotic symptoms (F30.2, F31.2, F31.5, F31.64, F32.3, F33.3)
              schizophrenia (F20.-)

     F25.0   **Schizoaffective disorder, bipolar type**
Cyclic schizophrenia
Schizoaffective disorder, manic type
Schizoaffective disorder, mixed type
Schizoaffective psychosis, bipolar type
Schizophreniform psychosis, manic type

     F25.1   **Schizoaffective disorder, depressive type**
Schizoaffective psychosis, depressive type
Schizophreniform psychosis, depressive type

     F25.8   **Other schizoaffective disorders**

     F25.9   **Schizoaffective disorder, unspecified**
Schizoaffective psychosis NOS

F28   **Other psychotic disorder not due to a substance or known physiological condition**
Chronic hallucinatory psychosis

● **F29**   **Unspecified psychosis not due to a substance or known physiological condition**
Psychosis NOS

   Excludes1   mental disorder NOS (F99)
              unspecified mental disorder due to known physiological condition (F09)

CHAPTER 5 (F01-F99)

MOOD [AFFECTIVE] DISORDERS (F30-F39)

● **F30**   **Manic episode**
     Elevated, expansive, or irritable mood

> **Includes**   bipolar disorder, single manic episode
>   mixed affective episode

> **Excludes1**   bipolar disorder (F31.-)
>   major depressive disorder, single episode (F32.-)
>   major depressive disorder, recurrent (F33.-)

     ● **F30.1**   **Manic episode without psychotic symptoms**

         F30.10   **Manic episode without psychotic symptoms, unspecified**

         F30.11   **Manic episode without psychotic symptoms, mild**

         F30.12   **Manic episode without psychotic symptoms, moderate**

         F30.13   **Manic episode, severe, without psychotic symptoms**

     F30.2   **Manic episode, severe with psychotic symptoms**
            Manic stupor
            Mania with mood-congruent psychotic symptoms
            Mania with mood-incongruent psychotic symptoms

     F30.3   **Manic episode in partial remission**

     F30.4   **Manic episode in full remission**

     F30.8   **Other manic episodes**
            Abnormality of mood resembling mania but less intense
            Hypomania

     F30.9   **Manic episode, unspecified**
            Mania NOS

● **F31**   **Bipolar disorder**
     Mood disorders with history of manic, mixed, or hypomanic episodes

> **Includes**   manic-depressive illness
>   manic-depressive psychosis
>   manic-depressive reaction

> **Excludes1**   bipolar disorder, single manic episode (F30.-)
>   major depressive disorder, single episode (F32.-)
>   major depressive disorder, recurrent (F33.-)

> **Excludes2**   cyclothymia (F34.0)

     F31.0   **Bipolar disorder, current episode hypomanic**

     ● **F31.1**   **Bipolar disorder, current episode manic without psychotic features**

         F31.10   **Bipolar disorder, current episode manic without psychotic features, unspecified**

         F31.11   **Bipolar disorder, current episode manic without psychotic features, mild**

         F31.12   **Bipolar disorder, current episode manic without psychotic features, moderate**

         F31.13   **Bipolar disorder, current episode manic without psychotic features, severe**

     F31.2   **Bipolar disorder, current episode manic severe with psychotic features**
            Bipolar disorder, current episode manic with mood-congruent psychotic symptoms
            Bipolar disorder, current episode manic with mood-incongruent psychotic symptoms

     ● **F31.3**   **Bipolar disorder, current episode depressed, mild or moderate severity**

         F31.30   **Bipolar disorder, current episode depressed, mild or moderate severity, unspecified**

         F31.31   **Bipolar disorder, current episode depressed, mild**

         F31.32   **Bipolar disorder, current episode depressed, moderate**

     F31.4   **Bipolar disorder, current episode depressed, severe, without psychotic features**

     F31.5   **Bipolar disorder, current episode depressed, severe, with psychotic features**
            Bipolar disorder, current episode depressed with mood-incongruent psychotic symptoms
            Bipolar disorder, current episode depressed with mood-congruent psychotic symptoms

● **F31.6**   **Bipolar disorder, current episode mixed**

     F31.60   **Bipolar disorder, current episode mixed, unspecified**

     F31.61   **Bipolar disorder, current episode mixed, mild**

     F31.62   **Bipolar disorder, current episode mixed, moderate**

     F31.63   **Bipolar disorder, current episode mixed, severe, without psychotic features**

     F31.64   **Bipolar disorder, current episode mixed, severe, with psychotic features**
            Bipolar disorder, current episode mixed with mood-congruent psychotic symptoms
            Bipolar disorder, current episode mixed with mood-incongruent psychotic symptoms

● **F31.7**   **Bipolar disorder, currently in remission**

     F31.70   **Bipolar disorder, currently in remission, most recent episode unspecified**

     F31.71   **Bipolar disorder, in partial remission, most recent episode hypomanic**

     F31.72   **Bipolar disorder, in full remission, most recent episode hypomanic**

     F31.73   **Bipolar disorder, in partial remission, most recent episode manic**

     F31.74   **Bipolar disorder, in full remission, most recent episode manic**

     F31.75   **Bipolar disorder, in partial remission, most recent episode depressed**

     F31.76   **Bipolar disorder, in full remission, most recent episode depressed**

     F31.77   **Bipolar disorder, in partial remission, most recent episode mixed**

     F31.78   **Bipolar disorder, in full remission, most recent episode mixed**

● **F31.8**   **Other bipolar disorders**

     F31.81   **Bipolar II disorder**

     F31.89   **Other bipolar disorder**
            Recurrent manic episodes NOS

     F31.9   **Bipolar disorder, unspecified**

● **F32**   **Major depressive disorder, single episode**

> **Includes**   single episode of agitated depression
>   single episode of depressive reaction
>   single episode of major depression
>   single episode of psychogenic depression
>   single episode of reactive depression
>   single episode of vital depression

> **Excludes1**   bipolar disorder (F31.-)
>   manic episode (F30.-)
>   recurrent depressive disorder (F33.-)

> **Excludes2**   adjustment disorder (F43.2)

     F32.0   **Major depressive disorder, single episode, mild**

     F32.1   **Major depressive disorder, single episode, moderate**

     F32.2   **Major depressive disorder, single episode, severe without psychotic features**

     F32.3   **Major depressive disorder, single episode, severe with psychotic features**
            Single episode of major depression with mood-congruent psychotic symptoms
            Single episode of major depression with mood-incongruent psychotic symptoms
            Single episode of major depression with psychotic symptoms
            Single episode of psychogenic depressive psychosis
            Single episode of psychotic depression
            Single episode of reactive depressive psychosis

     F32.4   **Major depressive disorder, single episode, in partial remission**

     F32.5   **Major depressive disorder, single episode, in full remission**

◀ New   ◀▦ Revised   ~~deleted~~ Deleted   Excludes 1   Excludes 2   Includes   Use additional   Code first   Code also   Unspecified

OGCR Official Guidelines   X Assign placeholder X   ● Use Additional Character(s)   ▶ Manifestation Code   **Coding Clinic**

F32.8   **Other depressive episodes**
     Atypical depression
     Post-schizophrenic depression
     Single episode of 'masked' depression NOS

F32.9   **Major depressive disorder, single episode, unspecified**
     Depression NOS
     Depressive disorder NOS
     Major depression NOS

● **F33**   **Major depressive disorder, recurrent**

     Includes   recurrent episodes of depressive reaction
               recurrent episodes of endogenous depression
               recurrent episodes of major depression
               recurrent episodes of psychogenic depression
               recurrent episodes of reactive depression
               recurrent episodes of seasonal depressive
                  disorder
               recurrent episodes of vital depression

     Excludes1   bipolar disorder (F31.-)
                  manic episode (F30.-)

F33.0   **Major depressive disorder, recurrent, mild**

F33.1   **Major depressive disorder, recurrent, moderate**

F33.2   **Major depressive disorder, recurrent severe without psychotic features**

F33.3   **Major depressive disorder, recurrent, severe with psychotic symptoms**
     Endogenous depression with psychotic symptoms
     Recurrent severe episodes of major depression with mood-congruent psychotic symptoms
     Recurrent severe episodes of major depression with mood-incongruent psychotic symptoms
     Recurrent severe episodes of major depression with psychotic symptoms
     Recurrent severe episodes of psychogenic depressive psychosis
     Recurrent severe episodes of psychotic depression
     Recurrent severe episodes of reactive depressive psychosis

● **F33.4**   **Major depressive disorder, recurrent, in remission**

     F33.40   **Major depressive disorder, recurrent, in remission, unspecified**

     F33.41   **Major depressive disorder, recurrent, in partial remission**

     F33.42   **Major depressive disorder, recurrent, in full remission**

F33.8   **Other recurrent depressive disorders**
     Recurrent brief depressive episodes

F33.9   **Major depressive disorder, recurrent, unspecified**
     Monopolar depression NOS

● **F34**   **Persistent mood [affective] disorders**

F34.0   **Cyclothymic disorder**
     Affective personality disorder
     Cycloid personality
     Cyclothymia
     Cyclothymic personality

F34.1   **Dysthymic disorder**
     Depressive neurosis
     Depressive personality disorder
     Dysthymia
     Neurotic depression
     Persistent anxiety depression

     Excludes2   anxiety depression (mild or not persistent) (F41.8)

F34.8   **Other persistent mood [affective] disorders**

F34.9   **Persistent mood [affective] disorder, unspecified**

F39   **Unspecified mood [affective] disorder**
     Affective psychosis NOS

ANXIETY, DISSOCIATIVE, STRESS-RELATED, SOMATOFORM AND OTHER NONPSYCHOTIC MENTAL DISORDERS (F40-F48)

● **F40**   **Phobic anxiety disorders**
Irrational fear with avoidance of the feared subject, activity, or situation even though the individual knows that the reaction is excessive.

● **F40.0**   **Agoraphobia**
Intense, irrational fear of open spaces

     F40.00   **Agoraphobia, unspecified**

     F40.01   **Agoraphobia with panic disorder**
         Panic disorder with agoraphobia

         Excludes1   panic disorder without agoraphobia (F41.0)

     F40.02   **Agoraphobia without panic disorder**

● **F40.1**   **Social phobias**
     Anthropophobia
     Social anxiety disorder of childhood
     Social neurosis

     F40.10   **Social phobia, unspecified**

     F40.11   **Social phobia, generalized**

● **F40.2**   **Specific (isolated) phobias**

     Excludes2   dysmorphophobia (nondelusional) (F45.22)
                  nosophobia (F45.22)

     ● **F40.21**   **Animal type phobia**

         F40.210   **Arachnophobia**
                 Fear of spiders

         F40.218   **Other animal type phobia**

     ● **F40.22**   **Natural environment type phobia**

         F40.220   **Fear of thunderstorms**

         F40.228   **Other natural environment type phobia**

     ● **F40.23**   **Blood, injection, injury type phobia**

         F40.230   **Fear of blood**

         F40.231   **Fear of injections and transfusions**

         F40.232   **Fear of other medical care**

         F40.233   **Fear of injury**

     ● **F40.24**   **Situational type phobia**

         F40.240   **Claustrophobia**
                 Fear of closed spaces

         F40.241   **Acrophobia**
                 Fear of heights

         F40.242   **Fear of bridges**

         F40.243   **Fear of flying**

         F40.248   **Other situational type phobia**

     ● **F40.29**   **Other specified phobia**

         F40.290   **Androphobia**
                 Fear of men

         F40.291   **Gynephobia**
                 Fear of women

         F40.298   **Other specified phobia**

     F40.8   **Other phobic anxiety disorders**
         Phobic anxiety disorder of childhood

     F40.9   **Phobic anxiety disorder, unspecified**
         Phobia NOS
         Phobic state NOS

● **F41**   **Other anxiety disorders**

     Excludes2   anxiety in:
                  acute stress reaction (F43.0)
                  transient adjustment reaction (F43.2)
                  neurasthenia (F48.8)
                  psychophysiologic disorders (F45.-)
                  separation anxiety (F93.0)

     F41.0   **Panic disorder [episodic paroxysmal anxiety] without agoraphobia**
         Panic attack
         Panic state

         Excludes1   panic disorder with agoraphobia (F40.01)

CHAPTER 5 (F01-F99)

F41.1 Generalized anxiety disorder
Anxiety neurosis
Anxiety reaction
Anxiety state
Overanxious disorder

> **Excludes2** neurasthenia (F48.8)

F41.3 Other mixed anxiety disorders

F41.8 Other specified anxiety disorders
Anxiety depression (mild or not persistent)
Anxiety hysteria
Mixed anxiety and depressive disorder

F41.9 Anxiety disorder, unspecified
Anxiety NOS

F42 Obsessive-compulsive disorder
Anxiety disorder with recurrent obsessions or compulsions
Anancastic neurosis
Obsessive-compulsive neurosis

> **Excludes2** obsessive-compulsive personality (disorder) (F60.5)
> obsessive-compulsive symptoms occurring in depression (F32-F33)
> obsessive-compulsive symptoms occurring in schizophrenia (F20.-)

●**F43 Reaction to severe stress and adjustment disorders**

F43.0 Acute stress reaction
Acute crisis reaction
Acute reaction to stress
Combat and operational stress reaction
Combat fatigue
Crisis state
Psychic shock

●**F43.1 Post-traumatic stress disorder (PTSD)**
Traumatic neurosis

F43.10 Post-traumatic stress disorder, unspecified

F43.11 Post-traumatic stress disorder, acute

F43.12 Post-traumatic stress disorder, chronic

●**F43.2 Adjustment disorders**
Culture shock
Grief reaction
Hospitalism in children

> **Excludes2** separation anxiety disorder of childhood (F93.0)

F43.20 Adjustment disorder, unspecified

F43.21 Adjustment disorder with depressed mood

F43.22 Adjustment disorder with anxiety

F43.23 Adjustment disorder with mixed anxiety and depressed mood

F43.24 Adjustment disorder with disturbance of conduct

F43.25 Adjustment disorder with mixed disturbance of emotions and conduct

F43.29 Adjustment disorder with other symptoms

F43.8 Other reactions to severe stress

F43.9 Reaction to severe stress, unspecified

●**F44 Dissociative and conversion disorders**

> **Includes** conversion hysteria
> conversion reaction
> hysteria
> hysterical psychosis

> **Excludes2** malingering [conscious simulation] (Z76.5)

F44.0 Dissociative amnesia
Sudden loss of memory for personal information

> **Excludes1** amnesia NOS (R41.3)
> anterograde amnesia (R41.1)
> retrograde amnesia (R41.2)

> **Excludes2** alcohol-or other psychoactive substance-induced amnestic disorder (F10, F13, F19 with .26, .96)
> amnestic disorder due to known physiological condition (F04)
> postictal amnesia in epilepsy (G40.-)

F44.1 Dissociative fugue
Characterized by episode of sudden, unexpected travel with amnesia for past and partial to total confusion about identity or assumption of new identity

> **Excludes2** postictal fugue in epilepsy (G40.-)

F44.2 Dissociative stupor
Profound diminution or absence of voluntary movement and responsiveness to external stimuli

> **Excludes1** catatonic stupor (R40.1)
> stupor NOS (R40.1)

> **Excludes2** catatonic disorder due to known physiological condition (F06.1)
> depressive stupor (F32, F33)
> manic stupor (F30, F31)

F44.4 Conversion disorder with motor symptom or deficit
Dissociative motor disorders
Psychogenic aphonia
Psychogenic dysphonia

F44.5 Conversion disorder with seizures or convulsions
Dissociative convulsions

F44.6 Conversion disorder with sensory symptom or deficit
Dissociative anesthesia and sensory loss
Psychogenic deafness

F44.7 Conversion disorder with mixed symptom presentation

●**F44.8 Other dissociative and conversion disorders**

F44.81 Dissociative identity disorder
Multiple personality disorder

F44.89 Other dissociative and conversion disorders
Ganser's syndrome
Psychogenic confusion
Psychogenic twilight state
Trance and possession disorders

F44.9 Dissociative and conversion disorder, unspecified
Dissociative disorder NOS

OGCR Section I.C.5.a

Pain disorders related to psychological factors

Assign code F45.41, for pain that is exclusively psychological. Code F45.41, Pain disorder exclusively related to psychological factors, should be used following the appropriate code from category G89, Pain, not elsewhere classified, if there is documentation of a psychological component for a patient with acute or chronic pain.
See Section I.C.6. Pain

●**F45 Somatoform disorders**
Mental disorders characterized by symptoms suggesting general medical condition

> **Excludes2** dissociative and conversion disorders (F44.-)
> factitious disorders (F68.1-)
> hair-plucking (F63.3)
> lalling (F80.0)
> lisping (F80.0)
> malingering [conscious simulation] (Z76.5)
> nail-biting (F98.8)
> psychological or behavioral factors associated with disorders or diseases classified elsewhere (F54)
> sexual dysfunction, not due to a substance or known physiological condition (F52.-)
> thumb-sucking (F98.8)
> tic disorders (in childhood and adolescence) (F95.-)
> Tourette's syndrome (F95.2)
> trichotillomania (F63.3)

F45.0 Somatization disorder
Briquet's disorder
Multiple psychosomatic disorder

F45.1 Undifferentiated somatoform disorder
Undifferentiated psychosomatic disorder

● **F45.2**   **Hypochondriacal disorders**
Persistent, unrealistic preoccupation with possibility of having serious disease

    Excludes2   delusional dysmorphophobia (F22)
fixed delusions about bodily functions or shape (F22)

   F45.20   **Hypochondriacal disorder, unspecified**

   F45.21   **Hypochondriasis**
Hypochondriacal neurosis

   F45.22   **Body dysmorphic disorder**
Dysmorphophobia (nondelusional)
Nosophobia

   F45.29   **Other hypochondriacal disorders**

● **F45.4**   **Pain disorders related to psychological factors**

    Excludes1   pain NOS (R52)

   F45.41   **Pain disorder exclusively related to psychological factors**
Somatoform pain disorder (persistent)

   F45.42   **Pain disorder with related psychological factors**
Code also associated acute or chronic pain (G89.-)

   F45.8   **Other somatoform disorders**
Psychogenic dysmenorrhea
Psychogenic dysphagia, including 'globus hystericus'
Psychogenic pruritus
Psychogenic torticollis
Somatoform autonomic dysfunction
Teeth grinding

    Excludes1   sleep related teeth grinding (G47.63)

   F45.9   **Somatoform disorder, unspecified**
Psychosomatic disorder NOS

● **F48**   **Other nonpsychotic mental disorders**

   F48.1   **Depersonalization-derealization syndrome**

   F48.2   **Pseudobulbar affect**
Involuntary emotional expression disorder

    Code first underlying cause, if known, such as:
amyotrophic lateral sclerosis (G12.21)
multiple sclerosis (G35)
sequelae of cerebrovascular disease (I69.-)
sequelae of traumatic intracranial injury (S06.-)

   F48.8   **Other specified nonpsychotic mental disorders**
Dhat syndrome
Neurasthenia
Occupational neurosis, including writer's cramp
Psychasthenia
Psychasthenic neurosis
Psychogenic syncope

   F48.9   **Nonpsychotic mental disorder, unspecified**
Neurosis NOS

BEHAVIORAL SYNDROMES ASSOCIATED WITH PHYSIOLOGICAL DISTURBANCES AND PHYSICAL FACTORS (F50-F59)

● **F50**   **Eating disorders**

    Excludes1   anorexia NOS (R63.0)
feeding difficulties (R63.3)
polyphagia (R63.2)

    Excludes2   feeding disorder in infancy or childhood (F98.2-)

● **F50.0**   **Anorexia nervosa**

    Excludes1   loss of appetite (R63.0)
psychogenic loss of appetite (F50.8)

   F50.00   **Anorexia nervosa, unspecified**

   F50.01   **Anorexia nervosa, restricting type**

   F50.02   **Anorexia nervosa, binge eating/purging type**

     Excludes1   bulimia nervosa (F50.2)

   F50.2   **Bulimia nervosa**
Bulimia NOS
Hyperorexia nervosa

    Excludes1   anorexia nervosa, binge eating/purging type (F50.02)

   F50.8   **Other eating disorders**
Pica in adults
Psychogenic loss of appetite

    Excludes2   pica of infancy and childhood (F98.3)

   F50.9   **Eating disorder, unspecified**
Atypical anorexia nervosa
Atypical bulimia nervosa

● **F51**   **Sleep disorders not due to a substance or known physiological condition**

    Excludes2   organic sleep disorders (G47.-)

● **F51.0**   **Insomnia not due to a substance or known physiological condition**

    Excludes2   alcohol related insomnia (F10.182, F10.282, F10.982)
drug-related insomnia (F11.182, F11.282, F11.982, F13.182, F13.282, F13.982, F14.182, F14.282, F14.982, F15.182, F15.282, F15.982, F19.182, F19.282, F19.982)
insomnia NOS (G47.0-)
insomnia due to known physiological condition (G47.0-)
organic insomnia (G47.0-)
sleep deprivation (Z72.820)

   F51.01   **Primary insomnia**
Idiopathic insomnia

   F51.02   **Adjustment insomnia**

   F51.03   **Paradoxical insomnia**

   F51.04   **Psychophysiologic insomnia**

   F51.05   **Insomnia due to other mental disorder**
Code also associated mental disorder

   F51.09   **Other insomnia not due to a substance or known physiological condition**

● **F51.1**   **Hypersomnia not due to a substance or known physiological condition**
Hypersomnia: Excessive sleeping/sleepiness

    Excludes2   alcohol related hypersomnia (F10.182, F10.282, F10.982)
drug-related hypersomnia (F11.182, F11.282, F11.982, F13.182, F13.282, F13.982, F14.182, F14.282, F14.982, F15.182, F15.282, F15.982, F19.182, F19.282, F19.982)
hypersomnia NOS (G47.10)
hypersomnia due to known physiological condition (G47.10)
idiopathic hypersomnia (G47.11, G47.12)
narcolepsy (G47.4-)

   F51.11   **Primary hypersomnia**

   F51.12   **Insufficient sleep syndrome**

     Excludes1   sleep deprivation (Z72.820)

   F51.13   **Hypersomnia due to other mental disorder**
Code also associated mental disorder

   F51.19   **Other hypersomnia not due to a substance or known physiological condition**

   F51.3   **Sleepwalking [somnambulism]**

   F51.4   **Sleep terrors [night terrors]**

   F51.5   **Nightmare disorder**
Dream anxiety disorder

   F51.8   **Other sleep disorders not due to a substance or known physiological condition**

   F51.9   **Sleep disorder not due to a substance or known physiological condition, unspecified**
Emotional sleep disorder NOS

CHAPTER 5 (F01-F99)

● **F52**   **Sexual dysfunction not due to a substance or known physiological condition**
> **Excludes2**   Dhat syndrome (F48.8)

F52.0   **Hypoactive sexual desire disorder**
Anhedonia (sexual)
Total loss of feeling of sexual pleasure
Lack or loss of sexual desire
> **Excludes1**   decreased libido (R68.82)

F52.1   **Sexual aversion disorder**
Sexual aversion and lack of sexual enjoyment

● **F52.2**   **Sexual arousal disorders**
Failure of genital response

     F52.21   **Male erectile disorder** ♂
Psychogenic impotence
> **Excludes1**   impotence of organic origin (N52.-)
> impotence NOS (N52.-)

     F52.22   **Female sexual arousal disorder** ♀
Frigidity

● **F52.3**   **Orgasmic disorder**
Inhibited orgasm
Psychogenic anorgasmy

     F52.31   **Female orgasmic disorder** ♀

     F52.32   **Male orgasmic disorder** ♂

F52.4   **Premature ejaculation** ♂

F52.5   **Vaginismus not due to a substance or known physiological condition** ♀
Psychogenic vaginismus
> **Excludes2**   vaginismus (due to a known physiological condition) (N94.2)

F52.6   **Dyspareunia not due to a substance or known physiological condition** ♀
Dyspareunia: Difficult or painful sexual intercourse
Psychogenic dyspareunia
> **Excludes2**   dyspareunia (due to a known physiological condition) (N94.1)

F52.8   **Other sexual dysfunction not due to a substance or known physiological condition**
Excessive sexual drive
Nymphomania
Satyriasis

F52.9   **Unspecified sexual dysfunction not due to a substance or known physiological condition**
Sexual dysfunction NOS

F53   **Puerperal psychosis** ♀
Postpartum depression
Acute mental illness with sudden onset following childbirth with symptoms of affective psychosis, disorientation, and confusion are prevalent
> **Excludes1**   mood disorders with psychotic features (F30.2, F31.2, F31.5, F31.64, F32.3, F33.3)
> postpartum dysphoria (O90.6)
> psychosis in schizophrenia, schizotypal, delusional, and other psychotic disorders (F20-F29)

▌ **F54**   *Psychological and behavioral factors associated with disorders or diseases classified elsewhere*
Psychological factors affecting physical conditions
Code first the associated physical disorder, such as:
> asthma (J45.-)
> dermatitis (L23-L25)
> gastric ulcer (K25.-)
> mucous colitis (K58.-)
> ulcerative colitis (K51.-)
> urticaria (L50.-)
> **Excludes2**   tension-type headache (G44.2)

● **F55**   **Abuse of non-psychoactive substances**
> **Excludes2**   abuse of psychoactive substances (F10-F19)

F55.0   **Abuse of antacids**

F55.1   **Abuse of herbal or folk remedies**

F55.2   **Abuse of laxatives**

F55.3   **Abuse of steroids or hormones**

F55.4   **Abuse of vitamins**

F55.8   **Abuse of other non-psychoactive substances**

F59   **Unspecified behavioral syndromes associated with physiological disturbances and physical factors**
Psychogenic physiological dysfunction NOS

DISORDERS OF ADULT PERSONALITY AND BEHAVIOR (F60-F69)

● **F60**   **Specific personality disorders**
Long-term patterns of thoughts and behaviors causing serious problems with relationships and work.

F60.0   **Paranoid personality disorder**
Hostile, devious, and combative response to disappointments
Expansive paranoid personality (disorder)
Fanatic personality (disorder)
Querulant personality (disorder)
Paranoid personality (disorder)
Sensitive paranoid personality (disorder)
> **Excludes2**   paranoia (F22)
> paranoia querulans (F22)
> paranoid psychosis (F22)
> paranoid schizophrenia (F20.0)
> paranoid state (F22)

F60.1   **Schizoid personality disorder**
Detachment from social relationships with minimal emotional experiences and expressions
> **Excludes2**   Asperger's syndrome (F84.5)
> delusional disorder (F22)
> schizoid disorder of childhood (F84.5)
> schizophrenia (F20.-)
> schizotypal disorder (F21)

F60.2   **Antisocial personality disorder**
Continuous and chronic antisocial behavior
Amoral personality (disorder)
Asocial personality (disorder)
Dissocial personality disorder
Psychopathic personality (disorder)
Sociopathic personality (disorder)
> **Excludes1**   conduct disorders (F91.-)
> **Excludes2**   borderline personality disorder (F60.3)

F60.3   **Borderline personality disorder**
Instability of mood, self-image or sense of self, and interpersonal relationships
Aggressive personality (disorder)
Emotionally unstable personality disorder
Explosive personality (disorder)
> **Excludes2**   antisocial personality disorder (F60.2)

F60.4   **Histrionic personality disorder**
Personality disorder with excessive emotional and attention-seeking behavior
Hysterical personality (disorder)
Psychoinfantile personality (disorder)

F60.5   **Obsessive-compulsive personality disorder**
Anankastic personality (disorder)
Compulsive personality (disorder)
Obsessional personality (disorder)
> **Excludes2**   obsessive-compulsive disorder (F42)

F60.6   **Avoidant personality disorder**
Anxious personality disorder

F60.7   **Dependent personality disorder**
Asthenic personality (disorder)
Inadequate personality (disorder)
Passive personality (disorder)

◄ New   ◀▏▏▏ Revised   ~~deleted~~ Deleted   Excludes 1   Excludes 2   Includes   Use additional   Code first   Code also   Unspecified
OGCR Official Guidelines   **X** Assign placeholder X   ● Use Additional Character(s)   ▌ Manifestation Code   **Coding Clinic**

● F60.8   **Other specific personality disorders**

     F60.81   **Narcissistic personality disorder**
          Vanity, conceit, egotism or indifference to plight
          of others

     F60.89   **Other specific personality disorders**
          Eccentric personality disorder
          'Haltlose' type personality disorder
          Immature personality disorder
          Passive-aggressive personality disorder
          Psychoneurotic personality disorder
          Self-defeating personality disorder

    F60.9   **Personality disorder, unspecified**
       Character disorder NOS
       Character neurosis NOS
       Pathological personality NOS

● F63   **Impulse disorders**

    Excludes2   habitual excessive use of alcohol or psychoactive
         substances (F10-F19)
         impulse disorders involving sexual behavior
         (F65.-)

    F63.0   **Pathological gambling**
       Compulsive gambling

       Excludes1   gambling and betting NOS (Z72.6)

       Excludes2   excessive gambling by manic patients
          (F30, F31)
          gambling in antisocial personality
          disorder (F60.2)

    F63.1   **Pyromania**
       Pathological fire-setting

       Excludes2   fire-setting (by) (in):
          adult with antisocial personality
          disorder (F60.2)
          alcohol or psychoactive substance
          intoxication (F10-F19)
          conduct disorders (F91.-)
          mental disorders due to known
          physiological condition (F01-F09)
          schizophrenia (F20.-)

    F63.2   **Kleptomania**
       Pathological stealing

       Excludes1   shoplifting as the reason for observation
          for suspected mental disorder
          (Z03.8)

       Excludes2   depressive disorder with stealing
          (F31-F33)
          stealing due to underlying mental
          condition-code to mental condition
          stealing in mental disorders due to
          known physiological condition
          (F01-F09)

    F63.3   **Trichotillomania**
       Hair plucking

       Excludes2   other stereotyped movement disorder
          (F98.4)

●   F63.8   **Other impulse disorders**

     F63.81   **Intermittent explosive disorder**

     F63.89   **Other impulse disorders**

    F63.9   **Impulse disorder, unspecified**
       Impulse control disorder NOS

● F64   **Gender identity disorders**

    F64.1   **Gender identity disorder in adolescence and adulthood**
       Dual role transvestism
       Transsexualism

       Use additional code to identify sex reassignment status
       (Z87.890)

       Excludes1   gender identity disorder in childhood
          (F64.2)

       Excludes2   fetishistic transvestism (F65.1)

    F64.2   **Gender identity disorder of childhood**   **P**

       Excludes1   gender identity disorder in adolescence
          and adulthood (F64.1)

       Excludes2   sexual maturation disorder (F66)

    F64.8   **Other gender identity disorders**

    F64.9   **Gender identity disorder, unspecified**
       Gender-role disorder NOS

● F65   **Paraphilias**

    F65.0   **Fetishism**
       Intense sexual urges and arousing fantasies using inanimate
       objects

    F65.1   **Transvestic fetishism**
       Intense sexual urges, arousal, or orgasm associated with
       fantasized/actual cross-dressing
       Fetishistic transvestism

    F65.2   **Exhibitionism**

    F65.3   **Voyeurism**
       Sexual urges or arousal involving real or fantasized
       observation of unsuspecting people who are naked,
       disrobing, or engaging in sexual activity

    F65.4   **Pedophilia**

●   F65.5   **Sadomasochism**

     F65.50   **Sadomasochism, unspecified**

     F65.51   **Sexual masochism**

     F65.52   **Sexual sadism**

●   F65.8   **Other paraphilias**

     F65.81   **Frotteurism**
          Sexual arousal or orgasm is achieved by rubbing
          up against another person (or fantasies of), in
          crowded place with unsuspecting victim

     F65.89   **Other paraphilias**
          Necrophilia

    F65.9   **Paraphilia, unspecified**
       Sexual deviation NOS

   F66   **Other sexual disorders**
       Sexual maturation disorder
       Sexual relationship disorder

● F68   **Other disorders of adult personality and behavior**

●   F68.1   **Factitious disorder**
       Compensation neurosis
       Elaboration of physical symptoms for psychological
       reasons
       Hospital hopper syndrome
       Münchhausen's syndrome
       Peregrinating patient

       Excludes2   factitial dermatitis (L98.1)
          person feigning illness (with obvious
          motivation) (Z76.5)

     F68.10   **Factitious disorder, unspecified**

     F68.11   **Factitious disorder with predominantly psychological signs and symptoms**

     F68.12   **Factitious disorder with predominantly physical signs and symptoms**

     F68.13   **Factitious disorder with combined psychological and physical signs and symptoms**

    F68.8   **Other specified disorders of adult personality and behavior**

   F69   **Unspecified disorder of adult personality and behavior**   **A**

INTELLECTUAL DISABILITIES (F70-F79)

Code first any associated physical or developmental disorders

    Excludes1   borderline intellectual functioning, IQ above 70 to
          84 (R41.83)

   F70   **Mild intellectual disabilities**
       IQ level 50-55 to approximately 70
       Mild mental subnormality

CHAPTER 5 (F01-F99)

F71   **Moderate intellectual disabilities**
IQ level 35-40 to 50-55
Moderate mental subnormality

F72   **Severe intellectual disabilities**
IQ 20-25 to 35-40
Severe mental subnormality

F73   **Profound intellectual disabilities**
IQ level below 20-25
Profound mental subnormality

F78   **Other intellectual disabilities**

F79   **Unspecified intellectual disabilities**
Mental deficiency NOS
Mental subnormality NOS

PERVASIVE AND SPECIFIC DEVELOPMENTAL DISORDERS (F80-F89)

● **F80**   **Specific developmental disorders of speech and language**

  F80.0   **Phonological disorder**
Communication disorder of unknown cause, characterized by failure to use age-appropriate sounds
Dyslalia
Functional speech articulation disorder
Lalling
Lisping
Phonological developmental disorder
Speech articulation developmental disorder

    Excludes1   speech articulation impairment due to aphasia NOS (R47.01)
speech articulation impairment due to apraxia (R48.2)

    Excludes2   speech articulation impairment due to hearing loss (F80.4)
speech articulation impairment due to intellectual disabilities (F70-F79)
speech articulation impairment with expressive language developmental disorder (F80.1)
speech articulation impairment with mixed receptive expressive language developmental disorder (F80.2)

  F80.1   **Expressive language disorder**
Developmental dysphasia or aphasia, expressive type

    Excludes1   mixed receptive-expressive language disorder (F80.2)
dysphasia and aphasia NOS (R47.-)

    Excludes2   acquired aphasia with epilepsy [Landau-Kleffner] (G40.80-)
intellectual disabilities (F70-F79)
pervasive developmental disorders (F84.-)
selective mutism (F94.0)

  F80.2   **Mixed receptive-expressive language disorder**
Developmental dysphasia or aphasia, receptive type
Developmental Wernicke's aphasia

    Excludes1   central auditory processing disorder (H93.25)
dysphasia or aphasia NOS (R47.-)
expressive language disorder (F80.1)
expressive type dysphasia or aphasia (F80.1)
word deafness (H93.25)

    Excludes2   acquired aphasia with epilepsy [Landau-Kleffner] (G40.80-)
intellectual disabilities (F70-F79)
pervasive developmental disorders (F84.-)
selective mutism (F94.0)

  F80.4   **Speech and language development delay due to hearing loss**
Code also type of hearing loss (H90.-, H91.-)

●   **F80.8**   **Other developmental disorders of speech or language**

    F80.81   **Childhood onset fluency disorder**
Cluttering NOS
Stuttering NOS

      Excludes1   adult onset fluency disorder (F98.5)
fluency disorder in conditions classified elsewhere (R47.82)
fluency disorder (stuttering) following cerebrovascular disease (I69. with final characters -23)

    F80.89   **Other developmental disorders of speech and language**

  F80.9   **Developmental disorder of speech and language, unspecified**
Communication disorder NOS
Language disorder NOS

● **F81**   **Specific developmental disorders of scholastic skills**

  F81.0   **Specific reading disorder**
'Backward reading'
Developmental dyslexia
Specific reading retardation

    Excludes1   alexia NOS (R48.0)
dyslexia NOS (R48.0)

  F81.2   **Mathematics disorder**
Developmental acalculia
Developmental arithmetical disorder
Developmental Gerstmann's syndrome

    Excludes1   acalculia NOS (R48.8)

    Excludes2   arithmetical difficulties associated with a reading disorder (F81.0)
arithmetical difficulties associated with a spelling disorder (F81.81)
arithmetical difficulties due to inadequate teaching (Z55.8)

●   **F81.8**   **Other developmental disorders of scholastic skills**

    F81.81   **Disorder of written expression**
Specific spelling disorder

    F81.89   **Other developmental disorders of scholastic skills**

  F81.9   **Developmental disorder of scholastic skills, unspecified**
Knowledge acquisition disability NOS
Learning disability NOS
Learning disorder NOS

F82   **Specific developmental disorder of motor function**
Clumsy child syndrome
Developmental coordination disorder
Developmental dyspraxia

    Excludes1   abnormalities of gait and mobility (R26.-)
lack of coordination (R27.-)

    Excludes2   lack of coordination secondary to intellectual disabilities (F70-F79)

◀ New   ◀▟ Revised   ~~deleted~~ Deleted   Excludes 1   Excludes 2   Includes   Use additional   Code first   Code also   Unspecified

OGCR Official Guidelines   X Assign placeholder X   ● Use Additional Character(s)   ▶ Manifestation Code   **Coding Clinic**

● **F84   Pervasive developmental disorders**
     Use additional code to identify any associated medical
     condition and intellectual disabilities.

    F84.0   Autistic disorder
       Infantile autism
       Infantile psychosis
       Kanner's syndrome
       Excludes1   Asperger's syndrome (F84.5)

    F84.2   Rett's syndrome
       Neurodevelopmental disorder
       Excludes1   Asperger's syndrome (F84.5)
                 Autistic disorder (F84.0)
                 other childhood disintegrative disorder
                   (F84.3)

    F84.3   Other childhood disintegrative disorder   P
       Dementia infantilis
       At least two years of normal development followed by
         significant loss of language abilities, social skills,
         bowel/bladder control, motor skills
       Disintegrative psychosis
       Heller's syndrome
       At least two years of normal development followed by
         significant loss of language abilities, social skills,
         bowel/bladder control, motor skills
       Symbiotic psychosis
       Abnormal relationship to mothering figure, characterized
         by intense separation anxiety, severe regression,
         giving up of useful speech, and autism
       Use additional code to identify any associated
       neurological condition.
       Excludes1   Asperger's syndrome (F84.5)
                 Autistic disorder (F84.0)
                 Rett's syndrome (F84.2)

    F84.5   Asperger's syndrome
       Developmental disorder
       Asperger's disorder
       Autistic psychopathy
       Schizoid disorder of childhood

    F84.8   Other pervasive developmental disorders
       Overactive disorder associated with intellectual
       disabilities and stereotyped movements

    F84.9   Pervasive developmental disorder, unspecified
       Atypical autism

F88   Other disorders of psychological development
       Developmental agnosia

F89   Unspecified disorder of psychological development
       Developmental disorder NOS

BEHAVIORAL AND EMOTIONAL DISORDERS WITH ONSET USUALLY OCCURRING IN CHILDHOOD AND ADOLESCENCE (F90-F98)

Note: Codes within categories F90-F98 may be used regardless
     of the age of a patient. These disorders generally have onset
     within the childhood or adolescent years, but may continue
     throughout life or not be diagnosed until adulthood.

● **F90   Attention-deficit hyperactivity disorders**
     Attention deficit disorder with hyperactivity=ADHD
     Includes   attention deficit disorder with hyperactivity
               attention deficit syndrome with hyperactivity
     Excludes2   anxiety disorders (F40.-, F41.-)
               mood [affective] disorders (F30-F39)
               pervasive developmental disorders (F84.-)
               schizophrenia (F20.-)

    F90.0   Attention-deficit hyperactivity disorder, predominantly inattentive type

    F90.1   Attention-deficit hyperactivity disorder, predominantly hyperactive type

    F90.2   Attention-deficit hyperactivity disorder, combined type

    F90.8   Attention-deficit hyperactivity disorder, other type

    F90.9   Attention-deficit hyperactivity disorder, unspecified type
       Attention-deficit hyperactivity disorder of childhood or
       adolescence NOS
       Attention-deficit hyperactivity disorder NOS

● **F91   Conduct disorders**
     Childhood/adolescence disruptive behavior disorder
     Excludes1   antisocial behavior (Z72.81-)
               antisocial personality disorder (F60.2)
     Excludes2   conduct problems associated with attention-
               deficit hyperactivity disorder (F90.-)
               mood [affective] disorders (F30-F39)
               pervasive developmental disorders (F84.-)
               schizophrenia (F20.-)

    F91.0   Conduct disorder confined to family context

    F91.1   Conduct disorder, childhood-onset type
       Unsocialized conduct disorder
       Conduct disorder, solitary aggressive type
       Unsocialized aggressive disorder

    F91.2   Conduct disorder, adolescent-onset type
       Socialized conduct disorder
       Conduct disorder, group type

    F91.3   Oppositional defiant disorder

    F91.8   Other conduct disorders

    F91.9   Conduct disorder, unspecified
       Behavioral disorder NOS
       Conduct disorder NOS
       Disruptive behavior disorder NOS

● **F93   Emotional disorders with onset specific to childhood**

    F93.0   Separation anxiety disorder of childhood   P
       Excludes2   mood [affective] disorders (F30-F39)
               nonpsychotic mental disorders (F40-F48)
               phobic anxiety disorder of childhood
                 (F40.8)
               social phobia (F40.1)

    F93.8   Other childhood emotional disorders   P
       Identity disorder
       Excludes2   gender identity disorder of childhood
                 (F64.2)

    F93.9   Childhood emotional disorder, unspecified   P

● **F94   Disorders of social functioning with onset specific to childhood and adolescence**

    F94.0   Selective mutism
       Elective mutism
       Excludes2   pervasive developmental disorders
                 (F84.-)
               schizophrenia (F20.-)
               specific developmental disorders of
                 speech and language (F80.-)
               transient mutism as part of separation
                 anxiety in young children (F93.0)

    F94.1   Reactive attachment disorder of childhood   P
       Use additional code to identify any associated failure to
       thrive or growth retardation
       Excludes1   disinhibited attachment disorder of
                 childhood (F94.2)
               normal variation in pattern of selective
                 attachment
       Excludes2   Asperger's syndrome (F84.5)
               maltreatment syndromes (T74.-)
               sexual or physical abuse in childhood,
                 resulting in psychosocial problems
                 (Z62.81-)

    F94.2   Disinhibited attachment disorder of childhood   P
       Affectionless psychopathy
       Institutional syndrome
       Excludes1   reactive attachment disorder of childhood
                 (F94.1)
       Excludes2   Asperger's syndrome (F84.5)
               attention-deficit hyperactivity disorders
                 (F90.-)
               hospitalism in children (F43.2-)

    F94.8   Other childhood disorders of social functioning   P

    F94.9   Childhood disorder of social functioning, unspecified   P

CHAPTER 5 (F01-F99)

Item 5–2 Enuresis: Bed wetting by children at night. Causes can be either psychological or medical (diabetes, urinary tract infections, or abnormalities). **Encopresis:** Overflow incontinence of bowels sometimes resulting from chronic constipation or fecal impaction. Check the documentation for additional diagnoses.

● **F95**   **Tic disorder**
        Involuntary twitch

     F95.0   **Transient tic disorder**

     F95.1   **Chronic motor or vocal tic disorder**

     F95.2   **Tourette's disorder**
          Combined vocal and multiple motor tic disorder [de la Tourette]
          Tourette's syndrome

     F95.8   **Other tic disorders**

     F95.9   **Tic disorder, `unspecified`**
          Tic NOS

● **F98**   **Other behavioral and emotional disorders with onset usually occurring in childhood and adolescence**
      `Excludes2`   breath-holding spells (R06.89)
          gender identity disorder of childhood (F64.2)
          Kleine-Levin syndrome (G47.13)
          obsessive-compulsive disorder (F42)
          sleep disorders not due to a substance or known physiological condition (F51.-)

     F98.0   **Enuresis not due to a substance or known physiological condition**
          Enuresis: Urinary incontinence
          Enuresis (primary) (secondary) of nonorganic origin
          Functional enuresis
          Psychogenic enuresis
          Urinary incontinence of nonorganic origin
      `Excludes1`   enuresis NOS (R32)

     F98.1   **Encopresis not due to a substance or known physiological condition**
          Encopresis: Fecal incontinence
          Functional encopresis
          Incontinence of feces of nonorganic origin
          Psychogenic encopresis
          Use additional code to identify the cause of any coexisting constipation.
      `Excludes1`   encopresis NOS (R15.-)

●   **F98.2**   **Other feeding disorders of infancy and childhood**
      `Excludes1`   feeding difficulties (R63.3)
      `Excludes2`   anorexia nervosa and other eating disorders (F50.-)
          feeding problems of newborn (P92.-)
          pica of infancy or childhood (F98.3)

        F98.21   **Rumination disorder of infancy**   **P**

        F98.29   **Other feeding disorders of infancy and early childhood**   **P**

     F98.3   **Pica of infancy and childhood**   **P**
          Craving and eating substances such as paint, clay, or dirt to replace a nutritional deficit in the body.

     F98.4   **Stereotyped movement disorders**
          Stereotype/habit disorder
      `Excludes1`   abnormal involuntary movements (R25.-)
      `Excludes2`   compulsions in obsessive-compulsive disorder (F42)
          hair plucking (F63.3)
          movement disorders of organic origin (G20-G25)
          nail-biting (F98.8)
          nose-picking (F98.8)
          stereotypies that are part of a broader psychiatric condition (F01-F95)
          thumb-sucking (F98.8)
          tic disorders (F95.-)
          trichotillomania (F63.3)

     F98.5   **Adult onset fluency disorder**
      `Excludes1`   childhood onset fluency disorder (F80.81)
          dysphasia (R47.02)
          fluency disorder in conditions classified elsewhere (R47.82)
          fluency disorder (stuttering) following cerebrovascular disease (I69. with final characters -23)
          tic disorders (F95.-)

     F98.8   **Other specified behavioral and emotional disorders with onset usually occurring in childhood and adolescence**   **P**
          Excessive masturbation
          Nail-biting
          Nose-picking
          Thumb-sucking

     F98.9   **`Unspecified` behavioral and emotional disorders with onset usually occurring in childhood and adolescence**   **P**

UNSPECIFIED MENTAL DISORDER (F99)

     F99   **Mental disorder, not otherwise specified**
          Mental illness NOS
      `Excludes1`   unspecified mental disorder due to known physiological condition (F09)

◀ New   ◀⁞⁞ Revised   ~~deleted~~ Deleted   `Excludes 1`   `Excludes 2`   `Includes`   `Use additional`   `Code first`   `Code also`   `Unspecified`

OGCR Official Guidelines   **X** Assign placeholder X   ● Use Additional Character(s)   ▶ Manifestation Code   **Coding Clinic**

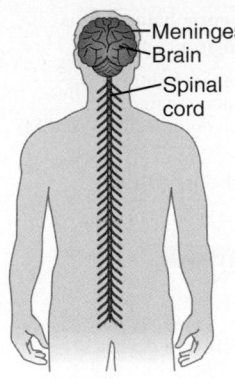

—Meninges
—Brain
—Spinal cord

Figure 6-1 The brain and spinal cord make up the central nervous system.

Item 6-1 The two major classifications of the nervous system are the peripheral nervous system and the central nervous system (CNS). The central nervous system is comprised of the brain and the spinal cord. The peripheral nervous system is comprised of the parasympathetic and sympathetic systems. **Encephalitis** is the swelling of the brain. **Meningitis** is swelling of the covering of the brain, the meninges. Types and causes of brain infections are:

Type	Cause
purulent	bacterial
aseptic/abacterial	viral
chronic meningitis	mycobacterial and fungal

CHAPTER 6

DISEASES OF THE NERVOUS SYSTEM (G00-G99)

Excludes2　certain conditions originating in the perinatal period (P04-P96)
certain infectious and parasitic diseases (A00-B99)
complications of pregnancy, childbirth and the puerperium (O00-O9A)
congenital malformations, deformations, and chromosomal abnormalities (Q00-Q99)
endocrine, nutritional and metabolic diseases (E00-E88)
injury, poisoning and certain other consequences of external causes (S00-T88)
neoplasms (C00-D49)
symptoms, signs and abnormal clinical and laboratory findings, not elsewhere classified (R00-R94)

This chapter contains the following blocks:

G00-G09	Inflammatory diseases of the central nervous system
G10-G14	Systemic atrophies primarily affecting the central nervous system
G20-G26	Extrapyramidal and movement disorders
G30-G32	Other degenerative diseases of the nervous system
G35-G37	Demyelinating diseases of the central nervous system
G40-G47	Episodic and paroxysmal disorders
G50-G59	Nerve, nerve root and plexus disorders
G60-G65	Polyneuropathies and other disorders of the peripheral nervous system
G70-G73	Diseases of myoneural junction and muscle
G80-G83	Cerebral palsy and other paralytic syndromes
G89-G99	Other disorders of the nervous system

INFLAMMATORY DISEASES OF THE CENTRAL NERVOUS SYSTEM (G00-G09)

● **G00　Bacterial meningitis, not elsewhere classified**
An infection of the cerebrospinal fluid surrounding the spinal cord and brain.

Includes　bacterial arachnoiditis
bacterial leptomeningitis
bacterial meningitis
bacterial pachymeningitis

Excludes1　bacterial:
meningoencephalitis (G04.2)
meningomyelitis (G04.2)

G00.0　Hemophilus meningitis
Meningitis due to Hemophilus influenzae

G00.1　Pneumococcal meningitis

G00.2　Streptococcal meningitis
Use additional code to further identify organism (B95.0-B95.5)

G00.3　Staphylococcal meningitis
Use additional code to further identify organism (B95.61-B95.8)

G00.8　Other bacterial meningitis
Meningitis due to Escherichia coli
Meningitis due to Friedländer bacillus
Meningitis due to Klebsiella
Use additional code to further identify organism (B96.-)

G00.9　Bacterial meningitis, unspecified
Meningitis due to gram-negative bacteria, unspecified
Purulent meningitis NOS
Pyogenic meningitis NOS
Suppurative meningitis NOS

▶ **G01　Meningitis in bacterial diseases classified elsewhere**
Code first underlying disease
Excludes1　meningitis (in):
gonococcal (A54.81)
leptospirosis (A27.81)
listeriosis (A32.11)
Lyme disease (A69.21)
meningococcal (A39.0)
neurosyphilis (A52.13)
tuberculosis (A17.0)
meningoencephalitis and meningomyelitis in bacterial diseases classified elsewhere (G05)

▶ **G02　Meningitis in other infectious and parasitic diseases classified elsewhere**
Code first underlying disease, such as:
African trypanosomiasis (B56.-)
poliovirus infection (A80.-)
Excludes1　candidal meningitis (B37.5)
coccidioidomycosis meningitis (B38.4)
cryptococcal meningitis (B45.1)
herpesviral [herpes simplex] meningitis (B00.3)
infectious mononucleosis complicated by meningitis (B27.- with fourth character 2)
measles complicated by meningitis (B05.1)
meningoencephalitis and meningomyelitis in other infectious and parasitic diseases classified elsewhere (G05)
mumps meningitis (B26.1)
rubella meningitis (B06.02)
varicella [chickenpox] meningitis (B01.0)
zoster meningitis (B02.1)

CHAPTER 6 (G00-G99)

● **G03 Meningitis due to other and unspecified causes**

> **Includes**   arachnoiditis NOS
> leptomeningitis NOS
> meningitis NOS
> pachymeningitis NOS

> **Excludes1**   meningoencephalitis (G04.-)
> meningomyelitis (G04.-)

G03.0 Nonpyogenic meningitis
   Aseptic meningitis
   Nonbacterial meningitis

G03.1 Chronic meningitis

G03.2 Benign recurrent meningitis [Mollaret]

G03.8 Meningitis due to other specified causes

G03.9 Meningitis, unspecified
   Arachnoiditis (spinal) NOS

● **G04 Encephalitis, myelitis and encephalomyelitis**

> **Includes**   acute ascending myelitis
> meningoencephalitis
> meningomyelitis

> **Excludes1**   encephalopathy NOS (G93.40)
> other noninfectious acute disseminated
> encephalomyelitis (noninfectious ADEM)
> (G04.81)

> **Excludes2**   acute transverse myelitis (G37.3-)
> alcoholic encephalopathy (G31.2)
> benign myalgic encephalomyelitis (G93.3)
> multiple sclerosis (G35)
> subacute necrotizing myelitis (G37.4)
> toxic encephalitis (G92)
> toxic encephalopathy (G92)

● **G04.0 Acute disseminated encephalitis and encephalomyelitis (ADEM)**

> **Excludes1**   acute necrotizing hemorrhagic
> encephalopathy (G04.3-)

G04.00 Acute disseminated encephalitis and encephalomyelitis, unspecified

▷ *G04.01 Postinfectious acute disseminated encephalitis and encephalomyelitis (postinfectious ADEM)*

> **Excludes1**   post chickenpox encephalitis
> (B01.1)
> post measles encephalitis (B05.0)
> post measles myelitis (B05.1)

G04.02 Postimmunization acute disseminated encephalitis, myelitis and encephalomyelitis
   Encephalitis, post immunization
   Encephalomyelitis, post immunization
   Use additional code to identify the vaccine
   (T50.A-, T50.B-, T50.Z-)

G04.1 Tropical spastic paraplegia

G04.2 Bacterial meningoencephalitis and meningomyelitis, not elsewhere classified

● **G04.3 Acute necrotizing hemorrhagic encephalopathy**
   Sudden and severe CNS disease with pathology of hemorrhages and necrosis of white matter

> **Excludes1**   acute disseminated encephalitis and
> encephalomyelitis (G04.0-)

G04.30 Acute necrotizing hemorrhagic encephalopathy, unspecified

▷ *G04.31 Postinfectious acute necrotizing hemorrhagic encephalopathy*

G04.32 Postimmunization acute necrotizing hemorrhagic encephalopathy
   Use additional code to identify vaccine
   (T50.A-, T50.B-, T50.Z-)

▷ *G04.39 Other acute necrotizing hemorrhagic encephalopathy*
   Code also underlying etiology, if applicable

● **G04.8 Other encephalitis, myelitis and encephalomyelitis**
   Code also any associated seizure (G40.-, R56.9)

G04.81 Other encephalitis and encephalomyelitis
   Noninfectious acute disseminated
   encephalomyelitis (noninfectious ADEM)

G04.89 Other myelitis

● **G04.9 Encephalitis, myelitis and encephalomyelitis, unspecified**

G04.90 Encephalitis and encephalomyelitis, unspecified
   Ventriculitis (cerebral) NOS

G04.91 Myelitis, unspecified

● **G05 Encephalitis, myelitis and encephalomyelitis in diseases classified elsewhere**

> *Code first underlying disease, such as:*
> human immunodeficiency virus [HIV] disease (B20)
> poliovirus (A80.-)
> suppurative otitis media (H66.01-H66.4)
> trichinellosis (B75)

> **Excludes1**   adenoviral encephalitis, myelitis and
> encephalomyelitis (A85.1)
> congenital toxoplasmosis encephalitis, myelitis
> and encephalomyelitis (P37.1)
> cytomegaloviral encephalitis, myelitis and
> encephalomyelitis (B25.8)
> encephalitis, myelitis and encephalomyelitis (in)
> measles (B05.0)
> encephalitis, myelitis and encephalomyelitis (in)
> systemic lupus erythematosus (M32.19)
> enteroviral encephalitis, myelitis and
> encephalomyelitis (A85.0)
> herpesviral [herpes simplex] encephalitis,
> myelitis and encephalomyelitis (B00.4)
> listerial encephalitis, myelitis and
> encephalomyelitis (A32.12)
> meningococcal encephalitis, myelitis and
> encephalomyelitis (A39.81)
> mumps encephalitis, myelitis and
> encephalomyelitis (B26.2)
> postchickenpox encephalitis, myelitis and
> encephalomyelitis (B01.1-)
> rubella encephalitis, myelitis and
> encephalomyelitis (B06.01)
> toxoplasmosis encephalitis, myelitis and
> encephalomyelitis (B58.2)
> zoster encephalitis, myelitis and
> encephalomyelitis (B02.0)

▷ *G05.3 Encephalitis and encephalomyelitis in diseases classified elsewhere*
   Meningoencephalitis in diseases classified elsewhere

▷ *G05.4 Myelitis in diseases classified elsewhere*
   Meningomyelitis in diseases classified elsewhere

● **G06 Intracranial and intraspinal abscess and granuloma**
   An accumulation of pus in either the brain or spinal cord
   Use additional code (B95-B97) to identify infectious agent.

G06.0 Intracranial abscess and granuloma
   Brain [any part] abscess (embolic)
   Cerebellar abscess (embolic)
   Cerebral abscess (embolic)
   Intracranial epidural abscess or granuloma
   Intracranial extradural abscess or granuloma
   Intracranial subdural abscess or granuloma
   Otogenic abscess (embolic)

> **Excludes1**   tuberculous intracranial abscess and
> granuloma (A17.81)

G06.1 Intraspinal abscess and granuloma
   Abscess (embolic) of spinal cord [any part]
   Intraspinal epidural abscess or granuloma
   Intraspinal extradural abscess or granuloma
   Intraspinal subdural abscess or granuloma

> **Excludes1**   tuberculous intraspinal abscess and
> granuloma (A17.81)

G06.2 Extradural and subdural abscess, unspecified

◀ New   ◀ Revised   ~~deleted~~ Deleted   Excludes 1   Excludes 2   Includes   Use additional   Code first   Code also   Unspecified

OGCR Official Guidelines   **X** Assign placeholder X   ● Use Additional Character(s)   ▷ Manifestation Code   **Coding Clinic**

▶ **G07   Intracranial and intraspinal abscess and granuloma in diseases classified elsewhere**

Code first underlying disease, such as:
schistosomiasis granuloma of brain (B65.-)

> **Excludes1**   abscess of brain:
> amebic (A06.6)
> chromomycotic (B43.1)
> gonococcal (A54.82)
> tuberculous (A17.81)
> tuberculoma of meninges (A17.1)

G08   Intracranial and intraspinal phlebitis and thrombophlebitis

Septic embolism of intracranial or intraspinal venous sinuses and veins
Septic endophlebitis of intracranial or intraspinal venous sinuses and veins
Septic phlebitis of intracranial or intraspinal venous sinuses and veins
Septic thrombophlebitis of intracranial or intraspinal venous sinuses and veins
Septic thrombosis of intracranial or intraspinal venous sinuses and veins

> **Excludes1**   intracranial phlebitis and thrombophlebitis complicating:
> abortion, ectopic or molar pregnancy (O00-O07, O08.7)
> pregnancy, childbirth and the puerperium (O22.5, O87.3)
> nonpyogenic intracranial phlebitis and thrombophlebitis (I67.6)

> **Excludes2**   intracranial phlebitis and thrombophlebitis complicating nonpyogenic intraspinal phlebitis and thrombophlebitis (G95.1)

G09   Sequelae of inflammatory diseases of central nervous system

Note: Category G09 is to be used to indicate conditions whose primary classification is to G00-G08 as the cause of sequelae, themselves classifiable elsewhere. The 'sequelae' include conditions specified as residuals.

Code first condition resulting from (sequela) of inflammatory diseases of central nervous system

SYSTEMIC ATROPHIES PRIMARILY AFFECTING THE CENTRAL NERVOUS SYSTEM (G10-G14)

G10   Huntington's disease
Genetic disease with degeneration of cells of the nervous system, including brain
Huntington's chorea
Huntington's dementia

● **G11   Hereditary ataxia**
Genetic neurological disorder affecting coordination

> **Excludes2**   cerebral palsy (G80.-)
> hereditary and idiopathic neuropathy (G60.-)
> metabolic disorders (E70-E88)

G11.0   Congenital nonprogressive ataxia

G11.1   Early-onset cerebellar ataxia
Early-onset cerebellar ataxia with essential tremor
Early-onset cerebellar ataxia with myoclonus [Hunt's ataxia]
Early-onset cerebellar ataxia with retained tendon reflexes
Friedreich's ataxia (autosomal recessive)
X-linked recessive spinocerebellar ataxia

G11.2   Late-onset cerebellar ataxia   A

G11.3   Cerebellar ataxia with defective DNA repair
Ataxia telangiectasia [Louis-Bar]

> **Excludes2**   Cockayne's syndrome (Q87.1)
> other disorders of purine and pyrimidine metabolism (E79.-)
> xeroderma pigmentosum (Q82.1)

G11.4   Hereditary spastic paraplegia

G11.8   Other hereditary ataxias

G11.9   Hereditary ataxia, unspecified
Hereditary cerebellar ataxia NOS
Hereditary cerebellar degeneration
Hereditary cerebellar disease
Hereditary cerebellar syndrome

● **G12   Spinal muscular atrophy and related syndromes**

G12.0   Infantile spinal muscular atrophy, type I [Werdnig-Hoffman]

G12.1   Other inherited spinal muscular atrophy
Adult form spinal muscular atrophy
Childhood form, type II spinal muscular atrophy
Distal spinal muscular atrophy
Juvenile form, type III spinal muscular atrophy [Kugelberg-Welander]
Progressive bulbar palsy of childhood [Fazio-Londe]
Scapuloperoneal form spinal muscular atrophy

● **G12.2   Motor neuron disease**
Progressive disease of motor neurons that carry impulses to muscles to move

G12.20   Motor neuron disease, unspecified

G12.21   Amyotrophic lateral sclerosis   A
Lou Gehrig's disease (ALS)
Progressive spinal muscle atrophy

G12.22   Progressive bulbar palsy

G12.29   Other motor neuron disease
Familial motor neuron disease
Primary lateral sclerosis

G12.8   Other spinal muscular atrophies and related syndromes

G12.9   Spinal muscular atrophy, unspecified

● **G13   Systemic atrophies primarily affecting central nervous system in diseases classified elsewhere**

▶ **G13.0   Paraneoplastic neuromyopathy and neuropathy**
Carcinomatous neuromyopathy
Sensorial paraneoplastic neuropathy [Denny Brown]
Code first underlying neoplasm (C00-D49)

▶ **G13.1   Other systemic atrophy primarily affecting central nervous system in neoplastic disease**
Paraneoplastic limbic encephalopathy
Code first underlying neoplasm (C00-D49)

▶ **G13.2   Systemic atrophy primarily affecting the central nervous system in myxedema**
Code first underlying disease, such as:
hypothyroidism (E03.-)
myxedematous congenital iodine deficiency (E00.1)

▶ **G13.8   Systemic atrophy primarily affecting central nervous system in other diseases classified elsewhere**
Code first underlying disease

G14   Postpolio syndrome

> **Includes**   Postpolio myelitic syndrome
> **Excludes1**   sequelae of poliomyelitis (B91)

EXTRAPYRAMIDAL AND MOVEMENT DISORDERS (G20-G26)

G20   Parkinson's disease
Progressive disease of the nervous system that affects muscle coordination
Hemiparkinsonism
Idiopathic Parkinsonism or Parkinson's disease
Paralysis agitans
Parkinsonism or Parkinson's disease NOS
Primary Parkinsonism or Parkinson's disease

> **Excludes1**   dementia with Parkinsonism (G31.83)

Item 6–2 Huntington's chorea is an inherited degenerative disorder of the central nervous system and is characterized by ceaseless, jerky movements and progressive cognitive and behavioral deterioration.

CHAPTER 6 (G00-G99)

● **G21   Secondary parkinsonism**
Symptoms of Parkinson's caused by medicines, illness, or other nervous system disorder

     Excludes1   dementia with Parkinsonism (G31.83)
                      Huntington's disease (G10)
                      Shy-Drager syndrome (G90.3)
                      syphilitic Parkinsonism (A52.19)

     G21.0   Malignant neuroleptic syndrome

          Use additional code for adverse effect, if applicable, to identify drug (T43.3X5, T43.4X5, T43.505, T43.595)

          Excludes1   neuroleptic induced parkinsonism (G21.11)

  ● **G21.1   Other drug-induced secondary parkinsonism**

          G21.11   Neuroleptic induced parkinsonism

             Use additional code for adverse effect, if applicable, to identify drug (T43.3X5, T43.4X5, T43.505, T43.595)

             Excludes1   malignant neuroleptic syndrome (G21.0)

          G21.19   Other drug induced secondary parkinsonism

             Use additional code for adverse effect, if applicable, to identify drug (T36-T50 with fifth or sixth character 5)

     G21.2   Secondary parkinsonism due to other external agents

          Code first (T51-T65) to identify external agent

     G21.3   Postencephalitic parkinsonism

     G21.4   Vascular parkinsonism

     G21.8   Other secondary parkinsonism

     G21.9   Secondary parkinsonism, unspecified

● **G23   Other degenerative diseases of basal ganglia**

     Excludes2   multi-system degeneration of the autonomic nervous system (G90.3)

     G23.0   Hallervorden-Spatz disease
          Pigmentary pallidal degeneration

     G23.1   Progressive supranuclear ophthalmoplegia [Steele-Richardson-Olszewski]
          Progressive supranuclear palsy

     G23.2   Striatonigral degeneration

     G23.8   Other specified degenerative diseases of basal ganglia
          Calcification of basal ganglia

     G23.9   Degenerative disease of basal ganglia, unspecified

● **G24   Dystonia**
Involuntary movements

     Includes   dyskinesia
     Excludes2   athetoid cerebral palsy (G80.3)

  ● **G24.0   Drug induced dystonia**

          Use additional code for adverse effect, if applicable, to identify drug (T36-T50 with fifth or sixth character 5)

          G24.01   Drug induced subacute dyskinesia
             Drug induced blepharospasm
             Drug induced orofacial dyskinesia
             Neuroleptic induced tardive dyskinesia
             Tardive dyskinesia

          G24.02   Drug induced acute dystonia
             Acute dystonic reaction to drugs
             Neuroleptic induced acute dystonia

          G24.09   Other drug induced dystonia

     G24.1   Genetic torsion dystonia
          Dystonia deformans progressiva
          Dystonia musculorum deformans
          Familial torsion dystonia
          Idiopathic familial dystonia
          Idiopathic (torsion) dystonia NOS
          (Schwalbe-) Ziehen-Oppenheim disease

     G24.2   Idiopathic nonfamilial dystonia

     G24.3   Spasmodic torticollis
Head tilts toward one side and chin is elevated and turned toward opposite side (wry neck)

          Excludes1   congenital torticollis (Q68.0)
                     hysterical torticollis (F44.4)
                     ocular torticollis (R29.891)
                     psychogenic torticollis (F45.8)
                     torticollis NOS (M43.6)
                     traumatic recurrent torticollis (S13.4)

     G24.4   Idiopathic orofacial dystonia
          Orofacial dyskinesia

          Excludes1   drug induced orofacial dyskinesia (G24.01)

     G24.5   Blepharospasm
Tonic spasm of orbicularis oculi muscle, producing closure of eyelids

          Excludes1   drug induced blepharospasm (G24.01)

     G24.8   Other dystonia
          Acquired torsion dystonia NOS

     G24.9   Dystonia, unspecified
          Dyskinesia NOS

● **G25   Other extrapyramidal and movement disorders**
Extrapyramidal: Other than pyramidal tracts

     Excludes2   sleep related movement disorders (G47.6-)

     G25.0   Essential tremor
          Familial tremor

          Excludes1   tremor NOS (R25.1)

     G25.1   Drug-induced tremor

          Use additional code for adverse effect, if applicable, to identify drug (T36-T50 with fifth or sixth character 5)

     G25.2   Other specified forms of tremor
          Intention tremor

     G25.3   Myoclonus
Shocklike contractions muscle(s)
          Drug-induced myoclonus
          Palatal myoclonus

          Use additional code for adverse effect, if applicable, to identify drug (T36-T50 with fifth or sixth character 5)

          Excludes1   facial myokymia (G51.4)
                     myoclonic epilepsy (G40.-)

     G25.4   Drug-induced chorea

          Use additional code for adverse effect, if applicable, to identify drug (T36-T50 with fifth or sixth character 5)

     G25.5   Other chorea
Continual, involuntary, jerky, movements
          Chorea NOS

          Excludes1   chorea NOS with heart involvement (I02.0)
                     Huntington's chorea (G10)
                     rheumatic chorea (I02.-)
                     Sydenham's chorea (I02.-)

  ● **G25.6   Drug induced tics and other tics of organic origin**

          G25.61   Drug induced tics

             Use additional code for adverse effect, if applicable, to identify drug (T36-T50 with fifth or sixth character 5)

          G25.69   Other tics of organic origin

             Excludes1   habit spasm (F95.9)
                       tic NOS (F95.9)
                       Tourette's syndrome (F95.2)

  ● **G25.7   Other and unspecified drug induced movement disorders**

          Use additional code for adverse effect, if applicable, to identify drug (T36-T50 with fifth or sixth character 5)

          G25.70   Drug induced movement disorder, unspecified

          G25.71   Drug induced akathisia
             Drug induced acathisia
             Neuroleptic induced acute akathisia

          G25.79   Other drug induced movement disorders

◀ New   ⇐ Revised   ~~deleted~~ Deleted   Excludes 1   Excludes 2   Includes   Use additional   Code first   Code also   Unspecified

OGCR Official Guidelines   **X** Assign placeholder X   ● Use Additional Character(s)   ▶ Manifestation Code   **Coding Clinic**

CHAPTER 6 (G00-G99)

● **G25.8 Other specified extrapyramidal and movement disorders**
    G25.81 Restless legs syndrome
    G25.82 Stiff-man syndrome
    G25.83 Benign shuddering attacks
    G25.89 Other specified extrapyramidal and movement disorders
G25.9 Extrapyramidal and movement disorder, unspecified

◗ *G26 Extrapyramidal and movement disorders in diseases classified elsewhere*
    Code first underlying disease

OTHER DEGENERATIVE DISEASES OF THE NERVOUS SYSTEM (G30-G32)

● **G30 Alzheimer's disease**
Progressive central neurodegenerative disorder
Includes   Alzheimer's dementia senile and presenile forms
Use additional code to identify:
    delirium, if applicable (F05)
    dementia with behavioral disturbance (F02.81)
    dementia without behavioral disturbance (F02.80)
Excludes1   senile degeneration of brain NEC (G31.1)
       senile dementia NOS (F03)
       senility NOS (R41.81)

G30.0 Alzheimer's disease with early onset
G30.1 Alzheimer's disease with late onset   **A**
G30.8 Other Alzheimer's disease
G30.9 Alzheimer's disease, unspecified
    Coding Clinic: 2012, Q4, P95

● **G31 Other degenerative diseases of nervous system, not elsewhere classified**
Use additional code to identify:
    dementia with behavioral disturbance (F02.81)
    dementia without behavioral disturbance (F02.80)
Excludes2   Reye's syndrome (G93.7)

● **G31.0 Frontotemporal dementia**
    G31.01 Pick's disease
       Primary progressive aphasia
       Progressive isolated aphasia
    G31.09 Other frontotemporal dementia
       Frontal dementia

G31.1 Senile degeneration of brain, not elsewhere classified
    Excludes1   Alzheimer's disease (G30.-)
         senility NOS (R41.81)

G31.2 Degeneration of nervous system due to alcohol
    Alcoholic cerebellar ataxia
    Alcoholic cerebellar degeneration
    Alcoholic cerebral degeneration
    Alcoholic encephalopathy
    Dysfunction of the autonomic nervous system due to alcohol
    Code also associated alcoholism (F10.-)

● **G31.8 Other specified degenerative diseases of nervous system**
    G31.81 Alpers' disease
       Rare neuronal degeneration of cerebral cortex disease of young children
       Grey-matter degeneration
    G31.82 Leigh's disease
       Rare neurometabolic disorder that affects central nervous system
       Subacute necrotizing encephalopathy
    G31.83 Dementia with Lewy bodies
       Closely allied to Parkinson's Disease
       Dementia with Parkinsonism
       Lewy body dementia
       Lewy body disease

    G31.84 Mild cognitive impairment, so stated
       Excludes1   age related cognitive decline (R41.81)
          altered mental status (R41.82)
          cerebral degeneration (G31.9)
          change in mental status (R41.82)
          cognitive deficits following (sequelae of) cerebral hemorrhage or infarction (I69.01, I69.11, I69.21, I69.31, I69.81, I69.91)
          cognitive impairment due to intracranial or head injury (S06.-)
          dementia (F01.-, F02.-, F03)
          mild memory disturbance (F06.8)
          neurologic neglect syndrome (R41.4)
          personality change, nonpsychotic (F68.8)

    G31.85 Corticobasal degeneration
    G31.89 Other specified degenerative diseases of nervous system
G31.9 Degenerative disease of nervous system, unspecified

● **G32 Other degenerative disorders of nervous system in diseases classified elsewhere**
◗ *G32.0 Subacute combined degeneration of spinal cord in diseases classified elsewhere*
    Dana-Putnam syndrome
    Sclerosis of spinal cord (combined) (dorsolateral) (posterolateral)
    Code first underlying disease, such as:
       anemia (D51.9)
       dietary (D51.3)
       pernicious (D51.0)
       vitamin B12 deficiency (E53.8)
    Excludes1   syphilitic combined degeneration of spinal cord (A52.11)

● **G32.8 Other specified degenerative disorders of nervous system in diseases classified elsewhere**
    Code first underlying disease, such as:
       amyloidosis cerebral degeneration (E85.-)
       cerebral degeneration (due to) hypothyroidism (E00.0-E03.9)
       cerebral degeneration (due to) neoplasm (C00-D49)
       cerebral degeneration (due to) vitamin B deficiency, except thiamine (E52-E53.-)
    Excludes1   superior hemorrhagic polioencephalitis [Wernicke's encephalopathy] (E51.2)

◗ *G32.81 Cerebellar ataxia in diseases classified elsewhere*
    Code first underlying disease, such as:
       celiac disease (with gluten ataxia) (K90.0)
       cerebellar ataxia (in) neoplastic disease (paraneoplastic cerebellar degeneration) (C00-D49)
       non-celiac gluten ataxia (M35.9)
    Excludes1   systemic atrophy primarily affecting the central nervous system in alcoholic cerebellar ataxia (G31.2)
          systemic atrophy primarily affecting the central nervous system in myxedema (G13.2)

◗ *G32.89 Other specified degenerative disorders of nervous system in diseases classified elsewhere*
    Degenerative encephalopathy in diseases classified elsewhere

Item 6–3   Multiple sclerosis (MS) is a nervous system disease affecting the brain and spinal cord by damaging the myelin sheath surrounding and protecting nerve cells. The damage slows down/blocks messages between the brain and body. Symptoms are: visual disturbances, muscle weakness, coordination and balance issues, numbness, prickling, thinking and memory problems. The cause is unknown, though it is thought that it may be an autoimmune disease. It affects women more than men, between 20 and 40 years of age. MS can be mild, but it may cause the loss of ability to write, walk, and speak. There is no cure, but medication may slow or control symptoms.

DEMYELINATING DISEASES OF THE CENTRAL NERVOUS SYSTEM (G35-G37)

G35   **Multiple sclerosis**
Destruction of central nervous system; four types: relapsing remitting, secondary progressive, primary progressive, and progressive relapsing
Disseminated multiple sclerosis
Generalized multiple sclerosis
Multiple sclerosis NOS
Multiple sclerosis of brain stem
Multiple sclerosis of cord

● G36   **Other acute disseminated demyelination**
    Excludes1   postinfectious encephalitis and encephalomyelitis NOS (G04.01)

  G36.0   **Neuromyelitis optica [Devic]**
      Inflammatory disorder in which immune system attacks optic nerves and spinal cord producing inflammation of optic nerve (optic neuritis) and spinal cord (myelitis)
      Demyelination in optic neuritis
      Excludes1   optic neuritis NOS (H46)

  G36.1   **Acute and subacute hemorrhagic leukoencephalitis [Hurst]**

  G36.8   **Other specified acute disseminated demyelination**

  G36.9   **Acute disseminated demyelination, unspecified**

● G37   **Other demyelinating diseases of central nervous system**
    Destruction of central nervous system

  G37.0   **Diffuse sclerosis of central nervous system**
      Periaxial encephalitis
      Schilder's disease
      Excludes1   X linked adrenoleukodystrophy (E71.52-)

  G37.1   **Central demyelination of corpus callosum**

  G37.2   **Central pontine myelinolysis**

  G37.3   **Acute transverse myelitis in demyelinating disease of central nervous system**
      Acute transverse myelitis NOS
      Acute transverse myelopathy
      Excludes1   multiple sclerosis (G35)
              neuromyelitis optica [Devic] (G36.0)

  G37.4   **Subacute necrotizing myelitis of central nervous system**

  G37.5   **Concentric sclerosis [Baló] of central nervous system**

  G37.8   **Other specified demyelinating diseases of central nervous system**

  G37.9   **Demyelinating disease of central nervous system, unspecified**

EPISODIC AND PAROXYSMAL DISORDERS (G40-G47)

● G40   **Epilepsy and recurrent seizures**
    Note: The following terms are to be considered equivalent to intractable: pharmacoresistant (pharmacologically resistant), treatment resistant, refractory (medically) and poorly controlled
    Excludes1   conversion disorder with seizures (F44.5)
          convulsions NOS (R56.9)
          hippocampal sclerosis (G93.81)
          mesial temporal sclerosis (G93.81)
          post traumatic seizures (R56.1)
          seizure (convulsive) NOS (R56.9)
          seizure of newborn (P90)
          temporal sclerosis (G93.81)
          Todd's paralysis (G83.8)

● G40.0   **Localization-related (focal) (partial) idiopathic epilepsy and epileptic syndromes with seizures of localized onset**
    Benign childhood epilepsy with centrotemporal EEG spikes
    Childhood epilepsy with occipital EEG paroxysms
    Excludes1   adult onset localization-related epilepsy (G40.1-, G40.2-)

● G40.00   **Localization-related (focal) (partial) idiopathic epilepsy and epileptic syndromes with seizures of localized onset, not intractable**
    Localization-related (focal) (partial) idiopathic epilepsy and epileptic syndromes with seizures of localized onset without intractability

  G40.001   **Localization-related (focal) (partial) idiopathic epilepsy and epileptic syndromes with seizures of localized onset, not intractable, with status epilepticus**

  G40.009   **Localization-related (focal) (partial) idiopathic epilepsy and epileptic syndromes with seizures of localized onset, not intractable, without status epilepticus**
      Localization-related (focal) (partial) idiopathic epilepsy and epileptic syndromes with seizures of localized onset NOS

● G40.01   **Localization-related (focal) (partial) idiopathic epilepsy and epileptic syndromes with seizures of localized onset, intractable**

  G40.011   **Localization-related (focal) (partial) idiopathic epilepsy and epileptic syndromes with seizures of localized onset, intractable, with status epilepticus**

  G40.019   **Localization-related (focal) (partial) idiopathic epilepsy and epileptic syndromes with seizures of localized onset, intractable, without status epilepticus**

◄ New   ⬅ Revised   ~~deleted~~ Deleted   Excludes 1   Excludes 2   Includes   Use additional   Code first   Code also   Unspecified
OGCR Official Guidelines   **X** Assign placeholder X   ● Use Additional Character(s)   ▶ Manifestation Code   **Coding Clinic**

● **G40.1** **Localization-related (focal) (partial) symptomatic epilepsy and epileptic syndromes with simple partial seizures**
　　Attacks without alteration of consciousness
　　Epilepsia partialis continua [Kozhevnikof]
　　Simple partial seizures developing into secondarily generalized seizures

　● **G40.10** **Localization-related (focal) (partial) symptomatic epilepsy and epileptic syndromes with simple partial seizures, not intractable**
　　　Localization-related (focal) (partial) symptomatic epilepsy and epileptic syndromes with simple partial seizures without intractability

　　G40.101 **Localization-related (focal) (partial) symptomatic epilepsy and epileptic syndromes with simple partial seizures, not intractable, with status epilepticus**

　　G40.109 **Localization-related (focal) (partial) symptomatic epilepsy and epileptic syndromes with simple partial seizures, not intractable, without status epilepticus**
　　　Localization-related (focal) (partial) symptomatic epilepsy and epileptic syndromes with simple partial seizures NOS

　● **G40.11** **Localization-related (focal) (partial) symptomatic epilepsy and epileptic syndromes with simple partial seizures, intractable**

　　G40.111 **Localization-related (focal) (partial) symptomatic epilepsy and epileptic syndromes with simple partial seizures, intractable, with status epilepticus**

　　G40.119 **Localization-related (focal) (partial) symptomatic epilepsy and epileptic syndromes with simple partial seizures, intractable, without status epilepticus**

● **G40.2** **Localization-related (focal) (partial) symptomatic epilepsy and epileptic syndromes with complex partial seizures**
　　Attacks with alteration of consciousness, often with automatisms
　　Complex partial seizures developing into secondarily generalized seizures

　● **G40.20** **Localization-related (focal) (partial) symptomatic epilepsy and epileptic syndromes with complex partial seizures, not intractable**
　　　Localization-related (focal) (partial) symptomatic epilepsy and epileptic syndromes with complex partial seizures without intractability

　　G40.201 **Localization-related (focal) (partial) symptomatic epilepsy and epileptic syndromes with complex partial seizures, not intractable, with status epilepticus**

　　G40.209 **Localization-related (focal) (partial) symptomatic epilepsy and epileptic syndromes with complex partial seizures, not intractable, without status epilepticus**
　　　Localization-related (focal) (partial) symptomatic epilepsy and epileptic syndromes with complex partial seizures NOS

　● **G40.21** **Localization-related (focal) (partial) symptomatic epilepsy and epileptic syndromes with complex partial seizures, intractable**

　　G40.211 **Localization-related (focal) (partial) symptomatic epilepsy and epileptic syndromes with complex partial seizures, intractable, with status epilepticus**

　　G40.219 **Localization-related (focal) (partial) symptomatic epilepsy and epileptic syndromes with complex partial seizures, intractable, without status epilepticus**

● **G40.3** **Generalized idiopathic epilepsy and epileptic syndromes**
　　Code also MERRF syndrome, if applicable (E88.42)

　● **G40.30** **Generalized idiopathic epilepsy and epileptic syndromes, not intractable**
　　　Generalized idiopathic epilepsy and epileptic syndromes without intractability

　　G40.301 **Generalized idiopathic epilepsy and epileptic syndromes, not intractable, with status epilepticus**

　　G40.309 **Generalized idiopathic epilepsy and epileptic syndromes, not intractable, without status epilepticus**
　　　Generalized idiopathic epilepsy and epileptic syndromes NOS

　● **G40.31** **Generalized idiopathic epilepsy and epileptic syndromes, intractable**

　　G40.311 **Generalized idiopathic epilepsy and epileptic syndromes, intractable, with status epilepticus**

　　G40.319 **Generalized idiopathic epilepsy and epileptic syndromes, intractable, without status epilepticus**

● **G40.A** **Absence epileptic syndrome**
　　Childhood absence epilepsy [pyknolepsy]
　　Juvenile absence epilepsy
　　Absence epileptic syndrome, NOS

　● **G40.A0** **Absence epileptic syndrome, not intractable**
　　　G40.A01 **Absence epileptic syndrome, not intractable, with status epilepticus**
　　　G40.A09 **Absence epileptic syndrome, not intractable, without status epilepticus**

　● **G40.A1** **Absence epileptic syndrome, intractable**
　　　G40.A11 **Absence epileptic syndrome, intractable, with status epilepticus**
　　　G40.A19 **Absence epileptic syndrome, intractable, without status epilepticus**

● **G40.B** **Juvenile myoclonic epilepsy [impulsive petit mal]**
　● **G40.B0** **Juvenile myoclonic epilepsy, not intractable**
　　　G40.B01 **Juvenile myoclonic epilepsy, not intractable, with status epilepticus**
　　　G40.B09 **Juvenile myoclonic epilepsy, not intractable, without status epilepticus**

　● **G40.B1** **Juvenile myoclonic epilepsy, intractable**
　　　G40.B11 **Juvenile myoclonic epilepsy, intractable, with status epilepticus**
　　　G40.B19 **Juvenile myoclonic epilepsy, intractable, without status epilepticus**

CHAPTER 6 (G00-G99)

● **G40.4   Other generalized epilepsy and epileptic syndromes**
Epilepsy with grand mal seizures on awakening
Epilepsy with myoclonic absences
Epilepsy with myoclonic-astatic seizures
Grand mal seizure NOS
Nonspecific atonic epileptic seizures
Nonspecific clonic epileptic seizures
Nonspecific myoclonic epileptic seizures
Nonspecific tonic epileptic seizures
Nonspecific tonic-clonic epileptic seizures
Symptomatic early myoclonic encephalopathy

● **G40.40   Other generalized epilepsy and epileptic syndromes, not intractable**
Other generalized epilepsy and epileptic syndromes without intractability
Other generalized epilepsy and epileptic syndromes NOS

    G40.401   Other generalized epilepsy and epileptic syndromes, not intractable, with status epilepticus

    G40.409   Other generalized epilepsy and epileptic syndromes, not intractable, without status epilepticus

● **G40.41   Other generalized epilepsy and epileptic syndromes, intractable**

    G40.411   Other generalized epilepsy and epileptic syndromes, intractable, with status epilepticus

    G40.419   Other generalized epilepsy and epileptic syndromes, intractable, without status epilepticus

● **G40.5   Epileptic seizures related to external causes**
Epileptic seizures related to alcohol
Epileptic seizures related to drugs
Epileptic seizures related to hormonal changes
Epileptic seizures related to sleep deprivation
Epileptic seizures related to stress

Code also, if applicable, associated epilepsy and recurrent seizures (G40.-)

Use additional code for adverse effect, if applicable, to identify drug (T36-T50 with fifth or sixth character 5)

● **G40.50   Epileptic seizures related to external causes, not intractable**

    G40.501   Epileptic seizures related to external causes, not intractable, with status epilepticus

    G40.509   Epileptic seizures related to external causes, not intractable, without status epilepticus
Epileptic seizures related to external causes, NOS

● **G40.8   Other epilepsy and recurrent seizures**
Epilepsies and epileptic syndromes undetermined as to whether they are focal or generalized
Landau-Kleffner syndrome

● **G40.80   Other epilepsy**

    G40.801   Other epilepsy, not intractable, with status epilepticus
Other epilepsy without intractability with status epilepticus

    G40.802   Other epilepsy, not intractable, without status epilepticus
Other epilepsy NOS
Other epilepsy without intractability without status epilepticus

    G40.803   Other epilepsy, intractable, with status epilepticus

    G40.804   Other epilepsy, intractable, without status epilepticus

● **G40.81   Lennox-Gastaut syndrome**

    G40.811   Lennox-Gastaut syndrome, not intractable, with status epilepticus

    G40.812   Lennox-Gastaut syndrome, not intractable, without status epilepticus

    G40.813   Lennox-Gastaut syndrome, intractable, with status epilepticus

    G40.814   Lennox-Gastaut syndrome, intractable, without status epilepticus

● **G40.82   Epileptic spasms**
Infantile spasms
Salaam attacks
West's syndrome

    G40.821   Epileptic spasms, not intractable, with status epilepticus

    G40.822   Epileptic spasms, not intractable, without status epilepticus

    G40.823   Epileptic spasms, intractable, with status epilepticus

    G40.824   Epileptic spasms, intractable, without status epilepticus

G40.89   Other seizures

> **Excludes1**   post traumatic seizures (R56.1)
> recurrent seizures NOS (G40.909)
> seizure NOS (R56.9)

● **G40.9   Epilepsy, unspecified**

● **G40.90   Epilepsy, unspecified, not intractable**
Epilepsy, unspecified, without intractability

    G40.901   Epilepsy, unspecified, not intractable, with status epilepticus

    G40.909   Epilepsy, unspecified, not intractable, without status epilepticus
Epilepsy NOS
Epileptic convulsions NOS
Epileptic fits NOS
Epileptic seizures NOS
Recurrent seizures NOS
Seizure disorder NOS

● **G40.91   Epilepsy, unspecified, intractable**
Intractable seizure disorder NOS

    G40.911   Epilepsy, unspecified, intractable, with status epilepticus

    G40.919   Epilepsy, unspecified, intractable, without status epilepticus

● **G43   Migraine**

Note: The following terms are to be considered equivalent to intractable: pharmacoresistant (pharmacologically resistant), treatment resistant, refractory (medically) and poorly controlled

Use additional code for adverse effect, if applicable, to identify drug (T36-T50 with fifth or sixth character 5)

> **Excludes1**   headache NOS (R51)
> lower half migraine (G44.00)

> **Excludes2**   headache syndromes (G44.-)

● **G43.0   Migraine without aura**
Neurological disorder, generally recurring headaches without early symptom (aura)
Common migraine

> **Excludes1**   chronic migraine without aura (G43.7-)

● **G43.00   Migraine without aura, not intractable**
Neurological disorder, generally recurring headaches without early symptom (aura); resistant to cure, relief, or control
Migraine without aura without mention of refractory migraine

    G43.001   Migraine without aura, not intractable, with status migrainosus

    G43.009   Migraine without aura, not intractable, without status migrainosus
Migraine without aura NOS

◀ New   ◀ Revised   ~~deleted~~ Deleted   Excludes 1   Excludes 2   Includes   Use additional   Code first   Code also   Unspecified
OGCR Official Guidelines   X Assign placeholder X   ● Use Additional Character(s)   ▶ Manifestation Code   **Coding Clinic**

Item 6-4 Migraine headache is described as an intense pulsing or throbbing pain in one area of the head. It can be accompanied by extreme sensitivity to light (photophobic) and sound and is three times more common in women than in men. Symptoms include nausea and vomiting. Research indicates migraine headaches are caused by inherited abnormalities in genes that control the activities of certain cell populations in the brain.

● **G43.01**   **Migraine without aura, intractable**
     Intractable migraine: Not easily cured or managed; relentless pain from a migraine
     Migraine without aura with refractory migraine

     G43.011   **Migraine without aura, intractable, with status migrainosus**

     G43.019   **Migraine without aura, intractable, without status migrainosus**

● **G43.1**   **Migraine with aura**
     Basilar migraine
     Classical migraine
     Migraine equivalents
     Migraine preceded or accompanied by transient focal neurological phenomena
     Migraine triggered seizures
     Migraine with acute-onset aura
     Migraine with aura without headache (migraine equivalents)
     Migraine with prolonged aura
     Migraine with typical aura
     Retinal migraine
     Code also any associated seizure (G40.-, R56.9)
     Excludes1   persistent migraine aura (G43.5-, G43.6-)

● **G43.10**   **Migraine with aura, not intractable**
     Migraine with aura without mention of refractory migraine

     G43.101   **Migraine with aura, not intractable, with status migrainosus**

     G43.109   **Migraine with aura, not intractable, without status migrainosus**
         Migraine with aura NOS

● **G43.11**   **Migraine with aura, intractable**
     Migraine with aura with refractory migraine

     G43.111   **Migraine with aura, intractable, with status migrainosus**

     G43.119   **Migraine with aura, intractable, without status migrainosus**

● **G43.4**   **Hemiplegic migraine**
     Inherited migraine disorder causing temporary paralysis of one side of body followed by severe headache and nausea
     Familial migraine
     Sporadic migraine

● **G43.40**   **Hemiplegic migraine, not intractable**
     Hemiplegic migraine without refractory migraine

     G43.401   **Hemiplegic migraine, not intractable, with status migrainosus**

     G43.409   **Hemiplegic migraine, not intractable, without status migrainosus**
         Hemiplegic migraine NOS

● **G43.41**   **Hemiplegic migraine, intractable**
     Hemiplegic migraine with refractory migraine

     G43.411   **Hemiplegic migraine, intractable, with status migrainosus**

     G43.419   **Hemiplegic migraine, intractable, without status migrainosus**

● **G43.5**   **Persistent migraine aura without cerebral infarction**

● **G43.50**   **Persistent migraine aura without cerebral infarction, not intractable**
     Persistent migraine aura without cerebral infarction, without refractory migraine

     G43.501   **Persistent migraine aura without cerebral infarction, not intractable, with status migrainosus**

     G43.509   **Persistent migraine aura without cerebral infarction, not intractable, without status migrainosus**
         Persistent migraine aura NOS

● **G43.51**   **Persistent migraine aura without cerebral infarction, intractable**
     Persistent migraine aura without cerebral infarction, with refractory migraine

     G43.511   **Persistent migraine aura without cerebral infarction, intractable, with status migrainosus**

     G43.519   **Persistent migraine aura without cerebral infarction, intractable, without status migrainosus**

● **G43.6**   **Persistent migraine aura with cerebral infarction**
     Visual, motor, or psychic disturbances, paresthesias, and related neurologic abnormalities accompanying migraine
     Code also the type of cerebral infarction (I63.-)

● **G43.60**   **Persistent migraine aura with cerebral infarction, not intractable**
     Persistent migraine aura with cerebral infarction, without refractory migraine

     G43.601   **Persistent migraine aura with cerebral infarction, not intractable, with status migrainosus**

     G43.609   **Persistent migraine aura with cerebral infarction, not intractable, without status migrainosus**

● **G43.61**   **Persistent migraine aura with cerebral infarction, intractable**
     Persistent migraine aura with cerebral infarction, with refractory migraine

     G43.611   **Persistent migraine aura with cerebral infarction, intractable, with status migrainosus**

     G43.619   **Persistent migraine aura with cerebral infarction, intractable, without status migrainosus**

● **G43.7**   **Chronic migraine without aura**
     Transformed migraine
     Excludes1   migraine without aura (G43.0-)

● **G43.70**   **Chronic migraine without aura, not intractable**
     Chronic migraine without aura, without refractory migraine

     G43.701   **Chronic migraine without aura, not intractable, with status migrainosus**

     G43.709   **Chronic migraine without aura, not intractable, without status migrainosus**
         Chronic migraine without aura NOS

● **G43.71**   **Chronic migraine without aura, intractable**
     Chronic migraine without aura, with refractory migraine

     G43.711   **Chronic migraine without aura, intractable, with status migrainosus**

     G43.719   **Chronic migraine without aura, intractable, without status migrainosus**

● **G43.A   Cyclical vomiting**
   G43.A0   Cyclical vomiting, not intractable
      Cyclical vomiting, without refractory migraine
   G43.A1   Cyclical vomiting, intractable
      Cyclical vomiting, with refractory migraine

● **G43.B   Ophthalmoplegic migraine**
   G43.B0   Ophthalmoplegic migraine, not intractable
      Ophthalmoplegic migraine, without refractory migraine
   G43.B1   Ophthalmoplegic migraine, intractable
      Ophthalmoplegic migraine, with refractory migraine

● **G43.C   Periodic headache syndromes in child or adult**
   G43.C0   Periodic headache syndromes in child or adult, not intractable
      Periodic headache syndromes in child or adult, without refractory migraine
   G43.C1   Periodic headache syndromes in child or adult, intractable
      Periodic headache syndromes in child or adult, with refractory migraine

● **G43.D   Abdominal migraine**
   G43.D0   Abdominal migraine, not intractable
      Abdominal migraine, without refractory migraine
   G43.D1   Abdominal migraine, intractable
      Abdominal migraine, with refractory migraine

● **G43.8   Other migraine**
  ● **G43.80   Other migraine, not intractable**
      Other migraine, without refractory migraine
    G43.801   Other migraine, not intractable, with status migrainosus
    G43.809   Other migraine, not intractable, without status migrainosus
  ● **G43.81   Other migraine, intractable**
      Other migraine, with refractory migraine
    G43.811   Other migraine, intractable, with status migrainosus
    G43.819   Other migraine, intractable, without status migrainosus
  ● **G43.82   Menstrual migraine, not intractable**
      Menstrual headache, not intractable
      Menstrual migraine, without refractory migraine
      Menstrually related migraine, not intractable
      Pre-menstrual headache, not intractable
      Pre-menstrual migraine, not intractable
      Pure menstrual migraine, not intractable
      Code also associated premenstrual tension syndrome (N94.3)
    G43.821   Menstrual migraine, not intractable, with status migrainosus ♀
    G43.829   Menstrual migraine, not intractable, without status migrainosus ♀
      Menstrual migraine NOS
  ● **G43.83   Menstrual migraine, intractable**
      Menstrual headache, intractable
      Menstrual migraine, with refractory migraine
      Menstrually related migraine, intractable
      Pre-menstrual headache, intractable
      Pre-menstrual migraine, intractable
      Pure menstrual migraine, intractable
      Code also associated premenstrual tension syndrome (N94.3)
    G43.831   Menstrual migraine, intractable, with status migrainosus ♀
    G43.839   Menstrual migraine, intractable, without status migrainosus ♀

● **G43.9   Migraine, unspecified**
  ● **G43.90   Migraine, unspecified, not intractable**
      Migraine, unspecified, without refractory migraine
    G43.901   Migraine, unspecified, not intractable, with status migrainosus
      Status migrainosus NOS
    G43.909   Migraine, unspecified, not intractable, without status migrainosus
      Migraine NOS
  ● **G43.91   Migraine, unspecified, intractable**
      Migraine, unspecified, with refractory migraine
    G43.911   Migraine, unspecified, intractable, with status migrainosus
    G43.919   Migraine, unspecified, intractable, without status migrainosus

● **G44   Other headache syndromes**
  Excludes1   headache NOS (R51)
  Excludes2   atypical facial pain (G50.1)
      headache due to lumbar puncture (G97.1)
      migraines (G43.-)
      trigeminal neuralgia (G50.0)
  ● **G44.0   Cluster headaches and other trigeminal autonomic cephalgias (TAC)**
    ● **G44.00   Cluster headache syndrome, unspecified**
        Ciliary neuralgia
        Cluster headache NOS
        Histamine cephalgia
        Lower half migraine
        Migrainous neuralgia
      G44.001   Cluster headache syndrome, unspecified, intractable
      G44.009   Cluster headache syndrome, unspecified, not intractable
        Cluster headache syndrome NOS
    ● **G44.01   Episodic cluster headache**
      G44.011   Episodic cluster headache, intractable
      G44.019   Episodic cluster headache, not intractable
        Episodic cluster headache NOS
    ● **G44.02   Chronic cluster headache**
      G44.021   Chronic cluster headache, intractable
      G44.029   Chronic cluster headache, not intractable
        Chronic cluster headache NOS
    ● **G44.03   Episodic paroxysmal hemicrania**
      Paroxysmal hemicrania NOS
      G44.031   Episodic paroxysmal hemicrania, intractable
      G44.039   Episodic paroxysmal hemicrania, not intractable
        Episodic paroxysmal hemicrania NOS
    ● **G44.04   Chronic paroxysmal hemicrania**
      Unilateral headache
      G44.041   Chronic paroxysmal hemicrania, intractable
      G44.049   Chronic paroxysmal hemicrania, not intractable
        Chronic paroxysmal hemicrania NOS

◄ New   ◄▪ Revised   d̶e̶l̶e̶t̶e̶d̶ Deleted   Excludes 1   Excludes 2   Includes   Use additional   Code first   Code also   Unspecified
OGCR Official Guidelines   X Assign placeholder X   ● Use Additional Character(s)   ▶ Manifestation Code   **Coding Clinic**

- **G44.05** **Short lasting unilateral neuralgiform headache with conjunctival injection and tearing (SUNCT)**
  - G44.051 **Short lasting unilateral neuralgiform headache with conjunctival injection and tearing (SUNCT), intractable**
  - G44.059 **Short lasting unilateral neuralgiform headache with conjunctival injection and tearing (SUNCT), not intractable**
    Short lasting unilateral neuralgiform headache with conjunctival injection and tearing (SUNCT) NOS
- **G44.09** **Other trigeminal autonomic cephalgias (TAC)**
  Cluster headaches
  - G44.091 **Other trigeminal autonomic cephalgias (TAC), intractable**
  - G44.099 **Other trigeminal autonomic cephalgias (TAC), not intractable**

G44.1 **Vascular headache, not elsewhere classified**
  Excludes2   cluster headache (G44.0)
  complicated headache syndromes (G44.5-)
  drug-induced headache (G44.4-)
  migraine (G43.-)
  other specified headache syndromes (G44.8-)
  post-traumatic headache (G44.3-)
  tension-type headache (G44.2-)

- **G44.2** **Tension-type headache**
  - **G44.20** **Tension-type headache, unspecified**
    - G44.201 **Tension-type headache, unspecified, intractable**
    - G44.209 **Tension-type headache, unspecified, not intractable**
      Tension headache NOS
  - **G44.21** **Episodic tension-type headache**
    - G44.211 **Episodic tension-type headache, intractable**
    - G44.219 **Episodic tension-type headache, not intractable**
      Episodic tension-type headache NOS
  - **G44.22** **Chronic tension-type headache**
    - G44.221 **Chronic tension-type headache, intractable**
    - G44.229 **Chronic tension-type headache, not intractable**
      Chronic tension-type headache NOS
- **G44.3** **Post-traumatic headache**
  - **G44.30** **Post-traumatic headache, unspecified**
    - G44.301 **Post-traumatic headache, unspecified, intractable**
    - G44.309 **Post-traumatic headache, unspecified, not intractable**
      Post-traumatic headache NOS
  - **G44.31** **Acute post-traumatic headache**
    - G44.311 **Acute post-traumatic headache, intractable**
    - G44.319 **Acute post-traumatic headache, not intractable**
      Acute post-traumatic headache NOS
  - **G44.32** **Chronic post-traumatic headache**
    - G44.321 **Chronic post-traumatic headache, intractable**
    - G44.329 **Chronic post-traumatic headache, not intractable**
      Chronic post-traumatic headache NOS

- **G44.4** **Drug-induced headache, not elsewhere classified**
  Medication overuse headache
  Use additional code for adverse effect, if applicable, to identify drug (T36-T50 with fifth or sixth character 5)
  - G44.40 **Drug-induced headache, not elsewhere classified, not intractable**
  - G44.41 **Drug-induced headache, not elsewhere classified, intractable**
- **G44.5** **Complicated headache syndromes**
  - G44.51 **Hemicrania continua**
    Persistent unilateral headache
  - G44.52 **New daily persistent headache (NDPH)**
  - G44.53 **Primary thunderclap headache**
  - G44.59 **Other complicated headache syndrome**
- **G44.8** **Other specified headache syndromes**
  - G44.81 **Hypnic headache**
    Benign primary headaches
  - G44.82 **Headache associated with sexual activity**
    Orgasmic headache
    Preorgasmic headache
  - G44.83 **Primary cough headache**
  - G44.84 **Primary exertional headache**
  - G44.85 **Primary stabbing headache**
  - G44.89 **Other headache syndrome**

- **G45** **Transient cerebral ischemic attacks and related syndromes**
  Excludes1   neonatal cerebral ischemia (P91.0)
  transient retinal artery occlusion (H34.0-)
  - G45.0 **Vertebro-basilar artery syndrome**
  - G45.1 **Carotid artery syndrome (hemispheric)**
  - G45.2 **Multiple and bilateral precerebral artery syndromes**
  - G45.3 **Amaurosis fugax**
    Transient visual loss in one eye
  - G45.4 **Transient global amnesia**
    Episode of short-term memory loss, nonrecurrent, lasting few hours
    Excludes1   amnesia NOS (R41.3)
  - G45.8 **Other transient cerebral ischemic attacks and related syndromes**
  - G45.9 **Transient cerebral ischemic attack, unspecified**
    Spasm of cerebral artery
    TIA
    Transient cerebral ischemia NOS

- **G46** **Vascular syndromes of brain in cerebrovascular diseases**
  Code first underlying cerebrovascular disease (I60-I69)
  - G46.0 **Middle cerebral artery syndrome**
  - G46.1 **Anterior cerebral artery syndrome**
  - G46.2 **Posterior cerebral artery syndrome**
  - G46.3 **Brain stem stroke syndrome**
    Benedikt syndrome
    Claude syndrome
    Foville syndrome
    Millard-Gubler syndrome
    Wallenberg syndrome
    Weber syndrome
  - G46.4 **Cerebellar stroke syndrome**
  - G46.5 **Pure motor lacunar syndrome**
    Occlusion of single deep penetrating artery
  - G46.6 **Pure sensory lacunar syndrome**
  - G46.7 **Other lacunar syndromes**
  - G46.8 **Other vascular syndromes of brain in cerebrovascular diseases**

CHAPTER 6 (G00-G99)

CHAPTER 6 (G00-G99)

● **G47   Sleep disorders**
     Excludes2   nightmares (F51.5)
                      nonorganic sleep disorders (F51.-)
                      sleep terrors (F51.4)
                      sleepwalking (F51.3)

     ● **G47.0   Insomnia**
         Excludes2   alcohol related insomnia (F10.182,
                             F10.282, F10.982)
                        drug-related insomnia (F11.182, F11.282,
                             F11.982, F13.182, F13.282, F13.982,
                             F14.182, F14.282, F14.982, F15.182,
                             F15.282, F15.982, F19.182, F19.282,
                             F19.982)
                        idiopathic insomnia (F51.01)
                        insomnia due to a mental disorder (F51.05)
                        insomnia not due to a substance or known
                             physiological condition (F51.0-)
                        nonorganic insomnia (F51.0-)
                        primary insomnia (F51.01)
                        sleep apnea (G47.3-)

         G47.00   Insomnia, unspecified
                  Insomnia NOS

         G47.01   Insomnia due to medical condition
                  Code also associated medical condition

         G47.09   Other insomnia

     ● **G47.1   Hypersomnia**
         Excludes2   alcohol-related hypersomnia (F10.182,
                             F10.282, F10.982)
                        drug-related hypersomnia (F11.182,
                             F11.282, F11.982, F13.182, F13.282,
                             F13.982, F14.182, F14.282, F14.982,
                             F15.182, F15.282, F15.982, F19.182,
                             F19.282, F19.982)
                        hypersomnia due to a mental disorder
                             (F51.13)
                        hypersomnia not due to a substance
                             or known physiological condition
                             (F51.1-)
                        primary hypersomnia (F51.11)
                        sleep apnea (G47.3-)

         G47.10   Hypersomnia, unspecified
                  Hypersomnia NOS

         G47.11   Idiopathic hypersomnia with long sleep time
                  Idiopathic hypersomnia NOS

         G47.12   Idiopathic hypersomnia without long sleep time

         G47.13   Recurrent hypersomnia
                  Kleine-Levin syndrome
                  Menstrual related hypersomnia

         G47.14   Hypersomnia due to medical condition
                  Code also associated medical condition

         G47.19   Other hypersomnia

     ● **G47.2   Circadian rhythm sleep disorders**
             Disorders of the sleep wake schedule
             Inversion of nyctohemeral rhythm
             Inversion of sleep rhythm

         **G47.20   Circadian rhythm sleep disorder, unspecified
                   type**
                  Sleep wake schedule disorder NOS

         **G47.21   Circadian rhythm sleep disorder, delayed sleep
                   phase type**
                  Delayed sleep phase syndrome

         **G47.22   Circadian rhythm sleep disorder, advanced
                   sleep phase type**

         **G47.23   Circadian rhythm sleep disorder, irregular sleep
                   wake type**
                  Irregular sleep-wake pattern

         **G47.24   Circadian rhythm sleep disorder, free running
                   type**

         G47.25   Circadian rhythm sleep disorder, jet lag type

         G47.26   Circadian rhythm sleep disorder, shift work type

         ▌ *G47.27   Circadian rhythm sleep disorder in conditions
                   classified elsewhere*
                  Code first underlying condition

         G47.29   Other circadian rhythm sleep disorder

     ● **G47.3   Sleep apnea**
         Characterized by episodes in which breathing stops during sleep
         Code also any associated underlying condition
         Excludes1   apnea NOS (R06.81)
                        Cheyne-Stokes breathing (R06.3)
                        pickwickian syndrome (E66.2)
                        sleep apnea of newborn (P28.3)

         G47.30   Sleep apnea, unspecified
                  Sleep apnea NOS

         G47.31   Primary central sleep apnea

         G47.32   High altitude periodic breathing

         G47.33   Obstructive sleep apnea (adult) (pediatric)
                  Excludes1   obstructive sleep apnea of
                                     newborn (P28.3)

         **G47.34   Idiopathic sleep related nonobstructive alveolar
                   hypoventilation**
                  Sleep related hypoxia

         **G47.35   Congenital central alveolar hypoventilation
                   syndrome**

         ▌ *G47.36   Sleep related hypoventilation in conditions
                   classified elsewhere*
                  Sleep related hypoxemia in conditions
                        classified elsewhere
                  Code first underlying condition

         ▌ *G47.37   Central sleep apnea in conditions classified
                   elsewhere*
                  Code first underlying condition

         G47.39   Other sleep apnea

     ● **G47.4   Narcolepsy and cataplexy**
         *Cataplexy is a disorder evidenced by seizures including
             minor slacking of the facial muscles to complete
             collapse and often affects people who have* **narcolepsy**,
             *a disorder in which there is great difficulty remaining
             awake during the daytime.*

         ● **G47.41   Narcolepsy**
                  G47.411   Narcolepsy with cataplexy
                  G47.419   Narcolepsy without cataplexy
                         Narcolepsy NOS

         ● **G47.42   Narcolepsy in conditions classified elsewhere**
                  Code first underlying condition

             ▌ *G47.421   Narcolepsy in conditions classified
                         elsewhere with cataplexy*

             ▌ *G47.429   Narcolepsy in conditions classified
                         elsewhere without cataplexy*

     ● **G47.5   Parasomnia**
         Excludes1   alcohol induced parasomnia (F10.182,
                             F10.282, F10.982)
                        drug induced parasomnia (F11.182,
                             F11.282, F11.982, F13.182, F13.282,
                             F13.982, F14.182, F14.282, F14.982,
                             F15.182, F15.282, F15.982, F19.182,
                             F19.282, F19.982)
                        parasomnia not due to a substance or
                             known physiological condition (F51.8)

         G47.50   Parasomnia, unspecified
                  Parasomnia NOS

         G47.51   Confusional arousals

         G47.52   REM sleep behavior disorder

         G47.53   Recurrent isolated sleep paralysis

         ▌ *G47.54   Parasomnia in conditions classified elsewhere*
                  Code first underlying condition

         G47.59   Other parasomnia

◀ New   ◀▦ Revised   ~~deleted~~ Deleted   Excludes 1   Excludes 2   Includes   Use additional   Code first   Code also   Unspecified

OGCR Official Guidelines   **X** Assign placeholder X   ● Use Additional Character(s)   ▌ Manifestation Code   **Coding Clinic**

Item 6-5 Trigeminal neuralgia, tic douloureux, is a pain syndrome diagnosed from the patient's history alone. The condition is characterized by pain and a brief facial spasm or tic. Pain is unilateral and follows the sensory distribution of cranial nerve V, typically radiating to the maxillary (V2) or mandibular (V3) area.

● G47.6　**Sleep related movement disorders**
> **Excludes2**　restless legs syndrome (G25.81)

　　G47.61　**Periodic limb movement disorder**
> Periodic limb movement disorder

　　G47.62　**Sleep related leg cramps**

　　G47.63　**Sleep related bruxism**
> **Excludes1**　psychogenic bruxism (F45.8)

　　G47.69　**Other sleep related movement disorders**

　G47.8　**Other sleep disorders**

　G47.9　**Sleep disorder, unspecified**
> Sleep disorder NOS

(See Plate 118 on page 54.)

NERVE, NERVE ROOT AND PLEXUS DISORDERS (G50-G59)

> **Excludes1**　current traumatic nerve, nerve root and plexus
> 　　disorders - see Injury, nerve by body region
> neuralgia NOS (M79.2)
> neuritis NOS (M79.2)
> peripheral neuritis in pregnancy (O26.82-)
> radiculitis NOS (M54.1-)

● G50　**Disorders of trigeminal nerve**
> **Includes**　disorders of 5th cranial nerve

　G50.0　**Trigeminal neuralgia**
> Syndrome of paroxysmal facial pain
> Tic douloureux

　G50.1　**Atypical facial pain**

　G50.8　**Other disorders of trigeminal nerve**

　G50.9　**Disorder of trigeminal nerve, unspecified**

● G51　**Facial nerve disorders**
> **Includes**　disorders of 7th cranial nerve

　G51.0　**Bell's palsy**
> Facial palsy

　G51.1　**Geniculate ganglionitis**
> *Rare disorder with symptoms of severe pain deep in ear,*
> *spreading to ear canal, outer ear, mastoid or eye regions*
> **Excludes1**　postherpetic geniculate ganglionitis
> 　　(B02.21)

　G51.2　**Melkersson's syndrome**
> Melkersson-Rosenthal syndrome

　G51.3　**Clonic hemifacial spasm**

　G51.4　**Facial myokymia**
> *Involuntary facial muscle movement*

　G51.8　**Other disorders of facial nerve**

　G51.9　**Disorder of facial nerve, unspecified**

● G52　**Disorders of other cranial nerves**
> **Excludes2**　disorders of acoustic [8th] nerve (H93.3)
> 　　disorders of optic [2nd] nerve (H46, H47.0)
> 　　paralytic strabismus due to nerve palsy
> 　　(H49.0-H49.2)

　G52.0　**Disorders of olfactory nerve**
> Disorders of 1st cranial nerve

　G52.1　**Disorders of glossopharyngeal nerve**
> Disorder of 9th cranial nerve
> Glossopharyngeal neuralgia

　G52.2　**Disorders of vagus nerve**
> Disorders of pneumogastric [10th] nerve

　G52.3　**Disorders of hypoglossal nerve**
> Disorders of 12th cranial nerve

　G52.7　**Disorders of multiple cranial nerves**
> Polyneuritis cranialis

　G52.8　**Disorders of other specified cranial nerves**

　G52.9　**Cranial nerve disorder, unspecified**

▷ G53　*Cranial nerve disorders in diseases classified elsewhere*
> *Code first* underlying disease, such as:
> neoplasm (C00-D49)
> **Excludes1**　multiple cranial nerve palsy in sarcoidosis
> 　　(D86.82)
> 　　multiple cranial nerve palsy in syphilis (A52.15)
> 　　postherpetic geniculate ganglionitis (B02.21)
> 　　postherpetic trigeminal neuralgia (B02.22)

● G54　**Nerve root and plexus disorders**
> *Raiculopathy (nerve root disorder) caused by pressure on nerve root,*
> *most common cause is herniation of intervertebral disk. Plexus*
> *disorders (plexopathies) are due to compression or injury.*
> **Excludes1**　current traumatic nerve root and plexus disorders
> 　　- see nerve injury by body region
> 　　intervertebral disc disorders (M50-M51)
> 　　neuralgia or neuritis NOS (M79.2)
> 　　neuritis or radiculitis brachial NOS (M54.13)
> 　　neuritis or radiculitis lumbar NOS (M54.16)
> 　　neuritis or radiculitis lumbosacral NOS (M54.17)
> 　　neuritis or radiculitis thoracic NOS (M54.14)
> 　　radiculitis NOS (M54.10)
> 　　radiculopathy NOS (M54.10)
> 　　spondylosis (M47.-)

　G54.0　**Brachial plexus disorders**
> Thoracic outlet syndrome

　G54.1　**Lumbosacral plexus disorders**

　G54.2　**Cervical root disorders, not elsewhere classified**

　G54.3　**Thoracic root disorders, not elsewhere classified**

　G54.4　**Lumbosacral root disorders, not elsewhere classified**

　G54.5　**Neuralgic amyotrophy**
> Parsonage-Aldren-Turner syndrome
> Shoulder-girdle neuritis
> **Excludes1**　neuralgic amyotrophy in diabetes
> 　　mellitus (E08-E13 with .44)

　G54.6　**Phantom limb syndrome with pain**
> *Sensations (cramping, itching) in a limb that no longer*
> *exists.*

　G54.7　**Phantom limb syndrome without pain**
> Phantom limb syndrome NOS

　G54.8　**Other nerve root and plexus disorders**

　G54.9　**Nerve root and plexus disorder, unspecified**

▷ G55　*Nerve root and plexus compressions in diseases classified*
elsewhere
> *Code first* underlying disease, such as:
> neoplasm (C00-D49)
> **Excludes1**　nerve root compression (due to) (in) ankylosing
> 　　spondylitis (M45.-)
> 　　nerve root compression (due to) (in)dorsopathies
> 　　(M53.-, M54.-)
> 　　nerve root compression (due to) (in)intervertebral
> 　　disc disorders (M50.1-, M51.1.-)
> 　　nerve root compression (due to) (in)
> 　　spondylopathies (M46.-, M48.-)

Item 6-6　The most common facial nerve disorder is **Bell's Palsy,** which occurs suddenly and results in facial drooping unilaterally. This disorder is the result of a reaction to a virus that causes the facial nerve in the ear to swell resulting in pressure in the bony canal.

CHAPTER 6 (G00-G99)

CHAPTER 6 (G00–G99)

(See Plates 472 and 473 on pages 56 and 57.)

- ● **G56   Mononeuropathies of upper limb**
  - **Excludes1**   current traumatic nerve disorder - see nerve injury by body region
  - ● **G56.0   Carpal tunnel syndrome**
    - G56.00   Carpal tunnel syndrome, unspecified upper limb
    - G56.01   Carpal tunnel syndrome, right upper limb
    - G56.02   Carpal tunnel syndrome, left upper limb
  - ● **G56.1   Other lesions of median nerve**
    - G56.10   Other lesions of median nerve, unspecified side
    - G56.11   Other lesions of median nerve, right upper limb
    - G56.12   Other lesions of median nerve, left upper limb
  - ● **G56.2   Lesion of ulnar nerve**
    - Tardy ulnar nerve palsy
    - G56.20   Lesion of ulnar nerve, unspecified upper limb
    - G56.21   Lesion of ulnar nerve, right upper limb
    - G56.22   Lesion of ulnar nerve, left upper limb
  - ● **G56.3   Lesion of radial nerve**
    - G56.30   Lesion of radial nerve, unspecified upper limb
    - G56.31   Lesion of radial nerve, right upper limb
    - G56.32   Lesion of radial nerve, left upper limb
  - ● **G56.4   Causalgia of upper limb**
    - *Intense burning pain and sensitivity to slight touch*
    - Complex regional pain syndrome II of upper limb
    - **Excludes1**   complex regional pain syndrome I of lower limb (G90.52-)
      - complex regional pain syndrome I of upper limb (G90.51-)
      - complex regional pain syndrome II of lower limb (G57.7-)
      - reflex sympathetic dystrophy of lower limb (G90.52-)
      - reflex sympathetic dystrophy (G90.51-)
    - G56.40   Causalgia of unspecified upper limb
    - G56.41   Causalgia of right upper limb
    - G56.42   Causalgia of left upper limb
  - ● **G56.8   Other specified mononeuropathies of upper limb**
    - *Disease of a single nerve*
    - Interdigital neuroma of upper limb
    - G56.80   Other specified mononeuropathies of unspecified upper limb
    - G56.81   Other specified mononeuropathies of right upper limb
    - G56.82   Other specified mononeuropathies of left upper limb
  - ● **G56.9   Unspecified mononeuropathy of upper limb**
    - *Disease of a single nerve*
    - G56.90   Unspecified mononeuropathy of unspecified upper limb
    - G56.91   Unspecified mononeuropathy of right upper limb
    - G56.92   Unspecified mononeuropathy of left upper limb
- ● **G57   Mononeuropathies of lower limb**
  - **Excludes1**   current traumatic nerve disorder - see nerve injury by body region

(See Plates 544 and 545 on pages 58 and 59.)

- ● **G57.0   Lesion of sciatic nerve**
  - **Excludes1**   sciatica NOS (M54.3-)
  - **Excludes2**   sciatica attributed to intervertebral disc disorder (M51.1.-)
  - G57.00   Lesion of sciatic nerve, unspecified lower limb
  - G57.01   Lesion of sciatic nerve, right lower limb
  - G57.02   Lesion of sciatic nerve, left lower limb
- ● **G57.1   Meralgia paresthetica**
  - *Numbness or pain in outer thigh caused by injury to nerve*
  - Lateral cutaneous nerve of thigh syndrome
  - G57.10   Meralgia paresthetica, unspecified lower limb
  - G57.11   Meralgia paresthetica, right lower limb
  - G57.12   Meralgia paresthetica, left lower limb
- ● **G57.2   Lesion of femoral nerve**
  - G57.20   Lesion of femoral nerve, unspecified lower limb
  - G57.21   Lesion of femoral nerve, right lower limb
  - G57.22   Lesion of femoral nerve, left lower limb
- ● **G57.3   Lesion of lateral popliteal nerve**
  - Peroneal nerve palsy
  - G57.30   Lesion of lateral popliteal nerve, unspecified lower limb
  - G57.31   Lesion of lateral popliteal nerve, right lower limb
  - G57.32   Lesion of lateral popliteal nerve, left lower limb
- ● **G57.4   Lesion of medial popliteal nerve**
  - G57.40   Lesion of medial popliteal nerve, unspecified lower limb
  - G57.41   Lesion of medial popliteal nerve, right lower limb
  - G57.42   Lesion of medial popliteal nerve, left lower limb
- ● **G57.5   Tarsal tunnel syndrome**
  - G57.50   Tarsal tunnel syndrome, unspecified lower limb
  - G57.51   Tarsal tunnel syndrome, right lower limb
  - G57.52   Tarsal tunnel syndrome, left lower limb
- ● **G57.6   Lesion of plantar nerve**
  - Morton's metatarsalgia
  - G57.60   Lesion of plantar nerve, unspecified lower limb
  - G57.61   Lesion of plantar nerve, right lower limb
  - G57.62   Lesion of plantar nerve, left lower limb
- ● **G57.7   Causalgia of lower limb**
  - Complex regional pain syndrome II of lower limb
  - **Excludes1**   complex regional pain syndrome I of lower limb (G90.52-)
    - complex regional pain syndrome I of upper limb (G90.51-)
    - complex regional pain syndrome II of upper limb (G56.4-)
    - reflex sympathetic dystrophy of lower limb (G90.52-)
    - reflex sympathetic dystrophy of upper limb (G90.51-)
  - G57.70   Causalgia of unspecified lower limb
  - G57.71   Causalgia of right lower limb
  - G57.72   Causalgia of left lower limb
- ● **G57.8   Other specified mononeuropathies of lower limb**
  - Interdigital neuroma of lower limb
  - G57.80   Other specified mononeuropathies of unspecified lower limb
  - G57.81   Other specified mononeuropathies of right lower limb
  - G57.82   Other specified mononeuropathies of left lower limb

● **G57.9   Unspecified mononeuropathy of lower limb**
    G57.90   Unspecified mononeuropathy of unspecified lower limb
    G57.91   Unspecified mononeuropathy of right lower limb
    G57.92   Unspecified mononeuropathy of left lower limb

● **G58   Other mononeuropathies**
    G58.0   Intercostal neuropathy
    G58.7   Mononeuritis multiplex
    G58.8   Other specified mononeuropathies
    G58.9   Mononeuropathy, unspecified

▶ *G59   Mononeuropathy in diseases classified elsewhere*
    Code first underlying disease
    Excludes1 diabetic mononeuropathy (E08-E13 with .41)
                syphilitic nerve paralysis (A52.19)
                syphilitic neuritis (A52.15)
                tuberculous mononeuropathy (A17.83)

POLYNEUROPATHIES AND OTHER DISORDERS OF THE PERIPHERAL NERVOUS SYSTEM (G60-G65)

    Excludes1 neuralgia NOS (M79.2)
                neuritis NOS (M79.2)
                peripheral neuritis in pregnancy (O26.82-)
                radiculitis NOS (M54.10)

● **G60   Hereditary and idiopathic neuropathy**
    G60.0   Hereditary motor and sensory neuropathy
        Charcot-Marie-Tooth disease
        Déjerine-Sottas disease
        Hereditary motor and sensory neuropathy, types I-IV
        Hypertrophic neuropathy of infancy
        Peroneal muscular atrophy (axonal type) (hypertrophic type)
        Roussy-Lévy syndrome
    G60.1   Refsum's disease
        Genetic disorder affecting fatty acid metabolism
        Infantile Refsum disease
    G60.2   Neuropathy in association with hereditary ataxia
    G60.3   Idiopathic progressive neuropathy
    G60.8   Other hereditary and idiopathic neuropathies
        Dominantly inherited sensory neuropathy
        Morvan's disease
        Nelaton's syndrome
        Recessively inherited sensory neuropathy
    G60.9   Hereditary and idiopathic neuropathy, unspecified

Item 6–7 The **peripheral nervous system** consists of 31 pairs of spinal nerves, 12 pairs of cranial nerves, and the autonomic nerves, which are divided into the parasympathetic and sympathetic nerves. The cranial nerves are: olfactory (I), optic (II), oculomotor (III), trochlear (IV), trigeminal (V), abducens (VI), facial (VII), vestibulocochlear (VIII), glossopharyngeal (IX), vagus (X), accessory (XI), and hypoglossal (XII).

● **G61   Inflammatory polyneuropathy**
    G61.0   Guillain-Barré syndrome
        Autoimmune disease affecting peripheral nervous system
        Acute (post-)infective polyneuritis
        Miller Fisher Syndrome
    G61.1   Serum neuropathy
        Use additional code for adverse effect, if applicable, to identify serum (T50.-)
●   **G61.8   Other inflammatory polyneuropathies**
        G61.81   Chronic inflammatory demyelinating polyneuritis
        G61.89   Other inflammatory polyneuropathies
    G61.9   Inflammatory polyneuropathy, unspecified

● **G62   Other and unspecified polyneuropathies**
    G62.0   Drug-induced polyneuropathy
        Use additional code for adverse effect, if applicable, to identify drug (T36-T50 with fifth or sixth character 5)
    G62.1   Alcoholic polyneuropathy
        Malfunction of many peripheral nerves throughout the body
    G62.2   Polyneuropathy due to other toxic agents
        Code first (T51-T65) to identify toxic agent
●   **G62.8   Other specified polyneuropathies**
        G62.81   Critical illness polyneuropathy
            Acute motor neuropathy
        G62.82   Radiation-induced polyneuropathy
            Use additional external cause code (W88-W90, X39.0-) to identify cause
        G62.89   Other specified polyneuropathies
    G62.9   Polyneuropathy, unspecified
        Neuropathy NOS

CHAPTER 6 (G00-G99)

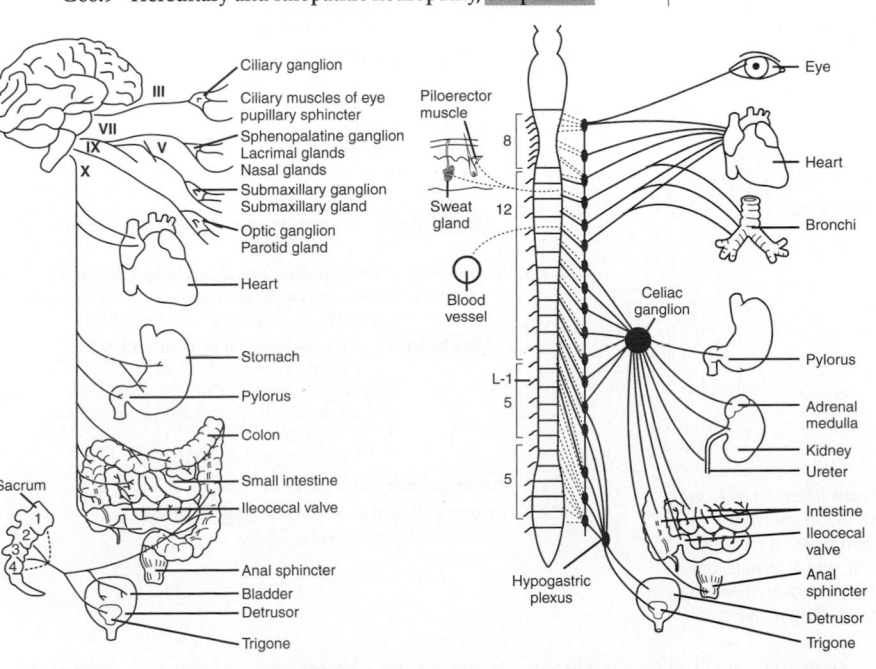

Figure 6-2   A. Parasympathetic nervous system. **B.** Sympathetic nervous system. (From Buck CJ: Step-by-Step Medical Coding, Philadelphia, WB Saunders, 1998)

CHAPTER 6 (G00-G99)

▶ **G63 Polyneuropathy in diseases classified elsewhere**

Code first underlying disease, such as:
    amyloidosis (E85.-)
    endocrine disease, except diabetes (E00-E07, E15-E16,
      E20-E34)
    metabolic diseases (E70-E88)
    neoplasm (C00-D49)
    nutritional deficiency (E40-E64)

    Excludes1 polyneuropathy (in):
               diabetes mellitus (E08-E13 with .42)
               diphtheria (A36.83)
               infectious mononucleosis (B27.0-B27.9 with 1)
               Lyme disease (A69.22)
               mumps (B26.84)
               postherpetic (B02.23)
               rheumatoid arthritis (M05.33)
               scleroderma (M34.83)
               systemic lupus erythematosus (M32.19)

    Coding Clinic: 2012, Q4, P100

G64 Other disorders of peripheral nervous system
    Disorder of peripheral nervous system NOS

● **G65 Sequelae of inflammatory and toxic polyneuropathies**

Code first condition resulting from (sequela) of inflammatory and toxic polyneuropathies

    G65.0 Sequelae of Guillain-Barré syndrome
    G65.1 Sequelae of other inflammatory polyneuropathy
    G65.2 Sequelae of toxic polyneuropathy

DISEASES OF MYONEURAL JUNCTION AND MUSCLE (G70-G73)

● **G70 Myasthenia gravis and other myoneural disorders**
    Excludes1 botulism (A05.1, A48.51-A48.52)
              transient neonatal myasthenia gravis (P94.0)

  ● **G70.0 Myasthenia gravis**
    Acquired and results in fatigable muscle weakness exacerbated by activity and improved with rest.

    G70.00 Myasthenia gravis without (acute) exacerbation
        Myasthenia gravis NOS

    G70.01 Myasthenia gravis with (acute) exacerbation
        Myasthenia gravis in crisis

    G70.1 Toxic myoneural disorders
    Dysfunction at junction of muscle and motor nerve (myoneural junction)
    Code first (T51-T65) to identify toxic agent

    G70.2 Congenital and developmental myasthenia

  ● **G70.8 Other specified myoneural disorders**
    G70.80 Lambert-Eaton syndrome, unspecified
        Lambert-Eaton syndrome NOS

    ▶ **G70.81 Lambert-Eaton syndrome in disease classified elsewhere**
        Code first underlying disease
        Excludes1 Lambert-Eaton syndrome in
                  neoplastic disease (G73.1)

    G70.89 Other specified myoneural disorders

    G70.9 Myoneural disorder, unspecified

● **G71 Primary disorders of muscles**
    Excludes2 arthrogryposis multiplex congenita (Q74.3)
             metabolic disorders (E70-E88)
             myositis (M60.-)

  G71.0 Muscular dystrophy
    Autosomal recessive, childhood type, muscular dystrophy resembling Duchenne or Becker muscular dystrophy
    Benign [Becker] muscular dystrophy
    Benign scapuloperoneal muscular dystrophy with early contractures [Emery-Dreifuss]
    Congenital muscular dystrophy NOS
    Congenital muscular dystrophy with specific morphological abnormalities of the muscle fiber
    Distal muscular dystrophy
    Facioscapulohumeral muscular dystrophy
    Limb-girdle muscular dystrophy
    Ocular muscular dystrophy
    Oculopharyngeal muscular dystrophy
    Scapuloperoneal muscular dystrophy
    Severe [Duchenne] muscular dystrophy

● **G71.1 Myotonic disorders**
    Inherited disorder that affects muscles tone

    G71.11 Myotonic muscular dystrophy
        Dystrophia myotonica [Steinert]
        Myotonia atrophica
        Myotonic dystrophy
        Proximal myotonic myopathy (PROMM)
        Steinert disease

    G71.12 Myotonia congenita
        Acetazolamide responsive myotonia congenita
        Dominant myotonia congenita [Thomsen disease]
        Myotonia levior
        Recessive myotonia congenita [Becker disease]

    G71.13 Myotonic chondrodystrophy
        Chondrodystrophic myotonia
        Congenital myotonic chondrodystrophy
        Schwartz-Jampel disease

    G71.14 Drug induced myotonia
        Use additional code for adverse effect, if applicable, to identify drug (T36-T50 with fifth or sixth character 5)

    G71.19 Other specified myotonic disorders
        Myotonia fluctuans
        Myotonia permanens
        Neuromyotonia [Isaacs]
        Paramyotonia congenita (of von Eulenburg)
        Pseudomyotonia
        Symptomatic myotonia

  G71.2 Congenital myopathies
    Central core disease
    Fiber-type disproportion
    Minicore disease
    Multicore disease
    Myotubular (centronuclear) myopathy
    Nemaline myopathy
    Excludes1 arthrogryposis multiplex congenita (Q74.3)

  G71.3 Mitochondrial myopathy, not elsewhere classified
    Myopathies associated with increased number of enlarged, often abnormal, mitochondria in muscle fibers
    Excludes1 Kearns-Sayre syndrome (H49.81)
             Leber's disease (H47.21)
             Leigh's encephalopathy (G31.82)
             mitochondrial metabolism disorders (E88.4.-)
             Reye's syndrome (G93.7)

  G71.8 Other primary disorders of muscles

  G71.9 Primary disorder of muscle, unspecified
    Hereditary myopathy NOS

Item 6–8 Muscular dystrophies (MD) are a group of rare inherited muscle diseases. Voluntary muscles become progressively weaker. In the late stages of MD, fat and connective tissue replace muscle fibers. In some types of muscular dystrophy, heart muscles, other involuntary muscles, and other organs are affected. **Myopathies** is a general term for neuromuscular diseases in which the muscle fibers dysfunction for any one of many reasons, resulting in muscular weakness.

◀ New   ◀▬ Revised   ~~deleted~~ Deleted   Excludes 1   Excludes 2   Includes   Use additional   Code first   Code also   Unspecified

OGCR Official Guidelines   **X** Assign placeholder X   ● Use Additional Character(s)   ▶ Manifestation Code   **Coding Clinic**

● **G72**   **Other and unspecified myopathies**

    Excludes1   arthrogryposis multiplex congenita (Q74.3)
                 dermatopolymyositis (M33.-)
                 ischemic infarction of muscle (M62.2-)
                 myositis (M60.-)
                 polymyositis (M33.2.-)

   G72.0   **Drug-induced myopathy**
        Use additional code for adverse effect, if applicable, to identify drug (T36-T50 with fifth or sixth character 5)

   G72.1   **Alcoholic myopathy**
        Use additional code to identify alcoholism (F10.-)

   G72.2   **Myopathy due to other toxic agents**
        Code first (T51-T65) to identify toxic agent

   G72.3   **Periodic paralysis**
        Familial periodic paralysis
        Hyperkalemic periodic paralysis (familial)
        Hypokalemic periodic paralysis (familial)
        Myotonic periodic paralysis (familial)
        Normokalemic paralysis (familial)
        Potassium sensitive periodic paralysis

      Excludes1   paramyotonia congenita (of von Eulenburg) (G71.19)

● **G72.4**   **Inflammatory and immune myopathies, not elsewhere classified**

    G72.41   **Inclusion body myositis [IBM]**

    G72.49   **Other inflammatory and immune myopathies, not elsewhere classified**
           Inflammatory myopathy NOS

● **G72.8**   **Other specified myopathies**

    G72.81   **Critical illness myopathy**
           Acute necrotizing myopathy
           Acute quadriplegic myopathy
           Intensive care (ICU) myopathy
           Myopathy of critical illness

    G72.89   **Other specified myopathies**

   G72.9   **Myopathy, unspecified**

● **G73**   **Disorders of myoneural junction and muscle in diseases classified elsewhere**

 ▸ *G73.1*   *Lambert-Eaton syndrome in neoplastic disease*
        Rare autoimmune disorder affecting calcium channels of nerve-muscle (neuromuscular) junction
        Code first underlying neoplasm (C00-D49)

      Excludes1   Lambert-Eaton syndrome not associated with neoplasm (G70.80-G70.81)

 ▸ *G73.3*   *Myasthenic syndromes in other diseases classified elsewhere*
        Code first underlying disease, such as:
           neoplasm (C00-D49)
           thyrotoxicosis (E05.-)

 ▸ *G73.7*   *Myopathy in diseases classified elsewhere*
        Code first underlying disease, such as:
           hyperparathyroidism (E21.0, E21.3)
           hypoparathyroidism (E20.-)
           glycogen storage disease (E74.0)
           lipid storage disorders (E75.-)

      Excludes1   myopathy in:
                 rheumatoid arthritis (M05.32)
                 sarcoidosis (D86.87)
                 scleroderma (M34.82)
                 sicca syndrome [Sjögren] (M35.03)
                 systemic lupus erythematosus (M32.19)

Item 6-9   **Hemiplegia** is complete paralysis of one side of the body—arm, leg, and trunk. **Hemiparesis** is a generalized weakness or incomplete paralysis of one side of the body. If most activities (eating, writing) are performed with the right hand, the right is the dominant side, and the left is the nondominant side. **Quadriplegia,** also called tetraplegia, is the complete paralysis of all four limbs. **Quadriparesis** is the incomplete paralysis of all four limbs. Nerve damage in C1–C4 is associated with lower limb paralysis, and C5–C7 damage is associated with upper limb paralysis. **Diplegia** is the paralysis of the upper limbs. **Monoplegia** is the complete paralysis of one limb.

CEREBRAL PALSY AND OTHER PARALYTIC SYNDROMES (G80-G83)

● **G80**   **Cerebral palsy**

    Excludes1   hereditary spastic paraplegia (G11.4)

   G80.0   **Spastic quadriplegic cerebral palsy**
        Congenital spastic paralysis (cerebral)

   G80.1   **Spastic diplegic cerebral palsy**
        Spastic cerebral palsy NOS

   G80.2   **Spastic hemiplegic cerebral palsy**

   G80.3   **Athetoid cerebral palsy**
        Result of damage to cerebellum or basal ganglia responsible for processing neuromuscular signals
        Double athetosis (syndrome)
        Dyskinetic cerebral palsy
        Dystonic cerebral palsy
        Vogt disease

   G80.4   **Ataxic cerebral palsy**
        Poor muscle tone and coordination

   G80.8   **Other cerebral palsy**
        Mixed cerebral palsy syndromes

   G80.9   **Cerebral palsy, unspecified**
        Cerebral palsy NOS

OGCR Section I.C.6.a.

Dominant/nondominant side

Codes from category G81, Hemiplegia and hemiparesis, and subcategories, G83.1, Monoplegia of lower limb, G83.2, Monoplegia of upper limb, and G83.3, Monoplegia, unspecified, identify whether the dominant and nondominant side is affected. Should the affected side be documented, but not specified as dominant or nondominant, and the classification system does not indicate a default, code selection is as follows:

- For ambidextrous patients, the default should be dominant.
- If the left side is affected, the default is non-dominant.
- If the right side is affected, the default is dominant.

● **G81**   **Hemiplegia and hemiparesis**

    Note: This category is to be used only when hemiplegia (complete)(incomplete) is reported without further specification, or is stated to be old or longstanding but of unspecified cause. The category is also for use in multiple coding to identify these types of hemiplegia resulting from any cause.

    Excludes1   congenital cerebral palsy (G80.-)
            hemiplegia and hemiparesis due to sequela of cerebrovascular disease (I69.05-, I69.15-, I69.25-, I69.35-, I69.85-, I69.95-)

    Coding Clinic: 2012, Q4, P106

● **G81.0**   **Flaccid hemiplegia**
        Paralysis of half of body with loss of tone of muscles of paralyzed part and absence of tendon reflexes

    G81.00   **Flaccid hemiplegia affecting unspecified side**

    G81.01   **Flaccid hemiplegia affecting right dominant side**

    G81.02   **Flaccid hemiplegia affecting left dominant side**

    G81.03   **Flaccid hemiplegia affecting right nondominant side**

    G81.04   **Flaccid hemiplegia affecting left nondominant side**

● **G81.1 Spastic hemiplegia**
*Paralysis of half of body with spasticity of muscles of
paralyzed part and increased tendon reflexes*

    G81.10 Spastic hemiplegia affecting unspecified side

    G81.11 Spastic hemiplegia affecting right dominant
side

    G81.12 Spastic hemiplegia affecting left dominant side

    G81.13 Spastic hemiplegia affecting right nondominant
side

    G81.14 Spastic hemiplegia affecting left nondominant
side

● **G81.9 Hemiplegia, unspecified**

    G81.90 Hemiplegia, unspecified affecting unspecified
side

    G81.91 Hemiplegia, unspecified affecting right
dominant side

    G81.92 Hemiplegia, unspecified affecting left
dominant side

    G81.93 Hemiplegia, unspecified affecting right
nondominant side

    G81.94 Hemiplegia, unspecified affecting left
nondominant side
        Coding Clinic: 2015, Q1, P26

● **G82 Paraplegia (paraparesis) and quadriplegia (quadriparesis)**
Note: This category is to be used only when the listed
conditions are reported without further specification, or
are stated to be old or longstanding but of unspecified
cause. The category is also for use in multiple coding to
identify these conditions resulting from any cause.

    Excludes1 congenital cerebral palsy (G80.-)
functional quadriplegia (R53.2)
hysterical paralysis (F44.4)

● **G82.2 Paraplegia**
Paralysis of both lower limbs NOS
Paraparesis (lower) NOS
Paraplegia (lower) NOS

    G82.20 Paraplegia, unspecified

    G82.21 Paraplegia, complete

    G82.22 Paraplegia, incomplete

● **G82.5 Quadriplegia**
Paralysis of all limbs; AKA tetraplegia

    G82.50 Quadriplegia, unspecified

    G82.51 Quadriplegia, C1-C4 complete

    G82.52 Quadriplegia, C1-C4 incomplete

    G82.53 Quadriplegia, C5-C7 complete

    G82.54 Quadriplegia, C5-C7 incomplete

● **G83 Other paralytic syndromes**
Note: This category is to be used only when the listed
conditions are reported without further specification, or
are stated to be old or longstanding but of unspecified
cause. The category is also for use in multiple coding to
identify these conditions resulting from any cause.

    Includes paralysis (complete) (incomplete), except as in
G80-G82

    G83.0 Diplegia of upper limbs
*Paralysis affecting limbs on both sides; AKA bilateral
paralysis*
Diplegia (upper)
Paralysis of both upper limbs

● **G83.1 Monoplegia of lower limb**
Paralysis of limb on one side
Paralysis of lower limb

    Excludes1 monoplegia of lower limbs due to sequela
of cerebrovascular disease (I69.04-,
I69.14-, I69.24-, I69.34-, I69.84-,
I69.94-)
        Coding Clinic: 2012, Q4, P106

    G83.10 Monoplegia of lower limb affecting unspecified
side

    G83.11 Monoplegia of lower limb affecting right
dominant side

    G83.12 Monoplegia of lower limb affecting left
dominant side

    G83.13 Monoplegia of lower limb affecting right
nondominant side

    G83.14 Monoplegia of lower limb affecting left
nondominant side

● **G83.2 Monoplegia of upper limb**
Paralysis of upper limb

    Excludes1 monoplegia of upper limbs due to
sequela of cerebrovascular disease
(I69.03-, I69.13-, I69.23-, I69.33-,
I69.83-, I69.93-)
        Coding Clinic: 2012, Q4, P106

    G83.20 Monoplegia of upper limb affecting unspecified
side

    G83.21 Monoplegia of upper limb affecting right
dominant side

    G83.22 Monoplegia of upper limb affecting left
dominant side

    G83.23 Monoplegia of upper limb affecting right
nondominant side

    G83.24 Monoplegia of upper limb affecting left
nondominant side

● **G83.3 Monoplegia, unspecified**
        Coding Clinic: 2012, Q4, P106

    G83.30 Monoplegia, unspecified affecting unspecified
side

    G83.31 Monoplegia, unspecified affecting right
dominant side

    G83.32 Monoplegia, unspecified affecting left
dominant side

    G83.33 Monoplegia, unspecified affecting right
nondominant side

    G83.34 Monoplegia, unspecified affecting left
nondominant side

    G83.4 Cauda equina syndrome
Aching pain due to compression of spinal nerve roots
Neurogenic bladder due to cauda equina syndrome

    Excludes1 cord bladder NOS (G95.89)
neurogenic bladder NOS (N31.9)

    G83.5 Locked-in state

● **G83.8 Other specified paralytic syndromes**

    Excludes1 paralytic syndromes due to current spinal
cord injury-code to spinal cord
injury (S14, S24, S34)

    G83.81 Brown-Séquard syndrome

    G83.82 Anterior cord syndrome

    G83.83 Posterior cord syndrome

    G83.84 Todd's paralysis (postepileptic)

    G83.89 Other specified paralytic syndromes

    G83.9 Paralytic syndrome, unspecified

◄ New   ◄▪▪▪ Revised   ~~deleted~~ Deleted   Excludes 1   Excludes 2   Includes   Use additional   Code first   Code also   Unspecified
    OGCR Official Guidelines   X Assign placeholder X   ● Use Additional Character(s)   ▶ Manifestation Code   **Coding Clinic**

OTHER DISORDERS OF THE NERVOUS SYSTEM (G89-G99)

● **G89   Pain, not elsewhere classified**

Code also related psychological factors associated with pain (F45.42)

| **Excludes1** | generalized pain NOS (R52) |
| pain disorders exclusively related to psychological factors (F45.41) |
| pain NOS (R52) |

Excludes2   atypical face pain (G50.1)
headache syndromes (G44.-)
localized pain, unspecified type - code to pain by site, such as:
   abdomen pain (R10.-)
   back pain (M54.9)
   breast pain (N64.4)
   chest pain (R07.1-R07.9)
   ear pain (H92.0-)
   eye pain (H57.1)
   headache (R51)
   joint pain (M25.5-)
   limb pain (M79.6-)
   lumbar region pain (M54.5)
   painful urination (R30.9)
   pelvic and perineal pain (R10.2)
   shoulder pain (M25.51-)
   spine pain (M54.-)
   throat pain (R07.0)
   tongue pain (K14.6)
   tooth pain (K08.8)
renal colic (N23)
migraines (G43.-)
myalgia (M79.1)
pain from prosthetic devices, implants, and grafts (T82.84, T83.84, T84.84, T85.84)
phantom limb syndrome with pain (G54.6)
vulvar vestibulitis (N94.810)
vulvodynia (N94.81-)

G89.0   Central pain syndrome

Neurological condition causing intractable pain resulting from damage to CNS
Déjérine-Roussy syndrome
Myelopathic pain syndrome
Thalamic pain syndrome (hyperesthetic)

● **G89.1   Acute pain, not elsewhere classified**

   G89.11   Acute pain due to trauma

   G89.12   Acute post-thoracotomy pain
     Post-thoracotomy pain NOS

   G89.18   Other acute postprocedural pain
     Postoperative pain NOS
     Postprocedural pain NOS

● **G89.2   Chronic pain, not elsewhere classified**

Excludes1   causalgia, lower limb (G57.7-)
causalgia, upper limb (G56.4-)
central pain syndrome (G89.0)
chronic pain syndrome (G89.4)
complex regional pain syndrome II, lower limb (G57.7-)
complex regional pain syndrome II, upper limb (G56.4-)
neoplasm related chronic pain (G89.3)
reflex sympathetic dystrophy (G90.5-)

   G89.21   Chronic pain due to trauma

   G89.22   Chronic post-thoracotomy pain

   G89.28   Other chronic postprocedural pain
     Other chronic postoperative pain

   G89.29   Other chronic pain

G89.3   Neoplasm related pain (acute) (chronic)
Cancer associated pain
Pain due to malignancy (primary) (secondary)
Tumor associated pain

G89.4   Chronic pain syndrome
Chronic pain associated with significant psychosocial dysfunction

● **G90   Disorders of autonomic nervous system**

Excludes1   dysfunction of the autonomic nervous system due to alcohol (G31.2)

● **G90.0   Idiopathic peripheral autonomic neuropathy**

   G90.01   Carotid sinus syncope
     Carotid sinus syndrome

   G90.09   Other idiopathic peripheral autonomic neuropathy
     Idiopathic peripheral autonomic neuropathy NOS

G90.1   Familial dysautonomia [Riley-Day]
Inherited disorder that affects nerve function

G90.2   Horner's syndrome
Due to damage of the sympathetic nervous system
Bernard(-Horner) syndrome
Cervical sympathetic dystrophy or paralysis

G90.3   Multi-system degeneration of the autonomic nervous system
Neurogenic orthostatic hypotension [Shy-Drager]

   Excludes1   orthostatic hypotension NOS (I95.1)

G90.4   Autonomic dysreflexia
Syndrome resulting from lesions of spinal cord
Use additional code to identify the cause, such as:
   fecal impaction (K56.41)
   pressure ulcer (pressure area) (L89.-)
   urinary tract infection (N39.0)

● **G90.5   Complex regional pain syndrome I (CRPS I)**
Reflex sympathetic dystrophy

   Excludes1   causalgia of lower limb (G57.7-)
causalgia of upper limb (G56.4-)
complex regional pain syndrome II of lower limb (G57.7-)
complex regional pain syndrome II of upper limb (G56.4-)

   G90.50   Complex regional pain syndrome I, unspecified

● **G90.51   Complex regional pain syndrome I of upper limb**

     G90.511   Complex regional pain syndrome I of right upper limb

     G90.512   Complex regional pain syndrome I of left upper limb

     G90.513   Complex regional pain syndrome I of upper limb, bilateral

     G90.519   Complex regional pain syndrome I of unspecified upper limb

● **G90.52   Complex regional pain syndrome I of lower limb**

     G90.521   Complex regional pain syndrome I of right lower limb

     G90.522   Complex regional pain syndrome I of left lower limb

     G90.523   Complex regional pain syndrome I of lower limb, bilateral

     G90.529   Complex regional pain syndrome I of unspecified lower limb

   G90.59   Complex regional pain syndrome I of other specified site

G90.8   Other disorders of autonomic nervous system

G90.9   Disorder of the autonomic nervous system, unspecified

● **G91   Hydrocephalus**
Dilatation of cerebral ventricles, accompanied by accumulation of cerebrospinal fluid

   Includes   acquired hydrocephalus

   Excludes1   Arnold-Chiari syndrome with hydrocephalus (Q07.-)
congenital hydrocephalus (Q03.-)
spina bifida with hydrocephalus (Q05.-)

G91.0   Communicating hydrocephalus
Secondary normal pressure hydrocephalus

G91.1   Obstructive hydrocephalus

CHAPTER 6 (G00-G99)

CHAPTER 6 (G00-G99)

G91.2 (Idiopathic) normal pressure hydrocephalus
Normal pressure hydrocephalus NOS

G91.3 Post-traumatic hydrocephalus, unspecified

▶**G91.4 *Hydrocephalus in diseases classified elsewhere***
Code first underlying condition, such as:
congenital syphilis (A50.4-)
neoplasm (C00-D49)

>**Excludes1** hydrocephalus due to congenital
toxoplasmosis (P37.1)

G91.8 Other hydrocephalus

G91.9 Hydrocephalus, unspecified

G92 Toxic encephalopathy
Disorder or disease of brain caused by chemicals
Toxic encephalitis
Toxic metabolic encephalopathy
Code first (T51-T65) to identify toxic agent

●**G93 Other disorders of brain**

G93.0 Cerebral cysts
Arachnoid cyst
Porencephalic cyst, acquired

>**Excludes1** acquired periventricular cysts of newborn
(P91.1)
congenital cerebral cysts (Q04.6)

G93.1 Anoxic brain damage, not elsewhere classified
*Permanent brain damage by lack of oxygen perfusion
through brain tissues.*

>**Excludes1** cerebral anoxia due to anesthesia during
labor and delivery (O74.3)
cerebral anoxia due to anesthesia during
the puerperium (O89.2)
neonatal anoxia (P84)

G93.2 Benign intracranial hypertension

>**Excludes1** hypertensive encephalopathy (I67.4)

G93.3 Postviral fatigue syndrome
Benign myalgic encephalomyelitis

>**Excludes1** chronic fatigue syndrome NOS (R53.82)

●**G93.4 Other and unspecified encephalopathy**

>**Excludes1** alcoholic encephalopathy (G31.2)
encephalopathy in diseases classified
elsewhere (G94)
hypertensive encephalopathy (I67.4)
toxic (metabolic) encephalopathy (G92)

G93.40 Encephalopathy, unspecified

G93.41 Metabolic encephalopathy
Septic encephalopathy

G93.49 Other encephalopathy
Encephalopathy NEC

G93.5 Compression of brain
Arnold-Chiari type 1 compression of brain
Compression of brain (stem)
Herniation of brain (stem)

>**Excludes1** diffuse traumatic compression of brain
(S06.2-)
focal traumatic compression of brain
(S06.3-)

G93.6 Cerebral edema

>**Excludes1** cerebral edema due to birth injury (P11.0)
traumatic cerebral edema (S06.1-)

G93.7 Reye's syndrome   P
*Life-threatening neurological condition, usually follows viral
illness*
Code first (T39.0-), if salicylates-induced

●**G93.8 Other specified disorders of brain**

G93.81 Temporal sclerosis
Hippocampal sclerosis
Mesial temporal sclerosis

G93.82 Brain death

G93.89 Other specified disorders of brain
Postradiation encephalopathy

G93.9 Disorder of brain, unspecified

▶**G94 *Other disorders of brain in diseases classified elsewhere***
Code first underlying disease

>**Excludes1** encephalopathy in congenital syphilis (A50.49)
encephalopathy in influenza (J09.X9, J10.81,
J11.81)
encephalopathy in syphilis (A52.19)
hydrocephalus in diseases classified elsewhere
(G91.4)

●**G95 Other and unspecified diseases of spinal cord**

>**Excludes2** myelitis (G04.-)

G95.0 Syringomyelia and syringobulbia

●**G95.1 Vascular myelopathies**

>**Excludes2** intraspinal phlebitis and
thrombophlebitis, except nonpyogenic (G08)

**G95.11 Acute infarction of spinal cord (embolic)
(nonembolic)**
Anoxia of spinal cord
Arterial thrombosis of spinal cord

G95.19 Other vascular myelopathies
Edema of spinal cord
Hematomyelia
Nonpyogenic intraspinal phlebitis and
thrombophlebitis
Subacute necrotic myelopathy

●**G95.2 Other and unspecified cord compression**

G95.20 Unspecified cord compression

G95.29 Other cord compression

●**G95.8 Other specified diseases of spinal cord**

>**Excludes1** neurogenic bladder NOS (N31.9)
neurogenic bladder due to cauda equina
syndrome (G83.4)
neuromuscular dysfunction of bladder
without spinal cord lesion (N31.-)

G95.81 Conus medullaris syndrome
*Damage to gray matter and/or nerve roots in lower
end of spinal cord*

G95.89 Other specified diseases of spinal cord
Cord bladder NOS
Drug-induced myelopathy
Radiation-induced myelopathy

>**Excludes1** myelopathy NOS (G95.9)

G95.9 Disease of spinal cord, unspecified
Myelopathy NOS

●**G96 Other disorders of central nervous system**

G96.0 Cerebrospinal fluid leak

>**Excludes1** cerebrospinal fluid leak from spinal
puncture (G97.0)

●**G96.1 Disorders of meninges, not elsewhere classified**

G96.11 Dural tear

>**Excludes1** accidental puncture or laceration
of dura during a procedure
(G97.41)

G96.12 Meningeal adhesions (cerebral) (spinal)

**G96.19 Other disorders of meninges, not elsewhere
classified**

G96.8 Other specified disorders of central nervous system

G96.9 Disorder of central nervous system, unspecified

●**G97 Intraoperative and postprocedural complications and disorders
of nervous system, not elsewhere classified**

>**Excludes2** intraoperative and postprocedural
cerebrovascular infarction (I97.81-, I97.82-)

G97.0 Cerebrospinal fluid leak from spinal puncture

G97.1 Other reaction to spinal and lumbar puncture
Headache due to lumbar puncture

G97.2 Intracranial hypotension following ventricular shunting

---

◀ New   ◀▥ Revised   ~~deleted~~ Deleted   Excludes 1   Excludes 2   Includes   Use additional   Code first   Code also   Unspecified

OGCR Official Guidelines   X Assign placeholder X   ● Use Additional Character(s)   ▶ Manifestation Code   **Coding Clinic**

● G97.3 **Intraoperative hemorrhage and hematoma of a nervous system organ or structure complicating a procedure**

>   **Excludes1** intraoperative hemorrhage and hematoma of a nervous system organ or structure due to accidental puncture and laceration during a procedure (G97.4-)

>   G97.31 **Intraoperative hemorrhage and hematoma of a nervous system organ or structure complicating a nervous system procedure**

>   G97.32 **Intraoperative hemorrhage and hematoma of a nervous system organ or structure complicating other procedure**

● G97.4 **Accidental puncture and laceration of a nervous system organ or structure during a procedure**

>   G97.41 **Accidental puncture or laceration of dura during a procedure**
>   Incidental (inadvertent) durotomy

>   G97.48 **Accidental puncture and laceration of other nervous system organ or structure during a nervous system procedure**

>   G97.49 **Accidental puncture and laceration of other nervous system organ or structure during other procedure**

● G97.5 **Postprocedural hemorrhage and hematoma of a nervous system organ or structure following a procedure**

>   G97.51 **Postprocedural hemorrhage and hematoma of a nervous system organ or structure following a nervous system procedure**

>   G97.52 **Postprocedural hemorrhage and hematoma of a nervous system organ or structure following other procedure**

● G97.8 **Other intraoperative and postprocedural complications and disorders of nervous system**

>   Use additional code to further specify disorder

>   G97.81 **Other intraoperative complications of nervous system**

>   G97.82 **Other postprocedural complications and disorders of nervous system**

● G98 **Other disorders of nervous system not elsewhere classified**

>   **Includes** nervous system disorder NOS

>   G98.0 **Neurogenic arthritis, not elsewhere classified**
>   Nonsyphilitic neurogenic arthropathy NEC
>   Nonsyphilitic neurogenic spondylopathy NEC

>   **Excludes1** spondylopathy (in):
>   syringomyelia and syringobulbia (G95.0)
>   tabes dorsalis (A52.11)

>   G98.8 **Other disorders of nervous system**
>   Nervous system disorder NOS

● G99 **Other disorders of nervous system in diseases classified elsewhere**

>   G99.0 *Autonomic neuropathy in diseases classified elsewhere*
>   *Code first* underlying disease, such as:
>   amyloidosis (E85.-)
>   gout (M1A.-, M10.-)
>   hyperthyroidism (E05.-)

>   **Excludes1** diabetic autonomic neuropathy (E08-E13 with .43)

>   G99.2 *Myelopathy in diseases classified elsewhere*
>   *Code first* underlying disease, such as:
>   neoplasm (C00-D49)

>   **Excludes1** myelopathy in:
>   intervertebral disease (M50.0-, M51.0-)
>   spondylosis (M47.0-, M47.1-)

>   G99.8 *Other specified disorders of nervous system in diseases classified elsewhere*
>   *Code first* underlying disorder, such as:
>   amyloidosis (E85.-)
>   avitaminosis (E56.9)

>   **Excludes1** nervous system involvement in:
>   cysticercosis (B69.0)
>   rubella (B06.0-)
>   syphilis (A52.1-)

CHAPTER 6 (G00-G99)

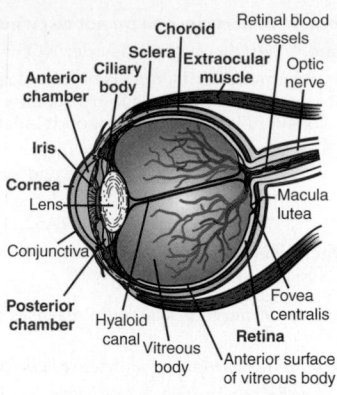

Figure 7–1 Eye and ocular adnexa. (From Buck CJ: Step-by-Step Medical Coding, ed 2011, Philadelphia, WB Saunders, 2011)

(See Plate 87 on page 63.)

CHAPTER 7

DISEASES OF THE EYE AND ADNEXA (H00-H59)

Note: Use an external cause code following the code for the eye condition, if applicable, to identify the cause of the eye condition

Excludes2   certain conditions originating in the perinatal period (P04-P96)

certain infectious and parasitic diseases (A00-B99)

complications of pregnancy, childbirth and the puerperium (O00-O9A)

congenital malformations, deformations, and chromosomal abnormalities (Q00-Q99)

diabetes mellitus related eye conditions (E09.3-, E10.3-, E11.3-, E13.3-)

endocrine, nutritional and metabolic diseases (E00-E88)

injury (trauma) of eye and orbit (S05.-)

injury, poisoning and certain other consequences of external causes (S00-T88)

neoplasms (C00-D49)

symptoms, signs and abnormal clinical and laboratory findings, not elsewhere classified (R00-R94)

syphilis related eye disorders (A50.01, A50.3-, A51.43, A52.71)

This chapter contains the following blocks:

H00-H05	Disorders of eyelid, lacrimal system and orbit
H10-H11	Disorders of conjunctiva
H15-H22	Disorders of sclera, cornea, iris and ciliary body
H25-H28	Disorders of lens
H30-H36	Disorders of choroid and retina
H40-H42	Glaucoma
H43-H44	Disorders of vitreous body and globe
H46-H47	Disorders of optic nerve and visual pathways
H49-H52	Disorders of ocular muscles, binocular movement, accommodation and refraction
H53-H54	Visual disturbances and blindness
H55-H57	Other disorders of eye and adnexa
H59	Intraoperative and postprocedural complications and disorders of eye and adnexa, not elsewhere classified

DISORDERS OF EYELID, LACRIMAL SYSTEM AND ORBIT (H00-H05)

Excludes2   open wound of eyelid (S01.1-)

superficial injury of eyelid (S00.1-, S00.2-)

● **H00   Hordeolum and chalazion**

Hordeolum: inflammatory staphylococcal infection of sebaceous glands of eyelids; AKA stye. Chalazion: eyelid mass

   ● **H00.0   Hordeolum (externum) (internum) of eyelid**

Bacterial infection (staphylococcus) of the sebaceous gland of the eyelid (stye)

     ● **H00.01   Hordeolum externum**

       Hordeolum NOS

       Stye

       H00.011   Hordeolum externum right upper eyelid

       H00.012   Hordeolum externum right lower eyelid

       H00.013   Hordeolum externum right eye, unspecified eyelid

       H00.014   Hordeolum externum left upper eyelid

       H00.015   Hordeolum externum left lower eyelid

       H00.016   Hordeolum externum left eye, unspecified eyelid

       H00.019   Hordeolum externum unspecified eye, unspecified eyelid

     ● **H00.02   Hordeolum internum**

       Infection of meibomian gland

       H00.021   Hordeolum internum right upper eyelid

       H00.022   Hordeolum internum right lower eyelid

       H00.023   Hordeolum internum right eye, unspecified eyelid

       H00.024   Hordeolum internum left upper eyelid

       H00.025   Hordeolum internum left lower eyelid

       H00.026   Hordeolum internum left eye, unspecified eyelid

       H00.029   Hordeolum internum unspecified eye, unspecified eyelid

     ● **H00.03   Abscess of eyelid**

       Furuncle of eyelid

       H00.031   Abscess of right upper eyelid

       H00.032   Abscess of right lower eyelid

       H00.033   Abscess of eyelid right eye, unspecified eyelid

       H00.034   Abscess of left upper eyelid

       H00.035   Abscess of left lower eyelid

       H00.036   Abscess of eyelid left eye, unspecified eyelid

       H00.039   Abscess of eyelid unspecified eye, unspecified eyelid

   ● **H00.1   Chalazion**

Often caused by accumulation of meibomian gland secretions resulting from a blockage of duct.

     Meibomian (gland) cyst

     Excludes2   infected meibomian gland (H00.02-)

     H00.11   Chalazion right upper eyelid

     H00.12   Chalazion right lower eyelid

     H00.13   Chalazion right eye, unspecified eyelid

     H00.14   Chalazion left upper eyelid

     H00.15   Chalazion left lower eyelid

     H00.16   Chalazion left eye, unspecified eyelid

     H00.19   Chalazion unspecified eye, unspecified eyelid

◀ New   ◀▬ Revised   ~~deleted~~ Deleted   Excludes 1   Excludes 2   Includes   Use additional   Code first   Code also   Unspecified

OGCR Official Guidelines   **X** Assign placeholder X   ● Use Additional Character(s)   ▶ Manifestation Code   **Coding Clinic**

● **H01   Other inflammation of eyelid**
   ● **H01.0   Blepharitis**
     Inflammation of eyelids
     Excludes1   blepharoconjunctivitis (H10.5-)
     ● **H01.00   Unspecified blepharitis**
       H01.001   Unspecified blepharitis right upper eyelid
       H01.002   Unspecified blepharitis right lower eyelid
       H01.003   Unspecified blepharitis right eye, unspecified eyelid
       H01.004   Unspecified blepharitis left upper eyelid
       H01.005   Unspecified blepharitis left lower eyelid
       H01.006   Unspecified blepharitis left eye, unspecified eyelid
       H01.009   Unspecified blepharitis unspecified eye, unspecified eyelid
     ● **H01.01   Ulcerative blepharitis**
       H01.011   Ulcerative blepharitis right upper eyelid
       H01.012   Ulcerative blepharitis right lower eyelid
       H01.013   Ulcerative blepharitis right eye, unspecified eyelid
       H01.014   Ulcerative blepharitis left upper eyelid
       H01.015   Ulcerative blepharitis left lower eyelid
       H01.016   Ulcerative blepharitis left eye, unspecified eyelid
       H01.019   Ulcerative blepharitis unspecified eye, unspecified eyelid
     ● **H01.02   Squamous blepharitis**
       H01.021   Squamous blepharitis right upper eyelid
       H01.022   Squamous blepharitis right lower eyelid
       H01.023   Squamous blepharitis right eye, unspecified eyelid
       H01.024   Squamous blepharitis left upper eyelid
       H01.025   Squamous blepharitis left lower eyelid
       H01.026   Squamous blepharitis left eye, unspecified eyelid
       H01.029   Squamous blepharitis unspecified eye, unspecified eyelid
   ● **H01.1   Noninfectious dermatoses of eyelid**
     ● **H01.11   Allergic dermatitis of eyelid**
       Contact dermatitis of eyelid
       H01.111   Allergic dermatitis of right upper eyelid
       H01.112   Allergic dermatitis of right lower eyelid
       H01.113   Allergic dermatitis of right eye, unspecified eyelid
       H01.114   Allergic dermatitis of left upper eyelid
       H01.115   Allergic dermatitis of left lower eyelid
       H01.116   Allergic dermatitis of left eye, unspecified eyelid
       H01.119   Allergic dermatitis of unspecified eye, unspecified eyelid

     ● **H01.12   Discoid lupus erythematosus of eyelid**
       H01.121   Discoid lupus erythematosus of right upper eyelid
       H01.122   Discoid lupus erythematosus of right lower eyelid
       H01.123   Discoid lupus erythematosus of right eye, unspecified eyelid
       H01.124   Discoid lupus erythematosus of left upper eyelid
       H01.125   Discoid lupus erythematosus of left lower eyelid
       H01.126   Discoid lupus erythematosus of left eye, unspecified eyelid
       H01.129   Discoid lupus erythematosus of unspecified eye, unspecified eyelid
     ● **H01.13   Eczematous dermatitis of eyelid**
       H01.131   Eczematous dermatitis of right upper eyelid
       H01.132   Eczematous dermatitis of right lower eyelid
       H01.133   Eczematous dermatitis of right eye, unspecified eyelid
       H01.134   Eczematous dermatitis of left upper eyelid
       H01.135   Eczematous dermatitis of left lower eyelid
       H01.136   Eczematous dermatitis of left eye, unspecified eyelid
       H01.139   Eczematous dermatitis of unspecified eye, unspecified eyelid
     ● **H01.14   Xeroderma of eyelid**
       Abnormally dry
       H01.141   Xeroderma of right upper eyelid
       H01.142   Xeroderma of right lower eyelid
       H01.143   Xeroderma of right eye, unspecified eyelid
       H01.144   Xeroderma of left upper eyelid
       H01.145   Xeroderma of left lower eyelid
       H01.146   Xeroderma of left eye, unspecified eyelid
       H01.149   Xeroderma of unspecified eye, unspecified eyelid
   H01.8   **Other specified inflammations of eyelid**
   H01.9   **Unspecified inflammation of eyelid**
     Inflammation of eyelid NOS

● **H02   Other disorders of eyelid**
   Turning inward (inversion) of eyelid margin and ingrowing eyelashes
   Excludes1   congenital malformations of eyelid (Q10.0-Q10.3)
   ● **H02.0   Entropion and trichiasis of eyelid**
     ● **H02.00   Unspecified entropion of eyelid**
       H02.001   Unspecified entropion of right upper eyelid
       H02.002   Unspecified entropion of right lower eyelid
       H02.003   Unspecified entropion of right eye, unspecified eyelid
       H02.004   Unspecified entropion of left upper eyelid

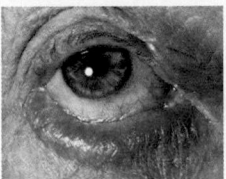

Figure 7-2   Right lower eyelid entropion. Note the inward rotation of the tarsal plate about the horizontal axis and the resultant contact between the mucocutaneous junction and ocular surface. (From Yanoff: Ophthalmology, ed 3, Mosby, Inc., 2008)

H02.005   **Unspecified** entropion of left lower eyelid

H02.006   **Unspecified** entropion of left eye, unspecified eyelid

H02.009   **Unspecified** entropion of unspecified eye, unspecified eyelid

● H02.01   Cicatricial entropion of eyelid
Scar

H02.011   Cicatricial entropion of right upper eyelid

H02.012   Cicatricial entropion of right lower eyelid

H02.013   Cicatricial entropion of right eye, **unspecified** eyelid

H02.014   Cicatricial entropion of left upper eyelid

H02.015   Cicatricial entropion of left lower eyelid

H02.016   Cicatricial entropion of left eye, **unspecified** eyelid

H02.019   Cicatricial entropion of **unspecified** eye, unspecified eyelid

● H02.02   Mechanical entropion of eyelid
Turning inward (inversion) of eyelid margin due to lack of support

H02.021   Mechanical entropion of right upper eyelid

H02.022   Mechanical entropion of right lower eyelid

H02.023   Mechanical entropion of right eye, **unspecified** eyelid

H02.024   Mechanical entropion of left upper eyelid

H02.025   Mechanical entropion of left lower eyelid

H02.026   Mechanical entropion of left eye, **unspecified** eyelid

H02.029   Mechanical entropion of **unspecified** eye, unspecified eyelid

● H02.03   Senile entropion of eyelid
Turning inward (inversion) of eyelid margin due to aging

H02.031   Senile entropion of right upper eyelid   **A**

H02.032   Senile entropion of right lower eyelid   **A**

H02.033   Senile entropion of right eye, **unspecified** eyelid   **A**

H02.034   Senile entropion of left upper eyelid **A**

H02.035   Senile entropion of left lower eyelid **A**

H02.036   Senile entropion of left eye, **unspecified** eyelid   **A**

H02.039   Senile entropion of unspecified eye, **unspecified** eyelid   **A**

● H02.04   Spastic entropion of eyelid
Turning inward (inversion) of eyelid margin caused by spasm of muscle

H02.041   Spastic entropion of right upper eyelid

H02.042   Spastic entropion of right lower eyelid

H02.043   Spastic entropion of right eye, **unspecified** eyelid

H02.044   Spastic entropion of left upper eyelid

H02.045   Spastic entropion of left lower eyelid

H02.046   Spastic entropion of left eye, **unspecified** eyelid

H02.049   Spastic entropion of unspecified eye, **unspecified** eyelid

● H02.05   Trichiasis without entropian
Ingrowing hairs of eyelashes

H02.051   Trichiasis without entropian right upper eyelid

H02.052   Trichiasis without entropian right lower eyelid

H02.053   Trichiasis without entropian right eye, **unspecified** eyelid

H02.054   Trichiasis without entropian left upper eyelid

H02.055   Trichiasis without entropian left lower eyelid

H02.056   Trichiasis without entropian left eye, **unspecified** eyelid

H02.059   Trichiasis without entropian **unspecified** eye, unspecified eyelid

● H02.1   Ectropion of eyelid
Eversion (pulling away) of eyelid

● H02.10   Unspecified ectropion of eyelid

H02.101   **Unspecified** ectropion of right upper eyelid

H02.102   **Unspecified** ectropion of right lower eyelid

H02.103   **Unspecified** ectropion of right eye, unspecified eyelid

H02.104   **Unspecified** ectropion of left upper eyelid

H02.105   **Unspecified** ectropion of left lower eyelid

H02.106   **Unspecified** ectropion of left eye, unspecified eyelid

H02.109   **Unspecified** ectropion of unspecified eye, unspecified eyelid

● H02.11   Cicatricial ectropion of eyelid
Pulling of eyelid down and away from eye due to scar or tightening

H02.111   Cicatricial ectropion of right upper eyelid

H02.112   Cicatricial ectropion of right lower eyelid

H02.113   Cicatricial ectropion of right eye, **unspecified** eyelid

H02.114   Cicatricial ectropion of left upper eyelid

H02.115   Cicatricial ectropion of left lower eyelid

H02.116   Cicatricial ectropion of left eye, **unspecified** eyelid

H02.119   Cicatricial ectropion of **unspecified** eye, unspecified eyelid

● H02.12   Mechanical ectropion of eyelid
Eversion (pulling away) of eyelid due to lack of support

H02.121   Mechanical ectropion of right upper eyelid

H02.122   Mechanical ectropion of right lower eyelid

H02.123   Mechanical ectropion of right eye, **unspecified** eyelid

H02.124   Mechanical ectropion of left upper eyelid

H02.125   Mechanical ectropion of left lower eyelid

H02.126   Mechanical ectropion of left eye, **unspecified** eyelid

H02.129   Mechanical ectropion of **unspecified** eye, unspecified eyelid

◀ New   ◀▨ Revised   ~~deleted~~ Deleted   Excludes 1   Excludes 2   Includes   Use additional   Code first   Code also   Unspecified

OGCR Official Guidelines   X Assign placeholder X   ● Use Additional Character(s)   ▶ Manifestation Code   **Coding Clinic**

● **H02.13   Senile ectropion of eyelid**
Eversion (pulling away) of eyelid due to age
H02.131   Senile ectropion of right upper eyelid   **A**
H02.132   Senile ectropion of right lower eyelid   **A**
H02.133   Senile ectropion of right eye, unspecified eyelid   **A**
H02.134   Senile ectropion of left upper eyelid **A**
H02.135   Senile ectropion of left lower eyelid **A**
H02.136   Senile ectropion of left eye, unspecified eyelid   **A**
H02.139   Senile ectropion of unspecified eye, unspecified eyelid   **A**

● **H02.14   Spastic ectropion of eyelid**
Eversion (pulling away) of eyelid due to tonic muscle spasm
H02.141   Spastic ectropion of right upper eyelid
H02.142   Spastic ectropion of right lower eyelid
H02.143   Spastic ectropion of right eye, unspecified eyelid
H02.144   Spastic ectropion of left upper eyelid
H02.145   Spastic ectropion of left lower eyelid
H02.146   Spastic ectropion of left eye, unspecified eyelid
H02.149   Spastic ectropion of unspecified eye, unspecified eyelid

● **H02.2   Lagophthalmos**
Condition in which eye cannot completely close
● **H02.20   Unspecified lagophthalmos**
H02.201   Unspecified lagophthalmos right upper eyelid
H02.202   Unspecified lagophthalmos right lower eyelid
H02.203   Unspecified lagophthalmos right eye, unspecified eyelid
H02.204   Unspecified lagophthalmos left upper eyelid
H02.205   Unspecified lagophthalmos left lower eyelid
H02.206   Unspecified lagophthalmos left eye, unspecified eyelid
H02.209   Unspecified lagophthalmos unspecified eye, unspecified eyelid

● **H02.21   Cicatricial lagophthalmos**
Upper or lower eyelid does not close due to scar or tightening
H02.211   Cicatricial lagophthalmos right upper eyelid
H02.212   Cicatricial lagophthalmos right lower eyelid
H02.213   Cicatricial lagophthalmos right eye, unspecified eyelid
H02.214   Cicatricial lagophthalmos left upper eyelid
H02.215   Cicatricial lagophthalmos left lower eyelid
H02.216   Cicatricial lagophthalmos left eye, unspecified eyelid
H02.219   Cicatricial lagophthalmos unspecified eye, unspecified eyelid

● **H02.22   Mechanical lagophthalmos**
Inability to close lids due to structural disorder
H02.221   Mechanical lagophthalmos right upper eyelid
H02.222   Mechanical lagophthalmos right lower eyelid
H02.223   Mechanical lagophthalmos right eye, unspecified eyelid
H02.224   Mechanical lagophthalmos left upper eyelid
H02.225   Mechanical lagophthalmos left lower eyelid
H02.226   Mechanical lagophthalmos left eye, unspecified eyelid
H02.229   Mechanical lagophthalmos unspecified eye, unspecified eyelid

● **H02.23   Paralytic lagophthalmos**
Eyelids do not close due to paralysis
H02.231   Paralytic lagophthalmos right upper eyelid
H02.232   Paralytic lagophthalmos right lower eyelid
H02.233   Paralytic lagophthalmos right eye, unspecified eyelid
H02.234   Paralytic lagophthalmos left upper eyelid
H02.235   Paralytic lagophthalmos left lower eyelid
H02.236   Paralytic lagophthalmos left eye, unspecified eyelid
H02.239   Paralytic lagophthalmos unspecified eye, unspecified eyelid

(See Plate 81, middle, on page 65.)

● **H02.3   Blepharochalasis**
Relaxation of skin of eyelid, due to atrophy of intercellular tissue
Pseudoptosis
H02.30   Blepharochalasis unspecified eye, unspecified eyelid
H02.31   Blepharochalasis right upper eyelid
H02.32   Blepharochalasis right lower eyelid
H02.33   Blepharochalasis right eye, unspecified eyelid
H02.34   Blepharochalasis left upper eyelid
H02.35   Blepharochalasis left lower eyelid
H02.36   Blepharochalasis left eye, unspecified eyelid

● **H02.4   Ptosis of eyelid**
Falling forward, drooping, sagging of eyelid
● **H02.40   Unspecified ptosis of eyelid**
H02.401   Unspecified ptosis of right eyelid
H02.402   Unspecified ptosis of left eyelid
H02.403   Unspecified ptosis of bilateral eyelids
H02.409   Unspecified ptosis of unspecified eyelid

● **H02.41   Mechanical ptosis of eyelid**
H02.411   Mechanical ptosis of right eyelid
H02.412   Mechanical ptosis of left eyelid
H02.413   Mechanical ptosis of bilateral eyelids
H02.419   Mechanical ptosis of unspecified eyelid

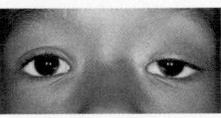

Figure 7-3 Ptosis of eyelid. (From Yanoff: Ophthalmology, ed 3, Mosby, Inc., 2008)

Item 7-1 Ptosis of eyelid is drooping of the upper eyelid over the pupil when the eyes are fully opened resulting from nerve or muscle damage, which may require surgical correction.

CHAPTER 7 (H00-H59)

CHAPTER 7 (H00-H59)

● H02.42   Myogenic ptosis of eyelid
    H02.421   Myogenic ptosis of right eyelid
    H02.422   Myogenic ptosis of left eyelid
    H02.423   Myogenic ptosis of bilateral eyelids
    H02.429   Myogenic ptosis of unspecified eyelid

● H02.43   Paralytic ptosis of eyelid
    Neurogenic ptosis of eyelid
    H02.431   Paralytic ptosis of right eyelid
    H02.432   Paralytic ptosis of left eyelid
    H02.433   Paralytic ptosis of bilateral eyelids
    H02.439   Paralytic ptosis unspecified eyelid

● H02.5   Other disorders affecting eyelid function
    Excludes2   blepharospasm (G24.5)
               organic tic (G25.69)
               psychogenic tic (F95.-)

● H02.51   Abnormal innervation syndrome
    H02.511   Abnormal innervation syndrome right upper eyelid
    H02.512   Abnormal innervation syndrome right lower eyelid
    H02.513   Abnormal innervation syndrome right eye, unspecified eyelid
    H02.514   Abnormal innervation syndrome left upper eyelid
    H02.515   Abnormal innervation syndrome left lower eyelid
    H02.516   Abnormal innervation syndrome left eye, unspecified eyelid
    H02.519   Abnormal innervation syndrome unspecified eye, unspecified eyelid

● H02.52   Blepharophimosis
    Drooping of eyelid with reduced lid size
    Ankyloblepharon
    H02.521   Blepharophimosis right upper eyelid
    H02.522   Blepharophimosis right lower eyelid
    H02.523   Blepharophimosis right eye, unspecified eyelid
    H02.524   Blepharophimosis left upper eyelid
    H02.525   Blepharophimosis left lower eyelid
    H02.526   Blepharophimosis left eye, unspecified eyelid
    H02.529   Blepharophimosis unspecified eye, unspecified lid

● H02.53   Eyelid retraction
    Eyelid lag
    H02.531   Eyelid retraction right upper eyelid
    H02.532   Eyelid retraction right lower eyelid
    H02.533   Eyelid retraction right eye, unspecified eyelid
    H02.534   Eyelid retraction left upper eyelid
    H02.535   Eyelid retraction left lower eyelid
    H02.536   Eyelid retraction left eye, unspecified eyelid
    H02.539   Eyelid retraction unspecified eye, unspecified lid

H02.59   Other disorders affecting eyelid function
    Deficient blink reflex
    Sensory disorders

● H02.6   Xanthelasma of eyelid
    Yellow-to-orange patches or pimples clustered together on eyelid
    H02.60   Xanthelasma of unspecified eye, unspecified eyelid
    H02.61   Xanthelasma of right upper eyelid
    H02.62   Xanthelasma of right lower eyelid
    H02.63   Xanthelasma of right eye, unspecified eyelid
    H02.64   Xanthelasma of left upper eyelid
    H02.65   Xanthelasma of left lower eyelid
    H02.66   Xanthelasma of left eye, unspecified eyelid

● H02.7   Other and unspecified degenerative disorders of eyelid and periocular area
    H02.70   Unspecified degenerative disorders of eyelid and periocular area

● H02.71   Chloasma of eyelid and periocular area
    Dyspigmentation of eyelid
    Hyperpigmentation of eyelid
    H02.711   Chloasma of right upper eyelid and periocular area
    H02.712   Chloasma of right lower eyelid and periocular area
    H02.713   Chloasma of right eye, unspecified eyelid and periocular area
    H02.714   Chloasma of left upper eyelid and periocular area
    H02.715   Chloasma of left lower eyelid and periocular area
    H02.716   Chloasma of left eye, unspecified eyelid and periocular area
    H02.719   Chloasma of unspecified eye, unspecified eyelid and periocular area

● H02.72   Madarosis of eyelid and periocular area
    Loss of eyelashes and/or eyebrows
    Hypotrichosis of eyelid
    H02.721   Madarosis of right upper eyelid and periocular area
    H02.722   Madarosis of right lower eyelid and periocular area
    H02.723   Madarosis of right eye, unspecified eyelid and periocular area
    H02.724   Madarosis of left upper eyelid and periocular area
    H02.725   Madarosis of left lower eyelid and periocular area
    H02.726   Madarosis of left eye, unspecified eyelid and periocular area
    H02.729   Madarosis of unspecified eye, unspecified eyelid and periocular area

● H02.73   Vitiligo of eyelid and periocular area
    Skin pigmentation disease characterized by white patches
    Hypopigmentation of eyelid
    H02.731   Vitiligo of right upper eyelid and periocular area
    H02.732   Vitiligo of right lower eyelid and periocular area
    H02.733   Vitiligo of right eye, unspecified eyelid and periocular area
    H02.734   Vitiligo of left upper eyelid and periocular area
    H02.735   Vitiligo of left lower eyelid and periocular area
    H02.736   Vitiligo of left eye, unspecified eyelid and periocular area
    H02.739   Vitiligo of unspecified eye, unspecified eyelid and periocular area

● H02.79   Other degenerative disorders of eyelid and periocular area

◀ New   ◀▥▥ Revised   ~~deleted~~ Deleted   Excludes 1   Excludes 2   Includes   Use additional   Code first   Code also   Unspecified

OGCR Official Guidelines   **X** Assign placeholder X   ● Use Additional Character(s)   ▶ Manifestation Code   **Coding Clinic**

● **H02.8   Other specified disorders of eyelid**
  ● **H02.81   Retained foreign body in eyelid**
    Use additional code to identify the type of retained foreign body (Z18.-)

    Excludes1   laceration of eyelid with foreign body (S01.12-)
         retained intraocular foreign body (H44.6-, H44.7-)
         superficial foreign body of eyelid and periocular area (S00.25-)

    H02.811   Retained foreign body in right upper eyelid
    H02.812   Retained foreign body in right lower eyelid
    H02.813   Retained foreign body in right eye, unspecified eyelid
    H02.814   Retained foreign body in left upper eyelid
    H02.815   Retained foreign body in left lower eyelid
    H02.816   Retained foreign body in left eye, unspecified eyelid
    H02.819   Retained foreign body in unspecified eye, unspecified eyelid

  ● **H02.82   Cysts of eyelid**
    Sebaceous cyst of eyelid
    H02.821   Cysts of right upper eyelid
    H02.822   Cysts of right lower eyelid
    H02.823   Cysts of right eye, unspecified eyelid
    H02.824   Cysts of left upper eyelid
    H02.825   Cysts of left lower eyelid
    H02.826   Cysts of left eye, unspecified eyelid
    H02.829   Cysts of unspecified eye, unspecified eyelid

  ● **H02.83   Dermatochalasis of eyelid**
    Skin is inelastic and hangs loosely in folds
    H02.831   Dermatochalasis of right upper eyelid
    H02.832   Dermatochalasis of right lower eyelid
    H02.833   Dermatochalasis of right eye, unspecified eyelid
    H02.834   Dermatochalasis of left upper eyelid
    H02.835   Dermatochalasis of left lower eyelid
    H02.836   Dermatochalasis of left eye, unspecified eyelid
    H02.839   Dermatochalasis of unspecified eye, unspecified eyelid

  ● **H02.84   Edema of eyelid**
    Hyperemia of eyelid
    H02.841   Edema of right upper eyelid
    H02.842   Edema of right lower eyelid
    H02.843   Edema of right eye, unspecified eyelid
    H02.844   Edema of left upper eyelid
    H02.845   Edema of left lower eyelid
    H02.846   Edema of left eye, unspecified eyelid
    H02.849   Edema of unspecified eye, unspecified eyelid

  ● **H02.85   Elephantiasis of eyelid**
    Massive secondary lymphedema with hypertrophy of skin and subcutaneous tissues (pachyderma)
    H02.851   Elephantiasis of right upper eyelid
    H02.852   Elephantiasis of right lower eyelid
    H02.853   Elephantiasis of right eye, unspecified eyelid
    H02.854   Elephantiasis of left upper eyelid
    H02.855   Elephantiasis of left lower eyelid

    H02.856   Elephantiasis of left eye, unspecified eyelid
    H02.859   Elephantiasis of unspecified eye, unspecified eyelid

  ● **H02.86   Hypertrichosis of eyelid**
    Excessive growth of hair
    H02.861   Hypertrichosis of right upper eyelid
    H02.862   Hypertrichosis of right lower eyelid
    H02.863   Hypertrichosis of right eye, unspecified eyelid
    H02.864   Hypertrichosis of left upper eyelid
    H02.865   Hypertrichosis of left lower eyelid
    H02.866   Hypertrichosis of left eye, unspecified eyelid
    H02.869   Hypertrichosis of unspecified eye, unspecified eyelid

  ● **H02.87   Vascular anomalies of eyelid**
    H02.871   Vascular anomalies of right upper eyelid
    H02.872   Vascular anomalies of right lower eyelid
    H02.873   Vascular anomalies of right eye, unspecified eyelid
    H02.874   Vascular anomalies of left upper eyelid
    H02.875   Vascular anomalies of left lower eyelid
    H02.876   Vascular anomalies of left eye, unspecified eyelid
    H02.879   Vascular anomalies of unspecified eye, unspecified eyelid

  H02.89   Other specified disorders of eyelid
    Hemorrhage of eyelid

  H02.9   Unspecified disorder of eyelid
    Disorder of eyelid NOS

● **H04   Disorders of lacrimal system**
  Excludes1   congenital malformations of lacrimal system (Q10.4-Q10.6)

  ● **H04.0   Dacryoadenitis**
    Inflammation of lacrimal gland
    ● **H04.00   Unspecified dacryoadenitis**
      H04.001   Unspecified dacryoadenitis, right lacrimal gland
      H04.002   Unspecified dacryoadenitis, left lacrimal gland
      H04.003   Unspecified dacryoadenitis, bilateral lacrimal glands
      H04.009   Unspecified dacryoadenitis, unspecified lacrimal gland

    ● **H04.01   Acute dacryoadenitis**
      H04.011   Acute dacryoadenitis, right lacrimal gland
      H04.012   Acute dacryoadenitis, left lacrimal gland
      H04.013   Acute dacryoadenitis, bilateral lacrimal glands
      H04.019   Acute dacryoadenitis, unspecified lacrimal gland

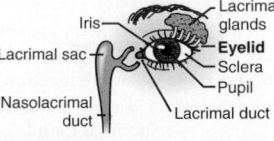

Figure 7-4   Lacrimal apparatus. (From Buck CJ: Step-by-Step Medical Coding, Philadelphia, WB Saunders, 2006, p 302)

(See Plate 82 on page 67.)

CHAPTER 7 (H00-H59)

● **H04.02**   **Chronic dacryoadenitis**
     H04.021   Chronic dacryoadenitis, right lacrimal gland
     H04.022   Chronic dacryoadenitis, left lacrimal gland
     H04.023   Chronic dacryoadenitis, bilateral lacrimal gland
     H04.029   Chronic dacryoadenitis, unspecified lacrimal gland

● **H04.03**   **Chronic enlargement of lacrimal gland**
     H04.031   Chronic enlargement of right lacrimal gland
     H04.032   Chronic enlargement of left lacrimal gland
     H04.033   Chronic enlargement of bilateral lacrimal glands
     H04.039   Chronic enlargement of unspecified lacrimal gland

● **H04.1**   **Other disorders of lacrimal gland**
   ● **H04.11**   **Dacryops**
       Watery eye or distention of lacrimal duct due to fluid
     H04.111   Dacryops of right lacrimal gland
     H04.112   Dacryops of left lacrimal gland
     H04.113   Dacryops of bilateral lacrimal glands
     H04.119   Dacryops of unspecified lacrimal gland

   ● **H04.12**   **Dry eye syndrome**
       Tear film insufficiency, NOS
     H04.121   Dry eye syndrome of right lacrimal gland
     H04.122   Dry eye syndrome of left lacrimal gland
     H04.123   Dry eye syndrome of bilateral lacrimal glands
     H04.129   Dry eye syndrome of unspecified lacrimal gland

   ● **H04.13**   **Lacrimal cyst**
       Lacrimal cystic degeneration
     H04.131   Lacrimal cyst right lacrimal gland
     H04.132   Lacrimal cyst left lacrimal gland
     H04.133   Lacrimal cyst bilateral lacrimal glands
     H04.139   Lacrimal cyst unspecified lacrimal gland

   ● **H04.14**   **Primary lacrimal gland atrophy**
     H04.141   Primary lacrimal gland atrophy, right lacrimal gland
     H04.142   Primary lacrimal gland atrophy, left lacrimal gland
     H04.143   Primary lacrimal gland atrophy, bilateral lacrimal glands
     H04.149   Primary lacrimal gland atrophy, unspecified lacrimal gland

   ● **H04.15**   **Secondary lacrimal gland atrophy**
     H04.151   Secondary lacrimal gland atrophy, right lacrimal gland
     H04.152   Secondary lacrimal gland atrophy, left lacrimal gland
     H04.153   Secondary lacrimal gland atrophy, bilateral lacrimal glands
     H04.159   Secondary lacrimal gland atrophy, unspecified lacrimal gland

   ● **H04.16**   **Lacrimal gland dislocation**
     H04.161   Lacrimal gland dislocation, right lacrimal gland
     H04.162   Lacrimal gland dislocation, left lacrimal gland

     H04.163   Lacrimal gland dislocation, bilateral lacrimal glands
     H04.169   Lacrimal gland dislocation, unspecified lacrimal gland

   H04.19   Other specified disorders of lacrimal gland

● **H04.2**   **Epiphora**
     Overflow of tears due to stricture of lacrimal passages; AKA lacrimation
   ● **H04.20**   **Unspecified epiphora**
     H04.201   Unspecified epiphora, right lacrimal gland
     H04.202   Unspecified epiphora, left lacrimal gland
     H04.203   Unspecified epiphora, bilateral lacrimal glands
     H04.209   Unspecified epiphora, unspecified lacrimal gland

   ● **H04.21**   **Epiphora due to excess lacrimation**
     H04.211   Epiphora due to excess lacrimation, right lacrimal gland
     H04.212   Epiphora due to excess lacrimation, left lacrimal gland
     H04.213   Epiphora due to excess lacrimation, bilateral lacrimal glands
     H04.219   Epiphora due to excess lacrimation, unspecified lacrimal gland

   ● **H04.22**   **Epiphora due to insufficient drainage**
     H04.221   Epiphora due to insufficient drainage, right lacrimal gland
     H04.222   Epiphora due to insufficient drainage, left lacrimal gland
     H04.223   Epiphora due to insufficient drainage, bilateral lacrimal glands
     H04.229   Epiphora due to insufficient drainage, unspecified lacrimal gland

● **H04.3**   **Acute and unspecified inflammation of lacrimal passages**
     Excludes1   neonatal dacryocystitis (P39.1)
   ● **H04.30**   **Unspecified dacryocystitis**
     H04.301   Unspecified dacryocystitis of right lacrimal passage
     H04.302   Unspecified dacryocystitis of left lacrimal passage
     H04.303   Unspecified dacryocystitis of bilateral lacrimal passages
     H04.309   Unspecified dacryocystitis of unspecified lacrimal passage

   ● **H04.31**   **Phlegmonous dacryocystitis**
       Cellulitis of lacrimal sac
     H04.311   Phlegmonous dacryocystitis of right lacrimal passage
     H04.312   Phlegmonous dacryocystitis of left lacrimal passage
     H04.313   Phlegmonous dacryocystitis of bilateral lacrimal passages
     H04.319   Phlegmonous dacryocystitis of unspecified lacrimal passage

   ● **H04.32**   **Acute dacryocystitis**
       Acute dacryopericystitis
     H04.321   Acute dacryocystitis of right lacrimal passage
     H04.322   Acute dacryocystitis of left lacrimal passage
     H04.323   Acute dacryocystitis of bilateral lacrimal passages
     H04.329   Acute dacryocystitis of unspecified lacrimal passage

◀ New   ◀▥ Revised   ~~deleted~~ Deleted   Excludes 1   Excludes 2   Includes   Use additional   Code first   Code also   Unspecified
OGCR Official Guidelines   **X** Assign placeholder X   ● Use Additional Character(s)   ▶ Manifestation Code   **Coding Clinic**

● **H04.33** Acute lacrimal canaliculitis
    H04.331 Acute lacrimal canaliculitis of right lacrimal passage
    H04.332 Acute lacrimal canaliculitis of left lacrimal passage
    H04.333 Acute lacrimal canaliculitis of bilateral lacrimal passages
    H04.339 Acute lacrimal canaliculitis of unspecified lacrimal passage

● **H04.4** Chronic inflammation of lacrimal passages
  ● **H04.41** Chronic dacryocystitis
    Inflammation of lacrimal sac
    H04.411 Chronic dacryocystitis of right lacrimal passage
    H04.412 Chronic dacryocystitis of left lacrimal passage
    H04.413 Chronic dacryocystitis of bilateral lacrimal passages
    H04.419 Chronic dacryocystitis of unspecified lacrimal passage

  ● **H04.42** Chronic lacrimal canaliculitis
    Inflammation of lacrimal ducts
    H04.421 Chronic lacrimal canaliculitis of right lacrimal passage
    H04.422 Chronic lacrimal canaliculitis of left lacrimal passage
    H04.423 Chronic lacrimal canaliculitis of bilateral lacrimal passages
    H04.429 Chronic lacrimal canaliculitis of unspecified lacrimal passage

  ● **H04.43** Chronic lacrimal mucocele
    Accumulation of mucous secretion
    H04.431 Chronic lacrimal mucocele of right lacrimal passage
    H04.432 Chronic lacrimal mucocele of left lacrimal passage
    H04.433 Chronic lacrimal mucocele of bilateral lacrimal passages
    H04.439 Chronic lacrimal mucocele of unspecified lacrimal passage

● **H04.5** Stenosis and insufficiency of lacrimal passages
  ● **H04.51** Dacryolith
    Concretion in lacrimal sac/duct; AKA lacrimal calculus
    H04.511 Dacryolith of right lacrimal passage
    H04.512 Dacryolith of left lacrimal passage
    H04.513 Dacryolith of bilateral lacrimal passages
    H04.519 Dacryolith of unspecified lacrimal passage

  ● **H04.52** Eversion of lacrimal punctum
    Turning out of lacrimal drainage opening
    H04.521 Eversion of right lacrimal punctum
    H04.522 Eversion of left lacrimal punctum
    H04.523 Eversion of bilateral lacrimal punctum
    H04.529 Eversion of unspecified lacrimal punctum

  ● **H04.53** Neonatal obstruction of nasolacrimal duct
    Excludes1 congenital stenosis and stricture of lacrimal duct (Q10.5)
    H04.531 Neonatal obstruction of right nasolacrimal duct   **N**
    H04.532 Neonatal obstruction of left nasolacrimal duct   **N**
    H04.533 Neonatal obstruction of bilateral nasolacrimal duct   **N**
    H04.539 Neonatal obstruction of unspecified nasolacrimal duct   **N**

● **H04.54** Stenosis of lacrimal canaliculi
    H04.541 Stenosis of right lacrimal canaliculi
    H04.542 Stenosis of left lacrimal canaliculi
    H04.543 Stenosis of bilateral lacrimal canaliculi
    H04.549 Stenosis of unspecified lacrimal canaliculi

● **H04.55** Acquired stenosis of nasolacrimal duct
    H04.551 Acquired stenosis of right nasolacrimal duct
    H04.552 Acquired stenosis of left nasolacrimal duct
    H04.553 Acquired stenosis of bilateral nasolacrimal duct
    H04.559 Acquired stenosis of unspecified nasolacrimal duct

● **H04.56** Stenosis of lacrimal punctum
    H04.561 Stenosis of right lacrimal punctum
    H04.562 Stenosis of left lacrimal punctum
    H04.563 Stenosis of bilateral lacrimal punctum
    H04.569 Stenosis of unspecified lacrimal punctum

● **H04.57** Stenosis of lacrimal sac
    H04.571 Stenosis of right lacrimal sac
    H04.572 Stenosis of left lacrimal sac
    H04.573 Stenosis of bilateral lacrimal sac
    H04.579 Stenosis of unspecified lacrimal sac

● **H04.6** Other changes of lacrimal passages
  ● **H04.61** Lacrimal fistula
    H04.611 Lacrimal fistula right lacrimal passage
    H04.612 Lacrimal fistula left lacrimal passage
    H04.613 Lacrimal fistula bilateral lacrimal passages
    H04.619 Lacrimal fistula unspecified lacrimal passage
  H04.69 Other changes of lacrimal passages

● **H04.8** Other disorders of lacrimal system
  ● **H04.81** Granuloma of lacrimal passages
    Inflammatory response due to infectious or noninfectious agents
    H04.811 Granuloma of right lacrimal passage
    H04.812 Granuloma of left lacrimal passage
    H04.813 Granuloma of bilateral lacrimal passages
    H04.819 Granuloma of unspecified lacrimal passage
  H04.89 Other disorders of lacrimal system

H04.9 Disorder of lacrimal system, unspecified

● **H05** Disorders of orbit
  Excludes1 congenital malformation of orbit (Q10.7)
  ● **H05.0** Acute inflammation of orbit
    H05.00 Unspecified acute inflammation of orbit
    ● **H05.01** Cellulitis of orbit
      Infection of soft tissue of orbit
      Abscess of orbit
      H05.011 Cellulitis of right orbit
      H05.012 Cellulitis of left orbit
      H05.013 Cellulitis of bilateral orbits
      H05.019 Cellulitis of unspecified orbit
    ● **H05.02** Osteomyelitis of orbit
      Infection of boney orbit of eye
      H05.021 Osteomyelitis of right orbit
      H05.022 Osteomyelitis of left orbit
      H05.023 Osteomyelitis of bilateral orbits
      H05.029 Osteomyelitis of unspecified orbit

● **H05.03** Periostitis of orbit
Inflammation of periosteum (membrane covering bone surface)
H05.031 Periostitis of right orbit
H05.032 Periostitis of left orbit
H05.033 Periostitis of bilateral orbits
H05.039 Periostitis of unspecified orbit

● **H05.04** Tenonitis of orbit
Inflammation of tenon capsule (space enclosing fascia of Tenon between eyeball and fat of orbit)
H05.041 Tenonitis of right orbit
H05.042 Tenonitis of left orbit
H05.043 Tenonitis of bilateral orbits
H05.049 Tenonitis of unspecified orbit

● **H05.1** Chronic inflammatory disorders of orbit
H05.10 Unspecified chronic inflammatory disorders of orbit

● **H05.11** Granuloma of orbit
Pseudotumor (inflammatory) of orbit
H05.111 Granuloma of right orbit
H05.112 Granuloma of left orbit
H05.113 Granuloma of bilateral orbits
H05.119 Granuloma of unspecified orbit

● **H05.12** Orbital myositis
Inflammation of extraocular muscles of orbit
H05.121 Orbital myositis, right orbit
H05.122 Orbital myositis, left orbit
H05.123 Orbital myositis, bilateral
H05.129 Orbital myositis, unspecified orbit

● **H05.2** Exophthalmic conditions
Bulging eyes
H05.20 Unspecified exophthalmos

● **H05.21** Displacement (lateral) of globe
H05.211 Displacement (lateral) of globe, right eye
H05.212 Displacement (lateral) of globe, left eye
H05.213 Displacement (lateral) of globe, bilateral
H05.219 Displacement (lateral) of globe, unspecified eye

● **H05.22** Edema of orbit
Orbital congestion
H05.221 Edema of right orbit
H05.222 Edema of left orbit
H05.223 Edema of bilateral orbit
H05.229 Edema of unspecified orbit

● **H05.23** Hemorrhage of orbit
H05.231 Hemorrhage of right orbit
H05.232 Hemorrhage of left orbit
H05.233 Hemorrhage of bilateral orbit
H05.239 Hemorrhage of unspecified orbit

● **H05.24** Constant exophthalmos
Constant bulging eyes, often symptom of Graves disease
H05.241 Constant exophthalmos, right eye
H05.242 Constant exophthalmos, left eye
H05.243 Constant exophthalmos, bilateral
H05.249 Constant exophthalmos, unspecified eye

● **H05.25** Intermittent exophthalmos
Intermittent bulging eye occurring with bending forward or sharp turning of head
H05.251 Intermittent exophthalmos, right eye
H05.252 Intermittent exophthalmos, left eye
H05.253 Intermittent exophthalmos, bilateral
H05.259 Intermittent exophthalmos, unspecified eye

● **H05.26** Pulsating exophthalmos
Bulging eyes with pulsation and bruit, often due to aneurysm pushing eye forward
H05.261 Pulsating exophthalmos, right eye
H05.262 Pulsating exophthalmos, left eye
H05.263 Pulsating exophthalmos, bilateral
H05.269 Pulsating exophthalmos, unspecified eye

● **H05.3** Deformity of orbit
Excludes1 congenital deformity of orbit (Q10.7)
hypertelorism (Q75.2)
H05.30 Unspecified deformity of orbit

● **H05.31** Atrophy of orbit
H05.311 Atrophy of right orbit
H05.312 Atrophy of left orbit
H05.313 Atrophy of bilateral orbit
H05.319 Atrophy of unspecified orbit

● **H05.32** Deformity of orbit due to bone disease
Code also associated bone disease
H05.321 Deformity of right orbit due to bone disease
H05.322 Deformity of left orbit due to bone disease
H05.323 Deformity of bilateral orbits due to bone disease
H05.329 Deformity of unspecified orbit due to bone disease

● **H05.33** Deformity of orbit due to trauma or surgery
H05.331 Deformity of right orbit due to trauma or surgery
H05.332 Deformity of left orbit due to trauma or surgery
H05.333 Deformity of bilateral orbits due to trauma or surgery
H05.339 Deformity of unspecified orbit due to trauma or surgery

● **H05.34** Enlargement of orbit
H05.341 Enlargement of right orbit
H05.342 Enlargement of left orbit
H05.343 Enlargement of bilateral orbits
H05.349 Enlargement of unspecified orbit

● **H05.35** Exostosis of orbit
H05.351 Exostosis of right orbit
H05.352 Exostosis of left orbit
H05.353 Exostosis of bilateral orbits
H05.359 Exostosis of unspecified orbit

● **H05.4** Enophthalmos
Recessed eyeball into orbit
H05.40 Unspecified enophthalmos
H05.401 Unspecified enophthalmos, right eye
H05.402 Unspecified enophthalmos, left eye
H05.403 Unspecified enophthalmos, bilateral
H05.409 Unspecified enophthalmos, unspecified eye

● **H05.41** Enophthalmos due to atrophy of orbital tissue

    H05.411   **Enophthalmos due to atrophy of orbital tissue, right eye**

    H05.412   **Enophthalmos due to atrophy of orbital tissue, left eye**

    H05.413   **Enophthalmos due to atrophy of orbital tissue, bilateral**

    H05.419   **Enophthalmos due to atrophy of orbital tissue, unspecified eye**

● **H05.42** Enophthalmos due to trauma or surgery

    H05.421   **Enophthalmos due to trauma or surgery, right eye**

    H05.422   **Enophthalmos due to trauma or surgery, left eye**

    H05.423   **Enophthalmos due to trauma or surgery, bilateral**

    H05.429   **Enophthalmos due to trauma or surgery, unspecified eye**

● **H05.5** Retained (old) foreign body following penetrating wound of orbit

    Retrobulbar foreign body

    Use additional code to identify the type of retained foreign body (Z18.-)

    Excludes1   current penetrating wound of orbit (S05.4-)

    Excludes2   retained foreign body of eyelid (H02.81-) retained intraocular foreign body (H44.6-, H44.7-)

    H05.50   **Retained (old) foreign body following penetrating wound of unspecified orbit**

    H05.51   **Retained (old) foreign body following penetrating wound of right orbit**

    H05.52   **Retained (old) foreign body following penetrating wound of left orbit**

    H05.53   **Retained (old) foreign body following penetrating wound of bilateral orbits**

● **H05.8** Other disorders of orbit

    ● **H05.81** Cyst of orbit

       Encephalocele of orbit

       H05.811   **Cyst of right orbit**

       H05.812   **Cyst of left orbit**

       H05.813   **Cyst of bilateral orbits**

       H05.819   **Cyst of unspecified orbit**

    ● **H05.82** Myopathy of extraocular muscles

       Weakness of muscles of eye

       H05.821   **Myopathy of extraocular muscles, right orbit**

       H05.822   **Myopathy of extraocular muscles, left orbit**

       H05.823   **Myopathy of extraocular muscles, bilateral**

       H05.829   **Myopathy of extraocular muscles, unspecified orbit**

    H05.89   **Other disorders of orbit**

    H05.9   **Unspecified disorder of orbit**

DISORDERS OF CONJUNCTIVA (H10-H11)

(See Plate 81, upper, on page 66.)

● **H10** Conjunctivitis

    Inflammation of membrane of the inside of the eyelid or on surface of eye (conjunctiva)

    Excludes1   keratoconjunctivitis (H16.2-)

    ● **H10.0** Mucopurulent conjunctivitis

       ● **H10.01** Acute follicular conjunctivitis

          H10.011   **Acute follicular conjunctivitis, right eye**

          H10.012   **Acute follicular conjunctivitis, left eye**

          H10.013   **Acute follicular conjunctivitis, bilateral**

          H10.019   **Acute follicular conjunctivitis, unspecified eye**

       ● **H10.02** Other mucopurulent conjunctivitis

          H10.021   **Other mucopurulent conjunctivitis, right eye**

          H10.022   **Other mucopurulent conjunctivitis, left eye**

          H10.023   **Other mucopurulent conjunctivitis, bilateral**

          H10.029   **Other mucopurulent conjunctivitis, unspecified eye**

    ● **H10.1** Acute atopic conjunctivitis

       Acute papillary conjunctivitis

       H10.10   **Acute atopic conjunctivitis, unspecified eye**

       H10.11   **Acute atopic conjunctivitis, right eye**

       H10.12   **Acute atopic conjunctivitis, left eye**

       H10.13   **Acute atopic conjunctivitis, bilateral**

    ● **H10.2** Other acute conjunctivitis

       ● **H10.21** Acute toxic conjunctivitis

          Acute chemical conjunctivitis

          Code first (T51-T65) to identify chemical and intent

          Excludes1   burn and corrosion of eye and adnexa (T26.-)

          H10.211   **Acute toxic conjunctivitis, right eye**

          H10.212   **Acute toxic conjunctivitis, left eye**

          H10.213   **Acute toxic conjunctivitis, bilateral**

          H10.219   **Acute toxic conjunctivitis, unspecified eye**

       ● **H10.22** Pseudomembranous conjunctivitis

          H10.221   **Pseudomembranous conjunctivitis, right eye**

          H10.222   **Pseudomembranous conjunctivitis, left eye**

          H10.223   **Pseudomembranous conjunctivitis, bilateral**

          H10.229   **Pseudomembranous conjunctivitis, unspecified eye**

       ● **H10.23** Serous conjunctivitis, except viral

          Excludes1   viral conjunctivitis (B30.-)

          H10.231   **Serous conjunctivitis, except viral, right eye**

          H10.232   **Serous conjunctivitis, except viral, left eye**

          H10.233   **Serous conjunctivitis, except viral, bilateral**

          H10.239   **Serous conjunctivitis, except viral, unspecified eye**

CHAPTER 7 (H00-H59)

● **H10.3**   **Unspecified acute conjunctivitis**

     Excludes1   ophthalmia neonatorum NOS (P39.1)

     H10.30   **Unspecified** acute conjunctivitis, unspecified eye

     H10.31   **Unspecified** acute conjunctivitis, right eye

     H10.32   **Unspecified** acute conjunctivitis, left eye

     H10.33   **Unspecified** acute conjunctivitis, bilateral

● **H10.4**   **Chronic conjunctivitis**

   ● **H10.40**   Unspecified chronic conjunctivitis

     H10.401   **Unspecified** chronic conjunctivitis, right eye

     H10.402   **Unspecified** chronic conjunctivitis, left eye

     H10.403   **Unspecified** chronic conjunctivitis, bilateral

     H10.409   **Unspecified** chronic conjunctivitis, unspecified eye

   ● **H10.41**   Chronic giant papillary conjunctivitis

     Inflammation of membrane of the inside of the eyelid or on surface of eye often associated with contact lens wear

     H10.411   Chronic giant papillary conjunctivitis, right eye

     H10.412   Chronic giant papillary conjunctivitis, left eye

     H10.413   Chronic giant papillary conjunctivitis, bilateral

     H10.419   Chronic giant papillary conjunctivitis, **unspecified** eye

   ● **H10.42**   Simple chronic conjunctivitis

     H10.421   Simple chronic conjunctivitis, right eye

     H10.422   Simple chronic conjunctivitis, left eye

     H10.423   Simple chronic conjunctivitis, bilateral

     H10.429   Simple chronic conjunctivitis, **unspecified** eye

   ● **H10.43**   Chronic follicular conjunctivitis

     Inflammation of membrane of the inside of the eyelid or on surface of eye due to topical medications or infection

     H10.431   Chronic follicular conjunctivitis, right eye

     H10.432   Chronic follicular conjunctivitis, left eye

     H10.433   Chronic follicular conjunctivitis, bilateral

     H10.439   Chronic follicular conjunctivitis, **unspecified** eye

   H10.44   Vernal conjunctivitis

     Affecting children, especially boys in which there are flattened papules with thick, gelatinous exudate on conjunctivae on inside of upper lid

     Excludes1   vernal keratoconjunctivitis with limbar and corneal involvement (H16.26-)

   H10.45   Other chronic allergic conjunctivitis

● **H10.5**   **Blepharoconjunctivitis**

     Inflammation of eyelids and conjunctiva

   ● **H10.50**   Unspecified blepharoconjunctivitis

     H10.501   **Unspecified** blepharoconjunctivitis, right eye

     H10.502   **Unspecified** blepharoconjunctivitis, left eye

     H10.503   **Unspecified** blepharoconjunctivitis, bilateral

     H10.509   **Unspecified** blepharoconjunctivitis, unspecified eye

   ● **H10.51**   Ligneous conjunctivitis

     H10.511   Ligneous conjunctivitis, right eye

     H10.512   Ligneous conjunctivitis, left eye

     H10.513   Ligneous conjunctivitis, bilateral

     H10.519   Ligneous conjunctivitis, **unspecified** eye

   ● **H10.52**   Angular blepharoconjunctivitis

     H10.521   Angular blepharoconjunctivitis, right eye

     H10.522   Angular blepharoconjunctivitis, left eye

     H10.523   Angular blepharoconjunctivitis, bilateral

     H10.529   Angular blepharoconjunctivitis, **unspecified** eye

   ● **H10.53**   Contact blepharoconjunctivitis

     H10.531   Contact blepharoconjunctivitis, right eye

     H10.532   Contact blepharoconjunctivitis, left eye

     H10.533   Contact blepharoconjunctivitis, bilateral

     H10.539   Contact blepharoconjunctivitis, **unspecified** eye

   ● **H10.8**   Other conjunctivitis

   ● **H10.81**   Pingueculitis

     Inflammation of a yellow, raised thickening on the white of the eye associated with chronic dry eyes

     Excludes1   pinguecula (H11.15-)

     H10.811   Pingueculitis, right eye

     H10.812   Pingueculitis, left eye

     H10.813   Pingueculitis, bilateral

     H10.819   Pingueculitis, **unspecified** eye

   H10.89   Other conjunctivitis

   H10.9   **Unspecified** conjunctivitis

● **H11**   **Other disorders of conjunctiva**

     Excludes1   keratoconjunctivitis (H16.2-)

   ● **H11.0**   Pterygium of eye

     Excludes1   pseudopterygium (H11.81-)

   ● **H11.00**   Unspecified pterygium of eye

     H11.001   **Unspecified** pterygium of right eye

     H11.002   **Unspecified** pterygium of left eye

     H11.003   **Unspecified** pterygium of eye, bilateral

     H11.009   **Unspecified** pterygium of unspecified eye

   ● **H11.01**   Amyloid pterygium

     H11.011   Amyloid pterygium of right eye

     H11.012   Amyloid pterygium of left eye

     H11.013   Amyloid pterygium of eye, bilateral

     H11.019   Amyloid pterygium of **unspecified** eye

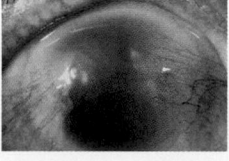

Figure 7-5   Double pterygium. Note both nasal and temporal pterygia in a 57-year-old farmer. (From Yanoff: Ophthalmology, ed 3, Mosby, Inc., 2008)

Item 7–2   **Pterygium** is Greek for batlike. The condition is characterized by a membrane that extends from the limbus to the center of the cornea and resembles a wing.

◀ New   ◀▥ Revised   ~~deleted~~ Deleted   Excludes 1   Excludes 2   Includes   Use additional   Code first   Code also   Unspecified

OGCR Official Guidelines   **X** Assign placeholder X   ● Use Additional Character(s)   ▶ Manifestation Code   **Coding Clinic**

● H11.02 Central pterygium of eye
  H11.021 Central pterygium of right eye
  H11.022 Central pterygium of left eye
  H11.023 Central pterygium of eye, bilateral
  H11.029 Central pterygium of unspecified eye

● H11.03 Double pterygium of eye
  H11.031 Double pterygium of right eye
  H11.032 Double pterygium of left eye
  H11.033 Double pterygium of eye, bilateral
  H11.039 Double pterygium of unspecified eye

● H11.04 Peripheral pterygium of eye, stationary
  H11.041 Peripheral pterygium, stationary, right eye
  H11.042 Peripheral pterygium, stationary, left eye
  H11.043 Peripheral pterygium, stationary, bilateral
  H11.049 Peripheral pterygium, stationary, unspecified eye

● H11.05 Peripheral pterygium of eye, progressive
  H11.051 Peripheral pterygium, progressive, right eye
  H11.052 Peripheral pterygium, progressive, left eye
  H11.053 Peripheral pterygium, progressive, bilateral
  H11.059 Peripheral pterygium, progressive, unspecified eye

● H11.06 Recurrent pterygium of eye
  H11.061 Recurrent pterygium of right eye
  H11.062 Recurrent pterygium of left eye
  H11.063 Recurrent pterygium of eye, bilateral
  H11.069 Recurrent pterygium of unspecified eye

● H11.1 Conjunctival degenerations and deposits
  Excludes2   pseudopterygium (H11.81)
  H11.10 Unspecified conjunctival degenerations

● H11.11 Conjunctival deposits
  H11.111 Conjunctival deposits, right eye
  H11.112 Conjunctival deposits, left eye
  H11.113 Conjunctival deposits, bilateral
  H11.119 Conjunctival deposits, unspecified eye

● H11.12 Conjunctival concretions
  White to yellow nodules within or beneath conjunctiva
  H11.121 Conjunctival concretions, right eye
  H11.122 Conjunctival concretions, left eye
  H11.123 Conjunctival concretions, bilateral
  H11.129 Conjunctival concretions, unspecified eye

● H11.13 Conjunctival pigmentations
  Conjunctival argyrosis [argyria]
  H11.131 Conjunctival pigmentations, right eye
  H11.132 Conjunctival pigmentations, left eye
  H11.133 Conjunctival pigmentations, bilateral
  H11.139 Conjunctival pigmentations, unspecified eye

● H11.14 Conjunctival xerosis, unspecified
  Excludes1   xerosis of conjunctiva due to vitamin A deficiency (E50.0, E50.1)
  H11.141 Conjunctival xerosis, unspecified, right eye
  H11.142 Conjunctival xerosis, unspecified, left eye
  H11.143 Conjunctival xerosis, unspecified, bilateral
  H11.149 Conjunctival xerosis, unspecified, unspecified eye

● H11.15 Pinguecula
  Yellowish spot near sclerocorneal junction, usually on nasal side; associated with aging
  Excludes1   pingueculitis (H10.81-)
  H11.151 Pinguecula, right eye
  H11.152 Pinguecula, left eye
  H11.153 Pinguecula, bilateral
  H11.159 Pinguecula, unspecified eye

● H11.2 Conjunctival scars
  ● H11.21 Conjunctival adhesions and strands (localized)
    H11.211 Conjunctival adhesions and strands (localized), right eye
    H11.212 Conjunctival adhesions and strands (localized), left eye
    H11.213 Conjunctival adhesions and strands (localized), bilateral
    H11.219 Conjunctival adhesions and strands (localized), unspecified eye

  ● H11.22 Conjunctival granuloma
    H11.221 Conjunctival granuloma, right eye
    H11.222 Conjunctival granuloma, left eye
    H11.223 Conjunctival granuloma, bilateral
    H11.229 Conjunctival granuloma, unspecified

  ● H11.23 Symblepharon
    Adhesion between tarsal conjunctiva and bulbar conjunctiva
    H11.231 Symblepharon, right eye
    H11.232 Symblepharon, left eye
    H11.233 Symblepharon, bilateral
    H11.239 Symblepharon, unspecified eye

  ● H11.24 Scarring of conjunctiva
    H11.241 Scarring of conjunctiva, right eye
    H11.242 Scarring of conjunctiva, left eye
    H11.243 Scarring of conjunctiva, bilateral
    H11.249 Scarring of conjunctiva, unspecified eye

● H11.3 Conjunctival hemorrhage
  Subconjunctival hemorrhage
  H11.30 Conjunctival hemorrhage, unspecified eye
  H11.31 Conjunctival hemorrhage, right eye
  H11.32 Conjunctival hemorrhage, left eye
  H11.33 Conjunctival hemorrhage, bilateral

● H11.4 Other conjunctival vascular disorders and cysts
  ● H11.41 Vascular abnormalities of conjunctiva
    Conjunctival aneurysm
    H11.411 Vascular abnormalities of conjunctiva, right eye
    H11.412 Vascular abnormalities of conjunctiva, left eye
    H11.413 Vascular abnormalities of conjunctiva, bilateral
    H11.419 Vascular abnormalities of conjunctiva, unspecified eye

● **H11.42** Conjunctival edema
    H11.421 Conjunctival edema, right eye
    H11.422 Conjunctival edema, left eye
    H11.423 Conjunctival edema, bilateral
    H11.429 Conjunctival edema, unspecified eye

● **H11.43** Conjunctival hyperemia
    H11.431 Conjunctival hyperemia, right eye
    H11.432 Conjunctival hyperemia, left eye
    H11.433 Conjunctival hyperemia, bilateral
    H11.439 Conjunctival hyperemia, unspecified eye

● **H11.44** Conjunctival cysts
    H11.441 Conjunctival cysts, right eye
    H11.442 Conjunctival cysts, left eye
    H11.443 Conjunctival cysts, bilateral
    H11.449 Conjunctival cysts, unspecified eye

● **H11.8** Other specified disorders of conjunctiva
  ● **H11.81** Pseudopterygium of conjunctiva
     Conjunctival scar attached to cornea
    H11.811 Pseudopterygium of conjunctiva, right eye
    H11.812 Pseudopterygium of conjunctiva, left eye
    H11.813 Pseudopterygium of conjunctiva, bilateral
    H11.819 Pseudopterygium of conjunctiva, unspecified eye

  ● **H11.82** Conjunctivochalasis
     Conjunctiva bulges over eyelid margin or covers lower punctum
    H11.821 Conjunctivochalasis, right eye
    H11.822 Conjunctivochalasis, left eye
    H11.823 Conjunctivochalasis, bilateral
    H11.829 Conjunctivochalasis, unspecified eye

  H11.89 Other specified disorders of conjunctiva

H11.9 Unspecified disorder of conjunctiva

DISORDERS OF SCLERA, CORNEA, IRIS AND CILIARY BODY (H15-H22)

● **H15** Disorders of sclera
  ● **H15.0** Scleritis
    Inflammation of the white (sclera and episclera) of the eye.
   ● **H15.00** Unspecified scleritis
     H15.001 Unspecified scleritis, right eye
     H15.002 Unspecified scleritis, left eye
     H15.003 Unspecified scleritis, bilateral
     H15.009 Unspecified scleritis, unspecified eye

   ● **H15.01** Anterior scleritis
     H15.011 Anterior scleritis, right eye
     H15.012 Anterior scleritis, left eye
     H15.013 Anterior scleritis, bilateral
     H15.019 Anterior scleritis, unspecified eye

   ● **H15.02** Brawny scleritis
     Swelling around the cornea that is gelantinous in appearance
     H15.021 Brawny scleritis, right eye
     H15.022 Brawny scleritis, left eye
     H15.023 Brawny scleritis, bilateral
     H15.029 Brawny scleritis, unspecified eye

   ● **H15.03** Posterior scleritis
     Sclerotenonitis
     H15.031 Posterior scleritis, right eye
     H15.032 Posterior scleritis, left eye
     H15.033 Posterior scleritis, bilateral
     H15.039 Posterior scleritis, unspecified eye

● **H15.04** Scleritis with corneal involvement
    H15.041 Scleritis with corneal involvement, right eye
    H15.042 Scleritis with corneal involvement, left eye
    H15.043 Scleritis with corneal involvement, bilateral
    H15.049 Scleritis with corneal involvement, unspecified eye

● **H15.05** Scleromalacia perforans
    Necrotic without inflammation; usually associated with rheumatoid arthritis
    H15.051 Scleromalacia perforans, right eye
    H15.052 Scleromalacia perforans, left eye
    H15.053 Scleromalacia perforans, bilateral
    H15.059 Scleromalacia perforans, unspecified eye

● **H15.09** Other scleritis
    Scleral abscess
    H15.091 Other scleritis, right eye
    H15.092 Other scleritis, left eye
    H15.093 Other scleritis, bilateral
    H15.099 Other scleritis, unspecified eye

● **H15.1** Episcleritis
   Inflammation of the white (sclera and episclera) of the eye.
  ● **H15.10** Unspecified episcleritis
     H15.101 Unspecified episcleritis, right eye
     H15.102 Unspecified episcleritis, left eye
     H15.103 Unspecified episcleritis, bilateral
     H15.109 Unspecified episcleritis, unspecified eye

  ● **H15.11** Episcleritis periodica fugax
     Transient, recurrent inflammation of portion of episclera (connective tissue on the surface of the sclera)
     H15.111 Episcleritis periodica fugax, right eye
     H15.112 Episcleritis periodica fugax, left eye
     H15.113 Episcleritis periodica fugax, bilateral
     H15.119 Episcleritis periodica fugax, unspecified eye

  ● **H15.12** Nodular episcleritis
     Characterized by tender, localized, moveable nodule within inflamed area
     H15.121 Nodular episcleritis, right eye
     H15.122 Nodular episcleritis, left eye
     H15.123 Nodular episcleritis, bilateral
     H15.129 Nodular episcleritis, unspecified eye

● **H15.8** Other disorders of sclera
   Excludes2   blue sclera (Q13.5)
           degenerative myopia (H44.2-)
  ● **H15.81** Equatorial staphyloma
     H15.811 Equatorial staphyloma, right eye
     H15.812 Equatorial staphyloma, left eye
     H15.813 Equatorial staphyloma, bilateral
     H15.819 Equatorial staphyloma, unspecified eye

  ● **H15.82** Localized anterior staphyloma
     H15.821 Localized anterior staphyloma, right eye
     H15.822 Localized anterior staphyloma, left eye
     H15.823 Localized anterior staphyloma, bilateral
     H15.829 Localized anterior staphyloma, unspecified eye

◀ New   ◀═ Revised   ~~deleted~~ Deleted   Excludes 1   Excludes 2   Includes   Use additional   Code first   Code also   Unspecified
OGCR Official Guidelines   **X** Assign placeholder X   ● Use Additional Character(s)   ▶ Manifestation Code   **Coding Clinic**

●H15.83   Staphyloma posticum
    H15.831   Staphyloma posticum, right eye
    H15.832   Staphyloma posticum, left eye
    H15.833   Staphyloma posticum, bilateral
    H15.839   Staphyloma posticum, unspecified eye

●H15.84   Scleral ectasia
    H15.841   Scleral ectasia, right eye
    H15.842   Scleral ectasia, left eye
    H15.843   Scleral ectasia, bilateral
    H15.849   Scleral ectasia, unspecified eye

●H15.85   Ring staphyloma
    H15.851   Ring staphyloma, right eye
    H15.852   Ring staphyloma, left eye
    H15.853   Ring staphyloma, bilateral
    H15.859   Ring staphyloma, unspecified eye

   H15.89   Other disorders of sclera
  H15.9   Unspecified disorder of sclera

●H16   **Keratitis**
   ●H16.0   Corneal ulcer
     ●H16.00   Unspecified corneal ulcer
       H16.001   Unspecified corneal ulcer, right eye
       H16.002   Unspecified corneal ulcer, left eye
       H16.003   Unspecified corneal ulcer, bilateral
       H16.009   Unspecified corneal ulcer, unspecified eye

     ●H16.01   Central corneal ulcer
       H16.011   Central corneal ulcer, right eye
       H16.012   Central corneal ulcer, left eye
       H16.013   Central corneal ulcer, bilateral
       H16.019   Central corneal ulcer, unspecified eye

     ●H16.02   Ring corneal ulcer
       H16.021   Ring corneal ulcer, right eye
       H16.022   Ring corneal ulcer, left eye
       H16.023   Ring corneal ulcer, bilateral
       H16.029   Ring corneal ulcer, unspecified eye

     ●H16.03   Corneal ulcer with hypopyon
       H16.031   Corneal ulcer with hypopyon, right eye
       H16.032   Corneal ulcer with hypopyon, left eye
       H16.033   Corneal ulcer with hypopyon, bilateral
       H16.039   Corneal ulcer with hypopyon, unspecified eye

●H16.04   Marginal corneal ulcer
    H16.041   Marginal corneal ulcer, right eye
    H16.042   Marginal corneal ulcer, left eye
    H16.043   Marginal corneal ulcer, bilateral
    H16.049   Marginal corneal ulcer, unspecified eye

●H16.05   Mooren's corneal ulcer
    H16.051   Mooren's corneal ulcer, right eye
    H16.052   Mooren's corneal ulcer, left eye
    H16.053   Mooren's corneal ulcer, bilateral
    H16.059   Mooren's corneal ulcer, unspecified eye

●H16.06   Mycotic corneal ulcer
    H16.061   Mycotic corneal ulcer, right eye
    H16.062   Mycotic corneal ulcer, left eye
    H16.063   Mycotic corneal ulcer, bilateral
    H16.069   Mycotic corneal ulcer, unspecified eye

●H16.07   Perforated corneal ulcer
    H16.071   Perforated corneal ulcer, right eye
    H16.072   Perforated corneal ulcer, left eye
    H16.073   Perforated corneal ulcer, bilateral
    H16.079   Perforated corneal ulcer, unspecified eye

●H16.1   Other and unspecified superficial keratitis without conjunctivitis
   ●H16.10   Unspecified superficial keratitis
     H16.101   Unspecified superficial keratitis, right eye
     H16.102   Unspecified superficial keratitis, left eye
     H16.103   Unspecified superficial keratitis, bilateral
     H16.109   Unspecified superficial keratitis, unspecified eye

   ●H16.11   Macular keratitis
     Areolar keratitis
     Nummular keratitis
     Stellate keratitis
     Striate keratitis
     H16.111   Macular keratitis, right eye
     H16.112   Macular keratitis, left eye
     H16.113   Macular keratitis, bilateral
     H16.119   Macular keratitis, unspecified eye

   ●H16.12   Filamentary keratitis
     H16.121   Filamentary keratitis, right eye
     H16.122   Filamentary keratitis, left eye
     H16.123   Filamentary keratitis, bilateral
     H16.129   Filamentary keratitis, unspecified eye

   ●H16.13   Photokeratitis
     Snow blindness
     Welders' keratitis
     H16.131   Photokeratitis, right eye
     H16.132   Photokeratitis, left eye
     H16.133   Photokeratitis, bilateral
     H16.139   Photokeratitis, unspecified eye

   ●H16.14   Punctate keratitis
     H16.141   Punctate keratitis, right eye
     H16.142   Punctate keratitis, left eye
     H16.143   Punctate keratitis, bilateral
     H16.149   Punctate keratitis, unspecified eye

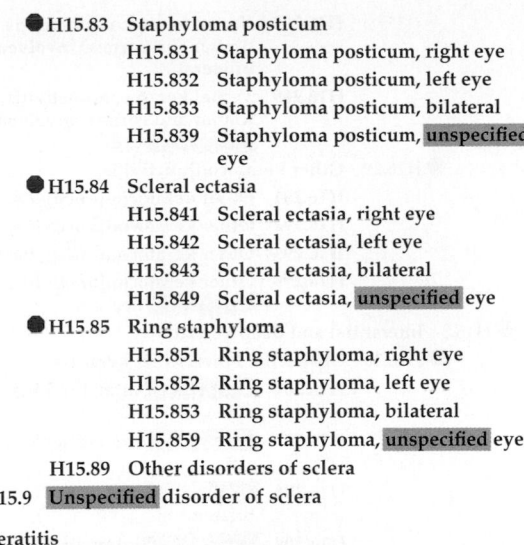

Figure 7-6   Corneal ulcers: marginal, ring, central corneal, rosacea, and Mooren's.

Marginal (catarrhal) ulcer   Ring ulcer   Central corneal ulcer   Rosacea ulcer   Mooren's (rodent) ulcer

Item 7–3   An infected ulcer is usually called a **serpiginous** or **hypopyon** ulcer which is a pus sac in the anterior chamber of the eye. **Marginal** ulcers are usually asymptomatic, not primary, and are often superficial and simple. More severe marginal ulcers spread to form a ring ulcer. **Ring** ulcers can extend around the entire corneal periphery. **Central corneal** ulcers develop when there is an abrasion to the epithelium and an infection develops in the eroded area. The **pyocyaneal** ulcer is the most serious corneal infection, which, if left untreated, can lead to loss of the eye.

CHAPTER 7 (H00-H59)

● **H16.2   Keratoconjunctivitis**
  ● **H16.20   Unspecified keratoconjunctivitis**
      Superficial keratitis with conjunctivitis NOS
    H16.201   Unspecified keratoconjunctivitis, right eye
    H16.202   Unspecified keratoconjunctivitis, left eye
    H16.203   Unspecified keratoconjunctivitis, bilateral
    H16.209   Unspecified keratoconjunctivitis, unspecified eye

  ● **H16.21   Exposure keratoconjunctivitis**
    H16.211   Exposure keratoconjunctivitis, right eye
    H16.212   Exposure keratoconjunctivitis, left eye
    H16.213   Exposure keratoconjunctivitis, bilateral
    H16.219   Exposure keratoconjunctivitis, unspecified eye

  ● **H16.22   Keratoconjunctivitis sicca, not specified as Sjögren's**
      Excludes1   Sjogren's syndrome (M35.01)
    H16.221   Keratoconjunctivitis sicca, not specified as Sjögren's, right eye
    H16.222   Keratoconjunctivitis sicca, not specified as Sjögren's, left eye
    H16.223   Keratoconjunctivitis sicca, not specified as Sjögren's, bilateral
    H16.229   Keratoconjunctivitis sicca, not specified as Sjögren's, unspecified eye

  ● **H16.23   Neurotrophic keratoconjunctivitis**
    H16.231   Neurotrophic keratoconjunctivitis, right eye
    H16.232   Neurotrophic keratoconjunctivitis, left eye
    H16.233   Neurotrophic keratoconjunctivitis, bilateral
    H16.239   Neurotrophic keratoconjunctivitis, unspecified eye

  ● **H16.24   Ophthalmia nodosa**
    H16.241   Ophthalmia nodosa, right eye
    H16.242   Ophthalmia nodosa, left eye
    H16.243   Ophthalmia nodosa, bilateral
    H16.249   Ophthalmia nodosa, unspecified eye

  ● **H16.25   Phlyctenular keratoconjunctivitis**
    H16.251   Phlyctenular keratoconjunctivitis, right eye
    H16.252   Phlyctenular keratoconjunctivitis, left eye
    H16.253   Phlyctenular keratoconjunctivitis, bilateral
    H16.259   Phlyctenular keratoconjunctivitis, unspecified eye

  ● **H16.26   Vernal keratoconjunctivitis, with limbar and corneal involvement**
      Excludes1   vernal conjunctivitis without limbar and corneal involvement (H10.44)
    H16.261   Vernal keratoconjunctivitis, with limbar and corneal involvement, right eye
    H16.262   Vernal keratoconjunctivitis, with limbar and corneal involvement, left eye
    H16.263   Vernal keratoconjunctivitis, with limbar and corneal involvement, bilateral
    H16.269   Vernal keratoconjunctivitis, with limbar and corneal involvement, unspecified eye

  ● **H16.29   Other keratoconjunctivitis**
    H16.291   Other keratoconjunctivitis, right eye
    H16.292   Other keratoconjunctivitis, left eye
    H16.293   Other keratoconjunctivitis, bilateral
    H16.299   Other keratoconjunctivitis, unspecified eye

● **H16.3   Interstitial and deep keratitis**
  ● **H16.30   Unspecified interstitial keratitis**
    H16.301   Unspecified interstitial keratitis, right eye
    H16.302   Unspecified interstitial keratitis, left eye
    H16.303   Unspecified interstitial keratitis, bilateral
    H16.309   Unspecified interstitial keratitis, unspecified eye

  ● **H16.31   Corneal abscess**
    H16.311   Corneal abscess, right eye
    H16.312   Corneal abscess, left eye
    H16.313   Corneal abscess, bilateral
    H16.319   Corneal abscess, unspecified eye

  ● **H16.32   Diffuse interstitial keratitis**
      Cogan's syndrome
    H16.321   Diffuse interstitial keratitis, right eye
    H16.322   Diffuse interstitial keratitis, left eye
    H16.323   Diffuse interstitial keratitis, bilateral
    H16.329   Diffuse interstitial keratitis, unspecified eye

  ● **H16.33   Sclerosing keratitis**
    H16.331   Sclerosing keratitis, right eye
    H16.332   Sclerosing keratitis, left eye
    H16.333   Sclerosing keratitis, bilateral
    H16.339   Sclerosing keratitis, unspecified eye

  ● **H16.39   Other interstitial and deep keratitis**
    H16.391   Other interstitial and deep keratitis, right eye
    H16.392   Other interstitial and deep keratitis, left eye
    H16.393   Other interstitial and deep keratitis, bilateral
    H16.399   Other interstitial and deep keratitis, unspecified eye

● **H16.4   Corneal neovascularization**
  ● **H16.40   Unspecified corneal neovascularization**
    H16.401   Unspecified corneal neovascularization, right eye
    H16.402   Unspecified corneal neovascularization, left eye
    H16.403   Unspecified corneal neovascularization, bilateral
    H16.409   Unspecified corneal neovascularization, unspecified eye

  ● **H16.41   Ghost vessels (corneal)**
    H16.411   Ghost vessels (corneal), right eye
    H16.412   Ghost vessels (corneal), left eye
    H16.413   Ghost vessels (corneal), bilateral
    H16.419   Ghost vessels (corneal), unspecified eye

◀ New   ◀▥ Revised   ~~deleted~~ Deleted   Excludes 1   Excludes 2   Includes   Use additional   Code first   Code also   Unspecified

OGCR Official Guidelines   X Assign placeholder X   ● Use Additional Character(s)   ▶ Manifestation Code   **Coding Clinic**

● H16.42 Pannus (corneal)
    H16.421 Pannus (corneal), right eye
    H16.422 Pannus (corneal), left eye
    H16.423 Pannus (corneal), bilateral
    H16.429 Pannus (corneal), unspecified eye
● H16.43 Localized vascularization of cornea
    H16.431 Localized vascularization of cornea, right eye
    H16.432 Localized vascularization of cornea, left eye
    H16.433 Localized vascularization of cornea, bilateral
    H16.439 Localized vascularization of cornea, unspecified eye
● H16.44 Deep vascularization of cornea
    H16.441 Deep vascularization of cornea, right eye
    H16.442 Deep vascularization of cornea, left eye
    H16.443 Deep vascularization of cornea, bilateral
    H16.449 Deep vascularization of cornea, unspecified eye

H16.8 Other keratitis
H16.9 Unspecified keratitis

● H17 Corneal scars and opacities
  ● H17.0 Adherent leukoma
    H17.00 Adherent leukoma, unspecified eye
    H17.01 Adherent leukoma, right eye
    H17.02 Adherent leukoma, left eye
    H17.03 Adherent leukoma, bilateral
  ● H17.1 Central corneal opacity
    H17.10 Central corneal opacity, unspecified eye
    H17.11 Central corneal opacity, right eye
    H17.12 Central corneal opacity, left eye
    H17.13 Central corneal opacity, bilateral
  ● H17.8 Other corneal scars and opacities
    ● H17.81 Minor opacity of cornea
      Corneal nebula
      H17.811 Minor opacity of cornea, right eye
      H17.812 Minor opacity of cornea, left eye
      H17.813 Minor opacity of cornea, bilateral
      H17.819 Minor opacity of cornea, unspecified eye
    ● H17.82 Peripheral opacity of cornea
      H17.821 Peripheral opacity of cornea, right eye
      H17.822 Peripheral opacity of cornea, left eye
      H17.823 Peripheral opacity of cornea, bilateral
      H17.829 Peripheral opacity of cornea, unspecified eye
    H17.89 Other corneal scars and opacities
  H17.9 Unspecified corneal scar and opacity

● H18 Other disorders of cornea
  ● H18.0 Corneal pigmentations and deposits
    ● H18.00 Unspecified corneal deposit
      H18.001 Unspecified corneal deposit, right eye
      H18.002 Unspecified corneal deposit, left eye
      H18.003 Unspecified corneal deposit, bilateral
      H18.009 Unspecified corneal deposit, unspecified eye
    ● H18.01 Anterior corneal pigmentations
      Staehli's line
      H18.011 Anterior corneal pigmentations, right eye
      H18.012 Anterior corneal pigmentations, left eye

      H18.013 Anterior corneal pigmentations, bilateral
      H18.019 Anterior corneal pigmentations, unspecified eye
    ● H18.02 Argentous corneal deposits
      H18.021 Argentous corneal deposits, right eye
      H18.022 Argentous corneal deposits, left eye
      H18.023 Argentous corneal deposits, bilateral
      H18.029 Argentous corneal deposits, unspecified eye
    ● H18.03 Corneal deposits in metabolic disorders
      Code also associated metabolic disorder
      H18.031 Corneal deposits in metabolic disorders, right eye
      H18.032 Corneal deposits in metabolic disorders, left eye
      H18.033 Corneal deposits in metabolic disorders, bilateral
      H18.039 Corneal deposits in metabolic disorders, unspecified eye
    ● H18.04 Kayser-Fleischer ring
      Code also associated Wilson's disease (E83.01)
      H18.041 Kayser-Fleischer ring, right eye
      H18.042 Kayser-Fleischer ring, left eye
      H18.043 Kayser-Fleischer ring, bilateral
      H18.049 Kayser-Fleischer ring, unspecified eye
    ● H18.05 Posterior corneal pigmentations
      Krukenberg's spindle
      H18.051 Posterior corneal pigmentations, right eye
      H18.052 Posterior corneal pigmentations, left eye
      H18.053 Posterior corneal pigmentations, bilateral
      H18.059 Posterior corneal pigmentations, unspecified eye
    ● H18.06 Stromal corneal pigmentations
      Hematocornea
      H18.061 Stromal corneal pigmentations, right eye
      H18.062 Stromal corneal pigmentations, left eye
      H18.063 Stromal corneal pigmentations, bilateral
      H18.069 Stromal corneal pigmentations, unspecified eye
  ● H18.1 Bullous keratopathy
    H18.10 Bullous keratopathy, unspecified eye
    H18.11 Bullous keratopathy, right eye
    H18.12 Bullous keratopathy, left eye
    H18.13 Bullous keratopathy, bilateral
  ● H18.2 Other and unspecified corneal edema
    H18.20 Unspecified corneal edema
    ● H18.21 Corneal edema secondary to contact lens
      Excludes2 other corneal disorders due to contact lens (H18.82-)
      H18.211 Corneal edema secondary to contact lens, right eye
      H18.212 Corneal edema secondary to contact lens, left eye
      H18.213 Corneal edema secondary to contact lens, bilateral
      H18.219 Corneal edema secondary to contact lens, unspecified eye

CHAPTER 7 (H00-H59)

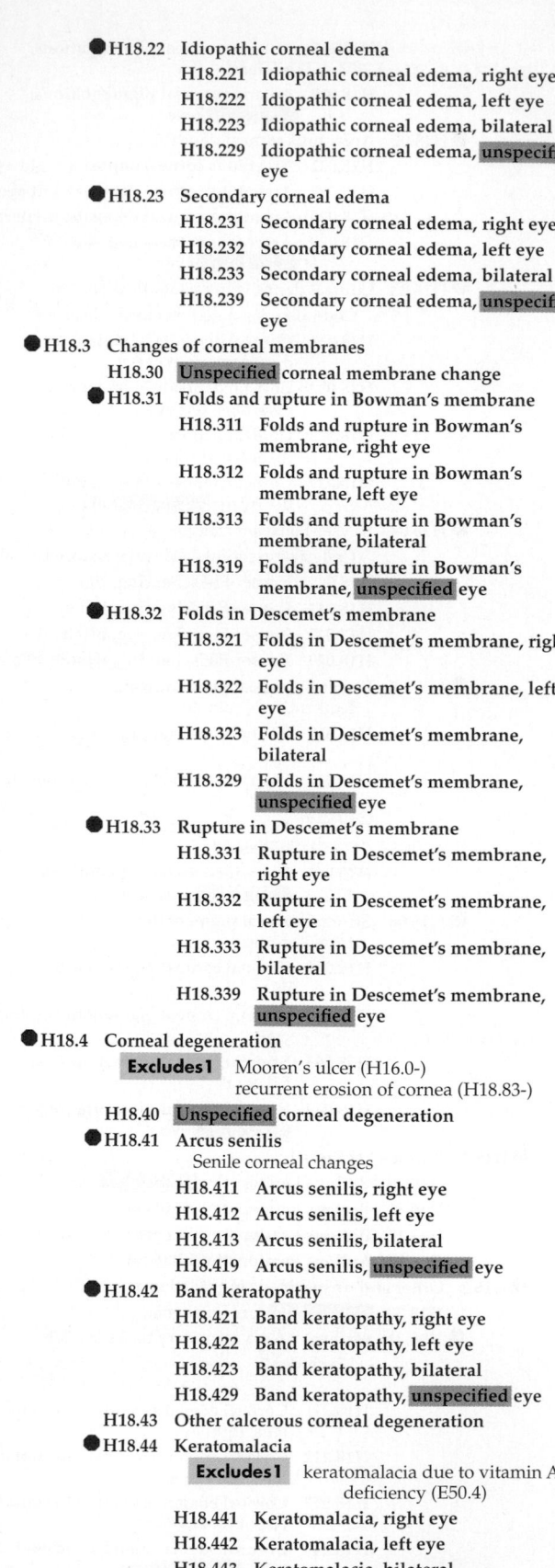

● H18.22 Idiopathic corneal edema
    H18.221 Idiopathic corneal edema, right eye
    H18.222 Idiopathic corneal edema, left eye
    H18.223 Idiopathic corneal edema, bilateral
    H18.229 Idiopathic corneal edema, unspecified eye

● H18.23 Secondary corneal edema
    H18.231 Secondary corneal edema, right eye
    H18.232 Secondary corneal edema, left eye
    H18.233 Secondary corneal edema, bilateral
    H18.239 Secondary corneal edema, unspecified eye

● H18.3 Changes of corneal membranes
    H18.30 Unspecified corneal membrane change
● H18.31 Folds and rupture in Bowman's membrane
    H18.311 Folds and rupture in Bowman's membrane, right eye
    H18.312 Folds and rupture in Bowman's membrane, left eye
    H18.313 Folds and rupture in Bowman's membrane, bilateral
    H18.319 Folds and rupture in Bowman's membrane, unspecified eye
● H18.32 Folds in Descemet's membrane
    H18.321 Folds in Descemet's membrane, right eye
    H18.322 Folds in Descemet's membrane, left eye
    H18.323 Folds in Descemet's membrane, bilateral
    H18.329 Folds in Descemet's membrane, unspecified eye
● H18.33 Rupture in Descemet's membrane
    H18.331 Rupture in Descemet's membrane, right eye
    H18.332 Rupture in Descemet's membrane, left eye
    H18.333 Rupture in Descemet's membrane, bilateral
    H18.339 Rupture in Descemet's membrane, unspecified eye

● H18.4 Corneal degeneration
    Excludes1 Mooren's ulcer (H16.0-)
            recurrent erosion of cornea (H18.83-)
    H18.40 Unspecified corneal degeneration
● H18.41 Arcus senilis
    Senile corneal changes
    H18.411 Arcus senilis, right eye
    H18.412 Arcus senilis, left eye
    H18.413 Arcus senilis, bilateral
    H18.419 Arcus senilis, unspecified eye
● H18.42 Band keratopathy
    H18.421 Band keratopathy, right eye
    H18.422 Band keratopathy, left eye
    H18.423 Band keratopathy, bilateral
    H18.429 Band keratopathy, unspecified eye
    H18.43 Other calcerous corneal degeneration
● H18.44 Keratomalacia
    Excludes1 keratomalacia due to vitamin A deficiency (E50.4)
    H18.441 Keratomalacia, right eye
    H18.442 Keratomalacia, left eye
    H18.443 Keratomalacia, bilateral
    H18.449 Keratomalacia, unspecified eye

● H18.45 Nodular corneal degeneration
    H18.451 Nodular corneal degeneration, right eye
    H18.452 Nodular corneal degeneration, left eye
    H18.453 Nodular corneal degeneration, bilateral
    H18.459 Nodular corneal degeneration, unspecified eye
● H18.46 Peripheral corneal degeneration
    H18.461 Peripheral corneal degeneration, right eye
    H18.462 Peripheral corneal degeneration, left eye
    H18.463 Peripheral corneal degeneration, bilateral
    H18.469 Peripheral corneal degeneration, unspecified eye
    H18.49 Other corneal degeneration
● H18.5 Hereditary corneal dystrophies
    H18.50 Unspecified hereditary corneal dystrophies
    H18.51 Endothelial corneal dystrophy
            Fuchs' dystrophy
    H18.52 Epithelial (juvenile) corneal dystrophy
    H18.53 Granular corneal dystrophy
    H18.54 Lattice corneal dystrophy
    H18.55 Macular corneal dystrophy
    H18.59 Other hereditary corneal dystrophies
● H18.6 Keratoconus
● H18.60 Keratoconus, unspecified
    H18.601 Keratoconus, unspecified, right eye
    H18.602 Keratoconus, unspecified, left eye
    H18.603 Keratoconus, unspecified, bilateral
    H18.609 Keratoconus, unspecified, unspecified eye
● H18.61 Keratoconus, stable
    H18.611 Keratoconus, stable, right eye
    H18.612 Keratoconus, stable, left eye
    H18.613 Keratoconus, stable, bilateral
    H18.619 Keratoconus, stable, unspecified eye
● H18.62 Keratoconus, unstable
    Acute hydrops
    H18.621 Keratoconus, unstable, right eye
    H18.622 Keratoconus, unstable, left eye
    H18.623 Keratoconus, unstable, bilateral
    H18.629 Keratoconus, unstable, unspecified eye

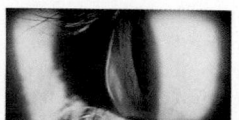

Figure 7-7 Lateral view of the displacement of the cone apex in keratoconus. (From Yanoff: Ophthalmology, ed 3, Mosby, Inc., 2008)

Item 7-4 Keratoconus results in corneal degeneration that begins in childhood, gradually changes the cornea from a round to cone shape, decreasing visual acuity. Treatment includes contact lenses. In severe cases the need for corneal transplant may be the treatment of choice; however, newer technologies may use high frequency radio energy to shrink the edges of the cornea, pulling the central area back to a more normal shape. It can help delay or avoid the need for a corneal transplantation.

CHAPTER 7 (H00-H59)

● H18.7   Other and unspecified corneal deformities

     Excludes1   congenital malformations of cornea (Q13.3-Q13.4)

     H18.70   Unspecified corneal deformity

   ● H18.71   Corneal ectasia

     H18.711   Corneal ectasia, right eye

     H18.712   Corneal ectasia, left eye

     H18.713   Corneal ectasia, bilateral

     H18.719   Corneal ectasia, unspecified eye

   ● H18.72   Corneal staphyloma

     H18.721   Corneal staphyloma, right eye

     H18.722   Corneal staphyloma, left eye

     H18.723   Corneal staphyloma, bilateral

     H18.729   Corneal staphyloma, unspecified eye

   ● H18.73   Descemetocele

     H18.731   Descemetocele, right eye

     H18.732   Descemetocele, left eye

     H18.733   Descemetocele, bilateral

     H18.739   Descemetocele, unspecified eye

   ● H18.79   Other corneal deformities

     H18.791   Other corneal deformities, right eye

     H18.792   Other corneal deformities, left eye

     H18.793   Other corneal deformities, bilateral

     H18.799   Other corneal deformities, unspecified eye

● H18.8   Other specified disorders of cornea

   ● H18.81   Anesthesia and hypoesthesia of cornea

     H18.811   Anesthesia and hypoesthesia of cornea, right eye

     H18.812   Anesthesia and hypoesthesia of cornea, left eye

     H18.813   Anesthesia and hypoesthesia of cornea, bilateral

     H18.819   Anesthesia and hypoesthesia of cornea, unspecified eye

   ● H18.82   Corneal disorder due to contact lens

     Excludes2   corneal edema due to contact lens (H18.21-)

     H18.821   Corneal disorder due to contact lens, right eye

     H18.822   Corneal disorder due to contact lens, left eye

     H18.823   Corneal disorder due to contact lens, bilateral

     H18.829   Corneal disorder due to contact lens, unspecified eye

   ● H18.83   Recurrent erosion of cornea

     H18.831   Recurrent erosion of cornea, right eye

     H18.832   Recurrent erosion of cornea, left eye

     H18.833   Recurrent erosion of cornea, bilateral

     H18.839   Recurrent erosion of cornea, unspecified eye

   ● H18.89   Other specified disorders of cornea

     H18.891   Other specified disorders of cornea, right eye

     H18.892   Other specified disorders of cornea, left eye

     H18.893   Other specified disorders of cornea, bilateral

     H18.899   Other specified disorders of cornea, unspecified eye

● H18.9   Unspecified disorder of cornea

● H20   Iridocyclitis

   ● H20.0   Acute and subacute iridocyclitis

     Acute anterior uveitis

     Acute cyclitis

     Acute iritis

     Subacute anterior uveitis

     Subacute cyclitis

     Subacute iritis

     Excludes1   iridocyclitis, iritis, uveitis (due to) (in) diabetes mellitus (E08-E13 with .39)

         iridocyclitis, iritis, uveitis (due to) (in) diphtheria (A36.89)

         iridocyclitis, iritis, uveitis (due to) (in) gonococcal (A54.32)

         iridocyclitis, iritis, uveitis (due to) (in) herpes (simplex) (B00.51)

         iridocyclitis, iritis, uveitis (due to) (in) herpes zoster (B02.32)

         iridocyclitis, iritis, uveitis (due to) (in) late congenital syphilis (A50.39)

         iridocyclitis, iritis, uveitis (due to) (in) late syphilis (A52.71)

         iridocyclitis, iritis, uveitis (due to) (in) sarcoidosis (D86.83)

         iridocyclitis, iritis, uveitis (due to) (in) syphilis (A51.43)

         iridocyclitis, iritis, uveitis (due to) (in) toxoplasmosis (B58.09)

         iridocyclitis, iritis, uveitis (due to) (in) tuberculosis (A18.54)

     H20.00   Unspecified acute and subacute iridocyclitis

   ● H20.01   Primary iridocyclitis

     H20.011   Primary iridocyclitis, right eye

     H20.012   Primary iridocyclitis, left eye

     H20.013   Primary iridocyclitis, bilateral

     H20.019   Primary iridocyclitis, unspecified eye

   ● H20.02   Recurrent acute iridocyclitis

     H20.021   Recurrent acute iridocyclitis, right eye

     H20.022   Recurrent acute iridocyclitis, left eye

     H20.023   Recurrent acute iridocyclitis, bilateral

     H20.029   Recurrent acute iridocyclitis, unspecified eye

   ● H20.03   Secondary infectious iridocyclitis

     H20.031   Secondary infectious iridocyclitis, right eye

     H20.032   Secondary infectious iridocyclitis, left eye

     H20.033   Secondary infectious iridocyclitis, bilateral

     H20.039   Secondary infectious iridocyclitis, unspecified eye

   ● H20.04   Secondary noninfectious iridocyclitis

     H20.041   Secondary noninfectious iridocyclitis, right eye

     H20.042   Secondary noninfectious iridocyclitis, left eye

     H20.043   Secondary noninfectious iridocyclitis, bilateral

     H20.049   Secondary noninfectious iridocyclitis, unspecified eye

   ● H20.05   Hypopyon

     H20.051   Hypopyon, right eye

     H20.052   Hypopyon, left eye

     H20.053   Hypopyon, bilateral

     H20.059   Hypopyon, unspecified eye

CHAPTER 7 (H00-H59)

● **H20.1**   **Chronic iridocyclitis**
     Use additional code for any associated cataract (H26.21-)
     Excludes2   posterior cyclitis (H30.2-)
     H20.10   Chronic iridocyclitis, unspecified eye
     H20.11   Chronic iridocyclitis, right eye
     H20.12   Chronic iridocyclitis, left eye
     H20.13   Chronic iridocyclitis, bilateral

● **H20.2**   **Lens-induced iridocyclitis**
     H20.20   Lens-induced iridocyclitis, unspecified eye
     H20.21   Lens-induced iridocyclitis, right eye
     H20.22   Lens-induced iridocyclitis, left eye
     H20.23   Lens-induced iridocyclitis, bilateral

● **H20.8**   **Other iridocyclitis**
     Excludes2   glaucomatocyclitis crises (H40.4-)
                 posterior cyclitis (H30.2-)
                 sympathetic uveitis (H44.13-)
    ● H20.81   Fuchs' heterochromic cyclitis
        H20.811   Fuchs' heterochromic cyclitis, right eye
        H20.812   Fuchs' heterochromic cyclitis, left eye
        H20.813   Fuchs' heterochromic cyclitis, bilateral
        H20.819   Fuchs' heterochromic cyclitis, unspecified eye
    ● H20.82   Vogt-Koyanagi syndrome
        H20.821   Vogt-Koyanagi syndrome, right eye
        H20.822   Vogt-Koyanagi syndrome, left eye
        H20.823   Vogt-Koyanagi syndrome, bilateral
        H20.829   Vogt-Koyanagi syndrome, unspecified eye

    H20.9   Unspecified iridocyclitis
       Uveitis NOS

● **H21**   **Other disorders of iris and ciliary body**
     Excludes2   sympathetic uveitis (H44.1-)
● **H21.0**   **Hyphema**
     Excludes1   traumatic hyphema (S05.1-)
     H21.00   Hyphema, unspecified eye
     H21.01   Hyphema, right eye
     H21.02   Hyphema, left eye
     H21.03   Hyphema, bilateral

● **H21.1**   **Other vascular disorders of iris and ciliary body**
     Neovascularization of iris or ciliary body
     Rubeosis iridis
     Rubeosis of iris
    ● H21.1X   Other vascular disorders of iris and ciliary body
        H21.1X1   Other vascular disorders of iris and ciliary body, right eye
        H21.1X2   Other vascular disorders of iris and ciliary body, left eye
        H21.1X3   Other vascular disorders of iris and ciliary body, bilateral
        H21.1X9   Other vascular disorders of iris and ciliary body, unspecified eye

● **H21.2**   **Degeneration of iris and ciliary body**
    ● H21.21   Degeneration of chamber angle
        H21.211   Degeneration of chamber angle, right eye
        H21.212   Degeneration of chamber angle, left eye
        H21.213   Degeneration of chamber angle, bilateral
        H21.219   Degeneration of chamber angle, unspecified eye

● **H21.22**   **Degeneration of ciliary body**
     H21.221   Degeneration of ciliary body, right eye
     H21.222   Degeneration of ciliary body, left eye
     H21.223   Degeneration of ciliary body, bilateral
     H21.229   Degeneration of ciliary body, unspecified eye

● **H21.23**   **Degeneration of iris (pigmentary)**
     Translucency of iris
     H21.231   Degeneration of iris (pigmentary), right eye
     H21.232   Degeneration of iris (pigmentary), left eye
     H21.233   Degeneration of iris (pigmentary), bilateral
     H21.239   Degeneration of iris (pigmentary), unspecified eye

● **H21.24**   **Degeneration of pupillary margin**
     H21.241   Degeneration of pupillary margin, right eye
     H21.242   Degeneration of pupillary margin, left eye
     H21.243   Degeneration of pupillary margin, bilateral
     H21.249   Degeneration of pupillary margin, unspecified eye

● **H21.25**   **Iridoschisis**
     H21.251   Iridoschisis, right eye
     H21.252   Iridoschisis, left eye
     H21.253   Iridoschisis, bilateral
     H21.259   Iridoschisis, unspecified eye

● **H21.26**   **Iris atrophy (essential) (progressive)**
     H21.261   Iris atrophy (essential) (progressive), right eye
     H21.262   Iris atrophy (essential) (progressive), left eye
     H21.263   Iris atrophy (essential) (progressive), bilateral
     H21.269   Iris atrophy (essential) (progressive), unspecified eye

● **H21.27**   **Miotic pupillary cyst**
     H21.271   Miotic pupillary cyst, right eye
     H21.272   Miotic pupillary cyst, left eye
     H21.273   Miotic pupillary cyst, bilateral
     H21.279   Miotic pupillary cyst, unspecified eye

    H21.29   Other iris atrophy

● **H21.3**   **Cyst of iris, ciliary body and anterior chamber**
     Excludes2   miotic pupillary cyst (H21.27-)
    ● H21.30   Idiopathic cysts of iris, ciliary body or anterior chamber
        Cyst of iris, ciliary body or anterior chamber NOS
        H21.301   Idiopathic cysts of iris, ciliary body or anterior chamber, right eye
        H21.302   Idiopathic cysts of iris, ciliary body or anterior chamber, left eye
        H21.303   Idiopathic cysts of iris, ciliary body or anterior chamber, bilateral
        H21.309   Idiopathic cysts of iris, ciliary body or anterior chamber, unspecified eye
    ● H21.31   Exudative cysts of iris or anterior chamber
        H21.311   Exudative cysts of iris or anterior chamber, right eye
        H21.312   Exudative cysts of iris or anterior chamber, left eye
        H21.313   Exudative cysts of iris or anterior chamber, bilateral
        H21.319   Exudative cysts of iris or anterior chamber, unspecified eye

◀ New   ◀▬ Revised   ~~deleted~~ Deleted   Excludes 1   Excludes 2   Includes   Use additional   Code first   Code also   Unspecified
OGCR Official Guidelines   **X** Assign placeholder X   ● Use Additional Character(s)   ▶ Manifestation Code   **Coding Clinic**

● **H21.32**   **Implantation cysts of iris, ciliary body or anterior chamber**
    H21.321   Implantation cysts of iris, ciliary body or anterior chamber, right eye
    H21.322   Implantation cysts of iris, ciliary body or anterior chamber, left eye
    H21.323   Implantation cysts of iris, ciliary body or anterior chamber, bilateral
    H21.329   Implantation cysts of iris, ciliary body or anterior chamber, unspecified eye

● **H21.33**   **Parasitic cyst of iris, ciliary body or anterior chamber**
    H21.331   Parasitic cyst of iris, ciliary body or anterior chamber, right eye
    H21.332   Parasitic cyst of iris, ciliary body or anterior chamber, left eye
    H21.333   Parasitic cyst of iris, ciliary body or anterior chamber, bilateral
    H21.339   Parasitic cyst of iris, ciliary body or anterior chamber, unspecified eye

● **H21.34**   **Primary cyst of pars plana**
    H21.341   Primary cyst of pars plana, right eye
    H21.342   Primary cyst of pars plana, left eye
    H21.343   Primary cyst of pars plana, bilateral
    H21.349   Primary cyst of pars plana, unspecified eye

● **H21.35**   **Exudative cyst of pars plana**
    H21.351   Exudative cyst of pars plana, right eye
    H21.352   Exudative cyst of pars plana, left eye
    H21.353   Exudative cyst of pars plana, bilateral
    H21.359   Exudative cyst of pars plana, unspecified eye

● **H21.4**   **Pupillary membranes**
    Iris bombé
    Pupillary occlusion
    Pupillary seclusion
    Excludes1   congenital pupillary membranes (Q13.8)
    H21.40   Pupillary membranes, unspecified eye
    H21.41   Pupillary membranes, right eye
    H21.42   Pupillary membranes, left eye
    H21.43   Pupillary membranes, bilateral

● **H21.5**   **Other and unspecified adhesions and disruptions of iris and ciliary body**
    Excludes1   corectopia (Q13.2)
   ● **H21.50**   **Unspecified adhesions of iris**
     Synechia (iris) NOS
     H21.501   Unspecified adhesions of iris, right eye
     H21.502   Unspecified adhesions of iris, left eye
     H21.503   Unspecified adhesions of iris, bilateral
     H21.509   Unspecified adhesions of iris and ciliary body, unspecified eye
   ● **H21.51**   **Anterior synechiae (iris)**
     H21.511   Anterior synechiae (iris), right eye
     H21.512   Anterior synechiae (iris), left eye
     H21.513   Anterior synechiae (iris), bilateral
     H21.519   Anterior synechiae (iris), unspecified eye
   ● **H21.52**   **Goniosynechiae**
     H21.521   Goniosynechiae, right eye
     H21.522   Goniosynechiae, left eye
     H21.523   Goniosynechiae, bilateral
     H21.529   Goniosynechiae, unspecified eye
   ● **H21.53**   **Iridodialysis**
     H21.531   Iridodialysis, right eye
     H21.532   Iridodialysis, left eye

     H21.533   Iridodialysis, bilateral
     H21.539   Iridodialysis, unspecified eye
   ● **H21.54**   **Posterior synechiae (iris)**
     H21.541   Posterior synechiae (iris), right eye
     H21.542   Posterior synechiae (iris), left eye
     H21.543   Posterior synechiae (iris), bilateral
     H21.549   Posterior synechiae (iris), unspecified eye
   ● **H21.55**   **Recession of chamber angle**
     H21.551   Recession of chamber angle, right eye
     H21.552   Recession of chamber angle, left eye
     H21.553   Recession of chamber angle, bilateral
     H21.559   Recession of chamber angle, unspecified eye
   ● **H21.56**   **Pupillary abnormalities**
     Deformed pupil
     Ectopic pupil
     Rupture of sphincter, pupil
     Excludes1   congenital deformity of pupil (Q13.2-)
     H21.561   Pupillary abnormality, right eye
     H21.562   Pupillary abnormality, left eye
     H21.563   Pupillary abnormality, bilateral
     H21.569   Pupillary abnormality, unspecified eye
● **H21.8**   **Other specified disorders of iris and ciliary body**
    H21.81   **Floppy iris syndrome**
     Intraoperative floppy iris syndrome (IFIS)
     Use additional code for adverse effect, if applicable, to identify drug (T36-T50 with fifth or sixth character 5)
    H21.82   **Plateau iris syndrome (post-iridectomy) (postprocedural)**
    H21.89   Other specified disorders of iris and ciliary body
  H21.9   Unspecified disorder of iris and ciliary body

▶ *H22*   *Disorders of iris and ciliary body in diseases classified elsewhere*
    Code first underlying disease, such as:
    gout (M1A.-, M10.-)
    leprosy (A30.-)
    parasitic disease (B89)

DISORDERS OF LENS (H25-H28)

● **H25**   **Age-related cataract**
    Senile cataract
    Excludes2   capsular glaucoma with pseudoexfoliation of lens (H40.1-)
  ● **H25.0**   **Age-related incipient cataract**
   ● **H25.01**   **Cortical age-related cataract**
     H25.011   Cortical age-related cataract, right eye   A
     H25.012   Cortical age-related cataract, left eye   A
     H25.013   Cortical age-related cataract, bilateral   A
     H25.019   Cortical age-related cataract, unspecified eye   A
   ● **H25.03**   **Anterior subcapsular polar age-related cataract**
     H25.031   Anterior subcapsular polar age-related cataract, right eye   A
     H25.032   Anterior subcapsular polar age-related cataract, left eye   A
     H25.033   Anterior subcapsular polar age-related cataract, bilateral   A
     H25.039   Anterior subcapsular polar age-related cataract, unspecified eye   A

CHAPTER 7 (H00-H59)

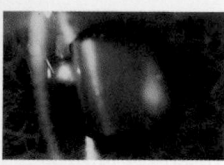

Figure 7-8 Age-related cataract. Nuclear sclerosis and cortical lens opacities are present. (From Yanoff: Ophthalmology, ed 3, Mosby, Inc., 2008)

Item 7–5 Senile cataracts are linked to the aging process. The most common area for the formation of a cataract is the cortical area of the lens. **Polar cataracts** can be either anterior or posterior. **Anterior polar cataracts** are more common and are small, white, capsular cataracts located on the anterior portion of the lens. **Total cataracts,** also called **complete** or **mature,** cause an opacity of all fibers of the lens. **Hypermature** describes a mature cataract with a swollen, milky cortex that covers the entire lens. **Immature**, also called **incipient,** cataracts have a clear cortex and are only slightly opaque. Treatment for all cataracts is the removal of the lens.

● **H25.04** Posterior subcapsular polar age-related cataract
   H25.041 Posterior subcapsular polar age-related cataract, right eye A
   H25.042 Posterior subcapsular polar age-related cataract, left eye A
   H25.043 Posterior subcapsular polar age-related cataract, bilateral A
   H25.049 Posterior subcapsular polar age-related cataract, unspecified eye A

● **H25.09** Other age-related incipient cataract
   Coronary age-related cataract
   Punctate age-related cataract
   Water clefts
   H25.091 Other age-related incipient cataract, right eye A
   H25.092 Other age-related incipient cataract, left eye A
   H25.093 Other age-related incipient cataract, bilateral A
   H25.099 Other age-related incipient cataract, unspecified eye A

● **H25.1** Age-related nuclear cataract
   Cataracta brunescens
   Nuclear sclerosis cataract
   H25.10 Age-related nuclear cataract, unspecified eye A
   H25.11 Age-related nuclear cataract, right eye A
   H25.12 Age-related nuclear cataract, left eye A
   H25.13 Age-related nuclear cataract, bilateral A

● **H25.2** Age-related cataract, morgagnian type
   Age-related hypermature cataract
   H25.20 Age-related cataract, morgagnian type, unspecified eye A
   H25.21 Age-related cataract, morgagnian type, right eye A
   H25.22 Age-related cataract, morgagnian type, left eye A
   H25.23 Age-related cataract, morgagnian type, bilateral A

● **H25.8** Other age-related cataract
  ● **H25.81** Combined forms of age-related cataract
   H25.811 Combined forms of age-related cataract, right eye A
   H25.812 Combined forms of age-related cataract, left eye A
   H25.813 Combined forms of age-related cataract, bilateral A
   H25.819 Combined forms of age-related cataract, unspecified eye A
   H25.89 Other age-related cataract A
  H25.9 Unspecified age-related cataract A

● **H26** Other cataract
  Excludes1 congenital cataract (Q12.0)
 ● **H26.0** Infantile and juvenile cataract
  ● **H26.00** Unspecified infantile and juvenile cataract
   H26.001 Unspecified infantile and juvenile cataract, right eye P
   H26.002 Unspecified infantile and juvenile cataract, left eye P
   H26.003 Unspecified infantile and juvenile cataract, bilateral P
   H26.009 Unspecified infantile and juvenile cataract, unspecified eye P

  ● **H26.01** Infantile and juvenile cortical, lamellar, or zonular cataract
   H26.011 Infantile and juvenile cortical, lamellar, or zonular cataract, right eye P
   H26.012 Infantile and juvenile cortical, lamellar, or zonular cataract, left eye P
   H26.013 Infantile and juvenile cortical, lamellar, or zonular cataract, bilateral P
   H26.019 Infantile and juvenile cortical, lamellar, or zonular cataract, unspecified eye P

  ● **H26.03** Infantile and juvenile nuclear cataract
   H26.031 Infantile and juvenile nuclear cataract, right eye P
   H26.032 Infantile and juvenile nuclear cataract, left eye P
   H26.033 Infantile and juvenile nuclear cataract, bilateral P
   H26.039 Infantile and juvenile nuclear cataract, unspecified eye P

  ● **H26.04** Anterior subcapsular polar infantile and juvenile cataract
   H26.041 Anterior subcapsular polar infantile and juvenile cataract, right eye P
   H26.042 Anterior subcapsular polar infantile and juvenile cataract, left eye P
   H26.043 Anterior subcapsular polar infantile and juvenile cataract, bilateral P
   H26.049 Anterior subcapsular polar infantile and juvenile cataract, unspecified eye P

  ● **H26.05** Posterior subcapsular polar infantile and juvenile cataract
   H26.051 Posterior subcapsular polar infantile and juvenile cataract, right eye P
   H26.052 Posterior subcapsular polar infantile and juvenile cataract, left eye P
   H26.053 Posterior subcapsular polar infantile and juvenile cataract, bilateral P
   H26.059 Posterior subcapsular polar infantile and juvenile cataract, unspecified eye P

  ● **H26.06** Combined forms of infantile and juvenile cataract
   H26.061 Combined forms of infantile and juvenile cataract, right eye P
   H26.062 Combined forms of infantile and juvenile cataract, left eye P
   H26.063 Combined forms of infantile and juvenile cataract bilateral P
   H26.069 Combined forms of infantile and juvenile cataract, unspecified eye P
   H26.09 Other infantile and juvenile cataract P

CHAPTER 7 (H00-H59)

◀ New ◀░ Revised ~~deleted~~ Deleted Excludes 1 Excludes 2 Includes Use additional Code first Code also Unspecified
OGCR Official Guidelines X Assign placeholder X ● Use Additional Character(s) ▶ Manifestation Code **Coding Clinic**

● **H26.1   Traumatic cataract**

Use additional code (Chapter 20) to identify external cause

● **H26.10   Unspecified traumatic cataract**

H26.101   Unspecified traumatic cataract, right eye

H26.102   Unspecified traumatic cataract, left eye

H26.103   Unspecified traumatic cataract, bilateral

H26.109   Unspecified traumatic cataract, unspecified eye

● **H26.11   Localized traumatic opacities**

H26.111   Localized traumatic opacities, right eye

H26.112   Localized traumatic opacities, left eye

H26.113   Localized traumatic opacities, bilateral

H26.119   Localized traumatic opacities, unspecified eye

● **H26.12   Partially resolved traumatic cataract**

H26.121   Partially resolved traumatic cataract, right eye

H26.122   Partially resolved traumatic cataract, left eye

H26.123   Partially resolved traumatic cataract, bilateral

H26.129   Partially resolved traumatic cataract, unspecified eye

● **H26.13   Total traumatic cataract**

H26.131   Total traumatic cataract, right eye

H26.132   Total traumatic cataract, left eye

H26.133   Total traumatic cataract, bilateral

H26.139   Total traumatic cataract, unspecified eye

● **H26.2   Complicated cataract**

H26.20   Unspecified complicated cataract

Cataracta complicata NOS

● **H26.21   Cataract with neovascularization**

Code also associated condition, such as: chronic iridocyclitis (H20.1-)

H26.211   Cataract with neovascularization, right eye

H26.212   Cataract with neovascularization, left eye

H26.213   Cataract with neovascularization, bilateral

H26.219   Cataract with neovascularization, unspecified eye

● **H26.22   Cataract secondary to ocular disorders (degenerative) (inflammatory)**

Code also associated ocular disorder

H26.221   Cataract secondary to ocular disorders (degenerative) (inflammatory), right eye

H26.222   Cataract secondary to ocular disorders (degenerative) (inflammatory), left eye

H26.223   Cataract secondary to ocular disorders (degenerative) (inflammatory), bilateral

H26.229   Cataract secondary to ocular disorders (degenerative) (inflammatory), unspecified eye

● **H26.23   Glaucomatous flecks (subcapsular)**

Code first underlying glaucoma (H40-H42)

H26.231   Glaucomatous flecks (subcapsular), right eye

H26.232   Glaucomatous flecks (subcapsular), left eye

H26.233   Glaucomatous flecks (subcapsular), bilateral

H26.239   Glaucomatous flecks (subcapsular), unspecified eye

● **H26.3   Drug-induced cataract**

Toxic cataract

Use additional code for adverse effect, if applicable, to identify drug (T36-T50 with fifth or sixth character 5)

H26.30   Drug-induced cataract, unspecified eye

H26.31   Drug-induced cataract, right eye

H26.32   Drug-induced cataract, left eye

H26.33   Drug-induced cataract, bilateral

● **H26.4   Secondary cataract**

H26.40   Unspecified secondary cataract

● **H26.41   Soemmering's ring**

H26.411   Soemmering's ring, right eye

H26.412   Soemmering's ring, left eye

H26.413   Soemmering's ring, bilateral

H26.419   Soemmering's ring, unspecified eye

● **H26.49   Other secondary cataract**

H26.491   Other secondary cataract, right eye

H26.492   Other secondary cataract, left eye

H26.493   Other secondary cataract, bilateral

H26.499   Other secondary cataract, unspecified eye

H26.8   Other specified cataract

H26.9   Unspecified cataract

● **H27   Other disorders of lens**

Excludes1   congenital lens malformations (Q12.-)
mechanical complications of intraocular lens implant (T85.2)
pseudophakia (Z96.1)

● **H27.0   Aphakia**

Acquired absence of lens
Acquired aphakia
Aphakia due to trauma

Excludes1   cataract extraction status (Z98.4-)
congenital absence of lens (Q12.3)
congenital aphakia (Q12.3)

H27.00   Aphakia, unspecified eye

H27.01   Aphakia, right eye

H27.02   Aphakia, left eye

H27.03   Aphakia, bilateral

● **H27.1   Dislocation of lens**

H27.10   Unspecified dislocation of lens

● **H27.11   Subluxation of lens**

H27.111   Subluxation of lens, right eye

H27.112   Subluxation of lens, left eye

H27.113   Subluxation of lens, bilateral

H27.119   Subluxation of lens, unspecified eye

● **H27.12   Anterior dislocation of lens**

H27.121   Anterior dislocation of lens, right eye

H27.122   Anterior dislocation of lens, left eye

H27.123   Anterior dislocation of lens, bilateral

H27.129   Anterior dislocation of lens, unspecified eye

● **H27.13   Posterior dislocation of lens**

H27.131   Posterior dislocation of lens, right eye

H27.132   Posterior dislocation of lens, left eye

H27.133   Posterior dislocation of lens, bilateral

H27.139   Posterior dislocation of lens, unspecified eye

H27.8   Other specified disorders of lens

H27.9   Unspecified disorder of lens

CHAPTER 7 (H00-H59)

▶ **H28**   *Cataract in diseases classified elsewhere*

> *Code first underlying disease, such as:*
>   hypoparathyroidism (E20.-)
>   myotonia (G71.1-)
>   myxedema (E03.-)
>   protein-calorie malnutrition (E40-E46)
>
> **Excludes1**   cataract in diabetes mellitus (E08.36, E09.36, E10.36, E11.36, E13.36)

DISORDERS OF CHOROID AND RETINA (H30-H36)

(See Plate 90 on page 64.)

● **H30**   Chorioretinal inflammation

   ● **H30.0**   Focal chorioretinal inflammation
       Focal chorioretinitis
       Focal choroiditis
       Focal retinitis
       Focal retinochoroiditis

     ● **H30.00**   Unspecified focal chorioretinal inflammation
         Focal chorioretinitis NOS
         Focal choroiditis NOS
         Focal retinitis NOS
         Focal retinochoroiditis NOS

       H30.001   Unspecified focal chorioretinal inflammation, right eye
       H30.002   Unspecified focal chorioretinal inflammation, left eye
       H30.003   Unspecified focal chorioretinal inflammation, bilateral
       H30.009   Unspecified focal chorioretinal inflammation, unspecified eye

     ● **H30.01**   Focal chorioretinal inflammation, juxtapapillary
       H30.011   Focal chorioretinal inflammation, juxtapapillary, right eye
       H30.012   Focal chorioretinal inflammation, juxtapapillary, left eye
       H30.013   Focal chorioretinal inflammation, juxtapapillary, bilateral
       H30.019   Focal chorioretinal inflammation, juxtapapillary, unspecified eye

     ● **H30.02**   Focal chorioretinal inflammation of posterior pole
       H30.021   Focal chorioretinal inflammation of posterior pole, right eye
       H30.022   Focal chorioretinal inflammation of posterior pole, left eye
       H30.023   Focal chorioretinal inflammation of posterior pole, bilateral
       H30.029   Focal chorioretinal inflammation of posterior pole, unspecified eye

     ● **H30.03**   Focal chorioretinal inflammation, peripheral
       H30.031   Focal chorioretinal inflammation, peripheral, right eye
       H30.032   Focal chorioretinal inflammation, peripheral, left eye
       H30.033   Focal chorioretinal inflammation, peripheral, bilateral
       H30.039   Focal chorioretinal inflammation, peripheral, unspecified eye

     ● **H30.04**   Focal chorioretinal inflammation, macular or paramacular
       H30.041   Focal chorioretinal inflammation, macular or paramacular, right eye
       H30.042   Focal chorioretinal inflammation, macular or paramacular, left eye
       H30.043   Focal chorioretinal inflammation, macular or paramacular, bilateral
       H30.049   Focal chorioretinal inflammation, macular or paramacular, unspecified eye

● **H30.1**   Disseminated chorioretinal inflammation
     Disseminated chorioretinitis
     Disseminated choroiditis
     Disseminated retinitis
     Disseminated retinochoroiditis

   Excludes2   exudative retinopathy (H35.02-)

   ● **H30.10**   Unspecified disseminated chorioretinal inflammation
       Disseminated chorioretinitis NOS
       Disseminated choroiditis NOS
       Disseminated retinitis NOS
       Disseminated retinochoroiditis NOS

     H30.101   Unspecified disseminated chorioretinal inflammation, right eye
     H30.102   Unspecified disseminated chorioretinal inflammation, left eye
     H30.103   Unspecified disseminated chorioretinal inflammation, bilateral
     H30.109   Unspecified disseminated chorioretinal inflammation, unspecified eye

   ● **H30.11**   Disseminated chorioretinal inflammation of posterior pole
     H30.111   Disseminated chorioretinal inflammation of posterior pole, right eye
     H30.112   Disseminated chorioretinal inflammation of posterior pole, left eye
     H30.113   Disseminated chorioretinal inflammation of posterior pole, bilateral
     H30.119   Disseminated chorioretinal inflammation of posterior pole, unspecified eye

   ● **H30.12**   Disseminated chorioretinal inflammation, peripheral
     H30.121   Disseminated chorioretinal inflammation, peripheral right eye
     H30.122   Disseminated chorioretinal inflammation, peripheral, left eye
     H30.123   Disseminated chorioretinal inflammation, peripheral, bilateral
     H30.129   Disseminated chorioretinal inflammation, peripheral, unspecified eye

   ● **H30.13**   Disseminated chorioretinal inflammation, generalized
     H30.131   Disseminated chorioretinal inflammation, generalized, right eye
     H30.132   Disseminated chorioretinal inflammation, generalized, left eye
     H30.133   Disseminated chorioretinal inflammation, generalized, bilateral
     H30.139   Disseminated chorioretinal inflammation, generalized, unspecified eye

   ● **H30.14**   Acute posterior multifocal placoid pigment epitheliopathy
     H30.141   Acute posterior multifocal placoid pigment epitheliopathy, right eye
     H30.142   Acute posterior multifocal placoid pigment epitheliopathy, left eye
     H30.143   Acute posterior multifocal placoid pigment epitheliopathy, bilateral
     H30.149   Acute posterior multifocal placoid pigment epitheliopathy, unspecified eye

---

◀ New   ◀▥ Revised   ~~deleted~~ Deleted   Excludes 1   Excludes 2   Includes   Use additional   Code first   Code also   Unspecified

OGCR Official Guidelines   X Assign placeholder X   ● Use Additional Character(s)   ▶ Manifestation Code   **Coding Clinic**

● H30.2   **Posterior cyclitis**
     Pars planitis
   H30.20   Posterior cyclitis, unspecified eye
   H30.21   Posterior cyclitis, right eye
   H30.22   Posterior cyclitis, left eye
   H30.23   Posterior cyclitis, bilateral

● H30.8   **Other chorioretinal inflammations**
  ● H30.81   **Harada's disease**
    H30.811   Harada's disease, right eye
    H30.812   Harada's disease, left eye
    H30.813   Harada's disease, bilateral
    H30.819   Harada's disease, unspecified eye
  ● H30.89   **Other chorioretinal inflammations**
    H30.891   Other chorioretinal inflammations, right eye
    H30.892   Other chorioretinal inflammations, left eye
    H30.893   Other chorioretinal inflammations, bilateral
    H30.899   Other chorioretinal inflammations, unspecified eye

● H30.9   **Unspecified chorioretinal inflammation**
     Chorioretinitis NOS
     Choroiditis NOS
     Neuroretinitis NOS
     Retinitis NOS
     Retinochoroiditis NOS
   H30.90   Unspecified chorioretinal inflammation, unspecified eye
   H30.91   Unspecified chorioretinal inflammation, right eye
   H30.92   Unspecified chorioretinal inflammation, left eye
   H30.93   Unspecified chorioretinal inflammation, bilateral

● H31   **Other disorders of choroid**
  ● H31.0   **Chorioretinal scars**
     Excludes2   postsurgical chorioretinal scars (H59.81-)
   ● H31.00   **Unspecified chorioretinal scars**
    H31.001   Unspecified chorioretinal scars, right eye
    H31.002   Unspecified chorioretinal scars, left eye
    H31.003   Unspecified chorioretinal scars, bilateral
    H31.009   Unspecified chorioretinal scars, unspecified eye
   ● H31.01   **Macula scars of posterior pole (postinflammatory) (post-traumatic)**
     Excludes1   postprocedural chorioretinal scar (H59.81-)
    H31.011   Macula scars of posterior pole (postinflammatory) (post-traumatic), right eye
    H31.012   Macula scars of posterior pole (postinflammatory) (post-traumatic), left eye
    H31.013   Macula scars of posterior pole (postinflammatory) (post-traumatic), bilateral
    H31.019   Macula scars of posterior pole (postinflammatory) (post-traumatic), unspecified eye

● H31.02   **Solar retinopathy**
   H31.021   Solar retinopathy, right eye
   H31.022   Solar retinopathy, left eye
   H31.023   Solar retinopathy, bilateral
   H31.029   Solar retinopathy, unspecified eye

● H31.09   **Other chorioretinal scars**
   H31.091   Other chorioretinal scars, right eye
   H31.092   Other chorioretinal scars, left eye
   H31.093   Other chorioretinal scars, bilateral
   H31.099   Other chorioretinal scars, unspecified eye

● H31.1   **Choroidal degeneration**
     Excludes2   angioid streaks of macula (H35.33)
  ● H31.10   **Unspecified choroidal degeneration**
     Choroidal sclerosis NOS
    H31.101   Choroidal degeneration, unspecified, right eye
    H31.102   Choroidal degeneration, unspecified, left eye
    H31.103   Choroidal degeneration, unspecified, bilateral
    H31.109   Choroidal degeneration, unspecified, unspecified eye
  ● H31.11   **Age-related choroidal atrophy**
    H31.111   Age-related choroidal atrophy, right eye   **A**
    H31.112   Age-related choroidal atrophy, left eye   **A**
    H31.113   Age-related choroidal atrophy, bilateral   **A**
    H31.119   Age-related choroidal atrophy, unspecified eye   **A**
  ● H31.12   **Diffuse secondary atrophy of choroid**
    H31.121   Diffuse secondary atrophy of choroid, right eye
    H31.122   Diffuse secondary atrophy of choroid, left eye
    H31.123   Diffuse secondary atrophy of choroid, bilateral
    H31.129   Diffuse secondary atrophy of choroid, unspecified eye

● H31.2   **Hereditary choroidal dystrophy**
     Excludes2   hyperornithinemia (E72.4)
                   ornithinemia (E72.4)
   H31.20   Hereditary choroidal dystrophy, unspecified
   H31.21   Choroideremia
   H31.22   Choroidal dystrophy (central areolar) (generalized) (peripapillary)
   H31.23   Gyrate atrophy, choroid
   H31.29   Other hereditary choroidal dystrophy

● H31.3   **Choroidal hemorrhage and rupture**
  ● H31.30   **Unspecified choroidal hemorrhage**
    H31.301   Unspecified choroidal hemorrhage, right eye
    H31.302   Unspecified choroidal hemorrhage, left eye
    H31.303   Unspecified choroidal hemorrhage, bilateral
    H31.309   Unspecified choroidal hemorrhage, unspecified eye

CHAPTER 7 (H00-H59)

● H31.31   Expulsive choroidal hemorrhage

     H31.311   Expulsive choroidal hemorrhage, right eye

     H31.312   Expulsive choroidal hemorrhage, left eye

     H31.313   Expulsive choroidal hemorrhage, bilateral

     H31.319   Expulsive choroidal hemorrhage, unspecified eye

● H31.32   Choroidal rupture

     H31.321   Choroidal rupture, right eye

     H31.322   Choroidal rupture, left eye

     H31.323   Choroidal rupture, bilateral

     H31.329   Choroidal rupture, unspecified eye

● H31.4   Choroidal detachment

   ● H31.40   Unspecified choroidal detachment

     H31.401   Unspecified choroidal detachment, right eye

     H31.402   Unspecified choroidal detachment, left eye

     H31.403   Unspecified choroidal detachment, bilateral

     H31.409   Unspecified choroidal detachment, unspecified eye

   ● H31.41   Hemorrhagic choroidal detachment

     H31.411   Hemorrhagic choroidal detachment, right eye

     H31.412   Hemorrhagic choroidal detachment, left eye

     H31.413   Hemorrhagic choroidal detachment, bilateral

     H31.419   Hemorrhagic choroidal detachment, unspecified eye

   ● H31.42   Serous choroidal detachment

     H31.421   Serous choroidal detachment, right eye

     H31.422   Serous choroidal detachment, left eye

     H31.423   Serous choroidal detachment, bilateral

     H31.429   Serous choroidal detachment, unspecified eye

   H31.8   Other specified disorders of choroid

   H31.9   Unspecified disorder of choroid

▶ H32   *Chorioretinal disorders in diseases classified elsewhere*

    Code first underlying disease, such as:
    congenital toxoplasmosis (P37.1)
    histoplasmosis (B39.-)
    leprosy (A30.-)

    Excludes1   chorioretinitis (in):
       toxoplasmosis (acquired) (B58.01)
       tuberculosis (A18.53)

● H33   Retinal detachments and breaks

    Excludes1   detachment of retinal pigment epithelium (H35.72-, H35.73-)

   ● H33.0   Retinal detachment with retinal break
     Rhegmatogenous retinal detachment

     Excludes1   serous retinal detachment (without retinal break) (H33.2-)

    ● H33.00   Unspecified retinal detachment with retinal break

     H33.001   Unspecified retinal detachment with retinal break, right eye

     H33.002   Unspecified retinal detachment with retinal break, left eye

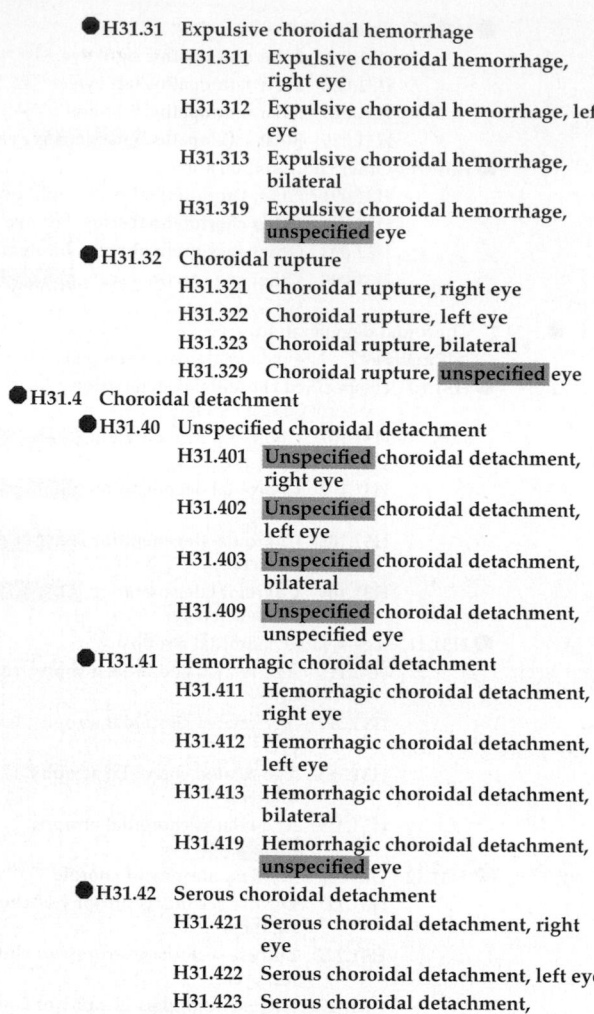

NON-RHEGMATOGENOUS RETINAL DETACHMENT
— Vitreous
— Retina
— Protein-rich fluid in sub-retinal space
Retinal pigment epithelium

VITREOUS DETACHMENT
— Vitreous
— Posterior hyaloid
Internal limiting membrane

RHEGMATOGENOUS RETINAL DETACHMENT
Blood
— Vitreous
— Posterior hyaloid
— Retina
— Retinal tear
— Liquified vitreous
Retinal pigment epithelium

Figure 7-9   Retinal detachment. (From Kumar: Robbins and Cotran: Pathologic Basis of Disease, ed 7, Saunders, 2005)

Item 7–6   Retinal detachments and defects are conditions of the eye in which the retina separates from the underlying tissue. Initial detachment may be localized, requiring rapid treatment (medical emergency) to avoid the entire retina from detaching which leads to vision loss and blindness.

     H33.003   Unspecified retinal detachment with retinal break, bilateral

     H33.009   Unspecified retinal detachment with retinal break, unspecified eye

   ● H33.01   Retinal detachment with single break

     H33.011   Retinal detachment with single break, right eye

     H33.012   Retinal detachment with single break, left eye

     H33.013   Retinal detachment with single break, bilateral

     H33.019   Retinal detachment with single break, unspecified eye

   ● H33.02   Retinal detachment with multiple breaks

     H33.021   Retinal detachment with multiple breaks, right eye

     H33.022   Retinal detachment with multiple breaks, left eye

     H33.023   Retinal detachment with multiple breaks, bilateral

     H33.029   Retinal detachment with multiple breaks, unspecified eye

   ● H33.03   Retinal detachment with giant retinal tear

     H33.031   Retinal detachment with giant retinal tear, right eye

     H33.032   Retinal detachment with giant retinal tear, left eye

     H33.033   Retinal detachment with giant retinal tear, bilateral

     H33.039   Retinal detachment with giant retinal tear, unspecified eye

◀ New   ◀ Revised   ~~deleted~~ Deleted   Excludes 1   Excludes 2   Includes   Use additional   Code first   Code also   Unspecified

OGCR Official Guidelines   X Assign placeholder X   ● Use Additional Character(s)   ▶ Manifestation Code   **Coding Clinic**

● **H33.04** Retinal detachment with retinal dialysis
     H33.041   Retinal detachment with retinal dialysis, right eye
     H33.042   Retinal detachment with retinal dialysis, left eye
     H33.043   Retinal detachment with retinal dialysis, bilateral
     H33.049   Retinal detachment with retinal dialysis, unspecified eye

● H33.05   Total retinal detachment
     H33.051   Total retinal detachment, right eye
     H33.052   Total retinal detachment, left eye
     H33.053   Total retinal detachment, bilateral
     H33.059   Total retinal detachment, unspecified eye

● **H33.1**   Retinoschisis and retinal cysts
     Excludes1   congenital retinoschisis (Q14.1)
              microcystoid degeneration of retina (H35.42-)

● H33.10   Unspecified retinoschisis
     H33.101   Unspecified retinoschisis, right eye
     H33.102   Unspecified retinoschisis, left eye
     H33.103   Unspecified retinoschisis, bilateral
     H33.109   Unspecified retinoschisis, unspecified eye

● H33.11   Cyst of ora serrata
     H33.111   Cyst of ora serrata, right eye
     H33.112   Cyst of ora serrata, left eye
     H33.113   Cyst of ora serrata, bilateral
     H33.119   Cyst of ora serrata, unspecified eye

● H33.12   Parasitic cyst of retina
     H33.121   Parasitic cyst of retina, right eye
     H33.122   Parasitic cyst of retina, left eye
     H33.123   Parasitic cyst of retina, bilateral
     H33.129   Parasitic cyst of retina, unspecified eye

● H33.19   Other retinoschisis and retinal cysts
         Pseudocyst of retina
     H33.191   Other retinoschisis and retinal cysts, right eye
     H33.192   Other retinoschisis and retinal cysts, left eye
     H33.193   Other retinoschisis and retinal cysts, bilateral
     H33.199   Other retinoschisis and retinal cysts, unspecified eye

● **H33.2**   Serous retinal detachment
         Retinal detachment NOS
         Retinal detachment without retinal break
     Excludes1   central serous chorioretinopathy (H35.71-)
     H33.20   Serous retinal detachment, unspecified eye
     H33.21   Serous retinal detachment, right eye
     H33.22   Serous retinal detachment, left eye
     H33.23   Serous retinal detachment, bilateral

● **H33.3**   Retinal breaks without detachment
     Excludes1   chorioretinal scars after surgery for detachment (H59.81-)
              peripheral retinal degeneration without break (H35.4-)

● H33.30   Unspecified retinal break
     H33.301   Unspecified retinal break, right eye
     H33.302   Unspecified retinal break, left eye
     H33.303   Unspecified retinal break, bilateral
     H33.309   Unspecified retinal break, unspecified eye

● H33.31   Horseshoe tear of retina without detachment
         Operculum of retina without detachment
     H33.311   Horseshoe tear of retina without detachment, right eye
     H33.312   Horseshoe tear of retina without detachment, left eye
     H33.313   Horseshoe tear of retina without detachment, bilateral
     H33.319   Horseshoe tear of retina without detachment, unspecified eye

● H33.32   Round hole of retina without detachment
     H33.321   Round hole, right eye
     H33.322   Round hole, left eye
     H33.323   Round hole, bilateral
     H33.329   Round hole, unspecified eye

● H33.33   Multiple defects of retina without detachment
     H33.331   Multiple defects of retina without detachment, right eye
     H33.332   Multiple defects of retina without detachment, left eye
     H33.333   Multiple defects of retina without detachment, bilateral
     H33.339   Multiple defects of retina without detachment, unspecified eye

● **H33.4**   Traction detachment of retina
         Proliferative vitreo-retinopathy with retinal detachment
     H33.40   Traction detachment of retina, unspecified eye
     H33.41   Traction detachment of retina, right eye
     H33.42   Traction detachment of retina, left eye
     H33.43   Traction detachment of retina, bilateral

   H33.8   Other retinal detachments

● **H34**   Retinal vascular occlusions
         Blockage in vessel of the retina
     Excludes1   amaurosis fugax (G45.3)

● **H34.0**   Transient retinal artery occlusion
     H34.00   Transient retinal artery occlusion, unspecified eye
     H34.01   Transient retinal artery occlusion, right eye
     H34.02   Transient retinal artery occlusion, left eye
     H34.03   Transient retinal artery occlusion, bilateral

● **H34.1**   Central retinal artery occlusion
     H34.10   Central retinal artery occlusion, unspecified eye
     H34.11   Central retinal artery occlusion, right eye
     H34.12   Central retinal artery occlusion, left eye
     H34.13   Central retinal artery occlusion, bilateral

● **H34.2**   Other retinal artery occlusions
   ● H34.21   Partial retinal artery occlusion
         Hollenhorst's plaque
         Retinal microembolism
     H34.211   Partial retinal artery occlusion, right eye
     H34.212   Partial retinal artery occlusion, left eye
     H34.213   Partial retinal artery occlusion, bilateral
     H34.219   Partial retinal artery occlusion, unspecified eye

CHAPTER 7 (H00-H59)

● H34.23   Retinal artery branch occlusion

    H34.231   Retinal artery branch occlusion, right eye

    H34.232   Retinal artery branch occlusion, left eye

    H34.233   Retinal artery branch occlusion, bilateral

    H34.239   Retinal artery branch occlusion, unspecified eye

● H34.8   Other retinal vascular occlusions

   ● H34.81   Central retinal vein occlusion

    H34.811   Central retinal vein occlusion, right eye

    H34.812   Central retinal vein occlusion, left eye

    H34.813   Central retinal vein occlusion, bilateral

    H34.819   Central retinal vein occlusion, unspecified eye

   ● H34.82   Venous engorgement
       Incipient retinal vein occlusion
       Partial retinal vein occlusion

    H34.821   Venous engorgement, right eye

    H34.822   Venous engorgement, left eye

    H34.823   Venous engorgement, bilateral

    H34.829   Venous engorgement, unspecified eye

   ● H34.83   Tributary (branch) retinal vein occlusion

    H34.831   Tributary (branch) retinal vein occlusion, right eye

    H34.832   Tributary (branch) retinal vein occlusion, left eye

    H34.833   Tributary (branch) retinal vein occlusion, bilateral

    H34.839   Tributary (branch) retinal vein occlusion, unspecified eye

  H34.9   Unspecified retinal vascular occlusion

● H35   Other retinal disorders

   Excludes2   diabetic retinal disorders (E08.311-E08.359, E09.311-E09.359, E10.311-E10.359, E11.311-E11.359, E13.311-E13.359)

   ● H35.0   Background retinopathy and retinal vascular changes
       Code also any associated hypertension (I10.-)

    H35.00   Unspecified background retinopathy

   ● H35.01   Changes in retinal vascular appearance
       Retinal vascular sheathing

    H35.011   Changes in retinal vascular appearance, right eye

    H35.012   Changes in retinal vascular appearance, left eye

    H35.013   Changes in retinal vascular appearance, bilateral

    H35.019   Changes in retinal vascular appearance, unspecified eye

OGCR Section I. C.9.a.5.

Hypertensive Retinopathy

Subcategory H35.0, Background retinopathy and retinal vascular changes, should be used with a code from category I10–I15, Hypertensive disease to include the systemic hypertension. The sequencing is based on the reason for the encounter.

● H35.02   Exudative retinopathy
       Coats retinopathy

    H35.021   Exudative retinopathy, right eye

    H35.022   Exudative retinopathy, left eye

    H35.023   Exudative retinopathy, bilateral

    H35.029   Exudative retinopathy, unspecified eye

● H35.03   Hypertensive retinopathy

    H35.031   Hypertensive retinopathy, right eye

    H35.032   Hypertensive retinopathy, left eye

    H35.033   Hypertensive retinopathy, bilateral

    H35.039   Hypertensive retinopathy, unspecified eye

● H35.04   Retinal micro-aneurysms, unspecified

    H35.041   Retinal micro-aneurysms, unspecified, right eye

    H35.042   Retinal micro-aneurysms, unspecified, left eye

    H35.043   Retinal micro-aneurysms, unspecified, bilateral

    H35.049   Retinal micro-aneurysms, unspecified, unspecified eye

● H35.05   Retinal neovascularization, unspecified

    H35.051   Retinal neovascularization, unspecified, right eye

    H35.052   Retinal neovascularization, unspecified, left eye

    H35.053   Retinal neovascularization, unspecified, bilateral

    H35.059   Retinal neovascularization, unspecified, unspecified eye

● H35.06   Retinal vasculitis
       Eales disease
       Retinal perivasculitis

    H35.061   Retinal vasculitis, right eye

    H35.062   Retinal vasculitis, left eye

    H35.063   Retinal vasculitis, bilateral

    H35.069   Retinal vasculitis, unspecified eye

● H35.07   Retinal telangiectasis

    H35.071   Retinal telangiectasis, right eye

    H35.072   Retinal telangiectasis, left eye

    H35.073   Retinal telangiectasis, bilateral

    H35.079   Retinal telangiectasis, unspecified eye

   H35.09   Other intraretinal microvascular abnormalities
       Retinal varices

  H35.1   Retinopathy of prematurity

   ● H35.10   Retinopathy of prematurity, unspecified
       Retinopathy of prematurity NOS

    H35.101   Retinopathy of prematurity, unspecified, right eye

    H35.102   Retinopathy of prematurity, unspecified, left eye

    H35.103   Retinopathy of prematurity, unspecified, bilateral

    H35.109   Retinopathy of prematurity, unspecified, unspecified eye

● H35.11   Retinopathy of prematurity, stage 0

    H35.111   Retinopathy of prematurity, stage 0, right eye

    H35.112   Retinopathy of prematurity, stage 0, left eye

    H35.113   Retinopathy of prematurity, stage 0, bilateral

    H35.119   Retinopathy of prematurity, stage 0, unspecified eye

◀ New   ◀ Revised   ~~deleted~~ Deleted   Excludes 1   Excludes 2   Includes   Use additional   Code first   Code also   Unspecified

OGCR Official Guidelines   **X** Assign placeholder X   ● Use Additional Character(s)   ▶ Manifestation Code   **Coding Clinic**

● H35.12 Retinopathy of prematurity, stage 1

   H35.121 Retinopathy of prematurity, stage 1, right eye

   H35.122 Retinopathy of prematurity, stage 1, left eye

   H35.123 Retinopathy of prematurity, stage 1, bilateral

   H35.129 Retinopathy of prematurity, stage 1, unspecified eye

● H35.13 Retinopathy of prematurity, stage 2

   H35.131 Retinopathy of prematurity, stage 2, right eye

   H35.132 Retinopathy of prematurity, stage 2, left eye

   H35.133 Retinopathy of prematurity, stage 2, bilateral

   H35.139 Retinopathy of prematurity, stage 2, unspecified eye

● H35.14 Retinopathy of prematurity, stage 3

   H35.141 Retinopathy of prematurity, stage 3, right eye

   H35.142 Retinopathy of prematurity, stage 3, left eye

   H35.143 Retinopathy of prematurity, stage 3, bilateral

   H35.149 Retinopathy of prematurity, stage 3, unspecified eye

● H35.15 Retinopathy of prematurity, stage 4

   H35.151 Retinopathy of prematurity, stage 4, right eye

   H35.152 Retinopathy of prematurity, stage 4, left eye

   H35.153 Retinopathy of prematurity, stage 4, bilateral

   H35.159 Retinopathy of prematurity, stage 4, unspecified eye

● H35.16 Retinopathy of prematurity, stage 5

   H35.161 Retinopathy of prematurity, stage 5, right eye

   H35.162 Retinopathy of prematurity, stage 5, left eye

   H35.163 Retinopathy of prematurity, stage 5, bilateral

   H35.169 Retinopathy of prematurity, stage 5, unspecified eye

● H35.17 Retrolental fibroplasia

   H35.171 Retrolental fibroplasia, right eye

   H35.172 Retrolental fibroplasia, left eye

   H35.173 Retrolental fibroplasia, bilateral

   H35.179 Retrolental fibroplasia, unspecified eye

● H35.2 Other non-diabetic proliferative retinopathy
         Proliferative vitreo-retinopathy

   Excludes 1 proliferative vitreo-retinopathy with retinal detachment (H33.4-)

   H35.20 Other non-diabetic proliferative retinopathy, unspecified eye

   H35.21 Other non-diabetic proliferative retinopathy, right eye

   H35.22 Other non-diabetic proliferative retinopathy, left eye

   H35.23 Other non-diabetic proliferative retinopathy, bilateral

Item 7–7 Macular degeneration is typically age-related, chronic, and is evidenced by deterioration of the macula (the part of the retina that provides for central field vision), resulting in blurred vision or a blind spot in the center of visual field while not affecting peripheral vision.

● H35.3 Degeneration of macula and posterior pole

   H35.30 Unspecified macular degeneration   A
           Age-related macular degeneration

   H35.31 Nonexudative age-related macular degeneration   A
           Atrophic age-related macular degeneration

   H35.32 Exudative age-related macular degeneration   A

   H35.33 Angioid streaks of macula

● H35.34 Macular cyst, hole, or pseudohole

   H35.341 Macular cyst, hole, or pseudohole, right eye

   H35.342 Macular cyst, hole, or pseudohole, left eye

   H35.343 Macular cyst, hole, or pseudohole, bilateral

   H35.349 Macular cyst, hole, or pseudohole, unspecified eye

● H35.35 Cystoid macular degeneration

   Excludes 1 cystoid macular edema following cataract surgery (H59.03-)

   H35.351 Cystoid macular degeneration, right eye

   H35.352 Cystoid macular degeneration, left eye

   H35.353 Cystoid macular degeneration, bilateral

   H35.359 Cystoid macular degeneration, unspecified eye

● H35.36 Drusen (degenerative) of macula

   H35.361 Drusen (degenerative) of macula, right eye

   H35.362 Drusen (degenerative) of macula, left eye

   H35.363 Drusen (degenerative) of macula, bilateral

   H35.369 Drusen (degenerative) of macula, unspecified eye

● H35.37 Puckering of macula

   H35.371 Puckering of macula, right eye

   H35.372 Puckering of macula, left eye

   H35.373 Puckering of macula, bilateral

   H35.379 Puckering of macula, unspecified eye

● H35.38 Toxic maculopathy

   Code first poisoning due to drug or toxin, if applicable (T36-T65 with fifth or sixth character 1-4 or 6)

   Use additional code for adverse effect, if applicable, to identify drug (T36-T50 with fifth or sixth character 5)

   H35.381 Toxic maculopathy, right eye

   H35.382 Toxic maculopathy, left eye

   H35.383 Toxic maculopathy, bilateral

   H35.389 Toxic maculopathy, unspecified eye

● H35.4   **Peripheral retinal degeneration**
     Excludes1   hereditary retinal degeneration
                 (dystrophy) (H35.5-)
                 peripheral retinal degeneration with
                 retinal break (H33.3-)

   H35.40   **Unspecified** peripheral retinal degeneration

● H35.41   **Lattice degeneration of retina**
         Palisade degeneration of retina

       H35.411   **Lattice degeneration of retina, right eye**

       H35.412   **Lattice degeneration of retina, left eye**

       H35.413   **Lattice degeneration of retina, bilateral**

       H35.419   **Lattice degeneration of retina, unspecified eye**

● H35.42   **Microcystoid degeneration of retina**

       H35.421   **Microcystoid degeneration of retina, right eye**

       H35.422   **Microcystoid degeneration of retina, left eye**

       H35.423   **Microcystoid degeneration of retina, bilateral**

       H35.429   **Microcystoid degeneration of retina, unspecified eye**

● H35.43   **Paving stone degeneration of retina**

       H35.431   **Paving stone degeneration of retina, right eye**

       H35.432   **Paving stone degeneration of retina, left eye**

       H35.433   **Paving stone degeneration of retina, bilateral**

       H35.439   **Paving stone degeneration of retina, unspecified eye**

● H35.44   **Age-related reticular degeneration of retina**

       H35.441   **Age-related reticular degeneration of retina, right eye**   A

       H35.442   **Age-related reticular degeneration of retina, left eye**   A

       H35.443   **Age-related reticular degeneration of retina, bilateral**   A

       H35.449   **Age-related reticular degeneration of retina, unspecified eye**   A

● H35.45   **Secondary pigmentary degeneration**

       H35.451   **Secondary pigmentary degeneration, right eye**

       H35.452   **Secondary pigmentary degeneration, left eye**

       H35.453   **Secondary pigmentary degeneration, bilateral**

       H35.459   **Secondary pigmentary degeneration, unspecified eye**

● H35.46   **Secondary vitreoretinal degeneration**

       H35.461   **Secondary vitreoretinal degeneration, right eye**

       H35.462   **Secondary vitreoretinal degeneration, left eye**

       H35.463   **Secondary vitreoretinal degeneration, bilateral**

       H35.469   **Secondary vitreoretinal degeneration, unspecified eye**

● H35.5   **Hereditary retinal dystrophy**
     Excludes1   dystrophies primarily involving Bruch's
                 membrane (H31.1-)

   H35.50   **Unspecified** hereditary retinal dystrophy

   H35.51   **Vitreoretinal dystrophy**

   H35.52   **Pigmentary retinal dystrophy**
         Albipunctate retinal dystrophy
         Retinitis pigmentosa
         Tapetoretinal dystrophy

   H35.53   **Other dystrophies primarily involving the sensory retina**
         Stargardt's disease

   H35.54   **Dystrophies primarily involving the retinal pigment epithelium**
         Vitelliform retinal dystrophy

● H35.6   **Retinal hemorrhage**

   H35.60   **Retinal hemorrhage, unspecified eye**

   H35.61   **Retinal hemorrhage, right eye**

   H35.62   **Retinal hemorrhage, left eye**

   H35.63   **Retinal hemorrhage, bilateral**

● H35.7   **Separation of retinal layers**
     Excludes1   retinal detachment (serous) (H33.2-)
                 rhegmatogenous retinal detachment
                 (H33.0-)

   H35.70   **Unspecified** separation of retinal layers

● H35.71   **Central serous chorioretinopathy**

       H35.711   **Central serous chorioretinopathy, right eye**

       H35.712   **Central serous chorioretinopathy, left eye**

       H35.713   **Central serous chorioretinopathy, bilateral**

       H35.719   **Central serous chorioretinopathy, unspecified eye**

● H35.72   **Serous detachment of retinal pigment epithelium**

       H35.721   **Serous detachment of retinal pigment epithelium, right eye**

       H35.722   **Serous detachment of retinal pigment epithelium, left eye**

       H35.723   **Serous detachment of retinal pigment epithelium, bilateral**

       H35.729   **Serous detachment of retinal pigment epithelium, unspecified eye**

● H35.73   **Hemorrhagic detachment of retinal pigment epithelium**

       H35.731   **Hemorrhagic detachment of retinal pigment epithelium, right eye**

       H35.732   **Hemorrhagic detachment of retinal pigment epithelium, left eye**

       H35.733   **Hemorrhagic detachment of retinal pigment epithelium, bilateral**

       H35.739   **Hemorrhagic detachment of retinal pigment epithelium, unspecified eye**

● H35.8   **Other specified retinal disorders**
     Excludes2   retinal hemorrhage (H35.6-)

   H35.81   **Retinal edema**
         Retinal cotton wool spots

   H35.82   **Retinal ischemia**

   H35.89   **Other specified retinal disorders**

● H35.9   **Unspecified** retinal disorder

▶ H36   *Retinal disorders in diseases classified elsewhere*
     Code first underlying disease, such as:
       lipid storage disorders (E75.-)
       sickle-cell disorders (D57.-)
     Excludes1   arteriosclerotic retinopathy (H35.0-)
                 diabetic retinopathy (E08.3-, E09.3-, E10.3-, E11.3-,
                 E13.3-)

◀ New   ◀◀◀ Revised   ~~deleted~~ Deleted   Excludes 1   Excludes 2   Includes   Use additional   Code first   Code also   Unspecified
OGCR Official Guidelines   X Assign placeholder X   ● Use Additional Character(s)   ▶ Manifestation Code   **Coding Clinic**

GLAUCOMA (H40-H42)

● **H40 Glaucoma**

Intraocular pressure (IOP) that is too high results from too much aqueous humor and because of excess production or inadequate drainage, optic nerve damage and vision loss may occur.

> **Excludes1** absolute glaucoma (H44.51-)
> congenital glaucoma (Q15.0)
> traumatic glaucoma due to birth injury (P15.3)

● **H40.0 Glaucoma suspect**

● **H40.00 Preglaucoma, unspecified**

H40.001 Preglaucoma, unspecified, right eye

H40.002 Preglaucoma, unspecified, left eye

H40.003 Preglaucoma, unspecified, bilateral

H40.009 Preglaucoma, unspecified, unspecified eye

● **H40.01 Open angle with borderline findings, low risk**
Open angle, low risk

H40.011 Open angle with borderline findings, low risk, right eye

H40.012 Open angle with borderline findings, low risk, left eye

H40.013 Open angle with borderline findings, low risk, bilateral

H40.019 Open angle with borderline findings, low risk, unspecified eye

● **H40.02 Open angle with borderline findings, high risk**
Open angle, high risk

H40.021 Open angle with borderline findings, high risk, right eye

H40.022 Open angle with borderline findings, high risk, left eye

H40.023 Open angle with borderline findings, high risk, bilateral

H40.029 Open angle with borderline findings, high risk, unspecified eye

● **H40.03 Anatomical narrow angle**
Primary angle closure suspect

H40.031 Anatomical narrow angle, right eye

H40.032 Anatomical narrow angle, left eye

H40.033 Anatomical narrow angle, bilateral

H40.039 Anatomical narrow angle, unspecified eye

● **H40.04 Steroid responder**

H40.041 Steroid responder, right eye

H40.042 Steroid responder, left eye

H40.043 Steroid responder, bilateral

H40.049 Steroid responder, unspecified eye

● **H40.05 Ocular hypertension**

H40.051 Ocular hypertension, right eye

H40.052 Ocular hypertension, left eye

H40.053 Ocular hypertension, bilateral

H40.059 Ocular hypertension, unspecified eye

● **H40.06 Primary angle closure without glaucoma damage**

H40.061 Primary angle closure without glaucoma damage, right eye

H40.062 Primary angle closure without glaucoma damage, left eye

H40.063 Primary angle closure without glaucoma damage, bilateral

H40.069 Primary angle closure without glaucoma damage, unspecified eye

● **H40.1 Open-angle glaucoma**

X● **H40.10 Unspecified open-angle glaucoma**

One of the following 7th characters is to be assigned to code H40.10 to designate the stage of glaucoma

0	stage unspecified
1	mild stage
2	moderate stage
3	severe stage
4	indeterminate stage

X● **H40.11 Primary open-angle glaucoma**
Chronic simple glaucoma

One of the following 7th characters is to be assigned to code H40.11 to designate the stage of glaucoma

0	stage unspecified
1	mild stage
2	moderate stage
3	severe stage
4	indeterminate stage

● **H40.12 Low-tension glaucoma**

One of the following 7th characters is to be assigned to each code in subcategory H40.12 to designate the stage of glaucoma

0	stage unspecified
1	mild stage
2	moderate stage
3	severe stage
4	indeterminate stage

● H40.121 Low-tension glaucoma, right eye

● H40.122 Low-tension glaucoma, left eye

● H40.123 Low-tension glaucoma, bilateral

● H40.129 Low-tension glaucoma, unspecified eye

● **H40.13 Pigmentary glaucoma**

One of the following 7th characters is to be assigned to each code in subcategory H40.13 to designate the stage of glaucoma

0	stage unspecified
1	mild stage
2	moderate stage
3	severe stage
4	indeterminate stage

● H40.131 Pigmentary glaucoma, right eye

● H40.132 Pigmentary glaucoma, left eye

● H40.133 Pigmentary glaucoma, bilateral

● H40.139 Pigmentary glaucoma, unspecified eye

● **H40.14 Capsular glaucoma with pseudoexfoliation of lens**

One of the following 7th characters is to be assigned to each code in subcategory H40.14 to designate the stage of glaucoma

0	stage unspecified
1	mild stage
2	moderate stage
3	severe stage
4	indeterminate stage

● H40.141 Capsular glaucoma with pseudoexfoliation of lens, right eye

● H40.142 Capsular glaucoma with pseudoexfoliation of lens, left eye

CHAPTER 7 (H00-H59)

● H40.143   Capsular glaucoma with pseudoexfoliation of lens, bilateral

● H40.149   Capsular glaucoma with pseudoexfoliation of lens, unspecified eye

● H40.15   Residual stage of open-angle glaucoma

     H40.151   Residual stage of open-angle glaucoma, right eye

     H40.152   Residual stage of open-angle glaucoma, left eye

     H40.153   Residual stage of open-angle glaucoma, bilateral

     H40.159   Residual stage of open-angle glaucoma, unspecified eye

● H40.2   Primary angle-closure glaucoma

     Excludes1   aqueous misdirection (H40.83-)
                  malignant glaucoma (H40.83-)

● H40.20   Unspecified primary angle-closure glaucoma

     One of the following 7th characters is to be assigned to code H40.20 to designate the stage of glaucoma

0	stage unspecified
1	mild stage
2	moderate stage
3	severe stage
4	indeterminate stage

● H40.21   Acute angle-closure glaucoma

     Acute angle-closure glaucoma attack
     Acute angle-closure glaucoma crisis

     H40.211   Acute angle-closure glaucoma, right eye

     H40.212   Acute angle-closure glaucoma, left eye

     H40.213   Acute angle-closure glaucoma, bilateral

     H40.219   Acute angle-closure glaucoma, unspecified eye

● H40.22   Chronic angle-closure glaucoma

     Chronic primary angle closure glaucoma

     One of the following 7th characters is to be assigned to each code in subcategory H40.22 to designate the stage of glaucoma

0	stage unspecified
1	mild stage
2	moderate stage
3	severe stage
4	indeterminate stage

● H40.221   Chronic angle-closure glaucoma, right eye

● H40.222   Chronic angle-closure glaucoma, left eye

● H40.223   Chronic angle-closure glaucoma, bilateral

● H40.229   Chronic angle-closure glaucoma, unspecified eye

● H40.23   Intermittent angle-closure glaucoma

     H40.231   Intermittent angle-closure glaucoma, right eye

     H40.232   Intermittent angle-closure glaucoma, left eye

     H40.233   Intermittent angle-closure glaucoma, bilateral

     H40.239   Intermittent angle-closure glaucoma, unspecified eye

● H40.24   Residual stage of angle-closure glaucoma

     H40.241   Residual stage of angle-closure glaucoma, right eye

     H40.242   Residual stage of angle-closure glaucoma, left eye

     H40.243   Residual stage of angle-closure glaucoma, bilateral

     H40.249   Residual stage of angle-closure glaucoma, unspecified eye

● H40.3   Glaucoma secondary to eye trauma

     Code also underlying condition

     One of the following 7th characters is to be assigned to each code in subcategory H40.3 to designate the stage of glaucoma

0	stage unspecified
1	mild stage
2	moderate stage
3	severe stage
4	indeterminate stage

X ● H40.30   Glaucoma secondary to eye trauma, unspecified eye

X ● H40.31   Glaucoma secondary to eye trauma, right eye

X ● H40.32   Glaucoma secondary to eye trauma, left eye

X ● H40.33   Glaucoma secondary to eye trauma, bilateral

● H40.4   Glaucoma secondary to eye inflammation

     Code also underlying condition

     One of the following 7th characters is to be assigned to each code in subcategory H40.4 to designate the stage of glaucoma

0	stage unspecified
1	mild stage
2	moderate stage
3	severe stage
4	indeterminate stage

X ● H40.40   Glaucoma secondary to eye inflammation, unspecified eye

X ● H40.41   Glaucoma secondary to eye inflammation, right eye

X ● H40.42   Glaucoma secondary to eye inflammation, left eye

X ● H40.43   Glaucoma secondary to eye inflammation, bilateral

● H40.5   Glaucoma secondary to other eye disorders

     Code also underlying eye disorder

     One of the following 7th characters is to be assigned to each code in subcategory H40.5 to designate the stage of glaucoma

0	stage unspecified
1	mild stage
2	moderate stage
3	severe stage
4	indeterminate stage

X ● H40.50   Glaucoma secondary to other eye disorders, unspecified eye

X ● H40.51   Glaucoma secondary to other eye disorders, right eye

X ● H40.52   Glaucoma secondary to other eye disorders, left eye

X ● H40.53   Glaucoma secondary to other eye disorders, bilateral

◀ New   ◀■ Revised   ~~deleted~~ Deleted   Excludes 1   Excludes 2   Includes   Use additional   Code first   Code also   Unspecified

OGCR Official Guidelines   X Assign placeholder X   ● Use Additional Character(s)   ▶ Manifestation Code   **Coding Clinic**

● H40.6 Glaucoma secondary to drugs

> Use additional code for adverse effect, if applicable, to identify drug (T36-T50 with fifth or sixth character 5)
>
> One of the following 7th characters is to be assigned to each code in subcategory H40.6 to designate the stage of glaucoma

0	stage unspecified
1	mild stage
2	moderate stage
3	severe stage
4	indeterminate stage

X● H40.60 Glaucoma secondary to drugs, unspecified eye
X● H40.61 Glaucoma secondary to drugs, right eye
X● H40.62 Glaucoma secondary to drugs, left eye
X● H40.63 Glaucoma secondary to drugs, bilateral

● H40.8 Other glaucoma
  ● H40.81 Glaucoma with increased episcleral venous pressure
    H40.811 Glaucoma with increased episcleral venous pressure, right eye
    H40.812 Glaucoma with increased episcleral venous pressure, left eye
    H40.813 Glaucoma with increased episcleral venous pressure, bilateral
    H40.819 Glaucoma with increased episcleral venous pressure, unspecified eye
  ● H40.82 Hypersecretion glaucoma
    H40.821 Hypersecretion glaucoma, right eye
    H40.822 Hypersecretion glaucoma, left eye
    H40.823 Hypersecretion glaucoma, bilateral
    H40.829 Hypersecretion glaucoma, unspecified eye
  ● H40.83 Aqueous misdirection
    Malignant glaucoma
    H40.831 Aqueous misdirection, right eye
    H40.832 Aqueous misdirection, left eye
    H40.833 Aqueous misdirection, bilateral
    H40.839 Aqueous misdirection, unspecified eye
  H40.89 Other specified glaucoma
  H40.9 Unspecified glaucoma

❱ H42 *Glaucoma in diseases classified elsewhere*
> *Code first* underlying condition, such as:
> amyloidosis (E85.-)
> aniridia (Q13.1)
> Lowe's syndrome (E72.03)
> Reiger's anomaly (Q13.81)
> specified metabolic disorder (E70-E88)
>
> **Excludes1** glaucoma (in):
>   diabetes mellitus (E08.39, E09.39, E10.39, E11.39, E13.39)
>   onchocerciasis (B73.02)
>   syphilis (A52.71)
>   tuberculous (A18.59)

DISORDERS OF VITREOUS BODY AND GLOBE (H43-H44)

● H43 Disorders of vitreous body
  ● H43.0 Vitreous prolapse
    Excludes1 vitreous syndrome following cataract surgery (H59.0-)
      traumatic vitreous prolapse (S05.2-)
    H43.00 Vitreous prolapse, unspecified eye
    H43.01 Vitreous prolapse, right eye
    H43.02 Vitreous prolapse, left eye
    H43.03 Vitreous prolapse, bilateral

● H43.1 Vitreous hemorrhage
  H43.10 Vitreous hemorrhage, unspecified eye
  H43.11 Vitreous hemorrhage, right eye
  H43.12 Vitreous hemorrhage, left eye
  H43.13 Vitreous hemorrhage, bilateral
● H43.2 Crystalline deposits in vitreous body
  H43.20 Crystalline deposits in vitreous body, unspecified eye
  H43.21 Crystalline deposits in vitreous body, right eye
  H43.22 Crystalline deposits in vitreous body, left eye
  H43.23 Crystalline deposits in vitreous body, bilateral
● H43.3 Other vitreous opacities
  ● H43.31 Vitreous membranes and strands
    H43.311 Vitreous membranes and strands, right eye
    H43.312 Vitreous membranes and strands, left eye
    H43.313 Vitreous membranes and strands, bilateral
    H43.319 Vitreous membranes and strands, unspecified eye
  ● H43.39 Other vitreous opacities
    Vitreous floaters
    Small clumps of cells that float in the vitreous of the eye, appearing as black specks or dots in the field of vision and common in the aging eye.
    H43.391 Other vitreous opacities, right eye
    H43.392 Other vitreous opacities, left eye
    H43.393 Other vitreous opacities, bilateral
    H43.399 Other vitreous opacities, unspecified eye
● H43.8 Other disorders of vitreous body
  Excludes1 proliferative vitreo-retinopathy with retinal detachment (H33.4)
  Excludes2 vitreous abscess (H44.02-)
  ● H43.81 Vitreous degeneration
    Vitreous detachment
    H43.811 Vitreous degeneration, right eye
    H43.812 Vitreous degeneration, left eye
    H43.813 Vitreous degeneration, bilateral
    H43.819 Vitreous degeneration, unspecified eye
  ● H43.82 Vitreomacular adhesion
    Vitreomacular traction
    H43.821 Vitreomacular adhesion, right eye   A
    H43.822 Vitreomacular adhesion, left eye   A
    H43.823 Vitreomacular adhesion, bilateral   A
    H43.829 Vitreomacular adhesion, unspecified eye   A
  H43.89 Other disorders of vitreous body
  H43.9 Unspecified disorder of vitreous body

● H44 Disorders of globe
  Includes disorders affecting multiple structures of eye
  ● H44.0 Purulent endophthalmitis
    Use additional code to identify organism
    Excludes1 bleb associated endophthalmitis (H59.4-)
    ● H44.00 Unspecified purulent endophthalmitis
      H44.001 Unspecified purulent endophthalmitis, right eye
      H44.002 Unspecified purulent endophthalmitis, left eye
      H44.003 Unspecified purulent endophthalmitis, bilateral
      H44.009 Unspecified purulent endophthalmitis, unspecified eye

CHAPTER 7 (H00-H59)

● **H44.01 Panophthalmitis (acute)**
    H44.011 Panophthalmitis (acute), right eye
    H44.012 Panophthalmitis (acute), left eye
    H44.013 Panophthalmitis (acute), bilateral
    H44.019 Panophthalmitis (acute), unspecified eye

● **H44.02 Vitreous abscess (chronic)**
    H44.021 Vitreous abscess (chronic), right eye
    H44.022 Vitreous abscess (chronic), left eye
    H44.023 Vitreous abscess (chronic), bilateral
    H44.029 Vitreous abscess (chronic), unspecified eye

● **H44.1 Other endophthalmitis**
    Excludes1 bleb associated endophthalmitis (H59.4-)
    Excludes2 ophthalmia nodosa (H16.2-)

● **H44.11 Panuveitis**
    H44.111 Panuveitis, right eye
    H44.112 Panuveitis, left eye
    H44.113 Panuveitis, bilateral
    H44.119 Panuveitis, unspecified eye

● **H44.12 Parasitic endophthalmitis, unspecified**
    H44.121 Parasitic endophthalmitis, unspecified, right eye
    H44.122 Parasitic endophthalmitis, unspecified, left eye
    H44.123 Parasitic endophthalmitis, unspecified, bilateral
    H44.129 Parasitic endophthalmitis, unspecified, unspecified eye

● **H44.13 Sympathetic uveitis**
    H44.131 Sympathetic uveitis, right eye
    H44.132 Sympathetic uveitis, left eye
    H44.133 Sympathetic uveitis, bilateral
    H44.139 Sympathetic uveitis, unspecified eye

    H44.19 Other endophthalmitis

● **H44.2 Degenerative myopia**
    Malignant myopia
    H44.20 Degenerative myopia, unspecified eye
    H44.21 Degenerative myopia, right eye
    H44.22 Degenerative myopia, left eye
    H44.23 Degenerative myopia, bilateral

● **H44.3 Other and unspecified degenerative disorders of globe**
    H44.30 Unspecified degenerative disorder of globe

● **H44.31 Chalcosis**
    H44.311 Chalcosis, right eye
    H44.312 Chalcosis, left eye
    H44.313 Chalcosis, bilateral
    H44.319 Chalcosis, unspecified eye

● **H44.32 Siderosis of eye**
    H44.321 Siderosis of eye, right eye
    H44.322 Siderosis of eye, left eye
    H44.323 Siderosis of eye, bilateral
    H44.329 Siderosis of eye, unspecified eye

● **H44.39 Other degenerative disorders of globe**
    H44.391 Other degenerative disorders of globe, right eye
    H44.392 Other degenerative disorders of globe, left eye
    H44.393 Other degenerative disorders of globe, bilateral
    H44.399 Other degenerative disorders of globe, unspecified eye

● **H44.4 Hypotony of eye**
    H44.40 Unspecified hypotony of eye

● **H44.41 Flat anterior chamber hypotony of eye**
    H44.411 Flat anterior chamber hypotony of right eye
    H44.412 Flat anterior chamber hypotony of left eye
    H44.413 Flat anterior chamber hypotony of eye, bilateral
    H44.419 Flat anterior chamber hypotony of unspecified eye

● **H44.42 Hypotony of eye due to ocular fistula**
    H44.421 Hypotony of right eye due to ocular fistula
    H44.422 Hypotony of left eye due to ocular fistula
    H44.423 Hypotony of eye due to ocular fistula, bilateral
    H44.429 Hypotony of unspecified eye due to ocular fistula

● **H44.43 Hypotony of eye due to other ocular disorders**
    H44.431 Hypotony of eye due to other ocular disorders, right eye
    H44.432 Hypotony of eye due to other ocular disorders, left eye
    H44.433 Hypotony of eye due to other ocular disorders, bilateral
    H44.439 Hypotony of eye due to other ocular disorders, unspecified eye

● **H44.44 Primary hypotony of eye**
    H44.441 Primary hypotony of right eye
    H44.442 Primary hypotony of left eye
    H44.443 Primary hypotony of eye, bilateral
    H44.449 Primary hypotony of unspecified eye

● **H44.5 Degenerated conditions of globe**
    H44.50 Unspecified degenerated conditions of globe

● **H44.51 Absolute glaucoma**
    H44.511 Absolute glaucoma, right eye
    H44.512 Absolute glaucoma, left eye
    H44.513 Absolute glaucoma, bilateral
    H44.519 Absolute glaucoma, unspecified eye

● **H44.52 Atrophy of globe**
    Phthisis bulbi
    H44.521 Atrophy of globe, right eye
    H44.522 Atrophy of globe, left eye
    H44.523 Atrophy of globe, bilateral
    H44.529 Atrophy of globe, unspecified eye

● **H44.53 Leucocoria**
    H44.531 Leucocoria, right eye
    H44.532 Leucocoria, left eye
    H44.533 Leucocoria, bilateral
    H44.539 Leucocoria, unspecified eye

● **H44.6 Retained (old) intraocular foreign body, magnetic**
    Use additional code to identify magnetic foreign body (Z18.11)
    Excludes1 current intraocular foreign body (S05.-)
    Excludes2 retained foreign body in eyelid (H02.81-)
    retained (old) foreign body following penetrating wound of orbit (H05.5-)
    retained (old) intraocular foreign body, nonmagnetic (H44.7-)

● **H44.60 Unspecified retained (old) intraocular foreign body, magnetic**
    H44.601 Unspecified retained (old) intraocular foreign body, magnetic, right eye
    H44.602 Unspecified retained (old) intraocular foreign body, magnetic, left eye

◀ New   ◀ Revised   ~~deleted~~ Deleted   Excludes 1   Excludes 2   Includes   Use additional   Code first   Code also   Unspecified
OGCR Official Guidelines   X Assign placeholder X   ● Use Additional Character(s)   ▶ Manifestation Code   **Coding Clinic**

H44.603 **Unspecified** retained (old) intraocular foreign body, magnetic, bilateral

H44.609 **Unspecified** retained (old) intraocular foreign body, magnetic, unspecified eye

● H44.61 Retained (old) magnetic foreign body in anterior chamber

H44.611 Retained (old) magnetic foreign body in anterior chamber, right eye

H44.612 Retained (old) magnetic foreign body in anterior chamber, left eye

H44.613 Retained (old) magnetic foreign body in anterior chamber, bilateral

H44.619 Retained (old) magnetic foreign body in anterior chamber, **unspecified** eye

● H44.62 Retained (old) magnetic foreign body in iris or ciliary body

H44.621 Retained (old) magnetic foreign body in iris or ciliary body, right eye

H44.622 Retained (old) magnetic foreign body in iris or ciliary body, left eye

H44.623 Retained (old) magnetic foreign body in iris or ciliary body, bilateral

H44.629 Retained (old) magnetic foreign body in iris or ciliary body, **unspecified** eye

● H44.63 Retained (old) magnetic foreign body in lens

H44.631 Retained (old) magnetic foreign body in lens, right eye

H44.632 Retained (old) magnetic foreign body in lens, left eye

H44.633 Retained (old) magnetic foreign body in lens, bilateral

H44.639 Retained (old) magnetic foreign body in lens, **unspecified** eye

● H44.64 Retained (old) magnetic foreign body in posterior wall of globe

H44.641 Retained (old) magnetic foreign body in posterior wall of globe, right eye

H44.642 Retained (old) magnetic foreign body in posterior wall of globe, left eye

H44.643 Retained (old) magnetic foreign body in posterior wall of globe, bilateral

H44.649 Retained (old) magnetic foreign body in posterior wall of globe, **unspecified** eye

● H44.65 Retained (old) magnetic foreign body in vitreous body

H44.651 Retained (old) magnetic foreign body in vitreous body, right eye

H44.652 Retained (old) magnetic foreign body in vitreous body, left eye

H44.653 Retained (old) magnetic foreign body in vitreous body, bilateral

H44.659 Retained (old) magnetic foreign body in vitreous body, **unspecified** eye

● H44.69 Retained (old) intraocular foreign body, magnetic, in other or multiple sites

H44.691 Retained (old) intraocular foreign body, magnetic, in other or multiple sites, right eye

H44.692 Retained (old) intraocular foreign body, magnetic, in other or multiple sites, left eye

H44.693 Retained (old) intraocular foreign body, magnetic, in other or multiple sites, bilateral

H44.699 Retained (old) intraocular foreign body, magnetic, in other or multiple sites, **unspecified** eye

● H44.7 Retained (old) intraocular foreign body, nonmagnetic

Use additional code to identify nonmagnetic foreign body (Z18.01-Z18.10, Z18.12, Z18.2-Z18.9)

Excludes1 current intraocular foreign body (S05.-)

Excludes2 retained foreign body in eyelid (H02.81-)
retained (old) foreign body following penetrating wound of orbit (H05.5-)
retained (old) intraocular foreign body, magnetic (H44.6-)

● H44.70 Unspecified retained (old) intraocular foreign body, nonmagnetic

H44.701 **Unspecified** retained (old) intraocular foreign body, nonmagnetic, right eye

H44.702 **Unspecified** retained (old) intraocular foreign body, nonmagnetic, left eye

H44.703 **Unspecified** retained (old) intraocular foreign body, nonmagnetic, bilateral

H44.709 **Unspecified** retained (old) intraocular foreign body, nonmagnetic, unspecified eye

Retained (old) intraocular foreign body NOS

● H44.71 Retained (nonmagnetic) (old) foreign body in anterior chamber

H44.711 Retained (nonmagnetic) (old) foreign body in anterior chamber, right eye

H44.712 Retained (nonmagnetic) (old) foreign body in anterior chamber, left eye

H44.713 Retained (nonmagnetic) (old) foreign body in anterior chamber, bilateral

H44.719 Retained (nonmagnetic) (old) foreign body in anterior chamber, **unspecified** eye

● H44.72 Retained (nonmagnetic) (old) foreign body in iris or ciliary body

H44.721 Retained (nonmagnetic) (old) foreign body in iris or ciliary body, right eye

H44.722 Retained (nonmagnetic) (old) foreign body in iris or ciliary body, left eye

H44.723 Retained (nonmagnetic) (old) foreign body in iris or ciliary body, bilateral

H44.729 Retained (nonmagnetic) (old) foreign body in iris or ciliary body, **unspecified** eye

● H44.73 Retained (nonmagnetic) (old) foreign body in lens

H44.731 Retained (nonmagnetic) (old) foreign body in lens, right eye

H44.732 Retained (nonmagnetic) (old) foreign body in lens, left eye

H44.733 Retained (nonmagnetic) (old) foreign body in lens, bilateral

H44.739 Retained (nonmagnetic) (old) foreign body in lens, **unspecified** eye

● H44.74 Retained (nonmagnetic) (old) foreign body in posterior wall of globe

H44.741 Retained (nonmagnetic) (old) foreign body in posterior wall of globe, right eye

H44.742 Retained (nonmagnetic) (old) foreign body in posterior wall of globe, left eye

H44.743 Retained (nonmagnetic) (old) foreign body in posterior wall of globe, bilateral

H44.749 Retained (nonmagnetic) (old) foreign body in posterior wall of globe, **unspecified** eye

CHAPTER 7 (H00-H59)

● **H44.75** Retained (nonmagnetic) (old) foreign body in vitreous body

H44.751 Retained (nonmagnetic) (old) foreign body in vitreous body, right eye

H44.752 Retained (nonmagnetic) (old) foreign body in vitreous body, left eye

H44.753 Retained (nonmagnetic) (old) foreign body in vitreous body, bilateral

H44.759 Retained (nonmagnetic) (old) foreign body in vitreous body, unspecified eye

● **H44.79** Retained (old) intraocular foreign body, nonmagnetic, in other or multiple sites

H44.791 Retained (old) intraocular foreign body, nonmagnetic, in other or multiple sites, right eye

H44.792 Retained (old) intraocular foreign body, nonmagnetic, in other or multiple sites, left eye

H44.793 Retained (old) intraocular foreign body, nonmagnetic, in other or multiple sites, bilateral

H44.799 Retained (old) intraocular foreign body, nonmagnetic, in other or multiple sites, unspecified eye

● **H44.8** Other disorders of globe

● **H44.81** Hemophthalmos

H44.811 Hemophthalmos, right eye

H44.812 Hemophthalmos, left eye

H44.813 Hemophthalmos, bilateral

H44.819 Hemophthalmos, unspecified eye

● **H44.82** Luxation of globe

H44.821 Luxation of globe, right eye

H44.822 Luxation of globe, left eye

H44.823 Luxation of globe, bilateral

H44.829 Luxation of globe, unspecified eye

H44.89 Other disorders of globe

H44.9 Unspecified disorder of globe

(See Plate 86 on page 55.)

DISORDERS OF OPTIC NERVE AND VISUAL PATHWAYS (H46-H47)

● **H46** Optic neuritis

Excludes2 ischemic optic neuropathy (H47.01-)
neuromyelitis optica [Devic] (G36.0)

● **H46.0** Optic papillitis

H46.00 Optic papillitis, unspecified eye

H46.01 Optic papillitis, right eye

H46.02 Optic papillitis, left eye

H46.03 Optic papillitis, bilateral

● **H46.1** Retrobulbar neuritis
Retrobulbar neuritis NOS

Excludes1 syphilitic retrobulbar neuritis (A52.15)

H46.10 Retrobulbar neuritis, unspecified eye

H46.11 Retrobulbar neuritis, right eye

H46.12 Retrobulbar neuritis, left eye

H46.13 Retrobulbar neuritis, bilateral

H46.2 Nutritional optic neuropathy

H46.3 Toxic optic neuropathy
Code first (T51-T65) to identify cause

H46.8 Other optic neuritis

H46.9 Unspecified optic neuritis

● **H47** Other disorders of optic [2nd] nerve and visual pathways

● **H47.0** Disorders of optic nerve, not elsewhere classified

● **H47.01** Ischemic optic neuropathy

H47.011 Ischemic optic neuropathy, right eye

H47.012 Ischemic optic neuropathy, left eye

H47.013 Ischemic optic neuropathy, bilateral

H47.019 Ischemic optic neuropathy, unspecified eye

● **H47.02** Hemorrhage in optic nerve sheath

H47.021 Hemorrhage in optic nerve sheath, right eye

H47.022 Hemorrhage in optic nerve sheath, left eye

H47.023 Hemorrhage in optic nerve sheath, bilateral

H47.029 Hemorrhage in optic nerve sheath, unspecified eye

● **H47.03** Optic nerve hypoplasia

H47.031 Optic nerve hypoplasia, right eye

H47.032 Optic nerve hypoplasia, left eye

H47.033 Optic nerve hypoplasia, bilateral

H47.039 Optic nerve hypoplasia, unspecified eye

● **H47.09** Other disorders of optic nerve, not elsewhere classified
Compression of optic nerve

H47.091 Other disorders of optic nerve, not elsewhere classified, right eye

H47.092 Other disorders of optic nerve, not elsewhere classified, left eye

H47.093 Other disorders of optic nerve, not elsewhere classified, bilateral

H47.099 Other disorders of optic nerve, not elsewhere classified, unspecified eye

● **H47.1** Papilledema

H47.10 Unspecified papilledema

H47.11 Papilledema associated with increased intracranial pressure

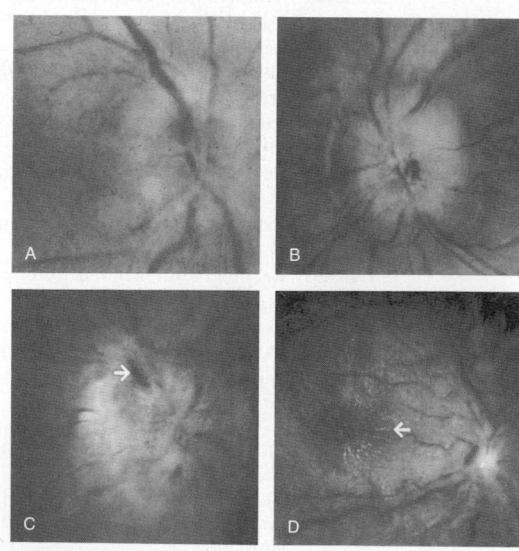

Figure 7-10 Papilledema. (From Behrma: Nelson Textbook of Pediatrics, ed 17, Saunders, 2004)

Item 7–8 Papilledema is swelling of the optic disc caused by increased intracranial pressure. It is most often bilateral and occurs quickly (hours) or over weeks of time. It is a common symptom of a brain tumor. The term should not be used to describe optic disc swelling with underlying infectious, infiltrative, or inflammatory etiologies.

◄ New   ◄▪▪ Revised   ~~deleted~~ Deleted   Excludes 1   Excludes 2   Includes   Use additional   Code first   Code also   Unspecified

OGCR Official Guidelines   X Assign placeholder X   ● Use Additional Character(s)   ▶ Manifestation Code   **Coding Clinic**

H47.12   Papilledema associated with decreased ocular pressure

H47.13   Papilledema associated with retinal disorder

● H47.14   Foster-Kennedy syndrome

    H47.141   Foster-Kennedy syndrome, right eye

    H47.142   Foster-Kennedy syndrome, left eye

    H47.143   Foster-Kennedy syndrome, bilateral

    H47.149   Foster-Kennedy syndrome, unspecified eye

● H47.2   Optic atrophy

    H47.20   Unspecified optic atrophy

   ● H47.21   Primary optic atrophy

      H47.211   Primary optic atrophy, right eye

      H47.212   Primary optic atrophy, left eye

      H47.213   Primary optic atrophy, bilateral

      H47.219   Primary optic atrophy, unspecified eye

   H47.22   Hereditary optic atrophy

      Leber's optic atrophy

   ● H47.23   Glaucomatous optic atrophy

      H47.231   Glaucomatous optic atrophy, right eye

      H47.232   Glaucomatous optic atrophy, left eye

      H47.233   Glaucomatous optic atrophy, bilateral

      H47.239   Glaucomatous optic atrophy, unspecified eye

   ● H47.29   Other optic atrophy

      Temporal pallor of optic disc

      H47.291   Other optic atrophy, right eye

      H47.292   Other optic atrophy, left eye

      H47.293   Other optic atrophy, bilateral

      H47.299   Other optic atrophy, unspecified eye

● H47.3   Other disorders of optic disc

   ● H47.31   Coloboma of optic disc

      H47.311   Coloboma of optic disc, right eye

      H47.312   Coloboma of optic disc, left eye

      H47.313   Coloboma of optic disc, bilateral

      H47.319   Coloboma of optic disc, unspecified eye

   ● H47.32   Drusen of optic disc

      H47.321   Drusen of optic disc, right eye

      H47.322   Drusen of optic disc, left eye

      H47.323   Drusen of optic disc, bilateral

      H47.329   Drusen of optic disc, unspecified eye

   ● H47.33   Pseudopapilledema of optic disc

      H47.331   Pseudopapilledema of optic disc, right eye

      H47.332   Pseudopapilledema of optic disc, left eye

      H47.333   Pseudopapilledema of optic disc, bilateral

      H47.339   Pseudopapilledema of optic disc, unspecified eye

   ● H47.39   Other disorders of optic disc

      H47.391   Other disorders of optic disc, right eye

      H47.392   Other disorders of optic disc, left eye

      H47.393   Other disorders of optic disc, bilateral

      H47.399   Other disorders of optic disc, unspecified eye

● H47.4   Disorders of optic chiasm

     Code also underlying condition

   H47.41   Disorders of optic chiasm in (due to) inflammatory disorders

   H47.42   Disorders of optic chiasm in (due to) neoplasm

   H47.43   Disorders of optic chiasm in (due to) vascular disorders

   H47.49   Disorders of optic chiasm in (due to) other disorders

● H47.5   Disorders of other visual pathways

     Disorders of optic tracts, geniculate nuclei and optic radiations

     Code also underlying condition

   ● H47.51   Disorders of visual pathways in (due to) inflammatory disorders

      H47.511   Disorders of visual pathways in (due to) inflammatory disorders, right side

      H47.512   Disorders of visual pathways in (due to) inflammatory disorders, left side

      H47.519   Disorders of visual pathways in (due to) inflammatory disorders, unspecified side

   ● H47.52   Disorders of visual pathways in (due to) neoplasm

      H47.521   Disorders of visual pathways in (due to) neoplasm, right side

      H47.522   Disorders of visual pathways in (due to) neoplasm, left side

      H47.529   Disorders of visual pathways in (due to) neoplasm, unspecified side

   ● H47.53   Disorders of visual pathways in (due to) vascular disorders

      H47.531   Disorders of visual pathways in (due to) vascular disorders, right side

      H47.532   Disorders of visual pathways in (due to) vascular disorders, left side

      H47.539   Disorders of visual pathways in (due to) vascular disorders, unspecified side

● H47.6   Disorders of visual cortex

     Code also underlying condition

     Excludes1   injury to visual cortex S04.04

   ● H47.61   Cortical blindness

      H47.611   Cortical blindness, right side of brain

      H47.612   Cortical blindness, left side of brain

      H47.619   Cortical blindness, unspecified side of brain

   ● H47.62   Disorders of visual cortex in (due to) inflammatory disorders

      H47.621   Disorders of visual cortex in (due to) inflammatory disorders, right side of brain

      H47.622   Disorders of visual cortex in (due to) inflammatory disorders, left side of brain

      H47.629   Disorders of visual cortex in (due to) inflammatory disorders, unspecified side of brain

   ● H47.63   Disorders of visual cortex in (due to) neoplasm

      H47.631   Disorders of visual cortex in (due to) neoplasm, right side of brain

      H47.632   Disorders of visual cortex in (due to) neoplasm, left side of brain

      H47.639   Disorders of visual cortex in (due to) neoplasm, unspecified side of brain

CHAPTER 7 (H00-H59)

CHAPTER 7 (H00-H59)

● H47.64   Disorders of visual cortex in (due to) vascular disorders

     H47.641   Disorders of visual cortex in (due to) vascular disorders, right side of brain

     H47.642   Disorders of visual cortex in (due to) vascular disorders, left side of brain

     H47.649   Disorders of visual cortex in (due to) vascular disorders, unspecified side of brain

H47.9   Unspecified disorder of visual pathways

DISORDERS OF OCULAR MUSCLES, BINOCULAR MOVEMENT, ACCOMMODATION AND REFRACTION (H49-H52)

Excludes2   nystagmus and other irregular eye movements (H55)

● H49   Paralytic strabismus

     Excludes2   internal ophthalmoplegia (H52.51-)
                 internuclear ophthalmoplegia (H51.2-)
                 progressive supranuclear ophthalmoplegia (G23.1)

● H49.0   Third [oculomotor] nerve palsy

     H49.00   Third [oculomotor] nerve palsy, unspecified eye

     H49.01   Third [oculomotor] nerve palsy, right eye

     H49.02   Third [oculomotor] nerve palsy, left eye

     H49.03   Third [oculomotor] nerve palsy, bilateral

● H49.1   Fourth [trochlear] nerve palsy

     H49.10   Fourth [trochlear] nerve palsy, unspecified eye

     H49.11   Fourth [trochlear] nerve palsy, right eye

     H49.12   Fourth [trochlear] nerve palsy, left eye

     H49.13   Fourth [trochlear] nerve palsy, bilateral

● H49.2   Sixth [abducent] nerve palsy

     H49.20   Sixth [abducent] nerve palsy, unspecified eye

     H49.21   Sixth [abducent] nerve palsy, right eye

     H49.22   Sixth [abducent] nerve palsy, left eye

     H49.23   Sixth [abducent] nerve palsy, bilateral

● H49.3   Total (external) ophthalmoplegia

     H49.30   Total (external) ophthalmoplegia, unspecified eye

     H49.31   Total (external) ophthalmoplegia, right eye

     H49.32   Total (external) ophthalmoplegia, left eye

     H49.33   Total (external) ophthalmoplegia, bilateral

● H49.4   Progressive external ophthalmoplegia

     Excludes1   Kearns-Sayre syndrome (H49.81-)

     H49.40   Progressive external ophthalmoplegia, unspecified eye

     H49.41   Progressive external ophthalmoplegia, right eye

     H49.42   Progressive external ophthalmoplegia, left eye

     H49.43   Progressive external ophthalmoplegia, bilateral

Item 7-9   Strabismus or esotropia (crossed eyes) is a condition of the extraocular eye muscles, resulting in an inability of the eyes to focus and also affects depth perception.

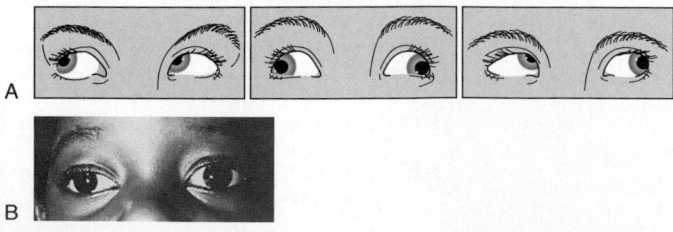

Figure 7-11   **A.** Image of strabismus. **B.** Exotropia. (**A** from Yanoff: Ophthalmology, ed 3, Mosby, Inc., 2008. **B** from Rakel: Textbook of Family Practice, ed 7, Saunders, 2007)

● H49.8   Other paralytic strabismus

     ● H49.81   Kearns-Sayre syndrome
              Progressive external ophthalmoplegia with pigmentary retinopathy

              Use additional code for other manifestation, such as:
              heart block (I45.9)

         H49.811   Kearns-Sayre syndrome, right eye

         H49.812   Kearns-Sayre syndrome, left eye

         H49.813   Kearns-Sayre syndrome, bilateral

         H49.819   Kearns-Sayre syndrome, unspecified eye

     ● H49.88   Other paralytic strabismus
              External ophthalmoplegia NOS

         H49.881   Other paralytic strabismus, right eye

         H49.882   Other paralytic strabismus, left eye

         H49.883   Other paralytic strabismus, bilateral

         H49.889   Other paralytic strabismus, unspecified eye

H49.9   Unspecified paralytic strabismus

● H50   Other strabismus

     ● H50.0   Esotropia
              Convergent concomitant strabismus

         Excludes1   intermittent esotropia (H50.31-, H50.32)

         H50.00   Unspecified esotropia

         ● H50.01   Monocular esotropia

              H50.011   Monocular esotropia, right eye

              H50.012   Monocular esotropia, left eye

         ● H50.02   Monocular esotropia with A pattern

              H50.021   Monocular esotropia with A pattern, right eye

              H50.022   Monocular esotropia with A pattern, left eye

         ● H50.03   Monocular esotropia with V pattern

              H50.031   Monocular esotropia with V pattern, right eye

              H50.032   Monocular esotropia with V pattern, left eye

         ● H50.04   Monocular esotropia with other noncomitancies

              H50.041   Monocular esotropia with other noncomitancies, right eye

              H50.042   Monocular esotropia with other noncomitancies, left eye

         H50.05   Alternating esotropia

         H50.06   Alternating esotropia with A pattern

         H50.07   Alternating esotropia with V pattern

         H50.08   Alternating esotropia with other noncomitancies

     ● H50.1   Exotropia
              Misalignment in which one eye deviates outward (away from nose) while the other fixates normally
              Divergent concomitant strabismus

         Excludes1   intermittent exotropia (H50.33-, H50.34)

         H50.10   Unspecified exotropia

         ● H50.11   Monocular exotropia

              H50.111   Monocular exotropia, right eye

              H50.112   Monocular exotropia, left eye

         ● H50.12   Monocular exotropia with A pattern

              H50.121   Monocular exotropia with A pattern, right eye

              H50.122   Monocular exotropia with A pattern, left eye

         ● H50.13   Monocular exotropia with V pattern

              H50.131   Monocular exotropia with V pattern, right eye

              H50.132   Monocular exotropia with V pattern, left eye

◄ New   ◀▥ Revised   ~~deleted~~ Deleted   Excludes 1   Excludes 2   Includes   Use additional   Code first   Code also   Unspecified

OGCR Official Guidelines   **X** Assign placeholder X   ● Use Additional Character(s)   ▶ Manifestation Code   **Coding Clinic**

● H50.14   Monocular exotropia with other noncomitancies
    H50.141   Monocular exotropia with other noncomitancies, right eye
    H50.142   Monocular exotropia with other noncomitancies, left eye
    H50.15   Alternating exotropia
    H50.16   Alternating exotropia with A pattern
    H50.17   Alternating exotropia with V pattern
    H50.18   Alternating exotropia with other noncomitancies
● H50.2   Vertical strabismus
    Hypertropia
    H50.21   Vertical strabismus, right eye
    H50.22   Vertical strabismus, left eye
● H50.3   Intermittent heterotropia
    Displacement of an organ or part of an organ from its normal position
    H50.30   Unspecified intermittent heterotropia
● H50.31   Intermittent monocular esotropia
    H50.311   Intermittent monocular esotropia, right eye
    H50.312   Intermittent monocular esotropia, left eye
    H50.32   Intermittent alternating esotropia
● H50.33   Intermittent monocular exotropia
    H50.331   Intermittent monocular exotropia, right eye
    H50.332   Intermittent monocular exotropia, left eye
    H50.34   Intermittent alternating exotropia
● H50.4   Other and unspecified heterotropia
    H50.40   Unspecified heterotropia
● H50.41   Cyclotropia
    H50.411   Cyclotropia, right eye
    H50.412   Cyclotropia, left eye
    H50.42   Monofixation syndrome
    H50.43   Accommodative component in esotropia
● H50.5   Heterophoria
    One or both eyes wander away from the position where both eyes are looking together in the same direction
    H50.50   Unspecified heterophoria
    H50.51   Esophoria
      Eye deviates inward (toward the nose)
    H50.52   Exophoria
      Eye deviates outward (toward the ear)
    H50.53   Vertical heterophoria
    H50.54   Cyclophoria
    H50.55   Alternating heterophoria
● H50.6   Mechanical strabismus
    H50.60   Mechanical strabismus, unspecified
● H50.61   Brown's sheath syndrome
    H50.611   Brown's sheath syndrome, right eye
    H50.612   Brown's sheath syndrome, left eye
    H50.69   Other mechanical strabismus
      Strabismus due to adhesions
      Traumatic limitation of duction of eye muscle
● H50.8   Other specified strabismus
● H50.81   Duane's syndrome
    H50.811   Duane's syndrome, right eye
    H50.812   Duane's syndrome, left eye
    H50.89   Other specified strabismus
    H50.9   Unspecified strabismus

● H51   Other disorders of binocular movement
    H51.0   Palsy (spasm) of conjugate gaze
● H51.1   Convergence insufficiency and excess
    H51.11   Convergence insufficiency
    H51.12   Convergence excess
● H51.2   Internuclear ophthalmoplegia
    H51.20   Internuclear ophthalmoplegia, unspecified eye
    H51.21   Internuclear ophthalmoplegia, right eye
    H51.22   Internuclear ophthalmoplegia, left eye
    H51.23   Internuclear ophthalmoplegia, bilateral
    H51.8   Other specified disorders of binocular movement
    H51.9   Unspecified disorder of binocular movement
● H52   Disorders of refraction and accommodation
● H52.0   Hypermetropia
    H52.00   Hypermetropia, unspecified eye
    H52.01   Hypermetropia, right eye
    H52.02   Hypermetropia, left eye
    H52.03   Hypermetropia, bilateral
● H52.1   Myopia
    Excludes1   degenerative myopia (H44.2-)
    H52.10   Myopia, unspecified eye
    H52.11   Myopia, right eye
    H52.12   Myopia, left eye
    H52.13   Myopia, bilateral
● H52.2   Astigmatism
● H52.20   Unspecified astigmatism
    H52.201   Unspecified astigmatism, right eye
    H52.202   Unspecified astigmatism, left eye
    H52.203   Unspecified astigmatism, bilateral
    H52.209   Unspecified astigmatism, unspecified eye
● H52.21   Irregular astigmatism
    H52.211   Irregular astigmatism, right eye
    H52.212   Irregular astigmatism, left eye
    H52.213   Irregular astigmatism, bilateral
    H52.219   Irregular astigmatism, unspecified eye
● H52.22   Regular astigmatism
    H52.221   Regular astigmatism, right eye
    H52.222   Regular astigmatism, left eye
    H52.223   Regular astigmatism, bilateral
    H52.229   Regular astigmatism, unspecified eye
● H52.3   Anisometropia and aniseikonia
    H52.31   Anisometropia
    H52.32   Aniseikonia
    H52.4   Presbyopia
● H52.5   Disorders of accommodation
● H52.51   Internal ophthalmoplegia (complete) (total)
    H52.511   Internal ophthalmoplegia (complete) (total), right eye
    H52.512   Internal ophthalmoplegia (complete) (total), left eye
    H52.513   Internal ophthalmoplegia (complete) (total), bilateral
    H52.519   Internal ophthalmoplegia (complete) (total), unspecified eye

Item 7–10   Disorders of refraction: **Hypermetropia**, or farsightedness, means focus at a distance is adequate but not on close objects. **Myopia** is near-sightedness or short-sightedness and means the focus on nearby objects is clear but distant objects appear blurred. **Astigmatism** is warping of the curvature of the cornea so light rays entering do not meet a single focal point, resulting in a distorted image. **Anisometropia** is unequal refractive power in which one eye may be myopic (near-sighted) and the other hyperopic (far-sighted). **Presbyopia** is the loss of focus on near objects, which occurs with age because the lens loses elasticity.

CHAPTER 7 (H00–H59)

● H52.52   Paresis of accommodation
      H52.521   Paresis of accommodation, right eye
      H52.522   Paresis of accommodation, left eye
      H52.523   Paresis of accommodation, bilateral
      H52.529   Paresis of accommodation, unspecified eye

● H52.53   Spasm of accommodation
      H52.531   Spasm of accommodation, right eye
      H52.532   Spasm of accommodation, left eye
      H52.533   Spasm of accommodation, bilateral
      H52.539   Spasm of accommodation, unspecified eye

H52.6   Other disorders of refraction

H52.7   Unspecified disorder of refraction

VISUAL DISTURBANCES AND BLINDNESS (H53-H54)

● H53   Visual disturbances

● H53.0   Amblyopia ex anopsia
     Excludes1   amblyopia due to vitamin A deficiency (E50.5)

   ● H53.00   Unspecified amblyopia
      H53.001   Unspecified amblyopia, right eye
      H53.002   Unspecified amblyopia, left eye
      H53.003   Unspecified amblyopia, bilateral
      H53.009   Unspecified amblyopia, unspecified eye

   ● H53.01   Deprivation amblyopia
      H53.011   Deprivation amblyopia, right eye
      H53.012   Deprivation amblyopia, left eye
      H53.013   Deprivation amblyopia, bilateral
      H53.019   Deprivation amblyopia, unspecified eye

   ● H53.02   Refractive amblyopia
      H53.021   Refractive amblyopia, right eye
      H53.022   Refractive amblyopia, left eye
      H53.023   Refractive amblyopia, bilateral
      H53.029   Refractive amblyopia, unspecified eye

   ● H53.03   Strabismic amblyopia
      Excludes1   strabismus (H50.-)
      H53.031   Strabismic amblyopia, right eye
      H53.032   Strabismic amblyopia, left eye
      H53.033   Strabismic amblyopia, bilateral
      H53.039   Strabismic amblyopia, unspecified eye

● H53.1   Subjective visual disturbances
     Excludes1   subjective visual disturbances due to vitamin A deficiency (E50.5)
               visual hallucinations (R44.1)

   H53.10   Unspecified subjective visual disturbances

   H53.11   Day blindness
        Hemeralopia

   ● H53.12   Transient visual loss
        Scintillating scotoma
      Excludes1   amaurosis fugax (G45.3-)
               transient retinal artery occlusion (H34.0-)
      H53.121   Transient visual loss, right eye
      H53.122   Transient visual loss, left eye
      H53.123   Transient visual loss, bilateral
      H53.129   Transient visual loss, unspecified eye

   ● H53.13   Sudden visual loss
      H53.131   Sudden visual loss, right eye
      H53.132   Sudden visual loss, left eye
      H53.133   Sudden visual loss, bilateral
      H53.139   Sudden visual loss, unspecified eye

   ● H53.14   Visual discomfort
        Asthenopia
        Photophobia
      H53.141   Visual discomfort, right eye
      H53.142   Visual discomfort, left eye
      H53.143   Visual discomfort, bilateral
      H53.149   Visual discomfort, unspecified

   H53.15   Visual distortions of shape and size
        Metamorphopsia

   H53.16   Psychophysical visual disturbances

   H53.19   Other subjective visual disturbances
        Visual halos

H53.2   Diplopia
     Double vision

● H53.3   Other and unspecified disorders of binocular vision
   H53.30   Unspecified disorder of binocular vision
   H53.31   Abnormal retinal correspondence
   H53.32   Fusion with defective stereopsis
   H53.33   Simultaneous visual perception without fusion
   H53.34   Suppression of binocular vision

● H53.4   Visual field defects
   H53.40   Unspecified visual field defects

   ● H53.41   Scotoma involving central area
        Central scotoma
      H53.411   Scotoma involving central area, right eye
      H53.412   Scotoma involving central area, left eye
      H53.413   Scotoma involving central area, bilateral
      H53.419   Scotoma involving central area, unspecified eye

   ● H53.42   Scotoma of blind spot area
        Enlarged blind spot
      H53.421   Scotoma of blind spot area, right eye
      H53.422   Scotoma of blind spot area, left eye
      H53.423   Scotoma of blind spot area, bilateral
      H53.429   Scotoma of blind spot area, unspecified eye

   ● H53.43   Sector or arcuate defects
        Arcuate scotoma
        Bjerrum scotoma
      H53.431   Sector or arcuate defects, right eye
      H53.432   Sector or arcuate defects, left eye
      H53.433   Sector or arcuate defects, bilateral
      H53.439   Sector or arcuate defects, unspecified eye

   ● H53.45   Other localized visual field defect
        Peripheral visual field defect
        Ring scotoma NOS
        Scotoma NOS
      H53.451   Other localized visual field defect, right eye
      H53.452   Other localized visual field defect, left eye
      H53.453   Other localized visual field defect, bilateral
      H53.459   Other localized visual field defect, unspecified eye

◄ New   ◄ Revised   ~~deleted~~ Deleted   Excludes 1   Excludes 2   Includes   Use additional   Code first   Code also   Unspecified

OGCR Official Guidelines   X Assign placeholder X   ● Use Additional Character(s)   ▶ Manifestation Code   Coding Clinic

● **H53.46** **Homonymous bilateral field defects**
Homonymous hemianopia
Homonymous hemianopsia
Quadrant anopia
Quadrant anopsia

H53.461 **Homonymous bilateral field defects, right side**

H53.462 **Homonymous bilateral field defects, left side**

H53.469 **Homonymous bilateral field defects, unspecified side**
Homonymous bilateral field defects NOS

H53.47 **Heteronymous bilateral field defects**
Heteronymous hemianop(s)ia

● **H53.48** **Generalized contraction of visual field**

H53.481 **Generalized contraction of visual field, right eye**

H53.482 **Generalized contraction of visual field, left eye**

H53.483 **Generalized contraction of visual field, bilateral**

H53.489 **Generalized contraction of visual field, unspecified eye**

● **H53.5** **Color vision deficiencies**
Color blindness

Excludes2   day blindness (H53.11)

H53.50 **Unspecified color vision deficiencies**
Color blindness NOS

H53.51 **Achromatopsia**

H53.52 **Acquired color vision deficiency**

H53.53 **Deuteranomaly**
Deuteranopia

H53.54 **Protanomaly**
Protanopia

H53.55 **Tritanomaly**
Tritanopia

H53.59 **Other color vision deficiencies**

● **H53.6** **Night blindness**

Excludes1   night blindness due to vitamin A deficiency (E50.5)

H53.60 **Unspecified night blindness**

H53.61 **Abnormal dark adaptation curve**

H53.62 **Acquired night blindness**

H53.63 **Congenital night blindness**

H53.69 **Other night blindness**

● **H53.7** **Vision sensitivity deficiencies**

H53.71 **Glare sensitivity**

H53.72 **Impaired contrast sensitivity**

H53.8 **Other visual disturbances**

H53.9 **Unspecified visual disturbance**

● **H54** **Blindness and low vision**

Note: For definition of visual impairment categories see table below.

Code first any associated underlying cause of the blindness

Excludes1   amaurosis fugax (G45.3)

H54.0 **Blindness, both eyes**
Visual impairment categories 3, 4, 5 in both eyes.

● **H54.1** **Blindness, one eye, low vision other eye**
Visual impairment categories 3, 4, 5 in one eye, with categories 1 or 2 in the other eye.

H54.10 **Blindness, one eye, low vision other eye, unspecified eyes**

H54.11 **Blindness, right eye, low vision left eye**

H54.12 **Blindness, left eye, low vision right eye**

H54.2 **Low vision, both eyes**
Visual impairment categories 1 or 2 in both eyes.

H54.3 **Unqualified visual loss, both eyes**
Visual impairment category 9 in both eyes.

● **H54.4** **Blindness, one eye**
Visual impairment categories 3, 4, 5 in one eye [normal vision in other eye]

H54.40 **Blindness, one eye, unspecified eye**

H54.41 **Blindness, right eye, normal vision left eye**

H54.42 **Blindness, left eye, normal vision right eye**

● **H54.5** **Low vision, one eye**
Visual impairment categories 1 or 2 in one eye [normal vision in other eye].

H54.50 **Low vision, one eye, unspecified eye**

H54.51 **Low vision, right eye, normal vision left eye**

H54.52 **Low vision, left eye, normal vision right eye**

● **H54.6** **Unqualified visual loss, one eye**
Visual impairment category 9 in one eye [normal vision in other eye].

H54.60 **Unqualified visual loss, one eye, unspecified**

H54.61 **Unqualified visual loss, right eye, normal vision left eye**

H54.62 **Unqualified visual loss, left eye, normal vision right eye**

H54.7 **Unspecified visual loss**
Visual impairment category 9 NOS

H54.8 **Legal blindness, as defined in USA**
Blindness NOS according to USA definition

Excludes1   legal blindness with specification of impairment level (H54.0-H54.7)

Note: The table below gives a classification of severity of visual impairment recommended by a WHO Study Group on the Prevention of Blindness, Geneva, 6-10 November 1972.

The term 'low vision' in category H54 comprises categories 1 and 2 of the table, the term 'blindness' categories 3, 4 and 5, and the term 'unqualified visual loss' category 9.

If the extent of the visual field is taken into account, patients with a field no greater than 10 but greater than 5 around central fixation should be placed in category 3 and patients with a field no greater than 5 around central fixation should be placed in category 4, even if the central acuity is not impaired.

Category of visual impairment	Visual acuity with best possible correction	
	Maximum less than:	**Minimum equal to or better than:**
	6/18	6/60
3/10 (0.3)	1/10 (0.1)	
20/70	20/200	
	6/60	3/60
1/10 (0.1)	1/20 (0.05)	
20/200	20/400	
	3/60	1/60 (finger counting at one meter)
1/20 (0.05)	1/50 (0.02)	
20/400	5/300 (20/1200)	
	1/60 (finger counting at one meter)	Light perception
1/50 (0.02)		
5/300		
	No light perception	
	Undetermined or unspecified	

CHAPTER 7 (H00-H59)

CHAPTER 7 (H00–H59)

OTHER DISORDERS OF EYE AND ADNEXA (H55–H57)

- H55   Nystagmus and other irregular eye movements
  - H55.0   Nystagmus
    - *Rapid, involuntary movements of the eyes in the horizontal or vertical direction.*
    - H55.00   Unspecified nystagmus
    - H55.01   Congenital nystagmus
    - H55.02   Latent nystagmus
    - H55.03   Visual deprivation nystagmus
    - H55.04   Dissociated nystagmus
    - H55.09   Other forms of nystagmus
  - H55.8   Other irregular eye movements
    - H55.81   Saccadic eye movements
    - H55.89   Other irregular eye movements

- H57   Other disorders of eye and adnexa
  - H57.0   Anomalies of pupillary function
    - H57.00   Unspecified anomaly of pupillary function
    - H57.01   Argyll Robertson pupil, atypical
      - **Excludes1**   syphilitic Argyll Robertson pupil (A52.19)
    - H57.02   Anisocoria
    - H57.03   Miosis
    - H57.04   Mydriasis
    - H57.05   Tonic pupil
      - H57.051   Tonic pupil, right eye
      - H57.052   Tonic pupil, left eye
      - H57.053   Tonic pupil, bilateral
      - H57.059   Tonic pupil, unspecified eye
    - H57.09   Other anomalies of pupillary function
  - H57.1   Ocular pain
    - H57.10   Ocular pain, unspecified eye
    - H57.11   Ocular pain, right eye
    - H57.12   Ocular pain, left eye
    - H57.13   Ocular pain, bilateral
  - H57.8   Other specified disorders of eye and adnexa
  - H57.9   Unspecified disorder of eye and adnexa

INTRAOPERATIVE AND POSTPROCEDURAL COMPLICATIONS AND DISORDERS OF EYE AND ADNEXA, NOT ELSEWHERE CLASSIFIED (H59)

- H59   Intraoperative and postprocedural complications and disorders of eye and adnexa, not elsewhere classified
  - **Excludes1**   mechanical complication of intraocular lens (T85.2)
    - mechanical complication of other ocular prosthetic devices, implants and grafts (T85.3)
    - pseudophakia (Z96.1)
    - secondary cataracts (H26.4-)
  - H59.0   Disorders of the eye following cataract surgery
    - H59.01   Keratopathy (bullous aphakic) following cataract surgery
      - Vitreal corneal syndrome
      - Vitreous (touch) syndrome
      - H59.011   Keratopathy (bullous aphakic) following cataract surgery, right eye
      - H59.012   Keratopathy (bullous aphakic) following cataract surgery, left eye
      - H59.013   Keratopathy (bullous aphakic) following cataract surgery, bilateral
      - H59.019   Keratopathy (bullous aphakic) following cataract surgery, unspecified eye

- H59.02   Cataract (lens) fragments in eye following cataract surgery
  - H59.021   Cataract (lens) fragments in eye following cataract surgery, right eye
  - H59.022   Cataract (lens) fragments in eye following cataract surgery, left eye
  - H59.023   Cataract (lens) fragments in eye following cataract surgery, bilateral
  - H59.029   Cataract (lens) fragments in eye following cataract surgery, unspecified eye
- H59.03   Cystoid macular edema following cataract surgery
  - H59.031   Cystoid macular edema following cataract surgery, right eye
  - H59.032   Cystoid macular edema following cataract surgery, left eye
  - H59.033   Cystoid macular edema following cataract surgery, bilateral
  - H59.039   Cystoid macular edema following cataract surgery, unspecified eye
- H59.09   Other disorders of the eye following cataract surgery
  - H59.091   Other disorders of the right eye following cataract surgery
  - H59.092   Other disorders of the left eye following cataract surgery
  - H59.093   Other disorders of the eye following cataract surgery, bilateral
  - H59.099   Other disorders of unspecified eye following cataract surgery
- H59.1   Intraoperative hemorrhage and hematoma of eye and adnexa complicating a procedure
  - **Excludes1**   intraoperative hemorrhage and hematoma of eye and adnexa due to accidental puncture or laceration during a procedure (H59.2-)
  - H59.11   Intraoperative hemorrhage and hematoma of eye and adnexa complicating an ophthalmic procedure
    - H59.111   Intraoperative hemorrhage and hematoma of right eye and adnexa complicating an ophthalmic procedure
    - H59.112   Intraoperative hemorrhage and hematoma of left eye and adnexa complicating an ophthalmic procedure
    - H59.113   Intraoperative hemorrhage and hematoma of eye and adnexa complicating an ophthalmic procedure, bilateral
    - H59.119   Intraoperative hemorrhage and hematoma of unspecified eye and adnexa complicating an ophthalmic procedure
  - H59.12   Intraoperative hemorrhage and hematoma of eye and adnexa complicating other procedure
    - H59.121   Intraoperative hemorrhage and hematoma of right eye and adnexa complicating other procedure
    - H59.122   Intraoperative hemorrhage and hematoma of left eye and adnexa complicating other procedure
    - H59.123   Intraoperative hemorrhage and hematoma of eye and adnexa complicating other procedure, bilateral
    - H59.129   Intraoperative hemorrhage and hematoma of unspecified eye and adnexa complicating other procedure

---

◀ New   ◀▨ Revised   ~~deleted~~ Deleted   Excludes 1   Excludes 2   Includes   Use additional   Code first   Code also   Unspecified

OGCR Official Guidelines   **X** Assign placeholder X   ● Use Additional Character(s)   ▶ Manifestation Code   **Coding Clinic**

- H59.2 Accidental puncture and laceration of eye and adnexa during a procedure
  - H59.21 Accidental puncture and laceration of eye and adnexa during an ophthalmic procedure
    - H59.211 Accidental puncture and laceration of right eye and adnexa during an ophthalmic procedure
    - H59.212 Accidental puncture and laceration of left eye and adnexa during an ophthalmic procedure
    - H59.213 Accidental puncture and laceration of eye and adnexa during an ophthalmic procedure, bilateral
    - H59.219 Accidental puncture and laceration of unspecified eye and adnexa during an ophthalmic procedure
  - H59.22 Accidental puncture and laceration of eye and adnexa during other procedure
    - H59.221 Accidental puncture and laceration of right eye and adnexa during other procedure
    - H59.222 Accidental puncture and laceration of left eye and adnexa during other procedure
    - H59.223 Accidental puncture and laceration of eye and adnexa during other procedure, bilateral
    - H59.229 Accidental puncture and laceration of unspecified eye and adnexa during other procedure
- H59.3 Postprocedural hemorrhage and hematoma of eye and adnexa following a procedure
  - H59.31 Postprocedural hemorrhage and hematoma of eye and adnexa following an ophthalmic procedure
    - H59.311 Postprocedural hemorrhage and hematoma of right eye and avdnexa following an ophthalmic procedure
    - H59.312 Postprocedural hemorrhage and hematoma of left eye and adnexa following an ophthalmic procedure
    - H59.313 Postprocedural hemorrhage and hematoma of eye and adnexa following an ophthalmic procedure, bilateral
    - H59.319 Postprocedural hemorrhage and hematoma of unspecified eye and adnexa following an ophthalmic procedure
- H59.32 Postprocedural hemorrhage and hematoma of eye and adnexa following other procedure
  - H59.321 Postprocedural hemorrhage and hematoma of right eye and adnexa following other procedure
  - H59.322 Postprocedural hemorrhage and hematoma of left eye and adnexa following other procedure
  - H59.323 Postprocedural hemorrhage and hematoma of eye and adnexa following other procedure, bilateral
  - H59.329 Postprocedural hemorrhage and hematoma of unspecified eye and adnexa following other procedure
- H59.4 Inflammation (infection) of postprocedural bleb
  Postprocedural blebitis

  Excludes1   filtering (vitreous) bleb after glaucoma surgery status (Z98.83)

  - H59.40 Inflammation (infection) of postprocedural bleb, unspecified
  - H59.41 Inflammation (infection) of postprocedural bleb, stage 1
  - H59.42 Inflammation (infection) of postprocedural bleb, stage 2
  - H59.43 Inflammation (infection) of postprocedural bleb, stage 3
    Bleb endophthalmitis
- H59.8 Other intraoperative and postprocedural complications and disorders of eye and adnexa, not elsewhere classified
  - H59.81 Chorioretinal scars after surgery for detachment
    - H59.811 Chorioretinal scars after surgery for detachment, right eye
    - H59.812 Chorioretinal scars after surgery for detachment, left eye
    - H59.813 Chorioretinal scars after surgery for detachment, bilateral
    - H59.819 Chorioretinal scars after surgery for detachment, unspecified eye
  - H59.88 Other intraoperative complications of eye and adnexa, not elsewhere classified
  - H59.89 Other postprocedural complications and disorders of eye and adnexa, not elsewhere classified

CHAPTER 7 (H00-H59)

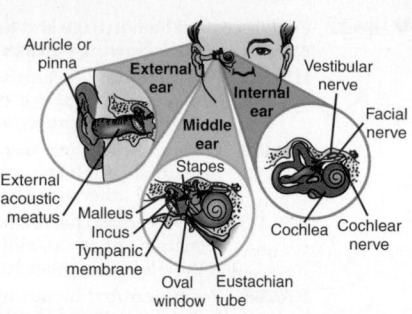

Figure 8-1 Auditory system. (From Buck CJ: Step-by-Step Medical Coding, ed 2010, Philadelphia, WB Saunders, 2010)

(See Plate 92 on page 68.)

CHAPTER 8

DISEASES OF THE EAR AND MASTOID PROCESS (H60-H95)

Note: Use an external cause code following the code for the ear condition, if applicable, to identify the cause of the ear condition

> **Excludes2** certain conditions originating in the perinatal period (P04-P96)
> certain infectious and parasitic diseases (A00-B99)
> complications of pregnancy, childbirth and the puerperium (O00-O9A)
> congenital malformations, deformations and chromosomal abnormalities (Q00-Q99)
> endocrine, nutritional and metabolic diseases (E00-E88)
> injury, poisoning and certain other consequences of external causes (S00-T88)
> neoplasms (C00-D49)
> symptoms, signs and abnormal clinical and laboratory findings, not elsewhere classified (R00-R94)

This chapter contains the following blocks:

H60-H62	Diseases of external ear
H65-H75	Diseases of middle ear and mastoid
H80-H83	Diseases of inner ear
H90-H94	Other disorders of ear
H95	Intraoperative and postprocedural complications and disorders of ear and mastoid process, not elsewhere classified

DISEASES OF EXTERNAL EAR (H60-H62)

● **H60   Otitis externa**

● H60.0   **Abscess of external ear**
Boil of external ear
Carbuncle of auricle or external auditory canal
Furuncle of external ear

H60.00   Abscess of external ear, unspecified ear
H60.01   Abscess of right external ear
H60.02   Abscess of left external ear
H60.03   Abscess of external ear, bilateral

● H60.1   **Cellulitis of external ear**
Cellulitis of auricle
Cellulitis of external auditory canal

H60.10   Cellulitis of external ear, unspecified ear
H60.11   Cellulitis of right external ear
H60.12   Cellulitis of left external ear
H60.13   Cellulitis of external ear, bilateral

● H60.2   Malignant otitis externa
H60.20   Malignant otitis externa, unspecified ear
H60.21   Malignant otitis externa, right ear
H60.22   Malignant otitis externa, left ear
H60.23   Malignant otitis externa, bilateral

● H60.3   Other infective otitis externa
● H60.31   Diffuse otitis externa
H60.311   Diffuse otitis externa, right ear
H60.312   Diffuse otitis externa, left ear
H60.313   Diffuse otitis externa, bilateral
H60.319   Diffuse otitis externa, unspecified ear

● H60.32   Hemorrhagic otitis externa
H60.321   Hemorrhagic otitis externa, right ear
H60.322   Hemorrhagic otitis externa, left ear
H60.323   Hemorrhagic otitis externa, bilateral
H60.329   Hemorrhagic otitis externa, unspecified ear

● H60.33   Swimmer's ear
H60.331   Swimmer's ear, right ear
H60.332   Swimmer's ear, left ear
H60.333   Swimmer's ear, bilateral
H60.339   Swimmer's ear, unspecified ear

● H60.39   Other infective otitis externa
H60.391   Other infective otitis externa, right ear
H60.392   Other infective otitis externa, left ear
H60.393   Other infective otitis externa, bilateral
H60.399   Other infective otitis externa, unspecified ear

● H60.4   **Cholesteatoma of external ear**
Keratosis obturans of external ear (canal)

> **Excludes2** cholesteatoma of middle ear (H71.-)
> recurrent cholesteatoma of postmastoidectomy cavity (H95.0-)

H60.40   Cholesteatoma of external ear, unspecified ear
H60.41   Cholesteatoma of right external ear
H60.42   Cholesteatoma of left external ear
H60.43   Cholesteatoma of external ear, bilateral

● H60.5   **Acute noninfective otitis externa**
● H60.50   Unspecified acute noninfective otitis externa
Acute otitis externa NOS
H60.501   Unspecified acute noninfective otitis externa, right ear
H60.502   Unspecified acute noninfective otitis externa, left ear
H60.503   Unspecified acute noninfective otitis externa, bilateral
H60.509   Unspecified acute noninfective otitis externa, unspecified ear

● H60.51   Acute actinic otitis externa
H60.511   Acute actinic otitis externa, right ear
H60.512   Acute actinic otitis externa, left ear
H60.513   Acute actinic otitis externa, bilateral
H60.519   Acute actinic otitis externa, unspecified ear

● H60.52   Acute chemical otitis externa
H60.521   Acute chemical otitis externa, right ear
H60.522   Acute chemical otitis externa, left ear
H60.523   Acute chemical otitis externa, bilateral
H60.529   Acute chemical otitis externa, unspecified ear

● H60.53   Acute contact otitis externa
H60.531   Acute contact otitis externa, right ear
H60.532   Acute contact otitis externa, left ear
H60.533   Acute contact otitis externa, bilateral
H60.539   Acute contact otitis externa, unspecified ear

◀ New   ◀▥ Revised   ~~deleted~~ Deleted   Excludes 1   Excludes 2   Includes   Use additional   Code first   Code also   Unspecified
OGCR Official Guidelines   X Assign placeholder X   ● Use Additional Character(s)   ▶ Manifestation Code   **Coding Clinic**

● **H60.54**   Acute eczematoid otitis externa
   H60.541   Acute eczematoid otitis externa, right ear
   H60.542   Acute eczematoid otitis externa, left ear
   H60.543   Acute eczematoid otitis externa, bilateral
   H60.549   Acute eczematoid otitis externa, unspecified ear

● **H60.55**   Acute reactive otitis externa
   H60.551   Acute reactive otitis externa, right ear
   H60.552   Acute reactive otitis externa, left ear
   H60.553   Acute reactive otitis externa, bilateral
   H60.559   Acute reactive otitis externa, unspecified ear

● **H60.59**   Other noninfective acute otitis externa
   H60.591   Other noninfective acute otitis externa, right ear
   H60.592   Other noninfective acute otitis externa, left ear
   H60.593   Other noninfective acute otitis externa, bilateral
   H60.599   Other noninfective acute otitis externa, unspecified ear

● **H60.6**   Unspecified chronic otitis externa
   H60.60   Unspecified chronic otitis externa, unspecified ear
   H60.61   Unspecified chronic otitis externa, right ear
   H60.62   Unspecified chronic otitis externa, left ear
   H60.63   Unspecified chronic otitis externa, bilateral

● **H60.8**   Other otitis externa
   ● **H60.8X**   Other otitis externa
     H60.8X1   Other otitis externa, right ear
     H60.8X2   Other otitis externa, left ear
     H60.8X3   Other otitis externa, bilateral
     H60.8X9   Other otitis externa, unspecified ear

● **H60.9**   Unspecified otitis externa
   H60.90   Unspecified otitis externa, unspecified ear
   H60.91   Unspecified otitis externa, right ear
   H60.92   Unspecified otitis externa, left ear
   H60.93   Unspecified otitis externa, bilateral

● **H61**   Other disorders of external ear
   ● **H61.0**   Chondritis and perichondritis of external ear
     Chondrodermatitis nodularis chronica helicis
     Perichondritis of auricle
     Perichondritis of pinna
     ● **H61.00**   Unspecified perichondritis of external ear
       H61.001   Unspecified perichondritis of right external ear
       H61.002   Unspecified perichondritis of left external ear
       H61.003   Unspecified perichondritis of external ear, bilateral
       H61.009   Unspecified perichondritis of external ear, unspecified ear
     ● **H61.01**   Acute perichondritis of external ear
       H61.011   Acute perichondritis of right external ear
       H61.012   Acute perichondritis of left external ear
       H61.013   Acute perichondritis of external ear, bilateral
       H61.019   Acute perichondritis of external ear, unspecified ear

● **H61.02**   Chronic perichondritis of external ear
   H61.021   Chronic perichondritis of right external ear
   H61.022   Chronic perichondritis of left external ear
   H61.023   Chronic perichondritis of external ear, bilateral
   H61.029   Chronic perichondritis of external ear, unspecified ear

● **H61.03**   Chondritis of external ear
   Chondritis of auricle
   Chondritis of pinna
   H61.031   Chondritis of right external ear
   H61.032   Chondritis of left external ear
     Coding Clinic: 2015, Q1, P18
   H61.033   Chondritis of external ear, bilateral
   H61.039   Chondritis of external ear, unspecified ear

● **H61.1**   Noninfective disorders of pinna
   Excludes2   cauliflower ear (M95.1-)
          gouty tophi of ear (M1A.-)
   ● **H61.10**   Unspecified noninfective disorders of pinna
     Disorder of pinna NOS
     H61.101   Unspecified noninfective disorders of pinna, right ear
     H61.102   Unspecified noninfective disorders of pinna, left ear
     H61.103   Unspecified noninfective disorders of pinna, bilateral
     H61.109   Unspecified noninfective disorders of pinna, unspecified ear
   ● **H61.11**   Acquired deformity of pinna
     Acquired deformity of auricle
     Excludes2   cauliflower ear (M95.1-)
     H61.111   Acquired deformity of pinna, right ear
     H61.112   Acquired deformity of pinna, left ear
     H61.113   Acquired deformity of pinna, bilateral
     H61.119   Acquired deformity of pinna, unspecified ear
   ● **H61.12**   Hematoma of pinna
     Hematoma of auricle
     H61.121   Hematoma of pinna, right ear
     H61.122   Hematoma of pinna, left ear
     H61.123   Hematoma of pinna, bilateral
     H61.129   Hematoma of pinna, unspecified ear
   ● **H61.19**   Other noninfective disorders of pinna
     H61.191   Noninfective disorders of pinna, right ear
     H61.192   Noninfective disorders of pinna, left ear
     H61.193   Noninfective disorders of pinna, bilateral
     H61.199   Noninfective disorders of pinna, unspecified ear

● **H61.2**   Impacted cerumen
   Wax in ear
   H61.20   Impacted cerumen, unspecified ear
   H61.21   Impacted cerumen, right ear
   H61.22   Impacted cerumen, left ear
   H61.23   Impacted cerumen, bilateral

CHAPTER 8 (H60-H95)

● **H61.3**   **Acquired stenosis of external ear canal**
Collapse of external ear canal
> **Excludes1**   postprocedural stenosis of external ear canal (H95.81-)

  ● **H61.30**   **Acquired stenosis of external ear canal, unspecified**
    H61.301   Acquired stenosis of right external ear canal, unspecified
    H61.302   Acquired stenosis of left external ear canal, unspecified
    H61.303   Acquired stenosis of external ear canal, unspecified, bilateral
    H61.309   Acquired stenosis of external ear canal, unspecified, unspecified ear

  ● **H61.31**   **Acquired stenosis of external ear canal secondary to trauma**
    H61.311   Acquired stenosis of right external ear canal secondary to trauma
    H61.312   Acquired stenosis of left external ear canal secondary to trauma
    H61.313   Acquired stenosis of external ear canal secondary to trauma, bilateral
    H61.319   Acquired stenosis of external ear canal secondary to trauma, unspecified ear

  ● **H61.32**   **Acquired stenosis of external ear canal secondary to inflammation and infection**
    H61.321   Acquired stenosis of right external ear canal secondary to inflammation and infection
    H61.322   Acquired stenosis of left external ear canal secondary to inflammation and infection
    H61.323   Acquired stenosis of external ear canal secondary to inflammation and infection, bilateral
    H61.329   Acquired stenosis of external ear canal secondary to inflammation and infection, unspecified ear

  ● **H61.39**   **Other acquired stenosis of external ear canal**
    H61.391   Other acquired stenosis of right external ear canal
    H61.392   Other acquired stenosis of left external ear canal
    H61.393   Other acquired stenosis of external ear canal, bilateral
    H61.399   Other acquired stenosis of external ear canal, unspecified ear

● **H61.8**   **Other specified disorders of external ear**
  ● **H61.81**   **Exostosis of external canal**
    H61.811   Exostosis of right external canal
    H61.812   Exostosis of left external canal
    H61.813   Exostosis of external canal, bilateral
    H61.819   Exostosis of external canal, unspecified ear

  ● **H61.89**   **Other specified disorders of external ear**
    H61.891   Other specified disorders of right external ear
    H61.892   Other specified disorders of left external ear
    H61.893   Other specified disorders of external ear, bilateral
    H61.899   Other specified disorders of external ear, unspecified ear

● **H61.9**   **Disorder of external ear, unspecified**
    H61.90   Disorder of external ear, unspecified, unspecified ear
    H61.91   Disorder of right external ear, unspecified
    H61.92   Disorder of left external ear, unspecified
    H61.93   Disorder of external ear, unspecified, bilateral

● **H62**   **Disorders of external ear in diseases classified elsewhere**
  ● **H62.4**   **Otitis externa in other diseases classified elsewhere**
> *Code first* underlying disease, such as:
>   erysipelas (A46)
>   impetigo (L01.0)
> **Excludes1**   otitis externa (in):
>   candidiasis (B37.84)
>   herpes viral [herpes simplex] (B00.1)
>   herpes zoster (B02.8)

    ▌*H62.40*   *Otitis externa in other diseases classified elsewhere, unspecified ear*
    ▌*H62.41*   *Otitis externa in other diseases classified elsewhere, right ear*
    ▌*H62.42*   *Otitis externa in other diseases classified elsewhere, left ear*
    ▌*H62.43*   *Otitis externa in other diseases classified elsewhere, bilateral*

  ● **H62.8**   **Other disorders of external ear in diseases classified elsewhere**
> *Code first* underlying disease, such as:
>   gout (M1A.-, M10.-)

  ● **H62.8X**   **Other disorders of external ear in diseases classified elsewhere**
    ▌*H62.8X1*   *Other disorders of right external ear in diseases classified elsewhere*
    ▌*H62.8X2*   *Other disorders of left external ear in diseases classified elsewhere*
    ▌*H62.8X3*   *Other disorders of external ear in diseases classified elsewhere, bilateral*
    ▌*H62.8X9*   *Other disorders of external ear in diseases classified elsewhere, unspecified ear*

DISEASES OF MIDDLE EAR AND MASTOID (H65-H75)

(See Plate 94 on page 69.)

● **H65**   **Nonsuppurative otitis media**
Bacterial or viral infection or inflammation of the middle ear; may result in fluid accumulation with pain and temporary hearing loss.
> **Includes**   nonsuppurative otitis media with myringitis

Use additional code for any associated perforated tympanic membrane (H72.-)
Use additional code to identify:
  exposure to environmental tobacco smoke (Z77.22)
  exposure to tobacco smoke in the perinatal period (P96.81)
  history of tobacco use (Z87.891)
  occupational exposure to environmental tobacco smoke (Z57.31)
  tobacco dependence (F17.-)
  tobacco use (Z72.0)

● **H65.0**   **Acute serous otitis media**
Acute and subacute secretory otitis
    H65.00   Acute serous otitis media, unspecified ear
    H65.01   Acute serous otitis media, right ear
    H65.02   Acute serous otitis media, left ear
    H65.03   Acute serous otitis media, bilateral
    H65.04   Acute serous otitis media, recurrent, right ear
    H65.05   Acute serous otitis media, recurrent, left ear
    H65.06   Acute serous otitis media, recurrent, bilateral
    H65.07   Acute serous otitis media, recurrent, unspecified ear

● **H65.1**   **Other acute nonsuppurative otitis media**
> **Excludes1**   otitic barotrauma (T70.0)
>   otitis media (acute) NOS (H66.9)

  ● **H65.11**   **Acute and subacute allergic otitis media (mucoid) (sanguinous) (serous)**
    H65.111   Acute and subacute allergic otitis media (mucoid) (sanguinous) (serous), right ear

◀ New   ◀═ Revised   ~~deleted~~ Deleted   Excludes 1   Excludes 2   Includes   Use additional   Code first   Code also   Unspecified
OGCR Official Guidelines   X Assign placeholder X   ● Use Additional Character(s)   ▌ Manifestation Code   **Coding Clinic**

     H65.112   Acute and subacute allergic otitis media (mucoid) (sanguinous) (serous), left ear

     H65.113   Acute and subacute allergic otitis media (mucoid) (sanguinous) (serous), bilateral

     H65.114   Acute and subacute allergic otitis media (mucoid) (sanguinous) (serous), recurrent, right ear

     H65.115   Acutc and subacute allergic otitis media (mucoid) (sanguinous) (serous), recurrent, left ear

     H65.116   Acute and subacute allergic otitis media (mucoid) (sanguinous) (serous), recurrent, bilateral

     H65.117   Acute and subacute allergic otitis media (mucoid) (sanguinous) (serous), recurrent, unspecified ear

     H65.119   Acute and subacute allergic otitis media (mucoid) (sanguinous) (serous), unspecified ear

● H65.19   **Other acute nonsuppurative otitis media**
    Acute and subacute mucoid otitis media
    Acute and subacute nonsuppurative otitis media NOS
    Acute and subacute sanguinous otitis media
    Acute and subacute seromucinous otitis media

     H65.191   Other acute nonsuppurative otitis media, right ear

     H65.192   Other acute nonsuppurative otitis media, left ear

     H65.193   Other acute nonsuppurative otitis media, bilateral

     H65.194   Other acute nonsuppurative otitis media, recurrent, right ear

     H65.195   Other acute nonsuppurative otitis media, recurrent, left ear

     H65.196   Other acute nonsuppurative otitis media, recurrent, bilateral

     H65.197   Other acute nonsuppurative otitis media recurrent, unspecified ear

     H65.199   Other acute nonsuppurative otitis media, unspecified ear

● H65.2   **Chronic serous otitis media**
    Chronic tubotympanal catarrh

    H65.20   Chronic serous otitis media, unspecified ear

    H65.21   Chronic serous otitis media, right ear

    H65.22   Chronic serous otitis media, left ear

    H65.23   Chronic serous otitis media, bilateral

● H65.3   **Chronic mucoid otitis media**
    Chronic mucinous otitis media
    Chronic secretory otitis media
    Chronic transudative otitis media
    Glue ear

    Excludes1   adhesive middle ear disease (H74.1)

    H65.30   Chronic mucoid otitis media, unspecified ear

    H65.31   Chronic mucoid otitis media, right ear

    H65.32   Chronic mucoid otitis media, left ear

    H65.33   Chronic mucoid otitis media, bilateral

● H65.4   **Other chronic nonsuppurative otitis media**

   ● H65.41   **Chronic allergic otitis media**

     H65.411   Chronic allergic otitis media, right ear

     H65.412   Chronic allergic otitis media, left ear

     H65.413   Chronic allergic otitis media, bilateral

     H65.419   Chronic allergic otitis media, unspecified ear

● H65.49   **Other chronic nonsuppurative otitis media**
    Chronic exudative otitis media
    Chronic nonsuppurative otitis media NOS
    Chronic otitis media with effusion (nonpurulent)
    Chronic seromucinous otitis media

     H65.491   Other chronic nonsuppurative otitis media, right ear

     H65.492   Other chronic nonsuppurative otitis media, left ear

     H65.493   Other chronic nonsuppurative otitis media, bilateral

     H65.499   Other chronic nonsuppurative otitis media, unspecified ear

● H65.9   **Unspecified nonsuppurative otitis media**
    Allergic otitis media NOS
    Catarrhal otitis media NOS
    Exudative otitis media NOS
    Mucoid otitis media NOS
    Otitis media with effusion (nonpurulent) NOS
    Secretory otitis media NOS
    Seromucinous otitis media NOS
    Serous otitis media NOS
    Transudative otitis media NOS

    H65.90   Unspecified nonsuppurative otitis media, unspecified ear

    H65.91   Unspecified nonsuppurative otitis media, right ear

    H65.92   Unspecified nonsuppurative otitis media, left ear

    H65.93   Unspecified nonsuppurative otitis media, bilateral

● H66   **Suppurative and unspecified otitis media**
    Suppurative: Discharging pus

    Includes   suppurative and unspecified otitis media with myringitis

    Use additional code to identify:
    exposure to environmental tobacco smoke (Z77.22)
    exposure to tobacco smoke in the perinatal period (P96.81)
    history of tobacco use (Z87.891)
    occupational exposure to environmental tobacco smoke (Z57.31)
    tobacco dependence (F17.-)
    tobacco use (Z72.0)

● H66.0   **Acute suppurative otitis media**

   ● H66.00   **Acute suppurative otitis media without spontaneous rupture of ear drum**

     H66.001   Acute suppurative otitis media without spontaneous rupture of ear drum, right ear

     H66.002   Acute suppurative otitis media without spontaneous rupture of ear drum, left ear

     H66.003   Acute suppurative otitis media without spontaneous rupture of ear drum, bilateral

     H66.004   Acute suppurative otitis media without spontaneous rupture of ear drum, recurrent, right ear

     H66.005   Acute suppurative otitis media without spontaneous rupture of ear drum, recurrent, left ear

     H66.006   Acute suppurative otitis media without spontaneous rupture of ear drum, recurrent, bilateral

     H66.007   Acute suppurative otitis media without spontaneous rupture of ear drum, recurrent, unspecified ear

     H66.009   Acute suppurative otitis media without spontaneous rupture of ear drum, unspecified ear

● **H66.01**   Acute suppurative otitis media with spontaneous rupture of ear drum

     H66.011   Acute suppurative otitis media with spontaneous rupture of ear drum, right ear

     H66.012   Acute suppurative otitis media with spontaneous rupture of ear drum, left ear

     H66.013   Acute suppurative otitis media with spontaneous rupture of ear drum, bilateral

     H66.014   Acute suppurative otitis media with spontaneous rupture of ear drum, recurrent, right ear

     H66.015   Acute suppurative otitis media with spontaneous rupture of ear drum, recurrent, left ear

     H66.016   Acute suppurative otitis media with spontaneous rupture of ear drum, recurrent, bilateral

     H66.017   Acute suppurative otitis media with spontaneous rupture of ear drum, recurrent, unspecified ear

     H66.019   Acute suppurative otitis media with spontaneous rupture of ear drum, unspecified ear

● **H66.1**   Chronic tubotympanic suppurative otitis media

     Benign chronic suppurative otitis media
     Chronic tubotympanic disease

     Use additional code for any associated perforated tympanic membrane (H72.-)

     H66.10   Chronic tubotympanic suppurative otitis media, unspecified

     H66.11   Chronic tubotympanic suppurative otitis media, right ear

     H66.12   Chronic tubotympanic suppurative otitis media, left ear

     H66.13   Chronic tubotympanic suppurative otitis media, bilateral

● **H66.2**   Chronic atticoantral suppurative otitis media

     Chronic atticoantral disease

     Use additional code for any associated perforated tympanic membrane (H72.-)

     H66.20   Chronic atticoantral suppurative otitis media, unspecified ear

     H66.21   Chronic atticoantral suppurative otitis media, right ear

     H66.22   Chronic atticoantral suppurative otitis media, left ear

     H66.23   Chronic atticoantral suppurative otitis media, bilateral

● **H66.3**   Other chronic suppurative otitis media

     Chronic suppurative otitis media NOS

     Use additional code for any associated perforated tympanic membrane (H72.-)

     Excludes1   tuberculous otitis media (A18.6)

     ● H66.3X   Other chronic suppurative otitis media

         H66.3X1   Other chronic suppurative otitis media, right ear

         H66.3X2   Other chronic suppurative otitis media, left ear

         H66.3X3   Other chronic suppurative otitis media, bilateral

         H66.3X9   Other chronic suppurative otitis media, unspecified ear

● **H66.4**   Suppurative otitis media, unspecified

     Purulent otitis media NOS

     Use additional code for any associated perforated tympanic membrane (H72.-)

     H66.40   Suppurative otitis media, unspecified, unspecified ear

     H66.41   Suppurative otitis media, unspecified, right ear

     H66.42   Suppurative otitis media, unspecified, left ear

     H66.43   Suppurative otitis media, unspecified, bilateral

● **H66.9**   Otitis media, unspecified

     Otitis media NOS
     Acute otitis media NOS
     Chronic otitis media NOS

     Use additional code for any associated perforated tympanic membrane (H72.-)

     H66.90   Otitis media, unspecified, unspecified ear

     H66.91   Otitis media, unspecified, right ear

     H66.92   Otitis media, unspecified, left ear

     H66.93   Otitis media, unspecified, bilateral

● **H67**   Otitis media in diseases classified elsewhere

     Code first underlying disease, such as:
     viral disease NEC (B00-B34)

     Use additional code for any associated perforated tympanic membrane (H72.-)

     Excludes1   otitis media in:
         influenza (J09.X9, J10.83, J11.83)
         measles (B05.3)
         scarlet fever (A38.0)
         tuberculosis (A18.6)

     ◗ *H67.1*   *Otitis media in diseases classified elsewhere, right ear*

     ◗ *H67.2*   *Otitis media in diseases classified elsewhere, left ear*

     ◗ *H67.3*   *Otitis media in diseases classified elsewhere, bilateral*

     ◗ *H67.9*   *Otitis media in diseases classified elsewhere, unspecified ear*

● **H68**   Eustachian salpingitis and obstruction

     ● **H68.0**   Eustachian salpingitis

         ● H68.00   Unspecified Eustachian salpingitis

             H68.001   Unspecified Eustachian salpingitis, right ear

             H68.002   Unspecified Eustachian salpingitis, left ear

             H68.003   Unspecified Eustachian salpingitis, bilateral

             H68.009   Unspecified Eustachian salpingitis, unspecified ear

         ● H68.01   Acute Eustachian salpingitis

             H68.011   Acute Eustachian salpingitis, right ear

             H68.012   Acute Eustachian salpingitis, left ear

             H68.013   Acute Eustachian salpingitis, bilateral

             H68.019   Acute Eustachian salpingitis, unspecified ear

         ● H68.02   Chronic Eustachian salpingitis

             H68.021   Chronic Eustachian salpingitis, right ear

             H68.022   Chronic Eustachian salpingitis, left ear

             H68.023   Chronic Eustachian salpingitis, bilateral

             H68.029   Chronic Eustachian salpingitis, unspecified ear

◀ New   ◀▥ Revised   ~~deleted~~ Deleted   Excludes 1   Excludes 2   Includes   Use additional   Code first   Code also   Unspecified

OGCR Official Guidelines   **X** Assign placeholder X   ● Use Additional Character(s)   ◗ Manifestation Code   **Coding Clinic**

● H68.1   Obstruction of Eustachian tube
    Stenosis of Eustachian tube
    Stricture of Eustachian tube

   ● H68.10   Unspecified obstruction of Eustachian tube

      H68.101   Unspecified obstruction of Eustachian tube, right ear

      H68.102   Unspecified obstruction of Eustachian tube, left ear

      H68.103   Unspecified obstruction of Eustachian tube, bilateral

      H68.109   Unspecified obstruction of Eustachian tube, unspecified ear

   ● H68.11   Osseous obstruction of Eustachian tube

      H68.111   Osseous obstruction of Eustachian tube, right ear

      H68.112   Osseous obstruction of Eustachian tube, left ear

      H68.113   Osseous obstruction of Eustachian tube, bilateral

      H68.119   Osseous obstruction of Eustachian tube, unspecified ear

   ● H68.12   Intrinsic cartilagenous obstruction of Eustachian tube

      H68.121   Intrinsic cartilagenous obstruction of Eustachian tube, right ear

      H68.122   Intrinsic cartilagenous obstruction of Eustachian tube, left ear

      H68.123   Intrinsic cartilagenous obstruction of Eustachian tube, bilateral

      H68.129   Intrinsic cartilagenous obstruction of Eustachian tube, unspecified ear

   ● H68.13   Extrinsic cartilagenous obstruction of Eustachian tube
      Compression of Eustachian tube

      H68.131   Extrinsic cartilagenous obstruction of Eustachian tube, right ear

      H68.132   Extrinsic cartilagenous obstruction of Eustachian tube, left ear

      H68.133   Extrinsic cartilagenous obstruction of Eustachian tube, bilateral

      H68.139   Extrinsic cartilagenous obstruction of Eustachian tube, unspecified ear

● H69   Other and unspecified disorders of Eustachian tube

   ● H69.0   Patulous Eustachian tube

      H69.00   Patulous Eustachian tube, unspecified ear

      H69.01   Patulous Eustachian tube, right ear

      H69.02   Patulous Eustachian tube, left ear

      H69.03   Patulous Eustachian tube, bilateral

   ● H69.8   Other specified disorders of Eustachian tube

      H69.80   Other specified disorders of Eustachian tube, unspecified ear

      H69.81   Other specified disorders of Eustachian tube, right ear

      H69.82   Other specified disorders of Eustachian tube, left ear

      H69.83   Other specified disorders of Eustachian tube, bilateral

   ● H69.9   Unspecified Eustachian tube disorder

      H69.90   Unspecified Eustachian tube disorder, unspecified ear

      H69.91   Unspecified Eustachian tube disorder, right ear

      H69.92   Unspecified Eustachian tube disorder, left ear

      H69.93   Unspecified Eustachian tube disorder, bilateral

● H70   Mastoiditis and related conditions

   ● H70.0   Acute mastoiditis
      Abscess of mastoid
      Empyema of mastoid

    ● H70.00   Acute mastoiditis without complications

      H70.001   Acute mastoiditis without complications, right ear

      H70.002   Acute mastoiditis without complications, left ear

      H70.003   Acute mastoiditis without complications, bilateral

      H70.009   Acute mastoiditis without complications, unspecified ear

    ● H70.01   Subperiosteal abscess of mastoid

      H70.011   Subperiosteal abscess of mastoid, right ear

      H70.012   Subperiosteal abscess of mastoid, left ear

      H70.013   Subperiosteal abscess of mastoid, bilateral

      H70.019   Subperiosteal abscess of mastoid, unspecified ear

    ● H70.09   Acute mastoiditis with other complications

      H70.091   Acute mastoiditis with other complications, right ear

      H70.092   Acute mastoiditis with other complications, left ear

      H70.093   Acute mastoiditis with other complications, bilateral

      H70.099   Acute mastoiditis with other complications, unspecified ear

   ● H70.1   Chronic mastoiditis
      Caries of mastoid
      Fistula of mastoid

      Excludes1   tuberculous mastoiditis (A18.03)

      H70.10   Chronic mastoiditis, unspecified ear

      H70.11   Chronic mastoiditis, right ear

      H70.12   Chronic mastoiditis, left ear

      H70.13   Chronic mastoiditis, bilateral

   ● H70.2   Petrositis
      Inflammation of petrous bone

    ● H70.20   Unspecified petrositis

      H70.201   Unspecified petrositis, right ear

      H70.202   Unspecified petrositis, left ear

      H70.203   Unspecified petrositis, bilateral

      H70.209   Unspecified petrositis, unspecified ear

    ● H70.21   Acute petrositis

      H70.211   Acute petrositis, right ear

      H70.212   Acute petrositis, left ear

      H70.213   Acute petrositis, bilateral

      H70.219   Acute petrositis, unspecified ear

    ● H70.22   Chronic petrositis

      H70.221   Chronic petrositis, right ear

      H70.222   Chronic petrositis, left ear

      H70.223   Chronic petrositis, bilateral

      H70.229   Chronic petrositis, unspecified ear

   ● H70.8   Other mastoiditis and related conditions

      Excludes1   preauricular sinus and cyst (Q18.1)
        sinus, fistula, and cyst of branchial cleft (Q18.0)

    ● H70.81   Postauricular fistula

      H70.811   Postauricular fistula, right ear

      H70.812   Postauricular fistula, left ear

      H70.813   Postauricular fistula, bilateral

      H70.819   Postauricular fistula, unspecified ear

N Newborn Age: 0   **P** Pediatric Age: 0–17   **M** Maternity DX: 12–55   **A** Adult Age: 15–124   ♀ Females Only   ♂ Males Only

933

Item 8–1   Mastoiditis is an infection of the portion of the temporal bone of the skull that is behind the ear (mastoid process) caused by an untreated otitis media, leading to an infection of the surrounding structures which may include the brain.

- **H70.89   Other mastoiditis and related conditions**
  - H70.891   Other mastoiditis and related conditions, right ear
  - H70.892   Other mastoiditis and related conditions, left ear
  - H70.893   Other mastoiditis and related conditions, bilateral
  - H70.899   Other mastoiditis and related conditions, unspecified ear
- **H70.9   Unspecified mastoiditis**
  - H70.90   Unspecified mastoiditis, unspecified ear
  - H70.91   Unspecified mastoiditis, right ear
  - H70.92   Unspecified mastoiditis, left ear
  - H70.93   Unspecified mastoiditis, bilateral

- **H71   Cholesteatoma of middle ear**

  Excludes2   cholesteatoma of external ear (H60.4-)
  recurrent cholesteatoma of postmastoidectomy cavity (H95.0-)

  - **H71.0   Cholesteatoma of attic**
    - H71.00   Cholesteatoma of attic, unspecified ear
    - H71.01   Cholesteatoma of attic, right ear
    - H71.02   Cholesteatoma of attic, left ear
    - H71.03   Cholesteatoma of attic, bilateral
  - **H71.1   Cholesteatoma of tympanum**
    - H71.10   Cholesteatoma of tympanum, unspecified ear
    - H71.11   Cholesteatoma of tympanum, right ear
    - H71.12   Cholesteatoma of tympanum, left ear
    - H71.13   Cholesteatoma of tympanum, bilateral
  - **H71.2   Cholesteatoma of mastoid**
    - H71.20   Cholesteatoma of mastoid, unspecified ear
    - H71.21   Cholesteatoma of mastoid, right ear
    - H71.22   Cholesteatoma of mastoid, left ear
    - H71.23   Cholesteatoma of mastoid, bilateral
  - **H71.3   Diffuse cholesteatosis**
    - H71.30   Diffuse cholesteatosis, unspecified ear
    - H71.31   Diffuse cholesteatosis, right ear
    - H71.32   Diffuse cholesteatosis, left ear
    - H71.33   Diffuse cholesteatosis, bilateral
  - **H71.9   Unspecified cholesteatoma**
    - H71.90   Unspecified cholesteatoma, unspecified ear
    - H71.91   Unspecified cholesteatoma, right ear
    - H71.92   Unspecified cholesteatoma, left ear
    - H71.93   Unspecified cholesteatoma, bilateral

(See Plate 93 on page 69.)

- **H72   Perforation of tympanic membrane**
  Hole or rupture in ear drum

  Includes   persistent post-traumatic perforation of ear drum
  postinflammatory perforation of ear drum

  Code first any associated otitis media (H65.-, H66.1-, H66.2-, H66.3-, H66.4-, H66.9-, H67.-)

  Excludes1   acute suppurative otitis media with rupture of the tympanic membrane (H66.01-)
  traumatic rupture of ear drum (S09.2-)

  - **H72.0   Central perforation of tympanic membrane**
    - H72.00   Central perforation of tympanic membrane, unspecified ear
    - H72.01   Central perforation of tympanic membrane, right ear

- H72.02   Central perforation of tympanic membrane, left ear
- H72.03   Central perforation of tympanic membrane, bilateral
- **H72.1   Attic perforation of tympanic membrane**
  Perforation of pars flaccida
  - H72.10   Attic perforation of tympanic membrane, unspecified ear
  - H72.11   Attic perforation of tympanic membrane, right ear
  - H72.12   Attic perforation of tympanic membrane, left ear
  - H72.13   Attic perforation of tympanic membrane, bilateral
- **H72.2   Other marginal perforations of tympanic membrane**
  - **H72.2X   Other marginal perforations of tympanic membrane**
    - H72.2X1   Other marginal perforations of tympanic membrane, right ear
    - H72.2X2   Other marginal perforations of tympanic membrane, left ear
    - H72.2X3   Other marginal perforations of tympanic membrane, bilateral
    - H72.2X9   Other marginal perforations of tympanic membrane, unspecified ear
- **H72.8   Other perforations of tympanic membrane**
  - **H72.81   Multiple perforations of tympanic membrane**
    - H72.811   Multiple perforations of tympanic membrane, right ear
    - H72.812   Multiple perforations of tympanic membrane, left ear
    - H72.813   Multiple perforations of tympanic membrane, bilateral
    - H72.819   Multiple perforations of tympanic membrane, unspecified ear
  - **H72.82   Total perforations of tympanic membrane**
    - H72.821   Total perforations of tympanic membrane, right ear
    - H72.822   Total perforations of tympanic membrane, left ear
    - H72.823   Total perforations of tympanic membrane, bilateral
    - H72.829   Total perforations of tympanic membrane, unspecified ear
- **H72.9   Unspecified perforation of tympanic membrane**
  - H72.90   Unspecified perforation of tympanic membrane, unspecified ear
  - H72.91   Unspecified perforation of tympanic membrane, right ear
  - H72.92   Unspecified perforation of tympanic membrane, left ear
  - H72.93   Unspecified perforation of tympanic membrane, bilateral

- **H73   Other disorders of tympanic membrane**
  - **H73.0   Acute myringitis**

    Excludes1   acute myringitis with otitis media (H65, H66)

    - **H73.00   Unspecified acute myringitis**
      Acute tympanitis NOS
      - H73.001   Acute myringitis, right ear
      - H73.002   Acute myringitis, left ear
      - H73.003   Acute myringitis, bilateral
      - H73.009   Acute myringitis, unspecified ear
    - **H73.01   Bullous myringitis**
      - H73.011   Bullous myringitis, right ear
      - H73.012   Bullous myringitis, left ear
      - H73.013   Bullous myringitis, bilateral
      - H73.019   Bullous myringitis, unspecified ear

◀ New   ◀▥ Revised   ~~deleted~~ Deleted   Excludes 1   Excludes 2   Includes   Use additional   Code first   Code also   Unspecified

OGCR Official Guidelines   **X** Assign placeholder X   ▶ Use Additional Character(s)   ▶ Manifestation Code   **Coding Clinic**

● H73.09   Other acute myringitis
   H73.091   Other acute myringitis, right ear
   H73.092   Other acute myringitis, left ear
   H73.093   Other acute myringitis, bilateral
   H73.099   Other acute myringitis, unspecified ear

● H73.1   Chronic myringitis
   Chronic tympanitis
   Excludes1   chronic myringitis with otitis media (H65, H66)
   H73.10   Chronic myringitis, unspecified ear
   H73.11   Chronic myringitis, right ear
   H73.12   Chronic myringitis, left ear
   H73.13   Chronic myringitis, bilateral

● H73.2   Unspecified myringitis
   H73.20   Unspecified myringitis, unspecified ear
   H73.21   Unspecified myringitis, right ear
   H73.22   Unspecified myringitis, left ear
   H73.23   Unspecified myringitis, bilateral

● H73.8   Other specified disorders of tympanic membrane
  ● H73.81   Atrophic flaccid tympanic membrane
    H73.811   Atrophic flaccid tympanic membrane, right ear
    H73.812   Atrophic flaccid tympanic membrane, left ear
    H73.813   Atrophic flaccid tympanic membrane, bilateral
    H73.819   Atrophic flaccid tympanic membrane, unspecified ear
  ● H73.82   Atrophic nonflaccid tympanic membrane
    H73.821   Atrophic nonflaccid tympanic membrane, right ear
    H73.822   Atrophic nonflaccid tympanic membrane, left ear
    H73.823   Atrophic nonflaccid tympanic membrane, bilateral
    H73.829   Atrophic nonflaccid tympanic membrane, unspecified ear
  ● H73.89   Other specified disorders of tympanic membrane
    H73.891   Other specified disorders of tympanic membrane, right ear
    H73.892   Other specified disorders of tympanic membrane, left ear
    H73.893   Other specified disorders of tympanic membrane, bilateral
    H73.899   Other specified disorders of tympanic membrane, unspecified ear

● H73.9   Unspecified disorder of tympanic membrane
   H73.90   Unspecified disorder of tympanic membrane, unspecified ear
   H73.91   Unspecified disorder of tympanic membrane, right ear
   H73.92   Unspecified disorder of tympanic membrane, left ear
   H73.93   Unspecified disorder of tympanic membrane, bilateral

● H74   Other disorders of middle ear mastoid
   Excludes2   mastoiditis (H70.-)
● H74.0   Tympanosclerosis
   H74.01   Tympanosclerosis, right ear
   H74.02   Tympanosclerosis, left ear
   H74.03   Tympanosclerosis, bilateral
   H74.09   Tympanosclerosis, unspecified ear

● H74.1   Adhesive middle ear disease
   Adhesive otitis
   Excludes1   glue ear (H65.3-)
   H74.11   Adhesive right middle ear disease
   H74.12   Adhesive left middle ear disease
   H74.13   Adhesive middle ear disease, bilateral
   H74.19   Adhesive middle ear disease, unspecified ear

● H74.2   Discontinuity and dislocation of ear ossicles
   H74.20   Discontinuity and dislocation of ear ossicles, unspecified ear
   H74.21   Discontinuity and dislocation of right ear ossicles
   H74.22   Discontinuity and dislocation of left ear ossicles
   H74.23   Discontinuity and dislocation of ear ossicles, bilateral

● H74.3   Other acquired abnormalities of ear ossicles
  ● H74.31   Ankylosis of ear ossicles
    H74.311   Ankylosis of ear ossicles, right ear
    H74.312   Ankylosis of ear ossicles, left ear
    H74.313   Ankylosis of ear ossicles, bilateral
    H74.319   Ankylosis of ear ossicles, unspecified ear
  ● H74.32   Partial loss of ear ossicles
    H74.321   Partial loss of ear ossicles, right ear
    H74.322   Partial loss of ear ossicles, left ear
    H74.323   Partial loss of ear ossicles, bilateral
    H74.329   Partial loss of ear ossicles, unspecified ear
  ● H74.39   Other acquired abnormalities of ear ossicles
    H74.391   Other acquired abnormalities of right ear ossicles
    H74.392   Other acquired abnormalities of left ear ossicles
    H74.393   Other acquired abnormalities of ear ossicles, bilateral
    H74.399   Other acquired abnormalities of ear ossicles, unspecified ear

● H74.4   Polyp of middle ear
   H74.40   Polyp of middle ear, unspecified ear
   H74.41   Polyp of right middle ear
   H74.42   Polyp of left middle ear
   H74.43   Polyp of middle ear, bilateral

● H74.8   Other specified disorders of middle ear and mastoid
  ● H74.8X   Other specified disorders of middle ear and mastoid
    H74.8X1   Other specified disorders of right middle ear and mastoid
    H74.8X2   Other specified disorders of left middle ear and mastoid
    H74.8X3   Other specified disorders of middle ear and mastoid, bilateral
    H74.8X9   Other specified disorders of middle ear and mastoid, unspecified ear

● H74.9   Unspecified disorder of middle ear and mastoid
   H74.90   Unspecified disorder of middle ear and mastoid, unspecified ear
   H74.91   Unspecified disorder of right middle ear and mastoid
   H74.92   Unspecified disorder of left middle ear and mastoid
   H74.93   Unspecified disorder of middle ear and mastoid, bilateral

CHAPTER 8 (H60-H95)

CHAPTER 8 (H60-H95)

● **H75**   **Other disorders of middle ear and mastoid in diseases classified elsewhere**

Code first underlying disease

● **H75.0**   **Mastoiditis in infectious and parasitic diseases classified elsewhere**

     Excludes1   mastoiditis (in):
                 syphilis (A52.77)
                 tuberculosis (A18.03)

▷ *H75.00*   *Mastoiditis in infectious and parasitic diseases classified elsewhere,* unspecified *ear*

▷ *H75.01*   *Mastoiditis in infectious and parasitic diseases classified elsewhere, right ear*

▷ *H75.02*   *Mastoiditis in infectious and parasitic diseases classified elsewhere, left ear*

▷ *H75.03*   *Mastoiditis in infectious and parasitic diseases classified elsewhere, bilateral*

● **H75.8**   **Other specified disorders of middle ear and mastoid in diseases classified elsewhere**

▷ *H75.80*   *Other specified disorders of middle ear and mastoid in diseases classified elsewhere,* unspecified *ear*

▷ *H75.81*   *Other specified disorders of right middle ear and mastoid in diseases classified elsewhere*

▷ *H75.82*   *Other specified disorders of left middle ear and mastoid in diseases classified elsewhere*

▷ *H75.83*   *Other specified disorders of middle ear and mastoid in diseases classified elsewhere, bilateral*

DISEASES OF INNER EAR (H80-H83)

(See Plate 95 on page 69.)

● **H80**   **Otosclerosis**

Inherited middle ear spongelike bone growth causing hearing loss

     Includes   Otospongiosis

● **H80.0**   **Otosclerosis involving oval window, nonobliterative**

H80.00   **Otosclerosis involving oval window, nonobliterative,** unspecified **ear**

H80.01   **Otosclerosis involving oval window, nonobliterative, right ear**

H80.02   **Otosclerosis involving oval window, nonobliterative, left ear**

H80.03   **Otosclerosis involving oval window, nonobliterative, bilateral**

● **H80.1**   **Otosclerosis involving oval window, obliterative**

H80.10   **Otosclerosis involving oval window, obliterative,** unspecified **ear**

H80.11   **Otosclerosis involving oval window, obliterative, right ear**

H80.12   **Otosclerosis involving oval window, obliterative, left ear**

H80.13   **Otosclerosis involving oval window, obliterative, bilateral**

● **H80.2**   **Cochlear otosclerosis**

     Otosclerosis involving otic capsule
     Otosclerosis involving round window

H80.20   **Cochlear otosclerosis,** unspecified **ear**

H80.21   **Cochlear otosclerosis, right ear**

H80.22   **Cochlear otosclerosis, left ear**

H80.23   **Cochlear otosclerosis, bilateral**

● **H80.8**   **Other otosclerosis**

H80.80   **Other otosclerosis,** unspecified **ear**

H80.81   **Other otosclerosis, right ear**

H80.82   **Other otosclerosis, left ear**

H80.83   **Other otosclerosis, bilateral**

● **H80.9**   **Unspecified otosclerosis**

H80.90   unspecified **otosclerosis, unspecified ear**

H80.91   unspecified **otosclerosis, right ear**

H80.92   unspecified **otosclerosis, left ear**

H80.93   unspecified **otosclerosis, bilateral**

● **H81**   **Disorders of vestibular function**

     Excludes1   epidemic vertigo (A88.1)
                 vertigo NOS (R42)

● **H81.0**   **Ménière's disease**

Vestibular disorder that produces recurring symptoms including severe and intermittent hearing loss including the feeling of ear pressure or pain.
     Labyrinthine hydrops
     Ménière's syndrome or vertigo

H81.01   **Ménière's disease, right ear**

H81.02   **Ménière's disease, left ear**

H81.03   **Ménière's disease, bilateral**

H81.09   **Ménière's disease,** unspecified **ear**

● **H81.1**   **Benign paroxysmal vertigo**

H81.10   **Benign paroxysmal vertigo,** unspecified **ear**

H81.11   **Benign paroxysmal vertigo, right ear**

H81.12   **Benign paroxysmal vertigo, left ear**

H81.13   **Benign paroxysmal vertigo, bilateral**

● **H81.2**   **Vestibular neuronitis**

H81.20   **Vestibular neuronitis,** unspecified **ear**

H81.21   **Vestibular neuronitis, right ear**

H81.22   **Vestibular neuronitis, left ear**

H81.23   **Vestibular neuronitis, bilateral**

● **H81.3**   **Other peripheral vertigo**

● **H81.31**   **Aural vertigo**

     H81.311   **Aural vertigo, right ear**

     H81.312   **Aural vertigo, left ear**

     H81.313   **Aural vertigo, bilateral**

     H81.319   **Aural vertigo,** unspecified **ear**

● **H81.39**   **Other peripheral vertigo**

     Lermoyez' syndrome
     Otogenic vertigo
     Peripheral vertigo NOS

     H81.391   **Other peripheral vertigo, right ear**

     H81.392   **Other peripheral vertigo, left ear**

     H81.393   **Other peripheral vertigo, bilateral**

     H81.399   **Other peripheral vertigo,** unspecified **ear**

● **H81.4**   **Vertigo of central origin**

     Central positional nystagmus

H81.41   **Vertigo of central origin, right ear**

H81.42   **Vertigo of central origin, left ear**

H81.43   **Vertigo of central origin, bilateral**

H81.49   **Vertigo of central origin,** unspecified **ear**

● **H81.8**   **Other disorders of vestibular function**

● **H81.8X**   **Other disorders of vestibular function**

     H81.8X1   **Other disorders of vestibular function, right ear**

     H81.8X2   **Other disorders of vestibular function, left ear**

     H81.8X3   **Other disorders of vestibular function, bilateral**

     H81.8X9   **Other disorders of vestibular function,** unspecified **ear**

◀ New   ⬅ Revised   ~~deleted~~ Deleted   Excludes 1   Excludes 2   Includes   Use additional   Code first   Code also   Unspecified

OGCR Official Guidelines   **X** Assign placeholder X   ● Use Additional Character(s)   ▷ Manifestation Code   **Coding Clinic**

● H81.9 **Unspecified disorder of vestibular function**
Vertiginous syndrome NOS

    H81.90 **Unspecified disorder of vestibular function, unspecified ear**

    H81.91 **Unspecified disorder of vestibular function, right ear**

    H81.92 **Unspecified disorder of vestibular function, left ear**

    H81.93 **Unspecified disorder of vestibular function, bilateral**

● H82 **Vertiginous syndromes in diseases classified elsewhere**
Code first underlying disease

    Excludes1 epidemic vertigo (A88.1)

▶ *H82.1 Vertiginous syndromes in diseases classified elsewhere, right ear*

▶ *H82.2 Vertiginous syndromes in diseases classified elsewhere, left ear*

▶ *H82.3 Vertiginous syndromes in diseases classified elsewhere, bilateral*

▶ *H82.9 Vertiginous syndromes in diseases classified elsewhere, unspecified ear*

● H83 **Other diseases of inner ear**

  ● H83.0 **Labyrinthitis**
    Balance disorder that follows URI or head injury.

    H83.01 **Labyrinthitis, right ear**

    H83.02 **Labyrinthitis, left ear**

    H83.03 **Labyrinthitis, bilateral**

    H83.09 **Labyrinthitis, unspecified ear**

  ● H83.1 **Labyrinthine fistula**

    H83.11 **Labyrinthine fistula, right ear**

    H83.12 **Labyrinthine fistula, left ear**

    H83.13 **Labyrinthine fistula, bilateral**

    H83.19 **Labyrinthine fistula, unspecified ear**

  ● H83.2 **Labyrinthine dysfunction**
Labyrinthine hypersensitivity
Labyrinthine hypofunction
Labyrinthine loss of function

    ● H83.2X **Labyrinthine dysfunction**

      H83.2X1 **Labyrinthine dysfunction, right ear**

      H83.2X2 **Labyrinthine dysfunction, left ear**

      H83.2X3 **Labyrinthine dysfunction, bilateral**

      H83.2X9 **Labyrinthine dysfunction, unspecified ear**

  ● H83.3 **Noise effects on inner ear**
Acoustic trauma of inner ear
Noise-induced hearing loss of inner ear

    ● H83.3X **Noise effects on inner ear**

      H83.3X1 **Noise effects on right inner ear**

      H83.3X2 **Noise effects on left inner ear**

      H83.3X3 **Noise effects on inner ear, bilateral**

      H83.3X9 **Noise effects on inner ear, unspecified ear**

  ● H83.8 **Other specified diseases of inner ear**

    ● H83.8X **Other specified diseases of inner ear**

      H83.8X1 **Other specified diseases of right inner ear**

      H83.8X2 **Other specified diseases of left inner ear**

      H83.8X3 **Other specified diseases of inner ear, bilateral**

      H83.8X9 **Other specified diseases of inner ear, unspecified ear**

  ● H83.9 **Unspecified disease of inner ear**

    H83.90 **Unspecified disease of inner ear, unspecified ear**

    H83.91 **Unspecified disease of right inner ear**

    H83.92 **Unspecified disease of left inner ear**

    H83.93 **Unspecified disease of inner ear, bilateral**

OTHER DISORDERS OF EAR (H90-H94)

● H90 **Conductive and sensorineural hearing loss**

    Excludes1 deaf nonspeaking NEC (H91.3)
deafness NOS (H91.9-)
hearing loss NOS (H91.9-)
noise-induced hearing loss (H83.3-)
ototoxic hearing loss (H91.0-)
sudden (idiopathic) hearing loss (H91.2-)

  H90.0 **Conductive hearing loss, bilateral**

  ● H90.1 **Conductive hearing loss, unilateral with unrestricted hearing on the contralateral side**

    H90.11 **Conductive hearing loss, unilateral, right ear, with unrestricted hearing on the contralateral side**

    H90.12 **Conductive hearing loss, unilateral, left ear, with unrestricted hearing on the contralateral side**

  H90.2 **Conductive hearing loss, unspecified**
Conductive deafness NOS

  H90.3 **Sensorineural hearing loss, bilateral**

  ● H90.4 **Sensorineural hearing loss, unilateral with unrestricted hearing on the contralateral side**

    H90.41 **Sensorineural hearing loss, unilateral, right ear, with unrestricted hearing on the contralateral side**

    H90.42 **Sensorineural hearing loss, unilateral, left ear, with unrestricted hearing on the contralateral side**

  H90.5 **Unspecified sensorineural hearing loss**
Central hearing loss NOS
Congenital deafness NOS
Neural hearing loss NOS
Perceptive hearing loss NOS
Sensorineural deafness NOS
Sensory hearing loss NOS

    Excludes1 abnormal auditory perception (H93.2-)
psychogenic deafness (F44.6)

  H90.6 **Mixed conductive and sensorineural hearing loss, bilateral**

  ● H90.7 **Mixed conductive and sensorineural hearing loss, unilateral with unrestricted hearing on the contralateral side**

    H90.71 **Mixed conductive and sensorineural hearing loss, unilateral, right ear, with unrestricted hearing on the contralateral side**

    H90.72 **Mixed conductive and sensorineural hearing loss, unilateral, left ear, with unrestricted hearing on the contralateral side**

  H90.8 **Mixed conductive and sensorineural hearing loss, unspecified**

● H91 **Other and unspecified hearing loss**

    Excludes1 abnormal auditory perception (H93.2-)
hearing loss as classified in H90.-
impacted cerumen (H61.2-)
noise-induced hearing loss (H83.3-)
psychogenic deafness (F44.6)
transient ischemic deafness (H93.01-)

  ● H91.0 **Ototoxic hearing loss**

    Code first poisoning due to drug or toxin, if applicable (T36-T65 with fifth or sixth character 1-4 or 6)

    Use additional code for adverse effect, if applicable, to identify drug (T36-T50 with fifth or sixth character 5)

    H91.01 **Ototoxic hearing loss, right ear**

    H91.02 **Ototoxic hearing loss, left ear**

    H91.03 **Ototoxic hearing loss, bilateral**

    H91.09 **Ototoxic hearing loss, unspecified ear**

CHAPTER 8 (H60-H95)

● **H91.1**   **Presbycusis**
Presbyacusia
    H91.10   Presbycusis, unspecified ear
    H91.11   Presbycusis, right ear
    H91.12   Presbycusis, left ear
    H91.13   Presbycusis, bilateral

● **H91.2**   **Sudden idiopathic hearing loss**
Sudden hearing loss NOS
    H91.20   Sudden idiopathic hearing loss, unspecified ear
    H91.21   Sudden idiopathic hearing loss, right ear
    H91.22   Sudden idiopathic hearing loss, left ear
    H91.23   Sudden idiopathic hearing loss, bilateral

  H91.3   **Deaf nonspeaking, not elsewhere classified**

● **H91.8**   **Other specified hearing loss**
  ● **H91.8X**   **Other specified hearing loss**
      H91.8X1   Other specified hearing loss, right ear
      H91.8X2   Other specified hearing loss, left ear
      H91.8X3   Other specified hearing loss, bilateral
      H91.8X9   Other specified hearing loss, unspecified ear

● **H91.9**   **Unspecified hearing loss**
Deafness NOS
High frequency deafness
Low frequency deafness
    H91.90   Unspecified hearing loss, unspecified ear
    H91.91   Unspecified hearing loss, right ear
    H91.92   Unspecified hearing loss, left ear
    H91.93   Unspecified hearing loss, bilateral

● **H92**   **Otalgia and effusion of ear**
  ● **H92.0**   **Otalgia**
    H92.01   Otalgia, right ear
    H92.02   Otalgia, left ear
    H92.03   Otalgia, bilateral
    H92.09   Otalgia, unspecified ear

  ● **H92.1**   **Otorrhea**
    Excludes1   leakage of cerebrospinal fluid through ear (G96.0)
    H92.10   Otorrhea, unspecified ear
    H92.11   Otorrhea, right ear
    H92.12   Otorrhea, left ear
    H92.13   Otorrhea, bilateral

  ● **H92.2**   **Otorrhagia**
    Excludes1   traumatic otorrhagia - code to injury
    H92.20   Otorrhagia, unspecified ear
    H92.21   Otorrhagia, right ear
    H92.22   Otorrhagia, left ear
    H92.23   Otorrhagia, bilateral

● **H93**   **Other disorders of ear, not elsewhere classified**
  ● **H93.0**   **Degenerative and vascular disorders of ear**
    Excludes1   presbycusis (H91.1)
    ● **H93.01**   **Transient ischemic deafness**
      H93.011   Transient ischemic deafness, right ear
      H93.012   Transient ischemic deafness, left ear
      H93.013   Transient ischemic deafness, bilateral
      H93.019   Transient ischemic deafness, unspecified ear
    ● **H93.09**   **Unspecified degenerative and vascular disorders of ear**
      H93.091   Unspecified degenerative and vascular disorders of right ear
      H93.092   Unspecified degenerative and vascular disorders of left ear
      H93.093   Unspecified degenerative and vascular disorders of ear, bilateral
      H93.099   Unspecified degenerative and vascular disorders of unspecified ear

● **H93.1**   **Tinnitus**
Perception of sound (ringing, buzzing, humming, whistling tunes, or singing)
    H93.11   Tinnitus, right ear
    H93.12   Tinnitus, left ear
    H93.13   Tinnitus, bilateral
    H93.19   Tinnitus, unspecified ear

● **H93.2**   **Other abnormal auditory perceptions**
    Excludes2   auditory hallucinations (R44.0)
  ● **H93.21**   **Auditory recruitment**
      H93.211   Auditory recruitment, right ear
      H93.212   Auditory recruitment, left ear
      H93.213   Auditory recruitment, bilateral
      H93.219   Auditory recruitment, unspecified ear
  ● **H93.22**   **Diplacusis**
      H93.221   Diplacusis, right ear
      H93.222   Diplacusis, left ear
      H93.223   Diplacusis, bilateral
      H93.229   Diplacusis, unspecified ear
  ● **H93.23**   **Hyperacusis**
      H93.231   Hyperacusis, right ear
      H93.232   Hyperacusis, left ear
      H93.233   Hyperacusis, bilateral
      H93.239   Hyperacusis, unspecified ear
  ● **H93.24**   **Temporary auditory threshold shift**
      H93.241   Temporary auditory threshold shift, right ear
      H93.242   Temporary auditory threshold shift, left ear
      H93.243   Temporary auditory threshold shift, bilateral
      H93.249   Temporary auditory threshold shift, unspecified ear
    H93.25   Central auditory processing disorder
      Congenital auditory imperception
      Word deafness
      Excludes1   mixed receptive-expressive language disorder (F80.2)
  ● **H93.29**   **Other abnormal auditory perceptions**
      H93.291   Other abnormal auditory perceptions, right ear
      H93.292   Other abnormal auditory perceptions, left ear
      H93.293   Other abnormal auditory perceptions, bilateral
      H93.299   Other abnormal auditory perceptions, unspecified ear

● **H93.3**   **Disorders of acoustic nerve**
Disorder of 8th cranial nerve
    Excludes1   acoustic neuroma (D33.3)
                syphilitic acoustic neuritis (A52.15)
  ● **H93.3X**   **Disorders of acoustic nerve**
      H93.3X1   Disorders of right acoustic nerve
      H93.3X2   Disorders of left acoustic nerve
      H93.3X3   Disorders of bilateral acoustic nerves
      H93.3X9   Disorders of unspecified acoustic nerve

● **H93.8**   **Other specified disorders of ear**
  ● **H93.8X**   **Other specified disorders of ear**
      H93.8X1   Other specified disorders of right ear
      H93.8X2   Other specified disorders of left ear
      H93.8X3   Other specified disorders of ear, bilateral
      H93.8X9   Other specified disorders of ear, unspecified ear

◄ New   ◄━ Revised   deleted Deleted   Excludes 1   Excludes 2   Includes   Use additional   Code first   Code also   Unspecified

OGCR Official Guidelines   **X** Assign placeholder X   ● Use Additional Character(s)   ▶ Manifestation Code   **Coding Clinic**

● **H93.9**   Unspecified disorder of ear
     H93.90   Unspecified disorder of ear, unspecified ear
     H93.91   Unspecified disorder of right ear
     H93.92   Unspecified disorder of left ear
     H93.93   Unspecified disorder of ear, bilateral

● **H94**   Other disorders of ear in diseases classified elsewhere

   ● **H94.0**   Acoustic neuritis in infectious and parasitic diseases classified elsewhere

       Code first underlying disease, such as:
       parasitic disease (B65-B89)

       Excludes1   acoustic neuritis (in):
               herpes zoster (B02.29)
               syphilis (A52.15)

     ▸ *H94.00*   *Acoustic neuritis in infectious and parasitic diseases classified elsewhere, unspecified ear*
     ▸ *H94.01*   *Acoustic neuritis in infectious and parasitic diseases classified elsewhere, right ear*
     ▸ *H94.02*   *Acoustic neuritis in infectious and parasitic diseases classified elsewhere, left ear*
     ▸ *H94.03*   *Acoustic neuritis in infectious and parasitic diseases classified elsewhere, bilateral*

   ● **H94.8**   Other specified disorders of ear in diseases classified elsewhere

       Code first underlying disease, such as:
       congenital syphilis (A50.0)

       Excludes1   aural myiasis (B87.4)
               syphilitic labyrinthitis (A52.79)

     ▸ *H94.80*   *Other specified disorders of ear in diseases classified elsewhere, unspecified ear*
     ▸ *H94.81*   *Other specified disorders of right ear in diseases classified elsewhere*
     ▸ *H94.82*   *Other specified disorders of left ear in diseases classified elsewhere*
     ▸ *H94.83*   *Other specified disorders of ear in diseases classified elsewhere, bilateral*

● **H95**   Intraoperative and postprocedural complications and disorders of ear and mastoid process, not elsewhere classified

   ● **H95.0**   Recurrent cholesteatoma of postmastoidectomy cavity
     H95.00   Recurrent cholesteatoma of postmastoidectomy cavity, unspecified ear
     H95.01   Recurrent cholesteatoma of postmastoidectomy cavity, right ear
     H95.02   Recurrent cholesteatoma of postmastoidectomy cavity, left ear
     H95.03   Recurrent cholesteatoma of postmastoidectomy cavity, bilateral ears

   ● **H95.1**   Other disorders of ear and mastoid process following mastoidectomy

     ● **H95.11**   Chronic inflammation of postmastoidectomy cavity
         H95.111   Chronic inflammation of postmastoidectomy cavity, right ear
         H95.112   Chronic inflammation of postmastoidectomy cavity, left ear
         H95.113   Chronic inflammation of postmastoidectomy cavity, bilateral ears
         H95.119   Chronic inflammation of postmastoidectomy cavity, unspecified ear

     ● **H95.12**   Granulation of postmastoidectomy cavity
         H95.121   Granulation of postmastoidectomy cavity, right ear
         H95.122   Granulation of postmastoidectomy cavity, left ear
         H95.123   Granulation of postmastoidectomy cavity, bilateral ears
         H95.129   Granulation of postmastoidectomy cavity, unspecified ear

● **H95.13**   Mucosal cyst of postmastoidectomy cavity
     H95.131   Mucosal cyst of postmastoidectomy cavity, right ear
     H95.132   Mucosal cyst of postmastoidectomy cavity, left ear
     H95.133   Mucosal cyst of postmastoidectomy cavity, bilateral ears
     H95.139   Mucosal cyst of postmastoidectomy cavity, unspecified ear

   ● **H95.19**   Other disorders following mastoidectomy
     H95.191   Other disorders following mastoidectomy, right ear
     H95.192   Other disorders following mastoidectomy, left ear
     H95.193   Other disorders following mastoidectomy, bilateral ears
     H95.199   Other disorders following mastoidectomy, unspecified ear

● **H95.2**   Intraoperative hemorrhage and hematoma of ear and mastoid process complicating a procedure

       Excludes1   intraoperative hemorrhage and hematoma of ear and mastoid process due to accidental puncture or laceration during a procedure (H95.3-)

     H95.21   Intraoperative hemorrhage and hematoma of ear and mastoid process complicating a procedure on the ear and mastoid process
     H95.22   Intraoperative hemorrhage and hematoma of ear and mastoid process complicating other procedure

● **H95.3**   Accidental puncture and laceration of ear and mastoid process during a procedure
     H95.31   Accidental puncture and laceration of the ear and mastoid process during a procedure on the ear and mastoid process
     H95.32   Accidental puncture and laceration of the ear and mastoid process during other procedure

● **H95.4**   Postprocedural hemorrhage and hematoma of ear and mastoid process following a procedure
     H95.41   Postprocedural hemorrhage and hematoma of ear and mastoid process following a procedure on the ear and mastoid process
     H95.42   Postprocedural hemorrhage and hematoma of ear and mastoid process following other procedure

● **H95.8**   Other intraoperative and postprocedural complications and disorders of the ear and mastoid process, not elsewhere classified

       Excludes2   postprocedural complications and disorders following mastoidectomy (H95.0-, H95.1-)

   ● **H95.81**   Postprocedural stenosis of external ear canal
         H95.811   Postprocedural stenosis of right external ear canal
         H95.812   Postprocedural stenosis of left external ear canal
         H95.813   Postprocedural stenosis of external ear canal, bilateral
         H95.819   Postprocedural stenosis of unspecified external ear canal

     H95.88   Other intraoperative complications and disorders of the ear and mastoid process, not elsewhere classified

       Use additional code, if applicable, to further specify disorder

     H95.89   Other postprocedural complications and disorders of the ear and mastoid process, not elsewhere classified

       Use additional code, if applicable, to further specify disorder

CHAPTER 8 (H60-H95)

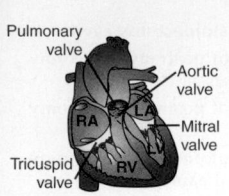

Pulmonary valve
Aortic valve
Mitral valve
Tricuspid valve
RA LA
RV

Figure 9-1 Cardiovascular valves.

Item 9–1 Rheumatic fever is the inflammation of the valve(s) of the heart, usually the mitral or aortic, which leads to valve damage. Rheumatic heart inflammations are usually **pericarditis** (sac surrounding heart), **endocarditis** (heart cavity), or **myocarditis** (heart muscle).

CHAPTER 9   DISEASES OF THE CIRCULATORY SYSTEM (I00-I99)

Excludes2   certain conditions originating in the perinatal period (P04-P96)
certain infectious and parasitic diseases (A00-B99)
complications of pregnancy, childbirth and the puerperium (O00-O9A)
congenital malformations, deformations, and chromosomal abnormalities (Q00-Q99)
endocrine, nutritional and metabolic diseases (E00-E88)
injury, poisoning and certain other consequences of external causes (S00-T88)
neoplasms (C00-D49)
symptoms, signs and abnormal clinical and laboratory findings, not elsewhere classified (R00-R94)
systemic connective tissue disorders (M30-M36)
transient cerebral ischemic attacks and related syndromes (G45.-)

This chapter contains the following blocks:

I00-I02	Acute rheumatic fever
I05-I09	Chronic rheumatic heart diseases
I10-I15	Hypertensive diseases
I20-I25	Ischemic heart diseases
I26-I28	Pulmonary heart disease and diseases of pulmonary circulation
I30-I52	Other forms of heart disease
I60-I69	Cerebrovascular diseases
I70-I79	Diseases of arteries, arterioles and capillaries
I80-I89	Diseases of veins, lymphatic vessels and lymph nodes, not elsewhere classified
I95-I99	Other and unspecified disorders of the circulatory system

ACUTE RHEUMATIC FEVER (I00-I02)

I00   Rheumatic fever without heart involvement
Includes   arthritis, rheumatic, acute or subacute
Excludes1   rheumatic fever with heart involvement (I01.0-I01.9)

● **I01   Rheumatic fever with heart involvement**
Excludes1   chronic diseases of rheumatic origin (I05-I09) unless rheumatic fever is also present or there is evidence of reactivation or activity of the rheumatic process.

I01.0   Acute rheumatic pericarditis
Any condition in I00 with pericarditis
Rheumatic pericarditis (acute)
Excludes1   acute pericarditis not specified as rheumatic (I30.-)

I01.1   Acute rheumatic endocarditis
Any condition in I00 with endocarditis or valvulitis
Acute rheumatic valvulitis

I01.2   Acute rheumatic myocarditis
Any condition in I00 with myocarditis

Item 9–2 Rheumatic chorea, also called Sydenham's, juvenile, minor, simple, or St. Vitus' dance, is a major symptom of rheumatic fever and is characterized by ceaseless, involuntary, jerky, purposeless movements.

I01.8   Other acute rheumatic heart disease
Any condition in I00 with other or multiple types of heart involvement
Acute rheumatic pancarditis

I01.9   Acute rheumatic heart disease, unspecified
Any condition in I00 with unspecified type of heart involvement
Rheumatic carditis, acute
Rheumatic heart disease, active or acute

● **I02   Rheumatic chorea**
Includes   Sydenham's chorea
Excludes1   chorea NOS (G25.5)
Huntington's chorea (G10)

I02.0   Rheumatic chorea with heart involvement
Chorea NOS with heart involvement
Rheumatic chorea with heart involvement of any type classifiable under I01.-

I02.9   Rheumatic chorea without heart involvement
Rheumatic chorea NOS

CHRONIC RHEUMATIC HEART DISEASES (I05-I09)

● **I05   Rheumatic mitral valve diseases**
Includes   conditions classifiable to both I05.0 and I05.2-I05.9, whether specified as rheumatic or not
Excludes1   mitral valve disease specified as nonrheumatic (I34.-)
mitral valve disease with aortic and/or tricuspid valve involvement (I08.-)

I05.0   Rheumatic mitral stenosis
Mitral (valve) obstruction (rheumatic)

I05.1   Rheumatic mitral insufficiency
Rheumatic mitral incompetence
Rheumatic mitral regurgitation
Excludes1   mitral insufficiency not specified as rheumatic (I34.0)

I05.2   Rheumatic mitral stenosis with insufficiency
Rheumatic mitral stenosis with incompetence or regurgitation

I05.8   Other rheumatic mitral valve diseases
Rheumatic mitral (valve) failure

I05.9   Rheumatic mitral valve disease, unspecified
Rheumatic mitral (valve) disorder (chronic) NOS

● **I06   Rheumatic aortic valve diseases**
Excludes1   aortic valve disease not specified as rheumatic (I35.-)
aortic valve disease with mitral and/or tricuspid valve involvement (I08.-)

I06.0   Rheumatic aortic stenosis
Rheumatic aortic (valve) obstruction

I06.1   Rheumatic aortic insufficiency
Rheumatic aortic incompetence
Rheumatic aortic regurgitation

(See Plate 244 on page 78.)

Item 9–3 Mitral stenosis is the narrowing of the mitral valve separating the left atrium from the left ventricle. **Mitral insufficiency** is the improper closure of the mitral valve which may lead to enlargement (hypertrophy) of the left atrium.

Item 9–4 Aortic stenosis is the narrowing of the aortic valve located between the left ventricle and the aorta. **Aortic insufficiency** is the improper closure of the aortic valve which may lead to enlargement (hypertrophy) of the left ventricle.

◀ New   ◀▥ Revised   ~~deleted~~ Deleted   Excludes 1   Excludes 2   Includes   Use additional   Code first   Code also   Unspecified

OGCR Official Guidelines   **X** Assign placeholder X   ● Use Additional Character(s)   ▶ Manifestation Code   **Coding Clinic**

CHAPTER 9 (I00-I99)

I06.2   **Rheumatic aortic stenosis with insufficiency**
Rheumatic aortic stenosis with incompetence or regurgitation

I06.8   **Other rheumatic aortic valve diseases**

I06.9   **Rheumatic aortic valve disease, unspecified**
Rheumatic aortic (valve) disease NOS

● **I07**   **Rheumatic tricuspid valve diseases**

> **Includes**   rheumatic tricuspid valve diseases specified as rheumatic or unspecified

> **Excludes1**   tricuspid valve disease specified as nonrheumatic (I36.-)
> tricuspid valve disease with aortic and/or mitral valve involvement (I08.-)

I07.0   **Rheumatic tricuspid stenosis**
Tricuspid (valve) stenosis (rheumatic)

I07.1   **Rheumatic tricuspid insufficiency**
Tricuspid (valve) insufficiency (rheumatic)

I07.2   **Rheumatic tricuspid stenosis and insufficiency**

I07.8   **Other rheumatic tricuspid valve diseases**

I07.9   **Rheumatic tricuspid valve disease, unspecified**
Rheumatic tricuspid valve disorder NOS

● **I08**   **Multiple valve diseases**

> **Includes**   multiple valve diseases specified as rheumatic or unspecified

> **Excludes1**   endocarditis, valve unspecified (I38)
> multiple valve disease specified a nonrheumatic (I34.-, I35.-, I36.-, I37.-, I38.-, Q22.-, Q23.-, Q24.8-)
> rheumatic valve disease NOS (I09.1)

I08.0   **Rheumatic disorders of both mitral and aortic valves**
Involvement of both mitral and aortic valves specified as rheumatic or unspecified

I08.1   **Rheumatic disorders of both mitral and tricuspid valves**

I08.2   **Rheumatic disorders of both aortic and tricuspid valves**

I08.3   **Combined rheumatic disorders of mitral, aortic and tricuspid valves**

I08.8   **Other rheumatic multiple valve diseases**

I08.9   **Rheumatic multiple valve disease, unspecified**

● **I09**   **Other rheumatic heart diseases**

I09.0   **Rheumatic myocarditis**

> **Excludes1**   myocarditis not specified as rheumatic (I51.4)

I09.1   **Rheumatic diseases of endocardium, valve unspecified**
Rheumatic endocarditis (chronic)
Rheumatic valvulitis (chronic)

> **Excludes1**   endocarditis, valve unspecified (I38)

I09.2   **Chronic rheumatic pericarditis**
Adherent pericardium, rheumatic
Chronic rheumatic mediastinopericarditis
Chronic rheumatic myopericarditis

> **Excludes1**   chronic pericarditis not specified as rheumatic (I31.-)

● **I09.8**   **Other specified rheumatic heart diseases**

I09.81   **Rheumatic heart failure**
Use additional code to identify type of heart failure (I50.-)

I09.89   **Other specified rheumatic heart diseases**
Rheumatic disease of pulmonary valve

I09.9   **Rheumatic heart disease, unspecified**
Rheumatic carditis

> **Excludes1**   rheumatoid carditis (M05.31)

Item 9–5 Hypertension is caused by high arterial blood pressure in the arteries. **Essential, primary,** or **idiopathic** hypertension occurs without identifiable organic cause. **Secondary** hypertension is that which has an organic cause. **Malignant** hypertension is severely elevated blood pressure. **Benign** hypertension is mildly elevated blood pressure.

HYPERTENSIVE DISEASES (I10-I15)

Use additional code to identify:
   exposure to environmental tobacco smoke (Z77.22)
   history of tobacco use (Z87.891)
   occupational exposure to environmental tobacco smoke (Z57.31)
   tobacco dependence (F17.-)
   tobacco use (Z72.0)

> **Excludes1**   hypertensive disease complicating pregnancy, childbirth and the puerperium (O10-O11, O13-O16)
> neonatal hypertension (P29.2)
> primary pulmonary hypertension (I27.0)

I10   **Essential (primary) hypertension**

> **Includes**   high blood pressure
> hypertension (arterial) (benign) (essential) (malignant) (primary) (systemic)

> **Excludes1**   hypertensive disease complicating pregnancy, childbirth and the puerperium (O10-O11, O13-O16)

> **Excludes2**   essential (primary) hypertension involving vessels of brain (I60-I69)
> essential (primary) hypertension involving vessels of eye (H35.0-)

● **I11**   **Hypertensive heart disease**

> **Includes**   any condition in I51.4-I51.9 due to hypertension

I11.0   **Hypertensive heart disease with heart failure**
Hypertensive heart failure
Use additional code to identify type of heart failure (I50.-)

I11.9   **Hypertensive heart disease without heart failure**
Hypertensive heart disease NOS

OGCR   Section I.C.9.a.2

Hypertensive Chronic Kidney Disease

Assign codes from category I12, Hypertensive chronic kidney disease, when both hypertension and a condition classifiable to category N18, Chronic kidney disease (CKD), are present. Unlike hypertension with heart disease, ICD-10-CM presumes a cause-and-effect relationship and classifies chronic kidney disease with hypertension as hypertensive chronic kidney disease.

The appropriate code from category N18 should be used as a secondary code with a code from category I12 to identify the stage of chronic kidney disease.

See Section I.C.14. Chronic kidney disease.

If a patient has hypertensive chronic kidney disease and acute renal failure, an additional code for the acute renal failure is required.

● **I12**   **Hypertensive chronic kidney disease**

> **Includes**   any condition in N18 and N26 - due to hypertension
> arteriosclerosis of kidney
> arteriosclerotic nephritis (chronic) (interstitial)
> hypertensive nephropathy
> nephrosclerosis

> **Excludes1**   hypertension due to kidney disease (I15.0, I15.1)
> renovascular hypertension (I15.0)
> secondary hypertension (I15.-)

> **Excludes2**   acute kidney failure (N17.-)

I12.0   **Hypertensive chronic kidney disease with stage 5 chronic kidney disease or end stage renal disease**
Use additional code to identify the stage of chronic kidney disease (N18.5, N18.6)

CHAPTER 9 (I00-I99)

CHAPTER 9 (I00-I99)

I12.9   **Hypertensive chronic kidney disease with stage 1 through stage 4 chronic kidney disease, or unspecified chronic kidney disease**
> Hypertensive chronic kidney disease NOS
> Hypertensive renal disease NOS
>
> Use additional code to identify the stage of chronic kidney disease (N18.1-N18.4, N18.9)

OGCR Section I.c.9.a.6

Hypertensive Heart and Chronic Kidney Disease

Assign codes from combination category I13, Hypertensive heart and chronic kidney disease, when both hypertensive kidney disease and hypertensive heart disease are stated in the diagnosis. Assume a relationship between the hypertension and the chronic kidney disease, whether or not the condition is so designated. If heart failure is present, assign an additional code from category I50 to identify the type of heart failure.

The appropriate code from category N18, Chronic kidney disease, should be used as a secondary code with a code from category I13 to identify the stage of chronic kidney disease.

See Section I.C.14. Chronic kidney disease.

The codes in category I13, Hypertensive heart and chronic kidney disease, are combination codes that include hypertension, heart disease and chronic kidney disease. The Includes note at I13 specifies that the conditions included at I11 and I12 are included together in I13. If a patient has hypertension, heart disease and chronic kidney disease then a code from I13 should be used, not individual codes for hypertension, heart disease and chronic kidney disease, or codes from I11 or I12.

For patients with both acute renal failure and chronic kidney disease an additional code for acute renal failure is required.

● **I13**   **Hypertensive heart and chronic kidney disease**
> **Includes**   any condition in I11.- with any condition in I12.-
> > cardiorenal disease
> > cardiovascular renal disease

     I13.0   **Hypertensive heart and chronic kidney disease with heart failure and stage 1 through stage 4 chronic kidney disease, or unspecified chronic kidney disease**
> > Use additional code to identify type of heart failure (I50.-)
> > Use additional code to identify stage of chronic kidney disease (N18.1-N18.4, N18.9)

●   **I13.1**   **Hypertensive heart and chronic kidney disease without heart failure**

        I13.10   **Hypertensive heart and chronic kidney disease without heart failure, with stage 1 through stage 4 chronic kidney disease, or unspecified chronic kidney disease**
> > > Hypertensive heart disease and hypertensive chronic kidney disease NOS
> > >
> > > Use additional code to identify the stage of chronic kidney disease (N18.1-N18.4, N18.9)

        I13.11   **Hypertensive heart and chronic kidney disease without heart failure, with stage 5 chronic kidney disease, or end stage renal disease**
> > > Use additional code to identify the stage of chronic kidney disease (N18.5, N18.6)

     I13.2   **Hypertensive heart and chronic kidney disease with heart failure and with stage 5 chronic kidney disease, or end stage renal disease**
> > Use additional code to identify type of heart failure (I50.-)
> > Use additional code to identify the stage of chronic kidney disease (N18.5, N18.6)

OGCR Section I.9.a.6

Hypertension, Secondary

Secondary hypertension is due to an underlying condition. Two codes are required: one to identify the underlying etiology and one from category I15 to identify the hypertension. Sequencing of codes is determined by the reason for admission/encounter.

● **I15**   **Secondary hypertension**
> Code also underlying condition
>
> **Excludes1**   postprocedural hypertension (I97.3)
> **Excludes2**   secondary hypertension involving vessels of brain (I60-I69)
> > secondary hypertension involving vessels of eye (H35.0-)

     I15.0   **Renovascular hypertension**
     I15.1   **Hypertension secondary to other renal disorders**
     I15.2   **Hypertension secondary to endocrine disorders**
     I15.8   **Other secondary hypertension**
     I15.9   **Secondary hypertension, unspecified**

ISCHEMIC HEART DISEASES (I20-I25)

Use additional code to identify presence of hypertension (I10-I15)

● **I20**   **Angina pectoris**
> *Chest pain/discomfort due to lack of oxygen to the heart muscle. Principal symptom of myocardial infarction.*
>
> Use additional code to identify:
> > exposure to environmental tobacco smoke (Z77.22)
> > history of tobacco use (Z87.891)
> > occupational exposure to environmental tobacco smoke (Z57.31)
> > tobacco dependence (F17.-)
> > tobacco use (Z72.0)
>
> **Excludes1**   angina pectoris with atherosclerotic heart disease of native coronary arteries (I25.1-)
> > atherosclerosis of coronary artery bypass graft(s) and coronary artery of transplanted heart with angina pectoris (I25.7-)
> > postinfarction angina (I23.7)

     I20.0   **Unstable angina**
> Accelerated angina
> Crescendo angina
> De novo effort angina
> Intermediate coronary syndrome
> Preinfarction syndrome
> Worsening effort angina

     I20.1   **Angina pectoris with documented spasm**
> Angiospastic angina
> Prinzmetal angina
> Spasm-induced angina
> Variant angina

     I20.8   **Other forms of angina pectoris**
> Angina equivalent
> Angina of effort
> Coronary slow flow syndrome
> Stenocardia
>
> Use additional code(s) for symptoms associated with angina equivalent

     I20.9   **Angina pectoris, unspecified**
> Angina NOS
> Anginal syndrome
> Cardiac angina
> Ischemic chest pain

OGCR See Section I.c.9.e.3

Acute myocardial infarction, unspecified

Code I21.3, ST elevation (STEMI) myocardial infarction of unspecified site, is the default for unspecified acute myocardial infarction. If only STEMI or transmural MI without the site is documented, assign I21.3.

I21   ST elevation (STEMI) and non-ST elevation (NSTEMI) myocardial infarction

> **Includes**   cardiac infarction
> coronary (artery) embolism
> coronary (artery) occlusion
> coronary (artery) rupture
> coronary (artery) thrombosis
> infarction of heart, myocardium, or ventricle
> myocardial infarction specified as acute or with a stated duration of 4 weeks (28 days) or less from onset

Use additional code, if applicable, to identify:
exposure to environmental tobacco smoke (Z77.22)
history of tobacco use (Z87.891)
occupational exposure to environmental tobacco smoke (Z57.31)
status post administration of tPA (rtPA) in a different facility within the last 24 hours prior to admission to current facility (Z92.82)
tobacco dependence (F17.-)
tobacco use (Z72.0)

> **Excludes2**   old myocardial infarction (I25.2)
> postmyocardial infarction syndrome (I24.1)
> subsequent myocardial infarction (I22.-)

Coding Clinic: 2013, Q1, P25-26; 2012, Q4, P103

● **I21.0   ST elevation (STEMI) myocardial infarction of anterior wall**
Coding Clinic: 2013, Q1, P26

    I21.01   ST elevation (STEMI) myocardial infarction involving left main coronary artery

    I21.02   ST elevation (STEMI) myocardial infarction involving left anterior descending coronary artery
ST elevation (STEMI) myocardial infarction involving diagonal coronary artery
Coding Clinic: 2013, Q1, P26

    I21.09   ST elevation (STEMI) myocardial infarction involving other coronary artery of anterior wall
Acute transmural myocardial infarction of anterior wall
Anteroapical transmural (Q wave) infarction (acute)
Anterolateral transmural (Q wave) infarction (acute)
Anteroseptal transmural (Q wave) infarction (acute)
Transmural (Q wave) infarction (acute) (of) anterior (wall) NOS
Coding Clinic: 2012, Q4, P102, 104

● **I21.1   ST elevation (STEMI) myocardial infarction of inferior wall**
Coding Clinic: 2013, Q1, P26

    I21.11   ST elevation (STEMI) myocardial infarction involving right coronary artery
Inferoposterior transmural (Q wave) infarction (acute)

    I21.19   ST elevation (STEMI) myocardial infarction involving other coronary artery of inferior wall
Acute transmural myocardial infarction of inferior wall
Inferolateral transmural (Q wave) infarction (acute)
Transmural (Q wave) infarction (acute) (of) diaphragmatic wall
Transmural (Q wave) infarction (acute) (of) inferior (wall) NOS

> **Excludes2**   ST elevation (STEMI) myocardial infarction involving left circumflex coronary artery (I21.21)

Coding Clinic: 2012, Q4, P97

● **I21.2   ST elevation (STEMI) myocardial infarction of other sites**
Coding Clinic: 2013, Q1, P26

    I21.21   ST elevation (STEMI) myocardial infarction involving left circumflex coronary artery
ST elevation (STEMI) myocardial infarction involving oblique marginal coronary artery

    I21.29   ST elevation (STEMI) myocardial infarction involving other sites
Acute transmural myocardial infarction of other sites
Apical-lateral transmural (Q wave) infarction (acute)
Basal-lateral transmural (Q wave) infarction (acute)
High lateral transmural (Q wave) infarction (acute)
Lateral (wall) NOS transmural (Q wave) infarction (acute)
Posterior (true) transmural (Q wave) infarction (acute)
Posterobasal transmural (Q wave) infarction (acute)
Posterolateral transmural (Q wave) infarction (acute)
Posteroseptal transmural (Q wave) infarction (acute)
Septal transmural (Q wave) infarction (acute) NOS

I21.3   ST elevation (STEMI) myocardial infarction of unspecified site
Acute transmural myocardial infarction of unspecified site
Myocardial infarction (acute) NOS
Transmural (Q wave) myocardial infarction NOS
Coding Clinic: 2013, Q1, P26

I21.4   Non-ST elevation (NSTEMI) myocardial infarction
Acute subendocardial myocardial infarction
Non-Q wave myocardial infarction NOS
Nontransmural myocardial infarction NOS
Coding Clinic: 2013, Q1, P26

● **I22 Subsequent ST elevation (STEMI) and non-ST elevation (NSTEMI) myocardial infarction**

Includes acute myocardial infarction occurring within four weeks (28 days) of a previous acute myocardial infarction, regardless of site
cardiac infarction
coronary (artery) embolism
coronary (artery) occlusion
coronary (artery) rupture
coronary (artery) thrombosis
infarction of heart, myocardium, or ventricle
recurrent myocardial infarction
reinfarction of myocardium
rupture of heart, myocardium, or ventricle

Use additional code, if applicable, to identify:
exposure to environmental tobacco smoke (Z77.22)
history of tobacco use (Z87.891)
occupational exposure to environmental tobacco smoke (Z57.31)
status post administration of tPA (rtPA) in a different facility within the last 24 hours prior to admission to current facility (Z92.82)
tobacco dependence (F17.-)
tobacco use (Z72.0)
Coding Clinic: 2013, Q1, P25; 2012, Q4, P103

I22.0 Subsequent ST elevation (STEMI) myocardial infarction of anterior wall
Subsequent acute transmural myocardial infarction of anterior wall
Subsequent transmural (Q wave) infarction (acute)(of) anterior (wall) NOS
Subsequent anteroapical transmural (Q wave) infarction (acute)
Subsequent anterolateral transmural (Q wave) infarction (acute)
Subsequent anteroseptal transmural (Q wave) infarction (acute)

I22.1 Subsequent ST elevation (STEMI) myocardial infarction of inferior wall
Subsequent acute transmural myocardial infarction of inferior wall
Subsequent transmural (Q wave) infarction (acute)(of) diaphragmatic wall
Subsequent transmural (Q wave) infarction (acute)(of) inferior (wall) NOS
Subsequent inferolateral transmural (Q wave) infarction (acute)
Subsequent inferoposterior transmural (Q wave) infarction (acute)
Coding Clinic: 2012, Q4, P97, 102, 104

I22.2 Subsequent non-ST elevation (NSTEMI) myocardial infarction
Subsequent acute subendocardial myocardial infarction
Subsequent non-Q wave myocardial infarction NOS
Subsequent nontransmural myocardial infarction NOS

I22.8 Subsequent ST elevation (STEMI) myocardial infarction of other sites
Subsequent acute transmural myocardial infarction of other sites
Subsequent apical-lateral transmural (Q wave) myocardial infarction (acute)
Subsequent basal-lateral transmural (Q wave) myocardial infarction (acute)
Subsequent high lateral transmural (Q wave) myocardial infarction (acute)
Subsequent transmural (Q wave) myocardial infarction (acute)(of) lateral (wall) NOS
Subsequent posterior (true) transmural (Q wave) myocardial infarction (acute)
Subsequent posterobasal transmural (Q wave) myocardial infarction (acute)
Subsequent posterolateral transmural (Q wave) myocardial infarction (acute)
Subsequent posteroseptal transmural (Q wave) myocardial infarction (acute)
Subsequent septal NOS transmural (Q wave) myocardial infarction (acute)

I22.9 Subsequent ST elevation (STEMI) myocardial infarction of unspecified site
Subsequent acute myocardial infarction of unspecified site
Subsequent myocardial infarction (acute) NOS

● **I23 Certain current complications following ST elevation (STEMI) and non-ST elevation (NSTEMI) myocardial infarction (within the 28 day period)**

I23.0 Hemopericardium as current complication following acute myocardial infarction A
Excludes1 hemopericardium not specified as current complication following acute myocardial infarction (I31.2)

I23.1 Atrial septal defect as current complication following acute myocardial infarction A
Excludes1 acquired atrial septal defect not specified as current complication following acute myocardial infarction (I51.0)

I23.2 Ventricular septal defect as current complication following acute myocardial infarction A
Excludes1 acquired ventricular septal defect not specified as current complication following acute myocardial infarction (I51.0)

I23.3 Rupture of cardiac wall without hemopericardium as current complication following acute myocardial infarction A

I23.4 Rupture of chordae tendineae as current complication following acute myocardial infarction
Excludes1 rupture of chordae tendineae not specified as current complication following acute myocardial infarction (I51.1)

I23.5 Rupture of papillary muscle as current complication following acute myocardial infarction
Excludes1 rupture of papillary muscle not specified as current complication following acute myocardial infarction (I51.2)

I23.6 Thrombosis of atrium, auricular appendage, and ventricle as current complications following acute myocardial infarction A
Excludes1 thrombosis of atrium, auricular appendage, and ventricle not specified as current complication following acute myocardial infarction (I51.3)

I23.7 Postinfarction angina A
I23.8 Other current complications following acute myocardial infarction A

● **I24 Other acute ischemic heart diseases**
Excludes1 angina pectoris (I20.-)
transient myocardial ischemia in newborn (P29.4)

I24.0 Acute coronary thrombosis not resulting in myocardial infarction
Acute coronary (artery) (vein) embolism not resulting in myocardial infarction
Acute coronary (artery) (vein) occlusion not resulting in myocardial infarction
Acute coronary (artery) (vein) thromboembolism not resulting in myocardial infarction
Excludes1 atherosclerotic heart disease (I25.1-)
Coding Clinic: 2013, Q1, P24

I24.1 Dressler's syndrome
Postmyocardial infarction syndrome
Excludes1 postinfarction angina (I23.7)

I24.8 Other forms of acute ischemic heart disease
I24.9 Acute ischemic heart disease, unspecified
Excludes1 ischemic heart disease (chronic) NOS (I25.9)

◄ New ◄ Revised ~~deleted~~ Deleted Excludes 1 Excludes 2 Includes Use additional Code first Code also Unspecified
OGCR Official Guidelines X Assign placeholder X ● Use Additional Character(s) ▶ Manifestation Code Coding Clinic

Item 9–6 Classification is based on the location of the atherosclerosis. **"Of native coronary artery"** indicates the atherosclerosis is within an original heart artery. **"Of autologous vein bypass graft"** indicates that the atherosclerosis is within a vein graft that was taken from within the patient. **"Of nonautologous biological bypass graft"** indicates the atherosclerosis is within a vessel grafted from other than the patient. **"Of artery bypass graft"** indicates the atherosclerosis is within an artery that was grafted from within the patient.

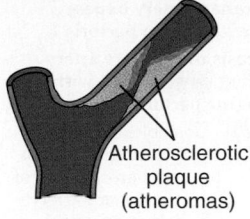

Figure 9-2 Atherosclerotic plaque.

Atherosclerotic plaque (atheromas)

● **I25   Chronic ischemic heart disease**

     Use additional code to identify:
       chronic total occlusion of coronary artery (I25.82)
       exposure to environmental tobacco smoke (Z77.22)
       history of tobacco use (Z87.891)
       occupational exposure to environmental tobacco smoke (Z57.31)
       tobacco dependence (F17.-)
       tobacco use (Z72.0)

OGCR See Section I.9.b.

Atherosclerotic Coronary Artery Disease and Angina

ICD-10-CM has combination codes for atherosclerotic heart disease with angina pectoris. The subcategories for these codes are I25.11, Atherosclerotic heart disease of native coronary artery with angina pectoris and I25.7, Atherosclerosis of coronary artery bypass graft(s) and coronary artery of transplanted heart with angina pectoris.

When using one of these combination codes it is not necessary to use an additional code for angina pectoris. A causal relationship can be assumed in a patient with both atherosclerosis and angina pectoris, unless the documentation indicates the angina is due to something other than the atherosclerosis.

If a patient with coronary artery disease is admitted due to an acute myocardial infarction (AMI), the AMI should be sequenced before the coronary artery disease.
See Section I.C.9. Acute myocardial infarction (AMI)

(See Plates 218 and 219 on pages 74 and 75.)

● **I25.1   Atherosclerotic heart disease of native coronary artery**
     Disease in which fatty deposits form on the walls of arteries
     Atherosclerotic cardiovascular disease
     Coronary (artery) atheroma
     Coronary (artery) atherosclerosis
     Coronary (artery) disease
     Coronary (artery) sclerosis

     Use additional code, if applicable, to identify:
       coronary atherosclerosis due to calcified coronary lesion (I25.84)
       coronary atherosclerosis due to lipid rich plaque (I25.83)

     Excludes2   atheroembolism (I75.-)
                  atherosclerosis of coronary artery bypass graft(s) and transplanted heart (I25.7-)

     I25.10   Atherosclerotic heart disease of native coronary artery without angina pectoris   A
         Atherosclerotic heart disease NOS
         Coding Clinic: 2012, Q4, P92

● **I25.11   Atherosclerotic heart disease of native coronary artery with angina pectoris**
     I25.110   Atherosclerotic heart disease of native coronary artery with unstable angina pectoris   A
         Excludes1   unstable angina without atherosclerotic heart disease (I20.0)

     I25.111   Atherosclerotic heart disease of native coronary artery with angina pectoris with documented spasm   A
         Excludes1   angina pectoris with documented spasm without atherosclerotic heart disease (I20.1)

     I25.118   Atherosclerotic heart disease of native coronary artery with other forms of angina pectoris   A
         Excludes1   other forms of angina pectoris without atherosclerotic heart disease (I20.8)

     I25.119   Atherosclerotic heart disease of native coronary artery with unspecified angina pectoris   A
         Atherosclerotic heart disease with angina NOS
         Atherosclerotic heart disease with ischemic chest pain
         Excludes1   unspecified angina pectoris without atherosclerotic heart disease (I20.9)

     I25.2   Old myocardial infarction
       Healed myocardial infarction
       Past myocardial infarction diagnosed by ECG or other investigation, but currently presenting no symptoms

     I25.3   Aneurysm of heart
       Mural aneurysm
       Ventricular aneurysm

● **I25.4   Coronary artery aneurysm and dissection**
     I25.41   Coronary artery aneurysm
         Coronary arteriovenous fistula, acquired
         Excludes1   congenital coronary (artery) aneurysm (Q24.5)

     I25.42   Coronary artery dissection

     I25.5   Ischemic cardiomyopathy
       Excludes2   coronary atherosclerosis (I25.1-, I25.7-)

     I25.6   Silent myocardial ischemia

● **I25.7   Atherosclerosis of coronary artery bypass graft(s) and coronary artery of transplanted heart with angina pectoris**

     Use additional code, if applicable, to identify:
       coronary atherosclerosis due to calcified coronary lesion (I25.84)
       coronary atherosclerosis due to lipid rich plaque (I25.83)

     Excludes1   atherosclerosis of bypass graft(s) of transplanted heart without angina pectoris (I25.812)
              atherosclerosis of coronary artery bypass graft(s) without angina pectoris (I25.810)
              atherosclerosis of native coronary artery of transplanted heart without angina pectoris (I25.811)
              embolism or thrombus of coronary artery bypass graft(s) (T82.8-)

CHAPTER 9 (I00-I99)

● **I25.70** **Atherosclerosis of coronary artery bypass graft(s), unspecified, with angina pectoris**

 I25.700 **Atherosclerosis of coronary artery bypass graft(s), unspecified, with unstable angina pectoris** A

  Excludes1 unstable angina pectoris without atherosclerosis of coronary artery bypass graft (I20.0)

 I25.701 **Atherosclerosis of coronary artery bypass graft(s), unspecified, with angina pectoris with documented spasm** A

  Excludes1 angina pectoris with documented spasm without atherosclerosis of coronary artery bypass graft (I20.1)

 I25.708 **Atherosclerosis of coronary artery bypass graft(s), unspecified, with other forms of angina pectoris** A

  Excludes1 other forms of angina pectoris without atherosclerosis of coronary artery bypass graft (I20.8)

 I25.709 **Atherosclerosis of coronary artery bypass graft(s), unspecified, with unspecified angina pectoris** A

  Excludes1 unspecified angina pectoris without atherosclerosis of coronary artery bypass graft (I20.9)

● **I25.71** **Atherosclerosis of autologous vein coronary artery bypass graft(s) with angina pectoris**

 I25.710 **Atherosclerosis of autologous vein coronary artery bypass graft(s) with unstable angina pectoris** A

  Excludes1 unstable angina without atherosclerosis of autologous vein coronary artery bypass graft(s) (I20.0)

 I25.711 **Atherosclerosis of autologous vein coronary artery bypass graft(s) with angina pectoris with documented spasm** A

  Excludes1 angina pectoris with documented spasm without atherosclerosis of autologous vein coronary artery bypass graft(s) (I20.1)

 I25.718 **Atherosclerosis of autologous vein coronary artery bypass graft(s) with other forms of angina pectoris** A

  Excludes1 other forms of angina pectoris without atherosclerosis of autologous vein coronary artery bypass graft(s) (I20.8)

 I25.719 **Atherosclerosis of autologous vein coronary artery bypass graft(s) with unspecified angina pectoris** A

  Excludes1 unspecified angina pectoris without atherosclerosis of autologous vein coronary artery bypass graft(s) (I20.9)

● **I25.72** **Atherosclerosis of autologous artery coronary artery bypass graft(s) with angina pectoris**

 Atherosclerosis of internal mammary artery graft with angina pectoris

 I25.720 **Atherosclerosis of autologous artery coronary artery bypass graft(s) with unstable angina pectoris** A

  Excludes1 unstable angina without atherosclerosis of autologous artery coronary artery bypass graft(s) (I20.0)

 I25.721 **Atherosclerosis of autologous artery coronary artery bypass graft(s) with angina pectoris with documented spasm** A

  Excludes1 angina pectoris with documented spasm without atherosclerosis of autologous artery coronary artery bypass graft(s) (I20.1)

 I25.728 **Atherosclerosis of autologous artery coronary artery bypass graft(s) with other forms of angina pectoris** A

  Excludes1 other forms of angina pectoris without atherosclerosis of autologous artery coronary artery bypass graft(s) (I20.8)

 I25.729 **Atherosclerosis of autologous artery coronary artery bypass graft(s) with unspecified angina pectoris** A

  Excludes1 unspecified angina pectoris without atherosclerosis of autologous artery coronary artery bypass graft(s) (I20.9)

◄ New   ◄▪▪▪ Revised   deleted Deleted   Excludes 1   Excludes 2   Includes   Use additional   Code first   Code also   Unspecified

OGCR Official Guidelines   X Assign placeholder X   ● Use Additional Character(s)   ▶ Manifestation Code   **Coding Clinic**

● **I25.73**   Atherosclerosis of nonautologous biological coronary artery bypass graft(s) with angina pectoris

     I25.730   Atherosclerosis of nonautologous biological coronary artery bypass graft(s) with unstable angina pectoris   **A**

         Excludes1   unstable angina without atherosclerosis of nonautologous biological coronary artery bypass graft(s) (I20.0)

     I25.731   Atherosclerosis of nonautologous biological coronary artery bypass graft(s) with angina pectoris with documented spasm   **A**

         Excludes1   angina pectoris with documented spasm without atherosclerosis of nonautologous biological coronary artery bypass graft(s) (I20.1)

     I25.738   Atherosclerosis of nonautologous biological coronary artery bypass graft(s) with other forms of angina pectoris   **A**

         Excludes1   other forms of angina pectoris without atherosclerosis of nonautologous biological coronary artery bypass graft(s) (I20.8)

     I25.739   Atherosclerosis of nonautologous biological coronary artery bypass graft(s) with unspecified angina pectoris   **A**

         Excludes1   unspecified angina pectoris without atherosclerosis of nonautologous biological coronary artery bypass graft(s) (I20.9)

● **I25.75**   Atherosclerosis of native coronary artery of transplanted heart with angina pectoris

     Excludes1   atherosclerosis of native coronary artery of transplanted heart without angina pectoris (I25.811)

     I25.750   Atherosclerosis of native coronary artery of transplanted heart with unstable angina

     I25.751   Atherosclerosis of native coronary artery of transplanted heart with angina pectoris with documented spasm

     I25.758   Atherosclerosis of native coronary artery of transplanted heart with other forms of angina pectoris

     I25.759   Atherosclerosis of native coronary artery of transplanted heart with unspecified angina pectoris

● **I25.76**   Atherosclerosis of bypass graft of coronary artery of transplanted heart with angina pectoris

     Excludes1   atherosclerosis of bypass graft of coronary artery of transplanted heart without angina pectoris (I25.812)

     I25.760   Atherosclerosis of bypass graft of coronary artery of transplanted heart with unstable angina   **A**

     I25.761   Atherosclerosis of bypass graft of coronary artery of transplanted heart with angina pectoris with documented spasm   **A**

     I25.768   Atherosclerosis of bypass graft of coronary artery of transplanted heart with other forms of angina pectoris   **A**

     I25.769   Atherosclerosis of bypass graft of coronary artery of transplanted heart with unspecified angina pectoris   **A**

● **I25.79**   Atherosclerosis of other coronary artery bypass graft(s) with angina pectoris   **A**

     I25.790   Atherosclerosis of other coronary artery bypass graft(s) with unstable angina pectoris

         Excludes1   unstable angina without atherosclerosis of other coronary artery bypass graft(s) (I20.0)

     I25.791   Atherosclerosis of other coronary artery bypass graft(s) with angina pectoris with documented spasm   **A**

         Excludes1   angina pectoris with documented spasm without atherosclerosis of other coronary artery bypass graft(s) (I20.1)

     I25.798   Atherosclerosis of other coronary artery bypass graft(s) with other forms of angina pectoris   **A**

         Excludes1   other forms of angina pectoris without atherosclerosis of other coronary artery bypass graft(s) (I20.8)

     I25.799   Atherosclerosis of other coronary artery bypass graft(s) with unspecified angina pectoris   **A**

         Excludes1   unspecified angina pectoris without atherosclerosis of other coronary artery bypass graft(s) (I20.9)

CHAPTER 9 (I00-I99)

- **I25.8**   **Other forms of chronic ischemic heart disease**
  - **I25.81**   **Atherosclerosis of other coronary vessels without angina pectoris**

    Use additional code, if applicable, to identify:
    coronary atherosclerosis due to calcified coronary lesion (I25.84)
    coronary atherosclerosis due to lipid rich plaque (I25.83)

    Excludes1   atherosclerotic heart disease of native coronary artery without angina pectoris (I25.10)

    - **I25.810**   **Atherosclerosis of coronary artery bypass graft(s) without angina pectoris**   A

      Atherosclerosis of coronary artery bypass graft NOS

      Excludes1   atherosclerosis of coronary bypass graft(s) with angina pectoris (I25.70- -I25.73-, I25.79-)

    - **I25.811**   **Atherosclerosis of native coronary artery of transplanted heart without angina pectoris**

      Atherosclerosis of native coronary artery of transplanted heart NOS

      Excludes1   atherosclerosis of native coronary artery of transplanted heart with angina pectoris (I25.75-)

    - **I25.812**   **Atherosclerosis of bypass graft of coronary artery of transplanted heart without angina pectoris**   A

      Atherosclerosis of bypass graft of transplanted heart NOS

      Excludes1   atherosclerosis of bypass graft of transplanted heart with angina pectoris (I25.76)

  - **I25.82**   **Chronic total occlusion of coronary artery**

    Complete occlusion of coronary artery
    Total occlusion of coronary artery

    Code first coronary atherosclerosis (I25.1-, I25.7-, I25.81-)

    Excludes1   acute coronary occlusion with myocardial infarction (I21.-, I22.-)
    acute coronary occlusion without myocardial infarction (I24.0)

  - **I25.83**   **Coronary atherosclerosis due to lipid rich plaque**   A

    Code first coronary atherosclerosis (I25.1-, I25.7-, I25.81-)

  - **I25.84**   **Coronary atherosclerosis due to calcified coronary lesion**

    Coronary atherosclerosis due to severely calcified coronary lesion

    Code first coronary atherosclerosis (I25.1-, I25.7-, I25.81-)

  - **I25.89**   **Other forms of chronic ischemic heart disease**
- **I25.9**   **Chronic ischemic heart disease, unspecified**

  Ischemic heart disease (chronic) NOS

Item 9-7   Pulmonary heart disease or **cor pulmonale** is right ventricle hypertrophy or RVH as a result of a respiratory disorder increasing back flow pressure to the right ventricle. Left untreated, cor pulmonale leads to right-heart failure and death.

PULMONARY HEART DISEASE AND DISEASES OF PULMONARY CIRCULATION (I26-I28)

- **I26**   **Pulmonary embolism**

  Includes   pulmonary (acute)(artery)(vein) infarction
  pulmonary (acute)(artery)(vein) thromboembolism
  pulmonary (acute)(artery)(vein) thrombosis

  Excludes2   chronic pulmonary embolism (I27.82)
  personal history of pulmonary embolism (Z86.711)
  pulmonary embolism due to trauma (T79.0, T79.1)
  pulmonary embolism due to complications of surgical and medical care (T80.0, T81.7-, T82.8-)
  pulmonary embolism complicating abortion, ectopic or molar pregnancy (O00-O07, O08.2)
  pulmonary embolism complicating pregnancy, childbirth and the puerperium (O88.-)
  septic (non-pulmonary) arterial embolism (I76)

  - **I26.0**   **Pulmonary embolism with acute cor pulmonale**
    - **I26.01**   **Septic pulmonary embolism with acute cor pulmonale**

      Code first underlying infection

    - **I26.02**   **Saddle embolus of pulmonary artery with acute cor pulmonale**
    - **I26.09**   **Other pulmonary embolism with acute cor pulmonale**

      Acute cor pulmonale NOS

  - **I26.9**   **Pulmonary embolism without acute cor pulmonale**
    - **I26.90**   **Septic pulmonary embolism without acute cor pulmonale**

      Code first underlying infection

    - **I26.92**   **Saddle embolus of pulmonary artery without acute cor pulmonale**
    - **I26.99**   **Other pulmonary embolism without acute cor pulmonale**

      Acute pulmonary embolism NOS
      Pulmonary embolism NOS

- **I27**   **Other pulmonary heart diseases**
  - **I27.0**   **Primary pulmonary hypertension**

    Excludes1   pulmonary hypertension NOS (I27.2)
    secondary pulmonary hypertension (I27.2)

  - **I27.1**   **Kyphoscoliotic heart disease**
  - **I27.2**   **Other secondary pulmonary hypertension**

    Pulmonary hypertension NOS

    Code also associated underlying condition

  - **I27.8**   **Other specified pulmonary heart diseases**
    - **I27.81**   **Cor pulmonale (chronic)**

      Cor pulmonale NOS

      Excludes1   acute cor pulmonale (I26.0-)

    - **I27.82**   **Chronic pulmonary embolism**

      Use additional code, if applicable, for associated long-term (current) use of anticoagulants (Z79.01)

      Excludes1   personal history of pulmonary embolism (Z86.711)

    - **I27.89**   **Other specified pulmonary heart diseases**

      Eisenmenger's complex
      Eisenmenger's syndrome

      Excludes1   Eisenmenger's defect (Q21.8)

  - **I27.9**   **Pulmonary heart disease, unspecified**

    Chronic cardiopulmonary disease

◀ New   ◀▦ Revised   ~~deleted~~ Deleted   Excludes 1   Excludes 2   Includes   Use additional   Code first   Code also   Unspecified

OGCR Official Guidelines   X Assign placeholder X   ● Use Additional Character(s)   ▶ Manifestation Code   **Coding Clinic**

● **I28** Other diseases of pulmonary vessels

I28.0 Arteriovenous fistula of pulmonary vessels

> **Excludes1** congenital arteriovenous fistula (Q25.72)

I28.1 Aneurysm of pulmonary artery

> **Excludes1** congenital aneurysm (Q25.79)
> congenital arteriovenous aneurysm (Q25.72)

I28.8 Other diseases of pulmonary vessels
Pulmonary arteritis
Pulmonary endarteritis
Rupture of pulmonary vessels
Stenosis of pulmonary vessels
Stricture of pulmonary vessels

I28.9 Disease of pulmonary vessels, unspecified

OTHER FORMS OF HEART DISEASE (I30-I52)

● **I30** Acute pericarditis

Inflammation of pericardium (sac surrounding the heart) caused by an infection.

> **Includes** acute mediastinopericarditis
> acute myopericarditis
> acute pericardial effusion
> acute pleuropericarditis
> acute pneumopericarditis

> **Excludes1** Dressler's syndrome (I24.1)
> rheumatic pericarditis (acute) (I01.0)

I30.0 Acute nonspecific idiopathic pericarditis

I30.1 Infective pericarditis
Pneumococcal pericarditis
Pneumopyopericardium
Purulent pericarditis
Pyopericarditis
Pyopericardium
Pyopneumopericardium
Staphylococcal pericarditis
Streptococcal pericarditis
Suppurative pericarditis
Viral pericarditis

> Use additional code (B95-B97) to identify infectious agent

I30.8 Other forms of acute pericarditis

I30.9 Acute pericarditis, unspecified

● **I31** Other diseases of pericardium

> **Excludes1** diseases of pericardium specified as rheumatic (I09.2)
> postcardiotomy syndrome (I97.0)
> traumatic injury to pericardium (S26.-)

I31.0 Chronic adhesive pericarditis
Accretio cordis
Adherent pericardium
Adhesive mediastinopericarditis

I31.1 Chronic constrictive pericarditis
Concretio cordis
Pericardial calcification

I31.2 Hemopericardium, not elsewhere classified

> **Excludes1** hemopericardium as current complication following acute myocardial infarction (I23.0)

I31.3 Pericardial effusion (noninflammatory)
Chylopericardium

> **Excludes1** acute pericardial effusion (I30.9)

I31.4 Cardiac tamponade

> *Code first underlying cause*

I31.8 Other specified diseases of pericardium
Epicardial plaques
Focal pericardial adhesions

I31.9 Disease of pericardium, unspecified
Pericarditis (chronic) NOS

▶ **I32** *Pericarditis in diseases classified elsewhere*

> *Code first underlying disease*

> **Excludes1** pericarditis (in):
> coxsackie (virus) (B33.23)
> gonococcal (A54.83)
> meningococcal (A39.53)
> rheumatoid (arthritis) (M05.31)
> syphilitic (A52.06)
> systemic lupus erythematosus (M32.12)
> tuberculosis (A18.84)

● **I33** Acute and subacute endocarditis

Inflammation/infection of lining of heart, affecting heart valves including replacement valves and is usually caused by a bacterial infection

> **Excludes1** acute rheumatic endocarditis (I01.1)
> endocarditis NOS (I38)

I33.0 Acute and subacute infective endocarditis
Bacterial endocarditis (acute) (subacute)
Infective endocarditis (acute) (subacute) NOS
Endocarditis lenta (acute) (subacute)
Malignant endocarditis (acute) (subacute)
Purulent endocarditis (acute) (subacute)
Septic endocarditis (acute) (subacute)
Ulcerative endocarditis (acute) (subacute)
Vegetative endocarditis (acute) (subacute)

> Use additional code (B95-B97) to identify infectious agent

I33.9 Acute and subacute endocarditis, unspecified
Acute endocarditis NOS
Acute myoendocarditis NOS
Acute periendocarditis NOS
Subacute endocarditis NOS
Subacute myoendocarditis NOS
Subacute periendocarditis NOS

● **I34** Nonrheumatic mitral valve disorders

> **Excludes1** mitral valve disease (I05.9)
> mitral valve failure (I05.8)
> mitral valve stenosis (I05.0)
> mitral valve disorder of unspecified cause with diseases of aortic and/or tricuspid valve(s) (I08.-)
> mitral valve disorder of unspecified cause with mitral stenosis or obstruction (I05.0)
> mitral valve disorder specified as congenital (Q23.2, Q23.3)
> mitral valve disorder specified as rheumatic (I05.-)

I34.0 Nonrheumatic mitral (valve) insufficiency
Nonrheumatic mitral (valve) incompetence NOS
Nonrheumatic mitral (valve) regurgitation NOS

I34.1 Nonrheumatic mitral (valve) prolapse
Floppy nonrheumatic mitral valve syndrome

> **Excludes1** Marfan's syndrome (Q87.4-)

I34.2 Nonrheumatic mitral (valve) stenosis

I34.8 Other nonrheumatic mitral valve disorders

I34.9 Nonrheumatic mitral valve disorder, unspecified

● **I35** Nonrheumatic aortic valve disorders

> **Excludes1** aortic valve disorder of unspecified cause but with diseases of mitral and/or tricuspid valve(s) (I08.-)
> aortic valve disorder specified as congenital (Q23.0, Q23.1)
> aortic valve disorder specified as rheumatic (I06.-)
> hypertrophic subaortic stenosis (I42.1)

I35.0 Nonrheumatic aortic (valve) stenosis

I35.1 Nonrheumatic aortic (valve) insufficiency
Nonrheumatic aortic (valve) incompetence NOS
Nonrheumatic aortic (valve) regurgitation NOS

I35.2 Nonrheumatic aortic (valve) stenosis with insufficiency

I35.8 Other nonrheumatic aortic valve disorders

I35.9 Nonrheumatic aortic valve disorder, unspecified

CHAPTER 9 (I00-I99)

N Newborn Age: 0 **P** Pediatric Age: 0–17 **M** Maternity DX: 12–55 **A** Adult Age: 15–124 ♀ Females Only ♂ Males Only

949

CHAPTER 9 (I00-I99)

● **I36** **Nonrheumatic tricuspid valve disorders**

Excludes1 tricuspid valve disorders of unspecified cause
(I07.-)
tricuspid valve disorders specified as congenital
(Q22.4, Q22.8, Q22.9)
tricuspid valve disorders specified as rheumatic
(I07.-)
tricuspid valve disorders with aortic and/or
mitral valve involvement (I08.-)

I36.0 **Nonrheumatic tricuspid (valve) stenosis**

I36.1 **Nonrheumatic tricuspid (valve) insufficiency**
Nonrheumatic tricuspid (valve) incompetence
Nonrheumatic tricuspid (valve) regurgitation

I36.2 **Nonrheumatic tricuspid (valve) stenosis with
insufficiency**

I36.8 **Other nonrheumatic tricuspid valve disorders**

I36.9 **Nonrheumatic tricuspid valve disorder, unspecified**

● **I37** **Nonrheumatic pulmonary valve disorders**

Excludes1 pulmonary valve disorder specified as congenital
(Q22.1, Q22.2, Q22.3)
pulmonary valve disorder specified as rheumatic
(I09.89)

I37.0 **Nonrheumatic pulmonary valve stenosis**

I37.1 **Nonrheumatic pulmonary valve insufficiency**
Nonrheumatic pulmonary valve incompetence
Nonrheumatic pulmonary valve regurgitation

I37.2 **Nonrheumatic pulmonary valve stenosis with
insufficiency**

I37.8 **Other nonrheumatic pulmonary valve disorders**

I37.9 **Nonrheumatic pulmonary valve disorder, unspecified**

I38 **Endocarditis, valve unspecified**

Includes endocarditis (chronic) NOS
valvular incompetence NOS
valvular insufficiency NOS
valvular regurgitation NOS
valvular stenosis NOS
valvulitis (chronic) NOS

Excludes1 congenital insufficiency of cardiac valve NOS
(Q24.8)
congenital stenosis of cardiac valve NOS (Q24.8)
endocardial fibroelastosis (I42.4)
endocarditis specified as rheumatic (I09.1)

▌ *I39* *Endocarditis and heart valve disorders in diseases classified
elsewhere*
Code first underlying disease, such as:
Q fever (A78)

Excludes1 endocardial involvement in:
candidiasis (B37.6)
gonococcal infection (A54.83)
Libman-Sacks disease (M32.11)
listerosis (A32.82)
meningococcal infection (A39.51)
rheumatoid arthritis (M05.31)
syphilis (A52.03)
tuberculosis (A18.84)
typhoid fever (A01.02)

● I40 **Acute myocarditis**
Inflammation of heart muscle due to infection (viral/bacterial).
Includes subacute myocarditis
Excludes1 acute rheumatic myocarditis (I01.2)

I40.0 **Infective myocarditis**
Septic myocarditis
Use additional code (B95-B97) to identify infectious
agent

I40.1 **Isolated myocarditis**
Fiedler's myocarditis
Giant cell myocarditis
Idiopathic myocarditis

I40.8 **Other acute myocarditis**

I40.9 **Acute myocarditis, unspecified**

▌ *I41* *Myocarditis in diseases classified elsewhere*
Code first underlying disease, such as:
typhus (A75.0-A75.9)

Excludes1 myocarditis (in):
Chagas' disease (chronic) (B57.2)
acute (B57.0)
coxsackie (virus) infection (B33.22)
diphtheritic (A36.81)
gonococcal (A54.83)
influenzal (J09.X9, J10.82, J11.82)
meningococcal (A39.52)
mumps (B26.82)
rheumatoid arthritis (M05.31)
sarcoid (D86.85)
syphilis (A52.06)
toxoplasmosis (B58.81)
tuberculous (A18.84)

● I42 **Cardiomyopathy**
*Disease of the heart muscle resulting in an abnormally enlarged,
weakened, thickened, and/or stiffened muscles*
Includes myocardiopathy
*Code first pre-existing cardiomyopathy complicating pregnancy and
puerperium (O99.4)*

Excludes1 ischemic cardiomyopathy (I25.5)
peripartum cardiomyopathy (O90.3)

Excludes2 ventricular hypertrophy (I51.7)

I42.0 **Dilated cardiomyopathy**
Congestive cardiomyopathy

I42.1 **Obstructive hypertrophic cardiomyopathy**
Hypertrophic subaortic stenosis (idiopathic)

I42.2 **Other hypertrophic cardiomyopathy**
Nonobstructive hypertrophic cardiomyopathy

I42.3 **Endomyocardial (eosinophilic) disease**
Endomyocardial (tropical) fibrosis
Löffler's endocarditis

I42.4 **Endocardial fibroelastosis**
Congenital cardiomyopathy
Elastomyofibrosis

I42.5 **Other restrictive cardiomyopathy**
Constrictive cardiomyopathy NOS

I42.6 **Alcoholic cardiomyopathy**
Code also presence of alcoholism (F10.-)

I42.7 **Cardiomyopathy due to drug and external agent**
*Code first poisoning due to drug or toxin, if applicable
(T36-T65 with fifth or sixth character 1-4 or 6)*
Use additional code for adverse effect, if applicable,
to identify drug (T36-T50 with fifth or sixth
character 5)

I42.8 **Other cardiomyopathies**

I42.9 **Cardiomyopathy, unspecified**
Cardiomyopathy (primary) (secondary) NOS

▌ *I43* *Cardiomyopathy in diseases classified elsewhere*
Code first underlying disease, such as:
amyloidosis (E85.-)
glycogen storage disease (E74.0)
gout (M10.0-)
thyrotoxicosis (E05.0-E05.9-)

Excludes1 cardiomyopathy (in):
coxsackie (virus) (B33.24)
diphtheria (A36.81)
sarcoidosis (D86.85)
tuberculosis (A18.84)

◄ New   ◄▌ Revised   ~~deleted~~ Deleted   Excludes 1   Excludes 2   Includes   Use additional   Code first   Code also   Unspecified

OGCR Official Guidelines   **X** Assign placeholder X   ● Use Additional Character(s)   ▌ Manifestation Code   **Coding Clinic**

● **I44** **Atrioventricular and left bundle-branch block**
Conduction problem resulting in arrhythmias/dysrhythmias due to a lack of electrical impulses being transmitted normally through the heart.

　I44.0 **Atrioventricular block, first degree**

　I44.1 **Atrioventricular block, second degree**
　　Atrioventricular block, type I and II
　　Möbitz block, type I and II
　　Second degree block, type I and II
　　Wenckebach's block

　I44.2 **Atrioventricular block, complete**
　　Complete heart block NOS
　　Third degree block

● **I44.3** **Other and unspecified atrioventricular block**
　　Atrioventricular block NOS

　　I44.30 Unspecified atrioventricular block

　　I44.39 Other atrioventricular block

　I44.4 **Left anterior fascicular block**

　I44.5 **Left posterior fascicular block**

● **I44.6** **Other and unspecified fascicular block**

　　I44.60 Unspecified fascicular block
　　　　Left bundle-branch hemiblock NOS

　　I44.69 Other fascicular block

　I44.7 **Left bundle-branch block, unspecified**

● **I45** **Other conduction disorders**

　I45.0 **Right fascicular block**

● **I45.1** **Other and unspecified right bundle-branch block**

　　I45.10 Unspecified right bundle-branch block
　　　　Right bundle-branch block NOS

　　I45.19 Other right bundle-branch block

　I45.2 **Bifascicular block**

　I45.3 **Trifascicular block**

　I45.4 **Nonspecific intraventricular block**
　　Bundle-branch block NOS

　I45.5 **Other specified heart block**
　　Sinoatrial block
　　Sinoauricular block
　　Excludes1 heart block NOS (I45.9)

　I45.6 **Pre-excitation syndrome**
　　Accelerated atrioventricular conduction
　　Accessory atrioventricular conduction
　　Anomalous atrioventricular excitation
　　Lown-Ganong-Levine syndrome
　　Pre-excitation atrioventricular conduction
　　Wolff-Parkinson-White syndrome

● **I45.8** **Other specified conduction disorders**

　　I45.81 **Long QT syndrome**

　　I45.89 **Other specified conduction disorders**
　　　　Atrioventricular [AV] dissociation
　　　　Interference dissociation
　　　　Isorhythmic dissociation
　　　　Nonparoxysmal AV nodal tachycardia
　　　　Coding Clinic: 2013, Q2, P32

　I45.9 **Conduction disorder, unspecified**
　　Heart block NOS
　　Stokes-Adams syndrome

● **I46** **Cardiac arrest**
　　Excludes1 cardiogenic shock (R57.0)

　I46.2 **Cardiac arrest due to underlying cardiac condition**
　　Code first underlying cardiac condition

　I46.8 **Cardiac arrest due to other underlying condition**
　　Code first underlying condition

　I46.9 **Cardiac arrest, cause unspecified**

● **I47** **Paroxysmal tachycardia**
Code first tachycardia complicating:
　　abortion or ectopic or molar pregnancy (O00-O07, O08.8)
　　obstetric surgery and procedures (O75.4)
　　Excludes1 tachycardia NOS (R00.0)
　　　　sinoauricular tachycardia NOS (R00.0)
　　　　sinus [sinusal] tachycardia NOS (R00.0)

　I47.0 **Re-entry ventricular arrhythmia**

　I47.1 **Supraventricular tachycardia**
　　Atrial (paroxysmal) tachycardia
　　Atrioventricular [AV] (paroxysmal) tachycardia
　　Atrioventricular re-entrant (nodal) tachycardia [AVNRT] [AVRT]
　　Junctional (paroxysmal) tachycardia
　　Nodal (paroxysmal) tachycardia

　I47.2 **Ventricular tachycardia**
　　Coding Clinic: 2013, Q3, P23

　I47.9 **Paroxysmal tachycardia, unspecified**
　　Bouveret (-Hoffman) syndrome

● **I48** **Atrial fibrillation and flutter**
Most common abnormal heart rhythm (arrhythmia) presenting as irregular, rapid beating (tachycardia) of the heart's upper chamber.

　I48.0 **Paroxysmal atrial fibrillation**

　I48.1 **Persistent atrial fibrillation**
　　Rapid contractions of the upper heart chamber

　I48.2 **Chronic atrial fibrillation**
　　Permanent atrial fibrillation

　I48.3 **Typical atrial flutter**
　　Type I atrial flutter

　I48.4 **Atypical atrial flutter**
　　Type II atrial flutter

● **I48.9** **Unspecified atrial fibrillation and atrial flutter**

　　I48.91 Unspecified atrial fibrillation

　　I48.92 Unspecified atrial flutter

● **I49** **Other cardiac arrhythmias**
Code first cardiac arrhythmia complicating:
　　abortion or ectopic or molar pregnancy (O00-O07, O08.8)
　　obstetric surgery and procedures (O75.4)
　　Excludes1 bradycardia NOS (R00.1)
　　　　neonatal dysrhythmia (P29.1-)
　　　　sinoatrial bradycardia (R00.1)
　　　　sinus bradycardia (R00.1)
　　　　vagal bradycardia (R00.1)

● **I49.0** **Ventricular fibrillation and flutter**

　　I49.01 **Ventricular fibrillation**

　　I49.02 **Ventricular flutter**

　I49.1 **Atrial premature depolarization**
　　Atrial premature beats

　I49.2 **Junctional premature depolarization**

　I49.3 **Ventricular premature depolarization**

● **I49.4** **Other and unspecified premature depolarization**

　　I49.40 Unspecified premature depolarization
　　　　Premature beats NOS

　　I49.49 **Other premature depolarization**
　　　　Ectopic beats
　　　　Extrasystoles
　　　　Extrasystolic arrhythmias
　　　　Premature contractions

　I49.5 **Sick sinus syndrome**
　　Tachycardia-bradycardia syndrome

　I49.8 **Other specified cardiac arrhythmias**
　　Coronary sinus rhythm disorder
　　Ectopic rhythm disorder
　　Nodal rhythm disorder

　I49.9 **Cardiac arrhythmia, unspecified**
　　Arrhythmia (cardiac) NOS

CHAPTER 9 (I00-I99)

Item 9–8 Congestive heart failure (CHF) is a condition in which the left ventricle of the heart cannot pump enough blood to the body. The blood flow from the heart slows or returns to the heart from the venous system back flow resulting in congestion (fluid accumulation) particularly in the abdomen. Most commonly, fluid collects in the lungs and results in shortness of breath, especially when in a reclining position.

● **I50 Heart failure**

Code first heart failure complicating abortion or ectopic or molar pregnancy (O00-O07, O08.8)
heart failure due to hypertension (I11.0)
heart failure due to hypertension with chronic kidney disease (I13.-)
heart failure following surgery (I97.13-)
obstetric surgery and procedures (O75.4)
rheumatic heart failure (I09.81)

Excludes1 cardiac arrest (I46.-)
neonatal cardiac failure (P29.0)

I50.1 Left ventricular failure
Cardiac asthma
Edema of lung with heart disease NOS
Edema of lung with heart failure
Left heart failure
Pulmonary edema with heart disease NOS
Pulmonary edema with heart failure

Excludes1 edema of lung without heart disease or heart failure (J81.-)
pulmonary edema without heart disease or failure (J81.-)

● **I50.2 Systolic (congestive) heart failure**

Excludes1 combined systolic (congestive) and diastolic (congestive) heart failure (I50.4-)

I50.20 Unspecified systolic (congestive) heart failure

I50.21 Acute systolic (congestive) heart failure
Presenting a short and relatively severe episode

I50.22 Chronic systolic (congestive) heart failure
Long-lasting, presenting over time

I50.23 Acute on chronic systolic (congestive) heart failure
Combination code. What was a chronic condition now has an acute exacerbation (to make more severe).

Coding Clinic: 2013, Q2, P33

● **I50.3 Diastolic (congestive) heart failure**

Excludes1 combined systolic (congestive) and diastolic (congestive) heart failure (I50.4-)

I50.30 Unspecified diastolic (congestive) heart failure

I50.31 Acute diastolic (congestive) heart failure

I50.32 Chronic diastolic (congestive) heart failure

I50.33 Acute on chronic diastolic (congestive) heart failure

● **I50.4 Combined systolic (congestive) and diastolic (congestive) heart failure**

I50.40 Unspecified combined systolic (congestive) and diastolic (congestive) heart failure

I50.41 Acute combined systolic (congestive) and diastolic (congestive) heart failure

I50.42 Chronic combined systolic (congestive) and diastolic (congestive) heart failure

I50.43 Acute on chronic combined systolic (congestive) and diastolic (congestive) heart failure

I50.9 Heart failure, unspecified
Biventricular (heart) failure NOS
Cardiac, heart or myocardial failure NOS
Congestive heart disease
Congestive heart failure NOS
Right ventricular failure (secondary to left heart failure)

Excludes1 fluid overload (E87.70)

Coding Clinic: 2012, Q4, P92

● **I51 Complications and ill-defined descriptions of heart disease**

Excludes1 any condition in I51.4-I51.9 due to hypertension (I11.-)
any condition in I51.4-I51.9 due to hypertension and chronic kidney disease (I13.-)
heart disease specified as rheumatic (I00-I09)

I51.0 Cardiac septal defect, acquired A
Acquired septal atrial defect (old)
Acquired septal auricular defect (old)
Acquired septal ventricular defect (old)

Excludes1 cardiac septal defect as current complication following acute myocardial infarction (I23.1, I23.2)

I51.1 Rupture of chordae tendineae, not elsewhere classified

Excludes1 rupture of chordae tendineae as current complication following acute myocardial infarction (I23.4)

I51.2 Rupture of papillary muscle, not elsewhere classified

Excludes1 rupture of papillary muscle as current complication following acute myocardial infarction (I23.5)

I51.3 Intracardiac thrombosis, not elsewhere classified
Apical thrombosis (old)
Atrial thrombosis (old)
Auricular thrombosis (old)
Mural thrombosis (old)
Ventricular thrombosis (old)

Excludes1 intracardiac thrombosis as current complication following acute myocardial infarction (I23.6)

Coding Clinic: 2013, Q1, P24

I51.4 Myocarditis, unspecified
Chronic (interstitial) myocarditis
Myocardial fibrosis
Myocarditis NOS

Excludes1 acute or subacute myocarditis (I40.-)

I51.5 Myocardial degeneration
Fatty degeneration of heart or myocardium
Myocardial disease
Senile degeneration of heart or myocardium

I51.7 Cardiomegaly
Cardiac dilatation
Cardiac hypertrophy
Ventricular dilatation

● **I51.8 Other ill-defined heart diseases**

I51.81 Takotsubo syndrome
Reversible left ventricular dysfunction following sudden emotional stress
Stress induced cardiomyopathy
Takotsubo cardiomyopathy
Transient left ventricular apical ballooning syndrome

I51.89 Other ill-defined heart diseases
Carditis (acute)(chronic)
Pancarditis (acute)(chronic)

I51.9 Heart disease, unspecified

▷ **I52 Other heart disorders in diseases classified elsewhere**

Code first underlying disease, such as:
congenital syphilis (A50.5)
mucopolysaccharidosis (E76.3)
schistosomiasis (B65.0-B65.9)

Excludes1 heart disease (in):
gonococcal infection (A54.83)
meningococcal infection (A39.50)
rheumatoid arthritis (M05.31)
syphilis (A52.06)

CEREBROVASCULAR DISEASES (I60-I69)

Use additional code to identify presence of:
　alcohol abuse and dependence (F10.-)
　exposure to environmental tobacco smoke (Z77.22)
　history of tobacco use (Z87.891)
　hypertension (I10-I15)
　occupational exposure to environmental tobacco smoke
　　(Z57.31)
　tobacco dependence (F17.-)
　tobacco use (Z72.0)

Excludes1　transient cerebral ischemic attacks and related
　　　　　　syndromes (G45.-)
　　　　　　traumatic intracranial hemorrhage (S06.-)

● **I60**　**Nontraumatic subarachnoid hemorrhage**

　Includes　ruptured cerebral aneurysm

　Excludes1　sequelae of subarachnoid hemorrhage (I69.0-)
　　　　　　syphilitic ruptured cerebral aneurysm (A52.05)

● **I60.0**　**Nontraumatic subarachnoid hemorrhage from carotid siphon and bifurcation**

　　I60.00　**Nontraumatic subarachnoid hemorrhage from unspecified carotid siphon and bifurcation**

　　I60.01　**Nontraumatic subarachnoid hemorrhage from right carotid siphon and bifurcation**

　　I60.02　**Nontraumatic subarachnoid hemorrhage from left carotid siphon and bifurcation**

● **I60.1**　**Nontraumatic subarachnoid hemorrhage from middle cerebral artery**

　　I60.10　**Nontraumatic subarachnoid hemorrhage from unspecified middle cerebral artery**

　　I60.11　**Nontraumatic subarachnoid hemorrhage from right middle cerebral artery**

　　I60.12　**Nontraumatic subarachnoid hemorrhage from left middle cerebral artery**

● **I60.2**　**Nontraumatic subarachnoid hemorrhage from anterior communicating artery**

　　I60.20　**Nontraumatic subarachnoid hemorrhage from unspecified anterior communicating artery**

　　I60.21　**Nontraumatic subarachnoid hemorrhage from right anterior communicating artery**

　　I60.22　**Nontraumatic subarachnoid hemorrhage from left anterior communicating artery**

● **I60.3**　**Nontraumatic subarachnoid hemorrhage from posterior communicating artery**

　　I60.30　**Nontraumatic subarachnoid hemorrhage from unspecified posterior communicating artery**

　　I60.31　**Nontraumatic subarachnoid hemorrhage from right posterior communicating artery**

　　I60.32　**Nontraumatic subarachnoid hemorrhage from left posterior communicating artery**

　I60.4　**Nontraumatic subarachnoid hemorrhage from basilar artery**

● **I60.5**　**Nontraumatic subarachnoid hemorrhage from vertebral artery**

　　I60.50　**Nontraumatic subarachnoid hemorrhage from unspecified vertebral artery**

　　I60.51　**Nontraumatic subarachnoid hemorrhage from right vertebral artery**

　　I60.52　**Nontraumatic subarachnoid hemorrhage from left vertebral artery**

　I60.6　**Nontraumatic subarachnoid hemorrhage from other intracranial arteries**

　I60.7　**Nontraumatic subarachnoid hemorrhage from unspecified intracranial artery**

　　　Ruptured (congenital) berry aneurysm
　　　Ruptured (congenital) cerebral aneurysm
　　　Subarachnoid hemorrhage (nontraumatic) from cerebral
　　　　artery NOS
　　　Subarachnoid hemorrhage (nontraumatic) from
　　　　communicating artery NOS

　　Excludes1　berry aneurysm, nonruptured (I67.1)

　I60.8　**Other nontraumatic subarachnoid hemorrhage**
　　　Meningeal hemorrhage
　　　Rupture of cerebral arteriovenous malformation

　I60.9　**Nontraumatic subarachnoid hemorrhage, unspecified**

● **I61**　**Nontraumatic intracerebral hemorrhage**

　Excludes1　sequelae of intracerebral hemorrhage (I69.1-)

　I61.0　**Nontraumatic intracerebral hemorrhage in hemisphere, subcortical**
　　　Deep intracerebral hemorrhage (nontraumatic)

　I61.1　**Nontraumatic intracerebral hemorrhage in hemisphere, cortical**
　　　Cerebral lobe hemorrhage (nontraumatic)
　　　Superficial intracerebral hemorrhage (nontraumatic)

　I61.2　**Nontraumatic intracerebral hemorrhage in hemisphere, unspecified**

　I61.3　**Nontraumatic intracerebral hemorrhage in brain stem**

　I61.4　**Nontraumatic intracerebral hemorrhage in cerebellum**

　I61.5　**Nontraumatic intracerebral hemorrhage, intraventricular**

　I61.6　**Nontraumatic intracerebral hemorrhage, multiple localized**

　I61.8　**Other nontraumatic intracerebral hemorrhage**

　I61.9　**Nontraumatic intracerebral hemorrhage, unspecified**

● **I62**　**Other and unspecified nontraumatic intracranial hemorrhage**

　Excludes1　sequelae of intracranial hemorrhage (I69.2)

● **I62.0**　**Nontraumatic subdural hemorrhage**

　　I62.00　**Nontraumatic subdural hemorrhage, unspecified**

　　I62.01　**Nontraumatic acute subdural hemorrhage**

　　I62.02　**Nontraumatic subacute subdural hemorrhage**

　　I62.03　**Nontraumatic chronic subdural hemorrhage**

　I62.1　**Nontraumatic extradural hemorrhage**
　　　Nontraumatic epidural hemorrhage

　I62.9　**Nontraumatic intracranial hemorrhage, unspecified**

(See Plate 141 on page 76.)

● **I63**　**Cerebral infarction**

　Includes　occlusion and stenosis of cerebral and precerebral
　　　　　arteries, resulting in cerebral infarction

　Use additional code, if applicable, to identify status post
　　administration of tPA (rtPA) in a different facility within
　　the last 24 hours prior to admission to current facility
　　(Z92.82)

　Excludes1　sequelae of cerebral infarction (I69.3-)

● **I63.0**　**Cerebral infarction due to thrombosis of precerebral arteries**

　　I63.00　**Cerebral infarction due to thrombosis of unspecified precerebral artery**

　　● **I63.01**　**Cerebral infarction due to thrombosis of vertebral artery**

　　　　I63.011　**Cerebral infarction due to thrombosis of right vertebral artery**

　　　　I63.012　**Cerebral infarction due to thrombosis of left vertebral artery**

　　　　I63.019　**Cerebral infarction due to thrombosis of unspecified vertebral artery**

　　I63.02　**Cerebral infarction due to thrombosis of basilar artery**

　　● **I63.03**　**Cerebral infarction due to thrombosis of carotid artery**

　　　　I63.031　**Cerebral infarction due to thrombosis of right carotid artery**

　　　　I63.032　**Cerebral infarction due to thrombosis of left carotid artery**

　　　　I63.039　**Cerebral infarction due to thrombosis of unspecified carotid artery**

　　I63.09　**Cerebral infarction due to thrombosis of other precerebral artery**

● **I63.1** Cerebral infarction due to embolism of precerebral arteries

    I63.10 Cerebral infarction due to embolism of unspecified precerebral artery

    ● **I63.11** Cerebral infarction due to embolism of vertebral artery

        I63.111 Cerebral infarction due to embolism of right vertebral artery

        I63.112 Cerebral infarction due to embolism of left vertebral artery

        I63.119 Cerebral infarction due to embolism of unspecified vertebral artery

    I63.12 Cerebral infarction due to embolism of basilar artery

    ● **I63.13** Cerebral infarction due to embolism of carotid artery

        I63.131 Cerebral infarction due to embolism of right carotid artery

        I63.132 Cerebral infarction due to embolism of left carotid artery

        I63.139 Cerebral infarction due to embolism of unspecified carotid artery

    I63.19 Cerebral infarction due to embolism of other precerebral artery

● **I63.2** Cerebral infarction due to unspecified occlusion or stenosis of precerebral arteries

    I63.20 Cerebral infarction due to unspecified occlusion or stenosis of unspecified precerebral arteries

    ● **I63.21** Cerebral infarction due to unspecified occlusion or stenosis of vertebral arteries

        I63.211 Cerebral infarction due to unspecified occlusion or stenosis of right vertebral arteries

        I63.212 Cerebral infarction due to unspecified occlusion or stenosis of left vertebral arteries

        I63.219 Cerebral infarction due to unspecified occlusion or stenosis of unspecified vertebral arteries

    I63.22 Cerebral infarction due to unspecified occlusion or stenosis of basilar arteries

    ● **I63.23** Cerebral infarction due to unspecified occlusion or stenosis of carotid arteries

        I63.231 Cerebral infarction due to unspecified occlusion or stenosis of right carotid arteries

        I63.232 Cerebral infarction due to unspecified occlusion or stenosis of left carotid arteries

        I63.239 Cerebral infarction due to unspecified occlusion or stenosis of unspecified carotid arteries

    I63.29 Cerebral infarction due to unspecified occlusion or stenosis of other precerebral arteries

● **I63.3** Cerebral infarction due to thrombosis of cerebral arteries

    I63.30 Cerebral infarction due to thrombosis of unspecified cerebral artery

    ● **I63.31** Cerebral infarction due to thrombosis of middle cerebral artery

        I63.311 Cerebral infarction due to thrombosis of right middle cerebral artery

        I63.312 Cerebral infarction due to thrombosis of left middle cerebral artery

        I63.319 Cerebral infarction due to thrombosis of unspecified middle cerebral artery

    ● **I63.32** Cerebral infarction due to thrombosis of anterior cerebral artery

        I63.321 Cerebral infarction due to thrombosis of right anterior cerebral artery

        I63.322 Cerebral infarction due to thrombosis of left anterior cerebral artery

        I63.329 Cerebral infarction due to thrombosis of unspecified anterior cerebral artery

    ● **I63.33** Cerebral infarction due to thrombosis of posterior cerebral artery

        I63.331 Cerebral infarction due to thrombosis of right posterior cerebral artery

        I63.332 Cerebral infarction due to thrombosis of left posterior cerebral artery

        I63.339 Cerebral infarction due to thrombosis of unspecified posterior cerebral artery

    ● **I63.34** Cerebral infarction due to thrombosis of cerebellar artery

        I63.341 Cerebral infarction due to thrombosis of right cerebellar artery

        I63.342 Cerebral infarction due to thrombosis of left cerebellar artery

        I63.349 Cerebral infarction due to thrombosis of unspecified cerebellar artery

    I63.39 Cerebral infarction due to thrombosis of other cerebral artery

● **I63.4** Cerebral infarction due to embolism of cerebral arteries

    I63.40 Cerebral infarction due to embolism of unspecified cerebral artery

    ● **I63.41** Cerebral infarction due to embolism of middle cerebral artery

        I63.411 Cerebral infarction due to embolism of right middle cerebral artery

        I63.412 Cerebral infarction due to embolism of left middle cerebral artery

        I63.419 Cerebral infarction due to embolism of unspecified middle cerebral artery

    ● **I63.42** Cerebral infarction due to embolism of anterior cerebral artery

        I63.421 Cerebral infarction due to embolism of right anterior cerebral artery

        I63.422 Cerebral infarction due to embolism of left anterior cerebral artery

        I63.429 Cerebral infarction due to embolism of unspecified anterior cerebral artery

    ● **I63.43** Cerebral infarction due to embolism of posterior cerebral artery

        I63.431 Cerebral infarction due to embolism of right posterior cerebral artery

        I63.432 Cerebral infarction due to embolism of left posterior cerebral artery

        I63.439 Cerebral infarction due to embolism of unspecified posterior cerebral artery

    ● **I63.44** Cerebral infarction due to embolism of cerebellar artery

        I63.441 Cerebral infarction due to embolism of right cerebellar artery

        I63.442 Cerebral infarction due to embolism of left cerebellar artery

        I63.449 Cerebral infarction due to embolism of unspecified cerebellar artery

    I63.49 Cerebral infarction due to embolism of other cerebral artery

◀ New   ◀▬ Revised   ~~deleted~~ Deleted   Excludes 1   Excludes 2   Includes   Use additional   Code first   Code also   Unspecified

954   OGCR Official Guidelines   X Assign placeholder X   ● Use Additional Character(s)   ▶ Manifestation Code   **Coding Clinic**

● **I63.5**   **Cerebral infarction due to unspecified occlusion or stenosis of cerebral arteries**

     I63.50   Cerebral infarction due to unspecified occlusion or stenosis of unspecified cerebral artery

   ● **I63.51**   Cerebral infarction due to unspecified occlusion or stenosis of middle cerebral artery

       I63.511   Cerebral infarction due to unspecified occlusion or stenosis of right middle cerebral artery

       I63.512   Cerebral infarction due to unspecified occlusion or stenosis of left middle cerebral artery

       I63.519   Cerebral infarction due to unspecified occlusion or stenosis of unspecified middle cerebral artery

   ● **I63.52**   Cerebral infarction due to unspecified occlusion or stenosis of anterior cerebral artery

       I63.521   Cerebral infarction due to unspecified occlusion or stenosis of right anterior cerebral artery

       I63.522   Cerebral infarction due to unspecified occlusion or stenosis of left anterior cerebral artery

       I63.529   Cerebral infarction due to unspecified occlusion or stenosis of unspecified anterior cerebral artery

   ● **I63.53**   Cerebral infarction due to unspecified occlusion or stenosis of posterior cerebral artery

       I63.531   Cerebral infarction due to unspecified occlusion or stenosis of right posterior cerebral artery

       I63.532   Cerebral infarction due to unspecified occlusion or stenosis of left posterior cerebral artery

       I63.539   Cerebral infarction due to unspecified occlusion or stenosis of unspecified posterior cerebral artery

   ● **I63.54**   Cerebral infarction due to unspecified occlusion or stenosis of cerebellar artery

       I63.541   Cerebral infarction due to unspecified occlusion or stenosis of right cerebellar artery

       I63.542   Cerebral infarction due to unspecified occlusion or stenosis of left cerebellar artery

       I63.549   Cerebral infarction due to unspecified occlusion or stenosis of unspecified cerebellar artery

     I63.59   Cerebral infarction due to unspecified occlusion or stenosis of other cerebral artery

   I63.6   Cerebral infarction due to cerebral venous thrombosis, nonpyogenic

   I63.8   Other cerebral infarction

   I63.9   Cerebral infarction, unspecified
      Stroke NOS
      Coding Clinic: 2015, Q1, P26

● **I65**   **Occlusion and stenosis of precerebral arteries, not resulting in cerebral infarction**

   Includes   embolism of precerebral artery
             narrowing of precerebral artery
             obstruction (complete) (partial) of precerebral artery
             thrombosis of precerebral artery

   Excludes1   insufficiency, NOS, of precerebral artery (G45.-)
             insufficiency of precerebral arteries causing cerebral infarction (I63.0-I63.2)

   ● **I65.0**   Occlusion and stenosis of vertebral artery

       I65.01   Occlusion and stenosis of right vertebral artery

       I65.02   Occlusion and stenosis of left vertebral artery

       I65.03   Occlusion and stenosis of bilateral vertebral arteries

       I65.09   Occlusion and stenosis of unspecified vertebral artery

   I65.1   Occlusion and stenosis of basilar artery

   ● **I65.2**   Occlusion and stenosis of carotid artery

       I65.21   Occlusion and stenosis of right carotid artery

       I65.22   Occlusion and stenosis of left carotid artery

       I65.23   Occlusion and stenosis of bilateral carotid arteries

       I65.29   Occlusion and stenosis of unspecified carotid artery

   I65.8   Occlusion and stenosis of other precerebral arteries

   I65.9   Occlusion and stenosis of unspecified precerebral artery
      Occlusion and stenosis of precerebral artery NOS

● **I66**   **Occlusion and stenosis of cerebral arteries, not resulting in cerebral infarction**

   Includes   embolism of cerebral artery
             narrowing of cerebral artery
             obstruction (complete) (partial) of cerebral artery
             thrombosis of cerebral artery

   Excludes1   occlusion and stenosis of cerebral artery causing cerebral infarction (I63.3-I63.5)

   ● **I66.0**   Occlusion and stenosis of middle cerebral artery

       I66.01   Occlusion and stenosis of right middle cerebral artery

       I66.02   Occlusion and stenosis of left middle cerebral artery

       I66.03   Occlusion and stenosis of bilateral middle cerebral arteries

       I66.09   Occlusion and stenosis of unspecified middle cerebral artery

   ● **I66.1**   Occlusion and stenosis of anterior cerebral artery

       I66.11   Occlusion and stenosis of right anterior cerebral artery

       I66.12   Occlusion and stenosis of left anterior cerebral artery

       I66.13   Occlusion and stenosis of bilateral anterior cerebral arteries

       I66.19   Occlusion and stenosis of unspecified anterior cerebral artery

   ● **I66.2**   Occlusion and stenosis of posterior cerebral artery

       I66.21   Occlusion and stenosis of right posterior cerebral artery

       I66.22   Occlusion and stenosis of left posterior cerebral artery

       I66.23   Occlusion and stenosis of bilateral posterior cerebral arteries

       I66.29   Occlusion and stenosis of unspecified posterior cerebral artery

   I66.3   Occlusion and stenosis of cerebellar arteries

   I66.8   Occlusion and stenosis of other cerebral arteries
      Occlusion and stenosis of perforating arteries

   I66.9   Occlusion and stenosis of unspecified cerebral artery

CHAPTER 9 (I00-I99)

● **I67** **Other cerebrovascular diseases**
> **Excludes1** sequelae of the listed conditions (I69.8)
> **I67.0** **Dissection of cerebral arteries, nonruptured**
>   **Excludes1** ruptured cerebral arteries (I60.7)
>
> **I67.1** **Cerebral aneurysm, nonruptured**
>   Cerebral aneurysm NOS
>   Cerebral arteriovenous fistula, acquired
>   Internal carotid artery aneurysm, intracranial portion
>   Internal carotid artery aneurysm, NOS
>   **Excludes1** congenital cerebral aneurysm, nonruptured (Q28.-)
>   ruptured cerebral aneurysm (I60.7)
>
> **I67.2** **Cerebral atherosclerosis** A
>   Atheroma of cerebral and precerebral arteries
>
> **I67.3** **Progressive vascular leukoencephalopathy**
>   Binswanger's disease
>
> **I67.4** **Hypertensive encephalopathy**
> **I67.5** **Moyamoya disease**
> **I67.6** **Nonpyogenic thrombosis of intracranial venous system**
>   Nonpyogenic thrombosis of cerebral vein
>   Nonpyogenic thrombosis of intracranial venous sinus
>   **Excludes1** nonpyogenic thrombosis of intracranial venous system causing infarction (I63.6)
>
> **I67.7** **Cerebral arteritis, not elsewhere classified**
>   Granulomatous angiitis of the nervous system
>   **Excludes1** allergic granulomatous angiitis (M30.1)
>
> ● **I67.8** **Other specified cerebrovascular diseases**
>   **I67.81** **Acute cerebrovascular insufficiency**
>   Acute cerebrovascular insufficiency unspecified as to location or reversibility
>   **I67.82** **Cerebral ischemia**
>   Chronic cerebral ischemia
>   **I67.83** **Posterior reversible encephalopathy syndrome**
>   PRES
> ● **I67.84** **Cerebral vasospasm and vasoconstriction**
>   **I67.841** **Reversible cerebrovascular vasoconstriction syndrome**
>   Call-Fleming syndrome
>   *Code first underlying condition, if applicable, such as eclampsia (O15.00-O15.9)*
>   **I67.848** **Other cerebrovascular vasospasm and vasoconstriction**
>   **I67.89** **Other cerebrovascular disease**
> **I67.9** **Cerebrovascular disease, unspecified**

● **I68** **Cerebrovascular disorders in diseases classified elsewhere**
> ▷ *I68.0* *Cerebral amyloid angiopathy*
>   *Code first underlying amyloidosis (E85.-)*
> ▷ *I68.2* *Cerebral arteritis in other diseases classified elsewhere*
>   *Code first underlying disease*
>   **Excludes1** cerebral arteritis (in):
>   listerosis (A32.89)
>   systemic lupus erythematosus (M32.19)
>   syphilis (A52.04)
>   tuberculosis (A18.89)
> ▷ *I68.8* *Other cerebrovascular disorders in diseases classified elsewhere*
>   *Code first underlying disease*
>   **Excludes1** syphilitic cerebral aneurysm (A52.05)

OGCR Section I.c.9.d.

Sequelae of Cerebrovascular Disease

1) Category I69, Sequelae of Cerebrovascular disease

Category I69 is used to indicate conditions classifiable to categories I60-I67 as the causes of sequela (neurologic deficits), themselves classified elsewhere. These "late effects" include neurologic deficits that persist after initial onset of conditions classifiable to categories I60-I67. The neurologic deficits caused by cerebrovascular disease may be present from the onset of may arise at any time after the onset of the condition classifiable to categories I60-I67.

Codes from category I69, Sequelae of cerebrovascular disease, that specify hemiplegia, hemiparesis and monoplegia identify whether the dominant or nondominant side is affected. Should the affected side be documented, but not specified as dominant or nondominant, and the classification system does not indicate a default, code selection is as follows:

For ambidextrous patients, the default should be dominant.

If the left side is affected, the default is non-dominant.

If the right side is affected, the default is dominant.

2) Codes from category I69 with codes from I60-I67

Codes from category I69 may be assigned on a health care record with codes from I60-I67, if the patient has a current cerebrovascular disease and deficits from an old cerebrovascular disease.

● **I69** **Sequelae of cerebrovascular disease**
> **Note:** Category I69 is to be used to indicate conditions in I60-I67 as the cause of sequelae. The 'sequelae' include conditions specified as such or as residuals which may occur at any time after the onset of the causal condition.
> **Excludes1** personal history of cerebral infarction without residual deficit (Z86.73)
>   personal history of prolonged reversible ischemic neurologic deficit (PRIND) (Z86.73)
>   personal history of reversible ischemic neurologcial deficit (RIND) (Z86.73)
>   sequelae of traumatic intracranial injury (S06.-)
>   transient ischemic attack (TIA) (G45.9)
> **Coding Clinic: 2012, Q4, P107**
> ● **I69.0** **Sequelae of nontraumatic subarachnoid hemorrhage**
>   **I69.00** **Unspecified sequelae of nontraumatic subarachnoid hemorrhage**
>   **I69.01** **Cognitive deficits following nontraumatic subarachnoid hemorrhage**
> ● **I69.02** **Speech and language deficits following nontraumatic subarachnoid hemorrhage**
>   **I69.020** **Aphasia following nontraumatic subarachnoid hemorrhage**
>   **I69.021** **Dysphasia following nontraumatic subarachnoid hemorrhage**
>   **I69.022** **Dysarthria following nontraumatic subarachnoid hemorrhage**
>   **I69.023** **Fluency disorder following nontraumatic subarachnoid hemorrhage**
>   Stuttering following nontraumatic subarachnoid hemorrhage
>   **I69.028** **Other speech and language deficits following nontraumatic subarachnoid hemorrhage**

◄ New ◄▦ Revised ~~deleted~~ Deleted | Excludes 1 | Excludes 2 | Includes | Use additional | Code first | Code also | Unspecified
OGCR Official Guidelines X Assign placeholder X ● Use Additional Character(s) ▷ Manifestation Code **Coding Clinic**

● I69.03   **Monoplegia of upper limb following nontraumatic subarachnoid hemorrhage**

I69.031   Monoplegia of upper limb following nontraumatic subarachnoid hemorrhage affecting right dominant side

I69.032   Monoplegia of upper limb following nontraumatic subarachnoid hemorrhage affecting left dominant side

I69.033   Monoplegia of upper limb following nontraumatic subarachnoid hemorrhage affecting right non-dominant side

I69.034   Monoplegia of upper limb following nontraumatic subarachnoid hemorrhage affecting left non-dominant side

I69.039   Monoplegia of upper limb following nontraumatic subarachnoid hemorrhage affecting unspecified side

● I69.04   **Monoplegia of lower limb following nontraumatic subarachnoid hemorrhage**

I69.041   Monoplegia of lower limb following nontraumatic subarachnoid hemorrhage affecting right dominant side

I69.042   Monoplegia of lower limb following nontraumatic subarachnoid hemorrhage affecting left dominant side

I69.043   Monoplegia of lower limb following nontraumatic subarachnoid hemorrhage affecting right non-dominant side

I69.044   Monoplegia of lower limb following nontraumatic subarachnoid hemorrhage affecting left non-dominant side

I69.049   Monoplegia of lower limb following nontraumatic subarachnoid hemorrhage affecting unspecified side

● I69.05   **Hemiplegia and hemiparesis following nontraumatic subarachnoid hemorrhage**

I69.051   Hemiplegia and hemiparesis following nontraumatic subarachnoid hemorrhage affecting right dominant side

I69.052   Hemiplegia and hemiparesis following nontraumatic subarachnoid hemorrhage affecting left dominant side

I69.053   Hemiplegia and hemiparesis following nontraumatic subarachnoid hemorrhage affecting right non-dominant side

I69.054   Hemiplegia and hemiparesis following nontraumatic subarachnoid hemorrhage affecting left non-dominant side

I69.059   Hemiplegia and hemiparesis following nontraumatic subarachnoid hemorrhage affecting unspecified side

● I69.06   **Other paralytic syndrome following nontraumatic subarachnoid hemorrhage**

Use additional code to identify type of paralytic syndrome, such as:
locked-in state (G83.5)
quadriplegia (G82.5-)

Excludes1   hemiplegia/hemiparesis following nontraumatic subarachnoid hemorrhage (I69.05-)
monoplegia of lower limb following nontraumatic subarachnoid hemorrhage (I69.04-)
monoplegia of upper limb following nontraumatic subarachnoid hemorrhage (I69.03-)

I69.061   Other paralytic syndrome following nontraumatic subarachnoid hemorrhage affecting right dominant side

I69.062   Other paralytic syndrome following nontraumatic subarachnoid hemorrhage affecting left dominant side

I69.063   Other paralytic syndrome following nontraumatic subarachnoid hemorrhage affecting right non-dominant side

I69.064   Other paralytic syndrome following nontraumatic subarachnoid hemorrhage affecting left non-dominant side

I69.065   Other paralytic syndrome following nontraumatic subarachnoid hemorrhage, bilateral

I69.069   Other paralytic syndrome following nontraumatic subarachnoid hemorrhage affecting unspecified side

● I69.09   **Other sequelae of nontraumatic subarachnoid hemorrhage**

I69.090   **Apraxia following nontraumatic subarachnoid hemorrhage**

I69.091   **Dysphagia following nontraumatic subarachnoid hemorrhage**

Use additional code to identify the type of dysphagia, if known (R13.1-)

I69.092   **Facial weakness following nontraumatic subarachnoid hemorrhage**

Facial droop following nontraumatic subarachnoid hemorrhage

I69.093   **Ataxia following nontraumatic subarachnoid hemorrhage**

I69.098   **Other sequelae following nontraumatic subarachnoid hemorrhage**

Alterations of sensation following nontraumatic subarachnoid hemorrhage

Disturbance of vision following nontraumatic subarachnoid hemorrhage

Use additional code to identify the sequelae

CHAPTER 9 (I00-I99)

● **I69.1   Sequelae of nontraumatic intracerebral hemorrhage**

    I69.10   Unspecified sequelae of nontraumatic intracerebral hemorrhage

    I69.11   Cognitive deficits following nontraumatic intracerebral hemorrhage

● **I69.12   Speech and language deficits following nontraumatic intracerebral hemorrhage**

        I69.120   Aphasia following nontraumatic intracerebral hemorrhage

        I69.121   Dysphasia following nontraumatic intracerebral hemorrhage

        I69.122   Dysarthria following nontraumatic intracerebral hemorrhage

        I69.123   Fluency disorder following nontraumatic intracerebral hemorrhage
                Stuttering following nontraumatic subarachnoid hemorrhage

        I69.128   Other speech and language deficits following nontraumatic intracerebral hemorrhage

● **I69.13   Monoplegia of upper limb following nontraumatic intracerebral hemorrhage**

        I69.131   Monoplegia of upper limb following nontraumatic intracerebral hemorrhage affecting right dominant side

        I69.132   Monoplegia of upper limb following nontraumatic intracerebral hemorrhage affecting left dominant side

        I69.133   Monoplegia of upper limb following nontraumatic intracerebral hemorrhage affecting right non-dominant side

        I69.134   Monoplegia of upper limb following nontraumatic intracerebral hemorrhage affecting left non-dominant side

        I69.139   Monoplegia of upper limb following nontraumatic intracerebral hemorrhage affecting unspecified side

● **I69.14   Monoplegia of lower limb following nontraumatic intracerebral hemorrhage**

        I69.141   Monoplegia of lower limb following nontraumatic intracerebral hemorrhage affecting right dominant side

        I69.142   Monoplegia of lower limb following nontraumatic intracerebral hemorrhage affecting left dominant side

        I69.143   Monoplegia of lower limb following nontraumatic intracerebral hemorrhage affecting right non-dominant side

        I69.144   Monoplegia of lower limb following nontraumatic intracerebral hemorrhage affecting left non-dominant side

        I69.149   Monoplegia of lower limb following nontraumatic intracerebral hemorrhage affecting unspecified side

● **I69.15   Hemiplegia and hemiparesis following nontraumatic intracerebral hemorrhage**

        I69.151   Hemiplegia and hemiparesis following nontraumatic intracerebral hemorrhage affecting right dominant side

        I69.152   Hemiplegia and hemiparesis following nontraumatic intracerebral hemorrhage affecting left dominant side

        I69.153   Hemiplegia and hemiparesis following nontraumatic intracerebral hemorrhage affecting right non-dominant side

        I69.154   Hemiplegia and hemiparesis following nontraumatic intracerebral hemorrhage affecting left non-dominant side

        I69.159   Hemiplegia and hemiparesis following nontraumatic intracerebral hemorrhage affecting unspecified side

● **I69.16   Other paralytic syndrome following nontraumatic intracerebral hemorrhage**

        Use additional code to identify type of paralytic syndrome, such as:
            locked-in state (G83.5)
            quadriplegia (G82.5-)

        **Excludes1   hemiplegia/hemiparesis following nontraumatic intracerebral hemorrhage (I69.15-)
                monoplegia of lower limb following nontraumatic intracerebral hemorrhage (I69.14-)
                monoplegia of upper limb following nontraumatic intracerebral hemorrhage (I69.13-)**

        I69.161   Other paralytic syndrome following nontraumatic intracerebral hemorrhage affecting right dominant side

        I69.162   Other paralytic syndrome following nontraumatic intracerebral hemorrhage affecting left dominant side

        I69.163   Other paralytic syndrome following nontraumatic intracerebral hemorrhage affecting right non-dominant side

        I69.164   Other paralytic syndrome following nontraumatic intracerebral hemorrhage affecting left non-dominant side

        I69.165   Other paralytic syndrome following nontraumatic intracerebral hemorrhage, bilateral

        I69.169   Other paralytic syndrome following nontraumatic intracerebral hemorrhage affecting unspecified side

◄ New   ◄◂◂ Revised   d̶e̶l̶e̶t̶e̶d̶ Deleted   Excludes 1   Excludes 2   Includes   Use additional   Code first   Code also   Unspecified
OGCR Official Guidelines   X Assign placeholder X   ● Use Additional Character(s)   ▶ Manifestation Code   **Coding Clinic**

● **I69.19**   **Other sequelae of nontraumatic intracerebral hemorrhage**

     I69.190   **Apraxia following nontraumatic intracerebral hemorrhage**

     I69.191   **Dysphagia following nontraumatic intracerebral hemorrhage**

         Use additional code to identify the type of dysphagia, if known (R13.1-)

     I69.192   **Facial weakness following nontraumatic intracerebral hemorrhage**

         Facial droop following nontraumatic intracerebral hemorrhage

     I69.193   **Ataxia following nontraumatic intracerebral hemorrhage**

     I69.198   **Other sequelae of nontraumatic intracerebral hemorrhage**

         Alteration of sensations following nontraumatic intracerebral hemorrhage

         Disturbance of vision following nontraumatic intracerebral hemorrhage

         Use additional code to identify the sequelae

● **I69.2**   **Sequelae of other nontraumatic intracranial hemorrhage**

     I69.20   **Unspecified sequelae of other nontraumatic intracranial hemorrhage**

     I69.21   **Cognitive deficits following other nontraumatic intracranial hemorrhage**

●   I69.22   **Speech and language deficits following other nontraumatic intracranial hemorrhage**

     I69.220   **Aphasia following other nontraumatic intracranial hemorrhage**

     I69.221   **Dysphasia following other nontraumatic intracranial hemorrhage**

     I69.222   **Dysarthria following other nontraumatic intracranial hemorrhage**

     I69.223   **Fluency disorder following other nontraumatic intracranial hemorrhage**

         Stuttering following nontraumatic subarachnoid hemorrhage

     I69.228   **Other speech and language deficits following other nontraumatic intracranial hemorrhage**

●   I69.23   **Monoplegia of upper limb following other nontraumatic intracranial hemorrhage**

     I69.231   **Monoplegia of upper limb following other nontraumatic intracranial hemorrhage affecting right dominant side**

     I69.232   **Monoplegia of upper limb following other nontraumatic intracranial hemorrhage affecting left dominant side**

     I69.233   **Monoplegia of upper limb following other nontraumatic intracranial hemorrhage affecting right non-dominant side**

     I69.234   **Monoplegia of upper limb following other nontraumatic intracranial hemorrhage affecting left non-dominant side**

     I69.239   **Monoplegia of upper limb following other nontraumatic intracranial hemorrhage affecting unspecified side**

● **I69.24**   **Monoplegia of lower limb following other nontraumatic intracranial hemorrhage**

     I69.241   **Monoplegia of lower limb following other nontraumatic intracranial hemorrhage affecting right dominant side**

     I69.242   **Monoplegia of lower limb following other nontraumatic intracranial hemorrhage affecting left dominant side**

     I69.243   **Monoplegia of lower limb following other nontraumatic intracranial hemorrhage affecting right non-dominant side**

     I69.244   **Monoplegia of lower limb following other nontraumatic intracranial hemorrhage affecting left non-dominant side**

     I69.249   **Monoplegia of lower limb following other nontraumatic intracranial hemorrhage affecting unspecified side**

● **I69.25**   **Hemiplegia and hemiparesis following other nontraumatic intracranial hemorrhage**

     I69.251   **Hemiplegia and hemiparesis following other nontraumatic intracranial hemorrhage affecting right dominant side**

     I69.252   **Hemiplegia and hemiparesis following other nontraumatic intracranial hemorrhage affecting left dominant side**

     I69.253   **Hemiplegia and hemiparesis following other nontraumatic intracranial hemorrhage affecting right non-dominant side**

     I69.254   **Hemiplegia and hemiparesis following other nontraumatic intracranial hemorrhage affecting left non-dominant side**

     I69.259   **Hemiplegia and hemiparesis following other nontraumatic intracranial hemorrhage affecting unspecified side**

● **I69.26**   **Other paralytic syndrome following other nontraumatic intracranial hemorrhage**

         Use additional code to identify type of paralytic syndrome, such as:
         locked-in state (G83.5)
         quadriplegia (G82.5-)

         Excludes1   hemiplegia/hemiparesis following other nontraumatic intracranial hemorrhage (I69.25-)
         monoplegia of lower limb following other nontraumatic intracranial hemorrhage (I69.24-)
         monoplegia of upper limb following other nontraumatic intracranial hemorrhage (I69.23-)

     I69.261   **Other paralytic syndrome following other nontraumatic intracranial hemorrhage affecting right dominant side**

     I69.262   **Other paralytic syndrome following other nontraumatic intracranial hemorrhage affecting left dominant side**

CHAPTER 9 (I00-I99)

CHAPTER 9 (I00-I99)

I69.263   Other paralytic syndrome following other nontraumatic intracranial hemorrhage affecting right non-dominant side

I69.264   Other paralytic syndrome following other nontraumatic intracranial hemorrhage affecting left non-dominant side

I69.265   Other paralytic syndrome following other nontraumatic intracranial hemorrhage, bilateral

I69.269   Other paralytic syndrome following other nontraumatic intracranial hemorrhage affecting unspecified side

● I69.29   Other sequelae of other nontraumatic intracranial hemorrhage

I69.290   Apraxia following other nontraumatic intracranial hemorrhage

I69.291   Dysphagia following other nontraumatic intracranial hemorrhage
    Use additional code to identify the type of dysphagia, if known (R13.1-)

I69.292   Facial weakness following other nontraumatic intracranial hemorrhage
    Facial droop following other nontraumatic intracranial hemorrhage

I69.293   Ataxia following other nontraumatic intracranial hemorrhage

I69.298   Other sequelae of other nontraumatic intracranial hemorrhage
    Alteration of sensation following other nontraumatic intracranial hemorrhage
    Disturbance of vision following other nontraumatic intracranial hemorrhage
    Use additional code to identify the sequelae

● I69.3   Sequelae of cerebral infarction
    Sequelae of stroke NOS
    Coding Clinic: 2012, Q4, P92, 95

I69.30   Unspecified sequelae of cerebral infarction

I69.31   Cognitive deficits following cerebral infarction

● I69.32   Speech and language deficits following cerebral infarction

I69.320   Aphasia following cerebral infarction

I69.321   Dysphasia following cerebral infarction
    Coding Clinic: 2012, Q4, P91

I69.322   Dysarthria following cerebral infarction

I69.323   Fluency disorder following cerebral infarction
    Stuttering following nontraumatic subarachnoid hemorrhage

I69.328   Other speech and language deficits following cerebral infarction

● I69.33   Monoplegia of upper limb following cerebral infarction

I69.331   Monoplegia of upper limb following cerebral infarction affecting right dominant side

I69.332   Monoplegia of upper limb following cerebral infarction affecting left dominant side

I69.333   Monoplegia of upper limb following cerebral infarction affecting right non-dominant side

I69.334   Monoplegia of upper limb following cerebral infarction affecting left non-dominant side

I69.339   Monoplegia of upper limb following cerebral infarction affecting unspecified side

● I69.34   Monoplegia of lower limb following cerebral infarction

I69.341   Monoplegia of lower limb following cerebral infarction affecting right dominant side

I69.342   Monoplegia of lower limb following cerebral infarction affecting left dominant side

I69.343   Monoplegia of lower limb following cerebral infarction affecting right non-dominant side

I69.344   Monoplegia of lower limb following cerebral infarction affecting left non-dominant side

I69.349   Monoplegia of lower limb following cerebral infarction affecting unspecified side

● I69.35   Hemiplegia and hemiparesis following cerebral infarction

I69.351   Hemiplegia and hemiparesis following cerebral infarction affecting right dominant side
    Coding Clinic: 2015, Q1, P25

I69.352   Hemiplegia and hemiparesis following cerebral infarction affecting left dominant side

I69.353   Hemiplegia and hemiparesis following cerebral infarction affecting right non-dominant side

I69.354   Hemiplegia and hemiparesis following cerebral infarction affecting left non-dominant side
    Coding Clinic: 2012, Q4, P91

I69.359   Hemiplegia and hemiparesis following cerebral infarction affecting unspecified side

● I69.36 Other paralytic syndrome following cerebral infarction
    Use additional code to identify type of paralytic syndrome, such as:
    locked-in state (G83.5)
    quadriplegia (G82.5-)

    Excludes1   hemiplegia/hemiparesis following cerebral infarction (I69.35-)
    monoplegia of lower limb following cerebral infarction (I69.34-)
    monoplegia of upper limb following cerebral infarction (I69.33-)

I69.361   Other paralytic syndrome following cerebral infarction affecting right dominant side

I69.362   Other paralytic syndrome following cerebral infarction affecting left dominant side

I69.363   Other paralytic syndrome following cerebral infarction affecting right non-dominant side

◀ New   ⬅ Revised   d̶e̶l̶e̶t̶e̶d̶ Deleted   Excludes 1   Excludes 2   Includes   Use additional   Code first   Code also   Unspecified
OGCR Official Guidelines   X Assign placeholder X   ● Use Additional Character(s)   ▌ Manifestation Code   Coding Clinic

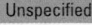

I69.364   Other paralytic syndrome following cerebral infarction affecting left non-dominant side

I69.365   Other paralytic syndrome following cerebral infarction, bilateral

I69.369   Other paralytic syndrome following cerebral infarction affecting unspecified side

● I69.39   Other sequelae of cerebral infarction

I69.390   Apraxia following cerebral infarction

I69.391   Dysphagia following cerebral infarction

> Use additional code to identify the type of dysphagia, if known (R13.1-)

I69.392   Facial weakness following cerebral infarction

> Facial droop following cerebral infarction

I69.393   Ataxia following cerebral infarction

I69.398   Other sequelae of cerebral infarction

> Alteration of sensation following cerebral infarction
> Disturbance of vision following cerebral infarction
> Use additional code to identify the sequelae

● I69.8   Sequelae of other cerebrovascular diseases

> **Excludes1**   sequelae of traumatic intracranial injury (S06.-)

I69.80   Unspecified sequelae of other cerebrovascular disease

I69.81   Cognitive deficits following other cerebrovascular disease

● I69.82   Speech and language deficits following other cerebrovascular disease

I69.820   Aphasia following other cerebrovascular disease

I69.821   Dysphasia following other cerebrovascular disease

I69.822   Dysarthria following other cerebrovascular disease

I69.823   Fluency disorder following other cerebrovascular disease

> Stuttering following nontraumatic subarachnoid hemorrhage

I69.828   Other speech and language deficits following other cerebrovascular disease

● I69.83   Monoplegia of upper limb following other cerebrovascular disease

I69.831   Monoplegia of upper limb following other cerebrovascular disease affecting right dominant side

I69.832   Monoplegia of upper limb following other cerebrovascular disease affecting left dominant side

I69.833   Monoplegia of upper limb following other cerebrovascular disease affecting right non-dominant side

I69.834   Monoplegia of upper limb following other cerebrovascular disease affecting left non-dominant side

I69.839   Monoplegia of upper limb following other cerebrovascular disease affecting unspecified side

● I69.84   Monoplegia of lower limb following other cerebrovascular disease

I69.841   Monoplegia of lower limb following other cerebrovascular disease affecting right dominant side

I69.842   Monoplegia of lower limb following other cerebrovascular disease affecting left dominant side

I69.843   Monoplegia of lower limb following other cerebrovascular disease affecting right non-dominant side

I69.844   Monoplegia of lower limb following other cerebrovascular disease affecting left non-dominant side

I69.849   Monoplegia of lower limb following other cerebrovascular disease affecting unspecified side

● I69.85   Hemiplegia and hemiparesis following other cerebrovascular disease

I69.851   Hemiplegia and hemiparesis following other cerebrovascular disease affecting right dominant side

I69.852   Hemiplegia and hemiparesis following other cerebrovascular disease affecting left dominant side

I69.853   Hemiplegia and hemiparesis following other cerebrovascular disease affecting right non-dominant side

I69.854   Hemiplegia and hemiparesis following other cerebrovascular disease affecting left non-dominant side

I69.859   Hemiplegia and hemiparesis following other cerebrovascular disease affecting unspecified side

● I69.86   Other paralytic syndrome following other cerebrovascular disease

> Use additional code to identify type of paralytic syndrome, such as:
> locked-in state (G83.5)
> quadriplegia (G82.5-)

> **Excludes1**   hemiplegia/hemiparesis following other cerebrovascular disease (I69.85-)
> monoplegia of lower limb following other cerebrovascular disease (I69.84-)
> monoplegia of upper limb following other cerebrovascular disease (I69.83-)

I69.861   Other paralytic syndrome following other cerebrovascular disease affecting right dominant side

I69.862   Other paralytic syndrome following other cerebrovascular disease affecting left dominant side

I69.863   Other paralytic syndrome following other cerebrovascular disease affecting right non-dominant side

I69.864   Other paralytic syndrome following other cerebrovascular disease affecting left non-dominant side

I69.865   Other paralytic syndrome following other cerebrovascular disease, bilateral

I69.869   Other paralytic syndrome following other cerebrovascular disease affecting unspecified side

CHAPTER 9 (I00–I99)

● **I69.89**   **Other sequelae of other cerebrovascular disease**

     I69.890   **Apraxia following other cerebrovascular disease**

     I69.891   **Dysphagia following other cerebrovascular disease**

         Use additional code to identify the type of dysphagia, if known (R13.1-)

     I69.892   **Facial weakness following other cerebrovascular disease**

         Facial droop following other cerebrovascular disease

     I69.893   **Ataxia following other cerebrovascular disease**

     I69.898   **Other sequelae of other cerebrovascular disease**

         Alteration of sensation following other cerebrovascular disease

         Disturbance of vision following other cerebrovascular disease

         Use additional code to identify the sequelae

● **I69.9**   **Sequelae of unspecified cerebrovascular diseases**

     Excludes1   sequelae of stroke (I69.3)

         sequelae of traumatic intracranial injury (S06.-)

     I69.90   **Unspecified sequelae of unspecified cerebrovascular disease**

     I69.91   **Cognitive deficits following unspecified cerebrovascular disease**

● **I69.92**   **Speech and language deficits following unspecified cerebrovascular disease**

     I69.920   **Aphasia following unspecified cerebrovascular disease**

     I69.921   **Dysphasia following unspecified cerebrovascular disease**

     I69.922   **Dysarthria following unspecified cerebrovascular disease**

     I69.923   **Fluency disorder following unspecified cerebrovascular disease**

         Stuttering following nontraumatic subarachnoid hemorrhage

     I69.928   **Other speech and language deficits following unspecified cerebrovascular disease**

● **I69.93**   **Monoplegia of upper limb following unspecified cerebrovascular disease**

     I69.931   **Monoplegia of upper limb following unspecified cerebrovascular disease affecting right dominant side**

     I69.932   **Monoplegia of upper limb following unspecified cerebrovascular disease affecting left dominant side**

     I69.933   **Monoplegia of upper limb following unspecified cerebrovascular disease affecting right non-dominant side**

     I69.934   **Monoplegia of upper limb following unspecified cerebrovascular disease affecting left non-dominant side**

     I69.939   **Monoplegia of upper limb following unspecified cerebrovascular disease affecting unspecified side**

● **I69.94**   **Monoplegia of lower limb following unspecified cerebrovascular disease**

     I69.941   **Monoplegia of lower limb following unspecified cerebrovascular disease affecting right dominant side**

     I69.942   **Monoplegia of lower limb following unspecified cerebrovascular disease affecting left dominant side**

     I69.943   **Monoplegia of lower limb following unspecified cerebrovascular disease affecting right non-dominant side**

     I69.944   **Monoplegia of lower limb following unspecified cerebrovascular disease affecting left non-dominant side**

     I69.949   **Monoplegia of lower limb following unspecified cerebrovascular disease affecting unspecified side**

● **I69.95**   **Hemiplegia and hemiparesis following unspecified cerebrovascular disease**

     I69.951   **Hemiplegia and hemiparesis following unspecified cerebrovascular disease affecting right dominant side**

     I69.952   **Hemiplegia and hemiparesis following unspecified cerebrovascular disease affecting left dominant side**

     I69.953   **Hemiplegia and hemiparesis following unspecified cerebrovascular disease affecting right non-dominant side**

     I69.954   **Hemiplegia and hemiparesis following unspecified cerebrovascular disease affecting left non-dominant side**

     I69.959   **Hemiplegia and hemiparesis following unspecified cerebrovascular disease affecting unspecified side**

● **I69.96**   **Other paralytic syndrome following unspecified cerebrovascular disease**

     Use additional code to identify type of paralytic syndrome, such as:

         locked-in state (G83.5)

         quadriplegia (G82.5-)

     Excludes1   hemiplegia/hemiparesis following unspecified cerebrovascular disease (I69.95-)

         monoplegia of lower limb following unspecified cerebrovascular disease (I69.94-)

         monoplegia of upper limb following unspecified cerebrovascular disease (I69.93-)

     I69.961   **Other paralytic syndrome following unspecified cerebrovascular disease affecting right dominant side**

     I69.962   **Other paralytic syndrome following unspecified cerebrovascular disease affecting left dominant side**

     I69.963   **Other paralytic syndrome following unspecified cerebrovascular disease affecting right non-dominant side**

     I69.964   **Other paralytic syndrome following unspecified cerebrovascular disease affecting left non-dominant side**

     I69.965   **Other paralytic syndrome following unspecified cerebrovascular disease, bilateral**

     I69.969   **Other paralytic syndrome following unspecified cerebrovascular disease affecting unspecified side**

◀ New   ◀◀ Revised   ~~deleted~~ Deleted   Excludes 1   Excludes 2   Includes   Use additional   Code first   Code also   Unspecified

OGCR Official Guidelines   **X** Assign placeholder X   ● Use Additional Character(s)   ▶ Manifestation Code   **Coding Clinic**

● **I69.99**   **Other sequelae of unspecified cerebrovascular disease**

     I69.990   **Apraxia following unspecified cerebrovascular disease**

     I69.991   **Dysphagia following unspecified cerebrovascular disease**

         Use additional code to identify the type of dysphagia, if known (R13.1-)

     I69.992   **Facial weakness following unspecified cerebrovascular disease**

         Facial droop following unspecified cerebrovascular disease

     I69.993   **Ataxia following unspecified cerebrovascular disease**

     I69.998   **Other sequelae following unspecified cerebrovascular disease**

         Alteration in sensation following unspecified cerebrovascular disease

         Disturbance of vision following unspecified cerebrovascular disease

         Use additional code to identify the sequelae

DISEASES OF ARTERIES, ARTERIOLES AND CAPILLARIES (I70-I79)

● **I70**   **Atherosclerosis**

     Includes   arteriolosclerosis
         arterial degeneration
         arteriosclerosis
         arteriosclerotic vascular disease
         arteriovascular degeneration
         atheroma
         endarteritis deformans or obliterans
         senile arteritis
         senile endarteritis
         vascular degeneration

     Use additional code to identify:
         exposure to environmental tobacco smoke (Z77.22)
         history of tobacco use (Z87.891)
         occupational exposure to environmental tobacco smoke (Z57.31)
         tobacco dependence (F17.-)
         tobacco use (Z72.0)

     Excludes2   arteriosclerotic cardiovascular disease (I25.1-)
         arteriosclerotic heart disease (I25.1-)
         atheroembolism (I75.-)
         cerebral atherosclerosis (I67.2)
         coronary atherosclerosis (I25.1-)
         mesenteric atherosclerosis (K55.1)
         precerebral atherosclerosis (I67.2)
         primary pulmonary atherosclerosis (I27.0)

   I70.0   **Atherosclerosis of aorta**   A

   I70.1   **Atherosclerosis of renal artery**   A
         Goldblatt's kidney

     Excludes2   atherosclerosis of renal arterioles (I12.-)

(See Plates 500, 501, and 502 on pages 60 – 62.)

● **I70.2**   **Atherosclerosis of native arteries of the extremities**
     Mönckeberg's (medial) sclerosis

     Use additional code, if applicable, to identify chronic total occlusion of artery of extremity (I70.92)

     Excludes2   atherosclerosis of bypass graft of extremities (I70.30-I70.79)

   ● **I70.20**   **Unspecified atherosclerosis of native arteries of extremities**

     I70.201   **Unspecified atherosclerosis of native arteries of extremities, right leg**   A

     I70.202   **Unspecified atherosclerosis of native arteries of extremities, left leg**   A

     I70.203   **Unspecified atherosclerosis of native arteries of extremities, bilateral legs** A

     I70.208   **Unspecified atherosclerosis of native arteries of extremities, other extremity**   A

     I70.209   **Unspecified atherosclerosis of native arteries of extremities, unspecified extremity**   A

   ● **I70.21**   **Atherosclerosis of native arteries of extremities with intermittent claudication**

     I70.211   **Atherosclerosis of native arteries of extremities with intermittent claudication, right leg**   A

     I70.212   **Atherosclerosis of native arteries of extremities with intermittent claudication, left leg**   A

     I70.213   **Atherosclerosis of native arteries of extremities with intermittent claudication, bilateral legs**   A

     I70.218   **Atherosclerosis of native arteries of extremities with intermittent claudication, other extremity**   A

     I70.219   **Atherosclerosis of native arteries of extremities with intermittent claudication, unspecified extremity**   A

   ● **I70.22**   **Atherosclerosis of native arteries of extremities with rest pain**

     Includes   any condition classifiable to I70.21-

     I70.221   **Atherosclerosis of native arteries of extremities with rest pain, right leg**   A

     I70.222   **Atherosclerosis of native arteries of extremities with rest pain, left leg**   A

     I70.223   **Atherosclerosis of native arteries of extremities with rest pain, bilateral legs**   A

     I70.228   **Atherosclerosis of native arteries of extremities with rest pain, other extremity**   A

     I70.229   **Atherosclerosis of native arteries of extremities with rest pain, unspecified extremity**   A

   ● **I70.23**   **Atherosclerosis of native arteries of right leg with ulceration**

     Includes   any condition classifiable to I70.211 and I70.221

     Use additional code to identify severity of ulcer (L97.-)

     I70.231   **Atherosclerosis of native arteries of right leg with ulceration of thigh**   A

     I70.232   **Atherosclerosis of native arteries of right leg with ulceration of calf**   A

     I70.233   **Atherosclerosis of native arteries of right leg with ulceration of ankle**   A

     I70.234   **Atherosclerosis of native arteries of right leg with ulceration of heel and midfoot**   A

         Atherosclerosis of native arteries of right leg with ulceration of plantar surface of midfoot

     I70.235   **Atherosclerosis of native arteries of right leg with ulceration of other part of foot**   A

         Atherosclerosis of native arteries of right leg extremities with ulceration of toe

     I70.238   **Atherosclerosis of native arteries of right leg with ulceration of other part of lower right leg**   A

     I70.239   **Atherosclerosis of native arteries of right leg with ulceration of unspecified site**   A

● **I70.24**   **Atherosclerosis of native arteries of left leg with ulceration**

> **Includes**   any condition classifiable to I70.212 and I70.222

> Use additional code to identify severity of ulcer (L97.-)

I70.241   Atherosclerosis of native arteries of left leg with ulceration of thigh   **A**

I70.242   Atherosclerosis of native arteries of left leg with ulceration of calf   **A**

I70.243   Atherosclerosis of native arteries of left leg with ulceration of ankle   **A**

I70.244   Atherosclerosis of native arteries of left leg with ulceration of heel and midfoot   **A**
> Atherosclerosis of native arteries of left leg with ulceration of plantar surface of midfoot

I70.245   Atherosclerosis of native arteries of left leg with ulceration of other part of foot   **A**
> Atherosclerosis of native arteries of left leg extremities with ulceration of toe

I70.248   Atherosclerosis of native arteries of left leg with ulceration of other part of lower left leg   **A**

I70.249   Atherosclerosis of native arteries of left leg with ulceration of unspecified site   **A**

I70.25   **Atherosclerosis of native arteries of other extremities with ulceration**   **A**

> **Includes**   any condition classifiable to I70.218 and I70.228

> Use additional code to identify the severity of the ulcer (L98.49-)

● **I70.26**   **Atherosclerosis of native arteries of extremities with gangrene**

> **Includes**   any condition classifiable to I70.21-, I70.22-, I70.23-, I70.24-, and I70.25-

> Use additional code to identify the severity of any ulcer (L97.-, L98.49-), if applicable

I70.261   Atherosclerosis of native arteries of extremities with gangrene, right leg   **A**

I70.262   Atherosclerosis of native arteries of extremities with gangrene, left leg   **A**

I70.263   Atherosclerosis of native arteries of extremities with gangrene, bilateral legs   **A**

I70.268   Atherosclerosis of native arteries of extremities with gangrene, other extremity   **A**

I70.269   Atherosclerosis of native arteries of extremities with gangrene, unspecified extremity   **A**

● **I70.29**   **Other atherosclerosis of native arteries of extremities**

I70.291   Other atherosclerosis of native arteries of extremities, right leg   **A**

I70.292   Other atherosclerosis of native arteries of extremities, left leg   **A**

I70.293   Other atherosclerosis of native arteries of extremities, bilateral legs   **A**

I70.298   Other atherosclerosis of native arteries of extremities, other extremity   **A**

I70.299   Other atherosclerosis of native arteries of extremities, unspecified extremity   **A**

● **I70.3**   **Atherosclerosis of unspecified type of bypass graft(s) of the extremities**

> Use additional code, if applicable, to identify chronic total occlusion of artery of extremity (I70.92)

> **Excludes1**   embolism or thrombus of bypass graft(s) of extremities (T82.8-)

● **I70.30**   **Unspecified atherosclerosis of unspecified type of bypass graft(s) of the extremities**

I70.301   Unspecified atherosclerosis of unspecified type of bypass graft(s) of the extremities, right leg   **A**

I70.302   Unspecified atherosclerosis of unspecified type of bypass graft(s) of the extremities, left leg   **A**

I70.303   Unspecified atherosclerosis of unspecified type of bypass graft(s) of the extremities, bilateral legs   **A**

I70.308   Unspecified atherosclerosis of unspecified type of bypass graft(s) of the extremities, other extremity   **A**

I70.309   Unspecified atherosclerosis of unspecified type of bypass graft(s) of the extremities, unspecified extremity   **A**

● **I70.31**   **Atherosclerosis of unspecified type of bypass graft(s) of the extremities with intermittent claudication**

I70.311   Atherosclerosis of unspecified type of bypass graft(s) of the extremities with intermittent claudication, right leg   **A**

I70.312   Atherosclerosis of unspecified type of bypass graft(s) of the extremities with intermittent claudication, left leg   **A**

I70.313   Atherosclerosis of unspecified type of bypass graft(s) of the extremities with intermittent claudication, bilateral legs   **A**

I70.318   Atherosclerosis of unspecified type of bypass graft(s) of the extremities with intermittent claudication, other extremity   **A**

I70.319   Atherosclerosis of unspecified type of bypass graft(s) of the extremities with intermittent claudication, unspecified extremity   **A**

● **I70.32**   **Atherosclerosis of unspecified type of bypass graft(s) of the extremities with rest pain**

> **Includes**   any condition classifiable to I70.31-

I70.321   Atherosclerosis of unspecified type of bypass graft(s) of the extremities with rest pain, right leg   **A**

I70.322   Atherosclerosis of unspecified type of bypass graft(s) of the extremities with rest pain, left leg   **A**

I70.323   Atherosclerosis of unspecified type of bypass graft(s) of the extremities with rest pain, bilateral legs   **A**

I70.328   Atherosclerosis of unspecified type of bypass graft(s) of the extremities with rest pain, other extremity   **A**

I70.329   Atherosclerosis of unspecified type of bypass graft(s) of the extremities with rest pain, unspecified extremity   **A**

◀ New   ⬅ Revised   ~~deleted~~ Deleted   Excludes 1   Excludes 2   Includes   Use additional   Code first   Code also   Unspecified

OGCR Official Guidelines   X Assign placeholder X   ● Use Additional Character(s)   ▶ Manifestation Code   **Coding Clinic**

● **I70.33**   **Atherosclerosis of unspecified type of bypass graft(s) of the right leg with ulceration**   **A**

> **Includes**   any condition classifiable to I70.311 and I70.321

> Use additional code to identify severity of ulcer (L97.-)

    I70.331   Atherosclerosis of unspecified type of bypass graft(s) of the right leg with ulceration of thigh   **A**

    I70.332   Atherosclerosis of unspecified type of bypass graft(s) of the right leg with ulceration of calf   **A**

    I70.333   Atherosclerosis of unspecified type of bypass graft(s) of the right leg with ulceration of ankle   **A**

    I70.334   Atherosclerosis of unspecified type of bypass graft(s) of the right leg with ulceration of heel and midfoot   **A**
> Atherosclerosis of unspecified type of bypass graft(s) of right leg with ulceration of plantar surface of midfoot

    I70.335   Atherosclerosis of unspecified type of bypass graft(s) of the right leg with ulceration of other part of foot   **A**
> Atherosclerosis of unspecified type of bypass graft(s) of the right leg with ulceration of toe

    I70.338   Atherosclerosis of unspecified type of bypass graft(s) of the right leg with ulceration of other part of lower leg   **A**

    I70.339   Atherosclerosis of unspecified type of bypass graft(s) of the right leg with ulceration of unspecified site   **A**

● **I70.34**   **Atherosclerosis of unspecified type of bypass graft(s) of the left leg with ulceration**

> **Includes**   any condition classifiable to I70.312 and I70.322

> Use additional code to identify severity of ulcer (L97.-)

    I70.341   Atherosclerosis of unspecified type of bypass graft(s) of the left leg with ulceration of thigh   **A**

    I70.342   Atherosclerosis of unspecified type of bypass graft(s) of the left leg with ulceration of calf   **A**

    I70.343   Atherosclerosis of unspecified type of bypass graft(s) of the left leg with ulceration of ankle   **A**

    I70.344   Atherosclerosis of unspecified type of bypass graft(s) of the left leg with ulceration of heel and midfoot   **A**
> Atherosclerosis of unspecified type of bypass graft(s) of left leg with ulceration of plantar surface of midfoot

    I70.345   Atherosclerosis of unspecified type of bypass graft(s) of the left leg with ulceration of other part of foot   **A**
> Atherosclerosis of unspecified type of bypass graft(s) of the left leg with ulceration of toe

    I70.348   Atherosclerosis of unspecified type of bypass graft(s) of the left leg with ulceration of other part of lower leg   **A**

    I70.349   Atherosclerosis of unspecified type of bypass graft(s) of the left leg with ulceration of unspecified site   **A**

I70.35   Atherosclerosis of unspecified type of bypass graft(s) of other extremity with ulceration   **A**

> **Includes**   any condition classifiable to I70.318 and I70.328

> Use additional code to identify severity of ulcer (L98.49-)

● **I70.36**   **Atherosclerosis of unspecified type of bypass graft(s) of the extremities with gangrene**

> **Includes**   any condition classifiable to I70.31-, I70.32-, I70.33-, I70.34-, I70.35

> Use additional code to identify the severity of any ulcer (L97.-, L98.49-), if applicable

    I70.361   Atherosclerosis of unspecified type of bypass graft(s) of the extremities with gangrene, right leg   **A**

    I70.362   Atherosclerosis of unspecified type of bypass graft(s) of the extremities with gangrene, left leg   **A**

    I70.363   Atherosclerosis of unspecified type of bypass graft(s) of the extremities with gangrene, bilateral legs   **A**

    I70.368   Atherosclerosis of unspecified type of bypass graft(s) of the extremities with gangrene, other extremity   **A**

    I70.369   Atherosclerosis of unspecified type of bypass graft(s) of the extremities with gangrene, unspecified extremity   **A**

● **I70.39**   **Other atherosclerosis of unspecified type of bypass graft(s) of the extremities**

    I70.391   Other atherosclerosis of unspecified type of bypass graft(s) of the extremities, right leg   **A**

    I70.392   Other atherosclerosis of unspecified type of bypass graft(s) of the extremities, left leg   **A**

    I70.393   Other atherosclerosis of unspecified type of bypass graft(s) of the extremities, bilateral legs   **A**

    I70.398   Other atherosclerosis of unspecified type of bypass graft(s) of the extremities, other extremity   **A**

    I70.399   Other atherosclerosis of unspecified type of bypass graft(s) of the extremities, unspecified extremity   **A**

● **I70.4**   **Atherosclerosis of autologous vein bypass graft(s) of the extremities**

> Use additional code, if applicable, to identify chronic total occlusion of artery of extremity (I70.92)

● **I70.40**   **Unspecified atherosclerosis of autologous vein bypass graft(s) of the extremities**

    I70.401   Unspecified atherosclerosis of autologous vein bypass graft(s) of the extremities, right leg   **A**

    I70.402   Unspecified atherosclerosis of autologous vein bypass graft(s) of the extremities, left leg   **A**

    I70.403   Unspecified atherosclerosis of autologous vein bypass graft(s) of the extremities, bilateral legs   **A**

    I70.408   Unspecified atherosclerosis of autologous vein bypass graft(s) of the extremities, other extremity   **A**

    I70.409   Unspecified atherosclerosis of autologous vein bypass graft(s) of the extremities, unspecified extremity   **A**

CHAPTER 9 (I00-I99)

● **I70.41** **Atherosclerosis of autologous vein bypass graft(s) of the extremities with intermittent claudication**

    I70.411 Atherosclerosis of autologous vein bypass graft(s) of the extremities with intermittent claudication, right leg   A

    I70.412 Atherosclerosis of autologous vein bypass graft(s) of the extremities with intermittent claudication, left leg   A

    I70.413 Atherosclerosis of autologous vein bypass graft(s) of the extremities with intermittent claudication, bilateral legs   A

    I70.418 Atherosclerosis of autologous vein bypass graft(s) of the extremities with intermittent claudication, other extremity

    I70.419 Atherosclerosis of autologous vein bypass graft(s) of the extremities with intermittent claudication, unspecified extremity   A

● **I70.42** **Atherosclerosis of autologous vein bypass graft(s) of the extremities with rest pain**

    Includes any condition classifiable to I70.41-

    I70.421 Atherosclerosis of autologous vein bypass graft(s) of the extremities with rest pain, right leg   A

    I70.422 Atherosclerosis of autologous vein bypass graft(s) of the extremities with rest pain, left leg   A

    I70.423 Atherosclerosis of autologous vein bypass graft(s) of the extremities with rest pain, bilateral legs   A

    I70.428 Atherosclerosis of autologous vein bypass graft(s) of the extremities with rest pain, other extremity   A

    I70.429 Atherosclerosis of autologous vein bypass graft(s) of the extremities with rest pain, unspecified extremity   A

● **I70.43** **Atherosclerosis of autologous vein bypass graft(s) of the right leg with ulceration**

    Includes any condition classifiable to I70.411 and I70.421

    Use additional code to identify severity of ulcer (L97.-)

    I70.431 Atherosclerosis of autologous vein bypass graft(s) of the right leg with ulceration of thigh   A

    I70.432 Atherosclerosis of autologous vein bypass graft(s) of the right leg with ulceration of calf   A

    I70.433 Atherosclerosis of autologous vein bypass graft(s) of the right leg with ulceration of ankle   A

    I70.434 Atherosclerosis of autologous vein bypass graft(s) of the right leg with ulceration of heel and midfoot   A
        Atherosclerosis of autologous vein bypass graft(s) of right leg with ulceration of plantar surface of midfoot

    I70.435 Atherosclerosis of autologous vein bypass graft(s) of the right leg with ulceration of other part of foot   A
        Atherosclerosis of autologous vein bypass graft(s) of right leg with ulceration of toe

    I70.438 Atherosclerosis of autologous vein bypass graft(s) of the right leg with ulceration of other part of lower leg   A

    I70.439 Atherosclerosis of autologous vein bypass graft(s) of the right leg with ulceration of unspecified site   A

● **I70.44** **Atherosclerosis of autologous vein bypass graft(s) of the left leg with ulceration**

    Includes any condition classifiable to I70.412 and I70.422

    Use additional code to identify severity of ulcer (L97.-)

    I70.441 Atherosclerosis of autologous vein bypass graft(s) of the left leg with ulceration of thigh   A

    I70.442 Atherosclerosis of autologous vein bypass graft(s) of the left leg with ulceration of calf   A

    I70.443 Atherosclerosis of autologous vein bypass graft(s) of the left leg with ulceration of ankle   A

    I70.444 Atherosclerosis of autologous vein bypass graft(s) of the left leg with ulceration of heel and midfoot   A
        Atherosclerosis of autologous vein bypass graft(s) of left leg with ulceration of plantar surface of midfoot

    I70.445 Atherosclerosis of autologous vein bypass graft(s) of the left leg with ulceration of other part of foot   A
        Atherosclerosis of autologous vein bypass graft(s) of left leg with ulceration of toe

    I70.448 Atherosclerosis of autologous vein bypass graft(s) of the left leg with ulceration of other part of lower leg   A

    I70.449 Atherosclerosis of autologous vein bypass graft(s) of the left leg with ulceration of unspecified site   A

  I70.45 **Atherosclerosis of autologous vein bypass graft(s) of other extremity with ulceration**   A

    Includes any condition classifiable to I70.418, I70.428, and I70.438

    Use additional code to identify severity of ulcer (L98.49-)

● **I70.46** **Atherosclerosis of autologous vein bypass graft(s) of the extremities with gangrene**

    Includes any condition classifiable to I70.41-, I70.42-, and I70.43-, I70.44-, I70.45

    Use additional code to identify the severity of any ulcer (L97.-, L98.49-), if applicable

    I70.461 Atherosclerosis of autologous vein bypass graft(s) of the extremities with gangrene, right leg   A

    I70.462 Atherosclerosis of autologous vein bypass graft(s) of the extremities with gangrene, left leg   A

    I70.463 Atherosclerosis of autologous vein bypass graft(s) of the extremities with gangrene, bilateral legs   A

    I70.468 Atherosclerosis of autologous vein bypass graft(s) of the extremities with gangrene, other extremity   A

    I70.469 Atherosclerosis of autologous vein bypass graft(s) of the extremities with gangrene, unspecified extremity   A

◀ New   ◀◀◀ Revised   ~~deleted~~ Deleted   Excludes 1   Excludes 2   Includes   Use additional   Code first   Code also   Unspecified

OGCR Official Guidelines   **X** Assign placeholder X   ● Use Additional Character(s)   ▶ Manifestation Code   **Coding Clinic**

● **I70.49**   Other atherosclerosis of autologous vein bypass graft(s) of the extremities

    I70.491   Other atherosclerosis of autologous vein bypass graft(s) of the extremities, right leg   A

    I70.492   Other atherosclerosis of autologous vein bypass graft(s) of the extremities, left leg   A

    I70.493   Other atherosclerosis of autologous vein bypass graft(s) of the extremities, bilateral legs   A

    I70.498   Other atherosclerosis of autologous vein bypass graft(s) of the extremities, other extremity   A

    I70.499   Other atherosclerosis of autologous vein bypass graft(s) of the extremities, unspecified extremity   A

● **I70.5**   Atherosclerosis of nonautologous biological bypass graft(s) of the extremities

    Use additional code, if applicable, to identify chronic total occlusion of artery of extremity (I70.92)

● **I70.50**   Unspecified atherosclerosis of nonautologous biological bypass graft(s) of the extremities

    I70.501   Unspecified atherosclerosis of nonautologous biological bypass graft(s) of the extremities, right leg   A

    I70.502   Unspecified atherosclerosis of nonautologous biological bypass graft(s) of the extremities, left leg   A

    I70.503   Unspecified atherosclerosis of nonautologous biological bypass graft(s) of the extremities, bilateral legs   A

    I70.508   Unspecified atherosclerosis of nonautologous biological bypass graft(s) of the extremities, other extremity   A

    I70.509   Unspecified atherosclerosis of nonautologous biological bypass graft(s) of the extremities, unspecified extremity   A

● **I70.51**   Atherosclerosis of nonautologous biological bypass graft(s) of the extremities intermittent claudication

    I70.511   Atherosclerosis of nonautologous biological bypass graft(s) of the extremities with intermittent claudication, right leg   A

    I70.512   Atherosclerosis of nonautologous biological bypass graft(s) of the extremities with intermittent claudication, left leg   A

    I70.513   Atherosclerosis of nonautologous biological bypass graft(s) of the extremities with intermittent claudication, bilateral legs   A

    I70.518   Atherosclerosis of nonautologous biological bypass graft(s) of the extremities with intermittent claudication, other extremity   A

    I70.519   Atherosclerosis of nonautologous biological bypass graft(s) of the extremities with intermittent claudication, unspecified extremity   A

● **I70.52**   Atherosclerosis of nonautologous biological bypass graft(s) of the extremities with rest pain

    Includes   any condition classifiable to I70.51-

    I70.521   Atherosclerosis of nonautologous biological bypass graft(s) of the extremities with rest pain, right leg   A

    I70.522   Atherosclerosis of nonautologous biological bypass graft(s) of the extremities with rest pain, left leg   A

    I70.523   Atherosclerosis of nonautologous biological bypass graft(s) of the extremities with rest pain, bilateral legs   A

    I70.528   Atherosclerosis of nonautologous biological bypass graft(s) of the extremities with rest pain, other extremity   A

    I70.529   Atherosclerosis of nonautologous biological bypass graft(s) of the extremities with rest pain, unspecified extremity   A

● **I70.53**   Atherosclerosis of nonautologous biological bypass graft(s) of the right leg with ulceration

    Includes   any condition classifiable to I70.511 and I70.521

    Use additional code to identify severity of ulcer (L97.-)

    I70.531   Atherosclerosis of nonautologous biological bypass graft(s) of the right leg with ulceration of thigh   A

    I70.532   Atherosclerosis of nonautologous biological bypass graft(s) of the right leg with ulceration of calf   A

    I70.533   Atherosclerosis of nonautologous biological bypass graft(s) of the right leg with ulceration of ankle   A

    I70.534   Atherosclerosis of nonautologous biological bypass graft(s) of the right leg with ulceration of heel and midfoot   A

      Atherosclerosis of nonautologous biological bypass graft(s) of right leg with ulceration of plantar surface of midfoot

    I70.535   Atherosclerosis of nonautologous biological bypass graft(s) of the right leg with ulceration of other part of foot   A

      Atherosclerosis of nonautologous biological bypass graft(s) of the right leg with ulceration of toe

    I70.538   Atherosclerosis of nonautologous biological bypass graft(s) of the right leg with ulceration of other part of lower leg   A

    I70.539   Atherosclerosis of nonautologous biological bypass graft(s) of the right leg with ulceration of unspecified site   A

● I70.54 **Atherosclerosis of nonautologous biological bypass graft(s) of the left leg with ulceration**
  Includes any condition classifiable to I70.512 and I70.522
  Use additional code to identify severity of ulcer (L97.-)

I70.541 Atherosclerosis of nonautologous biological bypass graft(s) of the left leg with ulceration of thigh A

I70.542 Atherosclerosis of nonautologous biological bypass graft(s) of the left leg with ulceration of calf A

I70.543 Atherosclerosis of nonautologous biological bypass graft(s) of the left leg with ulceration of ankle A

I70.544 Atherosclerosis of nonautologous biological bypass graft(s) of the left leg with ulceration of heel and midfoot A
  Atherosclerosis of nonautologous biological bypass graft(s) of left leg with ulceration of plantar surface of midfoot

I70.545 Atherosclerosis of nonautologous biological bypass graft(s) of the left leg with ulceration of other part of foot A
  Atherosclerosis of nonautologous biological bypass graft(s) of the left leg with ulceration of toe

I70.548 Atherosclerosis of nonautologous biological bypass graft(s) of the left leg with ulceration of other part of lower leg A

I70.549 Atherosclerosis of nonautologous biological bypass graft(s) of the left leg with ulceration of unspecified site A

I70.55 **Atherosclerosis of nonautologous biological bypass graft(s) of other extremity with ulceration** A
  Includes any condition classifiable to I70.518, I70.528, and I70.538
  Use additional code to identify severity of ulcer (L98.49)

● I70.56 **Atherosclerosis of nonautologous biological bypass graft(s) of the extremities with gangrene**
  Includes any condition classifiable to I70.51-, I70.52-, and I70.53-, I70.54-, I70.55
  Use additional code to identify the severity of any ulcer (L97.-, L98.49-), if applicable

I70.561 Atherosclerosis of nonautologous biological bypass graft(s) of the extremities with gangrene, right leg A

I70.562 Atherosclerosis of nonautologous biological bypass graft(s) of the extremities with gangrene, left leg A

I70.563 Atherosclerosis of nonautologous biological bypass graft(s) of the extremities with gangrene, bilateral legs A

I70.568 Atherosclerosis of nonautologous biological bypass graft(s) of the extremities with gangrene, other extremity A

I70.569 Atherosclerosis of nonautologous biological bypass graft(s) of the extremities with gangrene, unspecified extremity A

● I70.59 **Other atherosclerosis of nonautologous biological bypass graft(s) of the extremities**

I70.591 Other atherosclerosis of nonautologous biological bypass graft(s) of the extremities, right leg A

I70.592 Other atherosclerosis of nonautologous biological bypass graft(s) of the extremities, left leg A

I70.593 Other atherosclerosis of nonautologous biological bypass graft(s) of the extremities, bilateral legs A

I70.598 Other atherosclerosis of nonautologous biological bypass graft(s) of the extremities, other extremity A

I70.599 Other atherosclerosis of nonautologous biological bypass graft(s) of the extremities, unspecified extremity A

● I70.6 **Atherosclerosis of nonbiological bypass graft(s) of the extremities**
  Use additional code, if applicable, to identify chronic total occlusion of artery of extremity (I70.92)

● I70.60 **Unspecified atherosclerosis of nonbiological bypass graft(s) of the extremities**

I70.601 Unspecified atherosclerosis of nonbiological bypass graft(s) of the extremities, right leg A

I70.602 Unspecified atherosclerosis of nonbiological bypass graft(s) of the extremities, left leg A

I70.603 Unspecified atherosclerosis of nonbiological bypass graft(s) of the extremities, bilateral legs A

I70.608 Unspecified atherosclerosis of nonbiological bypass graft(s) of the extremities, other extremity A

I70.609 Unspecified atherosclerosis of nonbiological bypass graft(s) of the extremities, unspecified extremity A

● I70.61 **Atherosclerosis of nonbiological bypass graft(s) of the extremities with intermittent claudication**

I70.611 Atherosclerosis of nonbiological bypass graft(s) of the extremities with intermittent claudication, right leg A

I70.612 Atherosclerosis of nonbiological bypass graft(s) of the extremities with intermittent claudication, left leg A

I70.613 Atherosclerosis of nonbiological bypass graft(s) of the extremities with intermittent claudication, bilateral legs A

I70.618 Atherosclerosis of nonbiological bypass graft(s) of the extremities with intermittent claudication, other extremity A

I70.619 Atherosclerosis of nonbiological bypass graft(s) of the extremities with intermittent claudication, unspecified extremity A

CHAPTER 9 (I00-I99)

◄ New   ◄ Revised   deleted Deleted   Excludes 1   Excludes 2   Includes   Use additional   Code first   Code also   Unspecified
OGCR Official Guidelines   X Assign placeholder X   ● Use Additional Character(s)   ▶ Manifestation Code   **Coding Clinic**

● **I70.62**   **Atherosclerosis of nonbiological bypass graft(s) of the extremities with rest pain**
> **Includes**   any condition classifiable to I70.61-

   I70.621   **Atherosclerosis of nonbiological bypass graft(s) of the extremities with rest pain, right leg**   **A**

   I70.622   **Atherosclerosis of nonbiological bypass graft(s) of the extremities with rest pain, left leg**   **A**

   I70.623   **Atherosclerosis of nonbiological bypass graft(s) of the extremities with rest pain, bilateral legs**   **A**

   I70.628   **Atherosclerosis of nonbiological bypass graft(s) of the extremities with rest pain, other extremity**   **A**

   I70.629   **Atherosclerosis of nonbiological bypass graft(s) of the extremities with rest pain, unspecified extremity**   **A**

● **I70.63**   **Atherosclerosis of nonbiological bypass graft(s) of the right leg with ulceration**
> **Includes**   any condition classifiable to I70.611 and I70.621

> Use additional code to identify severity of ulcer (L97.-)

   I70.631   **Atherosclerosis of nonbiological bypass graft(s) of the right leg with ulceration of thigh**   **A**

   I70.632   **Atherosclerosis of nonbiological bypass graft(s) of the right leg with ulceration of calf**   **A**

   I70.633   **Atherosclerosis of nonbiological bypass graft(s) of the right leg with ulceration of ankle**   **A**

   I70.634   **Atherosclerosis of nonbiological bypass graft(s) of the right leg with ulceration of heel and midfoot**   **A**
> Atherosclerosis of nonbiological bypass graft(s) of right leg with ulceration of plantar surface of midfoot

   I70.635   **Atherosclerosis of nonbiological bypass graft(s) of the right leg with ulceration of other part of foot**   **A**
> Atherosclerosis of nonbiological bypass graft(s) of the right leg with ulceration of toe

   I70.638   **Atherosclerosis of nonbiological bypass graft(s) of the right leg with ulceration of other part of lower leg**   **A**

   I70.639   **Atherosclerosis of nonbiological bypass graft(s) of the right leg with ulceration of unspecified site**   **A**

● **I70.64**   **Atherosclerosis of nonbiological bypass graft(s) of the left leg with ulceration**
> **Includes**   any condition classifiable to I70.612 and I70.622

> Use additional code to identify severity of ulcer (L97.-)

   I70.641   **Atherosclerosis of nonbiological bypass graft(s) of the left leg with ulceration of thigh**   **A**

   I70.642   **Atherosclerosis of nonbiological bypass graft(s) of the left leg with ulceration of calf**   **A**

   I70.643   **Atherosclerosis of nonbiological bypass graft(s) of the left leg with ulceration of ankle**   **A**

   I70.644   **Atherosclerosis of nonbiological bypass graft(s) of the left leg with ulceration of heel and midfoot**   **A**
> Atherosclerosis of nonbiological bypass graft(s) of left leg with ulceration of plantar surface of midfoot

   I70.645   **Atherosclerosis of nonbiological bypass graft(s) of the left leg with ulceration of other part of foot**   **A**
> Atherosclerosis of nonbiological bypass graft(s) of the left leg with ulceration of toe

   I70.648   **Atherosclerosis of nonbiological bypass graft(s) of the left leg with ulceration of other part of lower leg**   **A**

   I70.649   **Atherosclerosis of nonbiological bypass graft(s) of the left leg with ulceration of unspecified site**   **A**

I70.65   **Atherosclerosis of nonbiological bypass graft(s) of other extremity with ulceration**   **A**
> **Includes**   any condition classifiable to I70.618 and I70.628

> Use additional code to identify severity of ulcer (L98.49-)

● **I70.66**   **Atherosclerosis of nonbiological bypass graft(s) of the extremities with gangrene**
> **Includes**   any condition classifiable to I70.61-, I70.62-, I70.63-, I70.64-, I70.65

> Use additional code to identify the severity of any ulcer (L97.-, L98.49-), if applicable

   I70.661   **Atherosclerosis of nonbiological bypass graft(s) of the extremities with gangrene, right leg**   **A**

   I70.662   **Atherosclerosis of nonbiological bypass graft(s) of the extremities with gangrene, left leg**   **A**

   I70.663   **Atherosclerosis of nonbiological bypass graft(s) of the extremities with gangrene, bilateral legs**   **A**

   I70.668   **Atherosclerosis of nonbiological bypass graft(s) of the extremities with gangrene, other extremity**   **A**

   I70.669   **Atherosclerosis of nonbiological bypass graft(s) of the extremities with gangrene, unspecified extremity**   **A**

● **I70.69**   **Other atherosclerosis of nonbiological bypass graft(s) of the extremities**

   I70.691   **Other atherosclerosis of nonbiological bypass graft(s) of the extremities, right leg**   **A**

   I70.692   **Other atherosclerosis of nonbiological bypass graft(s) of the extremities, left leg**   **A**

   I70.693   **Other atherosclerosis of nonbiological bypass graft(s) of the extremities, bilateral legs**   **A**

   I70.698   **Other atherosclerosis of nonbiological bypass graft(s) of the extremities, other extremity**   **A**

   I70.699   **Other atherosclerosis of nonbiological bypass graft(s) of the extremities, unspecified extremity**   **A**

CHAPTER 9 (I00-I99)

● **I70.7**   **Atherosclerosis of other type of bypass graft(s) of the extremities**

Use additional code, if applicable, to identify chronic total occlusion of artery of extremity (I70.92)

● **I70.70**   **Unspecified atherosclerosis of other type of bypass graft(s) of the extremities**

I70.701   Unspecified atherosclerosis of other type of bypass graft(s) of the extremities, right leg   **A**

I70.702   Unspecified atherosclerosis of other type of bypass graft(s) of the extremities, left leg   **A**

I70.703   Unspecified atherosclerosis of other type of bypass graft(s) of the extremities, bilateral legs   **A**

I70.708   Unspecified atherosclerosis of other type of bypass graft(s) of the extremities, other extremity   **A**

I70.709   Unspecified atherosclerosis of other type of bypass graft(s) of the extremities, unspecified extremity   **A**

● **I70.71**   **Atherosclerosis of other type of bypass graft(s) of the extremities with intermittent claudication**

I70.711   Atherosclerosis of other type of bypass graft(s) of the extremities with intermittent claudication, right leg   **A**

I70.712   Atherosclerosis of other type of bypass graft(s) of the extremities with intermittent claudication, left leg   **A**

I70.713   Atherosclerosis of other type of bypass graft(s) of the extremities with intermittent claudication, bilateral legs   **A**

I70.718   Atherosclerosis of other type of bypass graft(s) of the extremities with intermittent claudication, other extremity   **A**

I70.719   Atherosclerosis of other type of bypass graft(s) of the extremities with intermittent claudication, unspecified extremity   **A**

● **I70.72**   **Atherosclerosis of other type of bypass graft(s) of the extremities with rest pain**

Includes any condition classifiable to I70.71-

I70.721   Atherosclerosis of other type of bypass graft(s) of the extremities with rest pain, right leg   **A**

I70.722   Atherosclerosis of other type of bypass graft(s) of the extremities with rest pain, left leg   **A**

I70.723   Atherosclerosis of other type of bypass graft(s) of the extremities with rest pain, bilateral legs   **A**

I70.728   Atherosclerosis of other type of bypass graft(s) of the extremities with rest pain, other extremity   **A**

I70.729   Atherosclerosis of other type of bypass graft(s) of the extremities with rest pain, unspecified extremity   **A**

● **I70.73**   **Atherosclerosis of other type of bypass graft(s) of the right leg with ulceration**

Includes any condition classifiable to I70.711 and I70.721

Use additional code to identify severity of ulcer (L97.-)

I70.731   Atherosclerosis of other type of bypass graft(s) of the right leg with ulceration of thigh   **A**

I70.732   Atherosclerosis of other type of bypass graft(s) of the right leg with ulceration of calf   **A**

I70.733   Atherosclerosis of other type of bypass graft(s) of the right leg with ulceration of ankle   **A**

I70.734   Atherosclerosis of other type of bypass graft(s) of the right leg with ulceration of heel and midfoot   **A**

Atherosclerosis of other type of bypass graft(s) of right leg with ulceration of plantar surface of midfoot

I70.735   Atherosclerosis of other type of bypass graft(s) of the right leg with ulceration of other part of foot   **A**

Atherosclerosis of other type of bypass graft(s) of right leg with ulceration of toe

I70.738   Atherosclerosis of other type of bypass graft(s) of the right leg with ulceration of other part of lower leg   **A**

I70.739   Atherosclerosis of other type of bypass graft(s) of the right leg with ulceration of unspecified site   **A**

● **I70.74**   **Atherosclerosis of other type of bypass graft(s) of the left leg with ulceration**

Includes any condition classifiable to I70.712 and I70.722

Use additional code to identify severity of ulcer (L97.-)

I70.741   Atherosclerosis of other type of bypass graft(s) of the left leg with ulceration of thigh   **A**

I70.742   Atherosclerosis of other type of bypass graft(s) of the left leg with ulceration of calf   **A**

I70.743   Atherosclerosis of other type of bypass graft(s) of the left leg with ulceration of ankle   **A**

I70.744   Atherosclerosis of other type of bypass graft(s) of the left leg with ulceration of heel and midfoot   **A**

Atherosclerosis of other type of bypass graft(s) of left leg with ulceration of plantar surface of midfoot

I70.745   Atherosclerosis of other type of bypass graft(s) of the left leg with ulceration of other part of foot   **A**

Atherosclerosis of other type of bypass graft(s) of left leg with ulceration of toe

I70.748   Atherosclerosis of other type of bypass graft(s) of the left leg with ulceration of other part of lower leg   **A**

I70.749   Atherosclerosis of other type of bypass graft(s) of the left leg with ulceration of unspecified site   **A**

I70.75   Atherosclerosis of other type of bypass graft(s) of other extremity with ulceration   **A**

Includes any condition classifiable to I70.718 and I70.728

Use additional code to identify severity of ulcer (L98.49)

● **I70.76**   **Atherosclerosis of other type of bypass graft(s) of the extremities with gangrene**

Includes any condition classifiable to I70.71-, I70.72-, I70.73-, I70.74-, I70.75

Use additional code to identify the severity of any ulcer (L97.-, L98.49-), if applicable

I70.761   Atherosclerosis of other type of bypass graft(s) of the extremities with gangrene, right leg   **A**

◀ New   ◀▦ Revised   ~~deleted~~ Deleted   Excludes 1   Excludes 2   Includes   Use additional   Code first   Code also   Unspecified

OGCR Official Guidelines   **X** Assign placeholder X   ● Use Additional Character(s)   ▶ Manifestation Code   **Coding Clinic**

I70.762 Atherosclerosis of other type of bypass graft(s) of the extremities with gangrene, left leg A

I70.763 Atherosclerosis of other type of bypass graft(s) of the extremities with gangrene, bilateral legs A

I70.768 Atherosclerosis of other type of bypass graft(s) of the extremities with gangrene, other extremity A

I70.769 Atherosclerosis of other type of bypass graft(s) of the extremities with gangrene, unspecified extremity A

● I70.79 Other atherosclerosis of other type of bypass graft(s) of the extremities

I70.791 Other atherosclerosis of other type of bypass graft(s) of the extremities, right leg A

I70.792 Other atherosclerosis of other type of bypass graft(s) of the extremities, left leg A

I70.793 Other atherosclerosis of other type of bypass graft(s) of the extremities, bilateral legs A

I70.798 Other atherosclerosis of other type of bypass graft(s) of the extremities, other extremity A

I70.799 Other atherosclerosis of other type of bypass graft(s) of the extremities, unspecified extremity A

I70.8 Atherosclerosis of other arteries A

● I70.9 Other and unspecified atherosclerosis

I70.90 Unspecified atherosclerosis A

I70.91 Generalized atherosclerosis A

I70.92 Chronic total occlusion of artery of the extremities A
　　Complete occlusion of artery of the extremities
　　Total occlusion of artery of the extremities
　　Code first atherosclerosis of arteries of the extremities (I70.2-, I70.3-, I70.4-, I70.5-, I70.6-, I70.7-)

● I71 Aortic aneurysm and dissection

　Excludes1 aortic ectasia (I77.81-)
　　syphilitic aortic aneurysm (A52.01)
　　traumatic aortic aneurysm (S25.09, S35.09)

● I71.0 Dissection of aorta

I71.00 Dissection of unspecified site of aorta

I71.01 Dissection of thoracic aorta

I71.02 Dissection of abdominal aorta

I71.03 Dissection of thoracoabdominal aorta

I71.1 Thoracic aortic aneurysm, ruptured

I71.2 Thoracic aortic aneurysm, without rupture

I71.3 Abdominal aortic aneurysm, ruptured

I71.4 Abdominal aortic aneurysm, without rupture

I71.5 Thoracoabdominal aortic aneurysm, ruptured

I71.6 Thoracoabdominal aortic aneurysm, without rupture

I71.8 Aortic aneurysm of unspecified site, ruptured
　　Rupture of aorta NOS

I71.9 Aortic aneurysm of unspecified site, without rupture
　　Aneurysm of aorta
　　Dilatation of aorta
　　Hyaline necrosis of aorta

● I72 Other aneurysm

　Includes aneurysm (cirsoid) (false) (ruptured)
　Excludes2 acquired aneurysm (I77.0)
　　aneurysm (of) aorta (I71.-)
　　aneurysm (of) arteriovenous NOS (Q27.3-)
　　carotid artery dissection (I77.71)
　　cerebral (nonruptured) aneurysm (I67.1)
　　coronary aneurysm (I25.4)
　　coronary artery dissection (I25.42)
　　dissection of artery NEC (I77.79)
　　heart aneurysm (I25.3)
　　iliac artery dissection (I77.72)
　　pulmonary artery aneurysm (I28.1)
　　renal artery dissection (I77.73)
　　retinal aneurysm (H35.0)
　　ruptured cerebral aneurysm (I60.7)
　　varicose aneurysm (I77.0)
　　vertebral artery dissection (I77.74)

I72.0 Aneurysm of carotid artery
　　Aneurysm of common carotid artery
　　Aneurysm of external carotid artery
　　Aneurysm of internal carotid artery, extracranial portion

　Excludes1 aneurysm of internal carotid artery, intracranial portion (I67.1)
　　aneurysm of internal carotid artery NOS (I67.1)

I72.1 Aneurysm of artery of upper extremity

I72.2 Aneurysm of renal artery

I72.3 Aneurysm of iliac artery

I72.4 Aneurysm of artery of lower extremity

I72.8 Aneurysm of other specified arteries

I72.9 Aneurysm of unspecified site

● I73 Other peripheral vascular diseases

　Excludes2 chilblains (T69.1)
　　frostbite (T33-T34)
　　immersion hand or foot (T69.0-)
　　spasm of cerebral artery (G45.9)

● I73.0 Raynaud's syndrome
　　Diminishing oxygen supply to fingers, toes, nose, and ears when exposed to temperature changes or stress
　　Raynaud's disease
　　Raynaud's phenomenon (secondary)

I73.00 Raynaud's syndrome without gangrene

I73.01 Raynaud's syndrome with gangrene

I73.1 Thromboangiitis obliterans [Buerger's disease]
　　Inflammatory occlusive disease resulting in poor circulation to the legs, feet, and sometimes the hands due to progressive inflammatory narrowing and eventually obliteration of the small arteries

● I73.8 Other specified peripheral vascular diseases

　Excludes1 diabetic (peripheral) angiopathy (E08-E13 with .51-.52)

I73.81 Erythromelalgia

I73.89 Other specified peripheral vascular diseases
　　Acrocyanosis
　　Erythrocyanosis
　　Simple acroparesthesia [Schultze's type]
　　Vasomotor acroparesthesia [Nothnagel's type]

I73.9 Peripheral vascular disease, unspecified
　　Intermittent claudication
　　Peripheral angiopathy NOS
　　Spasm of artery

　Excludes1 atherosclerosis of the extremities (I70.2--I70.7-)

N Newborn Age: 0　**P** Pediatric Age: 0–17　**M** Maternity DX: 12–55　**A** Adult Age: 15–124　♀ Females Only　♂ Males Only

971

CHAPTER 9 (I00-I99)

CHAPTER 9 (I00-I99)

Item 9–9 An **embolus** is a mass of undissolved matter present in the blood that is transported by the blood current. A **thrombus** is a blood clot that occludes or shuts off a vessel. When a thrombus is dislodged, it becomes an embolus.

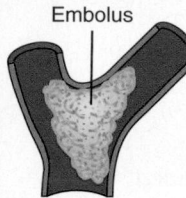

Embolus

Figure 9-3 An arterial embolus.

● **I74**   **Arterial embolism and thrombosis**

    Includes   embolic infarction
                   embolic occlusion
                   thrombotic infarction
                   thrombotic occlusion

    Code first embolism and thrombosis complicating abortion or ectopic or molar pregnancy (O00-O07, O08.2)
       embolism and thrombosis complicating pregnancy, childbirth and the puerperium (O88.-)

    Excludes2   atheroembolism (I75.-)
                 basilar embolism and thrombosis (I63.0-I63.2, I65.1)
                 carotid embolism and thrombosis (I63.0-I63.2, I65.2)
                 cerebral embolism and thrombosis (I63.3-I63.5, I66.-)
                 coronary embolism and thrombosis (I21-I25)
                 mesenteric embolism and thrombosis (K55.0)
                 ophthalmic embolism and thrombosis (H34.-)
                 precerebral embolism and thrombosis NOS (I63.0-I63.2, I65.9)
                 pulmonary embolism and thrombosis (I26.-)
                 renal embolism and thrombosis (N28.0)
                 retinal embolism and thrombosis (H34.-)
                 septic embolism and thrombosis (I76)
                 vertebral embolism and thrombosis (I63.0-I63.2, I65.0)

● **I74.0**   **Embolism and thrombosis of abdominal aorta**

    I74.01   **Saddle embolus of abdominal aorta**

    I74.09   **Other arterial embolism and thrombosis of abdominal aorta**
             Aortic bifurcation syndrome
             Aortoiliac obstruction
             Leriche's syndrome

● **I74.1**   **Embolism and thrombosis of other and unspecified parts of aorta**

    I74.10   **Embolism and thrombosis of unspecified parts of aorta**

    I74.11   **Embolism and thrombosis of thoracic aorta**

    I74.19   **Embolism and thrombosis of other parts of aorta**

    I74.2   **Embolism and thrombosis of arteries of the upper extremities**

    I74.3   **Embolism and thrombosis of arteries of the lower extremities**

    I74.4   **Embolism and thrombosis of arteries of extremities, unspecified**
           Peripheral arterial embolism NOS

    I74.5   **Embolism and thrombosis of iliac artery**

    I74.8   **Embolism and thrombosis of other arteries**

    I74.9   **Embolism and thrombosis of unspecified artery**

● **I75**   **Atheroembolism**

    Includes   atherothrombotic microembolism
                  cholesterol embolism

● **I75.0**   **Atheroembolism of extremities**

    ● **I75.01**   **Atheroembolism of upper extremity**

       I75.011   **Atheroembolism of right upper extremity**

       I75.012   **Atheroembolism of left upper extremity**

       I75.013   **Atheroembolism of bilateral upper extremities**

       I75.019   **Atheroembolism of unspecified upper extremity**

    ● **I75.02**   **Atheroembolism of lower extremity**

       I75.021   **Atheroembolism of right lower extremity**

       I75.022   **Atheroembolism of left lower extremity**

       I75.023   **Atheroembolism of bilateral lower extremities**

       I75.029   **Atheroembolism of unspecified lower extremity**

● **I75.8**   **Atheroembolism of other sites**

    I75.81   **Atheroembolism of kidney**
           Use additional code for any associated acute kidney failure and chronic kidney disease (N17.-, N18.-)

    I75.89   **Atheroembolism of other site**

I76   **Septic arterial embolism**
    Code first underlying infection, such as:
       infective endocarditis (I33.0)
       lung abscess (J85.-)
    Use additional code to identify the site of the embolism (I74.-)
    Excludes2   septic pulmonary embolism (I26.01, I26.90)

● **I77**   **Other disorders of arteries and arterioles**

    Excludes2   collagen (vascular) diseases (M30-M36)
                hypersensitivity angiitis (M31.0)
                pulmonary artery (I28.-)

    I77.0   **Arteriovenous fistula, acquired**
         Aneurysmal varix
         Arteriovenous aneurysm, acquired

      Excludes1   arteriovenous aneurysm NOS (Q27.3-)
                presence of arteriovenous shunt (fistula) for dialysis (Z99.2)
                traumatic - see injury of blood vessel by body region

      Excludes2   cerebral (I67.1)
                coronary (I25.4)

    I77.1   **Stricture of artery**
         Narrowing of artery

    I77.2   **Rupture of artery**
         Erosion of artery
         Fistula of artery
         Ulcer of artery

      Excludes1   traumatic rupture of artery - see injury of blood vessel by body region

    I77.3   **Arterial fibromuscular dysplasia**
         Fibromuscular hyperplasia (of) carotid artery
         Fibromuscular hyperplasia (of) renal artery

    I77.4   **Celiac artery compression syndrome**

    I77.5   **Necrosis of artery**

◀ New   ⬗ Revised   ~~deleted~~ Deleted   Excludes 1   Excludes 2   Includes   Use additional   Code first   Code also   Unspecified

OGCR Official Guidelines   X Assign placeholder X   ● Use Additional Character(s)   ▶ Manifestation Code   **Coding Clinic**

I77.6   Arteritis, unspecified
Aortitis NOS
Endarteritis NOS

> **Excludes1**   arteritis or endarteritis:
> aortic arch (M31.4)
> cerebral NEC (I67.7)
> coronary (I25.89)
> deformans (I70.-)
> giant cell (M31.5., M31.6)
> obliterans (I70.-)
> senile (I70.-)

● **I77.7**   Other arterial dissection

> **Excludes2**   dissection of aorta (I71.0-)
> dissection of coronary artery (I25.42)

    I77.71   Dissection of carotid artery

    I77.72   Dissection of iliac artery

    I77.73   Dissection of renal artery

    I77.74   Dissection of vertebral artery

    I77.79   Dissection of other artery

● **I77.8**   Other specified disorders of arteries and arterioles

    I77.81   Aortic ectasia
Ectasis aorta

> **Excludes1**   aortic aneurysm and dissection (I71.0-)

      I77.810   Thoracic aortic ectasia

      I77.811   Abdominal aortic ectasia

      I77.812   Thoracoabdominal aortic ectasia

      I77.819   Aortic ectasia, unspecified site

    I77.89   Other specified disorders of arteries and arterioles

I77.9   Disorder of arteries and arterioles, unspecified

● **I78**   Diseases of capillaries

I78.0   Hereditary hemorrhagic telangiectasia
Rendu-Osler-Weber disease

I78.1   Nevus, non-neoplastic
Araneus nevus   Spider nevus
Senile nevus   Stellar nevus

> **Excludes1**   nevus NOS (D22.-)
> vascular NOS (Q82.5)

> **Excludes2**   blue nevus (D22.-)
> flammeus nevus (Q82.5)
> hairy nevus (D22.-)
> melanocytic nevus (D22.-)
> pigmented nevus (D22.-)
> portwine nevus (Q82.5)
> sanguineous nevus (Q82.5)
> strawberry nevus (Q82.5)
> verrucous nevus (Q82.5)

I78.8   Other diseases of capillaries

I78.9   Disease of capillaries, unspecified

● **I79**   Disorders of arteries, arterioles and capillaries in diseases classified elsewhere

▷ *I79.0*   *Aneurysm of aorta in diseases classified elsewhere*

> *Code first underlying disease*

> **Excludes1**   syphilitic aneurysm (A52.01)

▷ *I79.1*   *Aortitis in diseases classified elsewhere*

> *Code first underlying disease*

> **Excludes1**   syphilitic aortitis (A52.02)

▷ *I79.8*   *Other disorders of arteries, arterioles and capillaries in diseases classified elsewhere*

> *Code first underlying disease, such as:*
> amyloidosis (E85.-)

> **Excludes1**   diabetic (peripheral) angiopathy (E08-E13 with .51-.52)
> syphilitic endarteritis (A52.09)
> tuberculous endarteritis (A18.89)

DISEASES OF VEINS, LYMPHATIC VESSELS AND LYMPH NODES, NOT ELSEWHERE CLASSIFIED (I80-I89)

● **I80**   Phlebitis and thrombophlebitis
Inflammation of a vein with infiltration of walls (phlebitis).

> **Includes**   endophlebitis
> inflammation, vein
> periphlebitis
> suppurative phlebitis

Code first phlebitis and thrombophlebitis complicating abortion, ectopic or molar pregnancy (O00-O07, O08.7)
phlebitis and thrombophlebitis complicating pregnancy, childbirth and the puerperium (O22.-, O87.-)

> **Excludes1**   venous embolism and thrombosis of lower extremities (I82.4-, I82.5-, I82.81-)

● **I80.0**   Phlebitis and thrombophlebitis of superficial vessels of lower extremities
Phlebitis and thrombophlebitis of femoropopliteal vein

    I80.00   Phlebitis and thrombophlebitis of superficial vessels of unspecified lower extremity

    I80.01   Phlebitis and thrombophlebitis of superficial vessels of right lower extremity

    I80.02   Phlebitis and thrombophlebitis of superficial vessels of left lower extremity

    I80.03   Phlebitis and thrombophlebitis of superficial vessels of lower extremities, bilateral

● **I80.1**   Phlebitis and thrombophlebitis of femoral vein

    I80.10   Phlebitis and thrombophlebitis of unspecified femoral vein

    I80.11   Phlebitis and thrombophlebitis of right femoral vein

    I80.12   Phlebitis and thrombophlebitis of left femoral vein

    I80.13   Phlebitis and thrombophlebitis of femoral vein, bilateral

● **I80.2**   Phlebitis and thrombophlebitis of other and unspecified deep vessels of lower extremities

  ● **I80.20**   Phlebitis and thrombophlebitis of unspecified deep vessels of lower extremities

      I80.201   Phlebitis and thrombophlebitis of unspecified deep vessels of right lower extremity

      I80.202   Phlebitis and thrombophlebitis of unspecified deep vessels of left lower extremity

      I80.203   Phlebitis and thrombophlebitis of unspecified deep vessels of lower extremities, bilateral

      I80.209   Phlebitis and thrombophlebitis of unspecified deep vessels of unspecified lower extremity

  ● **I80.21**   Phlebitis and thrombophlebitis of iliac vein

      I80.211   Phlebitis and thrombophlebitis of right iliac vein

      I80.212   Phlebitis and thrombophlebitis of left iliac vein

      I80.213   Phlebitis and thrombophlebitis of iliac vein, bilateral

      I80.219   Phlebitis and thrombophlebitis of unspecified iliac vein

  ● **I80.22**   Phlebitis and thrombophlebitis of popliteal vein

      I80.221   Phlebitis and thrombophlebitis of right popliteal vein

      I80.222   Phlebitis and thrombophlebitis of left popliteal vein

      I80.223   Phlebitis and thrombophlebitis of popliteal vein, bilateral

      I80.229   Phlebitis and thrombophlebitis of unspecified popliteal vein

CHAPTER 9 (I00-I99)

● I80.23 Phlebitis and thrombophlebitis of tibial vein

  I80.231 Phlebitis and thrombophlebitis of right tibial vein

  I80.232 Phlebitis and thrombophlebitis of left tibial vein

  I80.233 Phlebitis and thrombophlebitis of tibial vein, bilateral

  I80.239 Phlebitis and thrombophlebitis of unspecified tibial vein

● I80.29 Phlebitis and thrombophlebitis of other deep vessels of lower extremities

  I80.291 Phlebitis and thrombophlebitis of other deep vessels of right lower extremity

  I80.292 Phlebitis and thrombophlebitis of other deep vessels of left lower extremity

  I80.293 Phlebitis and thrombophlebitis of other deep vessels of lower extremity, bilateral

  I80.299 Phlebitis and thrombophlebitis of other deep vessels of unspecified lower extremity

I80.3 Phlebitis and thrombophlebitis of lower extremities, unspecified

I80.8 Phlebitis and thrombophlebitis of other sites

I80.9 Phlebitis and thrombophlebitis of unspecified site

I81 Portal vein thrombosis
  Portal (vein) obstruction
  Excludes2 hepatic vein thrombosis (I82.0)
    phlebitis of portal vein (K75.1)

● I82 Other venous embolism and thrombosis
  Code first venous embolism and thrombosis complicating:
  abortion, ectopic or molar pregnancy (O00-O07, O08.7)
  pregnancy, childbirth and the puerperium (O22.-, O87.-)
  Excludes2 venous embolism and thrombosis (of):
    cerebral (I63.6, I67.6)
    coronary (I21-I25)
    intracranial and intraspinal, septic or NOS (G08)
    intracranial, nonpyogenic (I67.6)
    intraspinal, nonpyogenic (G95.1)
    mesenteric (K55.0)
    portal (I81)
    pulmonary (I26.-)

I82.0 Budd-Chiari syndrome
  Hepatic vein thrombosis

I82.1 Thrombophlebitis migrans
  "White leg" is the other term to describe a migrating thrombus.

● I82.2 Embolism and thrombosis of vena cava and other thoracic veins

  ● I82.21 Embolism and thrombosis of superior vena cava

    I82.210 Acute embolism and thrombosis of superior vena cava
      Embolism and thrombosis of superior vena cava NOS

    I82.211 Chronic embolism and thrombosis of superior vena cava

  ● I82.22 Embolism and thrombosis of inferior vena cava

    I82.220 Acute embolism and thrombosis of inferior vena cava
      Embolism and thrombosis of inferior vena cava NOS

    I82.221 Chronic embolism and thrombosis of inferior vena cava

● I82.29 Embolism and thrombosis of other thoracic veins
  Embolism and thrombosis of brachiocephalic (innominate) vein

  I82.290 Acute embolism and thrombosis of other thoracic veins

  I82.291 Chronic embolism and thrombosis of other thoracic veins

I82.3 Embolism and thrombosis of renal vein

● I82.4 Acute embolism and thrombosis of deep veins of lower extremity

  I82.40 Acute embolism and thrombosis of unspecified deep veins of lower extremity
    Deep vein thrombosis NOS
    DVT NOS
    Excludes1 acute embolism and thrombosis of unspecified deep veins of distal lower extremity (I82.4Z-)
      acute embolism and thrombosis of unspecified deep veins of proximal lower extremity (I82.4Y-)

  I82.401 Acute embolism and thrombosis of unspecified deep veins of right lower extremity

  I82.402 Acute embolism and thrombosis of unspecified deep veins of left lower extremity

  I82.403 Acute embolism and thrombosis of unspecified deep veins of lower extremity, bilateral

  I82.409 Acute embolism and thrombosis of unspecified deep veins of unspecified lower extremity

● I82.41 Acute embolism and thrombosis of femoral vein

  I82.411 Acute embolism and thrombosis of right femoral vein

  I82.412 Acute embolism and thrombosis of left femoral vein

  I82.413 Acute embolism and thrombosis of femoral vein, bilateral

  I82.419 Acute embolism and thrombosis of unspecified femoral vein

● I82.42 Acute embolism and thrombosis of iliac vein

  I82.421 Acute embolism and thrombosis of right iliac vein

  I82.422 Acute embolism and thrombosis of left iliac vein

  I82.423 Acute embolism and thrombosis of iliac vein, bilateral

  I82.429 Acute embolism and thrombosis of unspecified iliac vein

● I82.43 Acute embolism and thrombosis of popliteal vein

  I82.431 Acute embolism and thrombosis of right popliteal vein

  I82.432 Acute embolism and thrombosis of left popliteal vein

  I82.433 Acute embolism and thrombosis of popliteal vein, bilateral

  I82.439 Acute embolism and thrombosis of unspecified popliteal vein

◀ New ◀▦ Revised ~~deleted~~ Deleted | Excludes 1 | Excludes 2 | Includes | Use additional | Code first | Code also | Unspecified

OGCR Official Guidelines   X Assign placeholder X   ● Use Additional Character(s)   ▶ Manifestation Code   **Coding Clinic**

● **I82.44**   **Acute embolism and thrombosis of tibial vein**

    I82.441   Acute embolism and thrombosis of right tibial vein

    I82.442   Acute embolism and thrombosis of left tibial vein

    I82.443   Acute embolism and thrombosis of tibial vein, bilateral

    I82.449   Acute embolism and thrombosis of unspecified tibial vein

● **I82.49**   **Acute embolism and thrombosis of other specified deep vein of lower extremity**

    I82.491   Acute embolism and thrombosis of other specified deep vein of right lower extremity

    I82.492   Acute embolism and thrombosis of other specified deep vein of left lower extremity

    I82.493   Acute embolism and thrombosis of other specified deep vein of lower extremity, bilateral

    I82.499   Acute embolism and thrombosis of other specified deep vein of unspecified lower extremity

● **I82.4Y**   **Acute embolism and thrombosis of unspecified deep veins of proximal lower extremity**

    Acute embolism and thrombosis of deep vein of thigh NOS

    Acute embolism and thrombosis of deep vein of upper leg NOS

    I82.4Y1   Acute embolism and thrombosis of unspecified deep veins of right proximal lower extremity

    I82.4Y2   Acute embolism and thrombosis of unspecified deep veins of left proximal lower extremity

    I82.4Y3   Acute embolism and thrombosis of unspecified deep veins of proximal lower extremity, bilateral

    I82.4Y9   Acute embolism and thrombosis of unspecified deep veins of unspecified proximal lower extremity

● **I82.4Z**   **Acute embolism and thrombosis of unspecified deep veins of distal lower extremity**

    Acute embolism and thrombosis of deep vein of calf NOS

    Acute embolism and thrombosis of deep vein of lower leg NOS

    I82.4Z1   Acute embolism and thrombosis of unspecified deep veins of right distal lower extremity

    I82.4Z2   Acute embolism and thrombosis of unspecified deep veins of left distal lower extremity

    I82.4Z3   Acute embolism and thrombosis of unspecified deep veins of distal lower extremity, bilateral

    I82.4Z9   Acute embolism and thrombosis of unspecified deep veins of unspecified distal lower extremity

● **I82.5**   **Chronic embolism and thrombosis of deep veins of lower extremity**

    Use additional code, if applicable, for associated long-term (current) use of anticoagulants (Z79.01)

    Excludes1   personal history of venous embolism and thrombosis (Z86.718)

● **I82.50**   **Chronic embolism and thrombosis of unspecified deep veins of lower extremity**

    Excludes1   chronic embolism and thrombosis of unspecified deep veins of distal lower extremity (I82.5Z-)

             chronic embolism and thrombosis of unspecified deep veins of proximal lower extremity (I82.5Y-)

    I82.501   Chronic embolism and thrombosis of unspecified deep veins of right lower extremity

    I82.502   Chronic embolism and thrombosis of unspecified deep veins of left lower extremity

    I82.503   Chronic embolism and thrombosis of unspecified deep veins of lower extremity, bilateral

    I82.509   Chronic embolism and thrombosis of unspecified deep veins of unspecified lower extremity

● **I82.51**   **Chronic embolism and thrombosis of femoral vein**

    I82.511   Chronic embolism and thrombosis of right femoral vein

    I82.512   Chronic embolism and thrombosis of left femoral vein

    I82.513   Chronic embolism and thrombosis of femoral vein, bilateral

    I82.519   Chronic embolism and thrombosis of unspecified femoral vein

● **I82.52**   **Chronic embolism and thrombosis of iliac vein**

    I82.521   Chronic embolism and thrombosis of right iliac vein

    I82.522   Chronic embolism and thrombosis of left iliac vein

    I82.523   Chronic embolism and thrombosis of iliac vein, bilateral

    I82.529   Chronic embolism and thrombosis of unspecified iliac vein

● **I82.53**   **Chronic embolism and thrombosis of popliteal vein**

    I82.531   Chronic embolism and thrombosis of right popliteal vein

    I82.532   Chronic embolism and thrombosis of left popliteal vein

    I82.533   Chronic embolism and thrombosis of popliteal vein, bilateral

    I82.539   Chronic embolism and thrombosis of unspecified popliteal vein

● **I82.54**   **Chronic embolism and thrombosis of tibial vein**

    I82.541   Chronic embolism and thrombosis of right tibial vein

    I82.542   Chronic embolism and thrombosis of left tibial vein

    I82.543   Chronic embolism and thrombosis of tibial vein, bilateral

    I82.549   Chronic embolism and thrombosis of unspecified tibial vein

Item 9–10 Varicose/Varicosities (varix = singular, varices = plural): Enlarged, engorged, tortuous, twisted vascular vessels (veins, arteries, lymphatics). As such, the condition can present in various parts of the body, although the most familiar locations are the lower extremities. A common complication of varices is thrombophlebitis. Varicosities of the anus and rectum are called hemorrhoids.

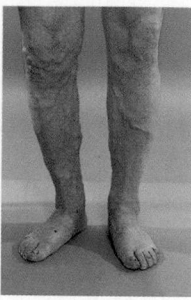

Figure 9-4 Varicose veins of the legs. (From Goldman: Cecil Medicine, ed 23, Saunders, 2008)

● **I82.59** Chronic embolism and thrombosis of other specified deep vein of lower extremity

     I82.591 Chronic embolism and thrombosis of other specified deep vein of right lower extremity

     I82.592 Chronic embolism and thrombosis of other specified deep vein of left lower extremity

     I82.593 Chronic embolism and thrombosis of other specified deep vein of lower extremity, bilateral

     I82.599 Chronic embolism and thrombosis of other specified deep vein of unspecified lower extremity

● **I82.5Y** Chronic embolism and thrombosis of unspecified deep veins of proximal lower extremity

     Chronic embolism and thrombosis of deep veins of thigh NOS

     Chronic embolism and thrombosis of deep veins of upper leg NOS

     I82.5Y1 Chronic embolism and thrombosis of unspecified deep veins of right proximal lower extremity

     I82.5Y2 Chronic embolism and thrombosis of unspecified deep veins of left proximal lower extremity

     I82.5Y3 Chronic embolism and thrombosis of unspecified deep veins of proximal lower extremity, bilateral

     I82.5Y9 Chronic embolism and thrombosis of unspecified deep veins of unspecified proximal lower extremity

● **I82.5Z** Chronic embolism and thrombosis of unspecified deep veins of distal lower extremity

     Chronic embolism and thrombosis of deep veins of calf NOS

     Chronic embolism and thrombosis of deep veins of lower leg NOS

     I82.5Z1 Chronic embolism and thrombosis of unspecified deep veins of right distal lower extremity

     I82.5Z2 Chronic embolism and thrombosis of unspecified deep veins of left distal lower extremity

     I82.5Z3 Chronic embolism and thrombosis of unspecified deep veins of distal lower extremity, bilateral

     I82.5Z9 Chronic embolism and thrombosis of unspecified deep veins of unspecified distal lower extremity

● **I82.6** Acute embolism and thrombosis of veins of upper extremity

   ● **I82.60** Acute embolism and thrombosis of unspecified veins of upper extremity

     I82.601 Acute embolism and thrombosis of unspecified veins of right upper extremity

     I82.602 Acute embolism and thrombosis of unspecified veins of left upper extremity

     I82.603 Acute embolism and thrombosis of unspecified veins of upper extremity, bilateral

     I82.609 Acute embolism and thrombosis of unspecified veins of unspecified upper extremity

   ● **I82.61** Acute embolism and thrombosis of superficial veins of upper extremity

     Acute embolism and thrombosis of antecubital vein

     Acute embolism and thrombosis of basilic vein

     Acute embolism and thrombosis of cephalic vein

     I82.611 Acute embolism and thrombosis of superficial veins of right upper extremity

     I82.612 Acute embolism and thrombosis of superficial veins of left upper extremity

     I82.613 Acute embolism and thrombosis of superficial veins of upper extremity, bilateral

     I82.619 Acute embolism and thrombosis of superficial veins of unspecified upper extremity

   ● **I82.62** Acute embolism and thrombosis of deep veins of upper extremity

     Acute embolism and thrombosis of brachial vein

     Acute embolism and thrombosis of radial vein

     Acute embolism and thrombosis of ulnar vein

     I82.621 Acute embolism and thrombosis of deep veins of right upper extremity

     I82.622 Acute embolism and thrombosis of deep veins of left upper extremity

     I82.623 Acute embolism and thrombosis of deep veins of upper extremity, bilateral

     I82.629 Acute embolism and thrombosis of deep veins of unspecified upper extremity

● **I82.7** Chronic embolism and thrombosis of veins of upper extremity

     Use additional code, if applicable, for associated long-term (current) use of anticoagulants (Z79.01)

     Excludes1 personal history of venous embolism and thrombosis (Z86.718)

   ● **I82.70** Chronic embolism and thrombosis of unspecified veins of upper extremity

     I82.701 Chronic embolism and thrombosis of unspecified veins of right upper extremity

     I82.702 Chronic embolism and thrombosis of unspecified veins of left upper extremity

     I82.703 Chronic embolism and thrombosis of unspecified veins of upper extremity, bilateral

     I82.709 Chronic embolism and thrombosis of unspecified veins of unspecified upper extremity

◀ New   ◀▥ Revised   ~~deleted~~ Deleted   Excludes 1   Excludes 2   Includes   Use additional   Code first   Code also   Unspecified

OGCR Official Guidelines   **X** Assign placeholder X   ● Use Additional Character(s)   ▌ Manifestation Code   **Coding Clinic**

● **I82.71**   Chronic embolism and thrombosis of superficial veins of upper extremity
     Chronic embolism and thrombosis of antecubital vein
     Chronic embolism and thrombosis of basilic vein
     Chronic embolism and thrombosis of cephalic vein

    I82.711   Chronic embolism and thrombosis of superficial veins of right upper extremity

    I82.712   Chronic embolism and thrombosis of superficial veins of left upper extremity

    I82.713   Chronic embolism and thrombosis of superficial veins of upper extremity, bilateral

    I82.719   Chronic embolism and thrombosis of superficial veins of ==unspecified== upper extremity

● **I82.72**   Chronic embolism and thrombosis of deep veins of upper extremity
     Chronic embolism and thrombosis of brachial vein
     Chronic embolism and thrombosis of radial vein
     Chronic embolism and thrombosis of ulnar vein

    I82.721   Chronic embolism and thrombosis of deep veins of right upper extremity

    I82.722   Chronic embolism and thrombosis of deep veins of left upper extremity

    I82.723   Chronic embolism and thrombosis of deep veins of upper extremity, bilateral

    I82.729   Chronic embolism and thrombosis of deep veins of ==unspecified== upper extremity

● **I82.A**   Embolism and thrombosis of axillary vein

 ● **I82.A1**   Acute embolism and thrombosis of axillary vein

    I82.A11   Acute embolism and thrombosis of right axillary vein

    I82.A12   Acute embolism and thrombosis of left axillary vein

    I82.A13   Acute embolism and thrombosis of axillary vein, bilateral

    I82.A19   Acute embolism and thrombosis of ==unspecified== axillary vein

 ● **I82.A2**   Chronic embolism and thrombosis of axillary vein

    I82.A21   Chronic embolism and thrombosis of right axillary vein

    I82.A22   Chronic embolism and thrombosis of left axillary vein

    I82.A23   Chronic embolism and thrombosis of axillary vein, bilateral

    I82.A29   Chronic embolism and thrombosis of ==unspecified== axillary vein

● **I82.B**   Embolism and thrombosis of subclavian vein

 ● **I82.B1**   Acute embolism and thrombosis of subclavian vein

    I82.B11   Acute embolism and thrombosis of right subclavian vein

    I82.B12   Acute embolism and thrombosis of left subclavian vein

    I82.B13   Acute embolism and thrombosis of subclavian vein, bilateral

    I82.B19   Acute embolism and thrombosis of ==unspecified== subclavian vein

 ● **I82.B2**   Chronic embolism and thrombosis of subclavian vein

    I82.B21   Chronic embolism and thrombosis of right subclavian vein

    I82.B22   Chronic embolism and thrombosis of left subclavian vein

    I82.B23   Chronic embolism and thrombosis of subclavian vein, bilateral

    I82.B29   Chronic embolism and thrombosis of ==unspecified== subclavian vein

● **I82.C**   Embolism and thrombosis of internal jugular vein

 ● **I82.C1**   Acute embolism and thrombosis of internal jugular vein

    I82.C11   Acute embolism and thrombosis of right internal jugular vein

    I82.C12   Acute embolism and thrombosis of left internal jugular vein

    I82.C13   Acute embolism and thrombosis of internal jugular vein, bilateral

    I82.C19   Acute embolism and thrombosis of ==unspecified== internal jugular vein

 ● **I82.C2**   Chronic embolism and thrombosis of internal jugular vein

    I82.C21   Chronic embolism and thrombosis of right internal jugular vein

    I82.C22   Chronic embolism and thrombosis of left internal jugular vein

    I82.C23   Chronic embolism and thrombosis of internal jugular vein, bilateral

    I82.C29   Chronic embolism and thrombosis of ==unspecified== internal jugular vein

● **I82.8**   Embolism and thrombosis of other specified veins
    Use additional code, if applicable, for associated long-term (current) use of anticoagulants (Z79.01)

 ● **I82.81**   Embolism and thrombosis of superficial veins of lower extremities
     Embolism and thrombosis of saphenous vein (greater) (lesser)

    I82.811   Embolism and thrombosis of superficial veins of right lower extremities

    I82.812   Embolism and thrombosis of superficial veins of left lower extremities

    I82.813   Embolism and thrombosis of superficial veins of lower extremities, bilateral

    I82.819   Embolism and thrombosis of superficial veins of ==unspecified== lower extremities

 ● **I82.89**   Embolism and thrombosis of other specified veins

    I82.890   Acute embolism and thrombosis of other specified veins

    I82.891   Chronic embolism and thrombosis of other specified veins

● **I82.9**   Embolism and thrombosis of unspecified vein

    I82.90   Acute embolism and thrombosis of ==unspecified== vein
     Embolism of vein NOS
     Thrombosis (vein) NOS

    I82.91   Chronic embolism and thrombosis of ==unspecified== vein

CHAPTER 9 (I00-I99)

● **I83**   **Varicose veins of lower extremities**
     Excludes1   varicose veins complicating pregnancy (O22.0-)
                varicose veins complicating the puerperium
                (O87.4)

● **I83.0**   **Varicose veins of lower extremities with ulcer**
     Use additional code to identify severity of ulcer (L97.-)

     ● **I83.00**   **Varicose veins of unspecified lower extremity with ulcer**

         I83.001   Varicose veins of unspecified lower extremity with ulcer of thigh   A

         I83.002   Varicose veins of unspecified lower extremity with ulcer of calf   A

         I83.003   Varicose veins of unspecified lower extremity with ulcer of ankle   A

         I83.004   Varicose veins of unspecified lower extremity with ulcer of heel and midfoot   A
                Varicose veins of unspecified lower extremity with ulcer of plantar surface of midfoot

         I83.005   Varicose veins of unspecified lower extremity with ulcer other part of foot   A
                Varicose veins of unspecified lower extremity with ulcer of toe

         I83.008   Varicose veins of unspecified lower extremity with ulcer other part of lower leg   A

         I83.009   Varicose veins of unspecified lower extremity with ulcer of unspecified site   A

     ● **I83.01**   **Varicose veins of right lower extremity with ulcer**

         I83.011   Varicose veins of right lower extremity with ulcer of thigh

         I83.012   Varicose veins of right lower extremity with ulcer of calf   A

         I83.013   Varicose veins of right lower extremity with ulcer of ankle   A

         I83.014   Varicose veins of right lower extremity with ulcer of heel and midfoot   A
                Varicose veins of right lower extremity with ulcer of plantar surface of midfoot

         I83.015   Varicose veins of right lower extremity with ulcer other part of foot   A
                Varicose veins of right lower extremity with ulcer of toe

         I83.018   Varicose veins of right lower extremity with ulcer other part of lower leg   A

         I83.019   Varicose veins of right lower extremity with ulcer of unspecified site   A

     ● **I83.02**   **Varicose veins of left lower extremity with ulcer**

         I83.021   Varicose veins of left lower extremity with ulcer of thigh   A

         I83.022   Varicose veins of left lower extremity with ulcer of calf   A

         I83.023   Varicose veins of left lower extremity with ulcer of ankle   A

         I83.024   Varicose veins of left lower extremity with ulcer of heel and midfoot   A
                Varicose veins of left lower extremity with ulcer of plantar surface of midfoot

         I83.025   Varicose veins of left lower extremity with ulcer other part of foot   A
                Varicose veins of left lower extremity with ulcer of toe

         I83.028   Varicose veins of left lower extremity with ulcer other part of lower leg   A

         I83.029   Varicose veins of left lower extremity with ulcer of unspecified site   A

● **I83.1**   **Varicose veins of lower extremities with inflammation**
     Stasis dermatitis

     I83.10   Varicose veins of unspecified lower extremity with inflammation   A

     I83.11   Varicose veins of right lower extremity with inflammation   A

     I83.12   Varicose veins of left lower extremity with inflammation   A

● **I83.2**   **Varicose veins of lower extremities with both ulcer and inflammation**
     Use additional code to identify severity of ulcer (L97.-)

     ● **I83.20**   **Varicose veins of unspecified lower extremity with both ulcer and inflammation**

         I83.201   Varicose veins of unspecified lower extremity with both ulcer of thigh and inflammation   A

         I83.202   Varicose veins of unspecified lower extremity with both ulcer of calf and inflammation   A

         I83.203   Varicose veins of unspecified lower extremity with both ulcer of ankle and inflammation   A

         I83.204   Varicose veins of unspecified lower extremity with both ulcer of heel and midfoot and inflammation   A
                Varicose veins of unspecified lower extremity with both ulcer of plantar surface of midfoot and inflammation

         I83.205   Varicose veins of unspecified lower extremity with both ulcer other part of foot and inflammation   A
                Varicose veins of unspecified lower extremity with both ulcer of toe and inflammation

         I83.208   Varicose veins of unspecified lower extremity with both ulcer of other part of lower extremity and inflammation   A

         I83.209   Varicose veins of unspecified lower extremity with both ulcer of unspecified site and inflammation   A

     ● **I83.21**   **Varicose veins of right lower extremity with both ulcer and inflammation**

         I83.211   Varicose veins of right lower extremity with both ulcer of thigh and inflammation   A

         I83.212   Varicose veins of right lower extremity with both ulcer of calf and inflammation   A

         I83.213   Varicose veins of right lower extremity with both ulcer of ankle and inflammation   A

         I83.214   Varicose veins of right lower extremity with both ulcer of heel and midfoot and inflammation   A
                Varicose veins of right lower extremity with both ulcer of plantar surface of midfoot and inflammation

◄ New   ◄ Revised   ~~deleted~~ Deleted   Excludes 1   Excludes 2   Includes   Use additional   Code first   Code also   Unspecified
OGCR Official Guidelines   X Assign placeholder X   ● Use Additional Character(s)   ▶ Manifestation Code   **Coding Clinic**

I83.215   Varicose veins of right lower extremity with both ulcer other part of foot and inflammation   **A**
     Varicose veins of right lower extremity with both ulcer of toe and inflammation

I83.218   Varicose veins of right lower extremity with both ulcer of other part of lower extremity and inflammation   **A**

I83.219   Varicose veins of right lower extremity with both ulcer of unspecified site and inflammation   **A**

● **I83.22**   Varicose veins of left lower extremity with both ulcer and inflammation

I83.221   Varicose veins of left lower extremity with both ulcer of thigh and inflammation   **A**

I83.222   Varicose veins of left lower extremity with both ulcer of calf and inflammation   **A**

I83.223   Varicose veins of left lower extremity with both ulcer of ankle and inflammation   **A**

I83.224   Varicose veins of left lower extremity with both ulcer of heel and midfoot and inflammation   **A**
     Varicose veins of left lower extremity with both ulcer of plantar surface of midfoot and inflammation

I83.225   Varicose veins of left lower extremity with both ulcer other part of foot and inflammation   **A**
     Varicose veins of left lower extremity with both ulcer of toe and inflammation

I83.228   Varicose veins of left lower extremity with both ulcer of other part of lower extremity and inflammation   **A**

I83.229   Varicose veins of left lower extremity with both ulcer of unspecified site and inflammation   **A**

● **I83.8**   Varicose veins of lower extremities with other complications

   ● **I83.81**   Varicose veins of lower extremities with pain

I83.811   Varicose veins of right lower extremities with pain   **A**

I83.812   Varicose veins of left lower extremities with pain   **A**

I83.813   Varicose veins of bilateral lower extremities with pain   **A**

I83.819   Varicose veins of unspecified lower extremities with pain   **A**

   ● **I83.89**   Varicose veins of lower extremities with other complications
     Varicose veins of lower extremities with edema
     Varicose veins of lower extremities with swelling

I83.891   Varicose veins of right lower extremities with other complications   **A**

I83.892   Varicose veins of left lower extremities with other complications   **A**

I83.893   Varicose veins of bilateral lower extremities with other complications   **A**

I83.899   Varicose veins of unspecified lower extremities with other complications   **A**

● **I83.9**   Asymptomatic varicose veins of lower extremities
     Phlebectasia of lower extremities
     Varicose veins of lower extremities
     Varix of lower extremities

I83.90   Asymptomatic varicose veins of unspecified lower extremity   **A**
     Varicose veins NOS

I83.91   Asymptomatic varicose veins of right lower extremity   **A**

I83.92   Asymptomatic varicose veins of left lower extremity   **A**

I83.93   Asymptomatic varicose veins of bilateral lower extremities   **A**

● **I85**   **Esophageal varices**
     Use additional code to identify:
     alcohol abuse and dependence (F10.-)

  ● **I85.0**   Esophageal varices
     Idiopathic esophageal varices
     Primary esophageal varices

I85.00   Esophageal varices without bleeding
     Esophageal varices NOS

I85.01   Esophageal varices with bleeding

  ● **I85.1**   Secondary esophageal varices
     Esophageal varices secondary to alcoholic liver disease
     Esophageal varices secondary to cirrhosis of liver
     Esophageal varices secondary to schistosomiasis
     Esophageal varices secondary to toxic liver disease
     Code first underlying disease

I85.10   Secondary esophageal varices without bleeding

I85.11   Secondary esophageal varices with bleeding

● **I86**   **Varicose veins of other sites**
     Excludes1   varicose veins of unspecified site (I83.9-)
     Excludes2   retinal varices (H35.0-)

I86.0   Sublingual varices

I86.1   Scrotal varices ♂
     Varicocele

I86.2   Pelvic varices

I86.3   Vulval varices ♀
     Excludes1   vulval varices complicating childbirth and the puerperium (O87.8)
          vulval varices complicating pregnancy (O22.1-)

I86.4   Gastric varices

I86.8   Varicose veins of other specified sites   **A**
     Varicose ulcer of nasal septum

● **I87**   **Other disorders of veins**

  ● **I87.0**   Postthrombotic syndrome
     Chronic venous hypertension due to deep vein thrombosis
     Postphlebitic syndrome
     Excludes1   chronic venous hypertension without deep vein thrombosis (I87.3-)

   ● **I87.00**   Postthrombotic syndrome without complications
     Asymptomatic Postthrombotic syndrome

I87.001   Postthrombotic syndrome without complications of right lower extremity

I87.002   Postthrombotic syndrome without complications of left lower extremity

I87.003   Postthrombotic syndrome without complications of bilateral lower extremity

I87.009   Postthrombotic syndrome without complications of unspecified extremity
     Postthrombotic syndrome NOS

CHAPTER 9 (I00–I99)

CHAPTER 9 (I00-I99)

● **I87.01**   **Postthrombotic syndrome with ulcer**
Use additional code to specify site and severity of ulcer (L97.-)

- **I87.011**   **Postthrombotic syndrome with ulcer of right lower extremity**
- **I87.012**   **Postthrombotic syndrome with ulcer of left lower extremity**
- **I87.013**   **Postthrombotic syndrome with ulcer of bilateral lower extremity**
- **I87.019**   **Postthrombotic syndrome with ulcer of unspecified lower extremity**

● **I87.02**   **Postthrombotic syndrome with inflammation**

- **I87.021**   **Postthrombotic syndrome with inflammation of right lower extremity**
- **I87.022**   **Postthrombotic syndrome with inflammation of left lower extremity**
- **I87.023**   **Postthrombotic syndrome with inflammation of bilateral lower extremity**
- **I87.029**   **Postthrombotic syndrome with inflammation of unspecified lower extremity**

● **I87.03**   **Postthrombotic syndrome with ulcer and inflammation**
Use additional code to specify site and severity of ulcer (L97.-)

- **I87.031**   **Postthrombotic syndrome with ulcer and inflammation of right lower extremity**
- **I87.032**   **Postthrombotic syndrome with ulcer and inflammation of left lower extremity**
- **I87.033**   **Postthrombotic syndrome with ulcer and inflammation of bilateral lower extremity**
- **I87.039**   **Postthrombotic syndrome with ulcer and inflammation of unspecified lower extremity**

● **I87.09**   **Postthrombotic syndrome with other complications**

- **I87.091**   **Postthrombotic syndrome with other complications of right lower extremity**
- **I87.092**   **Postthrombotic syndrome with other complications of left lower extremity**
- **I87.093**   **Postthrombotic syndrome with other complications of bilateral lower extremity**
- **I87.099**   **Postthrombotic syndrome with other complications of unspecified lower extremity**

I87.1   **Compression of vein**
Stricture of vein
Vena cava syndrome (inferior) (superior)

   Excludes2   compression of pulmonary vein (I28.8)

I87.2   **Venous insufficiency (chronic) (peripheral)**

● **I87.3**   **Chronic venous hypertension (idiopathic)**
Stasis edema

   Excludes1   chronic venous hypertension due to deep vein thrombosis (I87.0-)
varicose veins of lower extremities (I83.-)

● **I87.30**   **Chronic venous hypertension (idiopathic) without complications**
Asymptomatic chronic venous hypertension (idiopathic)

- **I87.301**   **Chronic venous hypertension (idiopathic) without complications of right lower extremity**
- **I87.302**   **Chronic venous hypertension (idiopathic) without complications of left lower extremity**
- **I87.303**   **Chronic venous hypertension (idiopathic) without complications of bilateral lower extremity**
- **I87.309**   **Chronic venous hypertension (idiopathic) without complications of unspecified lower extremity**
Chronic venous hypertension NOS

● **I87.31**   **Chronic venous hypertension (idiopathic) with ulcer**
Use additional code to specify site and severity of ulcer (L97.-)

- **I87.311**   **Chronic venous hypertension (idiopathic) with ulcer of right lower extremity**
- **I87.312**   **Chronic venous hypertension (idiopathic) with ulcer of left lower extremity**
- **I87.313**   **Chronic venous hypertension (idiopathic) with ulcer of bilateral lower extremity**
- **I87.319**   **Chronic venous hypertension (idiopathic) with ulcer of unspecified lower extremity**

● **I87.32**   **Chronic venous hypertension (idiopathic) with inflammation**

- **I87.321**   **Chronic venous hypertension (idiopathic) with inflammation of right lower extremity**
- **I87.322**   **Chronic venous hypertension (idiopathic) with inflammation of left lower extremity**
- **I87.323**   **Chronic venous hypertension (idiopathic) with inflammation of bilateral lower extremity**
- **I87.329**   **Chronic venous hypertension (idiopathic) with inflammation of unspecified lower extremity**

● **I87.33**   **Chronic venous hypertension (idiopathic) with ulcer and inflammation**
Use additional code to specify site and severity of ulcer (L97.-)

- **I87.331**   **Chronic venous hypertension (idiopathic) with ulcer and inflammation of right lower extremity**
- **I87.332**   **Chronic venous hypertension (idiopathic) with ulcer and inflammation of left lower extremity**
- **I87.333**   **Chronic venous hypertension (idiopathic) with ulcer and inflammation of bilateral lower extremity**
- **I87.339**   **Chronic venous hypertension (idiopathic) with ulcer and inflammation of unspecified lower extremity**

● **I87.39**   **Chronic venous hypertension (idiopathic) with other complications**

- **I87.391**   **Chronic venous hypertension (idiopathic) with other complications of right lower extremity**
- **I87.392**   **Chronic venous hypertension (idiopathic) with other complications of left lower extremity**
- **I87.393**   **Chronic venous hypertension (idiopathic) with other complications of bilateral lower extremity**
- **I87.399**   **Chronic venous hypertension (idiopathic) with other complications of unspecified lower extremity**

I87.8   **Other specified disorders of veins**
Phlebosclerosis
Venofibrosis

I87.9   **Disorder of vein, unspecified**

◄ New   ◄⁣⁣⁣⁣ Revised   ~~deleted~~ Deleted   Excludes 1   Excludes 2   Includes   Use additional   Code first   Code also   Unspecified
OGCR Official Guidelines   **X** Assign placeholder X   ● Use Additional Character(s)   ▶ Manifestation Code   **Coding Clinic**

● **I88** **Nonspecific lymphadenitis**

> **Excludes1** acute lymphadenitis, except mesenteric (L04.-)
> enlarged lymph nodes NOS (R59.-)
> human immunodeficiency virus [HIV] disease
> resulting in generalized lymphadenopathy
> (B20)

I88.0 **Nonspecific mesenteric lymphadenitis**
Mesenteric lymphadenitis (acute)(chronic)

I88.1 **Chronic lymphadenitis, except mesenteric**
Adenitis
Lymphadenitis

I88.8 **Other nonspecific lymphadenitis**

I88.9 **Nonspecific lymphadenitis, unspecified**
Lymphadenitis NOS

● **I89** **Other noninfective disorders of lymphatic vessels and lymph nodes**

> **Excludes1** chylocele, tunica vaginalis (nonfilarial) NOS
> (N50.8)
> enlarged lymph nodes NOS (R59.-)
> filarial chylocele (B74.-)
> hereditary lymphedema (Q82.0)

I89.0 **Lymphedema, not elsewhere classified**
Elephantiasis (nonfilarial) NOS
Lymphangiectasis
Obliteration, lymphatic vessel
Praecox lymphedema
Secondary lymphedema

> **Excludes1** postmastectomy lymphedema (I97.2)

I89.1 **Lymphangitis**
Chronic lymphangitis
Lymphangitis NOS
Subacute lymphangitis

> **Excludes1** acute lymphangitis (L03.-)

I89.8 **Other specified noninfective disorders of lymphatic vessels and lymph nodes**
Chylocele (nonfilarial)
Chylous ascites
Chylous cyst
Lipomelanotic reticulosis
Lymph node or vessel fistula
Lymph node or vessel infarction
Lymph node or vessel rupture

I89.9 **Noninfective disorder of lymphatic vessels and lymph nodes, unspecified**
Disease of lymphatic vessels NOS

OTHER AND UNSPECIFIED DISORDERS OF THE CIRCULATORY SYSTEM (I95-I99)

● **I95** **Hypotension**
Subnormal arterial blood pressure

> **Excludes1** cardiovascular collapse (R57.9)
> maternal hypotension syndrome (O26.5-)
> nonspecific low blood pressure reading NOS
> (R03.1)

I95.0 **Idiopathic hypotension**

I95.1 **Orthostatic hypotension**
Hypotension, postural
> *Moving from a sitting or reclining position to a standing position precipitates a sudden drop in blood pressure (hypotension).*

> **Excludes1** neurogenic orthostatic hypotension [Shy-Drager] (G90.3)
> orthostatic hypotension due to drugs
> (I95.2)

I95.2 **Hypotension due to drugs**
Orthostatic hypotension due to drugs
> Use additional code for adverse effect, if applicable, to identify drug (T36-T50 with fifth or sixth character 5)

I95.3 **Hypotension of hemodialysis**
Intra-dialytic hypotension

● **I95.8** **Other hypotension**

I95.81 **Postprocedural hypotension**

I95.89 **Other hypotension**
Chronic hypotension

I95.9 **Hypotension, unspecified**

I96 **Gangrene, not elsewhere classified**
Gangrenous cellulitis

> **Excludes1** gangrene in atherosclerosis of native arteries of
> the extremities (I70.26)
> gangrene of certain specified sites - *see*
> Alphabetical Index
> gangrene in diabetes mellitus (E08-E13)
> gangrene in hernia (K40.1, K40.4, K41.1, K41.4,
> K42.1, K43.1-, K44.1, K45.1, K46.1)
> gangrene in other peripheral vascular diseases
> (I73.-)
> gas gangrene (A48.0)
> pyoderma gangrenosum (L88)

Coding Clinic: 2013, Q2, P35

● **I97** **Intraoperative and postprocedural complications and disorders of circulatory system, not elsewhere classified**

> **Excludes2** postprocedural shock (T81.1-)

I97.0 **Postcardiotomy syndrome**

● **I97.1** **Other postprocedural cardiac functional disturbances**

> **Excludes2** acute pulmonary insufficiency following
> thoracic surgery (J95.1)
> intraoperative cardiac functional
> disturbances (I97.7-)

● **I97.11** **Postprocedural cardiac insufficiency**

I97.110 **Postprocedural cardiac insufficiency following cardiac surgery**

I97.111 **Postprocedural cardiac insufficiency following other surgery**

● **I97.12** **Postprocedural cardiac arrest**

I97.120 **Postprocedural cardiac arrest following cardiac surgery**

I97.121 **Postprocedural cardiac arrest following other surgery**

● **I97.13** **Postprocedural heart failure**
> Use additional code to identify the heart failure (I50.-)

I97.130 **Postprocedural heart failure following cardiac surgery**

I97.131 **Postprocedural heart failure following other surgery**

● **I97.19** **Other postprocedural cardiac functional disturbances**
> Use additional code, if applicable, to further specify disorder

I97.190 **Other postprocedural cardiac functional disturbances following cardiac surgery**

I97.191 **Other postprocedural cardiac functional disturbances following other surgery**

I97.2 **Postmastectomy lymphedema syndrome**   A
Elephantiasis due to mastectomy
Obliteration of lymphatic vessels

I97.3 **Postprocedural hypertension**

N Newborn Age: 0   **P** Pediatric Age: 0–17   **M** Maternity DX: 12–55   **A** Adult Age: 15–124   ♀ Females Only   ♂ Males Only

981

● **I97.4** **Intraoperative hemorrhage and hematoma of a circulatory system organ or structure complicating a procedure**

　　Excludes1　intraoperative hemorrhage and hematoma of a circulatory system organ or structure due to accidental puncture and laceration during a procedure (I97.5-)

　　Excludes2　intraoperative cerebrovascular hemorrhage complicating a procedure (G97.3-)

● **I97.41** **Intraoperative hemorrhage and hematoma of a circulatory system organ or structure complicating a circulatory system procedure**

　　I97.410 Intraoperative hemorrhage and hematoma of a circulatory system organ or structure complicating a cardiac catheterization

　　I97.411 Intraoperative hemorrhage and hematoma of a circulatory system organ or structure complicating a cardiac bypass

　　I97.418 Intraoperative hemorrhage and hematoma of a circulatory system organ or structure complicating other circulatory system procedure

　　I97.42 **Intraoperative hemorrhage and hematoma of a circulatory system organ or structure complicating other procedure**

● **I97.5** **Accidental puncture and laceration of a circulatory system organ or structure during a procedure**

　　Excludes2　accidental puncture and laceration of brain during a procedure (G97.4-)

　　I97.51 **Accidental puncture and laceration of a circulatory system organ or structure during a circulatory system procedure**

　　I97.52 **Accidental puncture and laceration of a circulatory system organ or structure during other procedure**

● **I97.6** **Postprocedural hemorrhage and hematoma of a circulatory system organ or structure following a procedure**

　　Excludes2　postprocedural cerebrovascular hemorrhage complicating a procedure (G97.5-)

● **I97.61** **Postprocedural hemorrhage and hematoma of a circulatory system organ or structure following a circulatory system procedure**

　　I97.610 Postprocedural hemorrhage and hematoma of a circulatory system organ or structure following a cardiac catheterization

　　I97.611 Postprocedural hemorrhage and hematoma of a circulatory system organ or structure following cardiac bypass

　　I97.618 Postprocedural hemorrhage and hematoma of a circulatory system organ or structure following other circulatory system procedure

　　I97.62 **Postprocedural hemorrhage and hematoma of a circulatory system organ or structure following other procedure**

● **I97.7** **Intraoperative cardiac functional disturbances**

　　Excludes2　acute pulmonary insufficiency following thoracic surgery (J95.1)
　　　　　　　　postprocedural cardiac functional disturbances (I97.1-)

● **I97.71** **Intraoperative cardiac arrest**

　　I97.710 Intraoperative cardiac arrest during cardiac surgery

　　I97.711 Intraoperative cardiac arrest during other surgery

● **I97.79** **Other intraoperative cardiac functional disturbances**

　　Use additional code, if applicable, to further specify disorder

　　I97.790 Other intraoperative cardiac functional disturbances during cardiac surgery

　　I97.791 Other intraoperative cardiac functional disturbances during other surgery

● **I97.8** **Other intraoperative and postprocedural complications and disorders of the circulatory system, not elsewhere classified**

　　Use additional code, if applicable, to further specify disorder

● **I97.81** **Intraoperative cerebrovascular infarction**

　　I97.810 Intraoperative cerebrovascular infarction during cardiac surgery

　　I97.811 Intraoperative cerebrovascular infarction during other surgery

● **I97.82** **Postprocedural cerebrovascular infarction**

　　I97.820 Postprocedural cerebrovascular infarction during cardiac surgery

　　I97.821 Postprocedural cerebrovascular infarction during other surgery

　　I97.88 **Other intraoperative complications of the circulatory system, not elsewhere classified**

　　I97.89 **Other postprocedural complications and disorders of the circulatory system, not elsewhere classified**

● **I99** **Other and unspecified disorders of circulatory system**

　　I99.8 **Other disorder of circulatory system**

　　I99.9 **Unspecified disorder of circulatory system**

◄ New　◄ Revised　deleted Deleted　Excludes 1　Excludes 2　Includes　Use additional　Code first　Code also　Unspecified

OGCR Official Guidelines　X Assign placeholder X　● Use Additional Character(s)　▶ Manifestation Code　**Coding Clinic**

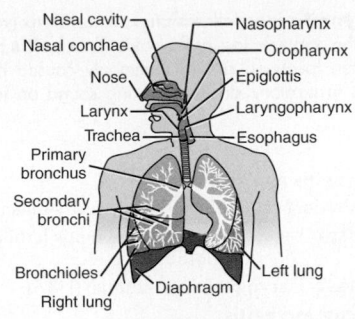

Figure 10–1 Respiratory system. (From Buck CJ: Step-by-Step Medical Coding, ed 2011, Philadelphia, WB Saunders, 2011)

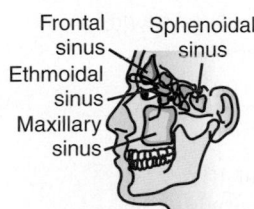

Figure 10-2 Paranasal sinuses. (From Buck CJ: Step-by-Step Medical Coding, ed 2011, Philadelphia, WB Saunders, 2011)

Item 10–1 Pharyngitis is painful inflammation of the pharynx (sore throat). Ninety percent of the infections are caused by a virus with the remaining being bacterial and rarely a fungus (candidiasis). Other irritants such as pollutants, chemicals, or smoke may cause similar symptoms.

OGCR See Section I.C., Chapter 10
Chronic Obstructive Pulmonary Disease (COPD) and Asthma

CHAPTER 10

DISEASES OF THE RESPIRATORY SYSTEM (J00-J99)

Note: When a respiratory condition is described as occurring in more than one site and is not specifically indexed, it should be classified to the lower anatomic site (e.g., tracheobronchitis to bronchitis in J40).

Use additional code, where applicable, to identify:
exposure to environmental tobacco smoke (Z77.22)
exposure to tobacco smoke in the perinatal period (P96.81)
history of tobacco use (Z87.891)
occupational exposure to environmental tobacco smoke (Z57.31)
tobacco dependence (F17.-)
tobacco use (Z72.0)

Excludes2   certain conditions originating in the perinatal period (P04-P96)
certain infectious and parasitic diseases (A00-B99)
complications of pregnancy, childbirth and the puerperium (O00-O99A)
congenital malformations, deformations and chromosomal abnormalities (Q00-Q99)
endocrine, nutritional and metabolic diseases (E00-E88)
injury, poisoning and certain other consequences of external causes (S00-T88)
neoplasms (C00-D49)
smoke inhalation (T59.81-)
symptoms, signs and abnormal clinical and laboratory findings, not elsewhere classified (R00-R94)

This chapter contains the following blocks:

J00-J06	Acute upper respiratory infections
J09-J18	Influenza and pneumonia
J20-J22	Other acute lower respiratory infections
J30-J39	Other diseases of upper respiratory tract
J40-J47	Chronic lower respiratory diseases
J60-J70	Lung diseases due to external agents
J80-J84	Other respiratory diseases principally affecting the interstitium
J85-J86	Suppurative and necrotic conditions of the lower respiratory tract
J90-J94	Other diseases of the pleura
J95	Intraoperative and postprocedural complications and disorders of respiratory system, not elsewhere classified
J96-J99	Other diseases of the respiratory system

ACUTE UPPER RESPIRATORY INFECTIONS (J00-J06)

Excludes1   chronic obstructive pulmonary disease with acute lower respiratory infection (J44.0)
influenza virus with other respiratory manifestations (J09.X2, J10.1, J11.1)

J00   **Acute nasopharyngitis [common cold]**
Acute rhinitis
Coryza (acute)
Infective nasopharyngitis NOS
Infective rhinitis
Nasal catarrh, acute
Nasopharyngitis NOS

Excludes1   acute pharyngitis (J02.-)
acute sore throat NOS (J02.9)
pharyngitis NOS (J02.9)
rhinitis NOS (J31.0)
sore throat NOS (J02.9)

Excludes2   allergic rhinitis (J30.1-J30.9)
chronic pharyngitis (J31.2)
chronic rhinitis (J31.0)
chronic sore throat (J31.2)
nasopharyngitis, chronic (J31.1)
vasomotor rhinitis (J30.0)

(See Plate 49 on page 72.)

● **J01**   **Acute sinusitis**
    Includes   acute abscess of sinus
acute empyema of sinus
acute infection of sinus
acute inflammation of sinus
acute suppuration of sinus

Use additional code (B95-B97) to identify infectious agent.
    Excludes1   sinusitis NOS (J32.9)
    Excludes2   chronic sinusitis (J32.0-J32.8)

● **J01.0**   **Acute maxillary sinusitis**
Acute antritis
    J01.00   **Acute maxillary sinusitis, unspecified**
    J01.01   **Acute recurrent maxillary sinusitis**

● **J01.1**   **Acute frontal sinusitis**
    J01.10   **Acute frontal sinusitis, unspecified**
    J01.11   **Acute recurrent frontal sinusitis**

● **J01.2**   **Acute ethmoidal sinusitis**
    J01.20   **Acute ethmoidal sinusitis, unspecified**
    J01.21   **Acute recurrent ethmoidal sinusitis**

● **J01.3**   **Acute sphenoidal sinusitis**
    J01.30   **Acute sphenoidal sinusitis, unspecified**
    J01.31   **Acute recurrent sphenoidal sinusitis**

● **J01.4**   **Acute pansinusitis**
    J01.40   **Acute pansinusitis, unspecified**
    J01.41   **Acute recurrent pansinusitis**

● **J01.8**   **Other acute sinusitis**

     J01.80   **Other acute sinusitis**
         Acute sinusitis involving more than one sinus but not pansinusitis

     J01.81   **Other acute recurrent sinusitis**
         Acute recurrent sinusitis involving more than one sinus but not pansinusitis

● **J01.9**   **Acute sinusitis, unspecified**

     J01.90   **Acute sinusitis, unspecified**

     J01.91   **Acute recurrent sinusitis, unspecified**

● **J02**   **Acute pharyngitis**

     Includes   acute sore throat

     Excludes1   acute laryngopharyngitis (J06.0)
         peritonsillar abscess (J36)
         pharyngeal abscess (J39.1)
         retropharyngeal abscess (J39.0)

     Excludes2   chronic pharyngitis (J31.2)

     J02.0   **Streptococcal pharyngitis**
         Septic pharyngitis
         Streptococcal sore throat

         Excludes2   scarlet fever (A38.-)

     J02.8   **Acute pharyngitis due to other specified organisms**
         Use additional code (B95-B97) to identify infectious agent

         Excludes1   pharyngitis due to coxsackie virus (B08.5)
              pharyngitis due to gonococcus (A54.5)
              acute pharyngitis due to herpes [simplex] virus (B00.2)
              acute pharyngitis due to infectious mononucleosis (B27.-)
              enteroviral vesicular pharyngitis (B08.5)

     J02.9   **Acute pharyngitis, unspecified**
         Gangrenous pharyngitis (acute)
         Infective pharyngitis (acute) NOS
         Pharyngitis (acute) NOS
         Sore throat (acute) NOS
         Suppurative pharyngitis (acute)
         Ulcerative pharyngitis (acute)

● **J03**   **Acute tonsillitis**

     Inflammation of pharyngeal tonsils caused by virus or bacteria

     Excludes1   acute sore throat (J02.-)
         hypertrophy of tonsils (J35.1)
         peritonsillar abscess (J36)
         sore throat NOS (J02.9)
         streptococcal sore throat (J02.0)

     Excludes2   chronic tonsillitis (J35.0)

●   J03.0   **Streptococcal tonsillitis**

     J03.00   **Acute streptococcal tonsillitis, unspecified**

     J03.01   **Acute recurrent streptococcal tonsillitis**

●   J03.8   **Acute tonsillitis due to other specified organisms**
         Use additional code (B95-B97) to identify infectious agent.

         Excludes1   diphtheritic tonsillitis (A36.0)
              herpesviral pharyngotonsillitis (B00.2)
              streptococcal tonsillitis (J03.0)
              tuberculous tonsillitis (A15.8)
              Vincent's tonsillitis (A69.1)

     J03.80   **Acute tonsillitis due to other specified organisms**

     J03.81   **Acute recurrent tonsillitis due to other specified organisms**

●   J03.9   **Acute tonsillitis, unspecified**
         Follicular tonsillitis (acute)
         Gangrenous tonsillitis (acute)
         Infective tonsillitis (acute)
         Tonsillitis (acute) NOS
         Ulcerative tonsillitis (acute)

     J03.90   **Acute tonsillitis, unspecified**

     J03.91   **Acute recurrent tonsillitis, unspecified**

Item 10–2   **Laryngitis** is an inflammation of the larynx (voice box) resulting in hoarse voice or the complete loss of the voice. **Tracheitis** is an inflammation of the trachea (often following a URI) commonly caused by *staphylococcus aureus* resulting in inspiratory stridor (crowing sound on inspiration) and a croup like cough.

● **J04**   **Acute laryngitis and tracheitis**
     Use additional code (B95-B97) to identify infectious agent.

     Excludes1   acute obstructive laryngitis [croup] and epiglottitis (J05.-)

     Excludes2   laryngismus (stridulus) (J38.5)

     J04.0   **Acute laryngitis**
         Edematous laryngitis (acute)
         Laryngitis (acute) NOS
         Subglottic laryngitis (acute)
         Suppurative laryngitis (acute)
         Ulcerative laryngitis (acute)

         Excludes1   acute obstructive laryngitis (J05.0)

         Excludes2   chronic laryngitis (J37.0)

●   J04.1   **Acute tracheitis**
         Acute viral tracheitis
         Catarrhal tracheitis (acute)
         Tracheitis (acute) NOS

         Excludes2   chronic tracheitis (J42)

     J04.10   **Acute tracheitis without obstruction**

     J04.11   **Acute tracheitis with obstruction**

     J04.2   **Acute laryngotracheitis**
         Laryngotracheitis NOS
         Tracheitis (acute) with laryngitis (acute)

         Excludes1   acute obstructive laryngotracheitis (J05.0)

         Excludes2   chronic laryngotracheitis (J37.1)

●   J04.3   **Supraglottitis, unspecified**

     J04.30   **Supraglottitis, unspecified, without obstruction**

     J04.31   **Supraglottitis, unspecified, with obstruction**

● **J05**   **Acute obstructive laryngitis [croup] and epiglottitis**
     Use additional code (B95-B97) to identify infectious agent.

     J05.0   **Acute obstructive laryngitis [croup]**
         Obstructive laryngitis (acute) NOS
         Obstructive laryngotracheitis NOS

     J05.1   **Acute epiglottitis**

         Excludes2   epiglottitis, chronic (J37.0)

     J05.10   **Acute epiglottitis without obstruction**
          Epiglottitis NOS

     J05.11   **Acute epiglottitis with obstruction**

● **J06**   **Acute upper respiratory infections of multiple and unspecified sites**

     Excludes1   acute respiratory infection NOS (J22)
         streptococcal pharyngitis (J02.0)

     J06.0   **Acute laryngopharyngitis**

     J06.9   **Acute upper respiratory infection, unspecified**
         Upper respiratory disease, acute
         Upper respiratory infection NOS

◀ New   ◀⁞⁞ Revised   ~~deleted~~ Deleted   Excludes 1   Excludes 2   Includes   Use additional   Code first   Code also   Unspecified

OGCR Official Guidelines   **X** Assign placeholder X   ● Use Additional Character(s)   ▶ Manifestation Code   **Coding Clinic**

INFLUENZA AND PNEUMONIA (J09-J18)

Excludes2   allergic or eosinophilic pneumonia (J82)
aspiration pneumonia NOS (J69.0)
meconium pneumonia (P24.01)
neonatal aspiration pneumonia (P24.-)
pneumonia due to solids and liquids (J69.-)
congenital pneumonia (P23.9)
lipid pneumonia (J69.1)
rheumatic pneumonia (I00)
ventilator associated pneumonia (J95.851)

● **J09**   **Influenza due to certain identified influenza viruses**

    Excludes1   influenza due to other influenza viruses (J10.-)
influenza due to unidentified influenza virus (J11.-)
seasonal influenza due to other identified influenza virus (J10.-)
seasonal influenza due to unidentified influenza virus (J11.-)

● **J09.X**   **Influenza due to identified novel influenza A virus**
Avian influenza
Bird influenza
Influenza A/H5N1
Influenza of other animal origin, not bird or swine
Swine influenza virus (viruses that normally cause infections in pigs)

   J09.X1   **Influenza due to identified novel influenza A virus with pneumonia**
Code also , if applicable, associated:
lung abscess (J85.1)
other specified type of pneumonia

   J09.X2   **Influenza due to identified novel influenza A virus with other respiratory manifestations**
Influenza due to identified novel influenza A virus NOS
Influenza due to identified novel influenza A virus with laryngitis
Influenza due to identified novel influenza A virus with pharyngitis
Influenza due to identified novel influenza A virus with upper respiratory symptoms
Use additional code, if applicable, for associated:
pleural effusion (J91.8)
sinusitis (J01.-)

   J09.X3   **Influenza due to identified novel influenza A virus with gastrointestinal manifestations**
Influenza due to identified novel influenza A virus gastroenteritis

     Excludes1   'intestinal flu' [viral gastroenteritis] (A08.-)

   J09.X9   **Influenza due to identified novel influenza A virus with other manifestations**
Influenza due to identified novel influenza A virus with encephalopathy
Influenza due to identified novel influenza A virus with myocarditis
Influenza due to identified novel influenza A virus with otitis media
Use additional code to identify manifestation

● **J10**   **Influenza due to other identified influenza virus**

    Excludes1   influenza due to avian influenza virus (J09.X-)
influenza due to swine flu (J09.X-)
influenza due to unidentified influenza virus (J11.-)

● **J10.0**   **Influenza due to other identified influenza virus with pneumonia**
Code also associated lung abscess, if applicable (J85.1)

   J10.00   **Influenza due to other identified influenza virus with unspecified type of pneumonia**

   J10.01   **Influenza due to other identified influenza virus with the same other identified influenza virus pneumonia**

   J10.08   **Influenza due to other identified influenza virus with other specified pneumonia**
Code also other specified type of pneumonia

   J10.1   **Influenza due to other identified influenza virus with other respiratory manifestations**
Influenza due to other identified influenza virus NOS
Influenza due to other identified influenza virus with laryngitis
Influenza due to other identified influenza virus with pharyngitis
Influenza due to other identified influenza virus with upper respiratory symptoms
Use additional code for associated pleural effusion, if applicable (J91.8)
Use additional code for associated sinusitis, if applicable (J01.-)

   J10.2   **Influenza due to other identified influenza virus with gastrointestinal manifestations**
Influenza due to other identified influenza virus gastroenteritis

     Excludes1   'intestinal flu' [viral gastroenteritis] (A08.-)

● **J10.8**   **Influenza due to other identified influenza virus with other manifestations**

   J10.81   **Influenza due to other identified influenza virus with encephalopathy**

   J10.82   **Influenza due to other identified influenza virus with myocarditis**

   J10.83   **Influenza due to other identified influenza virus with otitis media**
Use additional code for any associated perforated tympanic membrane (H72.-)

   J10.89   **Influenza due to other identified influenza virus with other manifestations**
Use additional codes to identify the manifestations

● **J11**   **Influenza due to unidentified influenza virus**

● **J11.0**   **Influenza due to unidentified influenza virus with pneumonia**
Code also associated lung abscess, if applicable (J85.1)

   J11.00   **Influenza due to unidentified influenza virus with unspecified type of pneumonia**
Influenza with pneumonia NOS

   J11.08   **Influenza due to unidentified influenza virus with specified pneumonia**
Code also other specified type of pneumonia

J11.1 Influenza due to unidentified influenza virus with other respiratory manifestations
Influenza NOS
Influenzal laryngitis NOS
Influenzal pharyngitis NOS
Influenza with upper respiratory symptoms NOS

Use additional code for associated pleural effusion, if applicable (J91.8)

Use additional code for associated sinusitis, if applicable (J01.-)

J11.2 Influenza due to unidentified influenza virus with gastrointestinal manifestations
Influenza gastroenteritis NOS

Excludes1 'intestinal flu' [viral gastroenteritis] (A08.-)

● **J11.8 Influenza due to unidentified influenza virus with other manifestations**

J11.81 Influenza due to unidentified influenza virus with encephalopathy
Influenzal encephalopathy NOS

J11.82 Influenza due to unidentified influenza virus with myocarditis
Influenzal myocarditis NOS

J11.83 Influenza due to unidentified influenza virus with otitis media
Influenzal otitis media NOS

Use additional code for any associated perforated tympanic membrane (H72.-)

J11.89 Influenza due to unidentified influenza virus with other manifestations

Use additional codes to identify the manifestations

● **J12 Viral pneumonia, not elsewhere classified**

Includes bronchopneumonia due to viruses other than influenza viruses

Code first associated influenza, if applicable (J09.X1, J10.0-, J11.0-)

Code also associated abscess, if applicable (J85.1)

Excludes1 aspiration pneumonia due to anesthesia during labor and delivery (O74.0)
aspiration pneumonia due to anesthesia during pregnancy (O29)
aspiration pneumonia due to anesthesia during puerperium (O89.0)
aspiration pneumonia due to solids and liquids (J69.-)
aspiration pneumonia NOS (J69.0)
congenital pneumonia (P23.0)
congenital rubella pneumonitis (P35.0)
interstitial pneumonia NOS (J84.9)
lipid pneumonia (J69.1)
neonatal aspiration pneumonia (P24.-)

J12.0 Adenoviral pneumonia

J12.1 Respiratory syncytial virus pneumonia

J12.2 Parainfluenza virus pneumonia

J12.3 Human metapneumovirus pneumonia

● **J12.8 Other viral pneumonia**

J12.81 Pneumonia due to SARS-associated coronavirus
Severe acute respiratory syndrome NOS

J12.89 Other viral pneumonia

J12.9 Viral pneumonia, unspecified

Item 10–3 Pneumonia is an infection of the lungs, caused by a variety of microorganisms, including viruses, most commonly the Streptococcus pneumoniae (pneumococcus) bacteria, fungi, and parasites. Pneumonia occurs when the immune system is weakened, often by a URI or influenza.

J13 Pneumonia due to Streptococcus pneumoniae
Bronchopneumonia due to S. pneumoniae

Code first associated influenza, if applicable (J09.X1, J10.0-, J11.0-)

Code also associated abscess, if applicable (J85.1)

Excludes1 congenital pneumonia due to S. pneumoniae (P23.6)
lobar pneumonia, unspecified organism (J18.1)
pneumonia due to other streptococci (J15.3-J15.4)

J14 Pneumonia due to Hemophilus influenzae
Bronchopneumonia due to H. influenzae

Code first associated influenza, if applicable (J09.X1, J10.0-, J11.0-)

Code also associated abscess, if applicable (J85.1)

Excludes1 congenital pneumonia due to H. influenzae (P23.6)

● **J15 Bacterial pneumonia, not elsewhere classified**

Includes bronchopneumonia due to bacteria other than S. pneumoniae and H. influenzae

Code first associated influenza, if applicable (J09.X1, J10.0-, J11.0-)

Code also associated abscess, if applicable (J85.1)

Excludes1 chlamydial pneumonia (J16.0)
congenital pneumonia (P23.-)
Legionnaires' disease (A48.1)
spirochetal pneumonia (A69.8)

J15.0 Pneumonia due to Klebsiella pneumoniae

J15.1 Pneumonia due to Pseudomonas

● **J15.2 Pneumonia due to staphylococcus**

J15.20 Pneumonia due to staphylococcus, unspecified

● **J15.21 Pneumonia due to staphylococcus aureus**

J15.211 Pneumonia due to Methicillin susceptible Staphylococcus aureus
MSSA pneumonia
Pneumonia due to Staphylococcus aureus NOS

J15.212 Pneumonia due to Methicillin resistant Staphylococcus aureus

J15.29 Pneumonia due to other staphylococcus

J15.3 Pneumonia due to streptococcus, group B

J15.4 Pneumonia due to other streptococci

Excludes1 pneumonia due to streptococcus, group B (J15.3)
pneumonia due to Streptococcus pneumoniae (J13)

J15.5 Pneumonia due to Escherichia coli

J15.6 Pneumonia due to other aerobic Gram-negative bacteria
Pneumonia due to Serratia marcescens

J15.7 Pneumonia due to Mycoplasma pneumoniae

J15.8 Pneumonia due to other specified bacteria

J15.9 Unspecified bacterial pneumonia
Pneumonia due to gram-positive bacteria

● **J16 Pneumonia due to other infectious organisms, not elsewhere classified**

Code first associated influenza, if applicable (J09.X1, J10.0-, J11.0-)

Code also associated abscess, if applicable (J85.1)

Excludes1 congenital pneumonia (P23.-)
ornithosis (A70)
pneumocystosis (B59)
pneumonia NOS (J18.9)

J16.0 Chlamydial pneumonia

J16.8 Pneumonia due to other specified infectious organisms

◀ New   ◀◀ Revised   ~~deleted~~ Deleted   Excludes 1   Excludes 2   Includes   Use additional   Code first   Code also   Unspecified

OGCR Official Guidelines   X Assign placeholder X   ● Use Additional Character(s)   ▌ Manifestation Code   **Coding Clinic**

▶ **J17**   *Pneumonia in diseases classified elsewhere*
     Code first underlying disease, such as:
       Q fever (A78)
       rheumatic fever (I00)
       schistosomiasis (B65.0-B65.9)

     Excludes1   candidial pneumonia (B37.1)
                chlamydial pneumonia (J16.0)
                gonorrheal pneumonia (A54.84)
                histoplasmosis pneumonia (B39.0-B39.2)
                measles pneumonia (B05.2)
                nocardiosis pneumonia (A43.0)
                pneumocystosis (B59)
                pneumonia due to Pneumocystis carinii (B59)
                pneumonia due to Pneumocystis jiroveci (B59)
                pneumonia in actinomycosis (A42.0)
                pneumonia in anthrax (A22.1)
                pneumonia in ascariasis (B77.81)
                pneumonia in aspergillosis (B44.0-B44.1)
                pneumonia in coccidioidomycosis (B38.0-B38.2)
                pneumonia in cytomegalovirus disease (B25.0)
                pneumonia in toxoplasmosis (B58.3)
                rubella pneumonia (B06.81)
                salmonella pneumonia (A02.22)
                spirochetal infection NEC with pneumonia
                   (A69.8)
                tularemia pneumonia (A21.2)
                typhoid fever with pneumonia (A01.03)
                varicella pneumonia (B01.2)
                whooping cough with pneumonia (A37 with
                   fifth-character 1)

● **J18**   **Pneumonia, unspecified organism**
     Code first associated influenza, if applicable (J09.X1, J10.0-, J11.0-)

     Excludes1   abscess of lung with pneumonia (J85.1)
                aspiration pneumonia due to anesthesia during
                   labor and delivery (O74.0)
                aspiration pneumonia due to anesthesia during
                   pregnancy (O29)
                aspiration pneumonia due to anesthesia during
                   puerperium (O89.0)
                aspiration pneumonia due to solids and liquids
                   (J69.-)
                aspiration pneumonia NOS (J69.0)
                congenital pneumonia (P23.0)
                drug-induced interstitial lung disorder
                   (J70.2-J70.4)
                interstitial pneumonia NOS (J84.9)
                lipid pneumonia (J69.1)
                neonatal aspiration pneumonia (P24.-)
                pneumonitis due to external agents (J67-J70)
                pneumonitis due to fumes and vapors (J68.0)
                usual interstitial pneumonia (J84.17)

    J18.0   **Bronchopneumonia, unspecified organism**

       Excludes1   hypostatic bronchopneumonia (J18.2)
                   lipid pneumonia (J69.1)

       Excludes2   acute bronchiolitis (J21.-)
                   chronic bronchiolitis (J44.9)

    J18.1   **Lobar pneumonia, unspecified organism**

    J18.2   **Hypostatic pneumonia, unspecified organism**
                Hypostatic bronchopneumonia
                Passive pneumonia

    J18.8   **Other pneumonia, unspecified organism**

    J18.9   **Pneumonia, unspecified organism**
           Coding Clinic: 2012, Q4, P94

OTHER ACUTE LOWER RESPIRATORY INFECTIONS (J20-J22)

     Excludes2   chronic obstructive pulmonary disease with acute
                   lower respiratory infection (J44.0)

● **J20**   **Acute bronchitis**
     Inflammation/irritation of the bronchial tubes lasting 2-3 weeks, most
       commonly caused by a virus.

     Includes   acute and subacute bronchitis (with)
                  bronchospasm
                acute and subacute bronchitis (with) tracheitis
                acute and subacute bronchitis (with)
                  tracheobronchitis, acute
                acute and subacute fibrinous bronchitis
                acute and subacute membranous bronchitis
                acute and subacute purulent bronchitis
                acute and subacute septic bronchitis

     Excludes1   bronchitis NOS (J40)
                tracheobronchitis NOS (J40)

     Excludes2   acute bronchitis with bronchiectasis (J47.0)
                acute bronchitis with chronic obstructive asthma
                  (J44.0)
                acute bronchitis with chronic obstructive
                  pulmonary disease (J44.0)
                allergic bronchitis NOS (J45.909-)
                bronchitis due to chemicals, fumes and vapors
                  (J68.0)
                chronic bronchitis NOS (J42)
                chronic mucopurulent bronchitis (J41.1)
                chronic obstructive bronchitis (J44.-)
                chronic obstructive tracheobronchitis (J44.-)
                chronic simple bronchitis (J41.0)
                chronic tracheobronchitis (J42)

    J20.0   **Acute bronchitis due to Mycoplasma pneumoniae**
    J20.1   **Acute bronchitis due to Hemophilus influenzae**
    J20.2   **Acute bronchitis due to streptococcus**
    J20.3   **Acute bronchitis due to coxsackievirus**
    J20.4   **Acute bronchitis due to parainfluenza virus**
    J20.5   **Acute bronchitis due to respiratory syncytial virus**
    J20.6   **Acute bronchitis due to rhinovirus**
    J20.7   **Acute bronchitis due to echovirus**
    J20.8   **Acute bronchitis due to other specified organisms**
    J20.9   **Acute bronchitis, unspecified**

● **J21**   **Acute bronchiolitis**
     Bronchiolitis obliterans with organizing pneumonia (BOOP)
       inflammation of bronchioles and surrounding tissue in lung.

     Includes   acute bronchiolitis with bronchospasm
     Excludes2   respiratory bronchiolitis interstitial lung disease
                  (J84.115)

    J21.0   **Acute bronchiolitis due to respiratory syncytial virus**
    J21.1   **Acute bronchiolitis due to human metapneumovirus**
    J21.8   **Acute bronchiolitis due to other specified organisms**
    J21.9   **Acute bronchiolitis, unspecified**
          Bronchiolitis (acute)

       Excludes1   chronic bronchiolitis (J44.-)

    J22   **Unspecified acute lower respiratory infection**
       Acute (lower) respiratory (tract) infection NOS

       Excludes1   upper respiratory infection (acute) (J06.9)

OTHER DISEASES OF UPPER RESPIRATORY TRACT (J30-J39)

● **J30   Vasomotor and allergic rhinitis**

Includes   spasmodic rhinorrhea

Excludes1   allergic rhinitis with asthma (bronchial) (J45.909)
rhinitis NOS (J31.0)

J30.0   Vasomotor rhinitis

J30.1   Allergic rhinitis due to pollen
Allergy NOS due to pollen
Hay fever
Pollinosis

J30.2   Other seasonal allergic rhinitis

J30.5   Allergic rhinitis due to food

● **J30.8   Other allergic rhinitis**

J30.81   Allergic rhinitis due to animal (cat) (dog) hair and dander

J30.89   Other allergic rhinitis
Perennial allergic rhinitis

J30.9   Allergic rhinitis, unspecified

● **J31   Chronic rhinitis, nasopharyngitis and pharyngitis**

Use additional code to identify:
exposure to environmental tobacco smoke (Z77.22)
exposure to tobacco smoke in the perinatal period (P96.81)
history of tobacco use (Z87.891)
occupational exposure to environmental tobacco smoke (Z57.31)
tobacco dependence (F17.-)
tobacco use (Z72.0)

J31.0   Chronic rhinitis
Atrophic rhinitis (chronic)
Granulomatous rhinitis (chronic)
Hypertrophic rhinitis (chronic)
Obstructive rhinitis (chronic)
Ozena
Purulent rhinitis (chronic)
Rhinitis (chronic) NOS
Ulcerative rhinitis (chronic)

Excludes1   allergic rhinitis (J30.1-J30.9)
vasomotor rhinitis (J30.0)

J31.1   Chronic nasopharyngitis

Excludes2   acute nasopharyngitis (J00)

J31.2   Chronic pharyngitis
Chronic sore throat
Atrophic pharyngitis (chronic)
Granular pharyngitis (chronic)
Hypertrophic pharyngitis (chronic)

Excludes2   acute pharyngitis (J02.9)

● **J32   Chronic sinusitis**

Includes   sinus abscess
sinus empyema
sinus infection
sinus suppuration

Use additional code to identify:
exposure to environmental tobacco smoke (Z77.22)
exposure to tobacco smoke in the perinatal period (P96.81)
history of tobacco use (Z87.891)
infectious agent (B95-B97)
occupational exposure to environmental tobacco smoke (Z57.31)
tobacco dependence (F17.-)
tobacco use (Z72.0)

Excludes2   acute sinusitis (J01.-)

J32.0   Chronic maxillary sinusitis
Antritis (chronic)
Maxillary sinusitis NOS

J32.1   Chronic frontal sinusitis
Frontal sinusitis NOS

Item 10–4   Nasal polyps are an abnormal growth of tissue (tumor) projecting from a mucous membrane and attached to the surface by a narrow elongated stalk (pedunculated). Nasal polyps usually originate in the ethmoid sinus but also may occur in the maxillary sinus. Symptoms are nasal block, sinusitis, anosmia, and secondary infections.

J32.2   Chronic ethmoidal sinusitis
Ethmoidal sinusitis NOS

Excludes1   Woakes' ethmoiditis (J33.1)

J32.3   Chronic sphenoidal sinusitis
Sphenoidal sinusitis NOS

J32.4   Chronic pansinusitis
Pansinusitis NOS

J32.8   Other chronic sinusitis
Sinusitis (chronic) involving more than one sinus but not pansinusitis

J32.9   Chronic sinusitis, unspecified
Sinusitis (chronic) NOS

● **J33   Nasal polyp**

Use additional code to identify:
exposure to environmental tobacco smoke (Z77.22)
exposure to tobacco smoke in the perinatal period (P96.81)
history of tobacco use (Z87.891)
occupational exposure to environmental tobacco smoke (Z57.31)
tobacco dependence (F17.-)
tobacco use (Z72.0)

Excludes1   adenomatous polyps (D14.0)

J33.0   Polyp of nasal cavity
Choanal polyp
Nasopharyngeal polyp

J33.1   Polypoid sinus degeneration
Woakes' syndrome or ethmoiditis

J33.8   Other polyp of sinus
Accessory polyp of sinus
Ethmoidal polyp of sinus
Maxillary polyp of sinus
Sphenoidal polyp of sinus

J33.9   Nasal polyp, unspecified

● **J34   Other and unspecified disorders of nose and nasal sinuses**

Excludes2   varicose ulcer of nasal septum (I86.8)

J34.0   Abscess, furuncle and carbuncle of nose
Cellulitis of nose
Necrosis of nose
Ulceration of nose

J34.1   Cyst and mucocele of nose and nasal sinus

J34.2   Deviated nasal septum
Deflection or deviation of septum (nasal) (acquired)

Excludes1   congenital deviated nasal septum (Q67.4)

J34.3   Hypertrophy of nasal turbinates

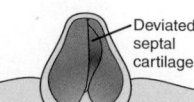
Deviated septal cartilage

Figure 10-3   Deviated nasal septum.

Item 10–5   A deviated nasal septum is the displacement of the septal cartilage that separates the nares. This displacement causes obstructed air flow through the nasal passages. A child can be born with this displacement (congenital), or the condition may be acquired through trauma, such as a sports injury. Symptoms include nasal block, sinusitis, and related secondary infections. Septoplasty is surgical repair of this condition.

◀ New   ◀|||| Revised   ~~deleted~~ Deleted   Excludes 1   Excludes 2   Includes   Use additional   Code first   Code also   Unspecified

OGCR Official Guidelines   X Assign placeholder X   ● Use Additional Character(s)   ▶ Manifestation Code   **Coding Clinic**

● **J34.8**   **Other specified disorders of nose and nasal sinuses**

   J34.81   **Nasal mucositis (ulcerative)**

      Code also type of associated therapy, such as:
        antineoplastic and immunosuppressive
         drugs (T45.1X-)
        radiological procedure and radiotherapy
         (Y84.2)

      Excludes2   gastrointestinal mucositis
             (ulcerative) (K92.81)
             mucositis (ulcerative) of vagina
               and vulva (N76.81)
             oral mucositis (ulcerative)
               (K12.3-)

   J34.89   **Other specified disorders of nose and nasal
        sinuses**
      Perforation of nasal septum NOS
      Rhinolith

J34.9   **Unspecified** **disorder of nose and nasal sinuses**

● **J35**   **Chronic diseases of tonsils and adenoids**
   Use additional code to identify:
     exposure to environmental tobacco smoke (Z77.22)
     exposure to tobacco smoke in the perinatal period (P96.81)
     history of tobacco use (Z87.891)
     occupational exposure to environmental tobacco smoke
       (Z57.31)
     tobacco dependence (F17.-)
     tobacco use (Z72.0)

 ● **J35.0**   **Chronic tonsillitis and adenoiditis**
     Excludes2   acute tonsillitis (J03.-)

   J35.01   **Chronic tonsillitis**
   J35.02   **Chronic adenoiditis**
   J35.03   **Chronic tonsillitis and adenoiditis**

  J35.1   **Hypertrophy of tonsils**
    Enlargement of tonsils
    Excludes1   hypertrophy of tonsils with tonsillitis
           (J35.0-)

  J35.2   **Hypertrophy of adenoids**
    Enlargement of adenoids
    Excludes1   hypertrophy of adenoids with adenoiditis
           (J35.0-)

  J35.3   **Hypertrophy of tonsils with hypertrophy of adenoids**
    Excludes1   hypertrophy of tonsils and adenoids with
           tonsillitis and adenoiditis (J35.03)

  J35.8   **Other chronic diseases of tonsils and adenoids**
    Adenoid vegetations
    Amygdalolith
    Calculus, tonsil
    Cicatrix of tonsil (and adenoid)
    Tonsillar tag
    Ulcer of tonsil

  J35.9   **Chronic disease of tonsils and adenoids, unspecified**
    Disease (chronic) of tonsils and adenoids NOS

J36   **Peritonsillar abscess**
   Includes   abscess of tonsil
         peritonsillar cellulitis
         quinsy
   Use additional code (B95-B97) to identify infectious agent.
   Excludes1   acute tonsillitis (J03.-)
         chronic tonsillitis (J35.0)
         retropharyngeal abscess (J39.0)
         tonsillitis NOS (J03.9-)

● **J37**   **Chronic laryngitis and laryngotracheitis**
   Use additional code to identify:
     exposure to environmental tobacco smoke (Z77.22)
     exposure to tobacco smoke in the perinatal period (P96.81)
     history of tobacco use (Z87.891)
     infectious agent (B95-B97)
     occupational exposure to environmental tobacco smoke
       (Z57.31)
     tobacco dependence (F17.-)
     tobacco use (Z72.0)

  J37.0   **Chronic laryngitis**
    Catarrhal laryngitis
    Hypertrophic laryngitis
    Sicca laryngitis
    Excludes2   acute laryngitis (J04.0)
         obstructive (acute) laryngitis (J05.0)

  J37.1   **Chronic laryngotracheitis**
    Laryngitis, chronic, with tracheitis (chronic)
    Tracheitis, chronic, with laryngitis
    Excludes1   chronic tracheitis (J42)
    Excludes2   acute laryngotracheitis (J04.2)
         acute tracheitis (J04.1)

● **J38**   **Diseases of vocal cords and larynx, not elsewhere classified**
   Use additional code to identify:
     exposure to environmental tobacco smoke (Z77.22)
     exposure to tobacco smoke in the perinatal period (P96.81)
     history of tobacco use (Z87.891)
     occupational exposure to environmental tobacco smoke
       (Z57.31)
     tobacco dependence (F17.-)
     tobacco use (Z72.0)
   Excludes1   congenital laryngeal stridor (P28.89)
         obstructive laryngitis (acute) (J05.0)
         postprocedural subglottic stenosis (J95.5)
         stridor (R06.1)
         ulcerative laryngitis (J04.0)

 ● **J38.0**   **Paralysis of vocal cords and larynx**
    Laryngoplegia
    Paralysis of glottis
   J38.00   **Paralysis of vocal cords and larynx, unspecified**
   J38.01   **Paralysis of vocal cords and larynx, unilateral**
   J38.02   **Paralysis of vocal cords and larynx, bilateral**

  J38.1   **Polyp of vocal cord and larynx**
    Excludes1   adenomatous polyps (D14.1)

  J38.2   **Nodules of vocal cords**
    Chorditis (fibrinous)(nodosa)(tuberosa)
    Singer's nodes
    Teacher's nodes

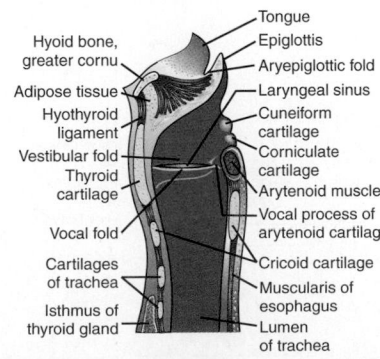

Figure 10-4   Coronal section of the larynx.

Item 10-6   The **larynx** extends from the tongue to the trachea and is divided into an upper and lower portion separated by folds. The framework of the larynx is cartilage composed of the single cricoid, thyroid, and epiglottic cartilages, and the paired arytenoid, cuneiform, and corniculate cartilages.

CHAPTER 10 (J00–J99)

J38.3   Other diseases of vocal cords
Abscess of vocal cords
Cellulitis of vocal cords
Granuloma of vocal cords
Leukokeratosis of vocal cords
Leukoplakia of vocal cords

J38.4   Edema of larynx
Edema (of) glottis
Subglottic edema
Supraglottic edema

> **Excludes1**   acute obstructive laryngitis [croup] (J05.0)
> edematous laryngitis (J04.0)

J38.5   Laryngeal spasm
Laryngismus (stridulus)

J38.6   Stenosis of larynx

J38.7   Other diseases of larynx
Abscess of larynx
Cellulitis of larynx
Disease of larynx NOS
Necrosis of larynx
Pachyderma of larynx
Perichondritis of larynx
Ulcer of larynx

● **J39   Other diseases of upper respiratory tract**

> **Excludes1**   acute respiratory infection NOS (J22)
> acute upper respiratory infection (J06.9)
> upper respiratory inflammation due to chemicals, gases, fumes or vapors (J68.2)

J39.0   Retropharyngeal and parapharyngeal abscess
Peripharyngeal abscess

> **Excludes1**   peritonsillar abscess (J36)

J39.1   Other abscess of pharynx
Cellulitis of pharynx
Nasopharyngeal abscess

J39.2   Other diseases of pharynx
Cyst of pharynx
Edema of pharynx

> **Excludes2**   chronic pharyngitis (J31.2)
> ulcerative pharyngitis (J02.9)

J39.3   Upper respiratory tract hypersensitivity reaction, site unspecified

> **Excludes1**   hypersensitivity reaction of upper respiratory tract, such as:
> extrinsic allergic alveolitis (J67.9)
> pneumoconiosis (J60-J67.9)

J39.8   Other specified diseases of upper respiratory tract

J39.9   Disease of upper respiratory tract, unspecified

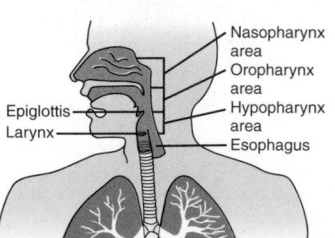

Nasopharynx area
Oropharynx area
Hypopharynx area
Esophagus
Epiglottis
Larynx

Figure 10-5   The pharynx.

Item 10–7 The **pharynx** is the passage for both food and air between the mouth and the esophagus and is divided into three areas: nasopharynx, oropharynx, and hypopharynx. The hypopharynx branches into the esophagus and the voice box.

Item 10–8 **Chronic bronchitis** is usually defined as being present in any patient who has persistent cough with sputum production for at least three months in at least two consecutive years. **Simple chronic bronchitis** is marked by a productive cough but no pathological airflow obstruction. **Chronic obstructive pulmonary disease (COPD)** is a group of conditions— bronchitis, emphysema, asthma, bronchiectasis, allergic alveolitis—marked by dyspnea. **Catarrhal** bronchitis is an acute form of bronchitis marked by profuse mucus and pus production (**mucopurulent** discharge). **Croupous** bronchitis, also known as pseudomembranous, fibrinous, plastic, exudative, or membranous, is marked by a violent cough and dyspnea.

CHRONIC LOWER RESPIRATORY DISEASES (J40-J47)

> **Excludes1**   bronchitis due to chemicals, gases, fumes and vapors (J68.0)

> **Excludes2**   cystic fibrosis (E84.-)

J40   Bronchitis, not specified as acute or chronic
Bronchitis NOS
Catarrhal bronchitis
Bronchitis with tracheitis NOS
Tracheobronchitis NOS

Use additional code to identify:
exposure to environmental tobacco smoke (Z77.22)
exposure to tobacco smoke in the perinatal period (P96.81)
history of tobacco use (Z87.891)
occupational exposure to environmental tobacco smoke (Z57.31)
tobacco dependence (F17.-)
tobacco use (Z72.0)

> **Excludes1**   acute bronchitis (J20.-)
> allergic bronchitis NOS (J45.909-)
> asthmatic bronchitis NOS (J45.9-)
> bronchitis due to chemicals, gases, fumes and vapors (J68.0)

● **J41   Simple and mucopurulent chronic bronchitis**

Use additional code to identify:
exposure to environmental tobacco smoke (Z77.22)
exposure to tobacco smoke in the perinatal period (P96.81)
history of tobacco use (Z87.891)
occupational exposure to environmental tobacco smoke (Z57.31)
tobacco dependence (F17.-)
tobacco use (Z72.0)

> **Excludes1**   chronic bronchitis NOS (J42)
> chronic obstructive bronchitis (J44.-)

J41.0   Simple chronic bronchitis

J41.1   Mucopurulent chronic bronchitis

J41.8   Mixed simple and mucopurulent chronic bronchitis

J42   Unspecified chronic bronchitis
Chronic bronchitis NOS
Chronic tracheitis
Chronic tracheobronchitis

Use additional code to identify:
exposure to environmental tobacco smoke (Z77.22)
exposure to tobacco smoke in the perinatal period (P96.81)
history of tobacco use (Z87.891)
occupational exposure to environmental tobacco smoke (Z57.31)
tobacco dependence (F17.-)
tobacco use (Z72.0)

> **Excludes1**   chronic asthmatic bronchitis (J44.-)
> chronic bronchitis with airways obstruction (J44.-)
> chronic emphysematous bronchitis (J44.-)
> chronic obstructive pulmonary disease NOS (J44.9)
> simple and mucopurulent chronic bronchitis (J41.-)

● **J43   Emphysema**

Use additional code to identify:

exposure to environmental tobacco smoke (Z77.22)

history of tobacco use (Z87.891)

occupational exposure to environmental tobacco smoke (Z57.31)

tobacco dependence (F17.-)

tobacco use (Z72.0)

Excludes1   compensatory emphysema (J98.3)

emphysema due to inhalation of chemicals, gases, fumes or vapors (J68.4)

emphysema with chronic (obstructive) bronchitis (J44.-)

emphysematous (obstructive) bronchitis (J44.-)

interstitial emphysema (J98.2)

mediastinal emphysema (J98.2)

neonatal interstitial emphysema (P25.0)

surgical (subcutaneous) emphysema (T81.82)

traumatic subcutaneous emphysema (T79.7)

J43.0   Unilateral pulmonary emphysema [MacLeod's syndrome]

Swyer-James syndrome

Unilateral emphysema

Unilateral hyperlucent lung

Unilateral pulmonary artery functional hypoplasia

Unilateral transparency of lung

J43.1   Panlobular emphysema

Panacinar emphysema

J43.2   Centrilobular emphysema

J43.8   Other emphysema

J43.9   Emphysema, unspecified

Bullous emphysema (lung)(pulmonary)

Emphysema (lung)(pulmonary) NOS

Emphysematous bleb

Vesicular emphysema (lung)(pulmonary)

● **J44   Other chronic obstructive pulmonary disease**

Includes   asthma with chronic obstructive pulmonary disease

chronic asthmatic (obstructive) bronchitis

chronic bronchitis with airways obstruction

chronic bronchitis with emphysema

chronic emphysematous bronchitis

chronic obstructive asthma

chronic obstructive bronchitis

chronic obstructive tracheobronchitis

Code also type of asthma, if applicable (J45.-)

Use additional code to identify:

exposure to environmental tobacco smoke (Z77.22)

history of tobacco use (Z87.891)

occupational exposure to environmental tobacco smoke (Z57.31)

tobacco dependence (F17.-)

tobacco use (Z72.0)

Excludes1   bronchiectasis (J47.-)

chronic bronchitis NOS (J42)

chronic simple and mucopurulent bronchitis (J41.-)

chronic tracheitis (J42)

chronic tracheobronchitis (J42)

emphysema without chronic bronchitis (J43.-)

lung diseases due to external agents (J60-J70)

J44.0   Chronic obstructive pulmonary disease with acute lower respiratory infection

Use additional code to identify the infection

J44.1   Chronic obstructive pulmonary disease with (acute) exacerbation

Decompensated COPD

Decompensated COPD with (acute) exacerbation

Excludes2   chronic obstructive pulmonary disease [COPD] with acute bronchitis (J44.0)

J44.9   Chronic obstructive pulmonary disease, unspecified

Chronic obstructive airway disease NOS

Chronic obstructive lung disease NOS

Item 10-9   Asthma is a bronchial condition marked by airway obstruction, hyper-responsiveness, and inflammation. **Extrinsic** asthma, also known as allergic asthma, is characterized by the same symptoms that occur with exposure to allergens and is divided into the following types: **atopic, occupational, and allergic bronchopulmonary aspergillosis. Intrinsic** asthma occurs in patients who have no history of allergy or sensitivities to allergens and is divided into the following types: **nonreaginic and pharmacologic. Status asthmaticus** is the most severe form of asthma attack and can last for days or weeks.

● **J45   Asthma**

Allergic (predominantly) asthma

Allergic bronchitis NOS

Allergic rhinitis with asthma

Atopic asthma

Extrinsic allergic asthma

Hay fever with asthma

Idiosyncratic asthma

Intrinsic nonallergic asthma

Nonallergic asthma

Use additional code to identify:

exposure to environmental tobacco smoke (Z77.22)

exposure to tobacco smoke in the perinatal period (P96.81)

history of tobacco use (Z87.891)

occupational exposure to environmental tobacco smoke (Z57.31)

tobacco dependence (F17.-)

tobacco use (Z72.0)

Excludes1   detergent asthma (J69.8)

eosinophilic asthma (J82)

lung diseases due to external agents (J60-J70)

miner's asthma (J60)

wheezing NOS (R06.2)

wood asthma (J67.8)

Excludes2   asthma with chronic obstructive pulmonary disease (J44.9)

chronic asthmatic (obstructive) bronchitis (J44.9)

chronic obstructive asthma (J44.9)

● **J45.2   Mild intermittent asthma**

J45.20   Mild intermittent asthma, uncomplicated

Mild intermittent asthma NOS

J45.21   Mild intermittent asthma with (acute) exacerbation

J45.22   Mild intermittent asthma with status asthmaticus

● **J45.3   Mild persistent asthma**

J45.30   Mild persistent asthma, uncomplicated

Mild persistent asthma NOS

J45.31   Mild persistent asthma with (acute) exacerbation

J45.32   Mild persistent asthma with status asthmaticus

● **J45.4   Moderate persistent asthma**

J45.40   Moderate persistent asthma, uncomplicated

Moderate persistent asthma NOS

J45.41   Moderate persistent asthma with (acute) exacerbation

J45.42   Moderate persistent asthma with status asthmaticus

● **J45.5   Severe persistent asthma**

J45.50   Severe persistent asthma, uncomplicated

Severe persistent asthma NOS

J45.51   Severe persistent asthma with (acute) exacerbation

J45.52   Severe persistent asthma with status asthmaticus

● **J45.9**   **Other and unspecified asthma**
   ● **J45.90**   **Unspecified asthma**
       Asthmatic bronchitis NOS
       Childhood asthma NOS
       Late onset asthma
      J45.901   **Unspecified asthma with (acute) exacerbation**
      J45.902   **Unspecified asthma with status asthmaticus**
      J45.909   **Unspecified asthma, uncomplicated**
         Asthma NOS
   ● **J45.99**   **Other asthma**
      J45.990   **Exercise induced bronchospasm**
      J45.991   **Cough variant asthma**
      J45.998   **Other asthma**

● **J47**   **Bronchiectasis**
   Includes   bronchiolectasis
   Use additional code to identify:
     exposure to environmental tobacco smoke (Z77.22)
     exposure to tobacco smoke in the perinatal period (P96.81)
     history of tobacco use (Z87.891)
     occupational exposure to environmental tobacco smoke (Z57.31)
     tobacco dependence (F17.-)
     tobacco use (Z72.0)
   Excludes1   congenital bronchiectasis (Q33.4)
         tuberculous bronchiectasis (current disease) (A15.0)
   J47.0   **Bronchiectasis with acute lower respiratory infection**
      Bronchiectasis with acute bronchitis
   J47.1   **Bronchiectasis with (acute) exacerbation**
   J47.9   **Bronchiectasis, uncomplicated**
      Bronchiectasis NOS

LUNG DISEASES DUE TO EXTERNAL AGENTS (J60-J70)

   Excludes2   asthma (J45.-)
         malignant neoplasm of bronchus and lung (C34.-)

J60   **Coalworker's pneumoconiosis**   **A**
     Anthracosilicosis
     Anthracosis
     Black lung disease
     Coalworker's lung
   Excludes1   coalworker pneumoconiosis with tuberculosis, any type in A15 (J65)

J61   **Pneumoconiosis due to asbestos and other mineral fibers**   **A**
     Asbestosis
   Excludes1   pleural plaque with asbestosis (J92.0)
         pneumoconiosis with tuberculosis, any type in A15 (J65)

● **J62**   **Pneumoconiosis due to dust containing silica**
   Includes   silicotic fibrosis (massive) of lung
   Excludes1   pneumoconiosis with tuberculosis, any type in A15 (J65)
   J62.0   **Pneumoconiosis due to talc dust**
   J62.8   **Pneumoconiosis due to other dust containing silica**
      Silicosis NOS

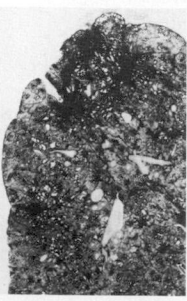

Figure 10-6 Progressive massive fibrosis superimposed on coal workers' pneumoconiosis. The large, blackened scars are located principally in the upper lobe. (From Cotran R, Kumar V, Collins T: Robbins Pathologic Basis of Disease, ed 8, Philadelphia, WB Saunders, 2009. Courtesy of Dr. Warner Laquer, Dr. Jerome Kleinerman, and the National Institute of Occupational Safety and Health, Morgantown, WV)

Item 10–10   **Pneumoconiosis** refers to a lung condition resulting from exposure to inorganic or organic airborne particles, such as coal dust or moldy hay, as well as chemical fumes and vapors, such as insecticides. In this condition, the lungs retain the airborne particles.

● **J63**   **Pneumoconiosis due to other inorganic dusts**
   Excludes1   pneumoconiosis with tuberculosis, any type in A15 (J65)
   J63.0   **Aluminosis (of lung)**
   J63.1   **Bauxite fibrosis (of lung)**
   J63.2   **Berylliosis**
   J63.3   **Graphite fibrosis (of lung)**
   J63.4   **Siderosis**
   J63.5   **Stannosis**
   J63.6   **Pneumoconiosis due to other specified inorganic dusts**

J64   **Unspecified pneumoconiosis**
   Excludes1   pneumonoconiosis with tuberculosis, any type in A15 (J65)

J65   **Pneumoconiosis associated with tuberculosis**
     Any condition in J60-J64 with tuberculosis, any type in A15
     Silicotuberculosis

● **J66**   **Airway disease due to specific organic dust**
   Excludes2   allergic alveolitis (J67.-)
         asbestosis (J61)
         bagassosis (J67.1)
         farmer's lung (J67.0)
         hypersensitivity pneumonitis due to organic dust (J67.-)
         reactive airways dysfunction syndrome (J68.3)
   J66.0   **Byssinosis**
      Airway disease due to cotton dust
   J66.1   **Flax-dressers' disease**
   J66.2   **Cannabinosis**
   J66.8   **Airway disease due to other specific organic dusts**

● **J67**   **Hypersensitivity pneumonitis due to organic dust**
   Includes   allergic alveolitis and pneumonitis due to inhaled organic dust and particles of fungal, actinomycetic or other origin
   Excludes1   pneumonitis due to inhalation of chemicals, gases, fumes or vapors (J68.0)
   J67.0   **Farmer's lung**
      Harvester's lung
      Haymaker's lung
      Moldy hay disease
   J67.1   **Bagassosis**
      Bagasse disease
      Bagasse pneumonitis
   J67.2   **Bird fancier's lung**
      Budgerigar fancier's disease or lung
      Pigeon fancier's disease or lung
   J67.3   **Suberosis**
      Corkhandler's disease or lung
      Corkworker's disease or lung
   J67.4   **Maltworker's lung**
      Alveolitis due to Aspergillus clavatus
   J67.5   **Mushroom-worker's lung**
   J67.6   **Maple-bark-stripper's lung**
      Alveolitis due to Cryptostroma corticale
      Cryptostromosis
   J67.7   **Air conditioner and humidifier lung**
      Allergic alveolitis due to fungal, thermophilic actinomycetes and other organisms growing in ventilation [air conditioning] systems

◀ New   ◀■ Revised   ~~deleted~~ Deleted   Excludes 1   Excludes 2   Includes   Use additional   Code first   Code also   Unspecified

OGCR Official Guidelines   **X** Assign placeholder X   ● Use Additional Character(s)   ▶ Manifestation Code   **Coding Clinic**

J67.8   **Hypersensitivity pneumonitis due to other organic dusts**
       Cheese-washer's lung
       Coffee-worker's lung
       Fish-meal worker's lung
       Furrier's lung
       Sequoiosis

J67.9   **Hypersensitivity pneumonitis due to unspecified organic dust**
       Allergic alveolitis (extrinsic) NOS
       Hypersensitivity pneumonitis NOS

● **J68**   **Respiratory conditions due to inhalation of chemicals, gases, fumes and vapors**
       Code first (T51-T65) to identify cause
       Use additional code to identify associated respiratory conditions, such as:
       acute respiratory failure (J96.0-)

J68.0   **Bronchitis and pneumonitis due to chemicals, gases, fumes and vapors**
       Chemical bronchitis (acute)

J68.1   **Pulmonary edema due to chemicals, gases, fumes and vapors**
       Chemical pulmonary edema (acute) (chronic)
       Excludes1   pulmonary edema (acute) (chronic) NOS (J81.-)

J68.2   **Upper respiratory inflammation due to chemicals, gases, fumes and vapors, not elsewhere classified**

J68.3   **Other acute and subacute respiratory conditions due to chemicals, gases, fumes and vapors**
       Reactive airways dysfunction syndrome

J68.4   **Chronic respiratory conditions due to chemicals, gases, fumes and vapors**
       Emphysema (diffuse) (chronic) due to inhalation of chemicals, gases, fumes and vapors
       Obliterative bronchiolitis (chronic) (subacute) due to inhalation of chemicals, gases, fumes and vapors
       Pulmonary fibrosis (chronic) due to inhalation of chemicals, gases, fumes and vapors
       Excludes1   chronic pulmonary edema due to chemicals, gases, fumes and vapors (J68.1)

J68.8   **Other respiratory conditions due to chemicals, gases, fumes and vapors**

J68.9   **Unspecified respiratory condition due to chemicals, gases, fumes and vapors**

● **J69**   **Pneumonitis due to solids and liquids**
       Excludes1   neonatal aspiration syndromes (P24.-)
                   postprocedural pneumonitis (J95.4)

J69.0   **Pneumonitis due to inhalation of food and vomit**
       Aspiration pneumonia NOS
       Aspiration pneumonia (due to) food (regurgitated)
       Aspiration pneumonia (due to) gastric secretions
       Aspiration pneumonia (due to) milk
       Aspiration pneumonia (due to) vomit
       Code also any associated foreign body in respiratory tract (T17.-)
       Excludes1   chemical pneumonitis due to anesthesia (J95.4)
                   obstetric aspiration pneumonitis (O74.0)

J69.1   **Pneumonitis due to inhalation of oils and essences**
       Exogenous lipoid pneumonia
       Lipid pneumonia NOS
       Code first (T51-T65) to identify substance
       Excludes1   endogenous lipoid pneumonia (J84.89)

J69.8   **Pneumonitis due to inhalation of other solids and liquids**
       Pneumonitis due to aspiration of blood
       Pneumonitis due to aspiration of detergent
       Code first (T51-T65) to identify substance

● **J70**   **Respiratory conditions due to other external agents**

J70.0   **Acute pulmonary manifestations due to radiation**
       Radiation pneumonitis
       Use additional code (W88-W90, X39.0-) to identify the external cause

J70.1   **Chronic and other pulmonary manifestations due to radiation**
       Fibrosis of lung following radiation
       Use additional code (W88-W90, X39.0-) to identify the external cause

J70.2   **Acute drug-induced interstitial lung disorders**
       Use additional code for adverse effect, if applicable, to identify drug (T36-T50 with fifth or sixth character 5)
       Excludes1   interstitial pneumonia NOS (J84.9)
                   lymphoid interstitial pneumonia (J84.2)

J70.3   **Chronic drug-induced interstitial lung disorders**
       Use additional code for adverse effect, if applicable, to identify drug (T36-T50 with fifth or sixth character 5)
       Excludes1   interstitial pneumonia NOS (J84.9)
                   lymphoid interstitial pneumonia (J84.2)

J70.4   **Drug-induced interstitial lung disorders, unspecified**
       Use additional code for adverse effect, if applicable, to identify drug (T36-T50 with fifth or sixth character 5)
       Excludes1   interstitial pneumonia NOS (J84.9)
                   lymphoid interstitial pneumonia (J84.2)

J70.5   **Respiratory conditions due to smoke inhalation**
       Smoke inhalation NOS
       Excludes1   smoke inhalation due to chemicals, gases, fumes and vapors (J68.9)

J70.8   **Respiratory conditions due to other specified external agents**
       Code first (T51-T65) to identify the external agent

J70.9   **Respiratory conditions due to unspecified external agent**
       Code first (T51-T65) to identify the external agent

OTHER RESPIRATORY DISEASES PRINCIPALLY AFFECTING THE INTERSTITIUM (J80-J84)

J80   **Acute respiratory distress syndrome**
       Acute respiratory distress syndrome in adult or child
       Adult hyaline membrane disease
       Excludes1   respiratory distress syndrome in newborn (perinatal) (P22.0)

● **J81**   **Pulmonary edema**
       Use additional code to identify:
       exposure to environmental tobacco smoke (Z77.22)
       history of tobacco use (Z87.891)
       occupational exposure to environmental tobacco smoke (Z57.31)
       tobacco dependence (F17.-)
       tobacco use (Z72.0)
       Excludes1   chemical (acute) pulmonary edema (J68.1)
                   hypostatic pneumonia (J18.2)
                   passive pneumonia (J18.2)
                   pulmonary edema due to external agents (J60-J70)
                   pulmonary edema with heart disease NOS (I50.1)
                   pulmonary edema with heart failure (I50.1)

J81.0   **Acute pulmonary edema**
       Acute edema of lung

J81.1   **Chronic pulmonary edema**
       Pulmonary congestion (chronic) (passive)
       Pulmonary edema NOS

J82   **Pulmonary eosinophilia, not elsewhere classified**
Allergic pneumonia
Eosinophilic asthma
Eosinophilic pneumonia
Löffler's pneumonia
Tropical (pulmonary) eosinophilia NOS

> **Excludes1**   pulmonary eosinophilia due to aspergillosis (B44.-)
> pulmonary eosinophilia due to drugs (J70.2-J70.4)
> pulmonary eosinophilia due to specified parasitic infection (B50-B83)
> pulmonary eosinophilia due to systemic connective tissue disorders (M30-M36)
> pulmonary infiltrate NOS (R91.8)

● **J84**   **Other interstitial pulmonary diseases**

> **Excludes1**   drug-induced interstitial lung disorders (J70.2-J70.4)
> interstitial emphysema (J98.2)
> lung diseases due to external agents (J60-J70)

● **J84.0**   **Alveolar and parieto-alveolar conditions**

    J84.01   **Alveolar proteinosis**

    J84.02   **Pulmonary alveolar microlithiasis**

▶ **J84.03**   *Idiopathic pulmonary hemosiderosis*
Essential brown induration of lung

> *Code first* underlying disease, such as:
> disorders of iron metabolism (E83.1-)

> **Excludes1**   acute idiopathic pulmonary hemorrhage in infants [AIPHI] (R04.81)

    J84.09   **Other alveolar and parieto-alveolar conditions**

● **J84.1**   **Other interstitial pulmonary diseases with fibrosis**

> **Excludes1**   pulmonary fibrosis (chronic) due to inhalation of chemicals, gases, fumes or vapors (J68.4)
> pulmonary fibrosis (chronic) following radiation (J70.1)

    J84.10   **Pulmonary fibrosis, unspecified**
Capillary fibrosis of lung
Cirrhosis of lung (chronic) NOS
Fibrosis of lung (atrophic) (chronic) (confluent) (massive) (perialveolar) (peribronchial) NOS
Induration of lung (chronic) NOS
Postinflammatory pulmonary fibrosis

    ● **J84.11**   **Idiopathic interstitial pneumonia**

> **Excludes1**   lymphoid interstitial pneumonia (J84.2)
> pneumocystis pneumonia (B59)

       J84.111   **Idiopathic interstitial pneumonia, not otherwise specified**

       J84.112   **Idiopathic pulmonary fibrosis**
Cryptogenic fibrosing alveolitis
Idiopathic fibrosing alveolitis

       J84.113   **Idiopathic non-specific interstitial pneumonitis**

> **Excludes1**   non-specific interstitial pneumonia NOS, or due to known underlying cause (J84.89)

       J84.114   **Acute interstitial pneumonitis**
Hamman-Rich syndrome

> **Excludes1**   pneumocystis pneumonia (B59)

       J84.115   **Respiratory bronchiolitis interstitial lung disease**

       J84.116   **Cryptogenic organizing pneumonia**

> **Excludes1**   organizing pneumonia NOS, or due to known underlying cause (J84.89)

       J84.117   **Desquamative interstitial pneumonia**

▶ **J84.17**   *Other interstitial pulmonary diseases with fibrosis in diseases classified elsewhere*
Interstitial pneumonia (nonspecific) (usual) due to collagen vascular disease
Interstitial pneumonia (nonspecific) (usual) in diseases classified elsewhere
Organizing pneumonia due to collagen vascular disease
Organizing pneumonia in diseases classified elsewhere

> *Code first* underlying disease, such as:
> progressive systemic sclerosis (M34.0)
> rheumatoid arthritis (M05.00-M06.9)
> systemic lupus erythematosis (M32.0-M32.9)

J84.2   **Lymphoid interstitial pneumonia**
Lymphoid interstitial pneumonitis

● **J84.8**   **Other specified interstitial pulmonary diseases**

> **Excludes1**   exogenous lipoid pneumonia (J69.1)
> unspecified lipoid pneumonia (J69.1)

    J84.81   **Lymphangioleiomyomatosis ♀**
Lymphangiomyomatosis

    J84.82   **Adult pulmonary Langerhans cell histiocytosis**   **A**
Adult PLCH

    J84.83   **Surfactant mutations of the lung**

    ● **J84.84**   **Other interstitial lung diseases of childhood**

       J84.841   **Neuroendocrine cell hyperplasia of infancy**

       J84.842   **Pulmonary interstitial glycogenosis**

       J84.843   **Alveolar capillary dysplasia with vein misalignment**

       J84.848   **Other interstitial lung diseases of childhood**

    J84.89   **Other specified interstitial pulmonary diseases**
Endogenous lipoid pneumonia
Interstitial pneumonitis
Non-specific interstitial pneumonitis NOS
Organizing pneumonia due to known underlying cause
Organizing pneumonia NOS

> *Code first*, if applicable:
> poisoning due to drug or toxin (T51-T65 with fifth or sixth character to indicate intent), for toxic pneumonopathy underlying cause of pneumonopathy, if known

> *Use additional code*, for adverse effect, to identify drug (T36-T50 with fifth or sixth character 5), if drug-induced

> **Excludes1**   cryptogenic organizing pneumonia (J84.116)
> idiopathic non-specific interstitial pneumonitis (J84.113)
> lipoid pneumonia, exogenous or unspecified (J69.1)
> lymphoid interstitial pneumonia (J84.2)

J84.9   **Interstitial pulmonary disease, unspecified**
Interstitial pneumonia NOS

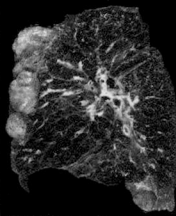

Figure 10-7   Bullous emphysema with large subpleural bullae *(upper left)*. (From Kumar: Robbins and Cotran: Pathologic Basis of Disease, ed 8, Saunders, An Imprint of Elsevier, 2009)

◀ New   ◀ Revised   ~~deleted~~ Deleted   Excludes 1   Excludes 2   Includes   Use additional   Code first   Code also   Unspecified
OGCR Official Guidelines   X Assign placeholder X   ● Use Additional Character(s)   ▶ Manifestation Code   **Coding Clinic**

Item 10–11 **Empyema** is a condition in which pus accumulates in a body cavity. Empyema **with fistula** occurs when the pus passes from one cavity to another organ or structure.

SUPPURATIVE AND NECROTIC CONDITIONS OF THE LOWER RESPIRATORY TRACT (J85-J86)

● **J85**   **Abscess of lung and mediastinum**
        Use additional code (B95-B97) to identify infectious agent.

    J85.0   **Gangrene and necrosis of lung**

    J85.1   **Abscess of lung with pneumonia**
           Code also the type of pneumonia

    J85.2   **Abscess of lung without pneumonia**
           Abscess of lung NOS

    J85.3   **Abscess of mediastinum**

● **J86**   **Pyothorax**
        Use additional code (B95-B97) to identify infectious agent.
        Excludes1   abscess of lung (J85.-)
                    pyothorax due to tuberculosis (A15.6)

    J86.0   **Pyothorax with fistula**
           Bronchocutaneous fistula
           Bronchopleural fistula
           Hepatopleural fistula
           Mediastinal fistula
           Pleural fistula
           Thoracic fistula
           Any condition classifiable to J86.9 with fistula

    J86.9   **Pyothorax without fistula**
           Abscess of pleura
           Abscess of thorax
           Empyema (chest) (lung) (pleura)
           Fibrinopurulent pleurisy
           Purulent pleurisy
           Pyopneumothorax
           Septic pleurisy
           Seropurulent pleurisy
           Suppurative pleurisy

OTHER DISEASES OF THE PLEURA (J90-J94)

J90   **Pleural effusion, not elsewhere classified**
        Encysted pleurisy
        Pleural effusion NOS
        Pleurisy with effusion (exudative) (serous)
        Excludes1   chylous (pleural) effusion (J94.0)
                    malignant pleural effusion (J91.0))
                    pleurisy NOS (R09.1)
                    tuberculous pleural effusion (A15.6)

● **J91**   **Pleural effusion in conditions classified elsewhere**
        Excludes2   pleural effusion in heart failure (I50.-)
                    pleural effusion in systemic lupus erythematosus
                      (M32.13)

  ▸ **J91.0**   *Malignant pleural effusion*
           Code first underlying neoplasm

  ▸ **J91.8**   *Pleural effusion in other conditions classified elsewhere*
           Code first underlying disease, such as:
              filariasis (B74.0-B74.9)
              influenza (J09.X2, J10.1, J11.1)

● **J92**   **Pleural plaque**
        Includes   pleural thickening
    J92.0   **Pleural plaque with presence of asbestos**
    J92.9   **Pleural plaque without asbestos**
           Pleural plaque NOS

● **J93**   **Pneumothorax and air leak**
        Collapsed lung
        Excludes1   congenital or perinatal pneumothorax (P25.1)
                    postprocedural air leak (J95.812)
                    postprocedural pneumothorax (J95.811)
                    traumatic pneumothorax (S27.0)
                    tuberculous (current disease) pneumothorax
                      (A15.-)
                    pyopneumothorax (J86.-)

    J93.0   **Spontaneous tension pneumothorax**
           Tension pneumothorax (most serious type) occurs when air (positive pressure) collects in the pleural space

●   **J93.1**   **Other spontaneous pneumothorax**
      J93.11   **Primary spontaneous pneumothorax**
      J93.12   **Secondary spontaneous pneumothorax**
             Code first underlying condition, such as:
               catamenial pneumothorax due to
                  endometriosis (N80.8)
               cystic fibrosis (E84.-)
               eosinophilic pneumonia (J82)
               lymphangioleiomyomatosis (J84.81)
               malignant neoplasm of bronchus and lung
                  (C34.-)
               Marfan's syndrome (Q87.4)
               pneumonia due to Pneumocystis carinii
                  (B59)
               secondary malignant neoplasm of lung
                  (C78.0-)
               spontaneous rupture of the esophagus
                  (K22.3)

● **J93.8**   **Other pneumothorax and air leak**
      J93.81   **Chronic pneumothorax**
      J93.82   **Other air leak**
             Persistent air leak
      J93.83   **Other pneumothorax**
             Acute pneumothorax
             Spontaneous pneumothorax NOS

    J93.9   **Pneumothorax, unspecified**
           Pneumothorax NOS

● **J94**   **Other pleural conditions**
        Excludes1   pleurisy NOS (R09.1)
                    traumatic hemopneumothorax (S27.2)
                    traumatic hemothorax (S27.1)
                    tuberculous pleural conditions (current disease)
                      (A15.-)

    J94.0   **Chylous effusion**
           Chyliform effusion
    J94.1   **Fibrothorax**
    J94.2   **Hemothorax**
           Hemopneumothorax
    J94.8   **Other specified pleural conditions**
           Hydropneumothorax
           Hydrothorax
    J94.9   **Pleural condition, unspecified**

CHAPTER 10 (J00-J99)

INTRAOPERATIVE AND POSTPROCEDURAL COMPLICATIONS AND DISORDERS OF RESPIRATORY SYSTEM, NOT ELSEWHERE CLASSIFIED (J95)

● **J95**   **Intraoperative and postprocedural complications and disorders of respiratory system, not elsewhere classified**

     Excludes2   aspiration pneumonia (J69.-)
           emphysema (subcutaneous) resulting from a procedure (T81.82)
           hypostatic pneumonia (J18.2)
           pulmonary manifestations due to radiation (J70.0- J70.1)

● **J95.0**   **Tracheostomy complications**

   J95.00   **Unspecified tracheostomy complication**

   J95.01   **Hemorrhage from tracheostomy stoma**

   J95.02   **Infection of tracheostomy stoma**

      Use additional code to identify type of infection, such as:
        cellulitis of neck (L03.8)
        sepsis (A40, A41.-)

   J95.03   **Malfunction of tracheostomy stoma**
      Mechanical complication of tracheostomy stoma
      Obstruction of tracheostomy airway
      Tracheal stenosis due to tracheostomy

   J95.04   **Tracheo-esophageal fistula following tracheostomy**

   J95.09   **Other tracheostomy complication**

J95.1   **Acute pulmonary insufficiency following thoracic surgery**

     Excludes2   functional disturbances following cardiac surgery (I97.0, I97.1-)

J95.2   **Acute pulmonary insufficiency following nonthoracic surgery**

     Excludes2   functional disturbances following cardiac surgery (I97.0, I97.1-)

J95.3   **Chronic pulmonary insufficiency following surgery**

     Excludes2   functional disturbances following cardiac surgery (I97.0, I97.1-)

J95.4   **Chemical pneumonitis due to anesthesia**
     Mendelson's syndrome
     Postprocedural aspiration pneumonia

     Use additional code for adverse effect, if applicable, to identify drug (T41.- with fifth or sixth character 5)

     Excludes1   aspiration pneumonitis due to anesthesia complicating labor and delivery (O74.0)
          aspiration pneumonitis due to anesthesia complicating pregnancy (O29)
          aspiration pneumonitis due to anesthesia complicating the puerperium (O89.01)

J95.5   **Postprocedural subglottic stenosis**

● **J95.6**   **Intraoperative hemorrhage and hematoma of a respiratory system organ or structure complicating a procedure**

     Excludes1   intraoperative hemorrhage and hematoma of a respiratory system organ or structure due to accidental puncture and laceration during procedure (J95.7-)

   J95.61   **Intraoperative hemorrhage and hematoma of a respiratory system organ or structure complicating a respiratory system procedure**

   J95.62   **Intraoperative hemorrhage and hematoma of a respiratory system organ or structure complicating other procedure**

● **J95.7**   **Accidental puncture and laceration of a respiratory system organ or structure during a procedure**

     Excludes2   postprocedural pneumothorax (J95.811)

   J95.71   **Accidental puncture and laceration of a respiratory system organ or structure during a respiratory system procedure**

   J95.72   **Accidental puncture and laceration of a respiratory system organ or structure during other procedure**

● **J95.8**   **Other intraoperative and postprocedural complications and disorders of respiratory system, not elsewhere classified**

   ● **J95.81**   **Postprocedural pneumothorax and air leak**

     J95.811   **Postprocedural pneumothorax**

     J95.812   **Postprocedural air leak**

   ● **J95.82**   **Postprocedural respiratory failure**

     Excludes1   Respiratory failure in other conditions (J96.-)

     J95.821   **Acute postprocedural respiratory failure**
        Postprocedural respiratory failure NOS

     J95.822   **Acute and chronic postprocedural respiratory failure**

   ● **J95.83**   **Postprocedural hemorrhage and hematoma of a respiratory system organ or structure following a procedure**

     J95.830   **Postprocedural hemorrhage and hematoma of a respiratory system organ or structure following a respiratory system procedure**

     J95.831   **Postprocedural hemorrhage and hematoma of a respiratory system organ or structure following other procedure**

   J95.84   **Transfusion-related acute lung injury (TRALI)**

   ● **J95.85**   **Complication of respirator [ventilator]**

     J95.850   **Mechanical complication of respirator**

       Excludes1   encounter for respirator [ventilator] dependence during power failure (Z99.12)

     J95.851   **Ventilator associated pneumonia**
       Ventilator associated pneumonitis

       Use additional code to identify the organism, if known (B95.-, B96.-, B97.-)

       Excludes1   ventilator lung in newborn (P27.8)

     J95.859   **Other complication of respirator [ventilator]**

   J95.88   **Other intraoperative complications of respiratory system, not elsewhere classified**

   J95.89   **Other postprocedural complications and disorders of respiratory system, not elsewhere classified**

     Use additional code to identify disorder, such as:
       aspiration pneumonia (J69.-)
       bacterial or viral pneumonia (J12-J18)

     Excludes2   acute pulmonary insufficiency following thoracic surgery (J95.1)
         postprocedural subglottic stenosis (J95.5)

OTHER DISEASES OF THE RESPIRATORY SYSTEM (J96-J99)

● **J96**   **Respiratory failure, not elsewhere classified**
     Excludes1   acute respiratory distress syndrome (J80)
                  cardiorespiratory failure (R09.2)
                  newborn respiratory distress syndrome (P22.0)
                  postprocedural respiratory failure (J95.82-)
                  respiratory arrest (R09.2)
                  respiratory arrest of newborn (P28.81)
                  respiratory failure of newborn (P28.5)

● **J96.0**   **Acute respiratory failure**
     J96.00   **Acute respiratory failure, unspecified whether with hypoxia or hypercapnia**
     J96.01   **Acute respiratory failure with hypoxia**
     J96.02   **Acute respiratory failure with hypercapnia**

● **J96.1**   **Chronic respiratory failure**
     J96.10   **Chronic respiratory failure, unspecified whether with hypoxia or hypercapnia**
               Coding Clinic: 2015, Q1, P21
     J96.11   **Chronic respiratory failure with hypoxia**
     J96.12   **Chronic respiratory failure with hypercapnia**

● **J96.2**   **Acute and chronic respiratory failure**
     Acute on chronic respiratory failure
     J96.20   **Acute and chronic respiratory failure, unspecified whether with hypoxia or hypercapnia**
     J96.21   **Acute and chronic respiratory failure with hypoxia**
     J96.22   **Acute and chronic respiratory failure with hypercapnia**

● **J96.9**   **Respiratory failure, unspecified**
     J96.90   **Respiratory failure, unspecified, unspecified whether with hypoxia or hypercapnia**
     J96.91   **Respiratory failure, unspecified with hypoxia**
     J96.92   **Respiratory failure, unspecified with hypercapnia**

● **J98**   **Other respiratory disorders**
     Use additional code to identify:
       exposure to environmental tobacco smoke (Z77.22)
       exposure to tobacco smoke in the perinatal period (P96.81)
       history of tobacco use (Z87.891)
       occupational exposure to environmental tobacco smoke (Z57.31)
       tobacco dependence (F17.-)
       tobacco use (Z72.0)
     Excludes1   newborn apnea (P28.4)
                  newborn sleep apnea (P28.3)
     Excludes2   apnea NOS (R06.81)
                  sleep apnea (G47.3-)

● **J98.0**   **Diseases of bronchus, not elsewhere classified**
     J98.01   **Acute bronchospasm**
         Excludes1   acute bronchiolitis with bronchospasm (J21.-)
                      acute bronchitis with bronchospasm (J20.-)
                      asthma (J45.-)
                      exercise induced bronchospasm (J45.990)
     J98.09   **Other diseases of bronchus, not elsewhere classified**
         Broncholithiasis
         Calcification of bronchus
         Stenosis of bronchus
         Tracheobronchial collapse
         Tracheobronchial dyskinesia
         Ulcer of bronchus

● **J98.1**   **Pulmonary collapse**
     Excludes1   therapeutic collapse of lung status (Z98.3)
     J98.11   **Atelectasis**
         Excludes1   newborn atelectasis
                      tuberculous atelectasis (current disease) (A15)
     J98.19   **Other pulmonary collapse**

   J98.2   **Interstitial emphysema**
     Mediastinal emphysema
     Excludes1   emphysema NOS (J43.9)
                  emphysema in newborn (P25.0)
                  surgical emphysema (subcutaneous) (T81.82)
                  traumatic subcutaneous emphysema (T79.7)

   J98.3   **Compensatory emphysema**

   J98.4   **Other disorders of lung**
     Calcification of lung
     Cystic lung disease (acquired)
     Lung disease NOS
     Pulmolithiasis
     Excludes1   acute interstitial pneumonitis (J84.114)
                  pulmonary insufficiency following surgery (J95.1-J95.2)

   J98.5   **Diseases of mediastinum, not elsewhere classified**
     Fibrosis of mediastinum
     Hernia of mediastinum
     Retraction of mediastinum
     Mediastinitis
     Excludes2   abscess of mediastinum (J85.3)

   J98.6   **Disorders of diaphragm**
     Diaphragmatitis
     Paralysis of diaphragm
     Relaxation of diaphragm
     Excludes1   congenital malformation of diaphragm NEC (Q79.1)
                  congenital diaphragmatic hernia (Q79.0)
     Excludes2   diaphragmatic hernia (K44.-)

   J98.8   **Other specified respiratory disorders**

   J98.9   **Respiratory disorder, unspecified**
     Respiratory disease (chronic) NOS

▹ **J99**   *Respiratory disorders in diseases classified elsewhere*
     Code first underlying disease, such as:
       amyloidosis (E85.-)
       ankylosing spondylitis (M45)
       congenital syphilis (A50.5)
       cryoglobulinemia (D89.1)
       early congenital syphilis (A50.0)
       schistosomiasis (B65.0-B65.9)
     Excludes1   respiratory disorders in:
                  amebiasis (A06.5)
                  blastomycosis (B40.0-B40.2)
                  candidiasis (B37.1)
                  coccidioidomycosis (B38.0-B38.2)
                  cystic fibrosis with pulmonary manifestations (E84.0)
                  dermatomyositis (M33.01, M33.11)
                  histoplasmosis (B39.0-B39.2)
                  late syphilis (A52.72, A52.73)
                  polymyositis (M33.21)
                  sicca syndrome (M35.02)
                  systemic lupus erythematosus (M32.13)
                  systemic sclerosis (M34.81)
                  Wegener's granulomatosis (M31.30-M31.31)

CHAPTER 10 (J00-J99)

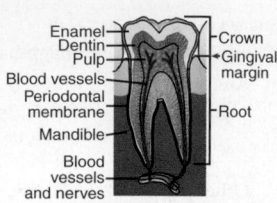

Figure 11-1 Anatomy of a tooth.

Item 11–1 Anodontia is the congenital absence of teeth. **Hypodontia** is partial anodontia. **Oligodontia** is the congenital absence of some teeth, whereas **supernumerary** is having more teeth than the normal number. **Mesiodens** are small extra teeth that often appear in pairs, although single small teeth are not uncommon.

CHAPTER 11

DISEASES OF THE DIGESTIVE SYSTEM (K00-K95)

> **Excludes2** certain conditions originating in the perinatal period (P04-P96)
> certain infectious and parasitic diseases (A00-B99)
> complications of pregnancy, childbirth and the puerperium (O00-O9A)
> congenital malformations, deformations and chromosomal abnormalities (Q00-Q99)
> endocrine, nutritional and metabolic diseases (E00-E88)
> injury, poisoning and certain other consequences of external causes (S00-T88)
> neoplasms (C00-D49)
> symptoms, signs and abnormal clinical and laboratory findings, not elsewhere classified (R00-R94)

This chapter contains the following blocks:

K00-K14	Diseases of oral cavity and salivary glands
K20-K31	Diseases of esophagus, stomach and duodenum
K35-K38	Diseases of appendix
K40-K46	Hernia
K50-K52	Noninfective enteritis and colitis
K55-K64	Other diseases of intestines
K65-K68	Diseases of peritoneum and retroperitoneum
K70-K77	Diseases of liver
K80-K87	Disorders of gallbladder, biliary tract and pancreas
K90-K95	Other diseases of the digestive system

DISEASES OF ORAL CAVITY AND SALIVARY GLANDS (K00-K14)

● **K00 Disorders of tooth development and eruption**
> **Excludes2** embedded and impacted teeth (K01.-)

K00.0 Anodontia
Hypodontia
Oligodontia
> **Excludes1** acquired absence of teeth (K08.1-)

K00.1 Supernumerary teeth
Distomolar
Fourth molar
Mesiodens
Paramolar
Supplementary teeth
> **Excludes2** supernumerary roots (K00.2)

K00.2 Abnormalities of size and form of teeth
Concrescence of teeth
Fusion of teeth
Gemination of teeth
Dens evaginatus
Dens in dente
Dens invaginatus
Enamel pearls
Macrodontia
Microdontia
Peg-shaped [conical] teeth
Supernumerary roots
Taurodontism
Tuberculum paramolare
> **Excludes1** abnormalities of teeth due to congenital syphilis (A50.5)
> tuberculum Carabelli, which is regarded as a normal variation and should not be coded

K00.3 Mottled teeth
Dental fluorosis
Mottling of enamel
Nonfluoride enamel opacities
> **Excludes2** deposits [accretions] on teeth (K03.6)

K00.4 Disturbances in tooth formation
Aplasia and hypoplasia of cementum
Dilaceration of tooth
Enamel hypoplasia (neonatal) (postnatal) (prenatal)
Regional odontodysplasia
Turner's tooth
> **Excludes1** Hutchinson's teeth and mulberry molars in congenital syphilis (A50.5)
> **Excludes2** mottled teeth (K00.3)

K00.5 Hereditary disturbances in tooth structure, not elsewhere classified
Amelogenesis imperfecta
Dentinogenesis imperfecta
Odontogenesis imperfecta
Dentinal dysplasia
Shell teeth

K00.6 Disturbances in tooth eruption
Dentia praecox
Natal tooth
Neonatal tooth
Premature eruption of tooth
Premature shedding of primary [deciduous] tooth
Prenatal teeth
Retained [persistent] primary tooth
> **Excludes2** embedded and impacted teeth (K01.-)

K00.7 Teething syndrome

K00.8 Other disorders of tooth development
Color changes during tooth formation
Intrinsic staining of teeth NOS
> **Excludes2** posteruptive color changes (K03.7)

K00.9 Disorder of tooth development, unspecified
Disorder of odontogenesis NOS

● **K01 Embedded and impacted teeth**
> **Excludes1** abnormal position of fully erupted teeth (M26.3-)

K01.0 Embedded teeth

K01.1 Impacted teeth

◀ New ◀▦ Revised d̶e̶l̶e̶t̶e̶d̶ Deleted Excludes 1 Excludes 2 Includes Use additional Code first Code also Unspecified
OGCR Official Guidelines X Assign placeholder X ● Use Additional Character(s) ▸ Manifestation Code **Coding Clinic**

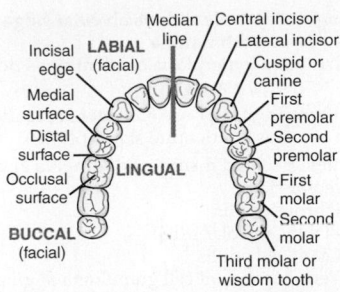

Figure 11-2 The permanent teeth within the dental arch.

Item 11–2 Each dental arch (jaw) normally contains 16 teeth. Tooth decay or **dental caries** is a disease of the enamel, dentin, and cementum of the tooth and can result in a cavity.

● K02   **Dental caries**
     Includes   dental cavities
                 tooth decay

    K02.3   **Arrested dental caries**
           Arrested coronal and root caries

● K02.5   **Dental caries on pit and fissure surface**
           Dental caries on chewing surface of tooth

        K02.51   **Dental caries on pit and fissure surface limited to enamel**
                 White spot lesions [initial caries] on pit and fissure surface of tooth

        K02.52   **Dental caries on pit and fissure surface penetrating into dentin**

        K02.53   **Dental caries on pit and fissure surface penetrating into pulp**

● K02.6   **Dental caries on smooth surface**

        K02.61   **Dental caries on smooth surface limited to enamel**
                 White spot lesions [initial caries] on smooth surface of tooth

        K02.62   **Dental caries on smooth surface penetrating into dentin**

        K02.63   **Dental caries on smooth surface penetrating into pulp**

    K02.7   **Dental root caries**

    K02.9   **Dental caries, unspecified**

● K03   **Other diseases of hard tissues of teeth**
     Excludes2   bruxism (F45.8)
                 dental caries (K02.-)
                 teeth-grinding NOS (F45.8)

    K03.0   **Excessive attrition of teeth**
           Approximal wear of teeth
           Occlusal wear of teeth

    K03.1   **Abrasion of teeth**
           Dentifrice abrasion of teeth
           Habitual abrasion of teeth
           Occupational abrasion of teeth
           Ritual abrasion of teeth
           Traditional abrasion of teeth
           Wedge defect NOS

    K03.2   **Erosion of teeth**
           Erosion of teeth due to diet
           Erosion of teeth due to drugs and medicaments
           Erosion of teeth due to persistent vomiting
           Erosion of teeth NOS
           Idiopathic erosion of teeth
           Occupational erosion of teeth

    K03.3   **Pathological resorption of teeth**
           Internal granuloma of pulp
           Resorption of teeth (external)

    K03.4   **Hypercementosis**
           Cementation hyperplasia

    K03.5   **Ankylosis of teeth**

    K03.6   **Deposits [accretions] on teeth**
           Betel deposits [accretions] on teeth
           Black deposits [accretions] on teeth
           Extrinsic staining of teeth NOS
           Green deposits [accretions] on teeth
           Materia alba deposits [accretions] on teeth
           Orange deposits [accretions] on teeth
           Staining of teeth NOS
           Subgingival dental calculus
           Supragingival dental calculus
           Tobacco deposits [accretions] on teeth

    K03.7   **Posteruptive color changes of dental hard tissues**
        Excludes2   deposits [accretions] on teeth (K03.6)

● K03.8   **Other specified diseases of hard tissues of teeth**

        K03.81   **Cracked tooth**
            Excludes1   asymptomatic craze lines in enamel - omit code
                    broken or fractured tooth due to trauma (S02.5)

        K03.89   **Other specified diseases of hard tissues of teeth**

    K03.9   **Disease of hard tissues of teeth, unspecified**

  K04   **Diseases of pulp and periapical tissues**

    K04.0   **Pulpitis**
           Acute pulpitis
           Chronic (hyperplastic) (ulcerative) pulpitis
           Irreversible pulpitis
           Reversible pulpitis

    K04.1   **Necrosis of pulp**
           Pulpal gangrene

    K04.2   **Pulp degeneration**
           Denticles
           Pulpal calcifications
           Pulpal stones

    K04.3   **Abnormal hard tissue formation in pulp**
           Secondary or irregular dentine

    K04.4   **Acute apical periodontitis of pulpal origin**
           Acute apical periodontitis NOS
         Excludes1   acute periodontitis (K05.2-)

    K04.5   **Chronic apical periodontitis**
           Apical or periapical granuloma
           Apical periodontitis NOS
         Excludes1   chronic periodontitis (K05.3-)

    K04.6   **Periapical abscess with sinus**
           Dental abscess with sinus
           Dentoalveolar abscess with sinus

    K04.7   **Periapical abscess without sinus**
           Dental abscess without sinus
           Dentoalveolar abscess without sinus
           Periapical abscess without sinus

    K04.8   **Radicular cyst**
           Apical (periodontal) cyst
           Periapical cyst
           Residual radicular cyst
         Excludes2   lateral periodontal cyst (K09.0)

● K04.9   **Other and unspecified diseases of pulp and periapical tissues**

        K04.90   **Unspecified diseases of pulp and periapical tissues**

        K04.99   **Other diseases of pulp and periapical tissues**

CHAPTER 11 (K00-K95)

Item 11-3 Acute gingivitis, also known as orilitis or ulitis, is the short-term, severe inflammation of the gums (gingiva) caused by bacteria. **Chronic gingivitis** is persistent inflammation of the gums. When the gingivitis moves into the periodontium it is called periodontitis, also known as paradentitis.

● **K05   Gingivitis and periodontal diseases**
    Use additional code to identify:
        alcohol abuse and dependence (F10.-)
        exposure to environmental tobacco smoke (Z77.22)
        exposure to tobacco smoke in the perinatal period (P96.81)
        history of tobacco use (Z87.891)
        occupational exposure to environmental tobacco smoke (Z57.31)
        tobacco dependence (F17.-)
        tobacco use (Z72.0)

● **K05.0   Acute gingivitis**
        Excludes1   acute necrotizing ulcerative gingivitis (A69.1)
                herpesviral [herpes simplex] gingivostomatitis (B00.2)

    K05.00   Acute gingivitis, plaque induced
            Acute gingivitis NOS

    K05.01   Acute gingivitis, non-plaque induced

● **K05.1   Chronic gingivitis**
        Desquamative gingivitis (chronic)
        Gingivitis (chronic) NOS
        Hyperplastic gingivitis (chronic)
        Simple marginal gingivitis (chronic)
        Ulcerative gingivitis (chronic)

    K05.10   Chronic gingivitis, plaque induced
            Chronic gingivitis NOS
            Gingivitis NOS

    K05.11   Chronic gingivitis, non-plaque induced

● **K05.2   Aggressive periodontitis**
        Acute pericoronitis
        Excludes1   acute apical periodontitis (K04.4)
                periapical abscess (K04.7)
                periapical abscess with sinus (K04.6)

    K05.20   Aggressive periodontitis, unspecified

    K05.21   Aggressive periodontitis, localized
            Periodontal abscess

    K05.22   Aggressive periodontitis, generalized

● **K05.3   Chronic periodontitis**
        Chronic pericoronitis
        Complex periodontitis
        Periodontitis NOS
        Simplex periodontitis
        Excludes1   chronic apical periodontitis (K04.5)

    K05.30   Chronic periodontitis, unspecified

    K05.31   Chronic periodontitis, localized

    K05.32   Chronic periodontitis, generalized

    K05.4   Periodontosis
            Juvenile periodontosis

    K05.5   Other periodontal diseases
            Excludes2   leukoplakia of gingiva (K13.21)

    K05.6   Periodontal disease, unspecified

● **K06   Other disorders of gingiva and edentulous alveolar ridge**
        Excludes2   acute gingivitis (K05.0)
                atrophy of edentulous alveolar ridge (K08.2)
                chronic gingivitis (K05.1)
                gingivitis NOS (K05.1)

    K06.0   Gingival recession
            Gingival recession (generalized) (localized) (postinfective) (postprocedural)

    K06.1   Gingival enlargement
            Gingival fibromatosis**

    K06.2   Gingival and edentulous alveolar ridge lesions associated with trauma
            Irritative hyperplasia of edentulous ridge [denture hyperplasia]
            Use additional code (Chapter 20) to identify external cause or denture status (Z97.2)

    K06.8   Other specified disorders of gingiva and edentulous alveolar ridge
            Fibrous epulis
            Flabby alveolar ridge
            Giant cell epulis
            Peripheral giant cell granuloma of gingiva
            Pyogenic granuloma of gingiva
            Excludes2   gingival cyst (K09.0)

    K06.9   Disorder of gingiva and edentulous alveolar ridge, unspecified

● **K08   Other disorders of teeth and supporting structures**
        Excludes2   dentofacial anomalies [including malocclusion] (M26.-)
                disorders of jaw (M27.-)

    K08.0   Exfoliation of teeth due to systemic causes
            Code also underlying systemic condition

● **K08.1   Complete loss of teeth**
        Acquired loss of teeth, complete
        Excludes1   congenital absence of teeth (K00.0)
                exfoliation of teeth due to systemic causes (K08.0)
                partial loss of teeth (K08.4-)

● **K08.10   Complete loss of teeth, unspecified cause**

    K08.101   Complete loss of teeth, unspecified cause, class I

    K08.102   Complete loss of teeth, unspecified cause, class II

    K08.103   Complete loss of teeth, unspecified cause, class III

    K08.104   Complete loss of teeth, unspecified cause, class IV

    K08.109   Complete loss of teeth, unspecified cause, unspecified class
            Edentulism NOS

● **K08.11   Complete loss of teeth due to trauma**

    K08.111   Complete loss of teeth due to trauma, class I

    K08.112   Complete loss of teeth due to trauma, class II

    K08.113   Complete loss of teeth due to trauma, class III

    K08.114   Complete loss of teeth due to trauma, class IV

    K08.119   Complete loss of teeth due to trauma, unspecified class

● **K08.12   Complete loss of teeth due to periodontal diseases**

    K08.121   Complete loss of teeth due to periodontal diseases, class I

    K08.122   Complete loss of teeth due to periodontal diseases, class II

    K08.123   Complete loss of teeth due to periodontal diseases, class III

    K08.124   Complete loss of teeth due to periodontal diseases, class IV

    K08.129   Complete loss of teeth due to periodontal diseases, unspecified class

CHAPTER 11 (K00-K95)

◀ New   ◀⁞ Revised   ~~deleted~~ Deleted   Excludes 1   Excludes 2   Includes   Use additional   Code first   Code also   Unspecified
        OGCR Official Guidelines   **X** Assign placeholder X   ● Use Additional Character(s)   ▶ Manifestation Code   **Coding Clinic**

● K08.13 Complete loss of teeth due to caries
    K08.131 Complete loss of teeth due to caries, class I
    K08.132 Complete loss of teeth due to caries, class II
    K08.133 Complete loss of teeth due to caries, class III
    K08.134 Complete loss of teeth due to caries, class IV
    K08.139 Complete loss of teeth due to caries, unspecified class

● K08.19 Complete loss of teeth due to other specified cause
    K08.191 Complete loss of teeth due to other specified cause, class I
    K08.192 Complete loss of teeth due to other specified cause, class II
    K08.193 Complete loss of teeth due to other specified cause, class III
    K08.194 Complete loss of teeth due to other specified cause, class IV
    K08.199 Complete loss of teeth due to other specified cause, unspecified class

● K08.2 Atrophy of edentulous alveolar ridge
    K08.20 Unspecified atrophy of edentulous alveolar ridge
        Atrophy of the mandible NOS
        Atrophy of the maxilla NOS
    K08.21 Minimal atrophy of the mandible
        Minimal atrophy of the edentulous mandible
    K08.22 Moderate atrophy of the mandible
        Moderate atrophy of the edentulous mandible
    K08.23 Severe atrophy of the mandible
        Severe atrophy of the edentulous mandible
    K08.24 Minimal atrophy of maxilla
        Minimal atrophy of the edentulous maxilla
    K08.25 Moderate atrophy of the maxilla
        Moderate atrophy of the edentulous maxilla
    K08.26 Severe atrophy of the maxilla
        Severe atrophy of the edentulous maxilla

K08.3 Retained dental root

● K08.4 Partial loss of teeth
    Acquired loss of teeth, partial

    Excludes1 complete loss of teeth (K08.1-)
              congenital absence of teeth (K00.0)

    Excludes2 exfoliation of teeth due to systemic causes (K08.0)

    ● K08.40 Partial loss of teeth, unspecified cause
        K08.401 Partial loss of teeth, unspecified cause, class I
        K08.402 Partial loss of teeth, unspecified cause, class II
        K08.403 Partial loss of teeth, unspecified cause, class III
        K08.404 Partial loss of teeth, unspecified cause, class IV
        K08.409 Partial loss of teeth, unspecified cause, unspecified class
            Tooth extraction status NOS

● K08.41 Partial loss of teeth due to trauma
    K08.411 Partial loss of teeth due to trauma, class I
    K08.412 Partial loss of teeth due to trauma, class II
    K08.413 Partial loss of teeth due to trauma, class III
    K08.414 Partial loss of teeth duc to trauma, class IV
    K08.419 Partial loss of teeth due to trauma, unspecified class

● K08.42 Partial loss of teeth due to periodontal diseases
    K08.421 Partial loss of teeth due to periodontal diseases, class I
    K08.422 Partial loss of teeth due to periodontal diseases, class II
    K08.423 Partial loss of teeth due to periodontal diseases, class III
    K08.424 Partial loss of teeth due to periodontal diseases, class IV
    K08.429 Partial loss of teeth due to periodontal diseases, unspecified class

● K08.43 Partial loss of teeth due to caries
    K08.431 Partial loss of teeth due to caries, class I
    K08.432 Partial loss of teeth due to caries, class II
    K08.433 Partial loss of teeth due to caries, class III
    K08.434 Partial loss of teeth due to caries, class IV
    K08.439 Partial loss of teeth due to caries, unspecified class

● K08.49 Partial loss of teeth due to other specified cause
    K08.491 Partial loss of teeth due to other specified cause, class I
    K08.492 Partial loss of teeth due to other specified cause, class II
    K08.493 Partial loss of teeth due to other specified cause, class III
    K08.494 Partial loss of teeth due to other specified cause, class IV
    K08.499 Partial loss of teeth due to other specified cause, unspecified class

● K08.5 Unsatisfactory restoration of tooth
    Defective bridge, crown, filling
    Defective dental restoration

    Excludes1 dental restoration status (Z98.811)
    Excludes2 endosseous dental implant failure (M27.6-)
              unsatisfactory endodontic treatment (M27.5-)

    K08.50 Unsatisfactory restoration of tooth, unspecified
        Defective dental restoration NOS
    K08.51 Open restoration margins of tooth
        Dental restoration failure of marginal integrity
        Open margin on tooth restoration
        Poor gingival margin to tooth restoration
    K08.52 Unrepairable overhanging of dental restorative materials
        Overhanging of tooth restoration

CHAPTER 11 (K00-K95)

● **K08.53　Fractured dental restorative material**

> **Excludes1**　cracked tooth (K03.81)
> traumatic fracture of tooth
> (S02.5)

K08.530　Fractured dental restorative material without loss of material

K08.531　Fractured dental restorative material with loss of material

K08.539　Fractured dental restorative material, unspecified

K08.54　Contour of existing restoration of tooth biologically incompatible with oral health
Dental restoration failure of periodontal anatomical integrity
Unacceptable contours of existing restoration of tooth
Unacceptable morphology of existing restoration of tooth

K08.55　Allergy to existing dental restorative material
Use additional code to identify the specific type of allergy

K08.56　Poor aesthetic of existing restoration of tooth
Dental restoration aesthetically inadequate or displeasing

K08.59　Other unsatisfactory restoration of tooth
Other defective dental restoration

K08.8　Other specified disorders of teeth and supporting structures
Enlargement of alveolar ridge NOS
Irregular alveolar process
Toothache NOS

K08.9　Disorder of teeth and supporting structures, unspecified

● **K09　Cysts of oral region, not elsewhere classified**

> **Includes**　lesions showing histological features both of aneurysmal cyst and of another fibro-osseous lesion

> **Excludes2**　cysts of jaw (M27.0-, M27.4-)
> radicular cyst (K04.8)

K09.0　Developmental odontogenic cysts
Dentigerous cyst
Eruption cyst
Follicular cyst
Gingival cyst
Lateral periodontal cyst
Primordial cyst

> **Excludes2**　keratocysts (D16.4, D16.5)
> odontogenic keratocystic tumors (D16.4, D16.5)

K09.1　Developmental (nonodontogenic) cysts of oral region
Cyst (of) incisive canal
Cyst (of) palatine of papilla
Globulomaxillary cyst
Median palatal cyst
Nasoalveolar cyst
Nasolabial cyst
Nasopalatine duct cyst

K09.8　Other cysts of oral region, not elsewhere classified
Dermoid cyst
Epidermoid cyst
Lymphoepithelial cyst
Epstein's pearl

K09.9　Cyst of oral region, unspecified

Item 11–4　**Atrophy** is wasting away of a tissue or organ, whereas **hypertrophy** is overdevelopment or enlargement of a tissue or organ. **Sialoadenitis** is salivary gland inflammation. **Parotitis** is the inflammation of the parotid gland. In the epidemic form, parotitis is also known as mumps. **Sialolithiasis** is the formation of calculus within a salivary gland. **Mucocele** is a polyp composed of mucus.

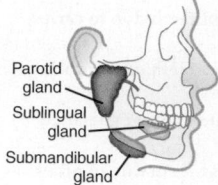

Figure 11-3　Major salivary glands.

Parotid gland
Sublingual gland
Submandibular gland

(See Plate 61 on page 73.)

● **K11　Diseases of salivary glands**
Use additional code to identify:
alcohol abuse and dependence (F10.-)
exposure to environmental tobacco smoke (Z77.22)
exposure to tobacco smoke in the perinatal period (P96.81)
history of tobacco use (Z87.891)
occupational exposure to environmental tobacco smoke (Z57.31)
tobacco dependence (F17.-)
tobacco use (Z72.0)

K11.0　Atrophy of salivary gland

K11.1　Hypertrophy of salivary gland

● **K11.2　Sialoadenitis**
Parotitis

> **Excludes1**　epidemic parotitis (B26.-)
> mumps (B26.-)
> uveoparotid fever [Heerfordt] (D86.89)

K11.20　Sialoadenitis, unspecified

K11.21　Acute sialoadenitis

> **Excludes1**　acute recurrent sialoadenitis (K11.22)

K11.22　Acute recurrent sialoadenitis

K11.23　Chronic sialoadenitis

K11.3　Abscess of salivary gland

K11.4　Fistula of salivary gland

> **Excludes1**　congenital fistula of salivary gland (Q38.4)

K11.5　Sialolithiasis
Calculus of salivary gland or duct
Stone of salivary gland or duct

K11.6　Mucocele of salivary gland
Mucous extravasation cyst of salivary gland
Mucous retention cyst of salivary gland
Ranula

K11.7　Disturbances of salivary secretion
Hypoptyalism
Ptyalism
Xerostomia

> **Excludes2**　dry mouth NOS (R68.2)

K11.8　Other diseases of salivary glands
Benign lymphoepithelial lesion of salivary gland
Mikulicz' disease
Necrotizing sialometaplasia
Sialectasia
Stenosis of salivary duct
Stricture of salivary duct

> **Excludes1**　sicca syndrome [Sjögren] (M35.0-)

K11.9　Disease of salivary gland, unspecified
Sialoadenopathy NOS

◀ New　◀▦ Revised　deleted Deleted　Excludes 1　Excludes 2　Includes　Use additional　Code first　Code also　Unspecified

OGCR Official Guidelines　X Assign placeholder X　● Use Additional Character(s)　▌ Manifestation Code　Coding Clinic

Item 11–5 Stomatitis is the inflammation of the oral mucosa. **Mucositis** is the inflammation of the mucous membranes lining the digestive tract from the mouth to the anus. It is a common side effect of chemotherapy and of radiotherapy that involves any part of the digestive tract.

● **K12   Stomatitis and related lesions**
　　　Use additional code to identify:
　　　　alcohol abuse and dependence (F10.-)
　　　　exposure to environmental tobacco smoke (Z77.22)
　　　　exposure to tobacco smoke in the perinatal period (P96.81)
　　　　history of tobacco use (Z87.891)
　　　　occupational exposure to environmental tobacco smoke
　　　　　(Z57.31)
　　　　tobacco dependence (F17.-)
　　　　tobacco use (Z72.0)
　　　Excludes1　cancrum oris (A69.0)
　　　　　　　cheilitis (K13.0)
　　　　　　　gangrenous stomatitis (A69.0)
　　　　　　　herpesviral [herpes simplex] gingivostomatitis
　　　　　　　　(B00.2)
　　　　　　　noma (A69.0)

　K12.0　Recurrent oral aphthae
　　　　Aphthous stomatitis (major) (minor)
　　　　Bednar's aphthae
　　　　Periadenitis mucosa necrotica recurrens
　　　　Recurrent aphthous ulcer
　　　　Stomatitis herpetiformis

　K12.1　Other forms of stomatitis
　　　　Stomatitis NOS
　　　　Denture stomatitis
　　　　Ulcerative stomatitis
　　　　Vesicular stomatitis
　　　　Excludes1　acute necrotizing ulcerative stomatitis
　　　　　　　　(A69.1)
　　　　　　　　Vincent's stomatitis (A69.1)

　K12.2　Cellulitis and abscess of mouth
　　　　Cellulitis of mouth (floor)
　　　　Submandibular abscess
　　　　Excludes2　abscess of salivary gland (K11.3)
　　　　　　　　abscess of tongue (K14.0)
　　　　　　　　periapical abscess (K04.6-K04.7)
　　　　　　　　periodontal abscess (K05.21)
　　　　　　　　peritonsillar abscess (J36)

● **K12.3　Oral mucositis (ulcerative)**
　　　　Mucositis (oral) (oropharyneal)
　　　　Excludes2　gastrointestinal mucositis (ulcerative)
　　　　　　　　(K92.81)
　　　　　　　　mucositis (ulcerative) of vagina and vulva
　　　　　　　　　(N76.81)
　　　　　　　　nasal mucositis (ulcerative) (J34.81)

　　K12.30　Oral mucositis (ulcerative), unspecified
　　**K12.31　Oral mucositis (ulcerative) due to antineoplastic
　　　　　therapy**
　　　　　Use additional code for adverse effect, if
　　　　　　applicable, to identify antineoplastic and
　　　　　　immunosuppressive drugs (T45.1X5)
　　　　　Use additional code for other antineoplastic
　　　　　　therapy, such as:
　　　　　　radiological procedure and radiotherapy
　　　　　　　(Y84.2)
　　K12.32　Oral mucositis (ulcerative) due to other drugs
　　　　　Use additional code for adverse effect, if
　　　　　　applicable, to identify drug (T36-T50 with
　　　　　　fifth or sixth character 5)
　　K12.33　Oral mucositis (ulcerative) due to radiation
　　　　　Use additional external cause code (W88-W90,
　　　　　　X39.0-) to identify cause
　　K12.39　Other oral mucositis (ulcerative)
　　　　　Viral oral mucositis (ulcerative)

● **K13   Other diseases of lip and oral mucosa**
　　　Includes　epithelial disturbances of tongue
　　　Use additional code to identify:
　　　　alcohol abuse and dependence (F10.-)
　　　　exposure to environmental tobacco smoke (Z77.22)
　　　　exposure to tobacco smoke in the perinatal period (P96.81)
　　　　history of tobacco use (Z87.891)
　　　　occupational exposure to environmental tobacco smoke
　　　　　(Z57.31)
　　　　tobacco dependence (F17.-)
　　　　tobacco use (Z72.0)
　　　Excludes2　certain disorders of gingiva and edentulous
　　　　　　　　alveolar ridge (K05-K06)
　　　　　　　cysts of oral region (K09.-)
　　　　　　　diseases of tongue (K14.-)
　　　　　　　stomatitis and related lesions (K12.-)

　K13.0　Diseases of lips

Abscess of lips	Exfoliative cheilitis
Angular cheilitis	Fistula of lips
Cellulitis of lips	Glandular cheilitis
Cheilitis NOS	Hypertrophy of lips
Cheilodynia	Perlèche NEC
Cheilosis	

　　　　Excludes1　ariboflavinosis (E53.0)
　　　　　　　cheilitis due to radiation-related disorders
　　　　　　　　(L55-L59)
　　　　　　　congenital fistula of lips (Q38.0)
　　　　　　　congenital hypertrophy of lips (Q18.6)
　　　　　　　Perlèche due to candidiasis (B37.83)
　　　　　　　Perlèche due to riboflavin deficiency
　　　　　　　　(E53.0)

　K13.1　Cheek and lip biting
● **K13.2　Leukoplakia and other disturbances of oral epithelium,
　　　　including tongue**
　　　　Excludes1　carcinoma in situ of oral epithelium
　　　　　　　　(D00.0-)
　　　　　　　hairy leukoplakia (K13.3)

　　K13.21　Leukoplakia of oral mucosa, including tongue
　　　　　*Considered precancerous and evidenced by
　　　　　　thickened white patches of epithelium on
　　　　　　mucous membranes*
　　　　　Leukokeratosis of oral mucosa
　　　　　Leukoplakia of gingiva, lips, tongue
　　　　　Excludes1　hairy leukoplakia (K13.3)
　　　　　　　　　leukokeratosis nicotina palati
　　　　　　　　　　(K13.24)

　　K13.22　Minimal keratinized residual ridge mucosa
　　　　　Minimal keratinization of alveolar ridge
　　　　　　mucosa

　　K13.23　Excessive keratinized residual ridge mucosa
　　　　　Excessive keratinization of alveolar ridge
　　　　　　mucosa

　　K13.24　Leukokeratosis nicotina palati
　　　　　Smoker's palate

　　**K13.29　Other disturbances of oral epithelium,
　　　　　including tongue**
　　　　　Erythroplakia of mouth or tongue
　　　　　Focal epithelial hyperplasia of mouth or
　　　　　　tongue
　　　　　Leukoedema of mouth or tongue
　　　　　Other oral epithelium disturbances

　K13.3　Hairy leukoplakia

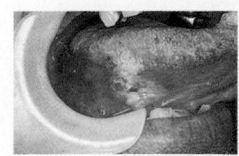

Figure 11-4　Oral leukoplakia and associated squamous carcinoma. (From Feldman: Sleisenger & Fordtran's Gastrointestinal and Liver Disease, ed 8, Saunders, An Imprint of Elsevier, 2006)

K13.4 Granuloma and granuloma-like lesions of oral mucosa
Eosinophilic granuloma
Granuloma pyogenicum
Verrucous xanthoma

K13.5 Oral submucous fibrosis
Submucous fibrosis of tongue

K13.6 Irritative hyperplasia of oral mucosa
Excludes2   irritative hyperplasia of edentulous ridge [denture hyperplasia] (K06.2)

● **K13.7 Other and unspecified lesions of oral mucosa**

(See Plate 58 on page 71.)

K13.70 Unspecified lesions of oral mucosa

K13.79 Other lesions of oral mucosa
Focal oral mucinosis

● **K14 Diseases of tongue**
Use additional code to identify:
alcohol abuse and dependence (F10.-)
exposure to environmental tobacco smoke (Z77.22)
history of tobacco use (Z87.891)
occupational exposure to environmental tobacco smoke (Z57.31)
tobacco dependence (F17.-)
tobacco use (Z72.0)
Excludes2   erythroplakia (K13.29)
focal epithelial hyperplasia (K13.29)
leukedema of tongue (K13.29)
leukoplakia of tongue (K13.21)
hairy leukoplakia (K13.3)
macroglossia (congenital) (Q38.2)
submucous fibrosis of tongue (K13.5)

K14.0 Glossitis
Abscess of tongue
Ulceration (traumatic) of tongue
Excludes1   atrophic glossitis (K14.4)

K14.1 Geographic tongue
Benign migratory glossitis
Glossitis areata exfoliativa

K14.2 Median rhomboid glossitis

K14.3 Hypertrophy of tongue papillae
Black hairy tongue
Coated tongue
Hypertrophy of foliate papillae
Lingua villosa nigra

K14.4 Atrophy of tongue papillae
Atrophic glossitis

K14.5 Plicated tongue
Fissured tongue   Scrotal tongue
Furrowed tongue
Excludes1   fissured tongue, congenital (Q38.3)

K14.6 Glossodynia
Glossopyrosis   Painful tongue

K14.8 Other diseases of tongue
Atrophy of tongue   Glossocele
Crenated tongue   Glossoptosis
Enlargement of tongue   Hypertrophy of tongue

K14.9 Disease of tongue, unspecified
Glossopathy NOS

DISEASES OF ESOPHAGUS, STOMACH AND DUODENUM (K20-K31)

Excludes2   hiatus hernia (K44.-)

● **K20 Esophagitis**
Use additional code to identify:
alcohol abuse and dependence (F10.-)
Excludes1   erosion of esophagus (K22.1-)
esophagitis with gastro-esophageal reflux disease (K21.0)
reflux esophagitis (K21.0)
ulcerative esophagitis (K22.1-)
Excludes2   eosinophilic gastritis or gastroenteritis (K52.81)

K20.0 Eosinophilic esophagitis

K20.8 Other esophagitis
Abscess of esophagus

K20.9 Esophagitis, unspecified
Esophagitis NOS

● **K21 Gastro-esophageal reflux disease**
Excludes1   newborn esophageal reflux (P78.83)

K21.0 Gastro-esophageal reflux disease with esophagitis
Reflux esophagitis

K21.9 Gastro-esophageal reflux disease without esophagitis
Esophageal reflux NOS

● **K22 Other diseases of esophagus**
Excludes2   esophageal varices (I85.-)

K22.0 Achalasia of cardia
Achalasia NOS
Cardiospasm
Excludes1   congenital cardiospasm (Q39.5)

● **K22.1 Ulcer of esophagus**
Barrett's ulcer
Erosion of esophagus
Fungal ulcer of esophagus
Peptic ulcer of esophagus
Ulcer of esophagus due to ingestion of chemicals
Ulcer of esophagus due to ingestion of drugs and medicaments
Ulcerative esophagitis
Code first poisoning due to drug or toxin, if applicable (T36-T65 with fifth or sixth character 1-4 or 6)
Use additional code for adverse effect, if applicable, to identify drug (T36-T50 with fifth or sixth character 5)
Excludes1   Barrett's esophagus (K22.87-)

K22.10 Ulcer of esophagus without bleeding
Ulcer of esophagus NOS

K22.11 Ulcer of esophagus with bleeding
Excludes2   bleeding esophageal varices (I85.01, I85.11)

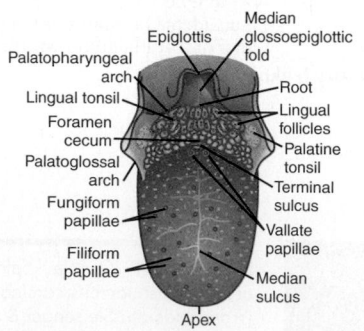

Figure 11-5   Structure of the tongue.

Item 11–6   **Esophageal reflux** is the return flow of the contents of the stomach to the esophagus and is referred to as GERD and/or "heartburn." **Gastroesophageal reflux** is the return flow of the contents of the stomach and duodenum to the esophagus. **Esophageal leukoplakia** are white areas on the mucous membrane of the esophagus for which no specific cause can be identified.

◀ New   ⬅ Revised   ~~deleted~~ Deleted   Excludes 1   Excludes 2   Includes   Use additional   Code first   Code also   Unspecified

OGCR Official Guidelines   **X** Assign placeholder X   ● Use Additional Character(s)   ▶ Manifestation Code   **Coding Clinic**

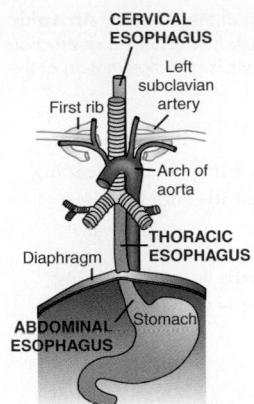

CERVICAL ESOPHAGUS
Left subclavian artery
First rib
Arch of aorta
THORACIC ESOPHAGUS
Diaphragm
ABDOMINAL ESOPHAGUS
Stomach

Figure 11-6 The esophagus is the muscular tube that connects the pharynx and the stomach. The 10 inch (25 cm) long esophagus is divided into three parts: **cervical, thoracic,** and **abdominal.**

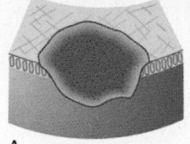
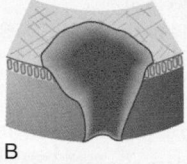
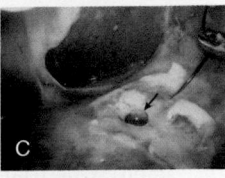

A   B   C

Figure 11-7 **A.** Ulcer. **B.** Perforated ulcer. **C.** Laparoscopic view of a perforated duodenal ulcer *(arrow)* with fibrinous exudate on the adjacent peritoneum. (**C** from Feldman: Sleisenger & Fordtran's Gastrointestinal and Liver Disease, ed 8, Saunders, An Imprint of Elsevier, 2006)

Item 11-8 Gastric ulcers are lesions of the stomach that result in the death of the tissue and a defect of the surface. **Perforated ulcers** are those in which the lesion penetrates the gastric wall, leaving a hole. **Peptic ulcers** are lesions of the stomach or the duodenum. **Peptic** refers to the gastric juice, pepsin.

K22.2 Esophageal obstruction
Compression of esophagus
Constriction of esophagus
Stenosis of esophagus
Stricture of esophagus
Excludes1 congenital stenosis or stricture of esophagus (Q39.3)

K22.3 Perforation of esophagus
Rupture of esophagus
Excludes1 traumatic perforation of (thoracic) esophagus (S27.8-)

K22.4 Dyskinesia of esophagus
Difficulty in moving
Corkscrew esophagus
Diffuse esophageal spasm
Spasm of esophagus
Excludes1 cardiospasm (K22.0)

K22.5 Diverticulum of esophagus, acquired
Esophageal pouch, acquired
Excludes1 diverticulum of esophagus (congenital) (Q39.6)

K22.6 Gastro-esophageal laceration-hemorrhage syndrome
Mallory-Weiss syndrome

● **K22.7 Barrett's esophagus**
Barrett's disease
Barrett's syndrome
Excludes1 Barrett's ulcer (K22.1)
malignant neoplasm of esophagus (C15.-)

K22.70 Barrett's esophagus without dysplasia
Barrett's esophagus NOS

● **K22.71 Barrett's esophagus with dysplasia**
K22.710 Barrett's esophagus with low grade dysplasia
K22.711 Barrett's esophagus with high grade dysplasia
K22.719 Barrett's esophagus with dysplasia, unspecified

K22.8 Other specified diseases of esophagus
Hemorrhage of esophagus NOS
Excludes2 esophageal varices (I85.-)
Paterson-Kelly syndrome (D50.1)

K22.9 Disease of esophagus, unspecified

▶ **K23 Disorders of esophagus in diseases classified elsewhere**
Code first underlying disease, such as:
congenital syphilis (A50.5)
Excludes1 late syphilis (A52.79)
megaesophagus due to Chagas' disease (B57.31)
tuberculosis (A18.83)

● **K25 Gastric ulcer**
Includes erosion (acute) of stomach
pylorus ulcer (peptic)
stomach ulcer (peptic)
Use additional code to identify:
alcohol abuse and dependence (F10.-)
Excludes1 acute gastritis (K29.0-)
peptic ulcer NOS (K27.-)

K25.0 Acute gastric ulcer with hemorrhage
K25.1 Acute gastric ulcer with perforation
K25.2 Acute gastric ulcer with both hemorrhage and perforation
K25.3 Acute gastric ulcer without hemorrhage or perforation
K25.4 Chronic or unspecified gastric ulcer with hemorrhage
K25.5 Chronic or unspecified gastric ulcer with perforation
K25.6 Chronic or unspecified gastric ulcer with both hemorrhage and perforation
K25.7 Chronic gastric ulcer without hemorrhage or perforation
K25.9 Gastric ulcer, unspecified as acute or chronic, without hemorrhage or perforation

● **K26 Duodenal ulcer**
Includes erosion (acute) of duodenum
duodenum ulcer (peptic)
postpyloric ulcer (peptic)
Use additional code to identify:
alcohol abuse and dependence (F10.-)
Excludes1 peptic ulcer NOS (K27.-)

K26.0 Acute duodenal ulcer with hemorrhage
K26.1 Acute duodenal ulcer with perforation
K26.2 Acute duodenal ulcer with both hemorrhage and perforation
K26.3 Acute duodenal ulcer without hemorrhage or perforation
K26.4 Chronic or unspecified duodenal ulcer with hemorrhage
K26.5 Chronic or unspecified duodenal ulcer with perforation
K26.6 Chronic or unspecified duodenal ulcer with both hemorrhage and perforation
K26.7 Chronic duodenal ulcer without hemorrhage or perforation
K26.9 Duodenal ulcer, unspecified as acute or chronic, without hemorrhage or perforation

Item 11-7 Achalasia is a condition in which the smooth muscle fibers of the esophagus do not relax. Most frequently, this condition occurs at the esophagogastric sphincter. **Cardiospasm,** also known as **megaesophagus,** is achalasia of the thoracic esophagus.

CHAPTER 11 (K00-K95)

CHAPTER 11 (K00-K95)

● **K27**   Peptic ulcer, site unspecified

> **Includes**   gastroduodenal ulcer NOS
>   peptic ulcer NOS

> Use additional code to identify:
>   alcohol abuse and dependence (F10.-)

> **Excludes1**   peptic ulcer of newborn (P78.82)

K27.0   Acute peptic ulcer, site unspecified, with hemorrhage

K27.1   Acute peptic ulcer, site unspecified, with perforation

K27.2   Acute peptic ulcer, site unspecified, with both hemorrhage and perforation

K27.3   Acute peptic ulcer, site unspecified, without hemorrhage or perforation

K27.4   Chronic or unspecified peptic ulcer, site unspecified, with hemorrhage

K27.5   Chronic or unspecified peptic ulcer, site unspecified, with perforation

K27.6   Chronic or unspecified peptic ulcer, site unspecified, with both hemorrhage and perforation

K27.7   Chronic peptic ulcer, site unspecified, without hemorrhage or perforation

K27.9   Peptic ulcer, site unspecified, unspecified as acute or chronic, without hemorrhage or perforation

● **K28**   Gastrojejunal ulcer

> **Includes**   anastomotic ulcer (peptic) or erosion
>   gastrocolic ulcer (peptic) or erosion
>   gastrointestinal ulcer (peptic) or erosion
>   gastrojejunal ulcer (peptic) or erosion
>   jejunal ulcer (peptic) or erosion
>   marginal ulcer (peptic) or erosion
>   stomal ulcer (peptic) or erosion

> Use additional code to identify:
>   alcohol abuse and dependence (F10.-)

> **Excludes1**   primary ulcer of small intestine (K63.3)

K28.0   Acute gastrojejunal ulcer with hemorrhage

K28.1   Acute gastrojejunal ulcer with perforation

K28.2   Acute gastrojejunal ulcer with both hemorrhage and perforation

K28.3   Acute gastrojejunal ulcer without hemorrhage or perforation

K28.4   Chronic or unspecified gastrojejunal ulcer with hemorrhage

K28.5   Chronic or unspecified gastrojejunal ulcer with perforation

K28.6   Chronic or unspecified gastrojejunal ulcer with both hemorrhage and perforation

K28.7   Chronic gastrojejunal ulcer without hemorrhage or perforation

K28.9   Gastrojejunal ulcer, unspecified as acute or chronic, without hemorrhage or perforation

● **K29**   Gastritis and duodenitis

> **Excludes1**   eosinophilic gastritis or gastroenteritis (K52.81)
>   Zollinger-Ellison syndrome (E16.4)

● **K29.0**   Acute gastritis

> Use additional code to identify:
>   alcohol abuse and dependence (F10.-)

> **Excludes1**   erosion (acute) of stomach (K25.-)

K29.00   Acute gastritis without bleeding

K29.01   Acute gastritis with bleeding

● **K29.2**   Alcoholic gastritis

> Use additional code to identify:
>   alcohol abuse and dependence (F10.-)

K29.20   Alcoholic gastritis without bleeding

K29.21   Alcoholic gastritis with bleeding

Item 11-9   **Gastritis** is a severe inflammation of the stomach. **Atrophic gastritis** is a chronic inflammation of the stomach that results in destruction of the cells of the mucosa of the stomach. Duodenitis is an inflammation of the duodenum, the first section of the small intestine.

● **K29.3**   Chronic superficial gastritis

K29.30   Chronic superficial gastritis without bleeding

K29.31   Chronic superficial gastritis with bleeding

● **K29.4**   Chronic atrophic gastritis

> Gastric atrophy

K29.40   Chronic atrophic gastritis without bleeding

K29.41   Chronic atrophic gastritis with bleeding

● **K29.5**   Unspecified chronic gastritis

> Chronic antral gastritis
> Chronic fundal gastritis

K29.50   Unspecified chronic gastritis without bleeding

K29.51   Unspecified chronic gastritis with bleeding

● **K29.6**   Other gastritis

> Giant hypertrophic gastritis
> Granulomatous gastritis
> Ménétrier's disease

K29.60   Other gastritis without bleeding

K29.61   Other gastritis with bleeding

● **K29.7**   Gastritis, unspecified

K29.70   Gastritis, unspecified, without bleeding

K29.71   Gastritis, unspecified, with bleeding

● **K29.8**   Duodenitis

K29.80   Duodenitis without bleeding

K29.81   Duodenitis with bleeding

● **K29.9**   Gastroduodenitis, unspecified

K29.90   Gastroduodenitis, unspecified, without bleeding

K29.91   Gastroduodenitis, unspecified, with bleeding

K30   Functional dyspepsia

> Indigestion

> **Excludes1**   dyspepsia NOS (R10.13)
>   heartburn (R12)
>   nervous dyspepsia (F45.8)
>   neurotic dyspepsia (F45.8)
>   psychogenic dyspepsia (F45.8)

● **K31**   Other diseases of stomach and duodenum

> Includes   functional disorders of stomach

> **Excludes2**   diabetic gastroparesis (E08.43, E09.43, E10.43, E11.43, E13.43)
>   diverticulum of duodenum (K57.00-K57.13)

K31.0   Acute dilatation of stomach

> Acute distention of stomach

K31.1   Adult hypertrophic pyloric stenosis   **A**

> Pyloric stenosis NOS

> **Excludes1**   congenital or infantile pyloric stenosis (Q40.0)

K31.2   Hourglass stricture and stenosis of stomach

> **Excludes1**   congenital hourglass stomach (Q40.2)
>   hourglass contraction of stomach (K31.89)

K31.3   Pylorospasm, not elsewhere classified

> **Excludes1**   congenital or infantile pylorospasm (Q40.0)
>   neurotic pylorospasm (F45.8)
>   psychogenic pylorospasm (F45.8)

K31.4   Gastric diverticulum

> **Excludes1**   congenital diverticulum of stomach (Q40.2)

◄ New   ◄═ Revised   ~~deleted~~ Deleted   Excludes 1   Excludes 2   Includes   Use additional   Code first   Code also   Unspecified

OGCR Official Guidelines   X Assign placeholder X   ● Use Additional Character(s)   ▶ Manifestation Code   **Coding Clinic**

Item 11–10 Achlorhydria, also known as gastric anacidity, is the absence of gastric acid.

K31.5 **Obstruction of duodenum**
  Constriction of duodenum
  Duodenal ileus (chronic)
  Stenosis of duodenum
    Narrowing
  Stricture of duodenum
    Narrowing
  Volvulus of duodenum
    Twisting/knotting
  Excludes1 congenital stenosis of duodenum (Q41.0)

K31.6 **Fistula of stomach and duodenum**
  Gastrocolic fistula
  Gastrojejunocolic fistula

K31.7 **Polyp of stomach and duodenum**
  Excludes1 adenomatous polyp of stomach (D13.1)

● **K31.8** **Other specified diseases of stomach and duodenum**
  ● **K31.81** **Angiodysplasia of stomach and duodenum**
      K31.811 **Angiodysplasia of stomach and duodenum with bleeding**
      K31.819 **Angiodysplasia of stomach and duodenum without bleeding**
        Angiodysplasia of stomach and duodenum NOS
    K31.82 **Dieulafoy lesion (hemorrhagic) of stomach and duodenum**
        Excludes2 Dieulafoy lesion of intestine (K63.81)
    K31.83 **Achlorhydria**
    K31.84 **Gastroparesis**
        Gastroparalysis
        Code first underlying disease, if known, such as:
        anorexia nervosa (F50.0-)
        diabetes mellitus (E08.43, E09.43, E10.43, E11.43, E13.43)
        scleroderma (M34.-)
    K31.89 **Other diseases of stomach and duodenum**
  K31.9 **Disease of stomach and duodenum, unspecified**

DISEASES OF APPENDIX (K35-K38)

● **K35** **Acute appendicitis**
  K35.2 **Acute appendicitis with generalized peritonitis**
      Appendicitis (acute) with generalized (diffuse) peritonitis following rupture or perforation of appendix
      Perforated appendix NOS
      Ruptured appendix NOS
  K35.3 **Acute appendicitis with localized peritonitis**
      Acute appendicitis with or without perforation or rupture NOS
      Acute appendicitis with or without perforation or rupture with localized peritonitis
      Acute appendicitis with peritoneal abscess
  ● **K35.8** **Other and unspecified acute appendicitis**
      K35.80 Unspecified **acute appendicitis**
          Acute appendicitis NOS
          Acute appendicitis without (localized) (generalized) peritonitis
      K35.89 **Other acute appendicitis**

  K36 **Other appendicitis**
      Chronic appendicitis
      Recurrent appendicitis

  K37 Unspecified **appendicitis**
      Excludes1 -unspecified appendicitis with peritonitis (K35.2-K35.3)

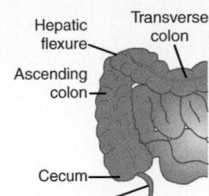

Figure 11-8 Acute appendicitis is the inflammation of the appendix, usually associated with obstruction. Most often this is a disease of adolescents and young adults.

● **K38** **Other diseases of appendix**
  K38.0 **Hyperplasia of appendix**
  K38.1 **Appendicular concretions**
      Fecalith of appendix
      Stercolith of appendix
  K38.2 **Diverticulum of appendix**
  K38.3 **Fistula of appendix**
  K38.8 **Other specified diseases of appendix**
      Intussusception of appendix
  K38.9 **Disease of appendix,** unspecified

HERNIA (K40-K46)

  Note: Hernia with both gangrene and obstruction is classified to hernia with gangrene.
  Includes acquired hernia
      congenital [except diaphragmatic or hiatus] hernia
      recurrent hernia

● **K40** **Inguinal hernia**
  Includes bubonocele
      direct inguinal hernia
      double inguinal hernia
      indirect inguinal hernia
      inguinal hernia NOS
      oblique inguinal hernia
      scrotal hernia
  ● **K40.0** **Bilateral inguinal hernia, with obstruction, without gangrene**
      Inguinal hernia (bilateral) causing obstruction without gangrene
      Incarcerated inguinal hernia (bilateral) without gangrene
      Irreducible inguinal hernia (bilateral) without gangrene
      Strangulated inguinal hernia (bilateral) without gangrene
      K40.00 **Bilateral inguinal hernia, with obstruction, without gangrene, not specified as recurrent**
          Bilateral inguinal hernia, with obstruction, without gangrene NOS
      K40.01 **Bilateral inguinal hernia, with obstruction, without gangrene, recurrent**

Item 11–11 Hernias of the groin are the most common type, accounting for 80 percent of all hernias. There are two major types of inguinal hernias: indirect (oblique) affecting men only and direct. **Indirect inguinal hernias** result when the intestines emerge through the abdominal wall in an indirect fashion through the inguinal canal. **Direct inguinal hernias** penetrate through the abdominal wall in a direct fashion. **Femoral hernias** occur at the femoral ring where the femoral vessels enter the thigh and is most common in women. An abdominal wall hernia is also called a ventral or epigastric hernia and occurs in both sexes. Classification is based on location of the hernia and whether there is obstruction or gangrene.
  Ventral, epigastric, or incisional hernia occurs on the abdominal surface caused by musculature weakness or a tear at a previous surgical site and is evidenced by a bulge that changes in size, becoming larger with exertion. An **incarcerated** hernia is one in which the intestines become trapped in the hernia. A **strangulated** hernia is one in which the blood supply to the intestines is lost. Hiatal hernia occurs when a loop of the stomach protrudes upward through the small opening in the diaphragm through which the esophagus passes, leaving the abdominal cavity and entering the chest. It occurs in both sexes.

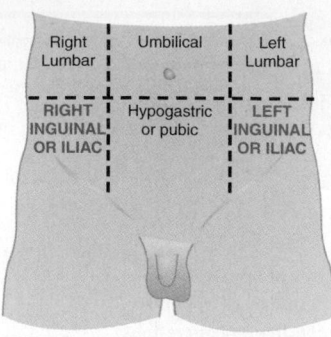

Right Lumbar	Umbilical	Left Lumbar
RIGHT INGUINAL OR ILIAC	Hypogastric or pubic	LEFT INGUINAL OR ILIAC

Figure 11-9   Inguinal hernias are those that are located in the inguinal or iliac areas of the abdomen.

● **K40.1**   **Bilateral inguinal hernia, with gangrene**
    K40.10   **Bilateral inguinal hernia, with gangrene, not specified as recurrent**
       Bilateral inguinal hernia, with gangrene NOS
    K40.11   **Bilateral inguinal hernia, with gangrene, recurrent**

● **K40.2**   **Bilateral inguinal hernia, without obstruction or gangrene**
    K40.20   **Bilateral inguinal hernia, without obstruction or gangrene, not specified as recurrent**
       Bilateral inguinal hernia NOS
    K40.21   **Bilateral inguinal hernia, without obstruction or gangrene, recurrent**

● **K40.3**   **Unilateral inguinal hernia, with obstruction, without gangrene**
       Inguinal hernia (unilateral) causing obstruction without gangrene
       Incarcerated inguinal hernia (unilateral) without gangrene
       Irreducible inguinal hernia (unilateral) without gangrene
       Strangulated inguinal hernia (unilateral) without gangrene
    K40.30   **Unilateral inguinal hernia, with obstruction, without gangrene, not specified as recurrent**
       Inguinal hernia, with obstruction NOS
       Unilateral inguinal hernia, with obstruction, without gangrene NOS
    K40.31   **Unilateral inguinal hernia, with obstruction, without gangrene, recurrent**

● **K40.4**   **Unilateral inguinal hernia, with gangrene**
    K40.40   **Unilateral inguinal hernia, with gangrene, not specified as recurrent**
       Inguinal hernia with gangrene NOS
       Unilateral inguinal hernia with gangrene NOS
    K40.41   **Unilateral inguinal hernia, with gangrene, recurrent**

● **K40.9**   **Unilateral inguinal hernia, without obstruction or gangrene**
    K40.90   **Unilateral inguinal hernia, without obstruction or gangrene, not specified as recurrent**
       Inguinal hernia NOS
       Unilateral inguinal hernia NOS
    K40.91   **Unilateral inguinal hernia, without obstruction or gangrene, recurrent**

● **K41**   **Femoral hernia**
● **K41.0**   **Bilateral femoral hernia, with obstruction, without gangrene**
       Femoral hernia (bilateral) causing obstruction, without gangrene
       Incarcerated femoral hernia (bilateral), without gangrene
       Irreducible femoral hernia (bilateral), without gangrene
       Strangulated femoral hernia (bilateral), without gangrene
    K41.00   **Bilateral femoral hernia, with obstruction, without gangrene, not specified as recurrent**
       Bilateral femoral hernia, with obstruction, without gangrene NOS
    K41.01   **Bilateral femoral hernia, with obstruction, without gangrene, recurrent**

● **K41.1**   **Bilateral femoral hernia, with gangrene**
    K41.10   **Bilateral femoral hernia, with gangrene, not specified as recurrent**
       Bilateral femoral hernia, with gangrene NOS
    K41.11   **Bilateral femoral hernia, with gangrene, recurrent**

● **K41.2**   **Bilateral femoral hernia, without obstruction or gangrene**
    K41.20   **Bilateral femoral hernia, without obstruction or gangrene, not specified as recurrent**
       Bilateral femoral hernia NOS
    K41.21   **Bilateral femoral hernia, without obstruction or gangrene, recurrent**

● **K41.3**   **Unilateral femoral hernia, with obstruction, without gangrene**
       Femoral hernia (unilateral) causing obstruction, without gangrene
       Incarcerated femoral hernia (unilateral), without gangrene
       Irreducible femoral hernia (unilateral), without gangrene
       Strangulated femoral hernia (unilateral), without gangrene
    K41.30   **Unilateral femoral hernia, with obstruction, without gangrene, not specified as recurrent**
       Femoral hernia, with obstruction NOS
       Unilateral femoral hernia, with obstruction NOS
    K41.31   **Unilateral femoral hernia, with obstruction, without gangrene, recurrent**

● **K41.4**   **Unilateral femoral hernia, with gangrene**
    K41.40   **Unilateral femoral hernia, with gangrene, not specified as recurrent**
       Femoral hernia, with gangrene NOS
       Unilateral femoral hernia, with gangrene NOS
    K41.41   **Unilateral femoral hernia, with gangrene, recurrent**

● **K41.9**   **Unilateral femoral hernia, without obstruction or gangrene**
    K41.90   **Unilateral femoral hernia, without obstruction or gangrene, not specified as recurrent**
       Femoral hernia NOS
       Unilateral femoral hernia NOS
    K41.91   **Unilateral femoral hernia, without obstruction or gangrene, recurrent**

● **K42**   **Umbilical hernia**
    Includes   paraumbilical hernia
    Excludes1   omphalocele (Q79.2)
    K42.0   **Umbilical hernia with obstruction, without gangrene**
       Umbilical hernia causing obstruction, without gangrene
       Incarcerated umbilical hernia, without gangrene
       Irreducible umbilical hernia, without gangrene
       Strangulated umbilical hernia, without gangrene

CHAPTER 11 (K00-K95)

◄ New   ⬅ Revised   ~~deleted~~ Deleted   Excludes 1   Excludes 2   Includes   Use additional   Code first   Code also   Unspecified
   OGCR Official Guidelines   **X** Assign placeholder X   ● Use Additional Character(s)   ▶ Manifestation Code   **Coding Clinic**

K42.1   **Umbilical hernia with gangrene**
Gangrenous umbilical hernia

K42.9   **Umbilical hernia without obstruction or gangrene**
Umbilical hernia NOS

● **K43**   **Ventral hernia**

K43.0   **Incisional hernia with obstruction, without gangrene**
Incisional hernia causing obstruction, without gangrene
Incarcerated incisional hernia, without gangrene
Irreducible incisional hernia, without gangrene
Strangulated incisional hernia, without gangrene

K43.1   **Incisional hernia with gangrene**
Gangrenous incisional hernia

K43.2   **Incisional hernia without obstruction or gangrene**
Incisional hernia NOS

K43.3   **Parastomal hernia with obstruction, without gangrene**
Incarcerated parastomal hernia, without gangrene
Irreducible parastomal hernia, without gangrene
Parastomal hernia causing obstruction, without gangrene
Strangulated parastomal hernia, without gangrene

K43.4   **Parastomal hernia with gangrene**
Gangrenous parastomal hernia

K43.5   **Parastomal hernia without obstruction or gangrene**
Parastomal hernia NOS

K43.6   **Other and unspecified ventral hernia with obstruction, without gangrene**
Epigastric hernia causing obstruction, without gangrene
Hypogastric hernia causing obstruction, without gangrene
Incarcerated epigastric hernia without gangrene
Incarcerated hypogastric hernia without gangrene
Incarcerated midline hernia without gangrene
Incarcerated spigelian hernia without gangrene
Incarcerated subxiphoid hernia without gangrene
Irreducible epigastric hernia without gangrene
Irreducible hypogastric hernia without gangrene
Irreducible midline hernia without gangrene
Irreducible spigelian hernia without gangrene
Irreducible subxiphoid hernia without gangrene
Midline hernia causing obstruction, without gangrene
Spigelian hernia causing obstruction, without gangrene
Strangulated epigastric hernia without gangrene
Strangulated hypogastric hernia without gangrene
Strangulated midline hernia without gangrene
Strangulated spigelian hernia without gangrene
Strangulated subxiphoid hernia without gangrene
Subxiphoid hernia causing obstruction, without gangrene

K43.7   **Other and unspecified ventral hernia with gangrene**
Any condition listed under K43.6 specified as gangrenous

K43.9   **Ventral hernia without obstruction or gangrene**
Epigastric hernia
Ventral hernia NOS

● **K44**   **Diaphragmatic hernia**

> **Includes**   hiatus hernia (esophageal) (sliding)
> paraesophageal hernia

> **Excludes1**   congenital diaphragmatic hernia (Q79.0)
> congenital hiatus hernia (Q40.1)

K44.0   **Diaphragmatic hernia with obstruction, without gangrene**
Diaphragmatic hernia causing obstruction
Incarcerated diaphragmatic hernia
Irreducible diaphragmatic hernia
Strangulated diaphragmatic hernia

K44.1   **Diaphragmatic hernia with gangrene**
Gangrenous diaphragmatic hernia

K44.9   **Diaphragmatic hernia without obstruction or gangrene**
Diaphragmatic hernia NOS

● **K45**   **Other abdominal hernia**

> **Includes**   abdominal hernia, specified site NEC
> lumbar hernia
> obturator hernia
> pudendal hernia
> retroperitoneal hernia
> sciatic hernia

K45.0   **Other specified abdominal hernia with obstruction, without gangrene**
Other specified abdominal hernia causing obstruction
Other specified incarcerated abdominal hernia
Other specified irreducible abdominal hernia
Other specified strangulated abdominal hernia

K45.1   **Other specified abdominal hernia with gangrene**
Any condition listed under K45 specified as gangrenous

K45.8   **Other specified abdominal hernia without obstruction or gangrene**

● **K46**   **Unspecified abdominal hernia**

> **Includes**   enterocele
> epiplocele
> hernia NOS
> interstitial hernia
> intestinal hernia
> intra-abdominal hernia

> **Excludes1**   vaginal enterocele (N81.5)

K46.0   **Unspecified abdominal hernia with obstruction, without gangrene**
Unspecified abdominal hernia causing obstruction
Unspecified incarcerated abdominal hernia
Unspecified irreducible abdominal hernia
Unspecified strangulated abdominal hernia

K46.1   **Unspecified abdominal hernia with gangrene**
Any condition listed under K46 specified as gangrenous

K46.9   **Unspecified abdominal hernia without obstruction or gangrene**
Abdominal hernia NOS

(See Plate 284 on page 77.)

NONINFECTIVE ENTERITIS AND COLITIS (K50-K52)

> **Includes**   noninfective inflammatory bowel disease
> **Excludes1**   irritable bowel syndrome (K58.-)
> megacolon (K59.3)

● **K50**   **Crohn's disease [regional enteritis]**

> **Includes**   granulomatous enteritis

Use additional code to identify manifestations, such as:
pyoderma gangrenosum (L88)

> **Excludes1**   ulcerative colitis (K51.-)

● **K50.0**   **Crohn's disease of small intestine**
Crohn's disease [regional enteritis] of duodenum
Crohn's disease [regional enteritis] of ileum
Crohn's disease [regional enteritis] of jejunum
Regional ileitis
Terminal ileitis

> **Excludes1**   Crohn's disease of both small and large intestine (K50.8-)

K50.00   **Crohn's disease of small intestine without complications**

Item 11-12 Crohn's disease, also known as **regional enteritis**, is a chronic inflammatory disease of the intestines. Classification is based on location in the small (duodenum, ileum, jejunum) or large (cecum, colon, rectum, anal canal) intestine.

● **K50.01**   **Crohn's disease of small intestine with complications**

     K50.011   Crohn's disease of small intestine with rectal bleeding

     K50.012   Crohn's disease of small intestine with intestinal obstruction

     K50.013   Crohn's disease of small intestine with fistula

     K50.014   Crohn's disease of small intestine with abscess
         Coding Clinic: 2012, Q4, P104

     K50.018   Crohn's disease of small intestine with other complication

     K50.019   Crohn's disease of small intestine with unspecified complications

● **K50.1**   **Crohn's disease of large intestine**
Crohn's disease [regional enteritis] of colon
Crohn's disease [regional enteritis] of large bowel
Crohn's disease [regional enteritis] of rectum
Granulomatous colitis
Regional colitis

    Excludes1   Crohn's disease of both small and large intestine (K50.8)

     K50.10   Crohn's disease of large intestine without complications

●   **K50.11**   **Crohn's disease of large intestine with complications**

     K50.111   Crohn's disease of large intestine with rectal bleeding

     K50.112   Crohn's disease of large intestine with intestinal obstruction

     K50.113   Crohn's disease of large intestine with fistula

     K50.114   Crohn's disease of large intestine with abscess
         Coding Clinic: 2012, Q4, P104

     K50.118   Crohn's disease of large intestine with other complication

     K50.119   Crohn's disease of large intestine with unspecified complications

● **K50.8**   **Crohn's disease of both small and large intestine**

     K50.80   Crohn's disease of both small and large intestine without complications

●   **K50.81**   Crohn's disease of both small and large intestine with complications

     K50.811   Crohn's disease of both small and large intestine with rectal bleeding

     K50.812   Crohn's disease of both small and large intestine with intestinal obstruction

     K50.813   Crohn's disease of both small and large intestine with fistula

     K50.814   Crohn's disease of both small and large intestine with abscess
         Coding Clinic: 2012, Q4, P104

     K50.818   Crohn's disease of both small and large intestine with other complication

     K50.819   Crohn's disease of both small and large intestine with unspecified complications

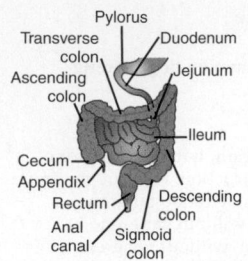

Figure 11-10   Small and large intestines.

● **K50.9**   **Crohn's disease, unspecified**

     K50.90   Crohn's disease, unspecified, without complications
Crohn's disease NOS
Regional enteritis NOS

●   **K50.91**   Crohn's disease, unspecified, with complications

     K50.911   Crohn's disease, unspecified, with rectal bleeding

     K50.912   Crohn's disease, unspecified, with intestinal obstruction

     K50.913   Crohn's disease, unspecified, with fistula

     K50.914   Crohn's disease, unspecified, with abscess
         Coding Clinic: 2012, Q4, P104

     K50.918   Crohn's disease, unspecified, with other complication

     K50.919   Crohn's disease, unspecified, with unspecified complications

● **K51**   **Ulcerative colitis**
Use additional code to identify manifestations, such as: pyoderma gangrenosum (L88)

    Excludes1   Crohn's disease [regional enteritis] (K50.-)

● **K51.0**   **Ulcerative (chronic) pancolitis**
Backwash ileitis

     K51.00   Ulcerative (chronic) pancolitis without complications
Ulcerative (chronic) pancolitis NOS

●   **K51.01**   Ulcerative (chronic) pancolitis with complications

     K51.011   Ulcerative (chronic) pancolitis with rectal bleeding

     K51.012   Ulcerative (chronic) pancolitis with intestinal obstruction

     K51.013   Ulcerative (chronic) pancolitis with fistula

     K51.014   Ulcerative (chronic) pancolitis with abscess

     K51.018   Ulcerative (chronic) pancolitis with other complication

     K51.019   Ulcerative (chronic) pancolitis with unspecified complications

Item 11-13 Ulcerative colitis attacks the colonic mucosa and forms abscesses. The disease involves the intestines. Classification is based on the location:

- Enterocolitis: large and small intestine
- Ileocolitis: ileum and colon
- Proctitis: rectum
- Proctosigmoiditis: sigmoid colon and rectum

◄ New   ◄═ Revised   ~~deleted~~ Deleted   Excludes 1   Excludes 2   Includes   Use additional   Code first   Code also   Unspecified

OGCR Official Guidelines   **X** Assign placeholder X   ● Use Additional Character(s)   ▶ Manifestation Code   **Coding Clinic**

● **K51.2   Ulcerative (chronic) proctitis**
   K51.20   Ulcerative (chronic) proctitis without complications
         Ulcerative (chronic) proctitis NOS
● **K51.21   Ulcerative (chronic) proctitis with complications**
      K51.211   Ulcerative (chronic) proctitis with rectal bleeding
      K51.212   Ulcerative (chronic) proctitis with intestinal obstruction
      K51.213   Ulcerative (chronic) proctitis with fistula
      K51.214   Ulcerative (chronic) proctitis with abscess
      K51.218   Ulcerative (chronic) proctitis with other complication
      K51.219   Ulcerative (chronic) proctitis with unspecified **complications**

● **K51.3   Ulcerative (chronic) rectosigmoiditis**
   K51.30   Ulcerative (chronic) rectosigmoiditis without complications
         Ulcerative (chronic) rectosigmoiditis NOS
● **K51.31   Ulcerative (chronic) rectosigmoiditis with complications**
      K51.311   Ulcerative (chronic) rectosigmoiditis with rectal bleeding
      K51.312   Ulcerative (chronic) rectosigmoiditis with intestinal obstruction
      K51.313   Ulcerative (chronic) rectosigmoiditis with fistula
      K51.314   Ulcerative (chronic) rectosigmoiditis with abscess
      K51.318   Ulcerative (chronic) rectosigmoiditis with other complication
      K51.319   Ulcerative (chronic) rectosigmoiditis with unspecified **complications**

● **K51.4   Inflammatory polyps of colon**
Excludes1	adenomatous polyp of colon (D12.6)
	polyposis of colon (D12.6)
	polyps of colon NOS (K63.5)

   K51.40   Inflammatory polyps of colon without complications
         Inflammatory polyps of colon NOS
● **K51.41   Inflammatory polyps of colon with complications**
      K51.411   Inflammatory polyps of colon with rectal bleeding
      K51.412   Inflammatory polyps of colon with intestinal obstruction
      K51.413   Inflammatory polyps of colon with fistula
      K51.414   Inflammatory polyps of colon with abscess
      K51.418   Inflammatory polyps of colon with other complication
      K51.419   Inflammatory polyps of colon with unspecified **complications**

● **K51.5   Left sided colitis**
         Left hemicolitis
   K51.50   Left sided colitis without complications
         Left sided colitis NOS
● **K51.51   Left sided colitis with complications**
      K51.511   Left sided colitis with rectal bleeding
      K51.512   Left sided colitis with intestinal obstruction
      K51.513   Left sided colitis with fistula
      K51.514   Left sided colitis with abscess
      K51.518   Left sided colitis with other complication
      K51.519   Left sided colitis with unspecified **complications**

● **K51.8   Other ulcerative colitis**
   K51.80   Other ulcerative colitis without complications
● **K51.81   Other ulcerative colitis with complications**
      K51.811   Other ulcerative colitis with rectal bleeding
      K51.812   Other ulcerative colitis with intestinal obstruction
      K51.813   Other ulcerative colitis with fistula
      K51.814   Other ulcerative colitis with abscess
      K51.818   Other ulcerative colitis with other complication
      K51.819   Other ulcerative colitis with unspecified **complications**

● **K51.9   Ulcerative colitis, unspecified**
   K51.90   Ulcerative colitis, unspecified, **without complications**
● **K51.91   Ulcerative colitis, unspecified, with complications**
      K51.911   Ulcerative colitis, unspecified **with rectal bleeding**
      K51.912   Ulcerative colitis, unspecified **with intestinal obstruction**
      K51.913   Ulcerative colitis, unspecified **with fistula**
      K51.914   Ulcerative colitis, unspecified **with abscess**
      K51.918   Ulcerative colitis, unspecified **with other complication**
      K51.919   Ulcerative colitis, unspecified **with unspecified complications**

● **K52   Other and unspecified noninfective gastroenteritis and colitis**
   K52.0   Gastroenteritis and colitis due to radiation
   K52.1   Toxic gastroenteritis and colitis
         Drug-induced gastroenteritis and colitis
         Code first (T51-T65) to identify toxic agent
         Use additional code for adverse effect, if applicable, to identify drug (T36-T50 with fifth or sixth character 5)
   K52.2   Allergic and dietetic gastroenteritis and colitis
         Food hypersensitivity gastroenteritis or colitis
         Use additional code to identify type of food allergy (Z91.01-, Z91.02-)
● **K52.8   Other specified noninfective gastroenteritis and colitis**
   K52.81   Eosinophilic gastritis or gastroenteritis
         Eosinophilic enteritis

Excludes1	eosinophilic esophagitis (K20.0)

   K52.82   Eosinophilic colitis
   K52.89   Other specified noninfective gastroenteritis and colitis
         Collagenous colitis
         Lymphocytic colitis
         Microscopic colitis (collagenous or lymphocytic)
   K52.9   Noninfective gastroenteritis and colitis, unspecified
         Colitis NOS   Ileitis NOS
         Enteritis NOS   Jejunitis NOS
         Gastroenteritis NOS   Sigmoiditis NOS

Excludes1	diarrhea NOS (R19.7)
	functional diarrhea (K59.1)
	infectious gastroenteritis and colitis NOS (A09)
	neonatal diarrhea (noninfective) (P78.3)
	psychogenic diarrhea (F45.8)

CHAPTER 11 (K00-K95)

OTHER DISEASES OF INTESTINES (K55-K64)

● **K55   Vascular disorders of intestine**

> **Excludes1**   necrotizing enterocolitis of newborn (P77.-)

     K55.0   Acute vascular disorders of intestine
         Acute fulminant ischemic colitis
         Acute intestinal infarction
         Acute small intestine ischemia
         Infarction of appendices epiploicae
         Mesenteric (artery) (vein) embolism
         Mesenteric (artery) (vein) infarction
         Mesenteric (artery) (vein) thrombosis
         Necrosis of intestine
         Subacute ischemic colitis

     K55.1   Chronic vascular disorders of intestine
         Chronic ischemic colitis
         Chronic ischemic enteritis
         Chronic ischemic enterocolitis
         Ischemic stricture of intestine
         Mesenteric atherosclerosis
         Mesenteric vascular insufficiency

     ● **K55.2   Angiodysplasia of colon**

         K55.20   Angiodysplasia of colon without hemorrhage

         K55.21   Angiodysplasia of colon with hemorrhage

     K55.8   Other vascular disorders of intestine

     K55.9   Vascular disorder of intestine, unspecified
         Ischemic colitis
         Ischemic enteritis
         Ischemic enterocolitis

● **K56   Paralytic ileus and intestinal obstruction without hernia**

> **Excludes1**   congenital stricture or stenosis of intestine
>   (Q41-Q42)
>   cystic fibrosis with meconium ileus (E84.11)
>   ischemic stricture of intestine (K55.1)
>   meconium ileus NOS (P76.0)
>   neonatal intestinal obstructions classifiable
>   to P76.-
>   obstruction of duodenum (K31.5)
>   postprocedural intestinal obstruction (K91.3)
>   stenosis of anus or rectum (K62.4)
>   intestinal obstruction with hernia (K40-K46)

     K56.0   Paralytic ileus
         Paralysis of bowel
         Paralysis of colon
         Paralysis of intestine

> **Excludes1**   gallstone ileus (K56.3)
>   ileus NOS (K56.7)
>   obstructive ileus NOS (K56.69)

     K56.1   Intussusception
         Intussusception or invagination of bowel
         Intussusception or invagination of colon
         Intussusception or invagination of intestine
         Intussusception or invagination of rectum

> **Excludes2**   intussusception of appendix (K38.8)

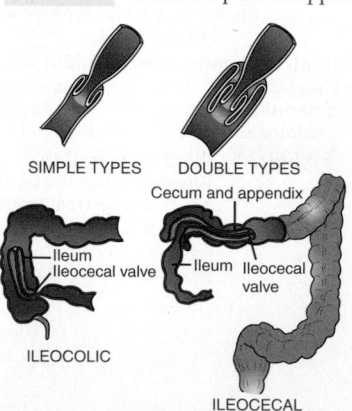

SIMPLE TYPES   DOUBLE TYPES

Cecum and appendix

Ileum
Ileocecal valve   Ileum   Ileocecal valve

ILEOCOLIC

ILEOCECAL

Figure 11-11   Types of intussusception.

Item 11–14   Intussusception is the prolapse (telescoping) of a part of the intestine into another adjacent part of the intestine. Intussusception may be enteric (ileoileal, jejunoileal, jejunojejunal), colic (colocolic), or intracolic (ileocecal, ileocolic).

Item 11–15   Volvulus is the twisting of a segment of the intestine, resulting in obstruction. Paralytic ileus is paralysis of the intestine. It need not be a complete paralysis, but it must prohibit the passage of food through the intestine and lead to intestinal blockage. It is a common aftermath of some types of surgery.

     K56.2   Volvulus
         Strangulation of colon or intestine
         Torsion of colon or intestine
         Twist of colon or intestine

> **Excludes2**   volvulus of duodenum (K31.5)

     K56.3   Gallstone ileus
         Obstruction of intestine by gallstone

     ● **K56.4   Other impaction of intestine**

         K56.41   Fecal impaction

> **Excludes1**   constipation (K59.0-)
>   incomplete defecation (R15.0)

         K56.49   Other impaction of intestine

     K56.5   Intestinal adhesions [bands] with obstruction (postprocedural) (postinfection)
         Abdominal hernia due to adhesions with obstruction
         Peritoneal adhesions [bands] with intestinal obstruction
         (postprocedural) (postinfection)

     ● **K56.6   Other and unspecified intestinal obstruction**

         K56.60   Unspecified intestinal obstruction Intestinal obstruction NOS

> **Excludes1**   intestinal obstruction due to specified condition-code to condition

         K56.69   Other intestinal obstruction
         Enterostenosis NOS
         Obstructive ileus NOS
         Occlusion of colon or intestine NOS
         Stenosis of colon or intestine NOS
         Stricture of colon or intestine NOS

> **Excludes1**   intestinal obstruction due to specified condition-code to condition

     K56.7   Ileus, unspecified

> **Excludes1**   obstructive ileus (K56.69)

● **K57   Diverticular disease of intestine**

> **Excludes1**   congenital diverticulum of intestine (Q43.8)
>   Meckel's diverticulum (Q43.0)

> **Excludes2**   diverticulum of appendix (K38.2)

     ● **K57.0   Diverticulitis of small intestine with perforation and abscess**
         Diverticulitis of small intestine with peritonitis

> **Excludes1**   diverticulitis of both small and large intestine with perforation and abscess (K57.4-)

         K57.00   Diverticulitis of small intestine with perforation and abscess without bleeding

         K57.01   Diverticulitis of small intestine with perforation and abscess with bleeding

◀ New   ◀ Revised   ~~deleted~~ Deleted   Excludes 1   Excludes 2   Includes   Use additional   Code first   Code also   Unspecified

OGCR Official Guidelines   **X** Assign placeholder X   ● Use Additional Character(s)   ▶ Manifestation Code   **Coding Clinic**

Item 11-16 **Diverticula** of the intestines are acquired herniations of the mucosa. Diverticulum (singular): Pocket or pouch that bulges outward through a weak spot (herniation) in the colon. Diverticula (plural). **Diverticulosis** is the condition of having diverticula. **Diverticulitis** is inflammation of these pouches or herniations. Classification is based on location (small intestine or colon) and whether it occurs with or without hemorrhage.

● K57.1   **Diverticular disease of small intestine without perforation or abscess**

> **Excludes1**   diverticular disease of both small and large intestine without perforation or abscess (K57.5-)

    K57.10   **Diverticulosis of small intestine without perforation or abscess without bleeding**
> Diverticular disease of small intestine NOS

    K57.11   **Diverticulosis of small intestine without perforation or abscess with bleeding**

    K57.12   **Diverticulitis of small intestine without perforation or abscess without bleeding**

    K57.13   **Diverticulitis of small intestine without perforation or abscess with bleeding**

● K57.2   **Diverticulitis of large intestine with perforation and abscess**
> Diverticulitis of colon with peritonitis

> **Excludes1**   diverticulitis of both small and large intestine with perforation and abscess (K57.4-)

    K57.20   **Diverticulitis of large intestine with perforation and abscess without bleeding**

    K57.21   **Diverticulitis of large intestine with perforation and abscess with bleeding**

● K57.3   **Diverticular disease of large intestine without perforation or abscess**

> **Excludes1**   diverticular disease of both small and large intestine without perforation or abscess (K57.5-)

    K57.30   **Diverticulosis of large intestine without perforation or abscess without bleeding**
> Diverticular disease of colon NOS

    K57.31   **Diverticulosis of large intestine without perforation or abscess with bleeding**

    K57.32   **Diverticulitis of large intestine without perforation or abscess without bleeding**

    K57.33   **Diverticulitis of large intestine without perforation or abscess with bleeding**

● K57.4   **Diverticulitis of both small and large intestine with perforation and abscess**
> Diverticulitis of both small and large intestine with peritonitis

    K57.40   **Diverticulitis of both small and large intestine with perforation and abscess without bleeding**

    K57.41   **Diverticulitis of both small and large intestine with perforation and abscess with bleeding**

● K57.5   **Diverticular disease of both small and large intestine without perforation or abscess**

    K57.50   **Diverticulosis of both small and large intestine without perforation or abscess without bleeding**
> Diverticular disease of both small and large intestine NOS

    K57.51   **Diverticulosis of both small and large intestine without perforation or abscess with bleeding**

    K57.52   **Diverticulitis of both small and large intestine without perforation or abscess without bleeding**

    K57.53   **Diverticulitis of both small and large intestine without perforation or abscess with bleeding**

● K57.8   **Diverticulitis of intestine, part unspecified, with perforation and abscess**
> Diverticulitis of intestine NOS with peritonitis

    K57.80   **Diverticulitis of intestine, part unspecified, with perforation and abscess without bleeding**

    K57.81   **Diverticulitis of intestine, part unspecified, with perforation and abscess with bleeding**

● K57.9   **Diverticular disease of intestine, part unspecified, without perforation or abscess**

    K57.90   **Diverticulosis of intestine, part unspecified, without perforation or abscess without bleeding**
> Diverticular disease of intestine NOS

    K57.91   **Diverticulosis of intestine, part unspecified, without perforation or abscess with bleeding**

    K57.92   **Diverticulitis of intestine, part unspecified, without perforation or abscess without bleeding**

    K57.93   **Diverticulitis of intestine, part unspecified, without perforation or abscess with bleeding**

● K58   **Irritable bowel syndrome**

> **Includes**   irritable colon
> spastic colon

    K58.0   **Irritable bowel syndrome with diarrhea**

    K58.9   **Irritable bowel syndrome without diarrhea**
> Irritable bowel syndrome NOS

● K59   **Other functional intestinal disorders**

> **Excludes1**   change in bowel habit NOS (R19.4)
> intestinal malabsorption (K90.-)
> psychogenic intestinal disorders (F45.8)

> **Excludes2**   functional disorders of stomach (K31.-)

● K59.0   **Constipation**

> **Excludes1**   fecal impaction (K56.41)
> incomplete defecation (R15.0)

    K59.00   **Constipation, unspecified**

    K59.01   **Slow transit constipation**

    K59.02   **Outlet dysfunction constipation**

    K59.09   **Other constipation**

    K59.1   **Functional diarrhea**

> **Excludes1**   diarrhea NOS (R19.7)
> irritable bowel syndrome with diarrhea (K58.0)

    K59.2   **Neurogenic bowel, not elsewhere classified**

    K59.3   **Megacolon, not elsewhere classified**
> Dilatation of colon
> Toxic megacolon
> *Code first (T51-T65) to identify toxic agent*

> **Excludes1**   congenital megacolon (aganglionic) (Q43.1)
> megacolon (due to) (in) Chagas' disease (B57.32)
> megacolon (due to) (in) Clostridium difficile (A04.7)
> megacolon (due to) (in) Hirschsprung's disease (Q43.1)

    K59.4   **Anal spasm**
> Proctalgia fugax

    K59.8   **Other specified functional intestinal disorders**
> Atony of colon Pseudo-obstruction (acute) (chronic) of intestine

    K59.9   **Functional intestinal disorder, unspecified**

CHAPTER 11 (K00-K95)

Item 11–17 A **fissure** is a groove in the surface, whereas a **fistula** is an abnormal passage. An **abscess** is an accumulation of pus in a tissue cavity resulting from a bacterial or parasitic infection.

● **K60   Fissure and fistula of anal and rectal regions**
      Excludes1 fissure and fistula of anal and rectal regions with abscess or cellulitis (K61.-)
      Excludes2 anal sphincter tear (healed) (nontraumatic) (old) (K62.81)
    K60.0   Acute anal fissure
    K60.1   Chronic anal fissure
    K60.2   Anal fissure, unspecified
    K60.3   Anal fistula
    K60.4   Rectal fistula
        Fistula of rectum to skin
        Excludes1 rectovaginal fistula (N82.3)
                       vesicorectal fistula (N32.1)
    K60.5   Anorectal fistula

● **K61   Abscess of anal and rectal regions**
      Includes   abscess of anal and rectal regions
                  cellulitis of anal and rectal regions
    K61.0   Anal abscess
        Perianal abscess
        Excludes1 intrasphincteric abscess (K61.4)
    K61.1   Rectal abscess
        Perirectal abscess
        Excludes1 ischiorectal abscess (K61.3)
        Coding Clinic: 2012, Q4, P104
    K61.2   Anorectal abscess
    K61.3   Ischiorectal abscess
        Abscess of ischiorectal fossa
    K61.4   Intrasphincteric abscess

● **K62   Other diseases of anus and rectum**
      Includes   anal canal
      Excludes2 colostomy and enterostomy malfunction (K94.0-, K91.4-)
                  fecal incontinence (R15.-)
                  hemorrhoids (K64.-)
    K62.0   Anal polyp
    K62.1   Rectal polyp
        Excludes1 adenomatous polyp (D12.8)
    K62.2   Anal prolapse
        Prolapse of anal canal
    K62.3   Rectal prolapse
        Prolapse of rectal mucosa
    K62.4   Stenosis of anus and rectum
        Stricture of anus (sphincter)
    K62.5   Hemorrhage of anus and rectum
        Excludes1 gastrointestinal bleeding NOS (K92.2)
                      melena (K92.1)
                      neonatal rectal hemorrhage (P54.2)
    K62.6   Ulcer of anus and rectum
        Solitary ulcer of anus and rectum
        Stercoral ulcer of anus and rectum
        Excludes1 fissure and fistula of anus and rectum (K60.-)
                      ulcerative colitis (K51.-)
    K62.7   Radiation proctitis
        Use additional code to identify the type of radiation (W90.-)

● **K62.8   Other specified diseases of anus and rectum**
      Excludes2 ulcerative proctitis (K51.2)
    K62.81   Anal sphincter tear (healed) (nontraumatic) (old)
        Tear of anus, nontraumatic
        Use additional code for any associated fecal incontinence (R15.-)
        Excludes2 anal fissure (K60.-)
                      anal sphincter tear (healed) (old) complicating delivery (O34.7-)
                      traumatic tear of anal sphincter (S31.831)
    K62.82   Dysplasia of anus
        Anal intraepithelial neoplasia I and II (AIN I and II) (histologically confirmed)
        Dysplasia of anus NOS
        Mild and moderate dysplasia of anus (histologically confirmed)
        Excludes1 abnormal results from anal cytologic examination without histologic confirmation (R85.61-)
                      anal intraepithelial neoplasia III (D01.3)
                      carcinoma in situ of anus (D01.3)
                      HGSIL of anus (R85.613)
                      severe dysplasia of anus (D01.3)
    K62.89   Other specified diseases of anus and rectum
        Proctitis NOS
        Use additional code for any associated fecal incontinence (R15.-)
    K62.9   Disease of anus and rectum, unspecified

● **K63   Other diseases of intestine**
    K63.0   Abscess of intestine
        Excludes1 abscess of intestine with Crohn's disease (K50.014, K50.114, K50.814, K50.914)
                      abscess of intestine with diverticular disease (K57.0, K57.2, K57.4, K57.8)
                      abscess of intestine with ulcerative colitis (K51.014, K51.214, K51.314, K51.414, K51.514, K51.814, K51.914)
        Excludes2 abscess of anal and rectal regions (K61.-)
                      abscess of appendix (K35.3)
    K63.1   Perforation of intestine (nontraumatic)
        Perforation (nontraumatic) of rectum
        Excludes1 perforation (nontraumatic) of duodenum (K26.-)
                      perforation (nontraumatic) of intestine with diverticular disease (K57.0, K57.2, K57.4, K57.8)
        Excludes2 perforation (nontraumatic) of appendix (K35.2, K35.3)
    K63.2   Fistula of intestine
        Excludes1 fistula of duodenum (K31.6)
                      fistula of intestine with Crohn's disease (K50.013, K50.113, K50.813, K50.913)
                      fistula of intestine with ulcerative colitis (K51.013, K51.213, K51.313, K51.413, K51.513, K51.813, K51.913)
        Excludes2 fistula of anal and rectal regions (K60.-)
                      fistula of appendix (K38.3)
                      intestinal-genital fistula, female (N82.2-N82.4)
                      vesicointestinal fistula (N32.1)

◀ New   ⬅ Revised   ~~deleted~~ Deleted   Excludes 1   Excludes 2   Includes   Use additional   Code first   Code also   Unspecified
OGCR Official Guidelines   X Assign placeholder X   ● Use Additional Character(s)   ▶ Manifestation Code   **Coding Clinic**

K63.3   **Ulcer of intestine**
Primary ulcer of small intestine
> **Excludes1**   duodenal ulcer (K26.-)
> gastrointestinal ulcer (K28.-)
> gastrojejunal ulcer (K28.-)
> jejunal ulcer (K28.-)
> peptic ulcer, site unspecified (K27.-)
> ulcer of intestine with perforation (K63.1)
> ulcer of anus or rectum (K62.6)
> ulcerative colitis (K51.-)

K63.4   **Enteroptosis**

K63.5   **Polyp of colon**
> **Excludes1**   adenomatous polyp of colon (D12.6)
> inflammatory polyp of colon (K51.4-)
> polyposis of colon (D12.6)

● **K63.8**   **Other specified diseases of intestine**

    K63.81   **Dieulafoy lesion of intestine**
> **Excludes2**   Dieulafoy lesion of stomach and
> duodenum (K31.82)

    K63.89   **Other specified diseases of intestine**
        Coding Clinic: 2013, Q2, P31

K63.9   **Disease of intestine, unspecified**

● **K64**   **Hemorrhoids and perianal venous thrombosis**
> **Includes**   piles
> **Excludes1**   hemorrhoids complicating childbirth and the
> puerperium (O87.2)
> hemorrhoids complicating pregnancy (O22.4)

K64.0   **First degree hemorrhoids**
Grade/stage I hemorrhoids
Hemorrhoids (bleeding) without prolapse outside of
anal canal

K64.1   **Second degree hemorrhoids**
Grade/stage II hemorrhoids
Hemorrhoids (bleeding) that prolapse with straining,
but retract spontaneously

K64.2   **Third degree hemorrhoids**
Grade/stage III hemorrhoids
Hemorrhoids (bleeding) that prolapse with straining
and require manual replacement back inside anal
canal

K64.3   **Fourth degree hemorrhoids**
Grade/stage IV hemorrhoids
Hemorrhoids (bleeding) with prolapsed tissue that
cannot be manually replaced

K64.4   **Residual hemorrhoidal skin tags**
External hemorrhoids, NOS
Skin tags of anus

K64.5   **Perianal venous thrombosis**
External hemorrhoids with thrombosis
Perianal hematoma
Thrombosed hemorrhoids NOS

K64.8   **Other hemorrhoids**
Internal hemorrhoids, without mention of degree
Prolapsed hemorrhoids, degree not specified

K64.9   **Unspecified hemorrhoids**
Hemorrhoids (bleeding) NOS
Hemorrhoids (bleeding) without mention of degree

Item 11-18   **Peritonitis** is an inflammation of the lining (peritoneum) of the abdominal cavity and surface of the intestines.

Item 11-19   **Retroperitoneal infections** occur between the posterior parietal peritoneum and posterior abdominal wall where the kidneys, adrenal glands, ureters, duodenum, ascending colon, descending colon, pancreas, and the large vessels and nerves are located.

DISEASES OF PERITONEUM AND RETROPERITONEUM (K65-K68)

● **K65**   **Peritonitis**
Use additional code (B95-B97), to identify infectious agent
> **Excludes1**   acute appendicitis with generalized peritonitis
> (K35.2)
> aseptic peritonitis (T81.6)
> benign paroxysmal peritonitis (E85.0)
> chemical peritonitis (T81.6)
> diverticulitis of both small and large intestine
> with peritonitis (K57.4-)
> diverticulitis of colon with peritonitis (K57.2-)
> diverticulitis of intestine, NOS, with peritonitis
> (K57.8-)
> diverticulitis of small intestine with peritonitis
> (K57.0-)
> gonococcal peritonitis (A54.85)
> neonatal peritonitis (P78.0-P78.1)
> pelvic peritonitis, female (N73.3-N73.5)
> periodic familial peritonitis (E85.0)
> peritonitis due to talc or other foreign substance
> (T81.6)
> peritonitis in chlamydia (A74.81)
> peritonitis in diphtheria (A36.89)
> peritonitis in syphilis (late) (A52.74)
> peritonitis in tuberculosis (A18.31)
> peritonitis with or following abortion or ectopic
> or molar pregnancy (O00-O07, O08.0)
> peritonitis with or following appendicitis (K35.-)
> peritonitis with or following diverticular disease
> of intestine (K57.-)
> puerperal peritonitis (O85)
> retroperitoneal infections (K68.-)

K65.0   **Generalized (acute) peritonitis**
Pelvic peritonitis (acute), male
Subphrenic peritonitis (acute)
Suppurative peritonitis (acute)

K65.1   **Peritoneal abscess**
Abdominopelvic abscess
Abscess (of) omentum
Abscess (of) peritoneum
Mesenteric abscess
Retrocecal abscess
Subdiaphragmatic abscess
Subhepatic abscess
Subphrenic abscess

K65.2   **Spontaneous bacterial peritonitis**
> **Excludes1**   bacterial peritonitis NOS (K65.9)

K65.3   **Choleperitonitis**
Peritonitis due to bile

K65.4   **Sclerosing mesenteritis**
Fat necrosis of peritoneum
(Idiopathic) sclerosing mesenteric fibrosis
Mesenteric lipodystrophy
Mesenteric panniculitis
Retractile mesenteritis

K65.8   **Other peritonitis**
Chronic proliferative peritonitis
Peritonitis due to urine

K65.9   **Peritonitis, unspecified**
Bacterial peritonitis NOS
Coding Clinic: 2013, Q2, P31

CHAPTER 11 (K00-K95)

CHAPTER 11 (K00-K95)

● **K66 Other disorders of peritoneum**

  Excludes2 ascites (R18.-)
            peritoneal effusion (chronic) (R18.8)

  K66.0 Peritoneal adhesions (postprocedural) (postinfection)
    Adhesions (of) abdominal (wall)
    Adhesions (of) diaphragm
    Adhesions (of) intestine
    Adhesions (of) male pelvis
    Adhesions (of) omentum
    Adhesions (of) stomach
    Adhesive bands
    Mesenteric adhesions

    Excludes1 female pelvic adhesions [bands] (N73.6)
              peritoneal adhesions with intestinal obstruction (K56.5)

  K66.1 Hemoperitoneum
    Excludes1 traumatic hemoperitoneum (S36.8-)

  K66.8 Other specified disorders of peritoneum

  K66.9 Disorder of peritoneum, unspecified

▌**K67 Disorders of peritoneum in infectious diseases classified elsewhere**

  Code first underlying disease, such as:
    congenital syphilis (A50.0)
    helminthiasis (B65.0-B83.9)

  Excludes1 peritonitis in chlamydia (A74.81)
            peritonitis in diphtheria (A36.89)
            peritonitis in gonococcal (A54.85)
            peritonitis in syphilis (late) (A52.74)
            peritonitis in tuberculosis (A18.31)

● **K68 Disorders of retroperitoneum**

  ● **K68.1 Retroperitoneal abscess**
    K68.11 Postprocedural retroperitoneal abscess
    K68.12 Psoas muscle abscess
    K68.19 Other retroperitoneal abscess

  K68.9 Other disorders of retroperitoneum

DISEASES OF LIVER (K70-K77)

  Excludes1 jaundice NOS (R17)
  Excludes2 hemochromatosis (E83.11-)
            Reye's syndrome (G93.7)
            viral hepatitis (B15-B19)
            Wilson's disease (E83.0)

● **K70 Alcoholic liver disease**

  Use additional code to identify:
    alcohol abuse and dependence (F10.-)

  K70.0 Alcoholic fatty liver   A

  ● **K70.1 Alcoholic hepatitis**
    K70.10 Alcoholic hepatitis without ascites   A
    K70.11 Alcoholic hepatitis with ascites   A

  K70.2 Alcoholic fibrosis and sclerosis of liver   A

  ● **K70.3 Alcoholic cirrhosis of liver**
    Alcoholic cirrhosis NOS
    K70.30 Alcoholic cirrhosis of liver without ascites   A
    K70.31 Alcoholic cirrhosis of liver with ascites   A

  ● **K70.4 Alcoholic hepatic failure**
    Acute alcoholic hepatic failure
    Alcoholic hepatic failure NOS
    Chronic alcoholic hepatic failure
    Subacute alcoholic hepatic failure
    K70.40 Alcoholic hepatic failure without coma   A
    K70.41 Alcoholic hepatic failure with coma   A

  K70.9 Alcoholic liver disease, unspecified   A

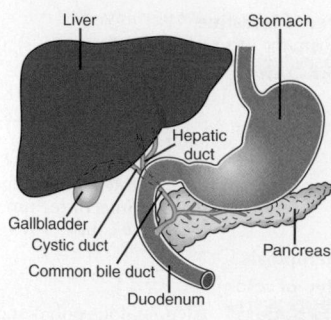

Figure 11-12 Liver and bile ducts.

● **K71 Toxic liver disease**

  Includes drug-induced idiosyncratic (unpredictable) liver disease
          drug-induced toxic (predictable) liver disease

  Code first poisoning due to drug or toxin, if applicable (T36-T65 with fifth or sixth character 1-4 or 6)

  Use additional code for adverse effect, if applicable, to identify drug (T36-T50 with fifth or sixth character 5)

  Excludes2 alcoholic liver disease (K70.-)
            Budd-Chiari syndrome (I82.0)

  K71.0 Toxic liver disease with cholestasis
    Cholestasis with hepatocyte injury
    'Pure' cholestasis

  ● **K71.1 Toxic liver disease with hepatic necrosis**
    Hepatic failure (acute) (chronic) due to drugs
    K71.10 Toxic liver disease with hepatic necrosis, without coma
    K71.11 Toxic liver disease with hepatic necrosis, with coma

  K71.2 Toxic liver disease with acute hepatitis

  K71.3 Toxic liver disease with chronic persistent hepatitis

  K71.4 Toxic liver disease with chronic lobular hepatitis

  ● **K71.5 Toxic liver disease with chronic active hepatitis**
    Toxic liver disease with lupoid hepatitis
    K71.50 Toxic liver disease with chronic active hepatitis without ascites
    K71.51 Toxic liver disease with chronic active hepatitis with ascites

  K71.6 Toxic liver disease with hepatitis, not elsewhere classified

  K71.7 Toxic liver disease with fibrosis and cirrhosis of liver

  K71.8 Toxic liver disease with other disorders of liver
    Toxic liver disease with focal nodular hyperplasia
    Toxic liver disease with hepatic granulomas
    Toxic liver disease with peliosis hepatis
    Toxic liver disease with veno-occlusive disease of liver

  K71.9 Toxic liver disease, unspecified

Item 11-20 Cirrhosis is the progressive fibrosis of the liver resulting in loss of liver function. The main causes of cirrhosis of the liver are alcohol abuse, chronic hepatitis (inflammation of the liver), biliary disease, and excessive amounts of iron. **Alcoholic cirrhosis of the liver** is also called portal, Laënnec's, or fatty nutritional cirrhosis.

1016

◀ New   ◀ᴵᴵᴵᴵ Revised   ~~deleted~~ Deleted   Excludes 1   Excludes 2   Includes   Use additional   Code first   Code also   Unspecified

OGCR Official Guidelines   X Assign placeholder X   ● Use Additional Character(s)   ▌ Manifestation Code   **Coding Clinic**

● **K72　Hepatic failure, not elsewhere classified**
- **Includes**　acute hepatitis NEC, with hepatic failure
  - fulminant hepatitis NEC, with hepatic failure
  - hepatic encephalopathy NOS
  - liver (cell) necrosis with hepatic failure
  - malignant hepatitis NEC, with hepatic failure
  - yellow liver atrophy or dystrophy
- **Excludes1**　alcoholic hepatic failure (K70.4)
  - hepatic failure with toxic liver disease (K71.1-)
  - icterus of newborn (P55-P59)
  - postprocedural hepatic failure (K91.82)
  - viral hepatitis with hepatic coma (B15-B19)
- **Excludes2**　hepatic failure complicating abortion or ectopic or molar pregnancy (O00-O07, O08.8)
  - hepatic failure complicating pregnancy, childbirth and the puerperium (O26.6-)

● **K72.0　Acute and subacute hepatic failure**
- **K72.00**　Acute and subacute hepatic failure without coma
- **K72.01**　Acute and subacute hepatic failure with coma

● **K72.1　Chronic hepatic failure**
- **K72.10**　Chronic hepatic failure without coma
- **K72.11**　Chronic hepatic failure with coma

● **K72.9　Hepatic failure, unspecified**
- **K72.90**　Hepatic failure, unspecified without coma
- **K72.91**　Hepatic failure, unspecified with coma
  - Hepatic coma NOS

● **K73　Chronic hepatitis, not elsewhere classified**
- **Excludes1**　alcoholic hepatitis (chronic) (K70.1-)
  - drug-induced hepatitis (chronic) (K71.-)
  - granulomatous hepatitis (chronic) NEC (K75.3)
  - reactive, nonspecific hepatitis (chronic) (K75.2)
  - viral hepatitis (chronic) (B15-B19)

K73.0　Chronic persistent hepatitis, not elsewhere classified
K73.1　Chronic lobular hepatitis, not elsewhere classified
K73.2　Chronic active hepatitis, not elsewhere classified
K73.8　Other chronic hepatitis, not elsewhere classified
K73.9　Chronic hepatitis, unspecified

● **K74　Fibrosis and cirrhosis of liver**
- Code also, if applicable, viral hepatitis (acute) (chronic) (B15-B19)
- **Excludes1**　alcoholic cirrhosis (of liver) (K70.3)
  - alcoholic fibrosis of liver (K70.2)
  - cardiac sclerosis of liver (K76.1)
  - cirrhosis (of liver) with toxic liver disease (K71.7)
  - congenital cirrhosis (of liver) (P78.81)
  - pigmentary cirrhosis (of liver) (E83.110)

K74.0　Hepatic fibrosis
K74.1　Hepatic sclerosis
K74.2　Hepatic fibrosis with hepatic sclerosis
K74.3　Primary biliary cirrhosis
- Chronic nonsuppurative destructive cholangitis
K74.4　Secondary biliary cirrhosis
K74.5　Biliary cirrhosis, unspecified
● **K74.6　Other and unspecified cirrhosis of liver**
- **K74.60**　Unspecified cirrhosis of liver
  - Cirrhosis (of liver) NOS
- **K74.69**　Other cirrhosis of liver
  - Cryptogenic cirrhosis (of liver)
  - Macronodular cirrhosis (of liver)
  - Micronodular cirrhosis (of liver)
  - Mixed type cirrhosis (of liver)
  - Portal cirrhosis (of liver)
  - Postnecrotic cirrhosis (of liver)

● **K75　Other inflammatory liver diseases**
- **Excludes2**　toxic liver disease (K71.-)

K75.0　Abscess of liver
- Cholangitic hepatic abscess
- Hematogenic hepatic abscess
- Hepatic abscess NOS
- Lymphogenic hepatic abscess
- Pylephlebitic hepatic abscess
- **Excludes1**　amebic liver abscess (A06.4)
  - cholangitis without liver abscess (K83.0)
  - pylephlebitis without liver abscess (K75.1)

K75.1　Phlebitis of portal vein
- Pylephlebitis
- **Excludes1**　pylephlebitic liver abscess (K75.0)

K75.2　Nonspecific reactive hepatitis
- **Excludes1**　acute or subacute hepatitis (K72.0-)
  - chronic hepatitis NEC (K73.-)
  - viral hepatitis (B15-B19)

K75.3　Granulomatous hepatitis, not elsewhere classified
- **Excludes1**　acute or subacute hepatitis (K72.0-)
  - chronic hepatitis NEC (K73.-)
  - viral hepatitis (B15-B19)

K75.4　Autoimmune hepatitis
- Lupoid hepatitis NEC
● **K75.8　Other specified inflammatory liver diseases**
- **K75.81**　Nonalcoholic steatohepatitis (NASH)
- **K75.89**　Other specified inflammatory liver diseases
K75.9　Inflammatory liver disease, unspecified
- Hepatitis NOS
- **Excludes1**　acute or subacute hepatitis (K72.0-)
  - chronic hepatitis NEC (K73.-)
  - viral hepatitis (B15-B19)

● **K76　Other diseases of liver**
- **Excludes2**　alcoholic liver disease (K70.-)
  - amyloid degeneration of liver (E85.-)
  - cystic disease of liver (congenital) (Q44.6)
  - hepatic vein thrombosis (I82.0)
  - hepatomegaly NOS (R16.0)
  - pigmentary cirrhosis (of liver) (E83.110)
  - portal vein thrombosis (I81)
  - toxic liver disease (K71.-)

K76.0　Fatty (change of) liver, not elsewhere classified
- Nonalcoholic fatty liver disease (NAFLD)
- **Excludes1**　nonalcoholic steatohepatitis (NASH) (K75.81)

K76.1　Chronic passive congestion of liver
- Cardiac cirrhosis
- Cardiac sclerosis
K76.2　Central hemorrhagic necrosis of liver
- **Excludes1**　liver necrosis with hepatic failure (K72.-)
K76.3　Infarction of liver
K76.4　Peliosis hepatis
- Hepatic angiomatosis
K76.5　Hepatic veno-occlusive disease
- **Excludes1**　Budd-Chiari syndrome (I82.0)
K76.6　Portal hypertension
- Use additional code for any associated complications, such as:
  - portal hypertensive gastropathy (K31.89)
K76.7　Hepatorenal syndrome
- **Excludes1**　hepatorenal syndrome following labor and delivery (O90.4)
  - postprocedural hepatorenal syndrome (K91.82)

CHAPTER 11 (K00-K95)

CHAPTER 11 (K00-K95)

● **K76.8**   **Other specified diseases of liver**

    K76.81   **Hepatopulmonary syndrome**

       Code first underlying liver disease, such as:
       alcoholic cirrhosis of liver (K70.3-)
       cirrhosis of liver without mention of alcohol
       (K74.6-)

    K76.89   **Other specified diseases of liver**
       Cyst (simple) of liver
       Focal nodular hyperplasia of liver
       Hepatoptosis

    K76.9   **Liver disease, unspecified**

▶ **K77**   *Liver disorders in diseases classified elsewhere*

       Code first underlying disease, such as:
       amyloidosis (E85.-)
       congenital syphilis (A50.0, A50.5)
       congenital toxoplasmosis (P37.1)
       schistosomiasis (B65.0-B65.9)

    Excludes1   alcoholic hepatitis (K70.1-)
       alcoholic liver disease (K70.-)
       cytomegaloviral hepatitis (B25.1)
       herpesviral [herpes simplex] hepatitis (B00.81)
       infectious mononucleosis with liver disease
       (B27.0-B27.9 with .9)
       mumps hepatitis (B26.81)
       sarcoidosis with liver disease (D86.89)
       secondary syphilis with liver disease (A51.45)
       syphilis (late) with liver disease (A52.74)
       toxoplasmosis (acquired) hepatitis (B58.1)
       tuberculosis with liver disease (A18.83)

DISORDERS OF GALLBLADDER, BILIARY TRACT AND PANCREAS (K80–K87)

● **K80**   **Cholelithiasis**
    Presence or formation of gallstones

    Excludes1   retained cholelithiasis following cholecystectomy
       (K91.86)

● **K80.0**   **Calculus of gallbladder with acute cholecystitis**
    Any condition listed in K80.2 with acute cholecystitis
    Check documentation for acute/chronic gallbladder/common bile duct either with or without obstruction.

    K80.00   **Calculus of gallbladder with acute cholecystitis without obstruction**

    K80.01   **Calculus of gallbladder with acute cholecystitis with obstruction**

● **K80.1**   **Calculus of gallbladder with other cholecystitis**

    K80.10   **Calculus of gallbladder with chronic cholecystitis without obstruction**
       Cholelithiasis with cholecystitis NOS

    K80.11   **Calculus of gallbladder with chronic cholecystitis with obstruction**

    K80.12   **Calculus of gallbladder with acute and chronic cholecystitis without obstruction**

    K80.13   **Calculus of gallbladder with acute and chronic cholecystitis with obstruction**

    K80.18   **Calculus of gallbladder with other cholecystitis without obstruction**

    K80.19   **Calculus of gallbladder with other cholecystitis with obstruction**

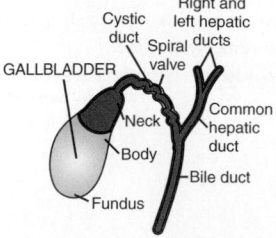

● **K80.2**   **Calculus of gallbladder without cholecystitis**
    Cholecystolithiasis without cholecystitis
    Cholelithiasis (without cholecystitis)
    Colic (recurrent) of gallbladder (without cholecystitis)
    Gallstone (impacted) of cystic duct (without cholecystitis)
    Gallstone (impacted) of gallbladder (without cholecystitis)

    K80.20   **Calculus of gallbladder without cholecystitis without obstruction**

    K80.21   **Calculus of gallbladder without cholecystitis with obstruction**

● **K80.3**   **Calculus of bile duct with cholangitis**
    Any condition listed in K80.5 with cholangitis

    K80.30   **Calculus of bile duct with cholangitis, unspecified, without obstruction**

    K80.31   **Calculus of bile duct with cholangitis, unspecified, with obstruction**

    K80.32   **Calculus of bile duct with acute cholangitis without obstruction**

    K80.33   **Calculus of bile duct with acute cholangitis with obstruction**

    K80.34   **Calculus of bile duct with chronic cholangitis without obstruction**

    K80.35   **Calculus of bile duct with chronic cholangitis with obstruction**

    K80.36   **Calculus of bile duct with acute and chronic cholangitis without obstruction**

    K80.37   **Calculus of bile duct with acute and chronic cholangitis with obstruction**

● **K80.4**   **Calculus of bile duct with cholecystitis**
    Any condition listed in K80.5 with cholecystitis (with cholangitis)

    K80.40   **Calculus of bile duct with cholecystitis, unspecified, without obstruction**

    K80.41   **Calculus of bile duct with cholecystitis, unspecified, with obstruction**

    K80.42   **Calculus of bile duct with acute cholecystitis without obstruction**

    K80.43   **Calculus of bile duct with acute cholecystitis with obstruction**

    K80.44   **Calculus of bile duct with chronic cholecystitis without obstruction**

    K80.45   **Calculus of bile duct with chronic cholecystitis with obstruction**

    K80.46   **Calculus of bile duct with acute and chronic cholecystitis without obstruction**

    K80.47   **Calculus of bile duct with acute and chronic cholecystitis with obstruction**

● **K80.5**   **Calculus of bile duct without cholangitis or cholecystitis**
    Choledocholithiasis (without cholangitis or cholecystitis)
    Gallstone (impacted) of bile duct NOS (without cholangitis or cholecystitis)
    Gallstone (impacted) of common duct (without cholangitis or cholecystitis)
    Gallstone (impacted) of hepatic duct (without cholangitis or cholecystitis)
    Hepatic cholelithiasis (without cholangitis or cholecystitis)
    Hepatic colic (recurrent) (without cholangitis or cholecystitis)

    K80.50   **Calculus of bile duct without cholangitis or cholecystitis without obstruction**

    K80.51   **Calculus of bile duct without cholangitis or cholecystitis with obstruction**

Figure 11-13   Gallbladder and bile ducts.

◀ New   ◀ Revised   ~~deleted~~ Deleted   Excludes 1   Excludes 2   Includes   Use additional   Code first   Code also   Unspecified
OGCR Official Guidelines   X Assign placeholder X   ● Use Additional Character(s)   ▶ Manifestation Code   **Coding Clinic**

● **K80.6** **Calculus of gallbladder and bile duct with cholecystitis**

   K80.60 Calculus of gallbladder and bile duct with cholecystitis unspecified, without obstruction

   K80.61 Calculus of gallbladder and bile duct with cholecystitis unspecified, with obstruction

   K80.62 Calculus of gallbladder and bile duct with acute cholecystitis without obstruction

   K80.63 Calculus of gallbladder and bile duct with acute cholecystitis with obstruction

   K80.64 Calculus of gallbladder and bile duct with chronic cholecystitis without obstruction

   K80.65 Calculus of gallbladder and bile duct with chronic cholecystitis with obstruction

   K80.66 Calculus of gallbladder and bile duct with acute and chronic cholecystitis without obstruction

   K80.67 Calculus of gallbladder and bile duct with acute and chronic cholecystitis with obstruction

● **K80.7** **Calculus of gallbladder and bile duct without cholecystitis**

   K80.70 Calculus of gallbladder and bile duct without cholecystitis without obstruction

   K80.71 Calculus of gallbladder and bile duct without cholecystitis with obstruction

● **K80.8** **Other cholelithiasis**

   K80.80 Other cholelithiasis without obstruction

   K80.81 Other cholelithiasis with obstruction

● **K81** **Cholecystitis**

   Chronic or acute inflammation of the gallbladder.

   Excludes1 cholecystitis with cholelithiasis (K80.-)

   K81.0 **Acute cholecystitis**
   Abscess of gallbladder
   Angiocholecystitis
   Emphysematous (acute) cholecystitis
   Empyema of gallbladder
   Gangrene of gallbladder
   Gangrenous cholecystitis
   Suppurative cholecystitis

   K81.1 **Chronic cholecystitis**

   K81.2 **Acute cholecystitis with chronic cholecystitis**

   K81.9 **Cholecystitis, unspecified**

● **K82** **Other diseases of gallbladder**

   Excludes1 nonvisualization of gallbladder (R93.2)
   postcholecystectomy syndrome (K91.5)

   K82.0 **Obstruction of gallbladder**
   Occlusion of cystic duct or gallbladder without cholelithiasis
   Stenosis of cystic duct or gallbladder without cholelithiasis
   Stricture of cystic duct or gallbladder without cholelithiasis

   Excludes1 obstruction of gallbladder with cholelithiasis (K80.-)

   K82.1 **Hydrops of gallbladder**
   Mucocele of gallbladder

   K82.2 **Perforation of gallbladder**
   Rupture of cystic duct or gallbladder

   K82.3 **Fistula of gallbladder**
   Cholecystocolic fistula
   Cholecystoduodenal fistula

   K82.4 **Cholesterolosis of gallbladder**
   Strawberry gallbladder

   Excludes1 cholesterolosis of gallbladder with cholecystitis (K81.-)
   cholesterolosis of gallbladder with cholelithiasis (K80.-)

K82.8 **Other specified diseases of gallbladder**
Adhesions of cystic duct or gallbladder
Atrophy of cystic duct or gallbladder
Cyst of cystic duct or gallbladder
Dyskinesia of cystic duct or gallbladder
Hypertrophy of cystic duct or gallbladder
Nonfunctioning of cystic duct or gallbladder
Ulcer of cystic duct or gallbladder

K82.9 **Disease of gallbladder, unspecified**

● **K83** **Other diseases of biliary tract**

   Excludes1 postcholecystectomy syndrome (K91.5)
   Excludes2 conditions involving the gallbladder (K81-K82)
   conditions involving the cystic duct (K81-K82)

   K83.0 **Cholangitis**
   Ascending cholangitis   Sclerosing cholangitis
   Cholangitis NOS   Secondary cholangitis
   Primary cholangitis   Stenosing cholangitis
   Recurrent cholangitis   Suppurative cholangitis

   Excludes1 cholangitic liver abscess (K75.0)
   cholangitis with choledocholithiasis (K80.3-, K80.4-)
   chronic nonsuppurative destructive cholangitis (K74.3)

   K83.1 **Obstruction of bile duct**
   Occlusion of bile duct without cholelithiasis
   Stenosis of bile duct without cholelithiasis
   Stricture of bile duct without cholelithiasis

   Excludes1 congenital obstruction of bile duct (Q44.3)
   obstruction of bile duct with cholelithiasis (K80.-)

   K83.2 **Perforation of bile duct**
   Rupture of bile duct

   K83.3 **Fistula of bile duct**
   Choledochoduodenal fistula

   K83.4 **Spasm of sphincter of Oddi**

   K83.5 **Biliary cyst**

   K83.8 **Other specified diseases of biliary tract**
   Adhesions of biliary tract
   Atrophy of biliary tract
   Hypertrophy of biliary tract
   Ulcer of biliary tract

   K83.9 **Disease of biliary tract, unspecified**

● **K85** **Acute pancreatitis**
   Inflammatory process in which pancreatic enzymes autodigest the gland.

   Includes abscess of pancreas
   acute necrosis of pancreas
   acute (recurrent) pancreatitis
   gangrene of (gangrenous) pancreas
   hemorrhagic pancreatitis
   infective necrosis of pancreas
   subacute pancreatitis
   suppurative pancreatitis

   K85.0 **Idiopathic acute pancreatitis**

   K85.1 **Biliary acute pancreatitis**
   Gallstone pancreatitis

   K85.2 **Alcohol induced acute pancreatitis**

   Excludes2 alcohol induced chronic pancreatitis (K86.0)

   K85.3 **Drug induced acute pancreatitis**

   Use additional code for adverse effect, if applicable, to identify drug (T36-T50 with fifth or sixth character 5)

   Use additional code to identify drug abuse and dependence (F11.-F17.-)

   K85.8 **Other acute pancreatitis**

   K85.9 **Acute pancreatitis, unspecified**
   Pancreatitis NOS

N Newborn Age: 0   **P** Pediatric Age: 0–17   **M** Maternity DX: 12–55   **A** Adult Age: 15–124   ♀ Females Only   ♂ Males Only

CHAPTER 11 (K00-K95)

1019

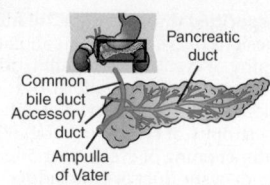

Figure 11-14 Pancreatic ductal system.

● K86   Other diseases of pancreas

> **Excludes2**   fibrocystic disease of pancreas (E84.-)
> islet cell tumor (of pancreas) (D13.7)
> pancreatic steatorrhea (K90.3)

K86.0   Alcohol-induced chronic pancreatitis

> Use additional code to identify:
> alcohol abuse and dependence (F10.-)
>
> > **Excludes2**   alcohol induced acute pancreatitis (K85.2)

K86.1   Other chronic pancreatitis

> Chronic pancreatitis NOS
> Infectious chronic pancreatitis
> Recurrent chronic pancreatitis
> Relapsing chronic pancreatitis

K86.2   Cyst of pancreas

K86.3   Pseudocyst of pancreas

K86.8   Other specified diseases of pancreas

> Aseptic pancreatic necrosis
> Atrophy of pancreas
> Calculus of pancreas
> Cirrhosis of pancreas
> Fibrosis of pancreas
> Pancreatic fat necrosis
> Pancreatic infantilism
> Pancreatic necrosis NOS

K86.9   Disease of pancreas, unspecified

▌K87   *Disorders of gallbladder, biliary tract and pancreas in diseases classified elsewhere*

> *Code first* underlying disease
>
> **Excludes1**   cytomegaloviral pancreatitis (B25.2)
> mumps pancreatitis (B26.3)
> syphilitic gallbladder (A52.74)
> syphilitic pancreas (A52.74)
> tuberculosis of gallbladder (A18.83)
> tuberculosis of pancreas (A18.83)

OTHER DISEASES OF THE DIGESTIVE SYSTEM (K90-K95)

● K90   Intestinal malabsorption

> **Excludes1**   intestinal malabsorption following gastrointestinal surgery (K91.2)

K90.0   Celiac disease

> Gluten-sensitive enteropathy
> Idiopathic steatorrhea
> Nontropical sprue
>
> Use additional code for associated disorders including:
> dermatitis herpetiformis (L13.0)
> gluten ataxia (G32.81)

K90.1   Tropical sprue

> Sprue NOS
> Tropical steatorrhea

K90.2   Blind loop syndrome, not elsewhere classified

> Blind loop syndrome NOS
>
> **Excludes1**   congenital blind loop syndrome (Q43.8)
> postsurgical blind loop syndrome (K91.2)

K90.3   Pancreatic steatorrhea

K90.4   Malabsorption due to intolerance, not elsewhere classified

> Malabsorption due to intolerance to carbohydrate
> Malabsorption due to intolerance to fat
> Malabsorption due to intolerance to protein
> Malabsorption due to intolerance to starch
>
> **Excludes2**   gluten-sensitive enteropathy (K90.0)
> lactose intolerance (E73.-)

● K90.8   Other intestinal malabsorption

K90.81   Whipple's disease

K90.89   Other intestinal malabsorption

K90.9   Intestinal malabsorption, unspecified

● K91   Intraoperative and postprocedural complications and disorders of digestive system, not elsewhere classified

> **Excludes2**   complications of artificial opening of digestive system (K94.-)
> complications of bariatric procedures (K95.-)
> gastrojejunal ulcer (K28.-)
> postprocedural (radiation) retroperitoneal abscess (K68.11)
> radiation colitis (K52.0)
> radiation gastroenteritis (K52.0)
> radiation proctitis (K62.7)

K91.0   Vomiting following gastrointestinal surgery

K91.1   Postgastric surgery syndromes

> Dumping syndrome
> Postgastrectomy syndrome
> Postvagotomy syndrome

K91.2   Postsurgical malabsorption, not elsewhere classified

> Postsurgical blind loop syndrome
>
> **Excludes1**   malabsorption osteomalacia in adults (M83.2)
> malabsorption osteoporosis, postsurgical (M80.8-, M81.8)

K91.3   Postprocedural intestinal obstruction

K91.5   Postcholecystectomy syndrome

● K91.6   Intraoperative hemorrhage and hematoma of a digestive system organ or structure complicating a procedure

> **Excludes1**   intraoperative hemorrhage and hematoma of a digestive system organ or structure due to accidental puncture and laceration during a procedure (K91.7-)

K91.61   Intraoperative hemorrhage and hematoma of a digestive system organ or structure complicating a digestive sytem procedure

K91.62   Intraoperative hemorrhage and hematoma of a digestive system organ or structure complicating other procedure

● K91.7   Accidental puncture and laceration of a digestive system organ or structure during a procedure

K91.71   Accidental puncture and laceration of a digestive system organ or structure during a digestive system procedure

K91.72   Accidental puncture and laceration of a digestive system organ or structure during other procedure

● K91.8   Other intraoperative and postprocedural complications and disorders of digestive system

K91.81   Other intraoperative complications of digestive system

K91.82   Postprocedural hepatic failure

K91.83   Postprocedural hepatorenal syndrome

● K91.84 **Postprocedural hemorrhage and hematoma of a digestive system organ or structure following a procedure**

    K91.840 **Postprocedural hemorrhage and hematoma of a digestive system organ or structure following a digestive system procedure**

    K91.841 **Postprocedural hemorrhage and hematoma of a digestive system organ or structure following other procedure**

● K91.85 **Complications of intestinal pouch**

    K91.850 **Pouchitis**

       Inflammation of internal ileoanal pouch

    K91.858 **Other complications of intestinal pouch**

K91.86 **Retained cholelithiasis following cholecystectomy**

K91.89 **Other postprocedural complications and disorders of digestive system**

    Use additional code, if applicable, to further specify disorder

    Excludes2 postprocedural retroperitoneal abscess (K68.11)

● K92 **Other diseases of digestive system**

    Excludes1 neonatal gastrointestinal hemorrhage (P54.0-P54.3)

K92.0 **Hematemesis**

K92.1 **Melena**

    Excludes1 occult blood in feces (R19.5)

K92.2 **Gastrointestinal hemorrhage, unspecified**

    Gastric hemorrhage NOS

    Intestinal hemorrhage NOS

    Excludes1 acute hemorrhagic gastritis (K29.01)

       hemorrhage of anus and rectum (K62.5)

       angiodysplasia of stomach with hemorrhage (K31.811)

       diverticular disease with hemorrhage (K57.-)

       gastritis and duodenitis with hemorrhage (K29.-)

       peptic ulcer with hemorrhage (K25-K28)

● K92.8 **Other specified diseases of the digestive system**

    K92.81 **Gastrointestinal mucositis (ulcerative)**

       Code also type of associated therapy, such as:

         antineoplastic and immunosuppressive drugs (T45.1X-)

         radiological procedure and radiotherapy (Y84.2)

       Excludes2 mucositis (ulcerative) of vagina and vulva (N76.81)

         nasal mucositis (ulcerative) (J34.81)

         oral mucositis (ulcerative) (K12.3-)

    K92.89 **Other specified diseases of the digestive system**

K92.9 **Disease of digestive system, unspecified**

● K94 **Complications of artificial openings of the digestive system**

  ● K94.0 **Colostomy complications**

    K94.00 **Colostomy complication, unspecified**

    K94.01 **Colostomy hemorrhage**

    K94.02 **Colostomy infection**

       Use additional code to specify type of infection, such as:

         cellulitis of abdominal wall (L03.311)

         sepsis (A40.-, A41.-)

    K94.03 **Colostomy malfunction**

       Mechanical complication of colostomy

    K94.09 **Other complications of colostomy**

● K94.1 **Enterostomy complications**

    K94.10 **Enterostomy complication, unspecified**

    K94.11 **Enterostomy hemorrhage**

    K94.12 **Enterostomy infection**

       Use additional code to specify type of infection, such as:

         cellulitis of abdominal wall (L03.311)

         sepsis (A40.-, A41.-)

    K94.13 **Enterostomy malfunction**

       Mechanical complication of enterostomy

    K94.19 **Other complications of enterostomy**

● K94.2 **Gastrostomy complications**

    K94.20 **Gastrostomy complication, unspecified**

    K94.21 **Gastrostomy hemorrhage**

    K94.22 **Gastrostomy infection**

       Use additional code to specify type of infection, such as:

         cellulitis of abdominal wall (L03.311)

         sepsis (A40.-, A41.-)

    K94.23 **Gastrostomy malfunction**

       Mechanical complication of gastrostomy

    K94.29 **Other complications of gastrostomy**

● K94.3 **Esophagostomy complications**

    K94.30 **Esophagostomy complications, unspecified**

    K94.31 **Esophagostomy hemorrhage**

    K94.32 **Esophagostomy infection**

       Use additional code to identify the infection

    K94.33 **Esophagostomy malfunction**

       Mechanical complication of esophagostomy

    K94.39 **Other complications of esophagostomy**

● K95 **Complications of bariatric procedures**

  ● K95.0 **Complications of gastric band procedure**

    K95.01 **Infection due to gastric band procedure**

       Use additional code to specify type of infection or organism, such as:

         bacterial and viral infectious agents (B95.-, B96.-)

         cellulitis of abdominal wall (L03.311)

         sepsis (A40.-, A41.-)

    K95.09 **Other complications of gastric band procedure**

       Use additional code, if applicable, to further specify complication

  ● K95.8 **Complications of other bariatric procedure**

    Excludes1 complications of gastric band surgery (K95.0-)

    K95.81 **Infection due to other bariatric procedure**

       Use additional code to specify type of infection or organism, such as:

         bacterial and viral infectious agents (B95.-, B96.-)

         cellulitis of abdominal wall (L03.311)

         sepsis (A40.-, A41.-)

    K95.89 **Other complications of other bariatric procedure**

       Use additional code, if applicable, to further specify complication

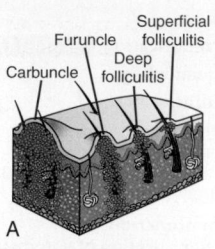
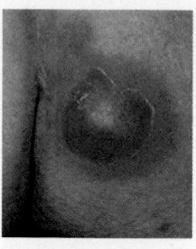

Figure 12-1 Furuncle, also known as a boil, is a staphylococcal infection. The organism enters the body through a hair follicle and so furuncles usually appear in hairy areas of the body. A cluster of furuncles is known as a carbuncle and involves infection into the deep subcutaneous fascia. These usually appear on the back and neck. (**B** from Habif: Clinical Dermatology, ed 5, Mosby, 2009)

CHAPTER 12

DISEASES OF THE SKIN AND SUBCUTANEOUS TISSUE (L00-L99)

> **Excludes2**   certain conditions originating in the perinatal period (P04-P96)
> certain infectious and parasitic diseases (A00-B99)
> complications of pregnancy, childbirth and the puerperium (O00-O9A)
> congenital malformations, deformations, and chromosomal abnormalities (Q00-Q99)
> endocrine, nutritional and metabolic diseases (E00-E88)
> lipomelanotic reticulosis (I89.8)
> neoplasms (C00-D49)
> symptoms, signs and abnormal clinical and laboratory findings, not elsewhere classified (R00-R94)
> systemic connective tissue disorders (M30-M36)
> viral warts (B07.-)

This chapter contains the following blocks:

L00-L08	Infections of the skin and subcutaneous tissue
L10-L14	Bullous disorders
L20-L30	Dermatitis and eczema
L40-L45	Papulosquamous disorders
L49-L54	Urticaria and erythema
L55-L59	Radiation-related disorders of the skin and subcutaneous tissue
L60-L75	Disorders of skin appendages
L76	Intraoperative and postprocedural complications of skin and subcutaneous tissue
L80-L99	Other disorders of the skin and subcutaneous tissue

INFECTIONS OF THE SKIN AND SUBCUTANEOUS TISSUE (L00-L08)

Use additional code (B95-B97) to identify infectious agent.

> **Excludes2**   hordeolum (H00.0)
> infective dermatitis (L30.3)
> local infections of skin classified in Chapter 1
> lupus panniculitis (L93.2)
> panniculitis NOS (M79.3)
> panniculitis of neck and back (M54.0-)
> Perlèche NOS (K13.0)
> Perlèche due to candidiasis (B37.0)
> Perlèche due to riboflavin deficiency (E53.0)
> pyogenic granuloma (L98.0)
> relapsing panniculitis [Weber-Christian] (M35.6)
> viral warts (B07.-)
> zoster (B02.-)

L00   **Staphylococcal scalded skin syndrome**
     Ritter's disease
     Use additional code to identify percentage of skin exfoliation (L49.-)

> **Excludes1**   bullous impetigo (L01.03)
> pemphigus neonatorum (L01.03)
> toxic epidermal necrolysis [Lyell] (L51.2)

● **L01**   **Impetigo**
     Contagious skin infection caused by a streptococcus or staphylococcus aureus, common skin infections among children.

> **Excludes1**   impetigo herpetiformis (L40.1)

   ● **L01.0**   **Impetigo**
       Impetigo contagiosa
       Impetigo vulgaris

     L01.00   **Impetigo, unspecified**
         Impetigo NOS

     L01.01   **Non-bullous impetigo**

     L01.02   **Bockhart's impetigo**
         Impetigo follicularis
         Perifolliculitis NOS
         Superficial pustular perifolliculitis

     L01.03   **Bullous impetigo**
         Impetigo neonatorum
         Pemphigus neonatorum
         Neonate = newborn

     L01.09   **Other impetigo**
         Ulcerative impetigo

   L01.1   **Impetiginization of other dermatoses**

● **L02**   **Cutaneous abscess, furuncle and carbuncle**
     Use additional code to identify organism (B95-B96)

> **Excludes2**   abscess of anus and rectal regions (K61.-)
> abscess of female genital organs (external) (N76.4)
> abscess of male genital organs (external) (N48.2, N49.-)

   ● **L02.0**   **Cutaneous abscess, furuncle and carbuncle of face**

> **Excludes2**   abscess of ear, external (H60.0)
> abscess of eyelid (H00.0)
> abscess of head [any part, except face] (L02.8)
> abscess of lacrimal gland (H04.0)
> abscess of lacrimal passages (H04.3)
> abscess of mouth (K12.2)
> abscess of nose (J34.0)
> abscess of orbit (H05.0)
> submandibular abscess (K12.2)

     L02.01   **Cutaneous abscess of face**

     L02.02   **Furuncle of face**
         Boil of face
         Folliculitis of face

     L02.03   **Carbuncle of face**

   ● **L02.1**   **Cutaneous abscess, furuncle and carbuncle of neck**

     L02.11   **Cutaneous abscess of neck**

     L02.12   **Furuncle of neck**
         Boil of neck
         Folliculitis of neck

     L02.13   **Carbuncle of neck**

   ● **L02.2**   **Cutaneous abscess, furuncle and carbuncle of trunk**

> **Excludes1**   non-newborn omphalitis (L08.82)
> omphalitis of newborn (P38.-)

> **Excludes2**   abscess of breast (N61)
> abscess of buttocks (L02.3)
> abscess of female external genital organs (N76.4)
> abscess of male external genital organs (N48.2, N49.-)
> abscess of hip (L02.4)

● L02.21   **Cutaneous abscess of trunk**
     L02.211   Cutaneous abscess of abdominal wall
     L02.212   Cutaneous abscess of back [any part, except buttock]
     L02.213   Cutaneous abscess of chest wall
     L02.214   Cutaneous abscess of groin
     L02.215   Cutaneous abscess of perineum
     L02.216   Cutaneous abscess of umbilicus
     L02.219   Cutaneous abscess of trunk, unspecified

● L02.22   **Furuncle of trunk**
     Boil of trunk
     Folliculitis of trunk
     L02.221   Furuncle of abdominal wall
     L02.222   Furuncle of back [any part, except buttock]
     L02.223   Furuncle of chest wall
     L02.224   Furuncle of groin
     L02.225   Furuncle of perineum
     L02.226   Furuncle of umbilicus
     L02.229   Furuncle of trunk, unspecified

● L02.23   **Carbuncle of trunk**
     L02.231   Carbuncle of abdominal wall
     L02.232   Carbuncle of back [any part, except buttock]
     L02.233   Carbuncle of chest wall
     L02.234   Carbuncle of groin
     L02.235   Carbuncle of perineum
     L02.236   Carbuncle of umbilicus
     L02.239   Carbuncle of trunk, unspecified

● L02.3   **Cutaneous abscess, furuncle and carbuncle of buttock**
     Excludes1   pilonidal cyst with abscess (L05.01)
     L02.31   **Cutaneous abscess of buttock**
         Cutaneous abscess of gluteal region
     L02.32   **Furuncle of buttock**
         Boil of buttock
         Folliculitis of buttock
         Furuncle of gluteal region
     L02.33   **Carbuncle of buttock**
         Carbuncle of gluteal region

● L02.4   **Cutaneous abscess, furuncle and carbuncle of limb**
     Excludes2   Cutaneous abscess, furuncle and carbuncle of groin (L02.214, L02.224, L02.234)
         Cutaneous abscess, furuncle and carbuncle of hand (L02.5-)
         Cutaneous abscess, furuncle and carbuncle of foot (L02.6-)
     L02.41   **Cutaneous abscess of limb**
     L02.411   Cutaneous abscess of right axilla
     L02.412   Cutaneous abscess of left axilla
     L02.413   Cutaneous abscess of right upper limb
     L02.414   Cutaneous abscess of left upper limb
     L02.415   Cutaneous abscess of right lower limb
     L02.416   Cutaneous abscess of left lower limb
     L02.419   Cutaneous abscess of limb, unspecified

● L02.42   **Furuncle of limb**
     Boil of limb
     Folliculitis of limb
     L02.421   Furuncle of right axilla
     L02.422   Furuncle of left axilla
     L02.423   Furuncle of right upper limb

     L02.424   Furuncle of left upper limb
     L02.425   Furuncle of right lower limb
     L02.426   Furuncle of left lower limb
     L02.429   Furuncle of limb, unspecified
● L02.43   **Carbuncle of limb**
     L02.431   Carbuncle of right axilla
     L02.432   Carbuncle of left axilla
     L02.433   Carbuncle of right upper limb
     L02.434   Carbuncle of left upper limb
     L02.435   Carbuncle of right lower limb
     L02.436   Carbuncle of left lower limb
     L02.439   Carbuncle of limb, unspecified

● L02.5   **Cutaneous abscess, furuncle and carbuncle of hand**
     ● L02.51   **Cutaneous abscess of hand**
     L02.511   Cutaneous abscess of right hand
     L02.512   Cutaneous abscess of left hand
     L02.519   Cutaneous abscess of unspecified hand
     ● L02.52   **Furuncle hand**
         Boil of hand
         Folliculitis of hand
     L02.521   Furuncle right hand
     L02.522   Furuncle left hand
     L02.529   Furuncle unspecified hand
     ● L02.53   **Carbuncle of hand**
     L02.531   Carbuncle of right hand
     L02.532   Carbuncle of left hand
     L02.539   Carbuncle of unspecified hand

● L02.6   **Cutaneous abscess, furuncle and carbuncle of foot**
     ● L02.61   **Cutaneous abscess of foot**
     L02.611   Cutaneous abscess of right foot
     L02.612   Cutaneous abscess of left foot
     L02.619   Cutaneous abscess of unspecified foot
     ● L02.62   **Furuncle of foot**
         Boil of foot
         Folliculitis of foot
     L02.621   Furuncle of right foot
     L02.622   Furuncle of left foot
     L02.629   Furuncle of unspecified foot
     ● L02.63   **Carbuncle of foot**
     L02.631   Carbuncle of right foot
     L02.632   Carbuncle of left foot
     L02.639   Carbuncle of unspecified foot

● L02.8   **Cutaneous abscess, furuncle and carbuncle of other sites**
     ● L02.81   **Cutaneous abscess of other sites**
     L02.811   Cutaneous abscess of head [any part, except face]
     L02.818   Cutaneous abscess of other sites
     ● L02.82   **Furuncle of other sites**
         Boil of other sites
         Folliculitis of other sites
     L02.821   Furuncle of head [any part, except face]
     L02.828   Furuncle of other sites
     ● L02.83   **Carbuncle of other sites**
     L02.831   Carbuncle of head [any part, except face]
     L02.838   Carbuncle of other sites

● L02.9   **Cutaneous abscess, furuncle and carbuncle, unspecified**
     L02.91   **Cutaneous abscess, unspecified**
     L02.92   **Furuncle, unspecified**
         Boil NOS
         Furunculosis NOS
     L02.93   **Carbuncle, unspecified**

CHAPTER 12 (L00–L99)

CHAPTER 12 (L00-L99)

Item 12-1 **Onychia** is an inflammation of the tissue surrounding the nail with pus accumulation and loss of the nail, resulting from microscopic pathogens entering through small wounds. **Paronychia** is a nail disease also known as felon or whitlow and is a bacterial or fungal infection.

● **L03**   **Cellulitis and acute lymphangitis**

     Excludes2   cellulitis of anal and rectal region (K61.-)
                cellulitis of external auditory canal (H60.1)
                cellulitis of eyelid (H00.0)
                cellulitis of female external genital organs (N76.4)
                cellulitis of lacrimal apparatus (H04.3)
                cellulitis of male external genital organs (N48.2, N49.-)
                cellulitis of mouth (K12.2)
                cellulitis of nose (J34.0)
                eosinophilic cellulitis [Wells] (L98.3)
                febrile neutrophilic dermatosis [Sweet] (L98.2)
                lymphangitis (chronic) (subacute) (I89.1)

● **L03.0**   **Cellulitis and acute lymphangitis of finger and toe**
         Infection of nail
         Onychia
         Paronychia
         Perionychia

   ● **L03.01**   **Cellulitis of finger**
                Felon
                Whitlow

              Excludes1   herpetic whitlow (B00.89)

         L03.011   **Cellulitis of right finger**
         L03.012   **Cellulitis of left finger**
         L03.019   **Cellulitis of unspecified finger**

   ● **L03.02**   **Acute lymphangitis of finger**
                Hangnail with lymphangitis of finger
         L03.021   **Acute lymphangitis of right finger**
         L03.022   **Acute lymphangitis of left finger**
         L03.029   **Acute lymphangitis of unspecified finger**

   ● **L03.03**   **Cellulitis of toe**
         L03.031   **Cellulitis of right toe**
         L03.032   **Cellulitis of left toe**
         L03.039   **Cellulitis of unspecified toe**

   ● **L03.04**   **Acute lymphangitis of toe**
                Hangnail with lymphangitis of toe
         L03.041   **Acute lymphangitis of right toe**
         L03.042   **Acute lymphangitis of left toe**
         L03.049   **Acute lymphangitis of unspecified toe**

● **L03.1**   **Cellulitis and acute lymphangitis of other parts of limb**

   ● **L03.11**   **Cellulitis of other parts of limb**

           Excludes2   cellulitis of fingers (L03.01-)
                      cellulitis of toes (L03.03-)
                      groin (L03.314)

         L03.111   **Cellulitis of right axilla**
         L03.112   **Cellulitis of left axilla**
         L03.113   **Cellulitis of right upper limb**
         L03.114   **Cellulitis of left upper limb**
         L03.115   **Cellulitis of right lower limb**
         L03.116   **Cellulitis of left lower limb**
         L03.119   **Cellulitis of unspecified part of limb**

   ● **L03.12**   **Acute lymphangitis of other parts of limb**

           Excludes2   acute lymphangitis of fingers (L03.2-)
                      acute lymphangitis of toes (L03.04-)
                      acute lymphangitis of groin (L03.324)

         L03.121   **Acute lymphangitis of right axilla**
         L03.122   **Acute lymphangitis of left axilla**

         L03.123   **Acute lymphangitis of right upper limb**
         L03.124   **Acute lymphangitis of left upper limb**
         L03.125   **Acute lymphangitis of right lower limb**
         L03.126   **Acute lymphangitis of left lower limb**
         L03.129   **Acute lymphangitis of unspecified part of limb**

● **L03.2**   **Cellulitis and acute lymphangitis of face and neck**

   ● **L03.21**   **Cellulitis and acute lymphangitis of face**

         L03.211   **Cellulitis of face**

              Excludes2   cellulitis of ear (H60.1-)
                        cellulitis of eyelid (H00.0-)
                        cellulitis of head (L03.81)
                        cellulitis of lacrimal apparatus (H04.3)
                        cellulitis of lip (K13.0)
                        cellulitis of mouth (K12.2)
                        cellulitis of nose (internal) (J34.0)
                        cellulitis of orbit (H05.0)
                        cellulitis of scalp (L03.81)

         L03.212   **Acute lymphangitis of face**

   ● **L03.22**   **Cellulitis and acute lymphangitis of neck**
         L03.221   **Cellulitis of neck**
         L03.222   **Acute lymphangitis of neck**

● **L03.3**   **Cellulitis and acute lymphangitis of trunk**

   ● **L03.31**   **Cellulitis of trunk**

           Excludes2   cellulitis of anal and rectal regions (K61.-)
                      cellulitis of breast NOS (N61)
                      cellulitis of female external genital organs (N76.4)
                      cellulitis of male external genital organs (N48.2, N49.-)
                      omphalitis of newborn (P38.-)
                      puerperal cellulitis of breast (O91.2)

         L03.311   **Cellulitis of abdominal wall**

              Excludes2   cellulitis of umbilicus (L03.316)
                        cellulitis of groin (L03.314)

         L03.312   **Cellulitis of back [any part except buttock]**
         L03.313   **Cellulitis of chest wall**
         L03.314   **Cellulitis of groin**
         L03.315   **Cellulitis of perineum**
         L03.316   **Cellulitis of umbilicus**
         L03.317   **Cellulitis of buttock**
         L03.319   **Cellulitis of trunk, unspecified**

Item 12-2 **Cellulitis** is an acute spreading bacterial infection below the surface of the skin characterized by redness (erythema), warmth, swelling, pain, fever, chills, and enlarged lymph nodes ("swollen glands").

● **L03.32   Acute lymphangitis of trunk**
 L03.321   Acute lymphangitis of abdominal wall
 L03.322   Acute lymphangitis of back [any part except buttock]
 L03.323   Acute lymphangitis of chest wall
 L03.324   Acute lymphangitis of groin
 L03.325   Acute lymphangitis of perineum
 L03.326   Acute lymphangitis of umbilicus
 L03.327   Acute lymphangitis of buttock
 L03.329   Acute lymphangitis of trunk, unspecified

● **L03.8   Cellulitis and acute lymphangitis of other sites**
 ● **L03.81   Cellulitis of other sites**
  L03.811   Cellulitis of head [any part, except face]
   Cellulitis of scalp
   Excludes2   cellulitis of face (L03.211)
  L03.818   Cellulitis of other sites
 ● **L03.89   Acute lymphangitis of other sites**
  L03.891   Acute lymphangitis of head [any part, except face]
  L03.898   Acute lymphangitis of other sites
● **L03.9   Cellulitis and acute lymphangitis, unspecified**
 L03.90   Cellulitis, unspecified
 L03.91   Acute lymphangitis, unspecified
  Excludes1   lymphangitis NOS (I89.1)

● **L04   Acute lymphadenitis**
 Short-term inflammation of lymph nodes which can be regionalized to involve a given area of the lymph system or systemic involving much of the body
 Includes   abscess (acute) of lymph nodes, except mesenteric
  acute lymphadenitis, except mesenteric
 Excludes1   chronic or subacute lymphadenitis, except mesenteric (I88.1)
  enlarged lymph nodes (R59.-)
  human immunodeficiency virus [HIV] disease resulting in generalized lymphadenopathy (B20)
  lymphadenitis NOS (I88.9)
  nonspecific mesenteric lymphadenitis (I88.0)
 L04.0   Acute lymphadenitis of face, head and neck
 L04.1   Acute lymphadenitis of trunk
 L04.2   Acute lymphadenitis of upper limb
  Acute lymphadenitis of axilla
  Acute lymphadenitis of shoulder
 L04.3   Acute lymphadenitis of lower limb
  Acute lymphadenitis of hip
  Excludes2   acute lymphadenitis of groin (L04.1)
 L04.8   Acute lymphadenitis of other sites
 L04.9   Acute lymphadenitis, unspecified

● **L05   Pilonidal cyst and sinus**
 ● **L05.0   Pilonidal cyst and sinus with abscess**
  L05.01   Pilonidal cyst with abscess
   Parasacral dimple with abscess
   Pilonidal abscess
   Pilonidal dimple with abscess
   Postanal dimple with abscess
  L05.02   Pilonidal sinus with abscess
   Coccygeal fistula with abscess
   Coccygeal sinus with abscess
   Pilonidal fistula with abscess

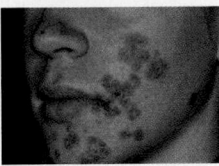

Figure 12-2   Impetigo. A thick, honey-yellow adherent crust covers the entire eroded surface. (From Habif: Clinical Dermatology, ed 4, Mosby, Inc., 2004)

Item 12-3   Abscess is a localized collection of pus in tissues or organs and is a sign of infection resulting in swelling and inflammation.

Item 12-4   Pilonidal cyst, also called a coccygeal cyst, is the result of a disorder called pilonidal disease. The cyst usually contains hair and pus.

● **L05.9   Pilonidal cyst and sinus without abscess**
 L05.91   Pilonidal cyst without abscess
  Parasacral dimple
  Pilonidal dimple
  Postanal dimple
  Pilonidal cyst NOS
 L05.92   Pilonidal sinus without abscess
  Coccygeal fistula
  Coccygeal sinus without abscess
  Pilonidal fistula

● **L08   Other local infections of skin and subcutaneous tissue**
 L08.0   Pyoderma
  Dermatitis gangrenosa
  Purulent dermatitis
  Septic dermatitis
  Suppurative dermatitis
  Excludes1   pyoderma gangrenosum (L88)
   pyoderma vegetans (L08.81)
 L08.1   Erythrasma
 ● **L08.8   Other specified local infections of the skin and subcutaneous tissue**
  L08.81   Pyoderma vegetans
   Excludes1   pyoderma gangrenosum (L88)
   pyoderma NOS (L08.0)
  L08.82   Omphalitis not of newborn
   Excludes1   omphalitis of newborn (P38.-)
  L08.89   Other specified local infections of the skin and subcutaneous tissue
 L08.9   Local infection of the skin and subcutaneous tissue, unspecified

BULLOUS DISORDERS (L10-L14)

 Excludes1   benign familial pemphigus [Hailey-Hailey] (Q82.8)
  staphylococcal scalded skin syndrome (L00)
  toxic epidermal necrolysis [Lyell] (L51.2)

● **L10   Pemphigus**
 Excludes1   pemphigus neonatorum (L01.03)
 L10.0   Pemphigus vulgaris
 L10.1   Pemphigus vegetans
 L10.2   Pemphigus foliaceus
 L10.3   Brazilian pemphigus [fogo selvagem]
 L10.4   Pemphigus erythematosus
  Senear-Usher syndrome
 L10.5   Drug-induced pemphigus
  Use additional code for adverse effect, if applicable, to identify drug (T36-T50 with fifth or sixth character 5)
 ● **L10.8   Other pemphigus**
  L10.81   Paraneoplastic pemphigus
  L10.89   Other pemphigus
 L10.9   Pemphigus, unspecified

CHAPTER 12 (L00-L99)

CHAPTER 12 (L00-L99)

Item 12–5 Dermatitis herpetiformis, also known as Duhring's disease, is a systemic disease characterized by small blisters (3 to 5 mm) and occasionally large bullae (> 5 mm).

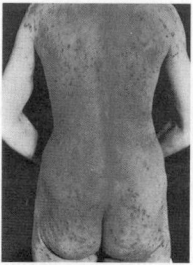

Figure 12-3 Dermatitis herpetiformis. (From Arnold HL, Odom RB, James WD: Andrews' Diseases of the Skin, Clinical Dermatology, ed 8, Philadelphia, WB Saunders, 1990)

● **L11 Other acantholytic disorders**
 L11.0 Acquired keratosis follicularis
   Excludes1 keratosis follicularis (congenital) [Darier-White] (Q82.8)
 L11.1 Transient acantholytic dermatosis [Grover]
 L11.8 Other specified acantholytic disorders
 L11.9 Acantholytic disorder, unspecified

● **L12 Pemphigoid**
  Excludes1 herpes gestationis (O26.4-)
       impetigo herpetiformis (L40.1)
 L12.0 Bullous pemphigoid
 L12.1 Cicatricial pemphigoid
   Benign mucous membrane pemphigoid
 L12.2 Chronic bullous disease of childhood **P**
   Juvenile dermatitis herpetiformis
 ● **L12.3 Acquired epidermolysis bullosa**
   Excludes1 epidermolysis bullosa (congenital) (Q81.-)
  L12.30 Acquired epidermolysis bullosa, unspecified
  L12.31 Epidermolysis bullosa due to drug
    Use additional code for adverse effect, if applicable, to identify drug (T36-T50 with fifth or sixth character 5)
  L12.35 Other acquired epidermolysis bullosa
 L12.8 Other pemphigoid
 L12.9 Pemphigoid, unspecified

● **L13 Other bullous disorders**
 L13.0 Dermatitis herpetiformis
   Duhring's disease
   Hydroa herpetiformis
   Excludes1 juvenile dermatitis herpetiformis (L12.2)
       senile dermatitis herpetiformis (L12.0)
 L13.1 Subcorneal pustular dermatitis
   Sneddon-Wilkinson disease
 L13.8 Other specified bullous disorders
 L13.9 Bullous disorder, unspecified

▶ *L14 Bullous disorders in diseases classified elsewhere*
  Code first underlying disease

Item 12–6 Seborrheic dermatitis is characterized by greasy, scaly, red patches and is associated with oily skin and scalp.

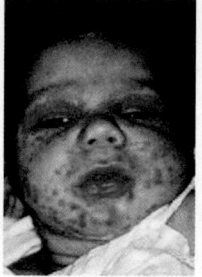

Figure 12-4 Seborrheic dermatitis. (From Cohen BA: Atlas of Pediatric Dermatology, St. Louis, Mosby, 1993)

Item 12–7 Atopic dermatitis, also known as atopic eczema, infantile eczema, disseminated neuro dermatitis, flexural eczema, and *prurigo diathesique* (Besnier), is characterized by intense itching and is often hereditary.

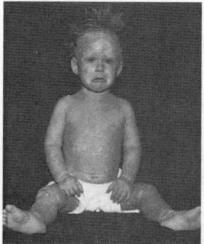

Figure 12-5 Atopic dermatitis. (From Moschella SL, Hurley HJ: Dermatology, ed 3, Philadelphia, WB Saunders, 1993)

DERMATITIS AND ECZEMA (L20-L30)

 Note: In this block the terms dermatitis and eczema are used synonymously and interchangeably.
  Excludes2 chronic (childhood) granulomatous disease (D71)
      dermatitis gangrenosa (L08.0)
      dermatitis herpetiformis (L13.0)
      dry skin dermatitis (L85.3)
      factitial dermatitis (L98.1)
      perioral dermatitis (L71.0)
      radiation-related disorders of the skin and subcutaneous tissue (L55-L59)
      stasis dermatitis (I83.1-I83.2)

● **L20 Atopic dermatitis**
 L20.0 Besnier's prurigo
 ● **L20.8 Other atopic dermatitis**
   Excludes2 circumscribed neurodermatitis (L28.0)
  L20.81 Atopic neurodermatitis
    Diffuse neurodermatitis
  L20.82 Flexural eczema
  L20.83 Infantile (acute) (chronic) eczema **P**
  L20.84 Intrinsic (allergic) eczema
  L20.89 Other atopic dermatitis
 L20.9 Atopic dermatitis, unspecified

● **L21 Seborrheic dermatitis**
  Excludes2 infective dermatitis (L30.3)
      seborrheic keratosis (L82.-)
 L21.0 Seborrhea capitis   **P**
   Cradle cap
 L21.1 Seborrheic infantile dermatitis **P**
 L21.8 Other seborrheic dermatitis
 L21.9 Seborrheic dermatitis, unspecified
   Seborrhea NOS

 L22 Diaper dermatitis
   Diaper erythema
   Diaper rash
   Psoriasiform diaper rash

◀ New ⬅ Revised ~~deleted~~ Deleted Excludes 1 Excludes 2 Includes Use additional Code first Code also Unspecified

OGCR Official Guidelines X Assign placeholder X ● Use Additional Character(s) ▶ Manifestation Code **Coding Clinic**

● **L23**   **Allergic contact dermatitis**

     Excludes1   allergy NOS (T78.40)
                  contact dermatitis NOS (L25.9)
                  dermatitis NOS (L30.9)

     Excludes2   dermatitis due to substances taken internally (L27.-)
                  dermatitis of eyelid (H01.1-)
                  diaper dermatitis (L22)
                  eczema of external ear (H60.5-)
                  irritant contact dermatitis (L24.-)
                  perioral dermatitis (L71.0)
                  radiation-related disorders of the skin and subcutaneous tissue (L55-L59)

L23.0   **Allergic contact dermatitis due to metals**
     Allergic contact dermatitis due to chromium
     Allergic contact dermatitis due to nickel

L23.1   **Allergic contact dermatitis due to adhesives**

L23.2   **Allergic contact dermatitis due to cosmetics**

L23.3   **Allergic contact dermatitis due to drugs in contact with skin**
     Use additional code for adverse effect, if applicable, to identify drug (T36-T50 with fifth or sixth character 5)
     Excludes2   dermatitis due to ingested drugs and medicaments (L27.0-L27.1)

L23.4   **Allergic contact dermatitis due to dyes**

L23.5   **Allergic contact dermatitis due to other chemical products**
     Allergic contact dermatitis due to cement
     Allergic contact dermatitis due to insecticide
     Allergic contact dermatitis due to plastic
     Allergic contact dermatitis due to rubber

L23.6   **Allergic contact dermatitis due to food in contact with the skin**
     Excludes2   dermatitis due to ingested food (L27.2)

L23.7   **Allergic contact dermatitis due to plants, except food**
     Excludes2   allergy NOS due to pollen (J30.1)

● **L23.8**   **Allergic contact dermatitis due to other agents**

     L23.81   **Allergic contact dermatitis due to animal (cat) (dog) dander**
         Allergic contact dermatitis due to animal (cat) (dog) hair

     L23.89   **Allergic contact dermatitis due to other agents**

L23.9   **Allergic contact dermatitis, unspecified cause**
     Allergic contact eczema NOS

● **L24**   **Irritant contact dermatitis**

     Excludes1   allergy NOS (T78.40)
                  contact dermatitis NOS (L25.9)
                  dermatitis NOS (L30.9)

     Excludes2   allergic contact dermatitis (L23.-)
                  dermatitis due to substances taken internally (L27.-)
                  dermatitis of eyelid (H01.1-)
                  diaper dermatitis (L22)
                  eczema of external ear (H60.5-)
                  perioral dermatitis (L71.0)
                  radiation-related disorders of the skin and subcutaneous tissue (L55-L59)

L24.0   **Irritant contact dermatitis due to detergents**

L24.1   **Irritant contact dermatitis due to oils and greases**

L24.2   **Irritant contact dermatitis due to solvents**
     Irritant contact dermatitis due to chlorocompound
     Irritant contact dermatitis due to cyclohexane
     Irritant contact dermatitis due to ester
     Irritant contact dermatitis due to glycol
     Irritant contact dermatitis due to hydrocarbon
     Irritant contact dermatitis due to ketone

L24.3   **Irritant contact dermatitis due to cosmetics**

L24.4   **Irritant contact dermatitis due to drugs in contact with skin**
     Use additional code for adverse effect, if applicable, to identify drug (T36-T50 with fifth or sixth character 5)

L24.5   **Irritant contact dermatitis due to other chemical products**
     Irritant contact dermatitis due to cement
     Irritant contact dermatitis due to insecticide
     Irritant contact dermatitis due to plastic
     Irritant contact dermatitis due to rubber

L24.6   **Irritant contact dermatitis due to food in contact with skin**
     Excludes2   dermatitis due to ingested food (L27.2)

L24.7   **Irritant contact dermatitis due to plants, except food**
     Excludes2   allergy NOS to pollen (J30.1)

● **L24.8**   **Irritant contact dermatitis due to other agents**

     L24.81   **Irritant contact dermatitis due to metals**
         Irritant contact dermatitis due to chromium
         Irritant contact dermatitis due to nickel

     L24.89   **Irritant contact dermatitis due to other agents**
         Irritant contact dermatitis due to dyes

L24.9   **Irritant contact dermatitis, unspecified cause**
     Irritant contact eczema NOS

● **L25**   **Unspecified contact dermatitis**

     Excludes1   allergic contact dermatitis (L23.-)
                  allergy NOS (T78.40)
                  dermatitis NOS (L30.9)
                  irritant contact dermatitis (L24.-)

     Excludes2   dermatitis due to ingested substances (L27.-)
                  dermatitis of eyelid (H01.1-)
                  eczema of external ear (H60.5-)
                  perioral dermatitis (L71.0)
                  radiation-related disorders of the skin and subcutaneous tissue (L55-L59)

L25.0   **Unspecified contact dermatitis due to cosmetics**

L25.1   **Unspecified contact dermatitis due to drugs in contact with skin**
     Use additional code for adverse effect, if applicable, to identify drug (T36-T50 with fifth or sixth character 5)
     Excludes2   dermatitis due to ingested drugs and medicaments (L27.0-L27.1)

L25.2   **Unspecified contact dermatitis due to dyes**

L25.3   **Unspecified contact dermatitis due to other chemical products**
     Unspecified contact dermatitis due to cement
     Unspecified contact dermatitis due to insecticide

L25.4   **Unspecified contact dermatitis due to food in contact with skin**
     Excludes2   dermatitis due to ingested food (L27.2)

L25.5   **Unspecified contact dermatitis due to plants, except food**
     Excludes1   nettle rash (L50.9)
     Excludes2   allergy NOS due to pollen (J30.1)

L25.8   **Unspecified contact dermatitis due to other agents**

L25.9   **Unspecified contact dermatitis, unspecified cause**
     Contact dermatitis (occupational) NOS
     Contact eczema (occupational) NOS

L26   **Exfoliative dermatitis**
     Hebra's pityriasis
     Excludes1   Ritter's disease (L00)

CHAPTER 12 (L00-L99)

● **L27**   **Dermatitis due to substances taken internally**
  - **Excludes1**   allergy NOS (T78.40)
  - **Excludes2**   adverse food reaction, except dermatitis (T78.0-T78.1)
    - contact dermatitis (L23-L25)
    - drug photoallergic response (L56.1)
    - drug phototoxic response (L56.0)
    - urticaria (L50.-)
  - **L27.0**   **Generalized skin eruption due to drugs and medicaments taken internally**
    - Use additional code for adverse effect, if applicable, to identify drug (T36-T50 with fifth or sixth character 5)
  - **L27.1**   **Localized skin eruption due to drugs and medicaments taken internally**
    - Use additional code for adverse effect, if applicable, to identify drug (T36-T50 with fifth or sixth character 5)
  - **L27.2**   **Dermatitis due to ingested food**
    - **Excludes2**   dermatitis due to food in contact with skin (L23.6, L24.6, L25.4)
  - **L27.8**   **Dermatitis due to other substances taken internally**
  - **L27.9**   **Dermatitis due to unspecified substance taken internally**

● **L28**   **Lichen simplex chronicus and prurigo**
  - **L28.0**   **Lichen simplex chronicus**
    - Circumscribed neurodermatitis
    - Lichen NOS
  - **L28.1**   **Prurigo nodularis**
  - **L28.2**   **Other prurigo**
    - Prurigo NOS   Prurigo mitis
    - Prurigo Hebra   Urticaria papulosa

● **L29**   **Pruritus**
  - **Excludes1**   neurotic excoriation (L98.1)
    - psychogenic pruritus (F45.8)
  - **L29.0**   **Pruritus ani**
  - **L29.1**   **Pruritus scroti** ♂
  - **L29.2**   **Pruritus vulvae** ♀
  - **L29.3**   **Anogenital pruritus, unspecified**
  - **L29.8**   **Other pruritus**
  - **L29.9**   **Pruritus, unspecified**
    - Itch NOS

● **L30**   **Other and unspecified dermatitis**
  - **Excludes2**   contact dermatitis (L23-L25)
    - dry skin dermatitis (L85.3)
    - small plaque parapsoriasis (L41.3)
    - stasis dermatitis (I83.1-.2)
  - **L30.0**   **Nummular dermatitis**
  - **L30.1**   **Dyshidrosis [pompholyx]**
  - **L30.2**   **Cutaneous autosensitization**
    - Candidid [levurid]   Eczematid
    - Dermatophytid
  - **L30.3**   **Infective dermatitis**
    - Infectious eczematoid dermatitis
  - **L30.4**   **Erythema intertrigo**
  - **L30.5**   **Pityriasis alba**
  - **L30.8**   **Other specified dermatitis**
  - **L30.9**   **Dermatitis, unspecified**
    - Eczema NOS

Item 12-8   **Psoriasis** is a chronic, recurrent inflammatory skin disease characterized by small patches covered with thick silvery scales. **Parapsoriasis** is a treatment-resistant erythroderma. **Pityriasis rosea** is characterized by a herald patch that is a single large lesion and that usually appears on the trunk and is followed by scattered, smaller lesions.

PAPULOSQUAMOUS DISORDERS (L40-L45)

● **L40**   **Psoriasis**
  - **L40.0**   **Psoriasis vulgaris**
    - Nummular psoriasis   Plaque psoriasis
  - **L40.1**   **Generalized pustular psoriasis**
    - Impetigo herpetiformis
    - Von Zumbusch's disease
  - **L40.2**   **Acrodermatitis continua**
  - **L40.3**   **Pustulosis palmaris et plantaris**
  - **L40.4**   **Guttate psoriasis**
  - ● **L40.5**   **Arthropathic psoriasis**
    - **L40.50**   **Arthropathic psoriasis, unspecified**
    - **L40.51**   **Distal interphalangeal psoriatic arthropathy**
    - **L40.52**   **Psoriatic arthritis mutilans**
    - **L40.53**   **Psoriatic spondylitis**
    - **L40.54**   **Psoriatic juvenile arthropathy**
    - **L40.59**   **Other psoriatic arthropathy**
  - **L40.8**   **Other psoriasis**
    - Flexural psoriasis
  - **L40.9**   **Psoriasis, unspecified**

● **L41**   **Parapsoriasis**
  - **Excludes1**   poikiloderma vasculare atrophicans (L94.5)
  - **L41.0**   **Pityriasis lichenoides et varioliformis acuta**
    - Mucha-Habermann disease
  - **L41.1**   **Pityriasis lichenoides chronica**
  - **L41.3**   **Small plaque parapsoriasis**
  - **L41.4**   **Large plaque parapsoriasis**
  - **L41.5**   **Retiform parapsoriasis**
  - **L41.8**   **Other parapsoriasis**
  - **L41.9**   **Parapsoriasis, unspecified**

   L42   **Pityriasis rosea**

● **L43**   **Lichen planus**
  - **Excludes1**   lichen planopilaris (L66.1)
  - **L43.0**   **Hypertrophic lichen planus**
  - **L43.1**   **Bullous lichen planus**
  - **L43.2**   **Lichenoid drug reaction**
    - Use additional code for adverse effect, if applicable, to identify drug (T36-T50 with fifth or sixth character 5)
  - **L43.3**   **Subacute (active) lichen planus**
    - Lichen planus tropicus
  - **L43.8**   **Other lichen planus**
  - **L43.9**   **Lichen planus, unspecified**

● **L44**   **Other papulosquamous disorders**
  - **L44.0**   **Pityriasis rubra pilaris**
  - **L44.1**   **Lichen nitidus**
  - **L44.2**   **Lichen striatus**
  - **L44.3**   **Lichen ruber moniliformis**
  - **L44.4**   **Infantile papular acrodermatitis [Gianotti-Crosti]**   P
  - **L44.8**   **Other specified papulosquamous disorders**
  - **L44.9**   **Papulosquamous disorder, unspecified**

▷ *L45*   *Papulosquamous disorders in diseases classified elsewhere*
  - *Code first underlying disease*

◀ New   ◀|||| Revised   ~~deleted~~ Deleted   Excludes 1   Excludes 2   Includes   Use additional   Code first   Code also   Unspecified

OGCR Official Guidelines   X Assign placeholder X   ● Use Additional Character(s)   ▷ Manifestation Code   **Coding Clinic**

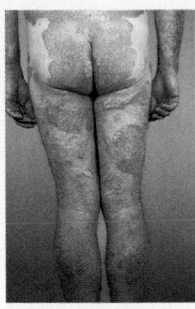

Figure 12-6 Erythematous plaques with silvery scales in a patient with psoriasis. (From Goldman: Cecil Textbook of Medicine, ed 22, Saunders, 2004)

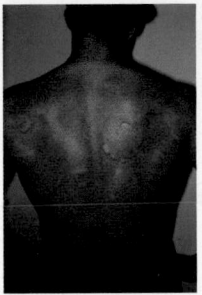

Figure 12-7 Urticaria (hives). *(Courtesy of David Effron, MD.)* (From Marx: Rosen's Emergency Medicine: Concepts and Clinical Practice, ed 6, Mosby, Inc., 2006)

URTICARIA AND ERYTHEMA (L49-L54)

> **Excludes1**   Lyme disease (A69.2-)
> rosacea (L71.-)

● **L49**   **Exfoliation due to erythematous conditions according to extent of body surface involved**

> *Code first erythematous condition causing exfoliation, such as:*
> Ritter's disease (L00)
> (Staphylococcal) scalded skin syndrome (L00)
> Stevens-Johnson syndrome (L51.1)
> Stevens-Johnson syndrome-toxic epidermal necrolysis overlap syndrome (L51.3)
> Toxic epidermal necrolysis (L51.2)

L49.0   **Exfoliation due to erythematous condition involving less than 10 percent of body surface**
> Exfoliation due to erythematous condition NOS

L49.1   **Exfoliation due to erythematous condition involving 10-19 percent of body surface**

L49.2   **Exfoliation due to erythematous condition involving 20-29 percent of body surface**

L49.3   **Exfoliation due to erythematous condition involving 30-39 percent of body surface**

L49.4   **Exfoliation due to erythematous condition involving 40-49 percent of body surface**

L49.5   **Exfoliation due to erythematous condition involving 50-59 percent of body surface**

L49.6   **Exfoliation due to erythematous condition involving 60-69 percent of body surface**

L49.7   **Exfoliation due to erythematous condition involving 70-79 percent of body surface**

L49.8   **Exfoliation due to erythematous condition involving 80-89 percent of body surface**

L49.9   **Exfoliation due to erythematous condition involving 90 or more percent of body surface**

● **L50**   **Urticaria**

> **Excludes1**   allergic contact dermatitis (L23.-)
> angioneurotic edema (T78.3)
> giant urticaria (T78.3)
> hereditary angio-edema (D84.1)
> Quincke's edema (T78.3)
> serum urticaria (T80.6-)
> solar urticaria (L56.3)
> urticaria neonatorum (P83.8)
> urticaria papulosa (L28.2)
> urticaria pigmentosa (Q82.2)

L50.0   **Allergic urticaria**

L50.1   **Idiopathic urticaria**

L50.2   **Urticaria due to cold and heat**

L50.3   **Dermatographic urticaria**

L50.4   **Vibratory urticaria**

L50.5   **Cholinergic urticaria**

L50.6   **Contact urticaria**

L50.8   **Other urticaria**
> Chronic urticaria
> Recurrent periodic urticaria

L50.9   **Urticaria, unspecified**

Item 12–9   **Urticaria** is a vascular reaction in which wheals surrounded by a red halo appear and cause severe itching. The causes of urticaria or hives are extensive and varied (e.g., food, heat, cold, drugs, stress, infections).

● **L51**   **Erythema multiforme**

> Use additional code for adverse effect, if applicable, to identify drug (T36-T50 with fifth or sixth character 5)
> Use additional code to identify associated manifestations, such as:
> arthropathy associated with dermatological disorders (M14.8-)
> conjunctival edema (H11.42)
> conjunctivitis (H10.22-)
> corneal scars and opacities (H17.-)
> corneal ulcer (H16.0-)
> edema of eyelid (H02.84)
> inflammation of eyelid (H01.8)
> keratoconjunctivitis sicca (H16.22-)
> mechanical lagophthalmos (H02.22-)
> stomatitis (K12.-)
> symblepharon (H11.23-)
> Use additional code to identify percentage of skin exfoliation (L49.-)

> **Excludes1**   staphylococcal scalded skin syndrome (L00)
> Ritter's disease (L00)

L51.0   **Nonbullous erythema multiforme**

L51.1   **Stevens-Johnson syndrome**

L51.2   **Toxic epidermal necrolysis [Lyell]**

L51.3   **Stevens-Johnson syndrome-toxic epidermal necrolysis overlap syndrome**
> SJS-TEN overlap syndrome

L51.8   **Other erythema multiforme**

L51.9   **Erythema multiforme, unspecified**
> Erythema iris
> Erythema multiforme major NOS
> Erythema multiforme minor NOS
> Herpes iris

L52   **Erythema nodosum**
> **Excludes1**   tuberculous erythema nodosum (A18.4)

● **L53**   **Other erythematous conditions**
> **Excludes1**   erythema ab igne (L59.0)
> erythema due to external agents in contact with skin (L23-L25)
> erythema intertrigo (L30.4)

L53.0   **Toxic erythema**
> *Code first poisoning due to drug or toxin, if applicable (T36-T65 with fifth or sixth character 1-4 or 6)*
> Use additional code for adverse effect, if applicable, to identify drug (T36-T50 with fifth or sixth character 5)
> **Excludes1**   neonatal erythema toxicum (P83.1)

L53.1   **Erythema annulare centrifugum**

L53.2   **Erythema marginatum**

L53.3   **Other chronic figurate erythema**

L53.8   Other specified erythematous conditions

L53.9   Erythematous condition, unspecified
Erythema NOS
Erythroderma NOS

▶ **L54   *Erythema in diseases classified elsewhere***
Code first underlying disease

RADIATION-RELATED DISORDERS OF THE SKIN AND SUBCUTANEOUS TISSUE (L55-L59)

● **L55   Sunburn**

L55.0   Sunburn of first degree

L55.1   Sunburn of second degree

L55.2   Sunburn of third degree

L55.9   Sunburn, unspecified

● **L56   Other acute skin changes due to ultraviolet radiation**
Use additional code to identify the source of the ultraviolet radiation (W89, X32)

L56.0   Drug phototoxic response
Use additional code for adverse effect, if applicable, to identify drug (T36-T50 with fifth or sixth character 5)

L56.1   Drug photoallergic response
Use additional code for adverse effect, if applicable, to identify drug (T36-T50 with fifth or sixth character 5)

L56.2   Photocontact dermatitis [berloque dermatitis]

L56.3   Solar urticaria

L56.4   Polymorphous light eruption

L56.5   Disseminated superficial actinic porokeratosis (DSAP)

L56.8   Other specified acute skin changes due to ultraviolet radiation

L56.9   Acute skin change due to ultraviolet radiation, unspecified

● **L57   Skin changes due to chronic exposure to nonionizing radiation**
Use additional code to identify the source of the ultraviolet radiation (W89, X32)

L57.0   Actinic keratosis
Keratosis NOS   Solar keratosis
Senile keratosis

L57.1   Actinic reticuloid

L57.2   Cutis rhomboidalis nuchae

L57.3   Poikiloderma of Civatte

L57.4   Cutis laxa senilis
Elastosis senilis

L57.5   Actinic granuloma

L57.8   Other skin changes due to chronic exposure to nonionizing radiation
Farmer's skin   Solar dermatitis
Sailor's skin

L57.9   Skin changes due to chronic exposure to nonionizing radiation, unspecified

● **L58   Radiodermatitis**
Use additional code to identify the source of the radiation (W88, W90)

L58.0   Acute radiodermatitis

L58.1   Chronic radiodermatitis

L58.9   Radiodermatitis, unspecified

● **L59   Other disorders of skin and subcutaneous tissue related to radiation**

L59.0   Erythema ab igne [dermatitis ab igne]

L59.8   Other specified disorders of the skin and subcutaneous tissue related to radiation

L59.9   Disorder of the skin and subcutaneous tissue related to radiation, unspecified

Item 12–10   Alopecia is lack of hair and takes many forms. The most common is male pattern alopecia, also known as **androgenetic alopecia.** **Telogen effluvium** is early and excessive loss of hair resulting from a trauma to the hair follicle (fever, drugs, surgery, etc.).

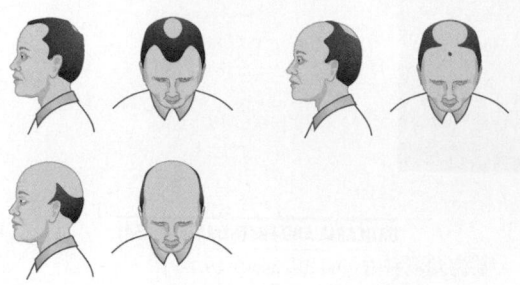

Figure 12-8   Male pattern alopecia.

DISORDERS OF SKIN APPENDAGES (L60-L75)

Excludes1   congenital malformations of integument (Q84.-)

● **L60   Nail disorders**

Excludes2   clubbing of nails (R68.3)
onychia and paronychia (L03.0-)

L60.0   Ingrowing nail

L60.1   Onycholysis

L60.2   Onychogryphosis

L60.3   Nail dystrophy

L60.4   Beau's lines

L60.5   Yellow nail syndrome

L60.8   Other nail disorders

L60.9   Nail disorder, unspecified

▶ **L62   *Nail disorders in diseases classified elsewhere***
Code first underlying disease, such as:
pachydermoperiostosis (M89.4-)

● **L63   Alopecia areata**

L63.0   Alopecia (capitis) totalis

L63.1   Alopecia universalis

L63.2   Ophiasis

L63.8   Other alopecia areata

L63.9   Alopecia areata, unspecified

● **L64   Androgenic alopecia**

Includes   male-pattern baldness

L64.0   Drug-induced androgenic alopecia
Use additional code for adverse effect, if applicable, to identify drug (T36-T50 with fifth or sixth character 5)

L64.8   Other androgenic alopecia

L64.9   Androgenic alopecia, unspecified

● **L65   Other nonscarring hair loss**
Use additional code for adverse effect, if applicable, to identify drug (T36-T50 with fifth or sixth character 5)

Excludes1   trichotillomania (F63.3)

L65.0   Telogen effluvium

L65.1   Anagen effluvium

L65.2   Alopecia mucinosa

L65.8   Other specified nonscarring hair loss

L65.9   Nonscarring hair loss, unspecified
Alopecia NOS

◀ New   ◀══ Revised   ~~deleted~~ Deleted   Excludes 1   Excludes 2   Includes   Use additional   Code first   Code also   Unspecified

OGCR Official Guidelines   X Assign placeholder X   ● Use Additional Character(s)   ▶ Manifestation Code   **Coding Clinic**

● **L66**   **Cicatricial alopecia [scarring hair loss]**
    L66.0   **Pseudopelade**
    L66.1   **Lichen planopilaris**
         Follicular lichen planus
    L66.2   **Folliculitis decalvans**
    L66.3   **Perifolliculitis capitis abscedens**
    L66.4   **Folliculitis ulerythematosa reticulata**
    L66.8   **Other cicatricial alopecia**
         Coding Clinic: 2015, Q1, P19
    L66.9   **Cicatricial alopecia, unspecified**

● **L67**   **Hair color and hair shaft abnormalities**
       Excludes1   monilethrix (Q84.1)
               pili annulati (Q84.1)
               telogen effluvium (L65.0)
    L67.0   **Trichorrhexis nodosa**
    L67.1   **Variations in hair color**
         Canities
         Greyness, hair (premature)
         Heterochromia of hair
         Poliosis circumscripta, acquired
         Poliosis NOS
    L67.8   **Other hair color and hair shaft abnormalities**
         Fragilitas crinium
    L67.9   **Hair color and hair shaft abnormality, unspecified**

● **L68**   **Hypertrichosis**
       Includes   excess hair
       Excludes1   congenital hypertrichosis (Q84.2)
               persistent lanugo (Q84.2)
    L68.0   **Hirsutism**
         Excessive growth of hair
    L68.1   **Acquired hypertrichosis lanuginosa**
    L68.2   **Localized hypertrichosis**
    L68.3   **Polytrichia**
    L68.8   **Other hypertrichosis**
    L68.9   **Hypertrichosis, unspecified**

● **L70**   **Acne**
       Excludes2   acne keloid (L73.0)
    L70.0   **Acne vulgaris**
    L70.1   **Acne conglobata**
    L70.2   **Acne varioliformis**
         Acne necrotica miliaris
    L70.3   **Acne tropica**
    L70.4   **Infantile acne**   P
    L70.5   **Acné excoriée des jeunes filles**
         Picker's acne
    L70.8   **Other acne**
    L70.9   **Acne, unspecified**

● **L71**   **Rosacea**
       Use additional code for adverse effect, if applicable, to identify drug (T36-T50 with fifth or sixth character 5)
    L71.0   **Perioral dermatitis**
    L71.1   **Rhinophyma**
    L71.8   **Other rosacea**
    L71.9   **Rosacea, unspecified**

● **L72**   **Follicular cysts of skin and subcutaneous tissue**
    L72.0   **Epidermal cyst**
   ● **L72.1**   **Pilar and trichodermal cyst**
      L72.11   **Pilar cyst**
      L72.12   **Trichodermal cyst**
            Trichilemmal (proliferating) cyst
    L72.3   **Sebaceous cyst**
         Excludes2   pilar cyst (L72.11)
                  trichilemmal (proliferating) cyst (L72.12)
    L72.2   **Steatocystoma multiplex**

    L72.8   **Other follicular cysts of the skin and subcutaneous tissue**
    L72.9   **Follicular cyst of the skin and subcutaneous tissue, unspecified**

● **L73**   **Other follicular disorders**
    L73.0   **Acne keloid**
    L73.1   **Pseudofolliculitis barbae**
    L73.2   **Hidradenitis suppurativa**
    L73.8   **Other specified follicular disorders**
         Sycosis barbae
    L73.9   **Follicular disorder, unspecified**

● **L74**   **Eccrine sweat disorders**
       Excludes2   generalized hyperhidrosis (R61)
    L74.0   **Miliaria rubra**
    L74.1   **Miliaria crystallina**
    L74.2   **Miliaria profunda**
         Miliaria tropicalis
    L74.3   **Miliaria, unspecified**
    L74.4   **Anhidrosis**
         Hypohidrosis
   ● **L74.5**   **Focal hyperhidrosis**
      ● **L74.51**   **Primary focal hyperhidrosis**
          L74.510   **Primary focal hyperhidrosis, axilla**
          L74.511   **Primary focal hyperhidrosis, face**
          L74.512   **Primary focal hyperhidrosis, palms**
          L74.513   **Primary focal hyperhidrosis, soles**
          L74.519   **Primary focal hyperhidrosis, unspecified**
      L74.52   **Secondary focal hyperhidrosis**
          Frey's syndrome
    L74.8   **Other eccrine sweat disorders**
    L74.9   **Eccrine sweat disorder, unspecified**
         Sweat gland disorder NOS

● **L75**   **Apocrine sweat disorders**
       Excludes1   dyshidrosis (L30.1)
               hidradenitis suppurativa (L73.2)
    L75.0   **Bromhidrosis**
    L75.1   **Chromhidrosis**
    L75.2   **Apocrine miliaria**
         Fox-Fordyce disease
    L75.8   **Other apocrine sweat disorders**
    L75.9   **Apocrine sweat disorder, unspecified**
         Intraoperative and postprocedural complications of skin and subcutaneous tissue (L76)

INTRAOPERATIVE AND POSTPROCEDURAL COMPLICATIONS OF SKIN AND SUBCUTANEOUS TISSUE (L76)

● **L76**   **Intraoperative and postprocedural complications of skin and subcutaneous tissue**
   ● **L76.0**   **Intraoperative hemorrhage and hematoma of skin and subcutaneous tissue complicating a procedure**
         Excludes1   intraoperative hemorrhage and hematoma of skin and subcutaneous tissue due to accidental puncture and laceration during a procedure (L76.1-)
      L76.01   **Intraoperative hemorrhage and hematoma of skin and subcutaneous tissue complicating a dermatologic procedure**
      L76.02   **Intraoperative hemorrhage and hematoma of skin and subcutaneous tissue complicating other procedure**

CHAPTER 12 (L00-L99)

● **L76.1** **Accidental puncture and laceration of skin and subcutaneous tissue during a procedure**

     L76.11 Accidental puncture and laceration of skin and subcutaneous tissue during a dermatologic procedure

     L76.12 Accidental puncture and laceration of skin and subcutaneous tissue during other procedure

● **L76.2** **Postprocedural hemorrhage and hematoma of skin and subcutaneous tissue following a procedure**

     L76.21 Postprocedural hemorrhage and hematoma of skin and subcutaneous tissue following a dermatologic procedure

     L76.22 Postprocedural hemorrhage and hematoma of skin and subcutaneous tissue following other procedure

● **L76.8** **Other intraoperative and postprocedural complications of skin and subcutaneous tissue**

     Use additional code, if applicable, to further specify disorder

     L76.81 Other intraoperative complications of skin and subcutaneous tissue

     L76.82 Other postprocedural complications of skin and subcutaneous tissue

OTHER DISORDERS OF THE SKIN AND SUBCUTANEOUS TISSUE (L80-L99)

L80 **Vitiligo**

     Excludes2   vitiligo of eyelids (H02.73-)
                        vitiligo of vulva (N90.89)

● **L81** **Other disorders of pigmentation**

     Excludes1   birthmark NOS (Q82.5)
                        Peutz-Jeghers syndrome (Q85.8)

     Excludes2   nevus - see Alphabetical Index

     L81.0 **Postinflammatory hyperpigmentation**

     L81.1 **Chloasma**

     L81.2 **Freckles**

     L81.3 **Café au lait spots**

     L81.4 **Other melanin hyperpigmentation**
            Lentigo

     L81.5 **Leukoderma, not elsewhere classified**

     L81.6 **Other disorders of diminished melanin formation**

     L81.7 **Pigmented purpuric dermatosis**
            Angioma serpiginosum

     L81.8 **Other specified disorders of pigmentation**
            Iron pigmentation
            Tattoo pigmentation

     L81.9 **Disorder of pigmentation, unspecified**

● **L82** **Seborrheic keratosis**

     Includes   dermatosis papulosa nigra
                   Leser-Trélat disease

     Excludes2   seborrheic dermatitis (L21.-)

     L82.0 **Inflamed seborrheic keratosis**

     L82.1 **Other seborrheic keratosis**
            Seborrheic keratosis NOS

L83 **Acanthosis nigricans**
     Confluent and reticulated papillomatosis

L84 **Corns and callosities**
     Callus
     Clavus

● **L85** **Other epidermal thickening**

     Excludes2   hypertrophic disorders of the skin (L91.-)

     L85.0 **Acquired ichthyosis**

          Excludes1   congenital ichthyosis (Q80.-)

     L85.1 **Acquired keratosis [keratoderma] palmaris et plantaris**

          Excludes1   inherited keratosis palmaris et plantaris (Q82.8)

     L85.2 **Keratosis punctata (palmaris et plantaris) L85.3**
            Xerosis cutis
            Dry skin dermatitis

     L85.8 **Other specified epidermal thickening**
            Cutaneous horn

     L85.9 **Epidermal thickening, unspecified**

▶ *L86*   *Keratoderma in diseases classified elsewhere*
     Firm horny papules that have a cobblestone appearance.

     Code first underlying disease, such as:
          Reiter's disease (M02.3-)

     Excludes1   gonococcal keratoderma (A54.89)
                       gonococcal keratosis (A54.89)
                       keratoderma due to vitamin A deficiency (E50.8)
                       keratosis due to vitamin A deficiency (E50.8)
                       xeroderma due to vitamin A deficiency (E50.8)

● **L87** **Transepidermal elimination disorders**

     Excludes1   granuloma annulare (perforating) (L92.0)

     L87.0 **Keratosis follicularis et parafollicularis in cutem penetrans**
            Kyrle disease
            Hyperkeratosis follicularis penetrans

     L87.1 **Reactive perforating collagenosis**

     L87.2 **Elastosis perforans serpiginosa**

     L87.8 **Other transepidermal elimination disorders**

     L87.9 **Transepidermal elimination disorder, unspecified**

● **L88** **Pyoderma gangrenosum**
     Phagedenic pyoderma

     Excludes1   dermatitis gangrenosa (L08.0)

OGCR Section I.B.14.

General Coding Guidelines

14. Documentation for BMI, Non-pressure ulcers and Pressure Ulcer Stages

For the Body Mass Index (BMI), depth of non-pressure chronic ulcers and pressure ulcer stage codes, code assignment may be based on medical record documentation from clinicians who are not the patient's provider (i.e., physician or other qualified healthcare practitioner legally accountable for establishing the patient's diagnosis), since this information is typically documented by other clinicians involved in the care of the patient (e.g., a dietitian often documents the BMI and nurses often documents the pressure ulcer stages). However, the associated diagnosis (such as overweight, obesity, or pressure ulcer) must be documented by the patient's provider. If there is conflicting medical record documentation, either from the same clinician or different clinicians, the patient's attending provider should be queried for clarification.

● **L89** **Pressure ulcer**

     Includes   bed sore   pressure area
                   decubitus ulcer   pressure sore
                   plaster ulcer

     Code first any associated gangrene (I96)

     Excludes2   decubitus (trophic) ulcer of cervix (uteri) (N86)
                       diabetic ulcers (E08.621, E08.622, E09.621, E09.622, E10.621, E10.622, E11.621, E11.622, E13.621, E13.622)
                       non-pressure chronic ulcer of skin (L97.-)
                       skin infections (L00-L08)
                       varicose ulcer (I83.0, I83.2)

     ● **L89.0** **Pressure ulcer of elbow**

         ● **L89.00** **Pressure ulcer of unspecified elbow**

             L89.000 **Pressure ulcer of unspecified elbow, unstageable**

             L89.001 **Pressure ulcer of unspecified elbow, stage 1**
                 Healing pressure ulcer of unspecified elbow, stage 1
                 Pressure pre-ulcer skin changes limited to persistent focal edema, unspecified elbow

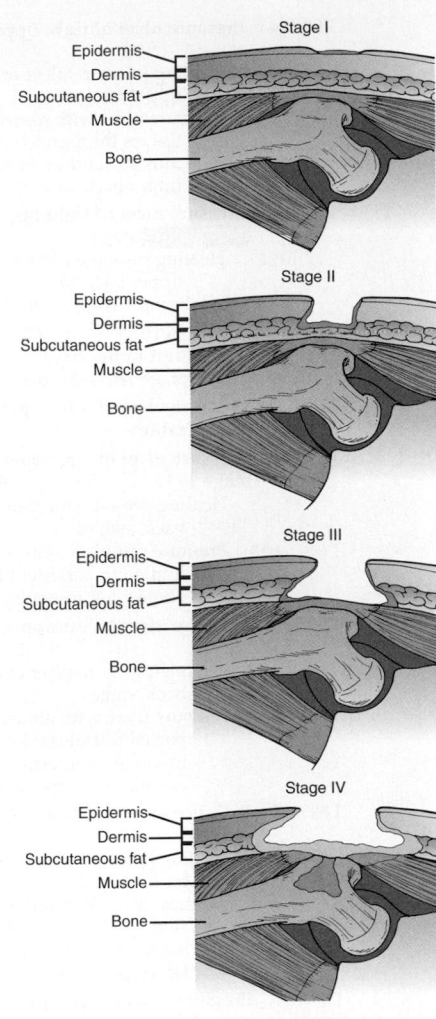

Figure 12-9 Stage I, II, III, and IV of pressure ulcers.

L89.002   **Pressure ulcer of unspecified elbow, stage 2**
Healing pressure ulcer of unspecified elbow, stage 2
Pressure ulcer with abrasion, blister, partial thickness skin loss involving epidermis and/or dermis, unspecified elbow

L89.003   **Pressure ulcer of unspecified elbow, stage 3**
Healing pressure ulcer of unspecified elbow, stage 3
Pressure ulcer with full thickness skin loss involving damage or necrosis of subcutaneous tissue, unspecified elbow

L89.004   **Pressure ulcer of unspecified elbow, stage 4**
Healing pressure ulcer of unspecified elbow, stage 4
Pressure ulcer with necrosis of soft tissues through to underlying muscle, tendon, or bone, unspecified elbow

L89.009   **Pressure ulcer of unspecified elbow, unspecified stage**
Healing pressure ulcer of elbow NOS
Healing pressure ulcer of unspecified elbow, unspecified stage

● **L89.01**   **Pressure ulcer of right elbow**

L89.010   **Pressure ulcer of right elbow, unstageable**

L89.011   **Pressure ulcer of right elbow, stage 1**
Healing pressure ulcer of right elbow, stage 1
Pressure pre-ulcer skin changes limited to persistent focal edema, right elbow

L89.012   **Pressure ulcer of right elbow, stage 2**
Healing pressure ulcer of right elbow, stage 2
Pressure ulcer with abrasion, blister, partial thickness skin loss involving epidermis and/or dermis, right elbow

L89.013   **Pressure ulcer of right elbow, stage 3**
Healing pressure ulcer of right elbow, stage 3
Pressure ulcer with full thickness skin loss involving damage or necrosis of subcutaneous tissue, right elbow

L89.014   **Pressure ulcer of right elbow, stage 4**
Healing pressure ulcer of right elbow, stage 4
Pressure ulcer with necrosis of soft tissues through to underlying muscle, tendon, or bone, right elbow

L89.019   **Pressure ulcer of right elbow, unspecified stage**
Healing pressure right of elbow NOS
Healing pressure ulcer of unspecified elbow, unspecified stage

● **L89.02**   **Pressure ulcer of left elbow**

L89.020   **Pressure ulcer of left elbow, unstageable**

L89.021   **Pressure ulcer of left elbow, stage 1**
Healing pressure ulcer of left elbow, stage 1
Pressure pre-ulcer skin changes limited to persistent focal edema, left elbow

L89.022   **Pressure ulcer of left elbow, stage 2**
Healing pressure ulcer of left elbow, stage 2
Pressure ulcer with abrasion, blister, partial thickness skin loss involving epidermis and/or dermis, left elbow

L89.023   **Pressure ulcer of left elbow, stage 3**
Healing pressure ulcer of left elbow, stage 3
Pressure ulcer with full thickness skin loss involving damage or necrosis of subcutaneous tissue, left elbow

L89.024   **Pressure ulcer of left elbow, stage 4**
Healing pressure ulcer of left elbow, stage 4
Pressure ulcer with necrosis of soft tissues through to underlying muscle, tendon, or bone, left elbow

L89.029   **Pressure ulcer of left elbow, unspecified stage**
Healing pressure ulcer of left of elbow NOS
Healing pressure ulcer of unspecified elbow, unspecified stage

CHAPTER 12 (L00-L99)

CHAPTER 12 (L00-L99)

● **L89.1**   **Pressure ulcer of back**

  ● **L89.10**   **Pressure ulcer of unspecified part of back**

      L89.100   **Pressure ulcer of** <mark>unspecified</mark> **part of back, unstageable**

      L89.101   **Pressure ulcer of** <mark>unspecified</mark> **part of back, stage 1**

          Healing pressure ulcer of unspecified part of back, stage 1

          Pressure pre-ulcer skin changes limited to persistent focal edema, unspecified part of back

      L89.102   **Pressure ulcer of** <mark>unspecified</mark> **part of back, stage 2**

          Healing pressure ulcer of unspecified part of back, stage 2

          Pressure ulcer with abrasion, blister, partial thickness skin loss involving epidermis and/or dermis, unspecified part of back

      L89.103   **Pressure ulcer of** <mark>unspecified</mark> **part of back, stage 3**

          Healing pressure ulcer of unspecified part of back, stage 3

          Pressure ulcer with full thickness skin loss involving damage or necrosis of subcutaneous tissue, unspecified part of back

      L89.104   **Pressure ulcer of** <mark>unspecified</mark> **part of back, stage 4**

          Healing pressure ulcer of unspecified part of back, stage 4

          Pressure ulcer with necrosis of soft tissues through to underlying muscle, tendon, or bone, unspecified part of back

      L89.109   **Pressure ulcer of** <mark>unspecified</mark> **part of back, unspecified stage**

          Healing pressure ulcer of unspecified part of back NOS

          Healing pressure ulcer of unspecified part of back, unspecified stage

  ● **L89.11**   **Pressure ulcer of right upper back**

          Pressure ulcer of right shoulder blade

      L89.110   **Pressure ulcer of right upper back, unstageable**

      L89.111   **Pressure ulcer of right upper back, stage 1**

          Healing pressure ulcer of right upper back, stage 1

          Pressure pre-ulcer skin changes limited to persistent focal edema, right upper back

      L89.112   **Pressure ulcer of right upper back, stage 2**

          Healing pressure ulcer of right upper back, stage 2

          Pressure ulcer with abrasion, blister, partial thickness skin loss involving epidermis and/or dermis, right upper back

      L89.113   **Pressure ulcer of right upper back, stage 3**

          Healing pressure ulcer of right upper back, stage 3

          Pressure ulcer with full thickness skin loss involving damage or necrosis of subcutaneous tissue, right upper back

      L89.114   **Pressure ulcer of right upper back, stage 4**

          Healing pressure ulcer of right upper back, stage 4

          Pressure ulcer with necrosis of soft tissues through to underlying muscle, tendon, or bone, right upper back

      L89.119   **Pressure ulcer of right upper back,** <mark>unspecified</mark> **stage**

          Healing pressure ulcer of right upper back NOS

          Healing pressure ulcer of right upper back, unspecified stage

  ● **L89.12**   **Pressure ulcer of left upper back**

          Pressure ulcer of left shoulder blade

      L89.120   **Pressure ulcer of left upper back, unstageable**

      L89.121   **Pressure ulcer of left upper back, stage 1**

          Healing pressure ulcer of left upper back, stage 1

          Pressure pre-ulcer skin changes limited to persistent focal edema, left upper back

      L89.122   **Pressure ulcer of left upper back, stage 2**

          Healing pressure ulcer of left upper back, stage 2

          Pressure ulcer with abrasion, blister, partial thickness skin loss involving epidermis and/or dermis, left upper back

      L89.123   **Pressure ulcer of left upper back, stage 3**

          Healing pressure ulcer of left upper back, stage 3

          Pressure ulcer with full thickness skin loss involving damage or necrosis of subcutaneous tissue, left upper back

      L89.124   **Pressure ulcer of left upper back, stage 4**

          Healing pressure ulcer of left upper back, stage 4

          Pressure ulcer with necrosis of soft tissues through to underlying muscle, tendon, or bone, left upper back

      L89.129   **Pressure ulcer of left upper back,** <mark>unspecified</mark> **stage**

          Healing pressure ulcer of left upper back NOS

          Healing pressure ulcer of left upper back, unspecified stage

  ● **L89.13**   **Pressure ulcer of right lower back**

      L89.130   **Pressure ulcer of right lower back, unstageable**

      L89.131   **Pressure ulcer of right lower back, stage 1**

          Healing pressure ulcer of right lower back, stage 1

          Pressure pre-ulcer skin changes limited to persistent focal edema, right lower back

      L89.132   **Pressure ulcer of right lower back, stage 2**

          Healing pressure ulcer of right lower back, stage 2

          Pressure ulcer with abrasion, blister, partial thickness skin loss involving epidermis and/or dermis, right lower back

◀ New   ◀▥ Revised   ~~deleted~~ Deleted   Excludes 1   Excludes 2   Includes   Use additional   Code first   Code also   <mark>Unspecified</mark>

OGCR Official Guidelines   X Assign placeholder X   ● Use Additional Character(s)   ▶ Manifestation Code   **Coding Clinic**

L89.133   Pressure ulcer of right lower back, stage 3
    Healing pressure ulcer of right lower back, stage 3
    Pressure ulcer with full thickness skin loss involving damage or necrosis of subcutaneous tissue, right lower back

L89.134   Pressure ulcer of right lower back, stage 4
    Healing pressure ulcer of right lower back, stage 4
    Pressure ulcer with necrosis of soft tissues through to underlying muscle, tendon, or bone, right lower back

L89.139   Pressure ulcer of right lower back, unspecified stage
    Healing pressure ulcer of right lower back NOS
    Healing pressure ulcer of right lower back, unspecified stage

● **L89.14   Pressure ulcer of left lower back**

L89.140   Pressure ulcer of left lower back, unstageable

L89.141   Pressure ulcer of left lower back, stage 1
    Healing pressure ulcer of left lower back, stage 1
    Pressure pre-ulcer skin changes limited to persistent focal edema, left lower back

L89.142   Pressure ulcer of left lower back, stage 2
    Healing pressure ulcer of left lower back, stage 2
    Pressure ulcer with abrasion, blister, partial thickness skin loss involving epidermis and/or dermis, left lower back

L89.143   Pressure ulcer of left lower back, stage 3
    Healing pressure ulcer of left lower back, stage 3
    Pressure ulcer with full thickness skin loss involving damage or necrosis of subcutaneous tissue, left lower back

L89.144   Pressure ulcer of left lower back, stage 4
    Healing pressure ulcer of left lower back, stage 4
    Pressure ulcer with necrosis of soft tissues through to underlying muscle, tendon, or bone, left lower back

L89.149   Pressure ulcer of left lower back, unspecified stage
    Healing pressure ulcer of left lower back NOS
    Healing pressure ulcer of left lower back, unspecified stage

● **L89.15   Pressure ulcer of sacral region**
    Pressure ulcer of coccyx
    Pressure ulcer of tailbone

L89.150   Pressure ulcer of sacral region, unstageable

L89.151   Pressure ulcer of sacral region, stage 1
    Healing pressure ulcer of sacral region, stage 1
    Pressure pre-ulcer skin changes limited to persistent focal edema, sacral region

L89.152   Pressure ulcer of sacral region, stage 2
    Healing pressure ulcer of sacral region, stage 2
    Pressure ulcer with abrasion, blister, partial thickness skin loss involving epidermis and/or dermis, sacral region

L89.153   Pressure ulcer of sacral region, stage 3
    Healing pressure ulcer of sacral region, stage 3
    Pressure ulcer with full thickness skin loss involving damage or necrosis of subcutaneous tissue, sacral region

L89.154   Pressure ulcer of sacral region, stage 4
    Healing pressure ulcer of sacral region, stage 4
    Pressure ulcer with necrosis of soft tissues through to underlying muscle, tendon, or bone, sacral region

L89.159   Pressure ulcer of sacral region, unspecified stage
    Healing pressure ulcer of sacral region NOS
    Healing pressure ulcer of sacral region, unspecified stage

● **L89.2   Pressure ulcer of hip**

● **L89.20   Pressure ulcer of unspecified hip**

L89.200   Pressure ulcer of unspecified hip, unstageable

L89.201   Pressure ulcer of unspecified hip, stage 1
    Healing pressure ulcer of unspecified hip back, stage 1
    Pressure pre-ulcer skin changes limited to persistent focal edema, unspecified hip

L89.202   Pressure ulcer of unspecified hip, stage 2
    Healing pressure ulcer of unspecified hip, stage 2
    Pressure ulcer with abrasion, blister, partial thickness skin loss involving epidermis and/or dermis, unspecified hip

L89.203   Pressure ulcer of unspecified hip, stage 3
    Healing pressure ulcer of unspecified hip, stage 3
    Pressure ulcer with full thickness skin loss involving damage or necrosis of subcutaneous tissue, unspecified hip

L89.204   Pressure ulcer of unspecified hip, stage 4
    Healing pressure ulcer of unspecified hip, stage 4
    Pressure ulcer with necrosis of soft tissues through to underlying muscle, tendon, or bone, unspecified hip

L89.209   Pressure ulcer of unspecified hip, unspecified stage
    Healing pressure ulcer of unspecified hip NOS
    Healing pressure ulcer of unspecified hip, unspecified stage

CHAPTER 12 (L00-L99)

● L89.21   **Pressure ulcer of right hip**

   L89.210   **Pressure ulcer of right hip, unstageable**

   L89.211   **Pressure ulcer of right hip, stage 1**
     Healing pressure ulcer of right hip back, stage 1
     Pressure pre-ulcer skin changes limited to persistent focal edema, right hip

   L89.212   **Pressure ulcer of right hip, stage 2**
     Healing pressure ulcer of right hip, stage 2
     Pressure ulcer with abrasion, blister, partial thickness skin loss involving epidermis and/or dermis, right hip

   L89.213   **Pressure ulcer of right hip, stage 3**
     Healing pressure ulcer of right hip, stage 3
     Pressure ulcer with full thickness skin loss involving damage or necrosis of subcutaneous tissue, right hip

   L89.214   **Pressure ulcer of right hip, stage 4**
     Healing pressure ulcer of right hip, stage 4
     Pressure ulcer with necrosis of soft tissues through to underlying muscle, tendon, or bone, right hip

   L89.219   **Pressure ulcer of right hip, unspecified stage**
     Healing pressure ulcer of right hip NOS
     Healing pressure ulcer of right hip, unspecified stage

● L89.22   **Pressure ulcer of left hip**

   L89.220   **Pressure ulcer of left hip, unstageable**

   L89.221   **Pressure ulcer of left hip, stage 1**
     Healing pressure ulcer of left hip back, stage 1
     Pressure pre-ulcer skin changes limited to persistent focal edema, left hip

   L89.222   **Pressure ulcer of left hip, stage 2**
     Healing pressure ulcer of left hip, stage 2
     Pressure ulcer with abrasion, blister, partial thickness skin loss involving epidermis and/or dermis, left hip

   L89.223   **Pressure ulcer of left hip, stage 3**
     Healing pressure ulcer of left hip, stage 3
     Pressure ulcer with full thickness skin loss involving damage or necrosis of subcutaneous tissue, left hip

   L89.224   **Pressure ulcer of left hip, stage 4**
     Healing pressure ulcer of left hip, stage 4
     Pressure ulcer with necrosis of soft tissues through to underlying muscle, tendon, or bone, left hip

   L89.229   **Pressure ulcer of left hip, unspecified stage**
     Healing pressure ulcer of left hip NOS
     Healing pressure ulcer of left hip, unspecified stage

● L89.3   **Pressure ulcer of buttock**

● L89.30   **Pressure ulcer of unspecified buttock**

   L89.300   **Pressure ulcer of unspecified buttock, unstageable**

   L89.301   **Pressure ulcer of unspecified buttock, stage 1**
     Healing pressure ulcer of unspecified buttock, stage 1
     Pressure pre-ulcer skin changes limited to persistent focal edema, unspecified buttock

   L89.302   **Pressure ulcer of unspecified buttock, stage 2**
     Healing pressure ulcer of unspecified buttock, stage 2
     Pressure ulcer with abrasion, blister, partial thickness skin loss involving epidermis and/or dermis, unspecified buttock

   L89.303   **Pressure ulcer of unspecified buttock, stage 3**
     Healing pressure ulcer of unspecified buttock, stage 3
     Pressure ulcer with full thickness skin loss involving damage or necrosis of subcutaneous tissue, unspecified buttock

   L89.304   **Pressure ulcer of unspecified buttock, stage 4**
     Healing pressure ulcer of unspecified buttock, stage 4
     Pressure ulcer with necrosis of soft tissues through to underlying muscle, tendon, or bone, unspecified buttock

   L89.309   **Pressure ulcer of unspecified buttock, unspecified stage**
     Healing pressure ulcer of unspecified buttock NOS
     Healing pressure ulcer of unspecified buttock, unspecified stage

● L89.31   **Pressure ulcer of right buttock**

   L89.310   **Pressure ulcer of right buttock, unstageable**

   L89.311   **Pressure ulcer of right buttock, stage 1**
     Healing pressure ulcer of right buttock, stage 1
     Pressure pre-ulcer skin changes limited to persistent focal edema, right buttock

   L89.312   **Pressure ulcer of right buttock, stage 2**
     Healing pressure ulcer of right buttock, stage 2
     Pressure ulcer with abrasion, blister, partial thickness skin loss involving epidermis and/or dermis, right buttock

   L89.313   **Pressure ulcer of right buttock, stage 3**
     Healing pressure ulcer of right buttock, stage 3
     Pressure ulcer with full thickness skin loss involving damage or necrosis of subcutaneous tissue, right buttock

   L89.314   **Pressure ulcer of right buttock, stage 4**
     Healing pressure ulcer of right buttock, stage 4
     Pressure ulcer with necrosis of soft tissues through to underlying muscle, tendon, or bone, right buttock

◄ New   ◄ Revised   ~~deleted~~ Deleted   Excludes 1   Excludes 2   Includes   Use additional   Code first   Code also   Unspecified

OGCR Official Guidelines   X Assign placeholder X   ● Use Additional Character(s)   ▶ Manifestation Code   **Coding Clinic**

L89.319   **Pressure ulcer of right buttock, unspecified stage**
Healing pressure ulcer of right buttock NOS
Healing pressure ulcer of right buttock, unspecified stage

● L89.32   **Pressure ulcer of left buttock**

L89.320   **Pressure ulcer of left buttock, unstageable**

L89.321   **Pressure ulcer of left buttock, stage 1**
Healing pressure ulcer of left buttock, stage 1
Pressure pre-ulcer skin changes limited to persistent focal edema, left buttock

L89.322   **Pressure ulcer of left buttock, stage 2**
Healing pressure ulcer of left buttock, stage 2
Pressure ulcer with abrasion, blister, partial thickness skin loss involving epidermis and/or dermis, left buttock

L89.323   **Pressure ulcer of left buttock, stage 3**
Healing pressure ulcer of left buttock, stage 3
Pressure ulcer with full thickness skin loss involving damage or necrosis of subcutaneous tissue, left buttock

L89.324   **Pressure ulcer of left buttock, stage 4**
Healing pressure ulcer of left buttock, stage 4
Pressure ulcer with necrosis of soft tissues through to underlying muscle, tendon, or bone, left buttock

L89.329   **Pressure ulcer of left buttock, unspecified stage**
Healing pressure ulcer of left buttock NOS
Healing pressure ulcer of left buttock, unspecified stage

● L89.4   **Pressure ulcer of contiguous site of back, buttock and hip**

L89.40   **Pressure ulcer of contiguous site of back, buttock and hip, unspecified stage**
Healing pressure ulcer of contiguous site of back, buttock and hip NOS
Healing pressure ulcer of contiguous site of back, buttock and hip, unspecified stage

L89.41   **Pressure ulcer of contiguous site of back, buttock and hip, stage 1**
Healing pressure ulcer of contiguous site of back, buttock and hip, stage 1
Pressure pre-ulcer skin changes limited to persistent focal edema, contiguous site of back, buttock and hip

L89.42   **Pressure ulcer of contiguous site of back, buttock and hip, stage 2**
Healing pressure ulcer of contiguous site of back, buttock and hip, stage 2
Pressure ulcer with abrasion, blister, partial thickness skin loss involving epidermis and/or dermis, contiguous site of back, buttock and hip

L89.43   **Pressure ulcer of contiguous site of back, buttock and hip, stage 3**
Healing pressure ulcer of contiguous site of back, buttock and hip, stage 3
Pressure ulcer with full thickness skin loss involving damage or necrosis of subcutaneous tissue, contiguous site of back, buttock and hip

L89.44   **Pressure ulcer of contiguous site of back, buttock and hip, stage 4**
Healing pressure ulcer of contiguous site of back, buttock and hip, stage 4
Pressure ulcer with necrosis of soft tissues through to underlying muscle, tendon, or bone, contiguous site of back, buttock and hip

L89.45   **Pressure ulcer of contiguous site of back, buttock and hip, unstageable**

● L89.5   **Pressure ulcer of ankle**

● L89.50   **Pressure ulcer of unspecified ankle**

L89.500   **Pressure ulcer of unspecified ankle, unstageable**

L89.501   **Pressure ulcer of unspecified ankle, stage 1**
Healing pressure ulcer of unspecified ankle, stage 1
Pressure pre-ulcer skin changes limited to persistent focal edema, unspecified ankle

L89.502   **Pressure ulcer of unspecified ankle, stage 2**
Healing pressure ulcer of unspecified ankle, stage 2
Pressure ulcer with abrasion, blister, partial thickness skin loss involving epidermis and/or dermis, unspecified ankle

L89.503   **Pressure ulcer of unspecified ankle, stage 3**
Healing pressure ulcer of unspecified ankle, stage 3
Pressure ulcer with full thickness skin loss involving damage or necrosis of subcutaneous tissue, unspecified ankle

L89.504   **Pressure ulcer of unspecified ankle, stage 4**
Healing pressure ulcer of unspecified ankle, stage 4
Pressure ulcer with necrosis of soft tissues through to underlying muscle, tendon, or bone, unspecified ankle

L89.509   **Pressure ulcer of unspecified ankle, unspecified stage**
Healing pressure ulcer of unspecified ankle NOS
Healing pressure ulcer of unspecified ankle, unspecified stage

● L89.51   **Pressure ulcer of right ankle**

L89.510   **Pressure ulcer of right ankle, unstageable**

L89.511   **Pressure ulcer of right ankle, stage 1**
Healing pressure ulcer of right ankle, stage 1
Pressure pre-ulcer skin changes limited to persistent focal edema, right ankle

L89.512   **Pressure ulcer of right ankle, stage 2**
Healing pressure ulcer of right ankle, stage 2
Pressure ulcer with abrasion, blister, partial thickness skin loss involving epidermis and/or dermis, right ankle

CHAPTER 12 (L00-L99)

L89.513   Pressure ulcer of right ankle, stage 3
Healing pressure ulcer of right ankle, stage 3
Pressure ulcer with full thickness skin loss involving damage or necrosis of subcutaneous tissue, right ankle

L89.514   Pressure ulcer of right ankle, stage 4
Healing pressure ulcer of right ankle, stage 4
Pressure ulcer with necrosis of soft tissues through to underlying muscle, tendon, or bone, right ankle

L89.519   Pressure ulcer of right ankle, unspecified stage
Healing pressure ulcer of right ankle NOS
Healing pressure ulcer of right ankle, unspecified stage

● **L89.52   Pressure ulcer of left ankle**

L89.520   Pressure ulcer of left ankle, unstageable

L89.521   Pressure ulcer of left ankle, stage 1
Healing pressure ulcer of left ankle, stage 1
Pressure pre-ulcer skin changes limited to persistent focal edema, left ankle

L89.522   Pressure ulcer of left ankle, stage 2
Healing pressure ulcer of left ankle, stage 2
Pressure ulcer with abrasion, blister, partial thickness skin loss involving epidermis and/or dermis, left ankle

L89.523   Pressure ulcer of left ankle, stage 3
Healing pressure ulcer of left ankle, stage 3
Pressure ulcer with full thickness skin loss involving damage or necrosis of subcutaneous tissue, left ankle

L89.524   Pressure ulcer of left ankle, stage 4
Healing pressure ulcer of left ankle, stage 4
Pressure ulcer with necrosis of soft tissues through to underlying muscle, tendon, or bone, left ankle

L89.529   Pressure ulcer of left ankle, unspecified stage
Healing pressure ulcer of left ankle NOS
Healing pressure ulcer of left ankle, unspecified stage

● **L89.6   Pressure ulcer of heel**

● **L89.60   Pressure ulcer of unspecified heel**

L89.600   Pressure ulcer of unspecified heel, unstageable

L89.601   Pressure ulcer of unspecified heel, stage 1
Healing pressure ulcer of unspecified heel, stage 1
Pressure pre-ulcer skin changes limited to persistent focal edema, unspecified heel

L89.602   Pressure ulcer of unspecified heel, stage 2
Healing pressure ulcer of unspecified heel, stage 2
Pressure ulcer with abrasion, blister, partial thickness skin loss involving epidermis and/or dermis, unspecified heel

L89.603   Pressure ulcer of unspecified heel, stage 3
Healing pressure ulcer of unspecified heel, stage 3
Pressure ulcer with full thickness skin loss involving damage or necrosis of subcutaneous tissue, unspecified heel

L89.604   Pressure ulcer of unspecified heel, stage 4
Healing pressure ulcer of unspecified heel, stage 4
Pressure ulcer with necrosis of soft tissues through to underlying muscle, tendon, or bone, unspecified heel

L89.609   Pressure ulcer of unspecified heel, unspecified stage
Healing pressure ulcer of unspecified heel NOS
Healing pressure ulcer of unspecified heel, unspecified stage

● **L89.61   Pressure ulcer of right heel**

L89.610   Pressure ulcer of right heel, unstageable

L89.611   Pressure ulcer of right heel, stage 1
Healing pressure ulcer of right heel, stage 1
Pressure pre-ulcer skin changes limited to persistent focal edema, right heel

L89.612   Pressure ulcer of right heel, stage 2
Healing pressure ulcer of right heel, stage 2
Pressure ulcer with abrasion, blister, partial thickness skin loss involving epidermis and/or dermis, right heel

L89.613   Pressure ulcer of right heel, stage 3
Healing pressure ulcer of right heel, stage 3
Pressure ulcer with full thickness skin loss involving damage or necrosis of subcutaneous tissue, right heel

L89.614   Pressure ulcer of right heel, stage 4
Healing pressure ulcer of right heel, stage 4
Pressure ulcer with necrosis of soft tissues through to underlying muscle, tendon, or bone, right heel

L89.619   Pressure ulcer of right heel, unspecified stage
Healing pressure ulcer of right heel NOS
Healing pressure ulcer of unspecified heel, right stage

● **L89.62   Pressure ulcer of left heel**

L89.620   Pressure ulcer of left heel, unstageable

L89.621   Pressure ulcer of left heel, stage 1
Healing pressure ulcer of left heel, stage 1
Pressure pre-ulcer skin changes limited to persistent focal edema, left heel

L89.622   Pressure ulcer of left heel, stage 2
Healing pressure ulcer of left heel, stage 2
Pressure ulcer with abrasion, blister, partial thickness skin loss involving epidermis and/or dermis, left heel

◀ New   ◀▥ Revised   ~~deleted~~ Deleted   Excludes 1   Excludes 2   Includes   Use additional   Code first   Code also   Unspecified

OGCR Official Guidelines   X Assign placeholder X   ● Use Additional Character(s)   ▶ Manifestation Code   **Coding Clinic**

L89.623   **Pressure ulcer of left heel, stage 3**
Healing pressure ulcer of left heel, stage 3
Pressure ulcer with full thickness skin loss involving damage or necrosis of subcutaneous tissue, left heel

L89.624   **Pressure ulcer of left heel, stage 4**
Healing pressure ulcer of left heel, stage 4
Pressure ulcer with necrosis of soft tissues through to underlying muscle, tendon, or bone, left heel

L89.629   **Pressure ulcer of left heel, unspecified stage**
Healing pressure ulcer of left heel NOS
Healing pressure ulcer of left heel, unspecified stage

● **L89.8**   **Pressure ulcer of other site**

   ● **L89.81**   **Pressure ulcer of head**
Pressure ulcer of face

     L89.810   **Pressure ulcer of head, unstageable**

     L89.811   **Pressure ulcer of head, stage 1**
Healing pressure ulcer of head, stage 1
Pressure pre-ulcer skin changes limited to persistent focal edema, head

     L89.812   **Pressure ulcer of head, stage 2**
Healing pressure ulcer of head, stage 2
Pressure ulcer with abrasion, blister, partial thickness skin loss involving epidermis and/or dermis, head

     L89.813   **Pressure ulcer of head, stage 3**
Healing pressure ulcer of head, stage 3
Pressure ulcer with full thickness skin loss involving damage or necrosis of subcutaneous tissue, head

     L89.814   **Pressure ulcer of head, stage 4**
Healing pressure ulcer of head, stage 4
Pressure ulcer with necrosis of soft tissues through to underlying muscle, tendon, or bone, head

     L89.819   **Pressure ulcer of head, unspecified stage**
Healing pressure ulcer of head NOS
Healing pressure ulcer of head, unspecified stage

   ● **L89.89**   **Pressure ulcer of other site**

     L89.890   **Pressure ulcer of other site, unstageable**

     L89.891   **Pressure ulcer of other site, stage 1**
Healing pressure ulcer of other site, stage 1
Pressure pre-ulcer skin changes limited to persistent focal edema, other site

     L89.892   **Pressure ulcer of other site, stage 2**
Healing pressure ulcer of other site, stage 2
Pressure ulcer with abrasion, blister, partial thickness skin loss involving epidermis and/or dermis, other site

L89.893   **Pressure ulcer of other site, stage 3**
Healing pressure ulcer of other site, stage 3
Pressure ulcer with full thickness skin loss involving damage or necrosis of subcutaneous tissue, other site

L89.894   **Pressure ulcer of other site, stage 4**
Healing pressure ulcer of other site, stage 4
Pressure ulcer with necrosis of soft tissues through to underlying muscle, tendon, or bone, other site

L89.899   **Pressure ulcer of other site, unspecified stage**
Healing pressure ulcer of other site NOS
Healing pressure ulcer of other site, unspecified stage

● **L89.9**   **Pressure ulcer of unspecified site**

   L89.90   **Pressure ulcer of unspecified site, unspecified stage**
Healing pressure ulcer of unspecified site NOS
Healing pressure ulcer of unspecified site, unspecified stage

   L89.91   **Pressure ulcer of unspecified site, stage 1**
Healing pressure ulcer of unspecified site, stage 1
Pressure pre-ulcer skin changes limited to persistent focal edema, unspecified site

   L89.92   **Pressure ulcer of unspecified site, stage 2**
Healing pressure ulcer of unspecified site, stage 2
Pressure ulcer with abrasion, blister, partial thickness skin loss involving epidermis and/or dermis, unspecified site

   L89.93   **Pressure ulcer of unspecified site, stage 3**
Healing pressure ulcer of unspecified site, stage 3
Pressure ulcer with full thickness skin loss involving damage or necrosis of subcutaneous tissue, unspecified site

   L89.94   **Pressure ulcer of unspecified site, stage 4**
Healing pressure ulcer of unspecified site, stage 4
Pressure ulcer with necrosis of soft tissues through to underlying muscle, tendon, or bone, unspecified site

   L89.95   **Pressure ulcer of unspecified site, unstageable**

● **L90**   **Atrophic disorders of skin**

   L90.0   **Lichen sclerosus et atrophicus**
> **Excludes2**   lichen sclerosus of external female genital organs (N90.4)
> lichen sclerosus of external male genital organs (N48.0)

   L90.1   **Anetoderma of Schweninger-Buzzi**

   L90.2   **Anetoderma of Jadassohn-Pellizzari**

   L90.3   **Atrophoderma of Pasini and Pierini**

   L90.4   **Acrodermatitis chronica atrophicans**

   L90.5   **Scar conditions and fibrosis of skin**
Adherent scar (skin)
Cicatrix
Disfigurement of skin due to scar
Fibrosis of skin NOS
Scar NOS
> **Excludes2**   hypertrophic scar (L91.0)
> keloid scar (L91.0)
Coding Clinic: 2015, Q1, P19

   L90.6   **Striae atrophicae**

   L90.8   **Other atrophic disorders of skin**

   L90.9   **Atrophic disorder of skin, unspecified**

CHAPTER 12 (L00-L99)

● **L91 Hypertrophic disorders of skin**

     L91.0 Keloid scar
         Hypertrophic scar
         Keloid
         Excludes2   acne keloid (L73.0)
                       scar NOS (L90.5)

     L91.8 Other hypertrophic disorders of the skin

     L91.9 Hypertrophic disorder of the skin, unspecified

● **L92 Granulomatous disorders of skin and subcutaneous tissue**

     Excludes2   actinic granuloma (L57.5)

     L92.0 Granuloma annulare
         Perforating granuloma annulare

     L92.1 Necrobiosis lipoidica, not elsewhere classified
         Excludes1   necrobiosis lipoidica associated with
                       diabetes mellitus (E08-E13 with .620)

     L92.2 Granuloma faciale [eosinophilic granuloma of skin]

     L92.3 Foreign body granuloma of the skin and subcutaneous tissue
         Use additional code to identify the type of retained foreign body (Z18.-)

     L92.8 Other granulomatous disorders of the skin and subcutaneous tissue

     L92.9 Granulomatous disorder of the skin and subcutaneous tissue, unspecified

● **L93 Lupus erythematosus**

     Use additional code for adverse effect, if applicable, to identify drug (T36-T50 with fifth or sixth character 5)
     Excludes1   lupus exedens (A18.4)
                   lupus vulgaris (A18.4)
                   scleroderma (M34.-)
                   systemic lupus erythematosus (M32.-)

     L93.0 Discoid lupus erythematosus
         Lupus erythematosus NOS

     L93.1 Subacute cutaneous lupus erythematosus

     L93.2 Other local lupus erythematosus
         Lupus erythematosus profundus
         Lupus panniculitis

● **L94 Other localized connective tissue disorders**

     Excludes1   systemic connective tissue disorders (M30-M36)

     L94.0 Localized scleroderma [morphea]
         Circumscribed scleroderma

     L94.1 Linear scleroderma
         En coup de sabre lesion

     L94.2 Calcinosis cutis

     L94.3 Sclerodactyly

     L94.4 Gottron's papules

     L94.5 Poikiloderma vasculare atrophicans

     L94.6 Ainhum

     L94.8 Other specified localized connective tissue disorders

     L94.9 Localized connective tissue disorder, unspecified

● **L95 Vasculitis limited to skin, not elsewhere classified**

     Excludes1   angioma serpiginosum (L81.7)
                   Henoch(-Schönlein) purpura (D69.0)
                   hypersensitivity angiitis (M31.0)
                   lupus panniculitis (L93.2)
                   panniculitis NOS (M79.3)
                   panniculitis of neck and back (M54.0-)
                   polyarteritis nodosa (M30.0)
                   relapsing panniculitis (M35.6)
                   rheumatoid vasculitis (M05.2)
                   serum sickness (T80.6-)
                   urticaria (L50.-)
                   Wegener's granulomatosis (M31.3-)

     L95.0 Livedoid vasculitis
         Atrophie blanche (en plaque)

     L95.1 Erythema elevatum diutinum

     L95.8 Other vasculitis limited to the skin

     L95.9 Vasculitis limited to the skin, unspecified

● **L97 Non-pressure chronic ulcer of lower limb, not elsewhere classified**

     Includes   chronic ulcer of skin of lower limb NOS
                 non-healing ulcer of skin
                 non-infected sinus of skin
                 trophic ulcer NOS
                 tropical ulcer NOS
                 ulcer of skin of lower limb NOS

     Code first any associated underlying condition, such as:
     any associated gangrene (I96)
     atherosclerosis of the lower extremities (I70.23-, I70.24-, I70.33-, I70.34-, I70.43-, I70.44-, I70.53-, I70.54-, I70.63-, I70.64-, I70.73-, I70.74-)
     chronic venous hypertension (I87.31-, I87.33-)
     diabetic ulcers (E08.621, E08.622, E09.621, E09.622, E10.621, E10.622, E11.621, E11.622, E13.621, E13.622)
     postphlebitic syndrome (I87.01-, I87.03-)
     postthrombotic syndrome (I87.01-, I87.03-)
     varicose ulcer (I83.0-, I83.2-)

     Excludes2   pressure ulcer (pressure area) (L89.-)
                   skin infections (L00-L08)
                   specific infections classified to A00-B99

● **L97.1 Non-pressure chronic ulcer of thigh**

     ● **L97.10 Non-pressure chronic ulcer of unspecified thigh**

         L97.101 Non-pressure chronic ulcer of unspecified thigh limited to breakdown of skin

         L97.102 Non-pressure chronic ulcer of unspecified thigh with fat layer exposed

         L97.103 Non-pressure chronic ulcer of unspecified thigh with necrosis of muscle

         L97.104 Non-pressure chronic ulcer of unspecified thigh with necrosis of bone

         L97.109 Non-pressure chronic ulcer of unspecified thigh with unspecified severity

     ● **L97.11 Non-pressure chronic ulcer of right thigh**

         L97.111 Non-pressure chronic ulcer of right thigh limited to breakdown of skin

         L97.112 Non-pressure chronic ulcer of right thigh with fat layer exposed

         L97.113 Non-pressure chronic ulcer of right thigh with necrosis of muscle

         L97.114 Non-pressure chronic ulcer of right thigh with necrosis of bone

         L97.119 Non-pressure chronic ulcer of right thigh with unspecified severity

---

Item 12-11 Scleroderma means hard skin. It is a group of diseases that causes abnormal growth of connective tissues that support the skin and organs. There are two types: localized scleroderma affecting the skin and systemic scleroderma affecting blood vessels and internal organs and the skin.

◄ New   ◄ Revised   ~~deleted~~ Deleted   Excludes 1   Excludes 2   Includes   Use additional   Code first   Code also   Unspecified

OGCR Official Guidelines   X Assign placeholder X   ● Use Additional Character(s)   ▸ Manifestation Code   **Coding Clinic**

● L97.12   Non-pressure chronic ulcer of left thigh

     L97.121   Non-pressure chronic ulcer of left thigh limited to breakdown of skin

     L97.122   Non-pressure chronic ulcer of left thigh with fat layer exposed

     L97.123   Non-pressure chronic ulcer of left thigh with necrosis of muscle

     L97.124   Non-pressure chronic ulcer of left thigh with necrosis of bone

     L97.129   Non-pressure chronic ulcer of left thigh with unspecified severity

● L97.2   Non-pressure chronic ulcer of calf

  ● L97.20   Non-pressure chronic ulcer of unspecified calf

     L97.201   Non-pressure chronic ulcer of unspecified calf limited to breakdown of skin

     L97.202   Non-pressure chronic ulcer of unspecified calf with fat layer exposed

     L97.203   Non-pressure chronic ulcer of unspecified calf with necrosis of muscle

     L97.204   Non-pressure chronic ulcer of unspecified calf with necrosis of bone

     L97.209   Non-pressure chronic ulcer of unspecified calf with unspecified severity

  ● L97.21   Non-pressure chronic ulcer of right calf

     L97.211   Non-pressure chronic ulcer of right calf limited to breakdown of skin

     L97.212   Non-pressure chronic ulcer of right calf with fat layer exposed

     L97.213   Non-pressure chronic ulcer of right calf with necrosis of muscle

     L97.214   Non-pressure chronic ulcer of right calf with necrosis of bone

     L97.219   Non-pressure chronic ulcer of right calf with unspecified severity

  ● L97.22   Non-pressure chronic ulcer of left calf

     L97.221   Non-pressure chronic ulcer of left calf limited to breakdown of skin

     L97.222   Non-pressure chronic ulcer of left calf with fat layer exposed

     L97.223   Non-pressure chronic ulcer of left calf with necrosis of muscle

     L97.224   Non-pressure chronic ulcer of left calf with necrosis of bone

     L97.229   Non-pressure chronic ulcer of left calf with unspecified severity

● L97.3   Non-pressure chronic ulcer of ankle

  ● L97.30   Non-pressure chronic ulcer of unspecified ankle

     L97.301   Non-pressure chronic ulcer of unspecified ankle limited to breakdown of skin

     L97.302   Non-pressure chronic ulcer of unspecified ankle with fat layer exposed

     L97.303   Non-pressure chronic ulcer of unspecified ankle with necrosis of muscle

     L97.304   Non-pressure chronic ulcer of unspecified ankle with necrosis of bone

     L97.309   Non-pressure chronic ulcer of unspecified ankle with unspecified severity

● L97.31   Non-pressure chronic ulcer of right ankle

     L97.311   Non-pressure chronic ulcer of right ankle limited to breakdown of skin

     L97.312   Non-pressure chronic ulcer of right ankle with fat layer exposed

     L97.313   Non-pressure chronic ulcer of right ankle with necrosis of muscle

     L97.314   Non-pressure chronic ulcer of right ankle with necrosis of bone

     L97.319   Non-pressure chronic ulcer of right ankle with unspecified severity

● L97.32   Non-pressure chronic ulcer of left ankle

     L97.321   Non-pressure chronic ulcer of left ankle limited to breakdown of skin

     L97.322   Non-pressure chronic ulcer of left ankle with fat layer exposed

     L97.323   Non-pressure chronic ulcer of left ankle with necrosis of muscle

     L97.324   Non-pressure chronic ulcer of left ankle with necrosis of bone

     L97.329   Non-pressure chronic ulcer of left ankle with unspecified severity

● L97.4   Non-pressure chronic ulcer of heel and midfoot

     Non-pressure chronic ulcer of plantar surface of midfoot

  ● L97.40   Non-pressure chronic ulcer of unspecified heel and midfoot

     L97.401   Non-pressure chronic ulcer of unspecified heel and midfoot limited to breakdown of skin

     L97.402   Non-pressure chronic ulcer of unspecified heel and midfoot with fat layer exposed

     L97.403   Non-pressure chronic ulcer of unspecified heel and midfoot with necrosis of muscle

     L97.404   Non-pressure chronic ulcer of unspecified heel and midfoot with necrosis of bone

     L97.409   Non-pressure chronic ulcer of unspecified heel and midfoot with unspecified severity

  ● L97.41   Non-pressure chronic ulcer of right heel and midfoot

     L97.411   Non-pressure chronic ulcer of right heel and midfoot limited to breakdown of skin

     L97.412   Non-pressure chronic ulcer of right heel and midfoot with fat layer exposed

     L97.413   Non-pressure chronic ulcer of right heel and midfoot with necrosis of muscle

     L97.414   Non-pressure chronic ulcer of right heel and midfoot with necrosis of bone

     L97.419   Non-pressure chronic ulcer of right heel and midfoot with unspecified severity

● **L97.42**   Non-pressure chronic ulcer of left heel and midfoot

     L97.421   Non-pressure chronic ulcer of left heel and midfoot limited to breakdown of skin

     L97.422   Non-pressure chronic ulcer of left heel and midfoot with fat layer exposed

     L97.423   Non-pressure chronic ulcer of left heel and midfoot with necrosis of muscle

     L97.424   Non-pressure chronic ulcer of left heel and midfoot with necrosis of bone

     L97.429   Non-pressure chronic ulcer of left heel and midfoot with unspecified severity

● **L97.5**   Non-pressure chronic ulcer of other part of foot
     Non-pressure chronic ulcer of toe

   ● **L97.50**   Non-pressure chronic ulcer of other part of unspecified foot

     L97.501   Non-pressure chronic ulcer of other part of unspecified foot limited to breakdown of skin

     L97.502   Non-pressure chronic ulcer of other part of unspecified foot with fat layer exposed

     L97.503   Non-pressure chronic ulcer of other part of unspecified foot with necrosis of muscle

     L97.504   Non-pressure chronic ulcer of other part of unspecified foot with necrosis of bone

     L97.509   Non-pressure chronic ulcer of other part of unspecified foot with unspecified severity

   ● **L97.51**   Non-pressure chronic ulcer of other part of right foot

     L97.511   Non-pressure chronic ulcer of other part of right foot limited to breakdown of skin

     L97.512   Non-pressure chronic ulcer of other part of right foot with fat layer exposed

     L97.513   Non-pressure chronic ulcer of other part of right foot with necrosis of muscle

     L97.514   Non-pressure chronic ulcer of other part of right foot with necrosis of bone

     L97.519   Non-pressure chronic ulcer of other part of right foot with unspecified severity

   ● **L97.52**   Non-pressure chronic ulcer of other part of left foot

     L97.521   Non-pressure chronic ulcer of other part of left foot limited to breakdown of skin

     L97.522   Non-pressure chronic ulcer of other part of left foot with fat layer exposed

     L97.523   Non-pressure chronic ulcer of other part of left foot with necrosis of muscle

     L97.524   Non-pressure chronic ulcer of other part of left foot with necrosis of bone

     L97.529   Non-pressure chronic ulcer of other part of left foot with unspecified severity

● **L97.8**   Non-pressure chronic ulcer of other part of lower leg

   ● **L97.80**   Non-pressure chronic ulcer of other part of unspecified lower leg

     L97.801   Non-pressure chronic ulcer of other part of unspecified lower leg limited to breakdown of skin

     L97.802   Non-pressure chronic ulcer of other part of unspecified lower leg with fat layer exposed

     L97.803   Non-pressure chronic ulcer of other part of unspecified lower leg with necrosis of muscle

     L97.804   Non-pressure chronic ulcer of other part of unspecified lower leg with necrosis of bone

     L97.809   Non-pressure chronic ulcer of other part of unspecified lower leg with unspecified severity

   ● **L97.81**   Non-pressure chronic ulcer of other part of right lower leg

     L97.811   Non-pressure chronic ulcer of other part of right lower leg limited to breakdown of skin

     L97.812   Non-pressure chronic ulcer of other part of right lower leg with fat layer exposed

     L97.813   Non-pressure chronic ulcer of other part of right lower leg with necrosis of muscle

     L97.814   Non-pressure chronic ulcer of other part of right lower leg with necrosis of bone

     L97.819   Non-pressure chronic ulcer of other part of right lower leg with unspecified severity

   ● **L97.82**   Non-pressure chronic ulcer of other part of left lower leg

     L97.821   Non-pressure chronic ulcer of other part of left lower leg limited to breakdown of skin

     L97.822   Non-pressure chronic ulcer of other part of left lower leg with fat layer exposed

     L97.823   Non-pressure chronic ulcer of other part of left lower leg with necrosis of muscle

     L97.824   Non-pressure chronic ulcer of other part of left lower leg with necrosis of bone

     L97.829   Non-pressure chronic ulcer of other part of left lower leg with unspecified severity

● **L97.9**   Non-pressure chronic ulcer of unspecified part of lower leg

   ● **L97.90**   Non-pressure chronic ulcer of unspecified part of unspecified lower leg

     L97.901   Non-pressure chronic ulcer of unspecified part of unspecified lower leg limited to breakdown of skin

     L97.902   Non-pressure chronic ulcer of unspecified part of unspecified lower leg with fat layer exposed

     L97.903   Non-pressure chronic ulcer of unspecified part of unspecified lower leg with necrosis of muscle

     L97.904   Non-pressure chronic ulcer of unspecified part of unspecified lower leg with necrosis of bone

     L97.909   Non-pressure chronic ulcer of unspecified part of unspecified lower leg with unspecified severity

◀ New   ◀▦ Revised   ~~deleted~~ Deleted   Excludes 1   Excludes 2   Includes   Use additional   Code first   Code also   Unspecified

OGCR Official Guidelines   **X** Assign placeholder X   ● Use Additional Character(s)   ▸ Manifestation Code   **Coding Clinic**

● **L97.91**   **Non-pressure chronic ulcer of unspecified part of right lower leg**

    L97.911   Non-pressure chronic ulcer of unspecified part of right lower leg limited to breakdown of skin

    L97.912   Non-pressure chronic ulcer of unspecified part of right lower leg with fat layer exposed

    L97.913   Non-pressure chronic ulcer of unspecified part of right lower leg with necrosis of muscle

    L97.914   Non-pressure chronic ulcer of unspecified part of right lower leg with necrosis of bone

    L97.919   Non-pressure chronic ulcer of unspecified part of right lower leg with unspecified severity

● **L97.92**   **Non-pressure chronic ulcer of unspecified part of left lower leg**

    L97.921   Non-pressure chronic ulcer of unspecified part of left lower leg limited to breakdown of skin

    L97.922   Non-pressure chronic ulcer of unspecified part of left lower leg with fat layer exposed

    L97.923   Non-pressure chronic ulcer of unspecified part of left lower leg with necrosis of muscle

    L97.924   Non-pressure chronic ulcer of unspecified part of left lower leg with necrosis of bone

    L97.929   Non-pressure chronic ulcer of unspecified part of left lower leg with unspecified severity

● **L98**   **Other disorders of skin and subcutaneous tissue, not elsewhere classified**

L98.0   **Pyogenic granuloma**

    Excludes2   pyogenic granuloma of gingiva (K06.8)
         pyogenic granuloma of maxillary alveolar ridge (K04.5)
         pyogenic granuloma of oral mucosa (K13.4)

L98.1   **Factitial dermatitis**
    Neurotic excoriation

L98.2   **Febrile neutrophilic dermatosis [Sweet]**

L98.3   **Eosinophilic cellulitis [Wells]**

● **L98.4**   **Non-pressure chronic ulcer of skin, not elsewhere classified**
    Chronic ulcer of skin NOS
    Tropical ulcer NOS
    Ulcer of skin NOS

    Excludes2   pressure ulcer (pressure area) (L89.-)
         gangrene (I96)
         skin infections (L00-L08)
         specific infections classified to A00-B99
         ulcer of lower limb NEC (L97.-)
         varicose ulcer (I83.0-I82.2)

● **L98.41**   **Non-pressure chronic ulcer of buttock**

    L98.411   Non-pressure chronic ulcer of buttock limited to breakdown of skin

    L98.412   Non-pressure chronic ulcer of buttock with fat layer exposed

    L98.413   Non-pressure chronic ulcer of buttock with necrosis of muscle

    L98.414   Non-pressure chronic ulcer of buttock with necrosis of bone

    L98.419   Non-pressure chronic ulcer of buttock with unspecified severity

● **L98.42**   **Non-pressure chronic ulcer of back**

    L98.421   Non-pressure chronic ulcer of back limited to breakdown of skin

    L98.422   Non-pressure chronic ulcer of back with fat layer exposed

    L98.423   Non-pressure chronic ulcer of back with necrosis of muscle

    L98.424   Non-pressure chronic ulcer of back with necrosis of bone

    L98.429   Non-pressure chronic ulcer of back with unspecified severity

● **L98.49**   **Non-pressure chronic ulcer of skin of other sites**
    Non-pressure chronic ulcer of skin NOS

    L98.491   Non-pressure chronic ulcer of skin of other sites limited to breakdown of skin

    L98.492   Non-pressure chronic ulcer of skin of other sites with fat layer exposed

    L98.493   Non-pressure chronic ulcer of skin of other sites with necrosis of muscle

    L98.494   Non-pressure chronic ulcer of skin of other sites with necrosis of bone

    L98.499   Non-pressure chronic ulcer of skin of other sites with unspecified severity

L98.5   **Mucinosis of the skin**
    Focal mucinosis
    Lichen myxedematosus
    Reticular erythematous mucinosis

    Excludes1   focal oral mucinosis (K13.79)
         myxedema (E03.9)

L98.6   **Other infiltrative disorders of the skin and subcutaneous tissue**

    Excludes1   hyalinosis cutis et mucosae (E78.89)

L98.8   **Other specified disorders of the skin and subcutaneous tissue**
    Coding Clinic: 2013, Q2, P32

L98.9   **Disorder of the skin and subcutaneous tissue, unspecified**

▶ *L99*   ***Other disorders of skin and subcutaneous tissue in diseases classified elsewhere***

    Code first underlying disease, such as:
    amyloidosis (E85.-)

    Excludes1   skin disorders in diabetes (E08-E13 with .62)
         skin disorders in gonorrhea (A54.89)
         skin disorders in syphilis (A51.31, A52.79)

CHAPTER 12 (L00-L99)

OGCR   Section I.C.a.-c.

a. Site and laterality

Most of the codes within Chapter 13 have site and laterality designations. The site represents the bone, joint or the muscle involved. For some conditions where more than one bone, joint or muscle is usually involved, such as osteoarthritis, there is a "multiple sites" code available. For categories where no multiple site code is provided and more than one bone, joint or muscle is involved, multiple codes should be used to indicate the different sites involved.

1) Bone versus joint

For certain conditions, the bone may be affected at the upper or lower end, (e.g., avascular necrosis of bone, M87, Osteoporosis, M80, M81). Though the portion of the bone affected may be at the joint, the site designation will be the bone, not the joint.

b. Acute traumatic versus chronic or recurrent musculoskeletal conditions

Many musculoskeletal conditions are a result of previous injury or trauma to a site, or are recurrent conditions. Bone, joint or muscle conditions that are the result of a healed injury are usually found in chapter 13. Recurrent bone, joint or muscle conditions are also usually found in chapter 13. Any current, acute injury should be coded to the appropriate injury code from chapter 19. Chronic or recurrent conditions should generally be coded with a code from chapter 13. If it is difficult to determine from the documentation in the record which code is best to describe a condition, query the provider.

c. Coding of Pathologic Fractures

7th character A is for use as long as the patient is receiving active treatment for the fracture. Examples of active treatment are: surgical treatment, emergency department encounter, evaluation and continuing treatment by the same or a different physician. While the patient may be seen by a new or different provider over the course of treatment for a pathological fracture, assignment of the 7th character is based on whether the patient is undergoing active treatment and not whether the provider is seeing the patient for the first time.

7th character, D is to be used for encounters after the patient has completed active treatment. The other 7th characters, listed under each subcategory in the Tabular List, are to be used for subsequent encounters for treatment of problems associated with the healing, such as malunions and nonunions, and sequelae. Care for complications of surgical treatment for fracture repairs during the healing or recovery phase should be coded with the appropriate complication codes.

See Section I.C.19. Coding of traumatic fractures.

CHAPTER 13

DISEASES OF THE MUSCULOSKELETAL SYSTEM AND CONNECTIVE TISSUE (M00-M99)

> **Note:** Use an external cause code following the code for the musculoskeletal condition, if applicable, to identify the cause of the musculoskeletal condition
>
> **Excludes2**   arthropathic psoriasis (L40.5-)
> certain conditions originating in the perinatal period (P04-P96)
> certain infectious and parasitic diseases (A00-B99)
> compartment syndrome (traumatic) (T79.A-)
> complications of pregnancy, childbirth and the puerperium (O00-O9A)
> congenital malformations, deformations, and chromosomal abnormalities (Q00-Q99)
> endocrine, nutritional and metabolic diseases (E00-E88)
> injury, poisoning and certain other consequences of external causes (S00-T88)
> neoplasms (C00-D49)
> symptoms, signs and abnormal clinical and laboratory findings, not elsewhere classified (R00-R94)

This chapter contains the following blocks:

M00-M02	Infectious arthropathies
M05-M14	Inflammatory polyarthropathies
M15-M19	Osteoarthritis
M20-M25	Other joint disorders
M26-M27	Dentofacial anomalies [including malocclusion] and other disorders of jaw
M30-M36	Systemic connective tissue disorders
M40-M43	Deforming dorsopathies
M45-M49	Spondylopathies
M50-M54	Other dorsopathies
M60-M63	Disorders of muscles
M65-M67	Disorders of synovium and tendon
M70-M79	Other soft tissue disorders
M80-M85	Disorders of bone density and structure
M86-M90	Other osteopathies
M91-M94	Chondropathies
M95	Other disorders of the musculoskeletal system and connective tissue
M96	Intraoperative and postprocedural complications and disorders of musculoskeletal system, not elsewhere classified
M99	Biomechanical lesions, not elsewhere classified

ARTHROPATHIES (M00-M25)

> **Includes**   Disorders affecting predominantly peripheral (limb) joints

INFECTIOUS ARTHROPATHIES (M00-M02)

> **Note:** This block comprises arthropathies due to microbiological agents.
>
> Distinction is made between the following types of etiological relationship:
>
> a) direct infection of joint, where organisms invade synovial tissue and microbial antigen is present in the joint;
>
> b) indirect infection, which may be of two types: a reactive arthropathy, where microbial infection of the body is established but neither organisms nor antigens can be identified in the joint, and a postinfective arthropathy, where microbial antigen is present but recovery of an organism is inconstant and evidence of local multiplication is lacking.

● **M00   Pyogenic arthritis**

  ● **M00.0   Staphylococcal arthritis and polyarthritis**

      Use additional code (B95.61-B95.8) to identify bacterial agent

      Excludes2   infection and inflammatory reaction due to internal joint prosthesis (T84.5-)

     M00.00   Staphylococcal arthritis, **unspecified** joint

   ● M00.01   Staphylococcal arthritis, shoulder

       M00.011   Staphylococcal arthritis, right shoulder

       M00.012   Staphylococcal arthritis, left shoulder

       M00.019   Staphylococcal arthritis, **unspecified** shoulder

   ● M00.02   Staphylococcal arthritis, elbow

       M00.021   Staphylococcal arthritis, right elbow

       M00.022   Staphylococcal arthritis, left elbow

       M00.029   Staphylococcal arthritis, **unspecified** elbow

   ● M00.03   Staphylococcal arthritis, wrist
      Staphylococcal arthritis of carpal bones

       M00.031   Staphylococcal arthritis, right wrist

       M00.032   Staphylococcal arthritis, left wrist

       M00.039   Staphylococcal arthritis, **unspecified** wrist

● **M00.04** **Staphylococcal arthritis, hand**
     Staphylococcal arthritis of metacarpus and phalanges
     M00.041   Staphylococcal arthritis, right hand
     M00.042   Staphylococcal arthritis, left hand
     M00.049   Staphylococcal arthritis, unspecified hand

● **M00.05** **Staphylococcal arthritis, hip**
     M00.051   Staphylococcal arthritis, right hip
     M00.052   Staphylococcal arthritis, left hip
     M00.059   Staphylococcal arthritis, unspecified hip

● **M00.06** **Staphylococcal arthritis, knee**
     M00.061   Staphylococcal arthritis, right knee
     M00.062   Staphylococcal arthritis, left knee
     M00.069   Staphylococcal arthritis, unspecified knee

● **M00.07** **Staphylococcal arthritis, ankle and foot**
     Staphylococcal arthritis, tarsus, metatarsus and phalanges
     M00.071   Staphylococcal arthritis, right ankle and foot
     M00.072   Staphylococcal arthritis, left ankle and foot
     M00.079   Staphylococcal arthritis, unspecified ankle and foot

     M00.08 **Staphylococcal arthritis, vertebrae**
     M00.09 **Staphylococcal polyarthritis**

● **M00.1** **Pneumococcal arthritis and polyarthritis**
     M00.10 **Pneumococcal arthritis, unspecified joint**

● **M00.11** **Pneumococcal arthritis, shoulder**
     M00.111   Pneumococcal arthritis, right shoulder
     M00.112   Pneumococcal arthritis, left shoulder
     M00.119   Pneumococcal arthritis, unspecified shoulder

● **M00.12** **Pneumococcal arthritis, elbow**
     M00.121   Pneumococcal arthritis, right elbow
     M00.122   Pneumococcal arthritis, left elbow
     M00.129   Pneumococcal arthritis, unspecified elbow

● **M00.13** **Pneumococcal arthritis, wrist**
     Pneumococcal arthritis of carpal bones
     M00.131   Pneumococcal arthritis, right wrist
     M00.132   Pneumococcal arthritis, left wrist
     M00.139   Pneumococcal arthritis, unspecified wrist

● **M00.14** **Pneumococcal arthritis, hand**
     Pneumococcal arthritis of metacarpus and phalanges
     M00.141   Pneumococcal arthritis, right hand
     M00.142   Pneumococcal arthritis, left hand
     M00.149   Pneumococcal arthritis, unspecified hand

● **M00.15** **Pneumococcal arthritis, hip**
     M00.151   Pneumococcal arthritis, right hip
     M00.152   Pneumococcal arthritis, left hip
     M00.159   Pneumococcal arthritis, unspecified hip

● **M00.16** **Pneumococcal arthritis, knee**
     M00.161   Pneumococcal arthritis, right knee
     M00.162   Pneumococcal arthritis, left knee
     M00.169   Pneumococcal arthritis, unspecified knee

● **M00.17** **Pneumococcal arthritis, ankle and foot**
     Pneumococcal arthritis, tarsus, metatarsus and phalanges
     M00.171   Pneumococcal arthritis, right ankle and foot
     M00.172   Pneumococcal arthritis, left ankle and foot
     M00.179   Pneumococcal arthritis, unspecified ankle and foot

     M00.18 **Pneumococcal arthritis, vertebrae**
     M00.19 **Pneumococcal polyarthritis**

● **M00.2** **Other streptococcal arthritis and polyarthritis**
     Use additional code (B95.0-B95.2, B95.4-B95.5) to identify bacterial agent
     M00.20 **Other streptococcal arthritis, unspecified joint**

● **M00.21** **Other streptococcal arthritis, shoulder**
     M00.211   Other streptococcal arthritis, right shoulder
     M00.212   Other streptococcal arthritis, left shoulder
     M00.219   Other streptococcal arthritis, unspecified shoulder

● **M00.22** **Other streptococcal arthritis, elbow**
     M00.221   Other streptococcal arthritis, right elbow
     M00.222   Other streptococcal arthritis, left elbow
     M00.229   Other streptococcal arthritis, unspecified elbow

● **M00.23** **Other streptococcal arthritis, wrist**
     Other streptococcal arthritis of carpal bones
     M00.231   Other streptococcal arthritis, right wrist
     M00.232   Other streptococcal arthritis, left wrist
     M00.239   Other streptococcal arthritis, unspecified wrist

● **M00.24** **Other streptococcal arthritis, hand**
     Other streptococcal arthritis metacarpus and phalanges
     M00.241   Other streptococcal arthritis, right hand
     M00.242   Other streptococcal arthritis, left hand
     M00.249   Other streptococcal arthritis, unspecified hand

● **M00.25** **Other streptococcal arthritis, hip**
     M00.251   Other streptococcal arthritis, right hip
     M00.252   Other streptococcal arthritis, left hip
     M00.259   Other streptococcal arthritis, unspecified hip

● **M00.26** **Other streptococcal arthritis, knee**
     M00.261   Other streptococcal arthritis, right knee
     M00.262   Other streptococcal arthritis, left knee
     M00.269   Other streptococcal arthritis, unspecified knee

● **M00.27** **Other streptococcal arthritis, ankle and foot**
     Other streptococcal arthritis, tarsus, metatarsus and phalanges
     M00.271   Other streptococcal arthritis, right ankle and foot
     M00.272   Other streptococcal arthritis, left ankle and foot
     M00.279   Other streptococcal arthritis, unspecified ankle and foot

     M00.28 **Other streptococcal arthritis, vertebrae**
     M00.29 **Other streptococcal polyarthritis**

CHAPTER 13 (M00-M99)

CHAPTER 13 (M00-M99)

● **M00.8   Arthritis and polyarthritis due to other bacteria**
     Use additional code (B96) to identify bacteria

     M00.80   Arthritis due to other bacteria, unspecified joint

●   **M00.81   Arthritis due to other bacteria, shoulder**

       M00.811   Arthritis due to other bacteria, right shoulder

       M00.812   Arthritis due to other bacteria, left shoulder

       M00.819   Arthritis due to other bacteria, unspecified shoulder

●   **M00.82   Arthritis due to other bacteria, elbow**

       M00.821   Arthritis due to other bacteria, right elbow

       M00.822   Arthritis due to other bacteria, left elbow

       M00.829   Arthritis due to other bacteria, unspecified elbow

●   **M00.83   Arthritis due to other bacteria, wrist**
       Arthritis due to other bacteria, carpal bones

       M00.831   Arthritis due to other bacteria, right wrist

       M00.832   Arthritis due to other bacteria, left wrist

       M00.839   Arthritis due to other bacteria, unspecified wrist

●   **M00.84   Arthritis due to other bacteria, hand**
       Arthritis due to other bacteria, metacarpus and phalanges

       M00.841   Arthritis due to other bacteria, right hand

       M00.842   Arthritis due to other bacteria, left hand

       M00.849   Arthritis due to other bacteria, unspecified hand

●   **M00.85   Arthritis due to other bacteria, hip**

       M00.851   Arthritis due to other bacteria, right hip

       M00.852   Arthritis due to other bacteria, left hip

       M00.859   Arthritis due to other bacteria, unspecified hip

●   **M00.86   Arthritis due to other bacteria, knee**

       M00.861   Arthritis due to other bacteria, right knee

       M00.862   Arthritis due to other bacteria, left knee

       M00.869   Arthritis due to other bacteria, unspecified knee

●   **M00.87   Arthritis due to other bacteria, ankle and foot**
       Arthritis due to other bacteria, tarsus, metatarsus, and phalanges

       M00.871   Arthritis due to other bacteria, right ankle and foot

       M00.872   Arthritis due to other bacteria, left ankle and foot

       M00.879   Arthritis due to other bacteria, unspecified ankle and foot

     M00.88   Arthritis due to other bacteria, vertebrae

     M00.89   Polyarthritis due to other bacteria

M00.9   Pyogenic arthritis, unspecified
     Infective arthritis NOS

● **M01   Direct infections of joint in infectious and parasitic diseases classified elsewhere**

     Code first underlying disease, such as:
     leprosy [Hansen's disease] (A30.-)
     mycoses (B35-B49)
     O'nyong-nyong fever (A92.1)
     paratyphoid fever (A01.1-A01.4)

     Excludes1   arthropathy in Lyme disease (A69.23)
                     gonococcal arthritis (A54.42)
                      meningococcal arthritis (A39.83)
                      mumps arthritis (B26.85)
                      postinfective arthropathy (M02.-)
                      postmeningococcal arthritis (A39.84)
                      reactive arthritis (M02.3)
                      rubella arthritis (B06.82)
                      sarcoidosis arthritis (D86.86)
                      typhoid fever arthritis (A01.04)
                      tuberculosis arthritis (A18.01-A18.02)

● **M01.X   Direct infection of joint in infectious and parasitic diseases classified elsewhere**

     M01.X0   Direct infection of unspecified joint in infectious and parasitic diseases classified elsewhere

●   **M01.X1   Direct infection of shoulder joint in infectious and parasitic diseases classified elsewhere**

       M01.X11   Direct infection of right shoulder in infectious and parasitic diseases classified elsewhere

       M01.X12   Direct infection of left shoulder in infectious and parasitic diseases classified elsewhere

       M01.X19   Direct infection of unspecified shoulder in infectious and parasitic diseases classified elsewhere

●   **M01.X2   Direct infection of elbow in infectious and parasitic diseases classified elsewhere**

       M01.X21   Direct infection of right elbow in infectious and parasitic diseases classified elsewhere

       M01.X22   Direct infection of left elbow in infectious and parasitic diseases classified elsewhere

       M01.X29   Direct infection of unspecified elbow in infectious and parasitic diseases classified elsewhere

●   **M01.X3   Direct infection of wrist in infectious and parasitic diseases classified elsewhere**
       Direct infection of carpal bones in infectious and parasitic diseases classified elsewhere

       M01.X31   Direct infection of right wrist in infectious and parasitic diseases classified elsewhere

       M01.X32   Direct infection of left wrist in infectious and parasitic diseases classified elsewhere

       M01.X39   Direct infection of unspecified wrist in infectious and parasitic diseases classified elsewhere

●   **M01.X4   Direct infection of hand in infectious and parasitic diseases classified elsewhere**
       Direct infection of metacarpus and phalanges in infectious and parasitic diseases classified elsewhere

       M01.X41   Direct infection of right hand in infectious and parasitic diseases classified elsewhere

       M01.X42   Direct infection of left hand in infectious and parasitic diseases classified elsewhere

       M01.X49   Direct infection of unspecified hand in infectious and parasitic diseases classified elsewhere

◄ New   ◄═ Revised   ~~deleted~~ Deleted   Excludes 1   Excludes 2   Includes   Use additional   Code first   Code also   Unspecified

OGCR Official Guidelines   X Assign placeholder X   ● Use Additional Character(s)   ▶ Manifestation Code   **Coding Clinic**

● **M01.X5** Direct infection of hip in infectious and parasitic diseases classified elsewhere

　▶ *M01.X51 Direct infection of right hip in infectious and parasitic diseases classified elsewhere*

　▶ *M01.X52 Direct infection of left hip in infectious and parasitic diseases classified elsewhere*

　▶ *M01.X59 Direct infection of unspecified hip in infectious and parasitic diseases classified elsewhere*

● **M01.X6** Direct infection of knee in infectious and parasitic diseases classified elsewhere

　▶ *M01.X61 Direct infection of right knee in infectious and parasitic diseases classified elsewhere*

　▶ *M01.X62 Direct infection of left knee in infectious and parasitic diseases classified elsewhere*

　▶ *M01.X69 Direct infection of unspecified knee in infectious and parasitic diseases classified elsewhere*

● **M01.X7** Direct infection of ankle and foot in infectious and parasitic diseases classified elsewhere
　　Direct infection of tarsus, metatarsus and phalanges in infectious and parasitic diseases classified elsewhere

　▶ *M01.X71 Direct infection of right ankle and foot in infectious and parasitic diseases classified elsewhere*

　▶ *M01.X72 Direct infection of left ankle and foot in infectious and parasitic diseases classified elsewhere*

　▶ *M01.X79 Direct infection of unspecified ankle and foot in infectious and parasitic diseases classified elsewhere*

　▶ *M01.X8 Direct infection of vertebrae in infectious and parasitic diseases classified elsewhere*

　▶ *M01.X9 Direct infection of multiple joints in infectious and parasitic diseases classified elsewhere*

● **M02** **Postinfective and reactive arthropathies**
　　Code first underlying disease, such as:
　　congenital syphilis [Clutton's joints] (A50.5)
　　enteritis due to Yersinia enterocolitica (A04.6)
　　infective endocarditis (I33.0)
　　viral hepatitis (B15-B19)

　　Excludes1　Behçet's disease (M35.2)
　　　　direct infections of joint in infectious and parasitic diseases classified elsewhere (M01.-)
　　　　postmeningococcal arthritis (A39.84)
　　　　mumps arthritis (B26.85)
　　　　rubella arthritis (B06.82)
　　　　syphilis arthritis (late) (A52.77)
　　　　rheumatic fever (I00)
　　　　tabetic arthropathy [Charcôt's] (A52.16)

● **M02.0** Arthropathy following intestinal bypass

　M02.00 Arthropathy following intestinal bypass, unspecified site

● **M02.01** Arthropathy following intestinal bypass, shoulder

　　M02.011 Arthropathy following intestinal bypass, right shoulder

　　M02.012 Arthropathy following intestinal bypass, left shoulder

　　M02.019 Arthropathy following intestinal bypass, unspecified shoulder

● **M02.02** Arthropathy following intestinal bypass, elbow

　　M02.021 Arthropathy following intestinal bypass, right elbow

　　M02.022 Arthropathy following intestinal bypass, left elbow

　　M02.029 Arthropathy following intestinal bypass, unspecified elbow

● **M02.03** Arthropathy following intestinal bypass, wrist
　　Arthropathy following intestinal bypass, carpal bones

　　M02.031 Arthropathy following intestinal bypass, right wrist

　　M02.032 Arthropathy following intestinal bypass, left wrist

　　M02.039 Arthropathy following intestinal bypass, unspecified wrist

● **M02.04** Arthropathy following intestinal bypass, hand
　　Arthropathy following intestinal bypass, metacarpals and phalanges

　　M02.041 Arthropathy following intestinal bypass, right hand

　　M02.042 Arthropathy following intestinal bypass, left hand

　　M02.049 Arthropathy following intestinal bypass, unspecified hand

● **M02.05** Arthropathy following intestinal bypass, hip

　　M02.051 Arthropathy following intestinal bypass, right hip

　　M02.052 Arthropathy following intestinal bypass, left hip

　　M02.059 Arthropathy following intestinal bypass, unspecified hip

● **M02.06** Arthropathy following intestinal bypass, knee

　　M02.061 Arthropathy following intestinal bypass, right knee

　　M02.062 Arthropathy following intestinal bypass, left knee

　　M02.069 Arthropathy following intestinal bypass, unspecified knee

● **M02.07** Arthropathy following intestinal bypass, ankle and foot
　　Arthropathy following intestinal bypass, tarsus, metatarsus and phalanges

　　M02.071 Arthropathy following intestinal bypass, right ankle and foot

　　M02.072 Arthropathy following intestinal bypass, left ankle and foot

　　M02.079 Arthropathy following intestinal bypass, unspecified ankle and foot

　M02.08 Arthropathy following intestinal bypass, vertebrae

　M02.09 Arthropathy following intestinal bypass, multiple sites

● **M02.1** Postdysenteric arthropathy

　　M02.10 Postdysenteric arthropathy, unspecified site

● **M02.11** Postdysenteric arthropathy, shoulder

　　M02.111 Postdysenteric arthropathy, right shoulder

　　M02.112 Postdysenteric arthropathy, left shoulder

　　M02.119 Postdysenteric arthropathy, unspecified shoulder

CHAPTER 13 (M00-M99)

- ● **M02.12**   Postdysenteric arthropathy, elbow
  - **M02.121**   Postdysenteric arthropathy, right elbow
  - **M02.122**   Postdysenteric arthropathy, left elbow
  - **M02.129**   Postdysenteric arthropathy, unspecified elbow
- ● **M02.13**   Postdysenteric arthropathy, wrist
  - Postdysenteric arthropathy, carpal bones
  - **M02.131**   Postdysenteric arthropathy, right wrist
  - **M02.132**   Postdysenteric arthropathy, left wrist
  - **M02.139**   Postdysenteric arthropathy, unspecified wrist
- ● **M02.14**   Postdysenteric arthropathy, hand
  - Postdysenteric arthropathy, metacarpus and phalanges
  - **M02.141**   Postdysenteric arthropathy, right hand
  - **M02.142**   Postdysenteric arthropathy, left hand
  - **M02.149**   Postdysenteric arthropathy, unspecified hand
- ● **M02.15**   Postdysenteric arthropathy, hip
  - **M02.151**   Postdysenteric arthropathy, right hip
  - **M02.152**   Postdysenteric arthropathy, left hip
  - **M02.159**   Postdysenteric arthropathy, unspecified hip
- ● **M02.16**   Postdysenteric arthropathy, knee
  - **M02.161**   Postdysenteric arthropathy, right knee
  - **M02.162**   Postdysenteric arthropathy, left knee
  - **M02.169**   Postdysenteric arthropathy, unspecified knee
- ● **M02.17**   Postdysenteric arthropathy, ankle and foot
  - Postdysenteric arthropathy, tarsus, metatarsus and phalanges
  - **M02.171**   Postdysenteric arthropathy, right ankle and foot
  - **M02.172**   Postdysenteric arthropathy, left ankle and foot
  - **M02.179**   Postdysenteric arthropathy, unspecified ankle and foot
  - **M02.18**   Postdysenteric arthropathy, vertebrae
  - **M02.19**   Postdysenteric arthropathy, multiple sites
- ● **M02.2**   Postimmunization arthropathy
  - **M02.20**   Postimmunization arthropathy, unspecified site
- ● **M02.21**   Postimmunization arthropathy, shoulder
  - **M02.211**   Postimmunization arthropathy, right shoulder
  - **M02.212**   Postimmunization arthropathy, left shoulder
  - **M02.219**   Postimmunization arthropathy, unspecified shoulder
- ● **M02.22**   Postimmunization arthropathy, elbow
  - **M02.221**   Postimmunization arthropathy, right elbow
  - **M02.222**   Postimmunization arthropathy, left elbow
  - **M02.229**   Postimmunization arthropathy, unspecified elbow
- ● **M02.23**   Postimmunization arthropathy, wrist
  - Postimmunization arthropathy, carpal bones
  - **M02.231**   Postimmunization arthropathy, right wrist
  - **M02.232**   Postimmunization arthropathy, left wrist
  - **M02.239**   Postimmunization arthropathy, unspecified wrist

- ● **M02.24**   Postimmunization arthropathy, hand
  - Postimmunization arthropathy, metacarpus and phalanges
  - **M02.241**   Postimmunization arthropathy, right hand
  - **M02.242**   Postimmunization arthropathy, left hand
  - **M02.249**   Postimmunization arthropathy, unspecified hand
- ● **M02.25**   Postimmunization arthropathy, hip
  - **M02.251**   Postimmunization arthropathy, right hip
  - **M02.252**   Postimmunization arthropathy, left hip
  - **M02.259**   Postimmunization arthropathy, unspecified hip
- ● **M02.26**   Postimmunization arthropathy, knee
  - **M02.261**   Postimmunization arthropathy, right knee
  - **M02.262**   Postimmunization arthropathy, left knee
  - **M02.269**   Postimmunization arthropathy, unspecified knee
- ● **M02.27**   Postimmunization arthropathy, ankle and foot
  - Postimmunization arthropathy, tarsus, metatarsus and phalanges
  - **M02.271**   Postimmunization arthropathy, right ankle and foot
  - **M02.272**   Postimmunization arthropathy, left ankle and foot
  - **M02.279**   Postimmunization arthropathy, unspecified ankle and foot
  - **M02.28**   Postimmunization arthropathy, vertebrae
  - **M02.29**   Postimmunization arthropathy, multiple sites
- ● **M02.3**   Reiter's disease
  - Reactive arthritis
  - **M02.30**   Reiter's disease, unspecified site
- ● **M02.31**   Reiter's disease, shoulder
  - **M02.311**   Reiter's disease, right shoulder
  - **M02.312**   Reiter's disease, left shoulder
  - **M02.319**   Reiter's disease, unspecified shoulder
- ● **M02.32**   Reiter's disease, elbow
  - **M02.321**   Reiter's disease, right elbow
  - **M02.322**   Reiter's disease, left elbow
  - **M02.329**   Reiter's disease, unspecified elbow
- ● **M02.33**   Reiter's disease, wrist
  - Reiter's disease, carpal bones
  - **M02.331**   Reiter's disease, right wrist
  - **M02.332**   Reiter's disease, left wrist
  - **M02.339**   Reiter's disease, unspecified wrist
- ● **M02.34**   Reiter's disease, hand
  - Reiter's disease, metacarpus and phalanges
  - **M02.341**   Reiter's disease, right hand
  - **M02.342**   Reiter's disease, left hand
  - **M02.349**   Reiter's disease, unspecified hand
- ● **M02.35**   Reiter's disease, hip
  - **M02.351**   Reiter's disease, right hip
  - **M02.352**   Reiter's disease, left hip
  - **M02.359**   Reiter's disease, unspecified hip
- ● **M02.36**   Reiter's disease, knee
  - **M02.361**   Reiter's disease, right knee
  - **M02.362**   Reiter's disease, left knee
  - **M02.369**   Reiter's disease, unspecified knee

◀ New   ◀◀ Revised   ~~deleted~~ Deleted   Excludes 1   Excludes 2   Includes   Use additional   Code first   Code also   Unspecified

OGCR Official Guidelines   **X** Assign placeholder X   ● Use Additional Character(s)   ▶ Manifestation Code   **Coding Clinic**

● M02.37 Reiter's disease, ankle and foot
   Reiter's disease, tarsus, metatarsus and phalanges
  M02.371 Reiter's disease, right ankle and foot
  M02.372 Reiter's disease, left ankle and foot
  M02.379 Reiter's disease, unspecified ankle and foot
 M02.38 Reiter's disease, vertebrae
 M02.39 Reiter's disease, multiple sites
● M02.8 Other reactive arthropathies
 M02.80 Other reactive arthropathies, unspecified site
● M02.81 Other reactive arthropathies, shoulder
  M02.811 Other reactive arthropathies, right shoulder
  M02.812 Other reactive arthropathies, left shoulder
  M02.819 Other reactive arthropathies, unspecified shoulder
● M02.82 Other reactive arthropathies, elbow
  M02.821 Other reactive arthropathies, right elbow
  M02.822 Other reactive arthropathies, left elbow
  M02.829 Other reactive arthropathies, unspecified elbow
● M02.83 Other reactive arthropathies, wrist
  Other reactive arthropathies, carpal bones
  M02.831 Other reactive arthropathies, right wrist
  M02.832 Other reactive arthropathies, left wrist
  M02.839 Other reactive arthropathies, unspecified wrist
● M02.84 Other reactive arthropathies, hand
  Other reactive arthropathies, metacarpus and phalanges
  M02.841 Other reactive arthropathies, right hand
  M02.842 Other reactive arthropathies, left hand
  M02.849 Other reactive arthropathies, unspecified hand
● M02.85 Other reactive arthropathies, hip
  M02.851 Other reactive arthropathies, right hip
  M02.852 Other reactive arthropathies, left hip
  M02.859 Other reactive arthropathies, unspecified hip
● M02.86 Other reactive arthropathies, knee
  M02.861 Other reactive arthropathies, right knee
  M02.862 Other reactive arthropathies, left knee
  M02.869 Other reactive arthropathies, unspecified knee
● M02.87 Other reactive arthropathies, ankle and foot
  Other reactive arthropathies, tarsus, metatarsus and phalanges
  M02.871 Other reactive arthropathies, right ankle and foot
  M02.872 Other reactive arthropathies, left ankle and foot
  M02.879 Other reactive arthropathies, unspecified ankle and foot
 ◗ M02.88 *Other reactive arthropathies, vertebrae*
 ◗ M02.89 *Other reactive arthropathies, multiple sites*
◗ *M02.9 Reactive arthropathy, unspecified*

Item 13–1 Rheumatoid arthritis (RA) is a chronic systemic inflammatory autoimmune disease of undetermined etiology involving primarily the synovial membranes and articular structures of multiple joints. It can also affect other organs, including the eyes, blood vessels, heart, and lungs. The disease is often progressive. In late stages, deformity, ankylosis, and other **inflammatory polyarthropathies** develop.

INFLAMMATORY POLYARTHROPATHIES (M05-M14)

● M05 Rheumatoid arthritis with rheumatoid factor
 Excludes1 rheumatic fever (I00)
    juvenile rheumatoid arthritis (M08.-)
    rheumatoid arthritis of spine (M45.-)
 ● M05.0 Felty's syndrome
  Rheumatoid arthritis with splenoadenomegaly and leukopenia
  M05.00 Felty's syndrome, unspecified site
 ● M05.01 Felty's syndrome, shoulder
   M05.011 Felty's syndrome, right shoulder
   M05.012 Felty's syndrome, left shoulder
   M05.019 Felty's syndrome, unspecified shoulder
 ● M05.02 Felty's syndrome, elbow
   M05.021 Felty's syndrome, right elbow
   M05.022 Felty's syndrome, left elbow
   M05.029 Felty's syndrome, unspecified elbow
 ● M05.03 Felty's syndrome, wrist
   Felty's syndrome, carpal bones
   M05.031 Felty's syndrome, right wrist
   M05.032 Felty's syndrome, left wrist
   M05.039 Felty's syndrome, unspecified wrist
 ● M05.04 Felty's syndrome, hand
   Felty's syndrome, metacarpus and phalanges
   M05.041 Felty's syndrome, right hand
   M05.042 Felty's syndrome, left hand
   M05.049 Felty's syndrome, unspecified hand
 ● M05.05 Felty's syndrome, hip
   M05.051 Felty's syndrome, right hip
   M05.052 Felty's syndrome, left hip
   M05.059 Felty's syndrome, unspecified hip
 ● M05.06 Felty's syndrome, knee
   M05.061 Felty's syndrome, right knee
   M05.062 Felty's syndrome, left knee
   M05.069 Felty's syndrome, unspecified knee
 ● M05.07 Felty's syndrome, ankle and foot
   Felty's syndrome, tarsus, metatarsus and phalanges
   M05.071 Felty's syndrome, right ankle and foot
   M05.072 Felty's syndrome, left ankle and foot
   M05.079 Felty's syndrome, unspecified ankle and foot
  M05.09 Felty's syndrome, multiple sites
 ● M05.1 Rheumatoid lung disease with rheumatoid arthritis
  M05.10 Rheumatoid lung disease with rheumatoid arthritis of unspecified site
 ● M05.11 Rheumatoid lung disease with rheumatoid arthritis of shoulder
   M05.111 Rheumatoid lung disease with rheumatoid arthritis of right shoulder
   M05.112 Rheumatoid lung disease with rheumatoid arthritis of left shoulder
   M05.119 Rheumatoid lung disease with rheumatoid arthritis of unspecified shoulder

CHAPTER 13 (M00-M99)

CHAPTER 13 (M00-M99)

● **M05.12** **Rheumatoid lung disease with rheumatoid arthritis of elbow**

     M05.121 Rheumatoid lung disease with rheumatoid arthritis of right elbow

     M05.122 Rheumatoid lung disease with rheumatoid arthritis of left elbow

     M05.129 Rheumatoid lung disease with rheumatoid arthritis of unspecified elbow

● **M05.13** **Rheumatoid lung disease with rheumatoid arthritis of wrist**

     Rheumatoid lung disease with rheumatoid arthritis, carpal bones

     M05.131 Rheumatoid lung disease with rheumatoid arthritis of right wrist

     M05.132 Rheumatoid lung disease with rheumatoid arthritis of left wrist

     M05.139 Rheumatoid lung disease with rheumatoid arthritis of unspecified wrist

● **M05.14** **Rheumatoid lung disease with rheumatoid arthritis of hand**

     Rheumatoid lung disease with rheumatoid arthritis, metacarpus and phalanges

     M05.141 Rheumatoid lung disease with rheumatoid arthritis of right hand

     M05.142 Rheumatoid lung disease with rheumatoid arthritis of left hand

     M05.149 Rheumatoid lung disease with rheumatoid arthritis of unspecified hand

● **M05.15** **Rheumatoid lung disease with rheumatoid arthritis of hip**

     M05.151 Rheumatoid lung disease with rheumatoid arthritis of right hip

     M05.152 Rheumatoid lung disease with rheumatoid arthritis of left hip

     M05.159 Rheumatoid lung disease with rheumatoid arthritis of unspecified hip

● **M05.16** **Rheumatoid lung disease with rheumatoid arthritis of knee**

     M05.161 Rheumatoid lung disease with rheumatoid arthritis of right knee

     M05.162 Rheumatoid lung disease with rheumatoid arthritis of left knee

     M05.169 Rheumatoid lung disease with rheumatoid arthritis of unspecified knee

● **M05.17** **Rheumatoid lung disease with rheumatoid arthritis of ankle and foot**

     Rheumatoid lung disease with rheumatoid arthritis, tarsus, metatarsus and phalanges

     M05.171 Rheumatoid lung disease with rheumatoid arthritis of right ankle and foot

     M05.172 Rheumatoid lung disease with rheumatoid arthritis of left ankle and foot

     M05.179 Rheumatoid lung disease with rheumatoid arthritis of unspecified ankle and foot

M05.19 **Rheumatoid lung disease with rheumatoid arthritis of multiple sites**

● **M05.2** **Rheumatoid vasculitis with rheumatoid arthritis**

     M05.20 Rheumatoid vasculitis with rheumatoid arthritis of unspecified site

● **M05.21** **Rheumatoid vasculitis with rheumatoid arthritis of shoulder**

     M05.211 Rheumatoid vasculitis with rheumatoid arthritis of right shoulder

     M05.212 Rheumatoid vasculitis with rheumatoid arthritis of left shoulder

     M05.219 Rheumatoid vasculitis with rheumatoid arthritis of unspecified shoulder

● **M05.22** **Rheumatoid vasculitis with rheumatoid arthritis of elbow**

     M05.221 Rheumatoid vasculitis with rheumatoid arthritis of right elbow

     M05.222 Rheumatoid vasculitis with rheumatoid arthritis of left elbow

     M05.229 Rheumatoid vasculitis with rheumatoid arthritis of unspecified elbow

● **M05.23** **Rheumatoid vasculitis with rheumatoid arthritis of wrist**

     Rheumatoid vasculitis with rheumatoid arthritis, carpal bones

     M05.231 Rheumatoid vasculitis with rheumatoid arthritis of right wrist

     M05.232 Rheumatoid vasculitis with rheumatoid arthritis of left wrist

     M05.239 Rheumatoid vasculitis with rheumatoid arthritis of unspecified wrist

● **M05.24** **Rheumatoid vasculitis with rheumatoid arthritis of hand**

     Rheumatoid vasculitis with rheumatoid arthritis, metacarpus and phalanges

     M05.241 Rheumatoid vasculitis with rheumatoid arthritis of right hand

     M05.242 Rheumatoid vasculitis with rheumatoid arthritis of left hand

     M05.249 Rheumatoid vasculitis with rheumatoid arthritis of unspecified hand

● **M05.25** **Rheumatoid vasculitis with rheumatoid arthritis of hip**

     M05.251 Rheumatoid vasculitis with rheumatoid arthritis of right hip

     M05.252 Rheumatoid vasculitis with rheumatoid arthritis of left hip

     M05.259 Rheumatoid vasculitis with rheumatoid arthritis of unspecified hip

● **M05.26** **Rheumatoid vasculitis with rheumatoid arthritis of knee**

     M05.261 Rheumatoid vasculitis with rheumatoid arthritis of right knee

     M05.262 Rheumatoid vasculitis with rheumatoid arthritis of left knee

     M05.269 Rheumatoid vasculitis with rheumatoid arthritis of unspecified knee

◄ New   ◄ Revised   deleted Deleted   Excludes 1   Excludes 2   Includes   Use additional   Code first   Code also   Unspecified

OGCR Official Guidelines   X Assign placeholder X   ● Use Additional Character(s)   ▶ Manifestation Code   **Coding Clinic**

● **M05.27** Rheumatoid vasculitis with rheumatoid arthritis of ankle and foot
　　　Rheumatoid vasculitis with rheumatoid arthritis, tarsus, metatarsus and phalanges

　　M05.271 Rheumatoid vasculitis with rheumatoid arthritis of right ankle and foot

　　M05.272 Rheumatoid vasculitis with rheumatoid arthritis of left ankle and foot

　　M05.279 Rheumatoid vasculitis with rheumatoid arthritis of unspecified ankle and foot

　M05.29 Rheumatoid vasculitis with rheumatoid arthritis of multiple sites

● **M05.3** Rheumatoid heart disease with rheumatoid arthritis
　　Rheumatoid carditis
　　Rheumatoid endocarditis
　　Rheumatoid myocarditis
　　Rheumatoid pericarditis

　M05.30 Rheumatoid heart disease with rheumatoid arthritis of unspecified site

● **M05.31** Rheumatoid heart disease with rheumatoid arthritis of shoulder

　　M05.311 Rheumatoid heart disease with rheumatoid arthritis of right shoulder

　　M05.312 Rheumatoid heart disease with rheumatoid arthritis of left shoulder

　　M05.319 Rheumatoid heart disease with rheumatoid arthritis of unspecified shoulder

● **M05.32** Rheumatoid heart disease with rheumatoid arthritis of elbow

　　M05.321 Rheumatoid heart disease with rheumatoid arthritis of right elbow

　　M05.322 Rheumatoid heart disease with rheumatoid arthritis of left elbow

　　M05.329 Rheumatoid heart disease with rheumatoid arthritis of unspecified elbow

● **M05.33** Rheumatoid heart disease with rheumatoid arthritis of wrist
　　　Rheumatoid heart disease with rheumatoid arthritis, carpal bones

　　M05.331 Rheumatoid heart disease with rheumatoid arthritis of right wrist

　　M05.332 Rheumatoid heart disease with rheumatoid arthritis of left wrist

　　M05.339 Rheumatoid heart disease with rheumatoid arthritis of unspecified wrist

● **M05.34** Rheumatoid heart disease with rheumatoid arthritis of hand
　　　Rheumatoid heart disease with rheumatoid arthritis, metacarpus and phalanges

　　M05.341 Rheumatoid heart disease with rheumatoid arthritis of right hand

　　M05.342 Rheumatoid heart disease with rheumatoid arthritis of left hand

　　M05.349 Rheumatoid heart disease with rheumatoid arthritis of unspecified hand

● **M05.35** Rheumatoid heart disease with rheumatoid arthritis of hip

　　M05.351 Rheumatoid heart disease with rheumatoid arthritis of right hip

　　M05.352 Rheumatoid heart disease with rheumatoid arthritis of left hip

　　M05.359 Rheumatoid heart disease with rheumatoid arthritis of unspecified hip

● **M05.36** Rheumatoid heart disease with rheumatoid arthritis of knee

　　M05.361 Rheumatoid heart disease with rheumatoid arthritis of right knee

　　M05.362 Rheumatoid heart disease with rheumatoid arthritis of left knee

　　M05.369 Rheumatoid heart disease with rheumatoid arthritis of unspecified knee

● **M05.37** Rheumatoid heart disease with rheumatoid arthritis of ankle and foot
　　　Rheumatoid heart disease with rheumatoid arthritis, tarsus, metatarsus and phalanges

　　M05.371 Rheumatoid heart disease with rheumatoid arthritis of right ankle and foot

　　M05.372 Rheumatoid heart disease with rheumatoid arthritis of left ankle and foot

　　M05.379 Rheumatoid heart disease with rheumatoid arthritis of unspecified ankle and foot

　M05.39 Rheumatoid heart disease with rheumatoid arthritis of multiple sites

● **M05.4** Rheumatoid myopathy with rheumatoid arthritis

　M05.40 Rheumatoid myopathy with rheumatoid arthritis of unspecified site

● **M05.41** Rheumatoid myopathy with rheumatoid arthritis of shoulder

　　M05.411 Rheumatoid myopathy with rheumatoid arthritis of right shoulder

　　M05.412 Rheumatoid myopathy with rheumatoid arthritis of left shoulder

　　M05.419 Rheumatoid myopathy with rheumatoid arthritis of unspecified shoulder

● **M05.42** Rheumatoid myopathy with rheumatoid arthritis of elbow

　　M05.421 Rheumatoid myopathy with rheumatoid arthritis of right elbow

　　M05.422 Rheumatoid myopathy with rheumatoid arthritis of left elbow

　　M05.429 Rheumatoid myopathy with rheumatoid arthritis of unspecified elbow

● **M05.43** Rheumatoid myopathy with rheumatoid arthritis of wrist
　　　Rheumatoid myopathy with rheumatoid arthritis, carpal bones

　　M05.431 Rheumatoid myopathy with rheumatoid arthritis of right wrist

　　M05.432 Rheumatoid myopathy with rheumatoid arthritis of left wrist

　　M05.439 Rheumatoid myopathy with rheumatoid arthritis of unspecified wrist

● **M05.44** Rheumatoid myopathy with rheumatoid arthritis of hand
　　　Rheumatoid myopathy with rheumatoid arthritis, metacarpus and phalanges

　　M05.441 Rheumatoid myopathy with rheumatoid arthritis of right hand

　　M05.442 Rheumatoid myopathy with rheumatoid arthritis of left hand

　　M05.449 Rheumatoid myopathy with rheumatoid arthritis of unspecified hand

● **M05.45** **Rheumatoid myopathy with rheumatoid arthritis of hip**

    M05.451 Rheumatoid myopathy with rheumatoid arthritis of right hip

    M05.452 Rheumatoid myopathy with rheumatoid arthritis of left hip

    M05.459 Rheumatoid myopathy with rheumatoid arthritis of `unspecified` hip

● **M05.46** **Rheumatoid myopathy with rheumatoid arthritis of knee**

    M05.461 Rheumatoid myopathy with rheumatoid arthritis of right knee

    M05.462 Rheumatoid myopathy with rheumatoid arthritis of left knee

    M05.469 Rheumatoid myopathy with rheumatoid arthritis of `unspecified` knee

● **M05.47** **Rheumatoid myopathy with rheumatoid arthritis of ankle and foot**

    Rheumatoid myopathy with rheumatoid arthritis, tarsus, metatarsus and phalanges

    M05.471 Rheumatoid myopathy with rheumatoid arthritis of right ankle and foot

    M05.472 Rheumatoid myopathy with rheumatoid arthritis of left ankle and foot

    M05.479 Rheumatoid myopathy with rheumatoid arthritis of `unspecified` ankle and foot

  M05.49 **Rheumatoid myopathy with rheumatoid arthritis of multiple sites**

● **M05.5** **Rheumatoid polyneuropathy with rheumatoid arthritis**

  M05.50 **Rheumatoid polyneuropathy with rheumatoid arthritis of `unspecified` site**

● **M05.51** **Rheumatoid polyneuropathy with rheumatoid arthritis of shoulder**

    M05.511 Rheumatoid polyneuropathy with rheumatoid arthritis of right shoulder

    M05.512 Rheumatoid polyneuropathy with rheumatoid arthritis of left shoulder

    M05.519 Rheumatoid polyneuropathy with rheumatoid arthritis of `unspecified` shoulder

● **M05.52** **Rheumatoid polyneuropathy with rheumatoid arthritis of elbow**

    M05.521 Rheumatoid polyneuropathy with rheumatoid arthritis of right elbow

    M05.522 Rheumatoid polyneuropathy with rheumatoid arthritis of left elbow

    M05.529 Rheumatoid polyneuropathy with rheumatoid arthritis of `unspecified` elbow

● **M05.53** **Rheumatoid polyneuropathy with rheumatoid arthritis of wrist**

    Rheumatoid polyneuropathy with rheumatoid arthritis, carpal bones

    M05.531 Rheumatoid polyneuropathy with rheumatoid arthritis of right wrist

    M05.532 Rheumatoid polyneuropathy with rheumatoid arthritis of left wrist

    M05.539 Rheumatoid polyneuropathy with rheumatoid arthritis of `unspecified` wrist

● **M05.54** **Rheumatoid polyneuropathy with rheumatoid arthritis of hand**

    Rheumatoid polyneuropathy with rheumatoid arthritis, metacarpus and phalanges

    M05.541 Rheumatoid polyneuropathy with rheumatoid arthritis of right hand

    M05.542 Rheumatoid polyneuropathy with rheumatoid arthritis of left hand

    M05.549 Rheumatoid polyneuropathy with rheumatoid arthritis of `unspecified` hand

● **M05.55** **Rheumatoid polyneuropathy with rheumatoid arthritis of hip**

    M05.551 Rheumatoid polyneuropathy with rheumatoid arthritis of right hip

    M05.552 Rheumatoid polyneuropathy with rheumatoid arthritis of left hip

    M05.559 Rheumatoid polyneuropathy with rheumatoid arthritis of `unspecified` hip

● **M05.56** **Rheumatoid polyneuropathy with rheumatoid arthritis of knee**

    M05.561 Rheumatoid polyneuropathy with rheumatoid arthritis of right knee

    M05.562 Rheumatoid polyneuropathy with rheumatoid arthritis of left knee

    M05.569 Rheumatoid polyneuropathy with rheumatoid arthritis of `unspecified` knee

● **M05.57** **Rheumatoid polyneuropathy with rheumatoid arthritis of ankle and foot**

    Rheumatoid polyneuropathy with rheumatoid arthritis, tarsus, metatarsus and phalanges

    M05.571 Rheumatoid polyneuropathy with rheumatoid arthritis of right ankle and foot

    M05.572 Rheumatoid polyneuropathy with rheumatoid arthritis of left ankle and foot

    M05.579 Rheumatoid polyneuropathy with rheumatoid arthritis of `unspecified` ankle and foot

  M05.59 **Rheumatoid polyneuropathy with rheumatoid arthritis of multiple sites**

● **M05.6** **Rheumatoid arthritis with involvement of other organs and systems**

  M05.60 **Rheumatoid arthritis of `unspecified` site with involvement of other organs and systems**

● **M05.61** **Rheumatoid arthritis of shoulder with involvement of other organs and systems**

    M05.611 Rheumatoid arthritis of right shoulder with involvement of other organs and systems

    M05.612 Rheumatoid arthritis of left shoulder with involvement of other organs and systems

    M05.619 Rheumatoid arthritis of `unspecified` shoulder with involvement of other organs and systems

● **M05.62** **Rheumatoid arthritis of elbow with involvement of other organs and systems**

    M05.621 Rheumatoid arthritis of right elbow with involvement of other organs and systems

    M05.622 Rheumatoid arthritis of left elbow with involvement of other organs and systems

    M05.629 Rheumatoid arthritis of `unspecified` elbow with involvement of other organs and systems

◄ New   ◄▥ Revised   ~~deleted~~ Deleted   Excludes 1   Excludes 2   Includes   Use additional   Code first   Code also   Unspecified

OGCR Official Guidelines   X Assign placeholder X   ● Use Additional Character(s)   ▸ Manifestation Code   **Coding Clinic**

● M05.63   Rheumatoid arthritis of wrist with involvement of other organs and systems
     Rheumatoid arthritis of carpal bones with involvement of other organs and systems

    M05.631   Rheumatoid arthritis of right wrist with involvement of other organs and systems

    M05.632   Rheumatoid arthritis of left wrist with involvement of other organs and systems

    M05.639   Rheumatoid arthritis of `unspecified` wrist with involvement of other organs and systems

● M05.64   Rheumatoid arthritis of hand with involvement of other organs and systems
     Rheumatoid arthritis of metacarpus and phalanges with involvement of other organs and systems

    M05.641   Rheumatoid arthritis of right hand with involvement of other organs and systems

    M05.642   Rheumatoid arthritis of left hand with involvement of other organs and systems

    M05.649   Rheumatoid arthritis of `unspecified` hand with involvement of other organs and systems

● M05.65   Rheumatoid arthritis of hip with involvement of other organs and systems

    M05.651   Rheumatoid arthritis of right hip with involvement of other organs and systems

    M05.652   Rheumatoid arthritis of left hip with involvement of other organs and systems

    M05.659   Rheumatoid arthritis of `unspecified` hip with involvement of other organs and systems

● M05.66   Rheumatoid arthritis of knee with involvement of other organs and systems

    M05.661   Rheumatoid arthritis of right knee with involvement of other organs and systems

    M05.662   Rheumatoid arthritis of left knee with involvement of other organs and systems

    M05.669   Rheumatoid arthritis of `unspecified` knee with involvement of other organs and systems

● M05.67   Rheumatoid arthritis of ankle and foot with involvement of other organs and systems
     Rheumatoid arthritis of tarsus, metatarsus and phalanges with involvement of other organs and systems

    M05.671   Rheumatoid arthritis of right ankle and foot with involvement of other organs and systems

    M05.672   Rheumatoid arthritis of left ankle and foot with involvement of other organs and systems

    M05.679   Rheumatoid arthritis of `unspecified` ankle and foot with involvement of other organs and systems

    M05.69   Rheumatoid arthritis of multiple sites with involvement of other organs and systems

● M05.7   Rheumatoid arthritis with rheumatoid factor without organ or systems involvement

    M05.70   Rheumatoid arthritis with rheumatoid factor of `unspecified` site without organ or systems involvement

● M05.71   Rheumatoid arthritis with rheumatoid factor of shoulder without organ or systems involvement

    M05.711   Rheumatoid arthritis with rheumatoid factor of right shoulder without organ or systems involvement

    M05.712   Rheumatoid arthritis with rheumatoid factor of left shoulder without organ or systems involvement

    M05.719   Rheumatoid arthritis with rheumatoid factor of `unspecified` shoulder without organ or systems involvement

● M05.72   Rheumatoid arthritis with rheumatoid factor of elbow without organ or systems involvement

    M05.721   Rheumatoid arthritis with rheumatoid factor of right elbow without organ or systems involvement

    M05.722   Rheumatoid arthritis with rheumatoid factor of left elbow without organ or systems involvement

    M05.729   Rheumatoid arthritis with rheumatoid factor of `unspecified` elbow without organ or systems involvement

● M05.73   Rheumatoid arthritis with rheumatoid factor of wrist without organ or systems involvement

    M05.731   Rheumatoid arthritis with rheumatoid factor of right wrist without organ or systems involvement

    M05.732   Rheumatoid arthritis with rheumatoid factor of left wrist without organ or systems involvement

    M05.739   Rheumatoid arthritis with rheumatoid factor of `unspecified` wrist without organ or systems involvement

● M05.74   Rheumatoid arthritis with rheumatoid factor of hand without organ or systems involvement

    M05.741   Rheumatoid arthritis with rheumatoid factor of right hand without organ or systems involvement

    M05.742   Rheumatoid arthritis with rheumatoid factor of left hand without organ or systems involvement

    M05.749   Rheumatoid arthritis with rheumatoid factor of `unspecified` hand without organ or systems involvement

● M05.75   Rheumatoid arthritis with rheumatoid factor of hip without organ or systems involvement

    M05.751   Rheumatoid arthritis with rheumatoid factor of right hip without organ or systems involvement

    M05.752   Rheumatoid arthritis with rheumatoid factor of left hip without organ or systems involvement

    M05.759   Rheumatoid arthritis with rheumatoid factor of `unspecified` hip without organ or systems involvement

CHAPTER 13 (M00-M99)

● M05.76   Rheumatoid arthritis with rheumatoid factor of knee without organ or systems involvement

     M05.761   Rheumatoid arthritis with rheumatoid factor of right knee without organ or systems involvement

     M05.762   Rheumatoid arthritis with rheumatoid factor of left knee without organ or systems involvement

     M05.769   Rheumatoid arthritis with rheumatoid factor of unspecified knee without organ or systems involvement

● M05.77   Rheumatoid arthritis with rheumatoid factor of ankle and foot without organ or systems involvement

     M05.771   Rheumatoid arthritis with rheumatoid factor of right ankle and foot without organ or systems involvement

     M05.772   Rheumatoid arthritis with rheumatoid factor of left ankle and foot without organ or systems involvement

     M05.779   Rheumatoid arthritis with rheumatoid factor of unspecified ankle and foot without organ or systems involvement

   M05.79   Rheumatoid arthritis with rheumatoid factor of multiple sites without organ or systems involvement

● M05.8   Other rheumatoid arthritis with rheumatoid factor

   M05.80   Other rheumatoid arthritis with rheumatoid factor of unspecified site

● M05.81   Other rheumatoid arthritis with rheumatoid factor of shoulder

     M05.811   Other rheumatoid arthritis with rheumatoid factor of right shoulder

     M05.812   Other rheumatoid arthritis with rheumatoid factor of left shoulder

     M05.819   Other rheumatoid arthritis with rheumatoid factor of unspecified shoulder

● M05.82   Other rheumatoid arthritis with rheumatoid factor of elbow

     M05.821   Other rheumatoid arthritis with rheumatoid factor of right elbow

     M05.822   Other rheumatoid arthritis with rheumatoid factor of left elbow

     M05.829   Other rheumatoid arthritis with rheumatoid factor of unspecified elbow

● M05.83   Other rheumatoid arthritis with rheumatoid factor of wrist

     M05.831   Other rheumatoid arthritis with rheumatoid factor of right wrist

     M05.832   Other rheumatoid arthritis with rheumatoid factor of left wrist

     M05.839   Other rheumatoid arthritis with rheumatoid factor of unspecified wrist

● M05.84   Other rheumatoid arthritis with rheumatoid factor of hand

     M05.841   Other rheumatoid arthritis with rheumatoid factor of right hand

     M05.842   Other rheumatoid arthritis with rheumatoid factor of left hand

     M05.849   Other rheumatoid arthritis with rheumatoid factor of unspecified hand

● M05.85   Other rheumatoid arthritis with rheumatoid factor of hip

     M05.851   Other rheumatoid arthritis with rheumatoid factor of right hip

     M05.852   Other rheumatoid arthritis with rheumatoid factor of left hip

     M05.859   Other rheumatoid arthritis with rheumatoid factor of unspecified hip

● M05.86   Other rheumatoid arthritis with rheumatoid factor of knee

     M05.861   Other rheumatoid arthritis with rheumatoid factor of right knee

     M05.862   Other rheumatoid arthritis with rheumatoid factor of left knee

     M05.869   Other rheumatoid arthritis with rheumatoid factor of unspecified knee

● M05.87   Other rheumatoid arthritis with rheumatoid factor of ankle and foot

     M05.871   Other rheumatoid arthritis with rheumatoid factor of right ankle and foot

     M05.872   Other rheumatoid arthritis with rheumatoid factor of left ankle and foot

     M05.879   Other rheumatoid arthritis with rheumatoid factor of unspecified ankle and foot

   M05.89   Other rheumatoid arthritis with rheumatoid factor of multiple sites

   M05.9   Rheumatoid arthritis with rheumatoid factor, unspecified

● M06   Other rheumatoid arthritis

 ● M06.0   Rheumatoid arthritis without rheumatoid factor

   M06.00   Rheumatoid arthritis without rheumatoid factor, unspecified site

 ● M06.01   Rheumatoid arthritis without rheumatoid factor, shoulder

     M06.011   Rheumatoid arthritis without rheumatoid factor, right shoulder

     M06.012   Rheumatoid arthritis without rheumatoid factor, left shoulder

     M06.019   Rheumatoid arthritis without rheumatoid factor, unspecified shoulder

 ● M06.02   Rheumatoid arthritis without rheumatoid factor, elbow

     M06.021   Rheumatoid arthritis without rheumatoid factor, right elbow

     M06.022   Rheumatoid arthritis without rheumatoid factor, left elbow

     M06.029   Rheumatoid arthritis without rheumatoid factor, unspecified elbow

 ● M06.03   Rheumatoid arthritis without rheumatoid factor, wrist

     M06.031   Rheumatoid arthritis without rheumatoid factor, right wrist

     M06.032   Rheumatoid arthritis without rheumatoid factor, left wrist

     M06.039   Rheumatoid arthritis without rheumatoid factor, unspecified wrist

 ● M06.04   Rheumatoid arthritis without rheumatoid factor, hand

     M06.041   Rheumatoid arthritis without rheumatoid factor, right hand

     M06.042   Rheumatoid arthritis without rheumatoid factor, left hand

     M06.049   Rheumatoid arthritis without rheumatoid factor, unspecified hand

◀ New   ◀◀ Revised   deleted Deleted   Excludes 1   Excludes 2   Includes   Use additional   Code first   Code also   Unspecified

OGCR Official Guidelines   X Assign placeholder X   ● Use Additional Character(s)   ▶ Manifestation Code   **Coding Clinic**

● M06.05 Rheumatoid arthritis without rheumatoid factor, hip

    M06.051 Rheumatoid arthritis without rheumatoid factor, right hip

    M06.052 Rheumatoid arthritis without rheumatoid factor, left hip

    M06.059 Rheumatoid arthritis without rheumatoid factor, unspecified hip

● M06.06 Rheumatoid arthritis without rheumatoid factor, knee

    M06.061 Rheumatoid arthritis without rheumatoid factor, right knee

    M06.062 Rheumatoid arthritis without rheumatoid factor, left knee

    M06.069 Rheumatoid arthritis without rheumatoid factor, unspecified knee

● M06.07 Rheumatoid arthritis without rheumatoid factor, ankle and foot

    M06.071 Rheumatoid arthritis without rheumatoid factor, right ankle and foot

    M06.072 Rheumatoid arthritis without rheumatoid factor, left ankle and foot

    M06.079 Rheumatoid arthritis without rheumatoid factor, unspecified ankle and foot

  M06.08 Rheumatoid arthritis without rheumatoid factor, vertebrae

  M06.09 Rheumatoid arthritis without rheumatoid factor, multiple sites

M06.1 Adult-onset Still's disease   A

    Excludes1 Still's disease NOS (M08.2-)

● M06.2 Rheumatoid bursitis

  M06.20 Rheumatoid bursitis, unspecified site

● M06.21 Rheumatoid bursitis, shoulder

    M06.211 Rheumatoid bursitis, right shoulder

    M06.212 Rheumatoid bursitis, left shoulder

    M06.219 Rheumatoid bursitis, unspecified shoulder

● M06.22 Rheumatoid bursitis, elbow

    M06.221 Rheumatoid bursitis, right elbow

    M06.222 Rheumatoid bursitis, left elbow

    M06.229 Rheumatoid bursitis, unspecified elbow

● M06.23 Rheumatoid bursitis, wrist

    M06.231 Rheumatoid bursitis, right wrist

    M06.232 Rheumatoid bursitis, left wrist

    M06.239 Rheumatoid bursitis, unspecified wrist

● M06.24 Rheumatoid bursitis, hand

    M06.241 Rheumatoid bursitis, right hand

    M06.242 Rheumatoid bursitis, left hand

    M06.249 Rheumatoid bursitis, unspecified hand

● M06.25 Rheumatoid bursitis, hip

    M06.251 Rheumatoid bursitis, right hip

    M06.252 Rheumatoid bursitis, left hip

    M06.259 Rheumatoid bursitis, unspecified hip

● M06.26 Rheumatoid bursitis, knee

    M06.261 Rheumatoid bursitis, right knee

    M06.262 Rheumatoid bursitis, left knee

    M06.269 Rheumatoid bursitis, unspecified knee

● M06.27 Rheumatoid bursitis, ankle and foot

    M06.271 Rheumatoid bursitis, right ankle and foot

    M06.272 Rheumatoid bursitis, left ankle and foot

    M06.279 Rheumatoid bursitis, unspecified ankle and foot

  M06.28 Rheumatoid bursitis, vertebrae

  M06.29 Rheumatoid bursitis, multiple sites

● M06.3 Rheumatoid nodule

  M06.30 Rheumatoid nodule, unspecified site

● M06.31 Rheumatoid nodule, shoulder

    M06.311 Rheumatoid nodule, right shoulder

    M06.312 Rheumatoid nodule, left shoulder

    M06.319 Rheumatoid nodule, unspecified shoulder

● M06.32 Rheumatoid nodule, elbow

    M06.321 Rheumatoid nodule, right elbow

    M06.322 Rheumatoid nodule, left elbow

    M06.329 Rheumatoid nodule, unspecified elbow

● M06.33 Rheumatoid nodule, wrist

    M06.331 Rheumatoid nodule, right wrist

    M06.332 Rheumatoid nodule, left wrist

    M06.339 Rheumatoid nodule, unspecified wrist

● M06.34 Rheumatoid nodule, hand

    M06.341 Rheumatoid nodule, right hand

    M06.342 Rheumatoid nodule, left hand

    M06.349 Rheumatoid nodule, unspecified hand

● M06.35 Rheumatoid nodule, hip

    M06.351 Rheumatoid nodule, right hip

    M06.352 Rheumatoid nodule, left hip

    M06.359 Rheumatoid nodule, unspecified hip

● M06.36 Rheumatoid nodule, knee

    M06.361 Rheumatoid nodule, right knee

    M06.362 Rheumatoid nodule, left knee

    M06.369 Rheumatoid nodule, unspecified knee

● M06.37 Rheumatoid nodule, ankle and foot

    M06.371 Rheumatoid nodule, right ankle and foot

    M06.372 Rheumatoid nodule, left ankle and foot

    M06.379 Rheumatoid nodule, unspecified ankle and foot

  M06.38 Rheumatoid nodule, vertebrae

  M06.39 Rheumatoid nodule, multiple sites

M06.4 Inflammatory polyarthropathy

    Excludes1 polyarthritis NOS (M13.0)

● M06.8 Other specified rheumatoid arthritis

  M06.80 Other specified rheumatoid arthritis, unspecified site

● M06.81 Other specified rheumatoid arthritis, shoulder

    M06.811 Other specified rheumatoid arthritis, right shoulder

    M06.812 Other specified rheumatoid arthritis, left shoulder

    M06.819 Other specified rheumatoid arthritis, unspecified shoulder

● **M06.82**   Other specified rheumatoid arthritis, elbow

     M06.821   Other specified rheumatoid arthritis, right elbow

     M06.822   Other specified rheumatoid arthritis, left elbow

     M06.829   Other specified rheumatoid arthritis, **unspecified** elbow

● **M06.83**   Other specified rheumatoid arthritis, wrist

     M06.831   Other specified rheumatoid arthritis, right wrist

     M06.832   Other specified rheumatoid arthritis, left wrist

     M06.839   Other specified rheumatoid arthritis, **unspecified** wrist

● **M06.84**   Other specified rheumatoid arthritis, hand

     M06.841   Other specified rheumatoid arthritis, right hand

     M06.842   Other specified rheumatoid arthritis, left hand

     M06.849   Other specified rheumatoid arthritis, **unspecified** hand

● **M06.85**   Other specified rheumatoid arthritis, hip

     M06.851   Other specified rheumatoid arthritis, right hip

     M06.852   Other specified rheumatoid arthritis, left hip

     M06.859   Other specified rheumatoid arthritis, **unspecified** hip

● **M06.86**   Other specified rheumatoid arthritis, knee

     M06.861   Other specified rheumatoid arthritis, right knee

     M06.862   Other specified rheumatoid arthritis, left knee

     M06.869   Other specified rheumatoid arthritis, **unspecified** knee

● **M06.87**   Other specified rheumatoid arthritis, ankle and foot

     M06.871   Other specified rheumatoid arthritis, right ankle and foot

     M06.872   Other specified rheumatoid arthritis, left ankle and foot

     M06.879   Other specified rheumatoid arthritis, **unspecified** ankle and foot

     M06.88   Other specified rheumatoid arthritis, vertebrae

     M06.89   Other specified rheumatoid arthritis, multiple sites

   M06.9   Rheumatoid arthritis, **unspecified**

● **M07**   **Enteropathic arthropathies**

     Code also associated enteropathy, such as:
        regional enteritis [Crohn's disease] (K50.-)
        ulcerative colitis (K51.-)

     Excludes1   psoriatic arthropathies (L40.5-)

● **M07.6**   Enteropathic arthropathies

     M07.60   Enteropathic arthropathies, **unspecified** site

● **M07.61**   Enteropathic arthropathies, shoulder

     M07.611   Enteropathic arthropathies, right shoulder

     M07.612   Enteropathic arthropathies, left shoulder

     M07.619   Enteropathic arthropathies, **unspecified** shoulder

● **M07.62**   Enteropathic arthropathies, elbow

     M07.621   Enteropathic arthropathies, right elbow

     M07.622   Enteropathic arthropathies, left elbow

     M07.629   Enteropathic arthropathies, **unspecified** elbow

● **M07.63**   Enteropathic arthropathies, wrist

     M07.631   Enteropathic arthropathies, right wrist

     M07.632   Enteropathic arthropathies, left wrist

     M07.639   Enteropathic arthropathies, **unspecified** wrist

● **M07.64**   Enteropathic arthropathies, hand

     M07.641   Enteropathic arthropathies, right hand

     M07.642   Enteropathic arthropathies, left hand

     M07.649   Enteropathic arthropathies, **unspecified** hand

● **M07.65**   Enteropathic arthropathies, hip

     M07.651   Enteropathic arthropathies, right hip

     M07.652   Enteropathic arthropathies, left hip

     M07.659   Enteropathic arthropathies, **unspecified** hip

● **M07.66**   Enteropathic arthropathies, knee

     M07.661   Enteropathic arthropathies, right knee

     M07.662   Enteropathic arthropathies, left knee

     M07.669   Enteropathic arthropathies, **unspecified** knee

● **M07.67**   Enteropathic arthropathies, ankle and foot

     M07.671   Enteropathic arthropathies, right ankle and foot

     M07.672   Enteropathic arthropathies, left ankle and foot

     M07.679   Enteropathic arthropathies, **unspecified** ankle and foot

     M07.68   Enteropathic arthropathies, vertebrae

     M07.69   Enteropathic arthropathies, multiple sites

● **M08**   **Juvenile arthritis**

     Code also any associated underlying condition, such as:
        regional enteritis [Crohn's disease] (K50.-)
        ulcerative colitis (K51.-)

     Excludes1   arthropathy in Whipple's disease (M14.8)
        Felty's syndrome (M05.0)
        juvenile dermatomyositis (M33.0-)
        psoriatic juvenile arthropathy (L40.54)

● **M08.0**   **Unspecified juvenile rheumatoid arthritis**

     Juvenile rheumatoid arthritis with or without rheumatoid factor

     M08.00   **Unspecified** juvenile rheumatoid arthritis of unspecified site

● **M08.01**   Unspecified juvenile rheumatoid arthritis, shoulder

     M08.011   **Unspecified** juvenile rheumatoid arthritis, right shoulder

     M08.012   **Unspecified** juvenile rheumatoid arthritis, left shoulder

     M08.019   **Unspecified** juvenile rheumatoid arthritis, unspecified shoulder

● **M08.02**   Unspecified juvenile rheumatoid arthritis of elbow

     M08.021   **Unspecified** juvenile rheumatoid arthritis, right elbow

     M08.022   **Unspecified** juvenile rheumatoid arthritis, left elbow

     M08.029   **Unspecified** juvenile rheumatoid arthritis, unspecified elbow

● **M08.03**   Unspecified juvenile rheumatoid arthritis, wrist

     M08.031   **Unspecified** juvenile rheumatoid arthritis, right wrist

     M08.032   **Unspecified** juvenile rheumatoid arthritis, left wrist

     M08.039   **Unspecified** juvenile rheumatoid arthritis, unspecified wrist

● **M08.04**   Unspecified juvenile rheumatoid arthritis, hand

      M08.041   Unspecified juvenile rheumatoid arthritis, right hand

      M08.042   Unspecified juvenile rheumatoid arthritis, left hand

      M08.049   Unspecified juvenile rheumatoid arthritis, unspecified hand

● **M08.05**   Unspecified juvenile rheumatoid arthritis, hip

      M08.051   Unspecified juvenile rheumatoid arthritis, right hip

      M08.052   Unspecified juvenile rheumatoid arthritis, left hip

      M08.059   Unspecified juvenile rheumatoid arthritis, unspecified hip

● **M08.06**   Unspecified juvenile rheumatoid arthritis, knee

      M08.061   Unspecified juvenile rheumatoid arthritis, right knee

      M08.062   Unspecified juvenile rheumatoid arthritis, left knee

      M08.069   Unspecified juvenile rheumatoid arthritis, unspecified knee

● **M08.07**   Unspecified juvenile rheumatoid arthritis, ankle and foot

      M08.071   Unspecified juvenile rheumatoid arthritis, right ankle and foot

      M08.072   Unspecified juvenile rheumatoid arthritis, left ankle and foot

      M08.079   Unspecified juvenile rheumatoid arthritis, unspecified ankle and foot

    M08.08   Unspecified juvenile rheumatoid arthritis, vertebrae

    M08.09   Unspecified juvenile rheumatoid arthritis, multiple sites

M08.1   Juvenile ankylosing spondylitis

     Excludes1   ankylosing spondylitis in adults (M45.0-)

● **M08.2**   Juvenile rheumatoid arthritis with systemic onset
     Still's disease NOS

     Excludes1   adult-onset Still's disease (M06.1-)

    M08.20   Juvenile rheumatoid arthritis with systemic onset, unspecified site

● **M08.21**   Juvenile rheumatoid arthritis with systemic onset, shoulder

      M08.211   Juvenile rheumatoid arthritis with systemic onset, right shoulder

      M08.212   Juvenile rheumatoid arthritis with systemic onset, left shoulder

      M08.219   Juvenile rheumatoid arthritis with systemic onset, unspecified shoulder

● **M08.22**   Juvenile rheumatoid arthritis with systemic onset, elbow

      M08.221   Juvenile rheumatoid arthritis with systemic onset, right elbow

      M08.222   Juvenile rheumatoid arthritis with systemic onset, left elbow

      M08.229   Juvenile rheumatoid arthritis with systemic onset, unspecified elbow

● **M08.23**   Juvenile rheumatoid arthritis with systemic onset, wrist

      M08.231   Juvenile rheumatoid arthritis with systemic onset, right wrist

      M08.232   Juvenile rheumatoid arthritis with systemic onset, left wrist

      M08.239   Juvenile rheumatoid arthritis with systemic onset, unspecified wrist

● **M08.24**   Juvenile rheumatoid arthritis with systemic onset, hand

      M08.241   Juvenile rheumatoid arthritis with systemic onset, right hand

      M08.242   Juvenile rheumatoid arthritis with systemic onset, left hand

      M08.249   Juvenile rheumatoid arthritis with systemic onset, unspecified hand

● **M08.25**   Juvenile rheumatoid arthritis with systemic onset, hip

      M08.251   Juvenile rheumatoid arthritis with systemic onset, right hip

      M08.252   Juvenile rheumatoid arthritis with systemic onset, left hip

      M08.259   Juvenile rheumatoid arthritis with systemic onset, unspecified hip

● **M08.26**   Juvenile rheumatoid arthritis with systemic onset, knee

      M08.261   Juvenile rheumatoid arthritis with systemic onset, right knee

      M08.262   Juvenile rheumatoid arthritis with systemic onset, left knee

      M08.269   Juvenile rheumatoid arthritis with systemic onset, unspecified knee

● **M08.27**   Juvenile rheumatoid arthritis with systemic onset, ankle and foot

      M08.271   Juvenile rheumatoid arthritis with systemic onset, right ankle and foot

      M08.272   Juvenile rheumatoid arthritis with systemic onset, left ankle and foot

      M08.279   Juvenile rheumatoid arthritis with systemic onset, unspecified ankle and foot

    M08.28   Juvenile rheumatoid arthritis with systemic onset, vertebrae

    M08.29   Juvenile rheumatoid arthritis with systemic onset, multiple sites

   M08.3   Juvenile rheumatoid polyarthritis (seronegative)

● **M08.4**   Pauciarticular juvenile rheumatoid arthritis

    M08.40   Pauciarticular juvenile rheumatoid arthritis, unspecified site

● **M08.41**   Pauciarticular juvenile rheumatoid arthritis, shoulder

      M08.411   Pauciarticular juvenile rheumatoid arthritis, right shoulder

      M08.412   Pauciarticular juvenile rheumatoid arthritis, left shoulder

      M08.419   Pauciarticular juvenile rheumatoid arthritis, unspecified shoulder

● **M08.42**   Pauciarticular juvenile rheumatoid arthritis, elbow

      M08.421   Pauciarticular juvenile rheumatoid arthritis, right elbow

      M08.422   Pauciarticular juvenile rheumatoid arthritis, left elbow

      M08.429   Pauciarticular juvenile rheumatoid arthritis, unspecified elbow

● **M08.43**   Pauciarticular juvenile rheumatoid arthritis, wrist

      M08.431   Pauciarticular juvenile rheumatoid arthritis, right wrist

      M08.432   Pauciarticular juvenile rheumatoid arthritis, left wrist

      M08.439   Pauciarticular juvenile rheumatoid arthritis, unspecified wrist

CHAPTER 13 (M00-M99)

● M08.44　Pauciarticular juvenile rheumatoid arthritis, hand

　　　M08.441　Pauciarticular juvenile rheumatoid arthritis, right hand

　　　M08.442　Pauciarticular juvenile rheumatoid arthritis, left hand

　　　M08.449　Pauciarticular juvenile rheumatoid arthritis, unspecified hand

● M08.45　Pauciarticular juvenile rheumatoid arthritis, hip

　　　M08.451　Pauciarticular juvenile rheumatoid arthritis, right hip

　　　M08.452　Pauciarticular juvenile rheumatoid arthritis, left hip

　　　M08.459　Pauciarticular juvenile rheumatoid arthritis, unspecified hip

● M08.46　Pauciarticular juvenile rheumatoid arthritis, knee

　　　M08.461　Pauciarticular juvenile rheumatoid arthritis, right knee

　　　M08.462　Pauciarticular juvenile rheumatoid arthritis, left knee

　　　M08.469　Pauciarticular juvenile rheumatoid arthritis, unspecified knee

● M08.47　Pauciarticular juvenile rheumatoid arthritis, ankle and foot

　　　M08.471　Pauciarticular juvenile rheumatoid arthritis, right ankle and foot

　　　M08.472　Pauciarticular juvenile rheumatoid arthritis, left ankle and foot

　　　M08.479　Pauciarticular juvenile rheumatoid arthritis, unspecified ankle and foot

　　M08.48　Pauciarticular juvenile rheumatoid arthritis, vertebrae

● M08.8　Other juvenile arthritis

　　M08.80　Other juvenile arthritis, unspecified site

● M08.81　Other juvenile arthritis, shoulder

　　　M08.811　Other juvenile arthritis, right shoulder

　　　M08.812　Other juvenile arthritis, left shoulder

　　　M08.819　Other juvenile arthritis, unspecified shoulder

● M08.82　Other juvenile arthritis, elbow

　　　M08.821　Other juvenile arthritis, right elbow

　　　M08.822　Other juvenile arthritis, left elbow

　　　M08.829　Other juvenile arthritis, unspecified elbow

● M08.83　Other juvenile arthritis, wrist

　　　M08.831　Other juvenile arthritis, right wrist

　　　M08.832　Other juvenile arthritis, left wrist

　　　M08.839　Other juvenile arthritis, unspecified wrist

● M08.84　Other juvenile arthritis, hand

　　　M08.841　Other juvenile arthritis, right hand

　　　M08.842　Other juvenile arthritis, left hand

　　　M08.849　Other juvenile arthritis, unspecified hand

● M08.85　Other juvenile arthritis, hip

　　　M08.851　Other juvenile arthritis, right hip

　　　M08.852　Other juvenile arthritis, left hip

　　　M08.859　Other juvenile arthritis, unspecified hip

● M08.86　Other juvenile arthritis, knee

　　　M08.861　Other juvenile arthritis, right knee

　　　M08.862　Other juvenile arthritis, left knee

　　　M08.869　Other juvenile arthritis, unspecified knee

● M08.87　Other juvenile arthritis, ankle and foot

　　　M08.871　Other juvenile arthritis, right ankle and foot

　　　M08.872　Other juvenile arthritis, left ankle and foot

　　　M08.879　Other juvenile arthritis, unspecified ankle and foot

　　M08.88　Other juvenile arthritis, other specified site
　　　　　　Other juvenile arthritis, vertebrae

　　M08.89　Other juvenile arthritis, multiple sites

● M08.9　Juvenile arthritis, unspecified

　　　Excludes1　juvenile rheumatoid arthritis, unspecified (M08.0-)

　　M08.90　Juvenile arthritis, unspecified, unspecified site

● M08.91　Juvenile arthritis, unspecified, shoulder

　　　M08.911　Juvenile arthritis, unspecified, right shoulder

　　　M08.912　Juvenile arthritis, unspecified, left shoulder

　　　M08.919　Juvenile arthritis, unspecified, unspecified shoulder

● M08.92　Juvenile arthritis, unspecified, elbow

　　　M08.921　Juvenile arthritis, unspecified, right elbow

　　　M08.922　Juvenile arthritis, unspecified, left elbow

　　　M08.929　Juvenile arthritis, unspecified, unspecified elbow

● M08.93　Juvenile arthritis, unspecified, wrist

　　　M08.931　Juvenile arthritis, unspecified, right wrist

　　　M08.932　Juvenile arthritis, unspecified, left wrist

　　　M08.939　Juvenile arthritis, unspecified, unspecified wrist

● M08.94　Juvenile arthritis, unspecified, hand

　　　M08.941　Juvenile arthritis, unspecified, right hand

　　　M08.942　Juvenile arthritis, unspecified, left hand

　　　M08.949　Juvenile arthritis, unspecified, unspecified hand

● M08.95　Juvenile arthritis, unspecified, hip

　　　M08.951　Juvenile arthritis, unspecified, right hip

　　　M08.952　Juvenile arthritis, unspecified, left hip

　　　M08.959　Juvenile arthritis, unspecified, unspecified hip

● M08.96　Juvenile arthritis, unspecified, knee

　　　M08.961　Juvenile arthritis, unspecified, right knee

　　　M08.962　Juvenile arthritis, unspecified, left knee

　　　M08.969　Juvenile arthritis, unspecified, unspecified knee

● M08.97　Juvenile arthritis, unspecified, ankle and foot

　　　M08.971　Juvenile arthritis, unspecified, right ankle and foot

　　　M08.972　Juvenile arthritis, unspecified, left ankle and foot

　　　M08.979　Juvenile arthritis, unspecified, unspecified ankle and foot

　　M08.98　Juvenile arthritis, unspecified, vertebrae

　　M08.99　Juvenile arthritis, unspecified, multiple sites

◀ New　　◀▦ Revised　　d̶e̶l̶e̶t̶e̶d̶ Deleted　　Excludes 1　　Excludes 2　　Includes　　Use additional　　Code first　　Code also　　Unspecified

OGCR Official Guidelines　　X Assign placeholder X　　● Use Additional Character(s)　　▶ Manifestation Code　　Coding Clinic

● **M1A Chronic gout**

         Use additional code to identify:

            Autonomic neuropathy in diseases classified elsewhere (G99.0)

            Calculus of urinary tract in diseases classified elsewhere (N22)

            Cardiomyopathy in diseases classified elsewhere (I43)

            Disorders of external ear in diseases classified elsewhere (H61.1-, H62.8-)

            Disorders of iris and ciliary body in diseases classified elsewhere (H22)

            Glomerular disorders in diseases classified elsewhere (N08)

         Excludes1   acute gout (M10.-)

                        gout NOS (M10.-)

         The appropriate 7th character is to be added to each code from category M1A

0	without tophus (tophi)
1	with tophus (tophi)

● **M1A.0 Idiopathic chronic gout**

         Chronic gouty bursitis

         Primary chronic gout

   X● **M1A.00 Idiopathic chronic gout, unspecified site**

     ● **M1A.01 Idiopathic chronic gout, shoulder**

         ● **M1A.011 Idiopathic chronic gout, right shoulder**

         ● **M1A.012 Idiopathic chronic gout, left shoulder**

         ● **M1A.019 Idiopathic chronic gout, unspecified shoulder**

     ● **M1A.02 Idiopathic chronic gout, elbow**

         ● **M1A.021 Idiopathic chronic gout, right elbow**

         ● **M1A.022 Idiopathic chronic gout, left elbow**

         ● **M1A.029 Idiopathic chronic gout, unspecified elbow**

     ● **M1A.03 Idiopathic chronic gout, wrist**

         ● **M1A.031 Idiopathic chronic gout, right wrist**

         ● **M1A.032 Idiopathic chronic gout, left wrist**

         ● **M1A.039 Idiopathic chronic gout, unspecified wrist**

     ● **M1A.04 Idiopathic chronic gout, hand**

         ● **M1A.041 Idiopathic chronic gout, right hand**

         ● **M1A.042 Idiopathic chronic gout, left hand**

         ● **M1A.049 Idiopathic chronic gout, unspecified hand**

     ● **M1A.05 Idiopathic chronic gout, hip**

         ● **M1A.051 Idiopathic chronic gout, right hip**

         ● **M1A.052 Idiopathic chronic gout, left hip**

         ● **M1A.059 Idiopathic chronic gout, unspecified hip**

     ● **M1A.06 Idiopathic chronic gout, knee**

         ● **M1A.061 Idiopathic chronic gout, right knee**

         ● **M1A.062 Idiopathic chronic gout, left knee**

         ● **M1A.069 Idiopathic chronic gout, unspecified knee**

     ● **M1A.07 Idiopathic chronic gout, ankle and foot**

         ● **M1A.071 Idiopathic chronic gout, right ankle and foot**

         ● **M1A.072 Idiopathic chronic gout, left ankle and foot**

         ● **M1A.079 Idiopathic chronic gout, unspecified ankle and foot**

   X● **M1A.08 Idiopathic chronic gout, vertebrae**

   X● **M1A.09 Idiopathic chronic gout, multiple sites**

● **M1A.1 Lead-induced chronic gout**

         Code first toxic effects of lead and its compounds (T56.0-)

   X● **M1A.10 Lead-induced chronic gout, unspecified site**

     ● **M1A.11 Lead-induced chronic gout, shoulder**

         ● **M1A.111 Lead-induced chronic gout, right shoulder**

         ● **M1A.112 Lead-induced chronic gout, left shoulder**

         ● **M1A.119 Lead-induced chronic gout, unspecified shoulder**

     ● **M1A.12 Lead-induced chronic gout, elbow**

         ● **M1A.121 Lead-induced chronic gout, right elbow**

         ● **M1A.122 Lead-induced chronic gout, left elbow**

         ● **M1A.129 Lead-induced chronic gout, unspecified elbow**

     ● **M1A.13 Lead-induced chronic gout, wrist**

         ● **M1A.131 Lead-induced chronic gout, right wrist**

         ● **M1A.132 Lead-induced chronic gout, left wrist**

         ● **M1A.139 Lead-induced chronic gout, unspecified wrist**

     ● **M1A.14 Lead-induced chronic gout, hand**

         ● **M1A.141 Lead-induced chronic gout, right hand**

         ● **M1A.142 Lead-induced chronic gout, left hand**

         ● **M1A.149 Lead-induced chronic gout, unspecified hand**

     ● **M1A.15 Lead-induced chronic gout, hip**

         ● **M1A.151 Lead-induced chronic gout, right hip**

         ● **M1A.152 Lead-induced chronic gout, left hip**

         ● **M1A.159 Lead-induced chronic gout, unspecified hip**

     ● **M1A.16 Lead-induced chronic gout, knee**

         ● **M1A.161 Lead-induced chronic gout, right knee**

         ● **M1A.162 Lead-induced chronic gout, left knee**

         ● **M1A.169 Lead-induced chronic gout, unspecified knee**

     ● **M1A.17 Lead-induced chronic gout, ankle and foot**

         ● **M1A.171 Lead-induced chronic gout, right ankle and foot**

         ● **M1A.172 Lead-induced chronic gout, left ankle and foot**

         ● **M1A.179 Lead-induced chronic gout, unspecified ankle and foot**

   X● **M1A.18 Lead-induced chronic gout, vertebrae**

   X● **M1A.19 Lead-induced chronic gout, multiple sites**

● **M1A.2 Drug-induced chronic gout**

         Use additional code for adverse effect, if applicable, to identify drug (T36-T50 with fifth or sixth character 5)

   X● **M1A.20 Drug-induced chronic gout, unspecified site**

     ● **M1A.21 Drug-induced chronic gout, shoulder**

         ● **M1A.211 Drug-induced chronic gout, right shoulder**

         ● **M1A.212 Drug-induced chronic gout, left shoulder**

         ● **M1A.219 Drug-induced chronic gout, unspecified shoulder**

     ● **M1A.22 Drug-induced chronic gout, elbow**

         ● **M1A.221 Drug-induced chronic gout, right elbow**

         ● **M1A.222 Drug-induced chronic gout, left elbow**

         ● **M1A.229 Drug-induced chronic gout, unspecified elbow**

● M1A.23 Drug-induced chronic gout, wrist
- ● M1A.231 Drug-induced chronic gout, right wrist
- ● M1A.232 Drug-induced chronic gout, left wrist
- ● M1A.239 Drug-induced chronic gout, unspecified wrist

● M1A.24 Drug-induced chronic gout, hand
- ● M1A.241 Drug-induced chronic gout, right hand
- ● M1A.242 Drug-induced chronic gout, left hand
- ● M1A.249 Drug-induced chronic gout, unspecified hand

● M1A.25 Drug-induced chronic gout, hip
- ● M1A.251 Drug-induced chronic gout, right hip
- ● M1A.252 Drug-induced chronic gout, left hip
- ● M1A.259 Drug-induced chronic gout, unspecified hip

● M1A.26 Drug-induced chronic gout, knee
- ● M1A.261 Drug-induced chronic gout, right knee
- ● M1A.262 Drug-induced chronic gout, left knee
- ● M1A.269 Drug-induced chronic gout, unspecified knee

● M1A.27 Drug-induced chronic gout, ankle and foot
- ● M1A.271 Drug-induced chronic gout, right ankle and foot
- ● M1A.272 Drug-induced chronic gout, left ankle and foot
- ● M1A.279 Drug-induced chronic gout, unspecified ankle and foot

X● M1A.28 Drug-induced chronic gout, vertebrae
X● M1A.29 Drug-induced chronic gout, multiple sites

● M1A.3 Chronic gout due to renal impairment
    Code first associated renal disease

X● M1A.30 Chronic gout due to renal impairment, unspecified site

● M1A.31 Chronic gout due to renal impairment, shoulder
- ● M1A.311 Chronic gout due to renal impairment, right shoulder
- ● M1A.312 Chronic gout due to renal impairment, left shoulder
- ● M1A.319 Chronic gout due to renal impairment, unspecified shoulder

● M1A.32 Chronic gout due to renal impairment, elbow
- ● M1A.321 Chronic gout due to renal impairment, right elbow
- ● M1A.322 Chronic gout due to renal impairment, left elbow
- ● M1A.329 Chronic gout due to renal impairment, unspecified elbow

● M1A.33 Chronic gout due to renal impairment, wrist
- ● M1A.331 Chronic gout due to renal impairment, right wrist
- ● M1A.332 Chronic gout due to renal impairment, left wrist
- ● M1A.339 Chronic gout due to renal impairment, unspecified wrist

● M1A.34 Chronic gout due to renal impairment, hand
- ● M1A.341 Chronic gout due to renal impairment, right hand
- ● M1A.342 Chronic gout due to renal impairment, left hand
- ● M1A.349 Chronic gout due to renal impairment, unspecified hand

● M1A.35 Chronic gout due to renal impairment, hip
- ● M1A.351 Chronic gout due to renal impairment, right hip
- ● M1A.352 Chronic gout due to renal impairment, left hip
- ● M1A.359 Chronic gout due to renal impairment, unspecified hip

● M1A.36 Chronic gout due to renal impairment, knee
- ● M1A.361 Chronic gout due to renal impairment, right knee
- ● M1A.362 Chronic gout due to renal impairment, left knee
- ● M1A.369 Chronic gout due to renal impairment, unspecified knee

● M1A.37 Chronic gout due to renal impairment, ankle and foot
- ● M1A.371 Chronic gout due to renal impairment, right ankle and foot
- ● M1A.372 Chronic gout due to renal impairment, left ankle and foot
- ● M1A.379 Chronic gout due to renal impairment, unspecified ankle and foot

X● M1A.38 Chronic gout due to renal impairment, vertebrae
X● M1A.39 Chronic gout due to renal impairment, multiple sites

● M1A.4 Other secondary chronic gout
    Code first associated condition

X● M1A.40 Other secondary chronic gout, unspecified site

● M1A.41 Other secondary chronic gout, shoulder
- ● M1A.411 Other secondary chronic gout, right shoulder
- ● M1A.412 Other secondary chronic gout, left shoulder
- ● M1A.419 Other secondary chronic gout, unspecified shoulder

● M1A.42 Other secondary chronic gout, elbow
- ● M1A.421 Other secondary chronic gout, right elbow
- ● M1A.422 Other secondary chronic gout, left elbow
- ● M1A.429 Other secondary chronic gout, unspecified elbow

● M1A.43 Other secondary chronic gout, wrist
- ● M1A.431 Other secondary chronic gout, right wrist
- ● M1A.432 Other secondary chronic gout, left wrist
- ● M1A.439 Other secondary chronic gout, unspecified wrist

● M1A.44 Other secondary chronic gout, hand
- ● M1A.441 Other secondary chronic gout, right hand
- ● M1A.442 Other secondary chronic gout, left hand
- ● M1A.449 Other secondary chronic gout, unspecified hand

● M1A.45 Other secondary chronic gout, hip
- ● M1A.451 Other secondary chronic gout, right hip
- ● M1A.452 Other secondary chronic gout, left hip
- ● M1A.459 Other secondary chronic gout, unspecified hip

● M1A.46 Other secondary chronic gout, knee
  ● M1A.461 Other secondary chronic gout, right knee
  ● M1A.462 Other secondary chronic gout, left knee
  ● M1A.469 Other secondary chronic gout, unspecified knee
● M1A.47 Other secondary chronic gout, ankle and foot
  ● M1A.471 Other secondary chronic gout, right ankle and foot
  ● M1A.472 Other secondary chronic gout, left ankle and foot
  ● M1A.479 Other secondary chronic gout, unspecified ankle and foot
X ● M1A.48 Other secondary chronic gout, vertebrae
X ● M1A.49 Other secondary chronic gout, multiple sites
X ● M1A.9 Chronic gout, unspecified

● M10 Gout
Accumulation of uric acid that results in swollen, red, hot, painful, stiff joints.
Acute gout
Gout attack
Gout flare
Gout NOS
Podagra
Use additional code to identify:
  Autonomic neuropathy in diseases classified elsewhere (G99.0)
  Calculus of urinary tract in diseases classified elsewhere (N22)
  Cardiomyopathy in diseases classified elsewhere (I43)
  Disorders of external ear in diseases classified elsewhere (H61.1-, H62.8-)
  Disorders of iris and ciliary body in diseases classified elsewhere (H22)
  Glomerular disorders in diseases classified elsewhere (N08)
Excludes 1 chronic gout (M1A.-)
● M10.0 Idiopathic gout
  Gouty bursitis
  Primary gout
  M10.00 Idiopathic gout, unspecified site
  ● M10.01 Idiopathic gout, shoulder
    M10.011 Idiopathic gout, right shoulder
    M10.012 Idiopathic gout, left shoulder
    M10.019 Idiopathic gout, unspecified shoulder
  ● M10.02 Idiopathic gout, elbow
    M10.021 Idiopathic gout, right elbow
    M10.022 Idiopathic gout, left elbow
    M10.029 Idiopathic gout, unspecified elbow
  ● M10.03 Idiopathic gout, wrist
    M10.031 Idiopathic gout, right wrist
    M10.032 Idiopathic gout, left wrist
    M10.039 Idiopathic gout, unspecified wrist
  ● M10.04 Idiopathic gout, hand
    M10.041 Idiopathic gout, right hand
    M10.042 Idiopathic gout, left hand
    M10.049 Idiopathic gout, unspecified hand
  ● M10.05 Idiopathic gout, hip
    M10.051 Idiopathic gout, right hip
    M10.052 Idiopathic gout, left hip
    M10.059 Idiopathic gout, unspecified hip
  ● M10.06 Idiopathic gout, knee
    M10.061 Idiopathic gout, right knee
    M10.062 Idiopathic gout, left knee
    M10.069 Idiopathic gout, unspecified knee

● M10.07 Idiopathic gout, ankle and foot
  M10.071 Idiopathic gout, right ankle and foot
  M10.072 Idiopathic gout, left ankle and foot
  M10.079 Idiopathic gout, unspecified ankle and foot
M10.08 Idiopathic gout, vertebrae
M10.09 Idiopathic gout, multiple sites
● M10.1 Lead-induced gout
Code first toxic effects of lead and its compounds (T56.0-)
M10.10 Lead-induced gout, unspecified site
● M10.11 Lead-induced gout, shoulder
  M10.111 Lead-induced gout, right shoulder
  M10.112 Lead-induced gout, left shoulder
  M10.119 Lead-induced gout, unspecified shoulder
● M10.12 Lead-induced gout, elbow
  M10.121 Lead-induced gout, right elbow
  M10.122 Lead-induced gout, left elbow
  M10.129 Lead-induced gout, unspecified elbow
● M10.13 Lead-induced gout, wrist
  M10.131 Lead-induced gout, right wrist
  M10.132 Lead-induced gout, left wrist
  M10.139 Lead-induced gout, unspecified wrist
● M10.14 Lead-induced gout, hand
  M10.141 Lead-induced gout, right hand
  M10.142 Lead-induced gout, left hand
  M10.149 Lead-induced gout, unspecified hand
● M10.15 Lead-induced gout, hip
  M10.151 Lead-induced gout, right hip
  M10.152 Lead-induced gout, left hip
  M10.159 Lead-induced gout, unspecified hip
● M10.16 Lead-induced gout, knee
  M10.161 Lead-induced gout, right knee
  M10.162 Lead-induced gout, left knee
  M10.169 Lead-induced gout, unspecified knee
● M10.17 Lead-induced gout, ankle and foot
  M10.171 Lead-induced gout, right ankle and foot
  M10.172 Lead-induced gout, left ankle and foot
  M10.179 Lead-induced gout, unspecified ankle and foot
M10.18 Lead-induced gout, vertebrae
M10.19 Lead-induced gout, multiple sites
● M10.2 Drug-induced gout
Use additional code for adverse effect, if applicable, to identify drug (T36-T50 with fifth or sixth character 5)
M10.20 Drug-induced gout, unspecified site
● M10.21 Drug-induced gout, shoulder
  M10.211 Drug-induced gout, right shoulder
  M10.212 Drug-induced gout, left shoulder
  M10.219 Drug-induced gout, unspecified shoulder
● M10.22 Drug-induced gout, elbow
  M10.221 Drug-induced gout, right elbow
  M10.222 Drug-induced gout, left elbow
  M10.229 Drug-induced gout, unspecified elbow
● M10.23 Drug-induced gout, wrist
  M10.231 Drug-induced gout, right wrist
  M10.232 Drug-induced gout, left wrist
  M10.239 Drug-induced gout, unspecified wrist

CHAPTER 13 (M00-M99)

CHAPTER 13 (M00-M99)

● M10.24 Drug-induced gout, hand
     M10.241 Drug-induced gout, right hand
     M10.242 Drug-induced gout, left hand
     M10.249 Drug-induced gout, unspecified hand

● M10.25 Drug-induced gout, hip
     M10.251 Drug-induced gout, right hip
     M10.252 Drug-induced gout, left hip
     M10.259 Drug-induced gout, unspecified hip

● M10.26 Drug-induced gout, knee
     M10.261 Drug-induced gout, right knee
     M10.262 Drug-induced gout, left knee
     M10.269 Drug-induced gout, unspecified knee

● M10.27 Drug-induced gout, ankle and foot
     M10.271 Drug-induced gout, right ankle and foot
     M10.272 Drug-induced gout, left ankle and foot
     M10.279 Drug-induced gout, unspecified ankle and foot

     M10.28 Drug-induced gout, vertebrae
     M10.29 Drug-induced gout, multiple sites

● M10.3 Gout due to renal impairment
     Code also associated renal disease
     M10.30 Gout due to renal impairment, unspecified site

● M10.31 Gout due to renal impairment, shoulder
     M10.311 Gout due to renal impairment, right shoulder
     M10.312 Gout due to renal impairment, left shoulder
     M10.319 Gout due to renal impairment, unspecified shoulder

● M10.32 Gout due to renal impairment, elbow
     M10.321 Gout due to renal impairment, right elbow
     M10.322 Gout due to renal impairment, left elbow
     M10.329 Gout due to renal impairment, unspecified elbow

● M10.33 Gout due to renal impairment, wrist
     M10.331 Gout due to renal impairment, right wrist
     M10.332 Gout due to renal impairment, left wrist
     M10.339 Gout due to renal impairment, unspecified wrist

● M10.34 Gout due to renal impairment, hand
     M10.341 Gout due to renal impairment, right hand
     M10.342 Gout due to renal impairment, left hand
     M10.349 Gout due to renal impairment, unspecified hand

● M10.35 Gout due to renal impairment, hip
     M10.351 Gout due to renal impairment, right hip
     M10.352 Gout due to renal impairment, left hip
     M10.359 Gout due to renal impairment, unspecified hip

● M10.36 Gout due to renal impairment, knee
     M10.361 Gout due to renal impairment, right knee
     M10.362 Gout due to renal impairment, left knee
     M10.369 Gout due to renal impairment, unspecified knee

● M10.37 Gout due to renal impairment, ankle and foot
     M10.371 Gout due to renal impairment, right ankle and foot
     M10.372 Gout due to renal impairment, left ankle and foot
     M10.379 Gout due to renal impairment, unspecified ankle and foot

     M10.38 Gout due to renal impairment, vertebrae
     M10.39 Gout due to renal impairment, multiple sites

● M10.4 Other secondary gout
     Code first associated condition
     M10.40 Other secondary gout, unspecified site

● M10.41 Other secondary gout, shoulder
     M10.411 Other secondary gout, right shoulder
     M10.412 Other secondary gout, left shoulder
     M10.419 Other secondary gout, unspecified shoulder

● M10.42 Other secondary gout, elbow
     M10.421 Other secondary gout, right elbow
     M10.422 Other secondary gout, left elbow
     M10.429 Other secondary gout, unspecified elbow

● M10.43 Other secondary gout, wrist
     M10.431 Other secondary gout, right wrist
     M10.432 Other secondary gout, left wrist
     M10.439 Other secondary gout, unspecified wrist

● M10.44 Other secondary gout, hand
     M10.441 Other secondary gout, right hand
     M10.442 Other secondary gout, left hand
     M10.449 Other secondary gout, unspecified hand

● M10.45 Other secondary gout, hip
     M10.451 Other secondary gout, right hip
     M10.452 Other secondary gout, left hip
     M10.459 Other secondary gout, unspecified hip

● M10.46 Other secondary gout, knee
     M10.461 Other secondary gout, right knee
     M10.462 Other secondary gout, left knee
     M10.469 Other secondary gout, unspecified knee

● M10.47 Other secondary gout, ankle and foot
     M10.471 Other secondary gout, right ankle and foot
     M10.472 Other secondary gout, left ankle and foot
     M10.479 Other secondary gout, unspecified ankle and foot

     M10.48 Other secondary gout, vertebrae
     M10.49 Other secondary gout, multiple sites

     M10.9 Gout, unspecified
         Gout NOS

● M11 Other crystal arthropathies
   ● M11.0 Hydroxyapatite deposition disease
     M11.00 Hydroxyapatite deposition disease, unspecified site

     ● M11.01 Hydroxyapatite deposition disease, shoulder
         M11.011 Hydroxyapatite deposition disease, right shoulder
         M11.012 Hydroxyapatite deposition disease, left shoulder
         M11.019 Hydroxyapatite deposition disease, unspecified shoulder

◄ New   ◄▦ Revised   ~~deleted~~ Deleted   Excludes 1   Excludes 2   Includes   Use additional   Code first   Code also   Unspecified
OGCR Official Guidelines   X Assign placeholder X   ● Use Additional Character(s)   ▶ Manifestation Code   **Coding Clinic**

● M11.02   Hydroxyapatite deposition disease, elbow
    M11.021   Hydroxyapatite deposition disease, right elbow
    M11.022   Hydroxyapatite deposition disease, left elbow
    M11.029   Hydroxyapatite deposition disease, unspecified elbow

● M11.03   Hydroxyapatite deposition disease, wrist
    M11.031   Hydroxyapatite deposition disease, right wrist
    M11.032   Hydroxyapatite deposition disease, left wrist
    M11.039   Hydroxyapatite deposition disease, unspecified wrist

● M11.04   Hydroxyapatite deposition disease, hand
    M11.041   Hydroxyapatite deposition disease, right hand
    M11.042   Hydroxyapatite deposition disease, left hand
    M11.049   Hydroxyapatite deposition disease, unspecified hand

● M11.05   Hydroxyapatite deposition disease, hip
    M11.051   Hydroxyapatite deposition disease, right hip
    M11.052   Hydroxyapatite deposition disease, left hip
    M11.059   Hydroxyapatite deposition disease, unspecified hip

● M11.06   Hydroxyapatite deposition disease, knee
    M11.061   Hydroxyapatite deposition disease, right knee
    M11.062   Hydroxyapatite deposition disease, left knee
    M11.069   Hydroxyapatite deposition disease, unspecified knee

● M11.07   Hydroxyapatite deposition disease, ankle and foot
    M11.071   Hydroxyapatite deposition disease, right ankle and foot
    M11.072   Hydroxyapatite deposition disease, left ankle and foot
    M11.079   Hydroxyapatite deposition disease, unspecified ankle and foot

    M11.08   Hydroxyapatite deposition disease, vertebrae
    M11.09   Hydroxyapatite deposition disease, multiple sites

● M11.1   Familial chondrocalcinosis
    M11.10   Familial chondrocalcinosis, unspecified site
● M11.11   Familial chondrocalcinosis, shoulder
    M11.111   Familial chondrocalcinosis, right shoulder
    M11.112   Familial chondrocalcinosis, left shoulder
    M11.119   Familial chondrocalcinosis, unspecified shoulder

● M11.12   Familial chondrocalcinosis, elbow
    M11.121   Familial chondrocalcinosis, right elbow
    M11.122   Familial chondrocalcinosis, left elbow
    M11.129   Familial chondrocalcinosis, unspecified elbow

● M11.13   Familial chondrocalcinosis, wrist
    M11.131   Familial chondrocalcinosis, right wrist
    M11.132   Familial chondrocalcinosis, left wrist
    M11.139   Familial chondrocalcinosis, unspecified wrist

● M11.14   Familial chondrocalcinosis, hand
    M11.141   Familial chondrocalcinosis, right hand
    M11.142   Familial chondrocalcinosis, left hand
    M11.149   Familial chondrocalcinosis, unspecified hand

● M11.15   Familial chondrocalcinosis, hip
    M11.151   Familial chondrocalcinosis, right hip
    M11.152   Familial chondrocalcinosis, left hip
    M11.159   Familial chondrocalcinosis, unspecified hip

● M11.16   Familial chondrocalcinosis, knee
    M11.161   Familial chondrocalcinosis, right knee
    M11.162   Familial chondrocalcinosis, left knee
    M11.169   Familial chondrocalcinosis, unspecified knee

● M11.17   Familial chondrocalcinosis, ankle and foot
    M11.171   Familial chondrocalcinosis, right ankle and foot
    M11.172   Familial chondrocalcinosis, left ankle and foot
    M11.179   Familial chondrocalcinosis, unspecified ankle and foot

    M11.18   Familial chondrocalcinosis, vertebrae
    M11.19   Familial chondrocalcinosis, multiple sites

● M11.2   Other chondrocalcinosis
    Chondrocalcinosis NOS
    M11.20   Other chondrocalcinosis, unspecified site
● M11.21   Other chondrocalcinosis, shoulder
    M11.211   Other chondrocalcinosis, right shoulder
    M11.212   Other chondrocalcinosis, left shoulder
    M11.219   Other chondrocalcinosis, unspecified shoulder

● M11.22   Other chondrocalcinosis, elbow
    M11.221   Other chondrocalcinosis, right elbow
    M11.222   Other chondrocalcinosis, left elbow
    M11.229   Other chondrocalcinosis, unspecified elbow

● M11.23   Other chondrocalcinosis, wrist
    M11.231   Other chondrocalcinosis, right wrist
    M11.232   Other chondrocalcinosis, left wrist
    M11.239   Other chondrocalcinosis, unspecified wrist

● M11.24   Other chondrocalcinosis, hand
    M11.241   Other chondrocalcinosis, right hand
    M11.242   Other chondrocalcinosis, left hand
    M11.249   Other chondrocalcinosis, unspecified hand

● M11.25   Other chondrocalcinosis, hip
    M11.251   Other chondrocalcinosis, right hip
    M11.252   Other chondrocalcinosis, left hip
    M11.259   Other chondrocalcinosis, unspecified hip

● M11.26   Other chondrocalcinosis, knee
    M11.261   Other chondrocalcinosis, right knee
    M11.262   Other chondrocalcinosis, left knee
    M11.269   Other chondrocalcinosis, unspecified knee

- M11.27 Other chondrocalcinosis, ankle and foot
  - M11.271 Other chondrocalcinosis, right ankle and foot
  - M11.272 Other chondrocalcinosis, left ankle and foot
  - M11.279 Other chondrocalcinosis, unspecified ankle and foot
  - M11.28 Other chondrocalcinosis, vertebrae
  - M11.29 Other chondrocalcinosis, multiple sites
- M11.8 Other specified crystal arthropathies
  - M11.80 Other specified crystal arthropathies, unspecified site
  - M11.81 Other specified crystal arthropathies, shoulder
    - M11.811 Other specified crystal arthropathies, right shoulder
    - M11.812 Other specified crystal arthropathies, left shoulder
    - M11.819 Other specified crystal arthropathies, unspecified shoulder
  - M11.82 Other specified crystal arthropathies, elbow
    - M11.821 Other specified crystal arthropathies, right elbow
    - M11.822 Other specified crystal arthropathies, left elbow
    - M11.829 Other specified crystal arthropathies, unspecified elbow
  - M11.83 Other specified crystal arthropathies, wrist
    - M11.831 Other specified crystal arthropathies, right wrist
    - M11.832 Other specified crystal arthropathies, left wrist
    - M11.839 Other specified crystal arthropathies, unspecified wrist
  - M11.84 Other specified crystal arthropathies, hand
    - M11.841 Other specified crystal arthropathies, right hand
    - M11.842 Other specified crystal arthropathies, left hand
    - M11.849 Other specified crystal arthropathies, unspecified hand
  - M11.85 Other specified crystal arthropathies, hip
    - M11.851 Other specified crystal arthropathies, right hip
    - M11.852 Other specified crystal arthropathies, left hip
    - M11.859 Other specified crystal arthropathies, unspecified hip
  - M11.86 Other specified crystal arthropathies, knee
    - M11.861 Other specified crystal arthropathies, right knee
    - M11.862 Other specified crystal arthropathies, left knee
    - M11.869 Other specified crystal arthropathies, unspecified knee
  - M11.87 Other specified crystal arthropathies, ankle and foot
    - M11.871 Other specified crystal arthropathies, right ankle and foot
    - M11.872 Other specified crystal arthropathies, left ankle and foot
    - M11.879 Other specified crystal arthropathies, unspecified ankle and foot
  - M11.88 Other specified crystal arthropathies, vertebrae
  - M11.89 Other specified crystal arthropathies, multiple sites
- M11.9 Crystal arthropathy, unspecified

- M12 Other and unspecified arthropathy
  - Excludes1 arthrosis (M15-M19)
    cricoarytenoid arthropathy (J38.7)
- M12.0 Chronic postrheumatic arthropathy [Jaccoud]
  - M12.00 Chronic postrheumatic arthropathy [Jaccoud], unspecified site
  - M12.01 Chronic postrheumatic arthropathy [Jaccoud], shoulder
    - M12.011 Chronic postrheumatic arthropathy [Jaccoud], right shoulder
    - M12.012 Chronic postrheumatic arthropathy [Jaccoud], left shoulder
    - M12.019 Chronic postrheumatic arthropathy [Jaccoud], unspecified shoulder
  - M12.02 Chronic postrheumatic arthropathy [Jaccoud], elbow
    - M12.021 Chronic postrheumatic arthropathy [Jaccoud], right elbow
    - M12.022 Chronic postrheumatic arthropathy [Jaccoud], left elbow
    - M12.029 Chronic postrheumatic arthropathy [Jaccoud], unspecified elbow
  - M12.03 Chronic postrheumatic arthropathy [Jaccoud], wrist
    - M12.031 Chronic postrheumatic arthropathy [Jaccoud], right wrist
    - M12.032 Chronic postrheumatic arthropathy [Jaccoud], left wrist
    - M12.039 Chronic postrheumatic arthropathy [Jaccoud], unspecified wrist
  - M12.04 Chronic postrheumatic arthropathy [Jaccoud], hand
    - M12.041 Chronic postrheumatic arthropathy [Jaccoud], right hand
    - M12.042 Chronic postrheumatic arthropathy [Jaccoud], left hand
    - M12.049 Chronic postrheumatic arthropathy [Jaccoud], unspecified hand
  - M12.05 Chronic postrheumatic arthropathy [Jaccoud], hip
    - M12.051 Chronic postrheumatic arthropathy [Jaccoud], right hip
    - M12.052 Chronic postrheumatic arthropathy [Jaccoud], left hip
    - M12.059 Chronic postrheumatic arthropathy [Jaccoud], unspecified hip
  - M12.06 Chronic postrheumatic arthropathy [Jaccoud], knee
    - M12.061 Chronic postrheumatic arthropathy [Jaccoud], right knee
    - M12.062 Chronic postrheumatic arthropathy [Jaccoud], left knee
    - M12.069 Chronic postrheumatic arthropathy [Jaccoud], unspecified knee
  - M12.07 Chronic postrheumatic arthropathy [Jaccoud], ankle and foot
    - M12.071 Chronic postrheumatic arthropathy [Jaccoud], right ankle and foot
    - M12.072 Chronic postrheumatic arthropathy [Jaccoud], left ankle and foot
    - M12.079 Chronic postrheumatic arthropathy [Jaccoud], unspecified ankle and foot
  - M12.08 Chronic postrheumatic arthropathy [Jaccoud], other specified site
    Chronic postrheumatic arthropathy [Jaccoud], vertebrae
  - M12.09 Chronic postrheumatic arthropathy [Jaccoud], multiple sites

◀ New ◀ Revised ~~deleted~~ Deleted Excludes 1 Excludes 2 Includes Use additional Code first Code also Unspecified

OGCR Official Guidelines X Assign placeholder X ● Use Additional Character(s) ▶ Manifestation Code Coding Clinic

● M12.1   **Kaschin-Beck disease**
     Osteochondroarthrosis deformans endemica
    M12.10   Kaschin-Beck disease, unspecified site
● M12.11   Kaschin-Beck disease, shoulder
       M12.111   Kaschin-Beck disease, right shoulder
       M12.112   Kaschin-Beck disease, left shoulder
       M12.119   Kaschin-Beck disease, unspecified shoulder
● M12.12   Kaschin-Beck disease, elbow
       M12.121   Kaschin-Beck disease, right elbow
       M12.122   Kaschin-Beck disease, left elbow
       M12.129   Kaschin-Beck disease, unspecified elbow
● M12.13   Kaschin-Beck disease, wrist
       M12.131   Kaschin-Beck disease, right wrist
       M12.132   Kaschin-Beck disease, left wrist
       M12.139   Kaschin-Beck disease, unspecified wrist
● M12.14   Kaschin-Beck disease, hand
       M12.141   Kaschin-Beck disease, right hand
       M12.142   Kaschin-Beck disease, left hand
       M12.149   Kaschin-Beck disease, unspecified hand
● M12.15   Kaschin-Beck disease, hip
       M12.151   Kaschin-Beck disease, right hip
       M12.152   Kaschin-Beck disease, left hip
       M12.159   Kaschin-Beck disease, unspecified hip
● M12.16   Kaschin-Beck disease, knee
       M12.161   Kaschin-Beck disease, right knee
       M12.162   Kaschin-Beck disease, left knee
       M12.169   Kaschin-Beck disease, unspecified knee
● M12.17   Kaschin-Beck disease, ankle and foot
       M12.171   Kaschin-Beck disease, right ankle and foot
       M12.172   Kaschin-Beck disease, left ankle and foot
       M12.179   Kaschin-Beck disease, unspecified ankle and foot
    M12.18   Kaschin-Beck disease, vertebrae
    M12.19   Kaschin-Beck disease, multiple sites
● M12.2   **Villonodular synovitis (pigmented)**
    M12.20   Villonodular synovitis (pigmented), unspecified site
● M12.21   Villonodular synovitis (pigmented), shoulder
       M12.211   Villonodular synovitis (pigmented), right shoulder
       M12.212   Villonodular synovitis (pigmented), left shoulder
       M12.219   Villonodular synovitis (pigmented), unspecified shoulder
● M12.22   Villonodular synovitis (pigmented), elbow
       M12.221   Villonodular synovitis (pigmented), right elbow
       M12.222   Villonodular synovitis (pigmented), left elbow
       M12.229   Villonodular synovitis (pigmented), unspecified elbow
● M12.23   Villonodular synovitis (pigmented), wrist
       M12.231   Villonodular synovitis (pigmented), right wrist
       M12.232   Villonodular synovitis (pigmented), left wrist
       M12.239   Villonodular synovitis (pigmented), unspecified wrist

● M12.24   Villonodular synovitis (pigmented), hand
       M12.241   Villonodular synovitis (pigmented), right hand
       M12.242   Villonodular synovitis (pigmented), left hand
       M12.249   Villonodular synovitis (pigmented), unspecified hand
● M12.25   Villonodular synovitis (pigmented), hip
       M12.251   Villonodular synovitis (pigmented), right hip
       M12.252   Villonodular synovitis (pigmented), left hip
       M12.259   Villonodular synovitis (pigmented), unspecified hip
● M12.26   Villonodular synovitis (pigmented), knee
       M12.261   Villonodular synovitis (pigmented), right knee
       M12.262   Villonodular synovitis (pigmented), left knee
       M12.269   Villonodular synovitis (pigmented), unspecified knee
● M12.27   Villonodular synovitis (pigmented), ankle and foot
       M12.271   Villonodular synovitis (pigmented), right ankle and foot
       M12.272   Villonodular synovitis (pigmented), left ankle and foot
       M12.279   Villonodular synovitis (pigmented), unspecified ankle and foot
    M12.28   Villonodular synovitis (pigmented), other specified site
      Villonodular synovitis (pigmented), vertebrae
    M12.29   Villonodular synovitis (pigmented), multiple sites
● M12.3   **Palindromic rheumatism**
    M12.30   Palindromic rheumatism, unspecified site
● M12.31   Palindromic rheumatism, shoulder
       M12.311   Palindromic rheumatism, right shoulder
       M12.312   Palindromic rheumatism, left shoulder
       M12.319   Palindromic rheumatism, unspecified shoulder
● M12.32   Palindromic rheumatism, elbow
       M12.321   Palindromic rheumatism, right elbow
       M12.322   Palindromic rheumatism, left elbow
       M12.329   Palindromic rheumatism, unspecified elbow
● M12.33   Palindromic rheumatism, wrist
       M12.331   Palindromic rheumatism, right wrist
       M12.332   Palindromic rheumatism, left wrist
       M12.339   Palindromic rheumatism, unspecified wrist
● M12.34   Palindromic rheumatism, hand
       M12.341   Palindromic rheumatism, right hand
       M12.342   Palindromic rheumatism, left hand
       M12.349   Palindromic rheumatism, unspecified hand
● M12.35   Palindromic rheumatism, hip
       M12.351   Palindromic rheumatism, right hip
       M12.352   Palindromic rheumatism, left hip
       M12.359   Palindromic rheumatism, unspecified hip

CHAPTER 13 (M00-M99)

● **M12.36** Palindromic rheumatism, knee
    M12.361 Palindromic rheumatism, right knee
    M12.362 Palindromic rheumatism, left knee
    M12.369 Palindromic rheumatism, unspecified knee
● **M12.37** Palindromic rheumatism, ankle and foot
    M12.371 Palindromic rheumatism, right ankle and foot
    M12.372 Palindromic rheumatism, left ankle and foot
    M12.379 Palindromic rheumatism, unspecified ankle and foot
    M12.38 Palindromic rheumatism, other specified site
       Palindromic rheumatism, vertebrae
    M12.39 Palindromic rheumatism, multiple sites
● **M12.4** Intermittent hydrarthrosis
    M12.40 Intermittent hydrarthrosis, unspecified site
● **M12.41** Intermittent hydrarthrosis, shoulder
    M12.411 Intermittent hydrarthrosis, right shoulder
    M12.412 Intermittent hydrarthrosis, left shoulder
    M12.419 Intermittent hydrarthrosis, unspecified shoulder
● **M12.42** Intermittent hydrarthrosis, elbow
    M12.421 Intermittent hydrarthrosis, right elbow
    M12.422 Intermittent hydrarthrosis, left elbow
    M12.429 Intermittent hydrarthrosis, unspecified elbow
● **M12.43** Intermittent hydrarthrosis, wrist
    M12.431 Intermittent hydrarthrosis, right wrist
    M12.432 Intermittent hydrarthrosis, left wrist
    M12.439 Intermittent hydrarthrosis, unspecified wrist
● **M12.44** Intermittent hydrarthrosis, hand
    M12.441 Intermittent hydrarthrosis, right hand
    M12.442 Intermittent hydrarthrosis, left hand
    M12.449 Intermittent hydrarthrosis, unspecified hand
● **M12.45** Intermittent hydrarthrosis, hip
    M12.451 Intermittent hydrarthrosis, right hip
    M12.452 Intermittent hydrarthrosis, left hip
    M12.459 Intermittent hydrarthrosis, unspecified hip
● **M12.46** Intermittent hydrarthrosis, knee
    M12.461 Intermittent hydrarthrosis, right knee
    M12.462 Intermittent hydrarthrosis, left knee
    M12.469 Intermittent hydrarthrosis, unspecified knee
● **M12.47** Intermittent hydrarthrosis, ankle and foot
    M12.471 Intermittent hydrarthrosis, right ankle and foot
    M12.472 Intermittent hydrarthrosis, left ankle and foot
    M12.479 Intermittent hydrarthrosis, unspecified ankle and foot
    M12.48 Intermittent hydrarthrosis, other site
    M12.49 Intermittent hydrarthrosis, multiple sites

● **M12.5** Traumatic arthropathy
    Excludes1 current injury-see Alphabetic Index
        post-traumatic osteoarthritis of first carpometacarpal joint (M18.2-M18.3)
        post-traumatic osteoarthritis of hip (M16.4-M16.5)
        post-traumatic osteoarthritis of knee (M17.2-M17.3)
        post-traumatic osteoarthritis NOS (M19.1-)
        post-traumatic osteoarthritis of other single joints (M19.1-)
    M12.50 Traumatic arthropathy, unspecified site
● **M12.51** Traumatic arthropathy, shoulder
    M12.511 Traumatic arthropathy, right shoulder
    M12.512 Traumatic arthropathy, left shoulder
    M12.519 Traumatic arthropathy, unspecified shoulder
● **M12.52** Traumatic arthropathy, elbow
    M12.521 Traumatic arthropathy, right elbow
    M12.522 Traumatic arthropathy, left elbow
    M12.529 Traumatic arthropathy, unspecified elbow
● **M12.53** Traumatic arthropathy, wrist
    M12.531 Traumatic arthropathy, right wrist
    M12.532 Traumatic arthropathy, left wrist
    M12.539 Traumatic arthropathy, unspecified wrist
● **M12.54** Traumatic arthropathy, hand
    M12.541 Traumatic arthropathy, right hand
    M12.542 Traumatic arthropathy, left hand
    M12.549 Traumatic arthropathy, unspecified hand
● **M12.55** Traumatic arthropathy, hip
    M12.551 Traumatic arthropathy, right hip
    M12.552 Traumatic arthropathy, left hip
        Coding Clinic: 2015, Q1, P17
    M12.559 Traumatic arthropathy, unspecified hip
● **M12.56** Traumatic arthropathy, knee
    M12.561 Traumatic arthropathy, right knee
    M12.562 Traumatic arthropathy, left knee
    M12.569 Traumatic arthropathy, unspecified knee
● **M12.57** Traumatic arthropathy, ankle and foot
    M12.571 Traumatic arthropathy, right ankle and foot
    M12.572 Traumatic arthropathy, left ankle and foot
    M12.579 Traumatic arthropathy, unspecified ankle and foot
    M12.58 Traumatic arthropathy, other specified site
       Traumatic arthropathy, vertebrae
    M12.59 Traumatic arthropathy, multiple sites
● **M12.8** Other specific arthropathies, not elsewhere classified
       Transient arthropathy
    M12.80 Other specific arthropathies, not elsewhere classified, unspecified site
● **M12.81** Other specific arthropathies, not elsewhere classified, shoulder
    M12.811 Other specific arthropathies, not elsewhere classified, right shoulder
    M12.812 Other specific arthropathies, not elsewhere classified, left shoulder
    M12.819 Other specific arthropathies, not elsewhere classified, unspecified shoulder

◄ New   ◄▯▯ Revised   ~~deleted~~ Deleted   Excludes 1   Excludes 2   Includes   Use additional   Code first   Code also   Unspecified
OGCR Official Guidelines   **X** Assign placeholder X   ● Use Additional Character(s)   ▶ Manifestation Code   **Coding Clinic**

● M12.82 Other specific arthropathies, not elsewhere classified, elbow

M12.821 Other specific arthropathies, not elsewhere classified, right elbow

M12.822 Other specific arthropathies, not elsewhere classified, left elbow

M12.829 Other specific arthropathies, not elsewhere classified, unspecified elbow

● M12.83 Other specific arthropathies, not elsewhere classified, wrist

M12.831 Other specific arthropathies, not elsewhere classified, right wrist

M12.832 Other specific arthropathies, not elsewhere classified, left wrist

M12.839 Other specific arthropathies, not elsewhere classified, unspecified wrist

● M12.84 Other specific arthropathies, not elsewhere classified, hand

M12.841 Other specific arthropathies, not elsewhere classified, right hand

M12.842 Other specific arthropathies, not elsewhere classified, left hand

M12.849 Other specific arthropathies, not elsewhere classified, unspecified hand

● M12.85 Other specific arthropathies, not elsewhere classified, hip

M12.851 Other specific arthropathies, not elsewhere classified, right hip

M12.852 Other specific arthropathies, not elsewhere classified, left hip

M12.859 Other specific arthropathies, not elsewhere classified, unspecified hip

● M12.86 Other specific arthropathies, not elsewhere classified, knee

M12.861 Other specific arthropathies, not elsewhere classified, right knee

M12.862 Other specific arthropathies, not elsewhere classified, left knee

M12.869 Other specific arthropathies, not elsewhere classified, unspecified knee

● M12.87 Other specific arthropathies, not elsewhere classified, ankle and foot

M12.871 Other specific arthropathies, not elsewhere classified, right ankle and foot

M12.872 Other specific arthropathies, not elsewhere classified, left ankle and foot

M12.879 Other specific arthropathies, not elsewhere classified, unspecified ankle and foot

M12.88 Other specific arthropathies, not elsewhere classified, other specified site

Other specific arthropathies, not elsewhere classified, vertebrae

M12.89 Other specific arthropathies, not elsewhere classified, multiple sites

M12.9 Arthropathy, unspecified

● M13 Other arthritis

Excludes1 arthrosis (M15-M19)
osteoarthritis (M15-M19)

M13.0 Polyarthritis, unspecified

● M13.1 Monoarthritis, not elsewhere classified

M13.10 Monoarthritis, not elsewhere classified, unspecified site

● M13.11 Monoarthritis, not elsewhere classified, shoulder

M13.111 Monoarthritis, not elsewhere classified, right shoulder

M13.112 Monoarthritis, not elsewhere classified, left shoulder

M13.119 Monoarthritis, not elsewhere classified, unspecified shoulder

● M13.12 Monoarthritis, not elsewhere classified, elbow

M13.121 Monoarthritis, not elsewhere classified, right elbow

M13.122 Monoarthritis, not elsewhere classified, left elbow

M13.129 Monoarthritis, not elsewhere classified, unspecified elbow

● M13.13 Monoarthritis, not elsewhere classified, wrist

M13.131 Monoarthritis, not elsewhere classified, right wrist

M13.132 Monoarthritis, not elsewhere classified, left wrist

M13.139 Monoarthritis, not elsewhere classified, unspecified wrist

● M13.14 Monoarthritis, not elsewhere classified, hand

M13.141 Monoarthritis, not elsewhere classified, right hand

M13.142 Monoarthritis, not elsewhere classified, left hand

M13.149 Monoarthritis, not elsewhere classified, unspecified hand

● M13.15 Monoarthritis, not elsewhere classified, hip

M13.151 Monoarthritis, not elsewhere classified, right hip

M13.152 Monoarthritis, not elsewhere classified, left hip

M13.159 Monoarthritis, not elsewhere classified, unspecified hip

● M13.16 Monoarthritis, not elsewhere classified, knee

M13.161 Monoarthritis, not elsewhere classified, right knee

M13.162 Monoarthritis, not elsewhere classified, left knee

M13.169 Monoarthritis, not elsewhere classified, unspecified knee

● M13.17 Monoarthritis, not elsewhere classified, ankle and foot

M13.171 Monoarthritis, not elsewhere classified, right ankle and foot

M13.172 Monoarthritis, not elsewhere classified, left ankle and foot

M13.179 Monoarthritis, not elsewhere classified, unspecified ankle and foot

● **M13.8**   **Other specified arthritis**
Allergic arthritis
> **Excludes1**   osteoarthritis (M15-M19)

     M13.80   Other specified arthritis, unspecified site
● **M13.81**   Other specified arthritis, shoulder
        M13.811   Other specified arthritis, right shoulder
        M13.812   Other specified arthritis, left shoulder
        M13.819   Other specified arthritis, unspecified shoulder
● **M13.82**   Other specified arthritis, elbow
        M13.821   Other specified arthritis, right elbow
        M13.822   Other specified arthritis, left elbow
        M13.829   Other specified arthritis, unspecified elbow
● **M13.83**   Other specified arthritis, wrist
        M13.831   Other specified arthritis, right wrist
        M13.832   Other specified arthritis, left wrist
        M13.839   Other specified arthritis, unspecified wrist
● **M13.84**   Other specified arthritis, hand
        M13.841   Other specified arthritis, right hand
        M13.842   Other specified arthritis, left hand
        M13.849   Other specified arthritis, unspecified hand
● **M13.85**   Other specified arthritis, hip
        M13.851   Other specified arthritis, right hip
        M13.852   Other specified arthritis, left hip
        M13.859   Other specified arthritis, unspecified hip
● **M13.86**   Other specified arthritis, knee
        M13.861   Other specified arthritis, right knee
        M13.862   Other specified arthritis, left knee
        M13.869   Other specified arthritis, unspecified knee
● **M13.87**   Other specified arthritis, ankle and foot
        M13.871   Other specified arthritis, right ankle and foot
        M13.872   Other specified arthritis, left ankle and foot
        M13.879   Other specified arthritis, unspecified ankle and foot
     M13.88   Other specified arthritis, other site
     M13.89   Other specified arthritis, multiple sites

● **M14**   **Arthropathies in other diseases classified elsewhere**
> **Excludes1**   arthropathy in:
>   diabetes mellitus (E08-E13 with .61-)
>   hematological disorders (M36.2-M36.3)
>   hypersensitivity reactions (M36.4)
>   neoplastic disease (M36.1)
>   neurosyphillis (A52.16)
>   sarcoidosis (D86.86)
>   enteropathic arthropathies (M07.0-)
>   juvenile psoriatic arthropathy (L40.54)
>   lipoid dermatoarthritis (E78.81)

● **M14.6**   **Charcôt's joint**
Neuropathic arthropathy
> **Excludes1**   Charcôt's joint in diabetes mellitus (E08-E13 with .610)
>   Charcôt's joint in tabes dorsalis (A52.16)

     M14.60   Charcôt's joint, unspecified site
● **M14.61**   Charcôt's joint, shoulder
        M14.611   Charcôt's joint, right shoulder
        M14.612   Charcôt's joint, left shoulder
        M14.619   Charcôt's joint, unspecified shoulder

● **M14.62**   Charcôt's joint, elbow
        M14.621   Charcôt's joint, right elbow
        M14.622   Charcôt's joint, left elbow
        M14.629   Charcôt's joint, unspecified elbow
● **M14.63**   Charcôt's joint, wrist
        M14.631   Charcôt's joint, right wrist
        M14.632   Charcôt's joint, left wrist
        M14.639   Charcôt's joint, unspecified wrist
● **M14.64**   Charcôt's joint, hand
        M14.641   Charcôt's joint, right hand
        M14.642   Charcôt's joint, left hand
        M14.649   Charcôt's joint, unspecified hand
● **M14.65**   Charcôt's joint, hip
        M14.651   Charcôt's joint, right hip
        M14.652   Charcôt's joint, left hip
        M14.659   Charcôt's joint, unspecified hip
● **M14.66**   Charcôt's joint, knee
        M14.661   Charcôt's joint, right knee
        M14.662   Charcôt's joint, left knee
        M14.669   Charcôt's joint, unspecified knee
● **M14.67**   Charcôt's joint, ankle and foot
        M14.671   Charcôt's joint, right ankle and foot
        M14.672   Charcôt's joint, left ankle and foot
        M14.679   Charcôt's joint, unspecified ankle and foot
     M14.68   Charcôt's joint, vertebrae
     M14.69   Charcôt's joint, multiple sites

● **M14.8**   **Arthropathies in other specified diseases classified elsewhere**
> *Code first* underlying disease, such as:
>   amyloidosis (E85.-)
>   erythema multiforme (L51.-)
>   erythema nodosum (L52)
>   hemochromatosis (E83.11-)
>   hyperparathyroidism (E21.-)
>   hypothyroidism (E00-E03)
>   sickle-cell disorders (D57.-)
>   thyrotoxicosis [hyperthyroidism] (E05.-)
>   Whipple's disease (K90.81)

▌ *M14.80*   *Arthropathies in other specified diseases classified elsewhere, unspecified site*
● **M14.81**   Arthropathies in other specified diseases classified elsewhere, shoulder
    ▌ *M14.811*   *Arthropathies in other specified diseases classified elsewhere, right shoulder*
    ▌ *M14.812*   *Arthropathies in other specified diseases classified elsewhere, left shoulder*
    ▌ *M14.819*   *Arthropathies in other specified diseases classified elsewhere, unspecified shoulder*
● **M14.82**   Arthropathies in other specified diseases classified elsewhere, elbow
    ▌ *M14.821*   *Arthropathies in other specified diseases classified elsewhere, right elbow*
    ▌ *M14.822*   *Arthropathies in other specified diseases classified elsewhere, left elbow*
    ▌ *M14.829*   *Arthropathies in other specified diseases classified elsewhere, unspecified elbow*

◄ New   ◄▥ Revised   ~~deleted~~ Deleted   Excludes 1   Excludes 2   Includes   Use additional   Code first   Code also   Unspecified

OGCR Official Guidelines   **X** Assign placeholder X   ● Use Additional Character(s)   ▌ Manifestation Code   **Coding Clinic**

● **M14.83** Arthropathies in other specified diseases classified elsewhere, wrist

   ▮ *M14.831*   *Arthropathies in other specified diseases classified elsewhere, right wrist*

   ▮ *M14.832*   *Arthropathies in other specified diseases classified elsewhere, left wrist*

   ▮ *M14.839*   *Arthropathies in other specified diseases classified elsewhere, unspecified wrist*

● **M14.84** Arthropathies in other specified diseases classified elsewhere, hand

   ▮ *M14.841*   *Arthropathies in other specified diseases classified elsewhere, right hand*

   ▮ *M14.842*   *Arthropathies in other specified diseases classified elsewhere, left hand*

   ▮ *M14.849*   *Arthropathies in other specified diseases classified elsewhere, unspecified hand*

● **M14.85** Arthropathies in other specified diseases classified elsewhere, hip

   ▮ *M14.851*   *Arthropathies in other specified diseases classified elsewhere, right hip*

   ▮ *M14.852*   *Arthropathies in other specified diseases classified elsewhere, left hip*

   ▮ *M14.859*   *Arthropathies in other specified diseases classified elsewhere, unspecified hip*

● **M14.86** Arthropathies in other specified diseases classified elsewhere, knee

   ▮ *M14.861*   *Arthropathies in other specified diseases classified elsewhere, right knee*

   ▮ *M14.862*   *Arthropathies in other specified diseases classified elsewhere, left knee*

   ▮ *M14.869*   *Arthropathies in other specified diseases classified elsewhere, unspecified knee*

● **M14.87** Arthropathies in other specified diseases classified elsewhere, ankle and foot

   ▮ *M14.871*   *Arthropathies in other specified diseases classified elsewhere, right ankle and foot*

   ▮ *M14.872*   *Arthropathies in other specified diseases classified elsewhere, left ankle and foot*

   ▮ *M14.879*   *Arthropathies in other specified diseases classified elsewhere, unspecified ankle and foot*

   ▮ *M14.88*   *Arthropathies in other specified diseases classified elsewhere, vertebrae*

   ▮ *M14.89*   *Arthropathies in other specified diseases classified elsewhere, multiple sites*

OSTEOARTHRITIS (M15-M19)

Osteoarthritis is the most common degenerative joint disease and form of arthritis that breaks down the cartilage causing pain, swelling, and reduced motion in the joints.

   Excludes2   osteoarthritis of spine (M47.-)

● **M15** Polyosteoarthritis

   Includes   arthritis of multiple sites

   Excludes1   bilateral involvement of single joint (M16-M19)

   M15.0 Primary generalized (osteo)arthritis

   M15.1 Heberden's nodes (with arthropathy)
       Interphalangeal distal osteoarthritis

   M15.2 Bouchard's nodes (with arthropathy)
       Juxtaphalangeal distal osteoarthritis

   M15.3 Secondary multiple arthritis
       Post-traumatic polyosteoarthritis

   M15.4 Erosive (osteo)arthritis

   M15.8 Other polyosteoarthritis

   M15.9 Polyosteoarthritis, unspecified
       Generalized osteoarthritis NOS

● **M16** Osteoarthritis of hip

   M16.0 Bilateral primary osteoarthritis of hip

  ● **M16.1** Unilateral primary osteoarthritis of hip
       Primary osteoarthritis of hip NOS

     M16.10 Unilateral primary osteoarthritis, unspecified hip

     M16.11 Unilateral primary osteoarthritis, right hip

     M16.12 Unilateral primary osteoarthritis, left hip

   M16.2 Bilateral osteoarthritis resulting from hip dysplasia

  ● **M16.3** Unilateral osteoarthritis resulting from hip dysplasia
       Dysplastic osteoarthritis of hip NOS

     M16.30 Unilateral osteoarthritis resulting from hip dysplasia, unspecified hip

     M16.31 Unilateral osteoarthritis resulting from hip dysplasia, right hip

     M16.32 Unilateral osteoarthritis resulting from hip dysplasia, left hip

   M16.4 Bilateral post-traumatic osteoarthritis of hip

  ● **M16.5** Unilateral post-traumatic osteoarthritis of hip
       Post-traumatic osteoarthritis of hip NOS

     M16.50 Unilateral post-traumatic osteoarthritis, unspecified hip

     M16.51 Unilateral post-traumatic osteoarthritis, right hip

     M16.52 Unilateral post-traumatic osteoarthritis, left hip

   M16.6 Other bilateral secondary osteoarthritis of hip

   M16.7 Other unilateral secondary osteoarthritis of hip
       Secondary osteoarthritis of hip NOS

   M16.9 Osteoarthritis of hip, unspecified

● **M17** Osteoarthritis of knee

   M17.0 Bilateral primary osteoarthritis of knee

  ● **M17.1** Unilateral primary osteoarthritis of knee
       Primary osteoarthritis of knee NOS

     M17.10 Unilateral primary osteoarthritis, unspecified knee

     M17.11 Unilateral primary osteoarthritis, right knee

     M17.12 Unilateral primary osteoarthritis, left knee

   M17.2 Bilateral post-traumatic osteoarthritis of knee

  ● **M17.3** Unilateral post-traumatic osteoarthritis of knee
       Post-traumatic osteoarthritis of knee NOS

     M17.30 Unilateral post-traumatic osteoarthritis, unspecified knee

     M17.31 Unilateral post-traumatic osteoarthritis, right knee

     M17.32 Unilateral post-traumatic osteoarthritis, left knee

   M17.4 Other bilateral secondary osteoarthritis of knee

   M17.5 Other unilateral secondary osteoarthritis of knee
       Secondary osteoarthritis of knee NOS

   M17.9 Osteoarthritis of knee, unspecified

● **M18** Osteoarthritis of first carpometacarpal joint

   M18.0 Bilateral primary osteoarthritis of first carpometacarpal joints

  ● **M18.1** Unilateral primary osteoarthritis of first carpometacarpal joint
       Primary osteoarthritis of first carpometacarpal joint NOS

     M18.10 Unilateral primary osteoarthritis of first carpometacarpal joint, unspecified hand

     M18.11 Unilateral primary osteoarthritis of first carpometacarpal joint, right hand

     M18.12 Unilateral primary osteoarthritis of first carpometacarpal joint, left hand

CHAPTER 13 (M00-M99)

CHAPTER 13 (M00-M99)

M18.2 **Bilateral post-traumatic osteoarthritis of first carpometacarpal joints**

● M18.3 **Unilateral post-traumatic osteoarthritis of first carpometacarpal joint**
Post-traumatic osteoarthritis of first carpometacarpal joint NOS

M18.30 Unilateral post-traumatic osteoarthritis of first carpometacarpal joint, unspecified hand

M18.31 Unilateral post-traumatic osteoarthritis of first carpometacarpal joint, right hand

M18.32 Unilateral post-traumatic osteoarthritis of first carpometacarpal joint, left hand

M18.4 **Other bilateral secondary osteoarthritis of first carpometacarpal joints**

● M18.5 **Other unilateral secondary osteoarthritis of first carpometacarpal joint**
Secondary osteoarthritis of first carpometacarpal joint NOS

M18.50 Other unilateral secondary osteoarthritis of first carpometacarpal joint, unspecified hand

M18.51 Other unilateral secondary osteoarthritis of first carpometacarpal joint, right hand

M18.52 Other unilateral secondary osteoarthritis of first carpometacarpal joint, left hand

M18.9 **Osteoarthritis of first carpometacarpal joint, unspecified**

● M19 **Other and unspecified osteoarthritis**
Excludes1 polyarthritis (M15.-)
Excludes2 arthrosis of spine (M47.-)
hallux rigidus (M20.2)
osteoarthritis of spine (M47.-)

● M19.0 **Primary osteoarthritis of other joints**

● M19.01 **Primary osteoarthritis, shoulder**
M19.011 Primary osteoarthritis, right shoulder
M19.012 Primary osteoarthritis, left shoulder
M19.019 Primary osteoarthritis, unspecified shoulder

● M19.02 **Primary osteoarthritis, elbow**
M19.021 Primary osteoarthritis, right elbow
M19.022 Primary osteoarthritis, left elbow
M19.029 Primary osteoarthritis, unspecified elbow

● M19.03 **Primary osteoarthritis, wrist**
M19.031 Primary osteoarthritis, right wrist
M19.032 Primary osteoarthritis, left wrist
M19.039 Primary osteoarthritis, unspecified wrist

● M19.04 **Primary osteoarthritis, hand**
Excludes2 primary osteoarthritis of first carpometacarpal joint (M18.0-, M18.1-)
M19.041 Primary osteoarthritis, right hand
M19.042 Primary osteoarthritis, left hand
M19.049 Primary osteoarthritis, unspecified hand

● M19.07 **Primary osteoarthritis ankle and foot**
M19.071 Primary osteoarthritis, right ankle and foot
M19.072 Primary osteoarthritis, left ankle and foot
M19.079 Primary osteoarthritis, unspecified ankle and foot

● M19.1 **Post-traumatic osteoarthritis of other joints**

● M19.11 **Post-traumatic osteoarthritis, shoulder**
M19.111 Post-traumatic osteoarthritis, right shoulder
M19.112 Post-traumatic osteoarthritis, left shoulder
M19.119 Post-traumatic osteoarthritis, unspecified shoulder

● M19.12 **Post-traumatic osteoarthritis, elbow**
M19.121 Post-traumatic osteoarthritis, right elbow
M19.122 Post-traumatic osteoarthritis, left elbow
M19.129 Post-traumatic osteoarthritis, unspecified elbow

● M19.13 **Post-traumatic osteoarthritis, wrist**
M19.131 Post-traumatic osteoarthritis, right wrist
M19.132 Post-traumatic osteoarthritis, left wrist
M19.139 Post-traumatic osteoarthritis, unspecified wrist

● M19.14 **Post-traumatic osteoarthritis, hand**
Excludes2 post-traumatic osteoarthritis of first carpometacarpal joint (M18.2-, M18.3-)
M19.141 Post-traumatic osteoarthritis, right hand
M19.142 Post-traumatic osteoarthritis, left hand
M19.149 Post-traumatic osteoarthritis, unspecified hand

● M19.17 **Post-traumatic osteoarthritis, ankle and foot**
M19.171 Post-traumatic osteoarthritis, right ankle and foot
M19.172 Post-traumatic osteoarthritis, left ankle and foot
M19.179 Post-traumatic osteoarthritis, unspecified ankle and foot

● M19.2 **Secondary osteoarthritis of other joints**

● M19.21 **Secondary osteoarthritis, shoulder**
M19.211 Secondary osteoarthritis, right shoulder
M19.212 Secondary osteoarthritis, left shoulder
M19.219 Secondary osteoarthritis, unspecified shoulder

● M19.22 **Secondary osteoarthritis, elbow**
M19.221 Secondary osteoarthritis, right elbow
M19.222 Secondary osteoarthritis, left elbow
M19.229 Secondary osteoarthritis, unspecified elbow

● M19.23 **Secondary osteoarthritis, wrist**
M19.231 Secondary osteoarthritis, right wrist
M19.232 Secondary osteoarthritis, left wrist
M19.239 Secondary osteoarthritis, unspecified wrist

● M19.24 **Secondary osteoarthritis, hand**
M19.241 Secondary osteoarthritis, right hand
M19.242 Secondary osteoarthritis, left hand
M19.249 Secondary osteoarthritis, unspecified hand

● M19.27 **Secondary osteoarthritis, ankle and foot**
M19.271 Secondary osteoarthritis, right ankle and foot
M19.272 Secondary osteoarthritis, left ankle and foot
M19.279 Secondary osteoarthritis, unspecified ankle and foot

◄ New   ◄▥ Revised   ~~deleted~~ Deleted   Excludes 1   Excludes 2   Includes   Use additional   Code first   Code also   Unspecified
OGCR Official Guidelines   X Assign placeholder X   ● Use Additional Character(s)   ▶ Manifestation Code   **Coding Clinic**

● **M19.9 Osteoarthritis, unspecified site**

     M19.90 Unspecified osteoarthritis, unspecified site
        Arthrosis NOS
        Arthritis NOS
        Osteoarthritis NOS

     M19.91 Primary osteoarthritis, unspecified site
        Primary osteoarthritis NOS

     M19.92 Post-traumatic osteoarthritis, unspecified site
        Post-traumatic osteoarthritis NOS

     M19.93 Secondary osteoarthritis, unspecified site
        Secondary osteoarthritis NOS

OTHER JOINT DISORDERS (M20-M25)

Excludes2   joints of the spine (M40-M54)

● **M20 Acquired deformities of fingers and toes**

     Excludes1   acquired absence of fingers and toes (Z89.-)
        congenital absence of fingers and toes (Q71.3-, Q72.3-)
        congenital deformities and malformations of fingers and toes (Q66.-, Q68-Q70, Q74.-)

● **M20.0 Deformity of finger(s)**

     Excludes1   clubbing of fingers (R68.3)
        palmar fascial fibromatosis [Dupuytren] (M72.0)
        trigger finger (M65.3)

    ● **M20.00 Unspecified deformity of finger(s)**

       M20.001 Unspecified deformity of right finger(s)

       M20.002 Unspecified deformity of left finger(s)

       M20.009 Unspecified deformity of unspecified finger(s)

    ● **M20.01 Mallet finger**

       M20.011 Mallet finger of right finger(s)

       M20.012 Mallet finger of left finger(s)

       M20.019 Mallet finger of unspecified finger(s)

    ● **M20.02 Boutonnière deformity**

       M20.021 Boutonnière deformity of right finger(s)

       M20.022 Boutonnière deformity of left finger(s)

       M20.029 Boutonnière deformity of unspecified finger(s)

    ● **M20.03 Swan-neck deformity**

       M20.031 Swan-neck deformity of right finger(s)

       M20.032 Swan-neck deformity of left finger(s)

       M20.039 Swan-neck deformity of unspecified finger(s)

    ● **M20.09 Other deformity of finger(s)**

       M20.091 Other deformity of right finger(s)

       M20.092 Other deformity of left finger(s)

       M20.099 Other deformity of finger(s), unspecified finger(s)

● **M20.1 Hallux valgus (acquired)**
    Bunion

     M20.10 Hallux valgus (acquired), unspecified foot

     M20.11 Hallux valgus (acquired), right foot

     M20.12 Hallux valgus (acquired), left foot

● **M20.2 Hallux rigidus**

     M20.20 Hallux rigidus, unspecified foot

     M20.21 Hallux rigidus, right foot

     M20.22 Hallux rigidus, left foot

● **M20.3 Hallux varus (acquired)**

     M20.30 Hallux varus (acquired), unspecified foot

     M20.31 Hallux varus (acquired), right foot

     M20.32 Hallux varus (acquired), left foot

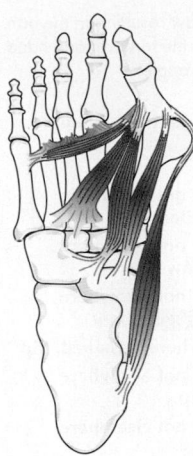

Figure 13-1   Hallux valgus or bunion.

Item 13-2   Hallux valgus or bunion is a sometimes painful structural deformity caused by an inflammation of the bursal sac at the base of the metatarsophalangeal joint (big toe). **Hallus varus** is a deviation of the great toe to the inner side of the foot or away from the next toe.

Item 13-3   Cubitus valgus is a deformity of the elbow resulting in an increased carrying angle in which the arm extends at the side and the palm faces forward, which results in the forearm and hand extended at a greater than 15 degrees.

● **M20.4 Other hammer toe(s) (acquired)**

     M20.40 Other hammer toe(s) (acquired), unspecified foot

     M20.41 Other hammer toe(s) (acquired), right foot

     M20.42 Other hammer toe(s) (acquired), left foot

● **M20.5 Other deformities of toe(s) (acquired)**

    ● **M20.5X Other deformities of toe(s) (acquired)**

       M20.5X1 Other deformities of toe(s) (acquired), right foot

       M20.5X2 Other deformities of toe(s) (acquired), left foot

       M20.5X9 Other deformities of toe(s) (acquired), unspecified foot

● **M20.6 Acquired deformities of toe(s), unspecified**

     M20.60 Acquired deformities of toe(s), unspecified, unspecified foot

     M20.61 Acquired deformities of toe(s), unspecified, right foot

     M20.62 Acquired deformities of toe(s), unspecified, left foot

● **M21 Other acquired deformities of limbs**

     Excludes1   acquired absence of limb (Z89.-)
        congenital absence of limbs (Q71-Q73)
        congenital deformities and malformations of limbs (Q65-Q66, Q68-Q74)

     Excludes2   acquired deformities of fingers or toes (M20.-)
        coxa plana (M91.2)

● **M21.0 Valgus deformity, not elsewhere classified**

     Excludes1   metatarsus valgus (Q66.6)
        talipes calcaneovalgus (Q66.4)

     M21.00 Valgus deformity, not elsewhere classified, unspecified site

CHAPTER 13 (M00-M99)

Item 13-4   Cubitus varus is a deformity of the elbow resulting in the arm extended at the side and the palm facing forward so that the forearm and hand are held at less than 5 degrees, decreasing the carrying angle.

● M21.02   Valgus deformity, not elsewhere classified, elbow
     Cubitus valgus
   M21.021   Valgus deformity, not elsewhere classified, right elbow
   M21.022   Valgus deformity, not elsewhere classified, left elbow
   M21.029   Valgus deformity, not elsewhere classified, unspecified elbow

● M21.05   Valgus deformity, not elsewhere classified, hip
   M21.051   Valgus deformity, not elsewhere classified, right hip
   M21.052   Valgus deformity, not elsewhere classified, left hip
   M21.059   Valgus deformity, not elsewhere classified, unspecified hip

● M21.06   Valgus deformity, not elsewhere classified, knee
     Genu valgum
     Knock knee
   M21.061   Valgus deformity, not elsewhere classified, right knee
   M21.062   Valgus deformity, not elsewhere classified, left knee
   M21.069   Valgus deformity, not elsewhere classified, unspecified knee

● M21.07   Valgus deformity, not elsewhere classified, ankle
   M21.071   Valgus deformity, not elsewhere classified, right ankle
   M21.072   Valgus deformity, not elsewhere classified, left ankle
   M21.079   Valgus deformity, not elsewhere classified, unspecified ankle

● M21.1   Varus deformity, not elsewhere classified
   Excludes1   metatarsus varus (Q66.2)
              tibia vara (M92.5)
   M21.10   Varus deformity, not elsewhere classified, unspecified site

● M21.12   Varus deformity, not elsewhere classified, elbow
     Cubitus varus, elbow
   M21.121   Varus deformity, not elsewhere classified, right elbow
   M21.122   Varus deformity, not elsewhere classified, left elbow
   M21.129   Varus deformity, not elsewhere classified, unspecified elbow

● M21.15   Varus deformity, not elsewhere classified, hip
   M21.151   Varus deformity, not elsewhere classified, right hip
   M21.152   Varus deformity, not elsewhere classified, left hip
   M21.159   Varus deformity, not elsewhere classified, unspecified

● M21.16   Varus deformity, not elsewhere classified, knee
     Bow leg
     Genu varum
   M21.161   Varus deformity, not elsewhere classified, right knee
   M21.162   Varus deformity, not elsewhere classified, left knee
   M21.169   Varus deformity, not elsewhere classified, unspecified knee

● M21.17   Varus deformity, not elsewhere classified, ankle
   M21.171   Varus deformity, not elsewhere classified, right ankle
   M21.172   Varus deformity, not elsewhere classified, left ankle
   M21.179   Varus deformity, not elsewhere classified, unspecified ankle

● M21.2   Flexion deformity
   M21.20   Flexion deformity, unspecified site
● M21.21   Flexion deformity, shoulder
   M21.211   Flexion deformity, right shoulder
   M21.212   Flexion deformity, left shoulder
   M21.219   Flexion deformity, unspecified shoulder
● M21.22   Flexion deformity, elbow
   M21.221   Flexion deformity, right elbow
   M21.222   Flexion deformity, left elbow
   M21.229   Flexion deformity, unspecified elbow
● M21.23   Flexion deformity, wrist
   M21.231   Flexion deformity, right wrist
   M21.232   Flexion deformity, left wrist
   M21.239   Flexion deformity, unspecified wrist
● M21.24   Flexion deformity, finger joints
   M21.241   Flexion deformity, right finger joints
   M21.242   Flexion deformity, left finger joints
   M21.249   Flexion deformity, unspecified finger joints
● M21.25   Flexion deformity, hip
   M21.251   Flexion deformity, right hip
   M21.252   Flexion deformity, left hip
   M21.259   Flexion deformity, unspecified hip
● M21.26   Flexion deformity, knee
   M21.261   Flexion deformity, right knee
   M21.262   Flexion deformity, left knee
   M21.269   Flexion deformity, unspecified knee
● M21.27   Flexion deformity, ankle and toes
   M21.271   Flexion deformity, right ankle and toes
   M21.272   Flexion deformity, left ankle and toes
   M21.279   Flexion deformity, unspecified ankle and toes

● M21.3   Wrist or foot drop (acquired)
● M21.33   Wrist drop (acquired)
   M21.331   Wrist drop, right wrist
   M21.332   Wrist drop, left wrist
   M21.339   Wrist drop, unspecified wrist
● M21.37   Foot drop (acquired)
   M21.371   Foot drop, right foot
   M21.372   Foot drop, left foot
   M21.379   Foot drop, unspecified foot

● M21.4   Flat foot [pes planus] (acquired)
   Excludes1   congenital pes planus (Q66.5-)
   M21.40   Flat foot [pes planus] (acquired), unspecified foot
   M21.41   Flat foot [pes planus] (acquired), right foot
   M21.42   Flat foot [pes planus] (acquired), left foot

● M21.5   Acquired clawhand, clubhand, clawfoot and clubfoot
   Excludes1   clubfoot, not specified as acquired (Q66.89)
● M21.51   Acquired clawhand
   M21.511   Acquired clawhand, right hand
   M21.512   Acquired clawhand, left hand
   M21.519   Acquired clawhand, unspecified hand

◀ New   ⬅ Revised   ~~deleted~~ Deleted   Excludes 1   Excludes 2   Includes   Use additional   Code first   Code also   Unspecified
OGCR Official Guidelines   **X** Assign placeholder X   ● Use Additional Character(s)   ▶ Manifestation Code   **Coding Clinic**

● **M21.52**   **Acquired clubhand**
   M21.521   Acquired clubhand, right hand
   M21.522   Acquired clubhand, left hand
   M21.529   Acquired clubhand, unspecified hand

● **M21.53**   **Acquired clawfoot**
   M21.531   Acquired clawfoot, right foot
   M21.532   Acquired clawfoot, left foot
   M21.539   Acquired clawfoot, unspecified foot

● **M21.54**   **Acquired clubfoot**
   M21.541   Acquired clubfoot, right foot
   M21.542   Acquired clubfoot, left foot
   M21.549   Acquired clubfoot, unspecified foot

● **M21.6**   **Other acquired deformities of foot**
   Excludes2   deformities of toe (acquired) (M20.1-M20.6)

● **M21.6X**   **Other acquired deformities of foot**
   M21.6X1   Other acquired deformities of right foot
   M21.6X2   Other acquired deformities of left foot
   M21.6X9   Other acquired deformities of unspecified foot

● **M21.7**   **Unequal limb length (acquired)**
   Note: The site used should correspond to the shorter limb.
   M21.70   Unequal limb length (acquired), unspecified site

● **M21.72**   **Unequal limb length (acquired), humerus**
   M21.721   Unequal limb length (acquired), right humerus
   M21.722   Unequal limb length (acquired), left humerus
   M21.729   Unequal limb length (acquired), unspecified humerus

● **M21.73**   **Unequal limb length (acquired), ulna and radius**
   M21.731   Unequal limb length (acquired), right ulna
   M21.732   Unequal limb length (acquired), left ulna
   M21.733   Unequal limb length (acquired), right radius
   M21.734   Unequal limb length (acquired), left radius
   M21.739   Unequal limb length (acquired), unspecified ulna and radius

● **M21.75**   **Unequal limb length (acquired), femur**
   M21.751   Unequal limb length (acquired), right femur
   M21.752   Unequal limb length (acquired), left femur
   M21.759   Unequal limb length (acquired), unspecified femur

● **M21.76**   **Unequal limb length (acquired), tibia and fibula**
   M21.761   Unequal limb length (acquired), right tibia
   M21.762   Unequal limb length (acquired), left tibia
   M21.763   Unequal limb length (acquired), right fibula
   M21.764   Unequal limb length (acquired), left fibula
   M21.769   Unequal limb length (acquired), unspecified tibia and fibula

● **M21.8**   **Other specified acquired deformities of limbs**
   Excludes2   coxa plana (M91.2)
   M21.80   Other specified acquired deformities of unspecified limb

● **M21.82**   **Other specified acquired deformities of upper arm**
   M21.821   Other specified acquired deformities of right upper arm
   M21.822   Other specified acquired deformities of left upper arm
   M21.829   Other specified acquired deformities of unspecified upper arm

● **M21.83**   **Other specified acquired deformities of forearm**
   M21.831   Other specified acquired deformities of right forearm
   M21.832   Other specified acquired deformities of left forearm
   M21.839   Other specified acquired deformities of unspecified forearm

● **M21.85**   **Other specified acquired deformities of thigh**
   M21.851   Other specified acquired deformities of right thigh
   M21.852   Other specified acquired deformities of left thigh
   M21.859   Other specified acquired deformities of unspecified thigh

● **M21.86**   **Other specified acquired deformities of lower leg**
   M21.861   Other specified acquired deformities of right lower leg
   M21.862   Other specified acquired deformities of left lower leg
   M21.869   Other specified acquired deformities of unspecified lower leg

● **M21.9**   **Unspecified acquired deformity of limb and hand**
   M21.90   Unspecified acquired deformity of unspecified limb

● **M21.92**   **Unspecified acquired deformity of upper arm**
   M21.921   Unspecified acquired deformity of right upper arm
   M21.922   Unspecified acquired deformity of left upper arm
   M21.929   Unspecified acquired deformity of unspecified upper arm

● **M21.93**   **Unspecified acquired deformity of forearm**
   M21.931   Unspecified acquired deformity of right forearm
   M21.932   Unspecified acquired deformity of left forearm
   M21.939   Unspecified acquired deformity of unspecified forearm

● **M21.94**   **Unspecified acquired deformity of hand**
   M21.941   Unspecified acquired deformity of hand, right hand
   M21.942   Unspecified acquired deformity of hand, left hand
   M21.949   Unspecified acquired deformity of hand, unspecified hand

● **M21.95**   **Unspecified acquired deformity of thigh**
   M21.951   Unspecified acquired deformity of right thigh
   M21.952   Unspecified acquired deformity of left thigh
   M21.959   Unspecified acquired deformity of unspecified thigh

CHAPTER 13 (M00-M99)

CHAPTER 13 (M00-M99)

● M21.96   Unspecified acquired deformity of lower leg

    M21.961   Unspecified acquired deformity of right lower leg

    M21.962   Unspecified acquired deformity of left lower leg

    M21.969   Unspecified acquired deformity of unspecified lower leg

● M22   Disorder of patella

    Excludes1   traumatic dislocation of patella (S83.0-)

   ● M22.0   Recurrent dislocation of patella

    M22.00   Recurrent dislocation of patella, unspecified knee

    M22.01   Recurrent dislocation of patella, right knee

    M22.02   Recurrent dislocation of patella, left knee

   ● M22.1   Recurrent subluxation of patella

     Incomplete dislocation of patella

    M22.10   Recurrent subluxation of patella, unspecified knee

    M22.11   Recurrent subluxation of patella, right knee

    M22.12   Recurrent subluxation of patella, left knee

   ● M22.2   Patellofemoral disorders

    ● M22.2X   Patellofemoral disorders

     M22.2X1   Patellofemoral disorders, right knee

     M22.2X2   Patellofemoral disorders, left knee

     M22.2X9   Patellofemoral disorders, unspecified knee

   ● M22.3   Other derangements of patella

    ● M22.3X   Other derangements of patella

     M22.3X1   Other derangements of patella, right knee

     M22.3X2   Other derangements of patella, left knee

     M22.3X9   Other derangements of patella, unspecified knee

   ● M22.4   Chondromalacia patellae

    M22.40   Chondromalacia patellae, unspecified knee

    M22.41   Chondromalacia patellae, right knee

    M22.42   Chondromalacia patellae, left knee

   ● M22.8   Other disorders of patella

    ● M22.8X   Other disorders of patella

     M22.8X1   Other disorders of patella, right knee

     M22.8X2   Other disorders of patella, left knee

     M22.8X9   Other disorders of patella, unspecified knee

   ● M22.9   Unspecified disorder of patella

    M22.90   Unspecified disorder of patella, unspecified knee

    M22.91   Unspecified disorder of patella, right knee

    M22.92   Unspecified disorder of patella, left knee

● M23   Internal derangement of knee

    Excludes1   ankylosis (M24.66)

     current injury - see injury of knee and lower leg (S80-S89)

     deformity of knee (M21.-)

     osteochondritis dissecans (M93.2)

     recurrent dislocation or subluxation of joints (M24.4)

     recurrent dislocation or subluxation of patella (M22.0-M22.1)

   ● M23.0   Cystic meniscus

    ● M23.00   Cystic meniscus, unspecified meniscus

     Cystic meniscus, unspecified lateral meniscus

     Cystic meniscus, unspecified medial meniscus

     M23.000   Cystic meniscus, unspecified lateral meniscus, right knee

     M23.001   Cystic meniscus, unspecified lateral meniscus, left knee

     M23.002   Cystic meniscus, unspecified lateral meniscus, unspecified knee

     M23.003   Cystic meniscus, unspecified medial meniscus, right knee

     M23.004   Cystic meniscus, unspecified medial meniscus, left knee

     M23.005   Cystic meniscus, unspecified medial meniscus, unspecified knee

     M23.006   Cystic meniscus, unspecified meniscus, right knee

     M23.007   Cystic meniscus, unspecified meniscus, left knee

     M23.009   Cystic meniscus, unspecified meniscus, unspecified knee

    ● M23.01   Cystic meniscus, anterior horn of medial meniscus

     M23.011   Cystic meniscus, anterior horn of medial meniscus, right knee

     M23.012   Cystic meniscus, anterior horn of medial meniscus, left knee

     M23.019   Cystic meniscus, anterior horn of medial meniscus, unspecified knee

    ● M23.02   Cystic meniscus, posterior horn of medial meniscus

     M23.021   Cystic meniscus, posterior horn of medial meniscus, right knee

     M23.022   Cystic meniscus, posterior horn of medial meniscus, left knee

     M23.029   Cystic meniscus, posterior horn of medial meniscus, unspecified knee

    ● M23.03   Cystic meniscus, other medial meniscus

     M23.031   Cystic meniscus, other medial meniscus, right knee

     M23.032   Cystic meniscus, other medial meniscus, left knee

     M23.039   Cystic meniscus, other medial meniscus, unspecified knee

    ● M23.04   Cystic meniscus, anterior horn of lateral meniscus

     M23.041   Cystic meniscus, anterior horn of lateral meniscus, right knee

     M23.042   Cystic meniscus, anterior horn of lateral meniscus, left knee

     M23.049   Cystic meniscus, anterior horn of lateral meniscus, unspecified knee

    ● M23.05   Cystic meniscus, posterior horn of lateral meniscus

     M23.051   Cystic meniscus, posterior horn of lateral meniscus, right knee

     M23.052   Cystic meniscus, posterior horn of lateral meniscus, left knee

     M23.059   Cystic meniscus, posterior horn of lateral meniscus, unspecified knee

    ● M23.06   Cystic meniscus, other lateral meniscus

     M23.061   Cystic meniscus, other lateral meniscus, right knee

     M23.062   Cystic meniscus, other lateral meniscus, left knee

     M23.069   Cystic meniscus, other lateral meniscus, unspecified knee

◀ New   ◀ Revised   ~~deleted~~ Deleted   Excludes 1   Excludes 2   Includes   Use additional   Code first   Code also   Unspecified

OGCR Official Guidelines   X Assign placeholder X   ● Use Additional Character(s)   ▶ Manifestation Code   **Coding Clinic**

(See Plate 509 on page 79.)

● M23.2 Derangement of meniscus due to old tear or injury
Old bucket-handle tear

● M23.20 Derangement of unspecified meniscus due to old tear or injury
Derangement of unspecified lateral meniscus due to old tear or injury
Derangement of unspecified medial meniscus due to old tear or injury

M23.200 Derangement of unspecified lateral meniscus due to old tear or injury, right knee

M23.201 Derangement of unspecified lateral meniscus due to old tear or injury, left knee

M23.202 Derangement of unspecified lateral meniscus due to old tear or injury, unspecified knee

M23.203 Derangement of unspecified medial meniscus due to old tear or injury, right knee

M23.204 Derangement of unspecified medial meniscus due to old tear or injury, left knee

M23.205 Derangement of unspecified medial meniscus due to old tear or injury, unspecified knee

M23.206 Derangement of unspecified meniscus due to old tear or injury, right knee

M23.207 Derangement of unspecified meniscus due to old tear or injury, left knee

M23.209 Derangement of unspecified meniscus due to old tear or injury, unspecified knee

● M23.21 Derangement of anterior horn of medial meniscus due to old tear or injury

M23.211 Derangement of anterior horn of medial meniscus due to old tear or injury, right knee

M23.212 Derangement of anterior horn of medial meniscus due to old tear or injury, left knee

M23.219 Derangement of anterior horn of medial meniscus due to old tear or injury, unspecified knee

● M23.22 Derangement of posterior horn of medial meniscus due to old tear or injury

M23.221 Derangement of posterior horn of medial meniscus due to old tear or injury, right knee

M23.222 Derangement of posterior horn of medial meniscus due to old tear or injury, left knee

M23.229 Derangement of posterior horn of medial meniscus due to old tear or injury, unspecified knee

● M23.23 Derangement of other medial meniscus due to old tear or injury

M23.231 Derangement of other medial meniscus due to old tear or injury, right knee

M23.232 Derangement of other medial meniscus due to old tear or injury, left knee

M23.239 Derangement of other medial meniscus due to old tear or injury, unspecified knee

● M23.24 Derangement of anterior horn of lateral meniscus due to old tear or injury

M23.241 Derangement of anterior horn of lateral meniscus due to old tear or injury, right knee

M23.242 Derangement of anterior horn of lateral meniscus due to old tear or injury, left knee

M23.249 Derangement of anterior horn of lateral meniscus due to old tear or injury, unspecified knee

● M23.25 Derangement of posterior horn of lateral meniscus due to old tear or injury

M23.251 Derangement of posterior horn of lateral meniscus due to old tear or injury, right knee

M23.252 Derangement of posterior horn of lateral meniscus due to old tear or injury, left knee

M23.259 Derangement of posterior horn of lateral meniscus due to old tear or injury, unspecified knee

● M23.26 Derangement of other lateral meniscus due to old tear or injury

M23.261 Derangement of other lateral meniscus due to old tear or injury, right knee

M23.262 Derangement of other lateral meniscus due to old tear or injury, left knee

M23.269 Derangement of other lateral meniscus due to old tear or injury, unspecified knee

● M23.3 Other meniscus derangements
Degenerate meniscus
Detached meniscus
Retained meniscus

● M23.30 Other meniscus derangements, unspecified meniscus
Other meniscus derangements, unspecified lateral meniscus
Other meniscus derangements, unspecified medial meniscus

M23.300 Other meniscus derangements, unspecified lateral meniscus, right knee

M23.301 Other meniscus derangements, unspecified lateral meniscus, left knee

M23.302 Other meniscus derangements, unspecified lateral meniscus, unspecified knee

M23.303 Other meniscus derangements, unspecified medial meniscus, right knee

M23.304 Other meniscus derangements, unspecified medial meniscus, left knee

M23.305 Other meniscus derangements, unspecified medial meniscus, unspecified knee

M23.306 Other meniscus derangements, unspecified meniscus, right knee

M23.307 Other meniscus derangements, unspecified meniscus, left knee

M23.309 Other meniscus derangements, unspecified meniscus, unspecified knee

CHAPTER 13 (M00-M99)

● M23.31 Other meniscus derangements, anterior horn of medial meniscus
   M23.311 Other meniscus derangements, anterior horn of medial meniscus, right knee
   M23.312 Other meniscus derangements, anterior horn of medial meniscus, left knee
   M23.319 Other meniscus derangements, anterior horn of medial meniscus, unspecified knee

● M23.32 Other meniscus derangements, posterior horn of medial meniscus
   M23.321 Other meniscus derangements, posterior horn of medial meniscus, right knee
   M23.322 Other meniscus derangements, posterior horn of medial meniscus, left knee
   M23.329 Other meniscus derangements, posterior horn of medial meniscus, unspecified knee

● M23.33 Other meniscus derangements, other medial meniscus
   M23.331 Other meniscus derangements, other medial meniscus, right knee
   M23.332 Other meniscus derangements, other medial meniscus, left knee
   M23.339 Other meniscus derangements, other medial meniscus, unspecified knee

● M23.34 Other meniscus derangements, anterior horn of lateral meniscus
   M23.341 Other meniscus derangements, anterior horn of lateral meniscus, right knee
   M23.342 Other meniscus derangements, anterior horn of lateral meniscus, left knee
   M23.349 Other meniscus derangements, anterior horn of lateral meniscus, unspecified knee

● M23.35 Other meniscus derangements, posterior horn of lateral meniscus
   M23.351 Other meniscus derangements, posterior horn of lateral meniscus, right knee
   M23.352 Other meniscus derangements, posterior horn of lateral meniscus, left knee
   M23.359 Other meniscus derangements, posterior horn of lateral meniscus, unspecified knee

● M23.36 Other meniscus derangements, other lateral meniscus
   M23.361 Other meniscus derangements, other lateral meniscus, right knee
   M23.362 Other meniscus derangements, other lateral meniscus, left knee
   M23.369 Other meniscus derangements, other lateral meniscus, unspecified knee

● M23.4 Loose body in knee
   M23.40 Loose body in knee, unspecified knee
   M23.41 Loose body in knee, right knee
   M23.42 Loose body in knee, left knee

● M23.5 Chronic instability of knee
   M23.50 Chronic instability of knee, unspecified knee
   M23.51 Chronic instability of knee, right knee
   M23.52 Chronic instability of knee, left knee

● M23.6 Other spontaneous disruption of ligament(s) of knee
  ● M23.60 Other spontaneous disruption of unspecified ligament of knee
   M23.601 Other spontaneous disruption of unspecified ligament of right knee
   M23.602 Other spontaneous disruption of unspecified ligament of left knee
   M23.609 Other spontaneous disruption of unspecified ligament of unspecified knee

  ● M23.61 Other spontaneous disruption of anterior cruciate ligament of knee
   M23.611 Other spontaneous disruption of anterior cruciate ligament of right knee
   M23.612 Other spontaneous disruption of anterior cruciate ligament of left knee
   M23.619 Other spontaneous disruption of anterior cruciate ligament of unspecified knee

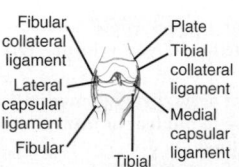

Figure 13-2 Collateral and cruciate ligament of knee. (From DeLee: DeLee and Drez's Orthopaedic Sports Medicine, ed 3, Saunders, 2009)

  ● M23.62 Other spontaneous disruption of posterior cruciate ligament of knee
   M23.621 Other spontaneous disruption of posterior cruciate ligament of right knee
   M23.622 Other spontaneous disruption of posterior cruciate ligament of left knee
   M23.629 Other spontaneous disruption of posterior cruciate ligament of unspecified knee

  ● M23.63 Other spontaneous disruption of medial collateral ligament of knee
   M23.631 Other spontaneous disruption of medial collateral ligament of right knee
   M23.632 Other spontaneous disruption of medial collateral ligament of left knee
   M23.639 Other spontaneous disruption of medial collateral ligament of unspecified knee

  ● M23.64 Other spontaneous disruption of lateral collateral ligament of knee
   M23.641 Other spontaneous disruption of lateral collateral ligament of right knee
   M23.642 Other spontaneous disruption of lateral collateral ligament of left knee
   M23.649 Other spontaneous disruption of lateral collateral ligament of unspecified knee

  ● M23.67 Other spontaneous disruption of capsular ligament of knee
   M23.671 Other spontaneous disruption of capsular ligament of right knee
   M23.672 Other spontaneous disruption of capsular ligament of left knee
   M23.679 Other spontaneous disruption of capsular ligament of unspecified knee

◀ New   ◀▦ Revised   ~~deleted~~ Deleted   Excludes 1   Excludes 2   Includes   Use additional   Code first   Code also   Unspecified
OGCR Official Guidelines   X Assign placeholder X   ● Use Additional Character(s)   ▶ Manifestation Code   **Coding Clinic**

● **M23.8**   **Other internal derangements of knee**
     Laxity of ligament of knee
     Snapping knee
  ● **M23.8X**   **Other internal derangements of knee**
     M23.8X1   Other internal derangements of right knee
     M23.8X2   Other internal derangements of left knee
     M23.8X9   Other internal derangements of unspecified knee

● **M23.9**   **Unspecified internal derangement of knee**
     M23.90   Unspecified internal derangement of unspecified knee
     M23.91   Unspecified internal derangement of right knee
     M23.92   Unspecified internal derangement of left knee

● **M24**   **Other specific joint derangements**
     Excludes1   current injury - see injury of joint by body region
     Excludes2   ganglion (M67.4)
                 snapping knee (M23.8-)
                 temporomandibular joint disorders (M26.6-)

● **M24.0**   **Loose body in joint**
     Excludes2   loose body in knee (M23.4)
     M24.00   Loose body in unspecified joint
  ● **M24.01**   **Loose body in shoulder**
     M24.011   Loose body in right shoulder
     M24.012   Loose body in left shoulder
     M24.019   Loose body in unspecified shoulder
  ● **M24.02**   **Loose body in elbow**
     M24.021   Loose body in right elbow
     M24.022   Loose body in left elbow
     M24.029   Loose body in unspecified elbow
  ● **M24.03**   **Loose body in wrist**
     M24.031   Loose body in right wrist
     M24.032   Loose body in left wrist
     M24.039   Loose body in unspecified wrist
  ● **M24.04**   **Loose body in finger joints**
     M24.041   Loose body in right finger joint(s)
     M24.042   Loose body in left finger joint(s)
     M24.049   Loose body in unspecified finger joint(s)
  ● **M24.05**   **Loose body in hip**
     M24.051   Loose body in right hip
     M24.052   Loose body in left hip
     M24.059   Loose body in unspecified hip
  ● **M24.07**   **Loose body in ankle and toe joints**
     M24.071   Loose body in right ankle
     M24.072   Loose body in left ankle
     M24.073   Loose body in unspecified ankle
     M24.074   Loose body in right toe joint(s)
     M24.075   Loose body in left toe joint(s)
     M24.076   Loose body in unspecified toe joints
     M24.08   Loose body, other site

● **M24.1**   **Other articular cartilage disorders**
     Excludes2   chondrocalcinosis (M11.1, M11.2-)
                 internal derangement of knee (M23.-)
                 metastatic calcification (E83.5)
                 ochronosis (E70.2)
     M24.10   Other articular cartilage disorders, unspecified site
  ● **M24.11**   **Other articular cartilage disorders, shoulder**
     M24.111   Other articular cartilage disorders, right shoulder
     M24.112   Other articular cartilage disorders, left shoulder
     M24.119   Other articular cartilage disorders, unspecified shoulder

● **M24.12**   **Other articular cartilage disorders, elbow**
     M24.121   Other articular cartilage disorders, right elbow
     M24.122   Other articular cartilage disorders, left elbow
     M24.129   Other articular cartilage disorders, unspecified elbow
● **M24.13**   **Other articular cartilage disorders, wrist**
     M24.131   Other articular cartilage disorders, right wrist
     M24.132   Other articular cartilage disorders, left wrist
     M24.139   Other articular cartilage disorders, unspecified wrist
● **M24.14**   **Other articular cartilage disorders, hand**
     M24.141   Other articular cartilage disorders, right hand
     M24.142   Other articular cartilage disorders, left hand
     M24.149   Other articular cartilage disorders, unspecified hand
● **M24.15**   **Other articular cartilage disorders, hip**
     M24.151   Other articular cartilage disorders, right hip
     M24.152   Other articular cartilage disorders, left hip
     M24.159   Other articular cartilage disorders, unspecified hip
● **M24.17**   **Other articular cartilage disorders, ankle and foot**
     M24.171   Other articular cartilage disorders, right ankle
     M24.172   Other articular cartilage disorders, left ankle
     M24.173   Other articular cartilage disorders, unspecified ankle
     M24.174   Other articular cartilage disorders, right foot
     M24.175   Other articular cartilage disorders, left foot
     M24.176   Other articular cartilage disorders, unspecified foot

● **M24.2**   **Disorder of ligament**
     Instability secondary to old ligament injury
     Ligamentous laxity NOS
     Excludes1   familial ligamentous laxity (M35.7)
     Excludes2   internal derangement of knee (M23.5-M23.89)
     M24.20   Disorder of ligament, unspecified site
  ● **M24.21**   **Disorder of ligament, shoulder**
     M24.211   Disorder of ligament, right shoulder
     M24.212   Disorder of ligament, left shoulder
     M24.219   Disorder of ligament, unspecified shoulder
  ● **M24.22**   **Disorder of ligament, elbow**
     M24.221   Disorder of ligament, right elbow
     M24.222   Disorder of ligament, left elbow
     M24.229   Disorder of ligament, unspecified elbow
  ● **M24.23**   **Disorder of ligament, wrist**
     M24.231   Disorder of ligament, right wrist
     M24.232   Disorder of ligament, left wrist
     M24.239   Disorder of ligament, unspecified wrist
  ● **M24.24**   **Disorder of ligament, hand**
     M24.241   Disorder of ligament, right hand
     M24.242   Disorder of ligament, left hand
     M24.249   Disorder of ligament, unspecified hand

● **M24.25** Disorder of ligament, hip
     M24.251 Disorder of ligament, right hip
     M24.252 Disorder of ligament, left hip
     M24.259 Disorder of ligament, unspecified hip

● **M24.27** Disorder of ligament, ankle and foot
     M24.271 Disorder of ligament, right ankle
     M24.272 Disorder of ligament, left ankle
     M24.273 Disorder of ligament, unspecified ankle
     M24.274 Disorder of ligament, right foot
     M24.275 Disorder of ligament, left foot
     M24.276 Disorder of ligament, unspecified foot

   M24.28 Disorder of ligament, vertebrae

● **M24.3** Pathological dislocation of joint, not elsewhere classified
     Excludes1   congenital dislocation or displacement of joint - see congenital malformations and deformations of the musculoskeletal system (Q65-Q79)
         current injury - see injury of joints and ligaments by body region
         recurrent dislocation of joint (M24.4-)

   M24.30 Pathological dislocation of unspecified joint, not elsewhere classified

● **M24.31** Pathological dislocation of shoulder, not elsewhere classified
     M24.311 Pathological dislocation of right shoulder, not elsewhere classified
     M24.312 Pathological dislocation of left shoulder, not elsewhere classified
     M24.319 Pathological dislocation of unspecified shoulder, not elsewhere classified

● **M24.32** Pathological dislocation of elbow, not elsewhere classified
     M24.321 Pathological dislocation of right elbow, not elsewhere classified
     M24.322 Pathological dislocation of left elbow, not elsewhere classified
     M24.329 Pathological dislocation of unspecified elbow, not elsewhere classified

● **M24.33** Pathological dislocation of wrist, not elsewhere classified
     M24.331 Pathological dislocation of right wrist, not elsewhere classified
     M24.332 Pathological dislocation of left wrist, not elsewhere classified
     M24.339 Pathological dislocation of unspecified wrist, not elsewhere classified

● **M24.34** Pathological dislocation of hand, not elsewhere classified
     M24.341 Pathological dislocation of right hand, not elsewhere classified
     M24.342 Pathological dislocation of left hand, not elsewhere classified
     M24.349 Pathological dislocation of unspecified hand, not elsewhere classified

● **M24.35** Pathological dislocation of hip, not elsewhere classified
     M24.351 Pathological dislocation of right hip, not elsewhere classified
     M24.352 Pathological dislocation of left hip, not elsewhere classified
     M24.359 Pathological dislocation of unspecified hip, not elsewhere classified

● **M24.36** Pathological dislocation of knee, not elsewhere classified
     M24.361 Pathological dislocation of right knee, not elsewhere classified
     M24.362 Pathological dislocation of left knee, not elsewhere classified
     M24.369 Pathological dislocation of unspecified knee, not elsewhere classified

● **M24.37** Pathological dislocation of ankle and foot, not elsewhere classified
     M24.371 Pathological dislocation of right ankle, not elsewhere classified
     M24.372 Pathological dislocation of left ankle, not elsewhere classified
     M24.373 Pathological dislocation of unspecified ankle, not elsewhere classified
     M24.374 Pathological dislocation of right foot, not elsewhere classified
     M24.375 Pathological dislocation of left foot, not elsewhere classified
     M24.376 Pathological dislocation of unspecified foot, not elsewhere classified

● **M24.4** Recurrent dislocation of joint
     Recurrent subluxation of joint
     Excludes2   recurrent dislocation of patella (M22.0-M22.1)
         recurrent vertebral dislocation (M43.3-, M43.4, M43.5-)

   M24.40 Recurrent dislocation, unspecified joint

● **M24.41** Recurrent dislocation, shoulder
     M24.411 Recurrent dislocation, right shoulder
     M24.412 Recurrent dislocation, left shoulder
     M24.419 Recurrent dislocation, unspecified shoulder

● **M24.42** Recurrent dislocation, elbow
     M24.421 Recurrent dislocation, right elbow
     M24.422 Recurrent dislocation, left elbow
     M24.429 Recurrent dislocation, unspecified elbow

● **M24.43** Recurrent dislocation, wrist
     M24.431 Recurrent dislocation, right wrist
     M24.432 Recurrent dislocation, left wrist
     M24.439 Recurrent dislocation, unspecified wrist

● **M24.44** Recurrent dislocation, hand and finger(s)
     M24.441 Recurrent dislocation, right hand
     M24.442 Recurrent dislocation, left hand
     M24.443 Recurrent dislocation, unspecified hand
     M24.444 Recurrent dislocation, right finger
     M24.445 Recurrent dislocation, left finger
     M24.446 Recurrent dislocation, unspecified finger

● **M24.45** Recurrent dislocation, hip
     M24.451 Recurrent dislocation, right hip
     M24.452 Recurrent dislocation, left hip
     M24.459 Recurrent dislocation, unspecified hip

● **M24.46** Recurrent dislocation, knee
     M24.461 Recurrent dislocation, right knee
     M24.462 Recurrent dislocation, left knee
     M24.469 Recurrent dislocation, unspecified knee

◀ New   ◀▥ Revised   ~~deleted~~ Deleted   Excludes 1   Excludes 2   Includes   Use additional   Code first   Code also   Unspecified
OGCR Official Guidelines   **X** Assign placeholder X   ● Use Additional Character(s)   ▶ Manifestation Code   **Coding Clinic**

● M24.47   Recurrent dislocation, ankle, foot and toes
    M24.471   Recurrent dislocation, right ankle
    M24.472   Recurrent dislocation, left ankle
    M24.473   Recurrent dislocation, unspecified ankle
    M24.474   Recurrent dislocation, right foot
    M24.475   Recurrent dislocation, left foot
    M24.476   Recurrent dislocation, unspecified foot
    M24.477   Recurrent dislocation, right toe(s)
    M24.478   Recurrent dislocation, left toe(s)
    M24.479   Recurrent dislocation, unspecified toe(s)

● M24.5   Contracture of joint
    Excludes1   contracture of muscle without contracture of joint (M62.4-)
       contracture of tendon (sheath) without contracture of joint (M62.4-)
       Dupuytren's contracture (M72.0)
    Excludes2   acquired deformities of limbs (M20-M21)
    M24.50   Contracture, unspecified joint
● M24.51   Contracture, shoulder
    M24.511   Contracture, right shoulder
    M24.512   Contracture, left shoulder
    M24.519   Contracture, unspecified shoulder
● M24.52   Contracture, elbow
    M24.521   Contracture, right elbow
    M24.522   Contracture, left elbow
    M24.529   Contracture, unspecified elbow
● M24.53   Contracture, wrist
    M24.531   Contracture, right wrist
    M24.532   Contracture, left wrist
    M24.539   Contracture, unspecified wrist
● M24.54   Contracture, hand
    M24.541   Contracture, right hand
    M24.542   Contracture, left hand
    M24.549   Contracture, unspecified hand
● M24.55   Contracture, hip
    M24.551   Contracture, right hip
    M24.552   Contracture, left hip
    M24.559   Contracture, unspecified hip
● M24.56   Contracture, knee
    M24.561   Contracture, right knee
    M24.562   Contracture, left knee
    M24.569   Contracture, unspecified knee
● M24.57   Contracture, ankle and foot
    M24.571   Contracture, right ankle
    M24.572   Contracture, left ankle
    M24.573   Contracture, unspecified ankle
    M24.574   Contracture, right foot
    M24.575   Contracture, left foot
    M24.576   Contracture, unspecified foot

● M24.6   Ankylosis of joint
    Excludes1   stiffness of joint without ankylosis (M25.6-)
    Excludes2   spine (M43.2-)
    M24.60   Ankylosis, unspecified joint
● M24.61   Ankylosis, shoulder
    M24.611   Ankylosis, right shoulder
    M24.612   Ankylosis, left shoulder
    M24.619   Ankylosis, unspecified shoulder
● M24.62   Ankylosis, elbow
    M24.621   Ankylosis, right elbow
    M24.622   Ankylosis, left elbow
    M24.629   Ankylosis, unspecified elbow

Item 13-5   **Ankylosis** or arthrokleisis is a consolidation of a joint due to disease, injury, or surgical procedure. Spondylosis is the degeneration of the vertebral processes and formation of osteophytes and commonly occurs with age. **Spondylitis** or ankylosing spondylitis is a type of arthritis that affects the spine or backbone causing back pain and stiffness.

● M24.63   Ankylosis, wrist
    M24.631   Ankylosis, right wrist
    M24.632   Ankylosis, left wrist
    M24.639   Ankylosis, unspecified wrist
● M24.64   Ankylosis, hand
    M24.641   Ankylosis, right hand
    M24.642   Ankylosis, left hand
    M24.649   Ankylosis, unspecified hand
● M24.65   Ankylosis, hip
    M24.651   Ankylosis, right hip
    M24.652   Ankylosis, left hip
    M24.659   Ankylosis, unspecified hip
● M24.66   Ankylosis, knee
    M24.661   Ankylosis, right knee
    M24.662   Ankylosis, left knee
    M24.669   Ankylosis, unspecified knee
● M24.67   Ankylosis, ankle and foot
    M24.671   Ankylosis, right ankle
    M24.672   Ankylosis, left ankle
    M24.673   Ankylosis, unspecified ankle
    M24.674   Ankylosis, right foot
    M24.675   Ankylosis, left foot
    M24.676   Ankylosis, unspecified foot

    M24.7   Protrusio acetabuli
● M24.8   Other specific joint derangements, not elsewhere classified
    Excludes2   iliotibial band syndrome (M76.3)
    M24.80   Other specific joint derangements of unspecified joint, not elsewhere classified
● M24.81   Other specific joint derangements of shoulder, not elsewhere classified
    M24.811   Other specific joint derangements of right shoulder, not elsewhere classified
    M24.812   Other specific joint derangements of left shoulder, not elsewhere classified
    M24.819   Other specific joint derangements of unspecified shoulder, not elsewhere classified
● M24.82   Other specific joint derangements of elbow, not elsewhere classified
    M24.821   Other specific joint derangements of right elbow, not elsewhere classified
    M24.822   Other specific joint derangements of left elbow, not elsewhere classified
    M24.829   Other specific joint derangements of unspecified elbow, not elsewhere classified
● M24.83   Other specific joint derangements of wrist, not elsewhere classified
    M24.831   Other specific joint derangements of right wrist, not elsewhere classified
    M24.832   Other specific joint derangements of left wrist, not elsewhere classified
    M24.839   Other specific joint derangements of unspecified wrist, not elsewhere classified

CHAPTER 13 (M00-M99)

● M24.84 Other specific joint derangements of hand, not elsewhere classified

    M24.841 Other specific joint derangements of right hand, not elsewhere classified

    M24.842 Other specific joint derangements of left hand, not elsewhere classified

    M24.849 Other specific joint derangements of unspecified hand, not elsewhere classified

● M24.85 Other specific joint derangements of hip, not elsewhere classified
    Irritable hip

    M24.851 Other specific joint derangements of right hip, not elsewhere classified

    M24.852 Other specific joint derangements of left hip, not elsewhere classified

    M24.859 Other specific joint derangements of unspecified hip, not elsewhere classified

● M24.87 Other specific joint derangements of ankle and foot, not elsewhere classified

    M24.871 Other specific joint derangements of right ankle, not elsewhere classified

    M24.872 Other specific joint derangements of left ankle, not elsewhere classified

    M24.873 Other specific joint derangements of unspecified ankle, not elsewhere classified

    M24.874 Other specific joint derangements of right foot, not elsewhere classified

    M24.875 Other specific joint derangements left foot, not elsewhere classified

    M24.876 Other specific joint derangements of unspecified foot, not elsewhere classified

  M24.9 Joint derangement, unspecified

● M25 Other joint disorder, not elsewhere classified

    Excludes2 abnormality of gait and mobility (R26.-)
      acquired deformities of limb (M20-M21)
      calcification of bursa (M71.4-)
      calcification of shoulder (joint) (M75.3)
      calcification of tendon (M65.2-)
      difficulty in walking (R26.2)
      temporomandibular joint disorder (M26.6-)

● M25.0 Hemarthrosis

    Excludes1 current injury - see injury of joint by body region
      hemophilic arthropathy (M36.2)

  M25.00 Hemarthrosis, unspecified joint

● M25.01 Hemarthrosis, shoulder
    M25.011 Hemarthrosis, right shoulder
    M25.012 Hemarthrosis, left shoulder
    M25.019 Hemarthrosis, unspecified shoulder

● M25.02 Hemarthrosis, elbow
    M25.021 Hemarthrosis, right elbow
    M25.022 Hemarthrosis, left elbow
    M25.029 Hemarthrosis, unspecified elbow

● M25.03 Hemarthrosis, wrist
    M25.031 Hemarthrosis, right wrist
    M25.032 Hemarthrosis, left wrist
    M25.039 Hemarthrosis, unspecified wrist

● M25.04 Hemarthrosis, hand
    M25.041 Hemarthrosis, right hand
    M25.042 Hemarthrosis, left hand
    M25.049 Hemarthrosis, unspecified hand

● M25.05 Hemarthrosis, hip
    M25.051 Hemarthrosis, right hip
    M25.052 Hemarthrosis, left hip
    M25.059 Hemarthrosis, unspecified hip

● M25.06 Hemarthrosis, knee
    M25.061 Hemarthrosis, right knee
    M25.062 Hemarthrosis, left knee
    M25.069 Hemarthrosis, unspecified knee

● M25.07 Hemarthrosis, ankle and foot
    M25.071 Hemarthrosis, right ankle
    M25.072 Hemarthrosis, left ankle
    M25.073 Hemarthrosis, unspecified ankle
    M25.074 Hemarthrosis, right foot
    M25.075 Hemarthrosis, left foot
    M25.076 Hemarthrosis, unspecified foot

  M25.08 Hemarthrosis, other specified site
    Hemarthrosis, vertebrae

● M25.1 Fistula of joint
  M25.10 Fistula, unspecified joint

● M25.11 Fistula, shoulder
    M25.111 Fistula, right shoulder
    M25.112 Fistula, left shoulder
    M25.119 Fistula, unspecified shoulder

● M25.12 Fistula, elbow
    M25.121 Fistula, right elbow
    M25.122 Fistula, left elbow
    M25.129 Fistula, unspecified elbow

● M25.13 Fistula, wrist
    M25.131 Fistula, right wrist
    M25.132 Fistula, left wrist
    M25.139 Fistula, unspecified wrist

● M25.14 Fistula, hand
    M25.141 Fistula, right hand
    M25.142 Fistula, left hand
    M25.149 Fistula, unspecified hand

● M25.15 Fistula, hip
    M25.151 Fistula, right hip
    M25.152 Fistula, left hip
    M25.159 Fistula, unspecified hip

● M25.16 Fistula, knee
    M25.161 Fistula, right knee
    M25.162 Fistula, left knee
    M25.169 Fistula, unspecified knee

● M25.17 Fistula, ankle and foot
    M25.171 Fistula, right ankle
    M25.172 Fistula, left ankle
    M25.173 Fistula, unspecified ankle
    M25.174 Fistula, right foot
    M25.175 Fistula, left foot
    M25.176 Fistula, unspecified foot

  M25.18 Fistula, other specified site
    Fistula, vertebrae

● M25.2 Flail joint
  M25.20 Flail joint, unspecified joint

● M25.21 Flail joint, shoulder
    M25.211 Flail joint, right shoulder
    M25.212 Flail joint, left shoulder
    M25.219 Flail joint, unspecified shoulder

● M25.22 Flail joint, elbow
    M25.221 Flail joint, right elbow
    M25.222 Flail joint, left elbow
    M25.229 Flail joint, unspecified elbow

● M25.23 Flail joint, wrist
    M25.231 Flail joint, right wrist
    M25.232 Flail joint, left wrist
    M25.239 Flail joint, unspecified wrist

◄ New ⟵ Revised ~~deleted~~ Deleted | Excludes 1 | Excludes 2 | Includes | Use additional | Code first | Code also | Unspecified

OGCR Official Guidelines X Assign placeholder X ● Use Additional Character(s) ▶ Manifestation Code **Coding Clinic**

● M25.24 Flail joint, hand
    M25.241 Flail joint, right hand
    M25.242 Flail joint, left hand
    M25.249 Flail joint, unspecified hand
● M25.25 Flail joint, hip
    M25.251 Flail joint, right hip
    M25.252 Flail joint, left hip
    M25.259 Flail joint, unspecified hip
● M25.26 Flail joint, knee
    M25.261 Flail joint, right knee
    M25.262 Flail joint, left knee
    M25.269 Flail joint, unspecified knee
● M25.27 Flail joint, ankle and foot
    M25.271 Flail joint, right ankle and foot
    M25.272 Flail joint, left ankle and foot
    M25.279 Flail joint, unspecified ankle and foot
    M25.28 Flail joint, other site
● M25.3 Other instability of joint
    Excludes1 instability of joint secondary to old ligament injury (M24.2-)
                        instability of joint secondary to removal of joint prosthesis (M96.8-)
    Excludes2 spinal instabilities (M53.2-)
    M25.30 Other instability, unspecified joint
● M25.31 Other instability, shoulder
    M25.311 Other instability, right shoulder
    M25.312 Other instability, left shoulder
    M25.319 Other instability, unspecified shoulder
● M25.32 Other instability, elbow
    M25.321 Other instability, right elbow
    M25.322 Other instability, left elbow
    M25.329 Other instability, unspecified elbow
● M25.33 Other instability, wrist
    M25.331 Other instability, right wrist
    M25.332 Other instability, left wrist
    M25.339 Other instability, unspecified wrist
● M25.34 Other instability, hand
    M25.341 Other instability, right hand
    M25.342 Other instability, left hand
    M25.349 Other instability, unspecified hand
● M25.35 Other instability, hip
    M25.351 Other instability, right hip
    M25.352 Other instability, left hip
    M25.359 Other instability, unspecified hip
● M25.36 Other instability, knee
    M25.361 Other instability, right knee
    M25.362 Other instability, left knee
    M25.369 Other instability, unspecified knee
● M25.37 Other instability, ankle and foot
    M25.371 Other instability, right ankle
    M25.372 Other instability, left ankle
    M25.373 Other instability, unspecified ankle
    M25.374 Other instability, right foot
    M25.375 Other instability, left foot
    M25.376 Other instability, unspecified foot
● M25.4 Effusion of joint
    Excludes1 hydrarthrosis in yaws (A66.6)
                        intermittent hydrarthrosis (M12.4-)
                        other infective (teno)synovitis (M65.1-)
    M25.40 Effusion, unspecified joint
● M25.41 Effusion, shoulder
    M25.411 Effusion, right shoulder
    M25.412 Effusion, left shoulder
    M25.419 Effusion, unspecified shoulder

● M25.42 Effusion, elbow
    M25.421 Effusion, right elbow
    M25.422 Effusion, left elbow
    M25.429 Effusion, unspecified elbow
● M25.43 Effusion, wrist
    M25.431 Effusion, right wrist
    M25.432 Effusion, left wrist
    M25.439 Effusion, unspecified wrist
● M25.44 Effusion, hand
    M25.441 Effusion, right hand
    M25.442 Effusion, left hand
    M25.449 Effusion, unspecified hand
● M25.45 Effusion, hip
    M25.451 Effusion, right hip
    M25.452 Effusion, left hip
    M25.459 Effusion, unspecified hip
● M25.46 Effusion, knee
    M25.461 Effusion, right knee
    M25.462 Effusion, left knee
    M25.469 Effusion, unspecified knee
● M25.47 Effusion, ankle and foot
    M25.471 Effusion, right ankle
    M25.472 Effusion, left ankle
    M25.473 Effusion, unspecified ankle
    M25.474 Effusion, right foot
    M25.475 Effusion, left foot
    M25.476 Effusion, unspecified foot
    M25.48 Effusion, other site
● M25.5 Pain in joint
    Excludes2 pain in hand (M79.64-)
                        pain in fingers (M79.64-)
                        pain in foot (M79.67-)
                        pain in limb (M79.6-)
                        pain in toes (M79.67-)
    M25.50 Pain in unspecified joint
● M25.51 Pain in shoulder
    M25.511 Pain in right shoulder
    M25.512 Pain in left shoulder
    M25.519 Pain in unspecified shoulder
● M25.52 Pain in elbow
    M25.521 Pain in right elbow
    M25.522 Pain in left elbow
    M25.529 Pain in unspecified elbow
● M25.53 Pain in wrist
    M25.531 Pain in right wrist
    M25.532 Pain in left wrist
    M25.539 Pain in unspecified wrist
● M25.55 Pain in hip
    M25.551 Pain in right hip
    M25.552 Pain in left hip
    M25.559 Pain in unspecified hip
● M25.56 Pain in knee
    M25.561 Pain in right knee
    M25.562 Pain in left knee
    M25.569 Pain in unspecified knee
● M25.57 Pain in ankle and joints of foot
    M25.571 Pain in right ankle and joints of right foot
    M25.572 Pain in left ankle and joints of left foot
    M25.579 Pain in unspecified ankle and joints of unspecified foot

● M25.6 Stiffness of joint, not elsewhere classified
  Excludes1 ankylosis of joint (M24.6-)
                contracture of joint (M24.5-)
  M25.60 Stiffness of unspecified joint, not elsewhere classified
  ● M25.61 Stiffness of shoulder, not elsewhere classified
    M25.611 Stiffness of right shoulder, not elsewhere classified
    M25.612 Stiffness of left shoulder, not elsewhere classified
    M25.619 Stiffness of unspecified shoulder, not elsewhere classified
  ● M25.62 Stiffness of elbow, not elsewhere classified
    M25.621 Stiffness of right elbow, not elsewhere classified
    M25.622 Stiffness of left elbow, not elsewhere classified
    M25.629 Stiffness of unspecified elbow, not elsewhere classified
  ● M25.63 Stiffness of wrist, not elsewhere classified
    M25.631 Stiffness of right wrist, not elsewhere classified
    M25.632 Stiffness of left wrist, not elsewhere classified
    M25.639 Stiffness of unspecified wrist, not elsewhere classified
  ● M25.64 Stiffness of hand, not elsewhere classified
    M25.641 Stiffness of right hand, not elsewhere classified
    M25.642 Stiffness of left hand, not elsewhere classified
    M25.649 Stiffness of unspecified hand, not elsewhere classified
  ● M25.65 Stiffness of hip, not elsewhere classified
    M25.651 Stiffness of right hip, not elsewhere classified
    M25.652 Stiffness of left hip, not elsewhere classified
    M25.659 Stiffness of unspecified hip, not elsewhere classified
  ● M25.66 Stiffness of knee, not elsewhere classified
    M25.661 Stiffness of right knee, not elsewhere classified
    M25.662 Stiffness of left knee, not elsewhere classified
    M25.669 Stiffness of unspecified knee, not elsewhere classified
  ● M25.67 Stiffness of ankle and foot, not elsewhere classified
    M25.671 Stiffness of right ankle, not elsewhere classified
    M25.672 Stiffness of left ankle, not elsewhere classified
    M25.673 Stiffness of unspecified ankle, not elsewhere classified
    M25.674 Stiffness of right foot, not elsewhere classified
    M25.675 Stiffness of left foot, not elsewhere classified
    M25.676 Stiffness of unspecified foot, not elsewhere classified
● M25.7 Osteophyte
  M25.70 Osteophyte, unspecified joint
  ● M25.71 Osteophyte, shoulder
    M25.711 Osteophyte, right shoulder
    M25.712 Osteophyte, left shoulder
    M25.719 Osteophyte, unspecified shoulder

● M25.72 Osteophyte, elbow
  M25.721 Osteophyte, right elbow
  M25.722 Osteophyte, left elbow
  M25.729 Osteophyte, unspecified elbow
● M25.73 Osteophyte, wrist
  M25.731 Osteophyte, right wrist
  M25.732 Osteophyte, left wrist
  M25.739 Osteophyte, unspecified wrist
● M25.74 Osteophyte, hand
  M25.741 Osteophyte, right hand
  M25.742 Osteophyte, left hand
  M25.749 Osteophyte, unspecified hand
● M25.75 Osteophyte, hip
  M25.751 Osteophyte, right hip
  M25.752 Osteophyte, left hip
  M25.759 Osteophyte, unspecified hip
● M25.76 Osteophyte, knee
  M25.761 Osteophyte, right knee
  M25.762 Osteophyte, left knee
  M25.769 Osteophyte, unspecified knee
● M25.77 Osteophyte, ankle and foot
  M25.771 Osteophyte, right ankle
  M25.772 Osteophyte, left ankle
  M25.773 Osteophyte, unspecified ankle
  M25.774 Osteophyte, right foot
  M25.775 Osteophyte, left foot
  M25.776 Osteophyte, unspecified foot
  M25.78 Osteophyte, vertebrae
● M25.8 Other specified joint disorders
  M25.80 Other specified joint disorders, unspecified joint
  ● M25.81 Other specified joint disorders, shoulder
    M25.811 Other specified joint disorders, right shoulder
    M25.812 Other specified joint disorders, left shoulder
    M25.819 Other specified joint disorders, unspecified shoulder
  ● M25.82 Other specified joint disorders, elbow
    M25.821 Other specified joint disorders, right elbow
    M25.822 Other specified joint disorders, left elbow
    M25.829 Other specified joint disorders, unspecified elbow
  ● M25.83 Other specified joint disorders, wrist
    M25.831 Other specified joint disorders, right wrist
    M25.832 Other specified joint disorders, left wrist
    M25.839 Other specified joint disorders, unspecified wrist
  ● M25.84 Other specified joint disorders, hand
    M25.841 Other specified joint disorders, right hand
    M25.842 Other specified joint disorders, left hand
    M25.849 Other specified joint disorders, unspecified hand
  ● M25.85 Other specified joint disorders, hip
    M25.851 Other specified joint disorders, right hip
    M25.852 Other specified joint disorders, left hip
    M25.859 Other specified joint disorders, unspecified hip

◀ New   ◀▥ Revised   ~~deleted~~ Deleted   Excludes 1   Excludes 2   Includes   Use additional   Code first   Code also   Unspecified
OGCR Official Guidelines   X Assign placeholder X   ● Use Additional Character(s)   ▶ Manifestation Code   Coding Clinic

● M25.86 Other specified joint disorders, knee
  M25.861 Other specified joint disorders, right knee
  M25.862 Other specified joint disorders, left knee
  M25.869 Other specified joint disorders, unspecified knee
● M25.87 Other specified joint disorders, ankle and foot
  M25.871 Other specified joint disorders, right ankle and foot
  M25.872 Other specified joint disorders, left ankle and foot
  M25.879 Other specified joint disorders, unspecified ankle and foot
M25.9 Joint disorder, unspecified

DENTOFACIAL ANOMALIES [INCLUDING MALOCCLUSION] AND OTHER DISORDERS OF JAW (M26-M27)

  Excludes1   hemifacial atrophy or hypertrophy (Q67.4)
              unilateral condylar hyperplasia or hypoplasia (M27.8)

● M26 Dentofacial anomalies [including malocclusion]
  ● M26.0 Major anomalies of jaw size
      Excludes1   acromegaly (E22.0)
                  Robin's syndrome (Q87.0)
    M26.00 Unspecified anomaly of jaw size
    M26.01 Maxillary hyperplasia
    M26.02 Maxillary hypoplasia
    M26.03 Mandibular hyperplasia
    M26.04 Mandibular hypoplasia
    M26.05 Macrogenia
    M26.06 Microgenia
    M26.07 Excessive tuberosity of jaw
            Entire maxillary tuberosity
    M26.09 Other specified anomalies of jaw size
  ● M26.1 Anomalies of jaw-cranial base relationship
    M26.10 Unspecified anomaly of jaw-cranial base relationship
    M26.11 Maxillary asymmetry
    M26.12 Other jaw asymmetry
    M26.19 Other specified anomalies of jaw-cranial base relationship
  ● M26.2 Anomalies of dental arch relationship
    M26.20 Unspecified anomaly of dental arch relationship
  ● M26.21 Malocclusion, Angle's class
    M26.211 Malocclusion, Angle's class I
             Neutro-occlusion
    M26.212 Malocclusion, Angle's class II
             Disto-occlusion Division I
             Disto-occlusion Division II
    M26.213 Malocclusion, Angle's class III
             Mesio-occlusion
    M26.219 Malocclusion, Angle's class, unspecified

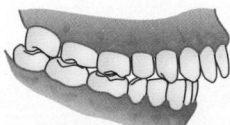

Figure 13-3 Dentofacial malocclusion.

Item 13–6 Hyperplasia is a condition of overdevelopment, whereas **hypoplasia** is a condition of underdevelopment. **Macrogenia** is overdevelopment of the chin, whereas **microgenia** is underdevelopment of the chin.

● M26.22 Open occlusal relationship
  M26.220 Open anterior occlusal relationship
           Anterior openbite
  M26.221 Open posterior occlusal relationship
           Posterior openbite
M26.23 Excessive horizontal overlap
        Excessive horizontal overjet
M26.24 Reverse articulation
        Crossbite (anterior) (posterior)
M26.25 Anomalies of interarch distance
M26.29 Other anomalies of dental arch relationship
        Midline deviation of dental arch
        Overbite (excessive) deep
        Overbite (excessive) horizontal
        Overbite (excessive) vertical
        Posterior lingual occlusion of mandibular teeth
● M26.3 Anomalies of tooth position of fully erupted tooth or teeth
    Excludes2   embedded and impacted teeth (K01.-)
  M26.30 Unspecified anomaly of tooth position of fully erupted tooth or teeth
          Abnormal spacing of fully erupted tooth or teeth NOS
          Displacement of fully erupted tooth or teeth NOS
          Transposition of fully erupted tooth or teeth NOS
  M26.31 Crowding of fully erupted teeth
  M26.32 Excessive spacing of fully erupted teeth
          Diastema of fully erupted tooth or teeth NOS
  M26.33 Horizontal displacement of fully erupted tooth or teeth
          Tipped tooth or teeth
          Tipping of fully erupted tooth
  M26.34 Vertical displacement of fully erupted tooth or teeth
          Extruded tooth
          Infraeruption of tooth or teeth
          Supraeruption of tooth or teeth
  M26.35 Rotation of fully erupted tooth or teeth
  M26.36 Insufficient interocclusal distance of fully erupted teeth (ridge)
          Lack of adequate intermaxillary vertical dimension of fully erupted teeth
  M26.37 Excessive interocclusal distance of fully erupted teeth
          Excessive intermaxillary vertical dimension of fully erupted teeth
          Loss of occlusal vertical dimension of fully erupted teeth
  M26.39 Other anomalies of tooth position of fully erupted tooth or teeth
M26.4 Malocclusion, unspecified
● M26.5 Dentofacial functional abnormalities
    Excludes1   bruxism (F45.8)
                teeth-grinding NOS (F45.8)
  M26.50 Dentofacial functional abnormalities, unspecified
  M26.51 Abnormal jaw closure
  M26.52 Limited mandibular range of motion
  M26.53 Deviation in opening and closing of the mandible
  M26.54 Insufficient anterior guidance
          Insufficient anterior occlusal guidance
  M26.55 Centric occlusion maximum intercuspation discrepancy
      Excludes1   centric occlusion NOS (M26.59)
  M26.56 Non-working side interference
          Balancing side interference
  M26.57 Lack of posterior occlusal support

CHAPTER 13 (M00-M99)

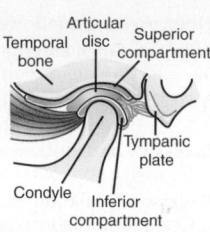

Figure 13-4 Temporomandibular joint.

Item 13–7 Dysfunction of the temporomandibular joint is termed **temporomandibular joint (TMJ) syndrome** and is characterized by pain and tenderness/spasm of the muscles of mastication, joint noise, and in the later stages, limited mandibular movement.

M26.59   **Other dentofacial functional abnormalities**
     Centric occlusion (of teeth) NOS
     Malocclusion due to abnormal swallowing
     Malocclusion due to mouth breathing
     Malocclusion due to tongue, lip or finger
       habits

● M26.6   **Temporomandibular joint disorders**

    Excludes2   current temporomandibular joint
           dislocation (S03.0)
          current temporomandibular joint sprain
           (S03.4)

   M26.60   **Temporomandibular joint disorder, unspecified**
   M26.61   **Adhesions and ankylosis of temporomandibular joint**
   M26.62   **Arthralgia of temporomandibular joint**
   M26.63   **Articular disc disorder of temporomandibular joint**
   M26.69   **Other specified disorders of temporomandibular joint**

● M26.7   **Dental alveolar anomalies**

   M26.70   **Unspecified alveolar anomaly**
   M26.71   **Alveolar maxillary hyperplasia**
   M26.72   **Alveolar mandibular hyperplasia**
   M26.73   **Alveolar maxillary hypoplasia**
   M26.74   **Alveolar mandibular hypoplasia**
   M26.79   **Other specified alveolar anomalies**

● M26.8   **Other dentofacial anomalies**

   M26.81   **Anterior soft tissue impingement**
       Anterior soft tissue impingement on teeth
   M26.82   **Posterior soft tissue impingement**
       Posterior soft tissue impingement on teeth
   M26.89   **Other dentofacial anomalies**

  M26.9   **Dentofacial anomaly, unspecified**

● M27   **Other diseases of jaws**

  M27.0   **Developmental disorders of jaws**
     Latent bone cyst of jaw
     Stafne's cyst
     Torus mandibularis
     Torus palatinus

  M27.1   **Giant cell granuloma, central**
     Giant cell granuloma NOS

    Excludes1   peripheral giant cell granuloma (K06.8)

  M27.2   **Inflammatory conditions of jaws**
     Osteitis of jaw(s)
     Osteomyelitis (neonatal) jaw(s)
     Osteoradionecrosis jaw(s)
     Periostitis jaw(s)
     Sequestrum of jaw bone

    Use additional code (W88-W90, X39.0) to identify
     radiation, if radiation-induced

    Excludes2   osteonecrosis of jaw due to drug
          (M87.180)

  M27.3   **Alveolitis of jaws**
     Alveolar osteitis
     Dry socket

● M27.4   **Other and unspecified cysts of jaw**

    Excludes1   cysts of oral region (K09.-)
          latent bone cyst of jaw (M27.0)
          Stafne's cyst (M27.0)

   M27.40   **Unspecified cyst of jaw**
       Cyst of jaw NOS

   M27.49   **Other cysts of jaw**
       Aneurysmal cyst of jaw
       Hemorrhagic cyst of jaw
       Traumatic cyst of jaw

● M27.5   **Periradicular pathology associated with previous endodontic treatment**

   M27.51   **Perforation of root canal space due to endodontic treatment**
   M27.52   **Endodontic overfill**
   M27.53   **Endodontic underfill**
   M27.59   **Other periradicular pathology associated with previous endodontic treatment**

● M27.6   **Endosseous dental implant failure**

   M27.61   **Osseointegration failure of dental implant**
       Hemorrhagic complications of dental implant
         placement
       Iatrogenic osseointegration failure of dental
         implant
       Osseointegration failure of dental implant due
         to complications of systemic disease
       Osseointegration failure of dental implant due
         to poor bone quality
       Pre-integration failure of dental implant NOS
       Pre-osseointegration failure of dental implant

   M27.62   **Post-osseointegration biological failure of dental implant**
       Failure of dental implant due to lack of
         attached gingiva
       Failure of dental implant due to occlusal
         trauma (caused by poor prosthetic design)
       Failure of dental implant due to parafunctional
         habits
       Failure of dental implant due to periodontal
         infection (peri–implantitis)
       Failure of dental implant due to poor oral
         hygiene
       Iatrogenic post-osseointegration failure of
         dental implant
       Post-osseointegration failure of dental implant
         due to complications of systemic disease

   M27.63   **Post-osseointegration mechanical failure of dental implant**
       Failure of dental prosthesis causing loss of
         dental implant
       Fracture of dental implant

    Excludes2   cracked tooth (K03.81)
          fractured dental restorative
            material with loss of
            material (K08.531)
          fractured dental restorative
            material without loss of
            material (K08.530)
          fractured tooth (S02.5)

   M27.69   **Other endosseous dental implant failure**
       Dental implant failure NOS

  M27.8   **Other specified diseases of jaws**
     Cherubism
     Exostosis
     Fibrous dysplasia
     Unilateral condylar hyperplasia
     Unilateral condylar hypoplasia

    Excludes1   jaw pain (R68.84)

  M27.9   **Disease of jaws, unspecified**

◀ New   ◀◀ Revised   ~~deleted~~ Deleted   Excludes 1   Excludes 2   Includes   Use additional   Code first   Code also   Unspecified

OGCR Official Guidelines   **X** Assign placeholder X   ● Use Additional Character(s)   ▶ Manifestation Code   **Coding Clinic**

CHAPTER 13 (M00-M99)

SYSTEMIC CONNECTIVE TISSUE DISORDERS (M30-M36)

Includes
autoimmune disease NOS
collagen (vascular) disease NOS
systemic autoimmune disease
systemic collagen (vascular) disease

Excludes1
autoimmune disease, single organ or single cell-
type - code to relevant condition category

● M30 Polyarteritis nodosa and related conditions

Excludes1 microscopic polyarteritis (M31.7)

M30.0 Polyarteritis nodosa

M30.1 Polyarteritis with lung involvement [Churg-Strauss]
Allergic granulomatous angiitis

M30.2 Juvenile polyarteritis

M30.3 Mucocutaneous lymph node syndrome [Kawasaki]

M30.8 Other conditions related to polyarteritis nodosa
Polyangiitis overlap syndrome

● M31 Other necrotizing vasculopathies

M31.0 Hypersensitivity angiitis
Goodpasture's syndrome

M31.1 Thrombotic microangiopathy
Thrombotic thrombocytopenic purpura

M31.2 Lethal midline granuloma

M31.3 Wegener's granulomatosis
Necrotizing respiratory granulomatosis

　　M31.30 Wegener's granulomatosis without renal
involvement
Wegener's granulomatosis NOS

　　M31.31 Wegener's granulomatosis with renal
involvement

M31.4 Aortic arch syndrome [Takayasu]

M31.5 Giant cell arteritis with polymyalgia rheumatica

M31.6 Other giant cell arteritis

M31.7 Microscopic polyangiitis
Microscopic polyarteritis
Excludes1 polyarteritis nodosa (M30.0)

M31.8 Other specified necrotizing vasculopathies
Hypocomplementemic vasculitis
Septic vasculitis

M31.9 Necrotizing vasculopathy, unspecified

● M32 Systemic lupus erythematosus (SLE)
Autoimmune inflammatory connective tissue disease of unknown
cause that occurs most often in women.

Excludes1 lupus erythematosus (discoid) (NOS) (L93.0)

M32.0 Drug-induced systemic lupus erythematosus
Use additional code for adverse effect, if applicable,
to identify drug (T36-T50 with fifth or sixth
character 5)

● M32.1 Systemic lupus erythematosus with organ or system
involvement

　　M32.10 Systemic lupus erythematosus, organ or system
involvement unspecified

　　M32.11 Endocarditis in systemic lupus erythematosus
Libman-Sacks disease

　　M32.12 Pericarditis in systemic lupus erythematosus
Lupus pericarditis

　　M32.13 Lung involvement in systemic lupus
erythematosus
Pleural effusion due to systemic lupus
erythematosus

　　M32.14 Glomerular disease in systemic lupus
erythematosus
Lupus renal disease NOS

　　M32.15 Tubulo-interstitial nephropathy in systemic
lupus erythematosus

　　M32.19 Other organ or system involvement in systemic
lupus erythematosus

M32.8 Other forms of systemic lupus erythematosus

M32.9 Systemic lupus erythematosus, unspecified
SLE NOS
Systemic lupus erythematosus NOS
Systemic lupus erythematosus without organ
involvement

● M33 Dermatopolymyositis

● M33.0 Juvenile dermatopolymyositis

　　M33.00 Juvenile dermatopolymyositis, organ
involvement unspecified

　　M33.01 Juvenile dermatopolymyositis with respiratory
involvement

　　M33.02 Juvenile dermatopolymyositis with myopathy

　　M33.09 Juvenile dermatopolymyositis with other organ
involvement

● M33.1 Other dermatopolymyositis

　　M33.10 Other dermatopolymyositis, organ involvement
unspecified

　　M33.11 Other dermatopolymyositis with respiratory
involvement

　　M33.12 Other dermatopolymyositis with myopathy

　　M33.19 Other dermatopolymyositis with other organ
involvement

● M33.2 Polymyositis

　　M33.20 Polymyositis, organ involvement unspecified

　　M33.21 Polymyositis with respiratory involvement

　　M33.22 Polymyositis with myopathy

　　M33.29 Polymyositis with other organ involvement

● M33.9 Dermatopolymyositis, unspecified

　　M33.90 Dermatopolymyositis, unspecified, organ
involvement unspecified

　　M33.91 Dermatopolymyositis, unspecified with
respiratory involvement

　　M33.92 Dermatopolymyositis, unspecified with
myopathy

　　M33.99 Dermatopolymyositis, unspecified with other
organ involvement

● M34 Systemic sclerosis [scleroderma]

Excludes1 circumscribed scleroderma (L94.0)
neonatal scleroderma (P83.8)

M34.0 Progressive systemic sclerosis

M34.1 CR(E)ST syndrome
Combination of calcinosis, Raynaud's phenomenon,
esophageal dysfunction, sclerodactyly,
telangiectasia

M34.2 Systemic sclerosis induced by drug and chemical
Code first poisoning due to drug or toxin, if applicable
(T36-T65 with fifth or sixth character 1-4 or 6)
Use additional code for adverse effect, if applicable,
to identify drug (T36-T50 with fifth or sixth
character 5)

● M34.8 Other forms of systemic sclerosis

　　M34.81 Systemic sclerosis with lung involvement

　　M34.82 Systemic sclerosis with myopathy

　　M34.83 Systemic sclerosis with polyneuropathy

　　M34.89 Other systemic sclerosis

M34.9 Systemic sclerosis, unspecified

● M35 Other systemic involvement of connective tissue
Excludes1 reactive perforating collagenosis (L87.1)

● M35.0 Sicca syndrome [Sjögren]

　　M35.00 Sicca syndrome, unspecified

　　M35.01 Sicca syndrome with keratoconjunctivitis

　　M35.02 Sicca syndrome with lung involvement

　　M35.03 Sicca syndrome with myopathy

　　M35.04 Sicca syndrome with tubulo-interstitial
nephropathy
Renal tubular acidosis in sicca syndrome

　　M35.09 Sicca syndrome with other organ involvement

CHAPTER 13 (M00-M99)

CHAPTER 13 (M00-M99)

Item 13-8 Polymyalgia rheumatica is a syndrome characterized by aching and morning stiffness and is related to aging and hereditary predisposition.

M35.1 Other overlap syndromes
Mixed connective tissue disease
> **Excludes1** polyangiitis overlap syndrome (M30.8)

M35.2 Behçet's disease

M35.3 Polymyalgia rheumatica
> **Excludes1** polymyalgia rheumatica with giant cell arteritis (M31.5)

M35.4 Diffuse (eosinophilic) fasciitis

M35.5 Multifocal fibrosclerosis

M35.6 Relapsing panniculitis [Weber-Christian]
> **Excludes1** lupus panniculitis (L93.2)
> panniculitis NOS (M79.3-)

M35.7 Hypermobility syndrome
Familial ligamentous laxity
> **Excludes1** Ehlers-Danlos syndrome (Q79.6)
> ligamentous laxity, NOS (M24.2-)

M35.8 Other specified systemic involvement of connective tissue

M35.9 Systemic involvement of connective tissue, unspecified
Autoimmune disease (systemic) NOS
Collagen (vascular) disease NOS

● **M36 Systemic disorders of connective tissue in diseases classified elsewhere**
> **Excludes2** arthropathies in diseases classified elsewhere (M14.-)

� *M36.0 Dermato(poly)myositis in neoplastic disease*
> *Code first underlying neoplasm (C00-D49)*

▷ *M36.1 Arthropathy in neoplastic disease*
> *Code first underlying neoplasm, such as:*
> leukemia (C91-C95)
> malignant histiocytosis (C96.A)
> multiple myeloma (C90.0)

▷ *M36.2 Hemophilic arthropathy*
Hemarthrosis in hemophilic arthropathy
> *Code first underlying disease, such as:*
> factor VIII deficiency (D66)
> with vascular defect (D68.0)
> factor IX deficiency (D67)
> hemophilia (classical) (D66)
> hemophilia B (D67)
> hemophilia C (D68.1)

▷ *M36.3 Arthropathy in other blood disorders*

▷ *M36.4 Arthropathy in hypersensitivity reactions classified elsewhere*
> *Code first underlying disease, such as:*
> Henoch (-Schönlein) purpura (D69.0)
> serum sickness (T80.6-)

▷ *M36.8 Systemic disorders of connective tissue in other diseases classified elsewhere*
> *Code first underlying disease, such as:*
> alkaptonuria (E70.2)
> hypogammaglobulinemia (D80.-)
> ochronosis (E70.2)

Item 13-9 Kyphosis is an abnormal curvature of the spine. **Senile kyphosis** is a result of disc degeneration causing ossification (turning to bone). **Adolescent** or **juvenile** kyphosis is also known as **Scheuermann's disease,** a condition in which the discs of the lower thoracic spine herniate, causing the disc space to narrow and the spine to tilt forward. This condition is attributed to poor posture. Lordosis or swayback is an abnormal curvature of the spine resulting in an inward curve of the lumbar spine just above the buttocks. Scoliosis causes a sideways curve to the spine. The curves are S- or C-shaped, and it is most commonly acquired in late childhood and early teen years, when growth is fast.

DORSOPATHIES (M40-M54)

DEFORMING DORSOPATHIES (M40-M43)

● **M40 Kyphosis and lordosis**
> **Excludes1** congenital kyphosis and lordosis (Q76.4)
> kyphoscoliosis (M41.-)
> postprocedural kyphosis and lordosis (M96.-)

● **M40.0 Postural kyphosis**
> **Excludes1** osteochondrosis of spine (M42.-)
M40.00 Postural kyphosis, site unspecified
M40.03 Postural kyphosis, cervicothoracic region
M40.04 Postural kyphosis, thoracic region
M40.05 Postural kyphosis, thoracolumbar region

● **M40.1 Other secondary kyphosis**
M40.10 Other secondary kyphosis, site unspecified
M40.12 Other secondary kyphosis, cervical region
M40.13 Other secondary kyphosis, cervicothoracic region
M40.14 Other secondary kyphosis, thoracic region
M40.15 Other secondary kyphosis, thoracolumbar region

● **M40.2 Other and unspecified kyphosis**
● **M40.20 Unspecified kyphosis**
M40.202 Unspecified kyphosis, cervical region
M40.203 Unspecified kyphosis, cervicothoracic region
M40.204 Unspecified kyphosis, thoracic region
M40.205 Unspecified kyphosis, thoracolumbar region
M40.209 Unspecified kyphosis, site unspecified

● **M40.29 Other kyphosis**
M40.292 Other kyphosis, cervical region
M40.293 Other kyphosis, cervicothoracic region
M40.294 Other kyphosis, thoracic region
M40.295 Other kyphosis, thoracolumbar region
M40.299 Other kyphosis, site unspecified

● **M40.3 Flatback syndrome**
M40.30 Flatback syndrome, site unspecified
M40.35 Flatback syndrome, thoracolumbar region
M40.36 Flatback syndrome, lumbar region
M40.37 Flatback syndrome, lumbosacral region

● **M40.4 Postural lordosis**
> *Abnormal increase in the normal curvature of the lumbar spine (sway back)*
> Acquired lordosis
M40.40 Postural lordosis, site unspecified
M40.45 Postural lordosis, thoracolumbar region
M40.46 Postural lordosis, lumbar region
M40.47 Postural lordosis, lumbosacral region

◀ New   ◀▪▪▪ Revised   ~~deleted~~ Deleted   Excludes 1   Excludes 2   Includes   Use additional   Code first   Code also   Unspecified
OGCR Official Guidelines   **X** Assign placeholder X   ● Use Additional Character(s)   ▷ Manifestation Code   **Coding Clinic**

● **M40.5   Lordosis, unspecified**
    M40.50   Lordosis, unspecified, site unspecified
    M40.55   Lordosis, unspecified, thoracolumbar region
    M40.56   Lordosis, unspecified, lumbar region
    M40.57   Lordosis, unspecified, lumbosacral region

● **M41   Scoliosis**
    Includes   kyphoscoliosis
    Excludes1   congenital scoliosis NOS (Q67.5)
                congenital scoliosis due to bony malformation
                   (Q76.3)
                postural congenital scoliosis (Q67.5)
                kyphoscoliotic heart disease (I27.1)
                postprocedural scoliosis (M96.-)

  ● **M41.0   Infantile idiopathic scoliosis**
    M41.00   Infantile idiopathic scoliosis, site unspecified
    M41.02   Infantile idiopathic scoliosis, cervical region
    M41.03   Infantile idiopathic scoliosis, cervicothoracic region
    M41.04   Infantile idiopathic scoliosis, thoracic region
    M41.05   Infantile idiopathic scoliosis, thoracolumbar region
    M41.06   Infantile idiopathic scoliosis, lumbar region
    M41.07   Infantile idiopathic scoliosis, lumbosacral region
    M41.08   Infantile idiopathic scoliosis, sacral and sacrococcygeal region

  ● **M41.1   Juvenile and adolescent idiopathic scoliosis**
    ● **M41.11   Juvenile idiopathic scoliosis**
        M41.112   Juvenile idiopathic scoliosis, cervical region
        M41.113   Juvenile idiopathic scoliosis, cervicothoracic region
        M41.114   Juvenile idiopathic scoliosis, thoracic region
        M41.115   Juvenile idiopathic scoliosis, thoracolumbar region
        M41.116   Juvenile idiopathic scoliosis, lumbar region
        M41.117   Juvenile idiopathic scoliosis, lumbosacral region
        M41.119   Juvenile idiopathic scoliosis, site unspecified

    ● **M41.12   Adolescent scoliosis**
        M41.122   Adolescent idiopathic scoliosis, cervical region
        M41.123   Adolescent idiopathic scoliosis, cervicothoracic region
        M41.124   Adolescent idiopathic scoliosis, thoracic region
        M41.125   Adolescent idiopathic scoliosis, thoracolumbar region
        M41.126   Adolescent idiopathic scoliosis, lumbar region
        M41.127   Adolescent idiopathic scoliosis, lumbosacral region
        M41.129   Adolescent idiopathic scoliosis, site unspecified

  ● **M41.2   Other idiopathic scoliosis**
    M41.20   Other idiopathic scoliosis, site unspecified
    M41.22   Other idiopathic scoliosis, cervical region
    M41.23   Other idiopathic scoliosis, cervicothoracic region
    M41.24   Other idiopathic scoliosis, thoracic region
    M41.25   Other idiopathic scoliosis, thoracolumbar region
    M41.26   Other idiopathic scoliosis, lumbar region
    M41.27   Other idiopathic scoliosis, lumbosacral region

● **M41.3   Thoracogenic scoliosis**
    M41.30   Thoracogenic scoliosis, site unspecified
    M41.34   Thoracogenic scoliosis, thoracic region
    M41.35   Thoracogenic scoliosis, thoracolumbar region

  ● **M41.4   Neuromuscular scoliosis**
    Scoliosis secondary to cerebral palsy, Friedreich's ataxia, poliomyelitis and other neuromuscular disorders
    Code also underlying condition
    M41.40   Neuromuscular scoliosis, site unspecified
    M41.41   Neuromuscular scoliosis, occipito-atlanto-axial region
    M41.42   Neuromuscular scoliosis, cervical region
    M41.43   Neuromuscular scoliosis, cervicothoracic region
    M41.44   Neuromuscular scoliosis, thoracic region
    M41.45   Neuromuscular scoliosis, thoracolumbar region
    M41.46   Neuromuscular scoliosis, lumbar region
    M41.47   Neuromuscular scoliosis, lumbosacral region

  ● **M41.5   Other secondary scoliosis**
    M41.50   Other secondary scoliosis, site unspecified
    M41.52   Other secondary scoliosis, cervical region
    M41.53   Other secondary scoliosis, cervicothoracic region
    M41.54   Other secondary scoliosis, thoracic region
    M41.55   Other secondary scoliosis, thoracolumbar region
    M41.56   Other secondary scoliosis, lumbar region
    M41.57   Other secondary scoliosis, lumbosacral region

  ● **M41.8   Other forms of scoliosis**
    M41.80   Other forms of scoliosis, site unspecified
    M41.82   Other forms of scoliosis, cervical region
    M41.83   Other forms of scoliosis, cervicothoracic region
    M41.84   Other forms of scoliosis, thoracic region
    M41.85   Other forms of scoliosis, thoracolumbar region
    M41.86   Other forms of scoliosis, lumbar region
    M41.87   Other forms of scoliosis, lumbosacral region

    M41.9   Scoliosis, unspecified

● **M42   Spinal osteochondrosis**
  ● **M42.0   Juvenile osteochondrosis of spine**
    Calvé's disease
    Scheuermann's disease
    Excludes1   postural kyphosis (M40.0)
    M42.00   Juvenile osteochondrosis of spine, site unspecified
    M42.01   Juvenile osteochondrosis of spine, occipito-atlanto-axial region
    M42.02   Juvenile osteochondrosis of spine, cervical region
    M42.03   Juvenile osteochondrosis of spine, cervicothoracic region
    M42.04   Juvenile osteochondrosis of spine, thoracic region
    M42.05   Juvenile osteochondrosis of spine, thoracolumbar region
    M42.06   Juvenile osteochondrosis of spine, lumbar region
    M42.07   Juvenile osteochondrosis of spine, lumbosacral region
    M42.08   Juvenile osteochondrosis of spine, sacral and sacrococcygeal region
    M42.09   Juvenile osteochondrosis of spine, multiple sites in spine

CHAPTER 13 (M00-M99)

● **M42.1   Adult osteochondrosis of spine**
     M42.10   Adult osteochondrosis of spine, site unspecified   **A**
     M42.11   Adult osteochondrosis of spine, occipitoatlanto-axial region   **A**
     M42.12   Adult osteochondrosis of spine, cervical region   **A**
     M42.13   Adult osteochondrosis of spine, cervicothoracic region   **A**
     M42.14   Adult osteochondrosis of spine, thoracic region   **A**
     M42.15   Adult osteochondrosis of spine, thoracolumbar region   **A**
     M42.16   Adult osteochondrosis of spine, lumbar region   **A**
     M42.17   Adult osteochondrosis of spine, lumbosacral region   **A**
     M42.18   Adult osteochondrosis of spine, sacral and sacrococcygeal region   **A**
     M42.19   Adult osteochondrosis of spine, multiple sites in spine   **A**
   M42.9   Spinal osteochondrosis, unspecified

● **M43   Other deforming dorsopathies**
   Excludes1   congenital spondylolysis and spondylolisthesis (Q76.2)
           hemivertebra (Q76.3-Q76.4)
           Klippel-Feil syndrome (Q76.1)
           lumbarization and sacralization (Q76.4)
           platyspondylisis (Q76.4)
           spina bifida occulta (Q76.0)
           spinal curvature in osteoporosis (M80.-)
           spinal curvature in Paget's disease of bone [osteitis deformans] (M88.-)

● **M43.0   Spondylolysis**
     Excludes1   congenital spondylolysis (Q76.2)
            spondylolisthesis (M43.1)
     M43.00   Spondylolysis, site unspecified
     M43.01   Spondylolysis, occipito-atlanto-axial region
     M43.02   Spondylolysis, cervical region
     M43.03   Spondylolysis, cervicothoracic region
     M43.04   Spondylolysis, thoracic region
     M43.05   Spondylolysis, thoracolumbar region
     M43.06   Spondylolysis, lumbar region
     M43.07   Spondylolysis, lumbosacral region
     M43.08   Spondylolysis, sacral and sacrococcygeal region
     M43.09   Spondylolysis, multiple sites in spine

● **M43.1   Spondylolisthesis**
     Excludes1   acute traumatic of lumbosacral region (S33.1)
            acute traumatic of sites other than lumbosacral - code to Fracture, vertebra, by region
            congenital spondylolisthesis (Q76.2)
     M43.10   Spondylolisthesis, site unspecified
     M43.11   Spondylolisthesis, occipito-atlanto-axial region
     M43.12   Spondylolisthesis, cervical region
     M43.13   Spondylolisthesis, cervicothoracic region
     M43.14   Spondylolisthesis, thoracic region
     M43.15   Spondylolisthesis, thoracolumbar region
     M43.16   Spondylolisthesis, lumbar region
     M43.17   Spondylolisthesis, lumbosacral region
     M43.18   Spondylolisthesis, sacral and sacrococcygeal region
     M43.19   Spondylolisthesis, multiple sites in spine

● **M43.2   Fusion of spine**
     Ankylosis of spinal joint
     Excludes1   ankylosing spondylitis (M45.0-)
            congenital fusion of spine (Q76.4)
     Excludes2   arthrodesis status (Z98.1)
            pseudoarthrosis after fusion or arthrodesis (M96.0)
     M43.20   Fusion of spine, site unspecified
     M43.21   Fusion of spine, occipito-atlanto-axial region
     M43.22   Fusion of spine, cervical region
     M43.23   Fusion of spine, cervicothoracic region
     M43.24   Fusion of spine, thoracic region
     M43.25   Fusion of spine, thoracolumbar region
     M43.26   Fusion of spine, lumbar region
     M43.27   Fusion of spine, lumbosacral region
     M43.28   Fusion of spine, sacral and sacrococcygeal region
   M43.3   Recurrent atlantoaxial dislocation with myelopathy
   M43.4   Other recurrent atlantoaxial dislocation

● **M43.5   Other recurrent vertebral dislocation**
     Excludes1   biomechanical lesions NEC (M99.-)
     ● **M43.5X   Other recurrent vertebral dislocation**
       M43.5X2   Other recurrent vertebral dislocation, cervical region
       M43.5X3   Other recurrent vertebral dislocation, cervicothoracic region
       M43.5X4   Other recurrent vertebral dislocation, thoracic region
       M43.5X5   Other recurrent vertebral dislocation, thoracolumbar region
       M43.5X6   Other recurrent vertebral dislocation, lumbar region
       M43.5X7   Other recurrent vertebral dislocation, lumbosacral region
       M43.5X8   Other recurrent vertebral dislocation, sacral and sacrococcygeal region
       M43.5X9   Other recurrent vertebral dislocation, site unspecified

   M43.6   Torticollis
     Excludes1   congenital (sternomastoid) torticollis (Q68.0)
            current injury - see Injury, of spine, by body region ocular torticollis (R29.891)
            psychogenic torticollis (F45.8)
            spasmodic torticollis (G24.3)
            torticollis due to birth injury (P15.2)

● **M43.8   Other specified deforming dorsopathies**
     Excludes2   kyphosis and lordosis (M40.-)
            scoliosis (M41.-)
     ● **M43.8X   Other specified deforming dorsopathies**
       M43.8X1   Other specified deforming dorsopathies, occipito-atlanto-axial region
       M43.8X2   Other specified deforming dorsopathies, cervical region
       M43.8X3   Other specified deforming dorsopathies, cervicothoracic region
       M43.8X4   Other specified deforming dorsopathies, thoracic region
       M43.8X5   Other specified deforming dorsopathies, thoracolumbar region
       M43.8X6   Other specified deforming dorsopathies, lumbar region
       M43.8X7   Other specified deforming dorsopathies, lumbosacral region

---

Item 13–10   Spondylolisthesis is a condition caused by the slipping forward of one disc over another.

◀ New   ⬅ Revised   ~~deleted~~ Deleted   Excludes 1   Excludes 2   Includes   Use additional   Code first   Code also   Unspecified

OGCR Official Guidelines   **X** Assign placeholder X   ● Use Additional Character(s)   ▷ Manifestation Code   **Coding Clinic**

M43.8X8   Other specified deforming dorsopathies, sacral and sacrococcygeal region

▶ M43.8X9   *Other specified deforming dorsopathies, site unspecified*

M43.9   Deforming dorsopathy, unspecified

     Curvature of spine NOS

SPONDYLOPATHIES (M45-M49)

● M45   Ankylosing spondylitis

     Rheumatoid arthritis of spine

     Excludes1   arthropathy in Reiter's disease (M02.3-)

                   juvenile (ankylosing) spondylitis (M08.1)

     Excludes2   Behçet's disease (M35.2)

M45.0   Ankylosing spondylitis of multiple sites in spine

M45.1   Ankylosing spondylitis of occipito-atlanto-axial region

M45.2   Ankylosing spondylitis of cervical region

M45.3   Ankylosing spondylitis of cervicothoracic region

M45.4   Ankylosing spondylitis of thoracic region

M45.5   Ankylosing spondylitis of thoracolumbar region

M45.6   Ankylosing spondylitis lumbar region

M45.7   Ankylosing spondylitis of lumbosacral region

M45.8   Ankylosing spondylitis sacral and sacrococcygeal region

M45.9   Ankylosing spondylitis of unspecified sites in spine

● M46   Other inflammatory spondylopathies

 ● M46.0   Spinal enthesopathy

     Disorder of ligamentous or muscular attachments of spine

     M46.00   Spinal enthesopathy, site unspecified

     M46.01   Spinal enthesopathy, occipito-atlanto-axial region

     M46.02   Spinal enthesopathy, cervical region

     M46.03   Spinal enthesopathy, cervicothoracic region

     M46.04   Spinal enthesopathy, thoracic region

     M46.05   Spinal enthesopathy, thoracolumbar region

     M46.06   Spinal enthesopathy, lumbar region

     M46.07   Spinal enthesopathy, lumbosacral region

     M46.08   Spinal enthesopathy, sacral and sacrococcygeal region

     M46.09   Spinal enthesopathy, multiple sites in spine

 M46.1   Sacroiliitis, not elsewhere classified

 ● M46.2   Osteomyelitis of vertebra

     M46.20   Osteomyelitis of vertebra, site unspecified

     M46.21   Osteomyelitis of vertebra, occipito-atlanto-axial region

     M46.22   Osteomyelitis of vertebra, cervical region

     M46.23   Osteomyelitis of vertebra, cervicothoracic region

     M46.24   Osteomyelitis of vertebra, thoracic region

     M46.25   Osteomyelitis of vertebra, thoracolumbar region

     M46.26   Osteomyelitis of vertebra, lumbar region

     M46.27   Osteomyelitis of vertebra, lumbosacral region

     M46.28   Osteomyelitis of vertebra, sacral and sacrococcygeal region

 ● M46.3   Infection of intervertebral disc (pyogenic)

     Use additional code (B95-B97) to identify infectious agent

     M46.30   Infection of intervertebral disc (pyogenic), site unspecified

     M46.31   Infection of intervertebral disc (pyogenic), occipito-atlanto-axial region

     M46.32   Infection of intervertebral disc (pyogenic), cervical region

     M46.33   Infection of intervertebral disc (pyogenic), cervicothoracic region

M46.34   Infection of intervertebral disc (pyogenic), thoracic region

M46.35   Infection of intervertebral disc (pyogenic), thoracolumbar region

M46.36   Infection of intervertebral disc (pyogenic), lumbar region

M46.37   Infection of intervertebral disc (pyogenic), lumbosacral region

M46.38   Infection of intervertebral disc (pyogenic), sacral and sacrococcygeal region

M46.39   Infection of intervertebral disc (pyogenic), multiple sites in spine

● M46.4   Discitis, unspecified

     M46.40   Discitis, unspecified, site unspecified

     M46.41   Discitis, unspecified, occipito-atlanto-axial region

     M46.42   Discitis, unspecified, cervical region

     M46.43   Discitis, unspecified, cervicothoracic region

     M46.44   Discitis, unspecified, thoracic region

     M46.45   Discitis, unspecified, thoracolumbar region

     M46.46   Discitis, unspecified, lumbar region

     M46.47   Discitis, unspecified, lumbosacral region

     M46.48   Discitis, unspecified, sacral and sacrococcygeal region

     M46.49   Discitis, unspecified, multiple sites in spine

● M46.5   Other infective spondylopathies

     M46.50   Other infective spondylopathies, site unspecified

     M46.51   Other infective spondylopathies, occipitoatlanto-axial region

     M46.52   Other infective spondylopathies, cervical region

     M46.53   Other infective spondylopathies, cervicothoracic region

     M46.54   Other infective spondylopathies, thoracic region

     M46.55   Other infective spondylopathies, thoracolumbar region

     M46.56   Other infective spondylopathies, lumbar region

     M46.57   Other infective spondylopathies, lumbosacral region

     M46.58   Other infective spondylopathies, sacral and sacrococcygeal region

     M46.59   Other infective spondylopathies, multiple sites in spine

● M46.8   Other specified inflammatory spondylopathies

     M46.80   Other specified inflammatory spondylopathies, site unspecified

     M46.81   Other specified inflammatory spondylopathies, occipito-atlanto-axial region

     M46.82   Other specified inflammatory spondylopathies, cervical region

     M46.83   Other specified inflammatory spondylopathies, cervicothoracic region

     M46.84   Other specified inflammatory spondylopathies, thoracic region

     M46.85   Other specified inflammatory spondylopathies, thoracolumbar region

     M46.86   Other specified inflammatory spondylopathies, lumbar region

     M46.87   Other specified inflammatory spondylopathies, lumbosacral region

     M46.88   Other specified inflammatory spondylopathies, sacral and sacrococcygeal region

     M46.89   Other specified inflammatory spondylopathies, multiple sites in spine

CHAPTER 13 (M00-M99)

CHAPTER 13 (M00-M99)

● M46.9   Unspecified inflammatory spondylopathy

    M46.90   Unspecified inflammatory spondylopathy, site unspecified

    M46.91   Unspecified inflammatory spondylopathy, occipito-atlanto-axial region

    M46.92   Unspecified inflammatory spondylopathy, cervical region

    M46.93   Unspecified inflammatory spondylopathy, cervicothoracic region

    M46.94   Unspecified inflammatory spondylopathy, thoracic region

    M46.95   Unspecified inflammatory spondylopathy, thoracolumbar region

    M46.96   Unspecified inflammatory spondylopathy, lumbar region

    M46.97   Unspecified inflammatory spondylopathy, lumbosacral region

    M46.98   Unspecified inflammatory spondylopathy, sacral and sacrococcygeal region

    M46.99   Unspecified inflammatory spondylopathy, multiple sites in spine

● M47   Spondylosis

    Includes   arthrosis or osteoarthritis of spine
                    degeneration of facet joints

   ● M47.0   Anterior spinal and vertebral artery compression syndromes

      ● M47.01   Anterior spinal artery compression syndromes

        M47.011   Anterior spinal artery compression syndromes, occipito-atlanto-axial region

        M47.012   Anterior spinal artery compression syndromes, cervical region

        M47.013   Anterior spinal artery compression syndromes, cervicothoracic region

        M47.014   Anterior spinal artery compression syndromes, thoracic region

        M47.015   Anterior spinal artery compression syndromes, thoracolumbar region

        M47.016   Anterior spinal artery compression syndromes, lumbar region

        M47.019   Anterior spinal artery compression syndromes, site unspecified

      ● M47.02   Vertebral artery compression syndromes

        M47.021   Vertebral artery compression syndromes, occipito-atlanto-axial region

        M47.022   Vertebral artery compression syndromes, cervical region

        M47.029   Vertebral artery compression syndromes, site unspecified

   ● M47.1   Other spondylosis with myelopathy

      Spondylogenic compression of spinal cord

      Excludes1   vertebral subluxation (M43.3-M43.59)

    M47.10   Other spondylosis with myelopathy, site unspecified

    M47.11   Other spondylosis with myelopathy, occipito-atlanto-axial region

    M47.12   Other spondylosis with myelopathy, cervical region

    M47.13   Other spondylosis with myelopathy, cervicothoracic region

    M47.14   Other spondylosis with myelopathy, thoracic region

    M47.15   Other spondylosis with myelopathy, thoracolumbar region

    M47.16   Other spondylosis with myelopathy, lumbar region

   ● M47.2   Other spondylosis with radiculopathy

    M47.20   Other spondylosis with radiculopathy, site unspecified

    M47.21   Other spondylosis with radiculopathy, occipito-atlanto-axial region

    M47.22   Other spondylosis with radiculopathy, cervical region

    M47.23   Other spondylosis with radiculopathy, cervicothoracic region

    M47.24   Other spondylosis with radiculopathy, thoracic region

    M47.25   Other spondylosis with radiculopathy, thoracolumbar region

    M47.26   Other spondylosis with radiculopathy, lumbar region

    M47.27   Other spondylosis with radiculopathy, lumbosacral region

    M47.28   Other spondylosis with radiculopathy, sacral and sacrococcygeal region

   ● M47.8   Other spondylosis

      ● M47.81   Spondylosis without myelopathy or radiculopathy

        M47.811   Spondylosis without myelopathy or radiculopathy, occipito-atlanto-axial region

        M47.812   Spondylosis without myelopathy or radiculopathy, cervical region

        M47.813   Spondylosis without myelopathy or radiculopathy, cervicothoracic region

        M47.814   Spondylosis without myelopathy or radiculopathy, thoracic region

        M47.815   Spondylosis without myelopathy or radiculopathy, thoracolumbar region

        M47.816   Spondylosis without myelopathy or radiculopathy, lumbar region

        M47.817   Spondylosis without myelopathy or radiculopathy, lumbosacral region

        M47.818   Spondylosis without myelopathy or radiculopathy, sacral and sacrococcygeal region

        M47.819   Spondylosis without myelopathy or radiculopathy, site unspecified

      ● M47.89   Other spondylosis

        M47.891   Other spondylosis, occipito-atlanto-axial region

        M47.892   Other spondylosis, cervical region

        M47.893   Other spondylosis, cervicothoracic region

        M47.894   Other spondylosis, thoracic region

        M47.895   Other spondylosis, thoracolumbar region

        M47.896   Other spondylosis, lumbar region

        M47.897   Other spondylosis, lumbosacral region

        M47.898   Other spondylosis, sacral and sacrococcygeal region

        M47.899   Other spondylosis, site unspecified

   M47.9   Spondylosis, unspecified

◄ New   ◄▥ Revised   ~~deleted~~ Deleted   Excludes 1   Excludes 2   Includes   Use additional   Code first   Code also   Unspecified

OGCR Official Guidelines   X Assign placeholder X   ● Use Additional Character(s)   ▶ Manifestation Code   **Coding Clinic**

● **M48 Other spondylopathies**
  ● **M48.0 Spinal stenosis**
      Caudal stenosis
      M48.00 Spinal stenosis, site unspecified
      M48.01 Spinal stenosis, occipito-atlanto-axial region
      M48.02 Spinal stenosis, cervical region
      M48.03 Spinal stenosis, cervicothoracic region
      M48.04 Spinal stenosis, thoracic region
      M48.05 Spinal stenosis, thoracolumbar region
      M48.06 Spinal stenosis, lumbar region
      M48.07 Spinal stenosis, lumbosacral region
      M48.08 Spinal stenosis, sacral and sacrococcygeal region
  ● **M48.1 Ankylosing hyperostosis [Forestier]**
      Diffuse idiopathic skeletal hyperostosis [DISH]
      M48.10 Ankylosing hyperostosis [Forestier], site unspecified
      M48.11 Ankylosing hyperostosis [Forestier], occipito-atlanto-axial region
      M48.12 Ankylosing hyperostosis [Forestier], cervical region
      M48.13 Ankylosing hyperostosis [Forestier], cervicothoracic region
      M48.14 Ankylosing hyperostosis [Forestier], thoracic region
      M48.15 Ankylosing hyperostosis [Forestier], thoracolumbar region
      M48.16 Ankylosing hyperostosis [Forestier], lumbar region
      M48.17 Ankylosing hyperostosis [Forestier], lumbosacral region
      M48.18 Ankylosing hyperostosis [Forestier], sacral and sacrococcygeal region
      M48.19 Ankylosing hyperostosis [Forestier], multiple sites in spine
  ● **M48.2 Kissing spine**
      M48.20 Kissing spine, site unspecified
      M48.21 Kissing spine, occipito-atlanto-axial region
      M48.22 Kissing spine, cervical region
      M48.23 Kissing spine, cervicothoracic region
      M48.24 Kissing spine, thoracic region
      M48.25 Kissing spine, thoracolumbar region
      M48.26 Kissing spine, lumbar region
      M48.27 Kissing spine, lumbosacral region
  ● **M48.3 Traumatic spondylopathy**
      M48.30 Traumatic spondylopathy, site unspecified
      M48.31 Traumatic spondylopathy, occipito-atlanto-axial region
      M48.32 Traumatic spondylopathy, cervical region
      M48.33 Traumatic spondylopathy, cervicothoracic region
      M48.34 Traumatic spondylopathy, thoracic region
      M48.35 Traumatic spondylopathy, thoracolumbar region
      M48.36 Traumatic spondylopathy, lumbar region
      M48.37 Traumatic spondylopathy, lumbosacral region
      M48.38 Traumatic spondylopathy, sacral and sacrococcygeal region

● **M48.4 Fatigue fracture of vertebra**
    Stress fracture of vertebra
    Excludes1 pathological fracture NOS (M84.4-)
                pathological fracture of vertebra due to neoplasm (M84.58)
                pathological fracture of vertebra due to other diagnosis (M84.68)
                pathological fracture of vertebra due to osteoporosis (M80.-)
                traumatic fracture of vertebrae (S12.0-S12.3-, S22.0-, S32.0-)

  The appropriate 7th character is to be added to each code from subcategory M48.4:

A	initial encounter for fracture
D	subsequent encounter for fracture with routine healing
G	subsequent encounter for fracture with delayed healing
S	sequela of fracture

  X● **M48.40 Fatigue fracture of vertebra, site unspecified**
  X● **M48.41 Fatigue fracture of vertebra, occipitoatlanto-axial region**
  X● **M48.42 Fatigue fracture of vertebra, cervical region**
  X● **M48.43 Fatigue fracture of vertebra, cervicothoracic region**
  X● **M48.44 Fatigue fracture of vertebra, thoracic region**
  X● **M48.45 Fatigue fracture of vertebra, thoracolumbar region**
  X● **M48.46 Fatigue fracture of vertebra, lumbar region**
  X● **M48.47 Fatigue fracture of vertebra, lumbosacral region**
  X● **M48.48 Fatigue fracture of vertebra, sacral and sacrococcygeal region**

● **M48.5 Collapsed vertebra, not elsewhere classified**
    Collapsed vertebra NOS
    Wedging of vertebra NOS
    Excludes1 current injury - see Injury of spine, by body region
                fatigue fracture of vertebra (M48.4)
                pathological fracture of vertebra due to neoplasm (M84.58)
                pathological fracture of vertebra due to other diagnosis (M84.68)
                pathological fracture of vertebra due to osteoporosis (M80.-)
                pathological fracture NOS (M84.4-)
                stress fracture of vertebra (M48.4-)
                traumatic fracture of vertebra (S12.-, S22.-, S32.-)

  The appropriate 7th character is to be added to each code from subcategory M48.5:

A	initial encounter for fracture
D	subsequent encounter for fracture with routine healing
G	subsequent encounter for fracture with delayed healing
S	sequela of fracture

  X● **M48.50 Collapsed vertebra, not elsewhere classified, site unspecified**
  X● **M48.51 Collapsed vertebra, not elsewhere classified, occipito-atlanto-axial region**
  X● **M48.52 Collapsed vertebra, not elsewhere classified, cervical region**
  X● **M48.53 Collapsed vertebra, not elsewhere classified, cervicothoracic region**

CHAPTER 13 (M00-M99)

X● **M48.54** Collapsed vertebra, not elsewhere classified, thoracic region

X● **M48.55** Collapsed vertebra, not elsewhere classified, thoracolumbar region

X● **M48.56** Collapsed vertebra, not elsewhere classified, lumbar region

X● **M48.57** Collapsed vertebra, not elsewhere classified, lumbosacral region

X● **M48.58** Collapsed vertebra, not elsewhere classified, sacral and sacrococcygeal region

● **M48.8** Other specified spondylopathies
Ossification of posterior longitudinal ligament

● **M48.8X** Other specified spondylopathies

M48.8X1 Other specified spondylopathies, occipito-atlanto-axial region

M48.8X2 Other specified spondylopathies, cervical region

M48.8X3 Other specified spondylopathies, cervicothoracic region

M48.8X4 Other specified spondylopathies, thoracic region

M48.8X5 Other specified spondylopathies, thoracolumbar region

M48.8X6 Other specified spondylopathies, lumbar region

M48.8X7 Other specified spondylopathies, lumbosacral region

M48.8X8 Other specified spondylopathies, sacral and sacrococcygeal region

M48.8X9 Other specified spondylopathies, site unspecified

M48.9 Spondylopathy, unspecified

● **M49** Spondylopathies in diseases classified elsewhere

Includes curvature of spine in diseases classified elsewhere
deformity of spine in diseases classified elsewhere
kyphosis in diseases classified elsewhere
scoliosis in diseases classified elsewhere
spondylopathy in diseases classified elsewhere

Code first underlying disease, such as:
brucellosis (A23.-)
Charcot-Marie-Tooth disease (G60.0)
enterobacterial infections (A01-A04)
osteitis fibrosa cystica (E21.0)

Excludes1 curvature of spine in tuberculosis [Pott's] (A18.01)
enteropathic arthropathies (M07.-)
gonococcal spondylitis (A54.41)
neuropathic [tabes dorsalis] spondylitis (A52.11)
neuropathic spondylopathy in syringomyelia (G95.0)
neuropathic spondylopathy in tabes dorsalis (A52.11)
nonsyphilitic neuropathic spondylopathy NEC (G98.0)
spondylitis in syphilis (acquired) (A52.77)
tuberculous spondylitis (A18.01)
typhoid fever spondylitis (A01.05)

● **M49.8** Spondylopathy in diseases classified elsewhere

▷ *M49.80* *Spondylopathy in diseases classified elsewhere, site unspecified*

▷ *M49.81* *Spondylopathy in diseases classified elsewhere, occipito-atlanto-axial region*

▷ *M49.82* *Spondylopathy in diseases classified elsewhere, cervical region*

▷ *M49.83* *Spondylopathy in diseases classified elsewhere, cervicothoracic region*

▷ *M49.84* *Spondylopathy in diseases classified elsewhere, thoracic region*

▷ *M49.85* *Spondylopathy in diseases classified elsewhere, thoracolumbar region*

▷ *M49.86* *Spondylopathy in diseases classified elsewhere, lumbar region*

▷ *M49.87* *Spondylopathy in diseases classified elsewhere, lumbosacral region*

▷ *M49.88* *Spondylopathy in diseases classified elsewhere, sacral and sacrococcygeal region*

▷ *M49.89* *Spondylopathy in diseases classified elsewhere, multiple sites in spine*

OTHER DORSOPATHIES (M50-M54)

Excludes1 current injury - see injury of spine by body region
discitis NOS (M46.4-)

● **M50** Cervical disc disorders

Note: Code to the most superior level of disorder.

Includes cervicothoracic disc disorders with cervicalgia
cervicothoracic disc disorders

● **M50.0** Cervical disc disorder with myelopathy

M50.00 Cervical disc disorder with myelopathy, unspecified cervical region

M50.01 Cervical disc disorder with myelopathy, high cervical region
C2-C3 disc disorder with myelopathy
C3-C4 disc disorder with myelopathy

M50.02 Cervical disc disorder with myelopathy, mid-cervical region
C4-C5 disc disorder with myelopathy
C5-C6 disc disorder with myelopathy
C6-C7 disc disorder with myelopathy

M50.03 Cervical disc disorder with myelopathy, cervicothoracic region
C7-T1 disc disorder with myelopathy

● **M50.1** Cervical disc disorder with radiculopathy

Excludes2 brachial radiculitis NOS (M54.13)

M50.10 Cervical disc disorder with radiculopathy, unspecified cervical region

M50.11 Cervical disc disorder with radiculopathy, high cervical region
C2-C3 disc disorder with radiculopathy
C3 radiculopathy due to disc disorder
C3-C4 disc disorder with radiculopathy
C4 radiculopathy due to disc disorder

M50.12 Cervical disc disorder with radiculopathy, mid-cervical region
C4-C5 disc disorder with radiculopathy
C5 radiculopathy due to disc disorder
C5-C6 disc disorder with radiculopathy
C6 radiculopathy due to disc disorder
C6-C7 disc disorder with radiculopathy
C7 radiculopathy due to disc disorder

M50.13 Cervical disc disorder with radiculopathy, cervicothoracic region
C7-T1 disc disorder with radiculopathy
C8 radiculopathy due to disc disorder

● **M50.2** Other cervical disc displacement

M50.20 Other cervical disc displacement, unspecified cervical region

M50.21 Other cervical disc displacement, high cervical region
Other C2-C3 cervical disc displacement
Other C3-C4 cervical disc displacement

M50.22 Other cervical disc displacement, mid-cervical region
Other C4-C5 cervical disc displacement
Other C5-C6 cervical disc displacement
Other C6-C7 cervical disc displacement

M50.23 Other cervical disc displacement, cervicothoracic region
Other C7-T1 cervical disc displacement

◄ New   ◄━ Revised   ~~deleted~~ Deleted   Excludes 1   Excludes 2   Includes   Use additional   Code first   Code also   Unspecified

OGCR Official Guidelines   X Assign placeholder X   ● Use Additional Character(s)   ▷ Manifestation Code   **Coding Clinic**

● **M50.3 Other cervical disc degeneration**

  M50.30 Other cervical disc degeneration, unspecified cervical region

  M50.31 Other cervical disc degeneration, high cervical region
      Other C2-C3 cervical disc degeneration
      Other C3-C4 cervical disc degeneration

  M50.32 Other cervical disc degeneration, mid-cervical region
      Other C4-C5 cervical disc degeneration
      Other C5-C6 cervical disc degeneration
      Other C6-C7 cervical disc degeneration

  M50.33 Other cervical disc degeneration, cervicothoracic region
      Other C7-T1 cervical disc degeneration

● **M50.8 Other cervical disc disorders**

  M50.80 Other cervical disc disorders, unspecified cervical region

  M50.81 Other cervical disc disorders, high cervical region
      Other C2-C3 cervical disc disorders
      Other C3-C4 cervical disc disorders

  M50.82 Other cervical disc disorders, mid-cervical region
      Other C4-C5 cervical disc disorders
      Other C5-C6 cervical disc disorders
      Other C6-C7 cervical disc disorders

  M50.83 Other cervical disc disorders, cervicothoracic region
      Other C7-T1 cervical disc disorders

● **M50.9 Cervical disc disorder, unspecified**

  M50.90 Cervical disc disorder, unspecified, unspecified cervical region

  M50.91 Cervical disc disorder, unspecified, high cervical region
      C2-C3 cervical disc disorder, unspecified
      C3-C4 cervical disc disorder, unspecified

  M50.92 Cervical disc disorder, unspecified, mid-cervical region
      C4-C5 cervical disc disorder, unspecified
      C5-C6 cervical disc disorder, unspecified
      C6-C7 cervical disc disorder, unspecified

  M50.93 Cervical disc disorder, unspecified, cervicothoracic region
      C7-T1 cervical disc disorder, unspecified

● **M51 Thoracic, thoracolumbar, and lumbosacral intervertebral disc disorders**

  Excludes2   cervical and cervicothoracic disc disorders (M50.-)
            sacral and sacrococcygeal disorders (M53.3)

● **M51.0 Thoracic, thoracolumbar and lumbosacral intervertebral disc disorders with myelopathy**

  M51.04 Intervertebral disc disorders with myelopathy, thoracic region

  M51.05 Intervertebral disc disorders with myelopathy, thoracolumbar region

  M51.06 Intervertebral disc disorders with myelopathy, lumbar region

● **M51.1 Thoracic, thoracolumbar and lumbosacral intervertebral disc disorders with radiculopathy**
  Sciatica due to intervertebral disc disorder

  Excludes1   lumbar radiculitis NOS (M54.16)
            sciatica NOS (M54.3)

  M51.14 Intervertebral disc disorders with radiculopathy, thoracic region

  M51.15 Intervertebral disc disorders with radiculopathy, thoracolumbar region

  M51.16 Intervertebral disc disorders with radiculopathy, lumbar region

  M51.17 Intervertebral disc disorders with radiculopathy, lumbosacral region

● **M51.2 Other thoracic, thoracolumbar and lumbosacral intervertebral disc displacement**
  Lumbago due to displacement of intervertebral disc

  M51.24 Other intervertebral disc displacement, thoracic region

  M51.25 Other intervertebral disc displacement, thoracolumbar region

  M51.26 Other intervertebral disc displacement, lumbar region

  M51.27 Other intervertebral disc displacement, lumbosacral region

● **M51.3 Other thoracic, thoracolumbar and lumbosacral intervertebral disc degeneration**
  Coding Clinic: 2013, Q3, P22

  M51.34 Other intervertebral disc degeneration, thoracic region

  M51.35 Other intervertebral disc degeneration, thoracolumbar region

  M51.36 Other intervertebral disc degeneration, lumbar region

  M51.37 Other intervertebral disc degeneration, lumbosacral region

● **M51.4 Schmorl's nodes**

  M51.44 Schmorl's nodes, thoracic region

  M51.45 Schmorl's nodes, thoracolumbar region

  M51.46 Schmorl's nodes, lumbar region

  M51.47 Schmorl's nodes, lumbosacral region

● **M51.8 Other thoracic, thoracolumbar and lumbosacral intervertebral disc disorders**

  M51.84 Other intervertebral disc disorders, thoracic region

  M51.85 Other intervertebral disc disorders, thoracolumbar region

  M51.86 Other intervertebral disc disorders, lumbar region

  M51.87 Other intervertebral disc disorders, lumbosacral region

  M51.9 Unspecified thoracic, thoracolumbar and lumbosacral intervertebral disc disorder

● **M53 Other and unspecified dorsopathies, not elsewhere classified**

  M53.0 Cervicocranial syndrome
      Posterior cervical sympathetic syndrome

  M53.1 Cervicobrachial syndrome

    Excludes2   cervical disc disorder (M50.-)
              thoracic outlet syndrome (G54.0)

● **M53.2 Spinal instabilities**

  ● M53.2X Spinal instabilities

    M53.2X1 Spinal instabilities, occipito-atlanto-axial region

    M53.2X2 Spinal instabilities, cervical region

    M53.2X3 Spinal instabilities, cervicothoracic region

    M53.2X4 Spinal instabilities, thoracic region

    M53.2X5 Spinal instabilities, thoracolumbar region

    M53.2X6 Spinal instabilities, lumbar region

    M53.2X7 Spinal instabilities, lumbosacral region

    M53.2X8 Spinal instabilities, sacral and sacrococcygeal region

    M53.2X9 Spinal instabilities, site unspecified

  M53.3 Sacrococcygeal disorders, not elsewhere classified
      Coccygodynia

● **M53.8 Other specified dorsopathies**

  M53.80 Other specified dorsopathies, site unspecified

  M53.81 Other specified dorsopathies, occipito-atlanto-axial region

  M53.82 Other specified dorsopathies, cervical region

CHAPTER 13 (M00-M99)

M53.83 Other specified dorsopathies, cervicothoracic region

M53.84 Other specified dorsopathies, thoracic region

M53.85 Other specified dorsopathies, thoracolumbar region

M53.86 Other specified dorsopathies, lumbar region

M53.87 Other specified dorsopathies, lumbosacral region

M53.88 Other specified dorsopathies, sacral and sacrococcygeal region

M53.9 Dorsopathy, unspecified

● M54 Dorsalgia

Excludes1 psychogenic dorsalgia (F45.41)

● M54.0 Panniculitis affecting regions of neck and back

Excludes1 lupus panniculitis (L93.2)
panniculitis NOS (M79.3)
relapsing [Weber-Christian] panniculitis (M35.6)

M54.00 Panniculitis affecting regions of neck and back, site unspecified

M54.01 Panniculitis affecting regions of neck and back, occipito-atlanto-axial region

M54.02 Panniculitis affecting regions of neck and back, cervical region

M54.03 Panniculitis affecting regions of neck and back, cervicothoracic region

M54.04 Panniculitis affecting regions of neck and back, thoracic region

M54.05 Panniculitis affecting regions of neck and back, thoracolumbar region

M54.06 Panniculitis affecting regions of neck and back, lumbar region

M54.07 Panniculitis affecting regions of neck and back, lumbosacral region

M54.08 Panniculitis affecting regions of neck and back, sacral and sacrococcygeal region

M54.09 Panniculitis affecting regions, neck and back, multiple sites in spine

● M54.1 Radiculopathy
Brachial neuritis or radiculitis NOS
Lumbar neuritis or radiculitis NOS
Lumbosacral neuritis or radiculitis NOS
Thoracic neuritis or radiculitis NOS
Radiculitis NOS

Excludes1 neuralgia and neuritis NOS (M79.2)
radiculopathy with cervical disc disorder (M50.1)
radiculopathy with lumbar and other intervertebral disc disorder (M51.1-)
radiculopathy with spondylosis (M47.2-)

M54.10 Radiculopathy, site unspecified

M54.11 Radiculopathy, occipito-atlanto-axial region

M54.12 Radiculopathy, cervical region

M54.13 Radiculopathy, cervicothoracic region

M54.14 Radiculopathy, thoracic region

M54.15 Radiculopathy, thoracolumbar region

M54.16 Radiculopathy, lumbar region

M54.17 Radiculopathy, lumbosacral region

M54.18 Radiculopathy, sacral and sacrococcygeal region

M54.2 Cervicalgia

Excludes1 cervicalgia due to intervertebral cervical disc disorder (M50.-)

● M54.3 Sciatica

Excludes1 lesion of sciatic nerve (G57.0)
sciatica due to intervertebral disc disorder (M51.1-)
sciatica with lumbago (M54.4-)

M54.30 Sciatica, unspecified side

M54.31 Sciatica, right side

M54.32 Sciatica, left side

● M54.4 Lumbago with sciatica

Excludes1 lumbago with sciatica due to intervertebral disc disorder (M51.1-)

M54.40 Lumbago with sciatica, unspecified side

M54.41 Lumbago with sciatica, right side

M54.42 Lumbago with sciatica, left side

M54.5 Low back pain
Loin pain
Lumbago NOS

Excludes1 low back strain (S39.012)
lumbago due to intervertebral disc displacement (M51.2-)
lumbago with sciatica (M54.4-)

M54.6 Pain in thoracic spine

Excludes1 pain in thoracic spine due to intervertebral disc disorder (M51.)

● M54.8 Other dorsalgia

Excludes1 dorsalgia in thoracic region (M54.6)
low back pain (M54.5)

M54.81 Occipital neuralgia

M54.89 Other dorsalgia

M54.9 Dorsalgia, unspecified
Backache NOS
Back pain NOS

SOFT TISSUE DISORDERS (M60-M79)

DISORDERS OF MUSCLES (M60-M63)

Excludes1 dermatopolymyositis (M33.-)
muscular dystrophies and myopathies (G71-G72)
myopathy in amyloidosis (E85.-)
myopathy in polyarteritis nodosa (M30.0)
myopathy in rheumatoid arthritis (M05.32)
myopathy in scleroderma (M34.-)
myopathy in Sjögren's syndrome (M35.03)
myopathy in systemic lupus erythematosus (M32.-)

● M60 Myositis

Excludes2 inclusion body myositis [IBM] (G72.41)

● M60.0 Infective myositis
Tropical pyomyositis
Use additional code (B95-B97) to identify infectious agent

● M60.00 Infective myositis, unspecified site

M60.000 Infective myositis, unspecified right arm
Infective myositis, right upper limb NOS

M60.001 Infective myositis, unspecified left arm
Infective myositis, left upper limb NOS

M60.002 Infective myositis, unspecified arm
Infective myositis, upper limb NOS

M60.003 Infective myositis, unspecified right leg
Infective myositis, right lower limb NOS

M60.004 Infective myositis, unspecified left leg
Infective myositis, left lower limb NOS

M60.005 Infective myositis, unspecified leg
Infective myositis, lower limb NOS

M60.009 Infective myositis, unspecified site

● M60.01 Infective myositis, shoulder

M60.011 Infective myositis, right shoulder

M60.012 Infective myositis, left shoulder

M60.019 Infective myositis, unspecified shoulder

◄ New   ⬅ Revised   ~~deleted~~ Deleted   Excludes 1   Excludes 2   Includes   Use additional   Code first   Code also   Unspecified

OGCR Official Guidelines   X Assign placeholder X   ● Use Additional Character(s)   ▌ Manifestation Code   **Coding Clinic**

● **M60.02** Infective myositis, upper arm
     M60.021 Infective myositis, right upper arm
     M60.022 Infective myositis, left upper arm
     M60.029 Infective myositis, unspecified upper arm

● **M60.03** Infective myositis, forearm
     M60.031 Infective myositis, right forearm
     M60.032 Infective myositis, left forearm
     M60.039 Infective myositis, unspecified forearm

● **M60.04** Infective myositis, hand and fingers
     M60.041 Infective myositis, right hand
     M60.042 Infective myositis, left hand
     M60.043 Infective myositis, unspecified hand
     M60.044 Infective myositis, right finger(s)
     M60.045 Infective myositis, left finger(s)
     M60.046 Infective myositis, unspecified finger(s)

● **M60.05** Infective myositis, thigh
     M60.051 Infective myositis, right thigh
     M60.052 Infective myositis, left thigh
     M60.059 Infective myositis, unspecified thigh

● **M60.06** Infective myositis, lower leg
     M60.061 Infective myositis, right lower leg
     M60.062 Infective myositis, left lower leg
     M60.069 Infective myositis, unspecified lower leg

● **M60.07** Infective myositis, ankle, foot and toes
     M60.070 Infective myositis, right ankle
     M60.071 Infective myositis, left ankle
     M60.072 Infective myositis, unspecified ankle
     M60.073 Infective myositis, right foot
     M60.074 Infective myositis, left foot
     M60.075 Infective myositis, unspecified foot
     M60.076 Infective myositis, right toe(s)
     M60.077 Infective myositis, left toe(s)
     M60.078 Infective myositis, unspecified toe(s)

     M60.08 Infective myositis, other site
     M60.09 Infective myositis, multiple sites

● **M60.1** Interstitial myositis
     M60.10 Interstitial myositis of unspecified site

● **M60.11** Interstitial myositis, shoulder
     M60.111 Interstitial myositis, right shoulder
     M60.112 Interstitial myositis, left shoulder
     M60.119 Interstitial myositis, unspecified shoulder

● **M60.12** Interstitial myositis, upper arm
     M60.121 Interstitial myositis, right upper arm
     M60.122 Interstitial myositis, left upper arm
     M60.129 Interstitial myositis, unspecified upper arm

● **M60.13** Interstitial myositis, forearm
     M60.131 Interstitial myositis, right forearm
     M60.132 Interstitial myositis, left forearm
     M60.139 Interstitial myositis, unspecified forearm

● **M60.14** Interstitial myositis, hand
     M60.141 Interstitial myositis, right hand
     M60.142 Interstitial myositis, left hand
     M60.149 Interstitial myositis, unspecified hand

● **M60.15** Interstitial myositis, thigh
     M60.151 Interstitial myositis, right thigh
     M60.152 Interstitial myositis, left thigh
     M60.159 Interstitial myositis, unspecified thigh

● **M60.16** Interstitial myositis, lower leg
     M60.161 Interstitial myositis, right lower leg
     M60.162 Interstitial myositis, left lower leg
     M60.169 Interstitial myositis, unspecified lower leg

● **M60.17** Interstitial myositis, ankle and foot
     M60.171 Interstitial myositis, right ankle and foot
     M60.172 Interstitial myositis, left ankle and foot
     M60.179 Interstitial myositis, unspecified ankle and foot

     M60.18 Interstitial myositis, other site
     M60.19 Interstitial myositis, multiple sites

● **M60.2** Foreign body granuloma of soft tissue, not elsewhere classified
     Use additional code to identify the type of retained foreign body (Z18.-)
     Excludes1   foreign body granuloma of skin and subcutaneous tissue (L92.3)

     M60.20 Foreign body granuloma of soft tissue, not elsewhere classified, unspecified site

● **M60.21** Foreign body granuloma of soft tissue, not elsewhere classified, shoulder
     M60.211 Foreign body granuloma of soft tissue, not elsewhere classified, right shoulder
     M60.212 Foreign body granuloma of soft tissue, not elsewhere classified, left shoulder
     M60.219 Foreign body granuloma of soft tissue, not elsewhere classified, unspecified shoulder

● **M60.22** Foreign body granuloma of soft tissue, not elsewhere classified, upper arm
     M60.221 Foreign body granuloma of soft tissue, not elsewhere classified, right upper arm
     M60.222 Foreign body granuloma of soft tissue, not elsewhere classified, left upper arm
     M60.229 Foreign body granuloma of soft tissue, not elsewhere classified, unspecified upper arm

● **M60.23** Foreign body granuloma of soft tissue, not elsewhere classified, forearm
     M60.231 Foreign body granuloma of soft tissue, not elsewhere classified, right forearm
     M60.232 Foreign body granuloma of soft tissue, not elsewhere classified, left forearm
     M60.239 Foreign body granuloma of soft tissue, not elsewhere classified, unspecified forearm

● **M60.24** Foreign body granuloma of soft tissue, not elsewhere classified, hand
     M60.241 Foreign body granuloma of soft tissue, not elsewhere classified, right hand
     M60.242 Foreign body granuloma of soft tissue, not elsewhere classified, left hand
     M60.249 Foreign body granuloma of soft tissue, not elsewhere classified, unspecified hand

CHAPTER 13 (M00-M99)

CHAPTER 13 (M00-M99)

● M60.25 Foreign body granuloma of soft tissue, not elsewhere classified, thigh

    M60.251 Foreign body granuloma of soft tissue, not elsewhere classified, right thigh

    M60.252 Foreign body granuloma of soft tissue, not elsewhere classified, left thigh

    M60.259 Foreign body granuloma of soft tissue, not elsewhere classified, unspecified thigh

● M60.26 Foreign body granuloma of soft tissue, not elsewhere classified, lower leg

    M60.261 Foreign body granuloma of soft tissue, not elsewhere classified, right lower leg

    M60.262 Foreign body granuloma of soft tissue, not elsewhere classified, left lower leg

    M60.269 Foreign body granuloma of soft tissue, not elsewhere classified, unspecified lower leg

● M60.27 Foreign body granuloma of soft tissue, not elsewhere classified, ankle and foot

    M60.271 Foreign body granuloma of soft tissue, not elsewhere classified, right ankle and foot

    M60.272 Foreign body granuloma of soft tissue, not elsewhere classified, left ankle and foot

    M60.279 Foreign body granuloma of soft tissue, not elsewhere classified, unspecified ankle and foot

    M60.28 Foreign body granuloma of soft tissue, not elsewhere classified, other site

● M60.8 Other myositis

    M60.80 Other myositis, unspecified site

● M60.81 Other myositis shoulder

    M60.811 Other myositis, right shoulder

    M60.812 Other myositis, left shoulder

    M60.819 Other myositis, unspecified shoulder

● M60.82 Other myositis, upper arm

    M60.821 Other myositis, right upper arm

    M60.822 Other myositis, left upper arm

    M60.829 Other myositis, unspecified upper arm

● M60.83 Other myositis, forearm

    M60.831 Other myositis, right forearm

    M60.832 Other myositis, left forearm

    M60.839 Other myositis, unspecified forearm

● M60.84 Other myositis, hand

    M60.841 Other myositis, right hand

    M60.842 Other myositis, left hand

    M60.849 Other myositis, unspecified hand

● M60.85 Other myositis, thigh

    M60.851 Other myositis, right thigh

    M60.852 Other myositis, left thigh

    M60.859 Other myositis, unspecified thigh

● M60.86 Other myositis, lower leg

    M60.861 Other myositis, right lower leg

    M60.862 Other myositis, left lower leg

    M60.869 Other myositis, unspecified lower leg

● M60.87 Other myositis, ankle and foot

    M60.871 Other myositis, right ankle and foot

    M60.872 Other myositis, left ankle and foot

    M60.879 Other myositis, unspecified ankle and foot

    M60.88 Other myositis, other site

    M60.89 Other myositis, multiple sites

    M60.9 Myositis, unspecified

● M61 Calcification and ossification of muscle

  ● M61.0 Myositis ossificans traumatica

    M61.00 Myositis ossificans traumatica, unspecified site

  ● M61.01 Myositis ossificans traumatica, shoulder

    M61.011 Myositis ossificans traumatica, right shoulder

    M61.012 Myositis ossificans traumatica, left shoulder

    M61.019 Myositis ossificans traumatica, unspecified shoulder

  ● M61.02 Myositis ossificans traumatica, upper arm

    M61.021 Myositis ossificans traumatica, right upper arm

    M61.022 Myositis ossificans traumatica, left upper arm

    M61.029 Myositis ossificans traumatica, unspecified upper arm

  ● M61.03 Myositis ossificans traumatica, forearm

    M61.031 Myositis ossificans traumatica, right forearm

    M61.032 Myositis ossificans traumatica, left forearm

    M61.039 Myositis ossificans traumatica, unspecified forearm

  ● M61.04 Myositis ossificans traumatica, hand

    M61.041 Myositis ossificans traumatica, right hand

    M61.042 Myositis ossificans traumatica, left hand

    M61.049 Myositis ossificans traumatica, unspecified hand

  ● M61.05 Myositis ossificans traumatica, thigh

    M61.051 Myositis ossificans traumatica, right thigh

    M61.052 Myositis ossificans traumatica, left thigh

    M61.059 Myositis ossificans traumatica, unspecified thigh

  ● M61.06 Myositis ossificans traumatica, lower leg

    M61.061 Myositis ossificans traumatica, right lower leg

    M61.062 Myositis ossificans traumatica, left lower leg

    M61.069 Myositis ossificans traumatica, unspecified lower leg

  ● M61.07 Myositis ossificans traumatica, ankle and foot

    M61.071 Myositis ossificans traumatica, right ankle and foot

    M61.072 Myositis ossificans traumatica, left ankle and foot

    M61.079 Myositis ossificans traumatica, unspecified ankle and foot

    M61.08 Myositis ossificans traumatica, other site

    M61.09 Myositis ossificans traumatica, multiple sites

◀ New   ◀▥ Revised   ~~deleted~~ Deleted   Excludes 1   Excludes 2   Includes   Use additional   Code first   Code also   Unspecified

OGCR Official Guidelines   X Assign placeholder X   ● Use Additional Character(s)   ▶ Manifestation Code   **Coding Clinic**

● **M61.1**   **Myositis ossificans progressiva**
     Fibrodysplasia ossificans progressiva
   M61.10   Myositis ossificans progressiva, unspecified site
● **M61.11**   Myositis ossificans progressiva, shoulder
     M61.111   Myositis ossificans progressiva, right shoulder
     M61.112   Myositis ossificans progressiva, left shoulder
     M61.119   Myositis ossificans progressiva, unspecified shoulder
● **M61.12**   Myositis ossificans progressiva, upper arm
     M61.121   Myositis ossificans progressiva, right upper arm
     M61.122   Myositis ossificans progressiva, left upper arm
     M61.129   Myositis ossificans progressiva, unspecified arm
● **M61.13**   Myositis ossificans progressiva, forearm
     M61.131   Myositis ossificans progressiva, right forearm
     M61.132   Myositis ossificans progressiva, left forearm
     M61.139   Myositis ossificans progressiva, unspecified forearm
● **M61.14**   Myositis ossificans progressiva, hand and finger(s)
     M61.141   Myositis ossificans progressiva, right hand
     M61.142   Myositis ossificans progressiva, left hand
     M61.143   Myositis ossificans progressiva, unspecified hand
     M61.144   Myositis ossificans progressiva, right finger(s)
     M61.145   Myositis ossificans progressiva, left finger(s)
     M61.146   Myositis ossificans progressiva, unspecified finger(s)
● **M61.15**   Myositis ossificans progressiva, thigh
     M61.151   Myositis ossificans progressiva, right thigh
     M61.152   Myositis ossificans progressiva, left thigh
     M61.159   Myositis ossificans progressiva, unspecified thigh
● **M61.16**   Myositis ossificans progressiva, lower leg
     M61.161   Myositis ossificans progressiva, right lower leg
     M61.162   Myositis ossificans progressiva, left lower leg
     M61.169   Myositis ossificans progressiva, unspecified lower leg
● **M61.17**   Myositis ossificans progressiva, ankle, foot and toe(s)
     M61.171   Myositis ossificans progressiva, right ankle
     M61.172   Myositis ossificans progressiva, left ankle
     M61.173   Myositis ossificans progressiva, unspecified ankle
     M61.174   Myositis ossificans progressiva, right foot
     M61.175   Myositis ossificans progressiva, left foot
     M61.176   Myositis ossificans progressiva, unspecified foot
     M61.177   Myositis ossificans progressiva, right toe(s)

     M61.178   Myositis ossificans progressiva, left toe(s)
     M61.179   Myositis ossificans progressiva, unspecified toe(s)
   M61.18   Myositis ossificans progressiva, other site
   M61.19   Myositis ossificans progressiva, multiple sites
● **M61.2**   **Paralytic calcification and ossification of muscle**
     Myositis ossificans associated with quadriplegia or paraplegia
   M61.20   Paralytic calcification and ossification of muscle, unspecified site
● **M61.21**   Paralytic calcification and ossification of muscle, shoulder
     M61.211   Paralytic calcification and ossification of muscle, right shoulder
     M61.212   Paralytic calcification and ossification of muscle, left shoulder
     M61.219   Paralytic calcification and ossification of muscle, unspecified shoulder
● **M61.22**   Paralytic calcification and ossification of muscle, upper arm
     M61.221   Paralytic calcification and ossification of muscle, right upper arm
     M61.222   Paralytic calcification and ossification of muscle, left upper arm
     M61.229   Paralytic calcification and ossification of muscle, unspecified upper arm
● **M61.23**   Paralytic calcification and ossification of muscle, forearm
     M61.231   Paralytic calcification and ossification of muscle, right forearm
     M61.232   Paralytic calcification and ossification of muscle, left forearm
     M61.239   Paralytic calcification and ossification of muscle, unspecified forearm
● **M61.24**   Paralytic calcification and ossification of muscle, hand
     M61.241   Paralytic calcification and ossification of muscle, right hand
     M61.242   Paralytic calcification and ossification of muscle, left hand
     M61.249   Paralytic calcification and ossification of muscle, unspecified hand
● **M61.25**   Paralytic calcification and ossification of muscle, thigh
     M61.251   Paralytic calcification and ossification of muscle, right thigh
     M61.252   Paralytic calcification and ossification of muscle, left thigh
     M61.259   Paralytic calcification and ossification of muscle, unspecified thigh
● **M61.26**   Paralytic calcification and ossification of muscle, lower leg
     M61.261   Paralytic calcification and ossification of muscle, right lower leg
     M61.262   Paralytic calcification and ossification of muscle, left lower leg
     M61.269   Paralytic calcification and ossification of muscle, unspecified lower leg
● **M61.27**   Paralytic calcification and ossification of muscle, ankle and foot
     M61.271   Paralytic calcification and ossification of muscle, right ankle and foot
     M61.272   Paralytic calcification and ossification of muscle, left ankle and foot
     M61.279   Paralytic calcification and ossification of muscle, unspecified ankle and foot
   M61.28   Paralytic calcification and ossification of muscle, other site
   M61.29   Paralytic calcification and ossification of muscle, multiple sites

CHAPTER 13 (M00-M99)

CHAPTER 13 (M00-M99)

● **M61.3** Calcification and ossification of muscles associated with burns

    Myositis ossificans associated with burns

  M61.30 Calcification and ossification of muscles associated with burns, unspecified site

● **M61.31** Calcification and ossification of muscles associated with burns, shoulder

    M61.311 Calcification and ossification of muscles associated with burns, right shoulder

    M61.312 Calcification and ossification of muscles associated with burns, left shoulder

    M61.319 Calcification and ossification of muscles associated with burns, unspecified shoulder

● **M61.32** Calcification and ossification of muscles associated with burns, upper arm

    M61.321 Calcification and ossification of muscles associated with burns, right upper arm

    M61.322 Calcification and ossification of muscles associated with burns, left upper arm

    M61.329 Calcification and ossification of muscles associated with burns, unspecified upper arm

● **M61.33** Calcification and ossification of muscles associated with burns, forearm

    M61.331 Calcification and ossification of muscles associated with burns, right forearm

    M61.332 Calcification and ossification of muscles associated with burns, left forearm

    M61.339 Calcification and ossification of muscles associated with burns, unspecified forearm

● **M61.34** Calcification and ossification of muscles associated with burns, hand

    M61.341 Calcification and ossification of muscles associated with burns, right hand

    M61.342 Calcification and ossification of muscles associated with burns, left hand

    M61.349 Calcification and ossification of muscles associated with burns, unspecified hand

● **M61.35** Calcification and ossification of muscles associated with burns, thigh

    M61.351 Calcification and ossification of muscles associated with burns, right thigh

    M61.352 Calcification and ossification of muscles associated with burns, left thigh

    M61.359 Calcification and ossification of muscles associated with burns, unspecified thigh

● **M61.36** Calcification and ossification of muscles associated with burns, lower leg

    M61.361 Calcification and ossification of muscles associated with burns, right lower leg

    M61.362 Calcification and ossification of muscles associated with burns, left lower leg

    M61.369 Calcification and ossification of muscles associated with burns, unspecified lower leg

● **M61.37** Calcification and ossification of muscles associated with burns, ankle and foot

    M61.371 Calcification and ossification of muscles associated with burns, right ankle and foot

    M61.372 Calcification and ossification of muscles associated with burns, left ankle and foot

    M61.379 Calcification and ossification of muscles associated with burns, unspecified ankle and foot

  M61.38 Calcification and ossification of muscles associated with burns, other site

  M61.39 Calcification and ossification of muscles associated with burns, multiple sites

● **M61.4** Other calcification of muscle

    Excludes1   calcific tendinitis NOS (M65.2-)
                calcific tendinitis of shoulder (M75.3)

  M61.40 Other calcification of muscle, unspecified site

● **M61.41** Other calcification of muscle, shoulder

    M61.411 Other calcification of muscle, right shoulder

    M61.412 Other calcification of muscle, left shoulder

    M61.419 Other calcification of muscle, unspecified shoulder

● **M61.42** Other calcification of muscle, upper arm

    M61.421 Other calcification of muscle, right upper arm

    M61.422 Other calcification of muscle, left upper arm

    M61.429 Other calcification of muscle, unspecified upper arm

● **M61.43** Other calcification of muscle, forearm

    M61.431 Other calcification of muscle, right forearm

    M61.432 Other calcification of muscle, left forearm

    M61.439 Other calcification of muscle, unspecified forearm

● **M61.44** Other calcification of muscle, hand

    M61.441 Other calcification of muscle, right hand

    M61.442 Other calcification of muscle, left hand

    M61.449 Other calcification of muscle, unspecified hand

● **M61.45** Other calcification of muscle, thigh

    M61.451 Other calcification of muscle, right thigh

    M61.452 Other calcification of muscle, left thigh

    M61.459 Other calcification of muscle, unspecified thigh

● **M61.46** Other calcification of muscle, lower leg

    M61.461 Other calcification of muscle, right lower leg

    M61.462 Other calcification of muscle, left lower leg

    M61.469 Other calcification of muscle, unspecified lower leg

● **M61.47** Other calcification of muscle, ankle and foot

    M61.471 Other calcification of muscle, right ankle and foot

    M61.472 Other calcification of muscle, left ankle and foot

    M61.479 Other calcification of muscle, unspecified ankle and foot

  M61.48 Other calcification of muscle, other site

  M61.49 Other calcification of muscle, multiple sites

◀ New   ◀═ Revised   ~~deleted~~ Deleted   Excludes 1   Excludes 2   Includes   Use additional   Code first   Code also   Unspecified

OGCR Official Guidelines   **X** Assign placeholder X   ● Use Additional Character(s)   ▶ Manifestation Code   **Coding Clinic**

● M61.5   Other ossification of muscle
    M61.50   Other ossification of muscle, unspecified site
    ● M61.51   Other ossification of muscle, shoulder
        M61.511   Other ossification of muscle, right shoulder
        M61.512   Other ossification of muscle, left shoulder
        M61.519   Other ossification of muscle, unspecified shoulder
    ● M61.52   Other ossification of muscle, upper arm
        M61.521   Other ossification of muscle, right upper arm
        M61.522   Other ossification of muscle, left upper arm
        M61.529   Other ossification of muscle, unspecified upper arm
    ● M61.53   Other ossification of muscle, forearm
        M61.531   Other ossification of muscle, right forearm
        M61.532   Other ossification of muscle, left forearm
        M61.539   Other ossification of muscle, unspecified forearm
    ● M61.54   Other ossification of muscle, hand
        M61.541   Other ossification of muscle, right hand
        M61.542   Other ossification of muscle, left hand
        M61.549   Other ossification of muscle, unspecified hand
    ● M61.55   Other ossification of muscle, thigh
        M61.551   Other ossification of muscle, right thigh
        M61.552   Other ossification of muscle, left thigh
        M61.559   Other ossification of muscle, unspecified thigh
    ● M61.56   Other ossification of muscle, lower leg
        M61.561   Other ossification of muscle, right lower leg
        M61.562   Other ossification of muscle, left lower leg
        M61.569   Other ossification of muscle, unspecified lower leg
    ● M61.57   Other ossification of muscle, ankle and foot
        M61.571   Other ossification of muscle, right ankle and foot
        M61.572   Other ossification of muscle, left ankle and foot
        M61.579   Other ossification of muscle, unspecified ankle and foot
    M61.58   Other ossification of muscle, other site
    M61.59   Other ossification of muscle, multiple sites
  M61.9   Calcification and ossification of muscle, unspecified

● M62   Other disorders of muscle
    Excludes1   alcoholic myopathy (G72.1)
        cramp and spasm (R25.2)
        drug-induced myopathy (G72.0)
        myalgia (M79.1)
        stiff-man syndrome (G25.82)
    Excludes2   nontraumatic hematoma of muscle (M79.81)
  ● M62.0   Separation of muscle (nontraumatic)
    Diastasis of muscle
    Excludes1   diastasis recti complicating pregnancy, labor and delivery (O71.8)
        traumatic separation of muscle - see strain of muscle by body region
    M62.00   Separation of muscle (nontraumatic), unspecified site

● M62.01   Separation of muscle (nontraumatic), shoulder
    M62.011   Separation of muscle (nontraumatic), right shoulder
    M62.012   Separation of muscle (nontraumatic), left shoulder
    M62.019   Separation of muscle (nontraumatic), unspecified shoulder
● M62.02   Separation of muscle (nontraumatic), upper arm
    M62.021   Separation of muscle (nontraumatic), right upper arm
    M62.022   Separation of muscle (nontraumatic), left upper arm
    M62.029   Separation of muscle (nontraumatic), unspecified upper arm
● M62.03   Separation of muscle (nontraumatic), forearm
    M62.031   Separation of muscle (nontraumatic), right forearm
    M62.032   Separation of muscle (nontraumatic), left forearm
    M62.039   Separation of muscle (nontraumatic), unspecified forearm
● M62.04   Separation of muscle (nontraumatic), hand
    M62.041   Separation of muscle (nontraumatic), right hand
    M62.042   Separation of muscle (nontraumatic), left hand
    M62.049   Separation of muscle (nontraumatic), unspecified hand
● M62.05   Separation of muscle (nontraumatic), thigh
    M62.051   Separation of muscle (nontraumatic), right thigh
    M62.052   Separation of muscle (nontraumatic), left thigh
    M62.059   Separation of muscle (nontraumatic), unspecified thigh
● M62.06   Separation of muscle (nontraumatic), lower leg
    M62.061   Separation of muscle (nontraumatic), right lower leg
    M62.062   Separation of muscle (nontraumatic), left lower leg
    M62.069   Separation of muscle (nontraumatic), unspecified lower leg
● M62.07   Separation of muscle (nontraumatic), ankle and foot
    M62.071   Separation of muscle (nontraumatic), right ankle and foot
    M62.072   Separation of muscle (nontraumatic), left ankle and foot
    M62.079   Separation of muscle (nontraumatic), unspecified ankle and foot
  M62.08   Separation of muscle (nontraumatic), other site
● M62.1   Other rupture of muscle (nontraumatic)
    Excludes1   traumatic rupture of muscle - see strain of muscle by body region
    Excludes2   rupture of tendon (M66.-)
  M62.10   Other rupture of muscle (nontraumatic), unspecified site
● M62.11   Other rupture of muscle (nontraumatic), shoulder
    M62.111   Other rupture of muscle (nontraumatic), right shoulder
    M62.112   Other rupture of muscle (nontraumatic), left shoulder
    M62.119   Other rupture of muscle (nontraumatic), unspecified shoulder

CHAPTER 13 (M00-M99)

CHAPTER 13 (M00-M99)

● M62.12   Other rupture of muscle (nontraumatic), upper arm

    M62.121   Other rupture of muscle (nontraumatic), right upper arm

    M62.122   Other rupture of muscle (nontraumatic), left upper arm

    M62.129   Other rupture of muscle (nontraumatic), unspecified upper arm

● M62.13   Other rupture of muscle (nontraumatic), forearm

    M62.131   Other rupture of muscle (nontraumatic), right forearm

    M62.132   Other rupture of muscle (nontraumatic), left forearm

    M62.139   Other rupture of muscle (nontraumatic), unspecified forearm

● M62.14   Other rupture of muscle (nontraumatic), hand

    M62.141   Other rupture of muscle (nontraumatic), right hand

    M62.142   Other rupture of muscle (nontraumatic), left hand

    M62.149   Other rupture of muscle (nontraumatic), unspecified hand

● M62.15   Other rupture of muscle (nontraumatic), thigh

    M62.151   Other rupture of muscle (nontraumatic), right thigh

    M62.152   Other rupture of muscle (nontraumatic), left thigh

    M62.159   Other rupture of muscle (nontraumatic), unspecified thigh

● M62.16   Other rupture of muscle (nontraumatic), lower leg

    M62.161   Other rupture of muscle (nontraumatic), right lower leg

    M62.162   Other rupture of muscle (nontraumatic), left lower leg

    M62.169   Other rupture of muscle (nontraumatic), unspecified lower leg

● M62.17   Other rupture of muscle (nontraumatic), ankle and foot

    M62.171   Other rupture of muscle (nontraumatic), right ankle and foot

    M62.172   Other rupture of muscle (nontraumatic), left ankle and foot

    M62.179   Other rupture of muscle (nontraumatic), unspecified ankle and foot

  M62.18   Other rupture of muscle (nontraumatic), other site

● M62.2   Nontraumatic ischemic infarction of muscle

    Excludes1   compartment syndrome (traumatic) (T79.A-)

              nontraumatic compartment syndrome (M79.A-)

              traumatic ischemia of muscle (T79.6)

              rhabdomyolysis (M62.82)

              Volkmann's ischemic contracture (T79.6)

  M62.20   Nontraumatic ischemic infarction of muscle, unspecified site

● M62.21   Nontraumatic ischemic infarction of muscle, shoulder

    M62.211   Nontraumatic ischemic infarction of muscle, right shoulder

    M62.212   Nontraumatic ischemic infarction of muscle, left shoulder

    M62.219   Nontraumatic ischemic infarction of muscle, unspecified shoulder

● M62.22   Nontraumatic ischemic infarction of muscle, upper arm

    M62.221   Nontraumatic ischemic infarction of muscle, right upper arm

    M62.222   Nontraumatic ischemic infarction of muscle, left upper arm

    M62.229   Nontraumatic ischemic infarction of muscle, unspecified upper arm

● M62.23   Nontraumatic ischemic infarction of muscle, forearm

    M62.231   Nontraumatic ischemic infarction of muscle, right forearm

    M62.232   Nontraumatic ischemic infarction of muscle, left forearm

    M62.239   Nontraumatic ischemic infarction of muscle, unspecified forearm

● M62.24   Nontraumatic ischemic infarction of muscle, hand

    M62.241   Nontraumatic ischemic infarction of muscle, right hand

    M62.242   Nontraumatic ischemic infarction of muscle, left hand

    M62.249   Nontraumatic ischemic infarction of muscle, unspecified hand

● M62.25   Nontraumatic ischemic infarction of muscle, thigh

    M62.251   Nontraumatic ischemic infarction of muscle, right thigh

    M62.252   Nontraumatic ischemic infarction of muscle, left thigh

    M62.259   Nontraumatic ischemic infarction of muscle, unspecified thigh

● M62.26   Nontraumatic ischemic infarction of muscle, lower leg

    M62.261   Nontraumatic ischemic infarction of muscle, right lower leg

    M62.262   Nontraumatic ischemic infarction of muscle, left lower leg

    M62.269   Nontraumatic ischemic infarction of muscle, unspecified lower leg

● M62.27   Nontraumatic ischemic infarction of muscle, ankle and foot

    M62.271   Nontraumatic ischemic infarction of muscle, right ankle and foot

    M62.272   Nontraumatic ischemic infarction of muscle, left ankle and foot

    M62.279   Nontraumatic ischemic infarction of muscle, unspecified ankle and foot

  M62.28   Nontraumatic ischemic infarction of muscle, other site

  M62.3   Immobility syndrome (paraplegic)

  M62.4   Contracture of muscle

CONTRACTURE OF TENDON (SHEATH)

Excludes1   contracture of joint (M24.5-)

  M62.40   Contracture of muscle, unspecified site

● M62.41   Contracture of muscle, shoulder

    M62.411   Contracture of muscle, right shoulder

    M62.412   Contracture of muscle, left shoulder

    M62.419   Contracture of muscle, unspecified shoulder

● M62.42   Contracture of muscle, upper arm

    M62.421   Contracture of muscle, right upper arm

    M62.422   Contracture of muscle, left upper arm

    M62.429   Contracture of muscle, unspecified upper arm

◀ New   ◀▏▏ Revised   ~~deleted~~ Deleted   Excludes 1   Excludes 2   Includes   Use additional   Code first   Code also   Unspecified

OGCR Official Guidelines   X Assign placeholder X   ● Use Additional Character(s)   ▶ Manifestation Code   **Coding Clinic**

● **M62.43** Contracture of muscle, forearm
    M62.431 Contracture of muscle, right forearm
    M62.432 Contracture of muscle, left forearm
    M62.439 Contracture of muscle, unspecified forearm

● **M62.44** Contracture of muscle, hand
    M62.441 Contracture of muscle, right hand
    M62.442 Contracture of muscle, left hand
    M62.449 Contracture of muscle, unspecified hand

● **M62.45** Contracture of muscle, thigh
    M62.451 Contracture of muscle, right thigh
    M62.452 Contracture of muscle, left thigh
    M62.459 Contracture of muscle, unspecified thigh

● **M62.46** Contracture of muscle, lower leg
    M62.461 Contracture of muscle, right lower leg
    M62.462 Contracture of muscle, left lower leg
    M62.469 Contracture of muscle, unspecified lower leg

● **M62.47** Contracture of muscle, ankle and foot
    M62.471 Contracture of muscle, right ankle and foot
    M62.472 Contracture of muscle, left ankle and foot
    M62.479 Contracture of muscle, unspecified ankle and foot

M62.48 Contracture of muscle, other site
M62.49 Contracture of muscle, multiple sites

● **M62.5** Muscle wasting and atrophy, not elsewhere classified
    Disuse atrophy NEC

    Excludes1 neuralgic amyotrophy (G54.5)
                progressive muscular atrophy (G12.29)

    Excludes2 pelvic muscle wasting (N81.84)

    M62.50 Muscle wasting and atrophy, not elsewhere classified, unspecified site

● **M62.51** Muscle wasting and atrophy, not elsewhere classified, shoulder
    M62.511 Muscle wasting and atrophy, not elsewhere classified, right shoulder
    M62.512 Muscle wasting and atrophy, not elsewhere classified, left shoulder
    M62.519 Muscle wasting and atrophy, not elsewhere classified, unspecified shoulder

● **M62.52** Muscle wasting and atrophy, not elsewhere classified, upper arm
    M62.521 Muscle wasting and atrophy, not elsewhere classified, right upper arm
    M62.522 Muscle wasting and atrophy, not elsewhere classified, left upper arm
    M62.529 Muscle wasting and atrophy, not elsewhere classified, unspecified upper arm

● **M62.53** Muscle wasting and atrophy, not elsewhere classified, forearm
    M62.531 Muscle wasting and atrophy, not elsewhere classified, right forearm
    M62.532 Muscle wasting and atrophy, not elsewhere classified, left forearm
    M62.539 Muscle wasting and atrophy, not elsewhere classified, unspecified forearm

● **M62.54** Muscle wasting and atrophy, not elsewhere classified, hand
    M62.541 Muscle wasting and atrophy, not elsewhere classified, right hand
    M62.542 Muscle wasting and atrophy, not elsewhere classified, left hand
    M62.549 Muscle wasting and atrophy, not elsewhere classified, unspecified hand

● **M62.55** Muscle wasting and atrophy, not elsewhere classified, thigh
    M62.551 Muscle wasting and atrophy, not elsewhere classified, right thigh
    M62.552 Muscle wasting and atrophy, not elsewhere classified, left thigh
    M62.559 Muscle wasting and atrophy, not elsewhere classified, unspecified thigh

● **M62.56** Muscle wasting and atrophy, not elsewhere classified, lower leg
    M62.561 Muscle wasting and atrophy, not elsewhere classified, right lower leg
    M62.562 Muscle wasting and atrophy, not elsewhere classified, left lower leg
    M62.569 Muscle wasting and atrophy, not elsewhere classified, unspecified lower leg

● **M62.57** Muscle wasting and atrophy, not elsewhere classified, ankle and foot
    M62.571 Muscle wasting and atrophy, not elsewhere classified, right ankle and foot
    M62.572 Muscle wasting and atrophy, not elsewhere classified, left ankle and foot
    M62.579 Muscle wasting and atrophy, not elsewhere classified, unspecified ankle and foot

M62.58 Muscle wasting and atrophy, not elsewhere classified, other site
M62.59 Muscle wasting and atrophy, not elsewhere classified, multiple sites

● **M62.8** Other specified disorders of muscle

    Excludes2 nontraumatic hematoma of muscle (M79.81)

    M62.81 Muscle weakness (generalized)
    M62.82 Rhabdomyolysis

        Excludes1 traumatic rhabdomyolysis (T79.6)

● **M62.83** Muscle spasm
    M62.830 Muscle spasm of back
    M62.831 Muscle spasm of calf
        Charley-horse
    M62.838 Other muscle spasm

    M62.89 Other specified disorders of muscle
        Muscle (sheath) hernia

M62.9 Disorder of muscle, unspecified

CHAPTER 13 (M00-M99)

● **M63 Disorders of muscle in diseases classified elsewhere**

Code first underlying disease, such as:

leprosy (A30.-)
neoplasm (C49.-, C79.89, D21.-, D48.1)
schistosomiasis (B65.-)
trichinellosis (B75)

Excludes1 myopathy in cysticercosis (B69.81)
myopathy in endocrine diseases (G73.7)
myopathy in metabolic diseases (G73.7)
myopathy in sarcoidosis (D86.87)
myopathy in secondary syphilis (A51.49)
myopathy in syphilis (late) (A52.78)
myopathy in toxoplasmosis (B58.82)
myopathy in tuberculosis (A18.09)

● **M63.8 Disorders of muscle in diseases classified elsewhere**

  ▌ *M63.80 Disorders of muscle in diseases classified elsewhere, unspecified site*

  ● *M63.81 Disorders of muscle in diseases classified elsewhere, shoulder*

    ▌ *M63.811 Disorders of muscle in diseases classified elsewhere, right shoulder*

    ▌ *M63.812 Disorders of muscle in diseases classified elsewhere, left shoulder*

    ▌ *M63.819 Disorders of muscle in diseases classified elsewhere, unspecified shoulder*

  ● *M63.82 Disorders of muscle in diseases classified elsewhere, upper arm*

    ▌ *M63.821 Disorders of muscle in diseases classified elsewhere, right upper arm*

    ▌ *M63.822 Disorders of muscle in diseases classified elsewhere, left upper arm*

    ▌ *M63.829 Disorders of muscle in diseases classified elsewhere, unspecified upper arm*

  ● *M63.83 Disorders of muscle in diseases classified elsewhere, forearm*

    ▌ *M63.831 Disorders of muscle in diseases classified elsewhere, right forearm*

    ▌ *M63.832 Disorders of muscle in diseases classified elsewhere, left forearm*

    ▌ *M63.839 Disorders of muscle in diseases classified elsewhere, unspecified forearm*

  ● *M63.84 Disorders of muscle in diseases classified elsewhere, hand*

    ▌ *M63.841 Disorders of muscle in diseases classified elsewhere, right hand*

    ▌ *M63.842 Disorders of muscle in diseases classified elsewhere, left hand*

    ▌ *M63.849 Disorders of muscle in diseases classified elsewhere, unspecified hand*

  ● *M63.85 Disorders of muscle in diseases classified elsewhere, thigh*

    ▌ *M63.851 Disorders of muscle in diseases classified elsewhere, right thigh*

    ▌ *M63.852 Disorders of muscle in diseases classified elsewhere, left thigh*

    ▌ *M63.859 Disorders of muscle in diseases classified elsewhere, unspecified thigh*

  ● *M63.86 Disorders of muscle in diseases classified elsewhere, lower leg*

    ▌ *M63.861 Disorders of muscle in diseases classified elsewhere, right lower leg*

    ▌ *M63.862 Disorders of muscle in diseases classified elsewhere, left lower leg*

    ▌ *M63.869 Disorders of muscle in diseases classified elsewhere, unspecified lower leg*

  ● *M63.87 Disorders of muscle in diseases classified elsewhere, ankle and foot*

    ▌ *M63.871 Disorders of muscle in diseases classified elsewhere, right ankle and foot*

    ▌ *M63.872 Disorders of muscle in diseases classified elsewhere, left ankle and foot*

    ▌ *M63.879 Disorders of muscle in diseases classified elsewhere, unspecified ankle and foot*

  ▌ *M63.88 Disorders of muscle in diseases classified elsewhere, other site*

  ▌ *M63.89 Disorders of muscle in diseases classified elsewhere, multiple sites*

DISORDERS OF SYNOVIUM AND TENDON (M65-M67)

● **M65 Synovitis and tenosynovitis**

Excludes1 chronic crepitant synovitis of hand and wrist (M70.0-)
current injury - see injury of ligament or tendon by body region
soft tissue disorders related to use, overuse and pressure (M70.-)

● **M65.0 Abscess of tendon sheath**

Use additional code (B95-B96) to identify bacterial agent

  M65.00 Abscess of tendon sheath, unspecified site

  ● M65.01 Abscess of tendon sheath, shoulder

    M65.011 Abscess of tendon sheath, right shoulder

    M65.012 Abscess of tendon sheath, left shoulder

    M65.019 Abscess of tendon sheath, unspecified shoulder

  ● M65.02 Abscess of tendon sheath, upper arm

    M65.021 Abscess of tendon sheath, right upper arm

    M65.022 Abscess of tendon sheath, left upper arm

    M65.029 Abscess of tendon sheath, unspecified upper arm

  ● M65.03 Abscess of tendon sheath, forearm

    M65.031 Abscess of tendon sheath, right forearm

    M65.032 Abscess of tendon sheath, left forearm

    M65.039 Abscess of tendon sheath, unspecified forearm

  ● M65.04 Abscess of tendon sheath, hand

    M65.041 Abscess of tendon sheath, right hand

    M65.042 Abscess of tendon sheath, left hand

    M65.049 Abscess of tendon sheath, unspecified hand

  ● M65.05 Abscess of tendon sheath, thigh

    M65.051 Abscess of tendon sheath, right thigh

    M65.052 Abscess of tendon sheath, left thigh

    M65.059 Abscess of tendon sheath, unspecified thigh

Item 13–11 Synovitis is an inflammation of a synovial membrane resulting in pain on motion and is characterized by fluctuating swelling due to effusion in a synovial sac. **Tenosynovitis** is an inflammation of a tendon sheath and occurs most commonly in the wrists, hands, and feet. Bursitis is inflammation of a bursa (fluid filled sac) caused by repetitive use, trauma, infection, or systemic inflammatory disease. Bursae act as protectors and facilitate movement between bones and overlapping muscles (deep bursae) or between bones and tendons/skin (superficial bursae).

◄ New   ⬅ Revised   ~~deleted~~ Deleted   Excludes 1   Excludes 2   Includes   Use additional   Code first   Code also   Unspecified

OGCR Official Guidelines   **X** Assign placeholder X   ● Use Additional Character(s)   ▌ Manifestation Code   **Coding Clinic**

● **M65.06**   Abscess of tendon sheath, lower leg
    M65.061   Abscess of tendon sheath, right lower leg
    M65.062   Abscess of tendon sheath, left lower leg
    M65.069   Abscess of tendon sheath, unspecified lower leg
● **M65.07**   Abscess of tendon sheath, ankle and foot
    M65.071   Abscess of tendon sheath, right ankle and foot
    M65.072   Abscess of tendon sheath, left ankle and foot
    M65.079   Abscess of tendon sheath, unspecified ankle and foot
    M65.08   Abscess of tendon sheath, other site
● **M65.1**   Other infective (teno)synovitis
    M65.10   Other infective (teno)synovitis, unspecified site
● **M65.11**   Other infective (teno)synovitis, shoulder
    M65.111   Other infective (teno)synovitis, right shoulder
    M65.112   Other infective (teno)synovitis, left shoulder
    M65.119   Other infective (teno)synovitis, unspecified shoulder
● **M65.12**   Other infective (teno)synovitis, elbow
    M65.121   Other infective (teno)synovitis, right elbow
    M65.122   Other infective (teno)synovitis, left elbow
    M65.129   Other infective (teno)synovitis, unspecified elbow
● **M65.13**   Other infective (teno)synovitis, wrist
    M65.131   Other infective (teno)synovitis, right wrist
    M65.132   Other infective (teno)synovitis, left wrist
    M65.139   Other infective (teno)synovitis, unspecified wrist
● **M65.14**   Other infective (teno)synovitis, hand
    M65.141   Other infective (teno)synovitis, right hand
    M65.142   Other infective (teno)synovitis, left hand
    M65.149   Other infective (teno)synovitis, unspecified hand
● **M65.15**   Other infective (teno)synovitis, hip
    M65.151   Other infective (teno)synovitis, right hip
    M65.152   Other infective (teno)synovitis, left hip
    M65.159   Other infective (teno)synovitis, unspecified hip
● **M65.16**   Other infective (teno)synovitis, knee
    M65.161   Other infective (teno)synovitis, right knee
    M65.162   Other infective (teno)synovitis, left knee
    M65.169   Other infective (teno)synovitis, unspecified knee
● **M65.17**   Other infective (teno)synovitis, ankle and foot
    M65.171   Other infective (teno)synovitis, right ankle and foot
    M65.172   Other infective (teno)synovitis, left ankle and foot
    M65.179   Other infective (teno)synovitis, unspecified ankle and foot
    M65.18   Other infective (teno)synovitis, other site
    M65.19   Other infective (teno)synovitis, multiple sites

● **M65.2**   Calcific tendinitis
    Excludes1   tendinitis as classified in M75-M77
              calcified tendinitis of shoulder (M75.3)
    M65.20   Calcific tendinitis, unspecified site
● **M65.22**   Calcific tendinitis, upper arm
    M65.221   Calcific tendinitis, right upper arm
    M65.222   Calcific tendinitis, left upper arm
    M65.229   Calcific tendinitis, unspecified upper arm
● **M65.23**   Calcific tendinitis, forearm
    M65.231   Calcific tendinitis, right forearm
    M65.232   Calcific tendinitis, left forearm
    M65.239   Calcific tendinitis, unspecified forearm
● **M65.24**   Calcific tendinitis, hand
    M65.241   Calcific tendinitis, right hand
    M65.242   Calcific tendinitis, left hand
    M65.249   Calcific tendinitis, unspecified hand
● **M65.25**   Calcific tendinitis, thigh
    M65.251   Calcific tendinitis, right thigh
    M65.252   Calcific tendinitis, left thigh
    M65.259   Calcific tendinitis, unspecified thigh
● **M65.26**   Calcific tendinitis, lower leg
    M65.261   Calcific tendinitis, right lower leg
    M65.262   Calcific tendinitis, left lower leg
    M65.269   Calcific tendinitis, unspecified lower leg
● **M65.27**   Calcific tendinitis, ankle and foot
    M65.271   Calcific tendinitis, right ankle and foot
    M65.272   Calcific tendinitis, left ankle and foot
    M65.279   Calcific tendinitis, unspecified ankle and foot
    M65.28   Calcific tendinitis, other site
    M65.29   Calcific tendinitis, multiple sites
● **M65.3**   Trigger finger
    Nodular tendinous disease
    M65.30   Trigger finger, unspecified finger
● **M65.31**   Trigger thumb
    M65.311   Trigger thumb, right thumb
    M65.312   Trigger thumb, left thumb
    M65.319   Trigger thumb, unspecified thumb
● **M65.32**   Trigger finger, index finger
    M65.321   Trigger finger, right index finger
    M65.322   Trigger finger, left index finger
    M65.329   Trigger finger, unspecified index finger
● **M65.33**   Trigger finger, middle finger
    M65.331   Trigger finger, right middle finger
    M65.332   Trigger finger, left middle finger
    M65.339   Trigger finger, unspecified middle finger
● **M65.34**   Trigger finger, ring finger
    M65.341   Trigger finger, right ring finger
    M65.342   Trigger finger, left ring finger
    M65.349   Trigger finger, unspecified ring finger
● **M65.35**   Trigger finger, little finger
    M65.351   Trigger finger, right little finger
    M65.352   Trigger finger, left little finger
    M65.359   Trigger finger, unspecified little finger
   M65.4   Radial styloid tenosynovitis [de Quervain]

CHAPTER 13 (M00-M99)

● M65.8 Other synovitis and tenosynovitis

    M65.80 Other synovitis and tenosynovitis, unspecified site

  ● M65.81 Other synovitis and tenosynovitis, shoulder

    M65.811 Other synovitis and tenosynovitis, right shoulder

    M65.812 Other synovitis and tenosynovitis, left shoulder

    M65.819 Other synovitis and tenosynovitis, unspecified shoulder

  ● M65.82 Other synovitis and tenosynovitis, upper arm

    M65.821 Other synovitis and tenosynovitis, right upper arm

    M65.822 Other synovitis and tenosynovitis, left upper arm

    M65.829 Other synovitis and tenosynovitis, unspecified upper arm

  ● M65.83 Other synovitis and tenosynovitis, forearm

    M65.831 Other synovitis and tenosynovitis, right forearm

    M65.832 Other synovitis and tenosynovitis, left forearm

    M65.839 Other synovitis and tenosynovitis, unspecified forearm

  ● M65.84 Other synovitis and tenosynovitis, hand

    M65.841 Other synovitis and tenosynovitis, right hand

    M65.842 Other synovitis and tenosynovitis, left hand

    M65.849 Other synovitis and tenosynovitis, unspecified hand

  ● M65.85 Other synovitis and tenosynovitis, thigh

    M65.851 Other synovitis and tenosynovitis, right thigh

    M65.852 Other synovitis and tenosynovitis, left thigh

    M65.859 Other synovitis and tenosynovitis, unspecified thigh

  ● M65.86 Other synovitis and tenosynovitis, lower leg

    M65.861 Other synovitis and tenosynovitis, right lower leg

    M65.862 Other synovitis and tenosynovitis, left lower leg

    M65.869 Other synovitis and tenosynovitis, unspecified lower leg

  ● M65.87 Other synovitis and tenosynovitis, ankle and foot

    M65.871 Other synovitis and tenosynovitis, right ankle and foot

    M65.872 Other synovitis and tenosynovitis, left ankle and foot

    M65.879 Other synovitis and tenosynovitis, unspecified ankle and foot

    M65.88 Other synovitis and tenosynovitis, other site

    M65.89 Other synovitis and tenosynovitis, multiple sites

  M65.9 Synovitis and tenosynovitis, unspecified

● M66 Spontaneous rupture of synovium and tendon

  Includes rupture that occurs when a normal force is applied to tissues that are inferred to have less than normal strength

  Excludes2 rotator cuff syndrome (M75.1-)

    rupture where an abnormal force is applied to normal tissue - see injury of tendon by body region

  M66.0 Rupture of popliteal cyst

● M66.1 Rupture of synovium

    Rupture of synovial cyst

    Excludes2 rupture of popliteal cyst (M66.0)

    M66.10 Rupture of synovium, unspecified joint

  ● M66.11 Rupture of synovium, shoulder

    M66.111 Rupture of synovium, right shoulder

    M66.112 Rupture of synovium, left shoulder

    M66.119 Rupture of synovium, unspecified shoulder

  ● M66.12 Rupture of synovium, elbow

    M66.121 Rupture of synovium, right elbow

    M66.122 Rupture of synovium, left elbow

    M66.129 Rupture of synovium, unspecified elbow

  ● M66.13 Rupture of synovium, wrist

    M66.131 Rupture of synovium, right wrist

    M66.132 Rupture of synovium, left wrist

    M66.139 Rupture of synovium, unspecified wrist

  ● M66.14 Rupture of synovium, hand and fingers

    M66.141 Rupture of synovium, right hand

    M66.142 Rupture of synovium, left hand

    M66.143 Rupture of synovium, unspecified hand

    M66.144 Rupture of synovium, right finger(s)

    M66.145 Rupture of synovium, left finger(s)

    M66.146 Rupture of synovium, unspecified finger(s)

  ● M66.15 Rupture of synovium, hip

    M66.151 Rupture of synovium, right hip

    M66.152 Rupture of synovium, left hip

    M66.159 Rupture of synovium, unspecified hip

  ● M66.17 Rupture of synovium, ankle, foot and toes

    M66.171 Rupture of synovium, right ankle

    M66.172 Rupture of synovium, left ankle

    M66.173 Rupture of synovium, unspecified ankle

    M66.174 Rupture of synovium, right foot

    M66.175 Rupture of synovium, left foot

    M66.176 Rupture of synovium, unspecified foot

    M66.177 Rupture of synovium, right toe(s)

    M66.178 Rupture of synovium, left toe(s)

    M66.179 Rupture of synovium, unspecified toe(s)

  M66.18 Rupture of synovium, other site

◀ New   ◀◀ Revised   ~~deleted~~ Deleted   Excludes 1   Excludes 2   Includes   Use additional   Code first   Code also   Unspecified

OGCR Official Guidelines   X Assign placeholder X   ● Use Additional Character(s)   ▶ Manifestation Code   Coding Clinic

● **M66.2 Spontaneous rupture of extensor tendons**

M66.20 Spontaneous rupture of extensor tendons, unspecified site

● M66.21 Spontaneous rupture of extensor tendons, shoulder

M66.211 Spontaneous rupture of extensor tendons, right shoulder

M66.212 Spontaneous rupture of extensor tendons, left shoulder

M66.219 Spontaneous rupture of extensor tendons, unspecified shoulder

● M66.22 Spontaneous rupture of extensor tendons, upper arm

M66.221 Spontaneous rupture of extensor tendons, right upper arm

M66.222 Spontaneous rupture of extensor tendons, left upper arm

M66.229 Spontaneous rupture of extensor tendons, unspecified upper arm

● M66.23 Spontaneous rupture of extensor tendons, forearm

M66.231 Spontaneous rupture of extensor tendons, right forearm

M66.232 Spontaneous rupture of extensor tendons, left forearm

M66.239 Spontaneous rupture of extensor tendons, unspecified forearm

● M66.24 Spontaneous rupture of extensor tendons, hand

M66.241 Spontaneous rupture of extensor tendons, right hand

M66.242 Spontaneous rupture of extensor tendons, left hand

M66.249 Spontaneous rupture of extensor tendons, unspecified hand

● M66.25 Spontaneous rupture of extensor tendons, thigh

M66.251 Spontaneous rupture of extensor tendons, right thigh

M66.252 Spontaneous rupture of extensor tendons, left thigh

M66.259 Spontaneous rupture of extensor tendons, unspecified thigh

● M66.26 Spontaneous rupture of extensor tendons, lower leg

M66.261 Spontaneous rupture of extensor tendons, right lower leg

M66.262 Spontaneous rupture of extensor tendons, left lower leg

M66.269 Spontaneous rupture of extensor tendons, unspecified lower leg

● M66.27 Spontaneous rupture of extensor tendons, ankle and foot

M66.271 Spontaneous rupture of extensor tendons, right ankle and foot

M66.272 Spontaneous rupture of extensor tendons, left ankle and foot

M66.279 Spontaneous rupture of extensor tendons, unspecified ankle and foot

M66.28 Spontaneous rupture of extensor tendons, other site

M66.29 Spontaneous rupture of extensor tendons, multiple sites

● **M66.3 Spontaneous rupture of flexor tendons**

M66.30 Spontaneous rupture of flexor tendons, unspecified site

● M66.31 Spontaneous rupture of flexor tendons, shoulder

M66.311 Spontaneous rupture of flexor tendons, right shoulder

M66.312 Spontaneous rupture of flexor tendons, left shoulder

M66.319 Spontaneous rupture of flexor tendons, unspecified shoulder

● M66.32 Spontaneous rupture of flexor tendons, upper arm

M66.321 Spontaneous rupture of flexor tendons, right upper arm

M66.322 Spontaneous rupture of flexor tendons, left upper arm

M66.329 Spontaneous rupture of flexor tendons, unspecified upper arm

● M66.33 Spontaneous rupture of flexor tendons, forearm

M66.331 Spontaneous rupture of flexor tendons, right forearm

M66.332 Spontaneous rupture of flexor tendons, left forearm

M66.339 Spontaneous rupture of flexor tendons, unspecified forearm

● M66.34 Spontaneous rupture of flexor tendons, hand

M66.341 Spontaneous rupture of flexor tendons, right hand

M66.342 Spontaneous rupture of flexor tendons, left hand

M66.349 Spontaneous rupture of flexor tendons, unspecified hand

● M66.35 Spontaneous rupture of flexor tendons, thigh

M66.351 Spontaneous rupture of flexor tendons, right thigh

M66.352 Spontaneous rupture of flexor tendons, left thigh

M66.359 Spontaneous rupture of flexor tendons, unspecified thigh

● M66.36 Spontaneous rupture of flexor tendons, lower leg

M66.361 Spontaneous rupture of flexor tendons, right lower leg

M66.362 Spontaneous rupture of flexor tendons, left lower leg

M66.369 Spontaneous rupture of flexor tendons, unspecified lower leg

● M66.37 Spontaneous rupture of flexor tendons, ankle and foot

M66.371 Spontaneous rupture of flexor tendons, right ankle and foot

M66.372 Spontaneous rupture of flexor tendons, left ankle and foot

M66.379 Spontaneous rupture of flexor tendons, unspecified ankle and foot

M66.38 Spontaneous rupture of flexor tendons, other site

M66.39 Spontaneous rupture of flexor tendons, multiple sites

CHAPTER 13 (M00-M99)

● **M66.8 Spontaneous rupture of other tendons**

  M66.80   Spontaneous rupture of other tendons, **unspecified** site

  ● M66.81   Spontaneous rupture of other tendons, shoulder

    M66.811   Spontaneous rupture of other tendons, right shoulder

    M66.812   Spontaneous rupture of other tendons, left shoulder

    M66.819   Spontaneous rupture of other tendons, **unspecified** shoulder

  ● M66.82   Spontaneous rupture of other tendons, upper arm

    M66.821   Spontaneous rupture of other tendons, right upper arm

    M66.822   Spontaneous rupture of other tendons, left upper arm

    M66.829   Spontaneous rupture of other tendons, **unspecified** upper arm

  ● M66.83   Spontaneous rupture of other tendons, forearm

    M66.831   Spontaneous rupture of other tendons, right forearm

    M66.832   Spontaneous rupture of other tendons, left forearm

    M66.839   Spontaneous rupture of other tendons, **unspecified** forearm

  ● M66.84   Spontaneous rupture of other tendons, hand

    M66.841   Spontaneous rupture of other tendons, right hand

    M66.842   Spontaneous rupture of other tendons, left hand

    M66.849   Spontaneous rupture of other tendons, **unspecified** hand

  ● M66.85   Spontaneous rupture of other tendons, thigh

    M66.851   Spontaneous rupture of other tendons, right thigh

    M66.852   Spontaneous rupture of other tendons, left thigh

    M66.859   Spontaneous rupture of other tendons, **unspecified** thigh

  ● M66.86   Spontaneous rupture of other tendons, lower leg

    M66.861   Spontaneous rupture of other tendons, right lower leg

    M66.862   Spontaneous rupture of other tendons, left lower leg

    M66.869   Spontaneous rupture of other tendons, **unspecified** lower leg

  ● M66.87   Spontaneous rupture of other tendons, ankle and foot

    M66.871   Spontaneous rupture of other tendons, right ankle and foot

    M66.872   Spontaneous rupture of other tendons, left ankle and foot

    M66.879   Spontaneous rupture of other tendons, **unspecified** ankle and foot

  M66.88   Spontaneous rupture of other tendons, other

  M66.89   Spontaneous rupture of other tendons, multiple sites

M66.9 Spontaneous rupture of unspecified tendon
    Rupture at musculotendinous junction, nontraumatic

● **M67   Other disorders of synovium and tendon**

  Excludes1   palmar fascial fibromatosis [Dupuytren] (M72.0)
                tendinitis NOS (M77.9-)
                xanthomatosis localized to tendons (E78.2)

  ● M67.0   Short Achilles tendon (acquired)

    M67.00   Short Achilles tendon (acquired), **unspecified** ankle

    M67.01   Short Achilles tendon (acquired), right ankle

    M67.02   Short Achilles tendon (acquired), left ankle

  ● M67.2   Synovial hypertrophy, not elsewhere classified

    Excludes1   villonodular synovitis (pigmented) (M12.2-)

    M67.20   Synovial hypertrophy, not elsewhere classified, **unspecified** site

  ● M67.21   Synovial hypertrophy, not elsewhere classified, shoulder

    M67.211   Synovial hypertrophy, not elsewhere classified, right shoulder

    M67.212   Synovial hypertrophy, not elsewhere classified, left shoulder

    M67.219   Synovial hypertrophy, not elsewhere classified, **unspecified** shoulder

  ● M67.22   Synovial hypertrophy, not elsewhere classified, upper arm

    M67.221   Synovial hypertrophy, not elsewhere classified, right upper arm

    M67.222   Synovial hypertrophy, not elsewhere classified, left upper arm

    M67.229   Synovial hypertrophy, not elsewhere classified, **unspecified** upper arm

  ● M67.23   Synovial hypertrophy, not elsewhere classified, forearm

    M67.231   Synovial hypertrophy, not elsewhere classified, right forearm

    M67.232   Synovial hypertrophy, not elsewhere classified, left forearm

    M67.239   Synovial hypertrophy, not elsewhere classified, **unspecified** forearm

  ● M67.24   Synovial hypertrophy, not elsewhere classified, hand

    M67.241   Synovial hypertrophy, not elsewhere classified, right hand

    M67.242   Synovial hypertrophy, not elsewhere classified, left hand

    M67.249   Synovial hypertrophy, not elsewhere classified, **unspecified** hand

  ● M67.25   Synovial hypertrophy, not elsewhere classified, thigh

    M67.251   Synovial hypertrophy, not elsewhere classified, right thigh

    M67.252   Synovial hypertrophy, not elsewhere classified, left thigh

    M67.259   Synovial hypertrophy, not elsewhere classified, **unspecified** thigh

  ● M67.26   Synovial hypertrophy, not elsewhere classified, lower leg

    M67.261   Synovial hypertrophy, not elsewhere classified, right lower leg

    M67.262   Synovial hypertrophy, not elsewhere classified, left lower leg

    M67.269   Synovial hypertrophy, not elsewhere classified, **unspecified** lower leg

● **M67.27**   Synovial hypertrophy, not elsewhere classified, ankle and foot
- **M67.271**   Synovial hypertrophy, not elsewhere classified, right ankle and foot
- **M67.272**   Synovial hypertrophy, not elsewhere classified, left ankle and foot
- **M67.279**   Synovial hypertrophy, not elsewhere classified, unspecified ankle and foot

M67.28   Synovial hypertrophy, not elsewhere classified, other site

M67.29   Synovial hypertrophy, not elsewhere classified, multiple sites

● **M67.3**   Transient synovitis
     Toxic synovitis

> **Excludes1**   palindromic rheumatism (M12.3-)

M67.30   Transient synovitis, unspecified site

● **M67.31**   Transient synovitis, shoulder
- **M67.311**   Transient synovitis, right shoulder
- **M67.312**   Transient synovitis, left shoulder
- **M67.319**   Transient synovitis, unspecified shoulder

● **M67.32**   Transient synovitis, elbow
- **M67.321**   Transient synovitis, right elbow
- **M67.322**   Transient synovitis, left elbow
- **M67.329**   Transient synovitis, unspecified elbow

● **M67.33**   Transient synovitis, wrist
- **M67.331**   Transient synovitis, right wrist
- **M67.332**   Transient synovitis, left wrist
- **M67.339**   Transient synovitis, unspecified wrist

● **M67.34**   Transient synovitis, hand
- **M67.341**   Transient synovitis, right hand
- **M67.342**   Transient synovitis, left hand
- **M67.349**   Transient synovitis, unspecified hand

● **M67.35**   Transient synovitis, hip
- **M67.351**   Transient synovitis, right hip
- **M67.352**   Transient synovitis, left hip
- **M67.359**   Transient synovitis, unspecified hip

● **M67.36**   Transient synovitis, knee
- **M67.361**   Transient synovitis, right knee
- **M67.362**   Transient synovitis, left knee
- **M67.369**   Transient synovitis, unspecified knee

● **M67.37**   Transient synovitis, ankle and foot
- **M67.371**   Transient synovitis, right ankle and foot
- **M67.372**   Transient synovitis, left ankle and foot
- **M67.379**   Transient synovitis, unspecified ankle and foot

M67.38   Transient synovitis, other site

M67.39   Transient synovitis, multiple sites

● **M67.4**   Ganglion
     Ganglion of joint or tendon (sheath)

> **Excludes1**   ganglion in yaws (A66.6)
> **Excludes2**   cyst of bursa (M71.2-M71.3)
>   cyst of synovium (M71.2-M71.3)

M67.40   Ganglion, unspecified site

● **M67.41**   Ganglion, shoulder
- **M67.411**   Ganglion, right shoulder
- **M67.412**   Ganglion, left shoulder
- **M67.419**   Ganglion, unspecified shoulder

● **M67.42**   Ganglion, elbow
- **M67.421**   Ganglion, right elbow
- **M67.422**   Ganglion, left elbow
- **M67.429**   Ganglion, unspecified elbow

● **M67.43**   Ganglion, wrist
- **M67.431**   Ganglion, right wrist
- **M67.432**   Ganglion, left wrist
- **M67.439**   Ganglion, unspecified wrist

● **M67.44**   Ganglion, hand
- **M67.441**   Ganglion, right hand
- **M67.442**   Ganglion, left hand
- **M67.449**   Ganglion, unspecified hand

● **M67.45**   Ganglion, hip
- **M67.451**   Ganglion, right hip
- **M67.452**   Ganglion, left hip
- **M67.459**   Ganglion, unspecified hip

● **M67.46**   Ganglion, knee
- **M67.461**   Ganglion, right knee
- **M67.462**   Ganglion, left knee
- **M67.469**   Ganglion, unspecified knee

● **M67.47**   Ganglion, ankle and foot
- **M67.471**   Ganglion, right ankle and foot
- **M67.472**   Ganglion, left ankle and foot
- **M67.479**   Ganglion, unspecified ankle and foot

M67.48   Ganglion, other site

M67.49   Ganglion, multiple sites

● **M67.5**   Plica syndrome
     Plica knee

M67.50   Plica syndrome, unspecified knee

M67.51   Plica syndrome, right knee

M67.52   Plica syndrome, left knee

● **M67.8**   Other specified disorders of synovium and tendon

M67.80   Other specified disorders of synovium and tendon, unspecified site

● **M67.81**   Other specified disorders of synovium and tendon, shoulder
- **M67.811**   Other specified disorders of synovium, right shoulder
- **M67.812**   Other specified disorders of synovium, left shoulder
- **M67.813**   Other specified disorders of tendon, right shoulder
- **M67.814**   Other specified disorders of tendon, left shoulder
- **M67.819**   Other specified disorders of synovium and tendon, unspecified shoulder

● **M67.82**   Other specified disorders of synovium and tendon, elbow
- **M67.821**   Other specified disorders of synovium, right elbow
- **M67.822**   Other specified disorders of synovium, left elbow
- **M67.823**   Other specified disorders of tendon, right elbow
- **M67.824**   Other specified disorders of tendon, left elbow
- **M67.829**   Other specified disorders of synovium and tendon, unspecified elbow

● **M67.83** Other specified disorders of synovium and tendon, wrist

     M67.831 Other specified disorders of synovium, right wrist

     M67.832 Other specified disorders of synovium, left wrist

     M67.833 Other specified disorders of tendon, right wrist

     M67.834 Other specified disorders of tendon, left wrist

     M67.839 Other specified disorders of synovium and tendon, unspecified forearm

● **M67.84** Other specified disorders of synovium and tendon, hand

     M67.841 Other specified disorders of synovium, right hand

     M67.842 Other specified disorders of synovium, left hand

     M67.843 Other specified disorders of tendon, right hand

     M67.844 Other specified disorders of tendon, left hand

     M67.849 Other specified disorders of synovium and tendon, unspecified hand

● **M67.85** Other specified disorders of synovium and tendon, hip

     M67.851 Other specified disorders of synovium, right hip

     M67.852 Other specified disorders of synovium, left hip

     M67.853 Other specified disorders of tendon, right hip

     M67.854 Other specified disorders of tendon, left hip

     M67.859 Other specified disorders of synovium and tendon, unspecified hip

● **M67.86** Other specified disorders of synovium and tendon, knee

     M67.861 Other specified disorders of synovium, right knee

     M67.862 Other specified disorders of synovium, left knee

     M67.863 Other specified disorders of tendon, right knee

     M67.864 Other specified disorders of tendon, left knee

     M67.869 Other specified disorders of synovium and tendon, unspecified knee

● **M67.87** Other specified disorders of synovium and tendon, ankle and foot

     M67.871 Other specified disorders of synovium, right ankle and foot

     M67.872 Other specified disorders of synovium, left ankle and foot

     M67.873 Other specified disorders of tendon, right ankle and foot

     M67.874 Other specified disorders of tendon, left ankle and foot

     M67.879 Other specified disorders of synovium and tendon, unspecified ankle and foot

     M67.88 Other specified disorders of synovium and tendon, other site

     M67.89 Other specified disorders of synovium and tendon, multiple sites

● **M67.9** Unspecified disorder of synovium and tendon

     M67.90 Unspecified disorder of synovium and tendon, unspecified site

● **M67.91** Unspecified disorder of synovium and tendon, shoulder

     M67.911 Unspecified disorder of synovium and tendon, right shoulder

     M67.912 Unspecified disorder of synovium and tendon, left shoulder

     M67.919 Unspecified disorder of synovium and tendon, unspecified shoulder

● **M67.92** Unspecified disorder of synovium and tendon, upper arm

     M67.921 Unspecified disorder of synovium and tendon, right upper arm

     M67.922 Unspecified disorder of synovium and tendon, left upper arm

     M67.929 Unspecified disorder of synovium and tendon, unspecified upper arm

● **M67.93** Unspecified disorder of synovium and tendon, forearm

     M67.931 Unspecified disorder of synovium and tendon, right forearm

     M67.932 Unspecified disorder of synovium and tendon, left forearm

     M67.939 Unspecified disorder of synovium and tendon, unspecified forearm

● **M67.94** Unspecified disorder of synovium and tendon, hand

     M67.941 Unspecified disorder of synovium and tendon, right hand

     M67.942 Unspecified disorder of synovium and tendon, left hand

     M67.949 Unspecified disorder of synovium and tendon, unspecified hand

● **M67.95** Unspecified disorder of synovium and tendon, thigh

     M67.951 Unspecified disorder of synovium and tendon, right thigh

     M67.952 Unspecified disorder of synovium and tendon, left thigh

     M67.959 Unspecified disorder of synovium and tendon, unspecified thigh

● **M67.96** Unspecified disorder of synovium and tendon, lower leg

     M67.961 Unspecified disorder of synovium and tendon, right lower leg

     M67.962 Unspecified disorder of synovium and tendon, left lower leg

     M67.969 Unspecified disorder of synovium and tendon, unspecified lower leg

● **M67.97** Unspecified disorder of synovium and tendon, ankle and foot

     M67.971 Unspecified disorder of synovium and tendon, right ankle and foot

     M67.972 Unspecified disorder of synovium and tendon, left ankle and foot

     M67.979 Unspecified disorder of synovium and tendon, unspecified ankle and foot

     M67.98 Unspecified disorder of synovium and tendon, other site

     M67.99 Unspecified disorder of synovium and tendon, multiple sites

◀ New   ◀▥ Revised   ~~deleted~~ Deleted   Excludes 1   Excludes 2   Includes   Use additional   Code first   Code also   Unspecified

OGCR Official Guidelines   X Assign placeholder X   ● Use Additional Character(s)   ▶ Manifestation Code   **Coding Clinic**

OTHER SOFT TISSUE DISORDERS (M70-M79)

● **M70   Soft tissue disorders related to use, overuse and pressure**

> **Includes**   soft tissue disorders of occupational origin
>
> Use additional external cause code to identify activity causing disorder (Y93.-)
>
> **Excludes1**   bursitis NOS (M71.9-)
>
> **Excludes2**   bursitis of shoulder (M75.5)
> enthesopathies (M76-M77)
> pressure ulcer (pressure area) (L89.-)

● **M70.0   Crepitant synovitis (acute) (chronic) of hand and wrist**

   ● **M70.03   Crepitant synovitis (acute) (chronic), wrist**

     M70.031   Crepitant synovitis (acute) (chronic), right wrist

     M70.032   Crepitant synovitis (acute) (chronic), left wrist

     M70.039   Crepitant synovitis (acute) (chronic), unspecified wrist

   ● **M70.04   Crepitant synovitis (acute) (chronic), hand**

     M70.041   Crepitant synovitis (acute) (chronic), right hand

     M70.042   Crepitant synovitis (acute) (chronic), left hand

     M70.049   Crepitant synovitis (acute) (chronic), unspecified hand

● **M70.1   Bursitis of hand**

   M70.10   Bursitis, unspecified hand

   M70.11   Bursitis, right hand

   M70.12   Bursitis, left hand

● **M70.2   Olecranon bursitis**

   M70.20   Olecranon bursitis, unspecified elbow

   M70.21   Olecranon bursitis, right elbow

   M70.22   Olecranon bursitis, left elbow

● **M70.3   Other bursitis of elbow**

   M70.30   Other bursitis of elbow, unspecified elbow

   M70.31   Other bursitis of elbow, right elbow

   M70.32   Other bursitis of elbow, left elbow

● **M70.4   Prepatellar bursitis**

   M70.40   Prepatellar bursitis, unspecified knee

   M70.41   Prepatellar bursitis, right knee

   M70.42   Prepatellar bursitis, left knee

● **M70.5   Other bursitis of knee**

   M70.50   Other bursitis of knee, unspecified knee

   M70.51   Other bursitis of knee, right knee

   M70.52   Other bursitis of knee, left knee

● **M70.6   Trochanteric bursitis**

> Trochanteric tendinitis

   M70.60   Trochanteric bursitis, unspecified hip

   M70.61   Trochanteric bursitis, right hip

   M70.62   Trochanteric bursitis, left hip

● **M70.7   Other bursitis of hip**

> Ischial bursitis

   M70.70   Other bursitis of hip, unspecified hip

   M70.71   Other bursitis of hip, right hip

   M70.72   Other bursitis of hip, left hip

● **M70.8   Other soft tissue disorders related to use, overuse and pressure**

   M70.80   Other soft tissue disorders related to use, overuse and pressure of unspecified site

   ● **M70.81   Other soft tissue disorders related to use, overuse and pressure of shoulder**

     M70.811   Other soft tissue disorders related to use, overuse and pressure, right shoulder

     M70.812   Other soft tissue disorders related to use, overuse and pressure, left shoulder

     M70.819   Other soft tissue disorders related to use, overuse and pressure, unspecified shoulder

   ● **M70.82   Other soft tissue disorders related to use, overuse and pressure of upper arm**

     M70.821   Other soft tissue disorders related to use, overuse and pressure, right upper arm

     M70.822   Other soft tissue disorders related to use, overuse and pressure, left upper arm

     M70.829   Other soft tissue disorders related to use, overuse and pressure, unspecified upper arms

   ● **M70.83   Other soft tissue disorders related to use, overuse and pressure of forearm**

     M70.831   Other soft tissue disorders related to use, overuse and pressure, right forearm

     M70.832   Other soft tissue disorders related to use, overuse and pressure, left forearm

     M70.839   Other soft tissue disorders related to use, overuse and pressure, unspecified forearm

   ● **M70.84   Other soft tissue disorders related to use, overuse and pressure of hand**

     M70.841   Other soft tissue disorders related to use, overuse and pressure, right hand

     M70.842   Other soft tissue disorders related to use, overuse and pressure, left hand

     M70.849   Other soft tissue disorders related to use, overuse and pressure, unspecified hand

   ● **M70.85   Other soft tissue disorders related to use, overuse and pressure of thigh**

     M70.851   Other soft tissue disorders related to use, overuse and pressure, right thigh

     M70.852   Other soft tissue disorders related to use, overuse and pressure, left thigh

     M70.859   Other soft tissue disorders related to use, overuse and pressure, unspecified thigh

   ● **M70.86   Other soft tissue disorders related to use, overuse and pressure lower leg**

     M70.861   Other soft tissue disorders related to use, overuse and pressure, right lower leg

     M70.862   Other soft tissue disorders related to use, overuse and pressure, left lower leg

     M70.869   Other soft tissue disorders related to use, overuse and pressure, unspecified leg

CHAPTER 13 (M00-M99)

● M70.87   Other soft tissue disorders related to use, overuse and pressure of ankle and foot

    M70.871   Other soft tissue disorders related to use, overuse and pressure, right ankle and foot

    M70.872   Other soft tissue disorders related to use, overuse and pressure, left ankle and foot

    M70.879   Other soft tissue disorders related to use, overuse and pressure, unspecified ankle and foot

   M70.88   Other soft tissue disorders related to use, overuse and pressure other site

   M70.89   Other soft tissue disorders related to use, overuse and pressure multiple sites

● M70.9   Unspecified soft tissue disorder related to use, overuse and pressure

   M70.90   Unspecified soft tissue disorder related to use, overuse and pressure of unspecified site

● M70.91   Unspecified soft tissue disorder related to use, overuse and pressure of shoulder

    M70.911   Unspecified soft tissue disorder related to use, overuse and pressure, right shoulder

    M70.912   Unspecified soft tissue disorder related to use, overuse and pressure, left shoulder

    M70.919   Unspecified soft tissue disorder related to use, overuse and pressure, unspecified shoulder

● M70.92   Unspecified soft tissue disorder related to use, overuse and pressure of upper arm

    M70.921   Unspecified soft tissue disorder related to use, overuse and pressure, right upper arm

    M70.922   Unspecified soft tissue disorder related to use, overuse and pressure, left upper arm

    M70.929   Unspecified soft tissue disorder related to use, overuse and pressure, unspecified upper arm

● M70.93   Unspecified soft tissue disorder related to use, overuse and pressure of forearm

    M70.931   Unspecified soft tissue disorder related to use, overuse and pressure, right forearm

    M70.932   Unspecified soft tissue disorder related to use, overuse and pressure, left forearm

    M70.939   Unspecified soft tissue disorder related to use, overuse and pressure, unspecified forearm

● M70.94   Unspecified soft tissue disorder related to use, overuse and pressure of hand

    M70.941   Unspecified soft tissue disorder related to use, overuse and pressure, right hand

    M70.942   Unspecified soft tissue disorder related to use, overuse and pressure, left hand

    M70.949   Unspecified soft tissue disorder related to use, overuse and pressure, unspecified hand

● M70.95   Unspecified soft tissue disorder related to use, overuse and pressure of thigh

    M70.951   Unspecified soft tissue disorder related to use, overuse and pressure, right thigh

    M70.952   Unspecified soft tissue disorder related to use, overuse and pressure, left thigh

    M70.959   Unspecified soft tissue disorder related to use, overuse and pressure, unspecified thigh

● M70.96   Unspecified soft tissue disorder related to use, overuse and pressure lower leg

    M70.961   Unspecified soft tissue disorder related to use, overuse and pressure, right lower leg

    M70.962   Unspecified soft tissue disorder related to use, overuse and pressure, left lower leg

    M70.969   Unspecified soft tissue disorder related to use, overuse and pressure, unspecified lower leg

● M70.97   Unspecified soft tissue disorder related to use, overuse and pressure of ankle and foot

    M70.971   Unspecified soft tissue disorder related to use, overuse and pressure, right ankle and foot

    M70.972   Unspecified soft tissue disorder related to use, overuse and pressure, left ankle and foot

    M70.979   Unspecified soft tissue disorder related to use, overuse and pressure, unspecified ankle and foot

   M70.98   Unspecified soft tissue disorder related to use, overuse and pressure other

   M70.99   Unspecified soft tissue disorder related to use, overuse and pressure multiple sites

● M71   Other bursopathies

   Excludes1   bunion (M20.1)
               bursitis related to use, overuse or pressure (M70.-)
               enthesopathies (M76-M77)

● M71.0   Abscess of bursa

    Use additional code (B95.-, B96.-) to identify causative organism

   M71.00   Abscess of bursa, unspecified site

● M71.01   Abscess of bursa, shoulder

    M71.011   Abscess of bursa, right shoulder

    M71.012   Abscess of bursa, left shoulder

    M71.019   Abscess of bursa, unspecified shoulder

● M71.02   Abscess of bursa, elbow

    M71.021   Abscess of bursa, right elbow

    M71.022   Abscess of bursa, left elbow

    M71.029   Abscess of bursa, unspecified elbow

● M71.03   Abscess of bursa, wrist

    M71.031   Abscess of bursa, right wrist

    M71.032   Abscess of bursa, left wrist

    M71.039   Abscess of bursa, unspecified wrist

● M71.04   Abscess of bursa, hand

    M71.041   Abscess of bursa, right hand

    M71.042   Abscess of bursa, left hand

    M71.049   Abscess of bursa, unspecified hand

◄ New   ◄▦ Revised   ~~deleted~~ Deleted   Excludes 1   Excludes 2   Includes   Use additional   Code first   Code also   Unspecified

OGCR Official Guidelines   X Assign placeholder X   ● Use Additional Character(s)   ▌ Manifestation Code   **Coding Clinic**

● M71.05   Abscess of bursa, hip
     M71.051   Abscess of bursa, right hip
     M71.052   Abscess of bursa, left hip
     M71.059   Abscess of bursa, unspecified hip
● M71.06   Abscess of bursa, knee
     M71.061   Abscess of bursa, right knee
     M71.062   Abscess of bursa, left knee
     M71.069   Abscess of bursa, unspecified knee
● M71.07   Abscess of bursa, ankle and foot
     M71.071   Abscess of bursa, right ankle and foot
     M71.072   Abscess of bursa, left ankle and foot
     M71.079   Abscess of bursa, unspecified ankle and foot
     M71.08   Abscess of bursa, other site
     M71.09   Abscess of bursa, multiple sites
● M71.1   Other infective bursitis
     Use additional code (B95.-, B96.-) to identify causative organism
     M71.10   Other infective bursitis, unspecified site
● M71.11   Other infective bursitis, shoulder
     M71.111   Other infective bursitis, right shoulder
     M71.112   Other infective bursitis, left shoulder
     M71.119   Other infective bursitis, unspecified shoulder
● M71.12   Other infective bursitis, elbow
     M71.121   Other infective bursitis, right elbow
     M71.122   Other infective bursitis, left elbow
     M71.129   Other infective bursitis, unspecified elbow
● M71.13   Other infective bursitis, wrist
     M71.131   Other infective bursitis, right wrist
     M71.132   Other infective bursitis, left wrist
     M71.139   Other infective bursitis, unspecified wrist
● M71.14   Other infective bursitis, hand
     M71.141   Other infective bursitis, right hand
     M71.142   Other infective bursitis, left hand
     M71.149   Other infective bursitis, unspecified hand
● M71.15   Other infective bursitis, hip
     M71.151   Other infective bursitis, right hip
     M71.152   Other infective bursitis, left hip
     M71.159   Other infective bursitis, unspecified hip
● M71.16   Other infective bursitis, knee
     M71.161   Other infective bursitis, right knee
     M71.162   Other infective bursitis, left knee
     M71.169   Other infective bursitis, unspecified knee
● M71.17   Other infective bursitis, ankle and foot
     M71.171   Other infective bursitis, right ankle and foot
     M71.172   Other infective bursitis, left ankle and foot
     M71.179   Other infective bursitis, unspecified ankle and foot
     M71.18   Other infective bursitis, other site
     M71.19   Other infective bursitis, multiple sites

● M71.2   Synovial cyst of popliteal space [Baker]
     Popliteal space = popliteal cavity, popliteal fossa. Depression in the posterior aspect of the knee (behind the knee).
     Excludes1   synovial cyst of popliteal space with rupture (M66.0)
     M71.20   Synovial cyst of popliteal space [Baker], unspecified knee
     M71.21   Synovial cyst of popliteal space [Baker], right knee
     M71.22   Synovial cyst of popliteal space [Baker], left knee
● M71.3   Other bursal cyst
     Synovial cyst NOS
     Excludes1   synovial cyst with rupture (M66.1-)
     M71.30   Other bursal cyst, unspecified site
● M71.31   Other bursal cyst, shoulder
     M71.311   Other bursal cyst, right shoulder
     M71.312   Other bursal cyst, left shoulder
     M71.319   Other bursal cyst, unspecified shoulder
● M71.32   Other bursal cyst, elbow
     M71.321   Other bursal cyst, right elbow
     M71.322   Other bursal cyst, left elbow
     M71.329   Other bursal cyst, unspecified elbow
● M71.33   Other bursal cyst, wrist
     M71.331   Other bursal cyst, right wrist
     M71.332   Other bursal cyst, left wrist
     M71.339   Other bursal cyst, unspecified wrist
● M71.34   Other bursal cyst, hand
     M71.341   Other bursal cyst, right hand
     M71.342   Other bursal cyst, left hand
     M71.349   Other bursal cyst, unspecified hand
● M71.35   Other bursal cyst, hip
     M71.351   Other bursal cyst, right hip
     M71.352   Other bursal cyst, left hip
     M71.359   Other bursal cyst, unspecified hip
● M71.37   Other bursal cyst, ankle and foot
     M71.371   Other bursal cyst, right ankle and foot
     M71.372   Other bursal cyst, left ankle and foot
     M71.379   Other bursal cyst, unspecified ankle and foot
     M71.38   Other bursal cyst, other site
     M71.39   Other bursal cyst, multiple sites
● M71.4   Calcium deposit in bursa
     Excludes2   calcium deposit in bursa of shoulder (M75.3)
     M71.40   Calcium deposit in bursa, unspecified site
● M71.42   Calcium deposit in bursa, elbow
     M71.421   Calcium deposit in bursa, right elbow
     M71.422   Calcium deposit in bursa, left elbow
     M71.429   Calcium deposit in bursa, unspecified elbow
● M71.43   Calcium deposit in bursa, wrist
     M71.431   Calcium deposit in bursa, right wrist
     M71.432   Calcium deposit in bursa, left wrist
     M71.439   Calcium deposit in bursa, unspecified wrist
● M71.44   Calcium deposit in bursa, hand
     M71.441   Calcium deposit in bursa, right hand
     M71.442   Calcium deposit in bursa, left hand
     M71.449   Calcium deposit in bursa, unspecified hand

CHAPTER 13 (M00-M99)

● M71.45   Calcium deposit in bursa, hip
  M71.451   Calcium deposit in bursa, right hip
  M71.452   Calcium deposit in bursa, left hip
  M71.459   Calcium deposit in bursa, unspecified hip
● M71.46   Calcium deposit in bursa, knee
  M71.461   Calcium deposit in bursa, right knee
  M71.462   Calcium deposit in bursa, left knee
  M71.469   Calcium deposit in bursa, unspecified knee
● M71.47   Calcium deposit in bursa, ankle and foot
  M71.471   Calcium deposit in bursa, right ankle and foot
  M71.472   Calcium deposit in bursa, left ankle and foot
  M71.479   Calcium deposit in bursa, unspecified ankle and foot
  M71.48   Calcium deposit in bursa, other site
  M71.49   Calcium deposit in bursa, multiple sites
● M71.5   Other bursitis, not elsewhere classified
  Excludes1   bursitis NOS (M71.9-)
  Excludes2   bursitis of shoulder (M75.5)
    bursitis of tibial collateral [Pellegrini-Stieda] (M76.4)
  M71.50   Other bursitis, not elsewhere classified, unspecified site
● M71.52   Other bursitis, not elsewhere classified, elbow
  M71.521   Other bursitis, not elsewhere classified, right elbow
  M71.522   Other bursitis, not elsewhere classified, left elbow
  M71.529   Other bursitis, not elsewhere classified, unspecified elbow
● M71.53   Other bursitis, not elsewhere classified, wrist
  M71.531   Other bursitis, not elsewhere classified, right wrist
  M71.532   Other bursitis, not elsewhere classified, left wrist
  M71.539   Other bursitis, not elsewhere classified, unspecified wrist
● M71.54   Other bursitis, not elsewhere classified, hand
  M71.541   Other bursitis, not elsewhere classified, right hand
  M71.542   Other bursitis, not elsewhere classified, left hand
  M71.549   Other bursitis, not elsewhere classified, unspecified hand
● M71.55   Other bursitis, not elsewhere classified, hip
  M71.551   Other bursitis, not elsewhere classified, right hip
  M71.552   Other bursitis, not elsewhere classified, left hip
  M71.559   Other bursitis, not elsewhere classified, unspecified hip
● M71.56   Other bursitis, not elsewhere classified, knee
  M71.561   Other bursitis, not elsewhere classified, right knee
  M71.562   Other bursitis, not elsewhere classified, left knee
  M71.569   Other bursitis, not elsewhere classified, unspecified knee

● M71.57   Other bursitis, not elsewhere classified, ankle and foot
  M71.571   Other bursitis, not elsewhere classified, right ankle and foot
  M71.572   Other bursitis, not elsewhere classified, left ankle and foot
  M71.579   Other bursitis, not elsewhere classified, unspecified ankle and foot
  M71.58   Other bursitis, not elsewhere classified, other site
● M71.8   Other specified bursopathies
  M71.80   Other specified bursopathies, unspecified site
● M71.81   Other specified bursopathies, shoulder
  M71.811   Other specified bursopathies, right shoulder
  M71.812   Other specified bursopathies, left shoulder
  M71.819   Other specified bursopathies, unspecified shoulder
● M71.82   Other specified bursopathies, elbow
  M71.821   Other specified bursopathies, right elbow
  M71.822   Other specified bursopathies, left elbow
  M71.829   Other specified bursopathies, unspecified elbow
● M71.83   Other specified bursopathies, wrist
  M71.831   Other specified bursopathies, right wrist
  M71.832   Other specified bursopathies, left wrist
  M71.839   Other specified bursopathies, unspecified wrist
● M71.84   Other specified bursopathies, hand
  M71.841   Other specified bursopathies, right hand
  M71.842   Other specified bursopathies, left hand
  M71.849   Other specified bursopathies, unspecified hand
● M71.85   Other specified bursopathies, hip
  M71.851   Other specified bursopathies, right hip
  M71.852   Other specified bursopathies, left hip
  M71.859   Other specified bursopathies, unspecified hip
● M71.86   Other specified bursopathies, knee
  M71.861   Other specified bursopathies, right knee
  M71.862   Other specified bursopathies, left knee
  M71.869   Other specified bursopathies, unspecified knee
● M71.87   Other specified bursopathies, ankle and foot
  M71.871   Other specified bursopathies, right ankle and foot
  M71.872   Other specified bursopathies, left ankle and foot
  M71.879   Other specified bursopathies, unspecified ankle and foot
  M71.88   Other specified bursopathies, other site
  M71.89   Other specified bursopathies, multiple sites
M71.9   Bursopathy, unspecified
  Bursitis NOS

◄ New   ◄⁞ Revised   d̶e̶l̶e̶t̶e̶d̶ Deleted   Excludes 1   Excludes 2   Includes   Use additional   Code first   Code also   Unspecified
OGCR Official Guidelines   X Assign placeholder X   ● Use Additional Character(s)   ▶ Manifestation Code   Coding Clinic

● **M72 Fibroblastic disorders**
  Excludes2 retroperitoneal fibromatosis (D48.3)
  M72.0 Palmar fascial fibromatosis [Dupuytren]   **A**
  M72.1 Knuckle pads
  M72.2 Plantar fascial fibromatosis
        Plantar fasciitis
  M72.4 Pseudosarcomatous fibromatosis
        Nodular fasciitis
  M72.6 Necrotizing fasciitis
        Use additional code (B95.-, B96.-) to identify causative
        organism
  M72.8 Other fibroblastic disorders
        Abscess of fascia
        Fasciitis NEC
        Other infective fasciitis
        Use additional code to (B95.-, B96.-) identify causative
        organism
        Excludes1 diffuse (eosinophilic) fasciitis (M35.4)
                   necrotizing fasciitis (M72.6)
                   nodular fasciitis (M72.4)
                   perirenal fasciitis NOS (N13.5)
                   perirenal fasciitis with infection (N13.6)
                   plantar fasciitis (M72.2)
  M72.9 Fibroblastic disorder, unspecified
        Fasciitis NOS
        Fibromatosis NOS

● **M75 Shoulder lesions**
  Excludes2 shoulder-hand syndrome (M89.0-)
● **M75.0 Adhesive capsulitis of shoulder**
        Frozen shoulder
        Periarthritis of shoulder
  M75.00 Adhesive capsulitis of unspecified shoulder
  M75.01 Adhesive capsulitis of right shoulder
  M75.02 Adhesive capsulitis of left shoulder
● **M75.1 Rotator cuff tear or rupture, not specified as traumatic**
        Rotator cuff syndrome
        Supraspinatus syndrome
        Supraspinatus tear or rupture, not specified as
              traumatic
        Excludes1 tear of rotator cuff, traumatic (S46.01-)
        Gradual onset due to repetitive stress to rotator cuff
   ● **M75.10 Unspecified rotator cuff tear or rupture, not
               specified as traumatic**
        **M75.100 Unspecified rotator cuff tear or
                  rupture of unspecified shoulder, not
                  specified as traumatic**
        **M75.101 Unspecified rotator cuff tear or
                  rupture of right shoulder, not
                  specified as traumatic**
        **M75.102 Unspecified rotator cuff tear or
                  rupture of left shoulder, not specified
                  as traumatic**
   ● **M75.11 Incomplete rotator cuff tear or rupture not
               specified as traumatic**
        **M75.110 Incomplete rotator cuff tear or rupture
                  of unspecified shoulder, not specified
                  as traumatic**
        **M75.111 Incomplete rotator cuff tear or rupture
                  of right shoulder, not specified as
                  traumatic**
        **M75.112 Incomplete rotator cuff tear or rupture
                  of left shoulder, not specified as
                  traumatic**

● **M75.12 Complete rotator cuff tear or rupture not
             specified as traumatic**
        **M75.120 Complete rotator cuff tear or rupture
                  of unspecified shoulder, not specified
                  as traumatic**
        **M75.121 Complete rotator cuff tear or rupture
                  of right shoulder, not specified as
                  traumatic**
        **M75.122 Complete rotator cuff tear or rupture
                  of left shoulder, not specified as
                  traumatic**
● **M75.2 Bicipital tendinitis**
  M75.20 Bicipital tendinitis, unspecified shoulder
  M75.21 Bicipital tendinitis, right shoulder
  M75.22 Bicipital tendinitis, left shoulder
● **M75.3 Calcific tendinitis of shoulder**
        Calcified bursa of shoulder
  M75.30 Calcific tendinitis of unspecified shoulder
  M75.31 Calcific tendinitis of right shoulder
  M75.32 Calcific tendinitis of left shoulder
● **M75.4 Impingement syndrome of shoulder**
  **M75.40 Impingement syndrome of unspecified
           shoulder**
  M75.41 Impingement syndrome of right shoulder
  M75.42 Impingement syndrome of left shoulder
● **M75.5 Bursitis of shoulder**
  M75.50 Bursitis of unspecified shoulder
  M75.51 Bursitis of right shoulder
  M75.52 Bursitis of left shoulder
● **M75.8 Other shoulder lesions**
  M75.80 Other shoulder lesions, unspecified shoulder
  M75.81 Other shoulder lesions, right shoulder
  M75.82 Other shoulder lesions, left shoulder
● **M75.9 Shoulder lesion, unspecified**
  **M75.90 Shoulder lesion, unspecified, unspecified
           shoulder**
  M75.91 Shoulder lesion, unspecified, right shoulder
  M75.92 Shoulder lesion, unspecified, left shoulder

● **M76 Enthesopathies, lower limb, excluding foot**
  Excludes2 bursitis due to use, overuse and pressure (M70.-)
             enthesopathies of ankle and foot (M77.5-)
● **M76.0 Gluteal tendinitis**
  M76.00 Gluteal tendinitis, unspecified hip
  M76.01 Gluteal tendinitis, right hip
  M76.02 Gluteal tendinitis, left hip
● **M76.1 Psoas tendinitis**
  M76.10 Psoas tendinitis, unspecified hip
  M76.11 Psoas tendinitis, right hip
  M76.12 Psoas tendinitis, left hip
● **M76.2 Iliac crest spur**
  M76.20 Iliac crest spur, unspecified hip
  M76.21 Iliac crest spur, right hip
  M76.22 Iliac crest spur, left hip
● **M76.3 Iliotibial band syndrome**
  M76.30 Iliotibial band syndrome, unspecified leg
  M76.31 Iliotibial band syndrome, right leg
  M76.32 Iliotibial band syndrome, left leg
● **M76.4 Tibial collateral bursitis [Pellegrini-Stieda]**
  **M76.40 Tibial collateral bursitis [Pellegrini-Stieda],
           unspecified leg**
  **M76.41 Tibial collateral bursitis [Pellegrini-Stieda],
           right leg**
  **M76.42 Tibial collateral bursitis [Pellegrini-Stieda], left
           leg**

CHAPTER 13 (M00-M99)

● **M76.5**   **Patellar tendinitis**
    M76.50   Patellar tendinitis, unspecified knee
    M76.51   Patellar tendinitis, right knee
    M76.52   Patellar tendinitis, left knee

● **M76.6**   **Achilles tendinitis**
    Achilles bursitis
    M76.60   Achilles tendinitis, unspecified leg
    M76.61   Achilles tendinitis, right leg
    M76.62   Achilles tendinitis, left leg

● **M76.7**   **Peroneal tendinitis**
    M76.70   Peroneal tendinitis, unspecified leg
    M76.71   Peroneal tendinitis, right leg
    M76.72   Peroneal tendinitis, left leg

● **M76.8**   **Other specified enthesopathies of lower limb, excluding foot**
    ● M76.81   Anterior tibial syndrome
      M76.811   Anterior tibial syndrome, right leg
      M76.812   Anterior tibial syndrome, left leg
      M76.819   Anterior tibial syndrome, unspecified leg
    ● M76.82   Posterior tibial tendinitis
      M76.821   Posterior tibial tendinitis, right leg
      M76.822   Posterior tibial tendinitis, left leg
      M76.829   Posterior tibial tendinitis, unspecified leg
    ● M76.89   Other specified enthesopathies of lower limb, excluding foot
      M76.891   Other specified enthesopathies of right lower limb, excluding foot
      M76.892   Other specified enthesopathies of left lower limb, excluding foot
      M76.899   Other specified enthesopathies of unspecified lower limb, excluding foot

● **M76.9**   Unspecified enthesopathy, lower limb, excluding foot

● **M77**   **Other enthesopathies**
    Excludes1   bursitis NOS (M71.9-)
    Excludes2   bursitis due to use, overuse and pressure (M70.-)
             osteophyte (M25.7)
             spinal enthesopathy (M46.0-)

● **M77.0**   **Medial epicondylitis**
    M77.00   Medial epicondylitis, unspecified elbow
    M77.01   Medial epicondylitis, right elbow
    M77.02   Medial epicondylitis, left elbow

● **M77.1**   **Lateral epicondylitis**
    Tennis elbow
    M77.10   Lateral epicondylitis, unspecified elbow
    M77.11   Lateral epicondylitis, right elbow
    M77.12   Lateral epicondylitis, left elbow

● **M77.2**   **Periarthritis of wrist**
    M77.20   Periarthritis, unspecified wrist
    M77.21   Periarthritis, right wrist
    M77.22   Periarthritis, left wrist

● **M77.3**   **Calcaneal spur**
    M77.30   Calcaneal spur, unspecified foot
    M77.31   Calcaneal spur, right foot
    M77.32   Calcaneal spur, left foot

● **M77.4**   **Metatarsalgia**
    Excludes1   Morton's metatarsalgia (G57.6)
    M77.40   Metatarsalgia, unspecified foot
    M77.41   Metatarsalgia, right foot
    M77.42   Metatarsalgia, left foot

● **M77.5**   **Other enthesopathy of foot**
    M77.50   Other enthesopathy of unspecified foot
    M77.51   Other enthesopathy of right foot
    M77.52   Other enthesopathy of left foot

● **M77.8**   **Other enthesopathies, not elsewhere classified**

● **M77.9**   **Enthesopathy, unspecified**
    Bone spur NOS
    Capsulitis NOS
    Periarthritis NOS
    Tendinitis NOS

● **M79**   **Other and unspecified soft tissue disorders, not elsewhere classified**
    Excludes1   psychogenic rheumatism (F45.8)
             soft tissue pain, psychogenic (F45.41)

M79.0   **Rheumatism, unspecified**
    Excludes1   fibromyalgia (M79.7)
             palindromic rheumatism (M12.3-)

M79.1   **Myalgia**
    Myofascial pain syndrome
    Excludes1   fibromyalgia (M79.7)
             myositis (M60.-)

M79.2   **Neuralgia and neuritis, unspecified**
    Excludes1   brachial radiculitis NOS (M54.1)
             lumbosacral radiculitis NOS (M54.1)
             mononeuropathies (G56-G58)
             radiculitis NOS (M54.1)
             sciatica (M54.3-M54.4)

M79.3   **Panniculitis, unspecified**
    Excludes1   lupus panniculitis (L93.2)
             neck and back panniculitis (M54.0-)
             relapsing [Weber-Christian] panniculitis (M35.6)

M79.4   **Hypertrophy of (infrapatellar) fat pad**

M79.5   **Residual foreign body in soft tissue**
    Excludes1   foreign body granuloma of skin and subcutaneous tissue (L92.3)
             foreign body granuloma of soft tissue (M60.2-)

● **M79.6**   **Pain in limb, hand, foot, fingers and toes**
    Excludes2   pain in joint (M25.5-)
    ● M79.60   Pain in limb, unspecified
      M79.601   Pain in right arm
         Pain in right upper limb NOS
      M79.602   Pain in left arm
         Pain in left upper limb NOS
      M79.603   Pain in arm, unspecified
         Pain in upper limb NOS
      M79.604   Pain in right leg
         Pain in right lower limb NOS
      M79.605   Pain in left leg
         Pain in left lower limb NOS
      M79.606   Pain in leg, unspecified
         Pain in lower limb NOS
      M79.609   Pain in unspecified limb
         Pain in limb NOS
    ● M79.62   Pain in upper arm
      Pain in axillary region
      M79.621   Pain in right upper arm
      M79.622   Pain in left upper arm
      M79.629   Pain in unspecified upper arm
    ● M79.63   Pain in forearm
      M79.631   Pain in right forearm
      M79.632   Pain in left forearm
      M79.639   Pain in unspecified forearm

◀ New   ◀▥ Revised   ~~deleted~~ Deleted   Excludes 1   Excludes 2   Includes   Use additional   Code first   Code also   Unspecified
OGCR Official Guidelines   **X** Assign placeholder X   ● Use Additional Character(s)   ▶ Manifestation Code   **Coding Clinic**

● M79.64 Pain in hand and fingers
    M79.641 Pain in right hand
    M79.642 Pain in left hand
    M79.643 Pain in unspecified hand
    M79.644 Pain in right finger(s)
    M79.645 Pain in left finger(s)
    M79.646 Pain in unspecified finger(s)
● M79.65 Pain in thigh
    M79.651 Pain in right thigh
    M79.652 Pain in left thigh
    M79.659 Pain in unspecified thigh
● M79.66 Pain in lower leg
    M79.661 Pain in right lower leg
    M79.662 Pain in left lower leg
    M79.669 Pain in unspecified lower leg
● M79.67 Pain in foot and toes
    M79.671 Pain in right foot
    M79.672 Pain in left foot
    M79.673 Pain in unspecified foot
    M79.674 Pain in right toe(s)
    M79.675 Pain in left toe(s)
    M79.676 Pain in unspecified toe(s)

M79.7 **Fibromyalgia**
    Fibromyositis
    Fibrositis
    Myofibrositis

● M79.A **Nontraumatic compartment syndrome**
    Code first, if applicable, associated postprocedural
       complication
    Excludes1 compartment syndrome NOS (T79.A-)
       fibromyalgia (M79.7) nontraumatic
         ischemic infarction of muscle
         (M62.2-)
       traumatic compartment syndrome
         (T79.A-)

● M79.A1 **Nontraumatic compartment syndrome of upper extremity**
    Nontraumatic compartment syndrome of
       shoulder, arm, forearm, wrist, hand, and
       fingers
    M79.A11 **Nontraumatic compartment syndrome of right upper extremity**
    M79.A12 **Nontraumatic compartment syndrome of left upper extremity**
    M79.A19 **Nontraumatic compartment syndrome of unspecified upper extremity**

● M79.A2 **Nontraumatic compartment syndrome of lower extremity**
    Nontraumatic compartment syndrome of hip,
       buttock, thigh, leg, foot, and toes
    M79.A21 **Nontraumatic compartment syndrome of right lower extremity**
    M79.A22 **Nontraumatic compartment syndrome of left lower extremity**
    M79.A29 **Nontraumatic compartment syndrome of unspecified lower extremity**

M79.A3 **Nontraumatic compartment syndrome of abdomen**

M79.A9 **Nontraumatic compartment syndrome of other sites**

● M79.8 **Other specified soft tissue disorders**
    M79.81 **Nontraumatic hematoma of soft tissue**
       Nontraumatic hematoma of muscle
       Nontraumatic seroma of muscle and soft tissue
    M79.89 **Other specified soft tissue disorders**
       Polyalgia

M79.9 **Soft tissue disorder, unspecified**

OGCR See Section I.C., Chapter 13.d.
Osteoporosis

OSTEOPATHIES AND CHONDROPATHIES (M80-M94)

DISORDERS OF BONE DENSITY AND STRUCTURE (M80-M85)

M80 **Osteoporosis with current pathological fracture**
    Excessive skeletal fragility (porous bone) resulting in bone fractures
    Includes osteoporosis with current fragility fracture
    Use additional code to identify major osseous defect, if
       applicable (M89.7-)
    Excludes1 collapsed vertebra NOS (M48.5)
       pathological fracture NOS (M84.4)
       wedging of vertebra NOS (M48.5)
    Excludes2 personal history of (healed) osteoporosis fracture
       (Z87.310)
    The appropriate 7th character is to be added to each code from
       category M80:

> A   initial encounter for fracture
>   *All encounters involving diagnosis and treatment*
> D   subsequent encounter for fracture with routine healing
> G   subsequent encounter for fracture with delayed
>   healing
>   *Encounters for attention to casting or fixation devices,*
>   *medication, and follow-up visits during the healing phase*
> K   subsequent encounter for fracture with nonunion
>   *Total failure of fracture healing*
> P   subsequent encounter for fracture with malunion
>   *Fracture ends do not heal together correctly.*
> S   sequela

● M80.0 **Age-related osteoporosis with current pathological fracture**
    Involutional osteoporosis with current pathological
       fracture
    Osteoporosis NOS with current pathological fracture
    Postmenopausal osteoporosis with current pathological
       fracture
    Senile osteoporosis with current pathological fracture
  X ● M80.00 **Age-related osteoporosis with current pathological fracture, unspecified site** A
  ● M80.01 **Age-related osteoporosis with current pathological fracture, shoulder**
    ● M80.011 **Age-related osteoporosis with current pathological fracture, right shoulder** A
    ● M80.012 **Age-related osteoporosis with current pathological fracture, left shoulder** A
    ● M80.019 **Age-related osteoporosis with current pathological fracture, unspecified shoulder** A
  ● M80.02 **Age-related osteoporosis with current pathological fracture, humerus**
    ● M80.021 **Age-related osteoporosis with current pathological fracture, right humerus** A
    ● M80.022 **Age-related osteoporosis with current pathological fracture, left humerus** A
    ● M80.029 **Age-related osteoporosis with current pathological fracture, unspecified humerus** A
  ● M80.03 **Age-related osteoporosis with current pathological fracture, forearm**
    Age-related osteoporosis with current
       pathological fracture of wrist
    ● M80.031 **Age-related osteoporosis with current pathological fracture, right forearm** A
    ● M80.032 **Age-related osteoporosis with current pathological fracture, left forearm** A
    ● M80.039 **Age-related osteoporosis with current pathological fracture, unspecified forearm** A

CHAPTER 13 (M00-M99)

CHAPTER 13 (M00-M99)

● M80.04   **Age-related osteoporosis with current pathological fracture, hand**
- ● M80.041   Age-related osteoporosis with current pathological fracture, right hand   A
- ● M80.042   Age-related osteoporosis with current pathological fracture, left hand   A
- ● M80.049   Age-related osteoporosis with current pathological fracture, unspecified hand   A

● M80.05   **Age-related osteoporosis with current pathological fracture, femur**
     Age-related osteoporosis with current pathological fracture of hip
- ● M80.051   Age-related osteoporosis with current pathological fracture, right femur   A
- ● M80.052   Age-related osteoporosis with current pathological fracture, left femur   A
- ● M80.059   Age-related osteoporosis with current pathological fracture, unspecified femur   A

● M80.06   **Age-related osteoporosis with current pathological fracture, lower leg**
- ● M80.061   Age-related osteoporosis with current pathological fracture, right lower leg A
- ● M80.062   Age-related osteoporosis with current pathological fracture, left lower leg   A
- ● M80.069   Age-related osteoporosis with current pathological fracture, unspecified lower leg   A

● M80.07   **Age-related osteoporosis with current pathological fracture, ankle and foot**
- ● M80.071   Age-related osteoporosis with current pathological fracture, right ankle and foot   A
- ● M80.072   Age-related osteoporosis with current pathological fracture, left ankle and foot   A
- ● M80.079   Age-related osteoporosis with current pathological fracture, unspecified ankle and foot   A

X ● M80.08   **Age-related osteoporosis with current pathological fracture, vertebra(e)**   A

● M80.8   **Other osteoporosis with current pathological fracture**
     Drug-induced osteoporosis with current pathological fracture
     Idiopathic osteoporosis with current pathological fracture
     Osteoporosis of disuse with current pathological fracture
     Postoophorectomy osteoporosis with current pathological fracture
     Postsurgical malabsorption osteoporosis with current pathological fracture
     Post-traumatic osteoporosis with current pathological fracture
     Use additional code for adverse effect, if applicable, to identify drug (T36-T50 with fifth or sixth character 5)

X ● M80.80   **Other osteoporosis with current pathological fracture, unspecified site**   A

● M80.81   **Other osteoporosis with pathological fracture, shoulder**
- ● M80.811   Other osteoporosis with current pathological fracture, right shoulder
- ● M80.812   Other osteoporosis with current pathological fracture, left shoulder
- ● M80.819   Other osteoporosis with current pathological fracture, unspecified shoulder

● M80.82   **Other osteoporosis with current pathological fracture, humerus**
- ● M80.821   Other osteoporosis with current pathological fracture, right humerus
- ● M80.822   Other osteoporosis with current pathological fracture, left humerus
- ● M80.829   Other osteoporosis with current pathological fracture, unspecified humerus

● M80.83   **Other osteoporosis with current pathological fracture, forearm**
     Other osteoporosis with current pathological fracture of wrist
- ● M80.831   Other osteoporosis with current pathological fracture, right forearm
- ● M80.832   Other osteoporosis with current pathological fracture, left forearm
- ● M80.839   Other osteoporosis with current pathological fracture, unspecified forearm

● M80.84   **Other osteoporosis with current pathological fracture, hand**
- ● M80.841   Other osteoporosis with current pathological fracture, right hand
- ● M80.842   Other osteoporosis with current pathological fracture, left hand
- ● M80.849   Other osteoporosis with current pathological fracture, unspecified hand

● M80.85   **Other osteoporosis with current pathological fracture, femur**
     Other osteoporosis with current pathological fracture of hip
- ● M80.851   Other osteoporosis with current pathological fracture, right femur
- ● M80.852   Other osteoporosis with current pathological fracture, left femur
- ● M80.859   Other osteoporosis with current pathological fracture, unspecified femur

● M80.86   **Other osteoporosis with current pathological fracture, lower leg**
- ● M80.861   Other osteoporosis with current pathological fracture, right lower leg
- ● M80.862   Other osteoporosis with current pathological fracture, left lower leg
- ● M80.869   Other osteoporosis with current pathological fracture, unspecified lower leg

● M80.87   **Other osteoporosis with current pathological fracture, ankle and foot**
- ● M80.871   Other osteoporosis with current pathological fracture, right ankle and foot
- ● M80.872   Other osteoporosis with current pathological fracture, left ankle and foot
- ● M80.879   Other osteoporosis with current pathological fracture, unspecified ankle and foot

X ● M80.88   **Other osteoporosis with current pathological fracture, vertebra(e)**

◀ New   ◀◀ Revised   ~~deleted~~ Deleted   Excludes 1   Excludes 2   Includes   Use additional   Code first   Code also   Unspecified
OGCR Official Guidelines   X Assign placeholder X   ● Use Additional Character(s)   ▶ Manifestation Code   **Coding Clinic**

● **M81   Osteoporosis without current pathological fracture**
    Use additional code to identify:
       major osseous defect, if applicable (M89.7-)
       personal history of (healed) osteoporosis fracture, if
          applicable (Z87.310)
    Excludes1   osteoporosis with current pathological fracture
               (M80.-)
               Sudeck's atrophy (M89.0)

   M81.0   Age-related osteoporosis without current pathological
        fracture   **A**
       Involutional osteoporosis without current pathological
          fracture
       Osteoporosis NOS
       Postmenopausal osteoporosis without current
          pathological fracture
       Senile osteoporosis without current pathological
          fracture

   M81.6   Localized osteoporosis [Lequesne]
      Excludes1   Sudeck's atrophy (M89.0)

   M81.8   Other osteoporosis without current pathological fracture
       Drug-induced osteoporosis without current
          pathological fracture
       Idiopathic osteoporosis without current pathological
          fracture
       Osteoporosis of disuse without current pathological
          fracture
       Postoophorectomy osteoporosis without current
          pathological fracture
       Postsurgical malabsorption osteoporosis without
          current pathological fracture
       Post-traumatic osteoporosis without current
          pathological fracture
       Use additional code for adverse effect, if applicable,
          to identify drug (T36-T50 with fifth or sixth
          character 5)

● **M83   Adult osteomalacia**
    Excludes1   infantile and juvenile osteomalacia (E55.0)
              renal osteodystrophy (N25.0)
              rickets (active) (E55.0)
              rickets (active) sequelae (E64.3)
              vitamin D-resistant osteomalacia (E83.3)
              vitamin D-resistant rickets (active) (E83.3)

   M83.0   Puerperal osteomalacia ♀   **M**
   M83.1   Senile osteomalacia   **A**
   M83.2   Adult osteomalacia due to malabsorption   **A**
       Postsurgical malabsorption osteomalacia in adults
   M83.3   Adult osteomalacia due to malnutrition   **A**
   M83.4   Aluminum bone disease
   M83.5   Other drug-induced osteomalacia in adults   **A**
       Use additional code for adverse effect, if applicable,
          to identify drug (T36-T50 with fifth or sixth
          character 5)
   M83.8   Other adult osteomalacia   **A**
   M83.9   Adult osteomalacia, unspecified   **A**

● **M84   Disorder of continuity of bone**
    Excludes2   traumatic fracture of bone-see fracture, by site

   ● **M84.3   Stress fracture**
      Fatigue fracture
      March fracture
      Stress fracture NOS
      Stress reaction
      Use additional external cause code(s) to identify the
         cause of the stress fracture
     Excludes1   pathological fracture NOS (M84.4.-)
               pathological fracture due to osteoporosis
                   (M80.-)
               traumatic fracture (S12.-, S22.-, S32.-, S42.-
                   , S52.-, S62.-, S72.-, S82.-, S92.-)
     Excludes2   personal history of (healed) stress
               (fatigue) fracture (Z87.312)
               stress fracture of vertebra (M48.4-)
     The appropriate 7th character is to be added to each
        code from subcategory M84.3:

A	initial encounter for fracture
D	subsequent encounter for fracture with routine healing
G	subsequent encounter for fracture with delayed healing
K	subsequent encounter for fracture with nonunion
P	subsequent encounter for fracture with malunion
S	sequela

   X ● **M84.30   Stress fracture, unspecified site**
   ● **M84.31   Stress fracture, shoulder**
      ● **M84.311   Stress fracture, right shoulder**
      ● **M84.312   Stress fracture, left shoulder**
      ● **M84.319   Stress fracture, unspecified shoulder**
   ● **M84.32   Stress fracture, humerus**
      ● **M84.321   Stress fracture, right humerus**
      ● **M84.322   Stress fracture, left humerus**
      ● **M84.329   Stress fracture, unspecified humerus**
   ● **M84.33   Stress fracture, ulna and radius**
      ● **M84.331   Stress fracture, right ulna**
      ● **M84.332   Stress fracture, left ulna**
      ● **M84.333   Stress fracture, right radius**
      ● **M84.334   Stress fracture, left radius**
      ● **M84.339   Stress fracture, unspecified ulna and
               radius**
   ● **M84.34   Stress fracture, hand and fingers**
      ● **M84.341   Stress fracture, right hand**
      ● **M84.342   Stress fracture, left hand**
      ● **M84.343   Stress fracture, unspecified hand**
      ● **M84.344   Stress fracture, right finger(s)**
      ● **M84.345   Stress fracture, left finger(s)**
      ● **M84.346   Stress fracture, unspecified finger(s)**
   ● **M84.35   Stress fracture, pelvis and femur**
      Stress fracture, hip
      ● **M84.350   Stress fracture, pelvis**
      ● **M84.351   Stress fracture, right femur**
      ● **M84.352   Stress fracture, left femur**
      ● **M84.353   Stress fracture, unspecified femur**
      ● **M84.359   Stress fracture, hip, unspecified**

CHAPTER 13 (M00-M99)

● M84.36 Stress fracture, tibia and fibula
    ● M84.361 Stress fracture, right tibia
    ● M84.362 Stress fracture, left tibia
    ● M84.363 Stress fracture, right fibula
    ● M84.364 Stress fracture, left fibula
    ● M84.369 Stress fracture, `unspecified` tibia and fibula
● M84.37 Stress fracture, ankle, foot and toes
    ● M84.371 Stress fracture, right ankle
    ● M84.372 Stress fracture, left ankle
    ● M84.373 Stress fracture, `unspecified` ankle
    ● M84.374 Stress fracture, right foot
    ● M84.375 Stress fracture, left foot
    ● M84.376 Stress fracture, `unspecified` foot
    ● M84.377 Stress fracture, right toe(s)
    ● M84.378 Stress fracture, left toe(s)
    ● M84.379 Stress fracture, `unspecified` toe(s)
X● M84.38 Stress fracture, other site
        Excludes2 stress fracture of vertebra (M48.4-)

● M84.4 Pathological fracture, not elsewhere classified
    Chronic fracture
    Pathological fracture NOS
    Excludes1 collapsed vertebra NEC (M48.5)
        pathological fracture in neoplastic disease (M84.5-)
        pathological fracture in osteoporosis (M80.-)
        pathological fracture in other disease (M84.6-)
        stress fracture (M84.3-)
        traumatic fracture (S12.-, S22.-, S32.-, S42.-, S52.-, S62.-, S72.-, S82.-, S92.-)
    Excludes2 personal history of (healed) pathological fracture (Z87.311)

The appropriate 7th character is to be added to each code from subcategory M84.4:

> A   initial encounter for fracture
> D   subsequent encounter for fracture with routine healing
> G   subsequent encounter for fracture with delayed healing
> K   subsequent encounter for fracture with nonunion
> P   subsequent encounter for fracture with malunion
> S   sequela

X● M84.40 Pathological fracture, `unspecified` site
● M84.41 Pathological fracture, shoulder
    ● M84.411 Pathological fracture, right shoulder
    ● M84.412 Pathological fracture, left shoulder
    ● M84.419 Pathological fracture, `unspecified` shoulder

● M84.42 Pathological fracture, humerus
    ● M84.421 Pathological fracture, right humerus
    ● M84.422 Pathological fracture, left humerus
    ● M84.429 Pathological fracture, `unspecified` humerus
● M84.43 Pathological fracture, ulna and radius
    ● M84.431 Pathological fracture, right ulna
    ● M84.432 Pathological fracture, left ulna
    ● M84.433 Pathological fracture, right radius
    ● M84.434 Pathological fracture, left radius
    ● M84.439 Pathological fracture, `unspecified` ulna and radius
● M84.44 Pathological fracture, hand and fingers
    ● M84.441 Pathological fracture, right hand
    ● M84.442 Pathological fracture, left hand
    ● M84.443 Pathological fracture, `unspecified` hand
    ● M84.444 Pathological fracture, right finger(s)
    ● M84.445 Pathological fracture, left finger(s)
    ● M84.446 Pathological fracture, `unspecified` finger(s)
● M84.45 Pathological fracture, femur and pelvis
    ● M84.451 Pathological fracture, right femur
    ● M84.452 Pathological fracture, left femur
    ● M84.453 Pathological fracture, `unspecified` femur
    ● M84.454 Pathological fracture, pelvis
    ● M84.459 Pathological fracture, hip, `unspecified`
● M84.46 Pathological fracture, tibia and fibula
    ● M84.461 Pathological fracture, right tibia
    ● M84.462 Pathological fracture, left tibia
    ● M84.463 Pathological fracture, right fibula
    ● M84.464 Pathological fracture, left fibula
    ● M84.469 Pathological fracture, `unspecified` tibia and fibula
● M84.47 Pathological fracture, ankle, foot and toes
    ● M84.471 Pathological fracture, right ankle
    ● M84.472 Pathological fracture, left ankle
    ● M84.473 Pathological fracture, `unspecified` ankle
    ● M84.474 Pathological fracture, right foot
    ● M84.475 Pathological fracture, left foot
    ● M84.476 Pathological fracture, `unspecified` foot
    ● M84.477 Pathological fracture, right toe(s)
    ● M84.478 Pathological fracture, left toe(s)
    ● M84.479 Pathological fracture, `unspecified` toe(s)
X● M84.48 Pathological fracture, other site

◄ New   ◄ Revised   ~~deleted~~ Deleted   Excludes 1   Excludes 2   Includes   Use additional   Code first   Code also   Unspecified
OGCR Official Guidelines   X Assign placeholder X   ● Use Additional Character(s)   ▶ Manifestation Code   **Coding Clinic**

OGCR Section I.a, Chapter 13.C.

Coding of Pathologic Fractures

7th character A is for use as long as the patient is receiving active treatment for the fracture. Examples of active treatment are: surgical treatment, emergency department encounter, evaluation and continuing treatment by the same or a different physician. While the patient may be seen by a new or different provider over the course of treatment for a pathological fracture, assignment of the 7th character is based on whether the patient is undergoing active treatment and not whether the provider is seeing the patient for the first time.3. 7th character, D is to be used for encounters after the patient has completed active treatment. The other 7th characters, listed under each subcategory in the Tabular List, are to be used for subsequent encounters for treatment of problems associated with the healing, such as malunions, nonunions, and sequelae.

Care for complications of surgical treatment for fracture repairs during the healing or recovery phase should be coded with the appropriate complication codes.

See Section I.C.19. Coding of traumatic fractures.

● **M84.5   Pathological fracture in neoplastic disease**
  Code also underlying neoplasm
  The appropriate 7th character is to be added to each code from subcategory M84.5:

A	initial encounter for fracture
D	subsequent encounter for fracture with routine healing
G	subsequent encounter for fracture with delayed healing
K	subsequent encounter for fracture with nonunion
P	subsequent encounter for fracture with malunion
S	sequela

  X ● **M84.50**   Pathological fracture in neoplastic disease, unspecified site
  ● **M84.51**   Pathological fracture in neoplastic disease, shoulder
    ● **M84.511**   Pathological fracture in neoplastic disease, right shoulder
    ● **M84.512**   Pathological fracture in neoplastic disease, left shoulder
    ● **M84.519**   Pathological fracture in neoplastic disease, unspecified shoulder
  ● **M84.52**   Pathological fracture in neoplastic disease, humerus
    ● **M84.521**   Pathological fracture in neoplastic disease, right humerus
    ● **M84.522**   Pathological fracture in neoplastic disease, left humerus
    ● **M84.529**   Pathological fracture in neoplastic disease, unspecified humerus
  ● **M84.53**   Pathological fracture in neoplastic disease, ulna and radius
    ● **M84.531**   Pathological fracture in neoplastic disease, right ulna
    ● **M84.532**   Pathological fracture in neoplastic disease, left ulna
    ● **M84.533**   Pathological fracture in neoplastic disease, right radius
    ● **M84.534**   Pathological fracture in neoplastic disease, left radius
    ● **M84.539**   Pathological fracture in neoplastic disease, unspecified ulna and radius
  ● **M84.54**   Pathological fracture in neoplastic disease, hand
    ● **M84.541**   Pathological fracture in neoplastic disease, right hand
    ● **M84.542**   Pathological fracture in neoplastic disease, left hand
    ● **M84.549**   Pathological fracture in neoplastic disease, unspecified hand

● **M84.55**   Pathological fracture in neoplastic disease, pelvis and femur
  ● **M84.550**   Pathological fracture in neoplastic disease, pelvis
  ● **M84.551**   Pathological fracture in neoplastic disease, right femur
  ● **M84.552**   Pathological fracture in neoplastic disease, left femur
  ● **M84.553**   Pathological fracture in neoplastic disease, unspecified femur
  ● **M84.559**   Pathological fracture in neoplastic disease, hip, unspecified
● **M84.56**   Pathological fracture in neoplastic disease, tibia and fibula
  ● **M84.561**   Pathological fracture in neoplastic disease, right tibia
  ● **M84.562**   Pathological fracture in neoplastic disease, left tibia
  ● **M84.563**   Pathological fracture in neoplastic disease, right fibula
  ● **M84.564**   Pathological fracture in neoplastic disease, left fibula
  ● **M84.569**   Pathological fracture in neoplastic disease, unspecified tibia and fibula
● **M84.57**   Pathological fracture in neoplastic disease, ankle and foot
  ● **M84.571**   Pathological fracture in neoplastic disease, right ankle
  ● **M84.572**   Pathological fracture in neoplastic disease, left ankle
  ● **M84.573**   Pathological fracture in neoplastic disease, unspecified ankle
  ● **M84.574**   Pathological fracture in neoplastic disease, right foot
  ● **M84.575**   Pathological fracture in neoplastic disease, left foot
  ● **M84.576**   Pathological fracture in neoplastic disease, unspecified foot
X ● **M84.58**   Pathological fracture in neoplastic disease, other specified site
    Pathological fracture in neoplastic disease, vertebrae
● **M84.6   Pathological fracture in other disease**
  Code also underlying condition
  Excludes1   pathological fracture in osteoporosis (M80.-)

  The appropriate 7th character is to be added to each code from subcategory M84.6:

A	initial encounter for fracture
D	subsequent encounter for fracture with routine healing
G	subsequent encounter for fracture with delayed healing
K	subsequent encounter for fracture with nonunion
P	subsequent encounter for fracture with malunion
S	sequela

  X ● **M84.60**   Pathological fracture in other disease, unspecified site
  ● **M84.61**   Pathological fracture in other disease, shoulder
    ● **M84.611**   Pathological fracture in other disease, right shoulder
    ● **M84.612**   Pathological fracture in other disease, left shoulder
    ● **M84.619**   Pathological fracture in other disease, unspecified shoulder

CHAPTER 13 (M00-M99)

● M84.62   Pathological fracture in other disease, humerus
- ● M84.621   Pathological fracture in other disease, right humerus
- ● M84.622   Pathological fracture in other disease, left humerus
- ● M84.629   Pathological fracture in other disease, unspecified humerus

● M84.63   Pathological fracture in other disease, ulna and radius
- ● M84.631   Pathological fracture in other disease, right ulna
- ● M84.632   Pathological fracture in other disease, left ulna
- ● M84.633   Pathological fracture in other disease, right radius
- ● M84.634   Pathological fracture in other disease, left radius
- ● M84.639   Pathological fracture in other disease, unspecified ulna and radius

● M84.64   Pathological fracture in other disease, hand
- ● M84.641   Pathological fracture in other disease, right hand
- ● M84.642   Pathological fracture in other disease, left hand
- ● M84.649   Pathological fracture in other disease, unspecified hand

● M84.65   Pathological fracture in other disease, pelvis and femur
- ● M84.650   Pathological fracture in other disease, pelvis
- ● M84.651   Pathological fracture in other disease, right femur
- ● M84.652   Pathological fracture in other disease, left femur
- ● M84.653   Pathological fracture in other disease, unspecified femur
- ● M84.659   Pathological fracture in other disease, hip, unspecified

● M84.66   Pathological fracture in other disease, tibia and fibula
- ● M84.661   Pathological fracture in other disease, right tibia
- ● M84.662   Pathological fracture in other disease, left tibia
- ● M84.663   Pathological fracture in other disease, right fibula
- ● M84.664   Pathological fracture in other disease, left fibula
- ● M84.669   Pathological fracture in other disease, unspecified tibia and fibula

● M84.67   Pathological fracture in other disease, ankle and foot
- ● M84.671   Pathological fracture in other disease, right ankle
- ● M84.672   Pathological fracture in other disease, left ankle
- ● M84.673   Pathological fracture in other disease, unspecified ankle
- ● M84.674   Pathological fracture in other disease, right foot
- ● M84.675   Pathological fracture in other disease, left foot
- ● M84.676   Pathological fracture in other disease, unspecified foot

X ● M84.68   Pathological fracture in other disease, other site

● M84.8   Other disorders of continuity of bone
    M84.80   Other disorders of continuity of bone, unspecified site
● M84.81   Other disorders of continuity of bone, shoulder
- M84.811   Other disorders of continuity of bone, right shoulder
- M84.812   Other disorders of continuity of bone, left shoulder
- M84.819   Other disorders of continuity of bone, unspecified shoulder

● M84.82   Other disorders of continuity of bone, humerus
- M84.821   Other disorders of continuity of bone, right humerus
- M84.822   Other disorders of continuity of bone, left humerus
- M84.829   Other disorders of continuity of bone, unspecified humerus

● M84.83   Other disorders of continuity of bone, ulna and radius
- M84.831   Other disorders of continuity of bone, right ulna
- M84.832   Other disorders of continuity of bone, left ulna
- M84.833   Other disorders of continuity of bone, right radius
- M84.834   Other disorders of continuity of bone, left radius
- M84.839   Other disorders of continuity of bone, unspecified ulna and radius

● M84.84   Other disorders of continuity of bone, hand
- M84.841   Other disorders of continuity of bone, right hand
- M84.842   Other disorders of continuity of bone, left hand
- M84.849   Other disorders of continuity of bone, unspecified hand

● M84.85   Other disorders of continuity of bone, pelvic region and thigh
- M84.851   Other disorders of continuity of bone, right pelvic region and thigh
- M84.852   Other disorders of continuity of bone, left pelvic region and thigh
- M84.859   Other disorders of continuity of bone, unspecified pelvic region and thigh

● M84.86   Other disorders of continuity of bone, tibia and fibula
- M84.861   Other disorders of continuity of bone, right tibia
- M84.862   Other disorders of continuity of bone, left tibia
- M84.863   Other disorders of continuity of bone, right fibula
- M84.864   Other disorders of continuity of bone, left fibula
- M84.869   Other disorders of continuity of bone, unspecified tibia and fibula

● M84.87   Other disorders of continuity of bone, ankle and foot
- M84.871   Other disorders of continuity of bone, right ankle and foot
- M84.872   Other disorders of continuity of bone, left ankle and foot
- M84.879   Other disorders of continuity of bone, unspecified ankle and foot

    M84.88   Other disorders of continuity of bone, other site

M84.9   Disorder of continuity of bone, unspecified

◀ New   ◀ Revised   ~~deleted~~ Deleted   Excludes 1   Excludes 2   Includes   Use additional   Code first   Code also   Unspecified
OGCR Official Guidelines   X Assign placeholder X   ● Use Additional Character(s)   ▶ Manifestation Code   **Coding Clinic**

● **M85 Other disorders of bone density and structure**

> **Excludes1**   osteogenesis imperfecta (Q78.0)
> osteopetrosis (Q78.2)
> osteopoikilosis (Q78.8)
> polyostotic fibrous dysplasia (Q78.1)

● **M85.0 Fibrous dysplasia (monostotic)**

> **Excludes2**   fibrous dysplasia of jaw (M27.8)

     M85.00   Fibrous dysplasia (monostotic), unspecified site

●   M85.01   Fibrous dysplasia (monostotic), shoulder

         M85.011   Fibrous dysplasia (monostotic), right shoulder

         M85.012   Fibrous dysplasia (monostotic), left shoulder

         M85.019   Fibrous dysplasia (monostotic), unspecified shoulder

●   M85.02   Fibrous dysplasia (monostotic), upper arm

         M85.021   Fibrous dysplasia (monostotic), right upper arm

         M85.022   Fibrous dysplasia (monostotic), left upper arm

         M85.029   Fibrous dysplasia (monostotic), unspecified upper arm

●   M85.03   Fibrous dysplasia (monostotic), forearm

         M85.031   Fibrous dysplasia (monostotic), right forearm

         M85.032   Fibrous dysplasia (monostotic), left forearm

         M85.039   Fibrous dysplasia (monostotic), unspecified forearm

●   M85.04   Fibrous dysplasia (monostotic), hand

         M85.041   Fibrous dysplasia (monostotic), right hand

         M85.042   Fibrous dysplasia (monostotic), left hand

         M85.049   Fibrous dysplasia (monostotic), unspecified hand

●   M85.05   Fibrous dysplasia (monostotic), thigh

         M85.051   Fibrous dysplasia (monostotic), right thigh

         M85.052   Fibrous dysplasia (monostotic), left thigh

         M85.059   Fibrous dysplasia (monostotic), unspecified thigh

●   M85.06   Fibrous dysplasia (monostotic), lower leg

         M85.061   Fibrous dysplasia (monostotic), right lower leg

         M85.062   Fibrous dysplasia (monostotic), left lower leg

         M85.069   Fibrous dysplasia (monostotic), unspecified lower leg

●   M85.07   Fibrous dysplasia (monostotic), ankle and foot

         M85.071   Fibrous dysplasia (monostotic), right ankle and foot

         M85.072   Fibrous dysplasia (monostotic), left ankle and foot

         M85.079   Fibrous dysplasia (monostotic), unspecified ankle and foot

     M85.08   Fibrous dysplasia (monostotic), other site

     M85.09   Fibrous dysplasia (monostotic), multiple sites

● **M85.1 Skeletal fluorosis**

     M85.10   Skeletal fluorosis, unspecified site

●   M85.11   Skeletal fluorosis, shoulder

         M85.111   Skeletal fluorosis, right shoulder

         M85.112   Skeletal fluorosis, left shoulder

         M85.119   Skeletal fluorosis, unspecified shoulder

●   M85.12   Skeletal fluorosis, upper arm

         M85.121   Skeletal fluorosis, right upper arm

         M85.122   Skeletal fluorosis, left upper arm

         M85.129   Skeletal fluorosis, unspecified upper arm

●   M85.13   Skeletal fluorosis, forearm

         M85.131   Skeletal fluorosis, right forearm

         M85.132   Skeletal fluorosis, left forearm

         M85.139   Skeletal fluorosis, unspecified forearm

●   M85.14   Skeletal fluorosis, hand

         M85.141   Skeletal fluorosis, right hand

         M85.142   Skeletal fluorosis, left hand

         M85.149   Skeletal fluorosis, unspecified hand

●   M85.15   Skeletal fluorosis, thigh

         M85.151   Skeletal fluorosis, right thigh

         M85.152   Skeletal fluorosis, left thigh

         M85.159   Skeletal fluorosis, unspecified thigh

●   M85.16   Skeletal fluorosis, lower leg

         M85.161   Skeletal fluorosis, right lower leg

         M85.162   Skeletal fluorosis, left lower leg

         M85.169   Skeletal fluorosis, unspecified lower leg

●   M85.17   Skeletal fluorosis, ankle and foot

         M85.171   Skeletal fluorosis, right ankle and foot

         M85.172   Skeletal fluorosis, left ankle and foot

         M85.179   Skeletal fluorosis, unspecified ankle and foot

     M85.18   Skeletal fluorosis, other site

     M85.19   Skeletal fluorosis, multiple sites

   M85.2   Hyperostosis of skull

● **M85.3 Osteitis condensans**

     M85.30   Osteitis condensans, unspecified site

●   M85.31   Osteitis condensans, shoulder

         M85.311   Osteitis condensans, right shoulder

         M85.312   Osteitis condensans, left shoulder

         M85.319   Osteitis condensans, unspecified shoulder

●   M85.32   Osteitis condensans, upper arm

         M85.321   Osteitis condensans, right upper arm

         M85.322   Osteitis condensans, left upper arm

         M85.329   Osteitis condensans, unspecified upper arm

●   M85.33   Osteitis condensans, forearm

         M85.331   Osteitis condensans, right forearm

         M85.332   Osteitis condensans, left forearm

         M85.339   Osteitis condensans, unspecified forearm

●   M85.34   Osteitis condensans, hand

         M85.341   Osteitis condensans, right hand

         M85.342   Osteitis condensans, left hand

         M85.349   Osteitis condensans, unspecified hand

●   M85.35   Osteitis condensans, thigh

         M85.351   Osteitis condensans, right thigh

         M85.352   Osteitis condensans, left thigh

         M85.359   Osteitis condensans, unspecified thigh

●   M85.36   Osteitis condensans, lower leg

         M85.361   Osteitis condensans, right lower leg

         M85.362   Osteitis condensans, left lower leg

         M85.369   Osteitis condensans, unspecified lower leg

CHAPTER 13 (M00-M99)

- M85.37 Osteitis condensans, ankle and foot
  - M85.371 Osteitis condensans, right ankle and foot
  - M85.372 Osteitis condensans, left ankle and foot
  - M85.379 Osteitis condensans, unspecified ankle and foot
  - M85.38 Osteitis condensans, other site
  - M85.39 Osteitis condensans, multiple sites
- M85.4 Solitary bone cyst
  - Excludes2   solitary cyst of jaw (M27.4)
  - M85.40 Solitary bone cyst, unspecified site
- M85.41 Solitary bone cyst, shoulder
  - M85.411 Solitary bone cyst, right shoulder
  - M85.412 Solitary bone cyst, left shoulder
  - M85.419 Solitary bone cyst, unspecified shoulder
- M85.42 Solitary bone cyst, humerus
  - M85.421 Solitary bone cyst, right humerus
  - M85.422 Solitary bone cyst, left humerus
  - M85.429 Solitary bone cyst, unspecified humerus
- M85.43 Solitary bone cyst, ulna and radius
  - M85.431 Solitary bone cyst, right ulna and radius
  - M85.432 Solitary bone cyst, left ulna and radius
  - M85.439 Solitary bone cyst, unspecified ulna and radius
- M85.44 Solitary bone cyst, hand
  - M85.441 Solitary bone cyst, right hand
  - M85.442 Solitary bone cyst, left hand
  - M85.449 Solitary bone cyst, unspecified hand
- M85.45 Solitary bone cyst, pelvis
  - M85.451 Solitary bone cyst, right pelvis
  - M85.452 Solitary bone cyst, left pelvis
  - M85.459 Solitary bone cyst, unspecified pelvis
- M85.46 Solitary bone cyst, tibia and fibula
  - M85.461 Solitary bone cyst, right tibia and fibula
  - M85.462 Solitary bone cyst, left tibia and fibula
  - M85.469 Solitary bone cyst, unspecified tibia and fibula
- M85.47 Solitary bone cyst, ankle and foot
  - M85.471 Solitary bone cyst, right ankle and foot
  - M85.472 Solitary bone cyst, left ankle and foot
  - M85.479 Solitary bone cyst, unspecified ankle and foot
  - M85.48 Solitary bone cyst, other site
- M85.5 Aneurysmal bone cyst
  - Excludes2   aneurysmal cyst of jaw (M27.4)
  - M85.50 Aneurysmal bone cyst, unspecified site
- M85.51 Aneurysmal bone cyst, shoulder
  - M85.511 Aneurysmal bone cyst, right shoulder
  - M85.512 Aneurysmal bone cyst, left shoulder
  - M85.519 Aneurysmal bone cyst, unspecified shoulder
- M85.52 Aneurysmal bone cyst, upper arm
  - M85.521 Aneurysmal bone cyst, right upper arm
  - M85.522 Aneurysmal bone cyst, left upper arm
  - M85.529 Aneurysmal bone cyst, unspecified upper arm

- M85.53 Aneurysmal bone cyst, forearm
  - M85.531 Aneurysmal bone cyst, right forearm
  - M85.532 Aneurysmal bone cyst, left forearm
  - M85.539 Aneurysmal bone cyst, unspecified forearm
- M85.54 Aneurysmal bone cyst, hand
  - M85.541 Aneurysmal bone cyst, right hand
  - M85.542 Aneurysmal bone cyst, left hand
  - M85.549 Aneurysmal bone cyst, unspecified hand
- M85.55 Aneurysmal bone cyst, thigh
  - M85.551 Aneurysmal bone cyst, right thigh
  - M85.552 Aneurysmal bone cyst, left thigh
  - M85.559 Aneurysmal bone cyst, unspecified thigh
- M85.56 Aneurysmal bone cyst, lower leg
  - M85.561 Aneurysmal bone cyst, right lower leg
  - M85.562 Aneurysmal bone cyst, left lower leg
  - M85.569 Aneurysmal bone cyst, unspecified lower leg
- M85.57 Aneurysmal bone cyst, ankle and foot
  - M85.571 Aneurysmal bone cyst, right ankle and foot
  - M85.572 Aneurysmal bone cyst, left ankle and foot
  - M85.579 Aneurysmal bone cyst, unspecified ankle and foot
  - M85.58 Aneurysmal bone cyst, other site
  - M85.59 Aneurysmal bone cyst, multiple sites
- M85.6 Other cyst of bone
  - Excludes1   cyst of jaw NEC (M27.4)
  - osteitis fibrosa cystica generalisata [von Recklinghausen's disease of bone] (E21.0)
  - M85.60 Other cyst of bone, unspecified site
- M85.61 Other cyst of bone, shoulder
  - M85.611 Other cyst of bone, right shoulder
  - M85.612 Other cyst of bone, left shoulder
  - M85.619 Other cyst of bone, unspecified shoulder
- M85.62 Other cyst of bone, upper arm
  - M85.621 Other cyst of bone, right upper arm
  - M85.622 Other cyst of bone, left upper arm
  - M85.629 Other cyst of bone, unspecified upper arm
- M85.63 Other cyst of bone, forearm
  - M85.631 Other cyst of bone, right forearm
  - M85.632 Other cyst of bone, left forearm
  - M85.639 Other cyst of bone, unspecified forearm
- M85.64 Other cyst of bone, hand
  - M85.641 Other cyst of bone, right hand
  - M85.642 Other cyst of bone, left hand
  - M85.649 Other cyst of bone, unspecified hand
- M85.65 Other cyst of bone, thigh
  - M85.651 Other cyst of bone, right thigh
  - M85.652 Other cyst of bone, left thigh
  - M85.659 Other cyst of bone, unspecified thigh
- M85.66 Other cyst of bone, lower leg
  - M85.661 Other cyst of bone, right lower leg
  - M85.662 Other cyst of bone, left lower leg
  - M85.669 Other cyst of bone, unspecified lower leg

CHAPTER 13 (M00-M99)

◀ New   ◀▥ Revised   ~~deleted~~ Deleted   Excludes 1   Excludes 2   Includes   Use additional   Code first   Code also   Unspecified

OGCR Official Guidelines   X Assign placeholder X   ● Use Additional Character(s)   ▶ Manifestation Code   **Coding Clinic**

● **M85.67**   Other cyst of bone, ankle and foot

     M85.671   Other cyst of bone, right ankle and foot

     M85.672   Other cyst of bone, left ankle and foot

     M85.679   Other cyst of bone, unspecified ankle and foot

   M85.68   Other cyst of bone, other site

   M85.69   Other cyst of bone, multiple sites

● **M85.8**   Other specified disorders of bone density and structure

     Hyperostosis of bones, except skull

     Osteosclerosis, acquired

     Excludes1   diffuse idiopathic skeletal hyperostosis [DISH] (M48.1)

                 osteosclerosis congenita (Q77.4)

                 osteosclerosis fragilitas (generalista) (Q78.2)

                 osteosclerosis myelofibrosis (D75.81)

   M85.80   Other specified disorders of bone density and structure, unspecified site

● **M85.81**   Other specified disorders of bone density and structure, shoulder

     M85.811   Other specified disorders of bone density and structure, right shoulder

     M85.812   Other specified disorders of bone density and structure, left shoulder

     M85.819   Other specified disorders of bone density and structure, unspecified shoulder

● **M85.82**   Other specified disorders of bone density and structure, upper arm

     M85.821   Other specified disorders of bone density and structure, right upper arm

     M85.822   Other specified disorders of bone density and structure, left upper arm

     M85.829   Other specified disorders of bone density and structure, unspecified upper arm

● **M85.83**   Other specified disorders of bone density and structure, forearm

     M85.831   Other specified disorders of bone density and structure, right forearm

     M85.832   Other specified disorders of bone density and structure, left forearm

     M85.839   Other specified disorders of bone density and structure, unspecified forearm

● **M85.84**   Other specified disorders of bone density and structure, hand

     M85.841   Other specified disorders of bone density and structure, right hand

     M85.842   Other specified disorders of bone density and structure, left hand

     M85.849   Other specified disorders of bone density and structure, unspecified hand

● **M85.85**   Other specified disorders of bone density and structure, thigh

     M85.851   Other specified disorders of bone density and structure, right thigh

     M85.852   Other specified disorders of bone density and structure, left thigh

     M85.859   Other specified disorders of bone density and structure, unspecified thigh

● **M85.86**   Other specified disorders of bone density and structure, lower leg

     M85.861   Other specified disorders of bone density and structure, right lower leg

     M85.862   Other specified disorders of bone density and structure, left lower leg

     M85.869   Other specified disorders of bone density and structure, unspecified lower leg

● **M85.87**   Other specified disorders of bone density and structure, ankle and foot

     M85.871   Other specified disorders of bone density and structure, right ankle and foot

     M85.872   Other specified disorders of bone density and structure, left ankle and foot

     M85.879   Other specified disorders of bone density and structure, unspecified ankle and foot

   M85.88   Other specified disorders of bone density and structure, other site

   M85.89   Other specified disorders of bone density and structure, multiple sites

   M85.9   Disorder of bone density and structure, unspecified

OTHER OSTEOPATHIES (M86-M90)

   Excludes1   postprocedural osteopathies (M96.-)

● **M86**   Osteomyelitis

     Use additional code (B95-B97) to identify infectious agent

     Use additional code to identify major osseous defect, if applicable (M89.7-)

     Excludes1   osteomyelitis due to:

                 echinococcus (B67.2)

                 gonococcus (A54.43)

                 salmonella (A02.24)

     Excludes2   ostemyelitis of:

                 orbit (H05.0-)

                 petrous bone (H70.2-)

                 vertebra (M46.2-)

● **M86.0**   Acute hematogenous osteomyelitis

   M86.00   Acute hematogenous osteomyelitis, unspecified site

● **M86.01**   Acute hematogenous osteomyelitis, shoulder

     M86.011   Acute hematogenous osteomyelitis, right shoulder

     M86.012   Acute hematogenous osteomyelitis, left shoulder

     M86.019   Acute hematogenous osteomyelitis, unspecified shoulder

● **M86.02**   Acute hematogenous osteomyelitis, humerus

     M86.021   Acute hematogenous osteomyelitis, right humerus

     M86.022   Acute hematogenous osteomyelitis, left humerus

     M86.029   Acute hematogenous osteomyelitis, unspecified humerus

● **M86.03**   Acute hematogenous osteomyelitis, radius and ulna

     M86.031   Acute hematogenous osteomyelitis, right radius and ulna

     M86.032   Acute hematogenous osteomyelitis, left radius and ulna

     M86.039   Acute hematogenous osteomyelitis, unspecified radius and ulna

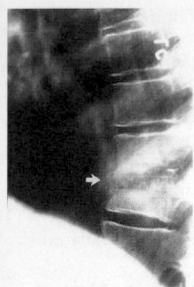

Figure 13-5 Osteomyelitis of the spine. A lateral view of the lower thoracic spine demonstrates destruction of the disk space *(arrow)* as well as destruction of the adjoining vertebral bodies. (From Mettler: Essentials of Radiology, ed 2, Saunders, An Imprint of Elsevier, 2005)

Item 13–12 Osteomyelitis is an inflammation of the bone. **Acute osteomyelitis** is a rapidly destructive, pus-producing infection capable of causing severe bone destruction. **Chronic osteomyelitis** can remain long after the initial acute episode has passed and may lead to a recurrence of the acute phase. **Brodie's abscess** is an encapsulated focal abscess that must be surgically drained. Periostitis is an inflammation of the periosteum, a dense membrane composed of fibrous connective tissue that closely wraps all bone, except those with articulating surfaces in joints, which are covered by synovial membranes.

● M86.04 Acute hematogenous osteomyelitis, hand
    M86.041 Acute hematogenous osteomyelitis, right hand
    M86.042 Acute hematogenous osteomyelitis, left hand
    M86.049 Acute hematogenous osteomyelitis, unspecified hand
● M86.05 Acute hematogenous osteomyelitis, femur
    M86.051 Acute hematogenous osteomyelitis, right femur
    M86.052 Acute hematogenous osteomyelitis, left femur
    M86.059 Acute hematogenous osteomyelitis, unspecified femur
● M86.06 Acute hematogenous osteomyelitis, tibia and fibula
    M86.061 Acute hematogenous osteomyelitis, right tibia and fibula
    M86.062 Acute hematogenous osteomyelitis, left tibia and fibula
    M86.069 Acute hematogenous osteomyelitis, unspecified tibia and fibula
● M86.07 Acute hematogenous osteomyelitis, ankle and foot
    M86.071 Acute hematogenous osteomyelitis, right ankle and foot
    M86.072 Acute hematogenous osteomyelitis, left ankle and foot
    M86.079 Acute hematogenous osteomyelitis, unspecified ankle and foot
    M86.08 Acute hematogenous osteomyelitis, other sites
    M86.09 Acute hematogenous osteomyelitis, multiple sites
● M86.1 Other acute osteomyelitis
    M86.10 Other acute osteomyelitis, unspecified site
● M86.11 Other acute osteomyelitis, shoulder
    M86.111 Other acute osteomyelitis, right shoulder
    M86.112 Other acute osteomyelitis, left shoulder
    M86.119 Other acute osteomyelitis, unspecified shoulder

● M86.12 Other acute osteomyelitis, humerus
    M86.121 Other acute osteomyelitis, right humerus
    M86.122 Other acute osteomyelitis, left humerus
    M86.129 Other acute osteomyelitis, unspecified humerus
● M86.13 Other acute osteomyelitis, radius and ulna
    M86.131 Other acute osteomyelitis, right radius and ulna
    M86.132 Other acute osteomyelitis, left radius and ulna
    M86.139 Other acute osteomyelitis, unspecified radius and ulna
● M86.14 Other acute osteomyelitis, hand
    M86.141 Other acute osteomyelitis, right hand
    M86.142 Other acute osteomyelitis, left hand
    M86.149 Other acute osteomyelitis, unspecified hand
● M86.15 Other acute osteomyelitis, femur
    M86.151 Other acute osteomyelitis, right femur
    M86.152 Other acute osteomyelitis, left femur
    M86.159 Other acute osteomyelitis, unspecified femur
● M86.16 Other acute osteomyelitis, tibia and fibula
    M86.161 Other acute osteomyelitis, right tibia and fibula
    M86.162 Other acute osteomyelitis, left tibia and fibula
    M86.169 Other acute osteomyelitis, unspecified tibia and fibula
● M86.17 Other acute osteomyelitis, ankle and foot
    M86.171 Other acute osteomyelitis, right ankle and foot
    M86.172 Other acute osteomyelitis, left ankle and foot
    M86.179 Other acute osteomyelitis, unspecified ankle and foot
    M86.18 Other acute osteomyelitis, other site
    M86.19 Other acute osteomyelitis, multiple sites
● M86.2 Subacute osteomyelitis
    M86.20 Subacute osteomyelitis, unspecified site
● M86.21 Subacute osteomyelitis, shoulder
    M86.211 Subacute osteomyelitis, right shoulder
    M86.212 Subacute osteomyelitis, left shoulder
    M86.219 Subacute osteomyelitis, unspecified shoulder
● M86.22 Subacute osteomyelitis, humerus
    M86.221 Subacute osteomyelitis, right humerus
    M86.222 Subacute osteomyelitis, left humerus
    M86.229 Subacute osteomyelitis, unspecified humerus
● M86.23 Subacute osteomyelitis, radius and ulna
    M86.231 Subacute osteomyelitis, right radius and ulna
    M86.232 Subacute osteomyelitis, left radius and ulna
    M86.239 Subacute osteomyelitis, unspecified radius and ulna
● M86.24 Subacute osteomyelitis, hand
    M86.241 Subacute osteomyelitis, right hand
    M86.242 Subacute osteomyelitis, left hand
    M86.249 Subacute osteomyelitis, unspecified hand

◀ New   ◀ Revised   ~~deleted~~ Deleted   Excludes 1   Excludes 2   Includes   Use additional   Code first   Code also   Unspecified
OGCR Official Guidelines   **X** Assign placeholder X   ● Use Additional Character(s)   ▶ Manifestation Code   **Coding Clinic**

● M86.25   Subacute osteomyelitis, femur

     M86.251   Subacute osteomyelitis, right femur

     M86.252   Subacute osteomyelitis, left femur

     M86.259   Subacute osteomyelitis, unspecified femur

● M86.26   Subacute osteomyelitis, tibia and fibula

     M86.261   Subacute osteomyelitis, right tibia and fibula

     M86.262   Subacute osteomyelitis, left tibia and fibula

     M86.269   Subacute osteomyelitis, unspecified tibia and fibula

● M86.27   Subacute osteomyelitis, ankle and foot

     M86.271   Subacute osteomyelitis, right ankle and foot

     M86.272   Subacute osteomyelitis, left ankle and foot

     M86.279   Subacute osteomyelitis, unspecified ankle and foot

   M86.28   Subacute osteomyelitis, other site

   M86.29   Subacute osteomyelitis, multiple sites

● M86.3   Chronic multifocal osteomyelitis

   M86.30   Chronic multifocal osteomyelitis, unspecified site

● M86.31   Chronic multifocal osteomyelitis, shoulder

     M86.311   Chronic multifocal osteomyelitis, right shoulder

     M86.312   Chronic multifocal osteomyelitis, left shoulder

     M86.319   Chronic multifocal osteomyelitis, unspecified shoulder

● M86.32   Chronic multifocal osteomyelitis, humerus

     M86.321   Chronic multifocal osteomyelitis, right humerus

     M86.322   Chronic multifocal osteomyelitis, left humerus

     M86.329   Chronic multifocal osteomyelitis, unspecified humerus

● M86.33   Chronic multifocal osteomyelitis, radius and ulna

     M86.331   Chronic multifocal osteomyelitis, right radius and ulna

     M86.332   Chronic multifocal osteomyelitis, left radius and ulna

     M86.339   Chronic multifocal osteomyelitis, unspecified radius and ulna

● M86.34   Chronic multifocal osteomyelitis, hand

     M86.341   Chronic multifocal osteomyelitis, right hand

     M86.342   Chronic multifocal osteomyelitis, left hand

     M86.349   Chronic multifocal osteomyelitis, unspecified hand

● M86.35   Chronic multifocal osteomyelitis, femur

     M86.351   Chronic multifocal osteomyelitis, right femur

     M86.352   Chronic multifocal osteomyelitis, left femur

     M86.359   Chronic multifocal osteomyelitis, unspecified femur

● M86.36   Chronic multifocal osteomyelitis, tibia and fibula

     M86.361   Chronic multifocal osteomyelitis, right tibia and fibula

     M86.362   Chronic multifocal osteomyelitis, left tibia and fibula

     M86.369   Chronic multifocal osteomyelitis, unspecified tibia and fibula

● M86.37   Chronic multifocal osteomyelitis, ankle and foot

     M86.371   Chronic multifocal osteomyelitis, right ankle and foot

     M86.372   Chronic multifocal osteomyelitis, left ankle and foot

     M86.379   Chronic multifocal osteomyelitis, unspecified ankle and foot

   M86.38   Chronic multifocal osteomyelitis, other site

   M86.39   Chronic multifocal osteomyelitis, multiple sites

● M86.4   Chronic osteomyelitis with draining sinus

   M86.40   Chronic osteomyelitis with draining sinus, unspecified site

● M86.41   Chronic osteomyelitis with draining sinus, shoulder

     M86.411   Chronic osteomyelitis with draining sinus, right shoulder

     M86.412   Chronic osteomyelitis with draining sinus, left shoulder

     M86.419   Chronic osteomyelitis with draining sinus, unspecified shoulder

● M86.42   Chronic osteomyelitis with draining sinus, humerus

     M86.421   Chronic osteomyelitis with draining sinus, right humerus

     M86.422   Chronic osteomyelitis with draining sinus, left humerus

     M86.429   Chronic osteomyelitis with draining sinus, unspecified humerus

● M86.43   Chronic osteomyelitis with draining sinus, radius and ulna

     M86.431   Chronic osteomyelitis with draining sinus, right radius and ulna

     M86.432   Chronic osteomyelitis with draining sinus, left radius and ulna

     M86.439   Chronic osteomyelitis with draining sinus, unspecified radius and ulna

● M86.44   Chronic osteomyelitis with draining sinus, hand

     M86.441   Chronic osteomyelitis with draining sinus, right hand

     M86.442   Chronic osteomyelitis with draining sinus, left hand

     M86.449   Chronic osteomyelitis with draining sinus, unspecified hand

● M86.45   Chronic osteomyelitis with draining sinus, femur

     M86.451   Chronic osteomyelitis with draining sinus, right femur

     M86.452   Chronic osteomyelitis with draining sinus, left femur

     M86.459   Chronic osteomyelitis with draining sinus, unspecified femur

● M86.46   Chronic osteomyelitis with draining sinus, tibia and fibula

     M86.461   Chronic osteomyelitis with draining sinus, right tibia and fibula

     M86.462   Chronic osteomyelitis with draining sinus, left tibia and fibula

     M86.469   Chronic osteomyelitis with draining sinus, unspecified tibia and fibula

● M86.47   Chronic osteomyelitis with draining sinus, ankle and foot

     M86.471   Chronic osteomyelitis with draining sinus, right ankle and foot

     M86.472   Chronic osteomyelitis with draining sinus, left ankle and foot

     M86.479   Chronic osteomyelitis with draining sinus, unspecified ankle and foot

CHAPTER 13 (M00-M99)

M86.48   Chronic osteomyelitis with draining sinus, other site

M86.49   Chronic osteomyelitis with draining sinus, multiple sites

● M86.5   Other chronic hematogenous osteomyelitis

    M86.50   Other chronic hematogenous osteomyelitis, unspecified site

● M86.51   Other chronic hematogenous osteomyelitis, shoulder

    M86.511   Other chronic hematogenous osteomyelitis, right shoulder

    M86.512   Other chronic hematogenous osteomyelitis, left shoulder

    M86.519   Other chronic hematogenous osteomyelitis, unspecified shoulder

● M86.52   Other chronic hematogenous osteomyelitis, humerus

    M86.521   Other chronic hematogenous osteomyelitis, right humerus

    M86.522   Other chronic hematogenous osteomyelitis, left humerus

    M86.529   Other chronic hematogenous osteomyelitis, unspecified humerus

● M86.53   Other chronic hematogenous osteomyelitis, radius and ulna

    M86.531   Other chronic hematogenous osteomyelitis, right radius and ulna

    M86.532   Other chronic hematogenous osteomyelitis, left radius and ulna

    M86.539   Other chronic hematogenous osteomyelitis, unspecified radius and ulna

● M86.54   Other chronic hematogenous osteomyelitis, hand

    M86.541   Other chronic hematogenous osteomyelitis, right hand

    M86.542   Other chronic hematogenous osteomyelitis, left hand

    M86.549   Other chronic hematogenous osteomyelitis, unspecified hand

● M86.55   Other chronic hematogenous osteomyelitis, femur

    M86.551   Other chronic hematogenous osteomyelitis, right femur

    M86.552   Other chronic hematogenous osteomyelitis, left femur

    M86.559   Other chronic hematogenous osteomyelitis, unspecified femur

● M86.56   Other chronic hematogenous osteomyelitis, tibia and fibula

    M86.561   Other chronic hematogenous osteomyelitis, right tibia and fibula

    M86.562   Other chronic hematogenous osteomyelitis, left tibia and fibula

    M86.569   Other chronic hematogenous osteomyelitis, unspecified tibia and fibula

● M86.57   Other chronic hematogenous osteomyelitis, ankle and foot

    M86.571   Other chronic hematogenous osteomyelitis, right ankle and foot

    M86.572   Other chronic hematogenous osteomyelitis, left ankle and foot

    M86.579   Other chronic hematogenous osteomyelitis, unspecified ankle and foot

M86.58   Other chronic hematogenous osteomyelitis, other site

M86.59   Other chronic hematogenous osteomyelitis, multiple sites

● M86.6   Other chronic osteomyelitis

    M86.60   Other chronic osteomyelitis, unspecified site

● M86.61   Other chronic osteomyelitis, shoulder

    M86.611   Other chronic osteomyelitis, right shoulder

    M86.612   Other chronic osteomyelitis, left shoulder

    M86.619   Other chronic osteomyelitis, unspecified shoulder

● M86.62   Other chronic osteomyelitis, humerus

    M86.621   Other chronic osteomyelitis, right humerus

    M86.622   Other chronic osteomyelitis, left humerus

    M86.629   Other chronic osteomyelitis, unspecified humerus

● M86.63   Other chronic osteomyelitis, radius and ulna

    M86.631   Other chronic osteomyelitis, right radius and ulna

    M86.632   Other chronic osteomyelitis, left radius and ulna

    M86.639   Other chronic osteomyelitis, unspecified radius and ulna

● M86.64   Other chronic osteomyelitis, hand

    M86.641   Other chronic osteomyelitis, right hand

    M86.642   Other chronic osteomyelitis, left hand

    M86.649   Other chronic osteomyelitis, unspecified hand

● M86.65   Other chronic osteomyelitis, thigh

    M86.651   Other chronic osteomyelitis, right thigh

    M86.652   Other chronic osteomyelitis, left thigh

    M86.659   Other chronic osteomyelitis, unspecified thigh

● M86.66   Other chronic osteomyelitis, tibia and fibula

    M86.661   Other chronic osteomyelitis, right tibia and fibula

    M86.662   Other chronic osteomyelitis, left tibia and fibula

    M86.669   Other chronic osteomyelitis, unspecified tibia and fibula

● M86.67   Other chronic osteomyelitis, ankle and foot

    M86.671   Other chronic osteomyelitis, right ankle and foot

    M86.672   Other chronic osteomyelitis, left ankle and foot

    M86.679   Other chronic osteomyelitis, unspecified ankle and foot

    M86.68   Other chronic osteomyelitis, other site

    M86.69   Other chronic osteomyelitis, multiple sites

● M86.8   Other osteomyelitis

    Brodie's abscess

● M86.8X   Other osteomyelitis

    M86.8X0   Other osteomyelitis, multiple sites

    M86.8X1   Other osteomyelitis, shoulder

    M86.8X2   Other osteomyelitis, upper arm

    M86.8X3   Other osteomyelitis, forearm

    M86.8X4   Other osteomyelitis, hand

    M86.8X5   Other osteomyelitis, thigh

    M86.8X6   Other osteomyelitis, lower leg

    M86.8X7   Other osteomyelitis, ankle and foot

    M86.8X8   Other osteomyelitis, other site

    M86.8X9   Other osteomyelitis, unspecified sites

M86.9   Osteomyelitis, unspecified

    Infection of bone NOS

    Periostitis without osteomyelitis

● M87 **Osteonecrosis**

> **Includes**   avascular necrosis of bone
>
> Use additional code to identify major osseous defect, if applicable (M89.7-)
>
> **Excludes1**   juvenile osteonecrosis (M91-M92)
>   osteochondropathies (M90-M93)

● M87.0 **Idiopathic aseptic necrosis of bone**

M87.00   Idiopathic aseptic necrosis of unspecified bone

● M87.01 **Idiopathic aseptic necrosis of shoulder**
> Idiopathic aseptic necrosis of clavicle and scapula

M87.011   Idiopathic aseptic necrosis of right shoulder

M87.012   Idiopathic aseptic necrosis of left shoulder

M87.019   Idiopathic aseptic necrosis of unspecified shoulder

● M87.02 **Idiopathic aseptic necrosis of humerus**

M87.021   Idiopathic aseptic necrosis of right humerus

M87.022   Idiopathic aseptic necrosis of left humerus

M87.029   Idiopathic aseptic necrosis of unspecified humerus

● M87.03 **Idiopathic aseptic necrosis of radius, ulna and carpus**

M87.031   Idiopathic aseptic necrosis of right radius

M87.032   Idiopathic aseptic necrosis of left radius

M87.033   Idiopathic aseptic necrosis of unspecified radius

M87.034   Idiopathic aseptic necrosis of right ulna

M87.035   Idiopathic aseptic necrosis of left ulna

M87.036   Idiopathic aseptic necrosis of unspecified ulna

M87.037   Idiopathic aseptic necrosis of right carpus

M87.038   Idiopathic aseptic necrosis of left carpus

M87.039   Idiopathic aseptic necrosis of unspecified carpus

● M87.04 **Idiopathic aseptic necrosis of hand and fingers**
> Idiopathic aseptic necrosis of metacarpals and phalanges of hands

M87.041   Idiopathic aseptic necrosis of right hand

M87.042   Idiopathic aseptic necrosis of left hand

M87.043   Idiopathic aseptic necrosis of unspecified hand

M87.044   Idiopathic aseptic necrosis of right finger(s)

M87.045   Idiopathic aseptic necrosis of left finger(s)

M87.046   Idiopathic aseptic necrosis of unspecified finger(s)

● M87.05 **Idiopathic aseptic necrosis of pelvis and femur**

M87.050   Idiopathic aseptic necrosis of pelvis

M87.051   Idiopathic aseptic necrosis of right femur

M87.052   Idiopathic aseptic necrosis of left femur

M87.059   Idiopathic aseptic necrosis of unspecified femur
> Idiopathic aseptic necrosis of hip NOS

● M87.06 **Idiopathic aseptic necrosis of tibia and fibula**

M87.061   Idiopathic aseptic necrosis of right tibia

M87.062   Idiopathic aseptic necrosis of left tibia

M87.063   Idiopathic aseptic necrosis of unspecified tibia

M87.064   Idiopathic aseptic necrosis of right fibula

M87.065   Idiopathic aseptic necrosis of left fibula

M87.066   Idiopathic aseptic necrosis of unspecified fibula

● M87.07 **Idiopathic aseptic necrosis of ankle, foot and toes**
> Idiopathic aseptic necrosis of metatarsus, tarsus, and phalanges of toes

M87.071   Idiopathic aseptic necrosis of right ankle

M87.072   Idiopathic aseptic necrosis of left ankle

M87.073   Idiopathic aseptic necrosis of unspecified ankle

M87.074   Idiopathic aseptic necrosis of right foot

M87.075   Idiopathic aseptic necrosis of left foot

M87.076   Idiopathic aseptic necrosis of unspecified foot

M87.077   Idiopathic aseptic necrosis of right toe(s)

M87.078   Idiopathic aseptic necrosis of left toe(s)

M87.079   Idiopathic aseptic necrosis of unspecified toe(s)

M87.08   Idiopathic aseptic necrosis of bone, other site

M87.09   Idiopathic aseptic necrosis of bone, multiple sites

● M87.1 **Osteonecrosis due to drugs**

> Use additional code for adverse effect, if applicable, to identify drug (T36-T50 with fifth or sixth character 5)

M87.10   Osteonecrosis due to drugs, unspecified bone

● M87.11 **Osteonecrosis due to drugs, shoulder**

M87.111   Osteonecrosis due to drugs, right shoulder

M87.112   Osteonecrosis due to drugs, left shoulder

M87.119   Osteonecrosis due to drugs, unspecified shoulder

● M87.12 **Osteonecrosis due to drugs, humerus**

M87.121   Osteonecrosis due to drugs, right humerus

M87.122   Osteonecrosis due to drugs, left humerus

M87.129   Osteonecrosis due to drugs, unspecified humerus

● M87.13 **Osteonecrosis due to drugs of radius, ulna and carpus**

M87.131   Osteonecrosis due to drugs of right radius

M87.132   Osteonecrosis due to drugs of left radius

M87.133   Osteonecrosis due to drugs of unspecified radius

M87.134   Osteonecrosis due to drugs of right ulna

M87.135   Osteonecrosis due to drugs of left ulna

    M87.136   Osteonecrosis due to drugs of ==unspecified== ulna

    M87.137   Osteonecrosis due to drugs of right carpus

    M87.138   Osteonecrosis due to drugs of left carpus

    M87.139   Osteonecrosis due to drugs of ==unspecified== carpus

● **M87.14**   Osteonecrosis due to drugs, hand and fingers

    M87.141   Osteonecrosis due to drugs, right hand

    M87.142   Osteonecrosis due to drugs, left hand

    M87.143   Osteonecrosis due to drugs, ==unspecified== hand

    M87.144   Osteonecrosis due to drugs, right finger(s)

    M87.145   Osteonecrosis due to drugs, left finger(s)

    M87.146   Osteonecrosis due to drugs, ==unspecified== finger(s)

● **M87.15**   Osteonecrosis due to drugs, pelvis and femur

    M87.150   Osteonecrosis due to drugs, pelvis

    M87.151   Osteonecrosis due to drugs, right femur

    M87.152   Osteonecrosis due to drugs, left femur

    M87.159   Osteonecrosis due to drugs, ==unspecified== femur

● **M87.16**   Osteonecrosis due to drugs, tibia and fibula

    M87.161   Osteonecrosis due to drugs, right tibia

    M87.162   Osteonecrosis due to drugs, left tibia

    M87.163   Osteonecrosis due to drugs, ==unspecified== tibia

    M87.164   Osteonecrosis due to drugs, right fibula

    M87.165   Osteonecrosis due to drugs, left fibula

    M87.166   Osteonecrosis due to drugs, ==unspecified== fibula

● **M87.17**   Osteonecrosis due to drugs, ankle, foot and toes

    M87.171   Osteonecrosis due to drugs, right ankle

    M87.172   Osteonecrosis due to drugs, left ankle

    M87.173   Osteonecrosis due to drugs, ==unspecified== ankle

    M87.174   Osteonecrosis due to drugs, right foot

    M87.175   Osteonecrosis due to drugs, left foot

    M87.176   Osteonecrosis due to drugs, ==unspecified== foot

    M87.177   Osteonecrosis due to drugs, right toe(s)

    M87.178   Osteonecrosis due to drugs, left toe(s)

    M87.179   Osteonecrosis due to drugs, ==unspecified== toe(s)

● **M87.18**   Osteonecrosis due to drugs, other site

    M87.180   Osteonecrosis due to drugs, jaw

    M87.188   Osteonecrosis due to drugs, other site

    M87.19   Osteonecrosis due to drugs, multiple sites

● **M87.2**   Osteonecrosis due to previous trauma

    M87.20   Osteonecrosis due to previous trauma, ==unspecified== bone

● **M87.21**   Osteonecrosis due to previous trauma, shoulder

    M87.211   Osteonecrosis due to previous trauma, right shoulder

    M87.212   Osteonecrosis due to previous trauma, left shoulder

    M87.219   Osteonecrosis due to previous trauma, ==unspecified== shoulder

● **M87.22**   Osteonecrosis due to previous trauma, humerus

    M87.221   Osteonecrosis due to previous trauma, right humerus

    M87.222   Osteonecrosis due to previous trauma, left humerus

    M87.229   Osteonecrosis due to previous trauma, ==unspecified== humerus

● **M87.23**   Osteonecrosis due to previous trauma of radius, ulna and carpus

    M87.231   Osteonecrosis due to previous trauma of right radius

    M87.232   Osteonecrosis due to previous trauma of left radius

    M87.233   Osteonecrosis due to previous trauma of ==unspecified== radius

    M87.234   Osteonecrosis due to previous trauma of right ulna

    M87.235   Osteonecrosis due to previous trauma of left ulna

    M87.236   Osteonecrosis due to previous trauma of ==unspecified== ulna

    M87.237   Osteonecrosis due to previous trauma of right carpus

    M87.238   Osteonecrosis due to previous trauma of left carpus

    M87.239   Osteonecrosis due to previous trauma of ==unspecified== carpus

● **M87.24**   Osteonecrosis due to previous trauma, hand and fingers

    M87.241   Osteonecrosis due to previous trauma, right hand

    M87.242   Osteonecrosis due to previous trauma, left hand

    M87.243   Osteonecrosis due to previous trauma, ==unspecified== hand

    M87.244   Osteonecrosis due to previous trauma, right finger(s)

    M87.245   Osteonecrosis due to previous trauma, left finger(s)

    M87.246   Osteonecrosis due to previous trauma, ==unspecified== finger(s)

● **M87.25**   Osteonecrosis due to previous trauma, pelvis and femur

    M87.250   Osteonecrosis due to previous trauma, pelvis

    M87.251   Osteonecrosis due to previous trauma, right femur

    M87.252   Osteonecrosis due to previous trauma, left femur

    M87.256   Osteonecrosis due to previous trauma, ==unspecified== femur

● **M87.26**   Osteonecrosis due to previous trauma, tibia and fibula

    M87.261   Osteonecrosis due to previous trauma, right tibia

    M87.262   Osteonecrosis due to previous trauma, left tibia

    M87.263   Osteonecrosis due to previous trauma, ==unspecified== tibia

    M87.264   Osteonecrosis due to previous trauma, right fibula

    M87.265   Osteonecrosis due to previous trauma, left fibula

    M87.266   Osteonecrosis due to previous trauma, ==unspecified== fibula

---

◄ New   ◄⁞⁞ Revised   ~~deleted~~ Deleted   Excludes 1   Excludes 2   Includes   Use additional   Code first   Code also   Unspecified

OGCR Official Guidelines   X Assign placeholder X   ● Use Additional Character(s)   ▶ Manifestation Code   **Coding Clinic**

● M87.27 Osteonecrosis due to previous trauma, ankle, foot and toes

    M87.271 Osteonecrosis due to previous trauma, right ankle

    M87.272 Osteonecrosis due to previous trauma, left ankle

    M87.273 Osteonecrosis due to previous trauma, unspecified ankle

    M87.274 Osteonecrosis due to previous trauma, right foot

    M87.275 Osteonecrosis due to previous trauma, left foot

    M87.276 Osteonecrosis due to previous trauma, unspecified foot

    M87.277 Osteonecrosis due to previous trauma, right toe(s)

    M87.278 Osteonecrosis due to previous trauma, left toe(s)

    M87.279 Osteonecrosis due to previous trauma, unspecified toe(s)

M87.28 Osteonecrosis due to previous trauma, other site

M87.29 Osteonecrosis due to previous trauma, multiple sites

● M87.3 Other secondary osteonecrosis

M87.30 Other secondary osteonecrosis, unspecified bone

● M87.31 Other secondary osteonecrosis, shoulder

    M87.311 Other secondary osteonecrosis, right shoulder

    M87.312 Other secondary osteonecrosis, left shoulder

    M87.319 Other secondary osteonecrosis, unspecified shoulder

● M87.32 Other secondary osteonecrosis, humerus

    M87.321 Other secondary osteonecrosis, right humerus

    M87.322 Other secondary osteonecrosis, left humerus

    M87.329 Other secondary osteonecrosis, unspecified humerus

● M87.33 Other secondary osteonecrosis of radius, ulna and carpus

    M87.331 Other secondary osteonecrosis of right radius

    M87.332 Other secondary osteonecrosis of left radius

    M87.333 Other secondary osteonecrosis of unspecified radius

    M87.334 Other secondary osteonecrosis of right ulna

    M87.335 Other secondary osteonecrosis of left ulna

    M87.336 Other secondary osteonecrosis of unspecified ulna

    M87.337 Other secondary osteonecrosis of right carpus

    M87.338 Other secondary osteonecrosis of left carpus

    M87.339 Other secondary osteonecrosis of unspecified carpus

● M87.34 Other secondary osteonecrosis, hand and fingers

    M87.341 Other secondary osteonecrosis, right hand

    M87.342 Other secondary osteonecrosis, left hand

    M87.343 Other secondary osteonecrosis, unspecified hand

    M87.344 Other secondary osteonecrosis, right finger(s)

    M87.345 Other secondary osteonecrosis, left finger(s)

    M87.346 Other secondary osteonecrosis, unspecified finger(s)

● M87.35 Other secondary osteonecrosis, pelvis and femur

    M87.350 Other secondary osteonecrosis, pelvis

    M87.351 Other secondary osteonecrosis, right femur

    M87.352 Other secondary osteonecrosis, left femur

    M87.353 Other secondary osteonecrosis, unspecified femur

● M87.36 Other secondary osteonecrosis, tibia and fibula

    M87.361 Other secondary osteonecrosis, right tibia

    M87.362 Other secondary osteonecrosis, left tibia

    M87.363 Other secondary osteonecrosis, unspecified tibia

    M87.364 Other secondary osteonecrosis, right fibula

    M87.365 Other secondary osteonecrosis, left fibula

    M87.366 Other secondary osteonecrosis, unspecified fibula

● M87.37 Other secondary osteonecrosis, ankle and foot

    M87.371 Other secondary osteonecrosis, right ankle

    M87.372 Other secondary osteonecrosis, left ankle

    M87.373 Other secondary osteonecrosis, unspecified ankle

    M87.374 Other secondary osteonecrosis, right foot

    M87.375 Other secondary osteonecrosis, left foot

    M87.376 Other secondary osteonecrosis, unspecified foot

    M87.377 Other secondary osteonecrosis, right toe(s)

    M87.378 Other secondary osteonecrosis, left toe(s)

    M87.379 Other secondary osteonecrosis, unspecified toe(s)

M87.38 Other secondary osteonecrosis, other site

M87.39 Other secondary osteonecrosis, multiple sites

● M87.8 Other osteonecrosis

M87.80 Other osteonecrosis, unspecified bone

● M87.81 Other osteonecrosis, shoulder

    M87.811 Other osteonecrosis, right shoulder

    M87.812 Other osteonecrosis, left shoulder

    M87.819 Other osteonecrosis, unspecified shoulder

● M87.82   Other osteonecrosis, humerus
    M87.821   Other osteonecrosis, right humerus
    M87.822   Other osteonecrosis, left humerus
    M87.829   Other osteonecrosis, unspecified humerus

● M87.83   Other osteonecrosis of radius, ulna and carpus
    M87.831   Other osteonecrosis of right radius
    M87.832   Other osteonecrosis of left radius
    M87.833   Other osteonecrosis of unspecified radius
    M87.834   Other osteonecrosis of right ulna
    M87.835   Other osteonecrosis of left ulna
    M87.836   Other osteonecrosis of unspecified ulna
    M87.837   Other osteonecrosis of right carpus
    M87.838   Other osteonecrosis of left carpus
    M87.839   Other osteonecrosis of unspecified carpus

● M87.84   Other osteonecrosis, hand and fingers
    M87.841   Other osteonecrosis, right hand
    M87.842   Other osteonecrosis, left hand
    M87.843   Other osteonecrosis, unspecified hand
    M87.844   Other osteonecrosis, right finger(s)
    M87.845   Other osteonecrosis, left finger(s)
    M87.849   Other osteonecrosis, unspecified finger(s)

● M87.85   Other osteonecrosis, pelvis and femur
    M87.850   Other osteonecrosis, pelvis
    M87.851   Other osteonecrosis, right femur
    M87.852   Other osteonecrosis, left femur
    M87.859   Other osteonecrosis, unspecified femur

● M87.86   Other osteonecrosis, tibia and fibula
    M87.861   Other osteonecrosis, right tibia
    M87.862   Other osteonecrosis, left tibia
    M87.863   Other osteonecrosis, unspecified tibia
    M87.864   Other osteonecrosis, right fibula
    M87.865   Other osteonecrosis, left fibula
    M87.869   Other osteonecrosis, unspecified fibula

● M87.87   Other osteonecrosis, ankle, foot and toes
    M87.871   Other osteonecrosis, right ankle
    M87.872   Other osteonecrosis, left ankle
    M87.873   Other osteonecrosis, unspecified ankle
    M87.874   Other osteonecrosis, right foot
    M87.875   Other osteonecrosis, left foot
    M87.876   Other osteonecrosis, unspecified foot
    M87.877   Other osteonecrosis, right toe(s)
    M87.878   Other osteonecrosis, left toe(s)
    M87.879   Other osteonecrosis, unspecified toe(s)

   M87.88   Other osteonecrosis, other site
   M87.89   Other osteonecrosis, multiple sites

M87.9   Osteonecrosis, unspecified
    Necrosis of bone NOS

● M88   Osteitis deformans [Paget's disease of bone]
Chronic disorder that results in enlarged and deformed bones. The excessive breakdown and formation of bone tissue causes bones to weaken and results in bone pain, arthritis, deformities, and fractures.

    Excludes1   osteitis deformans in neoplastic disease (M90.6)

M88.0   Osteitis deformans of skull
M88.1   Osteitis deformans of vertebrae

● M88.8   Osteitis deformans of other bones
   ● M88.81   Osteitis deformans of shoulder
     M88.811   Osteitis deformans of right shoulder
     M88.812   Osteitis deformans of left shoulder
     M88.819   Osteitis deformans of unspecified shoulder

   ● M88.82   Osteitis deformans of upper arm
     M88.821   Osteitis deformans of right upper arm
     M88.822   Osteitis deformans of left upper arm
     M88.829   Osteitis deformans of unspecified upper arm

   ● M88.83   Osteitis deformans of forearm
     M88.831   Osteitis deformans of right forearm
     M88.832   Osteitis deformans of left forearm
     M88.839   Osteitis deformans of unspecified forearm

   ● M88.84   Osteitis deformans of hand
     M88.841   Osteitis deformans of right hand
     M88.842   Osteitis deformans of left hand
     M88.849   Osteitis deformans of unspecified hand

   ● M88.85   Osteitis deformans of thigh
     M88.851   Osteitis deformans of right thigh
     M88.852   Osteitis deformans of left thigh
     M88.859   Osteitis deformans of unspecified thigh

   ● M88.86   Osteitis deformans of lower leg
     M88.861   Osteitis deformans of right lower leg
     M88.862   Osteitis deformans of left lower leg
     M88.869   Osteitis deformans of unspecified lower leg

   ● M88.87   Osteitis deformans of ankle and foot
     M88.871   Osteitis deformans of right ankle and foot
     M88.872   Osteitis deformans of left ankle and foot
     M88.879   Osteitis deformans of unspecified ankle and foot

   M88.88   Osteitis deformans of other bones
     Excludes2   osteitis deformans of skull (M88.0)
                osteitis deformans of vertebrae (M88.1)

   M88.89   Osteitis deformans of multiple sites
M88.9   Osteitis deformans of unspecified bone

◀ New   ◀▬ Revised   ~~deleted~~ Deleted   Excludes 1   Excludes 2   Includes   Use additional   Code first   Code also   Unspecified
OGCR Official Guidelines   **X** Assign placeholder X   ● Use Additional Character(s)   ▶ Manifestation Code   **Coding Clinic**

● M89 **Other disorders of bone**
  ● M89.0 **Algoneurodystrophy**
    Shoulder-hand syndrome
    Sudeck's atrophy
    Excludes1   causalgia, lower limb (G57.7-)
            causalgia, upper limb (G56.4-)
            complex regional pain syndrome II, lower
              limb (G57.7-)
            complex regional pain syndrome II,
              upper limb (G56.4-)
            reflex sympathetic dystrophy (G90.5-)
    M89.00   Algoneurodystrophy, unspecified site
   ● M89.01   Algoneurodystrophy, shoulder
      M89.011   Algoneurodystrophy, right shoulder
      M89.012   Algoneurodystrophy, left shoulder
      M89.019   Algoneurodystrophy, unspecified
             shoulder
   ● M89.02   Algoneurodystrophy, upper arm
      M89.021   Algoneurodystrophy, right upper arm
      M89.022   Algoneurodystrophy, left upper arm
      M89.029   Algoneurodystrophy, unspecified
             upper arm
   ● M89.03   Algoneurodystrophy, forearm
      M89.031   Algoneurodystrophy, right forearm
      M89.032   Algoneurodystrophy, left forearm
      M89.039   Algoneurodystrophy, unspecified
             forearm
   ● M89.04   Algoneurodystrophy, hand
      M89.041   Algoneurodystrophy, right hand
      M89.042   Algoneurodystrophy, left hand
      M89.049   Algoneurodystrophy, unspecified
             hand
   ● M89.05   Algoneurodystrophy, thigh
      M89.051   Algoneurodystrophy, right thigh
      M89.052   Algoneurodystrophy, left thigh
      M89.059   Algoneurodystrophy, unspecified
             thigh
   ● M89.06   Algoneurodystrophy, lower leg
      M89.061   Algoneurodystrophy, right lower leg
      M89.062   Algoneurodystrophy, left lower leg
      M89.069   Algoneurodystrophy, unspecified
             lower leg
   ● M89.07   Algoneurodystrophy, ankle and foot
      M89.071   Algoneurodystrophy, right ankle and
             foot
      M89.072   Algoneurodystrophy, left ankle and
             foot
      M89.079   Algoneurodystrophy, unspecified
             ankle and foot
    M89.08   Algoneurodystrophy, other site
    M89.09   Algoneurodystrophy, multiple sites
  ● M89.1 **Physeal arrest**
    Arrest of growth plate
    Epiphyseal arrest
    Growth plate arrest
   ● M89.12   Physeal arrest, humerus
      M89.121   Complete physeal arrest, right
             proximal humerus
      M89.122   Complete physeal arrest, left proximal
             humerus
      M89.123   Partial physeal arrest, right proximal
             humerus
      M89.124   Partial physeal arrest, left proximal
             humerus
      M89.125   Complete physeal arrest, right distal
             humerus

      M89.126   Complete physeal arrest, left distal
             humerus
      M89.127   Partial physeal arrest, right distal
             humerus
      M89.128   Partial physeal arrest, left distal
             humerus
      M89.129   Physeal arrest, humerus, unspecified
   ● M89.13   Physeal arrest, forearm
      M89.131   Complete physeal arrest, right distal
             radius
      M89.132   Complete physeal arrest, left distal
             radius
      M89.133   Partial physeal arrest, right distal
             radius
      M89.134   Partial physeal arrest, left distal
             radius
      M89.138   Other physeal arrest of forearm
      M89.139   Physeal arrest, forearm, unspecified
   ● M89.15   Physeal arrest, femur
      M89.151   Complete physeal arrest, right
             proximal femur
      M89.152   Complete physeal arrest, left proximal
             femur
      M89.153   Partial physeal arrest, right proximal
             femur
      M89.154   Partial physeal arrest, left proximal
             femur
      M89.155   Complete physeal arrest, right distal
             femur
      M89.156   Complete physeal arrest, left distal
             femur
      M89.157   Partial physeal arrest, right distal
             femur
      M89.158   Partial physeal arrest, left distal
             femur
      M89.159   Physeal arrest, femur, unspecified
   ● M89.16   Physeal arrest, lower leg
      M89.160   Complete physeal arrest, right
             proximal tibia
      M89.161   Complete physeal arrest, left proximal
             tibia
      M89.162   Partial physeal arrest, right proximal
             tibia
      M89.163   Partial physeal arrest, left proximal
             tibia
      M89.164   Complete physeal arrest, right distal
             tibia
      M89.165   Complete physeal arrest, left distal
             tibia
      M89.166   Partial physeal arrest, right distal
             tibia
      M89.167   Partial physeal arrest, left distal tibia
      M89.168   Other physeal arrest of lower leg
      M89.169   Physeal arrest, lower leg, unspecified
    M89.18   Physeal arrest, other site
  ● M89.2 **Other disorders of bone development and growth**
    M89.20   Other disorders of bone development and
          growth, unspecified site
   ● M89.21   Other disorders of bone development and
          growth, shoulder
      M89.211   Other disorders of bone development
             and growth, right shoulder
      M89.212   Other disorders of bone development
             and growth, left shoulder
      M89.219   Other disorders of bone development
             and growth, unspecified shoulder

CHAPTER 13 (M00-M99)

● **M89.22**   Other disorders of bone development and growth, humerus
    M89.221   Other disorders of bone development and growth, right humerus
    M89.222   Other disorders of bone development and growth, left humerus
    M89.229   Other disorders of bone development and growth, unspecified humerus

● **M89.23**   Other disorders of bone development and growth, ulna and radius
    M89.231   Other disorders of bone development and growth, right ulna
    M89.232   Other disorders of bone development and growth, left ulna
    M89.233   Other disorders of bone development and growth, right radius
    M89.234   Other disorders of bone development and growth, left radius
    M89.239   Other disorders of bone development and growth, unspecified ulna and radius

● **M89.24**   Other disorders of bone development and growth, hand
    M89.241   Other disorders of bone development and growth, right hand
    M89.242   Other disorders of bone development and growth, left hand
    M89.249   Other disorders of bone development and growth, unspecified hand

● **M89.25**   Other disorders of bone development and growth, femur
    M89.251   Other disorders of bone development and growth, right femur
    M89.252   Other disorders of bone development and growth, left femur
    M89.259   Other disorders of bone development and growth, unspecified femur

● **M89.26**   Other disorders of bone development and growth, tibia and fibula
    M89.261   Other disorders of bone development and growth, right tibia
    M89.262   Other disorders of bone development and growth, left tibia
    M89.263   Other disorders of bone development and growth, right fibula
    M89.264   Other disorders of bone development and growth, left fibula
    M89.269   Other disorders of bone development and growth, unspecified lower leg

● **M89.27**   Other disorders of bone development and growth, ankle and foot
    M89.271   Other disorders of bone development and growth, right ankle and foot
    M89.272   Other disorders of bone development and growth, left ankle and foot
    M89.279   Other disorders of bone development and growth, unspecified ankle and foot

   M89.28   Other disorders of bone development and growth, other site
   M89.29   Other disorders of bone development and growth, multiple sites

● **M89.3**   Hypertrophy of bone
   M89.30   Hypertrophy of bone, unspecified site

● **M89.31**   Hypertrophy of bone, shoulder
    M89.311   Hypertrophy of bone, right shoulder
    M89.312   Hypertrophy of bone, left shoulder
    M89.319   Hypertrophy of bone, unspecified shoulder

● **M89.32**   Hypertrophy of bone, humerus
    M89.321   Hypertrophy of bone, right humerus
    M89.322   Hypertrophy of bone, left humerus
    M89.329   Hypertrophy of bone, unspecified humerus

● **M89.33**   Hypertrophy of bone, ulna and radius
    M89.331   Hypertrophy of bone, right ulna
    M89.332   Hypertrophy of bone, left ulna
    M89.333   Hypertrophy of bone, right radius
    M89.334   Hypertrophy of bone, left radius
    M89.339   Hypertrophy of bone, unspecified ulna and radius

● **M89.34**   Hypertrophy of bone, hand
    M89.341   Hypertrophy of bone, right hand
    M89.342   Hypertrophy of bone, left hand
    M89.349   Hypertrophy of bone, unspecified hand

● **M89.35**   Hypertrophy of bone, femur
    M89.351   Hypertrophy of bone, right femur
    M89.352   Hypertrophy of bone, left femur
    M89.359   Hypertrophy of bone, unspecified femur

● **M89.36**   Hypertrophy of bone, tibia and fibula
    M89.361   Hypertrophy of bone, right tibia
    M89.362   Hypertrophy of bone, left tibia
    M89.363   Hypertrophy of bone, right fibula
    M89.364   Hypertrophy of bone, left fibula
    M89.369   Hypertrophy of bone, unspecified tibia and fibula

● **M89.37**   Hypertrophy of bone, ankle and foot
    M89.371   Hypertrophy of bone, right ankle and foot
    M89.372   Hypertrophy of bone, left ankle and foot
    M89.379   Hypertrophy of bone, unspecified ankle and foot

   M89.38   Hypertrophy of bone, other site
   M89.39   Hypertrophy of bone, multiple sites

● **M89.4**   Other hypertrophic osteoarthropathy
    Marie-Bamberger disease
    Pachydermoperiostosis
   M89.40   Other hypertrophic osteoarthropathy, unspecified site

● **M89.41**   Other hypertrophic osteoarthropathy, shoulder
    M89.411   Other hypertrophic osteoarthropathy, right shoulder
    M89.412   Other hypertrophic osteoarthropathy, left shoulder
    M89.419   Other hypertrophic osteoarthropathy, unspecified shoulder

● **M89.42**   Other hypertrophic osteoarthropathy, upper arm
    M89.421   Other hypertrophic osteoarthropathy, right upper arm
    M89.422   Other hypertrophic osteoarthropathy, left upper arm
    M89.429   Other hypertrophic osteoarthropathy, unspecified upper arm

● **M89.43**   Other hypertrophic osteoarthropathy, forearm
    M89.431   Other hypertrophic osteoarthropathy, right forearm
    M89.432   Other hypertrophic osteoarthropathy, left forearm
    M89.439   Other hypertrophic osteoarthropathy, unspecified forearm

◀ New   ◀▥ Revised   ~~deleted~~ Deleted   Excludes 1   Excludes 2   Includes   Use additional   Code first   Code also   Unspecified

1132   OGCR Official Guidelines   X Assign placeholder X   ● Use Additional Character(s)   ▶ Manifestation Code   **Coding Clinic**

● M89.44   Other hypertrophic osteoarthropathy, hand
    M89.441   Other hypertrophic osteoarthropathy, right hand
    M89.442   Other hypertrophic osteoarthropathy, left hand
    M89.449   Other hypertrophic osteoarthropathy, unspecified hand

● M89.45   Other hypertrophic osteoarthropathy, thigh
    M89.451   Other hypertrophic osteoarthropathy, right thigh
    M89.452   Other hypertrophic osteoarthropathy, left thigh
    M89.459   Other hypertrophic osteoarthropathy, unspecified thigh

● M89.46   Other hypertrophic osteoarthropathy, lower leg
    M89.461   Other hypertrophic osteoarthropathy, right lower leg
    M89.462   Other hypertrophic osteoarthropathy, left lower leg
    M89.469   Other hypertrophic osteoarthropathy, unspecified lower leg

● M89.47   Other hypertrophic osteoarthropathy, ankle and foot
    M89.471   Other hypertrophic osteoarthropathy, right ankle and foot
    M89.472   Other hypertrophic osteoarthropathy, left ankle and foot
    M89.479   Other hypertrophic osteoarthropathy, unspecified ankle and foot

    M89.48   Other hypertrophic osteoarthropathy, other site
    M89.49   Other hypertrophic osteoarthropathy, multiple sites

● M89.5   Osteolysis

    Use additional code to identify major osseous defect, if applicable (M89.7-)

    Excludes2   periprosthetic osteolysis of internal prosthetic joint (T84.05-)

    M89.50   Osteolysis, unspecified site

● M89.51   Osteolysis, shoulder
    M89.511   Osteolysis, right shoulder
    M89.512   Osteolysis, left shoulder
    M89.519   Osteolysis, unspecified shoulder

● M89.52   Osteolysis, upper arm
    M89.521   Osteolysis, right upper arm
    M89.522   Osteolysis, left upper arm
    M89.529   Osteolysis, unspecified upper arm

● M89.53   Osteolysis, forearm
    M89.531   Osteolysis, right forearm
    M89.532   Osteolysis, left forearm
    M89.539   Osteolysis, unspecified forearm

● M89.54   Osteolysis, hand
    M89.541   Osteolysis, right hand
    M89.542   Osteolysis, left hand
    M89.549   Osteolysis, unspecified hand

● M89.55   Osteolysis, thigh
    M89.551   Osteolysis, right thigh
    M89.552   Osteolysis, left thigh
    M89.559   Osteolysis, unspecified thigh

● M89.56   Osteolysis, lower leg
    M89.561   Osteolysis, right lower leg
    M89.562   Osteolysis, left lower leg
    M89.569   Osteolysis, unspecified lower leg

● M89.57   Osteolysis, ankle and foot
    M89.571   Osteolysis, right ankle and foot
    M89.572   Osteolysis, left ankle and foot
    M89.579   Osteolysis, unspecified ankle and foot

    M89.58   Osteolysis, other site
    M89.59   Osteolysis, multiple sites

● M89.6   Osteopathy after poliomyelitis

    Use additional code (B91) to identify previous poliomyelitis

    Excludes1   postpolio syndrome (G14)

    M89.60   Osteopathy after poliomyelitis, unspecified site

● M89.61   Osteopathy after poliomyelitis, shoulder
    M89.611   Osteopathy after poliomyelitis, right shoulder
    M89.612   Osteopathy after poliomyelitis, left shoulder
    M89.619   Osteopathy after poliomyelitis, unspecified shoulder

● M89.62   Osteopathy after poliomyelitis, upper arm
    M89.621   Osteopathy after poliomyelitis, right upper arm
    M89.622   Osteopathy after poliomyelitis, left upper arm
    M89.629   Osteopathy after poliomyelitis, unspecified upper arm

● M89.63   Osteopathy after poliomyelitis, forearm
    M89.631   Osteopathy after poliomyelitis, right forearm
    M89.632   Osteopathy after poliomyelitis, left forearm
    M89.639   Osteopathy after poliomyelitis, unspecified forearm

● M89.64   Osteopathy after poliomyelitis, hand
    M89.641   Osteopathy after poliomyelitis, right hand
    M89.642   Osteopathy after poliomyelitis, left hand
    M89.649   Osteopathy after poliomyelitis, unspecified hand

● M89.65   Osteopathy after poliomyelitis, thigh
    M89.651   Osteopathy after poliomyelitis, right thigh
    M89.652   Osteopathy after poliomyelitis, left thigh
    M89.659   Osteopathy after poliomyelitis, unspecified thigh

● M89.66   Osteopathy after poliomyelitis, lower leg
    M89.661   Osteopathy after poliomyelitis, right lower leg
    M89.662   Osteopathy after poliomyelitis, left lower leg
    M89.669   Osteopathy after poliomyelitis, unspecified lower leg

● M89.67   Osteopathy after poliomyelitis, ankle and foot
    M89.671   Osteopathy after poliomyelitis, right ankle and foot
    M89.672   Osteopathy after poliomyelitis, left ankle and foot
    M89.679   Osteopathy after poliomyelitis, unspecified ankle and foot

    M89.68   Osteopathy after poliomyelitis, other site
    M89.69   Osteopathy after poliomyelitis, multiple sites

CHAPTER 13 (M00-M99)

CHAPTER 13 (M00-M99)

● **M89.7 Major osseous defect**

Code first underlying disease, if known, such as:
aseptic necrosis of bone (M87.-)
malignant neoplasm of bone (C40.-)
osteolysis (M89.5)
osteomyelitis (M86.-)
osteonecrosis (M87.-)
osteoporosis (M80.-, M81.-)
periprosthetic osteolysis (T84.05-)

M89.70   Major osseous defect, unspecified site

● M89.71   Major osseous defect, shoulder region
    Major osseous defect clavicle or scapula

    M89.711   Major osseous defect, right shoulder region

    M89.712   Major osseous defect, left shoulder region

    M89.719   Major osseous defect, unspecified shoulder region

● M89.72   Major osseous defect, humerus

    M89.721   Major osseous defect, right humerus

    M89.722   Major osseous defect, left humerus

    M89.729   Major osseous defect, unspecified humerus

● M89.73   Major osseous defect, forearm
    Major osseous defect of radius and ulna

    M89.731   Major osseous defect, right forearm

    M89.732   Major osseous defect, left forearm

    M89.739   Major osseous defect, unspecified forearm

● M89.74   Major osseous defect, hand
    Major osseous defect of carpus, fingers, metacarpus

    M89.741   Major osseous defect, right hand

    M89.742   Major osseous defect, left hand

    M89.749   Major osseous defect, unspecified hand

● M89.75   Major osseous defect, pelvic region and thigh
    Major osseous defect of femur and pelvis

    M89.751   Major osseous defect, right pelvic region and thigh

    M89.752   Major osseous defect, left pelvic region and thigh

    M89.759   Major osseous defect, unspecified pelvic region and thigh

● M89.76   Major osseous defect, lower leg
    Major osseous defect of fibula and tibia

    M89.761   Major osseous defect, right lower leg

    M89.762   Major osseous defect, left lower leg

    M89.769   Major osseous defect, unspecified lower leg

● M89.77   Major osseous defect, ankle and foot
    Major osseous defect of metatarsus, tarsus, toes

    M89.771   Major osseous defect, right ankle and foot

    M89.772   Major osseous defect, left ankle and foot

    M89.779   Major osseous defect, unspecified ankle and foot

M89.78   Major osseous defect, other site

M89.79   Major osseous defect, multiple sites

● **M89.8 Other specified disorders of bone**
Infantile cortical hyperostoses
Post-traumatic subperiosteal ossification

● M89.8X   Other specified disorders of bone

    M89.8X0   Other specified disorders of bone, multiple sites

    M89.8X1   Other specified disorders of bone, shoulder

    M89.8X2   Other specified disorders of bone, upper arm

    M89.8X3   Other specified disorders of bone, forearm

    M89.8X4   Other specified disorders of bone, hand

    M89.8X5   Other specified disorders of bone, thigh

    M89.8X6   Other specified disorders of bone, lower leg

    M89.8X7   Other specified disorders of bone, ankle and foot

    M89.8X8   Other specified disorders of bone, other site

    M89.8X9   Other specified disorders of bone, unspecified site

M89.9   Disorder of bone, unspecified

● **M90 Osteopathies in diseases classified elsewhere**

Excludes1   osteochondritis, osteomyelitis, and osteopathy (in):
cryptococcosis (B45.3)
diabetes mellitus (E08-E13 with .61-)
gonococcal (A54.43)
neurogenic syphilis (A52.11)
renal osteodystrophy (N25.0)
salmonellosis (A02.24)
secondary syphilis (A51.46)
syphilis (late) (A52.77)

● **M90.5 Osteonecrosis in diseases classified elsewhere**

Code first underlying disease, such as:
caisson disease (T70.3)
hemoglobinopathy (D50-D64)

▌ *M90.50   Osteonecrosis in diseases classified elsewhere, unspecified site*

● M90.51   Osteonecrosis in diseases classified elsewhere, shoulder

    ▌ *M90.511   Osteonecrosis in diseases classified elsewhere, right shoulder*

    ▌ *M90.512   Osteonecrosis in diseases classified elsewhere, left shoulder*

    ▌ *M90.519   Osteonecrosis in diseases classified elsewhere, unspecified shoulder*

● M90.52   Osteonecrosis in diseases classified elsewhere, upper arm

    ▌ *M90.521   Osteonecrosis in diseases classified elsewhere, right upper arm*

    ▌ *M90.522   Osteonecrosis in diseases classified elsewhere, left upper arm*

    ▌ *M90.529   Osteonecrosis in diseases classified elsewhere, unspecified upper arm*

● M90.53   Osteonecrosis in diseases classified elsewhere, forearm

    ▌ *M90.531   Osteonecrosis in diseases classified elsewhere, right forearm*

    ▌ *M90.532   Osteonecrosis in diseases classified elsewhere, left forearm*

    ▌ *M90.539   Osteonecrosis in diseases classified elsewhere, unspecified forearm*

◀ New   ◀▬ Revised   ~~deleted~~ Deleted   Excludes 1   Excludes 2   Includes   Use additional   Code first   Code also   Unspecified

OGCR Official Guidelines   X Assign placeholder X   ● Use Additional Character(s)   ▌ Manifestation Code   **Coding Clinic**

● M90.54 **Osteonecrosis in diseases classified elsewhere, hand**

▶ *M90.541* *Osteonecrosis in diseases classified elsewhere, right hand*

▶ *M90.542* *Osteonecrosis in diseases classified elsewhere, left hand*

▶ *M90.549* *Osteonecrosis in diseases classified elsewhere, unspecified hand*

● M90.55 **Osteonecrosis in diseases classified elsewhere, thigh**

▶ *M90.551* *Osteonecrosis in diseases classified elsewhere, right thigh*

▶ *M90.552* *Osteonecrosis in diseases classified elsewhere, left thigh*

▶ *M90.559* *Osteonecrosis in diseases classified elsewhere, unspecified thigh*

● M90.56 **Osteonecrosis in diseases classified elsewhere, lower leg**

▶ *M90.561* *Osteonecrosis in diseases classified elsewhere, right lower leg*

▶ *M90.562* *Osteonecrosis in diseases classified elsewhere, left lower leg*

▶ *M90.569* *Osteonecrosis in diseases classified elsewhere, unspecified lower leg*

● M90.57 **Osteonecrosis in diseases classified elsewhere, ankle and foot**

▶ *M90.571* *Osteonecrosis in diseases classified elsewhere, right ankle and foot*

▶ *M90.572* *Osteonecrosis in diseases classified elsewhere, left ankle and foot*

▶ *M90.579* *Osteonecrosis in diseases classified elsewhere, unspecified ankle and foot*

▶ *M90.58* *Osteonecrosis in diseases classified elsewhere, other site*

▶ *M90.59* *Osteonecrosis in diseases classified elsewhere, multiple sites*

● M90.6 **Osteitis deformans in neoplastic diseases**

Osteitis deformans in malignant neoplasm of bone

Code first the neoplasm (C40.-, C41.-)

Excludes1 osteitis deformans [Paget's disease of bone] (M88.-)

▶ *M90.60* *Osteitis deformans in neoplastic diseases, unspecified site*

● M90.61 **Osteitis deformans in neoplastic diseases, shoulder**

▶ *M90.611* *Osteitis deformans in neoplastic diseases, right shoulder*

▶ *M90.612* *Osteitis deformans in neoplastic diseases, left shoulder*

▶ *M90.619* *Osteitis deformans in neoplastic diseases, unspecified shoulder*

● M90.62 **Osteitis deformans in neoplastic diseases, upper arm**

▶ *M90.621* *Osteitis deformans in neoplastic diseases, right upper arm*

▶ *M90.622* *Osteitis deformans in neoplastic diseases, left upper arm*

▶ *M90.629* *Osteitis deformans in neoplastic diseases, unspecified upper arm*

● M90.63 **Osteitis deformans in neoplastic diseases, forearm**

▶ *M90.631* *Osteitis deformans in neoplastic diseases, right forearm*

▶ *M90.632* *Osteitis deformans in neoplastic diseases, left forearm*

▶ *M90.639* *Osteitis deformans in neoplastic diseases, unspecified forearm*

● M90.64 **Osteitis deformans in neoplastic diseases, hand**

▶ *M90.641* *Osteitis deformans in neoplastic diseases, right hand*

▶ *M90.642* *Osteitis deformans in neoplastic diseases, left hand*

▶ *M90.649* *Osteitis deformans in neoplastic diseases, unspecified hand*

● M90.65 **Osteitis deformans in neoplastic diseases, thigh**

▶ *M90.651* *Osteitis deformans in neoplastic diseases, right thigh*

▶ *M90.652* *Osteitis deformans in neoplastic diseases, left thigh*

▶ *M90.659* *Osteitis deformans in neoplastic diseases, unspecified thigh*

● M90.66 **Osteitis deformans in neoplastic diseases, lower leg**

▶ *M90.661* *Osteitis deformans in neoplastic diseases, right lower leg*

▶ *M90.662* *Osteitis deformans in neoplastic diseases, left lower leg*

▶ *M90.669* *Osteitis deformans in neoplastic diseases, unspecified lower leg*

● M90.67 **Osteitis deformans in neoplastic diseases, ankle and foot**

▶ *M90.671* *Osteitis deformans in neoplastic diseases, right ankle and foot*

▶ *M90.672* *Osteitis deformans in neoplastic diseases, left ankle and foot*

▶ *M90.679* *Osteitis deformans in neoplastic diseases, unspecified ankle and foot*

▶ *M90.68* *Osteitis deformans in neoplastic diseases, other site*

▶ *M90.69* *Osteitis deformans in neoplastic diseases, multiple sites*

● M90.8 **Osteopathy in diseases classified elsewhere**

Code first underlying disease, such as:
rickets (E55.0)
vitamin-D-resistant rickets (E83.3)

▶ *M90.80* *Osteopathy in diseases classified elsewhere, unspecified site*

● M90.81 **Osteopathy in diseases classified elsewhere, shoulder**

▶ *M90.811* *Osteopathy in diseases classified elsewhere, right shoulder*

▶ *M90.812* *Osteopathy in diseases classified elsewhere, left shoulder*

▶ *M90.819* *Osteopathy in diseases classified elsewhere, unspecified shoulder*

● M90.82 **Osteopathy in diseases classified elsewhere, upper arm**

▶ *M90.821* *Osteopathy in diseases classified elsewhere, right upper arm*

▶ *M90.822* *Osteopathy in diseases classified elsewhere, left upper arm*

▶ *M90.829* *Osteopathy in diseases classified elsewhere, unspecified upper arm*

● M90.83 **Osteopathy in diseases classified elsewhere, forearm**

▶ *M90.831* *Osteopathy in diseases classified elsewhere, right forearm*

▶ *M90.832* *Osteopathy in diseases classified elsewhere, left forearm*

▶ *M90.839* *Osteopathy in diseases classified elsewhere, unspecified forearm*

CHAPTER 13 (M00-M99)

● **M90.84 Osteopathy in diseases classified elsewhere, hand**

▶ *M90.841 Osteopathy in diseases classified elsewhere, right hand*

▶ *M90.842 Osteopathy in diseases classified elsewhere, left hand*

▶ *M90.849 Osteopathy in diseases classified elsewhere, unspecified hand*

● **M90.85 Osteopathy in diseases classified elsewhere, thigh**

▶ *M90.851 Osteopathy in diseases classified elsewhere, right thigh*

▶ *M90.852 Osteopathy in diseases classified elsewhere, left thigh*

▶ *M90.859 Osteopathy in diseases classified elsewhere, unspecified thigh*

● **M90.86 Osteopathy in diseases classified elsewhere, lower leg**

▶ *M90.861 Osteopathy in diseases classified elsewhere, right lower leg*

▶ *M90.862 Osteopathy in diseases classified elsewhere, left lower leg*

▶ *M90.869 Osteopathy in diseases classified elsewhere, unspecified lower leg*

● **M90.87 Osteopathy in diseases classified elsewhere, ankle and foot**

▶ *M90.871 Osteopathy in diseases classified elsewhere, right ankle and foot*

▶ *M90.872 Osteopathy in diseases classified elsewhere, left ankle and foot*

▶ *M90.879 Osteopathy in diseases classified elsewhere, unspecified ankle and foot*

▶ *M90.88 Osteopathy in diseases classified elsewhere, other site*

▶ *M90.89 Osteopathy in diseases classified elsewhere, multiple sites*

CHONDROPATHIES (M91-M94)

Excludes1 postprocedural chondropathies (M96.-)

● **M91 Juvenile osteochondrosis of hip and pelvis**

Excludes1 slipped upper femoral epiphysis (nontraumatic) (M93.0)

M91.0 Juvenile osteochondrosis of pelvis
Osteochondrosis (juvenile) of acetabulum
Osteochondrosis (juvenile) of iliac crest [Buchanan]
Osteochondrosis (juvenile) of ischiopubic synchondrosis [van Neck]
Osteochondrosis (juvenile) of symphysis pubis [Pierson]

● **M91.1 Juvenile osteochondrosis of head of femur [Legg-Calvé-Perthes]**

M91.10 Juvenile osteochondrosis of head of femur [Legg-Calvé-Perthes], unspecified leg

M91.11 Juvenile osteochondrosis of head of femur [Legg-Calvé-Perthes], right leg

M91.12 Juvenile osteochondrosis of head of femur [Legg-Calvé-Perthes], left leg

● **M91.2 Coxa plana**
Hip deformity due to previous juvenile osteochondrosis

M91.20 Coxa plana, unspecified hip

M91.21 Coxa plana, right hip

M91.22 Coxa plana, left hip

● **M91.3 Pseudocoxalgia**

M91.30 Pseudocoxalgia, unspecified hip

M91.31 Pseudocoxalgia, right hip

M91.32 Pseudocoxalgia, left hip

● **M91.4 Coxa magna**

M91.40 Coxa magna, unspecified hip

M91.41 Coxa magna, right hip

M91.42 Coxa magna, left hip

● **M91.8 Other juvenile osteochondrosis of hip and pelvis**
Juvenile osteochondrosis after reduction of congenital dislocation of hip

M91.80 Other juvenile osteochondrosis of hip and pelvis, unspecified leg

M91.81 Other juvenile osteochondrosis of hip and pelvis, right leg

M91.82 Other juvenile osteochondrosis of hip and pelvis, left leg

● **M91.9 Juvenile osteochondrosis of hip and pelvis, unspecified**

M91.90 Juvenile osteochondrosis of hip and pelvis, unspecified, unspecified leg

M91.91 Juvenile osteochondrosis of hip and pelvis, unspecified, right leg

M91.92 Juvenile osteochondrosis of hip and pelvis, unspecified, left leg

● **M92 Other juvenile osteochondrosis**

● **M92.0 Juvenile osteochondrosis of humerus**
Osteochondrosis (juvenile) of capitulum of humerus [Panner]
Osteochondrosis (juvenile) of head of humerus [Haas]

M92.00 Juvenile osteochondrosis of humerus, unspecified arm

M92.01 Juvenile osteochondrosis of humerus, right arm

M92.02 Juvenile osteochondrosis of humerus, left arm

● **M92.1 Juvenile osteochondrosis of radius and ulna**
Osteochondrosis (juvenile) of lower ulna [Burns]
Osteochondrosis (juvenile) of radial head [Brailsford]

M92.10 Juvenile osteochondrosis of radius and ulna, unspecified arm

M92.11 Juvenile osteochondrosis of radius and ulna, right arm

M92.12 Juvenile osteochondrosis of radius and ulna, left arm

● **M92.2 Juvenile osteochondrosis, hand**

● **M92.20 Unspecified juvenile osteochondrosis, hand**

M92.201 Unspecified juvenile osteochondrosis, right hand

M92.202 Unspecified juvenile osteochondrosis, left hand

M92.209 Unspecified juvenile osteochondrosis, unspecified hand

● **M92.21 Osteochondrosis (juvenile) of carpal lunate [Kienböck]**

M92.211 Osteochondrosis (juvenile) of carpal lunate [Kienböck], right hand

M92.212 Osteochondrosis (juvenile) of carpal lunate [Kienböck], left hand

M92.219 Osteochondrosis (juvenile) of carpal lunate [Kienböck], unspecified hand

● **M92.22 Osteochondrosis (juvenile) of metacarpal heads [Mauclaire]**

M92.221 Osteochondrosis (juvenile) of metacarpal heads [Mauclaire], right hand

M92.222 Osteochondrosis (juvenile) of metacarpal heads [Mauclaire], left hand

M92.229 Osteochondrosis (juvenile) of metacarpal heads [Mauclaire], unspecified hand

◀ New   ⬅ Revised   ~~deleted~~ Deleted   Excludes 1   Excludes 2   Includes   Use additional   Code first   Code also   Unspecified

1136   **OGCR** Official Guidelines   **X** Assign placeholder X   ● Use Additional Character(s)   ▶ Manifestation Code   **Coding Clinic**

● **M92.29**   Other juvenile osteochondrosis, hand

     M92.291   Other juvenile osteochondrosis, right hand

     M92.292   Other juvenile osteochondrosis, left hand

     M92.299   Other juvenile osteochondrosis, unspecified hand

● **M92.3**   Other juvenile osteochondrosis, upper limb

     M92.30   Other juvenile osteochondrosis, unspecified upper limb

     M92.31   Other juvenile osteochondrosis, right upper limb

     M92.32   Other juvenile osteochondrosis, left upper limb

● **M92.4**   Juvenile osteochondrosis of patella

     Osteochondrosis (juvenile) of primary patellar center [Köhler]

     Osteochondrosis (juvenile) of secondary patellar center [Sinding Larsen]

     M92.40   Juvenile osteochondrosis of patella, unspecified knee

     M92.41   Juvenile osteochondrosis of patella, right knee

     M92.42   Juvenile osteochondrosis of patella, left knee

● **M92.5**   Juvenile osteochondrosis of tibia and fibula

     Osteochondrosis (juvenile) of proximal tibia [Blount]

     Osteochondrosis (juvenile) of tibial tubercle [Osgood-Schlatter]

     Tibia vara

     M92.50   Juvenile osteochondrosis of tibia and fibula, unspecified leg

     M92.51   Juvenile osteochondrosis of tibia and fibula, right leg

     M92.52   Juvenile osteochondrosis of tibia and fibula, left leg

● **M92.6**   Juvenile osteochondrosis of tarsus

     Osteochondrosis (juvenile) of calcaneum [Sever]

     Osteochondrosis (juvenile) of os tibiale externum [Haglund]

     Osteochondrosis (juvenile) of talus [Diaz]

     Osteochondrosis (juvenile) of tarsal navicular [Köhler]

     M92.60   Juvenile osteochondrosis of tarsus, unspecified ankle

     M92.61   Juvenile osteochondrosis of tarsus, right ankle

     M92.62   Juvenile osteochondrosis of tarsus, left ankle

● **M92.7**   Juvenile osteochondrosis of metatarsus

     Osteochondrosis (juvenile) of fifth metatarsus [Iselin]

     Osteochondrosis (juvenile) of second metatarsus [Freiberg]

     M92.70   Juvenile osteochondrosis of metatarsus, unspecified foot

     M92.71   Juvenile osteochondrosis of metatarsus, right foot

     M92.72   Juvenile osteochondrosis of metatarsus, left foot

M92.8   Other specified juvenile osteochondrosis

     Calcaneal apophysitis

M92.9   Juvenile osteochondrosis, unspecified

     Juvenile apophysitis NOS

     Juvenile epiphysitis NOS

     Juvenile osteochondritis NOS

     Juvenile osteochondrosis NOS

● **M93**   Other osteochondropathies

     Excludes2   osteochondrosis of spine (M42.-)

● **M93.0**   Slipped upper femoral epiphysis (nontraumatic)

     Use additional code for associated chondrolysis (M94.3)

     ● **M93.00**   Unspecified slipped upper femoral epiphysis (nontraumatic)

       M93.001   Unspecified slipped upper femoral epiphysis (nontraumatic), right hip

       M93.002   Unspecified slipped upper femoral epiphysis (nontraumatic), left hip

       M93.003   Unspecified slipped upper femoral epiphysis (nontraumatic), unspecified hip

     ● **M93.01**   Acute slipped upper femoral epiphysis (nontraumatic)

       M93.011   Acute slipped upper femoral epiphysis (nontraumatic), right hip

       M93.012   Acute slipped upper femoral epiphysis (nontraumatic), left hip

       M93.013   Acute slipped upper femoral epiphysis (nontraumatic), unspecified hip

     ● **M93.02**   Chronic slipped upper femoral epiphysis (nontraumatic)

       M93.021   Chronic slipped upper femoral epiphysis (nontraumatic), right hip

       M93.022   Chronic slipped upper femoral epiphysis (nontraumatic), left hip

       M93.023   Chronic slipped upper femoral epiphysis (nontraumatic), unspecified hip

     ● **M93.03**   Acute on chronic slipped upper femoral epiphysis (nontraumatic)

       M93.031   Acute on chronic slipped upper femoral epiphysis (nontraumatic), right hip

       M93.032   Acute on chronic slipped upper femoral epiphysis (nontraumatic), left hip

       M93.033   Acute on chronic slipped upper femoral epiphysis (nontraumatic), unspecified hip

M93.1   Kienböck's disease of adults   **A**

     Adult osteochondrosis of carpal lunates

● **M93.2**   Osteochondritis dissecans

     M93.20   Osteochondritis dissecans of unspecified site

     ● **M93.21**   Osteochondritis dissecans of shoulder

       M93.211   Osteochondritis dissecans, right shoulder

       M93.212   Osteochondritis dissecans, left shoulder

       M93.219   Osteochondritis dissecans, unspecified shoulder

     ● **M93.22**   Osteochondritis dissecans of elbow

       M93.221   Osteochondritis dissecans, right elbow

       M93.222   Osteochondritis dissecans, left elbow

       M93.229   Osteochondritis dissecans, unspecified elbow

     ● **M93.23**   Osteochondritis dissecans of wrist

       M93.231   Osteochondritis dissecans, right wrist

       M93.232   Osteochondritis dissecans, left wrist

       M93.239   Osteochondritis dissecans, unspecified wrist

CHAPTER 13 (M00-M99)

● M93.24 Osteochondritis dissecans of joints of hand

   M93.241 Osteochondritis dissecans, joints of right hand

   M93.242 Osteochondritis dissecans, joints of left hand

   M93.249 Osteochondritis dissecans, joints of unspecified hand

● M93.25 Osteochondritis dissecans of hip

   M93.251 Osteochondritis dissecans, right hip

   M93.252 Osteochondritis dissecans, left hip

   M93.259 Osteochondritis dissecans, unspecified hip

● M93.26 Osteochondritis dissecans knee

   M93.261 Osteochondritis dissecans, right knee

   M93.262 Osteochondritis dissecans, left knee

   M93.269 Osteochondritis dissecans, unspecified knee

● M93.27 Osteochondritis dissecans of ankle and joints of foot

   M93.271 Osteochondritis dissecans, right ankle and joints of right foot

   M93.272 Osteochondritis dissecans, left ankle and joints of left foot

   M93.279 Osteochondritis dissecans, unspecified ankle and joints of foot

   M93.28 Osteochondritis dissecans other site

   M93.29 Osteochondritis dissecans multiple sites

● M93.8 Other specified osteochondropathies

   M93.80 Other specified osteochondropathies of unspecified site

● M93.81 Other specified osteochondropathies of shoulder

   M93.811 Other specified osteochondropathies, right shoulder

   M93.812 Other specified osteochondropathies, left shoulder

   M93.819 Other specified osteochondropathies, unspecified shoulder

● M93.82 Other specified osteochondropathies of upper arm

   M93.821 Other specified osteochondropathies, right upper arm

   M93.822 Other specified osteochondropathies, left upper arm

   M93.829 Other specified osteochondropathies, unspecified upper arm

● M93.83 Other specified osteochondropathies of forearm

   M93.831 Other specified osteochondropathies, right forearm

   M93.832 Other specified osteochondropathies, left forearm

   M93.839 Other specified osteochondropathies, unspecified forearm

● M93.84 Other specified osteochondropathies of hand

   M93.841 Other specified osteochondropathies, right hand

   M93.842 Other specified osteochondropathies, left hand

   M93.849 Other specified osteochondropathies, unspecified hand

● M93.85 Other specified osteochondropathies of thigh

   M93.851 Other specified osteochondropathies, right thigh

   M93.852 Other specified osteochondropathies, left thigh

   M93.859 Other specified osteochondropathies, unspecified thigh

● M93.86 Other specified osteochondropathies lower leg

   M93.861 Other specified osteochondropathies, right lower leg

   M93.862 Other specified osteochondropathies, left lower leg

   M93.869 Other specified osteochondropathies, unspecified lower leg

● M93.87 Other specified osteochondropathies of ankle and foot

   M93.871 Other specified osteochondropathies, right ankle and foot

   M93.872 Other specified osteochondropathies, left ankle and foot

   M93.879 Other specified osteochondropathies, unspecified ankle and foot

   M93.88 Other specified osteochondropathies other

   M93.89 Other specified osteochondropathies multiple sites

M93.9 Osteochondropathy, unspecified

   Apophysitis NOS
   Epiphysitis NOS
   Osteochondritis NOS
   Osteochondrosis NOS

   M93.90 Osteochondropathy, unspecified of unspecified site

● M93.91 Osteochondropathy, unspecified of shoulder

   M93.911 Osteochondropathy, unspecified, right shoulder

   M93.912 Osteochondropathy, unspecified, left shoulder

   M93.919 Osteochondropathy, unspecified, unspecified shoulder

● M93.92 Osteochondropathy, unspecified of upper arm

   M93.921 Osteochondropathy, unspecified, right upper arm

   M93.922 Osteochondropathy, unspecified, left upper arm

   M93.929 Osteochondropathy, unspecified, unspecified upper arm

● M93.93 Osteochondropathy, unspecified of forearm

   M93.931 Osteochondropathy, unspecified, right forearm

   M93.932 Osteochondropathy, unspecified, left forearm

   M93.939 Osteochondropathy, unspecified, unspecified forearm

● M93.94 Osteochondropathy, unspecified of hand

   M93.941 Osteochondropathy, unspecified, right hand

   M93.942 Osteochondropathy, unspecified, left hand

   M93.949 Osteochondropathy, unspecified, unspecified hand

● M93.95 Osteochondropathy, unspecified of thigh

   M93.951 Osteochondropathy, unspecified, right thigh

   M93.952 Osteochondropathy, unspecified, left thigh

   M93.959 Osteochondropathy, unspecified, unspecified thigh

● M93.96 Osteochondropathy, unspecified lower leg

   M93.961 Osteochondropathy, unspecified, right lower leg

   M93.962 Osteochondropathy, unspecified, left lower leg

   M93.969 Osteochondropathy, unspecified, unspecified lower leg

◀ New   ◀ Revised   ~~deleted~~ Deleted   Excludes 1   Excludes 2   Includes   Use additional   Code first   Code also   Unspecified

OGCR Official Guidelines   X Assign placeholder X   ● Use Additional Character(s)   ▶ Manifestation Code   **Coding Clinic**

● M93.97 Osteochondropathy, unspecified of ankle and foot

    M93.971 Osteochondropathy, unspecified, right ankle and foot

    M93.972 Osteochondropathy, unspecified, left ankle and foot

    M93.979 Osteochondropathy, unspecified, unspecified ankle and foot

  M93.98 Osteochondropathy, unspecified other

  M93.99 Osteochondropathy, unspecified multiple sites

● M94 Other disorders of cartilage

  M94.0 Chondrocostal junction syndrome [Tietze]
    Costochondritis

  M94.1 Relapsing polychondritis

● M94.2 Chondromalacia

    Excludes1 chondromalacia patellae (M22.4)

  M94.20 Chondromalacia, unspecified site

● M94.21 Chondromalacia, shoulder

    M94.211 Chondromalacia, right shoulder

    M94.212 Chondromalacia, left shoulder

    M94.219 Chondromalacia, unspecified shoulder

● M94.22 Chondromalacia, elbow

    M94.221 Chondromalacia, right elbow

    M94.222 Chondromalacia, left elbow

    M94.229 Chondromalacia, unspecified elbow

● M94.23 Chondromalacia, wrist

    M94.231 Chondromalacia, right wrist

    M94.232 Chondromalacia, left wrist

    M94.239 Chondromalacia, unspecified wrist

● M94.24 Chondromalacia, joints of hand

    M94.241 Chondromalacia, joints of right hand

    M94.242 Chondromalacia, joints of left hand

    M94.249 Chondromalacia, joints of unspecified hand

● M94.25 Chondromalacia, hip

    M94.251 Chondromalacia, right hip

    M94.252 Chondromalacia, left hip

    M94.259 Chondromalacia, unspecified hip

● M94.26 Chondromalacia, knee

    M94.261 Chondromalacia, right knee

    M94.262 Chondromalacia, left knee

    M94.269 Chondromalacia, unspecified knee

● M94.27 Chondromalacia, ankle and joints of foot

    M94.271 Chondromalacia, right ankle and joints of right foot

    M94.272 Chondromalacia, left ankle and joints of left foot

    M94.279 Chondromalacia, unspecified ankle and joints of foot

  M94.28 Chondromalacia, other site

  M94.29 Chondromalacia, multiple sites

● M94.3 Chondrolysis

    Code first any associated slipped upper femoral epiphysis (nontraumatic) (M93.0-)

● M94.35 Chondrolysis, hip

    M94.351 Chondrolysis, right hip

    M94.352 Chondrolysis, left hip

    M94.359 Chondrolysis, unspecified hip

● M94.8 Other specified disorders of cartilage

● M94.8X Other specified disorders of cartilage

    M94.8X0 Other specified disorders of cartilage, multiple sites

    M94.8X1 Other specified disorders of cartilage, shoulder

    M94.8X2 Other specified disorders of cartilage, upper arm

    M94.8X3 Other specified disorders of cartilage, forearm

    M94.8X4 Other specified disorders of cartilage, hand

    M94.8X5 Other specified disorders of cartilage, thigh

    M94.8X6 Other specified disorders of cartilage, lower leg

    M94.8X7 Other specified disorders of cartilage, ankle and foot

    M94.8X8 Other specified disorders of cartilage, other site

    M94.8X9 Other specified disorders of cartilage, unspecified sites

  M94.9 Disorder of cartilage, unspecified

OTHER DISORDERS OF THE MUSCULOSKELETAL SYSTEM AND CONNECTIVE TISSUE (M95)

● M95 Other acquired deformities of musculoskeletal system and connective tissue

    Excludes2 acquired absence of limbs and organs (Z89-Z90)
    acquired deformities of limbs (M20-M21)
    congenital malformations and deformations of the musculoskeletal system (Q65-Q79)
    deforming dorsopathies (M40-M43)
    dentofacial anomalies [including malocclusion] (M26.-)
    postprocedural musculoskeletal disorders (M96.-)

  M95.0 Acquired deformity of nose

    Excludes2 deviated nasal septum (J34.2)

● M95.1 Cauliflower ear

    Excludes2 other acquired deformities of ear (H61.1)

  M95.10 Cauliflower ear, unspecified ear

  M95.11 Cauliflower ear, right ear

  M95.12 Cauliflower ear, left ear

  M95.2 Other acquired deformity of head

  M95.3 Acquired deformity of neck

  M95.4 Acquired deformity of chest and rib

  M95.5 Acquired deformity of pelvis

    Excludes1 maternal care for known or suspected disproportion (O33.-)

  M95.8 Other specified acquired deformities of musculoskeletal system

  M95.9 Acquired deformity of musculoskeletal system, unspecified

INTRAOPERATIVE AND POSTPROCEDURAL COMPLICATIONS AND DISORDERS OF MUSCULOSKELETAL SYSTEM, NOT ELSEWHERE CLASSIFIED (M96)

● M96 Intraoperative and postprocedural complications and disorders of musculoskeletal system, not elsewhere classified

    Excludes2 arthropathy following intestinal bypass (M02.0-)
    complications of internal orthopedic prosthetic devices, implants and grafts (T84.-)
    disorders associated with osteoporosis (M80)
    presence of functional implants and other devices (Z96-Z97)

  M96.0 Pseudarthrosis after fusion or arthrodesis

  M96.1 Postlaminectomy syndrome, not elsewhere classified

CHAPTER 13 (M00-M99)

M96.2 Postradiation kyphosis

M96.3 Postlaminectomy kyphosis

M96.4 Postsurgical lordosis

M96.5 Postradiation scoliosis

● M96.6 Fracture of bone following insertion of orthopedic implant, joint prosthesis, or bone plate
Intraoperative fracture of bone during insertion of orthopedic implant, joint prosthesis, or bone plate

Excludes2 complication of internal orthopedic devices, implants or grafts (T84.-)

● M96.62 Fracture of humerus following insertion of orthopedic implant, joint prosthesis, or bone plate

M96.621 Fracture of humerus following insertion of orthopedic implant, joint prosthesis, or bone plate, right arm

M96.622 Fracture of humerus following insertion of orthopedic implant, joint prosthesis, or bone plate, left arm

M96.629 Fracture of humerus following insertion of orthopedic implant, joint prosthesis, or bone plate, unspecified arm

● M96.63 Fracture of radius or ulna following insertion of orthopedic implant, joint prosthesis, or bone plate

M96.631 Fracture of radius or ulna following insertion of orthopedic implant, joint prosthesis, or bone plate, right arm

M96.632 Fracture of radius or ulna following insertion of orthopedic implant, joint prosthesis, or bone plate, left arm

M96.639 Fracture of radius or ulna following insertion of orthopedic implant, joint prosthesis, or bone plate, unspecified arm

M96.65 Fracture of pelvis following insertion of orthopedic implant, joint prosthesis, or bone plate

● M96.66 Fracture of femur following insertion of orthopedic implant, joint prosthesis, or bone plate

M96.661 Fracture of femur following insertion of orthopedic implant, joint prosthesis, or bone plate, right leg

M96.662 Fracture of femur following insertion of orthopedic implant, joint prosthesis, or bone plate, left leg

M96.669 Fracture of femur following insertion of orthopedic implant, joint prosthesis, or bone plate, unspecified leg

● M96.67 Fracture of tibia or fibula following insertion of orthopedic implant, joint prosthesis, or bone plate

M96.671 Fracture of tibia or fibula following insertion of orthopedic implant, joint prosthesis, or bone plate, right leg

M96.672 Fracture of tibia or fibula following insertion of orthopedic implant, joint prosthesis, or bone plate, left leg

M96.679 Fracture of tibia or fibula following insertion of orthopedic implant, joint prosthesis, or bone plate, unspecified leg

M96.69 Fracture of other bone following insertion of orthopedic implant, joint prosthesis, or bone plate

● M96.8 Other intraoperative and postprocedural complications and disorders of musculoskeletal system, not elsewhere classified

● M96.81 Intraoperative hemorrhage and hematoma of a musculoskeletal structure complicating a procedure

Excludes1 intraoperative hemorrhage and hematoma of a musculoskeletal structure due to accidental puncture and laceration during a procedure (M96.82-)

M96.810 Intraoperative hemorrhage and hematoma of a musculoskeletal structure complicating a musculoskeletal system procedure

M96.811 Intraoperative hemorrhage and hematoma of a musculoskeletal structure complicating other procedure

● M96.82 Accidental puncture and laceration of a musculoskeletal structure during a procedure

M96.820 Accidental puncture and laceration of a musculoskeletal structure during a musculoskeletal system procedure

M96.821 Accidental puncture and laceration of a musculoskeletal structure during other procedure

● M96.83 Postprocedural hemorrhage and hematoma of a musculoskeletal structure following a procedure

M96.830 Postprocedural hemorrhage and hematoma of a musculoskeletal structure following a musculoskeletal system procedure

M96.831 Postprocedural hemorrhage and hematoma of a musculoskeletal structure following other procedure

M96.89 Other intraoperative and postprocedural complications and disorders of the musculoskeletal system
Instability of joint secondary to removal of joint prosthesis
Use additional code, if applicable, to further specify disorder

BIOMECHANICAL LESIONS, NOT ELSEWHERE CLASSIFIED (M99)

● M99 Biomechanical lesions, not elsewhere classified
Note: This category should not be used if the condition can be classified elsewhere.

● M99.0 Segmental and somatic dysfunction

M99.00 Segmental and somatic dysfunction of head region

M99.01 Segmental and somatic dysfunction of cervical region

M99.02 Segmental and somatic dysfunction of thoracic region

M99.03 Segmental and somatic dysfunction of lumbar region

M99.04 Segmental and somatic dysfunction of sacral region

M99.05 Segmental and somatic dysfunction of pelvic region

M99.06 Segmental and somatic dysfunction of lower extremity

M99.07 Segmental and somatic dysfunction of upper extremity

M99.08 Segmental and somatic dysfunction of rib cage

M99.09 Segmental and somatic dysfunction of abdomen and other regions

◀ New   ⬅ Revised   d̶e̶l̶e̶t̶e̶d̶ Deleted   Excludes 1   Excludes 2   Includes   Use additional   Code first   Code also   Unspecified

OGCR Official Guidelines   X Assign placeholder X   ● Use Additional Character(s)   ▶ Manifestation Code   Coding Clinic

● **M99.1**   Subluxation complex (vertebral)

   M99.10   Subluxation complex (vertebral) of head region

   M99.11   Subluxation complex (vertebral) of cervical region

   M99.12   Subluxation complex (vertebral) of thoracic region

   M99.13   Subluxation complex (vertebral) of lumbar region

   M99.14   Subluxation complex (vertebral) of sacral region

   M99.15   Subluxation complex (vertebral) of pelvic region

   M99.16   Subluxation complex (vertebral) of lower extremity

   M99.17   Subluxation complex (vertebral) of upper extremity

   M99.18   Subluxation complex (vertebral) of rib cage

   M99.19   Subluxation complex (vertebral) of abdomen and other regions

● **M99.2**   Subluxation stenosis of neural canal

   M99.20   Subluxation stenosis of neural canal of head region

   M99.21   Subluxation stenosis of neural canal of cervical region

   M99.22   Subluxation stenosis of neural canal of thoracic region

   M99.23   Subluxation stenosis of neural canal of lumbar region

   M99.24   Subluxation stenosis of neural canal of sacral region

   M99.25   Subluxation stenosis of neural canal of pelvic region

   M99.26   Subluxation stenosis of neural canal of lower extremity

   M99.27   Subluxation stenosis of neural canal of upper extremity

   M99.28   Subluxation stenosis of neural canal of rib cage

   M99.29   Subluxation stenosis of neural canal of abdomen and other regions

● **M99.3**   Osseous stenosis of neural canal

   M99.30   Osseous stenosis of neural canal of head region

   M99.31   Osseous stenosis of neural canal of cervical region

   M99.32   Osseous stenosis of neural canal of thoracic region

   M99.33   Osseous stenosis of neural canal of lumbar region

   M99.34   Osseous stenosis of neural canal of sacral region

   M99.35   Osseous stenosis of neural canal of pelvic region

   M99.36   Osseous stenosis of neural canal of lower extremity

   M99.37   Osseous stenosis of neural canal of upper extremity

   M99.38   Osseous stenosis of neural canal of rib cage

   M99.39   Osseous stenosis of neural canal of abdomen and other regions

● **M99.4**   Connective tissue stenosis of neural canal

   M99.40   Connective tissue stenosis of neural canal of head region

   M99.41   Connective tissue stenosis of neural canal of cervical region

   M99.42   Connective tissue stenosis of neural canal of thoracic region

   M99.43   Connective tissue stenosis of neural canal of lumbar region

   M99.44   Connective tissue stenosis of neural canal of sacral region

   M99.45   Connective tissue stenosis of neural canal of pelvic region

   M99.46   Connective tissue stenosis of neural canal of lower extremity

   M99.47   Connective tissue stenosis of neural canal of upper extremity

   M99.48   Connective tissue stenosis of neural canal of rib cage

   M99.49   Connective tissue stenosis of neural canal of abdomen and other regions

● **M99.5**   Intervertebral disc stenosis of neural canal

   M99.50   Intervertebral disc stenosis of neural canal of head region

   M99.51   Intervertebral disc stenosis of neural canal of cervical region

   M99.52   Intervertebral disc stenosis of neural canal of thoracic region

   M99.53   Intervertebral disc stenosis of neural canal of lumbar region

   M99.54   Intervertebral disc stenosis of neural canal of sacral region

   M99.55   Intervertebral disc stenosis of neural canal of pelvic region

   M99.56   Intervertebral disc stenosis of neural canal of lower extremity

   M99.57   Intervertebral disc stenosis of neural canal of upper extremity

   M99.58   Intervertebral disc stenosis of neural canal of rib cage

   M99.59   Intervertebral disc stenosis of neural canal of abdomen and other regions

● **M99.6**   Osseous and subluxation stenosis of intervertebral foramina

   M99.60   Osseous and subluxation stenosis of intervertebral foramina of head region

   M99.61   Osseous and subluxation stenosis of intervertebral foramina of cervical region

   M99.62   Osseous and subluxation stenosis of intervertebral foramina of thoracic region

   M99.63   Osseous and subluxation stenosis of intervertebral foramina of lumbar region

   M99.64   Osseous and subluxation stenosis of intervertebral foramina of sacral region

   M99.65   Osseous and subluxation stenosis of intervertebral foramina of pelvic region

   M99.66   Osseous and subluxation stenosis of intervertebral foramina of lower extremity

   M99.67   Osseous and subluxation stenosis of intervertebral foramina of upper extremity

   M99.68   Osseous and subluxation stenosis of intervertebral foramina of rib cage

   M99.69   Osseous and subluxation stenosis of intervertebral foramina of abdomen and other regions

CHAPTER 13 (M00-M99)

● M99.7　Connective tissue and disc stenosis of intervertebral foramina

M99.70　Connective tissue and disc stenosis of intervertebral foramina of head region

M99.71　Connective tissue and disc stenosis of intervertebral foramina of cervical region

M99.72　Connective tissue and disc stenosis of intervertebral foramina of thoracic region

M99.73　Connective tissue and disc stenosis of intervertebral foramina of lumbar region

M99.74　Connective tissue and disc stenosis of intervertebral foramina of sacral region

M99.75　Connective tissue and disc stenosis of intervertebral foramina of pelvic region

M99.76　Connective tissue and disc stenosis of intervertebral foramina of lower extremity

M99.77　Connective tissue and disc stenosis of intervertebral foramina of upper extremity

M99.78　Connective tissue and disc stenosis of intervertebral foramina of rib cage

M99.79　Connective tissue and disc stenosis of intervertebral foramina of abdomen and other regions

● M99.8　Other biomechanical lesions

M99.80　Other biomechanical lesions of head region

M99.81　Other biomechanical lesions of cervical region

M99.82　Other biomechanical lesions of thoracic region

M99.83　Other biomechanical lesions of lumbar region

M99.84　Other biomechanical lesions of sacral region

M99.85　Other biomechanical lesions of pelvic region

M99.86　Other biomechanical lesions of lower extremity

M99.87　Other biomechanical lesions of upper extremity

M99.88　Other biomechanical lesions of rib cage

M99.89　Other biomechanical lesions of abdomen and other regions

M99.9　Biomechanical lesion, unspecified

◀ New　◀▥ Revised　d̶e̶l̶e̶t̶e̶d̶ Deleted　Excludes 1　Excludes 2　Includes　Use additional　Code first　Code also　Unspecified
OGCR Official Guidelines　X Assign placeholder X　● Use Additional Character(s)　▶ Manifestation Code　Coding Clinic

Item 14–1 Nephritis (inflammation) or **nephropathy** (disease) **with lesion of proliferative glomerulonephritis** results from a streptococcal infection.

Nephritis (inflammation) or **nephropathy** (disease) **with lesion of membranous glomerulonephritis** is characterized by deposits along the epithelial side of the basement membrane.

Nephritis (inflammation) or **nephropathy** (disease) **with lesion of membranoproliferative glomerulonephritis** is characterized by alterations in the basement membranes of the kidney and the glomerular cells.

Nephritis (inflammation) or **nephropathy** (disease) **with lesion of rapidly progressive glomerulonephritis** is characterized by rapid and progressive decline in renal function.

Nephritis (inflammation) or **nephropathy** (disease) **with lesion of renal cortical necrosis** is characterized by death of the cortical tissues.

Nephritis (inflammation) or **nephropathy** (disease) **with lesion of renal medullary necrosis** is characterized by death of the tissues that collect urine.

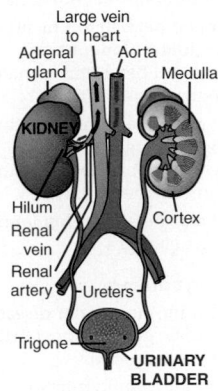

Figure 14-1   Kidneys within the urinary system.

Item 14–2 Glomerulonephritis is nephritis accompanied by inflammation of the glomeruli of the kidney, resulting in the degeneration of the glomeruli and the nephrons.

Acute glomerulonephritis primarily affects children and young adults and is usually a result of a streptococcal infection.

Proliferative glomerulonephritis is the acute form of the disease resulting from a streptococcal infection.

Rapidly progressive glomerulonephritis, also known as **crescentic** or **malignant glomerulonephritis**, is the acute form of the disease, which leads quickly to rapid and progressive decline in renal function.

CHAPTER 14

DISEASES OF THE GENITOURINARY SYSTEM (N00-N99)

Excludes2   certain conditions originating in the perinatal period (P04-P96)
certain infectious and parasitic diseases (A00-B99)
complications of pregnancy, childbirth and the puerperium (O00-O9A)
congenital malformations, deformations and chromosomal abnormalities (Q00-Q99)
endocrine, nutritional and metabolic diseases (E00-E88)
injury, poisoning and certain other consequences of external causes (S00-T88)
neoplasms (C00-D49)
symptoms, signs and abnormal clinical and laboratory findings, not elsewhere classified (R00-R94)

This chapter contains the following blocks:

N00-N08	Glomerular diseases
N10-N16	Renal tubulo-interstitial diseases
N17-N19	Acute kidney failure and chronic kidney disease
N20-N23	Urolithiasis
N25-N29	Other disorders of kidney and ureter
N30-N39	Other diseases of the urinary system
N40-N53	Diseases of male genital organs
N60-N65	Disorders of breast
N70-N77	Inflammatory diseases of female pelvic organs
N80-N98	Noninflammatory disorders of female genital tract
N99	Intraoperative and postprocedural complications and disorders of genitourinary system, not elsewhere classified

GLOMERULAR DISEASES (N00-N08)

Code also any associated kidney failure (N17-N19)

   Excludes1   hypertensive chronic kidney disease (I12.-)

● **N00**   **Acute nephritic syndrome**

   Includes   acute glomerular disease
acute glomerulonephritis
acute nephritis

   Excludes1   acute tubulo-interstitial nephritis (N10)
nephritic syndrome NOS (N05.-)

N00.0   **Acute nephritic syndrome with minor glomerular abnormality**
Acute nephritic syndrome with minimal change lesion

N00.1   **Acute nephritic syndrome with focal and segmental glomerular lesions**
Acute nephritic syndrome with focal and segmental hyalinosis
Acute nephritic syndrome with focal and segmental sclerosis
Acute nephritic syndrome with focal glomerulonephritis

N00.2   **Acute nephritic syndrome with diffuse membranous glomerulonephritis**

N00.3   **Acute nephritic syndrome with diffuse mesangial proliferative glomerulonephritis**

N00.4   **Acute nephritic syndrome with diffuse endocapillary proliferative glomerulonephritis**

N00.5   **Acute nephritic syndrome with diffuse mesangiocapillary glomerulonephritis**
Acute nephritic syndrome with membranoproliferative glomerulonephritis, types 1 and 3, or NOS

N00.6   **Acute nephritic syndrome with dense deposit disease**
Acute nephritic syndrome with membranoproliferative glomerulonephritis, type 2

N00.7   **Acute nephritic syndrome with diffuse crescentic glomerulonephritis**
Acute nephritic syndrome with extracapillary glomerulonephritis

N00.8   **Acute nephritic syndrome with other morphologic changes**
Acute nephritic syndrome with proliferative glomerulonephritis NOS

N00.9   **Acute nephritic syndrome with unspecified morphologic changes**

CHAPTER 14 (N00-N99)

● **N01**   **Rapidly progressive nephritic syndrome**

> **Includes**   rapidly progressive glomerular disease
> rapidly progressive glomerulonephritis
> rapidly progressive nephritis

> **Excludes1**   nephritic syndrome NOS (N05.-)

N01.0   **Rapidly progressive nephritic syndrome with minor glomerular abnormality**
> Rapidly progressive nephritic syndrome with minimal change lesion

N01.1   **Rapidly progressive nephritic syndrome with focal and segmental glomerular lesions**
> Rapidly progressive nephritic syndrome with focal and segmental hyalinosis
> Rapidly progressive nephritic syndrome with focal and segmental sclerosis
> Rapidly progressive nephritic syndrome with focal glomerulonephritis

N01.2   **Rapidly progressive nephritic syndrome with diffuse membranous glomerulonephritis**

N01.3   **Rapidly progressive nephritic syndrome with diffuse mesangial proliferative glomerulonephritis**

N01.4   **Rapidly progressive nephritic syndrome with diffuse endocapillary proliferative glomerulonephritis**

N01.5   **Rapidly progressive nephritic syndrome with diffuse mesangiocapillary glomerulonephritis**
> Rapidly progressive nephritic syndrome with membranoproliferative glomerulonephritis, types 1 and 3, or NOS

N01.6   **Rapidly progressive nephritic syndrome with dense deposit disease**
> Rapidly progressive nephritic syndrome with membranoproliferative glomerulonephritis, type 2

N01.7   **Rapidly progressive nephritic syndrome with diffuse crescentic glomerulonephritis**
> Rapidly progressive nephritic syndrome with extracapillary glomerulonephritis

N01.8   **Rapidly progressive nephritic syndrome with other morphologic changes**
> Rapidly progressive nephritic syndrome with proliferative glomerulonephritis NOS

N01.9   **Rapidly progressive nephritic syndrome with unspecified morphologic changes**

● **N02**   **Recurrent and persistent hematuria**

> **Excludes1**   acute cystitis with hematuria (N30.01)
> hematuria NOS (R31.9)
> hematuria not associated with specified morphologic lesions (R31.-)

N02.0   **Recurrent and persistent hematuria with minor glomerular abnormality**
> Recurrent and persistent hematuria with minimal change lesion

N02.1   **Recurrent and persistent hematuria with focal and segmental glomerular lesions**
> Recurrent and persistent hematuria with focal and segmental hyalinosis
> Recurrent and persistent hematuria with focal and segmental sclerosis
> Recurrent and persistent hematuria with focal glomerulonephritis

N02.2   **Recurrent and persistent hematuria with diffuse membranous glomerulonephritis**

N02.3   **Recurrent and persistent hematuria with diffuse mesangial proliferative glomerulonephritis**

N02.4   **Recurrent and persistent hematuria with diffuse endocapillary proliferative glomerulonephritis**

N02.5   **Recurrent and persistent hematuria with diffuse mesangiocapillary glomerulonephritis**
> Recurrent and persistent hematuria with membranoproliferative glomerulonephritis, types 1 and 3, or NOS

Item 14–3 Chronic glomerulonephritis (GN) persists over a period of years, with remissions and exacerbation.
Chronic GN with lesion of proliferative glomerulonephritis results from a streptococcal infection.
Chronic GN with lesion of membranous glomerulonephritis, also known as membranous nephropathy, is characterized by deposits along the epithelial side of the basement membrane.
Chronic GN with lesion of membrano-proliferative glomerulonephritis (MPGN) is a group of disorders characterized by alterations in the basement membranes of the kidney and the glomerular cells.
Chronic GN with lesion of rapidly progressive glomerulonephritis is characterized by necrosis, endothelial proliferation, and mesangial proliferation. The condition is marked by rapid and progressive decline in renal function.

N02.6   **Recurrent and persistent hematuria with dense deposit disease**
> Recurrent and persistent hematuria with membranoproliferative glomerulonephritis, type 2

N02.7   **Recurrent and persistent hematuria with diffuse crescentic glomerulonephritis**
> Recurrent and persistent hematuria with extracapillary glomerulonephritis

N02.8   **Recurrent and persistent hematuria with other morphologic changes**
> Recurrent and persistent hematuria with proliferative glomerulonephritis NOS

N02.9   **Recurrent and persistent hematuria with unspecified morphologic changes**

● **N03**   **Chronic nephritic syndrome**

> **Includes**   chronic glomerular disease
> chronic glomerulonephritis
> chronic nephritis

> **Excludes1**   chronic tubulo-interstitial nephritis (N11.-)
> diffuse sclerosing glomerulonephritis (N05.8-)
> nephritic syndrome NOS (N05.-)

N03.0   **Chronic nephritic syndrome with minor glomerular abnormality**
> Chronic nephritic syndrome with minimal change lesion

N03.1   **Chronic nephritic syndrome with focal and segmental glomerular lesions**
> Chronic nephritic syndrome with focal and segmental hyalinosis
> Chronic nephritic syndrome with focal and segmental sclerosis
> Chronic nephritic syndrome with focal glomerulonephritis

N03.2   **Chronic nephritic syndrome with diffuse membranous glomerulonephritis**

N03.3   **Chronic nephritic syndrome with diffuse mesangial proliferative glomerulonephritis**

N03.4   **Chronic nephritic syndrome with diffuse endocapillary proliferative glomerulonephritis**

N03.5   **Chronic nephritic syndrome with diffuse mesangiocapillary glomerulonephritis**
> Chronic nephritic syndrome with membranoproliferative glomerulonephritis, types 1 and 3, or NOS

N03.6   **Chronic nephritic syndrome with dense deposit disease**
> Chronic nephritic syndrome with membranoproliferative glomerulonephritis, type 2

N03.7   **Chronic nephritic syndrome with diffuse crescentic glomerulonephritis**
> Chronic nephritic syndrome with extracapillary glomerulonephritis

N03.8   **Chronic nephritic syndrome with other morphologic changes**
> Chronic nephritic syndrome with proliferative glomerulonephritis NOS

N03.9   **Chronic nephritic syndrome with unspecified morphologic changes**

◀ New   ⬅ Revised   ~~deleted~~ Deleted   Excludes 1   Excludes 2   Includes   Use additional   Code first   Code also   Unspecified

OGCR Official Guidelines   X Assign placeholder X   ● Use Additional Character(s)   ▶ Manifestation Code   **Coding Clinic**

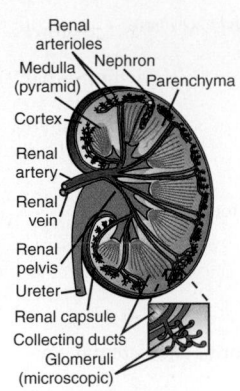

Renal arterioles
Medulla (pyramid)   Nephron
                              Parenchyma
Cortex
Renal artery
Renal vein
Renal pelvis
Ureter
Renal capsule
Collecting ducts
Glomeruli (microscopic)

Figure 14-2 Kidney cross section.

Item 14–4 Nephrotic syndrome (NS) is marked by massive proteinuria (protein in the urine) and water retention. Patients with NS are particularly vulnerable to staphylococcal and pneumococcal infections. NS with lesion of proliferative glomerulonephritis results from a streptococcal infection. NS with lesion of membranous glomerulonephritis results in thickening of the capillary walls. NS with lesion of minimal change glomerulonephritis is usually a benign disorder that occurs mostly in children and requires electron microscopy (biopsy) to verify changes in the glomeruli.

● **N04**   **Nephrotic syndrome**

    | **Includes** | congenital nephrotic syndrome
                      lipoid nephrosis

N04.0 **Nephrotic syndrome with minor glomerular abnormality**
    Nephrotic syndrome with minimal change lesion

N04.1 **Nephrotic syndrome with focal and segmental glomerular lesions**
    Nephrotic syndrome with focal and segmental hyalinosis
    Nephrotic syndrome with focal and segmental sclerosis
    Nephrotic syndrome with focal glomerulonephritis

N04.2 **Nephrotic syndrome with diffuse membranous glomerulonephritis**

N04.3 **Nephrotic syndrome with diffuse mesangial proliferative glomerulonephritis**

N04.4 **Nephrotic syndrome with diffuse endocapillary proliferative glomerulonephritis**

N04.5 **Nephrotic syndrome with diffuse mesangiocapillary glomerulonephritis**
    Nephrotic syndrome with membranoproliferative glomerulonephritis, types 1 and 3, or NOS

N04.6 **Nephrotic syndrome with dense deposit disease**
    Nephrotic syndrome with membranoproliferative glomerulonephritis, type 2

N04.7 **Nephrotic syndrome with diffuse crescentic glomerulonephritis**
    Nephrotic syndrome with extracapillary glomerulonephritis

N04.8 **Nephrotic syndrome with other morphologic changes**
    Nephrotic syndrome with proliferative glomerulonephritis NOS

N04.9 **Nephrotic syndrome with** unspecified **morphologic changes**

● **N05**   **Unspecified nephritic syndrome**

    | **Includes** | glomerular disease NOS
                      glomerulonephritis NOS
                      nephritis NOS
                      nephropathy NOS and renal disease NOS with morphological lesion specified in .0-.8

    | **Excludes1** | nephropathy NOS with no stated morphological lesion (N28.9)
                      renal disease NOS with no stated morphological lesion (N28.9)
                      tubulo-interstitial nephritis NOS (N12)

N05.0 Unspecified **nephritic syndrome with minor glomerular abnormality**
    Unspecified nephritic syndrome with minimal change lesion

N05.1 Unspecified **nephritic syndrome with focal and segmental glomerular lesions**
    Unspecified nephritic syndrome with focal and segmental hyalinosis
    Unspecified nephritic syndrome with focal and segmental sclerosis
    Unspecified nephritic syndrome with focal glomerulonephritis

N05.2 Unspecified **nephritic syndrome with diffuse membranous glomerulonephritis**

N05.3 Unspecified **nephritic syndrome with diffuse mesangial proliferative glomerulonephritis**

N05.4 Unspecified **nephritic syndrome with diffuse endocapillary proliferative glomerulonephritis**

N05.5 Unspecified **nephritic syndrome with diffuse mesangiocapillary glomerulonephritis**
    Unspecified nephritic syndrome with membranoproliferative glomerulonephritis, types 1 and 3, or NOS

N05.6 Unspecified **nephritic syndrome with dense deposit disease**
    Unspecified nephritic syndrome with membranoproliferative glomerulonephritis, type 2

N05.7 Unspecified **nephritic syndrome with diffuse crescentic glomerulonephritis**
    Unspecified nephritic syndrome with extracapillary glomerulonephritis

N05.8 Unspecified **nephritic syndrome with other morphologic changes**
    Unspecified nephritic syndrome with proliferative glomerulonephritis NOS

N05.9 Unspecified **nephritic syndrome with unspecified morphologic changes**

● **N06**   **Isolated proteinuria with specified morphological lesion**

    | **Excludes1** | proteinuria not associated with specific morphologic lesions (R80.0)

N06.0 **Isolated proteinuria with minor glomerular abnormality**
    Isolated proteinuria with minimal change lesion

N06.1 **Isolated proteinuria with focal and segmental glomerular lesions**
    Isolated proteinuria with focal and segmental hyalinosis
    Isolated proteinuria with focal and segmental sclerosis
    Isolated proteinuria with focal glomerulonephritis

N06.2 **Isolated proteinuria with diffuse membranous glomerulonephritis**

N06.3 **Isolated proteinuria with diffuse mesangial proliferative glomerulonephritis**

CHAPTER 14 (N00-N99)

N06.4   **Isolated proteinuria with diffuse endocapillary proliferative glomerulonephritis**

N06.5   **Isolated proteinuria with diffuse mesangiocapillary glomerulonephritis**
     Isolated proteinuria with membranoproliferative glomerulonephritis, types 1 and 3, or NOS

N06.6   **Isolated proteinuria with dense deposit disease**
     Isolated proteinuria with membranoproliferative glomerulonephritis, type 2

N06.7   **Isolated proteinuria with diffuse crescentic glomerulonephritis**
     Isolated proteinuria with extracapillary glomerulonephritis

N06.8   **Isolated proteinuria with other morphologic lesion**
     Isolated proteinuria with proliferative glomerulonephritis NOS

N06.9   **Isolated proteinuria with** `unspecified` **morphologic lesion**

● **N07**   **Hereditary nephropathy, not elsewhere classified**

     `Excludes2`   Alport's syndrome (Q87.81-)
          hereditary amyloid nephropathy (E85.-)
          nail patella syndrome (Q87.2)
          non-neuropathic heredofamilial amyloidosis (E85.-)

N07.0   **Hereditary nephropathy, not elsewhere classified with minor glomerular abnormality**
     Hereditary nephropathy, not elsewhere classified with minimal change lesion

N07.1   **Hereditary nephropathy, not elsewhere classified with focal and segmental glomerular lesions**
     Hereditary nephropathy, not elsewhere classified with focal and segmental hyalinosis
     Hereditary nephropathy, not elsewhere classified with focal and segmental sclerosis
     Hereditary nephropathy, not elsewhere classified with focal glomerulonephritis

N07.2   **Hereditary nephropathy, not elsewhere classified with diffuse membranous glomerulonephritis**

N07.3   **Hereditary nephropathy, not elsewhere classified with diffuse mesangial proliferative glomerulonephritis**

N07.4   **Hereditary nephropathy, not elsewhere classified with diffuse endocapillary proliferative glomerulonephritis**

N07.5   **Hereditary nephropathy, not elsewhere classified with diffuse mesangiocapillary glomerulonephritis**
     Hereditary nephropathy, not elsewhere classified with membranoproliferative glomerulonephritis, types 1 and 3, or NOS

N07.6   **Hereditary nephropathy, not elsewhere classified with dense deposit disease**
     Hereditary nephropathy, not elsewhere classified with membranoproliferative glomerulonephritis, type 2

N07.7   **Hereditary nephropathy, not elsewhere classified with diffuse crescentic glomerulonephritis**
     Hereditary nephropathy, not elsewhere classified with extracapillary glomerulonephritis

N07.8   **Hereditary nephropathy, not elsewhere classified with other morphologic lesions**
     Hereditary nephropathy, not elsewhere classified with proliferative glomerulonephritis NOS

N07.9   **Hereditary nephropathy, not elsewhere classified with** `unspecified` **morphologic lesions**

▶ **N08**   *Glomerular disorders in diseases classified elsewhere*
     Glomerulonephritis
     Nephritis
     Nephropathy
     Code first underlying disease, such as:
         amyloidosis (E85.-)
         congenital syphilis (A50.5)
         cryoglobulinemia (D89.1)
         disseminated intravascular coagulation (D65)
         gout (M1A.-, M10.-)
         microscopic polyangiitis (M31.7)
         multiple myeloma (C90.0-)
         sepsis (A40.0-A41.9)
         sickle-cell disease (D57.0-D57.8)

     `Excludes1`   glomerulonephritis, nephritis and nephropathy (in):
         antiglomerular basement membrane disease (M31.0)
         diabetes (E08-E13 with .21)
         gonococcal (A54.21)
         Goodpasture's syndrome (M31.0)
         hemolytic-uremic syndrome (D59.3)
         lupus (M32.14)
         mumps (B26.83)
         syphilis (A52.75)
         systemic lupus erythematosus (M32.14)
         Wegener's granulomatosis (M31.31)
       pyelonephritis in diseases classified elsewhere (N16)
       renal tubulo-interstitial disorders classified elsewhere (N16)

RENAL TUBULO-INTERSTITIAL DISEASES (N10-N16)

     `Includes`   pyelonephritis
     `Excludes1`   pyeloureteritis cystica (N28.85)

N10   **Acute tubulo-interstitial nephritis**
     Acute infectious interstitial nephritis
     Acute pyelitis
     Acute pyelonephritis
     Hemoglobin nephrosis
     Myoglobin nephrosis
     Use additional code (B95-B97), to identify infectious agent

● **N11**   **Chronic tubulo-interstitial nephritis**
     `Includes`   chronic infectious interstitial nephritis
         chronic pyelitis
         chronic pyelonephritis
     Use additional code (B95-B97), to identify infectious agent

N11.0   **Nonobstructive reflux-associated chronic pyelonephritis**
     Pyelonephritis (chronic) associated with (vesicoureteral) reflux

     `Excludes1`   vesicoureteral reflux NOS (N13.70)

N11.1   **Chronic obstructive pyelonephritis**
     Pyelonephritis (chronic) associated with anomaly of pelviureteric junction
     Pyelonephritis (chronic) associated with anomaly of pyeloureteric junction
     Pyelonephritis (chronic) associated with crossing of vessel
     Pyelonephritis (chronic) associated with kinking of ureter
     Pyelonephritis (chronic) associated with obstruction of ureter
     Pyelonephritis (chronic) associated with stricture of pelviureteric junction
     Pyelonephritis (chronic) associated with stricture of ureter

     `Excludes1`   calculous pyelonephritis (N20.9)
         obstructive uropathy (N13.-)

CHAPTER 14 (N00-N99)

◀ New   ◀━ Revised   ~~deleted~~ Deleted   `Excludes 1`   `Excludes 2`   `Includes`   `Use additional`   `Code first`   `Code also`   `Unspecified`

OGCR Official Guidelines   **X** Assign placeholder X   ● Use Additional Character(s)   ▶ Manifestation Code   **Coding Clinic**

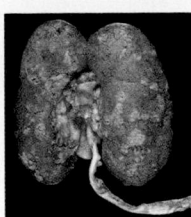

Figure 14-3   Acute pyelonephritis. Cortical surface exhibits grayish white areas of inflammation and abscess formation. (From Kumar: Robbins and Cotran: Pathologic Basis of Disease, ed 8, Saunders, An Imprint of Elsevier, 2009)

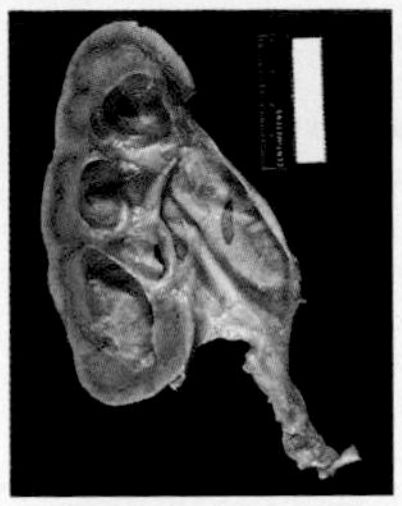

Figure 14-4   Hydronephrosis of the kidney, with marked dilatation of pelvis and calyces and thinning of renal parenchyma. (From Kumar: Robbins and Cotran: Pathologic Basis of Disease, ed 8, Saunders, An Imprint of Elsevier, 2009)

Item 14–5 Pyelonephritis is an infection of the kidneys and ureters and may be chronic or acute in one or both kidneys.

N11.8   **Other chronic tubulo-interstitial nephritis**
     Nonobstructive chronic pyelonephritis NOS

N11.9   **Chronic tubulo-interstitial nephritis, unspecified**
     Chronic interstitial nephritis NOS
     Chronic pyelitis NOS
     Chronic pyelonephritis NOS

N12   **Tubulo-interstitial nephritis, not specified as acute or chronic**
     Interstitial nephritis NOS
     Pyelitis NOS
     Pyelonephritis NOS
     Excludes1   calculous pyelonephritis (N20.9)

● **N13**   **Obstructive and reflux uropathy**
     Excludes2   calculus of kidney and ureter without hydronephrosis (N20.-)
           congenital obstructive defects of renal pelvis and ureter (Q62.0-Q62.3)
           hydronephrosis with ureteropelvic junction obstruction (Q62.1)
           obstructive pyelonephritis (N11.1)

N13.1   **Hydronephrosis with ureteral stricture, not elsewhere classified**
     Excludes1   hydronephrosis with ureteral stricture with infection (N13.6)

N13.2   **Hydronephrosis with renal and ureteral calculous obstruction**
     Excludes1   hydronephrosis with renal and ureteral calculous obstruction with infection (N13.6)

● **N13.3**   **Other and unspecified hydronephrosis**
     Excludes1   hydronephrosis with infection (N13.6)
   N13.30   Unspecified hydronephrosis
   N13.39   Other hydronephrosis

N13.4   **Hydroureter**
     Excludes1   congenital hydroureter (Q62.3-)
           hydroureter with infection (N13.6)
           vesicoureteral-reflux with hydroureter (N13.73-)

N13.5   **Crossing vessel and stricture of ureter without hydronephrosis**
     Kinking and stricture of ureter without hydronephrosis
     Excludes1   crossing vessel and stricture of ureter without hydronephrosis with infection (N13.6)

N13.6   **Pyonephrosis**
     Conditions in N13.1-N13.5 with infection
     Obstructive uropathy with infection
     Use additional code (B95-B97), to identify infectious agent

● **N13.7**   **Vesicoureteral-reflux**
     Excludes1   reflux-associated pyelonephritis (N11.0)
   N13.70   Vesicoureteral-reflux, unspecified
       Occurs when urine flows from bladder back into ureters
       Vesicoureteral-reflux NOS
   N13.71   Vesicoureteral-reflux without reflux nephropathy
 ● **N13.72**   Vesicoureteral-reflux with reflux nephropathy without hydroureter
     N13.721   Vesicoureteral-reflux with reflux nephropathy without hydroureter, unilateral
     N13.722   Vesicoureteral-reflux with reflux nephropathy without hydroureter, bilateral
     N13.729   Vesicoureteral-reflux with reflux nephropathy without hydroureter, unspecified
 ● **N13.73**   Vesicoureteral-reflux with reflux nephropathy with hydroureter
     N13.731   Vesicoureteral-reflux with reflux nephropathy with hydroureter, unilateral
     N13.732   Vesicoureteral-reflux with reflux nephropathy with hydroureter, bilateral
     N13.739   Vesicoureteral-reflux with reflux nephropathy with hydroureter, unspecified

N13.8   **Other obstructive and reflux uropathy**
     Urinary tract obstruction due to specified cause
     Code first, if applicable, any causal condition first, such as:
       enlarged prostate (N40.1)

N13.9   **Obstructive and reflux uropathy, unspecified**
     Urinary tract obstruction NOS

● **N14**   **Drug- and heavy-metal-induced tubulo-interstitial and tubular conditions**
     Code first poisoning due to drug or toxin, if applicable (T36-T65 with fifth or sixth character 1-4 or 6)
     Use additional code for adverse effect, if applicable, to identify drug (T36-T50 with fifth or sixth character 5)

N14.0   **Analgesic nephropathy**

N14.1   **Nephropathy induced by other drugs, medicaments and biological substances**

N14.2   **Nephropathy induced by unspecified drug, medicament or biological substance**

N14.3   **Nephropathy induced by heavy metals**

N14.4   **Toxic nephropathy, not elsewhere classified**

● **N15**   **Other renal tubulo-interstitial diseases**

N15.0   **Balkan nephropathy**
     Balkan endemic nephropathy

N15.1   **Renal and perinephric abscess**

N15.8   **Other specified renal tubulo-interstitial diseases**

N15.9   **Renal tubulo-interstitial disease, unspecified**
     Infection of kidney NOS
     Excludes1   urinary tract infection NOS (N39.0)

Item 14–6 Decreased blood flow is the usual cause of **acute renal failure** that offers a good prognosis for recovery.

    Chronic renal failure is usually the result of long-standing kidney disease and is a very serious condition that generally results in death.

▶ **N16** *Renal tubulo-interstitial disorders in diseases classified elsewhere*

    Pyelonephritis

    Tubulo-interstitial nephritis

    Code first underlying disease, such as:

      brucellosis (A23.0-A23.9)

      cryoglobulinemia (D89.1)

      glycogen storage disease (E74.0)

      leukemia (C91-C95)

      lymphoma (C81.0-C85.9, C96.0-C96.9)

      multiple myeloma (C90.0-)

      sepsis (A40.0-A41.9)

      Wilson's disease (E83.0)

    Excludes1   diphtheritic pyelonephritis and tubulo-interstitial nephritis (A36.84)

        pyelonephritis and tubulo-interstitial nephritis in candidiasis (B37.49)

        pyelonephritis and tubulo-interstitial nephritis in cystinosis (E72.04)

        pyelonephritis and tubulo-interstitial nephritis in salmonella infection (A02.25)

        pyelonephritis and tubulo-interstitial nephritis in sarcoidosis (D86.84)

        pyelonephritis and tubulo-interstitial nephritis in sicca syndrome [Sjogren's] (M35.04)

        pyelonephritis and tubulo-interstitial nephritis in systemic lupus erythematosus (M32.15)

        pyelonephritis and tubulo-interstitial nephritis in toxoplasmosis (B58.83)

        renal tubular degeneration in diabetes (E08-E13 with .29)

        syphilitic pyelonephritis and tubulo-interstitial nephritis (A52.75)

ACUTE KIDNEY FAILURE AND CHRONIC KIDNEY DISEASE (N17-N19)

    Excludes2   congenital renal failure (P96.0)

        drug- and heavy-metal-induced tubulo-interstitial and tubular conditions (N14.-)

        extrarenal uremia (R39.2)

        hemolytic-uremic syndrome (D59.3)

        hepatorenal syndrome (K76.7)

        postpartum hepatorenal syndrome (O90.4)

        posttraumatic renal failure (T79.5)

        prerenal uremia (R39.2)

        renal failure complicating abortion or ectopic or molar pregnancy (O00-O07, O08.4)

        renal failure following labor and delivery (O90.4)

        renal failure postprocedural (N99.0)

● **N17** **Acute kidney failure**

    Code also associated underlying condition

    Excludes1   posttraumatic renal failure (T79.5)

    N17.0 **Acute kidney failure with tubular necrosis**

      Acute tubular necrosis

      Renal tubular necrosis

      Tubular necrosis NOS

    N17.1 **Acute kidney failure with acute cortical necrosis**

      Acute cortical necrosis

      Cortical necrosis NOS

      Renal cortical necrosis

    N17.2 **Acute kidney failure with medullary necrosis**

      Medullary [papillary] necrosis NOS

      Acute medullary [papillary] necrosis

      Renal medullary [papillary] necrosis

    N17.8 **Other acute kidney failure**

    N17.9 **Acute kidney failure, unspecified**

      Acute kidney injury (nontraumatic)

      Excludes2   traumatic kidney injury (S37.0-)

● **N18** **Chronic kidney disease (CKD)**

    Code first any associated:

      diabetic chronic kidney disease (E08.22, E09.22, E10.22, E11.22, E13.22)

      hypertensive chronic kidney disease (I12.-, I13.-)

    Use additional code to identify kidney transplant status, if applicable, (Z94.0)

    N18.1 **Chronic kidney disease, stage 1**

    N18.2 **Chronic kidney disease, stage 2 (mild)**

    N18.3 **Chronic kidney disease, stage 3 (moderate)**

    N18.4 **Chronic kidney disease, stage 4 (severe)**

      Coding Clinic: 2013, Q1, P24

    N18.5 **Chronic kidney disease, stage 5**

      Excludes1   chronic kidney disease, stage 5 requiring chronic dialysis (N18.6)

    N18.6 **End stage renal disease**

      Chronic kidney disease requiring chronic dialysis

      Use additional code to identify dialysis status (Z99.2)

    N18.9 **Chronic kidney disease, unspecified**

      Chronic renal disease

      Chronic renal failure NOS

      Chronic renal insufficiency

      Chronic uremia

  N19 **Unspecified kidney failure**

    Uremia NOS

    Excludes1   acute kidney failure (N17.-)

        chronic kidney disease (N18.-)

        chronic uremia (N18.9)

        extrarenal uremia (R39.2)

        prerenal uremia (R39.2)

        renal insufficiency (acute) (N28.9)

        uremia of newborn (P96.0)

UROLITHIASIS (N20-N23)

● **N20** **Calculus of kidney and ureter**

    Calculous pyelonephritis

    Excludes1   nephrocalcinosis (E83.5)

        that with hydronephrosis (N13.2)

    N20.0 **Calculus of kidney**

      Nephrolithiasis NOS   Staghorn calculus

      Renal calculus   Stone in kidney

      Renal stone

    N20.1 **Calculus of ureter**

      Ureteric stone

    N20.2 **Calculus of kidney with calculus of ureter**

    N20.9 **Urinary calculus, unspecified**

● **N21** **Calculus of lower urinary tract**

    Includes   calculus of lower urinary tract with cystitis and urethritis

    N21.0 **Calculus in bladder**

      Calculus in diverticulum of bladder

      Urinary bladder stone

      Excludes2   staghorn calculus (N20.0)

    N21.1 **Calculus in urethra**

      Excludes2   calculus of prostate (N42.0)

    N21.8 **Other lower urinary tract calculus**

    N21.9 **Calculus of lower urinary tract, unspecified**

      Excludes1   calculus of urinary tract NOS (N20.9)

▶ **N22** *Calculus of urinary tract in diseases classified elsewhere*

    Code first underlying disease, such as:

      gout (M1A.-, M10.-)

      schistosomiasis (B65.0-B65.9)

  N23 **Unspecified renal colic**

◀ New   ◀▥ Revised   ~~deleted~~ Deleted   Excludes 1   Excludes 2   Includes   Use additional   Code first   Code also   Unspecified

OGCR Official Guidelines   **X** Assign placeholder X   ● Use Additional Character(s)   ▶ Manifestation Code   **Coding Clinic**

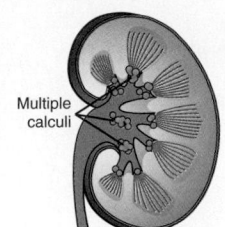

Figure 14-5   Multiple urinary calculi.

Multiple calculi

OTHER DISORDERS OF KIDNEY AND URETER (N25-N29)

> **Excludes2**   disorders of kidney and ureter with urolithiasis (N20-N23)

● **N25**   **Disorders resulting from impaired renal tubular function**
> **Excludes1**   metabolic disorders classifiable to E70-E88

N25.0   **Renal osteodystrophy**
Azotemic osteodystrophy
Phosphate-losing tubular disorders
Renal rickets
Renal short stature

N25.1   **Nephrogenic diabetes insipidus**
> **Excludes1**   diabetes insipidus NOS (E23.2)

● **N25.8**   **Other disorders resulting from impaired renal tubular function**

N25.81   **Secondary hyperparathyroidism of renal origin**
> **Excludes1**   secondary hyperparathyroidism, non-renal (E21.1)

N25.89   **Other disorders resulting from impaired renal tubular function**
Hypokalemic nephropathy
Lightwood-Albright syndrome
Renal tubular acidosis NOS

N25.9   **Disorder resulting from impaired renal tubular function, unspecified**

● **N26**   **Unspecified contracted kidney**
> **Excludes1**   contracted kidney due to hypertension (I12.-)
diffuse sclerosing glomerulonephritis (N05.8-)
hypertensive nephrosclerosis (arteriolar) (arteriosclerotic) (I12.-)
small kidney of unknown cause (N27.-)

N26.1   **Atrophy of kidney (terminal)**
N26.2   **Page kidney**
N26.9   **Renal sclerosis, unspecified**

● **N27**   **Small kidney of unknown cause**
> **Includes**   oligonephronia
N27.0   **Small kidney, unilateral**
N27.1   **Small kidney, bilateral**
N27.9   **Small kidney, unspecified**

● **N28**   **Other disorders of kidney and ureter, not elsewhere classified**
N28.0   **Ischemia and infarction of kidney**
Renal artery embolism
Renal artery obstruction
Renal artery occlusion
Renal artery thrombosis
Renal infarct
> **Excludes1**   atherosclerosis of renal artery (extrarenal part) (I70.1)
congenital stenosis of renal artery (Q27.1)
Goldblatt's kidney (I70.1)

N28.1   **Cyst of kidney, acquired**
Cyst (multiple)(solitary) of kidney, acquired
> **Excludes1**   cystic kidney disease (congenital) (Q61.-)

● **N28.8**   **Other specified disorders of kidney and ureter**
> **Excludes1**   hydroureter (N13.4)
ureteric stricture with hydronephrosis (N13.1)
ureteric stricture without hydronephrosis (N13.5)

N28.81   **Hypertrophy of kidney**
N28.82   **Megaloureter**
N28.83   **Nephroptosis**
N28.84   **Pyelitis cystica**
N28.85   **Pyeloureteritis cystica**
N28.86   **Ureteritis cystica**
N28.89   **Other specified disorders of kidney and ureter**

N28.9   **Disorder of kidney and ureter, unspecified**
Nephropathy NOS
Renal disease (acute) NOS
Renal insufficiency (acute)
> **Excludes1**   chronic renal insufficiency (N18.9)
unspecified nephritic syndrome (N05.-)

▶ **N29**   *Other disorders of kidney and ureter in diseases classified elsewhere*
Code first underlying disease, such as:
amyloidosis (E85.-)
nephrocalcinosis (E83.5)
schistosomiasis (B65.0-B65.9)
> **Excludes1**   disorders of kidney and ureter in:
cystinosis (E72.0)
gonorrhea (A54.21)
syphilis (A52.75)
tuberculosis (A18.11)

OTHER DISEASES OF THE URINARY SYSTEM (N30-N39)

> **Excludes1**   urinary infection (complicating):
abortion or ectopic or molar pregnancy (O00-O07, O08.8)
pregnancy, childbirth and the puerperium (O23.-, O75.3, O86.2-)

● **N30**   **Cystitis**
Infection of bladder and irritation in lower urinary tract
Use additional code to identify infectious agent (B95-B97)
> **Excludes1**   prostatocystitis (N41.3)

● **N30.0**   **Acute cystitis**
> **Excludes1**   irradiation cystitis (N30.4-)
trigonitis (N30.3-)

N30.00   **Acute cystitis without hematuria**
N30.01   **Acute cystitis with hematuria**

● **N30.1**   **Interstitial cystitis (chronic)**
Ongoing infection of kidney glomeruli and tubules
N30.10   **Interstitial cystitis (chronic) without hematuria**
N30.11   **Interstitial cystitis (chronic) with hematuria**

● **N30.2**   **Other chronic cystitis**
N30.20   **Other chronic cystitis without hematuria**
N30.21   **Other chronic cystitis with hematuria**

● **N30.3**   **Trigonitis**
Inflammation of triangular area of bladder (where the ureters and urethra come together)
Urethrotrigonitis
N30.30   **Trigonitis without hematuria**
N30.31   **Trigonitis with hematuria**

● **N30.4**   **Irradiation cystitis**
N30.40   **Irradiation cystitis without hematuria**
N30.41   **Irradiation cystitis with hematuria**

● **N30.8**   **Other cystitis**
Abscess of bladder
N30.80   **Other cystitis without hematuria**
N30.81   **Other cystitis with hematuria**

CHAPTER 14 (N00-N99)

● **N30.9**   **Cystitis, unspecified**
    N30.90   **Cystitis, unspecified without hematuria**
    N30.91   **Cystitis, unspecified with hematuria**

● **N31**   **Neuromuscular dysfunction of bladder, not elsewhere classified**
    Use additional code to identify any associated urinary
    incontinence (N39.3-N39.4-)
    Excludes1   cord bladder NOS (G95.89)
                 neurogenic bladder due to cauda equina
                     syndrome (G83.4)
                 neuromuscular dysfunction due to spinal cord
                     lesion (G95.89)

    N31.0   **Uninhibited neuropathic bladder, not elsewhere classified**

    N31.1   **Reflex neuropathic bladder, not elsewhere classified**

    N31.2   **Flaccid neuropathic bladder, not elsewhere classified**
        Atonic (motor) (sensory) neuropathic bladder
        Diminished tone of bladder muscle
        Autonomous neuropathic bladder
        Nonreflex neuropathic bladder

    N31.8   **Other neuromuscular dysfunction of bladder**

    N31.9   **Neuromuscular dysfunction of bladder, unspecified**
        Neurogenic bladder dysfunction NOS

● **N32**   **Other disorders of bladder**
    Excludes2   calculus of bladder (N21.0)
                 cystocele (N81.1-)
                 hernia or prolapse of bladder, female (N81.1-)

    N32.0   **Bladder-neck obstruction**
        Bladder-neck stenosis (acquired)
        Excludes1   congenital bladder-neck obstruction
                     (Q64.3-)

    N32.1   **Vesicointestinal fistula**
        Vesicorectal fistula

    N32.2   **Vesical fistula, not elsewhere classified**
        Excludes1   fistula between bladder and female
                     genital tract (N82.0-N82.1)

    N32.3   **Diverticulum of bladder**
        Formation of sac from a herniation of wall of bladder
        Excludes1   congenital diverticulum of bladder
                     (Q64.6)
                 diverticulitis of bladder (N30.8-)

● **N32.8**   **Other specified disorders of bladder**
    N32.81   **Overactive bladder**
        Detrusor muscle hyperactivity
        Excludes1   frequent urination due to
                     specified bladder condition-
                     code to condition

    N32.89   **Other specified disorders of bladder**
        Bladder hemorrhage
        Bladder hypertrophy
        Calcified bladder
        Contracted bladder

    N32.9   **Bladder disorder, unspecified**

◗ **N33**   *Bladder disorders in diseases classified elsewhere*
    Code first underlying disease, such as:
        schistosomiasis (B65.0-B65.9)
    Excludes1   bladder disorder in syphilis (A52.76)
                 bladder disorder in tuberculosis (A18.12)
                 candidal cystitis (B37.41)
                 chlamydial cystitis(A56.01)
                 cystitis in gonorrhea (A54.01)
                 cystitis in neurogenic bladder (N31.-)
                 diphtheritic cystitis (A36.85)
                 syphilitic cystitis (A52.76)
                 trichomonal cystitis (A59.03)

● **N34**   **Urethritis and urethral syndrome**
    Use additional code (B95-B97), to identify infectious agent
    Excludes2   Reiter's disease (M02.3-)
                 urethritis in diseases with a predominantly sexual
                     mode of transmission (A50-A64)
                 urethrotrigonitis (N30.3-)

    N34.0   **Urethral abscess**
        Abscess (of) Cowper's gland
        Abscess (of) Littré's gland
        Abscess (of) urethral (gland)
        Periurethral abscess
        Excludes1   urethral caruncle (N36.2)

    N34.1   **Nonspecific urethritis**
        Nongonococcal urethritis
        Nonvenereal urethritis

    N34.2   **Other urethritis**
        Inflammation of urethra
        Meatitis, urethral
        Postmenopausal urethritis
        Ulcer of urethra (meatus)
        Urethritis NOS

    N34.3   **Urethral syndrome, unspecified**

● **N35**   **Urethral stricture**
    Narrowing of lumen of urethra caused by scarring due to infection or
    injury
    Excludes1   congenital urethral stricture (Q64.3-)
                 postprocedural urethral stricture (N99.1-)

● **N35.0**   **Post-traumatic urethral stricture**
    Urethral stricture due to injury
    Excludes1   postprocedural urethral stricture (N99.1-)

   ● **N35.01**   **Post-traumatic urethral stricture, male**
      N35.010   **Post-traumatic urethral stricture,**
               male, meatal ♂
      N35.011   **Post-traumatic bulbous urethral**
               stricture
      N35.012   **Post-traumatic membranous urethral**
               stricture
      N35.013   **Post-traumatic anterior urethral**
               stricture
      N35.014   **Post-traumatic urethral stricture,**
               male, unspecified ♂

   ● **N35.02**   **Post-traumatic urethral stricture, female**
      N35.021   **Urethral stricture due to childbirth** ♀
      N35.028   **Other post-traumatic urethral**
               stricture, female ♀

   ● **N35.1**   **Postinfective urethral stricture, not elsewhere classified**
    Excludes1   urethral stricture associated with
                   schistosomiasis (B65.-, N29)
                 gonococcal urethral stricture (A54.01)
                 syphilitic urethral stricture (A52.76)

   ● **N35.11**   **Postinfective urethral stricture, not elsewhere**
               classified, male
      N35.111   **Postinfective urethral stricture, not**
               elsewhere classified, male, meatal ♂
      N35.112   **Postinfective bulbous urethral**
               stricture, not elsewhere classified
      N35.113   **Postinfective membranous urethral**
               stricture, not elsewhere classified
      N35.114   **Postinfective anterior urethral**
               stricture, not elsewhere classified
      N35.119   **Postinfective urethral stricture,**
               not elsewhere classified, male,
               unspecified ♂

    N35.12   **Postinfective urethral stricture, not elsewhere**
               classified, female ♀

    N35.8   **Other urethral stricture**
        Excludes1   postprocedural urethral stricture (N99.1-)

    N35.9   **Urethral stricture, unspecified**

◀ New   ⬅ Revised   ~~deleted~~ Deleted   Excludes 1   Excludes 2   Includes   Use additional   Code first   Code also   Unspecified

OGCR Official Guidelines   X Assign placeholder X   ● Use Additional Character(s)   ◗ Manifestation Code   **Coding Clinic**

● N36   **Other disorders of urethra**

    N36.0   **Urethral fistula**
        Urethroperineal fistula
        Urethrorectal fistula
        Urinary fistula NOS

        Excludes1   urethroscrotal fistula (N50.8)
                    urethrovaginal fistula (N82.1)
                    urethrovesicovaginal fistula (N82.1)

    N36.1   **Urethral diverticulum**

    N36.2   **Urethral caruncle**

●   N36.4   **Urethral functional and muscular disorders**
        Use additional code to identify associated urinary stress incontinence (N39.3)

        N36.41   **Hypermobility of urethra**

        N36.42   **Intrinsic sphincter deficiency (ISD)**

        N36.43   **Combined hypermobility of urethra and intrinsic sphincter deficiency**

        N36.44   **Muscular disorders of urethra**
                Bladder sphincter dyssynergy

    N36.5   **Urethral false passage**

    N36.8   **Other specified disorders of urethra**

    N36.9   **Urethral disorder, unspecified**

▶ N37   *Urethral disorders in diseases classified elsewhere*
        Code first underlying disease

        Excludes1   urethritis (in):
                    candidal infection (B37.41)
                    chlamydial (A56.01)
                    gonorrhea (A54.01)
                    syphilis (A52.76)
                    trichomonal infection (A59.03)
                    tuberculosis (A18.13)

● N39   **Other disorders of urinary system**

    Excludes2   hematuria NOS (R31.-)
               recurrent or persistent hematuria (N02.-)
               recurrent or persistent hematuria with specified morphological lesion (N02.-)
               proteinuria NOS (R80.-)

    N39.0   **Urinary tract infection, site not specified**
        Use additional code (B95-B97), to identify infectious agent

        Excludes1   candidiasis of urinary tract (B37.4-)
                    neonatal urinary tract infection (P39.3)
                    urinary tract infection of specified site, such as:
                        cystitis (N30.-)
                        urethritis (N34.-)
        Coding Clinic: 2012, Q4, P94

    N39.3   **Stress incontinence (female) (male)**
        Code also any associated overactive bladder (N32.81)
        Excludes1   mixed incontinence (N39.46)

●   N39.4   **Other specified urinary incontinence**
        Code also any associated overactive bladder (N32.81)

        Excludes1   enuresis NOS (R32)
                    functional urinary incontinence (R39.81)
                    urinary incontinence associated with cognitive impairment (R39.81)
                    urinary incontinence NOS (R32)
                    urinary incontinence of nonorganic origin (F98.0)

        N39.41   **Urge incontinence**
                Excludes1   mixed incontinence (N39.46)

        N39.42   **Incontinence without sensory awareness**

        N39.43   **Post-void dribbling**

        N39.44   **Nocturnal enuresis**

        N39.45   **Continuous leakage**

        N39.46   **Mixed incontinence**
                Urge and stress incontinence

        N39.49   **Other specified urinary incontinence**

        N39.490   **Overflow incontinence**

        N39.498   **Other specified urinary incontinence**
                Reflex incontinence
                Total incontinence

    N39.8   **Other specified disorders of urinary system**

    N39.9   **Disorder of urinary system, unspecified**

DISEASES OF MALE GENITAL ORGANS (N40-N53)

(See Plate 387 on page 53.)

● N40   **Enlarged prostate**

    Includes   adenofibromatous hypertrophy of prostate
               benign hypertrophy of the prostate
               Enlargement of prostate gland usually occurring with age and causing obstructed urine flow
               benign prostatic hyperplasia
               benign prostatic hypertrophy
               BPH
               nodular prostate
               polyp of prostate

    Excludes1   benign neoplasms of prostate (adenoma, benign) (fibroadenoma) (fibroma) (myoma) (D29.1)
               malignant neoplasm of prostate (C61)

    N40.0   **Enlarged prostate without lower urinary tract symptoms** ♂   A
        Enlarged prostate without LUTS
        Enlarged prostate NOS

    N40.1   **Enlarged prostate with lower urinary tract symptoms (LUTS)** ♂   A
        Enlarged prostate with LUTS
        Use additional code for associated symptoms, when specified:
            incomplete bladder emptying (R39.14)
            nocturia (R35.1)
            straining on urination (R39.16)
            urinary frequency (R35.0)
            urinary hesitancy (R39.11)
            urinary incontinence (N39.4-)
            urinary obstruction (N13.8)
            urinary retention (R33.8)
            urinary urgency (R39.15)
            weak urinary stream (R39.12)

    N40.2   **Nodular prostate without lower urinary tract symptoms** ♂   A
        Nodular prostate without LUTS

    N40.3   **Nodular prostate with lower urinary tract symptoms** ♂ A
        Use additional code for associated symptoms, when specified:
            incomplete bladder emptying (R39.14)
            nocturia (R35.1)
            straining on urination (R39.16)
            urinary frequency (R35.0)
            urinary hesitancy (R39.11)
            urinary incontinence (N39.4-)
            urinary obstruction (N13.8)
            urinary retention (R33.8)
            urinary urgency (R39.15)
            weak urinary stream (R39.12)

● N41   **Inflammatory diseases of prostate**
    Use additional code (B95-B97), to identify infectious agent

    N41.0   **Acute prostatitis** ♂   A

    N41.1   **Chronic prostatitis** ♂   A

    N41.2   **Abscess of prostate** ♂   A

    N41.3   **Prostatocystitis** ♂   A

    N41.4   **Granulomatous prostatitis** ♂   A

    N41.8   **Other inflammatory diseases of prostate** ♂   A

    N41.9   **Inflammatory disease of prostate, unspecified** ♂   A
        Prostatitis NOS

CHAPTER 14 (N00-N99)

CHAPTER 14 (N00-N99)

Item 14–7   **Hydrocele** is a sac of fluid accumulating in the testes membrane.

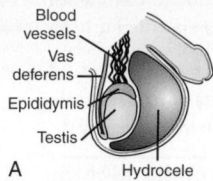
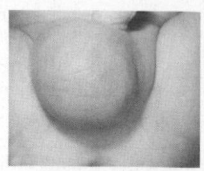

Figure 14-6   **A.** Hydrocele. **B.** Newborn with large right hydrocele. (**B** from Behrman: Nelson Textbook of Pediatrics, ed 18, Saunders, An Imprint of Elsevier, 2007)

● **N42**   **Other and unspecified disorders of prostate**

   N42.0   **Calculus of prostate** ♂   A
      Prostatic stone

   N42.1   **Congestion and hemorrhage of prostate** ♂   A
      Excludes1   enlarged prostate (N40.-)
                  hematuria (R31.-)
                  hyperplasia of prostate (N40.-)
                  inflammatory diseases of prostate (N41.-)

   N42.3   **Dysplasia of prostate** ♂
      Prostatic intraepithelial neoplasia I (PIN I)
      Prostatic intraepithelial neoplasia II (PIN II)
      Excludes1   prostatic intraepithelial neoplasia III (PIN III) (D07.5)

   ● **N42.8**   **Other specified disorders of prostate**

     N42.81   **Prostatodynia syndrome** ♂   A
        Painful prostate syndrome

     N42.82   **Prostatosis syndrome** ♂   A

     N42.83   **Cyst of prostate** ♂   A

     N42.89   **Other specified disorders of prostate** ♂   A

   N42.9   **Disorder of prostate, unspecified** ♂   A

● **N43**   **Hydrocele and spermatocele**

   Includes   hydrocele of spermatic cord, testis or tunica vaginalis

   Excludes1   congenital hydrocele (P83.5)

   N43.0   **Encysted hydrocele** ♂

   N43.1   **Infected hydrocele** ♂
      Use additional code (B95-B97), to identify infectious agent

   N43.2   **Other hydrocele** ♂

   N43.3   **Hydrocele, unspecified** ♂

   ● **N43.4**   **Spermatocele of epididymis**
      Spermatic cyst

     N43.40   **Spermatocele of epididymis, unspecified** ♂

     N43.41   **Spermatocele of epididymis, single** ♂

     N43.42   **Spermatocele of epididymis, multiple** ♂

● **N44**   **Noninflammatory disorders of testis**

   ● **N44.0**   **Torsion of testis**

     N44.00   **Torsion of testis, unspecified** ♂

     N44.01   **Extravaginal torsion of spermatic cord** ♂

     N44.02   **Intravaginal torsion of spermatic cord** ♂
        Torsion of spermatic cord NOS

     N44.03   **Torsion of appendix testis** ♂

     N44.04   **Torsion of appendix epididymis** ♂

   N44.1   **Cyst of tunica albuginea testis** ♂

   N44.2   **Benign cyst of testis** ♂

   N44.8   **Other noninflammatory disorders of the testis** ♂

Item 14-8 Male infertility is the inability of the female sex partner to conceive after one year of unprotected intercourse.
   Azoospermia is no sperm ejaculated and **oligospermia** is few sperm ejaculated—both resulting in infertility. Extratesticular causes such as injury, infections, radiation, and chemotherapy may also cause male infertility.

● **N45**   **Orchitis and epididymitis**
     Orchitis is inflammation of one or both of the testes as a result of mumps or other infection, trauma, or metastasis. **Epididymitis** *is inflammation of the tubular structure that connects the testicle with the vas deferens.*
     Use additional code (B95-B97), to identify infectious agent

   N45.1   **Epididymitis** ♂

   N45.2   **Orchitis** ♂

   N45.3   **Epididymo-orchitis** ♂

   N45.4   **Abscess of epididymis or testis** ♂

● **N46**   **Male infertility**

   Excludes1   vasectomy status (Z98.52)

   ● **N46.0**   **Azoospermia**
      Absolute male infertility
      Male infertility due to germinal (cell) aplasia
      Male infertility due to spermatogenic arrest (complete)

     N46.01   **Organic azoospermia** ♂   A
        Azoospermia NOS

     ● **N46.02**   **Azoospermia due to extratesticular causes**
        Code also associated cause

       N46.021   **Azoospermia due to drug therapy** ♂ A

       N46.022   **Azoospermia due to infection** ♂   A

       N46.023   **Azoospermia due to obstruction of efferent ducts** ♂   A

       N46.024   **Azoospermia due to radiation** ♂   A

       N46.025   **Azoospermia due to systemic disease** ♂   A

       N46.029   **Azoospermia due to other extratesticular causes** ♂   A

   ● **N46.1**   **Oligospermia**
      Male infertility due to germinal cell desquamation
      Male infertility due to hypospermatogenesis
      Male infertility due to incomplete spermatogenic arrest

     N46.11   **Organic oligospermia** ♂   A
        Oligospermia NOS

     ● **N46.12**   **Oligospermia due to extratesticular causes**
        Code also associated cause

       N46.121   **Oligospermia due to drug therapy** ♂ A

       N46.122   **Oligospermia due to infection** ♂   A

       N46.123   **Oligospermia due to obstruction of efferent ducts** ♂   A

       N46.124   **Oligospermia due to radiation** ♂   A

       N46.125   **Oligospermia due to systemic disease** ♂   A

       N46.129   **Oligospermia due to other extratesticular causes** ♂   A

   N46.8   **Other male infertility** ♂   A

   N46.9   **Male infertility, unspecified** ♂   A

● **N47**   **Disorders of prepuce**

   N47.0   **Adherent prepuce, newborn** ♂   N

   N47.1   **Phimosis** ♂

   N47.2   **Paraphimosis** ♂

   N47.3   **Deficient foreskin** ♂

   N47.4   **Benign cyst of prepuce** ♂

   N47.5   **Adhesions of prepuce and glans penis** ♂

◀ New   ◀◀ Revised   ~~deleted~~ Deleted   Excludes 1   Excludes 2   Includes   Use additional   Code first   Code also   Unspecified

OGCR Official Guidelines   **X** Assign placeholder X   ● Use Additional Character(s)   ▶ Manifestation Code   **Coding Clinic**

N47.6   **Balanoposthitis** ♂
     Use additional code (B95-B97), to identify infectious
       agent
     Excludes1   balanitis (N48.1)

N47.7   **Other inflammatory diseases of prepuce** ♂
     Use additional code (B95-B97), to identify infectious
       agent

N47.8   **Other disorders of prepuce** ♂

● **N48**   **Other disorders of penis**

N48.0   **Leukoplakia of penis** ♂
     Balanitis xerotica obliterans
     Kraurosis of penis
     Lichen sclerosus of external male genital organs
     Excludes1   carcinoma in situ of penis (D07.4)

N48.1   **Balanitis** ♂
     Use additional code (B95-B97), to identify infectious
       agent
     Excludes1   amebic balanitis (A06.8)
                 balanitis xerotica obliterans (N48.0)
                 candidal balanitis (B37.42)
                 gonococcal balanitis (A54.23)
                 herpesviral [herpes simplex] balanitis
                     (A60.01)

● **N48.2**   **Other inflammatory disorders of penis**
     Use additional code (B95-B97), to identify infectious
       agent
     Excludes1   balanitis (N48.1)
                 balanitis xerotica obliterans (N48.0)
                 balanoposthitis (N47.6)

N48.21   **Abscess of corpus cavernosum and penis** ♂

N48.22   **Cellulitis of corpus cavernosum and penis** ♂

N48.29   **Other inflammatory disorders of penis** ♂

● **N48.3**   **Priapism**
     Painful erection
     Code first underlying cause

N48.30   **Priapism, unspecified** ♂

N48.31   **Priapism due to trauma** ♂

▶ **N48.32**   *Priapism due to disease classified elsewhere* ♂

N48.33   **Priapism, drug-induced** ♂

N48.39   **Other priapism** ♂

N48.5   **Ulcer of penis** ♂

N48.6   **Induration penis plastica** ♂
     Peyronie's disease
     Plastic induration of penis

● **N48.8**   **Other specified disorders of penis**

N48.81   **Thrombosis of superficial vein of penis** ♂

N48.82   **Acquired torsion of penis** ♂
     Acquired torsion of penis NOS
     Excludes1   congenital torsion of penis
                   (Q55.63)

N48.83   **Acquired buried penis** ♂
     Excludes1   congenital hidden penis (Q55.64)

N48.89   **Other specified disorders of penis** ♂

N48.9   **Disorder of penis, unspecified** ♂

● **N49**   **Inflammatory disorders of male genital organs, not elsewhere classified**
     Use additional code (B95-B97), to identify infectious agent
     Excludes1   inflammation of penis (N48.1, N48.2-)
                 orchitis and epididymitis (N45.-)

N49.0   **Inflammatory disorders of seminal vesicle** ♂
     Vesiculitis NOS

N49.1   **Inflammatory disorders of spermatic cord, tunica vaginalis and vas deferens** ♂
     Vasitis

N49.2   **Inflammatory disorders of scrotum** ♂

N49.3   **Fournier gangrene** ♂

Item 14–9 Seminal vesiculitis is an inflammation of the seminal vesicle. Spermatocele is a benign cystic accumulation of sperm arising from the head of the epididymis. Torsion of the testis is a medical emergency occurring most commonly in boys 7 to 12 years of age and results from a congenital abnormality of the covering of the testis allowing the testis to twist within its sac and cutting off the blood supply to the testis.

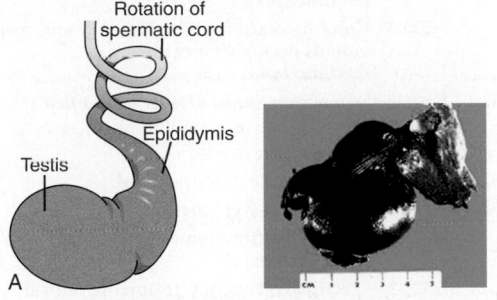

Figure 14-7   **A.** Torsion of testis. **B.** Torsion of the testis. (**B** from Kumar: Robbins and Cotran: Pathologic Basis of Disease, ed 8, Saunders, An Imprint of Elsevier, 2009)

N49.8   **Inflammatory disorders of other specified male genital organs** ♂
     Inflammation of multiple sites in male genital organs

N49.9   **Inflammatory disorder of unspecified male genital organ** ♂
     Abscess of unspecified male genital organ
     Boil of unspecified male genital organ
     Carbuncle of unspecified male genital organ
     Cellulitis of unspecified male genital organ

● **N50**   **Other and unspecified disorders of male genital organs**
     Excludes2   torsion of testis (N44.0-)

N50.0   **Atrophy of testis** ♂

N50.1   **Vascular disorders of male genital organs** ♂
     Hematocele, NOS, of male genital organs
     Hemorrhage of male genital organs
     Thrombosis of male genital organs

N50.3   **Cyst of epididymis** ♂

N50.8   **Other specified disorders of male genital organs** ♂
     Atrophy of scrotum, seminal vesicle, spermatic cord,
       tunica vaginalis and vas deferens
     Edema of scrotum, seminal vesicle, spermatic cord,
       testis, tunica vaginalis and vas deferens
     Hypertrophy of scrotum, seminal vesicle, spermatic
       cord, testis, tunica vaginalis and vas deferens
     Ulcer of scrotum, seminal vesicle, spermatic cord, testis,
       tunica vaginalis and vas deferens
     Chylocele, tunica vaginalis (nonfilarial) NOS
     Urethroscrotal fistula
     Stricture of spermatic cord, tunica vaginalis, and vas
       deferens

N50.9   **Disorder of male genital organs, unspecified** ♂

▶ **N51**   *Disorders of male genital organs in diseases classified elsewhere* ♂
     Code first underlying disease, such as:
     filariasis (B74.0-B74.9)
     Excludes1   amebic balanitis (A06.8)
                 candidal balanitis (B37.42)
                 gonococcal balanitis (A54.23)
                 gonococcal prostatitis (A54.22)
                 herpesviral [herpes simplex] balanitis (A60.01)
                 trichomonal prostatitis (A59.02)
                 tuberculous prostatitis (A18.14)

CHAPTER 14 (N00-N99)

CHAPTER 14 (N00-N99)

● **N52**   **Male erectile dysfunction**
> **Excludes1**   psychogenic impotence (F52.21)

  ● **N52.0**   **Vasculogenic erectile dysfunction**

     N52.01   Erectile dysfunction due to arterial insufficiency ♂   **A**

     N52.02   Corporo-venous occlusive erectile dysfunction ♂   **A**

     N52.03   Combined arterial insufficiency and corporo-venous occlusive erectile dysfunction ♂   **A**

  ▶ **N52.1**   *Erectile dysfunction due to diseases classified elsewhere* ♂   **A**
> *Code first underlying disease*

   N52.2   Drug-induced erectile dysfunction ♂   **A**

  ● **N52.3**   **Post-surgical erectile dysfunction**

     N52.31   Erectile dysfunction following radical prostatectomy ♂   **A**

     N52.32   Erectile dysfunction following radical cystectomy ♂   **A**

     N52.33   Erectile dysfunction following urethral surgery ♂   **A**

     N52.34   Erectile dysfunction following simple prostatectomy ♂   **A**

     N52.39   Other post-surgical erectile dysfunction ♂   **A**

   N52.8   Other male erectile dysfunction ♂   **A**

   N52.9   Male erectile dysfunction, unspecified ♂   **A**
> Impotence NOS

● **N53**   **Other male sexual dysfunction**
> **Excludes1**   psychogenic sexual dysfunction (F52.-)

  ● **N53.1**   **Ejaculatory dysfunction**
> **Excludes1**   premature ejaculation (F52.4)

     N53.11   Retarded ejaculation ♂

     N53.12   Painful ejaculation ♂

     N53.13   Anejaculatory orgasm ♂

     N53.14   Retrograde ejaculation ♂

     N53.19   Other ejaculatory dysfunction ♂
> Ejaculatory dysfunction NOS

   N53.8   Other male sexual dysfunction ♂

   N53.9   Unspecified male sexual dysfunction ♂

DISORDERS OF BREAST (N60-N65)

> **Excludes1**   disorders of breast associated with childbirth (O91-O92)

● **N60**   **Benign mammary dysplasia**
> *Benign lumpiness of breast*
> **Includes**   fibrocystic mastopathy

  ● **N60.0**   **Solitary cyst of breast**
> Cyst of breast

     N60.01   Solitary cyst of right breast

     N60.02   Solitary cyst of left breast

     N60.09   Solitary cyst of unspecified breast

  ● **N60.1**   **Diffuse cystic mastopathy**
> Cystic breast
> Fibrocystic disease of breast
> **Excludes1**   diffuse cystic mastopathy with epithelial proliferation (N60.3-)

     N60.11   Diffuse cystic mastopathy of right breast   **A**

     N60.12   Diffuse cystic mastopathy of left breast   **A**

     N60.19   Diffuse cystic mastopathy of unspecified breast   **A**

  ● **N60.2**   **Fibroadenosis of breast**
> Adenofibrosis of breast
> **Excludes2**   fibroadenoma of breast (D24.-)

     N60.21   Fibroadenosis of right breast

     N60.22   Fibroadenosis of left breast

     N60.29   Fibroadenosis of unspecified breast

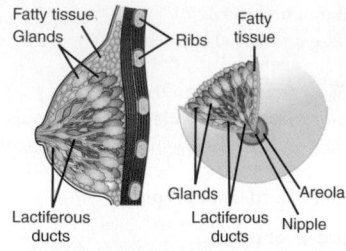

Figure 14-8   Breast.

  ● **N60.3**   **Fibrosclerosis of breast**
> Cystic mastopathy with epithelial proliferation

     N60.31   Fibrosclerosis of right breast

     N60.32   Fibrosclerosis of left breast

     N60.39   Fibrosclerosis of unspecified breast

  ● **N60.4**   **Mammary duct ectasia**

     N60.41   Mammary duct ectasia of right breast

     N60.42   Mammary duct ectasia of left breast

     N60.49   Mammary duct ectasia of unspecified breast

  ● **N60.8**   **Other benign mammary dysplasias**

     N60.81   Other benign mammary dysplasias of right breast

     N60.82   Other benign mammary dysplasias of left breast

     N60.89   Other benign mammary dysplasias of unspecified breast

  ● **N60.9**   **Unspecified benign mammary dysplasia**

     N60.91   Unspecified benign mammary dysplasia of right breast

     N60.92   Unspecified benign mammary dysplasia of left breast

     N60.99   Unspecified benign mammary dysplasia of unspecified breast

N61   **Inflammatory disorders of breast**
> Abscess (acute) (chronic) (nonpuerperal) of areola
> Abscess (acute) (chronic) (nonpuerperal) of breast
> Carbuncle of breast
> Infective mastitis (acute) (subacute) (nonpuerperal)
> Mastitis (acute) (subacute) (nonpuerperal) NOS
> **Excludes1**   inflammatory carcinoma of breast (C50.9)
>   inflammatory disorder of breast associated with childbirth (O91.-)
>   neonatal infective mastitis (P39.0)
>   thrombophlebitis of breast [Mondor's disease] (I80.8)

N62   **Hypertrophy of breast**
> Gynecomastia
> Hypertrophy of breast NOS
> Massive pubertal hypertrophy of breast
> **Excludes1**   breast engorgement of newborn (P83.4)
>   disproportion of reconstructed breast (N65.1)

N63   **Unspecified lump in breast**
> Nodule(s) NOS in breast

● **N64**   **Other disorders of breast**
> **Excludes2**   mechanical complication of breast prosthesis and implant (T85.4-)

   N64.0   Fissure and fistula of nipple

   N64.1   Fat necrosis of breast
> Fat necrosis (segmental) of breast
> *Code first breast necrosis due to breast graft (T85.89)*

   N64.2   Atrophy of breast

   N64.3   Galactorrhea not associated with childbirth
> *Excessive or spontaneous flow of milk*

   N64.4   Mastodynia

◀ New   ◀▥ Revised   ~~deleted~~ Deleted   Excludes 1   Excludes 2   Includes   Use additional   Code first   Code also   Unspecified

OGCR Official Guidelines   **X** Assign placeholder X   ● Use Additional Character(s)   ▶ Manifestation Code   **Coding Clinic**

- **N64.5**   Other signs and symptoms in breast
  - **Excludes2**   abnormal findings on diagnostic imaging of breast (R92.-)
  - **N64.51**   Induration of breast
  - **N64.52**   Nipple discharge
    - **Excludes1**   abnormal findings in nipple discharge (R89.-)
  - **N64.53**   Retraction of nipple
  - **N64.59**   Other signs and symptoms in breast
- **N64.8**   Other specified disorders of breast
  - **N64.81**   Ptosis of breast   A
    - **Excludes1**   ptosis of native breast in relation to reconstructed breast (N65.1)
  - **N64.82**   Hypoplasia of breast   A
    - Micromastia
    - **Excludes1**   congenital absence of breast (Q83.0)
    - hypoplasia of native breast in relation to reconstructed breast (N65.1)
  - **N64.89**   Other specified disorders of breast
    - Galactocele
    - Subinvolution of breast (postlactational)
  - **N64.9**   Disorder of breast, **unspecified**

- **N65**   Deformity and disproportion of reconstructed breast
  - **N65.0**   Deformity of reconstructed breast   A
    - Contour irregularity in reconstructed breast
    - Excess tissue in reconstructed breast
    - Misshapen reconstructed breast
  - **N65.1**   Disproportion of reconstructed breast   A
    - Breast asymmetry between native breast and reconstructed breast
    - Disproportion between native breast and reconstructed breast

---

INFLAMMATORY DISEASES OF FEMALE PELVIC ORGANS (N70-N77)

- **Excludes1**   inflammatory diseases of female pelvic organs complicating:
  - abortion or ectopic or molar pregnancy (O00-O07, O08.0)
  - pregnancy, childbirth and the puerperium (O23.-, O75.3, O85, O86.-)

(See Plate 360 on page 80.)

- **N70**   Salpingitis and oophoritis
  - *Oophoritis = inflammation of ovary*
  - *Salpingitis = inflammation of fallopian tube*
  - **Includes**   abscess (of) fallopian tube
    - abscess (of) ovary
    - pyosalpinx
    - salpingo-oophoritis
    - tubo-ovarian abscess
    - tubo-ovarian inflammatory disease
  - Use additional code (B95-B97), to identify infectious agent
  - **Excludes1**   gonococcal infection (A54.24)
    - tuberculous infection (A18.17)
  - **N70.0**   Acute salpingitis and oophoritis
    - **N70.01**   Acute salpingitis   ♀
    - **N70.02**   Acute oophoritis   ♀
    - **N70.03**   Acute salpingitis and oophoritis   ♀
  - **N70.1**   Chronic salpingitis and oophoritis
    - Hydrosalpinx
    - **N70.11**   Chronic salpingitis   ♀
    - **N70.12**   Chronic oophoritis   ♀
    - **N70.13**   Chronic salpingitis and oophoritis   ♀
  - **N70.9**   Salpingitis and oophoritis, unspecified
    - **N70.91**   Salpingitis, **unspecified**   ♀
    - **N70.92**   Oophoritis, **unspecified**   ♀
    - **N70.93**   Salpingitis and oophoritis, **unspecified**   ♀

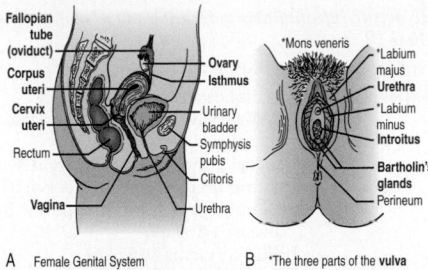

Figure 14-9   **A.** Female genital system. **B.** External female genital system. (From Buck CJ: Step-by-Step Medical Coding, ed 2011, Philadelphia, WB Saunders, 2011)

Item 14–10 Salpingitis is an infection of one or both fallopian tubes. **Oophoritis** is an infection of one or both ovaries.

- **N71**   Inflammatory disease of uterus, except cervix
  - **Includes**   endo (myo) metritis
    - metritis
    - myometritis
    - pyometra
    - uterine abscess
  - Use additional code (B95-B97), to identify infectious agent
  - **Excludes1**   hyperplastic endometritis (N85.0-)
    - infection of uterus following delivery (O85, O86.-)
  - **N71.0**   Acute inflammatory disease of uterus   ♀
  - **N71.1**   Chronic inflammatory disease of uterus   ♀
  - **N71.9**   Inflammatory disease of uterus, **unspecified**   ♀
- **N72**   Inflammatory disease of cervix uteri   ♀
  - **Includes**   cervicitis (with or without erosion or ectropion)
    - endocervicitis (with or without erosion or ectropion)
    - exocervicitis (with or without erosion or ectropion)
  - Use additional code (B95-B97), to identify infectious agent
  - **Excludes1**   erosion and ectropion of cervix without cervicitis (N86)
- **N73**   Other female pelvic inflammatory diseases
  - Use additional code (B95-B97), to identify infectious agent
  - **N73.0**   Acute parametritis and pelvic cellulitis   ♀
    - Abscess of broad ligament
    - Abscess of parametrium
    - Pelvic cellulitis, female
  - **N73.1**   Chronic parametritis and pelvic cellulitis   ♀
    - Any condition in N73.0 specified as chronic
    - **Excludes1**   tuberculous parametritis and pelvic cellultis (A18.17)
  - **N73.2**   **Unspecified** parametritis and pelvic cellulitis   ♀
    - Any condition in N73.0 unspecified whether acute or chronic
  - **N73.3**   Female acute pelvic peritonitis   ♀
  - **N73.4**   Female chronic pelvic peritonitis   ♀
    - **Excludes1**   tuberculous pelvic (female) peritonitis (A18.17)
  - **N73.5**   Female pelvic peritonitis, **unspecified**   ♀
  - **N73.6**   Female pelvic peritoneal adhesions (postinfective)   ♀
    - **Excludes2**   postprocedural pelvic peritoneal adhesions (N99.4)
  - **N73.8**   Other specified female pelvic inflammatory diseases   ♀
  - **N73.9**   Female pelvic inflammatory disease, **unspecified**   ♀
    - Female pelvic infection or inflammation NOS

CHAPTER 14 (N00-N99)

CHAPTER 14 (N00-N99)

▶ **N74**   *Female pelvic inflammatory disorders in diseases classified elsewhere* ♀

     Code first underlying disease

     Excludes1   chlamydial cervicitis (A56.02)
         chlamydial pelvic inflammatory disease (A56.11)
         gonococcal cervicitis (A54.03)
         gonococcal pelvic inflammatory disease (A54.24)
         herpesviral [herpes simplex] cervicitis (A60.03)
         herpesviral [herpes simplex] pelvic inflammatory disease (A60.09)
         syphilitic cervicitis (A52.76)
         syphilitic pelvic inflammatory disease (A52.76)
         trichomonal cervicitis (A59.09)
         tuberculous cervicitis (A18.16)
         tuberculous pelvic inflammatory disease (A18.17)

● **N75**   **Diseases of Bartholin's gland**

   N75.0   **Cyst of Bartholin's gland** ♀
       Cysts filled with liquid or semisolid material.

   N75.1   **Abscess of Bartholin's gland** ♀
       Localized collection of pus

   N75.8   **Other diseases of Bartholin's gland** ♀
       Bartholinitis

   N75.9   **Disease of Bartholin's gland, unspecified** ♀

● **N76**   **Other inflammation of vagina and vulva**

     Use additional code (B95-B97), to identify infectious agent

     Excludes2   senile (atrophic) vaginitis (N95.2)
         vulvar vestibulitis (N94.810)

   N76.0   **Acute vaginitis** ♀
       Acute vulvovaginitis
       Vaginitis NOS
       Vulvovaginitis NOS

   N76.1   **Subacute and chronic vaginitis** ♀
       Chronic vulvovaginitis
       Subacute vulvovaginitis

   N76.2   **Acute vulvitis** ♀
       Vulvitis NOS

   N76.3   **Subacute and chronic vulvitis** ♀

   N76.4   **Abscess of vulva** ♀
       Furuncle of vulva

   N76.5   **Ulceration of vagina** ♀

   N76.6   **Ulceration of vulva** ♀

 ● **N76.8**   **Other specified inflammation of vagina and vulva**

     N76.81   **Mucositis (ulcerative) of vagina and vulva** ♀

         Code also type of associated therapy, such as:
           antineoplastic and immunosuppressive drugs (T45.1X-)
           radiological procedure and radiotherapy (Y84.2)

         Excludes2   gastrointestinal mucositis (ulcerative) (K92.81)
           nasal mucositis (ulcerative) (J34.81)
           oral mucositis (ulcerative) (K12.3-)

     N76.89   **Other specified inflammation of vagina and vulva** ♀

● **N77**   **Vulvovaginal ulceration and inflammation in diseases classified elsewhere**

 ▶ **N77.0**   *Ulceration of vulva in diseases classified elsewhere* ♀

     Code first underlying disease, such as:
     Behçet's disease (M35.2)

     Excludes1   ulceration of vulva in gonococcal infection (A54.02)
         ulceration of vulva in herpesviral [herpes simplex] infection (A60.04)
         ulceration of vulva in syphilis (A51.0)
         ulceration of vulva in tuberculosis (A18.18)

▶ **N77.1**   *Vaginitis, vulvitis and vulvovaginitis in diseases classified elsewhere* ♀

     Code first underlying disease, such as:
     pinworm (B80)

     Excludes1   candidial vulvovaginitis (B37.3)
         chlamydial vulvovaginitis (A56.02)
         gonococcal vulvovaginitis (A54.02)
         herpesviral [herpes simplex] vulvovaginitis (A60.04)
         trichomonal vulvovaginitis (A59.01)
         tuberculous vulvovaginitis (A18.18)
         vulvovaginitis in early syphilis (A51.0)
         vulvovaginitis in late syphilis (A52.76)

NONINFLAMMATORY DISORDERS OF FEMALE GENITAL TRACT (N80-N98)

● **N80**   **Endometriosis**

   N80.0   **Endometriosis of uterus** ♀
       Adenomyosis

       Excludes1   stromal endometriosis (D39.0)

   N80.1   **Endometriosis of ovary** ♀

   N80.2   **Endometriosis of fallopian tube** ♀

   N80.3   **Endometriosis of pelvic peritoneum** ♀

   N80.4   **Endometriosis of rectovaginal septum and vagina** ♀

   N80.5   **Endometriosis of intestine** ♀

   N80.6   **Endometriosis in cutaneous scar** ♀

   N80.8   **Other endometriosis** ♀

   N80.9   **Endometriosis, unspecified** ♀

● **N81**   **Female genital prolapse**

     Excludes1   genital prolapse complicating pregnancy, labor or delivery (O34.5-)
         prolapse and hernia of ovary and fallopian tube (N83.4)
         prolapse of vaginal vault after hysterectomy (N99.3)

   N81.0   **Urethrocele** ♀

       Excludes1   urethrocele with cystocele (N81.1-)
         urethrocele with prolapse of uterus (N81.2-N81.4)

 ● **N81.1**   **Cystocele**
       Cystocele with urethrocele
       Cystourethrocele

       Excludes1   cystocele with prolapse of uterus (N81.2-N81.4)

     N81.10   **Cystocele, unspecified** ♀
         Prolapse of (anterior) vaginal wall NOS

     N81.11   **Cystocele, midline** ♀

     N81.12   **Cystocele, lateral** ♀
         Paravaginal cystocele

Item 14–11 Endometriosis is a condition for which no clear cause has been identified. Endometrial tissue is expelled from the uterus into the abdominal cavity and can implant onto a variety of organs. Classification is based on the site of implant of the endometrial tissue.

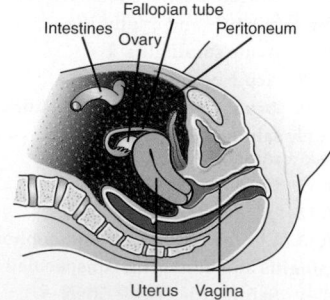

Figure 14-10   Sites of potential endometrial implants.

◀ New   ⬅ Revised   ~~deleted~~ Deleted   Excludes 1   Excludes 2   Includes   Use additional   Code first   Code also   Unspecified

OGCR Official Guidelines   **X** Assign placeholder X   ● Use Additional Character(s)   ▶ Manifestation Code   **Coding Clinic**

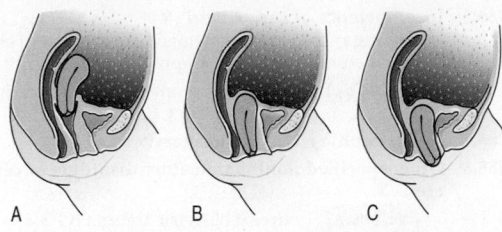

Figure 14-11   Three stages of uterine prolapse. **A.** Uterus is prolapsed. **B.** Vagina and uterus are prolapsed (incomplete uterovaginal prolapse). **C.** Vagina and uterus are completely prolapsed and are exposed through the external genitalia (complete uterovaginal prolapse).

N81.2   **Incomplete uterovaginal prolapse** ♀
     First degree uterine prolapse
     Prolapse of cervix NOS
     Second degree uterine prolapse
     Excludes1   cervical stump prolaspe (N81.85)

N81.3   **Complete uterovaginal prolapse** ♀
     Procidentia (uteri) NOS
     Third degree uterine prolapse

N81.4   **Uterovaginal prolapse, unspecified** ♀
     Prolapse of uterus NOS

N81.5   **Vaginal enterocele** ♀
     Excludes1   enterocele with prolapse of uterus
                   (N81.2-N81.4)

N81.6   **Rectocele** ♀
     Prolapse of posterior vaginal wall
     Use additional code for any associated fecal
         incontinence, if applicable (R15.-)
     Excludes2   perineocele (N81.81)
                   rectal prolapse (K62.3)
                   rectocele with prolapse of uterus
                   (N81.2-N81.4)

● **N81.8**   **Other female genital prolapse**

     N81.81   **Perineocele** ♀

     N81.82   **Incompetence or weakening of pubocervical tissue** ♀

     N81.83   **Incompetence or weakening of rectovaginal tissue** ♀

     N81.84   **Pelvic muscle wasting** ♀
           Disuse atrophy of pelvic muscles and anal
               sphincter

     N81.85   **Cervical stump prolapse** ♀

     N81.89   **Other female genital prolapse** ♀
           Deficient perineum
           Old laceration of muscles of pelvic floor

N81.9   **Female genital prolapse, unspecified** ♀

● **N82**   **Fistulae involving female genital tract**
     Excludes1   vesicointestinal fistulae (N32.1)

N82.0   **Vesicovaginal fistula** ♀

N82.1   **Other female urinary-genital tract fistulae** ♀
     Cervicovesical fistula
     Ureterovaginal fistula
     Urethrovaginal fistula
     Uteroureteric fistula
     Uterovesical fistula

N82.2   **Fistula of vagina to small intestine** ♀

N82.3   **Fistula of vagina to large intestine** ♀
     Rectovaginal fistula

N82.4   **Other female intestinal-genital tract fistulae** ♀
     Intestinouterine fistula

N82.5   **Female genital tract-skin fistulae** ♀
     Uterus to abdominal wall fistula
     Vaginoperineal fistula

N82.8   **Other female genital tract fistulae** ♀

N82.9   **Female genital tract fistula, unspecified** ♀

● **N83**   **Noninflammatory disorders of ovary, fallopian tube and broad ligament**
     Excludes2   hydrosalpinx (N70.1-)

N83.0   **Follicular cyst of ovary** ♀
     Cyst of graafian follicle
     Hemorrhagic follicular cyst (of ovary)

N83.1   **Corpus luteum cyst** ♀
     Hemorrhagic corpus luteum cyst

● **N83.2**   **Other and unspecified ovarian cysts**
     Excludes1   developmental ovarian cyst (Q50.1)
                   neoplastic ovarian cyst (D27.-)
                   polycystic ovarian syndrome (E28.2)
                   Stein-Leventhal syndrome (E28.2)

     N83.20   **Unspecified ovarian cysts** ♀

     N83.29   **Other ovarian cysts** ♀
           Retention cyst of ovary
           Simple cyst of ovary

● **N83.3**   **Acquired atrophy of ovary and fallopian tube**
     N83.31   **Acquired atrophy of ovary** ♀
     N83.32   **Acquired atrophy of fallopian tube** ♀
     N83.33   **Acquired atrophy of ovary and fallopian tube** ♀

N83.4   **Prolapse and hernia of ovary and fallopian tube** ♀

● **N83.5**   **Torsion of ovary, ovarian pedicle and fallopian tube**
     Torsion of accessory tube

     N83.51   **Torsion of ovary and ovarian pedicle** ♀

     N83.52   **Torsion of fallopian tube** ♀
           Torsion of hydatid of Morgagni

     N83.53   **Torsion of ovary, ovarian pedicle and fallopian tube** ♀

N83.6   **Hematosalpinx** ♀
     Excludes1   hematosalpinx (with) (in):
                   hematocolpos (N89.7)
                   hematometra (N85.7)
                   tubal pregnancy (O00.1)

N83.7   **Hematoma of broad ligament** ♀

N83.8   **Other noninflammatory disorders of ovary, fallopian tube and broad ligament** ♀
     Broad ligament laceration syndrome [Allen-Masters]

N83.9   **Noninflammatory disorder of ovary, fallopian tube and broad ligament, unspecified** ♀

● **N84**   **Polyp of female genital tract**
     Excludes1   adenomatous polyp (D28.-)
                   placental polyp (O90.89)

N84.0   **Polyp of corpus uteri** ♀
     Polyp of endometrium
     Polyp of uterus NOS
     Excludes1   polypoid endometrial hyperplasia
                   (N85.0-)

N84.1   **Polyp of cervix uteri** ♀
     Mucous polyp of cervix

N84.2   **Polyp of vagina** ♀

N84.3   **Polyp of vulva** ♀
     Polyp of labia

N84.8   **Polyp of other parts of female genital tract** ♀

N84.9   **Polyp of female genital tract, unspecified** ♀

● **N85**   **Other noninflammatory disorders of uterus, except cervix**
     Excludes1   endometriosis (N80.-)
                   inflammatory diseases of uterus (N71.-)
                   noninflammatory disorders of cervix, except
                      malposition (N86-N88)
                   polyp of corpus uteri (N84.0)
                   uterine prolapse (N81.-)

● **N85.0**   **Endometrial hyperplasia**

     N85.00   **Endometrial hyperplasia, unspecified** ♀
           Hyperplasia (adenomatous) (cystic)
               (glandular) of endometrium
           Hyperplastic endometritis

N85.01 Benign endometrial hyperplasia ♀
Endometrial hyperplasia (complex) (simple)
without atypia

N85.02 Endometrial intraepithelial neoplasia [EIN] ♀
Endometrial hyperplasia with atypia

> **Excludes1** malignant neoplasm of
> endometrium (with
> endometrial intraepithelial
> neoplasia [EIN]) (C54.1)

N85.2 Hypertrophy of uterus ♀
Bulky or enlarged uterus

> **Excludes1** puerperal hypertrophy of uterus (O90.89)

N85.3 Subinvolution of uterus ♀

> **Excludes1** puerperal subinvolution of uterus
> (O90.89)

N85.4 Malposition of uterus ♀
Anteversion of uterus
Retroflexion of uterus
Retroversion of uterus

> **Excludes1** malposition of uterus complicating
> pregnancy, labor or delivery (O34.5-,
> O65.5)

N85.5 Inversion of uterus ♀

> **Excludes1** current obstetric trauma (O71.2)
> postpartum inversion of uterus (O71.2)

N85.6 Intrauterine synechiae ♀

N85.7 Hematometra ♀
Hematosalpinx with hematometra

> **Excludes1** hematometra with hematocolpos (N89.7)

N85.8 Other specified noninflammatory disorders of uterus ♀
Atrophy of uterus, acquired
Fibrosis of uterus NOS

N85.9 Noninflammatory disorder of uterus, unspecified ♀
Disorder of uterus NOS

N86 Erosion and ectropion of cervix uteri ♀
Decubitus (trophic) ulcer of cervix
Eversion of cervix

> **Excludes1** erosion and ectropion of cervix with cervicitis
> (N72)

● **N87 Dysplasia of cervix uteri**

> **Excludes1** abnormal results from cervical cytologic
> examination without histologic confirmation
> (R87.61-)
> carcinoma in situ of cervix uteri (D06.-)
> cervical intraepithelial neoplasia III [CIN III]
> (D06.-)
> HGSIL of cervix (R87.613)
> severe dysplasia of cervix uteri (D06.-)

N87.0 Mild cervical dysplasia ♀
Cervical intraepithelial neoplasia I [CIN I]

N87.1 Moderate cervical dysplasia ♀
Cervical intraepithelial neoplasia II [CIN II]

N87.9 Dysplasia of cervix uteri, unspecified ♀
Anaplasia of cervix
Cervical atypism
Cervical dysplasia NOS

● **N88 Other noninflammatory disorders of cervix uteri**

> **Excludes2** inflammatory disease of cervix (N72)
> polyp of cervix (N84.1)

N88.0 Leukoplakia of cervix uteri ♀

N88.1 Old laceration of cervix uteri ♀
Adhesions of cervix

> **Excludes1** current obstetric trauma (O71.3)

N88.2 Stricture and stenosis of cervix uteri ♀

> **Excludes1** stricture and stenosis of cervix uteri
> complicating labor (O65.5)

N88.3 Incompetence of cervix uteri ♀
Investigation and management of (suspected) cervical
incompetence in a nonpregnant woman

> **Excludes1** cervical incompetence complicating
> pregnancy (O34.3-)

N88.4 Hypertrophic elongation of cervix uteri ♀

N88.8 Other specified noninflammatory disorders of cervix uteri ♀

> **Excludes1** current obstetric trauma (O71.3)

N88.9 Noninflammatory disorder of cervix uteri, unspecified ♀

● **N89 Other noninflammatory disorders of vagina**

> **Excludes1** abnormal results from vaginal cytologic
> examination without histologic confirmation
> (R87.62-)
> carcinoma in situ of vagina (D07.2)
> HGSIL of vagina (R87.623)
> inflammation of vagina (N76.-)
> senile (atrophic) vaginitis (N95.2)
> severe dysplasia of vagina (D07.2)
> trichomonal leukorrhea (A59.00)
> vaginal intraepithelial neoplasia [VAIN], grade
> III (D07.2)

N89.0 Mild vaginal dysplasia ♀
Vaginal intraepithelial neoplasia [VAIN], grade I

N89.1 Moderate vaginal dysplasia ♀
Vaginal intraepithelial neoplasia [VAIN], grade II

N89.3 Dysplasia of vagina, unspecified ♀

N89.4 Leukoplakia of vagina ♀

N89.5 Stricture and atresia of vagina ♀
Vaginal adhesions   Vaginal stenosis

> **Excludes1** congenital atresia or stricture (Q52.4)
> postprocedural adhesions of vagina
> (N99.2)

N89.6 Tight hymenal ring ♀
Rigid hymen   Tight introitus

> **Excludes1** imperforate hymen (Q52.3)

N89.7 Hematocolpos ♀
Hematocolpos with hematometra or hematosalpinx

N89.8 Other specified noninflammatory disorders of vagina ♀
Leukorrhea NOS
Old vaginal laceration
Pessary ulcer of vagina

> **Excludes1** current obstetric trauma (O70.-, O71.4,
> O71.7-O71.8)
> old laceration involving muscles of pelvic
> floor (N81.8)

N89.9 Noninflammatory disorder of vagina, unspecified ♀

● **N90 Other noninflammatory disorders of vulva and perineum**

> **Excludes1** anogenital (venereal) warts (A63.0)
> carcinoma in situ of vulva (D07.1)
> condyloma acuminatum (A63.0)
> current obstetric trauma (O70.-, O71.7-O71.8)
> inflammation of vulva (N76.-)
> severe dysplasia of vulva (D07.1)
> vulvar intraepithelial neoplasm III [VIN III]
> (D07.1)

N90.0 Mild vulvar dysplasia ♀
Vulvar intraepithelial neoplasia [VIN], grade I

N90.1 Moderate vulvar dysplasia ♀
Vulvar intraepithelial neoplasia [VIN], grade II

N90.3 Dysplasia of vulva, unspecified ♀

N90.4 Leukoplakia of vulva ♀
Dystrophy of vulva
Kraurosis of vulva
Lichen sclerosus of external female genital organs

N90.5 Atrophy of vulva ♀
Stenosis of vulva

N90.6 Hypertrophy of vulva ♀
Hypertrophy of labia

N90.7 Vulvar cyst ♀

◀ New   ◀▦ Revised   d̶e̶l̶e̶t̶e̶d̶ Deleted   Excludes 1   Excludes 2   Includes   Use additional   Code first   Code also   Unspecified

OGCR Official Guidelines   X Assign placeholder X   ● Use Additional Character(s)   ▌ Manifestation Code   **Coding Clinic**

● **N90.8** **Other specified noninflammatory disorders of vulva and perineum**

   ● **N90.81** **Female genital mutilation status**
      Female genital cutting status

      N90.810 **Female genital mutilation status, unspecified** ♀
         Female genital cutting status, unspecified
         Female genital mutilation status NOS

      N90.811 **Female genital mutilation Type I status** ♀
         Clitorectomy status
         Female genital cutting Type I status

      N90.812 **Female genital mutilation Type II status** ♀
         Clitorectomy with excision of labia minora status
         Female genital cutting Type II status

      N90.813 **Female genital mutilation Type III status** ♀
         Female genital cutting Type III status
         Infibulation status

      N90.818 **Other female genital mutilation status** ♀
         Female genital cutting Type IV status
         Female genital mutilation Type IV status
         Other female genital cutting status

   N90.89 **Other specified noninflammatory disorders of vulva and perineum** ♀
      Adhesions of vulva
      Hypertrophy of clitoris

● **N90.9** **Noninflammatory disorder of vulva and perineum, unspecified** ♀

● **N91** **Absent, scanty and rare menstruation**
   Excludes1 ovarian dysfunction (E28.-)

N91.0 **Primary amenorrhea** ♀

N91.1 **Secondary amenorrhea** ♀

N91.2 **Amenorrhea, unspecified** ♀

N91.3 **Primary oligomenorrhea** ♀

N91.4 **Secondary oligomenorrhea** ♀

N91.5 **Oligomenorrhea, unspecified** ♀
   Hypomenorrhea NOS

● **N92** **Excessive, frequent and irregular menstruation**
   Excludes1 postmenopausal bleeding (N95.0)
            precocious puberty (menstruation) (E30.1)

N92.0 **Excessive and frequent menstruation with regular cycle** ♀
   Heavy periods NOS   Polymenorrhea
   Menorrhagia NOS

N92.1 **Excessive and frequent menstruation with irregular cycle** ♀
   Irregular intermenstrual bleeding
   Irregular, shortened intervals between menstrual bleeding
   Menometrorrhagia
   Metrorrhagia

N92.2 **Excessive menstruation at puberty** ♀   P
   Excessive bleeding associated with onset of menstrual periods
   Pubertal menorrhagia
   Puberty bleeding

N92.3 **Ovulation bleeding** ♀
   Regular intermenstrual bleeding

N92.4 **Excessive bleeding in the premenopausal period** ♀
   Climacteric menorrhagia or metrorrhagia
   Menopausal menorrhagia or metrorrhagia
   Preclimacteric menorrhagia or metrorrhagia
   Premenopausal menorrhagia or metrorrhagia

N92.5 **Other specified irregular menstruation** ♀

N92.6 **Irregular menstruation, unspecified** ♀
   Irregular bleeding NOS
   Irregular periods NOS

   Excludes1 irregular menstruation with:
         lengthened intervals or scanty bleeding (N91.3-N91.5)
         shortened intervals or excessive bleeding (N92.1)

● **N93** **Other abnormal uterine and vaginal bleeding**
   Excludes1 neonatal vaginal hemorrhage (P54.6)
            precocious puberty (menstruation) (E30.1)
            pseudomenses (P54.6)

N93.0 **Postcoital and contact bleeding** ♀

N93.8 **Other specified abnormal uterine and vaginal bleeding** ♀
   Dysfunctional or functional uterine or vaginal bleeding NOS

N93.9 **Abnormal uterine and vaginal bleeding, unspecified** ♀

● **N94** **Pain and other conditions associated with female genital organs and menstrual cycle**

N94.0 **Mittelschmerz** ♀
   Ovulation pain

N94.1 **Dyspareunia** ♀
   Painful intercourse/coitus
   Excludes1 psychogenic dyspareunia (F52.6)

N94.2 **Vaginismus** ♀
   Vagina tightness
   Excludes1 psychogenic vaginismus (F52.5)

N94.3 **Premenstrual tension syndrome** ♀
   AKA: PMS
   Premenstrual dysphoric disorder
   Code also associated menstrual migraine (G43.82-, G43.83-)

N94.4 **Primary dysmenorrhea** ♀
   Lifelong painful menstruation

N94.5 **Secondary dysmenorrhea** ♀
   Later onset of painful menstruation

N94.6 **Dysmenorrhea, unspecified** ♀
   Excludes1 psychogenic dysmenorrhea (F45.8)

● **N94.8** **Other specified conditions associated with female genital organs and menstrual cycle**

   ● **N94.81** **Vulvodynia**

      N94.810 **Vulvar vestibulitis** ♀

      N94.818 **Other vulvodynia** ♀

      N94.819 **Vulvodynia, unspecified** ♀
         Vulvodynia NOS

   N94.89 **Other specified conditions associated with female genital organs and menstrual cycle** ♀

N94.9 **Unspecified condition associated with female genital organs and menstrual cycle** ♀

● **N95   Menopausal and other perimenopausal disorders**
Menopausal and other perimenopausal disorders due to
naturally occurring (age-related) menopause and
perimenopause

> **Excludes1**   excessive bleeding in the premenopausal period
> (N92.4)
> menopausal and perimenopausal disorders due
> to artificial or premature menopause (E89.4-,
> E28.31-)
> premature menopause (E28.31-)
>
> **Excludes2**   postmenopausal osteoporosis (M81.0-)
> postmenopausal osteoporosis with current
> pathological fracture (M80.0-)
> postmenopausal urethritis (N34.2)

N95.0   Postmenopausal bleeding ♀

N95.1   Menopausal and female climacteric states ♀
Symptoms such as flushing, sleeplessness, headache,
lack of concentration, associated with natural (age-
related) menopause

Use additional code for associated symptoms

> **Excludes1**   asymptomatic menopausal state (Z78.0)
> symptoms associated with artificial
> menopause (E89.41)
> symptoms associated with premature
> menopause (E28.310)

N95.2   Postmenopausal atrophic vaginitis ♀
Senile (atrophic) vaginitis

**N95.8   Other specified menopausal and perimenopausal
disorders** ♀

N95.9   Unspecified menopausal and perimenopausal disorder ♀

● **N96   Recurrent pregnancy loss** ♀
Investigation or care in a nonpregnant woman with history of
recurrent pregnancy loss

> **Excludes1**   recurrent pregnancy loss with current pregnancy
> (O26.2-)

● **N97   Female infertility**

> **Includes**   inability to achieve a pregnancy
> sterility, female NOS
>
> **Excludes1**   female infertility associated with:
> hypopituitarism (E23.0)
> Stein-Leventhal syndrome (E28.2)
>
> **Excludes2**   incompetence of cervix uteri (N88.3)

N97.0   Female infertility associated with anovulation ♀

N97.1   Female infertility of tubal origin ♀
Female infertility associated with congenital anomaly
of tube
Female infertility due to tubal block
Female infertility due to tubal occlusion
Female infertility due to tubal stenosis

N97.2   Female infertility of uterine origin ♀
Female infertility associated with congenital anomaly
of uterus
Female infertility due to nonimplantation of ovum

N97.8   Female infertility of other origin ♀

N97.9   Female infertility, unspecified ♀

● **N98   Complications associated with artificial fertilization**

N98.0   Infection associated with artificial insemination ♀

N98.1   Hyperstimulation of ovaries ♀
Hyperstimulation of ovaries NOS
Hyperstimulation of ovaries associated with induced
ovulation

**N98.2   Complications of attempted introduction of fertilized
ovum following in vitro fertilization** ♀

**N98.3   Complications of attempted introduction of embryo in
embryo transfer** ♀

**N98.8   Other complications associated with artificial
fertilization** ♀

**N98.9   Complication associated with artificial fertilization,
unspecified** ♀

INTRAOPERATIVE AND POSTPROCEDURAL COMPLICATIONS AND DISORDERS OF GENITOURINARY SYSTEM, NOT ELSEWHERE CLASSIFIED (N99)

● **N99   Intraoperative and postprocedural complications and disorders
of genitourinary system, not elsewhere classified**

> **Excludes2**   irradiation cystitis (N30.4-)
> postoophorectomy osteoporosis with current
> pathological fracture (M80.8-)
> postoophorectomy osteoporosis without current
> pathological fracture (M81.8)

N99.0   Postprocedural (acute) (chronic) kidney failure
Use additional code to type of kidney disease

● **N99.1   Postprocedural urethral stricture**
Postcatheterization urethral stricture

> ● **N99.11   Postprocedural urethral stricture, male**
>
> **N99.110   Postprocedural urethral stricture,
> male, meatal** ♂
>
> **N99.111   Postprocedural bulbous urethral
> stricture**
>
> **N99.112   Postprocedural membranous urethral
> stricture**
>
> **N99.113   Postprocedural anterior urethral
> stricture**
>
> **N99.114   Postprocedural urethral stricture,
> male, unspecified** ♂
>
> **N99.12   Postprocedural urethral stricture, female** ♀

N99.2   Postprocedural adhesions of vagina ♀

N99.3   Prolapse of vaginal vault after hysterectomy ♀

N99.4   Postprocedural pelvic peritoneal adhesions

> **Excludes2**   pelvic peritoneal adhesions NOS (N73.6)
> postinfective pelvic peritoneal adhesions
> (N73.6)

● **N99.5   Complications of stoma of urinary tract**

> **Excludes2**   mechanical complication of urinary
> (indwelling) catheter (T83.0-)

> ● **N99.51   Complication of cystostomy**
>
> **N99.510   Cystostomy hemorrhage**
>
> **N99.511   Cystostomy infection**
>
> **N99.512   Cystostomy malfunction**
>
> **N99.518   Other cystostomy complication**
>
> ● **N99.52   Complication of other external stoma of urinary
> tract**
>
> **N99.520   Hemorrhage of other external stoma
> of urinary tract**
>
> **N99.521   Infection of other external stoma of
> urinary tract**
>
> **N99.522   Malfunction of other external stoma
> of urinary tract**
>
> **N99.528   Other complication of other external
> stoma of urinary tract**
>
> ● **N99.53   Complication of other stoma of urinary tract**
>
> **N99.530   Hemorrhage of other stoma of urinary
> tract**
>
> **N99.531   Infection of other stoma of urinary
> tract**
>
> **N99.532   Malfunction of other stoma of urinary
> tract**
>
> **N99.538   Other complication of other stoma of
> urinary tract**

◄ New   ◄▥ Revised   ~~deleted~~ Deleted   Excludes 1   Excludes 2   Includes   Use additional   Code first   Code also   Unspecified
OGCR Official Guidelines   X Assign placeholder X   ● Use Additional Character(s)   ▶ Manifestation Code   **Coding Clinic**

● N99.6 **Intraoperative hemorrhage and hematoma of a genitourinary system organ or structure complicating a procedure**

    Excludes1 intraoperative hemorrhage and hematoma of a genitourinary system organ or structure due to accidental puncture or laceration during a procedure (N99.7-)

    N99.61 **Intraoperative hemorrhage and hematoma of a genitourinary system organ or structure complicating a genitourinary system procedure**

    N99.62 **Intraoperative hemorrhage and hematoma of a genitourinary system organ or structure complicating other procedure**

● N99.7 **Accidental puncture and laceration of a genitourinary system organ or structure during a procedure**

    N99.71 **Accidental puncture and laceration of a genitourinary system organ or structure during a genitourinary system procedure**

    N99.72 **Accidental puncture and laceration of a genitourinary system organ or structure during other procedure**

● N99.8 **Other intraoperative and postprocedural complications and disorders of genitourinary system**

    N99.81 **Other intraoperative complications of genitourinary system**

●   N99.82 **Postprocedural hemorrhage and hematoma of a genitourinary system organ or structure following a procedure**

    N99.820 **Postprocedural hemorrhage and hematoma of a genitourinary system organ or structure following a genitourinary system procedure**

    N99.821 **Postprocedural hemorrhage and hematoma of a genitourinary system organ or structure following other procedure**

    N99.83 **Residual ovary syndrome** ♀

    N99.89 **Other postprocedural complications and disorders of genitourinary system**

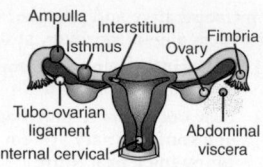

Figure 15-1 Implantation sites of ectopic pregnancy.

Item 15-1 Ectopic pregnancy most often occurs in the fallopian tube. Pregnancy outside the uterus may end in a lifethreatening rupture.

OGCR See Section I.C., Chapter 15
Pregnancy, Childbirth, and the Puerperium

(See Plate 375 on page 52.)

CHAPTER 15

PREGNANCY, CHILDBIRTH AND THE PUERPERIUM (O00-O9A)

Note: CODES FROM THIS CHAPTER ARE FOR USE ONLY ON MATERNAL RECORDS, NEVER ON NEWBORN RECORDS

Codes from this chapter are for use for conditions related to or aggravated by the pregnancy, childbirth, or by the puerperium (maternal causes or obstetric causes)

Trimesters are counted from the first day of the last menstrual period. They are defined as follows:

1st trimester - less than 14 weeks 0 days

2nd trimester - 14 weeks 0 days to less than 28 weeks 0 days

3rd trimester - 28 weeks 0 days until delivery

Use additional code from category Z3A, Weeks of gestation, to identify the specific week of the pregnancy

Excludes1 supervision of normal pregnancy (Z34.-)

Excludes2 mental and behavioral disorders associated with the puerperium (F53)
obstetrical tetanus (A34)
postpartum necrosis of pituitary gland (E23.0)
puerperal osteomalacia (M83.0)

This chapter contains the following blocks:

O00-O08	Pregnancy with abortive outcome
O09	Supervision of high risk pregnancy
O10-O16	Edema, proteinuria and hypertensive disorders in pregnancy, childbirth and the puerperium
O20-O29	Other maternal disorders predominantly related to pregnancy
O30-O48	Maternal care related to the fetus and amniotic cavity and possible delivery problems
O60-O77	Complications of labor and delivery
O80, O82	Encounter for delivery
O85-O92	Complications predominantly related to the puerperium
O94-O9A	Other obstetric conditions, not elsewhere classified

Item 15-2 A **hydatidiform** mole is an overproduction of placental tissue. The tumor secretes a hormone, chorionic gonadotropic hormone (CGH), that indicates a positive pregnancy test. There is no viable fetus. More than 80% of hydatidiform moles are noncancerous.

PREGNANCY WITH ABORTIVE OUTCOME (O00-O08)

Excludes1 continuing pregnancy in multiple gestation after abortion of one fetus or more (O31.1-, O31.3-)

● **O00 Ectopic pregnancy**

   Includes ruptured ectopic pregnancy

   Use additional code from category O08 to identify any associated complication

   O00.0 Abdominal pregnancy ♀   M

      Excludes1 maternal care for viable fetus in abdominal pregnancy (O36.7-)

   O00.1 Tubal pregnancy ♀   M
      Fallopian pregnancy
      Rupture of (fallopian) tube due to pregnancy
      Tubal abortion

   O00.2 Ovarian pregnancy ♀   M

   O00.8 Other ectopic pregnancy ♀   M
      Cervical pregnancy
      Cornual pregnancy
      Intraligamentous pregnancy
      Mural pregnancy

   O00.9 Ectopic pregnancy, unspecified ♀   M

● **O01 Hydatidiform mole**

   Use additional code from category O08 to identify any associated complication

   Excludes1 chorioadenoma (destruens) (D39.2)
      malignant hydatidiform mole (D39.2)

   O01.0 Classical hydatidiform mole ♀   M
      Complete hydatidiform mole

   O01.1 Incomplete and partial hydatidiform mole ♀   M

   O01.9 Hydatidiform mole, unspecified ♀   M
      Trophoblastic disease NOS
      Vesicular mole NOS

● **O02 Other abnormal products of conception**

   Use additional code from category O08 to identify any associated complication

   Excludes1 papyraceous fetus (O31.0-)

   O02.0 Blighted ovum and nonhydatidiform mole ♀   M
      Carneous mole   Molar pregnancy NEC
      Fleshy mole   Pathological ovum
      Intrauterine mole NOS

   O02.1 Missed abortion ♀   M
      Early fetal death, before completion of 20 weeks of gestation, with retention of dead fetus

      Excludes1 failed induced abortion (O07.-)
        fetal death (intrauterine) (late) (O36.4)
        missed abortion with blighted ovum (O02.0)
        missed abortion with hydatidiform mole (O01.-)
        missed abortion with nonhydatidiform (O02.0)
        missed abortion with other abnormal products of conception (O02.8-)
        missed delivery (O36.4)
        stillbirth (P95)

◄ New   ◄▮▮ Revised   ~~deleted~~ Deleted   Excludes 1   Excludes 2   Includes   Use additional   Code first   Code also   Unspecified

OGCR Official Guidelines   X Assign placeholder X   ● Use Additional Character(s)   ▶ Manifestation Code   **Coding Clinic**

● **O02.8　Other specified abnormal products of conception**

　　Excludes1　abnormal products of conception with
　　　　　　　blighted ovum (O02.0)
　　　　　　abnormal products of conception with
　　　　　　　hydatidiform mole (O01.-)
　　　　　　abnormal products of conception with
　　　　　　　nonhydatidiform mole (O02.0)

　　O02.81　**Inappropriate change in quantitative human
　　　　　chorionic gonadotropin (hCG) in early
　　　　　pregnancy ♀**　　　　　　　　　　　　　　**M**

　　　　　Biochemical pregnancy
　　　　　Chemical pregnancy
　　　　　Inappropriate level of quantitative human
　　　　　　chorionic gonadotropin (hCG) for
　　　　　　gestational age in early pregnancy

　　O02.89　**Other abnormal products of conception ♀**　**M**

　O02.9　**Abnormal product of conception, unspecified ♀**　**M**

● **O03　Spontaneous abortion**

　Note: Incomplete abortion includes retained products of
　　conception following spontaneous abortion.

　　Includes　miscarriage

　O03.0　**Genital tract and pelvic infection following incomplete
　　　　spontaneous abortion ♀**　　　　　　　　**M**

　　　　Endometritis following incomplete spontaneous
　　　　　abortion
　　　　Oophoritis following incomplete spontaneous abortion
　　　　Parametritis following incomplete spontaneous
　　　　　abortion
　　　　Pelvic peritonitis following incomplete spontaneous
　　　　　abortion
　　　　Salpingitis following incomplete spontaneous abortion
　　　　Salpingo-oophoritis following incomplete spontaneous
　　　　　abortion

　　　　Excludes1　sepsis following incomplete spontaneous
　　　　　　　　abortion (O03.37)
　　　　　　　urinary tract infection following
　　　　　　　　incomplete spontaneous abortion
　　　　　　　　(O03.38)

　O03.1　**Delayed or excessive hemorrhage following incomplete
　　　　spontaneous abortion ♀**　　　　　　　　**M**

　　　　Afibrinogenemia following incomplete spontaneous
　　　　　abortion
　　　　Defibrination syndrome following incomplete
　　　　　spontaneous abortion
　　　　Hemolysis following incomplete spontaneous abortion
　　　　Intravascular coagulation following incomplete
　　　　　spontaneous abortion

　O03.2　**Embolism following incomplete spontaneous
　　　　abortion ♀**　　　　　　　　　　　　　**M**

　　　　Air embolism following incomplete spontaneous
　　　　　abortion
　　　　Amniotic fluid embolism following incomplete
　　　　　spontaneous abortion
　　　　Blood-clot embolism following incomplete spontaneous
　　　　　abortion
　　　　Embolism NOS following incomplete spontaneous
　　　　　abortion
　　　　Fat embolism following incomplete spontaneous
　　　　　abortion
　　　　Pulmonary embolism following incomplete
　　　　　spontaneous abortion
　　　　Pyemic embolism following incomplete spontaneous
　　　　　abortion
　　　　Septic or septicopyemic embolism following incomplete
　　　　　spontaneous abortion
　　　　Soap embolism following incomplete spontaneous
　　　　　abortion

● **O03.3　Other and unspecified complications following
　　　　incomplete spontaneous abortion**

　　O03.30　**Unspecified complication following incomplete
　　　　　spontaneous abortion ♀**　　　　　　　**M**

　　O03.31　**Shock following incomplete spontaneous
　　　　　abortion ♀**　　　　　　　　　　　　**M**

　　　　　Circulatory collapse following incomplete
　　　　　　spontaneous abortion
　　　　　Shock (postprocedural) following incomplete
　　　　　　spontaneous abortion

　　　　　Excludes1　shock due to infection following
　　　　　　　　　incomplete spontaneous
　　　　　　　　　abortion (O03.37)

　　O03.32　**Renal failure following incomplete
　　　　　spontaneous abortion ♀**　　　　　　　**M**

　　　　　Kidney failure (acute) following incomplete
　　　　　　spontaneous abortion
　　　　　Oliguria following incomplete spontaneous
　　　　　　abortion
　　　　　Renal shutdown following incomplete
　　　　　　spontaneous abortion
　　　　　Renal tubular necrosis following incomplete
　　　　　　spontaneous abortion
　　　　　Uremia following incomplete spontaneous
　　　　　　abortion

　　O03.33　**Metabolic disorder following incomplete
　　　　　spontaneous abortion ♀**　　　　　　　**M**

　　O03.34　**Damage to pelvic organs following incomplete
　　　　　spontaneous abortion ♀**　　　　　　　**M**

　　　　　Laceration, perforation, tear or chemical
　　　　　　damage of bladder following incomplete
　　　　　　spontaneous abortion
　　　　　Laceration, perforation, tear or chemical
　　　　　　damage of bowel following incomplete
　　　　　　spontaneous abortion
　　　　　Laceration, perforation, tear or chemical
　　　　　　damage of broad ligament following
　　　　　　incomplete spontaneous abortion
　　　　　Laceration, perforation, tear or chemical
　　　　　　damage of cervix following incomplete
　　　　　　spontaneous abortion
　　　　　Laceration, perforation, tear or chemical
　　　　　　damage of periurethral tissue following
　　　　　　incomplete spontaneous abortion
　　　　　Laceration, perforation, tear or chemical
　　　　　　damage of uterus following incomplete
　　　　　　spontaneous abortion
　　　　　Laceration, perforation, tear or chemical
　　　　　　damage of vagina following incomplete
　　　　　　spontaneous abortion

　　O03.35　**Other venous complications following
　　　　　incomplete spontaneous abortion ♀**　　　**M**

　　O03.36　**Cardiac arrest following incomplete
　　　　　spontaneous abortion ♀**　　　　　　　**M**

　　O03.37　**Sepsis following incomplete spontaneous
　　　　　abortion ♀**　　　　　　　　　　　　**M**

　　　　　Use additional code to identify infectious
　　　　　　agent (B95-B97)

　　　　　Use additional code to identify severe sepsis, if
　　　　　　applicable (R65.2-)

　　　　　Excludes1　septic or septicopyemic
　　　　　　　　　embolism following
　　　　　　　　　incomplete spontaneous
　　　　　　　　　abortion (O03.2)

　　O03.38　**Urinary tract infection following incomplete
　　　　　spontaneous abortion ♀**　　　　　　　**M**

　　　　　Cystitis following incomplete spontaneous
　　　　　　abortion

　　O03.39　**Incomplete spontaneous abortion with other
　　　　　complications ♀**　　　　　　　　　　**M**

CHAPTER 15 (O00-O9A)

CHAPTER 15 (O00-O9A)

O03.4 Incomplete spontaneous abortion without complication ♀ M

O03.5 Genital tract and pelvic infection following complete or unspecified spontaneous abortion ♀ M

Endometritis following complete or unspecified spontaneous abortion

Oophoritis following complete or unspecified spontaneous abortion

Parametritis following complete or unspecified spontaneous abortion

Pelvic peritonitis following complete or unspecified spontaneous abortion

Salpingitis following complete or unspecified spontaneous abortion

Salpingo-oophoritis following complete or unspecified spontaneous abortion

> **Excludes1** sepsis following complete or unspecified spontaneous abortion (O03.87)
> urinary tract infection following complete or unspecified spontaneous abortion (O03.88)

O03.6 Delayed or excessive hemorrhage following complete or unspecified spontaneous abortion ♀ M

Afibrinogenemia following complete or unspecified spontaneous abortion

Defibrination syndrome following complete or unspecified spontaneous abortion

Hemolysis following complete or unspecified spontaneous abortion

Intravascular coagulation following complete or unspecified spontaneous abortion

O03.7 Embolism following complete or unspecified spontaneous abortion ♀ M

Air embolism following complete or unspecified spontaneous abortion

Amniotic fluid embolism following complete or unspecified spontaneous abortion

Blood-clot embolism following complete or unspecified spontaneous abortion

Embolism NOS following complete or unspecified spontaneous abortion

Fat embolism following complete or unspecified spontaneous abortion

Pulmonary embolism following complete or unspecified spontaneous abortion

Pyemic embolism following complete or unspecified spontaneous abortion

Septic or septicopyemic embolism following complete or unspecified spontaneous abortion

Soap embolism following complete or unspecified spontaneous abortion

● **O03.8** Other and unspecified complications following complete or unspecified spontaneous abortion

O03.80 Unspecified complication following complete or unspecified spontaneous abortion ♀ M

O03.81 Shock following complete or unspecified spontaneous abortion ♀ M

Circulatory collapse following complete or unspecified spontaneous abortion

Shock (postprocedural) following complete or unspecified spontaneous abortion

> **Excludes1** shock due to infection following complete or unspecified spontaneous abortion (O03.87)

O03.82 Renal failure following complete or unspecified spontaneous abortion ♀ M

Kidney failure (acute) following complete or unspecified spontaneous abortion

Oliguria following complete or unspecified spontaneous abortion

Renal shutdown following complete or unspecified spontaneous abortion

Renal tubular necrosis following complete or unspecified spontaneous abortion

Uremia following complete or unspecified spontaneous abortion

O03.83 Metabolic disorder following complete or unspecified spontaneous abortion ♀ M

O03.84 Damage to pelvic organs following complete or unspecified spontaneous abortion ♀ M

Laceration, perforation, tear or chemical damage of bladder following complete or unspecified spontaneous abortion

Laceration, perforation, tear or chemical damage of bowel following complete or unspecified spontaneous abortion

Laceration, perforation, tear or chemical damage of broad ligament following complete or unspecified spontaneous abortion

Laceration, perforation, tear or chemical damage of cervix following complete or unspecified spontaneous abortion

Laceration, perforation, tear or chemical damage of periurethral tissue following complete or unspecified spontaneous abortion

Laceration, perforation, tear or chemical damage of uterus following complete or unspecified spontaneous abortion

Laceration, perforation, tear or chemical damage of vagina following complete or unspecified spontaneous abortion

O03.85 Other venous complications following complete or unspecified spontaneous abortion ♀ M

O03.86 Cardiac arrest following complete or unspecified spontaneous abortion ♀ M

O03.87 Sepsis following complete or unspecified spontaneous abortion ♀ M

> Use additional code to identify infectious agent (B95-B97)
> Use additional code to identify severe sepsis, if applicable (R65.2-)
> **Excludes1** septic or septicopyemic embolism following complete or unspecified spontaneous abortion (O03.7)

O03.88 Urinary tract infection following complete or unspecified spontaneous abortion ♀ M

Cystitis following complete or unspecified spontaneous abortion

O03.89 Complete or unspecified spontaneous abortion with other complications ♀ M

O03.9 Complete or unspecified spontaneous abortion without complication ♀ M

Miscarriage NOS

Spontaneous abortion NOS

◀ New ⬅ Revised ~~deleted~~ Deleted | Excludes 1 | Excludes 2 | Includes | Use additional | Code first | Code also | Unspecified

OGCR Official Guidelines   X Assign placeholder X   ● Use Additional Character(s)   ▶ Manifestation Code   **Coding Clinic**

● **O04**   **Complications following (induced) termination of pregnancy**

     Includes   complications following (induced) termination of pregnancy

     Excludes1   encounter for elective termination of pregnancy, uncomplicated (Z33.2)

                failed attempted termination of pregnancy (O07.-)

     O04.5   **Genital tract and pelvic infection following (induced) termination of pregnancy ♀**   **M**

         Endometritis following (induced) termination of pregnancy

         Oophoritis following (induced) termination of pregnancy

         Parametritis following (induced) termination of pregnancy

         Pelvic peritonitis following (induced) termination of pregnancy

         Salpingitis following (induced) termination of pregnancy

         Salpingo-oophoritis following (induced) termination of pregnancy

         Excludes1   sepsis following (induced) termination of pregnancy (O04.87)

                 urinary tract infection following (induced) termination of pregnancy (O04.88)

     O04.6   **Delayed or excessive hemorrhage following (induced) termination of pregnancy ♀**   **M**

         Afibrinogenemia following (induced) termination of pregnancy

         Defibrination syndrome following (induced) termination of pregnancy

         Hemolysis following (induced) termination of pregnancy

         Intravascular coagulation following (induced) termination of pregnancy

     O04.7   **Embolism following (induced) termination of pregnancy ♀**   **M**

         Air embolism following (induced) termination of pregnancy

         Amniotic fluid embolism following (induced) termination of pregnancy

         Blood-clot embolism following (induced) termination of pregnancy

         Embolism NOS following (induced) termination of pregnancy

         Fat embolism following (induced) termination of pregnancy

         Pulmonary embolism following (induced) termination of pregnancy

         Pyemic embolism following (induced) termination of pregnancy

         Septic or septicopyemic embolism following (induced) termination of pregnancy

         Soap embolism following (induced) termination of pregnancy

● **O04.8**   **(Induced) termination of pregnancy with other and unspecified complications**

     O04.80   **(Induced) termination of pregnancy with unspecified complications ♀**   **M**

     O04.81   **Shock following (induced) termination of pregnancy ♀**   **M**

         Circulatory collapse following (induced) termination of pregnancy

         Shock (postprocedural) following (induced) termination of pregnancy

         Excludes1   shock due to infection following (induced) termination of pregnancy (O04.87)

     O04.82   **Renal failure following (induced) termination of pregnancy ♀**   **M**

         Kidney failure (acute) following (induced) termination of pregnancy

         Oliguria following (induced) termination of pregnancy

         Renal shutdown following (induced) termination of pregnancy

         Renal tubular necrosis following (induced) termination of pregnancy

         Uremia following (induced) termination of pregnancy

     O04.83   **Metabolic disorder following (induced) termination of pregnancy ♀**   **M**

     O04.84   **Damage to pelvic organs following (induced) termination of pregnancy ♀**   **M**

         Laceration, perforation, tear or chemical damage of bladder following (induced) termination of pregnancy

         Laceration, perforation, tear or chemical damage of bowel following (induced) termination of pregnancy

         Laceration, perforation, tear or chemical damage of broad ligament following (induced) termination of pregnancy

         Laceration, perforation, tear or chemical damage of cervix following (induced) termination of pregnancy

         Laceration, perforation, tear or chemical damage of periurethral tissue following (induced) termination of pregnancy

         Laceration, perforation, tear or chemical damage of uterus following (induced) termination of pregnancy

         Laceration, perforation, tear or chemical damage of vagina following (induced) termination of pregnancy

     O04.85   **Other venous complications following (induced) termination of pregnancy ♀**   **M**

     O04.86   **Cardiac arrest following (induced) termination of pregnancy ♀**   **M**

     O04.87   **Sepsis following (induced) termination of pregnancy ♀**   **M**

         Use additional code to identify infectious agent (B95-B97)

         Use additional code to identify severe sepsis, if applicable (R65.2-)

         Excludes1   septic or septicopyemic embolism following (induced) termination of pregnancy (O04.7)

     O04.88   **Urinary tract infection following (induced) termination of pregnancy ♀**   **M**

         Cystitis following (induced) termination of pregnancy

     O04.89   **(Induced) termination of pregnancy with other complications ♀**   **M**

CHAPTER 15 (O00-O9A)

● **O07 Failed attempted termination of pregnancy**

    Includes   failure of attempted induction of termination of
                       pregnancy
                       incomplete elective abortion

    Excludes1   incomplete spontaneous abortion (O03.0-)

**O07.0 Genital tract and pelvic infection following failed
attempted termination of pregnancy** ♀   **M**

    Endometritis following failed attempted termination of
      pregnancy
    Oophoritis following failed attempted termination of
      pregnancy
    Parametritis following failed attempted termination of
      pregnancy
    Pelvic peritonitis following failed attempted
      termination of pregnancy
    Salpingitis following failed attempted termination of
      pregnancy
    Salpingo-oophoritis following failed attempted
      termination of pregnancy

     Excludes1   sepsis following failed attempted
                      termination of pregnancy (O07.37)
                      urinary tract infection following failed
                      attempted termination of pregnancy
                      (O07.38)

**O07.1 Delayed or excessive hemorrhage following failed
attempted termination of pregnancy** ♀   **M**

    Afibrinogenemia following failed attempted
      termination of pregnancy
    Defibrination syndrome following failed attempted
      termination of pregnancy
    Hemolysis following failed attempted termination of
      pregnancy
    Intravascular coagulation following failed attempted
      termination of pregnancy

**O07.2 Embolism following failed attempted termination of
pregnancy** ♀   **M**

    Air embolism following failed attempted termination of
      pregnancy
    Amniotic fluid embolism following failed attempted
      termination of pregnancy
    Blood-clot embolism following failed attempted
      termination of pregnancy
    Embolism NOS following failed attempted termination
      of pregnancy
    Fat embolism following failed attempted termination of
      pregnancy
    Pulmonary embolism following failed attempted
      termination of pregnancy
    Pyemic embolism following failed attempted
      termination of pregnancy
    Septic or septicopyemic embolism following failed
      attempted termination of pregnancy
    Soap embolism following failed attempted termination
      of pregnancy

● **O07.3 Failed attempted termination of pregnancy with other
and unspecified complications**

**O07.30 Failed attempted termination of pregnancy with
unspecified complications** ♀   **M**

**O07.31 Shock following failed attempted termination
of pregnancy** ♀   **M**

    Circulatory collapse following failed attempted
      termination of pregnancy
    Shock (postprocedural) following failed
      attempted termination of pregnancy

     Excludes1   shock due to infection
                      following failed attempted
                      termination of pregnancy
                      (O07.37)

**O07.32 Renal failure following failed attempted
termination of pregnancy** ♀   **M**

    Kidney failure (acute) following failed
      attempted termination of pregnancy
    Oliguria following failed attempted
      termination of pregnancy
    Renal shutdown following failed attempted
      termination of pregnancy
    Renal tubular necrosis following failed
      attempted termination of pregnancy
    Uremia following failed attempted termination
      of pregnancy

**O07.33 Metabolic disorder following failed attempted
termination of pregnancy** ♀   **M**

**O07.34 Damage to pelvic organs following failed
attempted termination of pregnancy** ♀   **M**

    Laceration, perforation, tear or chemical
      damage of bladder following failed
      attempted termination of pregnancy
    Laceration, perforation, tear or chemical
      damage of bowel following failed
      attempted termination of pregnancy
    Laceration, perforation, tear or chemical
      damage of broad ligament following
      failed attempted termination of pregnancy
    Laceration, perforation, tear or chemical
      damage of cervix following failed
      attempted termination of pregnancy
    Laceration, perforation, tear or chemical
      damage of periurethral tissue following
      failed attempted termination of pregnancy
    Laceration, perforation, tear or chemical
      damage of uterus following failed
      attempted termination of pregnancy
    Laceration, perforation, tear or chemical
      damage of vagina following failed
      attempted termination of pregnancy

**O07.35 Other venous complications following failed
attempted termination of pregnancy** ♀   **M**

**O07.36 Cardiac arrest following failed attempted
termination of pregnancy** ♀   **M**

**O07.37 Sepsis following failed attempted termination
of pregnancy** ♀   **M**

    Use additional code (B95-B97), to identify
      infectious agent

    Use additional code (R65.2-) to identify severe
      sepsis, if applicable

     Excludes1   septic or septicopyemic
                      embolism following failed
                      attempted termination of
                      pregnancy (O07.2)

**O07.38 Urinary tract infection following failed
attempted termination of pregnancy** ♀   **M**

    Cystitis following failed attempted termination
      of pregnancy

**O07.39 Failed attempted termination of pregnancy with
other complications** ♀   **M**

**O07.4 Failed attempted termination of pregnancy without
complication** ♀   **M**

● **O08 Complications following ectopic and molar pregnancy**

    This category is for use with categories O00-O02 to identify any
    associated complications.

**O08.0 Genital tract and pelvic infection following ectopic and
molar pregnancy** ♀   **M**

    Endometritis following ectopic and molar pregnancy
    Oophoritis following ectopic and molar pregnancy
    Parametritis following ectopic and molar pregnancy
    Pelvic peritonitis following ectopic and molar
      pregnancy
    Salpingitis following ectopic and molar pregnancy
    Salpingo-oophoritis following ectopic and molar
      pregnancy

     Excludes1   sepsis following ectopic and molar
                      pregnancy (O08.82)
                      urinary tract infection (O08.83)

◀ New   ◀▥ Revised   ~~deleted~~ Deleted   Excludes 1   Excludes 2   Includes   Use additional   Code first   Code also   Unspecified

OGCR Official Guidelines   **X** Assign placeholder X   ● Use Additional Character(s)   ▶ Manifestation Code   **Coding Clinic**

O08.1   **Delayed or excessive hemorrhage following ectopic and molar pregnancy ♀**   M
     Afibrinogenemia following ectopic and molar pregnancy
     Defibrination syndrome following ectopic and molar pregnancy
     Hemolysis following ectopic and molar pregnancy
     Intravascular coagulation following ectopic and molar pregnancy

     Excludes1   delayed or excessive hemorrhage due to incomplete abortion (O03.1)

O08.2   **Embolism following ectopic and molar pregnancy ♀**   M
     Air embolism following ectopic and molar pregnancy
     Amniotic fluid embolism following ectopic and molar pregnancy
     Blood-clot embolism following ectopic and molar pregnancy
     Embolism NOS following ectopic and molar pregnancy
     Fat embolism following ectopic and molar pregnancy
     Pulmonary embolism following ectopic and molar pregnancy
     Pyemic embolism following ectopic and molar pregnancy
     Septic or septicopyemic embolism following ectopic and molar pregnancy
     Soap embolism following ectopic and molar pregnancy

O08.3   **Shock following ectopic and molar pregnancy ♀**   M
     Circulatory collapse following ectopic and molar pregnancy
     Shock (postprocedural) following ectopic and molar pregnancy

     Excludes1   shock due to infection following ectopic and molar pregnancy (O08.82)

O08.4   **Renal failure following ectopic and molar pregnancy ♀**   M
     Kidney failure (acute) following ectopic and molar pregnancy
     Oliguria following ectopic and molar pregnancy
     Renal shutdown following ectopic and molar pregnancy
     Renal tubular necrosis following ectopic and molar pregnancy
     Uremia following ectopic and molar pregnancy

O08.5   **Metabolic disorders following an ectopic and molar pregnancy ♀**   M

O08.6   **Damage to pelvic organs and tissues following an ectopic and molar pregnancy ♀**   M
     Laceration, perforation, tear or chemical damage of bladder following an ectopic and molar pregnancy
     Laceration, perforation, tear or chemical damage of bowel following an ectopic and molar pregnancy
     Laceration, perforation, tear or chemical damage of broad ligament following an ectopic and molar pregnancy
     Laceration, perforation, tear or chemical damage of cervix following an ectopic and molar pregnancy
     Laceration, perforation, tear or chemical damage of periurethral tissue following an ectopic and molar pregnancy
     Laceration, perforation, tear or chemical damage of uterus following an ectopic and molar pregnancy
     Laceration, perforation, tear or chemical damage of vagina following an ectopic and molar pregnancy

O08.7   **Other venous complications following an ectopic and molar pregnancy ♀**   M

● **O08.8**   **Other complications following an ectopic and molar pregnancy**
     O08.81   **Cardiac arrest following an ectopic and molar pregnancy ♀**   M
     O08.82   **Sepsis following ectopic and molar pregnancy ♀**   M
         Use additional code (B95-B97), to identify infectious agent
         Use additional code (R65.2-) to identify severe sepsis, if applicable
         Excludes1   septic or septicopyemic embolism following ectopic and molar pregnancy (O08.2)

     O08.83   **Urinary tract infection following an ectopic and molar pregnancy ♀**   M
         Cystitis following an ectopic and molar pregnancy

     O08.89   **Other complications following an ectopic and molar pregnancy ♀**   M

O08.9   **Unspecified complication following an ectopic and molar pregnancy ♀**   M

SUPERVISION OF HIGH RISK PREGNANCY (O09)

● **O09**   **Supervision of high risk pregnancy**
   ● **O09.0**   **Supervision of pregnancy with history of infertility**
     O09.00   **Supervision of pregnancy with history of infertility, unspecified trimester ♀**   M
     O09.01   **Supervision of pregnancy with history of infertility, first trimester ♀**   M
     O09.02   **Supervision of pregnancy with history of infertility, second trimester ♀**   M
     O09.03   **Supervision of pregnancy with history of infertility, third trimester ♀**   M

   ● **O09.1**   **Supervision of pregnancy with history of ectopic or molar pregnancy**
     O09.10   **Supervision of pregnancy with history of ectopic or molar pregnancy, unspecified trimester ♀**   M
     O09.11   **Supervision of pregnancy with history of ectopic or molar pregnancy, first trimester ♀**   M
     O09.12   **Supervision of pregnancy with history of ectopic or molar pregnancy, second trimester ♀**   M
     O09.13   **Supervision of pregnancy with history of ectopic or molar pregnancy, third trimester ♀**   M

   ● **O09.2**   **Supervision of pregnancy with other poor reproductive or obstetric history**
     Excludes2   pregnancy care for patient with history of recurrent pregnancy loss (O26.2-)

     ● **O09.21**   **Supervision of pregnancy with history of pre-term labor**
         O09.211   **Supervision of pregnancy with history of pre-term labor, first trimester ♀**   M
         O09.212   **Supervision of pregnancy with history of pre-term labor, second trimester ♀**   M
         O09.213   **Supervision of pregnancy with history of pre-term labor, third trimester ♀**   M
         O09.219   **Supervision of pregnancy with history of pre-term labor, unspecified trimester ♀**   M

● **O09.29** **Supervision of pregnancy with other poor reproductive or obstetric history**
Supervision of pregnancy with history of neonatal death
Supervision of pregnancy with history of stillbirth

     O09.291   Supervision of pregnancy with other poor reproductive or obstetric history, first trimester ♀   M

     O09.292   Supervision of pregnancy with other poor reproductive or obstetric history, second trimester ♀   M

     O09.293   Supervision of pregnancy with other poor reproductive or obstetric history, third trimester ♀   M

     O09.299   Supervision of pregnancy with other poor reproductive or obstetric history, unspecified trimester ♀   M

● **O09.3** **Supervision of pregnancy with insufficient antenatal care**
Supervision of concealed pregnancy
Supervision of hidden pregnancy

     O09.30   Supervision of pregnancy with insufficient antenatal care, unspecified trimester ♀   M

     O09.31   Supervision of pregnancy with insufficient antenatal care, first trimester ♀   M

     O09.32   Supervision of pregnancy with insufficient antenatal care, second trimester ♀   M

     O09.33   Supervision of pregnancy with insufficient antenatal care, third trimester ♀   M

● **O09.4** **Supervision of pregnancy with grand multiparity**

     O09.40   Supervision of pregnancy with grand multiparity, unspecified trimester ♀   M

     O09.41   Supervision of pregnancy with grand multiparity, first trimester ♀   M

     O09.42   Supervision of pregnancy with grand multiparity, second trimester ♀   M

     O09.43   Supervision of pregnancy with grand multiparity, third trimester ♀   M

● **O09.5** **Supervision of elderly primigravida and multigravida**
Pregnancy for a female 35 years and older at expected date of delivery

     ● O09.51   Supervision of elderly primigravida

         O09.511   Supervision of elderly primigravida, first trimester ♀   M

         O09.512   Supervision of elderly primigravida, second trimester ♀   M

         O09.513   Supervision of elderly primigravida, third trimester ♀   M

         O09.519   Supervision of elderly primigravida, unspecified trimester ♀   M

     ● O09.52   Supervision of elderly multigravida

         O09.521   Supervision of elderly multigravida, first trimester ♀   M

         O09.522   Supervision of elderly multigravida, second trimester ♀   M

         O09.523   Supervision of elderly multigravida, third trimester ♀   M

         O09.529   Supervision of elderly multigravida, unspecified trimester ♀   M

● **O09.6** **Supervision of young primigravida and multigravida**
Supervision of pregnancy for a female less than 16 years old at expected date of delivery

     ● O09.61   Supervision of young primigravida

         O09.611   Supervision of young primigravida, first trimester ♀   M

         O09.612   Supervision of young primigravida, second trimester ♀   M

         O09.613   Supervision of young primigravida, third trimester ♀   M

         O09.619   Supervision of young primigravida, unspecified trimester ♀   M

     ● O09.62   Supervision of young multigravida

         O09.621   Supervision of young multigravida, first trimester ♀   M

         O09.622   Supervision of young multigravida, second trimester ♀   M

         O09.623   Supervision of young multigravida, third trimester ♀   M

         O09.629   Supervision of young multigravida, unspecified trimester ♀   M

● **O09.7** **Supervision of high risk pregnancy due to social problems**

     O09.70   Supervision of high risk pregnancy due to social problems, unspecified trimester ♀   M

     O09.71   Supervision of high risk pregnancy due to social problems, first trimester ♀   M

     O09.72   Supervision of high risk pregnancy due to social problems, second trimester ♀   M

     O09.73   Supervision of high risk pregnancy due to social problems, third trimester ♀   M

● **O09.8** **Supervision of other high risk pregnancies**

     ● O09.81   Supervision of pregnancy resulting from assisted reproductive technology
Supervision of pregnancy resulting from in-vitro fertilization

         O09.811   Supervision of pregnancy resulting from assisted reproductive technology, first trimester ♀   M

         O09.812   Supervision of pregnancy resulting from assisted reproductive technology, second trimester ♀   M

         O09.813   Supervision of pregnancy resulting from assisted reproductive technology, third trimester ♀   M

         O09.819   Supervision of pregnancy resulting from assisted reproductive technology, unspecified trimester ♀   M

     ● O09.82   Supervision of pregnancy with history of in utero procedure during previous pregnancy

         O09.821   Supervision of pregnancy with history of in utero procedure during previous pregnancy, first trimester ♀   M

         O09.822   Supervision of pregnancy with history of in utero procedure during previous pregnancy, second trimester ♀   M

         O09.823   Supervision of pregnancy with history of in utero procedure during previous pregnancy, third trimester ♀   M

         O09.829   Supervision of pregnancy with history of in utero procedure during previous pregnancy, unspecified trimester ♀   M

            Excludes1   supervision of pregnancy affected by in utero procedure during current pregnancy (O35.7)

     ● O09.89   Supervision of other high risk pregnancies

         O09.891   Supervision of other high risk pregnancies, first trimester ♀   M

         O09.892   Supervision of other high risk pregnancies, second trimester ♀   M

         O09.893   Supervision of other high risk pregnancies, third trimester ♀   M

         O09.899   Supervision of other high risk pregnancies, unspecified trimester ♀   M

◀ New   ◀▥ Revised   ~~deleted~~ Deleted   Excludes 1   Excludes 2   Includes   Use additional   Code first   Code also   Unspecified
OGCR Official Guidelines   X Assign placeholder X   ● Use Additional Character(s)   ▶ Manifestation Code   **Coding Clinic**

● O09.9   Supervision of high risk pregnancy, unspecified
    O09.90   Supervision of high risk pregnancy, unspecified, unspecified trimester ♀   **M**
    O09.91   Supervision of high risk pregnancy, unspecified, first trimester ♀   **M**
    O09.92   Supervision of high risk pregnancy, unspecified, second trimester ♀   **M**
    O09.93   Supervision of high risk pregnancy, unspecified, third trimester ♀   **M**

EDEMA, PROTEINURIA AND HYPERTENSIVE DISORDERS IN PREGNANCY, CHILDBIRTH AND THE PUERPERIUM (O10-O16)

● O10   Pre-existing hypertension complicating pregnancy, childbirth and the puerperium

    Includes   pre-existing hypertension with pre-existing proteinuria complicating pregnancy, childbirth and the puerperium

    Excludes2   pre-existing hypertension with superimposed pre-eclampsia complicating pregnancy, childbirth and the puerperium (O11.-)

● O10.0   Pre-existing essential hypertension complicating pregnancy, childbirth and the puerperium
    Any condition in I10 specified as a reason for obstetric care during pregnancy, childbirth or the puerperium

  ● O10.01   Pre-existing essential hypertension complicating pregnancy
    O10.011   Pre-existing essential hypertension complicating pregnancy, first trimester ♀   **M**
    O10.012   Pre-existing essential hypertension complicating pregnancy, second trimester ♀   **M**
    O10.013   Pre-existing essential hypertension complicating pregnancy, third trimester ♀   **M**
    O10.019   Pre-existing essential hypertension complicating pregnancy, unspecified trimester ♀   **M**
  O10.02   Pre-existing essential hypertension complicating childbirth ♀   **M**
  O10.03   Pre-existing essential hypertension complicating the puerperium ♀   **M**

● O10.1   Pre-existing hypertensive heart disease complicating pregnancy, childbirth and the puerperium
    Any condition in I11 specified as a reason for obstetric care during pregnancy, childbirth or the puerperium
    Use additional code from I11 to identify the type of hypertensive heart disease

  ● O10.11   Pre-existing hypertensive heart disease complicating pregnancy
    O10.111   Pre-existing hypertensive heart disease complicating pregnancy, first trimester ♀   **M**
    O10.112   Pre-existing hypertensive heart disease complicating pregnancy, second trimester ♀   **M**
    O10.113   Pre-existing hypertensive heart disease complicating pregnancy, third trimester ♀   **M**
    O10.119   Pre-existing hypertensive heart disease complicating pregnancy, unspecified trimester ♀   **M**
  O10.12   Pre-existing hypertensive heart disease complicating childbirth ♀   **M**
  O10.13   Pre-existing hypertensive heart disease complicating the puerperium ♀   **M**

● O10.2   Pre-existing hypertensive chronic kidney disease complicating pregnancy, childbirth and the puerperium
    Any condition in I12 specified as a reason for obstetric care during pregnancy, childbirth or the puerperium
    Use additional code from I12 to identify the type of hypertensive chronic kidney disease

  ● O10.21   Pre-existing hypertensive chronic kidney disease complicating pregnancy
    O10.211   Pre-existing hypertensive chronic kidney disease complicating pregnancy, first trimester ♀   **M**
    O10.212   Pre-existing hypertensive chronic kidney disease complicating pregnancy, second trimester ♀   **M**
    O10.213   Pre-existing hypertensive chronic kidney disease complicating pregnancy, third trimester ♀   **M**
    O10.219   Pre-existing hypertensive chronic kidney disease complicating pregnancy, unspecified trimester ♀   **M**
  O10.22   Pre-existing hypertensive chronic kidney disease complicating childbirth ♀   **M**
  O10.23   Pre-existing hypertensive chronic kidney disease complicating the puerperium ♀   **M**

● O10.3   Pre-existing hypertensive heart and chronic kidney disease complicating pregnancy, childbirth and the puerperium
    Any condition in I13 specified as a reason for obstetric care during pregnancy, childbirth or the puerperium
    Use additional code from I13 to identify the type of hypertensive heart and chronic kidney disease

  ● O10.31   Pre-existing hypertensive heart and chronic kidney disease complicating pregnancy
    O10.311   Pre-existing hypertensive heart and chronic kidney disease complicating pregnancy, first trimester ♀   **M**
    O10.312   Pre-existing hypertensive heart and chronic kidney disease complicating pregnancy, second trimester ♀   **M**
    O10.313   Pre-existing hypertensive heart and chronic kidney disease complicating pregnancy, third trimester ♀   **M**
    O10.319   Pre-existing hypertensive heart and chronic kidney disease complicating pregnancy, unspecified trimester ♀   **M**
  O10.32   Pre-existing hypertensive heart and chronic kidney disease complicating childbirth ♀   **M**
  O10.33   Pre-existing hypertensive heart and chronic kidney disease complicating the puerperium ♀   **M**

● O10.4   Pre-existing secondary hypertension complicating pregnancy, childbirth and the puerperium
    Any condition in I15 specified as a reason for obstetric care during pregnancy, childbirth or the puerperium
    Use additional code from I15 to identify the type of secondary hypertension

  ● O10.41   Pre-existing secondary hypertension complicating pregnancy
    O10.411   Pre-existing secondary hypertension complicating pregnancy, first trimester ♀   **M**
    O10.412   Pre-existing secondary hypertension complicating pregnancy, second trimester ♀   **M**
    O10.413   Pre-existing secondary hypertension complicating pregnancy, third trimester ♀   **M**
    O10.419   Pre-existing secondary hypertension complicating pregnancy, unspecified trimester ♀   **M**

N Newborn Age: 0   **P** Pediatric Age: 0–17   **M** Maternity DX: 12–55   **A** Adult Age: 15–124   ♀ Females Only   ♂ Males Only

1169

    O10.42   Pre-existing secondary hypertension complicating childbirth ♀   **M**

    O10.43   Pre-existing secondary hypertension complicating the puerperium ♀   **M**

● O10.9   Unspecified pre-existing hypertension complicating pregnancy, childbirth and the puerperium

  ● O10.91   Unspecified pre-existing hypertension complicating pregnancy

    O10.911   `Unspecified` pre-existing hypertension complicating pregnancy, first trimester ♀   **M**

    O10.912   `Unspecified` pre-existing hypertension complicating pregnancy, second trimester ♀   **M**

    O10.913   `Unspecified` pre-existing hypertension complicating pregnancy, third trimester ♀   **M**

    O10.919   `Unspecified` pre-existing hypertension complicating pregnancy, unspecified trimester ♀   **M**

  O10.92   `Unspecified` pre-existing hypertension complicating childbirth ♀   **M**

  O10.93   `Unspecified` pre-existing hypertension complicating the puerperium ♀   **M**

● O11   Pre-existing hypertension with pre-eclampsia

  Includes   conditions in O10 complicated by pre-eclampsia pre-eclampsia superimposed pre-existing hypertension

  Use additional code from O10 to identify the type of hypertension

  O11.1   Pre-existing hypertension with pre-eclampsia, first trimester ♀   **M**

  O11.2   Pre-existing hypertension with pre-eclampsia, second trimester ♀   **M**

  O11.3   Pre-existing hypertension with pre-eclampsia, third trimester ♀   **M**

  O11.9   Pre-existing hypertension with pre-eclampsia, `unspecified` trimester ♀   **M**

● O12   Gestational [pregnancy-induced] edema and proteinuria without hypertension

  ● O12.0   Gestational edema

    O12.00   Gestational edema, `unspecified` trimester ♀   **M**

    O12.01   Gestational edema, first trimester ♀   **M**

    O12.02   Gestational edema, second trimester ♀   **M**

    O12.03   Gestational edema, third trimester ♀   **M**

  ● O12.1   Gestational proteinuria

    O12.10   Gestational proteinuria, `unspecified` trimester ♀   **M**

    O12.11   Gestational proteinuria, first trimester ♀   **M**

    O12.12   Gestational proteinuria, second trimester ♀   **M**

    O12.13   Gestational proteinuria, third trimester ♀   **M**

  ● O12.2   Gestational edema with proteinuria

    O12.20   Gestational edema with proteinuria, `unspecified` trimester ♀   **M**

    O12.21   Gestational edema with proteinuria, first trimester ♀   **M**

    O12.22   Gestational edema with proteinuria, second trimester ♀   **M**

    O12.23   Gestational edema with proteinuria, third trimester ♀   **M**

● O13   Gestational [pregnancy-induced] hypertension without significant proteinuria

  Includes   gestational hypertension NOS

  O13.1   Gestational [pregnancy-induced] hypertension without significant proteinuria, first trimester ♀   **M**

  O13.2   Gestational [pregnancy-induced] hypertension without significant proteinuria, second trimester ♀   **M**

  O13.3   Gestational [pregnancy-induced] hypertension without significant proteinuria, third trimester ♀   **M**

  O13.9   Gestational [pregnancy-induced] hypertension without significant proteinuria, `unspecified` trimester ♀   **M**

● O14   Pre-eclampsia

  Excludes1   pre-existing hypertension with pre-eclampsia (O11)

  ● O14.0   Mild to moderate pre-eclampsia

    O14.00   Mild to moderate pre-eclampsia, `unspecified` trimester ♀   **M**

    O14.02   Mild to moderate pre-eclampsia, second trimester ♀   **M**

    O14.03   Mild to moderate pre-eclampsia, third trimester ♀   **M**

  ● O14.1   Severe pre-eclampsia

  Excludes1   HELLP syndrome (O14.2-)

  H=hemolysis, EL=elevated liver enzymes, LP=low platelet count

    O14.10   Severe pre-eclampsia, `unspecified` trimester ♀   **M**

    O14.12   Severe pre-eclampsia, second trimester ♀   **M**

    O14.13   Severe pre-eclampsia, third trimester ♀   **M**

  ● O14.2   HELLP syndrome

  Severe pre-eclampsia with hemolysis, elevated liver enzymes and low platelet count (HELLP)

    O14.20   HELLP syndrome (HELLP), `unspecified` trimester ♀   **M**

    O14.22   HELLP syndrome (HELLP), second trimester ♀   **M**

    O14.23   HELLP syndrome (HELLP), third trimester ♀   **M**

  ● O14.9   Unspecified pre-eclampsia

    O14.90   `Unspecified` pre-eclampsia, unspecified trimester ♀   **M**

    O14.92   `Unspecified` pre-eclampsia, second trimester ♀   **M**

    O14.93   `Unspecified` pre-eclampsia, third trimester ♀   **M**

● O15   Eclampsia

  Includes   convulsions following conditions in O10-O14 and O16

  ● O15.0   Eclampsia in pregnancy

    O15.00   Eclampsia in pregnancy, `unspecified` trimester ♀   **M**

    O15.02   Eclampsia in pregnancy, second trimester ♀   **M**

    O15.03   Eclampsia in pregnancy, third trimester ♀   **M**

  O15.1   Eclampsia in labor ♀   **M**

  O15.2   Eclampsia in the puerperium ♀   **M**

  O15.9   Eclampsia, `unspecified` as to time period ♀   **M**
    Eclampsia NOS

● O16   Unspecified maternal hypertension

  O16.1   `Unspecified` maternal hypertension, first trimester ♀   **M**

  O16.2   `Unspecified` maternal hypertension, second trimester ♀   **M**

  O16.3   `Unspecified` maternal hypertension, third trimester ♀   **M**

  O16.9   `Unspecified` maternal hypertension, unspecified trimester ♀   **M**

◀ New   ◀▥ Revised   ~~deleted~~ Deleted   Excludes 1   Excludes 2   Includes   Use additional   Code first   Code also   Unspecified

OGCR Official Guidelines   X Assign placeholder X   ● Use Additional Character(s)   ▶ Manifestation Code   **Coding Clinic**

OTHER MATERNAL DISORDERS PREDOMINANTLY RELATED TO PREGNANCY (O20-O29)

Excludes2   maternal care related to the fetus and amniotic cavity and possible delivery problems (O30-O48)

maternal diseases classifiable elsewhere but complicating pregnancy, labor and delivery, and the puerperium (O98-O99)

● **O20**   **Hemorrhage in early pregnancy**

     Includes   hemorrhage before completion of 20 weeks gestation

     Excludes1   pregnancy with abortive outcome (O00-O08)

     O20.0   **Threatened abortion** ♀   **M**
         Hemorrhage specified as due to threatened abortion

     O20.8   **Other hemorrhage in early pregnancy** ♀   **M**

     O20.9   **Hemorrhage in early pregnancy, unspecified** ♀   **M**

● **O21**   **Excessive vomiting in pregnancy**

     O21.0   **Mild hyperemesis gravidarum** ♀   **M**
         Hyperemesis gravidarum, mild or unspecified, starting before the end of the 20th week of gestation

     O21.1   **Hyperemesis gravidarum with metabolic disturbance** ♀   **M**
         Hyperemesis gravidarum, starting before the end of the 20th week of gestation, with metabolic disturbance such as carbohydrate depletion
         Hyperemesis gravidarum, starting before the end of the 20th week of gestation, with metabolic disturbance such as dehydration
         Hyperemesis gravidarum, starting before the end of the 20th week of gestation, with metabolic disturbance such as electrolyte imbalance

     O21.2   **Late vomiting of pregnancy** ♀   **M**
         Excessive vomiting starting after 20 completed weeks of gestation

     O21.8   **Other vomiting complicating pregnancy** ♀   **M**
         Vomiting due to diseases classified elsewhere, complicating pregnancy
         Use additional code, to identify cause

     O21.9   **Vomiting of pregnancy, unspecified** ♀   **M**

● **O22**   **Venous complications and hemorrhoids in pregnancy**

     Excludes1   venous complications of:
         abortion NOS (O03.9)
         ectopic or molar pregnancy (O08.7)
         failed attempted abortion (O07.35)
         induced abortion (O04.85)
         spontaneous abortion (O03.89)

     Excludes2   obstetric pulmonary embolism (O88.-)
         venous complications and hemorrhoids of childbirth and the puerperium (O87.-)

     ● O22.0   **Varicose veins of lower extremity in pregnancy**
         Varicose veins NOS in pregnancy

         O22.00   **Varicose veins of lower extremity in pregnancy, unspecified trimester** ♀   **M**

         O22.01   **Varicose veins of lower extremity in pregnancy, first trimester** ♀   **M**

         O22.02   **Varicose veins of lower extremity in pregnancy, second trimester** ♀   **M**

         O22.03   **Varicose veins of lower extremity in pregnancy, third trimester** ♀   **M**

● **O22.1**   **Genital varices in pregnancy**
     Perineal varices in pregnancy
     Vaginal varices in pregnancy
     Vulval varices in pregnancy

     O22.10   **Genital varices in pregnancy, unspecified trimester** ♀   **M**

     O22.11   **Genital varices in pregnancy, first trimester** ♀ **M**

     O22.12   **Genital varices in pregnancy, second trimester** ♀

     O22.13   **Genital varices in pregnancy, third trimester** ♀ **M**

● **O22.2**   **Superficial thrombophlebitis in pregnancy**
     Phlebitis in pregnancy NOS
     Thrombophlebitis of legs in pregnancy
     Thrombosis in pregnancy NOS

     Use additional code to identify the superficial thrombophlebitis (I80.0-)

     O22.20   **Superficial thrombophlebitis in pregnancy, unspecified trimester** ♀   **M**

     O22.21   **Superficial thrombophlebitis in pregnancy, first trimester** ♀   **M**

     O22.22   **Superficial thrombophlebitis in pregnancy, second trimester** ♀

     O22.23   **Superficial thrombophlebitis in pregnancy, third trimester** ♀   **M**

● **O22.3**   **Deep phlebothrombosis in pregnancy**
     Deep vein thrombosis, antepartum

     Use additional code to identify the deep vein thrombosis (I82.4-, I82.5-, I82.62-. I82.72-)

     Use additional code, if applicable, for associated long-term (current) use of anticoagulants (Z79.01)

     O22.30   **Deep phlebothrombosis in pregnancy, unspecified trimester** ♀   **M**

     O22.31   **Deep phlebothrombosis in pregnancy, first trimester** ♀   **M**

     O22.32   **Deep phlebothrombosis in pregnancy, second trimester** ♀   **M**

     O22.33   **Deep phlebothrombosis in pregnancy, third trimester** ♀   **M**

● **O22.4**   **Hemorrhoids in pregnancy**

     O22.40   **Hemorrhoids in pregnancy, unspecified trimester** ♀   **M**

     O22.41   **Hemorrhoids in pregnancy, first trimester** ♀ **M**

     O22.42   **Hemorrhoids in pregnancy, second trimester** ♀

     O22.43   **Hemorrhoids in pregnancy, third trimester** ♀   **M**

● **O22.5**   **Cerebral venous thrombosis in pregnancy**
     Cerebrovenous sinus thrombosis in pregnancy

     O22.50   **Cerebral venous thrombosis in pregnancy, unspecified trimester** ♀   **M**

     O22.51   **Cerebral venous thrombosis in pregnancy, first trimester** ♀   **M**

     O22.52   **Cerebral venous thrombosis in pregnancy, second trimester** ♀   **M**

     O22.53   **Cerebral venous thrombosis in pregnancy, third trimester** ♀   **M**

● **O22.8**   **Other venous complications in pregnancy**

     ● O22.8X   **Other venous complications in pregnancy**

         O22.8X1   **Other venous complications in pregnancy, first trimester** ♀   **M**

         O22.8X2   **Other venous complications in pregnancy, second trimester** ♀   **M**

         O22.8X3   **Other venous complications in pregnancy, third trimester** ♀   **M**

         O22.8X9   **Other venous complications in pregnancy, unspecified trimester** ♀   **M**

CHAPTER 15 (O00-O9A)

● **O22.9**   **Venous complication in pregnancy, unspecified**
Gestational phlebitis NOS
Gestational phlebopathy NOS
Gestational thrombosis NOS

O22.90   Venous complication in pregnancy, unspecified, unspecified trimester ♀   M

O22.91   Venous complication in pregnancy, unspecified, first trimester ♀   M

O22.92   Venous complication in pregnancy, unspecified, second trimester ♀   M

O22.93   Venous complication in pregnancy, unspecified, third trimester ♀   M

● **O23**   **Infections of genitourinary tract in pregnancy**
Use additional code to identify organism (B95.-, B96.-)

Excludes2   gonococcal infections complicating pregnancy, childbirth and the puerperium (O98.2)
infections with a predominantly sexual mode of transmission NOS complicating pregnancy, childbirth and the puerperium (O98.3)
syphilis complicating pregnancy, childbirth and the puerperium (O98.1)
tuberculosis of genitourinary system complicating pregnancy, childbirth and the puerperium (O98.0)
venereal disease NOS complicating pregnancy, childbirth and the puerperium (O98.3)

● **O23.0**   **Infections of kidney in pregnancy**
Pyelonephritis in pregnancy

O23.00   Infections of kidney in pregnancy, unspecified trimester ♀   M

O23.01   Infections of kidney in pregnancy, first trimester ♀   M

O23.02   Infections of kidney in pregnancy, second trimester ♀   M

O23.03   Infections of kidney in pregnancy, third trimester ♀   M

● **O23.1**   **Infections of bladder in pregnancy**

O23.10   Infections of bladder in pregnancy, unspecified trimester ♀   M

O23.11   Infections of bladder in pregnancy, first trimester ♀   M

O23.12   Infections of bladder in pregnancy, second trimester ♀   M

O23.13   Infections of bladder in pregnancy, third trimester ♀   M

● **O23.2**   **Infections of urethra in pregnancy**

O23.20   Infections of urethra in pregnancy, unspecified trimester ♀   M

O23.21   Infections of urethra in pregnancy, first trimester ♀   M

O23.22   Infections of urethra in pregnancy, second trimester ♀   M

O23.23   Infections of urethra in pregnancy, third trimester ♀   M

● **O23.3**   **Infections of other parts of urinary tract in pregnancy**

O23.30   Infections of other parts of urinary tract in pregnancy, unspecified trimester ♀   M

O23.31   Infections of other parts of urinary tract in pregnancy, first trimester ♀   M

O23.32   Infections of other parts of urinary tract in pregnancy, second trimester ♀   M

O23.33   Infections of other parts of urinary tract in pregnancy, third trimester ♀   M

● **O23.4**   **Unspecified infection of urinary tract in pregnancy**

O23.40   Unspecified infection of urinary tract in pregnancy, unspecified trimester ♀   M

O23.41   Unspecified infection of urinary tract in pregnancy, first trimester ♀   M

O23.42   Unspecified infection of urinary tract in pregnancy, second trimester ♀   M

O23.43   Unspecified infection of urinary tract in pregnancy, third trimester ♀   M

● **O23.5**   **Infections of the genital tract in pregnancy**

● O23.51   Infection of cervix in pregnancy

O23.511   Infections of cervix in pregnancy, first trimester ♀   M

O23.512   Infections of cervix in pregnancy, second trimester ♀   M

O23.513   Infections of cervix in pregnancy, third trimester ♀   M

O23.519   Infections of cervix in pregnancy, unspecified trimester ♀   M

● O23.52   Salpingo-oophoritis in pregnancy
Oophoritis = inflammation of ovary
Salpingitis = inflammation of fallopian tube
Oophoritis in pregnancy
Salpingitis in pregnancy

O23.521   Salpingo-oophoritis in pregnancy, first trimester ♀   M

O23.522   Salpingo-oophoritis in pregnancy, second trimester ♀   M

O23.523   Salpingo-oophoritis in pregnancy, third trimester ♀   M

O23.529   Salpingo-oophoritis in pregnancy, unspecified trimester ♀   M

● O23.59   Infection of other part of genital tract in pregnancy

O23.591   Infection of other part of genital tract in pregnancy, first trimester ♀   M

O23.592   Infection of other part of genital tract in pregnancy, second trimester ♀   M

O23.593   Infection of other part of genital tract in pregnancy, third trimester ♀   M

O23.599   Infection of other part of genital tract in pregnancy, unspecified trimester ♀   M

● **O23.9**   **Unspecified genitourinary tract infection in pregnancy**
Genitourinary tract infection in pregnancy NOS

O23.90   Unspecified genitourinary tract infection in pregnancy, unspecified trimester ♀   M

O23.91   Unspecified genitourinary tract infection in pregnancy, first trimester ♀   M

O23.92   Unspecified genitourinary tract infection in pregnancy, second trimester ♀   M

O23.93   Unspecified genitourinary tract infection in pregnancy, third trimester ♀   M

◀ New   ◀▥ Revised   ~~deleted~~ Deleted   Excludes 1   Excludes 2   Includes   Use additional   Code first   Code also   Unspecified
OGCR Official Guidelines   X Assign placeholder X   ● Use Additional Character(s)   ▶ Manifestation Code   **Coding Clinic**

OGCR Section I.C.15.g.

g. Diabetes mellitus in pregnancy

Diabetes mellitus is a significant complicating factor in pregnancy. Pregnant women who are diabetic should be assigned a code from category O24, Diabetes mellitus in pregnancy, childbirth, and the puerperium, first, followed by the appropriate diabetes code(s) (E08-E13) from Chapter 4.

OGCR Section I.C.15.i.

i. Gestational (pregnancy induced) diabetes

Gestational (pregnancy induced) diabetes can occur during the second and third trimester of pregnancy in women who were not diabetic prior to pregnancy. Gestational diabetes can cause complications in the pregnancy similar to those of pre-existing diabetes mellitus. It also puts the woman at greater risk of developing diabetes after the pregnancy. Codes for gestational diabetes are in subcategory O24.4, Gestational diabetes mellitus. No other code from category O24, Diabetes mellitus in pregnancy, childbirth, and the puerperium, should be used with a code from O24.4

The codes under subcategory O24.4 include diet controlled and insulin controlled. If a patient with gestational diabetes is treated with both diet and insulin, only the code for insulin-controlled is required. Code Z79.4, Long-term (current) use of insulin, should not be assigned with codes from subcategory O24.4.

An abnormal glucose tolerance in pregnancy is assigned a code from subcategory O99.81, Abnormal glucose complicating pregnancy, childbirth, and the puerperium.

● O24   **Diabetes mellitus in pregnancy, childbirth, and the puerperium**
- ● O24.0   **Pre-existing diabetes mellitus, type 1, in pregnancy, childbirth and the puerperium**
  Juvenile onset diabetes mellitus, in pregnancy, childbirth and the puerperium
  Ketosis-prone diabetes mellitus in pregnancy, childbirth and the puerperium
  Use additional code from category E10 to further identify any manifestations
  - ● O24.01   Pre-existing diabetes mellitus, type 1, in pregnancy
    - O24.011   Pre-existing diabetes mellitus, type 1, in pregnancy, first trimester ♀   M
    - O24.012   Pre-existing diabetes mellitus, type 1, in pregnancy, second trimester ♀   M
    - O24.013   Pre-existing diabetes mellitus, type 1, in pregnancy, third trimester ♀   M
    - O24.019   Pre-existing diabetes mellitus, type 1, in pregnancy, unspecified trimester ♀   M
  - O24.02   Pre-existing diabetes mellitus, type 1, in childbirth ♀   M
  - O24.03   Pre-existing diabetes mellitus, type 1, in the puerperium ♀   M
- ● O24.1   **Pre-existing diabetes mellitus, type 2, in pregnancy, childbirth and the puerperium**
  Insulin-resistant diabetes mellitus in pregnancy, childbirth and the puerperium
  Use additional code (for):
  from category E11 to further identify any manifestations
  long-term (current) use of insulin (Z79.4)
  - ● O24.11   Pre-existing diabetes mellitus, type 2, in pregnancy
    - O24.111   Pre-existing diabetes mellitus, type 2, in pregnancy, first trimester ♀   M
    - O24.112   Pre-existing diabetes mellitus, type 2, in pregnancy, second trimester ♀   M
    - O24.113   Pre-existing diabetes mellitus, type 2, in pregnancy, third trimester ♀   M
    - O24.119   Pre-existing diabetes mellitus, type 2, in pregnancy, unspecified trimester ♀   M

- O24.12   Pre-existing diabetes mellitus, type 2, in childbirth ♀   M
- O24.13   Pre-existing diabetes mellitus, type 2, in the puerperium ♀   M
- ● O24.3   **Unspecified pre-existing diabetes mellitus in pregnancy, childbirth and the puerperium**
  Use additional code (for):
  from category E11 to further identify any manifestation
  long-term (current) use of insulin (Z79.4)
  - ● O24.31   Unspecified pre-existing diabetes mellitus in pregnancy
    - O24.311   Unspecified pre-existing diabetes mellitus in pregnancy, first trimester ♀   M
    - O24.312   Unspecified pre-existing diabetes mellitus in pregnancy, second trimester ♀   M
    - O24.313   Unspecified pre-existing diabetes mellitus in pregnancy, third trimester ♀   M
    - O24.319   Unspecified pre-existing diabetes mellitus in pregnancy, unspecified trimester ♀   M
  - O24.32   Unspecified pre-existing diabetes mellitus in childbirth ♀   M
  - O24.33   Unspecified pre-existing diabetes mellitus in the puerperium ♀   M
- ● O24.4   **Gestational diabetes mellitus**
  Diabetes mellitus arising in pregnancy
  Gestational diabetes mellitus NOS
  - ● O24.41   Gestational diabetes mellitus in pregnancy
    - O24.410   Gestational diabetes mellitus in pregnancy, diet controlled ♀   M
    - O24.414   Gestational diabetes mellitus in pregnancy, insulin controlled ♀   M
    - O24.419   Gestational diabetes mellitus in pregnancy, unspecified control ♀   M
  - ● O24.42   Gestational diabetes mellitus in childbirth
    - O24.420   Gestational diabetes mellitus in childbirth, diet controlled ♀   M
    - O24.424   Gestational diabetes mellitus in childbirth, insulin controlled ♀   M
    - O24.429   Gestational diabetes mellitus in childbirth, unspecified control ♀   M
  - ● O24.43   Gestational diabetes mellitus in the puerperium
    - O24.430   Gestational diabetes mellitus in the puerperium, diet controlled ♀   M
    - O24.434   Gestational diabetes mellitus in the puerperium, insulin controlled ♀   M
    - O24.439   Gestational diabetes mellitus in the puerperium, unspecified control ♀   M
- ● O24.8   **Other pre-existing diabetes mellitus in pregnancy, childbirth, and the puerperium**
  Use additional code (for):
  from categories E08, E09 and E13 to further identify any manifestation
  long-term (current) use of insulin (Z79.4)
  - ● O24.81   Other pre-existing diabetes mellitus in pregnancy
    - O24.811   Other pre-existing diabetes mellitus in pregnancy, first trimester ♀   M
    - O24.812   Other pre-existing diabetes mellitus in pregnancy, second trimester ♀   M
    - O24.813   Other pre-existing diabetes mellitus in pregnancy, third trimester ♀   M
    - O24.819   Other pre-existing diabetes mellitus in pregnancy, unspecified trimester ♀   M

CHAPTER 15 (O00-O9A)

O24.82   Other pre-existing diabetes mellitus in childbirth ♀   **M**

O24.83   Other pre-existing diabetes mellitus in the puerperium ♀   **M**

● O24.9   Unspecified diabetes mellitus in pregnancy, childbirth and the puerperium

> Use additional code for long-term (current) use of insulin (Z79.4)
> *Unknown whether patient was diabetic before pregnancy occurred*

   ● O24.91   Unspecified diabetes mellitus in pregnancy

       O24.911   Unspecified diabetes mellitus in pregnancy, first trimester ♀   **M**

       O24.912   Unspecified diabetes mellitus in pregnancy, second trimester ♀   **M**

       O24.913   Unspecified diabetes mellitus in pregnancy, third trimester ♀   **M**

       O24.919   Unspecified diabetes mellitus in pregnancy, unspecified trimester ♀   **M**

    O24.92   Unspecified diabetes mellitus in childbirth ♀   **M**

    O24.93   Unspecified diabetes mellitus in the puerperium ♀   **M**

● O25   Malnutrition in pregnancy, childbirth and the puerperium

  ● O25.1   Malnutrition in pregnancy

    O25.10   Malnutrition in pregnancy, unspecified trimester ♀   **M**

    O25.11   Malnutrition in pregnancy, first trimester ♀   **M**

    O25.12   Malnutrition in pregnancy, second trimester ♀ **M**

    O25.13   Malnutrition in pregnancy, third trimester ♀   **M**

   O25.2   Malnutrition in childbirth ♀   **M**

   O25.3   Malnutrition in the puerperium ♀   **M**

● O26   Maternal care for other conditions predominantly related to pregnancy

  ● O26.0   Excessive weight gain in pregnancy

> **Excludes2**   gestational edema (O12.0, O12.2)

    O26.00   Excessive weight gain in pregnancy, unspecified trimester ♀   **M**

    O26.01   Excessive weight gain in pregnancy, first trimester ♀   **M**

    O26.02   Excessive weight gain in pregnancy, second trimester ♀   **M**

    O26.03   Excessive weight gain in pregnancy, third trimester ♀   **M**

  ● O26.1   Low weight gain in pregnancy

    O26.10   Low weight gain in pregnancy, unspecified trimester ♀   **M**

    O26.11   Low weight gain in pregnancy, first trimester ♀   **M**

    O26.12   Low weight gain in pregnancy, second trimester ♀   **M**

    O26.13   Low weight gain in pregnancy, third trimester ♀   **M**

  ● O26.2   Pregnancy care for patient with recurrent pregnancy loss

    O26.20   Pregnancy care for patient with recurrent pregnancy loss, unspecified trimester ♀   **M**

    O26.21   Pregnancy care for patient with recurrent pregnancy loss, first trimester ♀   **M**

    O26.22   Pregnancy care for patient with recurrent pregnancy loss, second trimester ♀   **M**

    O26.23   Pregnancy care for patient with recurrent pregnancy loss, third trimester ♀   **M**

  ● O26.3   Retained intrauterine contraceptive device in pregnancy

    O26.30   Retained intrauterine contraceptive device in pregnancy, unspecified trimester ♀   **M**

    O26.31   Retained intrauterine contraceptive device in pregnancy, first trimester ♀   **M**

    O26.32   Retained intrauterine contraceptive device in pregnancy, second trimester ♀   **M**

    O26.33   Retained intrauterine contraceptive device in pregnancy, third trimester ♀   **M**

  ● O26.4   Herpes gestationis

    O26.40   Herpes gestationis, unspecified trimester ♀   **M**

    O26.41   Herpes gestationis, first trimester ♀   **M**

    O26.42   Herpes gestationis, second trimester ♀   **M**

    O26.43   Herpes gestationis, third trimester ♀   **M**

  ● O26.5   Maternal hypotension syndrome

> Supine hypotensive syndrome

    O26.50   Maternal hypotension syndrome, unspecified trimester ♀   **M**

    O26.51   Maternal hypotension syndrome, first trimester ♀   **M**

    O26.52   Maternal hypotension syndrome, second trimester ♀   **M**

    O26.53   Maternal hypotension syndrome, third trimester ♀   **M**

  ● O26.6   Liver and biliary tract disorders in pregnancy, childbirth and the puerperium

> Use additional code to identify the specific disorder
>
> **Excludes2**   hepatorenal syndrome following labor and delivery (O90.4)

   ● O26.61   Liver and biliary tract disorders in pregnancy

       O26.611   Liver and biliary tract disorders in pregnancy, first trimester ♀   **M**

       O26.612   Liver and biliary tract disorders in pregnancy, second trimester ♀   **M**

       O26.613   Liver and biliary tract disorders in pregnancy, third trimester ♀   **M**

       O26.619   Liver and biliary tract disorders in pregnancy, unspecified trimester ♀   **M**

    O26.62   Liver and biliary tract disorders in childbirth ♀   **M**

    O26.63   Liver and biliary tract disorders in the puerperium ♀   **M**

  ● O26.7   Subluxation of symphysis (pubis) in pregnancy, childbirth and the puerperium

> **Excludes1**   traumatic separation of symphysis (pubis) during childbirth (O71.6)

   ● O26.71   Subluxation of symphysis (pubis) in pregnancy

       O26.711   Subluxation of symphysis (pubis) in pregnancy, first trimester ♀   **M**

       O26.712   Subluxation of symphysis (pubis) in pregnancy, second trimester ♀   **M**

       O26.713   Subluxation of symphysis (pubis) in pregnancy, third trimester ♀   **M**

       O26.719   Subluxation of symphysis (pubis) in pregnancy, unspecified trimester ♀   **M**

    O26.72   Subluxation of symphysis (pubis) in childbirth ♀   **M**

    O26.73   Subluxation of symphysis (pubis) in the puerperium ♀   **M**

  ● O26.8   Other specified pregnancy related conditions

   ● O26.81   Pregnancy related exhaustion and fatigue

       O26.811   Pregnancy related exhaustion and fatigue, first trimester ♀   **M**

       O26.812   Pregnancy related exhaustion and fatigue, second trimester ♀   **M**

       O26.813   Pregnancy related exhaustion and fatigue, third trimester ♀   **M**

       O26.819   Pregnancy related exhaustion and fatigue, unspecified trimester ♀   **M**

◀ New   ⬅ Revised   ~~deleted~~ Deleted   Excludes 1   Excludes 2   Includes   Use additional   Code first   Code also   Unspecified

OGCR Official Guidelines   **X** Assign placeholder X   ● Use Additional Character(s)   ▶ Manifestation Code   **Coding Clinic**

● **O26.82**   **Pregnancy related peripheral neuritis**

    O26.821   Pregnancy related peripheral neuritis, first trimester ♀   M

    O26.822   Pregnancy related peripheral neuritis, second trimester ♀   M

    O26.823   Pregnancy related peripheral neuritis, third trimester ♀   M

    O26.829   Pregnancy related peripheral neuritis, unspecified trimester ♀   M

● **O26.83**   **Pregnancy related renal disease**

    Use additional code to identify the specific disorder

    O26.831   Pregnancy related renal disease, first trimester ♀   M

    O26.832   Pregnancy related renal disease, second trimester ♀   M

    O26.833   Pregnancy related renal disease, third trimester ♀   M

    O26.839   Pregnancy related renal disease, unspecified trimester ♀   M

● **O26.84**   **Uterine size-date discrepancy complicating pregnancy**

    Excludes1   encounter for suspected problem with fetal growth ruled out (Z03.74)

    O26.841   Uterine size-date discrepancy, first trimester ♀   M

    O26.842   Uterine size-date discrepancy, second trimester ♀   M

    O26.843   Uterine size-date discrepancy, third trimester ♀   M

    O26.849   Uterine size-date discrepancy, unspecified trimester ♀   M

● **O26.85**   **Spotting complicating pregnancy**

    O26.851   Spotting complicating pregnancy, first trimester ♀   M

    O26.852   Spotting complicating pregnancy, second trimester ♀   M

    O26.853   Spotting complicating pregnancy, third trimester ♀   M

    O26.859   Spotting complicating pregnancy, unspecified trimester ♀   M

   O26.86   Pruritic urticarial papules and plaques of pregnancy (PUPPP) ♀   M

    Polymorphic eruption of pregnancy

● **O26.87**   **Cervical shortening**

    Excludes1   encounter for suspected cervical shortening ruled out (Z03.75)

    O26.872   Cervical shortening, second trimester ♀   M

    O26.873   Cervical shortening, third trimester ♀   M

    O26.879   Cervical shortening, unspecified trimester ♀   M

● **O26.89**   **Other specified pregnancy related conditions**

    O26.891   Other specified pregnancy related conditions, first trimester ♀   M

    O26.892   Other specified pregnancy related conditions, second trimester ♀   M

    O26.893   Other specified pregnancy related conditions, third trimester ♀   M

    O26.899   Other specified pregnancy related conditions, unspecified trimester ♀   M

● **O26.9**   **Pregnancy related conditions, unspecified**

    O26.90   Pregnancy related conditions, unspecified, unspecified trimester ♀   M

    O26.91   Pregnancy related conditions, unspecified, first trimester ♀   M

    O26.92   Pregnancy related conditions, unspecified, second trimester ♀   M

    O26.93   Pregnancy related conditions, unspecified, third trimester ♀   M

● **O28**   **Abnormal findings on antenatal screening of mother**

    Excludes1   diagnostic findings classified elsewhere - see Alphabetical Index

   O28.0   Abnormal hematological finding on antenatal screening of mother ♀   M

   O28.1   Abnormal biochemical finding on antenatal screening of mother ♀   M

   O28.2   Abnormal cytological finding on antenatal screening of mother ♀   M

   O28.3   Abnormal ultrasonic finding on antenatal screening of mother ♀   M

   O28.4   Abnormal radiological finding on antenatal screening of mother ♀   M

   O28.5   Abnormal chromosomal and genetic finding on antenatal screening of mother ♀   M

   O28.8   Other abnormal findings on antenatal screening of mother ♀   M

   O28.9   Unspecified abnormal findings on antenatal screening of mother ♀   M

● **O29**   **Complications of anesthesia during pregnancy**

    Includes   maternal complications arising from the administration of a general, regional or local anesthetic, analgesic or other sedation during pregnancy

    Use additional code, if necessary, to identify the complication

    Excludes2   complications of anesthesia during labor and delivery (O74.-)

       complications of anesthesia during the puerperium (O89.-)

● **O29.0**   **Pulmonary complications of anesthesia during pregnancy**

   ● **O29.01**   **Aspiration pneumonitis due to anesthesia during pregnancy**

      Inhalation of stomach contents or secretions NOS due to anesthesia during pregnancy

      Mendelson's syndrome due to anesthesia during pregnancy

      O29.011   Aspiration pneumonitis due to anesthesia during pregnancy, first trimester ♀   M

      O29.012   Aspiration pneumonitis due to anesthesia during pregnancy, second trimester ♀   M

      O29.013   Aspiration pneumonitis due to anesthesia during pregnancy, third trimester ♀   M

      O29.019   Aspiration pneumonitis due to anesthesia during pregnancy, unspecified trimester ♀   M

● **O29.02**   **Pressure collapse of lung due to anesthesia during pregnancy**

     O29.021   Pressure collapse of lung due to anesthesia during pregnancy, first trimester ♀   M

     O29.022   Pressure collapse of lung due to anesthesia during pregnancy, second trimester ♀   M

     O29.023   Pressure collapse of lung due to anesthesia during pregnancy, third trimester ♀   M

     O29.029   Pressure collapse of lung due to anesthesia during pregnancy, unspecified trimester ♀   M

● **O29.09**   **Other pulmonary complications of anesthesia during pregnancy**

     O29.091   Other pulmonary complications of anesthesia during pregnancy, first trimester ♀   M

     O29.092   Other pulmonary complications of anesthesia during pregnancy, second trimester ♀   M

     O29.093   Other pulmonary complications of anesthesia during pregnancy, third trimester ♀   M

     O29.099   Other pulmonary complications of anesthesia during pregnancy, unspecified trimester ♀   M

● **O29.1**   **Cardiac complications of anesthesia during pregnancy**

   ● **O29.11**   **Cardiac arrest due to anesthesia during pregnancy**

     O29.111   Cardiac arrest due to anesthesia during pregnancy, first trimester ♀   M

     O29.112   Cardiac arrest due to anesthesia during pregnancy, second trimester ♀   M

     O29.113   Cardiac arrest due to anesthesia during pregnancy, third trimester ♀   M

     O29.119   Cardiac arrest due to anesthesia during pregnancy, unspecified trimester ♀   M

   ● **O29.12**   **Cardiac failure due to anesthesia during pregnancy**

     O29.121   Cardiac failure due to anesthesia during pregnancy, first trimester ♀   M

     O29.122   Cardiac failure due to anesthesia during pregnancy, second trimester ♀   M

     O29.123   Cardiac failure due to anesthesia during pregnancy, third trimester ♀   M

     O29.129   Cardiac failure due to anesthesia during pregnancy, unspecified trimester ♀   M

   ● **O29.19**   **Other cardiac complications of anesthesia during pregnancy**

     O29.191   Other cardiac complications of anesthesia during pregnancy, first trimester ♀   M

     O29.192   Other cardiac complications of anesthesia during pregnancy, second trimester ♀   M

     O29.193   Other cardiac complications of anesthesia during pregnancy, third trimester ♀   M

     O29.199   Other cardiac complications of anesthesia during pregnancy, unspecified trimester ♀   M

● **O29.2**   **Central nervous system complications of anesthesia during pregnancy**

   ● **O29.21**   **Cerebral anoxia due to anesthesia during pregnancy**

     O29.211   Cerebral anoxia due to anesthesia during pregnancy, first trimester ♀   M

     O29.212   Cerebral anoxia due to anesthesia during pregnancy, second trimester ♀   M

     O29.213   Cerebral anoxia due to anesthesia during pregnancy, third trimester ♀   M

     O29.219   Cerebral anoxia due to anesthesia during pregnancy, unspecified trimester ♀   M

   ● **O29.29**   **Other central nervous system complications of anesthesia during pregnancy**

     O29.291   Other central nervous system complications of anesthesia during pregnancy, first trimester ♀   M

     O29.292   Other central nervous system complications of anesthesia during pregnancy, second trimester ♀   M

     O29.293   Other central nervous system complications of anesthesia during pregnancy, third trimester ♀   M

     O29.299   Other central nervous system complications of anesthesia during pregnancy, unspecified trimester ♀   M

● **O29.3**   **Toxic reaction to local anesthesia during pregnancy**

   ● **O29.3X**   **Toxic reaction to local anesthesia during pregnancy**

     O29.3X1   Toxic reaction to local anesthesia during pregnancy, first trimester ♀   M

     O29.3X2   Toxic reaction to local anesthesia during pregnancy, second trimester ♀   M

     O29.3X3   Toxic reaction to local anesthesia during pregnancy, third trimester ♀   M

     O29.3X9   Toxic reaction to local anesthesia during pregnancy, unspecified trimester ♀   M

● **O29.4**   **Spinal and epidural anesthesia induced headache during pregnancy**

     O29.40   Spinal and epidural anesthesia induced headache during pregnancy, unspecified trimester ♀   M

     O29.41   Spinal and epidural anesthesia induced headache during pregnancy, first trimester ♀   M

     O29.42   Spinal and epidural anesthesia induced headache during pregnancy, second trimester ♀   M

     O29.43   Spinal and epidural anesthesia induced headache during pregnancy, third trimester ♀   M

● **O29.5**   **Other complications of spinal and epidural anesthesia during pregnancy**

   ● **O29.5X**   **Other complications of spinal and epidural anesthesia during pregnancy**

     O29.5X1   Other complications of spinal and epidural anesthesia during pregnancy, first trimester ♀   M

     O29.5X2   Other complications of spinal and epidural anesthesia during pregnancy, second trimester ♀   M

     O29.5X3   Other complications of spinal and epidural anesthesia during pregnancy, third trimester ♀   M

     O29.5X9   Other complications of spinal and epidural anesthesia during pregnancy, unspecified trimester ♀   M

◀ New   ◀ Revised   ~~deleted~~ Deleted   Excludes 1   Excludes 2   Includes   Use additional   Code first   Code also   Unspecified

OGCR Official Guidelines   X Assign placeholder X   ● Use Additional Character(s)   ▶ Manifestation Code   **Coding Clinic**

- O29.6   Failed or difficult intubation for anesthesia during pregnancy
  - O29.60   Failed or difficult intubation for anesthesia during pregnancy, unspecified trimester ♀   M
  - O29.61   Failed or difficult intubation for anesthesia during pregnancy, first trimester ♀   M
  - O29.62   Failed or difficult intubation for anesthesia during pregnancy, second trimester ♀   M
  - O29.63   Failed or difficult intubation for anesthesia during pregnancy, third trimester ♀   M
- O29.8   Other complications of anesthesia during pregnancy
  - O29.8X   Other complications of anesthesia during pregnancy
    - O29.8X1   Other complications of anesthesia during pregnancy, first trimester ♀   M
    - O29.8X2   Other complications of anesthesia during pregnancy, second trimester ♀   M
    - O29.8X3   Other complications of anesthesia during pregnancy, third trimester ♀   M
    - O29.8X9   Other complications of anesthesia during pregnancy, unspecified trimester ♀   M
- O29.9   Unspecified complication of anesthesia during pregnancy
  - O29.90   Unspecified complication of anesthesia during pregnancy, unspecified trimester ♀   M
  - O29.91   Unspecified complication of anesthesia during pregnancy, first trimester ♀   M
  - O29.92   Unspecified complication of anesthesia during pregnancy, second trimester ♀   M
  - O29.93   Unspecified complication of anesthesia during pregnancy, third trimester ♀   M

MATERNAL CARE RELATED TO THE FETUS AND AMNIOTIC CAVITY AND POSSIBLE DELIVERY PROBLEMS (O30-O48)

- O30   Multiple gestation
  Code also any complications specific to multiple gestation
  - O30.0   Twin pregnancy
    - O30.00   Twin pregnancy, unspecified number of placenta and unspecified number of amniotic sacs
      - O30.001   Twin pregnancy, unspecified number of placenta and unspecified number of amniotic sacs, first trimester ♀   M
      - O30.002   Twin pregnancy, unspecified number of placenta and unspecified number of amniotic sacs, second trimester ♀   M
      - O30.003   Twin pregnancy, unspecified number of placenta and unspecified number of amniotic sacs, third trimester ♀   M
      - O30.009   Twin pregnancy, unspecified number of placenta and unspecified number of amniotic sacs, unspecified trimester ♀   M
    - O30.01   Twin pregnancy, monochorionic/monoamniotic
      Twin pregnancy, one placenta, one amniotic sac
      Excludes1   conjoined twins (O30.02-)
      - O30.011   Twin pregnancy, monochorionic/monoamniotic, first trimester ♀   M
      - O30.012   Twin pregnancy, monochorionic/monoamniotic, second trimester ♀   M
      - O30.013   Twin pregnancy, monochorionic/monoamniotic, third trimester ♀   M
      - O30.019   Twin pregnancy, monochorionic/monoamniotic, unspecified trimester ♀   M

- O30.02   Conjoined twin pregnancy
  - O30.021   Conjoined twin pregnancy, first trimester ♀   M
  - O30.022   Conjoined twin pregnancy, second trimester ♀   M
  - O30.023   Conjoined twin pregnancy, third trimester ♀   M
  - O30.029   Conjoined twin pregnancy, unspecified trimester ♀   M
- O30.03   Twin pregnancy, monochorionic/diamniotic
  Twin pregnancy, one placenta, two amniotic sacs
  - O30.031   Twin pregnancy, monochorionic/diamniotic, first trimester ♀   M
  - O30.032   Twin pregnancy, monochorionic/diamniotic, second trimester ♀   M
  - O30.033   Twin pregnancy, monochorionic/diamniotic, third trimester ♀   M
  - O30.039   Twin pregnancy, monochorionic/diamniotic, unspecified trimester ♀   M
- O30.04   Twin pregnancy, dichorionic/diamniotic
  Twin pregnancy, two placentae, two amniotic sacs
  - O30.041   Twin pregnancy, dichorionic/diamniotic, first trimester ♀   M
  - O30.042   Twin pregnancy, dichorionic/diamniotic, second trimester ♀   M
  - O30.043   Twin pregnancy, dichorionic/diamniotic, third trimester ♀   M
  - O30.049   Twin pregnancy, dichorionic/diamniotic, unspecified trimester ♀   M
- O30.09   Twin pregnancy, unable to determine number of placenta and number of amniotic sacs
  - O30.091   Twin pregnancy, unable to determine number of placenta and number of amniotic sacs, first trimester ♀   M
  - O30.092   Twin pregnancy, unable to determine number of placenta and number of amniotic sacs, second trimester ♀   M
  - O30.093   Twin pregnancy, unable to determine number of placenta and number of amniotic sacs, third trimester ♀   M
  - O30.099   Twin pregnancy, unable to determine number of placenta and number of amniotic sacs, unspecified trimester ♀   M
- O30.1   Triplet pregnancy
  - O30.10   Triplet pregnancy, unspecified number of placenta and unspecified number of amniotic sacs
    - O30.101   Triplet pregnancy, unspecified number of placenta and unspecified number of amniotic sacs, first trimester ♀   M
    - O30.102   Triplet pregnancy, unspecified number of placenta and unspecified number of amniotic sacs, second trimester ♀   M
    - O30.103   Triplet pregnancy, unspecified number of placenta and unspecified number of amniotic sacs, third trimester ♀   M
    - O30.109   Triplet pregnancy, unspecified number of placenta and unspecified number of amniotic sacs, unspecified trimester ♀   M

● **O30.11** Triplet pregnancy with two or more monochorionic fetuses

     O30.111   Triplet pregnancy with two or more monochorionic fetuses, first trimester ♀   M

     O30.112   Triplet pregnancy with two or more monochorionic fetuses, second trimester ♀   M

     O30.113   Triplet pregnancy with two or more monochorionic fetuses, third trimester ♀   M

     O30.119   Triplet pregnancy with two or more monochorionic fetuses, unspecified trimester ♀   M

● **O30.12** Triplet pregnancy with two or more monoamniotic fetuses

     O30.121   Triplet pregnancy with two or more monoamniotic fetuses, first trimester ♀   M

     O30.122   Triplet pregnancy with two or more monoamniotic fetuses, second trimester ♀   M

     O30.123   Triplet pregnancy with two or more monoamniotic fetuses, third trimester ♀   M

     O30.129   Triplet pregnancy with two or more monoamniotic fetuses, unspecified trimester ♀   M

● **O30.19** Triplet pregnancy, unable to determine number of placenta and number of amniotic sacs

     O30.191   Triplet pregnancy, unable to determine number of placenta and number of amniotic sacs, first trimester ♀   M

     O30.192   Triplet pregnancy, unable to determine number of placenta and number of amniotic sacs, second trimester ♀   M

     O30.193   Triplet pregnancy, unable to determine number of placenta and number of amniotic sacs, third trimester ♀   M

     O30.199   Triplet pregnancy, unable to determine number of placenta and number of amniotic sacs, unspecified trimester ♀   M

● **O30.2**   Quadruplet pregnancy

   ● **O30.20** Quadruplet pregnancy, unspecified number of placenta and unspecified number of amniotic sacs

     O30.201   Quadruplet pregnancy, unspecified number of placenta and unspecified number of amniotic sacs, first trimester ♀   M

     O30.202   Quadruplet pregnancy, unspecified number of placenta and unspecified number of amniotic sacs, second trimester ♀   M

     O30.203   Quadruplet pregnancy, unspecified number of placenta and unspecified number of amniotic sacs, third trimester ♀   M

     O30.209   Quadruplet pregnancy, unspecified number of placenta and unspecified number of amniotic sacs, unspecified trimester ♀   M

● **O30.21** Quadruplet pregnancy with two or more monochorionic fetuses

     O30.211   Quadruplet pregnancy with two or more monochorionic fetuses, first trimester ♀   M

     O30.212   Quadruplet pregnancy with two or more monochorionic fetuses, second trimester ♀   M

     O30.213   Quadruplet pregnancy with two or more monochorionic fetuses, third trimester ♀   M

     O30.219   Quadruplet pregnancy with two or more monochorionic fetuses, unspecified trimester ♀   M

● **O30.22** Quadruplet pregnancy with two or more monoamniotic fetuses

     O30.221   Quadruplet pregnancy with two or more monoamniotic fetuses, first trimester ♀   M

     O30.222   Quadruplet pregnancy with two or more monoamniotic fetuses, second trimester ♀   M

     O30.223   Quadruplet pregnancy with two or more monoamniotic fetuses, third trimester ♀   M

     O30.229   Quadruplet pregnancy with two or more monoamniotic fetuses, unspecified trimester ♀   M

● **O30.29** Quadruplet pregnancy, unable to determine number of placenta and number of amniotic sacs

     O30.291   Quadruplet pregnancy, unable to determine number of placenta and number of amniotic sacs, first trimester ♀   M

     O30.292   Quadruplet pregnancy, unable to determine number of placenta and number of amniotic sacs, second trimester ♀   M

     O30.293   Quadruplet pregnancy, unable to determine number of placenta and number of amniotic sacs, third trimester ♀   M

     O30.299   Quadruplet pregnancy, unable to determine number of placenta and number of amniotic sacs, unspecified trimester ♀   M

● **O30.8**   Other specified multiple gestation

     Multiple gestation pregnancy greater then quadruplets

   ● **O30.80** Other specified multiple gestation, unspecified number of placenta and unspecified number of amniotic sacs

     O30.801   Other specified multiple gestation, unspecified number of placenta and unspecified number of amniotic sacs, first trimester ♀   M

     O30.802   Other specified multiple gestation, unspecified number of placenta and unspecified number of amniotic sacs, second trimester ♀   M

     O30.803   Other specified multiple gestation, unspecified number of placenta and unspecified number of amniotic sacs, third trimester ♀   M

     O30.809   Other specified multiple gestation, unspecified number of placenta and unspecified number of amniotic sacs, unspecified trimester ♀   M

◀ New   ◀ Revised   ~~deleted~~ Deleted   Excludes 1   Excludes 2   Includes   Use additional   Code first   Code also   Unspecified

OGCR Official Guidelines   X Assign placeholder X   ● Use Additional Character(s)   ▶ Manifestation Code   **Coding Clinic**

● O30.81   Other specified multiple gestation with two or more monochorionic fetuses

    O30.811   Other specified multiple gestation with two or more monochorionic fetuses, first trimester ♀   **M**

    O30.812   Other specified multiple gestation with two or more monochorionic fetuses, second trimester ♀   **M**

    O30.813   Other specified multiple gestation with two or more monochorionic fetuses, third trimester ♀   **M**

    O30.819   Other specified multiple gestation with two or more monochorionic fetuses, unspecified trimester ♀   **M**

● O30.82   Other specified multiple gestation with two or more monoamniotic fetuses

    O30.821   Other specified multiple gestation with two or more monoamniotic fetuses, first trimester ♀   **M**

    O30.822   Other specified multiple gestation with two or more monoamniotic fetuses, second trimester ♀   **M**

    O30.823   Other specified multiple gestation with two or more monoamniotic fetuses, third trimester ♀   **M**

    O30.829   Other specified multiple gestation with two or more monoamniotic fetuses, unspecified trimester ♀   **M**

● O30.89   Other specified multiple gestation, unable to determine number of placenta and number of amniotic sacs

    O30.891   Other specified multiple gestation, unable to determine number of placenta and number of amniotic sacs, first trimester ♀   **M**

    O30.892   Other specified multiple gestation, unable to determine number of placenta and number of amniotic sacs, second trimester ♀   **M**

    O30.893   Other specified multiple gestation, unable to determine number of placenta and number of amniotic sacs, third trimester ♀   **M**

    O30.899   Other specified multiple gestation, unable to determine number of placenta and number of amniotic sacs, unspecified trimester ♀   **M**

● O30.9   Multiple gestation, unspecified
    Multiple pregnancy NOS

    O30.90   Multiple gestation, unspecified, unspecified trimester ♀   **M**

    O30.91   Multiple gestation, unspecified, first trimester ♀   **M**

    O30.92   Multiple gestation, unspecified, second trimester ♀   **M**

    O30.93   Multiple gestation, unspecified, third trimester ♀   **M**

● O31   Complications specific to multiple gestation

    Excludes2   delayed delivery of second twin, triplet, etc. (O63.2)
       malpresentation of one fetus or more (O32.9)
       placental transfusion syndromes (O43.0-)

    Coding Clinic: 2012, Q4, P107

One of the following 7th characters is to be assigned to each code under category O31. 7th character 0 is for single gestations and multiple gestations where the fetus is unspecified. 7th characters 1 through 9 are for cases of multiple gestations to identify the fetus for which the code applies. The appropriate code from category O30, Multiple gestation, must also be assigned when assigning a code from category O31 that has a 7th character of 1 through 9.

0	not applicable or unspecified
1	fetus 1
2	fetus 2
3	fetus 3
4	fetus 4
5	fetus 5
9	other fetus

● O31.0   Papyraceous fetus
    Fetus compressus

   X ● O31.00   Papyraceous fetus, unspecified trimester ♀   **M**

   X ● O31.01   Papyraceous fetus, first trimester ♀   **M**

   X ● O31.02   Papyraceous fetus, second trimester ♀   **M**

   X ● O31.03   Papyraceous fetus, third trimester ♀   **M**

● O31.1   Continuing pregnancy after spontaneous abortion of one fetus or more

   X ● O31.10   Continuing pregnancy after spontaneous abortion of one fetus or more, unspecified trimester ♀   **M**

   X ● O31.11   Continuing pregnancy after spontaneous abortion of one fetus or more, first trimester ♀   **M**

   X ● O31.12   Continuing pregnancy after spontaneous abortion of one fetus or more, second trimester ♀   **M**

   X ● O31.13   Continuing pregnancy after spontaneous abortion of one fetus or more, third trimester ♀   **M**

● O31.2   Continuing pregnancy after intrauterine death of one fetus or more

   X ● O31.20   Continuing pregnancy after intrauterine death of one fetus or more, unspecified trimester ♀   **M**

   X ● O31.21   Continuing pregnancy after intrauterine death of one fetus or more, first trimester ♀   **M**

   X ● O31.22   Continuing pregnancy after intrauterine death of one fetus or more, second trimester ♀   **M**

   X ● O31.23   Continuing pregnancy after intrauterine death of one fetus or more, third trimester ♀   **M**

● O31.3   Continuing pregnancy after elective fetal reduction of one fetus or more
    Continuing pregnancy after selective termination of one fetus or more

   X ● O31.30   Continuing pregnancy after elective fetal reduction of one fetus or more, unspecified trimester ♀   **M**

   X ● O31.31   Continuing pregnancy after elective fetal reduction of one fetus or more, first trimester ♀   **M**

   X ● O31.32   Continuing pregnancy after elective fetal reduction of one fetus or more, second trimester ♀   **M**

   X ● O31.33   Continuing pregnancy after elective fetal reduction of one fetus or more, third trimester ♀   **M**

CHAPTER 15 (O00-O9A)

- ● **O31.8   Other complications specific to multiple gestation**
  - ● **O31.8X   Other complications specific to multiple gestation**
    - ● **O31.8X1   Other complications specific to multiple gestation, first trimester ♀ M**
    - ● **O31.8X2   Other complications specific to multiple gestation, second trimester ♀   M**
    - ● **O31.8X3   Other complications specific to multiple gestation, third trimester ♀ M**
    - ● **O31.8X9   Other complications specific to multiple gestation, unspecified trimester ♀   M**

● **O32   Maternal care for malpresentation of fetus**

> **Includes**   the listed conditions as a reason for observation, hospitalization or other obstetric care of the mother, or for cesarean delivery before onset of labor
>
> **Excludes1**   malpresentation of fetus with obstructed labor (O64.-)

Coding Clinic: 2012, Q4, P107

One of the following 7th characters is to be assigned to each code under category O32. 7th character 0 is for single gestations and multiple gestations where the fetus is unspecified. 7th characters 1 through 9 are for cases of multiple gestations to identify the fetus for which the code applies. The appropriate code from category O30, Multiple gestation, must also be assigned when assigning a code from category O32 that has a 7th character of 1 through 9.

0	not applicable or unspecified
1	fetus 1
2	fetus 2
3	fetus 3
4	fetus 4
5	fetus 5
9	other fetus

- X● **O32.0   Maternal care for unstable lie ♀   M**
- X● **O32.1   Maternal care for breech presentation ♀   M**
  Maternal care for buttocks presentation
  Maternal care for complete breech
  Maternal care for frank breech

  > **Excludes1**   footling presentation (O32.8) incomplete breech (O32.8)

- X● **O32.2   Maternal care for transverse and oblique lie ♀   M**
  Maternal care for oblique presentation
  Maternal care for transverse presentation
- X● **O32.3   Maternal care for face, brow and chin presentation ♀   M**
- X● **O32.4   Maternal care for high head at term ♀   M**
  Maternal care for failure of head to enter pelvic brim
- X● **O32.6   Maternal care for compound presentation ♀   M**
- X● **O32.8   Maternal care for other malpresentation of fetus ♀   M**
  Maternal care for footling presentation
  Maternal care for incomplete breech
- X● **O32.9   Maternal care for malpresentation of fetus, unspecified ♀   M**

● **O33   Maternal care for disproportion**

> **Includes**   the listed conditions as a reason for observation, hospitalization or other obstetric care of the mother, or for cesarean delivery before onset of labor
>
> **Excludes1**   disproportion with obstructed labor (O65-O66)

O33.0   Maternal care for disproportion due to deformity of maternal pelvic bones ♀   M
Maternal care for disproportion due to pelvic deformity causing disproportion NOS

O33.1   Maternal care for disproportion due to generally contracted pelvis ♀   M
Maternal care for disproportion due to contracted pelvis NOS causing disproportion

O33.2   Maternal care for disproportion due to inlet contraction of pelvis ♀   M
Maternal care for disproportion due to inlet contraction (pelvis) causing disproportion

X● **O33.3   Maternal care for disproportion due to outlet contraction of pelvis ♀   M**
Maternal care for disproportion due to mid-cavity contraction (pelvis)
Maternal care for disproportion due to outlet contraction (pelvis)

One of the following 7th characters is to be assigned to code O33.3. 7th character 0 is for single gestations and multiple gestations where the fetus is unspecified. 7th characters 1 through 9 are for cases of multiple gestations to identify the fetus for which the code applies. The appropriate code from category O30, Multiple gestation, must also be assigned when assigning code O33.3 with a 7th character of 1 through 9.

0	not applicable or unspecified
1	fetus 1
2	fetus 2
3	fetus 3
4	fetus 4
5	fetus 5
9	other fetus

X● **O33.4   Maternal care for disproportion of mixed maternal and fetal origin ♀   M**

One of the following 7th characters is to be assigned to code O33.4. 7th character 0 is for single gestations and multiple gestations where the fetus is unspecified. 7th characters 1 through 9 are for cases of multiple gestations to identify the fetus for which the code applies. The appropriate code from category O30, Multiple gestation, must also be assigned when assigning code O33.4 with a 7th character of 1 through 9.

0	not applicable or unspecified
1	fetus 1
2	fetus 2
3	fetus 3
4	fetus 4
5	fetus 5
9	other fetus

◀ New   ◀▥ Revised   ~~deleted~~ Deleted   Excludes 1   Excludes 2   Includes   Use additional   Code first   Code also   Unspecified
OGCR Official Guidelines   X Assign placeholder X   ● Use Additional Character(s)   ▶ Manifestation Code   **Coding Clinic**

X● **O33.5** **Maternal care for disproportion due to unusually large fetus ♀** M

> Maternal care for disproportion due to disproportion of fetal origin with normally formed fetus
>
> Maternal care for disproportion due to fetal disproportion NOS
>
> One of the following 7th characters is to be assigned to code O33.5. 7th character 0 is for single gestations and multiple gestations where the fetus is unspecified. 7th characters 1 through 9 are for cases of multiple gestations to identify the fetus for which the code applies. The appropriate code from category O30, Multiple gestation, must also be assigned when assigning code O33.5 with a 7th character of 1 through 9.

> | 0 | not applicable or unspecified |
> |---|---|
> | 1 | fetus 1 |
> | 2 | fetus 2 |
> | 3 | fetus 3 |
> | 4 | fetus 4 |
> | 5 | fetus 5 |
> | 9 | other fetus |

X● **O33.6** **Maternal care for disproportion due to hydrocephalic fetus ♀** M

> One of the following 7th characters is to be assigned to code O33.6. 7th character 0 is for single gestations and multiple gestations where the fetus is unspecified. 7th characters 1 through 9 are for cases of multiple gestations to identify the fetus for which the code applies. The appropriate code from category O30, Multiple gestation, must also be assigned when assigning code O33.6 with a 7th character of 1 through 9.

> | 0 | not applicable or unspecified |
> |---|---|
> | 1 | fetus 1 |
> | 2 | fetus 2 |
> | 3 | fetus 3 |
> | 4 | fetus 4 |
> | 5 | fetus 5 |
> | 9 | other fetus |

O33.7 **Maternal care for disproportion due to other fetal deformities ♀** M

> Maternal care for disproportion due to fetal ascites
>
> Maternal care for disproportion due to fetal hydrops
>
> Maternal care for disproportion due to fetal meningomyelocele
>
> Maternal care for disproportion due to fetal sacral teratoma
>
> Maternal care for disproportion due to fetal tumor
>
> **Excludes1** obstructed labor due to other fetal deformities (O66.3)

O33.8 **Maternal care for disproportion of other origin ♀** M

O33.9 **Maternal care for disproportion, unspecified ♀** M

> Maternal care for disproportion due to cephalopelvic disproportion NOS
>
> Maternal care for disproportion due to fetopelvic disproportion NOS

● **O34** **Maternal care for abnormality of pelvic organs**

> **Includes** the listed conditions as a reason for hospitalization or other obstetric care of the mother, or for cesarean delivery before onset of labor
>
> *Code first* any associated obstructed labor (O65.5)
>
> Use additional code for specific condition

● **O34.0** **Maternal care for congenital malformation of uterus**

> **O34.00** **Maternal care for unspecified congenital malformation of uterus, unspecified trimester ♀** M
>
> **O34.01** **Maternal care for unspecified congenital malformation of uterus, first trimester ♀** M
>
> **O34.02** **Maternal care for unspecified congenital malformation of uterus, second trimester ♀** M
>
> **O34.03** **Maternal care for unspecified congenital malformation of uterus, third trimester ♀** M

● **O34.1** **Maternal care for benign tumor of corpus uteri**

> **Excludes2** maternal care for benign tumor of cervix (O34.4-)
>
> maternal care for malignant neoplasm of uterus (O9A.1-)
>
> **O34.10** **Maternal care for benign tumor of corpus uteri, unspecified trimester ♀** M
>
> **O34.11** **Maternal care for benign tumor of corpus uteri, first trimester ♀** M
>
> **O34.12** **Maternal care for benign tumor of corpus uteri, second trimester ♀** M
>
> **O34.13** **Maternal care for benign tumor of corpus uteri, third trimester ♀** M

● **O34.2** **Maternal care due to uterine scar from previous surgery**

> **O34.21** **Maternal care for scar from previous cesarean delivery ♀** M
>
> **O34.29** **Maternal care due to uterine scar from other previous surgery ♀** M

● **O34.3** **Maternal care for cervical incompetence**

> Maternal care for cerclage with or without cervical incompetence
>
> Maternal care for Shirodkar suture with or without cervical incompetence
>
> **O34.30** **Maternal care for cervical incompetence, unspecified trimester ♀** M
>
> **O34.31** **Maternal care for cervical incompetence, first trimester ♀** M
>
> **O34.32** **Maternal care for cervical incompetence, second trimester ♀** M
>
> **O34.33** **Maternal care for cervical incompetence, third trimester ♀** M

● **O34.4** **Maternal care for other abnormalities of cervix**

> **O34.40** **Maternal care for other abnormalities of cervix, unspecified trimester ♀** M
>
> **O34.41** **Maternal care for other abnormalities of cervix, first trimester ♀** M
>
> **O34.42** **Maternal care for other abnormalities of cervix, second trimester ♀** M
>
> **O34.43** **Maternal care for other abnormalities of cervix, third trimester ♀** M

CHAPTER 15 (O00–O9A)

CHAPTER 15 (O00-O9A)

● **O34.5 Maternal care for other abnormalities of gravid uterus**
   ● **O34.51 Maternal care for incarceration of gravid uterus**
      O34.511 Maternal care for incarceration of gravid uterus, first trimester ♀   M
      O34.512 Maternal care for incarceration of gravid uterus, second trimester ♀   M
      O34.513 Maternal care for incarceration of gravid uterus, third trimester ♀   M
      O34.519 Maternal care for incarceration of gravid uterus, unspecified trimester ♀   M
   ● **O34.52 Maternal care for prolapse of gravid uterus**
      O34.521 Maternal care for prolapse of gravid uterus, first trimester ♀   M
      O34.522 Maternal care for prolapse of gravid uterus, second trimester ♀   M
      O34.523 Maternal care for prolapse of gravid uterus, third trimester ♀   M
      O34.529 Maternal care for prolapse of gravid uterus, unspecified trimester ♀   M
   ● **O34.53 Maternal care for retroversion of gravid uterus**
      O34.531 Maternal care for retroversion of gravid uterus, first trimester ♀   M
      O34.532 Maternal care for retroversion of gravid uterus, second trimester ♀   M
      O34.533 Maternal care for retroversion of gravid uterus, third trimester ♀   M
      O34.539 Maternal care for retroversion of gravid uterus, unspecified trimester ♀   M
   ● **O34.59 Maternal care for other abnormalities of gravid uterus**
      O34.591 Maternal care for other abnormalities of gravid uterus, first trimester ♀   M
      O34.592 Maternal care for other abnormalities of gravid uterus, second trimester ♀ M
      O34.593 Maternal care for other abnormalities of gravid uterus, third trimester ♀   M
      O34.599 Maternal care for other abnormalities of gravid uterus, unspecified trimester ♀   M
● **O34.6 Maternal care for abnormality of vagina**
   Excludes2   maternal care for vaginal varices in pregnancy (O22.1-)
      O34.60 Maternal care for abnormality of vagina, unspecified trimester ♀   M
      O34.61 Maternal care for abnormality of vagina, first trimester ♀   M
      O34.62 Maternal care for abnormality of vagina, second trimester ♀   M
      O34.63 Maternal care for abnormality of vagina, third trimester ♀   M
● **O34.7 Maternal care for abnormality of vulva and perineum**
   Excludes2   maternal care for perineal and vulval varices in pregnancy (O22.1-)
      O34.70 Maternal care for abnormality of vulva and perineum, unspecified trimester ♀   M
      O34.71 Maternal care for abnormality of vulva and perineum, first trimester ♀   M
      O34.72 Maternal care for abnormality of vulva and perineum, second trimester ♀   M
      O34.73 Maternal care for abnormality of vulva and perineum, third trimester ♀   M

● **O34.8 Maternal care for other abnormalities of pelvic organs**
      O34.80 Maternal care for other abnormalities of pelvic organs, unspecified trimester ♀   M
      O34.81 Maternal care for other abnormalities of pelvic organs, first trimester ♀   M
      O34.82 Maternal care for other abnormalities of pelvic organs, second trimester ♀   M
      O34.83 Maternal care for other abnormalities of pelvic organs, third trimester ♀   M
● **O34.9 Maternal care for abnormality of pelvic organ, unspecified**
      O34.90 Maternal care for abnormality of pelvic organ, unspecified, unspecified trimester ♀   M
      O34.91 Maternal care for abnormality of pelvic organ, unspecified, first trimester ♀   M
      O34.92 Maternal care for abnormality of pelvic organ, unspecified, second trimester ♀   M
      O34.93 Maternal care for abnormality of pelvic organ, unspecified, third trimester ♀   M

OGCR Section I.C.15.e.l.

Fetal Conditions Affecting the Management of the Mother

1) Code from categories O35 and O36

Codes from categories O35, Maternal care for known or suspected fetal abnormality and damage, and O36, Maternal care for other fetal problems, are assigned only when the fetal condition is actually responsible for modifying the management of the mother, i.e., by requiring diagnostic studies, additional observation, special care, or termination of pregnancy. The fact that the fetal condition exists does not justify assigning a code from this series to the mother's record.

2) In utero surgery

In cases when surgery is performed on the fetus, a diagnosis code from category O35, Maternal care for known or suspected fetal abnormality and damage, should be assigned identifying the fetal condition. Assign the appropriate procedure code for the procedure performed.

No code from Chapter 16, the perinatal codes, should be used on the mother's record to identify fetal conditions. Surgery performed in utero on a fetus is still to be coded as an obstetric encounter.

● **O35 Maternal care for known or suspected fetal abnormality and damage**

   Includes   the listed conditions in the fetus as a reason for hospitalization or other obstetric care to the mother, or for termination of pregnancy

   Code also any associated maternal condition

   Excludes1   encounter for suspected maternal and fetal conditions ruled out (Z03.7-)

   One of the following 7th characters is to be assigned to each code under category O35. 7th character 0 is for single gestations and multiple gestations where the fetus is unspecified. 7th characters 1 through 9 are for cases of multiple gestations to identify the fetus for which the code applies. The appropriate code from category O30, Multiple gestation, must also be assigned when assigning a code from category O35 that has a 7th character of 1 through 9.

0	not applicable or unspecified
1	fetus 1
2	fetus 2
3	fetus 3
4	fetus 4
5	fetus 5
9	other fetus

X● **O35.0 Maternal care for (suspected) central nervous system malformation in fetus ♀**   M
   Maternal care for fetal anencephaly
   Maternal care for fetal hydrocephalus
   Maternal care for fetal spina bifida
   Excludes2   chromosomal abnormality in fetus (O35.1)

X● **O35.1 Maternal care for (suspected) chromosomal abnormality in fetus ♀**   M

◀ New   ◀◀ Revised   ~~deleted~~ Deleted   Excludes 1   Excludes 2   Includes   Use additional   Code first   Code also   Unspecified

OGCR Official Guidelines   X Assign placeholder X   ● Use Additional Character(s)   ▶ Manifestation Code   **Coding Clinic**

X● **O35.2**   **Maternal care for (suspected) hereditary disease in fetus ♀**   **M**

     Excludes2   chromosomal abnormality in fetus (O35.1)

X● **O35.3**   **Maternal care for (suspected) damage to fetus from viral disease in mother ♀**   **M**

     Maternal care for damage to fetus from maternal cytomegalovirus infection

     Maternal care for damage to fetus from maternal rubella

X● **O35.4**   **Maternal care for (suspected) damage to fetus from alcohol ♀**   **M**

X● **O35.5**   **Maternal care for (suspected) damage to fetus by drugs ♀**   **M**

     Maternal care for damage to fetus from drug addiction

X● **O35.6**   **Maternal care for (suspected) damage to fetus by radiation ♀**   **M**

X● **O35.7**   **Maternal care for (suspected) damage to fetus by other medical procedures ♀**   **M**

     Maternal care for damage to fetus by amniocentesis

     Maternal care for damage to fetus by biopsy procedures

     Maternal care for damage to fetus by hematological investigation

     Maternal care for damage to fetus by intrauterine contraceptive device

     Maternal care for damage to fetus by intrauterine surgery

X● **O35.8**   **Maternal care for other (suspected) fetal abnormality and damage ♀**   **M**

     Maternal care for damage to fetus from maternal listeriosis

     Maternal care for damage to fetus from maternal toxoplasmosis

X● **O35.9**   **Maternal care for (suspected) fetal abnormality and damage, unspecified ♀**   **M**

● **O36**   **Maternal care for other fetal problems**

     Includes   the listed conditions in the fetus as a reason for hospitalization or other obstetric care of the mother, or for termination of pregnancy

     Excludes1   encounter for suspected maternal and fetal conditions ruled out (Z03.7-)

         placental transfusion syndromes (O43.0-)

     Excludes2   labor and delivery complicated by fetal stress (O77.-)

     One of the following 7th characters is to be assigned to each code under category O36. 7th character 0 is for single gestations and multiple gestations where the fetus is unspecified. 7th characters 1 through 9 are for cases of multiple gestations to identify the fetus for which the code applies. The appropriate code from category O30, Multiple gestation, must also be assigned when assigning a code from category O36 that has a 7th character of 1 through 9.

0	not applicable or unspecified
1	fetus 1
2	fetus 2
3	fetus 3
4	fetus 4
5	fetus 5
9	other fetus

● **O36.0**   **Maternal care for rhesus isoimmunization**

     Maternal care for Rh incompatibility (with hydrops fetalis)

   ● **O36.01**   **Maternal care for anti-D [Rh] antibodies**

     ● **O36.011**   **Maternal care for anti-D [Rh] antibodies, first trimester ♀**   **M**

     ● **O36.012**   **Maternal care for anti-D [Rh] antibodies, second trimester ♀**   **M**

     ● **O36.013**   **Maternal care for anti-D [Rh] antibodies, third trimester ♀**   **M**

     ● **O36.019**   **Maternal care for anti-D [Rh] antibodies, unspecified trimester ♀**   **M**

   ● **O36.09**   **Maternal care for other rhesus isoimmunization**

     ● **O36.091**   **Maternal care for other rhesus isoimmunization, first trimester ♀**   **M**

     ● **O36.092**   **Maternal care for other rhesus isoimmunization, second trimester ♀**   **M**

     ● **O36.093**   **Maternal care for other rhesus isoimmunization, third trimester ♀**   **M**

     ● **O36.099**   **Maternal care for other rhesus isoimmunization, unspecified trimester ♀**   **M**

● **O36.1**   **Maternal care for other isoimmunization**

     Maternal care for ABO isoimmunization

   ● **O36.11**   **Maternal care for Anti-A sensitization**

     Maternal care for isoimmunization NOS (with hydrops fetalis)

     ● **O36.111**   **Maternal care for Anti-A sensitization, first trimester ♀**   **M**

     ● **O36.112**   **Maternal care for Anti-A sensitization, second trimester ♀**   **M**

     ● **O36.113**   **Maternal care for Anti-A sensitization, third trimester ♀**   **M**

     ● **O36.119**   **Maternal care for Anti-A sensitization, unspecified trimester ♀**   **M**

   ● **O36.19**   **Maternal care for other isoimmunization**

     Maternal care for Anti-B sensitization

     ● **O36.191**   **Maternal care for other isoimmunization, first trimester ♀**   **M**

     ● **O36.192**   **Maternal care for other isoimmunization, second trimester ♀**   **M**

     ● **O36.193**   **Maternal care for other isoimmunization, third trimester ♀**   **M**

     ● **O36.199**   **Maternal care for other isoimmunization, unspecified trimester ♀**   **M**

● **O36.2**   **Maternal care for hydrops fetalis**

     Maternal care for hydrops fetalis NOS

     Maternal care for hydrops fetalis not associated with isoimmunization

     Excludes1   hydrops fetalis associated with ABO isoimmunization (O36.1-)

         hydrops fetalis associated with rhesus isoimmunization (O36.0-)

   ● **O36.20**   **Maternal care for hydrops fetalis, unspecified trimester ♀**   **M**

   ● **O36.21**   **Maternal care for hydrops fetalis, first trimester ♀**   **M**

   ● **O36.22**   **Maternal care for hydrops fetalis, second trimester ♀**   **M**

   ● **O36.23**   **Maternal care for hydrops fetalis, third trimester ♀**   **M**

● **O36.4**   **Maternal care for intrauterine death ♀**   **M**

     Maternal care for intrauterine fetal death NOS

     Maternal care for intrauterine fetal death after completion of 20 weeks of gestation

     Maternal care for late fetal death

     Maternal care for missed delivery

     Excludes1   missed abortion (O02.1)

         stillbirth (P95)

● **O36.5**   **Maternal care for known or suspected poor fetal growth**

   ● **O36.51**   **Maternal care for known or suspected placental insufficiency**

     ● **O36.511**   **Maternal care for known or suspected placental insufficiency, first trimester ♀**   **M**

     ● **O36.512**   **Maternal care for known or suspected placental insufficiency, second trimester ♀**   **M**

CHAPTER 15 (O00–O9A)

● O36.513   Maternal care for known or suspected placental insufficiency, third trimester ♀   M

● O36.519   Maternal care for known or suspected placental insufficiency, unspecified trimester ♀   M

● O36.59   Maternal care for other known or suspected poor fetal growth
     Maternal care for known or suspected light-for-dates NOS
     Maternal care for known or suspected small-for-dates NOS

     ● O36.591   Maternal care for other known or suspected poor fetal growth, first trimester ♀   M

     ● O36.592   Maternal care for other known or suspected poor fetal growth, second trimester ♀   M

     ● O36.593   Maternal care for other known or suspected poor fetal growth, third trimester ♀   M

     ● O36.599   Maternal care for other known or suspected poor fetal growth, unspecified trimester ♀   M

● O36.6   Maternal care for excessive fetal growth
     Maternal care for known or suspected large-for-dates

X ● O36.60   Maternal care for excessive fetal growth, unspecified trimester ♀   M

X ● O36.61   Maternal care for excessive fetal growth, first trimester ♀   M

X ● O36.62   Maternal care for excessive fetal growth, second trimester ♀   M

X ● O36.63   Maternal care for excessive fetal growth, third trimester ♀   M

● O36.7   Maternal care for viable fetus in abdominal pregnancy

X ● O36.70   Maternal care for viable fetus in abdominal pregnancy, unspecified trimester ♀   M

X ● O36.71   Maternal care for viable fetus in abdominal pregnancy, first trimester ♀   M

X ● O36.72   Maternal care for viable fetus in abdominal pregnancy, second trimester ♀   M

X ● O36.73   Maternal care for viable fetus in abdominal pregnancy, third trimester ♀   M

● O36.8   Maternal care for other specified fetal problems

X ● O36.80   Pregnancy with inconclusive fetal viability ♀ M
     Encounter to determine fetal viability of pregnancy

   ● O36.81   Decreased fetal movements

     ● O36.812   Decreased fetal movements, second trimester ♀   M

     ● O36.813   Decreased fetal movements, third trimester ♀   M

     ● O36.819   Decreased fetal movements, unspecified trimester ♀   M

   ● O36.82   Fetal anemia and thrombocytopenia

     ● O36.821   Fetal anemia and thrombocytopenia, first trimester ♀   M

     ● O36.822   Fetal anemia and thrombocytopenia, second trimester ♀   M

     ● O36.823   Fetal anemia and thrombocytopenia, third trimester ♀   M

     ● O36.829   Fetal anemia and thrombocytopenia, unspecified trimester ♀   M

   ● O36.89   Maternal care for other specified fetal problems

     ● O36.891   Maternal care for other specified fetal problems, first trimester ♀   M

     ● O36.892   Maternal care for other specified fetal problems, second trimester ♀   M

     ● O36.893   Maternal care for other specified fetal problems, third trimester ♀   M

     ● O36.899   Maternal care for other specified fetal problems, unspecified trimester ♀   M

● O36.9   Maternal care for fetal problem, unspecified

X ● O36.90   Maternal care for fetal problem, unspecified, unspecified trimester ♀   M

X ● O36.91   Maternal care for fetal problem, unspecified, first trimester ♀   M

X ● O36.92   Maternal care for fetal problem, unspecified, second trimester ♀   M

X ● O36.93   Maternal care for fetal problem, unspecified, third trimester ♀   M

● O40   **Polyhydramnios**
     Overabundance of amniotic fluid
     Includes   hydramnios
     Excludes1   encounter for suspected maternal and fetal conditions ruled out (Z03.7-)

One of the following 7th characters is to be assigned to each code under category O40. 7th character 0 is for single gestations and multiple gestations where the fetus is unspecified. 7th characters 1 through 9 are for cases of multiple gestations to identify the fetus for which the code applies. The appropriate code from category O30, Multiple gestation, must also be assigned when assigning a code from category O40 that has a 7th character of 1 through 9.

0	not applicable or unspecified
1	fetus 1
2	fetus 2
3	fetus 3
4	fetus 4
5	fetus 5
9	other fetus

X ● O40.1   Polyhydramnios, first trimester ♀   M
X ● O40.2   Polyhydramnios, second trimester ♀   M
X ● O40.3   Polyhydramnios, third trimester ♀   M
X ● O40.9   Polyhydramnios, unspecified trimester ♀   M

● O41   **Other disorders of amniotic fluid and membranes**
     Excludes1   encounter for suspected maternal and fetal conditions ruled out (Z03.7-)

One of the following 7th characters is to be assigned to each code under category O41. 7th character 0 is for single gestations and multiple gestations where the fetus is unspecified. 7th characters 1 through 9 are for cases of multiple gestations to identify the fetus for which the code applies. The appropriate code from category O30, Multiple gestation, must also be assigned when assigning a code from category O41 that has a 7th character of 1 through 9.

0	not applicable or unspecified
1	fetus 1
2	fetus 2
3	fetus 3
4	fetus 4
5	fetus 5
9	other fetus

● O41.0   Oligohydramnios
     Scant volume of amniotic fluid
     Oligohydramnios without rupture of membranes

X ● O41.00   Oligohydramnios, unspecified trimester ♀   M
X ● O41.01   Oligohydramnios, first trimester ♀   M
X ● O41.02   Oligohydramnios, second trimester ♀   M
X ● O41.03   Oligohydramnios, third trimester ♀   M

◀ New   ◀▥ Revised   ~~deleted~~ Deleted   Excludes 1   Excludes 2   Includes   Use additional   Code first   Code also   Unspecified

OGCR Official Guidelines   X Assign placeholder X   ● Use Additional Character(s)   ▶ Manifestation Code   **Coding Clinic**

● **O41.1**   Infection of amniotic sac and membranes
   ● **O41.10**   Infection of amniotic sac and membranes, unspecified
     ● **O41.101**   Infection of amniotic sac and membranes, unspecified, first trimester ♀   **M**
     ● **O41.102**   Infection of amniotic sac and membranes, unspecified, second trimester ♀   **M**
     ● **O41.103**   Infection of amniotic sac and membranes, unspecified, third trimester ♀   **M**
     ● **O41.109**   Infection of amniotic sac and membranes, unspecified, unspecified trimester ♀   **M**
   ● **O41.12**   Chorioamnionitis
     ● **O41.121**   Chorioamnionitis, first trimester ♀   **M**
     ● **O41.122**   Chorioamnionitis, second trimester ♀   **M**
     ● **O41.123**   Chorioamnionitis, third trimester ♀   **M**
     ● **O41.129**   Chorioamnionitis, unspecified trimester ♀   **M**
   ● **O41.14**   Placentitis
     ● **O41.141**   Placentitis, first trimester ♀   **M**
     ● **O41.142**   Placentitis, second trimester ♀   **M**
     ● **O41.143**   Placentitis, third trimester ♀   **M**
     ● **O41.149**   Placentitis, unspecified trimester ♀   **M**
● **O41.8**   Other specified disorders of amniotic fluid and membranes
   ● **O41.8X**   Other specified disorders of amniotic fluid and membranes
     ● **O41.8X1**   Other specified disorders of amniotic fluid and membranes, first trimester ♀   **M**
     ● **O41.8X2**   Other specified disorders of amniotic fluid and membranes, second trimester ♀   **M**
     ● **O41.8X3**   Other specified disorders of amniotic fluid and membranes, third trimester ♀   **M**
     ● **O41.8X9**   Other specified disorders of amniotic fluid and membranes, unspecified trimester ♀   **M**
● **O41.9**   Disorder of amniotic fluid and membranes, unspecified
   X ● **O41.90**   Disorder of amniotic fluid and membranes, unspecified, unspecified trimester ♀   **M**
   X ● **O41.91**   Disorder of amniotic fluid and membranes, unspecified, first trimester ♀   **M**
   X ● **O41.92**   Disorder of amniotic fluid and membranes, unspecified, second trimester ♀   **M**
   X ● **O41.93**   Disorder of amniotic fluid and membranes, unspecified, third trimester ♀   **M**

● **O42**   Premature rupture of membranes
   ● **O42.0**   Premature rupture of membranes, onset of labor within 24 hours of rupture
     O42.00   Premature rupture of membranes, onset of labor within 24 hours of rupture, unspecified weeks of gestation ♀   **M**
     ● **O42.01**   Preterm premature rupture of membranes, onset of labor within 24 hours of rupture
       Premature rupture of membranes before 37 completed weeks of gestation
       O42.011   Preterm premature rupture of membranes, onset of labor within 24 hours of rupture, first trimester ♀   **M**
       O42.012   Preterm premature rupture of membranes, onset of labor within 24 hours of rupture, second trimester ♀ **M**
       O42.013   Preterm premature rupture of membranes, onset of labor within 24 hours of rupture, third trimester ♀   **M**
       O42.019   Preterm premature rupture of membranes, onset of labor within 24 hours of rupture, unspecified trimester ♀   **M**
     O42.02   Full-term premature rupture of membranes, onset of labor within 24 hours of rupture ♀   **M**
       Premature rupture of membranes after 37 completed weeks of gestation
   ● **O42.1**   Premature rupture of membranes, onset of labor more than 24 hours following rupture
     O42.10   Premature rupture of membranes, onset of labor more than 24 hours following rupture, unspecified weeks of gestation ♀   **M**
     ● **O42.11**   Preterm premature rupture of membranes, onset of labor more than 24 hours following rupture
       Premature rupture of membranes before 37 completed weeks of gestation
       O42.111   Preterm premature rupture of membranes, onset of labor more than 24 hours following rupture, first trimester ♀   **M**
       O42.112   Preterm premature rupture of membranes, onset of labor more than 24 hours following rupture, second trimester ♀   **M**
       O42.113   Preterm premature rupture of membranes, onset of labor more than 24 hours following rupture, third trimester ♀   **M**
       O42.119   Preterm premature rupture of membranes, onset of labor more than 24 hours following rupture, unspecified trimester ♀   **M**
     O42.12   Full-term premature rupture of membranes, onset of labor more than 24 hours following rupture ♀   **M**
       Premature rupture of membranes after 37 completed weeks of gestation
   ● **O42.9**   Premature rupture of membranes, unspecified as to length of time between rupture and onset of labor
     O42.90   Premature rupture of membranes, unspecified as to length of time between rupture and onset of labor, unspecified weeks of gestation ♀   **M**
     ● **O42.91**   Preterm premature rupture of membranes, unspecified as to length of time between rupture and onset of labor
       Premature rupture of membranes before 37 completed weeks of gestation
       O42.911   Preterm premature rupture of membranes, unspecified as to length of time between rupture and onset of labor, first trimester ♀   **M**
       O42.912   Preterm premature rupture of membranes, unspecified as to length of time between rupture and onset of labor, second trimester ♀   **M**
       O42.913   Preterm premature rupture of membranes, unspecified as to length of time between rupture and onset of labor, third trimester ♀   **M**
       O42.919   Preterm premature rupture of membranes, unspecified as to length of time between rupture and onset of labor, unspecified trimester ♀   **M**
     O42.92   Full-term premature rupture of membranes, unspecified as to length of time between rupture and onset of labor ♀   **M**
       Premature rupture of membranes after 37 completed weeks of gestation

---

● **O43**   **Placental disorders**

     Excludes2   maternal care for poor fetal growth due to placental insufficiency (O36.5-)
                   placenta previa (O44.-)
                   placental polyp (O90.89)
                   placentitis (O41.14-)
                   premature separation of placenta [abruptio placentae] (O45.-)

    ● **O43.0**   **Placental transfusion syndromes**

       ● **O43.01**   **Fetomaternal placental transfusion syndrome**
               Maternofetal placental transfusion syndrome

          O43.011   Fetomaternal placental transfusion syndrome, first trimester ♀   **M**

          O43.012   Fetomaternal placental transfusion syndrome, second trimester ♀   **M**

          O43.013   Fetomaternal placental transfusion syndrome, third trimester ♀   **M**

          O43.019   Fetomaternal placental transfusion syndrome, unspecified trimester ♀   **M**

       ● **O43.02**   **Fetus-to-fetus placental transfusion syndrome**

          O43.021   Fetus-to-fetus placental transfusion syndrome, first trimester ♀   **M**

          O43.022   Fetus-to-fetus placental transfusion syndrome, second trimester ♀   **M**

          O43.023   Fetus-to-fetus placental transfusion syndrome, third trimester ♀   **M**

          O43.029   Fetus-to-fetus placental transfusion syndrome, unspecified trimester ♀   **M**

    ● **O43.1**   **Malformation of placenta**

       ● **O43.10**   **Malformation of placenta, unspecified**
               Abnormal placenta NOS

          O43.101   Malformation of placenta, unspecified, first trimester ♀   **M**

          O43.102   Malformation of placenta, unspecified, second trimester ♀   **M**

          O43.103   Malformation of placenta, unspecified, third trimester ♀   **M**

          O43.109   Malformation of placenta, unspecified, unspecified trimester ♀   **M**

       ● **O43.11**   **Circumvallate placenta**

          O43.111   Circumvallate placenta, first trimester ♀   **M**

          O43.112   Circumvallate placenta, second trimester ♀   **M**

          O43.113   Circumvallate placenta, third trimester ♀   **M**

          O43.119   Circumvallate placenta, unspecified trimester ♀   **M**

       ● **O43.12**   **Velamentous insertion of umbilical cord**

          O43.121   Velamentous insertion of umbilical cord, first trimester ♀   **M**

          O43.122   Velamentous insertion of umbilical cord, second trimester ♀   **M**

          O43.123   Velamentous insertion of umbilical cord, third trimester ♀   **M**

          O43.129   Velamentous insertion of umbilical cord, unspecified trimester ♀   **M**

       ● **O43.19**   **Other malformation of placenta**

          O43.191   Other malformation of placenta, first trimester ♀   **M**

          O43.192   Other malformation of placenta, second trimester ♀   **M**

          O43.193   Other malformation of placenta, third trimester ♀   **M**

          O43.199   Other malformation of placenta, unspecified trimester ♀   **M**

    ● **O43.2**   **Morbidly adherent placenta**
         Code also associated third stage postpartum hemorrhage, if applicable (O72.0)

      Excludes1   retained placenta (O73.-)

       ● **O43.21**   **Placenta accreta**

          O43.211   Placenta accreta, first trimester ♀   **M**

          O43.212   Placenta accreta, second trimester ♀   **M**

          O43.213   Placenta accreta, third trimester ♀   **M**

          O43.219   Placenta accreta, unspecified trimester ♀   **M**

       ● **O43.22**   **Placenta increta**

          O43.221   Placenta increta, first trimester ♀   **M**

          O43.222   Placenta increta, second trimester ♀   **M**

          O43.223   Placenta increta, third trimester ♀   **M**

          O43.229   Placenta increta, unspecified trimester ♀   **M**

       ● **O43.23**   **Placenta percreta**

          O43.231   Placenta percreta, first trimester ♀   **M**

          O43.232   Placenta percreta, second trimester ♀ **M**

          O43.233   Placenta percreta, third trimester ♀   **M**

          O43.239   Placenta percreta, unspecified trimester ♀   **M**

    ● **O43.8**   **Other placental disorders**

       ● **O43.81**   **Placental infarction**

          O43.811   Placental infarction, first trimester ♀ **M**

          O43.812   Placental infarction, second trimester ♀   **M**

          O43.813   Placental infarction, third trimester ♀   **M**

          O43.819   Placental infarction, unspecified trimester ♀   **M**

       ● **O43.89**   **Other placental disorders**
               Placental dysfunction

          O43.891   Other placental disorders, first trimester ♀   **M**

          O43.892   Other placental disorders, second trimester ♀   **M**

          O43.893   Other placental disorders, third trimester ♀   **M**

          O43.899   Other placental disorders, unspecified trimester ♀   **M**

    ● **O43.9**   **Unspecified placental disorder**

       O43.90   Unspecified placental disorder, unspecified trimester ♀   **M**

       O43.91   Unspecified placental disorder, first trimester ♀   **M**

       O43.92   Unspecified placental disorder, second trimester ♀   **M**

       O43.93   Unspecified placental disorder, third trimester ♀   **M**

● **O44**   **Placenta previa**

    ● **O44.0**   **Placenta previa specified as without hemorrhage**
         Low implantation of placenta specified as without hemorrhage

       O44.00   Placenta previa specified as without hemorrhage, unspecified trimester ♀   **M**

       O44.01   Placenta previa specified as without hemorrhage, first trimester ♀   **M**

       O44.02   Placenta previa specified as without hemorrhage, second trimester ♀   **M**

       O44.03   Placenta previa specified as without hemorrhage, third trimester ♀   **M**

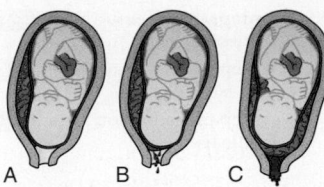

Figure 15-2 **A.** Marginal placento previa. **B.** Partial placenta previa. **C.** Total placento previa.

Item 15–3 Placenta previa is a condition in which the opening of the cervix is obstructed by the displaced placenta. The three types, marginal, partial, and total, are varying degrees of placenta displacement. Placenta abruption is the premature breaking away of the placenta from the site of the uterine implant before the delivery of the fetus.

- O44.1   **Placenta previa with hemorrhage**
  Low implantation of placenta, NOS or with hemorrhage
  Marginal placenta previa, NOS or with hemorrhage
  Partial placenta previa, NOS or with hemorrhage
  Total placenta previa, NOS or with hemorrhage
  > **Excludes1**   labor and delivery complicated by hemorrhage from vasa previa (O69.4)

  - O44.10   Placenta previa with hemorrhage, unspecified trimester ♀   M
  - O44.11   Placenta previa with hemorrhage, first trimester ♀   M
  - O44.12   Placenta previa with hemorrhage, second trimester ♀   M
  - O44.13   Placenta previa with hemorrhage, third trimester ♀   M

- O45   **Premature separation of placenta [abruptio placentae]**
  - O45.0   **Premature separation of placenta with coagulation defect**
    - O45.00   Premature separation of placenta with coagulation defect, unspecified
      - O45.001   Premature separation of placenta with coagulation defect, unspecified, first trimester ♀
      - O45.002   Premature separation of placenta with coagulation defect, unspecified, second trimester ♀   M
      - O45.003   Premature separation of placenta with coagulation defect, unspecified, third trimester ♀   M
      - O45.009   Premature separation of placenta with coagulation defect, unspecified, unspecified trimester ♀   M
    - O45.01   Premature separation of placenta with afibrinogenemia
      Premature separation of placenta with hypofibrinogenemia
      - O45.011   Premature separation of placenta with afibrinogenemia, first trimester ♀   M
      - O45.012   Premature separation of placenta with afibrinogenemia, second trimester ♀   M
      - O45.013   Premature separation of placenta with afibrinogenemia, third trimester ♀   M
      - O45.019   Premature separation of placenta with afibrinogenemia, unspecified trimester ♀   M

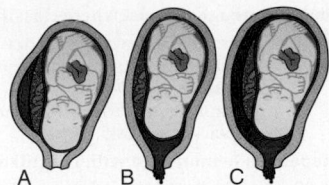

Figure 15-3 Abruptio placentae is classified according to the grade of separation of the placenta from the uterine wall. **A.** Mild separation in which hemorrhage is internal. **B.** Moderate separation in which there is external hemorrhage. **C.** Severe separation in which there is external hemorrhage and extreme separation.

- O45.02   Premature separation of placenta with disseminated intravascular coagulation
  - O45.021   Premature separation of placenta with disseminated intravascular coagulation, first trimester ♀   M
  - O45.022   Premature separation of placenta with disseminated intravascular coagulation, second trimester ♀   M
  - O45.023   Premature separation of placenta with disseminated intravascular coagulation, third trimester ♀   M
  - O45.029   Premature separation of placenta with disseminated intravascular coagulation, unspecified trimester ♀ M
- O45.09   Premature separation of placenta with other coagulation defect
  - O45.091   Premature separation of placenta with other coagulation defect, first trimester ♀   M
  - O45.092   Premature separation of placenta with other coagulation defect, second trimester ♀   M
  - O45.093   Premature separation of placenta with other coagulation defect, third trimester ♀   M
  - O45.099   Premature separation of placenta with other coagulation defect, unspecified trimester ♀   M
- O45.8   Other premature separation of placenta
  - O45.8X   Other premature separation of placenta
    - O45.8X1   Other premature separation of placenta, first trimester ♀   M
    - O45.8X2   Other premature separation of placenta, second trimester ♀   M
    - O45.8X3   Other premature separation of placenta, third trimester ♀   M
    - O45.8X9   Other premature separation of placenta, unspecified trimester ♀   M
- O45.9   Premature separation of placenta, unspecified
  Abruptio placentae NOS
  - O45.90   Premature separation of placenta, unspecified, unspecified trimester ♀   M
  - O45.91   Premature separation of placenta, unspecified, first trimester ♀   M
  - O45.92   Premature separation of placenta, unspecified, second trimester ♀   M
  - O45.93   Premature separation of placenta, unspecified, third trimester ♀   M

CHAPTER 15 (O00-O9A)

● **O46 Antepartum hemorrhage, not elsewhere classified**
     Excludes1   hemorrhage in early pregnancy (O20.-)
                    intrapartum hemorrhage NEC (O67.-)
                    placenta previa (O44.-)
                    premature separation of placenta [abruptio placentae] (O45.-)

   ● **O46.0 Antepartum hemorrhage with coagulation defect**
     ● **O46.00 Antepartum hemorrhage with coagulation defect, unspecified**
       O46.001   **Antepartum hemorrhage with coagulation defect, unspecified, first trimester** ♀   M
       O46.002   **Antepartum hemorrhage with coagulation defect, unspecified, second trimester** ♀   M
       O46.003   **Antepartum hemorrhage with coagulation defect, unspecified, third trimester** ♀   M
       O46.009   **Antepartum hemorrhage with coagulation defect, unspecified, unspecified trimester** ♀   M

     ● **O46.01 Antepartum hemorrhage with afibrinogenemia**
       Antepartum hemorrhage with hypofibrinogenemia
       O46.011   **Antepartum hemorrhage with afibrinogenemia, first trimester** ♀   M
       O46.012   **Antepartum hemorrhage with afibrinogenemia, second trimester** ♀ M
       O46.013   **Antepartum hemorrhage with afibrinogenemia, third trimester** ♀   M
       O46.019   **Antepartum hemorrhage with afibrinogenemia, unspecified trimester** ♀   M

     ● **O46.02 Antepartum hemorrhage with disseminated intravascular coagulation**
       O46.021   **Antepartum hemorrhage with disseminated intravascular coagulation, first trimester** ♀   M
       O46.022   **Antepartum hemorrhage with disseminated intravascular coagulation, second trimester** ♀   M
       O46.023   **Antepartum hemorrhage with disseminated intravascular coagulation, third trimester** ♀   M
       O46.029   **Antepartum hemorrhage with disseminated intravascular coagulation, unspecified trimester** ♀ M

     ● **O46.09 Antepartum hemorrhage with other coagulation defect**
       O46.091   **Antepartum hemorrhage with other coagulation defect, first trimester** ♀ M
       O46.092   **Antepartum hemorrhage with other coagulation defect, second trimester** ♀   M
       O46.093   **Antepartum hemorrhage with other coagulation defect, third trimester** ♀ M
       O46.099   **Antepartum hemorrhage with other coagulation defect, unspecified trimester** ♀   M

   ● **O46.8 Other antepartum hemorrhage**
     ● **O46.8x Other antepartum hemorrhage**
       O46.8x1   **Other antepartum hemorrhage, first trimester** ♀   M
       O46.8x2   **Other antepartum hemorrhage, second trimester** ♀   M
       O46.8x3   **Other antepartum hemorrhage, third trimester** ♀   M
       O46.8x9   **Other antepartum hemorrhage, unspecified trimester** ♀   M

   ● **O46.9 Antepartum hemorrhage, unspecified**
       O46.90   **Antepartum hemorrhage, unspecified, unspecified trimester** ♀   M

       O46.91   **Antepartum hemorrhage, unspecified, first trimester** ♀   M
       O46.92   **Antepartum hemorrhage, unspecified, second trimester** ♀   M
       O46.93   **Antepartum hemorrhage, unspecified, third trimester** ♀   M

● **O47 False labor**
     Includes   Braxton Hicks contractions
                threatened labor
     Excludes1   preterm labor (O60.-)

   ● **O47.0 False labor before 37 completed weeks of gestation**
       O47.00   **False labor before 37 completed weeks of gestation, unspecified trimester** ♀   M
       O47.02   **False labor before 37 completed weeks of gestation, second trimester** ♀   M
       O47.03   **False labor before 37 completed weeks of gestation, third trimester** ♀   M

     O47.1   **False labor at or after 37 completed weeks of gestation** ♀   M
     O47.9   **False labor, unspecified** ♀   M

● **O48 Late pregnancy**
     O48.0   **Post-term pregnancy** ♀   M
       Pregnancy over 40 completed weeks to 42 completed weeks gestation
     O48.1   **Prolonged pregnancy** ♀   M
       Pregnancy which has advanced beyond 42 completed weeks gestation

COMPLICATIONS OF LABOR AND DELIVERY (O60-O77)

● **O60 Preterm labor**
     Includes   onset (spontaneous) of labor before 37 completed weeks of gestation
     Excludes1   false labor (O47.0-)
                  threatened labor NOS (O47.0-)

   ● **O60.0 Preterm labor without delivery**
       O60.00   **Preterm labor without delivery, unspecified trimester** ♀   M
       O60.02   **Preterm labor without delivery, second trimester** ♀   M
       O60.03   **Preterm labor without delivery, third trimester** ♀   M

   ● **O60.1 Preterm labor with preterm delivery**
       One of the following 7th characters is to be assigned to each code under subcategory O60.1. 7th character 0 is for single gestations and multiple gestations where the fetus is unspecified. 7th characters 1 through 9 are for cases of multiple gestations to identify the fetus for which the code applies. The appropriate code from category O30, Multiple gestation, must also be assigned when assigning a code from subcategory O60.1 that has a 7th character of 1 through 9.

0	not applicable or unspecified
1	fetus 1
2	fetus 2
3	fetus 3
4	fetus 4
5	fetus 5
9	other fetus

     X ● O60.10   **Preterm labor with preterm delivery, unspecified trimester** ♀   M
                   Preterm labor with delivery NOS
     X ● O60.12   **Preterm labor second trimester with preterm delivery second trimester** ♀   M
     X ● O60.13   **Preterm labor second trimester with preterm delivery third trimester** ♀   M
     X ● O60.14   **Preterm labor third trimester with preterm delivery third trimester** ♀   M

◀ New   ◀|||| Revised   ~~deleted~~ Deleted   Excludes 1   Excludes 2   Includes   Use additional   Code first   Code also   Unspecified

OGCR Official Guidelines   X Assign placeholder X   ● Use Additional Character(s)   ▶ Manifestation Code   **Coding Clinic**

● **O60.2   Term delivery with preterm labor**

One of the following 7th characters is to be assigned to each code under subcategory O60.2. 7th character 0 is for single gestations and multiple gestations where the fetus is unspecified. 7th characters 1 through 9 are for cases of multiple gestations to identify the fetus for which the code applies. The appropriate code from category O30, Multiple gestation, must also be assigned when assigning a code from subcategory O60.2 that has a 7th character of 1 through 9.

0	not applicable or unspecified
1	fetus 1
2	fetus 2
3	fetus 3
4	fetus 4
5	fetus 5
9	other fetus

X● **O60.20   Term delivery with preterm labor, unspecified trimester** ♀   **M**

X● **O60.22   Term delivery with preterm labor, second trimester** ♀   **M**

X● **O60.23   Term delivery with preterm labor, third trimester** ♀   **M**

● **O61   Failed induction of labor**

O61.0   Failed medical induction of labor ♀   **M**
Failed induction (of labor) by oxytocin
Failed induction (of labor) by prostaglandins

O61.1   Failed instrumental induction of labor ♀   **M**
Failed mechanical induction (of labor)
Failed surgical induction (of labor)

O61.8   Other failed induction of labor ♀   **M**

O61.9   Failed induction of labor, unspecified ♀   **M**

● **O62   Abnormalities of forces of labor**

O62.0   Primary inadequate contractions ♀   **M**
Failure of cervical dilatation
Primary hypotonic uterine dysfunction
Uterine inertia during latent phase of labor

O62.1   Secondary uterine inertia ♀   **M**
Arrested active phase of labor
Secondary hypotonic uterine dysfunction

O62.2   Other uterine inertia ♀   **M**
Atony of uterus without hemorrhage
Atony of uterus NOS
Desultory labor
Hypotonic uterine dysfunction NOS
Irregular labor
Poor contractions
Slow slope active phase of labor
Uterine inertia NOS

> **Excludes1** atony of uterus with hemorrhage (postpartum) (O72.1)
> postpartum atony of uterus without hemorrhage (O75.89)

O62.3   Precipitate labor ♀   **M**

O62.4   Hypertonic, incoordinate, and prolonged uterine contractions ♀   **M**
Cervical spasm
Contraction ring dystocia
Dyscoordinate labor
Hour-glass contraction of uterus
Hypertonic uterine dysfunction
Incoordinate uterine action
Tetanic contractions
Uterine dystocia NOS
Uterine spasm

> **Excludes1** dystocia (fetal) (maternal) NOS (O66.9)

O62.8   Other abnormalities of forces of labor ♀   **M**

O62.9   Abnormality of forces of labor, unspecified ♀   **M**

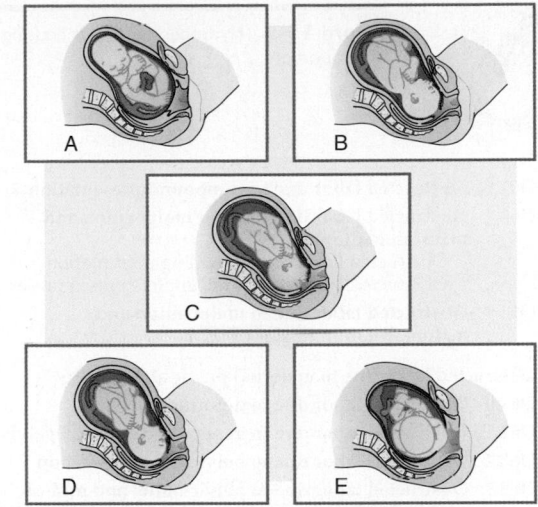

Figure 15-4 Five types of malposition and malpresentation of the fetus: **A.** Breech. **B.** Vertex. **C.** Face. **D.** Brow. **E.** Shoulder.

● **O63   Long labor**

O63.0   Prolonged first stage (of labor) ♀   **M**

O63.1   Prolonged second stage (of labor) ♀   **M**

O63.2   Delayed delivery of second twin, triplet, etc. ♀   **M**

O63.9   Long labor, unspecified ♀   **M**
Prolonged labor NOS

● **O64   Obstructed labor due to malposition and malpresentation of fetus**

One of the following 7th characters is to be assigned to each code under category O64. 7th character 0 is for single gestations and multiple gestations where the fetus is unspecified. 7th characters 1 through 9 are for cases of multiple gestations to identify the fetus for which the code applies. The appropriate code from category O30, Multiple gestation, must also be assigned when assigning a code from category O64 that has a 7th character of 1 through 9.

0	not applicable or unspecified
1	fetus 1
2	fetus 2
3	fetus 3
4	fetus 4
5	fetus 5
9	other fetus

X● **O64.0   Obstructed labor due to incomplete rotation of fetal head** ♀   **M**
Deep transverse arrest
Obstructed labor due to persistent occipitoiliac (position)
Obstructed labor due to persistent occipitoposterior (position)
Obstructed labor due to persistent occipitosacral (position)
Obstructed labor due to persistent occipitotransverse (position)

X● **O64.1   Obstructed labor due to breech presentation** ♀   **M**
Obstructed labor due to buttocks presentation
Obstructed labor due to complete breech presentation
Obstructed labor due to frank breech presentation

X● **O64.2   Obstructed labor due to face presentation** ♀   **M**
Obstructed labor due to chin presentation

X● **O64.3   Obstructed labor due to brow presentation** ♀   **M**

X● **O64.4   Obstructed labor due to shoulder presentation** ♀   **M**
Prolapsed arm

> **Excludes1** impacted shoulders (O66.0)
> shoulder dystocia (O66.0)

CHAPTER 15 (O00-O9A)

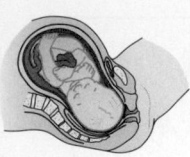

Figure 15-5 Hydrocephalic fetus causing disproportion.

X● **O64.5** Obstructed labor due to compound presentation ♀   M

X● **O64.8** Obstructed labor due to other malposition and malpresentation ♀   M
    Obstructed labor due to footling presentation
    Obstructed labor due to incomplete breech presentation

X● **O64.9** Obstructed labor due to malposition and malpresentation, unspecified ♀   M

● **O65** Obstructed labor due to maternal pelvic abnormality

    O65.0 Obstructed labor due to deformed pelvis ♀   M

    O65.1 Obstructed labor due to generally contracted pelvis ♀   M

    O65.2 Obstructed labor due to pelvic inlet contraction ♀   M

    O65.3 Obstructed labor due to pelvic outlet and mid-cavity contraction ♀   M

    O65.4 Obstructed labor due to fetopelvic disproportion, unspecified ♀   M
        Excludes1   dystocia due to abnormality of fetus (O66.2-O66.3)

    O65.5 Obstructed labor due to abnormality of maternal pelvic organs ♀   M
        Obstructed labor due to conditions listed in O34.-
        Use additional code to identify abnormality of pelvic organs O34.-

    O65.8 Obstructed labor due to other maternal pelvic abnormalities ♀   M

    O65.9 Obstructed labor due to maternal pelvic abnormality, unspecified ♀   M

● **O66** Other obstructed labor

    O66.0 Obstructed labor due to shoulder dystocia ♀   M
        Impacted shoulders

    O66.1 Obstructed labor due to locked twins ♀   M

    O66.2 Obstructed labor due to unusually large fetus ♀   M

    O66.3 Obstructed labor due to other abnormalities of fetus ♀ M
        Dystocia due to fetal ascites
        Dystocia due to fetal hydrops
        Dystocia due to fetal meningomyelocele
        Dystocia due to fetal sacral teratoma
        Dystocia due to fetal tumor
        Dystocia due to hydrocephalic fetus
        Use additional code to identify cause of obstruction

  ● **O66.4** Failed trial of labor

        O66.40 Failed trial of labor, unspecified ♀   M

        O66.41 Failed attempted vaginal birth after previous cesarean delivery ♀   M
            Code first rupture of uterus, if applicable (O71.0-, O71.1)

    O66.5 Attempted application of vacuum extractor and forceps ♀   M
        Attempted application of vacuum or forceps, with subsequent delivery by forceps or cesarean delivery

    O66.6 Obstructed labor due to other multiple fetuses ♀   M

    O66.8 Other specified obstructed labor ♀   M
        Use additional code to identify cause of obstruction

    O66.9 Obstructed labor, unspecified ♀   M
        Dystocia NOS
        Fetal dystocia NOS
        Maternal dystocia NOS

● **O67** Labor and delivery complicated by intrapartum hemorrhage, not elsewhere classified
    Excludes1   antepartum hemorrhage NEC (O46.-)
            placenta previa (O44.-)
            premature separation of placenta [abruptio placentae] (O45.-)
    Excludes2   postpartum hemorrhage (O72.-)

    O67.0 Intrapartum hemorrhage with coagulation defect ♀   M
        Intrapartum hemorrhage (excessive) associated with afibrinogenemia
        Intrapartum hemorrhage (excessive) associated with disseminated intravascular coagulation
        Intrapartum hemorrhage (excessive) associated with hyperfibrinolysis
        Intrapartum hemorrhage (excessive) associated with hypofibrinogenemia

    O67.8 Other intrapartum hemorrhage ♀   M
        Excessive intrapartum hemorrhage

    O67.9 Intrapartum hemorrhage, unspecified ♀   M

● **O68** Labor and delivery complicated by abnormality of fetal acid-base balance ♀   M
    Fetal acidemia complicating labor and delivery
    Fetal acidosis complicating labor and delivery
    Fetal alkalosis complicating labor and delivery
    Fetal metabolic acidemia complicating labor and delivery
    Excludes1   fetal stress NOS (O77.9)
            labor and delivery complicated by electrocardiographic evidence of fetal stress (O77.8)
            labor and delivery complicated by ultrasonic evidence of fetal stress (O77.8)
    Excludes2   abnormality in fetal heart rate or rhythm (O76)
            labor and delivery complicated by meconium in amniotic fluid (O77.0)

● **O69** Labor and delivery complicated by umbilical cord complications

    One of the following 7th characters is to be assigned to each code under category O69. 7th character 0 is for single gestations and multiple gestations where the fetus is unspecified. 7th characters 1 through 9 are for cases of multiple gestations to identify the fetus for which the code applies. The appropriate code from category O30, Multiple gestation, must also be assigned when assigning a code from category O69 that has a 7th character of 1 through 9.

0	not applicable or unspecified
1	fetus 1
2	fetus 2
3	fetus 3
4	fetus 4
5	fetus 5
9	other fetus

X● **O69.0** Labor and delivery complicated by prolapse of cord ♀ M

X● **O69.1** Labor and delivery complicated by cord around neck, with compression ♀   M
    Excludes1   labor and delivery complicated by cord around neck, without compression (O69.81)

X● **O69.2** Labor and delivery complicated by other cord entanglement, with compression ♀   M
    Labor and delivery complicated by compression of cord NOS
    Labor and delivery complicated by entanglement of cords of twins in monoamniotic sac
    Labor and delivery complicated by knot in cord
    Excludes1   labor and delivery complicated by other cord entanglement, without compression (O69.82)

◀ New   ◀▮▮ Revised   ~~deleted~~ Deleted   Excludes 1   Excludes 2   Includes   Use additional   Code first   Code also   Unspecified

OGCR Official Guidelines   **X** Assign placeholder X   ● Use Additional Character(s)   ▶ Manifestation Code   **Coding Clinic**

X ● O69.3   **Labor and delivery complicated by short cord** ♀   **M**

X ● O69.4   **Labor and delivery complicated by vasa previa** ♀   **M**
Labor and delivery complicated by hemorrhage from vasa previa

X ● O69.5   **Labor and delivery complicated by vascular lesion of cord** ♀   **M**
Labor and delivery complicated by cord bruising
Labor and delivery complicated by cord hematoma
Labor and delivery complicated by thrombosis of umbilical vessels

● O69.8   **Labor and delivery complicated by other cord complications**

X ● O69.81   **Labor and delivery complicated by cord around neck, without compression** ♀   **M**

X ● O69.82   **Labor and delivery complicated by other cord entanglement, without compression** ♀   **M**

X ● O69.89   **Labor and delivery complicated by other cord complications** ♀   **M**

X ● O69.9   **Labor and delivery complicated by cord complication, unspecified** ♀   **M**

● O70   **Perineal laceration during delivery**
Includes   episiotomy extended by laceration
Excludes1   obstetric high vaginal laceration alone (O71.4)

O70.0   **First degree perineal laceration during delivery** ♀   **M**
Perineal laceration, rupture or tear involving fourchette during delivery
Perineal laceration, rupture or tear involving labia during delivery
Perineal laceration, rupture or tear involving skin during delivery
Perineal laceration, rupture or tear involving vagina during delivery
Perineal laceration, rupture or tear involving vulva during delivery
Slight perineal laceration, rupture or tear during delivery

O70.1   **Second degree perineal laceration during delivery** ♀   **M**
Perineal laceration, rupture or tear during delivery as in O70.0, also involving pelvic floor
Perineal laceration, rupture or tear during delivery as in O70.0, also involving perineal muscles
Perineal laceration, rupture or tear during delivery as in O70.0, also involving vaginal muscles
Excludes1   perineal laceration involving anal sphincter (O70.2)

O70.2   **Third degree perineal laceration during delivery** ♀   **M**
Perineal laceration, rupture or tear during delivery as in O70.1, also involving anal sphincter
Perineal laceration, rupture or tear during delivery as in O70.1, also involving rectovaginal septum
Perineal laceration, rupture or tear during delivery as in O70.1, also involving sphincter NOS
Excludes1   anal sphincter tear during delivery without third degree perineal laceration (O70.4)
perineal laceration involving anal or rectal mucosa (O70.3)

O70.3   **Fourth degree perineal laceration during delivery** ♀   **M**
Perineal laceration, rupture or tear during delivery as in O70.2, also involving anal mucosa
Perineal laceration, rupture or tear during delivery as in O70.2, also involving rectal mucosa

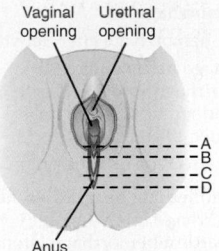

Figure 15-6   Perineal lacerations: **A.** First-degree is laceration of superficial tissues. **B.** Second-degree is limited to the pelvic floor and may involve the perineal or vaginal muscles. **C.** Third-degree involves the anal sphincter. **D.** Fourth-degree involves anal or rectal mucosa.

O70.4   **Anal sphincter tear complicating delivery, not associated with third degree laceration** ♀   **M**
Excludes1   anal sphincter tear with third degree perineal laceration (O70.2)

O70.9   **Perineal laceration during delivery, unspecified** ♀   **M**

● O71   **Other obstetric trauma**
Includes   obstetric damage from instruments

● O71.0   **Rupture of uterus (spontaneous) before onset of labor**
Excludes1   disruption of (current) cesarean delivery wound (O90.0)
laceration of uterus, NEC (O71.81)

O71.00   **Rupture of uterus before onset of labor, unspecified trimester** ♀   **M**

O71.02   **Rupture of uterus before onset of labor, second trimester** ♀   **M**

O71.03   **Rupture of uterus before onset of labor, third trimester** ♀   **M**

O71.1   **Rupture of uterus during labor** ♀   **M**
Rupture of uterus not stated as occurring before onset of labor
Excludes1   disruption of cesarean delivery wound (O90.0)
laceration of uterus, NEC (O71.81)

O71.2   **Postpartum inversion of uterus** ♀   **M**

O71.3   **Obstetric laceration of cervix** ♀   **M**
Annular detachment of cervix

O71.4   **Obstetric high vaginal laceration alone** ♀   **M**
Laceration of vaginal wall without perineal laceration
Excludes1   obstetric high vaginal laceration with perineal laceration (O70.-)

O71.5   **Other obstetric injury to pelvic organs** ♀   **M**
Obstetric injury to bladder
Obstetric injury to urethra
Excludes2   obstetric periurethral trauma (O71.82)

O71.6   **Obstetric damage to pelvic joints and ligaments** ♀   **M**
Obstetric avulsion of inner symphyseal cartilage
Obstetric damage to coccyx
Obstetric traumatic separation of symphysis (pubis)

O71.7   **Obstetric hematoma of pelvis** ♀   **M**
Obstetric hematoma of perineum
Obstetric hematoma of vagina
Obstetric hematoma of vulva

● O71.8   **Other specified obstetric trauma**

O71.81   **Laceration of uterus, not elsewhere classified** ♀   **M**

O71.82   **Other specified trauma to perineum and vulva** ♀   **M**
Obstetric periurethral trauma

O71.89   **Other specified obstetric trauma** ♀   **M**

O71.9   **Obstetric trauma, unspecified** ♀   **M**

CHAPTER 15 (O00-O9A)

● **O72   Postpartum hemorrhage**

> **Includes**   hemorrhage after delivery of fetus or infant

O72.0   **Third-stage hemorrhage** ♀   M
Hemorrhage associated with retained, trapped or adherent placenta
Retained placenta NOS

> Code also type of adherent placenta (O43.2-)

O72.1   **Other immediate postpartum hemorrhage** ♀   M
Hemorrhage following delivery of placenta
Postpartum hemorrhage (atonic) NOS
Uterine atony with hemorrhage

> **Excludes1**   uterine atony NOS (O62.2)
> uterine atony without hemorrhage (O62.2)
> postpartum atony of uterus without hemorrhage (O75.89)

O72.2   **Delayed and secondary postpartum hemorrhage** ♀   M
Hemorrhage associated with retained portions of placenta or membranes after the first 24 hours following delivery of placenta
Retained products of conception NOS, following delivery

O72.3   **Postpartum coagulation defects** ♀   M
Postpartum afibrinogenemia
Postpartum fibrinolysis

● **O73   Retained placenta and membranes, without hemorrhage**

> **Excludes1**   placenta accreta (O43.21-)
> placenta increta (O43.22-)
> placenta percreta (O43.23-)

O73.0   **Retained placenta without hemorrhage** ♀   M
Adherent placenta, without hemorrhage
Trapped placenta without hemorrhage

O73.1   **Retained portions of placenta and membranes, without hemorrhage** ♀   M
Retained products of conception following delivery, without hemorrhage

● **O74   Complications of anesthesia during labor and delivery**

> **Includes**   maternal complications arising from the administration of a general, regional or local anesthetic, analgesic or other sedation during labor and delivery

> Use additional code, if applicable, to identify specific complication

O74.0   **Aspiration pneumonitis due to anesthesia during labor and delivery** ♀   M
Inhalation of stomach contents or secretions NOS due to anesthesia during labor and delivery
Mendelson's syndrome due to anesthesia during labor and delivery

O74.1   **Other pulmonary complications of anesthesia during labor and delivery** ♀   M

O74.2   **Cardiac complications of anesthesia during labor and delivery** ♀   M

O74.3   **Central nervous system complications of anesthesia during labor and delivery** ♀   M

O74.4   **Toxic reaction to local anesthesia during labor and delivery** ♀   M

O74.5   **Spinal and epidural anesthesia-induced headache during labor and delivery** ♀   M

O74.6   **Other complications of spinal and epidural anesthesia during labor and delivery** ♀   M

O74.7   **Failed or difficult intubation for anesthesia during labor and delivery** ♀   M

O74.8   **Other complications of anesthesia during labor and delivery** ♀   M

O74.9   **Complication of anesthesia during labor and delivery, unspecified** ♀   M

● **O75   Other complications of labor and delivery, not elsewhere classified**

> **Excludes2**   puerperal (postpartum) infection (O86.-)
> puerperal (postpartum) sepsis (O85)

O75.0   **Maternal distress during labor and delivery** ♀   M

O75.1   **Shock during or following labor and delivery** ♀   M
Obstetric shock following labor and delivery

O75.2   **Pyrexia during labor, not elsewhere classified** ♀   M

O75.3   **Other infection during labor** ♀   M
Sepsis during labor

> Use additional code (B95-B97), to identify infectious agent

O75.4   **Other complications of obstetric surgery and procedures** ♀   M
Cardiac arrest following obstetric surgery or procedures
Cardiac failure following obstetric surgery or procedures
Cerebral anoxia following obstetric surgery or procedures
Pulmonary edema following obstetric surgery or procedures

> Use additional code to identify specific complication

> **Excludes2**   complications of anesthesia during labor and delivery (O74.-)
> disruption of obstetrical (surgical) wound (O90.0-O90.1)
> hematoma of obstetrical (surgical) wound (O90.2)
> infection of obstetrical (surgical) wound (O86.0)

O75.5   **Delayed delivery after artificial rupture of membranes** ♀   M

● O75.8   **Other specified complications of labor and delivery**

O75.81   **Maternal exhaustion complicating labor and delivery** ♀   M

O75.82   **Onset (spontaneous) of labor after 37 completed weeks of gestation but before 39 completed weeks gestation, with delivery by (planned) cesarean section** ♀   M
Delivery by (planned) cesarean section occurring after 37 completed weeks of gestation but before 39 completed weeks gestation due to (spontaneous) onset of labor

> *Code first to specify reason for planned cesarean section such as:*
> cephalopelvic disproportion (normally formed fetus) (O33.9)
> previous cesarean delivery (O34.21)

O75.89   **Other specified complications of labor and delivery** ♀   M

O75.9   **Complication of labor and delivery, unspecified** ♀   M

O76   **Abnormality in fetal heart rate and rhythm complicating labor and delivery** ♀   M
Depressed fetal heart rate tones complicating labor and delivery
Fetal bradycardia complicating labor and delivery
Fetal heart rate decelerations complicating labor and delivery
Fetal heart rate irregularity complicating labor and delivery
Fetal heart rate abnormal variability complicating labor and delivery
Fetal tachycardia complicating labor and delivery
Non-reassuring fetal heart rate or rhythm complicating labor and delivery

> **Excludes1**   fetal stress NOS (O77.9)
> labor and delivery complicated by electrocardiographic evidence of fetal stress (O77.8)
> labor and delivery complicated by ultrasonic evidence of fetal stress (O77.8)

> **Excludes2**   fetal metabolic acidemia (O68)
> other fetal stress (O77.0-O77.1)

◄ New   ◄▬ Revised   ~~deleted~~ Deleted   Excludes 1   Excludes 2   Includes   Use additional   Code first   Code also   Unspecified

OGCR Official Guidelines   **X** Assign placeholder X   ● Use Additional Character(s)   ▶ Manifestation Code   **Coding Clinic**

● **O77   Other fetal stress complicating labor and delivery**

O77.0   Labor and delivery complicated by meconium in amniotic fluid ♀   M

O77.1   Fetal stress in labor or delivery due to drug administration ♀   M

O77.8   Labor and delivery complicated by other evidence of fetal stress ♀   M

Labor and delivery complicated by electrocardiographic evidence of fetal stress

Labor and delivery complicated by ultrasonic evidence of fetal stress

> **Excludes1**   abnormality of fetal acid-base balance (O68)
> abnormality in fetal heart rate or rhythm (O76)
> fetal metabolic acidemia (O68)

O77.9   Labor and delivery complicated by fetal stress, unspecified ♀   M

> **Excludes1**   abnormality of fetal acid-base balance (O68)
> abnormality in fetal heart rate or rhythm (O76)
> fetal metabolic acidemia (O68)

OGCR   Section I.C., Chapter 15.m.

Normal Delivery, Code O80

1) Encounter for full term uncomplicated delivery

Code O80 should be assigned when a woman is admitted for a full-term normal delivery and delivers a single, healthy infant without any complications antepartum, during the delivery, or postpartum during the delivery episode. Code O80 is always a principal diagnosis. It is not to be used if any other code from chapter 15 is needed to describe a current complication of the antenatal, delivery, or perinatal period. Additional codes from other chapters may be used with code O80 if they are not related to or are in any way complicating the pregnancy.

2) Uncomplicated delivery with resolved antepartum complication

Code O80 may be used if the patient had a complication at some point during the pregnancy, but the complication is not present at the time of the admission for delivery.

3) Outcome of delivery for O80

Z37.0, Single live brith, is the only outcome of delivery code appropriate for use with O80.

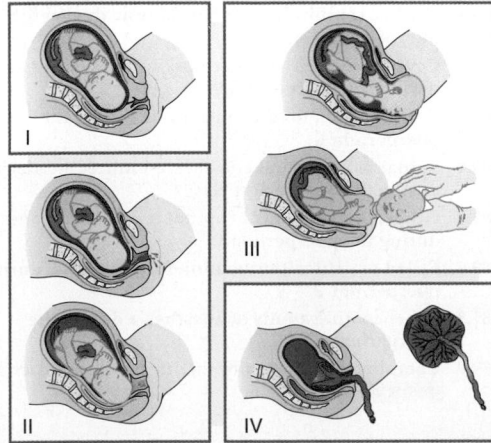

Figure 15-7   The four stages of normal delivery: **I.** Lightening, which occurs 2 to 4 weeks before birth, at which time the fetus turns with head toward the vagina. **II.** Regular contractions begin, the amniotic sac ruptures, and dilation is complete. **III.** Delivery of the head and rotation. **IV.** Expulsion of placenta.

ENCOUNTER FOR DELIVERY (O80-O82)

O80   Encounter for full-term uncomplicated delivery ♀   M

Delivery requiring minimal or no assistance, with or without episiotomy, without fetal manipulation [e.g., rotation version] or instrumentation [forceps] of a spontaneous, cephalic, vaginal, full-term, single, live-born infant. This code is for use as a single diagnosis code and is not to be used with any other code from chapter 15.

Use additional code to indicate outcome of delivery (Z37.0)

O82   Encounter for cesarean delivery without indication ♀   M

Use additional code to indicate outcome of delivery (Z37.0)

COMPLICATIONS PREDOMINANTLY RELATED TO THE PUERPERIUM (O85-O92)

> **Excludes2**   mental and behavioral disorders associated with the puerperium (F53)
> obstetrical tetanus (A34)
> puerperal osteomalacia (M83.0)

O85   Puerperal sepsis ♀   M

Postpartum sepsis

Puerperal peritonitis

Puerperal pyemia

Use additional code (B95-B97), to identify infectious agent

Use additional code (R65.2-) to identify severe sepsis, if applicable

> **Excludes1**   fever of unknown origin following delivery (O86.4)
> genital tract infection following delivery (O86.1-)
> obstetric pyemic and septic embolism (O88.3-)
> puerperal septic thrombophlebitis (O86.81)
> urinary tract infection following delivery (O86.2-)

> **Excludes2**   sepsis during labor (O75.3)

● **O86   Other puerperal infections**

Use additional code (B95-B97), to identify infectious agent

> **Excludes2**   infection during labor (O75.3)
> obstetrical tetanus (A34)

O86.0   Infection of obstetric surgical wound ♀   M

Infected cesarean delivery wound following delivery

Infected perineal repair following delivery

● **O86.1   Other infection of genital tract following delivery**

O86.11   Cervicitis following delivery ♀   M

O86.12   Endometritis following delivery ♀   M

O86.13   Vaginitis following delivery ♀   M

O86.19   Other infection of genital tract following delivery ♀   M

● **O86.2   Urinary tract infection following delivery**

O86.20   Urinary tract infection following delivery, unspecified ♀   M

Puerperal urinary tract infection NOS

O86.21   Infection of kidney following delivery ♀   M

O86.22   Infection of bladder following delivery ♀   M

Infection of urethra following delivery

O86.29   Other urinary tract infection following delivery ♀   M

O86.4   Pyrexia of unknown origin following delivery ♀   M

Puerperal infection NOS following delivery

Puerperal pyrexia NOS following delivery

> **Excludes2**   pyrexia during labor (O75.2)

● **O86.8   Other specified puerperal infections**

O86.81   Puerperal septic thrombophlebitis ♀   M

O86.89   Other specified puerperal infections ♀   M

CHAPTER 15 (O00-O9A)

● **O87   Venous complications and hemorrhoids in the puerperium**

> **Includes**   venous complications in labor, delivery and the puerperium

> **Excludes2**   obstetric embolism (O88.-)
> puerperal septic thrombophlebitis (O86.81)
> venous complications in pregnancy (O22.-)

O87.0   Superficial thrombophlebitis in the puerperium ♀   M
> Puerperal phlebitis NOS
> Puerperal thrombosis NOS

O87.1   Deep phlebothrombosis in the puerperium ♀   M
> Deep vein thrombosis, postpartum
> Pelvic thrombophlebitis, postpartum
> Use additional code to identify the deep vein thrombosis (I82.4-, I82.5-, I82.62-. I82.72-)
> Use additional code, if applicable, for associated long-term (current) use of anticoagulants (Z79.01)

O87.2   Hemorrhoids in the puerperium ♀   M

O87.3   Cerebral venous thrombosis in the puerperium ♀   M
> Cerebrovenous sinus thrombosis in the puerperium

O87.4   Varicose veins of lower extremity in the puerperium ♀   M

O87.8   Other venous complications in the puerperium ♀   M
> Genital varices in the puerperium

O87.9   Venous complication in the puerperium, unspecified ♀ M
> Puerperal phlebopathy NOS

O88   Obstetric embolism

> **Excludes1**   embolism complicating abortion NOS (O03.2)
> embolism complicating ectopic or molar pregnancy (O08.2)
> embolism complicating failed attempted abortion (O07.2)
> embolism complicating induced abortion (O04.7)
> embolism complicating spontaneous abortion (O03.2, O03.7)

● **O88.0   Obstetric air embolism**

● **O88.01   Obstetric air embolism in pregnancy**

O88.011   Air embolism in pregnancy, first trimester ♀   M

O88.012   Air embolism in pregnancy, second trimester ♀   M

O88.013   Air embolism in pregnancy, third trimester ♀   M

O88.019   Air embolism in pregnancy, unspecified trimester ♀   M

O88.02   Air embolism in childbirth ♀   M

O88.03   Air embolism in the puerperium ♀   M

● **O88.1   Amniotic fluid embolism**
> Anaphylactoid syndrome in pregnancy

● **O88.11   Amniotic fluid embolism in pregnancy**

O88.111   Amniotic fluid embolism in pregnancy, first trimester ♀   M

O88.112   Amniotic fluid embolism in pregnancy, second trimester ♀   M

O88.113   Amniotic fluid embolism in pregnancy, third trimester ♀   M

O88.119   Amniotic fluid embolism in pregnancy, unspecified trimester ♀   M

O88.12   Amniotic fluid embolism in childbirth ♀   M

O88.13   Amniotic fluid embolism in the puerperium ♀   M

● **O88.2   Obstetric thromboembolism**

● **O88.21   Thromboembolism in pregnancy**
> Obstetric (pulmonary) embolism NOS

O88.211   Thromboembolism in pregnancy, first trimester ♀   M

O88.212   Thromboembolism in pregnancy, second trimester ♀   M

O88.213   Thromboembolism in pregnancy, third trimester ♀   M

O88.219   Thromboembolism in pregnancy, unspecified trimester ♀   M

O88.22   Thromboembolism in childbirth ♀   M

O88.23   Thromboembolism in the puerperium ♀   M
> Puerperal (pulmonary) embolism NOS

● **O88.3   Obstetric pyemic and septic embolism**

● **O88.31   Pyemic and septic embolism in pregnancy**

O88.311   Pyemic and septic embolism in pregnancy, first trimester ♀   M

O88.312   Pyemic and septic embolism in pregnancy, second trimester ♀   M

O88.313   Pyemic and septic embolism in pregnancy, third trimester ♀   M

O88.319   Pyemic and septic embolism in pregnancy, unspecified trimester ♀   M

O88.32   Pyemic and septic embolism in childbirth ♀   M

O88.33   Pyemic and septic embolism in the puerperium ♀   M

● **O88.8   Other obstetric embolism**
> Obstetric fat embolism

● **O88.81   Other embolism in pregnancy**

O88.811   Other embolism in pregnancy, first trimester ♀   M

O88.812   Other embolism in pregnancy, second trimester ♀   M

O88.813   Other embolism in pregnancy, third trimester ♀   M

O88.819   Other embolism in pregnancy, unspecified trimester ♀   M

O88.82   Other embolism in childbirth ♀   M

O88.83   Other embolism in the puerperium ♀   M

● **O89   Complications of anesthesia during the puerperium**

> **Includes**   maternal complications arising from the administration of a general, regional or local anesthetic, analgesic or other sedation during the puerperium

> Use additional code, if applicable, to identify specific complication

● **O89.0   Pulmonary complications of anesthesia during the puerperium**

O89.01   Aspiration pneumonitis due to anesthesia during the puerperium ♀   M
> Inhalation of stomach contents or secretions NOS due to anesthesia during the puerperium
> Mendelson's syndrome due to anesthesia during the puerperium

O89.09   Other pulmonary complications of anesthesia during the puerperium ♀   M

O89.1   Cardiac complications of anesthesia during the puerperium ♀   M

O89.2   Central nervous system complications of anesthesia during the puerperium ♀   M

O89.3   Toxic reaction to local anesthesia during the puerperium ♀   M

O89.4   Spinal and epidural anesthesia-induced headache during the puerperium ♀   M

O89.5   Other complications of spinal and epidural anesthesia during the puerperium ♀   M

O89.6   Failed or difficult intubation for anesthesia during the puerperium ♀   M

O89.8   Other complications of anesthesia during the puerperium ♀   M

O89.9   Complication of anesthesia during the puerperium, unspecified ♀   M

◀ New   ◀▥ Revised   ~~deleted~~ Deleted   Excludes 1   Excludes 2   Includes   Use additional   Code first   Code also   Unspecified

OGCR Official Guidelines   **X** Assign placeholder X   ● Use Additional Character(s)   ▶ Manifestation Code   **Coding Clinic**

● **O90   Complications of the puerperium, not elsewhere classified**

O90.0   Disruption of cesarean delivery wound ♀   **M**
Dehiscence of cesarean delivery wound
> **Excludes1**   rupture of uterus (spontaneous) before
> onset of labor (O71.0-)
> rupture of uterus during labor (O71.1)

O90.1   Disruption of perineal obstetric wound ♀   **M**
Disruption of wound of episiotomy
Disruption of wound of perineal laceration
Secondary perineal tear

O90.2   Hematoma of obstetric wound ♀   **M**

O90.3   Peripartum cardiomyopathy ♀   **M**
Conditions in I42.- arising during pregnancy and the puerperium
> **Excludes1**   pre-existing heart disease complicating
> pregnancy and the puerperium
> (O99.4-)

O90.4   Postpartum acute kidney failure ♀   **M**
Hepatorenal syndrome following labor and delivery

O90.5   Postpartum thyroiditis ♀   **M**

O90.6   Postpartum mood disturbance ♀   **M**
Postpartum blues   Postpartum sadness
Postpartum dysphoria
> **Excludes1**   postpartum depression (F53)
> puerperal psychosis (F53)

● **O90.8   Other complications of the puerperium, not elsewhere classified**

O90.81   Anemia of the puerperium ♀   **M**
Postpartum anemia NOS
> **Excludes1**   pre-existing anemia complicating
> the puerperium (O99.03)

O90.89   Other complications of the puerperium, not elsewhere classified ♀   **M**
Placental polyp

O90.9   Complication of the puerperium, unspecified ♀   **M**

● **O91   Infections of breast associated with pregnancy, the puerperium and lactation**
Use additional code to identify infection

● **O91.0   Infection of nipple associated with pregnancy, the puerperium and lactation**

● **O91.01   Infection of nipple associated with pregnancy**
Gestational abscess of nipple

O91.011   Infection of nipple associated with pregnancy, first trimester ♀   **M**

O91.012   Infection of nipple associated with pregnancy, second trimester ♀   **M**

O91.013   Infection of nipple associated with pregnancy, third trimester ♀   **M**

O91.019   Infection of nipple associated with pregnancy, unspecified trimester ♀   **M**

O91.02   Infection of nipple associated with the puerperium ♀   **M**
Puerperal abscess of nipple

O91.03   Infection of nipple associated with lactation ♀ **M**
Abscess of nipple associated with lactation

● **O91.1   Abscess of breast associated with pregnancy, the puerperium and lactation**

● **O91.11   Abscess of breast associated with pregnancy**
Gestational mammary abscess
Gestational purulent mastitis
Gestational subareolar abscess

O91.111   Abscess of breast associated with pregnancy, first trimester ♀   **M**

O91.112   Abscess of breast associated with pregnancy, second trimester ♀   **M**

O91.113   Abscess of breast associated with pregnancy, third trimester ♀   **M**

O91.119   Abscess of breast associated with pregnancy, unspecified trimester ♀   **M**

O91.12   Abscess of breast associated with the puerperium ♀   **M**
Puerperal mammary abscess
Puerperal purulent mastitis
Puerperal subareolar abscess

O91.13   Abscess of breast associated with lactation ♀ **M**
Mammary abscess associated with lactation
Purulent mastitis associated with lactation
Subareolar abscess associated with lactation

● **O91.2   Nonpurulent mastitis associated with pregnancy, the puerperium and lactation**

● **O91.21   Nonpurulent mastitis associated with pregnancy**
Gestational interstitial mastitis
Gestational lymphangitis of breast
Gestational mastitis NOS
Gestational parenchymatous mastitis

O91.211   Nonpurulent mastitis associated with pregnancy, first trimester ♀   **M**

O91.212   Nonpurulent mastitis associated with pregnancy, second trimester ♀   **M**

O91.213   Nonpurulent mastitis associated with pregnancy, third trimester ♀   **M**

O91.219   Nonpurulent mastitis associated with pregnancy, unspecified trimester ♀ **M**

O91.22   Nonpurulent mastitis associated with the puerperium ♀   **M**
Puerperal interstitial mastitis
Puerperal lymphangitis of breast
Puerperal mastitis NOS
Puerperal parenchymatous mastitis

O91.23   Nonpurulent mastitis associated with lactation ♀   **M**
Interstitial mastitis associated with lactation
Lymphangitis of breast associated with lactation
Mastitis NOS associated with lactation
Parenchymatous mastitis associated with lactation

● **O92   Other disorders of breast and disorders of lactation associated with pregnancy and the puerperium**

● **O92.0   Retracted nipple associated with pregnancy, the puerperium, and lactation**

● **O92.01   Retracted nipple associated with pregnancy**

O92.011   Retracted nipple associated with pregnancy, first trimester ♀   **M**

O92.012   Retracted nipple associated with pregnancy, second trimester ♀   **M**

O92.013   Retracted nipple associated with pregnancy, third trimester ♀   **M**

O92.019   Retracted nipple associated with pregnancy, unspecified trimester ♀   **M**

O92.02   Retracted nipple associated with the puerperium ♀   **M**

O92.03   Retracted nipple associated with lactation ♀   **M**

● **O92.1   Cracked nipple associated with pregnancy, the puerperium, and lactation**
Fissure of nipple, gestational or puerperal

● **O92.11   Cracked nipple associated with pregnancy**

O92.111   Cracked nipple associated with pregnancy, first trimester ♀   **M**

O92.112   Cracked nipple associated with pregnancy, second trimester ♀   **M**

O92.113   Cracked nipple associated with pregnancy, third trimester ♀   **M**

O92.119   Cracked nipple associated with pregnancy, unspecified trimester ♀   **M**

O92.12   Cracked nipple associated with the puerperium ♀   **M**

O92.13   Cracked nipple associated with lactation ♀   **M**

● **O92.2** **Other and unspecified disorders of breast associated with pregnancy and the puerperium**
- **O92.20** Unspecified disorder of breast associated with pregnancy and the puerperium ♀   M
- **O92.29** Other disorders of breast associated with pregnancy and the puerperium ♀   M

O92.3 **Agalactia** ♀   M
Primary agalactia
> **Excludes1**   elective agalactia (O92.5)
> secondary agalactia (O92.5)
> therapeutic agalactia (O92.5)

O92.4 **Hypogalactia** ♀   M

O92.5 **Suppressed lactation** ♀   M
Elective agalactia   Therapeutic agalactia
Secondary agalactia
> **Excludes1**   primary agalactia (O92.3)

O92.6 **Galactorrhea** ♀   M

● **O92.7** **Other and unspecified disorders of lactation**
- **O92.70** Unspecified disorders of lactation ♀   M
- **O92.79** Other disorders of lactation ♀   M
Puerperal galactocele

OGCR Section I.C.2.I.3.

> Malignant neoplasm in a pregnant patient
>
> When a pregnant woman has a malignant neoplasm, a code from subcategory O9A.1-, Malignant neoplasm complicating pregnancy, childbirth, and the puerperium, should be sequenced first, followed by the appropriate code from Chapter 2 to indicate the type of neoplasm.

OTHER OBSTETRIC CONDITIONS, NOT ELSEWHERE CLASSIFIED (O94-O9A)

O94 **Sequelae of complication of pregnancy, childbirth, and the puerperium** ♀   M
> **Note:** This category is to be used to indicate conditions in O00-O77.-, O85-O94 and O98-O9A.- as the cause of late effects. The 'sequelae' include conditions specified as such, or as late effects, which may occur at any time after the puerperium.
>
> *Code first* condition resulting from (sequela) of complication of pregnancy, childbirth, and the puerperium

O98 **Maternal infectious and parasitic diseases classifiable elsewhere but complicating pregnancy, childbirth and the puerperium**
> **Includes**   the listed conditions when complicating the pregnant state, when aggravated by the pregnancy, or as a reason for obstetric care
>
> Use additional code (Chapter 1), to identify specific infectious or parasitic disease
>
> **Excludes2**   herpes gestationis (O26.4-)
> infectious carrier state (O99.82-, O99.83-)
> obstetrical tetanus (A34)
> puerperal infection (O86.-)
> puerperal sepsis (O85)
> when the reason for maternal care is that the disease is known or suspected to have affected the fetus (O35-O36)

● **O98.0** **Tuberculosis complicating pregnancy, childbirth and the puerperium**
Conditions in A15-A19
- ● **O98.01** Tuberculosis complicating pregnancy
  - **O98.011** Tuberculosis complicating pregnancy, first trimester ♀   M
  - **O98.012** Tuberculosis complicating pregnancy, second trimester ♀   M
  - **O98.013** Tuberculosis complicating pregnancy, third trimester ♀   M
  - **O98.019** Tuberculosis complicating pregnancy, unspecified trimester ♀   M
- **O98.02** Tuberculosis complicating childbirth ♀   M
- **O98.03** Tuberculosis complicating the puerperium ♀   M

● **O98.1** **Syphilis complicating pregnancy, childbirth and the puerperium**
Conditions in A50-A53
- ● **O98.11** Syphilis complicating pregnancy
  - **O98.111** Syphilis complicating pregnancy, first trimester ♀   M
  - **O98.112** Syphilis complicating pregnancy, second trimester ♀   M
  - **O98.113** Syphilis complicating pregnancy, third trimester ♀   M
  - **O98.119** Syphilis complicating pregnancy, unspecified trimester ♀   M
- **O98.12** Syphilis complicating childbirth ♀   M
- **O98.13** Syphilis complicating the puerperium ♀   M

● **O98.2** **Gonorrhea complicating pregnancy, childbirth and the puerperium**
Conditions in A54.-
- ● **O98.21** Gonorrhea complicating pregnancy
  - **O98.211** Gonorrhea complicating pregnancy, first trimester ♀   M
  - **O98.212** Gonorrhea complicating pregnancy, second trimester ♀   M
  - **O98.213** Gonorrhea complicating pregnancy, third trimester ♀   M
  - **O98.219** Gonorrhea complicating pregnancy, unspecified trimester ♀   M
- **O98.22** Gonorrhea complicating childbirth ♀   M
- **O98.23** Gonorrhea complicating the puerperium ♀   M

● **O98.3** **Other infections with a predominantly sexual mode of transmission complicating pregnancy, childbirth and the puerperium**
Conditions in A55-A64
- ● **O98.31** Other infections with a predominantly sexual mode of transmission complicating pregnancy
  - **O98.311** Other infections with a predominantly sexual mode of transmission complicating pregnancy, first trimester ♀   M
  - **O98.312** Other infections with a predominantly sexual mode of transmission complicating pregnancy, second trimester ♀   M
  - **O98.313** Other infections with a predominantly sexual mode of transmission complicating pregnancy, third trimester ♀   M
  - **O98.319** Other infections with a predominantly sexual mode of transmission complicating pregnancy, unspecified trimester ♀   M
- **O98.32** Other infections with a predominantly sexual mode of transmission complicating childbirth ♀   M
- **O98.33** Other infections with a predominantly sexual mode of transmission complicating the puerperium ♀   M

● **O98.4** **Viral hepatitis complicating pregnancy, childbirth and the puerperium**
Conditions in B15-B19
- ● **O98.41** Viral hepatitis complicating pregnancy
  - **O98.411** Viral hepatitis complicating pregnancy, first trimester ♀   M
  - **O98.412** Viral hepatitis complicating pregnancy, second trimester ♀   M
  - **O98.413** Viral hepatitis complicating pregnancy, third trimester ♀   M
  - **O98.419** Viral hepatitis complicating pregnancy, unspecified trimester ♀   M
- **O98.42** Viral hepatitis complicating childbirth ♀   M
- **O98.43** Viral hepatitis complicating the puerperium ♀   M

◀ New   ◀━ Revised   ~~deleted~~ Deleted   Excludes 1   Excludes 2   Includes   Use additional   Code first   Code also   Unspecified

1196   **OGCR** Official Guidelines   X Assign placeholder X   ● Use Additional Character(s)   ▌ Manifestation Code   **Coding Clinic**

● **O98.5 Other viral diseases complicating pregnancy, childbirth and the puerperium**
Conditions in A80-B09, B25-B34, R87.81-, R87.82-
Excludes:1 human immunodeficiency virus [HIV] disease complicating pregnancy, childbirth and the puerperium (O98.7-)

● **O98.51 Other viral diseases complicating pregnancy**
O98.511 Other viral diseases complicating pregnancy, first trimester ♀ M
O98.512 Other viral diseases complicating pregnancy, second trimester ♀ M
O98.513 Other viral diseases complicating pregnancy, third trimester ♀ M
O98.519 Other viral diseases complicating pregnancy, unspecified trimester ♀ M
O98.52 Other viral diseases complicating childbirth ♀ M
O98.53 Other viral diseases complicating the puerperium ♀ M

● **O98.6 Protozoal diseases complicating pregnancy, childbirth and the puerperium**
Conditions in B50-B64

● **O98.61 Protozoal diseases complicating pregnancy**
O98.611 Protozoal diseases complicating pregnancy, first trimester ♀ M
O98.612 Protozoal diseases complicating pregnancy, second trimester ♀ M
O98.613 Protozoal diseases complicating pregnancy, third trimester ♀ M
O98.619 Protozoal diseases complicating pregnancy, unspecified trimester ♀ M
O98.62 Protozoal diseases complicating childbirth ♀ M
O98.63 Protozoal diseases complicating the puerperium ♀ M

● **O98.7 Human immunodeficiency virus [HIV] disease complicating pregnancy, childbirth and the puerperium**
Use additional code to identify the type of HIV disease:
Acquired immune deficiency syndrome (AIDS) (B20)
Asymptomatic HIV status (Z21)
HIV positive NOS (Z21)
Symptomatic HIV disease (B20)

OGCR Section I.C.15.f.

HIV Infection in Pregnancy, Childbirth and the Puerperium

During pregnancy, childbirth or the puerperium, a patient admitted because of an HIV-related illness should receive a principal diagnosis from subcategory O98.7-. Human immunodeficiency [HIV] disease complicating pregnancy, childbirth and the puerperium, followed by the code(s) for the HIV-related illness(es).

Patients with asymptomatic HIV infection status admitted during pregnancy, childbirth, or the puerperium should receive codes of O98.7- and Z21, Asymptomatic human immunodeficiency virus [HIV] infection status.

● **O98.71 Human immunodeficiency virus [HIV] disease complicating pregnancy**
O98.711 Human immunodeficiency virus [HIV] disease complicating pregnancy, first trimester ♀ M
O98.712 Human immunodeficiency virus [HIV] disease complicating pregnancy, second trimester ♀ M
O98.713 Human immunodeficiency virus [HIV] disease complicating pregnancy, third trimester ♀ M
O98.719 Human immunodeficiency virus [HIV] disease complicating pregnancy, unspecified trimester ♀ M

O98.72 Human immunodeficiency virus [HIV] disease complicating childbirth ♀ M
O98.73 Human immunodeficiency virus [HIV] disease complicating the puerperium ♀ M

● **O98.8 Other maternal infectious and parasitic diseases complicating pregnancy, childbirth and the puerperium**

● **O98.81 Other maternal infectious and parasitic diseases complicating pregnancy**
O98.811 Other maternal infectious and parasitic diseases complicating pregnancy, first trimester ♀ M
O98.812 Other maternal infectious and parasitic diseases complicating pregnancy, second trimester ♀ M
O98.813 Other maternal infectious and parasitic diseases complicating pregnancy, third trimester ♀ M
O98.819 Other maternal infectious and parasitic diseases complicating pregnancy, unspecified trimester ♀ M
O98.82 Other maternal infectious and parasitic diseases complicating childbirth ♀ M
O98.83 Other maternal infectious and parasitic diseases complicating the puerperium ♀ M

● **O98.9 Unspecified maternal infectious and parasitic disease complicating pregnancy, childbirth and the puerperium**

● **O98.91 Unspecified maternal infectious and parasitic disease complicating pregnancy**
O98.911 Unspecified maternal infectious and parasitic disease complicating pregnancy, first trimester ♀ M
O98.912 Unspecified maternal infectious and parasitic disease complicating pregnancy, second trimester ♀ M
O98.913 Unspecified maternal infectious and parasitic disease complicating pregnancy, third trimester ♀ M
O98.919 Unspecified maternal infectious and parasitic disease complicating pregnancy, unspecified trimester ♀ M
O98.92 Unspecified maternal infectious and parasitic disease complicating childbirth ♀ M
O98.93 Unspecified maternal infectious and parasitic disease complicating the puerperium ♀ M

● **O99 Other maternal diseases classifiable elsewhere but complicating pregnancy, childbirth and the puerperium**
Includes: conditions which complicate the pregnant state, are aggravated by the pregnancy or are a main reason for obstetric care
Use additional code to identify specific condition
Excludes2 when the reason for maternal care is that the condition is known or suspected to have affected the fetus (O35-O36)

● **O99.0 Anemia complicating pregnancy, childbirth and the puerperium**
Conditions in D50-D64
Excludes1 anemia arising in the puerperium (O90.81)
postpartum anemia NOS (O90.81)

● **O99.01 Anemia complicating pregnancy**
O99.011 Anemia complicating pregnancy, first trimester ♀ M
O99.012 Anemia complicating pregnancy, second trimester ♀ M
O99.013 Anemia complicating pregnancy, third trimester ♀ M
O99.019 Anemia complicating pregnancy, unspecified trimester ♀ M

CHAPTER 15 (O00-O9A)

O99.02　Anemia complicating childbirth ♀　　　M

O99.03　Anemia complicating the puerperium ♀　　M

> **Excludes1**　postpartum anemia not pre-existing prior to delivery (O90.81)

● O99.1　Other diseases of the blood and blood-forming organs and certain disorders involving the immune mechanism complicating pregnancy, childbirth and the puerperium
Conditions in D65-D89

> **Excludes2**　hemorrhage with coagulation defects (O45.-, O46.0-, O67.0, O72.3)

● O99.11　Other diseases of the blood and blood-forming organs and certain disorders involving the immune mechanism complicating pregnancy

O99.111　Other diseases of the blood and blood-forming organs and certain disorders involving the immune mechanism complicating pregnancy, first trimester ♀　　M

O99.112　Other diseases of the blood and blood-forming organs and certain disorders involving the immune mechanism complicating pregnancy, second trimester ♀　　M

O99.113　Other diseases of the blood and blood-forming organs and certain disorders involving the immune mechanism complicating pregnancy, third trimester ♀　　M

O99.119　Other diseases of the blood and blood-forming organs and certain disorders involving the immune mechanism complicating pregnancy, unspecified trimester ♀　　M

O99.12　Other diseases of the blood and blood-forming organs and certain disorders involving the immune mechanism complicating childbirth ♀　　M

O99.13　Other diseases of the blood and blood-forming organs and certain disorders involving the immune mechanism complicating the puerperium ♀　　M

● O99.2　Endocrine, nutritional and metabolic diseases complicating pregnancy, childbirth and the puerperium
Conditions in E00-E88

> **Excludes2**　diabetes mellitus (O24.-)
> malnutrition (O25.-)
> postpartum thyroiditis (O90.5)

● O99.21　Obesity complicating pregnancy, childbirth, and the puerperium

> Use additional code to identify the type of obesity (E66.-)

O99.210　Obesity complicating pregnancy, unspecified trimester ♀　　M

O99.211　Obesity complicating pregnancy, first trimester ♀　　M

O99.212　Obesity complicating pregnancy, second trimester ♀　　M

O99.213　Obesity complicating pregnancy, third trimester ♀　　M

O99.214　Obesity complicating childbirth ♀　　M

O99.215　Obesity complicating the puerperium ♀　　M

● O99.28　Other endocrine, nutritional and metabolic diseases complicating pregnancy, childbirth and the puerperium

O99.280　Endocrine, nutritional and metabolic diseases complicating pregnancy, unspecified trimester ♀　　M

O99.281　Endocrine, nutritional and metabolic diseases complicating pregnancy, first trimester ♀　　M

O99.282　Endocrine, nutritional and metabolic diseases complicating pregnancy, second trimester ♀　　M

O99.283　Endocrine, nutritional and metabolic diseases complicating pregnancy, third trimester ♀　　M

O99.284　Endocrine, nutritional and metabolic diseases complicating childbirth ♀　M

O99.285　Endocrine, nutritional and metabolic diseases complicating the puerperium ♀　　M

● O99.3　Mental disorders and diseases of the nervous system complicating pregnancy, childbirth and the puerperium

● O99.31　Alcohol use complicating pregnancy, childbirth, and the puerperium

> Use additional code(s) from F10 to identify manifestations of the alcohol use

O99.310　Alcohol use complicating pregnancy, unspecified trimester ♀　　M

O99.311　Alcohol use complicating pregnancy, first trimester ♀　　M

O99.312　Alcohol use complicating pregnancy, second trimester ♀　　M

O99.313　Alcohol use complicating pregnancy, third trimester ♀　　M

O99.314　Alcohol use complicating childbirth ♀　　M

O99.315　Alcohol use complicating the puerperium ♀　　M

● O99.32　Drug use complicating pregnancy, childbirth, and the puerperium

> Use additional code(s) from F11-F16 and F18-F19 to identify manifestations of the drug use

O99.320　Drug use complicating pregnancy, unspecified trimester ♀　　M

O99.321　Drug use complicating pregnancy, first trimester ♀　　M

O99.322　Drug use complicating pregnancy, second trimester ♀　　M

O99.323　Drug use complicating pregnancy, third trimester ♀　　M

O99.324　Drug use complicating childbirth ♀　M

O99.325　Drug use complicating the puerperium ♀　　M

● O99.33　Smoking (tobacco) complicating pregnancy, childbirth, and the puerperium

> Use additional code from F17 to identify type of tobacco

O99.330　Smoking (tobacco) complicating pregnancy, unspecified trimester ♀　M

O99.331　Smoking (tobacco) complicating pregnancy, first trimester ♀　　M

O99.332　Smoking (tobacco) complicating pregnancy, second trimester ♀　　M

O99.333　Smoking (tobacco) complicating pregnancy, third trimester ♀　　M

O99.334　Smoking (tobacco) complicating childbirth ♀　　M

O99.335　Smoking (tobacco) complicating the puerperium ♀　　M

◄ New　◄▬ Revised　d̶e̶l̶e̶t̶e̶d̶ Deleted　Excludes 1　Excludes 2　Includes　Use additional　Code first　Code also　Unspecified
OGCR Official Guidelines　X Assign placeholder X　● Use Additional Character(s)　▶ Manifestation Code　Coding Clinic

● **O99.34   Other mental disorders complicating pregnancy, childbirth, and the puerperium**
Conditions in F01-F09 and F20-F99

> **Excludes2**   postpartum mood disturbance (O90.6)
> postnatal psychosis (F53)
> puerperal psychosis (F53)

O99.340   Other mental disorders complicating pregnancy, unspecified trimester ♀   **M**

O99.341   Other mental disorders complicating pregnancy, first trimester ♀   **M**

O99.342   Other mental disorders complicating pregnancy, second trimester ♀   **M**

O99.343   Other mental disorders complicating pregnancy, third trimester ♀   **M**

O99.344   Other mental disorders complicating childbirth ♀   **M**

O99.345   Other mental disorders complicating the puerperium ♀   **M**

● **O99.35   Diseases of the nervous system complicating pregnancy, childbirth, and the puerperium**
Conditions in G00-G99

> **Excludes2**   pregnancy related peripheral neuritis (O26.8-)

O99.350   Diseases of the nervous system complicating pregnancy, unspecified trimester ♀   **M**

O99.351   Diseases of the nervous system complicating pregnancy, first trimester ♀   **M**

O99.352   Diseases of the nervous system complicating pregnancy, second trimester ♀   **M**

O99.353   Diseases of the nervous system complicating pregnancy, third trimester ♀   **M**

O99.354   Diseases of the nervous system complicating childbirth ♀   **M**

O99.355   Diseases of the nervous system complicating the puerperium ♀   **M**

● **O99.4   Diseases of the circulatory system complicating pregnancy, childbirth and the puerperium**
Conditions in I00-I99

> **Excludes1**   peripartum cardiomyopathy (O90.3)
> **Excludes2**   hypertensive disorders (O10-O16)
> obstetric embolism (O88.-)
> venous complications and cerebrovenous sinus thrombosis in labor, childbirth and the puerperium (O87.-)
> venous complications and cerebrovenous sinus thrombosis in pregnancy (O22.-)

● **O99.41   Diseases of the circulatory system complicating pregnancy**

O99.411   Diseases of the circulatory system complicating pregnancy, first trimester ♀   **M**

O99.412   Diseases of the circulatory system complicating pregnancy, second trimester ♀   **M**

O99.413   Diseases of the circulatory system complicating pregnancy, third trimester ♀   **M**

O99.419   Diseases of the circulatory system complicating pregnancy, unspecified trimester ♀   **M**

O99.42   Diseases of the circulatory system complicating childbirth ♀   **M**

O99.43   Diseases of the circulatory system complicating the puerperium ♀   **M**

● **O99.5   Diseases of the respiratory system complicating pregnancy, childbirth and the puerperium**
Conditions in J00-J99

● **O99.51   Diseases of the respiratory system complicating pregnancy**

O99.511   Diseases of the respiratory system complicating pregnancy, first trimester ♀   **M**

O99.512   Diseases of the respiratory system complicating pregnancy, second trimester ♀   **M**

O99.513   Diseases of the respiratory system complicating pregnancy, third trimester ♀   **M**

O99.519   Diseases of the respiratory system complicating pregnancy, unspecified trimester ♀   **M**

O99.52   Diseases of the respiratory system complicating childbirth ♀   **M**

O99.53   Diseases of the respiratory system complicating the puerperium ♀   **M**

● **O99.6   Diseases of the digestive system complicating pregnancy, childbirth and the puerperium**
Conditions in K00-K93

> **Excludes2**   liver and biliary tract disorders in pregnancy, childbirth and the puerperium (O26.6-)

● **O99.61   Diseases of the digestive system complicating pregnancy**

O99.611   Diseases of the digestive system complicating pregnancy, first trimester ♀   **M**

O99.612   Diseases of the digestive system complicating pregnancy, second trimester ♀   **M**

O99.613   Diseases of the digestive system complicating pregnancy, third trimester ♀   **M**

O99.619   Diseases of the digestive system complicating pregnancy, unspecified trimester ♀   **M**

O99.62   Diseases of the digestive system complicating childbirth ♀   **M**

O99.63   Diseases of the digestive system complicating the puerperium ♀   **M**

● **O99.7   Diseases of the skin and subcutaneous tissue complicating pregnancy, childbirth and the puerperium**
Conditions in L00-L99

> **Excludes2**   herpes gestationis (O26.4)
> pruritic urticarial papules and plaques of pregnancy (PUPPP) (O26.86)

● **O99.71   Diseases of the skin and subcutaneous tissue complicating pregnancy**

O99.711   Diseases of the skin and subcutaneous tissue complicating pregnancy, first trimester ♀   **M**

O99.712   Diseases of the skin and subcutaneous tissue complicating pregnancy, second trimester ♀   **M**

O99.713   Diseases of the skin and subcutaneous tissue complicating pregnancy, third trimester ♀   **M**

O99.719   Diseases of the skin and subcutaneous tissue complicating pregnancy, unspecified trimester ♀   **M**

O99.72   Diseases of the skin and subcutaneous tissue complicating childbirth ♀   **M**

O99.73   Diseases of the skin and subcutaneous tissue complicating the puerperium ♀   **M**

CHAPTER 15 (O00-O9A)

● **O99.8** **Other specified diseases and conditions complicating pregnancy, childbirth and the puerperium**
Conditions in D00-D48, H00-H95, M00-N99, and Q00-Q99
Use additional code to identify condition
Excludes2 genitourinary infections in pregnancy (O23.-)
infection of genitourinary tract following delivery (O86.1-O86.3)
malignant neoplasm complicating pregnancy, childbirth and the puerperium (O9A.1-)
maternal care for known or suspected abnormality of maternal pelvic organs (O34.-)
postpartum acute kidney failure (O90.4)
traumatic injuries in pregnancy (O9A.2-)

● **O99.81** **Abnormal glucose complicating pregnancy, childbirth and the puerperium**
Excludes1 gestational diabetes (O24.4-)

    O99.810 **Abnormal glucose complicating pregnancy** ♀   **M**

    O99.814 **Abnormal glucose complicating childbirth** ♀   **M**

    O99.815 **Abnormal glucose complicating the puerperium** ♀   **M**

● **O99.82** **Streptococcus B carrier state complicating pregnancy, childbirth and the puerperium**

    O99.820 **Streptococcus B carrier state complicating pregnancy** ♀   **M**

    O99.824 **Streptococcus B carrier state complicating childbirth** ♀   **M**

    O99.825 **Streptococcus B carrier state complicating the puerperium** ♀   **M**

● **O99.83** **Other infection carrier state complicating pregnancy, childbirth and the puerperium**
Use additional code to identify the carrier state (Z22.-)

    O99.830 **Other infection carrier state complicating pregnancy** ♀   **M**

    O99.834 **Other infection carrier state complicating childbirth** ♀   **M**

    O99.835 **Other infection carrier state complicating the puerperium** ♀   **M**

● **O99.84** **Bariatric surgery status complicating pregnancy, childbirth and the puerperium**
Gastric banding status complicating pregnancy, childbirth and the puerperium
Gastric bypass status for obesity complicating pregnancy, childbirth and the puerperium
Obesity surgery status complicating pregnancy, childbirth and the puerperium

    O99.840 **Bariatric surgery status complicating pregnancy, unspecified trimester** ♀ **M**

    O99.841 **Bariatric surgery status complicating pregnancy, first trimester** ♀   **M**

    O99.842 **Bariatric surgery status complicating pregnancy, second trimester** ♀   **M**

    O99.843 **Bariatric surgery status complicating pregnancy, third trimester** ♀   **M**

    O99.844 **Bariatric surgery status complicating childbirth** ♀   **M**

    O99.845 **Bariatric surgery status complicating the puerperium** ♀   **M**

  O99.89 **Other specified diseases and conditions complicating pregnancy, childbirth and the puerperium** ♀   **M**

● **O9A** **Maternal malignant neoplasms, traumatic injuries and abuse classifiable elsewhere but complicating pregnancy, childbirth and the puerperium**

● **O9A.1** **Malignant neoplasm complicating pregnancy, childbirth and the puerperium**
Conditions in C00-C96
Use additional code to identify neoplasm
Excludes2 maternal care for benign tumor of corpus uteri (O34.1-)
maternal care for benign tumor of cervix (O34.4-)

● **O9A.11** **Malignant neoplasm complicating pregnancy**

    O9A.111 **Malignant neoplasm complicating pregnancy, first trimester** ♀   **M**

    O9A.112 **Malignant neoplasm complicating pregnancy, second trimester** ♀   **M**

    O9A.113 **Malignant neoplasm complicating pregnancy, third trimester** ♀   **M**

    O9A.119 **Malignant neoplasm complicating pregnancy, unspecified trimester** ♀ **M**

  O9A.12 **Malignant neoplasm complicating childbirth** ♀   **M**

  O9A.13 **Malignant neoplasm complicating the puerperium** ♀   **M**

● **O9A.2** **Injury, poisoning and certain other consequences of external causes complicating pregnancy, childbirth and the puerperium**
Conditions in S00-T88, except T74 and T76
Use additional code(s) to identify the injury or poisoning
Excludes2 physical, sexual and psychological abuse complicating pregnancy, childbirth and the puerperium (O9A.3-, O9A.4-, O9A.5-)

● **O9A.21** **Injury, poisoning and certain other consequences of external causes complicating pregnancy**

    O9A.211 **Injury, poisoning and certain other consequences of external causes complicating pregnancy, first trimester** ♀   **M**

    O9A.212 **Injury, poisoning and certain other consequences of external causes complicating pregnancy, second trimester** ♀   **M**

    O9A.213 **Injury, poisoning and certain other consequences of external causes complicating pregnancy, third trimester** ♀   **M**

    O9A.219 **Injury, poisoning and certain other consequences of external causes complicating pregnancy, unspecified trimester** ♀   **M**

  O9A.22 **Injury, poisoning and certain other consequences of external causes complicating childbirth** ♀   **M**

  O9A.23 **Injury, poisoning and certain other consequences of external causes complicating the puerperium** ♀   **M**

◀ New   ◀ Revised   ~~deleted~~ Deleted   Excludes 1   Excludes 2   Includes   Use additional   Code first   Code also   Unspecified
OGCR Official Guidelines   X Assign placeholder X   ● Use Additional Character(s)   ▶ Manifestation Code   **Coding Clinic**

● **O9A.3　Physical abuse complicating pregnancy, childbirth and the puerperium**
　　　Conditions in T74.11 or T76.11
　　　Use additional code (if applicable):
　　　　to identify any associated current injury due to physical abuse
　　　　to identify the perpetrator of abuse (Y07.-)
　　　Excludes2　sexual abuse complicating pregnancy, childbirth and the puerperium (O9A.4)

　● **O9A.31　Physical abuse complicating pregnancy**
　　　　O9A.311　Physical abuse complicating pregnancy, first trimester ♀　　**M**
　　　　O9A.312　Physical abuse complicating pregnancy, second trimester ♀　　**M**
　　　　O9A.313　Physical abuse complicating pregnancy, third trimester ♀　　**M**
　　　　O9A.319　Physical abuse complicating pregnancy, unspecified trimester ♀　**M**
　　O9A.32　Physical abuse complicating childbirth ♀　　**M**
　　O9A.33　Physical abuse complicating the puerperium ♀　　**M**

● **O9A.4　Sexual abuse complicating pregnancy, childbirth and the puerperium**
　　　Conditions in T74.21 or T76.21
　　　Use additional code (if applicable):
　　　　to identify any associated current injury due to sexual abuse
　　　　to identify the perpetrator of abuse (Y07.-)

　● **O9A.41　Sexual abuse complicating pregnancy**
　　　　O9A.411　Sexual abuse complicating pregnancy, first trimester ♀　　**M**
　　　　O9A.412　Sexual abuse complicating pregnancy, second trimester ♀　　**M**
　　　　O9A.413　Sexual abuse complicating pregnancy, third trimester ♀　　**M**
　　　　O9A.419　Sexual abuse complicating pregnancy, unspecified trimester ♀　**M**
　　O9A.42　Sexual abuse complicating childbirth ♀　　**M**
　　O9A.43　Sexual abuse complicating the puerperium ♀　**M**

● **O9A.5　Psychological abuse complicating pregnancy, childbirth and the puerperium**
　　　Conditions in T74.31 or T76.31
　　　Use additional code to identify the perpetrator of abuse (Y07.-)

　● **O9A.51　Psychological abuse complicating pregnancy**
　　　　O9A.511　Psychological abuse complicating pregnancy, first trimester ♀　　**M**
　　　　O9A.512　Psychological abuse complicating pregnancy, second trimester ♀　　**M**
　　　　O9A.513　Psychological abuse complicating pregnancy, third trimester ♀　　**M**
　　　　O9A.519　Psychological abuse complicating pregnancy, unspecified trimester ♀　**M**
　　O9A.52　Psychological abuse complicating childbirth ♀**M**
　　O9A.53　Psychological abuse complicating the puerperium ♀　　**M**

OGCR See Section I.C., Chapter 16
Newborn (Perinatal) Guidelines

CHAPTER 16

CERTAIN CONDITIONS ORIGINATING IN THE PERINATAL PERIOD (P00-P96)

Note: Codes from this chapter are for use on newborn records only, never on maternal records.

Includes   conditions that have their origin in the fetal or perinatal period (before birth through the first 28 days after birth) even if morbidity occurs later

Excludes2   congenital malformations, deformations and chromosomal abnormalities (Q00-Q99)
endocrine, nutritional and metabolic diseases (E00-E88)
injury, poisoning and certain other consequences of external causes (S00-T88)
neoplasms (C00-D49)
tetanus neonatorum (A33)

This chapter contains the following blocks:

P00-P04	Newborn affected by maternal factors and by complications of pregnancy, labor, and delivery
P05-P08	Disorders of newborns related to length of gestation and fetal growth
P09	Abnormal findings on neonatal screening
P10-P15	Birth trauma
P19-P29	Respiratory and cardiovascular disorders specific to the perinatal period
P35-P39	Infections specific to the perinatal period
P50-P61	Hemorrhagic and hematological disorders of newborn
P70-P74	Transitory endocrine and metabolic disorders specific to newborn
P76-P78	Digestive system disorders of newborn
P80-P83	Conditions involving the integument and temperature regulation of newborn
P84	Other problems with newborn
P90-P96	Other disorders originating in the perinatal period

NEWBORN AFFECTED BY MATERNAL FACTORS AND BY COMPLICATIONS OF PREGNANCY, LABOR, AND DELIVERY (P00–P04)

Note: These codes are for use when the listed maternal conditions are specified as the cause of confirmed morbidity or potential morbidity which have their origin in the perinatal period (before birth through the first 28 days after birth). Codes from these categories are also for use for newborns who are suspected of having an abnormal condition resulting from exposure from the mother or the birth process, but without signs or symptoms, and, which after examination and observation, is found not to exist. These codes may be used even if treatment is begun for a suspected condition that is ruled out.

● **P00**   **Newborn (suspected to be) affected by maternal conditions that may be unrelated to present pregnancy**

Code first any current condition in newborn

     Excludes2   newborn (suspected to be) affected by maternal complications of pregnancy (P01.-)
newborn affected by maternal endocrine and metabolic disorders (P70–P74)
newborn affected by noxious substances transmitted via placenta or breast milk (P04.-)

P00.0   **Newborn (suspected to be) affected by maternal hypertensive disorders**   N
Newborn (suspected to be) affected by maternal conditions classifiable to O10-O11, O13-O16

P00.1   **Newborn (suspected to be) affected by maternal renal and urinary tract diseases**   N
Newborn (suspected to be) affected by maternal conditions classifiable to N00-N39

P00.2   **Newborn (suspected to be) affected by maternal infectious and parasitic diseases**   N
Newborn (suspected to be) affected by maternal infectious disease classifiable to A00-B99, J09 and J10

     Excludes1   infections specific to the perinatal period (P35-P39)
maternal genital tract or other localized infections (P00.8)

P00.3   **Newborn (suspected to be) affected by other maternal circulatory and respiratory diseases**   N
Newborn (suspected to be) affected by maternal conditions classifiable to I00-I99, J00-J99, Q20-Q34 and not included in P00.0, P00.2

P00.4   **Newborn (suspected to be) affected by maternal nutritional disorders**   N
Newborn (suspected to be) affected by maternal disorders classifiable to E40-E64
Maternal malnutrition NOS

P00.5   **Newborn (suspected to be) affected by maternal injury**   N
Newborn (suspected to be) affected by maternal conditions classifiable to O9A.2-

P00.6   **Newborn (suspected to be) affected by surgical procedure on mother**   N
Newborn (suspected to be) affected by amniocentesis

     Excludes1   Cesarean delivery for present delivery (P03.4)
damage to placenta from amniocentesis, cesarean delivery or surgical induction (P02.1)
previous surgery to uterus or pelvic organs (P03.89)

     Excludes2   newborn affected by complication of (fetal) intrauterine procedure (P96.5)

P00.7   **Newborn (suspected to be) affected by other medical procedures on mother, not elsewhere classified**   N
Newborn (suspected to be) affected by radiation to mother

     Excludes1   damage to placenta from amniocentesis, cesarean delivery or surgical induction (P02.1)
newborn affected by other complications of labor and delivery (P03.-)

● **P00.8**   **Newborn (suspected to be) affected by other maternal conditions**

P00.81   **Newborn (suspected to be) affected by periodontal disease in mother**   N

P00.89   **Newborn (suspected to be) affected by other maternal conditions**   N
Newborn (suspected to be) affected by conditions classifiable to T80-T88
Newborn (suspected to be) affected by maternal genital tract or other localized infections
Newborn (suspected to be) affected by maternal systemic lupus erythematosus

P00.9   **Newborn (suspected to be) affected by unspecified maternal condition**   N

● **P01**   **Newborn (suspected to be) affected by maternal complications of pregnancy**

Code first any current condition in newborn

P01.0   **Newborn (suspected to be) affected by incompetent cervix**   N

P01.1   **Newborn (suspected to be) affected by premature rupture of membranes**   N

P01.2   **Newborn (suspected to be) affected by oligohydramnios**   N

     Excludes1   oligohydramnios due to premature rupture of membranes (P01.1)

P01.3   **Newborn (suspected to be) affected by polyhydramnios**   N
Excess of amniotic fluid, usually > 2000 mL
Newborn (suspected to be) affected by hydramnios

P01.4 Newborn (suspected to be) affected by ectopic pregnancy N
 Newborn (suspected to be) affected by abdominal pregnancy

P01.5 Newborn (suspected to be) affected by multiple pregnancy N
 Newborn (suspected to be) affected by triplet (pregnancy)
 Newborn (suspected to be) affected by twin (pregnancy)

P01.6 Newborn (suspected to be) affected by maternal death N

P01.7 Newborn (suspected to be) affected by malpresentation before labor N
 Newborn (suspected to be) affected by breech presentation before labor
 Newborn (suspected to be) affected by external version before labor
 Newborn (suspected to be) affected by face presentation before labor
 Newborn (suspected to be) affected by transverse lie before labor
 Newborn (suspected to be) affected by unstable lie before labor

P01.8 Newborn (suspected to be) affected by other maternal complications of pregnancy N

P01.9 Newborn (suspected to be) affected by maternal complication of pregnancy, unspecified N

● **P02 Newborn (suspected to be) affected by complications of placenta, cord and membranes**
 Code first any current condition in newborn

P02.0 Newborn (suspected to be) affected by placenta previa N

P02.1 Newborn (suspected to be) affected by other forms of placental separation and hemorrhage N
 Newborn (suspected to be) affected by abruptio placenta
 Newborn (suspected to be) affected by accidental hemorrhage
 Newborn (suspected to be) affected by antepartum hemorrhage
 Newborn (suspected to be) affected by damage to placenta from amniocentesis, cesarean delivery or surgical induction
 Newborn (suspected to be) affected by maternal blood loss
 Newborn (suspected to be) affected by premature separation of placenta

● **P02.2 Newborn (suspected to be) affected by other and unspecified morphological and functional abnormalities of placenta**

 P02.20 Newborn (suspected to be) affected by unspecified morphological and functional abnormalities of placenta N

 P02.29 Newborn (suspected to be) affected by other morphological and functional abnormalities of placenta N
 Newborn (suspected to be) affected by placental dysfunction
 Newborn (suspected to be) affected by placental infarction
 Newborn (suspected to be) affected by placental insufficiency

P02.3 Newborn (suspected to be) affected by placental transfusion syndromes N
 Newborn (suspected to be) affected by placental and cord abnormalities resulting in twin-to-twin or other transplacental transfusion

P02.4 Newborn (suspected to be) affected by prolapsed cord N

P02.5 Newborn (suspected to be) affected by other compression of umbilical cord N
 Newborn (suspected to be) affected by umbilical cord (tightly) around neck
 Newborn (suspected to be) affected by entanglement of umbilical cord
 Newborn (suspected to be) affected by knot in umbilical cord

● **P02.6 Newborn (suspected to be) affected by other and unspecified conditions of umbilical cord**

 P02.60 Newborn (suspected to be) affected by unspecified conditions of umbilical cord N

 P02.69 Newborn (suspected to be) affected by other conditions of umbilical cord N
 Newborn (suspected to be) affected by short umbilical cord
 Newborn (suspected to be) affected by vasa previa

 Excludes1 newborn affected by single umbilical artery (Q27.0)

P02.7 Newborn (suspected to be) affected by chorioamnionitis N
 Inflammation of chorion and amnion
 Newborn (suspected to be) affected by amnionitis
 Newborn (suspected to be) affected by membranitis
 Newborn (suspected to be) affected by placentitis

P02.8 Newborn (suspected to be) affected by other abnormalities of membranes N

P02.9 Newborn (suspected to be) affected by abnormality of membranes, unspecified N

● **P03 Newborn (suspected to be) affected by other complications of labor and delivery**
 Code first any current condition in newborn

P03.0 Newborn (suspected to be) affected by breech delivery and extraction N

P03.1 Newborn (suspected to be) affected by other malpresentation, malposition and disproportion during labor and delivery N
 Newborn (suspected to be) affected by contracted pelvis
 Newborn (suspected to be) affected by conditions classifiable to O64-O66
 Newborn (suspected to be) affected by persistent occipitoposterior
 Newborn (suspected to be) affected by transverse lie

P03.2 Newborn (suspected to be) affected by forceps delivery N

P03.3 Newborn (suspected to be) affected by delivery by vacuum extractor [ventouse] N

P03.4 Newborn (suspected to be) affected by Cesarean delivery N

P03.5 Newborn (suspected to be) affected by precipitate delivery N
 Newborn (suspected to be) affected by rapid second stage

P03.6 Newborn (suspected to be) affected by abnormal uterine contractions N
 Newborn (suspected to be) affected by conditions classifiable to O62.-, except O62.3
 Newborn (suspected to be) affected by hypertonic labor
 Newborn (suspected to be) affected by uterine inertia

● **P03.8 Newborn (suspected to be) affected by other specified complications of labor and delivery**

 ● **P03.81 Newborn (suspected to be) affected by abnormality in fetal (intrauterine) heart rate or rhythm**

 Excludes1 neonatal cardiac dysrhythmia (P29.1-)

 P03.810 Newborn (suspected to be) affected by abnormality in fetal (intrauterine) heart rate or rhythm before the onset of labor N

 P03.811 Newborn (suspected to be) affected by abnormality in fetal (intrauterine) heart rate or rhythm during labor N

 P03.819 Newborn (suspected to be) affected by abnormality in fetal (intrauterine) heart rate or rhythm, unspecified as to time of onset N

 P03.82 Meconium passage during delivery N

 Excludes1 meconium aspiration (P24.00, P24.01)
 meconium staining (P96.83)

CHAPTER 16 (P00-P96)

P03.89   **Newborn (suspected to be) affected by other specified complications of labor and delivery**   N
Newborn (suspected to be) affected by abnormality of maternal soft tissues
Newborn (suspected to be) affected by conditions classifiable to O60-O75 and by procedures used in labor and delivery not included in P02.- and P03.0-P03.6
Newborn (suspected to be) affected by induction of labor

P03.9   **Newborn (suspected to be) affected by complication of labor and delivery, unspecified**   N

● **P04**   **Newborn (suspected to be) affected by noxious substances transmitted via placenta or breast milk**

   Includes   nonteratogenic effects of substances transmitted via placenta

   Excludes2   congenital malformations (Q00-Q99)
neonatal jaundice from excessive hemolysis due to drugs or toxins transmitted from mother (P58.4)
newborn in contact with and (suspected) exposures hazardous to health not transmitted via placenta or breast milk (Z77.-)

P04.0   **Newborn (suspected to be) affected by maternal anesthesia and analgesia in pregnancy, labor and delivery**   N
Newborn (suspected to be) affected by reactions and intoxications from maternal opiates and tranquilizers administered during labor and delivery

P04.1   **Newborn (suspected to be) affected by other maternal medication**   N
Newborn (suspected to be) affected by cancer chemotherapy
Newborn (suspected to be) affected by cytotoxic drugs

   Excludes1   dysmorphism due to warfarin (Q86.2)
fetal hydantoin syndrome (Q86.1)
maternal use of drugs of addiction (P04.4-)

P04.2   **Newborn (suspected to be) affected by maternal use of tobacco**   N
Newborn (suspected to be) affected by exposure in utero to tobacco smoke

   Excludes2   newborn exposure to environmental tobacco smoke (P96.81)

P04.3   **Newborn (suspected to be) affected by maternal use of alcohol**   N

   Excludes1   fetal alcohol syndrome (Q86.0)

● **P04.4**   **Newborn (suspected to be) affected by maternal use of drugs of addiction**

P04.41   **Newborn (suspected to be) affected by maternal use of cocaine**   N
'Crack baby'

P04.49   **Newborn (suspected to be) affected by maternal use of other drugs of addiction**   N

   Excludes2   newborn (suspected to be) affected by maternal anesthesia and analgesia (P04.0)
withdrawal symptoms from maternal use of drugs of addiction (P96.1)

P04.5   **Newborn (suspected to be) affected by maternal use of nutritional chemical substances**   N

P04.6   **Newborn (suspected to be) affected by maternal exposure to environmental chemical substances**   N

P04.8   **Newborn (suspected to be) affected by other maternal noxious substances**   N

P04.9   **Newborn (suspected to be) affected by maternal noxious substance, unspecified**   N

OGCR   Section I.C.16.d.

Prematurity and Fetal Growth Retardation

Providers utilize different criteria in determining prematurity. A code for prematurity should not be assigned unless it is documented. Assignment of codes in categories P05, Disorders of newborn related to slow fetal growth and fetal malnutrition, and P07, Disorders of newborn related to short gestation and low birth weight, not elsewhere classified, should be based on the recorded birth weight and estimated gestational age. Codes from category P05 should not be assigned with codes from category P07.

When both birth weight and gestational age are available, two codes from category P07 should be assigned, with the code for birth weight sequenced before the code for gestational age.

A code from P05 and codes from P07.2 and P07.3 may be used to specify weeks of gestation as documented by the provider in the record.

DISORDERS OF NEWBORN RELATED TO LENGTH OF GESTATION AND FETAL GROWTH (P05-P08)

● **P05**   **Disorders of newborn related to slow fetal growth and fetal malnutrition**

● **P05.0**   **Newborn light for gestational age**
Newborn light-for-dates

P05.00   **Newborn light for gestational age, unspecified weight**   N

P05.01   **Newborn light for gestational age, less than 500 grams**   N

P05.02   **Newborn light for gestational age, 500-749 grams**   N

P05.03   **Newborn light for gestational age, 750-999 grams**   N

P05.04   **Newborn light for gestational age, 1000-1249 grams**   N

P05.05   **Newborn light for gestational age, 1250-1499 grams**   N

P05.06   **Newborn light for gestational age, 1500-1749 grams**   N

P05.07   **Newborn light for gestational age, 1750-1999 grams**   N

P05.08   **Newborn light for gestational age, 2000-2499 grams**   N

● **P05.1**   **Newborn small for gestational age**
Newborn small-and-light-for-dates
Newborn small-for-dates

P05.10   **Newborn small for gestational age, unspecified weight**   N

P05.11   **Newborn small for gestational age, less than 500 grams**   N

P05.12   **Newborn small for gestational age, 500-749 grams**   N

P05.13   **Newborn small for gestational age, 750-999 grams**   N

P05.14   **Newborn small for gestational age, 1000-1249 grams**   N

P05.15   **Newborn small for gestational age, 1250-1499 grams**   N

P05.16   **Newborn small for gestational age, 1500-1749 grams**   N

P05.17   **Newborn small for gestational age, 1750-1999 grams**   N

P05.18   **Newborn small for gestational age, 2000-2499 grams**   N

◀ New   ◀◀◀ Revised   ~~deleted~~ Deleted   Excludes 1   Excludes 2   Includes   Use additional   Code first   Code also   Unspecified

OGCR Official Guidelines   **X** Assign placeholder X   ● Use Additional Character(s)   ▶ Manifestation Code   **Coding Clinic**

P05.2 **Newborn affected by fetal (intrauterine) malnutrition not light or small for gestational age**　　N

Infant, not light or small for gestational age, showing signs of fetal malnutrition, such as dry, peeling skin and loss of subcutaneous tissue

> **Excludes1** newborn affected by fetal malnutrition with light for gestational age (P05.0-)
> newborn affected by fetal malnutrition with small for gestational age (P05.1-)

P05.9 **Newborn affected by slow intrauterine growth, unspecified**　　N

Newborn affected by fetal growth retardation NOS

● **P07** **Disorders of newborn related to short gestation and low birth weight, not elsewhere classified**

Note: When both birth weight and gestational age of the newborn are available, both should be coded with birth weight sequenced before gestational age.

> **Includes** the listed conditions, without further specification, as the cause of morbidity or additional care, in newborn

> **Excludes1** low birth weight due to slow fetal growth and fetal malnutrition (P05.-)

● **P07.0** **Extremely low birth weight newborn**

Newborn birth weight 999 g. or less

P07.00 **Extremely low birth weight newborn, unspecified weight**　　N

P07.01 **Extremely low birth weight newborn, less than 500 grams**　　N

P07.02 **Extremely low birth weight newborn, 500-749 grams**　　N

P07.03 **Extremely low birth weight newborn, 750-999 grams**　　N

● **P07.1** **Other low birth weight newborn**

Newborn birth weight 1000-2499 g.

P07.10 **Other low birth weight newborn, unspecified weight**　　N

P07.14 **Other low birth weight newborn, 1000-1249 grams**　　N

P07.15 **Other low birth weight newborn, 1250-1499 grams**　　N

P07.16 **Other low birth weight newborn, 1500-1749 grams**　　N

P07.17 **Other low birth weight newborn, 1750-1999 grams**　　N

P07.18 **Other low birth weight newborn, 2000-2499 grams**　　N

● **P07.2** **Extreme immaturity of newborn**

Less than 28 completed weeks (less than 196 completed days) of gestation

P07.20 **Extreme immaturity of newborn, unspecified weeks of gestation**　　N

Gestational age less than 28 completed weeks NOS

P07.21 **Extreme immaturity of newborn, gestational age less than 23 completed weeks**　　N

Extreme immaturity of newborn, gestational age less than 23 weeks, 0 days

P07.22 **Extreme immaturity of newborn, gestational age 23 completed weeks**　　N

Extreme immaturity of newborn, gestational age 23 weeks, 0 days through 23 weeks, 6 days

P07.23 **Extreme immaturity of newborn, gestational age 24 completed weeks**　　N

Extreme immaturity of newborn, gestational age 24 weeks, 0 days through 24 weeks, 6 days

P07.24 **Extreme immaturity of newborn, gestational age 25 completed weeks**　　N

Extreme immaturity of newborn, gestational age 25 weeks, 0 days through 25 weeks, 6 days

P07.25 **Extreme immaturity of newborn, gestational age 26 completed weeks**　　N

Extreme immaturity of newborn, gestational age 26 weeks, 0 days through 26 weeks, 6 days

P07.26 **Extreme immaturity of newborn, gestational age 27 completed weeks**　　N

Extreme immaturity of newborn, gestational age 27 weeks, 0 days through 27 weeks, 6 days

● **P07.3** **Preterm [premature] newborn [other]**

28 completed weeks or more but less than 37 completed weeks (196 completed days but less than 259 completed days) of gestation

Prematurity NOS

P07.30 **Preterm newborn, unspecified weeks of gestation**　　N

P07.31 **Preterm newborn, gestational age 28 completed weeks**　　N

Preterm newborn, gestational age 28 weeks, 0 days through 28 weeks, 6 days

P07.32 **Preterm newborn, gestational age 29 completed weeks**　　N

Preterm newborn, gestational age 29 weeks, 0 days through 29 weeks, 6 days

P07.33 **Preterm newborn, gestational age 30 completed weeks**　　N

Preterm newborn, gestational age 30 weeks, 0 days through 30 weeks, 6 days

P07.34 **Preterm newborn, gestational age 31 completed weeks**　　N

Preterm newborn, gestational age 31 weeks, 0 days through 31 weeks, 6 days

P07.35 **Preterm newborn, gestational age 32 completed weeks**　　N

Preterm newborn, gestational age 32 weeks, 0 days through 32 weeks, 6 days

P07.36 **Preterm newborn, gestational age 33 completed weeks**　　N

Preterm newborn, gestational age 33 weeks, 0 days through 33 weeks, 6 days

P07.37 **Preterm newborn, gestational age 34 completed weeks**　　N

Preterm newborn, gestational age 34 weeks, 0 days through 34 weeks, 6 days

P07.38 **Preterm newborn, gestational age 35 completed weeks**　　N

Preterm newborn, gestational age 35 weeks, 0 days through 35 weeks, 6 days

P07.39 **Preterm newborn, gestational age 36 completed weeks**　　N

Preterm newborn, gestational age 36 weeks, 0 days through 36 weeks, 6 days

CHAPTER 16 (P00-P96)

CHAPTER 16 (P00-P96)

● **P08** **Disorders of newborn related to long gestation and high birth weight**

Note: When both birth weight and gestational age of the newborn are available, priority of assignment should be given to birth weight.

> **Includes** the listed conditions, without further specification, as causes of morbidity or additional care, in newborn

P08.0 **Exceptionally large newborn baby**   N
Usually implies a birth weight of 4500 g. or more

> **Excludes1** syndrome of infant of diabetic mother (P70.1)
> syndrome of infant of mother with gestational diabetes (P70.0)

P08.1 **Other heavy for gestational age newborn**   N
Other newborn heavy- or large-for-dates regardless of period of gestation
Usually implies a birth weight of 4000 g. to 4499 g.

> **Excludes1** newborn with a birth weight of 4500 or more (P08.0)
> syndrome of infant of diabetic mother (P70.1)
> syndrome of infant of mother with gestational diabetes (P70.0)

● **P08.2** **Late newborn, not heavy for gestational age**

P08.21 **Post-term newborn**   N
Newborn with gestation period over 40 completed weeks to 42 completed weeks

P08.22 **Prolonged gestation of newborn**   N
Newborn with gestation period over 42 completed weeks (294 days or more), not heavy- or large-for-dates
Postmaturity NOS

Item 16–1 The **peripheral nervous system** consists of 31 pairs of spinal nerves, 12 pairs of cranial nerves, and the autonomic nerves, which are divided into the parasympathetic and sympathetic nerves. The cranial nerves are: olfactory (I), optic (II), oculomotor (III), trochlear (IV), trigeminal (V), abducens (VI), facial (VII), vestibulocochlear (VIII), glossopharyngeal (IX), vagus (X), accessory (XI), and hypoglossal (XII).

ABNORMAL FINDINGS ON NEONATAL SCREENING (P09)

P09 **Abnormal findings on neonatal screening**   N
Use additional code to identify signs, symptoms and conditions associated with the screening

> **Excludes2** nonspecific serologic evidence of human immunodeficiency virus [HIV] (R75)

BIRTH TRAUMA (P10-P15)

● **P10** **Intracranial laceration and hemorrhage due to birth injury**

> **Excludes1** intracranial hemorrhage of newborn NOS (P52.9)
> intracranial hemorrhage of newborn due to anoxia or hypoxia (P52.-)
> nontraumatic intracranial hemorrhage of newborn (P52.-)

P10.0 **Subdural hemorrhage due to birth injury**   N
Subdural hematoma (localized) due to birth injury

> **Excludes1** subdural hemorrhage accompanying tentorial tear (P10.4)

P10.1 **Cerebral hemorrhage due to birth injury**   N
P10.2 **Intraventricular hemorrhage due to birth injury**   N
P10.3 **Subarachnoid hemorrhage due to birth injury**   N
P10.4 **Tentorial tear due to birth injury**   N
Pertaining to tentorium of cerebellum (extension of dura mater that separates cerebellum from inferior portion of occipital lobes)

P10.8 **Other intracranial lacerations and hemorrhages due to birth injury**   N
P10.9 **Unspecified intracranial laceration and hemorrhage due to birth injury**   N

● **P11** **Other birth injuries to central nervous system**
P11.0 **Cerebral edema due to birth injury**   N
P11.1 **Other specified brain damage due to birth injury**   N
P11.2 **Unspecified brain damage due to birth injury**   N
P11.3 **Birth injury to facial nerve**   N
Facial palsy due to birth injury
P11.4 **Birth injury to other cranial nerves**   N

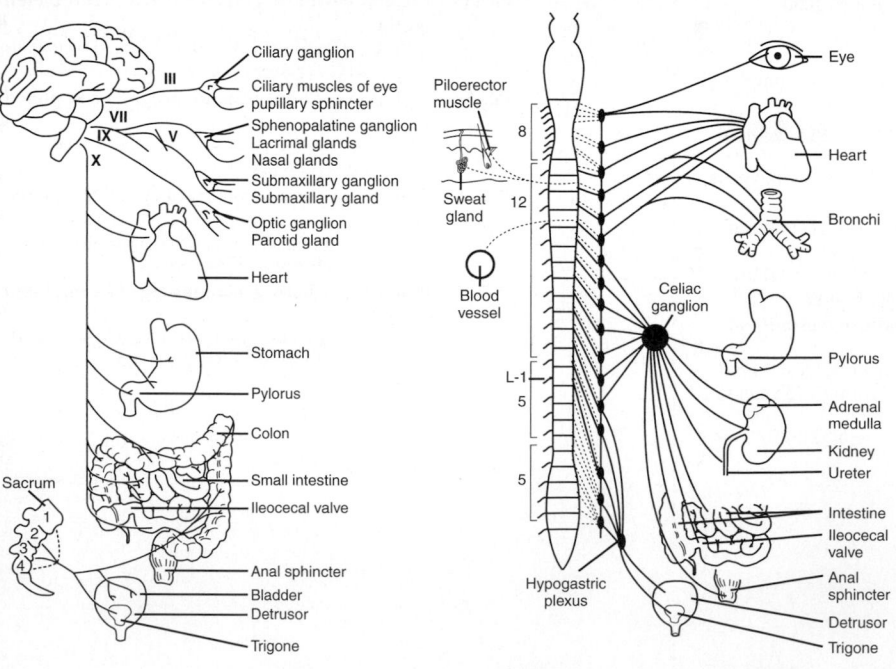

Figure 16-1 **A.** Parasympathetic nervous system. **B.** Sympathetic nervous system. (From Buck CJ: Step-by-Step Medical Coding, Philadelphia, WB Saunders, 1998)

◀ New   ◀▬ Revised   ~~deleted~~ Deleted   Excludes 1   Excludes 2   Includes   Use additional   Code first   Code also   Unspecified

OGCR Official Guidelines   **X** Assign placeholder X   ● Use Additional Character(s)   ▷ Manifestation Code   **Coding Clinic**

P11.5   **Birth injury to spine and spinal cord**   N
     Fracture of spine due to birth injury

P11.9   **Birth injury to central nervous system, unspecified**   N

● **P12**   **Birth injury to scalp**

P12.0   **Cephalhematoma due to birth injury**   N

P12.1   **Chignon (from vacuum extraction) due to birth injury**   N

P12.2   **Epicranial subaponeurotic hemorrhage due to birth injury**   N
     Subgaleal hemorrhage

P12.3   **Bruising of scalp due to birth injury**   N

P12.4   **Injury of scalp of newborn due to monitoring equipment**   N
     Sampling incision of scalp of newborn
     Scalp clip (electrode) injury of newborn

● P12.8   **Other birth injuries to scalp**

    P12.81   **Caput succedaneum**   N

    P12.89   **Other birth injuries to scalp**   N

P12.9   **Birth injury to scalp, unspecified**   N

● **P13**   **Birth injury to skeleton**

    Excludes2   birth injury to spine (P11.5)

P13.0   **Fracture of skull due to birth injury**   N

P13.1   **Other birth injuries to skull**   N
     Excludes1   cephalhematoma (P12.0)

P13.2   **Birth injury to femur**   N

P13.3   **Birth injury to other long bones**   N

P13.4   **Fracture of clavicle due to birth injury**   N

P13.8   **Birth injuries to other parts of skeleton**   N

P13.9   **Birth injury to skeleton, unspecified**   N

● **P14**   **Birth injury to peripheral nervous system**

P14.0   **Erb's paralysis due to birth injury**   N

P14.1   **Klumpke's paralysis due to birth injury**   N

P14.2   **Phrenic nerve paralysis due to birth injury**   N

P14.3   **Other brachial plexus birth injuries**   N

P14.8   **Birth injuries to other parts of peripheral nervous system**   N

P14.9   **Birth injury to peripheral nervous system, unspecified**   N

● **P15**   **Other birth injuries**

P15.0   **Birth injury to liver**   N
     Rupture of liver due to birth injury

P15.1   **Birth injury to spleen**   N
     Rupture of spleen due to birth injury

P15.2   **Sternomastoid injury due to birth injury**   N

P15.3   **Birth injury to eye**   N
     Subconjunctival hemorrhage due to birth injury
     Traumatic glaucoma due to birth injury

P15.4   **Birth injury to face**   N
     Facial congestion due to birth injury

P15.5   **Birth injury to external genitalia**   N

P15.6   **Subcutaneous fat necrosis due to birth injury**   N

P15.8   **Other specified birth injuries**   N

P15.9   **Birth injury, unspecified**   N

RESPIRATORY AND CARDIOVASCULAR DISORDERS SPECIFIC TO THE PERINATAL PERIOD (P19-P29)

● **P19**   **Metabolic acidemia in newborn**
    Includes   metabolic acidemia in newborn

P19.0   **Metabolic acidemia in newborn first noted before onset of labor**   N

P19.1   **Metabolic acidemia in newborn first noted during labor**   N

P19.2   **Metabolic acidemia noted at birth**   N

P19.9   **Metabolic acidemia, unspecified**   N

● **P22**   **Respiratory distress of newborn**
    Excludes1   respiratory arrest of newborn (P28.81)
             respiratory failure of newborn NOS (P28.5)

P22.0   **Respiratory distress syndrome of newborn**   N
     Cardiorespiratory distress syndrome of newborn
     Hyaline membrane disease
     Idiopathic respiratory distress syndrome [IRDS or RDS] of newborn
     Pulmonary hypoperfusion syndrome
     Respiratory distress syndrome, type I

P22.1   **Transient tachypnea of newborn**   N
     Idiopathic tachypnea of newborn
     Respiratory distress syndrome, type II
     Wet lung syndrome

P22.8   **Other respiratory distress of newborn**   N

P22.9   **Respiratory distress of newborn, unspecified**   N

● **P23**   **Congenital pneumonia**
    Includes   infective pneumonia acquired in utero or during birth
    Excludes1   neonatal pneumonia resulting from aspiration (P24.-)

P23.0   **Congenital pneumonia due to viral agent**   N
     Use additional code (B97) to identify organism
     Excludes1   congenital rubella pneumonitis (P35.0)

P23.1   **Congenital pneumonia due to Chlamydia**   N

P23.2   **Congenital pneumonia due to staphylococcus**   N

P23.3   **Congenital pneumonia due to streptococcus, group B**   N

P23.4   **Congenital pneumonia due to Escherichia coli**   N

P23.5   **Congenital pneumonia due to Pseudomonas**   N

P23.6   **Congenital pneumonia due to other bacterial agents**   N
     Congenital pneumonia due to Hemophilus influenzae
     Congenital pneumonia due to Klebsiella pneumoniae
     Congenital pneumonia due to Mycoplasma
     Congenital pneumonia due to Streptococcus, except group B
     Use additional code (B95-B96) to identify organism

P23.8   **Congenital pneumonia due to other organisms**   N

P23.9   **Congenital pneumonia, unspecified**   N

● **P24**   **Neonatal aspiration**
    Includes   aspiration in utero and during delivery

● P24.0   **Meconium aspiration**
    Excludes1   meconium passage (without aspiration) during delivery (P03.82)
            meconium staining (P96.83)

    P24.00   **Meconium aspiration without respiratory symptoms**   N
       Meconium aspiration NOS

    P24.01   **Meconium aspiration with respiratory symptoms**   N
       Meconium aspiration pneumonia
       Meconium aspiration pneumonitis
       Meconium aspiration syndrome NOS
       Use additional code to identify any secondary pulmonary hypertension, if applicable (I27.2)

● P24.1   **Neonatal aspiration of (clear) amniotic fluid and mucus**
     Neonatal aspiration of liquor (amnii)

    P24.10   **Neonatal aspiration of (clear) amniotic fluid and mucus without respiratory symptoms**   N
       Neonatal aspiration of amniotic fluid and mucus NOS

    P24.11   **Neonatal aspiration of (clear) amniotic fluid and mucus with respiratory symptoms**   N
       Neonatal aspiration of amniotic fluid and mucus with pneumonia
       Neonatal aspiration of amniotic fluid and mucus with pneumonitis
       Use additional code to identify any secondary pulmonary hypertension, if applicable (I27.2)

CHAPTER 16 (P00-P96)

● **P24.2** **Neonatal aspiration of blood**

P24.20 **Neonatal aspiration of blood without respiratory symptoms**   N
Neonatal aspiration of blood NOS

P24.21 **Neonatal aspiration of blood with respiratory symptoms**   N
Neonatal aspiration of blood with pneumonia
Neonatal aspiration of blood with pneumonitis
Use additional code to identify any secondary pulmonary hypertension, if applicable (I27.2)

● **P24.3** **Neonatal aspiration of milk and regurgitated food**
Neonatal aspiration of stomach contents

P24.30 **Neonatal aspiration of milk and regurgitated food without respiratory symptoms**   N
Neonatal aspiration of milk and regurgitated food NOS

P24.31 **Neonatal aspiration of milk and regurgitated food with respiratory symptoms**   N
Neonatal aspiration of milk and regurgitated food with pneumonia
Neonatal aspiration of milk and regurgitated food with pneumonitis
Use additional code to identify any secondary pulmonary hypertension, if applicable (I27.2)

● **P24.8** **Other neonatal aspiration**

P24.80 **Other neonatal aspiration without respiratory symptoms**   N
Neonatal aspiration NEC

P24.81 **Other neonatal aspiration with respiratory symptoms**   N
Neonatal aspiration pneumonia NEC
Neonatal aspiration with pneumonitis NEC
Neonatal aspiration with pneumonia NOS
Neonatal aspiration with pneumonitis NOS
Use additional code to identify any secondary pulmonary hypertension, if applicable (I27.2)

P24.9 **Neonatal aspiration, unspecified**   N

● **P25** **Interstitial emphysema and related conditions originating in the perinatal period**

P25.0 **Interstitial emphysema originating in the perinatal period**   N

P25.1 **Pneumothorax originating in the perinatal period**   N

P25.2 **Pneumomediastinum originating in the perinatal period**   N

P25.3 **Pneumopericardium originating in the perinatal period**   N

P25.8 **Other conditions related to interstitial emphysema originating in the perinatal period**   N

● **P26** **Pulmonary hemorrhage originating in the perinatal period**
Excludes1 acute idiopathic hemorrhage in infants over 28 days old (R04.81)

P26.0 **Tracheobronchial hemorrhage originating in the perinatal period**   N

P26.1 **Massive pulmonary hemorrhage originating in the perinatal period**   N

P26.8 **Other pulmonary hemorrhages originating in the perinatal period**   N

P26.9 **Unspecified pulmonary hemorrhage originating in the perinatal period**   N

● **P27** **Chronic respiratory disease originating in the perinatal period**
Excludes1 respiratory distress of newborn (P22.0-P22.9)

P27.0 **Wilson-Mikity syndrome**
Pulmonary dysmaturity

P27.1 **Bronchopulmonary dysplasia originating in the perinatal period**

P27.8 **Other chronic respiratory diseases originating in the perinatal period**
Congenital pulmonary fibrosis
Ventilator lung in newborn

P27.9 **Unspecified chronic respiratory disease originating in the perinatal period**

● **P28** **Other respiratory conditions originating in the perinatal period**
Excludes1 congenital malformations of the respiratory system (Q30-Q34)

P28.0 **Primary atelectasis of newborn**   N
Failure of lungs to expand properly at birth
Primary failure to expand terminal respiratory units
Pulmonary hypoplasia associated with short gestation
Pulmonary immaturity NOS

● **P28.1** **Other and unspecified atelectasis of newborn**

P28.10 **Unspecified atelectasis of newborn**   N
Atelectasis of newborn NOS

P28.11 **Resorption atelectasis without respiratory distress syndrome**   N
Excludes1 resorption atelectasis with respiratory distress syndrome (P22.0)

P28.19 **Other atelectasis of newborn**   N
Partial atelectasis of newborn
Secondary atelectasis of newborn

P28.2 **Cyanotic attacks of newborn**   N
Excludes1 apnea of newborn (P28.3-P28.4)

P28.3 **Primary sleep apnea of newborn**   N
Central sleep apnea of newborn
Obstructive sleep apnea of newborn
Sleep apnea of newborn NOS

P28.4 **Other apnea of newborn**   N
Apnea of prematurity
Obstructive apnea of newborn
Excludes1 obstructive sleep apnea of newborn (P28.3)

P28.5 **Respiratory failure of newborn**   N
Excludes1 respiratory arrest of newborn (P28.81)
respiratory distress of newborn (P22.0-)

● **P28.8** **Other specified respiratory conditions of newborn**

P28.81 **Respiratory arrest of newborn**   N

P28.89 **Other specified respiratory conditions of newborn**   N
Congenital laryngeal stridor
Sniffles in newborn
Snuffles in newborn
Excludes1 early congenital syphilitic rhinitis (A50.05)

P28.9 **Respiratory condition of newborn, unspecified**   N
Respiratory depression in newborn

● **P29** **Cardiovascular disorders originating in the perinatal period**
Excludes1 congenital malformations of the circulatory system (Q20-Q28)

P29.0 **Neonatal cardiac failure**   N

● **P29.1** **Neonatal cardiac dysrhythmia**

P29.11 **Neonatal tachycardia**   N
P29.12 **Neonatal bradycardia**   N

P29.2 **Neonatal hypertension**   N

P29.3 **Persistent fetal circulation**   N
Delayed closure of ductus arteriosus
(Persistent) pulmonary hypertension of newborn

P29.4 **Transient myocardial ischemia in newborn**   N

● **P29.8** **Other cardiovascular disorders originating in the perinatal period**

P29.81 **Cardiac arrest of newborn**   N

P29.89 **Other cardiovascular disorders originating in the perinatal period**   N

P29.9 **Cardiovascular disorder originating in the perinatal period, unspecified**   N

◀ New   ◀━ Revised   d̶e̶l̶e̶t̶e̶d̶ Deleted   Excludes 1   Excludes 2   Includes   Use additional   Code first   Code also   Unspecified
OGCR Official Guidelines   X Assign placeholder X   ● Use Additional Character(s)   ▌ Manifestation Code   **Coding Clinic**

CHAPTER 16 (P00-P96)

INFECTIONS SPECIFIC TO THE PERINATAL PERIOD (P35-P39)

Infections acquired in utero, during birth via the umbilicus, or during the first 28 days after birth

> **Excludes2**   asymptomatic human immunodeficiency virus [HIV] infection status (Z21)
> congenital gonococcal infection (A54.-)
> congenital pneumonia (P23.-)
> congenital syphilis (A50.-)
> human immunodeficiency virus [HIV] disease (B20)
> infant botulism (A48.51)
> infectious diseases not specific to the perinatal period (A00-B99, J09, J10.-)
> intestinal infectious disease (A00-A09)
> laboratory evidence of human immunodeficiency virus [HIV] (R75)
> tetanus neonatorum (A33)

● **P35   Congenital viral diseases**
> **Includes**   infections acquired in utero or during birth

P35.0   Congenital rubella syndrome   N
> Congenital rubella pneumonitis

P35.1   Congenital cytomegalovirus infection   N
> *Viruses transmitted by multiple routes that cause mild/ subclinical infection*

P35.2   Congenital herpesviral [herpes simplex] infection   N

P35.3   Congenital viral hepatitis   N

P35.8   Other congenital viral diseases   N
> Congenital varicella [chickenpox]

P35.9   Congenital viral disease, unspecified   N

● **P36   Bacterial sepsis of newborn**
> **Includes**   congenital sepsis

> Use additional code(s), if applicable, to identify severe sepsis (R65.2-) and associated acute organ dysfunction(s)

P36.0   Sepsis of newborn due to streptococcus, group B   N

● **P36.1   Sepsis of newborn due to other and unspecified streptococci**

    P36.10   Sepsis of newborn due to unspecified streptococci   N

    P36.19   Sepsis of newborn due to other streptococci   N

P36.2   Sepsis of newborn due to Staphylococcus aureus   N

● **P36.3   Sepsis of newborn due to other and unspecified staphylococci**

    P36.30   Sepsis of newborn due to unspecified staphylococci   N

    P36.39   Sepsis of newborn due to other staphylococci   N

P36.4   Sepsis of newborn due to Escherichia coli   N

P36.5   Sepsis of newborn due to anaerobes   N

P36.8   Other bacterial sepsis of newborn   N
> Use additional code from category B96 to identify organism

P36.9   Bacterial sepsis of newborn, unspecified   N

● **P37   Other congenital infectious and parasitic diseases**
> **Excludes2**   congenital syphilis (A50.-)
> infectious neonatal diarrhea (A00-A09)
> necrotizing enterocolitis in newborn (P77.-)
> noninfectious neonatal diarrhea (P78.3)
> ophthalmia neonatorum due to gonococcus (A54.31)
> tetanus neonatorum (A33)

P37.0   Congenital tuberculosis   N

P37.1   Congenital toxoplasmosis   N
> *Parasitic infection, often causing mild flu-like illness*
> Hydrocephalus due to congenital toxoplasmosis

P37.2   Neonatal (disseminated) listeriosis   N
> *Acquired transplacentally or during/after parturition in which symptoms are those of sepsis*

P37.3   Congenital falciparum malaria   N

P37.4   Other congenital malaria   N

P37.5   Neonatal candidiasis   N

P37.8   Other specified congenital infectious and parasitic diseases   N

P37.9   Congenital infectious or parasitic disease, unspecified   N

● **P38   Omphalitis of newborn**
> *Inflammation of umbilicus*
> **Excludes1**   omphalitis not of newborn (L08.82)
> tetanus omphalitis (A33)
> umbilical hemorrhage of newborn (P51.-)

P38.1   Omphalitis with mild hemorrhage   N

P38.9   Omphalitis without hemorrhage   N
> Omphalitis of newborn NOS

● **P39   Other infections specific to the perinatal period**
> Use additional code to identify organism or specific infection

P39.0   Neonatal infective mastitis   N
> **Excludes1**   breast engorgement of newborn (P83.4)
> noninfective mastitis of newborn (P83.4)

P39.1   Neonatal conjunctivitis and dacryocystitis   N
> Neonatal chlamydial conjunctivitis
> Ophthalmia neonatorum NOS
> *Neonate = newborn*
> **Excludes1**   gonococcal conjunctivitis (A54.31)

P39.2   Intra-amniotic infection affecting newborn, not elsewhere classified   N

P39.3   Neonatal urinary tract infection   N

P39.4   Neonatal skin infection   N
> Neonatal pyoderma
> **Excludes1**   pemphigus neonatorum (L00)
> staphylococcal scalded skin syndrome (L00)

P39.8   Other specified infections specific to the perinatal period   N

P39.9   Infection specific to the perinatal period, unspecified   N

HEMORRHAGIC AND HEMATOLOGICAL DISORDERS OF NEWBORN (P50-P61)

> **Excludes1**   congenital stenosis and stricture of bile ducts (Q44.3)
> Crigler-Najjar syndrome (E80.5)
> Dubin-Johnson syndrome (E80.6)
> Gilbert syndrome (E80.4)
> hereditary hemolytic anemias (D55-D58)

● **P50   Newborn affected by intrauterine (fetal) blood loss**
> **Excludes1**   congenital anemia from intrauterine (fetal) blood loss (P61.3)

P50.0   Newborn affected by intrauterine (fetal) blood loss from vasa previa   N

P50.1   Newborn affected by intrauterine (fetal) blood loss from ruptured cord   N

P50.2   Newborn affected by intrauterine (fetal) blood loss from placenta   N

P50.3   Newborn affected by hemorrhage into co-twin   N

P50.4   Newborn affected by hemorrhage into maternal circulation   N

P50.5   Newborn affected by intrauterine (fetal) blood loss from cut end of co-twin's cord   N

P50.8   Newborn affected by other intrauterine (fetal) blood loss   N

P50.9   Newborn affected by intrauterine (fetal) blood loss, unspecified   N
> Newborn affected by fetal hemorrhage NOS

CHAPTER 16 (P00-P96)

● **P51   Umbilical hemorrhage of newborn**

> **Excludes1**   omphalitis with mild hemorrhage (P38.1)
> umbilical hemorrhage from cut end of co-twins
> cord (P50.5)

     P51.0   Massive umbilical hemorrhage of newborn   N

     P51.8   Other umbilical hemorrhages of newborn   N
          Slipped umbilical ligature NOS

     P51.9   Umbilical hemorrhage of newborn, unspecified   N

● **P52   Intracranial nontraumatic hemorrhage of newborn**

> **Includes**   intracranial hemorrhage due to anoxia or hypoxia
>
> **Excludes1**   intracranial hemorrhage due to birth injury
> (P10.-)
> intracranial hemorrhage due to other injury
> (S06.-)

     P52.0   Intraventricular (nontraumatic) hemorrhage, grade 1, of newborn   N
          Subependymal hemorrhage (without intraventricular extension)
          Bleeding into germinal matrix

     P52.1   Intraventricular (nontraumatic) hemorrhage, grade 2, of newborn   N
          Subependymal hemorrhage with intraventricular extension
          Bleeding into ventricle

   ● **P52.2   Intraventricular (nontraumatic) hemorrhage, grade 3 and grade 4, of newborn**

          P52.21   Intraventricular (nontraumatic) hemorrhage, grade 3, of newborn   N
                 Subependymal hemorrhage with intraventricular extension with enlargement of ventricle

          P52.22   Intraventricular (nontraumatic) hemorrhage, grade 4, of newborn   N
                 Bleeding into cerebral cortex
                 Subependymal hemorrhage with intracerebral extension

     P52.3   Unspecified intraventricular (nontraumatic) hemorrhage of newborn   N

     P52.4   Intracerebral (nontraumatic) hemorrhage of newborn   N

     P52.5   Subarachnoid (nontraumatic) hemorrhage of newborn   N

     P52.6   Cerebellar (nontraumatic) and posterior fossa hemorrhage of newborn   N

     P52.8   Other intracranial (nontraumatic) hemorrhages of newborn   N

     P52.9   Intracranial (nontraumatic) hemorrhage of newborn, unspecified   N

   P53   Hemorrhagic disease of newborn   N
       Vitamin K deficiency of newborn

● **P54   Other neonatal hemorrhages**

> **Excludes1**   newborn affected by (intrauterine) blood loss
> (P50.-)
> pulmonary hemorrhage originating in the
> perinatal period (P26.-)

     P54.0   Neonatal hematemesis   N
          Vomiting of blood

> > **Excludes1**   neonatal hematemesis due to swallowed
> > maternal blood (P78.2)

     P54.1   Neonatal melena   N
          Dark-colored feces stained with blood pigments

> > **Excludes1**   neonatal melena due to swallowed
> > maternal blood (P78.2)

     P54.2   Neonatal rectal hemorrhage   N

     P54.3   Other neonatal gastrointestinal hemorrhage   N

     P54.4   Neonatal adrenal hemorrhage   N

     P54.5   Neonatal cutaneous hemorrhage   N
          Neonatal bruising
          Neonatal ecchymoses
          Neonatal petechiae
          Neonatal superficial hematomata

> > **Excludes2**   bruising of scalp due to birth injury
> > (P12.3)
> > cephalhematoma due to birth injury
> > (P12.0)

     P54.6   Neonatal vaginal hemorrhage ♀   N
          Neonatal pseudomenses

     P54.8   Other specified neonatal hemorrhages   N

     P54.9   Neonatal hemorrhage, unspecified   N

● **P55   Hemolytic disease of newborn**
       AKA erythroblastosis fetalis and is due to Rh isoimmunization, result of Rh blood factor incompatibilities between mother (Rh negative) and fetus (Rh positive)

     P55.0   Rh isoimmunization of newborn   N

     P55.1   ABO isoimmunization of newborn   N

     P55.8   Other hemolytic diseases of newborn   N

     P55.9   Hemolytic disease of newborn, unspecified   N

● **P56   Hydrops fetalis due to hemolytic disease**
       Caused by maternal sensitization to fetal blood group antigen

> **Excludes1**   hydrops fetalis NOS (P83.2)

     P56.0   Hydrops fetalis due to isoimmunization   N

   ● **P56.9   Hydrops fetalis due to other and unspecified hemolytic disease**

          P56.90   Hydrops fetalis due to unspecified hemolytic disease   N

          P56.99   Hydrops fetalis due to other hemolytic disease   N

● **P57   Kernicterus**
       High levels of bilirubin in blood, with severe neural symptoms

     P57.0   Kernicterus due to isoimmunization   N

     P57.8   Other specified kernicterus   N

> > **Excludes1**   Crigler-Najjar syndrome (E80.5)

     P57.9   Kernicterus, unspecified   N

● **P58   Neonatal jaundice due to other excessive hemolysis**

> **Excludes1**   jaundice due to isoimmunization (P55-P57)

     P58.0   Neonatal jaundice due to bruising   N

     P58.1   Neonatal jaundice due to bleeding   N

     P58.2   Neonatal jaundice due to infection   N

     P58.3   Neonatal jaundice due to polycythemia   N

   ● **P58.4   Neonatal jaundice due to drugs or toxins transmitted from mother or given to newborn**

> *Code first poisoning due to drug or toxin, if applicable (T36-T65 with fifth or sixth character 1-4 or 6)*
>
> Use additional code for adverse effect, if applicable, to identify drug (T36-T50 with fifth or sixth character 5)

          P58.41   Neonatal jaundice due to drugs or toxins transmitted from mother   N

          P58.42   Neonatal jaundice due to drugs or toxins given to newborn   N

     P58.5   Neonatal jaundice due to swallowed maternal blood   N

     P58.8   Neonatal jaundice due to other specified excessive hemolysis   N

     P58.9   Neonatal jaundice due to excessive hemolysis, unspecified   N

◄ New   ⇚ Revised   ~~deleted~~ Deleted   Excludes 1   Excludes 2   Includes   Use additional   Code first   Code also   Unspecified

OGCR Official Guidelines   X Assign placeholder X   ● Use Additional Character(s)   ▶ Manifestation Code   **Coding Clinic**

● **P59** Neonatal jaundice from other and unspecified causes

> **Excludes1** jaundice due to inborn errors of metabolism
> (E70-E88)
> kernicterus (P57.-)

P59.0 Neonatal jaundice associated with preterm delivery　N
Hyperbilirubinemia of prematurity
Jaundice due to delayed conjugation associated with
preterm delivery

P59.1 Inspissated bile syndrome　N

● **P59.2** Neonatal jaundice from other and unspecified
hepatocellular damage

> **Excludes1** congenital viral hepatitis (P35.3)

P59.20 Neonatal jaundice from unspecified
hepatocellular damage　N

P59.29 Neonatal jaundice from other hepatocellular
damage　N
Neonatal giant cell hepatitis
Neonatal (idiopathic) hepatitis

P59.3 Neonatal jaundice from breast milk inhibitor　N

P59.8 Neonatal jaundice from other specified causes　N

P59.9 Neonatal jaundice, unspecified　N
Neonatal physiological jaundice (intense)(prolonged)
NOS

P60 Disseminated intravascular coagulation of newborn　N
Defibrination syndrome of newborn

● **P61** Other perinatal hematological disorders

> **Excludes1** transient hypogammaglobulinemia of infancy
> (D80.7)

P61.0 Transient neonatal thrombocytopenia　N
*Lack of sufficient numbers of circulating thrombocytes
(platelets)*
Neonatal thrombocytopenia due to exchange
transfusion
Neonatal thrombocytopenia due to idiopathic maternal
thrombocytopenia
Neonatal thrombocytopenia due to isoimmunization

P61.1 Polycythemia neonatorum　N
Neonate = newborn

P61.2 Anemia of prematurity　N

P61.3 Congenital anemia from fetal blood loss　N

P61.4 Other congenital anemias, not elsewhere classified　N
Congenital anemia NOS

P61.5 Transient neonatal neutropenia　N
Low levels of granulocytic neutrophilic white blood cells

> **Excludes1** congenital neutropenia (nontransient)
> (D70.0)

P61.6 Other transient neonatal disorders of coagulation　N

P61.8 Other specified perinatal hematological disorders　N

P61.9 Perinatal hematological disorder, unspecified　N

TRANSITORY ENDOCRINE AND METABOLIC DISORDERS
SPECIFIC TO NEWBORN (P70-P74)

> **Includes** transitory endocrine and metabolic disturbances
> caused by the infant's response to maternal
> endocrine and metabolic factors, or its
> adjustment to extrauterine environment

● **P70** Transitory disorders of carbohydrate metabolism specific to
newborn

P70.0 Syndrome of infant of mother with gestational
diabetes　N
Newborn (with hypoglycemia) affected by maternal
gestational diabetes

> **Excludes1** newborn (with hypoglycemia) affected
> by maternal (pre-existing) diabetes
> mellitus (P70.1)
> syndrome of infant of a diabetic mother
> (P70.1)

P70.1 Syndrome of infant of a diabetic mother　N
Newborn (with hypoglycemia) affected by maternal
(pre-existing) diabetes mellitus

> **Excludes1** newborn (with hypoglycemia) affected by
> maternal gestational diabetes (P70.0)
> syndrome of infant of mother with
> gestational diabetes (P70.0)

P70.2 Neonatal diabetes mellitus　N

P70.3 Iatrogenic neonatal hypoglycemia　N

P70.4 Other neonatal hypoglycemia　N
Transitory neonatal hypoglycemia

P70.8 Other transitory disorders of carbohydrate metabolism
of newborn　N

P70.9 Transitory disorder of carbohydrate metabolism of
newborn, unspecified　N

● **P71** Transitory neonatal disorders of calcium and magnesium
metabolism

P71.0 Cow's milk hypocalcemia in newborn　N

P71.1 Other neonatal hypocalcemia　N

> **Excludes1** neonatal hypoparathyroidism (P71.4)

P71.2 Neonatal hypomagnesemia　N

P71.3 Neonatal tetany without calcium or magnesium
deficiency　N
Neonatal tetany NOS

P71.4 Transitory neonatal hypoparathyroidism　N

P71.8 Other transitory neonatal disorders of calcium and
magnesium metabolism　N

P71.9 Transitory neonatal disorder of calcium and magnesium
metabolism, unspecified　N

● **P72** Other transitory neonatal endocrine disorders

> **Excludes1** congenital hypothyroidism with or without goiter
> (E03.0-E03.1)
> dyshormogenetic goiter (E07.1)
> Pendred's syndrome (E07.1)

P72.0 Neonatal goiter, not elsewhere classified　N
Transitory congenital goiter with normal functioning

P72.1 Transitory neonatal hyperthyroidism　N
Neonatal thyrotoxicosis

P72.2 Other transitory neonatal disorders of thyroid function,
not elsewhere classified　N
Transitory neonatal hypothyroidism

P72.8 Other specified transitory neonatal endocrine
disorders　N

P72.9 Transitory neonatal endocrine disorder, unspecified　N

● **P74** Other transitory neonatal electrolyte and metabolic disturbances

P74.0 Late metabolic acidosis of newborn　N

> **Excludes1** (fetal) metabolic acidosis of newborn (P19)

P74.1 Dehydration of newborn　N

P74.2 Disturbances of sodium balance of newborn　N

P74.3 Disturbances of potassium balance of newborn　N

P74.4 Other transitory electrolyte disturbances of newborn　N

P74.5 Transitory tyrosinemia of newborn　N

P74.6 Transitory hyperammonemia of newborn　N

P74.8 Other transitory metabolic disturbances of newborn　N
Amino-acid metabolic disorders described as transitory

P74.9 Transitory metabolic disturbance of newborn,
unspecified　N

CHAPTER 16 (P00-P96)

DIGESTIVE SYSTEM DISORDERS OF NEWBORN (P76-P78)

● **P76**   **Other intestinal obstruction of newborn**

     P76.0   **Meconium plug syndrome**   N
           Fetal stool obstruction in large intestine, present at birth; may be symptom of organic disease.
           Meconium ileus NOS
           Excludes1   meconium ileus in cystic fibrosis (E84.11)

     P76.1   **Transitory ileus of newborn**   N
           Temporary obstruction of ileus (small intestine)
           Excludes1   Hirschsprung's disease (Q43.1)

     P76.2   **Intestinal obstruction due to inspissated milk**   N
           Being thickened, dried, or made less fluid

     P76.8   **Other specified intestinal obstruction of newborn**   N
           Excludes1   intestinal obstruction classifiable to K56.-

     P76.9   **Intestinal obstruction of newborn, unspecified**   N

● **P77**   **Necrotizing enterocolitis of newborn**

     P77.1   **Stage 1 necrotizing enterocolitis in newborn**   N
           Necrotizing enterocolitis without pneumatosis, without perforation

     P77.2   **Stage 2 necrotizing enterocolitis in newborn**   N
           Necrotizing enterocolitis with pneumatosis, without perforation

     P77.3   **Stage 3 necrotizing enterocolitis in newborn**   N
           Necrotizing enterocolitis with perforation
           Necrotizing enterocolitis with pneumatosis and perforation

     P77.9   **Necrotizing enterocolitis in newborn, unspecified**   N
           Necrotizing enterocolitis in newborn, NOS

● **P78**   **Other perinatal digestive system disorders**

     Excludes1   cystic fibrosis (E84.0-E84.9)
           neonatal gastrointestinal hemorrhages (P54.0-P54.3)

     P78.0   **Perinatal intestinal perforation**   N
           Meconium peritonitis

     P78.1   **Other neonatal peritonitis**   N
           Neonatal peritonitis NOS

     P78.2   **Neonatal hematemesis and melena due to swallowed maternal blood**   N

     P78.3   **Noninfective neonatal diarrhea**   N
           Neonatal diarrhea NOS

     ● **P78.8**   **Other specified perinatal digestive system disorders**
         P78.81   **Congenital cirrhosis (of liver)**   N
         P78.82   **Peptic ulcer of newborn**   N
         P78.83   **Newborn esophageal reflux**   N
            Neonatal esophageal reflux
         P78.89   **Other specified perinatal digestive system disorders**   N

     P78.9   **Perinatal digestive system disorder, unspecified**   N

CONDITIONS INVOLVING THE INTEGUMENT AND TEMPERATURE REGULATION OF NEWBORN (P80-P83)

● **P80**   **Hypothermia of newborn**

     P80.0   **Cold injury syndrome**   N
           Severe and usually chronic hypothermia associated with a pink flushed appearance, edema and neurological and biochemical abnormalities.
           Excludes1   mild hypothermia of newborn (P80.8)

     P80.8   **Other hypothermia of newborn**   N
           Mild hypothermia of newborn

     P80.9   **Hypothermia of newborn, unspecified**   N

● **P81**   **Other disturbances of temperature regulation of newborn**

     P81.0   **Environmental hyperthermia of newborn**   N

     P81.8   **Other specified disturbances of temperature regulation of newborn**   N

     P81.9   **Disturbance of temperature regulation of newborn, unspecified**   N
           Fever of newborn NOS

● **P83**   **Other conditions of integument specific to newborn**

     Excludes1   congenital malformations of skin and integument (Q80-Q84)
           hydrops fetalis due to hemolytic disease (P56.-)
           neonatal skin infection (P39.4)
           staphylococcal scalded skin syndrome (L00)

     Excludes2   cradle cap (L21.0)
           diaper [napkin] dermatitis (L22)

     P83.0   **Sclerema neonatorum**   N
           Neonate = newborn

     P83.1   **Neonatal erythema toxicum**   N
           Benign, generalized, transient pustules that become firm vesicles

     P83.2   **Hydrops fetalis not due to hemolytic disease**   N
           Severe, life-threatening problem of severe edema (swelling) as result of too much fluid leaving blood and entering tissue
           Hydrops fetalis NOS

     ● **P83.3**   **Other and unspecified edema specific to newborn**
         P83.30   **Unspecified edema specific to newborn**   N
         P83.39   **Other edema specific to newborn**   N

     P83.4   **Breast engorgement of newborn**   N
           Noninfective mastitis of newborn

     P83.5   **Congenital hydrocele** ♂

     P83.6   **Umbilical polyp of newborn**   N

     P83.8   **Other specified conditions of integument specific to newborn**   N
           Bronze baby syndrome
           Neonatal scleroderma
           Urticaria neonatorum

     P83.9   **Condition of the integument specific to newborn, unspecified**   N

OTHER PROBLEMS WITH NEWBORN (P84)

P84   **Other problems with newborn**   N
     Acidemia of newborn
     Acidosis of newborn
     Anoxia of newborn NOS
     Asphyxia of newborn NOS
     Hypercapnia of newborn
     Hypoxemia of newborn
     Hypoxia of newborn NOS
     Mixed metabolic and respiratory acidosis of newborn
     Excludes1   intracranial hemorrhage due to anoxia or hypoxia (P52.-)
           hypoxic ischemic encephalopathy [HIE] (P91.6-)
           late metabolic acidosis of newborn (P74.0)

OTHER DISORDERS ORIGINATING IN THE PERINATAL PERIOD (P90-P96)

P90   **Convulsions of newborn**   N
     Excludes1   benign myoclonic epilepsy in infancy (G40.3-)
           benign neonatal convulsions (familial) (G40.3-)

● **P91**   **Other disturbances of cerebral status of newborn**

     P91.0   **Neonatal cerebral ischemia**   N

     P91.1   **Acquired periventricular cysts of newborn**   N

     P91.2   **Neonatal cerebral leukomalacia**   N
           Degeneration of white matter adjacent to cerebral ventricles following cerebral hypoxia or brain ischemia in neonates
           Periventricular leukomalacia

     P91.3   **Neonatal cerebral irritability**   N

     P91.4   **Neonatal cerebral depression**   N

     P91.5   **Neonatal coma**   N

◄ New   ◄▥ Revised   ~~deleted~~ Deleted   Excludes 1   Excludes 2   Includes   Use additional   Code first   Code also   Unspecified

OGCR Official Guidelines   **X** Assign placeholder X   ● Use Additional Character(s)   ▶ Manifestation Code   **Coding Clinic**

● **P91.6 Hypoxic ischemic encephalopathy [HIE]**

    P91.60 Hypoxic ischemic encephalopathy [HIE], unspecified   N

    P91.61 Mild hypoxic ischemic encephalopathy [HIE]   N

    P91.62 Moderate hypoxic ischemic encephalopathy [HIE]   N

    P91.63 Severe hypoxic ischemic encephalopathy [HIE]   N

  P91.8 Other specified disturbances of cerebral status of newborn   N

  P91.9 Disturbance of cerebral status of newborn, unspecified   N

● **P92 Feeding problems of newborn**

    Excludes1   feeding problems in child over 28 days old (R63.3)

  ● **P92.0 Vomiting of newborn**

      Excludes1   vomiting of child over 28 days old (R11.-)

    P92.01 Bilious vomiting of newborn   N

        Excludes1   bilious vomiting in child over 28 days old (R11.14)

    P92.09 Other vomiting of newborn   N

        Excludes1   regurgitation of food in newborn (P92.1)

  P92.1 Regurgitation and rumination of newborn   N

  P92.2 Slow feeding of newborn   N

  P92.3 Underfeeding of newborn   N

  P92.4 Overfeeding of newborn   N

  P92.5 Neonatal difficulty in feeding at breast   N

  P92.6 Failure to thrive in newborn   N

    Excludes1   failure to thrive in child over 28 days old (R62.51)

  P92.8 Other feeding problems of newborn   N

  P92.9 Feeding problem of newborn, unspecified   N

● **P93 Reactions and intoxications due to drugs administered to newborn**

    Includes   reactions and intoxications due to drugs administered to fetus affecting newborn

    Excludes1   jaundice due to drugs or toxins transmitted from mother or given to newborn (P58.4-)

        reactions and intoxications from maternal opiates, tranquilizers and other medication (P04.0-P04.1, P04.4)

        withdrawal symptoms from maternal use of drugs of addiction (P96.1)

        withdrawal symptoms from therapeutic use of drugs in newborn (P96.2)

  P93.0 Grey baby syndrome   N

    Grey syndrome from chloramphenicol administration in newborn

  P93.8 Other reactions and intoxications due to drugs administered to newborn   N

    Use additional code for adverse effect, if applicable, to identify drug (T36-T50 with fifth or sixth character 5)

● **P94 Disorders of muscle tone of newborn**

  P94.0 Transient neonatal myasthenia gravis   N

    Excludes1   myasthenia gravis (G70.0)

  P94.1 Congenital hypertonia   N

  P94.2 Congenital hypotonia   N

    Floppy baby syndrome, unspecified

  P94.8 Other disorders of muscle tone of newborn   N

  P94.9 Disorder of muscle tone of newborn, unspecified   N

P95 Stillbirth   N

  Deadborn fetus NOS

  Fetal death of unspecified cause

  Stillbirth NOS

    Excludes1   maternal care for intrauterine death (O36.4)

        missed abortion (O02.1)

        outcome of delivery, stillbirth (Z37.1, Z37.3, Z37.4, Z37.7)

OGCR Section I.C.16.g.

Stillbirth

Code P95, Stillbirth, is only for use for institutions that maintain separate records for stillbirths. No other code should be used with P95. Code P95 should not be used on the mother's record.

● **P96 Other conditions originating in the perinatal period**

  P96.0 Congenital renal failure   N

    Uremia of newborn

  P96.1 Neonatal withdrawal symptoms from maternal use of drugs of addiction   N

    Drug withdrawal syndrome in infant of dependent mother

    Neonatal abstinence syndrome

    Excludes1   reactions and intoxications from maternal opiates and tranquilizers administered during labor and delivery (P04.0)

  P96.2 Withdrawal symptoms from therapeutic use of drugs in newborn   N

  P96.3 Wide cranial sutures of newborn   N

    Neonatal craniotabes

  P96.5 Complication to newborn due to (fetal) intrauterine procedure   N

    Excludes2   newborn (suspected to be) affected by amniocentesis (P00.6)

  ● **P96.8 Other specified conditions originating in the perinatal period**

    P96.81 Exposure to (parental) (environmental) tobacco smoke in the perinatal period

        Excludes2   newborn affected by in utero exposure to tobacco (P04.2)

           exposure to environmental tobacco smoke after the perinatal period (Z77.22)

    P96.82 Delayed separation of umbilical cord   N

    P96.83 Meconium staining   N

        Excludes1   meconium aspiration (P24.00, P24.01)

           meconium passage during delivery (P03.82)

    P96.89 Other specified conditions originating in the perinatal period   N

      Use additional code to specify condition

  P96.9 Condition originating in the perinatal period, unspecified   N

    Congenital debility NOS

CHAPTER 16 (P00-P96)

OGCR See Section I.C., Chapter 17

Congenital malformations, deformations, and chromosomal abnormalities

CHAPTER 17

CONGENITAL MALFORMATIONS, DEFORMATIONS AND CHROMOSOMAL ABNORMALITIES (Q00-Q99)

Note: Codes from this chapter are not for use on maternal or fetal records

Excludes2 inborn errors of metabolism (E70-E88)

This chapter contains the following blocks:

Q00-Q07	Congenital malformations of the nervous system
Q10-Q18	Congenital malformations of eye, ear, face and neck
Q20-Q28	Congenital malformations of the circulatory system
Q30-Q34	Congenital malformations of the respiratory system
Q35-Q37	Cleft lip and cleft palate
Q38-Q45	Other congenital malformations of the digestive system
Q50-Q56	Congenital malformations of genital organs
Q60-Q64	Congenital malformations of the urinary system
Q65-Q79	Congenital malformations and deformations of the musculoskeletal system
Q80-Q89	Other congenital malformations
Q90-Q99	Chromosomal abnormalities, not elsewhere classified

CONGENITAL MALFORMATIONS OF THE NERVOUS SYSTEM (Q00–Q07)

● **Q00 Anencephaly and similar malformations**

Q00.0 Anencephaly
Absence of skull with cerebral hemispheres missing or reduced to small masses attached to base of cranium
Acephaly
Acrania
Amyelencephaly
Hemianencephaly
Hemicephaly

Q00.1 Craniorachischisis
Developmental anomaly consisting of fissure of cranium and vertebral column

Q00.2 Iniencephaly
Developmental anomaly characterized by enlargement of foramen magnum and absence of laminae and spinous processes of cervical, dorsal

● **Q01 Encephalocele**
Sac-like protrusions of brain and membranes visible through an opening in skull

Includes Arnold-Chiari syndrome, type III
encephalocystocele
encephalomyelocele
hydroencephalocele
hydromeningocele, cranial
meningocele, cerebral
meningoencephalocele

Excludes1 Meckel-Gruber syndrome (Q61.9)

Q01.0 Frontal encephalocele

Q01.1 Nasofrontal encephalocele

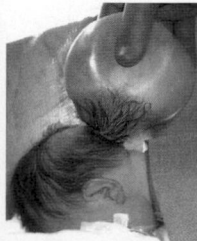

Figure 17-1 An infant with a large occipital encephalocele. The large skin-covered encephalocele is visible. (From Townsend: Sabiston Textbook of Surgery, ed 19, Saunders, An Imprint of Elsevier, 2012)

Q01.2 Occipital encephalocele

Q01.8 Encephalocele of other sites

Q01.9 Encephalocele, unspecified

● **Q02 Microcephaly**
Head size measures significantly below normal based on standardized charts

Includes hydromicrocephaly
micrencephalon

Excludes1 Meckel-Gruber syndrome (Q61.9)

● **Q03 Congenital hydrocephalus**
Accumulation of cerebrospinal fluid in ventricles resulting in swelling and enlargement

Includes hydrocephalus in newborn

Excludes1 Arnold-Chiari syndrome, type II (Q07.0-)
acquired hydrocephalus (G91.-)
hydrocephalus due to congenital toxoplasmosis (P37.1)
hydrocephalus with spina bifida (Q05.0-Q05.4)

Q03.0 Malformations of aqueduct of Sylvius
Anomaly of aqueduct of Sylvius
Obstruction of aqueduct of Sylvius, congenital
Stenosis of aqueduct of Sylvius

Q03.1 Atresia of foramina of Magendie and Luschka
Dandy-Walker syndrome

Q03.8 Other congenital hydrocephalus

Q03.9 Congenital hydrocephalus, unspecified

● **Q04 Other congenital malformations of brain**

Excludes1 cyclopia (Q87.0)
macrocephaly (Q75.3)

Q04.0 Congenital malformations of corpus callosum
Agenesis of corpus callosum

Q04.1 Arhinencephaly
Congenital absence of olfactory bulbs, tract, or nerves

Q04.2 Holoprosencephaly
Failure of cleavage of forebrain (prosencephalon) resulting in incomplete or absent cortical separation and deficits in midline facial development

Q04.3 Other reduction deformities of brain
Absence of part of brain   Agyria
Agenesis of part of brain
Cerebral cortex are not fully formed, brain surface is smooth
Aplasia of part of brain
Hydranencephaly
Hypoplasia of part of brain
Lissencephaly
Congenital malformation or absence of convolutions of cerebral cortex
Microgyria
Malformation of brain characterized by excessive number of small convolutions (gyri) on surface
Pachygyria
Reduction in number of sulci of cerebrum

Excludes1 congenital malformations of corpus callosum (Q04.0)

Q04.4 Septo-optic dysplasia of brain

Q04.5 Megalencephaly
Abnormally large brain

Q04.6 Congenital cerebral cysts
Porencephaly   Schizencephaly

Excludes1 acquired porencephalic cyst (G93.0)

Q04.8 Other specified congenital malformations of brain
Arnold-Chiari syndrome, type IV
Macrogyria

Q04.9 Congenital malformation of brain, unspecified
Congenital anomaly NOS of brain
Congenital deformity NOS of brain
Congenital disease or lesion NOS of brain
Multiple anomalies NOS of brain, congenital

◀ New   ◀ Revised   ~~deleted~~ Deleted   Excludes 1   Excludes 2   Includes   Use additional   Code first   Code also   Unspecified

OGCR Official Guidelines   X Assign placeholder X   ● Use Additional Character(s)   ▶ Manifestation Code   **Coding Clinic**

● **Q05　Spina bifida**
*Developmental anomaly characterized by defective closure of vertebral
arch, through which spinal cord and meninges may protrude*

Includes　　hydromeningocele (spinal)
　　　　　　　meningocele (spinal)
　　　　　　　meningomyelocele
　　　　　　　myelocele
　　　　　　　myelomeningocele
　　　　　　　rachischisis
　　　　　　　spina bifida (aperta)(cystica)
　　　　　　　syringomyelocele

Use additional code for any associated paraplegia (paraparesis)
(G82.2-)

Excludes1　　Arnold-Chiari syndrome, type II (Q07.0-)
　　　　　　　spina bifida occulta (Q76.0)

Q05.0　Cervical spina bifida with hydrocephalus

Q05.1　Thoracic spina bifida with hydrocephalus
　　　　Dorsal spina bifida with hydrocephalus
　　　　Thoracolumbar spina bifida with hydrocephalus

Q05.2　Lumbar spina bifida with hydrocephalus
　　　　Lumbosacral spina bifida with hydrocephalus

Q05.3　Sacral spina bifida with hydrocephalus

Q05.4　Unspecified spina bifida with hydrocephalus

Q05.5　Cervical spina bifida without hydrocephalus

Q05.6　Thoracic spina bifida without hydrocephalus
　　　　Dorsal spina bifida NOS
　　　　Thoracolumbar spina bifida NOS

Q05.7　Lumbar spina bifida without hydrocephalus
　　　　Lumbosacral spina bifida NOS

Q05.8　Sacral spina bifida without hydrocephalus

Q05.9　Spina bifida, unspecified

● **Q06　Other congenital malformations of spinal cord**

Q06.0　Amyelia
　　　　Congenital absence of spinal cord

Q06.1　Hypoplasia and dysplasia of spinal cord
　　　　Underdevelopment of spinal cord
　　　　Atelomyelia
　　　　　　Congenitally incomplete development of spinal cord
　　　　Myelatelia
　　　　Myelodysplasia of spinal cord
　　　　　　*Defective development of spinal cord, especially lower
　　　　　　segments*

Q06.2　Diastematomyelia
　　　　*Congenital anomaly, associated with spina bifida, in which
　　　　spinal cord is split into halves and surrounded by dural
　　　　sac*

Q06.3　Other congenital cauda equina malformations

Q06.4　Hydromyelia
　　　　*Dilation of central canal of spinal cord with increased fluid
　　　　accumulation*
　　　　Hydrorachis

Q06.8　Other specified congenital malformations of spinal cord

Q06.9　Congenital malformation of spinal cord, unspecified
　　　　Congenital anomaly NOS of spinal cord
　　　　Congenital deformity NOS of spinal cord
　　　　Congenital disease or lesion NOS of spinal cord

● **Q07　Other congenital malformations of nervous system**
Excludes2　　congenital central alveolar hypoventilation
　　　　　　　　syndrome (G47.35)
　　　　　　　familial dysautonomia [Riley-Day] (G90.1)
　　　　　　　neurofibromatosis (nonmalignant) (Q85.0-)

● **Q07.0　Arnold-Chiari syndrome**
　　　　*Herniation of cerebellar tonsils and vermis through foramen
　　　　magnum into spinal canal*
　　　　Arnold-Chiari syndrome, type II
　　　　Excludes1　　Arnold-Chiari syndrome, type III (Q01.-)
　　　　　　　　　　　Arnold-Chiari syndrome, type IV (Q04.8)

**Q07.00　Arnold-Chiari syndrome without spina bifida
　　　　　or hydrocephalus**

**Q07.01　Arnold-Chiari syndrome with spina
　　　　　bifida**

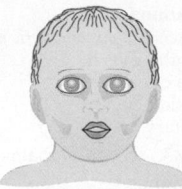

Figure 17-2　Bilateral congenital **hydrophthalmia,** in which the eyes
are very large in comparison to the other facial features due to glaucoma.

Q07.02　Arnold-Chiari syndrome with hydrocephalus

**Q07.03　Arnold-Chiari syndrome with spina
　　　　　bifida and hydrocephalus**

**Q07.8　Other specified congenital malformations of nervous
　　　　system**
　　　　Agenesis of nerve
　　　　Displacement of brachial plexus
　　　　Jaw-winking syndrome
　　　　Marcus Gunn's syndrome

Q07.9　Congenital malformation of nervous system, unspecified
　　　　Congenital anomaly NOS of nervous system
　　　　Congenital deformity NOS of nervous system
　　　　Congenital disease or lesion NOS of nervous system

CONGENITAL MALFORMATIONS OF EYE, EAR, FACE AND NECK (Q10-Q18)

Excludes2　　cleft lip and cleft palate (Q35-Q37)
　　　　　　　congenital malformation of cervical spine (Q05.0,
　　　　　　　　Q05.5, Q67.5, Q76.0-Q76.4)
　　　　　　　congenital malformation of larynx (Q31.-)
　　　　　　　congenital malformation of lip NEC (Q38.0)
　　　　　　　congenital malformation of nose (Q30.-)
　　　　　　　congenital malformation of parathyroid gland
　　　　　　　　(Q89.2)
　　　　　　　congenital malformation of thyroid gland (Q89.2)

● **Q10　Congenital malformations of eyelid, lacrimal apparatus and
　　　orbit**
Excludes1　　cryptophthalmos NOS (Q11.2)
　　　　　　　cryptophthalmos syndrome (Q87.0)

Q10.0　Congenital ptosis
　　　　*Prolapse or drooping of upper eyelid from paralysis of third
　　　　nerve or from sympathetic innervations*

Q10.1　Congenital ectropion
　　　　Outward turning of eyelid

Q10.2　Congenital entropion
　　　　Inward turning of eyelid

Q10.3　Other congenital malformations of eyelid
　　　　Ablepharon
　　　　Blepharophimosis, congenital
　　　　Coloboma of eyelid
　　　　Congenital absence or agenesis of cilia
　　　　Congenital absence or agenesis of eyelid
　　　　Congenital accessory eyelid
　　　　Congenital accessory eye muscle
　　　　Congenital malformation of eyelid NOS

Q10.4　Absence and agenesis of lacrimal apparatus
　　　　Congenital absence of punctum lacrimale

Q10.5　Congenital stenosis and stricture of lacrimal duct

Q10.6　Other congenital malformations of lacrimal apparatus
　　　　Congenital malformation of lacrimal apparatus NOS

Q10.7　Congenital malformation of orbit

● **Q11　Anophthalmos, microphthalmos and macrophthalmos**
　　　Absence of eye and optic pit

Q11.0　Cystic eyeball

Q11.1　Other anophthalmos
　　　　Anophthalmos NOS
　　　　Agenesis of eye
　　　　　　Absence of eye
　　　　Aplasia of eye

CHAPTER 17 (Q00-Q99)

Q11.2   **Microphthalmos**
Partial absence of eye and optic pit
Cryptophthalmos NOS
Dysplasia of eye
Hypoplasia of eye
Rudimentary eye
Excludes1   cryptophthalmos syndrome (Q87.0)

Q11.3   **Macrophthalmos**
Congenital enlargement of eyes
Excludes1   macrophthalmos in congenital glaucoma
(Q15.0)

● Q12   **Congenital lens malformations**

Q12.0   **Congenital cataract**

Q12.1   **Congenital displaced lens**

Q12.2   **Coloboma of lens**

Q12.3   **Congenital aphakia**

Q12.4   **Spherophakia**
Smaller, more spherical optic lens than normal

Q12.8   **Other congenital lens malformations**
Microphakia

Q12.9   **Congenital lens malformation, unspecified**

● Q13   **Congenital malformations of anterior segment of eye**

Q13.0   **Coloboma of iris**
Coloboma NOS

Q13.1   **Absence of iris**
Aniridia
Use additional code for associated glaucoma (H42)

Q13.2   **Other congenital malformations of iris**
Anisocoria, congenital
Atresia of pupil
Congenital malformation of iris NOS
Corectopia

Q13.3   **Congenital corneal opacity**

Q13.4   **Other congenital corneal malformations**
Congenital malformation of cornea NOS
Microcornea
Peter's anomaly

Q13.5   **Blue sclera**
Condition of unusual blueness of sclera; not harmful

● Q13.8   **Other congenital malformations of anterior segment of eye**

Q13.81   **Rieger's anomaly**
Use additional code for associated glaucoma (H42)

Q13.89   **Other congenital malformations of anterior segment of eye**

Q13.9   **Congenital malformation of anterior segment of eye, unspecified**

● Q14   **Congenital malformations of posterior segment of eye**
Excludes2   optic nerve hypoplasia (H47.03-)

Q14.0   **Congenital malformation of vitreous humor**
Congenital vitreous opacity

Q14.1   **Congenital malformation of retina**
Congenital retinal aneurysm

Q14.2   **Congenital malformation of optic disc**
Coloboma of optic disc

Q14.3   **Congenital malformation of choroid**

Q14.8   **Other congenital malformations of posterior segment of eye**
Coloboma of the fundus

Q14.9   **Congenital malformation of posterior segment of eye, unspecified**

● Q15   **Other congenital malformations of eye**
Excludes1   congenital nystagmus (H55.01)
ocular albinism (E70.31-)
optic nerve hypoplasia (H47.03-)
retinitis pigmentosa (H35.52)

Q15.0   **Congenital glaucoma**
Axenfeld's anomaly
Buphthalmos
*Congenital syndrome characterized by port-wine nevus
covering portions of face and cranium*
Glaucoma of childhood
Glaucoma of newborn
Hydrophthalmos
Keratoglobus, congenital, with glaucoma
Macrocornea with glaucoma
Macrophthalmos in congenital glaucoma
Megalocornea with glaucoma

Q15.8   **Other specified congenital malformations of eye**

Q15.9   **Congenital malformation of eye, unspecified**
Congenital anomaly of eye
Congenital deformity of eye

● Q16   **Congenital malformations of ear causing impairment of hearing**
Excludes1   congenital deafness (H90.-)

Q16.0   **Congenital absence of (ear) auricle**

Q16.1   **Congenital absence, atresia and stricture of auditory canal (external)**
Congenital atresia or stricture of osseous meatus

Q16.2   **Absence of eustachian tube**

Q16.3   **Congenital malformation of ear ossicles**
Congenital fusion of ear ossicles

Q16.4   **Other congenital malformations of middle ear**
Congenital malformation of middle ear NOS

Q16.5   **Congenital malformation of inner ear**
Congenital anomaly of membranous labyrinth
Congenital anomaly of organ of Corti

Q16.9   **Congenital malformation of ear causing impairment of hearing, unspecified**
Congenital absence of ear NOS

● Q17   **Other congenital malformations of ear**
Excludes1   congenital malformations of ear with impairment of hearing (Q16.0-Q16.9)
preauricular sinus (Q18.1)

Q17.0   **Accessory auricle**
Accessory tragus
Polyotia
Preauricular appendage or tag
Supernumerary ear
Supernumerary lobule

Q17.1   **Macrotia**
Enlarged ears

Q17.2   **Microtia**
An abnormally small or underdeveloped external ear

Q17.3   **Other misshapen ear**
Pointed ear

Q17.4   **Misplaced ear**
Low-set ears
Excludes1   cervical auricle (Q18.2)

Q17.5   **Prominent ear**
Bat ear

Q17.8   **Other specified congenital malformations of ear**
Congenital absence of lobe of ear

Q17.9   **Congenital malformation of ear, unspecified**
Congenital anomaly of ear NOS

◀ New   ◀▦ Revised   ~~deleted~~ Deleted   Excludes 1   Excludes 2   Includes   Use additional   Code first   Code also   Unspecified
OGCR Official Guidelines   **X** Assign placeholder X   ● Use Additional Character(s)   ▶ Manifestation Code   **Coding Clinic**

● **Q18 Other congenital malformations of face and neck**

> **Excludes1** cleft lip and cleft palate (Q35-Q37)
> conditions classified to Q67.0-Q67.4
> congenital malformations of skull and face bones
>   (Q75.-)
> cyclopia (Q87.0)
> dentofacial anomalies [including malocclusion]
>   (M26.-)
> malformation syndromes affecting facial
>   appearance (Q87.0)
> persistent thyroglossal duct (Q89.2)

Q18.0 Sinus, fistula and cyst of branchial cleft
Branchial vestige
Brachial remnants (cysts, fistula, skin tags) that are developmental anomalies

Q18.1 Preauricular sinus and cyst
Fistula of auricle, congenital
Cervicoaural fistula
Abnormal passage in neck originating from first branchial cleft

Q18.2 Other branchial cleft malformations
Branchial cleft malformation NOS
Cervical auricle
Otocephaly

Q18.3 Webbing of neck
Pterygium colli
Thick fold of skin on side of neck

Q18.4 Macrostomia
Results from failure of union of maxillary and mandibular processes, results in abnormally large mouth

Q18.5 Microstomia

Q18.6 Macrocheilia
Excessive size of lips
Hypertrophy of lip, congenital

Q18.7 Microcheilia
Abnormal smallness of lips

Q18.8 Other specified congenital malformations of face and neck
Medial cyst of face and neck
Medial fistula of face and neck
Medial sinus of face and neck

Q18.9 Congenital malformation of face and neck, unspecified
Congenital anomaly NOS of face and neck

CONGENITAL MALFORMATIONS OF THE CIRCULATORY SYSTEM (Q20-Q28)

● **Q20 Congenital malformations of cardiac chambers and connections**

> **Excludes1** dextrocardia with situs inversus (Q89.3)
> mirror-image atrial arrangement with situs
>   inversus (Q89.3)

Q20.0 Common arterial trunk
Persistent truncus arteriosus
> **Excludes1** aortic septal defect (Q21.4)

Q20.1 Double outlet right ventricle
Taussig-Bing syndrome

Q20.2 Double outlet left ventricle

Q20.3 Discordant ventriculoarterial connection
Dextrotransposition of aorta
Transposition of great vessels (complete)

Q20.4 Double inlet ventricle
Common ventricle
Cor triloculare biatriatum
Single ventricle

Q20.5 Discordant atrioventricular connection
Corrected transposition
Levotransposition
Ventricular inversion

Q20.6 Isomerism of atrial appendages
Isomerism of atrial appendages with asplenia or polysplenia

Q20.8 Other congenital malformations of cardiac chambers and connections
Cor binoculare

Q20.9 Congenital malformation of cardiac chambers and connections, unspecified

● **Q21 Congenital malformations of cardiac septa**
> **Excludes1** acquired cardiac septal defect (I51.0)

Q21.0 Ventricular septal defect
Roger's disease

Q21.1 Atrial septal defect
Coronary sinus defect
Patent or persistent foramen ovale
Patent or persistent ostium secundum defect (type II)
Patent or persistent sinus venosus defect

Q21.2 Atrioventricular septal defect
Common atrioventricular canal
Endocardial cushion defect
Ostium primum atrial septal defect (type I)

Q21.3 Tetralogy of Fallot
Ventricular septal defect with pulmonary stenosis or atresia, dextroposition of aorta and hypertrophy of right ventricle.

Q21.4 Aortopulmonary septal defect
Aortic septal defect
Aortopulmonary window

Q21.8 Other congenital malformations of cardiac septa
Eisenmenger's defect
Pentalogy of Fallot
> **Excludes1** Eisenmenger's complex (I27.8)
> Eisenmenger's syndrome (I27.8)

Q21.9 Congenital malformation of cardiac septum, unspecified
Septal (heart) defect NOS

● **Q22 Congenital malformations of pulmonary and tricuspid valves**

Q22.0 Pulmonary valve atresia

Q22.1 Congenital pulmonary valve stenosis

Q22.2 Congenital pulmonary valve insufficiency
Congenital pulmonary valve regurgitation

Q22.3 Other congenital malformations of pulmonary valve
Congenital malformation of pulmonary valve NOS
Supernumerary cusps of pulmonary valve

Q22.4 Congenital tricuspid stenosis
Congenital tricuspid atresia

Q22.5 Ebstein's anomaly
Malformation of tricuspid valve

Q22.6 Hypoplastic right heart syndrome

Q22.8 Other congenital malformations of tricuspid valve

Q22.9 Congenital malformation of tricuspid valve, unspecified

● **Q23 Congenital malformations of aortic and mitral valves**

Q23.0 Congenital stenosis of aortic valve
Congenital aortic atresia
Congenital aortic stenosis NOS
> **Excludes1** congenital stenosis of aortic valve in
>   hypoplastic left heart syndrome
>   (Q23.4)
> congenital subaortic stenosis (Q24.4)
> supravalvular aortic stenosis (congenital)
>   (Q25.3)

Q23.1 Congenital insufficiency of aortic valve
Bicuspid aortic valve
Congenital aortic insufficiency

Q23.2 Congenital mitral stenosis
Congenital mitral atresia

Q23.3 Congenital mitral insufficiency

Q23.4 Hypoplastic left heart syndrome

Q23.8 Other congenital malformations of aortic and mitral valves

Q23.9 Congenital malformation of aortic and mitral valves, unspecified

CHAPTER 17 (Q00-Q99)

CHAPTER 17 (Q00-Q99)

● **Q24 Other congenital malformations of heart**
    Excludes1   endocardial fibroelastosis (I42.4)

  Q24.0 Dextrocardia
    Heart is located in right hemithorax
    Excludes1   dextrocardia with situs inversus (Q89.3)
               isomerism of atrial appendages (with
                  asplenia or polysplenia) (Q20.6)
                mirror-image atrial arrangement with
                  situs inversus (Q89.3)

  Q24.1 Levocardia
    Normal position of heart but related structures on wrong side

  Q24.2 Cor triatriatum
    Congenital heart defect; left atrium is subdivided

  Q24.3 Pulmonary infundibular stenosis
    Subvalvular pulmonic stenosis

  Q24.4 Congenital subaortic stenosis

  Q24.5 Malformation of coronary vessels
    Congenital coronary (artery) aneurysm

  Q24.6 Congenital heart block

  Q24.8 Other specified congenital malformations of heart
    Congenital diverticulum of left ventricle
    Congenital malformation of myocardium
    Congenital malformation of pericardium
    Malposition of heart
    Uhl's disease

  Q24.9 Congenital malformation of heart, unspecified
    Congenital anomaly of heart
    Congenital disease of heart

● **Q25 Congenital malformations of great arteries**

  Q25.0 Patent ductus arteriosus
    Fetal blood vessel connecting left pulmonary artery directly
    to descending aorta
    Patent ductus Botallo
    Persistent ductus arteriosus

  Q25.1 Coarctation of aorta
    Coarctation of aorta (preductal) (postductal)

  Q25.2 Atresia of aorta

  Q25.3 Supravalvular aortic stenosis
    Excludes1   congenital aortic stenosis NOS (Q23.0)
               congenital stenosis of aortic valve (Q23.0)

  Q25.4 Other congenital malformations of aorta
    Absence of aorta
    Aneurysm of sinus of Valsalva (ruptured)
    Aplasia of aorta
    Congenital aneurysm of aorta
    Congenital malformations of aorta
    Congenital dilatation of aorta
    Double aortic arch [vascular ring of aorta]
    Hypoplasia of aorta
    Persistent convolutions of aortic arch
    Persistent right aortic arch
    Excludes1   hypoplasia of aorta in hypoplastic left
              heart syndrome (Q23.4)

  Q25.5 Atresia of pulmonary artery

  Q25.6 Stenosis of pulmonary artery
    Supravalvular pulmonary stenosis

● **Q25.7 Other congenital malformations of pulmonary artery**

    Q25.71 Coarctation of pulmonary artery

    Q25.72 Congenital pulmonary arteriovenous
            malformation
        Congenital pulmonary arteriovenous
            aneurysm

    Q25.79 Other congenital malformations of pulmonary
            artery
        Aberrant pulmonary artery
        Agenesis of pulmonary artery
        Congenital aneurysm of pulmonary artery
        Congenital anomaly of pulmonary artery
        Hypoplasia of pulmonary artery

  Q25.8 Other congenital malformations of other great arteries

  Q25.9 Congenital malformation of great arteries, unspecified

● **Q26 Congenital malformations of great veins**

  Q26.0 Congenital stenosis of vena cava
    Congenital stenosis of vena cava (inferior)(superior)

  Q26.1 Persistent left superior vena cava

  Q26.2 Total anomalous pulmonary venous connection
    Total anomalous pulmonary venous return [TAPVR],
       subdiaphragmatic
    Total anomalous pulmonary venous return [TAPVR],
       supradiaphragmatic

  Q26.3 Partial anomalous pulmonary venous connection
    Partial anomalous pulmonary venous return

  Q26.4 Anomalous pulmonary venous connection, unspecified

  Q26.5 Anomalous portal venous connection

  Q26.6 Portal vein-hepatic artery fistula

  Q26.8 Other congenital malformations of great veins
    Absence of vena cava (inferior) (superior)
    Azygos continuation of inferior vena cava
    Persistent left posterior cardinal vein
    Scimitar syndrome

  Q26.9 Congenital malformation of great vein, unspecified
    Congenital anomaly of vena cava (inferior) (superior)
    NOS

● **Q27 Other congenital malformations of peripheral vascular system**
    Excludes2   anomalies of cerebral and precerebral vessels
              (Q28.0-Q28.3)
              anomalies of coronary vessels (Q24.5)
              anomalies of pulmonary artery (Q25.5-Q25.7)
              congenital retinal aneurysm (Q14.1)
              hemangioma and lymphangioma (D18.-)

  Q27.0 Congenital absence and hypoplasia of umbilical artery
    Single umbilical artery

  Q27.1 Congenital renal artery stenosis

  Q27.2 Other congenital malformations of renal artery
    Congenital malformation of renal artery NOS
    Multiple renal arteries

● **Q27.3 Arteriovenous malformation (peripheral)**
    Arteriovenous aneurysm
    Excludes1   acquired arteriovenous aneurysm (I77.0)
    Excludes2   arteriovenous malformation of cerebral
              vessels (Q28.2)
              arteriovenous malformation of
              precerebral vessels (Q28.0)

    Q27.30 Arteriovenous malformation, site unspecified

    Q27.31 Arteriovenous malformation of vessel of upper
            limb

    Q27.32 Arteriovenous malformation of vessel of lower
            limb

    Q27.33 Arteriovenous malformation of digestive
            system vessel

    Q27.34 Arteriovenous malformation of renal vessel

    Q27.39 Arteriovenous malformation, other site

  Q27.4 Congenital phlebectasia

  Q27.8 Other specified congenital malformations of peripheral
    vascular system
    Absence of peripheral vascular system
    Atresia of peripheral vascular system
    Congenital aneurysm (peripheral)
    Congenital stricture, artery
    Congenital varix
    Excludes1   arteriovenous malformation (Q27.3-)

  Q27.9 Congenital malformation of peripheral vascular system,
    unspecified
    Anomaly of artery or vein NOS

◀ New   ⬅ Revised   ~~deleted~~ Deleted   Excludes 1   Excludes 2   Includes   Use additional   Code first   Code also   Unspecified

OGCR Official Guidelines   X Assign placeholder X   ● Use Additional Character(s)   ▶ Manifestation Code   **Coding Clinic**

● Q28   Other congenital malformations of circulatory system
    Excludes1   congenital aneurysm NOS (Q27.8)
                    congenital coronary aneurysm (Q24.5)
                    ruptured cerebral arteriovenous malformation
                        (I60.8)
                    ruptured malformation of precerebral vessels
                        (I72.0)

    Excludes2   congenital peripheral aneurysm (Q27.8)
                    congenital pulmonary aneurysm (Q25.79)
                    congenital retinal aneurysm (Q14.1)

    Q28.0   **Arteriovenous malformation of precerebral vessels**
            Congenital arteriovenous precerebral aneurysm
                (nonruptured)

    Q28.1   **Other malformations of precerebral vessels**
            Congenital malformation of precerebral vessels NOS
            Congenital precerebral aneurysm (nonruptured)

    Q28.2   **Arteriovenous malformation of cerebral vessels**
            Arteriovenous malformation of brain NOS
            Congenital arteriovenous cerebral aneurysm
                (nonruptured)

    Q28.3   **Other malformations of cerebral vessels**
            Congenital cerebral aneurysm (nonruptured)
            Congenital malformation of cerebral vessels NOS
            Developmental venous anomaly

    Q28.8   **Other specified congenital malformations of circulatory
            system**
            Congenital aneurysm, specified site NEC
            Spinal vessel anomaly

    Q28.9   **Congenital malformation of circulatory system,
            unspecified**

CONGENITAL MALFORMATIONS OF THE RESPIRATORY SYSTEM (Q30-Q34)

● Q30   Congenital malformations of nose
    Excludes1   congenital deviation of nasal septum (Q67.4)

    Q30.0   **Choanal atresia**
            Atresia of nares (anterior) (posterior)
            Congenital stenosis of nares (anterior) (posterior)

    Q30.1   **Agenesis and underdevelopment of nose**
            Congenital absent of nose

    Q30.2   **Fissured, notched and cleft nose**

    Q30.3   **Congenital perforated nasal septum**

    Q30.8   **Other congenital malformations of nose**
            Accessory nose
            Congenital anomaly of nasal sinus wall

    Q30.9   **Congenital malformation of nose, unspecified**

● Q31   Congenital malformations of larynx
    Excludes1   congenital laryngeal stridor NOS (P28.89)

    Q31.0   **Web of larynx**
            Glottic web of larynx
            Subglottic web of larynx
            Web of larynx NOS

    Q31.1   **Congenital subglottic stenosis**

    Q31.2   **Laryngeal hypoplasia**

    Q31.3   **Laryngocele**

    Q31.5   **Congenital laryngomalacia**

    Q31.8   **Other congenital malformations of larynx**
            Absence of larynx
            Agenesis of larynx
            Atresia of larynx
            Congenital cleft thyroid cartilage
            Congenital fissure of epiglottis
            Congenital stenosis of larynx NEC
            Posterior cleft of cricoid cartilage

    Q31.9   **Congenital malformation of larynx, unspecified**

● Q32   Congenital malformations of trachea and bronchus
    Excludes1   congenital bronchiectasis (Q33.4)

    Q32.0   **Congenital tracheomalacia**

    Q32.1   **Other congenital malformations of trachea**
            Atresia of trachea
            Congenital anomaly of tracheal cartilage
            Congenital dilatation of trachea
            Congenital malformation of trachea
            Congenital stenosis of trachea
            Congenital tracheocele

    Q32.2   **Congenital bronchomalacia**

    Q32.3   **Congenital stenosis of bronchus**

    Q32.4   **Other congenital malformations of bronchus**
            Absence of bronchus
            Agenesis of bronchus
            Atresia of bronchus
            Congenital diverticulum of bronchus
            Congenital malformation of bronchus NOS

● Q33   Congenital malformations of lung

    Q33.0   **Congenital cystic lung**
            Congenital cystic lung disease
            Congenital honeycomb lung
            Congenital polycystic lung disease
            Excludes1   cystic fibrosis (E84.0)
                            cystic lung disease, acquired or
                                unspecified (J98.4)

    Q33.1   **Accessory lobe of lung**
            Azygos lobe (fissured), lung

    Q33.2   **Sequestration of lung**

    Q33.3   **Agenesis of lung**
            Congenital absence of lung (lobe)

    Q33.4   **Congenital bronchiectasis**

    Q33.5   **Ectopic tissue in lung**

    Q33.6   **Congenital hypoplasia and dysplasia of lung**
            Excludes1   pulmonary hypoplasia associated with
                                short gestation (P28.0)

    Q33.8   **Other congenital malformations of lung**

    Q33.9   **Congenital malformation of lung, unspecified**

● Q34   Other congenital malformations of respiratory system
    Excludes2   congenital central alveolar hypoventilation
                        syndrome (G47.35)

    Q34.0   **Anomaly of pleura**

    Q34.1   **Congenital cyst of mediastinum**

    Q34.8   **Other specified congenital malformations of respiratory
            system**
            Atresia of nasopharynx

    Q34.9   **Congenital malformation of respiratory system,
            unspecified**
            Congenital absence of respiratory system
            Congenital anomaly of respiratory system NOS

CLEFT LIP AND CLEFT PALATE (Q35-Q37)

Use additional code to identify associated malformation of the
nose (Q30.2)

    Excludes1   Robin's syndrome (Q87.0)

● Q35   Cleft palate
    Includes   fissure of palate
                    palatoschisis
    Excludes1   cleft palate with cleft lip (Q37.-)

    Q35.1   **Cleft hard palate**

    Q35.3   **Cleft soft palate**

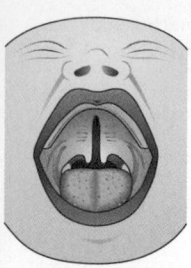

Figure 17-3   Cleft palate.

Q35.5   **Cleft hard palate with cleft soft palate**

Q35.7   **Cleft uvula**

Q35.9   **Cleft palate, unspecified**
        Cleft palate NOS

● **Q36**   **Cleft lip**
> **Includes**   cheiloschisis
>   congenital fissure of lip
>   harelip
>   labium leporinum
> **Excludes1**   cleft lip with cleft palate (Q37.-)

Q36.0   **Cleft lip, bilateral**

Q36.1   **Cleft lip, median**

Q36.9   **Cleft lip, unilateral**
        Cleft lip NOS

● **Q37**   **Cleft palate with cleft lip**
> **Includes**   cheilopalatoschisis

Q37.0   **Cleft hard palate with bilateral cleft lip**

Q37.1   **Cleft hard palate with unilateral cleft lip**
        Cleft hard palate with cleft lip NOS

Q37.2   **Cleft soft palate with bilateral cleft lip**

Q37.3   **Cleft soft palate with unilateral cleft lip**
        Cleft soft palate with cleft lip NOS

Q37.4   **Cleft hard and soft palate with bilateral cleft lip**

Q37.5   **Cleft hard and soft palate with unilateral cleft lip**
        Cleft hard and soft palate with cleft lip NOS

Q37.8   **Unspecified cleft palate with bilateral cleft lip**

Q37.9   **Unspecified cleft palate with unilateral cleft lip**
        Cleft palate with cleft lip NOS

OTHER CONGENITAL MALFORMATIONS OF THE DIGESTIVE SYSTEM (Q38-Q45)

● **Q38**   **Other congenital malformations of tongue, mouth and pharynx**
> **Excludes1**   dentofacial anomalies (M26.-)
>   macrostomia (Q18.4)
>   microstomia (Q18.5)

Q38.0   **Congenital malformations of lips, not elsewhere classified**
        Congenital fistula of lip
        Congenital malformation of lip NOS
        Van der Woude's syndrome
> **Excludes1**   cleft lip (Q36.-)
>   cleft lip with cleft palate (Q37.-)
>   macrocheilia (Q18.6)
>   microcheilia (Q18.7)

Q38.1   **Ankyloglossia**
        Restricted movement of tongue resulting in speech difficulty
        Tongue tie

Q38.2   **Macroglossia**
        Excessive size of tongue
        Congenital hypertrophy of tongue

Q38.3   **Other congenital malformations of tongue**
        Aglossia
        Bifid tongue
        Congenital adhesion of tongue
        Congenital fissure of tongue
        Congenital malformation of tongue NOS
        Double tongue
        Hypoglossia
        Hypoplasia of tongue
        Microglossia

Q38.4   **Congenital malformations of salivary glands and ducts**
        Atresia of salivary glands and ducts
        Congenital absence of salivary glands and ducts
        Congenital accessory salivary glands and ducts
        Congenital fistula of salivary gland

Q38.5   **Congenital malformations of palate, not elsewhere classified**
        Congenital absence of uvula
        Congenital malformation of palate NOS
        Congenital high arched palate
> **Excludes1**   cleft palate (Q35.-)
>   cleft palate with cleft lip (Q37.-)

Q38.6   **Other congenital malformations of mouth**
        Congenital malformation of mouth NOS

Q38.7   **Congenital pharyngeal pouch**
        Congenital diverticulum of pharynx
> **Excludes1**   pharyngeal pouch syndrome (D82.1)

Q38.8   **Other congenital malformations of pharynx**
        Congenital malformation of pharynx NOS
        Imperforate pharynx

● **Q39**   **Congenital malformations of esophagus**

Q39.0   **Atresia of esophagus without fistula**
        Atresia of esophagus NOS

Q39.1   **Atresia of esophagus with tracheo-esophageal fistula**
        Atresia of esophagus with broncho-esophageal fistula

Q39.2   **Congenital tracheo-esophageal fistula without atresia**
        Congenital tracheo-esophageal fistula NOS

Q39.3   **Congenital stenosis and stricture of esophagus**

Q39.4   **Esophageal web**

Q39.5   **Congenital dilatation of esophagus**
        Congenital cardiospasm

Q39.6   **Congenital diverticulum of esophagus**
        Congenital esophageal pouch

Q39.8   **Other congenital malformations of esophagus**
        Congenital absence of esophagus
        Congenital displacement of esophagus
        Congenital duplication of esophagus

Q39.9   **Congenital malformation of esophagus, unspecified**

● **Q40**   **Other congenital malformations of upper alimentary tract**

Q40.0   **Congenital hypertrophic pyloric stenosis**
        Congenital or infantile constriction
        Congenital or infantile hypertrophy
        Congenital or infantile spasm
        Congenital or infantile stenosis
        Congenital or infantile stricture

Q40.1   **Congenital hiatus hernia**
        Congenital displacement of cardia through esophageal hiatus
> **Excludes1**   congenital diaphragmatic hernia (Q79.0)

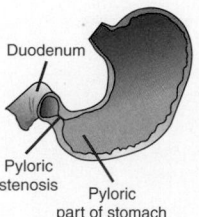

Duodenum

Pyloric stenosis

Pyloric part of stomach

Figure 17-4   Pyloric stenosis.

◀ New   ◀▪▪ Revised   ~~deleted~~ Deleted   Excludes 1   Excludes 2   Includes   Use additional   Code first   Code also   Unspecified

OGCR Official Guidelines   **X** Assign placeholder X   ● Use Additional Character(s)   ▶ Manifestation Code   **Coding Clinic**

Q40.2   **Other specified congenital malformations of stomach**
     Congenital displacement of stomach
     Congenital diverticulum of stomach
     Congenital hourglass stomach
     Congenital duplication of stomach
     Megalogastria
     Microgastria

Q40.3   **Congenital malformation of stomach, unspecified**

Q40.8   **Other specified congenital malformations of upper alimentary tract**

Q40.9   **Congenital malformation of upper alimentary tract, unspecified**
     Congenital anomaly of upper alimentary tract
     Congenital deformity of upper alimentary tract

● **Q41**   **Congenital absence, atresia and stenosis of small intestine**
     Includes   congenital obstruction, occlusion or stricture of small intestine or intestine NOS
     Excludes1   cystic fibrosis with intestinal manifestation (E84.11)
         meconium ileus NOS (without cystic fibrosis) (P76.0)

Q41.0   **Congenital absence, atresia and stenosis of duodenum**

Q41.1   **Congenital absence, atresia and stenosis of jejunum**
     Apple peel syndrome
     Imperforate jejunum

Q41.2   **Congenital absence, atresia and stenosis of ileum**

Q41.8   **Congenital absence, atresia and stenosis of other specified parts of small intestine**

Q41.9   **Congenital absence, atresia and stenosis of small intestine, part unspecified**
     Congenital absence, atresia and stenosis of intestine NOS

● **Q42**   **Congenital absence, atresia and stenosis of large intestine**
     Includes   congenital obstruction, occlusion and stricture of large intestine

Q42.0   **Congenital absence, atresia and stenosis of rectum with fistula**

Q42.1   **Congenital absence, atresia and stenosis of rectum without fistula**
     Imperforate rectum

Q42.2   **Congenital absence, atresia and stenosis of anus with fistula**

Q42.3   **Congenital absence, atresia and stenosis of anus without fistula**
     Imperforate anus

Q42.8   **Congenital absence, atresia and stenosis of other parts of large intestine**

Q42.9   **Congenital absence, atresia and stenosis of large intestine, part unspecified**

● **Q43**   **Other congenital malformations of intestine**

Q43.0   **Meckel's diverticulum (displaced) (hypertrophic)**
     Congenital abnormality in which a pouch remains on the lower end of the small intestine
     Persistent omphalomesenteric duct
     Persistent vitelline duct

Q43.1   **Hirschsprung's disease**
     Developmental disorder of enteric nervous system characterized by absence of ganglion cells in distal colon resulting in functional obstruction.
     Aganglionosis
     Congenital (aganglionic) megacolon

Q43.2   **Other congenital functional disorders of colon**
     Congenital dilatation of colon

Q43.3   **Congenital malformations of intestinal fixation**
     Congenital omental, anomalous adhesions [bands]
     Congenital peritoneal adhesions [bands]
     Incomplete rotation of cecum and colon
     Insufficient rotation of cecum and colon
     Jackson's membrane
     Malrotation of colon
     Rotation failure of cecum and colon
     Universal mesentery

Q43.4   **Duplication of intestine**

Q43.5   **Ectopic anus**
     Anal opening in abnormal location

Q43.6   **Congenital fistula of rectum and anus.**
     Excludes1   congenital fistula of anus with absence, atresia and stenosis (Q42.2)
         congenital fistula of rectum with absence, atresia and stenosis (Q42.0)
         congenital rectovaginal fistula (Q52.2)
         congenital urethrorectal fistula (Q64.73)
         pilonidal fistula or sinus (L05.-)

Q43.7   **Persistent cloaca**
     Malformation in which rectum, vagina, and urinary tract form one channel AKA congenital cloaca
     Cloaca NOS

Q43.8   **Other specified congenital malformations of intestine**
     Congenital blind loop syndrome
     Congenital diverticulitis, colon
     Congenital diverticulum, intestine
     Dolichocolon
     Megaloappendix
     Megaloduodenum
     Microcolon
     Transposition of appendix
     Transposition of colon
     Transposition of intestine

Q43.9   **Congenital malformation of intestine, unspecified**

● **Q44**   **Congenital malformations of gallbladder, bile ducts and liver**

Q44.0   **Agenesis, aplasia and hypoplasia of gallbladder**
     Congenital absence of gallbladder

Q44.1   **Other congenital malformations of gallbladder**
     Congenital malformation of gallbladder NOS
     Intrahepatic gallbladder

Q44.2   **Atresia of bile ducts**

Q44.3   **Congenital stenosis and stricture of bile ducts**

Q44.4   **Choledochal cyst**

Q44.5   **Other congenital malformations of bile ducts**
     Accessory hepatic duct
     Biliary duct duplication
     Congenital malformation of bile duct NOS
     Cystic duct duplication

Q44.6   **Cystic disease of liver**
     Fibrocystic disease of liver

Q44.7   **Other congenital malformations of liver**
     Accessory liver
     Alagille's syndrome
     Congenital absence of liver
     Congenital hepatomegaly
     Congenital malformation of liver NOS

● **Q45**   **Other congenital malformations of digestive system**
     Excludes2   congenital diaphragmatic hernia (Q79.0)
         congenital hiatus hernia (Q40.1)

Q45.0   **Agenesis, aplasia and hypoplasia of pancreas**
     Congenital absence of pancreas

Q45.1   **Annular pancreas**

Q45.2   **Congenital pancreatic cyst**

CHAPTER 17 (Q00–Q99)

Q45.3   **Other congenital malformations of pancreas and pancreatic duct**
> Accessory pancreas
> Congenital malformation of pancreas or pancreatic duct NOS
>
> > **Excludes1**   congenital diabetes mellitus (E10.-)
> >   cystic fibrosis (E84.0-E84.9)
> >   fibrocystic disease of pancreas (E84.-)
> >   neonatal diabetes mellitus (P70.2)

Q45.8   **Other specified congenital malformations of digestive system**
> Absence (complete) (partial) of alimentary tract NOS
> Duplication of digestive system
> Malposition, congenital of digestive system

Q45.9   **Congenital malformation of digestive system, unspecified**
> Congenital anomaly of digestive system
> Congenital deformity of digestive system

CONGENITAL MALFORMATIONS OF GENITAL ORGANS (Q50-Q56)

> **Excludes1**   androgen insensitivity syndrome (E34.5-)
>   syndromes associated with anomalies in
>   the number and form of chromosomes
>   (Q90-Q99)

● **Q50**   **Congenital malformations of ovaries, fallopian tubes and broad ligaments**

  ● **Q50.0**   **Congenital absence of ovary**
> > **Excludes1**   Turner's syndrome (Q96.-)

     Q50.01   **Congenital absence of ovary, unilateral** ♀

     Q50.02   **Congenital absence of ovary, bilateral** ♀

   Q50.1   **Developmental ovarian cyst** ♀

   Q50.2   **Congenital torsion of ovary** ♀

  ● **Q50.3**   **Other congenital malformations of ovary**

     Q50.31   **Accessory ovary** ♀

     Q50.32   **Ovarian streak** ♀
> *Inadequate ovaries with absent follicular and hormonal function*
> 46, XX with streak gonads

     Q50.39   **Other congenital malformation of ovary** ♀
> Congenital malformation of ovary NOS

   Q50.4   **Embryonic cyst of fallopian tube** ♀
> Fimbrial cyst

   Q50.5   **Embryonic cyst of broad ligament** ♀
> Epoophoron cyst
> Parovarian cyst

   Q50.6   **Other congenital malformations of fallopian tube and broad ligament** ♀
> Absence of fallopian tube and broad ligament
> Accessory fallopian tube and broad ligament
> Atresia of fallopian tube and broad ligament
> Congenital malformation of fallopian tube or broad ligament NOS

● **Q51**   **Congenital malformations of uterus and cervix**

   Q51.0   **Agenesis and aplasia of uterus** ♀
> Congenital absence of uterus

  ● **Q51.1**   **Doubling of uterus with doubling of cervix and vagina**

     Q51.10   **Doubling of uterus with doubling of cervix and vagina without obstruction** ♀
> Doubling of uterus with doubling of cervix and vagina NOS

     Q51.11   **Doubling of uterus with doubling of cervix and vagina with obstruction** ♀

   Q51.2   **Other doubling of uterus** ♀
> Doubling of uterus NOS
> Septate uterus, complete or partial

   Q51.3   **Bicornate uterus** ♀
> Bicornate uterus, complete or partial
> *Birth defect in which uterus has two separate 'horns' that form top of uterus*

   Q51.4   **Unicornate uterus** ♀
> Unicornate uterus with or without a separate uterine horn
> Uterus with only one functioning horn
> *Uterus with half being undeveloped*

   Q51.5   **Agenesis and aplasia of cervix** ♀
> Congenital absence of cervix

   Q51.6   **Embryonic cyst of cervix** ♀

   Q51.7   **Congenital fistulae between uterus and digestive and urinary tracts** ♀

  ● **Q51.8**   **Other congenital malformations of uterus and cervix**

    ● **Q51.81**   **Other congenital malformations of uterus**

       Q51.810   **Arcuate uterus** ♀
> Arcuatus uterus

       Q51.811   **Hypoplasia of uterus** ♀

       Q51.818   **Other congenital malformations of uterus** ♀
> Müllerian anomaly of uterus NEC

    ● **Q51.82**   **Other congenital malformations of cervix**

       Q51.820   **Cervical duplication** ♀

       Q51.821   **Hypoplasia of cervix** ♀

       Q51.828   **Other congenital malformations of cervix** ♀

   Q51.9   **Congenital malformation of uterus and cervix, unspecified** ♀

● **Q52**   **Other congenital malformations of female genitalia**

   Q52.0   **Congenital absence of vagina** ♀
> Vaginal agenesis, total or partial

  ● **Q52.1**   **Doubling of vagina**
> > **Excludes1**   doubling of vagina with doubling of uterus and cervix (Q51.1-)

     Q52.10   **Doubling of vagina, unspecified** ♀
> Septate vagina NOS

     Q52.11   **Transverse vaginal septum** ♀

     Q52.12   **Longitudinal vaginal septum** ♀
> Longitudinal vaginal septum with or without obstruction

   Q52.2   **Congenital rectovaginal fistula** ♀
> > **Excludes1**   cloaca (Q43.7)

   Q52.3   **Imperforate hymen** ♀
> *Membrane (hymen) completely closes vaginal orifice*

   Q52.4   **Other congenital malformations of vagina** ♀
> Canal of Nuck cyst, congenital
> Congenital malformation of vagina NOS
> Embryonic vaginal cyst
> Gartner's duct cyst

   Q52.5   **Fusion of labia** ♀

   Q52.6   **Congenital malformation of clitoris** ♀

  ● **Q52.7**   **Other and unspecified congenital malformations of vulva**

     Q52.70   **Unspecified congenital malformations of vulva** ♀
> Congenital malformation of vulva NOS

     Q52.71   **Congenital absence of vulva** ♀

     Q52.79   **Other congenital malformations of vulva** ♀
> Congenital cyst of vulva

   Q52.8   **Other specified congenital malformations of female genitalia** ♀

   Q52.9   **Congenital malformation of female genitalia, unspecified** ♀

◀ New   ◀▥ Revised   ~~deleted~~ Deleted   Excludes 1   Excludes 2   Includes   Use additional   Code first   Code also   Unspecified

OGCR Official Guidelines   **X** Assign placeholder X   ● Use Additional Character(s)   ▶ Manifestation Code   **Coding Clinic**

Item 17-1 Testes form in the abdomen of the male and only descend into the scrotum during normal embryonic development. "Ectopic" testes are out of their normal place or "retained" (left behind) in the abdomen. Crypto (hidden) orchism (testicle) is a major risk factor for testicular cancer.

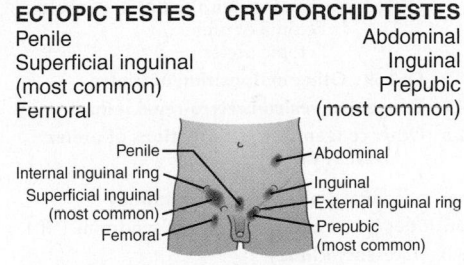

ECTOPIC TESTES	CRYPTORCHID TESTES
Penile	Abdominal
Superficial inguinal	Inguinal
(most common)	Prepubic
Femoral	(most common)

Figure 17-5 Undescended testes and the positions of the testes in various types of cryptorchidism or abnormal paths of descent.

- ● **Q53   Undescended and ectopic testicle**
  - ● Q53.0   Ectopic testis
    - Q53.00   Ectopic testis, <mark>unspecified</mark> ♂
    - Q53.01   Ectopic testis, unilateral ♂
    - Q53.02   Ectopic testes, bilateral ♂
  - ● Q53.1   Undescended testicle, unilateral
    - Q53.10   <mark>Unspecified</mark> undescended testicle, unilateral ♂
    - Q53.11   Abdominal testis, unilateral ♂
    - Q53.12   Ectopic perineal testis, unilateral ♂
  - ● Q53.2   Undescended testicle, bilateral
    - Q53.20   Undescended testicle, <mark>unspecified</mark>, bilateral ♂
    - Q53.21   Abdominal testis, bilateral ♂
    - Q53.22   Ectopic perineal testis, bilateral ♂
  - Q53.9   Undescended testicle, <mark>unspecified</mark> ♂
    - Cryptorchism NOS

- ● **Q54   Hypospadias**
  - *Birth defect of male; urethra opens in abnormal location on shaft*
  - **Excludes1**   epispadias (Q64.0)
  - Q54.0   Hypospadias, balanic ♂
    - Hypospadias, coronal
    - Hypospadias, glandular
  - Q54.1   Hypospadias, penile ♂
  - Q54.2   Hypospadias, penoscrotal ♂
  - Q54.3   Hypospadias, perineal ♂
  - Q54.4   Congenital chordee ♂
    - Chordee without hypospadias
  - Q54.8   Other hypospadias ♂
    - Hypospadias with intersex state
  - Q54.9   Hypospadias, <mark>unspecified</mark> ♂

- ● **Q55   Other congenital malformations of male genital organs**
  - **Excludes1**   congenital hydrocele (P83.5)
    - hypospadias (Q54.-)
  - Q55.0   Absence and aplasia of testis ♂
    - Monorchism
  - Q55.1   Hypoplasia of testis and scrotum ♂
    - Fusion of testes
  - ● Q55.2   Other and unspecified congenital malformations of testis and scrotum
    - Q55.20   <mark>Unspecified</mark> congenital malformations of testis and scrotum ♂
      - Congenital malformation of testis or scrotum NOS

- Q55.21   Polyorchism ♂
  - *Developmental anomaly characterized by presence of more than two testes*
- Q55.22   Retractile testis ♂
- Q55.23   Scrotal transposition ♂
- Q55.29   Other congenital malformations of testis and scrotum ♂
- Q55.3   Atresia of vas deferens ♂
  - *Code first any associated cystic fibrosis (E84.-)*
- Q55.4   Other congenital malformations of vas deferens, epididymis, seminal vesicles and prostate ♂
  - Absence or aplasia of prostate
  - Absence or aplasia of spermatic cord
  - Congenital malformation of vas deferens, epididymis, seminal vesicles or prostate NOS
- Q55.5   Congenital absence and aplasia of penis ♂
- ● Q55.6   Other congenital malformations of penis
  - Q55.61   Curvature of penis (lateral) ♂
  - Q55.62   Hypoplasia of penis ♂
    - *Underdevelopment penis*
    - Micropenis
  - Q55.63   Congenital torsion of penis ♂
    - **Excludes1**   acquired torsion of penis (N48.82)
  - Q55.64   Hidden penis ♂
    - Buried penis
    - Concealed penis
    - **Excludes1**   acquired buried penis (N48.83)
  - Q55.69   Other congenital malformation of penis ♂
    - Congenital malformation of penis NOS
- Q55.7   Congenital vasocutaneous fistula ♂
  - *Abnormal opening between vas deferens and skin*
- Q55.8   Other specified congenital malformations of male genital organs ♂
- Q55.9   Congenital malformation of male genital organ, <mark>unspecified</mark> ♂
  - Congenital anomaly of male genital organ
  - Congenital deformity of male genital organ

- ● **Q56   Indeterminate sex and pseudohermaphroditism**
  - *Internal reproductive organs are opposite external physical characteristics.*
  - **Excludes1**   46,XX true hermaphrodite (Q99.1)
    - androgen insensitivity syndrome (E34.5-)
    - chimera 46,XX/46,XY true hermaphrodite (Q99.0)
    - female pseudohermaphroditism with adrenocortical disorder (E25.-)
    - pseudohermaphroditism with specified chromosomal anomaly (Q96-Q99)
    - pure gonadal dysgenesis (Q99.1)
  - Q56.0   Hermaphroditism, not elsewhere classified
    - Ovotestis
  - Q56.1   Male pseudohermaphroditism, not elsewhere classified ♂
    - 46, XY with streak gonads
    - Male pseudohermaphroditism NOS
  - Q56.2   Female pseudohermaphroditism, not elsewhere classified ♀
    - Female pseudohermaphroditism NOS
  - Q56.3   Pseudohermaphroditism, <mark>unspecified</mark>
  - Q56.4   Indeterminate sex, <mark>unspecified</mark>
    - Ambiguous genitalia

CHAPTER 17 (Q00-Q99)

CONGENITAL MALFORMATIONS OF THE URINARY SYSTEM (Q60-Q64)

- **Q60 Renal agenesis and other reduction defects of kidney**
  - **Includes**   congenital absence of kidney
    congenital atrophy of kidney
    infantile atrophy of kidney
  - Q60.0 **Renal agenesis, unilateral**
  - Q60.1 **Renal agenesis, bilateral**
  - Q60.2 **Renal agenesis, unspecified**
  - Q60.3 **Renal hypoplasia, unilateral**
  - Q60.4 **Renal hypoplasia, bilateral**
  - Q60.5 **Renal hypoplasia, unspecified**
  - Q60.6 **Potter's syndrome**

- **Q61 Cystic kidney disease**
  - *Cysts that develop in failing kidney due to end-stage renal disease*
  - **Excludes1**   acquired cyst of kidney (N28.1)
    Potter's syndrome (Q60.6)
  - **● Q61.0 Congenital renal cyst**
    - Q61.00 **Congenital renal cyst, unspecified**
      Cyst of kidney NOS (congenital)
    - Q61.01 **Congenital single renal cyst**
    - Q61.02 **Congenital multiple renal cysts**
  - **● Q61.1 Polycystic kidney, infantile type**
    Polycystic kidney, autosomal recessive
    - Q61.11 **Cystic dilatation of collecting ducts**
    - Q61.19 **Other polycystic kidney, infantile type**
  - Q61.2 **Polycystic kidney, adult type**
    Polycystic kidney, autosomal dominant
  - Q61.3 **Polycystic kidney, unspecified**
  - Q61.4 **Renal dysplasia**
    Multicystic dysplastic kidney
    Multicystic kidney (development)
    Multicystic kidney disease
    Multicystic renal dysplasia
    - **Excludes1**   polycystic kidney disease (Q61.11-Q61.3)
  - Q61.5 **Medullary cystic kidney**
    Nephronopthisis
    Sponge kidney NOS
  - Q61.8 **Other cystic kidney diseases**
    Fibrocystic kidney
    Fibrocystic renal degeneration or disease
  - Q61.9 **Cystic kidney disease, unspecified**
    Meckel-Gruber syndrome

- **Q62 Congenital obstructive defects of renal pelvis and congenital malformations of ureter**
  - Q62.0 **Congenital hydronephrosis**
  - **● Q62.1 Congenital occlusion of ureter**
    Atresia and stenosis of ureter
    - Q62.10 **Congenital occlusion of ureter, unspecified**
    - Q62.11 **Congenital occlusion of ureteropelvic junction**
    - Q62.12 **Congenital occlusion of ureterovesical orifice**
  - Q62.2 **Congenital megaureter**
    Congenital dilatation of ureter
  - **● Q62.3 Other obstructive defects of renal pelvis and ureter**
    - Q62.31 **Congenital ureterocele, orthotopic**
    - Q62.32 **Cecoureterocele**
      Ectopic ureterocele
    - Q62.39 **Other obstructive defects of renal pelvis and ureter**
      Ureteropelvic junction obstruction NOS
  - Q62.4 **Agenesis of ureter**
    Congenital absence ureter
  - Q62.5 **Duplication of ureter**
    Accessory ureter
    Double ureter

- **● Q62.6 Malposition of ureter**
  - Q62.60 **Malposition of ureter, unspecified**
  - Q62.61 **Deviation of ureter**
  - Q62.62 **Displacement of ureter**
  - Q62.63 **Anomalous implantation of ureter**
    Ectopia of ureter
    Ectopic ureter
  - Q62.69 **Other malposition of ureter**
  - Q62.7 **Congenital vesico-uretero-renal reflux**
  - Q62.8 **Other congenital malformations of ureter**
    Anomaly of ureter NOS

- **● Q63 Other congenital malformations of kidney**
  - **Excludes1**   congenital nephrotic syndrome (N04.-)
  - Q63.0 **Accessory kidney**
  - Q63.1 **Lobulated, fused and horseshoe kidney**
  - Q63.2 **Ectopic kidney**
    Congenital displaced kidney
    Malrotation of kidney
  - Q63.3 **Hyperplastic and giant kidney**
    Compensatory hypertrophy of kidney
  - Q63.8 **Other specified congenital malformations of kidney**
    Congenital renal calculi
  - Q63.9 **Congenital malformation of kidney, unspecified**

- **● Q64 Other congenital malformations of urinary system**
  - Q64.0 **Epispadias ♂**
    Urethral opening somewhere on dorsum of penis
    - **Excludes1**   hypospadias (Q54.-)
  - **● Q64.1 Exstrophy of urinary bladder**
    Bladder is exposed, inside out, and protrudes through abdominal wall
    - Q64.10 **Exstrophy of urinary bladder, unspecified**
      Ectopia vesicae
    - Q64.11 **Supravesical fissure of urinary bladder**
    - Q64.12 **Cloacal exstrophy of urinary bladder**
    - Q64.19 **Other exstrophy of urinary bladder**
      Extroversion of bladder
  - Q64.2 **Congenital posterior urethral valves**
  - **● Q64.3 Other atresia and stenosis of urethra and bladder neck**
    - Q64.31 **Congenital bladder neck obstruction**
      Congenital obstruction of vesicourethral orifice
    - Q64.32 **Congenital stricture of urethra**
    - Q64.33 **Congenital stricture of urinary meatus**
    - Q64.39 **Other atresia and stenosis of urethra and bladder neck**
      Atresia and stenosis of urethra and bladder neck NOS
  - Q64.4 **Malformation of urachus**
    Cyst of urachus
    Patent urachus
    Prolapse of urachus
  - Q64.5 **Congenital absence of bladder and urethra**
  - Q64.6 **Congenital diverticulum of bladder**
  - **● Q64.7 Other and unspecified congenital malformations of bladder and urethra**
    - **Excludes1**   congenital prolapse of bladder (mucosa) (Q79.4)
    - Q64.70 **Unspecified congenital malformation of bladder and urethra**
      Malformation of bladder or urethra NOS
    - Q64.71 **Congenital prolapse of urethra**
    - Q64.72 **Congenital prolapse of urinary meatus**
    - Q64.73 **Congenital urethrorectal fistula**
    - Q64.74 **Double urethra**
    - Q64.75 **Double urinary meatus**
    - Q64.79 **Other congenital malformations of bladder and urethra**

◄ New   ◄ Revised   ~~deleted~~ Deleted   Excludes 1   Excludes 2   Includes   Use additional   Code first   Code also   Unspecified

OGCR Official Guidelines   X Assign placeholder X   ▶ Use Additional Character(s)   ▶ Manifestation Code   **Coding Clinic**

Q64.8   Other specified congenital malformations of urinary system

Q64.9   Congenital malformation of urinary system, unspecified
Congenital anomaly NOS of urinary system
Congenital deformity NOS of urinary system

CONGENITAL MALFORMATIONS AND DEFORMATIONS OF THE MUSCULOSKELETAL SYSTEM (Q65-Q79)

● **Q65   Congenital deformities of hip**
> **Excludes1**   clicking hip (R29.4)

● **Q65.0   Congenital dislocation of hip, unilateral**

Q65.00   Congenital dislocation of unspecified hip, unilateral

Q65.01   Congenital dislocation of right hip, unilateral

Q65.02   Congenital dislocation of left hip, unilateral

Q65.1   Congenital dislocation of hip, bilateral

Q65.2   Congenital dislocation of hip, unspecified

● **Q65.3   Congenital partial dislocation of hip, unilateral**

Q65.30   Congenital partial dislocation of unspecified hip, unilateral

Q65.31   Congenital partial dislocation of right hip, unilateral

Q65.32   Congenital partial dislocation of left hip, unilateral

Q65.4   Congenital partial dislocation of hip, bilateral

Q65.5   Congenital partial dislocation of hip, unspecified

Q65.6   Congenital unstable hip
Congenital dislocatable hip

● **Q65.8   Other congenital deformities of hip**

Q65.81   Congenital coxa valga

Q65.82   Congenital coxa vara

Q65.89   Other specified congenital deformities of hip
Anteversion of femoral neck
Congenital acetabular dysplasia

Q65.9   Congenital deformity of hip, unspecified

● **Q66   Congenital deformities of feet**
> **Excludes1**   reduction defects of feet (Q72.-)
> valgus deformities (acquired) (M21.0-)
> varus deformities (acquired) (M21.1-)

Q66.0   Congenital talipes equinovarus
Heel is turned inward from midline and foot is plantar flexed; AKA clubfoot

Q66.1   Congenital talipes calcaneovarus
Deformity of foot in which heel is turned toward midline of body and anterior of foot is elevated

Q66.2   Congenital metatarsus (primus) varus
Angulation of first metatarsal bone toward midline of body

Q66.3   Other congenital varus deformities of feet
Hallux varus, congenital

Q66.4   Congenital talipes calcaneovalgus

Item 17–2   Equinus foot is a term referring to the hoof of a horse. The deformity is usually congenital or spastic. Talipes equinovarus is referred to as clubfoot. The foot tends to be smaller than normal, with the heel pointing downward and the forefoot turning inward. The heel cord (Achilles tendon) is tight, causing the heel to be drawn up toward the leg.

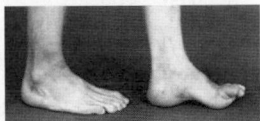

Figure 17-6   Supination and cavus deformity of forefoot. *(Courtesy Jay Cummings, MD.)* (From Canale: Campbell's Operative Orthopaedics, ed 11, Mosby, Inc., 2007)

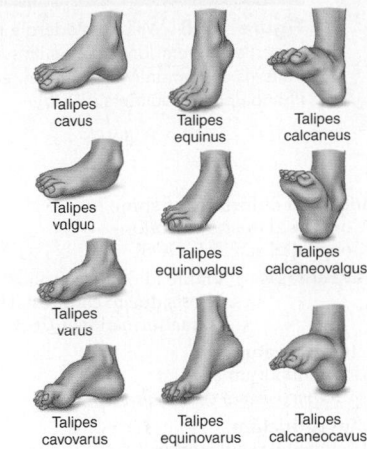

Figure 17-7   Talipes. (From Dorland: Dorland's Illustrated Medical Dictionary, ed 31, Saunders, 2007, p 1893)

● **Q66.5   Congenital pes planus**
Congenital flat foot
Congenital rigid flat foot
Congenital spastic (everted) flat foot
> **Excludes1**   pes planus, acquired (M21.4)

Q66.50   Congenital pes planus, unspecified foot

Q66.51   Congenital pes planus, right foot

Q66.52   Congenital pes planus, left foot

Q66.6   Other congenital valgus deformities of feet
Inward angulation
Congenital metatarsus valgus

Q66.7   Congenital pes cavus

● **Q66.8   Other congenital deformities of feet**

Q66.80   Congenital vertical talus deformity, unspecified foot

Q66.81   Congenital vertical talus deformity, right foot

Q66.82   Congenital vertical talus deformity, left foot

Q66.89   Other specified congenital deformities of feet
Congenital asymmetric talipes
Congenital clubfoot NOS
Congenital talipes NOS
Congenital tarsal coalition
Hammer toe, congenital

Q66.9   Congenital deformity of feet, unspecified

● **Q67   Congenital musculoskeletal deformities of head, face, spine and chest**
> **Excludes1**   congenital malformation syndromes classified to Q87.-
> Potter's syndrome (Q60.6)

Q67.0   Congenital facial asymmetry

Q67.1   Congenital compression facies

Q67.2   Dolichocephaly
Long head dimension

Q67.3   Plagiocephaly
Asymmetric shape of head resulting from irregular closure of cranial sutures

Q67.4   Other congenital deformities of skull, face and jaw
Congenital depressions in skull
Congenital hemifacial atrophy or hypertrophy
Deviation of nasal septum, congenital
Squashed or bent nose, congenital
> **Excludes1**   dentofacial anomalies [including malocclusion] (M26.-)
> syphilitic saddle nose (A50.5)

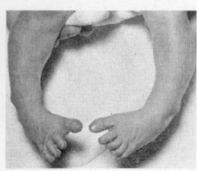

Figure 17-8 Mild to moderate inbowing of the lower leg. (From Jones KL: Smith's Recognizable Patterns of Human Malformation, ed 6, Philadelphia, Saunders, 2005)

CHAPTER 17 (Q00-Q99)

Q67.5 **Congenital deformity of spine**
Congenital postural scoliosis
Congenital scoliosis NOS
> **Excludes1** infantile idiopathic scoliosis (M41.0)
> scoliosis due to congenital bony
> malformation (Q76.3)

Q67.6 **Pectus excavatum**
Congenital funnel chest
Funnel-shaped chest depression

Q67.7 **Pectus carinatum**
Congenital pigeon chest

Q67.8 **Other congenital deformities of chest**
Congenital deformity of chest wall NOS

● Q68 **Other congenital musculoskeletal deformities**
> **Excludes1** reduction defects of limb(s) (Q71-Q73)
> **Excludes2** congenital myotonic chondrodystrophy (G71.13)

Q68.0 **Congenital deformity of sternocleidomastoid muscle**
Congenital contracture of sternocleidomastoid (muscle)
Congenital (sternomastoid) torticollis
Sternomastoid tumor (congenital)

Q68.1 **Congenital deformity of finger(s) and hand**
Congenital clubfinger
Spade-like hand (congenital)

Q68.2 **Congenital deformity of knee**
Congenital dislocation of knee
Congenital genu recurvatum
Hyperextension of knee resulting from hypermobility

Q68.3 **Congenital bowing of femur**
> **Excludes1** anteversion of femur (neck) (Q65.89)

Q68.4 **Congenital bowing of tibia and fibula**

Q68.5 **Congenital bowing of long bones of leg, unspecified**

Q68.6 **Discoid meniscus**

Q68.8 **Other specified congenital musculoskeletal deformities**
Congenital deformity of clavicle
Congenital deformity of elbow
Congenital deformity of forearm
Congenital deformity of scapula
Congenital deformity of wrist
Congenital dislocation of elbow
Congenital dislocation of shoulder
Congenital dislocation of wrist

● Q69 **Polydactyly**
AKA hyperdactyly, consists of supernumerary fingers or toes

Q69.0 **Accessory finger(s)**

Q69.1 **Accessory thumb(s)**

Q69.2 **Accessory toe(s)**
Accessory hallux

Q69.9 **Polydactyly, unspecified**
Supernumerary digit(s) NOS

● Q70 **Syndactyly**
Webbing between distal phalanges of adjacent digits

● Q70.0 **Fused fingers**
Complex syndactyly of fingers with synostosis
Q70.00 **Fused fingers, unspecified hand**
Q70.01 **Fused fingers, right hand**
Q70.02 **Fused fingers, left hand**
Q70.03 **Fused fingers, bilateral**

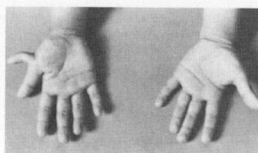

Figure 17-9 Polydactyly, congenital duplicated thumb. (From DeLee: DeLee and Drez's Orthopaedic Sports Medicine, ed 3, Saunders, An Imprint of Elsevier, 2009)

● Q70.1 **Webbed fingers**
Simple syndactyly of fingers without synostosis
Q70.10 **Webbed fingers, unspecified hand**
Q70.11 **Webbed fingers, right hand**
Q70.12 **Webbed fingers, left hand**
Q70.13 **Webbed fingers, bilateral**

● Q70.2 **Fused toes**
Complex syndactyly of toes with synostosis
Q70.20 **Fused toes, unspecified foot**
Q70.21 **Fused toes, right foot**
Q70.22 **Fused toes, left foot**
Q70.23 **Fused toes, bilateral**

● Q70.3 **Webbed toes**
Simple syndactyly of toes without synostosis
Q70.30 **Webbed toes, unspecified foot**
Q70.31 **Webbed toes, right foot**
Q70.32 **Webbed toes, left foot**
Q70.33 **Webbed toes, bilateral**

Q70.4 **Polysyndactyly, unspecified**
> **Excludes1** specified syndactyly of hand and
> feet - code to specified conditions
> (Q70.0- -Q70.3-)
Extra and webbed digits

Q70.9 **Syndactyly, unspecified**
Symphalangy NOS

● Q71 **Reduction defects of upper limb**
● Q71.0 **Congenital complete absence of upper limb**
Q71.00 **Congenital complete absence of unspecified upper limb**
Q71.01 **Congenital complete absence of right upper limb**
Q71.02 **Congenital complete absence of left upper limb**
Q71.03 **Congenital complete absence of upper limb, bilateral**

● Q71.1 **Congenital absence of upper arm and forearm with hand present**
Q71.10 **Congenital absence of unspecified upper arm and forearm with hand present**
Q71.11 **Congenital absence of right upper arm and forearm with hand present**
Q71.12 **Congenital absence of left upper arm and forearm with hand present**
Q71.13 **Congenital absence of upper arm and forearm with hand present, bilateral**

● Q71.2 **Congenital absence of both forearm and hand**
Q71.20 **Congenital absence of both forearm and hand, unspecified upper limb**
Q71.21 **Congenital absence of both forearm and hand, right upper limb**
Q71.22 **Congenital absence of both forearm and hand, left upper limb**
Q71.23 **Congenital absence of both forearm and hand, bilateral**

● Q71.3 **Congenital absence of hand and finger**
Q71.30 **Congenital absence of unspecified hand and finger**
Q71.31 **Congenital absence of right hand and finger**
Q71.32 **Congenital absence of left hand and finger**
Q71.33 **Congenital absence of hand and finger, bilateral**

◄ New   ◄▪▪ Revised   ̶d̶e̶l̶e̶t̶e̶d̶ Deleted   Excludes 1   Excludes 2   Includes   Use additional   Code first   Code also   Unspecified
OGCR Official Guidelines   **X** Assign placeholder X   ● Use Additional Character(s)   ▌ Manifestation Code   **Coding Clinic**

● **Q71.4** Longitudinal reduction defect of radius
   Clubhand (congenital)
   Radial clubhand

   Q71.40   Longitudinal reduction defect of unspecified radius

   Q71.41   Longitudinal reduction defect of right radius

   Q71.42   Longitudinal reduction defect of left radius

   Q71.43   Longitudinal reduction defect of radius, bilateral

● **Q71.5** Longitudinal reduction defect of ulna

   Q71.50   Longitudinal reduction defect of unspecified ulna

   Q71.51   Longitudinal reduction defect of right ulna

   Q71.52   Longitudinal reduction defect of left ulna

   Q71.53   Longitudinal reduction defect of ulna, bilateral

● **Q71.6** Lobster-claw hand

   Q71.60   Lobster-claw hand, unspecified hand

   Q71.61   Lobster-claw right hand

   Q71.62   Lobster-claw left hand

   Q71.63   Lobster-claw hand, bilateral

● **Q71.8** Other reduction defects of upper limb

   ● **Q71.81** Congenital shortening of upper limb

      Q71.811   Congenital shortening of right upper limb

      Q71.812   Congenital shortening of left upper limb

      Q71.813   Congenital shortening of upper limb, bilateral

      Q71.819   Congenital shortening of unspecified upper limb

   ● **Q71.89** Other reduction defects of upper limb

      Q71.891   Other reduction defects of right upper limb

      Q71.892   Other reduction defects of left upper limb

      Q71.893   Other reduction defects of upper limb, bilateral

      Q71.899   Other reduction defects of unspecified upper limb

● **Q71.9** Unspecified reduction defect of upper limb

   Q71.90   Unspecified reduction defect of unspecified upper limb

   Q71.91   Unspecified reduction defect of right upper limb

   Q71.92   Unspecified reduction defect of left upper limb

   Q71.93   Unspecified reduction defect of upper limb, bilateral

● **Q72** Reduction defects of lower limb

● **Q72.0** Congenital complete absence of lower limb

   Q72.00   Congenital complete absence of unspecified lower limb

   Q72.01   Congenital complete absence of right lower limb

   Q72.02   Congenital complete absence of left lower limb

   Q72.03   Congenital complete absence of lower limb, bilateral

● **Q72.1** Congenital absence of thigh and lower leg with foot present

   Q72.10   Congenital absence of unspecified thigh and lower leg with foot present

   Q72.11   Congenital absence of right thigh and lower leg with foot present

   Q72.12   Congenital absence of left thigh and lower leg with foot present

   Q72.13   Congenital absence of thigh and lower leg with foot present, bilateral

● **Q72.2** Congenital absence of both lower leg and foot

   Q72.20   Congenital absence of both lower leg and foot, unspecified lower limb

   Q72.21   Congenital absence of both lower leg and foot, right lower limb

   Q72.22   Congenital absence of both left lower leg and foot, left lower limb

   Q72.23   Congenital absence of both lower leg and foot, bilateral

● **Q72.3** Congenital absence of foot and toe(s)

   Q72.30   Congenital absence of unspecified foot and toe(s)

   Q72.31   Congenital absence of right foot and toe(s)

   Q72.32   Congenital absence of left foot and toe(s)

   Q72.33   Congenital absence of foot and toe(s), bilateral

● **Q72.4** Longitudinal reduction defect of femur
   Proximal femoral focal deficiency

   Q72.40   Longitudinal reduction defect of unspecified femur

   Q72.41   Longitudinal reduction defect of right femur

   Q72.42   Longitudinal reduction defect of left femur

   Q72.43   Longitudinal reduction defect of femur, bilateral

● **Q72.5** Longitudinal reduction defect of tibia

   Q72.50   Longitudinal reduction defect of unspecified tibia

   Q72.51   Longitudinal reduction defect of right tibia

   Q72.52   Longitudinal reduction defect of left tibia

   Q72.53   Longitudinal reduction defect of tibia, bilateral

● **Q72.6** Longitudinal reduction defect of fibula

   Q72.60   Longitudinal reduction defect of unspecified fibula

   Q72.61   Longitudinal reduction defect of right fibula

   Q72.62   Longitudinal reduction defect of left fibula

   Q72.63   Longitudinal reduction defect of fibula, bilateral

● **Q72.7** Split foot

   Q72.70   Split foot, unspecified lower limb

   Q72.71   Split foot, right lower limb

   Q72.72   Split foot, left lower limb

   Q72.73   Split foot, bilateral

● **Q72.8** Other reduction defects of lower limb

   ● **Q72.81** Congenital shortening of lower limb

      Q72.811   Congenital shortening of right lower limb

      Q72.812   Congenital shortening of left lower limb

      Q72.813   Congenital shortening of lower limb, bilateral

      Q72.819   Congenital shortening of unspecified lower limb

   ● **Q72.89** Other reduction defects of lower limb

      Q72.891   Other reduction defects of right lower limb

      Q72.892   Other reduction defects of left lower limb

      Q72.893   Other reduction defects of lower limb, bilateral

      Q72.899   Other reduction defects of unspecified lower limb

● **Q72.9** Unspecified reduction defect of lower limb

   Q72.90   Unspecified reduction defect of unspecified lower limb

   Q72.91   Unspecified reduction defect of right lower limb

   Q72.92   Unspecified reduction defect of left lower limb

   Q72.93   Unspecified reduction defect of lower limb, bilateral

CHAPTER 17 (Q00-Q99)

● **Q73**   **Reduction defects of unspecified limb**

   Q73.0   **Congenital absence of** unspecified **limb(s)**
       Amelia NOS

   Q73.1   **Phocomelia,** unspecified **limb(s)**
       Phocomelia NOS
       Absence/shortening of long bones primarily as a result of thalidomide

   Q73.8   **Other reduction defects of** unspecified **limb(s)**
       Longitudinal reduction deformity of unspecified limb(s)
       Ectromelia of limb NOS
       Gross hypoplasia or aplasia of one or more long bones of limb(s)
       Hemimelia of limb NOS
       Absence of one-half of long bone
       Reduction defect of limb NOS

● **Q74**   **Other congenital malformations of limb(s)**

   Excludes1   polydactyly (Q69.-)
         reduction defect of limb (Q71-Q73)
         syndactyly (Q70.-)

   Q74.0   **Other congenital malformations of upper limb(s), including shoulder girdle**
       Accessory carpal bones
       Cleidocranial dysostosis
       Congenital pseudarthrosis of clavicle
       Macrodactylia (fingers)
       Madelung's deformity
       Radioulnar synostosis
       Sprengel's deformity
       Triphalangeal thumb

   Q74.1   **Congenital malformation of knee**
       Congenital absence of patella
       Congenital dislocation of patella
       Congenital genu valgum
       Congenital genu varum
       Rudimentary patella

       Excludes1   congenital dislocation of knee (Q68.2)
            congenital genu recurvatum (Q68.2)
            nail patella syndrome (Q87.2)

   Q74.2   **Other congenital malformations of lower limb(s), including pelvic girdle**
       Congenital fusion of sacroiliac joint
       Congenital malformation of ankle joint
       Congenital malformation of sacroiliac joint

       Excludes1   anteversion of femur (neck) (Q65.89)

   Q74.3   **Arthrogryposis multiplex congenita**

   Q74.8   **Other specified congenital malformations of limb(s)**

   Q74.9   Unspecified **congenital malformation of limb(s)**
       Congenital anomaly of limb(s) NOS

● **Q75**   **Other congenital malformations of skull and face bones**

   Excludes1   congenital malformation of face NOS (Q18.-)
         congenital malformation syndromes classified to Q87.-
         dentofacial anomalies [including malocclusion] (M26.-)
         musculoskeletal deformities of head and face (Q67.0-Q67.4)
         skull defects associated with congenital anomalies of brain such as:
           anencephaly (Q00.0)
           encephalocele (Q01.-)
           hydrocephalus (Q03.-)
           microcephaly (Q02)

   Q75.0   **Craniosynostosis**
       Premature closure of sutures of skull
       Acrocephaly
       Imperfect fusion of skull
       Oxycephaly
       Trigonocephaly

   Q75.1   **Craniofacial dysostosis**
       Congenital deformity of head
       Crouzon's disease

Item 17–3   **Anencephalus** is a congenital deformity of the cranial vault. **Craniosynostosis,** also known as craniostenosis and stenocephaly, signifies any form of congenital deformity of the skull that results from the premature closing of the sutures of the skull. **Iniencephaly** is a deformity in which the head and neck are flexed backward to a great extent and the head is very large in comparison to the shortened body.

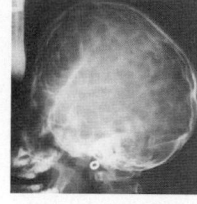

Figure 17-10   Generalized craniosynostosis in a 4-year-old girl without symptoms or signs of increased intracranial pressure. (From Bell WE, McCormick WF: Increased Intracranial Pressure in Children, ed 2, Philadelphia, WB Saunders, 1978, p 116)

   Q75.2   **Hypertelorism**

   Q75.3   **Macrocephaly**
       Unusually large size of head; AKA megalocephaly

   Q75.4   **Mandibulofacial dysostosis**
       Franceschetti syndrome
       Treacher Collins syndrome

   Q75.5   **Oculomandibular dysostosis**
       Ossification of occular and mandibular bones

   Q75.8   **Other specified congenital malformations of skull and face bones**
       Absence of skull bone, congenital
       Congenital deformity of forehead
       Platybasia

   Q75.9   **Congenital malformation of skull and face bones, unspecified**
       Congenital anomaly of face bones NOS
       Congenital anomaly of skull NOS

● **Q76**   **Congenital malformations of spine and bony thorax**

   Excludes1   congenital musculoskeletal deformities of spine and chest (Q67.5-Q67.8)

   Q76.0   **Spina bifida occulta**

       Excludes1   meningocele (spinal) (Q05.-)
            spina bifida (aperta) (cystica) (Q05.-)

   Q76.1   **Klippel-Feil syndrome**
       Cervical fusion syndrome

   Q76.2   **Congenital spondylolisthesis**
       Congenital spondylolysis

       Excludes1   spondylolisthesis (acquired) (M43.1-)
            spondylolysis (acquired) (M43.0-)

   Q76.3   **Congenital scoliosis due to congenital bony malformation**
       Hemivertebra fusion or failure of segmentation with scoliosis

● **Q76.4**   **Other congenital malformations of spine, not associated with scoliosis**

   ● **Q76.41**   **Congenital kyphosis**
       Abnormal increase in convexity curvature of thoracic spinal column; AKA humpback

       Q76.411   **Congenital kyphosis, occipito-atlanto-axial region**

       Q76.412   **Congenital kyphosis, cervical region**

       Q76.413   **Congenital kyphosis, cervicothoracic region**

       Q76.414   **Congenital kyphosis, thoracic region**

       Q76.415   **Congenital kyphosis, thoracolumbar region**

       Q76.419   **Congenital kyphosis, unspecified region**

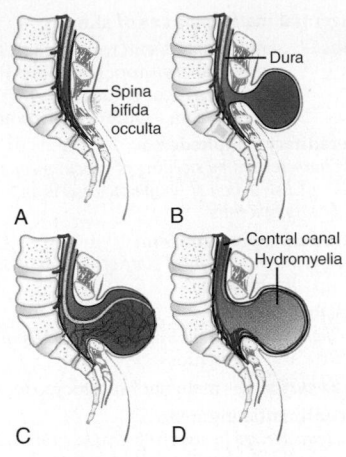

Figure 17-11 **A.** Spina bifida occulta. **B.** Meningocele.
C. Myelomeningocele. **D.** Myelocystocele (syringomyelocele)
or hydromyelia.

Item 17-4 **Spina bifida** is a midline spinal defect in which one or more vertebrae fail to fuse, leaving an opening in the vertebral canal. When the defect is not visible, it is called spina bifida occulta, and when it is visible, it is called spina bifida cystica.

● **Q76.42** **Congenital lordosis**
An abnormal increase in curvature of lumbar spine (sway back)

     Q76.425 **Congenital lordosis, thoracolumbar region**

     Q76.426 **Congenital lordosis, lumbar region**

     Q76.427 **Congenital lordosis, lumbosacral region**

     Q76.428 **Congenital lordosis, sacral and sacrococcygeal region**

     Q76.429 **Congenital lordosis, unspecified region**

   Q76.49 **Other congenital malformations of spine, not associated with scoliosis**
Congenital absence of vertebra NOS
Congenital fusion of spine NOS
Congenital malformation of lumbosacral (joint) (region) NOS
Congenital malformation of spine NOS
Hemivertebra NOS
Malformation of spine NOS
Platyspondylisis NOS
Supernumerary vertebra NOS

Q76.5 **Cervical rib**
Supernumerary rib in cervical region

Q76.6 **Other congenital malformations of ribs**
Accessory rib
Congenital absence of rib
Congenital fusion of ribs
Congenital malformation of ribs NOS

     Excludes1   short rib syndrome (Q77.2)

Q76.7 **Congenital malformation of sternum**
Congenital absence of sternum
Sternum bifidum

Q76.8 **Other congenital malformations of bony thorax**

Q76.9 **Congenital malformation of bony thorax, unspecified**

● **Q77** **Osteochondrodysplasia with defects of growth of tubular bones and spine**

     Excludes1   mucopolysaccharidosis (E76.0-E76.3)

     Excludes2   congenital myotonic chondrodystrophy (G71.13)

Q77.0 **Achondrogenesis**
Hypochondrogenesis

Q77.1 **Thanatophoric short stature**

Q77.2 **Short rib syndrome**
Asphyxiating thoracic dysplasia [Jeune]

Q77.3 **Chondrodysplasia punctata**
Benign cartilaginous neoplasms

     Excludes1   rhizomelic chondrodysplasia punctata (E71.43)

Q77.4 **Achondroplasia**
Disturbance of epiphyseal chondroblastic growth and maturation, results in dwarfism
Hypochondroplasia
Osteosclerosis congenita

Q77.5 **Diastrophic dysplasia**

Q77.6 **Chondroectodermal dysplasia**
Defective development of skin, hair, teeth, with polydactyly and defect of cardiac septum
Ellis-van Creveld syndrome

Q77.7 **Spondyloepiphyseal dysplasia**

Q77.8 **Other osteochondrodysplasia with defects of growth of tubular bones and spine**

Q77.9 **Osteochondrodysplasia with defects of growth of tubular bones and spine, unspecified**

● **Q78** **Other osteochondrodysplasias**
Disorder of development of bone and cartilage; common cause of dwarfism

     Excludes2   congenital myotonic chondrodystrophy (G71.13)

Q78.0 **Osteogenesis imperfecta**
Fragilitas ossium
Osteopsathyrosis

Q78.1 **Polyostotic fibrous dysplasia**
Albright(-McCune)(-Sternberg) syndrome

Q78.2 **Osteopetrosis**
Abnormally dense bone; AKA marble bones disease, ivory bones
Albers-Schönberg syndrome
Osteosclerosis NOS

Q78.3 **Progressive diaphyseal dysplasia**
Camurati-Engelmann syndrome

Q78.4 **Enchondromatosis**
Thinning of overlying cortex of bone and distorted length
Maffucci's syndrome
Ollier's disease

Q78.5 **Metaphyseal dysplasia**
Disturbance in enchondral bone growth, causing ends of shafts to remain larger than normal in circumference
Pyle's syndrome

Q78.6 **Multiple congenital exostoses**
Diaphyseal aclasis

Q78.8 **Other specified osteochondrodysplasias**
Osteopoikilosis

Q78.9 **Osteochondrodysplasia, unspecified**
Chondrodystrophy NOS
AKA skeletal dysplasia (dwarfism) caused by genetic mutations affecting hyaline cartilage capping long bones and vertebrae
Osteodystrophy NOS

CHAPTER 17 (Q00-Q99)

CHAPTER 17 (Q00-Q99)

● **Q79   Congenital malformations of musculoskeletal system, not elsewhere classified**

> **Excludes2**   congenital (sternomastoid) torticollis (Q68.0)

Q79.0   **Congenital diaphragmatic hernia**

> **Excludes1**   congenital hiatus hernia (Q40.1)

Q79.1   **Other congenital malformations of diaphragm**
Absence of diaphragm
Congenital malformation of diaphragm NOS
Eventration of diaphragm

Q79.2   **Exomphalos**
Abdominal hernia in which part of intestine protrudes at umbilicus; AKA exomphalos and exumbilication
Omphalocele

> **Excludes1**   umbilical hernia (K42.-)

Q79.3   **Gastroschisis**
Congenital fissure of anterior abdominal wall often with protrusion of small/large intestine

Q79.4   **Prune belly syndrome**
Congenital prolapse of bladder mucosa
Eagle-Barrett syndrome

● Q79.5   **Other congenital malformations of abdominal wall**

> **Excludes1**   umbilical hernia (K42.-)

Q79.51   **Congenital hernia of bladder**

Q79.59   **Other congenital malformations of abdominal wall**

Q79.6   **Ehlers-Danlos syndrome**
Group of inherited disorders of connective tissue; AKA cutis hyperelastica

Q79.8   **Other congenital malformations of musculoskeletal system**
Absence of muscle
Absence of tendon
Accessory muscle
Amyotrophia congenita
Congenital constricting bands
Congenital shortening of tendon
Poland syndrome

Q79.9   **Congenital malformation of musculoskeletal system, unspecified**
Congenital anomaly of musculoskeletal system NOS
Congenital deformity of musculoskeletal system NOS

OTHER CONGENITAL MALFORMATIONS (Q80-Q89)

● **Q80   Congenital ichthyosis**
Characterized by increased keratinization, resulting in noninflammatory scaling of skin

> **Excludes1**   Refsum's disease (G60.1)

Q80.0   **Ichthyosis vulgaris**

Q80.1   **X-linked ichthyosis**

Q80.2   **Lamellar ichthyosis**
Collodion baby

Q80.3   **Congenital bullous ichthyosiform erythroderma**

Q80.4   **Harlequin fetus**

Q80.8   **Other congenital ichthyosis**

Q80.9   **Congenital ichthyosis, unspecified**

● **Q81   Epidermolysis bullosa**
Loosening of epidermis

Q81.0   **Epidermolysis bullosa simplex**

> **Excludes1**   Cockayne's syndrome (Q87.1)

Q81.1   **Epidermolysis bullosa letalis**
Herlitz' syndrome

Q81.2   **Epidermolysis bullosa dystrophica**

Q81.8   **Other epidermolysis bullosa**

Q81.9   **Epidermolysis bullosa, unspecified**

● **Q82   Other congenital malformations of skin**

> **Excludes1**   acrodermatitis enteropathica (E83.2)
> congenital erythropoietic porphyria (E80.0)
> pilonidal cyst or sinus (L05.-)
> Sturge-Weber (-Dimitri) syndrome (Q85.8)

Q82.0   **Hereditary lymphedema**
Characterized by swelling of subcutaneous tissue caused by obstruction of lymphatic vessels and resulting edema of lymph fluid

Q82.1   **Xeroderma pigmentosum**
Dry, rough, discolored state of skin, and formation of scaly desquamation

Q82.2   **Mastocytosis**
Characterized by infiltrates of mast cells in tissues/organs
Urticaria pigmentosa

> **Excludes1**   malignant mastocytosis (C96.2)

Q82.3   **Incontinentia pigmenti**
Characterized by hyperpigmented cutaneous

Q82.4   **Ectodermal dysplasia (anhidrotic)**
Absence/deficiency of tissues/structures, including teeth, hair, nails, and certain glands

> **Excludes1**   Ellis-van Creveld syndrome (Q77.6)

Q82.5   **Congenital non-neoplastic nevus**
Birthmark NOS
Flammeus Nevus
Portwine Nevus
Sanguineous Nevus
Strawberry Nevus
Vascular Nevus NOS
Verrucous Nevus

> **Excludes2**   Café au lait spots (L81.3)
> lentigo (L81.4)
> nevus NOS (D22.-)
> araneus nevus (I78.1)
> melanocytic nevus (D22.-)
> pigmented nevus (D22.-)
> spider nevus (I78.1)
> stellar nevus (I78.1)

Q82.8   **Other specified congenital malformations of skin**
Abnormal palmar creases
Accessory skin tags
Benign familial pemphigus [Hailey-Hailey]
Congenital poikiloderma
Cutis laxa (hyperelastica)
Dermatoglyphic anomalies
Inherited keratosis palmaris et plantaris
Keratosis follicularis [Darier-White]

> **Excludes1**   Ehlers-Danlos syndrome (Q79.6)

Q82.9   **Congenital malformation of skin, unspecified**

● **Q83   Congenital malformations of breast**

> **Excludes2**   absence of pectoral muscle (Q79.8)
> hypoplasia of breast (N64.82)
> micromastia (N64.82)

Q83.0   **Congenital absence of breast with absent nipple**

Q83.1   **Accessory breast**
Supernumerary breast

Q83.2   **Absent nipple**

Q83.3   **Accessory nipple**
Supernumerary nipple

Q83.8   **Other congenital malformations of breast**

Q83.9   **Congenital malformation of breast, unspecified**

◀ New   ◀▥ Revised   ~~deleted~~ Deleted   Excludes 1   Excludes 2   Includes   Use additional   Code first   Code also   Unspecified

OGCR Official Guidelines   X Assign placeholder X   ● Use Additional Character(s)   ▶ Manifestation Code   **Coding Clinic**

● **Q84   Other congenital malformations of integument**

Q84.0   Congenital alopecia
Congenital atrichosis

Q84.1   Congenital morphological disturbances of hair, not elsewhere classified
Beaded hair
Monilethrix
Pili annulati

Excludes1   Menkes' kinky hair syndrome (E83.0)

Q84.2   Other congenital malformations of hair
Congenital hypertrichosis
Congenital malformation of hair NOS
Persistent lanugo

Q84.3   Anonychia
Absence of nail

Excludes1   nail patella syndrome (Q87.2)

Q84.4   Congenital leukonychia
Opaque, whitish discoloration of nails; AKA leukopathia unguium

Q84.5   Enlarged and hypertrophic nails
Congenital onychauxis
Pachyonychia

Q84.6   Other congenital malformations of nails
Congenital clubnail
Congenital koilonychia
Congenital malformation of nail NOS

Q84.8   Other specified congenital malformations of integument
Aplasia cutis congenita

Q84.9   Congenital malformation of integument, unspecified
Congenital anomaly of integument NOS
Congenital deformity of integument NOS

● **Q85   Phakomatoses, not elsewhere classified**

Excludes1   ataxia telangiectasia [Louis-Bar] (G11.3)
familial dysautonomia [Riley-Day] (G90.1)

● **Q85.0   Neurofibromatosis (nonmalignant)**
Developmental changes in nervous system and other structures, with formation of neurofibromas

Q85.00   Neurofibromatosis, unspecified

Q85.01   Neurofibromatosis, type 1
Von Recklinghausen disease

Q85.02   Neurofibromatosis, type 2
Acoustic neurofibromatosis

Q85.03   Schwannomatosis

Q85.09   Other neurofibromatosis

Q85.1   Tuberous sclerosis
Bourneville's disease
Epiloia

Q85.8   Other phakomatoses, not elsewhere classified
Peutz-Jeghers Syndrome
Sturge-Weber(-Dimitri) syndrome
von Hippel-Lindau syndrome

Excludes1   Meckel-Gruber syndrome (Q61.9)

Q85.9   Phakomatosis, unspecified
Hamartosis NOS

● **Q86   Congenital malformation syndromes due to known exogenous causes, not elsewhere classified**

Excludes2   iodine-deficiency-related hypothyroidism (E00-E02)
nonteratogenic effects of substances transmitted via placenta or breast milk (P04.-)

Q86.0   Fetal alcohol syndrome (dysmorphic)

Q86.1   Fetal hydantoin syndrome   **N**
Meadow's syndrome

Q86.2   Dysmorphism due to warfarin

Q86.8   Other congenital malformation syndromes due to known exogenous causes

● **Q87   Other specified congenital malformation syndromes affecting multiple systems**

Use additional code(s) to identify all associated manifestations

Q87.0   Congenital malformation syndromes predominantly affecting facial appearance
Acrocephalopolysyndactyly
Acrocephalosyndactyly [Apert]
Cryptophthalmos syndrome
Cyclopia
Goldenhar syndrome
Moebius syndrome
Oro-facial-digital syndrome
Robin syndrome
Whistling face

Q87.1   Congenital malformation syndromes predominantly associated with short stature
Aarskog syndrome
Cockayne syndrome
De Lange syndrome
Dubowitz syndrome
Noonan syndrome
Prader-Willi syndrome
Robinow-Silverman-Smith syndrome
Russell-Silver syndrome
Seckel syndrome

Excludes1   Ellis-van Creveld syndrome (Q77.6)
Smith-Lemli-Opitz syndrome (E78.72)

Q87.2   Congenital malformation syndromes predominantly involving limbs
Holt-Oram syndrome
Klippel-Trenaunay-Weber syndrome
Nail patella syndrome
Rubinstein-Taybi syndrome
Sirenomelia syndrome
Thrombocytopenia with absent radius [TAR] syndrome
VATER syndrome

Q87.3   Congenital malformation syndromes involving early overgrowth
Beckwith-Wiedemann syndrome
Sotos' syndrome
Weaver syndrome

● **Q87.4   Marfan's syndrome**

Q87.40   Marfan's syndrome, unspecified

● **Q87.41   Marfan's syndrome with cardiovascular manifestations**

Q87.410   Marfan's syndrome with aortic dilation

Q87.418   Marfan's syndrome with other cardiovascular manifestations

Q87.42   Marfan's syndrome with ocular manifestations

Q87.43   Marfan's syndrome with skeletal manifestation

Q87.5   Other congenital malformation syndromes with other skeletal changes

● **Q87.8   Other specified congenital malformation syndromes, not elsewhere classified**

Excludes1   Zellweger syndrome (E71.510)

Q87.81   Alport syndrome
Progressive sensorineural hearing loss, progressive pyelonephritis or glomerulonephritis, and ocular defects

Use additional code to identify stage of chronic kidney disease (N18.1-N18.6)

Q87.89   Other specified congenital malformation syndromes, not elsewhere classified
Laurence-Moon (-Bardet)-Biedl syndrome

CHAPTER 17 (Q00-Q99)

CHAPTER 17 (Q00-Q99)

● **Q89   Other congenital malformations, not elsewhere classified**

  ● **Q89.0   Congenital absence and malformations of spleen**

       Excludes1 isomerism of atrial appendages (with asplenia or polysplenia) (Q20.6)

      Q89.01   Asplenia (congenital)

      Q89.09   Congenital malformations of spleen
          Congenital splenomegaly

  Q89.1   Congenital malformations of adrenal gland

       Excludes1 adrenogenital disorders (E25.-)
          congenital adrenal hyperplasia (E25.0)

  Q89.2   Congenital malformations of other endocrine glands
      Congenital malformation of parathyroid or thyroid gland
      Persistent thyroglossal duct
      Thyroglossal cyst

       Excludes1 congenital goiter (E03.0)
          congenital hypothyroidism (E03.1)

  Q89.3   Situs inversus
      Lateral transposition of viscera of thorax and abdomen
      Dextrocardia with situs inversus
      Mirror-image atrial arrangement with situs inversus
      Situs inversus or transversus abdominalis
      Situs inversus or transversus thoracis
      Transposition of abdominal viscera
      Transposition of thoracic viscera

       Excludes1 dextrocardia NOS (Q24.0)

  Q89.4   Conjoined twins
      Craniopagus
      Dicephaly
      Pygopagus
      Thoracopagus

  Q89.7   Multiple congenital malformations, not elsewhere classified
      Multiple congenital anomalies NOS
      Multiple congenital deformities NOS

       Excludes1 congenital malformation syndromes affecting multiple systems (Q87.-)

  Q89.8   Other specified congenital malformations
      Use additional code(s) to identify all associated manifestations

  Q89.9   Congenital malformation, unspecified
      Congenital anomaly NOS
      Congenital deformity NOS

CHROMOSOMAL ABNORMALITIES, NOT ELSEWHERE CLASSIFIED (Q90-Q99)

    Excludes2 mitochondrial metabolic disorders (E88.4-)

● **Q90   Down syndrome**
    Use additional code(s) to identify any associated physical conditions and degree of intellectual disabilities (F70-F79)

  Q90.0   Trisomy 21, nonmosaicism (meiotic nondisjunction)
      Trisomy 21, nondisjunction, accounts for 95% of Downs syndrome cases

  Q90.1   Trisomy 21, mosaicism (mitotic nondisjunction)

  Q90.2   Trisomy 21, translocation

  Q90.9   Down syndrome, unspecified
      Trisomy 21 NOS

● **Q91   Trisomy 18 and Trisomy 13**

  Q91.0   Trisomy 18, nonmosaicism (meiotic nondisjunction)

  Q91.1   Trisomy 18, mosaicism (mitotic nondisjunction)

  Q91.2   Trisomy 18, translocation

  Q91.3   Trisomy 18, unspecified

  Q91.4   Trisomy 13, nonmosaicism (meiotic nondisjunction)

  Q91.5   Trisomy 13, mosaicism (mitotic nondisjunction)

  Q91.6   Trisomy 13, translocation

  Q91.7   Trisomy 13, unspecified

● **Q92   Other trisomies and partial trisomies of the autosomes, not elsewhere classified**

    Includes unbalanced translocations and insertions
    Excludes1 trisomies of chromosomes 13, 18, 21 (Q90-Q91)

  Q92.0   Whole chromosome trisomy, nonmosaicism (meiotic nondisjunction)

  Q92.1   Whole chromosome trisomy, mosaicism (mitotic nondisjunction)

  Q92.2   Partial trisomy
      Less than whole arm duplicated
      Whole arm or more duplicated

       Excludes1 partial trisomy due to unbalanced translocation (Q92.5)

  Q92.5   Duplications with other complex rearrangements
      Partial trisomy due to unbalanced translocations

      Code also any associated deletions due to unbalanced translocations, inversions and insertions (Q93.7)

  ● **Q92.6   Marker chromosomes**
      Trisomies due to dicentrics
      Trisomies due to extra rings
      Trisomies due to isochromosomes
      Individual with marker heterochromatin

      Q92.61   Marker chromosomes in normal individual

      Q92.62   Marker chromosomes in abnormal individual

  Q92.7   Triploidy and polyploidy

  Q92.8   Other specified trisomies and partial trisomies of autosomes
      Duplications identified by fluorescence in situ hybridization (FISH)
      Duplications identified by in situ hybridization (ISH)
      Duplications seen only at prometaphase

  Q92.9   Trisomy and partial trisomy of autosomes, unspecified

● **Q93   Monosomies and deletions from the autosomes, not elsewhere classified**

  Q93.0   Whole chromosome monosomy, nonmosaicism (meiotic nondisjunction)

  Q93.1   Whole chromosome monosomy, mosaicism (mitotic nondisjunction)

  Q93.2   Chromosome replaced with ring, dicentric or isochromosome

  Q93.3   Deletion of short arm of chromosome 4
      Wolff-Hirschorn syndrome

  Q93.4   Deletion of short arm of chromosome 5
      Cri-du-chat syndrome

  Q93.5   Other deletions of part of a chromosome
      Angelman syndrome

  Q93.7   Deletions with other complex rearrangements
      Deletions due to unbalanced translocations, inversions and insertions

      Code also any associated duplications due to unbalanced translocations, inversions and insertions (Q92.5)

  ● **Q93.8   Other deletions from the autosomes**

      Q93.81   Velo-cardio-facial syndrome
          Deletion 22q11.2

      Q93.88   Other microdeletions Miller-Dieker syndrome
          Smith-Magenis syndrome

      Q93.89   Other deletions from the autosomes
          Deletions identified by fluorescence in situ hybridization (FISH)
          Deletions identified by in situ hybridization (ISH)
          Deletions seen only at prometaphase

  Q93.9   Deletion from autosomes, unspecified

● **Q95**   **Balanced rearrangements and structural markers, not elsewhere classified**

     Includes   Robertsonian and balanced reciprocal translocations and insertions

     Q95.0   **Balanced translocation and insertion in normal individual**

     Q95.1   **Chromosome inversion in normal individual**

     Q95.2   **Balanced autosomal rearrangement in abnormal individual**

     Q95.3   **Balanced sex/autosomal rearrangement in abnormal individual**

     Q95.5   **Individual with autosomal fragile site**

     Q95.8   **Other balanced rearrangements and structural markers**

     Q95.9   **Balanced rearrangement and structural marker, unspecified**

● **Q96**   **Turner's syndrome**

     Caused by missing or incomplete X chromosome affecting growth and sexual development

     Excludes1   Noonan syndrome (Q87.1)

     Q96.0   **Karyotype 45, X ♀**

     Q96.1   **Karyotype 46, X iso (Xq) ♀**

           Karyotype 46, isochromosome Xq

     Q96.2   **Karyotype 46, X with abnormal sex chromosome, except iso (Xq) ♀**

           Karyotype 46, X with abnormal sex chromosome, except isochromosome Xq

     Q96.3   **Mosaicism, 45, X/46, XX or XY ♀**

     Q96.4   **Mosaicism, 45, X/other cell line(s) with abnormal sex chromosome ♀**

     Q96.8   **Other variants of Turner's syndrome ♀**

     Q96.9   **Turner's syndrome, unspecified ♀**

● **Q97**   **Other sex chromosome abnormalities, female phenotype, not elsewhere classified**

     Excludes1   Turner's syndrome (Q96.-)

     Q97.0   **Karyotype 47, XXX ♀**

     Q97.1   **Female with more than three X chromosomes ♀**

     Q97.2   **Mosaicism, lines with various numbers of X chromosomes ♀**

     Q97.3   **Female with 46, XY karyotype ♀**

     Q97.8   **Other specified sex chromosome abnormalities, female phenotype ♀**

     Q97.9   **Sex chromosome abnormality, female phenotype, unspecified ♀**

● **Q98**   **Other sex chromosome abnormalities, male phenotype, not elsewhere classified**

     Q98.0   **Klinefelter syndrome karyotype 47, XXY ♂**

     Q98.1   **Klinefelter syndrome, male with more than two X chromosomes ♂**

     Q98.3   **Other male with 46, XX karyotype ♂**

     Q98.4   **Klinefelter syndrome, unspecified ♂**

     Q98.5   **Karyotype 47, XYY**

     Q98.6   **Male with structurally abnormal sex chromosome ♂**

     Q98.7   **Male with sex chromosome mosaicism ♂**

     Q98.8   **Other specified sex chromosome abnormalities, male phenotype ♂**

     Q98.9   **Sex chromosome abnormality, male phenotype, unspecified ♂**

● **Q99**   **Other chromosome abnormalities, not elsewhere classified**

     Q99.0   **Chimera 46, XX/46, XY**

           Chimera 46, XX/46, XY true hermaphrodite

     Q99.1   **46, XX true hermaphrodite**

           46, XX with streak gonads

           46, XY with streak gonads

           Pure gonadal dysgenesis

     Q99.2   **Fragile X chromosome**

           Fragile X syndrome

     Q99.8   **Other specified chromosome abnormalities**

     Q99.9   **Chromosomal abnormality, unspecified**

CHAPTER 17 (Q00–Q99)

OGCR Section I.B.4.

Signs and symptoms

Codes that describe symptoms and signs, as opposed to diagnoses, are acceptable for reporting purposes when a related definitive diagnosis has not been established (confirmed) by the provider. Chapter 18 of ICD-10-CM, Symptoms, Signs, and Abnormal Clinical and Laboratory Findings, Not Elsewhere Classified (codes R00.0-R99) contains many, but not all codes for symptoms.

Section I.C.18.a. to c.

Symptoms, signs, and abnormal clinical and laboratory findings, not elsewhere classified.

Chapter 18 includes symptoms, signs, abnormal results of clinical or other investigative procedures, and ill-defined conditions regarding which no diagnosis classifiable elsewhere is recorded. Signs and symptoms that point to a specific diagnosis have been assigned to a category in other chapters of the classification.

a. Use of symptom codes

Codes that describe symptoms and signs are acceptable for reporting purposes when a related definitive diagnosis has not been established (confirmed) by the provider.

b. Use of a symptom code with a definitive diagnosis code

Codes for signs and symptoms may be reported in addition to a related definitive diagnosis when the sign or symptom is not routinely associated with that diagnosis, such as the various signs and symptoms associated with complex syndromes. The definitive diagnosis code should be sequenced before the symptom code.

Signs or symptoms that are associated routinely with a disease process should not be assigned as additional codes, unless otherwise instructed by the classification.

c. Combination codes that include symptoms

ICD-10-CM contains a number of combination codes that identify both the definitive diagnosis and common symptoms of that diagnosis. When using one of these combination codes, an additional code should not be assigned for the symptom.

CHAPTER 18

SYMPTOMS, SIGNS AND ABNORMAL CLINICAL AND LABORATORY FINDINGS, NOT ELSEWHERE CLASSIFIED (R00-R99)

Note: This chapter includes symptoms, signs, abnormal results of clinical or other investigative procedures, and ill-defined conditions regarding which no diagnosis classifiable elsewhere is recorded.

Signs and symptoms that point rather definitely to a given diagnosis have been assigned to a category in other chapters of the classification. In general, categories in this chapter include the less well-defined conditions and symptoms that, without the necessary study of the case to establish a final diagnosis, point perhaps equally to two or more diseases or to two or more systems of the body. Practically all categories in the chapter could be designated 'not otherwise specified', 'unknown etiology' or 'transient'. The Alphabetical Index should be consulted to determine which symptoms and signs are to be allocated here and which to other chapters. The residual subcategories, numbered .8, are generally provided for other relevant symptoms that cannot be allocated elsewhere in the classification.

The conditions and signs or symptoms included in categories R00-R94 consist of:
(a) cases for which no more specific diagnosis can be made even after all the facts bearing on the case have been investigated;
(b) signs or symptoms existing at the time of initial encounter that proved to be transient and whose causes could not be determined;
(c) provisional diagnosis in a patient who failed to return for further investigation or care;

(d) cases referred elsewhere for investigation or treatment before the diagnosis was made;
(e) cases in which a more precise diagnosis was not available for any other reason;
(f) certain symptoms, for which supplementary information is provided, that represent important problems in medical care in their own right.

Excludes2   abnormal findings on antenatal screening of mother (O28.-)
     certain conditions originating in the perinatal period (P04-P96)
     signs and symptoms classified in the body system chapters
     signs and symptoms of breast (N63, N64.5)

This chapter contains the following blocks:

R00-R09	Symptoms and signs involving the circulatory and respiratory systems
R10-R19	Symptoms and signs involving the digestive system and abdomen
R20-R23	Symptoms and signs involving the skin and subcutaneous tissue
R25-R29	Symptoms and signs involving the nervous and musculoskeletal systems
R30-R39	Symptoms and signs involving the genitourinary system
R40-R46	Symptoms and signs involving cognition, perception, emotional state and behavior
R47-R49	Symptoms and signs involving speech and voice
R50-R69	General symptoms and signs
R70-R79	Abnormal findings on examination of blood, without diagnosis
R80-R82	Abnormal findings on examination of urine, without diagnosis
R83-R89	Abnormal findings on examination of other body fluids, substances and tissues, without diagnosis
R90-R94	Abnormal findings on diagnostic imaging and in function studies, without diagnosis
R97	Abnormal tumor markers
R99	Ill-defined and unknown cause of mortality

SYMPTOMS AND SIGNS INVOLVING THE CIRCULATORY AND RESPIRATORY SYSTEMS (R00-R09)

● **R00**   **Abnormalities of heart beat**
    Excludes1   abnormalities originating in the perinatal period (P29.1-)
               specified arrhythmias (I47-I49)

  R00.0   **Tachycardia, unspecified**
      Rapid heart rate >100 beats
      Rapid heart beat
      Sinoauricular tachycardia NOS
      Sinus [sinusal] tachycardia NOS
      Excludes1   neonatal tachycardia (P29.11)
                paroxysmal tachycardia (I47.-)

  R00.1   **Bradycardia, unspecified**
      Slow heart rate, <60
      Sinoatrial bradycardia
      Sinus bradycardia
      Slow heart beat
      Vagal bradycardia
      Use additional code for adverse effect, if applicable, to identify drug (T36-T50 with fifth or sixth character 5)
      Excludes1   neonatal bradycardia (P29.12)

  R00.2   **Palpitations**
      Awareness of heart beat

  R00.8   **Other abnormalities of heart beat**

  R00.9   **Unspecified abnormalities of heart beat**

◀ New   ◀▥ Revised   ~~deleted~~ Deleted   Excludes 1   Excludes 2   Includes   Use additional   Code first   Code also   Unspecified

OGCR Official Guidelines   X Assign placeholder X   ● Use Additional Character(s)   ▶ Manifestation Code   **Coding Clinic**

● **R01**   **Cardiac murmurs and other cardiac sounds**
   Excludes1   cardiac murmurs and sounds originating in the perinatal period (P29.8)

   R01.0   **Benign and innocent cardiac murmurs**
     Functional cardiac murmur

   R01.1   **Cardiac murmur, unspecified**
     Cardiac bruit NOS
     Heart murmur NOS

   R01.2   **Other cardiac sounds**
     Cardiac dullness, increased or decreased
     Precordial friction

   OGCR   Section I.C.9.a.7.

   Hypertension, Transient

   Assign code R03.0, Elevated blood pressure reading without diagnosis of hypertension, unless patient has an established diagnosis of hypertension. Assign code O13.-, Gestational [pregnancy-induced] hypertension with significant proteinuria, or O14.-, Pre-eclampsia, for transient hypertension of pregnancy.

● **R03**   **Abnormal blood-pressure reading, without diagnosis**
   R03.0   **Elevated blood-pressure reading, without diagnosis of hypertension**
     Note: This category is to be used to record an episode of elevated blood pressure in a patient in whom no formal diagnosis of hypertension has been made, or as an isolated incidental finding.

   R03.1   **Nonspecific low blood-pressure reading**
     Excludes1   hypotension (I95.-)
       maternal hypotension syndrome (O26.5-)
       neurogenic orthostatic hypotension (G90.3)

● **R04**   **Hemorrhage from respiratory passages**
   R04.0   **Epistaxis**
     Hemorrhage from nose
     Nosebleed

   R04.1   **Hemorrhage from throat**
     Excludes2   hemoptysis (R04.2)

   R04.2   **Hemoptysis**
     Blood-stained sputum
     Cough with hemorrhage

   ● **R04.8**   **Hemorrhage from other sites in respiratory passages**
     R04.81   **Acute idiopathic pulmonary hemorrhage in infants**   **P**
       AIPHI
       Acute idiopathic hemorrhage in infants over 28 days old
       Excludes1   perinatal pulmonary hemorrhage (P26.-)
         von Willebrand's disease (D68.0)

     R04.89   **Hemorrhage from other sites in respiratory passages**
       Pulmonary hemorrhage NOS

   R04.9   **Hemorrhage from respiratory passages, unspecified**

   R05   **Cough**
     Excludes1   cough with hemorrhage (R04.2)
       smoker's cough (J41.0)

● **R06**   **Abnormalities of breathing**
   Excludes1   acute respiratory distress syndrome (J80)
     respiratory arrest (R09.2)
     respiratory arrest of newborn (P28.81)
     respiratory distress syndrome of newborn (P22.-)
     respiratory failure (J96.-)
     respiratory failure of newborn (P28.5)

● **R06.0**   **Dyspnea**
   Excludes1   tachypnea NOS (R06.82)
     transient tachypnea of newborn (P22.1)

   R06.00   **Dyspnea, unspecified**
   R06.01   **Orthopnea**
   R06.02   **Shortness of breath**
   R06.09   **Other forms of dyspnea**

   R06.1   **Stridor**
     Harsh, high-pitched breath sound
     Excludes1   congenital laryngeal stridor (P28.89)
       laryngismus (stridulus) (J38.5)

   R06.2   **Wheezing**
     Excludes1   Asthma (J45.-)

   R06.3   **Periodic breathing**
     Cheyne-Stokes breathing
     An abnormal pattern of breathing with gradually increasing and decreasing tidal volume with some periods of apnea

   R06.4   **Hyperventilation**
     Excludes1   psychogenic hyperventilation (F45.8)

   R06.5   **Mouth breathing**
     Excludes2   dry mouth NOS (R68.2)

   R06.6   **Hiccough**
     Excludes1   psychogenic hiccough (F45.8)

   R06.7   **Sneezing**

   ● **R06.8**   **Other abnormalities of breathing**
     R06.81   **Apnea, not elsewhere classified**
       Apnea NOS
       Excludes1   apnea (of) newborn (P28.4)
         sleep apnea (G47.3-)
         sleep apnea of newborn (primary) (P28.3)

     R06.82   **Tachypnea, not elsewhere classified**
       Tachypnea NOS
       Excludes1   transitory tachypnea of newborn (P22.1)

     R06.83   **Snoring**
     R06.89   **Other abnormalities of breathing**
       Breath-holding (spells)
       Sighing

   R06.9   **Unspecified abnormalities of breathing**

● **R07**   **Pain in throat and chest**
   Excludes1   epidemic myalgia (B33.0)
   Excludes2   jaw pain R68.84
     pain in breast (N64.4)

   R07.0   **Pain in throat**
     Excludes1   chronic sore throat (J31.2)
       sore throat (acute) NOS (J02.9)
     Excludes2   dysphagia (R13.1-)
       pain in neck (M54.2)

   R07.1   **Chest pain on breathing**
     Painful respiration

   R07.2   **Precordial pain**

   ● **R07.8**   **Other chest pain**
     R07.81   **Pleurodynia**
       Pleurodynia NOS
       Excludes1   epidemic pleurodynia (B33.0)

     R07.82   **Intercostal pain**
     R07.89   **Other chest pain**
       Anterior chest-wall pain NOS

   R07.9   **Chest pain, unspecified**

CHAPTER 18 (R00-R99)

CHAPTER 18 (R00-R99)

● **R09   Other symptoms and signs involving the circulatory and respiratory system**

> **Excludes1**   acute respiratory distress syndrome (J80)
> respiratory arrest of newborn (P28.81)
> respiratory distress syndrome of newborn (P22.0)
> respiratory failure (J96.-)
> respiratory failure of newborn (P28.5)

● **R09.0   Asphyxia and hypoxemia**

> **Excludes1**   asphyxia due to carbon monoxide (T58.-)
> asphyxia due to foreign body in respiratory tract (T17.-)
> birth (intrauterine) asphyxia (P84)
> hypercapnia (R06.4)
> hyperventilation (R06.4)
> traumatic asphyxia (T71.-)

R09.01   **Asphyxia**

R09.02   **Hypoxemia**

R09.1   **Pleurisy**
Occurs when double membrane (pleura) lining chest cavity and lung surface becomes inflamed causing sharp pain on inspiration/expiration.

> **Excludes1**   pleurisy with effusion (J90)

R09.2   **Respiratory arrest**
Cardiorespiratory failure

> **Excludes1**   cardiac arrest (I46.-)
> respiratory arrest of newborn (P28.81)
> respiratory distress of newborn (P22.0)
> respiratory failure (J96.-)
> respiratory failure of newborn (P28.5)
> respiratory insufficiency (R06.89)
> respiratory insufficiency of newborn (P28.5)

R09.3   **Abnormal sputum**
Abnormal amount of sputum
Abnormal color of sputum
Abnormal odor of sputum
Excessive sputum

> **Excludes1**   blood-stained sputum (R04.2)

● **R09.8   Other specified symptoms and signs involving the circulatory and respiratory systems**

R09.81   **Nasal congestion**

R09.82   **Postnasal drip**

R09.89   **Other specified symptoms and signs involving the circulatory and respiratory systems**
Bruit (arterial)
Abnormal chest percussion
Feeling of foreign body in throat
Friction sounds in chest
Chest tympany
Choking sensation
Rales
Wet rattling, clicking, crackling sounds on auscultation
Weak pulse

> **Excludes2**   foreign body in throat (T17.2-)
> wheezing (R06.2)

SYMPTOMS AND SIGNS INVOLVING THE DIGESTIVE SYSTEM AND ABDOMEN (R10-R19)

> **Excludes1**   congenital or infantile pylorospasm (Q40.0)
> gastrointestinal hemorrhage (K92.0-K92.2)
> intestinal obstruction (K56.-)
> newborn gastrointestinal hemorrhage (P54.0-P54.3)
> newborn intestinal obstruction (P76.-)
> pylorospasm (K31.3)
> signs and symptoms involving the urinary system (R30-R39)
> symptoms referable to female genital organs (N94.-)
> symptoms referable to male genital organs male (N48-N50)

● **R10   Abdominal and pelvic pain**

> **Excludes1**   renal colic (N23)
> **Excludes2**   dorsalgia (M54.-)
> flatulence and related conditions (R14.-)

R10.0   **Acute abdomen**
Severe abdominal pain (generalized) (with abdominal rigidity)

> **Excludes1**   abdominal rigidity NOS (R19.3)
> generalized abdominal pain NOS (R10.84)
> localized abdominal pain (R10.1-R10.3-)

● **R10.1   Pain localized to upper abdomen**

R10.10   **Upper abdominal pain, unspecified**

R10.11   **Right upper quadrant pain**

R10.12   **Left upper quadrant pain**

R10.13   **Epigastric pain**
Dyspepsia

> **Excludes1**   functional dyspepsia (K30)

R10.2   **Pelvic and perineal pain**

> **Excludes1**   vulvodynia (N94.81)

● **R10.3   Pain localized to other parts of lower abdomen**

R10.30   **Lower abdominal pain, unspecified**

R10.31   **Right lower quadrant pain**

R10.32   **Left lower quadrant pain**

R10.33   **Periumbilical pain**

● **R10.8   Other abdominal pain**

● **R10.81   Abdominal tenderness**
Abdominal tenderness NOS

R10.811   **Right upper quadrant abdominal tenderness**

R10.812   **Left upper quadrant abdominal tenderness**

R10.813   **Right lower quadrant abdominal tenderness**

R10.814   **Left lower quadrant abdominal tenderness**

R10.815   **Periumbilic abdominal tenderness**

R10.816   **Epigastric abdominal tenderness**

R10.817   **Generalized abdominal tenderness**

R10.819   **Abdominal tenderness, unspecified site**

● **R10.82   Rebound abdominal tenderness**

R10.821   **Right upper quadrant rebound abdominal tenderness**

R10.822   **Left upper quadrant rebound abdominal tenderness**

R10.823   **Right lower quadrant rebound abdominal tenderness**

R10.824   **Left lower quadrant rebound abdominal tenderness**

R10.825   **Periumbilic rebound abdominal tenderness**

R10.826   **Epigastric rebound abdominal tenderness**

R10.827   **Generalized rebound abdominal tenderness**

R10.829   **Rebound abdominal tenderness, unspecified site**

R10.83   **Colic**   P
Colic NOS
Infantile colic

> **Excludes1**   colic in adult and child over 12 months old (R10.84)

R10.84   **Generalized abdominal pain**

> **Excludes1**   generalized abdominal pain associated with acute abdomen (R10.0)

R10.9   **Unspecified abdominal pain**

◀ New   ◀▥ Revised   ~~deleted~~ Deleted   Excludes 1   Excludes 2   Includes   Use additional   Code first   Code also   Unspecified

OGCR Official Guidelines   X Assign placeholder X   ● Use Additional Character(s)   ▶ Manifestation Code   **Coding Clinic**

● **R11**   **Nausea and vomiting**
    Excludes1   cyclical vomiting associated with migraine
          (G43.A-)
        excessive vomiting in pregnancy (O21.-)
        hematemesis (K92.0)
        neonatal hematemesis (P54.0)
        newborn vomiting (P92.0-)
        psychogenic vomiting (F50.8)
        vomiting associated with bulimia nervosa (F50.2)
        vomiting following gastrointestinal surgery
          (K91.0)

● **R11.0**   **Nausea**
    Nausea NOS
    Nausea without vomiting

● **R11.1**   **Vomiting**
  R11.10   **Vomiting, unspecified**
      Vomiting NOS
  R11.11   **Vomiting without nausea**
  R11.12   **Projectile vomiting**
  R11.13   **Vomiting of fecal matter**
  R11.14   **Bilious vomiting**
      Bilious emesis

R11.2   **Nausea with vomiting, unspecified**
    Persistent nausea with vomiting NOS

R12   **Heartburn**
    Excludes1   dyspepsia NOS (R10.13)
        functional dyspepsia (K30)

● **R13**   **Aphagia and dysphagia**
  R13.0   **Aphagia**
    Inability to swallow
    Excludes1   psychogenic aphagia (F50.9)

● **R13.1**   **Dysphagia**
    Difficulty swallowing
    Code first, if applicable, dysphagia following cerebrovascular
      disease (I69. with final characters -91)
    Excludes1   psychogenic dysphagia (F45.8)
  R13.10   **Dysphagia, unspecified**
      Difficulty in swallowing NOS
  R13.11   **Dysphagia, oral phase**
  R13.12   **Dysphagia, oropharyngeal phase**
  R13.13   **Dysphagia, pharyngeal phase**
  R13.14   **Dysphagia, pharyngoesophageal phase**
  R13.19   **Other dysphagia**
      Cervical dysphagia
      Neurogenic dysphagia

● **R14**   **Flatulence and related conditions**
    Excludes1   psychogenic aerophagy (F45.8)
  R14.0   **Abdominal distension (gaseous)**
    Bloating
    Tympanites (abdominal) (intestinal)
  R14.1   **Gas pain**
  R14.2   **Eructation**
    Belching air from stomach through mouth
  R14.3   **Flatulence**

● **R15**   **Fecal incontinence**
    Includes   encopresis NOS
    Excludes1   fecal incontinence of nonorganic origin (F98.1)
  R15.0   **Incomplete defecation**
    Excludes1   constipation (K59.0-)
        fecal impaction (K56.41)
  R15.1   **Fecal smearing**
    Fecal soiling
  R15.2   **Fecal urgency**
  R15.9   **Full incontinence of feces**
    Fecal incontinence NOS

● **R16**   **Hepatomegaly and splenomegaly, not elsewhere classified**
    Enlargement of liver or spleen
  R16.0   **Hepatomegaly, not elsewhere classified**
    Hepatomegaly NOS
  R16.1   **Splenomegaly, not elsewhere classified**
    Splenomegaly NOS
  R16.2   **Hepatomegaly with splenomegaly, not elsewhere classified**
    Hepatosplenomegaly NOS

R17   **Unspecified jaundice**
    Excludes1   neonatal jaundice (P55, P57-P59)

● **R18**   **Ascites**
    Includes   fluid in peritoneal cavity
    Excludes1   ascites in alcoholic cirrhosis (K70.31)
        ascites in alcoholic hepatitis (K70.11)
        ascites in toxic liver disease with chronic active
          hepatitis (K71.51)
  R18.0   **Malignant ascites**
    Code first malignancy, such as:
      malignant neoplasm of ovary (C56.-)
      secondary malignant neoplasm of retroperitoneum
        and peritoneum (C78.6)
  R18.8   **Other ascites**
    Ascites NOS
    Peritoneal effusion (chronic)

● **R19**   **Other symptoms and signs involving the digestive system and abdomen**
    Excludes1   acute abdomen (R10.0)

● **R19.0**   **Intra-abdominal and pelvic swelling, mass and lump**
    Excludes1   abdominal distension (gaseous) (R14.-)
        ascites (R18.-)
  R19.00   **Intra-abdominal and pelvic swelling, mass and lump, unspecified site**
  R19.01   **Right upper quadrant abdominal swelling, mass and lump**
  R19.02   **Left upper quadrant abdominal swelling, mass and lump**
  R19.03   **Right lower quadrant abdominal swelling, mass and lump**
  R19.04   **Left lower quadrant abdominal swelling, mass and lump**
  R19.05   **Periumbilic swelling, mass or lump**
      Diffuse or generalized umbilical swelling or
        mass
  R19.06   **Epigastric swelling, mass or lump**
  R19.07   **Generalized intra-abdominal and pelvic swelling, mass and lump**
      Diffuse or generalized intra-abdominal
        swelling or mass NOS
      Diffuse or generalized pelvic swelling or mass
        NOS
  R19.09   **Other intra-abdominal and pelvic swelling, mass and lump**

● **R19.1**   **Abnormal bowel sounds**
  R19.11   **Absent bowel sounds**
  R19.12   **Hyperactive bowel sounds**
  R19.15   **Other abnormal bowel sounds**
      Abnormal bowel sounds NOS

R19.2   **Visible peristalsis**
    Hyperperistalsis

● **R19.3**   **Abdominal rigidity**
    Excludes1   abdominal rigidity with severe
        abdominal pain (R10.0)
  R19.30   **Abdominal rigidity, unspecified site**
  R19.31   **Right upper quadrant abdominal rigidity**

CHAPTER 18 (R00-R99)

CHAPTER 18 (R00-R99)

R19.32   Left upper quadrant abdominal rigidity
R19.33   Right lower quadrant abdominal rigidity
R19.34   Left lower quadrant abdominal rigidity
R19.35   Periumbilic abdominal rigidity
R19.36   Epigastric abdominal rigidity
R19.37   Generalized abdominal rigidity

R19.4   Change in bowel habit
> **Excludes1**   constipation (K59.0-)
>   functional diarrhea (K59.1)

R19.5   Other fecal abnormalities
Abnormal stool color
Bulky stools
Mucus in stools
Occult blood in feces
Occult blood in stools
> **Excludes1**   melena (K92.1)
>   neonatal melena (P54.1)

R19.6   Halitosis

R19.7   Diarrhea, unspecified
Diarrhea NOS
> **Excludes1**   functional diarrhea (K59.1)
>   neonatal diarrhea (P78.3)
>   psychogenic diarrhea (F45.8)

R19.8   Other specified symptoms and signs involving the digestive system and abdomen

SYMPTOMS AND SIGNS INVOLVING THE SKIN AND SUBCUTANEOUS TISSUE (R20-R23)

> **Excludes2**   symptoms relating to breast (N64.4-N64.5)

● **R20**   Disturbances of skin sensation
> **Excludes1**   dissociative anesthesia and sensory loss (F44.6)
>   psychogenic disturbances (F45.8)

R20.0   Anesthesia of skin
Loss of sensation

R20.1   Hypoesthesia of skin
Unpleasant abnormal sensation

R20.2   Paresthesia of skin
Abnormal touch sensation, including burning, prickling, often in absence of external stimulus
Formication   Tingling skin
Pins and needles
> **Excludes1**   acroparesthesia (I73.8)

R20.3   Hyperesthesia

R20.8   Other disturbances of skin sensation

R20.9   Unspecified disturbances of skin sensation

R21   Rash and other nonspecific skin eruption
> **Includes**   rash NOS
> **Excludes1**   specified type of rash- code to condition
>   vesicular eruption (R23.8)

● **R22**   Localized swelling, mass and lump of skin and subcutaneous tissue
> **Includes**   subcutaneous nodules (localized) (superficial)
> **Excludes1**   abnormal findings on diagnostic imaging (R90-R93)
>   edema (R60.-)
>   enlarged lymph nodes (R59.-)
>   localized adiposity (E65)
>   swelling of joint (M25.4-)

R22.0   Localized swelling, mass and lump, head

R22.1   Localized swelling, mass and lump, neck

R22.2   Localized swelling, mass and lump, trunk
> **Excludes1**   intra-abdominal or pelvic mass and lump (R19.0-)
>   intra-abdominal or pelvic swelling (R19.0-)
> **Excludes2**   breast mass and lump (N63)

● **R22.3**   Localized swelling, mass and lump, upper limb
R22.30   Localized swelling, mass and lump, unspecified upper limb
R22.31   Localized swelling, mass and lump, right upper limb
R22.32   Localized swelling, mass and lump, left upper limb
R22.33   Localized swelling, mass and lump, upper limb, bilateral

● **R22.4**   Localized swelling, mass and lump, lower limb
R22.40   Localized swelling, mass and lump, unspecified lower limb
R22.41   Localized swelling, mass and lump, right lower limb
R22.42   Localized swelling, mass and lump, left lower limb
R22.43   Localized swelling, mass and lump, lower limb, bilateral

R22.9   Localized swelling, mass and lump, unspecified

● **R23**   Other skin changes
R23.0   Cyanosis
> **Excludes1**   acrocyanosis (I73.8)
>   cyanotic attacks of newborn (P28.2)

R23.1   Pallor
Clammy skin

R23.2   Flushing
Excessive blushing
Code first, if applicable, menopausal and female climacteric states (N95.1)

R23.3   Spontaneous ecchymoses
Small hemorrhagic spot of skin; AKA black and blue spot
Petechiae
> **Excludes1**   ecchymoses of newborn (P54.5)
>   purpura (D69.-)

R23.4   Changes in skin texture
Desquamation of skin   Scaling of skin
Induration of skin
> **Excludes1**   epidermal thickening NOS (L85.9)

R23.8   Other skin changes

R23.9   Unspecified skin changes

SYMPTOMS AND SIGNS INVOLVING THE NERVOUS AND MUSCULOSKELETAL SYSTEMS (R25-R29)

● **R25**   Abnormal involuntary movements
> **Excludes1**   specific movement disorders (G20-G26)
>   stereotyped movement disorders (F98.4)
>   tic disorders (F95.-)

R25.0   Abnormal head movements

R25.1   Tremor, unspecified
> **Excludes1**   chorea NOS (G25.5)
>   essential tremor (G25.0)
>   hysterical tremor (F44.4)
>   intention tremor (G25.2)

R25.2   Cramp and spasm
> **Excludes2**   carpopedal spasm (R29.0)
>   charley-horse (M62.831)
>   infantile spasms (G40.4-)
>   muscle spasm of back (M62.830)
>   muscle spasm of calf (M62.831)

R25.3   Fasciculation
Twitching NOS

R25.8   Other abnormal involuntary movements

R25.9   Unspecified abnormal involuntary movements

◄ New   ◄▪ Revised   ~~deleted~~ Deleted   Excludes 1   Excludes 2   Includes   Use additional   Code first   Code also   Unspecified
 OGCR Official Guidelines   X Assign placeholder X   ● Use Additional Character(s)   ▶ Manifestation Code   **Coding Clinic**

● R26   **Abnormalities of gait and mobility**
     Excludes 1   ataxia NOS (R27.0)
                   hereditary ataxia (G11.-)
                    locomotor (syphilitic) ataxia (A52.11)
                    immobility syndrome (paraplegic) (M62.3)

     R26.0   **Ataxic gait**
             Staggering gait
     R26.1   **Paralytic gait**
             Spastic gait
     R26.2   **Difficulty in walking, not elsewhere classified**
             Excludes 1   falling (R29.6)
                           unsteadiness on feet (R26.81)
●   R26.8   **Other abnormalities of gait and mobility**
          R26.81   **Unsteadiness on feet**
          R26.89   **Other abnormalities of gait and mobility**
     R26.9   **Unspecified abnormalities of gait and mobility**

● R27   **Other lack of coordination**
     Excludes 1   ataxic gait (R26.0)
                    hereditary ataxia (G11.-)
                    vertigo NOS (R42)

     R27.0   **Ataxia, unspecified**
             Excludes 1   ataxia following cerebrovascular disease
                           (I69. with final characters -93)
     R27.8   **Other lack of coordination**
     R27.9   **Unspecified lack of coordination**

● R29   **Other symptoms and signs involving the nervous and musculoskeletal systems**
     R29.0   **Tetany**
             Hyperexcitability of nerves and muscles characterized by spasm, twitching, and cramps
             Carpopedal spasm
             Excludes 1   hysterical tetany (F44.5)
                         neonatal tetany (P71.3)
                         parathyroid tetany (E20.9)
                         post-thyroidectomy tetany (E89.2)
     R29.1   **Meningismus**
     R29.2   **Abnormal reflex**
             Excludes 2   abnormal pupillary reflex (H57.0)
                         hyperactive gag reflex (J39.2)
                         vasovagal reaction or syncope (R55)
     R29.3   **Abnormal posture**
     R29.4   **Clicking hip**
             Excludes 1   congenital deformities of hip (Q65.-)
     R29.5   **Transient paralysis**
             Code first any associated spinal cord injury (S14.0, S14.1-, S24.0, S24.1-, S34.0-, S34.1-)
             Excludes 1   transient ischemic attack (G45.9)
     R29.6   **Repeated falls**
             Falling
             Tendency to fall
             Excludes 2   at risk for falling (Z91.81)
                         history of falling (Z91.81)

             OGCR Section I.C.18.d.

             Repeated falls

             Code R29.6, Repeated falls, is for use for encounters when a patient has recently fallen and the reason for the fall is being investigated.

             Code Z91.81, History of falling, is for use when a patient has fallen in the past and is at risk for future falls. When appropriate, both codes R29.6 and Z91.81 may be assigned together.

● R29.8   **Other symptoms and signs involving the nervous and musculoskeletal systems**
    ● R29.81   **Other symptoms and signs involving the nervous system**
          R29.810   **Facial weakness**
                  Facial droop
                  Excludes 1   Bell's palsy (G51.0)
                             facial weakness following cerebrovascular disease (I69. with final characters -92)
          R29.818   **Other symptoms and signs involving the nervous system**
    ● R29.89   **Other symptoms and signs involving the musculoskeletal system**
             Excludes 2   pain in limb (M79.6-)
          R29.890   **Loss of height**
                  Excludes 1   osteoporosis (M80-M81)
          R29.891   **Ocular torticollis**
                  Excludes 1   congenital (sterno-mastoid) torticollis Q68.0
                             psychogenic torticollis (F45.8)
                             spasmodic torticollis (G24.3)
                             torticollis due to birth injury (P15.8)
                             torticollis NOS M43.6
          R29.898   **Other symptoms and signs involving the musculoskeletal system**
● R29.9   **Unspecified symptoms and signs involving the nervous and musculoskeletal systems**
          R29.90   **Unspecified symptoms and signs involving the nervous system**
          R29.91   **Unspecified symptoms and signs involving the musculoskeletal system**

SYMPTOMS AND SIGNS INVOLVING THE GENITOURINARY SYSTEM (R30-R39)

● R30   **Pain associated with micturition**
     Excludes 1   psychogenic pain associated with micturition (F45.8)
     R30.0   **Dysuria**
             Painful urination
             Strangury
     R30.1   **Vesical tenesmus**
             Straining to urinate
     R30.9   **Painful micturition, unspecified**
             Painful urination NOS

● R31   **Hematuria**
     Excludes 1   hematuria included with underlying conditions, such as:
                       acute cystitis with hematuria (N30.01)
                       recurrent and persistent hematuria in glomerular diseases (N02.-)
     R31.0   **Gross hematuria**
     R31.1   **Benign essential microscopic hematuria**
     R31.2   **Other microscopic hematuria**
     R31.9   **Hematuria, unspecified**

CHAPTER 18 (R00-R99)

R32   Unspecified urinary incontinence
Enuresis NOS

> **Excludes1** functional urinary incontinence (R39.81)
> nonorganic enuresis (F98.0)
> stress incontinence and other specified urinary
> incontinence (N39.3-N39.4-)
> urinary incontinence associated with cognitive
> impairment (R39.81)

● **R33   Retention of urine**

> **Excludes1** psychogenic retention of urine (F45.8)

R33.0   Drug induced retention of urine
Use additional code for adverse effect, if applicable,
to identify drug (T36-T50 with fifth or sixth
character 5)

R33.8   Other retention of urine
Code first, if applicable, any causal condition, such as:
enlarged prostate (N40.1)

R33.9   Retention of urine, unspecified

R34   Anuria and oliguria

> **Excludes1** anuria and oliguria complicating abortion or
> ectopic or molar pregnancy (O00-O07,
> O08.4)
> anuria and oliguria complicating pregnancy
> (O26.83-)
> anuria and oliguria complicating the puerperium
> (O90.4)

● **R35   Polyuria**
Passage of excessive volume of urine
Code first, if applicable, any causal condition, such as:
enlarged prostate (N40.1)

> **Excludes1** psychogenic polyuria (F45.8)

R35.0   Frequency of micturition
✱ *Discharge or passage of urine; AKA uresis*

R35.1   Nocturia
Urinary frequency at night

R35.8   Other polyuria
Polyuria NOS

● **R36   Urethral discharge**

R36.0   Urethral discharge without blood

R36.1   Hematospermia ♂
Presence of blood in semen

R36.9   Urethral discharge, unspecified
Penile discharge NOS
Urethrorrhea

R37   Sexual dysfunction, unspecified

● **R39   Other and unspecified symptoms and signs involving the
genitourinary system**

R39.0   Extravasation of urine
Leakage, discharge

● **R39.1   Other difficulties with micturition**
Code first, if applicable, any causal condition, such as:
enlarged prostate (N40.1)

R39.11   Hesitancy of micturition

R39.12   Poor urinary stream
Weak urinary steam

R39.13   Splitting of urinary stream

R39.14   Feeling of incomplete bladder emptying

R39.15   Urgency of urination

> **Excludes1** urge incontinence (N39.41,
> N39.46)

R39.16   Straining to void

R39.19   Other difficulties with micturition

R39.2   Extrarenal uremia
Prerenal uremia

> **Excludes1** uremia NOS (N19)

● **R39.8   Other symptoms and signs involving the genitourinary
system**

R39.81   Functional urinary incontinence
Urinary incontinence due to cognitive
impairment, or severe physical disability
or immobility

> **Excludes1** stress incontinence and
> other specified urinary
> incontinence (N39.3-N39.4-)
> urinary incontinence NOS (R32)

**R39.89   Other symptoms and signs involving the
genitourinary system**

**R39.9   Unspecified symptoms and signs involving the
genitourinary system**

SYMPTOMS AND SIGNS INVOLVING COGNITION, PERCEPTION, EMOTIONAL STATE AND BEHAVIOR (R40-R46)

> **Excludes1** symptoms and signs constituting part of a pattern
> of mental disorder (F01-F99)

● **R40   Somnolence, stupor and coma**

> **Excludes1** neonatal coma (P91.5)
> somnolence, stupor and coma in diabetes
> (E08-E13)
> somnolence, stupor and coma in hepatic failure
> (K72.-)
> somnolence, stupor and coma in hypoglycemia
> (nondiabetic) (E15)

R40.0   Somnolence
Drowsiness

> **Excludes1** coma (R40.2-)

R40.1   Stupor
Lowered level of consciousness
Catatonic stupor
Semicoma

> **Excludes1** catatonic schizophrenia (F20.2)
> coma (R40.2-)
> depressive stupor (F31-F33)
> dissociative stupor (F44.2)
> manic stupor (F30.2)

OGCR Section I.C.18.e.

Coma scale

The coma scale codes (R40.2-) can be used in conjunction with
traumatic brain injury codes, acute cerebrovascular disease or sequelae
of cerebrovascular disease codes. These codes are primarily for use
by trauma registries, but they may be used in any setting where this
information is collected. The coma scale codes should be sequenced
after the diagnosis code(s).

These codes, one from each subcategory, are needed to complete the
scale. The 7th character indicates when the scale was recorded. The 7th
character should match for all three codes.

At a minimum, report the initial score documented on presentation
at your facility. This may be a score from the emergency medicine
technician (EMT) or in the emergency department. If desired, a facility
may choose to capture multiple coma scale scores.

Assign code R40.24, Glasgow coma scale, total score, when only the total
score is documented in the medical record and not the individual score(s).

● **R40.2   Coma**
Code first any associated:
fracture of skull (S02.-)
intracranial injury (S06.-)

Note: One code from subcategories R40.21-R40-23 is
required to complete the coma scale

R40.20   Unspecified coma
Coma NOS
Unconsciousness NOS

◀ New   ◀▥ Revised   ~~deleted~~ Deleted   │ Excludes 1 │   │ Excludes 2 │   │ Includes │   │ Use additional │   │ Code first │   │ Code also │   │ Unspecified │

OGCR Official Guidelines   X Assign placeholder X   ● Use Additional Character(s)   ▶ Manifestation Code   **Coding Clinic**

● R40.21   Coma scale, eyes open

The following appropriate 7th character is to be added to subcategory R40.21-:

0	unspecified time
1	in the field [EMT or ambulance]
2	at arrival to emergency department
3	at hospital admission
4	24 hours or more after hospital admission

● R40.211   Coma scale, eyes open, never
● R40.212   Coma scale, eyes open, to pain
● R40.213   Coma scale, eyes open, to sound
● R40.214   Coma scale, eyes open, spontaneous

● R40.22   Coma scale, best verbal response

The following appropriate 7th character is to be added to subcategory R40.22-:

0	unspecified time
1	in the field [EMT or ambulance]
2	at arrival to emergency department
3	at hospital admission
4	24 hours or more after hospital admission

● R40.221   Coma scale, best verbal response, none
● R40.222   Coma scale, best verbal response, incomprehensible words
● R40.223   Coma scale, best verbal response, inappropriate words
● R40.224   Coma scale, best verbal response, confused conversation
● R40.225   Coma scale, best verbal response, oriented

Glasgow Coma Scale

Eye Opening Response	
• Spontaneous--open with blinking at baseline	4 points
• To verbal stimuli, command, speech	3 points
• To pain only (not applied to face)	2 points
• No response	1 point
Verbal Response	
• Oriented	5 points
• Confused conversation, but able to answer questions	4 points
• Inappropriate words	3 points
• Incomprehensible speech	2 points
• No response	1 point
Motor Response	
• Obeys commands for movement	6 points
• Purposeful movement to painful stimulus	5 points
• Withdraws in response to pain	4 points
• Flexion in response to pain (decorticate posturing)	3 points
• Extension response in response to pain (decerebrate posturing)	2 points
• No response	1 point
Categorization: Coma: No eye opening, no ability to follow commands, no word verbalizations (3-8)	
Head Injury Classification: Severe Head Injury--GCS score of 8 or less Moderate Head Injury--GCS score of 9 to 12 Mild head injury--GCS score of 13 to 15	
(Adapted from: Advanced Trauma Life Support: Course for Physicians, American College of Surgeons, 1993). http://www.bt.cdc.gov/masscasulatires/gscale.asp	

Figure 18-1

● R40.23   Coma scale, best motor response

The following appropriate 7th character is to be added to subcategory R40.23-:

0	unspecified time
1	in the field [EMT or ambulance]
2	at arrival to emergency department
3	at hospital admission
4	24 hours or more after hospital admission

● R40.231   Coma scale, best motor response, none
● R40.232   Coma scale, best motor response, extension
● R40.233   Coma scale, best motor response, abnormal
● R40.234   Coma scale, best motor response, flexion withdrawal
● R40.235   Coma scale, best motor response, localizes pain
● R40.236   Coma scale, best motor response, obeys commands

● R40.24   Glasgow coma scale, total score
Use codes R40.21- through R40.23- only when the individual score(s) are documented

R40.241   Glasgow coma scale score 13-15
R40.242   Glasgow coma scale score 9-12
R40.243   Glasgow coma scale score 3-8
R40.244   Other coma, without documented Glasgow coma scale score, or with partial score reported

R40.3   Persistent vegetative state
R40.4   Transient alteration of awareness

● R41   Other symptoms and signs involving cognitive functions and awareness

Excludes1   dissociative [conversion] disorders (F44.-)
mild cognitive impairment, so stated (G31.84)

R41.0   Disorientation, unspecified
Confusion NOS   Delirium NOS

R41.1   Anterograde amnesia
R41.2   Retrograde amnesia
R41.3   Other amnesia
Amnesia NOS
Memory loss NOS

Excludes1   amnestic disorder due to known physiologic condition (F04)
amnestic syndrome due to psychoactive substance use (F10-F19 with 5th character .6)
mild memory disturbance due to known physiological condition (F06.8)
transient global amnesia (G45.4)

R41.4   Neurologic neglect syndrome
Asomatognosia   Left-sided neglect
Hemi-akinesia   Sensory neglect
Hemi-inattention   Visuospatial neglect
Hemispatial neglect

Excludes1   visuospatial deficit (R41.842)

● R41.8   Other symptoms and signs involving cognitive functions and awareness

R41.81   Age-related cognitive decline   A
Senility NOS

R41.82   Altered mental status, unspecified
Change in mental status NOS

Excludes1   altered level of consciousness (R40.-)
altered mental status due to known condition - code to condition
delirium NOS (R41.0)

Coding Clinic: 2012, Q4, P98

R41.83 **Borderline intellectual functioning**
IQ level 71 to 84
Excludes1 intellectual disabilities (F70-F79)

● R41.84 **Other specified cognitive deficit**
R41.840 **Attention and concentration deficit**
Excludes1 attention-deficit hyperactivity disorders (F90.-)
R41.841 **Cognitive communication deficit**
R41.842 **Visuospatial deficit**
R41.843 **Psychomotor deficit**
R41.844 **Frontal lobe and executive function deficit**

R41.89 **Other symptoms and signs involving cognitive functions and awareness**
Anosognosia

R41.9 **Unspecified symptoms and signs involving cognitive functions and awareness**

R42 **Dizziness and giddiness**
Light-headedness
Vertigo NOS
Excludes1 vertiginous syndromes (H81.-)
vertigo from infrasound (T75.23)

● R43 **Disturbances of smell and taste**
R43.0 **Anosmia**
Absence of sense of smell; AKA anosphresia and olfactory anesthesia
R43.1 **Parosmia**
R43.2 **Parageusia**
Perversion of sense of taste or bad taste in mouth; AKA dysgeusia
R43.8 **Other disturbances of smell and taste**
Mixed disturbance of smell and taste
R43.9 **Unspecified disturbances of smell and taste**

● R44 **Other symptoms and signs involving general sensations and perceptions**
Excludes1 alcoholic hallucinations (F1.5)
hallucinations in drug psychosis (F11-F19 with .5)
hallucinations in mood disorders with psychotic symptoms (F30.2, F31.5, F32.3, F33.3)
hallucinations in schizophrenia, schizotypal and delusional disorders (F20-F29)
Excludes2 disturbances of skin sensation (R20.-)
R44.0 **Auditory hallucinations**
R44.1 **Visual hallucinations**
R44.2 **Other hallucinations**
R44.3 **Hallucinations, unspecified**
R44.8 **Other symptoms and signs involving general sensations and perceptions**
R44.9 **Unspecified symptoms and signs involving general sensations and perceptions**

● R45 **Symptoms and signs involving emotional state**
R45.0 **Nervousness**
Nervous tension
R45.1 **Restlessness and agitation**
R45.2 **Unhappiness**
R45.3 **Demoralization and apathy**
Excludes1 anhedonia (R45.84)
R45.4 **Irritability and anger**
R45.5 **Hostility**
R45.6 **Violent behavior**
R45.7 **State of emotional shock and stress, unspecified**

● R45.8 **Other symptoms and signs involving emotional state**
R45.81 **Low self-esteem**
R45.82 **Worries**
R45.83 **Excessive crying of child, adolescent or adult**
Excludes1 excessive crying of infant (baby) R68.11
R45.84 **Anhedonia**
Total loss of feeling of pleasure in pleasurable acts
● R45.85 **Homicidal and suicidal ideations**
Excludes1 suicide attempt (T14.91)
R45.850 **Homicidal ideations**
R45.851 **Suicidal ideations**
R45.86 **Emotional lability**
R45.87 **Impulsiveness**
R45.89 **Other symptoms and signs involving emotional state**

● R46 **Symptoms and signs involving appearance and behavior**
Excludes1 appearance and behavior in schizophrenia, schizotypal and delusional disorders (F20-F29)
mental and behavioral disorders (F01-F99)
R46.0 **Very low level of personal hygiene**
R46.1 **Bizarre personal appearance**
R46.2 **Strange and inexplicable behavior**
R46.3 **Overactivity**
R46.4 **Slowness and poor responsiveness**
Excludes1 stupor (R40.1)
R46.5 **Suspiciousness and marked evasiveness**
R46.6 **Undue concern and preoccupation with stressful events**
R46.7 **Verbosity and circumstantial detail obscuring reason for contact**
● R46.8 **Other symptoms and signs involving appearance and behavior**
R46.81 **Obsessive-compulsive behavior**
Excludes1 obsessive-compulsive disorder (F42)
R46.89 **Other symptoms and signs involving appearance and behavior**

SYMPTOMS AND SIGNS INVOLVING SPEECH AND VOICE (R47-R49)

● R47 **Speech disturbances, not elsewhere classified**
Excludes1 autism (F84.0)
cluttering (F80.81)
specific developmental disorders of speech and language (F80.-)
stuttering (F80.81)
● R47.0 **Dysphasia and aphasia**
R47.01 **Aphasia**
Excludes1 aphasia following cerebrovascular disease (I69. with final characters -20)
progressive isolated aphasia (G31.01)
R47.02 **Dysphasia**
Impairment in comprehension of speech, caused by left-sided brain damage
Excludes1 dysphasia following cerebrovascular disease (I69. with final characters -21)
R47.1 **Dysarthria and anarthria**
Motor speech disorder
Excludes1 dysarthria following cerebrovascular disease (I69. with final characters -22)

◀ New   ◀▪▪ Revised   ~~deleted~~ Deleted   Excludes 1   Excludes 2   Includes   Use additional   Code first   Code also   Unspecified
OGCR Official Guidelines   **X** Assign placeholder X   ● Use Additional Character(s)   ▶ Manifestation Code   **Coding Clinic**

● R47.8   **Other speech disturbances**

     Excludes1   dysarthria following cerebrovascular disease (I69. with final characters -28)

     R47.81   **Slurred speech**

▌   *R47.82*   *Fluency disorder in conditions classified elsewhere*

       Stuttering in conditions classified elsewhere

       Code first underlying disease or condition, such as:
       Parkinson's disease (G20)

       Excludes1   adult onset fluency disorder (F98.5)
             childhood onset fluency disorder (F80.81)
             fluency disorder (stuttering) following cerebrovascular disease (I69. with final characters -23)

     R47.89   **Other speech disturbances**

     R47.9   **Unspecified speech disturbances**

● R48   **Dyslexia and other symbolic dysfunctions, not elsewhere classified**

     Excludes1   specific developmental disorders of scholastic skills (F81.-)

     R48.0   **Dyslexia and alexia**

     R48.1   **Agnosia**

       Loss of ability to recognize objects, persons, sounds, shapes, or smells
       Astereognosia (astereognosis)
       Autotopagnosia

       Excludes1   visual object agnosia (R48.3)

     R48.2   **Apraxia**

       Loss of ability to execute or carry out learned purposeful movements

       Excludes1   apraxia following cerebrovascular disease (I69. with final characters -90)

     R48.3   **Visual agnosia**
       Prosopagnosia
       Simultanagnosia (asimultagnosia)

     R48.8   **Other symbolic dysfunctions**
       Acalculia
       Difficulty performing simple mathematical tasks resulting from neurological injury
       Agraphia

     R48.9   **Unspecified symbolic dysfunctions**

● R49   **Voice and resonance disorders**

     Excludes1   psychogenic voice and resonance disorders (F44.4)

     R49.0   **Dysphonia**
       Hoarseness

     R49.1   **Aphonia**
       Loss of voice

●   R49.2   **Hypernasality and hyponasality**

     R49.21   **Hypernasality**

     R49.22   **Hyponasality**

     R49.8   **Other voice and resonance disorders**

     R49.9   **Unspecified voice and resonance disorder**
       Change in voice NOS
       Resonance disorder NOS

GENERAL SYMPTOMS AND SIGNS (R50-R69)

● R50   **Fever of other and unknown origin**

     Excludes1   chills without fever (R68.83)
             febrile convulsions (R56.0-)
             fever of unknown origin during labor (O75.2)
             fever of unknown origin in newborn (P81.9)
             hypothermia due to illness (R68.0)
             malignant hyperthermia due to anesthesia (T88.3)
             puerperal pyrexia NOS (O86.4)

     R50.2   **Drug induced fever**

       Use additional code for adverse effect, if applicable, to identify drug (T36-T50 with fifth or sixth character 5)

       Excludes1   postvaccination (postimmunization) fever (R50.83)

●   R50.8   **Other specified fever**

▌   *R50.81*   *Fever presenting with conditions classified elsewhere*

       Code first underlying condition when associated fever is present, such as with:
       leukemia (C91-C95)
       neutropenia (D70.-)
       sickle-cell disease (D57.-)

     R50.82   **Postprocedural fever**

       Excludes1   postprocedural infection (T81.4)
             posttransfusion fever (R50.84)
             postvaccination (postimmunization) fever (R50.83)

     R50.83   **Postvaccination fever**
       Postimmunization fever

     R50.84   **Febrile nonhemolytic transfusion reaction**
       FNHTR
       Posttransfusion fever

     R50.9   **Fever, unspecified**
       Fever NOS
       Fever of unknown origin [FUO]
       Fever with chills
       Fever with rigors
       Hyperpyrexia NOS
       Persistent fever
       Pyrexia NOS

R51   **Headache**
     Facial pain NOS

     Excludes1   atypical face pain (G50.1)
             migraine and other headache syndromes (G43-G44)
             trigeminal neuralgia (G50.0)

R52   **Pain, unspecified**
     Acute pain NOS   Pain NOS
     Generalized pain NOS

     Excludes1   acute and chronic pain, not elsewhere classified (G89.-)
             localized pain, unspecified type - code to pain by site, such as:
             abdomen pain (R10.-)
             back pain (M54.9)
             breast pain (N64.4)
             chest pain (R07.1-R07.9)
             ear pain (H92.0-)
             eye pain (H57.1)
             headache (R51)
             joint pain (M25.5-)
             limb pain (M79.6-)
             lumbar region pain (M54.5)
             pelvic and perineal pain (R10.2)
             shoulder pain (M25.51-)
             spine pain (M54.-)
             throat pain (R07.0)
             tongue pain (K14.6)
             tooth pain (K08.8)
             renal colic (N23)
             pain disorders exclusively related to psychological factors (F45.41)

CHAPTER 18 (R00-R99)

● R53   **Malaise and fatigue**
    R53.0   **Neoplastic (malignant) related fatigue**
       Code first associated neoplasm
    R53.1   **Weakness**
       Asthenia NOS
       Excludes1   age-related weakness (R54)
                        muscle weakness (M62.8-)
                        senile asthenia (R54)
    R53.2   **Functional quadriplegia**
       Complete immobility due to severe physical disability
          or frailty
       Excludes1   frailty NOS (R54)
                        hysterical paralysis (F44.4)
                        immobility syndrome (M62.3)
                        neurologic quadriplegia (G82.5-)
                        quadriplegia (G82.50)
 ● R53.8   **Other malaise and fatigue**
       Excludes1   combat exhaustion and fatigue (F43.0)
                        congenital debility (P96.9)
                        exhaustion and fatigue due to depressive
                           episode (F32.-)
                        exhaustion and fatigue due to excessive
                           exertion (T73.3)
                        exhaustion and fatigue due to exposure
                           (T73.2)
                        exhaustion and fatigue due to heat (T67.-)
                        exhaustion and fatigue due to pregnancy
                           (O26.8-)
                        exhaustion and fatigue due to recurrent
                           depressive episode (F33)
                        exhaustion and fatigue due to senile
                           debility (R54)
      R53.81   **Other malaise**
          Chronic debility
          Debility NOS
          General physical deterioration
          Malaise NOS
          Nervous debility
          Excludes1   age-related physical debility
                          (R54)
      R53.82   **Chronic fatigue, unspecified**
          Chronic fatigue syndrome NOS
          Excludes1   postviral fatigue syndrome
                          (G93.3)
      R53.83   **Other fatigue**
          Fatigue NOS   Lethargy
          Lack of energy   Tiredness

R54   **Age-related physical debility**   **A**
    Frailty   Senile asthenia
    Old age   Senile debility
    Senescence
    Excludes1   age-related cognitive decline (R41.81)
                    senile psychosis (F03)
                    senility NOS (R41.81)

R55   **Syncope and collapse**
    Blackout
    Fainting
    Vasovagal attack
    Excludes1   cardiogenic shock (R57.0)
                    carotid sinus syncope (G90.01)
                    heat syncope (T67.1)
                    neurocirculatory asthenia (F45.8)
                    neurogenic orthostatic hypotension (G90.3)
                    orthostatic hypotension (I95.1)
                    postprocedural shock (T81.1-)
                    psychogenic syncope (F48.8)
                    shock NOS (R57.9)
                    shock complicating or following abortion or
                       ectopic or molar pregnancy (O00-O07, O08.3)
                    shock complicating or following labor and
                       delivery (O75.1)
                    Stokes-Adams attack (I45.9)
                    unconsciousness NOS (R40.2-)

● R56   **Convulsions, not elsewhere classified**
    Excludes1   dissociative convulsions and seizures (F44.5)
                    epileptic convulsions and seizures (G40.-)
                    newborn convulsions and seizures (P90)
 ● R56.0   **Febrile convulsions**
      R56.00   **Simple febrile convulsions**
          Febrile convulsion NOS
          Febrile seizure NOS
      R56.01   **Complex febrile convulsions**
          Atypical febrile seizure
          Complex febrile seizure
          Complicated febrile seizure
          Excludes1   status epilepticus (G40.901)
    R56.1   **Post traumatic seizures**
       Excludes1   post traumatic epilepsy (G40.-)
    R56.9   **Unspecified convulsions**
       Convulsion disorder   Recurrent convulsions
       Fit NOS   Seizure(s) (convulsive) NOS

● R57   **Shock, not elsewhere classified**
    Excludes1   anaphylactic shock NOS (T78.2)
                    anaphylactic reaction or shock due to adverse
                       food reaction (T78.0-)
                    anaphylactic shock due to adverse effect of
                       correct drug or medicament properly
                       administered (T88.6)
                    anaphylactic shock due to serum (T80.5-)
                    anesthetic shock (T88.3)
                    electric shock (T75.4)
                    obstetric shock (O75.1)
                    postprocedural shock (T81.1-)
                    psychic shock (F43.0)
                    septic shock (R65.21)
                    shock complicating or following ectopic or molar
                       pregnancy (O00-O07, O08.3)
                    shock due to lightning (T75.01)
                    traumatic shock (T79.4)
                    toxic shock syndrome (A48.3)
    R57.0   **Cardiogenic shock**
    R57.1   **Hypovolemic shock**
       Decreased blood volume (loss)
    R57.8   **Other shock**
    R57.9   **Shock, unspecified**
       Failure of peripheral circulation NOS
       Resulting in significant blood pressure drop

R58   **Hemorrhage, not elsewhere classified**
    Hemorrhage NOS
    Excludes1   hemorrhage included with underlying
                       conditions, such as:
                       acute duodenal ulcer with hemorrhage (K26.0)
                       acute gastritis with bleeding (K29.01)
                       ulcerative enterocolitis with rectal bleeding
                         (K51.01)

● R59   **Enlarged lymph nodes**
    Includes   swollen glands
    Excludes1   lymphadenitis NOS (I88.9)
                    acute lymphadenitis (L04.-)
                    chronic lymphadenitis (I88.1)
                    mesenteric (acute) (chronic) lymphadenitis (I88.0)
    R59.0   **Localized enlarged lymph nodes**
    R59.1   **Generalized enlarged lymph nodes**
       Lymphadenopathy NOS
    R59.9   **Enlarged lymph nodes, unspecified**

◀ New   ⬅ Revised   ~~deleted~~ Deleted   Excludes 1   Excludes 2   Includes   Use additional   Code first   Code also   Unspecified
OGCR Official Guidelines   **X** Assign placeholder X   ● Use Additional Character(s)   ▶ Manifestation Code   **Coding Clinic**

● **R60 Edema, not elsewhere classified**
  Excludes1 angioneurotic edema (T78.3)
     ascites (R18.-)
     cerebral edema (G93.6)
     cerebral edema due to birth injury (P11.0)
     edema of larynx (J38.4)
     edema of nasopharynx (J39.2)
     edema of pharynx (J39.2)
     gestational edema (O12.0-)
     hereditary edema (Q82.0)
     hydrops fetalis NOS (P83.2)
     hydrothorax (J94.8)
     nutritional edema (E40-E46)
     hydrops fetalis NOS (P83.2)
     newborn edema (P83.3)
     pulmonary edema (J81.-)

 R60.0 Localized edema

 R60.1 Generalized edema

 R60.9 Edema, unspecified
   Fluid retention NOS

R61 Generalized hyperhidrosis
  Excessive sweating
  Night sweats
  Secondary hyperhidrosis

  Code first, if applicable, menopausal and female climacteric states (N95.1)

  Excludes1 focal (primary) (secondary) hyperhidrosis (L74.5-)
     Frey's syndrome (L74.52)
     localized (primary) (secondary) hyperhidrosis (L74.5-)

● **R62 Lack of expected normal physiological development in childhood and adults**
  Excludes1 delayed puberty (E30.0)
     gonadal dysgenesis (Q99.1)
     hypopituitarism (E23.0)

 R62.0 Delayed milestone in childhood   **P**
   Delayed attainment of expected physiological developmental stage
   Late talker
   Late walker

● **R62.5 Other and unspecified lack of expected normal physiological development in childhood**
   Excludes1 HIV disease resulting in failure to thrive (B20)
      physical retardation due to malnutrition (E45)

  R62.50 Unspecified lack of expected normal physiological development in childhood **P**
    Infantilism NOS

  R62.51 Failure to thrive (child)   **P**
    Failure to gain weight
    Excludes1 failure to thrive in child under 28 days old (P92.6)

  R62.52 Short stature (child)   **P**
    Lack of growth Short stature NOS
    Physical retardation
    Excludes1 short stature due to endocrine disorder (E34.3)

  R62.59 Other lack of expected normal physiological development in childhood **P**

 R62.7 Adult failure to thrive   **A**

● **R63 Symptoms and signs concerning food and fluid intake**
  Excludes1 bulimia NOS (F50.2)
     eating disorders of nonorganic origin (F50.-)
     malnutrition (E40-E46)

 R63.0 Anorexia
   Loss of appetite
   Excludes1 anorexia nervosa (F50.0-)
      loss of appetite of nonorganic origin (F50.8)

 R63.1 Polydipsia
   Excessive thirst

 R63.2 Polyphagia
   Excessive eating Hyperalimentation NOS

 R63.3 Feeding difficulties
   Feeding problem (elderly) (infant) NOS
   Excludes1 feeding problems of newborn (P92.-)
      infant feeding disorder of nonorganic origin (F98.2-)

 R63.4 Abnormal weight loss

 R63.5 Abnormal weight gain
   Excludes1 excessive weight gain in pregnancy (O26.0-)
      obesity (E66.-)

 R63.6 Underweight
   Use additional code to identify body mass index (BMI), if known (Z68.-)
   Excludes1 abnormal weight loss (R63.4)
      anorexia nervosa (F50.0-)
      malnutrition (E40-E46)

 R63.8 Other symptoms and signs concerning food and fluid intake

R64 Cachexia
  Wasting syndrome
  Code first underlying condition, if known
  Excludes1 abnormal weight loss (R63.4)
     nutritional marasmus (E41)

OGCR Section I.C.18.g.

SIRS due to Non-Infectious Process

The systemic inflammatory response syndrome (SIRS) can develop as a result of certain non-infectious disease processes, such as trauma, malignant neoplasm, or pancreatitis. When SIRS is documented with a noninfectious condition, and no subsequent infection is documented, the code for the underlying condition, such as an injury, should be assigned, followed by code R65.10. Systemic inflammatory response syndrome (SIRS) of non-infectious origin without acute organ dysfunction, or code R65.11, Systemic inflammatory response syndrome (SIRS) of non-infectious origin with acute organ dysfunction. If an associated acute organ dysfunction is documented, the appropriate code(s) for the specific type of organ dysfunction(s) should be assigned in addition to code R65.11. If acute organ dysfunction is documented, but it cannot be determined if the acute organ dysfunction is associated with SIRS or due to another condition (e.g., directly due to the trauma), the provider should be queried.

● **R65 Symptoms and signs specifically associated with systemic inflammation and infection**

● **R65.1 Systemic inflammatory response syndrome (SIRS) of non-infectious origin**

   Code first underlying condition, such as:
   heatstroke (T67.0)
   injury and trauma (S00-T88)

   Excludes1 sepsis - code to infection
      severe sepsis (R65.2)

  R65.10 Systemic inflammatory response syndrome (SIRS) of non-infectious origin without acute organ dysfunction
    Systemic inflammatory response syndrome (SIRS) NOS

CHAPTER 18 (R00-R99)

R65.11   **Systemic inflammatory response syndrome (SIRS) of non-infectious origin with acute organ dysfunction**

> Use additional code to identify specific acute organ dysfunction, such as:
> acute kidney failure (N17.-)
> acute respiratory failure (J96.0-)
> critical illness myopathy (G72.81)
> critical illness polyneuropathy (G62.81)
> disseminated intravascular coagulopathy [DIC] (D65)
> encephalopathy (metabolic) (septic) (G93.41)
> hepatic failure (K72.0-)

● **R65.2**   **Severe sepsis**

> Infection with associated acute organ dysfunction
> Sepsis with acute organ dysfunction
> Sepsis with multiple organ dysfunction
> Systemic inflammatory response syndrome due to infectious process with acute organ dysfunction

> *Code first* underlying infection, such as:
> infection following a procedure (T81.4)
> infections following infusion, transfusion and therapeutic injection (T80.2-)
> puerperal sepsis (O85)
> sepsis following complete or unspecified spontaneous abortion (O03.87)
> sepsis following ectopic and molar pregnancy (O08.82)
> sepsis following incomplete spontaneous abortion (O03.37)
> sepsis following (induced) termination of pregnancy (O04.87)
> sepsis NOS (A41.9)

> Use additional code to identify specific acute organ dysfunction, such as:
> acute kidney failure (N17.-)
> acute respiratory failure (J96.0-)
> critical illness myopathy (G72.81)
> critical illness polyneuropathy (G62.81)
> disseminated intravascular coagulopathy [DIC] (D65)
> encephalopathy (metabolic) (septic) (G93.41)
> hepatic failure (K72.0-)

     R65.20   **Severe sepsis without septic shock**
> Severe sepsis NOS

     R65.21   **Severe sepsis with septic shock**

● **R68**   **Other general symptoms and signs**

     R68.0   **Hypothermia, not associated with low environmental temperature**

> **Excludes1**   hypothermia NOS (accidental) (T68)
> hypothermia due to anesthesia (T88.51)
> hypothermia due to low environmental temperature (T68)
> newborn hypothermia (P80.-)

● **R68.1**   **Nonspecific symptoms peculiar to infancy**

> **Excludes1**   colic, infantile (R10.83)
> neonatal cerebral irritability (P91.3)
> teething syndrome (K00.7)

     R68.11   **Excessive crying of infant (baby)**   **P**

> **Excludes1**   excessive crying of child, adolescent, or adult (R45.83)

     R68.12   **Fussy infant (baby)**   **P**
> Irritable infant

     R68.13   **Apparent life threatening event in infant (ALTE)**   **P**
> Apparent life threatening event in newborn
> *Code first* confirmed diagnosis, if known
> Use additional code(s) for associated signs and symptoms if no confirmed diagnosis established, or if signs and symptoms are not associated routinely with confirmed diagnosis, or provide additional information for cause of ALTE

     R68.19   **Other nonspecific symptoms peculiar to infancy**   **P**

     R68.2   **Dry mouth, unspecified**

> **Excludes1**   dry mouth due to dehydration (E86.0)
> dry mouth due to sicca syndrome [Sjögren] (M35.0-)
> salivary gland hyposecretion (K11.7)

     R68.3   **Clubbing of fingers**
> Clubbing of nails

> **Excludes1**   congenital clubfinger (Q68.1)

● **R68.8**   **Other general symptoms and signs**

     R68.81   **Early satiety**

     R68.82   **Decreased libido**   **A**
> Decreased sexual desire

     R68.83   **Chills (without fever)**
> Chills NOS

> **Excludes1**   chills with fever (R50.9)

     R68.84   **Jaw pain**
> Mandibular pain
> Maxilla pain

> **Excludes1**   temporomandibular joint arthralgia (M26.62)

     R68.89   **Other general symptoms and signs**

R69   **Illness, unspecified**
> Unknown and unspecified cases of morbidity

ABNORMAL FINDINGS ON EXAMINATION OF BLOOD, WITHOUT DIAGNOSIS (R70-R79)

> **Excludes1**   abnormalities (of)(on):
> abnormal findings on antenatal screening of mother (O28.-)
> coagulation hemorrhagic disorders (D65-D68)
> lipids (E78.-)
> platelets and thrombocytes (D69.-)
> white blood cells classified elsewhere (D70-D72)
> diagnostic abnormal findings classified elsewhere - see Alphabetical Index
> hemorrhagic and hematological disorders of newborn (P50-P61)

● **R70**   **Elevated erythrocyte sedimentation rate and abnormality of plasma viscosity**

     R70.0   **Elevated erythrocyte sedimentation rate**

     R70.1   **Abnormal plasma viscosity**

◀ New   ◀ Revised   ~~deleted~~ Deleted   Excludes 1   Excludes 2   Includes   Use additional   Code first   Code also   Unspecified

OGCR Official Guidelines   **X** Assign placeholder X   ● Use Additional Character(s)   ▶ Manifestation Code   **Coding Clinic**

● **R71**   **Abnormality of red blood cells**
> **Excludes1**   anemias (D50-D64)
> anemia of premature infant (P61.2)
> benign (familial) polycythemia (D75.0)
> congenital anemias (P61.2-P61.4)
> newborn anemia due to isoimmunization (P55.-)
> polycythemia neonatorum (P61.1)
> polycythemia NOS (D75.1)
> polycythemia vera (D45)
> secondary polycythemia (D75.1)

   R71.0   **Precipitous drop in hematocrit**
     Drop (precipitous) in hemoglobin
     Drop in hematocrit
       Blood volume that is red blood cells

   R71.8   **Other abnormality of red blood cells**
     Abnormal red-cell morphology NOS
     Abnormal red-cell volume NOS
     Anisocytosis
       Red blood cells of unequal size
     Poikilocytosis
       Red blood cells of abnormal shape

● **R73**   **Elevated blood glucose level**
> **Excludes1**   diabetes mellitus (E08-E13)
> diabetes mellitus in pregnancy, childbirth and the puerperium (O24.-)
> neonatal disorders (P70.0-P70.2)
> postsurgical hypoinsulinemia (E89.1)

●   **R73.0**   **Abnormal glucose**
> **Excludes1**   abnormal glucose in pregnancy (O99.81-)
> diabetes mellitus (E08-E13)
> dysmetabolic syndrome X (E88.81)
> gestational diabetes (O24.4-)
> glycosuria (R81)
> hypoglycemia (E16.2)

     R73.01   **Impaired fasting glucose**
       Elevated fasting glucose

     R73.02   **Impaired glucose tolerance (oral)**
       Elevated glucose tolerance

     R73.09   **Other abnormal glucose**
       Abnormal glucose NOS
       Abnormal non-fasting glucose tolerance
       Latent diabetes
       Prediabetes

   R73.9   **Hyperglycemia, unspecified**

● **R74**   **Abnormal serum enzyme levels**
   R74.0   **Nonspecific elevation of levels of transaminase and lactic acid dehydrogenase [LDH]**

   R74.8   **Abnormal levels of other serum enzymes**
     Abnormal level of acid phosphatase
     Abnormal level of alkaline phosphatase
     Abnormal level of amylase
     Abnormal level of lipase [triacylglycerol lipase]

   R74.9   **Abnormal serum enzyme level, unspecified**

OGCR Section I.C.1.2.e and f.
> Patients with inconclusive HIV serology
> e. Patients with inconclusive HIV serology, but no definitive diagnosis or manifestations of the illness, may be assigned code R75, Inconclusive laboratory evidence of human immunodeficiency virus [HIV].
> f. Previously diagnosed HIV-related illness
> Patients with any known prior diagnosis of an HIV-related illness should be coded to B20. Once a patient has developed an HIV-related illness, the patient should always be assigned code B20 on every subsequent admission/encounter. Patients previously diagnosed with any HIV illness (B20) should never be assigned to R75 or Z21, Asymptomatic human immunodeficiency virus [HIV] infection status.

● **R75**   **Inconclusive laboratory evidence of human immunodeficiency virus [HIV]**
   Nonconclusive HIV-test finding in infants
> **Excludes1**   asymptomatic human immunodeficiency virus [HIV] infection status (Z21)
> human immunodeficiency virus [HIV] disease (B20)

● **R76**   **Other abnormal immunological findings in serum**
   R76.0   **Raised antibody titer**
> **Excludes1**   isoimmunization in pregnancy (O36.0-O36.1)
> isoimmunization affecting newborn (P55.-)

●   **R76.1**   **Nonspecific reaction to test for tuberculosis**

     R76.11   **Nonspecific reaction to tuberculin skin test without active tuberculosis**
       Abnormal result of Mantoux test
       PPD positive
       Tuberculin (skin test) positive
       Tuberculin (skin test) reactor
> **Excludes1**   nonspecific reaction to cell mediated immunity measurement of gamma interferon antigen response without active tuberculosis (R76.12)

     R76.12   **Nonspecific reaction to cell mediated immunity measurement of gamma interferon antigen response without active tuberculosis**
       Nonspecific reaction to QuantiFERON-TB test (QFT) without active tuberculosis
> **Excludes1**   nonspecific reaction to tuberculin skin test without active tuberculosis (R76.11)
> positive tuberculin skin test (R76.11)

   R76.8   **Other specified abnormal immunological findings in serum**
     Raised level of immunoglobulins NOS

   R76.9   **Abnormal immunological finding in serum, unspecified**

● **R77**   **Other abnormalities of plasma proteins**
> **Excludes1**   disorders of plasma-protein metabolism (E88.0)

   R77.0   **Abnormality of albumin**

   R77.1   **Abnormality of globulin**
     Hyperglobulinemia NOS

   R77.2   **Abnormality of alphafetoprotein**

   R77.8   **Other specified abnormalities of plasma proteins**

   R77.9   **Abnormality of plasma protein, unspecified**

CHAPTER 18 (R00-R99)

CHAPTER 18 (R00-R99)

● **R78**   **Findings of drugs and other substances, not normally found in blood**

> Use additional code to identify any retained foreign body, if applicable (Z18.-)
>
> **Excludes1**   mental or behavioral disorders due to psychoactive substance use (F10-F19)

   R78.0   **Finding of alcohol in blood**

> Use additional external cause code (Y90.-), for detail regarding alcohol level.

   R78.1   **Finding of opiate drug in blood**

   R78.2   **Finding of cocaine in blood**

   R78.3   **Finding of hallucinogen in blood**

   R78.4   **Finding of other drugs of addictive potential in blood**

   R78.5   **Finding of other psychotropic drug in blood**

   R78.6   **Finding of steroid agent in blood**

●   **R78.7**   **Finding of abnormal level of heavy metals in blood**

     R78.71   **Abnormal lead level in blood**

> **Excludes1**   lead poisoning (T56.0-)

     R78.79   **Finding of abnormal level of heavy metals in blood**

●   **R78.8**   **Finding of other specified substances, not normally found in blood**

     R78.81   **Bacteremia**

> *Blood poisoning/bacteremia*
>
> **Excludes1**   sepsis-code to specified infection (A00-B99)

     R78.89   **Finding of other specified substances, not normally found in blood**

> Finding of abnormal level of lithium in blood

   R78.9   **Finding of unspecified substance, not normally found in blood**

● **R79**   **Other abnormal findings of blood chemistry**

> Use additional code to identify any retained foreign body, if applicable (Z18.-)
>
> **Excludes1**   abnormality of fluid, electrolyte or acid-base balance (E86-E87)
> asymptomatic hyperuricemia (E79.0)
> hyperglycemia NOS (R73.9)
> hypoglycemia NOS (E16.2)
> neonatal hypoglycemia (P70.3-P70.4)
> specific findings indicating disorder of amino-acid metabolism (E70-E72)
> specific findings indicating disorder of carbohydrate metabolism (E73-E74)
> specific findings indicating disorder of lipid metabolism (E75.-)

   R79.0   **Abnormal level of blood mineral**

> Abnormal blood level of cobalt
> Abnormal blood level of copper
> Abnormal blood level of iron
> Abnormal blood level of magnesium
> Abnormal blood level of mineral NEC
> Abnormal blood level of zinc
>
> **Excludes1**   abnormal level of lithium (R78.89)
> disorders of mineral metabolism (E83.-)
> neonatal hypomagnesemia (P71.2)
> nutritional mineral deficiency (E58-E61)

   R79.1   **Abnormal coagulation profile**

> Abnormal or prolonged bleeding time
> Abnormal or prolonged coagulation time
> Abnormal or prolonged partial thromboplastin time [PTT]
> Abnormal or prolonged prothrombin time [PT]
>
> **Excludes1**   coagulation defects (D68.-)

●   **R79.8**   **Other specified abnormal findings of blood chemistry**

     R79.81   **Abnormal blood-gas level**

     R79.82   **Elevated C-reactive protein (CRP)**

     R79.89   **Other specified abnormal findings of blood chemistry**

   R79.9   **Abnormal finding of blood chemistry, unspecified**

ABNORMAL FINDINGS ON EXAMINATION OF URINE, WITHOUT DIAGNOSIS (R80-R82)

> **Excludes1**   abnormal findings on antenatal screening of mother (O28.-)
> diagnostic abnormal findings classified elsewhere - see Alphabetical Index
> specific findings indicating disorder of amino-acid metabolism (E70-E72)
> specific findings indicating disorder of carbohydrate metabolism (E73-E74)

● **R80**   **Proteinuria**

> **Excludes1**   gestational proteinuria (O12.1-)

   R80.0   **Isolated proteinuria**

> Idiopathic proteinuria
>
> **Excludes1**   isolated proteinuria with specific morphological lesion (N06.-)

   R80.1   **Persistent proteinuria, unspecified**

   R80.2   **Orthostatic proteinuria, unspecified**

> Postural proteinuria

   R80.3   **Bence Jones proteinuria**

   R80.8   **Other proteinuria**

   R80.9   **Proteinuria, unspecified**

> Albuminuria NOS

   R81   **Glycosuria**

> **Excludes1**   renal glycosuria (E74.8)

● **R82**   **Other and unspecified abnormal findings in urine**

> **Includes**   chromoabnormalities in urine
>
> Use additional code to identify any retained foreign body, if applicable (Z18.-)
>
> **Excludes2**   hematuria (R31.-)

   R82.0   **Chyluria**

> *White milky urine*
>
> **Excludes1**   filarial chyluria (B74.-)

   R82.1   **Myoglobinuria**

> *Presence of myoglobin (iron containing protein) in urine*

   R82.2   **Biliuria**

> *Presence of bile pigments/salts in urine*

   R82.3   **Hemoglobinuria**

> *Presence of hemoglobin in urine*
>
> **Excludes1**   hemoglobinuria due to hemolysis from external causes NEC (D59.6)
> hemoglobinuria due to paroxysmal nocturnal [Marchiafava-Micheli] (D59.5)

   R82.4   **Acetonuria**

> Ketonuria

   R82.5   **Elevated urine levels of drugs, medicaments and biological substances**

> Elevated urine levels of catecholamines
> Elevated urine levels of indoleacetic acid
> Elevated urine levels of 17-ketosteroids
> Elevated urine levels of steroids

   R82.6   **Abnormal urine levels of substances chiefly nonmedicinal as to source**

> Abnormal urine level of heavy metals

   R82.7   **Abnormal findings on microbiological examination of urine**

> Positive culture findings of urine
>
> **Excludes1**   colonization status (Z22.-)

   R82.8   **Abnormal findings on cytological and histological examination of urine**

◀ New   ⬅ Revised   ~~deleted~~ Deleted   Excludes 1   Excludes 2   Includes   Use additional   Code first   Code also   Unspecified

1248   **OGCR** Official Guidelines   X Assign placeholder X   ● Use Additional Character(s)   ▶ Manifestation Code   **Coding Clinic**

● **R82.9**   **Other and unspecified abnormal findings in urine**

    R82.90   Unspecified abnormal findings in urine

    R82.91   Other chromoabnormalities of urine
       Chromoconversion (dipstick)
       Idiopathic dipstick converts positive for blood
         with no cellular forms in sediment

       Excludes1   hemoglobinuria (R82.3)
                  myoglobinuria (R82.1)

    R82.99   Other abnormal findings in urine
       Cells and casts in urine
       Crystalluria
       Melanuria

ABNORMAL FINDINGS ON EXAMINATION OF OTHER BODY FLUIDS, SUBSTANCES AND TISSUES, WITHOUT DIAGNOSIS (R83-R89)

   Excludes1   abnormal findings on antenatal screening of
           mother (O28.-)
         diagnostic abnormal findings classified elsewhere
           - see Alphabetical Index

   Excludes2   abnormal findings on examination of blood,
           without diagnosis (R70-R79)
         abnormal findings on examination of urine,
           without diagnosis (R80-R82)
         abnormal tumor markers (R97.-)

● **R83**   **Abnormal findings in cerebrospinal fluid**

    R83.0   Abnormal level of enzymes in cerebrospinal fluid

    R83.1   Abnormal level of hormones in cerebrospinal fluid

    R83.2   Abnormal level of other drugs, medicaments and biological substances in cerebrospinal fluid

    R83.3   Abnormal level of substances chiefly nonmedicinal as to source in cerebrospinal fluid

    R83.4   Abnormal immunological findings in cerebrospinal fluid

    R83.5   Abnormal microbiological findings in cerebrospinal fluid
       Positive culture findings in cerebrospinal fluid

       Excludes1   colonization status (Z22.-)

    R83.6   Abnormal cytological findings in cerebrospinal fluid

    R83.8   Other abnormal findings in cerebrospinal fluid
       Abnormal chromosomal findings in cerebrospinal fluid

    R83.9   Unspecified abnormal finding in cerebrospinal fluid

● **R84**   **Abnormal findings in specimens from respiratory organs and thorax**

   Includes   abnormal findings in bronchial washings
         abnormal findings in nasal secretions
         abnormal findings in pleural fluid
         abnormal findings in sputum
         abnormal findings in throat scrapings

   Excludes1   blood-stained sputum (R04.2)

    R84.0   Abnormal level of enzymes in specimens from respiratory organs and thorax

    R84.1   Abnormal level of hormones in specimens from respiratory organs and thorax

    R84.2   Abnormal level of other drugs, medicaments and biological substances in specimens from respiratory organs and thorax

    R84.3   Abnormal level of substances chiefly nonmedicinal as to source in specimens from respiratory organs and thorax

    R84.4   Abnormal immunological findings in specimens from respiratory organs and thorax

    R84.5   Abnormal microbiological findings in specimens from respiratory organs and thorax
       Positive culture findings in specimens from respiratory organs and thorax

       Excludes1   colonization status (Z22.-)

    R84.6   Abnormal cytological findings in specimens from respiratory organs and thorax

    R84.7   Abnormal histological findings in specimens from respiratory organs and thorax

    R84.8   Other abnormal findings in specimens from respiratory organs and thorax
       Abnormal chromosomal findings in specimens from respiratory organs and thorax

    R84.9   Unspecified abnormal finding in specimens from respiratory organs and thorax

● **R85**   **Abnormal findings in specimens from digestive organs and abdominal cavity**

   Includes   abnormal findings in peritoneal fluid
         abnormal findings in saliva

   Excludes1   cloudy peritoneal dialysis effluent (R88.0)
         fecal abnormalities (R19.5)

    R85.0   Abnormal level of enzymes in specimens from digestive organs and abdominal cavity

    R85.1   Abnormal level of hormones in specimens from digestive organs and abdominal cavity

    R85.2   Abnormal level of other drugs, medicaments and biological substances in specimens from digestive organs and abdominal cavity

    R85.3   Abnormal level of substances chiefly nonmedicinal as to source in specimens from digestive organs and abdominal cavity

    R85.4   Abnormal immunological findings in digestive organs and abdominal cavity

    R85.5   Abnormal microbiological findings in specimens from digestive organs and abdominal cavity
       Positive culture findings in specimens from digestive organs and abdominal cavity

       Excludes1   colonization status (Z22.-)

● **R85.6**   **Abnormal cytological findings in specimens from digestive organs and abdominal cavity**

  ● **R85.61**   Abnormal cytologic smear of anus

       Excludes1   abnormal cytological findings
              in specimens from other
              digestive organs and
              abdominal cavity (R85.69)
           carcinoma in situ of anus
              (histologically confirmed)
              (D01.3)
           anal intraepithelial neoplasia I
              [AIN I] (K62.82)
           anal intraepithelial neoplasia II
              [AIN II] (K62.82)
           anal intraepithelial neoplasia III
              [AIN III] (D01.3)
           dysplasia (mild) (moderate)
              of anus (histologically
              confirmed) (K62.82)
           severe dysplasia of anus
              (histologically confirmed)
              (D01.3)

       Excludes2   anal high risk human
              papillomavirus (HPV) DNA
              test positive (R85.81)
           anal low risk human
              papillomavirus (HPV) DNA
              test positive (R85.82)

     R85.610   Atypical squamous cells of undetermined significance on cytologic smear of anus (ASC-US)

     R85.611   Atypical squamous cells cannot exclude high grade squamous intraepithelial lesion on cytologic smear of anus (ASC-H)

     R85.612   Low grade squamous intraepithelial lesion on cytologic smear of anus (LGSIL)

     R85.613   High grade squamous intraepithelial lesion on cytologic smear of anus (HGSIL)

R85.614   Cytologic evidence of malignancy on smear of anus

R85.615   Unsatisfactory cytologic smear of anus

> Inadequate sample of cytologic smear of anus

R85.616   Satisfactory anal smear but lacking transformation zone

R85.618   Other abnormal cytological findings on specimens from anus

R85.619   Unspecified abnormal cytological findings in specimens from anus

> Abnormal anal cytology NOS
> Atypical glandular cells of anus NOS

R85.69   Abnormal cytological findings in specimens from other digestive organs and abdominal cavity

R85.7   Abnormal histological findings in specimens from digestive organs and abdominal cavity

●**R85.8**   Other abnormal findings in specimens from digestive organs and abdominal cavity

R85.81   Anal high risk human papillomavirus (HPV) DNA test positive

> **Excludes1**   anogenital warts due to human papillomavirus (HPV) (A63.0)
> condyloma acuminatum (A63.0)

R85.82   Anal low risk human papillomavirus (HPV) DNA test positive

> Use additional code for associated human papillomavirus (B97.7)

R85.89   Other abnormal findings in specimens from digestive organs and abdominal cavity

> Abnormal chromosomal findings in specimens from digestive organs and abdominal cavity

R85.9   Unspecified abnormal finding in specimens from digestive organs and abdominal cavity

●**R86**   Abnormal findings in specimens from male genital organs

> **Includes**   abnormal findings in prostatic secretions
> abnormal findings in semen, seminal fluid
> abnormal spermatozoa

> **Excludes1**   azoospermia (N46.0-)
> oligospermia (N46.1-)

R86.0   Abnormal level of enzymes in specimens from male genital organs ♂

R86.1   Abnormal level of hormones in specimens from male genital organs ♂

R86.2   Abnormal level of other drugs, medicaments and biological substances in specimens from male genital organs ♂

R86.3   Abnormal level of substances chiefly nonmedicinal as to source in specimens from male genital organs ♂

R86.4   Abnormal immunological findings in specimens from male genital organs ♂

R86.5   Abnormal microbiological findings in specimens from male genital organs ♂

> Positive culture findings in specimens from male genital organs

> **Excludes1**   colonization status (Z22.-)

R86.6   Abnormal cytological findings in specimens from male genital organs ♂

R86.7   Abnormal histological findings in specimens from male genital organs ♂

R86.8   Other abnormal findings in specimens from male genital organs ♂

> Abnormal chromosomal findings in specimens from male genital organs

R86.9   Unspecified abnormal finding in specimens from male genital organs ♂

●**R87**   Abnormal findings in specimens from female genital organs

> **Includes**   abnormal findings in secretion and smears from cervix uteri
> abnormal findings in secretion and smears from vagina
> abnormal findings in secretion and smears from vulva

R87.0   Abnormal level of enzymes in specimens from female genital organs ♀

R87.1   Abnormal level of hormones in specimens from female genital organs ♀

R87.2   Abnormal level of other drugs, medicaments and biological substances in specimens from female genital organs ♀

R87.3   Abnormal level of substances chiefly nonmedicinal as to source in specimens from female genital organs ♀

R87.4   Abnormal immunological findings in specimens from female genital organs ♀

R87.5   Abnormal microbiological findings in specimens from female genital organs ♀

> Positive culture findings in specimens from female genital organs

> **Excludes1**   colonization status (Z22.-)

●**R87.6**   Abnormal cytological findings in specimens from female genital organs

●**R87.61**   Abnormal cytological findings in specimens from cervix uteri

> **Excludes1**   abnormal cytological findings in specimens from other female genital organs (R87.69)
> abnormal cytological findings in specimens from vagina (R87.62-)
> carcinoma in situ of cervix uteri (histologically confirmed) (D06.-)
> cervical intraepithelial neoplasia I [CIN I] (N87.0)
> cervical intraepithelial neoplasia II [CIN II] (N87.1)
> cervical intraepithelial neoplasia III [CIN III] (D06.-)
> dysplasia (mild) (moderate) of cervix uteri (histologically confirmed) (N87.-)
> severe dysplasia of cervix uteri (histologically confirmed) (D06.-)

> **Excludes2**   cervical high risk human papillomavirus (HPV) DNA test positive (R87.810)
> cervical low risk human papillomavirus (HPV) DNA test positive (R87.820)

R87.610   Atypical squamous cells of undetermined significance on cytologic smear of cervix (ASC-US) ♀

R87.611   Atypical squamous cells cannot exclude high grade squamous intraepithelial lesion on cytologic smear of cervix (ASC-H) ♀

R87.612   Low grade squamous intraepithelial lesion on cytologic smear of cervix (LGSIL) ♀

R87.613   High grade squamous intraepithelial lesion on cytologic smear of cervix (HGSIL) ♀

R87.614   Cytologic evidence of malignancy on smear of cervix ♀

◀ New   ◀⚬⚬ Revised   ~~deleted~~ Deleted   Excludes 1   Excludes 2   Includes   Use additional   Code first   Code also   Unspecified

OGCR Official Guidelines   X Assign placeholder X   ● Use Additional Character(s)   ▶ Manifestation Code   **Coding Clinic**

R87.615 **Unsatisfactory cytologic smear of cervix** ♀

    Inadequate sample of cytologic smear of cervix

R87.616 **Satisfactory cervical smear but lacking transformation zone** ♀

R87.618 **Other abnormal cytological findings on specimens from cervix uteri** ♀

R87.619 Unspecified **abnormal cytological findings in specimens from cervix uteri** ♀

    Abnormal cervical cytology NOS

    Abnormal Papanicolaou smear of cervix NOS

    Abnormal thin preparation smear of cervix NOS

    Atypical endocervical cells of cervix NOS

    Atypical endometrial cells of cervix NOS

    Atypical glandular cells of cervix NOS

● R87.62 **Abnormal cytological findings in specimens from vagina**

    Use additional code to identify acquired absence of uterus and cervix, if applicable (Z90.71-)

    Excludes1   abnormal cytological findings in specimens from cervix uteri (R87.61-)

        abnormal cytological findings in specimens from other female genital organs (R87.69)

        carcinoma in situ of vagina (histologically confirmed) (D07.2)

        vaginal intraepithelial neoplasia I [VAIN I] (N89.0)

        vaginal intraepithelial neoplasia II [VAIN II] (N89.1)

        vaginal intraepithelial neoplasia III [VAIN III] (D07.2)

        dysplasia (mild) (moderate) of vagina (histologically confirmed) (N89.-)

        severe dysplasia of vagina (histologically confirmed) (D07.2)

    Excludes2   vaginal high risk human papillomavirus (HPV) DNA test positive (R87.811)

        vaginal low risk human papillomavirus (HPV) DNA test positive (R87.821)

R87.620 **Atypical squamous cells of undetermined significance on cytologic smear of vagina (ASC-US)** ♀

R87.621 **Atypical squamous cells cannot exclude high grade squamous intraepithelial lesion on cytologic smear of vagina (ASC-H)** ♀

R87.622 **Low grade squamous intraepithelial lesion on cytologic smear of vagina (LGSIL)** ♀

R87.623 **High grade squamous intraepithelial lesion on cytologic smear of vagina (HGSIL)** ♀

R87.624 **Cytologic evidence of malignancy on smear of vagina** ♀

R87.625 **Unsatisfactory cytologic smear of vagina** ♀

    Inadequate sample of cytologic smear of vagina

R87.628 **Other abnormal cytological findings on specimens from vagina** ♀

R87.629 Unspecified **abnormal cytological findings in specimens from vagina** ♀

    Abnormal Papanicolaou smear of vagina NOS

    Abnormal thin preparation smear of vagina NOS

    Abnormal vaginal cytology NOS

    Atypical endocervical cells of vagina NOS

    Atypical endometrial cells of vagina NOS

    Atypical glandular cells of vagina NOS

R87.69 **Abnormal cytological findings in specimens from other female genital organs** ♀

    Abnormal cytological findings in specimens from female genital organs NOS

    Excludes1   dysplasia of vulva (histologically confirmed) (N90.0-N90.3)

R87.7 **Abnormal histological findings in specimens from female genital organs** ♀

    Excludes1   carcinoma in situ (histologically confirmed) of female genital organs (D06-D07.3)

        cervical intraepithelial neoplasia I [CIN I] (N87.0)

        cervical intraepithelial neoplasia II [CIN II] (N87.1)

        cervical intraepithelial neoplasia III [CIN III] (D06.-)

        dysplasia (mild) (moderate) of cervix uteri (histologically confirmed) (N87.-)

        dysplasia (mild) (moderate) of vagina (histologically confirmed) (N89.-)

        vaginal intraepithelial neoplasia I [VAIN I] (N89.0)

        vaginal intraepithelial neoplasia II [VAIN II] (N89.1)

        vaginal intraepithelial neoplasia III [VAIN III] (D07.2)

        severe dysplasia of cervix uteri (histologically confirmed) (D06.-)

        severe dysplasia of vagina (histologically confirmed) (D07.2)

● R87.8 **Other abnormal findings in specimens from female genital organs**

● R87.81 **High risk human papillomavirus (HPV) DNA test positive from female genital organs**

    Excludes1   anogenital warts due to human papillomavirus (HPV) (A63.0)

        condyloma acuminatum (A63.0)

R87.810 **Cervical high risk human papillomavirus (HPV) DNA test positive** ♀

R87.811 **Vaginal high risk human papillomavirus (HPV) DNA test positive** ♀

● R87.82 **Low risk human papillomavirus (HPV) DNA test positive from female genital organs**

    Use additional code for associated human papillomavirus (B97.7)

R87.820 **Cervical low risk human papillomavirus (HPV) DNA test positive** ♀

R87.821 **Vaginal low risk human papillomavirus (HPV) DNA test positive** ♀

R87.89 **Other abnormal findings in specimens from female genital organs** ♀

    Abnormal chromosomal findings in specimens from female genital organs

R87.9 Unspecified **abnormal finding in specimens from female genital organs** ♀

CHAPTER 18 (R00-R99)

● **R88**   **Abnormal findings in other body fluids and substances**

     R88.0   Cloudy (hemodialysis) (peritoneal) dialysis effluent

     R88.8   Abnormal findings in other body fluids and substances

● **R89**   **Abnormal findings in specimens from other organs, systems and tissues**

     Includes   abnormal findings in nipple discharge

                   abnormal findings in synovial fluid

                   abnormal findings in wound secretions

     R89.0   Abnormal level of enzymes in specimens from other organs, systems and tissues

     R89.1   Abnormal level of hormones in specimens from other organs, systems and tissues

     R89.2   Abnormal level of other drugs, medicaments and biological substances in specimens from other organs, systems and tissues

     R89.3   Abnormal level of substances chiefly nonmedicinal as to source in specimens from other organs, systems and tissues

     R89.4   Abnormal immunological findings in specimens from other organs, systems and tissues

     R89.5   Abnormal microbiological findings in specimens from other organs, systems and tissues

          Positive culture findings in specimens from other organs, systems and tissues

          Excludes1   colonization status (Z22.-)

     R89.6   Abnormal cytological findings in specimens from other organs, systems and tissues

     R89.7   Abnormal histological findings in specimens from other organs, systems and tissues

     R89.8   Other abnormal findings in specimens from other organs, systems and tissues

          Abnormal chromosomal findings in specimens from other organs, systems and tissues

     R89.9   **Unspecified** abnormal finding in specimens from other organs, systems and tissues

---

ABNORMAL FINDINGS ON DIAGNOSTIC IMAGING AND IN FUNCTION STUDIES, WITHOUT DIAGNOSIS (R90-R94)

     Includes   nonspecific abnormal findings on diagnostic imaging by computerized axial tomography [CAT scan]

                   nonspecific abnormal findings on diagnostic imaging by magnetic resonance imaging [MRI][NMR]

                   nonspecific abnormal findings on diagnostic imaging by positron emission tomography [PET scan]

                   nonspecific abnormal findings on diagnostic imaging by thermography

                   nonspecific abnormal findings on diagnostic imaging by ultrasound [echogram]

                   nonspecific abnormal findings on diagnostic imaging by X-ray examination

     Excludes1   abnormal findings on antenatal screening of mother (O28.-)

                   diagnostic abnormal findings classified elsewhere - see Alphabetical Index

● **R90**   **Abnormal findings on diagnostic imaging of central nervous system**

     R90.0   Intracranial space-occupying lesion found on diagnostic imaging of central nervous system

  ● R90.8   Other abnormal findings on diagnostic imaging of central nervous system

          R90.81   Abnormal echoencephalogram

          R90.82   White matter disease, unspecified

          R90.89   Other abnormal findings on diagnostic imaging of central nervous system

                 Other cerebrovascular abnormality found on diagnostic imaging of central nervous system

● **R91**   **Abnormal findings on diagnostic imaging of lung**

     R91.1   Solitary pulmonary nodule

          Coin lesion lung

          Solitary pulmonary nodule, subsegmental branch of the bronchial tree

     R91.8   Other nonspecific abnormal finding of lung field

          Lung mass NOS found on diagnostic imaging of lung

          Pulmonary infiltrate NOS

          Shadow, lung

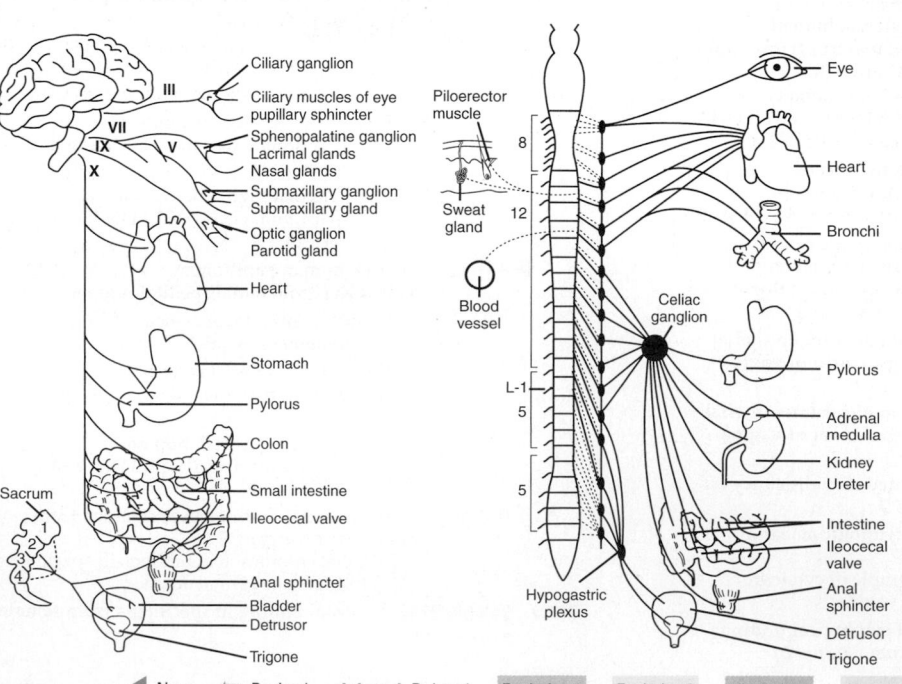

Figure 18-2   **A.** Parasympathetic nervous system. **B.** Sympathetic nervous system. (From Buck CJ: Step-by-Step Medical Coding, Philadelphia, WB Saunders, 1998)

◀ New   ◀▥ Revised   ~~deleted~~ Deleted   Excludes 1   Excludes 2   Includes   Use additional   Code first   Code also   Unspecified

OGCR Official Guidelines   X Assign placeholder X   ● Use Additional Character(s)   ▶ Manifestation Code   **Coding Clinic**

● **R92**   **Abnormal and inconclusive findings on diagnostic imaging of breast**

     R92.0   **Mammographic microcalcification found on diagnostic imaging of breast**

        Excludes2   mammographic calcification (calculus) found on diagnostic imaging of breast (R92.1)

     R92.1   **Mammographic calcification found on diagnostic imaging of breast**

        Mammographic calculus found on diagnostic imaging of breast

     R92.2   **Inconclusive mammogram**

        Dense breasts NOS
        Inconclusive mammogram NEC
        Inconclusive mammography due to dense breasts
        Inconclusive mammography NEC
        Coding Clinic: 2015, Q1, P24

     R92.8   **Other abnormal and inconclusive findings on diagnostic imaging of breast**

● **R93**   **Abnormal findings on diagnostic imaging of other body structures**

     R93.0   **Abnormal findings on diagnostic imaging of skull and head, not elsewhere classified**

        Excludes1   intracranial space-occupying lesion found on diagnostic imaging (R90.0)

     R93.1   **Abnormal findings on diagnostic imaging of heart and coronary circulation**

        Abnormal echocardiogram NOS
        Abnormal heart shadow

     R93.2   **Abnormal findings on diagnostic imaging of liver and biliary tract**

        Nonvisualization of gallbladder

     R93.3   **Abnormal findings on diagnostic imaging of other parts of digestive tract**

     R93.4   **Abnormal findings on diagnostic imaging of urinary organs**

        Filling defect of bladder found on diagnostic imaging
        Filling defect of kidney found on diagnostic imaging
        Filling defect of ureter found on diagnostic imaging

        Excludes1   hypertrophy of kidney (N28.81)

     R93.5   **Abnormal findings on diagnostic imaging of other abdominal regions, including retroperitoneum**

     R93.6   **Abnormal findings on diagnostic imaging of limbs**

        Excludes2   abnormal finding in skin and subcutaneous tissue (R93.8)

     R93.7   **Abnormal findings on diagnostic imaging of other parts of musculoskeletal system**

        Excludes2   abnormal findings on diagnostic imaging of skull (R93.0)

     R93.8   **Abnormal findings on diagnostic imaging of other specified body structures**

        Abnormal finding by radioisotope localization of placenta
        Abnormal radiological finding in skin and subcutaneous tissue
        Mediastinal shift

     R93.9   **Diagnostic imaging inconclusive due to excess body fat of patient**

Item 18–1 The **peripheral nervous system** consists of 31 pairs of spinal nerves, 12 pairs of cranial nerves, and the autonomic nerves, which are divided into the parasympathetic and sympathetic nerves. The cranial nerves are: olfactory (I), optic (II), oculomotor (III), trochlear (IV), trigeminal (V), abducens (VI), facial (VII), vestibulocochlear (VIII), glossopharyngeal (IX), vagus (X), accessory (XI), and hypoglossal (XII).

● **R94**   **Abnormal results of function studies**

     Includes   abnormal results of radionuclide [radioisotope] uptake studies
        abnormal results of scintigraphy

     ● **R94.0**   **Abnormal results of function studies of central nervous system**

        R94.01   **Abnormal electroencephalogram [EEG]**

        R94.02   **Abnormal brain scan**

        R94.09   **Abnormal results of other function studies of central nervous system**

     ● **R94.1**   **Abnormal results of function studies of peripheral nervous system and special senses**

        ● **R94.11**   **Abnormal results of function studies of eye**

          R94.110   **Abnormal electro-oculogram [EOG]**

          R94.111   **Abnormal electroretinogram [ERG]**
            Abnormal retinal function study

          R94.112   **Abnormal visually evoked potential [VEP]**

          R94.113   **Abnormal oculomotor study**

          R94.118   **Abnormal results of other function studies of eye**

        ● **R94.12**   **Abnormal results of function studies of ear and other special senses**

          R94.120   **Abnormal auditory function study**

          R94.121   **Abnormal vestibular function study**

          R94.128   **Abnormal results of other function studies of ear and other special senses**

        ● **R94.13**   **Abnormal results of function studies of peripheral nervous system**

          R94.130   **Abnormal response to nerve stimulation, unspecified**

          R94.131   **Abnormal electromyogram [EMG]**

            Excludes1   electromyogram of eye (R94.113)

          R94.138   **Abnormal results of other function studies of peripheral nervous system**

     R94.2   **Abnormal results of pulmonary function studies**

        Reduced ventilatory capacity
        Reduced vital capacity

     ● **R94.3**   **Abnormal results of cardiovascular function studies**

        R94.30   **Abnormal result of cardiovascular function study, unspecified**

        R94.31   **Abnormal electrocardiogram [ECG] [EKG]**

          Excludes1   long QT syndrome (I45.81)

        R94.39   **Abnormal result of other cardiovascular function study**

          Abnormal electrophysiological intracardiac studies
          Abnormal phonocardiogram
          Abnormal vectorcardiogram

     R94.4   **Abnormal results of kidney function studies**

        Abnormal renal function test

     R94.5   **Abnormal results of liver function studies**

     R94.6   **Abnormal results of thyroid function studies**

     R94.7   **Abnormal results of other endocrine function studies**

        Excludes2   abnormal glucose (R73.0-)

     R94.8   **Abnormal results of function studies of other organs and systems**

        Abnormal basal metabolic rate [BMR]
        Abnormal bladder function test
        Abnormal splenic function test

CHAPTER 18 (R00-R99)

CHAPTER 18 (R00-R99)

ABNORMAL TUMOR MARKERS (R97)

● **R97**   **Abnormal tumor markers**
      Elevated tumor associated antigens [TAA]
      Elevated tumor specific antigens [TSA]
    R97.0   **Elevated carcinoembryonic antigen [CEA]**
    R97.1   **Elevated cancer antigen 125 [CA 125] ♀**
    R97.2   **Elevated prostate specific antigen [PSA] ♂**   A
    R97.8   **Other abnormal tumor markers**

ILL-DEFINED AND UNKNOWN CAUSE OF MORTALITY (R99)

  R99   **Ill-defined and unknown cause of mortality**
      Death (unexplained) NOS
      Unspecified cause of mortality

OGCR Section I.C.18.h.

18.6 Death NOS

Code R99, Ill-defined and unknown cause of mortality, is only for use in the very limited circumstance when a patient who has already died is brought into the emergency department or other healthcare facility and is pronounced dead upon arrival. It does not represent the discharge disposition of death.

◄ New   ◄▥ Revised   ~~deleted~~ Deleted   Excludes 1   Excludes 2   Includes   Use additional   Code first   Code also   Unspecified
OGCR Official Guidelines   X Assign placeholder X   ● Use Additional Character(s)   ▶ Manifestation Code   **Coding Clinic**

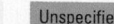

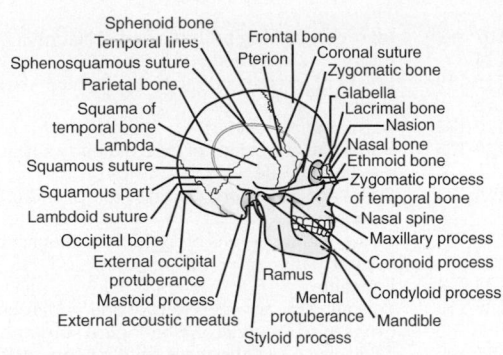

Figure 19-1 Lateral view of skull.

Figure 19-2 Frontal view of skull.

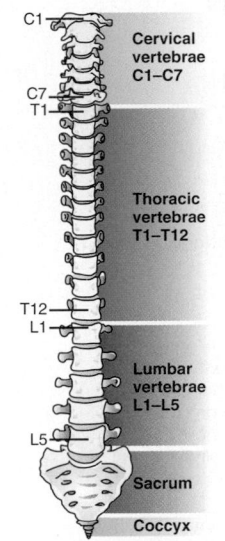

Figure 19-3 Anterior view of vertebral column.

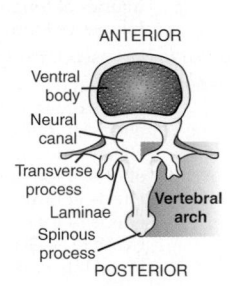

Figure 19-4 Vertebra viewed from above.

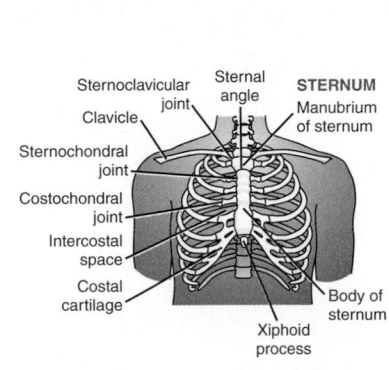

Figure 19-5 Anterior view of rib cage.

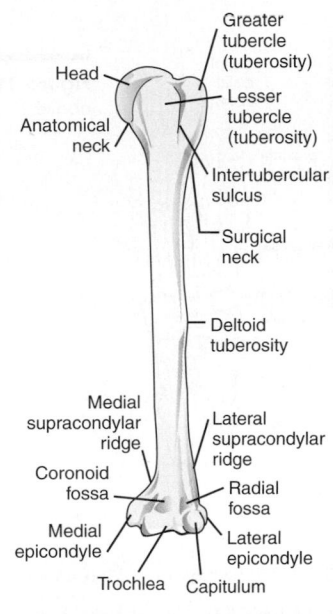

Figure 19-6 Anterior aspect of left humerus.

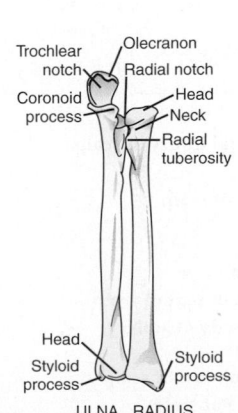

Figure 19-7 Anterior aspect of left radius and ulna.

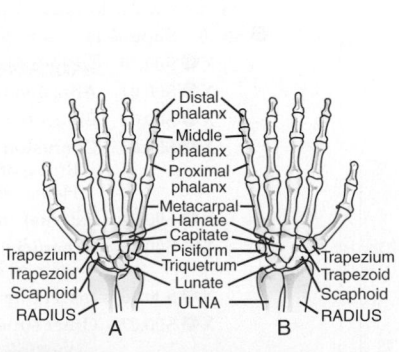

Figure 19-8 Right hand and wrist: **A.** Dorsal surface. **B.** Palmar surface.

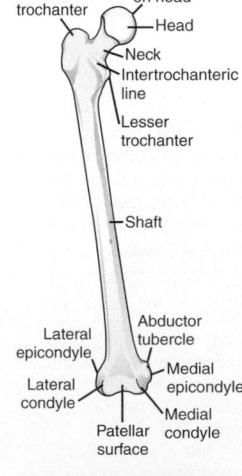

Figure 19-9 Anterior aspect of right femur.

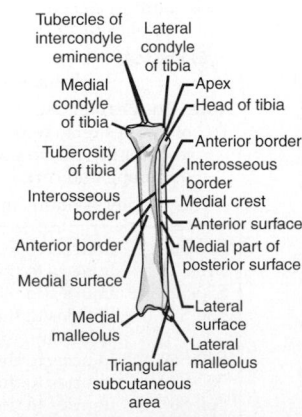

Figure 19-10 Anterior aspect of left tibia and fibula.

CHAPTER 19 (S00-T88)

N Newborn Age: 0   **P** Pediatric Age: 0–17   **M** Maternity DX: 12–55   **A** Adult Age: 15–124   ♀ Females Only   ♂ Males Only   1255

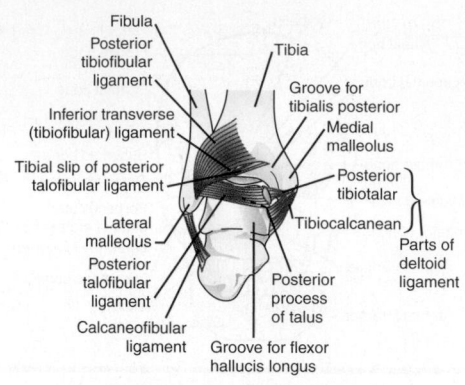

Figure 19-11   Posterior aspect of the left ankle joint.

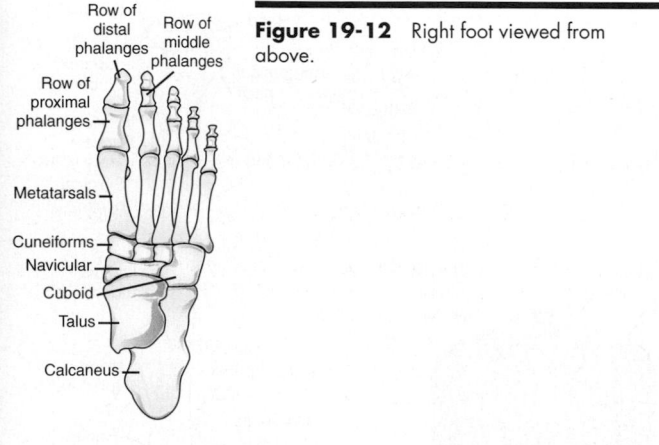

Figure 19-12   Right foot viewed from above.

OGCR See Section I.C., Chapter 19

CHAPTER 19

INJURY, POISONING AND CERTAIN OTHER CONSEQUENCES OF EXTERNAL CAUSES (S00-T88)

Note: Use secondary code(s) from Chapter 20, External causes of morbidity, to indicate cause of injury. Codes within the T section that include the external cause do not require an additional external cause code.

Use additional code to identify any retained foreign body, if applicable (Z18.-)

Excludes1   birth trauma (P10-P15)
                obstetric trauma (O70-O71)

Note: The chapter uses the S-section for coding different types of injuries related to single body regions and the T-section to cover injuries to unspecified body regions as well as poisoning and certain other consequences of external causes.

This chapter contains the following blocks:

S00-S09	Injuries to the head
S10-S19	Injuries to the neck
S20-S29	Injuries to the thorax
S30-S39	Injuries to the abdomen, lower back, lumbar spine, pelvis and external genitals
S40-S49	Injuries to the shoulder and upper arm
S50-S59	Injuries to the elbow and forearm
S60-S69	Injuries to the wrist, hand, and fingers
S70-S79	Injuries to the hip and thigh
S80-S89	Injuries to the knee and lower leg
S90-S99	Injuries to the ankle and foot

T07	Injuries involving multiple body regions
T14	Injury of unspecified body region
T15-T19	Effects of foreign body entering through natural orifice
T20-T32	Burns and corrosions
T20-T25	Burns and corrosions of external body surface, specified by site
T26-T28	Burns and corrosions confined to eye and internal organs
T30-T32	Burns and corrosions of multiple and unspecified body regions
T33-T34	Frostbite
T36-T50	Poisoning by, adverse effect of and underdosing of drugs, medicaments and biological substances
T51-T65	Toxic effects of substances chiefly nonmedicinal as to source
T66-T78	Other and unspecified effects of external causes
T79	Certain early complications of trauma
T80-T88	Complications of surgical and medical care, not elsewhere classified

INJURIES TO THE HEAD (S00-S09)

Includes   injuries of ear
              injuries of eye
              injuries of face [any part]
              injuries of gum
              injuries of jaw
              injuries of oral cavity
              injuries of palate
              injuries of periocular area
              injuries of scalp
              injuries of temporomandibular joint area
              injuries of tongue
              injuries of tooth

Code also for any associated infection

Excludes2   burns and corrosions (T20-T32)
               effects of foreign body in ear (T16)
               effects of foreign body in larynx (T17.3)
               effects of foreign body in mouth NOS (T18.0)
               effects of foreign body in nose (T17.0-T17.1)
               effects of foreign body in pharynx (T17.2)
               effects of foreign body on external eye (T15.-)
               frostbite (T33-T34)
               insect bite or sting, venomous (T63.4)

● **S00**   **Superficial injury of head**

Excludes1   diffuse cerebral contusion (S06.2-)
               focal cerebral contusion (S06.3-)
               injury of eye and orbit (S05.-)
               open wound of head (S01.-)

The appropriate 7th character is to be added to each code from category S00

A	initial encounter
	All encounters involving diagnosis and treatment
D	subsequent encounter
	Encounters during the healing phase
S	sequela

● **S00.0**   **Superficial injury of scalp**

X● **S00.00**   **Unspecified** superficial injury of scalp

X● **S00.01**   **Abrasion of scalp**

X● **S00.02**   **Blister (nonthermal) of scalp**

X● **S00.03**   **Contusion of scalp**
              Bruise of scalp
              Hematoma of scalp

X● **S00.04**   **External constriction of part of scalp**

X● **S00.05**   **Superficial foreign body of scalp**
              Splinter in the scalp

X● **S00.06**   **Insect bite (nonvenomous) of scalp**

X● **S00.07**   **Other superficial bite of scalp**

              Excludes1   open bite of scalp (S01.05)

◀ New   ◀━ Revised   ~~deleted~~ Deleted   Excludes 1   Excludes 2   Includes   Use additional   Code first   Code also   Unspecified

OGCR Official Guidelines   X Assign placeholder X   ● Use Additional Character(s)   ▶ Manifestation Code   **Coding Clinic**

● **S00.1**   **Contusion of eyelid and periocular area**
     Black eye
       Excludes2   contusion of eyeball and orbital tissues
             (S05.1)

X● **S00.10**   Contusion of unspecified eyelid and periocular
             area

X● **S00.11**   Contusion of right eyelid and periocular area

X● **S00.12**   Contusion of left eyelid and periocular area

● **S00.2**   **Other and unspecified superficial injuries of eyelid and periocular area**
       Excludes2   superficial injury of conjunctiva and
             cornea (S05.0-)

  ● **S00.20**   Unspecified superficial injury of eyelid and
             periocular area

    ● **S00.201**   Unspecified superficial injury of right
               eyelid and periocular area

    ● **S00.202**   Unspecified superficial injury of left
               eyelid and periocular area

    ● **S00.209**   Unspecified superficial injury of
               unspecified eyelid and periocular area

  ● **S00.21**   Abrasion of eyelid and periocular area

    ● **S00.211**   Abrasion of right eyelid and
               periocular area

    ● **S00.212**   Abrasion of left eyelid and periocular
               area

    ● **S00.219**   Abrasion of unspecified eyelid and
               periocular area

  ● **S00.22**   Blister (nonthermal) of eyelid and periocular
             area

    ● **S00.221**   Blister (nonthermal) of right eyelid
               and periocular area

    ● **S00.222**   Blister (nonthermal) of left eyelid and
               periocular area

    ● **S00.229**   Blister (nonthermal) of unspecified
               eyelid and periocular area

  ● **S00.24**   External constriction of eyelid and periocular
             area

    ● **S00.241**   External constriction of right eyelid
               and periocular area

    ● **S00.242**   External constriction of left eyelid
               and periocular area

    ● **S00.249**   External constriction of unspecified
               eyelid and periocular area

  ● **S00.25**   Superficial foreign body of eyelid and
             periocular area
        Splinter of eyelid and periocular area
          Excludes2   retained foreign body in eyelid
                 (H02.81-)

    ● **S00.251**   Superficial foreign body of right
               eyelid and periocular area

    ● **S00.252**   Superficial foreign body of left eyelid
               and periocular area

    ● **S00.259**   Superficial foreign body of
               unspecified eyelid and periocular area

  ● **S00.26**   Insect bite (nonvenomous) of eyelid and
             periocular area

    ● **S00.261**   Insect bite (nonvenomous) of right
               eyelid and periocular area

    ● **S00.262**   Insect bite (nonvenomous) of left
               eyelid and periocular area

    ● **S00.269**   Insect bite (nonvenomous) of
               unspecified eyelid and periocular area

● **S00.27**   **Other superficial bite of eyelid and periocular area**
       Excludes1   open bite of eyelid and
             periocular area (S01.15)

  ● **S00.271**   Other superficial bite of right eyelid
              and periocular area

  ● **S00.272**   Other superficial bite of left eyelid
              and periocular area

  ● **S00.279**   Other superficial bite of unspecified
              eyelid and periocular area

● **S00.3**   **Superficial injury of nose**

X● **S00.30**   Unspecified superficial injury of nose

X● **S00.31**   Abrasion of nose

X● **S00.32**   Blister (nonthermal) of nose

X● **S00.33**   Contusion of nose
       Bruise of nose
       Hematoma of nose

X● **S00.34**   External constriction of nose

X● **S00.35**   Superficial foreign body of nose
       Splinter in the nose

X● **S00.36**   Insect bite (nonvenomous) of nose

X● **S00.37**   Other superficial bite of nose
         Excludes1   open bite of nose (S01.25)

● **S00.4**   **Superficial injury of ear**

  ● **S00.40**   Unspecified superficial injury of ear

    ● **S00.401**   Unspecified superficial injury of right
              ear

    ● **S00.402**   Unspecified superficial injury of left
              ear

    ● **S00.409**   Unspecified superficial injury of
              unspecified ear

  ● **S00.41**   Abrasion of ear

    ● **S00.411**   Abrasion of right ear

    ● **S00.412**   Abrasion of left ear

    ● **S00.419**   Abrasion of unspecified ear

  ● **S00.42**   Blister (nonthermal) of ear

    ● **S00.421**   Blister (nonthermal) of right ear

    ● **S00.422**   Blister (nonthermal) of left ear

    ● **S00.429**   Blister (nonthermal) of unspecified
              ear

  ● **S00.43**   Contusion of ear
       Bruise of ear
       Hematoma of ear

    ● **S00.431**   Contusion of right ear

    ● **S00.432**   Contusion of left ear

    ● **S00.439**   Contusion of unspecified ear

  ● **S00.44**   External constriction of ear

    ● **S00.441**   External constriction of right ear

    ● **S00.442**   External constriction of left ear

    ● **S00.449**   External constriction of unspecified
              ear

  ● **S00.45**   Superficial foreign body of ear
       Splinter in the ear

    ● **S00.451**   Superficial foreign body of right ear

    ● **S00.452**   Superficial foreign body of left ear

    ● **S00.459**   Superficial foreign body of
              unspecified ear

  ● **S00.46**   Insect bite (nonvenomous) of ear

    ● **S00.461**   Insect bite (nonvenomous) of right
              ear

    ● **S00.462**   Insect bite (nonvenomous) of left ear

    ● **S00.469**   Insect bite (nonvenomous) of
              unspecified ear

CHAPTER 19 (S00-T88)

● S00.47   Other superficial bite of ear
       Excludes1   open bite of ear (S01.35)
  - ● S00.471   Other superficial bite of right ear
  - ● S00.472   Other superficial bite of left ear
  - ● S00.479   Other superficial bite of unspecified ear

● S00.5   Superficial injury of lip and oral cavity
  - ● S00.50   Unspecified superficial injury of lip and oral cavity
    - ● S00.501   Unspecified superficial injury of lip
    - ● S00.502   Unspecified superficial injury of oral cavity
  - ● S00.51   Abrasion of lip and oral cavity
    - ● S00.511   Abrasion of lip
    - ● S00.512   Abrasion of oral cavity
  - ● S00.52   Blister (nonthermal) of lip and oral cavity
    - ● S00.521   Blister (nonthermal) of lip
    - ● S00.522   Blister (nonthermal) of oral cavity
  - ● S00.53   Contusion of lip and oral cavity
    - ● S00.531   Contusion of lip
      Bruise of lip
      Hematoma of oral cavity
    - ● S00.532   Contusion of oral cavity
      Bruise of lip
      Hematoma of oral cavity
  - ● S00.54   External constriction of lip and oral cavity
    - ● S00.541   External constriction of lip
    - ● S00.542   External constriction of oral cavity
  - ● S00.55   Superficial foreign body of lip and oral cavity
    - ● S00.551   Superficial foreign body of lip
      Splinter of lip and oral cavity
    - ● S00.552   Superficial foreign body of oral cavity
      Splinter of lip and oral cavity
  - ● S00.56   Insect bite (nonvenomous) of lip and oral cavity
    - ● S00.561   Insect bite (nonvenomous) of lip
    - ● S00.562   Insect bite (nonvenomous) of oral cavity
  - ● S00.57   Other superficial bite of lip and oral cavity
    - ● S00.571   Other superficial bite of lip
           Excludes1   open bite of lip (S01.551)
    - ● S00.572   Other superficial bite of oral cavity
           Excludes1   open bite of oral cavity (S01.552)

● S00.8   Superficial injury of other parts of head
  - X ● S00.80   Unspecified superficial injury of other part of head
  - X ● S00.81   Abrasion of other part of head
  - X ● S00.82   Blister (nonthermal) of other part of head
  - X ● S00.83   Contusion of other part of head
    Bruise of other part of head
    Hematoma of other part of head
  - X ● S00.84   External constriction of other part of head
  - X ● S00.85   Superficial foreign body of other part of head
    Splinter in other part of head
  - X ● S00.86   Insect bite (nonvenomous) of other part of head
  - X ● S00.87   Other superficial bite of other part of head
         Excludes1   open bite of other part of head (S01.85)

● S00.9   Superficial injury of unspecified part of head
  - X ● S00.90   Unspecified superficial injury of unspecified part of head
  - X ● S00.91   Abrasion of unspecified part of head
  - X ● S00.92   Blister (nonthermal) of unspecified part of head
  - X ● S00.93   Contusion of unspecified part of head
    Bruise of head
    Hematoma of head

- X ● S00.94   External constriction of unspecified part of head
- X ● S00.95   Superficial foreign body of unspecified part of head
  Splinter of head
- X ● S00.96   Insect bite (nonvenomous) of unspecified part of head
- X ● S00.97   Other superficial bite of unspecified part of head
       Excludes1   open bite of head (S01.95)

● S01   Open wound of head
  Code also any associated:
     injury of cranial nerve (S04.-)
     injury of muscle and tendon of head (S09.1-)
     intracranial injury (S06.-)
     wound infection
       Excludes1   open skull fracture (S02.- with 7th character B)
       Excludes2   injury of eye and orbit (S05.-)
            traumatic amputation of part of head (S08.-)

  The appropriate 7th character is to be added to each code from category S01

A	initial encounter
D	subsequent encounter
S	sequela

● S01.0   Open wound of scalp
       Excludes1   avulsion of scalp (S08.0)
  - X ● S01.00   Unspecified open wound of scalp
  - X ● S01.01   Laceration without foreign body of scalp
  - X ● S01.02   Laceration with foreign body of scalp
    Coding Clinic: 2015, Q1, P5-7
  - X ● S01.03   Puncture wound without foreign body of scalp
  - X ● S01.04   Puncture wound with foreign body of scalp
  - X ● S01.05   Open bite of scalp
    Bite of scalp NOS
         Excludes1   superficial bite of scalp (S00.06, S00.07-)

● S01.1   Open wound of eyelid and periocular area
  Open wound of eyelid and periocular area with or without involvement of lacrimal passages
  - ● S01.10   Unspecified open wound of eyelid and periocular area
    - ● S01.101   Unspecified open wound of right eyelid and periocular area
    - ● S01.102   Unspecified open wound of left eyelid and periocular area
    - ● S01.109   Unspecified open wound of unspecified eyelid and periocular area
  - ● S01.11   Laceration without foreign body of eyelid and periocular area
    - ● S01.111   Laceration without foreign body of right eyelid and periocular area
    - ● S01.112   Laceration without foreign body of left eyelid and periocular area
    - ● S01.119   Laceration without foreign body of unspecified eyelid and periocular area
  - ● S01.12   Laceration with foreign body of eyelid and periocular area
    - ● S01.121   Laceration with foreign body of right eyelid and periocular area
    - ● S01.122   Laceration with foreign body of left eyelid and periocular area
    - ● S01.129   Laceration with foreign body of unspecified eyelid and periocular area

◀ New   ◀ Revised   ~~deleted~~ Deleted   Excludes 1   Excludes 2   Includes   Use additional   Code first   Code also   Unspecified

OGCR Official Guidelines   X Assign placeholder X   ● Use Additional Character(s)   ▶ Manifestation Code   **Coding Clinic**

● S01.13   Puncture wound without foreign body of eyelid and periocular area
    ● S01.131   Puncture wound without foreign body of right eyelid and periocular area
    ● S01.132   Puncture wound without foreign body of left eyelid and periocular area
    ● S01.139   Puncture wound without foreign body of unspecified eyelid and periocular area

● S01.14   Puncture wound with foreign body of eyelid and periocular area
    ● S01.141   Puncture wound with foreign body of right eyelid and periocular area
    ● S01.142   Puncture wound with foreign body of left eyelid and periocular area
    ● S01.149   Puncture wound with foreign body of unspecified eyelid and periocular area

● S01.15   Open bite of eyelid and periocular area
      Bite of eyelid and periocular area NOS
      Excludes1   superficial bite of eyelid and periocular area (S00.26, S00.27)
    ● S01.151   Open bite of right eyelid and periocular area
    ● S01.152   Open bite of left eyelid and periocular area
    ● S01.159   Open bite of unspecified eyelid and periocular area

● S01.2   Open wound of nose
   X ● S01.20   Unspecified open wound of nose
   X ● S01.21   Laceration without foreign body of nose
        Coding Clinic: 2015, Q1, P5-6
   X ● S01.22   Laceration with foreign body of nose
   X ● S01.23   Puncture wound without foreign body of nose
   X ● S01.24   Puncture wound with foreign body of nose
   X ● S01.25   Open bite of nose
        Bite of nose NOS
        Excludes1   superficial bite of nose (S00.36, S00.37)

● S01.3   Open wound of ear
   ● S01.30   Unspecified open wound of ear
    ● S01.301   Unspecified open wound of right ear
    ● S01.302   Unspecified open wound of left ear
    ● S01.309   Unspecified open wound of unspecified ear
   ● S01.31   Laceration without foreign body of ear
    ● S01.311   Laceration without foreign body of right ear
    ● S01.312   Laceration without foreign body of left ear
    ● S01.319   Laceration without foreign body of unspecified ear
   ● S01.32   Laceration with foreign body of ear
    ● S01.321   Laceration with foreign body of right ear
    ● S01.322   Laceration with foreign body of left ear
    ● S01.329   Laceration with foreign body of unspecified ear
   ● S01.33   Puncture wound without foreign body of ear
    ● S01.331   Puncture wound without foreign body of right ear
    ● S01.332   Puncture wound without foreign body of left ear
    ● S01.339   Puncture wound without foreign body of unspecified ear

● S01.34   Puncture wound with foreign body of ear
    ● S01.341   Puncture wound with foreign body of right ear
    ● S01.342   Puncture wound with foreign body of left ear
    ● S01.349   Puncture wound with foreign body of unspecified ear

● S01.35   Open bite of ear
      Bite of ear NOS
      Excludes1   superficial bite of ear (S00.46, S00.47)
    ● S01.351   Open bite of right ear
    ● S01.352   Open bite of left ear
    ● S01.359   Open bite of unspecified ear

● S01.4   Open wound of cheek and temporomandibular area
   ● S01.40   Unspecified open wound of cheek and temporomandibular area
    ● S01.401   Unspecified open wound of right cheek and temporomandibular area
    ● S01.402   Unspecified open wound of left cheek and temporomandibular area
    ● S01.409   Unspecified open wound of unspecified cheek and temporomandibular area
   ● S01.41   Laceration without foreign body of cheek and temporomandibular area
    ● S01.411   Laceration without foreign body of right cheek and temporomandibular area
        Coding Clinic: 2015, Q1, P5-7
    ● S01.412   Laceration without foreign body of left cheek and temporomandibular area
    ● S01.419   Laceration without foreign body of unspecified cheek and temporomandibular area
   ● S01.42   Laceration with foreign body of cheek and temporomandibular area
    ● S01.421   Laceration with foreign body of right cheek and temporomandibular area
    ● S01.422   Laceration with foreign body of left cheek and temporomandibular area
    ● S01.429   Laceration with foreign body of unspecified cheek and temporomandibular area
   ● S01.43   Puncture wound without foreign body of cheek and temporomandibular area
    ● S01.431   Puncture wound without foreign body of right cheek and temporomandibular area
    ● S01.432   Puncture wound without foreign body of left cheek and temporomandibular area
    ● S01.439   Puncture wound without foreign body of unspecified cheek and temporomandibular area
   ● S01.44   Puncture wound with foreign body of cheek and temporomandibular area
    ● S01.441   Puncture wound with foreign body of right cheek and temporomandibular area
    ● S01.442   Puncture wound with foreign body of left cheek and temporomandibular area
    ● S01.449   Puncture wound with foreign body of unspecified cheek and temporomandibular area

● **S01.45** **Open bite of cheek and temporomandibular area**
> Bite of cheek and temporomandibular area NOS
>
> **Excludes2**   superficial bite of cheek and temporomandibular area (S00.86, S00.87)

  ● **S01.451**   **Open bite of right cheek and temporomandibular area**
  ● **S01.452**   **Open bite of left cheek and temporomandibular area**
  ● **S01.459**   **Open bite of unspecified cheek and temporomandibular area**

● **S01.5** **Open wound of lip and oral cavity**
> **Excludes2**   tooth dislocation (S03.2)
> tooth fracture (S02.5)

  ● **S01.50**   **Unspecified open wound of lip and oral cavity**
    ● **S01.501**   **Unspecified open wound of lip**
    ● **S01.502**   **Unspecified open wound of oral cavity**
  ● **S01.51**   **Laceration of lip and oral cavity without foreign body**
    ● **S01.511**   **Laceration without foreign body of lip**
    ● **S01.512**   **Laceration without foreign body of oral cavity**
  ● **S01.52**   **Laceration of lip and oral cavity with foreign body**
    ● **S01.521**   **Laceration with foreign body of lip**
    ● **S01.522**   **Laceration with foreign body of oral cavity**
  ● **S01.53**   **Puncture wound of lip and oral cavity without foreign body**
    ● **S01.531**   **Puncture wound without foreign body of lip**
    ● **S01.532**   **Puncture wound without foreign body of oral cavity**
  ● **S01.54**   **Puncture wound of lip and oral cavity with foreign body**
    ● **S01.541**   **Puncture wound with foreign body of lip**
    ● **S01.542**   **Puncture wound with foreign body of oral cavity**
  ● **S01.55**   **Open bite of lip and oral cavity**
    ● **S01.551**   **Open bite of lip**
      > Bite of lip NOS
      >
      > **Excludes1**   superficial bite of lip (S00.571)
    ● **S01.552**   **Open bite of oral cavity**
      > Bite of oral cavity NOS
      >
      > **Excludes1**   superficial bite of oral cavity (S00.572)

● **S01.8** **Open wound of other parts of head**
  X ● **S01.80**   **Unspecified open wound of other part of head**
  X ● **S01.81**   **Laceration without foreign body of other part of head**
  X ● **S01.82**   **Laceration with foreign body of other part of head**
  X ● **S01.83**   **Puncture wound without foreign body of other part of head**
  X ● **S01.84**   **Puncture wound with foreign body of other part of head**
  X ● **S01.85**   **Open bite of other part of head**
    > Bite of other part of head NOS
    >
    > **Excludes1**   superficial bite of other part of head (S00.85)

● **S01.9** **Open wound of unspecified part of head**
  X ● **S01.90**   **Unspecified open wound of unspecified part of head**
  X ● **S01.91**   **Laceration without foreign body of unspecified part of head**
  X ● **S01.92**   **Laceration with foreign body of unspecified part of head**
  X ● **S01.93**   **Puncture wound without foreign body of unspecified part of head**
  X ● **S01.94**   **Puncture wound with foreign body of unspecified part of head**
  X ● **S01.95**   **Open bite of unspecified part of head**
    > Bite of head NOS
    >
    > **Excludes1**   superficial bite of head NOS (S00.97)

● **S02** **Fracture of skull and facial bones**
> **Note:** A fracture not indicated as open or closed should be coded to closed
>
> The appropriate 7th character is to be added to each code from category S02

A	initial encounter for closed fracture
B	initial encounter for open fracture
D	subsequent encounter for fracture with routine healing
G	subsequent encounter for fracture with delayed healing
K	subsequent encounter for fracture with nonunion
S	sequela

> Code also any associated intracranial injury (S06.-)

  X ● **S02.0**   **Fracture of vault of skull**
    > Fracture of frontal bone
    > Fracture of parietal bone
  ● **S02.1**   **Fracture of base of skull**
    > **Excludes1**   orbit NOS (S02.8)
    > **Excludes2**   orbital floor (S02.3-)

    X ● **S02.10**   **Unspecified fracture of base of skull**
    ● **S02.11**   **Fracture of occiput**
      ● **S02.110**   **Type I occipital condyle fracture**
      ● **S02.111**   **Type II occipital condyle fracture**
      ● **S02.112**   **Type III occipital condyle fracture**
      ● **S02.113**   **Unspecified occipital condyle fracture**
      ● **S02.118**   **Other fracture of occiput**
      ● **S02.119**   **Unspecified fracture of occiput**
    X ● **S02.19**   **Other fracture of base of skull**
      > Fracture of anterior fossa of base of skull
      > Fracture of ethmoid sinus
      > Fracture of frontal sinus
      > Fracture of middle fossa of base of skull
      > Fracture of orbital roof
      > Fracture of posterior fossa of base of skull
      > Fracture of sphenoid
      > Fracture of temporal bone

  X ● **S02.2**   **Fracture of nasal bones**
  X ● **S02.3**   **Fracture of orbital floor**
    > **Excludes1**   orbit NOS (S02.8)
    > **Excludes2**   orbital roof (S02.1-)

  ● **S02.4**   **Fracture of malar, maxillary and zygoma bones**
    > Fracture of superior maxilla
    > Fracture of upper jaw (bone)
    > Fracture of zygomatic process of temporal bone

    ● **S02.40**   **Fracture of malar, maxillary and zygoma bones, unspecified**
      ● **S02.400**   **Malar fracture unspecified**
      ● **S02.401**   **Maxillary fracture, unspecified**
      ● **S02.402**   **Zygomatic fracture, unspecified**

1260

◄ New   ◄▥ Revised   ~~deleted~~ Deleted   Excludes 1   Excludes 2   Includes   Use additional   Code first   Code also   Unspecified

OGCR Official Guidelines   **X** Assign placeholder X   ● Use Additional Character(s)   ▶ Manifestation Code   **Coding Clinic**

● **S02.41**   **LeFort fracture**
  ● **S02.411**   **LeFort I fracture**
  ● **S02.412**   **LeFort II fracture**
  ● **S02.413**   **LeFort III fracture**
X● **S02.42**   **Fracture of alveolus of maxilla**
X● **S02.5**   **Fracture of tooth (traumatic) Broken tooth**
  Excludes1   cracked tooth (nontraumatic) (K03.81)
● **S02.6**   **Fracture of mandible**
  Fracture of lower jaw (bone)
  ● **S02.60**   **Fracture of mandible of unspecified site**
    ● **S02.600**   **Fracture of unspecified part of body of mandible**
    ● **S02.609**   **Fracture of mandible, unspecified**
  X● **S02.61**   **Fracture of condylar process of mandible**
  X● **S02.62**   **Fracture of subcondylar process of mandible**
  X● **S02.63**   **Fracture of coronoid process of mandible**
  X● **S02.64**   **Fracture of ramus of mandible**
  X● **S02.65**   **Fracture of angle of mandible**
  X● **S02.66**   **Fracture of symphysis of mandible**
  X● **S02.67**   **Fracture of alveolus of mandible**
  X● **S02.69**   **Fracture of mandible of other specified site**
X● **S02.8**   **Fractures of other specified skull and facial bones**
  Fracture of orbit NOS
  Fracture of palate
  Excludes1   fracture of orbital floor (S02.3-)
              fracture of orbital roof (S02.1-)
● **S02.9**   **Fracture of unspecified skull and facial bones**
  X● **S02.91**   **Unspecified fracture of skull**
  X● **S02.92**   **Unspecified fracture of facial bones**

● **S03**   **Dislocation and sprain of joints and ligaments of head**
  Includes   avulsion of joint (capsule) or ligament of head
            laceration of cartilage, joint (capsule) or ligament of head
            sprain of cartilage, joint (capsule) or ligament of head
            traumatic hemarthrosis of joint or ligament of head
            traumatic rupture of joint or ligament of head
            traumatic subluxation of joint or ligament of head
            traumatic tear of joint or ligament of head
  Code also any associated open wound
  Excludes2   Strain of muscle or tendon of head (S09.1)
  The appropriate 7th character is to be added to each code from category S03

A	initial encounter
D	subsequent encounter
S	sequela

  X● **S03.0**   **Dislocation of jaw**
    Dislocation of jaw (cartilage) (meniscus)
    Dislocation of mandible
    Dislocation of temporomandibular (joint)
  X● **S03.1**   **Dislocation of septal cartilage of nose**
  X● **S03.2**   **Dislocation of tooth**
  X● **S03.4**   **Sprain of jaw**
    Sprain of temporomandibular (joint) (ligament)
  X● **S03.8**   **Sprain of joints and ligaments of other parts of head**
  X● **S03.9**   **Sprain of joints and ligaments of unspecified parts of head**

● **S04**   **Injury of cranial nerve**
  The selection of side should be based on the side of the body being affected
  Code first any associated intracranial injury (S06.-)
  Code also any associated:
    open wound of head (S01.-)
    skull fracture (S02.-)
  The appropriate 7th character is to be added to each code from category S04

A	initial encounter
D	subsequent encounter
S	sequela

  ● **S04.0**   **Injury of optic nerve and pathways**
    Use additional code to identify any visual field defect or blindness (H53.4-, H54)
    ● **S04.01**   **Injury of optic nerve**
      Injury of 2nd cranial nerve
      ● **S04.011**   **Injury of optic nerve, right eye**
      ● **S04.012**   **Injury of optic nerve, left eye**
      ● **S04.019**   **Injury of optic nerve, unspecified eye**
        Injury of optic nerve NOS
    X● **S04.02**   **Injury of optic chiasm**
    ● **S04.03**   **Injury of optic tract and pathways**
      Injury of optic radiation
      ● **S04.031**   **Injury of optic tract and pathways, right eye**
      ● **S04.032**   **Injury of optic tract and pathways, left eye**
      ● **S04.039**   **Injury of optic tract and pathways, unspecified eye**
        Injury of optic tract and pathways NOS
    ● **S04.04**   **Injury of visual cortex**
      ● **S04.041**   **Injury of visual cortex, right eye**
      ● **S04.042**   **Injury of visual cortex, left eye**
      ● **S04.049**   **Injury of visual cortex, unspecified eye**
        Injury of visual cortex NOS
  ● **S04.1**   **Injury of oculomotor nerve**
    Injury of 3rd cranial nerve
    X● **S04.10**   **Injury of oculomotor nerve, unspecified side**
    X● **S04.11**   **Injury of oculomotor nerve, right side**
    X● **S04.12**   **Injury of oculomotor nerve, left side**
  ● **S04.2**   **Injury of trochlear nerve**
    Injury of 4th cranial nerve
    X● **S04.20**   **Injury of trochlear nerve, unspecified side**
    X● **S04.21**   **Injury of trochlear nerve, right side**
    X● **S04.22**   **Injury of trochlear nerve, left side**
  ● **S04.3**   **Injury of trigeminal nerve**
    Injury of 5th cranial nerve
    X● **S04.30**   **Injury of trigeminal nerve, unspecified side**
    X● **S04.31**   **Injury of trigeminal nerve, right side**
    X● **S04.32**   **Injury of trigeminal nerve, left side**
  ● **S04.4**   **Injury of abducent nerve**
    Injury of 6th cranial nerve
    X● **S04.40**   **Injury of abducent nerve, unspecified side**
    X● **S04.41**   **Injury of abducent nerve, right side**
    X● **S04.42**   **Injury of abducent nerve, left side**
  ● **S04.5**   **Injury of facial nerve**
    Injury of 7th cranial nerve
    X● **S04.50**   **Injury of facial nerve, unspecified side**
    X● **S04.51**   **Injury of facial nerve, right side**
    X● **S04.52**   **Injury of facial nerve, left side**

CHAPTER 19 (S00–T88)

● **S04.6**   **Injury of acoustic nerve**
     Injury of auditory nerve
     Injury of 8th cranial nerve

X● **S04.60**   Injury of acoustic nerve, unspecified side

X● **S04.61**   Injury of acoustic nerve, right side

X● **S04.62**   Injury of acoustic nerve, left side

● **S04.7**   **Injury of accessory nerve**
     Injury of 11th cranial nerve

X● **S04.70**   Injury of accessory nerve, unspecified side

X● **S04.71**   Injury of accessory nerve, right side

X● **S04.72**   Injury of accessory nerve, left side

● **S04.8**   **Injury of other cranial nerves**

   ● **S04.81**   **Injury of olfactory [1st] nerve**

     ● **S04.811**   Injury of olfactory [1st] nerve, right side

     ● **S04.812**   Injury of olfactory [1st] nerve, left side

     ● **S04.819**   Injury of olfactory [1st] nerve, unspecified side

   ● **S04.89**   **Injury of other cranial nerves**
      Injury of vagus [10th] nerve

     ● **S04.891**   Injury of other cranial nerves, right side

     ● **S04.892**   Injury of other cranial nerves, left side

     ● **S04.899**   Injury of other cranial nerves, unspecified side

X● **S04.9**   **Injury of unspecified cranial nerve**

● **S05**   **Injury of eye and orbit**

   Includes   open wound of eye and orbit

   Excludes2   2nd cranial [optic] nerve injury (S04.0-)
         3rd cranial [oculomotor] nerve injury (S04.1-)
         open wound of eyelid and periocular area (S01.1-)
         orbital bone fracture (S02.1-, S02.3-, S02.8-)
         superficial injury of eyelid (S00.1-S00.2)

   The appropriate 7th character is to be added to each code from category S05

A	initial encounter
D	subsequent encounter
S	sequela

● **S05.0**   **Injury of conjunctiva and corneal abrasion without foreign body**

   Excludes1   foreign body in conjunctival sac (T15.1)
         foreign body in cornea (T15.0)

X● **S05.00**   Injury of conjunctiva and corneal abrasion without foreign body, unspecified eye

X● **S05.01**   Injury of conjunctiva and corneal abrasion without foreign body, right eye

X● **S05.02**   Injury of conjunctiva and corneal abrasion without foreign body, left eye

● **S05.1**   **Contusion of eyeball and orbital tissues**
     Traumatic hyphema

   Excludes2   black eye NOS (S00.1)
         contusion of eyelid and periocular area (S00.1)

X● **S05.10**   Contusion of eyeball and orbital tissues, unspecified eye

X● **S05.11**   Contusion of eyeball and orbital tissues, right eye

X● **S05.12**   Contusion of eyeball and orbital tissues, left eye

● **S05.2**   **Ocular laceration and rupture with prolapse or loss of intraocular tissue**

X● **S05.20**   Ocular laceration and rupture with prolapse or loss of intraocular tissue, unspecified eye

X● **S05.21**   Ocular laceration and rupture with prolapse or loss of intraocular tissue, right eye

X● **S05.22**   Ocular laceration and rupture with prolapse or loss of intraocular tissue, left eye

● **S05.3**   **Ocular laceration without prolapse or loss of intraocular tissue**
     Laceration of eye NOS

X● **S05.30**   Ocular laceration without prolapse or loss of intraocular tissue, unspecified eye

X● **S05.31**   Ocular laceration without prolapse or loss of intraocular tissue, right eye

X● **S05.32**   Ocular laceration without prolapse or loss of intraocular tissue, left eye

● **S05.4**   **Penetrating wound of orbit with or without foreign body**

   Excludes2   retained (old) foreign body following penetrating wound in orbit (H05.5-)

X● **S05.40**   Penetrating wound of orbit with or without foreign body, unspecified eye

X● **S05.41**   Penetrating wound of orbit with or without foreign body, right eye

X● **S05.42**   Penetrating wound of orbit with or without foreign body, left eye

● **S05.5**   **Penetrating wound with foreign body of eyeball**

   Excludes2   retained (old) intraocular foreign body (H44.6-, H44.7)

X● **S05.50**   Penetrating wound with foreign body of unspecified eyeball

X● **S05.51**   Penetrating wound with foreign body of right eyeball

X● **S05.52**   Penetrating wound with foreign body of left eyeball

● **S05.6**   **Penetrating wound without foreign body of eyeball**
     Ocular penetration NOS

X● **S05.60**   Penetrating wound without foreign body of unspecified eyeball

X● **S05.61**   Penetrating wound without foreign body of right eyeball

X● **S05.62**   Penetrating wound without foreign body of left eyeball

● **S05.7**   **Avulsion of eye**
     Traumatic enucleation

X● **S05.70**   Avulsion of unspecified eye

X● **S05.71**   Avulsion of right eye

X● **S05.72**   Avulsion of left eye

● **S05.8**   **Other injuries of eye and orbit**
     Lacrimal duct injury

   ● **S05.8X**   **Other injuries of eye and orbit**

     ● **S05.8X1**   Other injuries of right eye and orbit

     ● **S05.8X2**   Other injuries of left eye and orbit

     ● **S05.8X9**   Other injuries of unspecified eye and orbit

● **S05.9**   **Unspecified injury of eye and orbit**
     Injury of eye NOS

X● **S05.90**   Unspecified injury of unspecified eye and orbit

X● **S05.91**   Unspecified injury of right eye and orbit

X● **S05.92**   Unspecified injury of left eye and orbit

◀ New   ◀▥ Revised   ~~deleted~~ Deleted   Excludes 1   Excludes 2   Includes   Use additional   Code first   Code also   Unspecified

1262   **OGCR** Official Guidelines   X Assign placeholder X   ● Use Additional Character(s)   ▶ Manifestation Code   **Coding Clinic**

● **S06   Intracranial injury**

> **Includes**   traumatic brain injury

> Code also any associated:
> open wound of head (S01.-)
> skull fracture (S02.-)

> **Excludes1**   head injury NOS (S09.90)

> The appropriate 7th character is to be added to each code from
> category S06

> | A | initial encounter |
> |---|---|
> | D | subsequent encounter |
> | S | sequela |

● **S06.0   Concussion**
> Commotio cerebri

> **Excludes1**   concussion with other intracranial
> injuries classified in category S06-
> code to specified intracranial injury

● **S06.0X   Concussion**

● **S06.0X0   Concussion without loss of
consciousness**

● **S06.0X1   Concussion with loss of
consciousness of 30 minutes or less**

● **S06.0X2   Concussion with loss of
consciousness of 31 minutes to
59 minutes**

● **S06.0X3   Concussion with loss of
consciousness of 1 hour to 5 hours
59 minutes**

● **S06.0X4   Concussion with loss of
consciousness of 6 hours to 24 hours**

● **S06.0X5   Concussion with loss of
consciousness greater than 24 hours
with return to pre-existing conscious
level**

● **S06.0X6   Concussion with loss of
consciousness greater than 24 hours
without return to pre-existing
conscious level with patient surviving**

● **S06.0X7   Concussion with loss of
consciousness of any duration with
death due to brain injury prior to
regaining consciousness**

● **S06.0X8   Concussion with loss of
consciousness of any duration with
death due to other cause prior to
regaining consciousness**

● **S06.0X9   Concussion with loss of
consciousness of unspecified duration**
> Concussion NOS

● **S06.1   Traumatic cerebral edema**
> Diffuse traumatic cerebral edema
> Focal traumatic cerebral edema

● **S06.1X   Traumatic cerebral edema**

● **S06.1X0   Traumatic cerebral edema without
loss of consciousness**
> **Coding Clinic: 2015, Q1, P12**

● **S06.1X1   Traumatic cerebral edema with loss of
consciousness of 30 minutes or less**

● **S06.1X2   Traumatic cerebral edema with loss of
consciousness of 31 minutes to
59 minutes**

● **S06.1X3   Traumatic cerebral edema with loss of
consciousness of 1 hour to 5 hours
59 minutes**

● **S06.1X4   Traumatic cerebral edema with loss of
consciousness of 6 hours to 24 hours**

● **S06.1X5   Traumatic cerebral edema with loss of
consciousness greater than 24 hours
with return to pre-existing conscious
level**

● **S06.1X6   Traumatic cerebral edema with loss of
consciousness greater than 24 hours
without return to pre-existing
conscious level with patient surviving**

● **S06.1X7   Traumatic cerebral edema with loss of
consciousness of any duration with
death due to brain injury prior to
regaining consciousness**

● **S06.1X8   Traumatic cerebral edema with loss of
consciousness of any duration with
death due to other cause prior to
regaining consciousness**

● **S06.1X9   Traumatic cerebral edema with loss of
consciousness of unspecified duration**
> Traumatic cerebral edema NOS

● **S06.2   Diffuse traumatic brain injury**
> Diffuse axonal brain injury

> **Excludes1**   traumatic diffuse cerebral edema
> (S06.1X-)

● **S06.2X   Diffuse traumatic brain injury**

● **S06.2X0   Diffuse traumatic brain injury
without loss of consciousness**

● **S06.2X1   Diffuse traumatic brain injury with
loss of consciousness of 30 minutes or
less**

● **S06.2X2   Diffuse traumatic brain injury with
loss of consciousness of 31 minutes to
59 minutes**

● **S06.2X3   Diffuse traumatic brain injury with
loss of consciousness of 1 hour to
5 hours 59 minutes**

● **S06.2X4   Diffuse traumatic brain injury with
loss
of consciousness of 6 hours to
24 hours**

● **S06.2X5   Diffuse traumatic brain injury with
loss of consciousness greater than
24 hours with return to pre-existing
conscious levels**

● **S06.2X6   Diffuse traumatic brain injury with
loss of consciousness greater than
24 hours without return to pre-
existing conscious level with patient
surviving**

● **S06.2X7   Diffuse traumatic brain injury with
loss of consciousness of any duration
with death due to brain injury prior
to regaining consciousness**

● **S06.2X8   Diffuse traumatic brain injury with
loss of consciousness of any duration
with death due to other cause prior to
regaining consciousness**

● **S06.2X9   Diffuse traumatic brain injury with
loss of consciousness of unspecified
duration**
> Diffuse traumatic brain injury NOS

● **S06.3   Focal traumatic brain injury**
> **Excludes1**   any condition classifiable to S06.4-S06.6
> focal cerebral edema (S06.1)

● **S06.30   Unspecified focal traumatic brain injury**

● **S06.300   Unspecified focal traumatic brain
injury without loss of consciousness**

● **S06.301   Unspecified focal traumatic brain
injury with loss of consciousness of
30 minutes or less**

● **S06.302   Unspecified focal traumatic brain
injury with loss of consciousness of
31 minutes to 59 minutes**

● **S06.303   Unspecified focal traumatic brain
injury with loss of consciousness of
1 hour to 5 hours 59 minutes**

CHAPTER 19 (S00-T88)

● S06.304 Unspecified focal traumatic brain injury with loss of consciousness of 6 hours to 24 hours

● S06.305 Unspecified focal traumatic brain injury with loss of consciousness greater than 24 hours with return to pre-existing conscious level

● S06.306 Unspecified focal traumatic brain injury with loss of consciousness greater than 24 hours without return to pre-existing conscious level with patient surviving

● S06.307 Unspecified focal traumatic brain injury with loss of consciousness of any duration with death due to brain injury prior to regaining consciousness

● S06.308 Unspecified focal traumatic brain injury with loss of consciousness of any duration with death due to other cause prior to regaining consciousness

● S06.309 Unspecified focal traumatic brain injury with loss of consciousness of unspecified duration
　　　Unspecified focal traumatic brain injury NOS

● S06.31 Contusion and laceration of right cerebrum

● S06.310 Contusion and laceration of right cerebrum without loss of consciousness

● S06.311 Contusion and laceration of right cerebrum with loss of consciousness of 30 minutes or less

● S06.312 Contusion and laceration of right cerebrum with loss of consciousness of 31 minutes to 59 minutes

● S06.313 Contusion and laceration of right cerebrum with loss of consciousness of 1 hour to 5 hours 59 minutes

● S06.314 Contusion and laceration of right cerebrum with loss of consciousness of 6 hours to 24 hours

● S06.315 Contusion and laceration of right cerebrum with loss of consciousness greater than 24 hours with return to pre-existing conscious level

● S06.316 Contusion and laceration of right cerebrum with loss of consciousness greater than 24 hours without return to pre-existing conscious level with patient surviving

● S06.317 Contusion and laceration of right cerebrum with loss of consciousness of any duration with death due to brain injury prior to regaining consciousness

● S06.318 Contusion and laceration of right cerebrum with loss of consciousness of any duration with death due to other cause prior to regaining consciousness

● S06.319 Contusion and laceration of right cerebrum with loss of consciousness of unspecified duration
　　　Contusion and laceration of right cerebrum NOS

● S06.32 Contusion and laceration of left cerebrum

● S06.320 Contusion and laceration of left cerebrum without loss of consciousness

● S06.321 Contusion and laceration of left cerebrum with loss of consciousness of 30 minutes or less

● S06.322 Contusion and laceration of left cerebrum with loss of consciousness of 31 minutes to 59 minutes

● S06.323 Contusion and laceration of left cerebrum with loss of consciousness of 1 hour to 5 hours 59 minutes

● S06.324 Contusion and laceration of left cerebrum with loss of consciousness of 6 hours to 24 hours

● S06.325 Contusion and laceration of left cerebrum with loss of consciousness greater than 24 hours with return to pre-existing conscious level

● S06.326 Contusion and laceration of left cerebrum with loss of consciousness greater than 24 hours without return to pre-existing conscious level with patient surviving

● S06.327 Contusion and laceration of left cerebrum with loss of consciousness of any duration with death due to brain injury prior to regaining consciousness

● S06.328 Contusion and laceration of left cerebrum with loss of consciousness of any duration with death due to other cause prior to regaining consciousness

● S06.329 Contusion and laceration of left cerebrum with loss of consciousness of unspecified duration
　　　Contusion and laceration of left cerebrum NOS

● S06.33 Contusion and laceration of cerebrum, unspecified

● S06.330 Contusion and laceration of cerebrum, unspecified, without loss of consciousness

● S06.331 Contusion and laceration of cerebrum, unspecified, with loss of consciousness of 30 minutes or less

● S06.332 Contusion and laceration of cerebrum, unspecified, with loss of consciousness of 31 minutes to 59 minutes

● S06.333 Contusion and laceration of cerebrum, unspecified, with loss of consciousness of 1 hour to 5 hours 59 minutes

● S06.334 Contusion and laceration of cerebrum, unspecified, with loss of consciousness of 6 hours to 24 hours

● S06.335 Contusion and laceration of cerebrum, unspecified, with loss of consciousness greater than 24 hours with return to pre-existing conscious level

● S06.336 Contusion and laceration of cerebrum, unspecified, with loss of consciousness greater than 24 hours without return to pre-existing conscious level with patient surviving

- S06.337   Contusion and laceration of cerebrum, unspecified, with loss of consciousness of any duration with death due to brain injury prior to regaining consciousness
- S06.338   Contusion and laceration of cerebrum, unspecified, with loss of consciousness of any duration with death due to other cause prior to regaining consciousness
- S06.339   Contusion and laceration of cerebrum, unspecified, with loss of consciousness of unspecified duration
  Contusion and laceration of cerebrum NOS

- S06.34   **Traumatic hemorrhage of right cerebrum**
  Traumatic intracerebral hemorrhage and hematoma of right cerebrum

  - S06.340   Traumatic hemorrhage of right cerebrum without loss of consciousness
    Coding Clinic: 2015, Q1, P12
  - S06.341   Traumatic hemorrhage of right cerebrum with loss of consciousness of 30 minutes or less
  - S06.342   Traumatic hemorrhage of right cerebrum with loss of consciousness of 31 minutes to 59 minutes
  - S06.343   Traumatic hemorrhage of right cerebrum with loss of consciousness of 1 hours to 5 hours 59 minutes
  - S06.344   Traumatic hemorrhage of right cerebrum with loss of consciousness of 6 hours to 24 hours
  - S06.345   Traumatic hemorrhage of right cerebrum with loss of consciousness greater than 24 hours with return to pre-existing conscious level
  - S06.346   Traumatic hemorrhage of right cerebrum with loss of consciousness greater than 24 hours without return to pre-existing conscious level with patient surviving
  - S06.347   Traumatic hemorrhage of right cerebrum with loss of consciousness of any duration with death due to brain injury prior to regaining consciousness
  - S06.348   Traumatic hemorrhage of right cerebrum with loss of consciousness of any duration with death due to other cause prior to regaining consciousness
  - S06.349   Traumatic hemorrhage of right cerebrum with loss of consciousness of unspecified duration
    Traumatic hemorrhage of right cerebrum NOS

- S06.35   **Traumatic hemorrhage of left cerebrum**
  Traumatic intracerebral hemorrhage and hematoma of left cerebrum

  - S06.350   Traumatic hemorrhage of left cerebrum without loss of consciousness
  - S06.351   Traumatic hemorrhage of left cerebrum with loss of consciousness of 30 minutes or less
  - S06.352   Traumatic hemorrhage of left cerebrum with loss of consciousness of 31 minutes to 59 minutes
  - S06.353   Traumatic hemorrhage of left cerebrum with loss of consciousness of 1 hours to 5 hours 59 minutes

- S06.354   Traumatic hemorrhage of left cerebrum with loss of consciousness of 6 hours to 24 hours
- S06.355   Traumatic hemorrhage of left cerebrum with loss of consciousness greater than 24 hours with return to pre-existing conscious level
- S06.356   Traumatic hemorrhage of left cerebrum with loss of consciousness greater than 24 hours without return to pre-existing conscious level with patient surviving
- S06.357   Traumatic hemorrhage of left cerebrum with loss of consciousness of any duration with death due to brain injury prior to regaining consciousness
- S06.358   Traumatic hemorrhage of left cerebrum with loss of consciousness of any duration with death due to other cause prior to regaining consciousness
- S06.359   Traumatic hemorrhage of left cerebrum with loss of consciousness of unspecified duration
  Traumatic hemorrhage of left cerebrum NOS

- S06.36   **Traumatic hemorrhage of cerebrum, unspecified**
  Traumatic intracerebral hemorrhage and hematoma, unspecified

  - S06.360   Traumatic hemorrhage of cerebrum, unspecified, without loss of consciousness
  - S06.361   Traumatic hemorrhage of cerebrum, unspecified, with loss of consciousness of 30 minutes or less
  - S06.362   Traumatic hemorrhage of cerebrum, unspecified, with loss of consciousness of 31 minutes to 59 minutes
  - S06.363   Traumatic hemorrhage of cerebrum, unspecified, with loss of consciousness of 1 hours to 5 hours 59 minutes
  - S06.364   Traumatic hemorrhage of cerebrum, unspecified, with loss of consciousness of 6 hours to 24 hours
  - S06.365   Traumatic hemorrhage of cerebrum, unspecified, with loss of consciousness greater than 24 hours with return to pre-existing conscious level
  - S06.366   Traumatic hemorrhage of cerebrum, unspecified, with loss of consciousness greater than 24 hours without return to pre-existing conscious level with patient surviving
  - S06.367   Traumatic hemorrhage of cerebrum, unspecified, with loss of consciousness of any duration with death due to brain injury prior to regaining consciousness
  - S06.368   Traumatic hemorrhage of cerebrum, unspecified, with loss of consciousness of any duration with death due to other cause prior to regaining consciousness
  - S06.369   Traumatic hemorrhage of cerebrum, unspecified, with loss of consciousness of unspecified duration
    Traumatic hemorrhage of cerebrum NOS

● S06.37   Contusion, laceration, and hemorrhage of cerebellum
  ● S06.370   Contusion, laceration, and hemorrhage of cerebellum without loss of consciousness
  ● S06.371   Contusion, laceration, and hemorrhage of cerebellum with loss of consciousness of 30 minutes or less
  ● S06.372   Contusion, laceration, and hemorrhage of cerebellum with loss of consciousness of 31 minutes to 59 minutes
  ● S06.373   Contusion, laceration, and hemorrhage of cerebellum with loss of consciousness of 1 hour to 5 hours 59 minutes
  ● S06.374   Contusion, laceration, and hemorrhage of cerebellum with loss of consciousness of 6 hours to 24 hours
  ● S06.375   Contusion, laceration, and hemorrhage of cerebellum with loss of consciousness greater than 24 hours with return to pre-existing conscious level
  ● S06.376   Contusion, laceration, and hemorrhage of cerebellum with loss of consciousness greater than 24 hours without return to pre-existing conscious level with patient surviving
  ● S06.377   Contusion, laceration, and hemorrhage of cerebellum with loss of consciousness of any duration with death due to brain injury prior to regaining consciousness
  ● S06.378   Contusion, laceration, and hemorrhage of cerebellum with loss of consciousness of any duration with death due to other cause prior to regaining consciousness
  ● S06.379   Contusion, laceration, and hemorrhage of cerebellum with loss of consciousness of unspecified duration
              Contusion, laceration, and hemorrhage of cerebellum NOS

● S06.38   Contusion, laceration, and hemorrhage of brainstem
  ● S06.380   Contusion, laceration, and hemorrhage of brainstem without loss of consciousness
  ● S06.381   Contusion, laceration, and hemorrhage of brainstem with loss of consciousness of 30 minutes or less
  ● S06.382   Contusion, laceration, and hemorrhage of brainstem with loss of consciousness of 31 minutes to 59 minutes
  ● S06.383   Contusion, laceration, and hemorrhage of brainstem with loss of consciousness of 1 hour to 5 hours 59 minutes
  ● S06.384   Contusion, laceration, and hemorrhage of brainstem with loss of consciousness of 6 hours to 24 hours
  ● S06.385   Contusion, laceration, and hemorrhage of brainstem with loss of consciousness greater than 24 hours with return to pre-existing conscious level

  ● S06.386   Contusion, laceration, and hemorrhage of brainstem with loss of consciousness greater than 24 hours without return to pre-existing conscious level with patient surviving
  ● S06.387   Contusion, laceration, and hemorrhage of brainstem with loss of consciousness of any duration with death due to brain injury prior to regaining consciousness
  ● S06.388   Contusion, laceration, and hemorrhage of brainstem with loss of consciousness of any duration with death due to other cause prior to regaining consciousness
  ● S06.389   Contusion, laceration, and hemorrhage of brainstem with loss of consciousness of unspecified duration
              Contusion, laceration, and hemorrhage of brainstem NOS

● S06.4   Epidural hemorrhage
          Situated outside dura mater
          Extradural hemorrhage NOS
          Intracranial hemorrhage due to trauma
          Extradural hemorrhage (traumatic)
  ● S06.4X   Epidural hemorrhage
    ● S06.4X0   Epidural hemorrhage without loss of consciousness
    ● S06.4X1   Epidural hemorrhage with loss of consciousness of 30 minutes or less
    ● S06.4X2   Epidural hemorrhage with loss of consciousness of 31 minutes to 59 minutes
    ● S06.4X3   Epidural hemorrhage with loss of consciousness of 1 hour to 5 hours 59 minutes
    ● S06.4X4   Epidural hemorrhage with loss of consciousness of 6 hours to 24 hours
    ● S06.4X5   Epidural hemorrhage with loss of consciousness greater than 24 hours with return to pre-existing conscious level
    ● S06.4X6   Epidural hemorrhage with loss of consciousness greater than 24 hours without return to pre-existing conscious level with patient surviving
    ● S06.4X7   Epidural hemorrhage with loss of consciousness of any duration with death due to brain injury prior to regaining consciousness
    ● S06.4X8   Epidural hemorrhage with loss of consciousness of any duration with death due to other causes prior to regaining consciousness
    ● S06.4X9   Epidural hemorrhage with loss of consciousness of unspecified duration
                Epidural hemorrhage NOS

● S06.5   Traumatic subdural hemorrhage
  ● S06.5X   Traumatic subdural hemorrhage
    ● S06.5X0   Traumatic subdural hemorrhage without loss of consciousness
    ● S06.5X1   Traumatic subdural hemorrhage with loss of consciousness of 30 minutes or less
    ● S06.5X2   Traumatic subdural hemorrhage with loss of consciousness of 31 minutes to 59 minutes

◀ New   ◀ᴵᴵᴵ Revised   ̶d̶e̶l̶e̶t̶e̶d̶ Deleted   Excludes 1   Excludes 2   Includes   Use additional   Code first   Code also   Unspecified
OGCR Official Guidelines   X Assign placeholder X   ● Use Additional Character(s)   ▶ Manifestation Code   **Coding Clinic**

● S06.5X3   Traumatic subdural hemorrhage with loss of consciousness of 1 hour to 5 hours 59 minutes

● S06.5X4   Traumatic subdural hemorrhage with loss of consciousness of 6 hours to 24 hours

● S06.5X5   Traumatic subdural hemorrhage with loss of consciousness greater than 24 hours with loss of return to pre-existing conscious level

● S06.5X6   Traumatic subdural hemorrhage with loss of consciousness greater than 24 hours without return to pre-existing conscious level with patient surviving

● S06.5X7   Traumatic subdural hemorrhage with loss of consciousness of any duration with death due to brain injury before regaining consciousness

● S06.5X8   Traumatic subdural hemorrhage with loss of consciousness of any duration with death due to other cause before regaining consciousness

● S06.5X9   Traumatic subdural hemorrhage with loss of consciousness of unspecified duration
            Traumatic subdural hemorrhage NOS

● **S06.6   Traumatic subarachnoid hemorrhage**
            Between arachnoid and pia mater

  ● **S06.6X   Traumatic subarachnoid hemorrhage**

    ● S06.6X0   Traumatic subarachnoid hemorrhage without loss of consciousness

    ● S06.6X1   Traumatic subarachnoid hemorrhage with loss of consciousness of 30 minutes or less

    ● S06.6X2   Traumatic subarachnoid hemorrhage with loss of consciousness of 31 minutes to 59 minutes

    ● S06.6X3   Traumatic subarachnoid hemorrhage with loss of consciousness of 1 hour to 5 hours 59 minutes

    ● S06.6X4   Traumatic subarachnoid hemorrhage with loss of consciousness of 6 hours to 24 hours

    ● S06.6X5   Traumatic subarachnoid hemorrhage with loss of consciousness greater than 24 hours with return to pre-existing conscious level

    ● S06.6X6   Traumatic subarachnoid hemorrhage with loss of consciousness greater than 24 hours without return to pre-existing conscious level with patient surviving

    ● S06.6X7   Traumatic subarachnoid hemorrhage with loss of consciousness of any duration with death due to brain injury prior to regaining consciousness

    ● S06.6X8   Traumatic subarachnoid hemorrhage with loss of consciousness of any duration with death due to other cause prior to regaining consciousness

    ● S06.6X9   Traumatic subarachnoid hemorrhage with loss of consciousness of unspecified duration
                Traumatic subarachnoid hemorrhage NOS

● **S06.8   Other specified intracranial injuries**

  ● **S06.81   Injury of right internal carotid artery, intracranial portion, not elsewhere classified**

    ● S06.810   Injury of right internal carotid artery, intracranial portion, not elsewhere classified without loss of consciousness

    ● S06.811   Injury of right internal carotid artery, intracranial portion, not elsewhere classified with loss of consciousness of 30 minutes or less

    ● S06.812   Injury of right internal carotid artery, intracranial portion, not elsewhere classified with loss of consciousness of 31 minutes to 59 minutes

    ● S06.813   Injury of right internal carotid artery, intracranial portion, not elsewhere classified with loss of consciousness of 1 hour to 5 hours 59 minutes

    ● S06.814   Injury of right internal carotid artery, intracranial portion, not elsewhere classified with loss of consciousness of 6 hours to 24 hours

    ● S06.815   Injury of right internal carotid artery, intracranial portion, not elsewhere classified with loss of consciousness greater than 24 hours with return to pre-existing conscious level

    ● S06.816   Injury of right internal carotid artery, intracranial portion, not elsewhere classified with loss of consciousness greater than 24 hours without return to pre-existing conscious level with patient surviving

    ● S06.817   Injury of right internal carotid artery, intracranial portion, not elsewhere classified with loss of consciousness of any duration with death due to brain injury prior to regaining consciousness

    ● S06.818   Injury of right internal carotid artery, intracranial portion, not elsewhere classified with loss of consciousness of any duration with death due to other cause prior to regaining consciousness

    ● S06.819   Injury of right internal carotid artery, intracranial portion, not elsewhere classified with loss of consciousness of unspecified duration
                Injury of right internal carotid artery, intracranial portion, not elsewhere classified NOS

  ● **S06.82   Injury of left internal carotid artery, intracranial portion, not elsewhere classified**

    ● S06.820   Injury of left internal carotid artery, intracranial portion, not elsewhere classified without loss of consciousness

    ● S06.821   Injury of left internal carotid artery, intracranial portion, not elsewhere classified with loss of consciousness of 30 minutes or less

    ● S06.822   Injury of left internal carotid artery, intracranial portion, not elsewhere classified with loss of consciousness of 31 minutes to 59 minutes

CHAPTER 19 (S00-T88)

● S06.823　Injury of left internal carotid artery, intracranial portion, not elsewhere classified with loss of consciousness of 1 hour to 5 hours 59 minutes

● S06.824　Injury of left internal carotid artery, intracranial portion, not elsewhere classified with loss of consciousness of 6 hours to 24 hours

● S06.825　Injury of left internal carotid artery, intracranial portion, not elsewhere classified with loss of consciousness greater than 24 hours with return to pre-existing conscious level

● S06.826　Injury of left internal carotid artery, intracranial portion, not elsewhere classified with loss of consciousness greater than 24 hours without return to pre-existing conscious level with patient surviving

● S06.827　Injury of left internal carotid artery, intracranial portion, not elsewhere classified with loss of consciousness of any duration with death due to brain injury prior to regaining consciousness

● S06.828　Injury of left internal carotid artery, intracranial portion, not elsewhere classified with loss of consciousness of any duration with death due to other cause prior to regaining consciousness

● S06.829　Injury of left internal carotid artery, intracranial portion, not elsewhere classified with loss of consciousness of unspecified duration
　　　　　　　Injury of left internal carotid artery, intracranial portion, not elsewhere classified NOS

● S06.89　Other specified intracranial injury

● S06.890　Other specified intracranial injury without loss of consciousness

● S06.891　Other specified intracranial injury with loss of consciousness of 30 minutes or less

● S06.892　Other specified intracranial injury with loss of consciousness of 31 minutes to 59 minutes

● S06.893　Other specified intracranial injury with loss of consciousness of 1 hour to 5 hours 59 minutes

● S06.894　Other specified intracranial injury with loss of consciousness of 6 hours to 24 hours

● S06.895　Other specified intracranial injury with loss of consciousness greater than 24 hours with return to pre-existing conscious level

● S06.896　Other specified intracranial injury with loss of consciousness greater than 24 hours without return to pre-existing conscious level with patient surviving

● S06.897　Other specified intracranial injury with loss of consciousness of any duration with death due to brain injury prior to regaining consciousness

● S06.898　Other specified intracranial injury with loss of consciousness of any duration with death due to other cause prior to regaining consciousness

● S06.899　Other specified intracranial injury with loss of consciousness of unspecified duration

● S06.9　Unspecified intracranial injury
　　　　　Brain injury NOS
　　　　　Head injury NOS with loss of consciousness
　　　　　Excludes1　head injury NOS (S09.90)

● S06.9X　Unspecified intracranial injury

● S06.9X0　Unspecified intracranial injury without loss of consciousness

● S06.9X1　Unspecified intracranial injury with loss of consciousness of 30 minutes or less

● S06.9X2　Unspecified intracranial injury with loss of consciousness of 31 minutes to 59 minutes

● S06.9X3　Unspecified intracranial injury with loss of consciousness of 1 hour to 5 hours 59 minutes

● S06.9X4　Unspecified intracranial injury with loss of consciousness of 6 hours to 24 hours

● S06.9X5　Unspecified intracranial injury with loss of consciousness greater than 24 hours with return to pre-existing conscious level

● S06.9X6　Unspecified intracranial injury with loss of consciousness greater than 24 hours without return to pre-existing conscious level with patient surviving

● S06.9X7　Unspecified intracranial injury with loss of consciousness of any duration with death due to brain injury prior to regaining consciousness

● S06.9X8　Unspecified intracranial injury with loss of consciousness of any duration with death due to other cause prior to regaining consciousness

● S06.9X9　Unspecified intracranial injury with loss of consciousness of unspecified duration

● S07　Crushing injury of head
　　　Use additional code for all associated injuries, such as:
　　　　　intracranial injuries (S06.-)
　　　　　skull fractures (S02.-)
　　　The appropriate 7th character is to be added to each code from category S07

A	initial encounter
D	subsequent encounter
S	sequela

X ● S07.0　Crushing injury of face
X ● S07.1　Crushing injury of skull
X ● S07.8　Crushing injury of other parts of head
X ● S07.9　Crushing injury of head, part unspecified

●**S08**   **Avulsion and traumatic amputation of part of head**

An amputation not identified as partial or complete should be coded to complete

The appropriate 7th character is to be added to each code from category S08

A	initial encounter
D	subsequent encounter
S	sequela

X●**S08.0**   **Avulsion of scalp**

●**S08.1**   **Traumatic amputation of ear**

   ●**S08.11**   **Complete traumatic amputation of ear**

     ●**S08.111**   **Complete traumatic amputation of right ear**

     ●**S08.112**   **Complete traumatic amputation of left ear**

     ●**S08.119**   **Complete traumatic amputation of unspecified ear**

   ●**S08.12**   **Partial traumatic amputation of ear**

     ●**S08.121**   **Partial traumatic amputation of right ear**

     ●**S08.122**   **Partial traumatic amputation of left ear**

     ●**S08.129**   **Partial traumatic amputation of unspecified ear**

●**S08.8**   **Traumatic amputation of other parts of head**

   ●**S08.81**   **Traumatic amputation of nose**

     ●**S08.811**   **Complete traumatic amputation of nose**

     ●**S08.812**   **Partial traumatic amputation of nose**

   X●**S08.89**   **Traumatic amputation of other parts of head**

●**S09**   **Other and unspecified injuries of head**

The appropriate 7th character is to be added to each code from category S09

A	initial encounter
D	subsequent encounter
S	sequela

X●**S09.0**   **Injury of blood vessels of head, not elsewhere classified**

   Excludes1   injury of cerebral blood vessels (S06.-)
               injury of precerebral blood vessels (S15.-)

●**S09.1**   **Injury of muscle and tendon of head**

   Code also any associated open wound (S01.-)

   Excludes2   sprain to joints and ligament of head (S03.9)

   X●**S09.10**   **Unspecified injury of muscle and tendon of head**

     Injury of muscle and tendon of head NOS

   X●**S09.11**   **Strain of muscle and tendon of head**

   X●**S09.12**   **Laceration of muscle and tendon of head**

   X●**S09.19**   **Other specified injury of muscle and tendon of head**

●**S09.2**   **Traumatic rupture of ear drum**

   Excludes1   traumatic rupture of ear drum due to blast injury (S09.31-)

   X●**S09.20**   **Traumatic rupture of unspecified ear drum**

   X●**S09.21**   **Traumatic rupture of right ear drum**

   X●**S09.22**   **Traumatic rupture of left ear drum**

●**S09.3**   **Other specified and unspecified injury of middle and inner ear**

   Excludes1   injury to ear NOS (S09.91-)

   Excludes2   injury to external ear (S00.4-, S01.3-, S08.1-)

   ●**S09.30**   **Unspecified injury of middle and inner ear**

     ●**S09.301**   **Unspecified injury of right middle and inner ear**

     ●**S09.302**   **Unspecified injury of left middle and inner ear**

     ●**S09.309**   **Unspecified injury of unspecified middle and inner ear**

   ●**S09.31**   **Primary blast injury of ear**

     Blast injury of ear NOS

     ●**S09.311**   **Primary blast injury of right ear**

     ●**S09.312**   **Primary blast injury of left ear**

     ●**S09.313**   **Primary blast injury of ear, bilateral**

     ●**S09.319**   **Primary blast injury of unspecified ear**

   ●**S09.39**   **Other specified injury of middle and inner ear**

     Secondary blast injury to ear

     ●**S09.391**   **Other specified injury of right middle and inner ear**

     ●**S09.392**   **Other specified injury of left middle and inner ear**

     ●**S09.399**   **Other specified injury of unspecified middle and inner ear**

X●**S09.8**   **Other specified injuries of head**

●**S09.9**   **Unspecified injury of face and head**

   X●**S09.90**   **Unspecified injury of head**

     Head injury NOS

     Excludes1   brain injury NOS (S06.9-)
               head injury NOS with loss of consciousness (S06.9-)
               intracranial injury NOS (S06.9-)

   X●**S09.91**   **Unspecified injury of ear**

     Injury of ear NOS

   X●**S09.92**   **Unspecified injury of nose**

     Injury of nose NOS

   X●**S09.93**   **Unspecified injury of face**

     Injury of face NOS

INJURIES TO THE NECK (S10-S19)

Includes	injuries of nape
	injuries of supraclavicular region
	injuries of throat

Excludes2	burns and corrosions (T20-T32)
	effects of foreign body in esophagus (T18.1)
	effects of foreign body in larynx (T17.3)
	effects of foreign body in pharynx (T17.2)
	effects of foreign body in trachea (T17.4)
	frostbite (T33-T34)
	insect bite or sting, venomous (T63.4)

●**S10**   **Superficial injury of neck**

The appropriate 7th character is to be added to each code from category S10

A	initial encounter
D	subsequent encounter
S	sequela

X●**S10.0**   **Contusion of throat**

   Contusion of cervical esophagus
   Contusion of larynx
   Contusion of pharynx
   Contusion of trachea

CHAPTER 19 (S00-T88)

● S10.1   Other and unspecified superficial injuries of throat
  X● S10.10   Unspecified superficial injuries of throat
  X● S10.11   Abrasion of throat
  X● S10.12   Blister (nonthermal) of throat
  X● S10.14   External constriction of part of throat
  X● S10.15   Superficial foreign body of throat
        Splinter in the throat
  X● S10.16   Insect bite (nonvenomous) of throat
  X● S10.17   Other superficial bite of throat
        Excludes1   open bite of throat (S11.85)

● S10.8   Superficial injury of other specified parts of neck
  X● S10.80   Unspecified superficial injury of other specified part of neck
  X● S10.81   Abrasion of other specified part of neck
  X● S10.82   Blister (nonthermal) of other specified part of neck
  X● S10.83   Contusion of other specified part of neck
  X● S10.84   External constriction of other specified part of neck
  X● S10.85   Superficial foreign body of other specified part of neck
        Splinter in other part of neck
  X● S10.86   Insect bite of other specified part of neck
  X● S10.87   Other superficial bite of other specified part of neck
        Excludes1   open bite of other specified parts of neck (S11.85)

● S10.9   Superficial injury of unspecified part of neck
  X● S10.90   Unspecified superficial injury of unspecified part of neck
  X● S10.91   Abrasion of unspecified part of neck
  X● S10.92   Blister (nonthermal) of unspecified part of neck
  X● S10.93   Contusion of unspecified part of neck
  X● S10.94   External constriction of unspecified part of neck
  X● S10.95   Superficial foreign body of unspecified part of neck
  X● S10.96   Insect bite of unspecified part of neck
  X● S10.97   Other superficial bite of unspecified part of neck

● S11   Open wound of neck
  Code also any associated:
    spinal cord injury (S14.0, S14.1-)
    wound infection
    Excludes2   open fracture of vertebra (S12.- with 7th character B)
  The appropriate 7th character is to be added to each code from category S11

    A   initial encounter
    D   subsequent encounter
    S   sequela

● S11.0   Open wound of larynx and trachea
  ● S11.01   Open wound of larynx
      Excludes2   open wound of vocal cord (S11.03)
    ● S11.011   Laceration without foreign body of larynx
    ● S11.012   Laceration with foreign body of larynx
    ● S11.013   Puncture wound without foreign body of larynx
    ● S11.014   Puncture wound with foreign body of larynx
    ● S11.015   Open bite of larynx
        Bite of larynx NOS
    ● S11.019   Unspecified open wound of larynx

● S11.02   Open wound of trachea
  Open wound of cervical trachea
  Open wound of trachea NOS
  Excludes2   open wound of thoracic trachea (S27.5-)
  ● S11.021   Laceration without foreign body of trachea
  ● S11.022   Laceration with foreign body of trachea
  ● S11.023   Puncture wound without foreign body of trachea
  ● S11.024   Puncture wound with foreign body of trachea
  ● S11.025   Open bite of trachea
      Bite of trachea NOS
  ● S11.029   Unspecified open wound of trachea

● S11.03   Open wound of vocal cord
  ● S11.031   Laceration without foreign body of vocal cord
  ● S11.032   Laceration with foreign body of vocal cord
  ● S11.033   Puncture wound without foreign body of vocal cord
  ● S11.034   Puncture wound with foreign body of vocal cord
  ● S11.035   Open bite of vocal cord
      Bite of vocal cord NOS
  ● S11.039   Unspecified open wound of vocal cord

● S11.1   Open wound of thyroid gland
  X● S11.10   Unspecified open wound of thyroid gland
  X● S11.11   Laceration without foreign body of thyroid gland
  X● S11.12   Laceration with foreign body of thyroid gland
  X● S11.13   Puncture wound without foreign body of thyroid gland
  X● S11.14   Puncture wound with foreign body of thyroid gland
  X● S11.15   Open bite of thyroid gland
      Bite of thyroid gland NOS

● S11.2   Open wound of pharynx and cervical esophagus
  Excludes1   open wound of esophagus NOS (S27.8-)
  X● S11.20   Unspecified open wound of pharynx and cervical esophagus
  X● S11.21   Laceration without foreign body of pharynx and cervical esophagus
  X● S11.22   Laceration with foreign body of pharynx and cervical esophagus
  X● S11.23   Puncture wound without foreign body of pharynx and cervical esophagus
  X● S11.24   Puncture wound with foreign body of pharynx and cervical esophagus
  X● S11.25   Open bite of pharynx and cervical esophagus
      Bite of pharynx and cervical esophagus NOS

● S11.8   Open wound of other specified parts of neck
  X● S11.80   Unspecified open specified wound of other part of neck
  X● S11.81   Laceration without foreign body of other specified part of neck
  X● S11.82   Laceration with foreign body of other specified part of neck
  X● S11.83   Puncture wound without foreign body of other specified part of neck
  X● S11.84   Puncture wound with foreign body of other specified part of neck
  X● S11.85   Open bite of other specified part of neck
      Bite of other part of neck NOS
      Excludes1   superficial bite of other specified part of neck (S10.87)
  X● S11.89   Other open wound of other part of neck

◀ New   ◀ﷺ Revised   ~~deleted~~ Deleted   Excludes 1   Excludes 2   Includes   Use additional   Code first   Code also   Unspecified

OGCR Official Guidelines   X Assign placeholder X   ● Use Additional Character(s)   ▌ Manifestation Code   **Coding Clinic**

● **S11.9**   **Open wound of unspecified part of neck**
   X● **S11.90**   Unspecified open wound of ▢unspecified▢ part of neck
   X● **S11.91**   Laceration without foreign body of ▢unspecified▢ part of neck
   X● **S11.92**   Laceration with foreign body of ▢unspecified▢ part of neck
   X● **S11.93**   Puncture wound without foreign body of ▢unspecified▢ part of neck
   X● **S11.94**   Puncture wound with foreign body of ▢unspecified▢ part of neck
   X● **S11.95**   Open bite of ▢unspecified▢ part of neck
        Bite of neck NOS
        Excludes1   superficial bite of neck (S10.97)

● **S12**   **Fracture of cervical vertebra and other parts of neck**
   Note: A fracture not indicated as displaced or nondisplaced should be coded to displaced

   A fracture not indicated as open or closed should be coded to closed

   ▢**Includes**▢   fracture of cervical neural arch
                 fracture of cervical spine
                 fracture of cervical spinous process
                 fracture of cervical transverse process
                 fracture of cervical vertebral arch
                 fracture of neck

   Code first any associated cervical spinal cord injury (S14.0, S14.1-)

   The appropriate 7th character is to be added to all codes from subcategories S12.0-S12.6

> A   initial encounter for closed fracture
> B   initial encounter for open fracture
> D   subsequent encounter for fracture with routine healing
> G   subsequent encounter for fracture with delayed healing
> K   subsequent encounter for fracture with nonunion
> S   sequela

● **S12.0**   **Fracture of first cervical vertebra**
       Atlas
   ● **S12.00**   Unspecified fracture of first cervical vertebra
     ● **S12.000**   ▢Unspecified▢ displaced fracture of first cervical vertebra
     ● **S12.001**   ▢Unspecified▢ nondisplaced fracture of first cervical vertebra
   X● **S12.01**   Stable burst fracture of first cervical vertebra
   X● **S12.02**   Unstable burst fracture of first cervical vertebra
   ● **S12.03**   Posterior arch fracture of first cervical vertebra
     ● **S12.030**   Displaced posterior arch fracture of first cervical vertebra
     ● **S12.031**   Nondisplaced posterior arch fracture of first cervical vertebra
   ● **S12.04**   Lateral mass fracture of first cervical vertebra
     ● **S12.040**   Displaced lateral mass fracture of first cervical vertebra
     ● **S12.041**   Nondisplaced lateral mass fracture of first cervical vertebra
   ● **S12.09**   Other fracture of first cervical vertebra
     ● **S12.090**   Other displaced fracture of first cervical vertebra
     ● **S12.091**   Other nondisplaced fracture of first cervical vertebra

● **S12.1**   **Fracture of second cervical vertebra**
       Axis
   ● **S12.10**   Unspecified fracture of second cervical vertebra
     ● **S12.100**   ▢Unspecified▢ displaced fracture of second cervical vertebra
     ● **S12.101**   ▢Unspecified▢ nondisplaced fracture of second cervical vertebra

● **S12.11**   Type II dens fracture
     ● **S12.110**   Anterior displaced Type II dens fracture
     ● **S12.111**   Posterior displaced Type II dens fracture
     ● **S12.112**   Nondisplaced Type II dens fracture
● **S12.12**   Other dens fracture
     ● **S12.120**   Other displaced dens fracture
     ● **S12.121**   Other nondisplaced dens fracture
● **S12.13**   Unspecified traumatic spondylolisthesis of second cervical vertebra
     ● **S12.130**   ▢Unspecified▢ traumatic displaced spondylolisthesis of second cervical vertebra
     ● **S12.131**   ▢Unspecified▢ traumatic nondisplaced spondylolisthesis of second cervical vertebra
X● **S12.14**   Type III traumatic spondylolisthesis of second cervical vertebra
● **S12.15**   Other traumatic spondylolisthesis of second cervical vertebra
     ● **S12.150**   Other traumatic displaced spondylolisthesis of second cervical vertebra
     ● **S12.151**   Other traumatic nondisplaced spondylolisthesis of second cervical vertebra
● **S12.19**   Other fracture of second cervical vertebra
     ● **S12.190**   Other displaced fracture of second cervical vertebra
     ● **S12.191**   Other nondisplaced fracture of second cervical vertebra

● **S12.2**   **Fracture of third cervical vertebra**
   ● **S12.20**   Unspecified fracture of third cervical vertebra
     ● **S12.200**   ▢Unspecified▢ displaced fracture of third cervical vertebra
     ● **S12.201**   ▢Unspecified▢ nondisplaced fracture of third cervical vertebra
   ● **S12.23**   Unspecified traumatic spondylolisthesis of third cervical vertebra
     ● **S12.230**   ▢Unspecified▢ traumatic displaced spondylolisthesis of third cervical vertebra
     ● **S12.231**   ▢Unspecified▢ traumatic nondisplaced spondylolisthesis of third cervical vertebra
   X● **S12.24**   Type III traumatic spondylolisthesis of third cervical vertebra
   ● **S12.25**   Other traumatic spondylolisthesis of third cervical vertebra
     ● **S12.250**   Other traumatic displaced spondylolisthesis of third cervical vertebra
     ● **S12.251**   Other traumatic nondisplaced spondylolisthesis of third cervical vertebra
   ● **S12.29**   Other fracture of third cervical vertebra
     ● **S12.290**   Other displaced fracture of third cervical vertebra
     ● **S12.291**   Other nondisplaced fracture of third cervical vertebra

● **S12.3**   **Fracture of fourth cervical vertebra**
   ● **S12.30**   Unspecified fracture of fourth cervical vertebra
     ● **S12.300**   ▢Unspecified▢ displaced fracture of fourth cervical vertebra
     ● **S12.301**   ▢Unspecified▢ nondisplaced fracture of fourth cervical vertebra

● **S12.33**   Unspecified traumatic spondylolisthesis of fourth cervical vertebra

  ● **S12.330**   Unspecified traumatic displaced spondylolisthesis of fourth cervical vertebra

  ● **S12.331**   Unspecified traumatic nondisplaced spondylolisthesis of fourth cervical vertebra

X ● **S12.34**   Type III traumatic spondylolisthesis of fourth cervical vertebra

● **S12.35**   Other traumatic spondylolisthesis of fourth cervical vertebra

  ● **S12.350**   Other traumatic displaced spondylolisthesis of fourth cervical vertebra

  ● **S12.351**   Other traumatic nondisplaced spondylolisthesis of fourth cervical vertebra

● **S12.39**   Other fracture of fourth cervical vertebra

  ● **S12.390**   Other displaced fracture of fourth cervical vertebra

  ● **S12.391**   Other nondisplaced fracture of fourth cervical vertebra

● **S12.4**   **Fracture of fifth cervical vertebra**

● **S12.40**   Unspecified fracture of fifth cervical vertebra

  ● **S12.400**   Unspecified displaced fracture of fifth cervical vertebra

  ● **S12.401**   Unspecified nondisplaced fracture of fifth cervical vertebra

● **S12.43**   Unspecified traumatic spondylolisthesis of fifth cervical vertebra

  ● **S12.430**   Unspecified traumatic displaced spondylolisthesis of fifth cervical vertebra

  ● **S12.431**   Unspecified traumatic nondisplaced spondylolisthesis of fifth cervical vertebra

X ● **S12.44**   Type III traumatic spondylolisthesis of fifth cervical vertebra

● **S12.45**   Other traumatic spondylolisthesis of fifth cervical vertebra

  ● **S12.450**   Other traumatic displaced spondylolisthesis of fifth cervical vertebra

  ● **S12.451**   Other traumatic nondisplaced spondylolisthesis of fifth cervical vertebra

● **S12.49**   Other fracture of fifth cervical vertebra

  ● **S12.490**   Other displaced fracture of fifth cervical vertebra

  ● **S12.491**   Other nondisplaced fracture of fifth cervical vertebra

● **S12.5**   **Fracture of sixth cervical vertebra**

● **S12.50**   Unspecified fracture of sixth cervical vertebra

  ● **S12.500**   Unspecified displaced fracture of sixth cervical vertebra

  ● **S12.501**   Unspecified nondisplaced fracture of sixth cervical vertebra

● **S12.53**   Unspecified traumatic spondylolisthesis of sixth cervical vertebra

  ● **S12.530**   Unspecified traumatic displaced spondylolisthesis of sixth cervical vertebra

  ● **S12.531**   Unspecified traumatic nondisplaced spondylolisthesis of sixth cervical vertebra

X ● **S12.54**   Type III traumatic spondylolisthesis of sixth cervical vertebra

● **S12.55**   Other traumatic spondylolisthesis of sixth cervical vertebra

  ● **S12.550**   Other traumatic displaced spondylolisthesis of sixth cervical vertebra

  ● **S12.551**   Other traumatic nondisplaced spondylolisthesis of sixth cervical vertebra

● **S12.59**   Other fracture of sixth cervical vertebra

  ● **S12.590**   Other displaced fracture of sixth cervical vertebra

  ● **S12.591**   Other nondisplaced fracture of sixth cervical vertebra

● **S12.6**   **Fracture of seventh cervical vertebra**

● **S12.60**   Unspecified fracture of seventh cervical vertebra

  ● **S12.600**   Unspecified displaced fracture of seventh cervical vertebra

  ● **S12.601**   Unspecified nondisplaced fracture of seventh cervical vertebra

● **S12.63**   Unspecified traumatic spondylolisthesis of seventh cervical vertebra

  ● **S12.630**   Unspecified traumatic displaced spondylolisthesis of seventh cervical vertebra

  ● **S12.631**   Unspecified traumatic nondisplaced spondylolisthesis of seventh cervical vertebra

X ● **S12.64**   Type III traumatic spondylolisthesis of seventh cervical vertebra

● **S12.65**   Other traumatic spondylolisthesis of seventh cervical vertebra

  ● **S12.650**   Other traumatic displaced spondylolisthesis of seventh cervical vertebra

  ● **S12.651**   Other traumatic nondisplaced spondylolisthesis of seventh cervical vertebra

● **S12.69**   Other fracture of seventh cervical vertebra

  ● **S12.690**   Other displaced fracture of seventh cervical vertebra

  ● **S12.691**   Other nondisplaced fracture of seventh cervical vertebra

X ● **S12.8**   **Fracture of other parts of neck**

    Hyoid bone   Thyroid cartilage
    Larynx   Trachea

    The appropriate 7th character is to be added to code S12.8

A	initial encounter
D	subsequent encounter
S	sequela

X ● **S12.9**   **Fracture of neck, unspecified**

    Fracture of neck NOS
    Fracture of cervical spine NOS
    Fracture of cervical vertebra NOS

    The appropriate 7th character is to be added to code S12.9

A	initial encounter
D	subsequent encounter
S	sequela

◄ New   ◄ Revised   ~~deleted~~ Deleted   Excludes 1   Excludes 2   Includes   Use additional   Code first   Code also   Unspecified

OGCR Official Guidelines   X Assign placeholder X   ● Use Additional Character(s)   ▶ Manifestation Code   **Coding Clinic**

● **S13**   **Dislocation and sprain of joints and ligaments at neck level**

     Includes   avulsion of joint or ligament at neck level
                   laceration of cartilage, joint or ligament at neck level
                   sprain of cartilage, joint or ligament at neck level
                   traumatic hemarthrosis of joint or ligament at neck level
                   traumatic rupture of joint or ligament at neck level
                   traumatic subluxation of joint or ligament at neck level
                   traumatic tear of joint or ligament at neck level

     Code also any associated open wound

     Excludes2   strain of muscle or tendon at neck level (S16.1)

     The appropriate 7th character is to be added to each code from category S13

> A   initial encounter
> D   subsequent encounter
> S   sequela

X● **S13.0**   **Traumatic rupture of cervical intervertebral disc**

     Excludes1   rupture or displacement (nontraumatic) of cervical intervertebral disc NOS (M50.-)

● **S13.1**   **Subluxation and dislocation of cervical vertebrae**

     Code also any associated:
         open wound of neck (S11.-)
         spinal cord injury (S14.1-)

     Excludes2   fracture of cervical vertebrae (S12.0-S12.3-)

     ● **S13.10**   **Subluxation and dislocation of unspecified cervical vertebrae**

         ● **S13.100**   **Subluxation of unspecified cervical vertebrae**

         ● **S13.101**   **Dislocation of unspecified cervical vertebrae**

     ● **S13.11**   **Subluxation and dislocation of C_0/C_1 cervical vertebrae**

         Subluxation and dislocation of atlantooccipital joint
         Subluxation and dislocation of atloidooccipital joint
         Subluxation and dislocation of occipitoatloid joint

         ● **S13.110**   **Subluxation of C_0/C_1 cervical vertebrae**

         ● **S13.111**   **Dislocation of C_0/C_1 cervical vertebrae**

     ● **S13.12**   **Subluxation and dislocation of C_1/C_2 cervical vertebrae**

         Subluxation and dislocation of atlantoaxial joint

         ● **S13.120**   **Subluxation of C_1/C_2 cervical vertebrae**

         ● **S13.121**   **Dislocation of C_1/C_2 cervical vertebrae**

     ● **S13.13**   **Subluxation and dislocation of C_2/C_3 cervical vertebrae**

         ● **S13.130**   **Subluxation of C_2/C_3 cervical vertebrae**

         ● **S13.131**   **Dislocation of C_2/C_3 cervical vertebrae**

     ● **S13.14**   **Subluxation and dislocation of C_3/C_4 cervical vertebrae**

         ● **S13.140**   **Subluxation of C_3/C_4 cervical vertebrae**

         ● **S13.141**   **Dislocation of C_3/C_4 cervical vertebrae**

     ● **S13.15**   **Subluxation and dislocation of C_4/C_5 cervical vertebrae**

         ● **S13.150**   **Subluxation of C_4/C_5 cervical vertebrae**

         ● **S13.151**   **Dislocation of C_4/C_5 cervical vertebrae**

     ● **S13.16**   **Subluxation and dislocation of C_5/C_6 cervical vertebrae**

         ● **S13.160**   **Subluxation of C_5/C_6 cervical vertebrae**

         ● **S13.161**   **Dislocation of C_5/C_6 cervical vertebrae**

     ● **S13.17**   **Subluxation and dislocation of C_6/C_7 cervical vertebrae**

         ● **S13.170**   **Subluxation of C_6/C_7 cervical vertebrae**

         ● **S13.171**   **Dislocation of C_6/C_7 cervical vertebrae**

     ● **S13.18**   **Subluxation and dislocation of C_7/T_1 cervical vertebrae**

         ● **S13.180**   **Subluxation of C_7/T_1 cervical vertebrae**

         ● **S13.181**   **Dislocation of C_7/T_1 cervical vertebrae**

   ● **S13.2**   **Dislocation of other and unspecified parts of neck**

     X● **S13.20**   **Dislocation of unspecified parts of neck**

     X● **S13.29**   **Dislocation of other parts of neck**

X● **S13.4**   **Sprain of ligaments of cervical spine**

     Sprain of anterior longitudinal (ligament), cervical
     Sprain of atlanto-axial (joints)
     Sprain of atlanto-occipital (joints)
     Whiplash injury of cervical spine

X● **S13.5**   **Sprain of thyroid region**

     Sprain of cricoarytenoid (joint) (ligament)
     Sprain of cricothyroid (joint) (ligament)
     Sprain of thyroid cartilage

X● **S13.8**   **Sprain of joints and ligaments of other parts of neck**

X● **S13.9**   **Sprain of joints and ligaments of unspecified parts of neck**

● **S14**   **Injury of nerves and spinal cord at neck level**

     Note: Code to highest level of cervical cord injury

     Code also any associated:
         fracture of cervical vertebra (S12.0--S12.6.-)
         open wound of neck (S11.-)
         transient paralysis (R29.5)

     The appropriate 7th character is to be added to each code from category S14

> A   initial encounter
> D   subsequent encounter
> S   sequela

X● **S14.0**   **Concussion and edema of cervical spinal cord**

● **S14.1**   **Other and unspecified injuries of cervical spinal cord**

     ● **S14.10**   **Unspecified injury of cervical spinal cord**

         ● **S14.101**   **Unspecified injury at C_1 level of cervical spinal cord**

         ● **S14.102**   **Unspecified injury at C_2 level of cervical spinal cord**

         ● **S14.103**   **Unspecified injury at C_3 level of cervical spinal cord**

         ● **S14.104**   **Unspecified injury at C_4 level of cervical spinal cord**

         ● **S14.105**   **Unspecified injury at C_5 level of cervical spinal cord**

         ● **S14.106**   **Unspecified injury at C_6 level of cervical spinal cord**

         ● **S14.107**   **Unspecified injury at C_7 level of cervical spinal cord**

         ● **S14.108**   **Unspecified injury at C_8 level of cervical spinal cord**

         ● **S14.109**   **Unspecified injury at unspecified level of cervical spinal cord**

             Injury of cervical spinal cord NOS

CHAPTER 19 (S00-T88)

CHAPTER 19 (S00-T88)

- S14.11   Complete lesion of cervical spinal cord
  - S14.111   Complete lesion at C_1 level of cervical spinal cord
  - S14.112   Complete lesion at C_2 level of cervical spinal cord
  - S14.113   Complete lesion at C_3 level of cervical spinal cord
  - S14.114   Complete lesion at C_4 level of cervical spinal cord
  - S14.115   Complete lesion at C_5 level of cervical spinal cord
  - S14.116   Complete lesion at C_6 level of cervical spinal cord
  - S14.117   Complete lesion at C_7 level of cervical spinal cord
  - S14.118   Complete lesion at C_8 level of cervical spinal cord
  - S14.119   Complete lesion at `unspecified` level of cervical spinal cord
- S14.12   Central cord syndrome of cervical spinal cord
  - S14.121   Central cord syndrome at C_1 level of cervical spinal cord
  - S14.122   Central cord syndrome at C_2 level of cervical spinal cord
  - S14.123   Central cord syndrome at C_3 level of cervical spinal cord
  - S14.124   Central cord syndrome at C_4 level of cervical spinal cord
  - S14.125   Central cord syndrome at C_5 level of cervical spinal cord
  - S14.126   Central cord syndrome at C_6 level of cervical spinal cord
  - S14.127   Central cord syndrome at C_7 level of cervical spinal cord
  - S14.128   Central cord syndrome at C_8 level of cervical spinal cord
  - S14.129   Central cord syndrome at `unspecified` level of cervical spinal cord
- S14.13   Anterior cord syndrome of cervical spinal cord
  - S14.131   Anterior cord syndrome at C_1 level of cervical spinal cord
  - S14.132   Anterior cord syndrome at C_2 level of cervical spinal cord
  - S14.133   Anterior cord syndrome at C_3 level of cervical spinal cord
  - S14.134   Anterior cord syndrome at C_4 level of cervical spinal cord
  - S14.135   Anterior cord syndrome at C_5 level of cervical spinal cord
  - S14.136   Anterior cord syndrome at C_6 level of cervical spinal cord
  - S14.137   Anterior cord syndrome at C_7 level of cervical spinal cord
  - S14.138   Anterior cord syndrome at C_8 level of cervical spinal cord
  - S14.139   Anterior cord syndrome at `unspecified` level of cervical spinal cord
- S14.14   Brown-Séquard syndrome of cervical spinal cord
  - S14.141   Brown-Séquard syndrome at C_1 level of cervical spinal cord
  - S14.142   Brown-Séquard syndrome at C_2 level of cervical spinal cord
  - S14.143   Brown-Séquard syndrome at C_3 level of cervical spinal cord
  - S14.144   Brown-Séquard syndrome at C_4 level of cervical spinal cord
  - S14.145   Brown-Séquard syndrome at C_5 level of cervical spinal cord
  - S14.146   Brown-Séquard syndrome at C_6 level of cervical spinal cord
  - S14.147   Brown-Séquard syndrome at C_7 level of cervical spinal cord
  - S14.148   Brown-Séquard syndrome at C_8 level of cervical spinal cord
  - S14.149   Brown-Séquard syndrome at `unspecified` level of cervical spinal cord
- S14.15   Other incomplete lesions of cervical spinal cord

  Incomplete lesion of cervical spinal cord NOS

  Posterior cord syndrome of cervical spinal cord
  - S14.151   Other incomplete lesion at C_1 level of cervical spinal cord
  - S14.152   Other incomplete lesion at C_2 level of cervical spinal cord
  - S14.153   Other incomplete lesion at C_3 level of cervical spinal cord
  - S14.154   Other incomplete lesion at C_4 level of cervical spinal cord
  - S14.155   Other incomplete lesion at C_5 level of cervical spinal cord
  - S14.156   Other incomplete lesion at C_6 level of cervical spinal cord
  - S14.157   Other incomplete lesion at C_7 level of cervical spinal cord
  - S14.158   Other incomplete lesion at C_8 level of cervical spinal cord
  - S14.159   Other incomplete lesion at `unspecified` level of cervical spinal cord
- X ● S14.2   Injury of nerve root of cervical spine
- X ● S14.3   Injury of brachial plexus
- X ● S14.4   Injury of peripheral nerves of neck
- X ● S14.5   Injury of cervical sympathetic nerves
- X ● S14.8   Injury of other specified nerves of neck
- X ● S14.9   Injury of `unspecified` nerves of neck

- S15   Injury of blood vessels at neck level

  Code also any associated open wound (S11.-)

  The appropriate 7th character is to be added to each code from category S15

  > A   initial encounter
  > D   subsequent encounter
  > S   sequela

  - S15.0   Injury of carotid artery of neck

    Injury of carotid artery (common) (external) (internal, extracranial portion)

    Injury of carotid artery NOS

    Excludes1   injury of internal carotid artery, intracranial portion (S06.8)

    - S15.00   Unspecified injury of carotid artery
      - S15.001   `Unspecified` injury of right carotid artery
      - S15.002   `Unspecified` injury of left carotid artery
      - S15.009   `Unspecified` injury of unspecified carotid artery
    - S15.01   Minor laceration of carotid artery

      Incomplete transection of carotid artery

      Laceration of carotid artery NOS

      Superficial laceration of carotid artery
      - S15.011   Minor laceration of right carotid artery
      - S15.012   Minor laceration of left carotid artery
      - S15.019   Minor laceration of `unspecified` carotid artery

◀ New   ◀ Revised   ~~deleted~~ Deleted   Excludes 1   Excludes 2   Includes   Use additional   Code first   Code also   Unspecified

OGCR Official Guidelines   X Assign placeholder X   ● Use Additional Character(s)   ▶ Manifestation Code   **Coding Clinic**

● **S15.02**   **Major laceration of carotid artery**
     Complete transection of carotid artery
     Traumatic rupture of carotid artery
     ● **S15.021**   **Major laceration of right carotid artery**
     ● **S15.022**   **Major laceration of left carotid artery**
     ● **S15.029**   **Major laceration of unspecified carotid artery**
● **S15.09**   **Other specified injury of carotid artery**
     ● **S15.091**   **Other specified injury of right carotid artery**
     ● **S15.092**   **Other specified injury of left carotid artery**
     ● **S15.099**   **Other specified injury of unspecified carotid artery**

● **S15.1**   **Injury of vertebral artery**
   ● **S15.10**   **Unspecified injury of vertebral artery**
     ● **S15.101**   **Unspecified injury of right vertebral artery**
     ● **S15.102**   **Unspecified injury of left vertebral artery**
     ● **S15.109**   **Unspecified injury of unspecified vertebral artery**
   ● **S15.11**   **Minor laceration of vertebral artery**
     Incomplete transection of vertebral artery
     Laceration of vertebral artery NOS
     Superficial laceration of vertebral artery
     ● **S15.111**   **Minor laceration of right vertebral artery**
     ● **S15.112**   **Minor laceration of left vertebral artery**
     ● **S15.119**   **Minor laceration of unspecified vertebral artery**
   ● **S15.12**   **Major laceration of vertebral artery**
     Complete transection of vertebral artery
     Traumatic rupture of vertebral artery
     ● **S15.121**   **Major laceration of right vertebral artery**
     ● **S15.122**   **Major laceration of left vertebral artery**
     ● **S15.129**   **Major laceration of unspecified vertebral artery**
   ● **S15.19**   **Other specified injury of vertebral artery**
     ● **S15.191**   **Other specified injury of right vertebral artery**
     ● **S15.192**   **Other specified injury of left vertebral artery**
     ● **S15.199**   **Other specified injury of unspecified vertebral artery**

● **S15.2**   **Injury of external jugular vein**
   ● **S15.20**   **Unspecified injury of external jugular vein**
     ● **S15.201**   **Unspecified injury of right external jugular vein**
     ● **S15.202**   **Unspecified injury of left external jugular vein**
     ● **S15.209**   **Unspecified injury of unspecified external jugular vein**
   ● **S15.21**   **Minor laceration of external jugular vein**
     Incomplete transection of external jugular vein
     Laceration of external jugular vein NOS
     Superficial laceration of external jugular vein
     ● **S15.211**   **Minor laceration of right external jugular vein**
     ● **S15.212**   **Minor laceration of left external jugular vein**
     ● **S15.219**   **Minor laceration of unspecified external jugular vein**

● **S15.22**   **Major laceration of external jugular vein**
     Complete transection of external jugular vein
     Traumatic rupture of external jugular vein
     ● **S15.221**   **Major laceration of right external jugular vein**
     ● **S15.222**   **Major laceration of left external jugular vein**
     ● **S15.229**   **Major laceration of unspecified external jugular vein**
● **S15.29**   **Other specified injury of external jugular vein**
     ● **S15.291**   **Other specified injury of right external jugular vein**
     ● **S15.292**   **Other specified injury of left external jugular vein**
     ● **S15.299**   **Other specified injury of unspecified external jugular vein**

● **S15.3**   **Injury of internal jugular vein**
   ● **S15.30**   **Unspecified injury of internal jugular vein**
     ● **S15.301**   **Unspecified injury of right internal jugular vein**
     ● **S15.302**   **Unspecified injury of left internal jugular vein**
     ● **S15.309**   **Unspecified injury of unspecified internal jugular vein**
   ● **S15.31**   **Minor laceration of internal jugular vein**
     Incomplete transection of internal jugular vein
     Laceration of internal jugular vein NOS
     Superficial laceration of internal jugular vein
     ● **S15.311**   **Minor laceration of right internal jugular vein**
     ● **S15.312**   **Minor laceration of left internal jugular vein**
     ● **S15.319**   **Minor laceration of unspecified internal jugular vein**
   ● **S15.32**   **Major laceration of internal jugular vein**
     Complete transection of internal jugular vein
     Traumatic rupture of internal jugular vein
     ● **S15.321**   **Major laceration of right internal jugular vein**
     ● **S15.322**   **Major laceration of left internal jugular vein**
     ● **S15.329**   **Major laceration of unspecified internal jugular vein**
   ● **S15.39**   **Other specified injury of internal jugular vein**
     ● **S15.391**   **Other specified injury of right internal jugular vein**
     ● **S15.392**   **Other specified injury of left internal jugular vein**
     ● **S15.399**   **Other specified injury of unspecified internal jugular vein**

X● **S15.8**   **Injury of other specified blood vessels at neck level**
X● **S15.9**   **Injury of unspecified blood vessel at neck level**

● **S16**   **Injury of muscle, fascia and tendon at neck level**
     Code also any associated open wound (S11.-)
     Excludes2   sprain of joint or ligament at neck level (S13.9)
     The appropriate 7th character is to be added to each code from category S16

A	initial encounter
D	subsequent encounter
S	sequela

X● **S16.1**   **Strain of muscle, fascia and tendon at neck level**
X● **S16.2**   **Laceration of muscle, fascia and tendon at neck level**
X● **S16.8**   **Other specified injury of muscle, fascia and tendon at neck level**
X● **S16.9**   **Unspecified injury of muscle, fascia and tendon at neck level**

● **S17   Crushing injury of neck**
Use additional code for all associated injuries, such as:
  injury of blood vessels (S15.-)
  open wound of neck (S11.-)
  spinal cord injury (S14.0, S14.1-)
  vertebral fracture (S12.0--S12.3-)
The appropriate 7th character is to be added to each code from category S17

A	initial encounter
D	subsequent encounter
S	sequela

X● **S17.0   Crushing injury of larynx and trachea**
X● **S17.8   Crushing injury of other specified parts of neck**
X● **S17.9   Crushing injury of neck, part unspecified**

● **S19   Other and unspecified injuries of neck**
The appropriate 7th character is to be added to each code from category S19

A	initial encounter
D	subsequent encounter
S	sequela

● **S19.8   Other specified injuries of neck**
X● **S19.80   Other specified injuries of unspecified part of neck**
X● **S19.81   Other specified injuries of larynx**
X● **S19.82   Other specified injuries of cervical trachea**
    Excludes2   other specified injury of thoracic trachea (S27.5-)
X● **S19.83   Other specified injuries of vocal cord**
X● **S19.84   Other specified injuries of thyroid gland**
X● **S19.85   Other specified injuries of pharynx and cervical esophagus**
X● **S19.89   Other specified injuries of other specified part of neck**
X● **S19.9   Unspecified injury of neck**

INJURIES TO THE THORAX (S20-S29)

Includes   injuries of breast
          injuries of chest (wall)
          injuries of interscapular area
Excludes2   burns and corrosions (T20-T32)
          effects of foreign body in bronchus (T17.5)
          effects of foreign body in esophagus (T18.1)
          effects of foreign body in lung (T17.8)
          effects of foreign body in trachea (T17.4)
          frostbite (T33-T34)
          injuries of axilla
          injuries of clavicle
          injuries of scapular region
          injuries of shoulder
          insect bite or sting, venomous (T63.4)

● **S20   Superficial injury of thorax**
The appropriate 7th character is to be added to each code from category S20

A	initial encounter
D	subsequent encounter
S	sequela

● **S20.0   Contusion of breast**
X● **S20.00   Contusion of breast, unspecified breast**
X● **S20.01   Contusion of right breast**
X● **S20.02   Contusion of left breast**

● **S20.1   Other and unspecified superficial injuries of breast**
● **S20.10   Unspecified superficial injuries of breast**
● **S20.101   Unspecified superficial injuries of breast, right breast**
● **S20.102   Unspecified superficial injuries of breast, left breast**
● **S20.109   Unspecified superficial injuries of breast, unspecified breast**
● **S20.11   Abrasion of breast**
● **S20.111   Abrasion of breast, right breast**
● **S20.112   Abrasion of breast, left breast**
● **S20.119   Abrasion of breast, unspecified breast**
● **S20.12   Blister (nonthermal) of breast**
● **S20.121   Blister (nonthermal) of breast, right breast**
● **S20.122   Blister (nonthermal) of breast, left breast**
● **S20.129   Blister (nonthermal) of breast, unspecified breast**
● **S20.14   External constriction of part of breast**
● **S20.141   External constriction of part of breast, right breast**
● **S20.142   External constriction of part of breast, left breast**
● **S20.149   External constriction of part of breast, unspecified breast**
● **S20.15   Superficial foreign body of breast**
    Splinter in the breast
● **S20.151   Superficial foreign body of breast, right breast**
● **S20.152   Superficial foreign body of breast, left breast**
● **S20.159   Superficial foreign body of breast, unspecified breast**
● **S20.16   Insect bite (nonvenomous) of breast**
● **S20.161   Insect bite (nonvenomous) of breast, right breast**
● **S20.162   Insect bite (nonvenomous) of breast, left breast**
● **S20.169   Insect bite (nonvenomous) of breast, unspecified breast**
● **S20.17   Other superficial bite of breast**
    Excludes1   open bite of breast (S21.05-)
● **S20.171   Other superficial bite of breast, right breast**
● **S20.172   Other superficial bite of breast, left breast**
● **S20.179   Other superficial bite of breast, unspecified breast**
● **S20.2   Contusion of thorax**
X● **S20.20   Contusion of thorax, unspecified**
● **S20.21   Contusion of front wall of thorax**
● **S20.211   Contusion of right front wall of thorax**
● **S20.212   Contusion of left front wall of thorax**
● **S20.219   Contusion of unspecified front wall of thorax**
● **S20.22   Contusion of back wall of thorax**
● **S20.221   Contusion of right back wall of thorax**
● **S20.222   Contusion of left back wall of thorax**
● **S20.229   Contusion of unspecified back wall of thorax**

◄ New   ◄▬ Revised   ~~deleted~~ Deleted   Excludes 1   Excludes 2   Includes   Use additional   Code first   Code also   Unspecified
OGCR Official Guidelines   X Assign placeholder X   ● Use Additional Character(s)   ▶ Manifestation Code   Coding Clinic

CHAPTER 19 (S00-T88)

● S20.3   Other and unspecified superficial injuries of front wall of thorax
    ● S20.30   Unspecified superficial injuries of front wall of thorax
       ● S20.301   Unspecified superficial injuries of right front wall of thorax
       ● S20.302   Unspecified superficial injuries of left front wall of thorax
       ● S20.309   Unspecified superficial injuries of unspecified front wall of thorax
    ● S20.31   Abrasion of front wall of thorax
       ● S20.311   Abrasion of right front wall of thorax
       ● S20.312   Abrasion of left front wall of thorax
       ● S20.319   Abrasion of unspecified front wall of thorax
    ● S20.32   Blister (nonthermal) of front wall of thorax
       ● S20.321   Blister (nonthermal) of right front wall of thorax
       ● S20.322   Blister (nonthermal) of left front wall of thorax
       ● S20.329   Blister (nonthermal) of unspecified front wall of thorax
    ● S20.34   External constriction of front wall of thorax
       ● S20.341   External constriction of right front wall of thorax
       ● S20.342   External constriction of left front wall of thorax
       ● S20.349   External constriction of unspecified front wall of thorax
    ● S20.35   Superficial foreign body of front wall of thorax
       Splinter in front wall of thorax
       ● S20.351   Superficial foreign body of right front wall of thorax
       ● S20.352   Superficial foreign body of left front wall of thorax
       ● S20.359   Superficial foreign body of unspecified front wall of thorax
    ● S20.36   Insect bite (nonvenomous) of front wall of thorax
       ● S20.361   Insect bite (nonvenomous) of right front wall of thorax
       ● S20.362   Insect bite (nonvenomous) of left front wall of thorax
       ● S20.369   Insect bite (nonvenomous) of unspecified front wall of thorax
    ● S20.37   Other superficial bite of front wall of thorax
       Excludes1   open bite of front wall of thorax (S21.14)
       ● S20.371   Other superficial bite of right front wall of thorax
       ● S20.372   Other superficial bite of left front wall of thorax
       ● S20.379   Other superficial bite of unspecified front wall of thorax
● S20.4   Other and unspecified superficial injuries of back wall of thorax
    ● S20.40   Unspecified superficial injuries of back wall of thorax
       ● S20.401   Unspecified superficial injuries of right back wall of thorax
       ● S20.402   Unspecified superficial injuries of left back wall of thorax
       ● S20.409   Unspecified superficial injuries of unspecified back wall of thorax
    ● S20.41   Abrasion of back wall of thorax
       ● S20.411   Abrasion of right back wall of thorax
       ● S20.412   Abrasion of left back wall of thorax
       ● S20.419   Abrasion of unspecified back wall of thorax

Item 19-1   **Pneumothorax** is a collection of gas (positive air pressure) in the pleural space resulting in the lung collapsing. A tension pneumothorax is life-threatening and is a result of air in the pleural space causing a displacement in the mediastinal structures and cardiopulmonary function compromise. A traumatic pneumothorax results from blunt or penetrating injury that disrupts the parietal/visceral pleura. **Hemothorax** is blood or bloody fluid in the pleural cavity as a result of traumatic blood vessel rupture or inflammation of the lungs from pneumonia.

    ● S20.42   Blister (nonthermal) of back wall of thorax
       ● S20.421   Blister (nonthermal) of right back wall of thorax
       ● S20.422   Blister (nonthermal) of left back wall of thorax
       ● S20.429   Blister (nonthermal) of unspecified back wall of thorax
    ● S20.44   External constriction of back wall of thorax
       ● S20.441   External constriction of right back wall of thorax
       ● S20.442   External constriction of left back wall of thorax
       ● S20.449   External constriction of unspecified back wall of thorax
    ● S20.45   Superficial foreign body of back wall of thorax
       Splinter of back wall of thorax
       ● S20.451   Superficial foreign body of right back wall of thorax
       ● S20.452   Superficial foreign body of left back wall of thorax
       ● S20.459   Superficial foreign body of unspecified back wall of thorax
    ● S20.46   Insect bite (nonvenomous) of back wall of thorax
       ● S20.461   Insect bite (nonvenomous) of right back wall of thorax
       ● S20.462   Insect bite (nonvenomous) of left back wall of thorax
       ● S20.469   Insect bite (nonvenomous) of unspecified back wall of thorax
    ● S20.47   Other superficial bite of back wall of thorax
       Excludes1   open bite of back wall of thorax (S21.24)
       ● S20.471   Other superficial bite of right back wall of thorax
       ● S20.472   Other superficial bite of left back wall of thorax
       ● S20.479   Other superficial bite of unspecified back wall of thorax
● S20.9   Superficial injury of unspecified parts of thorax
       Excludes1   contusion of thorax NOS (S20.20)
    X ● S20.90   Unspecified superficial injury of unspecified parts of thorax
       Superficial injury of thoracic wall NOS
    X ● S20.91   Abrasion of unspecified parts of thorax
    X ● S20.92   Blister (nonthermal) of unspecified parts of thorax
    X ● S20.94   External constriction of unspecified parts of thorax
    X ● S20.95   Superficial foreign body of unspecified parts of thorax
       Splinter in thorax NOS
    X ● S20.96   Insect bite (nonvenomous) of unspecified parts of thorax
    X ● S20.97   Other superficial bite of unspecified parts of thorax
       Excludes1   open bite of thorax NOS (S21.95)

CHAPTER 19 (S00-T88)

● **S21**   **Open wound of thorax**

Code also any associated injury such as:
injury of heart (S26.-)
injury of intrathoracic organs (S27.-)
rib fracture (S22.3-, S22.4-)
spinal cord injury (S24.0-, S24.1-)
traumatic hemothorax (S27.1)
traumatic hemopneumothorax (S27.3)
traumatic pneumothorax (S27.0)
wound infection

> **Excludes1**   traumatic amputation (partial) of thorax (S28.1)

The appropriate 7th character is to be added to each code from category S21

> | | |
> |---|---|
> | A | initial encounter |
> | D | subsequent encounter |
> | S | sequela |

● **S21.0**   **Open wound of breast**

  ● **S21.00**   Unspecified open wound of breast

    ● **S21.001**   Unspecified open wound of right breast

    ● **S21.002**   Unspecified open wound of left breast

    ● **S21.009**   Unspecified open wound of unspecified breast

  ● **S21.01**   Laceration without foreign body of breast

    ● **S21.011**   Laceration without foreign body of right breast

    ● **S21.012**   Laceration without foreign body of left breast

    ● **S21.019**   Laceration without foreign body of unspecified breast

  ● **S21.02**   Laceration with foreign body of breast

    ● **S21.021**   Laceration with foreign body of right breast

    ● **S21.022**   Laceration with foreign body of left breast

    ● **S21.029**   Laceration with foreign body of unspecified breast

  ● **S21.03**   Puncture wound without foreign body of breast

    ● **S21.031**   Puncture wound without foreign body of right breast

    ● **S21.032**   Puncture wound without foreign body of left breast

    ● **S21.039**   Puncture wound without foreign body of unspecified breast

  ● **S21.04**   Puncture wound with foreign body of breast

    ● **S21.041**   Puncture wound with foreign body of right breast

    ● **S21.042**   Puncture wound with foreign body of left breast

    ● **S21.049**   Puncture wound with foreign body of unspecified breast

  ● **S21.05**   Open bite of breast

Bite of breast NOS

> **Excludes1**   superficial bite of breast (S20.17)

    ● **S21.051**   Open bite of right breast

    ● **S21.052**   Open bite of left breast

    ● **S21.059**   Open bite of unspecified breast

● **S21.1**   **Open wound of front wall of thorax without penetration into thoracic cavity**

Open wound of chest without penetration into thoracic cavity

  ● **S21.10**   Unspecified open wound of front wall of thorax without penetration into thoracic cavity

    ● **S21.101**   Unspecified open wound of right front wall of thorax without penetration into thoracic cavity

    ● **S21.102**   Unspecified open wound of left front wall of thorax without penetration into thoracic cavity

    ● **S21.109**   Unspecified open wound of unspecified front wall of thorax without penetration into thoracic cavity

  ● **S21.11**   Laceration without foreign body of front wall of thorax without penetration into thoracic cavity

    ● **S21.111**   Laceration without foreign body of right front wall of thorax without penetration into thoracic cavity

    ● **S21.112**   Laceration without foreign body of left front wall of thorax without penetration into thoracic cavity

    ● **S21.119**   Laceration without foreign body of unspecified front wall of thorax without penetration into thoracic cavity

  ● **S21.12**   Laceration with foreign body of front wall of thorax without penetration into thoracic cavity

    ● **S21.121**   Laceration with foreign body of right front wall of thorax without penetration into thoracic cavity

    ● **S21.122**   Laceration with foreign body of left front wall of thorax without penetration into thoracic cavity

    ● **S21.129**   Laceration with foreign body of unspecified front wall of thorax without penetration into thoracic cavity

  ● **S21.13**   Puncture wound without foreign body of front wall of thorax without penetration into thoracic cavity

    ● **S21.131**   Puncture wound without foreign body of right front wall of thorax without penetration into thoracic cavity

    ● **S21.132**   Puncture wound without foreign body of left front wall of thorax without penetration into thoracic cavity

    ● **S21.139**   Puncture wound without foreign body of unspecified front wall of thorax without penetration into thoracic cavity

  ● **S21.14**   Puncture wound with foreign body of front wall of thorax without penetration into thoracic cavity

    ● **S21.141**   Puncture wound with foreign body of right front wall of thorax without penetration into thoracic cavity

    ● **S21.142**   Puncture wound with foreign body of left front wall of thorax without penetration into thoracic cavity

    ● **S21.149**   Puncture wound with foreign body of unspecified front wall of thorax without penetration into thoracic cavity

◄ New   ◄━ Revised   ~~deleted~~ Deleted   Excludes 1   Excludes 2   Includes   Use additional   Code first   Code also   Unspecified

OGCR Official Guidelines   X Assign placeholder X   ● Use Additional Character(s)   ❱ Manifestation Code   **Coding Clinic**

● **S21.15**   **Open bite of front wall of thorax without penetration into thoracic cavity**
Bite of front wall of thorax NOS

> **Excludes1**   superficial bite of front wall of thorax (S20.37)

  ● **S21.151**   Open bite of right front wall of thorax without penetration into thoracic cavity

  ● **S21.152**   Open bite of left front wall of thorax without penetration into thoracic cavity

  ● **S21.159**   Open bite of unspecified front wall of thorax without penetration into thoracic cavity

● **S21.2**   **Open wound of back wall of thorax without penetration into thoracic cavity**

  ● **S21.20**   Unspecified open wound of back wall of thorax without penetration into thoracic cavity

    ● **S21.201**   Unspecified open wound of right back wall of thorax without penetration into thoracic cavity

    ● **S21.202**   Unspecified open wound of left back wall of thorax without penetration into thoracic cavity

    ● **S21.209**   Unspecified open wound of unspecified back wall of thorax without penetration into thoracic cavity

  ● **S21.21**   Laceration without foreign body of back wall of thorax without penetration into thoracic cavity

    ● **S21.211**   Laceration without foreign body of right back wall of thorax without penetration into thoracic cavity

    ● **S21.212**   Laceration without foreign body of left back wall of thorax without penetration into thoracic cavity

    ● **S21.219**   Laceration without foreign body of unspecified back wall of thorax without penetration into thoracic cavity

  ● **S21.22**   Laceration with foreign body of back wall of thorax without penetration into thoracic cavity

    ● **S21.221**   Laceration with foreign body of right back wall of thorax without penetration into thoracic cavity

    ● **S21.222**   Laceration with foreign body of left back wall of thorax without penetration into thoracic cavity

    ● **S21.229**   Laceration with foreign body of unspecified back wall of thorax without penetration into thoracic cavity

  ● **S21.23**   Puncture wound without foreign body of back wall of thorax without penetration into thoracic cavity

    ● **S21.231**   Puncture wound without foreign body of right back wall of thorax without penetration into thoracic cavity

    ● **S21.232**   Puncture wound without foreign body of left back wall of thorax without penetration into thoracic cavity

    ● **S21.239**   Puncture wound without foreign body of unspecified back wall of thorax without penetration into thoracic cavity

● **S21.24**   Puncture wound with foreign body of back wall of thorax without penetration into thoracic cavity

  ● **S21.241**   Puncture wound with foreign body of right back wall of thorax without penetration into thoracic cavity

  ● **S21.242**   Puncture wound with foreign body of left back wall of thorax without penetration into thoracic cavity

  ● **S21.249**   Puncture wound with foreign body of unspecified back wall of thorax without penetration into thoracic cavity

● **S21.25**   Open bite of back wall of thorax without penetration into thoracic cavity
Bite of back wall of thorax NOS

> **Excludes1**   superficial bite of back wall of thorax (S20.47)

  ● **S21.251**   Open bite of right back wall of thorax without penetration into thoracic cavity

  ● **S21.252**   Open bite of left back wall of thorax without penetration into thoracic cavity

  ● **S21.259**   Open bite of unspecified back wall of thorax without penetration into thoracic cavity

● **S21.3**   **Open wound of front wall of thorax with penetration into thoracic cavity**
Open wound of chest with penetration into thoracic cavity

  ● **S21.30**   Unspecified open wound of front wall of thorax with penetration into thoracic cavity

    ● **S21.301**   Unspecified open wound of right front wall of thorax with penetration into thoracic cavity

    ● **S21.302**   Unspecified open wound of left front wall of thorax with penetration into thoracic cavity

    ● **S21.309**   Unspecified open wound of unspecified front wall of thorax with penetration into thoracic cavity

  ● **S21.31**   Laceration without foreign body of front wall of thorax with penetration into thoracic cavity

    ● **S21.311**   Laceration without foreign body of right front wall of thorax with penetration into thoracic cavity

    ● **S21.312**   Laceration without foreign body of left front wall of thorax with penetration into thoracic cavity

    ● **S21.319**   Laceration without foreign body of unspecified front wall of thorax with penetration into thoracic cavity

  ● **S21.32**   Laceration with foreign body of front wall of thorax with penetration into thoracic cavity

    ● **S21.321**   Laceration with foreign body of right front wall of thorax with penetration into thoracic cavity

    ● **S21.322**   Laceration with foreign body of left front wall of thorax with penetration into thoracic cavity

    ● **S21.329**   Laceration with foreign body of unspecified front wall of thorax with penetration into thoracic cavity

● S21.33   Puncture wound without foreign body of front wall of thorax with penetration into thoracic cavity

   ● S21.331   Puncture wound without foreign body of right front wall of thorax with penetration into thoracic cavity

   ● S21.332   Puncture wound without foreign body of left front wall of thorax with penetration into thoracic cavity

   ● S21.339   Puncture wound without foreign body of unspecified front wall of thorax with penetration into thoracic cavity

● S21.34   Puncture wound with foreign body of front wall of thorax with penetration into thoracic cavity

   ● S21.341   Puncture wound with foreign body of right front wall of thorax with penetration into thoracic cavity

   ● S21.342   Puncture wound with foreign body of left front wall of thorax with penetration into thoracic cavity

   ● S21.349   Puncture wound with foreign body of unspecified front wall of thorax with penetration into thoracic cavity

● S21.35   Open bite of front wall of thorax with penetration into thoracic cavity

     Excludes1   superficial bite of front wall of thorax (S20.37)

   ● S21.351   Open bite of right front wall of thorax with penetration into thoracic cavity

   ● S21.352   Open bite of left front wall of thorax with penetration into thoracic cavity

   ● S21.359   Open bite of unspecified front wall of thorax with penetration into thoracic cavity

● S21.4   Open wound of back wall of thorax with penetration into thoracic cavity

  ● S21.40   Unspecified open wound of back wall of thorax with penetration into thoracic cavity

   ● S21.401   Unspecified open wound of right back wall of thorax with penetration into thoracic cavity

   ● S21.402   Unspecified open wound of left back wall of thorax with penetration into thoracic cavity

   ● S21.409   Unspecified open wound of unspecified back wall of thorax with penetration into thoracic cavity

  ● S21.41   Laceration without foreign body of back wall of thorax with penetration into thoracic cavity

   ● S21.411   Laceration without foreign body of right back wall of thorax with penetration into thoracic cavity

   ● S21.412   Laceration without foreign body of left back wall of thorax with penetration into thoracic cavity

   ● S21.419   Laceration without foreign body of unspecified back wall of thorax with penetration into thoracic cavity

● S21.42   Laceration with foreign body of back wall of thorax with penetration into thoracic cavity

   ● S21.421   Laceration with foreign body of right back wall of thorax with penetration into thoracic cavity

   ● S21.422   Laceration with foreign body of left back wall of thorax with penetration into thoracic cavity

   ● S21.429   Laceration with foreign body of unspecified back wall of thorax with penetration into thoracic cavity

● S21.43   Puncture wound without foreign body of back wall of thorax with penetration into thoracic cavity

   ● S21.431   Puncture wound without foreign body of right back wall of thorax with penetration into thoracic cavity

   ● S21.432   Puncture wound without foreign body of left back wall of thorax with penetration into thoracic cavity

   ● S21.439   Puncture wound without foreign body of unspecified back wall of thorax with penetration into thoracic cavity

● S21.44   Puncture wound with foreign body of back wall of thorax with penetration into thoracic cavity

   ● S21.441   Puncture wound with foreign body of right back wall of thorax with penetration into thoracic cavity

   ● S21.442   Puncture wound with foreign body of left back wall of thorax with penetration into thoracic cavity

   ● S21.449   Puncture wound with foreign body of unspecified back wall of thorax with penetration into thoracic cavity

● S21.45   Open bite of back wall of thorax with penetration into thoracic cavity

    Bite of back wall of thorax NOS

     Excludes1   superficial bite of back wall of thorax (S20.47)

   ● S21.451   Open bite of right back wall of thorax with penetration into thoracic cavity

   ● S21.452   Open bite of left back wall of thorax with penetration into thoracic cavity

   ● S21.459   Open bite of unspecified back wall of thorax with penetration into thoracic cavity

● S21.9   Open wound of unspecified part of thorax

    Open wound of thoracic wall NOS

  X● S21.90   Unspecified open wound of unspecified part of thorax

  X● S21.91   Laceration without foreign body of unspecified part of thorax

  X● S21.92   Laceration with foreign body of unspecified part of thorax

  X● S21.93   Puncture wound without foreign body of unspecified part of thorax

  X● S21.94   Puncture wound with foreign body of unspecified part of thorax

  X● S21.95   Open bite of unspecified part of thorax

     Excludes1   superficial bite of thorax (S20.97)

◄ New   ◄▬ Revised   ~~deleted~~ Deleted   Excludes 1   Excludes 2   Includes   Use additional   Code first   Code also   Unspecified

OGCR Official Guidelines   X Assign placeholder X   ● Use Additional Character(s)   ▶ Manifestation Code   **Coding Clinic**

● **S22**   **Fracture of rib(s), sternum and thoracic spine**

    Note: A fracture not indicated as displaced or nondisplaced should be coded to displaced

    A fracture not indicated as open or closed should be coded to closed

    | **Includes** | fracture of thoracic neural arch |
    fracture of thoracic spinous process
    fracture of thoracic transverse process
    fracture of thoracic vertebra
    fracture of thoracic vertebral arch

    Code first any associated:
    injury of intrathoracic organ (S27.-)
    spinal cord injury (S24.0-, S24.1-)

    Excludes1   transection of thorax (S28.1)

    Excludes2   fracture of clavicle (S42.0-)
    fracture of scapula (S42.1-)

    The appropriate 7th character is to be added to each code from category S22

    | A | initial encounter for closed fracture |
    B   initial encounter for open fracture
    D   subsequent encounter for fracture with routine healing
    G   subsequent encounter for fracture with delayed healing
    K   subsequent encounter for fracture with nonunion
    S   sequela

● **S22.0**   Fracture of thoracic vertebra

  ● **S22.00**   Fracture of unspecified thoracic vertebra

    ● **S22.000**   Wedge compression fracture of unspecified thoracic vertebra

    ● **S22.001**   Stable burst fracture of unspecified thoracic vertebra

    ● **S22.002**   Unstable burst fracture of unspecified thoracic vertebra

    ● **S22.008**   Other fracture of unspecified thoracic vertebra

    ● **S22.009**   Unspecified fracture of unspecified thoracic vertebra

  ● **S22.01**   Fracture of first thoracic vertebra

    ● **S22.010**   Wedge compression fracture of first thoracic vertebra

    ● **S22.011**   Stable burst fracture of first thoracic vertebra

    ● **S22.012**   Unstable burst fracture of first thoracic vertebra

    ● **S22.018**   Other fracture of first thoracic vertebra

    ● **S22.019**   Unspecified fracture of first thoracic vertebra

  ● **S22.02**   Fracture of second thoracic vertebra

    ● **S22.020**   Wedge compression fracture of second thoracic vertebra

    ● **S22.021**   Stable burst fracture of second thoracic vertebra

    ● **S22.022**   Unstable burst fracture of second thoracic vertebra

    ● **S22.028**   Other fracture of second thoracic vertebra

    ● **S22.029**   Unspecified fracture of second thoracic vertebra

  ● **S22.03**   Fracture of third thoracic vertebra

    ● **S22.030**   Wedge compression fracture of third thoracic vertebra

    ● **S22.031**   Stable burst fracture of third thoracic vertebra

    ● **S22.032**   Unstable burst fracture of third thoracic vertebra

    ● **S22.038**   Other fracture of third thoracic vertebra

    ● **S22.039**   Unspecified fracture of third thoracic vertebra

● **S22.04**   Fracture of fourth thoracic vertebra

    ● **S22.040**   Wedge compression fracture of fourth thoracic vertebra

    ● **S22.041**   Stable burst fracture of fourth thoracic vertebra

    ● **S22.042**   Unstable burst fracture of fourth thoracic vertebra

    ● **S22.048**   Other fracture of fourth thoracic vertebra

    ● **S22.049**   Unspecified fracture of fourth thoracic vertebra

● **S22.05**   Fracture of T_5-T_6 vertebra

    ● **S22.050**   Wedge compression fracture of T_5-T_6 vertebra

    ● **S22.051**   Stable burst fracture of T_5-T_6 vertebra

    ● **S22.052**   Unstable burst fracture of T_5-T_6 vertebra

    ● **S22.058**   Other fracture of T_5-T_6 vertebra

    ● **S22.059**   Unspecified fracture of T_5-T_6 vertebra

● **S22.06**   Fracture of T_7-T_8 vertebra

    ● **S22.060**   Wedge compression fracture of T_7-T_8 vertebra

    ● **S22.061**   Stable burst fracture of T_7-T_8 vertebra

    ● **S22.062**   Unstable burst fracture of T_7-T_8 vertebra

    ● **S22.068**   Other fracture of T_7-T_8 thoracic vertebra

    ● **S22.069**   Unspecified fracture of T_7-T_8 vertebra

● **S22.07**   Fracture of T_9-T_{10} vertebra

    ● **S22.070**   Wedge compression fracture of T_9-T_{10} vertebra

    ● **S22.071**   Stable burst fracture of T_9-T_{10} vertebra

    ● **S22.072**   Unstable burst fracture of T_9-T_{10} vertebra

    ● **S22.078**   Other fracture of T_9-T_{10} vertebra

    ● **S22.079**   Unspecified fracture of T_9-T_{10} vertebra

● **S22.08**   Fracture of T_{11}-T_{12} vertebra

    ● **S22.080**   Wedge compression fracture of T_{11}-T_{12} vertebra

    ● **S22.081**   Stable burst fracture of T_{11}-T_{12} vertebra

    ● **S22.082**   Unstable burst fracture of T_{11}-T_{12} vertebra

    ● **S22.088**   Other fracture of T_{11}-T_{12} vertebra

    ● **S22.089**   Unspecified fracture of T_{11}-T_{12} vertebra

● **S22.2**   Fracture of sternum

  X● **S22.20**   Unspecified fracture of sternum

  X● **S22.21**   Fracture of manubrium

  X● **S22.22**   Fracture of body of sternum

  X● **S22.23**   Sternal manubrial dissociation

  X● **S22.24**   Fracture of xiphoid process

● **S22.3**   Fracture of one rib

  X● **S22.31**   Fracture of one rib, right side

  X● **S22.32**   Fracture of one rib, left side

  X● **S22.39**   Fracture of one rib, unspecified side

● **S22.4**   Multiple fractures of ribs
    Fractures of two or more ribs

    Excludes1   flail chest (S22.5-)

  X● **S22.41**   Multiple fractures of ribs, right side

  X● **S22.42**   Multiple fractures of ribs, left side

  X● **S22.43**   Multiple fractures of ribs, bilateral

  X● **S22.49**   Multiple fractures of ribs, unspecified side

X● **S22.5**   Flail chest
    Unstable chest due to sternum and/or rib fracture

X● **S22.9**   Fracture of bony thorax, part unspecified

CHAPTER 19 (S00-T88)

● **S23 Dislocation and sprain of joints and ligaments of thorax**

> **Includes** avulsion of joint or ligament of thorax
> laceration of cartilage, joint or ligament of thorax
> sprain of cartilage, joint or ligament of thorax
> traumatic hemarthrosis of joint or ligament of thorax
> traumatic rupture of joint or ligament of thorax
> traumatic subluxation of joint or ligament of thorax
> traumatic tear of joint or ligament of thorax

Code also any associated open wound

> **Excludes2** dislocation, sprain of sternoclavicular joint (S43.2, S43.6)
> strain of muscle or tendon of thorax (S29.01-)

The appropriate 7th character is to be added to each code from category S23

> A   initial encounter
> D   subsequent encounter
> S   sequela

X ● **S23.0 Traumatic rupture of thoracic intervertebral disc**

> **Excludes1** rupture or displacement (nontraumatic) of thoracic intervertebral disc NOS (M51.- with fifth character 4)

● **S23.1 Subluxation and dislocation of thoracic vertebra**

> Code also any associated
> open wound of thorax (S21.-)
> spinal cord injury (S24.0-, S24.1-)
>
> **Excludes2** fracture of thoracic vertebrae (S22.0-)

● **S23.10 Subluxation and dislocation of unspecified thoracic vertebra**

> ● **S23.100 Subluxation of** unspecified **thoracic vertebra**
> ● **S23.101 Dislocation of** unspecified **thoracic vertebra**

● **S23.11 Subluxation and dislocation of T_1/T_2 thoracic vertebra**

> ● **S23.110 Subluxation of T_1/T_2 thoracic vertebra**
> ● **S23.111 Dislocation of T_1/T_2 thoracic vertebra**

● **S23.12 Subluxation and dislocation of T_2/T_3-T_3/T_4 thoracic vertebra**

> ● **S23.120 Subluxation of T_2/T_3 thoracic vertebra**
> ● **S23.121 Dislocation of T_2/T_3 thoracic vertebra**
> ● **S23.122 Subluxation of T_3/T_4 thoracic vertebra**
> ● **S23.123 Dislocation of T_3/T_4 thoracic vertebra**

● **S23.13 Subluxation and dislocation of T_4/T_5-T_5/T_6 thoracic vertebra**

> ● **S23.130 Subluxation of T_4/T_5 thoracic vertebra**
> ● **S23.131 Dislocation of T_4/T_5 thoracic vertebra**
> ● **S23.132 Subluxation of T_5/T_6 thoracic vertebra**
> ● **S23.133 Dislocation of T_5/T_6 thoracic vertebra**

● **S23.14 Subluxation and dislocation of T_6/T_7-T_7/T_8 thoracic vertebra**

> ● **S23.140 Subluxation of T_6/T_7 thoracic vertebra**
> ● **S23.141 Dislocation of T_6/T_7 thoracic vertebra**
> ● **S23.142 Subluxation of T_7/T_8 thoracic vertebra**
> ● **S23.143 Dislocation of T_7/T_8 thoracic vertebra**

● **S23.15 Subluxation and dislocation of T_8/T_9-T_9/T_{10} thoracic vertebra**

> ● **S23.150 Subluxation of T_8/T_9 thoracic vertebra**
> ● **S23.151 Dislocation of T_8/T_9 thoracic vertebra**
> ● **S23.152 Subluxation of T_9/T_{10} thoracic vertebra**
> ● **S23.153 Dislocation of T_9/T_{10} thoracic vertebra**

● **S23.16 Subluxation and dislocation of T_{10}/T_{11}-T_{11}/T_{12} thoracic vertebra**

> ● **S23.160 Subluxation of T_{10}/T_{11} thoracic vertebra**
> ● **S23.161 Dislocation of T_{10}/T_{11} thoracic vertebra**
> ● **S23.162 Subluxation of T_{11}/T_{12} thoracic vertebra**
> ● **S23.163 Dislocation of T_{11}/T_{12} thoracic vertebra**

● **S23.17 Subluxation and dislocation of T_{12}/L_1 thoracic vertebra**

> ● **S23.170 Subluxation of T_{12}/L_1 thoracic vertebra**
> ● **S23.171 Dislocation of T_{12}/L_1 thoracic vertebra**

● **S23.2 Dislocation of other and unspecified parts of thorax**

> X ● **S23.20 Dislocation of** unspecified **part of thorax**
> X ● **S23.29 Dislocation of other parts of thorax**

X ● **S23.3 Sprain of ligaments of thoracic spine**

● **S23.4 Sprain of ribs and sternum**

> X ● **S23.41 Sprain of ribs**
> ● **S23.42 Sprain of sternum**
>
> > ● **S23.420 Sprain of sternoclavicular (joint) (ligament)**
> > ● **S23.421 Sprain of chondrosternal joint**
> > ● **S23.428 Other sprain of sternum**
> > ● **S23.429** Unspecified **sprain of sternum**

X ● **S23.8 Sprain of other specified parts of thorax**

X ● **S23.9 Sprain of** unspecified **parts of thorax**

● **S24 Injury of nerves and spinal cord at thorax level**

> **Note:** Code to highest level of thoracic spinal cord injury.
>
> Injuries to the spinal cord (S24.0 and S24.1) refer to the cord level and not bone level injury, and can affect nerve roots at and below the level given.
>
> Code also any associated:
> fracture of thoracic vertebra (S22.0-)
> open wound of thorax (S21.-)
> transient paralysis (R29.5)
>
> **Excludes2** injury of brachial plexus (S14.3)

The appropriate 7th character is to be added to each code from category S24

> A   initial encounter
> D   subsequent encounter
> S   sequela

X ● **S24.0 Concussion and edema of thoracic spinal cord**

● **S24.1 Other and unspecified injuries of thoracic spinal cord**

> ● **S24.10 Unspecified injury of thoracic spinal cord**
>
> > ● **S24.101** Unspecified **injury at T_1 level of thoracic spinal cord**
> > ● **S24.102** Unspecified **injury at T_2-T_6 level of thoracic spinal cord**
> > ● **S24.103** Unspecified **injury at T_7-T_{10} level of thoracic spinal cord**
> > ● **S24.104** Unspecified **injury at T_{11}-T_{12} level of thoracic spinal cord**
> > ● **S24.109** Unspecified **injury at unspecified level of thoracic spinal cord**
> > Injury of thoracic spinal cord NOS
>
> ● **S24.11 Complete lesion of thoracic spinal cord**
>
> > ● **S24.111 Complete lesion at T_1 level of thoracic spinal cord**
> > ● **S24.112 Complete lesion at T_2-T_6 level of thoracic spinal cord**
> > ● **S24.113 Complete lesion at T_7-T_{10} level of thoracic spinal cord**
> > ● **S24.114 Complete lesion at T_{11}-T_{12} level of thoracic spinal cord**
> > ● **S24.119 Complete lesion at** unspecified **level of thoracic spinal cord**

◄ New   ◄ Revised   ~~deleted~~ Deleted   Excludes 1   Excludes 2   Includes   Use additional   Code first   Code also   Unspecified

OGCR Official Guidelines   X Assign placeholder X   ● Use Additional Character(s)   ▶ Manifestation Code   **Coding Clinic**

● S24.13   Anterior cord syndrome of thoracic spinal cord
    ● S24.131   Anterior cord syndrome at T_1 level of thoracic spinal cord
    ● S24.132   Anterior cord syndrome at T_2-T_6 level of thoracic spinal cord
    ● S24.133   Anterior cord syndrome at T_7-T_{10} level of thoracic spinal cord
    ● S24.134   Anterior cord syndrome at T_{11}-T_{12} level of thoracic spinal cord
    ● S24.139   Anterior cord syndrome at unspecified level of thoracic spinal cord

● S24.14   Brown-Séquard syndrome of thoracic spinal cord
    ● S24.141   Brown-Séquard syndrome at T_1 level of thoracic spinal cord
    ● S24.142   Brown-Séquard syndrome at T_2-T_6 level of thoracic spinal cord
    ● S24.143   Brown-Séquard syndrome at T_7-T_{10} level of thoracic spinal cord
    ● S24.144   Brown-Séquard syndrome at T_{11}-T_{12} level of thoracic spinal cord
    ● S24.149   Brown-Séquard syndrome at unspecified level of thoracic spinal cord

● S24.15   Other incomplete lesions of thoracic spinal cord
    Incomplete lesion of thoracic spinal cord NOS
    Posterior cord syndrome of thoracic spinal cord
    ● S24.151   Other incomplete lesion at T_1 level of thoracic spinal cord
    ● S24.152   Other incomplete lesion at T_2-T_6 level of thoracic spinal cord
    ● S24.153   Other incomplete lesion at T_7-T_{10} level of thoracic spinal cord
    ● S24.154   Other incomplete lesion at T_{11}-T_{12} level of thoracic spinal cord
    ● S24.159   Other incomplete lesion at unspecified level of thoracic spinal cord

X ● S24.2   Injury of nerve root of thoracic spine
X ● S24.3   Injury of peripheral nerves of thorax
X ● S24.4   Injury of thoracic sympathetic nervous system
    Injury of cardiac plexus
    Injury of esophageal plexus
    Injury of pulmonary plexus
    Injury of stellate ganglion
    Injury of thoracic sympathetic ganglion
X ● S24.8   Injury of other specified nerves of thorax
X ● S24.9   Injury of unspecified nerve of thorax

● S25   Injury of blood vessels of thorax
    The appropriate 7th character is to be added to each code from category S25

    | | |
    | A | initial encounter |
    | D | subsequent encounter |
    | S | sequela |

    Code also any associated open wound (S21.-)

● S25.0   Injury of thoracic aorta
    Injury of aorta NOS
X ● S25.00   Unspecified injury of thoracic aorta
X ● S25.01   Minor laceration of thoracic aorta
    Incomplete transection of thoracic aorta
    Laceration of thoracic aorta NOS
    Superficial laceration of thoracic aorta
X ● S25.02   Major laceration of thoracic aorta
    Complete transection of thoracic aorta
    Traumatic rupture of thoracic aorta
X ● S25.09   Other specified injury of thoracic aorta

● S25.1   Injury of innominate or subclavian artery
    ● S25.10   Unspecified injury of innominate or subclavian artery
        ● S25.101   Unspecified injury of right innominate or subclavian artery
        ● S25.102   Unspecified injury of left innominate or subclavian artery
        ● S25.109   Unspecified injury of unspecified innominate or subclavian artery
    ● S25.11   Minor laceration of innominate or subclavian artery
        Incomplete transection of innominate or subclavian artery
        Laceration of innominate or subclavian artery NOS
        Superficial laceration of innominate or subclavian artery
        ● S25.111   Minor laceration of right innominate or subclavian artery
        ● S25.112   Minor laceration of left innominate or subclavian artery
        ● S25.119   Minor laceration of unspecified innominate or subclavian artery
    ● S25.12   Major laceration of innominate or subclavian artery
        Complete transection of innominate or subclavian artery
        Traumatic rupture of innominate or subclavian artery
        ● S25.121   Major laceration of right innominate or subclavian artery
        ● S25.122   Major laceration of left innominate or subclavian artery
        ● S25.129   Major laceration of unspecified innominate or subclavian artery
    ● S25.19   Other specified injury of innominate or subclavian artery
        ● S25.191   Other specified injury of right innominate or subclavian artery
        ● S25.192   Other specified injury of left innominate or subclavian artery
        ● S25.199   Other specified injury of unspecified innominate or subclavian artery

● S25.2   Injury of superior vena cava
    Injury of vena cava NOS
X ● S25.20   Unspecified injury of superior vena cava
X ● S25.21   Minor laceration of superior vena cava
    Incomplete transection of superior vena cava
    Laceration of superior vena cava NOS
    Superficial laceration of superior vena cava
X ● S25.22   Major laceration of superior vena cava
    Complete transection of superior vena cava
    Traumatic rupture of superior vena cava
X ● S25.29   Other specified injury of superior vena cava

● S25.3   Injury of innominate or subclavian vein
    ● S25.30   Unspecified injury of innominate or subclavian vein
        ● S25.301   Unspecified injury of right innominate or subclavian vein
        ● S25.302   Unspecified injury of left innominate or subclavian vein
        ● S25.309   Unspecified injury of unspecified innominate or subclavian vein

- ● S25.31 **Minor laceration of innominate or subclavian vein**
  Incomplete transection of innominate or subclavian vein
  Laceration of innominate or subclavian vein NOS
  Superficial laceration of innominate or subclavian vein
  - ● S25.311 **Minor laceration of right innominate or subclavian vein**
  - ● S25.312 **Minor laceration of left innominate or subclavian vein**
  - ● S25.319 **Minor laceration of unspecified innominate or subclavian vein**
  - ● S25.32 **Major laceration of innominate or subclavian vein**
    Complete transection of innominate or subclavian vein
    Traumatic rupture of innominate or subclavian vein
  - ● S25.321 **Major laceration of right innominate or subclavian vein**
  - ● S25.322 **Major laceration of left innominate or subclavian vein**
  - ● S25.329 **Major laceration of unspecified innominate or subclavian vein**
- ● S25.39 **Other specified injury of innominate or subclavian vein**
  - ● S25.391 **Other specified injury of right innominate or subclavian vein**
  - ● S25.392 **Other specified injury of left innominate or subclavian vein**
  - ● S25.399 **Other specified injury of unspecified innominate or subclavian vein**
- ● S25.4 **Injury of pulmonary blood vessels**
  - ● S25.40 **Unspecified injury of pulmonary blood vessels**
    - ● S25.401 **Unspecified injury of right pulmonary blood vessels**
    - ● S25.402 **Unspecified injury of left pulmonary blood vessels**
    - ● S25.409 **Unspecified injury of unspecified pulmonary blood vessels**
  - ● S25.41 **Minor laceration of pulmonary blood vessels**
    Incomplete transection of pulmonary blood vessels
    Laceration of pulmonary blood vessels NOS
    Superficial laceration of pulmonary blood vessels
    - ● S25.411 **Minor laceration of right pulmonary blood vessels**
    - ● S25.412 **Minor laceration of left pulmonary blood vessels**
    - ● S25.419 **Minor laceration of unspecified pulmonary blood vessels**
  - ● S25.42 **Major laceration of pulmonary blood vessels**
    Complete transection of pulmonary blood vessels
    Traumatic rupture of pulmonary blood vessels
    - ● S25.421 **Major laceration of right pulmonary blood vessels**
    - ● S25.422 **Major laceration of left pulmonary blood vessels**
    - ● S25.429 **Major laceration of unspecified pulmonary blood vessels**

- ● S25.49 **Other specified injury of pulmonary blood vessels**
  - ● S25.491 **Other specified injury of right pulmonary blood vessels**
  - ● S25.492 **Other specified injury of left pulmonary blood vessels**
  - ● S25.499 **Other specified injury of unspecified pulmonary blood vessels**
- ● S25.5 **Injury of intercostal blood vessels**
  - ● S25.50 **Unspecified injury of intercostal blood vessels**
    - ● S25.501 **Unspecified injury of intercostal blood vessels, right side**
    - ● S25.502 **Unspecified injury of intercostal blood vessels, left side**
    - ● S25.509 **Unspecified injury of intercostal blood vessels, unspecified side**
  - ● S25.51 **Laceration of intercostal blood vessels**
    - ● S25.511 **Laceration of intercostal blood vessels, right side**
    - ● S25.512 **Laceration of intercostal blood vessels, left side**
    - ● S25.519 **Laceration of intercostal blood vessels, unspecified side**
  - ● S25.59 **Other specified injury of intercostal blood vessels**
    - ● S25.591 **Other specified injury of intercostal blood vessels, right side**
    - ● S25.592 **Other specified injury of intercostal blood vessels, left side**
    - ● S25.599 **Other specified injury of intercostal blood vessels, unspecified side**
- ● S25.8 **Injury of other blood vessels of thorax**
  Injury of azygos vein
  Injury of mammary artery or vein
  - ● S25.80 **Unspecified injury of other blood vessels of thorax**
    - ● S25.801 **Unspecified injury of other blood vessels of thorax, right side**
    - ● S25.802 **Unspecified injury of other blood vessels of thorax, left side**
    - ● S25.809 **Unspecified injury of other blood vessels of thorax, unspecified side**
  - ● S25.81 **Laceration of other blood vessels of thorax**
    - ● S25.811 **Laceration of other blood vessels of thorax, right side**
    - ● S25.812 **Laceration of other blood vessels of thorax, left side**
    - ● S25.819 **Laceration of other blood vessels of thorax, unspecified side**
  - ● S25.89 **Other specified injury of other blood vessels of thorax**
    - ● S25.891 **Other specified injury of other blood vessels of thorax, right side**
    - ● S25.892 **Other specified injury of other blood vessels of thorax, left side**
    - ● S25.899 **Other specified injury of other blood vessels of thorax, unspecified side**
- ● S25.9 **Injury of unspecified blood vessel of thorax**
  - X ● S25.90 **Unspecified injury of unspecified blood vessel of thorax**
  - X ● S25.91 **Laceration of unspecified blood vessel of thorax**
  - X ● S25.99 **Other specified injury of unspecified blood vessel of thorax**

◀ New ◀▥ Revised ~~deleted~~ Deleted | Excludes 1 | Excludes 2 | Includes | Use additional | Code first | Code also | Unspecified |

OGCR Official Guidelines X Assign placeholder X ● Use Additional Character(s) ▶ Manifestation Code **Coding Clinic**

Item 19–2 **Pneumothorax** is a collection of gas (positive air pressure) in the pleural space resulting in the lung collapsing. A tension pneumothorax is life-threatening and is a result of air in the pleural space causing a displacement in the mediastinal structures and cardiopulmonary function compromise. A traumatic pneumothorax results from blunt or penetrating injury that disrupts the parietal/visceral pleura. **Hemothorax** is blood or bloody fluid in the pleural cavity as a result of traumatic blood vessel rupture or inflammation of the lungs from pneumonia.

● S26 **Injury of heart**

The appropriate 7th character is to be added to each code from category S26

> A   initial encounter
> D   subsequent encounter
> S   sequela

Code also any associated:
open wound of thorax (S21.-)
traumatic hemopneumothorax (S27.2)
traumatic hemothorax (S27.1)
traumatic pneumothorax (S27.0)

● S26.0 **Injury of heart with hemopericardium**
Hemopericardium: effusion of blood within pericardium

X● S26.00 Unspecified injury of heart with hemopericardium

X● S26.01 Contusion of heart with hemopericardium

● S26.02 Laceration of heart with hemopericardium

   ● S26.020 **Mild laceration of heart with hemopericardium**
Laceration of heart without penetration of heart chamber

   ● S26.021 **Moderate laceration of heart with hemopericardium**
Laceration of heart with penetration of heart chamber

   ● S26.022 **Major laceration of heart with hemopericardium**
Laceration of heart with penetration of multiple heart chambers

X● S26.09 Other injury of heart with hemopericardium

● S26.1 **Injury of heart without hemopericardium**
Hemopericardium: effusion of blood within pericardium

X● S26.10 Unspecified injury of heart without hemopericardium

X● S26.11 Contusion of heart without hemopericardium

X● S26.12 Laceration of heart without hemopericardium

X● S26.19 Other injury of heart without hemopericardium

● S26.9 **Injury of heart, unspecified with or without hemopericardium**
Hemopericardium: effusion of blood within pericardium

X● S26.90 Unspecified injury of heart, unspecified with or without hemopericardium

X● S26.91 Contusion of heart, unspecified with or without hemopericardium

X● S26.92 Laceration of heart, unspecified with or without hemopericardium
Laceration of heart NOS

X● S26.99 Other injury of heart, unspecified with or without hemopericardium

● S27 **Injury of other and unspecified intrathoracic organs**
Code also any associated open wound of thorax (S21.-)
Excludes2 injury of cervical esophagus (S10-S19)
injury of trachea (cervical) (S10-S19)

The appropriate 7th character is to be added to each code from category S27

> A   initial encounter
> D   subsequent encounter
> S   sequela

X● S27.0 **Traumatic pneumothorax**
Excludes1 spontaneous pneumothorax (J93.-)

X● S27.1 **Traumatic hemothorax**

X● S27.2 **Traumatic hemopneumothorax**

● S27.3 **Other and unspecified injuries of lung**

  ● S27.30 **Unspecified injury of lung**

    ● S27.301 Unspecified injury of lung, unilateral

    ● S27.302 Unspecified injury of lung, bilateral

    ● S27.309 Unspecified injury of lung, unspecified

  ● S27.31 **Primary blast injury of lung**
Blast injury of lung NOS

    ● S27.311 Primary blast injury of lung, unilateral

    ● S27.312 Primary blast injury of lung, bilateral

    ● S27.319 Primary blast injury of lung, unspecified

  ● S27.32 **Contusion of lung**

    ● S27.321 Contusion of lung, unilateral

    ● S27.322 Contusion of lung, bilateral

    ● S27.329 Contusion of lung, unspecified

  ● S27.33 **Laceration of lung**

    ● S27.331 Laceration of lung, unilateral

    ● S27.332 Laceration of lung, bilateral

    ● S27.339 Laceration of lung, unspecified

  ● S27.39 **Other injuries of lung**
Secondary blast injury of lung

    ● S27.391 Other injuries of lung, unilateral

    ● S27.392 Other injuries of lung, bilateral

    ● S27.399 Other injuries of lung, unspecified

● S27.4 **Injury of bronchus**

  ● S27.40 **Unspecified injury of bronchus**

    ● S27.401 Unspecified injury of bronchus, unilateral

    ● S27.402 Unspecified injury of bronchus, bilateral

    ● S27.409 Unspecified injury of bronchus, unspecified

  ● S27.41 **Primary blast injury of bronchus**
Blast injury of bronchus NOS

    ● S27.411 Primary blast injury of bronchus, unilateral

    ● S27.412 Primary blast injury of bronchus, bilateral

    ● S27.419 Primary blast injury of bronchus, unspecified

  ● S27.42 **Contusion of bronchus**

    ● S27.421 Contusion of bronchus, unilateral

    ● S27.422 Contusion of bronchus, bilateral

    ● S27.429 Contusion of bronchus, unspecified

CHAPTER 19 (S00-T88)

● S27.43   Laceration of bronchus
    ● S27.431   Laceration of bronchus, unilateral
    ● S27.432   Laceration of bronchus, bilateral
    ● S27.439   Laceration of bronchus, unspecified
● S27.49   Other injury of bronchus
    Secondary blast injury of bronchus
    ● S27.491   Other injury of bronchus, unilateral
    ● S27.492   Other injury of bronchus, bilateral
    ● S27.499   Other injury of bronchus, unspecified

● S27.5   Injury of thoracic trachea
X ● S27.50   Unspecified injury of thoracic trachea
X ● S27.51   Primary blast injury of thoracic trachea
    Blast injury of thoracic trachea NOS
X ● S27.52   Contusion of thoracic trachea
X ● S27.53   Laceration of thoracic trachea
X ● S27.59   Other injury of thoracic trachea
    Secondary blast injury of thoracic trachea

● S27.6   Injury of pleura
X ● S27.60   Unspecified injury of pleura
X ● S27.63   Laceration of pleura
X ● S27.69   Other injury of pleura

● S27.8   Injury of other specified intrathoracic organs
  ● S27.80   Injury of diaphragm
    ● S27.802   Contusion of diaphragm
    ● S27.803   Laceration of diaphragm
    ● S27.808   Other injury of diaphragm
    ● S27.809   Unspecified injury of diaphragm
  ● S27.81   Injury of esophagus (thoracic part)
    ● S27.812   Contusion of esophagus (thoracic part)
    ● S27.813   Laceration of esophagus (thoracic part)
    ● S27.818   Other injury of esophagus (thoracic part)
    ● S27.819   Unspecified injury of esophagus (thoracic part)
  ● S27.89   Injury of other specified intrathoracic organs
    Injury of lymphatic thoracic duct
    Injury of thymus gland
    ● S27.892   Contusion of other specified intrathoracic organs
    ● S27.893   Laceration of other specified intrathoracic organs
    ● S27.898   Other injury of other specified intrathoracic organs
    ● S27.899   Unspecified injury of other specified intrathoracic organs
X ● S27.9   Injury of unspecified intrathoracic organ

● S28   Crushing injury of thorax, and traumatic amputation of part of thorax

    The appropriate 7th character is to be added to each code from category S28

    | A | initial encounter |
    | D | subsequent encounter |
    | S | sequela |

X ● S28.0   Crushed chest
    Use additional code for all associated injuries
    Excludes1   flail chest (S22.5)
X ● S28.1   Traumatic amputation (partial) of part of thorax, except breast

● S28.2   Traumatic amputation of breast
  ● S28.21   Complete traumatic amputation of breast
    Traumatic amputation of breast NOS
    ● S28.211   Complete traumatic amputation of right breast
    ● S28.212   Complete traumatic amputation of left breast
    ● S28.219   Complete traumatic amputation of unspecified breast
  ● S28.22   Partial traumatic amputation of breast
    ● S28.221   Partial traumatic amputation of right breast
    ● S28.222   Partial traumatic amputation of left breast
    ● S28.229   Partial traumatic amputation of unspecified breast

● S29   Other and unspecified injuries of thorax
    Code also any associated open wound (S21.-)
    The appropriate 7th character is to be added to each code from category S29

    | A | initial encounter |
    | D | subsequent encounter |
    | S | sequela |

● S29.0   Injury of muscle and tendon at thorax level
  ● S29.00   Unspecified injury of muscle and tendon of thorax
    ● S29.001   Unspecified injury of muscle and tendon of front wall of thorax
    ● S29.002   Unspecified injury of muscle and tendon of back wall of thorax
    ● S29.009   Unspecified injury of muscle and tendon of unspecified wall of thorax
  ● S29.01   Strain of muscle and tendon of thorax
    ● S29.011   Strain of muscle and tendon of front wall of thorax
    ● S29.012   Strain of muscle and tendon of back wall of thorax
    ● S29.019   Strain of muscle and tendon of unspecified wall of thorax
  ● S29.02   Laceration of muscle and tendon of thorax
    ● S29.021   Laceration of muscle and tendon of front wall of thorax
    ● S29.022   Laceration of muscle and tendon of back wall of thorax
    ● S29.029   Laceration of muscle and tendon of unspecified wall of thorax
  ● S29.09   Other injury of muscle and tendon of thorax
    ● S29.091   Other injury of muscle and tendon of front wall of thorax
    ● S29.092   Other injury of muscle and tendon of back wall of thorax
    ● S29.099   Other injury of muscle and tendon of unspecified wall of thorax
X ● S29.8   Other specified injuries of thorax
X ● S29.9   Unspecified injury of thorax

◀ New   ◀ Revised   ~~deleted~~ Deleted   Excludes 1   Excludes 2   Includes   Use additional   Code first   Code also   Unspecified
OGCR Official Guidelines   X Assign placeholder X   ● Use Additional Character(s)   ▶ Manifestation Code   **Coding Clinic**

INJURIES TO THE ABDOMEN, LOWER BACK, LUMBAR SPINE, PELVIS AND EXTERNAL GENITALS (S30-S39)

Includes   injuries to the abdominal wall
injuries to the anus
injuries to the buttock
injuries to the external genitalia
injuries to the flank
injuries to the groin

Excludes2   burns and corrosions (T20-T32)
effects of foreign body in anus and rectum (T18.5)
effects of foreign body in genitourinary tract (T19.-)
effects of foreign body in stomach, small intestine and colon (T18.2-T18.4)
frostbite (T33-T34)
insect bite or sting, venomous (T63.4)

● **S30**   **Superficial injury of abdomen, lower back, pelvis and external genitals**

Excludes2   superficial injury of hip (S70.-)

The appropriate 7th character is to be added to each code from category S30

> A   initial encounter
> D   subsequent encounter
> S   sequela

X ● **S30.0**   **Contusion of lower back and pelvis**
Contusion of buttock

X ● **S30.1**   **Contusion of abdominal wall**
Contusion of flank
Contusion of groin

● **S30.2**   **Contusion of external genital organs**

   ● **S30.20**   **Contusion of unspecified external genital organ**

     ● **S30.201**   **Contusion of unspecified external genital organ, male ♂**

     ● **S30.202**   **Contusion of unspecified external genital organ, female ♀**

   X ● **S30.21**   **Contusion of penis ♂**

   X ● **S30.22**   **Contusion of scrotum and testes ♂**

   X ● **S30.23**   **Contusion of vagina and vulva ♀**

X ● **S30.3**   **Contusion of anus**

● **S30.8**   **Other superficial injuries of abdomen, lower back, pelvis and external genitals**

   ● **S30.81**   **Abrasion of abdomen, lower back, pelvis and external genitals**

     ● **S30.810**   **Abrasion of lower back and pelvis**

     ● **S30.811**   **Abrasion of abdominal wall**

     ● **S30.812**   **Abrasion of penis ♂**

     ● **S30.813**   **Abrasion of scrotum and testes ♂**

     ● **S30.814**   **Abrasion of vagina and vulva ♀**

     ● **S30.815**   **Abrasion of unspecified external genital organs, male ♂**

     ● **S30.816**   **Abrasion of unspecified external genital organs, female ♀**

     ● **S30.817**   **Abrasion of anus**

   ● **S30.82**   **Blister (nonthermal) of abdomen, lower back, pelvis and external genitals**

     ● **S30.820**   **Blister (nonthermal) of lower back and pelvis**

     ● **S30.821**   **Blister (nonthermal) of abdominal wall**

     ● **S30.822**   **Blister (nonthermal) of penis ♂**

     ● **S30.823**   **Blister (nonthermal) of scrotum and testes ♂**

     ● **S30.824**   **Blister (nonthermal) of vagina and vulva ♀**

     ● **S30.825**   **Blister (nonthermal) of unspecified external genital organs, male ♂**

     ● **S30.826**   **Blister (nonthermal) of unspecified external genital organs, female ♀**

     ● **S30.827**   **Blister (nonthermal) of anus**

   ● **S30.84**   **External constriction of abdomen, lower back, pelvis and external genitals**

     ● **S30.840**   **External constriction of lower back and pelvis**

     ● **S30.841**   **External constriction of abdominal wall**

     ● **S30.842**   **External constriction of penis ♂**
Hair tourniquet syndrome of penis
Use additional cause code to identify the constricting item (W49.0-)

     ● **S30.843**   **External constriction of scrotum and testes ♂**

     ● **S30.844**   **External constriction of vagina and vulva ♀**

     ● **S30.845**   **External constriction of unspecified external genital organs, male ♂**

     ● **S30.846**   **External constriction of unspecified external genital organs, female ♀**

   ● **S30.85**   **Superficial foreign body of abdomen, lower back, pelvis and external genitals**
Splinter in the abdomen, lower back, pelvis and external genitals

     ● **S30.850**   **Superficial foreign body of lower back and pelvis**

     ● **S30.851**   **Superficial foreign body of abdominal wall**

     ● **S30.852**   **Superficial foreign body of penis ♂**

     ● **S30.853**   **Superficial foreign body of scrotum and testes ♂**

     ● **S30.854**   **Superficial foreign body of vagina and vulva ♀**

     ● **S30.855**   **Superficial foreign body of unspecified external genital organs, male ♂**

     ● **S30.856**   **Superficial foreign body of unspecified external genital organs, female ♀**

     ● **S30.857**   **Superficial foreign body of anus**

   ● **S30.86**   **Insect bite (nonvenomous) of abdomen, lower back, pelvis and external genitals**

     ● **S30.860**   **Insect bite (nonvenomous) of lower back and pelvis**

     ● **S30.861**   **Insect bite (nonvenomous) of abdominal wall**

     ● **S30.862**   **Insect bite (nonvenomous) of penis ♂**

     ● **S30.863**   **Insect bite (nonvenomous) of scrotum and testes ♂**

     ● **S30.864**   **Insect bite (nonvenomous) of vagina and vulva ♀**

     ● **S30.865**   **Insect bite (nonvenomous) of unspecified external genital organs, male ♂**

     ● **S30.866**   **Insect bite (nonvenomous) of unspecified external genital organs, female ♀**

     ● **S30.867**   **Insect bite (nonvenomous) of anus**

CHAPTER 19 (S00-T88)

● S30.87 **Other superficial bite of abdomen, lower back, pelvis and external genitals**

Excludes1 open bite of abdomen, lower back, pelvis and external genitals (S31.05, S31.15, S31.25, S31.35, S31.45, S31.55)

● S30.870 **Other superficial bite of lower back and pelvis**

● S30.871 **Other superficial bite of abdominal wall**

● S30.872 **Other superficial bite of penis ♂**

● S30.873 **Other superficial bite of scrotum and testes ♂**

● S30.874 **Other superficial bite of vagina and vulva ♀**

● S30.875 **Other superficial bite of unspecified external genital organs, male ♂**

● S30.876 **Other superficial bite of unspecified external genital organs, female ♀**

● S30.877 **Other superficial bite of anus**

● S30.9 **Unspecified superficial injury of abdomen, lower back, pelvis and external genitals**

X ● S30.91 **Unspecified superficial injury of lower back and pelvis**

X ● S30.92 **Unspecified superficial injury of abdominal wall**

X ● S30.93 **Unspecified superficial injury of penis ♂**

X ● S30.94 **Unspecified superficial injury of scrotum and testes ♂**

X ● S30.95 **Unspecified superficial injury of vagina and vulva ♀**

X ● S30.96 **Unspecified superficial injury of unspecified external genital organs, male ♂**

X ● S30.97 **Unspecified superficial injury of unspecified external genital organs, female ♀**

X ● S30.98 **Unspecified superficial injury of anus**

● S31 **Open wound of abdomen, lower back, pelvis and external genitals**

Code also any associated:
spinal cord injury (S24.0, S24.1-, S34.0-, S34.1-)
wound infection

Excludes1 traumatic amputation of part of abdomen, lower back and pelvis (S38.2-, S38.3)

Excludes2 open wound of hip (S71.00-S71.02)
open fracture of pelvis (S32.1--S32.9 with 7th character B)

The appropriate 7th character is to be added to each code from category S31

A	initial encounter
D	subsequent encounter
S	sequela

● S31.0 **Open wound of lower back and pelvis**

● S31.00 **Unspecified open wound of lower back and pelvis**

● S31.000 **Unspecified open wound of lower back and pelvis without penetration into retroperitoneum**
Unspecified open wound of lower back and pelvis NOS

● S31.001 **Unspecified open wound of lower back and pelvis with penetration into retroperitoneum**

● S31.01 **Laceration without foreign body of lower back and pelvis**

● S31.010 **Laceration without foreign body of lower back and pelvis without penetration into retroperitoneum**
Laceration without foreign body of lower back and pelvis NOS

● S31.011 **Laceration without foreign body of lower back and pelvis with penetration into retroperitoneum**

● S31.02 **Laceration with foreign body of lower back and pelvis**

● S31.020 **Laceration with foreign body of lower back and pelvis without penetration into retroperitoneum**
Laceration with foreign body of lower back and pelvis NOS

● S31.021 **Laceration with foreign body of lower back and pelvis with penetration into retroperitoneum**

● S31.03 **Puncture wound without foreign body of lower back and pelvis**

● S31.030 **Puncture wound without foreign body of lower back and pelvis without penetration into retroperitoneum**
Puncture wound without foreign body of lower back and pelvis NOS

● S31.031 **Puncture wound without foreign body of lower back and pelvis with penetration into retroperitoneum**

● S31.04 **Puncture wound with foreign body of lower back and pelvis**

● S31.040 **Puncture wound with foreign body of lower back and pelvis without penetration into retroperitoneum**
Puncture wound with foreign body of lower back and pelvis NOS

● S31.041 **Puncture wound with foreign body of lower back and pelvis with penetration into retroperitoneum**

● S31.05 **Open bite of lower back and pelvis**
Bite of lower back and pelvis NOS

Excludes1 superficial bite of lower back and pelvis (S30.860, S30.870)

● S31.050 **Open bite of lower back and pelvis without penetration into retroperitoneum**
Open bite of lower back and pelvis NOS

● S31.051 **Open bite of lower back and pelvis with penetration into retroperitoneum**

● S31.1 **Open wound of abdominal wall without penetration into peritoneal cavity**
Open wound of abdominal wall NOS

Excludes2 open wound of abdominal wall with penetration into peritoneal cavity (S31.6-)

● S31.10 **Unspecified open wound of abdominal wall without penetration into peritoneal cavity**

● S31.100 **Unspecified open wound of abdominal wall, right upper quadrant without penetration into peritoneal cavity**

● S31.101 **Unspecified open wound of abdominal wall, left upper quadrant without penetration into peritoneal cavity**

◄ New   ◄═ Revised   ~~deleted~~ Deleted   Excludes 1   Excludes 2   Includes   Use additional   Code first   Code also   Unspecified
OGCR Official Guidelines   X Assign placeholder X   ● Use Additional Character(s)   ▶ Manifestation Code   **Coding Clinic**

● S31.102   Unspecified open wound of abdominal wall, epigastric region without penetration into peritoneal cavity

● S31.103   Unspecified open wound of abdominal wall, right lower quadrant without penetration into peritoneal cavity

● S31.104   Unspecified open wound of abdominal wall, left lower quadrant without penetration into peritoneal cavity

● S31.105   Unspecified open wound of abdominal wall, periumbilic region without penetration into peritoneal cavity

● S31.109   Unspecified open wound of abdominal wall, unspecified quadrant without penetration into peritoneal cavity

     Unspecified open wound of abdominal wall NOS

● S31.11   Laceration without foreign body of abdominal wall without penetration into peritoneal cavity

● S31.110   Laceration without foreign body of abdominal wall, right upper quadrant without penetration into peritoneal cavity

● S31.111   Laceration without foreign body of abdominal wall, left upper quadrant without penetration into peritoneal cavity

● S31.112   Laceration without foreign body of abdominal wall, epigastric region without penetration into peritoneal cavity

● S31.113   Laceration without foreign body of abdominal wall, right lower quadrant without penetration into peritoneal cavity

● S31.114   Laceration without foreign body of abdominal wall, left lower quadrant without penetration into peritoneal cavity

● S31.115   Laceration without foreign body of abdominal wall, periumbilic region without penetration into peritoneal cavity

● S31.119   Laceration without foreign body of abdominal wall, unspecified quadrant without penetration into peritoneal cavity

● S31.12   Laceration with foreign body of abdominal wall without penetration into peritoneal cavity

● S31.120   Laceration of abdominal wall with foreign body, right upper quadrant without penetration into peritoneal cavity

● S31.121   Laceration of abdominal wall with foreign body, left upper quadrant without penetration into peritoneal cavity

● S31.122   Laceration of abdominal wall with foreign body, epigastric region without penetration into peritoneal cavity

● S31.123   Laceration of abdominal wall with foreign body, right lower quadrant without penetration into peritoneal cavity

● S31.124   Laceration of abdominal wall with foreign body, left lower quadrant without penetration into peritoneal cavity

● S31.125   Laceration of abdominal wall with foreign body, periumbilic region without penetration into peritoneal cavity

● S31.129   Laceration of abdominal wall with foreign body, unspecified quadrant without penetration into peritoneal cavity

● S31.13   Puncture wound of abdominal wall without foreign body without penetration into peritoneal cavity

● S31.130   Puncture wound of abdominal wall without foreign body, right upper quadrant without penetration into peritoneal cavity

● S31.131   Puncture wound of abdominal wall without foreign body, left upper quadrant without penetration into peritoneal cavity

● S31.132   Puncture wound of abdominal wall without foreign body, epigastric region without penetration into peritoneal cavity

● S31.133   Puncture wound of abdominal wall without foreign body, right lower quadrant without penetration into peritoneal cavity

● S31.134   Puncture wound of abdominal wall without foreign body, left lower quadrant without penetration into peritoneal cavity

● S31.135   Puncture wound of abdominal wall without foreign body, periumbilic region without penetration into peritoneal cavity

● S31.139   Puncture wound of abdominal wall without foreign body, unspecified quadrant without penetration into peritoneal cavity

● S31.14   Puncture wound of abdominal wall with foreign body without penetration into peritoneal cavity

● S31.140   Puncture wound of abdominal wall with foreign body, right upper quadrant without penetration into peritoneal cavity

● S31.141   Puncture wound of abdominal wall with foreign body, left upper quadrant without penetration into peritoneal cavity

● S31.142   Puncture wound of abdominal wall with foreign body, epigastric region without penetration into peritoneal cavity

● S31.143   Puncture wound of abdominal wall with foreign body, right lower quadrant without penetration into peritoneal cavity

● S31.144   Puncture wound of abdominal wall with foreign body, left lower quadrant without penetration into peritoneal cavity

● S31.145   Puncture wound of abdominal wall with foreign body, periumbilic region without penetration into peritoneal cavity

● S31.149   Puncture wound of abdominal wall with foreign body, unspecified quadrant without penetration into peritoneal cavity

CHAPTER 19 (S00-T88)

● **S31.15** **Open bite of abdominal wall without penetration into peritoneal cavity**
Bite of abdominal wall NOS

> **Excludes1**   superficial bite of abdominal wall (S30.871)

   ● **S31.150** Open bite of abdominal wall, right upper quadrant without penetration into peritoneal cavity

   ● **S31.151** Open bite of abdominal wall, left upper quadrant without penetration into peritoneal cavity

   ● **S31.152** Open bite of abdominal wall, epigastric region without penetration into peritoneal cavity

   ● **S31.153** Open bite of abdominal wall, right lower quadrant without penetration into peritoneal cavity

   ● **S31.154** Open bite of abdominal wall, left lower quadrant without penetration into peritoneal cavity

   ● **S31.155** Open bite of abdominal wall, periumbilic region without penetration into peritoneal cavity

   ● **S31.159** Open bite of abdominal wall, unspecified quadrant without penetration into peritoneal cavity

● **S31.2** **Open wound of penis**

  X ● **S31.20** Unspecified open wound of penis ♂

  X ● **S31.21** Laceration without foreign body of penis ♂

  X ● **S31.22** Laceration with foreign body of penis ♂

  X ● **S31.23** Puncture wound without foreign body of penis ♂

  X ● **S31.24** Puncture wound with foreign body of penis ♂

  X ● **S31.25** Open bite of penis ♂
Bite of penis NOS

> **Excludes1**   superficial bite of penis (S30.862, S30.872)

● **S31.3** **Open wound of scrotum and testes**

  X ● **S31.30** Unspecified open wound of scrotum and testes ♂

  X ● **S31.31** Laceration without foreign body of scrotum and testes ♂

  X ● **S31.32** Laceration with foreign body of scrotum and testes ♂

  X ● **S31.33** Puncture wound without foreign body of scrotum and testes ♂

  X ● **S31.34** Puncture wound with foreign body of scrotum and testes ♂

  X ● **S31.35** Open bite of scrotum and testes ♂
Bite of scrotum and testes NOS

> **Excludes1**   superficial bite of scrotum and testes (S30.863, S30.873)

● **S31.4** **Open wound of vagina and vulva**

> **Excludes1**   injury to vagina and vulva during delivery (O70.-, O71.4)

  X ● **S31.40** Unspecified open wound of vagina and vulva ♀

  X ● **S31.41** Laceration without foreign body of vagina and vulva ♀

  X ● **S31.42** Laceration with foreign body of vagina and vulva ♀

  X ● **S31.43** Puncture wound without foreign body of vagina and vulva ♀

  X ● **S31.44** Puncture wound with foreign body of vagina and vulva ♀

  X ● **S31.45** Open bite of vagina and vulva ♀
Bite of vagina and vulva NOS

> **Excludes1**   superficial bite of vagina and vulva (S30.864, S30.874)

● **S31.5** **Open wound of unspecified external genital organs**

> **Excludes1**   traumatic amputation of external genital organs (S38.21, S38.22)

  ● **S31.50** Unspecified open wound of unspecified external genital organs

   ● **S31.501** Unspecified open wound of unspecified external genital organs, male ♂

   ● **S31.502** Unspecified open wound of unspecified external genital organs, female ♀

  ● **S31.51** Laceration without foreign body of unspecified external genital organs

   ● **S31.511** Laceration without foreign body of unspecified external genital organs, male ♂

   ● **S31.512** Laceration without foreign body of unspecified external genital organs, female ♀

  ● **S31.52** Laceration with foreign body of unspecified external genital organs

   ● **S31.521** Laceration with foreign body of unspecified external genital organs, male ♂

   ● **S31.522** Laceration with foreign body of unspecified external genital organs, female ♀

  ● **S31.53** Puncture wound without foreign body of unspecified external genital organs

   ● **S31.531** Puncture wound without foreign body of unspecified external genital organs, male ♂

   ● **S31.532** Puncture wound without foreign body of unspecified external genital organs, female ♀

  ● **S31.54** Puncture wound with foreign body of unspecified external genital organs

   ● **S31.541** Puncture wound with foreign body of unspecified external genital organs, male ♂

   ● **S31.542** Puncture wound with foreign body of unspecified external genital organs, female ♀

  ● **S31.55** Open bite of unspecified external genital organs
Bite of unspecified external genital organs NOS

> **Excludes1**   superficial bite of unspecified external genital organs (S30.865, S30.866, S30.875, S30.876)

   ● **S31.551** Open bite of unspecified external genital organs, male ♂

   ● **S31.552** Open bite of unspecified external genital organs, female ♀

● **S31.6** **Open wound of abdominal wall with penetration into peritoneal cavity**

  ● **S31.60** Unspecified open wound of abdominal wall with penetration into peritoneal cavity

   ● **S31.600** Unspecified open wound of abdominal wall, right upper quadrant with penetration into peritoneal cavity

   ● **S31.601** Unspecified open wound of abdominal wall, left upper quadrant with penetration into peritoneal cavity

◀ New   ◀◀◀ Revised   ~~deleted~~ Deleted   Excludes 1   Excludes 2   Includes   Use additional   Code first   Code also   Unspecified

OGCR Official Guidelines   X Assign placeholder X   ● Use Additional Character(s)   ▶ Manifestation Code   **Coding Clinic**

● S31.602   Unspecified open wound of abdominal wall, epigastric region with penetration into peritoneal cavity

● S31.603   Unspecified open wound of abdominal wall, right lower quadrant with penetration into peritoneal cavity

● S31.604   Unspecified open wound of abdominal wall, left lower quadrant with penetration into peritoneal cavity

● S31.605   Unspecified open wound of abdominal wall, periumbilic region with penetration into peritoneal cavity

● S31.609   Unspecified open wound of abdominal wall, unspecified quadrant with penetration into peritoneal cavity

● S31.61   Laceration without foreign body of abdominal wall with penetration into peritoneal cavity

● S31.610   Laceration without foreign body of abdominal wall, right upper quadrant with penetration into peritoneal cavity

● S31.611   Laceration without foreign body of abdominal wall, left upper quadrant with penetration into peritoneal cavity

● S31.612   Laceration without foreign body of abdominal wall, epigastric region with penetration into peritoneal cavity

● S31.613   Laceration without foreign body of abdominal wall, right lower quadrant with penetration into peritoneal cavity

● S31.614   Laceration without foreign body of abdominal wall, left lower quadrant with penetration into peritoneal cavity

● S31.615   Laceration without foreign body of abdominal wall, periumbilic region with penetration into peritoneal cavity

● S31.619   Laceration without foreign body of abdominal wall, unspecified quadrant with penetration into peritoneal cavity

● S31.62   Laceration with foreign body of abdominal wall with penetration into peritoneal cavity

● S31.620   Laceration with foreign body of abdominal wall, right upper quadrant with penetration into peritoneal cavity

● S31.621   Laceration with foreign body of abdominal wall, left upper quadrant with penetration into peritoneal cavity

● S31.622   Laceration with foreign body of abdominal wall, epigastric region with penetration into peritoneal cavity

● S31.623   Laceration with foreign body of abdominal wall, right lower quadrant with penetration into peritoneal cavity

● S31.624   Laceration with foreign body of abdominal wall, left lower quadrant with penetration into peritoneal cavity

● S31.625   Laceration with foreign body of abdominal wall, periumbilic region with penetration into peritoneal cavity

● S31.629   Laceration with foreign body of abdominal wall, unspecified quadrant with penetration into peritoneal cavity

● S31.63   Puncture wound without foreign body of abdominal wall with penetration into peritoneal cavity

● S31.630   Puncture wound without foreign body of abdominal wall, right upper quadrant with penetration into peritoneal cavity

● S31.631   Puncture wound without foreign body of abdominal wall, left upper quadrant with penetration into peritoneal cavity

● S31.632   Puncture wound without foreign body of abdominal wall, epigastric region with penetration into peritoneal cavity

● S31.633   Puncture wound without foreign body of abdominal wall, right lower quadrant with penetration into peritoneal cavity

● S31.634   Puncture wound without foreign body of abdominal wall, left lower quadrant with penetration into peritoneal cavity

● S31.635   Puncture wound without foreign body of abdominal wall, periumbilic region with penetration into peritoneal cavity

● S31.639   Puncture wound without foreign body of abdominal wall, unspecified quadrant with penetration into peritoneal cavity

● S31.64   Puncture wound with foreign body of abdominal wall with penetration into peritoneal cavity

● S31.640   Puncture wound with foreign body of abdominal wall, right upper quadrant with penetration into peritoneal cavity

● S31.641   Puncture wound with foreign body of abdominal wall, left upper quadrant with penetration into peritoneal cavity

● S31.642   Puncture wound with foreign body of abdominal wall, epigastric region with penetration into peritoneal cavity

● S31.643   Puncture wound with foreign body of abdominal wall, right lower quadrant with penetration into peritoneal cavity

● S31.644   Puncture wound with foreign body of abdominal wall, left lower quadrant with penetration into peritoneal cavity

● S31.645   Puncture wound with foreign body of abdominal wall, periumbilic region with penetration into peritoneal cavity

● S31.649   Puncture wound with foreign body of abdominal wall, unspecified quadrant with penetration into peritoneal cavity

● **S31.65**   **Open bite of abdominal wall with penetration into peritoneal cavity**
> **Excludes1**   superficial bite of abdominal wall (S30.861, S30.871)

● **S31.650**   Open bite of abdominal wall, right upper quadrant with penetration into peritoneal cavity

● **S31.651**   Open bite of abdominal wall, left upper quadrant with penetration into peritoneal cavity

● **S31.652**   Open bite of abdominal wall, epigastric region with penetration into peritoneal cavity

● **S31.653**   Open bite of abdominal wall, right lower quadrant with penetration into peritoneal cavity

● **S31.654**   Open bite of abdominal wall, left lower quadrant with penetration into peritoneal cavity

● **S31.655**   Open bite of abdominal wall, periumbilic region with penetration into peritoneal cavity

● **S31.659**   Open bite of abdominal wall, unspecified quadrant with penetration into peritoneal cavity

● **S31.8**   **Open wound of other parts of abdomen, lower back and pelvis**

● **S31.80**   **Open wound of unspecified buttock**

● **S31.801**   Laceration without foreign body of unspecified buttock

● **S31.802**   Laceration with foreign body of unspecified buttock

● **S31.803**   Puncture wound without foreign body of unspecified buttock

● **S31.804**   Puncture wound with foreign body of unspecified buttock

● **S31.805**   Open bite of unspecified buttock
> Bite of buttock NOS
> **Excludes1**   superficial bite of buttock (S30.870)

● **S31.809**   Unspecified open wound of unspecified buttock

● **S31.81**   **Open wound of right buttock**

● **S31.811**   Laceration without foreign body of right buttock

● **S31.812**   Laceration with foreign body of right buttock

● **S31.813**   Puncture wound without foreign body of right buttock

● **S31.814**   Puncture wound with foreign body of right buttock

● **S31.815**   Open bite of right buttock
> Bite of right buttock NOS
> **Excludes1**   superficial bite of buttock (S30.870)

● **S31.819**   Unspecified open wound of right buttock

● **S31.82**   **Open wound of left buttock**

● **S31.821**   Laceration without foreign body of left buttock

● **S31.822**   Laceration with foreign body of left buttock

● **S31.823**   Puncture wound without foreign body of left buttock

● **S31.824**   Puncture wound with foreign body of left buttock

● **S31.825**   Open bite of left buttock
> Bite of left buttock NOS
> **Excludes1**   superficial bite of buttock (S30.870)

● **S31.829**   Unspecified open wound of left buttock

● **S31.83**   **Open wound of anus**

● **S31.831**   Laceration without foreign body of anus

● **S31.832**   Laceration with foreign body of anus

● **S31.833**   Puncture wound without foreign body of anus

● **S31.834**   Puncture wound with foreign body of anus

● **S31.835**   Open bite of anus
> Bite of anus NOS
> **Excludes1**   superficial bite of anus (S30.877)

● **S31.839**   Unspecified open wound of anus

● **S32**   **Fracture of lumbar spine and pelvis**
> **Note:** A fracture not indicated as displaced or nondisplaced should be coded to displaced
>
> A fracture not indicated as opened or closed should be coded to closed

> **Includes**   fracture of lumbosacral neural arch
> fracture of lumbosacral spinous process
> fracture of lumbosacral transverse process
> fracture of lumbosacral vertebra
> fracture of lumbosacral vertebral arch

Code first any associated spinal cord and spinal nerve injury (S34.-)

Excludes1   transection of abdomen (S38.3)

Excludes2   fracture of hip NOS (S72.0-)

The appropriate 7th character is to be added to each code from category S32

A	initial encounter for closed fracture
B	initial encounter for open fracture
D	subsequent encounter for fracture with routine healing
G	subsequent encounter for fracture with delayed healing
K	subsequent encounter for fracture with nonunion
S	sequela

● **S32.0**   **Fracture of lumbar vertebra**
> Fracture of lumbar spine NOS

● **S32.00**   **Fracture of unspecified lumbar vertebra**

● **S32.000**   Wedge compression fracture of unspecified lumbar vertebra

● **S32.001**   Stable burst fracture of unspecified lumbar vertebra

● **S32.002**   Unstable burst fracture of unspecified lumbar vertebra

● **S32.008**   Other fracture of unspecified lumbar vertebra

● **S32.009**   Unspecified fracture of unspecified lumbar vertebra

● **S32.01**   **Fracture of first lumbar vertebra**

● **S32.010**   Wedge compression fracture of first lumbar vertebra

● **S32.011**   Stable burst fracture of first lumbar vertebra

● **S32.012**   Unstable burst fracture of first lumbar vertebra

● **S32.018**   Other fracture of first lumbar vertebra

● **S32.019**   Unspecified fracture of first lumbar vertebra

◄ New   ◄▬ Revised   ~~deleted~~ Deleted   Excludes 1   Excludes 2   Includes   Use additional   Code first   Code also   Unspecified

OGCR Official Guidelines   X Assign placeholder X   ● Use Additional Character(s)   ▶ Manifestation Code   **Coding Clinic**

● **S32.02   Fracture of second lumbar vertebra**
- ● **S32.020   Wedge compression fracture of second lumbar vertebra**
- ● **S32.021   Stable burst fracture of second lumbar vertebra**
- ● **S32.022   Unstable burst fracture of second lumbar vertebra**
- ● **S32.028   Other fracture of second lumbar vertebra**
- ● **S32.029   Unspecified fracture of second lumbar vertebra**

● **S32.03   Fracture of third lumbar vertebra**
- ● **S32.030   Wedge compression fracture of third lumbar vertebra**
- ● **S32.031   Stable burst fracture of third lumbar vertebra**
- ● **S32.032   Unstable burst fracture of third lumbar vertebra**
- ● **S32.038   Other fracture of third lumbar vertebra**
- ● **S32.039   Unspecified fracture of third lumbar vertebra**

● **S32.04   Fracture of fourth lumbar vertebra**
- ● **S32.040   Wedge compression fracture of fourth lumbar vertebra**
- ● **S32.041   Stable burst fracture of fourth lumbar vertebra**
- ● **S32.042   Unstable burst fracture of fourth lumbar vertebra**
- ● **S32.048   Other fracture of fourth lumbar vertebra**
- ● **S32.049   Unspecified fracture of fourth lumbar vertebra**

● **S32.05   Fracture of fifth lumbar vertebra**
- ● **S32.050   Wedge compression fracture of fifth lumbar vertebra**
- ● **S32.051   Stable burst fracture of fifth lumbar vertebra**
- ● **S32.052   Unstable burst fracture of fifth lumbar vertebra**
- ● **S32.058   Other fracture of fifth lumbar vertebra**
- ● **S32.059   Unspecified fracture of fifth lumbar vertebra**

● **S32.1   Fracture of sacrum**
   For vertical fractures, code to most medial fracture extension
   Use two codes if both a vertical and transverse fracture are present
   Code also any associated fracture of pelvic ring (S32.8-)
- X● **S32.10   Unspecified fracture of sacrum**
- ● **S32.11   Zone I fracture of sacrum**
      Vertical sacral ala fracture of sacrum
  - ● **S32.110   Nondisplaced Zone I fracture of sacrum**
  - ● **S32.111   Minimally displaced Zone I fracture of sacrum**
  - ● **S32.112   Severely displaced Zone I fracture of sacrum**
  - ● **S32.119   Unspecified Zone I fracture of sacrum**
- ● **S32.12   Zone II fracture of sacrum**
      Vertical foraminal region fracture of sacrum
  - ● **S32.120   Nondisplaced Zone II fracture of sacrum**
  - ● **S32.121   Minimally displaced Zone II fracture of sacrum**
  - ● **S32.122   Severely displaced Zone II fracture of sacrum**
  - ● **S32.129   Unspecified Zone II fracture of sacrum**
- ● **S32.13   Zone III fracture of sacrum**
      Vertical fracture into spinal canal region of sacrum
  - ● **S32.130   Nondisplaced Zone III fracture of sacrum**
  - ● **S32.131   Minimally displaced Zone III fracture of sacrum**
  - ● **S32.132   Severely displaced Zone III fracture of sacrum**
  - ● **S32.139   Unspecified Zone III fracture of sacrum**
- X● **S32.14   Type 1 fracture of sacrum**
      Transverse flexion fracture of sacrum without displacement
- X● **S32.15   Type 2 fracture of sacrum**
      Transverse flexion fracture of sacrum with posterior displacement
- X● **S32.16   Type 3 fracture of sacrum**
      Transverse extension fracture of sacrum with anterior displacement
- X● **S32.17   Type 4 fracture of sacrum**
      Transverse segmental comminution of upper sacrum
- X● **S32.19   Other fracture of sacrum**

X● **S32.2   Fracture of coccyx**

● **S32.3   Fracture of ilium**
   Excludes1   fracture of ilium with associated disruption of pelvic ring (S32.8-)
- ● **S32.30   Unspecified fracture of ilium**
  - ● **S32.301   Unspecified fracture of right ilium**
  - ● **S32.302   Unspecified fracture of left ilium**
  - ● **S32.309   Unspecified fracture of unspecified ilium**
- ● **S32.31   Avulsion fracture of ilium**
  - ● **S32.311   Displaced avulsion fracture of right ilium**
  - ● **S32.312   Displaced avulsion fracture of left ilium**
  - ● **S32.313   Displaced avulsion fracture of unspecified ilium**
  - ● **S32.314   Nondisplaced avulsion fracture of right ilium**
  - ● **S32.315   Nondisplaced avulsion fracture of left ilium**
  - ● **S32.316   Nondisplaced avulsion fracture of unspecified ilium**
- ● **S32.39   Other fracture of ilium**
  - ● **S32.391   Other fracture of right ilium**
  - ● **S32.392   Other fracture of left ilium**
  - ● **S32.399   Other fracture of unspecified ilium**

● **S32.4   Fracture of acetabulum**
   Code also any associated fracture of pelvic ring (S32.8-)
- ● **S32.40   Unspecified fracture of acetabulum**
  - ● **S32.401   Unspecified fracture of right acetabulum**
  - ● **S32.402   Unspecified fracture of left acetabulum**
  - ● **S32.409   Unspecified fracture of unspecified acetabulum**

● **S32.41**   Fracture of anterior wall of acetabulum
- ● **S32.411**   Displaced fracture of anterior wall of right acetabulum
- ● **S32.412**   Displaced fracture of anterior wall of left acetabulum
- ● **S32.413**   Displaced fracture of anterior wall of unspecified acetabulum
- ● **S32.414**   Nondisplaced fracture of anterior wall of right acetabulum
- ● **S32.415**   Nondisplaced fracture of anterior wall of left acetabulum
- ● **S32.416**   Nondisplaced fracture of anterior wall of unspecified acetabulum

● **S32.42**   Fracture of posterior wall of acetabulum
- ● **S32.421**   Displaced fracture of posterior wall of right acetabulum
- ● **S32.422**   Displaced fracture of posterior wall of left acetabulum
- ● **S32.423**   Displaced fracture of posterior wall of unspecified acetabulum
- ● **S32.424**   Nondisplaced fracture of posterior wall of right acetabulum
- ● **S32.425**   Nondisplaced fracture of posterior wall of left acetabulum
- ● **S32.426**   Nondisplaced fracture of posterior wall of unspecified acetabulum

● **S32.43**   Fracture of anterior column [iliopubic] of acetabulum
- ● **S32.431**   Displaced fracture of anterior column [iliopubic] of right acetabulum
- ● **S32.432**   Displaced fracture of anterior column [iliopubic] of left acetabulum
- ● **S32.433**   Displaced fracture of anterior column [iliopubic] of unspecified acetabulum
- ● **S32.434**   Nondisplaced fracture of anterior column [iliopubic] of right acetabulum
- ● **S32.435**   Nondisplaced fracture of anterior column [iliopubic] of left acetabulum
- ● **S32.436**   Nondisplaced fracture of anterior column [iliopubic] of unspecified acetabulum

● **S32.44**   Fracture of posterior column [ilioischial] of acetabulum
- ● **S32.441**   Displaced fracture of posterior column [ilioischial] of right acetabulum
- ● **S32.442**   Displaced fracture of posterior column [ilioischial] of left acetabulum
- ● **S32.443**   Displaced fracture of posterior column [ilioischial] of unspecified acetabulum
- ● **S32.444**   Nondisplaced fracture of posterior column [ilioischial] of right acetabulum
- ● **S32.445**   Nondisplaced fracture of posterior column [ilioischial] of left acetabulum
- ● **S32.446**   Nondisplaced fracture of posterior column [ilioischial] of unspecified acetabulum

● **S32.45**   Transverse fracture of acetabulum
- ● **S32.451**   Displaced transverse fracture of right acetabulum
- ● **S32.452**   Displaced transverse fracture of left acetabulum
- ● **S32.453**   Displaced transverse fracture of unspecified acetabulum
- ● **S32.454**   Nondisplaced transverse fracture of right acetabulum

- ● **S32.455**   Nondisplaced transverse fracture of left acetabulum
- ● **S32.456**   Nondisplaced transverse fracture of unspecified acetabulum

● **S32.46**   Associated transverse-posterior fracture of acetabulum
- ● **S32.461**   Displaced associated transverse-posterior fracture of right acetabulum
- ● **S32.462**   Displaced associated transverse-posterior fracture of left acetabulum
- ● **S32.463**   Displaced associated transverse-posterior fracture of unspecified acetabulum
- ● **S32.464**   Nondisplaced associated transverse-posterior fracture of right acetabulum
- ● **S32.465**   Nondisplaced associated transverse-posterior fracture of left acetabulum
- ● **S32.466**   Nondisplaced associated transverse-posterior fracture of unspecified acetabulum

● **S32.47**   Fracture of medial wall of acetabulum
- ● **S32.471**   Displaced fracture of medial wall of right acetabulum
- ● **S32.472**   Displaced fracture of medial wall of left acetabulum
- ● **S32.473**   Displaced fracture of medial wall of unspecified acetabulum
- ● **S32.474**   Nondisplaced fracture of medial wall of right acetabulum
- ● **S32.475**   Nondisplaced fracture of medial wall of left acetabulum
- ● **S32.476**   Nondisplaced fracture of medial wall of unspecified acetabulum

● **S32.48**   Dome fracture of acetabulum
- ● **S32.481**   Displaced dome fracture of right acetabulum
- ● **S32.482**   Displaced dome fracture of left acetabulum
- ● **S32.483**   Displaced dome fracture of unspecified acetabulum
- ● **S32.484**   Nondisplaced dome fracture of right acetabulum
- ● **S32.485**   Nondisplaced dome fracture of left acetabulum
- ● **S32.486**   Nondisplaced dome fracture of unspecified acetabulum

● **S32.49**   Other fracture of acetabulum
- ● **S32.491**   Other fracture of right acetabulum
- ● **S32.492**   Other fracture of left acetabulum
- ● **S32.499**   Other fracture of unspecified acetabulum

● **S32.5**   Fracture of pubis
> **Excludes1**   fracture of pubis with associated disruption of pelvic ring (S32.8-)

● **S32.50**   Unspecified fracture of pubis
- ● **S32.501**   Unspecified fracture of right pubis
- ● **S32.502**   Unspecified fracture of left pubis
- ● **S32.509**   Unspecified fracture of unspecified pubis

● **S32.51**   Fracture of superior rim of pubis
- ● **S32.511**   Fracture of superior rim of right pubis
- ● **S32.512**   Fracture of superior rim of left pubis
- ● **S32.519**   Fracture of superior rim of unspecified pubis

◄ New   ◄══ Revised   ~~deleted~~ Deleted   Excludes 1   Excludes 2   Includes   Use additional   Code first   Code also   Unspecified

OGCR Official Guidelines   X Assign placeholder X   ● Use Additional Character(s)   ▶ Manifestation Code   **Coding Clinic**

● S32.59　　Other specified fracture of pubis
　　● S32.591　　Other specified fracture of right pubis
　　● S32.592　　Other specified fracture of left pubis
　　● S32.599　　Other specified fracture of unspecified pubis

● S32.6　　Fracture of ischium
　　Excludes1　　fracture of ischium with associated disruption of pelvic ring (S32.8-)

● S32.60　　Unspecified fracture of ischium
　　● S32.601　　Unspecified fracture of right ischium
　　● S32.602　　Unspecified fracture of left ischium
　　● S32.609　　Unspecified fracture of unspecified ischium

● S32.61　　Avulsion fracture of ischium
　　● S32.611　　Displaced avulsion fracture of right ischium
　　● S32.612　　Displaced avulsion fracture of left ischium
　　● S32.613　　Displaced avulsion fracture of unspecified ischium
　　● S32.614　　Nondisplaced avulsion fracture of right ischium
　　● S32.615　　Nondisplaced avulsion fracture of left ischium
　　● S32.616　　Nondisplaced avulsion fracture of unspecified ischium

● S32.69　　Other specified fracture of ischium
　　● S32.691　　Other specified fracture of right ischium
　　● S32.692　　Other specified fracture of left ischium
　　● S32.699　　Other specified fracture of unspecified ischium

● S32.8　　Fracture of other parts of pelvis
　　Code also any associated:
　　　　fracture of acetabulum (S32.4-)
　　　　sacral fracture (S32.1-)
　　● S32.81　　Multiple fractures of pelvis with disruption of pelvic ring
　　　　Multiple pelvic fractures with disruption of pelvic circle
　　　　● S32.810　　Multiple fractures of pelvis with stable disruption of pelvic ring
　　　　● S32.811　　Multiple fractures of pelvis with unstable disruption of pelvic ring
　X● S32.82　　Multiple fractures of pelvis without disruption of pelvic ring
　　　　Multiple pelvic fractures without disruption of pelvic circle
　X● S32.89　　Fracture of other parts of pelvis
　X● S32.9　　Fracture of unspecified parts of lumbosacral spine and pelvis
　　　　Fracture of lumbosacral spine NOS
　　　　Fracture of pelvis NOS
　　　　Coding Clinic: 2012, Q4, P93

● S33　　Dislocation and sprain of joints and ligaments of lumbar spine and pelvis
　　Includes　　avulsion of joint or ligament of lumbar spine and pelvis
　　　　laceration of cartilage, joint or ligament of lumbar spine and pelvis
　　　　sprain of cartilage, joint or ligament of lumbar spine and pelvis
　　　　traumatic hemarthrosis of joint or ligament of lumbar spine and pelvis
　　　　traumatic rupture of joint or ligament of lumbar spine and pelvis
　　　　traumatic subluxation of joint or ligament of lumbar spine and pelvis
　　　　traumatic tear of joint or ligament of lumbar spine and pelvis
　　Code also any associated open wound
　　Excludes1　　nontraumatic rupture or displacement of lumbar intervertebral disc NOS (M51.-)
　　　　obstetric damage to pelvic joints and ligaments (O71.6)
　　Excludes2　　dislocation and sprain of joints and ligaments of hip (S73.-)
　　　　strain of muscle of lower back and pelvis (S39.01-)
　　The appropriate 7th character is to be added to each code from category S33

A	initial encounter
D	subsequent encounter
S	sequela

　X● S33.0　　Traumatic rupture of lumbar intervertebral disc
　　Excludes1　　rupture or displacement (nontraumatic) of lumbar intervertebral disc NOS (M51.- with fifth character 6)

● S33.1　　Subluxation and dislocation of lumbar vertebra
　　Code also any associated:
　　　　open wound of abdomen, lower back and pelvis (S31)
　　　　spinal cord injury (S24.0, S24.1-, S34.0-, S34.1-)
　　Excludes2　　fracture of lumbar vertebrae (S32.0-)
　　● S33.10　　Subluxation and dislocation of unspecified lumbar vertebra
　　　　● S33.100　　Subluxation of unspecified lumbar vertebra
　　　　● S33.101　　Dislocation of unspecified lumbar vertebra
　　● S33.11　　Subluxation and dislocation of L_1/L_2 lumbar vertebra
　　　　● S33.110　　Subluxation of L_1/L_2 lumbar vertebra
　　　　● S33.111　　Dislocation of L_1/L_2 lumbar vertebra
　　● S33.12　　Subluxation and dislocation of L_2/L_3 lumbar vertebra
　　　　● S33.120　　Subluxation of L_2/L_3 lumbar vertebra
　　　　● S33.121　　Dislocation of L_2/L_3 lumbar vertebra
　　● S33.13　　Subluxation and dislocation of L_3/L_4 lumbar vertebra
　　　　● S33.130　　Subluxation of L_3/L_4 lumbar vertebra
　　　　● S33.131　　Dislocation of L_3/L_4 lumbar vertebra
　　● S33.14　　Subluxation and dislocation of L_4/L_5 lumbar vertebra
　　　　● S33.140　　Subluxation of L_4/L_5 lumbar vertebra
　　　　● S33.141　　Dislocation of L_4/L_5 lumbar vertebra

CHAPTER 19 (S00-T88)

X● **S33.2**   **Dislocation of sacroiliac and sacrococcygeal joint**

● **S33.3**   **Dislocation of other and unspecified parts of lumbar spine and pelvis**

    X● **S33.30**   Dislocation of unspecified parts of lumbar spine and pelvis

    X● **S33.39**   Dislocation of other parts of lumbar spine and pelvis

X● **S33.4**   **Traumatic rupture of symphysis pubis**

X● **S33.5**   **Sprain of ligaments of lumbar spine**

X● **S33.6**   **Sprain of sacroiliac joint**

X● **S33.8**   **Sprain of other parts of lumbar spine and pelvis**

X● **S33.9**   **Sprain of unspecified parts of lumbar spine and pelvis**

● **S34**   **Injury of lumbar and sacral spinal cord and nerves at abdomen, lower back and pelvis level**

    Note: Code to highest level of lumbar cord injury

       Injuries to the spinal cord (S34.0 and S34.1) refer to the cord level and not bone level injury, and can affect nerve roots at and below the level given.

       The appropriate 7th character is to be added to each code from category S34

A	initial encounter
D	subsequent encounter
S	sequela

    Code also any associated:
       fracture of vertebra (S22.0-, S32.0-)
       open wound of abdomen, lower back and pelvis (S31.-)
       transient paralysis (R29.5)

● **S34.0**   **Concussion and edema of lumbar and sacral spinal cord**

    X● **S34.01**   **Concussion and edema of lumbar spinal cord**

    X● **S34.02**   **Concussion and edema of sacral spinal cord**
         Concussion and edema of conus medullaris

● **S34.1**   **Other and unspecified injury of lumbar and sacral spinal cord**

    ● **S34.10**   **Unspecified injury to lumbar spinal cord**

       ● **S34.101**   Unspecified injury to L_1 level of lumbar spinal cord

       ● **S34.102**   Unspecified injury to L_2 level of lumbar spinal cord

       ● **S34.103**   Unspecified injury to L_3 level of lumbar spinal cord

       ● **S34.104**   Unspecified injury to L_4 level of lumbar spinal cord

       ● **S34.105**   Unspecified injury to L_5 level of lumbar spinal cord

       ● **S34.109**   Unspecified injury to unspecified level of lumbar spinal cord

    ● **S34.11**   **Complete lesion of lumbar spinal cord**

       ● **S34.111**   Complete lesion of L_1 level of lumbar spinal cord

       ● **S34.112**   Complete lesion of L_2 level of lumbar spinal cord

       ● **S34.113**   Complete lesion of L_3 level of lumbar spinal cord

       ● **S34.114**   Complete lesion of L_4 level of lumbar spinal cord

       ● **S34.115**   Complete lesion of L_5 level of lumbar spinal cord

       ● **S34.119**   Complete lesion of unspecified level of lumbar spinal cord

    ● **S34.12**   **Incomplete lesion of lumbar spinal cord**

       ● **S34.121**   Incomplete lesion of L_1 level of lumbar spinal cord

       ● **S34.122**   Incomplete lesion of L_2 level of lumbar spinal cord

       ● **S34.123**   Incomplete lesion of L_3 level of lumbar spinal cord

       ● **S34.124**   Incomplete lesion of L_4 level of lumbar spinal cord

       ● **S34.125**   Incomplete lesion of L_5 level of lumbar spinal cord

       ● **S34.129**   Incomplete lesion of unspecified level of lumbar spinal cord

    ● **S34.13**   **Other and unspecified injury to sacral spinal cord**
       Other injury to conus medullaris

       ● **S34.131**   **Complete lesion of sacral spinal cord**
         Complete lesion of conus medullaris

       ● **S34.132**   **Incomplete lesion of sacral spinal cord**
         Incomplete lesion of conus medullaris

       ● **S34.139**   **Unspecified injury to sacral spinal cord**
         Unspecified injury of conus medullaris

● **S34.2**   **Injury of nerve root of lumbar and sacral spine**

    X● **S34.21**   **Injury of nerve root of lumbar spine**

    X● **S34.22**   **Injury of nerve root of sacral spine**

X● **S34.3**   **Injury of cauda equina**

X● **S34.4**   **Injury of lumbosacral plexus**

X● **S34.5**   **Injury of lumbar, sacral and pelvic sympathetic nerves**
       Injury of celiac ganglion or plexus
       Injury of hypogastric plexus
       Injury of mesenteric plexus (inferior) (superior)
       Injury of splanchnic nerve

X● **S34.6**   **Injury of peripheral nerve(s) at abdomen, lower back and pelvis level**

X● **S34.8**   **Injury of other nerves at abdomen, lower back and pelvis level**

X● **S34.9**   **Injury of unspecified nerves at abdomen, lower back and pelvis level**

● **S35**   **Injury of blood vessels at abdomen, lower back and pelvis level**

    The appropriate 7th character is to be added to each code from category S35

A	initial encounter
D	subsequent encounter
S	sequela

    Code also any associated open wound (S31.-)

● **S35.0**   **Injury of abdominal aorta**

       Excludes1   injury of aorta NOS (S25.0)

    X● **S35.00**   **Unspecified injury of abdominal aorta**

    X● **S35.01**   **Minor laceration of abdominal aorta**
       Incomplete transection of abdominal aorta
       Laceration of abdominal aorta NOS
       Superficial laceration of abdominal aorta

    X● **S35.02**   **Major laceration of abdominal aorta**
       Complete transection of abdominal aorta
       Traumatic rupture of abdominal aorta

    X● **S35.09**   **Other injury of abdominal aorta**

● **S35.1**   **Injury of inferior vena cava**
       Injury of hepatic vein

       Excludes1   injury of vena cava NOS (S25.2)

    X● **S35.10**   **Unspecified injury of inferior vena cava**

    X● **S35.11**   **Minor laceration of inferior vena cava**
       Incomplete transection of inferior vena cava
       Laceration of inferior vena cava NOS
       Superficial laceration of inferior vena cava

    X● **S35.12**   **Major laceration of inferior vena cava**
       Complete transection of inferior vena cava
       Traumatic rupture of inferior vena cava

    X● **S35.19**   **Other injury of inferior vena cava**

◄ New   ◄|||| Revised   ~~deleted~~ Deleted   Excludes 1   Excludes 2   Includes   Use additional   Code first   Code also   Unspecified

OGCR Official Guidelines   X Assign placeholder X   ● Use Additional Character(s)   ▶ Manifestation Code   **Coding Clinic**

● **S35.2**   **Injury of celiac or mesenteric artery and branches**

   ● **S35.21**   **Injury of celiac artery**

     ● **S35.211**   **Minor laceration of celiac artery**
       Incomplete transection of celiac artery
       Laceration of celiac artery NOS
       Superficial laceration of celiac artery

     ● **S35.212**   **Major laceration of celiac artery**
       Complete transection of celiac artery
       Traumatic rupture of celiac artery

     ● **S35.218**   **Other injury of celiac artery**

     ● **S35.219**   **Unspecified injury of celiac artery**

   ● **S35.22**   **Injury of superior mesenteric artery**

     ● **S35.221**   **Minor laceration of superior mesenteric artery**
       Incomplete transection of superior mesenteric artery
       Laceration of superior mesenteric artery NOS
       Superficial laceration of superior mesenteric artery

     ● **S35.222**   **Major laceration of superior mesenteric artery**
       Complete transection of superior mesenteric artery
       Traumatic rupture of superior mesenteric artery

     ● **S35.228**   **Other injury of superior mesenteric artery**

     ● **S35.229**   **Unspecified injury of superior mesenteric artery**

   ● **S35.23**   **Injury of inferior mesenteric artery**

     ● **S35.231**   **Minor laceration of inferior mesenteric artery**
       Incomplete transection of inferior mesenteric artery
       Laceration of inferior mesenteric artery NOS
       Superficial laceration of inferior mesenteric artery

     ● **S35.232**   **Major laceration of inferior mesenteric artery**
       Complete transection of inferior mesenteric artery
       Traumatic rupture of inferior mesenteric artery

     ● **S35.238**   **Other injury of inferior mesenteric artery**

     ● **S35.239**   **Unspecified injury of inferior mesenteric artery**

   ● **S35.29**   **Injury of branches of celiac and mesenteric artery**
     Injury of gastric artery
     Injury of gastroduodenal artery
     Injury of hepatic artery
     Injury of splenic artery

     ● **S35.291**   **Minor laceration of branches of celiac and mesenteric artery**
       Incomplete transection of branches of celiac and mesenteric artery
       Laceration of branches of celiac and mesenteric artery NOS
       Superficial laceration of branches of celiac and mesenteric artery

     ● **S35.292**   **Major laceration of branches of celiac and mesenteric artery**
       Complete transection of branches of celiac and mesenteric artery
       Traumatic rupture of branches of celiac and mesenteric artery

     ● **S35.298**   **Other injury of branches of celiac and mesenteric artery**

     ● **S35.299**   **Unspecified injury of branches of celiac and mesenteric artery**

● **S35.3**   **Injury of portal or splenic vein and branches**

   ● **S35.31**   **Injury of portal vein**

     ● **S35.311**   **Laceration of portal vein**

     ● **S35.318**   **Other specified injury of portal vein**

     ● **S35.319**   **Unspecified injury of portal vein**

   ● **S35.32**   **Injury of splenic vein**

     ● **S35.321**   **Laceration of splenic vein**

     ● **S35.328**   **Other specified injury of splenic vein**

     ● **S35.329**   **Unspecified injury of splenic vein**

   ● **S35.33**   **Injury of superior mesenteric vein**

     ● **S35.331**   **Laceration of superior mesenteric vein**

     ● **S35.338**   **Other specified injury of superior mesenteric vein**

     ● **S35.339**   **Unspecified injury of superior mesenteric vein**

   ● **S35.34**   **Injury of inferior mesenteric vein**

     ● **S35.341**   **Laceration of inferior mesenteric vein**

     ● **S35.348**   **Other specified injury of inferior mesenteric vein**

     ● **S35.349**   **Unspecified injury of inferior mesenteric vein**

● **S35.4**   **Injury of renal blood vessels**

   ● **S35.40**   **Unspecified injury of renal blood vessel**

     ● **S35.401**   **Unspecified injury of right renal artery**

     ● **S35.402**   **Unspecified injury of left renal artery**

     ● **S35.403**   **Unspecified injury of unspecified renal artery**

     ● **S35.404**   **Unspecified injury of right renal vein**

     ● **S35.405**   **Unspecified injury of left renal vein**

     ● **S35.406**   **Unspecified injury of unspecified renal vein**

   ● **S35.41**   **Laceration of renal blood vessel**

     ● **S35.411**   **Laceration of right renal artery**

     ● **S35.412**   **Laceration of left renal artery**

     ● **S35.413**   **Laceration of unspecified renal artery**

     ● **S35.414**   **Laceration of right renal vein**

     ● **S35.415**   **Laceration of left renal vein**

     ● **S35.416**   **Laceration of unspecified renal vein**

   ● **S35.49**   **Other specified injury of renal blood vessel**

     ● **S35.491**   **Other specified injury of right renal artery**

     ● **S35.492**   **Other specified injury of left renal artery**

     ● **S35.493**   **Other specified injury of unspecified renal artery**

     ● **S35.494**   **Other specified injury of right renal vein**

     ● **S35.495**   **Other specified injury of left renal vein**

     ● **S35.496**   **Other specified injury of unspecified renal vein**

● **S35.5**   **Injury of iliac blood vessels**

   X ● **S35.50**   **Injury of unspecified iliac blood vessel(s)**

   ● **S35.51**   **Injury of iliac artery or vein**
     Injury of hypogastric artery or vein

     ● **S35.511**   **Injury of right iliac artery**

     ● **S35.512**   **Injury of left iliac artery**

     ● **S35.513**   **Injury of unspecified iliac artery**

     ● **S35.514**   **Injury of right iliac vein**

     ● **S35.515**   **Injury of left iliac vein**

     ● **S35.516**   **Injury of unspecified iliac vein**

CHAPTER 19 (S00-T88)

● **S35.53**   Injury of uterine artery or vein
   ● **S35.531**   Injury of right uterine artery ♀
   ● **S35.532**   Injury of left uterine artery ♀
   ● **S35.533**   Injury of unspecified uterine artery ♀
   ● **S35.534**   Injury of right uterine vein ♀
   ● **S35.535**   Injury of left uterine vein ♀
   ● **S35.536**   Injury of unspecified uterine vein ♀
  X● **S35.59**   Injury of other iliac blood vessels

● **S35.8**   Injury of other blood vessels at abdomen, lower back and pelvis level
   Injury of ovarian artery or vein
  ● **S35.8X**   Injury of other blood vessels at abdomen, lower back and pelvis level
   ● **S35.8X1**   Laceration of other blood vessels at abdomen, lower back and pelvis level
   ● **S35.8X8**   Other specified injury of other blood vessels at abdomen, lower back and pelvis level
   ● **S35.8X9**   Unspecified injury of other blood vessels at abdomen, lower back and pelvis level

● **S35.9**   Injury of unspecified blood vessel at abdomen, lower back and pelvis level
  X● **S35.90**   Unspecified injury of unspecified blood vessel at abdomen, lower back and pelvis level
  X● **S35.91**   Laceration of unspecified blood vessel at abdomen, lower back and pelvis level
  X● **S35.99**   Other specified injury of unspecified blood vessel at abdomen, lower back and pelvis level

● **S36**   **Injury of intra-abdominal organs**
   The appropriate 7th character is to be added to each code from category S36

> A   initial encounter
> D   subsequent encounter
> S   sequela

   Code also any associated open wound (S31.-)

● **S36.0**   Injury of spleen
  X● **S36.00**   Unspecified injury of spleen
  ● **S36.02**   Contusion of spleen
   ● **S36.020**   Minor contusion of spleen
      Contusion of spleen less than 2 cm
   ● **S36.021**   Major contusion of spleen
      Contusion of spleen greater than 2 cm
   ● **S36.029**   Unspecified contusion of spleen
      Coding Clinic: 2015, Q1, P11
  ● **S36.03**   Laceration of spleen
   ● **S36.030**   Superficial (capsular) laceration of spleen
      Laceration of spleen less than 1 cm
      Minor laceration of spleen
   ● **S36.031**   Moderate laceration of spleen
      Laceration of spleen 1 to 3 cm
      Coding Clinic: 2015, Q1, P11
   ● **S36.032**   Major laceration of spleen
      Avulsion of spleen
      Laceration of spleen greater than 3 cm
      Massive laceration of spleen
      Multiple moderate lacerations of spleen
      Stellate laceration of spleen
   ● **S36.039**   Unspecified laceration of spleen
  X● **S36.09**   Other injury of spleen

● **S36.1**   Injury of liver and gallbladder and bile duct
  ● **S36.11**   Injury of liver
   ● **S36.112**   Contusion of liver
   ● **S36.113**   Laceration of liver, unspecified degree
   ● **S36.114**   Minor laceration of liver
      Laceration involving capsule only, or, without significant involvement of hepatic parenchyma [i.e., less than 1 cm deep]
   ● **S36.115**   Moderate laceration of liver
      Laceration involving parenchyma but without major disruption of parenchyma [i.e., less than 10 cm long and less than 3 cm deep]
   ● **S36.116**   Major laceration of liver
      Laceration with significant disruption of hepatic parenchyma [i.e., greater than 10 cm long and 3 cm deep]
      Multiple moderate lacerations, with or without hematoma
      Stellate laceration of liver
   ● **S36.118**   Other injury of liver
   ● **S36.119**   Unspecified injury of liver
  ● **S36.12**   Injury of gallbladder
   ● **S36.122**   Contusion of gallbladder
   ● **S36.123**   Laceration of gallbladder
   ● **S36.128**   Other injury of gallbladder
   ● **S36.129**   Unspecified injury of gallbladder
  X● **S36.13**   Injury of bile duct

● **S36.2**   Injury of pancreas
  ● **S36.20**   Unspecified injury of pancreas
   ● **S36.200**   Unspecified injury of head of pancreas
   ● **S36.201**   Unspecified injury of body of pancreas
   ● **S36.202**   Unspecified injury of tail of pancreas
   ● **S36.209**   Unspecified injury of unspecified part of pancreas
  ● **S36.22**   Contusion of pancreas
   ● **S36.220**   Contusion of head of pancreas
   ● **S36.221**   Contusion of body of pancreas
   ● **S36.222**   Contusion of tail of pancreas
   ● **S36.229**   Contusion of unspecified part of pancreas
  ● **S36.23**   Laceration of pancreas, unspecified degree
   ● **S36.230**   Laceration of head of pancreas, unspecified degree
   ● **S36.231**   Laceration of body of pancreas, unspecified degree
   ● **S36.232**   Laceration of tail of pancreas, unspecified degree
   ● **S36.239**   Laceration of unspecified part of pancreas, unspecified degree
  ● **S36.24**   Minor laceration of pancreas
   ● **S36.240**   Minor laceration of head of pancreas
   ● **S36.241**   Minor laceration of body of pancreas
   ● **S36.242**   Minor laceration of tail of pancreas
   ● **S36.249**   Minor laceration of unspecified part of pancreas

◄ New   ◄ Revised   ~~deleted~~ Deleted   Excludes 1   Excludes 2   Includes   Use additional   Code first   Code also   Unspecified

OGCR Official Guidelines   X Assign placeholder X   ● Use Additional Character(s)   ▶ Manifestation Code   **Coding Clinic**

● S36.25   Moderate laceration of pancreas
    ● S36.250   Moderate laceration of head of pancreas
    ● S36.251   Moderate laceration of body of pancreas
    ● S36.252   Moderate laceration of tail of pancreas
    ● S36.259   Moderate laceration of unspecified part of pancreas

● S36.26   Major laceration of pancreas
    ● S36.260   Major laceration of head of pancreas
    ● S36.261   Major laceration of body of pancreas
    ● S36.262   Major laceration of tail of pancreas
    ● S36.269   Major laceration of unspecified part of pancreas

● S36.29   Other injury of pancreas
    ● S36.290   Other injury of head of pancreas
    ● S36.291   Other injury of body of pancreas
    ● S36.292   Other injury of tail of pancreas
    ● S36.299   Other injury of unspecified part of pancreas

● S36.3   Injury of stomach
    X ● S36.30   Unspecified injury of stomach
    X ● S36.32   Contusion of stomach
    X ● S36.33   Laceration of stomach
    X ● S36.39   Other injury of stomach

● S36.4   Injury of small intestine
    ● S36.40   Unspecified injury of small intestine
      ● S36.400   Unspecified injury of duodenum
      ● S36.408   Unspecified injury of other part of small intestine
      ● S36.409   Unspecified injury of unspecified part of small intestine

    ● S36.41   Primary blast injury of small intestine
      Blast injury of small intestine NOS
      S36.410   Primary blast injury of duodenum
      S36.418   Primary blast injury of other part of small intestine
      ● S36.419   Primary blast injury of unspecified part of small intestine

    ● S36.42   Contusion of small intestine
      ● S36.420   Contusion of duodenum
      ● S36.428   Contusion of other part of small intestine
      ● S36.429   Contusion of unspecified part of small intestine

    ● S36.43   Laceration of small intestine
      ● S36.430   Laceration of duodenum
      ● S36.438   Laceration of other part of small intestine
      ● S36.439   Laceration of unspecified part of small intestine

    ● S36.49   Other injury of small intestine
      ● S36.490   Other injury of duodenum
      ● S36.498   Other injury of other part of small intestine
      ● S36.499   Other injury of unspecified part of small intestine

● S36.5   Injury of colon
    Excludes2   injury of rectum (S36.6-)
    ● S36.50   Unspecified injury of colon
      ● S36.500   Unspecified injury of ascending [right] colon
      ● S36.501   Unspecified injury of transverse colon
      ● S36.502   Unspecified injury of descending [left] colon

      ● S36.503   Unspecified injury of sigmoid colon
      ● S36.508   Unspecified injury of other part of colon
      ● S36.509   Unspecified injury of unspecified part of colon

    ● S36.51   Primary blast injury of colon
      Blast injury of colon NOS
      ● S36.510   Primary blast injury of ascending [right] colon
      ● S36.511   Primary blast injury of transverse colon
      ● S36.512   Primary blast injury of descending [left] colon
      ● S36.513   Primary blast injury of sigmoid colon
      ● S36.518   Primary blast injury of other part of colon
      ● S36.519   Primary blast injury of unspecified part of colon

    ● S36.52   Contusion of colon
      ● S36.520   Contusion of ascending [right] colon
      ● S36.521   Contusion of transverse colon
      ● S36.522   Contusion of descending [left] colon
      ● S36.523   Contusion of sigmoid colon
      ● S36.528   Contusion of other part of colon
      ● S36.529   Contusion of unspecified part of colon

    ● S36.53   Laceration of colon
      ● S36.530   Laceration of ascending [right] colon
      ● S36.531   Laceration of transverse colon
      ● S36.532   Laceration of descending [left] colon
      ● S36.533   Laceration of sigmoid colon
      ● S36.538   Laceration of other part of colon
      S36.539   Laceration of unspecified part of colon

    ● S36.59   Other injury of colon
      Secondary blast injury of colon
      ● S36.590   Other injury of ascending [right] colon
      ● S36.591   Other injury of transverse colon
      ● S36.592   Other injury of descending [left] colon
      ● S36.593   Other injury of sigmoid colon
      ● S36.598   Other injury of other part of colon
      ● S36.599   Other injury of unspecified part of colon

● S36.6   Injury of rectum
    X ● S36.60   Unspecified injury of rectum
    X ● S36.61   Primary blast injury of rectum
      Blast injury of rectum NOS
    X ● S36.62   Contusion of rectum
    X ● S36.63   Laceration of rectum
    X ● S36.69   Other injury of rectum
      Secondary blast injury of rectum

● S36.8   Injury of other intra-abdominal organs
    X ● S36.81   Injury of peritoneum
    ● S36.89   Injury of other intra-abdominal organs
      Injury of retroperitoneum
      ● S36.892   Contusion of other intra-abdominal organs
      ● S36.893   Laceration of other intra-abdominal organs
      ● S36.898   Other injury of other intra-abdominal organs
      S36.899   Unspecified injury of other intra-abdominal organs

- S36.9   Injury of unspecified intra-abdominal organ
  - X● S36.90   Unspecified injury of unspecified intra-abdominal organ
  - X● S36.92   Contusion of unspecified intra-abdominal organ
  - X● S36.93   Laceration of unspecified intra-abdominal organ
  - X● S36.99   Other injury of unspecified intra-abdominal organ

● S37   Injury of urinary and pelvic organs

     Code also any associated open wound (S31.-)

     Excludes1   obstetric trauma to pelvic organs (O71.-)

     Excludes2   injury of peritoneum (S36.81)
                     injury of retroperitoneum (S36.89-)

     The appropriate 7th character is to be added to each code from category S37

> A   initial encounter
> D   subsequent encounter
> S   sequela

- S37.0   Injury of kidney
  - **Excludes2**   acute kidney injury (nontraumatic) (N17.9)
  - ● S37.00   Unspecified injury of kidney
    - ● S37.001   Unspecified injury of right kidney
    - ● S37.002   Unspecified injury of left kidney
    - ● S37.009   Unspecified injury of unspecified kidney
  - ● S37.01   Minor contusion of kidney
    - Contusion of kidney less than 2 cm
    - Contusion of kidney NOS
    - ● S37.011   Minor contusion of right kidney
    - ● S37.012   Minor contusion of left kidney
    - ● S37.019   Minor contusion of unspecified kidney
  - ● S37.02   Major contusion of kidney
    - Contusion of kidney greater than 2 cm
    - ● S37.021   Major contusion of right kidney
    - ● S37.022   Major contusion of left kidney
    - ● S37.029   Major contusion of unspecified kidney
  - ● S37.03   Laceration of kidney, unspecified degree
    - ● S37.031   Laceration of right kidney, unspecified degree
    - ● S37.032   Laceration of left kidney, unspecified degree
    - ● S37.039   Laceration of unspecified kidney, unspecified degree
  - ● S37.04   Minor laceration of kidney
    - Laceration of kidney less than 1 cm
    - ● S37.041   Minor laceration of right kidney
    - ● S37.042   Minor laceration of left kidney
    - ● S37.049   Minor laceration of unspecified kidney
  - ● S37.05   Moderate laceration of kidney
    - Laceration of kidney 1 to 3 cm
    - ● S37.051   Moderate laceration of right kidney
    - ● S37.052   Moderate laceration of left kidney
    - ● S37.059   Moderate laceration of unspecified kidney

- ● S37.06   Major laceration of kidney
  - Avulsion of kidney
  - Laceration of kidney greater than 3 cm
  - Massive laceration of kidney
  - Multiple moderate lacerations of kidney
  - Stellate laceration of kidney
  - ● S37.061   Major laceration of right kidney
  - ● S37.062   Major laceration of left kidney
  - ● S37.069   Major laceration of unspecified kidney
- ● S37.09   Other injury of kidney
  - ● S37.091   Other injury of right kidney
  - ● S37.092   Other injury of left kidney
  - ● S37.099   Other injury of unspecified kidney
- ● S37.1   Injury of ureter
  - X● S37.10   Unspecified injury of ureter
  - X● S37.12   Contusion of ureter
  - X● S37.13   Laceration of ureter
  - X● S37.19   Other injury of ureter
- ● S37.2   Injury of bladder
  - X● S37.20   Unspecified injury of bladder
  - X● S37.22   Contusion of bladder
  - X● S37.23   Laceration of bladder
  - X● S37.29   Other injury of bladder
- ● S37.3   Injury of urethra
  - X● S37.30   Unspecified injury of urethra
  - X● S37.32   Contusion of urethra
  - X● S37.33   Laceration of urethra
  - X● S37.39   Other injury of urethra
- ● S37.4   Injury of ovary
  - ● S37.40   Unspecified injury of ovary
    - ● S37.401   Unspecified injury of ovary, unilateral ♀
    - ● S37.402   Unspecified injury of ovary, bilateral ♀
    - ● S37.409   Unspecified injury of ovary, unspecified ♀
  - ● S37.42   Contusion of ovary
    - ● S37.421   Contusion of ovary, unilateral ♀
    - ● S37.422   Contusion of ovary, bilateral ♀
    - ● S37.429   Contusion of ovary, unspecified ♀
  - ● S37.43   Laceration of ovary
    - ● S37.431   Laceration of ovary, unilateral ♀
    - ● S37.432   Laceration of ovary, bilateral ♀
    - ● S37.439   Laceration of ovary, unspecified ♀
  - ● S37.49   Other injury of ovary
    - ● S37.491   Other injury of ovary, unilateral ♀
    - ● S37.492   Other injury of ovary, bilateral ♀
    - ● S37.499   Other injury of ovary, unspecified ♀
- ● S37.5   Injury of fallopian tube
  - ● S37.50   Unspecified injury of fallopian tube
    - ● S37.501   Unspecified injury of fallopian tube, unilateral ♀
    - ● S37.502   Unspecified injury of fallopian tube, bilateral ♀
    - ● S37.509   Unspecified injury of fallopian tube, unspecified ♀
  - ● S37.51   Primary blast injury of fallopian tube
    - Blast injury of fallopian tube NOS
    - ● S37.511   Primary blast injury of fallopian tube, unilateral ♀
    - ● S37.512   Primary blast injury of fallopian tube, bilateral ♀
    - ● S37.519   Primary blast injury of fallopian tube, unspecified ♀

◀ New   ◀▥ Revised   ~~deleted~~ Deleted   Excludes 1   Excludes 2   Includes   Use additional   Code first   Code also   Unspecified

OGCR Official Guidelines   X Assign placeholder X   ● Use Additional Character(s)   ▶ Manifestation Code   **Coding Clinic**

● S37.52   Contusion of fallopian tube
    ● S37.521   Contusion of fallopian tube, unilateral ♀
    ● S37.522   Contusion of fallopian tube, bilateral ♀
    ● S37.529   Contusion of fallopian tube, unspecified ♀
● S37.53   Laceration of fallopian tube
    ● S37.531   Laceration of fallopian tube, unilateral ♀
    ● S37.532   Laceration of fallopian tube, bilateral ♀
    ● S37.539   Laceration of fallopian tube, unspecified ♀
● S37.59   Other injury of fallopian tube
      Secondary blast injury of fallopian tube
    ● S37.591   Other injury of fallopian tube, unilateral ♀
    ● S37.592   Other injury of fallopian tube, bilateral ♀
    ● S37.599   Other injury of fallopian tube, unspecified ♀

● S37.6   Injury of uterus
    Excludes1   injury to gravid uterus (O9A.2-)
                 injury to uterus during delivery (O71.-)
  X● S37.60   Unspecified injury of uterus ♀
  X● S37.62   Contusion of uterus ♀
  X● S37.63   Laceration of uterus ♀
  X● S37.69   Other injury of uterus ♀
● S37.8   Injury of other urinary and pelvic organs
   ● S37.81   Injury of adrenal gland
    ● S37.812   Contusion of adrenal gland
    ● S37.813   Laceration of adrenal gland
    ● S37.818   Other injury of adrenal gland
    ● S37.819   Unspecified injury of adrenal gland
   ● S37.82   Injury of prostate
    ● S37.822   Contusion of prostate ♂
    ● S37.823   Laceration of prostate ♂
    ● S37.828   Other injury of prostate ♂
    ● S37.829   Unspecified injury of prostate ♂
   ● S37.89   Injury of other urinary and pelvic organ
    ● S37.892   Contusion of other urinary and pelvic organ
    ● S37.893   Laceration of other urinary and pelvic organ
    ● S37.898   Other injury of other urinary and pelvic organ
    ● S37.899   Unspecified injury of other urinary and pelvic organ
● S37.9   Injury of unspecified urinary and pelvic organ
  X● S37.90   Unspecified injury of unspecified urinary and pelvic organ
  X● S37.92   Contusion of unspecified urinary and pelvic organ
  X● S37.93   Laceration of unspecified urinary and pelvic organ
  X● S37.99   Other injury of unspecified urinary and pelvic organ

● S38   Crushing injury and traumatic amputation of abdomen, lower back, pelvis and external genitals
    An amputation not identified as partial or complete should be coded to complete
    The appropriate 7th character is to be added to each code from category S38

> A   initial encounter
> D   subsequent encounter
> S   sequela

● S38.0   Crushing injury of external genital organs
     Use additional code for any associated injuries
   ● S38.00   Crushing injury of unspecified external genital organs
    ● S38.001   Crushing injury of unspecified external genital organs, male ♂
    ● S38.002   Crushing injury of unspecified external genital organs, female ♀
  X● S38.01   Crushing injury of penis ♂
  X● S38.02   Crushing injury of scrotum and testis ♂
  X● S38.03   Crushing injury of vulva ♀
  X● S38.1   Crushing injury of abdomen, lower back, and pelvis
     Use additional code for all associated injuries, such as:
      fracture of thoracic or lumbar spine and pelvis (S22.0-, S32.-)
      injury to intra-abdominal organs (S36.-)
      injury to urinary and pelvic organs (S37.-)
      open wound of abdominal wall (S31.-)
      spinal cord injury (S34.0, S34.1-)
    Excludes2   crushing injury of external genital organs (S38.0-)
● S38.2   Traumatic amputation of external genital organs
   ● S38.21   Traumatic amputation of female external genital organs
      Traumatic amputation of clitoris
      Traumatic amputation of labium (majus) (minus)
      Traumatic amputation of vulva
    ● S38.211   Complete traumatic amputation of female external genital organs ♀
    ● S38.212   Partial traumatic amputation of female external genital organs ♀
   ● S38.22   Traumatic amputation of penis
    ● S38.221   Complete traumatic amputation of penis ♂
    ● S38.222   Partial traumatic amputation of penis ♂
   ● S38.23   Traumatic amputation of scrotum and testis
    ● S38.231   Complete traumatic amputation of scrotum and testis ♂
    ● S38.232   Partial traumatic amputation of scrotum and testis ♂
  X● S38.3   Transection (partial) of abdomen

● **S39   Other and unspecified injuries of abdomen, lower back, pelvis and external genitals**

    Code also any associated open wound (S31.-)

    Excludes2   sprain of joints and ligaments of lumbar spine and pelvis (S33.-)

    The appropriate 7th character is to be added to each code from category S39

> A   initial encounter
> D   subsequent encounter
> S   sequela

● **S39.0   Injury of muscle, fascia and tendon of abdomen, lower back and pelvis**

  ● S39.00   Unspecified injury of muscle, fascia and tendon of abdomen, lower back and pelvis

    ● S39.001   Unspecified injury of muscle, fascia and tendon of abdomen

    ● S39.002   Unspecified injury of muscle, fascia and tendon of lower back

    ● S39.003   Unspecified injury of muscle, fascia and tendon of pelvis

  ● S39.01   Strain of muscle, fascia and tendon of abdomen, lower back and pelvis

    ● S39.011   Strain of muscle, fascia and tendon of abdomen

    ● S39.012   Strain of muscle, fascia and tendon of lower back

    ● S39.013   Strain of muscle, fascia and tendon of pelvis

  ● S39.02   Laceration of muscle, fascia and tendon of abdomen, lower back and pelvis

    ● S39.021   Laceration of muscle, fascia and tendon of abdomen

    ● S39.022   Laceration of muscle, fascia and tendon of lower back

    ● S39.023   Laceration of muscle, fascia and tendon of pelvis

  ● S39.09   Other injury of muscle, fascia and tendon of abdomen, lower back and pelvis

    ● S39.091   Other injury of muscle, fascia and tendon of abdomen

    ● S39.092   Other injury of muscle, fascia and tendon of lower back

    ● S39.093   Other injury of muscle, fascia and tendon of pelvis

● **S39.8   Other specified injuries of abdomen, lower back, pelvis and external genitals**

  X● S39.81   Other specified injuries of abdomen

  X● S39.82   Other specified injuries of lower back

  X● S39.83   Other specified injuries of pelvis

  ● S39.84   Other specified injuries of external genitals

    ● S39.840   Fracture of corpus cavernosum penis ♂

    ● S39.848   Other specified injuries of external genitals

● **S39.9   Unspecified injury of abdomen, lower back, pelvis and external genitals**

  X● S39.91   Unspecified injury of abdomen

  X● S39.92   Unspecified injury of lower back

  X● S39.93   Unspecified injury of pelvis

  X● S39.94   Unspecified injury of external genitals

INJURIES TO THE SHOULDER AND UPPER ARM (S40-S49)

Includes	injuries of axilla injuries of scapular region
Excludes2	burns and corrosions (T20-T32)
	frostbite (T33-T34)
	injuries of elbow (S50-S59)
	insect bite or sting, venomous (T63.4)

● **S40   Superficial injury of shoulder and upper arm**

    The appropriate 7th character is to be added to each code from category S40

> A   initial encounter
> D   subsequent encounter
> S   sequela

● **S40.0   Contusion of shoulder and upper arm**

  ● S40.01   Contusion of shoulder

    ● S40.011   Contusion of right shoulder

    ● S40.012   Contusion of left shoulder

    ● S40.019   Contusion of unspecified shoulder

  ● S40.02   Contusion of upper arm

    ● S40.021   Contusion of right upper arm

    ● S40.022   Contusion of left upper arm

    ● S40.029   Contusion of unspecified upper arm

● **S40.2   Other superficial injuries of shoulder**

  ● S40.21   Abrasion of shoulder

    ● S40.211   Abrasion of right shoulder

    ● S40.212   Abrasion of left shoulder

    ● S40.219   Abrasion of unspecified shoulder

  ● S40.22   Blister (nonthermal) of shoulder

    ● S40.221   Blister (nonthermal) of right shoulder

    ● S40.222   Blister (nonthermal) of left shoulder

    ● S40.229   Blister (nonthermal) of unspecified shoulder

  ● S40.24   External constriction of shoulder

    ● S40.241   External constriction of right shoulder

    ● S40.242   External constriction of left shoulder

    ● S40.249   External constriction of unspecified shoulder

  ● S40.25   Superficial foreign body of shoulder

    Splinter in the shoulder

    ● S40.251   Superficial foreign body of right shoulder

    ● S40.252   Superficial foreign body of left shoulder

    ● S40.259   Superficial foreign body of unspecified shoulder

  ● S40.26   Insect bite (nonvenomous) of shoulder

    ● S40.261   Insect bite (nonvenomous) of right shoulder

    ● S40.262   Insect bite (nonvenomous) of left shoulder

    ● S40.269   Insect bite (nonvenomous) of unspecified shoulder

  ● S40.27   Other superficial bite of shoulder

    Excludes1   open bite of shoulder (S41.05)

    ● S40.271   Other superficial bite of right shoulder

    ● S40.272   Other superficial bite of left shoulder

    ● S40.279   Other superficial bite of unspecified shoulder

◄ New   ⇐ Revised   ~~deleted~~ Deleted   Excludes 1   Excludes 2   Includes   Use additional   Code first   Code also   Unspecified

OGCR Official Guidelines   X Assign placeholder X   ● Use Additional Character(s)   ▶ Manifestation Code   **Coding Clinic**

● S40.8   Other superficial injuries of upper arm
  ● S40.81   Abrasion of upper arm
    ● S40.811   Abrasion of right upper arm
    ● S40.812   Abrasion of left upper arm
    ● S40.819   Abrasion of unspecified upper arm
  ● S40.82   Blister (nonthermal) of upper arm
    ● S40.821   Blister (nonthermal) of right upper arm
    ● S40.822   Blister (nonthermal) of left upper arm
    ● S40.829   Blister (nonthermal) of unspecified upper arm
  ● S40.84   External constriction of upper arm
    ● S40.841   External constriction of right upper arm
    ● S40.842   External constriction of left upper arm
    ● S40.849   External constriction of unspecified upper arm
  ● S40.85   Superficial foreign body of upper arm
    Splinter in the upper arm
    ● S40.851   Superficial foreign body of right upper arm
    ● S40.852   Superficial foreign body of left upper arm
    ● S40.859   Superficial foreign body of unspecified upper arm
  ● S40.86   Insect bite (nonvenomous) of upper arm
    ● S40.861   Insect bite (nonvenomous) of right upper arm
    ● S40.862   Insect bite (nonvenomous) of left upper arm
    ● S40.869   Insect bite (nonvenomous) of unspecified upper arm
  ● S40.87   Other superficial bite of upper arm
    Excludes1   open bite of upper arm (S41.14)
    Excludes2   other superficial bite of shoulder (S40.27-)
    ● S40.871   Other superficial bite of right upper arm
    ● S40.872   Other superficial bite of left upper arm
    ● S40.879   Other superficial bite of unspecified upper arm
● S40.9   Unspecified superficial injury of shoulder and upper arm
  ● S40.91   Unspecified superficial injury of shoulder
    ● S40.911   Unspecified superficial injury of right shoulder
    ● S40.912   Unspecified superficial injury of left shoulder
    ● S40.919   Unspecified superficial injury of unspecified shoulder
  ● S40.92   Unspecified superficial injury of upper arm
    ● S40.921   Unspecified superficial injury of right upper arm
    ● S40.922   Unspecified superficial injury of left upper arm
    ● S40.929   Unspecified superficial injury of unspecified upper arm

● S41   Open wound of shoulder and upper arm
  Code also any associated wound infection
  Excludes1   traumatic amputation of shoulder and upper arm (S48.-)
  Excludes2   open fracture of shoulder and upper arm (S42.- with 7th character B or C)
  The appropriate 7th character is to be added to each code from category S41

A	initial encounter
D	subsequent encounter
S	sequela

  ● S41.0   Open wound of shoulder
    ● S41.00   Unspecified open wound of shoulder
      ● S41.001   Unspecified open wound of right shoulder
      ● S41.002   Unspecified open wound of left shoulder
      ● S41.009   Unspecified open wound of unspecified shoulder
    ● S41.01   Laceration without foreign body of shoulder
      ● S41.011   Laceration without foreign body of right shoulder
      ● S41.012   Laceration without foreign body of left shoulder
      ● S41.019   Laceration without foreign body of unspecified shoulder
    ● S41.02   Laceration with foreign body of shoulder
      ● S41.021   Laceration with foreign body of right shoulder
      ● S41.022   Laceration with foreign body of left shoulder
      ● S41.029   Laceration with foreign body of unspecified shoulder
    ● S41.03   Puncture wound without foreign body of shoulder
      ● S41.031   Puncture wound without foreign body of right shoulder
      ● S41.032   Puncture wound without foreign body of left shoulder
      ● S41.039   Puncture wound without foreign body of unspecified shoulder
    ● S41.04   Puncture wound with foreign body of shoulder
      ● S41.041   Puncture wound with foreign body of right shoulder
      ● S41.042   Puncture wound with foreign body of left shoulder
      ● S41.049   Puncture wound with foreign body of unspecified shoulder
    ● S41.05   Open bite of shoulder
    Bite of shoulder NOS
    Excludes1   superficial bite of shoulder (S40.27)
      ● S41.051   Open bite of right shoulder
      ● S41.052   Open bite of left shoulder
      ● S41.059   Open bite of unspecified shoulder
  ● S41.1   Open wound of upper arm
    ● S41.10   Unspecified open wound of upper arm
      ● S41.101   Unspecified open wound of right upper arm
      ● S41.102   Unspecified open wound of left upper arm
      ● S41.109   Unspecified open wound of unspecified upper arm

- ● **S41.11**   **Laceration without foreign body of upper arm**
  - ● **S41.111**   **Laceration without foreign body of right upper arm**
  - ● **S41.112**   **Laceration without foreign body of left upper arm**
  - ● **S41.119**   **Laceration without foreign body of unspecified upper arm**
- ● **S41.12**   **Laceration with foreign body of upper arm**
  - ● **S41.121**   **Laceration with foreign body of right upper arm**
  - ● **S41.122**   **Laceration with foreign body of left upper arm**
  - ● **S41.129**   **Laceration with foreign body of unspecified upper arm**
- ● **S41.13**   **Puncture wound without foreign body of upper arm**
  - ● **S41.131**   **Puncture wound without foreign body of right upper arm**
  - ● **S41.132**   **Puncture wound without foreign body of left upper arm**
  - ● **S41.139**   **Puncture wound without foreign body of unspecified upper arm**
- ● **S41.14**   **Puncture wound with foreign body of upper arm**
  - ● **S41.141**   **Puncture wound with foreign body of right upper arm**
  - ● **S41.142**   **Puncture wound with foreign body of left upper arm**
  - ● **S41.149**   **Puncture wound with foreign body of unspecified upper arm**
- ● **S41.15**   **Open bite of upper arm**
  Bite of upper arm NOS

  > **Excludes1**   superficial bite of upper arm (S40.87)

  - ● **S41.151**   **Open bite of right upper arm**
  - ● **S41.152**   **Open bite of left upper arm**
  - ● **S41.159**   **Open bite of unspecified upper arm**

- ● **S42**   **Fracture of shoulder and upper arm**

  Note: A fracture not indicated as displaced or nondisplaced should be coded to displaced

  A fracture not indicated as open or closed should be coded to closed

  > **Excludes1**   traumatic amputation of shoulder and upper arm (S48.-)

  The appropriate 7th character is to be added to all codes from category S42

A	initial encounter for closed fracture
B	initial encounter for open fracture
D	subsequent encounter for fracture with routine healing
G	subsequent encounter for fracture with delayed healing
K	subsequent encounter for fracture with nonunion
P	subsequent encounter for fracture with malunion
S	sequela

  - ● **S42.0**   **Fracture of clavicle**
    - ● **S42.00**   **Fracture of unspecified part of clavicle**
      - ● **S42.001**   **Fracture of unspecified part of right clavicle**
      - ● **S42.002**   **Fracture of unspecified part of left clavicle**
      - ● **S42.009**   **Fracture of unspecified part of unspecified clavicle**
        Coding Clinic: 2012, Q4, P3

- ● **S42.01**   **Fracture of sternal end of clavicle**
  - ● **S42.011**   **Anterior displaced fracture of sternal end of right clavicle**
  - ● **S42.012**   **Anterior displaced fracture of sternal end of left clavicle**
  - ● **S42.013**   **Anterior displaced fracture of sternal end of unspecified clavicle**
    Displaced fracture of sternal end of clavicle NOS
  - ● **S42.014**   **Posterior displaced fracture of sternal end of right clavicle**
  - ● **S42.015**   **Posterior displaced fracture of sternal end of left clavicle**
  - ● **S42.016**   **Posterior displaced fracture of sternal end of unspecified clavicle**
  - ● **S42.017**   **Nondisplaced fracture of sternal end of right clavicle**
  - ● **S42.018**   **Nondisplaced fracture of sternal end of left clavicle**
  - ● **S42.019**   **Nondisplaced fracture of sternal end of unspecified clavicle**
- ● **S42.02**   **Fracture of shaft of clavicle**
  - ● **S42.021**   **Displaced fracture of shaft of right clavicle**
  - ● **S42.022**   **Displaced fracture of shaft of left clavicle**
  - ● **S42.023**   **Displaced fracture of shaft of unspecified clavicle**
  - ● **S42.024**   **Nondisplaced fracture of shaft of right clavicle**
  - ● **S42.025**   **Nondisplaced fracture of shaft of left clavicle**
  - ● **S42.026**   **Nondisplaced fracture of shaft of unspecified clavicle**
- ● **S42.03**   **Fracture of lateral end of clavicle**
  Fracture of acromial end of clavicle
  - ● **S42.031**   **Displaced fracture of lateral end of right clavicle**
  - ● **S42.032**   **Displaced fracture of lateral end of left clavicle**
  - ● **S42.033**   **Displaced fracture of lateral end of unspecified clavicle**
  - ● **S42.034**   **Nondisplaced fracture of lateral end of right clavicle**
  - ● **S42.035**   **Nondisplaced fracture of lateral end of left clavicle**
  - ● **S42.036**   **Nondisplaced fracture of lateral end of unspecified clavicle**
- ● **S42.1**   **Fracture of scapula**
  - ● **S42.10**   **Fracture of unspecified part of scapula**
    - ● **S42.101**   **Fracture of unspecified part of scapula, right shoulder**
    - ● **S42.102**   **Fracture of unspecified part of scapula, left shoulder**
    - ● **S42.109**   **Fracture of unspecified part of scapula, unspecified shoulder**
  - ● **S42.11**   **Fracture of body of scapula**
    - ● **S42.111**   **Displaced fracture of body of scapula, right shoulder**
    - ● **S42.112**   **Displaced fracture of body of scapula, left shoulder**
    - ● **S42.113**   **Displaced fracture of body of scapula, unspecified shoulder**
    - ● **S42.114**   **Nondisplaced fracture of body of scapula, right shoulder**
    - ● **S42.115**   **Nondisplaced fracture of body of scapula, left shoulder**
    - ● **S42.116**   **Nondisplaced fracture of body of scapula, unspecified shoulder**

◀ New   ◀▥ Revised   ~~deleted~~ Deleted   Excludes 1   Excludes 2   Includes   Use additional   Code first   Code also   Unspecified

OGCR Official Guidelines   **X** Assign placeholder X   ● Use Additional Character(s)   ▶ Manifestation Code   **Coding Clinic**

● S42.12   Fracture of acromial process

   ● S42.121   Displaced fracture of acromial process, right shoulder

   ● S42.122   Displaced fracture of acromial process, left shoulder

   ● S42.123   Displaced fracture of acromial process, unspecified shoulder

   ● S42.124   Nondisplaced fracture of acromial process, right shoulder

   ● S42.125   Nondisplaced fracture of acromial process, left shoulder

   ● S42.126   Nondisplaced fracture, of acromial process, unspecified shoulder

● S42.13   Fracture of coracoid process

   ● S42.131   Displaced fracture of coracoid process, right shoulder

   ● S42.132   Displaced fracture of coracoid process, left shoulder

   ● S42.133   Displaced fracture of coracoid process, unspecified shoulder

   ● S42.134   Nondisplaced fracture of coracoid process, right shoulder

   ● S42.135   Nondisplaced fracture of coracoid process, left shoulder

   ● S42.136   Nondisplaced fracture of coracoid process, unspecified shoulder

● S42.14   Fracture of glenoid cavity of scapula

   ● S42.141   Displaced fracture of glenoid cavity of scapula, right shoulder

   ● S42.142   Displaced fracture of glenoid cavity of scapula, left shoulder

   ● S42.143   Displaced fracture of glenoid cavity of scapula, unspecified shoulder

   ● S42.144   Nondisplaced fracture of glenoid cavity of scapula, right shoulder

   ● S42.145   Nondisplaced fracture of glenoid cavity of scapula, left shoulder

   ● S42.146   Nondisplaced fracture of glenoid cavity of scapula, unspecified shoulder

● S42.15   Fracture of neck of scapula

   ● S42.151   Displaced fracture of neck of scapula, right shoulder

   ● S42.152   Displaced fracture of neck of scapula, left shoulder

   ● S42.153   Displaced fracture of neck of scapula, unspecified shoulder

   ● S42.154   Nondisplaced fracture of neck of scapula, right shoulder

   ● S42.155   Nondisplaced fracture of neck of scapula, left shoulder

   ● S42.156   Nondisplaced fracture of neck of scapula, unspecified shoulder

● S42.19   Fracture of other part of scapula

   ● S42.191   Fracture of other part of scapula, right shoulder

   ● S42.192   Fracture of other part of scapula, left shoulder

   ● S42.199   Fracture of other part of scapula, unspecified shoulder

● S42.2   Fracture of upper end of humerus

    Fracture of proximal end of humerus

   Excludes2   fracture of shaft of humerus (S42.3-)

          physeal fracture of upper end of humerus (S49.0-)

  ● S42.20   Unspecified fracture of upper end of humerus

   ● S42.201   Unspecified fracture of upper end of right humerus

   ● S42.202   Unspecified fracture of upper end of left humerus

   ● S42.209   Unspecified fracture of upper end of unspecified humerus

  ● S42.21   Unspecified fracture of surgical neck of humerus

    Fracture of neck of humerus NOS

   ● S42.211   Unspecified displaced fracture of surgical neck of right humerus

   ● S42.212   Unspecified displaced fracture of surgical neck of left humerus

   ● S42.213   Unspecified displaced fracture of surgical neck of unspecified humerus

   ● S42.214   Unspecified nondisplaced fracture of surgical neck of right humerus

   ● S42.215   Unspecified nondisplaced fracture of surgical neck of left humerus

   ● S42.216   Unspecified nondisplaced fracture of surgical neck of unspecified humerus

  ● S42.22   2-part fracture of surgical neck of humerus

   ● S42.221   2-part displaced fracture of surgical neck of right humerus

   ● S42.222   2-part displaced fracture of surgical neck of left humerus

   ● S42.223   2-part displaced fracture of surgical neck of unspecified humerus

   ● S42.224   2-part nondisplaced fracture of surgical neck of right humerus

   ● S42.225   2-part nondisplaced fracture of surgical neck of left humerus

   ● S42.226   2-part nondisplaced fracture of surgical neck of unspecified humerus

  ● S42.23   3-part fracture of surgical neck of humerus

   ● S42.231   3-part fracture of surgical neck of right humerus

   ● S42.232   3-part fracture of surgical neck of left humerus

   ● S42.239   3-part fracture of surgical neck of unspecified humerus

  ● S42.24   4-part fracture of surgical neck of humerus

   ● S42.241   4-part fracture of surgical neck of right humerus

   ● S42.242   4-part fracture of surgical neck of left humerus

   ● S42.249   4-part fracture of surgical neck of unspecified humerus

  ● S42.25   Fracture of greater tuberosity of humerus

   ● S42.251   Displaced fracture of greater tuberosity of right humerus

   ● S42.252   Displaced fracture of greater tuberosity of left humerus

   ● S42.253   Displaced fracture of greater tuberosity of unspecified humerus

   ● S42.254   Nondisplaced fracture of greater tuberosity of right humerus

   ● S42.255   Nondisplaced fracture of greater tuberosity of left humerus

   ● S42.256   Nondisplaced fracture of greater tuberosity of unspecified humerus

CHAPTER 19 (S00-T88)

● **S42.26**   Fracture of lesser tuberosity of humerus
  ● **S42.261**   Displaced fracture of lesser tuberosity of right humerus
  ● **S42.262**   Displaced fracture of lesser tuberosity of left humerus
  ● **S42.263**   Displaced fracture of lesser tuberosity of unspecified humerus
  ● **S42.264**   Nondisplaced fracture of lesser tuberosity of right humerus
  ● **S42.265**   Nondisplaced fracture of lesser tuberosity of left humerus
  ● **S42.266**   Nondisplaced fracture of lesser tuberosity of unspecified humerus
● **S42.27**   Torus fracture of upper end of humerus

The appropriate 7th character is to be added to all codes in subcategory S42.27

> A   initial encounter for closed fracture
> D   subsequent encounter for fracture with routine healing
> G   subsequent encounter for fracture with delayed healing
> K   subsequent encounter for fracture with nonunion
> P   subsequent encounter for fracture with malunion
> S   sequela

  ● **S42.271**   Torus fracture of upper end of right humerus
  ● **S42.272**   Torus fracture of upper end of left humerus
  ● **S42.279**   Torus fracture of upper end of unspecified humerus
● **S42.29**   Other fracture of upper end of humerus
    Fracture of anatomical neck of humerus
    Fracture of articular head of humerus
  ● **S42.291**   Other displaced fracture of upper end of right humerus
  ● **S42.292**   Other displaced fracture of upper end of left humerus
  ● **S42.293**   Other displaced fracture of upper end of unspecified humerus
  ● **S42.294**   Other nondisplaced fracture of upper end of right humerus
  ● **S42.295**   Other nondisplaced fracture of upper end of left humerus
  ● **S42.296**   Other nondisplaced fracture of upper end of unspecified humerus
● **S42.3**   Fracture of shaft of humerus
    Fracture of humerus NOS
    Fracture of upper arm NOS

    Excludes2   physeal fractures of upper end of humerus (S49.0-)
                   physeal fractures of lower end of humerus (S49.1-)

  ● **S42.30**   Unspecified fracture of shaft of humerus
    ● **S42.301**   Unspecified fracture of shaft of humerus, right arm
    ● **S42.302**   Unspecified fracture of shaft of humerus, left arm
    ● **S42.309**   Unspecified fracture of shaft of humerus, unspecified arm

● **S42.31**   Greenstick fracture of shaft of humerus

The appropriate 7th character is to be added to all codes in subcategory S42.31

> A   initial encounter for closed fracture
> D   subsequent encounter for fracture with routine healing
> G   subsequent encounter for fracture with delayed healing
> K   subsequent encounter for fracture with nonunion
> P   subsequent encounter for fracture with malunion
> S   sequela

  ● **S42.311**   Greenstick fracture of shaft of humerus, right arm
  ● **S42.312**   Greenstick fracture of shaft of humerus, left arm
  ● **S42.319**   Greenstick fracture of shaft of humerus, unspecified arm
● **S42.32**   Transverse fracture of shaft of humerus
  ● **S42.321**   Displaced transverse fracture of shaft of humerus, right arm
  ● **S42.322**   Displaced transverse fracture of shaft of humerus, left arm
  ● **S42.323**   Displaced transverse fracture of shaft of humerus, unspecified arm
  ● **S42.324**   Nondisplaced transverse fracture of shaft of humerus, right arm
  ● **S42.325**   Nondisplaced transverse fracture of shaft of humerus, left arm
  ● **S42.326**   Nondisplaced transverse fracture of shaft of humerus, unspecified arm
● **S42.33**   Oblique fracture of shaft of humerus
  ● **S42.331**   Displaced oblique fracture of shaft of humerus, right arm
  ● **S42.332**   Displaced oblique fracture of shaft of humerus, left arm
  ● **S42.333**   Displaced oblique fracture of shaft of humerus, unspecified arm
  ● **S42.334**   Nondisplaced oblique fracture of shaft of humerus, right arm
  ● **S42.335**   Nondisplaced oblique fracture of shaft of humerus, left arm
  ● **S42.336**   Nondisplaced oblique fracture of shaft of humerus, unspecified arm
● **S42.34**   Spiral fracture of shaft of humerus
  ● **S42.341**   Displaced spiral fracture of shaft of humerus, right arm
  ● **S42.342**   Displaced spiral fracture of shaft of humerus, left arm
  ● **S42.343**   Displaced spiral fracture of shaft of humerus, unspecified arm
  ● **S42.344**   Nondisplaced spiral fracture of shaft of humerus, right arm
  ● **S42.345**   Nondisplaced spiral fracture of shaft of humerus, left arm
  ● **S42.346**   Nondisplaced spiral fracture of shaft of humerus, unspecified arm

◀ New   ◀◀◀ Revised   ~~deleted~~ Deleted   Excludes 1   Excludes 2   Includes   Use additional   Code first   Code also   Unspecified
OGCR Official Guidelines   **X** Assign placeholder X   ● Use Additional Character(s)   ▶ Manifestation Code   **Coding Clinic**

● **S42.35**   Comminuted fracture of shaft of humerus
   ● **S42.351**   Displaced comminuted fracture of shaft of humerus, right arm
   ● **S42.352**   Displaced comminuted fracture of shaft of humerus, left arm
   ● **S42.353**   Displaced comminuted fracture of shaft of humerus, unspecified arm
   ● **S42.354**   Nondisplaced comminuted fracture of shaft of humerus, right arm
   ● **S42.355**   Nondisplaced comminuted fracture of shaft of humerus, left arm
   ● **S42.356**   Nondisplaced comminuted fracture of shaft of humerus, unspecified arm
● **S42.36**   Segmental fracture of shaft of humerus
   ● **S42.361**   Displaced segmental fracture of shaft of humerus, right arm
   ● **S42.362**   Displaced segmental fracture of shaft of humerus, left arm
   ● **S42.363**   Displaced segmental fracture of shaft of humerus, unspecified arm
   ● **S42.364**   Nondisplaced segmental fracture of shaft of humerus, right arm
   ● **S42.365**   Nondisplaced segmental fracture of shaft of humerus, left arm
   ● **S42.366**   Nondisplaced segmental fracture of shaft of humerus, unspecified arm
● **S42.39**   Other fracture of shaft of humerus
   ● **S42.391**   Other fracture of shaft of right humerus
   ● **S42.392**   Other fracture of shaft of left humerus
   ● **S42.399**   Other fracture of shaft of unspecified humerus
● **S42.4**   Fracture of lower end of humerus
     Fracture of distal end of humerus

> **Excludes2**   fracture of shaft of humerus (S42.3-)
>   physeal fracture of lower end of humerus (S49.1-)

● **S42.40**   Unspecified fracture of lower end of humerus
     Fracture of elbow NOS
   ● **S42.401**   Unspecified fracture of lower end of right humerus
   ● **S42.402**   Unspecified fracture of lower end of left humerus
   ● **S42.409**   Unspecified fracture of lower end of unspecified humerus
● **S42.41**   Simple supracondylar fracture without intercondylar fracture of humerus
   ● **S42.411**   Displaced simple supracondylar fracture without intercondylar fracture of right humerus
   ● **S42.412**   Displaced simple supracondylar fracture without intercondylar fracture of left humerus
   ● **S42.413**   Displaced simple supracondylar fracture without intercondylar fracture of unspecified humerus
   ● **S42.414**   Nondisplaced simple supracondylar fracture without intercondylar fracture of right humerus
   ● **S42.415**   Nondisplaced simple supracondylar fracture without intercondylar fracture of left humerus
   ● **S42.416**   Nondisplaced simple supracondylar fracture without intercondylar fracture of unspecified humerus

● **S42.42**   Comminuted supracondylar fracture without intercondylar fracture of humerus
   ● **S42.421**   Displaced comminuted supracondylar fracture without intercondylar fracture of right humerus
   ● **S42.422**   Displaced comminuted supracondylar fracture without intercondylar fracture of left humerus
   ● **S42.423**   Displaced comminuted supracondylar fracture without intercondylar fracture of unspecified humerus
   ● **S42.424**   Nondisplaced comminuted supracondylar fracture without intercondylar fracture of right humerus
   ● **S42.425**   Nondisplaced comminuted supracondylar fracture without intercondylar fracture of left humerus
   ● **S42.426**   Nondisplaced comminuted supracondylar fracture without intercondylar fracture of unspecified humerus
● **S42.43**   Fracture (avulsion) of lateral epicondyle of humerus
   ● **S42.431**   Displaced fracture (avulsion) of lateral epicondyle of right humerus
   ● **S42.432**   Displaced fracture (avulsion) of lateral epicondyle of left humerus
   ● **S42.433**   Displaced fracture (avulsion) of lateral epicondyle of unspecified humerus
   ● **S42.434**   Nondisplaced fracture (avulsion) of lateral epicondyle of right humerus
   ● **S42.435**   Nondisplaced fracture (avulsion) of lateral epicondyle of left humerus
   ● **S42.436**   Nondisplaced fracture (avulsion) of lateral epicondyle of unspecified humerus
● **S42.44**   Fracture (avulsion) of medial epicondyle of humerus
   ● **S42.441**   Displaced fracture (avulsion) of medial epicondyle of right humerus
   ● **S42.442**   Displaced fracture (avulsion) of medial epicondyle of left humerus
   ● **S42.443**   Displaced fracture (avulsion) of medial epicondyle of unspecified humerus
   ● **S42.444**   Nondisplaced fracture (avulsion) of medial epicondyle of right humerus
   ● **S42.445**   Nondisplaced fracture (avulsion) of medial epicondyle of left humerus
   ● **S42.446**   Nondisplaced fracture (avulsion) of medial epicondyle of unspecified humerus
   ● **S42.447**   Incarcerated fracture (avulsion) of medial epicondyle of right humerus
   ● **S42.448**   Incarcerated fracture (avulsion) of medial epicondyle of left humerus
   ● **S42.449**   Incarcerated fracture (avulsion) of medial epicondyle of unspecified humerus
● **S42.45**   Fracture of lateral condyle of humerus
     Fracture of capitellum of humerus
   ● **S42.451**   Displaced fracture of lateral condyle of right humerus
   ● **S42.452**   Displaced fracture of lateral condyle of left humerus
   ● **S42.453**   Displaced fracture of lateral condyle of unspecified humerus

- S42.454   Nondisplaced fracture of lateral condyle of right humerus
- S42.455   Nondisplaced fracture of lateral condyle of left humerus
- S42.456   Nondisplaced fracture of lateral condyle of unspecified humerus
- S42.46   Fracture of medial condyle of humerus
  Trochlea fracture of humerus
  - S42.461   Displaced fracture of medial condyle of right humerus
  - S42.462   Displaced fracture of medial condyle of left humerus
  - S42.463   Displaced fracture of medial condyle of unspecified humerus
  - S42.464   Nondisplaced fracture of medial condyle of right humerus
  - S42.465   Nondisplaced fracture of medial condyle of left humerus
  - S42.466   Nondisplaced fracture of medial condyle of unspecified humerus
- S42.47   Transcondylar fracture of humerus
  - S42.471   Displaced transcondylar fracture of right humerus
  - S42.472   Displaced transcondylar fracture of left humerus
  - S42.473   Displaced transcondylar fracture of unspecified humerus
  - S42.474   Nondisplaced transcondylar fracture of right humerus
  - S42.475   Nondisplaced transcondylar fracture of left humerus
  - S42.476   Nondisplaced transcondylar fracture of unspecified humerus
- S42.48   Torus fracture of lower end of humerus

  The appropriate 7th character is to be added to all codes in subcategory S42.48

A	initial encounter for closed fracture
D	subsequent encounter for fracture with routine healing
G	subsequent encounter for fracture with delayed healing
K	subsequent encounter for fracture with nonunion
P	subsequent encounter for fracture with malunion
S	sequela

  - S42.481   Torus fracture of lower end of right humerus
  - S42.482   Torus fracture of lower end of left humerus
  - S42.489   Torus fracture of lower end of unspecified humerus
- S42.49   Other fracture of lower end of humerus
  - S42.491   Other displaced fracture of lower end of right humerus
  - S42.492   Other displaced fracture of lower end of left humerus
  - S42.493   Other displaced fracture of lower end of unspecified humerus
  - S42.494   Other nondisplaced fracture of lower end of right humerus
  - S42.495   Other nondisplaced fracture of lower end of left humerus
  - S42.496   Other nondisplaced fracture of lower end of unspecified humerus

- S42.9   Fracture of shoulder girdle, part unspecified
  Fracture of shoulder NOS
  - X ● S42.90   Fracture of unspecified shoulder girdle, part unspecified
  - X ● S42.91   Fracture of right shoulder girdle, part unspecified
  - X ● S42.92   Fracture of left shoulder girdle, part unspecified

- S43   Dislocation and sprain of joints and ligaments of shoulder girdle

  Includes   avulsion of joint or ligament of shoulder girdle
  laceration of cartilage, joint or ligament of shoulder girdle
  sprain of cartilage, joint or ligament of shoulder girdle
  traumatic hemarthrosis of joint or ligament of shoulder girdle
  traumatic rupture of joint or ligament of shoulder girdle
  traumatic subluxation of joint or ligament of shoulder girdle
  traumatic tear of joint or ligament of shoulder girdle

  Code also any associated open wound

  Excludes2   strain of muscle, fascia and tendon of shoulder and upper arm (S46.-)

  The appropriate 7th character is to be added to each code from category S43

A	initial encounter
D	subsequent encounter
S	sequela

  - S43.0   Subluxation and dislocation of shoulder joint
    Dislocation of glenohumeral joint
    Subluxation of glenohumeral joint
    - S43.00   Unspecified subluxation and dislocation of shoulder joint
      Dislocation of humerus NOS
      Subluxation of humerus NOS
      - S43.001   Unspecified subluxation of right shoulder joint
      - S43.002   Unspecified subluxation of left shoulder joint
      - S43.003   Unspecified subluxation of unspecified shoulder joint
      - S43.004   Unspecified dislocation of right shoulder joint
      - S43.005   Unspecified dislocation of left shoulder joint
      - S43.006   Unspecified dislocation of unspecified shoulder joint
    - S43.01   Anterior subluxation and dislocation of humerus
      - S43.011   Anterior subluxation of right humerus
      - S43.012   Anterior subluxation of left humerus
      - S43.013   Anterior subluxation of unspecified humerus
      - S43.014   Anterior dislocation of right humerus
      - S43.015   Anterior dislocation of left humerus
      - S43.016   Anterior dislocation of unspecified humerus

◀ New   ◀░ Revised   ~~deleted~~ Deleted   Excludes 1   Excludes 2   Includes   Use additional   Code first   Code also   Unspecified
OGCR Official Guidelines   X Assign placeholder X   ● Use Additional Character(s)   ▶ Manifestation Code   **Coding Clinic**

● **S43.02**   **Posterior subluxation and dislocation of humerus**
- ● **S43.021**   Posterior subluxation of right humerus
- ● **S43.022**   Posterior subluxation of left humerus
- ● **S43.023**   Posterior subluxation of unspecified humerus
- ● **S43.024**   Posterior dislocation of right humerus
- ● **S43.025**   Posterior dislocation of left humerus
- ● **S43.026**   Posterior dislocation of unspecified humerus

● **S43.03**   **Inferior subluxation and dislocation of humerus**
- ● **S43.031**   Inferior subluxation of right humerus
- ● **S43.032**   Inferior subluxation of left humerus
- ● **S43.033**   Inferior subluxation of unspecified humerus
- ● **S43.034**   Inferior dislocation of right humerus
- ● **S43.035**   Inferior dislocation of left humerus
- ● **S43.036**   Inferior dislocation of unspecified humerus

● **S43.08**   **Other subluxation and dislocation of shoulder joint**
- ● **S43.081**   Other subluxation of right shoulder joint
- ● **S43.082**   Other subluxation of left shoulder joint
- ● **S43.083**   Other subluxation of unspecified shoulder joint
- ● **S43.084**   Other dislocation of right shoulder joint
- ● **S43.085**   Other dislocation of left shoulder joint
- ● **S43.086**   Other dislocation of unspecified shoulder joint

● **S43.1**   **Subluxation and dislocation of acromioclavicular joint**
- ● **S43.10**   Unspecified dislocation of acromioclavicular joint
  - ● **S43.101**   Unspecified dislocation of right acromioclavicular joint
  - ● **S43.102**   Unspecified dislocation of left acromioclavicular joint
  - ● **S43.109**   Unspecified dislocation of unspecified acromioclavicular joint
- ● **S43.11**   Subluxation of acromioclavicular joint
  - ● **S43.111**   Subluxation of right acromioclavicular joint
  - ● **S43.112**   Subluxation of left acromioclavicular joint
  - ● **S43.119**   Subluxation of unspecified acromioclavicular joint
- ● **S43.12**   Dislocation of acromioclavicular joint, 100%-200% displacement
  - ● **S43.121**   Dislocation of right acromioclavicular joint, 100%-200% displacement
  - ● **S43.122**   Dislocation of left acromioclavicular joint, 100%-200% displacement
  - ● **S43.129**   Dislocation of unspecified acromioclavicular joint, 100%-200% displacement
- ● **S43.13**   Dislocation of acromioclavicular joint, greater than 200% displacement
  - ● **S43.131**   Dislocation of right acromioclavicular joint, greater than 200% displacement
  - ● **S43.132**   Dislocation of left acromioclavicular joint, greater than 200% displacement
  - ● **S43.139**   Dislocation of unspecified acromioclavicular joint, greater than 200% displacement

- ● **S43.14**   Inferior dislocation of acromioclavicular joint
  - ● **S43.141**   Inferior dislocation of right acromioclavicular joint
  - ● **S43.142**   Inferior dislocation of left acromioclavicular joint
  - ● **S43.149**   Inferior dislocation of unspecified acromioclavicular joint
- ● **S43.15**   Posterior dislocation of acromioclavicular joint
  - ● **S43.151**   Posterior dislocation of right acromioclavicular joint
  - ● **S43.152**   Posterior dislocation of left acromioclavicular joint
  - ● **S43.159**   Posterior dislocation of unspecified acromioclavicular joint

● **S43.2**   **Subluxation and dislocation of sternoclavicular joint**
- ● **S43.20**   Unspecified subluxation and dislocation of sternoclavicular joint
  - ● **S43.201**   Unspecified subluxation of right sternoclavicular joint
  - ● **S43.202**   Unspecified subluxation of left sternoclavicular joint
  - ● **S43.203**   Unspecified subluxation of unspecified sternoclavicular joint
  - ● **S43.204**   Unspecified dislocation of right sternoclavicular joint
  - ● **S43.205**   Unspecified dislocation of left sternoclavicular joint
  - ● **S43.206**   Unspecified dislocation of unspecified sternoclavicular joint
- ● **S43.21**   Anterior subluxation and dislocation of sternoclavicular joint
  - ● **S43.211**   Anterior subluxation of right sternoclavicular joint
  - ● **S43.212**   Anterior subluxation of left sternoclavicular joint
  - ● **S43.213**   Anterior subluxation of unspecified sternoclavicular joint
  - ● **S43.214**   Anterior dislocation of right sternoclavicular joint
  - ● **S43.215**   Anterior dislocation of left sternoclavicular joint
  - ● **S43.216**   Anterior dislocation of unspecified sternoclavicular joint
- ● **S43.22**   Posterior subluxation and dislocation of sternoclavicular joint
  - ● **S43.221**   Posterior subluxation of right sternoclavicular joint
  - ● **S43.222**   Posterior subluxation of left sternoclavicular joint
  - ● **S43.223**   Posterior subluxation of unspecified sternoclavicular joint
  - ● **S43.224**   Posterior dislocation of right sternoclavicular joint
  - ● **S43.225**   Posterior dislocation of left sternoclavicular joint
  - ● **S43.226**   Posterior dislocation of unspecified sternoclavicular joint

● **S43.3**   **Subluxation and dislocation of other and unspecified parts of shoulder girdle**
- ● **S43.30**   Subluxation and dislocation of unspecified parts of shoulder girdle
  Dislocation of shoulder girdle NOS
  Subluxation of shoulder girdle NOS
  - ● **S43.301**   Subluxation of unspecified parts of right shoulder girdle
  - ● **S43.302**   Subluxation of unspecified parts of left shoulder girdle

- ● S43.303   Subluxation of `unspecified` parts of unspecified shoulder girdle
- ● S43.304   Dislocation of `unspecified` parts of right shoulder girdle
- ● S43.305   Dislocation of `unspecified` parts of left shoulder girdle
- ● S43.306   Dislocation of `unspecified` parts of unspecified shoulder girdle
- ● S43.31   Subluxation and dislocation of scapula
  - ● S43.311   Subluxation of right scapula
  - ● S43.312   Subluxation of left scapula
  - ● S43.313   Subluxation of `unspecified` scapula
  - ● S43.314   Dislocation of right scapula
  - ● S43.315   Dislocation of left scapula
  - ● S43.316   Dislocation of `unspecified` scapula
- ● S43.39   Subluxation and dislocation of other parts of shoulder girdle
  - ● S43.391   Subluxation of other parts of right shoulder girdle
  - ● S43.392   Subluxation of other parts of left shoulder girdle
  - ● S43.393   Subluxation of other parts of `unspecified` shoulder girdle
  - ● S43.394   Dislocation of other parts of right shoulder girdle
  - ● S43.395   Dislocation of other parts of left shoulder girdle
  - ● S43.396   Dislocation of other parts of `unspecified` shoulder girdle
- ● S43.4   Sprain of shoulder joint
  - ● S43.40   Unspecified sprain of shoulder joint
    - ● S43.401   `Unspecified` sprain of right shoulder joint
    - ● S43.402   `Unspecified` sprain of left shoulder joint
    - ● S43.409   `Unspecified` sprain of unspecified shoulder joint
  - ● S43.41   Sprain of coracohumeral (ligament)
    - ● S43.411   Sprain of right coracohumeral (ligament)
    - ● S43.412   Sprain of left coracohumeral (ligament)
    - ● S43.419   Sprain of `unspecified` coracohumeral (ligament)
  - ● S43.42   Sprain of rotator cuff capsule
    > **Excludes1**   rotator cuff syndrome (complete) (incomplete), not specified as traumatic (M75.1-)
    > **Excludes2**   injury of tendon of rotator cuff (S46.0-)
    > *Encounters during the healing phase*
    - ● S43.421   Sprain of right rotator cuff capsule
    - ● S43.422   Sprain of left rotator cuff capsule
    - ● S43.429   Sprain of `unspecified` rotator cuff capsule
  - ● S43.43   Superior glenoid labrum lesion
    SLAP lesion
    - ● S43.431   Superior glenoid labrum lesion of right shoulder
    - ● S43.432   Superior glenoid labrum lesion of left shoulder
    - ● S43.439   Superior glenoid labrum lesion of `unspecified` shoulder

- ● S43.49   Other sprain of shoulder joint
  - ● S43.491   Other sprain of right shoulder joint
  - ● S43.492   Other sprain of left shoulder joint
  - ● S43.499   Other sprain of `unspecified` shoulder joint
- ● S43.5   Sprain of acromioclavicular joint
  Sprain of acromioclavicular ligament
  - X ● S43.50   Sprain of `unspecified` acromioclavicular joint
  - X ● S43.51   Sprain of right acromioclavicular joint
  - X ● S43.52   Sprain of left acromioclavicular joint
- ● S43.6   Sprain of sternoclavicular joint
  - X ● S43.60   Sprain of `unspecified` sternoclavicular joint
  - X ● S43.61   Sprain of right sternoclavicular joint
  - X ● S43.62   Sprain of left sternoclavicular joint
- ● S43.8   Sprain of other specified parts of shoulder girdle
  - X ● S43.80   Sprain of other specified parts of `unspecified` shoulder girdle
  - X ● S43.81   Sprain of other specified parts of right shoulder girdle
  - X ● S43.82   Sprain of other specified parts of left shoulder girdle
- ● S43.9   Sprain of unspecified parts of shoulder girdle
  - X ● S43.90   Sprain of `unspecified` parts of unspecified shoulder girdle
    Sprain of shoulder girdle NOS
  - X ● S43.91   Sprain of `unspecified` parts of right shoulder girdle
  - X ● S43.92   Sprain of `unspecified` parts of left shoulder girdle

- ● S44   **Injury of nerves at shoulder and upper arm level**
  Code also any associated open wound (S41.-)
  > **Excludes2**   injury of brachial plexus (S14.3-)
  The appropriate 7th character is to be added to each code from category S44

A	initial encounter
D	subsequent encounter
S	sequela

  - ● S44.0   Injury of ulnar nerve at upper arm level
    > **Excludes1**   ulnar nerve NOS (S54.0)
    - X ● S44.00   Injury of ulnar nerve at upper arm level, `unspecified` arm
    - X ● S44.01   Injury of ulnar nerve at upper arm level, right arm
    - X ● S44.02   Injury of ulnar nerve at upper arm level, left arm
  - ● S44.1   Injury of median nerve at upper arm level
    > **Excludes1**   median nerve NOS (S54.1)
    - X ● S44.10   Injury of median nerve at upper arm level, `unspecified` arm
    - X ● S44.11   Injury of median nerve at upper arm level, right arm
    - X ● S44.12   Injury of median nerve at upper arm level, left arm
  - ● S44.2   Injury of radial nerve at upper arm level
    > **Excludes1**   radial nerve NOS (S54.2)
    - X ● S44.20   Injury of radial nerve at upper arm level, `unspecified` arm
    - X ● S44.21   Injury of radial nerve at upper arm level, right arm
    - X ● S44.22   Injury of radial nerve at upper arm level, left arm

1310

◀ New   ◀▥ Revised   ~~deleted~~ Deleted   Excludes 1   Excludes 2   Includes   Use additional   Code first   Code also   Unspecified

OGCR Official Guidelines   X Assign placeholder X   ● Use Additional Character(s)   ▶ Manifestation Code   **Coding Clinic**

● **S44.3   Injury of axillary nerve**
  X● **S44.30**   Injury of axillary nerve, unspecified arm
  X● **S44.31**   Injury of axillary nerve, right arm
  X● **S44.32**   Injury of axillary nerve, left arm
● **S44.4   Injury of musculocutaneous nerve**
  X● **S44.40**   Injury of musculocutaneous nerve, unspecified arm
  X● **S44.41**   Injury of musculocutaneous nerve, right arm
  X● **S44.42**   Injury of musculocutaneous nerve, left arm
● **S44.5   Injury of cutaneous sensory nerve at shoulder and upper arm level**
  X● **S44.50**   Injury of cutaneous sensory nerve at shoulder and upper arm level, unspecified arm
  X● **S44.51**   Injury of cutaneous sensory nerve at shoulder and upper arm level, right arm
  X● **S44.52**   Injury of cutaneous sensory nerve at shoulder and upper arm level, left arm
● **S44.8   Injury of other nerves at shoulder and upper arm level**
  ● **S44.8X**   Injury of other nerves at shoulder and upper arm level
    ● **S44.8X1**   Injury of other nerves at shoulder and upper arm level, right arm
    ● **S44.8X2**   Injury of other nerves at shoulder and upper arm level, left arm
    ● **S44.8X9**   Injury of other nerves at shoulder and upper arm level, unspecified arm
● **S44.9   Injury of unspecified nerve at shoulder and upper arm level**
  X● **S44.90**   Injury of unspecified nerve at shoulder and upper arm level, unspecified arm
  X● **S44.91**   Injury of unspecified nerve at shoulder and upper arm level, right arm
  X● **S44.92**   Injury of unspecified nerve at shoulder and upper arm level, left arm

● **S45   Injury of blood vessels at shoulder and upper arm level**
  Code also any associated open wound (S41.-)
  Excludes2   injury of subclavian artery (S25.1)
             injury of subclavian vein (S25.3)
  The appropriate 7th character is to be added to each code from category S45

A	initial encounter
D	subsequent encounter
S	sequela

● **S45.0   Injury of axillary artery**
  ● **S45.00**   Unspecified injury of axillary artery
    ● **S45.001**   Unspecified injury of axillary artery, right side
    ● **S45.002**   Unspecified injury of axillary artery, left side
    ● **S45.009**   Unspecified injury of axillary artery, unspecified side
  ● **S45.01**   Laceration of axillary artery
    ● **S45.011**   Laceration of axillary artery, right side
    ● **S45.012**   Laceration of axillary artery, left side
    ● **S45.019**   Laceration of axillary artery, unspecified side
  ● **S45.09**   Other specified injury of axillary artery
    ● **S45.091**   Other specified injury of axillary artery, right side
    ● **S45.092**   Other specified injury of axillary artery, left side
    ● **S45.099**   Other specified injury of axillary artery, unspecified side

● **S45.1   Injury of brachial artery**
  ● **S45.10**   Unspecified injury of brachial artery
    ● **S45.101**   Unspecified injury of brachial artery, right side
    ● **S45.102**   Unspecified injury of brachial artery, left side
    ● **S45.109**   Unspecified injury of brachial artery, unspecified side
  ● **S45.11**   Laceration of brachial artery
    ● **S45.111**   Laceration of brachial artery, right side
    ● **S45.112**   Laceration of brachial artery, left side
    ● **S45.119**   Laceration of brachial artery, unspecified side
  ● **S45.19**   Other specified injury of brachial artery
    ● **S45.191**   Other specified injury of brachial artery, right side
    ● **S45.192**   Other specified injury of brachial artery, left side
    ● **S45.199**   Other specified injury of brachial artery, unspecified side
● **S45.2   Injury of axillary or brachial vein**
  ● **S45.20**   Unspecified injury of axillary or brachial vein
    ● **S45.201**   Unspecified injury of axillary or brachial vein, right side
    ● **S45.202**   Unspecified injury of axillary or brachial vein, left side
    ● **S45.209**   Unspecified injury of axillary or brachial vein, unspecified side
  ● **S45.21**   Laceration of axillary or brachial vein
    ● **S45.211**   Laceration of axillary or brachial vein, right side
    ● **S45.212**   Laceration of axillary or brachial vein, left side
    ● **S45.219**   Laceration of axillary or brachial vein, unspecified side
  ● **S45.29**   Other specified injury of axillary or brachial vein
    ● **S45.291**   Other specified injury of axillary or brachial vein, right side
    ● **S45.292**   Other specified injury of axillary or brachial vein, left side
    ● **S45.299**   Other specified injury of axillary or brachial vein, unspecified side
● **S45.3   Injury of superficial vein at shoulder and upper arm level**
  ● **S45.30**   Unspecified injury of superficial vein at shoulder and upper arm level
    ● **S45.301**   Unspecified injury of superficial vein at shoulder and upper arm level, right arm
    ● **S45.302**   Unspecified injury of superficial vein at shoulder and upper arm level, left arm
    ● **S45.309**   Unspecified injury of superficial vein at shoulder and upper arm level, unspecified arm
  ● **S45.31**   Laceration of superficial vein at shoulder and upper arm level
    ● **S45.311**   Laceration of superficial vein at shoulder and upper arm level, right arm
    ● **S45.312**   Laceration of superficial vein at shoulder and upper arm level, left arm
    ● **S45.319**   Laceration of superficial vein at shoulder and upper arm level, unspecified arm

CHAPTER 19 (S00-T88)

● S45.39   Other specified injury of superficial vein at shoulder and upper arm level
  ● S45.391   Other specified injury of superficial vein at shoulder and upper arm level, right arm
  ● S45.392   Other specified injury of superficial vein at shoulder and upper arm level, left arm
  ● S45.399   Other specified injury of superficial vein at shoulder and upper arm level, unspecified arm

● S45.8   Injury of other specified blood vessels at shoulder and upper arm level
 ● S45.80   Unspecified injury of other specified blood vessels at shoulder and upper arm level
  ● S45.801   Unspecified injury of other specified blood vessels at shoulder and upper arm level, right arm
  ● S45.802   Unspecified injury of other specified blood vessels at shoulder and upper arm level, left arm
  ● S45.809   Unspecified injury of other specified blood vessels at shoulder and upper arm level, unspecified arm
 ● S45.81   Laceration of other specified blood vessels at shoulder and upper arm level
  ● S45.811   Laceration of other specified blood vessels at shoulder and upper arm level, right arm
  ● S45.812   Laceration of other specified blood vessels at shoulder and upper arm level, left arm
  ● S45.819   Laceration of other specified blood vessels at shoulder and upper arm level, unspecified arm
 ● S45.89   Other specified injury of other specified blood vessels at shoulder and upper arm level
  ● S45.891   Other specified injury of other specified blood vessels at shoulder and upper arm level, right arm
  ● S45.892   Other specified injury of other specified blood vessels at shoulder and upper arm level, left arm
  ● S45.899   Other specified injury of other specified blood vessels at shoulder and upper arm level, unspecified arm

● S45.9   Injury of unspecified blood vessel at shoulder and upper arm level
 ● S45.90   Unspecified injury of unspecified blood vessel at shoulder and upper arm level
  ● S45.901   Unspecified injury of unspecified blood vessel at shoulder and upper arm level, right arm
  ● S45.902   Unspecified injury of unspecified blood vessel at shoulder and upper arm level, left arm
  ● S45.909   Unspecified injury of unspecified blood vessel at shoulder and upper arm level, unspecified arm
 ● S45.91   Laceration of unspecified blood vessel at shoulder and upper arm level
  ● S45.911   Laceration of unspecified blood vessel at shoulder and upper arm level, right arm
  ● S45.912   Laceration of unspecified blood vessel at shoulder and upper arm level, left arm
  ● S45.919   Laceration of unspecified blood vessel at shoulder and upper arm level, unspecified arm

● S45.99   Other specified injury of unspecified blood vessel at shoulder and upper arm level
  ● S45.991   Other specified injury of unspecified blood vessel at shoulder and upper arm level, right arm
  ● S45.992   Other specified injury of unspecified blood vessel at shoulder and upper arm level, left arm
  ● S45.999   Other specified injury of unspecified blood vessel at shoulder and upper arm level, unspecified arm

● S46   Injury of muscle, fascia and tendon at shoulder and upper arm level

  Code also any associated open wound (S41.-)

  Excludes2   injury of muscle, fascia and tendon at elbow (S56.-)
              sprain of joints and ligaments of shoulder girdle (S43.9)

  The appropriate 7th character is to be added to each code from category S46

A	initial encounter
D	subsequent encounter
S	sequela

● S46.0   Injury of muscle(s) and tendon(s) of the rotator cuff of shoulder
 ● S46.00   Unspecified injury of muscle(s) and tendon(s) of the rotator cuff of shoulder
  ● S46.001   Unspecified injury of muscle(s) and tendon(s) of the rotator cuff of right shoulder
  ● S46.002   Unspecified injury of muscle(s) and tendon(s) of the rotator cuff of left shoulder
  ● S46.009   Unspecified injury of muscle(s) and tendon(s) of the rotator cuff of unspecified shoulder
 ● S46.01   Strain of muscle(s) and tendon(s) of the rotator cuff of shoulder
   Acute onset due to trauma to rotator cuff muscle/tendon
  ● S46.011   Strain of muscle(s) and tendon(s) of the rotator cuff of right shoulder
  ● S46.012   Strain of muscle(s) and tendon(s) of the rotator cuff of left shoulder
  ● S46.019   Strain of muscle(s) and tendon(s) of the rotator cuff of unspecified shoulder
 ● S46.02   Laceration of muscle(s) and tendon(s) of the rotator cuff of shoulder
  ● S46.021   Laceration of muscle(s) and tendon(s) of the rotator cuff of right shoulder
  ● S46.022   Laceration of muscle(s) and tendon(s) of the rotator cuff of left shoulder
  ● S46.029   Laceration of muscle(s) and tendon(s) of the rotator cuff of unspecified shoulder
 ● S46.09   Other injury of muscle(s) and tendon(s) of the rotator cuff of shoulder
  ● S46.091   Other injury of muscle(s) and tendon(s) of the rotator cuff of right shoulder
  ● S46.092   Other injury of muscle(s) and tendon(s) of the rotator cuff of left shoulder
  ● S46.099   Other injury of muscle(s) and tendon(s) of the rotator cuff of unspecified shoulder

◀ New   ◀⊪ Revised   ~~deleted~~ Deleted   Excludes 1   Excludes 2   Includes   Use additional   Code first   Code also   Unspecified
OGCR Official Guidelines   X Assign placeholder X   ● Use Additional Character(s)   ▶ Manifestation Code   **Coding Clinic**

● **S46.1　Injury of muscle, fascia and tendon of long head of biceps**
  ● **S46.10　Unspecified injury of muscle, fascia and tendon of long head of biceps**
    ● S46.101　Unspecified injury of muscle, fascia and tendon of long head of biceps, right arm
    ● S46.102　Unspecified injury of muscle, fascia and tendon of long head of biceps, left arm
    ● S46.109　Unspecified injury of muscle, fascia and tendon of long head of biceps, unspecified arm
  ● **S46.11　Strain of muscle, fascia and tendon of long head of biceps**
    ● S46.111　Strain of muscle, fascia and tendon of long head of biceps, right arm
    ● S46.112　Strain of muscle, fascia and tendon of long head of biceps, left arm
    ● S46.119　Strain of muscle, fascia and tendon of long head of biceps, unspecified arm
  ● **S46.12　Laceration of muscle, fascia and tendon of long head of biceps**
    ● S46.121　Laceration of muscle, fascia and tendon of long head of biceps, right arm
    ● S46.122　Laceration of muscle, fascia and tendon of long head of biceps, left arm
    ● S46.129　Laceration of muscle, fascia and tendon of long head of biceps, unspecified arm
  ● **S46.19　Other injury of muscle, fascia and tendon of long head of biceps**
    ● S46.191　Other injury of muscle, fascia and tendon of long head of biceps, right arm
    ● S46.192　Other injury of muscle, fascia and tendon of long head of biceps, left arm
    ● S46.199　Other injury of muscle, fascia and tendon of long head of biceps, unspecified arm
● **S46.2　Injury of muscle, fascia and tendon of other parts of biceps**
  ● **S46.20　Unspecified injury of muscle, fascia and tendon of other parts of biceps**
    ● S46.201　Unspecified injury of muscle, fascia and tendon of other parts of biceps, right arm
    ● S46.202　Unspecified injury of muscle, fascia and tendon of other parts of biceps, left arm
    ● S46.209　Unspecified injury of muscle, fascia and tendon of other parts of biceps, unspecified arm
  ● **S46.21　Strain of muscle, fascia and tendon of other parts of biceps**
    ● S46.211　Strain of muscle, fascia and tendon of other parts of biceps, right arm
    ● S46.212　Strain of muscle, fascia and tendon of other parts of biceps, left arm
    ● S46.219　Strain of muscle, fascia and tendon of other parts of biceps, unspecified arm

● **S46.22　Laceration of muscle, fascia and tendon of other parts of biceps**
    ● S46.221　Laceration of muscle, fascia and tendon of other parts of biceps, right arm
    ● S46.222　Laceration of muscle, fascia and tendon of other parts of biceps, left arm
    ● S46.229　Laceration of muscle, fascia and tendon of other parts of biceps, unspecified arm
  ● **S46.29　Other injury of muscle, fascia and tendon of other parts of biceps**
    ● S46.291　Other injury of muscle, fascia and tendon of other parts of biceps, right arm
    ● S46.292　Other injury of muscle, fascia and tendon of other parts of biceps, left arm
    ● S46.299　Other injury of muscle, fascia and tendon of other parts of biceps, unspecified arm
● **S46.3　Injury of muscle, fascia and tendon of triceps**
  ● **S46.30　Unspecified injury of muscle, fascia and tendon of triceps**
    ● S46.301　Unspecified injury of muscle, fascia and tendon of triceps, right arm
    ● S46.302　Unspecified injury of muscle, fascia and tendon of triceps, left arm
    ● S46.309　Unspecified injury of muscle, fascia and tendon of triceps, unspecified arm
  ● **S46.31　Strain of muscle, fascia and tendon of triceps**
    ● S46.311　Strain of muscle, fascia and tendon of triceps, right arm
    ● S46.312　Strain of muscle, fascia and tendon of triceps, left arm
    ● S46.319　Strain of muscle, fascia and tendon of triceps, unspecified arm
  ● **S46.32　Laceration of muscle, fascia and tendon of triceps**
    ● S46.321　Laceration of muscle, fascia and tendon of triceps, right arm
    ● S46.322　Laceration of muscle, fascia and tendon of triceps, left arm
    ● S46.329　Laceration of muscle, fascia and tendon of triceps, unspecified arm
  ● **S46.39　Other injury of muscle, fascia and tendon of triceps**
    ● S46.391　Other injury of muscle, fascia and tendon of triceps, right arm
    ● S46.392　Other injury of muscle, fascia and tendon of triceps, left arm
    ● S46.399　Other injury of muscle, fascia and tendon of triceps, unspecified arm
● **S46.8　Injury of other muscles, fascia and tendons at shoulder and upper arm level**
  ● **S46.80　Unspecified injury of other muscles, fascia and tendons at shoulder and upper arm level**
    ● S46.801　Unspecified injury of other muscles, fascia and tendons at shoulder and upper arm level, right arm
    ● S46.802　Unspecified injury of other muscles, fascia and tendons at shoulder and upper arm level, left arm
    ● S46.809　Unspecified injury of other muscles, fascia and tendons at shoulder and upper arm level, unspecified arm

CHAPTER 19 (S00-T88)

● S46.81   Strain of other muscles, fascia and tendons at shoulder and upper arm level

     ● S46.811   Strain of other muscles, fascia and tendons at shoulder and upper arm level, right arm

     ● S46.812   Strain of other muscles, fascia and tendons at shoulder and upper arm level, left arm

     ● S46.819   Strain of other muscles, fascia and tendons at shoulder and upper arm level, unspecified arm

● S46.82   Laceration of other muscles, fascia and tendons at shoulder and upper arm level

     ● S46.821   Laceration of other muscles, fascia and tendons at shoulder and upper arm level, right arm

     ● S46.822   Laceration of other muscles, fascia and tendons at shoulder and upper arm level, left arm

     ● S46.829   Laceration of other muscles, fascia and tendons at shoulder and upper arm level, unspecified arm

● S46.89   Other injury of other muscles, fascia and tendons at shoulder and upper arm level

     ● S46.891   Other injury of other muscles, fascia and tendons at shoulder and upper arm level, right arm

     ● S46.892   Other injury of other muscles, fascia and tendons at shoulder and upper arm level, left arm

     ● S46.899   Other injury of other muscles, fascia and tendons at shoulder and upper arm level, unspecified arm

● S46.9   Injury of unspecified muscle, fascia and tendon at shoulder and upper arm level

     ● S46.90   Unspecified injury of unspecified muscle, fascia and tendon at shoulder and upper arm level

         ● S46.901   Unspecified injury of unspecified muscle, fascia and tendon at shoulder and upper arm level, right arm

         ● S46.902   Unspecified injury of unspecified muscle, fascia and tendon at shoulder and upper arm level, left arm

         ● S46.909   Unspecified injury of unspecified muscle, fascia and tendon at shoulder and upper arm level, unspecified arm

     ● S46.91   Strain of unspecified muscle, fascia and tendon at shoulder and upper arm level

         ● S46.911   Strain of unspecified muscle, fascia and tendon at shoulder and upper arm level, right arm

         ● S46.912   Strain of unspecified muscle, fascia and tendon at shoulder and upper arm level, left arm

         ● S46.919   Strain of unspecified muscle, fascia and tendon at shoulder and upper arm level, unspecified arm

     ● S46.92   Laceration of unspecified muscle, fascia and tendon at shoulder and upper arm level

         ● S46.921   Laceration of unspecified muscle, fascia and tendon at shoulder and upper arm level, right arm

         ● S46.922   Laceration of unspecified muscle, fascia and tendon at shoulder and upper arm level, left arm

         ● S46.929   Laceration of unspecified muscle, fascia and tendon at shoulder and upper arm level, unspecified arm

● S46.99   Other injury of unspecified muscle, fascia and tendon at shoulder and upper arm level

     ● S46.991   Other injury of unspecified muscle, fascia and tendon at shoulder and upper arm level, right arm

     ● S46.992   Other injury of unspecified muscle, fascia and tendon at shoulder and upper arm level, left arm

     ● S46.999   Other injury of unspecified muscle, fascia and tendon at shoulder and upper arm level, unspecified arm

● **S47**   **Crushing injury of shoulder and upper arm**

     Use additional code for all associated injuries

     Excludes2   crushing injury of elbow (S57.0-)

     The appropriate 7th character is to be added to each code from category S47

A	initial encounter
D	subsequent encounter
S	sequela

X ● S47.1   Crushing injury of right shoulder and upper arm

X ● S47.2   Crushing injury of left shoulder and upper arm

X ● S47.9   Crushing injury of shoulder and upper arm, unspecified arm

● **S48**   **Traumatic amputation of shoulder and upper arm**

     An amputation not identified as partial or complete should be coded to complete

     Excludes1   traumatic amputation at elbow level (S58.0)

     The appropriate 7th character is to be added to each code from category S48

A	initial encounter
D	subsequent encounter
S	sequela

● S48.0   Traumatic amputation at shoulder joint

     ● S48.01   Complete traumatic amputation at shoulder joint

         ● S48.011   Complete traumatic amputation at right shoulder joint

         ● S48.012   Complete traumatic amputation at left shoulder joint

         ● S48.019   Complete traumatic amputation at unspecified shoulder joint

     ● S48.02   Partial traumatic amputation at shoulder joint

         ● S48.021   Partial traumatic amputation at right shoulder joint

         ● S48.022   Partial traumatic amputation at left shoulder joint

         ● S48.029   Partial traumatic amputation at unspecified shoulder joint

● S48.1   Traumatic amputation at level between shoulder and elbow

     ● S48.11   Complete traumatic amputation at level between shoulder and elbow

         ● S48.111   Complete traumatic amputation at level between right shoulder and elbow

         ● S48.112   Complete traumatic amputation at level between left shoulder and elbow

         ● S48.119   Complete traumatic amputation at level between unspecified shoulder and elbow

● **S48.12** Partial traumatic amputation at level between shoulder and elbow
  ● **S48.121** Partial traumatic amputation at level between right shoulder and elbow
  ● **S48.122** Partial traumatic amputation at level between left shoulder and elbow
  ● **S48.129** Partial traumatic amputation at level between unspecified shoulder and elbow
● **S48.9** Traumatic amputation of shoulder and upper arm, level unspecified
  ● **S48.91** Complete traumatic amputation of shoulder and upper arm, level unspecified
    ● **S48.911** Complete traumatic amputation of right shoulder and upper arm, level unspecified
    ● **S48.912** Complete traumatic amputation of left shoulder and upper arm, level unspecified
    ● **S48.919** Complete traumatic amputation of unspecified shoulder and upper arm, level unspecified
  ● **S48.92** Partial traumatic amputation of shoulder and upper arm, level unspecified
    ● **S48.921** Partial traumatic amputation of right shoulder and upper arm, level unspecified
    ● **S48.922** Partial traumatic amputation of left shoulder and upper arm, level unspecified
    ● **S48.929** Partial traumatic amputation of unspecified shoulder and upper arm, level unspecified

● **S49** Other and unspecified injuries of shoulder and upper arm

The appropriate 7th character is to be added to each code from subcategories S49.0 and S49.1

A	initial encounter for closed fracture
D	subsequent encounter for fracture with routine healing
G	subsequent encounter for fracture with delayed healing
K	subsequent encounter for fracture with nonunion
P	subsequent encounter for fracture with malunion
S	sequela

● **S49.0** Physeal fracture of upper end of humerus
  ● **S49.00** Unspecified physeal fracture of upper end of humerus
    ● **S49.001** Unspecified physeal fracture of upper end of humerus, right arm
    ● **S49.002** Unspecified physeal fracture of upper end of humerus, left arm
    ● **S49.009** Unspecified physeal fracture of upper end of humerus, unspecified arm
  ● **S49.01** Salter-Harris Type I physeal fracture of upper end of humerus
    ● **S49.011** Salter-Harris Type I physeal fracture of upper end of humerus, right arm
    ● **S49.012** Salter-Harris Type I physeal fracture of upper end of humerus, left arm
    ● **S49.019** Salter-Harris Type I physeal fracture of upper end of humerus, unspecified arm

Item 19-3 SALTER-HARRIS TYPE 1: epiphysis is completely separated from end of bone, or metaphysic growth plate remains attached to epiphysis
SALTER-HARRIS TYPE 2: epiphysis and growth plate are partially separated from metaphysis, which is cracked—most common type
SALTER-HARRIS TYPE 3: fracture occurring through epiphysis and separates part of epiphysis and growth plate from metaphysis fracture, usually at distal end of tibia
SALTER-HARRIS TYPE 4: fracture runs through epiphysis, across growth plate, into metaphysic, surgery is required to restore joint surface to normal and align growth plate

  ● **S49.02** Salter-Harris Type II physeal fracture of upper end of humerus
    ● **S49.021** Salter-Harris Type II physeal fracture of upper end of humerus, right arm
    ● **S49.022** Salter-Harris Type II physeal fracture of upper end of humerus, left arm
    ● **S49.029** Salter-Harris Type II physeal fracture of upper end of humerus, unspecified arm
  ● **S49.03** Salter-Harris Type III physeal fracture of upper end of humerus
    ● **S49.031** Salter Harris Type III physeal fracture of upper end of humerus, right arm
    ● **S49.032** Salter Harris Type III physeal fracture of upper end of humerus, left arm
    ● **S49.039** Salter Harris Type III physeal fracture of upper end of humerus, unspecified arm
  ● **S49.04** Salter-Harris Type IV physeal fracture of upper end of humerus
    ● **S49.041** Salter-Harris Type IV physeal fracture of upper end of humerus, right arm
    ● **S49.042** Salter-Harris Type IV physeal fracture of upper end of humerus, left arm
    ● **S49.049** Salter-Harris Type IV physeal fracture of upper end of humerus, unspecified arm
  ● **S49.09** Other physeal fracture of upper end of humerus
    ● **S49.091** Other physeal fracture of upper end of humerus, right arm
    ● **S49.092** Other physeal fracture of upper end of humerus, left arm
    ● **S49.099** Other physeal fracture of upper end of humerus, unspecified arm
● **S49.1** Physeal fracture of lower end of humerus
  ● **S49.10** Unspecified physeal fracture of lower end of humerus
    ● **S49.101** Unspecified physeal fracture of lower end of humerus, right arm
    ● **S49.102** Unspecified physeal fracture of lower end of humerus, left arm
    ● **S49.109** Unspecified physeal fracture of lower end of humerus, unspecified arm
  ● **S49.11** Salter-Harris Type I physeal fracture of lower end of humerus
    ● **S49.111** Salter-Harris Type I physeal fracture of lower end of humerus, right arm
    ● **S49.112** Salter-Harris Type I physeal fracture of lower end of humerus, left arm
    ● **S49.119** Salter-Harris Type I physeal fracture of lower end of humerus, unspecified arm

CHAPTER 19 (S00-T88)

● **S49.12**   **Salter-Harris Type II physeal fracture of lower end of humerus**
    ● **S49.121**   Salter-Harris Type II physeal fracture of lower end of humerus, right arm
    ● **S49.122**   Salter-Harris Type II physeal fracture of lower end of humerus, left arm
    ● **S49.129**   Salter-Harris Type II physeal fracture of lower end of humerus, unspecified arm

● **S49.13**   **Salter Harris Type III physeal fracture of lower end of humerus**
    ● **S49.131**   Salter Harris Type III physeal fracture of lower end of humerus, right arm
    ● **S49.132**   Salter Harris Type III physeal fracture of lower end of humerus, left arm
    ● **S49.139**   Salter Harris Type III physeal fracture of lower end of humerus, unspecified arm

● **S49.14**   **Salter-Harris Type IV physeal fracture of lower end of humerus**
    ● **S49.141**   Salter-Harris Type IV physeal fracture of lower end of humerus, right arm
    ● **S49.142**   Salter-Harris Type IV physeal fracture of lower end of humerus, left arm
    ● **S49.149**   Salter-Harris Type IV physeal fracture of lower end of humerus, unspecified arm

● **S49.19**   **Other physeal fracture of lower end of humerus**
    ● **S49.191**   Other physeal fracture of lower end of humerus, right arm
    ● **S49.192**   Other physeal fracture of lower end of humerus, left arm
    ● **S49.199**   Other physeal fracture of lower end of humerus, unspecified arm

● **S49.8**   **Other specified injuries of shoulder and upper arm**

The appropriate 7th character is to be added to each code in subcategory S49.8

A	initial encounter
D	subsequent encounter
S	sequela

X ● **S49.80**   Other specified injuries of shoulder and upper arm, unspecified arm
X ● **S49.81**   Other specified injuries of right shoulder and upper arm
X ● **S49.82**   Other specified injuries of left shoulder and upper arm

● **S49.9**   **Unspecified injury of shoulder and upper arm**

The appropriate 7th character is to be added to each code in subcategory S49.9

A	initial encounter
D	subsequent encounter
S	sequela

X ● **S49.90**   Unspecified injury of shoulder and upper arm, unspecified arm
X ● **S49.91**   Unspecified injury of right shoulder and upper arm
X ● **S49.92**   Unspecified injury of left shoulder and upper arm

INJURIES TO THE ELBOW AND FOREARM (S50-S59)

Excludes2   burns and corrosions (T20-T32)
           frostbite (T33-T34)
           injuries of wrist and hand (S60-S69)
           insect bite or sting, venomous (T63.4)

● **S50**   **Superficial injury of elbow and forearm**
Excludes2   superficial injury of wrist and hand (S60.-)

The appropriate 7th character is to be added to each code from category S50

A	initial encounter
D	subsequent encounter
S	sequela

● **S50.0**   **Contusion of elbow**
X ● **S50.00**   Contusion of unspecified elbow
X ● **S50.01**   Contusion of right elbow
X ● **S50.02**   Contusion of left elbow

● **S50.1**   **Contusion of forearm**
X ● **S50.10**   Contusion of unspecified forearm
X ● **S50.11**   Contusion of right forearm
X ● **S50.12**   Contusion of left forearm

● **S50.3**   **Other superficial injuries of elbow**
   ● **S50.31**   **Abrasion of elbow**
     ● **S50.311**   Abrasion of right elbow
     ● **S50.312**   Abrasion of left elbow
     ● **S50.319**   Abrasion of unspecified elbow
   ● **S50.32**   **Blister (nonthermal) of elbow**
     ● **S50.321**   Blister (nonthermal) of right elbow
     ● **S50.322**   Blister (nonthermal) of left elbow
     ● **S50.329**   Blister (nonthermal) of unspecified elbow
   ● **S50.34**   **External constriction of elbow**
     ● **S50.341**   External constriction of right elbow
     ● **S50.342**   External constriction of left elbow
     ● **S50.349**   External constriction of unspecified elbow
   ● **S50.35**   **Superficial foreign body of elbow**
       Splinter in the elbow
     ● **S50.351**   Superficial foreign body of right elbow
     ● **S50.352**   Superficial foreign body of left elbow
     ● **S50.359**   Superficial foreign body of unspecified elbow
   ● **S50.36**   **Insect bite (nonvenomous) of elbow**
     ● **S50.361**   Insect bite (nonvenomous) of right elbow
     ● **S50.362**   Insect bite (nonvenomous) of left elbow
     ● **S50.369**   Insect bite (nonvenomous) of unspecified elbow
   ● **S50.37**   **Other superficial bite of elbow**
       Excludes1   open bite of elbow (S51.04)
     ● **S50.371**   Other superficial bite of right elbow
     ● **S50.372**   Other superficial bite of left elbow
     ● **S50.379**   Other superficial bite of unspecified elbow

● **S50.8**   **Other superficial injuries of forearm**
   ● **S50.81**   **Abrasion of forearm**
     ● **S50.811**   Abrasion of right forearm
     ● **S50.812**   Abrasion of left forearm
     ● **S50.819**   Abrasion of unspecified forearm

◀ New   ◀≡ Revised   ~~deleted~~ Deleted   Excludes 1   Excludes 2   Includes   Use additional   Code first   Code also   Unspecified
OGCR Official Guidelines   **X** Assign placeholder X   ● Use Additional Character(s)   ▶ Manifestation Code   **Coding Clinic**

● **S50.82 Blister (nonthermal) of forearm**
    ● S50.821 Blister (nonthermal) of right forearm
    ● S50.822 Blister (nonthermal) of left forearm
    ● S50.829 Blister (nonthermal) of unspecified forearm
● **S50.84 External constriction of forearm**
    ● S50.841 External constriction of right forearm
    ● S50.842 External constriction of left forearm
    ● S50.849 External constriction of unspecified forearm
● **S50.85 Superficial foreign body of forearm**
    Splinter in the forearm
    ● S50.851 Superficial foreign body of right forearm
    ● S50.852 Superficial foreign body of left forearm
    ● S50.859 Superficial foreign body of unspecified forearm
● **S50.86 Insect bite (nonvenomous) of forearm**
    ● S50.861 Insect bite (nonvenomous) of right forearm
    ● S50.862 Insect bite (nonvenomous) of left forearm
    ● S50.869 Insect bite (nonvenomous) of unspecified forearm
● **S50.87 Other superficial bite of forearm**
    Excludes1 open bite of forearm (S51.84)
    ● S50.871 Other superficial bite of right forearm
    ● S50.872 Other superficial bite of left forearm
    ● S50.879 Other superficial bite of unspecified forearm
● **S50.9 Unspecified superficial injury of elbow and forearm**
  ● S50.90 Unspecified superficial injury of elbow
    ● S50.901 Unspecified superficial injury of right elbow
    ● S50.902 Unspecified superficial injury of left elbow
    ● S50.909 Unspecified superficial injury of unspecified elbow
  ● S50.91 Unspecified superficial injury of forearm
    ● S50.911 Unspecified superficial injury of right forearm
    ● S50.912 Unspecified superficial injury of left forearm
    ● S50.919 Unspecified superficial injury of unspecified forearm

● **S51 Open wound of elbow and forearm**
  Code also any associated wound infection
  Excludes1 open fracture of elbow and forearm (S52.- with open fracture 7th character)
        traumatic amputation of elbow and forearm (S58.-)
  Excludes2 open wound of wrist and hand (S61.-)
  The appropriate 7th character is to be added to each code from category S51

A	initial encounter
D	subsequent encounter
S	sequela

● **S51.0 Open wound of elbow**
  ● S51.00 Unspecified open wound of elbow
    ● S51.001 Unspecified open wound of right elbow
        Coding Clinic: 2012, Q4, P108
    ● S51.002 Unspecified open wound of left elbow
    ● S51.009 Unspecified open wound of unspecified elbow
        Open wound of elbow NOS

● **S51.01 Laceration without foreign body of elbow**
    ● S51.011 Laceration without foreign body of right elbow
    ● S51.012 Laceration without foreign body of left elbow
    ● S51.019 Laceration without foreign body of unspecified elbow
● **S51.02 Laceration with foreign body of elbow**
    ● S51.021 Laceration with foreign body of right elbow
    ● S51.022 Laceration with foreign body of left elbow
    ● S51.029 Laceration with foreign body of unspecified elbow
● **S51.03 Puncture wound without foreign body of elbow**
    ● S51.031 Puncture wound without foreign body of right elbow
    ● S51.032 Puncture wound without foreign body of left elbow
    ● S51.039 Puncture wound without foreign body of unspecified elbow
● **S51.04 Puncture wound with foreign body of elbow**
    ● S51.041 Puncture wound with foreign body of right elbow
    ● S51.042 Puncture wound with foreign body of left elbow
    ● S51.049 Puncture wound with foreign body of unspecified elbow
● **S51.05 Open bite of elbow**
    Bite of elbow NOS
    Excludes1 superficial bite of elbow (S50.36, S50.37)
    ● S51.051 Open bite, right elbow
    ● S51.052 Open bite, left elbow
    ● S51.059 Open bite, unspecified elbow
● **S51.8 Open wound of forearm**
  Excludes2 open wound of elbow (S51.0-)
  ● S51.80 Unspecified open wound of forearm
    ● S51.801 Unspecified open wound of right forearm
    ● S51.802 Unspecified open wound of left forearm
    ● S51.809 Unspecified open wound of unspecified forearm
        Open wound of forearm NOS
  ● S51.81 Laceration without foreign body of forearm
    ● S51.811 Laceration without foreign body of right forearm
    ● S51.812 Laceration without foreign body of left forearm
    ● S51.819 Laceration without foreign body of unspecified forearm
  ● S51.82 Laceration with foreign body of forearm
    ● S51.821 Laceration with foreign body of right forearm
    ● S51.822 Laceration with foreign body of left forearm
    ● S51.829 Laceration with foreign body of unspecified forearm
  ● S51.83 Puncture wound without foreign body of forearm
    ● S51.831 Puncture wound without foreign body of right forearm
    ● S51.832 Puncture wound without foreign body of left forearm
    ● S51.839 Puncture wound without foreign body of unspecified forearm

● **S51.84**   **Puncture wound with foreign body of forearm**
- ● **S51.841**   **Puncture wound with foreign body of right forearm**
- ● **S51.842**   **Puncture wound with foreign body of left forearm**
- ● **S51.849**   **Puncture wound with foreign body of** unspecified **forearm**

● **S51.85**   **Open bite of forearm**
     Bite of forearm NOS

     Excludes1   superficial bite of forearm (S50.86, S50.87)

- ● **S51.851**   **Open bite of right forearm**
- ● **S51.852**   **Open bite of left forearm**
- ● **S51.859**   **Open bite of** unspecified **forearm**

● **S52**   **Fracture of forearm**

     Note: A fracture not identified as displaced or nondisplaced should be coded to displaced

     A fracture not designated as open or closed should be coded to closed

     The open fracture designations are based on the Gustilo open fracture classification

     Excludes1   traumatic amputation of forearm (S58.-)
     Excludes2   fracture at wrist and hand level (S62.-)

     The appropriate 7th character is to be added to all codes from category S52

A	initial encounter for closed fracture
B	initial encounter for open fracture type I or II initial encounter for open fracture NOS
C	initial encounter for open fracture type IIIA, IIIB, or IIIC
D	subsequent encounter for closed fracture with routine healing
E	subsequent encounter for open fracture type I or II with routine healing
F	subsequent encounter for open fracture type IIIA, IIIB, or IIIC with routine healing
G	subsequent encounter for closed fracture with delayed healing
H	subsequent encounter for open fracture type I or II with delayed healing
J	subsequent encounter for open fracture type IIIA, IIIB, or IIIC with delayed healing
K	subsequent encounter for closed fracture with nonunion
M	subsequent encounter for open fracture type I or II with nonunion
N	subsequent encounter for open fracture type IIIA, IIIB, or IIIC with nonunion
P	subsequent encounter for closed fracture with malunion
Q	subsequent encounter for open fracture type I or II with malunion
R	subsequent encounter for open fracture type IIIA, IIIB, or IIIC with malunion
S	sequela

● **S52.0**   **Fracture of upper end of ulna**
     Fracture of proximal end of ulna

     Excludes2   fracture of elbow NOS (S42.40-)
                     fractures of shaft of ulna (S52.2-)

● **S52.00**   **Unspecified fracture of upper end of ulna**
- ● **S52.001**   Unspecified **fracture of upper end of right ulna**
- ● **S52.002**   Unspecified **fracture of upper end of left ulna**
- ● **S52.009**   Unspecified **fracture of upper end of unspecified ulna**

● **S52.01**   **Torus fracture of upper end of ulna**
     The appropriate 7th character is to be added to all codes in subcategory S52.01

A	initial encounter for closed fracture
D	subsequent encounter for fracture with routine healing
G	subsequent encounter for fracture with delayed healing
K	subsequent encounter for fracture with nonunion
P	subsequent encounter for fracture with malunion
S	sequela

- ● **S52.011**   **Torus fracture of upper end of right ulna**
- ● **S52.012**   **Torus fracture of upper end of left ulna**
- ● **S52.019**   **Torus fracture of upper end of** unspecified **ulna**

● **S52.02**   **Fracture of olecranon process without intraarticular extension of ulna**
- ● **S52.021**   **Displaced fracture of olecranon process without intraarticular extension of right ulna**
- ● **S52.022**   **Displaced fracture of olecranon process without intraarticular extension of left ulna**
- ● **S52.023**   **Displaced fracture of olecranon process without intraarticular extension of** unspecified **ulna**
- ● **S52.024**   **Nondisplaced fracture of olecranon process without intraarticular extension of right ulna**
- ● **S52.025**   **Nondisplaced fracture of olecranon process without intraarticular extension of left ulna**
- ● **S52.026**   **Nondisplaced fracture of olecranon process without intraarticular extension of** unspecified **ulna**

● **S52.03**   **Fracture of olecranon process with intraarticular extension of ulna**
- ● **S52.031**   **Displaced fracture of olecranon process with intraarticular extension of right ulna**
- ● **S52.032**   **Displaced fracture of olecranon process with intraarticular extension of left ulna**
- ● **S52.033**   **Displaced fracture of olecranon process with intraarticular extension of** unspecified **ulna**
- ● **S52.034**   **Nondisplaced fracture of olecranon process with intraarticular extension of right ulna**
- ● **S52.035**   **Nondisplaced fracture of olecranon process with intraarticular extension of left ulna**
- ● **S52.036**   **Nondisplaced fracture of olecranon process with intraarticular extension of** unspecified **ulna**

● **S52.04**   **Fracture of coronoid process of ulna**
- ● **S52.041**   **Displaced fracture of coronoid process of right ulna**
- ● **S52.042**   **Displaced fracture of coronoid process of left ulna**
- ● **S52.043**   **Displaced fracture of coronoid process of** unspecified **ulna**
- ● **S52.044**   **Nondisplaced fracture of coronoid process of right ulna**
- ● **S52.045**   **Nondisplaced fracture of coronoid process of left ulna**
- ● **S52.046**   **Nondisplaced fracture of coronoid process of** unspecified **ulna**

◄ New   ◄■ Revised   ~~deleted~~ Deleted   Excludes 1   Excludes 2   Includes   Use additional   Code first   Code also   Unspecified

OGCR Official Guidelines   **X** Assign placeholder X   ● Use Additional Character(s)   ▶ Manifestation Code   **Coding Clinic**

● **S52.09**　Other fracture of upper end of ulna
　● S52.091　Other fracture of upper end of right ulna
　● S52.092　Other fracture of upper end of left ulna
　● S52.099　Other fracture of upper end of unspecified ulna

● **S52.1**　Fracture of upper end of radius
　　Fracture of proximal end of radius
　　Excludes2　physeal fractures of upper end of radius (S59.2-)
　　　　　　　　　fracture of shaft of radius (S52.3-)

● **S52.10**　Unspecified fracture of upper end of radius
　● S52.101　Unspecified fracture of upper end of right radius
　● S52.102　Unspecified fracture of upper end of left radius
　● S52.109　Unspecified fracture of upper end of unspecified radius

● **S52.11**　Torus fracture of upper end of radius
　　The appropriate 7th character is to be added to all codes in subcategory S52.11

A	initial encounter for closed fracture
D	subsequent encounter for fracture with routine healing
G	subsequent encounter for fracture with delayed healing
K	subsequent encounter for fracture with nonunion
P	subsequent encounter for fracture with malunion
S	sequela

　● S52.111　Torus fracture of upper end of right radius
　● S52.112　Torus fracture of upper end of left radius
　● S52.119　Torus fracture of upper end of unspecified radius

● **S52.12**　Fracture of head of radius
　● S52.121　Displaced fracture of head of right radius
　● S52.122　Displaced fracture of head of left radius
　● S52.123　Displaced fracture of head of unspecified radius
　● S52.124　Nondisplaced fracture of head of right radius
　● S52.125　Nondisplaced fracture of head of left radius
　● S52.126　Nondisplaced fracture of head of unspecified radius

● **S52.13**　Fracture of neck of radius
　● S52.131　Displaced fracture of neck of right radius
　● S52.132　Displaced fracture of neck of left radius
　● S52.133　Displaced fracture of neck of unspecified radius
　● S52.134　Nondisplaced fracture of neck of right radius
　● S52.135　Nondisplaced fracture of neck of left radius
　● S52.136　Nondisplaced fracture of neck of unspecified radius

● **S52.18**　Other fracture of upper end of radius
　● S52.181　Other fracture of upper end of right radius
　● S52.182　Other fracture of upper end of left radius
　● S52.189　Other fracture of upper end of unspecified radius

● **S52.2**　Fracture of shaft of ulna
　● **S52.20**　Unspecified fracture of shaft of ulna
　　　Fracture of ulna NOS
　　● S52.201　Unspecified fracture of shaft of right ulna
　　● S52.202　Unspecified fracture of shaft of left ulna
　　● S52.209　Unspecified fracture of shaft of unspecified ulna

　● **S52.21**　Greenstick fracture of shaft of ulna
　　　The appropriate 7th character is to be added to all codes in subcategory S52.21

A	initial encounter for closed fracture
D	subsequent encounter for fracture with routine healing
G	subsequent encounter for fracture with delayed healing
K	subsequent encounter for fracture with nonunion
P	subsequent encounter for fracture with malunion
S	sequela

　　● S52.211　Greenstick fracture of shaft of right ulna
　　● S52.212　Greenstick fracture of shaft of left ulna
　　● S52.219　Greenstick fracture of shaft of unspecified ulna

　● **S52.22**　Transverse fracture of shaft of ulna
　　● S52.221　Displaced transverse fracture of shaft of right ulna
　　● S52.222　Displaced transverse fracture of shaft of left ulna
　　● S52.223　Displaced transverse fracture of shaft of unspecified ulna
　　● S52.224　Nondisplaced transverse fracture of shaft of right ulna
　　● S52.225　Nondisplaced transverse fracture of shaft of left ulna
　　● S52.226　Nondisplaced transverse fracture of shaft of unspecified ulna

　● **S52.23**　Oblique fracture of shaft of ulna
　　● S52.231　Displaced oblique fracture of shaft of right ulna
　　● S52.232　Displaced oblique fracture of shaft of left ulna
　　● S52.233　Displaced oblique fracture of shaft of unspecified ulna
　　● S52.234　Nondisplaced oblique fracture of shaft of right ulna
　　● S52.235　Nondisplaced oblique fracture of shaft of left ulna
　　● S52.236　Nondisplaced oblique fracture of shaft of unspecified ulna

CHAPTER 19 (S00-T88)

● **S52.24**   Spiral fracture of shaft of ulna
  ● **S52.241**   Displaced spiral fracture of shaft of ulna, right arm
  ● **S52.242**   Displaced spiral fracture of shaft of ulna, left arm
  ● **S52.243**   Displaced spiral fracture of shaft of ulna, unspecified arm
  ● **S52.244**   Nondisplaced spiral fracture of shaft of ulna, right arm
  ● **S52.245**   Nondisplaced spiral fracture of shaft of ulna, left arm
  ● **S52.246**   Nondisplaced spiral fracture of shaft of ulna, unspecified arm
● **S52.25**   Comminuted fracture of shaft of ulna
  ● **S52.251**   Displaced comminuted fracture of shaft of ulna, right arm
  ● **S52.252**   Displaced comminuted fracture of shaft of ulna, left arm
  ● **S52.253**   Displaced comminuted fracture of shaft of ulna, unspecified arm
  ● **S52.254**   Nondisplaced comminuted fracture of shaft of ulna, right arm
  ● **S52.255**   Nondisplaced comminuted fracture of shaft of ulna, left arm
  ● **S52.256**   Nondisplaced comminuted fracture of shaft of ulna, unspecified arm
● **S52.26**   Segmental fracture of shaft of ulna
  ● **S52.261**   Displaced segmental fracture of shaft of ulna, right arm
  ● **S52.262**   Displaced segmental fracture of shaft of ulna, left arm
  ● **S52.263**   Displaced segmental fracture of shaft of ulna, unspecified arm
  ● **S52.264**   Nondisplaced segmental fracture of shaft of ulna, right arm
  ● **S52.265**   Nondisplaced segmental fracture of shaft of ulna, left arm
  ● **S52.266**   Nondisplaced segmental fracture of shaft of ulna, unspecified arm
● **S52.27**   Monteggia's fracture of ulna
  Fracture of upper shaft of ulna with dislocation of radial head
  ● **S52.271**   Monteggia's fracture of right ulna
  ● **S52.272**   Monteggia's fracture of left ulna
  ● **S52.279**   Monteggia's fracture of unspecified ulna
● **S52.28**   Bent bone of ulna
  ● **S52.281**   Bent bone of right ulna
  ● **S52.282**   Bent bone of left ulna
  ● **S52.283**   Bent bone of unspecified ulna
● **S52.29**   Other fracture of shaft of ulna
  ● **S52.291**   Other fracture of shaft of right ulna
  ● **S52.292**   Other fracture of shaft of left ulna
  ● **S52.299**   Other fracture of shaft of unspecified ulna
● **S52.3**   Fracture of shaft of radius
 ● **S52.30**   Unspecified fracture of shaft of radius
  ● **S52.301**   Unspecified fracture of shaft of right radius
  ● **S52.302**   Unspecified fracture of shaft of left radius
  ● **S52.309**   Unspecified fracture of shaft of unspecified radius

● **S52.31**   Greenstick fracture of shaft of radius

The appropriate 7th character is to be added to all codes in subcategory S52.31

A	initial encounter for closed fracture
D	subsequent encounter for fracture with routine healing
G	subsequent encounter for fracture with delayed healing
K	subsequent encounter for fracture with nonunion
P	subsequent encounter for fracture with malunion
S	sequela

  ● **S52.311**   Greenstick fracture of shaft of radius, right arm
  ● **S52.312**   Greenstick fracture of shaft of radius, left arm
  ● **S52.319**   Greenstick fracture of shaft of radius, unspecified arm
● **S52.32**   Transverse fracture of shaft of radius
  ● **S52.321**   Displaced transverse fracture of shaft of right radius
  ● **S52.322**   Displaced transverse fracture of shaft of left radius
  ● **S52.323**   Displaced transverse fracture of shaft of unspecified radius
  ● **S52.324**   Nondisplaced transverse fracture of shaft of right radius
  ● **S52.325**   Nondisplaced transverse fracture of shaft of left radius
  ● **S52.326**   Nondisplaced transverse fracture of shaft of unspecified radius
● **S52.33**   Oblique fracture of shaft of radius
  ● **S52.331**   Displaced oblique fracture of shaft of right radius
  ● **S52.332**   Displaced oblique fracture of shaft of left radius
  ● **S52.333**   Displaced oblique fracture of shaft of unspecified radius
  ● **S52.334**   Nondisplaced oblique fracture of shaft of right radius
  ● **S52.335**   Nondisplaced oblique fracture of shaft of left radius
  ● **S52.336**   Nondisplaced oblique fracture of shaft of unspecified radius
● **S52.34**   Spiral fracture of shaft of radius
  ● **S52.341**   Displaced spiral fracture of shaft of radius, right arm
  ● **S52.342**   Displaced spiral fracture of shaft of radius, left arm
  ● **S52.343**   Displaced spiral fracture of shaft of radius, unspecified arm
  ● **S52.344**   Nondisplaced spiral fracture of shaft of radius, right arm
  ● **S52.345**   Nondisplaced spiral fracture of shaft of radius, left arm
  ● **S52.346**   Nondisplaced spiral fracture of shaft of radius, unspecified arm

◀ New   ⬅ Revised   ~~deleted~~ Deleted   Excludes 1   Excludes 2   Includes   Use additional   Code first   Code also   Unspecified

OGCR Official Guidelines   X Assign placeholder X   ● Use Additional Character(s)   ▶ Manifestation Code   **Coding Clinic**

● **S52.35   Comminuted fracture of shaft of radius**
  ● S52.351   Displaced comminuted fracture of shaft of radius, right arm
  ● S52.352   Displaced comminuted fracture of shaft of radius, left arm
  ● S52.353   Displaced comminuted fracture of shaft of radius, unspecified arm
  ● S52.354   Nondisplaced comminuted fracture of shaft of radius, right arm
  ● S52.355   Nondisplaced comminuted fracture of shaft of radius, left arm
  ● S52.356   Nondisplaced comminuted fracture of shaft of radius, unspecified arm
● **S52.36   Segmental fracture of shaft of radius**
  ● S52.361   Displaced segmental fracture of shaft of radius, right arm
  ● S52.362   Displaced segmental fracture of shaft of radius, left arm
  ● S52.363   Displaced segmental fracture of shaft of radius, unspecified arm
  ● S52.364   Nondisplaced segmental fracture of shaft of radius, right arm
  ● S52.365   Nondisplaced segmental fracture of shaft of radius, left arm
  ● S52.366   Nondisplaced segmental fracture of shaft of radius, unspecified arm
● **S52.37   Galeazzi's fracture**
       Fracture of lower shaft of radius with radioulnar joint dislocation
  ● S52.371   Galeazzi's fracture of right radius
  ● S52.372   Galeazzi's fracture of left radius
  ● S52.379   Galeazzi's fracture of unspecified radius
● **S52.38   Bent bone of radius**
  ● S52.381   Bent bone of right radius
  ● S52.382   Bent bone of left radius
  ● S52.389   Bent bone of unspecified radius
● **S52.39   Other fracture of shaft of radius**
  ● S52.391   Other fracture of shaft of radius, right arm
  ● S52.392   Other fracture of shaft of radius, left arm
  ● S52.399   Other fracture of shaft of radius, unspecified arm
● **S52.5   Fracture of lower end of radius**
     Fracture of distal end of radius
     Excludes2   physeal fractures of lower end of radius (S59.2-)
● **S52.50   Unspecified fracture of the lower end of radius**
  ● S52.501   Unspecified fracture of the lower end of right radius
  ● S52.502   Unspecified fracture of the lower end of left radius
  ● S52.509   Unspecified fracture of the lower end of unspecified radius
● **S52.51   Fracture of radial styloid process**
  ● S52.511   Displaced fracture of right radial styloid process
  ● S52.512   Displaced fracture of left radial styloid process
  ● S52.513   Displaced fracture of unspecified radial styloid process
  ● S52.514   Nondisplaced fracture of right radial styloid process
  ● S52.515   Nondisplaced fracture of left radial styloid process
  ● S52.516   Nondisplaced fracture of unspecified radial styloid process

● **S52.52   Torus fracture of lower end of radius**
       The appropriate 7th character is to be added to all codes in subcategory S52.52

A	initial encounter for closed fracture
D	subsequent encounter for fracture with routine healing
G	subsequent encounter for fracture with delayed healing
K	subsequent encounter for fracture with nonunion
P	subsequent encounter for fracture with malunion
S	sequela

  ● S52.521   Torus fracture of lower end of right radius
  ● S52.522   Torus fracture of lower end of left radius
  ● S52.529   Torus fracture of lower end of unspecified radius
● **S52.53   Colles' fracture**
  ● S52.531   Colles' fracture of right radius
  ● S52.532   Colles' fracture of left radius
  ● S52.539   Colles' fracture of unspecified radius
● **S52.54   Smith's fracture**
  ● S52.541   Smith's fracture of right radius
  ● S52.542   Smith's fracture of left radius
  ● S52.549   Smith's fracture of unspecified radius
● **S52.55   Other extraarticular fracture of lower end of radius**
  ● S52.551   Other extraarticular fracture of lower end of right radius
  ● S52.552   Other extraarticular fracture of lower end of left radius
  ● S52.559   Other extraarticular fracture of lower end of unspecified radius
● **S52.56   Barton's fracture**
  ● S52.561   Barton's fracture of right radius
  ● S52.562   Barton's fracture of left radius
  ● S52.569   Barton's fracture of unspecified radius
● **S52.57   Other intraarticular fracture of lower end of radius**
  ● S52.571   Other intraarticular fracture of lower end of right radius
  ● S52.572   Other intraarticular fracture of lower end of left radius
  ● S52.579   Other intraarticular fracture of lower end of unspecified radius
● **S52.59   Other fractures of lower end of radius**
  ● S52.591   Other fractures of lower end of right radius
  ● S52.592   Other fractures of lower end of left radius
  ● S52.599   Other fractures of lower end of unspecified radius
● **S52.6   Fracture of lower end of ulna**
● **S52.60   Unspecified fracture of lower end of ulna**
  ● S52.601   Unspecified fracture of lower end of right ulna
  ● S52.602   Unspecified fracture of lower end of left ulna
  ● S52.609   Unspecified fracture of lower end of unspecified ulna
● **S52.61   Fracture of ulna styloid process**
  ● S52.611   Displaced fracture of right ulna styloid process
  ● S52.612   Displaced fracture of left ulna styloid process

CHAPTER 19 (S00-T88)

● S52.613   Displaced fracture of unspecified ulna styloid process
● S52.614   Nondisplaced fracture of right ulna styloid process
● S52.615   Nondisplaced fracture of left ulna styloid process
● S52.616   Nondisplaced fracture of unspecified ulna styloid process
● S52.62   Torus fracture of lower end of ulna

The appropriate 7th character is to be added to all codes in subcategory S52.62

A	initial encounter for closed fracture
D	subsequent encounter for fracture with routine healing
G	subsequent encounter for fracture with delayed healing
K	subsequent encounter for fracture with nonunion
P	subsequent encounter for fracture with malunion
S	sequela

● S52.621   Torus fracture of lower end of right ulna
● S52.622   Torus fracture of lower end of left ulna
● S52.629   Torus fracture of lower end of unspecified ulna
● S52.69   Other fracture of lower end of ulna
● S52.691   Other fracture of lower end of right ulna
● S52.692   Other fracture of lower end of left ulna
● S52.699   Other fracture of lower end of unspecified ulna
● S52.9   Unspecified fracture of forearm
X● S52.90   Unspecified fracture of unspecified forearm
X● S52.91   Unspecified fracture of right forearm
X● S52.92   Unspecified fracture of left forearm

● S53   Dislocation and sprain of joints and ligaments of elbow

Includes   avulsion of joint or ligament of elbow
laceration of cartilage, joint or ligament of elbow
sprain of cartilage, joint or ligament of elbow
traumatic hemarthrosis of joint or ligament of elbow
traumatic rupture of joint or ligament of elbow
traumatic subluxation of joint or ligament of elbow
traumatic tear of joint or ligament of elbow

Code also any associated open wound

Excludes2   strain of muscle, fascia and tendon at forearm level (S56.-)

The appropriate 7th character is to be added to each code from category S53

A	initial encounter
D	subsequent encounter
S	sequela

● S53.0   Subluxation and dislocation of radial head
Dislocation of radiohumeral joint
Subluxation of radiohumeral joint

Excludes1   Monteggia's fracture-dislocation (S52.27-)

● S53.00   Unspecified subluxation and dislocation of radial head
● S53.001   Unspecified subluxation of right radial head
● S53.002   Unspecified subluxation of left radial head
● S53.003   Unspecified subluxation of unspecified radial head

● S53.004   Unspecified dislocation of right radial head
● S53.005   Unspecified dislocation of left radial head
● S53.006   Unspecified dislocation of unspecified radial head
● S53.01   Anterior subluxation and dislocation of radial head
Anteriomedial subluxation and dislocation of radial head
● S53.011   Anterior subluxation of right radial head
● S53.012   Anterior subluxation of left radial head
● S53.013   Anterior subluxation of unspecified radial head
● S53.014   Anterior dislocation of right radial head
● S53.015   Anterior dislocation of left radial head
● S53.016   Anterior dislocation of unspecified radial head
● S53.02   Posterior subluxation and dislocation of radial head
Posteriolateral subluxation and dislocation of radial head
● S53.021   Posterior subluxation of right radial head
● S53.022   Posterior subluxation of left radial head
● S53.023   Posterior subluxation of unspecified radial head
● S53.024   Posterior dislocation of right radial head
● S53.025   Posterior dislocation of left radial head
● S53.026   Posterior dislocation of unspecified radial head
● S53.03   Nursemaid's elbow
● S53.031   Nursemaid's elbow, right elbow
    Coding Clinic: 2015, Q1, P7-8
● S53.032   Nursemaid's elbow, left elbow
● S53.033   Nursemaid's elbow, unspecified elbow
● S53.09   Other subluxation and dislocation of radial head
● S53.091   Other subluxation of right radial head
● S53.092   Other subluxation of left radial head
● S53.093   Other subluxation of unspecified radial head
● S53.094   Other dislocation of right radial head
● S53.095   Other dislocation of left radial head
● S53.096   Other dislocation of unspecified radial head
● S53.1   Subluxation and dislocation of ulnohumeral joint
Subluxation and dislocation of elbow NOS

Excludes1   dislocation of radial head alone (S53.0-)

● S53.10   Unspecified subluxation and dislocation of ulnohumeral joint
● S53.101   Unspecified subluxation of right ulnohumeral joint
● S53.102   Unspecified subluxation of left ulnohumeral joint
● S53.103   Unspecified subluxation of unspecified ulnohumeral joint
● S53.104   Unspecified dislocation of right ulnohumeral joint
● S53.105   Unspecified dislocation of left ulnohumeral joint
● S53.106   Unspecified dislocation of unspecified ulnohumeral joint

◄ New   ◄ Revised   ~~deleted~~ Deleted   Excludes 1   Excludes 2   Includes   Use additional   Code first   Code also   Unspecified

OGCR Official Guidelines   X Assign placeholder X   ● Use Additional Character(s)   ▷ Manifestation Code   Coding Clinic

● S53.11   Anterior subluxation and dislocation of ulnohumeral joint
  ● S53.111   Anterior subluxation of right ulnohumeral joint
  ● S53.112   Anterior subluxation of left ulnohumeral joint
  ● S53.113   Anterior subluxation of unspecified ulnohumeral joint
  ● S53.114   Anterior dislocation of right ulnohumeral joint
          Coding Clinic: 2012, Q4, P108
  ● S53.115   Anterior dislocation of left ulnohumeral joint
  ● S53.116   Anterior dislocation of unspecified ulnohumeral joint

● S53.12   Posterior subluxation and dislocation of ulnohumeral joint
  ● S53.121   Posterior subluxation of right ulnohumeral joint
  ● S53.122   Posterior subluxation of left ulnohumeral joint
  ● S53.123   Posterior subluxation of unspecified ulnohumeral joint
  ● S53.124   Posterior dislocation of right ulnohumeral joint
  ● S53.125   Posterior dislocation of left ulnohumeral joint
  ● S53.126   Posterior dislocation of unspecified ulnohumeral joint

● S53.13   Medial subluxation and dislocation of ulnohumeral joint
  ● S53.131   Medial subluxation of right ulnohumeral joint
  ● S53.132   Medial subluxation of left ulnohumeral joint
  ● S53.133   Medial subluxation of unspecified ulnohumeral joint
  ● S53.134   Medial dislocation of right ulnohumeral joint
  ● S53.135   Medial dislocation of left ulnohumeral joint
  ● S53.136   Medial dislocation of unspecified ulnohumeral joint

● S53.14   Lateral subluxation and dislocation of ulnohumeral joint
  ● S53.141   Lateral subluxation of right ulnohumeral joint
  ● S53.142   Lateral subluxation of left ulnohumeral joint
  ● S53.143   Lateral subluxation of unspecified ulnohumeral joint
  ● S53.144   Lateral dislocation of right ulnohumeral joint
  ● S53.145   Lateral dislocation of left ulnohumeral joint
  ● S53.146   Lateral dislocation of unspecified ulnohumeral joint

● S53.19   Other subluxation and dislocation of ulnohumeral joint
  ● S53.191   Other subluxation of right ulnohumeral joint
  ● S53.192   Other subluxation of left ulnohumeral joint
  ● S53.193   Other subluxation of unspecified ulnohumeral joint
  ● S53.194   Other dislocation of right ulnohumeral joint
  ● S53.195   Other dislocation of left ulnohumeral joint
  ● S53.196   Other dislocation of unspecified ulnohumeral joint

● S53.2   Traumatic rupture of radial collateral ligament
    Excludes1   sprain of radial collateral ligament NOS (S53.43-)
  X● S53.20   Traumatic rupture of unspecified radial collateral ligament
  X● S53.21   Traumatic rupture of right radial collateral ligament
  X● S53.22   Traumatic rupture of left radial collateral ligament

● S53.3   Traumatic rupture of ulnar collateral ligament
    Excludes1   sprain of ulnar collateral ligament (S53.44-)
  X● S53.30   Traumatic rupture of unspecified ulnar collateral ligament
  X● S53.31   Traumatic rupture of right ulnar collateral ligament
  X● S53.32   Traumatic rupture of left ulnar collateral ligament

● S53.4   Sprain of elbow
    Excludes2   traumatic rupture of radial collateral ligament (S53.2-)
                traumatic rupture of ulnar collateral ligament (S53.3-)
  ● S53.40   Unspecified sprain of elbow
    ● S53.401   Unspecified sprain of right elbow
    ● S53.402   Unspecified sprain of left elbow
    ● S53.409   Unspecified sprain of unspecified elbow
            Sprain of elbow NOS
  ● S53.41   Radiohumeral (joint) sprain
    ● S53.411   Radiohumeral (joint) sprain of right elbow
    ● S53.412   Radiohumeral (joint) sprain of left elbow
    ● S53.419   Radiohumeral (joint) sprain of unspecified elbow
  ● S53.42   Ulnohumeral (joint) sprain
    ● S53.421   Ulnohumeral (joint) sprain of right elbow
    ● S53.422   Ulnohumeral (joint) sprain of left elbow
    ● S53.429   Ulnohumeral (joint) sprain of unspecified elbow
  ● S53.43   Radial collateral ligament sprain
    ● S53.431   Radial collateral ligament sprain of right elbow
    ● S53.432   Radial collateral ligament sprain of left elbow
    ● S53.439   Radial collateral ligament sprain of unspecified elbow
  ● S53.44   Ulnar collateral ligament sprain
    ● S53.441   Ulnar collateral ligament sprain of right elbow
    ● S53.442   Ulnar collateral ligament sprain of left elbow
    ● S53.449   Ulnar collateral ligament sprain of unspecified elbow

CHAPTER 19 (S00-T88)

CHAPTER 19 (S00-T88)

● S53.49   Other sprain of elbow
    ● S53.491   Other sprain of right elbow
    ● S53.492   Other sprain of left elbow
    ● S53.499   Other sprain of unspecified elbow

● **S54**   **Injury of nerves at forearm level**
     Code also any associated open wound (S51.-)
     Excludes2   injury of nerves at wrist and hand level (S64.-)
     The appropriate 7th character is to be added to each code from category S54

         A   initial encounter
         D   subsequent encounter
         S   sequela

● **S54.0**   **Injury of ulnar nerve at forearm level**
     Injury of ulnar nerve NOS
   X ● S54.00   Injury of ulnar nerve at forearm level, unspecified arm
   X ● S54.01   Injury of ulnar nerve at forearm level, right arm
   X ● S54.02   Injury of ulnar nerve at forearm level, left arm

● **S54.1**   **Injury of median nerve at forearm level**
     Injury of median nerve NOS
   X ● S54.10   Injury of median nerve at forearm level, unspecified arm
   X ● S54.11   Injury of median nerve at forearm level, right arm
   X ● S54.12   Injury of median nerve at forearm level, left arm

● **S54.2**   **Injury of radial nerve at forearm level**
     Injury of radial nerve NOS
   X ● S54.20   Injury of radial nerve at forearm level, unspecified arm
   X ● S54.21   Injury of radial nerve at forearm level, right arm
   X ● S54.22   Injury of radial nerve at forearm level, left arm

● **S54.3**   **Injury of cutaneous sensory nerve at forearm level**
   X ● S54.30   Injury of cutaneous sensory nerve at forearm level, unspecified arm
   X ● S54.31   Injury of cutaneous sensory nerve at forearm level, right arm
   X ● S54.32   Injury of cutaneous sensory nerve at forearm level, left arm

● **S54.8**   **Injury of other nerves at forearm level**
   ● S54.8X   Unspecified injury of other nerves at forearm level
    ● S54.8X1   Unspecified injury of other nerves at forearm level, right arm
    ● S54.8X2   Unspecified injury of other nerves at forearm level, left arm
    ● S54.8X9   Unspecified injury of other nerves at forearm level, unspecified arm

● **S54.9**   **Injury of unspecified nerve at forearm level**
   X ● S54.90   Injury of unspecified nerve at forearm level, unspecified arm
   X ● S54.91   Injury of unspecified nerve at forearm level, right arm
   X ● S54.92   Injury of unspecified nerve at forearm level, left arm

● **S55**   **Injury of blood vessels at forearm level**
     Code also any associated open wound (S51.-)
     Excludes2   injury of blood vessels at wrist and hand level (S65.-)
           injury of brachial vessels (S45.1-S45.2)
     The appropriate 7th character is to be added to each code from category S55

         A   initial encounter
         D   subsequent encounter
         S   sequela

● **S55.0**   **Injury of ulnar artery at forearm level**
   ● S55.00   Unspecified injury of ulnar artery at forearm level
    ● S55.001   Unspecified injury of ulnar artery at forearm level, right arm
    ● S55.002   Unspecified injury of ulnar artery at forearm level, left arm
    ● S55.009   Unspecified injury of ulnar artery at forearm level, unspecified arm
   ● S55.01   Laceration of ulnar artery at forearm level
    ● S55.011   Laceration of ulnar artery at forearm level, right arm
    ● S55.012   Laceration of ulnar artery at forearm level, left arm
    ● S55.019   Laceration of ulnar artery at forearm level, unspecified arm
   ● S55.09   Other specified injury of ulnar artery at forearm level
    ● S55.091   Other specified injury of ulnar artery at forearm level, right arm
    ● S55.092   Other specified injury of ulnar artery at forearm level, left arm
    ● S55.099   Other specified injury of ulnar artery at forearm level, unspecified arm

● **S55.1**   **Injury of radial artery at forearm level**
   ● S55.10   Unspecified injury of radial artery at forearm level
    ● S55.101   Unspecified injury of radial artery at forearm level, right arm
    ● S55.102   Unspecified injury of radial artery at forearm level, left arm
    ● S55.109   Unspecified injury of radial artery at forearm level, unspecified arm
   ● S55.11   Laceration of radial artery at forearm level
    ● S55.111   Laceration of radial artery at forearm level, right arm
    ● S55.112   Laceration of radial artery at forearm level, left arm
    ● S55.119   Laceration of radial artery at forearm level, unspecified arm
   ● S55.19   Other specified injury of radial artery at forearm level
    ● S55.191   Other specified injury of radial artery at forearm level, right arm
    ● S55.192   Other specified injury of radial artery at forearm level, left arm
    ● S55.199   Other specified injury of radial artery at forearm level, unspecified arm

● **S55.2**   **Injury of vein at forearm level**
   ● S55.20   Unspecified injury of vein at forearm level
    ● S55.201   Unspecified injury of vein at forearm level, right arm
    ● S55.202   Unspecified injury of vein at forearm level, left arm
    ● S55.209   Unspecified injury of vein at forearm level, unspecified arm

◄ New   ◄║║ Revised   ~~deleted~~ Deleted   Excludes 1   Excludes 2   Includes   Use additional   Code first   Code also   Unspecified
   OGCR Official Guidelines   **X** Assign placeholder X   ● Use Additional Character(s)   ▶ Manifestation Code   **Coding Clinic**

● **S55.21**   Laceration of vein at forearm level
- ● **S55.211**   Laceration of vein at forearm level, right arm
- ● **S55.212**   Laceration of vein at forearm level, left arm
- ● **S55.219**   Laceration of vein at forearm level, unspecified arm

● **S55.29**   Other specified injury of vein at forearm level
- ● **S55.291**   Other specified injury of vein at forearm level, right arm
- ● **S55.292**   Other specified injury of vein at forearm level, left arm
- ● **S55.299**   Other specified injury of vein at forearm level, unspecified arm

● **S55.8**   Injury of other blood vessels at forearm level
- ● **S55.80**   Unspecified injury of other blood vessels at forearm level
  - ● **S55.801**   Unspecified injury of other blood vessels at forearm level, right arm
  - ● **S55.802**   Unspecified injury of other blood vessels at forearm level, left arm
  - ● **S55.809**   Unspecified injury of other blood vessels at forearm level, unspecified arm
- ● **S55.81**   Laceration of other blood vessels at forearm level
  - ● **S55.811**   Laceration of other blood vessels at forearm level, right arm
  - ● **S55.812**   Laceration of other blood vessels at forearm level, left arm
  - ● **S55.819**   Laceration of other blood vessels at forearm level, unspecified arm
- ● **S55.89**   Other specified injury of other blood vessels at forearm level
  - ● **S55.891**   Other specified injury of other blood vessels at forearm level, right arm
  - ● **S55.892**   Other specified injury of other blood vessels at forearm level, left arm
  - ● **S55.899**   Other specified injury of other blood vessels at forearm level, unspecified arm

● **S55.9**   Injury of unspecified blood vessel at forearm level
- ● **S55.90**   Unspecified injury of unspecified blood vessel at forearm level
  - ● **S55.901**   Unspecified injury of unspecified blood vessel at forearm level, right arm
  - ● **S55.902**   Unspecified injury of unspecified blood vessel at forearm level, left arm
  - ● **S55.909**   Unspecified injury of unspecified blood vessel at forearm level, unspecified arm
- ● **S55.91**   Laceration of unspecified blood vessel at forearm level
  - ● **S55.911**   Laceration of unspecified blood vessel at forearm level, right arm
  - ● **S55.912**   Laceration of unspecified blood vessel at forearm level, left arm
  - ● **S55.919**   Laceration of unspecified blood vessel at forearm level, unspecified arm
- ● **S55.99**   Other specified injury of unspecified blood vessel at forearm level
  - ● **S55.991**   Other specified injury of unspecified blood vessel at forearm level, right arm
  - ● **S55.992**   Other specified injury of unspecified blood vessel at forearm level, left arm
  - ● **S55.999**   Other specified injury of unspecified blood vessel at forearm level, unspecified arm

● **S56**   Injury of muscle, fascia and tendon at forearm level

Code also any associated open wound (S51.-)

Excludes2   injury of muscle, fascia and tendon at or below wrist (S66.-)
     sprain of joints and ligaments of elbow (S53.4-)

The appropriate 7th character is to be added to each code from category S56

A	initial encounter
D	subsequent encounter
S	sequela

● **S56.0**   Injury of flexor muscle, fascia and tendon of thumb at forearm level
- ● **S56.00**   Unspecified injury of flexor muscle, fascia and tendon of thumb at forearm level
  - ● **S56.001**   Unspecified injury of flexor muscle, fascia and tendon of right thumb at forearm level
  - ● **S56.002**   Unspecified injury of flexor muscle, fascia and tendon of left thumb at forearm level
  - ● **S56.009**   Unspecified injury of flexor muscle, fascia and tendon of unspecified thumb at forearm level
- ● **S56.01**   Strain of flexor muscle, fascia and tendon of thumb at forearm level
  - ● **S56.011**   Strain of flexor muscle, fascia and tendon of right thumb at forearm level
  - ● **S56.012**   Strain of flexor muscle, fascia and tendon of left thumb at forearm level
  - ● **S56.019**   Strain of flexor muscle, fascia and tendon of unspecified thumb at forearm level
- ● **S56.02**   Laceration of flexor muscle, fascia and tendon of thumb at forearm level
  - ● **S56.021**   Laceration of flexor muscle, fascia and tendon of right thumb at forearm level
  - ● **S56.022**   Laceration of flexor muscle, fascia and tendon of left thumb at forearm level
  - ● **S56.029**   Laceration of flexor muscle, fascia and tendon of unspecified thumb at forearm level
- ● **S56.09**   Other injury of flexor muscle, fascia and tendon of thumb at forearm level
  - ● **S56.091**   Other injury of flexor muscle, fascia and tendon of right thumb at forearm level
  - ● **S56.092**   Other injury of flexor muscle, fascia and tendon of left thumb at forearm level
  - ● **S56.099**   Other injury of flexor muscle, fascia and tendon of unspecified thumb at forearm level

● **S56.1**   Injury of flexor muscle, fascia and tendon of other and unspecified finger at forearm level
- ● **S56.10**   Unspecified injury of flexor muscle, fascia and tendon of other and unspecified finger at forearm level
  - ● **S56.101**   Unspecified injury of flexor muscle, fascia and tendon of right index finger at forearm level
  - ● **S56.102**   Unspecified injury of flexor muscle, fascia and tendon of left index finger at forearm level
  - ● **S56.103**   Unspecified injury of flexor muscle, fascia and tendon of right middle finger at forearm level

● S56.104   Unspecified injury of flexor muscle, fascia and tendon of left middle finger at forearm level

● S56.105   Unspecified injury of flexor muscle, fascia and tendon of right ring finger at forearm level

● S56.106   Unspecified injury of flexor muscle, fascia and tendon of left ring finger at forearm level

● S56.107   Unspecified injury of flexor muscle, fascia and tendon of right little finger at forearm level

● S56.108   Unspecified injury of flexor muscle, fascia and tendon of left little finger at forearm level

● S56.109   Unspecified injury of flexor muscle, fascia and tendon of unspecified finger at forearm level

● S56.11   Strain of flexor muscle, fascia and tendon of other and unspecified finger at forearm level

● S56.111   Strain of flexor muscle, fascia and tendon of right index finger at forearm level

● S56.112   Strain of flexor muscle, fascia and tendon of left index finger at forearm level

● S56.113   Strain of flexor muscle, fascia and tendon of right middle finger at forearm level

● S56.114   Strain of flexor muscle, fascia and tendon of left middle finger at forearm level

● S56.115   Strain of flexor muscle, fascia and tendon of right ring finger at forearm level

● S56.116   Strain of flexor muscle, fascia and tendon of left ring finger at forearm level

● S56.117   Strain of flexor muscle, fascia and tendon of right little finger at forearm level

● S56.118   Strain of flexor muscle, fascia and tendon of left little finger at forearm level

● S56.119   Strain of flexor muscle, fascia and tendon of finger of unspecified finger at forearm level

● S56.12   Laceration of flexor muscle, fascia and tendon of other and unspecified finger at forearm level

● S56.121   Laceration of flexor muscle, fascia and tendon of right index finger at forearm level

● S56.122   Laceration of flexor muscle, fascia and tendon of left index finger at forearm level

● S56.123   Laceration of flexor muscle, fascia and tendon of right middle finger at forearm level

● S56.124   Laceration of flexor muscle, fascia and tendon of left middle finger at forearm level

● S56.125   Laceration of flexor muscle, fascia and tendon of right ring finger at forearm level

● S56.126   Laceration of flexor muscle, fascia and tendon of left ring finger at forearm level

● S56.127   Laceration of flexor muscle, fascia and tendon of right little finger at forearm level

● S56.128   Laceration of flexor muscle, fascia and tendon of left little finger at forearm level

● S56.129   Laceration of flexor muscle, fascia and tendon of unspecified finger at forearm level

● S56.19   Other injury of flexor muscle, fascia and tendon of other and unspecified finger at forearm level

● S56.191   Other injury of flexor muscle, fascia and tendon of right index finger at forearm level

● S56.192   Other injury of flexor muscle, fascia and tendon of left index finger at forearm level

● S56.193   Other injury of flexor muscle, fascia and tendon of right middle finger at forearm level

● S56.194   Other injury of flexor muscle, fascia and tendon of left middle finger at forearm level

● S56.195   Other injury of flexor muscle, fascia and tendon of right ring finger at forearm level

● S56.196   Other injury of flexor muscle, fascia and tendon of left ring finger at forearm level

● S56.197   Other injury of flexor muscle, fascia and tendon of right little finger at forearm level

● S56.198   Other injury of flexor muscle, fascia and tendon of left little finger at forearm level

● S56.199   Other injury of flexor muscle, fascia and tendon of unspecified finger at forearm level

● S56.2   Injury of other flexor muscle, fascia and tendon at forearm level

● S56.20   Unspecified injury of other flexor muscle, fascia and tendon at forearm level

● S56.201   Unspecified injury of other flexor muscle, fascia and tendon at forearm level, right arm

● S56.202   Unspecified injury of other flexor muscle, fascia and tendon at forearm level, left arm

● S56.209   Unspecified injury of other flexor muscle, fascia and tendon at forearm level, unspecified arm

● S56.21   Strain of other flexor muscle, fascia and tendon at forearm level

● S56.211   Strain of other flexor muscle, fascia and tendon at forearm level, right arm

● S56.212   Strain of other flexor muscle, fascia and tendon at forearm level, left arm

● S56.219   Strain of other flexor muscle, fascia and tendon at forearm level, unspecified arm

● S56.22   Laceration of other flexor muscle, fascia and tendon at forearm level

● S56.221   Laceration of other flexor muscle, fascia and tendon at forearm level, right arm

● S56.222   Laceration of other flexor muscle, fascia and tendon at forearm level, left arm

● S56.229   Laceration of other flexor muscle, fascia and tendon at forearm level, unspecified arm

◀ New   ◀▦ Revised   d̶e̶l̶e̶t̶e̶d̶ Deleted   Excludes 1   Excludes 2   Includes   Use additional   Code first   Code also   Unspecified
OGCR Official Guidelines   X Assign placeholder X   ● Use Additional Character(s)   ▸ Manifestation Code   **Coding Clinic**

● S56.29　Other injury of other flexor muscle, fascia and tendon at forearm level
   ● S56.291　Other injury of other flexor muscle, fascia and tendon at forearm level, right arm
   ● S56.292　Other injury of other flexor muscle, fascia and tendon at forearm level, left arm
   ● S56.299　Other injury of other flexor muscle, fascia and tendon at forearm level, unspecified arm

● S56.3　Injury of extensor or abductor muscles, fascia and tendons of thumb at forearm level
  ● S56.30　Unspecified injury of extensor or abductor muscles, fascia and tendons of thumb at forearm level
   ● S56.301　Unspecified injury of extensor or abductor muscles, fascia and tendons of right thumb at forearm level
   ● S56.302　Unspecified injury of extensor or abductor muscles, fascia and tendons of left thumb at forearm level
   ● S56.309　Unspecified injury of extensor or abductor muscles, fascia and tendons of unspecified thumb at forearm level

  ● S56.31　Strain of extensor or abductor muscles, fascia and tendons of thumb at forearm level
   ● S56.311　Strain of extensor or abductor muscles, fascia and tendons of right thumb at forearm level
   ● S56.312　Strain of extensor or abductor muscles, fascia and tendons of left thumb at forearm level
   ● S56.319　Strain of extensor or abductor muscles, fascia and tendons of unspecified thumb at forearm level

  ● S56.32　Laceration of extensor or abductor muscles, fascia and tendons of thumb at forearm level
   ● S56.321　Laceration of extensor or abductor muscles, fascia and tendons of right thumb at forearm level
   ● S56.322　Laceration of extensor or abductor muscles, fascia and tendons of left thumb at forearm level
   ● S56.329　Laceration of extensor or abductor muscles, fascia and tendons of unspecified thumb at forearm level

  ● S56.39　Other injury of extensor or abductor muscles, fascia and tendons of thumb at forearm level
   ● S56.391　Other injury of extensor or abductor muscles, fascia and tendons of right thumb at forearm level
   ● S56.392　Other injury of extensor or abductor muscles, fascia and tendons of left thumb at forearm level
   ● S56.399　Other injury of extensor or abductor muscles, fascia and tendons of unspecified thumb at forearm level

● S56.4　Injury of extensor muscle, fascia and tendon of other and unspecified finger at forearm level
  ● S56.40　Unspecified injury of extensor muscle, fascia and tendon of other and unspecified finger at forearm level
   ● S56.401　Unspecified injury of extensor muscle, fascia and tendon of right index finger at forearm level
   ● S56.402　Unspecified injury of extensor muscle, fascia and tendon of left index finger at forearm level
   ● S56.403　Unspecified injury of extensor muscle, fascia and tendon of right middle finger at forearm level
   ● S56.404　Unspecified injury of extensor muscle, fascia and tendon of left middle finger at forearm level
   ● S56.405　Unspecified injury of extensor muscle, fascia and tendon of right ring finger at forearm level
   ● S56.406　Unspecified injury of extensor muscle, fascia and tendon of left ring finger at forearm level
   ● S56.407　Unspecified injury of extensor muscle, fascia and tendon of right little finger at forearm level
   ● S56.408　Unspecified injury of extensor muscle, fascia and tendon of left little finger at forearm level
   ● S56.409　Unspecified injury of extensor muscle, fascia and tendon of unspecified finger at forearm level

  ● S56.41　Strain of extensor muscle, fascia and tendon of other and unspecified finger at forearm level
   ● S56.411　Strain of extensor muscle, fascia and tendon of right index finger at forearm level
   ● S56.412　Strain of extensor muscle, fascia and tendon of left index finger at forearm level
   ● S56.413　Strain of extensor muscle, fascia and tendon of right middle finger at forearm level
   ● S56.414　Strain of extensor muscle, fascia and tendon of left middle finger at forearm level
   ● S56.415　Strain of extensor muscle, fascia and tendon of right ring finger at forearm level
   ● S56.416　Strain of extensor muscle, fascia and tendon of left ring finger at forearm level
   ● S56.417　Strain of extensor muscle, fascia and tendon of right little finger at forearm level
   ● S56.418　Strain of extensor muscle, fascia and tendon of left little finger at forearm level
   ● S56.419　Strain of extensor muscle, fascia and tendon of finger, unspecified finger at forearm level

  ● S56.42　Laceration of extensor muscle, fascia and tendon of other and unspecified finger at forearm level
   ● S56.421　Laceration of extensor muscle, fascia and tendon of right index finger at forearm level
   ● S56.422　Laceration of extensor muscle, fascia and tendon of left index finger at forearm level
   ● S56.423　Laceration of extensor muscle, fascia and tendon of right middle finger at forearm level
   ● S56.424　Laceration of extensor muscle, fascia and tendon of left middle finger at forearm level
   ● S56.425　Laceration of extensor muscle, fascia and tendon of right ring finger at forearm level

● S56.426   Laceration of extensor muscle, fascia and tendon of left ring finger at forearm level

● S56.427   Laceration of extensor muscle, fascia and tendon of right little finger at forearm level

● S56.428   Laceration of extensor muscle, fascia and tendon of left little finger at forearm level

● S56.429   Laceration of extensor muscle, fascia and tendon of unspecified finger at forearm level

● S56.49   Other injury of extensor muscle, fascia and tendon of other and unspecified finger at forearm level

● S56.491   Other injury of extensor muscle, fascia and tendon of right index finger at forearm level

● S56.492   Other injury of extensor muscle, fascia and tendon of left index finger at forearm level

● S56.493   Other injury of extensor muscle, fascia and tendon of right middle finger at forearm level

● S56.494   Other injury of extensor muscle, fascia and tendon of left middle finger at forearm level

● S56.495   Other injury of extensor muscle, fascia and tendon of right ring finger at forearm level

● S56.496   Other injury of extensor muscle, fascia and tendon of left ring finger at forearm level

● S56.497   Other injury of extensor muscle, fascia and tendon of right little finger at forearm level

● S56.498   Other injury of extensor muscle, fascia and tendon of left little finger at forearm level

● S56.499   Other injury of extensor muscle, fascia and tendon of unspecified finger at forearm level

● S56.5   Injury of other extensor muscle, fascia and tendon at forearm level

● S56.50   Unspecified injury of other extensor muscle, fascia and tendon at forearm level

● S56.501   Unspecified injury of other extensor muscle, fascia and tendon at forearm level, right arm

● S56.502   Unspecified injury of other extensor muscle, fascia and tendon at forearm level, left arm

● S56.509   Unspecified injury of other extensor muscle, fascia and tendon at forearm level, unspecified arm

● S56.51   Strain of other extensor muscle, fascia and tendon at forearm level

● S56.511   Strain of other extensor muscle, fascia and tendon at forearm level, right arm

● S56.512   Strain of other extensor muscle, fascia and tendon at forearm level, left arm

● S56.519   Strain of other extensor muscle, fascia and tendon at forearm level, unspecified arm

● S56.52   Laceration of other extensor muscle, fascia and tendon at forearm level

● S56.521   Laceration of other extensor muscle, fascia and tendon at forearm level, right arm

● S56.522   Laceration of other extensor muscle, fascia and tendon at forearm level, left arm

● S56.529   Laceration of other extensor muscle, fascia and tendon at forearm level, unspecified arm

● S56.59   Other injury of other extensor muscle, fascia and tendon at forearm level

● S56.591   Other injury of other extensor muscle, fascia and tendon at forearm level, right arm

● S56.592   Other injury of other extensor muscle, fascia and tendon at forearm level, left arm

● S56.599   Other injury of other extensor muscle, fascia and tendon at forearm level, unspecified arm

● S56.8   Injury of other muscles, fascia and tendons at forearm level

● S56.80   Unspecified injury of other muscles, fascia and tendons at forearm level

● S56.801   Unspecified injury of other muscles, fascia and tendons at forearm level, right arm

● S56.802   Unspecified injury of other muscles, fascia and tendons at forearm level, left arm

● S56.809   Unspecified injury of other muscles, fascia and tendons at forearm level, unspecified arm

● S56.81   Strain of other muscles, fascia and tendons at forearm level

● S56.811   Strain of other muscles, fascia and tendons at forearm level, right arm

● S56.812   Strain of other muscles, fascia and tendons at forearm level, left arm

● S56.819   Strain of other muscles, fascia and tendons at forearm level, unspecified arm

● S56.82   Laceration of other muscles, fascia and tendons at forearm level

● S56.821   Laceration of other muscles, fascia and tendons at forearm level, right arm

● S56.822   Laceration of other muscles, fascia and tendons at forearm level, left arm

● S56.829   Laceration of other muscles, fascia and tendons at forearm level, unspecified arm

● S56.89   Other injury of other muscles, fascia and tendons at forearm level

● S56.891   Other injury of other muscles, fascia and tendons at forearm level, right arm

● S56.892   Other injury of other muscles, fascia and tendons at forearm level, left arm

● S56.899   Other injury of other muscles, fascia and tendons at forearm level, unspecified arm

◀ New   ◀▦ Revised   ~~deleted~~ Deleted   Excludes 1   Excludes 2   Includes   Use additional   Code first   Code also   Unspecified

OGCR Official Guidelines   X Assign placeholder X   ● Use Additional Character(s)   ▌ Manifestation Code   **Coding Clinic**

● S56.9   Injury of unspecified muscles, fascia and tendons at forearm level
  ● S56.90   Unspecified injury of unspecified muscles, fascia and tendons at forearm level
    ● S56.901   Unspecified injury of unspecified muscles, fascia and tendons at forearm level, right arm
    ● S56.902   Unspecified injury of unspecified muscles, fascia and tendons at forearm level, left arm
    ● S56.909   Unspecified injury of unspecified muscles, fascia and tendons at forearm level, unspecified arm
  ● S56.91   Strain of unspecified muscles, fascia and tendons at forearm level
    ● S56.911   Strain of unspecified muscles, fascia and tendons at forearm level, right arm
    ● S56.912   Strain of unspecified muscles, fascia and tendons at forearm level, left arm
    ● S56.919   Strain of unspecified muscles, fascia and tendons at forearm level, unspecified arm
  ● S56.92   Laceration of unspecified muscles, fascia and tendons at forearm level
    ● S56.921   Laceration of unspecified muscles, fascia and tendons at forearm level, right arm
    ● S56.922   Laceration of unspecified muscles, fascia and tendons at forearm level, left arm
    ● S56.929   Laceration of unspecified muscles, fascia and tendons at forearm level, unspecified arm
  ● S56.99   Other injury of unspecified muscles, fascia and tendons at forearm level
    ● S56.991   Other injury of unspecified muscles, fascia and tendons at forearm level, right arm
    ● S56.992   Other injury of unspecified muscles, fascia and tendons at forearm level, left arm
    ● S56.999   Other injury of unspecified muscles, fascia and tendons at forearm level, unspecified arm

● S57   **Crushing injury of elbow and forearm**
  Use additional code(s) for all associated injuries
  Excludes2   crushing injury of wrist and hand (S67.-)
  The appropriate 7th character is to be added to each code from category S57

A	initial encounter
D	subsequent encounter
S	sequela

  ● S57.0   **Crushing injury of elbow**
    X● S57.00   Crushing injury of unspecified elbow
    X● S57.01   Crushing injury of right elbow
    X● S57.02   Crushing injury of left elbow
  ● S57.8   **Crushing injury of forearm**
    X● S57.80   Crushing injury of unspecified forearm
    X● S57.81   Crushing injury of right forearm
    X● S57.82   Crushing injury of left forearm

● S58   **Traumatic amputation of elbow and forearm**
  An amputation not identified as partial or complete should be coded to complete
  Excludes1   traumatic amputation of wrist and hand (S68.-)
  The appropriate 7th character is to be added to each code from category S58

A	initial encounter
D	subsequent encounter
S	sequela

  ● S58.0   **Traumatic amputation at elbow level**
    ● S58.01   Complete traumatic amputation at elbow level
      ● S58.011   Complete traumatic amputation at elbow level, right arm
      ● S58.012   Complete traumatic amputation at elbow level, left arm
      ● S58.019   Complete traumatic amputation at elbow level, unspecified arm
    ● S58.02   Partial traumatic amputation at elbow level
      ● S58.021   Partial traumatic amputation at elbow level, right arm
      ● S58.022   Partial traumatic amputation at elbow level, left arm
      ● S58.029   Partial traumatic amputation at elbow level, unspecified arm
  ● S58.1   **Traumatic amputation at level between elbow and wrist**
    ● S58.11   Complete traumatic amputation at level between elbow and wrist
      ● S58.111   Complete traumatic amputation at level between elbow and wrist, right arm
      ● S58.112   Complete traumatic amputation at level between elbow and wrist, left arm
      ● S58.119   Complete traumatic amputation at level between elbow and wrist, unspecified arm
    ● S58.12   Partial traumatic amputation at level between elbow and wrist
      ● S58.121   Partial traumatic amputation at level between elbow and wrist, right arm
      ● S58.122   Partial traumatic amputation at level between elbow and wrist, left arm
      ● S58.129   Partial traumatic amputation at level between elbow and wrist, unspecified arm
  ● S58.9   **Traumatic amputation of forearm, level unspecified**
    Excludes1   traumatic amputation of wrist (S68.-)
    ● S58.91   Complete traumatic amputation of forearm, level unspecified
      ● S58.911   Complete traumatic amputation of right forearm, level unspecified
      ● S58.912   Complete traumatic amputation of left forearm, level unspecified
      ● S58.919   Complete traumatic amputation of unspecified forearm, level unspecified
    ● S58.92   Partial traumatic amputation of forearm, level unspecified
      ● S58.921   Partial traumatic amputation of right forearm, level unspecified
      ● S58.922   Partial traumatic amputation of left forearm, level unspecified
      ● S58.929   Partial traumatic amputation of unspecified forearm, level unspecified

CHAPTER 19 (S00-T88)

Item 19-4 SALTER-HARRIS TYPE 1: epiphysis is completely separated from end of bone, or metaphysic growth plate remains attached to epiphysis
SALTER-HARRIS TYPE 2: epiphysis and growth plate are partially separated from metaphysis, which is cracked—most common type
SALTER-HARRIS TYPE 3: fracture occurring through epiphysis and separates part of epiphysis and growth plate from metaphysis fracture, usually at distal end of tibia
SALTER-HARRIS TYPE 4: fracture runs through epiphysis, across growth plate, into metaphysic, surgery is required to restore joint surface to normal and align growth plate

● **S59   Other and unspecified injuries of elbow and forearm**
> **Excludes2**   other and unspecified injuries of wrist and hand (S69.-)

> The appropriate 7th character is to be added to each code from subcategories S59.0, S59.1, and S59.2

> | | |
> |---|---|
> | A | initial encounter for closed fracture |
> | D | subsequent encounter for fracture with routine healing |
> | G | subsequent encounter for fracture with delayed healing |
> | K | subsequent encounter for fracture with nonunion |
> | P | subsequent encounter for fracture with malunion |
> | S | sequela |

● **S59.0   Physeal fracture of lower end of ulna**
  ● **S59.00   Unspecified physeal fracture of lower end of ulna**
    ● S59.001   Unspecified physeal fracture of lower end of ulna, right arm
    ● S59.002   Unspecified physeal fracture of lower end of ulna, left arm
    ● S59.009   Unspecified physeal fracture of lower end of ulna, unspecified arm
  ● **S59.01   Salter-Harris Type I physeal fracture of lower end of ulna**
    ● S59.011   Salter-Harris Type I physeal fracture of lower end of ulna, right arm
    ● S59.012   Salter-Harris Type I physeal fracture of lower end of ulna, left arm
    ● S59.019   Salter-Harris Type I physeal fracture of lower end of ulna, unspecified arm
  ● **S59.02   Salter-Harris Type II physeal fracture of lower end of ulna**
    ● S59.021   Salter-Harris Type II physeal fracture of lower end of ulna, right arm
    ● S59.022   Salter-Harris Type II physeal fracture of lower end of ulna, left arm
    ● S59.029   Salter-Harris Type II physeal fracture of lower end of ulna, unspecified arm
  ● **S59.03   Salter-Harris Type III physeal fracture of lower end of ulna**
    ● S59.031   Salter-Harris Type III physeal fracture of lower end of ulna, right arm
    ● S59.032   Salter-Harris Type III physeal fracture of lower end of ulna, left arm
    ● S59.039   Salter-Harris Type III physeal fracture of lower end of ulna, unspecified arm
  ● **S59.04   Salter-Harris Type IV physeal fracture of lower end of ulna**
    ● S59.041   Salter-Harris Type IV physeal fracture of lower end of ulna, right arm
    ● S59.042   Salter-Harris Type IV physeal fracture of lower end of ulna, left arm
    ● S59.049   Salter-Harris Type IV physeal fracture of lower end of ulna, unspecified arm

  ● S59.09   Other physeal fracture of lower end of ulna
    ● S59.091   Other physeal fracture of lower end of ulna, right arm
    ● S59.092   Other physeal fracture of lower end of ulna, left arm
    ● S59.099   Other physeal fracture of lower end of ulna, unspecified arm
● **S59.1   Physeal fracture of upper end of radius**
  ● **S59.10   Unspecified physeal fracture of upper end of radius**
    ● S59.101   Unspecified physeal fracture of upper end of radius, right arm
    ● S59.102   Unspecified physeal fracture of upper end of radius, left arm
    ● S59.109   Unspecified physeal fracture of upper end of radius, unspecified arm
  ● **S59.11   Salter-Harris Type I physeal fracture of upper end of radius**
    ● S59.111   Salter-Harris Type I physeal fracture of upper end of radius, right arm
    ● S59.112   Salter-Harris Type I physeal fracture of upper end of radius, left arm
    ● S59.119   Salter-Harris Type I physeal fracture of upper end of radius, unspecified arm
  ● **S59.12   Salter-Harris Type II physeal fracture of upper end of radius**
    ● S59.121   Salter-Harris Type II physeal fracture of upper end of radius, right arm
    ● S59.122   Salter-Harris Type II physeal fracture of upper end of radius, left arm
    ● S59.129   Salter-Harris Type II physeal fracture of upper end of radius, unspecified arm
  ● **S59.13   Salter-Harris Type III physeal fracture of upper end of radius**
    ● S59.131   Salter-Harris Type III physeal fracture of upper end of radius, right arm
    ● S59.132   Salter-Harris Type III physeal fracture of upper end of radius, left arm
    ● S59.139   Salter-Harris Type III physeal fracture of upper end of radius, unspecified arm
  ● **S59.14   Salter-Harris Type IV physeal fracture of upper end of radius**
    ● S59.141   Salter-Harris Type IV physeal fracture of upper end of radius, right arm
    ● S59.142   Salter-Harris Type IV physeal fracture of upper end of radius, left arm
    ● S59.149   Salter-Harris Type IV physeal fracture of upper end of radius, unspecified arm
  ● S59.19   Other physeal fracture of upper end of radius
    ● S59.191   Other physeal fracture of upper end of radius, right arm
    ● S59.192   Other physeal fracture of upper end of radius, left arm
    ● S59.199   Other physeal fracture of upper end of radius, unspecified arm
● **S59.2   Physeal fracture of lower end of radius**
  ● **S59.20   Unspecified physeal fracture of lower end of radius**
    ● S59.201   Unspecified physeal fracture of lower end of radius, right arm
    ● S59.202   Unspecified physeal fracture of lower end of radius, left arm
    ● S59.209   Unspecified physeal fracture of lower end of radius, unspecified arm

◀ New   ◀▦ Revised   d̶e̶l̶e̶t̶e̶d̶ Deleted   Excludes 1   Excludes 2   Includes   Use additional   Code first   Code also   Unspecified
OGCR Official Guidelines   X Assign placeholder X   ● Use Additional Character(s)   ▶ Manifestation Code   **Coding Clinic**

● **S59.21**   Salter-Harris Type I physeal fracture of lower end of radius

  ● **S59.211**   Salter-Harris Type I physeal fracture of lower end of radius, right arm

  ● **S59.212**   Salter-Harris Type I physeal fracture of lower end of radius, left arm

  ● **S59.219**   Salter-Harris Type I physeal fracture of lower end of radius, unspecified arm

● **S59.22**   Salter-Harris Type II physeal fracture of lower end of radius

  ● **S59.221**   Salter-Harris Type II physeal fracture of lower end of radius, right arm

  ● **S59.222**   Salter-Harris Type II physeal fracture of lower end of radius, left arm

  ● **S59.229**   Salter-Harris Type II physeal fracture of lower end of radius, unspecified arm

● **S59.23**   Salter-Harris Type III physeal fracture of lower end of radius

  ● **S59.231**   Salter-Harris Type III physeal fracture of lower end of radius, right arm

  ● **S59.232**   Salter-Harris Type III physeal fracture of lower end of radius, left arm

  ● **S59.239**   Salter-Harris Type III physeal fracture of lower end of radius, unspecified arm

● **S59.24**   Salter-Harris Type IV physeal fracture of lower end of radius

  ● **S59.241**   Salter-Harris Type IV physeal fracture of lower end of radius, right arm

  ● **S59.242**   Salter-Harris Type IV physeal fracture of lower end of radius, left arm

  ● **S59.249**   Salter-Harris Type IV physeal fracture of lower end of radius, unspecified arm

● **S59.29**   Other physeal fracture of lower end of radius

  ● **S59.291**   Other physeal fracture of lower end of radius, right arm

  ● **S59.292**   Other physeal fracture of lower end of radius, left arm

  ● **S59.299**   Other physeal fracture of lower end of radius, unspecified arm

● **S59.8**   Other specified injuries of elbow and forearm

The appropriate 7th character is to be added to each code in subcategory S59.8

> A   initial encounter
> D   subsequent encounter
> S   sequela

● **S59.80**   Other specified injuries of elbow

  ● **S59.801**   Other specified injuries of right elbow

  ● **S59.802**   Other specified injuries of left elbow

  ● **S59.809**   Other specified injuries of unspecified elbow

● **S59.81**   Other specified injuries of forearm

  ● **S59.811**   Other specified injuries right forearm

  ● **S59.812**   Other specified injuries left forearm

  ● **S59.819**   Other specified injuries unspecified forearm

● **S59.9**   Unspecified injury of elbow and forearm

The appropriate 7th character is to be added to each code in subcategory S59.9

> A   initial encounter
> D   subsequent encounter
> S   sequela

● **S59.90**   Unspecified injury of elbow

  ● **S59.901**   Unspecified injury of right elbow

  ● **S59.902**   Unspecified injury of left elbow

  ● **S59.909**   Unspecified injury of unspecified elbow

● **S59.91**   Unspecified injury of forearm

  ● **S59.911**   Unspecified injury of right forearm

  ● **S59.912**   Unspecified injury of left forearm

  ● **S59.919**   Unspecified injury of unspecified forearm

INJURIES TO THE WRIST, HAND AND FINGERS (S60-S69)

Excludes2   burns and corrosions (T20-T32)
     frostbite (T33-T34)
     insect bite or sting, venomous (T63.4)

● **S60**   Superficial injury of wrist, hand and fingers

The appropriate 7th character is to be added to each code from category S60

> A   initial encounter
> D   subsequent encounter
> S   sequela

● **S60.0**   Contusion of finger without damage to nail

> **Excludes1**   contusion involving nail (matrix) (S60.1)

X ● **S60.00**   Contusion of unspecified finger without damage to nail
     Contusion of finger(s) NOS

● **S60.01**   Contusion of thumb without damage to nail

  ● **S60.011**   Contusion of right thumb without damage to nail

  ● **S60.012**   Contusion of left thumb without damage to nail

  ● **S60.019**   Contusion of unspecified thumb without damage to nail

● **S60.02**   Contusion of index finger without damage to nail

  ● **S60.021**   Contusion of right index finger without damage to nail

  ● **S60.022**   Contusion of left index finger without damage to nail

  ● **S60.029**   Contusion of unspecified index finger without damage to nail

● **S60.03**   Contusion of middle finger without damage to nail

  ● **S60.031**   Contusion of right middle finger without damage to nail

  ● **S60.032**   Contusion of left middle finger without damage to nail

  ● **S60.039**   Contusion of unspecified middle finger without damage to nail

● **S60.04**   Contusion of ring finger without damage to nail

  ● **S60.041**   Contusion of right ring finger without damage to nail

  ● **S60.042**   Contusion of left ring finger without damage to nail

  ● **S60.049**   Contusion of unspecified ring finger without damage to nail

CHAPTER 19 (S00-T88)

● **S60.05**   Contusion of little finger without damage to nail
- ● **S60.051**   Contusion of right little finger without damage to nail
- ● **S60.052**   Contusion of left little finger without damage to nail
- ● **S60.059**   Contusion of <mark>unspecified</mark> little finger without damage to nail

● **S60.1**   Contusion of finger with damage to nail
- X ● **S60.10**   Contusion of unspecified finger with damage to nail
- ● **S60.11**   Contusion of thumb with damage to nail
  - ● **S60.111**   Contusion of right thumb with damage to nail
  - ● **S60.112**   Contusion of left thumb with damage to nail
  - ● **S60.119**   Contusion of <mark>unspecified</mark> thumb with damage to nail
- ● **S60.12**   Contusion of index finger with damage to nail
  - ● **S60.121**   Contusion of right index finger with damage to nail
  - ● **S60.122**   Contusion of left index finger with damage to nail
  - ● **S60.129**   Contusion of <mark>unspecified</mark> index finger with damage to nail
- ● **S60.13**   Contusion of middle finger with damage to nail
  - ● **S60.131**   Contusion of right middle finger with damage to nail
  - ● **S60.132**   Contusion of left middle finger with damage to nail
  - ● **S60.139**   Contusion of <mark>unspecified</mark> middle finger with damage to nail
- ● **S60.14**   Contusion of ring finger with damage to nail
  - ● **S60.141**   Contusion of right ring finger with damage to nail
  - ● **S60.142**   Contusion of left ring finger with damage to nail
  - ● **S60.149**   Contusion of <mark>unspecified</mark> ring finger with damage to nail
- ● **S60.15**   Contusion of little finger with damage to nail
  - ● **S60.151**   Contusion of right little finger with damage to nail
  - ● **S60.152**   Contusion of left little finger with damage to nail
  - ● **S60.159**   Contusion of <mark>unspecified</mark> little finger with damage to nail

● **S60.2**   Contusion of wrist and hand
> **Excludes2**   contusion of fingers (S60.0-, S60.1-)
- ● **S60.21**   Contusion of wrist
  - ● **S60.211**   Contusion of right wrist
  - ● **S60.212**   Contusion of left wrist
  - ● **S60.219**   Contusion of <mark>unspecified</mark> wrist
- ● **S60.22**   Contusion of hand
  - ● **S60.221**   Contusion of right hand
  - ● **S60.222**   Contusion of left hand
  - ● **S60.229**   Contusion of <mark>unspecified</mark> hand

● **S60.3**   Other superficial injuries of thumb
- ● **S60.31**   Abrasion of thumb
  - ● **S60.311**   Abrasion of right thumb
  - ● **S60.312**   Abrasion of left thumb
  - ● **S60.319**   Abrasion of <mark>unspecified</mark> thumb
- ● **S60.32**   Blister (nonthermal) of thumb
  - ● **S60.321**   Blister (nonthermal) of right thumb
  - ● **S60.322**   Blister (nonthermal) of left thumb
  - ● **S60.329**   Blister (nonthermal) of <mark>unspecified</mark> thumb
- ● **S60.34**   External constriction of thumb
  Hair tourniquet syndrome of thumb
  Use additional cause code to identify the constricting item (W49.0-)
  - ● **S60.341**   External constriction of right thumb
  - ● **S60.342**   External constriction of left thumb
  - ● **S60.349**   External constriction of <mark>unspecified</mark> thumb
- ● **S60.35**   Superficial foreign body of thumb
  Splinter in the thumb
  - ● **S60.351**   Superficial foreign body of right thumb
  - ● **S60.352**   Superficial foreign body of left thumb
  - ● **S60.359**   Superficial foreign body of <mark>unspecified</mark> thumb
- ● **S60.36**   Insect bite (nonvenomous) of thumb
  - ● **S60.361**   Insect bite (nonvenomous) of right thumb
  - ● **S60.362**   Insect bite (nonvenomous) of left thumb
  - ● **S60.369**   Insect bite (nonvenomous) of <mark>unspecified</mark> thumb
- ● **S60.37**   Other superficial bite of thumb
  > **Excludes1**   open bite of thumb (S61.05-, S61.15-)
  - ● **S60.371**   Other superficial bite of right thumb
  - ● **S60.372**   Other superficial bite of left thumb
  - ● **S60.379**   Other superficial bite of <mark>unspecified</mark> thumb
- ● **S60.39**   Other superficial injuries of thumb
  - ● **S60.391**   Other superficial injuries of right thumb
  - ● **S60.392**   Other superficial injuries of left thumb
  - ● **S60.399**   Other superficial injuries of <mark>unspecified</mark> thumb

● **S60.4**   Other superficial injuries of other fingers
- ● **S60.41**   Abrasion of fingers
  - ● **S60.410**   Abrasion of right index finger
  - ● **S60.411**   Abrasion of left index finger
  - ● **S60.412**   Abrasion of right middle finger
  - ● **S60.413**   Abrasion of left middle finger
  - ● **S60.414**   Abrasion of right ring finger
  - ● **S60.415**   Abrasion of left ring finger
  - ● **S60.416**   Abrasion of right little finger
  - ● **S60.417**   Abrasion of left little finger
  - ● **S60.418**   Abrasion of other finger
    Abrasion of specified finger with unspecified laterality
  - ● **S60.419**   Abrasion of <mark>unspecified</mark> finger

◀ New   ◀▥ Revised   ~~deleted~~ Deleted   Excludes 1   Excludes 2   Includes   Use additional   Code first   Code also   Unspecified

OGCR Official Guidelines   **X** Assign placeholder X   ● Use Additional Character(s)   ▶ Manifestation Code   **Coding Clinic**

- ● S60.42 **Blister (nonthermal) of fingers**
  - ● S60.420 **Blister (nonthermal) of right index finger**
  - ● S60.421 **Blister (nonthermal) of left index finger**
  - ● S60.422 **Blister (nonthermal) of right middle finger**
  - ● S60.423 **Blister (nonthermal) of left middle finger**
  - ● S60.424 **Blister (nonthermal) of right ring finger**
  - ● S60.425 **Blister (nonthermal) of left ring finger**
  - ● S60.426 **Blister (nonthermal) of right little finger**
  - ● S60.427 **Blister (nonthermal) of left little finger**
  - ● S60.428 **Blister (nonthermal) of other finger**
    Blister (nonthermal) of specified finger with unspecified laterality
  - ● S60.429 **Blister (nonthermal) of unspecified finger**
- ● S60.44 **External constriction of fingers**
    Hair tourniquet syndrome of finger
    Use additional cause code to identify the constricting item (W49.0-)
  - ● S60.440 **External constriction of right index finger**
  - ● S60.441 **External constriction of left index finger**
  - ● S60.442 **External constriction of right middle finger**
  - ● S60.443 **External constriction of left middle finger**
  - ● S60.444 **External constriction of right ring finger**
  - ● S60.445 **External constriction of left ring finger**
  - ● S60.446 **External constriction of right little finger**
  - ● S60.447 **External constriction of left little finger**
  - ● S60.448 **External constriction of other finger**
    External constriction of specified finger with unspecified laterality
  - ● S60.449 **External constriction of unspecified finger**
- ● S60.45 **Superficial foreign body of fingers**
    Splinter in the finger(s)
  - ● S60.450 **Superficial foreign body of right index finger**
  - ● S60.451 **Superficial foreign body of left index finger**
  - ● S60.452 **Superficial foreign body of right middle finger**
  - ● S60.453 **Superficial foreign body of left middle finger**
  - ● S60.454 **Superficial foreign body of right ring finger**
  - ● S60.455 **Superficial foreign body of left ring finger**
  - ● S60.456 **Superficial foreign body of right little finger**

- ● S60.457 **Superficial foreign body of left little finger**
- ● S60.458 **Superficial foreign body of other finger**
    Superficial foreign body of specified finger with unspecified laterality
- ● S60.459 **Superficial foreign body of unspecified finger**
- ● S60.46 **Insect bite (nonvenomous) of fingers**
  - ● S60.460 **Insect bite (nonvenomous) of right index finger**
  - ● S60.461 **Insect bite (nonvenomous) of left index finger**
  - ● S60.462 **Insect bite (nonvenomous) of right middle finger**
  - ● S60.463 **Insect bite (nonvenomous) of left middle finger**
  - ● S60.464 **Insect bite (nonvenomous) of right ring finger**
  - ● S60.465 **Insect bite (nonvenomous) of left ring finger**
  - ● S60.466 **Insect bite (nonvenomous) of right little finger**
  - ● S60.467 **Insect bite (nonvenomous) of left little finger**
  - ● S60.468 **Insect bite (nonvenomous) of other finger**
    Insect bite (nonvenomous) of specified finger with unspecified laterality
  - ● S60.469 **Insect bite (nonvenomous) of unspecified finger**
- ● S60.47 **Other superficial bite of fingers**
    Excludes1 open bite of fingers (S61.25-, S61.35-)
  - ● S60.470 **Other superficial bite of right index finger**
  - ● S60.471 **Other superficial bite of left index finger**
  - ● S60.472 **Other superficial bite of right middle finger**
  - ● S60.473 **Other superficial bite of left middle finger**
  - ● S60.474 **Other superficial bite of right ring finger**
  - ● S60.475 **Other superficial bite of left ring finger**
  - ● S60.476 **Other superficial bite of right little finger**
  - ● S60.477 **Other superficial bite of left little finger**
  - ● S60.478 **Other superficial bite of other finger**
    Other superficial bite of specified finger with unspecified laterality
  - ● S60.479 **Other superficial bite of unspecified finger**
- ● S60.5 **Other superficial injuries of hand**
    Excludes2 superficial injuries of fingers (S60.3-, S60.4-)
  - ● S60.51 **Abrasion of hand**
    - ● S60.511 **Abrasion of right hand**
    - ● S60.512 **Abrasion of left hand**
    - ● S60.519 **Abrasion of unspecified hand**

CHAPTER 19 (S00-T88)

- ● S60.52   Blister (nonthermal) of hand
  - ● S60.521   Blister (nonthermal) of right hand
  - ● S60.522   Blister (nonthermal) of left hand
  - ● S60.529   Blister (nonthermal) of unspecified hand
- ● S60.54   External constriction of hand
  - ● S60.541   External constriction of right hand
  - ● S60.542   External constriction of left hand
  - ● S60.549   External constriction of unspecified hand
- ● S60.55   Superficial foreign body of hand
    Splinter in the hand
  - ● S60.551   Superficial foreign body of right hand
  - ● S60.552   Superficial foreign body of left hand
  - ● S60.559   Superficial foreign body of unspecified hand
- ● S60.56   Insect bite (nonvenomous) of hand
  - ● S60.561   Insect bite (nonvenomous) of right hand
  - ● S60.562   Insect bite (nonvenomous) of left hand
  - ● S60.569   Insect bite (nonvenomous) of unspecified hand
- ● S60.57   Other superficial bite of hand
    Excludes1   open bite of hand (S61.45-)
  - ● S60.571   Other superficial bite of hand of right hand
  - ● S60.572   Other superficial bite of hand of left hand
  - ● S60.579   Other superficial bite of hand of unspecified hand
- ● S60.8   Other superficial injuries of wrist
  - ● S60.81   Abrasion of wrist
    - ● S60.811   Abrasion of right wrist
    - ● S60.812   Abrasion of left wrist
    - ● S60.819   Abrasion of unspecified wrist
  - ● S60.82   Blister (nonthermal) of wrist
    - ● S60.821   Blister (nonthermal) of right wrist
    - ● S60.822   Blister (nonthermal) of left wrist
    - ● S60.829   Blister (nonthermal) of unspecified wrist
  - ● S60.84   External constriction of wrist
    - ● S60.841   External constriction of right wrist
    - ● S60.842   External constriction of left wrist
    - ● S60.849   External constriction of unspecified wrist
  - ● S60.85   Superficial foreign body of wrist
      Splinter in the wrist
    - ● S60.851   Superficial foreign body of right wrist
    - ● S60.852   Superficial foreign body of left wrist
    - ● S60.859   Superficial foreign body of unspecified wrist
  - ● S60.86   Insect bite (nonvenomous) of wrist
    - ● S60.861   Insect bite (nonvenomous) of right wrist
    - ● S60.862   Insect bite (nonvenomous) of left wrist
    - ● S60.869   Insect bite (nonvenomous) of unspecified wrist
  - ● S60.87   Other superficial bite of wrist
      Excludes1   open bite of wrist (S61.55)
    - ● S60.871   Other superficial bite of right wrist
    - ● S60.872   Other superficial bite of left wrist
    - ● S60.879   Other superficial bite of unspecified wrist

- ● S60.9   Unspecified superficial injury of wrist, hand and fingers
  - ● S60.91   Unspecified superficial injury of wrist
    - ● S60.911   Unspecified superficial injury of right wrist
    - ● S60.912   Unspecified superficial injury of left wrist
    - ● S60.919   Unspecified superficial injury of unspecified wrist
  - ● S60.92   Unspecified superficial injury of hand
    - ● S60.921   Unspecified superficial injury of right hand
    - ● S60.922   Unspecified superficial injury of left hand
    - ● S60.929   Unspecified superficial injury of unspecified hand
  - ● S60.93   Unspecified superficial injury of thumb
    - ● S60.931   Unspecified superficial injury of right thumb
    - ● S60.932   Unspecified superficial injury of left thumb
    - ● S60.939   Unspecified superficial injury of unspecified thumb
  - ● S60.94   Unspecified superficial injury of other fingers
    - ● S60.940   Unspecified superficial injury of right index finger
    - ● S60.941   Unspecified superficial injury of left index finger
    - ● S60.942   Unspecified superficial injury of right middle finger
    - ● S60.943   Unspecified superficial injury of left middle finger
    - ● S60.944   Unspecified superficial injury of right ring finger
    - ● S60.945   Unspecified superficial injury of left ring finger
    - ● S60.946   Unspecified superficial injury of right little finger
    - ● S60.947   Unspecified superficial injury of left little finger
    - ● S60.948   Unspecified superficial injury of other finger
        Unspecified superficial injury of specified finger with unspecified laterality
    - ● S60.949   Unspecified superficial injury of unspecified finger

- ● S61   **Open wound of wrist, hand and fingers**
    Code also any associated wound infection
    Excludes1   open fracture of wrist, hand and finger (S62.- with 7th character B)
                     traumatic amputation of wrist and hand (S68.-)
    The appropriate 7th character is to be added to each code from category S61

A	initial encounter
D	subsequent encounter
S	sequela

  - ● S61.0   Open wound of thumb without damage to nail
      Excludes1   open wound of thumb with damage to nail (S61.1-)
    - ● S61.00   Unspecified open wound of thumb without damage to nail
      - ● S61.001   Unspecified open wound of right thumb without damage to nail
      - ● S61.002   Unspecified open wound of left thumb without damage to nail
      - ● S61.009   Unspecified open wound of unspecified thumb without damage to nail

◀ New   ◀ Revised   deleted Deleted   Excludes 1   Excludes 2   Includes   Use additional   Code first   Code also   Unspecified

OGCR Official Guidelines   X Assign placeholder X   ● Use Additional Character(s)   ▶ Manifestation Code   **Coding Clinic**

- S61.01 Laceration without foreign body of thumb without damage to nail
  - S61.011 Laceration without foreign body of right thumb without damage to nail
  - S61.012 Laceration without foreign body of left thumb without damage to nail
  - S61.019 Laceration without foreign body of unspecified thumb without damage to nail
- S61.02 Laceration with foreign body of thumb without damage to nail
  - S61.021 Laceration with foreign body of right thumb without damage to nail
  - S61.022 Laceration with foreign body of left thumb without damage to nail
  - S61.029 Laceration with foreign body of unspecified thumb without damage to nail
- S61.03 Puncture wound without foreign body of thumb without damage to nail
  - S61.031 Puncture wound without foreign body of right thumb without damage to nail
  - S61.032 Puncture wound without foreign body of left thumb without damage to nail
  - S61.039 Puncture wound without foreign body of unspecified thumb without damage to nail
- S61.04 Puncture wound with foreign body of thumb without damage to nail
  - S61.041 Puncture wound with foreign body of right thumb without damage to nail
  - S61.042 Puncture wound with foreign body of left thumb without damage to nail
  - S61.049 Puncture wound with foreign body of unspecified thumb without damage to nail
- S61.05 Open bite of thumb without damage to nail
  Bite of thumb NOS
  Excludes1 superficial bite of thumb (S60.36-, S60.37-)
  - S61.051 Open bite of right thumb without damage to nail
  - S61.052 Open bite of left thumb without damage to nail
  - S61.059 Open bite of unspecified thumb without damage to nail
- S61.1 Open wound of thumb with damage to nail
  - S61.10 Unspecified open wound of thumb with damage to nail
    - S61.101 Unspecified open wound of right thumb with damage to nail
    - S61.102 Unspecified open wound of left thumb with damage to nail
    - S61.109 Unspecified open wound of unspecified thumb with damage to nail
  - S61.11 Laceration without foreign body of thumb with damage to nail
    - S61.111 Laceration without foreign body of right thumb with damage to nail
    - S61.112 Laceration without foreign body of left thumb with damage to nail
    - S61.119 Laceration without foreign body of unspecified thumb with damage to nail

- S61.12 Laceration with foreign body of thumb with damage to nail
  - S61.121 Laceration with foreign body of right thumb with damage to nail
  - S61.122 Laceration with foreign body of left thumb with damage to nail
  - S61.129 Laceration with foreign body of unspecified thumb with damage to nail
- S61.13 Puncture wound without foreign body of thumb with damage to nail
  - S61.131 Puncture wound without foreign body of right thumb with damage to nail
  - S61.132 Puncture wound without foreign body of left thumb with damage to nail
  - S61.139 Puncture wound without foreign body of unspecified thumb with damage to nail
- S61.14 Puncture wound with foreign body of thumb with damage to nail
  - S61.141 Puncture wound with foreign body of right thumb with damage to nail
  - S61.142 Puncture wound with foreign body of left thumb with damage to nail
  - S61.149 Puncture wound with foreign body of unspecified thumb with damage to nail
- S61.15 Open bite of thumb with damage to nail
  Bite of thumb with damage to nail NOS
  Excludes1 superficial bite of thumb (S60.36-, S60.37-)
  - S61.151 Open bite of right thumb with damage to nail
  - S61.152 Open bite of left thumb with damage to nail
  - S61.159 Open bite of unspecified thumb with damage to nail
- S61.2 Open wound of other finger without damage to nail
  Excludes1 open wound of finger involving nail (matrix) (S61.3-)
  Excludes2 open wound of thumb without damage to nail (S61.0-)
  - S61.20 Unspecified open wound of other finger without damage to nail
    - S61.200 Unspecified open wound of right index finger without damage to nail
    - S61.201 Unspecified open wound of left index finger without damage to nail
    - S61.202 Unspecified open wound of right middle finger without damage to nail
    - S61.203 Unspecified open wound of left middle finger without damage to nail
    - S61.204 Unspecified open wound of right ring finger without damage to nail
    - S61.205 Unspecified open wound of left ring finger without damage to nail
    - S61.206 Unspecified open wound of right little finger without damage to nail
    - S61.207 Unspecified open wound of left little finger without damage to nail
    - S61.208 Unspecified open wound of other finger without damage to nail
      Unspecified open wound of specified finger with unspecified laterality without damage to nail
    - S61.209 Unspecified open wound of unspecified finger without damage to nail

● S61.21   Laceration without foreign body of finger without damage to nail

  ● S61.210   Laceration without foreign body of right index finger without damage to nail

  ● S61.211   Laceration without foreign body of left index finger without damage to nail

  ● S61.212   Laceration without foreign body of right middle finger without damage to nail

  ● S61.213   Laceration without foreign body of left middle finger without damage to nail

  ● S61.214   Laceration without foreign body of right ring finger without damage to nail

  ● S61.215   Laceration without foreign body of left ring finger without damage to nail

  ● S61.216   Laceration without foreign body of right little finger without damage to nail

  ● S61.217   Laceration without foreign body of left little finger without damage to nail

  ● S61.218   Laceration without foreign body of other finger without damage to nail
             Laceration without foreign body of specified finger with unspecified laterality without damage to nail

  ● S61.219   Laceration without foreign body of unspecified finger without damage to nail

● S61.22   Laceration with foreign body of finger without damage to nail

  ● S61.220   Laceration with foreign body of right index finger without damage to nail

  ● S61.221   Laceration with foreign body of left index finger without damage to nail

  ● S61.222   Laceration with foreign body of right middle finger without damage to nail

  ● S61.223   Laceration with foreign body of left middle finger without damage to nail

  ● S61.224   Laceration with foreign body of right ring finger without damage to nail

  ● S61.225   Laceration with foreign body of left ring finger without damage to nail

  ● S61.226   Laceration with foreign body of right little finger without damage to nail

  ● S61.227   Laceration with foreign body of left little finger without damage to nail

  ● S61.228   Laceration with foreign body of other finger without damage to nail
             Laceration with foreign body of specified finger with unspecified laterality without damage to nail

  ● S61.229   Laceration with foreign body of unspecified finger without damage to nail

● S61.23   Puncture wound without foreign body of finger without damage to nail

  ● S61.230   Puncture wound without foreign body of right index finger without damage to nail

  ● S61.231   Puncture wound without foreign body of left index finger without damage to nail

  ● S61.232   Puncture wound without foreign body of right middle finger without damage to nail

  ● S61.233   Puncture wound without foreign body of left middle finger without damage to nail

  ● S61.234   Puncture wound without foreign body of right ring finger without damage to nail

  ● S61.235   Puncture wound without foreign body of left ring finger without damage to nail

  ● S61.236   Puncture wound without foreign body of right little finger without damage to nail

  ● S61.237   Puncture wound without foreign body of left little finger without damage to nail

  ● S61.238   Puncture wound without foreign body of other finger without damage to nail
             Puncture wound without foreign body of specified finger with unspecified laterality without damage to nail

  ● S61.239   Puncture wound without foreign body of unspecified finger without damage to nail

● S61.24   Puncture wound with foreign body of finger without damage to nail

  ● S61.240   Puncture wound with foreign body of right index finger without damage to nail

  ● S61.241   Puncture wound with foreign body of left index finger without damage to nail

  ● S61.242   Puncture wound with foreign body of right middle finger without damage to nail

  ● S61.243   Puncture wound with foreign body of left middle finger without damage to nail

  ● S61.244   Puncture wound with foreign body of right ring finger without damage to nail

  ● S61.245   Puncture wound with foreign body of left ring finger without damage to nail

  ● S61.246   Puncture wound with foreign body of right little finger without damage to nail

  ● S61.247   Puncture wound with foreign body of left little finger without damage to nail

  ● S61.248   Puncture wound with foreign body of other finger without damage to nail
             Puncture wound with foreign body of specified finger with unspecified laterality without damage to nail

  ● S61.249   Puncture wound with foreign body of unspecified finger without damage to nail

◄ New   ◄ Revised   deleted Deleted   Excludes 1   Excludes 2   Includes   Use additional   Code first   Code also   Unspecified

OGCR Official Guidelines   X Assign placeholder X   ● Use Additional Character(s)   ▶ Manifestation Code   **Coding Clinic**

● S61.25   **Open bite of finger without damage to nail**
Bite of finger without damage to nail NOS
> **Excludes1**   superficial bite of finger (S60.46-, S60.47-)

● S61.250   **Open bite of right index finger without damage to nail**

● S61.251   **Open bite of left index finger without damage to nail**

● S61.252   **Open bite of right middle finger without damage to nail**

● S61.253   **Open bite of left middle finger without damage to nail**

● S61.254   **Open bite of right ring finger without damage to nail**

● S61.255   **Open bite of left ring finger without damage to nail**

● S61.256   **Open bite of right little finger without damage to nail**

● S61.257   **Open bite of left little finger without damage to nail**

● S61.258   **Open bite of other finger without damage to nail**
> Open bite of specified finger with unspecified laterality without damage to nail

● S61.259   **Open bite of unspecified finger without damage to nail**

● S61.3   **Open wound of other finger with damage to nail**

● S61.30   **Unspecified open wound of finger with damage to nail**

● S61.300   **Unspecified open wound of right index finger with damage to nail**

● S61.301   **Unspecified open wound of left index finger with damage to nail**

● S61.302   **Unspecified open wound of right middle finger with damage to nail**

● S61.303   **Unspecified open wound of left middle finger with damage to nail**

● S61.304   **Unspecified open wound of right ring finger with damage to nail**

● S61.305   **Unspecified open wound of left ring finger with damage to nail**

● S61.306   **Unspecified open wound of right little finger with damage to nail**

● S61.307   **Unspecified open wound of left little finger with damage to nail**

● S61.308   **Unspecified open wound of other finger with damage to nail**
> Unspecified open wound of specified finger with unspecified laterality with damage to nail

● S61.309   **Unspecified open wound of unspecified finger with damage to nail**

● S61.31   **Laceration without foreign body of finger with damage to nail**

● S61.310   **Laceration without foreign body of right index finger with damage to nail**

● S61.311   **Laceration without foreign body of left index finger with damage to nail**

● S61.312   **Laceration without foreign body of right middle finger with damage to nail**

● S61.313   **Laceration without foreign body of left middle finger with damage to nail**

● S61.314   **Laceration without foreign body of right ring finger with damage to nail**

● S61.315   **Laceration without foreign body of left ring finger with damage to nail**

● S61.316   **Laceration without foreign body of right little finger with damage to nail**

● S61.317   **Laceration without foreign body of left little finger with damage to nail**

● S61.318   **Laceration without foreign body of other finger with damage to nail**
> Laceration without foreign body of specified finger with unspecified laterality with damage to nail

● S61.319   **Laceration without foreign body of unspecified finger with damage to nail**

● S61.32   **Laceration with foreign body of finger with damage to nail**

● S61.320   **Laceration with foreign body of right index finger with damage to nail**

● S61.321   **Laceration with foreign body of left index finger with damage to nail**

● S61.322   **Laceration with foreign body of right middle finger with damage to nail**

● S61.323   **Laceration with foreign body of left middle finger with damage to nail**

● S61.324   **Laceration with foreign body of right ring finger with damage to nail**

● S61.325   **Laceration with foreign body of left ring finger with damage to nail**

● S61.326   **Laceration with foreign body of right little finger with damage to nail**

● S61.327   **Laceration with foreign body of left little finger with damage to nail**

● S61.328   **Laceration with foreign body of other finger with damage to nail**
> Laceration with foreign body of specified finger with unspecified laterality with damage to nail

● S61.329   **Laceration with foreign body of unspecified finger with damage to nail**

● S61.33   **Puncture wound without foreign body of finger with damage to nail**

● S61.330   **Puncture wound without foreign body of right index finger with damage to nail**

● S61.331   **Puncture wound without foreign body of left index finger with damage to nail**

● S61.332   **Puncture wound without foreign body of right middle finger with damage to nail**

● S61.333   **Puncture wound without foreign body of left middle finger with damage to nail**

● S61.334   **Puncture wound without foreign body of right ring finger with damage to nail**

● S61.335   **Puncture wound without foreign body of left ring finger with damage to nail**

● S61.336   **Puncture wound without foreign body of right little finger with damage to nail**

● S61.337   **Puncture wound without foreign body of left little finger with damage to nail**

● S61.338 Puncture wound without foreign body of other finger with damage to nail

> Puncture wound without foreign body of specified finger with unspecified laterality with damage to nail

● S61.339 Puncture wound without foreign body of unspecified finger with damage to nail

● S61.34 Puncture wound with foreign body of finger with damage to nail

● S61.340 Puncture wound with foreign body of right index finger with damage to nail

● S61.341 Puncture wound with foreign body of left index finger with damage to nail

● S61.342 Puncture wound with foreign body of right middle finger with damage to nail

● S61.343 Puncture wound with foreign body of left middle finger with damage to nail

● S61.344 Puncture wound with foreign body of right ring finger with damage to nail

● S61.345 Puncture wound with foreign body of left ring finger with damage to nail

● S61.346 Puncture wound with foreign body of right little finger with damage to nail

● S61.347 Puncture wound with foreign body of left little finger with damage to nail

● S61.348 Puncture wound with foreign body of other finger with damage to nail

> Puncture wound with foreign body of specified finger with unspecified laterality with damage to nail

● S61.349 Puncture wound with foreign body of unspecified finger with damage to nail

● S61.35 Open bite of finger with damage to nail

> Bite of finger with damage to nail NOS

Excludes1 superficial bite of finger (S60.46-, S60.47-)

● S61.350 Open bite of right index finger with damage to nail

● S61.351 Open bite of left index finger with damage to nail

● S61.352 Open bite of right middle finger with damage to nail

● S61.353 Open bite of left middle finger with damage to nail

● S61.354 Open bite of right ring finger with damage to nail

● S61.355 Open bite of left ring finger with damage to nail

● S61.356 Open bite of right little finger with damage to nail

● S61.357 Open bite of left little finger with damage to nail

● S61.358 Open bite of other finger with damage to nail

> Open bite of specified finger with unspecified laterality with damage to nail

● S61.359 Open bite of unspecified finger with damage to nail

● S61.4 Open wound of hand

● S61.40 Unspecified open wound of hand

● S61.401 Unspecified open wound of right hand

● S61.402 Unspecified open wound of left hand

● S61.409 Unspecified open wound of unspecified hand

● S61.41 Laceration without foreign body of hand

● S61.411 Laceration without foreign body of right hand

● S61.412 Laceration without foreign body of left hand

● S61.419 Laceration without foreign body of unspecified hand

● S61.42 Laceration with foreign body of hand

● S61.421 Laceration with foreign body of right hand

● S61.422 Laceration with foreign body of left hand

● S61.429 Laceration with foreign body of unspecified hand

● S61.43 Puncture wound without foreign body of hand

● S61.431 Puncture wound without foreign body of right hand

● S61.432 Puncture wound without foreign body of left hand

● S61.439 Puncture wound without foreign body of unspecified hand

● S61.44 Puncture wound with foreign body of hand

● S61.441 Puncture wound with foreign body of right hand

● S61.442 Puncture wound with foreign body of left hand

● S61.449 Puncture wound with foreign body of unspecified hand

● S61.45 Open bite of hand

> Bite of hand NOS

Excludes1 superficial bite of hand (S60.56-, S60.57-)

● S61.451 Open bite of right hand

● S61.452 Open bite of left hand

● S61.459 Open bite of unspecified hand

● S61.5 Open wound of wrist

● S61.50 Unspecified open wound of wrist

● S61.501 Unspecified open wound of right wrist

● S61.502 Unspecified open wound of left wrist

● S61.509 Unspecified open wound of unspecified wrist

● S61.51 Laceration without foreign body of wrist

● S61.511 Laceration without foreign body of right wrist

● S61.512 Laceration without foreign body of left wrist

● S61.519 Laceration without foreign body of unspecified wrist

● S61.52 Laceration with foreign body of wrist

● S61.521 Laceration with foreign body of right wrist

● S61.522 Laceration with foreign body of left wrist

● S61.529 Laceration with foreign body of unspecified wrist

● **S61.53**   Puncture wound without foreign body of wrist
  ● S61.531   Puncture wound without foreign body of right wrist
  ● S61.532   Puncture wound without foreign body of left wrist
  ● S61.539   Puncture wound without foreign body of ==unspecified== wrist
● **S61.54**   Puncture wound with foreign body of wrist
  ● S61.541   Puncture wound with foreign body of right wrist
  ● S61.542   Puncture wound with foreign body of left wrist
  ● S61.549   Puncture wound with foreign body of ==unspecified== wrist
● **S61.55**   Open bite of wrist
           Bite of wrist NOS
    ==Excludes1==   superficial bite of wrist (S60.86-, S60.87-)
  ● S61.551   Open bite of right wrist
  ● S61.552   Open bite of left wrist
  ● S61.559   Open bite of ==unspecified== wrist

● **S62**   Fracture at wrist and hand level
    Note: A fracture not indicated as displaced or nondisplaced should be coded to displaced
         A fracture not indicated as open or closed should be coded to closed
    ==Excludes1==   traumatic amputation of wrist and hand (S68.-)
    ==Excludes2==   fracture of distal parts of ulna and radius (S52.-)
    The appropriate 7th character is to be added to each code from category S62

A	initial encounter for closed fracture
B	initial encounter for open fracture
D	subsequent encounter for fracture with routine healing
G	subsequent encounter for fracture with delayed healing
K	subsequent encounter for fracture with nonunion
P	subsequent encounter for fracture with malunion
S	sequela

● **S62.0**   Fracture of navicular [scaphoid] bone of wrist
  ● **S62.00**   Unspecified fracture of navicular [scaphoid] bone of wrist
    ● S62.001   ==Unspecified== fracture of navicular [scaphoid] bone of right wrist
    ● S62.002   ==Unspecified== fracture of navicular [scaphoid] bone of left wrist
                 Coding Clinic: 2012, Q4, P106
    ● S62.009   ==Unspecified== fracture of navicular [scaphoid] bone of unspecified wrist
  ● **S62.01**   Fracture of distal pole of navicular [scaphoid] bone of wrist
               Fracture of volar tuberosity of navicular [scaphoid] bone of wrist
    ● S62.011   Displaced fracture of distal pole of navicular [scaphoid] bone of right wrist
    ● S62.012   Displaced fracture of distal pole of navicular [scaphoid] bone of left wrist
    ● S62.013   Displaced fracture of distal pole of navicular [scaphoid] bone of ==unspecified== wrist
    ● S62.014   Nondisplaced fracture of distal pole of navicular [scaphoid] bone of right wrist
    ● S62.015   Nondisplaced fracture of distal pole of navicular [scaphoid] bone of left wrist
    ● S62.016   Nondisplaced fracture of distal pole of navicular [scaphoid] bone of ==unspecified== wrist

● **S62.02**   Fracture of middle third of navicular [scaphoid] bone of wrist
  ● S62.021   Displaced fracture of middle third of navicular [scaphoid] bone of right wrist
  ● S62.022   Displaced fracture of middle third of navicular [scaphoid] bone of left wrist
  ● S62.023   Displaced fracture of middle third of navicular [scaphoid] bone of ==unspecified== wrist
  ● S62.024   Nondisplaced fracture of middle third of navicular [scaphoid] bone of right wrist
  ● S62.025   Nondisplaced fracture of middle third of navicular [scaphoid] bone of left wrist
  ● S62.026   Nondisplaced fracture of middle third of navicular [scaphoid] bone of ==unspecified== wrist
● **S62.03**   Fracture of proximal third of navicular [scaphoid] bone of wrist
  ● S62.031   Displaced fracture of proximal third of navicular [scaphoid] bone of right wrist
  ● S62.032   Displaced fracture of proximal third of navicular [scaphoid] bone of left wrist
  ● S62.033   Displaced fracture of proximal third of navicular [scaphoid] bone of ==unspecified== wrist
  ● S62.034   Nondisplaced fracture of proximal third of navicular [scaphoid] bone of right wrist
  ● S62.035   Nondisplaced fracture of proximal third of navicular [scaphoid] bone of left wrist
  ● S62.036   Nondisplaced fracture of proximal third of navicular [scaphoid] bone of ==unspecified== wrist
● **S62.1**   Fracture of other and unspecified carpal bone(s)
    ==Excludes2==   fracture of scaphoid of wrist (S62.0-)
  ● **S62.10**   Fracture of unspecified carpal bone
               Fracture of wrist NOS
    ● S62.101   Fracture of ==unspecified== carpal bone, right wrist
    ● S62.102   Fracture of ==unspecified== carpal bone, left wrist
                 Coding Clinic: 2012, Q4, P95
    ● S62.109   Fracture of ==unspecified== carpal bone, unspecified wrist
  ● **S62.11**   Fracture of triquetrum [cuneiform] bone of wrist
    ● S62.111   Displaced fracture of triquetrum [cuneiform] bone, right wrist
    ● S62.112   Displaced fracture of triquetrum [cuneiform] bone, left wrist
    ● S62.113   Displaced fracture of triquetrum [cuneiform] bone, ==unspecified== wrist
    ● S62.114   Nondisplaced fracture of triquetrum [cuneiform] bone, right wrist
    ● S62.115   Nondisplaced fracture of triquetrum [cuneiform] bone, left wrist
    ● S62.116   Nondisplaced fracture of triquetrum [cuneiform] bone, ==unspecified== wrist
  ● **S62.12**   Fracture of lunate [semilunar]
    ● S62.121   Displaced fracture of lunate [semilunar], right wrist
    ● S62.122   Displaced fracture of lunate [semilunar], left wrist

● S62.123   Displaced fracture of lunate
             [semilunar], unspecified wrist
● S62.124   Nondisplaced fracture of lunate
             [semilunar], right wrist
● S62.125   Nondisplaced fracture of lunate
             [semilunar], left wrist
● S62.126   Nondisplaced fracture of lunate
             [semilunar], unspecified wrist
● S62.13   Fracture of capitate [os magnum] bone
● S62.131   Displaced fracture of capitate
             [os magnum] bone, right wrist
● S62.132   Displaced fracture of capitate
             [os magnum] bone, left wrist
● S62.133   Displaced fracture of capitate
             [os magnum] bone, unspecified wrist
● S62.134   Nondisplaced fracture of capitate
             [os magnum] bone, right wrist
● S62.135   Nondisplaced fracture of capitate
             [os magnum] bone, left wrist
● S62.136   Nondisplaced fracture of capitate
             [os magnum] bone, unspecified wrist
● S62.14   Fracture of body of hamate [unciform] bone
           Fracture of hamate [unciform] bone NOS
● S62.141   Displaced fracture of body of hamate
             [unciform] bone, right wrist
● S62.142   Displaced fracture of body of hamate
             [unciform] bone, left wrist
● S62.143   Displaced fracture of body of hamate
             [unciform] bone, unspecified wrist
● S62.144   Nondisplaced fracture of body of
             hamate [unciform] bone, right wrist
● S62.145   Nondisplaced fracture of body of
             hamate [unciform] bone, left wrist
● S62.146   Nondisplaced fracture of body of
             hamate [unciform] bone, unspecified
             wrist
● S62.15   Fracture of hook process of hamate [unciform]
           bone
           Fracture of unciform process of hamate
             [unciform] bone
● S62.151   Displaced fracture of hook process of
             hamate [unciform] bone, right wrist
● S62.152   Displaced fracture of hook process of
             hamate [unciform] bone, left wrist
● S62.153   Displaced fracture of hook process of
             hamate [unciform] bone, unspecified
             wrist
● S62.154   Nondisplaced fracture of hook process
             of hamate [unciform] bone, right wrist
● S62.155   Nondisplaced fracture of hook process
             of hamate [unciform] bone, left wrist
● S62.156   Nondisplaced fracture of hook
             process of hamate [unciform] bone,
             unspecified wrist
● S62.16   Fracture of pisiform
● S62.161   Displaced fracture of pisiform, right
             wrist
● S62.162   Displaced fracture of pisiform, left
             wrist
● S62.163   Displaced fracture of pisiform,
             unspecified wrist
● S62.164   Nondisplaced fracture of pisiform,
             right wrist
● S62.165   Nondisplaced fracture of pisiform,
             left wrist
● S62.166   Nondisplaced fracture of pisiform,
             unspecified wrist

● S62.17   Fracture of trapezium [larger multangular]
● S62.171   Displaced fracture of trapezium
             [larger multangular], right wrist
● S62.172   Displaced fracture of trapezium
             [larger multangular], left wrist
● S62.173   Displaced fracture of trapezium
             [larger multangular], unspecified
             wrist
● S62.174   Nondisplaced fracture of trapezium
             [larger multangular], right wrist
● S62.175   Nondisplaced fracture of trapezium
             [larger multangular], left wrist
● S62.176   Nondisplaced fracture of trapezium
             [larger multangular], unspecified
             wrist
● S62.18   Fracture of trapezoid [smaller multangular]
● S62.181   Displaced fracture of trapezoid
             [smaller multangular], right wrist
● S62.182   Displaced fracture of trapezoid
             [smaller multangular], left wrist
● S62.183   Displaced fracture of trapezoid
             [smaller multangular], unspecified
             wrist
● S62.184   Nondisplaced fracture of trapezoid
             [smaller multangular], right wrist
● S62.185   Nondisplaced fracture of trapezoid
             [smaller multangular], left wrist
● S62.186   Nondisplaced fracture of trapezoid
             [smaller multangular], unspecified
             wrist
● S62.2   Fracture of first metacarpal bone
● S62.20   Unspecified fracture of first metacarpal bone
● S62.201   Unspecified fracture of first
             metacarpal bone, right hand
● S62.202   Unspecified fracture of first
             metacarpal bone, left hand
● S62.209   Unspecified fracture of first
             metacarpal bone, unspecified hand
● S62.21   Bennett's fracture
● S62.211   Bennett's fracture, right hand
● S62.212   Bennett's fracture, left hand
● S62.213   Bennett's fracture, unspecified hand
● S62.22   Rolando's fracture
● S62.221   Displaced Rolando's fracture, right
             hand
● S62.222   Displaced Rolando's fracture, left
             hand
● S62.223   Displaced Rolando's fracture,
             unspecified hand
● S62.224   Nondisplaced Rolando's fracture,
             right hand
● S62.225   Nondisplaced Rolando's fracture, left
             hand
● S62.226   Nondisplaced Rolando's fracture,
             unspecified hand
● S62.23   Other fracture of base of first metacarpal bone
● S62.231   Other displaced fracture of base of
             first metacarpal bone, right hand
● S62.232   Other displaced fracture of base of
             first metacarpal bone, left hand
● S62.233   Other displaced fracture of base of
             first metacarpal bone, unspecified
             hand
● S62.234   Other nondisplaced fracture of base
             of first metacarpal bone, right hand
● S62.235   Other nondisplaced fracture of base
             of first metacarpal bone, left hand
● S62.236   Other nondisplaced fracture of base
             of first metacarpal bone, unspecified
             hand

◀ New   ◀▥ Revised   d̶e̶l̶e̶t̶e̶d̶ Deleted   Excludes 1   Excludes 2   Includes   Use additional   Code first   Code also   Unspecified
OGCR Official Guidelines   X Assign placeholder X   ● Use Additional Character(s)   ▶ Manifestation Code   Coding Clinic

● **S62.24**　Fracture of shaft of first metacarpal bone
　● **S62.241**　Displaced fracture of shaft of first metacarpal bone, right hand
　● **S62.242**　Displaced fracture of shaft of first metacarpal bone, left hand
　● **S62.243**　Displaced fracture of shaft of first metacarpal bone, unspecified hand
　● **S62.244**　Nondisplaced fracture of shaft of first metacarpal bone, right hand
　● **S62.245**　Nondisplaced fracture of shaft of first metacarpal bone, left hand
　● **S62.246**　Nondisplaced fracture of shaft of first metacarpal bone, unspecified hand
● **S62.25**　Fracture of neck of first metacarpal bone
　● **S62.251**　Displaced fracture of neck of first metacarpal bone, right hand
　● **S62.252**　Displaced fracture of neck of first metacarpal bone, left hand
　● **S62.253**　Displaced fracture of neck of first metacarpal bone, unspecified hand
　● **S62.254**　Nondisplaced fracture of neck of first metacarpal bone, right hand
　● **S62.255**　Nondisplaced fracture of neck of first metacarpal bone, left hand
　● **S62.256**　Nondisplaced fracture of neck of first metacarpal bone, unspecified hand
● **S62.29**　Other fracture of first metacarpal bone
　● **S62.291**　Other fracture of first metacarpal bone, right hand
　● **S62.292**　Other fracture of first metacarpal bone, left hand
　● **S62.299**　Other fracture of first metacarpal bone, unspecified hand
● **S62.3**　Fracture of other and unspecified metacarpal bone
　　Excludes2　fracture of first metacarpal bone (S62.2-)
　● **S62.30**　Unspecified fracture of other metacarpal bone
　　● **S62.300**　Unspecified fracture of second metacarpal bone, right hand
　　● **S62.301**　Unspecified fracture of second metacarpal bone, left hand
　　● **S62.302**　Unspecified fracture of third metacarpal bone, right hand
　　● **S62.303**　Unspecified fracture of third metacarpal bone, left hand
　　● **S62.304**　Unspecified fracture of fourth metacarpal bone, right hand
　　● **S62.305**　Unspecified fracture of fourth metacarpal bone, left hand
　　● **S62.306**　Unspecified fracture of fifth metacarpal bone, right hand
　　● **S62.307**　Unspecified fracture of fifth metacarpal bone, left hand
　　● **S62.308**　Unspecified fracture of other metacarpal bone
　　　　Unspecified fracture of specified metacarpal bone with unspecified laterality
　　● **S62.309**　Unspecified fracture of unspecified metacarpal bone
　● **S62.31**　Displaced fracture of base of other metacarpal bone
　　● **S62.310**　Displaced fracture of base of second metacarpal bone, right hand
　　● **S62.311**　Displaced fracture of base of second metacarpal bone, left hand
　　● **S62.312**　Displaced fracture of base of third metacarpal bone, right hand

● **S62.313**　Displaced fracture of base of third metacarpal bone, left hand
● **S62.314**　Displaced fracture of base of fourth metacarpal bone, right hand
● **S62.315**　Displaced fracture of base of fourth metacarpal bone, left hand
● **S62.316**　Displaced fracture of base of fifth metacarpal bone, right hand
● **S62.317**　Displaced fracture of base of fifth metacarpal bone, left hand
● **S62.318**　Displaced fracture of base of other metacarpal bone
　　Displaced fracture of base of specified metacarpal bone with unspecified laterality
● **S62.319**　Displaced fracture of base of unspecified metacarpal bone
● **S62.32**　Displaced fracture of shaft of other metacarpal bone
　● **S62.320**　Displaced fracture of shaft of second metacarpal bone, right hand
　● **S62.321**　Displaced fracture of shaft of second metacarpal bone, left hand
　● **S62.322**　Displaced fracture of shaft of third metacarpal bone, right hand
　● **S62.323**　Displaced fracture of shaft of third metacarpal bone, left hand
　● **S62.324**　Displaced fracture of shaft of fourth metacarpal bone, right hand
　● **S62.325**　Displaced fracture of shaft of fourth metacarpal bone, left hand
　● **S62.326**　Displaced fracture of shaft of fifth metacarpal bone, right hand
　● **S62.327**　Displaced fracture of shaft of fifth metacarpal bone, left hand
　● **S62.328**　Displaced fracture of shaft of other metacarpal bone
　　　Displaced fracture of shaft of specified metacarpal bone with unspecified laterality
　● **S62.329**　Displaced fracture of shaft of unspecified metacarpal bone
● **S62.33**　Displaced fracture of neck of other metacarpal bone
　● **S62.330**　Displaced fracture of neck of second metacarpal bone, right hand
　● **S62.331**　Displaced fracture of neck of second metacarpal bone, left hand
　● **S62.332**　Displaced fracture of neck of third metacarpal bone, right hand
　● **S62.333**　Displaced fracture of neck of third metacarpal bone, left hand
　● **S62.334**　Displaced fracture of neck of fourth metacarpal bone, right hand
　● **S62.335**　Displaced fracture of neck of fourth metacarpal bone, left hand
　● **S62.336**　Displaced fracture of neck of fifth metacarpal bone, right hand
　● **S62.337**　Displaced fracture of neck of fifth metacarpal bone, left hand
　● **S62.338**　Displaced fracture of neck of other metacarpal bone
　　　Displaced fracture of neck of specified metacarpal bone with unspecified laterality
　● **S62.339**　Displaced fracture of neck of unspecified metacarpal bone

CHAPTER 19 (S00-T88)

● S62.34   Nondisplaced fracture of base of other
           metacarpal bone
    ● S62.340   Nondisplaced fracture of base of
               second metacarpal bone, right hand
    ● S62.341   Nondisplaced fracture of base of
               second metacarpal bone, left hand
    ● S62.342   Nondisplaced fracture of base of third
               metacarpal bone, right hand
    ● S62.343   Nondisplaced fracture of base of third
               metacarpal bone, left hand
    ● S62.344   Nondisplaced fracture of base of
               fourth metacarpal bone, right hand
    ● S62.345   Nondisplaced fracture of base of
               fourth metacarpal bone, left hand
    ● S62.346   Nondisplaced fracture of base of fifth
               metacarpal bone, right hand
    ● S62.347   Nondisplaced fracture of base of fifth
               metacarpal bone, left hand
    ● S62.348   Nondisplaced fracture of base of
               other metacarpal bone
                   Nondisplaced fracture of base of
                   specified metacarpal bone with
                   unspecified laterality
    ● S62.349   Nondisplaced fracture of base of
               unspecified metacarpal bone
● S62.35   Nondisplaced fracture of shaft of other
           metacarpal bone
    ● S62.350   Nondisplaced fracture of shaft of
               second metacarpal bone, right hand
    ● S62.351   Nondisplaced fracture of shaft of
               second metacarpal bone, left hand
    ● S62.352   Nondisplaced fracture of shaft of
               third metacarpal bone, right hand
    ● S62.353   Nondisplaced fracture of shaft of
               third metacarpal bone, left hand
    ● S62.354   Nondisplaced fracture of shaft of
               fourth metacarpal bone, right hand
    ● S62.355   Nondisplaced fracture of shaft of
               fourth metacarpal bone, left hand
    ● S62.356   Nondisplaced fracture of shaft of fifth
               metacarpal bone, right hand
    ● S62.357   Nondisplaced fracture of shaft of fifth
               metacarpal bone, left hand
    ● S62.358   Nondisplaced fracture of shaft of
               other metacarpal bone
                   Nondisplaced fracture of shaft of
                   specified metacarpal bone with
                   unspecified laterality
    ● S62.359   Nondisplaced fracture of shaft of
               unspecified metacarpal bone
● S62.36   Nondisplaced fracture of neck of other
           metacarpal bone
    ● S62.360   Nondisplaced fracture of neck of
               second metacarpal bone, right hand
    ● S62.361   Nondisplaced fracture of neck of
               second metacarpal bone, left hand
    ● S62.362   Nondisplaced fracture of neck of
               third metacarpal bone, right hand
    ● S62.363   Nondisplaced fracture of neck of
               third metacarpal bone, left hand
    ● S62.364   Nondisplaced fracture of neck of
               fourth metacarpal bone, right hand
    ● S62.365   Nondisplaced fracture of neck of
               fourth metacarpal bone, left hand
    ● S62.366   Nondisplaced fracture of neck of fifth
               metacarpal bone, right hand
    ● S62.367   Nondisplaced fracture of neck of fifth
               metacarpal bone, left hand

● S62.368   Nondisplaced fracture of neck of
           other metacarpal bone
               Nondisplaced fracture of neck of
               specified metacarpal bone with
               unspecified laterality
    ● S62.369   Nondisplaced fracture of neck of
               unspecified metacarpal bone
● S62.39   Other fracture of other metacarpal bone
    ● S62.390   Other fracture of second metacarpal
               bone, right hand
    ● S62.391   Other fracture of second metacarpal
               bone, left hand
    ● S62.392   Other fracture of third metacarpal
               bone, right hand
    ● S62.393   Other fracture of third metacarpal
               bone, left hand
    ● S62.394   Other fracture of fourth metacarpal
               bone, right hand
    ● S62.395   Other fracture of fourth metacarpal
               bone, left hand
    ● S62.396   Other fracture of fifth metacarpal
               bone, right hand
    ● S62.397   Other fracture of fifth metacarpal
               bone, left hand
    ● S62.398   Other fracture of other metacarpal
               bone
                   Other fracture of specified
                   metacarpal bone with
                   unspecified laterality
    ● S62.399   Other fracture of unspecified
               metacarpal bone
● S62.5   Fracture of thumb
    ● S62.50   Fracture of unspecified phalanx of thumb
        ● S62.501   Fracture of unspecified phalanx of
                   right thumb
        ● S62.502   Fracture of unspecified phalanx of left
                   thumb
        ● S62.509   Fracture of unspecified phalanx of
                   unspecified thumb
    ● S62.51   Fracture of proximal phalanx of thumb
        ● S62.511   Displaced fracture of proximal
                   phalanx of right thumb
        ● S62.512   Displaced fracture of proximal
                   phalanx of left thumb
        ● S62.513   Displaced fracture of proximal
                   phalanx of unspecified thumb
        ● S62.514   Nondisplaced fracture of proximal
                   phalanx of right thumb
        ● S62.515   Nondisplaced fracture of proximal
                   phalanx of left thumb
        ● S62.516   Nondisplaced fracture of proximal
                   phalanx of unspecified thumb
    ● S62.52   Fracture of distal phalanx of thumb
        ● S62.521   Displaced fracture of distal phalanx
                   of right thumb
        ● S62.522   Displaced fracture of distal phalanx
                   of left thumb
        ● S62.523   Displaced fracture of distal phalanx
                   of unspecified thumb
        ● S62.524   Nondisplaced fracture of distal
                   phalanx of right thumb
        ● S62.525   Nondisplaced fracture of distal
                   phalanx of left thumb
        ● S62.526   Nondisplaced fracture of distal
                   phalanx of unspecified thumb

◀ New   ◀▦ Revised   ~~deleted~~ Deleted   Excludes 1   Excludes 2   Includes   Use additional   Code first   Code also   Unspecified

OGCR Official Guidelines   X Assign placeholder X   ● Use Additional Character(s)   ▶ Manifestation Code   Coding Clinic

- ● S62.6   Fracture of other and unspecified finger(s)
  - **Excludes2**   fracture of thumb (S62.5-)
  - ● S62.60   Fracture of unspecified phalanx of finger
    - ● S62.600   Fracture of unspecified phalanx of right index finger
    - ● S62.601   Fracture of unspecified phalanx of left index finger
    - ● S62.602   Fracture of unspecified phalanx of right middle finger
    - ● S62.603   Fracture of unspecified phalanx of left middle finger
    - ● S62.604   Fracture of unspecified phalanx of right ring finger
    - ● S62.605   Fracture of unspecified phalanx of left ring finger
    - ● S62.606   Fracture of unspecified phalanx of right little finger
    - ● S62.607   Fracture of unspecified phalanx of left little finger
    - ● S62.608   Fracture of unspecified phalanx of other finger
      Fracture of unspecified phalanx of specified finger with unspecified laterality
    - ● S62.609   Fracture of unspecified phalanx of unspecified finger
  - ● S62.61   Displaced fracture of proximal phalanx of finger
    - ● S62.610   Displaced fracture of proximal phalanx of right index finger
    - ● S62.611   Displaced fracture of proximal phalanx of left index finger
    - ● S62.612   Displaced fracture of proximal phalanx of right middle finger
    - ● S62.613   Displaced fracture of proximal phalanx of left middle finger
    - ● S62.614   Displaced fracture of proximal phalanx of right ring finger
    - ● S62.615   Displaced fracture of proximal phalanx of left ring finger
    - ● S62.616   Displaced fracture of proximal phalanx of right little finger
    - ● S62.617   Displaced fracture of proximal phalanx of left little finger
    - ● S62.618   Displaced fracture of proximal phalanx of other finger
      Displaced fracture of proximal phalanx of specified finger with unspecified laterality
    - ● S62.619   Displaced fracture of proximal phalanx of unspecified finger
  - ● S62.62   Displaced fracture of medial phalanx of finger
    - ● S62.620   Displaced fracture of medial phalanx of right index finger
    - ● S62.621   Displaced fracture of medial phalanx of left index finger
    - ● S62.622   Displaced fracture of medial phalanx of right middle finger
    - ● S62.623   Displaced fracture of medial phalanx of left middle finger
    - ● S62.624   Displaced fracture of medial phalanx of right ring finger
    - ● S62.625   Displaced fracture of medial phalanx of left ring finger
    - ● S62.626   Displaced fracture of medial phalanx of right little finger
    - ● S62.627   Displaced fracture of medial phalanx of left little finger
    - ● S62.628   Displaced fracture of medial phalanx of other finger
      Displaced fracture of medial phalanx of specified finger with unspecified laterality
    - ● S62.629   Displaced fracture of medial phalanx of unspecified finger
  - ● S62.63   Displaced fracture of distal phalanx of finger
    - ● S62.630   Displaced fracture of distal phalanx of right index finger
    - ● S62.631   Displaced fracture of distal phalanx of left index finger
    - ● S62.632   Displaced fracture of distal phalanx of right middle finger
    - ● S62.633   Displaced fracture of distal phalanx of left middle finger
    - ● S62.634   Displaced fracture of distal phalanx of right ring finger
    - ● S62.635   Displaced fracture of distal phalanx of left ring finger
    - ● S62.636   Displaced fracture of distal phalanx of right little finger
    - ● S62.637   Displaced fracture of distal phalanx of left little finger
    - ● S62.638   Displaced fracture of distal phalanx of other finger
      Displaced fracture of distal phalanx of specified finger with unspecified laterality
    - ● S62.639   Displaced fracture of distal phalanx of unspecified finger
  - ● S62.64   Nondisplaced fracture of proximal phalanx of finger
    - ● S62.640   Nondisplaced fracture of proximal phalanx of right index finger
    - ● S62.641   Nondisplaced fracture of proximal phalanx of left index finger
    - ● S62.642   Nondisplaced fracture of proximal phalanx of right middle finger
    - ● S62.643   Nondisplaced fracture of proximal phalanx of left middle finger
    - ● S62.644   Nondisplaced fracture of proximal phalanx of right ring finger
    - ● S62.645   Nondisplaced fracture of proximal phalanx of left ring finger
    - ● S62.646   Nondisplaced fracture of proximal phalanx of right little finger
    - ● S62.647   Nondisplaced fracture of proximal phalanx of left little finger
    - ● S62.648   Nondisplaced fracture of proximal phalanx of other finger
      Nondisplaced fracture of proximal phalanx of specified finger with unspecified laterality
    - ● S62.649   Nondisplaced fracture of proximal phalanx of unspecified finger
  - ● S62.65   Nondisplaced fracture of medial phalanx of finger
    - ● S62.650   Nondisplaced fracture of medial phalanx of right index finger
    - ● S62.651   Nondisplaced fracture of medial phalanx of left index finger
    - ● S62.652   Nondisplaced fracture of medial phalanx of right middle finger
    - ● S62.653   Nondisplaced fracture of medial phalanx of left middle finger
    - ● S62.654   Nondisplaced fracture of medial phalanx of right ring finger
    - ● S62.655   Nondisplaced fracture of medial phalanx of left ring finger

CHAPTER 19 (S00-T88)

- ● S62.656 Nondisplaced fracture of medial phalanx of right little finger
- ● S62.657 Nondisplaced fracture of medial phalanx of left little finger
- ● S62.658 Nondisplaced fracture of medial phalanx of other finger
    Nondisplaced fracture of medial phalanx of specified finger with unspecified laterality
- ● S62.659 Nondisplaced fracture of medial phalanx of unspecified finger
- ● S62.66 Nondisplaced fracture of distal phalanx of finger
    - ● S62.660 Nondisplaced fracture of distal phalanx of right index finger
    - ● S62.661 Nondisplaced fracture of distal phalanx of left index finger
    - ● S62.662 Nondisplaced fracture of distal phalanx of right middle finger
    - ● S62.663 Nondisplaced fracture of distal phalanx of left middle finger
    - ● S62.664 Nondisplaced fracture of distal phalanx of right ring finger
    - ● S62.665 Nondisplaced fracture of distal phalanx of left ring finger
    - ● S62.666 Nondisplaced fracture of distal phalanx of right little finger
    - ● S62.667 Nondisplaced fracture of distal phalanx of left little finger
    - ● S62.668 Nondisplaced fracture of distal phalanx of other finger
        Nondisplaced fracture of distal phalanx of specified finger with unspecified laterality
    - ● S62.669 Nondisplaced fracture of distal phalanx of unspecified finger
- ● S62.9 Unspecified fracture of wrist and hand
    - X ● S62.90 Unspecified fracture of unspecified wrist and hand
    - X ● S62.91 Unspecified fracture of right wrist and hand
    - X ● S62.92 Unspecified fracture of left wrist and hand

● S63 Dislocation and sprain of joints and ligaments at wrist and hand level

> **Includes** avulsion of joint or ligament at wrist and hand level
> laceration of cartilage, joint or ligament at wrist and hand level
> sprain of cartilage, joint or ligament at wrist and hand level
> traumatic hemarthrosis of joint or ligament at wrist and hand level
> traumatic rupture of joint or ligament at wrist and hand level
> traumatic subluxation of joint or ligament at wrist and hand level
> traumatic tear of joint or ligament at wrist and hand level

Code also any associated open wound

> **Excludes2** strain of muscle, fascia and tendon of wrist and hand (S66.-)

The appropriate 7th character is to be added to each code from category S63

A	initial encounter
D	subsequent encounter
S	sequela

- ● S63.0 Subluxation and dislocation of wrist and hand joints
    - ● S63.00 Unspecified subluxation and dislocation of wrist and hand
        Dislocation of carpal bone NOS
        Dislocation of distal end of radius NOS
        Subluxation of carpal bone NOS
        Subluxation of distal end of radius NOS

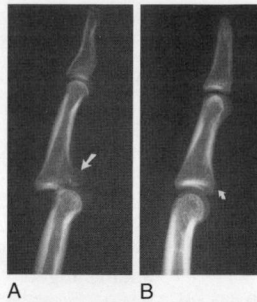

Figure 19-13 Dislocation including displacement and subluxation. (From Grainger & Allison's Diagnostic Radiology: A Textbook of Medical Imaging, ed 4, Churchill Livingstone, 2001)

- ● S63.001 Unspecified subluxation of right wrist and hand
- ● S63.002 Unspecified subluxation of left wrist and hand
- ● S63.003 Unspecified subluxation of unspecified wrist and hand
- ● S63.004 Unspecified dislocation of right wrist and hand
- ● S63.005 Unspecified dislocation of left wrist and hand
- ● S63.006 Unspecified dislocation of unspecified wrist and hand
- ● S63.01 Subluxation and dislocation of distal radioulnar joint
    - ● S63.011 Subluxation of distal radioulnar joint of right wrist
    - ● S63.012 Subluxation of distal radioulnar joint of left wrist
    - ● S63.013 Subluxation of distal radioulnar joint of unspecified wrist
    - ● S63.014 Dislocation of distal radioulnar joint of right wrist
    - ● S63.015 Dislocation of distal radioulnar joint of left wrist
    - ● S63.016 Dislocation of distal radioulnar joint of unspecified wrist
- ● S63.02 Subluxation and dislocation of radiocarpal joint
    - ● S63.021 Subluxation of radiocarpal joint of right wrist
    - ● S63.022 Subluxation of radiocarpal joint of left wrist
    - ● S63.023 Subluxation of radiocarpal joint of unspecified wrist
    - ● S63.024 Dislocation of radiocarpal joint of right wrist
    - ● S63.025 Dislocation of radiocarpal joint of left wrist
    - ● S63.026 Dislocation of radiocarpal joint of unspecified wrist
- ● S63.03 Subluxation and dislocation of midcarpal joint
    - ● S63.031 Subluxation of midcarpal joint of right wrist
    - ● S63.032 Subluxation of midcarpal joint of left wrist
    - ● S63.033 Subluxation of midcarpal joint of unspecified wrist
    - ● S63.034 Dislocation of midcarpal joint of right wrist
    - ● S63.035 Dislocation of midcarpal joint of left wrist
    - ● S63.036 Dislocation of midcarpal joint of unspecified wrist

◀ New   ◀▦ Revised   ~~deleted~~ Deleted   Excludes 1   Excludes 2   Includes   Use additional   Code first   Code also   Unspecified

OGCR Official Guidelines   X Assign placeholder X   ● Use Additional Character(s)   ▶ Manifestation Code   **Coding Clinic**

- ● S63.04 **Subluxation and dislocation of carpometacarpal joint of thumb**
    - **Excludes2** interphalangeal subluxation and dislocation of thumb (S63.1-)
    - ● S63.041 **Subluxation of carpometacarpal joint of right thumb**
    - ● S63.042 **Subluxation of carpometacarpal joint of left thumb**
    - ● S63.043 **Subluxation of carpometacarpal joint of unspecified thumb**
    - ● S63.044 **Dislocation of carpometacarpal joint of right thumb**
    - ● S63.045 **Dislocation of carpometacarpal joint of left thumb**
    - ● S63.046 **Dislocation of carpometacarpal joint of unspecified thumb**
- ● S63.05 **Subluxation and dislocation of other carpometacarpal joint**
    - **Excludes2** subluxation and dislocation of carpometacarpal joint of thumb (S63.04-)
    - ● S63.051 **Subluxation of other carpometacarpal joint of right hand**
    - ● S63.052 **Subluxation of other carpometacarpal joint of left hand**
    - ● S63.053 **Subluxation of other carpometacarpal joint of unspecified hand**
    - ● S63.054 **Dislocation of other carpometacarpal joint of right hand**
    - ● S63.055 **Dislocation of other carpometacarpal joint of left hand**
    - ● S63.056 **Dislocation of other carpometacarpal joint of unspecified hand**
- ● S63.06 **Subluxation and dislocation of metacarpal (bone), proximal end**
    - ● S63.061 **Subluxation of metacarpal (bone), proximal end of right hand**
    - ● S63.062 **Subluxation of metacarpal (bone), proximal end of left hand**
    - ● S63.063 **Subluxation of metacarpal (bone), proximal end of unspecified hand**
    - ● S63.064 **Dislocation of metacarpal (bone), proximal end of right hand**
    - ● S63.065 **Dislocation of metacarpal (bone), proximal end of left hand**
    - ● S63.066 **Dislocation of metacarpal (bone), proximal end of unspecified hand**
- ● S63.07 **Subluxation and dislocation of distal end of ulna**
    - ● S63.071 **Subluxation of distal end of right ulna**
    - ● S63.072 **Subluxation of distal end of left ulna**
    - ● S63.073 **Subluxation of distal end of unspecified ulna**
    - ● S63.074 **Dislocation of distal end of right ulna**
    - ● S63.075 **Dislocation of distal end of left ulna**
    - ● S63.076 **Dislocation of distal end of unspecified ulna**
- ● S63.09 **Other subluxation and dislocation of wrist and hand**
    - ● S63.091 **Other subluxation of right wrist and hand**
    - ● S63.092 **Other subluxation of left wrist and hand**
    - ● S63.093 **Other subluxation of unspecified wrist and hand**
    - ● S63.094 **Other dislocation of right wrist and hand**
    - ● S63.095 **Other dislocation of left wrist and hand**
    - ● S63.096 **Other dislocation of unspecified wrist and hand**
- ● S63.1 **Subluxation and dislocation of thumb**
    - ● S63.10 **Unspecified subluxation and dislocation of thumb**
        - ● S63.101 **Unspecified subluxation of right thumb**
        - ● S63.102 **Unspecified subluxation of left thumb**
        - ● S63.103 **Unspecified subluxation of unspecified thumb**
        - ● S63.104 **Unspecified dislocation of right thumb**
        - ● S63.105 **Unspecified dislocation of left thumb**
        - ● S63.106 **Unspecified dislocation of unspecified thumb**
    - ● S63.11 **Subluxation and dislocation of metacarpophalangeal joint of thumb**
        - ● S63.111 **Subluxation of metacarpophalangeal joint of right thumb**
        - ● S63.112 **Subluxation of metacarpophalangeal joint of left thumb**
        - ● S63.113 **Subluxation of metacarpophalangeal joint of unspecified thumb**
        - ● S63.114 **Dislocation of metacarpophalangeal joint of right thumb**
        - ● S63.115 **Dislocation of metacarpophalangeal joint of left thumb**
        - ● S63.116 **Dislocation of metacarpophalangeal joint of unspecified thumb**
    - ● S63.12 **Subluxation and dislocation of unspecified interphalangeal joint of thumb**
        - ● S63.121 **Subluxation of unspecified interphalangeal joint of right thumb**
        - ● S63.122 **Subluxation of unspecified interphalangeal joint of left thumb**
        - ● S63.123 **Subluxation of unspecified interphalangeal joint of unspecified thumb**
        - ● S63.124 **Dislocation of unspecified interphalangeal joint of right thumb**
        - ● S63.125 **Dislocation of unspecified interphalangeal joint of left thumb**
        - ● S63.126 **Dislocation of unspecified interphalangeal joint of unspecified thumb**
    - ● S63.13 **Subluxation and dislocation of proximal interphalangeal joint of thumb**
        - ● S63.131 **Subluxation of proximal interphalangeal joint of right thumb**
        - ● S63.132 **Subluxation of proximal interphalangeal joint of left thumb**
        - ● S63.133 **Subluxation of proximal interphalangeal joint of unspecified thumb**
        - ● S63.134 **Dislocation of proximal interphalangeal joint of right thumb**
        - ● S63.135 **Dislocation of proximal interphalangeal joint of left thumb**
        - ● S63.136 **Dislocation of proximal interphalangeal joint of unspecified thumb**

CHAPTER 19 (S00-T88)

- ● S63.14   Subluxation and dislocation of distal interphalangeal joint of thumb
  - ● S63.141   Subluxation of distal interphalangeal joint of right thumb
  - ● S63.142   Subluxation of distal interphalangeal joint of left thumb
  - ● S63.143   Subluxation of distal interphalangeal joint of unspecified thumb
  - ● S63.144   Dislocation of distal interphalangeal joint of right thumb
  - ● S63.145   Dislocation of distal interphalangeal joint of left thumb
  - ● S63.146   Dislocation of distal interphalangeal joint of unspecified thumb
- ● S63.2   Subluxation and dislocation of other finger(s)
  - **Excludes2**   subluxation and dislocation of thumb (S63.1-)
  - ● S63.20   Unspecified subluxation of other finger
    - ● S63.200   Unspecified subluxation of right index finger
    - ● S63.201   Unspecified subluxation of left index finger
    - ● S63.202   Unspecified subluxation of right middle finger
    - ● S63.203   Unspecified subluxation of left middle finger
    - ● S63.204   Unspecified subluxation of right ring finger
    - ● S63.205   Unspecified subluxation of left ring finger
    - ● S63.206   Unspecified subluxation of right little finger
    - ● S63.207   Unspecified subluxation of left little finger
    - ● S63.208   Unspecified subluxation of other finger
      - Unspecified subluxation of specified finger with unspecified laterality
    - ● S63.209   Unspecified subluxation of unspecified finger
  - ● S63.21   Subluxation of metacarpophalangeal joint of finger
    - ● S63.210   Subluxation of metacarpophalangeal joint of right index finger
    - ● S63.211   Subluxation of metacarpophalangeal joint of left index finger
    - ● S63.212   Subluxation of metacarpophalangeal joint of right middle finger
    - ● S63.213   Subluxation of metacarpophalangeal joint of left middle finger
    - ● S63.214   Subluxation of metacarpophalangeal joint of right ring finger
    - ● S63.215   Subluxation of metacarpophalangeal joint of left ring finger
    - ● S63.216   Subluxation of metacarpophalangeal joint of right little finger
    - ● S63.217   Subluxation of metacarpophalangeal joint of left little finger
    - ● S63.218   Subluxation of metacarpophalangeal joint of other finger
      - Subluxation of metacarpophalangeal joint of specified finger with unspecified laterality
    - ● S63.219   Subluxation of metacarpophalangeal joint of unspecified finger

- ● S63.22   Subluxation of unspecified interphalangeal joint of finger
  - ● S63.220   Subluxation of unspecified interphalangeal joint of right index finger
  - ● S63.221   Subluxation of unspecified interphalangeal joint of left index finger
  - ● S63.222   Subluxation of unspecified interphalangeal joint of right middle finger
  - ● S63.223   Subluxation of unspecified interphalangeal joint of left middle finger
  - ● S63.224   Subluxation of unspecified interphalangeal joint of right ring finger
  - ● S63.225   Subluxation of unspecified interphalangeal joint of left ring finger
  - ● S63.226   Subluxation of unspecified interphalangeal joint of right little finger
  - ● S63.227   Subluxation of unspecified interphalangeal joint of left little finger
  - ● S63.228   Subluxation of unspecified interphalangeal joint of other finger
    - Subluxation of unspecified interphalangeal joint of specified finger with unspecified laterality
  - ● S63.229   Subluxation of unspecified interphalangeal joint of unspecified finger
- ● S63.23   Subluxation of proximal interphalangeal joint of finger
  - ● S63.230   Subluxation of proximal interphalangeal joint of right index finger
  - ● S63.231   Subluxation of proximal interphalangeal joint of left index finger
  - ● S63.232   Subluxation of proximal interphalangeal joint of right middle finger
  - ● S63.233   Subluxation of proximal interphalangeal joint of left middle finger
  - ● S63.234   Subluxation of proximal interphalangeal joint of right ring finger
  - ● S63.235   Subluxation of proximal interphalangeal joint of left ring finger
  - ● S63.236   Subluxation of proximal interphalangeal joint of right little finger
  - ● S63.237   Subluxation of proximal interphalangeal joint of left little finger
  - ● S63.238   Subluxation of proximal interphalangeal joint of other finger
    - Subluxation of proximal interphalangeal joint of specified finger with unspecified laterality
  - ● S63.239   Subluxation of proximal interphalangeal joint of unspecified finger

◄ New   ◄▬ Revised   ~~deleted~~ Deleted   Excludes 1   Excludes 2   Includes   Use additional   Code first   Code also   Unspecified

OGCR Official Guidelines   X Assign placeholder X   ● Use Additional Character(s)   ▶ Manifestation Code   **Coding Clinic**

● S63.24   Subluxation of distal interphalangeal joint of finger
  ● S63.240   Subluxation of distal interphalangeal joint of right index finger
  ● S63.241   Subluxation of distal interphalangeal joint of left index finger
  ● S63.242   Subluxation of distal interphalangeal joint of right middle finger
  ● S63.243   Subluxation of distal interphalangeal joint of left middle finger
  ● S63.244   Subluxation of distal interphalangeal joint of right ring finger
  ● S63.245   Subluxation of distal interphalangeal joint of left ring finger
  ● S63.246   Subluxation of distal interphalangeal joint of right little finger
  ● S63.247   Subluxation of distal interphalangeal joint of left little finger
  ● S63.248   Subluxation of distal interphalangeal joint of other finger
        Subluxation of distal interphalangeal joint of specified finger with unspecified laterality
  ● S63.249   Subluxation of distal interphalangeal joint of unspecified finger
● S63.25   Unspecified dislocation of other finger
  ● S63.250   Unspecified dislocation of right index finger
  ● S63.251   Unspecified dislocation of left index finger
  ● S63.252   Unspecified dislocation of right middle finger
  ● S63.253   Unspecified dislocation of left middle finger
  ● S63.254   Unspecified dislocation of right ring finger
  ● S63.255   Unspecified dislocation of left ring finger
  ● S63.256   Unspecified dislocation of right little finger
  ● S63.257   Unspecified dislocation of left little finger
  ● S63.258   Unspecified dislocation of other finger
        Unspecified dislocation of specified finger with unspecified laterality
  ● S63.259   Unspecified dislocation of unspecified finger
        Unspecified dislocation of specified finger with unspecified laterality
● S63.26   Dislocation of metacarpophalangeal joint of finger
  ● S63.260   Dislocation of metacarpophalangeal joint of right index finger
  ● S63.261   Dislocation of metacarpophalangeal joint of left index finger
  ● S63.262   Dislocation of metacarpophalangeal joint of right middle finger
  ● S63.263   Dislocation of metacarpophalangeal joint of left middle finger
  ● S63.264   Dislocation of metacarpophalangeal joint of right ring finger
  ● S63.265   Dislocation of metacarpophalangeal joint of left ring finger

● S63.266   Dislocation of metacarpophalangeal joint of right little finger
● S63.267   Dislocation of metacarpophalangeal joint of left little finger
● S63.268   Dislocation of metacarpophalangeal joint of other finger
      Dislocation of metacarpophalangeal joint of specified finger with unspecified laterality
● S63.269   Dislocation of metacarpophalangeal joint of unspecified finger
● S63.27   Dislocation of unspecified interphalangeal joint of finger
  ● S63.270   Dislocation of unspecified interphalangeal joint of right index finger
  ● S63.271   Dislocation of unspecified interphalangeal joint of left index finger
  ● S63.272   Dislocation of unspecified interphalangeal joint of right middle finger
  ● S63.273   Dislocation of unspecified interphalangeal joint of left middle finger
  ● S63.274   Dislocation of unspecified interphalangeal joint of right ring finger
  ● S63.275   Dislocation of unspecified interphalangeal joint of left ring finger
  ● S63.276   Dislocation of unspecified interphalangeal joint of right little finger
  ● S63.277   Dislocation of unspecified interphalangeal joint of left little finger
  ● S63.278   Dislocation of unspecified interphalangeal joint of other finger
        Dislocation of unspecified interphalangeal joint of specified finger with unspecified laterality
  ● S63.279   Dislocation of unspecified interphalangeal joint of unspecified finger
        Dislocation of unspecified interphalangeal joint of specified finger without specified laterality
● S63.28   Dislocation of proximal interphalangeal joint of finger
  ● S63.280   Dislocation of proximal interphalangeal joint of right index finger
  ● S63.281   Dislocation of proximal interphalangeal joint of left index finger
  ● S63.282   Dislocation of proximal interphalangeal joint of right middle finger
  ● S63.283   Dislocation of proximal interphalangeal joint of left middle finger
  ● S63.284   Dislocation of proximal interphalangeal joint of right ring finger

CHAPTER 19 (S00-T88)

● S63.285   Dislocation of proximal interphalangeal joint of left ring finger

● S63.286   Dislocation of proximal interphalangeal joint of right little finger

● S63.287   Dislocation of proximal interphalangeal joint of left little finger

● S63.288   Dislocation of proximal interphalangeal joint of other finger

     Dislocation of proximal interphalangeal joint of specified finger with unspecified laterality

● S63.289   Dislocation of proximal interphalangeal joint of unspecified finger

● S63.29   Dislocation of distal interphalangeal joint of finger

● S63.290   Dislocation of distal interphalangeal joint of right index finger

● S63.291   Dislocation of distal interphalangeal joint of left index finger

● S63.292   Dislocation of distal interphalangeal joint of right middle finger

● S63.293   Dislocation of distal interphalangeal joint of left middle finger

● S63.294   Dislocation of distal interphalangeal joint of right ring finger

● S63.295   Dislocation of distal interphalangeal joint of left ring finger

● S63.296   Dislocation of distal interphalangeal joint of right little finger

● S63.297   Dislocation of distal interphalangeal joint of left little finger

● S63.298   Dislocation of distal interphalangeal joint of other finger

     Dislocation of distal interphalangeal joint of specified finger with unspecified laterality

● S63.299   Dislocation of distal interphalangeal joint of unspecified finger

● S63.3   Traumatic rupture of ligament of wrist

● S63.30   Traumatic rupture of unspecified ligament of wrist

● S63.301   Traumatic rupture of unspecified ligament of right wrist

● S63.302   Traumatic rupture of unspecified ligament of left wrist

● S63.309   Traumatic rupture of unspecified ligament of unspecified wrist

● S63.31   Traumatic rupture of collateral ligament of wrist

● S63.311   Traumatic rupture of collateral ligament of right wrist

● S63.312   Traumatic rupture of collateral ligament of left wrist

● S63.319   Traumatic rupture of collateral ligament of unspecified wrist

● S63.32   Traumatic rupture of radiocarpal ligament

● S63.321   Traumatic rupture of right radiocarpal ligament

● S63.322   Traumatic rupture of left radiocarpal ligament

● S63.329   Traumatic rupture of unspecified radiocarpal ligament

● S63.33   Traumatic rupture of ulnocarpal (palmar) ligament

● S63.331   Traumatic rupture of right ulnocarpal (palmar) ligament

● S63.332   Traumatic rupture of left ulnocarpal (palmar) ligament

● S63.339   Traumatic rupture of unspecified ulnocarpal (palmar) ligament

● S63.39   Traumatic rupture of other ligament of wrist

● S63.391   Traumatic rupture of other ligament of right wrist

● S63.392   Traumatic rupture of other ligament of left wrist

● S63.399   Traumatic rupture of other ligament of unspecified wrist

● S63.4   Traumatic rupture of ligament of finger at metacarpophalangeal and interphalangeal joint(s)

● S63.40   Traumatic rupture of unspecified ligament of finger at metacarpophalangeal and interphalangeal joint

● S63.400   Traumatic rupture of unspecified ligament of right index finger at metacarpophalangeal and interphalangeal joint

● S63.401   Traumatic rupture of unspecified ligament of left index finger at metacarpophalangeal and interphalangeal joint

● S63.402   Traumatic rupture of unspecified ligament of right middle finger at metacarpophalangeal and interphalangeal joint

● S63.403   Traumatic rupture of unspecified ligament of left middle finger at metacarpophalangeal and interphalangeal joint

● S63.404   Traumatic rupture of unspecified ligament of right ring finger at metacarpophalangeal and interphalangeal joint

● S63.405   Traumatic rupture of unspecified ligament of left ring finger at metacarpophalangeal and interphalangeal joint

● S63.406   Traumatic rupture of unspecified ligament of right little finger at metacarpophalangeal and interphalangeal joint

● S63.407   Traumatic rupture of unspecified ligament of left little finger at metacarpophalangeal and interphalangeal joint

● S63.408   Traumatic rupture of unspecified ligament of other finger at metacarpophalangeal and interphalangeal joint

     Traumatic rupture of unspecified ligament of specified finger with unspecified laterality at metacarpophalangeal and interphalangeal joint

● S63.409   Traumatic rupture of unspecified ligament of unspecified finger at metacarpophalangeal and interphalangeal joint

● S63.41 Traumatic rupture of collateral ligament of finger at metacarpophalangeal and interphalangeal joint

  ● S63.410 Traumatic rupture of collateral ligament of right index finger at metacarpophalangeal and interphalangeal joint

  ● S63.411 Traumatic rupture of collateral ligament of left index finger at metacarpophalangeal and interphalangeal joint

  ● S63.412 Traumatic rupture of collateral ligament of right middle finger at metacarpophalangeal and interphalangeal joint

  ● S63.413 Traumatic rupture of collateral ligament of left middle finger at metacarpophalangeal and interphalangeal joint

  ● S63.414 Traumatic rupture of collateral ligament of right ring finger at metacarpophalangeal and interphalangeal joint

  ● S63.415 Traumatic rupture of collateral ligament of left ring finger at metacarpophalangeal and interphalangeal joint

  ● S63.416 Traumatic rupture of collateral ligament of right little finger at metacarpophalangeal and interphalangeal joint

  ● S63.417 Traumatic rupture of collateral ligament of left little finger at metacarpophalangeal and interphalangeal joint

  ● S63.418 Traumatic rupture of collateral ligament of other finger at metacarpophalangeal and interphalangeal joint
    Traumatic rupture of collateral ligament of specified finger with unspecified laterality at metacarpophalangeal and interphalangeal joint

  ● S63.419 Traumatic rupture of collateral ligament of unspecified finger at metacarpophalangeal and interphalangeal joint

● S63.42 Traumatic rupture of palmar ligament of finger at metacarpophalangeal and interphalangeal joint

  ● S63.420 Traumatic rupture of palmar ligament of right index finger at metacarpophalangeal and interphalangeal joint

  ● S63.421 Traumatic rupture of palmar ligament of left index finger at metacarpophalangeal and interphalangeal joint

  ● S63.422 Traumatic rupture of palmar ligament of right middle finger at metacarpophalangeal and interphalangeal joint

  ● S63.423 Traumatic rupture of palmar ligament of left middle finger at metacarpophalangeal and interphalangeal joint

  ● S63.424 Traumatic rupture of palmar ligament of right ring finger at metacarpophalangeal and interphalangeal joint

  ● S63.425 Traumatic rupture of palmar ligament of left ring finger at metacarpophalangeal and interphalangeal joint

  ● S63.426 Traumatic rupture of palmar ligament of right little finger at metacarpophalangeal and interphalangeal joint

  ● S63.427 Traumatic rupture of palmar ligament of left little finger at metacarpophalangeal and interphalangeal joint

  ● S63.428 Traumatic rupture of palmar ligament of other finger at metacarpophalangeal and interphalangeal joint
    Traumatic rupture of palmar ligament of specified finger with unspecified laterality at metacarpophalangeal and interphalangeal joint

  ● S63.429 Traumatic rupture of palmar ligament of unspecified finger at metacarpophalangeal and interphalangeal joint

● S63.43 Traumatic rupture of volar plate of finger at metacarpophalangeal and interphalangeal joint

  ● S63.430 Traumatic rupture of volar plate of right index finger at metacarpophalangeal and interphalangeal joint

  ● S63.431 Traumatic rupture of volar plate of left index finger at metacarpophalangeal and interphalangeal joint

  ● S63.432 Traumatic rupture of volar plate of right middle finger at metacarpophalangeal and interphalangeal joint

  ● S63.433 Traumatic rupture of volar plate of left middle finger at metacarpophalangeal and interphalangeal joint

  ● S63.434 Traumatic rupture of volar plate of right ring finger at metacarpophalangeal and interphalangeal joint

  ● S63.435 Traumatic rupture of volar plate of left ring finger at metacarpophalangeal and interphalangeal joint

  ● S63.436 Traumatic rupture of volar plate of right little finger at metacarpophalangeal and interphalangeal joint

  ● S63.437 Traumatic rupture of volar plate of left little finger at metacarpophalangeal and interphalangeal joint

  ● S63.438 Traumatic rupture of volar plate of other finger at metacarpophalangeal and interphalangeal joint
    Traumatic rupture of volar plate of specified finger with unspecified laterality at metacarpophalangeal and interphalangeal joint

  ● S63.439 Traumatic rupture of volar plate of unspecified finger at metacarpophalangeal and interphalangeal joint

● S63.49   Traumatic rupture of other ligament of finger at metacarpophalangeal and interphalangeal joint

     ● S63.490   Traumatic rupture of other ligament of right index finger at metacarpophalangeal and interphalangeal joint

     ● S63.491   Traumatic rupture of other ligament of left index finger at metacarpophalangeal and interphalangeal joint

     ● S63.492   Traumatic rupture of other ligament of right middle finger at metacarpophalangeal and interphalangeal joint

     ● S63.493   Traumatic rupture of other ligament of left middle finger at metacarpophalangeal and interphalangeal joint

     ● S63.494   Traumatic rupture of other ligament of right ring finger at metacarpophalangeal and interphalangeal joint

     ● S63.495   Traumatic rupture of other ligament of left ring finger at metacarpophalangeal and interphalangeal joint

     ● S63.496   Traumatic rupture of other ligament of right little finger at metacarpophalangeal and interphalangeal joint

     ● S63.497   Traumatic rupture of other ligament of left little finger at metacarpophalangeal and interphalangeal joint

     ● S63.498   Traumatic rupture of other ligament of other finger at metacarpophalangeal and interphalangeal joint
          Traumatic rupture of ligament of specified finger with unspecified laterality at metacarpophalangeal and interphalangeal joint

     ● S63.499   Traumatic rupture of other ligament of unspecified finger at metacarpophalangeal and interphalangeal joint

● S63.5   Other and unspecified sprain of wrist

     ● S63.50   Unspecified sprain of wrist

         ● S63.501   Unspecified sprain of right wrist
         ● S63.502   Unspecified sprain of left wrist
         ● S63.509   Unspecified sprain of unspecified wrist

     ● S63.51   Sprain of carpal (joint)

         ● S63.511   Sprain of carpal joint of right wrist
         ● S63.512   Sprain of carpal joint of left wrist
         ● S63.519   Sprain of carpal joint of unspecified wrist

     ● S63.52   Sprain of radiocarpal joint
         Excludes1   traumatic rupture of radiocarpal ligament (S63.32-)

         ● S63.521   Sprain of radiocarpal joint of right wrist
         ● S63.522   Sprain of radiocarpal joint of left wrist
         ● S63.529   Sprain of radiocarpal joint of unspecified wrist

● S63.59   Other specified sprain of wrist

     ● S63.591   Other specified sprain of right wrist
     ● S63.592   Other specified sprain of left wrist
     ● S63.599   Other specified sprain of unspecified wrist

● S63.6   Other and unspecified sprain of finger(s)
     Excludes1   traumatic rupture of ligament of finger at metacarpophalangeal and interphalangeal joint(s) (S63.4-)

● S63.60   Unspecified sprain of thumb

     ● S63.601   Unspecified sprain of right thumb
     ● S63.602   Unspecified sprain of left thumb
     ● S63.609   Unspecified sprain of unspecified thumb

● S63.61   Unspecified sprain of other and unspecified finger(s)

     ● S63.610   Unspecified sprain of right index finger
     ● S63.611   Unspecified sprain of left index finger
     ● S63.612   Unspecified sprain of right middle finger
     ● S63.613   Unspecified sprain of left middle finger
     ● S63.614   Unspecified sprain of right ring finger
     ● S63.615   Unspecified sprain of left ring finger
     ● S63.616   Unspecified sprain of right little finger
     ● S63.617   Unspecified sprain of left little finger
     ● S63.618   Unspecified sprain of other finger
          Unspecified sprain of specified finger with unspecified laterality

     ● S63.619   Unspecified sprain of unspecified finger

● S63.62   Sprain of interphalangeal joint of thumb

     ● S63.621   Sprain of interphalangeal joint of right thumb
     ● S63.622   Sprain of interphalangeal joint of left thumb
     ● S63.629   Sprain of interphalangeal joint of unspecified thumb

● S63.63   Sprain of interphalangeal joint of other and unspecified finger(s)

     ● S63.630   Sprain of interphalangeal joint of right index finger
     ● S63.631   Sprain of interphalangeal joint of left index finger
     ● S63.632   Sprain of interphalangeal joint of right middle finger
     ● S63.633   Sprain of interphalangeal joint of left middle finger
     ● S63.634   Sprain of interphalangeal joint of right ring finger
     ● S63.635   Sprain of interphalangeal joint of left ring finger
     ● S63.636   Sprain of interphalangeal joint of right little finger
     ● S63.637   Sprain of interphalangeal joint of left little finger
     ● S63.638   Sprain of interphalangeal joint of other finger
     ● S63.639   Sprain of interphalangeal joint of unspecified finger

◀ New   ⬅ Revised   deleted Deleted   Excludes 1   Excludes 2   Includes   Use additional   Code first   Code also   Unspecified

OGCR Official Guidelines   X Assign placeholder X   ● Use Additional Character(s)   ▶ Manifestation Code   **Coding Clinic**

● S63.64   Sprain of metacarpophalangeal joint of thumb
    ● S63.641   Sprain of metacarpophalangeal joint of right thumb
    ● S63.642   Sprain of metacarpophalangeal joint of left thumb
    ● S63.649   Sprain of metacarpophalangeal joint of unspecified thumb
● S63.65   Sprain of metacarpophalangeal joint of other and unspecified finger(s)
    ● S63.650   Sprain of metacarpophalangeal joint of right index finger
    ● S63.651   Sprain of metacarpophalangeal joint of left index finger
    ● S63.652   Sprain of metacarpophalangeal joint of right middle finger
    ● S63.653   Sprain of metacarpophalangeal joint of left middle finger
    ● S63.654   Sprain of metacarpophalangeal joint of right ring finger
    ● S63.655   Sprain of metacarpophalangeal joint of left ring finger
    ● S63.656   Sprain of metacarpophalangeal joint of right little finger
    ● S63.657   Sprain of metacarpophalangeal joint of left little finger
    ● S63.658   Sprain of metacarpophalangeal joint of other finger
       Sprain of metacarpophalangeal joint of specified finger with unspecified laterality
    ● S63.659   Sprain of metacarpophalangeal joint of unspecified finger
● S63.68   Other sprain of thumb
    ● S63.681   Other sprain of right thumb
    ● S63.682   Other sprain of left thumb
    ● S63.689   Other sprain of unspecified thumb
● S63.69   Other sprain of other and unspecified finger(s)
    ● S63.690   Other sprain of right index finger
    ● S63.691   Other sprain of left index finger
    ● S63.692   Other sprain of right middle finger
    ● S63.693   Other sprain of left middle finger
    ● S63.694   Other sprain of right ring finger
    ● S63.695   Other sprain of left ring finger
    ● S63.696   Other sprain of right little finger
    ● S63.697   Other sprain of left little finger
    ● S63.698   Other sprain of other finger
       Other sprain of specified finger with unspecified laterality
    ● S63.699   Other sprain of unspecified finger
● S63.8   Sprain of other part of wrist and hand
    ● S63.8X   Sprain of other part of wrist and hand
       ● S63.8X1   Sprain of other part of right wrist and hand
       ● S63.8X2   Sprain of other part of left wrist and hand
       ● S63.8X9   Sprain of other part of unspecified wrist and hand
● S63.9   Sprain of unspecified part of wrist and hand
    X● S63.90   Sprain of unspecified part of unspecified wrist and hand
    X● S63.91   Sprain of unspecified part of right wrist and hand
    X● S63.92   Sprain of unspecified part of left wrist and hand

● S64   Injury of nerves at wrist and hand level
    The appropriate 7th character is to be added to each code from category S64

       A   initial encounter
       D   subsequent encounter
       S   sequela

    Code also any associated open wound (S61.-)
● S64.0   Injury of ulnar nerve at wrist and hand level
    X● S64.00   Injury of ulnar nerve at wrist and hand level of unspecified arm
    X● S64.01   Injury of ulnar nerve at wrist and hand level of right arm
    X● S64.02   Injury of ulnar nerve at wrist and hand level of left arm
● S64.1   Injury of median nerve at wrist and hand level
    X● S64.10   Injury of median nerve at wrist and hand level of unspecified arm
    X● S64.11   Injury of median nerve at wrist and hand level of right arm
    X● S64.12   Injury of median nerve at wrist and hand level of left arm
● S64.2   Injury of radial nerve at wrist and hand level
    X● S64.20   Injury of radial nerve at wrist and hand level of unspecified arm
    X● S64.21   Injury of radial nerve at wrist and hand level of right arm
    X● S64.22   Injury of radial nerve at wrist and hand level of left arm
● S64.3   Injury of digital nerve of thumb
    X● S64.30   Injury of digital nerve of unspecified thumb
    X● S64.31   Injury of digital nerve of right thumb
    X● S64.32   Injury of digital nerve of left thumb
● S64.4   Injury of digital nerve of other and unspecified finger
    X● S64.40   Injury of digital nerve of unspecified finger
    ● S64.49   Injury of digital nerve of other finger
       ● S64.490   Injury of digital nerve of right index finger
       ● S64.491   Injury of digital nerve of left index finger
       ● S64.492   Injury of digital nerve of right middle finger
       ● S64.493   Injury of digital nerve of left middle finger
       ● S64.494   Injury of digital nerve of right ring finger
       ● S64.495   Injury of digital nerve of left ring finger
       ● S64.496   Injury of digital nerve of right little finger
       ● S64.497   Injury of digital nerve of left little finger
       ● S64.498   Injury of digital nerve of other finger
          Injury of digital nerve of specified finger with unspecified laterality
● S64.8   Injury of other nerves at wrist and hand level
    ● S64.8X   Injury of other nerves at wrist and hand level

CHAPTER 19 (S00-T88)

- S64.8X1   Injury of other nerves at wrist and hand level of right arm
- S64.8X2   Injury of other nerves at wrist and hand level of left arm
- S64.8X9   Injury of other nerves at wrist and hand level of unspecified arm
- S64.9   Injury of unspecified nerve at wrist and hand level
  - X ● S64.90   Injury of unspecified nerve at wrist and hand level of unspecified arm
  - X ● S64.91   Injury of unspecified nerve at wrist and hand level of right arm
  - X ● S64.92   Injury of unspecified nerve at wrist and hand level of left arm

- ● S65   Injury of blood vessels at wrist and hand level

  The appropriate 7th character is to be added to each code from category S65

A	initial encounter
D	subsequent encounter
S	sequela

  Code also any associated open wound (S61.-)

  - ● S65.0   Injury of ulnar artery at wrist and hand level
    - ● S65.00   Unspecified injury of ulnar artery at wrist and hand level
      - ● S65.001   Unspecified injury of ulnar artery at wrist and hand level of right arm
      - ● S65.002   Unspecified injury of ulnar artery at wrist and hand level of left arm
      - ● S65.009   Unspecified injury of ulnar artery at wrist and hand level of unspecified arm
    - ● S65.01   Laceration of ulnar artery at wrist and hand level
      - ● S65.011   Laceration of ulnar artery at wrist and hand level of right arm
      - ● S65.012   Laceration of ulnar artery at wrist and hand level of left arm
      - ● S65.019   Laceration of ulnar artery at wrist and hand level of unspecified arm
    - ● S65.09   Other specified injury of ulnar artery at wrist and hand level
      - ● S65.091   Other specified injury of ulnar artery at wrist and hand level of right arm
      - ● S65.092   Other specified injury of ulnar artery at wrist and hand level of left arm
      - ● S65.099   Other specified injury of ulnar artery at wrist and hand level of unspecified arm
  - ● S65.1   Injury of radial artery at wrist and hand level
    - ● S65.10   Unspecified injury of radial artery at wrist and hand level
      - ● S65.101   Unspecified injury of radial artery at wrist and hand level of right arm
      - ● S65.102   Unspecified injury of radial artery at wrist and hand level of left arm
      - ● S65.109   Unspecified injury of radial artery at wrist and hand level of unspecified arm
    - ● S65.11   Laceration of radial artery at wrist and hand level
      - ● S65.111   Laceration of radial artery at wrist and hand level of right arm
      - ● S65.112   Laceration of radial artery at wrist and hand level of left arm
      - ● S65.119   Laceration of radial artery at wrist and hand level of unspecified arm

- ● S65.19   Other specified injury of radial artery at wrist and hand level
  - ● S65.191   Other specified injury of radial artery at wrist and hand level of right arm
  - ● S65.192   Other specified injury of radial artery at wrist and hand level of left arm
  - ● S65.199   Other specified injury of radial artery at wrist and hand level of unspecified arm
- ● S65.2   Injury of superficial palmar arch
  - ● S65.20   Unspecified injury of superficial palmar arch
    - ● S65.201   Unspecified injury of superficial palmar arch of right hand
    - ● S65.202   Unspecified injury of superficial palmar arch of left hand
    - ● S65.209   Unspecified injury of superficial palmar arch of unspecified hand
  - ● S65.21   Laceration of superficial palmar arch
    - ● S65.211   Laceration of superficial palmar arch of right hand
    - ● S65.212   Laceration of superficial palmar arch of left hand
    - ● S65.219   Laceration of superficial palmar arch of unspecified hand
  - ● S65.29   Other specified injury of superficial palmar arch
    - ● S65.291   Other specified injury of superficial palmar arch of right hand
    - ● S65.292   Other specified injury of superficial palmar arch of left hand
    - ● S65.299   Other specified injury of superficial palmar arch of unspecified hand
- ● S65.3   Injury of deep palmar arch
  - ● S65.30   Unspecified injury of deep palmar arch
    - ● S65.301   Unspecified injury of deep palmar arch of right hand
    - ● S65.302   Unspecified injury of deep palmar arch of left hand
    - ● S65.309   Unspecified injury of deep palmar arch of unspecified hand
  - ● S65.31   Laceration of deep palmar arch
    - ● S65.311   Laceration of deep palmar arch of right hand
    - ● S65.312   Laceration of deep palmar arch of left hand
    - ● S65.319   Laceration of deep palmar arch of unspecified hand
  - ● S65.39   Other specified injury of deep palmar arch
    - ● S65.391   Other specified injury of deep palmar arch of right hand
    - ● S65.392   Other specified injury of deep palmar arch of left hand
    - ● S65.399   Other specified injury of deep palmar arch of unspecified hand
- ● S65.4   Injury of blood vessel of thumb
  - ● S65.40   Unspecified injury of blood vessel of thumb
    - ● S65.401   Unspecified injury of blood vessel of right thumb
    - ● S65.402   Unspecified injury of blood vessel of left thumb
    - ● S65.409   Unspecified injury of blood vessel of unspecified thumb

◀ New   ◀█ Revised   ~~deleted~~ Deleted   Excludes 1   Excludes 2   Includes   Use additional   Code first   Code also   Unspecified

OGCR Official Guidelines   X Assign placeholder X   ● Use Additional Character(s)   ▶ Manifestation Code   **Coding Clinic**

● **S65.41**   Laceration of blood vessel of thumb
   ● **S65.411**   Laceration of blood vessel of right thumb
   ● **S65.412**   Laceration of blood vessel of left thumb
   ● **S65.419**   Laceration of blood vessel of unspecified thumb

● **S65.49**   Other specified injury of blood vessel of thumb
   ● **S65.491**   Other specified injury of blood vessel of right thumb
   ● **S65.492**   Other specified injury of blood vessel of left thumb
   ● **S65.499**   Other specified injury of blood vessel of unspecified thumb

● **S65.5**   Injury of blood vessel of other and unspecified finger
  ● **S65.50**   Unspecified injury of blood vessel of other and unspecified finger
   ● **S65.500**   Unspecified injury of blood vessel of right index finger
   ● **S65.501**   Unspecified injury of blood vessel of left index finger
   ● **S65.502**   Unspecified injury of blood vessel of right middle finger
   ● **S65.503**   Unspecified injury of blood vessel of left middle finger
   ● **S65.504**   Unspecified injury of blood vessel of right ring finger
   ● **S65.505**   Unspecified injury of blood vessel of left ring finger
   ● **S65.506**   Unspecified injury of blood vessel of right little finger
   ● **S65.507**   Unspecified injury of blood vessel of left little finger
   ● **S65.508**   Unspecified injury of blood vessel of other finger
       Unspecified injury of blood vessel of specified finger with unspecified laterality
   ● **S65.509**   Unspecified injury of blood vessel of unspecified finger

  ● **S65.51**   Laceration of blood vessel of other and unspecified finger
   ● **S65.510**   Laceration of blood vessel of right index finger
   ● **S65.511**   Laceration of blood vessel of left index finger
   ● **S65.512**   Laceration of blood vessel of right middle finger
   ● **S65.513**   Laceration of blood vessel of left middle finger
   ● **S65.514**   Laceration of blood vessel of right ring finger
   ● **S65.515**   Laceration of blood vessel of left ring finger
   ● **S65.516**   Laceration of blood vessel of right little finger
   ● **S65.517**   Laceration of blood vessel of left little finger
   ● **S65.518**   Laceration of blood vessel of other finger
       Laceration of blood vessel of specified finger with unspecified laterality
   ● **S65.519**   Laceration of blood vessel of unspecified finger

● **S65.59**   Other specified injury of blood vessel of other and unspecified finger
   ● **S65.590**   Other specified injury of blood vessel of right index finger
   ● **S65.591**   Other specified injury of blood vessel of left index finger
   ● **S65.592**   Other specified injury of blood vessel of right middle finger
   ● **S65.593**   Other specified injury of blood vessel of left middle finger
   ● **S65.594**   Other specified injury of blood vessel of right ring finger
   ● **S65.595**   Other specified injury of blood vessel of left ring finger
   ● **S65.596**   Other specified injury of blood vessel of right little finger
   ● **S65.597**   Other specified injury of blood vessel of left little finger
   ● **S65.598**   Other specified injury of blood vessel of other finger
       Other specified injury of blood vessel of specified finger with unspecified laterality
   ● **S65.599**   Other specified injury of blood vessel of unspecified finger

● **S65.8**   Injury of other blood vessels at wrist and hand level
  ● **S65.80**   Unspecified injury of other blood vessels at wrist and hand level
   ● **S65.801**   Unspecified injury of other blood vessels at wrist and hand level of right arm
   ● **S65.802**   Unspecified injury of other blood vessels at wrist and hand level of left arm
   ● **S65.809**   Unspecified injury of other blood vessels at wrist and hand level of unspecified arm

  ● **S65.81**   Laceration of other blood vessels at wrist and hand level
   ● **S65.811**   Laceration of other blood vessels at wrist and hand level of right arm
   ● **S65.812**   Laceration of other blood vessels at wrist and hand level of left arm
   ● **S65.819**   Laceration of other blood vessels at wrist and hand level of unspecified arm

  ● **S65.89**   Other specified injury of other blood vessels at wrist and hand level
   ● **S65.891**   Other specified injury of other blood vessels at wrist and hand level of right arm
   ● **S65.892**   Other specified injury of other blood vessels at wrist and hand level of left arm
   ● **S65.899**   Other specified injury of other blood vessels at wrist and hand level of unspecified arm

CHAPTER 19 (S00-T88)

● S65.9   Injury of unspecified blood vessel at wrist and hand level

  ● S65.90   Unspecified injury of unspecified blood vessel at wrist and hand level

    ● S65.901   Unspecified injury of unspecified blood vessel at wrist and hand level of right arm

    ● S65.902   Unspecified injury of unspecified blood vessel at wrist and hand level of left arm

    ● S65.909   Unspecified injury of unspecified blood vessel at wrist and hand level of unspecified arm

  ● S65.91   Laceration of unspecified blood vessel at wrist and hand level

    ● S65.911   Laceration of unspecified blood vessel at wrist and hand level of right arm

    ● S65.912   Laceration of unspecified blood vessel at wrist and hand level of left arm

    ● S65.919   Laceration of unspecified blood vessel at wrist and hand level of unspecified arm

  ● S65.99   Other specified injury of unspecified blood vessel at wrist and hand level

    ● S65.991   Other specified injury of unspecified blood vessel at wrist and hand of right arm

    ● S65.992   Other specified injury of unspecified blood vessel at wrist and hand of left arm

    ● S65.999   Other specified injury of unspecified blood vessel at wrist and hand of unspecified arm

● S66   Injury of muscle, fascia and tendon at wrist and hand level

  Code also any associated open wound (S61.-)

  Excludes2   sprain of joints and ligaments of wrist and hand (S63.-)

  The appropriate 7th character is to be added to each code from category S66

    A   initial encounter
    D   subsequent encounter
    S   sequela

  ● S66.0   Injury of long flexor muscle, fascia and tendon of thumb at wrist and hand level

    ● S66.00   Unspecified injury of long flexor muscle, fascia and tendon of thumb at wrist and hand level

      ● S66.001   Unspecified injury of long flexor muscle, fascia and tendon of right thumb at wrist and hand level

      ● S66.002   Unspecified injury of long flexor muscle, fascia and tendon of left thumb at wrist and hand level

      ● S66.009   Unspecified injury of long flexor muscle, fascia and tendon of unspecified thumb at wrist and hand level

    ● S66.01   Strain of long flexor muscle, fascia and tendon of thumb at wrist and hand level

      ● S66.011   Strain of long flexor muscle, fascia and tendon of right thumb at wrist and hand level

      ● S66.012   Strain of long flexor muscle, fascia and tendon of left thumb at wrist and hand level

      ● S66.019   Strain of long flexor muscle, fascia and tendon of unspecified thumb at wrist and hand level

    ● S66.02   Laceration of long flexor muscle, fascia and tendon of thumb at wrist and hand level

      ● S66.021   Laceration of long flexor muscle, fascia and tendon of right thumb at wrist and hand level

      ● S66.022   Laceration of long flexor muscle, fascia and tendon of left thumb at wrist and hand level

      ● S66.029   Laceration of long flexor muscle, fascia and tendon of unspecified thumb at wrist and hand level

    ● S66.09   Other specified injury of long flexor muscle, fascia and tendon of thumb at wrist and hand level

      ● S66.091   Other specified injury of long flexor muscle, fascia and tendon of right thumb at wrist and hand level

      ● S66.092   Other specified injury of long flexor muscle, fascia and tendon of left thumb at wrist and hand level

      ● S66.099   Other specified injury of long flexor muscle, fascia and tendon of unspecified thumb at wrist and hand level

  ● S66.1   Injury of flexor muscle, fascia and tendon of other and unspecified finger at wrist and hand level

    Excludes2   injury of long flexor muscle, fascia and tendon of thumb at wrist and hand level (S66.0-)

    ● S66.10   Unspecified injury of flexor muscle, fascia and tendon of other and unspecified finger at wrist and hand level

      ● S66.100   Unspecified injury of flexor muscle, fascia and tendon of right index finger at wrist and hand level

      ● S66.101   Unspecified injury of flexor muscle, fascia and tendon of left index finger at wrist and hand level

      ● S66.102   Unspecified injury of flexor muscle, fascia and tendon of right middle finger at wrist and hand level

      ● S66.103   Unspecified injury of flexor muscle, fascia and tendon of left middle finger at wrist and hand level

      ● S66.104   Unspecified injury of flexor muscle, fascia and tendon of right ring finger at wrist and hand level

      ● S66.105   Unspecified injury of flexor muscle, fascia and tendon of left ring finger at wrist and hand level

      ● S66.106   Unspecified injury of flexor muscle, fascia and tendon of right little finger at wrist and hand level

      ● S66.107   Unspecified injury of flexor muscle, fascia and tendon of left little finger at wrist and hand level

      ● S66.108   Unspecified injury of flexor muscle, fascia and tendon of other finger at wrist and hand level

        Unspecified injury of flexor muscle, fascia and tendon of specified finger with unspecified laterality at wrist and hand level

      ● S66.109   Unspecified injury of flexor muscle, fascia and tendon of unspecified finger at wrist and hand level

● S66.11   Strain of flexor muscle, fascia and tendon of other and unspecified finger at wrist and hand level
   ● S66.110   Strain of flexor muscle, fascia and tendon of right index finger at wrist and hand level
   ● S66.111   Strain of flexor muscle, fascia and tendon of left index finger at wrist and hand level
   ● S66.112   Strain of flexor muscle, fascia and tendon of right middle finger at wrist and hand level
   ● S66.113   Strain of flexor muscle, fascia and tendon of left middle finger at wrist and hand level
   ● S66.114   Strain of flexor muscle, fascia and tendon of right ring finger at wrist and hand level
   ● S66.115   Strain of flexor muscle, fascia and tendon of left ring finger at wrist and hand level
   ● S66.116   Strain of flexor muscle, fascia and tendon of right little finger at wrist and hand level
   ● S66.117   Strain of flexor muscle, fascia and tendon of left little finger at wrist and hand level
   ● S66.118   Strain of flexor muscle, fascia and tendon of other finger at wrist and hand level
              Strain of flexor muscle, fascia and tendon of specified finger with unspecified laterality at wrist and hand level
   ● S66.119   Strain of flexor muscle, fascia and tendon of unspecified finger at wrist and hand level
● S66.12   Laceration of flexor muscle, fascia and tendon of other and unspecified finger at wrist and hand level
   ● S66.120   Laceration of flexor muscle, fascia and tendon of right index finger at wrist and hand level
   ● S66.121   Laceration of flexor muscle, fascia and tendon of left index finger at wrist and hand level
   ● S66.122   Laceration of flexor muscle, fascia and tendon of right middle finger at wrist and hand level
   ● S66.123   Laceration of flexor muscle, fascia and tendon of left middle finger at wrist and hand level
   ● S66.124   Laceration of flexor muscle, fascia and tendon of right ring finger at wrist and hand level
   ● S66.125   Laceration of flexor muscle, fascia and tendon of left ring finger at wrist and hand level
   ● S66.126   Laceration of flexor muscle, fascia and tendon of right little finger at wrist and hand level
   ● S66.127   Laceration of flexor muscle, fascia and tendon of left little finger at wrist and hand level

● S66.128   Laceration of flexor muscle, fascia and tendon of other finger at wrist and hand level
              Laceration of flexor muscle, fascia and tendon of specified finger with unspecified laterality at wrist and hand level
   ● S66.129   Laceration of flexor muscle, fascia and tendon of unspecified finger at wrist and hand level
● S66.19   Other injury of flexor muscle, fascia and tendon of other and unspecified finger at wrist and hand level
   ● S66.190   Other injury of flexor muscle, fascia and tendon of right index finger at wrist and hand level
   ● S66.191   Other injury of flexor muscle, fascia and tendon of left index finger at wrist and hand level
   ● S66.192   Other injury of flexor muscle, fascia and tendon of right middle finger at wrist and hand level
   ● S66.193   Other injury of flexor muscle, fascia and tendon of left middle finger at wrist and hand level
   ● S66.194   Other injury of flexor muscle, fascia and tendon of right ring finger at wrist and hand level
   ● S66.195   Other injury of flexor muscle, fascia and tendon of left ring finger at wrist and hand level
   ● S66.196   Other injury of flexor muscle, fascia and tendon of right little finger at wrist and hand level
   ● S66.197   Other injury of flexor muscle, fascia and tendon of left little finger at wrist and hand level
   ● S66.198   Other injury of flexor muscle, fascia and tendon of other finger at wrist and hand level
              Other injury of flexor muscle, fascia and tendon of specified finger with unspecified laterality at wrist and hand level
   ● S66.199   Other injury of flexor muscle, fascia and tendon of unspecified finger at wrist and hand level
● S66.2   Injury of extensor muscle, fascia and tendon of thumb at wrist and hand level
   ● S66.20   Unspecified injury of extensor muscle, fascia and tendon of thumb at wrist and hand level
      ● S66.201   Unspecified injury of extensor muscle, fascia and tendon of right thumb at wrist and hand level
      ● S66.202   Unspecified injury of extensor muscle, fascia and tendon of left thumb at wrist and hand level
      ● S66.209   Unspecified injury of extensor muscle, fascia and tendon of unspecified thumb at wrist and hand level
   ● S66.21   Strain of extensor muscle, fascia and tendon of thumb at wrist and hand level
      ● S66.211   Strain of extensor muscle, fascia and tendon of right thumb at wrist and hand level
      ● S66.212   Strain of extensor muscle, fascia and tendon of left thumb at wrist and hand level
      ● S66.219   Strain of extensor muscle, fascia and tendon of unspecified thumb at wrist and hand level

● **S66.22** Laceration of extensor muscle, fascia and tendon of thumb at wrist and hand level

    ● **S66.221** Laceration of extensor muscle, fascia and tendon of right thumb at wrist and hand level

    ● **S66.222** Laceration of extensor muscle, fascia and tendon of left thumb at wrist and hand level

    ● **S66.229** Laceration of extensor muscle, fascia and tendon of unspecified thumb at wrist and hand level

● **S66.29** Other specified injury of extensor muscle, fascia and tendon of thumb at wrist and hand level

    ● **S66.291** Other specified injury of extensor muscle, fascia and tendon of right thumb at wrist and hand level

    ● **S66.292** Other specified injury of extensor muscle, fascia and tendon of left thumb at wrist and hand level

    ● **S66.299** Other specified injury of extensor muscle, fascia and tendon of unspecified thumb at wrist and hand level

● **S66.3** Injury of extensor muscle, fascia and tendon of other and unspecified finger at wrist and hand level

    Excludes2   injury of extensor muscle, fascia and tendon of thumb at wrist and hand level (S66.2-)

  ● **S66.30** Unspecified injury of extensor muscle, fascia and tendon of other and unspecified finger at wrist and hand level

    ● **S66.300** Unspecified injury of extensor muscle, fascia and tendon of right index finger at wrist and hand level

    ● **S66.301** Unspecified injury of extensor muscle, fascia and tendon of left index finger at wrist and hand level

    ● **S66.302** Unspecified injury of extensor muscle, fascia and tendon of right middle finger at wrist and hand level

    ● **S66.303** Unspecified injury of extensor muscle, fascia and tendon of left middle finger at wrist and hand level

    ● **S66.304** Unspecified injury of extensor muscle, fascia and tendon of right ring finger at wrist and hand level

    ● **S66.305** Unspecified injury of extensor muscle, fascia and tendon of left ring finger at wrist and hand level

    ● **S66.306** Unspecified injury of extensor muscle, fascia and tendon of right little finger at wrist and hand level

    ● **S66.307** Unspecified injury of extensor muscle, fascia and tendon of left little finger at wrist and hand level

    ● **S66.308** Unspecified injury of extensor muscle, fascia and tendon of other finger at wrist and hand level
        Unspecified injury of extensor muscle, fascia and tendon of specified finger with unspecified laterality at wrist and hand level

    ● **S66.309** Unspecified injury of extensor muscle, fascia and tendon of unspecified finger at wrist and hand level

● **S66.31** Strain of extensor muscle, fascia and tendon of other and unspecified finger at wrist and hand level

    ● **S66.310** Strain of extensor muscle, fascia and tendon of right index finger at wrist and hand level

    ● **S66.311** Strain of extensor muscle, fascia and tendon of left index finger at wrist and hand level

    ● **S66.312** Strain of extensor muscle, fascia and tendon of right middle finger at wrist and hand level

    ● **S66.313** Strain of extensor muscle, fascia and tendon of left middle finger at wrist and hand level

    ● **S66.314** Strain of extensor muscle, fascia and tendon of right ring finger at wrist and hand level

    ● **S66.315** Strain of extensor muscle, fascia and tendon of left ring finger at wrist and hand level

    ● **S66.316** Strain of extensor muscle, fascia and tendon of right little finger at wrist and hand level

    ● **S66.317** Strain of extensor muscle, fascia and tendon of left little finger at wrist and hand level

    ● **S66.318** Strain of extensor muscle, fascia and tendon of other finger at wrist and hand level
        Strain of extensor muscle, fascia and tendon of specified finger with unspecified laterality at wrist and hand level

    ● **S66.319** Strain of extensor muscle, fascia and tendon of unspecified finger at wrist and hand level

● **S66.32** Laceration of extensor muscle, fascia and tendon of other and unspecified finger at wrist and hand level

    ● **S66.320** Laceration of extensor muscle, fascia and tendon of right index finger at wrist and hand level

    ● **S66.321** Laceration of extensor muscle, fascia and tendon of left index finger at wrist and hand level

    ● **S66.322** Laceration of extensor muscle, fascia and tendon of right middle finger at wrist and hand level

    ● **S66.323** Laceration of extensor muscle, fascia and tendon of left middle finger at wrist and hand level

    ● **S66.324** Laceration of extensor muscle, fascia and tendon of right ring finger at wrist and hand level

    ● **S66.325** Laceration of extensor muscle, fascia and tendon of left ring finger at wrist and hand level

    ● **S66.326** Laceration of extensor muscle, fascia and tendon of right little finger at wrist and hand level

    ● **S66.327** Laceration of extensor muscle, fascia and tendon of left little finger at wrist and hand level

    ● **S66.328** Laceration of extensor muscle, fascia and tendon of other finger at wrist and hand level
        Laceration of extensor muscle, fascia and tendon of specified finger with unspecified laterality at wrist and hand level

    ● **S66.329** Laceration of extensor muscle, fascia and tendon of unspecified finger at wrist and hand level

◀ New   ◀▥ Revised   ~~deleted~~ Deleted   Excludes 1   Excludes 2   Includes   Use additional   Code first   Code also   Unspecified

OGCR Official Guidelines   **X** Assign placeholder X   ● Use Additional Character(s)   ▶ Manifestation Code   **Coding Clinic**

● **S66.39**   Other injury of extensor muscle, fascia and tendon of other and unspecified finger at wrist and hand level

    ● **S66.390**   Other injury of extensor muscle, fascia and tendon of right index finger at wrist and hand level

    ● **S66.391**   Other injury of extensor muscle, fascia and tendon of left index finger at wrist and hand level

    ● **S66.392**   Other injury of extensor muscle, fascia and tendon of right middle finger at wrist and hand level

    ● **S66.393**   Other injury of extensor muscle, fascia and tendon of left middle finger at wrist and hand level

    ● **S66.394**   Other injury of extensor muscle, fascia and tendon of right ring finger at wrist and hand level

    ● **S66.395**   Other injury of extensor muscle, fascia and tendon of left ring finger at wrist and hand level

    ● **S66.396**   Other injury of extensor muscle, fascia and tendon of right little finger at wrist and hand level

    ● **S66.397**   Other injury of extensor muscle, fascia and tendon of left little finger at wrist and hand level

    ● **S66.398**   Other injury of extensor muscle, fascia and tendon of other finger at wrist and hand level

         Other injury of extensor muscle, fascia and tendon of specified finger with unspecified laterality at wrist and hand level

    ● **S66.399**   Other injury of extensor muscle, fascia and tendon of unspecified finger at wrist and hand level

● **S66.4**   Injury of intrinsic muscle, fascia and tendon of thumb at wrist and hand level

    ● **S66.40**   Unspecified injury of intrinsic muscle, fascia and tendon of thumb at wrist and hand level

    ● **S66.401**   Unspecified injury of intrinsic muscle, fascia and tendon of right thumb at wrist and hand level

    ● **S66.402**   Unspecified injury of intrinsic muscle, fascia and tendon of left thumb at wrist and hand level

    ● **S66.409**   Unspecified injury of intrinsic muscle, fascia and tendon of unspecified thumb at wrist and hand level

    ● **S66.41**   Strain of intrinsic muscle, fascia and tendon of thumb at wrist and hand level

    ● **S66.411**   Strain of intrinsic muscle, fascia and tendon of right thumb at wrist and hand level

    ● **S66.412**   Strain of intrinsic muscle, fascia and tendon of left thumb at wrist and hand level

    ● **S66.419**   Strain of intrinsic muscle, fascia and tendon of unspecified thumb at wrist and hand level

● **S66.42**   Laceration of intrinsic muscle, fascia and tendon of thumb at wrist and hand level

    ● **S66.421**   Laceration of intrinsic muscle, fascia and tendon of right thumb at wrist and hand level

    ● **S66.422**   Laceration of intrinsic muscle, fascia and tendon of left thumb at wrist and hand level

    ● **S66.429**   Laceration of intrinsic muscle, fascia and tendon of unspecified thumb at wrist and hand level

● **S66.49**   Other specified injury of intrinsic muscle, fascia and tendon of thumb at wrist and hand level

    ● **S66.491**   Other specified injury of intrinsic muscle, fascia and tendon of right thumb at wrist and hand level

    ● **S66.492**   Other specified injury of intrinsic muscle, fascia and tendon of left thumb at wrist and hand level

    ● **S66.499**   Other specified injury of intrinsic muscle, fascia and tendon of unspecified thumb at wrist and hand level

● **S66.5**   Injury of intrinsic muscle, fascia and tendon of other and unspecified finger at wrist and hand level

    Excludes2   injury of intrinsic muscle, fascia and tendon of thumb at wrist and hand level (S66.4-)

    ● **S66.50**   Unspecified injury of intrinsic muscle, fascia and tendon of other and unspecified finger at wrist and hand level

    ● **S66.500**   Unspecified injury of intrinsic muscle, fascia and tendon of right index finger at wrist and hand level

    ● **S66.501**   Unspecified injury of intrinsic muscle, fascia and tendon of left index finger at wrist and hand level

    ● **S66.502**   Unspecified injury of intrinsic muscle, fascia and tendon of right middle finger at wrist and hand level

    ● **S66.503**   Unspecified injury of intrinsic muscle, fascia and tendon of left middle finger at wrist and hand level

    ● **S66.504**   Unspecified injury of intrinsic muscle, fascia and tendon of right ring finger at wrist and hand level

    ● **S66.505**   Unspecified injury of intrinsic muscle, fascia and tendon of left ring finger at wrist and hand level

    ● **S66.506**   Unspecified injury of intrinsic muscle, fascia and tendon of right little finger at wrist and hand level

    ● **S66.507**   Unspecified injury of intrinsic muscle, fascia and tendon of left little finger at wrist and hand level

    ● **S66.508**   Unspecified injury of intrinsic muscle, fascia and tendon of other finger at wrist and hand level

         Unspecified injury of intrinsic muscle, fascia and tendon of specified finger with unspecified laterality at wrist and hand level

    ● **S66.509**   Unspecified injury of intrinsic muscle, fascia and tendon of unspecified finger at wrist and hand level

● **S66.51** Strain of intrinsic muscle, fascia and tendon of other and unspecified finger at wrist and hand level

    ● **S66.510** Strain of intrinsic muscle, fascia and tendon of right index finger at wrist and hand level

    ● **S66.511** Strain of intrinsic muscle, fascia and tendon of left index finger at wrist and hand level

    ● **S66.512** Strain of intrinsic muscle, fascia and tendon of right middle finger at wrist and hand level

    ● **S66.513** Strain of intrinsic muscle, fascia and tendon of left middle finger at wrist and hand level

    ● **S66.514** Strain of intrinsic muscle, fascia and tendon of right ring finger at wrist and hand level

    ● **S66.515** Strain of intrinsic muscle, fascia and tendon of left ring finger at wrist and hand level

    ● **S66.516** Strain of intrinsic muscle, fascia and tendon of right little finger at wrist and hand level

    ● **S66.517** Strain of intrinsic muscle, fascia and tendon of left little finger at wrist and hand level

    ● **S66.518** Strain of intrinsic muscle, fascia and tendon of other finger at wrist and hand level

        Strain of intrinsic muscle, fascia and tendon of specified finger with unspecified laterality at wrist and hand level

    ● **S66.519** Strain of intrinsic muscle, fascia and tendon of unspecified finger at wrist and hand level

● **S66.52** Laceration of intrinsic muscle, fascia and tendon of other and unspecified finger at wrist and hand level

    ● **S66.520** Laceration of intrinsic muscle, fascia and tendon of right index finger at wrist and hand level

    ● **S66.521** Laceration of intrinsic muscle, fascia and tendon of left index finger at wrist and hand level

    ● **S66.522** Laceration of intrinsic muscle, fascia and tendon of right middle finger at wrist and hand level

    ● **S66.523** Laceration of intrinsic muscle, fascia and tendon of left middle finger at wrist and hand level

    ● **S66.524** Laceration of intrinsic muscle, fascia and tendon of right ring finger at wrist and hand level

    ● **S66.525** Laceration of intrinsic muscle, fascia and tendon of left ring finger at wrist and hand level

    ● **S66.526** Laceration of intrinsic muscle, fascia and tendon of right little finger at wrist and hand level

    ● **S66.527** Laceration of intrinsic muscle, fascia and tendon of left little finger at wrist and hand level

    ● **S66.528** Laceration of intrinsic muscle, fascia and tendon of other finger at wrist and hand level

        Laceration of intrinsic muscle, fascia and tendon of specified finger with unspecified laterality at wrist and hand level

    ● **S66.529** Laceration of intrinsic muscle, fascia and tendon of unspecified finger at wrist and hand level

● **S66.59** Other injury of intrinsic muscle, fascia and tendon of other and unspecified finger at wrist and hand level

    ● **S66.590** Other injury of intrinsic muscle, fascia and tendon of right index finger at wrist and hand level

    ● **S66.591** Other injury of intrinsic muscle, fascia and tendon of left index finger at wrist and hand level

    ● **S66.592** Other injury of intrinsic muscle, fascia and tendon of right middle finger at wrist and hand level

    ● **S66.593** Other injury of intrinsic muscle, fascia and tendon of left middle finger at wrist and hand level

    ● **S66.594** Other injury of intrinsic muscle, fascia and tendon of right ring finger at wrist and hand level

    ● **S66.595** Other injury of intrinsic muscle, fascia and tendon of left ring finger at wrist and hand level

    ● **S66.596** Other injury of intrinsic muscle, fascia and tendon of right little finger at wrist and hand level

    ● **S66.597** Other injury of intrinsic muscle, fascia and tendon of left little finger at wrist and hand level

    ● **S66.598** Other injury of intrinsic muscle, fascia and tendon of other finger at wrist and hand level

        Other injury of intrinsic muscle, fascia and tendon of specified finger with unspecified laterality at wrist and hand level

    ● **S66.599** Other injury of intrinsic muscle, fascia and tendon of unspecified finger at wrist and hand level

● **S66.8** Injury of other specified muscles, fascia and tendons at wrist and hand level

    ● **S66.80** Unspecified injury of other specified muscles, fascia and tendons at wrist and hand level

       ● **S66.801** Unspecified injury of other specified muscles, fascia and tendons at wrist and hand level, right hand

       ● **S66.802** Unspecified injury of other specified muscles, fascia and tendons at wrist and hand level, left hand

       ● **S66.809** Unspecified injury of other specified muscles, fascia and tendons at wrist and hand level, unspecified hand

    ● **S66.81** Strain of other specified muscles, fascia and tendons at wrist and hand level

       ● **S66.811** Strain of other specified muscles, fascia and tendons at wrist and hand level, right hand

       ● **S66.812** Strain of other specified muscles, fascia and tendons at wrist and hand level, left hand

       ● **S66.819** Strain of other specified muscles, fascia and tendons at wrist and hand level, unspecified hand

    ● **S66.82** Laceration of other specified muscles, fascia and tendons at wrist and hand level

       ● **S66.821** Laceration of other specified muscles, fascia and tendons at wrist and hand level, right hand

       ● **S66.822** Laceration of other specified muscles, fascia and tendons at wrist and hand level, left hand

       ● **S66.829** Laceration of other specified muscles, fascia and tendons at wrist and hand level, unspecified hand

◀ New   ◀ Revised   deleted Deleted   Excludes 1   Excludes 2   Includes   Use additional   Code first   Code also   Unspecified

OGCR Official Guidelines   X Assign placeholder X   ● Use Additional Character(s)   ❱ Manifestation Code   **Coding Clinic**

● **S66.89** Other injury of other specified muscles, fascia and tendons at wrist and hand level

　● **S66.891** Other injury of other specified muscles, fascia and tendons at wrist and hand level, right hand

　● **S66.892** Other injury of other specified muscles, fascia and tendons at wrist and hand level, left hand

　● **S66.899** Other injury of other specified muscles, fascia and tendons at wrist and hand level, unspecified hand

● **S66.9** Injury of unspecified muscle, fascia and tendon at wrist and hand level

　● **S66.90** Unspecified injury of unspecified muscle, fascia and tendon at wrist and hand level

　　● **S66.901** Unspecified injury of unspecified muscle, fascia and tendon at wrist and hand level, right hand

　　● **S66.902** Unspecified injury of unspecified muscle, fascia and tendon at wrist and hand level, left hand

　　● **S66.909** Unspecified injury of unspecified muscle, fascia and tendon at wrist and hand level, unspecified hand

　● **S66.91** Strain of unspecified muscle, fascia and tendon at wrist and hand level

　　● **S66.911** Strain of unspecified muscle, fascia and tendon at wrist and hand level, right hand

　　● **S66.912** Strain of unspecified muscle, fascia and tendon at wrist and hand level, left hand

　　● **S66.919** Strain of unspecified muscle, fascia and tendon at wrist and hand level, unspecified hand

　● **S66.92** Laceration of unspecified muscle, fascia and tendon at wrist and hand level

　　● **S66.921** Laceration of unspecified muscle, fascia and tendon at wrist and hand level, right hand

　　● **S66.922** Laceration of unspecified muscle, fascia and tendon at wrist and hand level, left hand

　　● **S66.929** Laceration of unspecified muscle, fascia and tendon at wrist and hand level, unspecified hand

　● **S66.99** Other injury of unspecified muscle, fascia and tendon at wrist and hand level

　　● **S66.991** Other injury of unspecified muscle, fascia and tendon at wrist and hand level, right hand

　　● **S66.992** Other injury of unspecified muscle, fascia and tendon at wrist and hand level, left hand

　　● **S66.999** Other injury of unspecified muscle, fascia and tendon at wrist and hand level, unspecified hand

● **S67** Crushing injury of wrist, hand and fingers

　Use additional code for all associated injuries, such as:
　　fracture of wrist and hand (S62.-)
　　open wound of wrist and hand (S61.-)

　The appropriate 7th character is to be added to each code from category S67

A	initial encounter
D	subsequent encounter
S	sequela

● **S67.0** Crushing injury of thumb

　X● **S67.00** Crushing injury of unspecified thumb

　X● **S67.01** Crushing injury of right thumb

　X● **S67.02** Crushing injury of left thumb

● **S67.1** Crushing injury of other and unspecified finger(s)

　Excludes2 crushing injury of thumb (S67.0-)

　X● **S67.10** Crushing injury of unspecified finger(s)

　● **S67.19** Crushing injury of other finger(s)

　　● **S67.190** Crushing injury of right index finger

　　● **S67.191** Crushing injury of left index finger

　　● **S67.192** Crushing injury of right middle finger

　　● **S67.193** Crushing injury of left middle finger

　　● **S67.194** Crushing injury of right ring finger

　　● **S67.195** Crushing injury of left ring finger

　　● **S67.196** Crushing injury of right little finger

　　● **S67.197** Crushing injury of left little finger

　　● **S67.198** Crushing injury of other finger
　　　　Crushing injury of specified finger with unspecified laterality

● **S67.2** Crushing injury of hand

　Excludes2 crushing injury of fingers (S67.1-)
　　　　crushing injury of thumb (S67.0-)

　X● **S67.20** Crushing injury of unspecified hand

　X● **S67.21** Crushing injury of right hand

　X● **S67.22** Crushing injury of left hand

● **S67.3** Crushing injury of wrist

　X● **S67.30** Crushing injury of unspecified wrist

　X● **S67.31** Crushing injury of right wrist

　X● **S67.32** Crushing injury of left wrist

● **S67.4** Crushing injury of wrist and hand

　Excludes1 crushing injury of hand alone (S67.2-)
　　　　crushing injury of wrist alone (S67.3-)

　Excludes2 crushing injury of fingers (S67.1-)
　　　　crushing injury of thumb (S67.0-)

　X● **S67.40** Crushing injury of unspecified wrist and hand

　X● **S67.41** Crushing injury of right wrist and hand

　X● **S67.42** Crushing injury of left wrist and hand

● **S67.9** Crushing injury of unspecified part(s) of wrist, hand and fingers

　X● **S67.90** Crushing injury of unspecified part(s) of unspecified wrist, hand and fingers

　X● **S67.91** Crushing injury of unspecified part(s) of right wrist, hand and fingers

　X● **S67.92** Crushing injury of unspecified part(s) of left wrist, hand and fingers

● **S68** Traumatic amputation of wrist, hand and fingers

　An amputation not identified as partial or complete should be coded to complete

　The appropriate 7th character is to be added to each code from category S68

A	initial encounter
D	subsequent encounter
S	sequela

● **S68.0** Traumatic metacarpophalangeal amputation of thumb
　Traumatic amputation of thumb NOS

　● **S68.01** Complete traumatic metacarpophalangeal amputation of thumb

　　● **S68.011** Complete traumatic metacarpophalangeal amputation of right thumb

　　● **S68.012** Complete traumatic metacarpophalangeal amputation of left thumb

　　● **S68.019** Complete traumatic metacarpophalangeal amputation of unspecified thumb

CHAPTER 19 (S00-T88)

● S68.02   Partial traumatic metacarpophalangeal amputation of thumb

    ● S68.021   Partial traumatic metacarpophalangeal amputation of right thumb

    ● S68.022   Partial traumatic metacarpophalangeal amputation of left thumb

    ● S68.029   Partial traumatic metacarpophalangeal amputation of unspecified thumb

● S68.1   Traumatic metacarpophalangeal amputation of other and unspecified finger

    Traumatic amputation of finger NOS

    Excludes2   traumatic metacarpophalangeal amputation of thumb (S68.0-)

   ● S68.11   Complete traumatic metacarpophalangeal amputation of other and unspecified finger

     ● S68.110   Complete traumatic metacarpophalangeal amputation of right index finger

     ● S68.111   Complete traumatic metacarpophalangeal amputation of left index finger

     ● S68.112   Complete traumatic metacarpophalangeal amputation of right middle finger

     ● S68.113   Complete traumatic metacarpophalangeal amputation of left middle finger

     ● S68.114   Complete traumatic metacarpophalangeal amputation of right ring finger

     ● S68.115   Complete traumatic metacarpophalangeal amputation of left ring finger

     ● S68.116   Complete traumatic metacarpophalangeal amputation of right little finger

     ● S68.117   Complete traumatic metacarpophalangeal amputation of left little finger

     ● S68.118   Complete traumatic metacarpophalangeal amputation of other finger

       Complete traumatic metacarpophalangeal amputation of specified finger with unspecified laterality

     ● S68.119   Complete traumatic metacarpophalangeal amputation of unspecified finger

   ● S68.12   Partial traumatic metacarpophalangeal amputation of other and unspecified finger

     ● S68.120   Partial traumatic metacarpophalangeal amputation of right index finger

     ● S68.121   Partial traumatic metacarpophalangeal amputation of left index finger

     ● S68.122   Partial traumatic metacarpophalangeal amputation of right middle finger

     ● S68.123   Partial traumatic metacarpophalangeal amputation of left middle finger

     ● S68.124   Partial traumatic metacarpophalangeal amputation of right ring finger

     ● S68.125   Partial traumatic metacarpophalangeal amputation of left ring finger

     ● S68.126   Partial traumatic metacarpophalangeal amputation of right little finger

     ● S68.127   Partial traumatic metacarpophalangeal amputation of left little finger

     ● S68.128   Partial traumatic metacarpophalangeal amputation of other finger

       Partial traumatic metacarpophalangeal amputation of specified finger with unspecified laterality

     ● S68.129   Partial traumatic metacarpophalangeal amputation of unspecified finger

● S68.4   Traumatic amputation of hand at wrist level

    Traumatic amputation of hand NOS

    Traumatic amputation of wrist

   ● S68.41   Complete traumatic amputation of hand at wrist level

     ● S68.411   Complete traumatic amputation of right hand at wrist level

     ● S68.412   Complete traumatic amputation of left hand at wrist level

     ● S68.419   Complete traumatic amputation of unspecified hand at wrist level

   ● S68.42   Partial traumatic amputation of hand at wrist level

     ● S68.421   Partial traumatic amputation of right hand at wrist level

     ● S68.422   Partial traumatic amputation of left hand at wrist level

     ● S68.429   Partial traumatic amputation of unspecified hand at wrist level

● S68.5   Traumatic transphalangeal amputation of thumb

    Traumatic interphalangeal joint amputation of thumb

   ● S68.51   Complete traumatic transphalangeal amputation of thumb

     ● S68.511   Complete traumatic transphalangeal amputation of right thumb

     ● S68.512   Complete traumatic transphalangeal amputation of left thumb

     ● S68.519   Complete traumatic transphalangeal amputation of unspecified thumb

   ● S68.52   Partial traumatic transphalangeal amputation of thumb

     ● S68.521   Partial traumatic transphalangeal amputation of right thumb

     ● S68.522   Partial traumatic transphalangeal amputation of left thumb

     ● S68.529   Partial traumatic transphalangeal amputation of unspecified thumb

- **S68.6**   Traumatic transphalangeal amputation of other and unspecified finger
  - **S68.61**   Complete traumatic transphalangeal amputation of other and unspecified finger(s)
    - **S68.610**   Complete traumatic transphalangeal amputation of right index finger
    - **S68.611**   Complete traumatic transphalangeal amputation of left index finger
    - **S68.612**   Complete traumatic transphalangeal amputation of right middle finger
    - **S68.613**   Complete traumatic transphalangeal amputation of left middle finger
    - **S68.614**   Complete traumatic transphalangeal amputation of right ring finger
    - **S68.615**   Complete traumatic transphalangeal amputation of left ring finger
    - **S68.616**   Complete traumatic transphalangeal amputation of right little finger
    - **S68.617**   Complete traumatic transphalangeal amputation of left little finger
    - **S68.618**   Complete traumatic transphalangeal amputation of other finger
      Complete traumatic transphalangeal amputation of specified finger with unspecified laterality
    - **S68.619**   Complete traumatic transphalangeal amputation of unspecified finger
  - **S68.62**   Partial traumatic transphalangeal amputation of other and unspecified finger
    - **S68.620**   Partial traumatic transphalangeal amputation of right index finger
    - **S68.621**   Partial traumatic transphalangeal amputation of left index finger
    - **S68.622**   Partial traumatic transphalangeal amputation of right middle finger
    - **S68.623**   Partial traumatic transphalangeal amputation of left middle finger
    - **S68.624**   Partial traumatic transphalangeal amputation of right ring finger
    - **S68.625**   Partial traumatic transphalangeal amputation of left ring finger
    - **S68.626**   Partial traumatic transphalangeal amputation of right little finger
    - **S68.627**   Partial traumatic transphalangeal amputation of left little finger
    - **S68.628**   Partial traumatic transphalangeal amputation of other finger
      Partial traumatic transphalangeal amputation of specified finger with unspecified laterality
    - **S68.629**   Partial traumatic transphalangeal amputation of unspecified finger
- **S68.7**   Traumatic transmetacarpal amputation of hand
  - **S68.71**   Complete traumatic transmetacarpal amputation of hand
    - **S68.711**   Complete traumatic transmetacarpal amputation of right hand
    - **S68.712**   Complete traumatic transmetacarpal amputation of left hand
    - **S68.719**   Complete traumatic transmetacarpal amputation of unspecified hand
  - **S68.72**   Partial traumatic transmetacarpal amputation of hand
    - **S68.721**   Partial traumatic transmetacarpal amputation of right hand
    - **S68.722**   Partial traumatic transmetacarpal amputation of left hand
    - **S68.729**   Partial traumatic transmetacarpal amputation of unspecified hand

- **S69**   Other and unspecified injuries of wrist, hand and finger(s)
  The appropriate 7th character is to be added to each code from category S69

A	initial encounter
D	subsequent encounter
S	sequela

  - **S69.8**   Other specified injuries of wrist, hand and finger(s)
    - X **S69.80**   Other specified injuries of unspecified wrist, hand and finger(s)
    - X **S69.81**   Other specified injuries of right wrist, hand and finger(s)
    - X **S69.82**   Other specified injuries of left wrist, hand and finger(s)
  - **S69.9**   Unspecified injury of wrist, hand and finger(s)
    - X **S69.90**   Unspecified injury of unspecified wrist, hand and finger(s)
    - X **S69.91**   Unspecified injury of right wrist, hand and finger(s)
    - X **S69.92**   Unspecified injury of left wrist, hand and finger(s)

INJURIES TO THE HIP AND THIGH (S70-S79)

Excludes2   burns and corrosions (T20-T32)
frostbite (T33-T34)
snake bite (T63.0-)
venomous insect bite or sting (T63.4-)

- **S70**   Superficial injury of hip and thigh
  The appropriate 7th character is to be added to each code from category S70

A	initial encounter
D	subsequent encounter
S	sequela

  - **S70.0**   Contusion of hip
    - X **S70.00**   Contusion of unspecified hip
    - X **S70.01**   Contusion of right hip
    - X **S70.02**   Contusion of left hip
  - **S70.1**   Contusion of thigh
    - X **S70.10**   Contusion of unspecified thigh
    - X **S70.11**   Contusion of right thigh
    - X **S70.12**   Contusion of left thigh
  - **S70.2**   Other superficial injuries of hip
    - **S70.21**   Abrasion of hip
      - **S70.211**   Abrasion, right hip
      - **S70.212**   Abrasion, left hip
      - **S70.219**   Abrasion, unspecified hip
    - **S70.22**   Blister (nonthermal) of hip
      - **S70.221**   Blister (nonthermal), right hip
      - **S70.222**   Blister (nonthermal), left hip
      - **S70.229**   Blister (nonthermal), unspecified hip
    - **S70.24**   External constriction of hip
      - **S70.241**   External constriction, right hip
      - **S70.242**   External constriction, left hip
      - **S70.249**   External constriction, unspecified hip
    - **S70.25**   Superficial foreign body of hip
      Splinter in the hip
      - **S70.251**   Superficial foreign body, right hip
      - **S70.252**   Superficial foreign body, left hip
      - **S70.259**   Superficial foreign body, unspecified hip

CHAPTER 19 (S00-T88)

CHAPTER 19 (S00-T88)

- S70.26 **Insect bite (nonvenomous) of hip**
  - S70.261 Insect bite (nonvenomous), right hip
  - S70.262 Insect bite (nonvenomous), left hip
  - S70.269 Insect bite (nonvenomous), unspecified hip
- S70.27 **Other superficial bite of hip**
  - **Excludes1** open bite of hip (S71.05-)
  - S70.271 Other superficial bite of hip, right hip
  - S70.272 Other superficial bite of hip, left hip
  - S70.279 Other superficial bite of hip, unspecified hip
- S70.3 **Other superficial injuries of thigh**
  - S70.31 **Abrasion of thigh**
    - S70.311 Abrasion, right thigh
    - S70.312 Abrasion, left thigh
    - S70.319 Abrasion, unspecified thigh
  - S70.32 **Blister (nonthermal) of thigh**
    - S70.321 Blister (nonthermal), right thigh
    - S70.322 Blister (nonthermal), left thigh
    - S70.329 Blister (nonthermal), unspecified thigh
  - S70.34 **External constriction of thigh**
    - S70.341 External constriction, right thigh
    - S70.342 External constriction, left thigh
    - S70.349 External constriction, unspecified thigh
  - S70.35 **Superficial foreign body of thigh**
    - Splinter in the thigh
    - S70.351 Superficial foreign body, right thigh
    - S70.352 Superficial foreign body, left thigh
    - S70.359 Superficial foreign body, unspecified thigh
  - S70.36 **Insect bite (nonvenomous) of thigh**
    - S70.361 Insect bite (nonvenomous), right thigh
    - S70.362 Insect bite (nonvenomous), left thigh
    - S70.369 Insect bite (nonvenomous), unspecified thigh
  - S70.37 **Other superficial bite of thigh**
    - **Excludes1** open bite of thigh (S71.15)
    - S70.371 Other superficial bite of right thigh
    - S70.372 Other superficial bite of left thigh
    - S70.379 Other superficial bite of unspecified thigh
- S70.9 **Unspecified superficial injury of hip and thigh**
  - S70.91 **Unspecified superficial injury of hip**
    - S70.911 Unspecified superficial injury of right hip
    - S70.912 Unspecified superficial injury of left hip
    - S70.919 Unspecified superficial injury of unspecified hip
  - S70.92 **Unspecified superficial injury of thigh**
    - S70.921 Unspecified superficial injury of right thigh
    - S70.922 Unspecified superficial injury of left thigh
    - S70.929 Unspecified superficial injury of unspecified thigh

- S71 **Open wound of hip and thigh**
  - Code also any associated wound infection
  - **Excludes1** open fracture of hip and thigh (S72.-)
    - traumatic amputation of hip and thigh (S78.-)
  - **Excludes2** bite of venomous animal (T63.-)
    - open wound of ankle, foot and toes (S91.-)
    - open wound of knee and lower leg (S81.-)
  - The appropriate 7th character is to be added to each code from category S71

A	initial encounter
D	subsequent encounter
S	sequela

  - S71.0 **Open wound of hip**
    - S71.00 **Unspecified open wound of hip**
      - S71.001 Unspecified open wound, right hip
      - S71.002 Unspecified open wound, left hip
      - S71.009 Unspecified open wound, unspecified hip
    - S71.01 **Laceration without foreign body of hip**
      - S71.011 Laceration without foreign body, right hip
      - S71.012 Laceration without foreign body, left hip
      - S71.019 Laceration without foreign body, unspecified hip
    - S71.02 **Laceration with foreign body of hip**
      - S71.021 Laceration with foreign body, right hip
      - S71.022 Laceration with foreign body, left hip
      - S71.029 Laceration with foreign body, unspecified hip
    - S71.03 **Puncture wound without foreign body of hip**
      - S71.031 Puncture wound without foreign body, right hip
      - S71.032 Puncture wound without foreign body, left hip
      - S71.039 Puncture wound without foreign body, unspecified hip
    - S71.04 **Puncture wound with foreign body of hip**
      - S71.041 Puncture wound with foreign body, right hip
      - S71.042 Puncture wound with foreign body, left hip
      - S71.049 Puncture wound with foreign body, unspecified hip
    - S71.05 **Open bite of hip**
      - Bite of hip NOS
      - **Excludes1** superficial bite of hip (S70.26, S70.27)
      - S71.051 Open bite, right hip
      - S71.052 Open bite, left hip
      - S71.059 Open bite, unspecified hip
  - S71.1 **Open wound of thigh**
    - S71.10 **Unspecified open wound of thigh**
      - S71.101 Unspecified open wound, right thigh
      - S71.102 Unspecified open wound, left thigh
      - S71.109 Unspecified open wound, unspecified thigh
    - S71.11 **Laceration without foreign body of thigh**
      - S71.111 Laceration without foreign body, right thigh
      - S71.112 Laceration without foreign body, left thigh
      - S71.119 Laceration without foreign body, unspecified thigh

◀ New   ◀▥ Revised   ̶d̶e̶l̶e̶t̶e̶d̶ Deleted   Excludes 1   Excludes 2   Includes   Use additional   Code first   Code also   Unspecified

OGCR Official Guidelines   X Assign placeholder X   ● Use Additional Character(s)   ▶ Manifestation Code   Coding Clinic

● S71.12   Laceration with foreign body of thigh
   ● S71.121   Laceration with foreign body, right thigh
   ● S71.122   Laceration with foreign body, left thigh
   ● S71.129   Laceration with foreign body, unspecified thigh
● S71.13   Puncture wound without foreign body of thigh
   ● S71.131   Puncture wound without foreign body, right thigh
   ● S71.132   Puncture wound without foreign body, left thigh
   ● S71.139   Puncture wound without foreign body, unspecified thigh
● S71.14   Puncture wound with foreign body of thigh
   ● S71.141   Puncture wound with foreign body, right thigh
   ● S71.142   Puncture wound with foreign body, left thigh
   ● S71.149   Puncture wound with foreign body, unspecified thigh
● S71.15   Open bite of thigh
    Bite of thigh NOS

    | **Excludes1** | superficial bite of thigh (S70.37-) |

   ● S71.151   Open bite, right thigh
   ● S71.152   Open bite, left thigh
   ● S71.159   Open bite, unspecified thigh

● **S72   Fracture of femur**
   Note: A fracture not indicated as displaced or nondisplaced should be coded to displaced
   A fracture not indicated as open or closed should be coded to closed
   The open fracture designations are based on the Gustilo open fracture classification

Excludes1	traumatic amputation of hip and thigh (S78.-)
Excludes2	fracture of lower leg and ankle (S82.-)
	fracture of foot (S92.-)
	periprosthetic fracture of prosthetic implant of hip (T84.040, T84.041)

   The appropriate 7th character is to be added to all codes from category S72

A	initial encounter for closed fracture
B	initial encounter for open fracture type I or II
	initial encounter for open fracture NOS
C	initial encounter for open fracture type IIIA, IIIB, or IIIC
D	subsequent encounter for closed fracture with routine healing
E	subsequent encounter for open fracture type I or II with routine healing
F	subsequent encounter for open fracture type IIIA, IIIB, or IIIC with routine healing
G	subsequent encounter for closed fracture with delayed healing
H	subsequent encounter for open fracture type I or II with delayed healing
J	subsequent encounter for open fracture type IIIA, IIIB, or IIIC with delayed healing
K	subsequent encounter for closed fracture with nonunion
M	subsequent encounter for open fracture type I or II with nonunion
N	subsequent encounter for open fracture type IIIA, IIIB, or IIIC with nonunion
P	subsequent encounter for closed fracture with malunion
Q	subsequent encounter for open fracture type I or II with malunion
R	subsequent encounter for open fracture type IIIA, IIIB, or IIIC with malunion
S	sequela

● S72.0   Fracture of head and neck of femur

   | **Excludes2** | physeal fracture of upper end of femur (S79.0-) |

   ● S72.00   Fracture of unspecified part of neck of femur
      Fracture of hip NOS
      Fracture of neck of femur NOS
     ● S72.001   Fracture of unspecified part of neck of right femur
     ● S72.002   Fracture of unspecified part of neck of left femur
        Coding Clinic: 2015, Q1, P17
     ● S72.009   Fracture of unspecified part of neck of unspecified femur
   ● S72.01   Unspecified intracapsular fracture of femur
      Subcapital fracture of femur
     ● S72.011   Unspecified intracapsular fracture of right femur
     ● S72.012   Unspecified intracapsular fracture of left femur
     ● S72.019   Unspecified intracapsular fracture of unspecified femur
   ● S72.02   Fracture of epiphysis (separation) (upper) of femur
      Transepiphyseal fracture of femur
      Fracture and separation across growth plate

     | **Excludes1** | capital femoral epiphyseal fracture (pediatric) of femur (S79.01-) |
     | | Salter-Harris Type I physeal fracture of upper end of femur (S79.01-) |

     ● S72.021   Displaced fracture of epiphysis (separation) (upper) of right femur
     ● S72.022   Displaced fracture of epiphysis (separation) (upper) of left femur
     ● S72.023   Displaced fracture of epiphysis (separation) (upper) of unspecified femur
     ● S72.024   Nondisplaced fracture of epiphysis (separation) (upper) of right femur
     ● S72.025   Nondisplaced fracture of epiphysis (separation) (upper) of left femur
     ● S72.026   Nondisplaced fracture of epiphysis (separation) (upper) of unspecified femur
   ● S72.03   Midcervical fracture of femur
      Transcervical fracture of femur NOS
     ● S72.031   Displaced midcervical fracture of right femur
     ● S72.032   Displaced midcervical fracture of left femur
     ● S72.033   Displaced midcervical fracture of unspecified femur
     ● S72.034   Nondisplaced midcervical fracture of right femur
     ● S72.035   Nondisplaced midcervical fracture of left femur
     ● S72.036   Nondisplaced midcervical fracture of unspecified femur

CHAPTER 19 (S00-T88)

● **S72.04**   **Fracture of base of neck of femur**
     Cervicotrochanteric fracture of femur
- ● S72.041   Displaced fracture of base of neck of right femur
- ● S72.042   Displaced fracture of base of neck of left femur
- ● S72.043   Displaced fracture of base of neck of unspecified femur
- ● S72.044   Nondisplaced fracture of base of neck of right femur
- ● S72.045   Nondisplaced fracture of base of neck of left femur
- ● S72.046   Nondisplaced fracture of base of neck of unspecified femur

● **S72.05**   **Unspecified fracture of head of femur**
     Fracture of head of femur NOS
- ● S72.051   Unspecified fracture of head of right femur
- ● S72.052   Unspecified fracture of head of left femur
- ● S72.059   Unspecified fracture of head of unspecified femur

● **S72.06**   **Articular fracture of head of femur**
- ● S72.061   Displaced articular fracture of head of right femur
- ● S72.062   Displaced articular fracture of head of left femur
- ● S72.063   Displaced articular fracture of head of unspecified femur
- ● S72.064   Nondisplaced articular fracture of head of right femur
- ● S72.065   Nondisplaced articular fracture of head of left femur
- ● S72.066   Nondisplaced articular fracture of head of unspecified femur

● **S72.09**   **Other fracture of head and neck of femur**
- ● S72.091   Other fracture of head and neck of right femur
- ● S72.092   Other fracture of head and neck of left femur
- ● S72.099   Other fracture of head and neck of unspecified femur

● **S72.1**   **Pertrochanteric fracture**
     Fracture extending close to, but not into, joint

  ● **S72.10**   **Unspecified trochanteric fracture of femur**
     Fracture of trochanter NOS
- ● S72.101   Unspecified trochanteric fracture of right femur
- ● S72.102   Unspecified trochanteric fracture of left femur
- ● S72.109   Unspecified trochanteric fracture of unspecified femur

  ● **S72.11**   **Fracture of greater trochanter of femur**
- ● S72.111   Displaced fracture of greater trochanter of right femur
- ● S72.112   Displaced fracture of greater trochanter of left femur
- ● S72.113   Displaced fracture of greater trochanter of unspecified femur
- ● S72.114   Nondisplaced fracture of greater trochanter of right femur
- ● S72.115   Nondisplaced fracture of greater trochanter of left femur
- ● S72.116   Nondisplaced fracture of greater trochanter of unspecified femur

  ● **S72.12**   **Fracture of lesser trochanter of femur**
- ● S72.121   Displaced fracture of lesser trochanter of right femur
- ● S72.122   Displaced fracture of lesser trochanter of left femur
- ● S72.123   Displaced fracture of lesser trochanter of unspecified femur
- ● S72.124   Nondisplaced fracture of lesser trochanter of right femur
- ● S72.125   Nondisplaced fracture of lesser trochanter of left femur
- ● S72.126   Nondisplaced fracture of lesser trochanter of unspecified femur

  ● **S72.13**   **Apophyseal fracture of femur**
     Pertaining to articulations between articular facets of adjacent vertebrae

     Excludes1   chronic (nontraumatic) slipped upper femoral epiphysis (M93.0-)
- ● S72.131   Displaced apophyseal fracture of right femur
- ● S72.132   Displaced apophyseal fracture of left femur
- ● S72.133   Displaced apophyseal fracture of unspecified femur
- ● S72.134   Nondisplaced apophyseal fracture of right femur
- ● S72.135   Nondisplaced apophyseal fracture of left femur
- ● S72.136   Nondisplaced apophyseal fracture of unspecified femur

  ● **S72.14**   **Intertrochanteric fracture of femur**
- ● S72.141   Displaced intertrochanteric fracture of right femur
- ● S72.142   Displaced intertrochanteric fracture of left femur
- ● S72.143   Displaced intertrochanteric fracture of unspecified femur
- ● S72.144   Nondisplaced intertrochanteric fracture of right femur
- ● S72.145   Nondisplaced intertrochanteric fracture of left femur
- ● S72.146   Nondisplaced intertrochanteric fracture of unspecified femur

● **S72.2**   **Subtrochanteric fracture of femur**
     Subtrochanteric: inferior to trochanter
- X● S72.21   Displaced subtrochanteric fracture of right femur
- X● S72.22   Displaced subtrochanteric fracture of left femur
- X● S72.23   Displaced subtrochanteric fracture of unspecified femur
- X● S72.24   Nondisplaced subtrochanteric fracture of right femur
- X● S72.25   Nondisplaced subtrochanteric fracture of left femur
- X● S72.26   Nondisplaced subtrochanteric fracture of unspecified femur

● **S72.3**   **Fracture of shaft of femur**

  ● **S72.30**   **Unspecified fracture of shaft of femur**
- ● S72.301   Unspecified fracture of shaft of right femur
- ● S72.302   Unspecified fracture of shaft of left femur
- ● S72.309   Unspecified fracture of shaft of unspecified femur

◀ New   ◀▪▪▪ Revised   ~~deleted~~ Deleted   Excludes 1   Excludes 2   Includes   Use additional   Code first   Code also   Unspecified

OGCR Official Guidelines   **X** Assign placeholder X   ● Use Additional Character(s)   ▶ Manifestation Code   **Coding Clinic**

● **S72.32**   Transverse fracture of shaft of femur
  ● S72.321   Displaced transverse fracture of shaft of right femur
  ● S72.322   Displaced transverse fracture of shaft of left femur
  ● S72.323   Displaced transverse fracture of shaft of unspecified femur
  ● S72.324   Nondisplaced transverse fracture of shaft of right femur
  ● S72.325   Nondisplaced transverse fracture of shaft of left femur
  ● S72.326   Nondisplaced transverse fracture of shaft of unspecified femur
● **S72.33**   Oblique fracture of shaft of femur
  ● S72.331   Displaced oblique fracture of shaft of right femur
  ● S72.332   Displaced oblique fracture of shaft of left femur
  ● S72.333   Displaced oblique fracture of shaft of unspecified femur
  ● S72.334   Nondisplaced oblique fracture of shaft of right femur
  ● S72.335   Nondisplaced oblique fracture of shaft of left femur
  ● S72.336   Nondisplaced oblique fracture of shaft of unspecified femur
● **S72.34**   Spiral fracture of shaft of femur
  ● S72.341   Displaced spiral fracture of shaft of right femur
  ● S72.342   Displaced spiral fracture of shaft of left femur
  ● S72.343   Displaced spiral fracture of shaft of unspecified femur
  ● S72.344   Nondisplaced spiral fracture of shaft of right femur
  ● S72.345   Nondisplaced spiral fracture of shaft of left femur
  ● S72.346   Nondisplaced spiral fracture of shaft of unspecified femur
● **S72.35**   Comminuted fracture of shaft of femur
  ● S72.351   Displaced comminuted fracture of shaft of right femur
  ● S72.352   Displaced comminuted fracture of shaft of left femur
  ● S72.353   Displaced comminuted fracture of shaft of unspecified femur
  ● S72.354   Nondisplaced comminuted fracture of shaft of right femur
  ● S72.355   Nondisplaced comminuted fracture of shaft of left femur
  ● S72.356   Nondisplaced comminuted fracture of shaft of unspecified femur
● **S72.36**   Segmental fracture of shaft of femur
  ● S72.361   Displaced segmental fracture of shaft of right femur
  ● S72.362   Displaced segmental fracture of shaft of left femur
  ● S72.363   Displaced segmental fracture of shaft of unspecified femur

  ● S72.364   Nondisplaced segmental fracture of shaft of right femur
  ● S72.365   Nondisplaced segmental fracture of shaft of left femur
  ● S72.366   Nondisplaced segmental fracture of shaft of unspecified femur
● **S72.39**   Other fracture of shaft of femur
  ● S72.391   Other fracture of shaft of right femur
  ● S72.392   Other fracture of shaft of left femur
  ● S72.399   Other fracture of shaft of unspecified femur
● **S72.4**   Fracture of lower end of femur
    Fracture of distal end of femur
    Excludes2   fracture of shaft of femur (S72.3-)
            physeal fracture of lower end of femur (S79.1-)
  ● **S72.40**   Unspecified fracture of lower end of femur
    ● S72.401   Unspecified fracture of lower end of right femur
    ● S72.402   Unspecified fracture of lower end of left femur
    ● S72.409   Unspecified fracture of lower end of unspecified femur
  ● **S72.41**   Unspecified condyle fracture of lower end of femur
      Condyle fracture of femur NOS
    ● S72.411   Displaced unspecified condyle fracture of lower end of right femur
    ● S72.412   Displaced unspecified condyle fracture of lower end of left femur
    ● S72.413   Displaced unspecified condyle fracture of lower end of unspecified femur
    ● S72.414   Nondisplaced unspecified condyle fracture of lower end of right femur
    ● S72.415   Nondisplaced unspecified condyle fracture of lower end of left femur
    ● S72.416   Nondisplaced unspecified condyle fracture of lower end of unspecified femur
  ● **S72.42**   Fracture of lateral condyle of femur
    ● S72.421   Displaced fracture of lateral condyle of right femur
    ● S72.422   Displaced fracture of lateral condyle of left femur
    ● S72.423   Displaced fracture of lateral condyle of unspecified femur
    ● S72.424   Nondisplaced fracture of lateral condyle of right femur
    ● S72.425   Nondisplaced fracture of lateral condyle of left femur
    ● S72.426   Nondisplaced fracture of lateral condyle of unspecified femur
  ● **S72.43**   Fracture of medial condyle of femur
    ● S72.431   Displaced fracture of medial condyle of right femur
    ● S72.432   Displaced fracture of medial condyle of left femur
    ● S72.433   Displaced fracture of medial condyle of unspecified femur

CHAPTER 19 (S00-T88)

● **S72.434**   Nondisplaced fracture of medial condyle of right femur

● **S72.435**   Nondisplaced fracture of medial condyle of left femur

● **S72.436**   Nondisplaced fracture of medial condyle of unspecified femur

● **S72.44**   Fracture of lower epiphysis (separation) of femur

     Excludes1   Salter-Harris Type I physeal fracture of lower end of femur (S79.11-)

● **S72.441**   Displaced fracture of lower epiphysis (separation) of right femur

● **S72.442**   Displaced fracture of lower epiphysis (separation) of left femur

● **S72.443**   Displaced fracture of lower epiphysis (separation) of unspecified femur

● **S72.444**   Nondisplaced fracture of lower epiphysis (separation) of right femur

● **S72.445**   Nondisplaced fracture of lower epiphysis (separation) of left femur

● **S72.446**   Nondisplaced fracture of lower epiphysis (separation) of unspecified femur

● **S72.45**   Supracondylar fracture without intracondylar extension of lower end of femur

     Supracondylar fracture of lower end of femur NOS

     Excludes1   supracondylar fracture with intracondylar extension of lower end of femur (S72.46-)

● **S72.451**   Displaced supracondylar fracture without intracondylar extension of lower end of right femur

● **S72.452**   Displaced supracondylar fracture without intracondylar extension of lower end of left femur

● **S72.453**   Displaced supracondylar fracture without intracondylar extension of lower end of unspecified femur

● **S72.454**   Nondisplaced supracondylar fracture without intracondylar extension of lower end of right femur

● **S72.455**   Nondisplaced supracondylar fracture without intracondylar extension of lower end of left femur

● **S72.456**   Nondisplaced supracondylar fracture without intracondylar extension of lower end of unspecified femur

● **S72.46**   Supracondylar fracture with intracondylar extension of lower end of femur

     Excludes1   supracondylar fracture without intracondylar extension of lower end of femur (S72.45-)

● **S72.461**   Displaced supracondylar fracture with intracondylar extension of lower end of right femur

● **S72.462**   Displaced supracondylar fracture with intracondylar extension of lower end of left femur

● **S72.463**   Displaced supracondylar fracture with intracondylar extension of lower end of unspecified femur

● **S72.464**   Nondisplaced supracondylar fracture with intracondylar extension of lower end of right femur

● **S72.465**   Nondisplaced supracondylar fracture with intracondylar extension of lower end of left femur

● **S72.466**   Nondisplaced supracondylar fracture with intracondylar extension of lower end of unspecified femur

● **S72.47**   Torus fracture of lower end of femur

     The appropriate 7th character is to be added to all codes in subcategory S72.47

A	initial encounter for closed fracture
D	subsequent encounter for fracture with routine healing
G	subsequent encounter for fracture with delayed healing
K	subsequent encounter for fracture with nonunion
P	subsequent encounter for fracture with malunion
S	sequela

● **S72.471**   Torus fracture of lower end of right femur

● **S72.472**   Torus fracture of lower end of left femur

● **S72.479**   Torus fracture of lower end of unspecified femur

● **S72.49**   Other fracture of lower end of femur

● **S72.491**   Other fracture of lower end of right femur

● **S72.492**   Other fracture of lower end of left femur

● **S72.499**   Other fracture of lower end of unspecified femur

● **S72.8**   Other fracture of femur

● **S72.8X**   Other fracture of femur

● **S72.8X1**   Other fracture of right femur

● **S72.8X2**   Other fracture of left femur

● **S72.8X9**   Other fracture of unspecified femur

● **S72.9**   Unspecified fracture of femur

     Fracture of thigh NOS

     Fracture of upper leg NOS

     Excludes1   fracture of hip NOS (S72.00-, S72.01-)

X ● **S72.90**   Unspecified fracture of unspecified femur

     Coding Clinic: 2012, Q4, P94

X ● **S72.91**   Unspecified fracture of right femur

X ● **S72.92**   Unspecified fracture of left femur

◀ New   ⬅ Revised   ~~deleted~~ Deleted   Excludes 1   Excludes 2   Includes   Use additional   Code first   Code also   Unspecified

OGCR Official Guidelines   X Assign placeholder X   ● Use Additional Character(s)   ❱ Manifestation Code   **Coding Clinic**

● **S73** **Dislocation and sprain of joint and ligaments of hip**

    Includes   avulsion of joint or ligament of hip
                    laceration of cartilage, joint or ligament of hip
                    sprain of cartilage, joint or ligament of hip
                    traumatic hemarthrosis of joint or ligament of hip
                    traumatic rupture of joint or ligament of hip
                    traumatic subluxation of joint or ligament of hip
                    traumatic tear of joint or ligament of hip

    Code also any associated open wound

    Excludes2   strain of muscle, fascia and tendon of hip and
                    thigh (S76.-)

    The appropriate 7th character is to be added to each code from
    category S73

        A   initial encounter
        D   subsequent encounter
        S   sequela

● **S73.0** **Subluxation and dislocation of hip**
        Out of position

      Excludes2   dislocation and subluxation of hip
                    prosthesis (T84.020, T84.021)

    ● **S73.00** **Unspecified subluxation and dislocation of hip**
            Dislocation of hip NOS
            Subluxation of hip NOS

        ● **S73.001** Unspecified subluxation of right hip
        ● **S73.002** Unspecified subluxation of left hip
        ● **S73.003** Unspecified subluxation of
                    unspecified hip
        ● **S73.004** Unspecified dislocation of right hip
        ● **S73.005** Unspecified dislocation of left hip
        ● **S73.006** Unspecified dislocation of unspecified
                    hip

    ● **S73.01** **Posterior subluxation and dislocation of hip**
        ● **S73.011** **Posterior subluxation of right hip**
        ● **S73.012** **Posterior subluxation of left hip**
        ● **S73.013** **Posterior subluxation of** unspecified
                    hip
        ● **S73.014** **Posterior dislocation of right hip**
        ● **S73.015** **Posterior dislocation of left hip**
        ● **S73.016** **Posterior dislocation of** unspecified
                    hip

    ● **S73.02** **Obturator subluxation and dislocation of hip**
        ● **S73.021** **Obturator subluxation of right hip**
        ● **S73.022** **Obturator subluxation of left hip**
        ● **S73.023** **Obturator subluxation of** unspecified
                    hip
        ● **S73.024** **Obturator dislocation of right hip**
        ● **S73.025** **Obturator dislocation of left hip**
        ● **S73.026** **Obturator dislocation of** unspecified
                    hip

    ● **S73.03** **Other anterior dislocation of hip**
        ● **S73.031** **Other anterior subluxation of right**
                    hip
        ● **S73.032** **Other anterior subluxation of left hip**
        ● **S73.033** **Other anterior subluxation of**
                    unspecified **hip**
        ● **S73.034** **Other anterior dislocation of right hip**
        ● **S73.035** **Other anterior dislocation of left hip**
        ● **S73.036** **Other anterior dislocation of**
                    unspecified **hip**

● **S73.04** **Central dislocation of hip**
    ● **S73.041** **Central subluxation of right hip**
    ● **S73.042** **Central subluxation of left hip**
    ● **S73.043** **Central subluxation of** unspecified
                hip
    ● **S73.044** **Central dislocation of right hip**
    ● **S73.045** **Central dislocation of left hip**
    ● **S73.046** **Central dislocation of** unspecified **hip**

● **S73.1** **Sprain of hip**
    ● **S73.10** **Unspecified sprain of hip**
        ● **S73.101** Unspecified **sprain of right hip**
        ● **S73.102** Unspecified **sprain of left hip**
        ● **S73.109** Unspecified **sprain of unspecified hip**
    ● **S73.11** **Iliofemoral ligament sprain of hip**
        ● **S73.111** **Iliofemoral ligament sprain of right**
                    hip
        ● **S73.112** **Iliofemoral ligament sprain of left hip**
        ● **S73.119** **Iliofemoral ligament sprain of**
                    unspecified **hip**
    ● **S73.12** **Ischiocapsular (ligament) sprain of hip**
        ● **S73.121** **Ischiocapsular ligament sprain of**
                    right hip
        ● **S73.122** **Ischiocapsular ligament sprain of left**
                    hip
        ● **S73.129** **Ischiocapsular ligament sprain of**
                    unspecified **hip**
    ● **S73.19** **Other sprain of hip**
        ● **S73.191** **Other sprain of right hip**
        ● **S73.192** **Other sprain of left hip**
        ● **S73.199** **Other sprain of** unspecified **hip**

● **S74** **Injury of nerves at hip and thigh level**
    Code also any associated open wound (S71.-)

    Excludes2   injury of nerves at ankle and foot level (S94.-)
                    injury of nerves at lower leg level (S84.-)

    The appropriate 7th character is to be added to each code from
    category S74

        A   initial encounter
        D   subsequent encounter
        S   sequela

● **S74.0** **Injury of sciatic nerve at hip and thigh level**
    X● **S74.00** **Injury of sciatic nerve at hip and thigh level,**
                    unspecified **leg**
    X● **S74.01** **Injury of sciatic nerve at hip and thigh level,**
                    right leg
    X● **S74.02** **Injury of sciatic nerve at hip and thigh level,**
                    left leg

● **S74.1** **Injury of femoral nerve at hip and thigh level**
    X● **S74.10** **Injury of femoral nerve at hip and thigh level,**
                    unspecified **leg**
    X● **S74.11** **Injury of femoral nerve at hip and thigh level,**
                    right leg
    X● **S74.12** **Injury of femoral nerve at hip and thigh level,**
                    left leg

● **S74.2** **Injury of cutaneous sensory nerve at hip and thigh level**
    X● **S74.20** **Injury of cutaneous sensory nerve at hip and**
                    thigh level, unspecified **leg**
    X● **S74.21** **Injury of cutaneous sensory nerve at hip and**
                    high level, right leg
    X● **S74.22** **Injury of cutaneous sensory nerve at hip and**
                    thigh level, left leg

CHAPTER 19 (S00-T88)

● S74.8 **Injury of other nerves at hip and thigh level**
  ● S74.8X **Injury of other nerves at hip and thigh level**
    ● S74.8X1 Injury of other nerves at hip and thigh level, right leg
    ● S74.8X2 Injury of other nerves at hip and thigh level, left leg
    ● S74.8X9 Injury of other nerves at hip and thigh level, unspecified leg
  ● S74.9 **Injury of unspecified nerve at hip and thigh level**
    X ● S74.90 Injury of unspecified nerve at hip and thigh level, unspecified leg
    X ● S74.91 Injury of unspecified nerve at hip and thigh level, right leg
    X ● S74.92 Injury of unspecified nerve at hip and thigh level, left leg

● S75 **Injury of blood vessels at hip and thigh level**
  Code also any associated open wound (S71.-)
  Excludes2 injury of blood vessels at lower leg level (S85.-)
    injury of popliteal artery (S85.0)
  The appropriate 7th character is to be added to each code from category S75

    A   initial encounter
    D   subsequent encounter
    S   sequela

  ● S75.0 **Injury of femoral artery**
    ● S75.00 **Unspecified injury of femoral artery**
      ● S75.001 Unspecified injury of femoral artery, right leg
      ● S75.002 Unspecified injury of femoral artery, left leg
      ● S75.009 Unspecified injury of femoral artery, unspecified leg
    ● S75.01 **Minor laceration of femoral artery**
      Incomplete transection of femoral artery
      Laceration of femoral artery NOS
      Superficial laceration of femoral artery
      ● S75.011 Minor laceration of femoral artery, right leg
      ● S75.012 Minor laceration of femoral artery, left leg
      ● S75.019 Minor laceration of femoral artery, unspecified leg
    ● S75.02 **Major laceration of femoral artery**
      Complete transection of femoral artery
      Traumatic rupture of femoral artery
      ● S75.021 Major laceration of femoral artery, right leg
      ● S75.022 Major laceration of femoral artery, left leg
      ● S75.029 Major laceration of femoral artery, unspecified leg
    ● S75.09 **Other specified injury of femoral artery**
      ● S75.091 Other specified injury of femoral artery, right leg
      ● S75.092 Other specified injury of femoral artery, left leg
      ● S75.099 Other specified injury of femoral artery, unspecified leg

● S75.1 **Injury of femoral vein at hip and thigh level**
  ● S75.10 **Unspecified injury of femoral vein at hip and thigh level**
    ● S75.101 Unspecified injury of femoral vein at hip and thigh level, right leg
    ● S75.102 Unspecified injury of femoral vein at hip and thigh level, left leg
    ● S75.109 Unspecified injury of femoral vein at hip and thigh level, unspecified leg
  ● S75.11 **Minor laceration of femoral vein at hip and thigh level**
    Incomplete transection of femoral vein at hip and thigh level
    Laceration of femoral vein at hip and thigh level NOS
    Superficial laceration of femoral vein at hip and thigh level
    ● S75.111 Minor laceration of femoral vein at hip and thigh level, right leg
    ● S75.112 Minor laceration of femoral vein at hip and thigh level, left leg
    ● S75.119 Minor laceration of femoral vein at hip and thigh level, unspecified leg
  ● S75.12 **Major laceration of femoral vein at hip and thigh level**
    Complete transection of femoral vein at hip and thigh level
    Traumatic rupture of femoral vein at hip and thigh level
    ● S75.121 Major laceration of femoral vein at hip and thigh level, right leg
    ● S75.122 Major laceration of femoral vein at hip and thigh level, left leg
    ● S75.129 Major laceration of femoral vein at hip and thigh level, unspecified leg
  ● S75.19 **Other specified injury of femoral vein at hip and thigh level**
    ● S75.191 Other specified injury of femoral vein at hip and thigh level, right leg
    ● S75.192 Other specified injury of femoral vein at hip and thigh level, left leg
    ● S75.199 Other specified injury of femoral vein at hip and thigh level, unspecified leg
● S75.2 **Injury of greater saphenous vein at hip and thigh level**
  Excludes1 greater saphenous vein NOS (S85.3)
  ● S75.20 **Unspecified injury of greater saphenous vein at hip and thigh level**
    ● S75.201 Unspecified injury of greater saphenous vein at hip and thigh level, right leg
    ● S75.202 Unspecified injury of greater saphenous vein at hip and thigh level, left leg
    ● S75.209 Unspecified injury of greater saphenous vein at hip and thigh level, unspecified leg
  ● S75.21 **Minor laceration of greater saphenous vein at hip and thigh level**
    Incomplete transection of greater saphenous vein at hip and thigh level
    Laceration of greater saphenous vein at hip and thigh level NOS
    Superficial laceration of greater saphenous vein at hip and thigh level
    ● S75.211 Minor laceration of greater saphenous vein at hip and thigh level, right leg
    ● S75.212 Minor laceration of greater saphenous vein at hip and thigh level, left leg
    ● S75.219 Minor laceration of greater saphenous vein at hip and thigh level, unspecified leg

◀ New ◀━ Revised ~~deleted~~ Deleted │ Excludes 1 │ │ Excludes 2 │ │ Includes │ │ Use additional │ │ Code first │ │ Code also │ │ Unspecified │
OGCR Official Guidelines X Assign placeholder X ● Use Additional Character(s) ▶ Manifestation Code **Coding Clinic**

● **S75.22**   Major laceration of greater saphenous vein at hip and thigh level

     Complete transection of greater saphenous vein at hip and thigh level

     Traumatic rupture of greater saphenous vein at hip and thigh level

     ● **S75.221**   Major laceration of greater saphenous vein at hip and thigh level, right leg

     ● **S75.222**   Major laceration of greater saphenous vein at hip and thigh level, left leg

     ● **S75.229**   Major laceration of greater saphenous vein at hip and thigh level, unspecified leg

● **S75.29**   Other specified injury of greater saphenous vein at hip and thigh level

     ● **S75.291**   Other specified injury of greater saphenous vein at hip and thigh level, right leg

     ● **S75.292**   Other specified injury of greater saphenous vein at hip and thigh level, left leg

     ● **S75.299**   Other specified injury of greater saphenous vein at hip and thigh level, unspecified leg

● **S75.8**   Injury of other blood vessels at hip and thigh level

   ● **S75.80**   Unspecified injury of other blood vessels at hip and thigh level

     ● **S75.801**   Unspecified injury of other blood vessels at hip and thigh level, right leg

     ● **S75.802**   Unspecified injury of other blood vessels at hip and thigh level, left leg

     ● **S75.809**   Unspecified injury of other blood vessels at hip and thigh level, unspecified leg

   ● **S75.81**   Laceration of other blood vessels at hip and thigh level

     ● **S75.811**   Laceration of other blood vessels at hip and thigh level, right leg

     ● **S75.812**   Laceration of other blood vessels at hip and thigh level, left leg

     ● **S75.819**   Laceration of other blood vessels at hip and thigh level, unspecified leg

   ● **S75.89**   Other specified injury of other blood vessels at hip and thigh level

     ● **S75.891**   Other specified injury of other blood vessels at hip and thigh level, right leg

     ● **S75.892**   Other specified injury of other blood vessels at hip and thigh level, left leg

     ● **S75.899**   Other specified injury of other blood vessels at hip and thigh level, unspecified leg

● **S75.9**   Injury of unspecified blood vessel at hip and thigh level

   ● **S75.90**   Unspecified injury of unspecified blood vessel at hip and thigh level

     ● **S75.901**   Unspecified injury of unspecified blood vessel at hip and thigh level, right leg

     ● **S75.902**   Unspecified injury of unspecified blood vessel at hip and thigh level, left leg

     ● **S75.909**   Unspecified injury of unspecified blood vessel at hip and thigh level, unspecified leg

● **S75.91**   Laceration of unspecified blood vessel at hip and thigh level

     ● **S75.911**   Laceration of unspecified blood vessel at hip and thigh level, right leg

     ● **S75.912**   Laceration of unspecified blood vessel at hip and thigh level, left leg

     ● **S75.919**   Laceration of unspecified blood vessel at hip and thigh level, unspecified leg

● **S75.99**   Other specified injury of unspecified blood vessel at hip and thigh level

     ● **S75.991**   Other specified injury of unspecified blood vessel at hip and thigh level, right leg

     ● **S75.992**   Other specified injury of unspecified blood vessel at hip and thigh level, left leg

     ● **S75.999**   Other specified injury of unspecified blood vessel at hip and thigh level, unspecified leg

● **S76**   Injury of muscle, fascia and tendon at hip and thigh level

   Code also any associated open wound (S71.-)

   Excludes2   injury of muscle, fascia and tendon at lower leg level (S86)

              sprain of joint and ligament of hip (S73.1)

   The appropriate 7th character is to be added to each code from category S76

> A   initial encounter
> D   subsequent encounter
> S   sequela

● **S76.0**   Injury of muscle, fascia and tendon of hip

   ● **S76.00**   Unspecified injury of muscle, fascia and tendon of hip

     ● **S76.001**   Unspecified injury of muscle, fascia and tendon of right hip

     ● **S76.002**   Unspecified injury of muscle, fascia and tendon of left hip

     ● **S76.009**   Unspecified injury of muscle, fascia and tendon of unspecified hip

   ● **S76.01**   Strain of muscle, fascia and tendon of hip

     ● **S76.011**   Strain of muscle, fascia and tendon of right hip

     ● **S76.012**   Strain of muscle, fascia and tendon of left hip

     ● **S76.019**   Strain of muscle, fascia and tendon of unspecified hip

   ● **S76.02**   Laceration of muscle, fascia and tendon of hip

     ● **S76.021**   Laceration of muscle, fascia and tendon of right hip

     ● **S76.022**   Laceration of muscle, fascia and tendon of left hip

     ● **S76.029**   Laceration of muscle, fascia and tendon of unspecified hip

   ● **S76.09**   Other specified injury of muscle, fascia and tendon of hip

     ● **S76.091**   Other specified injury of muscle, fascia and tendon of right hip

     ● **S76.092**   Other specified injury of muscle, fascia and tendon of left hip

     ● **S76.099**   Other specified injury of muscle, fascia and tendon of unspecified hip

● **S76.1**   Injury of quadriceps muscle, fascia and tendon
Injury of patellar ligament (tendon)

  ● **S76.10**   Unspecified injury of quadriceps muscle, fascia and tendon

    ● **S76.101**   ==Unspecified== injury of right quadriceps muscle, fascia and tendon

    ● **S76.102**   ==Unspecified== injury of left quadriceps muscle, fascia and tendon

    ● **S76.109**   ==Unspecified== injury of unspecified quadriceps muscle, fascia and tendon

  ● **S76.11**   Strain of quadriceps muscle, fascia and tendon

    ● **S76.111**   Strain of right quadriceps muscle, fascia and tendon

    ● **S76.112**   Strain of left quadriceps muscle, fascia and tendon

    ● **S76.119**   Strain of ==unspecified== quadriceps muscle, fascia and tendon

  ● **S76.12**   Laceration of quadriceps muscle, fascia and tendon

    ● **S76.121**   Laceration of right quadriceps muscle, fascia and tendon

    ● **S76.122**   Laceration of left quadriceps muscle, fascia and tendon

    ● **S76.129**   Laceration of ==unspecified== quadriceps muscle, fascia and tendon

  ● **S76.19**   Other specified injury of quadriceps muscle, fascia and tendon

    ● **S76.191**   Other specified injury of right quadriceps muscle, fascia and tendon

    ● **S76.192**   Other specified injury of left quadriceps muscle, fascia and tendon

    ● **S76.199**   Other specified injury of ==unspecified== quadriceps muscle, fascia and tendon

● **S76.2**   Injury of adductor muscle, fascia and tendon of thigh

  ● **S76.20**   Unspecified injury of adductor muscle, fascia and tendon of thigh

    ● **S76.201**   ==Unspecified== injury of adductor muscle, fascia and tendon of right thigh

    ● **S76.202**   ==Unspecified== injury of adductor muscle, fascia and tendon of left thigh

    ● **S76.209**   ==Unspecified== injury of adductor muscle, fascia and tendon of unspecified thigh

  ● **S76.21**   Strain of adductor muscle, fascia and tendon of thigh

    ● **S76.211**   Strain of adductor muscle, fascia and tendon of right thigh

    ● **S76.212**   Strain of adductor muscle, fascia and tendon of left thigh

    ● **S76.219**   Strain of adductor muscle, fascia and tendon of ==unspecified== thigh

  ● **S76.22**   Laceration of adductor muscle, fascia and tendon of thigh

    ● **S76.221**   Laceration of adductor muscle, fascia and tendon of right thigh

    ● **S76.222**   Laceration of adductor muscle, fascia and tendon of left thigh

    ● **S76.229**   Laceration of adductor muscle, fascia and tendon of ==unspecified== thigh

  ● **S76.29**   Other injury of adductor muscle, fascia and tendon of thigh

    ● **S76.291**   Other injury of adductor muscle, fascia and tendon of right thigh

    ● **S76.292**   Other injury of adductor muscle, fascia and tendon of left thigh

    ● **S76.299**   Other injury of adductor muscle, fascia and tendon of ==unspecified== thigh

● **S76.3**   Injury of muscle, fascia and tendon of the posterior muscle group at thigh level

  ● **S76.30**   Unspecified injury of muscle, fascia and tendon of the posterior muscle group at thigh level

    ● **S76.301**   ==Unspecified== injury of muscle, fascia and tendon of the posterior muscle group at thigh level, right thigh

    ● **S76.302**   ==Unspecified== injury of muscle, fascia and tendon of the posterior muscle group at thigh level, left thigh

    ● **S76.309**   ==Unspecified== injury of muscle, fascia and tendon of the posterior muscle group at thigh level, unspecified thigh

  ● **S76.31**   Strain of muscle, fascia and tendon of the posterior muscle group at thigh level

    ● **S76.311**   Strain of muscle, fascia and tendon of the posterior muscle group at thigh level, right thigh

    ● **S76.312**   Strain of muscle, fascia and tendon of the posterior muscle group at thigh level, left thigh

    ● **S76.319**   Strain of muscle, fascia and tendon of the posterior muscle group at thigh level, ==unspecified== thigh

  ● **S76.32**   Laceration of muscle, fascia and tendon of the posterior muscle group at thigh level

    ● **S76.321**   Laceration of muscle, fascia and tendon of the posterior muscle group at thigh level, right thigh

    ● **S76.322**   Laceration of muscle, fascia and tendon of the posterior muscle group at thigh level, left thigh

    ● **S76.329**   Laceration of muscle, fascia and tendon of the posterior muscle group at thigh level, ==unspecified== thigh

  ● **S76.39**   Other specified injury of muscle, fascia and tendon of the posterior muscle group at thigh level

    ● **S76.391**   Other specified injury of muscle, fascia and tendon of the posterior muscle group at thigh level, right thigh

    ● **S76.392**   Other specified injury of muscle, fascia and tendon of the posterior muscle group at thigh level, left thigh

    ● **S76.399**   Other specified injury of muscle, fascia and tendon of the posterior muscle group at thigh level, ==unspecified== thigh

◄ New   ◄ Revised   ~~deleted~~ Deleted   Excludes 1   Excludes 2   Includes   Use additional   Code first   Code also   Unspecified

OGCR Official Guidelines   X Assign placeholder X   ● Use Additional Character(s)   ▶ Manifestation Code   **Coding Clinic**

● S76.8   Injury of other specified muscles, fascia and tendons at thigh level

  ● S76.80   Unspecified injury of other specified muscles, fascia and tendons at thigh level

    ● S76.801   Unspecified injury of other specified muscles, fascia and tendons at thigh level, right thigh

    ● S76.802   Unspecified injury of other specified muscles, fascia and tendons at thigh level, left thigh

    ● S76.809   Unspecified injury of other specified muscles, fascia and tendons at thigh level, unspecified thigh

  ● S76.81   Strain of other specified specified muscles, fascia and tendons at thigh level

    ● S76.811   Strain of other specified muscles, fascia and tendons at thigh level, right thigh

    ● S76.812   Strain of other specified muscles, fascia and tendons at thigh level, left thigh

    ● S76.819   Strain of other specified muscles, fascia and tendons at thigh level, unspecified thigh

  ● S76.82   Laceration of other specified muscles, fascia and tendons at thigh level

    ● S76.821   Laceration of other specified muscles, fascia and tendons at thigh level, right thigh

    ● S76.822   Laceration of other specified muscles, fascia and tendons at thigh level, left thigh

    ● S76.829   Laceration of other specified muscles, fascia and tendons at thigh level, unspecified thigh

  ● S76.89   Other injury of other specified muscles, fascia and tendons at thigh level

    ● S76.891   Other injury of other specified muscles, fascia and tendons at thigh level, right thigh

    ● S76.892   Other injury of other specified muscles, fascia and tendons at thigh level, left thigh

    ● S76.899   Other injury of other specified muscles, fascia and tendons at thigh level, unspecified thigh

● S76.9   Injury of unspecified muscles, fascia and tendons at thigh level

  ● S76.90   Unspecified injury of unspecified muscles, fascia and tendons at thigh level

    ● S76.901   Unspecified injury of unspecified muscles, fascia and tendons at thigh level, right thigh

    ● S76.902   Unspecified injury of unspecified muscles, fascia and tendons at thigh level, left thigh

    ● S76.909   Unspecified injury of unspecified muscles, fascia and tendons at thigh level, unspecified thigh

  ● S76.91   Strain of unspecified muscles, fascia and tendons at thigh level

    ● S76.911   Strain of unspecified muscles, fascia and tendons at thigh level, right thigh

    ● S76.912   Strain of unspecified muscles, fascia and tendons at thigh level, left thigh

    ● S76.919   Strain of unspecified muscles, fascia and tendons at thigh level, unspecified thigh

  ● S76.92   Laceration of unspecified muscles, fascia and tendons at thigh level

    ● S76.921   Laceration of unspecified muscles, fascia and tendons at thigh level, right thigh

    ● S76.922   Laceration of unspecified muscles, fascia and tendons at thigh level, left thigh

    ● S76.929   Laceration of unspecified muscles, fascia and tendons at thigh level, unspecified thigh

  ● S76.99   Other specified injury of unspecified muscles, fascia and tendons at thigh level

    ● S76.991   Other specified injury of unspecified muscles, fascia and tendons at thigh level, right thigh

    ● S76.992   Other specified injury of unspecified muscles, fascia and tendons at thigh level, left thigh

    ● S76.999   Other specified injury of unspecified muscles, fascia and tendons at thigh level, unspecified thigh

● S77   Crushing injury of hip and thigh

  Use additional code(s) for all associated injuries

  Excludes2   crushing injury of ankle and foot (S97.-)
  crushing injury of lower leg (S87.-)

  The appropriate 7th character is to be added to each code from category S77

A	initial encounter
D	subsequent encounter
S	sequela

  ● S77.0   Crushing injury of hip

    X ● S77.00   Crushing injury of unspecified hip
    X ● S77.01   Crushing injury of right hip
    X ● S77.02   Crushing injury of left hip

  ● S77.1   Crushing injury of thigh

    X ● S77.10   Crushing injury of unspecified thigh
    X ● S77.11   Crushing injury of right thigh
    X ● S77.12   Crushing injury of left thigh

  ● S77.2   Crushing injury of hip with thigh

    X ● S77.20   Crushing injury of unspecified hip with thigh
    X ● S77.21   Crushing injury of right hip with thigh
    X ● S77.22   Crushing injury of left hip with thigh

● S78   Traumatic amputation of hip and thigh

  An amputation not identified as partial or complete should be coded to complete

  Excludes1   traumatic amputation of knee (S88.0-)

  The appropriate 7th character is to be added to each code from category S78

A	initial encounter
D	subsequent encounter
S	sequela

  ● S78.0   Traumatic amputation at hip joint

    ● S78.01   Complete traumatic amputation at hip joint

      ● S78.011   Complete traumatic amputation at right hip joint

      ● S78.012   Complete traumatic amputation at left hip joint

      ● S78.019   Complete traumatic amputation at unspecified hip joint

- S78.02   Partial traumatic amputation at hip joint
  - S78.021   Partial traumatic amputation at right hip joint
  - S78.022   Partial traumatic amputation at left hip joint
  - S78.029   Partial traumatic amputation at unspecified hip joint
- S78.1   Traumatic amputation at level between hip and knee
  - **Excludes1**   traumatic amputation of knee (S88.0-)
  - S78.11   Complete traumatic amputation at level between hip and knee
    - S78.111   Complete traumatic amputation at level between right hip and knee
    - S78.112   Complete traumatic amputation at level between left hip and knee
    - S78.119   Complete traumatic amputation at level between unspecified hip and knee
  - S78.12   Partial traumatic amputation at level between hip and knee
    - S78.121   Partial traumatic amputation at level between right hip and knee
    - S78.122   Partial traumatic amputation at level between left hip and knee
    - S78.129   Partial traumatic amputation at level between unspecified hip and knee
- S78.9   Traumatic amputation of hip and thigh, level unspecified
  - S78.91   Complete traumatic amputation of hip and thigh, level unspecified
    - S78.911   Complete traumatic amputation of right hip and thigh, level unspecified
    - S78.912   Complete traumatic amputation of left hip and thigh, level unspecified
    - S78.919   Complete traumatic amputation of unspecified hip and thigh, level unspecified
  - S78.92   Partial traumatic amputation of hip and thigh, level unspecified
    - S78.921   Partial traumatic amputation of right hip and thigh, level unspecified
    - S78.922   Partial traumatic amputation of left hip and thigh, level unspecified
    - S78.929   Partial traumatic amputation of unspecified hip and thigh, level unspecified

- S79   Other and unspecified injuries of hip and thigh
  - **Note:** A fracture not indicated as open or closed should be coded to closed
  - The appropriate 7th character is to be added to each code from subcategories S79.0 and S79.1

A	initial encounter for closed fracture
D	subsequent encounter for fracture with routine healing
G	subsequent encounter for fracture with delayed healing
K	subsequent encounter for fracture with nonunion
P	subsequent encounter for fracture with malunion
S	sequela

- S79.0   Physeal fracture of upper end of femur
  - **Excludes1**   apophyseal fracture of upper end of femur (S72.13-)
    - nontraumatic slipped upper femoral epiphysis (M93.0-)
  - S79.00   Unspecified physeal fracture of upper end of femur
    - S79.001   Unspecified physeal fracture of upper end of right femur
    - S79.002   Unspecified physeal fracture of upper end of left femur
    - S79.009   Unspecified physeal fracture of upper end of unspecified femur

Item 19–5   SALTER-HARRIS TYPE 1: epiphysis is completely separated from end of bone, or metaphysic growth plate remains attached to epiphysis

SALTER-HARRIS TYPE 2: epiphysis and growth plate are partially separated from metaphysis, which is cracked—most common type

SALTER-HARRIS TYPE 3: fracture occurring through epiphysis and separates part of epiphysis and growth plate from metaphysis fracture, usually at distal end of tibia

SALTER-HARRIS TYPE 4: fracture runs through epiphysis, across growth plate, into metaphysic, surgery is required to restore joint surface to normal and align growth plate

- S79.01   Salter-Harris Type I physeal fracture of upper end of femur
  - Acute on chronic slipped capital femoral epiphysis (traumatic)
  - Acute slipped capital femoral epiphysis (traumatic)
  - Capital femoral epiphyseal fracture
  - **Excludes1**   chronic slipped upper femoral epiphysis (nontraumatic) (M93.02-)
  - S79.011   Salter-Harris Type I physeal fracture of upper end of right femur
  - S79.012   Salter-Harris Type I physeal fracture of upper end of left femur
  - S79.019   Salter-Harris Type I physeal fracture of upper end of unspecified femur
- S79.09   Other physeal fracture of upper end of femur
  - S79.091   Other physeal fracture of upper end of right femur
  - S79.092   Other physeal fracture of upper end of left femur
  - S79.099   Other physeal fracture of upper end of unspecified femur
- S79.1   Physeal fracture of lower end of femur
  - S79.10   Unspecified physeal fracture of lower end of femur
    - S79.101   Unspecified physeal fracture of lower end of right femur
    - S79.102   Unspecified physeal fracture of lower end of left femur
    - S79.109   Unspecified physeal fracture of lower end of unspecified femur
  - S79.11   Salter-Harris Type I physeal fracture of lower end of femur
    - S79.111   Salter-Harris Type I physeal fracture of lower end of right femur
    - S79.112   Salter-Harris Type I physeal fracture of lower end of left femur
    - S79.119   Salter-Harris Type I physeal fracture of lower end of unspecified femur
  - S79.12   Salter-Harris Type II physeal fracture of lower end of femur
    - S79.121   Salter-Harris Type II physeal fracture of lower end of right femur
    - S79.122   Salter-Harris Type II physeal fracture of lower end of left femur
    - S79.129   Salter-Harris Type II physeal fracture of lower end of unspecified femur
  - S79.13   Salter-Harris Type III physeal fracture of lower end of femur
    - S79.131   Salter-Harris Type III physeal fracture of lower end of right femur
    - S79.132   Salter-Harris Type III physeal fracture of lower end of left femur
    - S79.139   Salter-Harris Type III physeal fracture of lower end of unspecified femur

◀ New   ◀▥ Revised   ~~deleted~~ Deleted   Excludes 1   Excludes 2   Includes   Use additional   Code first   Code also   Unspecified

OGCR Official Guidelines   X Assign placeholder X   ● Use Additional Character(s)   ▶ Manifestation Code   **Coding Clinic**

- **S79.14**   Salter-Harris Type IV physeal fracture of lower end of femur
  - **S79.141**   Salter-Harris Type IV physeal fracture of lower end of right femur
  - **S79.142**   Salter-Harris Type IV physeal fracture of lower end of left femur
  - **S79.149**   Salter-Harris Type IV physeal fracture of lower end of unspecified femur
- **S79.19**   Other physeal fracture of lower end of femur
  - **S79.191**   Other physeal fracture of lower end of right femur
  - **S79.192**   Other physeal fracture of lower end of left femur
  - **S79.199**   Other physeal fracture of lower end of unspecified femur

- **S79.8 Other specified injuries of hip and thigh**

  The appropriate 7th character is to be added to each code in subcategory S79.8

A	initial encounter
D	subsequent encounter
S	sequela

  - **S79.81**   Other specified injuries of hip
    - **S79.811**   Other specified injuries of right hip
    - **S79.812**   Other specified injuries of left hip
    - **S79.819**   Other specified injuries of unspecified hip
  - **S79.82**   Other specified injuries of thigh
    - **S79.821**   Other specified injuries of right thigh
    - **S79.822**   Other specified injuries of left thigh
    - **S79.829**   Other specified injuries of unspecified thigh

- **S79.9**   Unspecified injury of hip and thigh

  The appropriate 7th character is to be added to each code in subcategory S79.9

A	initial encounter
D	subsequent encounter
S	sequela

  - **S79.91**   Unspecified injury of hip
    - **S79.911**   Unspecified injury of right hip
    - **S79.912**   Unspecified injury of left hip
    - **S79.919**   Unspecified injury of unspecified hip
  - **S79.92**   Unspecified injury of thigh
    - **S79.921**   Unspecified injury of right thigh
    - **S79.922**   Unspecified injury of left thigh
    - **S79.929**   Unspecified injury of unspecified thigh

INJURIES TO THE KNEE AND LOWER LEG (S80-S89)

Excludes2   burns and corrosions (T20-T32)
frostbite (T33-T34)
injuries of ankle and foot, except fracture of ankle and malleolus (S90-S99)
insect bite or sting, venomous (T63.4)

- **S80**   **Superficial injury of knee and lower leg**

  Excludes2   superficial injury of ankle and foot (S90.-)

  The appropriate 7th character is to be added to each code from category S80

A	initial encounter
D	subsequent encounter
S	sequela

  - **S80.0**   Contusion of knee
    - X **S80.00**   Contusion of unspecified knee
    - X **S80.01**   Contusion of right knee
    - X **S80.02**   Contusion of left knee

- **S80.1**   Contusion of lower leg
  - X **S80.10**   Contusion of unspecified lower leg
  - X **S80.11**   Contusion of right lower leg
  - X **S80.12**   Contusion of left lower leg
- **S80.2**   Other superficial injuries of knee
  - **S80.21**   Abrasion of knee
    - **S80.211**   Abrasion, right knee
    - **S80.212**   Abrasion, left knee
    - **S80.219**   Abrasion, unspecified knee
  - **S80.22**   Blister (nonthermal) of knee
    - **S80.221**   Blister (nonthermal), right knee
    - **S80.222**   Blister (nonthermal), left knee
    - **S80.229**   Blister (nonthermal), unspecified knee
  - **S80.24**   External constriction of knee
    - **S80.241**   External constriction, right knee
    - **S80.242**   External constriction, left knee
    - **S80.249**   External constriction, unspecified knee
  - **S80.25**   Superficial foreign body of knee
    Splinter in the knee
    - **S80.251**   Superficial foreign body, right knee
    - **S80.252**   Superficial foreign body, left knee
    - **S80.259**   Superficial foreign body, unspecified knee
  - **S80.26**   Insect bite (nonvenomous) of knee
    - **S80.261**   Insect bite (nonvenomous), right knee
    - **S80.262**   Insect bite (nonvenomous), left knee
    - **S80.269**   Insect bite (nonvenomous), unspecified knee
  - **S80.27**   Other superficial bite of knee
    - **Excludes1**   open bite of knee (S81.05-)
    - **S80.271**   Other superficial bite of right knee
    - **S80.272**   Other superficial bite of left knee
    - **S80.279**   Other superficial bite of unspecified knee
- **S80.8**   Other superficial injuries of lower leg
  - **S80.81**   Abrasion of lower leg
    - **S80.811**   Abrasion, right lower leg
    - **S80.812**   Abrasion, left lower leg
    - **S80.819**   Abrasion, unspecified lower leg
  - **S80.82**   Blister (nonthermal) of lower leg
    - **S80.821**   Blister (nonthermal), right lower leg
    - **S80.822**   Blister (nonthermal), left lower leg
    - **S80.829**   Blister (nonthermal), unspecified lower leg
  - **S80.84**   External constriction of lower leg
    - **S80.841**   External constriction, right lower leg
    - **S80.842**   External constriction, left lower leg
    - **S80.849**   External constriction, unspecified lower leg
  - **S80.85**   Superficial foreign body of lower leg
    Splinter in the lower leg
    - **S80.851**   Superficial foreign body, right lower leg
    - **S80.852**   Superficial foreign body, left lower leg
    - **S80.859**   Superficial foreign body, unspecified lower leg

CHAPTER 19 (S00-T88)

- ● S80.86   Insect bite (nonvenomous) of lower leg
  - ● S80.861   Insect bite (nonvenomous), right lower leg
  - ● S80.862   Insect bite (nonvenomous), left lower leg
  - ● S80.869   Insect bite (nonvenomous), unspecified lower leg
- ● S80.87   Other superficial bite of lower leg
  - **Excludes1**   open bite of lower leg (S81.85-)
  - ● S80.871   Other superficial bite, right lower leg
  - ● S80.872   Other superficial bite, left lower leg
  - ● S80.879   Other superficial bite, unspecified lower leg
- ● S80.9   Unspecified superficial injury of knee and lower leg
  - ● S80.91   Unspecified superficial injury of knee
    - ● S80.911   Unspecified superficial injury of right knee
    - ● S80.912   Unspecified superficial injury of left knee
    - ● S80.919   Unspecified superficial injury of unspecified knee
  - ● S80.92   Unspecified superficial injury of lower leg
    - ● S80.921   Unspecified superficial injury of right lower leg
    - ● S80.922   Unspecified superficial injury of left lower leg
    - ● S80.929   Unspecified superficial injury of unspecified lower leg

- ● S81   **Open wound of knee and lower leg**
  - Code also any associated wound infection
  - **Excludes1**   open fracture of knee and lower leg (S82.-)
  -            traumatic amputation of lower leg (S88.-)
  - **Excludes2**   open wound of ankle and foot (S91.-)
  - The appropriate 7th character is to be added to each code from category S81

A	initial encounter
D	subsequent encounter
S	sequela

  - ● S81.0   Open wound of knee
    - ● S81.00   Unspecified open wound of knee
      - ● S81.001   Unspecified open wound, right knee
      - ● S81.002   Unspecified open wound, left knee
      - ● S81.009   Unspecified open wound, unspecified knee
    - ● S81.01   Laceration without foreign body of knee
      - ● S81.011   Laceration without foreign body, right knee
      - ● S81.012   Laceration without foreign body, left knee
      - ● S81.019   Laceration without foreign body, unspecified knee
    - ● S81.02   Laceration with foreign body of knee
      - ● S81.021   Laceration with foreign body, right knee
      - ● S81.022   Laceration with foreign body, left knee
      - ● S81.029   Laceration with foreign body, unspecified knee

- ● S81.03   Puncture wound without foreign body of knee
  - ● S81.031   Puncture wound without foreign body, right knee
  - ● S81.032   Puncture wound without foreign body, left knee
  - ● S81.039   Puncture wound without foreign body, unspecified knee
- ● S81.04   Puncture wound with foreign body of knee
  - ● S81.041   Puncture wound with foreign body, right knee
  - ● S81.042   Puncture wound with foreign body, left knee
  - ● S81.049   Puncture wound with foreign body, unspecified knee
- ● S81.05   Open bite of knee
  - Bite of knee NOS
  - **Excludes1**   superficial bite of knee (S80.27-)
  - ● S81.051   Open bite, right knee
  - ● S81.052   Open bite, left knee
  - ● S81.059   Open bite, unspecified knee
- ● S81.8   Open wound of lower leg
  - ● S81.80   Unspecified open wound of lower leg
    - ● S81.801   Unspecified open wound, right lower leg
    - ● S81.802   Unspecified open wound, left lower leg
    - ● S81.809   Unspecified open wound, unspecified lower leg
  - ● S81.81   Laceration without foreign body of lower leg
    - ● S81.811   Laceration without foreign body, right lower leg
    - ● S81.812   Laceration without foreign body, left lower leg
    - ● S81.819   Laceration without foreign body, unspecified lower leg
  - ● S81.82   Laceration with foreign body of lower leg
    - ● S81.821   Laceration with foreign body, right lower leg
    - ● S81.822   Laceration with foreign body, left lower leg
    - ● S81.829   Laceration with foreign body, unspecified lower leg
  - ● S81.83   Puncture wound without foreign body of lower leg
    - ● S81.831   Puncture wound without foreign body, right lower leg
    - ● S81.832   Puncture wound without foreign body, left lower leg
    - ● S81.839   Puncture wound without foreign body, unspecified lower leg
  - ● S81.84   Puncture wound with foreign body of lower leg
    - ● S81.841   Puncture wound with foreign body, right lower leg
    - ● S81.842   Puncture wound with foreign body, left lower leg
    - ● S81.849   Puncture wound with foreign body, unspecified lower leg
  - ● S81.85   Open bite of lower leg
    - Bite of lower leg NOS
    - **Excludes1**   superficial bite of lower leg (S80.86-, S80.87-)
    - ● S81.851   Open bite, right lower leg
    - ● S81.852   Open bite, left lower leg
    - ● S81.859   Open bite, unspecified lower leg

◀ New   ◀┉ Revised   ~~deleted~~ Deleted   Excludes 1   Excludes 2   Includes   Use additional   Code first   Code also   Unspecified

OGCR Official Guidelines   X Assign placeholder X   ● Use Additional Character(s)   ▸ Manifestation Code   **Coding Clinic**

● S82 **Fracture of lower leg, including ankle**

Note: A fracture not indicated as displaced or nondisplaced should be coded to displaced

A fracture not indicated as open or closed should be coded to closed

The open fracture designations are based on the Gustilo open fracture classification

Includes fracture of malleolus

Excludes1 traumatic amputation of lower leg (S88.-)

Excludes2 fracture of foot, except ankle (S92.-)
periprosthetic fracture of prosthetic implant of knee (T84.042, T84.043)

The appropriate 7th character is to be added to all codes from category S82

A	initial encounter for closed fracture
B	initial encounter for open fracture type I or II initial encounter for open fracture NOS
C	initial encounter for open fracture type IIIA, IIIB, or IIIC
D	subsequent encounter for closed fracture with routine healing
E	subsequent encounter for open fracture type I or II with routine healing
F	subsequent encounter for open fracture type IIIA, IIIB, or IIIC with routine healing
G	subsequent encounter for closed fracture with delayed healing
H	subsequent encounter for open fracture type I or II with delayed healing
J	subsequent encounter for open fracture type IIIA, IIIB, or IIIC with delayed healing
K	subsequent encounter for closed fracture with nonunion
M	subsequent encounter for open fracture type I or II with nonunion
N	subsequent encounter for open fracture type IIIA, IIIB, or IIIC with nonunion
P	subsequent encounter for closed fracture with malunion
Q	subsequent encounter for open fracture type I or II with malunion
R	subsequent encounter for open fracture type IIIA, IIIB, or IIIC with malunion
S	sequela

● S82.0 **Fracture of patella**
Knee cap

● S82.00 **Unspecified fracture of patella**

● S82.001 Unspecified fracture of right patella

● S82.002 Unspecified fracture of left patella

● S82.009 Unspecified fracture of unspecified patella

● S82.01 **Osteochondral fracture of patella**

● S82.011 Displaced osteochondral fracture of right patella

● S82.012 Displaced osteochondral fracture of left patella

● S82.013 Displaced osteochondral fracture of unspecified patella

● S82.014 Nondisplaced osteochondral fracture of right patella

● S82.015 Nondisplaced osteochondral fracture of left patella

● S82.016 Nondisplaced osteochondral fracture of unspecified patella

● S82.02 **Longitudinal fracture of patella**

● S82.021 Displaced longitudinal fracture of right patella

● S82.022 Displaced longitudinal fracture of left patella

● S82.023 Displaced longitudinal fracture of unspecified patella

● S82.024 Nondisplaced longitudinal fracture of right patella

● S82.025 Nondisplaced longitudinal fracture of left patella

● S82.026 Nondisplaced longitudinal fracture of unspecified patella

● S82.03 **Transverse fracture of patella**

● S82.031 Displaced transverse fracture of right patella

● S82.032 Displaced transverse fracture of left patella

● S82.033 Displaced transverse fracture of unspecified patella

● S82.034 Nondisplaced transverse fracture of right patella

● S82.035 Nondisplaced transverse fracture of left patella

● S82.036 Nondisplaced transverse fracture of unspecified patella

● S82.04 **Comminuted fracture of patella**

● S82.041 Displaced comminuted fracture of right patella

● S82.042 Displaced comminuted fracture of left patella

● S82.043 Displaced comminuted fracture of unspecified patella

● S82.044 Nondisplaced comminuted fracture of right patella

● S82.045 Nondisplaced comminuted fracture of left patella

● S82.046 Nondisplaced comminuted fracture of unspecified patella

● S82.09 **Other fracture of patella**

● S82.091 Other fracture of right patella

● S82.092 Other fracture of left patella

● S82.099 Other fracture of unspecified patella

● S82.1 **Fracture of upper end of tibia**
Fracture of proximal end of tibia

Excludes2 fracture of shaft of tibia (S82.2-)
physeal fracture of upper end of tibia (S89.0-)

● S82.10 **Unspecified fracture of upper end of tibia**

● S82.101 Unspecified fracture of upper end of right tibia

● S82.102 Unspecified fracture of upper end of left tibia

● S82.109 Unspecified fracture of upper end of unspecified tibia

● S82.11 **Fracture of tibial spine**

● S82.111 Displaced fracture of right tibial spine

● S82.112 Displaced fracture of left tibial spine

● S82.113 Displaced fracture of unspecified tibial spine

CHAPTER 19 (S00-T88)

● S82.114   Nondisplaced fracture of right tibial spine
● S82.115   Nondisplaced fracture of left tibial spine
● S82.116   Nondisplaced fracture of unspecified tibial spine
● S82.12   Fracture of lateral condyle of tibia
  ● S82.121   Displaced fracture of lateral condyle of right tibia
  ● S82.122   Displaced fracture of lateral condyle of left tibia
  ● S82.123   Displaced fracture of lateral condyle of unspecified tibia
  ● S82.124   Nondisplaced fracture of lateral condyle of right tibia
  ● S82.125   Nondisplaced fracture of lateral condyle of left tibia
  ● S82.126   Nondisplaced fracture of lateral condyle of unspecified tibia
● S82.13   Fracture of medial condyle of tibia
  ● S82.131   Displaced fracture of medial condyle of right tibia
  ● S82.132   Displaced fracture of medial condyle of left tibia
  ● S82.133   Displaced fracture of medial condyle of unspecified tibia
  ● S82.134   Nondisplaced fracture of medial condyle of right tibia
  ● S82.135   Nondisplaced fracture of medial condyle of left tibia
  ● S82.136   Nondisplaced fracture of medial condyle of unspecified tibia
● S82.14   Bicondylar fracture of tibia
  Fracture of tibial plateau NOS
  ● S82.141   Displaced bicondylar fracture of right tibia
  ● S82.142   Displaced bicondylar fracture of left tibia
  ● S82.143   Displaced bicondylar fracture of unspecified tibia
  ● S82.144   Nondisplaced bicondylar fracture of right tibia
  ● S82.145   Nondisplaced bicondylar fracture of left tibia
  ● S82.146   Nondisplaced bicondylar fracture of unspecified tibia
● S82.15   Fracture of tibial tuberosity
  ● S82.151   Displaced fracture of right tibial tuberosity
  ● S82.152   Displaced fracture of left tibial tuberosity
  ● S82.153   Displaced fracture of unspecified tibial tuberosity
  ● S82.154   Nondisplaced fracture of right tibial tuberosity
  ● S82.155   Nondisplaced fracture of left tibial tuberosity
  ● S82.156   Nondisplaced fracture of unspecified tibial tuberosity

● S82.16   Torus fracture of upper end of tibia
  The appropriate 7th character is to be added to all codes in subcategory S82.16

A	initial encounter for closed fracture
D	subsequent encounter for fracture with routine healing
G	subsequent encounter for fracture with delayed healing
K	subsequent encounter for fracture with nonunion
P	subsequent encounter for fracture with malunion
S	sequela

  ● S82.161   Torus fracture of upper end of right tibia
  ● S82.162   Torus fracture of upper end of left tibia
  ● S82.169   Torus fracture of upper end of unspecified tibia
● S82.19   Other fracture of upper end of tibia
  ● S82.191   Other fracture of upper end of right tibia
  ● S82.192   Other fracture of upper end of left tibia
  ● S82.199   Other fracture of upper end of unspecified tibia
● S82.2   Fracture of shaft of tibia
  ● S82.20   Unspecified fracture of shaft of tibia
    Fracture of tibia NOS
    ● S82.201   Unspecified fracture of shaft of right tibia
    ● S82.202   Unspecified fracture of shaft of left tibia
    ● S82.209   Unspecified fracture of shaft of unspecified tibia
  ● S82.22   Transverse fracture of shaft of tibia
    ● S82.221   Displaced transverse fracture of shaft of right tibia
    ● S82.222   Displaced transverse fracture of shaft of left tibia
    ● S82.223   Displaced transverse fracture of shaft of unspecified tibia
    ● S82.224   Nondisplaced transverse fracture of shaft of right tibia
    ● S82.225   Nondisplaced transverse fracture of shaft of left tibia
    ● S82.226   Nondisplaced transverse fracture of shaft of unspecified tibia
  ● S82.23   Oblique fracture of shaft of tibia
    ● S82.231   Displaced oblique fracture of shaft of right tibia
    ● S82.232   Displaced oblique fracture of shaft of left tibia
    ● S82.233   Displaced oblique fracture of shaft of unspecified tibia
    ● S82.234   Nondisplaced oblique fracture of shaft of right tibia
      Coding Clinic: 2015, Q1, P9-10
    ● S82.235   Nondisplaced oblique fracture of shaft of left tibia
    ● S82.236   Nondisplaced oblique fracture of shaft of unspecified tibia

◀ New   ◀▥ Revised   d̶e̶l̶e̶t̶e̶d̶ Deleted   Excludes 1   Excludes 2   Includes   Use additional   Code first   Code also   Unspecified
OGCR Official Guidelines   X Assign placeholder X   ● Use Additional Character(s)   ▶ Manifestation Code   **Coding Clinic**

● **S82.24** Spiral fracture of shaft of tibia
Toddler fracture
  ● S82.241 Displaced spiral fracture of shaft of right tibia
  ● S82.242 Displaced spiral fracture of shaft of left tibia
  ● S82.243 Displaced spiral fracture of shaft of unspecified tibia
  ● S82.244 Nondisplaced spiral fracture of shaft of right tibia
  ● S82.245 Nondisplaced spiral fracture of shaft of left tibia
  ● S82.246 Nondisplaced spiral fracture of shaft of unspecified tibia
● **S82.25** Comminuted fracture of shaft of tibia
  ● S82.251 Displaced comminuted fracture of shaft of right tibia
  ● S82.252 Displaced comminuted fracture of shaft of left tibia
  ● S82.253 Displaced comminuted fracture of shaft of unspecified tibia
  ● S82.254 Nondisplaced comminuted fracture of shaft of right tibia
  ● S82.255 Nondisplaced comminuted fracture of shaft of left tibia
  ● S82.256 Nondisplaced comminuted fracture of shaft of unspecified tibia
● **S82.26** Segmental fracture of shaft of tibia
  ● S82.261 Displaced segmental fracture of shaft of right tibia
  ● S82.262 Displaced segmental fracture of shaft of left tibia
  ● S82.263 Displaced segmental fracture of shaft of unspecified tibia
  ● S82.264 Nondisplaced segmental fracture of shaft of right tibia
  ● S82.265 Nondisplaced segmental fracture of shaft of left tibia
  ● S82.266 Nondisplaced segmental fracture of shaft of unspecified tibia
● **S82.29** Other fracture of shaft of tibia
  ● S82.291 Other fracture of shaft of right tibia
  ● S82.292 Other fracture of shaft of left tibia
  ● S82.299 Other fracture of shaft of unspecified tibia
● **S82.3** Fracture of lower end of tibia
  Excludes1 bimalleolar fracture of lower leg (S82.84-)
  fracture of medial malleolus alone (S82.5-)
  Maisonneuve's fracture (S82.86-)
  pilon fracture of distal tibia (S82.87-)
  trimalleolar fractures of lower leg (S82.85-)
● **S82.30** Unspecified fracture of lower end of tibia
  ● S82.301 Unspecified fracture of lower end of right tibia
  ● S82.302 Unspecified fracture of lower end of left tibia
  ● S82.309 Unspecified fracture of lower end of unspecified tibia

● **S82.31** Torus fracture of lower end of tibia
The appropriate 7th character is to be added to all codes in subcategory S82.31

A	initial encounter for closed fracture
D	subsequent encounter for fracture with routine healing
G	subsequent encounter for fracture with delayed healing
K	subsequent encounter for fracture with nonunion
P	subsequent encounter for fracture with malunion
S	sequela

  ● S82.311 Torus fracture of lower end of right tibia
  ● S82.312 Torus fracture of lower end of left tibia
  ● S82.319 Torus fracture of lower end of unspecified tibia
● **S82.39** Other fracture of lower end of tibia
  ● S82.391 Other fracture of lower end of right tibia
  ● S82.392 Other fracture of lower end of left tibia
    Coding Clinic: 2015, Q1, P25
  ● S82.399 Other fracture of lower end of unspecified tibia
● **S82.4** Fracture of shaft of fibula
  Excludes2 fracture of lateral malleolus alone (S82.6-)
● **S82.40** Unspecified fracture of shaft of fibula
  ● S82.401 Unspecified fracture of shaft of right fibula
  ● S82.402 Unspecified fracture of shaft of left fibula
  ● S82.409 Unspecified fracture of shaft of unspecified fibula
● **S82.42** Transverse fracture of shaft of fibula
  ● S82.421 Displaced transverse fracture of shaft of right fibula
  ● S82.422 Displaced transverse fracture of shaft of left fibula
  ● S82.423 Displaced transverse fracture of shaft of unspecified fibula
  ● S82.424 Nondisplaced transverse fracture of shaft of right fibula
  ● S82.425 Nondisplaced transverse fracture of shaft of left fibula
  ● S82.426 Nondisplaced transverse fracture of shaft of unspecified fibula
● **S82.43** Oblique fracture of shaft of fibula
  ● S82.431 Displaced oblique fracture of shaft of right fibula
  ● S82.432 Displaced oblique fracture of shaft of left fibula
  ● S82.433 Displaced oblique fracture of shaft of unspecified fibula
  ● S82.434 Nondisplaced oblique fracture of shaft of right fibula
  ● S82.435 Nondisplaced oblique fracture of shaft of left fibula
  ● S82.436 Nondisplaced oblique fracture of shaft of unspecified fibula

CHAPTER 19 (S00-T88)

- ● **S82.44**   Spiral fracture of shaft of fibula
  - ● **S82.441**   Displaced spiral fracture of shaft of right fibula
  - ● **S82.442**   Displaced spiral fracture of shaft of left fibula
  - ● **S82.443**   Displaced spiral fracture of shaft of unspecified fibula
  - ● **S82.444**   Nondisplaced spiral fracture of shaft of right fibula
  - ● **S82.445**   Nondisplaced spiral fracture of shaft of left fibula
  - ● **S82.446**   Nondisplaced spiral fracture of shaft of unspecified fibula
- ● **S82.45**   Comminuted fracture of shaft of fibula
  - ● **S82.451**   Displaced comminuted fracture of shaft of right fibula
  - ● **S82.452**   Displaced comminuted fracture of shaft of left fibula
  - ● **S82.453**   Displaced comminuted fracture of shaft of unspecified fibula
  - ● **S82.454**   Nondisplaced comminuted fracture of shaft of right fibula
  - ● **S82.455**   Nondisplaced comminuted fracture of shaft of left fibula
  - ● **S82.456**   Nondisplaced comminuted fracture of shaft of unspecified fibula
- ● **S82.46**   Segmental fracture of shaft of fibula
  - ● **S82.461**   Displaced segmental fracture of shaft of right fibula
  - ● **S82.462**   Displaced segmental fracture of shaft of left fibula
  - ● **S82.463**   Displaced segmental fracture of shaft of unspecified fibula
  - ● **S82.464**   Nondisplaced segmental fracture of shaft of right fibula
  - ● **S82.465**   Nondisplaced segmental fracture of shaft of left fibula
  - ● **S82.466**   Nondisplaced segmental fracture of shaft of unspecified fibula
- ● **S82.49**   Other fracture of shaft of fibula
  - ● **S82.491**   Other fracture of shaft of right fibula
  - ● **S82.492**   Other fracture of shaft of left fibula
  - ● **S82.499**   Other fracture of shaft of unspecified fibula
- ● **S82.5**   Fracture of medial malleolus
  - **Excludes1**   pilon fracture of distal tibia (S82.87-)
  -          Salter-Harris type III of lower end of tibia (S89.13-)
  -          Salter-Harris type IV of lower end of tibia (S89.14-)
  - X ● **S82.51**   Displaced fracture of medial malleolus of right tibia
  - X ● **S82.52**   Displaced fracture of medial malleolus of left tibia
  - X ● **S82.53**   Displaced fracture of medial malleolus of unspecified tibia
  - X ● **S82.54**   Nondisplaced fracture of medial malleolus of right tibia
  - X ● **S82.55**   Nondisplaced fracture of medial malleolus of left tibia
  - X ● **S82.56**   Nondisplaced fracture of medial malleolus of unspecified tibia

- ● **S82.6**   Fracture of lateral malleolus
  - **Excludes1**   pilon fracture of distal tibia (S82.87-)
  - X ● **S82.61**   Displaced fracture of lateral malleolus of right fibula
  - X ● **S82.62**   Displaced fracture of lateral malleolus of left fibula
  - X ● **S82.63**   Displaced fracture of lateral malleolus of unspecified fibula
  - X ● **S82.64**   Nondisplaced fracture of lateral malleolus of right fibula
  - X ● **S82.65**   Nondisplaced fracture of lateral malleolus of left fibula
  - X ● **S82.66**   Nondisplaced fracture of lateral malleolus of unspecified fibula
- ● **S82.8**   Other fractures of lower leg
  - ● **S82.81**   Torus fracture of upper end of fibula
    - The appropriate 7th character is to be added to all codes in subcategory S82.81

A	initial encounter for closed fracture
D	subsequent encounter for fracture with routine healing
G	subsequent encounter for fracture with delayed healing
K	subsequent encounter for fracture with nonunion
P	subsequent encounter for fracture with malunion
S	sequela

    - ● **S82.811**   Torus fracture of upper end of right fibula
    - ● **S82.812**   Torus fracture of upper end of left fibula
    - ● **S82.819**   Torus fracture of upper end of unspecified fibula
  - ● **S82.82**   Torus fracture of lower end of fibula
    - The appropriate 7th character is to be added to all codes in subcategory S82.82

A	initial encounter for closed fracture
D	subsequent encounter for fracture with routine healing
G	subsequent encounter for fracture with delayed healing
K	subsequent encounter for fracture with nonunion
P	subsequent encounter for fracture with malunion
S	sequela

    - ● **S82.821**   Torus fracture of lower end of right fibula
    - ● **S82.822**   Torus fracture of lower end of left fibula
    - ● **S82.829**   Torus fracture of lower end of unspecified fibula
  - ● **S82.83**   Other fracture of upper and lower end of fibula
    - ● **S82.831**   Other fracture of upper and lower end of right fibula
    - ● **S82.832**   Other fracture of upper and lower end of left fibula
      - Coding Clinic: 2015, Q1, P9-10
    - ● **S82.839**   Other fracture of upper and lower end of unspecified fibula

◀ New   ◀░ Revised   ~~deleted~~ Deleted   **Excludes 1**   Excludes 2   Includes   Use additional   Code first   Code also   Unspecified

OGCR Official Guidelines   X Assign placeholder X   ● Use Additional Character(s)   ▶ Manifestation Code   **Coding Clinic**

● **S82.84** **Bimalleolar fracture of lower leg**
　● **S82.841** **Displaced bimalleolar fracture of right lower leg**
　● **S82.842** **Displaced bimalleolar fracture of left lower leg**
　● **S82.843** **Displaced bimalleolar fracture of unspecified lower leg**
　● **S82.844** **Nondisplaced bimalleolar fracture of right lower leg**
　● **S82.845** **Nondisplaced bimalleolar fracture of left lower leg**
　● **S82.846** **Nondisplaced bimalleolar fracture of unspecified lower leg**

● **S82.85** **Trimalleolar fracture of lower leg**
　● **S82.851** **Displaced trimalleolar fracture of right lower leg**
　● **S82.852** **Displaced trimalleolar fracture of left lower leg**
　● **S82.853** **Displaced trimalleolar fracture of unspecified lower leg**
　● **S82.854** **Nondisplaced trimalleolar fracture of right lower leg**
　● **S82.855** **Nondisplaced trimalleolar fracture of left lower leg**
　● **S82.856** **Nondisplaced trimalleolar fracture of unspecified lower leg**

● **S82.86** **Maisonneuve's fracture**
　● **S82.861** **Displaced Maisonneuve's fracture of right leg**
　● **S82.862** **Displaced Maisonneuve's fracture of left leg**
　● **S82.863** **Displaced Maisonneuve's fracture of unspecified leg**
　● **S82.864** **Nondisplaced Maisonneuve's fracture of right leg**
　● **S82.865** **Nondisplaced Maisonneuve's fracture of left leg**
　● **S82.866** **Nondisplaced Maisonneuve's fracture of unspecified leg**

● **S82.87** **Pilon fracture of tibia**
　● **S82.871** **Displaced pilon fracture of right tibia**
　● **S82.872** **Displaced pilon fracture of left tibia**
　● **S82.873** **Displaced pilon fracture of unspecified tibia**
　● **S82.874** **Nondisplaced pilon fracture of right tibia**
　● **S82.875** **Nondisplaced pilon fracture of left tibia**
　● **S82.876** **Nondisplaced pilon fracture of unspecified tibia**

● **S82.89** **Other fractures of lower leg**
　　Fracture of ankle NOS
　● **S82.891** **Other fracture of right lower leg**
　● **S82.892** **Other fracture of left lower leg**
　● **S82.899** **Other fracture of unspecified lower leg**

● **S82.9** **Unspecified fracture of lower leg**
　X● **S82.90** **Unspecified fracture of unspecified lower leg**
　X● **S82.91** **Unspecified fracture of right lower leg**
　X● **S82.92** **Unspecified fracture of left lower leg**

● **S83** **Dislocation and sprain of joints and ligaments of knee**
　Includes　avulsion of joint or ligament of knee
　　　　laceration of cartilage, joint or ligament of knee
　　　　sprain of cartilage, joint or ligament of knee
　　　　traumatic hemarthrosis of joint or ligament of knee
　　　　traumatic rupture of joint or ligament of knee
　　　　traumatic subluxation of joint or ligament of knee
　　　　traumatic tear of joint or ligament of knee

Code also any associated open wound

　Excludes1　derangement of patella (M22.0-M22.3)
　　　　injury of patellar ligament (tendon) (S76.1-)
　　　　internal derangement of knee (M23.-)
　　　　old dislocation of knee (M24.36)
　　　　pathological dislocation of knee (M24.36)
　　　　recurrent dislocation of knee (M22.0)

　Excludes2　strain of muscle, fascia and tendon of lower leg (S86.-)

The appropriate 7th character is to be added to each code from category S83

A	initial encounter
D	subsequent encounter
S	sequela

● **S83.0** **Subluxation and dislocation of patella**
　● **S83.00** **Unspecified subluxation and dislocation of patella**
　　● **S83.001** **Unspecified subluxation of right patella**
　　● **S83.002** **Unspecified subluxation of left patella**
　　● **S83.003** **Unspecified subluxation of unspecified patella**
　　● **S83.004** **Unspecified dislocation of right patella**
　　● **S83.005** **Unspecified dislocation of left patella**
　　● **S83.006** **Unspecified dislocation of unspecified patella**

　● **S83.01** **Lateral subluxation and dislocation of patella**
　　● **S83.011** **Lateral subluxation of right patella**
　　● **S83.012** **Lateral subluxation of left patella**
　　● **S83.013** **Lateral subluxation of unspecified patella**
　　● **S83.014** **Lateral dislocation of right patella**
　　● **S83.015** **Lateral dislocation of left patella**
　　● **S83.016** **Lateral dislocation of unspecified patella**

　● **S83.09** **Other subluxation and dislocation of patella**
　　● **S83.091** **Other subluxation of right patella**
　　● **S83.092** **Other subluxation of left patella**
　　● **S83.093** **Other subluxation of unspecified patella**
　　● **S83.094** **Other dislocation of right patella**
　　● **S83.095** **Other dislocation of left patella**
　　● **S83.096** **Other dislocation of unspecified patella**

● **S83.1** **Subluxation and dislocation of knee**
　Excludes2　instability of knee prosthesis (T84.022, T84.023)
　● **S83.10** **Unspecified subluxation and dislocation of knee**
　　● **S83.101** **Unspecified subluxation of right knee**
　　● **S83.102** **Unspecified subluxation of left knee**
　　● **S83.103** **Unspecified subluxation of unspecified knee**

CHAPTER 19 (S00-T88)

● S83.104   Unspecified dislocation of right knee

● S83.105   Unspecified dislocation of left knee

● S83.106   Unspecified dislocation of unspecified knee

● S83.11   **Anterior subluxation and dislocation of proximal end of tibia**
Posterior subluxation and dislocation of distal end of femur

   ● S83.111   Anterior subluxation of proximal end of tibia, right knee

   ● S83.112   Anterior subluxation of proximal end of tibia, left knee

   ● S83.113   Anterior subluxation of proximal end of tibia, unspecified knee

   ● S83.114   Anterior dislocation of proximal end of tibia, right knee

   ● S83.115   Anterior dislocation of proximal end of tibia, left knee

   ● S83.116   Anterior dislocation of proximal end of tibia, unspecified knee

● S83.12   **Posterior subluxation and dislocation of proximal end of tibia**
Anterior dislocation of distal end of femur

   ● S83.121   Posterior subluxation of proximal end of tibia, right knee

   ● S83.122   Posterior subluxation of proximal end of tibia, left knee

   ● S83.123   Posterior subluxation of proximal end of tibia, unspecified knee

   ● S83.124   Posterior dislocation of proximal end of tibia, right knee

   ● S83.125   Posterior dislocation of proximal end of tibia, left knee

   ● S83.126   Posterior dislocation of proximal end of tibia, unspecified knee

● S83.13   **Medial subluxation and dislocation of proximal end of tibia**

   ● S83.131   Medial subluxation of proximal end of tibia, right knee

   ● S83.132   Medial subluxation of proximal end of tibia, left knee

   ● S83.133   Medial subluxation of proximal end of tibia, unspecified knee

   ● S83.134   Medial dislocation of proximal end of tibia, right knee

   ● S83.135   Medial dislocation of proximal end of tibia, left knee

   ● S83.136   Medial dislocation of proximal end of tibia, unspecified knee

● S83.14   **Lateral subluxation and dislocation of proximal end of tibia**

   ● S83.141   Lateral subluxation of proximal end of tibia, right knee

   ● S83.142   Lateral subluxation of proximal end of tibia, left knee

   ● S83.143   Lateral subluxation of proximal end of tibia, unspecified knee

   ● S83.144   Lateral dislocation of proximal end of tibia, right knee

   ● S83.145   Lateral dislocation of proximal end of tibia, left knee

   ● S83.146   Lateral dislocation of proximal end of tibia, unspecified knee

● S83.19   **Other subluxation and dislocation of knee**

   ● S83.191   Other subluxation of right knee

   ● S83.192   Other subluxation of left knee

   ● S83.193   Other subluxation of unspecified knee

   ● S83.194   Other dislocation of right knee

   ● S83.195   Other dislocation of left knee

   ● S83.196   Other dislocation of unspecified knee

● S83.2   **Tear of meniscus, current injury**
    Excludes1   old bucket-handle tear (M23.2)

● S83.20   **Tear of unspecified meniscus, current injury**
Tear of meniscus of knee NOS

   ● S83.200   Bucket-handle tear of unspecified meniscus, current injury, right knee

   ● S83.201   Bucket-handle tear of unspecified meniscus, current injury, left knee

   ● S83.202   Bucket-handle tear of unspecified meniscus, current injury, unspecified knee

   ● S83.203   Other tear of unspecified meniscus, current injury, right knee

   ● S83.204   Other tear of unspecified meniscus, current injury, left knee

   ● S83.205   Other tear of unspecified meniscus, current injury, unspecified knee

   ● S83.206   Unspecified tear of unspecified meniscus, current injury, right knee

   ● S83.207   Unspecified tear of unspecified meniscus, current injury, left knee

   ● S83.209   Unspecified tear of unspecified meniscus, current injury, unspecified knee

● S83.21   **Bucket-handle tear of medial meniscus, current injury**

   ● S83.211   Bucket-handle tear of medial meniscus, current injury, right knee

   ● S83.212   Bucket-handle tear of medial meniscus, current injury, left knee

   ● S83.219   Bucket-handle tear of medial meniscus, current injury, unspecified knee

● S83.22   **Peripheral tear of medial meniscus, current injury**

   ● S83.221   Peripheral tear of medial meniscus, current injury, right knee

   ● S83.222   Peripheral tear of medial meniscus, current injury, left knee

   ● S83.229   Peripheral tear of medial meniscus, current injury, unspecified knee

● S83.23   **Complex tear of medial meniscus, current injury**

   ● S83.231   Complex tear of medial meniscus, current injury, right knee

   ● S83.232   Complex tear of medial meniscus, current injury, left knee

   ● S83.239   Complex tear of medial meniscus, current injury, unspecified knee

● S83.24   **Other tear of medial meniscus, current injury**

   ● S83.241   Other tear of medial meniscus, current injury, right knee

   ● S83.242   Other tear of medial meniscus, current injury, left knee

   ● S83.249   Other tear of medial meniscus, current injury, unspecified knee

◀ New   ◀━ Revised   ~~deleted~~ Deleted   Excludes 1   Excludes 2   Includes   Use additional   Code first   Code also   Unspecified
OGCR Official Guidelines   **X** Assign placeholder X   ● Use Additional Character(s)   ▌ Manifestation Code   **Coding Clinic**

● S83.25   Bucket-handle tear of lateral meniscus, current injury
    ● S83.251   Bucket-handle tear of lateral meniscus, current injury, right knee
    ● S83.252   Bucket-handle tear of lateral meniscus, current injury, left knee
    ● S83.259   Bucket-handle tear of lateral meniscus, current injury, unspecified knee

● S83.26   Peripheral tear of lateral meniscus, current injury
    ● S83.261   Peripheral tear of lateral meniscus, current injury, right knee
    ● S83.262   Peripheral tear of lateral meniscus, current injury, left knee
    ● S83.269   Peripheral tear of lateral meniscus, current injury, unspecified knee

● S83.27   Complex tear of lateral meniscus, current injury
    ● S83.271   Complex tear of lateral meniscus, current injury, right knee
    ● S83.272   Complex tear of lateral meniscus, current injury, left knee
    ● S83.279   Complex tear of lateral meniscus, current injury, unspecified knee

● S83.28   Other tear of lateral meniscus, current injury
    ● S83.281   Other tear of lateral meniscus, current injury, right knee
    ● S83.282   Other tear of lateral meniscus, current injury, left knee
    ● S83.289   Other tear of lateral meniscus, current injury, unspecified knee

● S83.3   Tear of articular cartilage of knee, current
    X ● S83.30   Tear of articular cartilage of unspecified knee, current
    X ● S83.31   Tear of articular cartilage of right knee, current
    X ● S83.32   Tear of articular cartilage of left knee, current

● S83.4   Sprain of collateral ligament of knee
    ● S83.40   Sprain of unspecified collateral ligament of knee
        ● S83.401   Sprain of unspecified collateral ligament of right knee
        ● S83.402   Sprain of unspecified collateral ligament of left knee
        ● S83.409   Sprain of unspecified collateral ligament of unspecified knee
    ● S83.41   Sprain of medial collateral ligament of knee
        Sprain of tibial collateral ligament
        ● S83.411   Sprain of medial collateral ligament of right knee
        ● S83.412   Sprain of medial collateral ligament of left knee
        ● S83.419   Sprain of medial collateral ligament of unspecified knee
    ● S83.42   Sprain of lateral collateral ligament of knee
        Sprain of fibular collateral ligament
        ● S83.421   Sprain of lateral collateral ligament of right knee
        ● S83.422   Sprain of lateral collateral ligament of left knee
        ● S83.429   Sprain of lateral collateral ligament of unspecified knee

● S83.5   Sprain of cruciate ligament of knee
    ● S83.50   Sprain of unspecified cruciate ligament of knee
        ● S83.501   Sprain of unspecified cruciate ligament of right knee
        ● S83.502   Sprain of unspecified cruciate ligament of left knee
        ● S83.509   Sprain of unspecified cruciate ligament of unspecified knee

● S83.51   Sprain of anterior cruciate ligament of knee
    ● S83.511   Sprain of anterior cruciate ligament of right knee
    ● S83.512   Sprain of anterior cruciate ligament of left knee
    ● S83.519   Sprain of anterior cruciate ligament of unspecified knee

● S83.52   Sprain of posterior cruciate ligament of knee
    ● S83.521   Sprain of posterior cruciate ligament of right knee
    ● S83.522   Sprain of posterior cruciate ligament of left knee
    ● S83.529   Sprain of posterior cruciate ligament of unspecified knee

● S83.6   Sprain of the superior tibiofibular joint and ligament
    X ● S83.60   Sprain of the superior tibiofibular joint and ligament, unspecified knee
    X ● S83.61   Sprain of the superior tibiofibular joint and ligament, right knee
    X ● S83.62   Sprain of the superior tibiofibular joint and ligament, left knee

● S83.8   Sprain of other specified parts of knee
    ● S83.8X   Sprain of other specified parts of knee
        ● S83.8X1   Sprain of other specified parts of right knee
        ● S83.8X2   Sprain of other specified parts of left knee
        ● S83.8X9   Sprain of other specified parts of unspecified knee

● S83.9   Sprain of unspecified site of knee
    X ● S83.90   Sprain of unspecified site of unspecified knee
    X ● S83.91   Sprain of unspecified site of right knee
    X ● S83.92   Sprain of unspecified site of left knee

● S84   **Injury of nerves at lower leg level**
    Code also any associated open wound (S81.-)
    Excludes2   injury of nerves at ankle and foot level (S94.-)
    The appropriate 7th character is to be added to each code from category S84

A	initial encounter
D	subsequent encounter
S	sequela

● S84.0   Injury of tibial nerve at lower leg level
    X ● S84.00   Injury of tibial nerve at lower leg level, unspecified leg
    X ● S84.01   Injury of tibial nerve at lower leg level, right leg
    X ● S84.02   Injury of tibial nerve at lower leg level, left leg

● S84.1   Injury of peroneal nerve at lower leg level
    X ● S84.10   Injury of peroneal nerve at lower leg level, unspecified leg
    X ● S84.11   Injury of peroneal nerve at lower leg level, right leg
    X ● S84.12   Injury of peroneal nerve at lower leg level, left leg

● S84.2   Injury of cutaneous sensory nerve at lower leg level
    X ● S84.20   Injury of cutaneous sensory nerve at lower leg level, unspecified leg
    X ● S84.21   Injury of cutaneous sensory nerve at lower leg level, right leg
    X ● S84.22   Injury of cutaneous sensory nerve at lower leg level, left leg

● S84.8   Injury of other nerves at lower leg level
    ● S84.80   Injury of other nerves at lower leg level
        ● S84.801   Injury of other nerves at lower leg level, right leg
        ● S84.802   Injury of other nerves at lower leg level, left leg
        ● S84.809   Injury of other nerves at lower leg level, unspecified leg

● S84.9 Injury of unspecified nerve at lower leg level
  X ● S84.90 Injury of unspecified nerve at lower leg level, unspecified leg
  X ● S84.91 Injury of unspecified nerve at lower leg level, right leg
  X ● S84.92 Injury of unspecified nerve at lower leg level, left leg

● S85 Injury of blood vessels at lower leg level
  Code also any associated open wound (S81.-)
  Excludes2 injury of blood vessels at ankle and foot level (S95.-)

  The appropriate 7th character is to be added to each code from category S85

A	initial encounter
D	subsequent encounter
S	sequela

● S85.0 Injury of popliteal artery
  ● S85.00 Unspecified injury of popliteal artery
    ● S85.001 Unspecified injury of popliteal artery, right leg
    ● S85.002 Unspecified injury of popliteal artery, left leg
    ● S85.009 Unspecified injury of popliteal artery, unspecified leg
  ● S85.01 Laceration of popliteal artery
    ● S85.011 Laceration of popliteal artery, right leg
    ● S85.012 Laceration of popliteal artery, left leg
    ● S85.019 Laceration of popliteal artery, unspecified leg
  ● S85.09 Other specified injury of popliteal artery
    ● S85.091 Other specified injury of popliteal artery, right leg
    ● S85.092 Other specified injury of popliteal artery, left leg
    ● S85.099 Other specified injury of popliteal artery, unspecified leg

● S85.1 Injury of tibial artery
  ● S85.10 Unspecified injury of unspecified tibial artery
    Injury of tibial artery NOS
    ● S85.101 Unspecified injury of unspecified tibial artery, right leg
    ● S85.102 Unspecified injury of unspecified tibial artery, left leg
    ● S85.109 Unspecified injury of unspecified tibial artery, unspecified leg
  ● S85.11 Laceration of unspecified tibial artery
    ● S85.111 Laceration of unspecified tibial artery, right leg
    ● S85.112 Laceration of unspecified tibial artery, left leg
    ● S85.119 Laceration of unspecified tibial artery, unspecified leg
  ● S85.12 Other specified injury of unspecified tibial artery
    ● S85.121 Other specified injury of unspecified tibial artery, right leg
    ● S85.122 Other specified injury of unspecified tibial artery, left leg
    ● S85.129 Other specified injury of unspecified tibial artery, unspecified leg
  ● S85.13 Unspecified injury of anterior tibial artery
    ● S85.131 Unspecified injury of anterior tibial artery, right leg
    ● S85.132 Unspecified injury of anterior tibial artery, left leg
    ● S85.139 Unspecified injury of anterior tibial artery, unspecified leg

● S85.14 Laceration of anterior tibial artery
  ● S85.141 Laceration of anterior tibial artery, right leg
  ● S85.142 Laceration of anterior tibial artery, left leg
  ● S85.149 Laceration of anterior tibial artery, unspecified leg
● S85.15 Other specified injury of anterior tibial artery
  ● S85.151 Other specified injury of anterior tibial artery, right leg
  ● S85.152 Other specified injury of anterior tibial artery, left leg
  ● S85.159 Other specified injury of anterior tibial artery, unspecified leg
● S85.16 Unspecified injury of posterior tibial artery
  ● S85.161 Unspecified injury of posterior tibial artery, right leg
  ● S85.162 Unspecified injury of posterior tibial artery, left leg
  ● S85.169 Unspecified injury of posterior tibial artery, unspecified leg
● S85.17 Laceration of posterior tibial artery
  ● S85.171 Laceration of posterior tibial artery, right leg
  ● S85.172 Laceration of posterior tibial artery, left leg
  ● S85.179 Laceration of posterior tibial artery, unspecified leg
● S85.18 Other specified injury of posterior tibial artery
  ● S85.181 Other specified injury of posterior tibial artery, right leg
  ● S85.182 Other specified injury of posterior tibial artery, left leg
  ● S85.189 Other specified injury of posterior tibial artery, unspecified leg

● S85.2 Injury of peroneal artery
  ● S85.20 Unspecified injury of peroneal artery
    ● S85.201 Unspecified injury of peroneal artery, right leg
    ● S85.202 Unspecified injury of peroneal artery, left leg
    ● S85.209 Unspecified injury of peroneal artery, unspecified leg
  ● S85.21 Laceration of peroneal artery
    ● S85.211 Laceration of peroneal artery, right leg
    ● S85.212 Laceration of peroneal artery, left leg
    ● S85.219 Laceration of peroneal artery, unspecified leg
  ● S85.29 Other specified injury of peroneal artery
    ● S85.291 Other specified injury of peroneal artery, right leg
    ● S85.292 Other specified injury of peroneal artery, left leg
    ● S85.299 Other specified injury of peroneal artery, unspecified leg

● S85.3 Injury of greater saphenous vein at lower leg level
  Injury of greater saphenous vein NOS
  Injury of saphenous vein NOS
  ● S85.30 Unspecified injury of greater saphenous vein at lower leg level
    ● S85.301 Unspecified injury of greater saphenous vein at lower leg level, right leg
    ● S85.302 Unspecified injury of greater saphenous vein at lower leg level, left leg
    ● S85.309 Unspecified injury of greater saphenous vein at lower leg level, unspecified leg

◄ New ◄ Revised ~~deleted~~ Deleted Excludes 1 Excludes 2 Includes Use additional Code first Code also Unspecified
OGCR Official Guidelines X Assign placeholder X ● Use Additional Character(s) ▶ Manifestation Code **Coding Clinic**

- ● S85.31   Laceration of greater saphenous vein at lower leg level
  - ● S85.311   Laceration of greater saphenous vein at lower leg level, right leg
  - ● S85.312   Laceration of greater saphenous vein at lower leg level, left leg
  - ● S85.319   Laceration of greater saphenous vein at lower leg level, unspecified leg
- ● S85.39   Other specified injury of greater saphenous vein at lower leg level
  - ● S85.391   Other specified injury of greater saphenous vein at lower leg level, right leg
  - ● S85.392   Other specified injury of greater saphenous vein at lower leg level, left leg
  - ● S85.399   Other specified injury of greater saphenous vein at lower leg level, unspecified leg
- ● S85.4   Injury of lesser saphenous vein at lower leg level
  - ● S85.40   Unspecified injury of lesser saphenous vein at lower leg level
    - ● S85.401   Unspecified injury of lesser saphenous vein at lower leg level, right leg
    - ● S85.402   Unspecified injury of lesser saphenous vein at lower leg level, left leg
    - ● S85.409   Unspecified injury of lesser saphenous vein at lower leg level, unspecified leg
  - ● S85.41   Laceration of lesser saphenous vein at lower leg level
    - ● S85.411   Laceration of lesser saphenous vein at lower leg level, right leg
    - ● S85.412   Laceration of lesser saphenous vein at lower leg level, left leg
    - ● S85.419   Laceration of lesser saphenous vein at lower leg level, unspecified leg
  - ● S85.49   Other specified injury of lesser saphenous vein at lower leg level
    - ● S85.491   Other specified injury of lesser saphenous vein at lower leg level, right leg
    - ● S85.492   Other specified injury of lesser saphenous vein at lower leg level, left leg
    - ● S85.499   Other specified injury of lesser saphenous vein at lower leg level, unspecified leg
- ● S85.5   Injury of popliteal vein
  - ● S85.50   Unspecified injury of popliteal vein
    - ● S85.501   Unspecified injury of popliteal vein, right leg
    - ● S85.502   Unspecified injury of popliteal vein, left leg
    - ● S85.509   Unspecified injury of popliteal vein, unspecified leg
  - ● S85.51   Laceration of popliteal vein
    - ● S85.511   Laceration of popliteal vein, right leg
    - ● S85.512   Laceration of popliteal vein, left leg
    - ● S85.519   Laceration of popliteal vein, unspecified leg

- ● S85.59   Other specified injury of popliteal vein
  - ● S85.591   Other specified injury of popliteal vein, right leg
  - ● S85.592   Other specified injury of popliteal vein, left leg
  - ● S85.599   Other specified injury of popliteal vein, unspecified leg
- ● S85.8   Injury of other blood vessels at lower leg level
  - ● S85.80   Unspecified injury of other blood vessels at lower leg level
    - ● S85.801   Unspecified injury of other blood vessels at lower leg level, right leg
    - ● S85.802   Unspecified injury of other blood vessels at lower leg level, left leg
    - ● S85.809   Unspecified injury of other blood vessels at lower leg level, unspecified leg
  - ● S85.81   Laceration of other blood vessels at lower leg level
    - ● S85.811   Laceration of other blood vessels at lower leg level, right leg
    - ● S85.812   Laceration of other blood vessels at lower leg level, left leg
    - ● S85.819   Laceration of other blood vessels at lower leg level, unspecified leg
  - ● S85.89   Other specified injury of other blood vessels at lower leg level
    - ● S85.891   Other specified injury of other blood vessels at lower leg level, right leg
    - ● S85.892   Other specified injury of other blood vessels at lower leg level, left leg
    - ● S85.899   Other specified injury of other blood vessels at lower leg level, unspecified leg
- ● S85.9   Injury of unspecified blood vessel at lower leg level
  - ● S85.90   Unspecified injury of unspecified blood vessel at lower leg level
    - ● S85.901   Unspecified injury of unspecified blood vessel at lower leg level, right leg
    - ● S85.902   Unspecified injury of unspecified blood vessel at lower leg level, left leg
    - ● S85.909   Unspecified injury of unspecified blood vessel at lower leg level, unspecified leg
  - ● S85.91   Laceration of unspecified blood vessel at lower leg level
    - ● S85.911   Laceration of unspecified blood vessel at lower leg level, right leg
    - ● S85.912   Laceration of unspecified blood vessel at lower leg level, left leg
    - ● S85.919   Laceration of unspecified blood vessel at lower leg level, unspecified leg
  - ● S85.99   Other specified injury of unspecified blood vessel at lower leg level
    - ● S85.991   Other specified injury of unspecified blood vessel at lower leg level, right leg
    - ● S85.992   Other specified injury of unspecified blood vessel at lower leg level, left leg
    - ● S85.999   Other specified injury of unspecified blood vessel at lower leg level, unspecified leg

CHAPTER 19 (S00-T88)

● **S86**   **Injury of muscle, fascia and tendon at lower leg level**
    Code also any associated open wound (S81.-)
      Excludes2   injury of muscle, fascia and tendon at ankle
                 (S96.-)
                 injury of patellar ligament (tendon) (S76.1-)
                 sprain of joints and ligaments of knee (S83.-)
    The appropriate 7th character is to be added to each code from
      category S86

> A   initial encounter
> D   subsequent encounter
> S   sequela

  ● **S86.0**   **Injury of Achilles tendon**
    ● **S86.00**   Unspecified injury of Achilles tendon
      ● **S86.001**   Unspecified injury of right Achilles tendon
      ● **S86.002**   Unspecified injury of left Achilles tendon
      ● **S86.009**   Unspecified injury of unspecified Achilles tendon
    ● **S86.01**   Strain of Achilles tendon
      ● **S86.011**   Strain of right Achilles tendon
      ● **S86.012**   Strain of left Achilles tendon
      ● **S86.019**   Strain of unspecified Achilles tendon
    ● **S86.02**   Laceration of Achilles tendon
      ● **S86.021**   Laceration of right Achilles tendon
      ● **S86.022**   Laceration of left Achilles tendon
      ● **S86.029**   Laceration of unspecified Achilles tendon
    ● **S86.09**   Other specified injury of Achilles tendon
      ● **S86.091**   Other specified injury of right Achilles tendon
      ● **S86.092**   Other specified injury of left Achilles tendon
      ● **S86.099**   Other specified injury of unspecified Achilles tendon
  ● **S86.1**   **Injury of other muscle(s) and tendon(s) of posterior muscle group at lower leg level**
    ● **S86.10**   Unspecified injury of other muscle(s) and tendon(s) of posterior muscle group at lower leg level
      ● **S86.101**   Unspecified injury of other muscle(s) and tendon(s) of posterior muscle group at lower leg level, right leg
      ● **S86.102**   Unspecified injury of other muscle(s) and tendon(s) of posterior muscle group at lower leg level, left leg
      ● **S86.109**   Unspecified injury of other muscle(s) and tendon(s) of posterior muscle group at lower leg level, unspecified leg
    ● **S86.11**   Strain of other muscle(s) and tendon(s) of posterior muscle group at lower leg level
      ● **S86.111**   Strain of other muscle(s) and tendon(s) of posterior muscle group at lower leg level, right leg
      ● **S86.112**   Strain of other muscle(s) and tendon(s) of posterior muscle group at lower leg level, left leg
      ● **S86.119**   Strain of other muscle(s) and tendon(s) of posterior muscle group at lower leg level, unspecified leg

    ● **S86.12**   Laceration of other muscle(s) and tendon(s) of posterior muscle group at lower leg level
      ● **S86.121**   Laceration of other muscle(s) and tendon(s) of posterior muscle group at lower leg level, right leg
      ● **S86.122**   Laceration of other muscle(s) and tendon(s) of posterior muscle group at lower leg level, left leg
      ● **S86.129**   Laceration of other muscle(s) and tendon(s) of posterior muscle group at lower leg level, unspecified leg
    ● **S86.19**   Other injury of other muscle(s) and tendon(s) of posterior muscle group at lower leg level
      ● **S86.191**   Other injury of other muscle(s) and tendon(s) of posterior muscle group at lower leg level, right leg
      ● **S86.192**   Other injury of other muscle(s) and tendon(s) of posterior muscle group at lower leg level, left leg
      ● **S86.199**   Other injury of other muscle(s) and tendon(s) of posterior muscle group at lower leg level, unspecified leg
  ● **S86.2**   **Injury of muscle(s) and tendon(s) of anterior muscle group at lower leg level**
    ● **S86.20**   Unspecified injury of muscle(s) and tendon(s) of anterior muscle group at lower leg level
      ● **S86.201**   Unspecified injury of muscle(s) and tendon(s) of anterior muscle group at lower leg level, right leg
      ● **S86.202**   Unspecified injury of muscle(s) and tendon(s) of anterior muscle group at lower leg level, left leg
      ● **S86.209**   Unspecified injury of muscle(s) and tendon(s) of anterior muscle group at lower leg level, unspecified leg
    ● **S86.21**   Strain of muscle(s) and tendon(s) of anterior muscle group at lower leg level
      ● **S86.211**   Strain of muscle(s) and tendon(s) of anterior muscle group at lower leg level, right leg
      ● **S86.212**   Strain of muscle(s) and tendon(s) of anterior muscle group at lower leg level, left leg
      ● **S86.219**   Strain of muscle(s) and tendon(s) of anterior muscle group at lower leg level, unspecified leg
    ● **S86.22**   Laceration of muscle(s) and tendon(s) of anterior muscle group at lower leg level
      ● **S86.221**   Laceration of muscle(s) and tendon(s) of anterior muscle group at lower leg level, right leg
      ● **S86.222**   Laceration of muscle(s) and tendon(s) of anterior muscle group at lower leg level, left leg
      ● **S86.229**   Laceration of muscle(s) and tendon(s) of anterior muscle group at lower leg level, unspecified leg
    ● **S86.29**   Other injury of muscle(s) and tendon(s) of anterior muscle group at lower leg level
      ● **S86.291**   Other injury of muscle(s) and tendon(s) of anterior muscle group at lower leg level, right leg
      ● **S86.292**   Other injury of muscle(s) and tendon(s) of anterior muscle group at lower leg level, left leg
      ● **S86.299**   Other injury of muscle(s) and tendon(s) of anterior muscle group at lower leg level, unspecified leg

◄ New   ◀══ Revised   ~~deleted~~ Deleted   Excludes 1   Excludes 2   Includes   Use additional   Code first   Code also   Unspecified

1384   **OGCR** Official Guidelines   X Assign placeholder X   ● Use Additional Character(s)   ▶ Manifestation Code   **Coding Clinic**

● S86.3   Injury of muscle(s) and tendon(s) of peroneal muscle group at lower leg level

  ● S86.30   Unspecified injury of muscle(s) and tendon(s) of peroneal muscle group at lower leg level

    ● S86.301   Unspecified injury of muscle(s) and tendon(s) of peroneal muscle group at lower leg level, right leg

    ● S86.302   Unspecified injury of muscle(s) and tendon(s) of peroneal muscle group at lower leg level, left leg

    ● S86.309   Unspecified injury of muscle(s) and tendon(s) of peroneal muscle group at lower leg level, unspecified leg

  ● S86.31   Strain of muscle(s) and tendon(s) of peroneal muscle group at lower leg level

    ● S86.311   Strain of muscle(s) and tendon(s) of peroneal muscle group at lower leg level, right leg

    ● S86.312   Strain of muscle(s) and tendon(s) of peroneal muscle group at lower leg level, left leg

    ● S86.319   Strain of muscle(s) and tendon(s) of peroneal muscle group at lower leg level, unspecified leg

  ● S86.32   Laceration of muscle(s) and tendon(s) of peroneal muscle group at lower leg level

    ● S86.321   Laceration of muscle(s) and tendon(s) of peroneal muscle group at lower leg level, right leg

    ● S86.322   Laceration of muscle(s) and tendon(s) of peroneal muscle group at lower leg level, left leg

    ● S86.329   Laceration of muscle(s) and tendon(s) of peroneal muscle group at lower leg level, unspecified leg

  ● S86.39   Other injury of muscle(s) and tendon(s) of peroneal muscle group at lower leg level

    ● S86.391   Other injury of muscle(s) and tendon(s) of peroneal muscle group at lower leg level, right leg

    ● S86.392   Other injury of muscle(s) and tendon(s) of peroneal muscle group at lower leg level, left leg

    ● S86.399   Other injury of muscle(s) and tendon(s) of peroneal muscle group at lower leg level, unspecified leg

● S86.8   Injury of other muscles and tendons at lower leg level

  ● S86.80   Unspecified injury of other muscles and tendons at lower leg level

    ● S86.801   Unspecified injury of other muscle(s) and tendon(s) at lower leg level, right leg

    ● S86.802   Unspecified injury of other muscle(s) and tendon(s) at lower leg level, left leg

    ● S86.809   Unspecified injury of other muscle(s) and tendon(s) at lower leg level, unspecified leg

  ● S86.81   Strain of other muscles and tendons at lower leg level

    ● S86.811   Strain of other muscle(s) and tendon(s) at lower leg level, right leg

    ● S86.812   Strain of other muscle(s) and tendon(s) at lower leg level, left leg

    ● S86.819   Strain of other muscle(s) and tendon(s) at lower leg level, unspecified leg

● S86.82   Laceration of other muscles and tendons at lower leg level

    ● S86.821   Laceration of other muscle(s) and tendon(s) at lower leg level, right leg

    ● S86.822   Laceration of other muscle(s) and tendon(s) at lower leg level, left leg

    ● S86.829   Laceration of other muscle(s) and tendon(s) at lower leg level, unspecified leg

  ● S86.89   Other injury of other muscles and tendons at lower leg level

    ● S86.891   Other injury of other muscles and tendons at lower leg level, right leg

    ● S86.892   Other injury of other muscles and tendons at lower leg level, left leg

    ● S86.899   Other injury of other muscle(s) and tendon(s) at lower leg level, unspecified leg

● S86.9   Injury of unspecified muscle and tendon at lower leg level

  ● S86.90   Unspecified injury of unspecified muscle and tendon at lower leg level

    ● S86.901   Unspecified injury of unspecified muscle(s) and tendon(s) at lower leg level, right leg

    ● S86.902   Unspecified injury of unspecified muscle(s) and tendon(s) at lower leg level, left leg

    ● S86.909   Unspecified injury of unspecified muscle(s) and tendon(s) at lower leg level, unspecified leg

  ● S86.91   Strain of unspecified muscle and tendon at lower leg level

    ● S86.911   Strain of unspecified muscle(s) and tendon(s) at lower leg level, right leg

    ● S86.912   Strain of unspecified muscle(s) and tendon(s) at lower leg level, left leg

    ● S86.919   Strain of unspecified muscle(s) and tendon(s) at lower leg level, unspecified leg

  ● S86.92   Laceration of unspecified muscle and tendon at lower leg level

    ● S86.921   Laceration of unspecified muscle(s) and tendon(s) at lower leg level, right leg

    ● S86.922   Laceration of unspecified muscle(s) and tendon(s) at lower leg level, left leg

    ● S86.929   Laceration of unspecified muscle(s) and tendon(s) at lower leg level, unspecified leg

  ● S86.99   Other injury of unspecified muscle and tendon at lower leg level

    ● S86.991   Other injury of unspecified muscle(s) and tendon(s) at lower leg level, right leg

    ● S86.992   Other injury of unspecified muscle(s) and tendon(s) at lower leg level, left leg

    ● S86.999   Other injury of unspecified muscle(s) and tendon(s) at lower leg level, unspecified leg

● **S87**   **Crushing injury of lower leg**
     Use additional code(s) for all associated injuries
     Excludes2   crushing injury of ankle and foot (S97.-)
     The appropriate 7th character is to be added to each code from category S87

> A   initial encounter
> D   subsequent encounter
> S   sequela

   ● **S87.0**   **Crushing injury of knee**
     X● **S87.00**   Crushing injury of unspecified knee
     X● **S87.01**   Crushing injury of right knee
     X● **S87.02**   Crushing injury of left knee
   ● **S87.8**   **Crushing injury of lower leg**
     X● **S87.80**   Crushing injury of unspecified lower leg
     X● **S87.81**   Crushing injury of right lower leg
     X● **S87.82**   Crushing injury of left lower leg

● **S88**   **Traumatic amputation of lower leg**
     An amputation not identified as partial or complete should be coded to complete
     Excludes1   traumatic amputation of ankle and foot (S98.-)
     The appropriate 7th character is to be added to each code from category S88

> A   initial encounter
> D   subsequent encounter
> S   sequela

   ● **S88.0**   **Traumatic amputation at knee level**
     ● **S88.01**   Complete traumatic amputation at knee level
       ● **S88.011**   Complete traumatic amputation at knee level, right lower leg
       ● **S88.012**   Complete traumatic amputation at knee level, left lower leg
       ● **S88.019**   Complete traumatic amputation at knee level, unspecified lower leg
     ● **S88.02**   Partial traumatic amputation at knee level
       ● **S88.021**   Partial traumatic amputation at knee level, right lower leg
       ● **S88.022**   Partial traumatic amputation at knee level, left lower leg
       ● **S88.029**   Partial traumatic amputation at knee level, unspecified lower leg
   ● **S88.1**   **Traumatic amputation at level between knee and ankle**
     ● **S88.11**   Complete traumatic amputation at level between knee and ankle
       ● **S88.111**   Complete traumatic amputation at level between knee and ankle, right lower leg
       ● **S88.112**   Complete traumatic amputation at level between knee and ankle, left lower leg
       ● **S88.119**   Complete traumatic amputation at level between knee and ankle, unspecified lower leg
     ● **S88.12**   Partial traumatic amputation at level between knee and ankle
       ● **S88.121**   Partial traumatic amputation at level between knee and ankle, right lower leg
       ● **S88.122**   Partial traumatic amputation at level between knee and ankle, left lower leg
       ● **S88.129**   Partial traumatic amputation at level between knee and ankle, unspecified lower leg

● **S88.9**   **Traumatic amputation of lower leg, level unspecified**
   ● **S88.91**   Complete traumatic amputation of lower leg, level unspecified
     ● **S88.911**   Complete traumatic amputation of right lower leg, level unspecified
     ● **S88.912**   Complete traumatic amputation of left lower leg, level unspecified
     ● **S88.919**   Complete traumatic amputation of unspecified lower leg, level unspecified
   ● **S88.92**   Partial traumatic amputation of lower leg, level unspecified
     ● **S88.921**   Partial traumatic amputation of right lower leg, level unspecified
     ● **S88.922**   Partial traumatic amputation of left lower leg, level unspecified
     ● **S88.929**   Partial traumatic amputation of unspecified lower leg, level unspecified

● **S89**   **Other and unspecified injuries of lower leg**
     Note: A fracture not indicated as open or closed should be coded to closed
     Excludes2   other and unspecified injuries of ankle and foot (S99.-)
     The appropriate 7th character is to be added to each code from subcategories S89.0, S89.1, S89.2, and S89.3

> A   initial encounter for closed fracture
> D   subsequent encounter for fracture with routine healing
> G   subsequent encounter for fracture with delayed healing
> K   subsequent encounter for fracture with nonunion
> P   subsequent encounter for fracture with malunion
> S   sequela

   ● **S89.0**   **Physeal fracture of upper end of tibia**
     ● **S89.00**   Unspecified physeal fracture of upper end of tibia
       ● **S89.001**   Unspecified physeal fracture of upper end of right tibia
       ● **S89.002**   Unspecified physeal fracture of upper end of left tibia
       ● **S89.009**   Unspecified physeal fracture of upper end of unspecified tibia
     ● **S89.01**   Salter-Harris Type I physeal fracture of upper end of tibia
       ● **S89.011**   Salter-Harris Type I physeal fracture of upper end of right tibia
       ● **S89.012**   Salter-Harris Type I physeal fracture of upper end of left tibia
       ● **S89.019**   Salter-Harris Type I physeal fracture of upper end of unspecified tibia
     ● **S89.02**   Salter-Harris Type II physeal fracture of upper end of tibia
       ● **S89.021**   Salter-Harris Type II physeal fracture of upper end of right tibia
       ● **S89.022**   Salter-Harris Type II physeal fracture of upper end of left tibia
       ● **S89.029**   Salter-Harris Type II physeal fracture of upper end of unspecified tibia
     ● **S89.03**   Salter-Harris Type III physeal fracture of upper end of tibia
       ● **S89.031**   Salter-Harris Type III physeal fracture of upper end of right tibia
       ● **S89.032**   Salter-Harris Type III physeal fracture of upper end of left tibia
       ● **S89.039**   Salter-Harris Type III physeal fracture of upper end of unspecified tibia

◀ New   ◀▬ Revised   ~~deleted~~ Deleted   Excludes 1   Excludes 2   Includes   Use additional   Code first   Code also   Unspecified
OGCR Official Guidelines   **X** Assign placeholder X   ● Use Additional Character(s)   ❭ Manifestation Code   **Coding Clinic**

● S89.04 Salter-Harris Type IV physeal fracture of upper end of tibia
  ● S89.041 Salter-Harris Type IV physeal fracture of upper end of right tibia
  ● S89.042 Salter-Harris Type IV physeal fracture of upper end of left tibia
  ● S89.049 Salter-Harris Type IV physeal fracture of upper end of unspecified tibia
● S89.09 Other physeal fracture of upper end of tibia
  ● S89.091 Other physeal fracture of upper end of right tibia
  ● S89.092 Other physeal fracture of upper end of left tibia
  ● S89.099 Other physeal fracture of upper end of unspecified tibia
● S89.1 Physeal fracture of lower end of tibia
  ● S89.10 Unspecified physeal fracture of lower end of tibia
    ● S89.101 Unspecified physeal fracture of lower end of right tibia
    ● S89.102 Unspecified physeal fracture of lower end of left tibia
    ● S89.109 Unspecified physeal fracture of lower end of unspecified tibia
  ● S89.11 Salter-Harris Type I physeal fracture of lower end of tibia
    ● S89.111 Salter-Harris Type I physeal fracture of lower end of right tibia
    ● S89.112 Salter-Harris Type I physeal fracture of lower end of left tibia
    ● S89.119 Salter-Harris Type I physeal fracture of lower end of unspecified tibia
  ● S89.12 Salter-Harris Type II physeal fracture of lower end of tibia
    ● S89.121 Salter-Harris Type II physeal fracture of lower end of right tibia
    ● S89.122 Salter-Harris Type II physeal fracture of lower end of left tibia
    ● S89.129 Salter-Harris Type II physeal fracture of lower end of unspecified tibia
  ● S89.13 Salter-Harris Type III physeal fracture of lower end of tibia
    Excludes1 fracture of medial malleolus (adult) (S82.5-)
    ● S89.131 Salter-Harris Type III physeal fracture of lower end of right tibia
    ● S89.132 Salter-Harris Type III physeal fracture of lower end of left tibia
    ● S89.139 Salter-Harris Type III physeal fracture of lower end of unspecified tibia
  ● S89.14 Salter-Harris Type IV physeal fracture of lower end of tibia
    Excludes1 fracture of medial malleolus (adult) (S82.5-)
    ● S89.141 Salter-Harris Type IV physeal fracture of lower end of right tibia
    ● S89.142 Salter-Harris Type IV physeal fracture of lower end of left tibia
    ● S89.149 Salter-Harris Type IV physeal fracture of lower end of unspecified tibia
  ● S89.19 Other physeal fracture of lower end of tibia
    ● S89.191 Other physeal fracture of lower end of right tibia
    ● S89.192 Other physeal fracture of lower end of left tibia
    ● S89.199 Other physeal fracture of lower end of unspecified tibia

● S89.2 Physeal fracture of upper end of fibula
  ● S89.20 Unspecified physeal fracture of upper end of fibula
    ● S89.201 Unspecified physeal fracture of upper end of right fibula
    ● S89.202 Unspecified physeal fracture of upper end of left fibula
    ● S89.209 Unspecified physeal fracture of upper end of unspecified fibula
  ● S89.21 Salter-Harris Type I physeal fracture of upper end of fibula
    ● S89.211 Salter-Harris Type I physeal fracture of upper end of right fibula
    ● S89.212 Salter-Harris Type I physeal fracture of upper end of left fibula
    ● S89.219 Salter-Harris Type I physeal fracture of upper end of unspecified fibula
  ● S89.22 Salter-Harris Type II physeal fracture of upper end of fibula
    ● S89.221 Salter-Harris Type II physeal fracture of upper end of right fibula
    ● S89.222 Salter-Harris Type II physeal fracture of upper end of left fibula
    ● S89.229 Salter-Harris Type II physeal fracture of upper end of unspecified fibula
  ● S89.29 Other physeal fracture of upper end of fibula
    ● S89.291 Other physeal fracture of upper end of right fibula
    ● S89.292 Other physeal fracture of upper end of left fibula
    ● S89.299 Other physeal fracture of upper end of unspecified fibula
● S89.3 Physeal fracture of lower end of fibula
  ● S89.30 Unspecified physeal fracture of lower end of fibula
    ● S89.301 Unspecified physeal fracture of lower end of right fibula
    ● S89.302 Unspecified physeal fracture of lower end of left fibula
    ● S89.309 Unspecified physeal fracture of lower end of unspecified fibula
  ● S89.31 Salter-Harris Type I physeal fracture of lower end of fibula
    ● S89.311 Salter-Harris Type I physeal fracture of lower end of right fibula
    ● S89.312 Salter-Harris Type I physeal fracture of lower end of left fibula
    ● S89.319 Salter-Harris Type I physeal fracture of lower end of unspecified fibula
  ● S89.32 Salter-Harris Type II physeal fracture of lower end of fibula
    ● S89.321 Salter-Harris Type II physeal fracture of lower end of right fibula
    ● S89.322 Salter-Harris Type II physeal fracture of lower end of left fibula
    ● S89.329 Salter-Harris Type II physeal fracture of lower end of unspecified fibula
  ● S89.39 Other physeal fracture of lower end of fibula
    ● S89.391 Other physeal fracture of lower end of right fibula
    ● S89.392 Other physeal fracture of lower end of left fibula
    ● S89.399 Other physeal fracture of lower end of unspecified fibula

CHAPTER 19 (S00-T88)

● **S89.8**   Other specified injuries of lower leg

The appropriate 7th character is to be added to each code in subcategory S89.8

> A   initial encounter
> D   subsequent encounter
> S   sequela

X● **S89.80**   Other specified injuries of unspecified lower leg

X● **S89.81**   Other specified injuries of right lower leg

X● **S89.82**   Other specified injuries of left lower leg

● **S89.9**   Unspecified injury of lower leg

The appropriate 7th character is to be added to each code in subcategory S89.9

> A   initial encounter
> D   subsequent encounter
> S   sequela

X● **S89.90**   Unspecified injury of unspecified lower leg

X● **S89.91**   Unspecified injury of right lower leg

X● **S89.92**   Unspecified injury of left lower leg

INJURIES TO THE ANKLE AND FOOT (S90-S99)

Excludes2   burns and corrosions (T20-T32)
                fracture of ankle and malleolus (S82.-)
                frostbite (T33-T34)
                insect bite or sting, venomous (T63.4)

● **S90**   Superficial injury of ankle, foot and toes

The appropriate 7th character is to be added to each code from category S90

> A   initial encounter
> D   subsequent encounter
> S   sequela

● **S90.0**   Contusion of ankle

X● **S90.00**   Contusion of unspecified ankle

X● **S90.01**   Contusion of right ankle

X● **S90.02**   Contusion of left ankle

● **S90.1**   Contusion of toe without damage to nail

● **S90.11**   Contusion of great toe without damage to nail

● **S90.111**   Contusion of right great toe without damage to nail

● **S90.112**   Contusion of left great toe without damage to nail

● **S90.119**   Contusion of unspecified great toe without damage to nail

● **S90.12**   Contusion of lesser toe without damage to nail

● **S90.121**   Contusion of right lesser toe(s) without damage to nail

● **S90.122**   Contusion of left lesser toe(s) without damage to nail

● **S90.129**   Contusion of unspecified lesser toe(s) without damage to nail
         Contusion of toe NOS

● **S90.2**   Contusion of toe with damage to nail

● **S90.21**   Contusion of great toe with damage to nail

● **S90.211**   Contusion of right great toe with damage to nail

● **S90.212**   Contusion of left great toe with damage to nail

● **S90.219**   Contusion of unspecified great toe with damage to nail

● **S90.22**   Contusion of lesser toe with damage to nail

● **S90.221**   Contusion of right lesser toe(s) with damage to nail

● **S90.222**   Contusion of left lesser toe(s) with damage to nail

● **S90.229**   Contusion of unspecified lesser toe(s) with damage to nail

● **S90.3**   Contusion of foot

Excludes2   contusion of toes (S90.1-, S90.2-)

X● **S90.30**   Contusion of unspecified foot
         Contusion of foot NOS

X● **S90.31**   Contusion of right foot

X● **S90.32**   Contusion of left foot

● **S90.4**   Other superficial injuries of toe

● **S90.41**   Abrasion of toe

● **S90.411**   Abrasion, right great toe

● **S90.412**   Abrasion, left great toe

● **S90.413**   Abrasion, unspecified great toe

● **S90.414**   Abrasion, right lesser toe(s)

● **S90.415**   Abrasion, left lesser toe(s)

● **S90.416**   Abrasion, unspecified lesser toe(s)

● **S90.42**   Blister (nonthermal) of toe

● **S90.421**   Blister (nonthermal), right great toe

● **S90.422**   Blister (nonthermal), left great toe

● **S90.423**   Blister (nonthermal), unspecified great toe

● **S90.424**   Blister (nonthermal), right lesser toe(s)

● **S90.425**   Blister (nonthermal), left lesser toe(s)

● **S90.426**   Blister (nonthermal), unspecified lesser toe(s)

● **S90.44**   External constriction of toe
         Hair tourniquet syndrome of toe

● **S90.441**   External constriction, right great toe

● **S90.442**   External constriction, left great toe

● **S90.443**   External constriction, unspecified great toe

● **S90.444**   External constriction, right lesser toe(s)

● **S90.445**   External constriction, left lesser toe(s)

● **S90.446**   External constriction, unspecified lesser toe(s)

● **S90.45**   Superficial foreign body of toe
         Splinter in the toe

● **S90.451**   Superficial foreign body, right great toe

● **S90.452**   Superficial foreign body, left great toe

● **S90.453**   Superficial foreign body, unspecified great toe

● **S90.454**   Superficial foreign body, right lesser toe(s)

● **S90.455**   Superficial foreign body, left lesser toe(s)

● **S90.456**   Superficial foreign body, unspecified lesser toe(s)

● **S90.46**   Insect bite (nonvenomous) of toe

● **S90.461**   Insect bite (nonvenomous), right great toe

● **S90.462**   Insect bite (nonvenomous), left great toe

● **S90.463**   Insect bite (nonvenomous), unspecified great toe

● **S90.464**   Insect bite (nonvenomous), right lesser toe(s)

● **S90.465**   Insect bite (nonvenomous), left lesser toe(s)

● **S90.466**   Insect bite (nonvenomous), unspecified lesser toe(s)

◀ New   ◀▦ Revised   ~~deleted~~ Deleted   Excludes 1   Excludes 2   Includes   Use additional   Code first   Code also   Unspecified

OGCR Official Guidelines   **X** Assign placeholder X   ● Use Additional Character(s)   ▶ Manifestation Code   **Coding Clinic**

● S90.47   Other superficial bite of toe
     Excludes1   open bite of toe (S91.15-, S91.25-)
   ● S90.471   Other superficial bite of right great toe
   ● S90.472   Other superficial bite of left great toe
   ● S90.473   Other superficial bite of unspecified great toe
   ● S90.474   Other superficial bite of right lesser toe(s)
   ● S90.475   Other superficial bite of left lesser toe(s)
   ● S90.476   Other superficial bite of unspecified lesser toe(s)

● S90.5   Other superficial injuries of ankle
   ● S90.51   Abrasion of ankle
     ● S90.511   Abrasion, right ankle
     ● S90.512   Abrasion, left ankle
     ● S90.519   Abrasion, unspecified ankle
   ● S90.52   Blister (nonthermal) of ankle
     ● S90.521   Blister (nonthermal), right ankle
     ● S90.522   Blister (nonthermal), left ankle
     ● S90.529   Blister (nonthermal), unspecified ankle
   ● S90.54   External constriction of ankle
     ● S90.541   External constriction, right ankle
     ● S90.542   External constriction, left ankle
     ● S90.549   External constriction, unspecified ankle
   ● S90.55   Superficial foreign body of ankle
     Splinter in the ankle
     ● S90.551   Superficial foreign body, right ankle
     ● S90.552   Superficial foreign body, left ankle
     ● S90.559   Superficial foreign body, unspecified ankle
   ● S90.56   Insect bite (nonvenomous) of ankle
     ● S90.561   Insect bite (nonvenomous), right ankle
     ● S90.562   Insect bite (nonvenomous), left ankle
     ● S90.569   Insect bite (nonvenomous), unspecified ankle
   ● S90.57   Other superficial bite of ankle
     Excludes1   open bite of ankle (S91.05-)
     ● S90.571   Other superficial bite of ankle, right ankle
     ● S90.572   Other superficial bite of ankle, left ankle
     ● S90.579   Other superficial bite of ankle, unspecified ankle

● S90.8   Other superficial injuries of foot
   ● S90.81   Abrasion of foot
     ● S90.811   Abrasion, right foot
     ● S90.812   Abrasion, left foot
     ● S90.819   Abrasion, unspecified foot
   ● S90.82   Blister (nonthermal) of foot
     ● S90.821   Blister (nonthermal), right foot
     ● S90.822   Blister (nonthermal), left foot
     ● S90.829   Blister (nonthermal), unspecified foot
   ● S90.84   External constriction of foot
     ● S90.841   External constriction, right foot
     ● S90.842   External constriction, left foot
     ● S90.849   External constriction, unspecified foot

   ● S90.85   Superficial foreign body of foot
     Splinter in the foot
     ● S90.851   Superficial foreign body, right foot
     ● S90.852   Superficial foreign body, left foot
     ● S90.859   Superficial foreign body, unspecified foot
   ● S90.86   Insect bite (nonvenomous) of foot
     ● S90.861   Insect bite (nonvenomous), right foot
     ● S90.862   Insect bite (nonvenomous), left foot
     ● S90.869   Insect bite (nonvenomous), unspecified foot
   ● S90.87   Other superficial bite of foot
     Excludes1   open bite of foot (S91.35-)
     ● S90.871   Other superficial bite of right foot
     ● S90.872   Other superficial bite of left foot
     ● S90.879   Other superficial bite of unspecified foot

● S90.9   Unspecified superficial injury of ankle, foot and toe
   ● S90.91   Unspecified superficial injury of ankle
     ● S90.911   Unspecified superficial injury of right ankle
     ● S90.912   Unspecified superficial injury of left ankle
     ● S90.919   Unspecified superficial injury of unspecified ankle
   ● S90.92   Unspecified superficial injury of foot
     ● S90.921   Unspecified superficial injury of right foot
     ● S90.922   Unspecified superficial injury of left foot
     ● S90.929   Unspecified superficial injury of unspecified foot
   S90.93   Unspecified superficial injury of toes
     ● S90.931   Unspecified superficial injury of right great toe
     ● S90.932   Unspecified superficial injury of left great toe
     ● S90.933   Unspecified superficial injury of unspecified great toe
     ● S90.934   Unspecified superficial injury of right lesser toe(s)
     ● S90.935   Unspecified superficial injury of left lesser toe(s)
     ● S90.936   Unspecified superficial injury of unspecified lesser toe(s)

● S91   Open wound of ankle, foot and toes
     Code also any associated wound infection
     Excludes1   open fracture of ankle, foot and toes (S92.-with 7th character B)
            traumatic amputation of ankle and foot (S98.-)
     The appropriate 7th character is to be added to each code from category S91

A	initial encounter
D	subsequent encounter
S	sequela

● S91.0   Open wound of ankle
   ● S91.00   Unspecified open wound of ankle
     ● S91.001   Unspecified open wound, right ankle
     ● S91.002   Unspecified open wound, left ankle
     ● S91.009   Unspecified open wound, unspecified ankle

CHAPTER 19 (S00-T88)

● **S91.01**   Laceration without foreign body of ankle
- ● **S91.011**   Laceration without foreign body, right ankle
- ● **S91.012**   Laceration without foreign body, left ankle
- ● **S91.019**   Laceration without foreign body, unspecified ankle

● **S91.02**   Laceration with foreign body of ankle
- ● **S91.021**   Laceration with foreign body, right ankle
- ● **S91.022**   Laceration with foreign body, left ankle
- ● **S91.029**   Laceration with foreign body, unspecified ankle

● **S91.03**   Puncture wound without foreign body of ankle
- ● **S91.031**   Puncture wound without foreign body, right ankle
- ● **S91.032**   Puncture wound without foreign body, left ankle
- ● **S91.039**   Puncture wound without foreign body, unspecified ankle

● **S91.04**   Puncture wound with foreign body of ankle
- ● **S91.041**   Puncture wound with foreign body, right ankle
- ● **S91.042**   Puncture wound with foreign body, left ankle
- ● **S91.049**   Puncture wound with foreign body, unspecified ankle

● **S91.05**   Open bite of ankle
> **Excludes1**   superficial bite of ankle (S90.56-, S90.57-)
- ● **S91.051**   Open bite, right ankle
- ● **S91.052**   Open bite, left ankle
- ● **S91.059**   Open bite, unspecified ankle

● **S91.1**   Open wound of toe without damage to nail
- ● **S91.10**   Unspecified open wound of toe without damage to nail
  - ● **S91.101**   Unspecified open wound of right great toe without damage to nail
  - ● **S91.102**   Unspecified open wound of left great toe without damage to nail
  - ● **S91.103**   Unspecified open wound of unspecified great toe without damage to nail
  - ● **S91.104**   Unspecified open wound of right lesser toe(s) without damage to nail
  - ● **S91.105**   Unspecified open wound of left lesser toe(s) without damage to nail
  - ● **S91.106**   Unspecified open wound of unspecified lesser toe(s) without damage to nail
  - ● **S91.109**   Unspecified open wound of unspecified toe(s) without damage to nail

- ● **S91.11**   Laceration without foreign body of toe without damage to nail
  - ● **S91.111**   Laceration without foreign body of right great toe without damage to nail
  - ● **S91.112**   Laceration without foreign body of left great toe without damage to nail
  - ● **S91.113**   Laceration without foreign body of unspecified great toe without damage to nail
  - ● **S91.114**   Laceration without foreign body of right lesser toe(s) without damage to nail
  - ● **S91.115**   Laceration without foreign body of left lesser toe(s) without damage to nail
  - ● **S91.116**   Laceration without foreign body of unspecified lesser toe(s) without damage to nail
  - ● **S91.119**   Laceration without foreign body of unspecified toe without damage to nail

- ● **S91.12**   Laceration with foreign body of toe without damage to nail
  - ● **S91.121**   Laceration with foreign body of right great toe without damage to nail
  - ● **S91.122**   Laceration with foreign body of left great toe without damage to nail
  - ● **S91.123**   Laceration with foreign body of unspecified great toe without damage to nail
  - ● **S91.124**   Laceration with foreign body of right lesser toe(s) without damage to nail
  - ● **S91.125**   Laceration with foreign body of left lesser toe(s) without damage to nail
  - ● **S91.126**   Laceration with foreign body of unspecified lesser toe(s) without damage to nail
  - ● **S91.129**   Laceration with foreign body of unspecified toe(s) without damage to nail

- ● **S91.13**   Puncture wound without foreign body of toe without damage to nail
  - ● **S91.131**   Puncture wound without foreign body of right great toe without damage to nail
  - ● **S91.132**   Puncture wound without foreign body of left great toe without damage to nail
  - ● **S91.133**   Puncture wound without foreign body of unspecified great toe without damage to nail
  - ● **S91.134**   Puncture wound without foreign body of right lesser toe(s) without damage to nail
  - ● **S91.135**   Puncture wound without foreign body of left lesser toe(s) without damage to nail
  - ● **S91.136**   Puncture wound without foreign body of unspecified lesser toe(s) without damage to nail
  - ● **S91.139**   Puncture wound without foreign body of unspecified toe(s) without damage to nail

- ● **S91.14**   Puncture wound with foreign body of toe without damage to nail
  - ● **S91.141**   Puncture wound with foreign body of right great toe without damage to nail
  - ● **S91.142**   Puncture wound with foreign body of left great toe without damage to nail
  - ● **S91.143**   Puncture wound with foreign body of unspecified great toe without damage to nail
  - ● **S91.144**   Puncture wound with foreign body of right lesser toe(s) without damage to nail
  - ● **S91.145**   Puncture wound with foreign body of left lesser toe(s) without damage to nail
  - ● **S91.146**   Puncture wound with foreign body of unspecified lesser toe(s) without damage to nail
  - ● **S91.149**   Puncture wound with foreign body of unspecified toe(s) without damage to nail

◄ New   ◄▪▪▪ Revised   ~~deleted~~ Deleted   Excludes 1   Excludes 2   Includes   Use additional   Code first   Code also   Unspecified

OGCR Official Guidelines   **X** Assign placeholder X   ● Use Additional Character(s)   ▶ Manifestation Code   **Coding Clinic**

● S91.15   Open bite of toe without damage to nail
      Bite of toe NOS
      Excludes1   superficial bite of toe (S90.46-, S90.47-)

     ● S91.151   Open bite of right great toe without damage to nail

     ● S91.152   Open bite of left great toe without damage to nail

     ● S91.153   Open bite of unspecified great toe without damage to nail

     ● S91.154   Open bite of right lesser toe(s) without damage to nail

     ● S91.155   Open bite of left lesser toe(s) without damage to nail

     ● S91.156   Open bite of unspecified lesser toe(s) without damage to nail

     ● S91.159   Open bite of unspecified toe(s) without damage to nail

● S91.2   Open wound of toe with damage to nail

   ● S91.20   Unspecified open wound of toe with damage to nail

     ● S91.201   Unspecified open wound of right great toe with damage to nail

     ● S91.202   Unspecified open wound of left great toe with damage to nail

     ● S91.203   Unspecified open wound of unspecified great toe with damage to nail

     ● S91.204   Unspecified open wound of right lesser toe(s) with damage to nail

     ● S91.205   Unspecified open wound of left lesser toe(s) with damage to nail

     ● S91.206   Unspecified open wound of unspecified lesser toe(s) with damage to nail

     ● S91.209   Unspecified open wound of unspecified toe(s) with damage to nail

   ● S91.21   Laceration without foreign body of toe with damage to nail

     ● S91.211   Laceration without foreign body of right great toe with damage to nail

     ● S91.212   Laceration without foreign body of left great toe with damage to nail

     ● S91.213   Laceration without foreign body of unspecified great toe with damage to nail

     ● S91.214   Laceration without foreign body of right lesser toe(s) with damage to nail

     ● S91.215   Laceration without foreign body of left lesser toe(s) with damage to nail

     ● S91.216   Laceration without foreign body of unspecified lesser toe(s) with damage to nail

     ● S91.219   Laceration without foreign body of unspecified toe(s) with damage to nail

   ● S91.22   Laceration with foreign body of toe with damage to nail

     ● S91.221   Laceration with foreign body of right great toe with damage to nail

     ● S91.222   Laceration with foreign body of left great toe with damage to nail

     ● S91.223   Laceration with foreign body of unspecified great toe with damage to nail

     ● S91.224   Laceration with foreign body of right lesser toe(s) with damage to nail

     ● S91.225   Laceration with foreign body of left lesser toe(s) with damage to nail

     ● S91.226   Laceration with foreign body of unspecified lesser toe(s) with damage to nail

     ● S91.229   Laceration with foreign body of unspecified toe(s) with damage to nail

   ● S91.23   Puncture wound without foreign body of toe with damage to nail

     ● S91.231   Puncture wound without foreign body of right great toe with damage to nail

     ● S91.232   Puncture wound without foreign body of left great toe with damage to nail

     ● S91.233   Puncture wound without foreign body of unspecified great toe with damage to nail

     ● S91.234   Puncture wound without foreign body of right lesser toe(s) with damage to nail

     ● S91.235   Puncture wound without foreign body of left lesser toe(s) with damage to nail

     ● S91.236   Puncture wound without foreign body of unspecified lesser toe(s) with damage to nail

     ● S91.239   Puncture wound without foreign body of unspecified toe(s) with damage to nail

   ● S91.24   Puncture wound with foreign body of toe with damage to nail

     ● S91.241   Puncture wound with foreign body of right great toe with damage to nail

     ● S91.242   Puncture wound with foreign body of left great toe with damage to nail

     ● S91.243   Puncture wound with foreign body of unspecified great toe with damage to nail

     ● S91.244   Puncture wound with foreign body of right lesser toe(s) with damage to nail

     ● S91.245   Puncture wound with foreign body of left lesser toe(s) with damage to nail

     ● S91.246   Puncture wound with foreign body of unspecified lesser toe(s) with damage to nail

     ● S91.249   Puncture wound with foreign body of unspecified toe(s) with damage to nail

   ● S91.25   Open bite of toe with damage to nail
      Bite of toe with damage to nail NOS
      Excludes1   superficial bite of toe (S90.46-, S90.47-)

     ● S91.251   Open bite of right great toe with damage to nail

     ● S91.252   Open bite of left great toe with damage to nail

     ● S91.253   Open bite of unspecified great toe with damage to nail

     ● S91.254   Open bite of right lesser toe(s) with damage to nail

     ● S91.255   Open bite of left lesser toe(s) with damage to nail

     ● S91.256   Open bite of unspecified lesser toe(s) with damage to nail

     ● S91.259   Open bite of unspecified toe(s) with damage to nail

CHAPTER 19 (S00-T88)

- ● S91.3   **Open wound of foot**
  - ● S91.30   Unspecified open wound of foot
    - ● S91.301   Unspecified open wound, right foot
    - ● S91.302   Unspecified open wound, left foot
    - ● S91.309   Unspecified open wound, unspecified foot
  - ● S91.31   Laceration without foreign body of foot
    - ● S91.311   Laceration without foreign body, right foot
    - ● S91.312   Laceration without foreign body, left foot
    - ● S91.319   Laceration without foreign body, unspecified foot
  - ● S91.32   Laceration with foreign body of foot
    - ● S91.321   Laceration with foreign body, right foot
    - ● S91.322   Laceration with foreign body, left foot
    - ● S91.329   Laceration with foreign body, unspecified foot
  - ● S91.33   Puncture wound without foreign body of foot
    - ● S91.331   Puncture wound without foreign body, right foot
    - ● S91.332   Puncture wound without foreign body, left foot
    - ● S91.339   Puncture wound without foreign body, unspecified foot
  - ● S91.34   Puncture wound with foreign body of foot
    - ● S91.341   Puncture wound with foreign body, right foot
    - ● S91.342   Puncture wound with foreign body, left foot
    - ● S91.349   Puncture wound with foreign body, unspecified foot
  - ● S91.35   Open bite of foot
    - **Excludes1**   superficial bite of foot (S90.86-, S90.87-)
    - ● S91.351   Open bite, right foot
    - ● S91.352   Open bite, left foot
    - ● S91.359   Open bite, unspecified foot

- ● S92   **Fracture of foot and toe, except ankle**
  - **Note:** A fracture not indicated as displaced or nondisplaced should be coded to displaced
  - A fracture not indicated as open or closed should be coded to closed
  - **Excludes1**   traumatic amputation of ankle and foot (S98.-)
  - **Excludes2**   fracture of ankle (S82.-)
  -                fracture of malleolus (S82.-)
  - The appropriate 7th character is to be added to each code from category S92

A	initial encounter for closed fracture
B	initial encounter for open fracture
D	subsequent encounter for fracture with routine healing
G	subsequent encounter for fracture with delayed healing
K	subsequent encounter for fracture with nonunion
P	subsequent encounter for fracture with malunion
S	sequela

  - ● S92.0   **Fracture of calcaneus**
    - Heel bone   Os calcis
    - ● S92.00   Unspecified fracture of calcaneus
      - ● S92.001   Unspecified fracture of right calcaneus
      - ● S92.002   Unspecified fracture of left calcaneus
      - ● S92.009   Unspecified fracture of unspecified calcaneus

  - ● S92.01   Fracture of body of calcaneus
    - ● S92.011   Displaced fracture of body of right calcaneus
    - ● S92.012   Displaced fracture of body of left calcaneus
    - ● S92.013   Displaced fracture of body of unspecified calcaneus
    - ● S92.014   Nondisplaced fracture of body of right calcaneus
    - ● S92.015   Nondisplaced fracture of body of left calcaneus
    - ● S92.016   Nondisplaced fracture of body of unspecified calcaneus
  - ● S92.02   Fracture of anterior process of calcaneus
    - ● S92.021   Displaced fracture of anterior process of right calcaneus
    - ● S92.022   Displaced fracture of anterior process of left calcaneus
    - ● S92.023   Displaced fracture of anterior process of unspecified calcaneus
    - ● S92.024   Nondisplaced fracture of anterior process of right calcaneus
    - ● S92.025   Nondisplaced fracture of anterior process of left calcaneus
    - ● S92.026   Nondisplaced fracture of anterior process of unspecified calcaneus
  - ● S92.03   Avulsion fracture of tuberosity of calcaneus
    - ● S92.031   Displaced avulsion fracture of tuberosity of right calcaneus
    - ● S92.032   Displaced avulsion fracture of tuberosity of left calcaneus
    - ● S92.033   Displaced avulsion fracture of tuberosity of unspecified calcaneus
    - ● S92.034   Nondisplaced avulsion fracture of tuberosity of right calcaneus
    - ● S92.035   Nondisplaced avulsion fracture of tuberosity of left calcaneus
    - ● S92.036   Nondisplaced avulsion fracture of tuberosity of unspecified calcaneus
  - ● S92.04   Other fracture of tuberosity of calcaneus
    - ● S92.041   Displaced other fracture of tuberosity of right calcaneus
    - ● S92.042   Displaced other fracture of tuberosity of left calcaneus
    - ● S92.043   Displaced other fracture of tuberosity of unspecified calcaneus
    - ● S92.044   Nondisplaced other fracture of tuberosity of right calcaneus
    - ● S92.045   Nondisplaced other fracture of tuberosity of left calcaneus
    - ● S92.046   Nondisplaced other fracture of tuberosity of unspecified calcaneus
  - ● S92.05   Other extraarticular fracture of calcaneus
    - ● S92.051   Displaced other extraarticular fracture of right calcaneus
    - ● S92.052   Displaced other extraarticular fracture of left calcaneus
    - ● S92.053   Displaced other extraarticular fracture of unspecified calcaneus
    - ● S92.054   Nondisplaced other extraarticular fracture of right calcaneus
    - ● S92.055   Nondisplaced other extraarticular fracture of left calcaneus
    - ● S92.056   Nondisplaced other extraarticular fracture of unspecified calcaneus

- ● S92.06　Intraarticular fracture of calcaneus
  - ● S92.061　Displaced intraarticular fracture of right calcaneus
  - ● S92.062　Displaced intraarticular fracture of left calcaneus
  - ● S92.063　Displaced intraarticular fracture of unspecified calcaneus
  - ● S92.064　Nondisplaced intraarticular fracture of right calcaneus
  - ● S92.065　Nondisplaced intraarticular fracture of left calcaneus
  - ● S92.066　Nondisplaced intraarticular fracture of unspecified calcaneus
- ● S92.1　Fracture of talus
  - Astragalus
  - ● S92.10　Unspecified fracture of talus
    - ● S92.101　Unspecified fracture of right talus
    - ● S92.102　Unspecified fracture of left talus
    - ● S92.109　Unspecified fracture of unspecified talus
  - ● S92.11　Fracture of neck of talus
    - ● S92.111　Displaced fracture of neck of right talus
    - ● S92.112　Displaced fracture of neck of left talus
    - ● S92.113　Displaced fracture of neck of unspecified talus
    - ● S92.114　Nondisplaced fracture of neck of right talus
    - ● S92.115　Nondisplaced fracture of neck of left talus
    - ● S92.116　Nondisplaced fracture of neck of unspecified talus
  - ● S92.12　Fracture of body of talus
    - ● S92.121　Displaced fracture of body of right talus
    - ● S92.122　Displaced fracture of body of left talus
    - ● S92.123　Displaced fracture of body of unspecified talus
    - ● S92.124　Nondisplaced fracture of body of right talus
    - ● S92.125　Nondisplaced fracture of body of left talus
    - ● S92.126　Nondisplaced fracture of body of unspecified talus
  - ● S92.13　Fracture of posterior process of talus
    - ● S92.131　Displaced fracture of posterior process of right talus
    - ● S92.132　Displaced fracture of posterior process of left talus
    - ● S92.133　Displaced fracture of posterior process of unspecified talus
    - ● S92.134　Nondisplaced fracture of posterior process of right talus
    - ● S92.135　Nondisplaced fracture of posterior process of left talus
    - ● S92.136　Nondisplaced fracture of posterior process of unspecified talus
  - ● S92.14　Dome fracture of talus
    - **Excludes1**　osteochondritis dissecans (M93.2)
    - ● S92.141　Displaced dome fracture of right talus
    - ● S92.142　Displaced dome fracture of left talus
    - ● S92.143　Displaced dome fracture of unspecified talus
    - ● S92.144　Nondisplaced dome fracture of right talus
    - ● S92.145　Nondisplaced dome fracture of left talus
    - ● S92.146　Nondisplaced dome fracture of unspecified talus
  - ● S92.15　Avulsion fracture (chip fracture) of talus
    - ● S92.151　Displaced avulsion fracture (chip fracture) of right talus
    - ● S92.152　Displaced avulsion fracture (chip fracture) of left talus
    - ● S92.153　Displaced avulsion fracture (chip fracture) of unspecified talus
    - ● S92.154　Nondisplaced avulsion fracture (chip fracture) of right talus
    - ● S92.155　Nondisplaced avulsion fracture (chip fracture) of left talus
    - ● S92.156　Nondisplaced avulsion fracture (chip fracture) of unspecified talus
  - ● S92.19　Other fracture of talus
    - ● S92.191　Other fracture of right talus
    - ● S92.192　Other fracture of left talus
    - ● S92.199　Other fracture of unspecified talus
- ● S92.2　Fracture of other and unspecified tarsal bone(s)
  - ● S92.20　Fracture of unspecified tarsal bone(s)
    - ● S92.201　Fracture of unspecified tarsal bone(s) of right foot
    - ● S92.202　Fracture of unspecified tarsal bone(s) of left foot
    - ● S92.209　Fracture of unspecified tarsal bone(s) of unspecified foot
  - ● S92.21　Fracture of cuboid bone
    - ● S92.211　Displaced fracture of cuboid bone of right foot
    - ● S92.212　Displaced fracture of cuboid bone of left foot
    - ● S92.213　Displaced fracture of cuboid bone of unspecified foot
    - ● S92.214　Nondisplaced fracture of cuboid bone of right foot
    - ● S92.215　Nondisplaced fracture of cuboid bone of left foot
    - ● S92.216　Nondisplaced fracture of cuboid bone of unspecified foot
  - ● S92.22　Fracture of lateral cuneiform
    - ● S92.221　Displaced fracture of lateral cuneiform of right foot
    - ● S92.222　Displaced fracture of lateral cuneiform of left foot
    - ● S92.223　Displaced fracture of lateral cuneiform of unspecified foot
    - ● S92.224　Nondisplaced fracture of lateral cuneiform of right foot
    - ● S92.225　Nondisplaced fracture of lateral cuneiform of left foot
    - ● S92.226　Nondisplaced fracture of lateral cuneiform of unspecified foot
  - ● S92.23　Fracture of intermediate cuneiform
    - ● S92.231　Displaced fracture of intermediate cuneiform of right foot
    - ● S92.232　Displaced fracture of intermediate cuneiform of left foot
    - ● S92.233　Displaced fracture of intermediate cuneiform of unspecified foot
    - ● S92.234　Nondisplaced fracture of intermediate cuneiform of right foot
    - ● S92.235　Nondisplaced fracture of intermediate cuneiform of left foot
    - ● S92.236　Nondisplaced fracture of intermediate cuneiform of unspecified foot

CHAPTER 19 (S00-T88)

● S92.24   Fracture of medial cuneiform
     ● S92.241   Displaced fracture of medial cuneiform of right foot
     ● S92.242   Displaced fracture of medial cuneiform of left foot
     ● S92.243   Displaced fracture of medial cuneiform of unspecified foot
     ● S92.244   Nondisplaced fracture of medial cuneiform of right foot
     ● S92.245   Nondisplaced fracture of medial cuneiform of left foot
     ● S92.246   Nondisplaced fracture of medial cuneiform of unspecified foot

● S92.25   Fracture of navicular [scaphoid] of foot
     ● S92.251   Displaced fracture of navicular [scaphoid] of right foot
     ● S92.252   Displaced fracture of navicular [scaphoid] of left foot
     ● S92.253   Displaced fracture of navicular [scaphoid] of unspecified foot
     ● S92.254   Nondisplaced fracture of navicular [scaphoid] of right foot
     ● S92.255   Nondisplaced fracture of navicular [scaphoid] of left foot
     ● S92.256   Nondisplaced fracture of navicular [scaphoid] of unspecified foot

● S92.3   Fracture of metatarsal bone(s)
   ● S92.30   Fracture of unspecified metatarsal bone(s)
     ● S92.301   Fracture of unspecified metatarsal bone(s), right foot
     ● S92.302   Fracture of unspecified metatarsal bone(s), left foot
     ● S92.309   Fracture of unspecified metatarsal bone(s), unspecified foot

   ● S92.31   Fracture of first metatarsal bone
     ● S92.311   Displaced fracture of first metatarsal bone, right foot
     ● S92.312   Displaced fracture of first metatarsal bone, left foot
     ● S92.313   Displaced fracture of first metatarsal bone, unspecified foot
     ● S92.314   Nondisplaced fracture of first metatarsal bone, right foot
     ● S92.315   Nondisplaced fracture of first metatarsal bone, left foot
     ● S92.316   Nondisplaced fracture of first metatarsal bone, unspecified foot

   ● S92.32   Fracture of second metatarsal bone
     ● S92.321   Displaced fracture of second metatarsal bone, right foot
     ● S92.322   Displaced fracture of second metatarsal bone, left foot
     ● S92.323   Displaced fracture of second metatarsal bone, unspecified foot
     ● S92.324   Nondisplaced fracture of second metatarsal bone, right foot
     ● S92.325   Nondisplaced fracture of second metatarsal bone, left foot
     ● S92.326   Nondisplaced fracture of second metatarsal bone, unspecified foot

   ● S92.33   Fracture of third metatarsal bone
     ● S92.331   Displaced fracture of third metatarsal bone, right foot
     ● S92.332   Displaced fracture of third metatarsal bone, left foot
     ● S92.333   Displaced fracture of third metatarsal bone, unspecified foot
     ● S92.334   Nondisplaced fracture of third metatarsal bone, right foot

● S92.335   Nondisplaced fracture of third metatarsal bone, left foot
● S92.336   Nondisplaced fracture of third metatarsal bone, unspecified foot

● S92.34   Fracture of fourth metatarsal bone
     ● S92.341   Displaced fracture of fourth metatarsal bone, right foot
     ● S92.342   Displaced fracture of fourth metatarsal bone, left foot
     ● S92.343   Displaced fracture of fourth metatarsal bone, unspecified foot
     ● S92.344   Nondisplaced fracture of fourth metatarsal bone, right foot
     ● S92.345   Nondisplaced fracture of fourth metatarsal bone, left foot
     ● S92.346   Nondisplaced fracture of fourth metatarsal bone, unspecified foot

● S92.35   Fracture of fifth metatarsal bone
     ● S92.351   Displaced fracture of fifth metatarsal bone, right foot
     ● S92.352   Displaced fracture of fifth metatarsal bone, left foot
     ● S92.353   Displaced fracture of fifth metatarsal bone, unspecified foot
     ● S92.354   Nondisplaced fracture of fifth metatarsal bone, right foot
     ● S92.355   Nondisplaced fracture of fifth metatarsal bone, left foot
     ● S92.356   Nondisplaced fracture of fifth metatarsal bone, unspecified foot

● S92.4   Fracture of great toe
   ● S92.40   Unspecified fracture of great toe
     ● S92.401   Displaced unspecified fracture of right great toe
     ● S92.402   Displaced unspecified fracture of left great toe
     ● S92.403   Displaced unspecified fracture of unspecified great toe
     ● S92.404   Nondisplaced unspecified fracture of right great toe
     ● S92.405   Nondisplaced unspecified fracture of left great toe
     ● S92.406   Nondisplaced unspecified fracture of unspecified great toe

   ● S92.41   Fracture of proximal phalanx of great toe
     ● S92.411   Displaced fracture of proximal phalanx of right great toe
     ● S92.412   Displaced fracture of proximal phalanx of left great toe
     ● S92.413   Displaced fracture of proximal phalanx of unspecified great toe
     ● S92.414   Nondisplaced fracture of proximal phalanx of right great toe
     ● S92.415   Nondisplaced fracture of proximal phalanx of left great toe
     ● S92.416   Nondisplaced fracture of proximal phalanx of unspecified great toe

   ● S92.42   Fracture of distal phalanx of great toe
     ● S92.421   Displaced fracture of distal phalanx of right great toe
     ● S92.422   Displaced fracture of distal phalanx of left great toe
     ● S92.423   Displaced fracture of distal phalanx of unspecified great toe
     ● S92.424   Nondisplaced fracture of distal phalanx of right great toe
     ● S92.425   Nondisplaced fracture of distal phalanx of left great toe
     ● S92.426   Nondisplaced fracture of distal phalanx of unspecified great toe

◀ New   ◀▥ Revised   ~~deleted~~ Deleted   Excludes 1   Excludes 2   Includes   Use additional   Code first   Code also   Unspecified

OGCR Official Guidelines   X Assign placeholder X   ● Use Additional Character(s)   ▶ Manifestation Code   **Coding Clinic**

● **S92.49**   Other fracture of great toe
   ● **S92.491**   Other fracture of right great toe
   ● **S92.492**   Other fracture of left great toe
   ● **S92.499**   Other fracture of unspecified great toe

● **S92.5**   Fracture of lesser toe(s)
  ● **S92.50**   Unspecified fracture of lesser toe(s)
   ● **S92.501**   Displaced unspecified fracture of right lesser toe(s)
   ● **S92.502**   Displaced unspecified fracture of left lesser toe(s)
   ● **S92.503**   Displaced unspecified fracture of unspecified lesser toe(s)
   ● **S92.504**   Nondisplaced unspecified fracture of right lesser toe(s)
   ● **S92.505**   Nondisplaced unspecified fracture of left lesser toe(s)
   ● **S92.506**   Nondisplaced unspecified fracture of unspecified lesser toe(s)
  ● **S92.51**   Fracture of proximal phalanx of lesser toe(s)
   ● **S92.511**   Displaced fracture of proximal phalanx of right lesser toe(s)
   ● **S92.512**   Displaced fracture of proximal phalanx of left lesser toe(s)
   ● **S92.513**   Displaced fracture of proximal phalanx of unspecified lesser toe(s)
   ● **S92.514**   Nondisplaced fracture of proximal phalanx of right lesser toe(s)
   ● **S92.515**   Nondisplaced fracture of proximal phalanx of left lesser toe(s)
   ● **S92.516**   Nondisplaced fracture of proximal phalanx of unspecified lesser toe(s)
  ● **S92.52**   Fracture of medial phalanx of lesser toe(s)
   ● **S92.521**   Displaced fracture of medial phalanx of right lesser toe(s)
   ● **S92.522**   Displaced fracture of medial phalanx of left lesser toe(s)
   ● **S92.523**   Displaced fracture of medial phalanx of unspecified lesser toe(s)
   ● **S92.524**   Nondisplaced fracture of medial phalanx of right lesser toe(s)
   ● **S92.525**   Nondisplaced fracture of medial phalanx of left lesser toe(s)
   ● **S92.526**   Nondisplaced fracture of medial phalanx of unspecified lesser toe(s)
  ● **S92.53**   Fracture of distal phalanx of lesser toe(s)
   ● **S92.531**   Displaced fracture of distal phalanx of right lesser toe(s)
   ● **S92.532**   Displaced fracture of distal phalanx of left lesser toe(s)
   ● **S92.533**   Displaced fracture of distal phalanx of unspecified lesser toe(s)
   ● **S92.534**   Nondisplaced fracture of distal phalanx of right lesser toe(s)
   ● **S92.535**   Nondisplaced fracture of distal phalanx of left lesser toe(s)
   ● **S92.536**   Nondisplaced fracture of distal phalanx of unspecified lesser toe(s)
  ● **S92.59**   Other fracture of lesser toe(s)
   ● **S92.591**   Other fracture of right lesser toe(s)
   ● **S92.592**   Other fracture of left lesser toe(s)
   ● **S92.599**   Other fracture of unspecified lesser toe(s)

● **S92.9**   Unspecified fracture of foot and toe
  ● **S92.90**   Unspecified fracture of foot
   ● **S92.901**   Unspecified fracture of right foot
   ● **S92.902**   Unspecified fracture of left foot
   ● **S92.909**   Unspecified fracture of unspecified foot

● **S92.91**   Unspecified fracture of toe
  ● **S92.911**   Unspecified fracture of right toe(s)
  ● **S92.912**   Unspecified fracture of left toe(s)
  ● **S92.919**   Unspecified fracture of unspecified toe(s)

● **S93**   Dislocation and sprain of joints and ligaments at ankle, foot and toe level

   Includes   avulsion of joint or ligament of ankle, foot and toe
        laceration of cartilage, joint or ligament of ankle, foot and toe
        sprain of cartilage, joint or ligament of ankle, foot and toe
        traumatic hemarthrosis of joint or ligament of ankle, foot and toe
        traumatic rupture of joint or ligament of ankle, foot and toe
        traumatic subluxation of joint or ligament of ankle, foot and toe
        traumatic tear of joint or ligament of ankle, foot and toe

   Code also any associated open wound

   Excludes2   strain of muscle and tendon of ankle and foot (S96.-)

   The appropriate 7th character is to be added to each code from category S93

> A   initial encounter
> D   subsequent encounter
> S   sequela

● **S93.0**   Subluxation and dislocation of ankle joint
   Subluxation and dislocation of astragalus
   Subluxation and dislocation of fibula, lower end
   Subluxation and dislocation of talus
   Subluxation and dislocation of tibia, lower end
  X● **S93.01**   Subluxation of right ankle joint
  X● **S93.02**   Subluxation of left ankle joint
  X● **S93.03**   Subluxation of unspecified ankle joint
  X● **S93.04**   Dislocation of right ankle joint
  X● **S93.05**   Dislocation of left ankle joint
  X● **S93.06**   Dislocation of unspecified ankle joint

● **S93.1**   Subluxation and dislocation of toe
  ● **S93.10**   Unspecified subluxation and dislocation of toe
   Dislocation of toe NOS
   Subluxation of toe NOS
   ● **S93.101**   Unspecified subluxation of right toe(s)
   ● **S93.102**   Unspecified subluxation of left toe(s)
   ● **S93.103**   Unspecified subluxation of unspecified toe(s)
   ● **S93.104**   Unspecified dislocation of right toe(s)
   ● **S93.105**   Unspecified dislocation of left toe(s)
   ● **S93.106**   Unspecified dislocation of unspecified toe(s)
  ● **S93.11**   Dislocation of interphalangeal joint
   ● **S93.111**   Dislocation of interphalangeal joint of right great toe
   ● **S93.112**   Dislocation of interphalangeal joint of left great toe
   ● **S93.113**   Dislocation of interphalangeal joint of unspecified great toe
   ● **S93.114**   Dislocation of interphalangeal joint of right lesser toe(s)
   ● **S93.115**   Dislocation of interphalangeal joint of left lesser toe(s)
   ● **S93.116**   Dislocation of interphalangeal joint of unspecified lesser toe(s)
   ● **S93.119**   Dislocation of interphalangeal joint of unspecified toe(s)

● S93.12 Dislocation of metatarsophalangeal joint
　● S93.121 Dislocation of metatarsophalangeal joint of right great toe
　● S93.122 Dislocation of metatarsophalangeal joint of left great toe
　● S93.123 Dislocation of metatarsophalangeal joint of unspecified great toe
　● S93.124 Dislocation of metatarsophalangeal joint of right lesser toe(s)
　● S93.125 Dislocation of metatarsophalangeal joint of left lesser toe(s)
　● S93.126 Dislocation of metatarsophalangeal joint of unspecified lesser toe(s)
　● S93.129 Dislocation of metatarsophalangeal joint of unspecified toe(s)
● S93.13 Subluxation of interphalangeal joint
　● S93.131 Subluxation of interphalangeal joint of right great toe
　● S93.132 Subluxation of interphalangeal joint of left great toe
　● S93.133 Subluxation of interphalangeal joint of unspecified great toe
　● S93.134 Subluxation of interphalangeal joint of right lesser toe(s)
　● S93.135 Subluxation of interphalangeal joint of left lesser toe(s)
　● S93.136 Subluxation of interphalangeal joint of unspecified lesser toe(s)
　● S93.139 Subluxation of interphalangeal joint of unspecified toe(s)
● S93.14 Subluxation of metatarsophalangeal joint
　● S93.141 Subluxation of metatarsophalangeal joint of right great toe
　● S93.142 Subluxation of metatarsophalangeal joint of left great toe
　● S93.143 Subluxation of metatarsophalangeal joint of unspecified great toe
　● S93.144 Subluxation of metatarsophalangeal joint of right lesser toe(s)
　● S93.145 Subluxation of metatarsophalangeal joint of left lesser toe(s)
　● S93.146 Subluxation of metatarsophalangeal joint of unspecified lesser toe(s)
　● S93.149 Subluxation of metatarsophalangeal joint of unspecified toe(s)
● S93.3 Subluxation and dislocation of foot
　Excludes2 dislocation of toe (S93.1-)
● S93.30 Unspecified subluxation and dislocation of foot
　Dislocation of foot NOS
　Subluxation of foot NOS
　● S93.301 Unspecified subluxation of right foot
　● S93.302 Unspecified subluxation of left foot
　● S93.303 Unspecified subluxation of unspecified foot
　● S93.304 Unspecified dislocation of right foot
　● S93.305 Unspecified dislocation of left foot
　● S93.306 Unspecified dislocation of unspecified foot
● S93.31 Subluxation and dislocation of tarsal joint
　● S93.311 Subluxation of tarsal joint of right foot
　● S93.312 Subluxation of tarsal joint of left foot
　● S93.313 Subluxation of tarsal joint of unspecified foot
　● S93.314 Dislocation of tarsal joint of right foot
　● S93.315 Dislocation of tarsal joint of left foot
　● S93.316 Dislocation of tarsal joint of unspecified foot

● S93.32 Subluxation and dislocation of tarsometatarsal joint
　● S93.321 Subluxation of tarsometatarsal joint of right foot
　● S93.322 Subluxation of tarsometatarsal joint of left foot
　● S93.323 Subluxation of tarsometatarsal joint of unspecified foot
　● S93.324 Dislocation of tarsometatarsal joint of right foot
　● S93.325 Dislocation of tarsometatarsal joint of left foot
　● S93.326 Dislocation of tarsometatarsal joint of unspecified foot
● S93.33 Other subluxation and dislocation of foot
　● S93.331 Other subluxation of right foot
　● S93.332 Other subluxation of left foot
　● S93.333 Other subluxation of unspecified foot
　● S93.334 Other dislocation of right foot
　● S93.335 Other dislocation of left foot
　● S93.336 Other dislocation of unspecified foot
● S93.4 Sprain of ankle
　Injury to ligaments when one or more is stretched/torn
　Excludes2 injury of Achilles tendon (S86.0-)
● S93.40 Sprain of unspecified ligament of ankle
　Sprain of ankle NOS
　Sprained ankle NOS
　● S93.401 Sprain of unspecified ligament of right ankle
　● S93.402 Sprain of unspecified ligament of left ankle
　● S93.409 Sprain of unspecified ligament of unspecified ankle
● S93.41 Sprain of calcaneofibular ligament
　● S93.411 Sprain of calcaneofibular ligament of right ankle
　● S93.412 Sprain of calcaneofibular ligament of left ankle
　● S93.419 Sprain of calcaneofibular ligament of unspecified ankle
● S93.42 Sprain of deltoid ligament
　● S93.421 Sprain of deltoid ligament of right ankle
　● S93.422 Sprain of deltoid ligament of left ankle
　● S93.429 Sprain of deltoid ligament of unspecified ankle
● S93.43 Sprain of tibiofibular ligament
　● S93.431 Sprain of tibiofibular ligament of right ankle
　● S93.432 Sprain of tibiofibular ligament of left ankle
　● S93.439 Sprain of tibiofibular ligament of unspecified ankle
● S93.49 Sprain of other ligament of ankle
　Sprain of internal collateral ligament
　Sprain of talofibular ligament
　● S93.491 Sprain of other ligament of right ankle
　● S93.492 Sprain of other ligament of left ankle
　● S93.499 Sprain of other ligament of unspecified ankle

◀ New　⬅ Revised　~~deleted~~ Deleted　Excludes 1　Excludes 2　Includes　Use additional　Code first　Code also　Unspecified

OGCR Official Guidelines　X Assign placeholder X　● Use Additional Character(s)　▶ Manifestation Code　**Coding Clinic**

● **S93.5 Sprain of toe**
  ● **S93.50 Unspecified sprain of toe**
    ● **S93.501 Unspecified sprain of right great toe**
    ● **S93.502 Unspecified sprain of left great toe**
    ● **S93.503 Unspecified sprain of unspecified great toe**
    ● **S93.504 Unspecified sprain of right lesser toe(s)**
    ● **S93.505 Unspecified sprain of left lesser toe(s)**
    ● **S93.506 Unspecified sprain of unspecified lesser toe(s)**
    ● **S93.509 Unspecified sprain of unspecified toe(s)**
  ● **S93.51 Sprain of interphalangeal joint of toe**
    ● **S93.511 Sprain of interphalangeal joint of right great toe**
    ● **S93.512 Sprain of interphalangeal joint of left great toe**
    ● **S93.513 Sprain of interphalangeal joint of unspecified great toe**
    ● **S93.514 Sprain of interphalangeal joint of right lesser toe(s)**
    ● **S93.515 Sprain of interphalangeal joint of left lesser toe(s)**
    ● **S93.516 Sprain of interphalangeal joint of unspecified lesser toe(s)**
    ● **S93.519 Sprain of interphalangeal joint of unspecified toe(s)**
  ● **S93.52 Sprain of metatarsophalangeal joint of toe**
    ● **S93.521 Sprain of metatarsophalangeal joint of right great toe**
    ● **S93.522 Sprain of metatarsophalangeal joint of left great toe**
    ● **S93.523 Sprain of metatarsophalangeal joint of unspecified great toe**
    ● **S93.524 Sprain of metatarsophalangeal joint of right lesser toe(s)**
    ● **S93.525 Sprain of metatarsophalangeal joint of left lesser toe(s)**
    ● **S93.526 Sprain of metatarsophalangeal joint of unspecified lesser toe(s)**
    ● **S93.529 Sprain of metatarsophalangeal joint of unspecified toe(s)**
● **S93.6 Sprain of foot**
  Excludes2 sprain of metatarsophalangeal joint of toe (S93.52-)
             sprain of toe (S93.5-)
  ● **S93.60 Unspecified sprain of foot**
    ● **S93.601 Unspecified sprain of right foot**
    ● **S93.602 Unspecified sprain of left foot**
    ● **S93.609 Unspecified sprain of unspecified foot**
  ● **S93.61 Sprain of tarsal ligament of foot**
    ● **S93.611 Sprain of tarsal ligament of right foot**
    ● **S93.612 Sprain of tarsal ligament of left foot**
    ● **S93.619 Sprain of tarsal ligament of unspecified foot**
  ● **S93.62 Sprain of tarsometatarsal ligament of foot**
    ● **S93.621 Sprain of tarsometatarsal ligament of right foot**
    ● **S93.622 Sprain of tarsometatarsal ligament of left foot**
    ● **S93.629 Sprain of tarsometatarsal ligament of unspecified foot**
  ● **S93.69 Other sprain of foot**
    ● **S93.691 Other sprain of right foot**
    ● **S93.692 Other sprain of left foot**
    ● **S93.699 Other sprain of unspecified foot**

● **S94 Injury of nerves at ankle and foot level**
  The appropriate 7th character is to be added to each code from category S94

A	initial encounter
D	subsequent encounter
S	sequela

  Code also any associated open wound (S91.-)
● **S94.0 Injury of lateral plantar nerve**
  X● **S94.00 Injury of lateral plantar nerve, unspecified leg**
  X● **S94.01 Injury of lateral plantar nerve, right leg**
  X● **S94.02 Injury of lateral plantar nerve, left leg**
● **S94.1 Injury of medial plantar nerve**
  X● **S94.10 Injury of medial plantar nerve, unspecified leg**
  X● **S94.11 Injury of medial plantar nerve, right leg**
  X● **S94.12 Injury of medial plantar nerve, left leg**
● **S94.2 Injury of deep peroneal nerve at ankle and foot level**
  Injury of terminal, lateral branch of deep peroneal nerve
  X● **S94.20 Injury of deep peroneal nerve at ankle and foot level, unspecified leg**
  X● **S94.21 Injury of deep peroneal nerve at ankle and foot level, right leg**
  X● **S94.22 Injury of deep peroneal nerve at ankle and foot level, left leg**
● **S94.3 Injury of cutaneous sensory nerve at ankle and foot level**
  X● **S94.30 Injury of cutaneous sensory nerve at ankle and foot level, unspecified leg**
  X● **S94.31 Injury of cutaneous sensory nerve at ankle and foot level, right leg**
  X● **S94.32 Injury of cutaneous sensory nerve at ankle and foot level, left leg**
● **S94.8 Injury of other nerves at ankle and foot level**
  ● **S94.8X Injury of other nerves at ankle and foot level**
    ● **S94.8X1 Injury of other nerves at ankle and foot level, right leg**
    ● **S94.8X2 Injury of other nerves at ankle and foot level, left leg**
    ● **S94.8X9 Injury of other nerves at ankle and foot level, unspecified leg**
● **S94.9 Injury of unspecified nerve at ankle and foot level**
  X● **S94.90 Injury of unspecified nerve at ankle and foot level, unspecified leg**
  X● **S94.91 Injury of unspecified nerve at ankle and foot level, right leg**
  X● **S94.92 Injury of unspecified nerve at ankle and foot level, left leg**

● **S95 Injury of blood vessels at ankle and foot level**
  Code also any associated open wound (S91.-)
  Excludes2 injury of posterior tibial artery and vein (S85.1-, S85.8-)
  The appropriate 7th character is to be added to each code from category S95

A	initial encounter
D	subsequent encounter
S	sequela

● **S95.0 Injury of dorsal artery of foot**
  ● **S95.00 Unspecified injury of dorsal artery of foot**
    ● **S95.001 Unspecified injury of dorsal artery of right foot**
    ● **S95.002 Unspecified injury of dorsal artery of left foot**
    ● **S95.009 Unspecified injury of dorsal artery of unspecified foot**

- S95.01   Laceration of dorsal artery of foot
  - S95.011   Laceration of dorsal artery of right foot
  - S95.012   Laceration of dorsal artery of left foot
  - S95.019   Laceration of dorsal artery of unspecified foot
- S95.09   Other specified injury of dorsal artery of foot
  - S95.091   Other specified injury of dorsal artery of right foot
  - S95.092   Other specified injury of dorsal artery of left foot
  - S95.099   Other specified injury of dorsal artery of unspecified foot
- S95.1   Injury of plantar artery of foot
  - S95.10   Unspecified injury of plantar artery of foot
    - S95.101   Unspecified injury of plantar artery of right foot
    - S95.102   Unspecified injury of plantar artery of left foot
    - S95.109   Unspecified injury of plantar artery of unspecified foot
  - S95.11   Laceration of plantar artery of foot
    - S95.111   Laceration of plantar artery of right foot
    - S95.112   Laceration of plantar artery of left foot
    - S95.119   Laceration of plantar artery of unspecified foot
  - S95.19   Other specified injury of plantar artery of foot
    - S95.191   Other specified injury of plantar artery of right foot
    - S95.192   Other specified injury of plantar artery of left foot
    - S95.199   Other specified injury of plantar artery of unspecified foot
- S95.2   Injury of dorsal vein of foot
  - S95.20   Unspecified injury of dorsal vein of foot
    - S95.201   Unspecified injury of dorsal vein of right foot
    - S95.202   Unspecified injury of dorsal vein of left foot
    - S95.209   Unspecified injury of dorsal vein of unspecified foot
  - S95.21   Laceration of dorsal vein of foot
    - S95.211   Laceration of dorsal vein of right foot
    - S95.212   Laceration of dorsal vein of left foot
    - S95.219   Laceration of dorsal vein of unspecified foot
  - S95.29   Other specified injury of dorsal vein of foot
    - S95.291   Other specified injury of dorsal vein of right foot
    - S95.292   Other specified injury of dorsal vein of left foot
    - S95.299   Other specified injury of dorsal vein of unspecified foot

- S95.8   Injury of other blood vessels at ankle and foot level
  - S95.80   Unspecified injury of other blood vessels at ankle and foot level
    - S95.801   Unspecified injury of other blood vessels at ankle and foot level, right leg
    - S95.802   Unspecified injury of other blood vessels at ankle and foot level, left leg
    - S95.809   Unspecified injury of other blood vessels at ankle and foot level, unspecified leg
  - S95.81   Laceration of other blood vessels at ankle and foot level
    - S95.811   Laceration of other blood vessels at ankle and foot level, right leg
    - S95.812   Laceration of other blood vessels at ankle and foot level, left leg
    - S95.819   Laceration of other blood vessels at ankle and foot level, unspecified leg
  - S95.89   Other specified injury of other blood vessels at ankle and foot level
    - S95.891   Other specified injury of other blood vessels at ankle and foot level, right leg
    - S95.892   Other specified injury of other blood vessels at ankle and foot level, left leg
    - S95.899   Other specified injury of other blood vessels at ankle and foot level, unspecified leg
- S95.9   Injury of unspecified blood vessel at ankle and foot level
  - S95.90   Unspecified injury of unspecified blood vessel at ankle and foot level
    - S95.901   Unspecified injury of unspecified blood vessel at ankle and foot level, right leg
    - S95.902   Unspecified injury of unspecified blood vessel at ankle and foot level, left leg
    - S95.909   Unspecified injury of unspecified blood vessel at ankle and foot level, unspecified leg
  - S95.91   Laceration of unspecified blood vessel at ankle and foot level
    - S95.911   Laceration of unspecified blood vessel at ankle and foot level, right leg
    - S95.912   Laceration of unspecified blood vessel at ankle and foot level, left leg
    - S95.919   Laceration of unspecified blood vessel at ankle and foot level, unspecified leg
  - S95.99   Other specified injury of unspecified blood vessel at ankle and foot level
    - S95.991   Other specified injury of unspecified blood vessel at ankle and foot level, right leg
    - S95.992   Other specified injury of unspecified blood vessel at ankle and foot level, left leg
    - S95.999   Other specified injury of unspecified blood vessel at ankle and foot level, unspecified leg

◀ New   ◀▥ Revised   ~~deleted~~ Deleted   Excludes 1   Excludes 2   Includes   Use additional   Code first   Code also   Unspecified

OGCR Official Guidelines   X Assign placeholder X   ● Use Additional Character(s)   ▸ Manifestation Code   **Coding Clinic**

● **S96**   **Injury of muscle and tendon at ankle and foot level**

     Code also any associated open wound (S91.-)

     Excludes2   injury of Achilles tendon (S86.0-)
                     sprain of joints and ligaments of ankle and foot
                     (S93.-)

     The appropriate 7th character is to be added to each code from
     category S96

> A   initial encounter
> D   subsequent encounter
> S   sequela

● **S96.0**   **Injury of muscle and tendon of long flexor muscle of toe at ankle and foot level**

   ● **S96.00**   Unspecified injury of muscle and tendon of long flexor muscle of toe at ankle and foot level

     ● **S96.001**   Unspecified injury of muscle and tendon of long flexor muscle of toe at ankle and foot level, right foot

     ● **S96.002**   Unspecified injury of muscle and tendon of long flexor muscle of toe at ankle and foot level, left foot

     ● **S96.009**   Unspecified injury of muscle and tendon of long flexor muscle of toe at ankle and foot level, unspecified foot

   ● **S96.01**   Strain of muscle and tendon of long flexor muscle of toe at ankle and foot level

     ● **S96.011**   Strain of muscle and tendon of long flexor muscle of toe at ankle and foot level, right foot

     ● **S96.012**   Strain of muscle and tendon of long flexor muscle of toe at ankle and foot level, left foot

     ● **S96.019**   Strain of muscle and tendon of long flexor muscle of toe at ankle and foot level, unspecified foot

   ● **S96.02**   Laceration of muscle and tendon of long flexor muscle of toe at ankle and foot level

     ● **S96.021**   Laceration of muscle and tendon of long flexor muscle of toe at ankle and foot level, right foot

     ● **S96.022**   Laceration of muscle and tendon of long flexor muscle of toe at ankle and foot level, left foot

     ● **S96.029**   Laceration of muscle and tendon of long flexor muscle of toe at ankle and foot level, unspecified foot

   ● **S96.09**   Other injury of muscle and tendon of long flexor muscle of toe at ankle and foot level

     ● **S96.091**   Other injury of muscle and tendon of long flexor muscle of toe at ankle and foot level, right foot

     ● **S96.092**   Other injury of muscle and tendon of long flexor muscle of toe at ankle and foot level, left foot

     ● **S96.099**   Other injury of muscle and tendon of long flexor muscle of toe at ankle and foot level, unspecified foot

● **S96.1**   **Injury of muscle and tendon of long extensor muscle of toe at ankle and foot level**

   ● **S96.10**   Unspecified injury of muscle and tendon of long extensor muscle of toe at ankle and foot level

     ● **S96.101**   Unspecified injury of muscle and tendon of long extensor muscle of toe at ankle and foot level, right foot

     ● **S96.102**   Unspecified injury of muscle and tendon of long extensor muscle of toe at ankle and foot level, left foot

     ● **S96.109**   Unspecified injury of muscle and tendon of long extensor muscle of toe at ankle and foot level, unspecified foot

● **S96.11**   **Strain of muscle and tendon of long extensor muscle of toe at ankle and foot level**

   ● **S96.111**   Strain of muscle and tendon of long extensor muscle of toe at ankle and foot level, right foot

   ● **S96.112**   Strain of muscle and tendon of long extensor muscle of toe at ankle and foot level, left foot

   ● **S96.119**   Strain of muscle and tendon of long extensor muscle of toe at ankle and foot level, unspecified foot

● **S96.12**   Laceration of muscle and tendon of long extensor muscle of toe at ankle and foot level

   ● **S96.121**   Laceration of muscle and tendon of long extensor muscle of toe at ankle and foot level, right foot

   ● **S96.122**   Laceration of muscle and tendon of long extensor muscle of toe at ankle and foot level, left foot

   ● **S96.129**   Laceration of muscle and tendon of long extensor muscle of toe at ankle and foot level, unspecified foot

● **S96.19**   Other specified injury of muscle and tendon of long extensor muscle of toe at ankle and foot level

   ● **S96.191**   Other specified injury of muscle and tendon of long extensor muscle of toe at ankle and foot level, right foot

   ● **S96.192**   Other specified injury of muscle and tendon of long extensor muscle of toe at ankle and foot level, left foot

   ● **S96.199**   Other specified injury of muscle and tendon of long extensor muscle of toe at ankle and foot level, unspecified foot

● **S96.2**   **Injury of intrinsic muscle and tendon at ankle and foot level**

   ● **S96.20**   Unspecified injury of intrinsic muscle and tendon at ankle and foot level

     ● **S96.201**   Unspecified injury of intrinsic muscle and tendon at ankle and foot level, right foot

     ● **S96.202**   Unspecified injury of intrinsic muscle and tendon at ankle and foot level, left foot

     ● **S96.209**   Unspecified injury of intrinsic muscle and tendon at ankle and foot level, unspecified foot

   ● **S96.21**   Strain of intrinsic muscle and tendon at ankle and foot level

     ● **S96.211**   Strain of intrinsic muscle and tendon at ankle and foot level, right foot

     ● **S96.212**   Strain of intrinsic muscle and tendon at ankle and foot level, left foot

     ● **S96.219**   Strain of intrinsic muscle and tendon at ankle and foot level, unspecified foot

   ● **S96.22**   Laceration of intrinsic muscle and tendon at ankle and foot level

     ● **S96.221**   Laceration of intrinsic muscle and tendon at ankle and foot level, right foot

     ● **S96.222**   Laceration of intrinsic muscle and tendon at left ankle and foot level, left foot

     ● **S96.229**   Laceration of intrinsic muscle and tendon at ankle and foot level, unspecified foot

CHAPTER 19 (S00-T88)

● S96.29   Other specified injury of intrinsic muscle and tendon at ankle and foot level
   ● S96.291   Other specified injury of intrinsic muscle and tendon at ankle and foot level, right foot
   ● S96.292   Other specified injury of intrinsic muscle and tendon at ankle and foot level, left foot
   ● S96.299   Other specified injury of intrinsic muscle and tendon at ankle and foot level, unspecified foot

● S96.8   Injury of other specified muscles and tendons at ankle and foot level
  ● S96.80   Unspecified injury of other specified muscles and tendons at ankle and foot level
   ● S96.801   Unspecified injury of other specified muscles and tendons at ankle and foot level, right foot
   ● S96.802   Unspecified injury of other specified muscles and tendons at ankle and foot level, left foot
   ● S96.809   Unspecified injury of other specified muscles and tendons at ankle and foot level, unspecified foot
  ● S96.81   Strain of other specified muscles and tendons at ankle and foot level
   ● S96.811   Strain of other specified muscles and tendons at ankle and foot level, right foot
   ● S96.812   Strain of other specified muscles and tendons at ankle and foot level, left foot
   ● S96.819   Strain of other specified muscles and tendons at ankle and foot level, unspecified foot
  ● S96.82   Laceration of other specified muscles and tendons at ankle and foot level
   ● S96.821   Laceration of other specified muscles and tendons at ankle and foot level, right foot
   ● S96.822   Laceration of other specified muscles and tendons at ankle and foot level, left foot
   ● S96.829   Laceration of other specified muscles and tendons at ankle and foot level, unspecified foot
  ● S96.89   Other specified injury of other specified muscles and tendons at ankle and foot level
   ● S96.891   Other specified injury of other specified muscles and tendons at ankle and foot level, right foot
   ● S96.892   Other specified injury of other specified muscles and tendons at ankle and foot level, left foot
   ● S96.899   Other specified injury of other specified muscles and tendons at ankle and foot level, unspecified foot

● S96.9   Injury of unspecified muscle and tendon at ankle and foot level
  ● S96.90   Unspecified injury of unspecified muscle and tendon at ankle and foot level
   ● S96.901   Unspecified injury of unspecified muscle and tendon at ankle and foot level, right foot
   ● S96.902   Unspecified injury of unspecified muscle and tendon at ankle and foot level, left foot
   ● S96.909   Unspecified injury of unspecified muscle and tendon at ankle and foot level, unspecified foot

  ● S96.91   Strain of unspecified muscle and tendon at ankle and foot level
   ● S96.911   Strain of unspecified muscle and tendon at ankle and foot level, right foot
   ● S96.912   Strain of unspecified muscle and tendon at ankle and foot level, left foot
   ● S96.919   Strain of unspecified muscle and tendon at ankle and foot level, unspecified foot
  ● S96.92   Laceration of unspecified muscle and tendon at ankle and foot level
   ● S96.921   Laceration of unspecified muscle and tendon at ankle and foot level, right foot
   ● S96.922   Laceration of unspecified muscle and tendon at ankle and foot level, left foot
   ● S96.929   Laceration of unspecified muscle and tendon at ankle and foot level, unspecified foot
  ● S96.99   Other specified injury of unspecified muscle and tendon at ankle and foot level
   ● S96.991   Other specified injury of unspecified muscle and tendon at ankle and foot level, right foot
   ● S96.992   Other specified injury of unspecified muscle and tendon at ankle and foot level, left foot
   ● S96.999   Other specified injury of unspecified muscle and tendon at ankle and foot level, unspecified foot

● S97   **Crushing injury of ankle and foot**
   Use additional code(s) for all associated injuries
   The appropriate 7th character is to be added to each code from category S97

A	initial encounter
D	subsequent encounter
S	sequela

  ● S97.0   Crushing injury of ankle
   X ● S97.00   Crushing injury of unspecified ankle
   X ● S97.01   Crushing injury of right ankle
   X ● S97.02   Crushing injury of left ankle
  ● S97.1   Crushing injury of toe
   ● S97.10   Crushing injury of unspecified toe(s)
    ● S97.101   Crushing injury of unspecified right toe(s)
    ● S97.102   Crushing injury of unspecified left toe(s)
    ● S97.109   Crushing injury of unspecified toe(s)
     Crushing injury of toe NOS
   ● S97.11   Crushing injury of great toe
    ● S97.111   Crushing injury of right great toe
    ● S97.112   Crushing injury of left great toe
    ● S97.119   Crushing injury of unspecified great toe
   ● S97.12   Crushing injury of lesser toe(s)
    ● S97.121   Crushing injury of right lesser toe(s)
    ● S97.122   Crushing injury of left lesser toe(s)
    ● S97.129   Crushing injury of lesser toe(s), unspecified toe(s)
  ● S97.8   Crushing injury of foot
   X ● S97.80   Crushing injury of foot, unspecified side
     Crushing injury of foot NOS
   X ● S97.81   Crushing injury of right foot
   X ● S97.82   Crushing injury of left foot

◀ New   ⬅ Revised   ~~deleted~~ Deleted   Excludes 1   Excludes 2   Includes   Use additional   Code first   Code also   Unspecified

OGCR Official Guidelines   X Assign placeholder X   ● Use Additional Character(s)   ▶ Manifestation Code   **Coding Clinic**

● **S98   Traumatic amputation of ankle and foot**
     An amputation not identified as partial or complete should be
     coded to complete
     The appropriate 7th character is to be added to each code from
     category S98

A	initial encounter
D	subsequent encounter
S	sequela

 ● **S98.0   Traumatic amputation of foot at ankle level**
   ● **S98.01   Complete traumatic amputation of foot at ankle level**
      ● S98.011   Complete traumatic amputation of right foot at ankle level
      ● S98.012   Complete traumatic amputation of left foot at ankle level
      ● S98.019   Complete traumatic amputation of unspecified foot at ankle level
   ● **S98.02   Partial traumatic amputation of foot at ankle level**
      ● S98.021   Partial traumatic amputation of right foot at ankle level
      ● S98.022   Partial traumatic amputation of left foot at ankle level
      ● S98.029   Partial traumatic amputation of unspecified foot at ankle level

 ● **S98.1   Traumatic amputation of one toe**
   ● **S98.11   Complete traumatic amputation of great toe**
      ● S98.111   Complete traumatic amputation of right great toe
      ● S98.112   Complete traumatic amputation of left great toe
      ● S98.119   Complete traumatic amputation of unspecified great toe
   ● **S98.12   Partial traumatic amputation of great toe**
      ● S98.121   Partial traumatic amputation of right great toe
      ● S98.122   Partial traumatic amputation of left great toe
      ● S98.129   Partial traumatic amputation of unspecified great toe
   ● **S98.13   Complete traumatic amputation of one lesser toe**
       Traumatic amputation of toe NOS
      ● S98.131   Complete traumatic amputation of one right lesser toe
      ● S98.132   Complete traumatic amputation of one left lesser toe
      ● S98.139   Complete traumatic amputation of one unspecified lesser toe
   ● **S98.14   Partial traumatic amputation of one lesser toe**
      ● S98.141   Partial traumatic amputation of one right lesser toe
      ● S98.142   Partial traumatic amputation of one left lesser toe
      ● S98.149   Partial traumatic amputation of one unspecified lesser toe

 ● **S98.2   Traumatic amputation of two or more lesser toes**
   ● **S98.21   Complete traumatic amputation of two or more lesser toes**
      ● S98.211   Complete traumatic amputation of two or more right lesser toes
      ● S98.212   Complete traumatic amputation of two or more left lesser toes
      ● S98.219   Complete traumatic amputation of two or more unspecified lesser toes

   ● **S98.22   Partial traumatic amputation of two or more lesser toes**
      ● S98.221   Partial traumatic amputation of two or more right lesser toes
      ● S98.222   Partial traumatic amputation of two or more left lesser toes
      ● S98.229   Partial traumatic amputation of two or more unspecified lesser toes

 ● **S98.3   Traumatic amputation of midfoot**
   ● **S98.31   Complete traumatic amputation of midfoot**
      ● S98.311   Complete traumatic amputation of right midfoot
      ● S98.312   Complete traumatic amputation of left midfoot
      ● S98.319   Complete traumatic amputation of unspecified midfoot
   ● **S98.32   Partial traumatic amputation of midfoot**
      ● S98.321   Partial traumatic amputation of right midfoot
      ● S98.322   Partial traumatic amputation of left midfoot
      ● S98.329   Partial traumatic amputation of unspecified midfoot

 ● **S98.9   Traumatic amputation of foot, level unspecified**
   ● **S98.91   Complete traumatic amputation of foot, level unspecified**
      ● S98.911   Complete traumatic amputation of right foot, level unspecified
      ● S98.912   Complete traumatic amputation of left foot, level unspecified
      ● S98.919   Complete traumatic amputation of unspecified foot, level unspecified
   ● **S98.92   Partial traumatic amputation of foot, level unspecified**
      ● S98.921   Partial traumatic amputation of right foot, level unspecified
      ● S98.922   Partial traumatic amputation of left foot, level unspecified
      ● S98.929   Partial traumatic amputation of unspecified foot, level unspecified

● **S99   Other and unspecified injuries of ankle and foot**
     The appropriate 7th character is to be added to each code from
     category S99

A	initial encounter
D	subsequent encounter
S	sequela

 ● **S99.8   Other specified injuries of ankle and foot**
   ● **S99.81   Other specified injuries of ankle**
      ● S99.811   Other specified injuries of right ankle
      ● S99.812   Other specified injuries of left ankle
      ● S99.819   Other specified injuries of unspecified ankle
   ● **S99.82   Other specified injuries of foot**
      ● S99.821   Other specified injuries of right foot
      ● S99.822   Other specified injuries of left foot
      ● S99.829   Other specified injuries of unspecified foot

 ● **S99.9   Unspecified injury of ankle and foot**
   ● **S99.91   Unspecified injury of ankle**
      ● S99.911   Unspecified injury of right ankle
      ● S99.912   Unspecified injury of left ankle
      ● S99.919   Unspecified injury of unspecified ankle
   ● **S99.92   Unspecified injury of foot**
      ● S99.921   Unspecified injury of right foot
      ● S99.922   Unspecified injury of left foot
      ● S99.929   Unspecified injury of unspecified foot

CHAPTER 19 (S00-T88)

CHAPTER 19 (S00-T88)

INJURY, POISONING AND CERTAIN OTHER CONSEQUENCES OF EXTERNAL CAUSES (T07-T88)

INJURIES INVOLVING MULTIPLE BODY REGIONS (T07)

Excludes1   burns and corrosions (T20-T32)
                frostbite (T33-T34)
                insect bite or sting, venomous (T63.4)
                sunburn (L55.-)

T07   Unspecified multiple injuries

       Excludes1   injury NOS (T14)

INJURY OF UNSPECIFIED BODY REGION (T14)

● **T14**   Injury of unspecified body region

       Excludes1   multiple unspecified injuries (T07)

       T14.8   Other injury of unspecified body region
              Abrasion NOS   Fracture NOS
              Contusion NOS   Skin injury NOS
              Crush injury NOS   Vascular injury NOS

      ● **T14.9**   Unspecified injury

          T14.90   Injury, unspecified
                  Injury NOS

          T14.91   Suicide attempt
                  Attempted suicide NOS

EFFECTS OF FOREIGN BODY ENTERING THROUGH NATURAL ORIFICE (T15-T19)

       Excludes2   foreign body accidentally left in operation wound (T81.5-)
                foreign body in penetrating wound - see open wound by body region
                residual foreign body in soft tissue (M79.5)
                splinter, without open wound - see superficial injury by body region

● **T15**   Foreign body on external eye

       Excludes2   foreign body in penetrating wound of orbit and eye ball (S05.4-, S05.5-)
                open wound of eyelid and periocular area (S01.1-)
                retained foreign body in eyelid (H02.8-)
                retained (old) foreign body in penetrating wound of orbit and eye ball (H05.5-, H44.6-, H44.7-)
                superficial foreign body of eyelid and periocular area (S00.25-)

       The appropriate 7th character is to be added to each code from category T15

A	initial encounter
D	subsequent encounter
S	sequela

      ● **T15.0**   Foreign body in cornea

     X ● **T15.00**   Foreign body in cornea, unspecified eye

     X ● **T15.01**   Foreign body in cornea, right eye

     X ● **T15.02**   Foreign body in cornea, left eye

      ● **T15.1**   Foreign body in conjunctival sac

     X ● **T15.10**   Foreign body in conjunctival sac, unspecified eye

     X ● **T15.11**   Foreign body in conjunctival sac, right eye

     X ● **T15.12**   Foreign body in conjunctival sac, left eye

      ● **T15.8**   Foreign body in other and multiple parts of external eye
              Foreign body in lacrimal punctum

     X ● **T15.80**   Foreign body in other and multiple parts of external eye, unspecified eye

     X ● **T15.81**   Foreign body in other and multiple parts of external eye, right eye

     X ● **T15.82**   Foreign body in other and multiple parts of external eye, left eye

● **T15.9**   Foreign body on external eye, part unspecified

     X ● **T15.90**   Foreign body on external eye, part unspecified, unspecified eye

     X ● **T15.91**   Foreign body on external eye, part unspecified, right eye

     X ● **T15.92**   Foreign body on external eye, part unspecified, left eye

● **T16**   Foreign body in ear

       Includes   foreign body in auditory canal

       The appropriate 7th character is to be added to each code from category T16

A	initial encounter
D	subsequent encounter
S	sequela

     X ● **T16.1**   Foreign body in right ear

     X ● **T16.2**   Foreign body in left ear

     X ● **T16.9**   Foreign body in ear, unspecified ear

● **T17**   Foreign body in respiratory tract

       The appropriate 7th character is to be added to each code from category T17

A	initial encounter
D	subsequent encounter
S	sequela

     X ● **T17.0**   Foreign body in nasal sinus

     X ● **T17.1**   Foreign body in nostril
             Foreign body in nose NOS

      ● **T17.2**   Foreign body in pharynx
             Foreign body in nasopharynx
             Foreign body in throat NOS

      ● **T17.20**   Unspecified foreign body in pharynx

         ● **T17.200**   Unspecified foreign body in pharynx causing asphyxiation

         ● **T17.208**   Unspecified foreign body in pharynx causing other injury

      ● **T17.21**   Gastric contents in pharynx
              Aspiration of gastric contents into pharynx
              Vomitus in pharynx

         ● **T17.210**   Gastric contents in pharynx causing asphyxiation

         ● **T17.218**   Gastric contents in pharynx causing other injury

      ● **T17.22**   Food in pharynx
              Bones in pharynx
              Seeds in pharynx

         ● **T17.220**   Food in pharynx causing asphyxiation

         ● **T17.228**   Food in pharynx causing other injury

      ● **T17.29**   Other foreign object in pharynx

         ● **T17.290**   Other foreign object in pharynx causing asphyxiation

         ● **T17.298**   Other foreign object in pharynx causing other injury

      ● **T17.3**   Foreign body in larynx

      ● **T17.30**   Unspecified foreign body in larynx

         ● **T17.300**   Unspecified foreign body in larynx causing asphyxiation

         ● **T17.308**   Unspecified foreign body in larynx causing other injury

      ● **T17.31**   Gastric contents in larynx
              Aspiration of gastric contents into larynx
              Vomitus in larynx

         ● **T17.310**   Gastric contents in larynx causing asphyxiation

         ● **T17.318**   Gastric contents in larynx causing other injury

◀ New   ◀▬ Revised   ~~deleted~~ Deleted   Excludes 1   Excludes 2   Includes   Use additional   Code first   Code also   Unspecified

OGCR Official Guidelines   X Assign placeholder X   ● Use Additional Character(s)   ▶ Manifestation Code   **Coding Clinic**

● **T17.32**   **Food in larynx**
     Bones in larynx
     Seeds in larynx
  ● **T17.320**   **Food in larynx causing asphyxiation**
  ● **T17.328**   **Food in larynx causing other injury**
● **T17.39**   **Other foreign object in larynx**
  ● **T17.390**   **Other foreign object in larynx causing asphyxiation**
  ● **T17.398**   **Other foreign object in larynx causing other injury**

● **T17.4**   **Foreign body in trachea**
 ● **T17.40**   **Unspecified foreign body in trachea**
  ● **T17.400**   Unspecified **foreign body in trachea causing asphyxiation**
  ● **T17.408**   Unspecified **foreign body in trachea causing other injury**
 ● **T17.41**   **Gastric contents in trachea**
     Aspiration of gastric contents into trachea
     Vomitus in trachea
  ● **T17.410**   **Gastric contents in trachea causing asphyxiation**
  ● **T17.418**   **Gastric contents in trachea causing other injury**
 ● **T17.42**   **Food in trachea**
     Bones in trachea
     Seeds in trachea
  ● **T17.420**   **Food in trachea causing asphyxiation**
  ● **T17.428**   **Food in trachea causing other injury**
 ● **T17.49**   **Other foreign object in trachea**
  ● **T17.490**   **Other foreign object in trachea causing asphyxiation**
  ● **T17.498**   **Other foreign object in trachea causing other injury**

● **T17.5**   **Foreign body in bronchus**
 ● **T17.50**   **Unspecified foreign body in bronchus**
  ● **T17.500**   Unspecified **foreign body in bronchus causing asphyxiation**
  ● **T17.508**   Unspecified **foreign body in bronchus causing other injury**
 ● **T17.51**   **Gastric contents in bronchus**
     Aspiration of gastric contents into bronchus
     Vomitus in bronchus
  ● **T17.510**   **Gastric contents in bronchus causing asphyxiation**
  ● **T17.518**   **Gastric contents in bronchus causing other injury**
 ● **T17.52**   **Food in bronchus**
     Bones in bronchus
     Seeds in bronchus
  ● **T17.520**   **Food in bronchus causing asphyxiation**
  ● **T17.528**   **Food in bronchus causing other injury**
 ● **T17.59**   **Other foreign object in bronchus**
  ● **T17.590**   **Other foreign object in bronchus causing asphyxiation**
  ● **T17.598**   **Other foreign object in bronchus causing other injury**

● **T17.8**   **Foreign body in other parts of respiratory tract**
     Foreign body in bronchioles
     Foreign body in lung
 ● **T17.80**   **Unspecified foreign body in other parts of respiratory tract**
  ● **T17.800**   Unspecified **foreign body in other parts of respiratory tract causing asphyxiation**
  ● **T17.808**   Unspecified **foreign body in other parts of respiratory tract causing other injury**
 ● **T17.81**   **Gastric contents in other parts of respiratory tract**
     Aspiration of gastric contents into other parts of respiratory tract
     Vomitus in other parts of respiratory tract
  ● **T17.810**   **Gastric contents in other parts of respiratory tract causing asphyxiation**
  ● **T17.818**   **Gastric contents in other parts of respiratory tract causing other injury**
 ● **T17.82**   **Food in other parts of respiratory tract**
     Bones in other parts of respiratory tract
     Seeds in other parts of respiratory tract
  ● **T17.820**   **Food in other parts of respiratory tract causing asphyxiation**
  ● **T17.828**   **Food in other parts of respiratory tract causing other injury**
 ● **T17.89**   **Other foreign object in other parts of respiratory tract**
  ● **T17.890**   **Other foreign object in other parts of respiratory tract causing asphyxiation**
  ● **T17.898**   **Other foreign object in other parts of respiratory tract causing other injury**

● **T17.9**   **Foreign body in respiratory tract, part unspecified**
 ● **T17.90**   **Unspecified foreign body in respiratory tract, part unspecified**
  ● **T17.900**   Unspecified **foreign body in respiratory tract, part unspecified causing asphyxiation**
  ● **T17.908**   Unspecified **foreign body in respiratory tract, part unspecified causing other injury**
 ● **T17.91**   **Gastric contents in respiratory tract, part unspecified**
     Aspiration of gastric contents into respiratory tract, part unspecified
     Vomitus in trachea respiratory tract, part unspecified
  ● **T17.910**   **Gastric contents in respiratory tract, part** unspecified **causing asphyxiation**
  ● **T17.918**   **Gastric contents in respiratory tract, part** unspecified **causing other injury**
 ● **T17.92**   **Food in respiratory tract, part unspecified**
     Bones in respiratory tract, part unspecified
     Seeds in respiratory tract, part unspecified
  ● **T17.920**   **Food in respiratory tract, part** unspecified **causing asphyxiation**
  ● **T17.928**   **Food in respiratory tract, part** unspecified **causing other injury**
 ● **T17.99**   **Other foreign object in respiratory tract, part unspecified**
  ● **T17.990**   **Other foreign object in respiratory tract, part** unspecified **in causing asphyxiation**
  ● **T17.998**   **Other foreign object in respiratory tract, part** unspecified **causing other injury**

CHAPTER 19 (S00-T88)

CHAPTER 19 (S00-T88)

● **T18**   **Foreign body in alimentary tract**
   Excludes2   foreign body in pharynx (T17.2-)
   The appropriate 7th character is to be added to each code from
     category T18

> A   initial encounter
> D   subsequent encounter
> S   sequela

X● **T18.0**   **Foreign body in mouth**
X● **T18.1**   **Foreign body in esophagus**
   Excludes2   foreign body in respiratory tract (T17.-)
  ● **T18.10**   **Unspecified foreign body in esophagus**
    ● **T18.100**   **Unspecified foreign body in esophagus causing compression of trachea**
       Unspecified foreign body in esophagus causing obstruction of respiration
    ● **T18.108**   **Unspecified foreign body in esophagus causing other injury**
  ● **T18.11**   **Gastric contents in esophagus**
      Vomitus in esophagus
    ● **T18.110**   **Gastric contents in esophagus causing compression of trachea**
       Gastric contents in esophagus causing obstruction of respiration
    ● **T18.118**   **Gastric contents in esophagus causing other injury**
  ● **T18.12**   **Food in esophagus**
      Bones in esophagus
      Seeds in esophagus
    ● **T18.120**   **Food in esophagus causing compression of trachea**
       Food in esophagus causing obstruction of respiration
    ● **T18.128**   **Food in esophagus causing other injury**
  ● **T18.19**   **Other foreign object in esophagus**
    ● **T18.190**   **Other foreign object in esophagus causing compression of trachea**
       Other foreign body in esophagus causing obstruction of respiration
       Coding Clinic: 2015, Q1, P24
    ● **T18.198**   **Other foreign object in esophagus causing other injury**
       Coding Clinic: 2015, Q1, P24
X● **T18.2**   **Foreign body in stomach**
X● **T18.3**   **Foreign body in small intestine**
X● **T18.4**   **Foreign body in colon**
X● **T18.5**   **Foreign body in anus and rectum**
      Foreign body in rectosigmoid (junction)
X● **T18.8**   **Foreign body in other parts of alimentary tract**
X● **T18.9**   **Foreign body of alimentary tract, part unspecified**
      Foreign body in digestive system NOS
      Swallowed foreign body NOS

● **T19**   **Foreign body in genitourinary tract**
   Excludes2   complications due to implanted mesh (T83.7-)
      mechanical complications of contraceptive device (intrauterine) (vaginal) (T83.3-)
      presence of contraceptive device (intrauterine) (vaginal) (Z97.5)
   The appropriate 7th character is to be added to each code from
     category T19

> A   initial encounter
> D   subsequent encounter
> S   sequela

X● **T19.0**   **Foreign body in urethra**
X● **T19.1**   **Foreign body in bladder**
X● **T19.2**   **Foreign body in vulva and vagina** ♀
X● **T19.3**   **Foreign body in uterus** ♀
X● **T19.4**   **Foreign body in penis** ♂
X● **T19.8**   **Foreign body in other parts of genitourinary tract**
X● **T19.9**   **Foreign body in genitourinary tract, part unspecified**

BURNS AND CORROSIONS (T20-T32)

Includes   burns (thermal) from electrical heating appliances
      burns (thermal) from electricity
      burns (thermal) from flame
      burns (thermal) from friction
      burns (thermal) from hot air and hot gases
      burns (thermal) from hot objects
      burns (thermal) from lightning
      burns (thermal) from radiation chemical
      burn [corrosion] (external) (internal) scalds

Excludes2   erythema [dermatitis] ab igne (L59.0)
      radiation-related disorders of the skin and subcutaneous tissue (L55-L59)
      sunburn (L55.-)

OGCR Section I.C.19.d.

Burns and Corrosions
The ICD-10-CM makes a distinction between burn and corrosions. The burn codes are for thermal burns, except sunburns, that come from a heat source, such as a fire or hot appliance. The burn codes are also for burns resulting from electricity and radiation. Corrosions are burns due to chemicals. The guidelines for burns and corrosions are the same.

Current burns (T20-T25) are classified by depth, extent and by agent (X code). Burns are classified by depth as first degree (erythema), second degree (blistering), and third degree (full-thickness involvement). Burns of the eye and internal organs (T26-T28) are classified by site, but not by degree.

1) Sequencing of burn and related condition codes
Sequence first the code that reflects the highest degree of burn when more than one burn is present.

a. When the reason for the admission or encounter is for treatment of external multiple burns, sequence first the code that reflects the burn of the highest degree.

b. When a patient has both internal and external burns, the circumstances of admission govern the selection of the principal diagnosis or first-listed diagnosis.

c. When a patient is admitted for burn injuries and other related conditions such as smoke inhalation and/or respiratory failure, the circumstances of admission govern the selection of the principal or first-listed diagnosis.

2) Burns of the same local site
Classify burns of the same local site (three-character category level, T20-T28) but of different degrees to the subcategory identifying the highest degree recorded in the diagnosis.

◀ New   ⇐ Revised   ~~deleted~~ Deleted   Excludes 1   Excludes 2   Includes   Use additional   Code first   Code also   Unspecified
OGCR Official Guidelines   **X** Assign placeholder X   ● Use Additional Character(s)   ▶ Manifestation Code   **Coding Clinic**

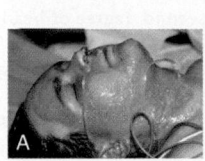
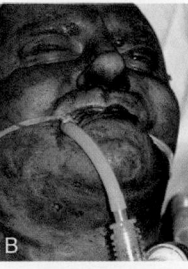

Figure 19-14 **A.** Second-degree burn. **B.** Third-degree burn. (From Cummings: Otolaryngology: Head & Neck Surgery, ed 4, Mosby, 2005)

BURNS AND CORROSIONS OF EXTERNAL BODY SURFACE, SPECIFIED BY SITE (T20-T25)

Includes   burns and corrosions of first degree [erythema]
burns and corrosions of second degree [blisters] [epidermal loss]
burns and corrosions of third degree [deep necrosis of underlying tissue] [full-thickness skin loss]

Use additional code from category T31 or T32 to identify extent of body surface involved

● **T20   Burn and corrosion of head, face, and neck**

Excludes2   burn and corrosion of ear drum (T28.41, T28.91)
burn and corrosion of eye and adnexa (T26.-)
burn and corrosion of mouth and pharynx (T28.0)

The appropriate 7th character is to be added to each code from category T20

> A   initial encounter
> D   subsequent encounter
> S   sequela

● **T20.0   Burn of unspecified degree of head, face, and neck**

Use additional external cause code to identify the source, place and intent of the burn (X00-X19, X75-X77, X96-X98, Y92)

X● **T20.00**   Burn of unspecified degree of head, face, and neck, unspecified site

● **T20.01**   Burn of unspecified degree of ear [any part, except ear drum]

Excludes2   burn of ear drum (T28.41-)

● **T20.011**   Burn of unspecified degree of right ear [any part, except ear drum]

● **T20.012**   Burn of unspecified degree of left ear [any part, except ear drum]

● **T20.019**   Burn of unspecified degree of unspecified ear [any part, except ear drum]

X● **T20.02**   Burn of unspecified degree of lip(s)

X● **T20.03**   Burn of unspecified degree of chin

X● **T20.04**   Burn of unspecified degree of nose (septum)

X● **T20.05**   Burn of unspecified degree of scalp [any part]

X● **T20.06**   Burn of unspecified degree of forehead and cheek

X● **T20.07**   Burn of unspecified degree of neck

X● **T20.09**   Burn of unspecified degree of multiple sites of head, face, and neck

● **T20.1   Burn of first degree of head, face, and neck**

Use additional external cause code to identify the source, place and intent of the burn (X00-X19, X75-X77, X96-X98, Y92)

X● **T20.10**   Burn of first degree of head, face, and neck, unspecified site

● **T20.11**   Burn of first degree of ear [any part, except ear drum]

Excludes2   burn of ear drum (T28.41-)

● **T20.111**   Burn of first degree of right ear [any part, except ear drum]

● **T20.112**   Burn of first degree of left ear [any part, except ear drum]

● **T20.119**   Burn of first degree of unspecified ear [any part, except ear drum]

X● **T20.12**   Burn of first degree of lip(s)

X● **T20.13**   Burn of first degree of chin

X● **T20.14**   Burn of first degree of nose (septum)

X● **T20.15**   Burn of first degree of scalp [any part]

X● **T20.16**   Burn of first degree of forehead and cheek

X● **T20.17**   Burn of first degree of neck

X● **T20.19**   Burn of first degree of multiple sites of head, face, and neck

● **T20.2   Burn of second degree of head, face, and neck**

Use additional external cause code to identify the source, place and intent of the burn (X00-X19, X75-X77, X96-X98, Y92)

X● **T20.20**   Burn of second degree of head, face, and neck, unspecified site

● **T20.21**   Burn of second degree of ear [any part, except ear drum]

Excludes2   burn of ear drum (T28.41-)

● **T20.211**   Burn of second degree of right ear [any part, except ear drum]

● **T20.212**   Burn of second degree of left ear [any part, except ear drum]

● **T20.219**   Burn of second degree of unspecified ear [any part, except ear drum]

X● **T20.22**   Burn of second degree of lip(s)

X● **T20.23**   Burn of second degree of chin

X● **T20.24**   Burn of second degree of nose (septum)

X● **T20.25**   Burn of second degree of scalp [any part]
Coding Clinic: 2015, Q1, P19

X● **T20.26**   Burn of second degree of forehead and cheek

X● **T20.27**   Burn of second degree of neck

X● **T20.29**   Burn of second degree of multiple sites of head, face, and neck

● **T20.3   Burn of third degree of head, face, and neck**

Use additional external cause code to identify the source, place and intent of the burn (X00-X19, X75-X77, X96-X98, Y92)

X● **T20.30**   Burn of third degree of head, face, and neck, unspecified site

● **T20.31**   Burn of third degree of ear [any part, except ear drum]

Excludes2   burn of ear drum (T28.41-)

● **T20.311**   Burn of third degree of right ear [any part, except ear drum]

● **T20.312**   Burn of third degree of left ear [any part, except ear drum]
Coding Clinic: 2015, Q1, P18

● **T20.319**   Burn of third degree of unspecified ear [any part, except ear drum]

X● T20.32   Burn of third degree of lip(s)

X● T20.33   Burn of third degree of chin

X● T20.34   Burn of third degree of nose (septum)

X● T20.35   Burn of third degree of scalp [any part]

X● T20.36   Burn of third degree of forehead and cheek

X● T20.37   Burn of third degree of neck

X● T20.39   Burn of third degree of multiple sites of head, face, and neck

● T20.4   Corrosion of unspecified degree of head, face, and neck

     Code first (T51-T65) to identify chemical and intent

     Use additional external cause code to identify place (Y92)

X● T20.40   Corrosion of unspecified degree of head, face, and neck, unspecified site

● T20.41   Corrosion of unspecified degree of ear [any part, except ear drum]

     Excludes2   corrosion of ear drum (T28.91-)

    ● T20.411   Corrosion of unspecified degree of right ear [any part, except ear drum]

    ● T20.412   Corrosion of unspecified degree of left ear [any part, except ear drum]

    ● T20.419   Corrosion of unspecified degree of unspecified ear [any part, except ear drum]

X● T20.42   Corrosion of unspecified degree of lip(s)

X● T20.43   Corrosion of unspecified degree of chin

X● T20.44   Corrosion of unspecified degree of nose (septum)

X● T20.45   Corrosion of unspecified degree of scalp [any part]

X● T20.46   Corrosion of unspecified degree of forehead and cheek

X● T20.47   Corrosion of unspecified degree of neck

X● T20.49   Corrosion of unspecified degree of multiple sites of head, face, and neck

● T20.5   Corrosion of first degree of head, face, and neck

     Code first (T51-T65) to identify chemical and intent

     Use additional external cause code to identify place (Y92)

X● T20.50   Corrosion of first degree of head, face, and neck, unspecified site

● T20.51   Corrosion of first degree of ear [any part, except ear drum]

     Excludes2   corrosion of ear drum (T28.91-)

    ● T20.511   Corrosion of first degree of right ear [any part, except ear drum]

    ● T20.512   Corrosion of first degree of left ear [any part, except ear drum]

    ● T20.519   Corrosion of first degree of unspecified ear [any part, except ear drum]

X● T20.52   Corrosion of first degree of lip(s)

X● T20.53   Corrosion of first degree of chin

X● T20.54   Corrosion of first degree of nose (septum)

X● T20.55   Corrosion of first degree of scalp [any part]

X● T20.56   Corrosion of first degree of forehead and cheek

X● T20.57   Corrosion of first degree of neck

X● T20.59   Corrosion of first degree of multiple sites of head, face, and neck

● T20.6   Corrosion of second degree of head, face, and neck

     Code first (T51-T65) to identify chemical and intent

     Use additional external cause code to identify place (Y92)

X● T20.60   Corrosion of second degree of head, face, and neck, unspecified site

● T20.61   Corrosion of second degree of ear [any part, except ear drum]

     Excludes2   corrosion of ear drum (T28.91-)

    ● T20.611   Corrosion of second degree of right ear [any part, except ear drum]

    ● T20.612   Corrosion of second degree of left ear [any part, except ear drum]

    ● T20.619   Corrosion of second degree of unspecified ear [any part, except ear drum]

X● T20.62   Corrosion of second degree of lip(s)

X● T20.63   Corrosion of second degree of chin

X● T20.64   Corrosion of second degree of nose (septum)

X● T20.65   Corrosion of second degree of scalp [any part]

X● T20.66   Corrosion of second degree of forehead and cheek

X● T20.67   Corrosion of second degree of neck

X● T20.69   Corrosion of second degree of multiple sites of head, face, and neck

● T20.7   Corrosion of third degree of head, face, and neck

     Code first (T51-T65) to identify chemical and intent

     Use additional external cause code to identify place (Y92)

X● T20.70   Corrosion of third degree of head, face, and neck, unspecified site

● T20.71   Corrosion of third degree of ear [any part, except ear drum]

     Excludes2   corrosion of ear drum (T28.91-)

    ● T20.711   Corrosion of third degree of right ear [any part, except ear drum]

    ● T20.712   Corrosion of third degree of left ear [any part, except ear drum]

    ● T20.719   Corrosion of third degree of unspecified ear [any part, except ear drum]

X● T20.72   Corrosion of third degree of lip(s)

X● T20.73   Corrosion of third degree of chin

X● T20.74   Corrosion of third degree of nose (septum)

X● T20.75   Corrosion of third degree of scalp [any part]

X● T20.76   Corrosion of third degree of forehead and cheek

X● T20.77   Corrosion of third degree of neck

X● T20.79   Corrosion of third degree of multiple sites of head, face, and neck

● **T21**   **Burn and corrosion of trunk**

> **Includes**   burns and corrosion of hip region
> **Excludes2**   burns and corrosion of axilla (T22.- with fifth
>   character 4)
>   burns and corrosion of scapular region
>   (T22.- with fifth character 6)
>   burns and corrosion of shoulder (T22.- with fifth
>   character 5)

> The appropriate 7th character is to be added to each code from
> category T21

> | A | initial encounter |
> |---|---|
> | D | subsequent encounter |
> | S | sequela |

● **T21.0**   **Burn of unspecified degree of trunk**

> Use additional external cause code to identify the
> source, place and intent of the burn (X00-X19,
> X75-X77, X96-X98, Y92)

  X● **T21.00**   **Burn of unspecified degree of trunk, unspecified site**

  X● **T21.01**   **Burn of unspecified degree of chest wall**
> Burn of of unspecified degree of breast

  X● **T21.02**   **Burn of unspecified degree of abdominal wall**
> Burn of unspecified degree of flank
> Burn of unspecified degree of groin

  X● **T21.03**   **Burn of unspecified degree of upper back**
> Burn of unspecified degree of interscapular region

  X● **T21.04**   **Burn of unspecified degree of lower back**

  X● **T21.05**   **Burn of unspecified degree of buttock**
> Burn of unspecified degree of anus

  X● **T21.06**   **Burn of unspecified degree of male genital region ♂**
> Burn of unspecified degree of penis
> Burn of unspecified degree of scrotum
> Burn of unspecified degree of testis

  X● **T21.07**   **Burn of unspecified degree of female genital region ♀**
> Burn of unspecified degree of labium (majus) (minus)
> Burn of unspecified degree of perineum
> Burn of unspecified degree of vulva
>> **Excludes2**   burn of vagina (T28.3)

  X● **T21.09**   **Burn of unspecified degree of other site of trunk**

● **T21.1**   **Burn of first degree of trunk**

> Use additional external cause code to identify the
> source, place and intent of the burn (X00-X19,
> X75-X77, X96-X98, Y92)

  X● **T21.10**   **Burn of first degree of trunk, unspecified site**

  X● **T21.11**   **Burn of first degree of chest wall**
> Burn of first degree of breast

  X● **T21.12**   **Burn of first degree of abdominal wall**
> Burn of first degree of flank
> Burn of first degree of groin

  X● **T21.13**   **Burn of first degree of upper back**
> Burn of first degree of interscapular region

  X● **T21.14**   **Burn of first degree of lower back**

  X● **T21.15**   **Burn of first degree of buttock**
> Burn of first degree of anus

  X● **T21.16**   **Burn of first degree of male genital region ♂**
> Burn of first degree of penis
> Burn of first degree of scrotum
> Burn of first degree of testis

  X● **T21.17**   **Burn of first degree of female genital region ♀**
> Burn of first degree of labium (majus) (minus)
> Burn of first degree of perineum
> Burn of first degree of vulva
>> **Excludes2**   burn of vagina (T28.3)

  X● **T21.19**   **Burn of first degree of other site of trunk**

● **T21.2**   **Burn of second degree of trunk**

> Use additional external cause code to identify the
> place and intent of the burn (X00-X19,
> X75-X77, X96-X98, Y92)

  X● **T21.20**   **Burn of second degree of trunk, unspecified site**

  X● **T21.21**   **Burn of second degree of chest wall**
> Burn of second degree of breast

  X● **T21.22**   **Burn of second degree of abdominal wall**
> Burn of second degree of flank
> Burn of second degree of groin

  X● **T21.23**   **Burn of second degree of upper back**
> Burn of second degree of interscapular region

  X● **T21.24**   **Burn of second degree of lower back**

  X● **T21.25**   **Burn of second degree of buttock**
> Burn of second degree of anus

  X● **T21.26**   **Burn of second degree of male genital region ♂**
> Burn of second degree of penis
> Burn of second degree of scrotum
> Burn of second degree of testis

  X● **T21.27**   **Burn of second degree of female genital region ♀**
> Burn of second degree of labium (majus) (minus)
> Burn of second degree of perineum
> Burn of second degree of vulva
>> **Excludes2**   burn of vagina (T28.3)

  X● **T21.29**   **Burn of second degree of other site of trunk**

● **T21.3**   **Burn of third degree of trunk**

> Use additional external cause code to identify the
> source, place and intent of the burn (X00-X19,
> X75-X77, X96-X98, Y92)

  X● **T21.30**   **Burn of third degree of trunk, unspecified site**

  X● **T21.31**   **Burn of third degree of chest wall**
> Burn of third degree of breast

  X● **T21.32**   **Burn of third degree of abdominal wall**
> Burn of third degree of flank
> Burn of third degree of groin

  X● **T21.33**   **Burn of third degree of upper back**
> Burn of third degree of interscapular region

  X● **T21.34**   **Burn of third degree of lower back**

  X● **T21.35**   **Burn of third degree of buttock**
> Burn of third degree of anus

  X● **T21.36**   **Burn of third degree of male genital region ♂**
> Burn of third degree of penis
> Burn of third degree of scrotum
> Burn of third degree of testis

  X● **T21.37**   **Burn of third degree of female genital region ♀**
> Burn of third degree of labium (majus) (minus)
> Burn of third degree of perineum
> Burn of third degree of vulva
>> **Excludes2**   burn of vagina (T28.3)

  X● **T21.39**   **Burn of third degree of other site of trunk**

● **T21.4**   **Corrosion of unspecified degree of trunk**

> *Code first (T51-T65) to identify chemical and intent*
> Use additional external cause code to identify
> place (Y92)

  X● **T21.40**   **Corrosion of unspecified degree of trunk, unspecified site**

  X● **T21.41**   **Corrosion of unspecified degree of chest wall**
> Corrosion of unspecified degree of breast

  X● **T21.42**   **Corrosion of unspecified degree of abdominal wall**
> Corrosion of unspecified degree of flank
> Corrosion of unspecified degree of groin

  X● **T21.43**   **Corrosion of unspecified degree of upper back**
> Corrosion of unspecified degree of interscapular region

CHAPTER 19 (S00-T88)

X● **T21.44** **Corrosion of unspecified degree of lower back**

X● **T21.45** **Corrosion of unspecified degree of buttock**
Corrosion of unspecified degree of anus

X● **T21.46** **Corrosion of unspecified degree of male genital region** ♂
Corrosion of unspecified degree of penis
Corrosion of unspecified degree of scrotum
Corrosion of unspecified degree of testis

X● **T21.47** **Corrosion of unspecified degree of female genital region** ♀
Corrosion of unspecified degree of labium (majus) (minus)
Corrosion of unspecified degree of perineum
Corrosion of unspecified degree of vulva

Excludes2 corrosion of vagina (T28.8)

X● **T21.49** **Corrosion of unspecified degree of other site of trunk**

● **T21.5** **Corrosion of first degree of trunk**
Code first (T51-T65) to identify chemical and intent
Use additional external cause code to identify place (Y92)

X● **T21.50** **Corrosion of first degree of trunk, unspecified site**

X● **T21.51** **Corrosion of first degree of chest wall**
Corrosion of first degree of breast

X● **T21.52** **Corrosion of first degree of abdominal wall**
Corrosion of first degree of flank
Corrosion of first degree of groin

X● **T21.53** **Corrosion of first degree of upper back**
Corrosion of first degree of interscapular region

X● **T21.54** **Corrosion of first degree of lower back**

X● **T21.55** **Corrosion of first degree of buttock**
Corrosion of first degree of anus

X● **T21.56** **Corrosion of first degree of male genital region** ♂
Corrosion of first degree of penis
Corrosion of first degree of scrotum
Corrosion of first degree of testis

X● **T21.57** **Corrosion of first degree of female genital region** ♀
Corrosion of first degree of labium (majus) (minus)
Corrosion of first degree of perineum
Corrosion of first degree of vulva

Excludes2 corrosion of vagina (T28.8)

X● **T21.59** **Corrosion of first degree of other site of trunk**

● **T21.6** **Corrosion of second degree of trunk**
Code first (T51-T65) to identify chemical and intent
Use additional external cause code to identify place (Y92)

X● **T21.60** **Corrosion of second degree of trunk, unspecified site**

X● **T21.61** **Corrosion of second degree of chest wall**
Corrosion of second degree of breast

X● **T21.62** **Corrosion of second degree of abdominal wall**
Corrosion of second degree of flank
Corrosion of second degree of groin

X● **T21.63** **Corrosion of second degree of upper back**
Corrosion of second degree of interscapular region

X● **T21.64** **Corrosion of second degree of lower back**

X● **T21.65** **Corrosion of second degree of buttock**
Corrosion of second degree of anus

X● **T21.66** **Corrosion of second degree of male genital region** ♂
Corrosion of second degree of penis
Corrosion of second degree of scrotum
Corrosion of second degree of testis

X● **T21.67** **Corrosion of second degree of female genital region** ♀
Corrosion of second degree of labium (majus) (minus)
Corrosion of second degree of perineum
Corrosion of second degree of vulva

Excludes2 corrosion of vagina (T28.8)

X● **T21.69** **Corrosion of second degree of other site of trunk**

● **T21.7** **Corrosion of third degree of trunk**
Code first (T51-T65) to identify chemical and intent
Use additional external cause code to identify place (Y92)

X● **T21.70** **Corrosion of third degree of trunk, unspecified site**

X● **T21.71** **Corrosion of third degree of chest wall**
Corrosion of third degree of breast

X● **T21.72** **Corrosion of third degree of abdominal wall**
Corrosion of third degree of flank
Corrosion of third degree of groin

X● **T21.73** **Corrosion of third degree of upper back**
Corrosion of third degree of interscapular region

X● **T21.74** **Corrosion of third degree of lower back**

X● **T21.75** **Corrosion of third degree of buttock**
Corrosion of third degree of anus

X● **T21.76** **Corrosion of third degree of male genital region** ♂
Corrosion of third degree of penis
Corrosion of third degree of scrotum
Corrosion of third degree of testis

X● **T21.77** **Corrosion of third degree of female genital region** ♀
Corrosion of third degree of labium (majus) (minus)
Corrosion of third degree of perineum
Corrosion of third degree of vulva

Excludes2 corrosion of vagina (T28.8)

X● **T21.79** **Corrosion of third degree of other site of trunk**

● **T22** **Burn and corrosion of shoulder and upper limb, except wrist and hand**

Excludes2 burn and corrosion of interscapular region (T21.-)
burn and corrosion of wrist and hand (T23.-)

The appropriate 7th character is to be added to each code from category T22

A	initial encounter
D	subsequent encounter
S	sequela

● **T22.0** **Burn of unspecified degree of shoulder and upper limb, except wrist and hand**
Use additional external cause code to identify the source, place and intent of the burn (X00-X19, X75-X77, X96-X98, Y92)

X● **T22.00** **Burn of unspecified degree of shoulder and upper limb, except wrist and hand, unspecified site**

● **T22.01** **Burn of unspecified degree of forearm**

● **T22.011** **Burn of unspecified degree of right forearm**

● **T22.012** **Burn of unspecified degree of left forearm**

● **T22.019** **Burn of unspecified degree of unspecified forearm**

● **T22.02** **Burn of unspecified degree of elbow**

● **T22.021** **Burn of unspecified degree of right elbow**

● **T22.022** **Burn of unspecified degree of left elbow**

● **T22.029** **Burn of unspecified degree of unspecified elbow**

◄ New ◄◄◄ Revised ~~deleted~~ Deleted Excludes 1 Excludes 2 Includes Use additional Code first Code also Unspecified
OGCR Official Guidelines X Assign placeholder X ● Use Additional Character(s) ▶ Manifestation Code **Coding Clinic**

● T22.03   Burn of unspecified degree of upper arm
  ● T22.031   Burn of unspecified degree of right upper arm
  ● T22.032   Burn of unspecified degree of left upper arm
  ● T22.039   Burn of unspecified degree of unspecified upper arm
● T22.04   Burn of unspecified degree of axilla
  ● T22.041   Burn of unspecified degree of right axilla
  ● T22.042   Burn of unspecified degree of left axilla
  ● T22.049   Burn of unspecified degree of unspecified axilla
● T22.05   Burn of unspecified degree of shoulder
  ● T22.051   Burn of unspecified degree of right shoulder
  ● T22.052   Burn of unspecified degree of left shoulder
  ● T22.059   Burn of unspecified degree of unspecified shoulder
● T22.06   Burn of unspecified degree of scapular region
  ● T22.061   Burn of unspecified degree of right scapular region
  ● T22.062   Burn of unspecified degree of left scapular region
  ● T22.069   Burn of unspecified degree of unspecified scapular region
● T22.09   Burn of unspecified degree of multiple sites of shoulder and upper limb, except wrist and hand
  ● T22.091   Burn of unspecified degree of multiple sites of right shoulder and upper limb, except wrist and hand
  ● T22.092   Burn of unspecified degree of multiple sites of left shoulder and upper limb, except wrist and hand
  ● T22.099   Burn of unspecified degree of multiple sites of unspecified shoulder and upper limb, except wrist and hand
● T22.1   Burn of first degree of shoulder and upper limb, except wrist and hand

> Use additional external cause code to identify the source, place and intent of the burn (X00-X19, X75-X77, X96-X98, Y92)

  X ● T22.10   Burn of first degree of shoulder and upper limb, except wrist and hand, unspecified site
  ● T22.11   Burn of first degree of forearm
    ● T22.111   Burn of first degree of right forearm
    ● T22.112   Burn of first degree of left forearm
    ● T22.119   Burn of first degree of unspecified forearm
  ● T22.12   Burn of first degree of elbow
    ● T22.121   Burn of first degree of right elbow
    ● T22.122   Burn of first degree of left elbow
    ● T22.129   Burn of first degree of unspecified elbow
  ● T22.13   Burn of first degree of upper arm
    ● T22.131   Burn of first degree of right upper arm
    ● T22.132   Burn of first degree of left upper arm
    ● T22.139   Burn of first degree of unspecified upper arm
  ● T22.14   Burn of first degree of axilla
    ● T22.141   Burn of first degree of right axilla
    ● T22.142   Burn of first degree of left axilla
    ● T22.149   Burn of first degree of unspecified axilla

● T22.15   Burn of first degree of shoulder
  ● T22.151   Burn of first degree of right shoulder
  ● T22.152   Burn of first degree of left shoulder
  ● T22.159   Burn of first degree of unspecified shoulder
● T22.16   Burn of first degree of scapular region
  ● T22.161   Burn of first degree of right scapular region
  ● T22.162   Burn of first degree of left scapular region
  ● T22.169   Burn of first degree of unspecified scapular region
● T22.19   Burn of first degree of multiple sites of shoulder and upper limb, except wrist and hand
  ● T22.191   Burn of first degree of multiple sites of right shoulder and upper limb, except wrist and hand
  ● T22.192   Burn of first degree of multiple sites of left shoulder and upper limb, except wrist and hand
  ● T22.199   Burn of first degree of multiple sites of unspecified shoulder and upper limb, except wrist and hand
● T22.2   Burn of second degree of shoulder and upper limb, except wrist and hand

> Use additional external cause code to identify the source, place and intent of the burn (X00-X19, X75-X77, X96-X98, Y92)

  X ● T22.20   Burn of second degree of shoulder and upper limb, except wrist and hand, unspecified site
  ● T22.21   Burn of second degree of forearm
    ● T22.211   Burn of second degree of right forearm
    ● T22.212   Burn of second degree of left forearm
    ● T22.219   Burn of second degree of unspecified forearm
  ● T22.22   Burn of second degree of elbow
    ● T22.221   Burn of second degree of right elbow
    ● T22.222   Burn of second degree of left elbow
    ● T22.229   Burn of second degree of unspecified elbow
  ● T22.23   Burn of second degree of upper arm
    ● T22.231   Burn of second degree of right upper arm
    ● T22.232   Burn of second degree of left upper arm
    ● T22.239   Burn of second degree of unspecified upper arm
  ● T22.24   Burn of second degree of axilla
    ● T22.241   Burn of second degree of right axilla
    ● T22.242   Burn of second degree of left axilla
    ● T22.249   Burn of second degree of unspecified axilla
  ● T22.25   Burn of second degree of shoulder
    ● T22.251   Burn of second degree of right shoulder
    ● T22.252   Burn of second degree of left shoulder
    ● T22.259   Burn of second degree of unspecified shoulder
  ● T22.26   Burn of second degree of scapular region
    ● T22.261   Burn of second degree of right scapular region
    ● T22.262   Burn of second degree of left scapular region
    ● T22.269   Burn of second degree of unspecified scapular region

CHAPTER 19 (S00-T88)

● T22.29   Burn of second degree of multiple sites of shoulder and upper limb, except wrist and hand
   ● T22.291   Burn of second degree of multiple sites of right shoulder and upper limb, except wrist and hand
   ● T22.292   Burn of second degree of multiple sites of left shoulder and upper limb, except wrist and hand
   ● T22.299   Burn of second degree of multiple sites of unspecified shoulder and upper limb, except wrist and hand

● T22.3   Burn of third degree of shoulder and upper limb, except wrist and hand
   Use additional external cause code to identify the source, place and intent of the burn (X00-X19, X75-X77, X96-X98, Y92)
  X ● T22.30   Burn of third degree of shoulder and upper limb, except wrist and hand, unspecified site
  ● T22.31   Burn of third degree of forearm
   ● T22.311   Burn of third degree of right forearm
   ● T22.312   Burn of third degree of left forearm
   ● T22.319   Burn of third degree of unspecified forearm
  ● T22.32   Burn of third degree of elbow
   ● T22.321   Burn of third degree of right elbow
   ● T22.322   Burn of third degree of left elbow
   ● T22.329   Burn of third degree of unspecified elbow
  ● T22.33   Burn of third degree of upper arm
   ● T22.331   Burn of third degree of right upper arm
   ● T22.332   Burn of third degree of left upper arm
   ● T22.339   Burn of third degree of unspecified upper arm
  ● T22.34   Burn of third degree of axilla
   ● T22.341   Burn of third degree of right axilla
   ● T22.342   Burn of third degree of left axilla
   ● T22.349   Burn of third degree of unspecified axilla
  ● T22.35   Burn of third degree of shoulder
   ● T22.351   Burn of third degree of right shoulder
   ● T22.352   Burn of third degree of left shoulder
   ● T22.359   Burn of third degree of unspecified shoulder
  ● T22.36   Burn of third degree of scapular region
   ● T22.361   Burn of third degree of right scapular region
   ● T22.362   Burn of third degree of left scapular region
   ● T22.369   Burn of third degree of unspecified scapular region
  ● T22.39   Burn of third degree of multiple sites of shoulder and upper limb, except wrist and hand
   ● T22.391   Burn of third degree of multiple sites of right shoulder and upper limb, except wrist and hand
   ● T22.392   Burn of third degree of multiple sites of left shoulder and upper limb, except wrist and hand
   ● T22.399   Burn of third degree of multiple sites of unspecified shoulder and upper limb, except wrist and hand

● T22.4   Corrosion of unspecified degree of shoulder and upper limb, except wrist and hand
   Code first (T51-T65) to identify chemical and intent
   Use additional external cause code to identify place (Y92)
  X ● T22.40   Corrosion of unspecified degree of shoulder and upper limb, except wrist and hand, unspecified site
  ● T22.41   Corrosion of unspecified degree of forearm
   ● T22.411   Corrosion of unspecified degree of right forearm
   ● T22.412   Corrosion of unspecified degree of left forearm
   ● T22.419   Corrosion of unspecified degree of unspecified forearm
  ● T22.42   Corrosion of unspecified degree of elbow
   ● T22.421   Corrosion of unspecified degree of right elbow
   ● T22.422   Corrosion of unspecified degree of left elbow
   ● T22.429   Corrosion of unspecified degree of unspecified elbow
  ● T22.43   Corrosion of unspecified degree of upper arm
   ● T22.431   Corrosion of unspecified degree of right upper arm
   ● T22.432   Corrosion of unspecified degree of left upper arm
   ● T22.439   Corrosion of unspecified degree of unspecified upper arm
  ● T22.44   Corrosion of unspecified degree of axilla
   ● T22.441   Corrosion of unspecified degree of right axilla
   ● T22.442   Corrosion of unspecified degree of left axilla
   ● T22.449   Corrosion of unspecified degree of unspecified axilla
  ● T22.45   Corrosion of unspecified degree of shoulder
   ● T22.451   Corrosion of unspecified degree of right shoulder
   ● T22.452   Corrosion of unspecified degree of left shoulder
   ● T22.459   Corrosion of unspecified degree of unspecified shoulder
  ● T22.46   Corrosion of unspecified degree of scapular region
   ● T22.461   Corrosion of unspecified degree of right scapular region
   ● T22.462   Corrosion of unspecified degree of left scapular region
   ● T22.469   Corrosion of unspecified degree of unspecified scapular region
  ● T22.49   Corrosion of unspecified degree of multiple sites of shoulder and upper limb, except wrist and hand
   ● T22.491   Corrosion of unspecified degree of multiple sites of right shoulder and upper limb, except wrist and hand
   ● T22.492   Corrosion of unspecified degree of multiple sites of left shoulder and upper limb, except wrist and hand
   ● T22.499   Corrosion of unspecified degree of multiple sites of unspecified shoulder and upper limb, except wrist and hand

CHAPTER 19 (S00-T88)

◀ New   ◀━ Revised   ~~deleted~~ Deleted   Excludes 1   Excludes 2   Includes   Use additional   Code first   Code also   Unspecified

OGCR Official Guidelines   X Assign placeholder X   ● Use Additional Character(s)   ▶ Manifestation Code   **Coding Clinic**

● **T22.5**   **Corrosion of first degree of shoulder and upper limb, except wrist and hand**

Code first (T51-T65) to identify chemical and intent

Use additional external cause code to identify place (Y92)

X ● **T22.50**   Corrosion of first degree of shoulder and upper limb, except wrist and hand unspecified site

● **T22.51**   Corrosion of first degree of forearm

    ● **T22.511**   Corrosion of first degree of right forearm

    ● **T22.512**   Corrosion of first degree of left forearm

    ● **T22.519**   Corrosion of first degree of unspecified forearm

● **T22.52**   Corrosion of first degree of elbow

    ● **T22.521**   Corrosion of first degree of right elbow

    ● **T22.522**   Corrosion of first degree of left elbow

    ● **T22.529**   Corrosion of first degree of unspecified elbow

● **T22.53**   Corrosion of first degree of upper arm

    ● **T22.531**   Corrosion of first degree of right upper arm

    ● **T22.532**   Corrosion of first degree of left upper arm

    ● **T22.539**   Corrosion of first degree of unspecified upper arm

● **T22.54**   Corrosion of first degree of axilla

    ● **T22.541**   Corrosion of first degree of right axilla

    ● **T22.542**   Corrosion of first degree of left axilla

    ● **T22.549**   Corrosion of first degree of unspecified axilla

● **T22.55**   Corrosion of first degree of shoulder

    ● **T22.551**   Corrosion of first degree of right shoulder

    ● **T22.552**   Corrosion of first degree of left shoulder

    ● **T22.559**   Corrosion of first degree of unspecified shoulder

● **T22.56**   Corrosion of first degree of scapular region

    ● **T22.561**   Corrosion of first degree of right scapular region

    ● **T22.562**   Corrosion of first degree of left scapular region

    ● **T22.569**   Corrosion of first degree of unspecified scapular region

● **T22.59**   Corrosion of first degree of multiple sites of shoulder and upper limb, except wrist and hand

    ● **T22.591**   Corrosion of first degree of multiple sites of right shoulder and upper limb, except wrist and hand

    ● **T22.592**   Corrosion of first degree of multiple sites of left shoulder and upper limb, except wrist and hand

    ● **T22.599**   Corrosion of first degree of multiple sites of unspecified shoulder and upper limb, except wrist and hand

● **T22.6**   **Corrosion of second degree of shoulder and upper limb, except wrist and hand**

Code first (T51-T65) to identify chemical and intent

Use additional external cause code to identify place (Y92)

X ● **T22.60**   Corrosion of second degree of shoulder and upper limb, except wrist and hand, unspecified site

● **T22.61**   Corrosion of second degree of forearm

    ● **T22.611**   Corrosion of second degree of right forearm

    ● **T22.612**   Corrosion of second degree of left forearm

    ● **T22.619**   Corrosion of second degree of unspecified forearm

● **T22.62**   Corrosion of second degree of elbow

    ● **T22.621**   Corrosion of second degree of right elbow

    ● **T22.622**   Corrosion of second degree of left elbow

    ● **T22.629**   Corrosion of second degree of unspecified elbow

● **T22.63**   Corrosion of second degree of upper arm

    ● **T22.631**   Corrosion of second degree of right upper arm

    ● **T22.632**   Corrosion of second degree of left upper arm

    ● **T22.639**   Corrosion of second degree of unspecified upper arm

● **T22.64**   Corrosion of second degree of axilla

    ● **T22.641**   Corrosion of second degree of right axilla

    ● **T22.642**   Corrosion of second degree of left axilla

    ● **T22.649**   Corrosion of second degree of unspecified axilla

● **T22.65**   Corrosion of second degree of shoulder

    ● **T22.651**   Corrosion of second degree of right shoulder

    ● **T22.652**   Corrosion of second degree of left shoulder

    ● **T22.659**   Corrosion of second degree of unspecified shoulder

● **T22.66**   Corrosion of second degree of scapular region

    ● **T22.661**   Corrosion of second degree of right scapular region

    ● **T22.662**   Corrosion of second degree of left scapular region

    ● **T22.669**   Corrosion of second degree of unspecified scapular region

● **T22.69**   Corrosion of second degree of multiple sites of shoulder and upper limb, except wrist and hand

    ● **T22.691**   Corrosion of second degree of multiple sites of right shoulder and upper limb, except wrist and hand

    ● **T22.692**   Corrosion of second degree of multiple sites of left shoulder and upper limb, except wrist and hand

    ● **T22.699**   Corrosion of second degree of multiple sites of unspecified shoulder and upper limb, except wrist and hand

CHAPTER 19 (S00-T88)

● **T22.7 Corrosion of third degree of shoulder and upper limb, except wrist and hand**

Code first (T51-T65) to identify chemical and intent

Use additional external cause code to identify place (Y92)

X ● **T22.70** Corrosion of third degree of shoulder and upper limb, except wrist and hand, unspecified site

● **T22.71** Corrosion of third degree of forearm

     ● **T22.711** Corrosion of third degree of right forearm

     ● **T22.712** Corrosion of third degree of left forearm

     ● **T22.719** Corrosion of third degree of unspecified forearm

● **T22.72** Corrosion of third degree of elbow

     ● **T22.721** Corrosion of third degree of right elbow

     ● **T22.722** Corrosion of third degree of left elbow

     ● **T22.729** Corrosion of third degree of unspecified elbow

● **T22.73** Corrosion of third degree of upper arm

     ● **T22.731** Corrosion of third degree of right upper arm

     ● **T22.732** Corrosion of third degree of left upper arm

     ● **T22.739** Corrosion of third degree of unspecified upper arm

● **T22.74** Corrosion of third degree of axilla

     ● **T22.741** Corrosion of third degree of right axilla

     ● **T22.742** Corrosion of third degree of left axilla

     ● **T22.749** Corrosion of third degree of unspecified axilla

● **T22.75** Corrosion of third degree of shoulder

     ● **T22.751** Corrosion of third degree of right shoulder

     ● **T22.752** Corrosion of third degree of left shoulder

     ● **T22.759** Corrosion of third degree of unspecified shoulder

● **T22.76** Corrosion of third degree of scapular region

     ● **T22.761** Corrosion of third degree of right scapular region

     ● **T22.762** Corrosion of third degree of left scapular region

     ● **T22.769** Corrosion of third degree of unspecified scapular region

● **T22.79** Corrosion of third degree of multiple sites of shoulder and upper limb, except wrist and hand

     ● **T22.791** Corrosion of third degree of multiple sites of right shoulder and upper limb, except wrist and hand

     ● **T22.792** Corrosion of third degree of multiple sites of left shoulder and upper limb, except wrist and hand

     ● **T22.799** Corrosion of third degree of multiple sites of unspecified shoulder and upper limb, except wrist and hand

● **T23 Burn and corrosion of wrist and hand**

The appropriate 7th character is to be added to each code from category T23

A	initial encounter
D	subsequent encounter
S	sequela

● **T23.0 Burn of unspecified degree of wrist and hand**

Use additional external cause code to identify the source, place and intent of the burn (X00-X19, X75-X77, X96-X98, Y92)

● **T23.00** Burn of unspecified degree of hand, unspecified site

     ● **T23.001** Burn of unspecified degree of right hand, unspecified site

     ● **T23.002** Burn of unspecified degree of left hand, unspecified site

     ● **T23.009** Burn of unspecified degree of unspecified hand, unspecified site

● **T23.01** Burn of unspecified degree of thumb (nail)

     ● **T23.011** Burn of unspecified degree of right thumb (nail)

     ● **T23.012** Burn of unspecified degree of left thumb (nail)

     ● **T23.019** Burn of unspecified degree of unspecified thumb (nail)

● **T23.02** Burn of unspecified degree of single finger (nail) except thumb

     ● **T23.021** Burn of unspecified degree of single right finger (nail) except thumb

     ● **T23.022** Burn of unspecified degree of single left finger (nail) except thumb

     ● **T23.029** Burn of unspecified degree of unspecified single finger (nail) except thumb

● **T23.03** Burn of unspecified degree of multiple fingers (nail), not including thumb

     ● **T23.031** Burn of unspecified degree of multiple right fingers (nail), not including thumb

     ● **T23.032** Burn of unspecified degree of multiple left fingers (nail), not including thumb

     ● **T23.039** Burn of unspecified degree of unspecified multiple fingers (nail), not including thumb

● **T23.04** Burn of unspecified degree of multiple fingers (nail), including thumb

     ● **T23.041** Burn of unspecified degree of multiple right fingers (nail), including thumb

     ● **T23.042** Burn of unspecified degree of multiple left fingers (nail), including thumb

     ● **T23.049** Burn of unspecified degree of unspecified multiple fingers (nail), including thumb

● **T23.05** Burn of unspecified degree of palm

     ● **T23.051** Burn of unspecified degree of right palm

     ● **T23.052** Burn of unspecified degree of left palm

     ● **T23.059** Burn of unspecified degree of unspecified palm

◄ New   ◄ Revised   ~~deleted~~ Deleted   Excludes 1   Excludes 2   Includes   Use additional   Code first   Code also   Unspecified

OGCR Official Guidelines   X Assign placeholder X   ● Use Additional Character(s)   ▶ Manifestation Code   **Coding Clinic**

● **T23.06** Burn of unspecified degree of back of hand
  ● **T23.061** Burn of unspecified degree of back of right hand
  ● **T23.062** Burn of unspecified degree of back of left hand
  ● **T23.069** Burn of unspecified degree of back of unspecified hand
● **T23.07** Burn of unspecified degree of wrist
  ● **T23.071** Burn of unspecified degree of right wrist
  ● **T23.072** Burn of unspecified degree of left wrist
  ● **T23.079** Burn of unspecified degree of unspecified wrist
● **T23.09** Burn of unspecified degree of multiple sites of wrist and hand
  ● **T23.091** Burn of unspecified degree of multiple sites of right wrist and hand
  ● **T23.092** Burn of unspecified degree of multiple sites of left wrist and hand
  ● **T23.099** Burn of unspecified degree of multiple sites of unspecified wrist and hand
● **T23.1** Burn of first degree of wrist and hand
  Use additional external cause code to identify the source, place and intent of the burn (X00-X19, X75-X77, X96-X98, Y92)
  ● **T23.10** Burn of first degree of hand, unspecified site
    ● **T23.101** Burn of first degree of right hand, unspecified site
    ● **T23.102** Burn of first degree of left hand, unspecified site
    ● **T23.109** Burn of first degree of unspecified hand, unspecified site
  ● **T23.11** Burn of first degree of thumb (nail)
    ● **T23.111** Burn of first degree of right thumb (nail)
    ● **T23.112** Burn of first degree of left thumb (nail)
    ● **T23.119** Burn of first degree of unspecified thumb (nail)
  ● **T23.12** Burn of first degree of single finger (nail) except thumb
    ● **T23.121** Burn of first degree of single right finger (nail) except thumb
    ● **T23.122** Burn of first degree of single left finger (nail) except thumb
    ● **T23.129** Burn of first degree of unspecified single finger (nail) except thumb
  ● **T23.13** Burn of first degree of multiple fingers (nail), not including thumb
    ● **T23.131** Burn of first degree of multiple right fingers (nail), not including thumb
    ● **T23.132** Burn of first degree of multiple left fingers (nail), not including thumb
    ● **T23.139** Burn of first degree of unspecified multiple fingers (nail), not including thumb
  ● **T23.14** Burn of first degree of multiple fingers (nail), including thumb
    ● **T23.141** Burn of first degree of multiple right fingers (nail), including thumb
    ● **T23.142** Burn of first degree of multiple left fingers (nail), including thumb
    ● **T23.149** Burn of first degree of unspecified multiple fingers (nail), including thumb

● **T23.15** Burn of first degree of palm
  ● **T23.151** Burn of first degree of right palm
  ● **T23.152** Burn of first degree of left palm
  ● **T23.159** Burn of first degree of unspecified palm
● **T23.16** Burn of first degree of back of hand
  ● **T23.161** Burn of first degree of back of right hand
  ● **T23.162** Burn of first degree of back of left hand
  ● **T23.169** Burn of first degree of back of unspecified hand
● **T23.17** Burn of first degree of wrist
  ● **T23.171** Burn of first degree of right wrist
  ● **T23.172** Burn of first degree of left wrist
  ● **T23.179** Burn of first degree of unspecified wrist
● **T23.19** Burn of first degree of multiple sites of wrist and hand
  ● **T23.191** Burn of first degree of multiple sites of right wrist and hand
  ● **T23.192** Burn of first degree of multiple sites of left wrist and hand
  ● **T23.199** Burn of first degree of multiple sites of unspecified wrist and hand
● **T23.2** Burn of second degree of wrist and hand
  Use additional external cause code to identify the source, place and intent of the burn (X00-X19, X75-X77, X96-X98, Y92)
  ● **T23.20** Burn of second degree of hand, unspecified site
    ● **T23.201** Burn of second degree of right hand, unspecified site
    ● **T23.202** Burn of second degree of left hand, unspecified site
    ● **T23.209** Burn of second degree of unspecified hand, unspecified site
  ● **T23.21** Burn of second degree of thumb (nail)
    ● **T23.211** Burn of second degree of right thumb (nail)
    ● **T23.212** Burn of second degree of left thumb (nail)
    ● **T23.219** Burn of second degree of unspecified thumb (nail)
  ● **T23.22** Burn of second degree of single finger (nail) except thumb
    ● **T23.221** Burn of second degree of single right finger (nail) except thumb
    ● **T23.222** Burn of second degree of single left finger (nail) except thumb
    ● **T23.229** Burn of second degree of unspecified single finger (nail) except thumb
  ● **T23.23** Burn of second degree of multiple fingers (nail), not including thumb
    ● **T23.231** Burn of second degree of multiple right fingers (nail), not including thumb
    ● **T23.232** Burn of second degree of multiple left fingers (nail), not including thumb
    ● **T23.239** Burn of second degree of unspecified multiple fingers (nail), not including thumb
  ● **T23.24** Burn of second degree of multiple fingers (nail), including thumb
    ● **T23.241** Burn of second degree of multiple right fingers (nail), including thumb
    ● **T23.242** Burn of second degree of multiple left fingers (nail), including thumb
    ● **T23.249** Burn of second degree of unspecified multiple fingers (nail), including thumb

CHAPTER 19 (S00-T88)

● **T23.25** Burn of second degree of palm
  ● **T23.251** Burn of second degree of right palm
  ● **T23.252** Burn of second degree of left palm
  ● **T23.259** Burn of second degree of unspecified palm
● **T23.26** Burn of second degree of back of hand
  ● **T23.261** Burn of second degree of back of right hand
  ● **T23.262** Burn of second degree of back of left hand
  ● **T23.269** Burn of second degree of back of unspecified hand
● **T23.27** Burn of second degree of wrist
  ● **T23.271** Burn of second degree of right wrist
  ● **T23.272** Burn of second degree of left wrist
  ● **T23.279** Burn of second degree of unspecified wrist
● **T23.29** Burn of second degree of multiple sites of wrist and hand
  ● **T23.291** Burn of second degree of multiple sites of right wrist and hand
  ● **T23.292** Burn of second degree of multiple sites of left wrist and hand
  ● **T23.299** Burn of second degree of multiple sites of unspecified wrist and hand
● **T23.3** Burn of third degree of wrist and hand
  Use additional external cause code to identify the source, place and intent of the burn (X00-X19, X75-X77, X96-X98, Y92)
  ● **T23.30** Burn of third degree of hand, unspecified site
    ● **T23.301** Burn of third degree of right hand, unspecified site
        Coding Clinic: 2015, Q1, P19
    ● **T23.302** Burn of third degree of left hand, unspecified site
    ● **T23.309** Burn of third degree of unspecified hand, unspecified site
  ● **T23.31** Burn of third degree of thumb (nail)
    ● **T23.311** Burn of third degree of right thumb (nail)
    ● **T23.312** Burn of third degree of left thumb (nail)
    ● **T23.319** Burn of third degree of unspecified thumb (nail)
  ● **T23.32** Burn of third degree of single finger (nail) except thumb
    ● **T23.321** Burn of third degree of single right finger (nail) except thumb
    ● **T23.322** Burn of third degree of single left finger (nail) except thumb
    ● **T23.329** Burn of third degree of unspecified single finger (nail) except thumb
  ● **T23.33** Burn of third degree of multiple fingers (nail), not including thumb
    ● **T23.331** Burn of third degree of multiple right fingers (nail), not including thumb
    ● **T23.332** Burn of third degree of multiple left fingers (nail), not including thumb
    ● **T23.339** Burn of third degree of unspecified multiple fingers (nail), not including thumb
  ● **T23.34** Burn of third degree of multiple fingers (nail), including thumb
    ● **T23.341** Burn of third degree of multiple right fingers (nail), including thumb
    ● **T23.342** Burn of third degree of multiple left fingers (nail), including thumb
    ● **T23.349** Burn of third degree of unspecified multiple fingers (nail), including thumb

● **T23.35** Burn of third degree of palm
  ● **T23.351** Burn of third degree of right palm
  ● **T23.352** Burn of third degree of left palm
  ● **T23.359** Burn of third degree of unspecified palm
● **T23.36** Burn of third degree of back of hand
  ● **T23.361** Burn of third degree of back of right hand
  ● **T23.362** Burn of third degree of back of left hand
  ● **T23.369** Burn of third degree of back of unspecified hand
● **T23.37** Burn of third degree of wrist
  ● **T23.371** Burn of third degree of right wrist
  ● **T23.372** Burn of third degree of left wrist
  ● **T23.379** Burn of third degree of unspecified wrist
● **T23.39** Burn of third degree of multiple sites of wrist and hand
  ● **T23.391** Burn of third degree of multiple sites of right wrist and hand
  ● **T23.392** Burn of third degree of multiple sites of left wrist and hand
  ● **T23.399** Burn of third degree of multiple sites of unspecified wrist and hand
● **T23.4** Corrosion of unspecified degree of wrist and hand
  Code first (T51-T65) to identify chemical and intent
  Use additional external cause code to identify place (Y92)
  ● **T23.40** Corrosion of unspecified degree of hand, unspecified site
    ● **T23.401** Corrosion of unspecified degree of right hand, unspecified site
    ● **T23.402** Corrosion of unspecified degree of left hand, unspecified site
    ● **T23.409** Corrosion of unspecified degree of unspecified hand, unspecified site
  ● **T23.41** Corrosion of unspecified degree of thumb (nail)
    ● **T23.411** Corrosion of unspecified degree of right thumb (nail)
    ● **T23.412** Corrosion of unspecified degree of left thumb (nail)
    ● **T23.419** Corrosion of unspecified degree of unspecified thumb (nail)
  ● **T23.42** Corrosion of unspecified degree of single finger (nail) except thumb
    ● **T23.421** Corrosion of unspecified degree of single right finger (nail) except thumb
    ● **T23.422** Corrosion of unspecified degree of single left finger (nail) except thumb
    ● **T23.429** Corrosion of unspecified degree of unspecified single finger (nail) except thumb
  ● **T23.43** Corrosion of unspecified degree of multiple fingers (nail), not including thumb
    ● **T23.431** Corrosion of unspecified degree of multiple right fingers (nail), not including thumb
    ● **T23.432** Corrosion of unspecified degree of multiple left fingers (nail), not including thumb
    ● **T23.439** Corrosion of unspecified degree of unspecified multiple fingers (nail), not including thumb

◄ New   ◀▏ Revised   ~~deleted~~ Deleted   Excludes 1   Excludes 2   Includes   Use additional   Code first   Code also   Unspecified
OGCR Official Guidelines   **X** Assign placeholder X   ● Use Additional Character(s)   ▶ Manifestation Code   **Coding Clinic**

● **T23.44** Corrosion of unspecified degree of multiple fingers (nail), including thumb
- ● **T23.441** Corrosion of unspecified degree of multiple right fingers (nail), including thumb
- ● **T23.442** Corrosion of unspecified degree of multiple left fingers (nail), including thumb
- ● **T23.449** Corrosion of unspecified degree of unspecified multiple fingers (nail), including thumb

● **T23.45** Corrosion of unspecified degree of palm
- ● **T23.451** Corrosion of unspecified degree of right palm
- ● **T23.452** Corrosion of unspecified degree of left palm
- ● **T23.459** Corrosion of unspecified degree of unspecified palm

● **T23.46** Corrosion of unspecified degree of back of hand
- ● **T23.461** Corrosion of unspecified degree of back of right hand
- ● **T23.462** Corrosion of unspecified degree of back of left hand
- ● **T23.469** Corrosion of unspecified degree of back of unspecified hand

● **T23.47** Corrosion of unspecified degree of wrist
- ● **T23.471** Corrosion of unspecified degree of right wrist
- ● **T23.472** Corrosion of unspecified degree of left wrist
- ● **T23.479** Corrosion of unspecified degree of unspecified wrist

● **T23.49** Corrosion of unspecified degree of multiple sites of wrist and hand
- ● **T23.491** Corrosion of unspecified degree of multiple sites of right wrist and hand
- ● **T23.492** Corrosion of unspecified degree of multiple sites of left wrist and hand
- ● **T23.499** Corrosion of unspecified degree of multiple sites of unspecified wrist and hand

● **T23.5** Corrosion of first degree of wrist and hand
  Code first (T51-T65) *to identify chemical and intent*
  Use additional external cause code to identify place (Y92)

● **T23.50** Corrosion of first degree of hand, unspecified site
- ● **T23.501** Corrosion of first degree of right hand, unspecified site
- ● **T23.502** Corrosion of first degree of left hand, unspecified site
- ● **T23.509** Corrosion of first degree of unspecified hand, unspecified site

● **T23.51** Corrosion of first degree of thumb (nail)
- ● **T23.511** Corrosion of first degree of right thumb (nail)
- ● **T23.512** Corrosion of first degree of left thumb (nail)
- ● **T23.519** Corrosion of first degree of unspecified thumb (nail)

● **T23.52** Corrosion of first degree of single finger (nail) except thumb
- ● **T23.521** Corrosion of first degree of single right finger (nail) except thumb
- ● **T23.522** Corrosion of first degree of single left finger (nail) except thumb
- ● **T23.529** Corrosion of first degree of unspecified single finger (nail) except thumb

● **T23.53** Corrosion of first degree of multiple fingers (nail), not including thumb
- ● **T23.531** Corrosion of first degree of multiple right fingers (nail), not including thumb
- ● **T23.532** Corrosion of first degree of multiple left fingers (nail), not including thumb
- ● **T23.539** Corrosion of first degree of unspecified multiple fingers (nail), not including thumb

● **T23.54** Corrosion of first degree of multiple fingers (nail), including thumb
- ● **T23.541** Corrosion of first degree of multiple right fingers (nail), including thumb
- ● **T23.542** Corrosion of first degree of multiple left fingers (nail), including thumb
- ● **T23.549** Corrosion of first degree of unspecified multiple fingers (nail), including thumb

● **T23.55** Corrosion of first degree of palm
- ● **T23.551** Corrosion of first degree of right palm
- ● **T23.552** Corrosion of first degree of left palm
- ● **T23.559** Corrosion of first degree of unspecified palm

● **T23.56** Corrosion of first degree of back of hand
- ● **T23.561** Corrosion of first degree of back of right hand
- ● **T23.562** Corrosion of first degree of back of left hand
- ● **T23.569** Corrosion of first degree of back of unspecified hand

● **T23.57** Corrosion of first degree of wrist
- ● **T23.571** Corrosion of first degree of right wrist
- ● **T23.572** Corrosion of first degree of left wrist
- ● **T23.579** Corrosion of first degree of unspecified wrist

● **T23.59** Corrosion of first degree of multiple sites of wrist and hand
- ● **T23.591** Corrosion of first degree of multiple sites of right wrist and hand
- ● **T23.592** Corrosion of first degree of multiple sites of left wrist and hand
- ● **T23.599** Corrosion of first degree of multiple sites of unspecified wrist and hand

● **T23.6** Corrosion of second degree of wrist and hand
  Code first (T51-T65) *to identify chemical and intent*
  Use additional external cause code to identify place (Y92)

● **T23.60** Corrosion of second degree of hand, unspecified site
- ● **T23.601** Corrosion of second degree of right hand, unspecified site
- ● **T23.602** Corrosion of second degree of left hand, unspecified site
- ● **T23.609** Corrosion of second degree of unspecified hand, unspecified site

● **T23.61** Corrosion of second degree of thumb (nail)
- ● **T23.611** Corrosion of second degree of right thumb (nail)
- ● **T23.612** Corrosion of second degree of left thumb (nail)
- ● **T23.619** Corrosion of second degree of unspecified thumb (nail)

● **T23.62** Corrosion of second degree of single finger (nail) except thumb
- ● **T23.621** Corrosion of second degree of single right finger (nail) except thumb
- ● **T23.622** Corrosion of second degree of single left finger (nail) except thumb
- ● **T23.629** Corrosion of second degree of unspecified single finger (nail) except thumb

CHAPTER 19 (S00-T88)

CHAPTER 19 (S00-T88)

● T23.63   Corrosion of second degree of multiple fingers (nail), not including thumb
     ● T23.631   Corrosion of second degree of multiple right fingers (nail), not including thumb
     ● T23.632   Corrosion of second degree of multiple left fingers (nail), not including thumb
     ● T23.639   Corrosion of second degree of unspecified multiple fingers (nail), not including thumb

● T23.64   Corrosion of second degree of multiple fingers (nail), including thumb
     ● T23.641   Corrosion of second degree of multiple right fingers (nail), including thumb
     ● T23.642   Corrosion of second degree of multiple left fingers (nail), including thumb
     ● T23.649   Corrosion of second degree of unspecified multiple fingers (nail), including thumb

● T23.65   Corrosion of second degree of palm
     ● T23.651   Corrosion of second degree of right palm
     ● T23.652   Corrosion of second degree of left palm
     ● T23.659   Corrosion of second degree of unspecified palm

● T23.66   Corrosion of second degree of back of hand
     ● T23.661   Corrosion of second degree back of right hand
     ● T23.662   Corrosion of second degree back of left hand
     ● T23.669   Corrosion of second degree back of unspecified hand

● T23.67   Corrosion of second degree of wrist
     ● T23.671   Corrosion of second degree of right wrist
     ● T23.672   Corrosion of second degree of left wrist
     ● T23.679   Corrosion of second degree of unspecified wrist

● T23.69   Corrosion of second degree of multiple sites of wrist and hand
     ● T23.691   Corrosion of second degree of multiple sites of right wrist and hand
     ● T23.692   Corrosion of second degree of multiple sites of left wrist and hand
     ● T23.699   Corrosion of second degree of multiple sites of unspecified wrist and hand

● T23.7   Corrosion of third degree of wrist and hand
     Code first (T51-T65) *to identify chemical and intent*
     Use additional external cause code to identify place (Y92)

● T23.70   Corrosion of third degree of hand, unspecified site
     ● T23.701   Corrosion of third degree of right hand, unspecified site
     ● T23.702   Corrosion of third degree of left hand, unspecified site
     ● T23.709   Corrosion of third degree of unspecified hand, unspecified site

● T23.71   Corrosion of third degree of thumb (nail)
     ● T23.711   Corrosion of third degree of right thumb (nail)
     ● T23.712   Corrosion of third degree of left thumb (nail)
     ● T23.719   Corrosion of third degree of unspecified thumb (nail)

● T23.72   Corrosion of third degree of single finger (nail) except thumb
     ● T23.721   Corrosion of third degree of single right finger (nail) except thumb
     ● T23.722   Corrosion of third degree of single left finger (nail) except thumb
     ● T23.729   Corrosion of third degree of unspecified single finger (nail) except thumb

● T23.73   Corrosion of third degree of multiple fingers (nail), not including thumb
     ● T23.731   Corrosion of third degree of multiple right fingers (nail), not including thumb
     ● T23.732   Corrosion of third degree of multiple left fingers (nail), not including thumb
     ● T23.739   Corrosion of third degree of unspecified multiple fingers (nail), not including thumb

● T23.74   Corrosion of third degree of multiple fingers (nail), including thumb
     ● T23.741   Corrosion of third degree of multiple right fingers (nail), including thumb
     ● T23.742   Corrosion of third degree of multiple left fingers (nail), including thumb
     ● T23.749   Corrosion of third degree of unspecified multiple fingers (nail), including thumb

● T23.75   Corrosion of third degree of palm
     ● T23.751   Corrosion of third degree of right palm
     ● T23.752   Corrosion of third degree of left palm
     ● T23.759   Corrosion of third degree of unspecified palm

● T23.76   Corrosion of third degree of back of hand
     ● T23.761   Corrosion of third degree of back of right hand
     ● T23.762   Corrosion of third degree of back of left hand
     ● T23.769   Corrosion of third degree of back of unspecified hand

● T23.77   Corrosion of third degree of wrist
     ● T23.771   Corrosion of third degree of right wrist
     ● T23.772   Corrosion of third degree of left wrist
     ● T23.779   Corrosion of third degree of unspecified wrist

● T23.79   Corrosion of third degree of multiple sites of wrist and hand
     ● T23.791   Corrosion of third degree of multiple sites of right wrist and hand
     ● T23.792   Corrosion of third degree of multiple sites of left wrist and hand
     ● T23.799   Corrosion of third degree of multiple sites of unspecified wrist and hand

◄ New   ⇐ Revised   ~~deleted~~ Deleted   Excludes 1   Excludes 2   Includes   Use additional   Code first   Code also   Unspecified
OGCR Official Guidelines   X Assign placeholder X   ● Use Additional Character(s)   ▶ Manifestation Code   **Coding Clinic**

● T24 **Burn and corrosion of lower limb, except ankle and foot**

> **Excludes2** burn and corrosion of ankle and foot (T25.-)
> burn and corrosion of hip region (T21.-)

> The appropriate 7th character is to be added to each code from category T24

> | A | initial encounter |
> |---|---|
> | D | subsequent encounter |
> | S | sequela |

● T24.0 **Burn of unspecified degree of lower limb, except ankle and foot**

> Use additional external cause code to identify the source, place and intent of the burn (X00-X19, X75-X77, X96-X98, Y92)

● T24.00 Burn of unspecified degree of unspecified site of lower limb, except ankle and foot

● T24.001 Burn of unspecified degree of unspecified site of right lower limb, except ankle and foot

● T24.002 Burn of unspecified degree of unspecified site of left lower limb, except ankle and foot

● T24.009 Burn of unspecified degree of unspecified site of unspecified lower limb, except ankle and foot

● T24.01 Burn of unspecified degree of thigh

● T24.011 Burn of unspecified degree of right thigh

● T24.012 Burn of unspecified degree of left thigh

● T24.019 Burn of unspecified degree of unspecified thigh

● T24.02 Burn of unspecified degree of knee

● T24.021 Burn of unspecified degree of right knee

● T24.022 Burn of unspecified degree of left knee

● T24.029 Burn of unspecified degree of unspecified knee

● T24.03 Burn of unspecified degree of lower leg

● T24.031 Burn of unspecified degree of right lower leg

● T24.032 Burn of unspecified degree of left lower leg

● T24.039 Burn of unspecified degree of unspecified lower leg

● T24.09 Burn of unspecified degree of multiple sites of lower limb, except ankle and foot

● T24.091 Burn of unspecified degree of multiple sites of right lower limb, except ankle and foot

● T24.092 Burn of unspecified degree of multiple sites of left lower limb, except ankle and foot

● T24.099 Burn of unspecified degree of multiple sites of unspecified lower limb, except ankle and foot

● T24.1 **Burn of first degree of lower limb, except ankle and foot**

> Use additional external cause code to identify the source, place and intent of the burn (X00-X19, X75-X77, X96-X98, Y92)

● T24.10 Burn of first degree of unspecified site of lower limb, except ankle and foot

● T24.101 Burn of first degree of unspecified site of right lower limb, except ankle and foot

● T24.102 Burn of first degree of unspecified site of left lower limb, except ankle and foot

● T24.109 Burn of first degree of unspecified site of unspecified lower limb, except ankle and foot

● T24.11 Burn of first degree of thigh

● T24.111 Burn of first degree of right thigh

● T24.112 Burn of first degree of left thigh

● T24.119 Burn of first degree of unspecified thigh

● T24.12 Burn of first degree of knee

● T24.121 Burn of first degree of right knee

● T24.122 Burn of first degree of left knee

● T24.129 Burn of first degree of unspecified knee

● T24.13 Burn of first degree of lower leg

● T24.131 Burn of first degree of right lower leg

● T24.132 Burn of first degree of left lower leg

● T24.139 Burn of first degree of unspecified lower leg

● T24.19 Burn of first degree of multiple sites of lower limb, except ankle and foot

● T24.191 Burn of first degree of multiple sites of right lower limb, except ankle and foot

● T24.192 Burn of first degree of multiple sites of left lower limb, except ankle and foot

● T24.199 Burn of first degree of multiple sites of unspecified lower limb, except ankle and foot

● T24.2 **Burn of second degree of lower limb, except ankle and foot**

> Use additional external cause code to identify the source, place and intent of the burn (X00-X19, X75-X77, X96-X98, Y92)

● T24.20 Burn of second degree of unspecified site of lower limb, except ankle and foot

● T24.201 Burn of second degree of unspecified site of right lower limb, except ankle and foot

● T24.202 Burn of second degree of unspecified site of left lower limb, except ankle and foot

● T24.209 Burn of second degree of unspecified site of unspecified lower limb, except ankle and foot

● T24.21 Burn of second degree of thigh

● T24.211 Burn of second degree of right thigh

● T24.212 Burn of second degree of left thigh

● T24.219 Burn of second degree of unspecified thigh

● T24.22 Burn of second degree of knee

● T24.221 Burn of second degree of right knee

● T24.222 Burn of second degree of left knee

● T24.229 Burn of second degree of unspecified knee

● T24.23 Burn of second degree of lower leg

● T24.231 Burn of second degree of right lower leg

● T24.232 Burn of second degree of left lower leg

● T24.239 Burn of second degree of unspecified lower leg

● T24.29 Burn of second degree of multiple sites of lower limb, except ankle and foot

● T24.291 Burn of second degree of multiple sites of right lower limb, except ankle and foot

● T24.292 Burn of second degree of multiple sites of left lower limb, except ankle and foot

● T24.299 Burn of second degree of multiple sites of unspecified lower limb, except ankle and foot

● T24.3   Burn of third degree of lower limb, except ankle and foot

    Use additional external cause code to identify the source, place and intent of the burn (X00-X19, X75-X77, X96-X98, Y92)

  ● T24.30   Burn of third degree of unspecified site of lower limb, except ankle and foot

    ● T24.301   Burn of third degree of unspecified site of right lower limb, except ankle and foot

    ● T24.302   Burn of third degree of unspecified site of left lower limb, except ankle and foot

    ● T24.309   Burn of third degree of unspecified site of unspecified lower limb, except ankle and foot

  ● T24.31   Burn of third degree of thigh

    ● T24.311   Burn of third degree of right thigh

    ● T24.312   Burn of third degree of left thigh

    ● T24.319   Burn of third degree of unspecified thigh

  ● T24.32   Burn of third degree of knee

    ● T24.321   Burn of third degree of right knee

    ● T24.322   Burn of third degree of left knee

    ● T24.329   Burn of third degree of unspecified knee

  ● T24.33   Burn of third degree of lower leg

    ● T24.331   Burn of third degree of right lower leg

    ● T24.332   Burn of third degree of left lower leg

    ● T24.339   Burn of third degree of unspecified lower leg

  ● T24.39   Burn of third degree of multiple sites of lower limb, except ankle and foot

    ● T24.391   Burn of third degree of multiple sites of right lower limb, except ankle and foot

    ● T24.392   Burn of third degree of multiple sites of left lower limb, except ankle and foot

    ● T24.399   Burn of third degree of multiple sites of unspecified lower limb, except ankle and foot

● T24.4   Corrosion of unspecified degree of lower limb, except ankle and foot

    Code first (T51-T65) to identify chemical and intent

    Use additional external cause code to identify place (Y92)

  ● T24.40   Corrosion of unspecified degree of unspecified site of lower limb, except ankle and foot

    ● T24.401   Corrosion of unspecified degree of unspecified site of right lower limb, except ankle and foot

    ● T24.402   Corrosion of unspecified degree of unspecified site of left lower limb, except ankle and foot

    ● T24.409   Corrosion of unspecified degree of unspecified site of unspecified lower limb, except ankle and foot

  ● T24.41   Corrosion of unspecified degree of thigh

    ● T24.411   Corrosion of unspecified degree of right thigh

    ● T24.412   Corrosion of unspecified degree of left thigh

    ● T24.419   Corrosion of unspecified degree of unspecified thigh

● T24.42   Corrosion of unspecified degree of knee

    ● T24.421   Corrosion of unspecified degree of right knee

    ● T24.422   Corrosion of unspecified degree of left knee

    ● T24.429   Corrosion of unspecified degree of unspecified knee

● T24.43   Corrosion of unspecified degree of lower leg

    ● T24.431   Corrosion of unspecified degree of right lower leg

    ● T24.432   Corrosion of unspecified degree of left lower leg

    ● T24.439   Corrosion of unspecified degree of unspecified lower leg

● T24.49   Corrosion of unspecified degree of multiple sites of lower limb, except ankle and foot

    ● T24.491   Corrosion of unspecified degree of multiple sites of right lower limb, except ankle and foot

    ● T24.492   Corrosion of unspecified degree of multiple sites of left lower limb, except ankle and foot

    ● T24.499   Corrosion of unspecified degree of multiple sites of unspecified lower limb, except ankle and foot

● T24.5   Corrosion of first degree of lower limb, except ankle and foot

    Code first (T51-T65) to identify chemical and intent

    Use additional external cause code to identify place (Y92)

  ● T24.50   Corrosion of first degree of unspecified site of lower limb, except ankle and foot

    ● T24.501   Corrosion of first degree of unspecified site of right lower limb, except ankle and foot

    ● T24.502   Corrosion of first degree of unspecified site of left lower limb, except ankle and foot

    ● T24.509   Corrosion of first degree of unspecified site of unspecified lower limb, except ankle and foot

  ● T24.51   Corrosion of first degree of thigh

    ● T24.511   Corrosion of first degree of right thigh

    ● T24.512   Corrosion of first degree of left thigh

    ● T24.519   Corrosion of first degree of unspecified thigh

  ● T24.52   Corrosion of first degree of knee

    ● T24.521   Corrosion of first degree of right knee

    ● T24.522   Corrosion of first degree of left knee

    ● T24.529   Corrosion of first degree of unspecified knee

  ● T24.53   Corrosion of first degree of lower leg

    ● T24.531   Corrosion of first degree of right lower leg

    ● T24.532   Corrosion of first degree of left lower leg

    ● T24.539   Corrosion of first degree of unspecified lower leg

  ● T24.59   Corrosion of first degree of multiple sites of lower limb, except ankle and foot

    ● T24.591   Corrosion of first degree of multiple sites of right lower limb, except ankle and foot

    ● T24.592   Corrosion of first degree of multiple sites of left lower limb, except ankle and foot

    ● T24.599   Corrosion of first degree of multiple sites of unspecified lower limb, except ankle and foot

◀ New   ◀ Revised   ~~deleted~~ Deleted   Excludes 1   Excludes 2   Includes   Use additional   Code first   Code also   Unspecified

OGCR Official Guidelines   X Assign placeholder X   ● Use Additional Character(s)   ▶ Manifestation Code   **Coding Clinic**

● **T24.6**   **Corrosion of second degree of lower limb, except ankle and foot**

> *Code first (T51-T65) to identify chemical and intent*
> Use additional external cause code to identify place (Y92)

● **T24.60**   Corrosion of second degree of unspecified site of lower limb, except ankle and foot

● **T24.601**   Corrosion of second degree of unspecified site of right lower limb, except ankle and foot

● **T24.602**   Corrosion of second degree of unspecified site of left lower limb, except ankle and foot

● **T24.609**   Corrosion of second degree of unspecified site of unspecified lower limb, except ankle and foot

● **T24.61**   Corrosion of second degree of thigh

● **T24.611**   Corrosion of second degree of right thigh

● **T24.612**   Corrosion of second degree of left thigh

● **T24.619**   Corrosion of second degree of unspecified thigh

● **T24.62**   Corrosion of second degree of knee

● **T24.621**   Corrosion of second degree of right knee

● **T24.622**   Corrosion of second degree of left knee

● **T24.629**   Corrosion of second degree of unspecified knee

● **T24.63**   Corrosion of second degree of lower leg

● **T24.631**   Corrosion of second degree of right lower leg

● **T24.632**   Corrosion of second degree of left lower leg

● **T24.639**   Corrosion of second degree of unspecified lower leg

● **T24.69**   Corrosion of second degree of multiple sites of lower limb, except ankle and foot

● **T24.691**   Corrosion of second degree of multiple sites of right lower limb, except ankle and foot

● **T24.692**   Corrosion of second degree of multiple sites of left lower limb, except ankle and foot

● **T24.699**   Corrosion of second degree of multiple sites of unspecified lower limb, except ankle and foot

● **T24.7**   **Corrosion of third degree of lower limb, except ankle and foot**

> *Code first (T51-T65) to identify chemical and intent*
> Use additional external cause code to identify place (Y92)

● **T24.70**   Corrosion of third degree of unspecified site of lower limb, except ankle and foot

● **T24.701**   Corrosion of third degree of unspecified site of right lower limb, except ankle and foot

● **T24.702**   Corrosion of third degree of unspecified site of left lower limb, except ankle and foot

● **T24.709**   Corrosion of third degree of unspecified site of unspecified lower limb, except ankle and foot

● **T24.71**   Corrosion of third degree of thigh

● **T24.711**   Corrosion of third degree of right thigh

● **T24.712**   Corrosion of third degree of left thigh

● **T24.719**   Corrosion of third degree of unspecified thigh

● **T24.72**   Corrosion of third degree of knee

● **T24.721**   Corrosion of third degree of right knee

● **T24.722**   Corrosion of third degree of left knee

● **T24.729**   Corrosion of third degree of unspecified knee

● **T24.73**   Corrosion of third degree of lower leg

● **T24.731**   Corrosion of third degree of right lower leg

● **T24.732**   Corrosion of third degree of left lower leg

● **T24.739**   Corrosion of third degree of unspecified lower leg

● **T24.79**   Corrosion of third degree of multiple sites of lower limb, except ankle and foot

● **T24.791**   Corrosion of third degree of multiple sites of right lower limb, except ankle and foot

● **T24.792**   Corrosion of third degree of multiple sites of left lower limb, except ankle and foot

● **T24.799**   Corrosion of third degree of multiple sites of unspecified lower limb, except ankle and foot

● **T25**   **Burn and corrosion of ankle and foot**

> The appropriate 7th character is to be added to each code from category T25

A	initial encounter
D	subsequent encounter
S	sequela

● **T25.0**   **Burn of unspecified degree of ankle and foot**

> Use additional external cause code to identify the source, place and intent of the burn (X00-X19, X75-X77, X96-X98, Y92)

● **T25.01**   Burn of unspecified degree of ankle

● **T25.011**   Burn of unspecified degree of right ankle

● **T25.012**   Burn of unspecified degree of left ankle

● **T25.019**   Burn of unspecified degree of unspecified ankle

● **T25.02**   Burn of unspecified degree of foot

> **Excludes2**   burn of unspecified degree of toe(s) (nail) (T25.03-)

● **T25.021**   Burn of unspecified degree of right foot

● **T25.022**   Burn of unspecified degree of left foot

● **T25.029**   Burn of unspecified degree of unspecified foot

● **T25.03**   Burn of unspecified degree of toe(s) (nail)

● **T25.031**   Burn of unspecified degree of right toe(s) (nail)

● **T25.032**   Burn of unspecified degree of left toe(s) (nail)

● **T25.039**   Burn of unspecified degree of unspecified toe(s) (nail)

● **T25.09** Burn of unspecified degree of multiple sites of ankle and foot

   ● **T25.091** Burn of unspecified degree of multiple sites of right ankle and foot

   ● **T25.092** Burn of unspecified degree of multiple sites of left ankle and foot

   ● **T25.099** Burn of unspecified degree of multiple sites of unspecified ankle and foot

● **T25.1** Burn of first degree of ankle and foot

Use additional external cause code to identify the source, place and intent of the burn (X00-X19, X75-X77, X96-X98, Y92)

 ● **T25.11** Burn of first degree of ankle

   ● **T25.111** Burn of first degree of right ankle

   ● **T25.112** Burn of first degree of left ankle

   ● **T25.119** Burn of first degree of unspecified ankle

 ● **T25.12** Burn of first degree of foot

     Excludes2   burn of first degree of toe(s) (nail) (T25.13-)

   ● **T25.121** Burn of first degree of right foot

   ● **T25.122** Burn of first degree of left foot

   ● **T25.129** Burn of first degree of unspecified foot

 ● **T25.13** Burn of first degree of toe(s) (nail)

   ● **T25.131** Burn of first degree of right toe(s) (nail)

   ● **T25.132** Burn of first degree of left toe(s) (nail)

   ● **T25.139** Burn of first degree of unspecified toe(s) (nail)

 ● **T25.19** Burn of first degree of multiple sites of ankle and foot

   ● **T25.191** Burn of first degree of multiple sites of right ankle and foot

   ● **T25.192** Burn of first degree of multiple sites of left ankle and foot

   ● **T25.199** Burn of first degree of multiple sites of unspecified ankle and foot

● **T25.2** Burn of second degree of ankle and foot

Use additional external cause code to identify the source, place and intent of the burn (X00-X19, X75-X77, X96-X98, Y92)

 ● **T25.21** Burn of second degree of ankle

   ● **T25.211** Burn of second degree of right ankle

   ● **T25.212** Burn of second degree of left ankle

   ● **T25.219** Burn of second degree of unspecified ankle

 ● **T25.22** Burn of second degree of foot

     Excludes2   burn of second degree of toe(s) (nail) (T25.23-)

   ● **T25.221** Burn of second degree of right foot

   ● **T25.222** Burn of second degree of left foot

   ● **T25.229** Burn of second degree of unspecified foot

 ● **T25.23** Burn of second degree of toe(s) (nail)

   ● **T25.231** Burn of second degree of right toe(s) (nail)

   ● **T25.232** Burn of second degree of left toe(s) (nail)

   ● **T25.239** Burn of second degree of unspecified toe(s) (nail)

● **T25.29** Burn of second degree of multiple sites of ankle and foot

   ● **T25.291** Burn of second degree of multiple sites of right ankle and foot

   ● **T25.292** Burn of second degree of multiple sites of left ankle and foot

   ● **T25.299** Burn of second degree of multiple sites of unspecified ankle and foot

● **T25.3** Burn of third degree of ankle and foot

Use additional external cause code to identify the source, place and intent of the burn (X00-X19, X75-X77, X96-X98, Y92)

 ● **T25.31** Burn of third degree of ankle

   ● **T25.311** Burn of third degree of right ankle

   ● **T25.312** Burn of third degree of left ankle

   ● **T25.319** Burn of third degree of unspecified ankle

 ● **T25.32** Burn of third degree of foot

     Excludes2   burn of third degree of toe(s) (nail) (T25.33-)

   ● **T25.321** Burn of third degree of right foot

   ● **T25.322** Burn of third degree of left foot

   ● **T25.329** Burn of third degree of unspecified foot

 ● **T25.33** Burn of third degree of toe(s) (nail)

   ● **T25.331** Burn of third degree of right toe(s) (nail)

   ● **T25.332** Burn of third degree of left toe(s) (nail)

   ● **T25.339** Burn of third degree of unspecified toe(s) (nail)

 ● **T25.39** Burn of third degree of multiple sites of ankle and foot

   ● **T25.391** Burn of third degree of multiple sites of right ankle and foot

   ● **T25.392** Burn of third degree of multiple sites of left ankle and foot

   ● **T25.399** Burn of third degree of multiple sites of unspecified ankle and foot

● **T25.4** Corrosion of unspecified degree of ankle and foot

Code first (T51-T65) to identify chemical and intent

Use additional external cause code to identify place (Y92)

 ● **T25.41** Corrosion of unspecified degree of ankle

   ● **T25.411** Corrosion of unspecified degree of right ankle

   ● **T25.412** Corrosion of unspecified degree of left ankle

   ● **T25.419** Corrosion of unspecified degree of unspecified ankle

 ● **T25.42** Corrosion of unspecified degree of foot

     Excludes2   corrosion of unspecified degree of toe(s) (nail) (T25.43-)

   ● **T25.421** Corrosion of unspecified degree of right foot

   ● **T25.422** Corrosion of unspecified degree of left foot

   ● **T25.429** Corrosion of unspecified degree of unspecified foot

 ● **T25.43** Corrosion of unspecified degree of toe(s) (nail)

   ● **T25.431** Corrosion of unspecified degree of right toe(s) (nail)

   ● **T25.432** Corrosion of unspecified degree of left toe(s) (nail)

   ● **T25.439** Corrosion of unspecified degree of unspecified toe(s) (nail)

◀ New   ◀ Revised   ~~deleted~~ Deleted   Excludes 1   Excludes 2   Includes   Use additional   Code first   Code also   Unspecified

OGCR Official Guidelines   **X** Assign placeholder X   ● Use Additional Character(s)   ▶ Manifestation Code   **Coding Clinic**

● **T25.49**   **Corrosion of unspecified degree of multiple sites of ankle and foot**
  - ● **T25.491**   Corrosion of unspecified degree of multiple sites of right ankle and foot
  - ● **T25.492**   Corrosion of unspecified degree of multiple sites of left ankle and foot
  - ● **T25.499**   Corrosion of unspecified degree of multiple sites of unspecified ankle and foot

● **T25.5**   **Corrosion of first degree of ankle and foot**
  Code first (T51-T65) to identify chemical and intent
  Use additional external cause code to identify place (Y92)

  - ● **T25.51**   **Corrosion of first degree of ankle**
    - ● **T25.511**   Corrosion of first degree of right ankle
    - ● **T25.512**   Corrosion of first degree of left ankle
    - ● **T25.519**   Corrosion of first degree of unspecified ankle
  - ● **T25.52**   **Corrosion of first degree of foot**
    - **Excludes2**   corrosion of first degree of toe(s) (nail) (T25.53-)
    - ● **T25.521**   Corrosion of first degree of right foot
    - ● **T25.522**   Corrosion of first degree of left foot
    - ● **T25.529**   Corrosion of first degree of unspecified foot
  - ● **T25.53**   **Corrosion of first degree of toe(s) (nail)**
    - ● **T25.531**   Corrosion of first degree of right toe(s) (nail)
    - ● **T25.532**   Corrosion of first degree of left toe(s) (nail)
    - ● **T25.539**   Corrosion of first degree of unspecified toe(s) (nail)
  - ● **T25.59**   **Corrosion of first degree of multiple sites of ankle and foot**
    - ● **T25.591**   Corrosion of first degree of multiple sites of right ankle and foot
    - ● **T25.592**   Corrosion of first degree of multiple sites of left ankle and foot
    - ● **T25.599**   Corrosion of first degree of multiple sites of unspecified ankle and foot

● **T25.6**   **Corrosion of second degree of ankle and foot**
  Code first (T51-T65) to identify chemical and intent
  Use additional external cause code to identify place (Y92)

  - ● **T25.61**   **Corrosion of second degree of ankle**
    - ● **T25.611**   Corrosion of second degree of right ankle
    - ● **T25.612**   Corrosion of second degree of left ankle
    - ● **T25.619**   Corrosion of second degree of unspecified ankle
  - ● **T25.62**   **Corrosion of second degree of foot**
    - **Excludes2**   corrosion of second degree of toe(s) (nail) (T25.63-)
    - ● **T25.621**   Corrosion of second degree of right foot
    - ● **T25.622**   Corrosion of second degree of left foot
    - ● **T25.629**   Corrosion of second degree of unspecified foot
  - ● **T25.63**   **Corrosion of second degree of toe(s) (nail)**
    - ● **T25.631**   Corrosion of second degree of right toe(s) (nail)
    - ● **T25.632**   Corrosion of second degree of left toe(s) (nail)
    - ● **T25.639**   Corrosion of second degree of unspecified toe(s) (nail)

● **T25.69**   **Corrosion of second degree of multiple sites of ankle and foot**
  - ● **T25.691**   Corrosion of second degree of right ankle and foot
  - ● **T25.692**   Corrosion of second degree of left ankle and foot
  - ● **T25.699**   Corrosion of second degree of unspecified ankle and foot

● **T25.7**   **Corrosion of third degree of ankle and foot**
  Code first (T51-T65) to identify chemical and intent
  Use additional external cause code to identify place (Y92)

  - ● **T25.71**   **Corrosion of third degree of ankle**
    - ● **T25.711**   Corrosion of third degree of right ankle
    - ● **T25.712**   Corrosion of third degree of left ankle
    - ● **T25.719**   Corrosion of third degree of unspecified ankle
  - ● **T25.72**   **Corrosion of third degree of foot**
    - **Excludes2**   corrosion of third degree of toe(s) (nail) (T25.73-)
    - ● **T25.721**   Corrosion of third degree of right foot
    - ● **T25.722**   Corrosion of third degree of left foot
    - ● **T25.729**   Corrosion of third degree of unspecified foot
  - ● **T25.73**   **Corrosion of third degree of toe(s) (nail)**
    - ● **T25.731**   Corrosion of third degree of right toe(s) (nail)
    - ● **T25.732**   Corrosion of third degree of left toe(s) (nail)
    - ● **T25.739**   Corrosion of third degree of unspecified toe(s) (nail)
  - ● **T25.79**   **Corrosion of third degree of multiple sites of ankle and foot**
    - ● **T25.791**   Corrosion of third degree of multiple sites of right ankle and foot
    - ● **T25.792**   Corrosion of third degree of multiple sites of left ankle and foot
    - ● **T25.799**   Corrosion of third degree of multiple sites of unspecified ankle and foot

BURNS AND CORROSIONS CONFINED TO EYE AND INTERNAL ORGANS (T26-T28)

● **T26**   **Burn and corrosion confined to eye and adnexa**
  The appropriate 7th character is to be added to each code from category T26

A	initial encounter
D	subsequent encounter
S	sequela

  - ● **T26.0**   **Burn of eyelid and periocular area**
    Use additional external cause code to identify the source, place and intent of the burn (X00-X19, X75-X77, X96-X98, Y92)
    - X● **T26.00**   Burn of unspecified eyelid and periocular area
    - X● **T26.01**   Burn of right eyelid and periocular area
    - X● **T26.02**   Burn of left eyelid and periocular area
  - ● **T26.1**   **Burn of cornea and conjunctival sac**
    Use additional external cause code to identify the source, place and intent of the burn (X00-X19, X75-X77, X96-X98, Y92)
    - X● **T26.10**   Burn of cornea and conjunctival sac, unspecified eye
    - X● **T26.11**   Burn of cornea and conjunctival sac, right eye
    - X● **T26.12**   Burn of cornea and conjunctival sac, left eye

CHAPTER 19 (S00-T88)

● **T26.2**   **Burn with resulting rupture and destruction of eyeball**

Use additional external cause code to identify the source, place and intent of the burn (X00-X19, X75-X77, X96-X98, Y92)

X● **T26.20**   Burn with resulting rupture and destruction of <mark>unspecified</mark> eyeball

X● **T26.21**   Burn with resulting rupture and destruction of right eyeball

X● **T26.22**   Burn with resulting rupture and destruction of left eyeball

● **T26.3**   **Burns of other specified parts of eye and adnexa**

Use additional external cause code to identify the source, place and intent of the burn (X00-X19, X75-X77, X96-X98, Y92)

X● **T26.30**   Burns of other specified parts of <mark>unspecified</mark> eye and adnexa

X● **T26.31**   Burns of other specified parts of right eye and adnexa

X● **T26.32**   Burns of other specified parts of left eye and adnexa

● **T26.4**   **Burn of eye and adnexa, part unspecified**

Use additional external cause code to identify the source, place and intent of the burn (X00-X19, X75-X77, X96-X98, Y92)

X● **T26.40**   Burn of unspecified eye and adnexa, part <mark>unspecified</mark>

X● **T26.41**   Burn of right eye and adnexa, part <mark>unspecified</mark>

X● **T26.42**   Burn of left eye and adnexa, part <mark>unspecified</mark>

● **T26.5**   **Corrosion of eyelid and periocular area**

Code first (T51-T65) to identify chemical and intent

Use additional external cause code to identify place (Y92)

X● **T26.50**   Corrosion of <mark>unspecified</mark> eyelid and periocular area

X● **T26.51**   Corrosion of right eyelid and periocular area

X● **T26.52**   Corrosion of left eyelid and periocular area

● **T26.6**   **Corrosion of cornea and conjunctival sac**

Code first (T51-T65) to identify chemical and intent

Use additional external cause code to identify place (Y92)

X● **T26.60**   Corrosion of cornea and conjunctival sac, <mark>unspecified</mark> eye

X● **T26.61**   Corrosion of cornea and conjunctival sac, right eye

X● **T26.62**   Corrosion of cornea and conjunctival sac, left eye

● **T26.7**   **Corrosion with resulting rupture and destruction of eyeball**

Code first (T51-T65) to identify chemical and intent

Use additional external cause code to identify place (Y92)

X● **T26.70**   Corrosion with resulting rupture and destruction of <mark>unspecified</mark> eyeball

X● **T26.71**   Corrosion with resulting rupture and destruction of right eyeball

X● **T26.72**   Corrosion with resulting rupture and destruction of left eyeball

● **T26.8**   **Corrosions of other specified parts of eye and adnexa**

Code first (T51-T65) to identify chemical and intent

Use additional external cause code to identify place (Y92)

X● **T26.80**   Corrosions of other specified parts of <mark>unspecified</mark> eye and adnexa

X● **T26.81**   Corrosions of other specified parts of right eye and adnexa

X● **T26.82**   Corrosions of other specified parts of left eye and adnexa

● **T26.9**   **Corrosion of eye and adnexa, part unspecified**

Code first (T51-T65) to identify chemical and intent

Use additional external cause code to identify place (Y92)

X● **T26.90**   Corrosion of unspecified eye and adnexa, part <mark>unspecified</mark>

X● **T26.91**   Corrosion of right eye and adnexa, part <mark>unspecified</mark>

X● **T26.92**   Corrosion of left eye and adnexa, part <mark>unspecified</mark>

● **T27**   **Burn and corrosion of respiratory tract**

Use additional external cause code to identify the source and intent of the burn (X00-X19, X75-X77, X96-X98)

Use additional external cause code to identify place (Y92)

The appropriate 7th character is to be added to each code from category T27

A	initial encounter
D	subsequent encounter
S	sequela

X● **T27.0**   Burn of larynx and trachea

X● **T27.1**   Burn involving larynx and trachea with lung

X● **T27.2**   Burn of other parts of respiratory tract

Burn of thoracic cavity

X● **T27.3**   Burn of respiratory tract, part <mark>unspecified</mark>

Code first (T51-T65) to identify chemical and intent for codes T27.4-T27.7

X● **T27.4**   Corrosion of larynx and trachea

X● **T27.5**   Corrosion involving larynx and trachea with lung

X● **T27.6**   Corrosion of other parts of respiratory tract

X● **T27.7**   Corrosion of respiratory tract, part <mark>unspecified</mark>

● **T28**   **Burn and corrosion of other internal organs**

Use additional external cause code to identify the source and intent of the burn (X00-X19, X75-X77, X96-X98)

Use additional external cause code to identify place (Y92)

The appropriate 7th character is to be added to each code from category T28

A	initial encounter
D	subsequent encounter
S	sequela

X● **T28.0**   Burn of mouth and pharynx

X● **T28.1**   Burn of esophagus

X● **T28.2**   Burn of other parts of alimentary tract

X● **T28.3**   Burn of internal genitourinary organs

X● **T28.4**   Burns of other and unspecified internal organs

    X● **T28.40**   Burn of <mark>unspecified</mark> internal organ

    ● **T28.41**   Burn of ear drum

      ● **T28.411**   Burn of right ear drum

      ● **T28.412**   Burn of left ear drum

      ● **T28.419**   Burn of <mark>unspecified</mark> ear drum

    X● **T28.49**   Burn of other internal organ

Code first (T51-T65) to identify chemical and intent for T28.5-T28.9-

X● **T28.5**   Corrosion of mouth and pharynx

X● **T28.6**   Corrosion of esophagus

X● **T28.7**   Corrosion of other parts of alimentary tract

X● **T28.8**   Corrosion of internal genitourinary organs

● **T28.9**   Corrosions of other and unspecified internal organs

    X● **T28.90**   Corrosions of <mark>unspecified</mark> internal organs

    ● **T28.91**   Corrosions of ear drum

      ● **T28.911**   Corrosions of right ear drum

      ● **T28.912**   Corrosions of left ear drum

      ● **T28.919**   Corrosions of <mark>unspecified</mark> ear drum

    X● **T28.99**   Corrosions of other internal organs

◀ New   ◀▬ Revised   ~~deleted~~ Deleted   Excludes 1   Excludes 2   Includes   Use additional   Code first   Code also   Unspecified

OGCR Official Guidelines   X Assign placeholder X   ● Use Additional Character(s)   ▶ Manifestation Code   **Coding Clinic**

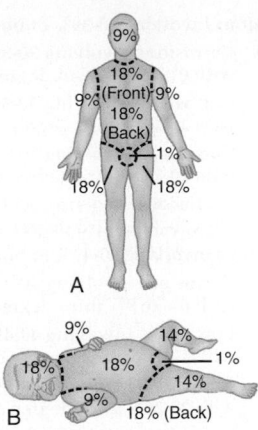

Figure 19-15 Rule of nines: percentages of total body area. (From Marx: Rosen's Emergency Medicine: Concepts and Clinical Practice, ed 6, Mosby, 2006)

OGCR Section I.C.19.d.5.

Assign separate code for each burn site
When coding burns, assign separate codes for each burn site. Category T30, Burn and corrosion, body region unspecified is extremely vague and should rarely be used.

OGCR See Section I.C.19.d.

BURNS AND CORROSIONS OF MULTIPLE AND UNSPECIFIED BODY REGIONS (T30-T32)

● **T30**   **Burn and corrosion, body region unspecified**

     T30.0   **Burn of** unspecified **body region, unspecified degree**
          This code is not for inpatient use. Code to specified site and degree of burns
          Burn NOS
          Multiple burns NOS

     T30.4   **Corrosion of** unspecified **body region, unspecified degree**
          This code is not for inpatient use. Code to specified site and degree of corrosion
          Corrosion NOS
          Multiple corrosion NOS

● **T31**   **Burns classified according to extent of body surface involved**

     Note: This category is to be used as the primary code only when the site of the burn is unspecified. It should be used as a supplementary code with categories T20-T25 when the site is specified.

     T31.0   **Burns involving less than 10% of body surface**

●   **T31.1**   **Burns involving 10-19% of body surface**

       T31.10   **Burns involving 10-19% of body surface with 0% to 9% third degree burns**
            Burns involving 10-19% of body surface NOS

       T31.11   **Burns involving 10-19% of body surface with 10-19% third degree burns**

●   **T31.2**   **Burns involving 20-29% of body surface**

       T31.20   **Burns involving 20-29% of body surface with 0% to 9% third degree burns**
            Burns involving 20-29% of body surface NOS

       T31.21   **Burns involving 20-29% of body surface with 10-19% third degree burns**

       T31.22   **Burns involving 20-29% of body surface with 20-29% third degree burns**

● **T31.3**   **Burns involving 30-39% of body surface**

     T31.30   **Burns involving 30-39% of body surface with 0% to 9% third degree burns**
          Burns involving 30-39% of body surface NOS

     T31.31   **Burns involving 30-39% of body surface with 10-19% third degree burns**

     T31.32   **Burns involving 30-39% of body surface with 20-29% third degree burns**

     T31.33   **Burns involving 30-39% of body surface with 30-39% third degree burns**

● **T31.4**   **Burns involving 40-49% of body surface**

     T31.40   **Burns involving 40-49% of body surface with 0% to 9% third degree burns**
          Burns involving 40-49% of body surface NOS

     T31.41   **Burns involving 40-49% of body surface with 10-19% third degree burns**

     T31.42   **Burns involving 40-49% of body surface with 20-29% third degree burns**

     T31.43   **Burns involving 40-49% of body surface with 30-39% third degree burns**

     T31.44   **Burns involving 40-49% of body surface with 40-49% third degree burns**

● **T31.5**   **Burns involving 50-59% of body surface**

     T31.50   **Burns involving 50-59% of body surface with 0% to 9% third degree burns**
          Burns involving 50-59% of body surface NOS

     T31.51   **Burns involving 50-59% of body surface with 10-19% third degree burns**

     T31.52   **Burns involving 50-59% of body surface with 20-29% third degree burns**

     T31.53   **Burns involving 50-59% of body surface with 30-39% third degree burns**

     T31.54   **Burns involving 50-59% of body surface with 40-49% third degree burns**

     T31.55   **Burns involving 50-59% of body surface with 50-59% third degree burns**

● **T31.6**   **Burns involving 60-69% of body surface**

     T31.60   **Burns involving 60-69% of body surface with 0% to 9% third degree burns**
          Burns involving 60-69% of body surface NOS

     T31.61   **Burns involving 60-69% of body surface with 10-19% third degree burns**

     T31.62   **Burns involving 60-69% of body surface with 20-29% third degree burns**

     T31.63   **Burns involving 60-69% of body surface with 30-39% third degree burns**

     T31.64   **Burns involving 60-69% of body surface with 40-49% third degree burns**

     T31.65   **Burns involving 60-69% of body surface with 50-59% third degree burns**

     T31.66   **Burns involving 60-69% of body surface with 60-69% third degree burns**

● **T31.7**   **Burns involving 70-79% of body surface**

     T31.70   **Burns involving 70-79% of body surface with 0% to 9% third degree burns**
          Burns involving 70-79% of body surface NOS

     T31.71   **Burns involving 70-79% of body surface with 10-19% third degree burns**

     T31.72   **Burns involving 70-79% of body surface with 20-29% third degree burns**

     T31.73   **Burns involving 70-79% of body surface with 30-39% third degree burns**

     T31.74   **Burns involving 70-79% of body surface with 40-49% third degree burns**

     T31.75   **Burns involving 70-79% of body surface with 50-59% third degree burns**

     T31.76   **Burns involving 70-79% of body surface with 60-69% third degree burns**

     T31.77   **Burns involving 70-79% of body surface with 70-79% third degree burns**

CHAPTER 19 (S00-T88)

● **T31.8** Burns involving 80-89% of body surface

T31.80 Burns involving 80-89% of body surface with 0% to 9% third degree burns
>>> Burns involving 80-89% of body surface NOS

T31.81 Burns involving 80-89% of body surface with 10-19% third degree burns

T31.82 Burns involving 80-89% of body surface with 20-29% third degree burns

T31.83 Burns involving 80-89% of body surface with 30-39% third degree burns

T31.84 Burns involving 80-89% of body surface with 40-49% third degree burns

T31.85 Burns involving 80-89% of body surface with 50-59% third degree burns

T31.86 Burns involving 80-89% of body surface with 60-69% third degree burns

T31.87 Burns involving 80-89% of body surface with 70-79% third degree burns

T31.88 Burns involving 80-89% of body surface with 80-89% third degree burns

● **T31.9** Burns involving 90% or more of body surface

T31.90 Burns involving 90% or more of body surface with 0% to 9% third degree burns
>>> Burns involving 90% or more of body surface NOS

T31.91 Burns involving 90% or more of body surface with 10-19% third degree burns

T31.92 Burns involving 90% or more of body surface with 20-29% third degree burns

T31.93 Burns involving 90% or more of body surface with 30-39% third degree burns

T31.94 Burns involving 90% or more of body surface with 40-49% third degree burns

T31.95 Burns involving 90% or more of body surface with 50-59% third degree burns

T31.96 Burns involving 90% or more of body surface with 60-69% third degree burns

T31.97 Burns involving 90% or more of body surface with 70-79% third degree burns

T31.98 Burns involving 90% or more of body surface with 80-89% third degree burns

T31.99 Burns involving 90% or more of body surface with 90% or more third degree burns

● **T32** Corrosions classified according to extent of body surface involved

Note: This category is to be used as the primary code only when the site of the corrosion is unspecified. It may be used as a supplementary code with categories T20-T25 when the site is specified.

T32.0 Corrosions involving less than 10% of body surface

● **T32.1** Corrosions involving 10-19% of body surface

T32.10 Corrosions involving 10-19% of body surface with 0% to 9% third degree corrosion
>>> Corrosions involving 10-19% of body surface NOS

T32.11 Corrosions involving 10-19% of body surface with 10-19% third degree corrosion

● **T32.2** Corrosions involving 20-29% of body surface

T32.20 Corrosions involving 20-29% of body surface with 0% to 9% third degree corrosion

T32.21 Corrosions involving 20-29% of body surface with 10-19% third degree corrosion

T32.22 Corrosions involving 20-29% of body surface with 20-29% third degree corrosion

● **T32.3** Corrosions involving 30-39% of body surface

T32.30 Corrosions involving 30-39% of body surface with 0% to 9% third degree corrosion

T32.31 Corrosions involving 30-39% of body surface with 10-19% third degree corrosion

T32.32 Corrosions involving 30-39% of body surface with 20-29% third degree corrosion

T32.33 Corrosions involving 30-39% of body surface with 30-39% third degree corrosion

● **T32.4** Corrosions involving 40-49% of body surface

T32.40 Corrosions involving 40-49% of body surface with 0% to 9% third degree corrosion

T32.41 Corrosions involving 40-49% of body surface with 10-19% third degree corrosion

T32.42 Corrosions involving 40-49% of body surface with 20-29% third degree corrosion

T32.43 Corrosions involving 40-49% of body surface with 30-39% third degree corrosion

T32.44 Corrosions involving 40-49% of body surface with 40-49% third degree corrosion

● **T32.5** Corrosions involving 50-59% of body surface

T32.50 Corrosions involving 50-59% of body surface with 0% to 9% third degree corrosion

T32.51 Corrosions involving 50-59% of body surface with 10-19% third degree corrosion

T32.52 Corrosions involving 50-59% of body surface with 20-29% third degree corrosion

T32.53 Corrosions involving 50-59% of body surface with 30-39% third degree corrosion

T32.54 Corrosions involving 50-59% of body surface with 40-49% third degree corrosion

T32.55 Corrosions involving 50-59% of body surface with 50-59% third degree corrosion

● **T32.6** Corrosions involving 60-69% of body surface

T32.60 Corrosions involving 60-69% of body surface with 0% to 9% third degree corrosion

T32.61 Corrosions involving 60-69% of body surface with 10-19% third degree corrosion

T32.62 Corrosions involving 60-69% of body surface with 20-29% third degree corrosion

T32.63 Corrosions involving 60-69% of body surface with 30-39% third degree corrosion

T32.64 Corrosions involving 60-69% of body surface with 40-49% third degree corrosion

T32.65 Corrosions involving 60-69% of body surface with 50-59% third degree corrosion

T32.66 Corrosions involving 60-69% of body surface with 60-69% third degree corrosion

● **T32.7** Corrosions involving 70-79% of body surface

T32.70 Corrosions involving 70-79% of body surface with 0% to 9% third degree corrosion

T32.71 Corrosions involving 70-79% of body surface with 10-19% third degree corrosion

T32.72 Corrosions involving 70-79% of body surface with 20-29% third degree corrosion

T32.73 Corrosions involving 70-79% of body surface with 30-39% third degree corrosion

T32.74 Corrosions involving 70-79% of body surface with 40-49% third degree corrosion

T32.75 Corrosions involving 70-79% of body surface with 50-59% third degree corrosion

T32.76 Corrosions involving 70-79% of body surface with 60-69% third degree corrosion

T32.77 Corrosions involving 70-79% of body surface with 70-79% third degree corrosion

◀ New   ◀▦ Revised   ~~deleted~~ Deleted   Excludes 1   Excludes 2   Includes   Use additional   Code first   Code also   Unspecified

OGCR Official Guidelines   X Assign placeholder X   ● Use Additional Character(s)   ▌ Manifestation Code   **Coding Clinic**

- T32.8   Corrosions involving 80-89% of body surface
  - T32.80   Corrosions involving 80-89% of body surface with 0% to 9% third degree corrosion
  - T32.81   Corrosions involving 80-89% of body surface with 10-19% third degree corrosion
  - T32.82   Corrosions involving 80-89% of body surface with 20-29% third degree corrosion
  - T32.83   Corrosions involving 80-89% of body surface with 30-39% third degree corrosion
  - T32.84   Corrosions involving 80-89% of body surface with 40-49% third degree corrosion
  - T32.85   Corrosions involving 80-89% of body surface with 50-59% third degree corrosion
  - T32.86   Corrosions involving 80-89% of body surface with 60-69% third degree corrosion
  - T32.87   Corrosions involving 80-89% of body surface with 70-79% third degree corrosion
  - T32.88   Corrosions involving 80-89% of body surface with 80-89% third degree corrosion
- T32.9   Corrosions involving 90% or more of body surface
  - T32.90   Corrosions involving 90% or more of body surface with 0% to 9% third degree corrosion
  - T32.91   Corrosions involving 90% or more of body surface with 10-19% third degree corrosion
  - T32.92   Corrosions involving 90% or more of body surface with 20-29% third degree corrosion
  - T32.93   Corrosions involving 90% or more of body surface with 30-39% third degree corrosion
  - T32.94   Corrosions involving 90% or more of body surface with 40-49% third degree corrosion
  - T32.95   Corrosions involving 90% or more of body surface with 50-59% third degree corrosion
  - T32.96   Corrosions involving 90% or more of body surface with 60-69% third degree corrosion
  - T32.97   Corrosions involving 90% or more of body surface with 70-79% third degree corrosion
  - T32.98   Corrosions involving 90% or more of body surface with 80-89% third degree corrosion
  - T32.99   Corrosions involving 90% or more of body surface with 90% or more third degree corrosion

FROSTBITE (T33-T34)

Excludes2   hypothermia and other effects of reduced temperature (T68, T69.-)

- T33   **Superficial frostbite**

  Includes   frostbite with partial thickness skin loss

  The appropriate 7th character is to be added to each code from category T33

A	initial encounter
D	subsequent encounter
S	sequela

  - T33.0   Superficial frostbite of head
    - T33.01   Superficial frostbite of ear
      - T33.011   Superficial frostbite of right ear
      - T33.012   Superficial frostbite of left ear
      - T33.019   Superficial frostbite of unspecified ear
    - X● T33.02   Superficial frostbite of nose
    - X● T33.09   Superficial frostbite of other part of head
  - X● T33.1   Superficial frostbite of neck
  - X● T33.2   Superficial frostbite of thorax
  - X● T33.3   Superficial frostbite of abdominal wall, lower back and pelvis
  - T33.4   Superficial frostbite of arm

    Excludes2   superficial frostbite of wrist and hand (T33.5-)

    - X● T33.40   Superficial frostbite of unspecified arm
    - X● T33.41   Superficial frostbite of right arm
    - X● T33.42   Superficial frostbite of left arm

- T33.5   Superficial frostbite of wrist, hand, and fingers
  - T33.51   Superficial frostbite of wrist
    - T33.511   Superficial frostbite of right wrist
    - T33.512   Superficial frostbite of left wrist
    - T33.519   Superficial frostbite of unspecified wrist
  - T33.52   Superficial frostbite of hand

    Excludes2   superficial frostbite of fingers (T33.53-)

    - T33.521   Superficial frostbite of right hand
    - T33.522   Superficial frostbite of left hand
    - T33.529   Superficial frostbite of unspecified hand
  - T33.53   Superficial frostbite of finger(s)
    - T33.531   Superficial frostbite of right finger(s)
    - T33.532   Superficial frostbite of left finger(s)
    - T33.539   Superficial frostbite of unspecified finger(s)
- T33.6   Superficial frostbite of hip and thigh
  - X● T33.60   Superficial frostbite of unspecified hip and thigh
  - X● T33.61   Superficial frostbite of right hip and thigh
  - X● T33.62   Superficial frostbite of left hip and thigh
- T33.7   Superficial frostbite of knee and lower leg

  Excludes2   superficial frostbite of ankle and foot (T33.8-)

  - X● T33.70   Superficial frostbite of unspecified knee and lower leg
  - X● T33.71   Superficial frostbite of right knee and lower leg
  - X● T33.72   Superficial frostbite of left knee and lower leg
- T33.8   Superficial frostbite of ankle, foot, and toe(s)
  - T33.81   Superficial frostbite of ankle
    - T33.811   Superficial frostbite of right ankle
    - T33.812   Superficial frostbite of left ankle
    - T33.819   Superficial frostbite of unspecified ankle
  - T33.82   Superficial frostbite of foot
    - T33.821   Superficial frostbite of right foot
    - T33.822   Superficial frostbite of left foot
    - T33.829   Superficial frostbite of unspecified foot
  - T33.83   Superficial frostbite of toe(s)
    - T33.831   Superficial frostbite of right toe(s)
    - T33.832   Superficial frostbite of left toe(s)
    - T33.839   Superficial frostbite of unspecified toe(s)
- T33.9   Superficial frostbite of other and unspecified sites
  - X● T33.90   Superficial frostbite of unspecified sites

    Superficial frostbite NOS
  - X● T33.99   Superficial frostbite of other sites

    Superficial frostbite of leg NOS

    Superficial frostbite of trunk NOS

- T34   **Frostbite with tissue necrosis**

  The appropriate 7th character is to be added to each code from category T34

A	initial encounter
D	subsequent encounter
S	sequela

  - T34.0   Frostbite with tissue necrosis of head
    - T34.01   Frostbite with tissue necrosis of ear
      - T34.011   Frostbite with tissue necrosis of right ear
      - T34.012   Frostbite with tissue necrosis of left ear
      - T34.019   Frostbite with tissue necrosis of unspecified ear

X● T34.02   Frostbite with tissue necrosis of nose

X● T34.09   Frostbite with tissue necrosis of other part of head

X● T34.1   Frostbite with tissue necrosis of neck

X● T34.2   Frostbite with tissue necrosis of thorax

X● T34.3   Frostbite with tissue necrosis of abdominal wall, lower back and pelvis

● T34.4   Frostbite with tissue necrosis of arm

> **Excludes2**   frostbite with tissue necrosis of wrist and hand (T34.5-)

X● T34.40   Frostbite with tissue necrosis of unspecified arm

X● T34.41   Frostbite with tissue necrosis of right arm

X● T34.42   Frostbite with tissue necrosis of left arm

● T34.5   Frostbite with tissue necrosis of wrist, hand, and finger(s)

   ● T34.51   Frostbite with tissue necrosis of wrist

     ● T34.511   Frostbite with tissue necrosis of right wrist

     ● T34.512   Frostbite with tissue necrosis of left wrist

     ● T34.519   Frostbite with tissue necrosis of unspecified wrist

   ● T34.52   Frostbite with tissue necrosis of hand

> **Excludes2**   frostbite with tissue necrosis of finger(s) (T34.53-)

     ● T34.521   Frostbite with tissue necrosis of right hand

     ● T34.522   Frostbite with tissue necrosis of left hand

     ● T34.529   Frostbite with tissue necrosis of unspecified hand

   ● T34.53   Frostbite with tissue necrosis of finger(s)

     ● T34.531   Frostbite with tissue necrosis of right finger(s)

     ● T34.532   Frostbite with tissue necrosis of left finger(s)

     ● T34.539   Frostbite with tissue necrosis of unspecified finger(s)

● T34.6   Frostbite with tissue necrosis of hip and thigh

X● T34.60   Frostbite with tissue necrosis of unspecified hip and thigh

X● T34.61   Frostbite with tissue necrosis of right hip and thigh

X● T34.62   Frostbite with tissue necrosis of left hip and thigh

● T34.7   Frostbite with tissue necrosis of knee and lower leg

> **Excludes2**   frostbite with tissue necrosis of ankle and foot (T34.8-)

X● T34.70   Frostbite with tissue necrosis of unspecified knee and lower leg

X● T34.71   Frostbite with tissue necrosis of right knee and lower leg

X● T34.72   Frostbite with tissue necrosis of left knee and lower leg

● T34.8   Frostbite with tissue necrosis of ankle, foot, and toe(s)

   ● T34.81   Frostbite with tissue necrosis of ankle

     ● T34.811   Frostbite with tissue necrosis of right ankle

     ● T34.812   Frostbite with tissue necrosis of left ankle

     ● T34.819   Frostbite with tissue necrosis of unspecified ankle

   ● T34.82   Frostbite with tissue necrosis of foot

     ● T34.821   Frostbite with tissue necrosis of right foot

     ● T34.822   Frostbite with tissue necrosis of left foot

     ● T34.829   Frostbite with tissue necrosis of unspecified foot

   ● T34.83   Frostbite with tissue necrosis of toe(s)

     ● T34.831   Frostbite with tissue necrosis of right toe(s)

     ● T34.832   Frostbite with tissue necrosis of left toe(s)

     ● T34.839   Frostbite with tissue necrosis of unspecified toe(s)

● T34.9   Frostbite with tissue necrosis of other and unspecified sites

X● T34.90   Frostbite with tissue necrosis of unspecified sites

     Frostbite with tissue necrosis NOS

X● T34.99   Frostbite with tissue necrosis of other sites

     Frostbite with tissue necrosis of leg NOS

     Frostbite with tissue necrosis of trunk NOS

OGCR See Section I.C.19.e.

Adverse Effects, Poisoning, Underdosing and Toxic Effects

POISONING BY, ADVERSE EFFECTS OF AND UNDERDOSING OF DRUGS, MEDICAMENTS AND BIOLOGICAL SUBSTANCES (T36-T50)

> **Includes**   adverse effect of correct substance properly administered
>
> poisoning by overdose of substance
>
> poisoning by wrong substance given or taken in error
>
> underdosing by (inadvertently) (deliberately) taking less substance than prescribed or instructed

Code first, for adverse effects, the nature of the adverse effect, such as:
adverse effect NOS (T88.7)
aspirin gastritis (K29.-)
blood disorders (D56-D76)
contact dermatitis (L23-L25)
dermatitis due to substances taken internally (L27.-)
nephropathy (N14.0-N14.2)

Note: The drug giving rise to the adverse effect should be identified by use of codes from categories T36-T50 with fifth or sixth character 5.

Use additional code(s) to specify:
manifestations of poisoning
underdosing or failure in dosage during medical and surgical care (Y63.6, Y63.8-Y63.9)
underdosing of medication regimen (Z91.12-, Z91.13-)

> **Excludes1**   toxic reaction to local anesthesia in pregnancy (O29.3-)

> **Excludes2**   abuse and dependence of psychoactive substances (F10-F19)
>
> abuse of non-dependence-producing substances (F55.-)
>
> drug reaction and poisoning affecting newborn (P00-P96)
>
> pathological drug intoxication (inebriation) (F10-F19)

● T36   **Poisoning by, adverse effect of and underdosing of systemic antibiotics**

> **Excludes1**   antineoplastic antibiotics (T45.1-)
>
> locally applied antibiotic NEC (T49.0)
>
> topically used antibiotic for ear, nose and throat (T49.6)
>
> topically used antibiotic for eye (T49.5)

The appropriate 7th character is to be added to each code from category T36

A	initial encounter
D	subsequent encounter
S	sequela

● T36.0   **Poisoning by, adverse effect of and underdosing of penicillins**

   ● T36.0X   **Poisoning by, adverse effect of and underdosing of penicillins**

     ● T36.0X1   **Poisoning by penicillins, accidental (unintentional)**

       Poisoning by penicillins NOS

● T36.0X2   Poisoning by penicillins, intentional self-harm

● T36.0X3   Poisoning by penicillins, assault

● T36.0X4   Poisoning by penicillins, undetermined

● T36.0X5   Adverse effect of penicillins

● T36.0X6   Underdosing of penicillins

● T36.1   Poisoning by, adverse effect of and underdosing of cephalosporins and other betalactam antibiotics

   ● T36.1X   Poisoning by, adverse effect of and underdosing of cephalosporins and other beta-lactam antibiotics

     ● T36.1X1   Poisoning by cephalosporins and other beta-lactam antibiotics, accidental (unintentional)
         Poisoning by cephalosporins and other beta-lactam antibiotics NOS

     ● T36.1X2   Poisoning by cephalosporins and other beta-lactam antibiotics, intentional self-harm

     ● T36.1X3   Poisoning by cephalosporins and other beta-lactam antibiotics, assault

     ● T36.1X4   Poisoning by cephalosporins and other beta-lactam antibiotics, undetermined

     ● T36.1X5   Adverse effect of cephalosporins and other beta-lactam antibiotics

     ● T36.1X6   Underdosing of cephalosporins and other beta-lactam antibiotics

● T36.2   Poisoning by, adverse effect of and underdosing of chloramphenicol group

   ● T36.2X   Poisoning by, adverse effect of and underdosing of chloramphenicol group

     ● T36.2X1   Poisoning by chloramphenicol group, accidental (unintentional)
         Poisoning by chloramphenicol group NOS

     ● T36.2X2   Poisoning by chloramphenicol group, intentional self-harm

     ● T36.2X3   Poisoning by chloramphenicol group, assault

     ● T36.2X4   Poisoning by chloramphenicol group, undetermined

     ● T36.2X5   Adverse effect of chloramphenicol group

     ● T36.2X6   Underdosing of chloramphenicol group

● T36.3   Poisoning by, adverse effect of and underdosing of macrolides

   ● T36.3X   Poisoning by, adverse effect of and underdosing of macrolides

     ● T36.3X1   Poisoning by macrolides, accidental (unintentional)
         Poisoning by macrolides NOS

     ● T36.3X2   Poisoning by macrolides, intentional self-harm

     ● T36.3X3   Poisoning by macrolides, assault

     ● T36.3X4   Poisoning by macrolides, undetermined

     ● T36.3X5   Adverse effect of macrolides

     ● T36.3X6   Underdosing of macrolides

● T36.4   Poisoning by, adverse effect of and underdosing of tetracyclines

   ● T36.4X   Poisoning by, adverse effect of and underdosing of tetracyclines

     ● T36.4X1   Poisoning by tetracyclines, accidental (unintentional)
         Poisoning by tetracyclines NOS

     ● T36.4X2   Poisoning by tetracyclines, intentional self-harm

     ● T36.4X3   Poisoning by tetracyclines, assault

     ● T36.4X4   Poisoning by tetracyclines, undetermined

     ● T36.4X5   Adverse effect of tetracyclines

     ● T36.4X6   Underdosing of tetracyclines

● T36.5   Poisoning by, adverse effect of and underdosing of aminoglycosides
     Poisoning by, adverse effect of and underdosing of streptomycin

   ● T36.5X   Poisoning by, adverse effect of and underdosing of aminoglycosides

     ● T36.5X1   Poisoning by aminoglycosides, accidental (unintentional)
         Poisoning by aminoglycosides NOS

     ● T36.5X2   Poisoning by aminoglycosides, intentional self-harm

     ● T36.5X3   Poisoning by aminoglycosides, assault

     ● T36.5X4   Poisoning by aminoglycosides, undetermined

     ● T36.5X5   Adverse effect of aminoglycosides

     ● T36.5X6   Underdosing of aminoglycosides

● T36.6   Poisoning by, adverse effect of and underdosing of rifampicins

   ● T36.6X   Poisoning by, adverse effect of and underdosing of rifampicins

     ● T36.6X1   Poisoning by rifampicins, accidental (unintentional)
         Poisoning by rifampicins NOS

     ● T36.6X2   Poisoning by rifampicins, intentional self-harm

     ● T36.6X3   Poisoning by rifampicins, assault

     ● T36.6X4   Poisoning by rifampicins, undetermined

     ● T36.6X5   Adverse effect of rifampicins

     ● T36.6X6   Underdosing of rifampicins

● T36.7   Poisoning by, adverse effect of and underdosing of antifungal antibiotics, systemically used

   ● T36.7X   Poisoning by, adverse effect of and underdosing of antifungal antibiotics, systemically used

     ● T36.7X1   Poisoning by antifungal antibiotics, systemically used, accidental (unintentional)
         Poisoning by antifungal antibiotics, systemically used NOS

     ● T36.7X2   Poisoning by antifungal antibiotics, systemically used, intentional self-harm

     ● T36.7X3   Poisoning by antifungal antibiotics, systemically used, assault

     ● T36.7X4   Poisoning by antifungal antibiotics, systemically used, undetermined

     ● T36.7X5   Adverse effect of antifungal antibiotics, systemically used

     ● T36.7X6   Underdosing of antifungal antibiotics, systemically used

CHAPTER 19 (S00-T88)

CHAPTER 19 (S00-T88)

- **T36.8**   Poisoning by, adverse effect of and underdosing of other systemic antibiotics
  - **T36.8X**   Poisoning by, adverse effect of and underdosing of other systemic antibiotics
    - **T36.8X1**   Poisoning by other systemic antibiotics, accidental (unintentional)
      Poisoning by other systemic antibiotics NOS
    - **T36.8X2**   Poisoning by other systemic antibiotics, intentional self-harm
    - **T36.8X3**   Poisoning by other systemic antibiotics, assault
    - **T36.8X4**   Poisoning by other systemic antibiotics, undetermined
    - **T36.8X5**   Adverse effect of other systemic antibiotics
    - **T36.8X6**   Underdosing of other systemic antibiotics
- **T36.9**   Poisoning by, adverse effect of and underdosing of unspecified systemic antibiotic
  - X **T36.91**   Poisoning by unspecified systemic antibiotic, accidental (unintentional)
    Poisoning by systemic antibiotic NOS
  - X **T36.92**   Poisoning by unspecified systemic antibiotic, intentional self-harm
  - X **T36.93**   Poisoning by unspecified systemic antibiotic, assault
  - X **T36.94**   Poisoning by unspecified systemic antibiotic, undetermined
  - X **T36.95**   Adverse effect of unspecified systemic antibiotic
  - X **T36.96**   Underdosing of unspecified systemic antibiotic

- **T37**   Poisoning by, adverse effect of and underdosing of other systemic anti-infectives and antiparasitics

  Excludes1   anti-infectives topically used for ear, nose and throat (T49.6-)
  anti-infectives topically used for eye (T49.5-)
  locally applied anti-infectives NEC (T49.0-)

  The appropriate 7th character is to be added to each code from category T37

A	initial encounter
D	subsequent encounter
S	sequela

  - **T37.0**   Poisoning by, adverse effect of and underdosing of sulfonamides
    - **T37.0X**   Poisoning by, adverse effect of and underdosing of sulfonamides
      - **T37.0X1**   Poisoning by sulfonamides, accidental (unintentional)
        Poisoning by sulfonamides NOS
      - **T37.0X2**   Poisoning by sulfonamides, intentional self-harm
      - **T37.0X3**   Poisoning by sulfonamides, assault
      - **T37.0X4**   Poisoning by sulfonamides, undetermined
      - **T37.0X5**   Adverse effect of sulfonamides
      - **T37.0X6**   Underdosing of sulfonamides
  - **T37.1**   Poisoning by, adverse effect of and underdosing of antimycobacterial drugs

    Excludes1   rifampicins (T36.6-) streptomycin (T36.5-)

    - **T37.1X**   Poisoning by, adverse effect of and underdosing of antimycobacterial drugs
      - **T37.1X1**   Poisoning by antimycobacterial drugs, accidental (unintentional)
        Poisoning by antimycobacterial drugs NOS
      - **T37.1X2**   Poisoning by antimycobacterial drugs, intentional self-harm

- **T37.1X3**   Poisoning by antimycobacterial drugs, assault
- **T37.1X4**   Poisoning by antimycobacterial drugs, undetermined
- **T37.1X5**   Adverse effect of antimycobacterial drugs
- **T37.1X6**   Underdosing of antimycobacterial drugs
- **T37.2**   Poisoning by, adverse effect of and underdosing of antimalarials and drugs acting on other blood protozoa

  Excludes1   hydroxyquinoline derivatives (T37.8-)

  - **T37.2X**   Poisoning by, adverse effect of and underdosing of antimalarials and drugs acting on other blood protozoa
    - **T37.2X1**   Poisoning by antimalarials and drugs acting on other blood protozoa, accidental (unintentional)
      Poisoning by antimalarials and drugs acting on other blood protozoa NOS
    - **T37.2X2**   Poisoning by antimalarials and drugs acting on other blood protozoa, intentional self-harm
    - **T37.2X3**   Poisoning by antimalarials and drugs acting on other blood protozoa, assault
    - **T37.2X4**   Poisoning by antimalarials and drugs acting on other blood protozoa, undetermined
    - **T37.2X5**   Adverse effect of antimalarials and drugs acting on other blood protozoa
    - **T37.2X6**   Underdosing of antimalarials and drugs acting on other blood protozoa
- **T37.3**   Poisoning by, adverse effect of and underdosing of other antiprotozoal drugs
  - **T37.3X**   Poisoning by, adverse effect of and underdosing of other antiprotozoal drugs
    - **T37.3X1**   Poisoning by other antiprotozoal drugs, accidental (unintentional)
      Poisoning by other antiprotozoal drugs NOS
    - **T37.3X2**   Poisoning by other antiprotozoal drugs, intentional self-harm
    - **T37.3X3**   Poisoning by other antiprotozoal drugs, assault
    - **T37.3X4**   Poisoning by other antiprotozoal drugs, undetermined
    - **T37.3X5**   Adverse effect of other antiprotozoal drugs
    - **T37.3X6**   Underdosing of other antiprotozoal drugs
- **T37.4**   Poisoning by, adverse effect of and underdosing of anthelminthics
  - **T37.4X**   Poisoning by, adverse effect of and underdosing of anthelminthics
    - **T37.4X1**   Poisoning by anthelminthics, accidental (unintentional)
      Poisoning by anthelminthics NOS
    - **T37.4X2**   Poisoning by anthelminthics, intentional self-harm
    - **T37.4X3**   Poisoning by anthelminthics, assault
    - **T37.4X4**   Poisoning by anthelminthics, undetermined
    - **T37.4X5**   Adverse effect of anthelminthics
    - **T37.4X6**   Underdosing of anthelminthics

◀ New   ⬅ Revised   ~~deleted~~ Deleted   Excludes 1   Excludes 2   Includes   Use additional   Code first   Code also   Unspecified

OGCR Official Guidelines   **X** Assign placeholder X   ● Use Additional Character(s)   ▶ Manifestation Code   **Coding Clinic**

● **T37.5** **Poisoning by, adverse effect of and underdosing of antiviral drugs**
> **Excludes1**   amantadine (T42.8-)
> cytarabine (T45.1-)

● **T37.5X** **Poisoning by, adverse effect of and underdosing of antiviral drugs**

● **T37.5X1** **Poisoning by antiviral drugs, accidental (unintentional)**
> Poisoning by antiviral drugs NOS

● **T37.5X2** **Poisoning by antiviral drugs, intentional self-harm**

● **T37.5X3** **Poisoning by antiviral drugs, assault**

● **T37.5X4** **Poisoning by antiviral drugs, undetermined**

● **T37.5X5** **Adverse effect of antiviral drugs**

● **T37.5X6** **Underdosing of antiviral drugs**

● **T37.8** **Poisoning by, adverse effect of and underdosing of other specified systemic anti-infectives and antiparasitics**
> Poisoning by, adverse effect of and underdosing of hydroxyquinoline derivatives
> **Excludes1**   antimalarial drugs (T37.2-)

● **T37.8X** **Poisoning by, adverse effect of and underdosing of other specified systemic anti-infectives and antiparasitics**

● **T37.8X1** **Poisoning by other specified systemic anti-infectives and antiparasitics, accidental (unintentional)**
> Poisoning by other specified systemic anti-infectives and antiparasitics NOS

● **T37.8X2** **Poisoning by other specified systemic anti-infectives and antiparasitics, intentional self-harm**

● **T37.8X3** **Poisoning by other specified systemic anti-infectives and antiparasitics, assault**

● **T37.8X4** **Poisoning by other specified systemic anti-infectives and antiparasitics, undetermined**

● **T37.8X5** **Adverse effect of other specified systemic anti-infectives and antiparasitics**

● **T37.8X6** **Underdosing of other specified systemic anti-infectives and antiparasitics**

● **T37.9** **Poisoning by, adverse effect of and underdosing of unspecified systemic anti-infective and antiparasitics**

X● **T37.91** **Poisoning by unspecified systemic anti-infective and antiparasitics, accidental (unintentional)**
> Poisoning by, adverse effect of and underdosing of systemic anti-infective and antiparasitics NOS

X● **T37.92** **Poisoning by unspecified systemic anti-infective and antiparasitics, intentional self-harm**

X● **T37.93** **Poisoning by unspecified systemic anti-infective and antiparasitics, assault**

X● **T37.94** **Poisoning by unspecified systemic anti-infective and antiparasitics, undetermined**

X● **T37.95** **Adverse effect of unspecified systemic anti-infective and antiparasitic**

X● **T37.96** **Underdosing of unspecified systemic anti-infectives and antiparasitics**

● **T38** **Poisoning by, adverse effect of and underdosing of hormones and their synthetic substitutes and antagonists, not elsewhere classified**
> **Excludes1**   mineralocorticoids and their antagonists (T50.0-)
> oxytocic hormones (T48.0-)
> parathyroid hormones and derivatives (T50.9-)

The appropriate 7th character is to be added to each code from category T38

> A   initial encounter
> D   subsequent encounter
> S   sequela

● **T38.0** **Poisoning by, adverse effect of and underdosing of glucocorticoids and synthetic analogues**
> **Excludes1**   glucocorticoids, topically used (T49.-)

● **T38.0X** **Poisoning by, adverse effect of and underdosing of glucocorticoids and synthetic analogues**

● **T38.0X1** **Poisoning by glucocorticoids and synthetic analogues, accidental (unintentional)**
> Poisoning by glucocorticoids and synthetic analogues NOS

● **T38.0X2** **Poisoning by glucocorticoids and synthetic analogues, intentional self-harm**

● **T38.0X3** **Poisoning by glucocorticoids and synthetic analogues, assault**

● **T38.0X4** **Poisoning by glucocorticoids and synthetic analogues, undetermined**

● **T38.0X5** **Adverse effect of glucocorticoids and synthetic analogues**

● **T38.0X6** **Underdosing of glucocorticoids and synthetic analogues**

● **T38.1** **Poisoning by, adverse effect of and underdosing of thyroid hormones and substitutes**

● **T38.1X** **Poisoning by, adverse effect of and underdosing of thyroid hormones and substitutes**

● **T38.1X1** **Poisoning by thyroid hormones and substitutes, accidental (unintentional)**
> Poisoning by thyroid hormones and substitutes NOS

● **T38.1X2** **Poisoning by thyroid hormones and substitutes, intentional self-harm**

● **T38.1X3** **Poisoning by thyroid hormones and substitutes, assault**

● **T38.1X4** **Poisoning by thyroid hormones and substitutes, undetermined**

● **T38.1X5** **Adverse effect of thyroid hormones and substitutes**

● **T38.1X6** **Underdosing of thyroid hormones and substitutes**

● **T38.2** **Poisoning by, adverse effect of and underdosing of antithyroid drugs**

● **T38.2X** **Poisoning by, adverse effect of and underdosing of antithyroid drugs**

● **T38.2X1** **Poisoning by antithyroid drugs, accidental (unintentional)**
> Poisoning by antithyroid drugs NOS

● **T38.2X2** **Poisoning by antithyroid drugs, intentional self-harm**

● **T38.2X3** **Poisoning by antithyroid drugs, assault**

● **T38.2X4** **Poisoning by antithyroid drugs, undetermined**

● **T38.2X5** **Adverse effect of antithyroid drugs**

● **T38.2X6** **Underdosing of antithyroid drugs**

CHAPTER 19 (S00-T88)

● T38.3   **Poisoning by, adverse effect of and underdosing of insulin and oral hypoglycemic [antidiabetic] drugs**

   ● T38.3X   **Poisoning by, adverse effect of and underdosing of insulin and oral hypoglycemic [antidiabetic] drugs**

      ● T38.3X1   **Poisoning by insulin and oral hypoglycemic [antidiabetic] drugs, accidental (unintentional)**
          Poisoning by insulin and oral hypoglycemic [antidiabetic] drugs NOS

      ● T38.3X2   **Poisoning by insulin and oral hypoglycemic [antidiabetic] drugs, intentional self-harm**

      ● T38.3X3   **Poisoning by insulin and oral hypoglycemic [antidiabetic] drugs, assault**

      ● T38.3X4   **Poisoning by insulin and oral hypoglycemic [antidiabetic] drugs, undetermined**

      ● T38.3X5   **Adverse effect of insulin and oral hypoglycemic [antidiabetic] drugs**

      ● T38.3X6   **Underdosing of insulin and oral hypoglycemic [antidiabetic] drugs**

● T38.4   **Poisoning by, adverse effect of and underdosing of oral contraceptives**
    Poisoning by, adverse effect of and underdosing of multiple- and single-ingredient oral contraceptive preparations

   ● T38.4X   **Poisoning by, adverse effect of and underdosing of oral contraceptives**

      ● T38.4X1   **Poisoning by oral contraceptives, accidental (unintentional)**
          Poisoning by oral contraceptives NOS

      ● T38.4X2   **Poisoning by oral contraceptives, intentional self-harm**

      ● T38.4X3   **Poisoning by oral contraceptives, assault**

      ● T38.4X4   **Poisoning by oral contraceptives, undetermined**

      ● T38.4X5   **Adverse effect of oral contraceptives**

      ● T38.4X6   **Underdosing of oral contraceptives**

● T38.5   **Poisoning by, adverse effect of and underdosing of other estrogens and progestogens**
    Poisoning by, adverse effect of and underdosing of estrogens and progestogens mixtures and substitutes

   ● T38.5X   **Poisoning by, adverse effect of and underdosing of other estrogens and progestogens**

      ● T38.5X1   **Poisoning by other estrogens and progestogens, accidental (unintentional)**
          Poisoning by other estrogens and progestogens NOS

      ● T38.5X2   **Poisoning by other estrogens and progestogens, intentional self-harm**

      ● T38.5X3   **Poisoning by other estrogens and progestogens, assault**

      ● T38.5X4   **Poisoning by other estrogens and progestogens, undetermined**

      ● T38.5X5   **Adverse effect of other estrogens and progestogens**

      ● T38.5X6   **Underdosing of other estrogens and progestogens**

● T38.6   **Poisoning by, adverse effect of and underdosing of antigonadotrophins, antiestrogens, antiandrogens, not elsewhere classified**
    Poisoning by, adverse effect of and underdosing of tamoxifen

   ● T38.6X   **Poisoning by, adverse effect of and underdosing of antigonadotrophins, antiestrogens, antiandrogens, not elsewhere classified**

      ● T38.6X1   **Poisoning by antigonadotrophins, antiestrogens, antiandrogens, not elsewhere classified, accidental (unintentional)**
          Poisoning by antigonadotrophins, antiestrogens, antiandrogens, not elsewhere classified NOS

      ● T38.6X2   **Poisoning by antigonadotrophins, antiestrogens, antiandrogens, not elsewhere classified, intentional self-harm**

      ● T38.6X3   **Poisoning by antigonadotrophins, antiestrogens, antiandrogens, not elsewhere classified, assault**

      ● T38.6X4   **Poisoning by antigonadotrophins, antiestrogens, antiandrogens, not elsewhere classified, undetermined**

      ● T38.6X5   **Adverse effect of antigonadotrophins, antiestrogens, antiandrogens, not elsewhere classified**

      ● T38.6X6   **Underdosing of antigonadotrophins, antiestrogens, antiandrogens, not elsewhere classified**

● T38.7   **Poisoning by, adverse effect of and underdosing of androgens and anabolic congeners**

   ● T38.7X   **Poisoning by, adverse effect of and underdosing of androgens and anabolic congeners**

      ● T38.7X1   **Poisoning by androgens and anabolic congeners, accidental (unintentional)**
          Poisoning by androgens and anabolic congeners NOS

      ● T38.7X2   **Poisoning by androgens and anabolic congeners, intentional self-harm**

      ● T38.7X3   **Poisoning by androgens and anabolic congeners, assault**

      ● T38.7X4   **Poisoning by androgens and anabolic congeners, undetermined**

      ● T38.7X5   **Adverse effect of androgens and anabolic congeners**

      ● T38.7X6   **Underdosing of androgens and anabolic congeners**

● T38.8   **Poisoning by, adverse effect of and underdosing of other and unspecified hormones and synthetic substitutes**

   ● T38.80   **Poisoning by, adverse effect of and underdosing of unspecified hormones and synthetic substitutes**

      ● T38.801   **Poisoning by unspecified hormones and synthetic substitutes, accidental (unintentional)**
          Poisoning by unspecified hormones and synthetic substitutes NOS

      ● T38.802   **Poisoning by unspecified hormones and synthetic substitutes, intentional self-harm**

      ● T38.803   **Poisoning by unspecified hormones and synthetic substitutes, assault**

      ● T38.804   **Poisoning by unspecified hormones and synthetic substitutes, undetermined**

      ● T38.805   **Adverse effect of unspecified hormones and synthetic substitutes**

      ● T38.806   **Underdosing of unspecified hormones and synthetic substitutes**

◀ New   ◀▥ Revised   ~~deleted~~ Deleted   Excludes 1   Excludes 2   Includes   Use additional   Code first   Code also   Unspecified

OGCR Official Guidelines   **X** Assign placeholder X   ● Use Additional Character(s)   ▶ Manifestation Code   **Coding Clinic**

- **T38.81** **Poisoning by, adverse effect of and underdosing of anterior pituitary [adenohypophyseal] hormones**
  - **T38.811** Poisoning by anterior pituitary [adenohypophyseal] hormones, accidental (unintentional)
    - Poisoning by anterior pituitary [adenohypophyseal] hormones NOS
  - **T38.812** Poisoning by anterior pituitary [adenohypophyseal] hormones, intentional self-harm
  - **T38.813** Poisoning by anterior pituitary [adenohypophyseal] hormones, assault
  - **T38.814** Poisoning by anterior pituitary [adenohypophyseal] hormones, undetermined
  - **T38.815** Adverse effect of anterior pituitary [adenohypophyseal] hormones
  - **T38.816** Underdosing of anterior pituitary [adenohypophyseal] hormones
- **T38.89** **Poisoning by, adverse effect of and underdosing of other hormones and synthetic substitutes**
  - **T38.891** Poisoning by other hormones and synthetic substitutes, accidental (unintentional)
    - Poisoning by other hormones and synthetic substitutes NOS
  - **T38.892** Poisoning by other hormones and synthetic substitutes, intentional self-harm
  - **T38.893** Poisoning by other hormones and synthetic substitutes, assault
  - **T38.894** Poisoning by other hormones and synthetic substitutes, undetermined
  - **T38.895** Adverse effect of other hormones and synthetic substitutes
  - **T38.896** Underdosing of other hormones and synthetic substitutes
- **T38.9** **Poisoning by, adverse effect of and underdosing of other and unspecified hormone antagonists**
  - **T38.90** **Poisoning by, adverse effect of and underdosing of unspecified hormone antagonists**
    - **T38.901** Poisoning by unspecified hormone antagonists, accidental (unintentional)
      - Poisoning by unspecified hormone antagonists NOS
    - **T38.902** Poisoning by unspecified hormone antagonists, intentional self-harm
    - **T38.903** Poisoning by unspecified hormone antagonists, assault
    - **T38.904** Poisoning by unspecified hormone antagonists, undetermined
    - **T38.905** Adverse effect of unspecified hormone antagonists
    - **T38.906** Underdosing of unspecified hormone antagonists

- **T38.99** **Poisoning by, adverse effect of and underdosing of other hormone antagonists**
  - **T38.991** Poisoning by other hormone antagonists, accidental (unintentional)
    - Poisoning by other hormone antagonists NOS
  - **T38.992** Poisoning by other hormone antagonists, intentional self-harm
  - **T38.993** Poisoning by other hormone antagonists, assault
  - **T38.994** Poisoning by other hormone antagonists, undetermined
  - **T38.995** Adverse effect of other hormone antagonists
  - **T38.996** Underdosing of other hormone antagonists
- **T39** **Poisoning by, adverse effect of and underdosing of nonopioid analgesics, antipyretics and antirheumatics**
  - The appropriate 7th character is to be added to each code from category T39

A	initial encounter
D	subsequent encounter
S	sequela

  - **T39.0** **Poisoning by, adverse effect of and underdosing of salicylates**
    - **T39.01** **Poisoning by, adverse effect of and underdosing of aspirin**
      - Poisoning by, adverse effect of and underdosing of acetylsalicylic acid
      - **T39.011** Poisoning by aspirin, accidental (unintentional)
      - **T39.012** Poisoning by aspirin, intentional self-harm
      - **T39.013** Poisoning by aspirin, assault
      - **T39.014** Poisoning by aspirin, undetermined
      - **T39.015** Adverse effect of aspirin
      - **T39.016** Underdosing of aspirin
    - **T39.09** **Poisoning by, adverse effect of and underdosing of other salicylates**
      - **T39.091** Poisoning by salicylates, accidental (unintentional)
        - Poisoning by salicylates NOS
      - **T39.092** Poisoning by salicylates, intentional self-harm
      - **T39.093** Poisoning by salicylates, assault
      - **T39.094** Poisoning by salicylates, undetermined
      - **T39.095** Adverse effect of salicylates
      - **T39.096** Underdosing of salicylates
  - **T39.1** **Poisoning by, adverse effect of and underdosing of 4-Aminophenol derivatives**
    - **T39.1X** **Poisoning by, adverse effect of and underdosing of 4-Aminophenol derivatives**
      - **T39.1X1** Poisoning by 4-Aminophenol derivatives, accidental (unintentional)
        - Poisoning by 4-Aminophenol derivatives NOS
      - **T39.1X2** Poisoning by 4-Aminophenol derivatives, intentional self-harm
      - **T39.1X3** Poisoning by 4-Aminophenol derivatives, assault
      - **T39.1X4** Poisoning by 4-Aminophenol derivatives, undetermined
      - **T39.1X5** Adverse effect of 4-Aminophenol derivatives
      - **T39.1X6** Underdosing of 4-Aminophenol derivatives

CHAPTER 19 (S00-T88)

● T39.2   Poisoning by, adverse effect of and underdosing of pyrazolone derivatives

    ● T39.2X   Poisoning by, adverse effect of and underdosing of pyrazolone derivatives

       ● T39.2X1   Poisoning by pyrazolone derivatives, accidental (unintentional)
          Poisoning by pyrazolone derivatives NOS

       ● T39.2X2   Poisoning by pyrazolone derivatives, intentional self-harm

       ● T39.2X3   Poisoning by pyrazolone derivatives, assault

       ● T39.2X4   Poisoning by pyrazolone derivatives, undetermined

       ● T39.2X5   Adverse effect of pyrazolone derivatives

       ● T39.2X6   Underdosing of pyrazolone derivatives

● T39.3   Poisoning by, adverse effect of and underdosing of other nonsteroidal anti-inflammatory drugs [NSAID]

    ● T39.31   Poisoning by, adverse effect of and underdosing of propionic acid derivatives
       Poisoning by, adverse effect of and underdosing of fenoprofen
       Poisoning by, adverse effect of and underdosing of flurbiprofen
       Poisoning by, adverse effect of and underdosing of ibuprofen
       Poisoning by, adverse effect of and underdosing of ketoprofen
       Poisoning by, adverse effect of and underdosing of naproxen
       Poisoning by, adverse effect of and underdosing of oxaprozin

       ● T39.311   Poisoning by propionic acid derivatives, accidental (unintentional)

       ● T39.312   Poisoning by propionic acid derivatives, intentional self-harm

       ● T39.313   Poisoning by propionic acid derivatives, assault

       ● T39.314   Poisoning by propionic acid derivatives, undetermined

       ● T39.315   Adverse effect of propionic acid derivatives

       ● T39.316   Underdosing of propionic acid derivatives

    ● T39.39   Poisoning by, adverse effect of and underdosing of other nonsteroidal anti-inflammatory drugs [NSAID]

       ● T39.391   Poisoning by other nonsteroidal anti-inflammatory drugs [NSAID], accidental (unintentional)
          Poisoning by other nonsteroidal anti-inflammatory drugs NOS

       ● T39.392   Poisoning by other nonsteroidal anti-inflammatory drugs [NSAID], intentional self-harm

       ● T39.393   Poisoning by other nonsteroidal anti-inflammatory drugs [NSAID], assault

       ● T39.394   Poisoning by other nonsteroidal anti-inflammatory drugs [NSAID], undetermined

       ● T39.395   Adverse effect of other nonsteroidal anti-inflammatory drugs [NSAID]

       ● T39.396   Underdosing of other nonsteroidal anti-inflammatory drugs [NSAID]

● T39.4   Poisoning by, adverse effect of and underdosing of antirheumatics, not elsewhere classified

    Excludes1   poisoning by, adverse effect of and underdosing of glucocorticoids (T38.0-)
       poisoning by, adverse effect of and underdosing of salicylates (T39.0-)

    ● T39.4X   Poisoning by, adverse effect of and underdosing of antirheumatics, not elsewhere classified

       ● T39.4X1   Poisoning by antirheumatics, not elsewhere classified, accidental (unintentional)
          Poisoning by antirheumatics, not elsewhere classified NOS

       ● T39.4X2   Poisoning by antirheumatics, not elsewhere classified, intentional self-harm

       ● T39.4X3   Poisoning by antirheumatics, not elsewhere classified, assault

       ● T39.4X4   Poisoning by antirheumatics, not elsewhere classified, undetermined

       ● T39.4X5   Adverse effect of antirheumatics, not elsewhere classified

       ● T39.4X6   Underdosing of antirheumatics, not elsewhere classified

● T39.8   Poisoning by, adverse effect of and underdosing of other nonopioid analgesics and antipyretics, not elsewhere classified

    ● T39.8X   Poisoning by, adverse effect of and underdosing of other nonopioid analgesics and antipyretics, not elsewhere classified

       ● T39.8X1   Poisoning by other nonopioid analgesics and antipyretics, not elsewhere classified, accidental (unintentional)
          Poisoning by other nonopioid analgesics and antipyretics, not elsewhere classified NOS

       ● T39.8X2   Poisoning by other nonopioid analgesics and antipyretics, not elsewhere classified, intentional self-harm

       ● T39.8X3   Poisoning by other nonopioid analgesics and antipyretics, not elsewhere classified, assault

       ● T39.8X4   Poisoning by other nonopioid analgesics and antipyretics, not elsewhere classified, undetermined

       ● T39.8X5   Adverse effect of other nonopioid analgesics and antipyretics, not elsewhere classified

       ● T39.8X6   Underdosing of other nonopioid analgesics and antipyretics, not elsewhere classified

● T39.9   Poisoning by, adverse effect of and underdosing of unspecified nonopioid analgesic, antipyretic and antirheumatic

    X ● T39.91   Poisoning by unspecified nonopioid analgesic, antipyretic and antirheumatic, accidental (unintentional)
       Poisoning by nonopioid analgesic, antipyretic and antirheumatic NOS

    X ● T39.92   Poisoning by unspecified nonopioid analgesic, antipyretic and antirheumatic, intentional self-harm

    X ● T39.93   Poisoning by unspecified nonopioid analgesic, antipyretic and antirheumatic, assault

    X ● T39.94   Poisoning by unspecified nonopioid analgesic, antipyretic and antirheumatic, undetermined

    X ● T39.95   Adverse effect of unspecified nonopioid analgesic, antipyretic and antirheumatic

    X ● T39.96   Underdosing of unspecified nonopioid analgesic, antipyretic and antirheumatic

◀ New   ◀▥ Revised   ~~deleted~~ Deleted   Excludes 1   Excludes 2   Includes   Use additional   Code first   Code also   Unspecified

OGCR Official Guidelines   X Assign placeholder X   ● Use Additional Character(s)   ▶ Manifestation Code   **Coding Clinic**

● T40   **Poisoning by, adverse effect of and underdosing of narcotics and psychodysleptics [hallucinogens]**

     Excludes2   drug dependence and related mental and behavioral disorders due to psychoactive substance use (F10.-F19.-)

     The appropriate 7th character is to be added to each code from category T40.

     | | |
     A   initial encounter
     D   subsequent encounter
     S   sequela

● T40.0   **Poisoning by, adverse effect of and underdosing of opium**

   ● T40.0X   **Poisoning by, adverse effect of and underdosing of opium**

     T40.0X1   **Poisoning by opium, accidental (unintentional)**
       Poisoning by opium NOS

     ● T40.0X2   **Poisoning by opium, intentional self-harm**

     ● T40.0X3   **Poisoning by opium, assault**

     ● T40.0X4   **Poisoning by opium, undetermined**

     ● T40.0X5   **Adverse effect of opium**

     ● T40.0X6   **Underdosing of opium**

● T40.1   **Poisoning by and adverse effect of heroin**

   ● T40.1X   **Poisoning by and adverse effect of heroin**

     ● T40.1X1   **Poisoning by heroin, accidental (unintentional)**
       Poisoning by heroin NOS

     ● T40.1X2   **Poisoning by heroin, intentional self-harm**

     ● T40.1X3   **Poisoning by heroin, assault**

     ● T40.1X4   **Poisoning by heroin, undetermined**

● T40.2   **Poisoning by, adverse effect of and underdosing of other opioids**

   ● T40.2X   **Poisoning by, adverse effect of and underdosing of other opioids**

     ● T40.2X1   **Poisoning by other opioids, accidental (unintentional)**
       Poisoning by other opioids NOS

     ● T40.2X2   **Poisoning by other opioids, intentional self-harm**

     ● T40.2X3   **Poisoning by other opioids, assault**

     ● T40.2X4   **Poisoning by other opioids, undetermined**

     ● T40.2X5   **Adverse effect of other opioids**

     ● T40.2X6   **Underdosing of other opioids**

● T40.3   **Poisoning by, adverse effect of and underdosing of methadone**

   ● T40.3X   **Poisoning by, adverse effect of and underdosing of methadone**

     ● T40.3X1   **Poisoning by methadone, accidental (unintentional)**
       Poisoning by methadone NOS

     ● T40.3X2   **Poisoning by methadone, intentional self-harm**

     ● T40.3X3   **Poisoning by methadone, assault**

     ● T40.3X4   **Poisoning by methadone, undetermined**

     ● T40.3X5   **Adverse effect of methadone**

     ● T40.3X6   **Underdosing of methadone**

● T40.4   **Poisoning by, adverse effect of and underdosing of other synthetic narcotics**

   ● T40.4X   **Poisoning by, adverse effect of and underdosing of other synthetic narcotics**

     ● T40.4X1   **Poisoning by other synthetic narcotics, accidental (unintentional)**
       Poisoning by other synthetic narcotics NOS

     ● T40.4X2   **Poisoning by other synthetic narcotics, intentional self-harm**

     ● T40.4X3   **Poisoning by other synthetic narcotics, assault**

     ● T40.4X4   **Poisoning by other synthetic narcotics, undetermined**

     ● T40.4X5   **Adverse effect of other synthetic narcotics**

     ● T40.4X6   **Underdosing of other synthetic narcotics**

● T40.5   **Poisoning by, adverse effect of and underdosing of cocaine**

   ● T40.5X   **Poisoning by, adverse effect of and underdosing of cocaine**

     ● T40.5X1   **Poisoning by cocaine, accidental (unintentional)**
       Poisoning by cocaine NOS

     ● T40.5X2   **Poisoning by cocaine, intentional self-harm**

     ● T40.5X3   **Poisoning by cocaine, assault**

     ● T40.5X4   **Poisoning by cocaine, undetermined**

     ● T40.5X5   **Adverse effect of cocaine**

     ● T40.5X6   **Underdosing of cocaine**

● T40.6   **Poisoning by, adverse effect of and underdosing of other and unspecified narcotics**

   ● T40.60   **Poisoning by, adverse effect of and underdosing of unspecified narcotics**

     ● T40.601   **Poisoning by unspecified narcotics, accidental (unintentional)**
       Poisoning by narcotics NOS

     ● T40.602   **Poisoning by unspecified narcotics, intentional self-harm**

     ● T40.603   **Poisoning by unspecified narcotics, assault**

     ● T40.604   **Poisoning by unspecified narcotics, undetermined**

     ● T40.605   **Adverse effect of unspecified narcotics**

     ● T40.606   **Underdosing of unspecified narcotics**

   ● T40.69   **Poisoning by, adverse effect of and underdosing of other narcotics**

     ● T40.691   **Poisoning by other narcotics, accidental (unintentional)**
       Poisoning by other narcotics NOS

     ● T40.692   **Poisoning by other narcotics, intentional self-harm**

     ● T40.693   **Poisoning by other narcotics, assault**

     ● T40.694   **Poisoning by other narcotics, undetermined**

     ● T40.695   **Adverse effect of other narcotics**

     ● T40.696   **Underdosing of other narcotics**

CHAPTER 19 (S00-T88)

● T40.7 **Poisoning by, adverse effect of and underdosing of cannabis (derivatives)**

  ● T40.7X **Poisoning by, adverse effect of and underdosing of cannabis (derivatives)**

    ● T40.7X1 **Poisoning by cannabis (derivatives), accidental (unintentional)**
      Poisoning by cannabis NOS

    ● T40.7X2 **Poisoning by cannabis (derivatives), intentional self-harm**

    ● T40.7X3 **Poisoning by cannabis (derivatives), assault**

    ● T40.7X4 **Poisoning by cannabis (derivatives), undetermined**

    ● T40.7X5 **Adverse effect of cannabis (derivatives)**

    ● T40.7X6 **Underdosing of cannabis (derivatives)**

● T40.8 **Poisoning by and adverse effect of lysergide [LSD]**

  ● T40.8X **Poisoning by and adverse effect of lysergide [LSD]**

    ● T40.8X1 **Poisoning by lysergide [LSD], accidental (unintentional)**
      Poisoning by lysergide [LSD] NOS

    ● T40.8X2 **Poisoning by lysergide [LSD], intentional self-harm**

    ● T40.8X3 **Poisoning by lysergide [LSD], assault**

    ● T40.8X4 **Poisoning by lysergide [LSD], undetermined**

● T40.9 **Poisoning by, adverse effect of and underdosing of other and unspecified psychodysleptics [hallucinogens]**

  ● T40.90 **Poisoning by, adverse effect of and underdosing of unspecified psychodysleptics [hallucinogens]**

    ● T40.901 **Poisoning by unspecified psychodysleptics [hallucinogens], accidental (unintentional)**

    ● T40.902 **Poisoning by unspecified psychodysleptics [hallucinogens], intentional self-harm**

    ● T40.903 **Poisoning by unspecified psychodysleptics [hallucinogens], assault**

    ● T40.904 **Poisoning by unspecified psychodysleptics [hallucinogens], undetermined**

    ● T40.905 **Adverse effect of unspecified psychodysleptics [hallucinogens]**

    ● T40.906 **Underdosing of unspecified psychodysleptics**

  ● T40.99 **Poisoning by, adverse effect of and underdosing of other psychodysleptics [hallucinogens]**

    ● T40.991 **Poisoning by other psychodysleptics [hallucinogens], accidental (unintentional)**
      Poisoning by other psychodysleptics [hallucinogens] NOS

    ● T40.992 **Poisoning by other psychodysleptics [hallucinogens], intentional self-harm**

    ● T40.993 **Poisoning by other psychodysleptics [hallucinogens], assault**

    ● T40.994 **Poisoning by other psychodysleptics [hallucinogens], undetermined**

    ● T40.995 **Adverse effect of other psychodysleptics [hallucinogens]**

    ● T40.996 **Underdosing of other psychodysleptics**

● T41 **Poisoning by, adverse effect of and underdosing of anesthetics and therapeutic gases**

  Excludes1 benzodiazepines (T42.4-)
    cocaine (T40.5-)
    complications of anesthesia during pregnancy (O29.-)
    complications of anesthesia during labor and delivery (O74.-)
    complications of anesthesia during the puerperium (O89.-) opioids (T40.0-T40.2-)

The appropriate 7th character is to be added to each code from category T41

A	initial encounter
D	subsequent encounter
S	sequela

● T41.0 **Poisoning by, adverse effect of and underdosing of inhaled anesthetics**

  Excludes1 oxygen (T41.5-)

  ● T41.0X **Poisoning by, adverse effect of and underdosing of inhaled anesthetics**

    ● T41.0X1 **Poisoning by inhaled anesthetics, accidental (unintentional)**
      Poisoning by inhaled anesthetics NOS

    ● T41.0X2 **Poisoning by inhaled anesthetics, intentional self-harm**

    ● T41.0X3 **Poisoning by inhaled anesthetics, assault**

    ● T41.0X4 **Poisoning by inhaled anesthetics, undetermined**

    ● T41.0X5 **Adverse effect of inhaled anesthetics**

    ● T41.0X6 **Underdosing of inhaled anesthetics**

● T41.1 **Poisoning by, adverse effect of and underdosing of intravenous anesthetics**
  Poisoning by, adverse effect of and underdosing of thiobarbiturates

  ● T41.1X **Poisoning by, adverse effect of and underdosing of intravenous anesthetics**

    ● T41.1X1 **Poisoning by intravenous anesthetics, accidental (unintentional)**
      Poisoning by intravenous anesthetics NOS

    ● T41.1X2 **Poisoning by intravenous anesthetics, intentional self-harm**

    ● T41.1X3 **Poisoning by intravenous anesthetics, assault**

    ● T41.1X4 **Poisoning by intravenous anesthetics, undetermined**

    ● T41.1X5 **Adverse effect of intravenous anesthetics**

    ● T41.1X6 **Underdosing of intravenous anesthetics**

● T41.2 **Poisoning by, adverse effect of and underdosing of other and unspecified general anesthetics**

  ● T41.20 **Poisoning by, adverse effect of and underdosing of unspecified general anesthetics**

    ● T41.201 **Poisoning by unspecified general anesthetics, accidental (unintentional)**
      Poisoning by general anesthetics NOS

    ● T41.202 **Poisoning by unspecified general anesthetics, intentional self-harm**

    ● T41.203 **Poisoning by unspecified general anesthetics, assault**

    ● T41.204 **Poisoning by unspecified general anesthetics, undetermined**

    ● T41.205 **Adverse effect of unspecified general anesthetics**

    ● T41.206 **Underdosing of unspecified general anesthetics**

● **T41.29**   **Poisoning by, adverse effect of and underdosing of other general anesthetics**

     ● **T41.291**   **Poisoning by other general anesthetics, accidental (unintentional)**
         Poisoning by other general anesthetics NOS

     ● **T41.292**   **Poisoning by other general anesthetics, intentional self-harm**

     ● **T41.293**   **Poisoning by other general anesthetics, assault**

     ● **T41.294**   **Poisoning by other general anesthetics, undetermined**

     ● **T41.295**   **Adverse effect of other general anesthetics**

     ● **T41.296**   **Underdosing of other general anesthetics**

● **T41.3**   **Poisoning by, adverse effect of and underdosing of local anesthetics**
   Cocaine (topical)

     Excludes2   poisoning by cocaine used as a central nervous system stimulant (T40.5X1-T40.5X4)

     ● **T41.3X**   **Poisoning by, adverse effect of and underdosing of local anesthetics**

         ● **T41.3X1**   **Poisoning by local anesthetics, accidental (unintentional)**
            Poisoning by local anesthetics NOS

         ● **T41.3X2**   **Poisoning by local anesthetics, intentional self-harm**

         ● **T41.3X3**   **Poisoning by local anesthetics, assault**

         ● **T41.3X4**   **Poisoning by local anesthetics, undetermined**

         ● **T41.3X5**   **Adverse effect of local anesthetics**

         ● **T41.3X6**   **Underdosing of local anesthetics**

● **T41.4**   **Poisoning by, adverse effect of and underdosing of unspecified anesthetic**

   X ● **T41.41**   **Poisoning by unspecified anesthetic, accidental (unintentional)**
       Poisoning by anesthetic NOS

   X ● **T41.42**   **Poisoning by unspecified anesthetic, intentional self-harm**

   X ● **T41.43**   **Poisoning by unspecified anesthetic, assault**

   X ● **T41.44**   **Poisoning by unspecified anesthetic, undetermined**

   X ● **T41.45**   **Adverse effect of unspecified anesthetic**

   X ● **T41.46**   **Underdosing of unspecified anesthetics**

● **T41.5**   **Poisoning by, adverse effect of and underdosing of therapeutic gases**

     ● **T41.5X**   **Poisoning by, adverse effect of and underdosing of therapeutic gases**

         ● **T41.5X1**   **Poisoning by therapeutic gases, accidental (unintentional)**
            Poisoning by therapeutic gases NOS

         ● **T41.5X2**   **Poisoning by therapeutic gases, intentional self-harm**

         ● **T41.5X3**   **Poisoning by therapeutic gases, assault**

         ● **T41.5X4**   **Poisoning by therapeutic gases, undetermined**

         ● **T41.5X5**   **Adverse effect of therapeutic gases**

         ● **T41.5X6**   **Underdosing of therapeutic gases**

● **T42**   **Poisoning by, adverse effect of and underdosing of antiepileptic, sedative-hypnotic and antiparkinsonism drugs**

    Excludes2   drug dependence and related mental and behavioral disorders due to psychoactive substance use (F10.--F19.-)

   The appropriate 7th character is to be added to each code from category T42

     A   initial encounter
     D   subsequent encounter
     S   sequela

● **T42.0**   **Poisoning by, adverse effect of and underdosing of hydantoin derivatives**

     ● **T42.0X**   **Poisoning by, adverse effect of and underdosing of hydantoin derivatives**

         ● **T42.0X1**   **Poisoning by hydantoin derivatives, accidental (unintentional)**
            Poisoning by hydantoin derivatives NOS

         ● **T42.0X2**   **Poisoning by hydantoin derivatives, intentional self-harm**

         ● **T42.0X3**   **Poisoning by hydantoin derivatives, assault**

         ● **T42.0X4**   **Poisoning by hydantoin derivatives, undetermined**

         ● **T42.0X5**   **Adverse effect of hydantoin derivatives**

         ● **T42.0X6**   **Underdosing of hydantoin derivatives**

● **T42.1**   **Poisoning by, adverse effect of and underdosing of iminostilbenes**
   Poisoning by, adverse effect of and underdosing of carbamazepine

     ● **T42.1X**   **Poisoning by, adverse effect of and underdosing of iminostilbenes**

         ● **T42.1X1**   **Poisoning by iminostilbenes, accidental (unintentional)**
            Poisoning by iminostilbenes NOS

         ● **T42.1X2**   **Poisoning by iminostilbenes, intentional self-harm**

         ● **T42.1X3**   **Poisoning by iminostilbenes, assault**

         ● **T42.1X4**   **Poisoning by iminostilbenes, undetermined**

         ● **T42.1X5**   **Adverse effect of iminostilbenes**

         ● **T42.1X6**   **Underdosing of iminostilbenes**

● **T42.2**   **Poisoning by, adverse effect of and underdosing of succinimides and oxazolidinediones**

     ● **T42.2X**   **Poisoning by, adverse effect of and underdosing of succinimides and oxazolidinediones**

         ● **T42.2X1**   **Poisoning by succinimides and oxazolidinediones, accidental (unintentional)**
            Poisoning by succinimides and oxazolidinediones NOS

         ● **T42.2X2**   **Poisoning by succinimides and oxazolidinediones, intentional self-harm**

         ● **T42.2X3**   **Poisoning by succinimides and oxazolidinediones, assault**

         ● **T42.2X4**   **Poisoning by succinimides and oxazolidinediones, undetermined**

         ● **T42.2X5**   **Adverse effect of succinimides and oxazolidinediones**

         ● **T42.2X6**   **Underdosing of succinimides and oxazolidinediones**

CHAPTER 19 (S00-T88)

CHAPTER 19 (S00-T88)

● T42.3   Poisoning by, adverse effect of and underdosing of barbiturates

    Excludes1   poisoning by, adverse effect of and underdosing of thiobarbiturates (T41.1-)

   ● T42.3X   Poisoning by, adverse effect of and underdosing of barbiturates

     ● T42.3X1   Poisoning by barbiturates, accidental (unintentional)

       Poisoning by barbiturates NOS

     ● T42.3X2   Poisoning by barbiturates, intentional self-harm

     ● T42.3X3   Poisoning by barbiturates, assault

     ● T42.3X4   Poisoning by barbiturates, undetermined

     ● T42.3X5   Adverse effect of barbiturates

     ● T42.3X6   Underdosing of barbiturates

● T42.4   Poisoning by, adverse effect of and underdosing of benzodiazepines

   ● T42.4X   Poisoning by, adverse effect of and underdosing of benzodiazepines

     ● T42.4X1   Poisoning by benzodiazepines, accidental (unintentional)

       Poisoning by benzodiazepines NOS

     ● T42.4X2   Poisoning by benzodiazepines, intentional self-harm

     ● T42.4X3   Poisoning by benzodiazepines, assault

     ● T42.4X4   Poisoning by benzodiazepines, undetermined

     ● T42.4X5   Adverse effect of benzodiazepines

     ● T42.4X6   Underdosing of benzodiazepines

● T42.5   Poisoning by, adverse effect of and underdosing of mixed antiepileptics

   ● T42.5X   Poisoning by, adverse effect of and underdosing of antiepileptics

     ● T42.5X1   Poisoning by mixed antiepileptics, accidental (unintentional)

       Poisoning by mixed antiepileptics NOS

     ● T42.5X2   Poisoning by mixed antiepileptics, intentional self-harm

     ● T42.5X3   Poisoning by mixed antiepileptics, assault

     ● T42.5X4   Poisoning by mixed antiepileptics, undetermined

     ● T42.5X5   Adverse effect of mixed antiepileptics

     ● T42.5X6   Underdosing of mixed antiepileptics

● T42.6   Poisoning by, adverse effect of and underdosing of other antiepileptic and sedative-hypnotic drugs

    Poisoning by, adverse effect of and underdosing of methaqualone

    Poisoning by, adverse effect of and underdosing of valproic acid

    Excludes1   poisoning by, adverse effect of and underdosing of carbamazepine (T42.1-)

   ● T42.6X   Poisoning by, adverse effect of and underdosing of other antiepileptic and sedative-hypnotic drugs

     ● T42.6X1   Poisoning by other antiepileptic and sedative-hypnotic drugs, accidental (unintentional)

       Poisoning by other antiepileptic and sedative-hypnotic drugs NOS

     ● T42.6X2   Poisoning by other antiepileptic and sedative-hypnotic drugs, intentional self-harm

     ● T42.6X3   Poisoning by other antiepileptic and sedative-hypnotic drugs, assault

     ● T42.6X4   Poisoning by other antiepileptic and sedative-hypnotic drugs, undetermined

     ● T42.6X5   Adverse effect of other antiepileptic and sedative-hypnotic drugs

     ● T42.6X6   Underdosing of other antiepileptic and sedative-hypnotic drugs

● T42.7   Poisoning by, adverse effect of and underdosing of unspecified antiepileptic and sedative-hypnotic drugs

   X ● T42.71   Poisoning by unspecified antiepileptic and sedative-hypnotic drugs, accidental (unintentional)

       Poisoning by antiepileptic and sedative-hypnotic drugs NOS

   X ● T42.72   Poisoning by unspecified antiepileptic and sedative-hypnotic drugs, intentional self-harm

   X ● T42.73   Poisoning by unspecified antiepileptic and sedative-hypnotic drugs, assault

   X ● T42.74   Poisoning by unspecified antiepileptic and sedative-hypnotic drugs, undetermined

   X ● T42.75   Adverse effect of unspecified antiepileptic and sedative-hypnotic drugs

   X ● T42.76   Underdosing of unspecified antiepileptic and sedative-hypnotic drugs

● T42.8   Poisoning by, adverse effect of and underdosing of antiparkinsonism drugs and other central muscle-tone depressants

    Poisoning by, adverse effect of and underdosing of amantadine

   ● T42.8X   Poisoning by, adverse effect of and underdosing of antiparkinsonism drugs and other central muscle-tone depressants

     ● T42.8X1   Poisoning by antiparkinsonism drugs and other central muscle-tone depressants, accidental (unintentional)

       Poisoning by antiparkinsonism drugs and other central muscle-tone depressants NOS

     ● T42.8X2   Poisoning by antiparkinsonism drugs and other central muscle-tone depressants, intentional self-harm

     ● T42.8X3   Poisoning by antiparkinsonism drugs and other central muscle-tone depressants, assault

     ● T42.8X4   Poisoning by antiparkinsonism drugs and other central muscle-tone depressants, undetermined

     ● T42.8X5   Adverse effect of antiparkinsonism drugs and other central muscle-tone depressants

     ● T42.8X6   Underdosing of antiparkinsonism drugs and other central muscle-tone depressants

◄ New   ◄◄◄ Revised   ~~deleted~~ Deleted   Excludes 1   Excludes 2   Includes   Use additional   Code first   Code also   Unspecified

OGCR Official Guidelines   **X** Assign placeholder X   ● Use Additional Character(s)   ▶ Manifestation Code   **Coding Clinic**

- T43   Poisoning by, adverse effect of and underdosing of psychotropic drugs, not elsewhere classified

  Excludes1   appetite depressants (T50.5-)
  barbiturates (T42.3-)
  benzodiazepines (T42.4-)
  methaqualone (T42.6-)
  psychodysleptics [hallucinogens] (T40.7-T40.9-)

  Excludes2   drug dependence and related mental and behavioral disorders due to psychoactive substance use (F10.--F19.-)

  The appropriate 7th character is to be added to each code from category T43

A	initial encounter
D	subsequent encounter
S	sequela

- T43.0   Poisoning by, adverse effect of and underdosing of tricyclic and tetracyclic antidepressants

  - T43.01   Poisoning by, adverse effect of and underdosing of tricyclic antidepressants

    - T43.011   Poisoning by tricyclic antidepressants, accidental (unintentional)
      Poisoning by tricyclic antidepressants NOS

    - T43.012   Poisoning by tricyclic antidepressants, intentional self-harm

    - T43.013   Poisoning by tricyclic antidepressants, assault

    - T43.014   Poisoning by tricyclic antidepressants, undetermined

    - T43.015   Adverse effect of tricyclic antidepressants

    - T43.016   Underdosing of tricyclic antidepressants

  - T43.02   Poisoning by, adverse effect of and underdosing of tetracyclic antidepressants

    - T43.021   Poisoning by tetracyclic antidepressants, accidental (unintentional)
      Poisoning by tetracyclic antidepressants NOS

    - T43.022   Poisoning by tetracyclic antidepressants, intentional self-harm

    - T43.023   Poisoning by tetracyclic antidepressants, assault

    - T43.024   Poisoning by tetracyclic antidepressants, undetermined

    - T43.025   Adverse effect of tetracyclic antidepressants

    - T43.026   Underdosing of tetracyclic antidepressants

- T43.1   Poisoning by, adverse effect of and underdosing of monoamine-oxidase-inhibitor antidepressants

  - T43.1X   Poisoning by, adverse effect of and underdosing of monoamine-oxidase-inhibitor antidepressants

    - T43.1X1   Poisoning by monoamine-oxidase-inhibitor antidepressants, accidental (unintentional)
      Poisoning by monoamine-oxidase-inhibitor antidepressants NOS

    - T43.1X2   Poisoning by monoamine-oxidase-inhibitor antidepressants, intentional self-harm

    - T43.1X3   Poisoning by monoamine-oxidase-inhibitor antidepressants, assault

    - T43.1X4   Poisoning by monoamine-oxidase-inhibitor antidepressants, undetermined

    - T43.1X5   Adverse effect of monoamine-oxidase-inhibitor antidepressants

    - T43.1X6   Underdosing of monoamine-oxidase-inhibitor antidepressants

- T43.2   Poisoning by, adverse effect of and underdosing of other and unspecified antidepressants

  - T43.20   Poisoning by, adverse effect of and underdosing of unspecified antidepressants

    - T43.201   Poisoning by unspecified antidepressants, accidental (unintentional)
      Poisoning by antidepressants NOS

    - T43.202   Poisoning by unspecified antidepressants, intentional self-harm

    - T43.203   Poisoning by unspecified antidepressants, assault

    - T43.204   Poisoning by unspecified antidepressants, undetermined

    - T43.205   Adverse effect of unspecified antidepressants

    - T43.206   Underdosing of unspecified antidepressants

  - T43.21   Poisoning by, adverse effect of and underdosing of selective serotonin and norepinephrine reuptake inhibitors
    Poisoning by, adverse effect of and underdosing of SSNRI antidepressants

    - T43.211   Poisoning by selective serotonin and norepinephrine reuptake inhibitors, accidental (unintentional)

    - T43.212   Poisoning by selective serotonin and norepinephrine reuptake inhibitors, intentional self-harm

    - T43.213   Poisoning by selective serotonin and norepinephrine reuptake inhibitors, assault

    - T43.214   Poisoning by selective serotonin and norepinephrine reuptake inhibitors, undetermined

    - T43.215   Adverse effect of selective serotonin and norepinephrine reuptake inhibitors

    - T43.216   Underdosing of selective serotonin and norepinephrine reuptake inhibitors

  - T43.22   Poisoning by, adverse effect of and underdosing of selective serotonin reuptake inhibitors
    Poisoning by, adverse effect of and underdosing of SSRI antidepressants

    - T43.221   Poisoning by selective serotonin reuptake inhibitors, accidental (unintentional)

    - T43.222   Poisoning by selective serotonin reuptake inhibitors, intentional self-harm

    - T43.223   Poisoning by selective serotonin reuptake inhibitors, assault

    - T43.224   Poisoning by selective serotonin reuptake inhibitors, undetermined

    - T43.225   Adverse effect of selective serotonin reuptake inhibitors

    - T43.226   Underdosing of selective serotonin reuptake inhibitors

● T43.29 Poisoning by, adverse effect of and underdosing of other antidepressants

   ● T43.291 Poisoning by other antidepressants, accidental (unintentional)
      Poisoning by other antidepressants NOS

   ● T43.292 Poisoning by other antidepressants, intentional self-harm

   ● T43.293 Poisoning by other antidepressants, assault

   ● T43.294 Poisoning by other antidepressants, undetermined

   ● T43.295 Adverse effect of other antidepressants

   ● T43.296 Underdosing of other antidepressants

● T43.3 Poisoning by, adverse effect of and underdosing of phenothiazine antipsychotics and neuroleptics

  ● T43.3X Poisoning by, adverse effect of and underdosing of phenothiazine antipsychotics and neuroleptics

   ● T43.3X1 Poisoning by phenothiazine antipsychotics and neuroleptics, accidental (unintentional)
      Poisoning by phenothiazine antipsychotics and neuroleptics NOS

   ● T43.3X2 Poisoning by phenothiazine antipsychotics and neuroleptics, intentional self-harm

   ● T43.3X3 Poisoning by phenothiazine antipsychotics and neuroleptics, assault

   ● T43.3X4 Poisoning by phenothiazine antipsychotics and neuroleptics, undetermined

   ● T43.3X5 Adverse effect of phenothiazine antipsychotics and neuroleptics

   ● T43.3X6 Underdosing of phenothiazine antipsychotics and neuroleptics

● T43.4 Poisoning by, adverse effect of and underdosing of butyrophenone and thiothixene neuroleptics

  ● T43.4X Poisoning by, adverse effect of and underdosing of butyrophenone and thiothixene neuroleptics

   ● T43.4X1 Poisoning by butyrophenone and thiothixene neuroleptics, accidental (unintentional)
      Poisoning by butyrophenone and thiothixene neuroleptics NOS

   ● T43.4X2 Poisoning by butyrophenone and thiothixene neuroleptics, intentional self-harm

   ● T43.4X3 Poisoning by butyrophenone and thiothixene neuroleptics, assault

   ● T43.4X4 Poisoning by butyrophenone and thiothixene neuroleptics, undetermined

   ● T43.4X5 Adverse effect of butyrophenone and thiothixene neuroleptics

   ● T43.4X6 Underdosing of butyrophenone and thiothixene neuroleptics

● T43.5 Poisoning by, adverse effect of and underdosing of other and unspecified antipsychotics and neuroleptics

  Excludes1 poisoning by, adverse effect of and underdosing of rauwolfia (T46.5-)

  ● T43.50 Poisoning by, adverse effect of and underdosing of unspecified antipsychotics and neuroleptics

   ● T43.501 Poisoning by unspecified antipsychotics and neuroleptics, accidental (unintentional)
      Poisoning by antipsychotics and neuroleptics NOS

   ● T43.502 Poisoning by unspecified antipsychotics and neuroleptics, intentional self-harm

   ● T43.503 Poisoning by unspecified antipsychotics and neuroleptics, assault

   ● T43.504 Poisoning by unspecified antipsychotics and neuroleptics, undetermined

   ● T43.505 Adverse effect of unspecified antipsychotics and neuroleptics

   ● T43.506 Underdosing of unspecified antipsychotics and neuroleptics

  ● T43.59 Poisoning by, adverse effect of and underdosing of other antipsychotics and neuroleptics

   ● T43.591 Poisoning by other antipsychotics and neuroleptics, accidental (unintentional)
      Poisoning by other antipsychotics and neuroleptics NOS

   ● T43.592 Poisoning by other antipsychotics and neuroleptics, intentional self-harm

   ● T43.593 Poisoning by other antipsychotics and neuroleptics, assault

   ● T43.594 Poisoning by other antipsychotics and neuroleptics, undetermined

   ● T43.595 Adverse effect of other antipsychotics and neuroleptics

   ● T43.596 Underdosing of other antipsychotics and neuroleptics

● T43.6 Poisoning by, adverse effect of and underdosing of psychostimulants

  Excludes1 poisoning by, adverse effect of and underdosing of cocaine (T40.5-)

  ● T43.60 Poisoning by, adverse effect of and underdosing of unspecified psychostimulant

   ● T43.601 Poisoning by unspecified psychostimulants, accidental (unintentional)
      Poisoning by psychostimulants NOS

   ● T43.602 Poisoning by unspecified psychostimulants, intentional self-harm

   ● T43.603 Poisoning by unspecified psychostimulants, assault

   ● T43.604 Poisoning by unspecified psychostimulants, undetermined

   ● T43.605 Adverse effect of unspecified psychostimulants

   ● T43.606 Underdosing of unspecified psychostimulants

◀ New ⬅ Revised ~~deleted~~ Deleted | Excludes 1 | Excludes 2 | Includes | Use additional | Code first | Code also | Unspecified

OGCR Official Guidelines   X Assign placeholder X   ● Use Additional Character(s)   ▶ Manifestation Code   **Coding Clinic**

● T43.61   Poisoning by, adverse effect of and underdosing of caffeine

  ● T43.611   Poisoning by caffeine, accidental (unintentional)
      Poisoning by caffeine NOS

  ● T43.612   Poisoning by caffeine, intentional self-harm

  ● T43.613   Poisoning by caffeine, assault

  ● T43.614   Poisoning by caffeine, undetermined

  ● T43.615   Adverse effect of caffeine

  ● T43.616   Underdosing of caffeine

● T43.62   Poisoning by, adverse effect of and underdosing of amphetamines
    Poisoning by, adverse effect of and underdosing of methamphetamines

  ● T43.621   Poisoning by amphetamines, accidental (unintentional)
      Poisoning by amphetamines NOS

  ● T43.622   Poisoning by amphetamines, intentional self-harm

  ● T43.623   Poisoning by amphetamines, assault

  ● T43.624   Poisoning by amphetamines, undetermined

  ● T43.625   Adverse effect of amphetamines

  ● T43.626   Underdosing of amphetamines

● T43.63   Poisoning by, adverse effect of and underdosing of methylphenidate

  ● T43.631   Poisoning by methylphenidate, accidental (unintentional)
      Poisoning by methylphenidate NOS

  ● T43.632   Poisoning by methylphenidate, intentional self-harm

  ● T43.633   Poisoning by methylphenidate, assault

  ● T43.634   Poisoning by methylphenidate, undetermined

  ● T43.635   Adverse effect of methylphenidate

  ● T43.636   Underdosing of methylphenidate

● T43.69   Poisoning by, adverse effect of and underdosing of other psychostimulants

  ● T43.691   Poisoning by other psychostimulants, accidental (unintentional)
      Poisoning by other psychostimulants NOS

  ● T43.692   Poisoning by other psychostimulants, intentional self-harm

  ● T43.693   Poisoning by other psychostimulants, assault

  ● T43.694   Poisoning by other psychostimulants, undetermined

  ● T43.695   Adverse effect of other psychostimulants

  ● T43.696   Underdosing of other psychostimulants

● T43.8   Poisoning by, adverse effect of and underdosing of other psychotropic drugs

  ● T43.8X   Poisoning by, adverse effect of and underdosing of other psychotropic drugs

  ● T43.8X1   Poisoning by other psychotropic drugs, accidental (unintentional)
      Poisoning by other psychotropic drugs NOS

  ● T43.8X2   Poisoning by other psychotropic drugs, intentional self-harm

  ● T43.8X3   Poisoning by other psychotropic drugs, assault

  ● T43.8X4   Poisoning by other psychotropic drugs, undetermined

  ● T43.8X5   Adverse effect of other psychotropic drugs

  ● T43.8X6   Underdosing of other psychotropic drugs

● T43.9   Poisoning by, adverse effect of and underdosing of unspecified psychotropic drug

  X● T43.91   Poisoning by unspecified psychotropic drug, accidental (unintentional)
      Poisoning by psychotropic drug NOS

  X● T43.92   Poisoning by unspecified psychotropic drug, intentional self-harm

  X● T43.93   Poisoning by unspecified psychotropic drug, assault

  X● T43.94   Poisoning by unspecified psychotropic drug, undetermined

  X● T43.95   Adverse effect of unspecified psychotropic drug

  X● T43.96   Underdosing of unspecified psychotropic drug

● T44   Poisoning by, adverse effect of and underdosing of drugs primarily affecting the autonomic nervous system

  The appropriate 7th character is to be added to each code from category T44

A	initial encounter
D	subsequent encounter
S	sequela

● T44.0   Poisoning by, adverse effect of and underdosing of anticholinesterase agents

  ● T44.0X   Poisoning by, adverse effect of and underdosing of anticholinesterase agents

  ● T44.0X1   Poisoning by anticholinesterase agents, accidental (unintentional)
      Poisoning by anticholinesterase agents NOS

  ● T44.0X2   Poisoning by anticholinesterase agents, intentional self-harm

  ● T44.0X3   Poisoning by anticholinesterase agents, assault

  ● T44.0X4   Poisoning by anticholinesterase agents, undetermined

  ● T44.0X5   Adverse effect of anticholinesterase agents

  ● T44.0X6   Underdosing of anticholinesterase agents

● T44.1   Poisoning by, adverse effect of and underdosing of other parasympathomimetics [cholinergics]

  ● T44.1X   Poisoning by, adverse effect of and underdosing of other parasympathomimetics [cholinergics]

  ● T44.1X1   Poisoning by other parasympathomimetics [cholinergics], accidental (unintentional)
      Poisoning by other parasympathomimetics [cholinergics] NOS

  ● T44.1X2   Poisoning by other parasympathomimetics [cholinergics], intentional self-harm

  ● T44.1X3   Poisoning by other parasympathomimetics [cholinergics], assault

  ● T44.1X4   Poisoning by other parasympathomimetics [cholinergics], undetermined

  ● T44.1X5   Adverse effect of other parasympathomimetics [cholinergics]

  ● T44.1X6   Underdosing of other parasympathomimetics

CHAPTER 19 (S00-T88)

● **T44.2** Poisoning by, adverse effect of and underdosing of ganglionic blocking drugs

　● **T44.2X** Poisoning by, adverse effect of and underdosing of ganglionic blocking drugs

　　● **T44.2X1** Poisoning by ganglionic blocking drugs, accidental (unintentional)
　　　　Poisoning by ganglionic blocking drugs NOS

　　● **T44.2X2** Poisoning by ganglionic blocking drugs, intentional self-harm

　　● **T44.2X3** Poisoning by ganglionic blocking drugs, assault

　　● **T44.2X4** Poisoning by ganglionic blocking drugs, undetermined

　　● **T44.2X5** Adverse effect of ganglionic blocking drugs

　　● **T44.2X6** Underdosing of ganglionic blocking drugs

● **T44.3** Poisoning by, adverse effect of and underdosing of other parasympatholytics [anticholinergics and antimuscarinics] and spasmolytics
　　Poisoning by, adverse effect of and underdosing of papaverine

　● **T44.3X** Poisoning by, adverse effect of and underdosing of other parasympatholytics [anticholinergics and antimuscarinics] and spasmolytics

　　● **T44.3X1** Poisoning by other parasympatholytics [anticholinergics and antimuscarinics] and spasmolytics, accidental (unintentional)
　　　　Poisoning by other parasympatholytics [anticholinergics and antimuscarinics] and spasmolytics NOS

　　● **T44.3X2** Poisoning by other parasympatholytics [anticholinergics and antimuscarinics] and spasmolytics, intentional self-harm

　　● **T44.3X3** Poisoning by other parasympatholytics [anticholinergics and antimuscarinics] and spasmolytics, assault

　　● **T44.3X4** Poisoning by other parasympatholytics [anticholinergics and antimuscarinics] and spasmolytics, undetermined

　　● **T44.3X5** Adverse effect of other parasympatholytics [anticholinergics and antimuscarinics] and spasmolytics

　　● **T44.3X6** Underdosing of other parasympatholytics [anticholinergics and antimuscarinics] and spasmolytics

● **T44.4** Poisoning by, adverse effect of and underdosing of predominantly alpha-adrenoreceptor agonists
　　Poisoning by, adverse effect of and underdosing of metaraminol

　● **T44.4X** Poisoning by, adverse effect of and underdosing of predominantly alpha-adrenoreceptor agonists

　　● **T44.4X1** Poisoning by predominantly alpha-adrenoreceptor agonists, accidental (unintentional)
　　　　Poisoning by predominantly alpha-adrenoreceptor agonists NOS

　　● **T44.4X2** Poisoning by predominantly alpha-adrenoreceptor agonists, intentional self-harm

　　● **T44.4X3** Poisoning by predominantly alpha-adrenoreceptor agonists, assault

　　● **T44.4X4** Poisoning by predominantly alpha-adrenoreceptor agonists, undetermined

　　● **T44.4X5** Adverse effect of predominantly alpha-adrenoreceptor agonists

　　● **T44.4X6** Underdosing of predominantly alpha-adrenoreceptor agonists

● **T44.5** Poisoning by, adverse effect of and underdosing of predominantly beta-adrenoreceptor agonists

　　Excludes 1　poisoning by, adverse effect of and underdosing of beta-adrenoreceptor agonists used in asthma therapy (T48.6-)

　● **T44.5X** Poisoning by, adverse effect of and underdosing of predominantly beta-adrenoreceptor agonists

　　● **T44.5X1** Poisoning by predominantly beta-adrenoreceptor agonists, accidental (unintentional)
　　　　Poisoning by predominantly beta-adrenoreceptor agonists NOS

　　● **T44.5X2** Poisoning by predominantly beta-adrenoreceptor agonists, intentional self-harm

　　● **T44.5X3** Poisoning by predominantly beta-adrenoreceptor agonists, assault

　　● **T44.5X4** Poisoning by predominantly beta-adrenoreceptor agonists, undetermined

　　● **T44.5X5** Adverse effect of predominantly beta-adrenoreceptor agonists

　　● **T44.5X6** Underdosing of predominantly beta-adrenoreceptor agonists

● **T44.6** Poisoning by, adverse effect of and underdosing of alpha-adrenoreceptor antagonists

　　Excludes 1　poisoning by, adverse effect of and underdosing of ergot alkaloids (T48.0)

　● **T44.6X** Poisoning by, adverse effect of and underdosing of alpha-adrenoreceptor antagonists

　　● **T44.6X1** Poisoning by alpha-adrenoreceptor antagonists, accidental (unintentional)
　　　　Poisoning by alpha-adrenoreceptor antagonists NOS

　　● **T44.6X2** Poisoning by alpha-adrenoreceptor antagonists, intentional self-harm

　　● **T44.6X3** Poisoning by alpha-adrenoreceptor antagonists, assault

　　● **T44.6X4** Poisoning by alpha-adrenoreceptor antagonists, undetermined

　　● **T44.6X5** Adverse effect of alpha-adrenoreceptor antagonists

　　● **T44.6X6** Underdosing of alpha-adrenoreceptor antagonists

● **T44.7** Poisoning by, adverse effect of and underdosing of beta-adrenoreceptor antagonists

　● **T44.7X** Poisoning by, adverse effect of and underdosing of beta-adrenoreceptor antagonists

　　● **T44.7X1** Poisoning by beta-adrenoreceptor antagonists, accidental (unintentional)
　　　　Poisoning by beta-adrenoreceptor antagonists NOS

　　● **T44.7X2** Poisoning by beta-adrenoreceptor antagonists, intentional self-harm

　　● **T44.7X3** Poisoning by beta-adrenoreceptor antagonists, assault

　　● **T44.7X4** Poisoning by beta-adrenoreceptor antagonists, undetermined

　　● **T44.7X5** Adverse effect of beta-adrenoreceptor antagonists

　　● **T44.7X6** Underdosing of beta-adrenoreceptor antagonists

◀ New　◀◀ Revised　~~deleted~~ Deleted　| Excludes 1 |　| Excludes 2 |　| Includes |　| Use additional |　| Code first |　| Code also |　| Unspecified |

OGCR Official Guidelines　**X** Assign placeholder X　● Use Additional Character(s)　▶ Manifestation Code　**Coding Clinic**

● **T44.8**   **Poisoning by, adverse effect of and underdosing of centrally-acting and adrenergic-neuron-blocking agents**

> **Excludes1**   poisoning by, adverse effect of and underdosing of clonidine (T46.5)
> poisoning by, adverse effect of and underdosing of guanethidine (T46.5)

● **T44.8X**   **Poisoning by, adverse effect of and underdosing of centrally-acting and adrenergic-neuron-blocking agents**

● **T44.8X1**   **Poisoning by centrally-acting and adrenergic-neuron-blocking agents, accidental (unintentional)**
> Poisoning by centrally-acting and adrenergic-neuron-blocking agents NOS

● **T44.8X2**   **Poisoning by centrally-acting and adrenergic-neuron-blocking agents, intentional self-harm**

● **T44.8X3**   **Poisoning by centrally-acting and adrenergic-neuron-blocking agents, assault**

● **T44.8X4**   **Poisoning by centrally-acting and adrenergic-neuron-blocking agents, undetermined**

● **T44.8X5**   **Adverse effect of centrally-acting and adrenergic-neuron-blocking agents**

● **T44.8X6**   **Underdosing of centrally-acting and adrenergic-neuron-blocking agents**

● **T44.9**   **Poisoning by, adverse effect of and underdosing of other and unspecified drugs primarily affecting the autonomic nervous system**
> Poisoning by, adverse effect of and underdosing of drug stimulating both alpha and beta-adrenoreceptors

● **T44.90**   **Poisoning by, adverse effect of and underdosing of unspecified drugs primarily affecting the autonomic nervous system**

● **T44.901**   **Poisoning by unspecified drugs primarily affecting the autonomic nervous system, accidental (unintentional)**
> Poisoning by unspecified drugs primarily affecting the autonomic nervous system NOS

● **T44.902**   **Poisoning by unspecified drugs primarily affecting the autonomic nervous system, intentional self-harm**

● **T44.903**   **Poisoning by unspecified drugs primarily affecting the autonomic nervous system, assault**

● **T44.904**   **Poisoning by unspecified drugs primarily affecting the autonomic nervous system, undetermined**

● **T44.905**   **Adverse effect of unspecified drugs primarily affecting the autonomic nervous system**

● **T44.906**   **Underdosing of unspecified drugs primarily affecting the autonomic nervous system**

● **T44.99**   **Poisoning by, adverse effect of and underdosing of other drugs primarily affecting the autonomic nervous system**

● **T44.991**   **Poisoning by other drug primarily affecting the autonomic nervous system, accidental (unintentional)**
> Poisoning by other drugs primarily affecting the autonomic nervous system NOS

● **T44.992**   **Poisoning by other drug primarily affecting the autonomic nervous system, intentional self-harm**

● **T44.993**   **Poisoning by other drug primarily affecting the autonomic nervous system, assault**

● **T44.994**   **Poisoning by other drug primarily affecting the autonomic nervous system, undetermined**

● **T44.995**   **Adverse effect of other drug primarily affecting the autonomic nervous system**

● **T44.996**   **Underdosing of other drug primarily affecting the autonomic nervous system**

● **T45**   **Poisoning by, adverse effect of and underdosing of primarily systemic and hematological agents, not elsewhere classified**

> The appropriate 7th character is to be added to each code from category T45

> | A | initial encounter |
> |---|---|
> | D | subsequent encounter |
> | S | sequela |

● **T45.0**   **Poisoning by, adverse effect of and underdosing of antiallergic and antiemetic drugs**

> **Excludes1**   poisoning by, adverse effect of and underdosing of phenothiazine-based neuroleptics (T43.3)

● **T45.0X**   **Poisoning by, adverse effect of and underdosing of antiallergic and antiemetic drugs**

● **T45.0X1**   **Poisoning by antiallergic and antiemetic drugs, accidental (unintentional)**
> Poisoning by antiallergic and antiemetic drugs NOS

● **T45.0X2**   **Poisoning by antiallergic and antiemetic drugs, intentional self-harm**

● **T45.0X3**   **Poisoning by antiallergic and antiemetic drugs, assault**

● **T45.0X4**   **Poisoning by antiallergic and antiemetic drugs, undetermined**

● **T45.0X5**   **Adverse effect of antiallergic and antiemetic drugs**

● **T45.0X6**   **Underdosing of antiallergic and antiemetic drugs**

● **T45.1**   **Poisoning by, adverse effect of and underdosing of antineoplastic and immunosuppressive drugs**

> **Excludes1**   poisoning by, adverse effect of and underdosing of tamoxifen (T38.6)

● **T45.1X**   **Poisoning by, adverse effect of and underdosing of antineoplastic and immunosuppressive drugs**

● **T45.1X1**   **Poisoning by antineoplastic and immunosuppressive drugs, accidental (unintentional)**
> Poisoning by antineoplastic and immunosuppressive drugs NOS

● **T45.1X2**   **Poisoning by antineoplastic and immunosuppressive drugs, intentional self-harm**

● **T45.1X3**   **Poisoning by antineoplastic and immunosuppressive drugs, assault**

● **T45.1X4**   **Poisoning by antineoplastic and immunosuppressive drugs, undetermined**

● **T45.1X5**   **Adverse effect of antineoplastic and immunosuppressive drugs**

● **T45.1X6**   **Underdosing of antineoplastic and immunosuppressive drugs**

CHAPTER 19 (S00-T88)

● T45.2　Poisoning by, adverse effect of and underdosing of vitamins

　Excludes2　poisoning by, adverse effect of and underdosing of nicotinic acid (derivatives) (T46.7)

　　　poisoning by, adverse effect of and underdosing of iron (T45.4)

　　　poisoning by, adverse effect of and underdosing of vitamin K (T45.7)

　● T45.2X　Poisoning by, adverse effect of and underdosing of vitamins

　　● T45.2X1　Poisoning by vitamins, accidental (unintentional)
　　　　Poisoning by vitamins NOS

　　● T45.2X2　Poisoning by vitamins, intentional self-harm

　　● T45.2X3　Poisoning by vitamins, assault

　　● T45.2X4　Poisoning by vitamins, undetermined

　　● T45.2X5　Adverse effect of vitamins

　　● T45.2X6　Underdosing of vitamins
　　　　Excludes1　vitamin deficiencies (E50-E56)

● T45.3　Poisoning by, adverse effect of and underdosing of enzymes

　● T45.3X　Poisoning by, adverse effect of and underdosing of enzymes

　　● T45.3X1　Poisoning by enzymes, accidental (unintentional)
　　　　Poisoning by enzymes NOS

　　● T45.3X2　Poisoning by enzymes, intentional self-harm

　　● T45.3X3　Poisoning by enzymes, assault

　　● T45.3X4　Poisoning by enzymes, undetermined

　　● T45.3X5　Adverse effect of enzymes

　　● T45.3X6　Underdosing of enzymes

● T45.4　Poisoning by, adverse effect of and underdosing of iron and its compounds

　● T45.4X　Poisoning by, adverse effect of and underdosing of iron and its compounds

　　● T45.4X1　Poisoning by iron and its compounds, accidental (unintentional)
　　　　Poisoning by iron and its compounds NOS

　　● T45.4X2　Poisoning by iron and its compounds, intentional self-harm

　　● T45.4X3　Poisoning by iron and its compounds, assault

　　● T45.4X4　Poisoning by iron and its compounds, undetermined

　　● T45.4X5　Adverse effect of iron and its compounds

　　● T45.4X6　Underdosing of iron and its compounds
　　　　Excludes1　iron deficiency (E61.1)

● T45.5　Poisoning by, adverse effect of and underdosing of anticoagulants and antithrombotic drugs

　● T45.51　Poisoning by, adverse effect of and underdosing of anticoagulants

　　　T45.511　Poisoning by anticoagulants, accidental (unintentional)
　　　　Poisoning by anticoagulants NOS

　　● T45.512　Poisoning by anticoagulants, intentional self-harm

　　● T45.513　Poisoning by anticoagulants, assault

　　● T45.514　Poisoning by anticoagulants, undetermined

　　● T45.515　Adverse effect of anticoagulants
　　　　Coding Clinic: 2013, Q2, P35

　　● T45.516　Underdosing of anticoagulants

● T45.52　Poisoning by, adverse effect of and underdosing of antithrombotic drugs
　Poisoning by, adverse effect of and underdosing of antiplatelet drugs

　　Excludes2　poisoning by, adverse effect of and underdosing of aspirin (T39.01-)

　　　poisoning by, adverse effect of and underdosing of acetylsalicylic acid (T39.01-)

　● T45.521　Poisoning by antithrombotic drugs, accidental (unintentional)
　　　Poisoning by antithrombotic drug NOS

　● T45.522　Poisoning by antithrombotic drugs, intentional self-harm

　● T45.523　Poisoning by antithrombotic drugs, assault

　● T45.524　Poisoning by antithrombotic drugs, undetermined

　● T45.525　Adverse effect of antithrombotic drugs

　● T45.526　Underdosing of antithrombotic drugs

● T45.6　Poisoning by, adverse effect of and underdosing of fibrinolysis-affecting drugs

　● T45.60　Poisoning by, adverse effect of and underdosing of unspecified fibrinolysis-affecting drugs

　　● T45.601　Poisoning by unspecified fibrinolysis-affecting drugs, accidental (unintentional)
　　　　Poisoning by fibrinolysis-affecting drug NOS

　　● T45.602　Poisoning by unspecified fibrinolysis-affecting drugs, intentional self-harm

　　● T45.603　Poisoning by unspecified fibrinolysis-affecting drugs, assault

　　● T45.604　Poisoning by unspecified fibrinolysis-affecting drugs, undetermined

　　● T45.605　Adverse effect of unspecified fibrinolysis-affecting drugs

　　● T45.606　Underdosing of unspecified fibrinolysis-affecting drugs

　● T45.61　Poisoning by, adverse effect of and underdosing of thrombolytic drugs

　　● T45.611　Poisoning by thrombolytic drug, accidental (unintentional)
　　　　Poisoning by thrombolytic drug NOS

　　● T45.612　Poisoning by thrombolytic drug, intentional self-harm

　　● T45.613　Poisoning by thrombolytic drug, assault

　　● T45.614　Poisoning by thrombolytic drug, undetermined

　　● T45.615　Adverse effect of thrombolytic drugs

　　● T45.616　Underdosing of thrombolytic drugs

　● T45.62　Poisoning by, adverse effect of and underdosing of hemostatic drugs

　　● T45.621　Poisoning by hemostatic drug, accidental (unintentional)
　　　　Poisoning by hemostatic drug NOS

　　● T45.622　Poisoning by hemostatic drug, intentional self-harm

　　● T45.623　Poisoning by hemostatic drug, assault

　　● T45.624　Poisoning by hemostatic drug, undetermined

　　● T45.625　Adverse effect of hemostatic drug

　　● T45.626　Underdosing of hemostatic drugs

● T45.69   Poisoning by, adverse effect of and underdosing of other fibrinolysis-affecting drugs

    ● T45.691   Poisoning by other fibrinolysis-affecting drugs, accidental (unintentional)
         Poisoning by other fibrinolysis-affecting drug NOS

    ● T45.692   Poisoning by other fibrinolysis-affecting drugs, intentional self-harm

    ● T45.693   Poisoning by other fibrinolysis-affecting drugs, assault

    ● T45.694   Poisoning by other fibrinolysis-affecting drugs, undetermined

    ● T45.695   Adverse effect of other fibrinolysis-affecting drugs

    ● T45.696   Underdosing of other fibrinolysis-affecting drugs

● T45.7   Poisoning by, adverse effect of and underdosing of anticoagulant antagonists, vitamin K and other coagulants

  ● T45.7X   Poisoning by, adverse effect of and underdosing of anticoagulant antagonists, vitamin K and other coagulants

    ● T45.7X1   Poisoning by anticoagulant antagonists, vitamin K and other coagulants, accidental (unintentional)
         Poisoning by anticoagulant antagonists, vitamin K and other coagulants NOS

    ● T45.7X2   Poisoning by anticoagulant antagonists, vitamin K and other coagulants, intentional self-harm

    ● T45.7X3   Poisoning by anticoagulant antagonists, vitamin K and other coagulants, assault

    ● T45.7X4   Poisoning by anticoagulant antagonists, vitamin K and other coagulants, undetermined

    ● T45.7X5   Adverse effect of anticoagulant antagonists, vitamin K and other coagulants

    ● T45.7X6   Underdosing of anticoagulant antagonist, vitamin K and other coagulants

         Excludes1   vitamin K deficiency (E56.1)

● T45.8   Poisoning by, adverse effect of and underdosing of other primarily systemic and hematological agents

     Poisoning by, adverse effect of and underdosing of liver preparations and other antianemic agents
     Poisoning by, adverse effect of and underdosing of natural blood and blood products
     Poisoning by, adverse effect of and underdosing of plasma substitute

     Excludes2   poisoning by, adverse effect of and underdosing of immunoglobulin (T50.Z1)
         poisoning by, adverse effect of and underdosing of iron (T45.4)
         transfusion reactions (T80.-)

  ● T45.8X   Poisoning by, adverse effect of and underdosing of other primarily systemic and hematological agents

    ● T45.8X1   Poisoning by other primarily systemic and hematological agents, accidental (unintentional)
         Poisoning by other primarily systemic and hematological agents NOS

    ● T45.8X2   Poisoning by other primarily systemic and hematological agents, intentional self-harm

    ● T45.8X3   Poisoning by other primarily systemic and hematological agents, assault

    ● T45.8X4   Poisoning by other primarily systemic and hematological agents, undetermined

    ● T45.8X5   Adverse effect of other primarily systemic and hematological agents

    ● T45.8X6   Underdosing of other primarily systemic and hematological agents

● T45.9   Poisoning by, adverse effect of and underdosing of unspecified primarily systemic and hematological agent

  X ● T45.91   Poisoning by unspecified primarily systemic and hematological agent, accidental (unintentional)
         Poisoning by primarily systemic and hematological agent NOS

  X ● T45.92   Poisoning by unspecified primarily systemic and hematological agent, intentional self-harm

  X ● T45.93   Poisoning by unspecified primarily systemic and hematological agent, assault

  X ● T45.94   Poisoning by unspecified primarily systemic and hematological agent, undetermined

  X ● T45.95   Adverse effect of unspecified primarily systemic and hematological agent

  X ● T45.96   Underdosing of unspecified primarily systemic and hematological agent

● T46   Poisoning by, adverse effect of and underdosing of agents primarily affecting the cardiovascular system

     Excludes1   poisoning by, adverse effect of and underdosing of metaraminol (T44.4)

     The appropriate 7th character is to be added to each code from category T46

     | | |
     A   initial encounter
     D   subsequent encounter
     S   sequela

● T46.0   Poisoning by, adverse effect of and underdosing of cardiac-stimulant glycosides and drugs of similar action

  ● T46.0X   Poisoning by, adverse effect of and underdosing of cardiac-stimulant glycosides and drugs of similar action

    ● T46.0X1   Poisoning by cardiac-stimulant glycosides and drugs of similar action, accidental (unintentional)
         Poisoning by cardiac-stimulant glycosides and drugs of similar action NOS

    ● T46.0X2   Poisoning by cardiac-stimulant glycosides and drugs of similar action, intentional self-harm

    ● T46.0X3   Poisoning by cardiac-stimulant glycosides and drugs of similar action, assault

    ● T46.0X4   Poisoning by cardiac-stimulant glycosides and drugs of similar action, undetermined

    ● T46.0X5   Adverse effect of cardiac-stimulant glycosides and drugs of similar action

    ● T46.0X6   Underdosing of cardiac-stimulant glycosides and drugs of similar action

● T46.1   Poisoning by, adverse effect of and underdosing of calcium-channel blockers

  ● T46.1X   Poisoning by, adverse effect of and underdosing of calcium-channel blockers

    ● T46.1X1   Poisoning by calcium-channel blockers, accidental (unintentional)
         Poisoning by calcium-channel blockers NOS

    ● T46.1X2   Poisoning by calcium-channel blockers, intentional self-harm

    ● T46.1X3   Poisoning by calcium-channel blockers, assault

● **T46.1X4**   **Poisoning by calcium-channel blockers, undetermined**

● **T46.1X5**   **Adverse effect of calcium-channel blockers**

● **T46.1X6**   **Underdosing of calcium-channel blockers**

● **T46.2**   **Poisoning by, adverse effect of and underdosing of other antidysrhythmic drugs, not elsewhere classified**

    Excludes1   poisoning by, adverse effect of and underdosing of beta-adrenoreceptor antagonists (T44.7-)

● **T46.2X**   **Poisoning by, adverse effect of and underdosing of other antidysrhythmic drugs**

● **T46.2X1**   **Poisoning by other antidysrhythmic drugs, accidental (unintentional)**
      Poisoning by other antidysrhythmic drugs NOS

● **T46.2X2**   **Poisoning by other antidysrhythmic drugs, intentional self-harm**

● **T46.2X3**   **Poisoning by other antidysrhythmic drugs, assault**

● **T46.2X4**   **Poisoning by other antidysrhythmic drugs, undetermined**

● **T46.2X5**   **Adverse effect of other antidysrhythmic drugs**

● **T46.2X6**   **Underdosing of other antidysrhythmic drugs**

● **T46.3**   **Poisoning by, adverse effect of and underdosing of coronary vasodilators**
      Poisoning by, adverse effect of and underdosing of dipyridamole

    Excludes1   poisoning by, adverse effect of and underdosing of calcium-channel blockers (T46.1)

● **T46.3X**   **Poisoning by, adverse effect of and underdosing of coronary vasodilators**

● **T46.3X1**   **Poisoning by coronary vasodilators, accidental (unintentional)**
      Poisoning by coronary vasodilators NOS

● **T46.3X2**   **Poisoning by coronary vasodilators, intentional self-harm**

● **T46.3X3**   **Poisoning by coronary vasodilators, assault**

● **T46.3X4**   **Poisoning by coronary vasodilators, undetermined**

● **T46.3X5**   **Adverse effect of coronary vasodilators**

● **T46.3X6**   **Underdosing of coronary vasodilators**

● **T46.4**   **Poisoning by, adverse effect of and underdosing of angiotensin-converting-enzyme inhibitors**

● **T46.4X**   **Poisoning by, adverse effect of and underdosing of angiotensin-converting-enzyme inhibitors**

● **T46.4X1**   **Poisoning by angiotensin-converting-enzyme inhibitors, accidental (unintentional)**
      Poisoning by angiotensin-converting-enzyme inhibitors NOS

● **T46.4X2**   **Poisoning by angiotensin-converting-enzyme inhibitors, intentional self-harm**

● **T46.4X3**   **Poisoning by angiotensin-converting-enzyme inhibitors, assault**

● **T46.4X4**   **Poisoning by angiotensin-converting-enzyme inhibitors, undetermined**

● **T46.4X5**   **Adverse effect of angiotensin-converting-enzyme inhibitors**

● **T46.4X6**   **Underdosing of angiotensin-converting-enzyme inhibitors**

● **T46.5**   **Poisoning by, adverse effect of and underdosing of other antihypertensive drugs**

    Excludes2   poisoning by, adverse effect of and underdosing of beta-adrenoreceptor antagonists (T44.7)
      poisoning by, adverse effect of and underdosing of calcium-channel blockers (T46.1)
      poisoning by, adverse effect of and underdosing of diuretics (T50.0-T50.2)

● **T46.5X**   **Poisoning by, adverse effect of and underdosing of other antihypertensive drugs**

● **T46.5X1**   **Poisoning by other antihypertensive drugs, accidental (unintentional)**
      Poisoning by other antihypertensive drugs NOS

● **T46.5X2**   **Poisoning by other antihypertensive drugs, intentional self-harm**

● **T46.5X3**   **Poisoning by other antihypertensive drugs, assault**

● **T46.5X4**   **Poisoning by other antihypertensive drugs, undetermined**

● **T46.5X5**   **Adverse effect of other antihypertensive drugs**

● **T46.5X6**   **Underdosing of other antihypertensive drugs**

● **T46.6**   **Poisoning by, adverse effect of and underdosing of antihyperlipidemic and antiarteriosclerotic drugs**

● **T46.6X**   **Poisoning by, adverse effect of and underdosing of antihyperlipidemic and antiarteriosclerotic drugs**

● **T46.6X1**   **Poisoning by antihyperlipidemic and antiarteriosclerotic drugs, accidental (unintentional)**
      Poisoning by antihyperlipidemic and antiarteriosclerotic drugs NOS

● **T46.6X2**   **Poisoning by antihyperlipidemic and antiarteriosclerotic drugs, intentional self-harm**

● **T46.6X3**   **Poisoning by antihyperlipidemic and antiarteriosclerotic drugs, assault**

● **T46.6X4**   **Poisoning by antihyperlipidemic and antiarteriosclerotic drugs, undetermined**

● **T46.6X5**   **Adverse effect of antihyperlipidemic and antiarteriosclerotic drugs**

● **T46.6X6**   **Underdosing of antihyperlipidemic and antiarteriosclerotic drugs**

● **T46.7**   **Poisoning by, adverse effect of and underdosing of peripheral vasodilators**
      Poisoning by, adverse effect of and underdosing of nicotinic acid (derivatives)

    Excludes1   poisoning by, adverse effect of and underdosing of papaverine (T44.3)

● **T46.7X**   **Poisoning by, adverse effect of and underdosing of peripheral vasodilators**

● **T46.7X1**   **Poisoning by peripheral vasodilators, accidental (unintentional)**
      Poisoning by peripheral vasodilators NOS

● **T46.7X2**   **Poisoning by peripheral vasodilators, intentional self-harm**

● **T46.7X3**   **Poisoning by peripheral vasodilators, assault**

● **T46.7X4**   **Poisoning by peripheral vasodilators, undetermined**

● **T46.7X5**   **Adverse effect of peripheral vasodilators**

● **T46.7X6**   **Underdosing of peripheral vasodilators**

◀ New   ⬅ Revised   ~~deleted~~ Deleted   Excludes 1   Excludes 2   Includes   Use additional   Code first   Code also   Unspecified

OGCR Official Guidelines   **X** Assign placeholder X   ● Use Additional Character(s)   ▶ Manifestation Code   **Coding Clinic**

● **T46.8**   Poisoning by, adverse effect of and underdosing of antivaricose drugs, including sclerosing agents

   ● **T46.8X**   Poisoning by, adverse effect of and underdosing of antivaricose drugs, including sclerosing agents

     ● **T46.8X1**   Poisoning by antivaricose drugs, including sclerosing agents, accidental (unintentional)

         Poisoning by antivaricose drugs, including sclerosing agents NOS

     ● **T46.8X2**   Poisoning by antivaricose drugs, including sclerosing agents, intentional self-harm

     ● **T46.8X3**   Poisoning by antivaricose drugs, including sclerosing agents, assault

     ● **T46.8X4**   Poisoning by antivaricose drugs, including sclerosing agents, undetermined

     ● **T46.8X5**   Adverse effect of antivaricose drugs, including sclerosing agents

     ● **T46.8X6**   Underdosing of antivaricose drugs, including sclerosing agents

● **T46.9**   Poisoning by, adverse effect of and underdosing of other and unspecified agents primarily affecting the cardiovascular system

   ● **T46.90**   Poisoning by, adverse effect of and underdosing of unspecified agents primarily affecting the cardiovascular system

     ● **T46.901**   Poisoning by unspecified agents primarily affecting the cardiovascular system, accidental (unintentional)

     ● **T46.902**   Poisoning by unspecified agents primarily affecting the cardiovascular system, intentional self-harm

     ● **T46.903**   Poisoning by unspecified agents primarily affecting the cardiovascular system, assault

     ● **T46.904**   Poisoning by unspecified agents primarily affecting the cardiovascular system, undetermined

     ● **T46.905**   Adverse effect of unspecified agents primarily affecting the cardiovascular system

     ● **T46.906**   Underdosing of unspecified agents primarily affecting the cardiovascular system

   ● **T46.99**   Poisoning by, adverse effect of and underdosing of other agents primarily affecting the cardiovascular system

     ● **T46.991**   Poisoning by other agents primarily affecting the cardiovascular system, accidental (unintentional)

     ● **T46.992**   Poisoning by other agents primarily affecting the cardiovascular system, intentional self-harm

     ● **T46.993**   Poisoning by other agents primarily affecting the cardiovascular system, assault

     ● **T46.994**   Poisoning by other agents primarily affecting the cardiovascular system, undetermined

     ● **T46.995**   Adverse effect of other agents primarily affecting the cardiovascular system

     ● **T46.996**   Underdosing of other agents primarily affecting the cardiovascular system

● **T47**   Poisoning by, adverse effect of and underdosing of agents primarily affecting the gastrointestinal system

   The appropriate 7th character is to be added to each code from category T47

A	initial encounter
D	subsequent encounter
S	sequela

● **T47.0**   Poisoning by, adverse effect of and underdosing of histamine H2-receptor blockers

   ● **T47.0X**   Poisoning by, adverse effect of and underdosing of histamine H2-receptor blockers

     ● **T47.0X1**   Poisoning by histamine H2-receptor blockers, accidental (unintentional)

         Poisoning by histamine H2-receptor blockers NOS

     ● **T47.0X2**   Poisoning by histamine H2-receptor blockers, intentional self-harm

     ● **T47.0X3**   Poisoning by histamine H2-receptor blockers, assault

     ● **T47.0X4**   Poisoning by histamine H2-receptor blockers, undetermined

     ● **T47.0X5**   Adverse effect of histamine H2-receptor blockers

     ● **T47.0X6**   Underdosing of histamine H2-receptor blockers

● **T47.1**   Poisoning by, adverse effect of and underdosing of other antacids and anti-gastric-secretion drugs

   ● **T47.1X**   Poisoning by, adverse effect of and underdosing of other antacids and anti-gastric-secretion drugs

     ● **T47.1X1**   Poisoning by other antacids and anti-gastric-secretion drugs, accidental (unintentional)

         Poisoning by other antacids and anti-gastric-secretion drugs NOS

     ● **T47.1X2**   Poisoning by other antacids and anti-gastric-secretion drugs, intentional self-harm

     ● **T47.1X3**   Poisoning by other antacids and anti-gastric-secretion drugs, assault

     ● **T47.1X4**   Poisoning by other antacids and anti-gastric-secretion drugs, undetermined

     ● **T47.1X5**   Adverse effect of other antacids and anti-gastric-secretion drugs

     ● **T47.1X6**   Underdosing of other antacids and anti-gastric-secretion drugs

● **T47.2**   Poisoning by, adverse effect of and underdosing of stimulant laxatives

   ● **T47.2X**   Poisoning by, adverse effect of and underdosing of stimulant laxatives

     ● **T47.2X1**   Poisoning by stimulant laxatives, accidental (unintentional)

         Poisoning by stimulant laxatives NOS

     ● **T47.2X2**   Poisoning by stimulant laxatives, intentional self-harm

     ● **T47.2X3**   Poisoning by stimulant laxatives, assault

     ● **T47.2X4**   Poisoning by stimulant laxatives, undetermined

     ● **T47.2X5**   Adverse effect of stimulant laxatives

     ● **T47.2X6**   Underdosing of stimulant laxatives

CHAPTER 19 (S00-T88)

● T47.3   **Poisoning by, adverse effect of and underdosing of saline and osmotic laxatives**
  ● T47.3X   **Poisoning by and adverse effect of saline and osmotic laxatives**
    ● T47.3X1   **Poisoning by saline and osmotic laxatives, accidental (unintentional)**
       Poisoning by saline and osmotic laxatives NOS
    ● T47.3X2   **Poisoning by saline and osmotic laxatives, intentional self-harm**
    ● T47.3X3   **Poisoning by saline and osmotic laxatives, assault**
    ● T47.3X4   **Poisoning by saline and osmotic laxatives, undetermined**
    ● T47.3X5   **Adverse effect of saline and osmotic laxatives**
    ● T47.3X6   **Underdosing of saline and osmotic laxatives**

● T47.4   **Poisoning by, adverse effect of and underdosing of other laxatives**
  ● T47.4X   **Poisoning by, adverse effect of and underdosing of other laxatives**
    ● T47.4X1   **Poisoning by other laxatives, accidental (unintentional)**
       Poisoning by other laxatives NOS
    ● T47.4X2   **Poisoning by other laxatives, intentional self-harm**
    ● T47.4X3   **Poisoning by other laxatives, assault**
    ● T47.4X4   **Poisoning by other laxatives, undetermined**
    ● T47.4X5   **Adverse effect of other laxatives**
    ● T47.4X6   **Underdosing of other laxatives**

● T47.5   **Poisoning by, adverse effect of and underdosing of digestants**
  ● T47.5X   **Poisoning by, adverse effect of and underdosing of digestants**
    ● T47.5X1   **Poisoning by digestants, accidental (unintentional)**
       Poisoning by digestants NOS
    ● T47.5X2   **Poisoning by digestants, intentional self-harm**
    ● T47.5X3   **Poisoning by digestants, assault**
    ● T47.5X4   **Poisoning by digestants, undetermined**
    ● T47.5X5   **Adverse effect of digestants**
    ● T47.5X6   **Underdosing of digestants**

● T47.6   **Poisoning by, adverse effect of and underdosing of antidiarrheal drugs**
   Excludes2   poisoning by, adverse effect of and underdosing of systemic antibiotics and other anti-infectives (T36-T37)
  ● T47.6X   **Poisoning by, adverse effect of and underdosing of antidiarrheal drugs**
    ● T47.6X1   **Poisoning by antidiarrheal drugs, accidental (unintentional)**
       Poisoning by antidiarrheal drugs NOS
    ● T47.6X2   **Poisoning by antidiarrheal drugs, intentional self-harm**
    ● T47.6X3   **Poisoning by antidiarrheal drugs, assault**
    ● T47.6X4   **Poisoning by antidiarrheal drugs, undetermined**
    ● T47.6X5   **Adverse effect of antidiarrheal drugs**
    ● T47.6X6   **Underdosing of antidiarrheal drugs**

● T47.7   **Poisoning by, adverse effect of and underdosing of emetics**
  ● T47.7X   **Poisoning by, adverse effect of and underdosing of emetics**
    ● T47.7X1   **Poisoning by emetics, accidental (unintentional)**
       Poisoning by emetics NOS
    ● T47.7X2   **Poisoning by emetics, intentional self-harm**
    ● T47.7X3   **Poisoning by emetics, assault**
    ● T47.7X4   **Poisoning by emetics, undetermined**
    ● T47.7X5   **Adverse effect of emetics**
    ● T47.7X6   **Underdosing of emetics**

● T47.8   **Poisoning by, adverse effect of and underdosing of other agents primarily affecting gastrointestinal system**
  ● T47.8X   **Poisoning by, adverse effect of and underdosing of other agents primarily affecting gastrointestinal system**
    ● T47.8X1   **Poisoning by other agents primarily affecting gastrointestinal system, accidental (unintentional)**
       Poisoning by other agents primarily affecting gastrointestinal system NOS
    ● T47.8X2   **Poisoning by other agents primarily affecting gastrointestinal system, intentional self-harm**
    ● T47.8X3   **Poisoning by other agents primarily affecting gastrointestinal system, assault**
    ● T47.8X4   **Poisoning by other agents primarily affecting gastrointestinal system, undetermined**
    ● T47.8X5   **Adverse effect of other agents primarily affecting gastrointestinal system**
    ● T47.8X6   **Underdosing of other agents primarily affecting gastrointestinal system**

● T47.9   **Poisoning by, adverse effect of and underdosing of unspecified agents primarily affecting the gastrointestinal system**
  X ● T47.91   **Poisoning by unspecified agents primarily affecting the gastrointestinal system, accidental (unintentional)**
       Poisoning by agents primarily affecting the gastrointestinal system NOS
  X ● T47.92   **Poisoning by unspecified agents primarily affecting the gastrointestinal system, intentional self-harm**
  X ● T47.93   **Poisoning by unspecified agents primarily affecting the gastrointestinal system, assault**
  X ● T47.94   **Poisoning by unspecified agents primarily affecting the gastrointestinal system, undetermined**
  X ● T47.95   **Adverse effect of unspecified agents primarily affecting the gastrointestinal system**
  X ● T47.96   **Underdosing of unspecified agents primarily affecting the gastrointestinal system**

◄ New   ◄ Revised   ~~deleted~~ Deleted   Excludes 1   Excludes 2   Includes   Use additional   Code first   Code also   Unspecified
OGCR Official Guidelines   X Assign placeholder X   ● Use Additional Character(s)   ▷ Manifestation Code   **Coding Clinic**

● T48 **Poisoning by, adverse effect of and underdosing of agents primarily acting on smooth and skeletal muscles and the respiratory system**

The appropriate 7th character is to be added to each code from category T48

A	initial encounter
D	subsequent encounter
S	sequela

● T48.0 **Poisoning by, adverse effect of and underdosing of oxytocic drugs**

Excludes1   poisoning by, adverse effect of and underdosing of estrogens, progestogens and antagonists (T38.4-T38.6)

● T48.0X **Poisoning by, adverse effect of and underdosing of oxytocic drugs**

● T48.0X1 **Poisoning by oxytocic drugs, accidental (unintentional)**
Poisoning by oxytocic drugs NOS

● T48.0X2 **Poisoning by oxytocic drugs, intentional self-harm**

● T48.0X3 **Poisoning by oxytocic drugs, assault**

● T48.0X4 **Poisoning by oxytocic drugs, undetermined**

● T48.0X5 **Adverse effect of oxytocic drugs**

● T48.0X6 **Underdosing of oxytocic drugs**

● T48.1 **Poisoning by, adverse effect of and underdosing of skeletal muscle relaxants [neuromuscular blocking agents]**

● T48.1X **Poisoning by, adverse effect of and underdosing of skeletal muscle relaxants [neuromuscular blocking agents]**

● T48.1X1 **Poisoning by skeletal muscle relaxants [neuromuscular blocking agents], accidental (unintentional)**
Poisoning by skeletal muscle relaxants [neuromuscular blocking agents] NOS

● T48.1X2 **Poisoning by skeletal muscle relaxants [neuromuscular blocking agents], intentional self-harm**

● T48.1X3 **Poisoning by skeletal muscle relaxants [neuromuscular blocking agents], assault**

● T48.1X4 **Poisoning by skeletal muscle relaxants [neuromuscular blocking agents], undetermined**

● T48.1X5 **Adverse effect of skeletal muscle relaxants [neuromuscular blocking agents]**

● T48.1X6 **Underdosing of skeletal muscle relaxants [neuromuscular blocking agents]**

● T48.2 **Poisoning by, adverse effect of and underdosing of other and unspecified drugs acting on muscles**

● T48.20 **Poisoning by, adverse effect of and underdosing of unspecified drugs acting on muscles**

● T48.201 **Poisoning by unspecified drugs acting on muscles, accidental (unintentional)**
Poisoning by unspecified drugs acting on muscles NOS

● T48.202 **Poisoning by unspecified drugs acting on muscles, intentional self-harm**

● T48.203 **Poisoning by unspecified drugs acting on muscles, assault**

● T48.204 **Poisoning by unspecified drugs acting on muscles, undetermined**

● T48.205 **Adverse effect of unspecified drugs acting on muscles**

● T48.206 **Underdosing of unspecified drugs acting on muscles**

● T48.29 **Poisoning by, adverse effect of and underdosing of other drugs acting on muscles**

● T48.291 **Poisoning by other drugs acting on muscles, accidental (unintentional)**
Poisoning by other drugs acting on muscles NOS

● T48.292 **Poisoning by other drugs acting on muscles, intentional self-harm**

● T48.293 **Poisoning by other drugs acting on muscles, assault**

● T48.294 **Poisoning by other drugs acting on muscles, undetermined**

● T48.295 **Adverse effect of other drugs acting on muscles**

● T48.296 **Underdosing of other drugs acting on muscles**

● T48.3 **Poisoning by, adverse effect of and underdosing of antitussives**

● T48.3X **Poisoning by, adverse effect of and underdosing of antitussives**

● T48.3X1 **Poisoning by antitussives, accidental (unintentional)**
Poisoning by antitussives NOS

● T48.3X2 **Poisoning by antitussives, intentional self-harm**

● T48.3X3 **Poisoning by antitussives, assault**

● T48.3X4 **Poisoning by antitussives, undetermined**

● T48.3X5 **Adverse effect of antitussives**

● T48.3X6 **Underdosing of antitussives**

● T48.4 **Poisoning by, adverse effect of and underdosing of expectorants**

● T48.4X **Poisoning by, adverse effect of and underdosing of expectorants**

● T48.4X1 **Poisoning by expectorants, accidental (unintentional)**
Poisoning by expectorants NOS

● T48.4X2 **Poisoning by expectorants, intentional self-harm**

● T48.4X3 **Poisoning by expectorants, assault**

● T48.4X4 **Poisoning by expectorants, undetermined**

● T48.4X5 **Adverse effect of expectorants**

● T48.4X6 **Underdosing of expectorants**

● T48.5 **Poisoning by, adverse effect of and underdosing of other anti-common-cold drugs**
Poisoning by, adverse effect of and underdosing of decongestants

Excludes2   poisoning by, adverse effect of and underdosing of antipyretics, NEC (T39.9-)
poisoning by, adverse effect of and underdosing of non-steroidal antiinflammatory drugs (T39.3-)
poisoning by, adverse effect of and underdosing of salicylates (T39.0-)

● T48.5X **Poisoning by, adverse effect of and underdosing of other anti-common-cold drugs**

● T48.5X1 **Poisoning by other anti-common-cold drugs, accidental (unintentional)**
Poisoning by other anti-common-cold drugs NOS

● T48.5X2 **Poisoning by other anti-common-cold drugs, intentional self-harm**

● T48.5X3 **Poisoning by other anti-common-cold drugs, assault**

● T48.5X4 **Poisoning by other anti-common-cold drugs, undetermined**

● T48.5X5 **Adverse effect of other anti-common-cold drugs**

● T48.5X6 **Underdosing of other anti-common-cold drugs**

● **T48.6   Poisoning by, adverse effect of and underdosing of antiasthmatics, not elsewhere classified**
Poisoning by, adverse effect of and underdosing of beta-adrenoreceptor agonists used in asthma therapy

<u>Excludes1</u>   poisoning by, adverse effect of and underdosing of beta-adrenoreceptor agonists not used in asthma therapy (T44.5)
poisoning by, adverse effect of and underdosing of anterior pituitary [adenohypophyseal] hormones (T38.8)

● **T48.6X   Poisoning by, adverse effect of and underdosing of antiasthmatics**

   ● **T48.6X1   Poisoning by antiasthmatics, accidental (unintentional)**
      Poisoning by antiasthmatics NOS

   ● **T48.6X2   Poisoning by antiasthmatics, intentional self-harm**

   ● **T48.6X3   Poisoning by antiasthmatics, assault**

   ● **T48.6X4   Poisoning by antiasthmatics, undetermined**

   ● **T48.6X5   Adverse effect of antiasthmatics**

   ● **T48.6X6   Underdosing of antiasthmatics**

● **T48.9   Poisoning by, adverse effect of and underdosing of other and unspecified agents primarily acting on the respiratory system**

  ● **T48.90   Poisoning by, adverse effect of and underdosing of unspecified agents primarily acting on the respiratory system**

   ● **T48.901   Poisoning by unspecified agents primarily acting on the respiratory system, accidental (unintentional)**

   ● **T48.902   Poisoning by unspecified agents primarily acting on the respiratory system, intentional self-harm**

   ● **T48.903   Poisoning by unspecified agents primarily acting on the respiratory system, assault**

   ● **T48.904   Poisoning by unspecified agents primarily acting on the respiratory system, undetermined**

   ● **T48.905   Adverse effect of unspecified agents primarily acting on the respiratory system**

   ● **T48.906   Underdosing of unspecified agents primarily acting on the respiratory system**

  ● **T48.99   Poisoning by, adverse effect of and underdosing of other agents primarily acting on the respiratory system**

   ● **T48.991   Poisoning by other agents primarily acting on the respiratory system, accidental (unintentional)**

   ● **T48.992   Poisoning by other agents primarily acting on the respiratory system, intentional self-harm**

   ● **T48.993   Poisoning by other agents primarily acting on the respiratory system, assault**

   ● **T48.994   Poisoning by other agents primarily acting on the respiratory system, undetermined**

   ● **T48.995   Adverse effect of other agents primarily acting on the respiratory system**

   ● **T48.996   Underdosing of other agents primarily acting on the respiratory system**

● **T49   Poisoning by, adverse effect of and underdosing of topical agents primarily affecting skin and mucous membrane and by ophthalmological, otorhinorlaryngological and dental drugs**

<u>Includes</u>   poisoning by, adverse effect of and underdosing of glucocorticoids, topically used

The appropriate 7th character is to be added to each code from category T49

A	initial encounter
D	subsequent encounter
S	sequela

● **T49.0   Poisoning by, adverse effect of and underdosing of local antifungal, anti-infective and anti-inflammatory drugs**

  ● **T49.0X   Poisoning by, adverse effect of and underdosing of local antifungal, anti-infective and anti-inflammatory drugs**

   ● **T49.0X1   Poisoning by local antifungal, anti-infective and anti-inflammatory drugs, accidental (unintentional)**
      Poisoning by local antifungal, anti-infective and anti-inflammatory drugs NOS

   ● **T49.0X2   Poisoning by local antifungal, anti-infective and anti-inflammatory drugs, intentional self-harm**

   ● **T49.0X3   Poisoning by local antifungal, anti-infective and anti-inflammatory drugs, assault**

   ● **T49.0X4   Poisoning by local antifungal, anti-infective and anti-inflammatory drugs, undetermined**

   ● **T49.0X5   Adverse effect of local antifungal, anti-infective and anti-inflammatory drugs**

   ● **T49.0X6   Underdosing of local antifungal, anti-infective and anti-inflammatory drugs**

● **T49.1   Poisoning by, adverse effect of and underdosing of antipruritics**

  ● **T49.1X   Poisoning by, adverse effect of and underdosing of antipruritics**

   ● **T49.1X1   Poisoning by antipruritics, accidental (unintentional)**
      Poisoning by antipruritics NOS

   ● **T49.1X2   Poisoning by antipruritics, intentional self-harm**

   ● **T49.1X3   Poisoning by antipruritics, assault**

   ● **T49.1X4   Poisoning by antipruritics, undetermined**

   ● **T49.1X5   Adverse effect of antipruritics**

   ● **T49.1X6   Underdosing of antipruritics**

● **T49.2   Poisoning by, adverse effect of and underdosing of local astringents and local detergents**

  ● **T49.2X   Poisoning by, adverse effect of and underdosing of local astringents and local detergents**

   ● **T49.2X1   Poisoning by local astringents and local detergents, accidental (unintentional)**
      Poisoning by local astringents and local detergents NOS

   ● **T49.2X2   Poisoning by local astringents and local detergents, intentional self-harm**

   ● **T49.2X3   Poisoning by local astringents and local detergents, assault**

   ● **T49.2X4   Poisoning by local astringents and local detergents, undetermined**

   ● **T49.2X5   Adverse effect of local astringents and local detergents**

   ● **T49.2X6   Underdosing of local astringents and local detergents**

◀ New   ◀▬ Revised   ~~deleted~~ Deleted   Excludes 1   Excludes 2   Includes   Use additional   Code first   Code also   Unspecified
OGCR Official Guidelines   X Assign placeholder X   ● Use Additional Character(s)   ▶ Manifestation Code   **Coding Clinic**

● T49.3   Poisoning by, adverse effect of and underdosing of emollients, demulcents and protectants
   ● T49.3X   Poisoning by, adverse effect of and underdosing of emollients, demulcents and protectants
     ● T49.3X1   Poisoning by emollients, demulcents and protectants, accidental (unintentional)
       Poisoning by emollients, demulcents and protectants NOS
     ● T49.3X2   Poisoning by emollients, demulcents and protectants, intentional self-harm
     ● T49.3X3   Poisoning by emollients, demulcents and protectants, assault
     ● T49.3X4   Poisoning by emollients, demulcents and protectants, undetermined
     ● T49.3X5   Adverse effect of emollients, demulcents and protectants
     ● T49.3X6   Underdosing of emollients, demulcents and protectants

● T49.4   Poisoning by, adverse effect of and underdosing of keratolytics, keratoplastics, and other hair treatment drugs and preparations
   ● T49.4X   Poisoning by, adverse effect of and underdosing of keratolytics, keratoplastics, and other hair treatment drugs and preparations
     ● T49.4X1   Poisoning by keratolytics, keratoplastics, and other hair treatment drugs and preparations, accidental (unintentional)
       Poisoning by keratolytics, keratoplastics, and other hair treatment drugs and preparations NOS
     ● T49.4X2   Poisoning by keratolytics, keratoplastics, and other hair treatment drugs and preparations, intentional self-harm
     ● T49.4X3   Poisoning by keratolytics, keratoplastics, and other hair treatment drugs and preparations, assault
     ● T49.4X4   Poisoning by keratolytics, keratoplastics, and other hair treatment drugs and preparations, undetermined
     ● T49.4X5   Adverse effect of keratolytics, keratoplastics, and other hair treatment drugs and preparations
     ● T49.4X6   Underdosing of keratolytics, keratoplastics, and other hair treatment drugs and preparations

● T49.5   Poisoning by, adverse effect of and underdosing of ophthalmological drugs and preparations
   ● T49.5X   Poisoning by, adverse effect of and underdosing of ophthalmological drugs and preparations
     ● T49.5X1   Poisoning by ophthalmological drugs and preparations, accidental (unintentional)
       Poisoning by ophthalmological drugs and preparations NOS
     ● T49.5X2   Poisoning by ophthalmological drugs and preparations, intentional self-harm
     ● T49.5X3   Poisoning by ophthalmological drugs and preparations, assault
     ● T49.5X4   Poisoning by ophthalmological drugs and preparations, undetermined
     ● T49.5X5   Adverse effect of ophthalmological drugs and preparations
     ● T49.5X6   Underdosing of ophthalmological drugs and preparations

● T49.6   Poisoning by, adverse effect of and underdosing of otorhinolaryngological drugs and preparations
   ● T49.6X   Poisoning by, adverse effect of and underdosing of otorhinolaryngological drugs and preparations
     ● T49.6X1   Poisoning by otorhinolaryngological drugs and preparations, accidental (unintentional)
       Poisoning by otorhinolaryngological drugs and preparations NOS
     ● T49.6X2   Poisoning by otorhinolaryngological drugs and preparations, intentional self-harm
     ● T49.6X3   Poisoning by otorhinolaryngological drugs and preparations, assault
     ● T49.6X4   Poisoning by otorhinolaryngological drugs and preparations, undetermined
     ● T49.6X5   Adverse effect of otorhinolaryngological drugs and preparations
     ● T49.6X6   Underdosing of otorhinolaryngological drugs and preparations

● T49.7   Poisoning by, adverse effect of and underdosing of dental drugs, topically applied
   ● T49.7X   Poisoning by, adverse effect of and underdosing of dental drugs, topically applied
     ● T49.7X1   Poisoning by dental drugs, topically applied, accidental (unintentional)
       Poisoning by dental drugs, topically applied NOS
     ● T49.7X2   Poisoning by dental drugs, topically applied, intentional self-harm
     ● T49.7X3   Poisoning by dental drugs, topically applied, assault
     ● T49.7X4   Poisoning by dental drugs, topically applied, undetermined
     ● T49.7X5   Adverse effect of dental drugs, topically applied
     ● T49.7X6   Underdosing of dental drugs, topically applied

● T49.8   Poisoning by, adverse effect of and underdosing of other topical agents
     Poisoning by, adverse effect of and underdosing of spermicides
   ● T49.8X   Poisoning by, adverse effect of and underdosing of other topical agents
     ● T49.8X1   Poisoning by other topical agents, accidental (unintentional)
       Poisoning by other topical agents NOS
     ● T49.8X2   Poisoning by other topical agents, intentional self-harm
     ● T49.8X3   Poisoning by other topical agents, assault
     ● T49.8X4   Poisoning by other topical agents, undetermined
     ● T49.8X5   Adverse effect of other topical agents
     ● T49.8X6   Underdosing of other topical agents

● T49.9   Poisoning by, adverse effect of and underdosing of unspecified topical agent
   X ● T49.91   Poisoning by unspecified topical agent, accidental (unintentional)
   X ● T49.92   Poisoning by unspecified topical agent, intentional self-harm
   X ● T49.93   Poisoning by unspecified topical agent, assault
   X ● T49.94   Poisoning by unspecified topical agent, undetermined
   X ● T49.95   Adverse effect of unspecified topical agent
   X ● T49.96   Underdosing of unspecified topical agent

● T50   Poisoning by, adverse effect of and underdosing of diuretics and other and unspecified drugs, medicaments and biological substances

> The appropriate 7th character is to be added to each code from category T50

A	initial encounter
D	subsequent encounter
S	sequela

● T50.0   Poisoning by, adverse effect of and underdosing of mineralocorticoids and their antagonists

    ● T50.0X   Poisoning by, adverse effect of and underdosing of mineralocorticoids and their antagonists

       ● T50.0X1   Poisoning by mineralocorticoids and their antagonists, accidental (unintentional)
> Poisoning by mineralocorticoids and their antagonists NOS

       ● T50.0X2   Poisoning by mineralocorticoids and their antagonists, intentional self-harm

       ● T50.0X3   Poisoning by mineralocorticoids and their antagonists, assault

       ● T50.0X4   Poisoning by mineralocorticoids and their antagonists, undetermined

       ● T50.0X5   Adverse effect of mineralocorticoids and their antagonists

       ● T50.0X6   Underdosing of mineralocorticoids and their antagonists

● T50.1   Poisoning by, adverse effect of and underdosing of loop [high-ceiling] diuretics

    ● T50.1X   Poisoning by, adverse effect of and underdosing of loop [high-ceiling] diuretics

       ● T50.1X1   Poisoning by loop [high-ceiling] diuretics, accidental (unintentional)
> Poisoning by loop [high-ceiling] diuretics NOS

       ● T50.1X2   Poisoning by loop [high-ceiling] diuretics, intentional self-harm

       ● T50.1X3   Poisoning by loop [high-ceiling] diuretics, assault

       ● T50.1X4   Poisoning by loop [high-ceiling] diuretics, undetermined

       ● T50.1X5   Adverse effect of loop [high-ceiling] diuretics

       ● T50.1X6   Underdosing of loop [high-ceiling] diuretics

● T50.2   Poisoning by, adverse effect of and underdosing of carbonic-anhydrase inhibitors, benzothiadiazides and other diuretics
> Poisoning by, adverse effect of and underdosing of acetazolamide

    ● T50.2X   Poisoning by, adverse effect of and underdosing of carbonic-anhydrase inhibitors, benzothiadiazides and other diuretics

       ● T50.2X1   Poisoning by carbonic-anhydrase inhibitors, benzothiadiazides and other diuretics, accidental (unintentional)
> Poisoning by carbonic-anhydrase inhibitors, benzothiadiazides and other diuretics NOS

       ● T50.2X2   Poisoning by carbonic-anhydrase inhibitors, benzothiadiazides and other diuretics, intentional self-harm

       ● T50.2X3   Poisoning by carbonic-anhydrase inhibitors, benzothiadiazides and other diuretics, assault

       ● T50.2X4   Poisoning by carbonic-anhydrase inhibitors, benzothiadiazides and other diuretics, undetermined

       ● T50.2X5   Adverse effect of carbonic-anhydrase inhibitors, benzothiadiazides and other diuretics

       ● T50.2X6   Underdosing of carbonic-anhydrase inhibitors, benzothiadiazides and other diuretics

● T50.3   Poisoning by, adverse effect of and underdosing of electrolytic, caloric and water-balance agents
> Poisoning by, adverse effect of and underdosing of oral rehydration salts

    ● T50.3X   Poisoning by, adverse effect of and underdosing of electrolytic, caloric and water-balance agents

       ● T50.3X1   Poisoning by electrolytic, caloric and water-balance agents, accidental (unintentional)
> Poisoning by electrolytic, caloric and water-balance agents NOS

       ● T50.3X2   Poisoning by electrolytic, caloric and water-balance agents, intentional self-harm

       ● T50.3X3   Poisoning by electrolytic, caloric and water-balance agents, assault

       ● T50.3X4   Poisoning by electrolytic, caloric and water-balance agents, undetermined

       ● T50.3X5   Adverse effect of electrolytic, caloric and water-balance agents

       ● T50.3X6   Underdosing of electrolytic, caloric and water-balance agents

● T50.4   Poisoning by, adverse effect of and underdosing of drugs affecting uric acid metabolism

    ● T50.4X   Poisoning by, adverse effect of and underdosing of drugs affecting uric acid metabolism

       ● T50.4X1   Poisoning by drugs affecting uric acid metabolism, accidental (unintentional)
> Poisoning by drugs affecting uric acid metabolism NOS

       ● T50.4X2   Poisoning by drugs affecting uric acid metabolism, intentional self-harm

       ● T50.4X3   Poisoning by drugs affecting uric acid metabolism, assault

       ● T50.4X4   Poisoning by drugs affecting uric acid metabolism, undetermined

       ● T50.4X5   Adverse effect of drugs affecting uric acid metabolism

       ● T50.4X6   Underdosing of drugs affecting uric acid metabolism

● T50.5   Poisoning by, adverse effect of and underdosing of appetite depressants

    ● T50.5X   Poisoning by, adverse effect of and underdosing of appetite depressants

       ● T50.5X1   Poisoning by appetite depressants, accidental (unintentional)
> Poisoning by appetite depressants NOS

       ● T50.5X2   Poisoning by appetite depressants, intentional self-harm

       ● T50.5X3   Poisoning by appetite depressants, assault

       ● T50.5X4   Poisoning by appetite depressants, undetermined

       ● T50.5X5   Adverse effect of appetite depressants

       ● T50.5X6   Underdosing of appetite depressants

◀ New   ◀◀ Revised   ~~deleted~~ Deleted   Excludes 1   Excludes 2   Includes   Use additional   Code first   Code also   Unspecified

OGCR Official Guidelines   X Assign placeholder X   ● Use Additional Character(s)   ▌ Manifestation Code   **Coding Clinic**

● T50.6 Poisoning by, adverse effect of and underdosing of antidotes and chelating agents
   Poisoning by, adverse effect of and underdosing of alcohol deterrents
   ● T50.6X Poisoning by, adverse effect of and underdosing of antidotes and chelating agents
      ● T50.6X1 Poisoning by antidotes and chelating agents, accidental (unintentional)
         Poisoning by antidotes and chelating agents NOS
      ● T50.6X2 Poisoning by antidotes and chelating agents, intentional self-harm
      ● T50.6X3 Poisoning by antidotes and chelating agents, assault
      ● T50.6X4 Poisoning by antidotes and chelating agents, undetermined
      ● T50.6X5 Adverse effect of antidotes and chelating agents
      ● T50.6X6 Underdosing of antidotes and chelating agents

● T50.7 Poisoning by, adverse effect of and underdosing of analeptics and opioid receptor antagonists
   ● T50.7X Poisoning by, adverse effect of and underdosing of analeptics and opioid receptor antagonists
      ● T50.7X1 Poisoning by analeptics and opioid receptor antagonists, accidental (unintentional)
         Poisoning by analeptics and opioid receptor antagonists NOS
      ● T50.7X2 Poisoning by analeptics and opioid receptor antagonists, intentional self-harm
      ● T50.7X3 Poisoning by analeptics and opioid receptor antagonists, assault
      ● T50.7X4 Poisoning by analeptics and opioid receptor antagonists, undetermined
      ● T50.7X5 Adverse effect of analeptics and opioid receptor antagonists
      ● T50.7X6 Underdosing of analeptics and opioid receptor antagonists

● T50.8 Poisoning by, adverse effect of and underdosing of diagnostic agents
   ● T50.8X Poisoning by, adverse effect of and underdosing of diagnostic agents
      ● T50.8X1 Poisoning by diagnostic agents, accidental (unintentional)
         Poisoning by diagnostic agents NOS
      ● T50.8X2 Poisoning by diagnostic agents, intentional self-harm
      ● T50.8X3 Poisoning by diagnostic agents, assault
      ● T50.8X4 Poisoning by diagnostic agents, undetermined
      ● T50.8X5 Adverse effect of diagnostic agents
      ● T50.8X6 Underdosing of diagnostic agents

● T50.A Poisoning by, adverse effect of and underdosing of bacterial vaccines
   ● T50.A1 Poisoning by, adverse effect of and underdosing of pertussis vaccine, including combinations with a pertussis component
      ● T50.A11 Poisoning by pertussis vaccine, including combinations with a pertussis component, accidental (unintentional)
      ● T50.A12 Poisoning by pertussis vaccine, including combinations with a pertussis component, intentional self-harm

● T50.A13 Poisoning by pertussis vaccine, including combinations with a pertussis component, assault
● T50.A14 Poisoning by pertussis vaccine, including combinations with a pertussis component, undetermined
● T50.A15 Adverse effect of pertussis vaccine, including combinations with a pertussis component
● T50.A16 Underdosing of pertussis vaccine, including combinations with a pertussis component

● T50.A2 Poisoning by, adverse effect of and underdosing of mixed bacterial vaccines without a pertussis component
   ● T50.A21 Poisoning by mixed bacterial vaccines without a pertussis component, accidental (unintentional)
   ● T50.A22 Poisoning by mixed bacterial vaccines without a pertussis component, intentional self-harm
   ● T50.A23 Poisoning by mixed bacterial vaccines without a pertussis component, assault
   ● T50.A24 Poisoning by mixed bacterial vaccines without a pertussis component, undetermined
   ● T50.A25 Adverse effect of mixed bacterial vaccines without a pertussis component
   ● T50.A26 Underdosing of mixed bacterial vaccines without a pertussis component

● T50.A9 Poisoning by, adverse effect of and underdosing of other bacterial vaccines
   ● T50.A91 Poisoning by other bacterial vaccines, accidental (unintentional)
   ● T50.A92 Poisoning by other bacterial vaccines, intentional self-harm
   ● T50.A93 Poisoning by other bacterial vaccines, assault
   ● T50.A94 Poisoning by other bacterial vaccines, undetermined
   ● T50.A95 Adverse effect of other bacterial vaccines
   ● T50.A96 Underdosing of other bacterial vaccines

● T50.B Poisoning by, adverse effect of and underdosing of viral vaccines
   ● T50.B1 Poisoning by, adverse effect of and underdosing of smallpox vaccines
      ● T50.B11 Poisoning by smallpox vaccines, accidental (unintentional)
      ● T50.B12 Poisoning by smallpox vaccines, intentional self-harm
      ● T50.B13 Poisoning by smallpox vaccines, assault
      ● T50.B14 Poisoning by smallpox vaccines, undetermined
      ● T50.B15 Adverse effect of smallpox vaccines
      ● T50.B16 Underdosing of smallpox vaccines

   ● T50.B9 Poisoning by, adverse effect of and underdosing of other viral vaccines
      ● T50.B91 Poisoning by other viral vaccines, accidental (unintentional)
      ● T50.B92 Poisoning by other viral vaccines, intentional self-harm
      ● T50.B93 Poisoning by other viral vaccines, assault

CHAPTER 19 (S00–T88)

● T50.B94   Poisoning by other viral vaccines, undetermined
● T50.B95   Adverse effect of other viral vaccines
● T50.B96   Underdosing of other viral vaccines
● T50.Z   Poisoning by, adverse effect of and underdosing of other vaccines and biological substances
  ● T50.Z1   Poisoning by, adverse effect of and underdosing of immunoglobulin
    ● T50.Z11   Poisoning by immunoglobulin, accidental (unintentional)
    ● T50.Z12   Poisoning by immunoglobulin, intentional self-harm
    ● T50.Z13   Poisoning by immunoglobulin, assault
    ● T50.Z14   Poisoning by immunoglobulin, undetermined
    ● T50.Z15   Adverse effect of immunoglobulin
    ● T50.Z16   Underdosing of immunoglobulin
  ● T50.Z9   Poisoning by, adverse effect of and underdosing of other vaccines and biological substances
    ● T50.Z91   Poisoning by other vaccines and biological substances, accidental (unintentional)
    ● T50.Z92   Poisoning by other vaccines and biological substances, intentional self-harm
    ● T50.Z93   Poisoning by other vaccines and biological substances, assault
    ● T50.Z94   Poisoning by other vaccines and biological substances, undetermined
    ● T50.Z95   Adverse effect of other vaccines and biological substances
    ● T50.Z96   Underdosing of other vaccines and biological substances
● T50.9   Poisoning by, adverse effect of and underdosing of other and unspecified drugs, medicaments and biological substances
  ● T50.90   Poisoning by, adverse effect of and underdosing of unspecified drugs, medicaments and biological substances
    ● T50.901   Poisoning by unspecified drugs, medicaments and biological substances, accidental (unintentional)
      Coding Clinic: 2015, Q1, P21
    ● T50.902   Poisoning by unspecified drugs, medicaments and biological substances, intentional self-harm
    ● T50.903   Poisoning by unspecified drugs, medicaments and biological substances, assault
    ● T50.904   Poisoning by unspecified drugs, medicaments and biological substances, undetermined
    ● T50.905   Adverse effect of unspecified drugs, medicaments and biological substances
    ● T50.906   Underdosing of unspecified drugs, medicaments and biological substances
  ● T50.99   Poisoning by, adverse effect of and underdosing of other drugs, medicaments and biological substances
    ● T50.991   Poisoning by other drugs, medicaments and biological substances, accidental (unintentional)
    ● T50.992   Poisoning by other drugs, medicaments and biological substances, intentional self-harm

● T50.993   Poisoning by other drugs, medicaments and biological substances, assault
● T50.994   Poisoning by other drugs, medicaments and biological substances, undetermined
● T50.995   Adverse effect of other drugs, medicaments and biological substances
● T50.996   Underdosing of other drugs, medicaments and biological substances

---

TOXIC EFFECTS OF SUBSTANCES CHIEFLY NONMEDICINAL AS TO SOURCE (T51-T65)

Note: When no intent is indicated code to accidental. Undetermined intent is only for use when there is specific documentation in the record that the intent of the toxic effect cannot be determined.

Use additional code(s): for all associated manifestations of toxic effect, such as:
respiratory conditions due to external agents (J60-J70)
personal history of foreign body fully removed (Z87.821)
to identify any retained foreign body, if applicable (Z18.-)

Excludes1   contact with and (suspected) exposure to toxic substances (Z77.-)

● **T51   Toxic effect of alcohol**

The appropriate 7th character is to be added to each code from category T51

A	initial encounter
D	subsequent encounter
S	sequela

● T51.0   Toxic effect of ethanol
  Toxic effect of ethyl alcohol
  Excludes2   acute alcohol intoxication or 'hangover' effects (F10.129, F10.229, F10.929)
    drunkenness (F10.129, F10.229, F10.929)
    pathological alcohol intoxication (F10.129, F10.229, F10.929)
  ● T51.0X   Toxic effect of ethanol
    ● T51.0X1   Toxic effect of ethanol, accidental (unintentional)
      Toxic effect of ethanol NOS
    ● T51.0X2   Toxic effect of ethanol, intentional self-harm
    ● T51.0X3   Toxic effect of ethanol, assault
    ● T51.0X4   Toxic effect of ethanol, undetermined
● T51.1   Toxic effect of methanol
  Toxic effect of methyl alcohol
  ● T51.1X   Toxic effect of methanol
    ● T51.1X1   Toxic effect of methanol, accidental (unintentional)
      Toxic effect of methanol NOS
    ● T51.1X2   Toxic effect of methanol, intentional self-harm
    ● T51.1X3   Toxic effect of methanol, assault
    ● T51.1X4   Toxic effect of methanol, undetermined
● T51.2   Toxic effect of 2-Propanol
  Toxic effect of isopropyl alcohol
  ● T51.2X   Toxic effect of 2-Propanol
    ● T51.2X1   Toxic effect of 2-Propanol, accidental (unintentional)
      Toxic effect of 2-Propanol NOS
    ● T51.2X2   Toxic effect of 2-Propanol, intentional self-harm
    ● T51.2X3   Toxic effect of 2-Propanol, assault
    ● T51.2X4   Toxic effect of 2-Propanol, undetermined

◀ New   ⬅ Revised   ~~deleted~~ Deleted   Excludes 1   Excludes 2   Includes   Use additional   Code first   Code also   Unspecified
OGCR Official Guidelines   **X** Assign placeholder X   ● Use Additional Character(s)   ▶ Manifestation Code   **Coding Clinic**

● **T51.3**   **Toxic effect of fusel oil**
Toxic effect of amyl alcohol
Toxic effect of butyl [1-butanol] alcohol
Toxic effect of propyl [1-propanol] alcohol
     ● **T51.3X**   **Toxic effect of fusel oil**
         ● **T51.3X1**   **Toxic effect of fusel oil, accidental (unintentional)**
             Toxic effect of fusel oil NOS
         ● **T51.3X2**   **Toxic effect of fusel oil, intentional self-harm**
         ● **T51.3X3**   **Toxic effect of fusel oil, assault**
         ● **T51.3X4**   **Toxic effect of fusel oil, undetermined**

● **T51.8**   **Toxic effect of other alcohols**
     ● **T51.8X**   **Toxic effect of other alcohols**
         ● **T51.8X1**   **Toxic effect of other alcohols, accidental (unintentional)**
             Toxic effect of other alcohols NOS
         ● **T51.8X2**   **Toxic effect of other alcohols, intentional self-harm**
         ● **T51.8X3**   **Toxic effect of other alcohols, assault**
         ● **T51.8X4**   **Toxic effect of other alcohols, undetermined**

● **T51.9**   **Toxic effect of unspecified alcohol**
     X ● **T51.91**   **Toxic effect of unspecified alcohol, accidental (unintentional)**
     X ● **T51.92**   **Toxic effect of unspecified alcohol, intentional self-harm**
     X ● **T51.93**   **Toxic effect of unspecified alcohol, assault**
     X ● **T51.94**   **Toxic effect of unspecified alcohol, undetermined**

● **T52**   **Toxic effect of organic solvents**
     Excludes1   halogen derivatives of aliphatic and aromatic hydrocarbons (T53.-)
     The appropriate 7th character is to be added to each code from category T52

A	initial encounter
D	subsequent encounter
S	sequela

● **T52.0**   **Toxic effects of petroleum products**
Toxic effects of gasoline [petrol]
Toxic effects of kerosene [paraffin oil]
Toxic effects of paraffin wax
Toxic effects of ether petroleum
Toxic effects of naphtha petroleum
Toxic effects of spirit petroleum
     ● **T52.0X**   **Toxic effects of petroleum products**
         ● **T52.0X1**   **Toxic effect of petroleum products, accidental (unintentional)**
             Toxic effects of petroleum products NOS
         ● **T52.0X2**   **Toxic effect of petroleum products, intentional self-harm**
         ● **T52.0X3**   **Toxic effect of petroleum products, assault**
         ● **T52.0X4**   **Toxic effect of petroleum products, undetermined**

● **T52.1**   **Toxic effects of benzene**
     Excludes1   homologues of benzene (T52.2)
             nitroderivatives and aminoderivatives of benzene and its homologues (T65.3)
     ● **T52.1X**   **Toxic effects of benzene**
         ● **T52.1X1**   **Toxic effect of benzene, accidental (unintentional)**
             Toxic effects of benzene NOS
         ● **T52.1X2**   **Toxic effect of benzene, intentional self-harm**
         ● **T52.1X3**   **Toxic effect of benzene, assault**
         ● **T52.1X4**   **Toxic effect of benzene, undetermined**

● **T52.2**   **Toxic effects of homologues of benzene**
Toxic effects of toluene [methylbenzene]
Toxic effects of xylene [dimethylbenzene]
     ● **T52.2X**   **Toxic effects of homologues of benzene**
         ● **T52.2X1**   **Toxic effect of homologues of benzene, accidental (unintentional)**
             Toxic effects of homologues of benzene NOS
         ● **T52.2X2**   **Toxic effect of homologues of benzene, intentional self-harm**
         ● **T52.2X3**   **Toxic effect of homologues of benzene, assault**
         ● **T52.2X4**   **Toxic effect of homologues of benzene, undetermined**

● **T52.3**   **Toxic effects of glycols**
     ● **T52.3X**   **Toxic effects of glycols**
         ● **T52.3X1**   **Toxic effect of glycols, accidental (unintentional)**
             Toxic effects of glycols NOS
         ● **T52.3X2**   **Toxic effect of glycols, intentional self-harm**
         ● **T52.3X3**   **Toxic effect of glycols, assault**
         ● **T52.3X4**   **Toxic effect of glycols, undetermined**

● **T52.4**   **Toxic effects of ketones**
     ● **T52.4X**   **Toxic effects of ketones**
         ● **T52.4X1**   **Toxic effect of ketones, accidental (unintentional)**
             Toxic effects of ketones NOS
         ● **T52.4X2**   **Toxic effect of ketones, intentional self-harm**
         ● **T52.4X3**   **Toxic effect of ketones, assault**
         ● **T52.4X4**   **Toxic effect of ketones, undetermined**

● **T52.8**   **Toxic effects of other organic solvents**
     ● **T52.8X**   **Toxic effects of other organic solvents**
         ● **T52.8X1**   **Toxic effect of other organic solvents, accidental (unintentional)**
             Toxic effects of other organic solvents NOS
         ● **T52.8X2**   **Toxic effect of other organic solvents, intentional self-harm**
         ● **T52.8X3**   **Toxic effect of other organic solvents, assault**
         ● **T52.8X4**   **Toxic effect of other organic solvents, undetermined**

● **T52.9**   **Toxic effects of unspecified organic solvent**
     X ● **T52.91**   **Toxic effect of unspecified organic solvent, accidental (unintentional)**
     X ● **T52.92**   **Toxic effect of unspecified organic solvent, intentional self-harm**
     X ● **T52.93**   **Toxic effect of unspecified organic solvent, assault**
     X ● **T52.94**   **Toxic effect of unspecified organic solvent, undetermined**

● **T53**   **Toxic effect of halogen derivatives of aliphatic and aromatic hydrocarbons**
     The appropriate 7th character is to be added to each code from category T53

A	initial encounter
D	subsequent encounter
S	sequela

● **T53.0**   **Toxic effects of carbon tetrachloride**
Toxic effects of tetrachloromethane
     ● **T53.0X**   **Toxic effects of carbon tetrachloride**
         ● **T53.0X1**   **Toxic effect of carbon tetrachloride, accidental (unintentional)**
             Toxic effects of carbon tetrachloride NOS
         ● **T53.0X2**   **Toxic effect of carbon tetrachloride, intentional self-harm**

CHAPTER 19 (S00-T88)

● **T53.0X3** Toxic effect of carbon tetrachloride, assault

● **T53.0X4** Toxic effect of carbon tetrachloride, undetermined

● **T53.1** Toxic effects of chloroform
Toxic effects of trichloromethane

● **T53.1X** Toxic effects of chloroform

● **T53.1X1** Toxic effect of chloroform, accidental (unintentional)
Toxic effects of chloroform NOS

● **T53.1X2** Toxic effect of chloroform, intentional self-harm

● **T53.1X3** Toxic effect of chloroform, assault

● **T53.1X4** Toxic effect of chloroform, undetermined

● **T53.2** Toxic effects of trichloroethylene
Toxic effects of trichloroethene

● **T53.2X** Toxic effects of trichloroethylene

● **T53.2X1** Toxic effect of trichloroethylene, accidental (unintentional)
Toxic effects of trichloroethylene NOS

● **T53.2X2** Toxic effect of trichloroethylene, intentional self-harm

● **T53.2X3** Toxic effect of trichloroethylene, assault

● **T53.2X4** Toxic effect of trichloroethylene, undetermined

● **T53.3** Toxic effects of tetrachloroethylene
Toxic effects of perchloroethylene
Toxic effect of tetrachloroethene

● **T53.3X** Toxic effects of tetrachloroethylene

● **T53.3X1** Toxic effect of tetrachloroethylene, accidental (unintentional)
Toxic effects of tetrachloroethylene NOS

● **T53.3X2** Toxic effect of tetrachloroethylene, intentional self-harm

● **T53.3X3** Toxic effect of tetrachloroethylene, assault

● **T53.3X4** Toxic effect of tetrachloroethylene, undetermined

● **T53.4** Toxic effects of dichloromethane
Toxic effects of methylene chloride

● **T53.4X** Toxic effects of dichloromethane

● **T53.4X1** Toxic effect of dichloromethane, accidental (unintentional)
Toxic effects of dichloromethane NOS

● **T53.4X2** Toxic effect of dichloromethane, intentional self-harm

● **T53.4X3** Toxic effect of dichloromethane, assault

● **T53.4X4** Toxic effect of dichloromethane, undetermined

● **T53.5** Toxic effects of chlorofluorocarbons

● **T53.5X** Toxic effects of chlorofluorocarbons

● **T53.5X1** Toxic effect of chlorofluorocarbons, accidental (unintentional)
Toxic effects of chlorofluorocarbons NOS

● **T53.5X2** Toxic effect of chlorofluorocarbons, intentional self-harm

● **T53.5X3** Toxic effect of chlorofluorocarbons, assault

● **T53.5X4** Toxic effect of chlorofluorocarbons, undetermined

● **T53.6** Toxic effects of other halogen derivatives of aliphatic hydrocarbons

● **T53.6X** Toxic effects of other halogen derivatives of aliphatic hydrocarbons

● **T53.6X1** Toxic effect of other halogen derivatives of aliphatic hydrocarbons, accidental (unintentional)
Toxic effects of other halogen derivatives of aliphatic hydrocarbons NOS

● **T53.6X2** Toxic effect of other halogen derivatives of aliphatic hydrocarbons, intentional self-harm

● **T53.6X3** Toxic effect of other halogen derivatives of aliphatic hydrocarbons, assault

● **T53.6X4** Toxic effect of other halogen derivatives of aliphatic hydrocarbons, undetermined

● **T53.7** Toxic effects of other halogen derivatives of aromatic hydrocarbons

● **T53.7X** Toxic effects of other halogen derivatives of aromatic hydrocarbons

● **T53.7X1** Toxic effect of other halogen derivatives of aromatic hydrocarbons, accidental (unintentional)
Toxic effects of other halogen derivatives of aromatic hydrocarbons NOS

● **T53.7X2** Toxic effect of other halogen derivatives of aromatic hydrocarbons, intentional self-harm

● **T53.7X3** Toxic effect of other halogen derivatives of aromatic hydrocarbons, assault

● **T53.7X4** Toxic effect of other halogen derivatives of aromatic hydrocarbons, undetermined

● **T53.9** Toxic effects of unspecified halogen derivatives of aliphatic and aromatic hydrocarbons

X ● **T53.91** Toxic effect of unspecified halogen derivatives of aliphatic and aromatic hydrocarbons, accidental (unintentional)

X ● **T53.92** Toxic effect of unspecified halogen derivatives of aliphatic and aromatic hydrocarbons, intentional self-harm

X ● **T53.93** Toxic effect of unspecified halogen derivatives of aliphatic and aromatic hydrocarbons, assault

X ● **T53.94** Toxic effect of unspecified halogen derivatives of aliphatic and aromatic hydrocarbons, undetermined

● **T54** **Toxic effect of corrosive substances**
The appropriate 7th character is to be added to each code from category T54

A	initial encounter
D	subsequent encounter
S	sequela

● **T54.0** Toxic effects of phenol and phenol homologues

● **T54.0X** Toxic effects of phenol and phenol homologues

● **T54.0X1** Toxic effect of phenol and phenol homologues, accidental (unintentional)
Toxic effects of phenol and phenol homologues NOS

● **T54.0X2** Toxic effect of phenol and phenol homologues, intentional self-harm

● **T54.0X3** Toxic effect of phenol and phenol homologues, assault

● **T54.0X4** Toxic effect of phenol and phenol homologues, undetermined

◀ New   ◀▬ Revised   ~~deleted~~ Deleted   Excludes 1   Excludes 2   Includes   Use additional   Code first   Code also   Unspecified
OGCR Official Guidelines   X Assign placeholder X   ● Use Additional Character(s)   ▶ Manifestation Code   **Coding Clinic**

● **T54.1**   **Toxic effects of other corrosive organic compounds**
    ● **T54.1X**   Toxic effects of other corrosive organic compounds
       ● **T54.1X1**   Toxic effect of other corrosive organic compounds, accidental (unintentional)
           Toxic effects of other corrosive organic compounds NOS
       ● **T54.1X2**   Toxic effect of other corrosive organic compounds, intentional self-harm
       ● **T54.1X3**   Toxic effect of other corrosive organic compounds, assault
       ● **T54.1X4**   Toxic effect of other corrosive organic compounds, undetermined

● **T54.2**   **Toxic effects of corrosive acids and acid-like substances**
     Toxic effects of hydrochloric acid
     Toxic effects of sulfuric acid
    ● **T54.2X**   Toxic effects of corrosive acids and acid-like substances
       ● **T54.2X1**   Toxic effect of corrosive acids and acid-like substances, accidental (unintentional)
           Toxic effects of corrosive acids and acid-like substances NOS
       ● **T54.2X2**   Toxic effect of corrosive acids and acid-like substances, intentional self-harm
       ● **T54.2X3**   Toxic effect of corrosive acids and acid-like substances, assault
       ● **T54.2X4**   Toxic effect of corrosive acids and acid-like substances, undetermined

● **T54.3**   **Toxic effects of corrosive alkalis and alkali-like substances**
     Toxic effects of potassium hydroxide
     Toxic effects of sodium hydroxide
    ● **T54.3X**   Toxic effects of corrosive alkalis and alkali-like substances
       ● **T54.3X1**   Toxic effect of corrosive alkalis and alkali-like substances, accidental (unintentional)
           Toxic effects of corrosive alkalis and alkali-like substances NOS
       ● **T54.3X2**   Toxic effect of corrosive alkalis and alkali-like substances, intentional self-harm
       ● **T54.3X3**   Toxic effect of corrosive alkalis and alkali-like substances, assault
       ● **T54.3X4**   Toxic effect of corrosive alkalis and alkali-like substances, undetermined

● **T54.9**   **Toxic effects of unspecified corrosive substance**
   X ● **T54.91**   Toxic effect of unspecified corrosive substance, accidental (unintentional)
   X ● **T54.92**   Toxic effect of unspecified corrosive substance, intentional self-harm
   X ● **T54.93**   Toxic effect of unspecified corrosive substance, assault
   X ● **T54.94**   Toxic effect of unspecified corrosive substance, undetermined

● **T55**   **Toxic effect of soaps and detergents**
    The appropriate 7th character is to be added to each code from category T55

A	initial encounter
D	subsequent encounter
S	sequela

   ● **T55.0**   **Toxic effect of soaps**
    ● **T55.0X**   Toxic effect of soaps
       ● **T55.0X1**   Toxic effect of soaps, accidental (unintentional)
           Toxic effect of soaps NOS
       ● **T55.0X2**   Toxic effect of soaps, intentional self-harm
       ● **T55.0X3**   Toxic effect of soaps, assault
       ● **T55.0X4**   Toxic effect of soaps, undetermined

   ● **T55.1**   **Toxic effect of detergents**
    ● **T55.1X**   Toxic effect of detergents
       ● **T55.1X1**   Toxic effect of detergents, accidental (unintentional)
           Toxic effect of detergents NOS
       ● **T55.1X2**   Toxic effect of detergents, intentional self-harm
       ● **T55.1X3**   Toxic effect of detergents, assault
       ● **T55.1X4**   Toxic effect of detergents, undetermined

● **T56**   **Toxic effect of metals**
   Includes   toxic effects of fumes and vapors of metals
           toxic effects of metals from all sources, except medicinal substances

   Use additional code to identify any retained metal foreign body, if applicable (Z18.0-, T18.1-)

   Excludes1   arsenic and its compounds (T57.0)
           manganese and its compounds (T57.2)

   The appropriate 7th character is to be added to each code from category T56

A	initial encounter
D	subsequent encounter
S	sequela

   ● **T56.0**   **Toxic effects of lead and its compounds**
    ● **T56.0X**   Toxic effects of lead and its compounds
       ● **T56.0X1**   Toxic effect of lead and its compounds, accidental (unintentional)
           Toxic effects of lead and its compounds NOS
       ● **T56.0X2**   Toxic effect of lead and its compounds, intentional self-harm
       ● **T56.0X3**   Toxic effect of lead and its compounds, assault
       ● **T56.0X4**   Toxic effect of lead and its compounds, undetermined

   ● **T56.1**   **Toxic effects of mercury and its compounds**
    ● **T56.1X**   Toxic effects of mercury and its compounds
       ● **T56.1X1**   Toxic effect of mercury and its compounds, accidental (unintentional)
           Toxic effects of mercury and its compounds NOS
       ● **T56.1X2**   Toxic effect of mercury and its compounds, intentional self-harm
       ● **T56.1X3**   Toxic effect of mercury and its compounds, assault
       ● **T56.1X4**   Toxic effect of mercury and its compounds, undetermined

CHAPTER 19 (S00-T88)

● T56.2   Toxic effects of chromium and its compounds
   ● T56.2X   Toxic effects of chromium and its compounds
     ● T56.2X1   Toxic effect of chromium and its compounds, accidental (unintentional)
         Toxic effects of chromium and its compounds NOS
     ● T56.2X2   Toxic effect of chromium and its compounds, intentional self-harm
     ● T56.2X3   Toxic effect of chromium and its compounds, assault
     ● T56.2X4   Toxic effect of chromium and its compounds, undetermined

● T56.3   Toxic effects of cadmium and its compounds
   ● T56.3X   Toxic effects of cadmium and its compounds
     ● T56.3X1   Toxic effect of cadmium and its compounds, accidental (unintentional)
         Toxic effects of cadmium and its compounds NOS
     ● T56.3X2   Toxic effect of cadmium and its compounds, intentional self-harm
     ● T56.3X3   Toxic effect of cadmium and its compounds, assault
     ● T56.3X4   Toxic effect of cadmium and its compounds, undetermined

● T56.4   Toxic effects of copper and its compounds
   ● T56.4X   Toxic effects of copper and its compounds
     ● T56.4X1   Toxic effect of copper and its compounds, accidental (unintentional)
         Toxic effects of copper and its compounds NOS
     ● T56.4X2   Toxic effect of copper and its compounds, intentional self-harm
     ● T56.4X3   Toxic effect of copper and its compounds, assault
     ● T56.4X4   Toxic effect of copper and its compounds, undetermined

● T56.5   Toxic effects of zinc and its compounds
   ● T56.5X   Toxic effects of zinc and its compounds
     ● T56.5X1   Toxic effect of zinc and its compounds, accidental (unintentional)
         Toxic effects of zinc and its compounds NOS
     ● T56.5X2   Toxic effect of zinc and its compounds, intentional self-harm
     ● T56.5X3   Toxic effect of zinc and its compounds, assault
     ● T56.5X4   Toxic effect of zinc and its compounds, undetermined

● T56.6   Toxic effects of tin and its compounds
   ● T56.6X   Toxic effects of tin and its compounds
     ● T56.6X1   Toxic effect of tin and its compounds, accidental (unintentional)
         Toxic effects of tin and its compounds NOS
     ● T56.6X2   Toxic effect of tin and its compounds, intentional self-harm
     ● T56.6X3   Toxic effect of tin and its compounds, assault
     ● T56.6X4   Toxic effect of tin and its compounds, undetermined

● T56.7   Toxic effects of beryllium and its compounds
   ● T56.7X   Toxic effects of beryllium and its compounds
     ● T56.7X1   Toxic effect of beryllium and its compounds, accidental (unintentional)
         Toxic effects of beryllium and its compounds NOS
     ● T56.7X2   Toxic effect of beryllium and its compounds, intentional self-harm
     ● T56.7X3   Toxic effect of beryllium and its compounds, assault
     ● T56.7X4   Toxic effect of beryllium and its compounds, undetermined

● T56.8   Toxic effects of other metals
   ● T56.81   Toxic effect of thallium
     ● T56.811   Toxic effect of thallium, accidental (unintentional)
         Toxic effect of thallium NOS
     ● T56.812   Toxic effect of thallium, intentional self-harm
     ● T56.813   Toxic effect of thallium, assault
     ● T56.814   Toxic effect of thallium, undetermined
   ● T56.89   Toxic effects of other metals
     ● T56.891   Toxic effect of other metals, accidental (unintentional)
         Toxic effects of other metals NOS
     ● T56.892   Toxic effect of other metals, intentional self-harm
     ● T56.893   Toxic effect of other metals, assault
     ● T56.894   Toxic effect of other metals, undetermined

● T56.9   Toxic effects of unspecified metal
   X● T56.91   Toxic effect of unspecified metal, accidental (unintentional)
   X● T56.92   Toxic effect of unspecified metal, intentional self-harm
   X● T56.93   Toxic effect of unspecified metal, assault
   X● T56.94   Toxic effect of unspecified metal, undetermined

● T57   Toxic effect of other inorganic substances
   The appropriate 7th character is to be added to each code from category T57

     A   initial encounter
     D   subsequent encounter
     S   sequela

● T57.0   Toxic effect of arsenic and its compounds
   ● T57.0X   Toxic effect of arsenic and its compounds
     ● T57.0X1   Toxic effect of arsenic and its compounds, accidental (unintentional)
         Toxic effect of arsenic and its compounds NOS
     ● T57.0X2   Toxic effect of arsenic and its compounds, intentional self-harm
     ● T57.0X3   Toxic effect of arsenic and its compounds, assault
     ● T57.0X4   Toxic effect of arsenic and its compounds, undetermined

- T57.1   Toxic effect of phosphorus and its compounds
  - **Excludes1**   organophosphate insecticides (T60.0)
  - T57.1X   Toxic effect of phosphorus and its compounds
    - T57.1X1   Toxic effect of phosphorus and its compounds, accidental (unintentional)
      - Toxic effect of phosphorus and its compounds NOS
    - T57.1X2   Toxic effect of phosphorus and its compounds, intentional self-harm
    - T57.1X3   Toxic effect of phosphorus and its compounds, assault
    - T57.1X4   Toxic effect of phosphorus and its compounds, undetermined
- T57.2   Toxic effect of manganese and its compounds
  - T57.2X   Toxic effect of manganese and its compounds
    - T57.2X1   Toxic effect of manganese and its compounds, accidental (unintentional)
      - Toxic effect of manganese and its compounds NOS
    - T57.2X2   Toxic effect of manganese and its compounds, intentional self-harm
    - T57.2X3   Toxic effect of manganese and its compounds, assault
    - T57.2X4   Toxic effect of manganese and its compounds, undetermined
- T57.3   Toxic effect of hydrogen cyanide
  - T57.3X   Toxic effect of hydrogen cyanide
    - T57.3X1   Toxic effect of hydrogen cyanide, accidental (unintentional)
      - Toxic effect of hydrogen cyanide NOS
    - T57.3X2   Toxic effect of hydrogen cyanide, intentional self-harm
    - T57.3X3   Toxic effect of hydrogen cyanide, assault
    - T57.3X4   Toxic effect of hydrogen cyanide, undetermined
- T57.8   Toxic effect of other specified inorganic substances
  - T57.8X   Toxic effect of other specified inorganic substances
    - T57.8X1   Toxic effect of other specified inorganic substances, accidental (unintentional)
      - Toxic effect of other specified inorganic substances NOS
    - T57.8X2   Toxic effect of other specified inorganic substances, intentional self-harm
    - T57.8X3   Toxic effect of other specified inorganic substances, assault
    - T57.8X4   Toxic effect of other specified inorganic substances, undetermined
- T57.9   Toxic effect of unspecified inorganic substance
  - X● T57.91   Toxic effect of unspecified inorganic substance, accidental (unintentional)
  - X● T57.92   Toxic effect of unspecified inorganic substance, intentional self-harm
  - X● T57.93   Toxic effect of unspecified inorganic substance, assault
  - X● T57.94   Toxic effect of unspecified inorganic substance, undetermined

- T58   Toxic effect of carbon monoxide
  - **Includes**   asphyxiation from carbon monoxide
    - toxic effect of carbon monoxide from all sources
  - The appropriate 7th character is to be added to each code from category T58

A	initial encounter
D	subsequent encounter
S	sequela

  - T58.0   Toxic effect of carbon monoxide from motor vehicle exhaust
    - Toxic effect of exhaust gas from gas engine
    - Toxic effect of exhaust gas from motor pump
    - X● T58.01   Toxic effect of carbon monoxide from motor vehicle exhaust, accidental (unintentional)
    - X● T58.02   Toxic effect of carbon monoxide from motor vehicle exhaust, intentional self-harm
    - X● T58.03   Toxic effect of carbon monoxide from motor vehicle exhaust, assault
    - X● T58.04   Toxic effect of carbon monoxide from motor vehicle exhaust, undetermined
  - T58.1   Toxic effect of carbon monoxide from utility gas
    - Toxic effect of acetylene
    - Toxic effect of gas NOS used for lighting, heating, cooking
    - Toxic effect of water gas
    - X● T58.11   Toxic effect of carbon monoxide from utility gas, accidental (unintentional)
    - X● T58.12   Toxic effect of carbon monoxide from utility gas, intentional self-harm
    - X● T58.13   Toxic effect of carbon monoxide from utility gas, assault
    - X● T58.14   Toxic effect of carbon monoxide from utility gas, undetermined
  - T58.2   Toxic effect of carbon monoxide from incomplete combustion of other domestic fuels
    - Toxic effect of carbon monoxide from incomplete combustion of coal, coke, kerosene, wood
    - T58.2X   Toxic effect of carbon monoxide from incomplete combustion of other domestic fuels
      - T58.2X1   Toxic effect of carbon monoxide from incomplete combustion of other domestic fuels, accidental (unintentional)
      - T58.2X2   Toxic effect of carbon monoxide from incomplete combustion of other domestic fuels, intentional self-harm
      - T58.2X3   Toxic effect of carbon monoxide from incomplete combustion of other domestic fuels, assault
      - T58.2X4   Toxic effect of carbon monoxide from incomplete combustion of other domestic fuels, undetermined
  - T58.8   Toxic effect of carbon monoxide from other source
    - Toxic effect of carbon monoxide from blast furnace gas
    - Toxic effect of carbon monoxide from fuels in industrial use
    - Toxic effect of carbon monoxide from kiln vapor
    - T58.8X   Toxic effect of carbon monoxide from other source
      - T58.8X1   Toxic effect of carbon monoxide from other source, accidental (unintentional)
      - T58.8X2   Toxic effect of carbon monoxide from other source, intentional self-harm
      - T58.8X3   Toxic effect of carbon monoxide from other source, assault
      - T58.8X4   Toxic effect of carbon monoxide from other source, undetermined

CHAPTER 19 (S00-T88)

CHAPTER 19 (S00-T88)

● T58.9   Toxic effect of carbon monoxide from unspecified source
  X ● T58.91   Toxic effect of carbon monoxide from unspecified source, accidental (unintentional)
  X ● T58.92   Toxic effect of carbon monoxide from unspecified source, intentional self-harm
  X ● T58.93   Toxic effect of carbon monoxide from unspecified source, assault
  X ● T58.94   Toxic effect of carbon monoxide from unspecified source, undetermined

● T59   Toxic effect of other gases, fumes and vapors
    Includes   aerosol propellants
    Excludes1   chlorofluorocarbons (T53.5)

    The appropriate 7th character is to be added to each code from category T59

    A   initial encounter
    D   subsequent encounter
    S   sequela

● T59.0   Toxic effect of nitrogen oxides
  ● T59.0X   Toxic effect of nitrogen oxides
    ● T59.0X1   Toxic effect of nitrogen oxides, accidental (unintentional)
                Toxic effect of nitrogen oxides NOS
    ● T59.0X2   Toxic effect of nitrogen oxides, intentional self-harm
    ● T59.0X3   Toxic effect of nitrogen oxides, assault
    ● T59.0X4   Toxic effect of nitrogen oxides, undetermined

● T59.1   Toxic effect of sulfur dioxide
  ● T59.1X   Toxic effect of sulfur dioxide
    ● T59.1X1   Toxic effect of sulfur dioxide, accidental (unintentional)
                Toxic effect of sulfur dioxide NOS
    ● T59.1X2   Toxic effect of sulfur dioxide, intentional self-harm
    ● T59.1X3   Toxic effect of sulfur dioxide, assault
    ● T59.1X4   Toxic effect of sulfur dioxide, undetermined

● T59.2   Toxic effect of formaldehyde
  ● T59.2X   Toxic effect of formaldehyde
    ● T59.2X1   Toxic effect of formaldehyde, accidental (unintentional)
                Toxic effect of formaldehyde NOS
    ● T59.2X2   Toxic effect of formaldehyde, intentional self-harm
    ● T59.2X3   Toxic effect of formaldehyde, assault
    ● T59.2X4   Toxic effect of formaldehyde, undetermined

● T59.3   Toxic effect of lacrimogenic gas
            Toxic effect of tear gas
  ● T59.3X   Toxic effect of lacrimogenic gas
    ● T59.3X1   Toxic effect of lacrimogenic gas, accidental (unintentional)
                Toxic effect of lacrimogenic gas NOS
    ● T59.3X2   Toxic effect of lacrimogenic gas, intentional self-harm
    ● T59.3X3   Toxic effect of lacrimogenic gas, assault
    ● T59.3X4   Toxic effect of lacrimogenic gas, undetermined

● T59.4   Toxic effect of chlorine gas
  ● T59.4X   Toxic effect of chlorine gas
    ● T59.4X1   Toxic effect of chlorine gas, accidental (unintentional)
                Toxic effect of chlorine gas NOS
    ● T59.4X2   Toxic effect of chlorine gas, intentional self-harm
    ● T59.4X3   Toxic effect of chlorine gas, assault
    ● T59.4X4   Toxic effect of chlorine gas, undetermined

● T59.5   Toxic effect of fluorine gas and hydrogen fluoride
  ● T59.5X   Toxic effect of fluorine gas and hydrogen fluoride
    ● T59.5X1   Toxic effect of fluorine gas and hydrogen fluoride, accidental (unintentional)
                Toxic effect of fluorine gas and hydrogen fluoride NOS
    ● T59.5X2   Toxic effect of fluorine gas and hydrogen fluoride, intentional self-harm
    ● T59.5X3   Toxic effect of fluorine gas and hydrogen fluoride, assault
    ● T59.5X4   Toxic effect of fluorine gas and hydrogen fluoride, undetermined

● T59.6   Toxic effect of hydrogen sulfide
  ● T59.6X   Toxic effect of hydrogen sulfide
    ● T59.6X1   Toxic effect of hydrogen sulfide, accidental (unintentional)
                Toxic effect of hydrogen sulfide NOS
    ● T59.6X2   Toxic effect of hydrogen sulfide, intentional self-harm
    ● T59.6X3   Toxic effect of hydrogen sulfide, assault
    ● T59.6X4   Toxic effect of hydrogen sulfide, undetermined

● T59.7   Toxic effect of carbon dioxide
  ● T59.7X   Toxic effect of carbon dioxide
    ● T59.7X1   Toxic effect of carbon dioxide, accidental (unintentional)
                Toxic effect of carbon dioxide NOS
    ● T59.7X2   Toxic effect of carbon dioxide, intentional self-harm
    ● T59.7X3   Toxic effect of carbon dioxide, assault
    ● T59.7X4   Toxic effect of carbon dioxide, undetermined

● T59.8   Toxic effect of other specified gases, fumes and vapors
  ● T59.81   Toxic effect of smoke
             Smoke inhalation
             Excludes2   toxic effect of cigarette (tobacco) smoke (T65.22-)
    ● T59.811   Toxic effect of smoke, accidental (unintentional)
                Toxic effect of smoke NOS
    ● T59.812   Toxic effect of smoke, intentional self-harm
    ● T59.813   Toxic effect of smoke, assault
    ● T59.814   Toxic effect of smoke, undetermined
  ● T59.89   Toxic effect of other specified gases, fumes and vapors
    ● T59.891   Toxic effect of other specified gases, fumes and vapors, accidental (unintentional)
    ● T59.892   Toxic effect of other specified gases, fumes and vapors, intentional self-harm
    ● T59.893   Toxic effect of other specified gases, fumes and vapors, assault
    ● T59.894   Toxic effect of other specified gases, fumes and vapors, undetermined

◀ New   ◀▦ Revised   ~~deleted~~ Deleted   Excludes 1   Excludes 2   Includes   Use additional   Code first   Code also   Unspecified

OGCR Official Guidelines   X Assign placeholder X   ● Use Additional Character(s)   ▌ Manifestation Code   **Coding Clinic**

● **T59.9**   Toxic effect of unspecified gases, fumes and vapors

   X● **T59.91**   Toxic effect of unspecified gases, fumes and vapors, accidental (unintentional)

   X● **T59.92**   Toxic effect of unspecified gases, fumes and vapors, intentional self-harm

   X● **T59.93**   Toxic effect of unspecified gases, fumes and vapors, assault

   X● **T59.94**   Toxic effect of unspecified gases, fumes and vapors, undetermined

● **T60**   Toxic effect of pesticides

   Includes   toxic effect of wood preservatives

   The appropriate 7th character is to be added to each code from category T60

> A   initial encounter
> D   subsequent encounter
> S   sequela

● **T60.0**   Toxic effect of organophosphate and carbamate insecticides

   ● **T60.0X**   Toxic effect of organophosphate and carbamate insecticides

     ● **T60.0X1**   Toxic effect of organophosphate and carbamate insecticides, accidental (unintentional)
       Toxic effect of organophosphate and carbamate insecticides NOS

     ● **T60.0X2**   Toxic effect of organophosphate and carbamate insecticides, intentional self-harm

     ● **T60.0X3**   Toxic effect of organophosphate and carbamate insecticides, assault

     ● **T60.0X4**   Toxic effect of organophosphate and carbamate insecticides, undetermined

● **T60.1**   Toxic effect of halogenated insecticides

   Excludes1   chlorinated hydrocarbon (T53.-)

   ● **T60.1X**   Toxic effect of halogenated insecticides

     ● **T60.1X1**   Toxic effect of halogenated insecticides, accidental (unintentional)
       Toxic effect of halogenated insecticides NOS

     ● **T60.1X2**   Toxic effect of halogenated insecticides, intentional self-harm

     ● **T60.1X3**   Toxic effect of halogenated insecticides, assault

     ● **T60.1X4**   Toxic effect of halogenated insecticides, undetermined

● **T60.2**   Toxic effect of other insecticides

   ● **T60.2X**   Toxic effect of other insecticides

     ● **T60.2X1**   Toxic effect of other insecticides, accidental (unintentional)
       Toxic effect of other insecticides NOS

     ● **T60.2X2**   Toxic effect of other insecticides, intentional self-harm

     ● **T60.2X3**   Toxic effect of other insecticides, assault

     ● **T60.2X4**   Toxic effect of other insecticides, undetermined

● **T60.3**   Toxic effect of herbicides and fungicides

   ● **T60.3X**   Toxic effect of herbicides and fungicides

     ● **T60.3X1**   Toxic effect of herbicides and fungicides, accidental (unintentional)
       Toxic effect of herbicides and fungicides NOS

     ● **T60.3X2**   Toxic effect of herbicides and fungicides, intentional self-harm

     ● **T60.3X3**   Toxic effect of herbicides and fungicides, assault

     ● **T60.3X4**   Toxic effect of herbicides and fungicides, undetermined

● **T60.4**   Toxic effect of rodenticides

   Excludes1   strychnine and its salts (T65.1)
       thallium (T56.81-)

   ● **T60.4X**   Toxic effect of rodenticides

     ● **T60.4X1**   Toxic effect of rodenticides, accidental (unintentional)
       Toxic effect of rodenticides NOS

     ● **T60.4X2**   Toxic effect of rodenticides, intentional self-harm

     ● **T60.4X3**   Toxic effect of rodenticides, assault

     ● **T60.4X4**   Toxic effect of rodenticides, undetermined

● **T60.8**   Toxic effect of other pesticides

   ● **T60.8X**   Toxic effect of other pesticides

     ● **T60.8X1**   Toxic effect of other pesticides, accidental (unintentional)
       Toxic effect of other pesticides NOS

     ● **T60.8X2**   Toxic effect of other pesticides, intentional self-harm

     ● **T60.8X3**   Toxic effect of other pesticides, assault

     ● **T60.8X4**   Toxic effect of other pesticides, undetermined

● **T60.9**   Toxic effect of unspecified pesticide

   X● **T60.91**   Toxic effect of unspecified pesticide, accidental (unintentional)

   X● **T60.92**   Toxic effect of unspecified pesticide, intentional self-harm

   X● **T60.93**   Toxic effect of unspecified pesticide, assault

   X● **T60.94**   Toxic effect of unspecified pesticide, undetermined

● **T61**   Toxic effect of noxious substances eaten as seafood

   Excludes1   allergic reaction to food, such as:
       anaphylactic reaction or shock due to adverse food reaction (T78.0-)
       bacterial foodborne intoxications (A05.-)
       dermatitis (L23.6, L25.4, L27.2)
       gastroenteritis (noninfective) (K52.2)
       toxic effect of aflatoxin and other mycotoxins (T64)
       toxic effect of cyanides (T65.0-)
       toxic effect of harmful algae bloom (T65.82-)
       toxic effect of hydrogen cyanide (T57.3-)
       toxic effect of mercury (T56.1-)
       toxic effect of red tide (T65.82-)

   The appropriate 7th character is to be added to each code from category T61

> A   initial encounter
> D   subsequent encounter
> S   sequela

● **T61.0**   Ciguatera fish poisoning

   X● **T61.01**   Ciguatera fish poisoning, accidental (unintentional)

   X● **T61.02**   Ciguatera fish poisoning, intentional self-harm

   X● **T61.03**   Ciguatera fish poisoning, assault

   X● **T61.04**   Ciguatera fish poisoning, undetermined

● **T61.1**   Scombroid fish poisoning
   Histamine-like syndrome

   X● **T61.11**   Scombroid fish poisoning, accidental (unintentional)

   X● **T61.12**   Scombroid fish poisoning, intentional self-harm

   X● **T61.13**   Scombroid fish poisoning, assault

   X● **T61.14**   Scombroid fish poisoning, undetermined

CHAPTER 19 (S00-T88)

● **T61.7** **Other fish and shellfish poisoning**
  ● **T61.77** **Other fish poisoning**
    ● **T61.771** Other fish poisoning, accidental (unintentional)
    ● **T61.772** Other fish poisoning, intentional self-harm
    ● **T61.773** Other fish poisoning, assault
    ● **T61.774** Other fish poisoning, undetermined
  ● **T61.78** **Other shellfish poisoning**
    ● **T61.781** Other shellfish poisoning, accidental (unintentional)
    ● **T61.782** Other shellfish poisoning, intentional self-harm
    ● **T61.783** Other shellfish poisoning, assault
    ● **T61.784** Other shellfish poisoning, undetermined
● **T61.8** **Toxic effect of other seafood**
  ● **T61.8X** **Toxic effect of other seafood**
    ● **T61.8X1** Toxic effect of other seafood, accidental (unintentional)
    ● **T61.8X2** Toxic effect of other seafood, intentional self-harm
    ● **T61.8X3** Toxic effect of other seafood, assault
    ● **T61.8X4** Toxic effect of other seafood, undetermined
● **T61.9** **Toxic effect of unspecified seafood**
  X ● **T61.91** Toxic effect of unspecified seafood, accidental (unintentional)
  X ● **T61.92** Toxic effect of unspecified seafood, intentional self-harm
  X ● **T61.93** Toxic effect of unspecified seafood, assault
  X ● **T61.94** Toxic effect of unspecified seafood, undetermined

● **T62** **Toxic effect of other noxious substances eaten as food**

Excludes1 allergic reaction to food, such as:
    anaphylactic shock (reaction) due to adverse food reaction (T78.0-)
    dermatitis (L23.6, L25.4, L27.2)
    gastroenteritis (noninfective) (K52.2)
    bacterial food borne intoxications (A05.-)
  toxic effect of aflatoxin and other mycotoxins (T64)
  toxic effect of cyanides (T65.0-)
  toxic effect of hydrogen cyanide (T57.3-)
  toxic effect of mercury (T56.1-)

The appropriate 7th character is to be added to each code from category T62

A	initial encounter
D	subsequent encounter
S	sequela

● **T62.0** **Toxic effect of ingested mushrooms**
  ● **T62.0X** **Toxic effect of ingested mushrooms**
    ● **T62.0X1** Toxic effect of ingested mushrooms, accidental (unintentional)
      Toxic effect of ingested mushrooms NOS
    ● **T62.0X2** Toxic effect of ingested mushrooms, intentional self-harm
    ● **T62.0X3** Toxic effect of ingested mushrooms, assault
    ● **T62.0X4** Toxic effect of ingested mushrooms, undetermined

● **T62.1** **Toxic effect of ingested berries**
  ● **T62.1X** **Toxic effect of ingested berries**
    ● **T62.1X1** Toxic effect of ingested berries, accidental (unintentional)
      Toxic effect of ingested berries NOS
    ● **T62.1X2** Toxic effect of ingested berries, intentional self-harm
    ● **T62.1X3** Toxic effect of ingested berries, assault
    ● **T62.1X4** Toxic effect of ingested berries, undetermined
● **T62.2** **Toxic effect of other ingested (parts of) plant(s)**
  ● **T62.2X** **Toxic effect of other ingested (parts of) plant(s)**
    ● **T62.2X1** Toxic effect of other ingested (parts of) plant(s), accidental (unintentional)
      Toxic effect of other ingested (parts of) plant(s) NOS
    ● **T62.2X2** Toxic effect of other ingested (parts of) plant(s), intentional self-harm
    ● **T62.2X3** Toxic effect of other ingested (parts of) plant(s), assault
    ● **T62.2X4** Toxic effect of other ingested (parts of) plant(s), undetermined
● **T62.8** **Toxic effect of other specified noxious substances eaten as food**
  ● **T62.8X** **Toxic effect of other specified noxious substances eaten as food**
    ● **T62.8X1** Toxic effect of other specified noxious substances eaten as food, accidental (unintentional)
      Toxic effect of other specified noxious substances eaten as food NOS
    ● **T62.8X2** Toxic effect of other specified noxious substances eaten as food, intentional self-harm
    ● **T62.8X3** Toxic effect of other specified noxious substances eaten as food, assault
    ● **T62.8X4** Toxic effect of other specified noxious substances eaten as food, undetermined
● **T62.9** **Toxic effect of unspecified noxious substance eaten as food**
  X ● **T62.91** Toxic effect of unspecified noxious substance eaten as food, accidental (unintentional)
    Toxic effect of unspecified noxious substance eaten as food NOS
  X ● **T62.92** Toxic effect of unspecified noxious substance eaten as food, intentional self-harm
  X ● **T62.93** Toxic effect of unspecified noxious substance eaten as food, assault
  X ● **T62.94** Toxic effect of unspecified noxious substance eaten as food, undetermined

● **T63** **Toxic effect of contact with venomous animals and plants**

Includes bite or touch of venomous animal
    pricked or stuck by thorn or leaf

Excludes2 ingestion of toxic animal or plant (T61.-, T62.-)

The appropriate 7th character is to be added to each code from category T63

A	initial encounter
D	subsequent encounter
S	sequela

● **T63.0** **Toxic effect of snake venom**
  ● **T63.00** **Toxic effect of unspecified snake venom**
    ● **T63.001** Toxic effect of unspecified snake venom, accidental (unintentional)
      Toxic effect of unspecified snake venom NOS
    ● **T63.002** Toxic effect of unspecified snake venom, intentional self-harm
    ● **T63.003** Toxic effect of unspecified snake venom, assault
    ● **T63.004** Toxic effect of unspecified snake venom, undetermined

◀ New   ◀▥ Revised   ~~deleted~~ Deleted   Excludes 1   Excludes 2   Includes   Use additional   Code first   Code also   Unspecified
OGCR Official Guidelines   X Assign placeholder X   ● Use Additional Character(s)   ▌ Manifestation Code   **Coding Clinic**

● T63.01　Toxic effect of rattlesnake venom
　● T63.011　Toxic effect of rattlesnake venom, accidental (unintentional)
　　　　　　Toxic effect of rattlesnake venom NOS
　● T63.012　Toxic effect of rattlesnake venom, intentional self-harm
　● T63.013　Toxic effect of rattlesnake venom, assault
　● T63.014　Toxic effect of rattlesnake venom, undetermined
● T63.02　Toxic effect of coral snake venom
　● T63.021　Toxic effect of coral snake venom, accidental (unintentional)
　　　　　　Toxic effect of coral snake venom NOS
　● T63.022　Toxic effect of coral snake venom, intentional self-harm
　● T63.023　Toxic effect of coral snake venom, assault
　● T63.024　Toxic effect of coral snake venom, undetermined
● T63.03　Toxic effect of taipan venom
　● T63.031　Toxic effect of taipan venom, accidental (unintentional)
　　　　　　Toxic effect of taipan venom NOS
　● T63.032　Toxic effect of taipan venom, intentional self-harm
　● T63.033　Toxic effect of taipan venom, assault
　● T63.034　Toxic effect of taipan venom, undetermined
● T63.04　Toxic effect of cobra venom
　● T63.041　Toxic effect of cobra venom, accidental (unintentional)
　　　　　　Toxic effect of cobra venom NOS
　● T63.042　Toxic effect of cobra venom, intentional self-harm
　● T63.043　Toxic effect of cobra venom, assault
　● T63.044　Toxic effect of cobra venom, undetermined
● T63.06　Toxic effect of venom of other North and South American snake
　● T63.061　Toxic effect of venom of other North and South American snake, accidental (unintentional)
　　　　　　Toxic effect of venom of other North and South American snake NOS
　● T63.062　Toxic effect of venom of other North and South American snake, intentional self-harm
　● T63.063　Toxic effect of venom of other North and South American snake, assault
　● T63.064　Toxic effect of venom of other North and South American snake, undetermined
● T63.07　Toxic effect of venom of other Australian snake
　● T63.071　Toxic effect of venom of other Australian snake, accidental (unintentional)
　　　　　　Toxic effect of venom of other Australian snake NOS
　● T63.072　Toxic effect of venom of other Australian snake, intentional self-harm
　● T63.073　Toxic effect of venom of other Australian snake, assault
　● T63.074　Toxic effect of venom of other Australian snake, undetermined

● T63.08　Toxic effect of venom of other African and Asian snake
　● T63.081　Toxic effect of venom of other African and Asian snake, accidental (unintentional)
　　　　　　Toxic effect of venom of other African and Asian snake NOS
　● T63.082　Toxic effect of venom of other African and Asian snake, intentional self-harm
　● T63.083　Toxic effect of venom of other African and Asian snake, assault
　● T63.084　Toxic effect of venom of other African and Asian snake, undetermined
● T63.09　Toxic effect of venom of other snake
　● T63.091　Toxic effect of venom of other snake, accidental (unintentional)
　　　　　　Toxic effect of venom of other snake NOS
　● T63.092　Toxic effect of venom of other snake, intentional self-harm
　● T63.093　Toxic effect of venom of other snake, assault
　● T63.094　Toxic effect of venom of other snake, undetermined
● T63.1　Toxic effect of venom of other reptiles
　● T63.11　Toxic effect of venom of gila monster
　　● T63.111　Toxic effect of venom of gila monster, accidental (unintentional)
　　　　　　　Toxic effect of venom of gila monster NOS
　　● T63.112　Toxic effect of venom of gila monster, intentional self-harm
　　● T63.113　Toxic effect of venom of gila monster, assault
　　● T63.114　Toxic effect of venom of gila monster, undetermined
　● T63.12　Toxic effect of venom of other venomous lizard
　　● T63.121　Toxic effect of venom of other venomous lizard, accidental (unintentional)
　　　　　　　Toxic effect of venom of other venomous lizard NOS
　　● T63.122　Toxic effect of venom of other venomous lizard, intentional self-harm
　　● T63.123　Toxic effect of venom of other venomous lizard, assault
　　● T63.124　Toxic effect of venom of other venomous lizard, undetermined
　● T63.19　Toxic effect of venom of other reptiles
　　● T63.191　Toxic effect of venom of other reptiles, accidental (unintentional)
　　　　　　　Toxic effect of venom of other reptiles NOS
　　● T63.192　Toxic effect of venom of other reptiles, intentional self-harm
　　● T63.193　Toxic effect of venom of other reptiles, assault
　　● T63.194　Toxic effect of venom of other reptiles, undetermined
● T63.2　Toxic effect of venom of scorpion
　● T63.2X　Toxic effect of venom of scorpion
　　● T63.2X1　Toxic effect of venom of scorpion, accidental (unintentional)
　　　　　　　Toxic effect of venom of scorpion NOS
　　● T63.2X2　Toxic effect of venom of scorpion, intentional self-harm
　　● T63.2X3　Toxic effect of venom of scorpion, assault
　　● T63.2X4　Toxic effect of venom of scorpion, undetermined

CHAPTER 19 (S00-T88)

● **T63.3**   Toxic effect of venom of spider

  ● **T63.30**   Toxic effect of unspecified spider venom

    ● **T63.301**   Toxic effect of unspecified spider venom, accidental (unintentional)

    ● **T63.302**   Toxic effect of unspecified spider venom, intentional self-harm

    ● **T63.303**   Toxic effect of unspecified spider venom, assault

    ● **T63.304**   Toxic effect of unspecified spider venom, undetermined

  ● **T63.31**   Toxic effect of venom of black widow spider

    ● **T63.311**   Toxic effect of venom of black widow spider, accidental (unintentional)

    ● **T63.312**   Toxic effect of venom of black widow spider, intentional self-harm

    ● **T63.313**   Toxic effect of venom of black widow spider, assault

    ● **T63.314**   Toxic effect of venom of black widow spider, undetermined

  ● **T63.32**   Toxic effect of venom of tarantula

    ● **T63.321**   Toxic effect of venom of tarantula, accidental (unintentional)

    ● **T63.322**   Toxic effect of venom of tarantula, intentional self-harm

    ● **T63.323**   Toxic effect of venom of tarantula, assault

    ● **T63.324**   Toxic effect of venom of tarantula, undetermined

  ● **T63.33**   Toxic effect of venom of brown recluse spider

    ● **T63.331**   Toxic effect of venom of brown recluse spider, accidental (unintentional)

    ● **T63.332**   Toxic effect of venom of brown recluse spider, intentional self-harm

    ● **T63.333**   Toxic effect of venom of brown recluse spider, assault

    ● **T63.334**   Toxic effect of venom of brown recluse spider, undetermined

  ● **T63.39**   Toxic effect of venom of other spider

    ● **T63.391**   Toxic effect of venom of other spider, accidental (unintentional)

    ● **T63.392**   Toxic effect of venom of other spider, intentional self-harm

    ● **T63.393**   Toxic effect of venom of other spider, assault

    ● **T63.394**   Toxic effect of venom of other spider, undetermined

● **T63.4**   Toxic effect of venom of other arthropods

  ● **T63.41**   Toxic effect of venom of centipedes and venomous millipedes

    ● **T63.411**   Toxic effect of venom of centipedes and venomous millipedes, accidental (unintentional)

    ● **T63.412**   Toxic effect of venom of centipedes and venomous millipedes, intentional self-harm

    ● **T63.413**   Toxic effect of venom of centipedes and venomous millipedes, assault

    ● **T63.414**   Toxic effect of venom of centipedes and venomous millipedes, undetermined

  ● **T63.42**   Toxic effect of venom of ants

    ● **T63.421**   Toxic effect of venom of ants, accidental (unintentional)

    ● **T63.422**   Toxic effect of venom of ants, intentional self-harm

    ● **T63.423**   Toxic effect of venom of ants, assault

    ● **T63.424**   Toxic effect of venom of ants, undetermined

● **T63.43**   Toxic effect of venom of caterpillars

    ● **T63.431**   Toxic effect of venom of caterpillars, accidental (unintentional)

    ● **T63.432**   Toxic effect of venom of caterpillars, intentional self-harm

    ● **T63.433**   Toxic effect of venom of caterpillars, assault

    ● **T63.434**   Toxic effect of venom of caterpillars, undetermined

  ● **T63.44**   Toxic effect of venom of bees

    ● **T63.441**   Toxic effect of venom of bees, accidental (unintentional)

    ● **T63.442**   Toxic effect of venom of bees, intentional self-harm

    ● **T63.443**   Toxic effect of venom of bees, assault

    ● **T63.444**   Toxic effect of venom of bees, undetermined

  ● **T63.45**   Toxic effect of venom of hornets

    ● **T63.451**   Toxic effect of venom of hornets, accidental (unintentional)

    ● **T63.452**   Toxic effect of venom of hornets, intentional self-harm

    ● **T63.453**   Toxic effect of venom of hornets, assault

    ● **T63.454**   Toxic effect of venom of hornets, undetermined

  ● **T63.46**   Toxic effect of venom of wasps
     Toxic effect of yellow jacket

    ● **T63.461**   Toxic effect of venom of wasps, accidental (unintentional)

    ● **T63.462**   Toxic effect of venom of wasps, intentional self-harm

    ● **T63.463**   Toxic effect of venom of wasps, assault

    ● **T63.464**   Toxic effect of venom of wasps, undetermined

  ● **T63.48**   Toxic effect of venom of other arthropod

    ● **T63.481**   Toxic effect of venom of other arthropod, accidental (unintentional)

    ● **T63.482**   Toxic effect of venom of other arthropod, intentional self-harm

    ● **T63.483**   Toxic effect of venom of other arthropod, assault

    ● **T63.484**   Toxic effect of venom of other arthropod, undetermined

● **T63.5**   Toxic effect of contact with venomous fish

   Excludes2   poisoning by ingestion of fish (T61.-)

  ● **T63.51**   Toxic effect of contact with stingray

    ● **T63.511**   Toxic effect of contact with stingray, accidental (unintentional)

    ● **T63.512**   Toxic effect of contact with stingray, intentional self-harm

    ● **T63.513**   Toxic effect of contact with stingray, assault

    ● **T63.514**   Toxic effect of contact with stingray, undetermined

  ● **T63.59**   Toxic effect of contact with other venomous fish

    ● **T63.591**   Toxic effect of contact with other venomous fish, accidental (unintentional)

    ● **T63.592**   Toxic effect of contact with other venomous fish, intentional self-harm

    ● **T63.593**   Toxic effect of contact with other venomous fish, assault

    ● **T63.594**   Toxic effect of contact with other venomous fish, undetermined

◄ New   ⬅ Revised   ~~deleted~~ Deleted   Excludes 1   Excludes 2   Includes   Use additional   Code first   Code also   Unspecified

OGCR Official Guidelines   X Assign placeholder X   ● Use Additional Character(s)   ▶ Manifestation Code   **Coding Clinic**

● **T63.6**   Toxic effect of contact with other venomous marine animals
> **Excludes1**   sea-snake venom (T63.09)
> **Excludes2**   poisoning by ingestion of shellfish (T61.78-)

● **T63.61**   Toxic effect of contact with Portugese Man-o-war
> Toxic effect of contact with bluebottle

  ● **T63.611**   Toxic effect of contact with Portugese Man-o-war, accidental (unintentional)

  ● **T63.612**   Toxic effect of contact with Portugese Man-o-war, intentional self-harm

  ● **T63.613**   Toxic effect of contact with Portugese Man-o-war, assault

  ● **T63.614**   Toxic effect of contact with Portugese Man-o-war, undetermined

● **T63.62**   Toxic effect of contact with other jellyfish

  ● **T63.621**   Toxic effect of contact with other jellyfish, accidental (unintentional)

  ● **T63.622**   Toxic effect of contact with other jellyfish, intentional self-harm

  ● **T63.623**   Toxic effect of contact with other jellyfish, assault

  ● **T63.624**   Toxic effect of contact with other jellyfish, undetermined

● **T63.63**   Toxic effect of contact with sea anemone

  ● **T63.631**   Toxic effect of contact with sea anemone, accidental (unintentional)

  ● **T63.632**   Toxic effect of contact with sea anemone, intentional self-harm

  ● **T63.633**   Toxic effect of contact with sea anemone, assault

  ● **T63.634**   Toxic effect of contact with sea anemone, undetermined

● **T63.69**   Toxic effect of contact with other venomous marine animals

  ● **T63.691**   Toxic effect of contact with other venomous marine animals, accidental (unintentional)

  ● **T63.692**   Toxic effect of contact with other venomous marine animals, intentional self-harm

  ● **T63.693**   Toxic effect of contact with other venomous marine animals, assault

  ● **T63.694**   Toxic effect of contact with other venomous marine animals, undetermined

● **T63.7**   Toxic effect of contact with venomous plant

● **T63.71**   Toxic effect of contact with venomous marine plant

  ● **T63.711**   Toxic effect of contact with venomous marine plant, accidental (unintentional)

  ● **T63.712**   Toxic effect of contact with venomous marine plant, intentional self-harm

  ● **T63.713**   Toxic effect of contact with venomous marine plant, assault

  ● **T63.714**   Toxic effect of contact with venomous marine plant, undetermined

● **T63.79**   Toxic effect of contact with other venomous plant

  ● **T63.791**   Toxic effect of contact with other venomous plant, accidental (unintentional)

  ● **T63.792**   Toxic effect of contact with other venomous plant, intentional self-harm

  ● **T63.793**   Toxic effect of contact with other venomous plant, assault

  ● **T63.794**   Toxic effect of contact with other venomous plant, undetermined

● **T63.8**   Toxic effect of contact with other venomous animals

● **T63.81**   Toxic effect of contact with venomous frog
> **Excludes1**   contact with nonvenomous frog (W62.0)

  ● **T63.811**   Toxic effect of contact with venomous frog, accidental (unintentional)

  ● **T63.812**   Toxic effect of contact with venomous frog, intentional self-harm

  ● **T63.813**   Toxic effect of contact with venomous frog, assault

  ● **T63.814**   Toxic effect of contact with venomous frog, undetermined

● **T63.82**   Toxic effect of contact with venomous toad
> **Excludes1**   contact with nonvenomous toad (W62.1)

  ● **T63.821**   Toxic effect of contact with venomous toad, accidental (unintentional)

  ● **T63.822**   Toxic effect of contact with venomous toad, intentional self-harm

  ● **T63.823**   Toxic effect of contact with venomous toad, assault

  ● **T63.824**   Toxic effect of contact with venomous toad, undetermined

● **T63.83**   Toxic effect of contact with other venomous amphibian
> **Excludes1**   contact with nonvenomous amphibian (W62.9)

  ● **T63.831**   Toxic effect of contact with other venomous amphibian, accidental (unintentional)

  ● **T63.832**   Toxic effect of contact with other venomous amphibian, intentional self-harm

  ● **T63.833**   Toxic effect of contact with other venomous amphibian, assault

  ● **T63.834**   Toxic effect of contact with other venomous amphibian, undetermined

● **T63.89**   Toxic effect of contact with other venomous animals

  ● **T63.891**   Toxic effect of contact with other venomous animals, accidental (unintentional)

  ● **T63.892**   Toxic effect of contact with other venomous animals, intentional self-harm

  ● **T63.893**   Toxic effect of contact with other venomous animals, assault

  ● **T63.894**   Toxic effect of contact with other venomous animals, undetermined

● **T63.9**   Toxic effect of contact with unspecified venomous animal

X ● **T63.91**   Toxic effect of contact with unspecified venomous animal, accidental (unintentional)

X ● **T63.92**   Toxic effect of contact with unspecified venomous animal, intentional self-harm

X ● **T63.93**   Toxic effect of contact with unspecified venomous animal, assault

X ● **T63.94**   Toxic effect of contact with unspecified venomous animal, undetermined

CHAPTER 19 (S00-T88)

● **T64 Toxic effect of aflatoxin and other mycotoxin food contaminants**

The appropriate 7th character is to be added to each code from category T64

> A   initial encounter
> D   subsequent encounter
> S   sequela

● **T64.0 Toxic effect of aflatoxin**

X● **T64.01** Toxic effect of aflatoxin, accidental (unintentional)

X● **T64.02** Toxic effect of aflatoxin, intentional self-harm

X● **T64.03** Toxic effect of aflatoxin, assault

X● **T64.04** Toxic effect of aflatoxin, undetermined

● **T64.8 Toxic effect of other mycotoxin food contaminants**

X● **T64.81** Toxic effect of other mycotoxin food contaminants, accidental (unintentional)

X● **T64.82** Toxic effect of other mycotoxin food contaminants, intentional self-harm

X● **T64.83** Toxic effect of other mycotoxin food contaminants, assault

X● **T64.84** Toxic effect of other mycotoxin food contaminants, undetermined

● **T65 Toxic effect of other and unspecified substances**

The appropriate 7th character is to be added to each code from category T65

> A   initial encounter
> D   subsequent encounter
> S   sequela

● **T65.0 Toxic effect of cyanides**

Excludes1 hydrogen cyanide (T57.3-)

● **T65.0X Toxic effect of cyanides**

● **T65.0X1** Toxic effect of cyanides, accidental (unintentional)
Toxic effect of cyanides NOS

● **T65.0X2** Toxic effect of cyanides, intentional self-harm

● **T65.0X3** Toxic effect of cyanides, assault

● **T65.0X4** Toxic effect of cyanides, undetermined

● **T65.1 Toxic effect of strychnine and its salts**

● **T65.1X Toxic effect of strychnine and its salts**

● **T65.1X1** Toxic effect of strychnine and its salts, accidental (unintentional)
Toxic effect of strychnine and its salts NOS

● **T65.1X2** Toxic effect of strychnine and its salts, intentional self-harm

● **T65.1X3** Toxic effect of strychnine and its salts, assault

● **T65.1X4** Toxic effect of strychnine and its salts, undetermined

● **T65.2 Toxic effect of tobacco and nicotine**

Excludes2 nicotine dependence (F17.-)

● **T65.21 Toxic effect of chewing tobacco**

● **T65.211** Toxic effect of chewing tobacco, accidental (unintentional)
Toxic effect of chewing tobacco NOS

● **T65.212** Toxic effect of chewing tobacco, intentional self-harm

● **T65.213** Toxic effect of chewing tobacco, assault

● **T65.214** Toxic effect of chewing tobacco, undetermined

● **T65.22 Toxic effect of tobacco cigarettes**
Toxic effect of tobacco smoke
Use additional code for exposure to second hand tobacco smoke (Z57.31, Z77.22)

● **T65.221** Toxic effect of tobacco cigarettes, accidental (unintentional)
Toxic effect of tobacco cigarettes NOS

● **T65.222** Toxic effect of tobacco cigarettes, intentional self-harm

● **T65.223** Toxic effect of tobacco cigarettes, assault

● **T65.224** Toxic effect of tobacco cigarettes, undetermined

● **T65.29 Toxic effect of other tobacco and nicotine**

● **T65.291** Toxic effect of other tobacco and nicotine, accidental (unintentional)
Toxic effect of other tobacco and nicotine NOS

● **T65.292** Toxic effect of other tobacco and nicotine, intentional self-harm

● **T65.293** Toxic effect of other tobacco and nicotine, assault

● **T65.294** Toxic effect of other tobacco and nicotine, undetermined

● **T65.3 Toxic effect of nitroderivatives and aminoderivatives of benzene and its homologues**
Toxic effect of anilin [benzenamine]
Toxic effect of nitrobenzene
Toxic effect of trinitrotoluene

● **T65.3X Toxic effect of nitroderivatives and aminoderivatives of benzene and its homologues**

● **T65.3X1** Toxic effect of nitroderivatives and aminoderivatives of benzene and its homologues, accidental (unintentional)
Toxic effect of nitroderivatives and aminoderivatives of benzene and its homologues NOS

● **T65.3X2** Toxic effect of nitroderivatives and aminoderivatives of benzene and its homologues, intentional self-harm

● **T65.3X3** Toxic effect of nitroderivatives and aminoderivatives of benzene and its homologues, assault

● **T65.3X4** Toxic effect of nitroderivatives and aminoderivatives of benzene and its homologues, undetermined

● **T65.4 Toxic effect of carbon disulfide**

● **T65.4X Toxic effect of carbon disulfide**

● **T65.4X1** Toxic effect of carbon disulfide, accidental (unintentional)
Toxic effect of carbon disulfide NOS

● **T65.4X2** Toxic effect of carbon disulfide, intentional self-harm

● **T65.4X3** Toxic effect of carbon disulfide, assault

● **T65.4X4** Toxic effect of carbon disulfide, undetermined

◄ New   ◄░ Revised   d̶e̶l̶e̶t̶e̶d̶ Deleted   Excludes 1   Excludes 2   Includes   Use additional   Code first   Code also   Unspecified

OGCR Official Guidelines   X Assign placeholder X   ● Use Additional Character(s)   ▸ Manifestation Code   Coding Clinic

CHAPTER 19 (S00-T88)

● **T65.5**   **Toxic effect of nitroglycerin and other nitric acids and esters**
    Toxic effect of 1,2,3-Propanetriol trinitrate
   ● **T65.5X**   **Toxic effect of nitroglycerin and other nitric acids and esters**
     ● **T65.5X1**   **Toxic effect of nitroglycerin and other nitric acids and esters, accidental (unintentional)**
       Toxic effect of nitroglycerin and other nitric acids and esters NOS
     ● **T65.5X2**   **Toxic effect of nitroglycerin and other nitric acids and esters, intentional self-harm**
     ● **T65.5X3**   **Toxic effect of nitroglycerin and other nitric acids and esters, assault**
     ● **T65.5X4**   **Toxic effect of nitroglycerin and other nitric acids and esters, undetermined**

● **T65.6**   **Toxic effect of paints and dyes, not elsewhere classified**
   ● **T65.6X**   **Toxic effect of paints and dyes, not elsewhere classified**
     ● **T65.6X1**   **Toxic effect of paints and dyes, not elsewhere classified, accidental (unintentional)**
       Toxic effect of paints and dyes NOS
     ● **T65.6X2**   **Toxic effect of paints and dyes, not elsewhere classified, intentional self-harm**
     ● **T65.6X3**   **Toxic effect of paints and dyes, not elsewhere classified, assault**
     ● **T65.6X4**   **Toxic effect of paints and dyes, not elsewhere classified, undetermined**

● **T65.8**   **Toxic effect of other specified substances**
   ● **T65.81**   **Toxic effect of latex**
     ● **T65.811**   **Toxic effect of latex, accidental (unintentional)**
       Toxic effect of latex NOS
     ● **T65.812**   **Toxic effect of latex, intentional self-harm**
     ● **T65.813**   **Toxic effect of latex, assault**
     ● **T65.814**   **Toxic effect of latex, undetermined**
   ● **T65.82**   **Toxic effect of harmful algae and algae toxins**
     Toxic effect of (harmful) algae bloom NOS
     Toxic effect of blue-green algae bloom
     Toxic effect of brown tide
     Toxic effect of cyanobacteria bloom
     Toxic effect of Florida red tide
     Toxic effect of pfiesteria piscicida
     Toxic effect of red tide
     ● **T65.821**   **Toxic effect of harmful algae and algae toxins, accidental (unintentional)**
       Toxic effect of harmful algae and algae toxins NOS
     ● **T65.822**   **Toxic effect of harmful algae and algae toxins, intentional self-harm**
     ● **T65.823**   **Toxic effect of harmful algae and algae toxins, assault**
     ● **T65.824**   **Toxic effect of harmful algae and algae toxins, undetermined**
   ● **T65.83**   **Toxic effect of fiberglass**
     ● **T65.831**   **Toxic effect of fiberglass, accidental (unintentional)**
       Toxic effect of fiberglass NOS
     ● **T65.832**   **Toxic effect of fiberglass, intentional self-harm**
     ● **T65.833**   **Toxic effect of fiberglass, assault**
     ● **T65.834**   **Toxic effect of fiberglass, undetermined**

● **T65.89**   **Toxic effect of other specified substances**
   ● **T65.891**   **Toxic effect of other specified substances, accidental (unintentional)**
     Toxic effect of other specified substances NOS
   ● **T65.892**   **Toxic effect of other specified substances, intentional self-harm**
   ● **T65.893**   **Toxic effect of other specified substances, assault**
   ● **T65.894**   **Toxic effect of other specified substances, undetermined**

● **T65.9**   **Toxic effect of unspecified substance**
   X● **T65.91**   **Toxic effect of unspecified substance, accidental (unintentional)**
     Poisoning NOS
   X● **T65.92**   **Toxic effect of unspecified substance, intentional self-harm**
   X● **T65.93**   **Toxic effect of unspecified substance, assault**
   X● **T65.94**   **Toxic effect of unspecified substance, undetermined**

OTHER AND UNSPECIFIED EFFECTS OF EXTERNAL CAUSES (T66-T78)

● **T66**   **Radiation sickness, unspecified**
   Excludes1   specified adverse effects of radiation, such as:
     burns (T20-T31)
     leukemia (C91-C95)
     radiation gastroenteritis and colitis (K52.0)
     radiation pneumonitis (J70.0)
     radiation related disorders of the skin and subcutaneous tissue (L55-L59)
     sunburn (L55.-)

   The appropriate 7th character is to be added to code T66

A	initial encounter
D	subsequent encounter
S	sequela

● **T67**   **Effects of heat and light**
   Excludes1   erythema [dermatitis] ab igne (L59.0)
     malignant hyperpyrexia due to anesthesia (T88.3)
     radiation-related disorders of the skin and subcutaneous tissue (L55-L59)
   Excludes2   burns (T20-T31)
     sunburn (L55.-)
     sweat disorder due to heat (L74-L75)

   The appropriate 7th character is to be added to each code from category T67

A	initial encounter
D	subsequent encounter
S	sequela

X● **T67.0**   **Heatstroke and sunstroke**
   Heat apoplexy
   Heat pyrexia
   Siriasis
   Thermoplegia
   Use additional code(s) to identify any associated complications of heatstroke, such as:
     coma and stupor (R40.-)
     systemic inflammatory response syndrome (R65.1-)

X● **T67.1**   **Heat syncope**
   Heat collapse

X● **T67.2**   **Heat cramp**

X● **T67.3**   **Heat exhaustion, anhydrotic**
   Heat prostration due to water depletion
   Excludes1   heat exhaustion due to salt depletion (T67.4)

X● **T67.4**   **Heat exhaustion due to salt depletion**
   Heat prostration due to salt (and water) depletion

CHAPTER 19 (S00-T88)

X● **T67.5** Heat exhaustion, unspecified
Heat prostration NOS

X● **T67.6** Heat fatigue, transient

X● **T67.7** Heat edema

X● **T67.8** Other effects of heat and light

X● **T67.9** Effect of heat and light, unspecified

● **T68** Hypothermia
Accidental hypothermia
Hypothermia NOS

Use additional code to identify source of exposure:
Exposure to excessive cold of man-made origin (W93)
Exposure to excessive cold of natural origin (X31)

Excludes1 hypothermia following anesthesia (T88.51)
hypothermia not associated with low
environmental temperature (R68.0)
hypothermia of newborn (P80.-)

Excludes2 frostbite (T33-T34)

The appropriate 7th character is to be added to code T68

A	initial encounter
D	subsequent encounter
S	sequela

● **T69** Other effects of reduced temperature
Use additional code to identify source of exposure:
Exposure to excessive cold of man-made origin (W93)
Exposure to excessive cold of natural origin (X31)

Excludes2 frostbite (T33-T34)

The appropriate 7th character is to be added to each code from
category T69

A	initial encounter
D	subsequent encounter
S	sequela

● **T69.0** Immersion hand and foot

● **T69.01** Immersion hand

● **T69.011** Immersion hand, right hand

● **T69.012** Immersion hand, left hand

● **T69.019** Immersion hand, unspecified hand

● **T69.02** Immersion foot
Trench foot

● **T69.021** Immersion foot, right foot

● **T69.022** Immersion foot, left foot

● **T69.029** Immersion foot, unspecified foot

X● **T69.1** Chilblains

X● **T69.8** Other specified effects of reduced temperature

X● **T69.9** Effect of reduced temperature, unspecified

● **T70** Effects of air pressure and water pressure
The appropriate 7th character is to be added to each code from
category T70

A	initial encounter
D	subsequent encounter
S	sequela

X● **T70.0** Otitic barotrauma
Aero-otitis media
Effects of change in ambient atmospheric pressure or
water pressure on ears

X● **T70.1** Sinus barotrauma
Aerosinusitis
Effects of change in ambient atmospheric pressure on
sinuses

● **T70.2** Other and unspecified effects of high altitude

Excludes2 polycythemia due to high altitude (D75.1)

X● **T70.20** Unspecified effects of high altitude

X● **T70.29** Other effects of high altitude
Alpine sickness
Anoxia due to high altitude
Barotrauma NOS
Hypobaropathy
Mountain sickness

X● **T70.3** Caisson disease [decompression sickness]
Compressed-air disease
Diver's palsy or paralysis

X● **T70.4** Effects of high-pressure fluids
Hydraulic jet injection (industrial)
Pneumatic jet injection (industrial)
Traumatic jet injection (industrial)

X● **T70.8** Other effects of air pressure and water pressure

X● **T70.9** Effect of air pressure and water pressure, unspecified

● **T71** Asphyxiation
Mechanical suffocation
Traumatic suffocation

Excludes1 acute respiratory distress (syndrome) (J80)
anoxia due to high altitude (T70.2)
asphyxia NOS (R09.01)
asphyxia from carbon monoxide (T58.-)
asphyxia from inhalation of food or foreign body
(T17.-)
asphyxia from other gases, fumes and vapors
(T59.-)
respiratory distress (syndrome) in newborn
(P22.-)

The appropriate 7th character is to be added to each code from
category T71

A	initial encounter
D	subsequent encounter
S	sequela

● **T71.1** Asphyxiation due to mechanical threat to breathing
Suffocation due to mechanical threat to breathing

● **T71.11** Asphyxiation due to smothering under pillow

● **T71.111** Asphyxiation due to smothering
under pillow, accidental
Asphyxiation due to smothering
under pillow NOS

● **T71.112** Asphyxiation due to smothering
under pillow, intentional self-harm

● **T71.113** Asphyxiation due to smothering
under pillow, assault

● **T71.114** Asphyxiation due to smothering
under pillow, undetermined

● **T71.12** Asphyxiation due to plastic bag

● **T71.121** Asphyxiation due to plastic bag,
accidental
Asphyxiation due to plastic bag
NOS

● **T71.122** Asphyxiation due to plastic bag,
intentional self-harm

● **T71.123** Asphyxiation due to plastic bag,
assault

● **T71.124** Asphyxiation due to plastic bag,
undetermined

◄ New ◄▦ Revised ~~deleted~~ Deleted | Excludes 1 | Excludes 2 | Includes | Use additional | Code first | Code also | Unspecified

OGCR Official Guidelines X Assign placeholder X ● Use Additional Character(s) ▌ Manifestation Code **Coding Clinic**

● **T71.13 Asphyxiation due to being trapped in bed linens**

  ● **T71.131 Asphyxiation due to being trapped in bed linens, accidental**
    Asphyxiation due to being trapped in bed linens NOS

  ● **T71.132 Asphyxiation due to being trapped in bed linens, intentional self-harm**

  ● **T71.133 Asphyxiation due to being trapped in bed linens, assault**

  ● **T71.134 Asphyxiation due to being trapped in bed linens, undetermined**

● **T71.14 Asphyxiation due to smothering under another person's body (in bed)**

  ● **T71.141 Asphyxiation due to smothering under another person's body (in bed), accidental**
    Asphyxiation due to smothering under another person's body (in bed) NOS

  ● **T71.143 Asphyxiation due to smothering under another person's body (in bed), assault**

  ● **T71.144 Asphyxiation due to smothering under another person's body (in bed), undetermined**

● **T71.15 Asphyxiation due to smothering in furniture**

  ● **T71.151 Asphyxiation due to smothering in furniture, accidental**
    Asphyxiation due to smothering in furniture NOS

  ● **T71.152 Asphyxiation due to smothering in furniture, intentional self-harm**

  ● **T71.153 Asphyxiation due to smothering in furniture, assault**

  ● **T71.154 Asphyxiation due to smothering in furniture, undetermined**

● **T71.16 Asphyxiation due to hanging**
  Hanging by window shade cord
  Use additional code for any associated injuries, such as:
  crushing injury of neck (S17.-)
  fracture of cervical vertebrae (S12.0-S12.2-)
  open wound of neck (S11.-)

  ● **T71.161 Asphyxiation due to hanging, accidental**
    Asphyxiation due to hanging NOS
    Hanging NOS

  ● **T71.162 Asphyxiation due to hanging, intentional self-harm**

  ● **T71.163 Asphyxiation due to hanging, assault**

  ● **T71.164 Asphyxiation due to hanging, undetermined**

● **T71.19 Asphyxiation due to mechanical**
  Threat to breathing due to other causes

  ● **T71.191 Asphyxiation due to mechanical threat to breathing due to other causes, accidental**
    Asphyxiation due to other causes NOS

  ● **T71.192 Asphyxiation due to mechanical threat to breathing due to other causes, intentional self-harm**

  ● **T71.193 Asphyxiation due to mechanical threat to breathing due to other causes, assault**

  ● **T71.194 Asphyxiation due to mechanical threat to breathing due to other causes, undetermined**

● **T71.2 Asphyxiation due to systemic oxygen deficiency due to low oxygen content in ambient air**
  Suffocation due to systemic oxygen deficiency due to low oxygen content in ambient air

X ● **T71.20 Asphyxiation due to systemic oxygen deficiency due to low oxygen content in ambient air due to unspecified cause**

X ● **T71.21 Asphyxiation due to cave-in or falling earth**
  Use additional code for any associated cataclysm (X34-X38)

● **T71.22 Asphyxiation due to being trapped in a car trunk**

  ● **T71.221 Asphyxiation due to being trapped in a car trunk, accidental**

  ● **T71.222 Asphyxiation due to being trapped in a car trunk, intentional self-harm**

  ● **T71.223 Asphyxiation due to being trapped in a car trunk, assault**

  ● **T71.224 Asphyxiation due to being trapped in a car trunk, undetermined**

● **T71.23 Asphyxiation due to being trapped in a (discarded) refrigerator**

  ● **T71.231 Asphyxiation due to being trapped in a (discarded) refrigerator, accidental**

  ● **T71.232 Asphyxiation due to being trapped in a (discarded) refrigerator, intentional self-harm**

  ● **T71.233 Asphyxiation due to being trapped in a (discarded) refrigerator, assault**

  ● **T71.234 Asphyxiation due to being trapped in a (discarded) refrigerator, undetermined**

X ● **T71.29 Asphyxiation due to being trapped in other low oxygen environment**

X ● **T71.9 Asphyxiation due to unspecified cause**
  Suffocation (by strangulation) due to unspecified cause
  Suffocation NOS
  Systemic oxygen deficiency due to low oxygen content in ambient air due to unspecified cause
  Systemic oxygen deficiency due to mechanical threat to breathing due to unspecified cause
  Traumatic asphyxia NOS

● **T73 Effects of other deprivation**
  The appropriate 7th character is to be added to each code from category T73

A	initial encounter
D	subsequent encounter
S	sequela

X ● **T73.0 Starvation**
  Deprivation of food

X ● **T73.1 Deprivation of water**

X ● **T73.2 Exhaustion due to exposure**

X ● **T73.3 Exhaustion due to excessive exertion**
  Exhaustion due to overexertion

X ● **T73.8 Other effects of deprivation**

X ● **T73.9 Effect of deprivation, unspecified**

CHAPTER 19 (S00–T88)

● **T74** **Adult and child abuse, neglect and other maltreatment, confirmed**

> Use additional code, if applicable, to identify any associated current injury
> external cause code to identify perpetrator, if known (Y07.-)
>
> **Excludes1**   abuse and maltreatment in pregnancy (O9A.3-, O9A.4-, O9A.5-)
>   adult and child maltreatment, suspected (T76.-)
>
> The appropriate 7th character is to be added to each code from category T74
>
> | A | initial encounter |
> |---|---|
> | D | subsequent encounter |
> | S | sequela |

  ● **T74.0** **Neglect or abandonment, confirmed**
    X● **T74.01**   Adult neglect or abandonment, confirmed   A
    X● **T74.02**   Child neglect or abandonment, confirmed   P
  ● **T74.1** **Physical abuse, confirmed**
       Excludes2   sexual abuse (T74.2-)
    X● **T74.11**   Adult physical abuse, confirmed   A
    X● **T74.12**   Child physical abuse, confirmed   P
         Excludes2   shaken infant syndrome (T74.4)
  ● **T74.2** **Sexual abuse, confirmed**
     Rape, confirmed
     Sexual assault, confirmed
    X● **T74.21**   Adult sexual abuse, confirmed   A
    X● **T74.22**   Child sexual abuse, confirmed   P
  ● **T74.3** **Psychological abuse, confirmed**
    X● **T74.31**   Adult psychological abuse, confirmed   A
    X● **T74.32**   Child psychological abuse, confirmed   P
  X● **T74.4** **Shaken infant syndrome**   P
  ● **T74.9** **Unspecified maltreatment, confirmed**
    X● **T74.91**   Unspecified adult maltreatment, confirmed   A
    X● **T74.92**   Unspecified child maltreatment, confirmed   P

● **T75** **Other and unspecified effects of other external causes**

> **Excludes1**   adverse effects NEC (T78.-)
> **Excludes2**   burns (electric) (T20-T31)
>
> The appropriate 7th character is to be added to each code from category T75
>
> | A | initial encounter |
> |---|---|
> | D | subsequent encounter |
> | S | sequela |

  ● **T75.0** **Effects of lightning**
     Struck by lightning
    X● **T75.00**   Unspecified effects of lightning
         Struck by lightning NOS
    X● **T75.01**   Shock due to being struck by lightning
    X● **T75.09**   Other effects of lightning
         Use additional code for other effects of lightning
  X● **T75.1** **Unspecified effects of drowning and nonfatal submersion**
     Immersion
      Excludes1   specified effects of drowning code to effects

---

  ● **T75.2** **Effects of vibration**
    X● **T75.20**   Unspecified effects of vibration
    X● **T75.21**   Pneumatic hammer syndrome
    X● **T75.22**   Traumatic vasospastic syndrome
    X● **T75.23**   Vertigo from infrasound
         Excludes1   vertigo NOS (R42)
    X● **T75.29**   Other effects of vibration
  X● **T75.3** **Motion sickness**
     Airsickness   Travel sickness
     Seasickness
     Use additional external cause code to identify vehicle or type of motion (Y92.81-, Y93.5-)
  X● **T75.4** **Electrocution**
     Shock from electric current
     Shock from electroshock gun (taser)
  ● **T75.8** **Other specified effects of external causes**
    X● **T75.81**   Effects of abnormal gravitation [G] forces
    X● **T75.82**   Effects of weightlessness
    X● **T75.89**   Other effects of external causes

● **T76** **Adult and child abuse, neglect and other maltreatment, suspected**

> Use additional code, if applicable, to identify any associated current injury
>
> **Excludes1**   adult and child maltreatment, confirmed (T74.-)
>   suspected abuse and maltreatment in pregnancy (O9A.3-, O9A.4-, O9A.5-)
>   suspected adult physical abuse, ruled out (Z04.71)
>   suspected adult sexual abuse, ruled out (Z04.41)
>   suspected child physical abuse, ruled out (Z04.72)
>   suspected child sexual abuse, ruled out (Z04.42)
>
> The appropriate 7th character is to be added to each code from category T76
>
> | A | initial encounter |
> |---|---|
> | D | subsequent encounter |
> | S | sequela |

  ● **T76.0** **Neglect or abandonment, suspected**
    X● **T76.01**   Adult neglect or abandonment, suspected   A
    X● **T76.02**   Child neglect or abandonment, suspected   P
  ● **T76.1** **Physical abuse, suspected**
    X● **T76.11**   Adult physical abuse, suspected   A
    X● **T76.12**   Child physical abuse, suspected   P
  ● **T76.2** **Sexual abuse, suspected**
     Rape, suspected
     Sexual abuse, suspected
      Excludes1   alleged abuse, ruled out (Z04.7)
    X● **T76.21**   Adult sexual abuse, suspected   A
    X● **T76.22**   Child sexual abuse, suspected   P
  ● **T76.3** **Psychological abuse, suspected**
    X● **T76.31**   Adult psychological abuse, suspected   A
    X● **T76.32**   Child psychological abuse, suspected   P
  ● **T76.9** **Unspecified maltreatment, suspected**
    X● **T76.91**   Unspecified adult maltreatment, suspected   A
    X● **T76.92**   Unspecified child maltreatment, suspected   P

◄ New   ⬅ Revised   ~~deleted~~ Deleted   Excludes 1   Excludes 2   Includes   Use additional   Code first   Code also   Unspecified

OGCR Official Guidelines   **X** Assign placeholder X   ● Use Additional Character(s)   ⧫ Manifestation Code   **Coding Clinic**

● **T78**   **Adverse effects, not elsewhere classified**

    Excludes2   complications of surgical and medical care NEC (T80-T88)

    The appropriate 7th character is to be added to each code from category T78

        A   initial encounter
        D   subsequent encounter
        S   sequela

● **T78.0**   **Anaphylactic reaction due to food**
       Anaphylactic reaction due to adverse food reaction
       Anaphylactic shock or reaction due to nonpoisonous foods
       Anaphylactoid reaction due to food

   X● **T78.00**   **Anaphylactic reaction due to unspecified food**

   X● **T78.01**   **Anaphylactic reaction due to peanuts**

   X● **T78.02**   **Anaphylactic reaction due to shellfish (crustaceans)**

   X● **T78.03**   **Anaphylactic reaction due to other fish**

   X● **T78.04**   **Anaphylactic reaction due to fruits and vegetables**

   X● **T78.05**   **Anaphylactic reaction due to tree nuts and seeds**

        Excludes1   anaphylactic reaction due to peanuts (T78.01)

   X● **T78.06**   **Anaphylactic reaction due to food additives**

   X● **T78.07**   **Anaphylactic reaction due to milk and dairy products**

   X● **T78.08**   **Anaphylactic reaction due to eggs**

   X● **T78.09**   **Anaphylactic reaction due to other food products**

X● **T78.1**   **Other adverse food reactions, not elsewhere classified**
       Use additional code to identify the type of reaction

    Excludes1   anaphylactic reaction or shock due to adverse food reaction (T78.0-)
           anaphylactic reaction due to food (T78.0-)
           bacterial food borne intoxications (A05.-)

    Excludes2   allergic and dietetic gastroenteritis and colitis (K52.2)
           allergic rhinitis due to food (J30.5)
           dermatitis due to food in contact with skin (L23.6, L24.6, L25.4)
           dermatitis due to ingested food (L27.2)

X● **T78.2**   **Anaphylactic shock, unspecified**
       Occurs when allergic response triggers large quantities of histamines, prostaglandins, leukotrienes resulting in systemic vasodilation
       Allergic shock
       Anaphylactic reaction
       Anaphylaxis

    Excludes1   anaphylactic reaction or shock due to adverse effect of correct medicinal substance properly administered (T88.6)
           anaphylactic reaction or shock due to adverse food reaction (T78.0-)
           anaphylactic reaction or shock due to serum (T80.5-)

X● **T78.3**   **Angioneurotic edema**
       Allergic angioedema
       Giant urticaria
       Vascular disorder resulting from abnormalities of autonomic nervous system fibers supplying blood vessels
       Quincke's edema

    Excludes1   serum urticaria (T80.6-)
           urticaria (L50.-)

● **T78.4**   **Other and unspecified allergy**

    Excludes1   specified types of allergic reaction such as:
           allergic diarrhea (K52.2)
           allergic gastroenteritis and colitis (K52.2)
           dermatitis (L23-L25, L27.-)
           hay fever (J30.1)

   X● **T78.40**   **Allergy, unspecified**
         Allergic reaction NOS
         Hypersensitivity NOS

   X● **T78.41**   **Arthus phenomenon**
         Arthus reaction

   X● **T78.49**   **Other allergy**

X● **T78.8**   **Other adverse effects, not elsewhere classified**

CERTAIN EARLY COMPLICATIONS OF TRAUMA (T79)

● **T79**   **Certain early complications of trauma, not elsewhere classified**

    Excludes2   acute respiratory distress syndrome (J80)
           complications occurring during or following medical procedures (T80-T88)
           complications of surgical and medical care NEC (T80-T88)
           newborn respiratory distress syndrome (P22.0)

    The appropriate 7th character is to be added to each code from category T79

        A   initial encounter
        D   subsequent encounter
        S   sequela

X● **T79.0**   **Air embolism (traumatic)**

    Excludes1   air embolism complicating abortion or ectopic or molar pregnancy (O00-O07, O08.2)
           air embolism complicating pregnancy, childbirth and the puerperium (O88.0)
           air embolism following infusion, transfusion, and therapeutic injection (T80.0)
           air embolism following procedure NEC (T81.7-)

X● **T79.1**   **Fat embolism (traumatic)**

    Excludes1   fat embolism complicating:
           abortion or ectopic or molar pregnancy (O00-O07, O08.2)
           pregnancy, childbirth and the puerperium (O88.8)

X● **T79.2**   **Traumatic secondary and recurrent hemorrhage and seroma**

CHAPTER 19 (S00-T88)

X● **T79.4 Traumatic shock**
Shock (immediate) (delayed) following injury

> **Excludes1**   anaphylactic shock due to adverse food
> reaction (T78.0-)
> anaphylactic shock due to correct
> medicinal substance properly
> administered (T88.6)
> anaphylactic shock due to serum (T80.5-)
> anaphylactic shock NOS (T78.2)
> anesthetic shock (T88.2)
> electric shock (T75.4)
> nontraumatic shock NEC (R57.-)
> obstetric shock (O75.1)
> postprocedural shock (T81.1-)
> septic shock (R65.21)
> shock complicating abortion or ectopic or
> molar pregnancy (O00-O07, O08.3)
> shock due to lightning (T75.01)
> shock NOS (R57.9)

X● **T79.5 Traumatic anuria**
Crush syndrome
Renal failure following crushing

X● **T79.6 Traumatic ischemia of muscle**
Traumatic rhabdomyolysis
Volkmann's ischemic contracture

> **Excludes2**   anterior tibial syndrome (M76.8)
> compartment syndrome (traumatic)
> (T79.A-)
> nontraumatic ischemia of muscle (M62.2-)

X● **T79.7 Traumatic subcutaneous emphysema**

> **Excludes1**   emphysema NOS (J43)
> emphysema (subcutaneous) resulting
> from a procedure (T81.82)

● **T79.A Traumatic compartment syndrome**

> **Excludes1**   fibromyalgia (M79.7)
> nontraumatic compartment syndrome
> (M79.A-)
> traumatic ischemic infarction of muscle
> (T79.6)

   X● **T79.A0 Compartment syndrome, unspecified**
Compartment syndrome NOS

   ● **T79.A1 Traumatic compartment syndrome of upper
extremity**
Traumatic compartment syndrome of shoulder,
arm, forearm, wrist, hand, and fingers

     ● **T79.A11 Traumatic compartment syndrome of
right upper extremity**

     ● **T79.A12 Traumatic compartment syndrome of
left upper extremity**

     ● **T79.A19 Traumatic compartment syndrome of
unspecified upper extremity**

   ● **T79.A2 Traumatic compartment syndrome of lower
extremity**
Traumatic compartment syndrome of hip,
buttock, thigh, leg, foot, and toes

     ● **T79.A21 Traumatic compartment syndrome of
right lower extremity**

     ● **T79.A22 Traumatic compartment syndrome of
left lower extremity**

     ● **T79.A29 Traumatic compartment syndrome of
unspecified lower extremity**

   X● **T79.A3 Traumatic compartment syndrome of abdomen**

   X● **T79.A9 Traumatic compartment syndrome of other sites**

X● **T79.8 Other early complications of trauma**

X● **T79.9 Unspecified early complication of trauma**

COMPLICATIONS OF SURGICAL AND MEDICAL CARE, NOT ELSEWHERE CLASSIFIED (T80-T88)

Use additional code for adverse effect, if applicable, to identify
drug (T36-T50 with fifth or sixth character 5)

Use additional code(s) to identify the specified condition
resulting from the complication.

Use additional code to identify devices involved and details of
circumstances (Y62-Y82)

> **Excludes2**   any encounters with medical care for
> postprocedural conditions in which no
> complications are present, such as:
> artificial opening status (Z93.-)
> closure of external stoma (Z43.-)
> fitting and adjustment of external prosthetic
> device (Z44.-)
> burns and corrosions from local applications and
> irradiation (T20-T32)
> complications of surgical procedures during
> pregnancy, childbirth and the puerperium
> (O00-O9A)
> mechanical complication of respirator [ventilator]
> (J95.850)
> poisoning and toxic effects of drugs and
> chemicals (T36-T65 with fifth or sixth
> character 1-4 or 6)
> postprocedural fever (R50.82)
> specified complications classified elsewhere, such
> as:
> cerebrospinal fluid leak from spinal puncture
> (G97.0)
> colostomy malfunction (K94.0-)
> disorders of fluid and electrolyte imbalance
> (E86-E87)
> functional disturbances following cardiac
> surgery (I97.0-I97.1)
> intraoperative and postprocedural
> complications of specified body systems
> (D78.-, E36.-, E89.-, G97.3-, G97.4, H59.3-,
> H59.-, H95.2-, H95.3, I97.4-, I97.5, J95.6-,
> J95.7, K91.6-, L76.-, M96.-, N99.-)
> ostomy complications (J95.0-, K94.-, N99.5-)
> postgastric surgery syndromes (K91.1)
> postlaminectomy syndrome NEC (M96.1)
> postmastectomy lymphedema syndrome
> (I97.2)
> postsurgical blind-loop syndrome (K91.2)
> ventilator associated pneumonia (J95.851)

● **T80 Complications following infusion, transfusion and therapeutic
injection**

> **Includes**   complications following perfusion
> **Excludes2**   bone marrow transplant rejection (T86.01)
> febrile nonhemolytic transfusion reaction (R50.84)
> fluid overload due to transfusion (E87.71)
> posttransfusion purpura (D69.51)
> transfusion associated circulatory overload
> (TACO) (E87.71)
> transfusion (red blood cell) associated
> hemochromatosis (E83.111)
> transfusion related acute lung injury (TRALI)
> (J95.84)

The appropriate 7th character is to be added to each code from
category T80

> A   initial encounter
> D   subsequent encounter
> S   sequela

X● **T80.0 Air embolism following infusion, transfusion and
therapeutic injection**

◀ New   ◀═ Revised   ~~deleted~~ Deleted   Excludes 1   Excludes 2   Includes   Use additional   Code first   Code also   Unspecified

OGCR Official Guidelines   X Assign placeholder X   ● Use Additional Character(s)   ▶ Manifestation Code   **Coding Clinic**

X● **T80.1**   **Vascular complications following infusion, transfusion and therapeutic injection**

Use additional code to identify the vascular complication

Excludes2   extravasation of vesicant agent (T80.81-)
infiltration of vesicant agent (T80.81-)
vascular complications specified as due to prosthetic devices, implants and grafts (T82.8- T83.8, T84.8-, T85.8)
postprocedural vascular complications (T81.7-)

● **T80.2**   **Infections following infusion, transfusion and therapeutic injection**

Use additional code to identify the specific infection, such as:
sepsis (A41.9)

Use additional code (R65.2-) to identify severe sepsis, if applicable

Excludes2   infections specified as due to prosthetic devices, implants and grafts (T82.6-T82.7, T83.5-T83.6, T84.5-T84.7, T85.7)
postprocedural infections (T81.4)

● **T80.21**   **Infection due to central venous catheter**

● **T80.211**   **Bloodstream infection due to central venous catheter**

Catheter-related bloodstream infection (CRBSI) NOS
Central line-associated bloodstream infection (CLABSI)
Bloodstream infection due to Hickman catheter
Bloodstream infection due to peripherally inserted central catheter (PICC)
Bloodstream infection due to portacath (port-a-cath)
Bloodstream infection due to triple lumen catheter
Bloodstream infection due to umbilical venous catheter

● **T80.212**   **Local infection due to central venous catheter**

Exit or insertion site infection
Local infection due to Hickman catheter
Local infection due to peripherally inserted central catheter (PICC)
Local infection due to portacath (port-a-cath)
Local infection due to triple lumen catheter
Local infection due to umbilical venous catheter
Port or reservoir infection
Tunnel infection

● **T80.218**   **Other infection due to central venous catheter**

Other central line-associated infection
Other infection due to Hickman catheter
Other infection due to peripherally inserted central catheter (PICC)
Other infection due to portacath (port-a-cath)
Other infection due to triple lumen catheter
Other infection due to umbilical venous catheter

● **T80.219**   **Unspecified infection due to central venous catheter**

Central line-associated infection NOS
Unspecified infection due to Hickman catheter
Unspecified infection due to peripherally inserted central catheter (PICC)
Unspecified infection due to portacath (port-a-cath)
Unspecified infection due to triple lumen catheter
Unspecified infection due to umbilical venous catheter

X● **T80.22**   **Acute infection following transfusion, infusion, or injection of blood and blood products**

X● **T80.29**   **Infection following other infusion, transfusion and therapeutic injection**

● **T80.3**   **ABO incompatibility reaction due to transfusion of blood or blood products**

Excludes1   minor blood group antigens reactions (Duffy) (E) (K(ell)) (Kidd) (Lewis) (M) (N) (P) (S) (T80.A)

X● **T80.30**   **ABO incompatibility reaction due to transfusion of blood or blood products, unspecified**

ABO incompatibility blood transfusion NOS
Reaction to ABO incompatibility from transfusion NOS

● **T80.31**   **ABO incompatibility with hemolytic transfusion reaction**

● **T80.310**   **ABO incompatibility with acute hemolytic transfusion reaction**

ABO incompatibility with hemolytic transfusion reaction less than 24 hours after transfusion
Acute hemolytic transfusion reaction (AHTR) due to ABO incompatibility

● **T80.311**   **ABO incompatibility with delayed hemolytic transfusion reaction**

ABO incompatibility with hemolytic transfusion reaction 24 hours or more after transfusion
Delayed hemolytic transfusion reaction (DHTR) due to ABO incompatibility

● **T80.319**   **ABO incompatibility with hemolytic transfusion reaction, unspecified**

ABO incompatibility with hemolytic transfusion reaction at unspecified time after transfusion
Hemolytic transfusion reaction (HTR) due to ABO incompatibility NOS

X● **T80.39**   **Other ABO incompatibility reaction due to transfusion of blood or blood products**

Delayed serologic transfusion reaction (DSTR) from ABO incompatibility
Other ABO incompatible blood transfusion
Other reaction to ABO incompatible blood transfusion

● **T80.4**   **Rh incompatibility reaction due to transfusion of blood or blood products**

Reaction due to incompatibility of Rh antigens (C) (c) (D) (E) (e)

X● **T80.40**   **Rh incompatibility reaction due to transfusion of blood or blood products, unspecified**

Reaction due to Rh factor in transfusion NOS
Rh incompatible blood transfusion NOS

CHAPTER 19 (S00-T88)

● **T80.41 Rh incompatibility with hemolytic transfusion reaction**

   ● **T80.410 Rh incompatibility with acute hemolytic transfusion reaction**

     Acute hemolytic transfusion reaction (AHTR) due to Rh incompatibility

     Rh incompatibility with hemolytic transfusion reaction less than 24 hours after transfusion

   ● **T80.411 Rh incompatibility with delayed hemolytic transfusion reaction**

     Delayed hemolytic transfusion reaction (DHTR) due to Rh incompatibility

     Rh incompatibility with hemolytic transfusion reaction 24 hours or more after transfusion

   ● **T80.419 Rh incompatibility with hemolytic transfusion reaction, unspecified**

     Rh incompatibility with hemolytic transfusion reaction at unspecified time after transfusion

     Hemolytic transfusion reaction (HTR) due to Rh incompatibility NOS

X ● **T80.49 Other Rh incompatibility reaction due to transfusion of blood or blood products**

   Delayed serologic transfusion reaction (DSTR) from Rh incompatibility

   Other reaction to Rh incompatible blood transfusion

● **T80.A Non-ABO incompatibility reaction due to transfusion of blood or blood products**

   Reaction due to incompatibility of minor antigens (Duffy) (Kell) (Kidd) (Lewis) (M) (N) (P) (S)

X ● **T80.A0 Non-ABO incompatibility reaction due to transfusion of blood or blood products, unspecified**

   Non-ABO antigen incompatibility reaction from transfusion NOS

● **T80.A1 Non-ABO incompatibility with hemolytic transfusion reaction**

   ● **T80.A10 Non-ABO incompatibility with acute hemolytic transfusion reaction**

     Acute hemolytic transfusion reaction (AHTR) due to non-ABO incompatibility

     Non-ABO incompatibility with hemolytic transfusion reaction less than 24 hours after transfusion

   ● **T80.A11 Non-ABO incompatibility with delayed hemolytic transfusion reaction**

     Delayed hemolytic transfusion reaction (DHTR) due to non-ABO incompatibility

     Non-ABO incompatibility with hemolytic transfusion reaction 24 or more hours after transfusion

   ● **T80.A19 Non-ABO incompatibility with hemolytic transfusion reaction, unspecified**

     Hemolytic transfusion reaction (HTR) due to non-ABO incompatibility NOS

     Non-ABO incompatibility with hemolytic transfusion reaction at unspecified time after transfusion

X ● **T80.A9 Other non-ABO incompatibility reaction due to transfusion of blood or blood products**

   Delayed serologic transfusion reaction (DSTR) from non-ABO incompatibility

   Other reaction to non-ABO incompatible blood transfusion

● **T80.5 Anaphylactic reaction due to serum**

   Allergic reaction due to serum

   Anaphylactic shock due to serum

   Anaphylactoid reaction due to serum

   Anaphylaxis due to serum

   Excludes1 ABO incompatibility reaction due to transfusion of blood or blood products (T80.3-)

     allergic reaction or shock NOS (T78.2)

     anaphylactic reaction or shock NOS (T78.2)

     anaphylactic reaction or shock due to adverse effect of correct medicinal substance properly administered (T88.6)

     other serum reaction (T80.6-)

X ● **T80.51 Anaphylactic reaction due to administration of blood and blood products**

X ● **T80.52 Anaphylactic reaction due to vaccination**

X ● **T80.59 Anaphylactic reaction due to other serum**

● **T80.6 Other serum reactions**

   Intoxication by serum   Serum sickness

   Protein sickness   Serum urticaria

   Serum rash

   Excludes2 serum hepatitis (B16.-)

X ● **T80.61 Other serum reaction due to administration of blood and blood products**

X ● **T80.62 Other serum reaction due to vaccination**

X ● **T80.69 Other serum reaction due to other serum**

● **T80.8 Other complications following infusion, transfusion and therapeutic injection**

   ● **T80.81 Extravasation of vesicant agent**

     Infiltration of vesicant agent

     ● **T80.810 Extravasation of vesicant antineoplastic chemotherapy**

       Infiltration of vesicant antineoplastic chemotherapy

     ● **T80.818 Extravasation of other vesicant agent**

       Infiltration of other vesicant agent

X ● **T80.89 Other complications following infusion, transfusion and therapeutic injection**

   Delayed serologic transfusion reaction (DSTR), unspecified incompatibility

   Use additional code to identify graft-versus-host reaction, if applicable, (D89.81-)

● **T80.9 Unspecified complication following infusion, transfusion and therapeutic injection**

X ● **T80.90 Unspecified complication following infusion and therapeutic injection**

   ● **T80.91 Hemolytic transfusion reaction, unspecified incompatibility**

     Excludes1 ABO incompatibility with hemolytic transfusion reaction (T80.31-)

       Non-ABO incompatibility with hemolytic transfusion reaction (T80.A1-)

       Rh incompatibility with hemolytic transfusion reaction (T80.41-)

     ● **T80.910 Acute hemolytic transfusion reaction, unspecified incompatibility**

     ● **T80.911 Delayed hemolytic transfusion reaction, unspecified incompatibility**

     ● **T80.919 Hemolytic transfusion reaction, unspecified incompatibility, unspecified as acute or delayed**

       Hemolytic transfusion reaction NOS

X ● **T80.92 Unspecified transfusion reaction**

   Transfusion reaction NOS

◄ New ◄▬ Revised ~~deleted~~ Deleted   Excludes 1   Excludes 2   Includes   Use additional   Code first   Code also   Unspecified

OGCR Official Guidelines   X Assign placeholder X   ● Use Additional Character(s)   ▌ Manifestation Code   **Coding Clinic**

● **T81**   **Complications of procedures, not elsewhere classified**

Use additional code for adverse effect, if applicable, to identify drug (T36-T50 with fifth or sixth character 5)

Excludes2   complications following immunization (T88.0-T88.1)

complications following infusion, transfusion and therapeutic injection (T80.-)

complications of transplanted organs and tissue (T86.-)

poisoning and toxic effects of drugs and chemicals (T36-T65 with fifth or sixth character 1-4 or 6)

specified complications classified elsewhere, such as:

complication of prosthetic devices, implants and grafts (T82-T85)

dermatitis due to drugs and medicaments (L23.3, L24.4, L25.1, L27.0-L27.1)

endosseous dental implant failure (M27.6-)

floppy iris syndrome (IFIS) (intraoperative) H21.81

intraoperative and postprocedural complications of specific body system (D78.-, E36.-, E89.-, G97.3-, G97.4, H59.3-, H59.-, H95.2-, H95.3, I97.4-, I97.5, J95, K91.-, L76.-, M96.-, N99.-)

ostomy complications (J95.0-, K94.-, N99.5-)

plateau iris syndrome (post-iridectomy) (postprocedural) H21.82

The appropriate 7th character is to be added to each code from category T81

A	initial encounter
D	subsequent encounter
S	sequela

● **T81.1**   **Postprocedural shock**

Shock during or resulting from a procedure, not elsewhere classified

Excludes1   anaphylactic shock NOS (T78.2)

anaphylactic shock due to correct substance properly administered (T88.6)

anaphylactic shock due to serum (T80.5-)

anesthetic shock (T88.2)

electric shock (T75.4)

obstetric shock (O75.1)

septic shock (R65.21)

shock following abortion or ectopic or molar pregnancy (O00-O07, O08.3)

traumatic shock (T79.4)

X● **T81.10**   **Postprocedural shock unspecified**

Collapse NOS during or resulting from a procedure, not elsewhere classified

Postprocedural failure of peripheral circulation

Postprocedural shock NOS

X● **T81.11**   **Postprocedural cardiogenic shock**

X● **T81.12**   **Postprocedural septic shock**

Postprocedural endotoxic shock during or resulting from a procedure, not elsewhere classified

Postprocedural gram-negative shock during or resulting from a procedure, not elsewhere classified

Code first underlying infection

Use additional code, to identify any associated acute organ dysfunction, if applicable

X● **T81.19**   **Other postprocedural shock**

Postprocedural hypovolemic shock

● **T81.3**   **Disruption of wound, not elsewhere classified**

Disruption of any suture materials or other closure methods

Excludes1   breakdown (mechanical) of permanent sutures (T85.612)

displacement of permanent sutures (T85.622)

disruption of cesarean delivery wound (O90.0)

disruption of perineal obstetric wound (O90.1)

mechanical complication of permanent sutures NEC (T85.692)

X● **T81.30**   **Disruption of wound, unspecified**

Disruption of wound NOS

X● **T81.31**   **Disruption of external operation (surgical) wound, not elsewhere classified**

Excludes1   dehiscence of amputation stump (T87.81)

Dehiscence of operation wound NOS

Disruption of operation wound NOS

Disruption or dehiscence of closure of cornea

Disruption or dehiscence of closure of mucosa

Disruption or dehiscence of closure of skin and subcutaneous tissue

Full-thickness skin disruption or dehiscence

Superficial disruption or dehiscence of operation wound

Coding Clinic: 2015, Q1, P20

X● **T81.32**   **Disruption of internal operation (surgical) wound, not elsewhere classified**

Deep disruption or dehiscence of operation wound NOS

Disruption or dehiscence of closure of internal organ or other internal tissue

Disruption or dehiscence of closure of muscle or muscle flap

Disruption or dehiscence of closure of ribs or rib cage

Disruption or dehiscence of closure of skull or craniotomy

Disruption or dehiscence of closure of sternum or sternotomy

Disruption or dehiscence of closure of tendon or ligament

Disruption or dehiscence of closure of superficial or muscular fascia

X● **T81.33**   **Disruption of traumatic injury wound repair**

Disruption or dehiscence of closure of traumatic laceration (external) (internal)

X● **T81.4**   **Infection following a procedure**

Intra-abdominal abscess following a procedure

Postprocedural infection, not elsewhere classified

Sepsis following a procedure

Stitch abscess following a procedure

Subphrenic abscess following a procedure

Wound abscess following a procedure

Use additional code to identify infection

Use additional code (R65.2-) to identify severe sepsis, if applicable

Excludes1   obstetric surgical wound infection (O86.0)

postprocedural fever NOS (R50.82)

postprocedural retroperitoneal abscess (K68.11)

Excludes2   bleb associated endophthalmitis (H59.4-)

infection due to infusion, transfusion and therapeutic injection (T80.2-)

infection due to prosthetic devices, implants and grafts (T82.6-T82.7, T83.5-T83.6, T84.5-T84.7, T85.7)

CHAPTER 19 (S00-T88)

●T81.5　Complications of foreign body accidentally left in body following procedure

　●T81.50　Unspecified complication of foreign body accidentally left in body following procedure

　　●T81.500　Unspecified complication of foreign body accidentally left in body following surgical operation

　　●T81.501　Unspecified complication of foreign body accidentally left in body following infusion or transfusion

　　●T81.502　Unspecified complication of foreign body accidentally left in body following kidney dialysis

　　●T81.503　Unspecified complication of foreign body accidentally left in body following injection or immunization

　　●T81.504　Unspecified complication of foreign body accidentally left in body following endoscopic examination

　　●T81.505　Unspecified complication of foreign body accidentally left in body following heart catheterization

　　●T81.506　Unspecified complication of foreign body accidentally left in body following aspiration, puncture or other catheterization

　　●T81.507　Unspecified complication of foreign body accidentally left in body following removal of catheter or packing

　　●T81.508　Unspecified complication of foreign body accidentally left in body following other procedure

　　●T81.509　Unspecified complication of foreign body accidentally left in body following unspecified procedure

　●T81.51　Adhesions due to foreign body accidentally left in body following procedure

　　●T81.510　Adhesions due to foreign body accidentally left in body following surgical operation

　　●T81.511　Adhesions due to foreign body accidentally left in body following infusion or transfusion

　　●T81.512　Adhesions due to foreign body accidentally left in body following kidney dialysis

　　●T81.513　Adhesions due to foreign body accidentally left in body following injection or immunization

　　●T81.514　Adhesions due to foreign body accidentally left in body following endoscopic examination

　　●T81.515　Adhesions due to foreign body accidentally left in body following heart catheterization

　　●T81.516　Adhesions due to foreign body accidentally left in body following aspiration, puncture or other catheterization

　　●T81.517　Adhesions due to foreign body accidentally left in body following removal of catheter or packing

　　●T81.518　Adhesions due to foreign body accidentally left in body following other procedure

　　●T81.519　Adhesions due to foreign body accidentally left in body following unspecified procedure

　●T81.52　Obstruction due to foreign body accidentally left in body following procedure

　　●T81.520　Obstruction due to foreign body accidentally left in body following surgical operation

　　●T81.521　Obstruction due to foreign body accidentally left in body following infusion or transfusion

　　●T81.522　Obstruction due to foreign body accidentally left in body following kidney dialysis

　　●T81.523　Obstruction due to foreign body accidentally left in body following injection or immunization

　　●T81.524　Obstruction due to foreign body accidentally left in body following endoscopic examination

　　●T81.525　Obstruction due to foreign body accidentally left in body following heart catheterization

　　●T81.526　Obstruction due to foreign body accidentally left in body following aspiration, puncture or other catheterization

　　●T81.527　Obstruction due to foreign body accidentally left in body following removal of catheter or packing

　　●T81.528　Obstruction due to foreign body accidentally left in body following other procedure

　　●T81.529　Obstruction due to foreign body accidentally left in body following unspecified procedure

　●T81.53　Perforation due to foreign body accidentally left in body following procedure

　　●T81.530　Perforation due to foreign body accidentally left in body following surgical operation

　　●T81.531　Perforation due to foreign body accidentally left in body following infusion or transfusion

　　●T81.532　Perforation due to foreign body accidentally left in body following kidney dialysis

　　●T81.533　Perforation due to foreign body accidentally left in body following injection or immunization

　　●T81.534　Perforation due to foreign body accidentally left in body following endoscopic examination

　　●T81.535　Perforation due to foreign body accidentally left in body following heart catheterization

　　●T81.536　Perforation due to foreign body accidentally left in body following aspiration, puncture or other catheterization

　　●T81.537　Perforation due to foreign body accidentally left in body following removal of catheter or packing

　　●T81.538　Perforation due to foreign body accidentally left in body following other procedure

　　●T81.539　Perforation due to foreign body accidentally left in body following unspecified procedure

◄ New　◄ Revised　deleted Deleted　Excludes 1　Excludes 2　Includes　Use additional　Code first　Code also　Unspecified

OGCR Official Guidelines　X Assign placeholder X　● Use Additional Character(s)　▶ Manifestation Code　Coding Clinic

- **T81.59**   **Other complications of foreign body accidentally left in body following procedure**
  - **Excludes2**   obstruction or perforation due to prosthetic devices and implants intentionally left in body (T82.0-T82.5, T83.0-T83.4, T83.7, T84.0-T84.4, T85.0-T85.6)
  - **T81.590**   **Other complications of foreign body accidentally left in body following surgical operation**
  - **T81.591**   **Other complications of foreign body accidentally left in body following infusion or transfusion**
  - **T81.592**   **Other complications of foreign body accidentally left in body following kidney dialysis**
  - **T81.593**   **Other complications of foreign body accidentally left in body following injection or immunization**
  - **T81.594**   **Other complications of foreign body accidentally left in body following endoscopic examination**
  - **T81.595**   **Other complications of foreign body accidentally left in body following heart catheterization**
  - **T81.596**   **Other complications of foreign body accidentally left in body following aspiration, puncture or other catheterization**
  - **T81.597**   **Other complications of foreign body accidentally left in body following removal of catheter or packing**
  - **T81.598**   **Other complications of foreign body accidentally left in body following other procedure**
  - **T81.599**   **Other complications of foreign body accidentally left in body following unspecified procedure**
- **T81.6**   **Acute reaction to foreign substance accidentally left during a procedure**
  - **Excludes2**   complications of foreign body accidentally left in body cavity or operation wound following procedure (T81.5-)
  - X● **T81.60**   **Unspecified acute reaction to foreign substance accidentally left during a procedure**
  - X● **T81.61**   **Aseptic peritonitis due to foreign substance accidentally left during a procedure**
    Chemical peritonitis
  - X● **T81.69**   **Other acute reaction to foreign substance accidentally left during a procedure**
- **T81.7**   **Vascular complications following a procedure, not elsewhere classified**
  Air embolism following procedure NEC
  Phlebitis or thrombophlebitis resulting from a procedure
  - **Excludes1**   embolism complicating abortion or ectopic or molar pregnancy (O00-O07, O08.2)
    embolism complicating pregnancy, childbirth and the puerperium (O88.-)
    traumatic embolism (T79.0)
  - **Excludes2**   embolism due to prosthetic devices, implants and grafts (T82.8, T83.8, T84.8-, T85.8)
    embolism following infusion, transfusion and therapeutic injection (T80.0)

- **T81.71**   **Complication of artery following a procedure, not elsewhere classified**
  - **T81.710**   **Complication of mesenteric artery following a procedure, not elsewhere classified**
  - **T81.711**   **Complication of renal artery following a procedure, not elsewhere classified**
  - **T81.718**   **Complication of other artery following a procedure, not elsewhere classified**
  - **T81.719**   **Complication of unspecified artery following a procedure, not elsewhere classified**
- X● **T81.72**   **Complication of vein following a procedure, not elsewhere classified**
- **T81.8**   **Other complications of procedures, not elsewhere classified**
  - **Excludes2**   hypothermia following anesthesia (T88.51)
    malignant hyperpyrexia due to anesthesia (T88.3)
  - X● **T81.81**   **Complication of inhalation therapy**
  - X● **T81.82**   **Emphysema (subcutaneous) resulting from a procedure**
  - X● **T81.83**   **Persistent postprocedural fistula**
  - X● **T81.89**   **Other complications of procedures, not elsewhere classified**
    Use additional code to specify complication, such as:
    postprocedural delirium (F05)
- X● **T81.9**   **Unspecified complication of procedure**
- ● **T82**   **Complications of cardiac and vascular prosthetic devices, implants and grafts**
  - **Excludes2**   failure and rejection of transplanted organs and tissue (T86.-)
    The appropriate 7th character is to be added to each code from category T82

A	initial encounter
D	subsequent encounter
S	sequela

  - ● **T82.0**   **Mechanical complication of heart valve prosthesis**
    Mechanical complication of artificial heart valve
    - **Excludes1**   mechanical complication of biological heart valve graft (T82.22-)
    - X● **T82.01**   **Breakdown (mechanical) of heart valve prosthesis**
    - X● **T82.02**   **Displacement of heart valve prosthesis**
      Malposition of heart valve prosthesis
    - X● **T82.03**   **Leakage of heart valve prosthesis**
    - X● **T82.09**   **Other mechanical complication of heart valve prosthesis**
      Obstruction (mechanical) of heart valve prosthesis
      Perforation of heart valve prosthesis
      Protrusion of heart valve prosthesis
  - ● **T82.1**   **Mechanical complication of cardiac electronic device**
    - ● **T82.11**   **Breakdown (mechanical) of cardiac electronic device**
      - **T82.110**   **Breakdown (mechanical) of cardiac electrode**
      - **T82.111**   **Breakdown (mechanical) of cardiac pulse generator (battery)**
      - **T82.118**   **Breakdown (mechanical) of other cardiac electronic device**
      - **T82.119**   **Breakdown (mechanical) of unspecified cardiac electronic device**

- T82.12 **Displacement of cardiac electronic device**
  Malposition of cardiac electronic device
  - T82.120 **Displacement of cardiac electrode**
  - T82.121 **Displacement of cardiac pulse generator (battery)**
  - T82.128 **Displacement of other cardiac electronic device**
  - T82.129 **Displacement of unspecified cardiac electronic device**
- T82.19 **Other mechanical complication of cardiac electronic device**
  Leakage of cardiac electronic device
  Obstruction of cardiac electronic device
  Perforation of cardiac electronic device
  Protrusion of cardiac electronic device
  - T82.190 **Other mechanical complication of cardiac electrode**
  - T82.191 **Other mechanical complication of cardiac pulse generator (battery)**
  - T82.198 **Other mechanical complication of other cardiac electronic device**
  - T82.199 **Other mechanical complication of unspecified cardiac device**

- T82.2 **Mechanical complication of coronary artery bypass graft and biological heart valve graft**
  > **Excludes1**   mechanical complication of artificial heart valve prosthesis (T82.0-)
  - T82.21 **Mechanical complication of coronary artery bypass graft**
    - T82.211 **Breakdown (mechanical) of coronary artery bypass graft**
    - T82.212 **Displacement of coronary artery bypass graft**
      Malposition of coronary artery bypass graft
    - T82.213 **Leakage of coronary artery bypass graft**
    - T82.218 **Other mechanical complication of coronary artery bypass graft**
      Obstruction, mechanical of coronary artery bypass graft
      Perforation of coronary artery bypass graft
      Protrusion of coronary artery bypass graft
  - T82.22 **Mechanical complication of biological heart valve graft**
    - T82.221 **Breakdown (mechanical) of biological heart valve graft**
    - T82.222 **Displacement of biological heart valve graft**
      Malposition of biological heart valve graft
    - T82.223 **Leakage of biological heart valve graft**
    - T82.228 **Other mechanical complication of biological heart valve graft**
      Obstruction of biological heart valve graft
      Perforation of biological heart valve graft
      Protrusion of biological heart valve graft

- T82.3 **Mechanical complication of other vascular grafts**
  - T82.31 **Breakdown (mechanical) of other vascular grafts**
    - T82.310 **Breakdown (mechanical) of aortic (bifurcation) graft (replacement)**
    - T82.311 **Breakdown (mechanical) of carotid arterial graft (bypass)**
    - T82.312 **Breakdown (mechanical) of femoral arterial graft (bypass)**
    - T82.318 **Breakdown (mechanical) of other vascular grafts**
    - T82.319 **Breakdown (mechanical) of unspecified vascular grafts**
  - T82.32 **Displacement of other vascular grafts**
    Malposition of other vascular grafts
    - T82.320 **Displacement of aortic (bifurcation) graft (replacement)**
    - T82.321 **Displacement of carotid arterial graft (bypass)**
    - T82.322 **Displacement of femoral arterial graft (bypass)**
    - T82.328 **Displacement of other vascular grafts**
    - T82.329 **Displacement of unspecified vascular grafts**
  - T82.33 **Leakage of other vascular grafts**
    - T82.330 **Leakage of aortic (bifurcation) graft (replacement)**
    - T82.331 **Leakage of carotid arterial graft (bypass)**
    - T82.332 **Leakage of femoral arterial graft (bypass)**
    - T82.338 **Leakage of other vascular grafts**
    - T82.339 **Leakage of unspecified vascular graft**
  - T82.39 **Other mechanical complication of other vascular grafts**
    Obstruction (mechanical) of other vascular grafts
    Perforation of other vascular grafts
    Protrusion of other vascular grafts
    - T82.390 **Other mechanical complication of aortic (bifurcation) graft (replacement)**
    - T82.391 **Other mechanical complication of carotid arterial graft (bypass)**
    - T82.392 **Other mechanical complication of femoral arterial graft (bypass)**
    - T82.398 **Other mechanical complication of other vascular grafts**
    - T82.399 **Other mechanical complication of unspecified vascular grafts**

- T82.4 **Mechanical complication of vascular dialysis catheter**
  Mechanical complication of hemodialysis catheter
  > **Excludes1**   mechanical complication of intraperitoneal dialysis catheter (T85.62)
  - X T82.41 **Breakdown (mechanical) of vascular dialysis catheter**
  - X T82.42 **Displacement of vascular dialysis catheter**
    Malposition of vascular dialysis catheter
  - X T82.43 **Leakage of vascular dialysis catheter**
  - X T82.49 **Other complication of vascular dialysis catheter**
    Obstruction (mechanical) of vascular dialysis catheter
    Perforation of vascular dialysis catheter
    Protrusion of vascular dialysis catheter

◀ New   ◀━ Revised   ~~deleted~~ Deleted   Excludes 1   Excludes 2   Includes   Use additional   Code first   Code also   Unspecified

OGCR Official Guidelines   X Assign placeholder X   ● Use Additional Character(s)   ▶ Manifestation Code   **Coding Clinic**

● T82.5 Mechanical complication of other cardiac and vascular devices and implants

> Excludes2   mechanical complication of epidural and subdural infusion catheter (T85.61)

● T82.51 Breakdown (mechanical) of other cardiac and vascular devices and implants

● T82.510 Breakdown (mechanical) of surgically created arteriovenous fistula

● T82.511 Breakdown (mechanical) of surgically created arteriovenous shunt

● T82.512 Breakdown (mechanical) of artificial heart

● T82.513 Breakdown (mechanical) of balloon (counterpulsation) device

● T82.514 Breakdown (mechanical) of infusion catheter

● T82.515 Breakdown (mechanical) of umbrella device

● T82.518 Breakdown (mechanical) of other cardiac and vascular devices and implants

● T82.519 Breakdown (mechanical) of unspecified cardiac and vascular devices and implants

● T82.52 Displacement of other cardiac and vascular devices and implants

> Malposition of other cardiac and vascular devices and implants

● T82.520 Displacement of surgically created arteriovenous fistula

● T82.521 Displacement of surgically created arteriovenous shunt

● T82.522 Displacement of artificial heart

● T82.523 Displacement of balloon (counterpulsation) device

● T82.524 Displacement of infusion catheter

● T82.525 Displacement of umbrella device

● T82.528 Displacement of other cardiac and vascular devices and implants

● T82.529 Displacement of unspecified cardiac and vascular devices and implants

● T82.53 Leakage of other cardiac and vascular devices and implants

● T82.530 Leakage of surgically created arteriovenous fistula

● T82.531 Leakage of surgically created arteriovenous shunt

● T82.532 Leakage of artificial heart

● T82.533 Leakage of balloon (counterpulsation) device

● T82.534 Leakage of infusion catheter

● T82.535 Leakage of umbrella device

● T82.538 Leakage of other cardiac and vascular devices and implants

● T82.539 Leakage of unspecified cardiac and vascular devices and implants

● T82.59 Other mechanical complication of other cardiac and vascular devices and implants

> Obstruction (mechanical) of other cardiac and vascular devices and implants
> Perforation of other cardiac and vascular devices and implants
> Protrusion of other cardiac and vascular devices and implants

● T82.590 Other mechanical complication of surgically created arteriovenous fistula

● T82.591 Other mechanical complication of surgically created arteriovenous shunt

● T82.592 Other mechanical complication of artificial heart

● T82.593 Other mechanical complication of balloon (counterpulsation) device

● T82.594 Other mechanical complication of infusion catheter

● T82.595 Other mechanical complication of umbrella device

● T82.598 Other mechanical complication of other cardiac and vascular devices and implants

● T82.599 Other mechanical complication of unspecified cardiac and vascular devices and implants

X ● T82.6 Infection and inflammatory reaction due to cardiac valve prosthesis

> Use additional code to identify infection

X ● T82.7 Infection and inflammatory reaction due to other cardiac and vascular devices, implants and grafts

> Use additional code to identify infection

● T82.8 Other specified complications of cardiac and vascular prosthetic devices, implants and grafts

● T82.81 Embolism of cardiac and vascular prosthetic devices, implants and grafts

● T82.817 Embolism of cardiac prosthetic devices, implants and grafts
  Coding Clinic: 2015, Q1, P20

● T82.818 Embolism of vascular prosthetic devices, implants and grafts

● T82.82 Fibrosis of cardiac and vascular prosthetic devices, implants and grafts

● T82.827 Fibrosis of cardiac prosthetic devices, implants and grafts

● T82.828 Fibrosis of vascular prosthetic devices, implants and grafts

● T82.83 Hemorrhage of cardiac and vascular prosthetic devices, implants and grafts

● T82.837 Hemorrhage of cardiac prosthetic devices, implants and grafts

● T82.838 Hemorrhage of vascular prosthetic devices, implants and grafts

● T82.84 Pain from cardiac and vascular prosthetic devices, implants and grafts

● T82.847 Pain from cardiac prosthetic devices, implants and grafts

● T82.848 Pain from vascular prosthetic devices, implants and grafts

● T82.85 Stenosis of cardiac and vascular prosthetic devices, implants and grafts

● T82.857 Stenosis of cardiac prosthetic devices, implants and grafts

● T82.858 Stenosis of vascular prosthetic devices, implants and grafts

● T82.86 Thrombosis of cardiac and vascular prosthetic devices, implants and grafts

● T82.867 Thrombosis of cardiac prosthetic devices, implants and grafts

● T82.868 Thrombosis of vascular prosthetic devices, implants and grafts

● T82.89 Other specified complication of cardiac and vascular prosthetic devices, implants and grafts

● T82.897 Other specified complication of cardiac prosthetic devices, implants and grafts

● T82.898 Other specified complication of vascular prosthetic devices, implants and grafts

X ● T82.9 Unspecified complication of cardiac and vascular prosthetic device, implant and graft

CHAPTER 19 (S00-T88)

● **T83**   **Complications of genitourinary prosthetic devices, implants and grafts**

    Excludes2   failure and rejection of transplanted organs and tissue (T86.-)

    The appropriate 7th character is to be added to each code from category T83

A	initial encounter
D	subsequent encounter
S	sequela

● **T83.0**   **Mechanical complication of urinary (indwelling) catheter**

    Excludes2   complications of stoma of urinary tract (N99.5-)

  ● **T83.01**   **Breakdown (mechanical) of urinary (indwelling) catheter**

    ● **T83.010**   **Breakdown (mechanical) of cystostomy catheter**

    ● **T83.018**   **Breakdown (mechanical) of other indwelling urethral catheter**

  ● **T83.02**   **Displacement of urinary (indwelling) catheter**

    Malposition of urinary (indwelling) catheter

    ● **T83.020**   **Displacement of cystostomy catheter**

    ● **T83.028**   **Displacement of other indwelling urethral catheter**

  ● **T83.03**   **Leakage of urinary (indwelling) catheter**

    ● **T83.030**   **Leakage of cystostomy catheter**

    ● **T83.038**   **Leakage of other indwelling urethral catheter**

  ● **T83.09**   **Other mechanical complication of urinary (indwelling) catheter**

    Obstruction (mechanical) of urinary (indwelling) catheter

    Perforation of urinary (indwelling) catheter

    Protrusion of urinary (indwelling) catheter

    ● **T83.090**   **Other mechanical complication of cystostomy catheter**

    ● **T83.098**   **Other mechanical complication of other indwelling urethral catheter**

● **T83.1**   **Mechanical complication of other urinary devices and implants**

  ● **T83.11**   **Breakdown (mechanical) of other urinary devices and implants**

    ● **T83.110**   **Breakdown (mechanical) of urinary electronic stimulator device**

    ● **T83.111**   **Breakdown (mechanical) of urinary sphincter implant**

    ● **T83.112**   **Breakdown (mechanical) of urinary stent**

    ● **T83.118**   **Breakdown (mechanical) of other urinary devices and implants**

  ● **T83.12**   **Displacement of other urinary devices and implants**

    Malposition of other urinary devices and implants

    ● **T83.120**   **Displacement of urinary electronic stimulator device**

    ● **T83.121**   **Displacement of urinary sphincter implant**

    ● **T83.122**   **Displacement of urinary stent**

    ● **T83.128**   **Displacement of other urinary devices and implants**

● **T83.19**   **Other mechanical complication of other urinary devices and implants**

    Leakage of other urinary devices and implants

    Obstruction (mechanical) of other urinary devices and implants

    Perforation of other urinary devices and implants

    Protrusion of other urinary devices and implants

  ● **T83.190**   **Other mechanical complication of urinary electronic stimulator device**

  ● **T83.191**   **Other mechanical complication of urinary sphincter implant**

  ● **T83.192**   **Other mechanical complication of urinary stent**

  ● **T83.198**   **Other mechanical complication of other urinary devices and implants**

● **T83.2**   **Mechanical complication of graft of urinary organ**

  X● **T83.21**   **Breakdown (mechanical) of graft of urinary organ**

  X● **T83.22**   **Displacement of graft of urinary organ**

    Malposition of graft of urinary organ

  X● **T83.23**   **Leakage of graft of urinary organ**

  X● **T83.29**   **Other mechanical complication of graft of urinary organ**

    Obstruction (mechanical) of graft of urinary organ

    Perforation of graft of urinary organ

    Protrusion of graft of urinary organ

● **T83.3**   **Mechanical complication of intrauterine contraceptive device**

  X● **T83.31**   **Breakdown (mechanical) of intrauterine contraceptive device ♀**

  X● **T83.32**   **Displacement of intrauterine contraceptive device ♀**

    Malposition of intrauterine contraceptive device

  X● **T83.39**   **Other mechanical complication of intrauterine contraceptive device ♀**

    Leakage of intrauterine contraceptive device

    Obstruction (mechanical) of intrauterine contraceptive device

    Perforation of intrauterine contraceptive device

    Protrusion of intrauterine contraceptive device

● **T83.4**   **Mechanical complication of other prosthetic devices, implants and grafts of genital tract**

  ● **T83.41**   **Breakdown (mechanical) of other prosthetic devices, implants and grafts of genital tract**

    ● **T83.410**   **Breakdown (mechanical) of penile (implanted) prosthesis ♂**

    ● **T83.418**   **Breakdown (mechanical) of other prosthetic devices, implants and grafts of genital tract**

  ● **T83.42**   **Displacement of other prosthetic devices, implants and grafts of genital tract**

    Malposition of other prosthetic devices, implants and grafts of genital tract

    ● **T83.420**   **Displacement of penile (implanted) prosthesis ♂**

    ● **T83.428**   **Displacement of other prosthetic devices, implants and grafts of genital tract**

◀ New   ⬅ Revised   ~~deleted~~ Deleted   Excludes 1   Excludes 2   Includes   Use additional   Code first   Code also   Unspecified

OGCR Official Guidelines   X Assign placeholder X   ● Use Additional Character(s)   ▶ Manifestation Code   **Coding Clinic**

● T83.49　Other mechanical complication of other prosthetic devices, implants and grafts of genital tract
　　　　Leakage of other prosthetic devices, implants and grafts of genital tract
　　　　Obstruction, mechanical of other prosthetic devices, implants and grafts of genital tract
　　　　Perforation of other prosthetic devices, implants and grafts of genital tract
　　　　Protrusion of other prosthetic devices, implants and grafts of genital tract

　　● T83.490　Other mechanical complication of penile (implanted) prosthesis ♂

　　● T83.498　Other mechanical complication of other prosthetic devices, implants and grafts of genital tract

● T83.5　Infection and inflammatory reaction due to prosthetic device, implant and graft in urinary system
　　　Use additional code to identify infection

　X ● T83.51　Infection and inflammatory reaction due to indwelling urinary catheter
　　　　Excludes2　complications of stoma of urinary tract (N99.5-)

　X ● T83.59　Infection and inflammatory reaction due to prosthetic device, implant and graft in urinary system

X ● T83.6　Infection and inflammatory reaction due to prosthetic device, implant and graft in genital tract
　　　Use additional code to identify infection

● T83.7　Complications due to implanted mesh and other prosthetic materials

　● T83.71　Erosion of implanted mesh and other prosthetic materials to surrounding organ or tissue

　　● T83.711　Erosion of implanted vaginal mesh and other prosthetic materials to surrounding organ or tissue
　　　　　　Erosion of implanted vaginal mesh and other prosthetic materials into pelvic floor muscles

　　● T83.718　Erosion of other implanted mesh and other prosthetic materials to surrounding organ or tissue

　● T83.72　Exposure of implanted mesh and other prosthetic materials into surrounding organ or tissue

　　● T83.721　Exposure of implanted vaginal mesh and other prosthetic materials into vagina
　　　　　　Exposure of implanted vaginal mesh and other prosthetic materials through vaginal wall

　　● T83.728　Exposure of other implanted mesh and other prosthetic materials to surrounding organ or tissue

● T83.8　Other specified complications of genitourinary prosthetic devices, implants and grafts

　X ● T83.81　Embolism of genitourinary prosthetic devices, implants and grafts

　X ● T83.82　Fibrosis of genitourinary prosthetic devices, implants and grafts

　X ● T83.83　Hemorrhage of genitourinary prosthetic devices, implants and grafts

　X ● T83.84　Pain from genitourinary prosthetic devices, implants and grafts

　X ● T83.85　Stenosis of genitourinary prosthetic devices, implants and grafts

　X ● T83.86　Thrombosis of genitourinary prosthetic devices, implants and grafts

　X ● T83.89　Other specified complication of genitourinary prosthetic devices, implants and grafts

X ● T83.9　Unspecified complication of genitourinary prosthetic device, implant and graft

● T84　Complications of internal orthopedic prosthetic devices, implants and grafts
　　Excludes2　failure and rejection of transplanted organs and tissues (T86.-)
　　　　　　fracture of bone following insertion of orthopedic implant, joint prosthesis or bone plate (M96.6)

The appropriate 7th character is to be added to each code from category T84

A	initial encounter
D	subsequent encounter
S	sequela

● T84.0　Mechanical complication of internal joint prosthesis

　● T84.01　Broken internal joint prosthesis
　　　　Breakage (fracture) of prosthetic joint
　　　　Broken prosthetic joint implant
　　　　Excludes1　periprosthetic joint implant fracture (T84.04)

　　● T84.010　Broken internal right hip prosthesis
　　● T84.011　Broken internal left hip prosthesis
　　● T84.012　Broken internal right knee prosthesis
　　● T84.013　Broken internal left knee prosthesis
　　● T84.018　Broken internal joint prosthesis, other site
　　　　　　Use additional code to identify the joint (Z96.6-)
　　● T84.019　Broken internal joint prosthesis, unspecified site

　● T84.02　Dislocation of internal joint prosthesis
　　　　Instability of internal joint prosthesis
　　　　Subluxation of internal joint prosthesis

　　● T84.020　Dislocation of internal right hip prosthesis
　　● T84.021　Dislocation of internal left hip prosthesis
　　● T84.022　Instability of internal right knee prosthesis
　　● T84.023　Instability of internal left knee prosthesis
　　● T84.028　Dislocation of other internal joint prosthesis
　　　　　　Use additional code to identify the joint (Z96.6-)
　　● T84.029　Dislocation of unspecified internal joint prosthesis

　● T84.03　Mechanical loosening of internal prosthetic joint
　　　　Aseptic loosening of prosthetic joint

　　● T84.030　Mechanical loosening of internal right hip prosthetic joint
　　● T84.031　Mechanical loosening of internal left hip prosthetic joint
　　● T84.032　Mechanical loosening of internal right knee prosthetic joint
　　● T84.033　Mechanical loosening of internal left knee prosthetic joint
　　● T84.038　Mechanical loosening of other internal prosthetic joint
　　　　　　Use additional code to identify the joint (Z96.6-)
　　● T84.039　Mechanical loosening of unspecified internal prosthetic joint

● **T84.04** **Periprosthetic fracture around internal prosthetic joint**
  Excludes2 breakage (fracture) of prosthetic joint (T84.01)
  ● **T84.040** **Periprosthetic fracture around internal prosthetic right hip joint**
  ● **T84.041** **Periprosthetic fracture around internal prosthetic left hip joint**
  ● **T84.042** **Periprosthetic fracture around internal prosthetic right knee joint**
  ● **T84.043** **Periprosthetic fracture around internal prosthetic left knee joint**
  ● **T84.048** **Periprosthetic fracture around other internal prosthetic joint**
    Use additional code to identify the joint (Z96.6-)
  ● **T84.049** **Periprosthetic fracture around unspecified internal prosthetic joint**

● **T84.05** **Periprosthetic osteolysis of internal prosthetic joint**
  Use additional code to identify major osseous defect, if applicable (M89.7-)
  ● **T84.050** **Periprosthetic osteolysis of internal prosthetic right hip joint**
  ● **T84.051** **Periprosthetic osteolysis of internal prosthetic left hip joint**
  ● **T84.052** **Periprosthetic osteolysis of internal prosthetic right knee joint**
  ● **T84.053** **Periprosthetic osteolysis of internal prosthetic left knee joint**
  ● **T84.058** **Periprosthetic osteolysis of other internal prosthetic joint**
    Use additional code to identify the joint (Z96.6-)
  ● **T84.059** **Periprosthetic osteolysis of unspecified internal prosthetic joint**

● **T84.06** **Wear of articular bearing surface of internal prosthetic joint**
  ● **T84.060** **Wear of articular bearing surface of internal prosthetic right hip joint**
  ● **T84.061** **Wear of articular bearing surface of internal prosthetic left hip joint**
  ● **T84.062** **Wear of articular bearing surface of internal prosthetic right knee joint**
  ● **T84.063** **Wear of articular bearing surface of internal prosthetic left knee joint**
  ● **T84.068** **Wear of articular bearing surface of other internal prosthetic joint**
    Use additional code to identify the joint (Z96.6-)
  ● **T84.069** **Wear of articular bearing surface of unspecified internal prosthetic joint**

● **T84.09** **Other mechanical complication of internal joint prosthesis**
  Prosthetic joint implant failure NOS
  ● **T84.090** **Other mechanical complication of internal right hip prosthesis**
  ● **T84.091** **Other mechanical complication of internal left hip prosthesis**
  ● **T84.092** **Other mechanical complication of internal right knee prosthesis**
  ● **T84.093** **Other mechanical complication of internal left knee prosthesis**
  ● **T84.098** **Other mechanical complication of other internal joint prosthesis**
    Use additional code to identify the joint (Z96.6-)
  ● **T84.099** **Other mechanical complication of unspecified internal joint prosthesis**

● **T84.1** **Mechanical complication of internal fixation device of bones of limb**
  Excludes2 mechanical complication of internal fixation device of bones of feet (T84.2-)
    mechanical complication of internal fixation device of bones of fingers (T84.2-)
    mechanical complication of internal fixation device of bones of hands (T84.2-)
    mechanical complication of internal fixation device of bones of toes (T84.2-)
  ● **T84.11** **Breakdown (mechanical) of internal fixation device of bones of limb**
    ● **T84.110** **Breakdown (mechanical) of internal fixation device of right humerus**
    ● **T84.111** **Breakdown (mechanical) of internal fixation device of left humerus**
    ● **T84.112** **Breakdown (mechanical) of internal fixation device of bone of right forearm**
    ● **T84.113** **Breakdown (mechanical) of internal fixation device of bone of left forearm**
    ● **T84.114** **Breakdown (mechanical) of internal fixation device of right femur**
    ● **T84.115** **Breakdown (mechanical) of internal fixation device of left femur**
    ● **T84.116** **Breakdown (mechanical) of internal fixation device of bone of right lower leg**
    ● **T84.117** **Breakdown (mechanical) of internal fixation device of bone of left lower leg**
    ● **T84.119** **Breakdown (mechanical) of internal fixation device of unspecified bone of limb**
  ● **T84.12** **Displacement of internal fixation device of bones of limb**
    Malposition of internal fixation device of bones of limb
    ● **T84.120** **Displacement of internal fixation device of right humerus**
    ● **T84.121** **Displacement of internal fixation device of left humerus**
    ● **T84.122** **Displacement of internal fixation device of bone of right forearm**
    ● **T84.123** **Displacement of internal fixation device of bone of left forearm**
    ● **T84.124** **Displacement of internal fixation device of right femur**
    ● **T84.125** **Displacement of internal fixation device of left femur**
    ● **T84.126** **Displacement of internal fixation device of bone of right lower leg**
    ● **T84.127** **Displacement of internal fixation device of bone of left lower leg**
    ● **T84.129** **Displacement of internal fixation device of unspecified bone of limb**

◄ New ◄ Revised ~~deleted~~ Deleted Excludes 1 Excludes 2 Includes Use additional Code first Code also Unspecified
OGCR Official Guidelines X Assign placeholder X ● Use Additional Character(s)) Manifestation Code **Coding Clinic**

● **T84.19**   **Other mechanical complication of internal fixation device of bones of limb**
     Obstruction (mechanical) of internal fixation device of bones of limb
     Perforation of internal fixation device of bones of limb
     Protrusion of internal fixation device of bones of limb

     ● **T84.190**   Other mechanical complication of internal fixation device of right humerus

     ● **T84.191**   Other mechanical complication of internal fixation device of left humerus

     ● **T84.192**   Other mechanical complication of internal fixation device of bone of right forearm

     ● **T84.193**   Other mechanical complication of internal fixation device of bone of left forearm

     ● **T84.194**   Other mechanical complication of internal fixation device of right femur

     ● **T84.195**   Other mechanical complication of internal fixation device of left femur

     ● **T84.196**   Other mechanical complication of internal fixation device of bone of right lower leg

     ● **T84.197**   Other mechanical complication of internal fixation device of bone of left lower leg

     ● **T84.199**   Other mechanical complication of internal fixation device of unspecified bone of limb

● **T84.2**   **Mechanical complication of internal fixation device of other bones**

     ● **T84.21**   **Breakdown (mechanical) of internal fixation device of other bones**

       ● **T84.210**   Breakdown (mechanical) of internal fixation device of bones of hand and fingers

       ● **T84.213**   Breakdown (mechanical) of internal fixation device of bones of foot and toes

       ● **T84.216**   Breakdown (mechanical) of internal fixation device of vertebrae

       ● **T84.218**   Breakdown (mechanical) of internal fixation device of other bones

     ● **T84.22**   **Displacement of internal fixation device of other bones**
       Malposition of internal fixation device of other bones

       ● **T84.220**   Displacement of internal fixation device of bones of hand and fingers

       ● **T84.223**   Displacement of internal fixation device of bones of foot and toes

       ● **T84.226**   Displacement of internal fixation device of vertebrae

       ● **T84.228**   Displacement of internal fixation device of other bones

     ● **T84.29**   **Other mechanical complication of internal fixation device of other bones**
       Obstruction (mechanical) of internal fixation device of other bones
       Perforation of internal fixation device of other bones
       Protrusion of internal fixation device of other bones

       ● **T84.290**   Other mechanical complication of internal fixation device of bones of hand and fingers

       ● **T84.293**   Other mechanical complication of internal fixation device of bones of foot and toes

       ● **T84.296**   Other mechanical complication of internal fixation device of vertebrae

       ● **T84.298**   Other mechanical complication of internal fixation device of other bones

● **T84.3**   **Mechanical complication of other bone devices, implants and grafts**

     Excludes2   other complications of bone graft (T86.83-)

     ● **T84.31**   **Breakdown (mechanical) of other bone devices, implants and grafts**

       ● **T84.310**   Breakdown (mechanical) of electronic bone stimulator

       ● **T84.318**   Breakdown (mechanical) of other bone devices, implants and grafts

     ● **T84.32**   **Displacement of other bone devices, implants and grafts**
       Malposition of other bone devices, implants and grafts

       ● **T84.320**   Displacement of electronic bone stimulator

       ● **T84.328**   Displacement of other bone devices, implants and grafts

     ● **T84.39**   **Other mechanical complication of other bone devices, implants and grafts**
       Obstruction (mechanical) of other bone devices, implants and grafts
       Perforation of other bone devices, implants and grafts
       Protrusion of other bone devices, implants and grafts

       ● **T84.390**   Other mechanical complication of electronic bone stimulator

       ● **T84.398**   Other mechanical complication of other bone devices, implants and grafts

● **T84.4**   **Mechanical complication of other internal orthopedic devices, implants and grafts**

     ● **T84.41**   **Breakdown (mechanical) of other internal orthopedic devices, implants and grafts**

       ● **T84.410**   Breakdown (mechanical) of muscle and tendon graft

       ● **T84.418**   Breakdown (mechanical) of other internal orthopedic devices, implants and grafts

     ● **T84.42**   **Displacement of other internal orthopedic devices, implants and grafts**
       Malposition of other internal orthopedic devices, implants and grafts

       ● **T84.420**   Displacement of muscle and tendon graft

       ● **T84.428**   Displacement of other internal orthopedic devices, implants and grafts

     ● **T84.49**   **Other mechanical complication of other internal orthopedic devices, implants and grafts**
       Mechanical complication of other internal orthopedic devices, implants and grafts NOS
       Obstruction (mechanical) of other internal orthopedic devices, implants and grafts
       Perforation of other internal orthopedic devices, implants and grafts
       Protrusion of other internal orthopedic devices, implants and grafts

       ● **T84.490**   Other mechanical complication of muscle and tendon graft

       ● **T84.498**   Other mechanical complication of other internal orthopedic devices, implants and grafts

● **T84.5**   **Infection and inflammatory reaction due to internal joint prosthesis**

> Use additional code to identify infection
> *Coding Clinic: 2015, Q1, P16*

    X● **T84.50**   Infection and inflammatory reaction due to unspecified internal joint prosthesis
> *Coding Clinic: 2015, Q1, P3*

    X● **T84.51**   Infection and inflammatory reaction due to internal right hip prosthesis

    X● **T84.52**   Infection and inflammatory reaction due to internal left hip prosthesis
> *Coding Clinic: 2015, Q1, P16-17*

    X● **T84.53**   Infection and inflammatory reaction due to internal right knee prosthesis

    X● **T84.54**   Infection and inflammatory reaction due to internal left knee prosthesis

    X● **T84.59**   Infection and inflammatory reaction due to other internal joint prosthesis

● **T84.6**   **Infection and inflammatory reaction due to internal fixation device**

> Use additional code to identify infection

    X● **T84.60**   Infection and inflammatory reaction due to internal fixation device of unspecified site

    ● **T84.61**   Infection and inflammatory reaction due to internal fixation device of arm

       ● **T84.610**   Infection and inflammatory reaction due to internal fixation device of right humerus

       ● **T84.611**   Infection and inflammatory reaction due to internal fixation device of left humerus

       ● **T84.612**   Infection and inflammatory reaction due to internal fixation device of right radius

       ● **T84.613**   Infection and inflammatory reaction due to internal fixation device of left radius

       ● **T84.614**   Infection and inflammatory reaction due to internal fixation device of right ulna

       ● **T84.615**   Infection and inflammatory reaction due to internal fixation device of left ulna

       ● **T84.619**   Infection and inflammatory reaction due to internal fixation device of unspecified bone of arm

    ● **T84.62**   Infection and inflammatory reaction due to internal fixation device of leg

       ● **T84.620**   Infection and inflammatory reaction due to internal fixation device of right femur

       ● **T84.621**   Infection and inflammatory reaction due to internal fixation device of left femur

       ● **T84.622**   Infection and inflammatory reaction due to internal fixation device of right tibia

       ● **T84.623**   Infection and inflammatory reaction due to internal fixation device of left tibia

       ● **T84.624**   Infection and inflammatory reaction due to internal fixation device of right fibula

       ● **T84.625**   Infection and inflammatory reaction due to internal fixation device of left fibula

       ● **T84.629**   Infection and inflammatory reaction due to internal fixation device of unspecified bone of leg

    X● **T84.63**   Infection and inflammatory reaction due to internal fixation device of spine

    X● **T84.69**   Infection and inflammatory reaction due to internal fixation device of other site

● **T84.7**   **Infection and inflammatory reaction due to other internal orthopedic prosthetic devices, implants and grafts**

> Use additional code to identify infection

● **T84.8**   **Other specified complications of internal orthopedic prosthetic devices, implants and grafts**

    X● **T84.81**   Embolism due to internal orthopedic prosthetic devices, implants and grafts

    X● **T84.82**   Fibrosis due to internal orthopedic prosthetic devices, implants and grafts

    X● **T84.83**   Hemorrhage due to internal orthopedic prosthetic devices, implants and grafts

    X● **T84.84**   Pain due to internal orthopedic prosthetic devices, implants and grafts

    X● **T84.85**   Stenosis due to internal orthopedic prosthetic devices, implants and grafts

    X● **T84.86**   Thrombosis due to internal orthopedic prosthetic devices, implants and grafts

    X● **T84.89**   Other specified complication of internal orthopedic prosthetic devices, implants and grafts

X● **T84.9**   **Unspecified complication of internal orthopedic prosthetic device, implant and graft**

● **T85**   **Complications of other internal prosthetic devices, implants and grafts**

> **Excludes2**   failure and rejection of transplanted organs and tissue (T86.-)

> The appropriate 7th character is to be added to each code from category T85

> | | |
> |---|---|
> | A | initial encounter |
> | D | subsequent encounter |
> | S | sequela |

● **T85.0**   **Mechanical complication of ventricular intracranial (communicating) shunt**

    X● **T85.01**   Breakdown (mechanical) of ventricular intracranial (communicating) shunt

    X● **T85.02**   Displacement of ventricular intracranial (communicating) shunt
> Malposition of ventricular intracranial (communicating) shunt

    X● **T85.03**   Leakage of ventricular intracranial (communicating) shunt

    X● **T85.09**   Other mechanical complication of ventricular intracranial (communicating) shunt
> Obstruction (mechanical) of ventricular intracranial (communicating) shunt
> Perforation of ventricular intracranial (communicating) shunt
> Protrusion of ventricular intracranial (communicating) shunt

● **T85.1**   **Mechanical complication of implanted electronic stimulator of nervous system**

    ● **T85.11**   Breakdown (mechanical) of implanted electronic stimulator of nervous system

       ● **T85.110**   Breakdown (mechanical) of implanted electronic neurostimulator (electrode) of brain

       ● **T85.111**   Breakdown (mechanical) of implanted electronic neurostimulator (electrode) of peripheral nerve

       ● **T85.112**   Breakdown (mechanical) of implanted electronic neurostimulator (electrode) of spinal cord

       ● **T85.118**   Breakdown (mechanical) of other implanted electronic stimulator of nervous system

◀ New   ⬅ Revised   ~~deleted~~ Deleted   Excludes 1   Excludes 2   Includes   Use additional   Code first   Code also   Unspecified

OGCR Official Guidelines   **X** Assign placeholder X   ● Use Additional Character(s)   ▶ Manifestation Code   **Coding Clinic**

● **T85.12**   **Displacement of implanted electronic stimulator of nervous system**
Malposition of implanted electronic stimulator of nervous system

   ● **T85.120**   **Displacement of implanted electronic neurostimulator (electrode) of brain**

   ● **T85.121**   **Displacement of implanted electronic neurostimulator (electrode) of peripheral nerve**

   ● **T85.122**   **Displacement of implanted electronic neurostimulator (electrode) of spinal cord**

   ● **T85.128**   **Displacement of other implanted electronic stimulator of nervous system**

● **T85.19**   **Other mechanical complication of implanted electronic stimulator of nervous system**
Leakage of implanted electronic stimulator of nervous system
Obstruction (mechanical) of implanted electronic stimulator of nervous system
Perforation of implanted electronic stimulator of nervous system
Protrusion of implanted electronic stimulator of nervous system

   ● **T85.190**   **Other mechanical complication of implanted electronic neurostimulator (electrode) of brain**

   ● **T85.191**   **Other mechanical complication of implanted electronic neurostimulator (electrode) of peripheral nerve**

   ● **T85.192**   **Other mechanical complication of implanted electronic neurostimulator (electrode) of spinal cord**

   ● **T85.199**   **Other mechanical complication of other implanted electronic stimulator of nervous system**

● **T85.2**   **Mechanical complication of intraocular lens**

   X● **T85.21**   **Breakdown (mechanical) of intraocular lens**

   X● **T85.22**   **Displacement of intraocular lens**
Malposition of intraocular lens

   X● **T85.29**   **Other mechanical complication of intraocular lens**
Obstruction (mechanical) of intraocular lens
Perforation of intraocular lens
Protrusion of intraocular lens

● **T85.3**   **Mechanical complication of other ocular prosthetic devices, implants and grafts**

   Excludes2   other complications of corneal graft (T86.84-)

   ● **T85.31**   **Breakdown (mechanical) of other ocular prosthetic devices, implants and grafts**

     ● **T85.310**   **Breakdown (mechanical) of prosthetic orbit of right eye**

     ● **T85.311**   **Breakdown (mechanical) of prosthetic orbit of left eye**

     ● **T85.318**   **Breakdown (mechanical) of other ocular prosthetic devices, implants and grafts**

   ● **T85.32**   **Displacement of other ocular prosthetic devices, implants and grafts**
Malposition of other ocular prosthetic devices, implants and grafts

     ● **T85.320**   **Displacement of prosthetic orbit of right eye**

     ● **T85.321**   **Displacement of prosthetic orbit of left eye**

     ● **T85.328**   **Displacement of other ocular prosthetic devices, implants and grafts**

● **T85.39**   **Other mechanical complication of other ocular prosthetic devices, implants and grafts**
Obstruction (mechanical) of other ocular prosthetic devices, implants and grafts
Perforation of other ocular prosthetic devices, implants and grafts
Protrusion of other ocular prosthetic devices, implants and grafts

   ● **T85.390**   **Other mechanical complication of prosthetic orbit of right eye**

   ● **T85.391**   **Other mechanical complication of prosthetic orbit of left eye**

   ● **T85.398**   **Other mechanical complication of other ocular prosthetic devices, implants and grafts**

● **T85.4**   **Mechanical complication of breast prosthesis and implant**

   X● **T85.41**   **Breakdown (mechanical) of breast prosthesis and implant**

   X● **T85.42**   **Displacement of breast prosthesis and implant**
Malposition of breast prosthesis and implant

   X● **T85.43**   **Leakage of breast prosthesis and implant**

   X● **T85.44**   **Capsular contracture of breast implant**

   X● **T85.49**   **Other mechanical complication of breast prosthesis and implant**
Obstruction (mechanical) of breast prosthesis and implant
Perforation of breast prosthesis and implant
Protrusion of breast prosthesis and implant

● **T85.5**   **Mechanical complication of gastrointestinal prosthetic devices, implants and grafts**

   ● **T85.51**   **Breakdown (mechanical) of gastrointestinal prosthetic devices, implants and grafts**

     ● **T85.510**   **Breakdown (mechanical) of bile duct prosthesis**

     ● **T85.511**   **Breakdown (mechanical) of esophageal anti-reflux device**

     ● **T85.518**   **Breakdown (mechanical) of other gastrointestinal prosthetic devices, implants and grafts**

   ● **T85.52**   **Displacement of gastrointestinal prosthetic devices, implants and grafts**
Malposition of gastrointestinal prosthetic devices, implants and grafts

     ● **T85.520**   **Displacement of bile duct prosthesis**

     ● **T85.521**   **Displacement of esophageal anti-reflux device**

     ● **T85.528**   **Displacement of other gastrointestinal prosthetic devices, implants and grafts**

   ● **T85.59**   **Other mechanical complication of gastrointestinal prosthetic devices, implants and**
Obstruction, mechanical of gastrointestinal prosthetic devices, implants and grafts
Perforation of gastrointestinal prosthetic devices, implants and grafts
Protrusion of gastrointestinal prosthetic devices, implants and grafts

     ● **T85.590**   **Other mechanical complication of bile duct prosthesis**

     ● **T85.591**   **Other mechanical complication of esophageal anti-reflux device**

     ● **T85.598**   **Other mechanical complication of other gastrointestinal prosthetic devices, implants and grafts**

CHAPTER 19 (S00-T88)

● **T85.6** **Mechanical complication of other specified internal and external prosthetic devices, implants and grafts**

● **T85.61** **Breakdown (mechanical) of other specified internal prosthetic devices, implants and grafts**

● **T85.610** **Breakdown (mechanical) of epidural and subdural infusion catheter**

● **T85.611** **Breakdown (mechanical) of intraperitoneal dialysis catheter**

> **Excludes1** mechanical complication of vascular dialysis catheter (T82.4-)

● **T85.612** **Breakdown (mechanical) of permanent sutures**

> **Excludes1** mechanical complication of permanent (wire) suture used in bone repair (T84.1-T84.2)

● **T85.613** **Breakdown (mechanical) of artificial skin graft and decellularized allodermis**

> Failure of artificial skin graft and decellularized allodermis
> Non-adherence of artificial skin graft and decellularized allodermis
> Poor incorporation of artificial skin graft and decellularized allodermis
> Shearing of artificial skin graft and decellularized allodermis

● **T85.614** **Breakdown (mechanical) of insulin pump**

● **T85.618** **Breakdown (mechanical) of other specified internal prosthetic devices, implants and grafts**

● **T85.62** **Displacement of other specified internal prosthetic devices, implants and grafts**

> Malposition of other specified internal prosthetic devices, implants and grafts

● **T85.620** **Displacement of epidural and subdural infusion catheter**

● **T85.621** **Displacement of intraperitoneal dialysis catheter**

> **Excludes1** mechanical complication of vascular dialysis catheter (T82.4-)

● **T85.622** **Displacement of permanent sutures**

> **Excludes1** mechanical complication of permanent (wire) suture used in bone repair (T84.1-T84.2)

● **T85.623** **Displacement of artificial skin graft and decellularized allodermis**

> Dislodgement of artificial skin graft and decellularized allodermis
> Displacement of artificial skin graft and decellularized allodermis

● **T85.624** **Displacement of insulin pump**

● **T85.628** **Displacement of other specified internal prosthetic devices, implants and grafts**

> **Coding Clinic: 2015, Q1, P15**

● **T85.63** **Leakage of other specified internal prosthetic devices, implants and grafts**

● **T85.630** **Leakage of epidural and subdural infusion catheter**

● **T85.631** **Leakage of intraperitoneal dialysis catheter**

> **Excludes1** mechanical complication of vascular dialysis catheter (T82.4)

● **T85.633** **Leakage of insulin pump**

● **T85.638** **Leakage of other specified internal prosthetic devices, implants and grafts**

● **T85.69** **Other mechanical complication of other specified internal prosthetic devices, implants and grafts**

> Obstruction, mechanical of other specified internal prosthetic devices, implants and grafts
> Perforation of other specified internal prosthetic devices, implants and grafts
> Protrusion of other specified internal prosthetic devices, implants and grafts

● **T85.690** **Other mechanical complication of epidural and subdural infusion catheter**

● **T85.691** **Other mechanical complication of intraperitoneal dialysis catheter**

> **Excludes1** mechanical complication of vascular dialysis catheter (T82.4)

● **T85.692** **Other mechanical complication of permanent sutures**

> **Excludes1** mechanical complication of permanent (wire) suture used in bone repair (T84.1-T84.2)

● **T85.693** **Other mechanical complication of artificial skin graft and decellularized allodermis**

● **T85.694** **Other mechanical complication of insulin pump**

● **T85.698** **Other mechanical complication of other specified internal prosthetic devices, implants and grafts**

> Mechanical complication of nonabsorbable surgical material NOS

● **T85.7** **Infection and inflammatory reaction due to other internal prosthetic devices, implants and grafts**

> Use additional code to identify infection

X● **T85.71** **Infection and inflammatory reaction due to peritoneal dialysis catheter**

X● **T85.72** **Infection and inflammatory reaction due to insulin pump**

X● **T85.79** **Infection and inflammatory reaction due to other internal prosthetic devices, implants and grafts**

◀ New   ⇐ Revised   ~~deleted~~ Deleted   Excludes 1   Excludes 2   Includes   Use additional   Code first   Code also   Unspecified

OGCR Official Guidelines   **X** Assign placeholder X   ● Use Additional Character(s)   ▶ Manifestation Code   **Coding Clinic**

● **T85.8**   **Other specified complications of internal prosthetic devices, implants and grafts, not elsewhere classified**

   X● **T85.81**   Embolism due to internal prosthetic devices, implants and grafts, not elsewhere classified

   X● **T85.82**   Fibrosis due to internal prosthetic devices, implants and grafts, not elsewhere classified

   X● **T85.83**   Hemorrhage due to internal prosthetic devices, implants and grafts, not elsewhere classified

   X● **T85.84**   Pain due to internal prosthetic devices, implants and grafts, not elsewhere classified

   X● **T85.85**   Stenosis due to internal prosthetic devices, implants and grafts, not elsewhere classified

   X● **T85.86**   Thrombosis due to internal prosthetic devices, implants and grafts, not elsewhere classified

   X● **T85.89**   Other specified complication of internal prosthetic devices, implants and grafts, not elsewhere classified

  X● **T85.9**   **Unspecified** complication of internal prosthetic device, implant and graft

     Complication of internal prosthetic device, implant and graft NOS

● **T86**   **Complications of transplanted organs and tissue**

   Use additional code to identify other transplant complications, such as:

     graft-versus-host disease (D89.81-)

     malignancy associated with organ transplant (C80.2)

     post-transplant lymphoproliferative disorders (PTLD) (D47.Z1)

  ● **T86.0**   **Complications of bone marrow transplant**

    T86.00   **Unspecified** complication of bone marrow transplant

    T86.01   Bone marrow transplant rejection

    T86.02   Bone marrow transplant failure

    T86.03   Bone marrow transplant infection

    T86.09   Other complications of bone marrow transplant

  ● **T86.1**   **Complications of kidney transplant**

    T86.10   **Unspecified** complication of kidney transplant

    T86.11   Kidney transplant rejection

    T86.12   Kidney transplant failure
      Coding Clinic: 2013, Q1, P24

    T86.13   Kidney transplant infection
      Use additional code to specify infection

    T86.19   Other complication of kidney transplant

● **T86.2**   **Complications of heart transplant**

    Excludes1   complication of:
      artificial heart device (T82.5)
      heart-lung transplant (T86.3)

   T86.20   **Unspecified** complication of heart transplant

   T86.21   Heart transplant rejection

   T86.22   Heart transplant failure

   T86.23   Heart transplant infection
     Use additional code to specify infection

  ● **T86.29**   Other complications of heart transplant

    T86.290   Cardiac allograft vasculopathy

      Excludes1   atherosclerosis of coronary arteries (I25.75-, I25.76-, I25.81-)

    T86.298   Other complications of heart transplant

● **T86.3**   **Complications of heart-lung transplant**

   T86.30   **Unspecified** complication of heart-lung transplant

   T86.31   Heart-lung transplant rejection

   T86.32   Heart-lung transplant failure

   T86.33   Heart-lung transplant infection
     Use additional code to specify infection

   T86.39   Other complications of heart-lung transplant

● **T86.4**   **Complications of liver transplant**

   T86.40   **Unspecified** complication of liver transplant

   T86.41   Liver transplant rejection

   T86.42   Liver transplant failure

   T86.43   Liver transplant infection
     Use additional code to identify infection, such as:
      Cytomegalovirus (CMV) infection (B25.-)

   T86.49   Other complications of liver transplant

● **T86.5**   **Complications of stem cell transplant**
   Complications from stem cells from peripheral blood
   Complications from stem cells from umbilical cord

● **T86.8**   **Complications of other transplanted organs and tissues**

  ● **T86.81**   **Complications of lung transplant**

    Excludes1   complication of heart-lung transplant (T86.3-)

    T86.810   Lung transplant rejection

    T86.811   Lung transplant failure

    T86.812   Lung transplant infection
      Use additional code to specify infection

    T86.818   Other complications of lung transplant

    T86.819   **Unspecified** complication of lung transplant

  ● **T86.82**   **Complications of skin graft (allograft) (autograft)**

    Excludes2   complication of artificial skin graft (T85.693)

    T86.820   Skin graft (allograft) rejection

    T86.821   Skin graft (allograft) (autograft) failure

    T86.822   Skin graft (allograft) (autograft) infection
      Use additional code to specify infection

    T86.828   Other complications of skin graft (allograft) (autograft)

    T86.829   **Unspecified** complication of skin graft (allograft) (autograft)

OGCR Section I.C.19.g.3.

Organ Transplant Complications

Transplant Complications

(a) Transplant complications other than kidney

Codes under category T86, Complications of transplanted organs and tissues, are for use for both complications and rejection of transplanted organs. A transplant complication code is only assigned if the complication affects the function of the transplanted organ. Two codes are required to fully describe a transplant complication: the appropriate code from category T86 and a secondary code that identifies the complication.

Pre-existing conditions or conditions that develop after the transplant are not coded as complications unless they affect the function of the transplanted organs.

See I.C.21 for transplant organ removal status

See I.C.2 for malignant neoplasm associated with transplanted organ.

CHAPTER 19 (S00-T88)

● T86.83   **Complications of bone graft**
    Excludes2   mechanical complications of bone graft (T84.3-)
   T86.830   **Bone graft rejection**
   T86.831   **Bone graft failure**
   T86.832   **Bone graft infection**
      Use additional code to specify infection
   T86.838   **Other complications of bone graft**
   T86.839   **Unspecified complication of bone graft**

● T86.84   **Complications of corneal transplant**
    Excludes2   mechanical complications of corneal graft (T85.3-)
   T86.840   **Corneal transplant rejection**
   T86.841   **Corneal transplant failure**
   T86.842   **Corneal transplant infection**
      Use additional code to specify infection
   T86.848   **Other complications of corneal transplant**
   T86.849   **Unspecified complication of corneal transplant**

● T86.85   **Complication of intestine transplant**
   T86.850   **Intestine transplant rejection**
   T86.851   **Intestine transplant failure**
   T86.852   **Intestine transplant infection**
      Use additional code to specify infection
   T86.858   **Other complications of intestine transplant**
   T86.859   **Unspecified complication of intestine transplant**

● T86.89   **Complications of other transplanted tissue**
    Transplant failure or rejection of pancreas
   T86.890   **Other transplanted tissue rejection**
   T86.891   **Other transplanted tissue failure**
   T86.892   **Other transplanted tissue infection**
      Use additional code to specify infection
   T86.898   **Other complications of other transplanted tissue**
   T86.899   **Unspecified complication of other transplanted tissue**

● T86.9   **Complication of unspecified transplanted organ and tissue**
   T86.90   **Unspecified complication of unspecified transplanted organ and tissue**
   T86.91   **Unspecified transplanted organ and tissue rejection**
   T86.92   **Unspecified transplanted organ and tissue failure**
   T86.93   **Unspecified transplanted organ and tissue infection**
      Use additional code to specify infection
   T86.99   **Other complications of unspecified transplanted organ and tissue**

● T87   **Complications peculiar to reattachment and amputation**
  ● T87.0   **Complications of reattached (part of) upper extremity**
   ● T87.0X   **Complications of reattached (part of) upper extremity**
     T87.0X1   **Complications of reattached (part of) right upper extremity**
     T87.0X2   **Complications of reattached (part of) left upper extremity**
     T87.0X9   **Complications of reattached (part of) unspecified upper extremity**

  ● T87.1   **Complications of reattached (part of) lower extremity**
   ● T87.1X   **Complications of reattached (part of) lower extremity**
     T87.1X1   **Complications of reattached (part of) right lower extremity**
     T87.1X2   **Complications of reattached (part of) left lower extremity**
     T87.1X9   **Complications of reattached (part of) unspecified lower extremity**

  T87.2   **Complications of other reattached body part**

  ● T87.3   **Neuroma of amputation stump**
   T87.30   **Neuroma of amputation stump, unspecified extremity**
   T87.31   **Neuroma of amputation stump, right upper extremity**
   T87.32   **Neuroma of amputation stump, left upper extremity**
   T87.33   **Neuroma of amputation stump, right lower extremity**
   T87.34   **Neuroma of amputation stump, left lower extremity**

  ● T87.4   **Infection of amputation stump**
   T87.40   **Infection of amputation stump, unspecified extremity**
   T87.41   **Infection of amputation stump, right upper extremity**
   T87.42   **Infection of amputation stump, left upper extremity**
   T87.43   **Infection of amputation stump, right lower extremity**
   T87.44   **Infection of amputation stump, left lower extremity**

  ● T87.5   **Necrosis of amputation stump**
   T87.50   **Necrosis of amputation stump, unspecified extremity**
   T87.51   **Necrosis of amputation stump, right upper extremity**
   T87.52   **Necrosis of amputation stump, left upper extremity**
   T87.53   **Necrosis of amputation stump, right lower extremity**
   T87.54   **Necrosis of amputation stump, left lower extremity**

  ● T87.8   **Other complications of amputation stump**
   T87.81   **Dehiscence of amputation stump**
   T87.89   **Other complications of amputation stump**
     Amputation stump contracture
     Amputation stump contracture of next proximal joint
     Amputation stump flexion
     Amputation stump edema
     Amputation stump hematoma
     Excludes2   phantom limb syndrome (G54.6-G54.7)

  T87.9   **Unspecified complications of amputation stump**

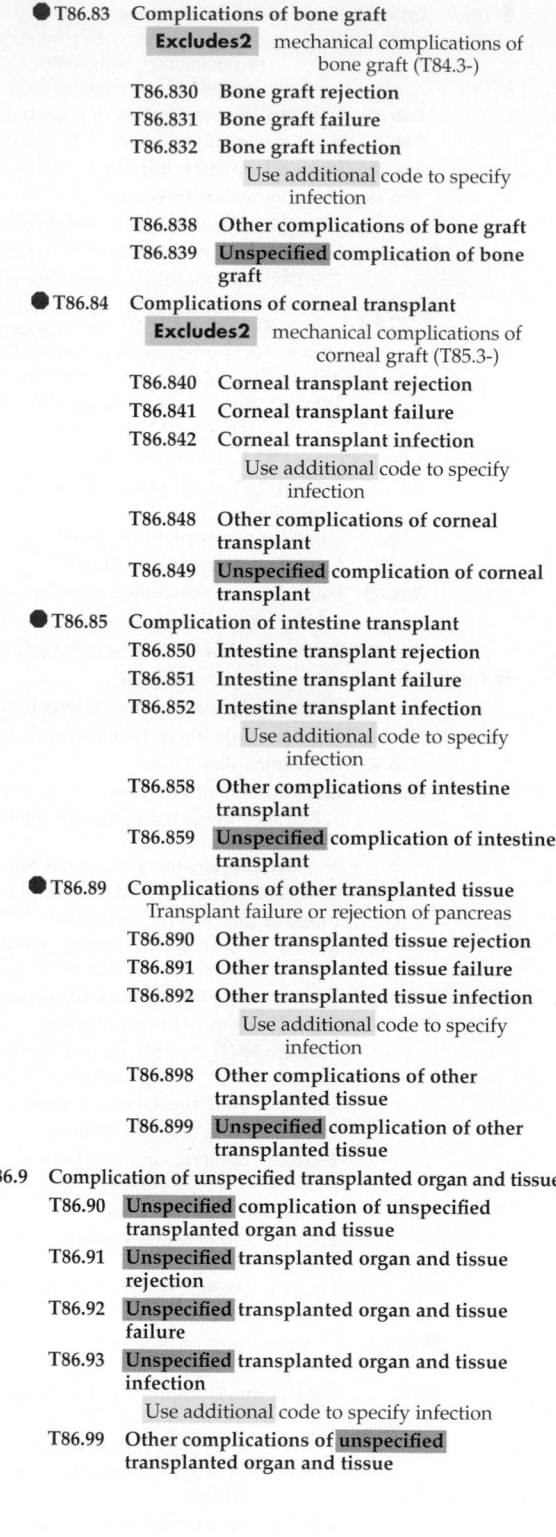

◀ New   ◀▥ Revised   ~~deleted~~ Deleted   Excludes 1   Excludes 2   Includes   Use additional   Code first   Code also   Unspecified

OGCR Official Guidelines   X Assign placeholder X   ● Use Additional Character(s)   ▶ Manifestation Code   **Coding Clinic**

CHAPTER 19 (S00-T88)

● T88   **Other complications of surgical and medical care, not elsewhere classified**

> **Excludes2**   complication following infusion, transfusion and therapeutic injection (T80.-)
> complication following procedure NEC (T81.-)
> complications of anesthesia in labor and delivery (O74.-)
> complications of anesthesia in pregnancy (O29.-)
> complications of anesthesia in puerperium (O89.-)
> complications of devices, implants and grafts (T82-T85)
> complications of obstetric surgery and procedure (O75.4)
> dermatitis due to drugs and medicaments (L23.3, L24.4, L25.1, L27.0-L27.1)
> poisoning and toxic effects of drugs and chemicals (T36-T65 with fifth or sixth character 1-4 or 6)
> specified complications classified elsewhere

The appropriate 7th character is to be added to each code from category T88

> A   initial encounter
> D   subsequent encounter
> S   sequela

X ● **T88.0**   **Infection following immunization**
Sepsis following immunization

X ● **T88.1**   **Other complications following immunization, not elsewhere classified**
Generalized vaccinia
Rash following immunization

> **Excludes1**   vaccinia not from vaccine (B08.011)
> **Excludes2**   anaphylactic shock due to serum (T80.5-)
> other serum reactions (T80.6-)
> postimmunization arthropathy (M02.2)
> postimmunization encephalitis (G04.02)
> postimmunization fever (R50.83)

X ● **T88.2**   **Shock due to anesthesia**
Use additional code for adverse effect, if applicable, to identify drug (T41.- with fifth or sixth character 5)

> **Excludes1**   complications of anesthesia (in):
> labor and delivery (O74.-)
> pregnancy (O29.-)
> puerperium (O89.-)
> postprocedural shock NOS (T81.1-)

X ● **T88.3**   **Malignant hyperthermia due to anesthesia**
Use additional code for adverse effect, if applicable, to identify drug (T41.- with fifth or sixth character 5)

X ● **T88.4**   **Failed or difficult intubation**

X ● **T88.5**   **Other complications of anesthesia**
Use additional code for adverse effect, if applicable, to identify drug (T41.- with fifth or sixth character 5)

X ● **T88.51**   **Hypothermia following anesthesia**

X ● **T88.52**   **Failed moderate sedation during procedure**
Failed conscious sedation during procedure

> **Excludes2**   personal history of failed moderate sedation (Z92.83)

X ● **T88.59**   **Other complications of anesthesia**

X ● **T88.6**   **Anaphylactic reaction due to adverse effect of correct drug or medicament properly administered**
Anaphylactic shock due to adverse effect of correct drug or medicament properly administered
Anaphylactoid reaction NOS
Use additional code for adverse effect, if applicable, to identify drug (T36-T50 with fifth or sixth character 5)

> **Excludes1**   anaphylactic reaction due to serum (T80.5-)
> anaphylactic shock or reaction due to adverse food reaction (T78.0-)

X ● **T88.7**   **Unspecified adverse effect of drug or medicament**
Drug hypersensitivity NOS
Drug reaction NOS
Use additional code for adverse effect, if applicable, to identify drug (T36-T50 with fifth or sixth character 5)

> **Excludes1**   specified adverse effects of drugs and medicaments (A00-R94 and T80-T88.6, T88.8)

X ● **T88.8**   **Other specified complications of surgical and medical care, not elsewhere classified**
Use additional code to identify the complication

X ● **T88.9**   **Complication of surgical and medical care, unspecified**

CHAPTER 20

EXTERNAL CAUSES OF MORBIDITY (V00-Y99)

Note: This chapter permits the classification of environmental events and circumstances as the cause of injury, and other adverse effects. Where a code from this section is applicable, it is intended that it shall be used secondary to a code from another chapter of the Classification indicating the nature of the condition. Most often, the condition will be classifiable to Chapter 19, Injury, poisoning and certain other consequences of external causes (S00-T88). Other conditions that may be stated to be due to external causes are classified in Chapters I to XVIII. For these conditions, codes from Chapter 20 should be used to provide additional information as to the cause of the condition.

This chapter contains the following blocks:

V00-X58	Accidents
V00-V99	Transport accidents
V00-V09	Pedestrian injured in transport accident
V10-V19	Pedal cycle rider injured in transport accident
V20-V29	Motorcycle rider injured in transport accident
V30-V39	Occupant of three-wheeled motor vehicle injured in transport accident
V40-V49	Car occupant injured in transport accident
V50-V59	Occupant of pick-up truck or van injured in transport accident
V60-V69	Occupant of heavy transport vehicle injured in transport accident
V70-V79	Bus occupant injured in transport accident
V80-V89	Other land transport accidents
V90-V94	Water transport accidents
V95-V97	Air and space transport accidents
V98-V99	Other and unspecified transport accidents
W00-X58	Other external causes of accidental injury
W00-W19	Slipping, tripping, stumbling and falls
W20-W49	Exposure to inanimate mechanical forces
W50-W64	Exposure to animate mechanical forces
W65-W74	Accidental non-transport drowning and submersion
W85-W99	Exposure to electric current, radiation and extreme ambient air temperature and pressure
X00-X08	Exposure to smoke, fire and flames
X10-X19	Contact with heat and hot substances
X30-X39	Exposure to forces of nature
X52, X58	Accidental exposure to other specified factors
X71-X83	Intentional self-harm
X92-Y08	Assault
Y21-Y33	Event of undetermined intent
Y35-Y38	Legal intervention, operations of war, military operations, and terrorism
Y62-Y84	Complications of medical and surgical care
Y62-Y69	Misadventures to patients during surgical and medical care
Y70-Y82	Medical devices associated with adverse incidents in diagnostic and therapeutic use
Y83-Y84	Surgical and other medical procedures as the cause of abnormal reaction of the patient, or of later complication, without mention of misadventure at the time of the procedure
Y90-Y99	Supplementary factors related to causes of morbidity classified elsewhere

Note: This section is structured in 12 groups. Those relating to land transport accidents (V01-V89) reflect the victim's mode of transport and are subdivided to identify the victim's 'counterpart' or the type of event. The vehicle of which the injured person is an occupant is identified in the first two characters since it is seen as the most important factor to identify for prevention purposes. A transport accident is one in which the vehicle involved must be moving or running or in use for transport purposes at the time of the accident.

Use additional code to identify:
Airbag injury (W22.1)
Type of street or road (Y92.4-)
Use of cellular telephone and other electronic equipment at the time of the transport accident (Y93.C-)

Excludes1 agricultural vehicles in stationary use or maintenance (W31.-)
assault by crashing of motor vehicle (Y03.-)
automobile or motor cycle in stationary use or maintenance - code to type of accident
crashing of motor vehicle, undetermined intent (Y32)
intentional self-harm by crashing of motor vehicle (X82)

Excludes2 transport accidents due to cataclysm (X34-X38)

Note: Definitions of transport vehicles:

(a) A transport accident is any accident involving a device designed primarily for, or used at the time primarily for, conveying persons or good from one place to another.

(b) A public highway [trafficway] or street is the entire width between property lines (or other boundary lines) of land open to the public as a matter of right or custom for purposes of moving persons or property from one place to another. A roadway is that part of the public highway designed, improved and customarily used for vehicular traffic.

(c) A traffic accident is any vehicle accident occurring on the public highway [i.e., originating on, terminating on, or involving a vehicle partially on the highway]. A vehicle accident is assumed to have occurred on the public highway unless another place is specified, except in the case of accidents involving only off-road motor vehicles, which are classified as nontraffic accidents unless the contrary is stated.

(d) A nontraffic accident is any vehicle accident that occurs entirely in any place other than a public highway.

(e) A pedestrian is any person involved in an accident who was not at the time of the accident riding in or on a motor vehicle, railway train, streetcar or animal-drawn or other vehicle, or on a pedal cycle or animal. This includes, a person changing a tire or working on a parked car. It also includes the use of a pedestrian conveyance such as a baby carriage, ice-skates, roller skates, a skateboard, nonmotorized or motorized wheelchair, motorized mobility scooter, or nonmotorized scooter.

(f) A driver is an occupant of a transport vehicle who is operating or intending to operate it.

(g) A passenger is any occupant of a transport vehicle other than the driver, except a person traveling on the outside of the vehicle.

(h) A person on the outside of a vehicle is any person being transported by a vehicle but not occupying the space normally reserved for the driver or passengers, or the space intended for the transport of property. This includes the body, bumper, fender, roof, running board or step of a vehicle.

◀ New ◀▮▮▮ Revised ~~deleted~~ Deleted | Excludes 1 | Excludes 2 | Includes | Use additional | Code first | Code also | Unspecified

OGCR Official Guidelines X Assign placeholder X ● Use Additional Character(s) ▶ Manifestation Code **Coding Clinic**

(i) A pedal cycle is any land transport vehicle operated solely by nonmotorized pedals including a bicycle or tricycle.

(j) A pedal cyclist is any person riding a pedal cycle or in a sidecar or trailer attached to a pedal cycle.

(k) A motorcycle is a two-wheeled motor vehicle with one or two riding saddles and sometimes with a third wheel for the support of a sidecar. The sidecar is considered part of the motorcycle.

(l) A motorcycle rider is any person riding a motorcycle or in a sidecar or trailer attached to the motorcycle.

(m) A three-wheeled motor vehicle is a motorized tricycle designed primarily for on-road use. This includes a motor-driven tricycle, a motorized rickshaw, or a three-wheeled motor car.

(n) A car [automobile] is a four-wheeled motor vehicle designed primarily for carrying up to 7 persons. A trailer being towed by the car is considered part of the car.

(o) A pick-up truck or van is a four or six-wheeled motor vehicle designed for carrying passengers as well as property or cargo weighing less than the local limit for classification as a heavy goods vehicle, and not requiring a special driver's license. This includes a minivan and a sport-utility vehicle (SUV).

(p) A heavy transport vehicle is a motor vehicle designed primarily for carrying property, meeting local criteria for classification as a heavy goods vehicle in terms of weight and requiring a special driver's license.

(q) A bus (coach) is a motor vehicle designed or adapted primarily for carrying more than 10 passengers, and requiring a special driver's license.

(r) A railway train or railway vehicle is any device, with or without freight or passenger cars coupled to it, designed for traffic on a railway track. This includes subterranean (subways) or elevated trains.

(s) A streetcar is a device designed and used primarily for transporting passengers within a municipality, running on rails, usually subject to normal traffic control signals, and operated principally on a right-of-way that forms part of the roadway. This includes a tram or trolley that runs on rails. A trailer being towed by a streetcar is considered part of the streetcar.

(t) A special vehicle mainly used on industrial premises is a motor vehicle designed primarily for use within the buildings and premises of industrial or commercial establishments. This includes battery-powered trucks, forklifts, coal-cars in a coal mine, logging cars and trucks used in mines or quarries.

(u) A special vehicle mainly used in agriculture is a motor vehicle designed specifically for use in farming and agriculture (horticulture), to work the land, tend and harvest crops and transport materials on the farm. This includes harvesters, farm machinery and tractor and trailers.

(v) A special construction vehicle is a motor vehicle designed specifically for use on construction and demolition sites. This includes bulldozers, diggers, earth levellers, dump trucks, backhoes, front-end loaders, pavers, and mechanical shovels.

(w) A special all-terrain vehicle is a motor vehicle of special design to enable it to negotiate over rough or soft terrain, snow or sand. This includes snow mobiles, all-terrain vehicles (ATV), and dune buggies. It does not include passenger vehicle designated as sport utility vehicles (SUV).

(x) A watercraft is any device designed for transporting passengers or goods on water. This includes motor or sail boats, ships, and hovercraft.

(y) An aircraft is any device for transporting passengers or goods in the air. This includes hot-air balloons, gliders, helicopters and airplanes.

(z) A military vehicle is any motorized vehicle operating on a public roadway owned by the military and being operated by a member of the military.

PEDESTRIAN INJURED IN TRANSPORT ACCIDENT (V00-V09)

Includes   person changing tire on transport vehicle
person examining engine of vehicle broken down in (on side of) road

Excludes1   fall due to non-transport collision with other person (W03)
pedestrian on foot falling (slipping) on ice and snow (W00.-)
struck or bumped by another person (W51)

● **V00**   **Pedestrian conveyance accident**
Use additional place of occurrence and activity external cause codes, if known (Y92.-, Y93.-)

Excludes1   collision with another person without fall (W51)
fall due to person on foot colliding with another person on foot (W03)
fall from non-moving wheelchair, nonmotorized scooter and motorized mobility scooter without collision (W05.-)
pedestrian (conveyance) collision with other land transport vehicle (V01-V09)
pedestrian on foot falling (slipping) on ice and snow (W00.-)

The appropriate 7th character is to be added to each code from category V00

A	initial encounter
D	subsequent encounter
S	sequela

● **V00.0**   **Pedestrian on foot injured in collision with pedestrian conveyance**

X● **V00.01**   **Pedestrian on foot injured in collision with roller-skater**

X● **V00.02**   **Pedestrian on foot injured in collision with skateboarder**

X● **V00.09**   **Pedestrian on foot injured in collision with other pedestrian conveyance**

● **V00.1**   **Rolling-type pedestrian conveyance accident**

Excludes1   accident with babystroller (V00.82-)
accident with wheelchair (powered) (V00.81-)
accident with motorized mobility scooter (V00.83-)

● **V00.11**   **In-line roller-skate accident**

● **V00.111**   **Fall from in-line roller-skates**

● **V00.112**   **In-line roller-skater colliding with stationary object**

● **V00.118**   **Other in-line roller-skate accident**

Excludes1   roller-skater collision with other land transport vehicle (V01-V09 with 5th character 1)

● **V00.12**   **Non-in-line roller-skate accident**

● **V00.121**   **Fall from non-in-line roller-skates**

● **V00.122**   **Non-in-line roller-skater colliding with stationary object**

● **V00.128**   **Other non-in-line roller-skating accident**

Excludes1   roller-skater collision with other land transport vehicle (V01-V09 with 5th character 1)

N Newborn Age: 0   **P** Pediatric Age: 0–17   **M** Maternity DX: 12–55   **A** Adult Age: 15–124   ♀ Females Only   ♂ Males Only

1489

- ● **V00.13**   **Skateboard accident**
  - ● **V00.131**   **Fall from skateboard**
  - ● **V00.132**   **Skateboarder colliding with stationary object**
  - ● **V00.138**   **Other skateboard accident**
    - **Excludes1**   skateboarder collision with other land transport vehicle (V01-V09 with 5th character 2)
- ● **V00.14**   **Scooter (nonmotorized) accident**
  - **Excludes1**   motorscooter accident (V20-V29)
  - ● **V00.141**   **Fall from scooter (nonmotorized)**
  - ● **V00.142**   **Scooter (nonmotorized) colliding with stationary object**
  - ● **V00.148**   **Other scooter (nonmotorized) accident**
    - **Excludes1**   scooter (non-motorized) collision with other land transport vehicle (V01-V09 with fifth character 9)
- ● **V00.15**   **Heelies accident**
  - Rolling shoe
  - Wheeled shoe
  - Wheelies accident
  - ● **V00.151**   **Fall from heelies**
  - ● **V00.152**   **Heelies colliding with stationary object**
  - ● **V00.158**   **Other heelies accident**
- ● **V00.18**   **Accident on other rolling-type pedestrian conveyance**
  - ● **V00.181**   **Fall from other rolling-type pedestrian conveyance**
  - ● **V00.182**   **Pedestrian on other rolling-type pedestrian conveyance colliding with stationary object**
  - ● **V00.188**   **Other accident on other rolling-type pedestrian conveyance**
- ● **V00.2**   **Gliding-type pedestrian conveyance accident**
  - ● **V00.21**   **Ice-skates accident**
    - ● **V00.211**   **Fall from ice-skates**
    - ● **V00.212**   **Ice-skater colliding with stationary object**
    - ● **V00.218**   **Other ice-skates accident**
      - **Excludes1**   ice-skater collision with other land transport vehicle (V01-V09 with 5th digit 9)
  - ● **V00.22**   **Sled accident**
    - ● **V00.221**   **Fall from sled**
    - ● **V00.222**   **Sledder colliding with stationary object**
    - ● **V00.228**   **Other sled accident**
      - **Excludes1**   sled collision with other land transport vehicle (V01-V09 with 5th digit 9)

- ● **V00.28**   **Other gliding-type pedestrian conveyance accident**
  - ● **V00.281**   **Fall from other gliding-type pedestrian conveyance**
  - ● **V00.282**   **Pedestrian on other gliding-type pedestrian conveyance colliding with stationary object**
  - ● **V00.288**   **Other accident on other gliding-type pedestrian conveyance**
    - **Excludes1**   gliding-type pedestrian conveyance collision with other land transport vehicle (V01-V09 with 5th digit 9)
- ● **V00.3**   **Flat-bottomed pedestrian conveyance accident**
  - ● **V00.31**   **Snowboard accident**
    - ● **V00.311**   **Fall from snowboard**
    - ● **V00.312**   **Snowboarder colliding with stationary object**
    - ● **V00.318**   **Other snowboard accident**
      - **Excludes1**   snowboarder collision with other land transport vehicle (V01-V09 with 5th digit 9)
  - ● **V00.32**   **Snow-ski accident**
    - ● **V00.321**   **Fall from snow-skis**
      - **Coding Clinic: 2015, Q1, P12**
    - ● **V00.322**   **Snow-skier colliding with stationary object**
    - ● **V00.328**   **Other snow-ski accident**
      - **Excludes1**   snow-skier collision with other land transport vehicle (V01-V09 with 5th digit 9)
  - ● **V00.38**   **Other flat-bottomed pedestrian conveyance accident**
    - ● **V00.381**   **Fall from other flat-bottomed pedestrian conveyance**
    - ● **V00.382**   **Pedestrian on other flat-bottomed pedestrian conveyance colliding with stationary object**
    - ● **V00.388**   **Other accident on other flat-bottomed pedestrian conveyance**
- ● **V00.8**   **Accident on other pedestrian conveyance**
  - ● **V00.81**   **Accident with wheelchair (powered)**
    - ● **V00.811**   **Fall from moving wheelchair (powered)**
      - **Excludes1**   fall from non-moving wheelchair (W05.0)
    - ● **V00.812**   **Wheelchair (powered) colliding with stationary object**
    - ● **V00.818**   **Other accident with wheelchair (powered)**
  - ● **V00.82**   **Accident with babystroller**
    - ● **V00.821**   **Fall from babystroller**
    - ● **V00.822**   **Babystroller colliding with stationary object**
    - ● **V00.828**   **Other accident with babystroller**

◀ New   ◀▥ Revised   ~~deleted~~ Deleted   **Excludes 1**   Excludes 2   Includes   Use additional   Code first   Code also   **Unspecified**

OGCR Official Guidelines   X Assign placeholder X   ● Use Additional Character(s)   ▶ Manifestation Code   **Coding Clinic**

- **V00.83**   **Accident with motorized mobility scooter**
  - **V00.831**   **Fall from motorized mobility scooter**

    Excludes1   fall from non-moving motorized mobility scooter (W05.2)
  - **V00.832**   **Motorized mobility scooter colliding with stationary object**
  - **V00.838**   **Other accident with motorized mobility scooter**
- **V00.89**   **Accident on other pedestrian conveyance**
  - **V00.891**   **Fall from other pedestrian conveyance**
  - **V00.892**   **Pedestrian on other pedestrian conveyance colliding with stationary object**
  - **V00.898**   **Other accident on other pedestrian conveyance**

    Excludes1   other pedestrian (conveyance) collision with other land transport vehicle (V01-V09 with 5th digit 9)

- **V01**   **Pedestrian injured in collision with pedal cycle**

  The appropriate 7th character is to be added to each code from category V01

A	initial encounter
D	subsequent encounter
S	sequela

  - **V01.0**   **Pedestrian injured in collision with pedal cycle in nontraffic accident**
    - X● **V01.00**   **Pedestrian on foot injured in collision with pedal cycle in nontraffic accident**

      Pedestrian NOS injured in collision with pedal cycle in nontraffic accident
    - X● **V01.01**   **Pedestrian on roller-skates injured in collision with pedal cycle in nontraffic accident**
    - X● **V01.02**   **Pedestrian on skateboard injured in collision with pedal cycle in nontraffic accident**
    - X● **V01.09**   **Pedestrian with other conveyance injured in collision with pedal cycle in nontraffic accident**

      Pedestrian with babystroller injured in collision with pedal cycle in nontraffic accident

      Pedestrian in wheelchair (powered) injured in collision with pedal cycle in nontraffic accident

      Pedestrian in motorized mobility scooter injured in collision with pedal cycle in nontraffic accident

      Pedestrian on ice-skates injured in collision with pedal cycle in nontraffic accident

      Pedestrian on nonmotorized scooter injured in collision with pedal cycle in nontraffic accident

      Pedestrian on sled injured in collision with pedal cycle in nontraffic accident

      Pedestrian on snowboard injured in collision with pedal cycle in nontraffic accident

      Pedestrian on snow-skis injured in collision with pedal cycle in nontraffic accident

- **V01.1**   **Pedestrian injured in collision with pedal cycle in traffic accident**
  - X● **V01.10**   **Pedestrian on foot injured in collision with pedal cycle in traffic accident**

    Pedestrian NOS injured in collision with pedal cycle in traffic accident
  - X● **V01.11**   **Pedestrian on roller-skates injured in collision with pedal cycle in traffic accident**
  - X● **V01.12**   **Pedestrian on skateboard injured in collision with pedal cycle in traffic accident**
  - X● **V01.19**   **Pedestrian with other conveyance injured in collision with pedal cycle in traffic accident**

    Pedestrian with babystroller injured in collision with pedal cycle in traffic accident

    Pedestrian in wheelchair (powered) injured in collision with pedal cycle in traffic accident

    Pedestrian in motorized mobility scooter injured in collision with pedal cycle in traffic accident

    Pedestrian on ice-skates injured in collision with pedal cycle in traffic accident

    Pedestrian on nonmotorized scooter injured in collision with pedal cycle in traffic accident

    Pedestrian on sled injured in collision with pedal cycle in traffic accident

    Pedestrian on snowboard injured in collision with pedal cycle in traffic accident

    Pedestrian on snow-skis injured in collision with pedal cycle in traffic accident

- **V01.9**   **Pedestrian injured in collision with pedal cycle, unspecified whether traffic or nontraffic accident**
  - X● **V01.90**   **Pedestrian on foot injured in collision with pedal cycle, unspecified whether traffic or nontraffic accident**

    Pedestrian NOS injured in collision with pedal cycle, unspecified whether traffic or nontraffic accident
  - X● **V01.91**   **Pedestrian on roller-skates injured in collision with pedal cycle, unspecified whether traffic or nontraffic accident**
  - X● **V01.92**   **Pedestrian on skateboard injured in collision with pedal cycle, unspecified whether traffic or nontraffic accident**
  - X● **V01.99**   **Pedestrian with other conveyance injured in collision with pedal cycle, unspecified whether traffic or nontraffic accident**

    Pedestrian with babystroller injured in collision with pedal cycle, unspecified whether traffic or nontraffic accident

    Pedestrian in wheelchair (powered) injured in collision with pedal cycle, unspecified whether traffic or nontraffic accident

    Pedestrian in motorized mobility scooter injured in collision with pedal cycle, unspecified whether traffic or nontraffic accident

    Pedestrian on ice-skates injured in collision with pedal cycle unspecified, whether traffic or nontraffic accident

    Pedestrian on nonmotorized scooter injured in collision with pedal cycle, unspecified whether traffic or nontraffic accident

    Pedestrian on sled injured in collision with pedal cycle unspecified, whether traffic or nontraffic accident

    Pedestrian on snowboard injured in collision with pedal cycle, unspecified whether traffic or nontraffic accident

    Pedestrian on snow-skis injured in collision with pedal cycle, unspecified whether traffic or nontraffic accident

CHAPTER 20 (V01-Y99)

● **V02**   **Pedestrian injured in collision with two- or three-wheeled motor vehicle**

The appropriate 7th character is to be added to each code from category V02

A	initial encounter
D	subsequent encounter
S	sequela

● **V02.0**   **Pedestrian injured in collision with two- or three-wheeled motor vehicle in nontraffic accident**

    X● **V02.00**   **Pedestrian on foot injured in collision with two- or three-wheeled motor vehicle in nontraffic accident**

       Pedestrian NOS injured in collision with two- or three-wheeled motor vehicle in nontraffic accident

    X● **V02.01**   **Pedestrian on roller-skates injured in collision with two- or three-wheeled motor vehicle in nontraffic accident**

    X● **V02.02**   **Pedestrian on skateboard injured in collision with two- or three-wheeled motor vehicle in nontraffic accident**

    X● **V02.09**   **Pedestrian with other conveyance injured in collision with two- or three-wheeled motor vehicle in nontraffic accident**

       Pedestrian with babystroller injured in collision with two- or three-wheeled motor vehicle in nontraffic accident

       Pedestrian on ice-skates injured in collision with two- or three-wheeled motor vehicle in nontraffic accident

       Pedestrian in wheelchair (powered) injured in collision with two- or three-wheeled motor vehicle in nontraffic accident

       Pedestrian in motorized mobility scooter injured in collision with two- or three-wheeled motor vehicle in nontraffic accident

       Pedestrian on nonmotorized scooter injured in collision with two- or three-wheeled motor vehicle in nontraffic accident

       Pedestrian on sled injured in collision with two- or three-wheeled motor vehicle in nontraffic accident

       Pedestrian on snowboard injured in collision with two- or three-wheeled motor vehicle in nontraffic accident

       Pedestrian on snow-skis injured in collision with two- or three-wheeled motor vehicle in nontraffic accident

● **V02.1**   **Pedestrian injured in collision with two- or three-wheeled motor vehicle in traffic accident**

    X● **V02.10**   **Pedestrian on foot injured in collision with two- or three-wheeled motor vehicle in traffic accident**

       Pedestrian NOS injured in collision with two- or three-wheeled motor vehicle in traffic accident

    X● **V02.11**   **Pedestrian on roller-skates injured in collision with two- or three-wheeled motor vehicle in traffic accident**

    X● **V02.12**   **Pedestrian on skateboard injured in collision with two- or three-wheeled motor vehicle in traffic accident**

    X● **V02.19**   **Pedestrian with other conveyance injured in collision with two- or three-wheeled motor vehicle in traffic accident**

       Pedestrian with babystroller injured in collision with two- or three-wheeled motor vehicle in traffic accident

       Pedestrian in wheelchair (powered) injured in collision with two- or three-wheeled motor vehicle in traffic accident

       Pedestrian in motorized mobility scooter injured in collision with two- or three-wheeled motor vehicle in traffic accident

       Pedestrian on ice-skates injured in collision with two- or three-wheeled motor vehicle in traffic accident

       Pedestrian on nonmotorized scooter injured in collision with two- or three-wheeled motor vehicle in traffic accident

       Pedestrian on sled injured in collision with two- or three-wheeled motor vehicle in traffic accident

       Pedestrian on snowboard injured in collision with two- or three-wheeled motor vehicle in traffic accident

       Pedestrian on snow-skis injured in collision with two- or three-wheeled motor vehicle in traffic accident

● **V02.9**   **Pedestrian injured in collision with two- or three-wheeled motor vehicle, unspecified whether traffic or nontraffic accident**

    X● **V02.90**   **Pedestrian on foot injured in collision with two- or three-wheeled motor vehicle, unspecified whether traffic or nontraffic accident**

       Pedestrian NOS injured in collision with two- or three-wheeled motor vehicle, unspecified whether traffic or nontraffic accident

    X● **V02.91**   **Pedestrian on roller-skates injured in collision with two- or three-wheeled motor vehicle, unspecified whether traffic or nontraffic accident**

    X● **V02.92**   **Pedestrian on skateboard injured in collision with two- or three-wheeled motor vehicle, unspecified whether traffic or nontraffic accident**

    X● **V02.99**   **Pedestrian with other conveyance injured in collision with two- or three-wheeled motor vehicle, unspecified whether traffic or nontraffic accident**

       Pedestrian with babystroller injured in collision with two- or three-wheeled motor vehicle, unspecified whether traffic or nontraffic accident

       Pedestrian in wheelchair (powered) injured in collision with two- or three-wheeled motor vehicle, unspecified whether traffic or nontraffic accident

       Pedestrian in motorized mobility scooter injured in collision with two- or three-wheeled motor vehicle, unspecified whether traffic or nontraffic accident

       Pedestrian on ice-skates injured in collision with two- or three-wheeled motor vehicle, unspecified whether traffic or nontraffic accident

       Pedestrian on nonmotorized scooter injured in collision with two- or three-wheeled motor vehicle, unspecified whether traffic or nontraffic accident

       Pedestrian on sled injured in collision with two- or three-wheeled motor vehicle, unspecified whether traffic or nontraffic accident

       Pedestrian on snowboard injured in collision with two- or three-wheeled motor vehicle, unspecified whether traffic or nontraffic accident

       Pedestrian on snow-skis injured in collision with two- or three-wheeled motor vehicle, unspecified whether traffic or nontraffic accident

◄ New   ◄▌ Revised   ~~deleted~~ Deleted   Excludes 1   Excludes 2   Includes   Use additional   Code first   Code also   Unspecified

OGCR Official Guidelines   X Assign placeholder X   ● Use Additional Character(s)   ▶ Manifestation Code   **Coding Clinic**

● V03 Pedestrian injured in collision with car, pick-up truck or van

The appropriate 7th character is to be added to each code from category V03

A	initial encounter
D	subsequent encounter
S	sequela

● V03.0 Pedestrian injured in collision with car, pick-up truck or van in nontraffic accident

X● V03.00 Pedestrian on foot injured in collision with car, pick-up truck or van in nontraffic accident

Pedestrian NOS injured in collision with car, pick-up truck or van in nontraffic accident

X● V03.01 Pedestrian on roller-skates injured in collision with car, pick-up truck or van in nontraffic accident

X● V03.02 Pedestrian on skateboard injured in collision with car, pick-up truck or van in nontraffic accident

X● V03.09 Pedestrian with other conveyance injured in collision with car, pick-up truck or van in nontraffic accident

Pedestrian with babystroller injured in collision with car, pick-up truck or van in nontraffic accident

Pedestrian in wheelchair (powered) injured in collision with car, pick-up truck or van in nontraffic accident

Pedestrian in motorized mobility scooter injured in collision with car, pick-up truck or van in nontraffic accident

Pedestrian on ice-skates injured in collision with car, pick-up truck or van in nontraffic accident

Pedestrian on nonmotorized scooter injured in collision with car, pick-up truck or van in nontraffic accident

Pedestrian on sled injured in collision with car, pick-up truck or van in nontraffic accident

Pedestrian on snowboard injured in collision with car, pick-up truck or van in nontraffic accident

Pedestrian on snow-skis injured in collision with car, pick-up truck or van in nontraffic accident

● V03.1 Pedestrian injured in collision with car, pick-up truck or van in traffic accident

X● V03.10 Pedestrian on foot injured in collision with car, pick-up truck or van in traffic accident

Pedestrian NOS injured in collision with car, pick-up truck or van in traffic accident

X● V03.11 Pedestrian on roller-skates injured in collision with car, pick-up truck or van in traffic accident

X● V03.12 Pedestrian on skateboard injured in collision with car, pick-up truck or van in traffic accident

X● V03.19 Pedestrian with other conveyance injured in collision with car, pick-up truck or van in traffic accident

Pedestrian with babystroller injured in collision with car, pick-up truck or van in traffic accident

Pedestrian in wheelchair (powered) injured in collision with car, pick-up truck or van in traffic accident

Pedestrian in motorized mobility scooter injured in collision with car, pick-up truck or van in traffic accident

Pedestrian on ice-skates injured in collision with car, pick-up truck or van in traffic accident

Pedestrian on nonmotorized scooter injured in collision with car, pick-up truck or van in traffic accident

Pedestrian on sled injured in collision with car, pick-up truck or van in traffic accident

Pedestrian on snowboard injured in collision with car, pick-up truck or van in traffic accident

Pedestrian on snow-skis injured in collision with car, pick-up truck or van in traffic accident

● V03.9 Pedestrian injured in collision with car, pick-up truck or van, unspecified whether traffic or nontraffic accident

X● V03.90 Pedestrian on foot injured in collision with car, pick-up truck or van, unspecified whether traffic or nontraffic accident

Pedestrian NOS injured in collision with car, pick-up truck or van, unspecified whether traffic or nontraffic accident

X● V03.91 Pedestrian on roller-skates injured in collision with car, pick-up truck or van, unspecified whether traffic or nontraffic accident

X● V03.92 Pedestrian on skateboard injured in collision with car, pick-up truck or van, unspecified whether traffic or nontraffic accident

X● V03.99 Pedestrian with other conveyance injured in collision with car, pick-up truck or van, unspecified whether traffic or nontraffic accident

Pedestrian with babystroller injured in collision with car, pick-up truck or van, unspecified whether traffic or nontraffic accident

Pedestrian in wheelchair (powered) injured in collision with car, pick-up truck or van, unspecified whether traffic or nontraffic accident

Pedestrian in motorized mobility scooter injured in collision with car, pick-up truck or van, unspecified whether traffic or nontraffic accident

Pedestrian on ice-skates injured in collision with car, pick-up truck or van, unspecified whether traffic or nontraffic accident

Pedestrian on nonmotorized scooter injured in collision with car, pick-up truck or van, unspecified whether traffic or nontraffic accident

Pedestrian on sled injured in collision with car, pick-up truck or van in nontraffic accident

Pedestrian on snowboard injured in collision with car, pick-up truck or van, unspecified whether traffic or nontraffic accident

Pedestrian on snow-skis injured in collision with car, pick-up truck or van, unspecified whether traffic or nontraffic accident

● **V04**   **Pedestrian injured in collision with heavy transport vehicle or bus**

> | Excludes1 | pedestrian injured in collision with military vehicle (V09.01, V09.21) |
> |---|---|

> The appropriate 7th character is to be added to each code from category V04
>
> | A | initial encounter |
> |---|---|
> | D | subsequent encounter |
> | S | sequela |

● **V04.0**   **Pedestrian injured in collision with heavy transport vehicle or bus in nontraffic accident**

   X● **V04.00**   **Pedestrian on foot injured in collision with heavy transport vehicle or bus in nontraffic accident**

      Pedestrian NOS injured in collision with heavy transport vehicle or bus in nontraffic accident

   X● **V04.01**   **Pedestrian on roller-skates injured in collision with heavy transport vehicle or bus in nontraffic accident**

   X● **V04.02**   **Pedestrian on skateboard injured in collision with heavy transport vehicle or bus in nontraffic accident**

   X● **V04.09**   **Pedestrian with other conveyance injured in collision with heavy transport vehicle or bus in nontraffic accident**

      Pedestrian with babystroller injured in collision with heavy transport vehicle or bus in nontraffic accident

      Pedestrian in wheelchair (powered) injured in collision with heavy transport vehicle or bus in nontraffic accident

      Pedestrian in motorized mobility scooter injured in collision with heavy transport vehicle or bus in nontraffic accident

      Pedestrian on ice-skates injured in collision with heavy transport vehicle or bus in nontraffic accident

      Pedestrian on nonmotorized scooter injured in collision with heavy transport vehicle or bus in nontraffic accident

      Pedestrian on sled injured in collision with heavy transport vehicle or bus in nontraffic accident

      Pedestrian on snowboard injured in collision with heavy transport vehicle or bus in nontraffic accident

      Pedestrian on snow-skis injured in collision with heavy transport vehicle or bus in nontraffic accident

● **V04.1**   **Pedestrian injured in collision with heavy transport vehicle or bus in traffic accident**

   X● **V04.10**   **Pedestrian on foot injured in collision with heavy transport vehicle or bus in traffic accident**

      Pedestrian NOS injured in collision with heavy transport vehicle or bus in traffic accident

   X● **V04.11**   **Pedestrian on roller-skates injured in collision with heavy transport vehicle or bus in traffic accident**

   X● **V04.12**   **Pedestrian on skateboard injured in collision with heavy transport vehicle or bus in traffic accident**

   X● **V04.19**   **Pedestrian with other conveyance injured in collision with heavy transport vehicle or bus in traffic accident**

      Pedestrian with babystroller injured in collision with heavy transport vehicle or bus in traffic accident

      Pedestrian in wheelchair (powered) injured in collision with heavy transport vehicle or bus in traffic accident

      Pedestrian in motorized mobility scooter injured in collision with heavy transport vehicle or bus in traffic accident

      Pedestrian on ice-skates injured in collision with heavy transport vehicle or bus in traffic accident

      Pedestrian on nonmotorized scooter injured in collision with heavy transport vehicle or bus in traffic accident

      Pedestrian on sled injured in collision with heavy transport vehicle or bus in traffic accident

      Pedestrian on snowboard injured in collision with heavy transport vehicle or bus in traffic accident

      Pedestrian on snow-skis injured in collision with heavy transport vehicle or bus in traffic accident

● **V04.9**   **Pedestrian injured in collision with heavy transport vehicle or bus, unspecified whether traffic or nontraffic accident**

   X● **V04.90**   **Pedestrian on foot injured in collision with heavy transport vehicle or bus, unspecified whether traffic or nontraffic accident**

      Pedestrian NOS injured in collision with heavy transport vehicle or bus, unspecified whether traffic or nontraffic accident

   X● **V04.91**   **Pedestrian on roller-skates injured in collision with heavy transport vehicle or bus, unspecified whether traffic or nontraffic accident**

   X● **V04.92**   **Pedestrian on skateboard injured in collision with heavy transport vehicle or bus, unspecified whether traffic or nontraffic accident**

   X● **V04.99**   **Pedestrian with other conveyance injured in collision with heavy transport vehicle or bus, unspecified whether traffic or nontraffic accident**

      Pedestrian with babystroller injured in collision with heavy transport vehicle or bus, unspecified whether traffic or nontraffic accident

      Pedestrian in wheelchair (powered) injured in collision with heavy transport vehicle or bus, unspecified whether traffic or nontraffic accident

      Pedestrian in motorized mobility scooter injured in collision with heavy transport vehicle or bus, unspecified whether traffic or nontraffic accident

      Pedestrian on ice-skates injured in collision with heavy transport vehicle or bus, unspecified whether traffic or nontraffic accident

      Pedestrian on nonmotorized scooter injured in collision with heavy transport vehicle or bus, unspecified whether traffic or nontraffic accident

      Pedestrian on sled injured in collision with heavy transport vehicle or bus, unspecified whether traffic or nontraffic accident

      Pedestrian on snowboard injured in collision with heavy transport vehicle or bus, unspecified whether traffic or nontraffic accident

      Pedestrian on snow-skis injured in collision with heavy transport vehicle or bus, unspecified whether traffic or nontraffic accident

◀ New   ◀▥ Revised   ~~deleted~~ Deleted   Excludes 1   Excludes 2   Includes   Use additional   Code first   Code also   Unspecified

OGCR Official Guidelines   X Assign placeholder X   ● Use Additional Character(s)   ▶ Manifestation Code   **Coding Clinic**

● **V05**   **Pedestrian injured in collision with railway train or railway vehicle**

The appropriate 7th character is to be added to each code from category V05

> A   initial encounter
> D   subsequent encounter
> S   sequela

● **V05.0**   **Pedestrian injured in collision with railway train or railway vehicle in nontraffic accident**

X● **V05.00**   **Pedestrian on foot injured in collision with railway train or railway vehicle in nontraffic accident**

Pedestrian NOS injured in collision with railway train or railway vehicle in nontraffic accident

X● **V05.01**   **Pedestrian on roller-skates injured in collision with railway train or railway vehicle in nontraffic accident**

X● **V05.02**   **Pedestrian on skateboard injured in collision with railway train or railway vehicle in nontraffic accident**

X● **V05.09**   **Pedestrian with other conveyance injured in collision with railway train or railway vehicle in nontraffic accident**

Pedestrian with babystroller injured in collision with railway train or railway vehicle in nontraffic accident

Pedestrian in wheelchair (powered) injured in collision with railway train or railway vehicle in nontraffic accident

Pedestrian in motorized mobility scooter injured in collision with railway train or railway vehicle in nontraffic accident

Pedestrian on ice-skates injured in collision with railway train or railway vehicle in nontraffic accident

Pedestrian on nonmotorized scooter injured in collision with railway train or railway vehicle in nontraffic accident

Pedestrian on sled injured in collision with railway train or railway vehicle in nontraffic accident

Pedestrian on snowboard injured in collision with railway train or railway vehicle in nontraffic accident

Pedestrian on snow-skis injured in collision with railway train or railway vehicle in nontraffic accident

● **V05.1**   **Pedestrian injured in collision with railway train or railway vehicle in traffic accident**

X● **V05.10**   **Pedestrian on foot injured in collision with railway train or railway vehicle in traffic accident**

Pedestrian NOS injured in collision with railway train or railway vehicle in traffic accident

X● **V05.11**   **Pedestrian on roller-skates injured in collision with railway train or railway vehicle in traffic accident**

X● **V05.12**   **Pedestrian on skateboard injured in collision with railway train or railway vehicle in traffic accident**

X● **V05.19**   **Pedestrian with other conveyance injured in collision with railway train or railway vehicle in traffic accident**

Pedestrian with babystroller injured in collision with railway train or railway vehicle in traffic accident

Pedestrian in wheelchair (powered) injured in collision with railway train or railway vehicle in traffic accident

Pedestrian in motorized mobility scooter injured in collision with railway train or railway vehicle in traffic accident

Pedestrian on ice-skates injured in collision with railway train or railway vehicle in traffic accident

Pedestrian on nonmotorized scooter injured in collision with railway train or railway vehicle in traffic accident

Pedestrian on sled injured in collision with railway train or railway vehicle in traffic accident

Pedestrian on snowboard injured in collision with railway train or railway vehicle in traffic accident

Pedestrian on snow-skis injured in collision with railway train or railway vehicle in traffic accident

● **V05.9**   **Pedestrian injured in collision with railway train or railway vehicle, unspecified whether traffic or nontraffic accident**

X● **V05.90**   **Pedestrian on foot injured in collision with railway train or railway vehicle, unspecified whether traffic or nontraffic accident**

Pedestrian NOS injured in collision with railway train or railway vehicle, unspecified whether traffic or nontraffic accident

X● **V05.91**   **Pedestrian on roller-skates injured in collision with railway train or railway vehicle, unspecified whether traffic or nontraffic accident**

X● **V05.92**   **Pedestrian on skateboard injured in collision with railway train or railway vehicle, unspecified whether traffic or nontraffic accident**

X● **V05.99**   **Pedestrian with other conveyance injured in collision with railway train or railway vehicle, unspecified whether traffic or nontraffic accident**

Pedestrian with babystroller injured in collision with railway train or railway vehicle, unspecified whether traffic or nontraffic

Pedestrian in wheelchair (powered) injured in collision with railway train or railway vehicle, unspecified whether traffic or nontraffic

Pedestrian in motorized mobility scooter injured in collision with railway train or railway vehicle, unspecified whether traffic or nontraffic

Pedestrian on ice-skates injured in collision with railway train or railway vehicle, unspecified whether traffic or nontraffic

Pedestrian on nonmotorized scooter injured in collision with railway train or railway vehicle, unspecified whether traffic or nontraffic

Pedestrian on sled injured in collision with railway train or railway vehicle, unspecified whether traffic or nontraffic

Pedestrian on snowboard injured in collision with railway train or railway vehicle, unspecified whether traffic or nontraffic

Pedestrian on snow-skis injured in collision with railway train or railway vehicle, unspecified whether traffic or nontraffic

CHAPTER 20 (V01-Y99)

● **V06   Pedestrian injured in collision with other nonmotor vehicle**

> **Includes**   collision with animal-drawn vehicle, animal being ridden, nonpowered streetcar

> **Excludes1**   pedestrian injured in collision with pedestrian conveyance (V00.0-)

The appropriate 7th character is to be added to each code from category V06

> A   initial encounter
> D   subsequent encounter
> S   sequela

● **V06.0   Pedestrian injured in collision with other nonmotor vehicle in nontraffic accident**

X● **V06.00   Pedestrian on foot injured in collision with other nonmotor vehicle in nontraffic accident**
> Pedestrian NOS injured in collision with other nonmotor vehicle in nontraffic accident

X● **V06.01   Pedestrian on roller-skates injured in collision with other nonmotor vehicle in nontraffic accident**

X● **V06.02   Pedestrian on skateboard injured in collision with other nonmotor vehicle in nontraffic accident**

X● **V06.09   Pedestrian with other conveyance injured in collision with other nonmotor vehicle in nontraffic accident**
> Pedestrian with babystroller injured in collision with other nonmotor vehicle in nontraffic accident
> Pedestrian in wheelchair (powered) injured in collision with other nonmotor vehicle in nontraffic accident
> Pedestrian in motorized mobility scooter injured in collision with other nonmotor vehicle in nontraffic accident
> Pedestrian on ice-skates injured in collision with other nonmotor vehicle in nontraffic accident
> Pedestrian on nonmotorized scooter injured in collision with other nonmotor vehicle in nontraffic accident
> Pedestrian on sled injured in collision with other nonmotor vehicle in nontraffic accident
> Pedestrian on snowboard injured in collision with other nonmotor vehicle in nontraffic accident
> Pedestrian on snow-skis injured in collision with other nonmotor vehicle in nontraffic accident

● **V06.1   Pedestrian injured in collision with other nonmotor vehicle in traffic accident**

X● **V06.10   Pedestrian on foot injured in collision with other nonmotor vehicle in traffic accident**
> Pedestrian NOS injured in collision with other nonmotor vehicle in traffic accident

X● **V06.11   Pedestrian on roller-skates injured in collision with other nonmotor vehicle in traffic accident**

X● **V06.12   Pedestrian on skateboard injured in collision with other nonmotor vehicle in traffic accident**

X● **V06.19   Pedestrian with other conveyance injured in collision with other nonmotor vehicle in traffic accident**
> Pedestrian with babystroller injured in collision with other nonmotor vehicle in nontraffic accident
> Pedestrian in wheelchair (powered) injured in collision with other nonmotor vehicle in traffic accident
> Pedestrian in motorized mobility scooter injured in collision with other nonmotor vehicle in traffic accident
> Pedestrian on ice-skates injured in collision with other nonmotor vehicle in traffic accident
> Pedestrian on nonmotorized scooter injured in collision with other nonmotor vehicle in traffic accident
> Pedestrian on sled injured in collision with other nonmotor vehicle in traffic accident
> Pedestrian on snowboard injured in collision with other nonmotor vehicle in traffic accident
> Pedestrian on snow-skis injured in collision with other nonmotor vehicle in traffic accident

● **V06.9   Pedestrian injured in collision with other nonmotor vehicle, unspecified whether traffic or nontraffic accident**

X● **V06.90   Pedestrian on foot injured in collision with other nonmotor vehicle, unspecified whether traffic or nontraffic accident**
> Pedestrian NOS injured in collision with other nonmotor vehicle, unspecified whether traffic or nontraffic accident

X● **V06.91   Pedestrian on roller-skates injured in collision with other nonmotor vehicle, unspecified whether traffic or nontraffic accident**

X● **V06.92   Pedestrian on skateboard injured in collision with other nonmotor vehicle, unspecified whether traffic or nontraffic accident**

X● **V06.99   Pedestrian with other conveyance injured in collision with other nonmotor vehicle, unspecified whether traffic or nontraffic accident**
> Pedestrian with babystroller injured in collision with other nonmotor vehicle, unspecified whether traffic or nontraffic accident
> Pedestrian in wheelchair (powered) injured in collision with other nonmotor vehicle, unspecified whether traffic or nontraffic accident
> Pedestrian in motorized mobility scooter injured in collision with other nonmotor vehicle, unspecified whether traffic or nontraffic accident
> Pedestrian on ice-skates injured in collision with other nonmotor vehicle, unspecified whether traffic or nontraffic accident
> Pedestrian on nonmotorized scooter injured in collision with other nonmotor vehicle, unspecified whether traffic or nontraffic accident
> Pedestrian on sled injured in collision with other nonmotor vehicle, unspecified whether traffic or nontraffic accident
> Pedestrian on snowboard injured in collision with other nonmotor vehicle, unspecified whether traffic or nontraffic accident
> Pedestrian on snow-skis injured in collision with other nonmotor vehicle, unspecified whether traffic or nontraffic accident

◀ New   ◀▬ Revised   ~~deleted~~ Deleted   Excludes 1   Excludes 2   Includes   Use additional   Code first   Code also   Unspecified

OGCR Official Guidelines   X Assign placeholder X   ● Use Additional Character(s)   ▶ Manifestation Code   **Coding Clinic**

● **V09**   **Pedestrian injured in other and unspecified transport accidents**
> The appropriate 7th character is to be added to each code from category V09

> | A | initial encounter |
> |---|---|
> | D | subsequent encounter |
> | S | sequela |

   ● **V09.0**   **Pedestrian injured in nontraffic accident involving other and unspecified motor vehicles**

     X● **V09.00**   Pedestrian injured in nontraffic accident involving unspecified motor vehicles

     X● **V09.01**   Pedestrian injured in nontraffic accident involving military vehicle

     X● **V09.09**   Pedestrian injured in nontraffic accident involving other motor vehicles
> Pedestrian injured in nontraffic accident by special vehicle

   X● **V09.1**   Pedestrian injured in unspecified nontraffic accident

   ● **V09.2**   **Pedestrian injured in traffic accident involving other and unspecified motor vehicles**

     X● **V09.20**   Pedestrian injured in traffic accident involving unspecified motor vehicles

     X● **V09.21**   Pedestrian injured in traffic accident involving military vehicle

     X● **V09.29**   Pedestrian injured in traffic accident involving other motor vehicles

   X● **V09.3**   Pedestrian injured in unspecified traffic accident

   X● **V09.9**   Pedestrian injured in unspecified transport accident

PEDAL CYCLE RIDER INJURED IN TRANSPORT ACCIDENT (V10-V19)

> | **Includes** | any non-motorized vehicle, excluding an animal-drawn vehicle, or a sidecar or trailer attached to the pedal cycle |
> |---|---|
> | **Excludes2** | rupture of pedal cycle tire (W37.0) |

● **V10**   **Pedal cycle rider injured in collision with pedestrian or animal**
> | **Excludes1** | pedal cycle rider collision with animal-drawn vehicle or animal being ridden (V16.-) |
> |---|---|

> The appropriate 7th character is to be added to each code from category V10

> | A | initial encounter |
> |---|---|
> | D | subsequent encounter |
> | S | sequela |

   X● **V10.0**   Pedal cycle driver injured in collision with pedestrian or animal in nontraffic accident

   X● **V10.1**   Pedal cycle passenger injured in collision with pedestrian or animal in nontraffic accident

   X● **V10.2**   Unspecified pedal cyclist injured in collision with pedestrian or animal in nontraffic accident

   X● **V10.3**   Person boarding or alighting a pedal cycle injured in collision with pedestrian or animal

   X● **V10.4**   Pedal cycle driver injured in collision with pedestrian or animal in traffic accident

   X● **V10.5**   Pedal cycle passenger injured in collision with pedestrian or animal in traffic accident

   X● **V10.9**   Unspecified pedal cyclist injured in collision with pedestrian or animal in traffic accident

● **V11**   **Pedal cycle rider injured in collision with other pedal cycle**
> The appropriate 7th character is to be added to each code from category V11

> | A | initial encounter |
> |---|---|
> | D | subsequent encounter |
> | S | sequela |

   X● **V11.0**   Pedal cycle driver injured in collision with other pedal cycle in nontraffic accident

   X● **V11.1**   Pedal cycle passenger injured in collision with other pedal cycle in nontraffic accident

   X● **V11.2**   Unspecified pedal cyclist injured in collision with other pedal cycle in nontraffic accident

   X● **V11.3**   Person boarding or alighting a pedal cycle injured in collision with other pedal cycle

   X● **V11.4**   Pedal cycle driver injured in collision with other pedal cycle in traffic accident

   X● **V11.5**   Pedal cycle passenger injured in collision with other pedal cycle in traffic accident

   X● **V11.9**   Unspecified pedal cyclist injured in collision with other pedal cycle in traffic accident

● **V12**   **Pedal cycle rider injured in collision with two- or three-wheeled motor vehicle**
> The appropriate 7th character is to be added to each code from category V12

> | A | initial encounter |
> |---|---|
> | D | subsequent encounter |
> | S | sequela |

   X● **V12.0**   Pedal cycle driver injured in collision with two- or three-wheeled motor vehicle in nontraffic accident

   X● **V12.1**   Pedal cycle passenger injured in collision with two- or three-wheeled motor vehicle in nontraffic accident

   X● **V12.2**   Unspecified pedal cyclist injured in collision with two- or three-wheeled motor vehicle in nontraffic accident

   X● **V12.3**   Person boarding or alighting a pedal cycle injured in collision with two- or three-wheeled motor vehicle

   X● **V12.4**   Pedal cycle driver injured in collision with two- or three-wheeled motor vehicle in traffic accident

   X● **V12.5**   Pedal cycle passenger injured in collision with two- or three-wheeled motor vehicle in traffic accident

   X● **V12.9**   Unspecified pedal cyclist injured in collision with two- or three-wheeled motor vehicle in traffic accident

● **V13**   **Pedal cycle rider injured in collision with car, pick-up truck or van**
> The appropriate 7th character is to be added to each code from category V13

> | A | initial encounter |
> |---|---|
> | D | subsequent encounter |
> | S | sequela |

   X● **V13.0**   Pedal cycle driver injured in collision with car, pick-up truck or van in nontraffic accident

   X● **V13.1**   Pedal cycle passenger injured in collision with car, pick-up truck or van in nontraffic accident

   X● **V13.2**   Unspecified pedal cyclist injured in collision with car, pick-up truck or van in nontraffic accident

   X● **V13.3**   Person boarding or alighting a pedal cycle injured in collision with car, pick-up truck or van

   X● **V13.4**   Pedal cycle driver injured in collision with car, pick-up truck or van in traffic accident

   X● **V13.5**   Pedal cycle passenger injured in collision with car, pick-up truck or van in traffic accident

   X● **V13.9**   Unspecified pedal cyclist injured in collision with car, pick-up truck or van in traffic accident

CHAPTER 20 (V01-Y99)

● **V14 Pedal cycle rider injured in collision with heavy transport vehicle or bus**

> **Excludes1**   pedal cycle rider injured in collision with military vehicle (V19.81)

> The appropriate 7th character is to be added to each code from category V14

> | | |
> |---|---|
> | A | initial encounter |
> | D | subsequent encounter |
> | S | sequela |

X● **V14.0** Pedal cycle driver injured in collision with heavy transport vehicle or bus in nontraffic accident

X● **V14.1** Pedal cycle passenger injured in collision with heavy transport vehicle or bus in nontraffic accident

X● **V14.2** Unspecified pedal cyclist injured in collision with heavy transport vehicle or bus in nontraffic accident

X● **V14.3** Person boarding or alighting a pedal cycle injured in collision with heavy transport vehicle or bus

X● **V14.4** Pedal cycle driver injured in collision with heavy transport vehicle or bus in traffic accident

X● **V14.5** Pedal cycle passenger injured in collision with heavy transport vehicle or bus in traffic accident

X● **V14.9** Unspecified pedal cyclist injured in collision with heavy transport vehicle or bus in traffic accident

● **V15 Pedal cycle rider injured in collision with railway train or railway vehicle**

> The appropriate 7th character is to be added to each code from category V15

> | | |
> |---|---|
> | A | initial encounter |
> | D | subsequent encounter |
> | S | sequela |

X● **V15.0** Pedal cycle driver injured in collision with railway train or railway vehicle in nontraffic accident

X● **V15.1** Pedal cycle passenger injured in collision with railway train or railway vehicle in nontraffic accident

X● **V15.2** Unspecified pedal cyclist injured in collision with railway train or railway vehicle in nontraffic accident

X● **V15.3** Person boarding or alighting a pedal cycle injured in collision with railway train or railway vehicle

X● **V15.4** Pedal cycle driver injured in collision with railway train or railway vehicle in traffic accident

X● **V15.5** Pedal cycle passenger injured in collision with railway train or railway vehicle in traffic accident

X● **V15.9** Unspecified pedal cyclist injured in collision with railway train or railway vehicle in traffic accident

● **V16 Pedal cycle rider injured in collision with other nonmotor vehicle**

> **Includes**   collision with animal-drawn vehicle, animal being ridden, streetcar

> The appropriate 7th character is to be added to each code from category V16

> | | |
> |---|---|
> | A | initial encounter |
> | D | subsequent encounter |
> | S | sequela |

X● **V16.0** Pedal cycle driver injured in collision with other nonmotor vehicle in nontraffic accident

X● **V16.1** Pedal cycle passenger injured in collision with other nonmotor vehicle in nontraffic accident

X● **V16.2** Unspecified pedal cyclist injured in collision with other nonmotor vehicle in nontraffic accident

X● **V16.3** Person boarding or alighting a pedal cycle injured in collision with other nonmotor vehicle in nontraffic accident

X● **V16.4** Pedal cycle driver injured in collision with other nonmotor vehicle in traffic accident

X● **V16.5** Pedal cycle passenger injured in collision with other nonmotor vehicle in traffic accident

X● **V16.9** Unspecified pedal cyclist injured in collision with other nonmotor vehicle in traffic accident

● **V17 Pedal cycle rider injured in collision with fixed or stationary object**

> The appropriate 7th character is to be added to each code from category V17

> | | |
> |---|---|
> | A | initial encounter |
> | D | subsequent encounter |
> | S | sequela |

X● **V17.0** Pedal cycle driver injured in collision with fixed or stationary object in nontraffic accident

X● **V17.1** Pedal cycle passenger injured in collision with fixed or stationary object in nontraffic accident

X● **V17.2** Unspecified pedal cyclist injured in collision with fixed or stationary object in nontraffic accident

X● **V17.3** Person boarding or alighting a pedal cycle injured in collision with fixed or stationary object

X● **V17.4** Pedal cycle driver injured in collision with fixed or stationary object in traffic accident

X● **V17.5** Pedal cycle passenger injured in collision with fixed or stationary object in traffic accident

X● **V17.9** Unspecified pedal cyclist injured in collision with fixed or stationary object in traffic accident

● **V18 Pedal cycle rider injured in noncollision transport accident**

> **Includes**   fall or thrown from pedal cycle (without antecedent collision)
> overturning pedal cycle NOS
> overturning pedal cycle without collision

> The appropriate 7th character is to be added to each code from category V18

> | | |
> |---|---|
> | A | initial encounter |
> | D | subsequent encounter |
> | S | sequela |

X● **V18.0** Pedal cycle driver injured in noncollision transport accident in nontraffic accident

X● **V18.1** Pedal cycle passenger injured in noncollision transport accident in nontraffic accident

X● **V18.2** Unspecified pedal cyclist injured in noncollision transport accident in nontraffic accident

X● **V18.3** Person boarding or alighting a pedal cycle injured in noncollision transport accident

X● **V18.4** Pedal cycle driver injured in noncollision transport accident in traffic accident

X● **V18.5** Pedal cycle passenger injured in noncollision transport accident in traffic accident

X● **V18.9** Unspecified pedal cyclist injured in noncollision transport accident in traffic accident

● **V19 Pedal cycle rider injured in other and unspecified transport accidents**

> The appropriate 7th character is to be added to each code from category V19

> | | |
> |---|---|
> | A | initial encounter |
> | D | subsequent encounter |
> | S | sequela |

● **V19.0** Pedal cycle driver injured in collision with other and unspecified motor vehicles in nontraffic accident

    X● **V19.00** Pedal cycle driver injured in collision with unspecified motor vehicles in nontraffic accident

    X● **V19.09** Pedal cycle driver injured in collision with other motor vehicles in nontraffic accident

◀ New   ◀◀ Revised   ~~deleted~~ Deleted   Excludes 1   Excludes 2   Includes   Use additional   Code first   Code also   Unspecified

OGCR Official Guidelines   **X** Assign placeholder X   ● Use Additional Character(s)   ▶ Manifestation Code   **Coding Clinic**

- **V19.1** Pedal cycle passenger injured in collision with other and unspecified motor vehicles in nontraffic accident
  - X● **V19.10** Pedal cycle passenger injured in collision with unspecified motor vehicles in nontraffic accident
  - X● **V19.19** Pedal cycle passenger injured in collision with other motor vehicles in nontraffic accident
- **V19.2** Unspecified pedal cyclist injured in collision with other and unspecified motor vehicles in nontraffic accident
  - X● **V19.20** Unspecified pedal cyclist injured in collision with unspecified motor vehicles in nontraffic accident
    Pedal cycle collision NOS, nontraffic
  - X● **V19.29** Unspecified pedal cyclist injured in collision with other motor vehicles in nontraffic accident
- X● **V19.3** Pedal cyclist (driver) (passenger) injured in unspecified nontraffic accident
  Pedal cycle accident NOS, nontraffic
  Pedal cyclist injured in nontraffic accident NOS
- **V19.4** Pedal cycle driver injured in collision with other and unspecified motor vehicles in traffic accident
  - X● **V19.40** Pedal cycle driver injured in collision with unspecified motor vehicles in traffic accident
  - X● **V19.49** Pedal cycle driver injured in collision with other motor vehicles in traffic accident
- **V19.5** Pedal cycle passenger injured in collision with other and unspecified motor vehicles in traffic accident
  - X● **V19.50** Pedal cycle passenger injured in collision with unspecified motor vehicles in traffic accident
  - X● **V19.59** Pedal cycle passenger injured in collision with other motor vehicles in traffic accident
- **V19.6** Unspecified pedal cyclist injured in collision with other and unspecified motor vehicles in traffic accident
  - X● **V19.60** Unspecified pedal cyclist injured in collision with unspecified motor vehicles in traffic accident
    Pedal cycle collision NOS (traffic)
  - X● **V19.69** Unspecified pedal cyclist injured in collision with other motor vehicles in traffic accident
- **V19.8** Pedal cyclist (driver) (passenger) injured in other specified transport accidents
  - X● **V19.81** Pedal cyclist (driver) (passenger) injured in transport accident with military vehicle
  - X● **V19.88** Pedal cyclist (driver) (passenger) injured in other specified transport accidents
- X● **V19.9** Pedal cyclist (driver) (passenger) injured in unspecified traffic accident
  Pedal cycle accident NOS

MOTORCYCLE RIDER INJURED IN TRANSPORT ACCIDENT (V20-V29)

Includes	moped motorcycle with sidecar motorized bicycle motor scooter
Excludes1	three-wheeled motor vehicle (V30-V39)

- ● **V20** Motorcycle rider injured in collision with pedestrian or animal

Excludes1	motorcycle rider collision with animal-drawn vehicle or animal being ridden (V26.-)

  The appropriate 7th character is to be added to each code from category V20

A	initial encounter
D	subsequent encounter
S	sequela

  - X● **V20.0** Motorcycle driver injured in collision with pedestrian or animal in nontraffic accident
  - X● **V20.1** Motorcycle passenger injured in collision with pedestrian or animal in nontraffic accident
  - X● **V20.2** Unspecified motorcycle rider injured in collision with pedestrian or animal in nontraffic accident
  - X● **V20.3** Person boarding or alighting a motorcycle injured in collision with pedestrian or animal

- X● **V20.4** Motorcycle driver injured in collision with pedestrian or animal in traffic accident
- X● **V20.5** Motorcycle passenger injured in collision with pedestrian or animal in traffic accident
- X● **V20.9** Unspecified motorcycle rider injured in collision with pedestrian or animal in traffic accident

- ● **V21** Motorcycle rider injured in collision with pedal cycle

  The appropriate 7th character is to be added to each code from category V21

A	initial encounter
D	subsequent encounter
S	sequela

  - X● **V21.0** Motorcycle driver injured in collision with pedal cycle in nontraffic accident
  - X● **V21.1** Motorcycle passenger injured in collision with pedal cycle in nontraffic accident
  - X● **V21.2** Unspecified motorcycle rider injured in collision with pedal cycle in nontraffic accident
  - X● **V21.3** Person boarding or alighting a motorcycle injured in collision with pedal cycle
  - X● **V21.4** Motorcycle driver injured in collision with pedal cycle in traffic accident
  - X● **V21.5** Motorcycle passenger injured in collision with pedal cycle in traffic accident
  - X● **V21.9** Unspecified motorcycle rider injured in collision with pedal cycle in traffic accident

- ● **V22** Motorcycle rider injured in collision with two- or three-wheeled motor vehicle

  The appropriate 7th character is to be added to each code from category V22

A	initial encounter
D	subsequent encounter
S	sequela

  - X● **V22.0** Motorcycle driver injured in collision with two- or three-wheeled motor vehicle in nontraffic accident
  - X● **V22.1** Motorcycle passenger injured in collision with two- or three-wheeled motor vehicle in nontraffic accident
  - X● **V22.2** Unspecified motorcycle rider injured in collision with two- or three-wheeled motor vehicle in nontraffic accident
  - X● **V22.3** Person boarding or alighting a motorcycle injured in collision with two- or three-wheeled motor vehicle
  - X● **V22.4** Motorcycle driver injured in collision with two- or three-wheeled motor vehicle in traffic accident
  - X● **V22.5** Motorcycle passenger injured in collision with two- or three-wheeled motor vehicle in traffic accident
  - X● **V22.9** Unspecified motorcycle rider injured in collision with two- or three-wheeled motor vehicle in traffic accident

- ● **V23** Motorcycle rider injured in collision with car, pick-up truck or van

  The appropriate 7th character is to be added to each code from category V23

A	initial encounter
D	subsequent encounter
S	sequela

  - X● **V23.0** Motorcycle driver injured in collision with car, pick-up truck or van in nontraffic accident
  - X● **V23.1** Motorcycle passenger injured in collision with car, pick-up truck or van in nontraffic accident
  - X● **V23.2** Unspecified motorcycle rider injured in collision with car, pick-up truck or van in nontraffic accident
  - X● **V23.3** Person boarding or alighting a motorcycle injured in collision with car, pick-up truck or van
  - X● **V23.4** Motorcycle driver injured in collision with car, pick-up truck or van in traffic accident

X● **V23.5** Motorcycle passenger injured in collision with car, pick-up truck or van in traffic accident

X● **V23.9** Unspecified motorcycle rider injured in collision with car, pick-up truck or van in traffic accident

● **V24** Motorcycle rider injured in collision with heavy transport vehicle or bus

> **Excludes1** motorcycle rider injured in collision with military vehicle (V29.81)

> The appropriate 7th character is to be added to each code from category V24

> | A | initial encounter |
> |---|---|
> | D | subsequent encounter |
> | S | sequela |

X● **V24.0** Motorcycle driver injured in collision with heavy transport vehicle or bus in nontraffic accident

X● **V24.1** Motorcycle passenger injured in collision with heavy transport vehicle or bus in nontraffic accident

X● **V24.2** Unspecified motorcycle rider injured in collision with heavy transport vehicle or bus in nontraffic accident

X● **V24.3** Person boarding or alighting a motorcycle injured in collision with heavy transport vehicle or bus

X● **V24.4** Motorcycle driver injured in collision with heavy transport vehicle or bus in traffic accident

X● **V24.5** Motorcycle passenger injured in collision with heavy transport vehicle or bus in traffic accident

X● **V24.9** Unspecified motorcycle rider injured in collision with heavy transport vehicle or bus in traffic accident

● **V25** Motorcycle rider injured in collision with railway train or railway vehicle

> The appropriate 7th character is to be added to each code from category V25

> | A | initial encounter |
> |---|---|
> | D | subsequent encounter |
> | S | sequela |

X● **V25.0** Motorcycle driver injured in collision with railway train or railway vehicle in nontraffic accident

X● **V25.1** Motorcycle passenger injured in collision with railway train or railway vehicle in nontraffic accident

X● **V25.2** Unspecified motorcycle rider injured in collision with railway train or railway vehicle in nontraffic accident

X● **V25.3** Person boarding or alighting a motorcycle injured in collision with railway train or railway vehicle

X● **V25.4** Motorcycle driver injured in collision with railway train or railway vehicle in traffic accident

X● **V25.5** Motorcycle passenger injured in collision with railway train or railway vehicle in traffic accident

X● **V25.9** Unspecified motorcycle rider injured in collision with railway train or railway vehicle in traffic accident

● **V26** Motorcycle rider injured in collision with other nonmotor vehicle

> **Includes** collision with animal-drawn vehicle, animal being ridden, streetcar

> The appropriate 7th character is to be added to each code from category V26

> | A | initial encounter |
> |---|---|
> | D | subsequent encounter |
> | S | sequela |

X● **V26.0** Motorcycle driver injured in collision with other nonmotor vehicle in nontraffic accident

X● **V26.1** Motorcycle passenger injured in collision with other nonmotor vehicle in nontraffic accident

X● **V26.2** Unspecified motorcycle rider injured in collision with other nonmotor vehicle in nontraffic accident

X● **V26.3** Person boarding or alighting a motorcycle injured in collision with other nonmotor vehicle

X● **V26.4** Motorcycle driver injured in collision with other nonmotor vehicle in traffic accident

X● **V26.5** Motorcycle passenger injured in collision with other nonmotor vehicle in traffic accident

X● **V26.9** Unspecified motorcycle rider injured in collision with other nonmotor vehicle in traffic accident

● **V27** Motorcycle rider injured in collision with fixed or stationary object

> The appropriate 7th character is to be added to each code from category V27

> | A | initial encounter |
> |---|---|
> | D | subsequent encounter |
> | S | sequela |

X● **V27.0** Motorcycle driver injured in collision with fixed or stationary object in nontraffic accident

X● **V27.1** Motorcycle passenger injured in collision with fixed or stationary object in nontraffic accident

X● **V27.2** Unspecified motorcycle rider injured in collision with fixed or stationary object in nontraffic accident

X● **V27.3** Person boarding or alighting a motorcycle injured in collision with fixed or stationary object

X● **V27.4** Motorcycle driver injured in collision with fixed or stationary object in traffic accident

X● **V27.5** Motorcycle passenger injured in collision with fixed or stationary object in traffic accident

X● **V27.9** Unspecified motorcycle rider injured in collision with fixed or stationary object in traffic accident

● **V28** Motorcycle rider injured in noncollision transport accident

> **Includes** fall or thrown from motorcycle (without antecedent collision)
> overturning motorcycle NOS
> overturning motorcycle without collision

> The appropriate 7th character is to be added to each code from category V28

> | A | initial encounter |
> |---|---|
> | D | subsequent encounter |
> | S | sequela |

X● **V28.0** Motorcycle driver injured in noncollision transport accident in nontraffic accident

X● **V28.1** Motorcycle passenger injured in noncollision transport accident in nontraffic accident

X● **V28.2** Unspecified motorcycle rider injured in noncollision transport accident in nontraffic accident

X● **V28.3** Person boarding or alighting a motorcycle injured in noncollision transport accident

X● **V28.4** Motorcycle driver injured in noncollision transport accident in traffic accident

X● **V28.5** Motorcycle passenger injured in noncollision transport accident in traffic accident

X● **V28.9** Unspecified motorcycle rider injured in noncollision transport accident in traffic accident

● **V29** Motorcycle rider injured in other and unspecified transport accidents

> The appropriate 7th character is to be added to each code from category V29

> | A | initial encounter |
> |---|---|
> | D | subsequent encounter |
> | S | sequela |

● **V29.0** Motorcycle driver injured in collision with other and unspecified motor vehicles in nontraffic accident

   X● **V29.00** Motorcycle driver injured in collision with unspecified motor vehicles in nontraffic accident

   X● **V29.09** Motorcycle driver injured in collision with other motor vehicles in nontraffic accident

◀ New   ◀━ Revised   ~~deleted~~ Deleted   Excludes 1   Excludes 2   Includes   Use additional   Code first   Code also   Unspecified

OGCR Official Guidelines   X Assign placeholder X   ● Use Additional Character(s)   ▌ Manifestation Code   **Coding Clinic**

● **V29.1** Motorcycle passenger injured in collision with other and unspecified motor vehicles in nontraffic accident

   X● **V29.10** Motorcycle passenger injured in collision with unspecified motor vehicles in nontraffic accident

   X● **V29.19** Motorcycle passenger injured in collision with other motor vehicles in nontraffic accident

● **V29.2** Unspecified motorcycle rider injured in collision with other and unspecified motor vehicles in nontraffic accident

   X● **V29.20** Unspecified motorcycle rider injured in collision with unspecified motor vehicles in nontraffic accident
       Motorcycle collision NOS, nontraffic

   X● **V29.29** Unspecified motorcycle rider injured in collision with other motor vehicles in nontraffic accident

X● **V29.3** Motorcycle rider (driver) (passenger) injured in unspecified nontraffic accident
      Motorcycle accident NOS, nontraffic
      Motorcycle rider injured in nontraffic accident NOS

● **V29.4** Motorcycle driver injured in collision with other and unspecified motor vehicles in traffic accident

   X● **V29.40** Motorcycle driver injured in collision with unspecified motor vehicles in traffic accident

   X● **V29.49** Motorcycle driver injured in collision with other motor vehicles in traffic accident

● **V29.5** Motorcycle passenger injured in collision with other and unspecified motor vehicles in traffic accident

   X● **V29.50** Motorcycle passenger injured in collision with unspecified motor vehicles in traffic accident

   X● **V29.59** Motorcycle passenger injured in collision with other motor vehicles in traffic accident

● **V29.6** Unspecified motorcycle rider injured in collision with other and unspecified motor vehicles in traffic accident

   X● **V29.60** Unspecified motorcycle rider injured in collision with unspecified motor vehicles in traffic accident
       Motorcycle collision NOS (traffic)

   X● **V29.69** Unspecified motorcycle rider injured in collision with other motor vehicles in traffic accident

● **V29.8** Motorcycle rider (driver) (passenger) injured in other specified transport accidents

   X● **V29.81** Motorcycle rider (driver) (passenger) injured in transport accident with military vehicle

   X● **V29.88** Motorcycle rider (driver) (passenger) injured in other specified transport accidents

X● **V29.9** Motorcycle rider (driver) (passenger) injured in unspecified traffic accident
      Motorcycle accident NOS

OCCUPANT OF THREE-WHEELED MOTOR VEHICLE INJURED IN TRANSPORT ACCIDENT (V30-V39)

Includes   motorized tricycle
           motorized rickshaw
           three-wheeled motor car

Excludes1   all-terrain vehicles (V86.-)
            motorcycle with sidecar (V20-V29)
            vehicle designed primarily for off-road use (V86.-)

● **V30** Occupant of three-wheeled motor vehicle injured in collision with pedestrian or animal

   Excludes1   three-wheeled motor vehicle collision with animal-drawn vehicle or animal being ridden (V36.-)

   The appropriate 7th character is to be added to each code from category V30

A	initial encounter
D	subsequent encounter
S	sequela

   X● **V30.0** Driver of three-wheeled motor vehicle injured in collision with pedestrian or animal in nontraffic accident

   X● **V30.1** Passenger in three-wheeled motor vehicle injured in collision with pedestrian or animal in nontraffic accident

   X● **V30.2** Person on outside of three-wheeled motor vehicle injured in collision with pedestrian or animal in nontraffic accident

   X● **V30.3** Unspecified occupant of three-wheeled motor vehicle injured in collision with pedestrian or animal in nontraffic accident

   X● **V30.4** Person boarding or alighting a three-wheeled motor vehicle injured in collision with pedestrian or animal

   X● **V30.5** Driver of three-wheeled motor vehicle injured in collision with pedestrian or animal in traffic accident

   X● **V30.6** Passenger in three-wheeled motor vehicle injured in collision with pedestrian or animal in traffic accident

   X● **V30.7** Person on outside of three-wheeled motor vehicle injured in collision with pedestrian or animal in traffic accident

   X● **V30.9** Unspecified occupant of three-wheeled motor vehicle injured in collision with pedestrian or animal in traffic accident

● **V31** Occupant of three-wheeled motor vehicle injured in collision with pedal cycle

   The appropriate 7th character is to be added to each code from category V31

A	initial encounter
D	subsequent encounter
S	sequela

   X● **V31.0** Driver of three-wheeled motor vehicle injured in collision with pedal cycle in nontraffic accident

   X● **V31.1** Passenger in three-wheeled motor vehicle injured in collision with pedal cycle in nontraffic accident

   X● **V31.2** Person on outside of three-wheeled motor vehicle injured in collision with pedal cycle in nontraffic accident

   X● **V31.3** Unspecified occupant of three-wheeled motor vehicle injured in collision with pedal cycle in nontraffic accident

   X● **V31.4** Person boarding or alighting a three-wheeled motor vehicle injured in collision with pedal cycle

   X● **V31.5** Driver of three-wheeled motor vehicle injured in collision with pedal cycle in traffic accident

   X● **V31.6** Passenger in three-wheeled motor vehicle injured in collision with pedal cycle in traffic accident

   X● **V31.7** Person on outside of three-wheeled motor vehicle injured in collision with pedal cycle in traffic accident

   X● **V31.9** Unspecified occupant of three-wheeled motor vehicle injured in collision with pedal cycle in traffic accident

● **V32 Occupant of three-wheeled motor vehicle injured in collision with two- or three-wheeled motor vehicle**

The appropriate 7th character is to be added to each code from category V32

A	initial encounter
D	subsequent encounter
S	sequela

X● **V32.0** Driver of three-wheeled motor vehicle injured in collision with two- or three-wheeled motor vehicle in nontraffic accident

X● **V32.1** Passenger in three-wheeled motor vehicle injured in collision with two- or three-wheeled motor vehicle in nontraffic accident

X● **V32.2** Person on outside of three-wheeled motor vehicle injured in collision with two- or three-wheeled motor vehicle in nontraffic accident

X● **V32.3** Unspecified occupant of three-wheeled motor vehicle injured in collision with two- or three-wheeled motor vehicle in nontraffic accident

X● **V32.4** Person boarding or alighting a three-wheeled motor vehicle injured in collision with two- or three-wheeled motor vehicle

X● **V32.5** Driver of three-wheeled motor vehicle injured in collision with two- or three-wheeled motor vehicle in traffic accident

X● **V32.6** Passenger in three-wheeled motor vehicle injured in collision with two- or three-wheeled motor vehicle in traffic accident

X● **V32.7** Person on outside of three-wheeled motor vehicle injured in collision with two- or three-wheeled motor vehicle in traffic accident

X● **V32.9** Unspecified occupant of three-wheeled motor vehicle injured in collision with two- or three-wheeled motor vehicle in traffic accident

● **V33 Occupant of three-wheeled motor vehicle injured in collision with car, pick-up truck or van**

The appropriate 7th character is to be added to each code from category V33

A	initial encounter
D	subsequent encounter
S	sequela

X● **V33.0** Driver of three-wheeled motor vehicle injured in collision with car, pick-up truck or van in nontraffic accident

X● **V33.1** Passenger in three-wheeled motor vehicle injured in collision with car, pick-up truck or van in nontraffic accident

X● **V33.2** Person on outside of three-wheeled motor vehicle injured in collision with car, pick-up truck or van in nontraffic accident

X● **V33.3** Unspecified occupant of three-wheeled motor vehicle injured in collision with car, pick-up truck or van in nontraffic accident

X● **V33.4** Person boarding or alighting a three-wheeled motor vehicle injured in collision with car, pick-up truck or van

X● **V33.5** Driver of three-wheeled motor vehicle injured in collision with car, pick-up truck or van in traffic accident

X● **V33.6** Passenger in three-wheeled motor vehicle injured in collision with car, pick-up truck or van in traffic accident

X● **V33.7** Person on outside of three-wheeled motor vehicle injured in collision with car, pick-up truck or van in traffic accident

X● **V33.9** Unspecified occupant of three-wheeled motor vehicle injured in collision with car, pick-up truck or van in traffic accident

● **V34 Occupant of three-wheeled motor vehicle injured in collision with heavy transport vehicle or bus**

Excludes 1   occupant of three-wheeled motor vehicle injured in collision with military vehicle (V39.81)

The appropriate 7th character is to be added to each code from category V34

A	initial encounter
D	subsequent encounter
S	sequela

X● **V34.0** Driver of three-wheeled motor vehicle injured in collision with heavy transport vehicle or bus in nontraffic accident

X● **V34.1** Passenger in three-wheeled motor vehicle injured in collision with heavy transport vehicle or bus in nontraffic accident

X● **V34.2** Person on outside of three-wheeled motor vehicle injured in collision with heavy transport vehicle or bus in nontraffic accident

X● **V34.3** Unspecified occupant of three-wheeled motor vehicle injured in collision with heavy transport vehicle or bus in nontraffic accident

X● **V34.4** Person boarding or alighting a three-wheeled motor vehicle injured in collision with heavy transport vehicle or bus

X● **V34.5** Driver of three-wheeled motor vehicle injured in collision with heavy transport vehicle or bus in traffic accident

X● **V34.6** Passenger in three-wheeled motor vehicle injured in collision with heavy transport vehicle or bus in traffic accident

X● **V34.7** Person on outside of three-wheeled motor vehicle injured in collision with heavy transport vehicle or bus in traffic accident

X● **V34.9** Unspecified occupant of three-wheeled motor vehicle injured in collision with heavy transport vehicle or bus in traffic accident

● **V35 Occupant of three-wheeled motor vehicle injured in collision with railway train or railway vehicle**

The appropriate 7th character is to be added to each code from category V35

A	initial encounter
D	subsequent encounter
S	sequela

X● **V35.0** Driver of three-wheeled motor vehicle injured in collision with railway train or railway vehicle in nontraffic accident

X● **V35.1** Passenger in three-wheeled motor vehicle injured in collision with railway train or railway vehicle in nontraffic accident

X● **V35.2** Person on outside of three-wheeled motor vehicle injured in collision with railway train or railway vehicle in nontraffic accident

X● **V35.3** Unspecified occupant of three-wheeled motor vehicle injured in collision with railway train or railway vehicle in nontraffic accident

X● **V35.4** Person boarding or alighting a three-wheeled motor vehicle injured in collision with railway train or railway vehicle

X● **V35.5** Driver of three-wheeled motor vehicle injured in collision with railway train or railway vehicle in traffic accident

X● **V35.6** Passenger in three-wheeled motor vehicle injured in collision with railway train or railway vehicle in traffic accident

X● **V35.7** Person on outside of three-wheeled motor vehicle injured in collision with railway train or railway vehicle in traffic accident

X● **V35.9** Unspecified occupant of three-wheeled motor vehicle injured in collision with railway train or railway vehicle in traffic accident

◀ New   ◀▥ Revised   ~~deleted~~ Deleted   Excludes 1   Excludes 2   Includes   Use additional   Code first   Code also   Unspecified

OGCR Official Guidelines   X Assign placeholder X   ● Use Additional Character(s)   ▶ Manifestation Code   **Coding Clinic**

● V36   **Occupant of three-wheeled motor vehicle injured in collision with other nonmotor vehicle**

> **Includes**   collision with animal-drawn vehicle, animal being ridden, streetcar

> The appropriate 7th character is to be added to each code from category V36

> | A | initial encounter |
> |---|---|
> | D | subsequent encounter |
> | S | sequela |

X● **V36.0**   Driver of three-wheeled motor vehicle injured in collision with other nonmotor vehicle in nontraffic accident

X● **V36.1**   Passenger in three-wheeled motor vehicle injured in collision with other nonmotor vehicle in nontraffic accident

X● **V36.2**   Person on outside of three-wheeled motor vehicle injured in collision with other nonmotor vehicle in nontraffic accident

X● **V36.3**   Unspecified occupant of three-wheeled motor vehicle injured in collision with other nonmotor vehicle in nontraffic accident

X● **V36.4**   Person boarding or alighting a three-wheeled motor vehicle injured in collision with other nonmotor vehicle

X● **V36.5**   Driver of three-wheeled motor vehicle injured in collision with other nonmotor vehicle in traffic accident

X● **V36.6**   Passenger in three-wheeled motor vehicle injured in collision with other nonmotor vehicle in traffic accident

X● **V36.7**   Person on outside of three-wheeled motor vehicle injured in collision with other nonmotor vehicle in traffic accident

X● **V36.9**   Unspecified occupant of three-wheeled motor vehicle injured in collision with other nonmotor vehicle in traffic accident

● V37   **Occupant of three-wheeled motor vehicle injured in collision with fixed or stationary object**

> The appropriate 7th character is to be added to each code from category V37

> | A | initial encounter |
> |---|---|
> | D | subsequent encounter |
> | S | sequela |

X● **V37.0**   Driver of three-wheeled motor vehicle injured in collision with fixed or stationary object in nontraffic accident

X● **V37.1**   Passenger in three-wheeled motor vehicle injured in collision with fixed or stationary object in nontraffic accident

X● **V37.2**   Person on outside of three-wheeled motor vehicle injured in collision with fixed or stationary object in nontraffic accident

X● **V37.3**   Unspecified occupant of three-wheeled motor vehicle injured in collision with fixed or stationary object in nontraffic accident

X● **V37.4**   Person boarding or alighting a three-wheeled motor vehicle injured in collision with fixed or stationary object

X● **V37.5**   Driver of three-wheeled motor vehicle injured in collision with fixed or stationary object in traffic accident

X● **V37.6**   Passenger in three-wheeled motor vehicle injured in collision with fixed or stationary object in traffic accident

X● **V37.7**   Person on outside of three-wheeled motor vehicle injured in collision with fixed or stationary object in traffic accident

X● **V37.9**   Unspecified occupant of three-wheeled motor vehicle injured in collision with fixed or stationary object in traffic accident

● V38   **Occupant of three-wheeled motor vehicle injured in noncollision transport accident**

> **Includes**   fall or thrown from three-wheeled motor vehicle
> overturning of three-wheeled motor vehicle NOS
> overturning of three-wheeled motor vehicle without collision

> The appropriate 7th character is to be added to each code from category V38

> | A | initial encounter |
> |---|---|
> | D | subsequent encounter |
> | S | sequela |

X● **V38.0**   Driver of three-wheeled motor vehicle injured in noncollision transport accident in nontraffic accident

X● **V38.1**   Passenger in three-wheeled motor vehicle injured in noncollision transport accident in nontraffic accident

X● **V38.2**   Person on outside of three-wheeled motor vehicle injured in noncollision transport accident in nontraffic accident

X● **V38.3**   Unspecified occupant of three-wheeled motor vehicle injured in noncollision transport accident in nontraffic accident

X● **V38.4**   Person boarding or alighting a three-wheeled motor vehicle injured in noncollision transport accident

X● **V38.5**   Driver of three-wheeled motor vehicle injured in noncollision transport accident in traffic accident

X● **V38.6**   Passenger in three-wheeled motor vehicle injured in noncollision transport accident in traffic accident

X● **V38.7**   Person on outside of three-wheeled motor vehicle injured in noncollision transport accident in traffic accident

X● **V38.9**   Unspecified occupant of three-wheeled motor vehicle injured in noncollision transport accident in traffic accident

● V39   **Occupant of three-wheeled motor vehicle injured in other and unspecified transport accidents**

> The appropriate 7th character is to be added to each code from category V39

> | A | initial encounter |
> |---|---|
> | D | subsequent encounter |
> | S | sequela |

● **V39.0**   Driver of three-wheeled motor vehicle injured in collision with other and unspecified motor vehicles in nontraffic accident

X● **V39.00**   Driver of three-wheeled motor vehicle injured in collision with unspecified motor vehicles in nontraffic accident

X● **V39.09**   Driver of three-wheeled motor vehicle injured in collision with other motor vehicles in nontraffic accident

● **V39.1**   Passenger in three-wheeled motor vehicle injured in collision with other and unspecified motor vehicles in nontraffic accident

X● **V39.10**   Passenger in three-wheeled motor vehicle injured in collision with unspecified motor vehicles in nontraffic accident

X● **V39.19**   Passenger in three-wheeled motor vehicle injured in collision with other motor vehicles in nontraffic accident

● **V39.2**   Unspecified occupant of three-wheeled motor vehicle injured in collision with other and unspecified motor vehicles in nontraffic accident

X● **V39.20**   Unspecified occupant of three-wheeled motor vehicle injured in collision with unspecified motor vehicles in nontraffic accident

> Collision NOS involving three-wheeled motor vehicle, nontraffic

X● **V39.29**   Unspecified occupant of three-wheeled motor vehicle injured in collision with other motor vehicles in nontraffic accident

X● **V39.3** Occupant (driver) (passenger) of three-wheeled motor vehicle injured in unspecified nontraffic accident

     Accident NOS involving three-wheeled motor vehicle, nontraffic

     Occupant of three-wheeled motor vehicle injured in nontraffic accident NOS

● **V39.4** Driver of three-wheeled motor vehicle injured in collision with other and unspecified motor vehicles in traffic accident

   X● **V39.40** Driver of three-wheeled motor vehicle injured in collision with unspecified motor vehicles in traffic accident

   X● **V39.49** Driver of three-wheeled motor vehicle injured in collision with other motor vehicles in traffic accident

● **V39.5** Passenger in three-wheeled motor vehicle injured in collision with other and unspecified motor vehicles in traffic accident

   X● **V39.50** Passenger in three-wheeled motor vehicle injured in collision with unspecified motor vehicles in traffic accident

   X● **V39.59** Passenger in three-wheeled motor vehicle injured in collision with other motor vehicles in traffic accident

● **V39.6** Unspecified occupant of three-wheeled motor vehicle injured in collision with other and unspecified motor vehicles in traffic accident

   X● **V39.60** Unspecified occupant of three-wheeled motor vehicle injured in collision with unspecified motor vehicles in traffic accident

     Collision NOS involving three-wheeled motor vehicle (traffic)

   X● **V39.69** Unspecified occupant of three-wheeled motor vehicle injured in collision with other motor vehicles in traffic accident

● **V39.8** Occupant (driver) (passenger) of three-wheeled motor vehicle injured in other specified transport accidents

   X● **V39.81** Occupant (driver) (passenger) of three-wheeled motor vehicle injured in transport accident with military vehicle

   X● **V39.89** Occupant (driver) (passenger) of three-wheeled motor vehicle injured in other specified transport accidents

X● **V39.9** Occupant (driver) (passenger) of three-wheeled motor vehicle injured in unspecified traffic accident

     Accident NOS involving three-wheeled motor vehicle

CAR OCCUPANT INJURED IN TRANSPORT ACCIDENT (V40-V49)

Includes   a four-wheeled motor vehicle designed primarily for carrying passengers

         automobile (pulling a trailer or camper)

Excludes1   bus (V50-V59)

         minibus (V50-V59)

         minivan (V50-V59)

         motorcoach (V70-V79)

         pick-up truck (V50-V59)

         sport utility vehicle (SUV) (V50-V59)

● **V40** Car occupant injured in collision with pedestrian or animal

   Excludes1   car collision with animal-drawn vehicle or animal being ridden (V46.-)

The appropriate 7th character is to be added to each code from category V40

A	initial encounter
D	subsequent encounter
S	sequela

X● **V40.0** Car driver injured in collision with pedestrian or animal in nontraffic accident

X● **V40.1** Car passenger injured in collision with pedestrian or animal in nontraffic accident

X● **V40.2** Person on outside of car injured in collision with pedestrian or animal in nontraffic accident

X● **V40.3** Unspecified car occupant injured in collision with pedestrian or animal in nontraffic accident

X● **V40.4** Person boarding or alighting a car injured in collision with pedestrian or animal

X● **V40.5** Car driver injured in collision with pedestrian or animal in traffic accident

X● **V40.6** Car passenger injured in collision with pedestrian or animal in traffic accident

X● **V40.7** Person on outside of car injured in collision with pedestrian or animal in traffic accident

X● **V40.9** Unspecified car occupant injured in collision with pedestrian or animal in traffic accident

● **V41** Car occupant injured in collision with pedal cycle

The appropriate 7th character is to be added to each code from category V41

A	initial encounter
D	subsequent encounter
S	sequela

X● **V41.0** Car driver injured in collision with pedal cycle in nontraffic accident

X● **V41.1** Car passenger injured in collision with pedal cycle in nontraffic accident

X● **V41.2** Person on outside of car injured in collision with pedal cycle in nontraffic accident

X● **V41.3** Unspecified car occupant injured in collision with pedal cycle in nontraffic accident

X● **V41.4** Person boarding or alighting a car injured in collision with pedal cycle

X● **V41.5** Car driver injured in collision with pedal cycle in traffic accident

X● **V41.6** Car passenger injured in collision with pedal cycle in traffic accident

X● **V41.7** Person on outside of car injured in collision with pedal cycle in traffic accident

X● **V41.9** Unspecified car occupant injured in collision with pedal cycle in traffic accident

● **V42** Car occupant injured in collision with two- or three-wheeled motor vehicle

The appropriate 7th character is to be added to each code from category V42

A	initial encounter
D	subsequent encounter
S	sequela

X● **V42.0** Car driver injured in collision with two- or three-wheeled motor vehicle in nontraffic accident

X● **V42.1** Car passenger injured in collision with two- or three-wheeled motor vehicle in nontraffic accident

X● **V42.2** Person on outside of car injured in collision with two- or three-wheeled motor vehicle in nontraffic accident

X● **V42.3** Unspecified car occupant injured in collision with two- or three-wheeled motor vehicle in nontraffic accident

X● **V42.4** Person boarding or alighting a car injured in collision with two- or three-wheeled motor vehicle

X● **V42.5** Car driver injured in collision with two- or three-wheeled motor vehicle in traffic accident

X● **V42.6** Car passenger injured in collision with two- or three-wheeled motor vehicle in traffic accident

X● **V42.7** Person on outside of car injured in collision with two- or three-wheeled motor vehicle in traffic accident

X● **V42.9** Unspecified car occupant injured in collision with two- or three-wheeled motor vehicle in traffic accident

◀ New   ◀◀ Revised   ~~deleted~~ Deleted   Excludes 1   Excludes 2   Includes   Use additional   Code first   Code also   Unspecified

OGCR Official Guidelines   X Assign placeholder X   ● Use Additional Character(s)   ▶ Manifestation Code   **Coding Clinic**

● **V43** Car occupant injured in collision with car, pick-up truck or van

The appropriate 7th character is to be added to each code from category V43

> A   initial encounter
> D   subsequent encounter
> S   sequela

● **V43.0** Car driver injured in collision with car, pick-up truck or van in nontraffic accident

X● **V43.01** Car driver injured in collision with sport utility vehicle in nontraffic accident

X● **V43.02** Car driver injured in collision with other type car in nontraffic accident

X● **V43.03** Car driver injured in collision with pick-up truck in nontraffic accident

X● **V43.04** Car driver injured in collision with van in nontraffic accident

● **V43.1** Car passenger injured in collision with car, pick-up truck or van in nontraffic accident

X● **V43.11** Car passenger injured in collision with sport utility vehicle in nontraffic accident

X● **V43.12** Car passenger injured in collision with other type car in nontraffic accident

X● **V43.13** Car passenger injured in collision with pick-up in nontraffic accident

X● **V43.14** Car passenger injured in collision with van in nontraffic accident

● **V43.2** Person on outside of car injured in collision with car, pick-up truck or van in nontraffic accident

X● **V43.21** Person on outside of car injured in collision with sport utility vehicle in nontraffic accident

X● **V43.22** Person on outside of car injured in collision with other type car in nontraffic accident

X● **V43.23** Person on outside of car injured in collision with pick-up truck in nontraffic accident

X● **V43.24** Person on outside of car injured in collision with van in nontraffic accident

● **V43.3** Unspecified car occupant injured in collision with car, pick-up truck or van in nontraffic accident

X● **V43.31** Unspecified car occupant injured in collision with sport utility vehicle in nontraffic accident

X● **V43.32** Unspecified car occupant injured in collision with other type car in nontraffic accident

X● **V43.33** Unspecified car occupant injured in collision with pick-up truck in nontraffic accident

X● **V43.34** Unspecified car occupant injured in collision with van in nontraffic accident

● **V43.4** Person boarding or alighting a car injured in collision with car, pick-up truck or van

X● **V43.41** Person boarding or alighting a car injured in collision with sport utility vehicle

X● **V43.42** Person boarding or alighting a car injured in collision with other type car

X● **V43.43** Person boarding or alighting a car injured in collision with pick-up truck

X● **V43.44** Person boarding or alighting a car injured in collision with van

● **V43.5** Car driver injured in collision with car, pick-up truck or van in traffic accident

X● **V43.51** Car driver injured in collision with sport utility vehicle in traffic accident

X● **V43.52** Car driver injured in collision with other type car in traffic accident

X● **V43.53** Car driver injured in collision with pick-up truck in traffic accident

X● **V43.54** Car driver injured in collision with van in traffic accident

● **V43.6** Car passenger injured in collision with car, pick-up truck or van in traffic accident

X● **V43.61** Car passenger injured in collision with sport utility vehicle in traffic accident
      Coding Clinic: 2015, Q1, P5-7

X● **V43.62** Car passenger injured in collision with other type car in traffic accident

X● **V43.63** Car passenger injured in collision with pick-up truck in traffic accident

X● **V43.64** Car passenger injured in collision with van in traffic accident

● **V43.7** Person on outside of car injured in collision with car, pick-up truck or van in traffic accident

X● **V43.71** Person on outside of car injured in collision with sport utility vehicle in traffic accident

X● **V43.72** Person on outside of car injured in collision with other type car in traffic accident

X● **V43.73** Person on outside of car injured in collision with pick-up truck in traffic accident

X● **V43.74** Person on outside of car injured in collision with van in traffic accident

● **V43.9** Unspecified car occupant injured in collision with car, pick-up truck or van in traffic accident

X● **V43.91** Unspecified car occupant injured in collision with sport utility vehicle in traffic accident

X● **V43.92** Unspecified car occupant injured in collision with other type car in traffic accident

X● **V43.93** Unspecified car occupant injured in collision with pick-up truck in traffic accident

X● **V43.94** Unspecified car occupant injured in collision with van in traffic accident

● **V44** Car occupant injured in collision with heavy transport vehicle or bus

> **Excludes1**   car occupant injured in collision with military vehicle (V49.81)

The appropriate 7th character is to be added to each code from category V44

> A   initial encounter
> D   subsequent encounter
> S   sequela

X● **V44.0** Car driver injured in collision with heavy transport vehicle or bus in nontraffic accident

X● **V44.1** Car passenger injured in collision with heavy transport vehicle or bus in nontraffic accident

X● **V44.2** Person on outside of car injured in collision with heavy transport vehicle or bus in nontraffic accident

X● **V44.3** Unspecified car occupant injured in collision with heavy transport vehicle or bus in nontraffic accident

X● **V44.4** Person boarding or alighting a car injured in collision with heavy transport vehicle or bus

X● **V44.5** Car driver injured in collision with heavy transport vehicle or bus in traffic accident

X● **V44.6** Car passenger injured in collision with heavy transport vehicle or bus in traffic accident

X● **V44.7** Person on outside of car injured in collision with heavy transport vehicle or bus in traffic accident

X● **V44.9** Unspecified car occupant injured in collision with heavy transport vehicle or bus in traffic accident

CHAPTER 20 (V01-Y99)

● **V45　Car occupant injured in collision with railway train or railway vehicle**

> The appropriate 7th character is to be added to each code from category V45

> | A | initial encounter |
> |---|---|
> | D | subsequent encounter |
> | S | sequela |

X● **V45.0** Car driver injured in collision with railway train or railway vehicle in nontraffic accident

X● **V45.1** Car passenger injured in collision with railway train or railway vehicle in nontraffic accident

X● **V45.2** Person on outside of car injured in collision with railway train or railway vehicle in nontraffic accident

X● **V45.3** Unspecified car occupant injured in collision with railway train or railway vehicle in nontraffic accident

X● **V45.4** Person boarding or alighting a car injured in collision with railway train or railway vehicle

X● **V45.5** Car driver injured in collision with railway train or railway vehicle in traffic accident

X● **V45.6** Car passenger injured in collision with railway train or railway vehicle in traffic accident

X● **V45.7** Person on outside of car injured in collision with railway train or railway vehicle in traffic accident

X● **V45.9** Unspecified car occupant injured in collision with railway train or railway vehicle in traffic accident

● **V46　Car occupant injured in collision with other nonmotor vehicle**

> **Includes** collision with animal-drawn vehicle, animal being ridden, streetcar

> The appropriate 7th character is to be added to each code from category V46

> | A | initial encounter |
> |---|---|
> | D | subsequent encounter |
> | S | sequela |

X● **V46.0** Car driver injured in collision with other nonmotor vehicle in nontraffic accident

X● **V46.1** Car passenger injured in collision with other nonmotor vehicle in nontraffic accident

X● **V46.2** Person on outside of car injured in collision with other nonmotor vehicle in nontraffic accident

X● **V46.3** Unspecified car occupant injured in collision with other nonmotor vehicle in nontraffic accident

X● **V46.4** Person boarding or alighting a car injured in collision with other nonmotor vehicle

X● **V46.5** Car driver injured in collision with other nonmotor vehicle in traffic accident

X● **V46.6** Car passenger injured in collision with other nonmotor vehicle in traffic accident

X● **V46.7** Person on outside of car injured in collision with other nonmotor vehicle in traffic accident

X● **V46.9** Unspecified car occupant injured in collision with other nonmotor vehicle in traffic accident

● **V47　Car occupant injured in collision with fixed or stationary object**

> The appropriate 7th character is to be added to each code from category V47

> | A | initial encounter |
> |---|---|
> | D | subsequent encounter |
> | S | sequela |

● **V47.0** Car driver injured in collision with fixed or stationary object in nontraffic accident

X● **V47.01** Driver of sport utility vehicle injured in collision with fixed or stationary object in nontraffic accident

X● **V47.02** Driver of other type car injured in collision with fixed or stationary object in nontraffic accident

● **V47.1** Car passenger injured in collision with fixed or stationary object in nontraffic accident

X● **V47.11** Passenger of sport utility vehicle injured in collision with fixed or stationary object in nontraffic accident

X● **V47.12** Passenger of other type car injured in collision with fixed or stationary object in nontraffic accident

X● **V47.2** Person on outside of car injured in collision with fixed or stationary object in nontraffic accident

● **V47.3** Unspecified car occupant injured in collision with fixed or stationary object in nontraffic accident

X● **V47.31** Unspecified occupant of sport utility vehicle injured in collision with fixed or stationary object in nontraffic accident

X● **V47.32** Unspecified occupant of other type car injured in collision with fixed or stationary object in nontraffic accident

X● **V47.4** Person boarding or alighting a car injured in collision with fixed or stationary object

● **V47.5** Car driver injured in collision with fixed or stationary object in traffic accident

X● **V47.51** Driver of sport utility vehicle injured in collision with fixed or stationary object in traffic accident

X● **V47.52** Driver of other type car injured in collision with fixed or stationary object in traffic accident

● **V47.6** Car passenger injured in collision with fixed or stationary object in traffic accident

X● **V47.61** Passenger of sport utility vehicle injured in collision with fixed or stationary object in traffic accident

X● **V47.62** Passenger of other type car injured in collision with fixed or stationary object in traffic accident

X● **V47.7** Person on outside of car injured in collision with fixed or stationary object in traffic accident

● **V47.9** Unspecified car occupant injured in collision with fixed or stationary object in traffic accident

X● **V47.91** Unspecified occupant of sport utility vehicle injured in collision with fixed or stationary object in traffic accident

X● **V47.92** Unspecified occupant of other type car injured in collision with fixed or stationary object in traffic accident

● **V48　Car occupant injured in noncollision transport accident**

> **Includes** overturning car NOS
> overturning car without collision

> The appropriate 7th character is to be added to each code from category V48

> | A | initial encounter |
> |---|---|
> | D | subsequent encounter |
> | S | sequela |

X● **V48.0** Car driver injured in noncollision transport accident in nontraffic accident

X● **V48.1** Car passenger injured in noncollision transport accident in nontraffic accident

X● **V48.2** Person on outside of car injured in noncollision transport accident in nontraffic accident

X● **V48.3** Unspecified car occupant injured in noncollision transport accident in nontraffic accident

X● **V48.4** Person boarding or alighting a car injured in noncollision transport accident

X● **V48.5** Car driver injured in noncollision transport accident in traffic accident

X● **V48.6** Car passenger injured in noncollision transport accident in traffic accident

X● **V48.7** Person on outside of car injured in noncollision transport accident in traffic accident

X● **V48.9** Unspecified car occupant injured in noncollision transport accident in traffic accident

◄ New　◄ Revised　deleted Deleted　Excludes 1　Excludes 2　Includes　Use additional　Code first　Code also　Unspecified

OGCR Official Guidelines　**X** Assign placeholder X　● Use Additional Character(s)　▸ Manifestation Code　**Coding Clinic**

● **V49**   **Car occupant injured in other and unspecified transport accidents**

> The appropriate 7th character is to be added to each code from category V49

> | A | initial encounter |
> |---|---|
> | D | subsequent encounter |
> | S | sequela |

- ● **V49.0**   Driver injured in collision with other and unspecified motor vehicles in nontraffic accident
  - X● **V49.00**   Driver injured in collision with unspecified motor vehicles in nontraffic accident
  - X● **V49.09**   Driver injured in collision with other motor vehicles in nontraffic accident
- ● **V49.1**   Passenger injured in collision with other and unspecified motor vehicles in nontraffic accident
  - X● **V49.10**   Passenger injured in collision with unspecified motor vehicles in nontraffic accident
  - X● **V49.19**   Passenger injured in collision with other motor vehicles in nontraffic accident
- ● **V49.2**   Unspecified car occupant injured in collision with other and unspecified motor vehicles in nontraffic accident
  - X● **V49.20**   Unspecified car occupant injured in collision with unspecified motor vehicles in nontraffic accident
    Car collision NOS, nontraffic
  - X● **V49.29**   Unspecified car occupant injured in collision with other motor vehicles in nontraffic accident
- X● **V49.3**   Car occupant (driver) (passenger) injured in unspecified nontraffic accident
    Car accident NOS, nontraffic
    Car occupant injured in nontraffic accident NOS
- ● **V49.4**   Driver injured in collision with other and unspecified motor vehicles in traffic accident
  - X● **V49.40**   Driver injured in collision with unspecified motor vehicles in traffic accident
  - X● **V49.49**   Driver injured in collision with other motor vehicles in traffic accident
- ● **V49.5**   Passenger injured in collision with other and unspecified motor vehicles in traffic accident
  - X● **V49.50**   Passenger injured in collision with unspecified motor vehicles in traffic accident
  - X● **V49.59**   Passenger injured in collision with other motor vehicles in traffic accident
- ● **V49.6**   Unspecified car occupant injured in collision with other and unspecified motor vehicles in traffic accident
  - X● **V49.60**   Unspecified car occupant injured in collision with unspecified motor vehicles in traffic accident
    Car collision NOS (traffic)
  - X● **V49.69**   Unspecified car occupant injured in collision with other motor vehicles in traffic accident
- ● **V49.8**   Car occupant (driver) (passenger) injured in other specified transport accidents
  - X● **V49.81**   Car occupant (driver) (passenger) injured in transport accident with military vehicle
  - X● **V49.88**   Car occupant (driver) (passenger) injured in other specified transport accidents
- X● **V49.9**   Car occupant (driver) (passenger) injured in unspecified traffic accident
    Car accident NOS
    Coding Clinic: 2015, Q1, P11

OCCUPANT OF PICK-UP TRUCK OR VAN INJURED IN TRANSPORT ACCIDENT (V50-V59)

Includes	a four- or six-wheel motor vehicle designed primarily for carrying passengers and property but weighing less than the local limit for classification as a heavy goods vehicle
	minibus
	minivan
	sport utility vehicle (SUV)
	truck
	van

Excludes1	heavy transport vehicle (V60-V69)

● **V50**   **Occupant of pick-up truck or van injured in collision with pedestrian or animal**

> | **Excludes1** | pick-up truck or van collision with animal-drawn vehicle or animal being ridden (V56.-) |
> |---|---|

> The appropriate 7th character is to be added to each code from category V50

> | A | initial encounter |
> |---|---|
> | D | subsequent encounter |
> | S | sequela |

- X● **V50.0**   Driver of pick-up truck or van injured in collision with pedestrian or animal in nontraffic accident
- X● **V50.1**   Passenger in pick-up truck or van injured in collision with pedestrian or animal in nontraffic accident
- X● **V50.2**   Person on outside of pick-up truck or van injured in collision with pedestrian or animal in nontraffic accident
- X● **V50.3**   Unspecified occupant of pick-up truck or van injured in collision with pedestrian or animal in nontraffic accident
- X● **V50.4**   Person boarding or alighting a pick-up truck or van injured in collision with pedestrian or animal
- X● **V50.5**   Driver of pick-up truck or van injured in collision with pedestrian or animal in traffic accident
- X● **V50.6**   Passenger in pick-up truck or van injured in collision with pedestrian or animal in traffic accident
- X● **V50.7**   Person on outside of pick-up truck or van injured in collision with pedestrian or animal in traffic accident
- X● **V50.9**   Unspecified occupant of pick-up truck or van injured in collision with pedestrian or animal in traffic accident

● **V51**   **Occupant of pick-up truck or van injured in collision with pedal cycle**

> The appropriate 7th character is to be added to each code from category V51

> | A | initial encounter |
> |---|---|
> | D | subsequent encounter |
> | S | sequela |

- X● **V51.0**   Driver of pick-up truck or van injured in collision with pedal cycle in nontraffic accident
- X● **V51.1**   Passenger in pick-up truck or van injured in collision with pedal cycle in nontraffic accident
- X● **V51.2**   Person on outside of pick-up truck or van injured in collision with pedal cycle in nontraffic accident
- X● **V51.3**   Unspecified occupant of pick-up truck or van injured in collision with pedal cycle in nontraffic accident
- X● **V51.4**   Person boarding or alighting a pick-up truck or van injured in collision with pedal cycle
- X● **V51.5**   Driver of pick-up truck or van injured in collision with pedal cycle in traffic accident
- X● **V51.6**   Passenger in pick-up truck or van injured in collision with pedal cycle in traffic accident
- X● **V51.7**   Person on outside of pick-up truck or van injured in collision with pedal cycle in traffic accident
- X● **V51.9**   Unspecified occupant of pick-up truck or van injured in collision with pedal cycle in traffic accident

CHAPTER 20 (V01-Y99)

● **V52** Occupant of pick-up truck or van injured in collision with two- or three-wheeled motor vehicle

> The appropriate 7th character is to be added to each code from category V52

> | A | initial encounter |
> |---|---|
> | D | subsequent encounter |
> | S | sequela |

X● **V52.0** Driver of pick-up truck or van injured in collision with two- or three-wheeled motor vehicle in nontraffic accident

X● **V52.1** Passenger in pick-up truck or van injured in collision with two- or three-wheeled motor vehicle in nontraffic accident

X● **V52.2** Person on outside of pick-up truck or van injured in collision with two- or three-wheeled motor vehicle in nontraffic accident

X● **V52.3** Unspecified occupant of pick-up truck or van injured in collision with two- or three-wheeled motor vehicle in nontraffic accident

X● **V52.4** Person boarding or alighting a pick-up truck or van injured in collision with two- or three-wheeled motor vehicle

X● **V52.5** Driver of pick-up truck or van injured in collision with two- or three-wheeled motor vehicle in traffic accident

X● **V52.6** Passenger in pick-up truck or van injured in collision with two- or three-wheeled motor vehicle in traffic accident

X● **V52.7** Person on outside of pick-up truck or van injured in collision with two- or three-wheeled motor vehicle in traffic accident

X● **V52.9** Unspecified occupant of pick-up truck or van injured in collision with two- or three-wheeled motor vehicle in traffic accident

● **V53** Occupant of pick-up truck or van injured in collision with car, pick-up truck or van

> The appropriate 7th character is to be added to each code from category V53

> | A | initial encounter |
> |---|---|
> | D | subsequent encounter |
> | S | sequela |

X● **V53.0** Driver of pick-up truck or van injured in collision with car, pick-up truck or van in nontraffic accident

X● **V53.1** Passenger in pick-up truck or van injured in collision with car, pick-up truck or van in nontraffic accident

X● **V53.2** Person on outside of pick-up truck or van injured in collision with car, pick-up truck or van in nontraffic accident

X● **V53.3** Unspecified occupant of pick-up truck or van injured in collision with car, pick-up truck or van in nontraffic accident

X● **V53.4** Person boarding or alighting a pick-up truck or van injured in collision with car, pick-up truck or van

X● **V53.5** Driver of pick-up truck or van injured in collision with car, pick-up truck or van in traffic accident

X● **V53.6** Passenger in pick-up truck or van injured in collision with car, pick-up truck or van in traffic accident

X● **V53.7** Person on outside of pick-up truck or van injured in collision with car, pick-up truck or van in traffic accident

X● **V53.9** Unspecified occupant of pick-up truck or van injured in collision with car, pick-up truck or van in traffic accident

● **V54** Occupant of pick-up truck or van injured in collision with heavy transport vehicle or bus

> **Excludes1** occupant of pick-up truck or van injured in collision with military vehicle (V59.81)

> The appropriate 7th character is to be added to each code from category V54

> | A | initial encounter |
> |---|---|
> | D | subsequent encounter |
> | S | sequela |

X● **V54.0** Driver of pick-up truck or van injured in collision with heavy transport vehicle or bus in nontraffic accident

X● **V54.1** Passenger in pick-up truck or van injured in collision with heavy transport vehicle or bus in nontraffic accident

X● **V54.2** Person on outside of pick-up truck or van injured in collision with heavy transport vehicle or bus in nontraffic accident

X● **V54.3** Unspecified occupant of pick-up truck or van injured in collision with heavy transport vehicle or bus in nontraffic accident

X● **V54.4** Person boarding or alighting a pick-up truck or van injured in collision with heavy transport vehicle or bus

X● **V54.5** Driver of pick-up truck or van injured in collision with heavy transport vehicle or bus in traffic accident

X● **V54.6** Passenger in pick-up truck or van injured in collision with heavy transport vehicle or bus in traffic accident

X● **V54.7** Person on outside of pick-up truck or van injured in collision with heavy transport vehicle or bus in traffic accident

X● **V54.9** Unspecified occupant of pick-up truck or van injured in collision with heavy transport vehicle or bus in traffic accident

● **V55** Occupant of pick-up truck or van injured in collision with railway train or railway vehicle

> The appropriate 7th character is to be added to each code from category V55

> | A | initial encounter |
> |---|---|
> | D | subsequent encounter |
> | S | sequela |

X● **V55.0** Driver of pick-up truck or van injured in collision with railway train or railway vehicle in nontraffic accident

X● **V55.1** Passenger in pick-up truck or van injured in collision with railway train or railway vehicle in nontraffic accident

X● **V55.2** Person on outside of pick-up truck or van injured in collision with railway train or railway vehicle in nontraffic accident

X● **V55.3** Unspecified occupant of pick-up truck or van injured in collision with railway train or railway vehicle in nontraffic accident

X● **V55.4** Person boarding or alighting a pick-up truck or van injured in collision with railway train or railway vehicle

X● **V55.5** Driver of pick-up truck or van injured in collision with railway train or railway vehicle in traffic accident

X● **V55.6** Passenger in pick-up truck or van injured in collision with railway train or railway vehicle in traffic accident

X● **V55.7** Person on outside of pick-up truck or van injured in collision with railway train or railway vehicle in traffic accident

X● **V55.9** Unspecified occupant of pick-up truck or van injured in collision with railway train or railway vehicle in traffic accident

◄ New   ◄▥ Revised   ~~deleted~~ Deleted   Excludes 1   Excludes 2   Includes   Use additional   Code first   Code also   Unspecified

OGCR Official Guidelines   X Assign placeholder X   ● Use Additional Character(s)   ▶ Manifestation Code   **Coding Clinic**

● **V56** **Occupant of pick-up truck or van injured in collision with other nonmotor vehicle**

> **Includes** collision with animal-drawn vehicle, animal being ridden, streetcar

> The appropriate 7th character is to be added to each code from category V56

> | | |
> |---|---|
> | A | initial encounter |
> | D | subsequent encounter |
> | S | sequela |

X● **V56.0** Driver of pick-up truck or van injured in collision with other nonmotor vehicle in nontraffic accident

X● **V56.1** Passenger in pick-up truck or van injured in collision with other nonmotor vehicle in nontraffic accident

X● **V56.2** Person on outside of pick-up truck or van injured in collision with other nonmotor vehicle in nontraffic accident

X● **V56.3** Unspecified occupant of pick-up truck or van injured in collision with other nonmotor vehicle in nontraffic accident

X● **V56.4** Person boarding or alighting a pick-up truck or van injured in collision with other nonmotor vehicle

X● **V56.5** Driver of pick-up truck or van injured in collision with other nonmotor vehicle in traffic accident

X● **V56.6** Passenger in pick-up truck or van injured in collision with other nonmotor vehicle in traffic accident

X● **V56.7** Person on outside of pick-up truck or van injured in collision with other nonmotor vehicle in traffic accident

X● **V56.9** Unspecified occupant of pick-up truck or van injured in collision with other nonmotor vehicle in traffic accident

● **V57** **Occupant of pick-up truck or van injured in collision with fixed or stationary object**

> The appropriate 7th character is to be added to each code from category V57

> | | |
> |---|---|
> | A | initial encounter |
> | D | subsequent encounter |
> | S | sequela |

X● **V57.0** Driver of pick-up truck or van injured in collision with fixed or stationary object in nontraffic accident

X● **V57.1** Passenger in pick-up truck or van injured in collision with fixed or stationary object in nontraffic accident

X● **V57.2** Person on outside of pick-up truck or van injured in collision with fixed or stationary object in nontraffic accident

X● **V57.3** Unspecified occupant of pick-up truck or van injured in collision with fixed or stationary object in nontraffic accident

X● **V57.4** Person boarding or alighting a pick-up truck or van injured in collision with fixed or stationary object

X● **V57.5** Driver of pick-up truck or van injured in collision with fixed or stationary object in traffic accident

X● **V57.6** Passenger in pick-up truck or van injured in collision with fixed or stationary object in traffic accident

X● **V57.7** Person on outside of pick-up truck or van injured in collision with fixed or stationary object in traffic accident

X● **V57.9** Unspecified occupant of pick-up truck or van injured in collision with fixed or stationary object in traffic accident

● **V58** **Occupant of pick-up truck or van injured in noncollision transport accident**

> **Includes** overturning pick-up truck or van NOS overturning pick-up truck or van without collision

> The appropriate 7th character is to be added to each code from category V58

> | | |
> |---|---|
> | A | initial encounter |
> | D | subsequent encounter |
> | S | sequela |

X● **V58.0** Driver of pick-up truck or van injured in noncollision transport accident in nontraffic accident

X● **V58.1** Passenger in pick-up truck or van injured in noncollision transport accident in nontraffic accident

X● **V58.2** Person on outside of pick-up truck or van injured in noncollision transport accident in nontraffic accident

X● **V58.3** Unspecified occupant of pick-up truck or van injured in noncollision transport accident in nontraffic accident

X● **V58.4** Person boarding or alighting a pick-up truck or van injured in noncollision transport accident

X● **V58.5** Driver of pick-up truck or van injured in noncollision transport accident in traffic accident

X● **V58.6** Passenger in pick-up truck or van injured in noncollision transport accident in traffic accident

X● **V58.7** Person on outside of pick-up truck or van injured in noncollision transport accident in traffic accident

X● **V58.9** Unspecified occupant of pick-up truck or van injured in noncollision transport accident in traffic accident

● **V59** **Occupant of pick-up truck or van injured in other and unspecified transport accidents**

> The appropriate 7th character is to be added to each code from category V59

> | | |
> |---|---|
> | A | initial encounter |
> | D | subsequent encounter |
> | S | sequela |

● **V59.0** Driver of pick-up truck or van injured in collision with other and unspecified motor vehicles in nontraffic accident

  X● **V59.00** Driver of pick-up truck or van injured in collision with unspecified motor vehicles in nontraffic accident

  X● **V59.09** Driver of pick-up truck or van injured in collision with other motor vehicles in nontraffic accident

● **V59.1** Passenger in pick-up truck or van injured in collision with other and unspecified motor vehicles in nontraffic accident

  X● **V59.10** Passenger in pick-up truck or van injured in collision with unspecified motor vehicles in nontraffic accident

  X● **V59.19** Passenger in pick-up truck or van injured in collision with other motor vehicles in nontraffic accident

● V59.2   Unspecified occupant of pick-up truck or van injured in collision with other and unspecified motor vehicles in nontraffic accident

    X ● V59.20   Unspecified occupant of pick-up truck or van injured in collision with unspecified motor vehicles in nontraffic accident

        Collision NOS involving pick-up truck or van, nontraffic

    X ● V59.29   Unspecified occupant of pick-up truck or van injured in collision with other motor vehicles in nontraffic accident

X ● V59.3   Occupant (driver) (passenger) of pick-up truck or van injured in unspecified nontraffic accident

       Accident NOS involving pick-up truck or van, nontraffic

       Occupant of pick-up truck or van injured in nontraffic accident NOS

● V59.4   Driver of pick-up truck or van injured in collision with other and unspecified motor vehicles in traffic accident

    X ● V59.40   Driver of pick-up truck or van injured in collision with unspecified motor vehicles in traffic accident

    X ● V59.49   Driver of pick-up truck or van injured in collision with other motor vehicles in traffic accident

● V59.5   Passenger in pick-up truck or van injured in collision with other and unspecified motor vehicles in traffic accident

    X ● V59.50   Passenger in pick-up truck or van injured in collision with unspecified motor vehicles in traffic accident

    X ● V59.59   Passenger in pick-up truck or van injured in collision with other motor vehicles in traffic accident

● V59.6   Unspecified occupant of pick-up truck or van injured in collision with other and unspecified motor vehicles in traffic accident

    X ● V59.60   Unspecified occupant of pick-up truck or van injured in collision with unspecified motor vehicles in traffic accident

        Collision NOS involving pick-up truck or van (traffic)

    X ● V59.69   Unspecified occupant of pick-up truck or van injured in collision with other motor vehicles in traffic accident

● V59.8   Occupant (driver) (passenger) of pick-up truck or van injured in other specified transport accidents

    X ● V59.81   Occupant (driver) (passenger) of pick-up truck or van injured in transport accident with military vehicle

    X ● V59.88   Occupant (driver) (passenger) of pick-up truck or van injured in other specified transport accidents

X ● V59.9   Occupant (driver) (passenger) of pick-up truck or van injured in unspecified traffic accident

       Accident NOS involving pick-up truck or van

OCCUPANT OF HEAVY TRANSPORT VEHICLE INJURED IN TRANSPORT ACCIDENT (V60-V69)

Includes	18 wheeler
	armored car
	panel truck
Excludes1	bus
	motorcoach

● V60   Occupant of heavy transport vehicle injured in collision with pedestrian or animal

    Excludes1   heavy transport vehicle collision with animal-drawn vehicle or animal being ridden (V66.-)

    The appropriate 7th character is to be added to each code from category V60

    A   initial encounter
    D   subsequent encounter
    S   sequela

    X ● V60.0   Driver of heavy transport vehicle injured in collision with pedestrian or animal in nontraffic accident

    X ● V60.1   Passenger in heavy transport vehicle injured in collision with pedestrian or animal in nontraffic accident

    X ● V60.2   Person on outside of heavy transport vehicle injured in collision with pedestrian or animal in nontraffic accident

    X ● V60.3   Unspecified occupant of heavy transport vehicle injured in collision with pedestrian or animal in nontraffic accident

    X ● V60.4   Person boarding or alighting a heavy transport vehicle injured in collision with pedestrian or animal

    X ● V60.5   Driver of heavy transport vehicle injured in collision with pedestrian or animal in traffic accident

    X ● V60.6   Passenger in heavy transport vehicle injured in collision with pedestrian or animal in traffic accident

    X ● V60.7   Person on outside of heavy transport vehicle injured in collision with pedestrian or animal in traffic accident

    X ● V60.9   Unspecified occupant of heavy transport vehicle injured in collision with pedestrian or animal in traffic accident

● V61   Occupant of heavy transport vehicle injured in collision with pedal cycle

    The appropriate 7th character is to be added to each code from category V61

    A   initial encounter
    D   subsequent encounter
    S   sequela

    X ● V61.0   Driver of heavy transport vehicle injured in collision with pedal cycle in nontraffic accident

    X ● V61.1   Passenger in heavy transport vehicle injured in collision with pedal cycle in nontraffic accident

    X ● V61.2   Person on outside of heavy transport vehicle injured in collision with pedal cycle in nontraffic accident

    X ● V61.3   Unspecified occupant of heavy transport vehicle injured in collision with pedal cycle in nontraffic accident

    X ● V61.4   Person boarding or alighting a heavy transport vehicle injured in collision with pedal cycle while boarding or alighting

    X ● V61.5   Driver of heavy transport vehicle injured in collision with pedal cycle in traffic accident

    X ● V61.6   Passenger in heavy transport vehicle injured in collision with pedal cycle in traffic accident

    X ● V61.7   Person on outside of heavy transport vehicle injured in collision with pedal cycle in traffic accident

    X ● V61.9   Unspecified occupant of heavy transport vehicle injured in collision with pedal cycle in traffic accident

CHAPTER 20 (V01-Y99)

● V62   **Occupant of heavy transport vehicle injured in collision with two- or three-wheeled motor vehicle**

> The appropriate 7th character is to be added to each code from category V62

> | | |
> |---|---|
> | A | initial encounter |
> | D | subsequent encounter |
> | S | sequela |

X● V62.0   Driver of heavy transport vehicle injured in collision with two- or three-wheeled motor vehicle in nontraffic accident

X● V62.1   Passenger in heavy transport vehicle injured in collision with two- or three-wheeled motor vehicle in nontraffic accident

X● V62.2   Person on outside of heavy transport vehicle injured in collision with two- or three-wheeled motor vehicle in nontraffic accident

X● V62.3   Unspecified occupant of heavy transport vehicle injured in collision with two- or three-wheeled motor vehicle in nontraffic accident

X● V62.4   Person boarding or alighting a heavy transport vehicle injured in collision with two- or three-wheeled motor vehicle

X● V62.5   Driver of heavy transport vehicle injured in collision with two- or three-wheeled motor vehicle in traffic accident

X● V62.6   Passenger in heavy transport vehicle injured in collision with two- or three-wheeled motor vehicle in traffic accident

X● V62.7   Person on outside of heavy transport vehicle injured in collision with two- or three-wheeled motor vehicle in traffic accident

X● V62.9   Unspecified occupant of heavy transport vehicle injured in collision with two- or three-wheeled motor vehicle in traffic accident

● V63   **Occupant of heavy transport vehicle injured in collision with car, pick-up truck or van**

> The appropriate 7th character is to be added to each code from category V63

> | | |
> |---|---|
> | A | initial encounter |
> | D | subsequent encounter |
> | S | sequela |

X● V63.0   Driver of heavy transport vehicle injured in collision with car, pick-up truck or van in nontraffic accident

X● V63.1   Passenger in heavy transport vehicle injured in collision with car, pick-up truck or van in nontraffic accident

X● V63.2   Person on outside of heavy transport vehicle injured in collision with car, pick-up truck or van in nontraffic accident

X● V63.3   Unspecified occupant of heavy transport vehicle injured in collision with car, pick-up truck or van in nontraffic accident

X● V63.4   Person boarding or alighting a heavy transport vehicle injured in collision with car, pick-up truck or van

X● V63.5   Driver of heavy transport vehicle injured in collision with car, pick-up truck or van in traffic accident

X● V63.6   Passenger in heavy transport vehicle injured in collision with car, pick-up truck or van in traffic accident

X● V63.7   Person on outside of heavy transport vehicle injured in collision with car, pick-up truck or van in traffic accident

X● V63.9   Unspecified occupant of heavy transport vehicle injured in collision with car, pick-up truck or van in traffic accident

● V64   **Occupant of heavy transport vehicle injured in collision with heavy transport vehicle or bus**

> **Excludes1**   occupant of heavy transport vehicle injured in collision with military vehicle (V69.81)

> The appropriate 7th character is to be added to each code from category V64

> | | |
> |---|---|
> | A | initial encounter |
> | D | subsequent encounter |
> | S | sequela |

X● V64.0   Driver of heavy transport vehicle injured in collision with heavy transport vehicle or bus in nontraffic accident

X● V64.1   Passenger in heavy transport vehicle injured in collision with heavy transport vehicle or bus in nontraffic accident

X● V64.2   Person on outside of heavy transport vehicle injured in collision with heavy transport vehicle or bus in nontraffic accident

X● V64.3   Unspecified occupant of heavy transport vehicle injured in collision with heavy transport vehicle or bus in nontraffic accident

X● V64.4   Person boarding or alighting a heavy transport vehicle injured in collision with heavy transport vehicle or bus while boarding or alighting

X● V64.5   Driver of heavy transport vehicle injured in collision with heavy transport vehicle or bus in traffic accident

X● V64.6   Passenger in heavy transport vehicle injured in collision with heavy transport vehicle or bus in traffic accident

X● V64.7   Person on outside of heavy transport vehicle injured in collision with heavy transport vehicle or bus in traffic accident

X● V64.9   Unspecified occupant of heavy transport vehicle injured in collision with heavy transport vehicle or bus in traffic accident

● V65   **Occupant of heavy transport vehicle injured in collision with railway train or railway vehicle**

> The appropriate 7th character is to be added to each code from category V65

> | | |
> |---|---|
> | A | initial encounter |
> | D | subsequent encounter |
> | S | sequela |

X● V65.0   Driver of heavy transport vehicle injured in collision with railway train or railway vehicle in nontraffic accident

X● V65.1   Passenger in heavy transport vehicle injured in collision with railway train or railway vehicle in nontraffic accident

X● V65.2   Person on outside of heavy transport vehicle injured in collision with railway train or railway vehicle in nontraffic accident

X● V65.3   Unspecified occupant of heavy transport vehicle injured in collision with railway train or railway vehicle in nontraffic accident

X● V65.4   Person boarding or alighting a heavy transport vehicle injured in collision with railway train or railway vehicle

X● V65.5   Driver of heavy transport vehicle injured in collision with railway train or railway vehicle in traffic accident

X● V65.6   Passenger in heavy transport vehicle injured in collision with railway train or railway vehicle in traffic accident

X● V65.7   Person on outside of heavy transport vehicle injured in collision with railway train or railway vehicle in traffic accident

X● V65.9   Unspecified occupant of heavy transport vehicle injured in collision with railway train or railway vehicle in traffic accident

CHAPTER 20 (V01-Y99)

● **V66**   **Occupant of heavy transport vehicle injured in collision with other nonmotor vehicle**

     Includes   collision with animal-drawn vehicle, animal being ridden, streetcar

     The appropriate 7th character is to be added to each code from category V66

        A   initial encounter
        D   subsequent encounter
        S   sequela

X● **V66.0**   Driver of heavy transport vehicle injured in collision with other nonmotor vehicle in nontraffic accident

X● **V66.1**   Passenger in heavy transport vehicle injured in collision with other nonmotor vehicle in nontraffic accident

X● **V66.2**   Person on outside of heavy transport vehicle injured in collision with other nonmotor vehicle in nontraffic accident

X● **V66.3**   Unspecified occupant of heavy transport vehicle injured in collision with other nonmotor vehicle in nontraffic accident

X● **V66.4**   Person boarding or alighting a heavy transport vehicle injured in collision with other nonmotor vehicle

X● **V66.5**   Driver of heavy transport vehicle injured in collision with other nonmotor vehicle in traffic accident

X● **V66.6**   Passenger in heavy transport vehicle injured in collision with other nonmotor vehicle in traffic accident

X● **V66.7**   Person on outside of heavy transport vehicle injured in collision with other nonmotor vehicle in traffic accident

X● **V66.9**   Unspecified occupant of heavy transport vehicle injured in collision with other nonmotor vehicle in traffic accident

● **V67**   **Occupant of heavy transport vehicle injured in collision with fixed or stationary object**

     The appropriate 7th character is to be added to each code from category V67

        A   initial encounter
        D   subsequent encounter
        S   sequela

X● **V67.0**   Driver of heavy transport vehicle injured in collision with fixed or stationary object in nontraffic accident

X● **V67.1**   Passenger in heavy transport vehicle injured in collision with fixed or stationary object in nontraffic accident

X● **V67.2**   Person on outside of heavy transport vehicle injured in collision with fixed or stationary object in nontraffic accident

X● **V67.3**   Unspecified occupant of heavy transport vehicle injured in collision with fixed or stationary object in nontraffic accident

X● **V67.4**   Person boarding or alighting a heavy transport vehicle injured in collision with fixed or stationary object

X● **V67.5**   Driver of heavy transport vehicle injured in collision with fixed or stationary object in traffic accident

X● **V67.6**   Passenger in heavy transport vehicle injured in collision with fixed or stationary object in traffic accident

X● **V67.7**   Person on outside of heavy transport vehicle injured in collision with fixed or stationary object in traffic accident

X● **V67.9**   Unspecified occupant of heavy transport vehicle injured in collision with fixed or stationary object in traffic accident

● **V68**   **Occupant of heavy transport vehicle injured in noncollision transport accident**

     Includes   overturning heavy transport vehicle NOS
                   overturning heavy transport vehicle without collision

     The appropriate 7th character is to be added to each code from category V68

        A   initial encounter
        D   subsequent encounter
        S   sequela

X● **V68.0**   Driver of heavy transport vehicle injured in noncollision transport accident in nontraffic accident

X● **V68.1**   Passenger in heavy transport vehicle injured in noncollision transport accident in nontraffic accident

X● **V68.2**   Person on outside of heavy transport vehicle injured in noncollision transport accident in nontraffic accident

X● **V68.3**   Unspecified occupant of heavy transport vehicle injured in noncollision transport accident in nontraffic accident

X● **V68.4**   Person boarding or alighting a heavy transport vehicle injured in noncollision transport accident

X● **V68.5**   Driver of heavy transport vehicle injured in noncollision transport accident in traffic accident

X● **V68.6**   Passenger in heavy transport vehicle injured in noncollision transport accident in traffic accident

X● **V68.7**   Person on outside of heavy transport vehicle injured in noncollision transport accident in traffic accident

X● **V68.9**   Unspecified occupant of heavy transport vehicle injured in noncollision transport accident in traffic accident

● **V69**   **Occupant of heavy transport vehicle injured in other and unspecified transport accidents**

     The appropriate 7th character is to be added to each code from category V69

        A   initial encounter
        D   subsequent encounter
        S   sequela

● **V69.0**   Driver of heavy transport vehicle injured in collision with other and unspecified motor vehicles in nontraffic accident

    X● **V69.00**   Driver of heavy transport vehicle injured in collision with unspecified motor vehicles in nontraffic accident

    X● **V69.09**   Driver of heavy transport vehicle injured in collision with other motor vehicles in nontraffic accident

● **V69.1**   Passenger in heavy transport vehicle injured in collision with other and unspecified motor vehicles in nontraffic accident

    X● **V69.10**   Passenger in heavy transport vehicle injured in collision with unspecified motor vehicles in nontraffic accident

    X● **V69.19**   Passenger in heavy transport vehicle injured in collision with other motor vehicles in nontraffic accident

● **V69.2**   Unspecified occupant of heavy transport vehicle injured in collision with other and unspecified motor vehicles in nontraffic accident

    X● **V69.20**   Unspecified occupant of heavy transport vehicle injured in collision with unspecified motor vehicles in nontraffic accident

        Collision NOS involving heavy transport vehicle, nontraffic

    X● **V69.29**   Unspecified occupant of heavy transport vehicle injured in collision with other motor vehicles in nontraffic accident

◀ New   ⬅ Revised   ~~deleted~~ Deleted   Excludes 1   Excludes 2   Includes   Use additional   Code first   Code also   Unspecified

OGCR Official Guidelines   X Assign placeholder X   ● Use Additional Character(s)   ▌ Manifestation Code   **Coding Clinic**

X● **V69.3** **Occupant (driver) (passenger) of heavy transport vehicle injured in unspecified nontraffic accident**
     Accident NOS involving heavy transport vehicle, nontraffic
     Occupant of heavy transport vehicle injured in nontraffic accident NOS

● **V69.4** **Driver of heavy transport vehicle injured in collision with other and unspecified motor vehicles in traffic accident**

   X● **V69.40** Driver of heavy transport vehicle injured in collision with unspecified motor vehicles in traffic accident

   X● **V69.49** Driver of heavy transport vehicle injured in collision with other motor vehicles in traffic accident

● **V69.5** **Passenger in heavy transport vehicle injured in collision with other and unspecified motor vehicles in traffic accident**

   X● **V69.50** Passenger in heavy transport vehicle injured in collision with unspecified motor vehicles in traffic accident

   X● **V69.59** Passenger in heavy transport vehicle injured in collision with other motor vehicles in traffic accident

● **V69.6** **Unspecified occupant of heavy transport vehicle injured in collision with other and unspecified motor vehicles in traffic accident**

   X● **V69.60** Unspecified occupant of heavy transport vehicle injured in collision with unspecified motor vehicles in traffic accident
       Collision NOS involving heavy transport vehicle (traffic)

   X● **V69.69** Unspecified occupant of heavy transport vehicle injured in collision with other motor vehicles in traffic accident

● **V69.8** **Occupant (driver) (passenger) of heavy transport vehicle injured in other specified transport accidents**

   X● **V69.81** Occupant (driver) (passenger) of heavy transport vehicle injured in transport accidents with military vehicle

   X● **V69.88** Occupant (driver) (passenger) of heavy transport vehicle injured in other specified transport accidents

X● **V69.9** **Occupant (driver) (passenger) of heavy transport vehicle injured in unspecified traffic accident**
     Accident NOS involving heavy transport vehicle

BUS OCCUPANT INJURED IN TRANSPORT ACCIDENT (V70-V79)

Includes	motorcoach
Excludes1	minibus (V50-V59)

● **V70** **Bus occupant injured in collision with pedestrian or animal**

   Excludes1   bus collision with animal-drawn vehicle or animal being ridden (V76.-)

   The appropriate 7th character is to be added to each code from category V70

A	initial encounter
D	subsequent encounter
S	sequela

X● **V70.0** Driver of bus injured in collision with pedestrian or animal in nontraffic accident

X● **V70.1** Passenger on bus injured in collision with pedestrian or animal in nontraffic accident

X● **V70.2** Person on outside of bus injured in collision with pedestrian or animal in nontraffic accident

X● **V70.3** Unspecified occupant of bus injured in collision with pedestrian or animal in nontraffic accident

X● **V70.4** Person boarding or alighting from bus injured in collision with pedestrian or animal

X● **V70.5** Driver of bus injured in collision with pedestrian or animal in traffic accident

X● **V70.6** Passenger on bus injured in collision with pedestrian or animal in traffic accident

X● **V70.7** Person on outside of bus injured in collision with pedestrian or animal in traffic accident

X● **V70.9** Unspecified occupant of bus injured in collision with pedestrian or animal in traffic accident

● **V71** **Bus occupant injured in collision with pedal cycle**

   The appropriate 7th character is to be added to each code from category V71

A	initial encounter
D	subsequent encounter
S	sequela

X● **V71.0** Driver of bus injured in collision with pedal cycle in nontraffic accident

X● **V71.1** Passenger on bus injured in collision with pedal cycle in nontraffic accident

X● **V71.2** Person on outside of bus injured in collision with pedal cycle in nontraffic accident

X● **V71.3** Unspecified occupant of bus injured in collision with pedal cycle in nontraffic accident

X● **V71.4** Person boarding or alighting from bus injured in collision with pedal cycle

X● **V71.5** Driver of bus injured in collision with pedal cycle in traffic accident

X● **V71.6** Passenger on bus injured in collision with pedal cycle in traffic accident

X● **V71.7** Person on outside of bus injured in collision with pedal cycle in traffic accident

X● **V71.9** Unspecified occupant of bus injured in collision with pedal cycle in traffic accident

● **V72** **Bus occupant injured in collision with two- or three-wheeled motor vehicle**

   The appropriate 7th character is to be added to each code from category V72

A	initial encounter
D	subsequent encounter
S	sequela

X● **V72.0** Driver of bus injured in collision with two- or three-wheeled motor vehicle in nontraffic accident

X● **V72.1** Passenger on bus injured in collision with two- or three-wheeled motor vehicle in nontraffic accident

X● **V72.2** Person on outside of bus injured in collision with two- or three-wheeled motor vehicle in nontraffic accident

X● **V72.3** Unspecified occupant of bus injured in collision with two- or three-wheeled motor vehicle in nontraffic accident

X● **V72.4** Person boarding or alighting from bus injured in collision with two- or three-wheeled motor vehicle

X● **V72.5** Driver of bus injured in collision with two- or three-wheeled motor vehicle in traffic accident

X● **V72.6** Passenger on bus injured in collision with two- or three-wheeled motor vehicle in traffic accident

X● **V72.7** Person on outside of bus injured in collision with two- or three-wheeled motor vehicle in traffic accident

X● **V72.9** Unspecified occupant of bus injured in collision with two- or three-wheeled motor vehicle in traffic accident

CHAPTER 20 (V01-Y99)

CHAPTER 20 (V01-Y99)

● **V73** **Bus occupant injured in collision with car, pick-up truck or van**

The appropriate 7th character is to be added to each code from category V73

A	initial encounter
D	subsequent encounter
S	sequela

X● **V73.0** Driver of bus injured in collision with car, pick-up truck or van in nontraffic accident

X● **V73.1** Passenger on bus injured in collision with car, pick-up truck or van in nontraffic accident

X● **V73.2** Person on outside of bus injured in collision with car, pick-up truck or van in nontraffic accident

X● **V73.3** Unspecified occupant of bus injured in collision with car, pick-up truck or van in nontraffic accident

X● **V73.4** Person boarding or alighting from bus injured in collision with car, pick-up truck or van

X● **V73.5** Driver of bus injured in collision with car, pick-up truck or van in traffic accident

X● **V73.6** Passenger on bus injured in collision with car, pick-up truck or van in traffic accident

X● **V73.7** Person on outside of bus injured in collision with car, pick-up truck or van in traffic accident

X● **V73.9** Unspecified occupant of bus injured in collision with car, pick-up truck or van in traffic accident

● **V74** **Bus occupant injured in collision with heavy transport vehicle or bus**

Excludes1 bus occupant injured in collision with military vehicle (V79.81)

The appropriate 7th character is to be added to each code from category V74

A	initial encounter
D	subsequent encounter
S	sequela

X● **V74.0** Driver of bus injured in collision with heavy transport vehicle or bus in nontraffic accident

X● **V74.1** Passenger on bus injured in collision with heavy transport vehicle or bus in nontraffic accident

X● **V74.2** Person on outside of bus injured in collision with heavy transport vehicle or bus in nontraffic accident

X● **V74.3** Unspecified occupant of bus injured in collision with heavy transport vehicle or bus in nontraffic accident

X● **V74.4** Person boarding or alighting from bus injured in collision with heavy transport vehicle or bus

X● **V74.5** Driver of bus injured in collision with heavy transport vehicle or bus in traffic accident

X● **V74.6** Passenger on bus injured in collision with heavy transport vehicle or bus in traffic accident

X● **V74.7** Person on outside of bus injured in collision with heavy transport vehicle or bus in traffic accident

X● **V74.9** Unspecified occupant of bus injured in collision with heavy transport vehicle or bus in traffic accident

● **V75** **Bus occupant injured in collision with railway train or railway vehicle**

The appropriate 7th character is to be added to each code from category V75

A	initial encounter
D	subsequent encounter
S	sequela

X● **V75.0** Driver of bus injured in collision with railway train or railway vehicle in nontraffic accident

X● **V75.1** Passenger on bus injured in collision with railway train or railway vehicle in nontraffic accident

X● **V75.2** Person on outside of bus injured in collision with railway train or railway vehicle in nontraffic accident

X● **V75.3** Unspecified occupant of bus injured in collision with railway train or railway vehicle in nontraffic accident

X● **V75.4** Person boarding or alighting from bus injured in collision with railway train or railway vehicle

X● **V75.5** Driver of bus injured in collision with railway train or railway vehicle in traffic accident

X● **V75.6** Passenger on bus injured in collision with railway train or railway vehicle in traffic accident

X● **V75.7** Person on outside of bus injured in collision with railway train or railway vehicle in traffic accident

X● **V75.9** Unspecified occupant of bus injured in collision with railway train or railway vehicle in traffic accident

● **V76** **Bus occupant injured in collision with other nonmotor vehicle**

Includes collision with animal-drawn vehicle, animal being ridden, streetcar

The appropriate 7th character is to be added to each code from category V76

A	initial encounter
D	subsequent encounter
S	sequela

X● **V76.0** Driver of bus injured in collision with other nonmotor vehicle in nontraffic accident

X● **V76.1** Passenger on bus injured in collision with other nonmotor vehicle in nontraffic accident

X● **V76.2** Person on outside of bus injured in collision with other nonmotor vehicle in nontraffic accident

X● **V76.3** Unspecified occupant of bus injured in collision with other nonmotor vehicle in nontraffic accident

X● **V76.4** Person boarding or alighting from bus injured in collision with other nonmotor vehicle

X● **V76.5** Driver of bus injured in collision with other nonmotor vehicle in traffic accident

X● **V76.6** Passenger on bus injured in collision with other nonmotor vehicle in traffic accident

X● **V76.7** Person on outside of bus injured in collision with other nonmotor vehicle in traffic accident

X● **V76.9** Unspecified occupant of bus injured in collision with other nonmotor vehicle in traffic accident

● **V77** **Bus occupant injured in collision with fixed or stationary object**

The appropriate 7th character is to be added to each code from category V77

A	initial encounter
D	subsequent encounter
S	sequela

X● **V77.0** Driver of bus injured in collision with fixed or stationary object in nontraffic accident

X● **V77.1** Passenger on bus injured in collision with fixed or stationary object in nontraffic accident

X● **V77.2** Person on outside of bus injured in collision with fixed or stationary object in nontraffic accident

X● **V77.3** Unspecified occupant of bus injured in collision with fixed or stationary object in nontraffic accident

X● **V77.4** Person boarding or alighting from bus injured in collision with fixed or stationary object

X● **V77.5** Driver of bus injured in collision with fixed or stationary object in traffic accident

X● **V77.6** Passenger on bus injured in collision with fixed or stationary object in traffic accident

X● **V77.7** Person on outside of bus injured in collision with fixed or stationary object in traffic accident

X● **V77.9** Unspecified occupant of bus injured in collision with fixed or stationary object in traffic accident

◀ New   ⬅ Revised   ~~deleted~~ Deleted   Excludes 1   Excludes 2   Includes   Use additional   Code first   Code also   Unspecified

OGCR Official Guidelines   X Assign placeholder X   ● Use Additional Character(s)   ▶ Manifestation Code   **Coding Clinic**

● **V78   Bus occupant injured in noncollision transport accident**

> | Includes | overturning bus NOS |
> | --- | --- |
> | | overturning bus without collision |

> The appropriate 7th character is to be added to each code from category V78

> | A | initial encounter |
> | --- | --- |
> | D | subsequent encounter |
> | S | sequela |

X● **V78.0   Driver of bus injured in noncollision transport accident in nontraffic accident**

X● **V78.1   Passenger on bus injured in noncollision transport accident in nontraffic accident**

X● **V78.2   Person on outside of bus injured in noncollision transport accident in nontraffic accident**

X● **V78.3   Unspecified occupant of bus injured in noncollision transport accident in nontraffic accident**

X● **V78.4   Person boarding or alighting from bus injured in noncollision transport accident**

X● **V78.5   Driver of bus injured in noncollision transport accident in traffic accident**

X● **V78.6   Passenger on bus injured in noncollision transport accident in traffic accident**

X● **V78.7   Person on outside of bus injured in noncollision transport accident in traffic accident**

X● **V78.9   Unspecified occupant of bus injured in noncollision transport accident in traffic accident**

● **V79   Bus occupant injured in other and unspecified transport accidents**

> The appropriate 7th character is to be added to each code from category V79

> | A | initial encounter |
> | --- | --- |
> | D | subsequent encounter |
> | S | sequela |

● **V79.0   Driver of bus injured in collision with other and unspecified motor vehicles in nontraffic accident**

   X● **V79.00   Driver of bus injured in collision with unspecified motor vehicles in nontraffic accident**

   X● **V79.09   Driver of bus injured in collision with other motor vehicles in nontraffic accident**

● **V79.1   Passenger on bus injured in collision with other and unspecified motor vehicles in nontraffic accident**

   X● **V79.10   Passenger on bus injured in collision with unspecified motor vehicles in nontraffic accident**

   X● **V79.19   Passenger on bus injured in collision with other motor vehicles in nontraffic accident**

● **V79.2   Unspecified bus occupant injured in collision with other and unspecified motor vehicles in nontraffic accident**

   X● **V79.20   Unspecified bus occupant injured in collision with unspecified motor vehicles in nontraffic accident**
> Bus collision NOS, nontraffic

   X● **V79.29   Unspecified bus occupant injured in collision with other motor vehicles in nontraffic accident**

X● **V79.3   Bus occupant (driver) (passenger) injured in unspecified nontraffic accident**
> Bus accident NOS, nontraffic
> Bus occupant injured in nontraffic accident NOS

● **V79.4   Driver of bus injured in collision with other and unspecified motor vehicles in traffic accident**

   X● **V79.40   Driver of bus injured in collision with unspecified motor vehicles in traffic accident**

   X● **V79.49   Driver of bus injured in collision with other motor vehicles in traffic accident**

● **V79.5   Passenger on bus injured in collision with other and unspecified motor vehicles in traffic accident**

   X● **V79.50   Passenger on bus injured in collision with unspecified motor vehicles in traffic accident**

   X● **V79.59   Passenger on bus injured in collision with other motor vehicles in traffic accident**

● **V79.6   Unspecified bus occupant injured in collision with other and unspecified motor vehicles in traffic accident**

   X● **V79.60   Unspecified bus occupant injured in collision with unspecified motor vehicles in traffic accident**
> Bus collision NOS (traffic)

   X● **V79.69   Unspecified bus occupant injured in collision with other motor vehicles in traffic accident**

● **V79.8   Bus occupant (driver) (passenger) injured in other specified transport accidents**

   X● **V79.81   Bus occupant (driver) (passenger) injured in transport accidents with military vehicle**

   X● **V79.88   Bus occupant (driver) (passenger) injured in other specified transport accidents**

X● **V79.9   Bus occupant (driver) (passenger) injured in unspecified traffic accident**
> Bus accident NOS

OTHER LAND TRANSPORT ACCIDENTS (V80-V89)

● **V80   Animal-rider or occupant of animal-drawn vehicle injured in transport accident**

> The appropriate 7th character is to be added to each code from category V80

> | A | initial encounter |
> | --- | --- |
> | D | subsequent encounter |
> | S | sequela |

● **V80.0   Animal-rider or occupant of animal drawn vehicle injured by fall from or being thrown from animal or animal-drawn vehicle in noncollision accident**

   ● **V80.01   Animal-rider injured by fall from or being thrown from animal in noncollision accident**

     ● **V80.010   Animal-rider injured by fall from or being thrown from horse in noncollision accident**

     ● **V80.018   Animal-rider injured by fall from or being thrown from other animal in noncollision accident**

   X● **V80.02   Occupant of animal-drawn vehicle injured by fall from or being thrown from animal-drawn vehicle in noncollision accident**
> Overturning animal-drawn vehicle NOS
> Overturning animal-drawn vehicle without collision

● **V80.1   Animal-rider or occupant of animal-drawn vehicle injured in collision with pedestrian or animal**

> | Excludes1 | animal-rider or animal-drawn vehicle collision with animal-drawn vehicle or animal being ridden (V80.7) |
> | --- | --- |

   X● **V80.11   Animal-rider injured in collision with pedestrian or animal**

   X● **V80.12   Occupant of animal-drawn vehicle injured in collision with pedestrian or animal**

CHAPTER 20 (V01-Y99)

● **V80.2**   Animal-rider or occupant of animal-drawn vehicle injured in collision with pedal cycle

   X● **V80.21**   Animal-rider injured in collision with pedal cycle

   X● **V80.22**   Occupant of animal-drawn vehicle injured in collision with pedal cycle

● **V80.3**   Animal-rider or occupant of animal-drawn vehicle injured in collision with two- or three-wheeled motor vehicle

   X● **V80.31**   Animal-rider injured in collision with two- or three-wheeled motor vehicle

   X● **V80.32**   Occupant of animal-drawn vehicle injured in collision with two- or three-wheeled motor vehicle

● **V80.4**   Animal-rider or occupant of animal-drawn vehicle injured in collision with car, pick-up truck, van, heavy transport vehicle or bus

> **Excludes1**   animal-rider injured in collision with military vehicle (V80.910)
> occupant of animal-drawn vehicle injured in collision with military vehicle (V80.920)

   X● **V80.41**   Animal-rider injured in collision with car, pick-up truck, van, heavy transport vehicle or bus

   X● **V80.42**   Occupant of animal-drawn vehicle injured in collision with car, pick-up truck, van, heavy transport vehicle or bus

● **V80.5**   Animal-rider or occupant of animal-drawn vehicle injured in collision with other specified motor vehicle

   X● **V80.51**   Animal-rider injured in collision with other specified motor vehicle

   X● **V80.52**   Occupant of animal-drawn vehicle injured in collision with other specified motor vehicle

● **V80.6**   Animal-rider or occupant of animal-drawn vehicle injured in collision with railway train or railway vehicle

   X● **V80.61**   Animal-rider injured in collision with railway train or railway vehicle

   X● **V80.62**   Occupant of animal-drawn vehicle injured in collision with railway train or railway vehicle

● **V80.7**   Animal-rider or occupant of animal-drawn vehicle injured in collision with other nonmotor vehicles

   ● **V80.71**   Animal-rider or occupant of animal-drawn vehicle injured in collision with animal being ridden

     ● **V80.710**   Animal-rider injured in collision with other animal being ridden

     ● **V80.711**   Occupant of animal-drawn vehicle injured in collision with animal being ridden

   ● **V80.72**   Animal-rider or occupant of animal-drawn vehicle injured in collision with other animal-drawn vehicle

     ● **V80.720**   Animal-rider injured in collision with animal-drawn vehicle

     ● **V80.721**   Occupant of animal-drawn vehicle injured in collision with other animal-drawn vehicle

   ● **V80.73**   Animal-rider or occupant of animal-drawn vehicle injured in collision with streetcar

     ● **V80.730**   Animal-rider injured in collision with streetcar

     ● **V80.731**   Occupant of animal-drawn vehicle injured in collision with streetcar

● **V80.79**   Animal-rider or occupant of animal-drawn vehicle injured in collision with other nonmotor vehicles

     ● **V80.790**   Animal-rider injured in collision with other nonmotor vehicles

     ● **V80.791**   Occupant of animal-drawn vehicle injured in collision with other nonmotor vehicles

● **V80.8**   Animal-rider or occupant of animal-drawn vehicle injured in collision with fixed or stationary object

   X● **V80.81**   Animal-rider injured in collision with fixed or stationary object

   X● **V80.82**   Occupant of animal-drawn vehicle injured in collision with fixed or stationary object

● **V80.9**   Animal-rider or occupant of animal-drawn vehicle injured in other and unspecified transport accidents

   ● **V80.91**   Animal-rider injured in other and unspecified transport accidents

     ● **V80.910**   Animal-rider injured in transport accident with military vehicle

     ● **V80.918**   Animal-rider injured in other transport accident

     ● **V80.919**   Animal-rider injured in unspecified transport accident
        Animal rider accident NOS

   ● **V80.92**   Occupant of animal-drawn vehicle injured in other and unspecified transport accidents

     ● **V80.920**   Occupant of animal-drawn vehicle injured in transport accident with military vehicle

     ● **V80.928**   Occupant of animal-drawn vehicle injured in other transport accident

     ● **V80.929**   Occupant of animal-drawn vehicle injured in unspecified transport accident
        Animal-drawn vehicle accident NOS

● **V81**   Occupant of railway train or railway vehicle injured in transport accident

> **Includes**   derailment of railway train or railway vehicle
> person on outside of train

> **Excludes1**   streetcar (V82.-)

The appropriate 7th character is to be added to each code from category V81

A	initial encounter
D	subsequent encounter
S	sequela

   X● **V81.0**   Occupant of railway train or railway vehicle injured in collision with motor vehicle in nontraffic accident

> **Excludes1**   occupant of railway train or railway vehicle injured due to collision with military vehicle (V81.83)

   X● **V81.1**   Occupant of railway train or railway vehicle injured in collision with motor vehicle in traffic accident

> **Excludes1**   occupant of railway train or railway vehicle injured due to collision with military vehicle (V81.83)

   X● **V81.2**   Occupant of railway train or railway vehicle injured in collision with or hit by rolling stock

   X● **V81.3**   Occupant of railway train or railway vehicle injured in collision with other object
        Railway collision NOS

   X● **V81.4**   Person injured while boarding or alighting from railway train or railway vehicle

   X● **V81.5**   Occupant of railway train or railway vehicle injured by fall in railway train or railway vehicle

   X● **V81.6**   Occupant of railway train or railway vehicle injured by fall from railway train or railway vehicle

◀ New   ⬅ Revised   ~~deleted~~ Deleted   Excludes 1   Excludes 2   Includes   Use additional   Code first   Code also   Unspecified

OGCR Official Guidelines   **X** Assign placeholder X   ● Use Additional Character(s)   ▶ Manifestation Code   **Coding Clinic**

X● **V81.7** Occupant of railway train or railway vehicle injured in derailment without antecedent collision

● **V81.8** Occupant of railway train or railway vehicle injured in other specified railway accidents

X● **V81.81** Occupant of railway train or railway vehicle injured due to explosion or fire on train

X● **V81.82** Occupant of railway train or railway vehicle injured due to object falling onto train
Occupant of railway train or railway vehicle injured due to falling earth onto train
Occupant of railway train or railway vehicle injured due to falling rocks onto train
Occupant of railway train or railway vehicle injured due to falling snow onto train
Occupant of railway train or railway vehicle injured due to falling trees onto train

X● **V81.83** Occupant of railway train or railway vehicle injured due to collision with military vehicle

X● **V81.89** Occupant of railway train or railway vehicle injured due to other specified railway accident

X● **V81.9** Occupant of railway train or railway vehicle injured in unspecified railway accident
Railway accident NOS

● **V82** Occupant of powered streetcar injured in transport accident

Includes   interurban electric car
person on outside of streetcar
tram (car)
trolley (car)

Excludes1   bus (V70-V79)
motorcoach (V70-V79)
nonpowered streetcar (V76.-)
train (V81.-)

The appropriate 7th character is to be added to each code from category V82

A   initial encounter
D   subsequent encounter
S   sequela

X● **V82.0** Occupant of streetcar injured in collision with motor vehicle in nontraffic accident

X● **V82.1** Occupant of streetcar injured in collision with motor vehicle in traffic accident

X● **V82.2** Occupant of streetcar injured in collision with or hit by rolling stock

X● **V82.3** Occupant of streetcar injured in collision with other object
Excludes1   collision with animal-drawn vehicle or animal being ridden (V82.8)

X● **V82.4** Person injured while boarding or alighting from streetcar

X● **V82.5** Occupant of streetcar injured by fall in streetcar
Excludes1   fall in streetcar:
while boarding or alighting (V82.4)
with antecedent collision (V82.0-V82.3)

X● **V82.6** Occupant of streetcar injured by fall from streetcar
Excludes1   fall from streetcar:
while boarding or alighting (V82.4)
with antecedent collision (V82.0-V82.3)

X● **V82.7** Occupant of streetcar injured in derailment without antecedent collision
Excludes1   occupant of streetcar injured in derailment with antecedent collision (V82.0-V82.3)

X● **V82.8** Occupant of streetcar injured in other specified transport accidents
Streetcar collision with military vehicle
Streetcar collision with train or nonmotor vehicles

X● **V82.9** Occupant of streetcar injured in unspecified traffic accident
Streetcar accident NOS

● **V83** Occupant of special vehicle mainly used on industrial premises injured in transport accident

Includes   battery-powered airport passenger vehicle
battery-powered truck (baggage) (mail)
coal-car in mine
forklift (truck)
logging car
self-propelled industrial truck
station baggage truck (powered)
tram, truck, or tub (powered) in mine or quarry

Excludes1   special construction vehicles (V85.-)
special industrial vehicle in stationary use or maintenance (W31.-)

The appropriate 7th character is to be added to each code from category V83

A   initial encounter
D   subsequent encounter
S   sequela

X● **V83.0** Driver of special industrial vehicle injured in traffic accident

X● **V83.1** Passenger of special industrial vehicle injured in traffic accident

X● **V83.2** Person on outside of special industrial vehicle injured in traffic accident

X● **V83.3** Unspecified occupant of special industrial vehicle injured in traffic accident

X● **V83.4** Person injured while boarding or alighting from special industrial vehicle

X● **V83.5** Driver of special industrial vehicle injured in nontraffic accident

X● **V83.6** Passenger of special industrial vehicle injured in nontraffic accident

X● **V83.7** Person on outside of special industrial vehicle injured in nontraffic accident

X● **V83.9** Unspecified occupant of special industrial vehicle injured in nontraffic accident
Special-industrial-vehicle accident NOS

● **V84** Occupant of special vehicle mainly used in agriculture injured in transport accident

Includes   self-propelled farm machinery
tractor (and trailer)

Excludes1   animal-powered farm machinery accident (W30.8-)
contact with combine harvester (W30.0)
special agricultural vehicle in stationary use or maintenance (W30.-)

The appropriate 7th character is to be added to each code from category V84

A   initial encounter
D   subsequent encounter
S   sequela

X● **V84.0** Driver of special agricultural vehicle injured in traffic accident

X● **V84.1** Passenger of special agricultural vehicle injured in traffic accident

X● **V84.2** Person on outside of special agricultural vehicle injured in traffic accident

X● **V84.3** Unspecified occupant of special agricultural vehicle injured in traffic accident

X● **V84.4** Person injured while boarding or alighting from special agricultural vehicle

X● **V84.5** Driver of special agricultural vehicle injured in nontraffic accident

X● **V84.6** Passenger of special agricultural vehicle injured in nontraffic accident

X● **V84.7** Person on outside of special agricultural vehicle injured in nontraffic accident

X● **V84.9** Unspecified occupant of special agricultural vehicle injured in nontraffic accident
Special-agricultural vehicle accident NOS

CHAPTER 20 (V01-Y99)

●V85 Occupant of special construction vehicle injured in transport accident

> **Includes**   bulldozer
> digger
> dump truck
> earth-leveller
> mechanical shovel
> road-roller

> **Excludes1**   special industrial vehicle (V83.-)
> special construction vehicle in stationary use or maintenance (W31.-)

The appropriate 7th character is to be added to each code from category V85

> A   initial encounter
> D   subsequent encounter
> S   sequela

X● **V85.0 Driver of special construction vehicle injured in traffic accident**

X● **V85.1 Passenger of special construction vehicle injured in traffic accident**

X● **V85.2 Person on outside of special construction vehicle injured in traffic accident**

X● **V85.3 Unspecified occupant of special construction vehicle injured in traffic accident**

X● **V85.4 Person injured while boarding or alighting from special construction vehicle**

X● **V85.5 Driver of special construction vehicle injured in nontraffic accident**

X● **V85.6 Passenger of special construction vehicle injured in nontraffic accident**

X● **V85.7 Person on outside of special construction vehicle injured in nontraffic accident**

X● **V85.9 Unspecified occupant of special construction vehicle injured in nontraffic accident**
> Special-construction-vehicle accident NOS

●V86 Occupant of special all-terrain or other off-road motor vehicle, injured in transport accident

> **Excludes1**   special all-terrain vehicle in stationary use or maintenance (W31.-)
> sport-utility vehicle (V50-V59)
> three-wheeled motor vehicle designed for on-road use (V30-V39)

The appropriate 7th character is to be added to each code from category V86

> A   initial encounter
> D   subsequent encounter
> S   sequela

●**V86.0 Driver of special all-terrain or other off-road motor vehicle injured in traffic accident**

X● **V86.01 Driver of ambulance or fire engine injured in traffic accident**

X● **V86.02 Driver of snowmobile injured in traffic accident**

X● **V86.03 Driver of dune buggy injured in traffic accident**

X● **V86.04 Driver of military vehicle injured in traffic accident**

X● **V86.09 Driver of other off-road special all-terrain or other off-road vehicle injured in traffic accident**
> Driver of dirt bike injured in traffic accident
> Driver of go cart injured in traffic accident
> Driver of golf cart injured in traffic accident

●**V86.1 Passenger of special all-terrain or other off-road motor vehicle injured in traffic accident**

X● **V86.11 Passenger of ambulance or fire engine injured in traffic accident**

X● **V86.12 Passenger of snowmobile injured in traffic accident**

X● **V86.13 Passenger of dune buggy injured in traffic accident**

X● **V86.14 Passenger of military vehicle injured in traffic accident**

X● **V86.19 Passenger of other off-road special all-terrain or other off-road off-road motor vehicle injured in traffic accident**
> Passenger of dirt bike injured in traffic accident
> Passenger of go cart injured in traffic accident
> Passenger of golf cart injured in traffic accident

●**V86.2 Person on outside of special all-terrain or other off-road motor vehicle injured in traffic accident**

X● **V86.21 Person on outside of ambulance or fire engine injured in traffic accident**

X● **V86.22 Person on outside of snowmobile injured in traffic accident**

X● **V86.23 Person on outside of dune buggy injured in traffic accident**

X● **V86.24 Person on outside of military vehicle injured in traffic accident**

X● **V86.29 Person on outside of other special all-terrain or other off-road motor vehicle injured in traffic accident**
> Person on outside of dirt bike injured in traffic accident
> Person on outside of go cart in traffic accident
> Person on outside of golf cart injured in traffic accident

●**V86.3 Unspecified occupant of special all-terrain or other off-road motor vehicle injured in traffic accident**

X● **V86.31 Unspecified occupant of ambulance or fire engine injured in traffic accident**

X● **V86.32 Unspecified occupant of snowmobile injured in traffic accident**

X● **V86.33 Unspecified occupant of dune buggy injured in traffic accident**

X● **V86.34 Unspecified occupant of military vehicle injured in traffic accident**

X● **V86.39 Unspecified occupant of other special all-terrain or other off-road motor vehicle injured in traffic accident**
> Unspecified occupant of dirt bike injured in traffic accident
> Unspecified occupant of go cart injured in traffic accident
> Unspecified occupant of golf cart injured in traffic accident

●**V86.4 Person injured while boarding or alighting from special all-terrain or other off-road motor vehicle**

X● **V86.41 Person injured while boarding or alighting from ambulance or fire engine**

X● **V86.42 Person injured while boarding or alighting from snowmobile**

X● **V86.43 Person injured while boarding or alighting from dune buggy**

X● **V86.44 Person injured while boarding or alighting from military vehicle**

X● **V86.49 Person injured while boarding or alighting from other special all-terrain or other off-road motor vehicle**
> Person injured while boarding or alighting from dirt bike
> Person injured while boarding or alighting from go cart
> Person injured while boarding or alighting from golf cart

◀ New   ⬅ Revised   ~~deleted~~ Deleted   Excludes 1   Excludes 2   Includes   Use additional   Code first   Code also   Unspecified

OGCR Official Guidelines   X Assign placeholder X   ● Use Additional Character(s)   ▶ Manifestation Code   **Coding Clinic**

● **V86.5**   **Driver of special all-terrain or other off-road motor vehicle injured in nontraffic accident**

   X● **V86.51**   Driver of ambulance or fire engine injured in nontraffic accident

   X● **V86.52**   Driver of snowmobile injured in nontraffic accident

   X● **V86.53**   Driver of dune buggy injured in nontraffic accident

   X● **V86.54**   Driver of military vehicle injured in nontraffic accident

   X● **V86.59**   Driver of other off-road special all-terrain or other off-road motor vehicle injured in nontraffic accident

        Driver of dirt bike injured in nontraffic accident

        Driver of go cart injured in nontraffic accident

        Driver of golf cart injured in nontraffic accident

● **V86.6**   **Passenger of special all-terrain or other off-road motor vehicle injured in nontraffic accident**

   X● **V86.61**   Passenger of ambulance or fire engine injured in nontraffic accident

   X● **V86.62**   Passenger of snowmobile injured in nontraffic accident

   X● **V86.63**   Passenger of dune buggy injured in nontraffic accident

   X● **V86.64**   Passenger of military vehicle injured in nontraffic accident

   X● **V86.69**   Passenger of other special all-terrain or other off-road vehicle injured in nontraffic accident

        Passenger of dirt bike injured in nontraffic accident

        Passenger of go cart injured in nontraffic accident

        Passenger of golf cart injured in nontraffic accident

● **V86.7**   **Person on outside of special all-terrain or other off-road motor vehicle injured in nontraffic accident**

   X● **V86.71**   Person on outside of ambulance or fire engine injured in nontraffic accident

   X● **V86.72**   Person on outside of snowmobile injured in nontraffic accident

   X● **V86.73**   Person on outside of dune buggy injured in nontraffic accident

   X● **V86.74**   Person on outside of military vehicle injured in nontraffic accident

   X● **V86.79**   Person on outside of other special all-terrain or other off-road motor vehicles injured in nontraffic accident

        Person on outside of dirt bike injured in nontraffic accident

        Person on outside of go cart injured in nontraffic accident

        Person on outside of golf cart injured in nontraffic accident

● **V86.9**   **Unspecified occupant of special all-terrain or other off-road motor vehicle injured in nontraffic accident**

   X● **V86.91**   Unspecified occupant of ambulance or fire engine injured in nontraffic accident

   X● **V86.92**   Unspecified occupant of snowmobile injured in nontraffic accident

   X● **V86.93**   Unspecified occupant of dune buggy injured in nontraffic accident

   X● **V86.94**   Unspecified occupant of military vehicle injured in nontraffic accident

   X● **V86.99**   Unspecified occupant of other off-road special all-terrain or other off-road motor vehicle injured in nontraffic accident

        All-terrain motor-vehicle accident NOS

        Off-road motor-vehicle accident NOS

        Other motor-vehicle accident NOS

        Unspecified occupant of dirt bike injured in nontraffic accident

        Unspecified occupant of go cart injured in nontraffic accident

        Unspecified occupant of golf cart injured in nontraffic accident

        Unspecified occupant of race car injured in nontraffic accident

● **V87**   **Traffic accident of specified type but victim's mode of transport unknown**

   Excludes1   collision involving:
        pedal cycle (V10-V19)
        pedestrian (V01-V09)

   The appropriate 7th character is to be added to each code from category V87

     A   initial encounter
     D   subsequent encounter
     S   sequela

   X● **V87.0**   Person injured in collision between car and two- or three-wheeled powered vehicle (traffic)

   X● **V87.1**   Person injured in collision between other motor vehicle and two- or three-wheeled motor vehicle (traffic)

   X● **V87.2**   Person injured in collision between car and pick-up truck or van (traffic)

   X● **V87.3**   Person injured in collision between car and bus (traffic)

   X● **V87.4**   Person injured in collision between car and heavy transport vehicle (traffic)

   X● **V87.5**   Person injured in collision between heavy transport vehicle and bus (traffic)

   X● **V87.6**   Person injured in collision between railway train or railway vehicle and car (traffic)

   X● **V87.7**   Person injured in collision between other specified motor vehicles (traffic)

   X● **V87.8**   Person injured in other specified noncollision transport accidents involving motor vehicle (traffic)

   X● **V87.9**   Person injured in other specified (collision) (noncollision) transport accidents involving nonmotor vehicle (traffic)

● **V88**   **Nontraffic accident of specified type but victim's mode of transport unknown**

   Excludes1   collision involving:
        pedal cycle (V10-V19)
        pedestrian (V01-V09)

   The appropriate 7th character is to be added to each code from category V88

     A   initial encounter
     D   subsequent encounter
     S   sequela

   X● **V88.0**   Person injured in collision between car and two- or three-wheeled motor vehicle, nontraffic

   X● **V88.1**   Person injured in collision between other motor vehicle and two- or three-wheeled motor vehicle, nontraffic

   X● **V88.2**   Person injured in collision between car and pick-up truck or van, nontraffic

CHAPTER 20 (V01-Y99)

X● **V88.3 Person injured in collision between car and bus, nontraffic**

X● **V88.4 Person injured in collision between car and heavy transport vehicle, nontraffic**

X● **V88.5 Person injured in collision between heavy transport vehicle and bus, nontraffic**

X● **V88.6 Person injured in collision between railway train or railway vehicle and car, nontraffic**

X● **V88.7 Person injured in collision between other specified motor vehicle, nontraffic**

X● **V88.8 Person injured in other specified noncollision transport accidents involving motor vehicle, nontraffic**

X● **V88.9 Person injured in other specified (collision) (noncollision) transport accidents involving nonmotor vehicle, nontraffic**

● **V89 Motor- or nonmotor-vehicle accident, type of vehicle unspecified**

The appropriate 7th character is to be added to each code from category V89

A   initial encounter
D   subsequent encounter
S   sequela

X● **V89.0 Person injured in unspecified motor-vehicle accident, nontraffic**
Motor-vehicle accident NOS, nontraffic

X● **V89.1 Person injured in unspecified nonmotor-vehicle accident, nontraffic**
Nonmotor-vehicle accident NOS (nontraffic)

X● **V89.2 Person injured in unspecified motor-vehicle accident, traffic**
Motor-vehicle accident [MVA] NOS
Road (traffic) accident [RTA] NOS

X● **V89.3 Person injured in unspecified nonmotor-vehicle accident, traffic**
Nonmotor-vehicle traffic accident NOS

X● **V89.9 Person injured in unspecified vehicle accident**
Collision NOS

WATER TRANSPORT ACCIDENTS (V90-V94)

● **V90 Drowning and submersion due to accident to watercraft**
Excludes1   civilian water transport accident involving military watercraft (V94.81-)
fall into water not from watercraft (W16.-)
military watercraft accident in military or war operations (Y36.0-, Y37.0-)
water-transport–related drowning or submersion without accident to watercraft (V92.-)

The appropriate 7th character is to be added to each code from category V90

A   initial encounter
D   subsequent encounter
S   sequela

● **V90.0 Drowning and submersion due to watercraft overturning**

X● **V90.00 Drowning and submersion due to merchant ship overturning**

X● **V90.01 Drowning and submersion due to passenger ship overturning**
Drowning and submersion due to ferry-boat overturning
Drowning and submersion due to liner overturning

X● **V90.02 Drowning and submersion due to fishing boat overturning**

X● **V90.03 Drowning and submersion due to other powered watercraft overturning**
Drowning and submersion due to hovercraft (on open water) overturning
Drowning and submersion due to jet ski overturning

X● **V90.04 Drowning and submersion due to sailboat overturning**

X● **V90.05 Drowning and submersion due to canoe or kayak overturning**

X● **V90.06 Drowning and submersion due to (nonpowered) inflatable craft overturning**

X● **V90.08 Drowning and submersion due to other unpowered watercraft overturning**
Drowning and submersion due to windsurfer overturning

X● **V90.09 Drowning and submersion due to unspecified watercraft overturning**
Drowning and submersion due to boat NOS overturning
Drowning and submersion due to ship NOS overturning
Drowning and submersion due to watercraft NOS overturning

● **V90.1 Drowning and submersion due to watercraft sinking**

X● **V90.10 Drowning and submersion due to merchant ship sinking**

X● **V90.11 Drowning and submersion due to passenger ship sinking**
Drowning and submersion due to ferry-boat sinking
Drowning and submersion due to liner sinking

X● **V90.12 Drowning and submersion due to fishing boat sinking**

X● **V90.13 Drowning and submersion due to other powered watercraft sinking**
Drowning and submersion due to hovercraft (on open water) sinking
Drowning and submersion due to jet ski sinking

X● **V90.14 Drowning and submersion due to sailboat sinking**

X● **V90.15 Drowning and submersion due to canoe or kayak sinking**

X● **V90.16 Drowning and submersion due to (nonpowered) inflatable craft sinking**

X● **V90.18 Drowning and submersion due to other unpowered watercraft sinking**

X● **V90.19 Drowning and submersion due to unspecified watercraft sinking**
Drowning and submersion due to boat NOS sinking
Drowning and submersion due to ship NOS sinking
Drowning and submersion due to watercraft NOS sinking

◄ New   ⬅ Revised   ~~deleted~~ Deleted   Excludes 1   Excludes 2   Includes   Use additional   Code first   Code also   Unspecified
OGCR Official Guidelines   X Assign placeholder X   ● Use Additional Character(s)   ▶ Manifestation Code   Coding Clinic

● **V90.2   Drowning and submersion due to falling or jumping from burning watercraft**

   X● **V90.20   Drowning and submersion due to falling or jumping from burning merchant ship**

   X● **V90.21   Drowning and submersion due to falling or jumping from burning passenger ship**
       Drowning and submersion due to falling or jumping from burning ferry-boat
       Drowning and submersion due to falling or jumping from burning liner

   X● **V90.22   Drowning and submersion due to falling or jumping from burning fishing boat**

   X● **V90.23   Drowning and submersion due to falling or jumping from other burning powered watercraft**
       Drowning and submersion due to falling and jumping from burning hovercraft (on open water)
       Drowning and submersion due to falling and jumping from burning jet ski

   X● **V90.24   Drowning and submersion due to falling or jumping from burning sailboat**

   X● **V90.25   Drowning and submersion due to falling or jumping from burning canoe or kayak**

   X● **V90.26   Drowning and submersion due to falling or jumping from burning (nonpowered) inflatable craft**

   X● **V90.27   Drowning and submersion due to falling or jumping from burning water-skis**

   X● **V90.28   Drowning and submersion due to falling or jumping from other burning unpowered watercraft**
       Drowning and submersion due to falling and jumping from burning surf-board
       Drowning and submersion due to falling and jumping from burning windsurfer

   X● **V90.29   Drowning and submersion due to falling or jumping from unspecified burning watercraft**
       Drowning and submersion due to falling or jumping from burning boat NOS
       Drowning and submersion due to falling or jumping from burning ship NOS
       Drowning and submersion due to falling or jumping from burning watercraft NOS

● **V90.3   Drowning and submersion due to falling or jumping from crushed watercraft**

   X● **V90.30   Drowning and submersion due to falling or jumping from crushed merchant ship**

   X● **V90.31   Drowning and submersion due to falling or jumping from crushed passenger ship**
       Drowning and submersion due to falling and jumping from crushed ferry-boat
       Drowning and submersion due to falling and jumping from crushed liner

   X● **V90.32   Drowning and submersion due to falling or jumping from crushed fishing boat**

   X● **V90.33   Drowning and submersion due to falling or jumping from other crushed powered watercraft**
       Drowning and submersion due to falling and jumping from crushed hovercraft
       Drowning and submersion due to falling and jumping from crushed jet ski

   X● **V90.34   Drowning and submersion due to falling or jumping from crushed sailboat**

   X● **V90.35   Drowning and submersion due to falling or jumping from crushed canoe or kayak**

   X● **V90.36   Drowning and submersion due to falling or jumping from crushed (nonpowered) inflatable craft**

   X● **V90.37   Drowning and submersion due to falling or jumping from crushed water-skis**

   X● **V90.38   Drowning and submersion due to falling or jumping from other crushed unpowered watercraft**
       Drowning and submersion due to falling and jumping from crushed surf-board
       Drowning and submersion due to falling and jumping from crushed windsurfer

   X● **V90.39   Drowning and submersion due to falling or jumping from crushed unspecified watercraft**
       Drowning and submersion due to falling and jumping from crushed boat NOS
       Drowning and submersion due to falling and jumping from crushed ship NOS
       Drowning and submersion due to falling and jumping from crushed watercraft NOS

● **V90.8   Drowning and submersion due to other accident to watercraft**

   X● **V90.80   Drowning and submersion due to other accident to merchant ship**

   X● **V90.81   Drowning and submersion due to other accident to passenger ship**
       Drowning and submersion due to other accident to ferry-boat
       Drowning and submersion due to other accident to liner

   X● **V90.82   Drowning and submersion due to other accident to fishing boat**

   X● **V90.83   Drowning and submersion due to other accident to other powered watercraft**
       Drowning and submersion due to other accident to hovercraft (on open water)
       Drowning and submersion due to other accident to jet ski

   X● **V90.84   Drowning and submersion due to other accident to sailboat**

   X● **V90.85   Drowning and submersion due to other accident to canoe or kayak**

   X● **V90.86   Drowning and submersion due to other accident to (nonpowered) inflatable craft**

   X● **V90.87   Drowning and submersion due to other accident to water-skis**

   X● **V90.88   Drowning and submersion due to other accident to other unpowered watercraft**
       Drowning and submersion due to other accident to surf-board
       Drowning and submersion due to other accident to windsurfer

   X● **V90.89   Drowning and submersion due to other accident to unspecified watercraft**
       Drowning and submersion due to other accident to boat NOS
       Drowning and submersion due to other accident to ship NOS
       Drowning and submersion due to other accident to watercraft NOS

CHAPTER 20 (V01-Y99)

● **V91**   **Other injury due to accident to watercraft**

> **Includes**   any injury except drowning and submersion as a result of an accident to watercraft
>
> **Excludes1**   civilian water transport accident involving military watercraft (V94.81-)
> military watercraft accident in military or war operations (Y36, Y37.-)
>
> **Excludes2**   drowning and submersion due to accident to watercraft (V90.-)
>
> The appropriate 7th character is to be added to each code from category V91

> A   initial encounter
> D   subsequent encounter
> S   sequela

● **V91.0**   **Burn due to watercraft on fire**

> **Excludes1**   burn from localized fire or explosion on board ship without accident to watercraft (V93.-)

X● **V91.00**   **Burn due to merchant ship on fire**

X● **V91.01**   **Burn due to passenger ship on fire**
> Burn due to ferry-boat on fire
> Burn due to liner on fire

X● **V91.02**   **Burn due to fishing boat on fire**

X● **V91.03**   **Burn due to other powered watercraft on fire**
> Burn due to hovercraft (on open water) on fire
> Burn due to jet ski on fire

X● **V91.04**   **Burn due to sailboat on fire**

X● **V91.05**   **Burn due to canoe or kayak on fire**

X● **V91.06**   **Burn due to (nonpowered) inflatable craft on fire**

X● **V91.07**   **Burn due to water-skis on fire**

X● **V91.08**   **Burn due to other unpowered watercraft on fire**

X● **V91.09**   **Burn due to unspecified watercraft on fire**
> Burn due to boat NOS on fire
> Burn due to ship NOS on fire
> Burn due to watercraft NOS on fire

● **V91.1**   **Crushed between watercraft and other watercraft or other object due to collision**
> Crushed by lifeboat after abandoning ship in a collision
>
> **Note:** Select the specified type of watercraft that the victim was on at the time of the collision.

X● **V91.10**   **Crushed between merchant ship and other watercraft or other object due to collision**

X● **V91.11**   **Crushed between passenger ship and other watercraft or other object due to collision**
> Crushed between ferry-boat and other watercraft or other object due to collision
> Crushed between liner and other watercraft or other object due to collision

X● **V91.12**   **Crushed between fishing boat and other watercraft or other object due to collision**

X● **V91.13**   **Crushed between other powered watercraft and other watercraft or other object due to collision**
> Crushed between hovercraft (on open water) and other watercraft or other object due to collision
> Crushed between jet ski and other watercraft or other object due to collision

X● **V91.14**   **Crushed between sailboat and other watercraft or other object due to collision**

X● **V91.15**   **Crushed between canoe or kayak and other watercraft or other object due to collision**

X● **V91.16**   **Crushed between (nonpowered) inflatable craft and other watercraft or other object due to collision**

X● **V91.18**   **Crushed between other unpowered watercraft and other watercraft or other object due to collision**
> Crushed between surfboard and other watercraft or other object due to collision
> Crushed between windsurfer and other watercraft or other object due to collision

X● **V91.19**   **Crushed between unspecified watercraft and other watercraft or other object due to collision**
> Crushed between boat NOS and other watercraft or other object due to collision
> Crushed between ship NOS and other watercraft or other object due to collision
> Crushed between watercraft NOS and other watercraft or other object due to collision

● **V91.2**   **Fall due to collision between watercraft and other watercraft or other object**
> Fall while remaining on watercraft after collision
>
> **Note:** Select the specified type of watercraft that the victim was on at the time of the collision.
>
> **Excludes1**   crushed between watercraft and other watercraft and other object due to collision (V91.1-)
> drowning and submersion due to falling from crushed watercraft (V90.3-)

X● **V91.20**   **Fall due to collision between merchant ship and other watercraft or other object**

X● **V91.21**   **Fall due to collision between passenger ship and other watercraft or other object**
> Fall due to collision between ferry-boat and other watercraft or other object
> Fall due to collision between liner and other watercraft or other object

X● **V91.22**   **Fall due to collision between fishing boat and other watercraft or other object**

X● **V91.23**   **Fall due to collision between other powered watercraft and other watercraft or other object**
> Fall due to collision between hovercraft (on open water) and other watercraft or other object
> Fall due to collision between jet ski and other watercraft or other object

X● **V91.24**   **Fall due to collision between sailboat and other watercraft or other object**

X● **V91.25**   **Fall due to collision between canoe or kayak and other watercraft or other object**

X● **V91.26**   **Fall due to collision between (nonpowered) inflatable craft and other watercraft or other object**

X● **V91.29**   **Fall due to collision between unspecified watercraft and other watercraft or other object**
> Fall due to collision between boat NOS and other watercraft or other object
> Fall due to collision between ship NOS and other watercraft or other object
> Fall due to collision between watercraft NOS and other watercraft or other object

---

◄ New   ◄═ Revised   ~~deleted~~ Deleted   Excludes 1   Excludes 2   Includes   Use additional   Code first   Code also   Unspecified

OGCR Official Guidelines   **X** Assign placeholder X   ● Use Additional Character(s)   ▶ Manifestation Code   **Coding Clinic**

● **V91.3**   **Hit or struck by falling object due to accident to watercraft**
> Hit or struck by falling object (part of damaged watercraft or other object) after falling or jumping from damaged watercraft
>
> **Excludes2**   drowning or submersion due to fall or jumping from damaged watercraft (V90.2-, V90.3-)

X● **V91.30**   **Hit or struck by falling object due to accident to merchant ship**

X● **V91.31**   **Hit or struck by falling object due to accident to passenger ship**
> Hit or struck by falling object due to accident to ferry-boat
> Hit or struck by falling object due to accident to liner

X● **V91.32**   **Hit or struck by falling object due to accident to fishing boat**

X● **V91.33**   **Hit or struck by falling object due to accident to other powered watercraft**
> Hit or struck by falling object due to accident to hovercraft (on open water)
> Hit or struck by falling object due to accident to jet ski

X● **V91.34**   **Hit or struck by falling object due to accident to sailboat**

X● **V91.35**   **Hit or struck by falling object due to accident to canoe or kayak**

X● **V91.36**   **Hit or struck by falling object due to accident to (nonpowered) inflatable craft**

X● **V91.37**   **Hit or struck by falling object due to accident to water-skis**
> Hit by water-skis after jumping off of waterskis

X● **V91.38**   **Hit or struck by falling object due to accident to other unpowered watercraft**
> Hit or struck by surf-board after falling off damaged surf-board
> Hit or struck by object after falling off damaged windsurfer

X● **V91.39**   **Hit or struck by falling object due to accident to unspecified watercraft**
> Hit or struck by falling object due to accident to boat NOS
> Hit or struck by falling object due to accident to ship NOS
> Hit or struck by falling object due to accident to watercraft NOS

● **V91.8**   **Other injury due to other accident to watercraft**

X● **V91.80**   **Other injury due to other accident to merchant ship**

X● **V91.81**   **Other injury due to other accident to passenger ship**
> Other injury due to other accident to ferry-boat
> Other injury due to other accident to liner

X● **V91.82**   **Other injury due to other accident to fishing boat**

X● **V91.83**   **Other injury due to other accident to other powered watercraft**
> Other injury due to other accident to hovercraft (on open water)
> Other injury due to other accident to jet ski

X● **V91.84**   **Other injury due to other accident to sailboat**

X● **V91.85**   **Other injury due to other accident to canoe or kayak**

X● **V91.86**   **Other injury due to other accident to (nonpowered) inflatable craft**

X● **V91.87**   **Other injury due to other accident to water-skis**

X● **V91.88**   **Other injury due to other accident to other unpowered watercraft**
> Other injury due to other accident to surf-board
> Other injury due to other accident to windsurfer

X● **V91.89**   **Other injury due to other accident to unspecified watercraft**
> Other injury due to other accident to boat NOS
> Other injury due to other accident to ship NOS
> Other injury due to other accident to watercraft NOS

● **V92**   **Drowning and submersion due to accident on board watercraft, without accident to watercraft**
> **Excludes1**   civilian water transport accident involving military watercraft (V94.81-)
> drowning or submersion due to accident to watercraft (V90-V91)
> drowning or submersion of diver who voluntarily jumps from boat not involved in an accident (W16.711, W16.721)
> fall into water without watercraft (W16.-)
> military watercraft accident in military or war operations (Y36, Y37)

> The appropriate 7th character is to be added to each code from category V92

> | | |
> |---|---|
> | A | initial encounter |
> | D | subsequent encounter |
> | S | sequela |

● **V92.0**   **Drowning and submersion due to fall off watercraft**
> Drowning and submersion due to fall from gangplank of watercraft
> Drowning and submersion due to fall overboard watercraft
>
> **Excludes2**   hitting head on object or bottom of body of water due to fall from watercraft (V94.0-)

X● **V92.00**   **Drowning and submersion due to fall off merchant ship**

X● **V92.01**   **Drowning and submersion due to fall off passenger ship**
> Drowning and submersion due to fall off ferry-boat
> Drowning and submersion due to fall off liner

X● **V92.02**   **Drowning and submersion due to fall off fishing boat**

X● **V92.03**   **Drowning and submersion due to fall off other powered watercraft**
> Drowning and submersion due to fall off hovercraft (on open water)
> Drowning and submersion due to fall off jet ski

X● **V92.04**   **Drowning and submersion due to fall off sailboat**

X● **V92.05**   **Drowning and submersion due to fall off canoe or kayak**

X● **V92.06**   **Drowning and submersion due to fall off (nonpowered) inflatable craft**

X● **V92.07** **Drowning and submersion due to fall off water-skis**

> **Excludes1** drowning and submersion due to falling off burning water-skis (V90.27)
> drowning and submersion due to falling off crushed water-skis (V90.37)
> hit by boat while water-skiing NOS (V94.X)

X● **V92.08** **Drowning and submersion due to fall off other unpowered watercraft**

> Drowning and submersion due to fall off surf-board
> Drowning and submersion due to fall off windsurfer

> **Excludes1** drowning and submersion due to fall off burning unpowered watercraft (V90.28)
> drowning and submersion due to fall off crushed unpowered watercraft (V90.38)
> drowning and submersion due to fall off damaged unpowered watercraft (V90.88)
> drowning and submersion due to rider of nonpowered watercraft being hit by other watercraft (V94.-)
> other injury due to rider of nonpowered watercraft being hit by other watercraft (V94.-)

X● **V92.09** **Drowning and submersion due to fall off unspecified watercraft**

> Drowning and submersion due to fall off boat NOS
> Drowning and submersion due to fall off ship
> Drowning and submersion due to fall off watercraft NOS

● **V92.1** **Drowning and submersion due to being thrown overboard by motion of watercraft**

> **Excludes1** drowning and submersion due to fall off surf-board (V92.08)
> drowning and submersion due to fall off water-skis (V92.07)
> drowning and submersion due to fall off windsurfer (V92.08)

X● **V92.10** **Drowning and submersion due to being thrown overboard by motion of merchant ship**

X● **V92.11** **Drowning and submersion due to being thrown overboard by motion of passenger ship**

> Drowning and submersion due to being thrown overboard by motion of ferry-boat
> Drowning and submersion due to being thrown overboard by motion of liner

X● **V92.12** **Drowning and submersion due to being thrown overboard by motion of fishing boat**

X● **V92.13** **Drowning and submersion due to being thrown overboard by motion of other powered watercraft**

> Drowning and submersion due to being thrown overboard by motion of hovercraft

X● **V92.14** **Drowning and submersion due to being thrown overboard by motion of sailboat**

X● **V92.15** **Drowning and submersion due to being thrown overboard by motion of canoe or kayak**

X● **V92.16** **Drowning and submersion due to being thrown overboard by motion of (nonpowered) inflatable craft**

X● **V92.19** **Drowning and submersion due to being thrown overboard by motion of unspecified watercraft**

> Drowning and submersion due to being thrown overboard by motion of boat NOS
> Drowning and submersion due to being thrown overboard by motion of ship NOS
> Drowning and submersion due to being thrown overboard by motion of watercraft NOS

● **V92.2** **Drowning and submersion due to being washed overboard from watercraft**

> *Code first* any associated cataclysm (X37.0-)

X● **V92.20** **Drowning and submersion due to being washed overboard from merchant ship**

X● **V92.21** **Drowning and submersion due to being washed overboard from passenger ship**

> Drowning and submersion due to being washed overboard from ferry-boat
> Drowning and submersion due to being washed overboard from liner

X● **V92.22** **Drowning and submersion due to being washed overboard from fishing boat**

X● **V92.23** **Drowning and submersion due to being washed overboard from other powered watercraft**

> Drowning and submersion due to being washed overboard from hovercraft (on open water)
> Drowning and submersion due to being washed overboard from jet ski

X● **V92.24** **Drowning and submersion due to being washed overboard from sailboat**

X● **V92.25** **Drowning and submersion due to being washed overboard from canoe or kayak**

X● **V92.26** **Drowning and submersion due to being washed overboard from (nonpowered) inflatable craft**

X● **V92.27** **Drowning and submersion due to being washed overboard from water-skis**

> **Excludes1** drowning and submersion due to fall off water-skis (V92.07)

X● **V92.28** **Drowning and submersion due to being washed overboard from other unpowered watercraft**

> Drowning and submersion due to being washed overboard from surf-board
> Drowning and submersion due to being washed overboard from windsurfer

X● **V92.29** **Drowning and submersion due to being washed overboard from unspecified watercraft**

> Drowning and submersion due to being washed overboard from boat NOS
> Drowning and submersion due to being washed overboard from ship NOS
> Drowning and submersion due to being washed overboard from watercraft NOS

◄ New ◄⋯ Revised ~~deleted~~ Deleted | Excludes 1 | Excludes 2 | Includes | Use additional | Code first | Code also | Unspecified
OGCR Official Guidelines X Assign placeholder X ● Use Additional Character(s) ▶ Manifestation Code **Coding Clinic**

● V93　Other injury due to accident on board watercraft, without accident to watercraft

> **Excludes1**　civilian water transport accident involving military watercraft (V94.81-)
> other injury due to accident to watercraft (V91.-)
> military watercraft accident in military or war operations (Y36, Y37.-)

> **Excludes2**　drowning and submersion due to accident on board watercraft, without accident to watercraft (V92.)

The appropriate 7th character is to be added to each code from category V93

> A　initial encounter
> D　subsequent encounter
> S　sequela

● V93.0　Burn due to localized fire on board watercraft

> **Excludes1**　burn due to watercraft on fire (V91.0-)

X● V93.00　Burn due to localized fire on board merchant vessel

X● V93.01　Burn due to localized fire on board passenger vessel
> Burn due to localized fire on board ferry-boat
> Burn due to localized fire on board liner

X● V93.02　Burn due to localized fire on board fishing boat

X● V93.03　Burn due to localized fire on board other powered watercraft
> Burn due to localized fire on board hovercraft
> Burn due to localized fire on board jet ski

X● V93.04　Burn due to localized fire on board sailboat

X● V93.09　Burn due to localized fire on board unspecified watercraft
> Burn due to localized fire on board boat NOS
> Burn due to localized fire on board ship NOS
> Burn due to localized fire on board watercraft NOS

● V93.1　Other burn on board watercraft
> Burn due to source other than fire on board watercraft

> **Excludes1**　burn due to watercraft on fire (V91.0-)

X● V93.10　Other burn on board merchant vessel

X● V93.11　Other burn on board passenger vessel
> Other burn on board ferry-boat
> Other burn on board liner

X● V93.12　Other burn on board fishing boat

X● V93.13　Other burn on board other powered watercraft
> Other burn on board hovercraft
> Other burn on board jet ski

X● V93.14　Other burn on board sailboat

X● V93.19　Other burn on board unspecified watercraft
> Other burn on board boat NOS
> Other burn on board ship NOS
> Other burn on board watercraft NOS

● V93.2　Heat exposure on board watercraft

> **Excludes1**　exposure to man-made heat not aboard watercraft (W92)
> exposure to natural heat while on board watercraft (X30)
> exposure to sunlight while on board watercraft (X32)

> **Excludes2**　burn due to fire on board watercraft (V93.0-)

X● V93.20　Heat exposure on board merchant ship

X● V93.21　Heat exposure on board passenger ship
> Heat exposure on board ferry-boat
> Heat exposure on board liner

X● V93.22　Heat exposure on board fishing boat

X● V93.23　Heat exposure on board other powered watercraft
> Heat exposure on board hovercraft

X● V93.24　Heat exposure on board sailboat

X● V93.29　Heat exposure on board unspecified watercraft
> Heat exposure on board boat NOS
> Heat exposure on board ship NOS
> Heat exposure on board watercraft NOS

● V93.3　Fall on board watercraft

> **Excludes1**　fall due to collision of watercraft (V91.2-)

X● V93.30　Fall on board merchant ship

X● V93.31　Fall on board passenger ship
> Fall on board ferry-boat
> Fall on board liner

X● V93.32　Fall on board fishing boat

X● V93.33　Fall on board other powered watercraft
> Fall on board hovercraft (on open water)
> Fall on board jet ski

X● V93.34　Fall on board sailboat

X● V93.35　Fall on board canoe or kayak

X● V93.36　Fall on board (nonpowered) inflatable craft

X● V93.38　Fall on board other unpowered watercraft

X● V93.39　Fall on board unspecified watercraft
> Fall on board boat NOS
> Fall on board ship NOS
> Fall on board watercraft NOS

● V93.4　Struck by falling object on board watercraft
> Hit by falling object on board watercraft

> **Excludes1**　struck by falling object due to accident to watercraft (V91.3)

X● V93.40　Struck by falling object on merchant ship

X● V93.41　Struck by falling object on passenger ship
> Struck by falling object on ferry-boat
> Struck by falling object on liner

X● V93.42　Struck by falling object on fishing boat

X● V93.43　Struck by falling object on other powered watercraft
> Struck by falling object on hovercraft

X● V93.44　Struck by falling object on sailboat

X● V93.48　Struck by falling object on other unpowered watercraft

X● V93.49　Struck by falling object on unspecified watercraft

● V93.5　Explosion on board watercraft
> Boiler explosion on steamship

> **Excludes2**　fire on board watercraft (V93.0-)

X● V93.50　Explosion on board merchant ship

X● V93.51　Explosion on board passenger ship
> Explosion on board ferry-boat
> Explosion on board liner

X● V93.52　Explosion on board fishing boat

X● V93.53　Explosion on board other powered watercraft
> Explosion on board hovercraft
> Explosion on board jet ski

X● V93.54　Explosion on board sailboat

X● V93.59　Explosion on board unspecified watercraft
> Explosion on board boat NOS
> Explosion on board ship NOS
> Explosion on board watercraft NOS

● V93.6   **Machinery accident on board watercraft**

    Excludes1   machinery explosion on board watercraft (V93.4-)

                    machinery fire on board watercraft (V93.0-)

   X● V93.60   **Machinery accident on board merchant ship**

   X● V93.61   **Machinery accident on board passenger ship**

           Machinery accident on board ferry-boat

           Machinery accident on board liner

   X● V93.62   **Machinery accident on board fishing boat**

   X● V93.63   **Machinery accident on board other powered watercraft**

           Machinery accident on board hovercraft

   X● V93.64   **Machinery accident on board sailboat**

   X● V93.69   **Machinery accident on board unspecified watercraft**

           Machinery accident on board boat NOS

           Machinery accident on board ship NOS

           Machinery accident on board watercraft NOS

● V93.8   **Other injury due to other accident on board watercraft**

       Accidental poisoning by gases or fumes on watercraft

   X● V93.80   **Other injury due to other accident on board merchant ship**

   X● V93.81   **Other injury due to other accident on board passenger ship**

           Other injury due to other accident on board ferry-boat

           Other injury due to other accident on board liner

   X● V93.82   **Other injury due to other accident on board fishing boat**

   X● V93.83   **Other injury due to other accident on board other powered watercraft**

           Other injury due to other accident on board hovercraft

           Other injury due to other accident on board jet ski

   X● V93.84   **Other injury due to other accident on board sailboat**

   X● V93.85   **Other injury due to other accident on board canoe or kayak**

   X● V93.86   **Other injury due to other accident on board (nonpowered) inflatable craft**

   X● V93.87   **Other injury due to other accident on board water-skis**

           Hit or struck by object while waterskiing

   X● V93.88   **Other injury due to other accident on board other unpowered watercraft**

           Hit or struck by object while surfing

           Hit or struck by object while on board windsurfer

   X● V93.89   **Other injury due to other accident on board unspecified watercraft**

           Other injury due to other accident on board boat NOS

           Other injury due to other accident on board ship NOS

           Other injury due to other accident on board watercraft NOS

● V94   **Other and unspecified water transport accidents**

    Excludes1   military watercraft accidents in military or war operations (Y36, Y37)

      The appropriate 7th character is to be added to each code from category V94

       A   initial encounter
       D   subsequent encounter
       S   sequela

   X● V94.0   **Hitting object or bottom of body of water due to fall from watercraft**

       Excludes2   drowning and submersion due to fall from watercraft (V92.0-)

 ● V94.1   **Bather struck by watercraft**

       Swimmer hit by watercraft

   X● V94.11   **Bather struck by powered watercraft**

   X● V94.12   **Bather struck by nonpowered watercraft**

 ● V94.2   **Rider of nonpowered watercraft struck by other watercraft**

   X● V94.21   **Rider of nonpowered watercraft struck by other nonpowered watercraft**

           Canoer hit by other nonpowered watercraft

           Surfer hit by other nonpowered watercraft

           Windsurfer hit by other nonpowered watercraft

   X● V94.22   **Rider of nonpowered watercraft struck by powered watercraft**

           Canoer hit by motorboat

           Surfer hit by motorboat

           Windsurfer hit by motorboat

 ● V94.3   **Injury to rider of (inflatable) watercraft being pulled behind other watercraft**

   X● V94.31   **Injury to rider of (inflatable) recreational watercraft being pulled behind other watercraft**

           Injury to rider of inner-tube pulled behind motor boat

   X● V94.32   **Injury to rider of non-recreational watercraft being pulled behind other watercraft**

           Injury to occupant of dingy being pulled behind boat or ship

           Injury to occupant of life-raft being pulled behind boat or ship

   X● V94.4   **Injury to barefoot water-skier**

       Injury to person being pulled behind boat or ship

 ● V94.8   **Other water transport accident**

   ● V94.81   **Water transport accident involving military watercraft**

      ● V94.810   **Civilian watercraft involved in water transport accident with military watercraft**

           Passenger on civilian watercraft injured due to accident with military watercraft

      ● V94.811   **Civilian in water injured by military watercraft**

      ● V94.818   **Other water transport accident involving military watercraft**

   X● V94.89   **Other water transport accident**

  X● V94.9   **Unspecified water transport accident**

       Water transport accident NOS

◀ New   ◀ Revised   ~~deleted~~ Deleted   Excludes 1   Excludes 2   Includes   Use additional   Code first   Code also   Unspecified

OGCR Official Guidelines   X Assign placeholder X   ● Use Additional Character(s)   ▶ Manifestation Code   **Coding Clinic**

AIR AND SPACE TRANSPORT ACCIDENTS (V95-V97)

Excludes1   military aircraft accidents in military or war operations (Y36, Y37)

● **V95**   **Accident to powered aircraft causing injury to occupant**

The appropriate 7th character is to be added to each code from category V95

> A   initial encounter
> D   subsequent encounter
> S   sequela

● **V95.0**   Helicopter accident injuring occupant

X● **V95.00**   Unspecified helicopter accident injuring occupant

X● **V95.01**   Helicopter crash injuring occupant

X● **V95.02**   Forced landing of helicopter injuring occupant

X● **V95.03**   Helicopter collision injuring occupant
> Helicopter collision with any object, fixed, movable or moving

X● **V95.04**   Helicopter fire injuring occupant

X● **V95.05**   Helicopter explosion injuring occupant

X● **V95.09**   Other helicopter accident injuring occupant

● **V95.1**   Ultralight, microlight or powered-glider accident injuring occupant

X● **V95.10**   Unspecified ultralight, microlight or powered-glider accident injuring occupant

X● **V95.11**   Ultralight, microlight or powered-glider crash injuring occupant

X● **V95.12**   Forced landing of ultralight, microlight or powered-glider injuring occupant

X● **V95.13**   Ultralight, microlight or powered-glider collision injuring occupant
> Ultralight, microlight or powered-glider collision with any object, fixed, movable or moving

X● **V95.14**   Ultralight, microlight or powered-glider fire injuring occupant

X● **V95.15**   Ultralight, microlight or powered-glider explosion injuring occupant

X● **V95.19**   Other ultralight, microlight or powered-glider accident injuring occupant

● **V95.2**   Other private fixed-wing aircraft accident injuring occupant

X● **V95.20**   Unspecified accident to other private fixed-wing aircraft, injuring occupant

X● **V95.21**   Other private fixed-wing aircraft crash injuring occupant

X● **V95.22**   Forced landing of other private fixed-wing aircraft injuring occupant

X● **V95.23**   Other private fixed-wing aircraft collision injuring occupant
> Other private fixed-wing aircraft collision with any object, fixed, movable or moving

X● **V95.24**   Other private fixed-wing aircraft fire injuring occupant

X● **V95.25**   Other private fixed-wing aircraft explosion injuring occupant

X● **V95.29**   Other accident to other private fixed-wing aircraft injuring occupant

● **V95.3**   Commercial fixed-wing aircraft accident injuring occupant

X● **V95.30**   Unspecified accident to commercial fixed-wing aircraft injuring occupant

X● **V95.31**   Commercial fixed-wing aircraft crash injuring occupant

X● **V95.32**   Forced landing of commercial fixed-wing aircraft injuring occupant

X● **V95.33**   Commercial fixed-wing aircraft collision injuring occupant
> Commercial fixed-wing aircraft collision with any object, fixed, movable or moving

X● **V95.34**   Commercial fixed-wing aircraft fire injuring occupant

X● **V95.35**   Commercial fixed-wing aircraft explosion injuring occupant

X● **V95.39**   Other accident to commercial fixed-wing aircraft injuring occupant

● **V95.4**   Spacecraft accident injuring occupant

X● **V95.40**   Unspecified spacecraft accident injuring occupant

X● **V95.41**   Spacecraft crash injuring occupant

X● **V95.42**   Forced landing of spacecraft injuring occupant

X● **V95.43**   Spacecraft collision injuring occupant
> Spacecraft collision with any object, fixed, moveable or moving

X● **V95.44**   Spacecraft fire injuring occupant

X● **V95.45**   Spacecraft explosion injuring occupant

X● **V95.49**   Other spacecraft accident injuring occupant

X● **V95.8**   Other powered aircraft accidents injuring occupant

X● **V95.9**   Unspecified aircraft accident injuring occupant
> Aircraft accident NOS
> Air transport accident NOS

● **V96**   **Accident to nonpowered aircraft causing injury to occupant**

The appropriate 7th character is to be added to each code from category V96

> A   initial encounter
> D   subsequent encounter
> S   sequela

● **V96.0**   Balloon accident injuring occupant

X● **V96.00**   Unspecified balloon accident injuring occupant

X● **V96.01**   Balloon crash injuring occupant

X● **V96.02**   Forced landing of balloon injuring occupant

X● **V96.03**   Balloon collision injuring occupant
> Balloon collision with any object, fixed, moveable or moving

X● **V96.04**   Balloon fire injuring occupant

X● **V96.05**   Balloon explosion injuring occupant

X● **V96.09**   Other balloon accident injuring occupant

● **V96.1**   Hang-glider accident injuring occupant

X● **V96.10**   Unspecified hang-glider accident injuring occupant

X● **V96.11**   Hang-glider crash injuring occupant

X● **V96.12**   Forced landing of hang-glider injuring occupant

X● **V96.13**   Hang-glider collision injuring occupant
> Hang-glider collision with any object, fixed, moveable or moving

X● **V96.14**   Hang-glider fire injuring occupant

X● **V96.15**   Hang-glider explosion injuring occupant

X● **V96.19**   Other hang-glider accident injuring occupant

- ● V96.2   Glider (nonpowered) accident injuring occupant
  - X ● V96.20   Unspecified glider (nonpowered) accident injuring occupant
  - X ● V96.21   Glider (nonpowered) crash injuring occupant
  - X ● V96.22   Forced landing of glider (nonpowered) injuring occupant
  - X ● V96.23   Glider (nonpowered) collision injuring occupant
    Glider (nonpowered) collision with any object, fixed, moveable or moving
  - X ● V96.24   Glider (nonpowered) fire injuring occupant
  - X ● V96.25   Glider (nonpowered) explosion injuring occupant
  - X ● V96.29   Other glider (nonpowered) accident injuring occupant
- X ● V96.8   Other nonpowered-aircraft accidents injuring occupant
    Kite carrying a person accident injuring occupant
- X ● V96.9   Unspecified nonpowered-aircraft accident injuring occupant
    Nonpowered-aircraft accident NOS

- ● V97   Other specified air transport accidents
    The appropriate 7th character is to be added to each code from category V97

A	initial encounter
D	subsequent encounter
S	sequela

  - X ● V97.0   Occupant of aircraft injured in other specified air transport accidents
      Fall in, on or from aircraft in air transport accident
      Excludes1   accident while boarding or alighting aircraft (V97.1)
  - X ● V97.1   Person injured while boarding or alighting from aircraft
  - ● V97.2   Parachutist accident
    - X ● V97.21   Parachutist entangled in object
        Parachutist landing in tree
    - X ● V97.22   Parachutist injured on landing
    - X ● V97.29   Other parachutist accident
  - ● V97.3   Person on ground injured in air transport accident
    - X ● V97.31   Hit by object falling from aircraft
        Hit by crashing aircraft
        Injured by aircraft hitting house
        Injured by aircraft hitting car
    - X ● V97.32   Injured by rotating propeller
    - X ● V97.33   Sucked into jet engine
    - X ● V97.39   Other injury to person on ground due to air transport accident
  - ● V97.8   Other air transport accidents, not elsewhere classified
      Excludes1   aircraft accident NOS (V95.9)
          exposure to changes in air pressure during ascent or descent (W94.-)
    - ● V97.81   Air transport accident involving military aircraft
      - ● V97.810   Civilian aircraft involved in air transport accident with military aircraft
          Passenger in civilian aircraft injured due to accident with military aircraft
      - ● V97.811   Civilian injured by military aircraft
      - ● V97.818   Other air transport accident involving military aircraft
    - X ● V97.89   Other air transport accidents, not elsewhere classified
        Injury from machinery on aircraft

OTHER AND UNSPECIFIED TRANSPORT ACCIDENTS (V98-V99)

Excludes1   vehicle accident, type of vehicle unspecified (V89.-)

- ● V98   Other specified transport accidents
    The appropriate 7th character is to be added to each code from category V98

A	initial encounter
D	subsequent encounter
S	sequela

  - X ● V98.0   Accident to, on or involving cable-car, not on rails
      Caught or dragged by cable-car, not on rails
      Fall or jump from cable-car, not on rails
      Object thrown from or in cable-car, not on rails
  - X ● V98.1   Accident to, on or involving land-yacht
  - X ● V98.2   Accident to, on or involving ice yacht
  - X ● V98.3   Accident to, on or involving ski lift
      Accident to, on or involving ski chair-lift
      Accident to, on or involving ski-lift with gondola
  - X ● V98.8   Other specified transport accidents

- X ● V99   Unspecified transport accident
    The appropriate 7th character is to be added to code V99

A	initial encounter
D	subsequent encounter
S	sequela

OTHER EXTERNAL CAUSES OF ACCIDENTAL INJURY (W00-X58)

SLIPPING, TRIPPING, STUMBLING AND FALLS (W00-W19)

Excludes1   assault involving a fall (Y01-Y02)
      fall from animal (V80.-)
      fall (in) (from) machinery (in operation) (W28-W31)
      fall (in) (from) transport vehicle (V01-V99)
      intentional self-harm involving a fall (X80-X81)
Excludes2   at risk for fall (history of fall) Z91.81
      fall (in) (from) burning building (X00.-)
      fall into fire (X00-X04, X08-X09)

- ● W00   Fall due to ice and snow
    Includes   pedestrian on foot falling (slipping) on ice and snow
    Excludes1   fall on (from) ice and snow involving pedestrian conveyance (V00.-)
        fall from stairs and steps not due to ice and snow (W10.-)
    The appropriate 7th character is to be added to each code from category W00

A	initial encounter
D	subsequent encounter
S	sequela

  - X ● W00.0   Fall on same level due to ice and snow
  - X ● W00.1   Fall from stairs and steps due to ice and snow
  - X ● W00.2   Other fall from one level to another due to ice and snow
  - X ● W00.9   Unspecified fall due to ice and snow

◀ New   ⬅ Revised   ~~deleted~~ Deleted   Excludes 1   Excludes 2   Includes   Use additional   Code first   Code also   Unspecified

OGCR Official Guidelines   **X** Assign placeholder X   ● Use Additional Character(s)   ▶ Manifestation Code   **Coding Clinic**

● **W01 Fall on same level from slipping, tripping and stumbling**

Includes	fall on moving sidewalk
Excludes1	fall due to bumping (striking) against object (W18.0-)

              fall in shower or bathtub (W18.2-)
              fall on same level NOS (W18.30)
              fall on same level from slipping, tripping and stumbling due to ice or snow (W00.0)
              fall off or from toilet (W18.1-)
              slipping, tripping and stumbling NOS (W18.40)
              slipping, tripping and stumbling without falling (W18.4-)

The appropriate 7th character is to be added to each code from category W01

A	initial encounter
D	subsequent encounter
S	sequela

X● **W01.0 Fall on same level from slipping, tripping and stumbling without subsequent striking against object**
        Falling over animal

● **W01.1 Fall on same level from slipping, tripping and stumbling with subsequent striking against object**

  X● **W01.10 Fall on same level from slipping, tripping and stumbling with subsequent striking against unspecified object**

  ● **W01.11 Fall on same level from slipping, tripping and stumbling with subsequent striking against sharp object**

    ● **W01.110 Fall on same level from slipping, tripping and stumbling with subsequent striking against sharp glass**

    ● **W01.111 Fall on same level from slipping, tripping and stumbling with subsequent striking against power tool or machine**

    ● **W01.118 Fall on same level from slipping, tripping and stumbling with subsequent striking against other sharp object**

    ● **W01.119 Fall on same level from slipping, tripping and stumbling with subsequent striking against unspecified sharp object**

  ● **W01.19 Fall on same level from slipping, tripping and stumbling with subsequent striking against other object**

    ● **W01.190 Fall on same level from slipping, tripping and stumbling with subsequent striking against furniture**

    ● **W01.198 Fall on same level from slipping, tripping and stumbling with subsequent striking against other object**

X● **W03 Other fall on same level due to collision with another person**
    Fall due to non-transport collision with other person

Excludes1	collision with another person without fall (W51)

          crushed or pushed by a crowd or human stampede (W52)
          fall involving pedestrian conveyance (V00-V09)
          fall due to ice or snow (W00)
          fall on same level NOS (W18.30)

The appropriate 7th character is to be added to code W03

A	initial encounter
D	subsequent encounter
S	sequela

Coding Clinic: 2015, Q1, P9-10; 2012, Q4, P108

X● **W04 Fall while being carried or supported by other persons**
    Accidentally dropped while being carried

The appropriate 7th character is to be added to code W04

A	initial encounter
D	subsequent encounter
S	sequel

● **W05 Fall from non-moving wheelchair, nonmotorized scooter and motorized mobility scooter**

Excludes1	fall from moving wheelchair (powered) (V00.811)

          fall from moving motorized mobility scooter (V00.831)
          fall from nonmotorized scooter (V00.141)

The appropriate 7th character is to be added to each code from category W05

A	initial encounter
D	subsequent encounter
S	sequela

X● **W05.0 Fall from non-moving wheelchair**
X● **W05.1 Fall from non-moving nonmotorized scooter**
X● **W05.2 Fall from non-moving motorized mobility scooter**

X● **W06 Fall from bed**
The appropriate 7th character is to be added to code W06

A	initial encounter
D	subsequent encounter
S	sequela

X● **W07 Fall from chair**
The appropriate 7th character is to be added to code W07

A	initial encounter
D	subsequent encounter
S	sequela

X● **W08 Fall from other furniture**
The appropriate 7th character is to be added to code W08

A	initial encounter
D	subsequent encounter
S	sequela

CHAPTER 20 (V01-Y99)

●W09　Fall on and from playground equipment

> **Excludes1**　fall involving recreational machinery (W31)
>
> The appropriate 7th character is to be added to each code from category W09
>
> | | |
> |---|---|
> | A | initial encounter |
> | D | subsequent encounter |
> | S | sequela |

X● **W09.0　Fall on or from playground slide**
X● **W09.1　Fall from playground swing**
X● **W09.2　Fall on or from jungle gym**
X● **W09.8　Fall on or from other playground equipment**

●W10　Fall on and from stairs and steps

> **Excludes1**　fall from stairs and steps due to ice and snow (W00.1)
>
> The appropriate 7th character is to be added to each code from category W10
>
> | | |
> |---|---|
> | A | initial encounter |
> | D | subsequent encounter |
> | S | sequela |

X● **W10.0　Fall (on) (from) escalator**
X● **W10.1　Fall (on) (from) sidewalk curb**
X● **W10.2　Fall (on) (from) incline**
　　　　　　Fall (on) (from) ramp
X● **W10.8　Fall (on) (from) other stairs and steps**
X● **W10.9　Fall (on) (from) unspecified stairs and steps**

X● **W11　Fall on and from ladder**

> The appropriate 7th character is to be added to code W11
>
> | | |
> |---|---|
> | A | initial encounter |
> | D | subsequent encounter |
> | S | sequela |

X● **W12　Fall on and from scaffolding**

> The appropriate 7th character is to be added to code W12
>
> | | |
> |---|---|
> | A | initial encounter |
> | D | subsequent encounter |
> | S | sequela |

●W13　Fall from, out of or through building or structure

> The appropriate 7th character is to be added to each code from category W13
>
> | | |
> |---|---|
> | A | initial encounter |
> | D | subsequent encounter |
> | S | sequela |

X● **W13.0　Fall from, out of or through balcony**
　　　　　　Fall from, out of or through railing
X● **W13.1　Fall from, out of or through bridge**
X● **W13.2　Fall from, out of or through roof**
X● **W13.3　Fall through floor**
X● **W13.4　Fall from, out of or through window**

> **Excludes2**　fall with subsequent striking against sharp glass (W01.110)

X● **W13.8　Fall from, out of or through other building or structure**
　　　　　　Fall from, out of or through viaduct
　　　　　　Fall from, out of or through wall
　　　　　　Fall from, out of or through flag-pole
X● **W13.9　Fall from, out of or through building, not otherwise specified**

> **Excludes1**　collapse of a building or structure (W20.-)
> fall or jump from burning building or structure (X00.-)

X● **W14　Fall from tree**

> The appropriate 7th character is to be added to code W14
>
> | | |
> |---|---|
> | A | initial encounter |
> | D | subsequent encounter |
> | S | sequela |

X● **W15　Fall from cliff**

> The appropriate 7th character is to be added to code W15
>
> | | |
> |---|---|
> | A | initial encounter |
> | D | subsequent encounter |
> | S | sequela |

●W16　Fall, jump or diving into water

> **Excludes1**　accidental non-watercraft drowning and submersion not involving fall (W65-W74)
> effects of air pressure from diving (W94.-)
> fall into water from watercraft (V90-V94)
> hitting an object or against bottom when falling from watercraft (V94.0)
>
> **Excludes2**　striking or hitting diving board (W21.4)
>
> The appropriate 7th character is to be added to each code from category W16
>
> | | |
> |---|---|
> | A | initial encounter |
> | D | subsequent encounter |
> | S | sequela |

● **W16.0　Fall into swimming pool**
　　　　　Fall into swimming pool NOS

> **Excludes1**　fall into empty swimming pool (W17.3)

● **W16.01　Fall into swimming pool striking water surface**

● **W16.011　Fall into swimming pool striking water surface causing drowning and submersion**

> **Excludes1**　drowning and submersion while in swimming pool without fall (W67)

● **W16.012　Fall into swimming pool striking water surface causing other injury**

● **W16.02　Fall into swimming pool striking bottom**

● **W16.021　Fall into swimming pool striking bottom causing drowning and submersion**

> **Excludes1**　drowning and submersion while in swimming pool without fall (W67)

● **W16.022　Fall into swimming pool striking bottom causing other injury**

● **W16.03　Fall into swimming pool striking wall**

● **W16.031　Fall into swimming pool striking wall causing drowning and submersion**

> **Excludes1**　drowning and submersion while in swimming pool without fall (W67)

● **W16.032　Fall into swimming pool striking wall causing other injury**

◄ New　⬅ Revised　~~deleted~~ Deleted　Excludes 1　Excludes 2　Includes　Use additional　Code first　Code also　Unspecified
OGCR Official Guidelines　**X** Assign placeholder X　● Use Additional Character(s)　▷ Manifestation Code　**Coding Clinic**

● **W16.1   Fall into natural body of water**
     Fall into lake
     Fall into open sea
     Fall into river
     Fall into stream

   ● **W16.11   Fall into natural body of water striking water surface**

     ● **W16.111   Fall into natural body of water striking water surface causing drowning and submersion**
        Excludes1   drowning and submersion while in natural body of water without fall (W69)

     ● **W16.112   Fall into natural body of water striking water surface causing other injury**

   ● **W16.12   Fall into natural body of water striking bottom**

     ● **W16.121   Fall into natural body of water striking bottom causing drowning and submersion**
        Excludes1   drowning and submersion while in natural body of water without fall (W69)

     ● **W16.122   Fall into natural body of water striking bottom causing other injury**

   ● **W16.13   Fall into natural body of water striking side**

     ● **W16.131   Fall into natural body of water striking side causing drowning and submersion**
        Excludes1   drowning and submersion while in natural body of water without fall (W69)

     ● **W16.132   Fall into natural body of water striking side causing other injury**

● **W16.2   Fall in (into) filled bathtub or bucket of water**

   ● **W16.21   Fall in (into) filled bathtub**
     Excludes1   fall into empty bathtub (W18.2)

     ● **W16.211   Fall in (into) filled bathtub causing drowning and submersion**
        Excludes1   drowning and submersion while in filled bathtub without fall (W65)

     ● **W16.212   Fall in (into) filled bathtub causing other injury**

   ● **W16.22   Fall in (into) bucket of water**

     ● **W16.221   Fall in (into) bucket of water causing drowning and submersion**

     ● **W16.222   Fall in (into) bucket of water causing other injury**

● **W16.3   Fall into other water**
     Fall into fountain
     Fall into reservoir

   ● **W16.31   Fall into other water striking water surface**

     ● **W16.311   Fall into other water striking water surface causing drowning and submersion**
        Excludes1   drowning and submersion while in other water without fall (W73)

     ● **W16.312   Fall into other water striking water surface causing other injury**

   ● **W16.32   Fall into other water striking bottom**

     ● **W16.321   Fall into other water striking bottom causing drowning and submersion**
        Excludes1   drowning and submersion while in other water without fall (W73)

     ● **W16.322   Fall into other water striking bottom causing other injury**

   ● **W16.33   Fall into other water striking wall**

     ● **W16.331   Fall into other water striking wall causing drowning and submersion**
        Excludes1   drowning and submersion while in other water without fall (W73)

     ● **W16.332   Fall into other water striking wall causing other injury**

● **W16.4   Fall into unspecified water**

   X● **W16.41   Fall into unspecified water causing drowning and submersion**

   X● **W16.42   Fall into unspecified water causing other injury**

● **W16.5   Jumping or diving into swimming pool**

   ● **W16.51   Jumping or diving into swimming pool striking water surface**

     ● **W16.511   Jumping or diving into swimming pool striking water surface causing drowning and submersion**
        Excludes1   drowning and submersion while in swimming pool without jumping or diving (W67)

     ● **W16.512   Jumping or diving into swimming pool striking water surface causing other injury**

   ● **W16.52   Jumping or diving into swimming pool striking bottom**

     ● **W16.521   Jumping or diving into swimming pool striking bottom causing drowning and submersion**
        Excludes1   drowning and submersion while in swimming pool without jumping or diving (W67)

     ● **W16.522   Jumping or diving into swimming pool striking bottom causing other injury**

   ● **W16.53   Jumping or diving into swimming pool striking wall**

     ● **W16.531   Jumping or diving into swimming pool striking wall causing drowning and submersion**
        Excludes1   drowning and submersion while in swimming pool without jumping or diving (W67)

     ● **W16.532   Jumping or diving into swimming pool striking wall causing other injury**

CHAPTER 20 (V01-Y99)

CHAPTER 20 (V01-Y99)

● **W16.6 Jumping or diving into natural body of water**
Jumping or diving into lake
Jumping or diving into open sea
Jumping or diving into river
Jumping or diving into stream

  ● **W16.61 Jumping or diving into natural body of water striking water surface**

    ● **W16.611 Jumping or diving into natural body of water striking water surface causing drowning and submersion**

       Excludes1 drowning and submersion while in natural body of water without jumping or diving (W69)

    ● **W16.612 Jumping or diving into natural body of water striking water surface causing other injury**

  ● **W16.62 Jumping or diving into natural body of water striking bottom**

    ● **W16.621 Jumping or diving into natural body of water striking bottom causing drowning and submersion**

       Excludes1 drowning and submersion while in natural body of water without jumping or diving (W69)

    ● **W16.622 Jumping or diving into natural body of water striking bottom causing other injury**

● **W16.7 Jumping or diving from boat**

   Excludes1 fall from boat into water - see watercraft accident (V90-V94)

  ● **W16.71 Jumping or diving from boat striking water surface**

    ● **W16.711 Jumping or diving from boat striking water surface causing drowning and submersion**

    ● **W16.712 Jumping or diving from boat striking water surface causing other injury**

  ● **W16.72 Jumping or diving from boat striking bottom**

    ● **W16.721 Jumping or diving from boat striking bottom causing drowning and submersion**

    ● **W16.722 Jumping or diving from boat striking bottom causing other injury**

● **W16.8 Jumping or diving into other water**
Jumping or diving into fountain
Jumping or diving into reservoir

  ● **W16.81 Jumping or diving into other water striking water surface**

    ● **W16.811 Jumping or diving into other water striking water surface causing drowning and submersion**

       Excludes1 drowning and submersion while in other water without jumping or diving (W73)

    ● **W16.812 Jumping or diving into other water striking water surface causing other injury**

  ● **W16.82 Jumping or diving into other water striking bottom**

    ● **W16.821 Jumping or diving into other water striking bottom causing drowning and submersion**

       Excludes1 drowning and submersion while in other water without jumping or diving (W73)

    ● **W16.822 Jumping or diving into other water striking bottom causing other injury**

  ● **W16.83 Jumping or diving into other water striking wall**

    ● **W16.831 Jumping or diving into other water striking wall causing drowning and submersion**

       Excludes1 drowning and submersion while in other water without jumping or diving (W73)

    ● **W16.832 Jumping or diving into other water striking wall causing other injury**

● **W16.9 Jumping or diving into unspecified water**

  X● **W16.91 Jumping or diving into unspecified water causing drowning and submersion**

  X● **W16.92 Jumping or diving into unspecified water causing other injury**

● **W17 Other fall from one level to another**

The appropriate 7th character is to be added to each code from category W17

A	initial encounter
D	subsequent encounter
S	sequela

X● **W17.0 Fall into well**

X● **W17.1 Fall into storm drain or manhole**

X● **W17.2 Fall into hole**
Fall into pit

X● **W17.3 Fall into empty swimming pool**

   Excludes1 fall into filled swimming pool (W16.0-)

X● **W17.4 Fall from dock**

● **W17.8 Other fall from one level to another**

  X● **W17.81 Fall down embankment (hill)**

  X● **W17.82 Fall from (out of) grocery cart**
Fall due to grocery cart tipping over

  X● **W17.89 Other fall from one level to another**
Fall from cherry picker
Fall from lifting device
Fall from mobile elevated work platform [MEWP]
Fall from sky lift

◄ New   ◄ Revised   ~~deleted~~ Deleted   Excludes 1   Excludes 2   Includes   Use additional   Code first   Code also   Unspecified

OGCR Official Guidelines   X Assign placeholder X   ● Use Additional Character(s)   ▶ Manifestation Code   **Coding Clinic**

● **W18   Other slipping, tripping and stumbling and falls**

The appropriate 7th character is to be added to each code from category W18

A	initial encounter
D	subsequent encounter
S	sequela

● **W18.0   Fall due to bumping against object**

Striking against object with subsequent fall

Excludes1   fall on same level due to slipping, tripping, or stumbling with subsequent striking against object (W01.1-)

X● **W18.00   Striking against unspecified object with subsequent fall**

X● **W18.01   Striking against sports equipment with subsequent fall**

X● **W18.02   Striking against glass with subsequent fall**

X● **W18.09   Striking against other object with subsequent fall**

● **W18.1   Fall from or off toilet**

X● **W18.11   Fall from or off toilet without subsequent striking against object**

Fall from (off) toilet NOS

X● **W18.12   Fall from or off toilet with subsequent striking against object**

X● **W18.2   Fall in (into) shower or empty bathtub**

Excludes1   fall in full bathtub causing drowning or submersion (W16.21-)

● **W18.3   Other and unspecified fall on same level**

X● **W18.30   Fall on same level, unspecified**

X● **W18.31   Fall on same level due to stepping on an object**

Fall on same level due to stepping on an animal

Excludes1   slipping, tripping and stumbling without fall due to stepping on animal (W18.41)

X● **W18.39   Other fall on same level**

● **W18.4   Slipping, tripping and stumbling without falling**

Excludes1   collision with another person without fall (W51)

X● **W18.40   Slipping, tripping and stumbling without falling, unspecified**

X● **W18.41   Slipping, tripping and stumbling without falling due to stepping on object**

Slipping, tripping and stumbling without falling due to stepping on animal

Excludes1   slipping, tripping and stumbling with fall due to stepping on animal (W18.31)

X● **W18.42   Slipping, tripping and stumbling without falling due to stepping into hole or opening**

X● **W18.43   Slipping, tripping and stumbling without falling due to stepping from one level to another**

X● **W18.49   Other slipping, tripping and stumbling without falling**

X● **W19   Unspecified fall**

Accidental fall NOS

The appropriate 7th character is to be added to code W19

A	initial encounter
D	subsequent encounter
S	sequela

Coding Clinic: 2012, Q4, P95

EXPOSURE TO INANIMATE MECHANICAL FORCES (W20-W49)

Excludes1   assault (X92-Y08)

contact or collision with animals or persons (W50-W64)

exposure to inanimate mechanical forces involving military or war operations (Y36.-, Y37.-)

intentional self-harm (X71-X83)

● **W20   Struck by thrown, projected or falling object**

Code first any associated:

cataclysm (X34-X39)

lightning strike (T75.00)

Excludes1   falling object in machinery accident (W24, W28-W31)

falling object in transport accident (V01-V99)

object set in motion by explosion (W35-W40)

object set in motion by firearm (W32-W34)

struck by thrown sports equipment (W21.-)

The appropriate 7th character is to be added to each code from category W20

A	initial encounter
D	subsequent encounter
S	sequela

X● **W20.0   Struck by falling object in cave-in**

Excludes2   asphyxiation due to cave-in (T71.21)

X● **W20.1   Struck by object due to collapse of building**

Excludes1   struck by object due to collapse of burning building (X00.2, X02.2)

X● **W20.8   Other cause of strike by thrown, projected or falling object**

Excludes1   struck by thrown sports equipment (W21.-)

● **W21   Striking against or struck by sports equipment**

Excludes1   assault with sports equipment (Y08.0-)

striking against or struck by sports equipment with subsequent fall (W18.01)

The appropriate 7th character is to be added to each code from category W21

A	initial encounter
D	subsequent encounter
S	sequela

● **W21.0   Struck by hit or thrown ball**

X● **W21.00   Struck by hit or thrown ball, unspecified type**

X● **W21.01   Struck by football**

X● **W21.02   Struck by soccer ball**

X● **W21.03   Struck by baseball**

X● **W21.04   Struck by golf ball**

X● **W21.05   Struck by basketball**

X● **W21.06   Struck by volleyball**

X● **W21.07   Struck by softball**

X● **W21.09   Struck by other hit or thrown ball**

● **W21.1   Struck by bat, racquet or club**

X● **W21.11   Struck by baseball bat**

X● **W21.12   Struck by tennis racquet**

X● **W21.13   Struck by golf club**

X● **W21.19   Struck by other bat, racquet or club**

● **W21.2   Struck by hockey stick or puck**

CHAPTER 20 (V01–Y99)

● W21.21   Struck by hockey stick
   ● W21.210   Struck by ice hockey stick
   ● W21.211   Struck by field hockey stick
● W21.22   Struck by hockey puck
   ● W21.220   Struck by ice hockey puck
   ● W21.221   Struck by field hockey puck
● W21.3   Struck by sports foot wear
 X ● W21.31   Struck by shoe cleats
    Stepped on by shoe cleats
 X ● W21.32   Struck by skate blades
    Skated over by skate blades
 X ● W21.39   Struck by other sports foot wear
X ● W21.4   Striking against diving board
   Use additional code for subsequent falling into water, if applicable (W16.-)
● W21.8   Striking against or struck by other sports equipment
 X ● W21.81   Striking against or struck by football helmet
 X ● W21.89   Striking against or struck by other sports equipment
X ● W21.9   Striking against or struck by unspecified sports equipment

● W22   Striking against or struck by other objects
   Excludes1   striking against or struck by object with subsequent fall (W18.09)

   The appropriate 7th character is to be added to each code from category W22

A	initial encounter
D	subsequent encounter
S	sequela

● W22.0   Striking against stationary object
   Excludes1   striking against stationary sports equipment (W21.8)
 X ● W22.01   Walked into wall
 X ● W22.02   Walked into lamppost
 X ● W22.03   Walked into furniture
 ● W22.04   Striking against wall of swimming pool
   ● W22.041   Striking against wall of swimming pool causing drowning and submersion
     Excludes1   drowning and submersion while swimming without striking against wall (W67)
   ● W22.042   Striking against wall of swimming pool causing other injury
 X ● W22.09   Striking against other stationary object
● W22.1   Striking against or struck by automobile airbag
 X ● W22.10   Striking against or struck by unspecified automobile airbag
 X ● W22.11   Striking against or struck by driver side automobile airbag
 X ● W22.12   Striking against or struck by front passenger side automobile airbag
 X ● W22.19   Striking against or struck by other automobile airbag
X ● W22.8   Striking against or struck by other objects
   Striking against or struck by object NOS
   Excludes1   struck by thrown, projected or falling object (W20.-)

● W23   Caught, crushed, jammed or pinched in or between objects
   Excludes1   injury caused by cutting or piercing instruments (W25-W27)
     injury caused by firearms malfunction (W32.1, W33.1-, W34.1-)
     injury caused by lifting and transmission devices (W24.-)
     injury caused by machinery (W28-W31)
     injury caused by nonpowered hand tools (W27.-)
     injury caused by transport vehicle being used as a means of transportation (V01-V99)
     injury caused by struck by thrown, projected or falling object (W20.-)
   The appropriate 7th character is to be added to each code from category W23

A	initial encounter
D	subsequent encounter
S	sequela

X ● W23.0   Caught, crushed, jammed, or pinched between moving objects
X ● W23.1   Caught, crushed, jammed, or pinched between stationary objects

● W24   Contact with lifting and transmission devices, not elsewhere classified
   Excludes1   transport accidents (V01-V99)
   The appropriate 7th character is to be added to each code from category W24

A	initial encounter
D	subsequent encounter
S	sequela

X ● W24.0   Contact with lifting devices, not elsewhere classified
   Contact with chain hoist
   Contact with drive belt
   Contact with pulley (block)
X ● W24.1   Contact with transmission devices, not elsewhere classified
   Contact with transmission belt or cable

X ● W25   Contact with sharp glass
   Code first any associated:
   injury due to flying glass from explosion or firearm discharge (W32-W40)
   transport accident (V00-V99)
   Excludes1   fall on same level due to slipping, tripping and stumbling with subsequent striking against sharp glass (W01.10)
     striking against sharp glass with subsequent fall (W18.02)
   The appropriate 7th character is to be added to code W25

A	initial encounter
D	subsequent encounter
S	sequela

● W26   Contact with knife, sword or dagger
   The appropriate 7th character is to be added to each code from category W26

A	initial encounter
D	subsequent encounter
S	sequela

X ● W26.0   Contact with knife
   Excludes1   contact with electric knife (W29.1)
X ● W26.1   Contact with sword or dagger

◄ New   ◄ Revised   ~~deleted~~ Deleted   Excludes 1   Excludes 2   Includes   Use additional   Code first   Code also   Unspecified

OGCR Official Guidelines   X Assign placeholder X   ● Use Additional Character(s)   ▌ Manifestation Code   **Coding Clinic**

● W27 **Contact with nonpowered hand tool**
> The appropriate 7th character is to be added to each code from category W27

> | | |
> |---|---|
> | A | initial encounter |
> | D | subsequent encounter |
> | S | sequela |

X● **W27.0 Contact with workbench tool**
Contact with auger
Contact with axe
Contact with chisel
Contact with handsaw
Contact with screwdriver

X● **W27.1 Contact with garden tool**
Contact with hoe
Contact with nonpowered lawn mower
Contact with pitchfork
Contact with rake

X● **W27.2 Contact with scissors**

X● **W27.3 Contact with needle (sewing)**
> **Excludes1**   contact with hypodermic needle (W46.-)

X● **W27.4 Contact with kitchen utensil**
Contact with fork
Contact with ice-pick
Contact with can-opener NOS

X● **W27.5 Contact with paper-cutter**

X● **W27.8 Contact with other nonpowered hand tool**
Contact with nonpowered sewing machine
Contact with shovel

X● **W28 Contact with powered lawn mower**
Powered lawn mower (commercial) (residential)
> **Excludes1**   contact with nonpowered lawn mower (W27.1)
> **Excludes2**   exposure to electric current (W86.-)

> The appropriate 7th character is to be added to code W28

> | | |
> |---|---|
> | A | initial encounter |
> | D | subsequent encounter |
> | S | sequela |

● W29 **Contact with other powered hand tools and household machinery**
> **Excludes1**   contact with commercial machinery (W31.82)
> contact with hot household appliance (X15)
> contact with nonpowered hand tool (W27.-)
> exposure to electric current (W86)

> The appropriate 7th character is to be added to each code from category W29

> | | |
> |---|---|
> | A | initial encounter |
> | D | subsequent encounter |
> | S | sequela |

X● **W29.0 Contact with powered kitchen appliance**
Contact with blender
Contact with can-opener
Contact with garbage disposal
Contact with mixer

X● **W29.1 Contact with electric knife**

X● **W29.2 Contact with other powered household machinery**
Contact with electric fan
Contact with powered dryer (clothes) (powered) (spin)
Contact with washing-machine
Contact with sewing machine

X● **W29.3 Contact with powered garden and outdoor hand tools and machinery**
Contact with chainsaw
Contact with edger
Contact with garden cultivator (tiller)
Contact with hedge trimmer
Contact with other powered garden tool
> **Excludes1**   contact with powered lawn mower (W28)

X● **W29.4 Contact with nail gun**

X● **W29.8 Contact with other powered powered hand tools and household machinery**
Contact with do-it-yourself tool NOS

● W30 **Contact with agricultural machinery**
> | **Includes** | animal-powered farm machine |
> |---|---|
> | **Excludes1** | agricultural transport vehicle accident (V01-V99) |
> | | explosion of grain store (W40.8) |
> | | exposure to electric current (W86.-) |

> The appropriate 7th character is to be added to each code from category W30

> | | |
> |---|---|
> | A | initial encounter |
> | D | subsequent encounter |
> | S | sequela |

X● **W30.0 Contact with combine harvester**
Contact with reaper
Contact with thresher

X● **W30.1 Contact with power take-off devices (PTO)**

X● **W30.2 Contact with hay derrick**

X● **W30.3 Contact with grain storage elevator**
> **Excludes1**   explosion of grain store (W40.8)

● **W30.8 Contact with other specified agricultural machinery**

X● **W30.81 Contact with agricultural transport vehicle in stationary use**
Contact with agricultural transport vehicle under repair, not on public roadway
> **Excludes1**   agricultural transport vehicle accident (V01-V99)

X● **W30.89 Contact with other specified agricultural machinery**

X● **W30.9 Contact with unspecified agricultural machinery**
Contact with farm machinery NOS

● W31 **Contact with other and unspecified machinery**
> **Excludes1**   contact with agricultural machinery (W30.-)
> contact with machinery in transport under own power or being towed by a vehicle (V01-V99)
> exposure to electric current (W86)

> The appropriate 7th character is to be added to each code from category W31

> | | |
> |---|---|
> | A | initial encounter |
> | D | subsequent encounter |
> | S | sequela |

X● **W31.0 Contact with mining and earth-drilling machinery**
Contact with bore or drill (land) (seabed)
Contact with shaft hoist
Contact with shaft lift
Contact with undercutter

X● **W31.1 Contact with metalworking machines**
Contact with abrasive wheel
Contact with forging machine
Contact with lathe
Contact with mechanical shears
Contact with metal drilling machine
Contact with milling machine
Contact with power press
Contact with rolling-mill
Contact with metal sawing machine

X● **W31.2 Contact with powered woodworking and forming machines**
Contact with band saw
Contact with bench saw
Contact with circular saw
Contact with molding machine
Contact with overhead plane
Contact with powered saw
Contact with radial saw
Contact with sander
> **Excludes1**   nonpowered woodworking tools (W27.0)

CHAPTER 20 (V01-Y99)

X● **W31.3** **Contact with prime movers**
Contact with gas turbine
Contact with internal combustion engine
Contact with steam engine
Contact with water driven turbine

● **W31.8** **Contact with other specified machinery**

X● **W31.81** **Contact with recreational machinery**
Contact with roller-coaster

X● **W31.82** **Contact with other commercial machinery**
Contact with commercial electric fan
Contact with commercial kitchen appliances
Contact with commercial powered dryer
(clothes) (powered) (spin)
Contact with commercial washing-machine
Contact with commercial sewing machine

Excludes1   contact with household
machinery (W29.-)
contact with powered lawn
mower (W28)

X● **W31.83** **Contact with special construction vehicle in stationary use**
Contact with special construction vehicle
under repair, not on public roadway

Excludes1   special construction vehicle
accident (V01-V99)

X● **W31.89** **Contact with other specified machinery**

X● **W31.9** **Contact with** unspecified **machinery**
Contact with machinery NOS

● **W32** **Accidental handgun discharge and malfunction**

Includes   accidental discharge and malfunction of gun for
single hand use
accidental discharge and malfunction of pistol
accidental discharge and malfunction of revolver
handgun discharge and malfunction NOS

Excludes1   accidental airgun discharge and malfunction
(W34.010, W34.110)
accidental BB gun discharge and malfunction
(W34.010, W34.110)
accidental pellet gun discharge and malfunction
(W34.010, W34.110)
accidental shotgun discharge and malfunction
(W33.01, W33.11)
assault by handgun discharge (X93)
handgun discharge involving legal intervention
(Y35.0-)
handgun discharge involving military or war
operations (Y36.4-)
intentional self-harm by handgun discharge (X72)
Very pistol discharge and malfunction (W34.09,
W34.19)

The appropriate 7th character is to be added to each code from
category W32

A	initial encounter
D	subsequent encounter
S	sequela

X● **W32.0** **Accidental handgun discharge**

X● **W32.1** **Accidental handgun malfunction**
Injury due to explosion of handgun (parts)
Injury due to malfunction of mechanism or component
of handgun
Injury due to recoil of handgun
Powder burn from handgun

● **W33** **Accidental rifle, shotgun and larger firearm discharge and malfunction**

Includes   rifle, shotgun and larger firearm discharge and
malfunction NOS

Excludes1   accidental airgun discharge and malfunction
(W34.010, W34.110)
accidental BB gun discharge and malfunction
(W34.010, W34.110)
accidental handgun discharge and malfunction
(W32.-)
accidental pellet gun discharge and malfunction
(W34.010, W34.110)
assault by rifle, shotgun and larger firearm
discharge (X94)
firearm discharge involving legal intervention
(Y35.0-)
firearm discharge involving military or war
operations (Y36.4-)
intentional self-harm by rifle, shotgun and larger
firearm discharge (X73)

The appropriate 7th character is to be added to each code from
category W33

A	initial encounter
D	subsequent encounter
S	sequela

● **W33.0** **Accidental rifle, shotgun and larger firearm discharge**

X● **W33.00** **Accidental discharge of** unspecified **larger firearm**
Discharge of unspecified larger firearm NOS

X● **W33.01** **Accidental discharge of shotgun**
Discharge of shotgun NOS

X● **W33.02** **Accidental discharge of hunting rifle**
Discharge of hunting rifle NOS

X● **W33.03** **Accidental discharge of machine gun**
Discharge of machine gun NOS

X● **W33.09** **Accidental discharge of other larger firearm**
Discharge of other larger firearm NOS

● **W33.1** **Accidental rifle, shotgun and larger firearm malfunction**
Injury due to explosion of rifle, shotgun and larger
firearm (parts)
Injury due to malfunction of mechanism or component
of rifle, shotgun and larger firearm
Injury due to piercing, cutting, crushing or pinching
due to (by) slide trigger mechanism, scope or other
gun part
Injury due to recoil of rifle, shotgun and larger firearm
Powder burn from rifle, shotgun and larger firearm

X● **W33.10** **Accidental malfunction of** unspecified **larger firearm**
Malfunction of unspecified larger firearm NOS

X● **W33.11** **Accidental malfunction of shotgun**
Malfunction of shotgun NOS

X● **W33.12** **Accidental malfunction of hunting rifle**
Malfunction of hunting rifle NOS

X● **W33.13** **Accidental malfunction of machine gun**
Malfunction of machine gun NOS

X● **W33.19** **Accidental malfunction of other larger firearm**
Malfunction of other larger firearm NOS

◀ New   ◀■ Revised   ~~deleted~~ Deleted   Excludes 1   Excludes 2   Includes   Use additional   Code first   Code also   Unspecified

OGCR Official Guidelines   X Assign placeholder X   ● Use Additional Character(s)   ▶ Manifestation Code   **Coding Clinic**

● **W34 Accidental discharge and malfunction from other and unspecified firearms and guns**

The appropriate 7th character is to be added to each code from category W34

> A   initial encounter
> D   subsequent encounter
> S   sequela

● **W34.0 Accidental discharge from other and unspecified firearms and guns**

X● **W34.00 Accidental discharge from unspecified firearms or gun**
Discharge from firearm NOS
Gunshot wound NOS
Shot NOS
Coding Clinic: 2015, Q1, P17

● **W34.01 Accidental discharge of gas, air or spring-operated guns**

● **W34.010 Accidental discharge of airgun**
Accidental discharge of BB gun
Accidental discharge of pellet gun

● **W34.011 Accidental discharge of paintball gun**
Accidental injury due to paintball discharge

● **W34.018 Accidental discharge of other gas, air or spring-operated gun**

X● **W34.09 Accidental discharge from other specified firearms**
Accidental discharge from Very pistol [flare]

● **W34.1 Accidental malfunction from other and unspecified firearms and guns**

X● **W34.10 Accidental malfunction from unspecified firearms or gun**
Firearm malfunction NOS

● **W34.11 Accidental malfunction of gas, air or spring-operated guns**

● **W34.110 Accidental malfunction of airgun**
Accidental malfunction of BB gun
Accidental malfunction of pellet gun

● **W34.111 Accidental malfunction of paintball gun**
Accidental injury due to paintball gun malfunction

● **W34.118 Accidental malfunction of other gas, air or spring-operated gun**

X● **W34.19 Accidental malfunction from other specified firearms**
Accidental malfunction from Very pistol [flare]

X● **W35 Explosion and rupture of boiler**

Excludes1   explosion and rupture of boiler on watercraft (V93.4)

The appropriate 7th character is to be added to code W35

> A   initial encounter
> D   subsequent encounter
> S   sequela

● **W36 Explosion and rupture of gas cylinder**

The appropriate 7th character is to be added to each code from category W36

> A   initial encounter
> D   subsequent encounter
> S   sequela

X● **W36.1 Explosion and rupture of aerosol can**
X● **W36.2 Explosion and rupture of air tank**
X● **W36.3 Explosion and rupture of pressurized-gas tank**
X● **W36.8 Explosion and rupture of other gas cylinder**
X● **W36.9 Explosion and rupture of unspecified gas cylinder**

● **W37 Explosion and rupture of pressurized tire, pipe or hose**

The appropriate 7th character is to be added to each code from category W37

> A   initial encounter
> D   subsequent encounter
> S   sequela

X● **W37.0 Explosion of bicycle tire**
X● **W37.8 Explosion and rupture of other pressurized tire, pipe or hose**

X● **W38 Explosion and rupture of other specified pressurized devices**

The appropriate 7th character is to be added to code W38

> A   initial encounter
> D   subsequent encounter
> S   sequela

X● **W39 Discharge of firework**

The appropriate 7th character is to be added to code W39

> A   initial encounter
> D   subsequent encounter
> S   sequela

● **W40 Explosion of other materials**

Excludes1   assault by explosive material (X96)
explosion involving legal intervention (Y35.1-)
explosion involving military or war operations (Y36.0-, Y36.2-)
intentional self-harm by explosive material (X75)

The appropriate 7th character is to be added to each code from category W40

> A   initial encounter
> D   subsequent encounter
> S   sequela

X● **W40.0 Explosion of blasting material**
Explosion of blasting cap
Explosion of detonator
Explosion of dynamite
Explosion of explosive (any) used in blasting operations

X● **W40.1 Explosion of explosive gases**
Explosion of acetylene
Explosion of butane
Explosion of coal gas
Explosion in mine NOS
Explosion of explosive gas
Explosion of fire damp
Explosion of gasoline fumes
Explosion of methane
Explosion of propane

X● **W40.8 Explosion of other specified explosive materials**
Explosion in dump NOS
Explosion in factory NOS
Explosion in grain store
Explosion in munitions

Excludes1   explosion involving legal intervention (Y35.1-)
explosion involving military or war operations (Y36.0-, Y36.2-)

X● **W40.9 Explosion of unspecified explosive materials**
Explosion NOS

● **W42 Exposure to noise**

The appropriate 7th character is to be added to each code from category W42

> A   initial encounter
> D   subsequent encounter
> S   sequela

X● **W42.0 Exposure to supersonic waves**
X● **W42.9 Exposure to other noise**
Exposure to sound waves NOS

CHAPTER 20 (V01-Y99)

● **W45   Foreign body or object entering through skin**

> **Excludes2**   contact with hand tools (nonpowered) (powered) (W27-W29)
> contact with knife, sword or dagger (W26.-)
> contact with sharp glass (W25.-)
> struck by objects (W20-W22)

The appropriate 7th character is to be added to each code from category W45

A	initial encounter
D	subsequent encounter
S	sequela

X ● **W45.0   Nail entering through skin**

X ● **W45.1   Paper entering through skin**
> Paper cut

X ● **W45.2   Lid of can entering through skin**

X ● **W45.8   Other foreign body or object entering through skin**
> Splinter in skin NOS

● **W46   Contact with hypodermic needle**

The appropriate 7th character is to be added to each code from category W46

A	initial encounter
D	subsequent encounter
S	sequela

X ● **W46.0   Contact with hypodermic needle**
> Hypodermic needle stick NOS

X ● **W46.1   Contact with contaminated hypodermic needle**

● **W49   Exposure to other inanimate mechanical forces**

> **Includes**   exposure to abnormal gravitational [G] forces
> exposure to inanimate mechanical forces NEC

> **Excludes1**   exposure to inanimate mechanical forces involving military or war operations (Y36.-, Y37.-)

The appropriate 7th character is to be added to each code from category W49

A	initial encounter
D	subsequent encounter
S	sequela

● **W49.0   Item causing external constriction**

X ● **W49.01   Hair causing external constriction**

X ● **W49.02   String or thread causing external constriction**

X ● **W49.03   Rubber band causing external constriction**

X ● **W49.04   Ring or other jewelry causing external constriction**

X ● **W49.09   Other item causing external constriction**

X ● **W49.9   Exposure to other inanimate mechanical forces**

EXPOSURE TO ANIMATE MECHANICAL FORCES (W50-W64)

> **Excludes1**   toxic effect of contact with venomous animals and plants (T63.-)

● **W50   Accidental hit, strike, kick, twist, bite or scratch by another person**

> **Includes**   hit, strike, kick, twist, bite, or scratch by another person NOS

> **Excludes1**   assault by bodily force (Y04)
> struck by objects (W20-W22)

The appropriate 7th character is to be added to each code from category W50

A	initial encounter
D	subsequent encounter
S	sequela

X ● **W50.0   Accidental hit or strike by another person**
> Hit or strike by another person NOS

X ● **W50.1   Accidental kick by another person**
> Kick by another person NOS

X ● **W50.2   Accidental twist by another person**
> Twist by another person NOS
> **Coding Clinic: 2015, Q1, P8**

X ● **W50.3   Accidental bite by another person**
> Human bite
> Bite by another person NOS

X ● **W50.4   Accidental scratch by another person**
> Scratch by another person NOS

X ● **W51   Accidental striking against or bumped into by another person**

> **Excludes1**   assault by striking against or bumping into by another person (Y04.2)
> fall due to collision with another person (W03)

The appropriate 7th character is to be added to code W51

A	initial encounter
D	subsequent encounter
S	sequela

X ● **W52   Crushed, pushed or stepped on by crowd or human stampede**
> Crushed, pushed or stepped on by crowd or human stampede with or without fall

The appropriate 7th character is to be added to code W52

A	initial encounter
D	subsequent encounter
S	sequela

● **W53   Contact with rodent**

> **Includes**   contact with saliva, feces or urine of rodent

The appropriate 7th character is to be added to each code from category W53

A	initial encounter
D	subsequent encounter
S	sequela

● **W53.0   Contact with mouse**

X ● **W53.01   Bitten by mouse**

X ● **W53.09   Other contact with mouse**

● **W53.1   Contact with rat**

X ● **W53.11   Bitten by rat**

X ● **W53.19   Other contact with rat**

● **W53.2   Contact with squirrel**

X ● **W53.21   Bitten by squirrel**

X ● **W53.29   Other contact with squirrel**

● **W53.8   Contact with other rodent**

X ● **W53.81   Bitten by other rodent**

X ● **W53.89   Other contact with other rodent**

● **W54   Contact with dog**

> **Includes**   contact with saliva, feces or urine of dog

The appropriate 7th character is to be added to each code from category W54

A	initial encounter
D	subsequent encounter
S	sequela

X ● **W54.0   Bitten by dog**

X ● **W54.1   Struck by dog**
> Knocked over by dog

X ● **W54.8   Other contact with dog**

◀ New   ◀═ Revised   ~~deleted~~ Deleted   Excludes 1   Excludes 2   Includes   Use additional   Code first   Code also   Unspecified

OGCR Official Guidelines   X Assign placeholder X   ● Use Additional Character(s)   ▶ Manifestation Code   **Coding Clinic**

● **W55 Contact with other mammals**

Includes	contact with saliva, feces or urine of mammal
Excludes1	animal being ridden - see transport accidents
	bitten or struck by dog (W54)
	bitten or struck by rodent (W53.-)
	contact with marine mammals (W56.X-)

The appropriate 7th character is to be added to each code from category W55

> A   initial encounter
> D   subsequent encounter
> S   sequela

● **W55.0 Contact with cat**
X● W55.01 **Bitten by cat**
X● W55.03 **Scratched by cat**
X● W55.09 **Other contact with cat**

● **W55.1 Contact with horse**
X● W55.11 **Bitten by horse**
X● W55.12 **Struck by horse**
X● W55.19 **Other contact with horse**

● **W55.2 Contact with cow**
    Contact with bull
X● W55.21 **Bitten by cow**
X● W55.22 **Struck by cow**
    Gored by bull
X● W55.29 **Other contact with cow**

● **W55.3 Contact with other hoof stock**
    Contact with goats
    Contact with sheep
X● W55.31 **Bitten by other hoof stock**
X● W55.32 **Struck by other hoof stock**
    Gored by goat
    Gored by ram
X● W55.39 **Other contact with other hoof stock**

● **W55.4 Contact with pig**
X● W55.41 **Bitten by pig**
X● W55.42 **Struck by pig**
X● W55.49 **Other contact with pig**

● **W55.5 Contact with raccoon**
X● W55.51 **Bitten by raccoon**
X● W55.52 **Struck by raccoon**
X● W55.59 **Other contact with raccoon**

● **W55.8 Contact with other mammals**
X● W55.81 **Bitten by other mammals**
X● W55.82 **Struck by other mammals**
X● W55.89 **Other contact with other mammals**

● **W56 Contact with nonvenomous marine animal**

Excludes1	contact with venomous marine animal (T63.-)

The appropriate 7th character is to be added to each code from category W56

> A   initial encounter
> D   subsequent encounter
> S   sequela

● **W56.0 Contact with dolphin**
X● W56.01 **Bitten by dolphin**
X● W56.02 **Struck by dolphin**
X● W56.09 **Other contact with dolphin**

● **W56.1 Contact with sea lion**
X● W56.11 **Bitten by sea lion**
X● W56.12 **Struck by sea lion**
X● W56.19 **Other contact with sea lion**

● **W56.2 Contact with orca**
    Contact with killer whale
X● W56.21 **Bitten by orca**
X● W56.22 **Struck by orca**
X● W56.29 **Other contact with orca**

● **W56.3 Contact with other marine mammals**
X● W56.31 **Bitten by other marine mammals**
X● W56.32 **Struck by other marine mammals**
X● W56.39 **Other contact with other marine mammals**

● **W56.4 Contact with shark**
X● W56.41 **Bitten by shark**
X● W56.42 **Struck by shark**
X● W56.49 **Other contact with shark**

● **W56.5 Contact with other fish**
X● W56.51 **Bitten by other fish**
X● W56.52 **Struck by other fish**
X● W56.59 **Other contact with other fish**

● **W56.8 Contact with other nonvenomous marine animals**
X● W56.81 **Bitten by other nonvenomous marine animals**
X● W56.82 **Struck by other nonvenomous marine animals**
X● W56.89 **Other contact with other nonvenomous marine animals**

X● **W57 Bitten or stung by nonvenomous insect and other nonvenomous arthropods**

Excludes1	contact with venomous insects and arthropods (T63.2-, T63.3-, T63.4-)

The appropriate 7th character is to be added to code W57

> A   initial encounter
> D   subsequent encounter
> S   sequela

● **W58 Contact with crocodile or alligator**

The appropriate 7th character is to be added to each code from category W58

> A   initial encounter
> D   subsequent encounter
> S   sequela

● **W58.0 Contact with alligator**
X● W58.01 **Bitten by alligator**
X● W58.02 **Struck by alligator**
X● W58.03 **Crushed by alligator**
X● W58.09 **Other contact with alligator**

● **W58.1 Contact with crocodile**
X● W58.11 **Bitten by crocodile**
X● W58.12 **Struck by crocodile**
X● W58.13 **Crushed by crocodile**
X● W58.19 **Other contact with crocodile**

● **W59 Contact with other nonvenomous reptiles**

Excludes1	contact with venomous reptile (T63.0-, T63.1-)

The appropriate 7th character is to be added to each code from category W59

> A   initial encounter
> D   subsequent encounter
> S   sequela

● **W59.0 Contact with nonvenomous lizards**
X● W59.01 **Bitten by nonvenomous lizards**
X● W59.02 **Struck by nonvenomous lizards**
X● W59.09 **Other contact with nonvenomous lizards**
    Exposure to nonvenomous lizards

CHAPTER 20 (V01-Y99)

● W59.1   Contact with nonvenomous snakes
   X● W59.11   Bitten by nonvenomous snake
   X● W59.12   Struck by nonvenomous snake
   X● W59.13   Crushed by nonvenomous snake
   X● W59.19   Other contact with nonvenomous snake
● W59.2   Contact with turtles
   Excludes1   contact with tortoises (W59.8-)
   X● W59.21   Bitten by turtle
   X● W59.22   Struck by turtle
   X● W59.29   Other contact with turtle
       Exposure to turtles
● W59.8   Contact with other nonvenomous reptiles
   X● W59.81   Bitten by other nonvenomous reptiles
   X● W59.82   Struck by other nonvenomous reptiles
   X● W59.83   Crushed by other nonvenomous reptiles
   X● W59.89   Other contact with other nonvenomous reptiles

X● W60   Contact with nonvenomous plant thorns and spines and sharp leaves
   Excludes1   contact with venomous plants (T63.X7-)
   The appropriate 7th character is to be added to code W60

A	initial encounter
D	subsequent encounter
S	sequela

● W61   Contact with birds (domestic) (wild)
   Includes   contact with excreta of birds
   The appropriate 7th character is to be added to each code from category W61

A	initial encounter
D	subsequent encounter
S	sequela

● W61.0   Contact with parrot
   X● W61.01   Bitten by parrot
   X● W61.02   Struck by parrot
   X● W61.09   Other contact with parrot
       Exposure to parrots
● W61.1   Contact with macaw
   X● W61.11   Bitten by macaw
   X● W61.12   Struck by macaw
   X● W61.19   Other contact with macaw
       Exposure to macaws
● W61.2   Contact with other psittacines
   X● W61.21   Bitten by other psittacines
   X● W61.22   Struck by other psittacines
   X● W61.29   Other contact with other psittacines
       Exposure to other psittacines
● W61.3   Contact with chicken
   X● W61.32   Struck by chicken
   X● W61.33   Pecked by chicken
   X● W61.39   Other contact with chicken
       Exposure to chickens
● W61.4   Contact with turkey
   X● W61.42   Struck by turkey
   X● W61.43   Pecked by turkey
   X● W61.49   Other contact with turkey
● W61.5   Contact with goose
   X● W61.51   Bitten by goose
   X● W61.52   Struck by goose
   X● W61.59   Other contact with goose

● W61.6   Contact with duck
   X● W61.61   Bitten by duck
   X● W61.62   Struck by duck
   X● W61.69   Other contact with duck
● W61.9   Contact with other birds
   X● W61.91   Bitten by other birds
   X● W61.92   Struck by other birds
   X● W61.99   Other contact with other birds
       Contact with bird NOS

● W62   Contact with nonvenomous amphibians
   Excludes1   contact with venomous amphibians (T63.81-R63.83)
   The appropriate 7th character is to be added to each code from category W62

A	initial encounter
D	subsequent encounter
S	sequela

X● W62.0   Contact with nonvenomous frogs
X● W62.1   Contact with nonvenomous toads
X● W62.9   Contact with other nonvenomous amphibians

X● W64   Exposure to other animate mechanical forces
   Includes   exposure to nonvenomous animal NOS
   Excludes1   contact with venomous animal (T63.-)
   The appropriate 7th character is to be added to code W64

A	initial encounter
D	subsequent encounter
S	sequela

ACCIDENTAL NON-TRANSPORT DROWNING AND SUBMERSION (W65-W74)

   Excludes1   accidental drowning and submersion due to fall into water (W16.-)
       accidental drowning and submersion due to water transport accident (V90.-, V92.-)
   Excludes2   accidental drowning and submersion due to cataclysm (X34-X39)

X● W65   Accidental drowning and submersion while in bathtub
   Excludes1   accidental drowning and submersion due to fall in (into) bathtub (W16.211)
   The appropriate 7th character is to be added to code W65

A	initial encounter
D	subsequent encounter
S	sequela

X● W67   Accidental drowning and submersion while in swimming pool
   Excludes1   accidental drowning and submersion due to fall into swimming pool (W16.011, W16.021, W16.031)
       accidental drowning and submersion due to striking into wall of swimming pool (W22.041)
   The appropriate 7th character is to be added to code W67

A	initial encounter
D	subsequent encounter
S	sequela

◀ New   ◀▥ Revised   ~~deleted~~ Deleted   Excludes 1   Excludes 2   Includes   Use additional   Code first   Code also   Unspecified

OGCR Official Guidelines   **X** Assign placeholder X   ● Use Additional Character(s)   ▶ Manifestation Code   **Coding Clinic**

X● **W69 Accidental drowning and submersion while in natural water**
Accidental drowning and submersion while in lake
Accidental drowning and submersion while in open sea
Accidental drowning and submersion while in river
Accidental drowning and submersion while in stream

> **Excludes1**   accidental drowning and submersion due to fall into natural body of water (W16.111, W16.121, W16.131)

The appropriate 7th character is to be added to code W69

A	initial encounter
D	subsequent encounter
S	sequela

X● **W73 Other specified cause of accidental non-transport drowning and submersion**
Accidental drowning and submersion while in quenching tank
Accidental drowning and submersion while in reservoir

> **Excludes1**   accidental drowning and submersion due to fall into other water (W16.311, W16.321, W16.331)

The appropriate 7th character is to be added to code W73

A	initial encounter
D	subsequent encounter
S	sequela

X● **W74 Unspecified cause of accidental drowning and submersion**
Drowning NOS

The appropriate 7th character is to be added to code W74

A	initial encounter
D	subsequent encounter
S	sequela

EXPOSURE TO ELECTRIC CURRENT, RADIATION AND EXTREME AMBIENT AIR TEMPERATURE AND PRESSURE (W85-W99)

> **Excludes1**   exposure to:
> failure in dosage of radiation or temperature during surgical and medical care (Y63.2-Y63.5)
> lightning (T75.0-)
> natural cold (X31)
> natural heat (X30)
> natural radiation NOS (X39)
> radiological procedure and radiotherapy (Y84.2)
> sunlight (X32)

X● **W85 Exposure to electric transmission lines**
Broken power line

The appropriate 7th character is to be added to code W85

A	initial encounter
D	subsequent encounter
S	sequela

● **W86 Exposure to other specified electric current**

The appropriate 7th character is to be added to each code from category W86

A	initial encounter
D	subsequent encounter
S	sequela

X● **W86.0 Exposure to domestic wiring and appliances**
X● **W86.1 Exposure to industrial wiring, appliances and electrical machinery**
Exposure to conductors
Exposure to control apparatus
Exposure to electrical equipment and machinery
Exposure to transformers

X● **W86.8 Exposure to other electric current**
Exposure to wiring and appliances in or on farm (not farmhouse)
Exposure to wiring and appliances outdoors
Exposure to wiring and appliances in or on public building
Exposure to wiring and appliances in or on residential institutions
Exposure to wiring and appliances in or on schools

● **W88 Exposure to ionizing radiation**

> **Excludes1**   exposure to sunlight (X32)

The appropriate 7th character is to be added to each code from category W88

A	initial encounter
D	subsequent encounter
S	sequela

X● **W88.0 Exposure to X-rays**
X● **W88.1 Exposure to radioactive isotopes**
X● **W88.8 Exposure to other ionizing radiation**

● **W89 Exposure to man-made visible and ultraviolet light**

> **Includes**   exposure to welding light (arc)
> **Excludes2**   exposure to sunlight (X32)

The appropriate 7th character is to be added to each code from category W89

A	initial encounter
D	subsequent encounter
S	sequela

X● **W89.0 Exposure to welding light (arc)**
X● **W89.1 Exposure to tanning bed**
X● **W89.8 Exposure to other man-made visible and ultraviolet light**
X● **W89.9 Exposure to unspecified man-made visible and ultraviolet light**

● **W90 Exposure to other nonionizing radiation**

> **Excludes1**   exposure to sunlight (X32)

The appropriate 7th character is to be added to each code from category W90

A	initial encounter
D	subsequent encounter
S	sequela

X● **W90.0 Exposure to radiofrequency**
X● **W90.1 Exposure to infrared radiation**
X● **W90.2 Exposure to laser radiation**
X● **W90.8 Exposure to other nonionizing radiation**

X● **W92 Exposure to excessive heat of man-made origin**
The appropriate 7th character is to be added to code W92

A	initial encounter
D	subsequent encounter
S	sequela

● **W93** **Exposure to excessive cold of man-made origin**

The appropriate 7th character is to be added to each code from category W93

> A   initial encounter
> D   subsequent encounter
> S   sequela

● **W93.0** **Contact with or inhalation of dry ice**
X ● **W93.01** **Contact with dry ice**
X ● **W93.02** **Inhalation of dry ice**
● **W93.1** **Contact with or inhalation of liquid air**
X ● **W93.11** **Contact with liquid air**
Contact with liquid hydrogen
Contact with liquid nitrogen
X ● **W93.12** **Inhalation of liquid air**
Inhalation of liquid hydrogen
Inhalation of liquid nitrogen
X ● **W93.2** **Prolonged exposure in deep freeze unit or refrigerator**
X ● **W93.8** **Exposure to other excessive cold of man-made origin**

● **W94** **Exposure to high and low air pressure and changes in air pressure**

The appropriate 7th character is to be added to each code from category W94

> A   initial encounter
> D   subsequent encounter
> S   sequela

X ● **W94.0** **Exposure to prolonged high air pressure**
● **W94.1** **Exposure to prolonged low air pressure**
X ● **W94.11** **Exposure to residence or prolonged visit at high altitude**
X ● **W94.12** **Exposure to other prolonged low air pressure**
● **W94.2** **Exposure to rapid changes in air pressure during ascent**
X ● **W94.21** **Exposure to reduction in atmospheric pressure while surfacing from deep-water diving**
X ● **W94.22** **Exposure to reduction in atmospheric pressure while surfacing from underground**
X ● **W94.23** **Exposure to sudden change in air pressure in aircraft during ascent**
X ● **W94.29** **Exposure to other rapid changes in air pressure during ascent**
● **W94.3** **Exposure to rapid changes in air pressure during descent**
X ● **W94.31** **Exposure to sudden change in air pressure in aircraft during descent**
X ● **W94.32** **Exposure to high air pressure from rapid descent in water**
X ● **W94.39** **Exposure to other rapid changes in air pressure during descent**

X ● **W99** **Exposure to other man-made environmental factors**

The appropriate 7th character is to be added to code W99

> A   initial encounter
> D   subsequent encounter
> S   sequela

EXPOSURE TO SMOKE, FIRE AND FLAMES (X00-X08)

Excludes1   arson (X97)
Excludes2   explosions (W35-W40)
lightning (T75.0-)
transport accident (V01-V99)

● **X00** **Exposure to uncontrolled fire in building or structure**
Includes   conflagration in building or structure
Code first any associated cataclysm
Excludes2   exposure to ignition or melting of nightwear (X05)
exposure to ignition or melting of other clothing and apparel (X06.-)
exposure to other specified smoke, fire and flames (X08.-)

The appropriate 7th character is to be added to each code from category X00

> A   initial encounter
> D   subsequent encounter
> S   sequela

X ● **X00.0** **Exposure to flames in uncontrolled fire in building or structure**
Coding Clinic: 2015, Q1, P19
X ● **X00.1** **Exposure to smoke in uncontrolled fire in building or structure**
X ● **X00.2** **Injury due to collapse of burning building or structure in uncontrolled fire**
Excludes1   injury due to collapse of building not on fire (W20.1)
X ● **X00.3** **Fall from burning building or structure in uncontrolled fire**
X ● **X00.4** **Hit by object from burning building or structure in uncontrolled fire**
X ● **X00.5** **Jump from burning building or structure in uncontrolled fire**
X ● **X00.8** **Other exposure to uncontrolled fire in building or structure**

● **X01** **Exposure to uncontrolled fire, not in building or structure**
Includes   exposure to forest fire

The appropriate 7th character is to be added to each code from category X01

> A   initial encounter
> D   subsequent encounter
> S   sequela

X ● **X01.0** **Exposure to flames in uncontrolled fire, not in building or structure**
X ● **X01.1** **Exposure to smoke in uncontrolled fire, not in building or structure**
X ● **X01.3** **Fall due to uncontrolled fire, not in building or structure**
X ● **X01.4** **Hit by object due to uncontrolled fire, not in building or structure**
X ● **X01.8** **Other exposure to uncontrolled fire, not in building or structure**

◀ New   ◀▥ Revised   ~~deleted~~ Deleted   Excludes 1   Excludes 2   Includes   Use additional   Code first   Code also   Unspecified

OGCR Official Guidelines   X Assign placeholder X   ● Use Additional Character(s)   ▌ Manifestation Code   Coding Clinic

● **X02**   **Exposure to controlled fire in building or structure**

     Includes   exposure to fire in fireplace exposure to fire in stove

     The appropriate 7th character is to be added to each code from category X02

A	initial encounter
D	subsequent encounter
S	sequela

X●**X02.0**   **Exposure to flames in controlled fire in building or structure**

X●**X02.1**   **Exposure to smoke in controlled fire in building or structure**

X●**X02.2**   **Injury due to collapse of burning building or structure in controlled fire**

      Excludes1   injury due to collapse of building not on fire (W20.1)

X●**X02.3**   **Fall from burning building or structure in controlled fire**

X●**X02.4**   **Hit by object from burning building or structure in controlled fire**

X●**X02.5**   **Jump from burning building or structure in controlled fire**

X●**X02.8**   **Other exposure to controlled fire in building or structure**

● **X03**   **Exposure to controlled fire, not in building or structure**

     Includes   exposure to bon fire exposure to camp fire exposure to trash fire

     The appropriate 7th character is to be added to each code from category X03

A	initial encounter
D	subsequent encounter
S	sequela

X●**X03.0**   **Exposure to flames in controlled fire, not in building or structure**
     Coding Clinic: 2015, Q1, P19

X●**X03.1**   **Exposure to smoke in controlled fire, not in building or structure**

X●**X03.3**   **Fall due to controlled fire, not in building or structure**

X●**X03.4**   **Hit by object due to controlled fire, not in building or structure**

X●**X03.8**   **Other exposure to controlled fire, not in building or structure**

X●**X04**   **Exposure to ignition of highly flammable material**
     Exposure to ignition of gasoline
     Exposure to ignition of kerosene
     Exposure to ignition of petrol

     Excludes2   exposure to ignition or melting of nightwear (X05)
                   exposure to ignition or melting of other clothing and apparel (X06)

     The appropriate 7th character is to be added to code X04

A	initial encounter
D	subsequent encounter
S	sequela

X●**X05**   **Exposure to ignition or melting of nightwear**

     Excludes2   exposure to uncontrolled fire in building or structure (X00.-)
                   exposure to uncontrolled fire, not in building or structure (X01.-)
                   exposure to controlled fire in building or structure (X02.-)
                   exposure to controlled fire, not in building or structure (X03.-)
                   exposure to ignition of highly flammable materials (X04.-)

     The appropriate 7th character is to be added to code X05

A	initial encounter
D	subsequent encounter
S	sequela

● **X06**   **Exposure to ignition or melting of other clothing and apparel**

     Excludes2   exposure to uncontrolled fire in building or structure (X00.-)
                   exposure to uncontrolled fire, not in building or structure (X01.-)
                   exposure to controlled fire in building or structure (X02.-)
                   exposure to controlled fire, not in building or structure (X03.-)
                   exposure to ignition of highly flammable materials (X04.-)

     The appropriate 7th character is to be added to each code from category X06

A	initial encounter
D	subsequent encounter
S	sequela

X●**X06.0**   **Exposure to ignition of plastic jewelry**

X●**X06.1**   **Exposure to melting of plastic jewelry**

X●**X06.2**   **Exposure to ignition of other clothing and apparel**

X●**X06.3**   **Exposure to melting of other clothing and apparel**

● **X08**   **Exposure to other specified smoke, fire and flames**

     The appropriate 7th character is to be added to each code from category X08

A	initial encounter
D	subsequent encounter
S	sequela

● **X08.0**   **Exposure to bed fire**
     Exposure to mattress fire

X●**X08.00**   **Exposure to bed fire due to unspecified burning material**

X●**X08.01**   **Exposure to bed fire due to burning cigarette**
        Coding Clinic: 2015, Q1, P19

X●**X08.09**   **Exposure to bed fire due to other burning material**

● **X08.1**   **Exposure to sofa fire**

X●**X08.10**   **Exposure to sofa fire due to unspecified burning material**

X●**X08.11**   **Exposure to sofa fire due to burning cigarette**

X●**X08.19**   **Exposure to sofa fire due to other burning material**

● **X08.2**   **Exposure to other furniture fire**

X●**X08.20**   **Exposure to other furniture fire due to unspecified burning material**

X●**X08.21**   **Exposure to other furniture fire due to burning cigarette**

X●**X08.29**   **Exposure to other furniture fire due to other burning material**

X●**X08.8**   **Exposure to other specified smoke, fire and flames**

CHAPTER 20 (V01-Y99)

CONTACT WITH HEAT AND HOT SUBSTANCES (X10-X19)

Excludes1 exposure to excessive natural heat (X30)
exposure to fire and flames (X00-X09)

● **X10 Contact with hot drinks, food, fats and cooking oils**

The appropriate 7th character is to be added to each code from category X10

> A initial encounter
> D subsequent encounter
> S sequela

X● **X10.0 Contact with hot drinks**
X● **X10.1 Contact with hot food**
X● **X10.2 Contact with fats and cooking oils**

● **X11 Contact with hot tap-water**

Includes contact with boiling tap-water
contact with boiling water NOS

Excludes1 contact with water heated on stove (X12)

The appropriate 7th character is to be added to each code from category X11

> A initial encounter
> D subsequent encounter
> S sequela

X● **X11.0 Contact with hot water in bath or tub**

Excludes1 contact with running hot water in bath or tub (X11.1)

X● **X11.1 Contact with running hot water**
Contact with hot water running out of hose
Contact with hot water running out of tap

X● **X11.8 Contact with other hot tap-water**
Contact with hot water in bucket
Contact with hot tap-water NOS

X● **X12 Contact with other hot fluids**
Contact with water heated on stove

Excludes1 hot (liquid) metals (X18)

The appropriate 7th character is to be added to code X12

> A initial encounter
> D subsequent encounter
> S sequela

● **X13 Contact with steam and other hot vapors**

The appropriate 7th character is to be added to each code from category X13

> A initial encounter
> D subsequent encounter
> S sequela

X● **X13.0 Inhalation of steam and other hot vapors**
X● **X13.1 Other contact with steam and other hot vapors**

● **X14 Contact with hot air and other hot gases**

The appropriate 7th character is to be added to each code from category X14

> A initial encounter
> D subsequent encounter
> S sequela

X● **X14.0 Inhalation of hot air and gases**
X● **X14.1 Other contact with hot air and other hot gases**

● **X15 Contact with hot household appliances**

Excludes1 contact with heating appliances (X16)
contact with powered household appliances (W29.-)
exposure to controlled fire in building or structure due to household appliance (X02.8)
exposure to household appliances electrical current (W86.0)

The appropriate 7th character is to be added to each code from category X15

> A initial encounter
> D subsequent encounter
> S sequela

X● **X15.0 Contact with hot stove (kitchen)**
X● **X15.1 Contact with hot toaster**
X● **X15.2 Contact with hotplate**
X● **X15.3 Contact with hot saucepan or skillet**
X● **X15.8 Contact with other hot household appliances**
Contact with cooker
Contact with kettle
Contact with light bulbs

X● **X16 Contact with hot heating appliances, radiators and pipes**

Excludes1 contact with powered appliances (W29.-)
exposure to controlled fire in building or structure due to appliance (X02.8)
exposure to industrial appliances electrical current (W86.1)

The appropriate 7th character is to be added to code X16

> A initial encounter
> D subsequent encounter
> S sequela

X● **X17 Contact with hot engines, machinery and tools**

Excludes1 contact with hot heating appliances, radiators and pipes (X16)
contact with hot household appliances (X15)

The appropriate 7th character is to be added to code X17

> A initial encounter
> D subsequent encounter
> S sequela

X● **X18 Contact with other hot metals**
Contact with liquid metal

The appropriate 7th character is to be added to code X18

> A initial encounter
> D subsequent encounter
> S sequela

X● **X19 Contact with other heat and hot substances**

Excludes1 objects that are not normally hot, e.g., an object made hot by a house fire (X00-X09)

The appropriate 7th character is to be added to code X19

> A initial encounter
> D subsequent encounter
> S sequela

◄ New ◄ Revised ~~deleted~~ Deleted Excludes 1 Excludes 2 Includes Use additional Code first Code also Unspecified

OGCR Official Guidelines X Assign placeholder X ● Use Additional Character(s) ▌ Manifestation Code **Coding Clinic**

EXPOSURE TO FORCES OF NATURE (X30-X39)

X● **X30**   **Exposure to excessive natural heat**
Exposure to excessive heat as the cause of sunstroke
Exposure to heat NOS

> **Excludes1**   excessive heat of man-made origin (W92)
> exposure to man-made radiation (W89)
> exposure to sunlight (X32)
> exposure to tanning bed (W89)

The appropriate 7th character is to be added to code X30

A	initial encounter
D	subsequent encounter
S	sequela

X● **X31**   **Exposure to excessive natural cold**
Excessive cold as the cause of chilblains NOS
Excessive cold as the cause of immersion foot or hand
Exposure to cold NOS
Exposure to weather conditions

> **Excludes1**   cold of man-made origin (W93.-)
> contact with or inhalation of dry ice (W93.-)
> contact with or inhalation of liquefied gas (W93.-)

The appropriate 7th character is to be added to code X31

A	initial encounter
D	subsequent encounter
S	sequela

X● **X32**   **Exposure to sunlight**

> **Excludes1**   radiation-related disorders of the skin and
> subcutaneous tissue (L55-L59)
> man-made radiation (tanning bed) (W89)

The appropriate 7th character is to be added to code X32

A	initial encounter
D	subsequent encounter
S	sequela

X● **X34**   **Earthquake**

> **Excludes2**   tidal wave (tsunami) due to earthquake (X37.41)

The appropriate 7th character is to be added to code X34

A	initial encounter
D	subsequent encounter
S	sequela

X● **X35**   **Volcanic eruption**

> **Excludes2**   tidal wave (tsunami) due to volcanic eruption
> (X37.41)

The appropriate 7th character is to be added to code X35

A	initial encounter
D	subsequent encounter
S	sequela

● **X36**   **Avalanche, landslide and other earth movements**

> **Includes**   victim of mudslide of cataclysmic nature
> **Excludes1**   earthquake (X34)
> **Excludes2**   transport accident involving collision with
> avalanche or landslide not in motion
> (V01-V99)

The appropriate 7th character is to be added to each code from
category X36

A	initial encounter
D	subsequent encounter
S	sequela

X● **X36.0**   **Collapse of dam or man-made structure causing earth movement**

X● **X36.1**   **Avalanche, landslide, or mudslide**

● **X37**   **Cataclysmic storm**
The appropriate 7th character is to be added to each code from
category X37

A	initial encounter
D	subsequent encounter
S	sequela

X● **X37.0**   **Hurricane**
Storm surge   Typhoon

X● **X37.1**   **Tornado**
Cyclone   Twister

X● **X37.2**   **Blizzard (snow) (ice)**

X● **X37.3**   **Dust storm**

● **X37.4**   **Tidalwave**

X● **X37.41**   **Tidal wave due to earthquake or volcanic eruption**
Tidal wave NOS
Tsunami

X● **X37.42**   **Tidal wave due to storm**

X● **X37.43**   **Tidal wave due to landslide**

X● **X37.8**   **Other cataclysmic storms**
Cloudburst
Torrential rain

> **Excludes2**   flood (X38)

X● **X37.9**   **Unspecified cataclysmic storm**
Storm NOS

> **Excludes1**   collapse of dam or man-made structure
> causing earth movement (X39.0)

X● **X38**   **Flood**
Flood arising from remote storm
Flood of cataclysmic nature arising from melting snow
Flood resulting directly from storm

> **Excludes1**   collapse of dam or man-made structure causing
> earth movement (X39.0)
> tidal wave NOS (X37.41)
> tidal wave caused by storm (X37.2)

The appropriate 7th character is to be added to code X38

A	initial encounter
D	subsequent encounter
S	sequela

● **X39**   **Exposure to other forces of nature**
The appropriate 7th character is to be added to each code from
category X39

A	initial encounter
D	subsequent encounter
S	sequela

● **X39.0**   **Exposure to natural radiation**

> **Excludes1**   contact with and (suspected) exposure to
> radon and other naturally occuring
> radiation (Z77.122)
> exposure to man-made radiation
> (W88-W90)
> exposure to sunlight (X32)

X● **X39.01**   **Exposure to radon**

X● **X39.08**   **Exposure to other natural radiation**

X● **X39.8**   **Other exposure to forces of nature**

ACCIDENTAL EXPOSURE TO OTHER SPECIFIED FACTORS (X52, X58)

X● X52   Prolonged stay in weightless environment
     Weightlessness in spacecraft (simulator)

     The appropriate 7th character is to be added to code X52

> A   initial encounter
> D   subsequent encounter
> S   sequela

X● X58   Exposure to other specified factors
     Accident NOS
     Exposure NOS

     The appropriate 7th character is to be added to code X58

> A   initial encounter
> D   subsequent encounter
> S   sequela

INTENTIONAL SELF-HARM (X71-X83)

Purposely self-inflicted injury
Suicide (attempted)

● X71   Intentional self-harm by drowning and submersion

     The appropriate 7th character is to be added to each code from category X71

> A   initial encounter
> D   subsequent encounter
> S   sequela

     X● X71.0   Intentional self-harm by drowning and submersion while in bathtub

     X● X71.1   Intentional self-harm by drowning and submersion while in swimming pool

     X● X71.2   Intentional self-harm by drowning and submersion after jump into swimming pool

     X● X71.3   Intentional self-harm by drowning and submersion in natural water

     X● X71.8   Other intentional self-harm by drowning and submersion

     X● X71.9   Intentional self-harm by drowning and submersion, unspecified

X● X72   Intentional self-harm by handgun discharge
     Intentional self-harm by gun for single hand use
     Intentional self-harm by pistol
     Intentional self-harm by revolver

> **Excludes1**   Very pistol (X74.8)

     The appropriate 7th character is to be added to code X72

> A   initial encounter
> D   subsequent encounter
> S   sequela

● X73   Intentional self-harm by rifle, shotgun and larger firearm discharge

> **Excludes1**   airgun (X74.01)

     The appropriate 7th character is to be added to each code from category X73

> A   initial encounter
> D   subsequent encounter
> S   sequela

     X● X73.0   Intentional self-harm by shotgun discharge

     X● X73.1   Intentional self-harm by hunting rifle discharge

     X● X73.2   Intentional self-harm by machine gun discharge

     X● X73.8   Intentional self-harm by other larger firearm discharge

     X● X73.9   Intentional self-harm by unspecified larger firearm discharge

● X74   Intentional self-harm by other and unspecified firearm and gun discharge

     The appropriate 7th character is to be added to each code from category X74

> A   initial encounter
> D   subsequent encounter
> S   sequela

     ● X74.0   Intentional self-harm by gas, air or spring-operated guns

         X● X74.01   Intentional self-harm by airgun
         Intentional self-harm by BB gun discharge
         Intentional self-harm by pellet gun discharge

         X● X74.02   Intentional self-harm by paintball gun

         X● X74.09   Intentional self-harm by other gas, air or spring-operated gun

     X● X74.8   Intentional self-harm by other firearm discharge
     Intentional self-harm by Very pistol [flare] discharge

     X● X74.9   Intentional self-harm by unspecified firearm discharge

X● X75   Intentional self-harm by explosive material

     The appropriate 7th character is to be added to code X75

> A   initial encounter
> D   subsequent encounter
> S   sequela

X● X76   Intentional self-harm by smoke, fire and flames

     The appropriate 7th character is to be added to code X76

> A   initial encounter
> D   subsequent encounter
> S   sequela

● X77   Intentional self-harm by steam, hot vapors and hot objects

     The appropriate 7th character is to be added to each code from category X77

> A   initial encounter
> D   subsequent encounter
> S   sequela

     X● X77.0   Intentional self-harm by steam or hot vapors

     X● X77.1   Intentional self-harm by hot tap water

     X● X77.2   Intentional self-harm by other hot fluids

     X● X77.3   Intentional self-harm by hot household appliances

     X● X77.8   Intentional self-harm by other hot objects

     X● X77.9   Intentional self-harm by unspecified hot objects

● X78   Intentional self-harm by sharp object

     The appropriate 7th character is to be added to each code from category X78

> A   initial encounter
> D   subsequent encounter
> S   sequela

     X● X78.0   Intentional self-harm by sharp glass

     X● X78.1   Intentional self-harm by knife

     X● X78.2   Intentional self-harm by sword or dagger

     X● X78.8   Intentional self-harm by other sharp object

     X● X78.9   Intentional self-harm by unspecified sharp object

X● X79   Intentional self-harm by blunt object

     The appropriate 7th character is to be added to code X79

> A   initial encounter
> D   subsequent encounter
> S   sequela

◀ New   ⬅ Revised   ~~deleted~~ Deleted   Excludes 1   Excludes 2   Includes   Use additional   Code first   Code also   Unspecified

OGCR Official Guidelines   X Assign placeholder X   ● Use Additional Character(s)   ▶ Manifestation Code   **Coding Clinic**

X● **X80**   **Intentional self-harm by jumping from a high place**
Intentional fall from one level to another

The appropriate 7th character is to be added to code X80

> A   initial encounter
> D   subsequent encounter
> S   sequela

● **X81**   **Intentional self-harm by jumping or lying in front of moving object**

The appropriate 7th character is to be added to each code from category X81

> A   initial encounter
> D   subsequent encounter
> S   sequela

   X● **X81.0**   **Intentional self-harm by jumping or lying in front of motor vehicle**

   X● **X81.1**   **Intentional self-harm by jumping or lying in front of (subway) train**

   X● **X81.8**   **Intentional self-harm by jumping or lying in front of other moving object**

● **X82**   **Intentional self-harm by crashing of motor vehicle**

The appropriate 7th character is to be added to each code from category X82

> A   initial encounter
> D   subsequent encounter
> S   sequela

   X● **X82.0**   **Intentional collision of motor vehicle with other motor vehicle**

   X● **X82.1**   **Intentional collision of motor vehicle with train**

   X● **X82.2**   **Intentional collision of motor vehicle with tree**

   X● **X82.8**   **Other intentional self-harm by crashing of motor vehicle**

● **X83**   **Intentional self-harm by other specified means**

> **Excludes1**   intentional self-harm by poisoning or contact with toxic substance - see Table of Drugs and Chemicals

The appropriate 7th character is to be added to each code from category X83

> A   initial encounter
> D   subsequent encounter
> S   sequela

   X● **X83.0**   **Intentional self-harm by crashing of aircraft**

   X● **X83.1**   **Intentional self-harm by electrocution**

   X● **X83.2**   **Intentional self-harm by exposure to extremes of cold**

   X● **X83.8**   **Intentional self-harm by other specified means**

ASSAULT (X92-Y08)

> **Includes**   homicide injuries inflicted by another person with intent to injure or kill, by any means

> **Excludes1**   injuries due to legal intervention (Y35.-)
> injuries due to operations of war (Y36.-)
> injuries due to terrorism (Y38.-)

● **X92**   **Assault by drowning and submersion**

The appropriate 7th character is to be added to each code from category X92

> A   initial encounter
> D   subsequent encounter
> S   sequela

   X● **X92.0**   **Assault by drowning and submersion while in bathtub**

   X● **X92.1**   **Assault by drowning and submersion while in swimming pool**

   X● **X92.2**   **Assault by drowning and submersion after push into swimming pool**

   X● **X92.3**   **Assault by drowning and submersion in natural water**

   X● **X92.8**   **Other assault by drowning and submersion**

   X● **X92.9**   **Assault by drowning and submersion, unspecified**

X● **X93**   **Assault by handgun discharge**
Assault by discharge of gun for single hand use
Assault by discharge of pistol
Assault by discharge of revolver

> **Excludes1**   Very pistol (X95.8)

The appropriate 7th character is to be added to code X93

> A   initial encounter
> D   subsequent encounter
> S   sequela

● **X94**   **Assault by rifle, shotgun and larger firearm discharge**

> **Excludes1**   airgun (X95.01)

The appropriate 7th character is to be added to each code from category X94

> A   initial encounter
> D   subsequent encounter
> S   sequela

   X● **X94.0**   **Assault by shotgun**

   X● **X94.1**   **Assault by hunting rifle**

   X● **X94.2**   **Assault by machine gun**

   X● **X94.8**   **Assault by other larger firearm discharge**

   X● **X94.9**   **Assault by unspecified larger firearm discharge**

● **X95**   **Assault by other and unspecified firearm and gun discharge**

The appropriate 7th character is to be added to each code from category X95

> A   initial encounter
> D   subsequent encounter
> S   sequela

   ● **X95.0**   **Assault by gas, air or spring-operated guns**

     X● **X95.01**   **Assault by airgun discharge**
Assault by BB gun discharge
Assault by pellet gun discharge

     X● **X95.02**   **Assault by paintball gun discharge**

     X● **X95.09**   **Assault by other gas, air or spring-operated gun**

   X● **X95.8**   **Assault by other firearm discharge**
Assault by very pistol [flare] discharge

   X● **X95.9**   **Assault by unspecified firearm discharge**

● **X96**   **Assault by explosive material**

> **Excludes1**   incendiary device (X97)
> terrorism involving explosive material (Y38.2-)

The appropriate 7th character is to be added to each code from category X96

> A   initial encounter
> D   subsequent encounter
> S   sequela

   X● **X96.0**   **Assault by antipersonnel bomb**

> **Excludes1**   antipersonnel bomb use in military or war (Y36.2-)

   X● **X96.1**   **Assault by gasoline bomb**

   X● **X96.2**   **Assault by letter bomb**

   X● **X96.3**   **Assault by fertilizer bomb**

   X● **X96.4**   **Assault by pipe bomb**

   X● **X96.8**   **Assault by other specified explosive**

   X● **X96.9**   **Assault by unspecified explosive**

CHAPTER 20 (V01-Y99)

X● **X97** **Assault by smoke, fire and flames**
Assault by arson
Assault by cigarettes
Assault by incendiary device
The appropriate 7th character is to be added to code X97

A	initial encounter
D	subsequent encounter
S	sequela

● **X98** **Assault by steam, hot vapors and hot objects**
The appropriate 7th character is to be added to each code from category X98

A	initial encounter
D	subsequent encounter
S	sequela

X● **X98.0** **Assault by steam or hot vapors**
X● **X98.1** **Assault by hot tap water**
X● **X98.2** **Assault by hot fluids**
X● **X98.3** **Assault by hot household appliances**
X● **X98.8** **Assault by other hot objects**
X● **X98.9** **Assault by** unspecified **hot objects**

● **X99** **Assault by sharp object**
Excludes1 assault by strike by sports equipment (Y08.0-)
The appropriate 7th character is to be added to each code from category X99

A	initial encounter
D	subsequent encounter
S	sequela

X● **X99.0** **Assault by sharp glass**
X● **X99.1** **Assault by knife**
X● **X99.2** **Assault by sword or dagger**
X● **X99.8** **Assault by other sharp object**
X● **X99.9** **Assault by** unspecified **sharp object**
Assault by stabbing NOS

X● **Y00** **Assault by blunt object**
Excludes1 assault by strike by sports equipment (Y08.0)
The appropriate 7th character is to be added to code Y00

A	initial encounter
D	subsequent encounter
S	sequela

X● **Y01** **Assault by pushing from high place**
The appropriate 7th character is to be added to code Y01

A	initial encounter
D	subsequent encounter
S	sequela

● **Y02** **Assault by pushing or placing victim in front of moving object**
The appropriate 7th character is to be added to each code from category Y02

A	initial encounter
D	subsequent encounter
S	sequela

X● **Y02.0** **Assault by pushing or placing victim in front of motor vehicle**
X● **Y02.1** **Assault by pushing or placing victim in front of (subway) train**
X● **Y02.8** **Assault by pushing or placing victim in front of other moving object**

● **Y03** **Assault by crashing of motor vehicle**
The appropriate 7th character is to be added to each code from category Y03

A	initial encounter
D	subsequent encounter
S	sequela

X● **Y03.0** **Assault by being hit or run over by motor vehicle**
X● **Y03.8** **Other assault by crashing of motor vehicle**

● **Y04** **Assault by bodily force**
Excludes1 assault by:
submersion (X92.-)
use of weapon (X93-X95, X99, Y00)
The appropriate 7th character is to be added to each code from category Y04

A	initial encounter
D	subsequent encounter
S	sequela

X● **Y04.0** **Assault by unarmed brawl or fight**
X● **Y04.1** **Assault by human bite**
X● **Y04.2** **Assault by strike against or bumped into by another person**
X● **Y04.8** **Assault by other bodily force**
Assault by bodily force NOS

OGCR Section I.C.19.f.

Adult and child abuse, neglect and other maltreatment
Sequence first the appropriate code from categories T74.- or T76.- for abuse, neglect and other maltreatment, followed by any accompanying mental health or injury code(s).

If the documentation in the medical record states abuse or neglect it is coded as confirmed. It is coded as suspected if it is documented as suspected.

For cases of confirmed abuse or neglect an external cause code from the assault section (X92-Y08) should be added to identify the cause of any physical injuries. A perpetrator code (Y07) should be added when the perpetrator of the abuse is known. For suspected cases of abuse or neglect, do not report external cause or perpetrator code.

If a suspected case of abuse, neglect or mistreatment is ruled out during an encounter code Z04.71, Encounter for examination and observation following alleged physical adult abuse, ruled out, or code Z04.72, Encounter for examination and observation following alleged child physical abuse, ruled out, should be used, not a code from T76.

If a suspected case of alleged rape or sexual abuse is ruled out during an encounter code Z04.41, Encounter for examination and observation following alleged physical adult abuse, ruled out, or code Z04.42, Encounter for examination and observation following alleged rape or sexual abuse, ruled out, should be used, not a code from T76.

● **Y07** **Perpetrator of assault, maltreatment and neglect**
Note: Codes from this category are for use only in cases of confirmed abuse (T74.-)
Selection of the correct perpetrator code is based on the relationship between the perpetrator and the victim
Includes perpetrator of abandonment
perpetrator of emotional neglect
perpetrator of mental cruelty
perpetrator of physical abuse
perpetrator of physical neglect
perpetrator of sexual abuse
perpetrator of torture

● **Y07.0** **Spouse or partner, perpetrator of maltreatment and neglect**
Spouse or partner, perpetrator of maltreatment and neglect against spouse or partner

Y07.01 **Husband, perpetrator of maltreatment and neglect**

Y07.02 **Wife, perpetrator of maltreatment and neglect**

◀ New   ⬅ Revised   ~~deleted~~ Deleted   Excludes 1   Excludes 2   Includes   Use additional   Code first   Code also   Unspecified
OGCR Official Guidelines   **X** Assign placeholder X   ● Use Additional Character(s)   ▶ Manifestation Code   **Coding Clinic**

Y07.03   Male partner, perpetrator of maltreatment and neglect

Y07.04   Female partner, perpetrator of maltreatment and neglect

● Y07.1   Parent (adoptive) (biological), perpetrator of maltreatment and neglect

       Y07.11   Biological father, perpetrator of maltreatment and neglect

       Y07.12   Biological mother, perpetrator of maltreatment and neglect

       Y07.13   Adoptive father, perpetrator of maltreatment and neglect

       Y07.14   Adoptive mother, perpetrator of maltreatment and neglect

● Y07.4   Other family member, perpetrator of maltreatment and neglect

   ● Y07.41   Sibling, perpetrator of maltreatment and neglect

       Excludes1   stepsibling, perpetrator of maltreatment and neglect (Y07.435, Y07.436)

       Y07.410   Brother, perpetrator of maltreatment and neglect

       Y07.411   Sister, perpetrator of maltreatment and neglect

   ● Y07.42   Foster parent, perpetrator of maltreatment and neglect

       Y07.420   Foster father, perpetrator of maltreatment and neglect

       Y07.421   Foster mother, perpetrator of maltreatment and neglect

   ● Y07.43   Stepparent or stepsibling, perpetrator of maltreatment and neglect

       Y07.430   Stepfather, perpetrator of maltreatment and neglect

       Y07.432   Male friend of parent (co-residing in household), perpetrator of maltreatment and neglect

       Y07.433   Stepmother, perpetrator of maltreatment and neglect

       Y07.434   Female friend of parent (co-residing in household), perpetrator of maltreatment and neglect

       Y07.435   Stepbrother, perpetrator or maltreatment and neglect

       Y07.436   Stepsister, perpetrator of maltreatment and neglect

   ● Y07.49   Other family member, perpetrator of maltreatment and neglect

       Y07.490   Male cousin, perpetrator of maltreatment and neglect

       Y07.491   Female cousin, perpetrator of maltreatment and neglect

       Y07.499   Other family member, perpetrator of maltreatment and neglect

● Y07.5   Non-family member, perpetrator of maltreatment and neglect

       Y07.50   Unspecified non-family member, perpetrator of maltreatment and neglect

   ● Y07.51   Daycare provider, perpetrator of maltreatment and neglect

       Y07.510   At-home childcare provider, perpetrator of maltreatment and neglect

       Y07.511   Daycare center childcare provider, perpetrator of maltreatment and neglect

       Y07.512   At-home adultcare provider, perpetrator of maltreatment and neglect

       Y07.513   Adultcare center provider, perpetrator of maltreatment and neglect

       Y07.519   Unspecified daycare provider, perpetrator of maltreatment and neglect

   ● Y07.52   Healthcare provider, perpetrator of maltreatment and neglect

       Y07.521   Mental health provider, perpetrator of maltreatment and neglect

       Y07.528   Other therapist or healthcare provider, perpetrator of maltreatment and neglect

         Nurse perpetrator of maltreatment and neglect

         Occupational therapist perpetrator of maltreatment and neglect

         Physical therapist perpetrator of maltreatment and neglect

         Speech therapist perpetrator of maltreatment and neglect

       Y07.529   Unspecified healthcare provider, perpetrator of maltreatment and neglect

       Y07.53   Teacher or instructor, perpetrator of maltreatment and neglect

         Coach, perpetrator of maltreatment and neglect

       Y07.59   Other non-family member, perpetrator of maltreatment and neglect

● Y07.9   Unspecified perpetrator of maltreatment and neglect

● Y08   **Assault by other specified means**

     The appropriate 7th character is to be added to each code from category Y08

     | | |
     A   initial encounter
     D   subsequent encounter
     S   sequela

   ● Y08.0   Assault by strike by sport equipment

     X ● Y08.01   Assault by strike by hockey stick

     X ● Y08.02   Assault by strike by baseball bat

     X ● Y08.09   Assault by strike by other specified type of sport equipment

   ● Y08.8   Assault by other specified means

     X ● Y08.81   Assault by crashing of aircraft

     X ● Y08.89   Assault by other specified means

● Y09   **Assault by unspecified means**

     Assassination (attempted) NOS

     Homicide (attempted) NOS

     Manslaughter (attempted) NOS

     Murder (attempted) NOS

EVENT OF UNDETERMINED INTENT (Y21-Y33)

     Undetermined intent is only for use when there is specific documentation in the record that the intent of the injury cannot be determined. If no such documentation is present, code to accidental (unintentional)

● Y21   **Drowning and submersion, undetermined intent**

     The appropriate 7th character is to be added to each code from category Y21

     A   initial encounter
     D   subsequent encounter
     S   sequela

     X ● Y21.0   Drowning and submersion while in bathtub, undetermined intent

     X ● Y21.1   Drowning and submersion after fall into bathtub, undetermined intent

X● **Y21.2**   Drowning and submersion while in swimming pool, undetermined intent

X● **Y21.3**   Drowning and submersion after fall into swimming pool, undetermined intent

X● **Y21.4**   Drowning and submersion in natural water, undetermined intent

X● **Y21.8**   Other drowning and submersion, undetermined intent

X● **Y21.9**   Unspecified drowning and submersion, undetermined intent

X● **Y22**   **Handgun discharge, undetermined intent**
> Discharge of gun for single hand use, undetermined intent
> Discharge of pistol, undetermined intent
> Discharge of revolver, undetermined intent
>
> **Excludes2**   very pistol (Y24.8)
>
> The appropriate 7th character is to be added to code Y22

A	initial encounter
D	subsequent encounter
S	sequela

● **Y23**   **Rifle, shotgun and larger firearm discharge, undetermined intent**
> **Excludes2**   airgun (Y24.0)
>
> The appropriate 7th character is to be added to each code from category Y23

A	initial encounter
D	subsequent encounter
S	sequela

X● **Y23.0**   Shotgun discharge, undetermined intent

X● **Y23.1**   Hunting rifle discharge, undetermined intent

X● **Y23.2**   Military firearm discharge, undetermined intent

X● **Y23.3**   Machine gun discharge, undetermined intent

X● **Y23.8**   Other larger firearm discharge, undetermined intent

X● **Y23.9**   Unspecified larger firearm discharge, undetermined intent

● **Y24**   **Other and unspecified firearm discharge, undetermined intent**
> The appropriate 7th character is to be added to each code from category Y24

A	initial encounter
D	subsequent encounter
S	sequela

X● **Y24.0**   **Airgun discharge, undetermined intent**
> BB gun discharge, undetermined intent
> Pellet gun discharge, undetermined intent

X● **Y24.8**   **Other firearm discharge, undetermined intent**
> Paintball gun discharge, undetermined intent
> Very pistol [flare] discharge, undetermined intent

X● **Y24.9**   Unspecified firearm discharge, undetermined intent

X● **Y25**   **Contact with explosive material, undetermined intent**
> The appropriate 7th character is to be added to code Y25

A	initial encounter
D	subsequent encounter
S	sequela

X● **Y26**   **Exposure to smoke, fire and flames, undetermined intent**
> The appropriate 7th character is to be added to code Y26

A	initial encounter
D	subsequent encounter
S	sequela

● **Y27**   **Contact with steam, hot vapors and hot objects, undetermined intent**
> The appropriate 7th character is to be added to each code from category Y27

A	initial encounter
D	subsequent encounter
S	sequela

X● **Y27.0**   Contact with steam and hot vapors, undetermined intent

X● **Y27.1**   Contact with hot tap water, undetermined intent

X● **Y27.2**   Contact with hot fluids, undetermined intent

X● **Y27.3**   Contact with hot household appliance, undetermined intent

X● **Y27.8**   Contact with other hot objects, undetermined intent

X● **Y27.9**   Contact with unspecified hot objects, undetermined intent

● **Y28**   **Contact with sharp object, undetermined intent**
> The appropriate 7th character is to be added to each code from category Y28

A	initial encounter
D	subsequent encounter
S	sequela

X● **Y28.0**   Contact with sharp glass, undetermined intent

X● **Y28.1**   Contact with knife, undetermined intent

X● **Y28.2**   Contact with sword or dagger, undetermined intent

X● **Y28.8**   Contact with other sharp object, undetermined intent

X● **Y28.9**   Contact with unspecified sharp object, undetermined intent

X● **Y29**   **Contact with blunt object, undetermined intent**
> The appropriate 7th character is to be added to code Y29

A	initial encounter
D	subsequent encounter
S	sequela

X● **Y30**   **Falling, jumping or pushed from a high place, undetermined intent**
> Victim falling from one level to another, undetermined intent
> The appropriate 7th character is to be added to code Y30

A	initial encounter
D	subsequent encounter
S	sequela

X● **Y31**   **Falling, lying or running before or into moving object, undetermined intent**
> The appropriate 7th character is to be added to code Y31

A	initial encounter
D	subsequent encounter
S	sequela

X● **Y32**   **Crashing of motor vehicle, undetermined intent**
> The appropriate 7th character is to be added to code Y32

A	initial encounter
D	subsequent encounter
S	sequela

X● **Y33**   **Other specified events, undetermined intent**
> The appropriate 7th character is to be added to code Y33

A	initial encounter
D	subsequent encounter
S	sequela

◄ New   ◄ Revised   ~~deleted~~ Deleted   Excludes 1   Excludes 2   Includes   Use additional   Code first   Code also   Unspecified

OGCR Official Guidelines   X Assign placeholder X   ● Use Additional Character(s)   ▸ Manifestation Code   **Coding Clinic**

LEGAL INTERVENTION, OPERATIONS OF WAR, MILITARY OPERATIONS, AND TERRORISM (Y35-Y38)

● Y35   Legal intervention

> **Includes**   any injury sustained as a result of an encounter with any law enforcement official, serving in any capacity at the time of the encounter, whether on-duty or off-duty. Includes: injury to law enforcement official, suspect and bystander

The appropriate 7th character is to be added to each code from category Y35

> A   initial encounter
> D   subsequent encounter
> S   sequela

● Y35.0   Legal intervention involving firearm discharge

  ● Y35.00   Legal intervention involving unspecified firearm discharge
    Legal intervention involving gunshot wound
    Legal intervention involving shot NOS

    ● Y35.001   Legal intervention involving unspecified firearm discharge, law enforcement official injured

    ● Y35.002   Legal intervention involving unspecified firearm discharge, bystander injured

    ● Y35.003   Legal intervention involving unspecified firearm discharge, suspect injured

  ● Y35.01   Legal intervention involving injury by machine gun

    ● Y35.011   Legal intervention involving injury by machine gun, law enforcement official injured

    ● Y35.012   Legal intervention involving injury by machine gun, bystander injured

    ● Y35.013   Legal intervention involving injury by machine gun, suspect injured

  ● Y35.02   Legal intervention involving injury by handgun

    ● Y35.021   Legal intervention involving injury by handgun, law enforcement official injured

    ● Y35.022   Legal intervention involving injury by handgun, bystander injured

    ● Y35.023   Legal intervention involving injury by handgun, suspect injured

  ● Y35.03   Legal intervention involving injury by rifle pellet

    ● Y35.031   Legal intervention involving injury by rifle pellet, law enforcement official injured

    ● Y35.032   Legal intervention involving injury by rifle pellet, bystander injured

    ● Y35.033   Legal intervention involving injury by rifle pellet, suspect injured

  ● Y35.04   Legal intervention involving injury by rubber bullet

    ● Y35.041   Legal intervention involving injury by rubber bullet, law enforcement official injured

    ● Y35.042   Legal intervention involving injury by rubber bullet, bystander injured

    ● Y35.043   Legal intervention involving injury by rubber bullet, suspect injured

  ● Y35.09   Legal intervention involving other firearm discharge

    ● Y35.091   Legal intervention involving other firearm discharge, law enforcement official injured

    ● Y35.092   Legal intervention involving other firearm discharge, bystander injured

    ● Y35.093   Legal intervention involving other firearm discharge, suspect injured

● Y35.1   Legal intervention involving explosives

  ● Y35.10   Legal intervention involving unspecified explosives

    ● Y35.101   Legal intervention involving unspecified explosives, law enforcement official injured

    ● Y35.102   Legal intervention involving unspecified explosives, bystander injured

    ● Y35.103   Legal intervention involving unspecified explosives, suspect injured

  ● Y35.11   Legal intervention involving injury by dynamite

    ● Y35.111   Legal intervention involving injury by dynamite, law enforcement official injured

    ● Y35.112   Legal intervention involving injury by dynamite, bystander injured

    ● Y35.113   Legal intervention involving injury by dynamite, suspect injured

  ● Y35.12   Legal intervention involving injury by explosive shell

    ● Y35.121   Legal intervention involving injury by explosive shell, law enforcement official injured

    ● Y35.122   Legal intervention involving injury by explosive shell, bystander injured

    ● Y35.123   Legal intervention involving injury by explosive shell, suspect injured

  ● Y35.19   Legal intervention involving other explosives
    Legal intervention involving injury by grenade
    Legal intervention involving injury by mortar bomb

    ● Y35.191   Legal intervention involving other explosives, law enforcement official injured

    ● Y35.192   Legal intervention involving other explosives, bystander injured

    ● Y35.193   Legal intervention involving other explosives, suspect injured

● Y35.2   Legal intervention involving gas
  Legal intervention involving asphyxiation by gas
  Legal intervention involving poisoning by gas

  ● Y35.20   Legal intervention involving unspecified gas

    ● Y35.201   Legal intervention involving unspecified gas, law enforcement official injured

    ● Y35.202   Legal intervention involving unspecified gas, bystander injured

    ● Y35.203   Legal intervention involving unspecified gas, suspect injured

  ● Y35.21   Legal intervention involving injury by tear gas

    ● Y35.211   Legal intervention involving injury by tear gas, law enforcement official injured

    ● Y35.212   Legal intervention involving injury by tear gas, bystander injured

    ● Y35.213   Legal intervention involving injury by tear gas, suspect injured

● Y35.29   Legal intervention involving other gas
  ● Y35.291   Legal intervention involving other gas, law enforcement official injured
  ● Y35.292   Legal intervention involving other gas, bystander injured
  ● Y35.293   Legal intervention involving other gas, suspect injured
● Y35.3   Legal intervention involving blunt objects
  Legal intervention involving being hit or struck by blunt object
  ● Y35.30   Legal intervention involving unspecified blunt objects
    ● Y35.301   Legal intervention involving unspecified blunt objects, law enforcement official injured
    ● Y35.302   Legal intervention involving unspecified blunt objects, bystander injured
    ● Y35.303   Legal intervention involving unspecified blunt objects, suspect injured
  ● Y35.31   Legal intervention involving baton
    ● Y35.311   Legal intervention involving baton, law enforcement official injured
    ● Y35.312   Legal intervention involving baton, bystander injured
    ● Y35.313   Legal intervention involving baton, suspect injured
  ● Y35.39   Legal intervention involving other blunt objects
    ● Y35.391   Legal intervention involving other blunt objects, law enforcement official injured
    ● Y35.392   Legal intervention involving other blunt objects, bystander injured
    ● Y35.393   Legal intervention involving other blunt objects, suspect injured
● Y35.4   Legal intervention involving sharp objects
  Legal intervention involving being cut by sharp objects
  Legal intervention involving being stabbed by sharp objects
  ● Y35.40   Legal intervention involving unspecified sharp objects
    ● Y35.401   Legal intervention involving unspecified sharp objects, law enforcement official injured
    ● Y35.402   Legal intervention involving unspecified sharp objects, bystander injured
    ● Y35.403   Legal intervention involving unspecified sharp objects, suspect injured
  ● Y35.41   Legal intervention involving bayonet
    ● Y35.411   Legal intervention involving bayonet, law enforcement official injured
    ● Y35.412   Legal intervention involving bayonet, bystander injured
    ● Y35.413   Legal intervention involving bayonet, suspect injured
  ● Y35.49   Legal intervention involving other sharp objects
    ● Y35.491   Legal intervention involving other sharp objects, law enforcement official injured
    ● Y35.492   Legal intervention involving other sharp objects, bystander injured
    ● Y35.493   Legal intervention involving other sharp objects, suspect injured

● Y35.8   Legal intervention involving other specified means
  ● Y35.81   Legal intervention involving manhandling
    ● Y35.811   Legal intervention involving manhandling, law enforcement official injured
    ● Y35.812   Legal intervention involving manhandling, bystander injured
    ● Y35.813   Legal intervention involving manhandling, suspect injured
  ● Y35.89   Legal intervention involving other specified means
    ● Y35.891   Legal intervention involving other specified means, law enforcement official injured
    ● Y35.892   Legal intervention involving other specified means, bystander injured
    ● Y35.893   Legal intervention involving other specified means, suspect injured
● Y35.9   Legal intervention, means unspecified
  X ● Y35.91   Legal intervention, means unspecified, law enforcement official injured
  X ● Y35.92   Legal intervention, means unspecified, bystander injured
  X ● Y35.93   Legal intervention, means unspecified, suspect injured

● Y36   Operations of war
  Includes   injuries to military personnel and civilians caused by war, civil insurrection, and peacekeeping missions

  Excludes1   injury to military personnel occurring during peacetime military operations (Y37.-)
    military vehicles involved in transport accidents with non-military vehicle during peacetime (V09.01, V09.21, V19.81, V29.81, V39.81, V49.81, V59.81, V69.81, V79.81)

  The appropriate 7th character is to be added to each code from category Y36

A	initial encounter
D	subsequent encounter
S	sequela

● Y36.0   War operations involving explosion of marine weapons
  Weapons and military watercraft
  ● Y36.00   War operations involving explosion of unspecified marine weapon
    War operations involving underwater blast NOS
    ● Y36.000   War operations involving explosion of unspecified marine weapon, military personnel
    ● Y36.001   War operations involving explosion of unspecified marine weapon, civilian
  ● Y36.01   War operations involving explosion of depth-charge
    ● Y36.010   War operations involving explosion of depth-charge, military personnel
    ● Y36.011   War operations involving explosion of depth-charge, civilian
  ● Y36.02   War operations involving explosion of marine mine
    War operations involving explosion of marine mine, at sea or in harbor
    ● Y36.020   War operations involving explosion of marine mine, military personnel
    ● Y36.021   War operations involving explosion of marine mine, civilian

◄ New   ◄▥ Revised   ~~deleted~~ Deleted   Excludes 1   Excludes 2   Includes   Use additional   Code first   Code also   Unspecified

OGCR Official Guidelines   X Assign placeholder X   ● Use Additional Character(s)   ▸ Manifestation Code   **Coding Clinic**

● **Y36.03**   **War operations involving explosion of sea-based artillery shell**

     ● **Y36.030**   War operations involving explosion of sea-based artillery shell, military personnel

     ● **Y36.031**   War operations involving explosion of sea-based artillery shell, civilian

● **Y36.04**   **War operations involving explosion of torpedo**

     ● **Y36.040**   War operations involving explosion of torpedo, military personnel

     ● **Y36.041**   War operations involving explosion of torpedo, civilian

● **Y36.05**   **War operations involving accidental detonation of onboard marine weapons**

     ● **Y36.050**   War operations involving accidental detonation of onboard marine weapons, military personnel

     ● **Y36.051**   War operations involving accidental detonation of onboard marine weapons, civilian

● **Y36.09**   **War operations involving explosion of other marine weapons**

     ● **Y36.090**   War operations involving explosion of other marine weapons, military personnel

     ● **Y36.091**   War operations involving explosion of other marine weapons, civilian

● **Y36.1**   **War operations involving destruction of aircraft**

     ● **Y36.10**   **War operations involving unspecified destruction of aircraft**

         ● **Y36.100**   War operations involving `unspecified` destruction of aircraft, military personnel

         ● **Y36.101**   War operations involving `unspecified` destruction of aircraft, civilian

     ● **Y36.11**   **War operations involving destruction of aircraft due to enemy fire or explosives**

         War operations involving destruction of aircraft due to air to air missile

         War operations involving destruction of aircraft due to explosive placed on aircraft

         War operations involving destruction of aircraft due to rocket propelled grenade [RPG]

         War operations involving destruction of aircraft due to small arms fire

         War operations involving destruction of aircraft due to surface to air missile

         ● **Y36.110**   War operations involving destruction of aircraft due to enemy fire or explosives, military personnel

         ● **Y36.111**   War operations involving destruction of aircraft due to enemy fire or explosives, civilian

     ● **Y36.12**   **War operations involving destruction of aircraft due to collision with other aircraft**

         ● **Y36.120**   War operations involving destruction of aircraft due to collision with other aircraft, military personnel

         ● **Y36.121**   War operations involving destruction of aircraft due to collision with other aircraft, civilian

     ● **Y36.13**   **War operations involving destruction of aircraft due to onboard fire**

         ● **Y36.130**   War operations involving destruction of aircraft due to onboard fire, military personnel

         ● **Y36.131**   War operations involving destruction of aircraft due to onboard fire, civilian

● **Y36.14**   **War operations involving destruction of aircraft due to accidental detonation of onboard munitions and explosives**

     ● **Y36.140**   War operations involving destruction of aircraft due to accidental detonation of onboard munitions and explosives, military personnel

     ● **Y36.141**   War operations involving destruction of aircraft due to accidental detonation of onboard munitions and explosives, civilian

● **Y36.19**   **War operations involving other destruction of aircraft**

     ● **Y36.190**   War operations involving other destruction of aircraft, military personnel

     ● **Y36.191**   War operations involving other destruction of aircraft, civilian

● **Y36.2**   **War operations involving other explosions and fragments**

     Excludes1   war operations involving explosion of aircraft (Y36.1-)

         war operations involving explosion of marine weapons (Y36.0-)

         war operations involving explosion of nuclear weapons (Y36.5-)

         war operations involving explosion occurring after cessation of hostilities (Y36.8-)

     ● **Y36.20**   **War operations involving unspecified explosion and fragments**

         War operations involving air blast NOS

         War operations involving blast NOS

         War operations involving blast fragments NOS

         War operations involving blast wave NOS

         War operations involving blast wind NOS

         War operations involving explosion NOS

         War operations involving explosion of bomb NOS

         ● **Y36.200**   War operations involving `unspecified` explosion and fragments, military personnel

         ● **Y36.201**   War operations involving `unspecified` explosion and fragments, civilian

     ● **Y36.21**   **War operations involving explosion of aerial bomb**

         ● **Y36.210**   War operations involving explosion of aerial bomb, military personnel

         ● **Y36.211**   War operations involving explosion of aerial bomb, civilian

     ● **Y36.22**   **War operations involving explosion of guided missile**

         ● **Y36.220**   War operations involving explosion of guided missile, military personnel

         ● **Y36.221**   War operations involving explosion of guided missile, civilian

     ● **Y36.23**   **War operations involving explosion of improvised explosive device [IED]**

         War operations involving explosion of person-borne improvised explosive device [IED]

         War operations involving explosion of vehicle-borne improvised explosive device [IED]

         War operations involving explosion of roadside improvised explosive device [IED]

         ● **Y36.230**   War operations involving explosion of improvised explosive device [IED], military personnel

         ● **Y36.231**   War operations involving explosion of improvised explosive device [IED], civilian

CHAPTER 20 (V01-Y99)

● Y36.24   War operations involving explosion due to accidental detonation and discharge of own munitions or munitions launch device

    ● Y36.240   War operations involving explosion due to accidental detonation and discharge of own munitions or munitions launch device, military personnel

    ● Y36.241   War operations involving explosion due to accidental detonation and discharge of own munitions or munitions launch device, civilian

● Y36.25   War operations involving fragments from munitions

    ● Y36.250   War operations involving fragments from munitions, military personnel

    ● Y36.251   War operations involving fragments from munitions, civilian

● Y36.26   War operations involving fragments of improvised explosive device [IED]

    War operations involving fragments of person-borne improvised explosive device [IED]

    War operations involving fragments of vehicle-borne improvised explosive device [IED]

    War operations involving fragments of roadside improvised explosive device [IED]

    ● Y36.260   War operations involving fragments of improvised explosive device [IED], military personnel

    ● Y36.261   War operations involving fragments of improvised explosive device [IED], civilian

● Y36.27   War operations involving fragments from weapons

    ● Y36.270   War operations involving fragments from weapons, military personnel

    ● Y36.271   War operations involving fragments from weapons, civilian

● Y36.29   War operations involving other explosions and fragments

    War operations involving explosion of grenade

    War operations involving explosions of land mine

    War operations involving shrapnel NOS

    ● Y36.290   War operations involving other explosions and fragments, military personnel

    ● Y36.291   War operations involving other explosions and fragments, civilian

● Y36.3   War operations involving fires, conflagrations and hot substances

    War operations involving smoke, fumes, and heat from fires, conflagrations and hot substances

    Excludes1   war operations involving fires and conflagrations aboard military aircraft (Y36.1-)

         war operations involving fires and conflagrations aboard military watercraft (Y36.0-)

         war operations involving fires and conflagrations caused indirectly by conventional weapons (Y36.2-)

         war operations involving fires and thermal effects of nuclear weapons (Y36.53-)

    ● Y36.30   War operations involving unspecified fire, conflagration and hot substance

        ● Y36.300   War operations involving unspecified fire, conflagration and hot substance, military personnel

        ● Y36.301   War operations involving unspecified fire, conflagration and hot substance, civilian

● Y36.31   War operations involving gasoline bomb

    War operations involving incendiary bomb

    War operations involving petrol bomb

    ● Y36.310   War operations involving gasoline bomb, military personnel

    ● Y36.311   War operations involving gasoline bomb, civilian

● Y36.32   War operations involving incendiary bullet

    ● Y36.320   War operations involving incendiary bullet, military personnel

    ● Y36.321   War operations involving incendiary bullet, civilian

● Y36.33   War operations involving flamethrower

    ● Y36.330   War operations involving flamethrower, military personnel

    ● Y36.331   War operations involving flamethrower, civilian

● Y36.39   War operations involving other fires, conflagrations and hot substances

    ● Y36.390   War operations involving other fires, conflagrations and hot substances, military personnel

    ● Y36.391   War operations involving other fires, conflagrations and hot substances, civilian

● Y36.4   War operations involving firearm discharge and other forms of conventional warfare

    ● Y36.41   War operations involving rubber bullets

        ● Y36.410   War operations involving rubber bullets, military personnel

        ● Y36.411   War operations involving rubber bullets, civilian

    ● Y36.42   War operations involving firearms pellets

        ● Y36.420   War operations involving firearms pellets, military personnel

        ● Y36.421   War operations involving firearms pellets, civilian

    ● Y36.43   War operations involving other firearms discharge

        War operations involving bullets NOS

        Excludes1   war operations involving munitions fragments (Y36.25-)

             war operations involving incendiary bullets (Y36.32-)

        ● Y36.430   War operations involving other firearms discharge, military personnel

        ● Y36.431   War operations involving other firearms discharge, civilian

    ● Y36.44   War operations involving unarmed hand to hand combat

        Excludes1   war operations involving combat using blunt or piercing object (Y36.45-)

             war operations involving intentional restriction of air and airway (Y36.46-)

             war operations involving unintentional restriction of air and airway (Y36.47-)

        ● Y36.440   War operations involving unarmed hand to hand combat, military personnel

        ● Y36.441   War operations involving unarmed hand to hand combat, civilian

◄ New   ◄■ Revised   ~~deleted~~ Deleted   Excludes 1   Excludes 2   Includes   Use additional   Code first   Code also   Unspecified

OGCR Official Guidelines   X Assign placeholder X   ● Use Additional Character(s)   ▶ Manifestation Code   **Coding Clinic**

● Y36.45   War operations involving combat using blunt
            or piercing object
      ● Y36.450   War operations involving combat
                   using blunt or piercing object,
                   military personnel
      ● Y36.451   War operations involving combat
                   using blunt or piercing object,
                   civilian

● Y36.46   War operations involving intentional restriction
            of air and airway
      ● Y36.460   War operations involving intentional
                   restriction of air and airway, military
                   personnel
      ● Y36.461   War operations involving intentional
                   restriction of air and airway, civilian

● Y36.47   War operations involving unintentional
            restriction of air and airway
      ● Y36.470   War operations involving
                   unintentional restriction of air and
                   airway, military personnel
      ● Y36.471   War operations involving
                   unintentional restriction of air and
                   airway, civilian

● Y36.49   War operations involving other forms of
            conventional warfare
      ● Y36.490   War operations involving other forms
                   of conventional warfare, military
                   personnel
      ● Y36.491   War operations involving other forms
                   of conventional warfare, civilian

● Y36.5   War operations involving nuclear weapons
            War operations involving dirty bomb NOS
      ● Y36.50   War operations involving unspecified effect of
                  nuclear weapon
            ● Y36.500   War operations involving unspecified
                         effect of nuclear weapon, military
                         personnel
            ● Y36.501   War operations involving unspecified
                         effect of nuclear weapon, civilian

      ● Y36.51   War operations involving direct blast effect of
                  nuclear weapon
                  War operations involving blast pressure of
                      nuclear weapon
            ● Y36.510   War operations involving direct blast
                         effect of nuclear weapon, military
                         personnel
            ● Y36.511   War operations involving direct blast
                         effect of nuclear weapon, civilian

      ● Y36.52   War operations involving indirect blast effect of
                  nuclear weapon
                  War operations involving being thrown by
                      blast of nuclear weapon
                  War operations involving being struck or
                      crushed by blast debris of nuclear weapon
            ● Y36.520   War operations involving indirect
                         blast effect of nuclear weapon,
                         military personnel
            ● Y36.521   War operations involving indirect
                         blast effect of nuclear weapon,
                         civilian

      ● Y36.53   War operations involving thermal radiation
                  effect of nuclear weapon
                  War operations involving direct heat from
                      nuclear weapon
                  War operation involving fireball effects from
                      nuclear weapon
            ● Y36.530   War operations involving thermal
                         radiation effect of nuclear weapon,
                         military personnel
            ● Y36.531   War operations involving thermal
                         radiation effect of nuclear weapon,
                         civilian

● Y36.54   War operation involving nuclear radiation
            effects of nuclear weapon
            War operation involving acute radiation
                exposure from nuclear weapon
            War operation involving exposure to
                immediate ionizing radiation from
                nuclear weapon
            War operation involving fallout exposure from
                nuclear weapon
            War operation involving secondary effects of
                nuclear weapons
      ● Y36.540   War operation involving nuclear
                   radiation effects of nuclear weapon,
                   military personnel
      ● Y36.541   War operation involving nuclear
                   radiation effects of nuclear weapon,
                   civilian

● Y36.59   War operation involving other effects of nuclear
            weapons
      ● Y36.590   War operation involving other
                   effects of nuclear weapons, military
                   personnel
      ● Y36.591   War operation involving other effects
                   of nuclear weapons, civilian

● Y36.6   War operations involving biological weapons
      ● Y36.6X   War operations involving biological weapons
            ● Y36.6X0   War operations involving biological
                         weapons, military personnel
            ● Y36.6X1   War operations involving biological
                         weapons, civilian

● Y36.7   War operations involving chemical weapons and other
            forms of unconventional warfare

            | Excludes1 | war operations involving incendiary
                          devices (Y36.3-, Y36.5-) |

      ● Y36.7X   War operations involving chemical weapons
                  and other forms of unconventional warfare
            ● Y36.7X0   War operations involving chemical
                         weapons and other forms of
                         unconventional warfare, military
                         personnel
            ● Y36.7X1   War operations involving chemical
                         weapons and other forms of
                         unconventional warfare, civilian

● Y36.8   War operations occurring after cessation of hostilities
            War operations classifiable to categories Y36.0-Y36.8 but
                occurring after cessation of hostilities
      ● Y36.81   Explosion of mine placed during war
                  operations but exploding after cessation of
                  hostilities
            ● Y36.810   Explosion of mine placed during
                         war operations but exploding after
                         cessation of hostilities, military
                         personnel
            ● Y36.811   Explosion of mine placed during
                         war operations but exploding after
                         cessation of hostilities, civilian

      ● Y36.82   Explosion of bomb placed during war
                  operations but exploding after cessation of
                  hostilities
            ● Y36.820   Explosion of bomb placed during
                         war operations but exploding after
                         cessation of hostilities, military
                         personnel
            ● Y36.821   Explosion of bomb placed during
                         war operations but exploding after
                         cessation of hostilities, civilian

CHAPTER 20 (V01-Y99)

● Y36.88   Other war operations occurring after cessation of hostilities

    ● Y36.880   Other war operations occurring after cessation of hostilities, military personnel

    ● Y36.881   Other war operations occurring after cessation of hostilities, civilian

● Y36.89   Unspecified war operations occurring after cessation of hostilities

    ● Y36.890   Unspecified war operations occurring after cessation of hostilities, military personnel

    ● Y36.891   Unspecified war operations occurring after cessation of hostilities, civilian

● Y36.9   Other and unspecified war operations

   X ● Y36.90   War operations, unspecified

   X ● Y36.91   War operations involving unspecified weapon of mass destruction [WMD]

   X ● Y36.92   War operations involving friendly fire

● Y37   **Military operations**

    Includes   Injuries to military personnel and civilians occurring during peacetime on military property and during routine military exercises and operations

    Excludes1   military aircraft involved in aircraft accident with civilian aircraft (V97.81-)

        military vehicles involved in transport accident with civilian vehicle (V09.01, V09.21, V19.81, V29.81, V39.81, V49.81, V59.81, V69.81, V79.81)

        military watercraft involved in water transport accident with civilian watercraft (V94.81-)

        war operations (Y36.-)

    The appropriate 7th character is to be added to each code from category Y37

      A   initial encounter
      D   subsequent encounter
      S   sequela

● Y37.0   Military operations involving explosion of marine weapons

   ● Y37.00   Military operations involving explosion of unspecified marine weapon

       Military operations involving underwater blast NOS

     ● Y37.000   Military operations involving explosion of unspecified marine weapon, military personnel

     ● Y37.001   Military operations involving explosion of unspecified marine weapon, civilian

   ● Y37.01   Military operations involving explosion of depth-charge

     ● Y37.010   Military operations involving explosion of depth-charge, military personnel

     ● Y37.011   Military operations involving explosion of depth-charge, civilian

   ● Y37.02   Military operations involving explosion of marine mine

       Military operations involving explosion of marine mine, at sea or in harbor

     ● Y37.020   Military operations involving explosion of marine mine, military personnel

     ● Y37.021   Military operations involving explosion of marine mine, civilian

● Y37.03   Military operations involving explosion of sea-based artillery shell

    ● Y37.030   Military operations involving explosion of sea-based artillery shell, military personnel

    ● Y37.031   Military operations involving explosion of sea-based artillery shell, civilian

● Y37.04   Military operations involving explosion of torpedo

    ● Y37.040   Military operations involving explosion of torpedo, military personnel

    ● Y37.041   Military operations involving explosion of torpedo, civilian

● Y37.05   Military operations involving accidental detonation of onboard marine weapons

    ● Y37.050   Military operations involving accidental detonation of onboard marine weapons, military personnel

    ● Y37.051   Military operations involving accidental detonation of onboard marine weapons, civilian

● Y37.09   Military operations involving explosion of other marine weapons

    ● Y37.090   Military operations involving explosion of other marine weapons, military personnel

    ● Y37.091   Military operations involving explosion of other marine weapons, civilian

● Y37.1   Military operations involving destruction of aircraft

   ● Y37.10   Military operations involving unspecified destruction of aircraft

     ● Y37.100   Military operations involving unspecified destruction of aircraft, military personnel

     ● Y37.101   Military operations involving unspecified destruction of aircraft, civilian

   ● Y37.11   Military operations involving destruction of aircraft due to enemy fire or explosives

       Military operations involving destruction of aircraft due to air to air missile

       Military operations involving destruction of aircraft due to explosive placed on aircraft

       Military operations involving destruction of aircraft due to rocket propelled grenade [RPG]

       Military operations involving destruction of aircraft due to small arms fire

       Military operations involving destruction of aircraft due to surface to air missile

     ● Y37.110   Military operations involving destruction of aircraft due to enemy fire or explosives, military personnel

     ● Y37.111   Military operations involving destruction of aircraft due to enemy fire or explosives, civilian

   ● Y37.12   Military operations involving destruction of aircraft due to collision with other aircraft

     ● Y37.120   Military operations involving destruction of aircraft due to collision with other aircraft, military personnel

     ● Y37.121   Military operations involving destruction of aircraft due to collision with other aircraft, civilian

◀ New   ◀▥ Revised   ~~deleted~~ Deleted   Excludes 1   Excludes 2   Includes   Use additional   Code first   Code also   Unspecified

1556   **OGCR** Official Guidelines   X Assign placeholder X   ● Use Additional Character(s)   ▶ Manifestation Code   **Coding Clinic**

● Y37.13   Military operations involving destruction of aircraft due to onboard fire

    ● Y37.130   Military operations involving destruction of aircraft due to onboard fire, military personnel

    ● Y37.131   Military operations involving destruction of aircraft due to onboard fire, civilian

● Y37.14   Military operations involving destruction of aircraft due to accidental detonation of onboard munitions and explosives

    ● Y37.140   Military operations involving destruction of aircraft due to accidental detonation of onboard munitions and explosives, military personnel

    ● Y37.141   Military operations involving destruction of aircraft due to accidental detonation of onboard munitions and explosives, civilian

● Y37.19   Military operations involving other destruction of aircraft

    ● Y37.190   Military operations involving other destruction of aircraft, military personnel

    ● Y37.191   Military operations involving other destruction of aircraft, civilian

● Y37.2   Military operations involving other explosions and fragments

> **Excludes1**   military operations involving explosion of aircraft (Y37.1-)
> military operations involving explosion of marine weapons (Y37.0-)
> military operations involving explosion of nuclear weapons (Y37.5-)

● Y37.20   Military operations involving unspecified explosion and fragments

Military operations involving air blast NOS
Military operations involving blast NOS
Military operations involving blast fragments NOS
Military operations involving blast wave NOS
Military operations involving blast wind NOS
Military operations involving explosion NOS
Military operations involving explosion of bomb NOS

    ● Y37.200   Military operations involving unspecified explosion and fragments, military personnel

    ● Y37.201   Military operations involving unspecified explosion and fragments, civilian

● Y37.21   Military operations involving explosion of aerial bomb

    ● Y37.210   Military operations involving explosion of aerial bomb, military personnel

    ● Y37.211   Military operations involving explosion of aerial bomb, civilian

● Y37.22   Military operations involving explosion of guided missile

    ● Y37.220   Military operations involving explosion of guided missile, military personnel

    ● Y37.221   Military operations involving explosion of guided missile, civilian

● Y37.23   Military operations involving explosion of improvised explosive device [IED]

Military operations involving explosion of person-borne improvised explosive device [IED]
Military operations involving explosion of vehicle-borne improvised explosive device [IED]
Military operations involving explosion of roadside improvised explosive device [IED]

    ● Y37.230   Military operations involving explosion of improvised explosive device [IED], military personnel

    ● Y37.231   Military operations involving explosion of improvised explosive device [IED], civilian

● Y37.24   Military operations involving explosion due to accidental detonation and discharge of own munitions or munitions launch device

    ● Y37.240   Military operations involving explosion due to accidental detonation and discharge of own munitions or munitions launch device, military personnel

    ● Y37.241   Military operations involving explosion due to accidental detonation and discharge of own munitions or munitions launch device, civilian

● Y37.25   Military operations involving fragments from munitions

    ● Y37.250   Military operations involving fragments from munitions, military personnel

    ● Y37.251   Military operations involving fragments from munitions, civilian

● Y37.26   Military operations involving fragments of improvised explosive device [IED]

Military operations involving fragments of person-borne improvised explosive device [IED]
Military operations involving fragments of vehicle-borne improvised explosive device [IED]
Military operations involving fragments of roadside improvised explosive device [IED]

    ● Y37.260   Military operations involving fragments of improvised explosive device [IED], military personnel

    ● Y37.261   Military operations involving fragments of improvised explosive device [IED], civilian

● Y37.27   Military operations involving fragments from weapons

    ● Y37.270   Military operations involving fragments from weapons, military personnel

    ● Y37.271   Military operations involving fragments from weapons, civilian

● Y37.29   Military operations involving other explosions and fragments

Military operations involving explosion of grenade
Military operations involving explosions of land mine
Military operations involving shrapnel NOS

    ● Y37.290   Military operations involving other explosions and fragments, military personnel

    ● Y37.291   Military operations involving other explosions and fragments, civilian

CHAPTER 20 (V01-Y99)

● **Y37.3** **Military operations involving fires, conflagrations and hot substances**
Military operations involving smoke, fumes, and heat from fires, conflagrations and hot substances
Excludes1 military operations involving fires and conflagrations aboard military aircraft (Y37.1-)
military operations involving fires and conflagrations aboard military watercraft (Y37.0-)
military operations involving fires and conflagrations caused indirectly by conventional weapons (Y37.2-)
military operations involving fires and thermal effects of nuclear weapons (Y36.53-)

● **Y37.30** **Military operations involving unspecified fire, conflagration and hot substance**
● **Y37.300** **Military operations involving unspecified fire, conflagration and hot substance, military personnel**
● **Y37.301** **Military operations involving unspecified fire, conflagration and hot substance, civilian**

● **Y37.31** **Military operations involving gasoline bomb**
Military operations involving incendiary bomb
Military operations involving petrol bomb
● **Y37.310** **Military operations involving gasoline bomb, military personnel**
● **Y37.311** **Military operations involving gasoline bomb, civilian**

● **Y37.32** **Military operations involving incendiary bullet**
● **Y37.320** **Military operations involving incendiary bullet, military personnel**
● **Y37.321** **Military operations involving incendiary bullet, civilian**

● **Y37.33** **Military operations involving flamethrower**
● **Y37.330** **Military operations involving flamethrower, military personnel**
● **Y37.331** **Military operations involving flamethrower, civilian**

● **Y37.39** **Military operations involving other fires, conflagrations and hot substances**
● **Y37.390** **Military operations involving other fires, conflagrations and hot substances, military personnel**
● **Y37.391** **Military operations involving other fires, conflagrations and hot substances, civilian**

● **Y37.4** **Military operations involving firearm discharge and other forms of conventional warfare**
● **Y37.41** **Military operations involving rubber bullets**
● **Y37.410** **Military operations involving rubber bullets, military personnel**
● **Y37.411** **Military operations involving rubber bullets, civilian**

● **Y37.42** **Military operations involving firearms pellets**
● **Y37.420** **Military operations involving firearms pellets, military personnel**
● **Y37.421** **Military operations involving firearms pellets, civilian**

● **Y37.43** **Military operations involving other firearms discharge**
Military operations involving bullets NOS
Excludes1 military operations involving munitions fragments (Y37.25-)
military operations involving incendiary bullets (Y37.32-)
● **Y37.430** **Military operations involving other firearms discharge, military personnel**
● **Y37.431** **Military operations involving other firearms discharge, civilian**

● **Y37.44** **Military operations involving unarmed hand to hand combat**
Excludes1 military operations involving combat using blunt or piercing object (Y37.45-)
military operations involving intentional restriction of air and airway (Y37.46-)
military operations involving unintentional restriction of air and airway (Y37.47-)
● **Y37.440** **Military operations involving unarmed hand to hand combat, military personnel**
● **Y37.441** **Military operations involving unarmed hand to hand combat, civilian**

● **Y37.45** **Military operations involving combat using blunt or piercing object**
● **Y37.450** **Military operations involving combat using blunt or piercing object, military personnel**
● **Y37.451** **Military operations involving combat using blunt or piercing object, civilian**

● **Y37.46** **Military operations involving intentional restriction of air and airway**
● **Y37.460** **Military operations involving intentional restriction of air and airway, military personnel**
● **Y37.461** **Military operations involving intentional restriction of air and airway, civilian**

● **Y37.47** **Military operations involving unintentional restriction of air and airway**
● **Y37.470** **Military operations involving unintentional restriction of air and airway, military personnel**
● **Y37.471** **Military operations involving unintentional restriction of air and airway, civilian**

● **Y37.49** **Military operations involving other forms of conventional warfare**
● **Y37.490** **Military operations involving other forms of conventional warfare, military personnel**
● **Y37.491** **Military operations involving other forms of conventional warfare, civilian**

◄ New ◀ Revised ~~deleted~~ Deleted | Excludes 1 | Excludes 2 | Includes | Use additional | Code first | Code also | Unspecified |
OGCR Official Guidelines X Assign placeholder X ● Use Additional Character(s) ▌ Manifestation Code **Coding Clinic**

● **Y37.5 Military operations involving nuclear weapons**
Military operation involving dirty bomb NOS

  ● **Y37.50 Military operations involving unspecified effect of nuclear weapon**

    ● **Y37.500 Military operations involving unspecified effect of nuclear weapon, military personnel**

    ● **Y37.501 Military operations involving unspecified effect of nuclear weapon, civilian**

  ● **Y37.51 Military operations involving direct blast effect of nuclear weapon**
Military operations involving blast pressure of nuclear weapon

    ● **Y37.510 Military operations involving direct blast effect of nuclear weapon, military personnel**

    ● **Y37.511 Military operations involving direct blast effect of nuclear weapon, civilian**

  ● **Y37.52 Military operations involving indirect blast effect of nuclear weapon**
Military operations involving being thrown by blast of nuclear weapon
Military operations involving being struck or crushed by blast debris of nuclear weapon

    ● **Y37.520 Military operations involving indirect blast effect of nuclear weapon, military personnel**

    ● **Y37.521 Military operations involving indirect blast effect of nuclear weapon, civilian**

  ● **Y37.53 Military operations involving thermal radiation effect of nuclear weapon**
Military operations involving direct heat from nuclear weapon
Military operation involving fireball effects from nuclear weapon

    ● **Y37.530 Military operations involving thermal radiation effect of nuclear weapon, military personnel**

    ● **Y37.531 Military operations involving thermal radiation effect of nuclear weapon, civilian**

  ● **Y37.54 Military operation involving nuclear radiation effects of nuclear weapon**
Military operation involving acute radiation exposure from nuclear weapon
Military operation involving exposure to immediate ionizing radiation from nuclear weapon
Military operation involving fallout exposure from nuclear weapon
Military operation involving secondary effects of nuclear weapons

    ● **Y37.540 Military operation involving nuclear radiation effects of nuclear weapon, military personnel**

    ● **Y37.541 Military operation involving nuclear radiation effects of nuclear weapon, civilian**

  ● **Y37.59 Military operation involving other effects of nuclear weapons**

    ● **Y37.590 Military operation involving other effects of nuclear weapons, military personnel**

    ● **Y37.591 Military operation involving other effects of nuclear weapons, civilian**

● **Y37.6 Military operations involving biological weapons**

  ● **Y37.6X Military operations involving biological weapons**

    ● **Y37.6X0 Military operations involving biological weapons, military personnel**

    ● **Y37.6X1 Military operations involving biological weapons, civilian**

● **Y37.7 Military operations involving chemical weapons and other forms of unconventional warfare**

  Excludes1   military operations involving incendiary devices (Y36.3-, Y36.5-)

  ● **Y37.7X Military operations involving chemical weapons and other forms of unconventional warfare**

    ● **Y37.7X0 Military operations involving chemical weapons and other forms of unconventional warfare, military personnel**

    ● **Y37.7X1 Military operations involving chemical weapons and other forms of unconventional warfare, civilian**

● **Y37.9 Other and unspecified military operations**

  X● **Y37.90 Military operations, unspecified**

  X● **Y37.91 Military operations involving unspecified weapon of mass destruction [WMD]**

  X● **Y37.92 Military operations involving friendly fire**

● **Y38 Terrorism**
These codes are for use to identify injuries resulting from the unlawful use of force or violence against persons or property to intimidate or coerce a government, the civilian population, or any segment thereof, in furtherance of political or social objective

Use additional code for place of occurrence (Y92.-)

The appropriate 7th character is to be added to each code from category Y38

A	initial encounter
D	subsequent encounter
S	sequela

● **Y38.0 Terrorism involving explosion of marine weapons**
Terrorism involving depth-charge
Terrorism involving marine mine
Terrorism involving mine NOS, at sea or in harbor
Terrorism involving sea-based artillery shell
Terrorism involving torpedo
Terrorism involving underwater blast

  ● **Y38.0X Terrorism involving explosion of marine weapons**

    ● **Y38.0X1 Terrorism involving explosion of marine weapons, public safety official injured**

    ● **Y38.0X2 Terrorism involving explosion of marine weapons, civilian injured**

    ● **Y38.0X3 Terrorism involving explosion of marine weapons, terrorist injured**

● **Y38.1 Terrorism involving destruction of aircraft**
Terrorism involving aircraft burned
Terrorism involving aircraft exploded
Terrorism involving aircraft being shot down
Terrorism involving aircraft used as a weapon

  ● **Y38.1X Terrorism involving destruction of aircraft**

    ● **Y38.1X1 Terrorism involving destruction of aircraft, public safety official injured**

    ● **Y38.1X2 Terrorism involving destruction of aircraft, civilian injured**

    ● **Y38.1X3 Terrorism involving destruction of aircraft, terrorist injured**

CHAPTER 20 (V01-Y99)

- ● Y38.2 **Terrorism involving other explosions and fragments**
  Terrorism involving antipersonnel (fragments) bomb
  Terrorism involving blast NOS
  Terrorism involving explosion NOS
  Terrorism involving explosion of breech block
  Terrorism involving explosion of cannon block
  Terrorism involving explosion (fragments) of artillery shell
  Terrorism involving explosion (fragments) of bomb
  Terrorism involving explosion (fragments) of grenade
  Terrorism involving explosion (fragments) of guided missile
  Terrorism involving explosion (fragments) of land mine
  Terrorism involving explosion of mortar bomb
  Terrorism involving explosion of munitions
  Terrorism involving explosion (fragments) of rocket
  Terrorism involving explosion (fragments) of shell
  Terrorism involving shrapnel
  Terrorism involving mine NOS, on land
  Excludes1 terrorism involving explosion of nuclear weapon (Y38.5)
  terrorism involving suicide bomber (Y38.81)
  - ● Y38.2X **Terrorism involving other explosions and fragments**
    - ● Y38.2X1 **Terrorism involving other explosions and fragments, public safety official injured**
    - ● Y38.2X2 **Terrorism involving other explosions and fragments, civilian injured**
    - ● Y38.2X3 **Terrorism involving other explosions and fragments, terrorist injured**
- ● Y38.3 **Terrorism involving fires, conflagration and hot substances**
  Terrorism involving conflagration NOS
  Terrorism involving fire NOS
  Terrorism involving petrol bomb
  Excludes1 terrorism involving fire or heat of nuclear weapon (Y38.5)
  - ● Y38.3X **Terrorism involving fires, conflagration and hot substances**
    - ● Y38.3X1 **Terrorism involving fires, conflagration and hot substances, public safety official injured**
    - ● Y38.3X2 **Terrorism involving fires, conflagration and hot substances, civilian injured**
    - ● Y38.3X3 **Terrorism involving fires, conflagration and hot substances, terrorist injured**
- ● Y38.4 **Terrorism involving firearms**
  Terrorism involving carbine bullet
  Terrorism involving machine gun bullet
  Terrorism involving pellets (shotgun)
  Terrorism involving pistol bullet
  Terrorism involving rifle bullet
  Terrorism involving rubber (rifle) bullet
  - ● Y38.4X **Terrorism involving firearms**
    - ● Y38.4X1 **Terrorism involving firearms, public safety official injured**
    - ● Y38.4X2 **Terrorism involving firearms, civilian injured**
    - ● Y38.4X3 **Terrorism involving firearms, terrorist injured**

- ● Y38.5 **Terrorism involving nuclear weapons**
  Terrorism involving blast effects of nuclear weapon
  Terrorism involving exposure to ionizing radiation from nuclear weapon
  Terrorism involving fireball effect of nuclear weapon
  Terrorism involving heat from nuclear weapon
  - ● Y38.5X **Terrorism involving nuclear weapons**
    - ● Y38.5X1 **Terrorism involving nuclear weapons, public safety official injured**
    - ● Y38.5X2 **Terrorism involving nuclear weapons, civilian injured**
    - ● Y38.5X3 **Terrorism involving nuclear weapons, terrorist injured**
- ● Y38.6 **Terrorism involving biological weapons**
  Terrorism involving anthrax
  Terrorism involving cholera
  A serious, often deadly, infectious disease of small intestine
  Terrorism involving smallpox
  - ● Y38.6X **Terrorism involving biological weapons**
    - ● Y38.6X1 **Terrorism involving biological weapons, public safety official injured**
    - ● Y38.6X2 **Terrorism involving biological weapons, civilian injured**
    - ● Y38.6X3 **Terrorism involving biological weapons, terrorist injured**
- ● Y38.7 **Terrorism involving chemical weapons**
  Terrorism involving gases, fumes, chemicals
  Terrorism involving hydrogen cyanide
  Terrorism involving phosgene
  Terrorism involving sarin
  - ● Y38.7X **Terrorism involving chemical weapons**
    - ● Y38.7X1 **Terrorism involving chemical weapons, public safety official injured**
    - ● Y38.7X2 **Terrorism involving chemical weapons, civilian injured**
    - ● Y38.7X3 **Terrorism involving chemical weapons, terrorist injured**
- ● Y38.8 **Terrorism involving other and unspecified means**
  - ● Y38.80 **Terrorism involving unspecified means**
    Terrorism NOS
  - ● Y38.81 **Terrorism involving suicide bomber**
    - ● Y38.811 **Terrorism involving suicide bomber, public safety official injured**
    - ● Y38.812 **Terrorism involving suicide bomber, civilian injured**
  - ● Y38.89 **Terrorism involving other means**
    Terrorism involving drowning and submersion
    Terrorism involving lasers
    Terrorism involving piercing or stabbing instruments
    - ● Y38.891 **Terrorism involving other means, public safety official injured**
    - ● Y38.892 **Terrorism involving other means, civilian injured**
    - ● Y38.893 **Terrorism involving other means, terrorist injured**
- ● Y38.9 **Terrorism, secondary effects**
  Note: This code is for use to identify conditions occurring subsequent to a terrorist attack not those that are due to the initial terrorist attack.
  - ● Y38.9X **Terrorism, secondary effects**
    - ● Y38.9X1 **Terrorism, secondary effects, public safety official injured**
    - ● Y38.9X2 **Terrorism, secondary effects, civilian injured categories**

◄ New ◄▬ Revised ~~deleted~~ Deleted | Excludes 1 | Excludes 2 | Includes | Use additional | Code first | Code also | Unspecified |
OGCR Official Guidelines X Assign placeholder X ● Use Additional Character(s) ▶ Manifestation Code **Coding Clinic**

COMPLICATIONS OF MEDICAL AND SURGICAL CARE (Y62-Y84)

| **Includes** | complications of medical devices surgical and medical procedures as the cause of abnormal reaction of the patient, or of later complication, without mention of misadventure at the time of the procedure |

MISADVENTURES TO PATIENTS DURING SURGICAL AND MEDICAL CARE (Y62-Y69)

| **Excludes2** | breakdown or malfunctioning of medical device (during procedure) (after implantation) (ongoing use) (Y70-Y82) |
| | surgical and medical procedures as the cause of abnormal reaction of the patient, without mention of misadventure at the time of the procedure (Y83-Y84) |

● Y62   Failure of sterile precautions during surgical and medical care

Y62.0   Failure of sterile precautions during surgical operation

Y62.1   Failure of sterile precautions during infusion or transfusion

Y62.2   Failure of sterile precautions during kidney dialysis and other perfusion

Y62.3   Failure of sterile precautions during injection or immunization

Y62.4   Failure of sterile precautions during endoscopic examination

Y62.5   Failure of sterile precautions during heart catheterization

Y62.6   Failure of sterile precautions during aspiration, puncture and other catheterization

Y62.8   Failure of sterile precautions during other surgical and medical care

Y62.9   Failure of sterile precautions during unspecified surgical and medical care

● Y63   Failure in dosage during surgical and medical care

| **Excludes2** | accidental overdose of drug or wrong drug given in error (T36-T50) |

Y63.0   Excessive amount of blood or other fluid given during transfusion or infusion

Y63.1   Incorrect dilution of fluid used during infusion

Y63.2   Overdose of radiation given during therapy

Y63.3   Inadvertent exposure of patient to radiation during medical care

Y63.4   Failure in dosage in electroshock or insulin-shock therapy

Y63.5   Inappropriate temperature in local application and packing

Y63.6   Underdosing and nonadministration of necessary drug, medicament or biological substance

Y63.8   Failure in dosage during other surgical and medical care

Y63.9   Failure in dosage during unspecified surgical and medical care

● Y64   Contaminated medical or biological substances

Y64.0   Contaminated medical or biological substance, transfused or infused

Y64.1   Contaminated medical or biological substance, injected or used for immunization

Y64.8   Contaminated medical or biological substance administered by other means

Y64.9   Contaminated medical or biological substance administered by unspecified means
         Administered contaminated medical or biological substance NOS

● Y65   Other misadventures during surgical and medical care

Y65.0   Mismatched blood in transfusion

Y65.1   Wrong fluid used in infusion

Y65.2   Failure in suture or ligature during surgical operation

Y65.3   Endotracheal tube wrongly placed during anesthetic procedure

Y65.4   Failure to introduce or to remove other tube or instrument

● Y65.5   Performance of wrong procedure (operation)

● Y65.51   Performance of wrong procedure (operation) on correct patient
             Wrong device implanted into correct surgical site

| **Excludes1** | performance of correct procedure (operation) on wrong side or body part (Y65.53) |

● Y65.52   Performance of procedure (operation) on patient not scheduled for surgery
             Performance of procedure (operation) intended for another patient
             Performance of procedure (operation) on wrong patient

● Y65.53   Performance of correct procedure (operation) on wrong side or body part
             Performance of correct procedure (operation) on wrong side
             Performance of correct procedure (operation) on wrong site

Y65.8   Other specified misadventures during surgical and medical care

Y66   Nonadministration of surgical and medical care
         Premature cessation of surgical and medical care

| **Excludes1** | DNR status (Z66) |
| | palliative care (Z51.5) |

Y69   Unspecified misadventure during surgical and medical care

MEDICAL DEVICES ASSOCIATED WITH ADVERSE INCIDENTS IN DIAGNOSTIC AND THERAPEUTIC USE (Y70-Y82)

| **Includes** | breakdown or malfunction of medical devices (during use) (after implantation) (ongoing use) |

| **Excludes1** | misadventure to patients during surgical and medical care, classifiable to (Y62-Y69) |
| | later complications following use of medical devices without breakdown or malfunctioning of device (Y83-Y84) |

● Y70   Anesthesiology devices associated with adverse incidents

Y70.0   Diagnostic and monitoring anesthesiology devices associated with adverse incidents

Y70.1   Therapeutic (nonsurgical) and rehabilitative anesthesiology devices associated with adverse incidents

Y70.2   Prosthetic and other implants, materials and accessory anesthesiology devices associated with adverse incidents

Y70.3   Surgical instruments, materials and anesthesiology devices (including sutures) associated with adverse incidents

Y70.8   Miscellaneous anesthesiology devices associated with adverse incidents, not elsewhere classified

CHAPTER 20 (V01-Y99)

● Y71 **Cardiovascular devices associated with adverse incidents**

   Y71.0 Diagnostic and monitoring cardiovascular devices associated with adverse incidents

   Y71.1 Therapeutic (nonsurgical) and rehabilitative cardiovascular devices associated with adverse incidents

   Y71.2 Prosthetic and other implants, materials and accessory cardiovascular devices associated with adverse incidents

   Y71.3 Surgical instruments, materials and cardiovascular devices (including sutures) associated with adverse incidents

   Y71.8 Miscellaneous cardiovascular devices associated with adverse incidents, not elsewhere classified

● Y72 **Otorhinolaryngological devices associated with adverse incidents**

   Y72.0 Diagnostic and monitoring otorhinolaryngological devices associated with adverse incidents

   Y72.1 Therapeutic (nonsurgical) and rehabilitative otorhinolaryngological devices associated with adverse incidents

   Y72.2 Prosthetic and other implants, materials and accessory otorhinolaryngological devices associated with adverse incidents

   Y72.3 Surgical instruments, materials and otorhinolaryngological devices (including sutures) associated with adverse incidents

   Y72.8 Miscellaneous otorhinolaryngological devices associated with adverse incidents, not elsewhere classified

● Y73 **Gastroenterology and urology devices associated with adverse incidents**

   Y73.0 Diagnostic and monitoring gastroenterology and urology devices associated with adverse incidents

   Y73.1 Therapeutic (nonsurgical) and rehabilitative gastroenterology and urology devices associated with adverse incidents

   Y73.2 Prosthetic and other implants, materials and accessory gastroenterology and urology devices associated with adverse incidents

   Y73.3 Surgical instruments, materials and gastroenterology and urology devices (including sutures) associated with adverse incidents

   Y73.8 Miscellaneous gastroenterology and urology devices associated with adverse incidents, not elsewhere classified

● Y74 **General hospital and personal-use devices associated with adverse incidents**

   Y74.0 Diagnostic and monitoring general hospital and personal-use devices associated with adverse incidents

   Y74.1 Therapeutic (nonsurgical) and rehabilitative general hospital and personal-use devices associated with adverse incidents

   Y74.2 Prosthetic and other implants, materials and accessory general hospital and personal-use devices associated with adverse incidents

   Y74.3 Surgical instruments, materials and general hospital and personal-use devices (including sutures) associated with adverse incidents

   Y74.8 Miscellaneous general hospital and personal-use devices associated with adverse incidents, not elsewhere classified

● Y75 **Neurological devices associated with adverse incidents**

   Y75.0 Diagnostic and monitoring neurological devices associated with adverse incidents

   Y75.1 Therapeutic (nonsurgical) and rehabilitative neurological devices associated with adverse incidents

   Y75.2 Prosthetic and other implants, materials and neurological devices associated with adverse incidents

   Y75.3 Surgical instruments, materials and neurological devices (including sutures) associated with adverse incidents

   Y75.8 Miscellaneous neurological devices associated with adverse incidents, not elsewhere classified

● Y76 **Obstetric and gynecological devices associated with adverse incidents**

   Y76.0 Diagnostic and monitoring obstetric and gynecological devices associated with adverse incidents ♀

   Y76.1 Therapeutic (nonsurgical) and rehabilitative obstetric and gynecological devices associated with adverse incidents ♀

   Y76.2 Prosthetic and other implants, materials and accessory obstetric and gynecological devices associated with adverse incidents ♀

   Y76.3 Surgical instruments, materials and obstetric and gynecological devices (including sutures) associated with adverse incidents ♀

   Y76.8 Miscellaneous obstetric and gynecological devices associated with adverse incidents, not elsewhere classified ♀

● Y77 **Ophthalmic devices associated with adverse incidents**

   Y77.0 Diagnostic and monitoring ophthalmic devices associated with adverse incidents

   Y77.1 Therapeutic (nonsurgical) and rehabilitative ophthalmic devices associated with adverse incidents

   Y77.2 Prosthetic and other implants, materials and accessory ophthalmic devices associated with adverse incidents

   Y77.3 Surgical instruments, materials and ophthalmic devices (including sutures) associated with adverse incidents

   Y77.8 Miscellaneous ophthalmic devices associated with adverse incidents, not elsewhere classified

● Y78 **Radiological devices associated with adverse incidents**

   Y78.0 Diagnostic and monitoring radiological devices associated with adverse incidents

   Y78.1 Therapeutic (nonsurgical) and rehabilitative radiological devices associated with adverse incidents

   Y78.2 Prosthetic and other implants, materials and accessory radiological devices associated with adverse incidents

   Y78.3 Surgical instruments, materials and radiological devices (including sutures) associated with adverse incidents

   Y78.8 Miscellaneous radiological devices associated with adverse incidents, not elsewhere classified

● Y79 **Orthopedic devices associated with adverse incidents**

   Y79.0 Diagnostic and monitoring orthopedic devices associated with adverse incidents

   Y79.1 Therapeutic (nonsurgical) and rehabilitative orthopedic devices associated with adverse incidents

   Y79.2 Prosthetic and other implants, materials and accessory orthopedic devices associated with adverse incidents

   Y79.3 Surgical instruments, materials and orthopedic devices (including sutures) associated with adverse incidents

   Y79.8 Miscellaneous orthopedic devices associated with adverse incidents, not elsewhere classified

◀ New   ◀▥ Revised   d̶e̶l̶e̶t̶e̶d̶ Deleted   Excludes 1   Excludes 2   Includes   Use additional   Code first   Code also   Unspecified

OGCR Official Guidelines   X Assign placeholder X   ● Use Additional Character(s)   ▶ Manifestation Code   **Coding Clinic**

● Y80   Physical medicine devices associated with adverse incidents

Y80.0   Diagnostic and monitoring physical medicine devices associated with adverse incidents

Y80.1   Therapeutic (nonsurgical) and rehabilitative physical medicine devices associated with adverse incidents

Y80.2   Prosthetic and other implants, materials and accessory physical medicine devices associated with adverse incidents

Y80.3   Surgical instruments, materials and physical medicine devices (including sutures) associated with adverse incidents

Y80.8   Miscellaneous physical medicine devices associated with adverse incidents, not elsewhere classified

● Y81   General- and plastic-surgery devices associated with adverse incidents

Y81.0   Diagnostic and monitoring general- and plastic-surgery devices associated with adverse incidents

Y81.1   Therapeutic (nonsurgical) and rehabilitative general- and plastic-surgery devices associated with adverse incidents

Y81.2   Prosthetic and other implants, materials and accessory general- and plastic-surgery devices associated with adverse incidents

Y81.3   Surgical instruments, materials and general- and plastic-surgery devices (including sutures) associated with adverse incidents

Y81.8   Miscellaneous general- and plastic-surgery devices associated with adverse incidents, not elsewhere classified

● Y82   Other and unspecified medical devices associated with adverse incidents

Y82.8   Other medical devices associated with adverse incidents

Y82.9   Unspecified medical devices associated with adverse incidents

---

SURGICAL AND OTHER MEDICAL PROCEDURES AS THE CAUSE OF ABNORMAL REACTION OF THE PATIENT, OR OF LATER COMPLICATION, WITHOUT MENTION OF MISADVENTURE AT THE TIME OF THE PROCEDURE (Y83-Y84)

> **Excludes1**   misadventures to patients during surgical and medical care, classifiable to (Y62-Y69)

● Y83   Surgical operation and other surgical procedures as the cause of abnormal reaction of the patient, or of later complication, without mention of misadventure at the time of the procedure

Y83.0   Surgical operation with transplant of whole organ as the cause of abnormal reaction of the patient, or of later complication, without mention of misadventure at the time of the procedure

Y83.1   Surgical operation with implant of artificial internal device as the cause of abnormal reaction of the patient, or of later complication, without mention of misadventure at the time of the procedure

Y83.2   Surgical operation with anastomosis, bypass or graft as the cause of abnormal reaction of the patient, or of later complication, without mention of misadventure at the time of the procedure

Y83.3   Surgical operation with formation of external stoma as the cause of abnormal reaction of the patient, or of later complication, without mention of misadventure at the time of the procedure

Y83.4   Other reconstructive surgery as the cause of abnormal reaction of the patient, or of later complication, without mention of misadventure at the time of the procedure

Y83.5   Amputation of limb(s) as the cause of abnormal reaction of the patient, or of later complication, without mention of misadventure at the time of the procedure

Y83.6   Removal of other organ (partial) (total) as the cause of abnormal reaction of the patient, or of later complication, without mention of misadventure at the time of the procedure

Y83.8   Other surgical procedures as the cause of abnormal reaction of the patient, or of later complication, without mention of misadventure at the time of the procedure

Y83.9   Surgical procedure, unspecified as the cause of abnormal reaction of the patient, or of later complication, without mention of misadventure at the time of the procedure

● Y84   Other medical procedures as the cause of abnormal reaction of the patient, or of later complication, without mention of misadventure at the time of the procedure

Y84.0   Cardiac catheterization as the cause of abnormal reaction of the patient, or of later complication, without mention of misadventure at the time of the procedure

Y84.1   Kidney dialysis as the cause of abnormal reaction of the patient, or of later complication, without mention of misadventure at the time of the procedure

Y84.2   Radiological procedure and radiotherapy as the cause of abnormal reaction of the patient, or of later complication, without mention of misadventure at the time of the procedure

Y84.3   Shock therapy as the cause of abnormal reaction of the patient, or of later complication, without mention of misadventure at the time of the procedure

Y84.4   Aspiration of fluid as the cause of abnormal reaction of the patient, or of later complication, without mention of misadventure at the time of the procedure

Y84.5   Insertion of gastric or duodenal sound as the cause of abnormal reaction of the patient, or of later complication, without mention of misadventure at the time of the procedure

Y84.6   Urinary catheterization as the cause of abnormal reaction of the patient, or of later complication, without mention of misadventure at the time of the procedure

Y84.7   Blood-sampling as the cause of abnormal reaction of the patient, or of later complication, without mention of misadventure at the time of the procedure

Y84.8   Other medical procedures as the cause of abnormal reaction of the patient, or of later complication, without mention of misadventure at the time of the procedure

Y84.9   Medical procedure, unspecified as the cause of abnormal reaction of the patient, or of later complication, without mention of misadventure at the time of the procedure

---

SUPPLEMENTARY FACTORS RELATED TO CAUSES OF MORBIDITY CLASSIFIED ELSEWHERE (Y90-Y99)

Note: These categories may be used to provide supplementary information concerning causes of morbidity. They are not to be used for single-condition coding.

● Y90   Evidence of alcohol involvement determined by blood alcohol level

Code first any associated alcohol related disorders (F10)

Y90.0   Blood alcohol level of less than 20 mg/100 ml

Y90.1   Blood alcohol level of 20-39 mg/100 ml

Y90.2   Blood alcohol level of 40-59 mg/100 ml

Y90.3   Blood alcohol level of 60-79 mg/100 ml

Y90.4   Blood alcohol level of 80-99 mg/100 ml

Y90.5   Blood alcohol level of 100-119 mg/100 ml

Y90.6   Blood alcohol level of 120-199 mg/100 ml

Y90.7   Blood alcohol level of 200-239 mg/100 ml

Y90.8   Blood alcohol level of 240 mg/100 ml or more

Y90.9   Presence of alcohol in blood, level not specified

OGCR Section I.C.20.b.

20.9 Place of Occurrence

Place of Occurrence Guideline

Codes from category Y92, Place of occurrence of the external cause, are secondary codes for use after other external cause codes to identify the location of the patient at the time of injury or other condition.

Generally, a place of occurrence code is assigned only once, at the initial encounter for treatment. However, in the rare instance that a new injury occurs during hospitalization, an additional place of occurrence code may be assigned. No 7th characters are used for Y92. Only one code from Y92 should be recorded on a medical record. A place of occurrence code should be used in conjunction with an activity code, Y93.

Do not use place of occurrence code Y92.9 if the place is not stated or is not applicable.

● **Y92　Place of occurrence of the external cause**

The following category is for use, when relevant, to identify the place of occurrence of the external cause. Use in conjunction with an activity code.

Place of occurrence should be recorded only at the initial encounter for treatment

● **Y92.0　Non-institutional (private) residence as the place of occurrence of the external cause**

Excludes1　abandoned or derelict house (Y92.89)
home under construction but not yet occupied (Y92.6-)
institutional place of residence (Y92.1-)

● **Y92.00　Unspecified non-institutional (private) residence as the place of occurrence of the external cause**

Y92.000　Kitchen of unspecified non-institutional (private) residence as the place of occurrence of the external cause

Y92.001　Dining room of unspecified non-institutional (private) residence as the place of occurrence of the external cause

Y92.002　Bathroom of unspecified non-institutional (private) residence single-family (private) house as the place of occurrence of the external cause

Y92.003　Bedroom of unspecified non-institutional (private) residence as the place of occurrence of the external cause

Y92.007　Garden or yard of unspecified non-institutional (private) residence as the place of occurrence of the external cause

Y92.008　Other place in unspecified non-institutional (private) residence as the place of occurrence of the external cause

Y92.009　Unspecified place in unspecified non-institutional (private) residence as the place of occurrence of the external cause
Home (NOS) as the place of occurrence of the external cause

● **Y92.01　Single-family non-institutional (private) house as the place of occurrence of the external cause**
Farmhouse as the place of occurrence of the external cause

Excludes1　barn (Y92.71)
chicken coop or hen house (Y92.72)
farm field (Y92.73)
orchard (Y92.74)
single family mobile home or trailer (Y92.02-)
slaughter house (Y92.86)

Y92.010　Kitchen of single-family (private) house as the place of occurrence of the external cause

Y92.011　Dining room of single-family (private) house as the place of occurrence of the external cause

Y92.012　Bathroom of single-family (private) house as the place of occurrence of the external cause

Y92.013　Bedroom of single-family (private) house as the place of occurrence of the external cause

Y92.014　Private driveway to single-family (private) house as the place of occurrence of the external cause

Y92.015　Private garage of single-family (private) house as the place of occurrence of the external cause

Y92.016　Swimming pool in single-family (private) house or garden as the place of occurrence of the external cause

Y92.017　Garden or yard in single-family (private) house as the place of occurrence of the external cause

Y92.018　Other place in single-family (private) house as the place of occurrence of the external cause

Y92.019　Unspecified place in single-family (private) house as the place of occurrence of the external cause

● **Y92.02　Mobile home as the place of occurrence of the external cause**

Y92.020　Kitchen in mobile home as the place of occurrence of the external cause

Y92.021　Dining room in mobile home as the place of occurrence of the external cause

Y92.022　Bathroom in mobile home as the place of occurrence of the external cause

Y92.023　Bedroom in mobile home as the place of occurrence of the external cause

Y92.024　Driveway of mobile home as the place of occurrence of the external cause

Y92.025　Garage of mobile home as the place of occurrence of the external cause

Y92.026　Swimming pool of mobile home as the place of occurrence of the external cause

Y92.027　Garden or yard of mobile home as the place of occurrence of the external cause

Y92.028　Other place in mobile home as the place of occurrence of the external cause

Y92.029　Unspecified place in mobile home as the place of occurrence of the external cause

● **Y92.03**   **Apartment as the place of occurrence of the external cause**
Condominium as the place of occurrence of the external cause
Co-op apartment as the place of occurrence of the external cause

   Y92.030   Kitchen in apartment as the place of occurrence of the external cause

   Y92.031   Bathroom in apartment as the place of occurrence of the external cause

   Y92.032   Bedroom in apartment as the place of occurrence of the external cause

   Y92.038   Other place in apartment as the place of occurrence of the external cause

   Y92.039   Unspecified place in apartment as the place of occurrence of the external cause

● **Y92.04**   **Boarding-house as the place of occurrence of the external cause**

   Y92.040   Kitchen in boarding-house as the place of occurrence of the external cause

   Y92.041   Bathroom in boarding-house as the place of occurrence of the external cause

   Y92.042   Bedroom in boarding-house as the place of occurrence of the external cause

   Y92.043   Driveway of boarding-house as the place of occurrence of the external cause

   Y92.044   Garage of boarding-house as the place of occurrence of the external cause

   Y92.045   Swimming pool of boarding-house as the place of occurrence of the external cause

   Y92.046   Garden or yard of boarding-house as the place of occurrence of the external cause

   Y92.048   Other place in boarding-house as the place of occurrence of the external cause

   Y92.049   Unspecified place in boarding-house as the place of occurrence of the external cause

● **Y92.09**   **Other non-institutional residence as the place of occurrence of the external cause**

   Y92.090   Kitchen in other non-institutional residence as the place of occurrence of the external cause

   Y92.091   Bathroom in other non-institutional residence as the place of occurrence of the external cause

   Y92.092   Bedroom in other non-institutional residence as the place of occurrence of the external cause

   Y92.093   Driveway of other non-institutional residence as the place of occurrence of the external cause

   Y92.094   Garage of other non-institutional residence as the place of occurrence of the external cause

   Y92.095   Swimming pool of other non-institutional residence as the place of occurrence of the external cause

   Y92.096   Garden or yard of other non-institutional residence as the place of occurrence of the external cause

   Y92.098   Other place in other non-institutional residence as the place of occurrence of the external cause

   Y92.099   Unspecified place in other non-institutional residence as the place of occurrence of the external cause

● **Y92.1**   **Institutional (nonprivate) residence as the place of occurrence of the external cause**

   Y92.10   Unspecified residential institution as the place of occurrence of the external cause

● **Y92.11**   **Children's home and orphanage as the place of occurrence of the external cause**

   Y92.110   Kitchen in children's home and orphanage as the place of occurrence of the external cause

   Y92.111   Bathroom in children's home and orphanage as the place of occurrence of the external cause

   Y92.112   Bedroom in children's home and orphanage as the place of occurrence of the external cause

   Y92.113   Driveway of children's home and orphanage as the place of occurrence of the external cause

   Y92.114   Garage of children's home and orphanage as the place of occurrence of the external cause

   Y92.115   Swimming pool of children's home and orphanage as the place of occurrence of the external cause

   Y92.116   Garden or yard of children's home and orphanage as the place of occurrence of the external cause

   Y92.118   Other place in children's home and orphanage as the place of occurrence of the external cause

   Y92.119   Unspecified place in children's home and orphanage as the place of occurrence of the external cause

● **Y92.12**   **Nursing home as the place of occurrence of the external cause**
Home for the sick as the place of occurrence of the external cause
Hospice as the place of occurrence of the external cause

   Y92.120   Kitchen in nursing home as the place of occurrence of the external cause

   Y92.121   Bathroom in nursing home as the place of occurrence of the external cause

   Y92.122   Bedroom in nursing home as the place of occurrence of the external cause

   Y92.123   Driveway of nursing home as the place of occurrence of the external cause

   Y92.124   Garage of nursing home as the place of occurrence of the external cause

   Y92.125   Swimming pool of nursing home as the place of occurrence of the external cause

   Y92.126   Garden or yard of nursing home as the place of occurrence of the external cause

   Y92.128   Other place in nursing home as the place of occurrence of the external cause

   Y92.129   Unspecified place in nursing home as the place of occurrence of the external cause

● Y92.13   Military base as the place of occurrence of the external cause
            Excludes1   military training grounds (Y92.83)

Y92.130   Kitchen on military base as the place of occurrence of the external cause

Y92.131   Mess hall on military base as the place of occurrence of the external cause

Y92.133   Barracks on military base as the place of occurrence of the external cause

Y92.135   Garage on military base as the place of occurrence of the external cause

Y92.136   Swimming pool on military base as the place of occurrence of the external cause

Y92.137   Garden or yard on military base as the place of occurrence of the external cause

Y92.138   Other place on military base as the place of occurrence of the external cause

Y92.139   Unspecified place military base as the place of occurrence of the external cause

● Y92.14   Prison as the place of occurrence of the external cause

Y92.140   Kitchen in prison as the place of occurrence of the external cause

Y92.141   Dining room in prison as the place of occurrence of the external cause

Y92.142   Bathroom in prison as the place of occurrence of the external cause

Y92.143   Cell of prison as the place of occurrence of the external cause

Y92.146   Swimming pool of prison as the place of occurrence of the external cause

Y92.147   Courtyard of prison as the place of occurrence of the external cause

Y92.148   Other place in prison as the place of occurrence of the external cause

Y92.149   Unspecified place in prison as the place of occurrence of the external cause

● Y92.15   Reform school as the place of occurrence of the external cause

Y92.150   Kitchen in reform school as the place of occurrence of the external cause

Y92.151   Dining room in reform school as the place of occurrence of the external cause

Y92.152   Bathroom in reform school as the place of occurrence of the external cause

Y92.153   Bedroom in reform school as the place of occurrence of the external cause

Y92.154   Driveway of reform school as the place of occurrence of the external cause

Y92.155   Garage of reform school as the place of occurrence of the external cause

Y92.156   Swimming pool of reform school as the place of occurrence of the external cause

Y92.157   Garden or yard of reform school as the place of occurrence of the external cause

Y92.158   Other place in reform school as the place of occurrence of the external cause

Y92.159   Unspecified place in reform school as the place of occurrence of the external cause

● Y92.16   School dormitory as the place of occurrence of the external cause
            Excludes1   reform school as the place of occurrence of the external cause (Y92.15-)
                             school buildings and grounds as the place of occurrence of the external cause (Y92.2-)
                             school sports and athletic areas as the place of occurrence of the external cause (Y92.3-)

Y92.160   Kitchen in school dormitory as the place of occurrence of the external cause

Y92.161   Dining room in school dormitory as the place of occurrence of the external cause

Y92.162   Bathroom in school dormitory as the place of occurrence of the external cause

Y92.163   Bedroom in school dormitory as the place of occurrence of the external cause

Y92.168   Other place in school dormitory as the place of occurrence of the external cause

Y92.169   Unspecified place in school dormitory as the place of occurrence of the external cause

● Y92.19   Other specified residential institution as the place of occurrence of the external cause

Y92.190   Kitchen in other specified residential institution as the place of occurrence of the external cause

Y92.191   Dining room in other specified residential institution as the place of occurrence of the external cause

Y92.192   Bathroom in other specified residential institution as the place of occurrence of the external cause

Y92.193   Bedroom in other specified residential institution as the place of occurrence of the external cause

Y92.194   Driveway of other specified residential institution as the place of occurrence of the external cause

Y92.195   Garage of other specified residential institution as the place of occurrence of the external cause

Y92.196   Pool of other specified residential institution as the place of occurrence of the external cause

Y92.197   Garden or yard of other specified residential institution as the place of occurrence of the external cause

Y92.198   Other place in other specified residential institution as the place of occurrence of the external cause

Y92.199   Unspecified place in other specified residential institution as the place of occurrence of the external cause

◀ New   ◀▦ Revised   ~~deleted~~ Deleted   Excludes 1   Excludes 2   Includes   Use additional   Code first   Code also   Unspecified
OGCR Official Guidelines   X Assign placeholder X   ● Use Additional Character(s)   ▶ Manifestation Code   **Coding Clinic**

● **Y92.2**   **School, other institution and public administrative area as the place of occurrence of the external cause**

Building and adjacent grounds used by the general public or by a particular group of the public

Excludes1   building under construction as the place of occurrence of the external cause (Y92.6)

residential institution as the place of occurrence of the external cause (Y92.1)

school dormitory as the place of occurrence of the external cause (Y92.16-)

sports and athletics area of schools as the place of occurrence of the external cause (Y92.3-)

● **Y92.21**   **School (private) (public) (state) as the place of occurrence of the external cause**

Y92.210   Daycare center as the place of occurrence of the external cause

Y92.211   Elementary school as the place of occurrence of the external cause

Kindergarten as the place of occurrence of the external cause

Y92.212   Middle school as the place of occurrence of the external cause

Y92.213   High school as the place of occurrence of the external cause

Coding Clinic: 2012, Q4, P108

Y92.214   College as the place of occurrence of the external cause

University as the place of occurrence of the external cause

Y92.215   Trade school as the place of occurrence of the external cause

Y92.218   Other school as the place of occurrence of the external cause

Y92.219   Unspecified school as the place of occurrence of the external cause

Y92.22   **Religious institution as the place of occurrence of the external cause**

Church as the place of occurrence of the external cause

Mosque as the place of occurrence of the external cause

Synagogue as the place of occurrence of the external cause

● **Y92.23**   **Hospital as the place of occurrence of the external cause**

Excludes1   ambulatory (outpatient) health services establishments (Y92.53-)

home for the sick as the place of occurrence of the external cause (Y92.12-)

hospice as the place of occurrence of the external cause (Y92.12-)

nursing home as the place of occurrence of the external cause (Y92.12-)

Y92.230   Patient room in hospital as the place of occurrence of the external cause

Y92.231   Patient bathroom in hospital as the place of occurrence of the external cause

Y92.232   Corridor of hospital as the place of occurrence of the external cause

Y92.233   Cafeteria of hospital as the place of occurrence of the external cause

Y92.234   Operating room of hospital as the place of occurrence of the external cause

Y92.238   Other place in hospital as the place of occurrence of the external cause

Y92.239   Unspecified place in hospital as the place of occurrence of the external cause

● **Y92.24**   **Public administrative building as the place of occurrence of the external cause**

Y92.240   Courthouse as the place of occurrence of the external cause

Y92.241   Library as the place of occurrence of the external cause

Y92.242   Post office as the place of occurrence of the external cause

Y92.243   City hall as the place of occurrence of the external cause

Y92.248   Other public administrative building as the place of occurrence of the external cause

● **Y92.25**   **Cultural building as the place of occurrence of the external cause**

Y92.250   Art gallery as the place of occurrence of the external cause

Y92.251   Museum as the place of occurrence of the external cause

Y92.252   Music hall as the place of occurrence of the external cause

Y92.253   Opera house as the place of occurrence of the external cause

Y92.254   Theater (live) as the place of occurrence of the external cause

Y92.258   Other cultural public building as the place of occurrence of the external cause

Y92.26   **Movie house or cinema as the place of occurrence of the external cause**

Y92.29   **Other specified public building as the place of occurrence of the external cause**

Assembly hall as the place of occurrence of the external cause

Clubhouse as the place of occurrence of the external cause

● **Y92.3**   **Sports and athletics area as the place of occurrence of the external cause**

● **Y92.31**   **Athletic court as the place of occurrence of the external cause**

Excludes1   tennis court in private home or garden (Y92.09)

Y92.310   Basketball court as the place of occurrence of the external cause

Y92.311   Squash court as the place of occurrence of the external cause

Y92.312   Tennis court as the place of occurrence of the external cause

Y92.318   Other athletic court as the place of occurrence of the external cause

● **Y92.32**   **Athletic field as the place of occurrence of the external cause**

Y92.320   Baseball field as the place of occurrence of the external cause

Y92.321   Football field as the place of occurrence of the external cause

Y92.322   Soccer field as the place of occurrence of the external cause

Y92.328   Other athletic field as the place of occurrence of the external cause

Cricket field as the place of occurrence of the external cause

Hockey field as the place of occurrence of the external cause

● **Y92.33**   **Skating rink as the place of occurrence of the external cause**

     Y92.330   **Ice skating rink (indoor) (outdoor) as the place of occurrence of the external cause**

     Y92.331   **Roller skating rink as the place of occurrence of the external cause**

   Y92.34   **Swimming pool (public) as the place of occurrence of the external cause**

     Excludes1   swimming pool in private home or garden (Y92.016)

   Y92.39   **Other specified sports and athletic area as the place of occurrence of the external cause**

     Golf-course as the place of occurrence of the external cause

     Gymnasium as the place of occurrence of the external cause

     Riding-school as the place of occurrence of the external cause

     Stadium as the place of occurrence of the external cause

● **Y92.4**   **Street, highway and other paved roadways as the place of occurrence of the external cause**

     Excludes1   private driveway of residence (Y92.014, Y92.024, Y92.043, Y92.093, Y92.113, Y92.123, Y92.154, Y92.194)

   ● **Y92.41**   **Street and highway as the place of occurrence of the external cause**

     Y92.410   **Unspecified street and highway as the place of occurrence of the external cause**

       Road NOS as the place of occurrence of the external cause

     Y92.411   **Interstate highway as the place of occurrence of the external cause**

       Freeway as the place of occurrence of the external cause

       Motorway as the place of occurrence of the external cause

     Y92.412   **Parkway as the place of occurrence of the external cause**

     Y92.413   **State road as the place of occurrence of the external cause**

     Y92.414   **Local residential or business street as the place of occurrence of the external cause**

     Y92.415   **Exit ramp or entrance ramp of street or highway as the place of occurrence of the external cause**

   ● **Y92.48**   **Other paved roadways as the place of occurrence of the external cause**

     Y92.480   **Sidewalk as the place of occurrence of the external cause**

     Y92.481   **Parking lot as the place of occurrence of the external cause**

     Y92.482   **Bike path as the place of occurrence of the external cause**

     Y92.488   **Other paved roadways as the place of occurrence of the external cause**

● **Y92.5**   **Trade and service area as the place of occurrence of the external cause**

     Excludes1   garage in private home (Y92.015) schools and other public administration buildings (Y92.2-)

   ● **Y92.51**   **Private commercial establishments as the place of occurrence of the external cause**

     Y92.510   **Bank as the place of occurrence of the external cause**

     Y92.511   **Restaurant or café as the place of occurrence of the external cause**

     Y92.512   **Supermarket, store or market as the place of occurrence of the external cause**

     Y92.513   **Shop (commercial) as the place of occurrence of the external cause**

   ● **Y92.52**   **Service areas as the place of occurrence of the external cause**

     Y92.520   **Airport as the place of occurrence of the external cause**

     Y92.521   **Bus station as the place of occurrence of the external cause**

     Y92.522   **Railway station as the place of occurrence of the external cause**

     Y92.523   **Highway rest stop as the place of occurrence of the external cause**

     Y92.524   **Gas station as the place of occurrence of the external cause**

       Petroleum station as the place of occurrence of the external cause

       Service station as the place of occurrence of the external cause

   ● **Y92.53**   **Ambulatory health services establishments as the place of occurrence of the external cause**

     Y92.530   **Ambulatory surgery center as the place of occurrence of the external cause**

       Outpatient surgery center, including that connected with a hospital as the place of occurrence of the external cause

       Same day surgery center, including that connected with a hospital as the place of occurrence of the external cause

     Y92.531   **Health care provider office as the place of occurrence of the external cause**

       Physician office as the place of occurrence of the external cause

     Y92.532   **Urgent care center as the place of occurrence of the external cause**

     Y92.538   **Other ambulatory health services establishments as the place of occurrence of the external cause**

   Y92.59   **Other trade areas as the place of occurrence of the external cause**

     Office building as the place of occurrence of the external cause

     Casino as the place of occurrence of the external cause

     Garage (commercial) as the place of occurrence of the external cause

     Hotel as the place of occurrence of the external cause

     Radio or television station as the place of occurrence of the external cause

     Shopping mall as the place of occurrence of the external cause

     Warehouse as the place of occurrence of the external cause

◀ New   ⬛ Revised   ~~deleted~~ Deleted   Excludes 1   Excludes 2   Includes   Use additional   Code first   Code also   Unspecified

OGCR Official Guidelines   X Assign placeholder X   ● Use Additional Character(s)   ▶ Manifestation Code   **Coding Clinic**

● **Y92.6**   **Industrial and construction area as the place of occurrence of the external cause**

     Y92.61   **Building [any] under construction as the place of occurrence of the external cause**

     Y92.62   **Dock or shipyard as the place of occurrence of the external cause**

         Dockyard as the place of occurrence of the external cause

         Dry dock as the place of occurrence of the external cause

         Shipyard as the place of occurrence of the external cause

     Y92.63   **Factory as the place of occurrence of the external cause**

         Factory building as the place of occurrence of the external cause

         Factory premises as the place of occurrence of the external cause

         Industrial yard as the place of occurrence of the external cause

     Y92.64   **Mine or pit as the place of occurrence of the external cause**

         Mine as the place of occurrence of the external cause

     Y92.65   **Oil rig as the place of occurrence of the external cause**

         Pit (coal) (gravel) (sand) as the place of occurrence of the external cause

     Y92.69   **Other specified industrial and construction area as the place of occurrence of the external cause**

         Gasworks as the place of occurrence of the external cause

         Power-station (coal) (nuclear) (oil) as the place of occurrence of the external cause

         Tunnel under construction as the place of occurrence of the external cause

         Workshop as the place of occurrence of the external cause

● **Y92.7**   **Farm as the place of occurrence of the external cause**

     Ranch as the place of occurrence of the external cause

     Excludes1   farmhouse and home premises of farm (Y92.01-)

     Y92.71   **Barn as the place of occurrence of the external cause**

     Y92.72   **Chicken coop as the place of occurrence of the external cause**

         Hen house as the place of occurrence of the external cause

     Y92.73   **Farm field as the place of occurrence of the external cause**

     Y92.74   **Orchard as the place of occurrence of the external cause**

     Y92.79   **Other farm location as the place of occurrence of the external cause**

● **Y92.8**   **Other places as the place of occurrence of the external cause**

     ● **Y92.81**   **Transport vehicle as the place of occurrence of the external cause**

         Excludes1   transport accidents (V00-V99)

         Y92.810   Car as the place of occurrence of the external cause

         Y92.811   Bus as the place of occurrence of the external cause

         Y92.812   Truck as the place of occurrence of the external cause

         Y92.813   Airplane as the place of occurrence of the external cause

         Y92.814   Boat as the place of occurrence of the external cause

         Y92.815   Train as the place of occurrence of the external cause

         Y92.816   Subway car as the place of occurrence of the external cause

         Y92.818   Other transport vehicle as the place of occurrence of the external cause

     ● **Y92.82**   **Wilderness area**

         Y92.820   Desert as the place of occurrence of the external cause

         Y92.821   Forest as the place of occurrence of the external cause

         Y92.828   Other wilderness area as the place of occurrence of the external cause

             Swamp as the place of occurrence of the external cause

             Mountain as the place of occurrence of the external cause

             Marsh as the place of occurrence of the external cause

             Prairie as the place of occurrence of the external cause

     ● **Y92.83**   **Recreation area as the place of occurrence of the external cause**

         Y92.830   Public park as the place of occurrence of the external cause

         Y92.831   Amusement park as the place of occurrence of the external cause

         Y92.832   Beach as the place of occurrence of the external cause

             Seashore as the place of occurrence of the external cause

         Y92.833   Campsite as the place of occurrence of the external cause

         Y92.834   Zoological garden (zoo) as the place of occurrence of the external cause

         Y92.838   Other recreation area as the place of occurrence of the external cause

     Y92.84   **Military training ground as the place of occurrence of the external cause**

     Y92.85   **Railroad track as the place of occurrence of the external cause**

     Y92.86   **Slaughter house as the place of occurrence of the external cause**

     Y92.89   **Other specified places as the place of occurrence of the external cause**

         Derelict house as the place of occurrence of the external cause

● **Y92.9**   **Unspecified place or not applicable**

CHAPTER 20 (V01-Y99)

CHAPTER 20 (V01-Y99)

OGCR See Section I.C.20.c.

Activity code

● Y93　Activity codes

Note: Category Y93 is provided for use to indicate the activity of the person seeking healthcare for an injury or health condition, such as a heart attack while shoveling snow, which resulted from, or was contributed to, by the activity. These codes are appropriate for use for both acute injuries, such as those from chapter 19, and conditions that are due to the long-term, cumulative effects of an activity, such as those from chapter 13. They are also appropriate for use with external cause codes for cause and intent if identifying the activity provides additional information on the event. These codes should be used in conjunction with codes for external cause status (Y99) and place of occurrence (Y92).

This section contains the following broad activity categories:

Y93.0	Activities involving walking and running
Y93.1	Activities involving water and water craft
Y93.2	Activities involving ice and snow
Y93.3	Activities involving climbing, rappelling, and jumping off
Y93.4	Activities involving dancing and other rhythmic movement
Y93.5	Activities involving other sports and athletics played individually
Y93.6	Activities involving other sports and athletics played as a team or group
Y93.7	Activities involving other specified sports and athletics
Y93.A	Activities involving other cardiorespiratory exercise
Y93.B	Activities involving other muscle strengthening exercises
Y93.C	Activities involving computer technology and electronic devices
Y93.D	Activities involving arts and handcrafts
Y93.E	Activities involving personal hygiene and interior property and clothing maintenance
Y93.F	Activities involving caregiving
Y93.G	Activities involving food preparation, cooking and grilling
Y93.H	Activities involving exterior property and land maintenance, building and construction
Y93.I	Activities involving roller coasters and other types of external motion
Y93.J	Activities involving playing musical instrument
Y93.K	Activities involving animal care
Y93.8	Activities, other specified
Y93.9	Activity, unspecified

● Y93.0　**Activities involving walking and running**

　　Excludes1　Activity, walking an animal (Y93.K1)
　　　　　　Activity, walking or running on a treadmill (Y93.A1)

Y93.01　**Activity, walking, marching and hiking**
　　Activity, walking, marching and hiking on level or elevated terrain
　　Excludes1　activity, mountain climbing (Y93.31)

Y93.02　**Activity, running**

● Y93.1　**Activities involving water and water craft**

　　Excludes1　activities involving ice (Y93.2-)

Y93.11　**Activity, swimming**

Y93.12　**Activity, springboard and platform diving**

Y93.13　**Activity, water polo**

Y93.14　**Activity, water aerobics and water exercise**

Y93.15　**Activity, underwater diving and snorkeling**
　　Activity, SCUBA diving

Y93.16　**Activity, rowing, canoeing, kayaking, rafting and tubing**
　　Activity, canoeing, kayaking, rafting and tubing in calm and turbulent water

Y93.17　**Activity, water skiing and wake boarding**

Y93.18　**Activity, surfing, windsurfing and boogie boarding**
　　Activity, water sliding

Y93.19　**Activity, other involving water and watercraft**
　　Activity involving water NOS
　　Activity, parasailing
　　Activity, water survival training and testing

● Y93.2　**Activities involving ice and snow**

　　Excludes1　activity, shoveling ice and snow (Y93.H1)

Y93.21　**Activity, ice skating**
　　Activity, figure skating (singles) (pairs)
　　Activity, ice dancing
　　Excludes1　activity, ice hockey (Y93.22)

Y93.22　**Activity, ice hockey**

Y93.23　**Activity, snow (alpine) (downhill) skiing, snow boarding, sledding, tobogganing and snow tubing**
　　Excludes1　activity, cross country skiing (Y93.24)

Y93.24　**Activity, cross country skiing**
　　Activity, nordic skiing

Y93.29　**Activity, other activity involving ice and snow**
　　Activity, activity involving ice and snow NOS

● Y93.3　**Activities involving climbing, rappelling and jumping off**

　　Excludes1　activity, hiking on level or elevated terrain (Y93.01)
　　　　　　activity, jumping rope (Y93.56)
　　　　　　activity, trampoline jumping (Y93.44)

Y93.31　**Activity, mountain climbing, rock climbing and wall climbing**

Y93.32　**Activity, rappelling**

Y93.33　**Activity, BASE jumping**
　　Activity, building, Antenna, Span, Earth jumping

Y93.34　**Activity, bungee jumping**

Y93.35　**Activity, hang gliding**

Y93.39　**Activity, other activity involving climbing, rappelling and jumping off**

● Y93.4　**Activities involving dancing and other rhythmic movement**

　　Excludes1　activity, martial arts (Y93.75)

Y93.41　**Activity, dancing**
　　Coding Clinic: 2012, Q4, P108

Y93.42　**Activity, yoga**

Y93.43　**Activity, gymnastics**
　　Activity, rhythmic gymnastics
　　Excludes1　activity, trampolining (Y93.44)

Y93.44　**Activity, trampolining**

Y93.45　**Activity, cheerleading**

Y93.49　**Activity, other involving dancing and other rhythmic movements**

◀ New　◀▦ Revised　d̶e̶l̶e̶t̶e̶d̶ Deleted　Excludes 1　Excludes 2　Includes　Use additional　Code first　Code also　Unspecified
OGCR Official Guidelines　X Assign placeholder X　● Use Additional Character(s)　▶ Manifestation Code　Coding Clinic

● **Y93.5** **Activities involving other sports and athletics played individually**

> **Excludes1**   activity, dancing (Y93.41)
> activity, gymnastic (Y93.43)
> activity, trampolining (Y93.44)
> activity, yoga (Y93.42)

Y93.51 **Activity, roller skating (inline) and skateboarding**

Y93.52 **Activity, horseback riding**

Y93.53 **Activity, golf**

Y93.54 **Activity, bowling**

Y93.55 **Activity, bike riding**

Y93.56 **Activity, jumping rope**

Y93.57 **Activity, non-running track and field events**

> **Excludes1**   activity, running (any form) (Y93.02)

Y93.59 **Activity, other involving other sports and athletics played individually**

> **Excludes1**   activities involving climbing, rappelling, and jumping (Y93.3-)
> activities involving ice and snow (Y93.2-)
> activities involving walking and running (Y93.0-)
> activities involving water and watercraft (Y93.1-)

● **Y93.6** **Activities involving other sports and athletics played as a team or group**

> **Excludes1**   activity, ice hockey (Y93.22)
> activity, water polo (Y93.13)

Y93.61 **Activity, American tackle football**
Activity, football NOS

Y93.62 **Activity, American flag or touch football**

Y93.63 **Activity, rugby**

Y93.64 **Activity, baseball**
Activity, softball

Y93.65 **Activity, lacrosse and field hockey**
Coding Clinic: 2015, Q1, P9

Y93.66 **Activity, soccer**

Y93.67 **Activity, basketball**

Y93.68 **Activity, volleyball (beach) (court)**

Y93.6A **Activity, physical games generally associated with school recess, summer camp and children**   P
Activity, capture the flag
Activity, dodge ball
Activity, four square
Activity, kickball

Y93.69 **Activity, other involving other sports and athletics played as a team or group**
Cricket

● **Y93.7** **Activities involving other specified sports and athletics**

Y93.71 **Activity, boxing**

Y93.72 **Activity, wrestling**

Y93.73 **Activity, racquet and hand sports**
Activity, handball
Activity, racquetball
Activity, squash
Activity, tennis

Y93.74 **Activity, frisbee**
Activity, ultimate frisbee

Y93.75 **Activity, martial arts**
Activity, combatives

Y93.79 **Activity, other specified sports and athletics**

> **Excludes1**   sports and athletics activities specified in categories Y93.0-Y93.6

● **Y93.A** **Activities involving other cardiorespiratory exercise**
Activities involving physical training

Y93.A1 **Activity, exercise machines primarily for cardiorespiratory conditioning**
Activity, elliptical and stepper machines
Activity, stationary bike
Activity, treadmill

Y93.A2 **Activity, calisthenics**
Activity, jumping jacks
Activity, warm up and cool down

Y93.A3 **Activity, aerobic and step exercise**

Y93.A4 **Activity, circuit training**

Y93.A5 **Activity, obstacle course**
Activity, challenge course
Activity, confidence course

Y93.A6 **Activity, grass drills**
Activity, guerilla drills

Y93.A9 **Activity, other involving other cardiorespiratory exercise**

> **Excludes1**   activities involving cardiorespiratory exercise specified in categories Y93.0-Y93.7

● **Y93.B** **Activity involving other muscle strengthening exercises**

Y93.B1 **Activity, exercise machines primarily for muscle strengthening**

Y93.B2 **Activity, push-ups, pull-ups, sit-ups**

Y93.B3 **Activity, free weights**
Activity, barbells
Activity, dumbbells

Y93.B4 **Activity, pilates**

Y93.B9 **Activity, other involving other muscle strengthening exercises**

> **Excludes1**   activities involving muscle strengthening specified in categories Y93.0-Y93.A

● **Y93.C** **Activities involving computer technology and electronic devices**

> **Excludes1**   activity, electronic musical keyboard or instruments (Y93.J-)

Y93.C1 **Activity, computer keyboarding**
Activity, electronic game playing using keyboard or other stationary device

Y93.C2 **Activity, hand held interactive electronic device**
Activity, cellular telephone and communication device
Activity, electronic game playing using interactive device

> **Excludes1**   activity, electronic game playing using keyboard or other stationary device (Y93.C1)

Y93.C9 **Activity, other involving computer technology and electronic devices**

● **Y93.D** **Activities involving arts and handcrafts**

> **Excludes1**   activities involving playing musical instrument (Y93.J-)

Y93.D1 **Knitting and crocheting**

Y93.D2 **Sewing**

Y93.D3 **Furniture building and finishing**
Furniture repair

Y93.D9 **Activity, other involving arts and handcrafts**

CHAPTER 20 (V01-Y99)

● **Y93.E** **Activities involving personal hygiene and interior property and clothing maintenance**

> Excludes1   activities involving cooking and grilling (Y93.G-)
> activities involving exterior property and land maintenance, building and construction (Y93.H-)
> activity involving caregiving (Y93.F-)
> activity, dishwashing (Y93.G1)
> activity, food preparation (Y93.G1)
> activity, gardening (Y93.H2)

     Y93.E1   **Activity, personal bathing and showering**

     Y93.E2   **Activity, laundry**

     Y93.E3   **Activity, vacuuming**

     Y93.E4   **Activity, ironing**

     Y93.E5   **Activity, floor mopping and cleaning**

     Y93.E6   **Activity, residential relocation**
> Activity, packing up and unpacking involved in moving to a new residence

     Y93.E8   **Activity, other personal hygiene activity**

     Y93.E9   **Activity, other household maintenance**

● **Y93.F** **Activities involving person providing caregiving**
> Activity involving the provider of caregiving

     Y93.F1   **Activity, caregiving involving bathing**

     Y93.F2   **Activity, caregiving involving lifting**

     Y93.F9   **Activity, other caregiving**

● **Y93.G** **Activities involving food preparation, cooking and grilling**

     Y93.G1   **Activity, food preparation and clean up**
> Activity, dishwashing

     Y93.G2   **Activity, grilling and smoking food**

     Y93.G3   **Activity, cooking and baking**
> Activity, use of stove, oven and microwave oven

     Y93.G9   **Activity, other activity involving cooking and grilling**

● **Y93.H** **Activities involving property and land maintenance, building and construction**

     Y93.H1   **Activity, digging, shoveling and raking**
> Activity, dirt digging
> Activity, raking leaves
> Activity, snow shoveling

     Y93.H2   **Activity, gardening and landscaping**
> Activity, pruning, trimming shrubs, weeding

     Y93.H3   **Activity, building and construction**

     Y93.H9   **Activity, other activity involving property and land maintenance, building and construction**

● **Y93.I** **Activities involving roller coasters and other types of external motion**

     Y93.I1   **Activity, rollercoaster riding**

     Y93.I9   **Activity, other involving external motion**

● **Y93.J** **Activities involving playing musical instrument**
> Activity involving playing electric musical instrument

     Y93.J1   **Activity, piano playing**
> Activity, musical keyboard (electronic) playing

     Y93.J2   **Activity, drum and other percussion instrument playing**

     Y93.J3   **Activity, string instrument playing**

     Y93.J4   **Activity, winds and brass instrument playing**

● **Y93.K** **Activities involving animal care**

> Excludes1   activity, horseback riding (Y93.52)

     Y93.K1   **Activity, walking an animal**

     Y93.K2   **Activity, milking an animal**

     Y93.K3   **Activity, grooming and shearing an animal**

     Y93.K9   **Activity, other activity involving animal care**

● **Y93.8** **Other activity**

     Y93.81   **Activity, refereeing a sports activity**

     Y93.82   **Activity, spectator at an event**

     Y93.83   **Activity, rough housing and horseplay**
> **Coding Clinic: 2015, Q1, P8**

     Y93.84   **Activity, sleeping**

     Y93.89   **Activity, other specified**

● **Y93.9** **Activity, unspecified**

Y95   **Nosocomial condition**

● **Y99**   **External cause status**

> **Note:** A single code from category Y99 should be used in conjunction with the external cause code(s) assigned to a record to indicate the status of the person at the time the event occurred.

     Y99.0   **Civilian activity done for income or pay**
> Civilian activity done for financial or other compensation

> Excludes1   military activity (Y99.1)
> volunteer activity (Y99.2)

     Y99.1   **Military activity**

> Excludes1   activity of off duty military personnel (Y99.8)

     Y99.2   **Volunteer activity**

> Excludes1   activity of child or other family member assisting in compensated work of other family member (Y99.8)

     Y99.8   **Other external cause status**
> Activity NEC
> Activity of child or other family member assisting in compensated work of other family member
> Hobby not done for income
> Leisure activity
> Off-duty activity of military personnel
> Recreation or sport not for income or while a student
> Student activity

> Excludes1   civilian activity done for income or compensation (Y99.0)
> military activity (Y99.1)

> **Coding Clinic: 2012, Q4, P108**

     Y99.9   **Unspecified external cause status**

◀ New   ◀▥ Revised   ~~deleted~~ Deleted   Excludes 1   Excludes 2   Includes   Use additional   Code first   Code also   Unspecified

OGCR Official Guidelines   X Assign placeholder X   ● Use Additional Character(s)   ▶ Manifestation Code   **Coding Clinic**

OGCR See Section I.C.21.

CHAPTER 21

FACTORS INFLUENCING HEALTH STATUS AND CONTACT WITH HEALTH SERVICES (Z00-Z99)

Note: Z codes represent reasons for encounters. A corresponding procedure code must accompany a Z code if a procedure is performed. Categories Z00-Z99 are provided for occasions when circumstances other than a disease, injury or external cause classifiable to categories A00-Y89 are recorded as 'diagnoses' or 'problems.' This can arise in two main ways:

(a) When a person who may or may not be sick encounters the health services for some specific purpose, such as to receive limited care or service for a current condition, to donate an organ or tissue, to receive prophylactic vaccination (immunization), or to discuss a problem which is in itself not a disease or injury.

(b) When some circumstance or problem is present which influences the person's health status but is not in itself a current illness or injury.

This chapter contains the following blocks:

Z00-Z13	Persons encountering health services for examination
Z14-Z15	Genetic carrier and genetic susceptibility to disease
Z16	Resistance to antimicrobial drugs
Z17	Estrogen receptor status
Z18	Retained foreign body fragments
Z20-Z28	Persons with potential health hazards related to communicable diseases
Z30-Z39	Persons encountering health services in circumstances related to reproduction
Z40-Z53	Encounters for other specific health care
Z55-Z65	Persons with potential health hazards related to socioeconomic and psychosocial circumstances
Z66	Do not resuscitate status
Z67	Blood type
Z68	Body mass index (BMI)
Z69-Z76	Persons encountering health services in other circumstances
Z77-Z99	Persons with potential health hazards related to family and personal history and certain conditions influencing health status

PERSONS ENCOUNTERING HEALTH SERVICES FOR EXAMINATIONS (Z00-Z13)

Note: Nonspecific abnormal findings disclosed at the time of these examinations are classified to categories R70-R94.

Excludes1   examinations related to pregnancy and reproduction (Z30-Z36, Z39.-)

● **Z00**   **Encounter for general examination without complaint, suspected or reported diagnosis**

     Excludes1   encounter for examination for administrative purposes (Z02.-)

     Excludes2   encounter for pre-procedural examinations (Z01.81-)
                  special screening examinations (Z11-Z13)

● **Z00.0**   **Encounter for general adult medical examination**
     Encounter for adult periodic examination (annual) (physical) and any associated laboratory and radiologic examinations

     Excludes1   encounter for examination of sign or symptom - code to sign or symptom
                  general health check-up of infant or child (Z00.12.-)

     Z00.00   **Encounter for general adult medical examination without abnormal findings**   **A**
         Encounter for adult health check-up NOS

     Z00.01   **Encounter for general adult medical examination with abnormal findings**   **A**
         Use additional code to identify abnormal findings

● **Z00.1**   **Encounter for newborn, infant and child health examinations**

● **Z00.11**   **Newborn health examination**
     Health check for child under 29 days old
     Use additional code to identify any abnormal findings

     Excludes1   health check for child over 28 days old (Z00.12-)

     Z00.110   **Health examination for newborn under 8 days old**   **N**
         Health check for newborn under 8 days old

     Z00.111   **Health examination for newborn 8 to 28 days old**   **N**
         Health check for newborn 8 to 28 days old
         Newborn weight check

● **Z00.12**   **Encounter for routine child health examination**
     Encounter for development testing of infant or child
     Health check (routine) for child over 28 days old

     Excludes1   health check for child under 29 days old (Z00.11-)
                  health supervision of foundling or other healthy infant or child (Z76.1-Z76.2)
                  newborn health examination (Z00.11-)

     Z00.121   **Encounter for routine child health examination with abnormal findings**   **P**
         Use additional code to identify abnormal findings

     Z00.129   **Encounter for routine child health examination without abnormal findings**   **P**
         Encounter for routine child health examination NOS

Z00.2   **Encounter for examination for period of rapid growth in childhood**   **P**

Z00.3   **Encounter for examination for adolescent development state**   **P**
     Encounter for puberty development state

Z00.5   **Encounter for examination of potential donor of organ and tissue**

Z00.6   **Encounter for examination for normal comparison and control in clinical research program**
     Examination of participant or control in clinical research program

● **Z00.7**   **Encounter for examination for period of delayed growth in childhood**

     Z00.70   **Encounter for examination for period of delayed growth in childhood without abnormal findings**   **P**

     Z00.71   **Encounter for examination for period of delayed growth in childhood with abnormal findings**   **P**
         Use additional code to identify abnormal findings

Z00.8   **Encounter for other general examination**
     Encounter for health examination in population surveys

CHAPTER 21 (Z00-Z99)

CHAPTER 21 (Z00-Z99)

● **Z01   Encounter for other special examination without complaint, suspected or reported diagnosis**

> **Includes**   routine examination of specific system
>
> **Note:** Codes from category Z01 represent the reason for the encounter. A separate procedure code is required to identify any examinations or procedures performed.
>
> **Excludes1**   encounter for examination for administrative purposes (Z02.-)
> encounter for examination for suspected conditions, proven not to exist (Z03.-)
> encounter for laboratory and radiologic examinations as a component of general medical examinations (Z00.0-)
> encounter for laboratory, radiologic and imaging examinations for sign(s) and symptom(s) - code to the sign(s) or symptom(s)
>
> **Excludes2**   screening examinations (Z11-Z13)

● **Z01.0   Encounter for examination of eyes and vision**

> **Excludes1**   examination for driving license (Z02.4)

> **Z01.00   Encounter for examination of eyes and vision without abnormal findings**
> Encounter for examination of eyes and vision NOS

> **Z01.01   Encounter for examination of eyes and vision with abnormal findings**
> Use additional code to identify abnormal findings

● **Z01.1   Encounter for examination of ears and hearing**

> **Z01.10   Encounter for examination of ears and hearing without abnormal findings**
> Encounter for examination of ears and hearing NOS

> ● **Z01.11   Encounter for examination of ears and hearing with abnormal findings**
>
> > **Z01.110   Encounter for hearing examination following failed hearing screening**
> >
> > **Z01.118   Encounter for examination of ears and hearing with other abnormal findings**
> > Use additional code to identify abnormal findings

> **Z01.12   Encounter for hearing conservation and treatment**

● **Z01.2   Encounter for dental examination and cleaning**

> **Z01.20   Encounter for dental examination and cleaning without abnormal findings**
> Encounter for dental examination and cleaning NOS

> **Z01.21   Encounter for dental examination and cleaning with abnormal findings**
> Use additional code to identify abnormal findings

● **Z01.3   Encounter for examination of blood pressure**

> **Z01.30   Encounter for examination of blood pressure without abnormal findings**
> Encounter for examination of blood pressure NOS

> **Z01.31   Encounter for examination of blood pressure with abnormal findings**
> Use additional code to identify abnormal findings

● **Z01.4   Encounter for gynecological examination**

> **Excludes2**   pregnancy examination or test (Z32.0-)
> routine examination for contraceptive maintenance (Z30.4-)

● **Z01.41   Encounter for routine gynecological examination**
> Encounter for general gynecological examination with or without cervical smear
> Encounter for gynecological examination (general) (routine) NOS
> Encounter for pelvic examination (annual) (periodic)
> Use additional code:
> for screening for human papillomavirus, if applicable (Z11.51)
> for screening vaginal pap smear, if applicable (Z12.72)
> to identify acquired absence of uterus, if applicable (Z90.71-)
>
> > **Excludes1**   gynecologic examination status-post hysterectomy for malignant condition (Z08)
> > screening cervical pap smear not a part of a routine gynecological examination (Z12.4)
>
> > **Z01.411   Encounter for gynecological examination (general) (routine) with abnormal findings ♀**
> >
> > **Z01.419   Encounter for gynecological examination (general) (routine) without abnormal findings ♀**
> > Use additional code to identify abnormal findings

> **Z01.42   Encounter for cervical smear to confirm findings of recent normal smear following initial abnormal smear ♀**

● **Z01.8   Encounter for other specified special examinations**

> ● **Z01.81   Encounter for preprocedural examinations**
> Encounter for preoperative examinations
> Encounter for radiological and imaging examinations as part of preprocedural examination
>
> > **Z01.810   Encounter for preprocedural cardiovascular examination**
> >
> > **Z01.811   Encounter for preprocedural respiratory examination**
> >
> > **Z01.812   Encounter for preprocedural laboratory examination**
> > Blood and urine tests prior to treatment or procedure
> >
> > **Z01.818   Encounter for other preprocedural examination**
> > Encounter for preprocedural examination NOS
> > Encounter for examinations prior to antineoplastic chemotherapy

> **Z01.82   Encounter for allergy testing**
>
> > **Excludes1**   encounter for antibody response examination (Z01.84)

> **Z01.83   Encounter for blood typing**
> Encounter for Rh typing

> **Z01.84   Encounter for antibody response examination**
> Encounter for immunity status testing
>
> > **Excludes1**   encounter for allergy testing (Z01.82)

> **Z01.89   Encounter for other specified special examinations**

◄ New   ◄▥ Revised   ~~deleted~~ Deleted   Excludes 1   Excludes 2   Includes   Use additional   Code first   Code also   Unspecified

OGCR Official Guidelines   X Assign placeholder X   ● Use Additional Character(s)   ▶ Manifestation Code   **Coding Clinic**

● **Z02**   **Encounter for administrative examination**

Z02.0   **Encounter for examination for admission to educational institution**

Encounter for examination for admission to preschool (education)

Encounter for examination for re-admission to school following illness or medical treatment

Z02.1   **Encounter for pre-employment examination**

Z02.2   **Encounter for examination for admission to residential institution**

Excludes1   examination for admission to prison (Z02.89)

Z02.3   **Encounter for examination for recruitment to armed forces**

Z02.4   **Encounter for examination for driving license**

Z02.5   **Encounter for examination for participation in sport**

Excludes1   blood-alcohol and blood-drug test (Z02.83)

Z02.6   **Encounter for examination for insurance purposes**

● **Z02.7**   **Encounter for issue of medical certificate**

Excludes1   encounter for general medical examination (Z00-Z01, Z02.0-Z02.6, Z02.8-Z02.9)

Z02.71   **Encounter for disability determination**

Encounter for issue of medical certificate of incapacity

Encounter for issue of medical certificate of invalidity

Z02.79   **Encounter for issue of other medical certificate**

● **Z02.8**   **Encounter for other administrative examinations**

Z02.81   **Encounter for paternity testing**

Z02.82   **Encounter for adoption services**

Z02.83   **Encounter for blood-alcohol and blood-drug test**

Use additional code for findings of alcohol or drugs in blood (R78.-)

Z02.89   **Encounter for other administrative examinations**

Encounter for examination for admission to prison

Encounter for examination for admission to summer camp

Encounter for immigration examination

Encounter for naturalization examination

Encounter for premarital examination

Excludes1   health supervision of foundling or other healthy infant or child (Z76.1-Z76.2)

Z02.9   **Encounter for administrative examinations, unspecified**

OGCR Section II.C.21.c.6.

21.2.2. Observation

There are two observation Z code categories. They are for use in very limited circumstances when a person is being observed for a suspected condition that is ruled out. The observation codes are not for use if an injury or illnesses or any signs or symptoms related to the suspected condition are present. In such cases the diagnosis/symptom code is used with the corresponding external cause code.

The observation codes are to be used as principal diagnosis only. Additional codes may be used in addition to the observation code but only if they are unrelated to the suspected condition being observed.

Codes from subcategory Z03.7 Encounter for suspected maternal and fetal conditions ruled out, may either be used as a first listed or as an additional code assignment depending on the case. They are for use in very limited circumstances on a maternal record when an encounter is for a suspected maternal or fetal condition that is ruled out during that encounter (for example, a maternal or fetal condition may be suspected due to an abnormal test result). These codes should not be used when the condition is confirmed. In those cases, the confirmed condition should be coded. In addition, these codes are not for use if an illness or any signs or symptoms related to the suspected condition or problem are present. In such cases the diagnosis/symptom code is used.

Additional codes may be used in addition to the code from subcategory Z03.7, but only if they are unrelated to the suspected condition being evaluated.

Codes from subcategory Z03.7 may not be used for encounters for antenatal screening of mother. *See Section I.C.21. Screening.*

For encounters for suspected fetal condition that are inconclusive following testing and evaluation, assign the appropriate code from category O35, O36, O40 or O41.

The observation Z code categories:

Z03   Encounter for medical observation for suspected diseases and conditions ruled out

Z04   Encounter for examination and observation for other reasons

Except: Z04.9, Encounter for examination and observation for unspecified reason

● **Z03**   **Encounter for medical observation for suspected diseases and conditions ruled out**

This category is to be used when a person without a diagnosis is suspected of having an abnormal condition, without signs or symptoms, which requires study, but after examination and observation, is ruled out. This category is also for use for administrative and legal observation status.

Excludes1   contact with and (suspected) exposures hazardous to health (Z77.-)

newborn observation for suspected condition, ruled out (P00-P04)

person with feared complaint in whom no diagnosis is made (Z71.1)

signs or symptoms under study - code to signs or symptoms

Z03.6   **Encounter for observation for suspected toxic effect from ingested substance ruled out**

Encounter for observation for suspected adverse effect from drug

Encounter for observation for suspected poisoning

CHAPTER 21 (Z00-Z99)

● **Z03.7** **Encounter for suspected maternal and fetal conditions ruled out**

Encounter for suspected maternal and fetal conditions not found

Excludes1 known or suspected fetal anomalies affecting management of mother, not ruled out (O26.-, O35.-, O36.-, O40.-, O41.-)

Z03.71 **Encounter for suspected problem with amniotic cavity and membrane ruled out ♀** **M**

Encounter for suspected oligohydramnios ruled out

Encounter for suspected polyhydramnios ruled out

Z03.72 **Encounter for suspected placental problem ruled out ♀** **M**

Z03.73 **Encounter for suspected fetal anomaly ruled out ♀** **M**

Z03.74 **Encounter for suspected problem with fetal growth ruled out ♀** **M**

Z03.75 **Encounter for suspected cervical shortening ruled out ♀** **M**

Z03.79 **Encounter for other suspected maternal and fetal conditions ruled out ♀** **M**

● **Z03.8** **Encounter for observation for other suspected diseases and conditions ruled out**

● **Z03.81** **Encounter for observation for suspected exposure to biological agents ruled out**

Z03.810 **Encounter for observation for suspected exposure to anthrax ruled out**

Z03.818 **Encounter for observation for suspected exposure to other biological agents ruled out**

Z03.89 **Encounter for observation for other suspected diseases and conditions ruled out**

● **Z04** **Encounter for examination and observation for other reasons**

Includes encounter for examination for medicolegal reasons

This category is to be used when a person without a diagnosis is suspected of having an abnormal condition, without signs or symptoms, which requires study, but after examination and observation, is ruled-out. This category is also for use for administrative and legal observation status.

Z04.1 **Encounter for examination and observation following transport accident**

Excludes1 encounter for examination and observation following work accident (Z04.2)

Z04.2 **Encounter for examination and observation following work accident**

Z04.3 **Encounter for examination and observation following other accident**

● **Z04.4** **Encounter for examination and observation following alleged rape**

Encounter for examination and observation of victim following alleged rape

Encounter for examination and observation of victim following alleged sexual abuse

Z04.41 **Encounter for examination and observation following alleged adult rape** **A**

Suspected adult rape, ruled out

Suspected adult sexual abuse, ruled out

Z04.42 **Encounter for examination and observation following alleged child rape** **P**

Suspected child rape, ruled out

Suspected child sexual abuse, ruled out

Z04.6 **Encounter for general psychiatric examination, requested by authority**

● **Z04.7** **Encounter for examination and observation following alleged physical abuse**

Z04.71 **Encounter for examination and observation following alleged adult physical abuse** **A**

Suspected adult physical abuse, ruled out

Excludes1 confirmed case of adult physical abuse (T74.-)

encounter for examination and observation following alleged adult sexual abuse (Z04.41)

suspected case of adult physical abuse, not ruled out (T76.-)

Z04.72 **Encounter for examination and observation following alleged child physical abuse** **P**

Suspected child physical abuse, ruled out

Excludes1 confirmed case of child physical abuse (T74.-)

encounter for examination and observation following alleged child sexual abuse (Z04.42)

suspected case of child physical abuse, not ruled out (T76.-)

Z04.8 **Encounter for examination and observation for other specified reasons**

Encounter for examination and observation for request for expert evidence

Z04.9 **Encounter for examination and observation for unspecified reason**

Encounter for observation NOS

OGCR See Section II.C.21.c.7.

The follow-up codes are used to explain continuing surveillance following completed treatment of a disease, condition, or injury. They imply that the condition has been fully treated and no longer exists. They should not be confused with aftercare codes, or injury codes with 7th character "D," that explain ongoing care of a healing condition or its sequelae. Follow-up codes may be used in conjunction with history codes to provide the full picture of the healed condition and its treatment. The follow-up code is sequenced first, followed by the history code.

A follow-up code may be used to explain multiple visits. Should a condition be found to have recurred on the follow-up visit, then the diagnosis code for the condition should be assigned in place of the follow-up code.

The follow-up Z code categories:

Z08 Encounter for follow-up examination after completed treatment for malignant neoplasm

Z09 Encounter for follow-up examination after completed treatment for conditions other than malignant neoplasm

Z39 Encounter for maternal postpartum care and examination

Z08 **Encounter for follow-up examination after completed treatment for malignant neoplasm**

Medical surveillance following completed treatment

Use additional code to identify any acquired absence of organs (Z90.-)

Use additional code to identify the personal history of malignant neoplasm (Z85.-)

Excludes1 aftercare following medical care (Z43-Z49, Z51)

Z09 **Encounter for follow-up examination after completed treatment for conditions other than malignant neoplasm**

Medical surveillance following completed treatment

Use additional code to identify any applicable history of disease code (Z86.-. Z87.-)

Excludes1 aftercare following medical care (Z43-Z49, Z51)

surveillance of contraception (Z30.4-)

surveillance of prosthetic and other medical devices (Z44-Z46)

Coding Clinic: 2015, Q1, P8

◄ New ⬅ Revised ~~deleted~~ Deleted Excludes 1 Excludes 2 Includes Use additional Code first Code also **Unspecified**

OGCR Official Guidelines X Assign placeholder X ● Use Additional Character(s) ▸ Manifestation Code **Coding Clinic**

CHAPTER 21 (Z00-Z99)

● **Z11   Encounter for screening for infectious and parasitic diseases**
Screening is the testing for disease or disease precursors in asymptomatic individuals so that early detection and treatment can be provided for those who test positive for the disease.

> **Excludes1**   encounter for diagnostic examination - code to sign or symptom

Z11.0   Encounter for screening for intestinal infectious diseases

OGCR Section II.C.21.c.5.

Screening

Screening is the testing for disease or disease precursors in seemingly well individuals so that early detection and treatment can be provided for those who test positive for the disease (e.g., screening mammogram).

The testing of a person to rule out or confirm a suspected diagnosis because the patient has some sign or symptom is a diagnostic examination, not a screening. In these cases, the sign or symptom is used to explain the reason for the test.

A screening code may be a first listed code if the reason for the visit is specifically the screening exam. It may also be used as an additional code if the screening is done during an office visit for other health problems. A screening code is not necessary if the screening is inherent to a routine examination, such as a pap smear done during a routine pelvic examination.

Should a condition be discovered during the screening then the code for the condition may be assigned as an additional diagnosis.

The Z code indicates that a screening exam is planned. A procedure code is required to confirm that the screening was performed.

The screening Z codes /categories:

Z11   Encounter for screening for infectious and parasitic diseases

Z12   Encounter for screening for malignant neoplasms

Z13   Encounter for screening for other diseases and disorders
   Except: Z13.9, Encounter for screening, unspecified

Z36   Encounter for antenatal screening for mother

Z11.1   Encounter for screening for respiratory tuberculosis

Z11.2   Encounter for screening for other bacterial diseases

Z11.3   Encounter for screening for infections with a predominantly sexual mode of transmission

> **Excludes2**   encounter for screening for human immunodeficiency virus [HIV] (Z11.4)
> encounter for screening for human papillomavirus (Z11.51)

Z11.4   Encounter for screening for human immunodeficiency virus [HIV]

● **Z11.5   Encounter for screening for other viral diseases**

> **Excludes2**   encounter for screening for viral intestinal disease (Z11.0)

Z11.51   Encounter for screening for human papillomavirus (HPV)

Z11.59   Encounter for screening for other viral diseases

Z11.6   Encounter for screening for other protozoal diseases and helminthiases
Diseases or infestations caused by parasitic worms

> **Excludes2**   encounter for screening for protozoal intestinal disease (Z11.0)

Z11.8   Encounter for screening for other infectious and parasitic diseases
Encounter for screening for chlamydia
Encounter for screening for rickettsial
Encounter for screening for spirochetal
Encounter for screening for mycoses

Z11.9   Encounter for screening for infectious and parasitic diseases, unspecified

● **Z12   Encounter for screening for malignant neoplasms**
Screening is the testing for disease or disease precursors in asymptomatic individuals so that early detection and treatment can be provided for those who test positive for the disease.
Use additional code to identify any family history of malignant neoplasm (Z80.-)

> **Excludes1**   encounter for diagnostic examination - code to sign or symptom

Z12.0   Encounter for screening for malignant neoplasm of stomach

● **Z12.1   Encounter for screening for malignant neoplasm of intestinal tract**

Z12.10   Encounter for screening for malignant neoplasm of intestinal tract, unspecified

Z12.11   Encounter for screening for malignant neoplasm of colon
Encounter for screening colonoscopy NOS

Z12.12   Encounter for screening for malignant neoplasm of rectum

Z12.13   Encounter for screening for malignant neoplasm of small intestine

Z12.2   Encounter for screening for malignant neoplasm of respiratory organs

● **Z12.3   Encounter for screening for malignant neoplasm of breast**

Z12.31   Encounter for screening mammogram for malignant neoplasm of breast

> **Excludes1**   inconclusive mammogram (R92.2)
> **Coding Clinic: 2015, Q1, P24**

Z12.39   Encounter for other screening for malignant neoplasm of breast

Z12.4   Encounter for screening for malignant neoplasm of cervix ♀
Encounter for screening pap smear for malignant neoplasm of cervix

> **Excludes1**   encounter for screening for human papillomavirus (Z11.51)
> when screening is part of general gynecological examination (Z01.4-)

Z12.5   Encounter for screening for malignant neoplasm of prostate ♂

Z12.6   Encounter for screening for malignant neoplasm of bladder

● **Z12.7   Encounter for screening for malignant neoplasm of other genitourinary organs**

Z12.71   Encounter for screening for malignant neoplasm of testis ♂

Z12.72   Encounter for screening for malignant neoplasm of vagina ♀
Vaginal pap smear status - post hysterectomy for non-malignant condition
Use additional code to identify acquired absence of uterus (Z90.71-)

> **Excludes1**   vaginal pap smear status - post hysterectomy for malignant conditions (Z08)

Z12.73   Encounter for screening for malignant neoplasm of ovary ♀

Z12.79   Encounter for screening for malignant neoplasm of other genitourinary organs

● **Z12.8   Encounter for screening for malignant neoplasm of other sites**

Z12.81   Encounter for screening for malignant neoplasm of oral cavity

Z12.82   Encounter for screening for malignant neoplasm of nervous system

Z12.83
ICD-10-CM

Z12.83 Encounter for screening for malignant neoplasm of skin

Z12.89 Encounter for screening for malignant neoplasm of other sites

Z12.9 Encounter for screening for malignant neoplasm, site unspecified

● Z13 Encounter for screening for other diseases and disorders
Screening is the testing for disease or disease precursors in asymptomatic individuals so that early detection and treatment can be provided for those who test positive for the disease.
Excludes1 encounter for diagnostic examination - code to sign or symptom

Z13.0 Encounter for screening for diseases of the blood and blood-forming organs and certain disorders involving the immune mechanism

Z13.1 Encounter for screening for diabetes mellitus

● Z13.2 Encounter for screening for nutritional, metabolic and other endocrine disorders

   Z13.21 Encounter for screening for nutritional disorder

   ● Z13.22 Encounter for screening for metabolic disorder

      Z13.220 Encounter for screening for lipoid disorders
Encounter for screening for cholesterol level
Encounter for screening for hypercholesterolemia
Encounter for screening for hyperlipidemia

      Z13.228 Encounter for screening for other metabolic disorders

   Z13.29 Encounter for screening for other suspected endocrine disorder
Excludes1 encounter for screening for diabetes mellitus (Z13.1)

Z13.4 Encounter for screening for certain developmental disorders in childhood   P
Encounter for screening for developmental handicaps in early childhood
Excludes1 routine development testing of infant or child (Z00.1-)

Z13.5 Encounter for screening for eye and ear disorders
Excludes2 encounter for general hearing examination (Z01.1-)
encounter for general vision examination (Z01.0-)

Z13.6 Encounter for screening for cardiovascular disorders

● Z13.7 Encounter for screening for genetic and chromosomal anomalies
Excludes1 genetic testing for procreative management (Z31.4-)

   Z13.71 Encounter for nonprocreative screening for genetic disease carrier status

   Z13.79 Encounter for other screening for genetic and chromosomal anomalies

● Z13.8 Encounter for screening for other specified diseases and disorders
Excludes2 screening for malignant neoplasms (Z12.-)

   ● Z13.81 Encounter for screening for digestive system disorders

      Z13.810 Encounter for screening for upper gastrointestinal disorder

      Z13.811 Encounter for screening for lower gastrointestinal disorder
Excludes1 encounter for screening for intestinal infectious disease (Z11.0)

      Z13.818 Encounter for screening for other digestive system disorders

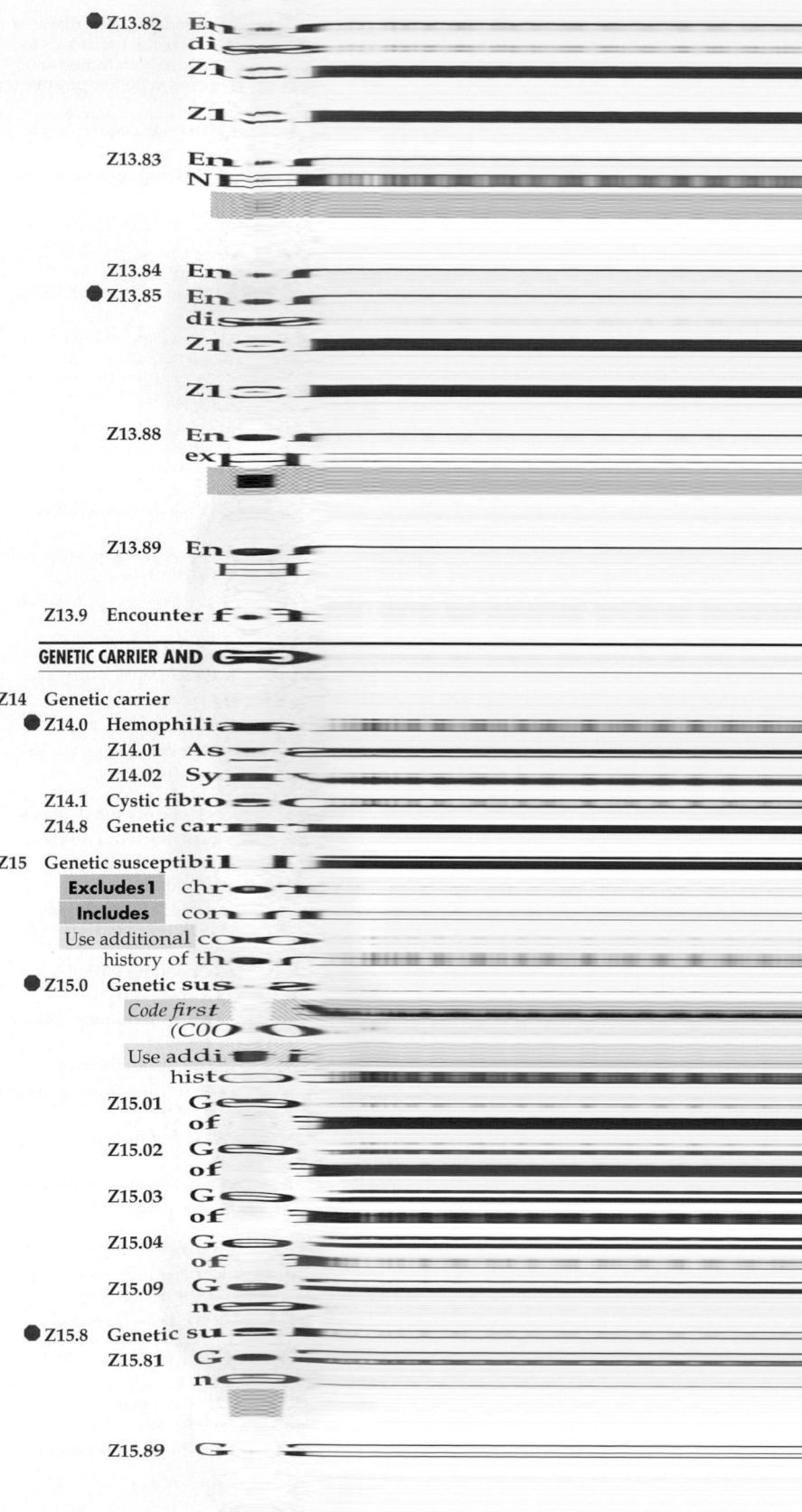

● Z13.82 En...

Z13.83 En... N...

Z13.84 En...
● Z13.85 En...

Z13.88 En... ex...

Z13.89 En...

Z13.9 Encounter f...

GENETIC CARRIER AND ...

● Z14 Genetic carrier
  ● Z14.0 Hemophilia...
    Z14.01 As...
    Z14.02 Sy...
  Z14.1 Cystic fibro...
  Z14.8 Genetic car...

● Z15 Genetic susceptibil...
  Excludes1 chr...
  Includes con...
  Use additional c... history of th...
  ● Z15.0 Genetic sus...
    Code first (CO...
    Use additi... hist...
    Z15.01 G... of...
    Z15.02 G... of...
    Z15.03 G... of...
    Z15.04 G... of...
    Z15.09 G... n...
  ● Z15.8 Genetic su...
    Z15.81 G... n...
    Z15.89 G...

◄ New ◄ Revised deleted Deleted Excludes 1 Excludes 2 Includes Use additi...
OGCR Official Guidelines X Assign placeholder X ● Use Additional Character(s)
1578

CHAPTER 21 (Z00-Z99)

PERSONS ENCOUNTERING HEALTH SERVICES IN CIRCUMSTANCES RELATED TO REPRODUCTION (Z30-Z39)

● **Z30   Encounter for contraceptive management**
- ● **Z30.0   Encounter for general counseling and advice on contraception**
  - ● **Z30.01   Encounter for initial prescription of contraceptives**
    - **Excludes 1**   encounter for surveillance of contraceptives (Z30.4-)
    - **Z30.011   Encounter for initial prescription of contraceptive pills** ♀
    - **Z30.012   Encounter for prescription of emergency contraception** ♀
      Encounter for postcoital contraception
    - **Z30.013   Encounter for initial prescription of injectable contraceptive** ♀
    - **Z30.014   Encounter for initial prescription of intrauterine contraceptive device** ♀
      - **Excludes 1**   encounter for insertion of intrauterine contraceptive device (Z30.430, Z30.432)
    - **Z30.018   Encounter for initial prescription of other contraceptives** ♀
    - **Z30.019   Encounter for initial prescription of contraceptives, unspecified** ♀
  - **Z30.02   Counseling and instruction in natural family planning to avoid pregnancy**
  - **Z30.09   Encounter for other general counseling and advice on contraception**
    Encounter for family planning advice NOS
- **Z30.2   Encounter for sterilization**
- ● **Z30.4   Encounter for surveillance of contraceptives**
  - **Z30.40   Encounter for surveillance of contraceptives, unspecified**
  - **Z30.41   Encounter for surveillance of contraceptive pills** ♀
    Encounter for repeat prescription for contraceptive pill
  - **Z30.42   Encounter for surveillance of injectable contraceptive** ♀
  - ● **Z30.43   Encounter for surveillance of intrauterine contraceptive device**
    - **Z30.430   Encounter for insertion of intrauterine contraceptive device** ♀
    - **Z30.431   Encounter for routine checking of intrauterine contraceptive device** ♀
    - **Z30.432   Encounter for removal of intrauterine contraceptive device** ♀
    - **Z30.433   Encounter for removal and reinsertion of intrauterine contraceptive device** ♀
      Encounter for replacement of intrauterine contraceptive device
  - **Z30.49   Encounter for surveillance of other contraceptives** ♀
- **Z30.8   Encounter for other contraceptive management**
  Encounter for postvasectomy sperm count
  Encounter for routine examination for contraceptive maintenance
  - **Excludes 1**   sperm count following sterilization reversal (Z31.42)
    sperm count for fertility testing (Z31.41)
- **Z30.9   Encounter for contraceptive management, unspecified**

● **Z31   Encounter for procreative management**
- **Excludes 1**   complications associated with artificial fertilization (N98.-)
  female infertility (N97.-)
  male infertility (N46.-)
- **Z31.0   Encounter for reversal of previous sterilization**
- ● **Z31.4   Encounter for procreative investigation and testing**
  - **Excludes 1**   postvasectomy sperm count (Z30.8)
  - **Z31.41   Encounter for fertility testing**
    Encounter for fallopian tube patency testing
    Encounter for sperm count for fertility testing
  - **Z31.42   Aftercare following sterilization reversal**
    Sperm count following sterilization reversal
  - ● **Z31.43   Encounter for genetic testing of female for procreative management**
    Use additional code for recurrent pregnancy loss, if applicable (N96, O26.2-)
    - **Excludes 1**   nonprocreative genetic testing (Z13.7-)
    - **Z31.430   Encounter of female for testing for genetic disease carrier status for procreative management** ♀
    - **Z31.438   Encounter for other genetic testing of female for procreative management** ♀
  - ● **Z31.44   Encounter for genetic testing of male for procreative management**
    - **Excludes 1**   nonprocreative genetic testing (Z13.7-)
    - **Z31.440   Encounter of male for testing for genetic disease carrier status for procreative management** ♂
    - **Z31.441   Encounter for testing of male partner of patient with recurrent pregnancy loss** ♂   **A**
    - **Z31.448   Encounter for other genetic testing of male for procreative management** ♂   **A**
  - **Z31.49   Encounter for other procreative investigation and testing**
- **Z31.5   Encounter for genetic counseling**
- ● **Z31.6   Encounter for general counseling and advice on procreation**
  - **Z31.61   Procreative counseling and advice using natural family planning**
  - **Z31.62   Encounter for fertility preservation counseling**
    Encounter for fertility preservation counseling prior to cancer therapy
    Encounter for fertility preservation counseling prior to surgical removal of gonads
  - **Z31.69   Encounter for other general counseling and advice on procreation**
- ● **Z31.8   Encounter for other procreative management**
  - **Z31.81   Encounter for male factor infertility in female patient** ♀
  - **Z31.82   Encounter for Rh incompatibility status** ♀
  - **Z31.83   Encounter for assisted reproductive fertility procedure cycle** ♀
    Patient undergoing in vitro fertilization cycle
    Use additional code to identify the type of infertility
    - **Excludes 1**   pre-cycle diagnosis and testing - code to reason for encounter
  - **Z31.84   Encounter for fertility preservation procedure**
    Encounter for fertility preservation procedure prior to cancer therapy
    Encounter for fertility preservation procedure prior to surgical removal of gonads
  - **Z31.89   Encounter for other procreative management**
- **Z31.9   Encounter for procreative management, unspecified**

CHAPTER 21 (Z00-Z99)

CHAPTER 21 (Z00-Z99)

● **Z32** Encounter for pregnancy test and childbirth and childcare instruction
  ● **Z32.0** Encounter for pregnancy test
    Z32.00 Encounter for pregnancy test, result unknown ♀
      Encounter for pregnancy test NOS
    Z32.01 Encounter for pregnancy test, result positive ♀ **M**
    Z32.02 Encounter for pregnancy test, result negative ♀
  Z32.2 Encounter for childbirth instruction
  Z32.3 Encounter for childcare instruction
    Encounter for prenatal or postpartum childcare instruction

● **Z33** Pregnant state
  Z33.1 Pregnant state, incidental ♀ **M**
    Pregnant state NOS
    Excludes1 complications of pregnancy (O00-O9A)
  Z33.2 Encounter for elective termination of pregnancy ♀ **M**
    Excludes1 early fetal death with retention of dead fetus (O02.1)
      late fetal death (O36.4)
      spontaneous abortion (O03)

● **Z34** Encounter for supervision of normal pregnancy
  Excludes1 any complication of pregnancy (O00-O9A)
    encounter for pregnancy test (Z32.0-)
    encounter for supervision of high risk pregnancy (O09.-)
  ● **Z34.0** Encounter for supervision of normal first pregnancy
    Z34.00 Encounter for supervision of normal first pregnancy, unspecified trimester ♀ **M**
    Z34.01 Encounter for supervision of normal first pregnancy, first trimester ♀ **M**
    Z34.02 Encounter for supervision of normal first pregnancy, second trimester ♀ **M**
    Z34.03 Encounter for supervision of normal first pregnancy, third trimester ♀ **M**
  ● **Z34.8** Encounter for supervision of other normal pregnancy
    Z34.80 Encounter for supervision of other normal pregnancy, unspecified trimester ♀ **M**
    Z34.81 Encounter for supervision of other normal pregnancy, first trimester ♀ **M**
    Z34.82 Encounter for supervision of other normal pregnancy, second trimester ♀ **M**
    Z34.83 Encounter for supervision of other normal pregnancy, third trimester ♀ **M**
  ● **Z34.9** Encounter for supervision of normal pregnancy, unspecified
    Z34.90 Encounter for supervision of normal pregnancy, unspecified, unspecified trimester ♀ **M**
    Z34.91 Encounter for supervision of normal pregnancy, unspecified, first trimester ♀ **M**
    Z34.92 Encounter for supervision of normal pregnancy, unspecified, second trimester ♀ **M**
    Z34.93 Encounter for supervision of normal pregnancy, unspecified, third trimester ♀ **M**

● **Z36** Encounter for antenatal screening of mother ♀ **M**
  Excludes1 abnormal findings on antenatal screening of mother (O28.-)
    diagnostic examination - code to sign or symptom
    encounter for suspected maternal and fetal conditions ruled out (Z03.7-)
    suspected fetal condition affecting management of pregnancy - code to condition in Chapter 15
  Excludes2 genetic counseling and testing (Z31.43-, Z31.5)
    routine prenatal care (Z34)

● **Z3A** Weeks of gestation
  Note: Codes from category Z3A are for use, only on the maternal record, to indicate the weeks of gestation of the pregnancy.
  Code first complications of pregnancy, childbirth and the puerperium (O00-O9A)
  Coding Clinic: 2013, Q2, P33
  ● **Z3A.0** Weeks of gestation of pregnancy, unspecified or less than 10 weeks
    Z3A.00 Weeks of gestation of pregnancy not specified ♀ **M**
    Z3A.01 Less than 8 weeks gestation of pregnancy ♀ **M**
    Z3A.08 8 weeks gestation of pregnancy ♀ **M**
    Z3A.09 9 weeks gestation of pregnancy ♀ **M**
  ● **Z3A.1** Weeks of gestation of pregnancy, weeks 10-19
    Z3A.10 10 weeks gestation of pregnancy ♀ **M**
    Z3A.11 11 weeks gestation of pregnancy ♀ **M**
    Z3A.12 12 weeks gestation of pregnancy ♀ **M**
    Z3A.13 13 weeks gestation of pregnancy ♀ **M**
    Z3A.14 14 weeks gestation of pregnancy ♀ **M**
    Z3A.15 15 weeks gestation of pregnancy ♀ **M**
    Z3A.16 16 weeks gestation of pregnancy ♀ **M**
    Z3A.17 17 weeks gestation of pregnancy ♀ **M**
    Z3A.18 18 weeks gestation of pregnancy ♀ **M**
    Z3A.19 19 weeks gestation of pregnancy ♀ **M**
  ● **Z3A.2** Weeks of gestation of pregnancy, weeks 20-29
    Z3A.20 20 weeks gestation of pregnancy ♀ **M**
    Z3A.21 21 weeks gestation of pregnancy ♀ **M**
    Z3A.22 22 weeks gestation of pregnancy ♀ **M**
    Z3A.23 23 weeks gestation of pregnancy ♀ **M**
    Z3A.24 24 weeks gestation of pregnancy ♀ **M**
    Z3A.25 25 weeks gestation of pregnancy ♀ **M**
    Z3A.26 26 weeks gestation of pregnancy ♀ **M**
    Z3A.27 27 weeks gestation of pregnancy ♀ **M**
    Z3A.28 28 weeks gestation of pregnancy ♀ **M**
    Z3A.29 29 weeks gestation of pregnancy ♀ **M**
  ● **Z3A.3** Weeks of gestation of pregnancy, weeks 30-39
    Z3A.30 30 weeks gestation of pregnancy ♀ **M**
    Z3A.31 31 weeks gestation of pregnancy ♀ **M**
    Z3A.32 32 weeks gestation of pregnancy ♀ **M**
    Z3A.33 33 weeks gestation of pregnancy ♀ **M**
    Z3A.34 34 weeks gestation of pregnancy ♀ **M**
    Z3A.35 35 weeks gestation of pregnancy ♀ **M**
    Z3A.36 36 weeks gestation of pregnancy ♀ **M**
    Z3A.37 37 weeks gestation of pregnancy ♀ **M**
    Z3A.38 38 weeks gestation of pregnancy ♀ **M**
    Z3A.39 39 weeks gestation of pregnancy ♀ **M**
  ● **Z3A.4** Weeks of gestation of pregnancy, weeks 40 or greater
    Z3A.40 40 weeks gestation of pregnancy ♀ **M**
    Z3A.41 41 weeks gestation of pregnancy ♀ **M**
    Z3A.42 42 weeks gestation of pregnancy ♀ **M**
    Z3A.49 Greater than 42 weeks gestation of pregnancy ♀ **M**

◀ New   ◀ Revised   ~~deleted~~ Deleted   Excludes 1   Excludes 2   Includes   Use additional   Code first   Code also   Unspecified
  OGCR Official Guidelines   **X** Assign placeholder X   ● Use Additional Character(s)   ▶ Manifestation Code   **Coding Clinic**

● **Z37　Outcome of delivery**
This category is intended for use as an additional code to
identify the outcome of delivery on the mother's record. It
is not for use on the newborn record.

> **Excludes1**　stillbirth (P95)

Z37.0　Single live birth ♀　　　　　　　　　　　　　M
Z37.1　Single stillbirth ♀　　　　　　　　　　　　　M
Z37.2　Twins, both liveborn ♀　　　　　　　　　　　M
Z37.3　Twins, one liveborn and one stillborn ♀　　　M
Z37.4　Twins, both stillborn ♀　　　　　　　　　　　M
● **Z37.5**　Other multiple births, all liveborn
　　Z37.50　Multiple births, unspecified, all liveborn ♀　M
　　Z37.51　Triplets, all liveborn ♀　　　　　　　　M
　　Z37.52　Quadruplets, all liveborn ♀　　　　　　M
　　Z37.53　Quintuplets, all liveborn ♀　　　　　　M
　　Z37.54　Sextuplets, all liveborn ♀　　　　　　　M
　　Z37.59　Other multiple births, all liveborn ♀　　M
● **Z37.6**　Other multiple births, some liveborn
　　Z37.60　Multiple births, unspecified, some liveborn ♀　M
　　Z37.61　Triplets, some liveborn ♀　　　　　　　M
　　Z37.62　Quadruplets, some liveborn ♀　　　　　M
　　Z37.63　Quintuplets, some liveborn ♀　　　　　M
　　Z37.64　Sextuplets, some liveborn ♀　　　　　　M
　　Z37.69　Other multiple births, some liveborn ♀　M
Z37.7　Other multiple births, all stillborn ♀　　　　M
Z37.9　Outcome of delivery, unspecified ♀　　　　　M
　　　　　Multiple birth NOS
　　　　　Single birth NOS

● **Z38　Liveborn infants according to place of birth and type of delivery**
This category is for use as the principal code on the initial
record of a newborn baby. It is to be used for the initial
birth record only. It is not to be used on the mother's
record.

● **Z38.0**　Single liveborn infant, born in hospital
　　　Single liveborn infant, born in birthing center or other
　　　health care facility
　　Z38.00　Single liveborn infant, delivered vaginally　N
　　Z38.01　Single liveborn infant, delivered by cesarean　N
Z38.1　Single liveborn infant, born outside hospital　　N
Z38.2　Single liveborn infant, unspecified as to place of birth　N
　　　Single liveborn infant NOS
● **Z38.3**　Twin liveborn infant, born in hospital
　　Z38.30　Twin liveborn infant, delivered vaginally　N
　　Z38.31　Twin liveborn infant, delivered by cesarean　N
Z38.4　Twin liveborn infant, born outside hospital　　N
Z38.5　Twin liveborn infant, unspecified as to place of birth　N
● **Z38.6**　Other multiple liveborn infant, born in hospital
　　Z38.61　Triplet liveborn infant, delivered vaginally　N
　　Z38.62　Triplet liveborn infant, delivered by cesarean　N
　　Z38.63　Quadruplet liveborn infant, delivered vaginally　N
　　Z38.64　Quadruplet liveborn infant, delivered by cesarean　N
　　Z38.65　Quintuplet liveborn infant, delivered vaginally　N
　　Z38.66　Quintuplet liveborn infant, delivered by cesarean　N
　　Z38.68　Other multiple liveborn infant, delivered vaginally　N
　　Z38.69　Other multiple liveborn infant, delivered by cesarean　N
Z38.7　Other multiple liveborn infant, born outside hospital　N
Z38.8　Other multiple liveborn infant, unspecified as to place of birth　N

● **Z39　Encounter for maternal postpartum care and examination**
Z39.0　Encounter for care and examination of mother immediately after delivery ♀　　　　　　M
　　　Care and observation in uncomplicated cases when the
　　　delivery occurs outside a healthcare facility

> **Excludes1**　care for postpartum complication - see
> 　　　　　Alphabetic index

Z39.1　Encounter for care and examination of lactating mother ♀　　　　　　　　　　　　　　M
　　　Encounter for supervision of lactation

> **Excludes1**　disorders of lactation (O92.-)

Z39.2　Encounter for routine postpartum follow-up ♀　M

ENCOUNTERS FOR OTHER SPECIFIC HEALTH CARE (Z40-Z53)

Categories Z40-Z53 are intended for use to indicate a reason
for care. They may be used for patients who have already been
treated for a disease or injury, but who are receiving aftercare or
prophylactic care, or care to consolidate the treatment, or to deal
with a residual state

> **Excludes2**　follow-up examination for medical surveillance
> 　　　　　after treatment (Z08-Z09)

● **Z40　Encounter for prophylactic surgery**

> **Excludes1**　organ donations (Z52.-)
> 　　　　　therapeutic organ removal - code to condition

● **Z40.0**　Encounter for prophylactic surgery for risk factors related to malignant neoplasms
　　　Admission for prophylactic organ removal
　　　Use additional code to identify risk factor
　　Z40.00　Encounter for prophylactic removal of unspecified organ
　　Z40.01　Encounter for prophylactic removal of breast
　　Z40.02　Encounter for prophylactic removal of ovary ♀
　　Z40.09　Encounter for prophylactic removal of other organ
Z40.8　Encounter for other prophylactic surgery
Z40.9　Encounter for prophylactic surgery, unspecified

● **Z41　Encounter for procedures for purposes other than remedying health state**
Z41.1　Encounter for cosmetic surgery
　　　Encounter for cosmetic breast implant
　　　Encounter for cosmetic procedure

> **Excludes1**　encounter for plastic and reconstructive
> 　　　　　surgery following medical procedure
> 　　　　　or healed injury (Z42.-)
> 　　　　　encounter for post-mastectomy breast
> 　　　　　implantation (Z42.1)

Z41.2　Encounter for routine and ritual male circumcision ♂
Z41.3　Encounter for ear piercing
Z41.8　Encounter for other procedures for purposes other than remedying health state
Z41.9　Encounter for procedure for purposes other than remedying health state, unspecified

● **Z42　Encounter for plastic and reconstructive surgery following medical procedure or healed injury**

> **Excludes1**　encounter for cosmetic plastic surgery (Z41.1)
> 　　　　　encounter for plastic surgery for treatment of
> 　　　　　current injury - code to relevent injury

Z42.1　Encounter for breast reconstruction following mastectomy　　　　　　　　　　　　A

> **Excludes1**　deformity and disproportion of
> 　　　　　reconstructed breast (N65.1-)

Z42.8　Encounter for other plastic and reconstructive surgery following medical procedure or healed injury

CHAPTER 21 (Z00-Z99)

● **Z43**   **Encounter for attention to artificial openings**

    Includes   closure of artificial openings
                passage of sounds or bougies through artificial
                   openings
                reforming artificial openings
                removal of catheter from artificial openings
                toilet or cleansing of artificial openings

    Excludes1   artificial opening status only, without need for
                  care (Z93.-)
                  complications of external stoma (J95.0-, K94.-,
                  N99.5-)

    Excludes2   fitting and adjustment of prosthetic and other
                  devices (Z44-Z46)

   Z43.0   **Encounter for attention to tracheostomy**

   Z43.1   **Encounter for attention to gastrostomy**

   Z43.2   **Encounter for attention to ileostomy**

   Z43.3   **Encounter for attention to colostomy**

   Z43.4   **Encounter for attention to other artificial openings of digestive tract**

   Z43.5   **Encounter for attention to cystostomy**

   Z43.6   **Encounter for attention to other artificial openings of urinary tract**
         Encounter for attention to nephrostomy
         Encounter for attention to ureterostomy
         Encounter for attention to urethrostomy

   Z43.7   **Encounter for attention to artificial vagina**

   Z43.8   **Encounter for attention to other artificial openings**

   Z43.9   **Encounter for attention to** unspecified **artificial opening**

● **Z44**   **Encounter for fitting and adjustment of external prosthetic device**

    Includes   removal or replacement of external prosthetic
                device

    Excludes1   malfunction or other complications of device - see
                  Alphabetical Index presence of prosthetic
                  device (Z97.-)

 ● **Z44.0**   **Encounter for fitting and adjustment of artificial arm**

  ● **Z44.00**   **Encounter for fitting and adjustment of unspecified artificial arm**

     Z44.001   **Encounter for fitting and adjustment of** unspecified **right artificial arm**

     Z44.002   **Encounter for fitting and adjustment of** unspecified **left artificial arm**

     Z44.009   **Encounter for fitting and adjustment of** unspecified **artificial arm, unspecified arm**

  ● **Z44.01**   **Encounter for fitting and adjustment of complete artificial arm**

     Z44.011   **Encounter for fitting and adjustment of complete right artificial arm**

     Z44.012   **Encounter for fitting and adjustment of complete left artificial arm**

     Z44.019   **Encounter for fitting and adjustment of complete artificial arm,** unspecified **arm**

  ● **Z44.02**   **Encounter for fitting and adjustment of partial artificial arm**

     Z44.021   **Encounter for fitting and adjustment of partial artificial right arm**

     Z44.022   **Encounter for fitting and adjustment of partial artificial left arm**

     Z44.029   **Encounter for fitting and adjustment of partial artificial arm,** unspecified **arm**

 ● **Z44.1**   **Encounter for fitting and adjustment of artificial leg**

  ● **Z44.10**   **Encounter for fitting and adjustment of unspecified artificial leg**

     Z44.101   **Encounter for fitting and adjustment of** unspecified **right artificial leg**

     Z44.102   **Encounter for fitting and adjustment of** unspecified **left artificial leg**

     Z44.109   **Encounter for fitting and adjustment of** unspecified **artificial leg, unspecified leg**

  ● **Z44.11**   **Encounter for fitting and adjustment of complete artificial leg**

     Z44.111   **Encounter for fitting and adjustment of complete right artificial leg**

     Z44.112   **Encounter for fitting and adjustment of complete left artificial leg**

     Z44.119   **Encounter for fitting and adjustment of complete artificial leg,** unspecified **leg**

  ● **Z44.12**   **Encounter for fitting and adjustment of partial artificial leg**

     Z44.121   **Encounter for fitting and adjustment of partial artificial right leg**

     Z44.122   **Encounter for fitting and adjustment of partial artificial left leg**

     Z44.129   **Encounter for fitting and adjustment of partial artificial leg,** unspecified **leg**

 ● **Z44.2**   **Encounter for fitting and adjustment of artificial eye**

    Excludes1   mechanical complication of ocular
                  prosthesis (T85.3)

   Z44.20   **Encounter for fitting and adjustment of artificial eye,** unspecified

   Z44.21   **Encounter for fitting and adjustment of artificial right eye**

   Z44.22   **Encounter for fitting and adjustment of artificial left eye**

 ● **Z44.3**   **Encounter for fitting and adjustment of external breast prosthesis**

    Excludes1   complications of breast implant (T85.4-)
                  encounter for adjustment or removal of
                  breast implant (Z45.81-)
                  encounter for initial breast implant
                  insertion for cosmetic breast
                  augmentation (Z41.1)
                  encounter for breast reconstruction
                  following mastectomy (Z42.1)

   Z44.30   **Encounter for fitting and adjustment of external breast prosthesis,** unspecified **breast ♀**

   Z44.31   **Encounter for fitting and adjustment of external right breast prosthesis ♀**

   Z44.32   **Encounter for fitting and adjustment of external left breast prosthesis ♀**

   Z44.8   **Encounter for fitting and adjustment of other external prosthetic devices**

   Z44.9   **Encounter for fitting and adjustment of** unspecified **external prosthetic device**

◀ New   ⇐ Revised   ~~deleted~~ Deleted   Excludes 1   Excludes 2   Includes   Use additional   Code first   Code also   Unspecified

OGCR Official Guidelines   X Assign placeholder X   ● Use Additional Character(s)   ▶ Manifestation Code   **Coding Clinic**

● **Z45   Encounter for adjustment and management of implanted device**

Includes	removal or replacement of implanted device
Excludes1	malfunction or other complications of device - see Alphabetical Index
	presence of prosthetic and other devices (Z95-Z97)
Excludes2	encounter for fitting and adjustment of non-implanted device (Z46.-)

● **Z45.0   Encounter for adjustment and management of cardiac device**

● **Z45.01   Encounter for adjustment and management of cardiac pacemaker**

Excludes1	encounter for adjustment and management of automatic implantable cardiac defibrillator with synchronous cardiac pacemaker (Z45.02)

Z45.010   Encounter for checking and testing of cardiac pacemaker pulse generator [battery]
Encounter for replacing cardiac pacemaker pulse generator [battery]

Z45.018   Encounter for adjustment and management of other part of cardiac pacemaker

Z45.02   Encounter for adjustment and management of automatic implantable cardiac defibrillator
Encounter for adjustment and management of automatic implantable cardiac defibrillator with synchronous cardiac pacemaker

Z45.09   Encounter for adjustment and management of other cardiac device

Z45.1   Encounter for adjustment and management of infusion pump

Z45.2   Encounter for adjustment and management of vascular access device
Encounter for adjustment and management of vascular catheters

Excludes1	encounter for adjustment and management of renal dialysis catheter (Z49.01)

● **Z45.3   Encounter for adjustment and management of implanted devices of the special senses**

Z45.31   Encounter for adjustment and management of implanted visual substitution device

● **Z45.32   Encounter for adjustment and management of implanted hearing device**

Excludes1	encounter for fitting and adjustment of hearing aide (Z46.1)

Z45.320   Encounter for adjustment and management of bone conduction device

Z45.321   Encounter for adjustment and management of cochlear device

Z45.328   Encounter for adjustment and management of other implanted hearing device

● **Z45.4   Encounter for adjustment and management of implanted nervous system device**

Z45.41   Encounter for adjustment and management of cerebrospinal fluid drainage device
Encounter for adjustment and management of cerebral ventricular (communicating) shunt

Z45.42   Encounter for adjustment and management of neuropacemaker (brain) (peripheral nerve) (spinal cord)

Z45.49   Encounter for adjustment and management of other implanted nervous system device

● **Z45.8   Encounter for adjustment and management of other implanted devices**

● **Z45.81   Encounter for adjustment or removal of breast implant**
Encounter for elective implant exchange (different material) (different size)
Encounter removal of tissue expander without synchronous insertion of permanent implant

Excludes1	complications of breast implant (T85.4-)
	encounter for initial breast implant insertion for cosmetic breast augmentation (Z41.1)
	encounter for breast reconstruction following mastectomy (Z42.1)

Z45.811   Encounter for adjustment or removal of right breast implant ♀

Z45.812   Encounter for adjustment or removal of left breast implant ♀

Z45.819   Encounter for adjustment or removal of unspecified breast implant ♀

Z45.82   Encounter for adjustment or removal of myringotomy device (stent) (tube)

Z45.89   Encounter for adjustment and management of other implanted devices

Z45.9   Encounter for adjustment and management of unspecified implanted device

● **Z46   Encounter for fitting and adjustment of other devices**

Includes	removal or replacement of other device
Excludes1	malfunction or other complications of device - see Alphabetical Index
Excludes2	encounter for fitting and management of implanted devices (Z45.-)
	issue of repeat prescription only (Z76.0)
	presence of prosthetic and other devices (Z95-Z97)

Z46.0   Encounter for fitting and adjustment of spectacles and contact lenses

Z46.1   Encounter for fitting and adjustment of hearing aid

Excludes1	encounter for adjustment and management of implanted hearing device (Z45.32-)

Z46.2   Encounter for fitting and adjustment of other devices related to nervous system and special senses

Excludes2	encounter for adjustment and management of implanted nervous system device (Z45.4-)
	encounter for adjustment and management of implanted visual substitution device (Z45.31)

Z46.3   Encounter for fitting and adjustment of dental prosthetic device
Encounter for fitting and adjustment of dentures

Z46.4   Encounter for fitting and adjustment of orthodontic device

CHAPTER 21 (Z00-Z99)

CHAPTER 21 (Z00-Z99)

● **Z46.5** **Encounter for fitting and adjustment of other gastrointestinal appliance and device**

    Excludes1 encounter for attention to artificial openings of digestive tract (Z43.1-Z43.4)

  Z46.51 Encounter for fitting and adjustment of gastric lap band

  Z46.59 Encounter for fitting and adjustment of other gastrointestinal appliance and device

Z46.6 **Encounter for fitting and adjustment of urinary device**

    Excludes2 attention to artificial openings of urinary tract (Z43.5, Z43.6)

● **Z46.8** **Encounter for fitting and adjustment of other specified devices**

  Z46.81 Encounter for fitting and adjustment of insulin pump

    Encounter for insulin pump instruction and training

    Encounter for insulin pump titration

  Z46.82 Encounter for fitting and adjustment of non-vascular catheter

  Z46.89 Encounter for fitting and adjustment of other specified devices

    Encounter for fitting and adjustment of wheelchair

Z46.9 **Encounter for fitting and adjustment of unspecified device**

● **Z47** **Orthopedic aftercare**

    Excludes1 aftercare for healing fracture - code to fracture with 7th character D

Z47.1 **Aftercare following joint replacement surgery**

    Use additional code to identify the joint (Z96.6-)

Z47.2 **Encounter for removal of internal fixation device**

    Excludes1 encounter for adjustment of internal fixation device for fracture treatment - code to fracture with appropriate 7th character

      encounter for removal of external fixation device - code to fracture with 7th character D

      infection or inflammatory reaction to internal fixation device (T84.6-)

      mechanical complication of internal fixation device (T84.1-)

● **Z47.3** **Aftercare following explantation of joint prosthesis**

    Aftercare following explantation of joint prosthesis, staged procedure

    Encounter for joint prosthesis insertion following prior explantation of joint prosthesis

    Coding Clinic: 2015, Q1, P17

  Z47.31 Aftercare following explantation of shoulder joint prosthesis

    Excludes1 acquired absence of shoulder joint following prior explantation of shoulder joint prosthesis (Z89.23-)

      shoulder joint prosthesis explantation status (Z89.23-)

  Z47.32 Aftercare following explantation of hip joint prosthesis

    Excludes1 acquired absence of hip joint following prior explantation of hip joint prosthesis (Z89.62-)

      hip joint prosthesis explantation status (Z89.62-)

    Coding Clinic: 2015, Q1, P17

  Z47.33 Aftercare following explantation of knee joint prosthesis

    Excludes1 acquired absence of knee joint following prior explantation of knee prosthesis (Z89.52-)

      knee joint prosthesis explantation status (Z89.52-)

● **Z47.8** **Encounter for other orthopedic aftercare**

  Z47.81 Encounter for orthopedic aftercare following surgical amputation

    Use additional code to identify the limb amputated (Z89.-)

  Z47.82 Encounter for orthopedic aftercare following scoliosis surgery

  Z47.89 Encounter for other orthopedic aftercare

    Coding Clinic: 2015, Q1, P8

● **Z48** **Encounter for other postprocedural aftercare**

    Excludes1 encounter for follow-up examination after completed treatment (Z08-Z09)

    Excludes2 encounter for attention to artificial openings (Z43.-)

      encounter for fitting and adjustment of prosthetic and other devices (Z44-Z46)

● **Z48.0** **Encounter for attention to dressings, sutures and drains**

    Excludes1 encounter for planned postprocedural wound closure (Z48.1)

  Z48.00 Encounter for change or removal of nonsurgical wound dressing

    Encounter for change or removal of wound dressing NOS

  Z48.01 Encounter for change or removal of surgical wound dressing

  Z48.02 Encounter for removal of sutures

    Encounter for removal of staples

    Coding Clinic: 2015, Q1, P6

  Z48.03 Encounter for change or removal of drains

Z48.1 **Encounter for planned postprocedural wound closure**

    Excludes1 encounter for attention to dressings and sutures (Z48.0-)

● **Z48.2** **Encounter for aftercare following organ transplant**

  Z48.21 Encounter for aftercare following heart transplant

  Z48.22 Encounter for aftercare following kidney transplant

  Z48.23 Encounter for aftercare following liver transplant

  Z48.24 Encounter for aftercare following lung transplant

  ● **Z48.28** Encounter for aftercare following multiple organ transplant

    Z48.280 Encounter for aftercare following heart-lung transplant

    Z48.288 Encounter for aftercare following multiple organ transplant

  ● **Z48.29** Encounter for aftercare following other organ transplant

    Z48.290 Encounter for aftercare following bone marrow transplant

    Z48.298 Encounter for aftercare following other organ transplant

Z48.3 **Aftercare following surgery for neoplasm**

    Use additional code to identify the neoplasm

◄ New   ⬅ Revised   ~~deleted~~ Deleted   Excludes 1   Excludes 2   Includes   Use additional   Code first   Code also   Unspecified

OGCR Official Guidelines   X Assign placeholder X   ● Use Additional Character(s)   ▶ Manifestation Code   **Coding Clinic**

● **Z48.8   Encounter for other specified postprocedural aftercare**

● **Z48.81   Encounter for surgical aftercare following surgery on specified body systems**

These codes identify the body system requiring aftercare. They are for use in conjunction with other aftercare codes to fully explain the aftercare encounter. The condition treated should also be coded if still present.

Excludes1   aftercare for injury - code the injury with 7th character D
aftercare following surgery for neoplasm (Z48.3)

Excludes2   aftercare following organ transplant (Z48.2-)
orthopedic aftercare (Z47.-)

Z48.810   Encounter for surgical aftercare following surgery on the sense organs

Z48.811   Encounter for surgical aftercare following surgery on the nervous system

Excludes2   encounter for surgical aftercare following surgery on the sense organs (Z48.810)

Z48.812   Encounter for surgical aftercare following surgery on the circulatory system
Coding Clinic: 2012, Q4, P96

Z48.813   Encounter for surgical aftercare following surgery on the respiratory system

Z48.814   Encounter for surgical aftercare following surgery on the teeth or oral cavity

Z48.815   Encounter for surgical aftercare following surgery on the digestive system

Z48.816   Encounter for surgical aftercare following surgery on the genitourinary system

Excludes1   encounter for aftercare following sterilization reversal (Z31.42)

Z48.817   Encounter for surgical aftercare following surgery on the skin and subcutaneous tissue
Coding Clinic: 2015, Q1, P6

Z48.89   Encounter for other specified surgical aftercare

● **Z49   Encounter for care involving renal dialysis**

Code also associated end stage renal disease (N18.6)

● **Z49.0   Preparatory care for renal dialysis**

Encounter for dialysis instruction and training

Z49.01   Encounter for fitting and adjustment of extracorporeal dialysis catheter

Removal or replacement of renal dialysis catheter
Toilet or cleansing of renal dialysis catheter

Z49.02   Encounter for fitting and adjustment of peritoneal dialysis catheter

● **Z49.3   Encounter for adequacy testing for dialysis**

Z49.31   Encounter for adequacy testing for hemodialysis

Z49.32   Encounter for adequacy testing for peritoneal dialysis

Encounter for peritoneal equilibration test

● **Z51   Encounter for other aftercare**

Code also condition requiring care

Excludes1   follow-up examination after treatment (Z08-Z09)

Z51.0   Encounter for antineoplastic radiation therapy

● **Z51.1   Encounter for antineoplastic chemotherapy and immunotherapy**

Excludes2   encounter for chemotherapy and immunotherapy for nonneoplastic condition-code to condition

Z51.11   Encounter for antineoplastic chemotherapy

Z51.12   Encounter for antineoplastic immunotherapy

Z51.5   Encounter for palliative care

● **Z51.8   Encounter for other specified aftercare**

Excludes1   holiday relief care (Z75.5)

Z51.81   Encounter for therapeutic drug level monitoring

Code also any long-term (current) drug therapy (Z79.-)

Excludes1   encounter for blood-drug test for administrative or medicolegal reasons (Z02.83)

Z51.89   Encounter for other specified aftercare
Coding Clinic: 2012, Q4, P96-97

● **Z52   Donors of organs and tissues**

Includes   autologous and other living donors

Excludes1   cadaveric donor - omit code
examination of potential donor (Z00.5)

Coding Clinic: 2012, Q4, P100

● **Z52.0   Blood donor**

● **Z52.00   Unspecified blood donor**

Z52.000   Unspecified donor, whole blood

Z52.001   Unspecified donor, stem cells

Z52.008   Unspecified donor, other blood

● **Z52.01   Autologous blood donor**

Z52.010   Autologous donor, whole blood

Z52.011   Autologous donor, stem cells

Z52.018   Autologous donor, other blood

● **Z52.09   Other blood donor**

Volunteer donor

Z52.090   Other blood donor, whole blood

Z52.091   Other blood donor, stem cells

Z52.098   Other blood donor, other blood

● **Z52.1   Skin donor**

Z52.10   Skin donor, unspecified

Z52.11   Skin donor, autologous

Z52.19   Skin donor, other

● **Z52.2   Bone donor**

Z52.20   Bone donor, unspecified

Z52.21   Bone donor, autologous

Z52.29   Bone donor, other

Z52.3   Bone marrow donor

Z52.4   Kidney donor

Z52.5   Cornea donor

Z52.6   Liver donor
Coding Clinic: 2012, Q4, P100

CHAPTER 21 (Z00-Z99)

● Z52.8   Donor of other specified organs or tissues
    ● Z52.81   Egg (Oocyte) donor
        Z52.810   Egg (Oocyte) donor under age 35, anonymous recipient ♀
               Egg donor under age 35 NOS
        Z52.811   Egg (Oocyte) donor under age 35, designated recipient ♀
        Z52.812   Egg (Oocyte) donor age 35 and over, anonymous recipient ♀
               Egg donor age 35 and over NOS
        Z52.813   Egg (Oocyte) donor age 35 and over, designated recipient ♀
        Z52.819   Egg (Oocyte) donor, unspecified ♀
    Z52.89   Donor of other specified organs or tissues
  Z52.9   Donor of unspecified organ or tissue
      Donor NOS

● Z53   Persons encountering health services for specific procedures and treatment, not carried out
  ● Z53.0   Procedure and treatment not carried out because of contraindication
    Z53.01   Procedure and treatment not carried out due to patient smoking
    Z53.09   Procedure and treatment not carried out because of other contraindication
  Z53.1   Procedure and treatment not carried out because of patient's decision for reasons of belief and group pressure
  ● Z53.2   Procedure and treatment not carried out because of patient's decision for other and unspecified reasons
    Z53.20   Procedure and treatment not carried out because of patient's decision for unspecified reasons
    Z53.21   Procedure and treatment not carried out due to patient leaving prior to being seen by health care provider
    Z53.29   Procedure and treatment not carried out because of patient's decision for other reasons
  Z53.8   Procedure and treatment not carried out for other reasons
  Z53.9   Procedure and treatment not carried out, unspecified reason

PERSONS WITH POTENTIAL HEALTH HAZARDS RELATED TO SOCIOECONOMIC AND PSYCHOSOCIAL CIRCUMSTANCES (Z55-Z65)

● Z55   Problems related to education and literacy
    Excludes1   disorders of psychological development (F80-F89)
  Z55.0   Illiteracy and low-level literacy
  Z55.1   Schooling unavailable and unattainable
  Z55.2   Failed school examinations
  Z55.3   Underachievement in school
  Z55.4   Educational maladjustment and discord with teachers and classmates
  Z55.8   Other problems related to education and literacy
      Problems related to inadequate teaching
  Z55.9   Problems related to education and literacy, unspecified
      Academic problems NOS

● Z56   Problems related to employment and unemployment
    Excludes2   occupational exposure to risk factors (Z57.-)
                problems related to housing and economic circumstances (Z59.-)
  Z56.0   Unemployment, unspecified
  Z56.1   Change of job
  Z56.2   Threat of job loss
  Z56.3   Stressful work schedule

  Z56.4   Discord with boss and workmates
  Z56.5   Uncongenial work environment
      Difficult conditions at work
  Z56.6   Other physical and mental strain related to work
  ● Z56.8   Other problems related to employment
    Z56.81   Sexual harassment on the job
    Z56.82   Military deployment status
        Individual (civilian or military) currently deployed in theater or in support of military war, peacekeeping and humanitarian operations
    Z56.89   Other problems related to employment
  Z56.9   Unspecified problems related to employment
      Occupational problems NOS

● Z57   Occupational exposure to risk factors
  Z57.0   Occupational exposure to noise
  Z57.1   Occupational exposure to radiation
  Z57.2   Occupational exposure to dust
  ● Z57.3   Occupational exposure to other air contaminants
    Z57.31   Occupational exposure to environmental tobacco smoke
        Excludes2   exposure to environmental tobacco smoke (Z77.22)
    Z57.39   Occupational exposure to other air contaminants
  Z57.4   Occupational exposure to toxic agents in agriculture
      Occupational exposure to solids, liquids, gases or vapors in agriculture
  Z57.5   Occupational exposure to toxic agents in other industries
      Occupational exposure to solids, liquids, gases or vapors in other industries
  Z57.6   Occupational exposure to extreme temperature
  Z57.7   Occupational exposure to vibration
  Z57.8   Occupational exposure to other risk factors
  Z57.9   Occupational exposure to unspecified risk factor

● Z59   Problems related to housing and economic circumstances
    Excludes2   problems related to upbringing (Z62.-)
  Z59.0   Homelessness
  Z59.1   Inadequate housing
      Lack of heating
      Restriction of space
      Technical defects in home preventing adequate care
      Unsatisfactory surroundings
    Excludes1   problems related to the natural and physical environment (Z77.1-)
  Z59.2   Discord with neighbors, lodgers and landlord
  Z59.3   Problems related to living in residential institution
      Boarding-school resident
    Excludes1   institutional upbringing (Z62.2)
  Z59.4   Lack of adequate food and safe drinking water
      Inadequate drinking water supply
    Excludes1   effects of hunger (T73.0)
                inappropriate diet or eating habits (Z72.4)
                malnutrition (E40-E46)
  Z59.5   Extreme poverty
  Z59.6   Low income
  Z59.7   Insufficient social insurance and welfare support
  Z59.8   Other problems related to housing and economic circumstances
      Foreclosure on loan
      Isolated dwelling
      Problems with creditors
  Z59.9   Problem related to housing and economic circumstances, unspecified

A

◀ New   ⬅ Revised   ~~deleted~~ Deleted   Excludes 1   Excludes 2   Includes   Use additional   Code first   Code also   Unspecified

OGCR Official Guidelines   X Assign placeholder X   ● Use Additional Character(s)   ▶ Manifestation Code   **Coding Clinic**

● Z60   **Problems related to social environment**

    Z60.0   **Problems of adjustment to life-cycle transitions**
           Empty nest syndrome
           Phase of life problem
           Problem with adjustment to retirement [pension]

    Z60.2   **Problems related to living alone**

    Z60.3   **Acculturation difficulty**
           Problem with migration
           Problem with social transplantation

    Z60.4   **Social exclusion and rejection**
           Exclusion and rejection on the basis of personal characteristics, such as unusual physical appearance, illness or behavior.

           `Excludes1` target of adverse discrimination such as for racial or religious reasons (Z60.5)

    Z60.5   **Target of (perceived) adverse discrimination and persecution**

           `Excludes1` social exclusion and rejection (Z60.4)

    Z60.8   **Other problems related to social environment**

    Z60.9   **Problem related to social environment, `unspecified`**

● Z62   **Problems related to upbringing**

    `Includes` current and past negative life events in childhood
           current and past problems of a child related to upbringing

    `Excludes2` maltreatment syndrome (T74.-)
           problems related to housing and economic circumstances (Z59.-)

    Z62.0   **Inadequate parental supervision and control**

    Z62.1   **Parental overprotection**

  ● **Z62.2**   **Upbringing away from parents**

           `Excludes1` problems with boarding school (Z59.3)

      Z62.21   **Child in welfare custody**   **P**
           Child in care of non-parental family member
           Child in foster care

           `Excludes2` problem for parent due to child in welfare custody (Z63.5)

      Z62.22   **Institutional upbringing**
           Child living in orphanage or group home

      Z62.29   **Other upbringing away from parents**

    Z62.3   **Hostility towards and scapegoating of child**   **P**

    Z62.6   **Inappropriate (excessive) parental pressure**

  ● **Z62.8**   **Other specified problems related to upbringing**

    ● **Z62.81**   **Personal history of abuse in childhood**

      Z62.810   **Personal history of physical and sexual abuse in childhood**

           `Excludes1` current child physical abuse (T74.12, T76.12)
                  current child sexual abuse (T74.22, T76.22)

      Z62.811   **Personal history of psychological abuse in childhood**

           `Excludes1` current child psychological abuse (T74.32, T76.32)

      Z62.812   **Personal history of neglect in childhood**

           `Excludes1` current child neglect (T74.02, T76.02)

      Z62.819   **Personal history of `unspecified` abuse in childhood**

           `Excludes1` current child abuse NOS (T74.92, T76.92)

      Z62.82   **Parent-child conflict**

      Z62.820   **Parent-biological child conflict**
           Parent-child problem NOS

      Z62.821   **Parent-adopted child conflict**

      Z62.822   **Parent-foster child conflict**

  ● **Z62.89**   **Other specified problems related to upbringing**

      Z62.890   **Parent-child estrangement NEC**

      Z62.891   **Sibling rivalry**

      Z62.898   **Other specified problems related to upbringing**

    Z62.9   **Problem related to upbringing, `unspecified`**

● Z63   **Other problems related to primary support group, including family circumstances**

    `Excludes2` maltreatment syndrome (T74.-, T76)
           parent-child problems (Z62.-)
           problems related to negative life events in childhood (Z62.-)
           problems related to upbringing (Z62.-)

    Z63.0   **Problems in relationship with spouse or partner**

           `Excludes1` counseling for spousal or partner abuse problems (Z69.1)
                  counseling related to sexual attitude, behavior, and orientation (Z70.-)

    Z63.1   **Problems in relationship with in-laws**

  ● **Z63.3**   **Absence of family member**

           `Excludes1` absence of family member due to disappearance and death (Z63.4)
                  absence of family member due to separation and divorce (Z63.5)

      Z63.31   **Absence of family member due to military deployment**
           Individual or family affected by other family member being on military deployment

           `Excludes1` family disruption due to return of family member from military deployment (Z63.71)

      Z63.32   **Other absence of family member**

    Z63.4   **Disappearance and death of family member**
           Assumed death of family member
           Bereavement

    Z63.5   **Disruption of family by separation and divorce**
           Marital estrangement

    Z63.6   **Dependent relative needing care at home**

  ● **Z63.7**   **Other stressful life events affecting family and household**

      Z63.71   **Stress on family due to return of family member from military deployment**
           Individual or family affected by family member having returned from military deployment (current or past conflict)

      Z63.72   **Alcoholism and drug addiction in family**

      Z63.79   **Other stressful life events affecting family and household**
           Anxiety (normal) about sick person in family
           Health problems within family
           Ill or disturbed family member
           Isolated family

    Z63.8   **Other specified problems related to primary support group**
           Family discord NOS
           Family estrangement NOS
           High expressed emotional level within family
           Inadequate family support NOS
           Inadequate or distorted communication within family

    Z63.9   **Problem related to primary support group, `unspecified`**
           Relationship disorder NOS

● **Z64** **Problems related to certain psychosocial circumstances**
     Z64.0 **Problems related to unwanted pregnancy ♀**   **M**
     Z64.1 **Problems related to multiparity ♀**
     Z64.4 **Discord with counselors**
          Discord with probation officer
          Discord with social worker

● **Z65** **Problems related to other psychosocial circumstances**
     Z65.0 **Conviction in civil and criminal proceedings without imprisonment**
     Z65.1 **Imprisonment and other incarceration**
     Z65.2 **Problems related to release from prison**
     Z65.3 **Problems related to other legal circumstances**
          Arrest
          Child custody or support proceedings
          Litigation
          Prosecution
     Z65.4 **Victim of crime and terrorism**
          Victim of torture
     Z65.5 **Exposure to disaster, war and other hostilities**
          Excludes1   target of perceived discrimination or persecution (Z60.5)
     Z65.8 **Other specified problems related to psychosocial circumstances**
     Z65.9 **Problem related to unspecified psychosocial circumstances**

DO NOT RESUSCITATE STATUS (Z66)

Z66 **Do not resuscitate**
     DNR status

BLOOD TYPE (Z67)

● **Z67** **Blood type**
   ● **Z67.1** **Type A blood**
         Z67.10   Type A blood, Rh positive
         Z67.11   Type A blood, Rh negative
   ● **Z67.2** **Type B blood**
         Z67.20   Type B blood, Rh positive
         Z67.21   Type B blood, Rh negative
   ● **Z67.3** **Type AB blood**
         Z67.30   Type AB blood, Rh positive
         Z67.31   Type AB blood, Rh negative
   ● **Z67.4** **Type O blood**
         Z67.40   Type O blood, Rh positive
         Z67.41   Type O blood, Rh negative
   ● **Z67.9** **Unspecified blood type**
         Z67.90   Unspecified blood type, Rh positive
         Z67.91   Unspecified blood type, Rh negative

BODY MASS INDEX [BMI] (Z68)

OGCR Section I.B.14.

General Coding Guidelines

14. Documentation for BMI, Non-pressure ulcers and Pressure Ulcer Stages

For the Body Mass Index (BMI), depth of non-pressure chronic ulcers and pressure ulcer stage codes, code assignment may be based on medical record documentation from clinicians who are not the patient's provider (i.e., physician or other qualified healthcare practitioner legally accountable for establishing the patient's diagnosis), since this information is typically documented by other clinicians involved in the care of the patient (e.g., a dietitian often documents the BMI and nurses often documents the pressure ulcer stages). However, the associated diagnosis (such as overweight, obesity, or pressure ulcer) must be documented by the patient's provider. If there is conflicting medical record documentation, either from the same clinician or different clinicians, the patient's attending provider should be queried for clarification.

The BMI codes should only be reported as secondary diagnoses.

● **Z68** **Body mass index [BMI]**
     Kilograms per meters squared
     Note: BMI adult codes are for use for persons 21 years of age or older.
          BMI pediatric codes are for use for persons 2-20 years of age. These percentiles are based on the growth charts published by the Centers for Disease Control and Prevention (CDC)
     Z68.1 **Body mass index (BMI) 19 or less, adult**   **A**
   ● **Z68.2** **Body mass index (BMI) 20-29, adult**
         Z68.20   Body mass index (BMI) 20.0-20.9, adult   **A**
         Z68.21   Body mass index (BMI) 21.0-21.9, adult   **A**
         Z68.22   Body mass index (BMI) 22.0-22.9, adult   **A**
         Z68.23   Body mass index (BMI) 23.0-23.9, adult   **A**
         Z68.24   Body mass index (BMI) 24.0-24.9, adult   **A**
         Z68.25   Body mass index (BMI) 25.0-25.9, adult   **A**
         Z68.26   Body mass index (BMI) 26.0-26.9, adult   **A**
         Z68.27   Body mass index (BMI) 27.0-27.9, adult   **A**
         Z68.28   Body mass index (BMI) 28.0-28.9, adult   **A**
         Z68.29   Body mass index (BMI) 29.0-29.9, adult   **A**
   ● **Z68.3** **Body mass index (BMI) 30-39, adult**
         Z68.30   Body mass index (BMI) 30.0-30.9, adult   **A**
         Z68.31   Body mass index (BMI) 31.0-31.9, adult   **A**
         Z68.32   Body mass index (BMI) 32.0-32.9, adult   **A**
         Z68.33   Body mass index (BMI) 33.0-33.9, adult   **A**
         Z68.34   Body mass index (BMI) 34.0-34.9, adult   **A**
         Z68.35   Body mass index (BMI) 35.0-35.9, adult   **A**
         Z68.36   Body mass index (BMI) 36.0-36.9, adult   **A**
         Z68.37   Body mass index (BMI) 37.0-37.9, adult   **A**
         Z68.38   Body mass index (BMI) 38.0-38.9, adult   **A**
         Z68.39   Body mass index (BMI) 39.0-39.9, adult   **A**
   ● **Z68.4** **Body mass index (BMI) 40 or greater, adult**
         Z68.41 Body mass index (BMI) 40.0-44.9, adult   **A**
         Z68.42 Body mass index (BMI) 45.0-49.9, adult   **A**
         Z68.43 Body mass index (BMI) 50-59.9, adult   **A**
         Z68.44 Body mass index (BMI) 60.0-69.9, adult   **A**
         Z68.45 Body mass index (BMI) 70 or greater, adult   **A**
   ● **Z68.5** **Body mass index (BMI) pediatric**
         Z68.51   Body mass index (BMI) pediatric, less than 5th percentile for age   **P**
         Z68.52   Body mass index (BMI) pediatric, 5th percentile to less than 85th percentile for age   **P**
         Z68.53   Body mass index (BMI) pediatric, 85th percentile to less than 95th percentile for age   **P**
         Z68.54   Body mass index (BMI) pediatric, greater than or equal to 95th percentile for age   **P**

PERSONS ENCOUNTERING HEALTH SERVICES IN OTHER CIRCUMSTANCES (Z69-Z76)

● **Z69** **Encounter for mental health services for victim and perpetrator of abuse**
     Includes   counseling for victims and perpetrators of abuse
   ● **Z69.0** **Encounter for mental health services for child abuse problems**
     ● **Z69.01** **Encounter for mental health services for parental child abuse**
         Z69.010   Encounter for mental health services for victim of parental child abuse   **P**
         Z69.011   Encounter for mental health services for perpetrator of parental child abuse
           Excludes1   encounter for mental health services for non-parental child abuse (Z69.02-)

◄ New   ◄▬ Revised   ~~deleted~~ Deleted   Excludes 1   Excludes 2   Includes   Use additional   Code first   Code also   Unspecified
OGCR Official Guidelines   **X** Assign placeholder X   ● Use Additional Character(s)   ▌ Manifestation Code   **Coding Clinic**

●Z69.02   Encounter for mental health services for non-parental child abuse

     Z69.020   Encounter for mental health services for victim of non-parental child abuse   **P**

     Z69.021   Encounter for mental health services for perpetrator of non- parental child abuse

●Z69.1   Encounter for mental health services for spousal or partner abuse problems

     Z69.11   Encounter for mental health services for victim of spousal or partner abuse

     Z69.12   Encounter for mental health services for perpetrator of spousal or partner abuse

●Z69.8   Encounter for mental health services for victim or perpetrator of other abuse

     Z69.81   Encounter for mental health services for victim of other abuse
         Encounter for rape victim counseling

     Z69.82   Encounter for mental health services for perpetrator of other abuse

●Z70   Counseling related to sexual attitude, behavior and orientation

     Includes   encounter for mental health services for sexual attitude, behavior and orientation

     Excludes2   contraceptive or procreative counseling (Z30-Z31)

Z70.0   Counseling related to sexual attitude

Z70.1   Counseling related to patient's sexual behavior and orientation
     Patient concerned regarding impotence
     Patient concerned regarding non-responsiveness
     Patient concerned regarding promiscuity
     Patient concerned regarding sexual orientation

Z70.2   Counseling related to sexual behavior and orientation of third party
     Advice sought regarding sexual behavior and orientation of child
     Advice sought regarding sexual behavior and orientation of partner
     Advice sought regarding sexual behavior and orientation of spouse

Z70.3   Counseling related to combined concerns regarding sexual attitude, behavior and orientation

Z70.8   Other sex counseling
     Encounter for sex education

Z70.9   Sex counseling, unspecified

●Z71   Persons encountering health services for other counseling and medical advice, not elsewhere classified

     Excludes2   contraceptive or procreation counseling (Z30-Z31)
         sex counseling (Z70.-)

Z71.0   Person encountering health services to consult on behalf of another person
     Person encountering health services to seek advice or treatment for non-attending third party

     Excludes2   anxiety (normal) about sick person in family (Z63.7)
         expectant (adoptive) parent(s) pre-birth pediatrician visit (Z76.81)

Z71.1   Person with feared health complaint in whom no diagnosis is made
     Person encountering health services with feared condition which was not demonstrated
     Person encountering health services in which problem was normal state
     'Worried well'

     Excludes1   medical observation for suspected diseases and conditions proven not to exist (Z03.-)

Z71.2   Person consulting for explanation of examination or test findings

Z71.3   Dietary counseling and surveillance
     Use additional code for any associated underlying medical condition
     Use additional code to identify body mass index (BMI), if known (Z68.-)

●Z71.4   Alcohol abuse counseling and surveillance
     Use additional code for alcohol abuse or dependence (F10.-)

     Z71.41   Alcohol abuse counseling and surveillance of alcoholic

     Z71.42   Counseling for family member of alcoholic
         Counseling for significant other, partner, or friend of alcoholic

●Z71.5   Drug abuse counseling and surveillance
     Use additional code for drug abuse or dependence (F11-F16, F18-F19)

     Z71.51   Drug abuse counseling and surveillance of drug abuser

     Z71.52   Counseling for family member of drug abuser
         Counseling for significant other, partner, or friend of drug abuser

Z71.6   Tobacco abuse counseling
     Use additional code for nicotine dependence (F17.-)

Z71.7   Human immunodeficiency virus [HIV] counseling

●Z71.8   Other specified counseling

     Excludes2   counseling for contraception (Z30.0-)
         counseling for genetics (Z31.5)
         counseling for procreative management (Z31.6-)

     Z71.81   Spiritual or religious counseling

     Z71.89   Other specified counseling

Z71.9   Counseling, unspecified
     Encounter for medical advice NOS

●Z72   Problems related to lifestyle

     Excludes2   problems related to life-management difficulty (Z73.-)
         problems related to socioeconomic and psychosocial circumstances (Z55-Z65)

Z72.0   Tobacco use
     Tobacco use NOS

     Excludes1   history of tobacco dependence (Z87.891)
         nicotine dependence (F17.2-)
         tobacco dependence (F17.2-)
         tobacco use during pregnancy (O99.33-)

Z72.3   Lack of physical exercise

Z72.4   Inappropriate diet and eating habits

     Excludes1   behavioral eating disorders of infancy or childhood (F98.2.-F98.3)
         eating disorders (F50.-)
         lack of adequate food (Z59.4)
         malnutrition and other nutritional deficiencies (E40-E64)

●Z72.5   High risk sexual behavior
     Promiscuity

     Excludes1   paraphilias (F65)

     Z72.51   High risk heterosexual behavior

     Z72.52   High risk homosexual behavior

     Z72.53   High risk bisexual behavior

Z72.6   Gambling and betting

     Excludes1   compulsive or pathological gambling (F63.0)

CHAPTER 21 (Z00-Z99)

● Z72.8   **Other problems related to lifestyle**
    ● Z72.81   **Antisocial behavior**
       Excludes1   conduct disorders (F91.-)
       Z72.810   **Child and adolescent antisocial behavior**   P
          Antisocial behavior (child) (adolescent) without manifest psychiatric disorder
          Delinquency NOS
          Group delinquency
          Offenses in the context of gang membership
          Stealing in company with others
          Truancy from school
       Z72.811   **Adult antisocial behavior**   A
          Adult antisocial behavior without manifest psychiatric disorder
    ● Z72.82   **Problems related to sleep**
       Z72.820   **Sleep deprivation**
          Lack of adequate sleep
          Excludes1   insomnia (G47.0-)
       Z72.821   **Inadequate sleep hygiene**
          Bad sleep habits
          Irregular sleep habits
          Unhealthy sleep wake schedule
          Excludes1   insomnia (F51.0-, G47.0-)
      Z72.89   **Other problems related to lifestyle**
         Self-damaging behavior
    Z72.9   **Problem related to lifestyle, unspecified**

● Z73   **Problems related to life management difficulty**
    Excludes2   problems related to socioeconomic and psychosocial circumstances (Z55-Z65)
    Z73.0   **Burn-out**
    Z73.1   **Type A behavior pattern**
    Z73.2   **Lack of relaxation and leisure**
    Z73.3   **Stress, not elsewhere classified**
       Physical and mental strain NOS
       Excludes1   stress related to employment or unemployment (Z56.-)
    Z73.4   **Inadequate social skills, not elsewhere classified**
    Z73.5   **Social role conflict, not elsewhere classified**
    Z73.6   **Limitation of activities due to disability**
       Excludes1   care-provider dependency (Z74.-)
    ● Z73.8   **Other problems related to life management difficulty**
      ● Z73.81   **Behavioral insomnia of childhood**
         Z73.810   **Behavioral insomnia of childhood, sleep-onset association type**   P
         Z73.811   **Behavioral insomnia of childhood, limit setting type**   P
         Z73.812   **Behavioral insomnia of childhood, combined type**   P
         Z73.819   **Behavioral insomnia of childhood, unspecified type**   P
      Z73.82   **Dual sensory impairment**
      Z73.89   **Other problems related to life management difficulty**
    Z73.9   **Problem related to life management difficulty, unspecified**

● Z74   **Problems related to care provider dependency**
    Excludes2   dependence on enabling machines or devices NEC (Z99.-)
    ● Z74.0   **Reduced mobility**
      Z74.01   **Bed confinement status**
        Bedridden
      Z74.09   **Other reduced mobility**
        Chairridden
        Reduced mobility NOS
        Excludes2   wheelchair dependence (Z99.3)

Z74.1   **Need for assistance with personal care**
Z74.2   **Need for assistance at home and no other household member able to render care**
Z74.3   **Need for continuous supervision**
Z74.8   **Other problems related to care provider dependency**
Z74.9   **Problem related to care provider dependency, unspecified**

● Z75   **Problems related to medical facilities and other health care**
    Z75.0   **Medical services not available in home**
       Excludes1   no other household member able to render care (Z74.2)
    Z75.1   **Person awaiting admission to adequate facility elsewhere**
    Z75.2   **Other waiting period for investigation and treatment**
    Z75.3   **Unavailability and inaccessibility of health care facilities**
       Excludes1   bed unavailable (Z75.1)
    Z75.4   **Unavailability and inaccessibility of other helping agencies**
    Z75.5   **Holiday relief care**
    Z75.8   **Other problems related to medical facilities and other health care**
    Z75.9   **Unspecified problem related to medical facilities and other health care**

● Z76   **Persons encountering health services in other circumstances**
    Z76.0   **Encounter for issue of repeat prescription**
       Encounter for issue of repeat prescription for appliance
       Encounter for issue of repeat prescription for medicaments
       Encounter for issue of repeat prescription for spectacles
       Excludes2   issue of medical certificate (Z02.7) repeat prescription for contraceptive (Z30.4-)
    Z76.1   **Encounter for health supervision and care of foundling**
    Z76.2   **Encounter for health supervision and care of other healthy infant and child**   P
       Encounter for medical or nursing care or supervision of healthy infant under circumstances such as adverse socioeconomic conditions at home
       Encounter for medical or nursing care or supervision of healthy infant under circumstances such as awaiting foster or adoptive placement
       Encounter for medical or nursing care or supervision of healthy infant under circumstances such as maternal illness
       Encounter for medical or nursing care or supervision of healthy infant under circumstances such as number of children at home preventing or interfering with normal care
    Z76.3   **Healthy person accompanying sick person**
    Z76.4   **Other boarder to healthcare facility**
       Excludes1   homelessness (Z59.0)
    Z76.5   **Malingerer [conscious simulation]**
       Person feigning illness (with obvious motivation)
       Excludes1   factitious disorder (F68.1-) peregrinating patient (F68.1-)
    ● Z76.8   **Persons encountering health services in other specified circumstances**
      Z76.81   **Expectant parent(s) prebirth pediatrician visit**
        Pre-adoption pediatrician visit for adoptive parent(s)
      Z76.82   **Awaiting organ transplant status**
        Patient waiting for organ availability
      Z76.89   **Persons encountering health services in other specified circumstances**
        Persons encountering health services NOS

◀ New   ◀▥ Revised   ~~deleted~~ Deleted   Excludes 1   Excludes 2   Includes   Use additional   Code first   Code also   Unspecified

OGCR Official Guidelines   **X** Assign placeholder X   ● Use Additional Character(s)   ▶ Manifestation Code   **Coding Clinic**

CHAPTER 21 (Z00-Z99)

PERSONS WITH POTENTIAL HEALTH HAZARDS RELATED TO FAMILY AND PERSONAL HISTORY AND CERTAIN CONDITIONS INFLUENCING HEALTH STATUS (Z77-Z99)

Code also any follow-up examination (Z08-Z09)

● **Z77** **Other contact with and (suspected) exposures hazardous to health**

> **Includes** contact with and (suspected) exposures to potential hazards to health

> **Excludes2** contact with and (suspected) exposure to communicable diseases (Z20.-)
> exposure to (parental) (environmental) tobacco smoke in the perinatal period (P96.81)
> newborn (suspected to be) affected by noxious substances transmitted via placenta or breast milk (P04.-)
> occupational exposure to risk factors (Z57.-)
> retained foreign body (Z18.-)
> retained foreign body fully removed (Z87.821)
> toxic effects of substances chiefly nonmedicinal as to source (T51-T65)

● **Z77.0** **Contact with and (suspected) exposure to hazardous, chiefly nonmedicinal, chemicals**

  ● **Z77.01** **Contact with and (suspected) exposure to hazardous metals**

    Z77.010 **Contact with and (suspected) exposure to arsenic**

    Z77.011 **Contact with and (suspected) exposure to lead**

    Z77.012 **Contact with and (suspected) exposure to uranium**

> **Excludes1** retained depleted uranium fragments (Z18.01)

    Z77.018 **Contact with and (suspected) exposure to other hazardous metals**
> Contact with and (suspected) exposure to chromium compounds
> Contact with and (suspected) exposure to nickel dust

  ● **Z77.02** **Contact with and (suspected) exposure to hazardous aromatic compounds**

    Z77.020 **Contact with and (suspected) exposure to aromatic amines**

    Z77.021 **Contact with and (suspected) exposure to benzene**

    Z77.028 **Contact with and (suspected) exposure to other hazardous aromatic compounds**
> Aromatic dyes NOS
> Polycyclic aromatic hydrocarbons

  ● **Z77.09** **Contact with and (suspected) exposure to other hazardous, chiefly nonmedicinal, chemicals**

    Z77.090 **Contact with and (suspected) exposure to asbestos**

    Z77.098 **Contact with and (suspected) exposure to other hazardous, chiefly nonmedicinal, chemicals**
> Dyes NOS

● **Z77.1** **Contact with and (suspected) exposure to environmental pollution and hazards in the physical environment**

  ● **Z77.11** **Contact with and (suspected) exposure to environmental pollution**

    Z77.110 **Contact with and (suspected) exposure to air pollution**

    Z77.111 **Contact with and (suspected) exposure to water pollution**

    Z77.112 **Contact with and (suspected) exposure to soil pollution**

    Z77.118 **Contact with and (suspected) exposure to other environmental pollution**

  ● **Z77.12** **Contact with and (suspected) exposure to hazards in the physical environment**

    Z77.120 **Contact with and (suspected) exposure to mold (toxic)**

    Z77.121 **Contact with and (suspected) exposure to harmful algae and algae toxins**
> Contact with and (suspected) exposure to (harmful) algae bloom NOS
> Contact with and (suspected) exposure to blue-green algae bloom
> Contact with and (suspected) exposure to brown tide
> Contact with and (suspected) exposure to cyanobacteria bloom
> Contact with and (suspected) exposure to Florida red tide
> Contact with and (suspected) exposure to pfiesteria piscicida
> Contact with and (suspected) exposure to red tide

    Z77.122 **Contact with and (suspected) exposure to noise**

    Z77.123 **Contact with and (suspected) exposure to radon and other naturally occuring radiation**

> **Excludes2** radiation exposure as the cause of a confirmed condition (W88-W90, X39.0-)
> radiation sickness NOS (T66)

    Z77.128 **Contact with and (suspected) exposure to other hazards in the physical environment**

● **Z77.2** **Contact with and (suspected) exposure to other hazardous substances**

  Z77.21 **Contact with and (suspected) exposure to potentially hazardous body fluids**

  Z77.22 **Contact with and (suspected) exposure to environmental tobacco smoke (acute) (chronic)**
> Exposure to second hand tobacco smoke (acute) (chronic)
> Passive smoking (acute) (chronic)

> **Excludes1** nicotine dependence (F17.-)
> tobacco use (Z72.0)

> **Excludes2** occupational exposure to environmental tobacco smoke (Z57.31)

  Z77.29 **Contact with and (suspected) exposure to other hazardous substances**

Z77.9 **Other contact with and (suspected) exposures hazardous to health**

CHAPTER 21 (Z00-Z99)

● **Z78**   **Other specified health status**

    Excludes2 asymptomatic human immunodeficiency virus [HIV] infection status (Z21)
         postprocedural status (Z93-Z99)
         sex reassignment status (Z87.890)

    Z78.0 **Asymptomatic menopausal state** ♀   **A**
        Menopausal state NOS
        Postmenopausal status NOS
        Excludes2 symptomatic menopausal state (N95.1)

    Z78.1 **Physical restraint status**
        Excludes1 physical restraint due to a procedure - omit code

    Z78.9 **Other specified health status**

● **Z79**   **Long term (current) drug therapy**

    Includes long term (current) drug use for prophylactic purposes

    Code also any therapeutic drug level monitoring (Z51.81)

    Excludes2 drug abuse and dependence (F11-F19)
         drug use complicating pregnancy, childbirth, and the puerperium (O99.32-)

  ● **Z79.0** **Long term (current) use of anticoagulants and antithrombotics/antiplatelets**
      Excludes2 long term (current) use of aspirin (Z79.82)

      Z79.01 **Long term (current) use of anticoagulants**

      Z79.02 **Long term (current) use of antithrombotics/antiplatelets**

    Z79.1 **Long term (current) use of non-steroidal anti-inflammatories (NSAID)**
      Excludes2 long term (current) use of aspirin (Z79.82)

    Z79.2 **Long term (current) use of antibiotics**

    Z79.3 **Long term (current) use of hormonal contraceptives**
      Long term (current) use of birth control pill or patch

    Z79.4 **Long term (current) use of insulin**

  ● **Z79.5** **Long term (current) use of steroids**

      Z79.51 **Long term (current) use of inhaled steroids**

      Z79.52 **Long term (current) use of systemic steroids**

  ● **Z79.8** **Other long term (current) drug therapy**

    ● **Z79.81** **Long term (current) use of agents affecting estrogen receptors and estrogen levels**

        Code first, if applicable:
        malignant neoplasm of breast (C50.-)
        malignant neoplasm of prostate (C61)

        Use additional code, if applicable, to identify:
        estrogen receptor positive status (Z17.0)
        family history of breast cancer (Z80.3)
        genetic susceptibility to malignant neoplasm (cancer) (Z15.0-)
        personal history of breast cancer (Z85.3)
        personal history of prostate cancer (Z85.46)
        postmenopausal status (Z78.0)

        Excludes1 hormone replacement therapy (postmenopausal) (Z79.890)

      Z79.810 **Long term (current) use of selective estrogen receptor modulators (SERMs)**
        Long term (current) use of raloxifene (Evista)
        Long term (current) use of tamoxifen (Nolvadex)
        Long term (current) use of toremifene (Fareston)

      Z79.811 **Long term (current) use of aromatase inhibitors**
        Long term (current) use of anastrozole (Arimidex)
        Long term (current) use of exemestane (Aromasin)
        Long term (current) use of letrozole (Femara)

      Z79.818 **Long term (current) use of other agents affecting estrogen receptors and estrogen levels**
        Long term (current) use of estrogen receptor downregulators
        Long term (current) use of fulvestrant (Faslodex)
        Long term (current) use of gonadotropin-releasing hormone (GnRH) agonist
        Long term (current) use of goserelin acetate (Zoladex)
        Long term (current) use of leuprolide acetate (leuprorelin) (Lupron)
        Long term (current) use of megestrol acetate (Megace)

    Z79.82 **Long term (current) use of aspirin**

    Z79.83 **Long term (current) use of bisphosphonates**

  ● **Z79.89** **Other long term (current) drug therapy**

      Z79.890 **Hormone replacement therapy (postmenopausal)** ♀

      Z79.891 **Long term (current) use of opiate analgesic**
        Long term (current) use of methadone for pain management
        Excludes1 methadone use NOS (F11.2-)
            use of methadone for treatment of heroin addiction (F11.2-)

      Z79.899 **Other long term (current) drug therapy**

● **Z80**   **Family history of primary malignant neoplasm**

    Z80.0 **Family history of malignant neoplasm of digestive organs**
      Conditions classifiable to C15-C26

    Z80.1 **Family history of malignant neoplasm of trachea, bronchus and lung**
      Conditions classifiable to C33-C34

    Z80.2 **Family history of malignant neoplasm of other respiratory and intrathoracic organs**
      Conditions classifiable to C30-C32, C37-C39

    Z80.3 **Family history of malignant neoplasm of breast**
      Conditions classifiable to C50.-

  ● **Z80.4** **Family history of malignant neoplasm of genital organs**
      Conditions classifiable to C51-C63

      Z80.41 **Family history of malignant neoplasm of ovary**

      Z80.42 **Family history of malignant neoplasm of prostate**

      Z80.43 **Family history of malignant neoplasm of testis**

      Z80.49 **Family history of malignant neoplasm of other genital organs**

  ● **Z80.5** **Family history of malignant neoplasm of urinary tract**
      Conditions classifiable to C64-C68

      Z80.51 **Family history of malignant neoplasm of kidney**

      Z80.52 **Family history of malignant neoplasm of bladder**

      Z80.59 **Family history of malignant neoplasm of other urinary tract organ**

    Z80.6 **Family history of leukemia**
      Conditions classifiable to C91-C95

◀ New   ⬅ Revised   ~~deleted~~ Deleted   Excludes 1   Excludes 2   Includes   Use additional   Code first   Code also   Unspecified

OGCR Official Guidelines   **X** Assign placeholder X   ● Use Additional Character(s)   ❱ Manifestation Code   **Coding Clinic**

Z80.7   **Family history of other malignant neoplasms of lymphoid, hematopoietic and related tissues**
Conditions classifiable to C81-C90, C96.-

Z80.8   **Family history of malignant neoplasm of other organs or systems**
Conditions classifiable to C00-C14, C40-C49, C69-C79

Z80.9   **Family history of malignant neoplasm, unspecified**
Conditions classifiable to C80.1

● **Z81**   **Family history of mental and behavioral disorders**

Z81.0   **Family history of intellectual disabilities**
Conditions classifiable to F70-F79

Z81.1   **Family history of alcohol abuse and dependence**
Conditions classifiable to F10.-

Z81.2   **Family history of tobacco abuse and dependence**
Conditions classifiable to F17.-

Z81.3   **Family history of other psychoactive substance abuse and dependence**
Conditions classifiable to F11-F16, F18-F19

Z81.4   **Family history of other substance abuse and dependence**
Conditions classifiable to F55

Z81.8   **Family history of other mental and behavioral disorders**
Conditions classifiable elsewhere in F01-F99

● **Z82**   **Family history of certain disabilities and chronic diseases (leading to disablement)**

Z82.0   **Family history of epilepsy and other diseases of the nervous system**
Conditions classifiable to G00-G99

Z82.1   **Family history of blindness and visual loss**
Conditions classifiable to H54.-

Z82.2   **Family history of deafness and hearing loss**
Conditions classifiable to H90-H91

Z82.3   **Family history of stroke**
Conditions classifiable to I60-I64

● **Z82.4**   **Family history of ischemic heart disease and other diseases of the circulatory system**
Conditions classifiable to I00-I52, I65-I99

Z82.41   **Family history of sudden cardiac death**

Z82.49   **Family history of ischemic heart disease and other diseases of the circulatory system**

Z82.5   **Family history of asthma and other chronic lower respiratory diseases**
Conditions classifiable to J40-J47

    Excludes2   family history of other diseases of the respiratory system (Z83.6)

● **Z82.6**   **Family history of arthritis and other diseases of the musculoskeletal system and connective tissue**
Conditions classifiable to M00-M99

Z82.61   **Family history of arthritis**

Z82.62   **Family history of osteoporosis**

Z82.69   **Family history of other diseases of the musculoskeletal system and connective tissue**

● **Z82.7**   **Family history of congenital malformations, deformations and chromosomal abnormalities**
Conditions classifiable to Q00-Q99

Z82.71   **Family history of polycystic kidney**

Z82.79   **Family history of other congenital malformations, deformations and chromosomal abnormalities**

Z82.8   **Family history of other disabilities and chronic diseases leading to disablement, not elsewhere classified**

● **Z83**   **Family history of other specific disorders**

    Excludes2   contact with and (suspected) exposure to communicable disease in the family (Z20.-)

Z83.0   **Family history of human immunodeficiency virus [HIV] disease**
Conditions classifiable to B20

Z83.1   **Family history of other infectious and parasitic diseases**
Conditions classifiable to A00-B19, B25-B94, B99

Z83.2   **Family history of diseases of the blood and blood-forming organs and certain disorders involving the immune mechanism**
Conditions classifiable to D50-D89

Z83.3   **Family history of diabetes mellitus**
Conditions classifiable to E08-E13

● **Z83.4**   **Family history of other endocrine, nutritional and metabolic diseases**
Conditions classifiable to E00-E07, E15-E88

Z83.41   **Family history of multiple endocrine neoplasia [MEN] syndrome**

Z83.49   **Family history of other endocrine, nutritional and metabolic diseases**

● **Z83.5**   **Family history of eye and ear disorders**

● **Z83.51**   **Family history of eye disorders**
Conditions classifiable to H00-H53, H55-H59

    Excludes2   family history of blindness and visual loss (Z82.1)

Z83.511   **Family history of glaucoma**

Z83.518   **Family history of other specified eye disorder**

Z83.52   **Family history of ear disorders**
Conditions classifiable to H60-H83, H92-H95

    Excludes2   family history of deafness and hearing loss (Z82.2)

Z83.6   **Family history of other diseases of the respiratory system**
Conditions classifiable to J00-J39, J60-J99

    Excludes2   family history of asthma and other chronic lower respiratory diseases (Z82.5)

● **Z83.7**   **Family history of diseases of the digestive system**
Conditions classifiable to K00-K93

Z83.71   **Family history of colonic polyps**

    Excludes1   family history of malignant neoplasm of digestive organs (Z80.0)

Z83.79   **Family history of other diseases of the digestive system**

● **Z84**   **Family history of other conditions**

Z84.0   **Family history of diseases of the skin and subcutaneous tissue**
Conditions classifiable to L00-L99

Z84.1   **Family history of disorders of kidney and ureter**
Conditions classifiable to N00-N29

Z84.2   **Family history of other diseases of the genitourinary system**
Conditions classifiable to N30-N99

Z84.3   **Family history of consanguinity**

● **Z84.8**   **Family history of other specified conditions**

Z84.81   **Family history of carrier of genetic disease**

Z84.89   **Family history of other specified conditions**

CHAPTER 21 (Z00-Z99)

CHAPTER 21 (Z00-Z99)

● **Z85　Personal history of malignant neoplasm**
　　Code first any follow-up examination after treatment of malignant
　　　neoplasm (Z08)
　　Use additional code to identify:
　　　alcohol use and dependence (F10.-)
　　　exposure to environmental tobacco smoke (Z77.22)
　　　history of tobacco use (Z87.891)
　　　occupational exposure to environmental tobacco smoke
　　　　(Z57.31)
　　　tobacco dependence (F17.-)
　　　tobacco use (Z72.0)
　　Excludes2　personal history of benign neoplasm (Z86.01-)
　　　　　　　personal history of carcinoma-in-situ (Z86.00-)

● **Z85.0　Personal history of malignant neoplasm of digestive
　　　organs**
　　　**Z85.00　Personal history of malignant neoplasm of
　　　　　unspecified digestive organ**
　　　**Z85.01　Personal history of malignant neoplasm of
　　　　　esophagus**
　　　　　Conditions classifiable to C15
● 　　**Z85.02　Personal history of malignant neoplasm of
　　　　　stomach**
　　　　　**Z85.020　Personal history of malignant
　　　　　　carcinoid tumor of stomach**
　　　　　　Conditions classifiable to C7A.092
　　　　　**Z85.028　Personal history of other malignant
　　　　　　neoplasm of stomach**
　　　　　　Conditions classifiable to C16
● 　　**Z85.03　Personal history of malignant neoplasm of
　　　　　large intestine**
　　　　　**Z85.030　Personal history of malignant
　　　　　　carcinoid tumor of large intestine**
　　　　　　Conditions classifiable to C7A.022-
　　　　　　C7A.025, C7A.029
　　　　　**Z85.038　Personal history of other malignant
　　　　　　neoplasm of large intestine**
　　　　　　Conditions classifiable to C18
● 　　**Z85.04　Personal history of malignant neoplasm of
　　　　　rectum, rectosigmoid junction, and anus**
　　　　　**Z85.040　Personal history of malignant
　　　　　　carcinoid tumor of rectum**
　　　　　　Conditions classifiable to C7A.026
　　　　　**Z85.048　Personal history of other malignant
　　　　　　neoplasm of rectum, rectosigmoid
　　　　　　junction, and anus**
　　　　　　Conditions classifiable to C19-C21
　　　Z85.05　Personal history of malignant neoplasm of liver
　　　　　Conditions classifiable to C22
● 　　**Z85.06　Personal history of malignant neoplasm of
　　　　　small intestine**
　　　　　**Z85.060　Personal history of malignant
　　　　　　carcinoid tumor of small intestine**
　　　　　　Conditions classifiable to C7A.01-
　　　　　**Z85.068　Personal history of other malignant
　　　　　　neoplasm of small intestine**
　　　　　　Conditions classifiable to C17
　　　**Z85.07　Personal history of malignant neoplasm of
　　　　　pancreas**
　　　　　Conditions classifiable to C25
　　　**Z85.09　Personal history of malignant neoplasm of
　　　　　other digestive organs**

● **Z85.1　Personal history of malignant neoplasm of trachea,
　　　bronchus and lung**
● 　　**Z85.11　Personal history of malignant neoplasm of
　　　　　bronchus and lung**
　　　　　**Z85.110　Personal history of malignant
　　　　　　carcinoid tumor of bronchus and lung**
　　　　　　Conditions classifiable to C7A.090
　　　　　**Z85.118　Personal history of other malignant
　　　　　　neoplasm of bronchus and lung**
　　　　　　Conditions classifiable to C34
　　　**Z85.12　Personal history of malignant neoplasm of
　　　　　trachea**
　　　　　Conditions classifiable to C33
● **Z85.2　Personal history of malignant neoplasm of other
　　　respiratory and intrathoracic organs**
　　　**Z85.20　Personal history of malignant neoplasm of
　　　　　unspecified respiratory organ**
　　　**Z85.21　Personal history of malignant neoplasm of
　　　　　larynx**
　　　　　Conditions classifiable to C32
　　　**Z85.22　Personal history of malignant neoplasm of
　　　　　nasal cavities, middle ear, and accessory sinuses**
　　　　　Conditions classifiable to C30-C31
● 　　**Z85.23　Personal history of malignant neoplasm of
　　　　　thymus**
　　　　　**Z85.230　Personal history of malignant
　　　　　　carcinoid tumor of thymus**
　　　　　　Conditions classifiable to C7A.091
　　　　　**Z85.238　Personal history of other malignant
　　　　　　neoplasm of thymus**
　　　　　　Conditions classifiable to C37
　　　**Z85.29　Personal history of malignant neoplasm of
　　　　　other respiratory and intrathoracic organs**
　　Z85.3　Personal history of malignant neoplasm of breast
　　　　　Conditions classifiable to C50.-
● **Z85.4　Personal history of malignant neoplasm of genital
　　　organs**
　　　　　Conditions classifiable to C51-C63
　　　**Z85.40　Personal history of malignant neoplasm of
　　　　　unspecified female genital organ ♀**
　　　**Z85.41　Personal history of malignant neoplasm of
　　　　　cervix uteri ♀**
　　　**Z85.42　Personal history of malignant neoplasm of
　　　　　other parts of uterus ♀**
　　　**Z85.43　Personal history of malignant neoplasm of
　　　　　ovary ♀**
　　　**Z85.44　Personal history of malignant neoplasm of
　　　　　other female genital organs ♀**
　　　**Z85.45　Personal history of malignant neoplasm of
　　　　　unspecified male genital organ ♂**
　　　**Z85.46　Personal history of malignant neoplasm of
　　　　　prostate ♂**
　　　**Z85.47　Personal history of malignant neoplasm of
　　　　　testis ♂**
　　　**Z85.48　Personal history of malignant neoplasm of
　　　　　epididymis ♂**
　　　**Z85.49　Personal history of malignant neoplasm of
　　　　　other male genital organs ♂**

◀ New　　◀▬ Revised　　~~deleted~~ Deleted　　Excludes 1　　Excludes 2　　Includes　　Use additional　　Code first　　Code also　　Unspecified
OGCR Official Guidelines　　**X** Assign placeholder X　　● Use Additional Character(s)　　▶ Manifestation Code　　**Coding Clinic**

● **Z85.5** **Personal history of malignant neoplasm of urinary tract**
Conditions classifiable to C64-C68

    Z85.50 **Personal history of malignant neoplasm of unspecified urinary tract organ**

    Z85.51 **Personal history of malignant neoplasm of bladder**

    ● **Z85.52** **Personal history of malignant neoplasm of kidney**

        Excludes1 personal history of malignant neoplasm of renal pelvis (Z85.53)

        Z85.520 **Personal history of malignant carcinoid tumor of kidney**
Conditions classifiable to C7A.093

        Z85.528 **Personal history of other malignant neoplasm of kidney**
Conditions classifiable to C64

    Z85.53 **Personal history of malignant neoplasm of renal pelvis**

    Z85.54 **Personal history of malignant neoplasm of ureter**

    Z85.59 **Personal history of malignant neoplasm of other urinary tract organ**

● **Z85.6** **Personal history of leukemia**
Conditions classifiable to C91-C95

    Excludes1 leukemia in remission C91.0-C95.9 with 5th character 1

● **Z85.7** **Personal history of other malignant neoplasms of lymphoid, hematopoietic and related tissues**

    Z85.71 **Personal history of Hodgkin lymphoma**
Conditions classifiable to C81

    Z85.72 **Personal history of non-Hodgkin lymphomas**
Conditions classifiable to C82-C85

    Z85.79 **Personal history of other malignant neoplasms of lymphoid, hematopoietic and related tissues**
Conditions classifiable to C88-C90, C96

        Excludes1 multiple myeloma in remission (C90.01)
plasma cell leukemia in remission (C90.11)
plasmacytoma in remission (C90.21)

● **Z85.8** **Personal history of malignant neoplasms of other organs and systems**
Conditions classifiable to C00-C14, C40-C49, C69-C79, C7A.098

    ● **Z85.81** **Personal history of malignant neoplasm of lip, oral cavity, and pharynx**

        Z85.810 **Personal history of malignant neoplasm of tongue**

        Z85.818 **Personal history of malignant neoplasm of other sites of lip, oral cavity, and pharynx**

        Z85.819 **Personal history of malignant neoplasm of unspecified site of lip, oral cavity, and pharynx**

    ● **Z85.82** **Personal history of malignant neoplasm of skin**

        Z85.820 **Personal history of malignant melanoma of skin**
Conditions classifiable to C43

        Z85.821 **Personal history of Merkel cell carcinoma**
Conditions classifiable to C4A

        Z85.828 **Personal history of other malignant neoplasm of skin**
Conditions classifiable to C44

● **Z85.83** **Personal history of malignant neoplasm of bone and soft tissue**

    Z85.830 **Personal history of malignant neoplasm of bone**

    Z85.831 **Personal history of malignant neoplasm of soft tissue**

        Excludes2 personal history of malignant neoplasm of skin (Z85.82-)

● **Z85.84** **Personal history of malignant neoplasm of eye and nervous tissue**

    Z85.840 **Personal history of malignant neoplasm of eye**

    Z85.841 **Personal history of malignant neoplasm of brain**

    Z85.848 **Personal history of malignant neoplasm of other parts of nervous tissue**

● **Z85.85** **Personal history of malignant neoplasm of endocrine glands**

    Z85.850 **Personal history of malignant neoplasm of thyroid**

    Z85.858 **Personal history of malignant neoplasm of other endocrine glands**

    Z85.89 **Personal history of malignant neoplasm of other organs and systems**

Z85.9 **Personal history of malignant neoplasm, unspecified**
Conditions classifiable to C7A.00, C80.1

● **Z86** **Personal history of certain other diseases**
Code first any follow-up examination after treatment (Z09)

    ● **Z86.0** **Personal history of in-situ and benign neoplasms and neoplasms of uncertain behavior**

        Excludes2 personal history of malignant neoplasms (Z85.-)

    ● **Z86.00** **Personal history of in-situ neoplasm**

        Z86.000 **Personal history of in-situ neoplasm of breast**

        Z86.001 **Personal history of in-situ neoplasm of cervix uteri ♀**

        Z86.008 **Personal history of in-situ neoplasm of other site**

    ● **Z86.01** **Personal history of benign neoplasm**

        Z86.010 **Personal history of colonic polyps**

        Z86.011 **Personal history of benign neoplasm of the brain**

        Z86.012 **Personal history of benign carcinoid tumor**

        Z86.018 **Personal history of other benign neoplasm**

    Z86.03 **Personal history of neoplasm of uncertain behavior**

    ● **Z86.1** **Personal history of infectious and parasitic diseases**
Conditions classifiable to A00-B89, B99

        Excludes1 personal history of infectious diseases specific to a body system sequelae of infectious and parasitic diseases (B90-B94)

    Z86.11 **Personal history of tuberculosis**

    Z86.12 **Personal history of poliomyelitis**

    Z86.13 **Personal history of malaria**

    Z86.14 **Personal history of Methicillin resistant Staphylococcus aureus infection**
Personal history of MRSA infection

    Z86.19 **Personal history of other infectious and parasitic diseases**

CHAPTER 21 (Z00-Z99)

Z86.2   Personal history of diseases of the blood and blood-forming organs and certain disorders involving the immune mechanism
Conditions classifiable to D50-D89

● **Z86.3   Personal history of endocrine, nutritional and metabolic diseases**
Conditions classifiable to E00-E88

     Z86.31   Personal history of diabetic foot ulcer
         Excludes2   current diabetic foot ulcer (E08.621, E09.621, E10.621, E11.621, E13.621)

     Z86.32   Personal history of gestational diabetes ♀
         Personal history of conditions classifiable to O24.4-
         Excludes1   gestational diabetes mellitus in current pregnancy (O24.4-)

     Z86.39   Personal history of other endocrine, nutritional and metabolic disease

● **Z86.5   Personal history of mental and behavioral disorders**
Conditions classifiable to F40-F59

     Z86.51   Personal history of combat and operational stress reaction   A

     Z86.59   Personal history of other mental and behavioral disorders

● **Z86.6   Personal history of diseases of the nervous system and sense organs**
Conditions classifiable to G00-G99, H00-H95

     Z86.61   Personal history of infections of the central nervous system
         Personal history of encephalitis
         Personal history of meningitis

     Z86.69   Personal history of other diseases of the nervous system and sense organs

● **Z86.7   Personal history of diseases of the circulatory system**
Conditions classifiable to I00-I99
     Excludes2   old myocardial infarction (I25.2)
         personal history of anaphylactic shock (Z87.892)
         postmyocardial infarction syndrome (I24.1)

     ● **Z86.71   Personal history of venous thrombosis and embolism**

         Z86.711   Personal history of pulmonary embolism

         Z86.718   Personal history of other venous thrombosis and embolism

     Z86.72   Personal history of thrombophlebitis

     Z86.73   Personal history of transient ischemic attack (TIA), and cerebral infarction without residual deficits
         Personal history of prolonged reversible ischemic neurological deficit (PRIND)
         Personal history of stroke NOS without residual deficits
         Excludes1   personal history of traumatic brain injury (Z87.820)
                 sequelae of cerebrovascular disease (I69.-)
         Coding Clinic: 2012, Q4, P3

     Z86.74   Personal history of sudden cardiac arrest
         Personal history of sudden cardiac death successfully resuscitated

     Z86.79   Personal history of other diseases of the circulatory system

● **Z87   Personal history of other diseases and conditions**
Code first any follow-up examination after treatment (Z09)

     ● **Z87.0   Personal history of diseases of the respiratory system**
Conditions classifiable to J00-J99

         Z87.01   Personal history of pneumonia (recurrent)

         Z87.09   Personal history of other diseases of the respiratory system

     ● **Z87.1   Personal history of diseases of the digestive system**
Conditions classifiable to K00-K93

         Z87.11   Personal history of peptic ulcer disease

         Z87.19   Personal history of other diseases of the digestive system

     Z87.2   Personal history of diseases of the skin and subcutaneous tissue
Conditions classifiable to L00-L99
         Excludes2   personal history of diabetic foot ulcer (Z86.31)

     ● **Z87.3   Personal history of diseases of the musculoskeletal system and connective tissue**
Conditions classifiable to M00-M99
         Excludes2   personal history of (healed) traumatic fracture (Z87.81)

       ● **Z87.31   Personal history of (healed) nontraumatic fracture**

         Z87.310   Personal history of (healed) osteoporosis fracture
            Personal history of (healed) fragility fracture
            Personal history of (healed) collapsed vertebra due to osteoporosis

         Z87.311   Personal history of (healed) other pathological fracture
            Personal history of (healed) collapsed vertebra NOS
            Excludes2   personal history of osteoporosis fracture (Z87.310)

         Z87.312   Personal history of (healed) stress fracture
            Personal history of (healed) fatigue fracture

       Z87.39   Personal history of other diseases of the musculoskeletal system and connective tissue

     ● **Z87.4   Personal history of diseases of genitourinary system**
Conditions classifiable to N00-N99

       ● **Z87.41   Personal history of dysplasia of the female genital tract**
         Excludes1   personal history of malignant neoplasm of female genital tract (Z85.40-Z85.44)

         Z87.410   Personal history of cervical dysplasia ♀

         Z87.411   Personal history of vaginal dysplasia ♀

         Z87.412   Personal history of vulvar dysplasia ♀

       Z87.42   Personal history of other diseases of the female genital tract ♀

◀ New   ◀▥ Revised   ~~deleted~~ Deleted   Excludes 1   Excludes 2   Includes   Use additional   Code first   Code also   Unspecified
OGCR Official Guidelines   X Assign placeholder X   ● Use Additional Character(s)   ▌ Manifestation Code   Coding Clinic

● **Z87.43   Personal history of diseases of male genital organs**

    Z87.430   **Personal history of prostatic dysplasia** ♂

        Excludes1   personal history of malignant neoplasm of prostate (Z85.46)

    Z87.438   **Personal history of other diseases of male genital organs** ♂

● **Z87.44   Personal history of diseases of urinary system**

    Excludes1   personal history of malignant neoplasm of cervix uteri (Z85.41)

    Z87.440   **Personal history of urinary (tract) infections**

    Z87.441   **Personal history of nephrotic syndrome**

    Z87.442   **Personal history of urinary calculi**
        Personal history of kidney stones

    Z87.448   **Personal history of other diseases of urinary system**

● **Z87.5   Personal history of complications of pregnancy, childbirth and the puerperium**
    Conditions classifiable to O00-O9A

    Excludes2   recurrent pregnancy loss (N96)

    Z87.51   **Personal history of pre-term labor** ♀

        Excludes1   current pregnancy with history of pre-term labor (O09.21-)

    Z87.59   **Personal history of other complications of pregnancy, childbirth and the puerperium** ♀
        Personal history of trophoblastic disease

● **Z87.7   Personal history of (corrected) congenital malformations**
    Conditions classifiable to Q00-Q89 that have been repaired or corrected

    Excludes1   congenital malformations that have been partially corrected or repair but which still require medical treatment - code to condition

    Excludes2   other postprocedural states (Z98.-)
        personal history of medical treatment (Z92.-)
        presence of cardiac and vascular implants and grafts (Z95.-)
        presence of other devices (Z97.-)
        presence of other functional implants (Z96.-)
        transplanted organ and tissue status (Z94.-)

  ● **Z87.71   Personal history of (corrected) congenital malformations of genitourinary system**

    Z87.710   **Personal history of (corrected) hypospadias** ♂

    Z87.718   **Personal history of other specified (corrected) congenital malformations of genitourinary system**

  ● **Z87.72   Personal history of (corrected) congenital malformations of nervous system and sense organs**

    Z87.720   **Personal history of (corrected) congenital malformations of eye**

    Z87.721   **Personal history of (corrected) congenital malformations of ear**

    Z87.728   **Personal history of other specified (corrected) congenital malformations of nervous system and sense organs**

  ● **Z87.73   Personal history of (corrected) congenital malformations of digestive system**

    Z87.730   **Personal history of (corrected) cleft lip and palate**

    Z87.738   **Personal history of other specified (corrected) congenital malformations of digestive system**

    Z87.74   **Personal history of (corrected) congenital malformations of heart and circulatory system**

    Z87.75   **Personal history of (corrected) congenital malformations of respiratory system**

    Z87.76   **Personal history of (corrected) congenital malformations of integument, limbs and musculoskeletal system**

  ● **Z87.79   Personal history of other (corrected) congenital malformations**

    Z87.790   **Personal history of (corrected) congenital malformations of face and neck**

    Z87.798   **Personal history of other (corrected) congenital malformations**

● **Z87.8   Personal history of other specified conditions**

    Excludes2   personal history of self harm (Z91.5)

    Z87.81   **Personal history of (healed) traumatic fracture**

        Excludes2   personal history of (healed) nontraumatic fracture (Z87.31-)

  ● **Z87.82   Personal history of other (healed) physical injury and trauma**
    Conditions classifiable to S00-T88, except traumatic fractures

    Z87.820   **Personal history of traumatic brain injury**

        Excludes1   personal history of transient ischemic attack (TIA), and cerebral infarction without residual deficits (Z86.73)

    Z87.821   **Personal history of retained foreign body fully removed**

    Z87.828   **Personal history of other (healed) physical injury and trauma**

  ● **Z87.89   Personal history of other specified conditions**

    Z87.890   **Personal history of sex reassignment**

    Z87.891   **Personal history of nicotine dependence**

        Excludes1   current nicotine dependence (F17.2-)

    Z87.892   **Personal history of anaphylaxis**

        Code also allergy status such as:
        allergy status to drugs, medicaments and biological substances (Z88.-)
        allergy status, other than to drugs and biological substances (Z91.0-)

    Z87.898   **Personal history of other specified conditions**
        Coding Clinic: 2013, Q1, P21

CHAPTER 21 (Z00-Z99)

● **Z88   Allergy status to drugs, medicaments and biological substances**
　　　Excludes2　allergy status, other than to drugs and biological
　　　　　　　　substances (Z91.0-)
　　Z88.0   Allergy status to penicillin
　　Z88.1   Allergy status to other antibiotic agents status
　　Z88.2   Allergy status to sulfonamides status
　　Z88.3   Allergy status to other anti-infective agents status
　　Z88.4   Allergy status to anesthetic agent status
　　Z88.5   Allergy status to narcotic agent status
　　Z88.6   Allergy status to analgesic agent status
　　Z88.7   Allergy status to serum and vaccine status
　　Z88.8   Allergy status to other drugs, medicaments and
　　　　　biological substances status
　　Z88.9   Allergy status to unspecified drugs, medicaments and
　　　　　biological substances status

● **Z89   Acquired absence of limb**
　　　Includes   amputation status
　　　　　　　postprocedural loss of limb
　　　　　　　post-traumatic loss of limb
　　　Excludes1   acquired deformities of limbs (M20-M21)
　　　　　　　congenital absence of limbs (Q71-Q73)
　● **Z89.0   Acquired absence of thumb and other finger(s)**
　　● **Z89.01   Acquired absence of thumb**
　　　　Z89.011   Acquired absence of right thumb
　　　　Z89.012   Acquired absence of left thumb
　　　　**Z89.019   Acquired absence of unspecified
　　　　　　　thumb**
　　● **Z89.02   Acquired absence of other finger(s)**
　　　　Excludes2   acquired absence of thumb
　　　　　　　(Z89.01-)
　　　　Z89.021   Acquired absence of right finger(s)
　　　　Z89.022   Acquired absence of left finger(s)
　　　　**Z89.029   Acquired absence of unspecified
　　　　　　　finger(s)**
　● **Z89.1   Acquired absence of hand and wrist**
　　● **Z89.11   Acquired absence of hand**
　　　　Z89.111   Acquired absence of right hand
　　　　Z89.112   Acquired absence of left hand
　　　　Z89.119   Acquired absence of unspecified hand
　　● **Z89.12   Acquired absence of wrist**
　　　　Disarticulation at wrist
　　　　Z89.121   Acquired absence of right wrist
　　　　Z89.122   Acquired absence of left wrist
　　　　Z89.129   Acquired absence of unspecified wrist
　● **Z89.2   Acquired absence of upper limb above wrist**
　　● **Z89.20   Acquired absence of upper limb, unspecified
　　　　　level**
　　　　**Z89.201   Acquired absence of right upper limb,
　　　　　　　unspecified level**
　　　　**Z89.202   Acquired absence of left upper limb,
　　　　　　　unspecified level**
　　　　**Z89.209   Acquired absence of unspecified
　　　　　　　upper limb, unspecified level**
　　　　　　Acquired absence of arm NOS
　　● **Z89.21   Acquired absence of upper limb below elbow**
　　　　**Z89.211   Acquired absence of right upper limb
　　　　　　　below elbow**
　　　　**Z89.212   Acquired absence of left upper limb
　　　　　　　below elbow**
　　　　**Z89.219   Acquired absence of unspecified
　　　　　　　upper limb below elbow**

　　● **Z89.22   Acquired absence of upper limb above elbow**
　　　　Disarticulation at elbow
　　　　**Z89.221   Acquired absence of right upper limb
　　　　　　　above elbow**
　　　　**Z89.222   Acquired absence of left upper limb
　　　　　　　above elbow**
　　　　**Z89.229   Acquired absence of unspecified
　　　　　　　upper limb above elbow**
　　● **Z89.23   Acquired absence of shoulder**
　　　　Acquired absence of shoulder joint following
　　　　　explantation of shoulder joint prosthesis,
　　　　　with or without presence of antibiotic-
　　　　　impregnated cement spacer
　　　　Z89.231   Acquired absence of right shoulder
　　　　Z89.232   Acquired absence of left shoulder
　　　　**Z89.239   Acquired absence of unspecified
　　　　　　　shoulder**
　● **Z89.4   Acquired absence of toe(s), foot, and ankle**
　　● **Z89.41   Acquired absence of great toe**
　　　　Z89.411   Acquired absence of right great toe
　　　　Z89.412   Acquired absence of left great toe
　　　　**Z89.419   Acquired absence of unspecified great
　　　　　　　toe**
　　● **Z89.42   Acquired absence of other toe(s)**
　　　　Excludes2   acquired absence of great toe
　　　　　　　(Z89.41-)
　　　　Z89.421   Acquired absence of other right toe(s)
　　　　Z89.422   Acquired absence of other left toe(s)
　　　　**Z89.429   Acquired absence of other toe(s),
　　　　　　　unspecified side**
　　● **Z89.43   Acquired absence of foot**
　　　　Z89.431   Acquired absence of right foot
　　　　Z89.432   Acquired absence of left foot
　　　　Z89.439   Acquired absence of unspecified foot
　　● **Z89.44   Acquired absence of ankle**
　　　　Disarticulation of ankle
　　　　Z89.441   Acquired absence of right ankle
　　　　Z89.442   Acquired absence of left ankle
　　　　**Z89.449   Acquired absence of unspecified
　　　　　　　ankle**
　● **Z89.5   Acquired absence of leg below knee**
　　● **Z89.51   Acquired absence of leg below knee**
　　　　**Z89.511   Acquired absence of right leg below
　　　　　　　knee**
　　　　**Z89.512   Acquired absence of left leg below
　　　　　　　knee**
　　　　**Z89.519   Acquired absence of unspecified leg
　　　　　　　below knee**
　　● **Z89.52   Acquired absence of knee**
　　　　Acquired absence of knee joint following
　　　　　explantation of knee joint prosthesis,
　　　　　with or without presence of antibiotic-
　　　　　impregnated cement spacer
　　　　Z89.521   Acquired absence of right knee
　　　　Z89.522   Acquired absence of left knee
　　　　Z89.529   Acquired absence of unspecified knee

◄ New　◄▦ Revised　~~deleted~~ Deleted　Excludes 1　Excludes 2　Includes　Use additional　Code first　Code also　Unspecified

OGCR Official Guidelines　X Assign placeholder X　● Use Additional Character(s)　▶ Manifestation Code　Coding Clinic

● **Z89.6** **Acquired absence of leg above knee**
  ● **Z89.61** **Acquired absence of leg above knee**
          Acquired absence of leg NOS
          Disarticulation at knee
          Z89.611 **Acquired absence of right leg above knee**
          Z89.612 **Acquired absence of left leg above knee**
          Z89.619 **Acquired absence of** unspecified **leg above knee**
  ● **Z89.62** **Acquired absence of hip**
          Acquired absence of hip joint following explantation of hip joint prosthesis, with or without presence of antibiotic-impregnated cement spacer
          Disarticulation at hip
          Z89.621 **Acquired absence of right hip joint**
          Z89.622 **Acquired absence of left hip joint**
          Z89.629 **Acquired absence of** unspecified **hip joint**
  Z89.9 **Acquired absence of limb,** unspecified

● **Z90** **Acquired absence of organs, not elsewhere classified**
      Includes   postprocedural or post-traumatic loss of body part NEC
      Excludes1   congenital absence - see Alphabetical Index
      Excludes2   postprocedural absence of endocrine glands (E89.-)
  ● **Z90.0** **Acquired absence of part of head and neck**
      Z90.01 **Acquired absence of eye**
      Z90.02 **Acquired absence of larynx**
      Z90.09 **Acquired absence of other part of head and neck**
              Acquired absence of nose
              Excludes2 teeth (K08.1)
  ● **Z90.1** **Acquired absence of breast and nipple**
      Z90.10 **Acquired absence of** unspecified **breast and nipple**
      Z90.11 **Acquired absence of right breast and nipple**
      Z90.12 **Acquired absence of left breast and nipple**
      Z90.13 **Acquired absence of bilateral breasts and nipples**
  Z90.2 **Acquired absence of lung [part of]**
  Z90.3 **Acquired absence of stomach [part of]**
  ● **Z90.4** **Acquired absence of other specified parts of digestive tract**
      ● **Z90.41** **Acquired absence of pancreas**
              Use additional code to identify any associated:
              insulin use (Z79.4)
              diabetes mellitus, postpancreatectomy (E13.-)
              Z90.410 **Acquired total absence of pancreas**
                      Acquired absence of pancreas NOS
              Z90.411 **Acquired partial absence of pancreas**
      Z90.49 **Acquired absence of other specified parts of digestive tract**
  Z90.5 **Acquired absence of kidney**
  Z90.6 **Acquired absence of other parts of urinary tract**
          Acquired absence of bladder

● **Z90.7** **Acquired absence of genital organ(s)**
      Excludes1   personal history of sex reassignment (Z87.890)
      Excludes2   female genital mutilation status (N90.81-)
  ● **Z90.71** **Acquired absence of cervix and uterus**
          Z90.710 **Acquired absence of both cervix and uterus ♀**
                  Acquired absence of uterus NOS
                  Status post total hysterectomy
          Z90.711 **Acquired absence of uterus with remaining cervical stump ♀**
                  Status post partial hysterectomy with remaining cervical stump
          Z90.712 **Acquired absence of cervix with remaining uterus ♀**
  ● **Z90.72** **Acquired absence of ovaries**
          Z90.721 **Acquired absence of ovaries, unilateral ♀**
          Z90.722 **Acquired absence of ovaries, bilateral ♀**
      Z90.79 **Acquired absence of other genital organ(s)**
  ● **Z90.8** **Acquired absence of other organs**
      Z90.81 **Acquired absence of spleen**
      Z90.89 **Acquired absence of other organs**

● **Z91** **Personal risk factors, not elsewhere classified**
      Excludes2   contact with and (suspected) exposures hazardous to health (Z77.-)
              exposure to pollution and other problems related to physical environment (Z77.1-)
              occupational exposure to risk factors (Z57.-)
              personal history of physical injury and trauma (Z87.81, Z87.82-)
  ● **Z91.0** **Allergy status, other than to drugs and biological substances**
      Excludes2   allergy status to drugs, medicaments, and biological substances (Z88.-)
      ● **Z91.01** **Food allergy status**
          Excludes2 food additives allergy status (Z91.02)
          Z91.010 **Allergy to peanuts**
          Z91.011 **Allergy to milk products**
                  Excludes1 lactose intolerance (E73.-)
          Z91.012 **Allergy to eggs**
          Z91.013 **Allergy to seafood**
                  Allergy to shellfish
                  Allergy to octopus or squid ink
          Z91.018 **Allergy to other foods**
                  Allergy to nuts other than peanuts
      Z91.02 **Food additives allergy status**
      ● **Z91.03** **Insect allergy status**
          Z91.030 **Bee allergy status**
          Z91.038 **Other insect allergy status**
      ● **Z91.04** **Nonmedicinal substance allergy status**
          Z91.040 **Latex allergy status**
                  Latex sensitivity status
          Z91.041 **Radiographic dye allergy status**
                  Allergy status to contrast media used for diagnostic X-ray procedure
          Z91.048 **Other nonmedicinal substance allergy status**
      Z91.09 **Other allergy status, other than to drugs and biological substances**

CHAPTER 21 (Z00-Z99)

CHAPTER 21 (Z00-Z99)

● **Z91.1**   **Patient's noncompliance with medical treatment and regimen**

     Z91.11   **Patient's noncompliance with dietary regimen**

●   **Z91.12**   **Patient's intentional underdosing of medication regimen**

        Code first underdosing of medication (T36-T50) with fifth or sixth character 6

        Excludes1   adverse effect of prescribed drug taken as directed - code to adverse effect
               poisoning (overdose) - code to poisoning

        Z91.120   **Patient's intentional underdosing of medication regimen due to financial hardship**

        Z91.128   **Patient's intentional underdosing of medication regimen for other reason**

●   **Z91.13**   **Patient's unintentional underdosing of medication regimen**

        Code first underdosing of medication (T36-T50) with fifth or sixth character 6

        Excludes1   adverse effect of prescribed drug taken as directed - code to adverse effect
               poisoning (overdose) - code to poisoning

        Z91.130   **Patient's unintentional underdosing of medication regimen due to age-related debility**

        Z91.138   **Patient's unintentional underdosing of medication regimen for other reason**

     Z91.14   **Patient's other noncompliance with medication regimen**
        Patient's underdosing of medication NOS

     Z91.15   **Patient's noncompliance with renal dialysis**

     Z91.19   **Patient's noncompliance with other medical treatment and regimen**

● **Z91.4**   **Personal history of psychological trauma, not elsewhere classified**

●   **Z91.41**   **Personal history of adult abuse**

        Excludes2   personal history of abuse in childhood (Z62.81-)

        Z91.410   **Personal history of adult physical and sexual abuse**   **A**

           Excludes1   current adult physical abuse (T74.11, T76.11)
                 current adult sexual abuse (T74.21, T76.11)

        Z91.411   **Personal history of adult psychological abuse**   **A**

        Z91.412   **Personal history of adult neglect**   **A**

           Excludes1   current adult neglect (T74.01, T76.01)

        Z91.419   **Personal history of unspecified adult abuse**   **A**

     Z91.49   **Other personal history of psychological trauma, not elsewhere classified**

Z91.5   **Personal history of self-harm**
     Personal history of parasuicide
     Personal history of self-poisoning
     Personal history of suicide attempt

● **Z91.8**   **Other specified personal risk factors, not elsewhere classified**

     Z91.81   **History of falling**
        At risk for falling

     Z91.82   **Personal history of military deployment**   **A**
        Individual (civilian or military) with past history of military war, peacekeeping and humanitarian deployment (current or past conflict)
        Returned from military deployment

▶   **Z91.83**   *Wandering in diseases classified elsewhere*

        Code first underlying disorder such as:
        Alzheimer's disease (G30.-)
        autism or pervasive developmental disorder (F84.-)
        intellectual disabilities (F70-F79)
        unspecified dementia with behavioral disturbance (F03.9-)

     Z91.89   **Other specified personal risk factors, not elsewhere classified**

● **Z92**   **Personal history of medical treatment**

     Excludes2   postprocedural states (Z98.-)

     Z92.0   **Personal history of contraception**

        Excludes1   counseling or management of current contraceptive practices (Z30.-)
               long term (current) use of contraception (Z79.3)
               presence of (intrauterine) contraceptive device (Z97.5)

●   **Z92.2**   **Personal history of drug therapy**

        Excludes2   long term (current) drug therapy (Z79.-)

        Z92.21   **Personal history of antineoplastic chemotherapy**

        Z92.22   **Personal history of monoclonal drug therapy**

        Z92.23   **Personal history of estrogen therapy**

●   **Z92.24**   **Personal history of steroid therapy**

           Z92.240   **Personal history of inhaled steroid therapy**

           Z92.241   **Personal history of systemic steroid therapy**
              Personal history of steroid therapy NOS

        Z92.25   **Personal history of immunosupression therapy**

           Excludes2   personal history of steroid therapy (Z92.24)

        Z92.29   **Personal history of other drug therapy**

     Z92.3   **Personal history of irradiation**
        Personal history of exposure to therapeutic radiation

        Excludes1   exposure to radiation in the physical environment (Z77.12)
               occupational exposure to radiation (Z57.1)

●   **Z92.8**   **Personal history of other medical treatment**

        Z92.81   **Personal history of extracorporeal membrane oxygenation (ECMO)**

        Z92.82   **Status post administration of tPA (rtPA) in a different facility within the last 24 hours prior to admission to current facility**

           Code first condition requiring tPA administration, such as:
           acute cerebral infarction (I63.-)
           acute myocardial infarction (I21.-, I22.-)

        Z92.83   **Personal history of failed moderate sedation**
           Personal history of failed conscious sedation

           Excludes2   failed moderate sedation during procedure (T88.52)

        Z92.89   **Personal history of other medical treatment**

▶ New   ◀▥ Revised   ~~deleted~~ Deleted   Excludes 1   Excludes 2   Includes   Use additional   Code first   Code also   Unspecified

1602   OGCR Official Guidelines   X Assign placeholder X   ● Use Additional Character(s)   ▶ Manifestation Code   **Coding Clinic**

● **Z93   Artificial opening status**

> **Excludes1**   artificial openings requiring attention or
> management (Z43.-)
> complications of external stoma (J95.0-, K94.-,
> N99.5-)

Z93.0   **Tracheostomy status**

Z93.1   **Gastrostomy status**

Z93.2   **Ileostomy status**

Z93.3   **Colostomy status**

Z93.4   **Other artificial openings of gastrointestinal tract status**

● Z93.5   **Cystostomy status**

    Z93.50   **Unspecified cystostomy status**

    Z93.51   **Cutaneous-vesicostomy status**

    Z93.52   **Appendico-vesicostomy status**

    Z93.59   **Other cystostomy status**

Z93.6   **Other artificial openings of urinary tract status**
> Nephrostomy status
> Ureterostomy status
> Urethrostomy status

Z93.8   **Other artificial opening status**

Z93.9   **Artificial opening status, unspecified**

● **Z94   Transplanted organ and tissue status**

> **Includes**   organ or tissue replaced by heterogenous or
> homogenous transplant

> **Excludes1**   complications of transplanted organ or tissue -
> see Alphabetical Index

> **Excludes2**   presence of vascular grafts (Z95.-)

Z94.0   **Kidney transplant status**

Z94.1   **Heart transplant status**

> **Excludes1**   artificial heart status (Z95.812)
> heart-valve replacement status
> (Z95.2-Z95.4)

Z94.2   **Lung transplant status**

Z94.3   **Heart and lungs transplant status**

Z94.4   **Liver transplant status**

Z94.5   **Skin transplant status**
> Autogenous skin transplant status

Z94.6   **Bone transplant status**

Z94.7   **Corneal transplant status**

● Z94.8   **Other transplanted organ and tissue status**

    Z94.81   **Bone marrow transplant status**

    Z94.82   **Intestine transplant status**

    Z94.83   **Pancreas transplant status**

    Z94.84   **Stem cells transplant status**

    Z94.89   **Other transplanted organ and tissue status**

Z94.9   **Transplanted organ and tissue status, unspecified**

● **Z95   Presence of cardiac and vascular implants and grafts**

> **Excludes1**   complications of cardiac and vascular devices,
> implants and grafts (T82.-)

Z95.0   **Presence of cardiac pacemaker**

> **Excludes1**   adjustment or management of cardiac
> pacemaker (Z45.0)
> presence of automatic (implantable)
> cardiac defibrillator with
> synchronous cardiac pacemaker
> (Z95.810)

Z95.1   **Presence of aortocoronary bypass graft**

Z95.2   **Presence of prosthetic heart valve**
> Presence of heart valve NOS

Z95.3   **Presence of xenogenic heart valve**

Z95.4   **Presence of other heart-valve replacement**

Z95.5   **Presence of coronary angioplasty implant and graft**

> **Excludes1**   coronary angioplasty status without
> implant and graft (Z98.61)

● Z95.8   **Presence of other cardiac and vascular implants and grafts**

● Z95.81   **Presence of other cardiac implants and grafts**

    Z95.810   **Presence of automatic (implantable) cardiac defibrillator**
> Presence of automatic (implantable) cardiac defibrillator with synchronous cardiac pacemaker

    Z95.811   **Presence of heart assist device**

    Z95.812   **Presence of fully implantable artificial heart**

    Z95.818   **Presence of other cardiac implants and grafts**

● Z95.82   **Presence of other vascular implants and grafts**

    Z95.820   **Peripheral vascular angioplasty status with implants and grafts**

> **Excludes1**   peripheral vascular
> angioplasty
> without implant
> and graft (Z98.62)

    Z95.828   **Presence of other vascular implants and grafts**
> Presence of intravascular prosthesis NEC

Z95.9   **Presence of cardiac and vascular implant and graft, unspecified**

● **Z96   Presence of other functional implants**

> **Excludes2**   complications of internal prosthetic devices,
> implants and grafts (T82-T85)
> fitting and adjustment of prosthetic and other
> devices (Z44-Z46)

Z96.0   **Presence of urogenital implants**

Z96.1   **Presence of intraocular lens**
> Presence of pseudophakia

● Z96.2   **Presence of otological and audiological implants**

    Z96.20   **Presence of otological and audiological implant, unspecified**

    Z96.21   **Cochlear implant status**

    Z96.22   **Myringotomy tube(s) status**

    Z96.29   **Presence of other otological and audiological implants**
> Presence of bone-conduction hearing device
> Presence of eustachian tube stent
> Stapes replacement

Z96.3   **Presence of artificial larynx**

● Z96.4   **Presence of endocrine implants**

    Z96.41   **Presence of insulin pump (external) (internal)**

    Z96.49   **Presence of other endocrine implants**

Z96.5   **Presence of tooth-root and mandibular implants**

● Z96.6   **Presence of orthopedic joint implants**

    Z96.60   **Presence of unspecified orthopedic joint implant**

● Z96.61   **Presence of artificial shoulder joint**

    Z96.611   **Presence of right artificial shoulder joint**

    Z96.612   **Presence of left artificial shoulder joint**

    Z96.619   **Presence of unspecified artificial shoulder joint**

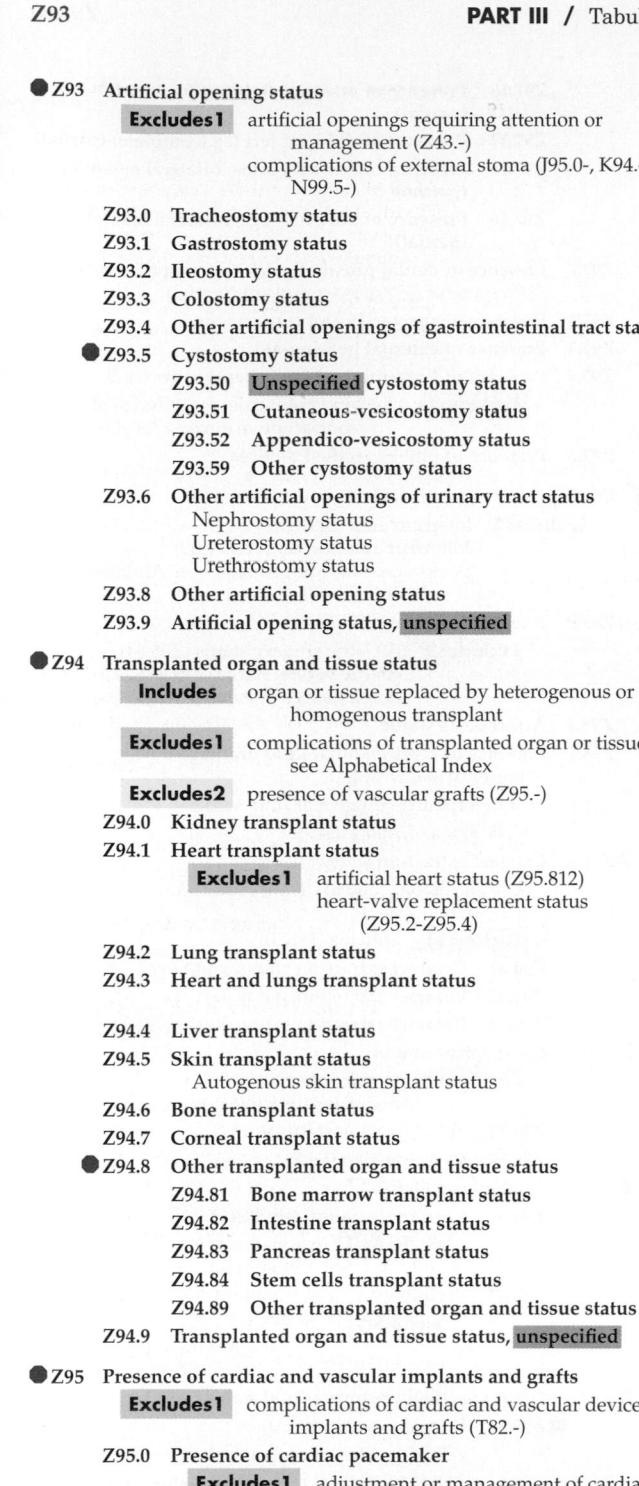

● **Z96.62**   Presence of artificial elbow joint
    Z96.621   Presence of right artificial elbow joint
    Z96.622   Presence of left artificial elbow joint
    Z96.629   Presence of unspecified artificial elbow joint

● **Z96.63**   Presence of artificial wrist joint
    Z96.631   Presence of right artificial wrist joint
    Z96.632   Presence of left artificial wrist joint
    Z96.639   Presence of unspecified artificial wrist joint

● **Z96.64**   Presence of artificial hip joint
    Hip-joint replacement (partial) (total)
    Z96.641   Presence of right artificial hip joint
    Z96.642   Presence of left artificial hip joint
      Coding Clinic: 2015, Q1, P16
    Z96.643   Presence of artificial hip joint, bilateral
    Z96.649   Presence of unspecified artificial hip joint

● **Z96.65**   Presence of artificial knee joint
    Z96.651   Presence of right artificial knee joint
    Z96.652   Presence of left artificial knee joint
    Z96.653   Presence of artificial knee joint, bilateral
    Z96.659   Presence of unspecified artificial knee joint

● **Z96.66**   Presence of artificial ankle joint
    Z96.661   Presence of right artificial ankle joint
    Z96.662   Presence of left artificial ankle joint
    Z96.669   Presence of unspecified artificial ankle joint

● **Z96.69**   Presence of other orthopedic joint implants
    Z96.691   Finger-joint replacement of right hand
    Z96.692   Finger-joint replacement of left hand
    Z96.693   Finger-joint replacement, bilateral
    Z96.698   Presence of other orthopedic joint implants

 Z96.7   Presence of other bone and tendon implants
    Presence of skull plate

● **Z96.8**   Presence of other specified functional implants
    Z96.81   Presence of artificial skin
    Z96.89   Presence of other specified functional implants

 Z96.9   Presence of functional implant, unspecified

● **Z97**   **Presence of other devices**
    Excludes1   complications of internal prosthetic devices, implants and grafts (T82-T85)
               fitting and adjustment of prosthetic and other devices (Z44-Z46)
    Excludes2   presence of cerebrospinal fluid drainage device (Z98.2)

 Z97.0   Presence of artificial eye

● **Z97.1**   Presence of artificial limb (complete) (partial)
    Z97.10   Presence of artificial limb (complete) (partial), unspecified
    Z97.11   Presence of artificial right arm (complete) (partial)
    Z97.12   Presence of artificial left arm (complete) (partial)

    Z97.13   Presence of artificial right leg (complete) (partial)
    Z97.14   Presence of artificial left leg (complete) (partial)
    Z97.15   Presence of artificial arms, bilateral (complete) (partial)
    Z97.16   Presence of artificial legs, bilateral (complete) (partial)

 Z97.2   Presence of dental prosthetic device (complete) (partial)
    Presence of dentures (complete) (partial)

 Z97.3   Presence of spectacles and contact lenses

 Z97.4   Presence of external hearing-aid

 Z97.5   Presence of (intrauterine) contraceptive device ♀
    Excludes1   checking, reinsertion or removal of contraceptive device (Z30.43)

 Z97.8   Presence of other specified devices

● **Z98**   **Other postprocedural states**
    Excludes2   aftercare (Z43-Z49, Z51)
               follow-up medical care (Z08-Z09)
               postprocedural complication - see Alphabetical Index

 Z98.0   Intestinal bypass and anastomosis status
    Excludes2   bariatric surgery status (Z98.84)
               gastric bypass status (Z98.84)
               obesity surgery status (Z98.84)

 Z98.1   Arthrodesis status

 Z98.2   Presence of cerebrospinal fluid drainage device
    Presence of CSF shunt

 Z98.3   Post therapeutic collapse of lung status
    Code first underlying disease

● **Z98.4**   Cataract extraction status
    Use additional code to identify intraocular lens implant status (Z96.1)
    Excludes1   aphakia (H27.0)
    Z98.41   Cataract extraction status, right eye
    Z98.42   Cataract extraction status, left eye
    Z98.49   Cataract extraction status, unspecified eye

● **Z98.5**   Sterilization status
    Excludes1   female infertility (N97.-)
               male infertility (N46.-)
    Z98.51   Tubal ligation status ♀
    Z98.52   Vasectomy status ♂   **A**

● **Z98.6**   Angioplasty status
    Z98.61   Coronary angioplasty status
       Excludes1   coronary angioplasty status with implant and graft (Z95.5)
    Z98.62   Peripheral vascular angioplasty status
       Excludes1   peripheral vascular angioplasty status with implant and graft (Z95.820)

● **Z98.8**   Other specified postprocedural states
    ● Z98.81   Dental procedure status
      Z98.810   Dental sealant status
      Z98.811   Dental restoration status
         Dental crown status
         Dental fillings status
      Z98.818   Other dental procedure status
    Z98.82   Breast implant status
      Excludes1   breast implant removal status (Z98.86)

◀ New   ⫷ Revised   ~~deleted~~ Deleted   Excludes 1   Excludes 2   Includes   Use additional   Code first   Code also   Unspecified
OGCR Official Guidelines   X Assign placeholder X   ● Use Additional Character(s)   ▶ Manifestation Code   **Coding Clinic**

Z98.83   **Filtering (vitreous) bleb after glaucoma surgery status**

> **Excludes1**   inflammation (infection) of postprocedural bleb (H59.4-)

Z98.84   **Bariatric surgery status**
Gastric banding status
Gastric bypass status for obesity
Obesity surgery status

> **Excludes1**   bariatric surgery status complicating pregnancy, childbirth, or the puerperium (O99.84)

> **Excludes2**   intestinal bypass and anastomosis status (Z98.0)

Z98.85   **Transplanted organ removal status**
Transplanted organ previously removed due to complication, failure, rejection or infection

> **Excludes1**   encounter for removal of transplanted organ -code to complication of transplanted organ (T86.-)

Z98.86   **Personal history of breast implant removal**

● Z98.87   **Personal history of in utero procedure**

Z98.870   **Personal history of in utero procedure during pregnancy** ♀

> **Excludes2**   complications from in utero procedure for current pregnancy (O35.7)
> supervision of current pregnancy with history of in utero procedure during previous pregnancy (O09.82-)

Z98.871   **Personal history of in utero procedure while a fetus**

Z98.89   **Other specified postprocedural states**
Personal history of surgery, not elsewhere classified

● Z99   **Dependence on enabling machines and devices, not elsewhere classified**

> **Excludes1**   cardiac pacemaker status (Z95.0)

Z99.0   **Dependence on aspirator**

● Z99.1   **Dependence on respirator**
Dependence on ventilator

Z99.11   **Dependence on respirator [ventilator] status**
Coding Clinic: 2015, Q1, P21

Z99.12   **Encounter for respirator [ventilator] dependence during power failure**

> **Excludes1**   mechanical complication of respirator [ventilator] (J95.850)

Z99.2   **Dependence on renal dialysis**
Hemodialysis status
Peritoneal dialysis status
Presence of arteriovenous shunt for dialysis
Renal dialysis status NOS

> **Excludes1**   encounter for fitting and adjustment of dialysis catheter (Z49.0-)
> noncompliance with renal dialysis (Z91.15)

Z99.3   **Dependence on wheelchair**
Wheelchair confinement status

Code first cause of dependence, such as:
muscular dystrophy (G71.0)
obesity (E66.-)

● Z99.8   **Dependence on other enabling machines and devices**

Z99.81   **Dependence on supplemental oxygen**
Dependence on long-term oxygen

Z99.89   **Dependence on other enabling machines and devices**
Dependence on machine or device NOS

CHAPTER 21 (Z00-Z99)

Trust Carol J. Buck and Elsevier
to take you through the levels of coding success

Step 4:
Professional Resources

Step 3:
Certify

With the resources you need for every level of coding success, Carol J. Buck and Elsevier are with you every step of your coding career. From beginning to advanced, from the classroom to the workplace, from application to certification, the Step Series products are your guides to greater opportunities and successful career advancement.

Step 2:
Practice

Step 1:
Learn

Keep climbing with the most trusted names in medical coding.

Author and Educator
Carol J. Buck,
MS, CPC, CCS-P

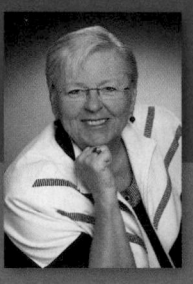

Lead Technical Collaborator
Jackie L. Grass,
CPC

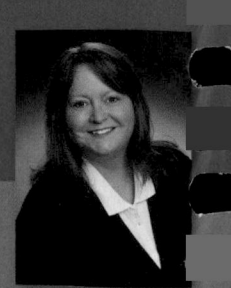

Trust Elsevier
to provide your complete curriculum solution!

Content

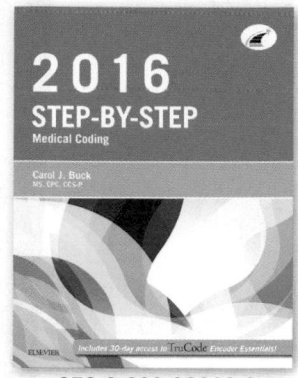

978-0-323-38919-8

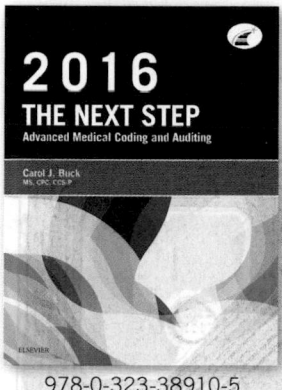

978-0-323-38910-5

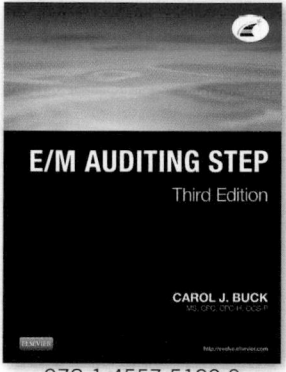

978-1-4557-5199-0

Study Tools

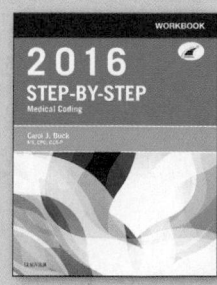

978-0-323-38921-1

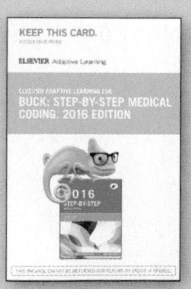

978-0-323-40124-1

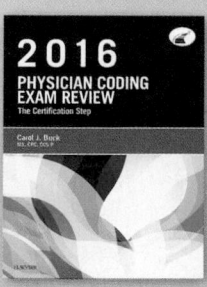

978-0-323-22750-6

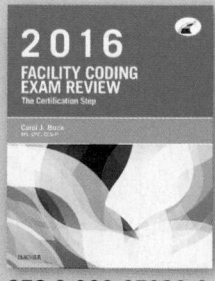

978-0-323-27982-6

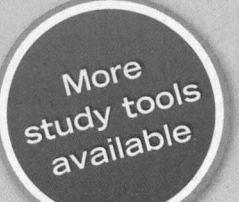

evolve

More study tools available

Simulations

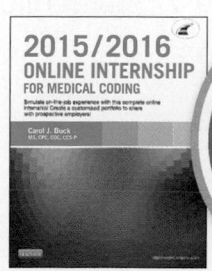

978-0-323-39250-1

Create a customized portfolio to show employers

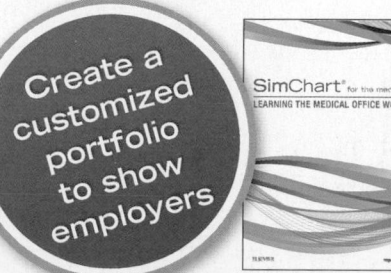

978-0-323-39423-9

Courses

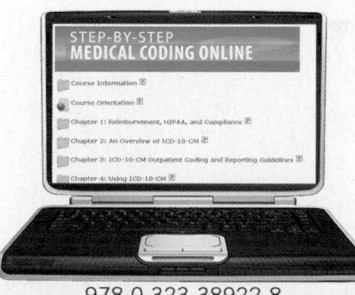

978-0-323-38922-8

Learn more at Elsevieradvantage.com!

CAMPBELL UNIVERSITY LIBRARY
BUIES CREEK   NORTH CAROLINA

REF RB115 .B835 2016 MED
Buck, Carol J.,
2016 ICD-10-CM for physicians